BRENNER & RECTOR'S THE KIDNEY

Tenth Edition

VOLUME 2

Karl Skorecki, MD, FRCP(C), FASN
Annie Chutick Professor and Chair in Medicine (Nephrology)
Technion—Israel Institute of Technology
Director of Medical and Research Development
Rambam Health Care Campus
Haifa, Israel

Glenn M. Chertow, MD
Norman S. Coplon/Satellite Healthcare Professor of Medicine
Chief, Division of Nephrology
Stanford University School of Medicine
Palo Alto, California

Philip A. Marsden, MD
Professor of Medicine
Elisabeth Hofmann Chair in Translational Research
Oreopoulos-Baxter Division Director of Nephrology
Vice Chair Research, Department of Medicine
University of Toronto
Toronto, Ontario, Canada

Maarten W. Taal, MBChB, MMed, MD, FCP(SA), FRCP
Professor of Medicine
Division of Medical Sciences and Graduate Entry Medicine
University of Nottingham
Honorary Consultant Nephrologist
Department of Renal Medicine
Royal Derby Hospital
Derby, United Kingdom

Alan S.L. Yu, MD
Harry Statland and Solon Summerfield Professor of Medicine
Director, Division of Nephrology and Hypertension and The Kidney Institute
University of Kansas Medical Center
Kansas City, Kansas

SPECIAL ASSISTANT TO THE EDITORS
Walter G. Wasser, MD
Attending Physician, Division of Nephrology
Mayanei HaYeshua Medical Center
Bnei Brak, Israel;
Rambam Health Care Campus
Haifa, Israel

ELSEVIER

ELSEVIER

1600 John F. Kennedy Blvd.
Ste 1800
Philadelphia, PA 19103-2899

BRENNER AND RECTOR'S THE KIDNEY, TENTH EDITION ISBN: 978-1-4557-4836-5
Copyright © 2016 by Elsevier, Inc. All rights reserved. Volume 1 part number 9996096807
Volume 2 part number 9996096866

No part of this publication may be reproduced or transmitted in any form or by any means, electronic or mechanical, including photocopying, recording, or any information storage and retrieval system, without permission in writing from the publisher. Details on how to seek permission, further information about the Publisher's permissions policies and our arrangements with organizations such as the Copyright Clearance Center and the Copyright Licensing Agency, can be found at our website: www.elsevier.com/permissions.

This book and the individual contributions contained in it are protected under copyright by the Publisher (other than as may be noted herein).

Notices

Knowledge and best practice in this field are constantly changing. As new research and experience broaden our understanding, changes in research methods, professional practices, or medical treatment may become necessary.

Practitioners and researchers must always rely on their own experience and knowledge in evaluating and using any information, methods, compounds, or experiments described herein. In using such information or methods they should be mindful of their own safety and the safety of others, including parties for whom they have a professional responsibility.

With respect to any drug or pharmaceutical products identified, readers are advised to check the most current information provided (i) on procedures featured or (ii) by the manufacturer of each product to be administered, to verify the recommended dose or formula, the method and duration of administration, and contraindications. It is the responsibility of practitioners, relying on their own experience and knowledge of their patients, to make diagnoses, to determine dosages and the best treatment for each individual patient, and to take all appropriate safety precautions.

To the fullest extent of the law, neither the Publisher nor the authors, contributors, or editors, assume any liability for any injury and/or damage to persons or property as a matter of products liability, negligence or otherwise, or from any use or operation of any methods, products, instructions, or ideas contained in the material herein.

Previous editions copyrighted 2012, 2008, 2004, 2000, 1996, 1991, 1986, 1981, 1976.

Library of Congress Cataloging-in-Publication Data

Brenner & Rector's the kidney / [edited by] Karl Skorecki, Glenn M. Chertow, Philip A. Marsden, Maarten W. Taal, Alan S.L. Yu ; special assistant to the editors, Walter G. Wasser.—10th edition.
   p. ; cm.
  Brenner and Rector's the kidney
  Kidney
  Includes bibliographical references and index.
  ISBN 978-1-4557-4836-5 (hardcover : alk. paper)
  I. Skorecki, Karl, editor. II. Chertow, Glenn M., editor. III. Marsden, Philip A., editor.
IV. Taal, Maarten W., editor. V. Yu, Alan S. L., editor. VI. Title: Brenner and Rector's the kidney. VII. Title: Kidney.
  [DNLM: 1. Kidney Diseases. 2. Kidney—physiology. 3. Kidney—physiopathology. WJ 300]
  RC902
  616.6′1—dc23
                                                          2015033607

Content Strategist: Kellie Heap
Senior Content Development Specialist: Joan Ryan
Publishing Services Manager: Jeffrey Patterson
Senior Project Manager: Mary Pohlman
Senior Book Designer: Margaret Reid

Printed in United States of America.

Last digit is the print number: 9 8 7 6 5 4 3 2 1

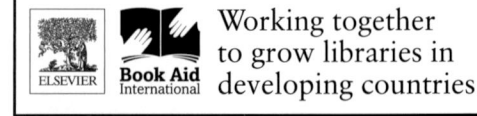

*Dedicated to our patients and to our students
—who provide us with the inspiration to learn,
teach, and discover.*

Contributors

Andrew Advani, BSc, MBChB(Hons), PhD, FRCP(UK)
Assistant Professor of Medicine
University of Toronto
St. Michael's Hospital
Toronto, Ontario, Canada
Chapter 13, Vasoactive Molecules and the Kidney

Michael Allon, MD
Professor of Medicine
Division of Nephrology
University of Alabama at Birmingham
Birmingham, Alabama
Chapter 70, Interventional Nephrology

Amanda Hyre Anderson, PhD, MPH
Assistant Professor of Epidemiology
Center for Clinical Epidemiology and Biostatistics
Perelman School of Medicine
University of Pennsylvania
Philadelphia, Pennsylvania
Chapter 21, Demographics of Kidney Disease

Gerald B. Appel, MD
Professor of Medicine
Director of Clinical Nephrology
Division of Nephrology
Columbia University Medical Center
New York, New York
Chapter 33, Secondary Glomerular Disease

Suheir Assady, MD, PhD
Director, Department of Nephrology and Hypertension
Rambam Health Care Campus
Haifa, Israel
Chapter 79, Near and Middle East

Anthony Atala, MD
Director, Wake Forest Institute for Regenerative Medicine
William H. Boyce Professor and Chair
Department of Urology
Wake Forest School of Medicine
Winston-Salem, North Carolina
Chapter 86, Tissue Engineering, Stem Cells, and Cell Therapy in Nephrology

Paul Ayoub, MD
Specialized Medicine
University of Montréal
Montréal, Quebec, Canada
Chapter 69, Elimination Enhancement of Poisons

Kara N. Babaian, MD
Assistant Professor of Clinical Urology
Department of Urology
University of California, Irvine
Orange, California
Chapter 41, Kidney Cancer

Colin Baigent, FFPH, FRCP
Professor of Epidemiology
Clinical Trial Service Unit
Nuffield Department of Population Health
Oxford, United Kingdom
Chapter 56, Cardiovascular Aspects of Kidney Disease

Sevcan A. Bakkaloglu, MD
Professor of Pediatrics
Head, Division of Pediatric Nephrology and Rheumatology
Gazi University School of Medicine
Ankara, Turkey
Chapter 74, Diseases of the Kidney and Urinary Tract in Children

George L. Bakris, MD
Professor of Medicine
Department of Medicine
University of Chicago Medicine
ASH Comprehensive Hypertension Center
Chicago, Illinois
Chapter 47, Primary and Secondary Hypertension

Gavin J. Becker, MD, FRACP
Professor
Department of Nephrology
Royal Melbourne Hospital and University of Melbourne
Melbourne, Victoria, Australia
Chapter 82, Oceania Region

Rachel Becker-Cohen, MD
Pediatric Nephrology
Shaare Zedek Medical Center
The Hebrew University School of Medicine
Jerusalem, Israel
Chapter 76, Renal Replacement Therapy (Dialysis and Transplantation) in Pediatric End-Stage Kidney Disease

Theresa J. Berndt
Department of Medicine
Division of Nephrology and Hypertension
Mayo Clinic College of Medicine
Mayo Clinic
Rochester, Minnesota
Chapter 7, The Regulation of Calcium, Magnesium, and Phosphate Excretion by the Kidney

Jeffrey S. Berns, MD
Professor of Medicine
Perelman School of Medicine
University of Pennsylvania
Philadelphia, Pennyslvania
  Chapter 21, *Demographics of Kidney Disease*

Prof John F. Bertram, BSc(Hons), PhD, FASN, DSc
Professor of Anatomy and Developmental Biology
Monash University
Clayton, Victoria, Australia
  Chapter 23, *Nephron Endowment and Developmental Programming of Blood Pressure and Renal Function*

Vivek Bhalla, MD
Assistant Professor of Medicine/Nephrology
Stanford University School of Medicine
Stanford, California
  Chapter 12, *Aldosterone and Mineralocorticoid Receptors: Renal and Extrarenal Roles*

Daniel G. Bichet, MD
Professor of Medicine and Physiology
University of Montréal
Nephrologist
Department of Medicine
Hôpital du Sacré-Coeur de Montréal
Montréal, Quebec, Canada
  Chapter 45, *Inherited Disorders of the Renal Tubule*

Alain Bonnardeaux, MD, PhD
Full Professor of Medicine
University of Montréal
Nephrologist
Hôpital Maisonneuve-Rosemont
Montréal, Quebec, Canada
  Chapter 45, *Inherited Disorders of the Renal Tubule*

William D. Boswell, Jr., MD, FACR
Professor and Chairman
Department of Radiology
City of Hope National Medical Center
Duarte, California
  Chapter 28, *Diagnostic Kidney Imaging*

Barry M. Brenner, MD, AM(Hon), DSc(Hon), DMSc(Hon), MD(Hon), Dipl(Hon), FRCP(London, Hon)
Samuel A. Levine Distinguished Professor of Medicine
Harvard Medical School
Director Emeritus, Renal Division, and Senior Physician
Department of Medicine
Brigham and Women's Hospital
Boston, Massachusetts
  Chapter 3, *The Renal Circulations and Glomerular Ultrafiltration*

Richard M. Breyer, PhD
Professor of Medicine
Professor of Biochemistry
Ruth King Scoville Chair in Medicine
Professor of Pharmacology
Vanderbilt University
Nashville, Tennessee
  Chapter 14, *Arachidonic Acid Metabolites and the Kidney*

Dennis Brown, PhD
Department of Medicine
Harvard Medical School
Center for Systems Biology
Program in Membrane Biology and Division of Nephrology
Massachusetts General Hospital
Boston, Massachussets
  Chapter 11, *The Cell Biology of Vasopressin Action*

Carlo Brugnara, MD
Professor of Pathology
Harvard Medical School
Director, Hematology Laboratory
Boston Children's Hospital
Boston, Massachusetts
  Chapter 57, *Hematologic Aspects of Kidney Disease*

Stéphan Busque, MD
Professor of Surgery (Abdominal Transplantation)
Director, Adult Kidney and Pancreas Transplant Program
Stanford University
Stanford, California
  Chapter 72, *Clinical Management of the Adult Kidney Transplant Recipient*

Juan Jesús Carrero, Pharm, PhD, MBA
Associate Professor
Karolinska Institutet
Stockholm, Sweden
  Chapter 58, *Endocrine Aspects of Chronic Kidney Disease*

Daniel Cattran, MD, FRCP(C), FACP
Professor of Medicine
University of Toronto
Senior Scientist
Toronto General Research Institute
Toronto General Hospital
Toronto, Ontario, Canada
  Chapter 34, *Overview of Therapy for Glomerular Disease*

James C. M. Chan, MD
Professor of Pediatrics
Tufts University School of Medicine
Director of Research
The Barbara Bush Children's Hospital
Maine Medical Center
Portland, Maine
  Chapter 75, *Fluid, Electrolyte, and Acid-Base Disorders in Children*

CONTRIBUTORS

Anil Chandraker, MD
Associate Professor of Medicine
Harvard Medical School
Brigham and Women's Hospital
Schuster Family Transplantation Research Center
Boston, Massachusetts
Chapter 71, Transplantation Immunobiology

Katrina Chau, MBBS, FRACP
Department of Nephrology
University of British Columbia
Vancouver, British Columbia, Canada;
Department of Nephrology
Liverpool Hospital
Sydney, Australia
Chapter 26, Laboratory Assessment of Kidney Disease: Glomerular Filtration Rate, Urinalysis, and Proteinuria

Glenn M. Chertow, MD, MPH
Norman S. Coplon/Satellite Healthcare
Professor of Medicine
Department of Medicine, Division of Nephrology
Stanford University School of Medicine
Palo Alto, California
Chapter 84, Health Disparities in Nephrology

Devasmita Choudhury, MD
Associate Professor of Medicine
University of Virginia School of Medicine
Virginia Tech-Carilion School of Medicine
Chief of Nephrology
Director of Dialysis and Interventional Nephrology
Salem Veterans Affairs Medical Center
Salem, Virginia
Chapter 24, Aging and Kidney Disease

John F. Collins, MBChB, FRACP
Clinical Associate Professor of Renal Medicine
Auckland City Hospital
Auckland, New Zealand
Chapter 82, Oceania Region

H. Terence Cook, MB, BS, FRCPath
Professor, Department of Medicine
Centre for Complement and Inflammation Research
Imperial College London
Hammersmith Hospital
London, United Kingdom
Chapter 29, The Kidney Biopsy

Ricardo Correa-Rotter, MD
Head, Department of Nephrology and Mineral Metabolism
Instituto Nacional de Ciencias Médicas y Nutrición Salvador Zubirán
Mexico City, Mexico
Chapter 66, Peritoneal Dialysis

Shawn E. Cowper, MD
Associate Professor of Dermatology and Pathology
Yale University
New Haven, Connecticut
Chapter 60, Dermatologic Conditions in Kidney Disease

Paolo Cravedi, MD, PhD
IRCCS-Istituto di Ricerche Farmacologiche Mario Negri
Centro Anna Maria Astori, Science and Technology Park Kilometro Rosso
Bergamo, Italy
Chapter 35, Microvascular and Macrovascular Diseases of the Kidney

Vivette D'Agati, MD
Professor of Pathology
Columbia University College of Physicians and Surgeons
Director, Renal Pathology Laboratory
Columbia University Medical Center
New York, New York
Chapter 33, Secondary Glomerular Disease

Mogamat Razeen Davids, MD
Division of Nephrology
Stellenbosch University and Tygerberg Hospital
Cape Town, South Africa
Chapter 27, Interpretation of Electrolyte and Acid-Base Parameters in Blood and Urine

Scott E. Delacroix, Jr., MD
Assistant Professor of Urology
Director of Urologic Oncology
Department of Oncology
Louisiana State University School of Medicine
New Orleans, Louisiana
Chapter 41, Kidney Cancer

Bradley M. Denker, MD
Associate Professor of Medicine
Harvard Medical School
Clinical Chief, Renal Division
Beth Israel Deaconess Medical Center
Boston, Massachusetts
Chapter 68, Plasmapheresis

Thomas A. Depner, MD
Professor of Medicine
Department of Internal Medicine/Nephrology
University of California Davis Health System
Sacramento, California
Chapter 65, Hemodialysis

Thomas D. DuBose, Jr., MD
Professor Emeritus of Medicine
Department of Internal Medicine
Wake Forest School of Medicine
Winston-Salem, North Carolina
Chapter 17, Disorders of Acid-Base Balance

Vinay A. Duddalwar, MD, FRCR
Associate Professor of Clinical Radiology and Urology
Section Chief, Abdominal Imaging
Medical Director, Imaging
USC Norris Comprehensive Cancer Center and Hospital
University of Southern California
Keck School of Medicine
Los Angeles, California
  Chapter 28, Diagnostic Kidney Imaging

Kai-Uwe Eckardt, MD
Professor of Medicine
Chair of Nephrology and Hypertension
Friedrich-Alexander University Erlangen-Nürnberg
Erlangen, Germany
  Chapter 57, Hematologic Aspects of Kidney Disease

Meghan J. Elliott, MD
Nephrology Resident
Department of Medicine
University of Calgary
Calgary, Alberta, Canada
  Chapter 85, Care of the Older Adult with Chronic Kidney Disease

William J. Elliott, MD, PhD
Professor of Preventive Medicine
Internal Medicine and Pharmacology
Pacific Northwest University of Health Sciences
Yakima, Washington
  Chapter 47, Primary and Secondary Hypertension

David H. Ellison, MD
Professor of Internal Medicine
Oregon Health & Science University
Portland, Oregon
  Chapter 51, Diuretics

Michael Emmett, MD
Chief of Internal Medicine
Department of Internal Medicine
Baylor University Medical Center
Dallas, Texas;
Professor of Medicine
Internal Medicine
Texas A&M College of Medicine
Baylor University Medical Center
Denton, Texas;
Clinical Professor of Medicine
University of Texas Southwestern Medical School
Dallas, Texas
  Chapter 25, Approach to the Patient with Kidney Disease

Ronald J. Falk, MD
Chair, Department of Medicine
Director, UNC Kidney Center
The University of North Carolina
Chapel Hill, North Carolina
  Chapter 32, Primary Glomerular Disease

Harold I. Feldman, MD, MSCE
Professor of Epidemiology and Medicine
Perelman School of Medicine
University of Pennsylvania
Philadelphia, Pennsylvania
  Chapter 21, Demographics of Kidney Disease

Bo Feldt-Rasmussen, MD, DMSc
Professor and Head of Clinic
Department of Nephrology
Rigshospitalet University of Copenhagen
Copenhagen, Denmark
  Chapter 39, Diabetic Nephropathy

Robert A. Fenton, PhD
Professor of Molecular Cell Biology
Department of Biomedicine
Aarhus University
Aarhus, Denmark
  Chapter 2, Anatomy of the Kidney
  Chapter 10, Urine Concentration and Dilution
  Chapter 11, The Cell Biology of Vasopressin Action

Andrew Z. Fenves, MD, FACP, FASN
Inpatient Clinical Educator
Massachusetts General Hospital
Associate Professor of Medicine
Harvard Medical School
Boston, Massachusetts
  Chapter 25, Approach to the Patient with Kidney Disease

Kevin W. Finkel, MD, FACP, FASN, FCCM
Department of Internal Medicine
Director, Division of Renal Diseases and Hypertension
University of Texas Health Science Center at Houston
Department of Internal Medicine
Section of Nephrology
The University of Texas MD Anderson Cancer Center
Houston, Texas
  Chapter 42, Onco-Nephrology: Kidney Disease in Patients with Cancer

Paola Fioretto, MD
Associate Professor
Department of Medical and Surgical Sciences
University of Padova Medical School
Padova, Italy
  Chapter 39, Diabetic Nephropathy

Damian G. Fogarty, BSc, MD, FRCP
Consultant Nephrologist
Regional Nephrology and Transplant Unit
Belfast City Hospital at the Belfast Health and Social Care Trust
Belfast, Northern Ireland
  Chapter 62, A Stepped Care Approach to the Management of Chronic Kidney Disease

Denis Fouque, MD, PhD
Professor of Nephrology
Chief, Division of Nephrology
Université Claude Bernard and Centre Hospitalier Lyon Sud
Lyon, France
Chapter 61, Dietary Approaches to Kidney Diseases

Yaacov Frishberg, MD
Director, Pediatric Nephrology
Shaare Zedek Medical Center
The Hebrew University School of Medicine
Jerusalem, Israel
Chapter 76, Renal Replacement Therapy (Dialysis and Transplantation) in Pediatric End-Stage Kidney Disease

Jørgen Frøkiaer, MD, DMSci
Head of Department of Nuclear Medicine and Molecular Imaging
Department of Clinical Medicine
Aarhus University and Aarhus University Hospital
Aarhus, Denmark
Chapter 38, Urinary Tract Obstruction

John W. Funder, MD, PhD, FRCP, FRACP
Distinguished Scholar
Steroid Biology
Hudson Institute of Medical Research
Clayton, Victoria, Australia
Chapter 12, Aldosterone and Mineralocorticoid Receptors: Renal and Extrarenal Roles

Marc Ghannoum, MD
Associate Professor
Specialized Medicine
University of Montréal
Verdun Hospital
Montréal, Quebec, Canada
Chapter 69, Elimination Enhancement of Poisons

Richard E. Gilbert, MBBS, PhD, FRACP, FRCPC, FACP, FASN
Professor of Medicine
University of Toronto
St. Michael's Hospital
Toronto, Ontario, Canada
Chapter 13, Vasoactive Molecules and the Kidney

Paul Goodyer, MD
Professor of Pediatrics
McGill University
Montréal, Quebec, Canada
Chapter 23, Nephron Endowment and Developmental Programming of Blood Pressure and Renal Function

Yoshio N. Hall, MD, MS
Associate Professor of Medicine
Department of Medicine, Division of Nephrology
University of Washington
Seattle, Washington
Chapter 84, Health Disparities in Nephrology

Mitchell L. Halperin, MD
Division of Nephrology
St. Michael's Hospital
University of Toronto
Toronto, Canada
Chapter 27, Interpretation of Electrolyte and Acid-Base Parameters in Blood and Urine

Donna S. Hanes, MD, FACP
Clinical Associate Professor of Medicine
Clerkship Director, Internal Medicine
University of Maryland Medical Systems
Baltimore, Maryland
Chapter 50, Antihypertensive Therapy

Chuan-Ming Hao, MD
Professor
Medicine/Nephrology
Huashan Hospital Fudan University
Shanghai, China
Chapter 81, The Far East

David C. H. Harris, MD, BS, FRACP
Associate Dean and Head of School
Sydney Medical School—Westmead
The University of Sydney
Sydney, New South Wales, Australia
Chapter 82, Oceania Region

Peter C. Harris, PhD
Professor of Biochemistry/Molecular Biology
Professor of Medicine
Nephrology and Hypertension
Mayo Clinic
Rochester, Minnesota
Chapter 46, Cystic Diseases of the Kidney

Raymond C. Harris, MD
Ann and Roscoe Robinson Professor of Medicine
Chief, Division of Nephrology and Hypertension
Vanderbilt University School of Medicine
Nashville, Tennessee
Chapter 14, Arachidonic Acid Metabolites and the Kidney

Richard Haynes, DM, FRCP
Associate Professor
Clinical Trial Service Unit and Epidemiological Studies Unit
Nuffield Department of Population Health
Honorary Consultant in Nephrology
Oxford Kidney Unit
Churchill Hospital
Oxford, United Kingdom
Chapter 56, Cardiovascular Aspects of Kidney Disease

Brenda R. Hemmelgarn, MD, PhD
Professor of Medicine
University of Calgary
Calgary, Alberta, Canada
Chapter 85, Care of the Older Adult with Chronic Kidney Disease

Friedhelm Hildebrandt, MD
Warren E. Grupe Professor of Pediatrics
Harvard Medical School
Investigator, Howard Hughes Medical Institute
Chief, Division of Nephrology
Boston Children's Hospital
Boston, Massachusetts
 Chapter 43, *Genetic Basis of Kidney Disease*

Michelle A. Hladunewich, MD, MSc
Associate Professor of Medicine
University of Toronto
Scientist, Sunnybrook Research Institute
Sunnybrook Health Sciences Centre
Toronto, Ontario, Canada
 Chapter 34, *Overview of Therapy for Glomerular Disease*

Kevin Ho, MD
Associate Professor of Medicine & Clinical and
 Translational Science
Renal-Electrolyte Division
University of Pittsburgh
Pittsburgh, Pennsylvania
 Chapter 87, *Quality Improvement Initiatives in Kidney Disease*

Ewout J. Hoorn, MD, PhD
Associate Professor
Department of Internal Medicine, Division of Nephrology
 and Transplantation
Erasmus Medical Center
Rotterdam, The Netherlands
 Chapter 51, *Diuretics*

Thomas H. Hostetter, MD
Professor of Medicine
Case Western Reserve University School of Medicine
Vice Chairman, Research Services
University Hospitals Case Medical Center
Cleveland, Ohio
 Chapter 54, *The Pathophysiology of Uremia*

Fan-Fan Hou, MD
Director of Guangdong Provincial Institute of Nephrology
Chief and Professor of Division of Nephrology
Nanfang Hospital
Professor of Medicine
Southern Medical University
Guangzhou, China
 Chapter 81, *The Far East*

Chi-yuan Hsu, MD
Professor and Division Chief
Division of Nephrology
University of California, San Francisco
San Francisco, California
 Chapter 20, *Epidemiology of Kidney Disease*

Raymond K. Hsu, MD
Assistant Professor of Medicine
Division of Nephrology
University of California, San Francisco
San Francisco, California
 Chapter 20, *Epidemiology of Kidney Disease*

Holly Hutton, MBBS, FRACP
Department of Nephrology
University of British Columbia
Vancouver, British Columbia, Canada;
Department of Nephrology
Monash Health
Clayton, Victoria, Australia
 Chapter 26, *Laboratory Assessment of Kidney Disease:*
 Glomerular Filtration Rate, Urinalysis, and Proteinuria

Hossein Jadvar, MD, PhD, MPH, MBA, FACNM
Associate Professor of Radiology
Associate Professor of Biomedical Engineering
University of Southern California
Keck School of Medicine
Los Angeles, California
 Chapter 28, *Diagnostic Kidney Imaging*

J. Charles Jennette, MD
Kenneth M. Brinkhous Distinguished Professor and Chair
Department of Pathology and Laboratory Medicine
The University of North Carolina
Chapel Hill, North Carolina
 Chapter 32, *Primary Glomerular Disease*

Eric Jonasch, MD
Associate Professor
Department of Genitourinary Medical Oncology
Division of Cancer Medicine
The University of Texas MD Anderson Cancer Center
Houston, Texas
 Chapter 41, *Kidney Cancer*

Kamel S. Kamel, MD
Division of Nephrology
St. Michael's Hospital
University of Toronto
Toronto, Canada
 Chapter 27, *Interpretation of Electrolyte and Acid-Base*
 Parameters in Blood and Urine

S. Ananth Karumanchi, MD
Professor
Department of Medicine, Obstetrics, and Gynecology
Harvard Medical School
Howard Hughes Medical Institute and Beth Israel
 Deaconess Medical Center
Boston, Massachusetts
 Chapter 49, *Hypertension and Kidney Disease in Pregnancy*

Frieder Keller, MD
Professor of Nephrology
Department of Internal Medicine 1
Ulm University
Ulm, Germany
 Chapter 64, *Drug Dosing Considerations in Patients with*
 Acute Kidney Injury and Chronic Kidney Disease

Carolyn J. Kelly, MD
Professor of Medicine
Associate Dean for Admissions and Student Affairs
University of California, San Diego School of Medicine
La Jolla, California
Chapter 36, Tubulointerstitial Diseases

David K. Klassen, MD
Professor of Medicine
Division of Nephrology, Department of Medicine
University of Maryland School of Medicine
Baltimore, Maryland
Chapter 50, Antihypertensive Therapy

Christine J. Ko, MD
Associate Professor of Dermatology and Pathology
Yale University
New Haven, Connecticut
Chapter 60, Dermatologic Conditions in Kidney Disease

Harbir Singh Kohli, MD, DM
Professor, Nephrology
Post Graduate Institute of Medical Education and Research
Chandigarh, India
Chapter 80, Indian Subcontinent

Curtis K. Kost, Jr., RPh, PhD
Associate Professor
Basic Biomedical Sciences
Sanford School of Medicine
University of South Dakota
Vermillion, South Dakota
Chapter 3, The Renal Circulations and Glomerular Ultrafiltration

Jay L. Koyner, MD
Assistant Professor of Medicine
Division of Nephrology
University of Chicago Medicine
Chicago, Illinois
Chapter 30, Biomarkers in Acute and Chronic Kidney Diseases

L. Spencer Krane, MD
Wake Forest Institute for Regenerative Medicine
Department of Urology
Wake Forest University School of Medicine
Winston-Salem, North Carolina
Chapter 86, Tissue Engineering, Stem Cells, and Cell Therapy in Nephrology

Jordan Kreidberg, MD, PhD
Associate Professor of Pediatrics
Division of Nephrology
Boston Children's Hospital
Harvard Medical School
Boston, Massachusetts
Chapter 1, Embryology of the Kidney

Rajiv Kumar, MBBS
Department of Medicine, Division of Nephrology and Hypertension
Department of Biochemistry and Molecular Biology
Mayo Clinic College of Medicine
Mayo Clinic
Rochester, Minnesota
Chapter 7, The Regulation of Calcium, Magnesium, and Phosphate Excretion by the Kidney

Martin J. Landray, PhD, FRCP, FASN
Professor of Medicine and Epidemiology
Clinical Trial Service Unit and Big Data Institute
Nuffield Department of Population Health
Oxford, United Kingdom
Chapter 56, Cardiovascular Aspects of Kidney Disease

Harold E. Layton, PhD
Professor, Department of Mathematics
Duke University
Durham, North Carolina
Chapter 10, Urine Concentration and Dilution

Timmy Lee, MD, MSPH
Associate Professor of Medicine
Division of Nephrology
University of Alabama at Birmingham
Birmingham, Alabama
Chapter 70, Interventional Nephrology

Colin R. Lenihan, MB BCh BAO, PhD
Clinical Assistant Professor of Medicine
Division of Nephrology
Stanford University
Stanford, California
Chapter 72, Clinical Management of the Adult Kidney Transplant Recipient

Moshe Levi, MD
Professor of Medicine, Bioengineering, Physiology, and Biophysics
Division of Renal Diseases and Hypertension
University of Colorado AMC
Aurora, Colorado
Chapter 24, Aging and Kidney Disease

Adeera Levin, BSc, MD, FRCPC
Professor of Medicine (Nephrology)
University of British Columbia
Vancouver, British Columbia, Canada;
Director
BC Provincial Renal Agency
British Columbia, Canada
Chapter 26, Laboratory Assessment of Kidney Disease: Glomerular Filtration Rate, Urinalysis, and Proteinuria

Shih-Hua Lin, MD
Division of Nephrology
Department of Medicine
Tri-Service General Hospital
National Defense Medical Center
Taipei, Taiwan, R.O.C.
  Chapter 27, Interpretation of Electrolyte and Acid-Base Parameters in Blood and Urine

Bengt Lindholm, MD, PhD
Adjunct Professor
Karolinska Institutet
Stockholm, Sweden
  Chapter 58, Endocrine Aspects of Chronic Kidney Disease

Kathleen Liu, MD, PhD, MAS
Associate Professor
Departments of Medicine and Anesthesia
University of California, San Francisco
San Francisco, California
  Chapter 67, Critical Care Nephrology

Valerie A. Luyckx, MBBCh, MSc
Associate Professor of Nephrology
University of Alberta
Edmonton, Alberta, Canada
  Chapter 23, Nephron Endowment and Developmental Programming of Blood Pressure and Renal Function

David A. Maddox, PhD, FASN
Professor of Internal Medicine and Basic Biomedical Sciences
Sanford School of Medicine
University of South Dakota
Coordinator, Research and Development (retired)
VA Medical Center
Sioux Falls VA Health Care System
Sioux Falls, South Dakota
  Chapter 3, The Renal Circulations and Glomerular Ultrafiltration

Yoshiro Maezawa, MD, PhD
Assistant Professor
Clinical Cell Biology and Medicine
Chiba University Graduate School of Medicine
Chiba, Japan
  Chapter 1, Embryology of the Kidney

Karine Mardini, B.Pharm
Department of Pharmacy
University of Montréal
Montréal, Quebec, Canada
  Chapter 69, Elimination Enhancement of Poisons

Peter W. Mathieson, MB, ChB(Hons), PhD, FRCP, FMedSci
President
President's Office
The University of Hong Kong
Hong Kong, China
  Chapter 4, The Podocyte

Gary R. Matzke, PharmD
Professor and Founding Director, ACCP/ASHP/VCU Congressional Health Care Policy Fellow Program
Virginia Commonwealth University School of Pharmacy
Department of Pharmacotherapy and Outcomes Sciences
Richmond, Virginia
  Chapter 64, Drug Dosing Considerations in Patients with Acute Kidney Injury and Chronic Kidney Disease

Ivan D. Maya, MD
Associate Professor of Medicine
Department of Medicine
University of Central Florida
Orlando, Florida
  Chapter 70, Interventional Nephrology

Sharon E. Maynard, MD
Associate Professor
Department of Medicine
Lehigh Valley Health Network
University of South Florida
Morsani College of Medicine
Allentown, Pennsylvania
  Chapter 49, Hypertension and Kidney Disease in Pregnancy

Alicia A. McDonough, PhD
Professor of Cell and Neurobiology
Keck School of Medicine
University of Southern California
Los Angeles, California
  Chapter 5, Metabolic Basis of Solute Transport

Rajnish Mehrotra, MD
Section Head, Nephrology
Harborview Medical Center
Division of Nephrology
University of Washington
Seattle, Washington
  Chapter 66, Peritoneal Dialysis

Timothy W. Meyer, MD
Professor of Medicine
Stanford University
Stanford, California;
Staff Physician
Department of Medicine
VA Palo Alto Health Care System
Palo Alto, California
  Chapter 54, The Pathophysiology of Uremia

William E. Mitch, MD
Professor of Medicine and Nephrology
Baylor College of Medicine
Houston, Texas
  Chapter 61, Dietary Approaches to Kidney Diseases

Orson W. Moe, MD
Professor of Internal Medicine, Division of Nephrology
University of Texas Southwestern Medical Center
Director
Charles and Jane Pak Center for Mineral Metabolism and Clinical Research
University of Texas Southwestern Medical Center
Dallas, Texas
  Chapter 8, Renal Handling of Organic Solutes
  Chapter 40, Urolithiasis

Sharon M. Moe, MD
Stuart A. Kleit Professor of Medicine
Professor of Anatomy and Cell Biology
Director, Division of Nephrology
Indiana University School of Medicine
Indianapolis, Indiana
  Chapter 55, Chronic Kidney Disease–Mineral Bone Disorder

Bruce A. Molitoris, MD
Professor of Medicine
Division of Nephrology, Department of Medicine
Director, Indiana Center for Biologic Microscopy
Indiana University School of Medicine
Indianapolis, Indiana
  Chapter 31, Acute Kidney Injury

Alvin H. Moss, MD
Professor of Medicine
Department of Medicine, Section of Nephrology
West Virginia University
Director
Center for Health Ethics and Law
West Virginia University
Medical Director
Supportive Care Service
West Virginia University Hospital
Morgantown, West Virginia
  Chapter 83, Ethical Dilemmas Facing Nephrology: Past, Present, and Future

David B. Mount, MD, FRCPC
Assistant Professor of Medicine
Harvard Medical School
Associate Division Chief, Renal Division
Brigham and Women's Hospital
Attending Physician, Renal Division
VA Boston Healthcare System
Boston, Massachusetts
  Chapter 6, Transport of Sodium, Chloride, and Potassium
  Chapter 18, Disorders of Potassium Balance

Karen A. Munger, PhD
Associate Professor of Internal Medicine
Sanford School of Medicine
University of South Dakota
Coordinator, Research and Development
VA Medical Center
Sioux Falls VA Health Care System
Sioux Falls, South Dakota
  Chapter 3, The Renal Circulations and Glomerular Ultrafiltration

Patrick H. Nachman, MD
Professor of Medicine
Division of Nephrology and Hypertension
Department of Medicine
UNC Kidney Center
The University of North Carolina
Chapel Hill, North Carolina
  Chapter 32, Primary Glomerular Disease

Saraladevi Naicker, MD, PhD
Professor
Department of Internal Medicine
University of the Witwatersrand
Johannesburg, South Africa
  Chapter 78, Africa

Sagren Naidoo, MD
Consultant Nephrologist
Department of Internal Medicine
Division of Nephrology
Charlotte Maxeke Johannesburg Academic Hospital
University of the Witwatersrand
Johannesburg, South Africa
  Chapter 78, Africa

Eric G. Neilson, MD
Vice President for Medical Affairs
Lewis Landsberg Dean
Professor of Medicine and Cell and Molecular Biology
Northwestern University Feinberg School of Medicine
Chicago, Illinois
  Chapter 36, Tubulointerstitial Diseases

Lindsay E. Nicolle, MD
Professor, Department of Internal Medicine and Medical Microbiology
University of Manitoba
Winnipeg, Manitoba, Canada
  Chapter 37, Urinary Tract Infection in Adults

Ann M. O'Hare, MD, MA
Associate Professor of Medicine
University of Washington
Staff Physician
Department of Medicine
Department of Veterans Affairs
Seattle, Washington
  Chapter 85, Care of the Older Adult with Chronic Kidney Disease

Daniel B. Ornt, MD
Clinical Professor
Department of Medicine
University of Rochester Medical Center
Vice President and Dean
College of Health Sciences and Technology
Rochester Institute of Technology
Rochester, New York
  Chapter 65, Hemodialysis

Manuel Palacín, PhD
Full Professor, Biochemistry and Molecular Biology
Universitat de Barcelona
Group Leader
CIBERER (The Spanish Network Center for Rare Diseases)
Group Leader
Molecular Medicine Program
Institute for Research in Biomedicine of Barcelona
Barcelona, Spain
   Chapter 8, Renal Handling of Organic Solutes

Paul M. Palevsky, MD
Chief, Renal Section, VA Pittsburgh Healthcare System
Professor of Medicine and Clinical and Translational Science
Renal-Electrolyte Division, Department of Medicine
University of Pittsburgh School of Medicine
Pittsburgh, Pennsylvania
   Chapter 31, Acute Kidney Injury

Suzanne L. Palmer, MD, FACP
Professor of Clinical Radiology and Medicine
Chief, Body Imaging Division
University of Southern California
Keck School of Medicine
Keck Hospital of USC
Los Angeles, California
   Chapter 28, Diagnostic Kidney Imaging

Chirag R. Parikh, MD, PhD, FACP
Associate Professor of Medicine
Director, Program of Applied Translational Research
Yale University and Veterans Affairs Medical Center
New Haven, Connecticut
   Chapter 30, Biomarkers in Acute and Chronic Kidney Diseases

Hans-Henrik Parving, MD, DMSc
Professor and Chief Physician
Department of Medical Endocrinology
Rigshospitalet Copenhagen
University of Copenhagen
Copenhagen, Denmark
   Chapter 39, Diabetic Nephropathy

Jaakko Patrakka, MD, PhD
Assistant Professor
Department of Medical Biochemistry and Biophysics
Karolinska Institute, Nephrology Fellow
Division of Nephrology
Karolinska University Hospital
Stockholm, Sweden
   Chapter 44, Inherited Disorders of the Glomerulus

David Pearce, MD
Professor of Medicine and Cellular and Molecular Pharmacology
University of California at San Francisco
Chief, Division of Nephrology
San Francisco General Hospital
San Francisco, California
   Chapter 12, Aldosterone and Mineralocorticoid Receptors: Renal and Extrarenal Roles

Aldo J. Peixoto, MD
Professor of Medicine
Department of Medicine
Section of Nephrology
Yale University School of Medicine
New Haven, Connecticut
   Chapter 47, Primary and Secondary Hypertension

William F. Pendergraft, III, MD, PhD
Assistant Professor of Medicine
Division of Nephrology and Hypertension
Department of Medicine
UNC Kidney Center
The University of North Carolina
Chapel Hill, North Carolina;
Visiting Postdoctoral Scholar, Hacohen Group
Broad Institute of Harvard and MIT
Cambridge, Massachusetts
   Chapter 32, Primary Glomerular Disease

Norberto Perico, MD
IRCCS-Istituto di Ricerche Farmacologiche Mario Negri
Bergamo, Italy
   Chapter 53, Mechanisms and Consequences of Proteinuria

Jeppe Praetorius, MD, PhD, DMSc
Professor of Medical Cell Biology
Department of Biomedicine
Aarhus University
Aarhus, Denmark
   Chapter 2, Anatomy of the Kidney

Susan E. Quaggin, MD
Professor and Chief, Division of Nephrology and Hypertension
Department of Medicine
Director, Feinberg Cardiovascular Research Institute
Feinberg School of Medicine
Northwestern University
Chicago, Illinois
   Chapter 1, Embryology of the Kidney

L. Darryl Quarles, MD
UTMG Endowed Professor of Nephrology
Director, Division of Nephrology
Associate Dean for Research, College of Medicine
University of Tennessee Health Science Center
Memphis, Tennessee
   Chapter 63, Therapeutic Approach to Chronic Kidney Disease–Mineral Bone Disorder

Jai Radhakrishnan, MD, MS
Professor of Medicine
Columbia University Medical Center
Associate Division Chief for Clinical Affairs
Division of Nephrology
New York Presbyterian Hospital
New York, New York
 Chapter 33, Secondary Glomerular Disease

Rawi Ramadan, MD
Director, Medical Transplantation Unit
Department of Nephrology and Hypertension
Rambam Health Care Campus
Haifa, Israel
 Chapter 79, Near and Middle East

Heather N. Reich, MD CM, PhD, FRCP(C)
Associate Professor of Medicine
University of Toronto
Clinician Scientist and Staff Nephrologist
Medicine
University Health Network
Toronto, Ontario, Canada
 Chapter 34, Overview of Therapy for Glomerular Disease

Andrea Remuzzi, MD
University of Bergamo
IRCCS-Istituto di Ricerche Farmacologiche Mario Negri
Bergamo, Italy
 Chapter 53, Mechanisms and Consequences of Proteinuria

Giuseppe Remuzzi, MD, FRCP
IRCCS-Istituto di Ricerche Farmacologiche Mario Negri
Centro Anna Maria Astori, Science and Technology Park
 Kilometro Rosso
Unit of Nephrology and Dialysis
Azienda Ospedaliera Papa Giovanni XXIII
University of Milan
Bergamo, Italy
 *Chapter 35, Microvascular and Macrovascular Diseases
 of the Kidney*
 Chapter 53, Mechanisms and Consequences of Proteinuria

Leonardo V. Riella, MD, PhD, FASN
Assistant Professor of Medicine
Department of Medicine, Renal Division
Harvard Medical School
Brigham and Women's Hospital
Schuster Family Transplantation Research Center
Boston, Massachusetts
 Chapter 71, Transplantation Immunobiology
 Chapter 77, Latin America

Miquel C. Riella, MD, PhD
Professor of Medicine
Evangelic School of Medicine
Catholic University of Parana
Curitiba, Brazil
 Chapter 77, Latin America

Choni Rinat, MD
Pediatric Nephrology
Shaare Zedek Medical Center
The Hebrew University School of Medicine
Jerusalem, Israel
 *Chapter 76, Renal Replacement Therapy (Dialysis and
 Transplantation) in Pediatric End-Stage Kidney Disease*

Norman D. Rosenblum, MD, FRCPC
Staff Nephrologist and Senior Scientist
The Hospital for Sick Children, Toronto
Professor of Pediatrics, Physiology, and Laboratory
 Medicine and Pathobiology
Canada Research Chair in Developmental Nephrology
University of Toronto
Toronto, Ontario, Canada
 *Chapter 73, Malformation of the Kidney: Structural and
 Functional Consequences*

Peter Rossing, MD, DMSc
Professor and Chief Physician
Steno Diabetes Center
University of Copenhagen
Copenhagen, Denmark;
Aarhus University
Aarhus, Denmark
 Chapter 39, Diabetic Nephropathy

Dvora Rubinger, MD
Associate Professor of Medicine
Department of Nephrology
Hadassah Hebrew University Medical Center
Jerusalem, Israel
 Chapter 79, Near and Middle East

Piero Ruggenenti, MD
IRCCS-Istituto di Ricerche Farmacologiche Mario Negri
Centro Anna Maria Astori, Science and Technology Park
 Kilometro Rosso
Unit of Nephrology and Dialysis
Azienda Ospedaliera Papa Giovanni XXIII
Bergamo, Italy
 *Chapter 35, Microvascular and Macrovascular Diseases
 of the Kidney*

Ernesto Sabath, MD
Renal Department
Hospital General de Querétaro
Queretaro, Mexico
 Chapter 68, Plasamapheresis

Khashayar Sakhaee, MD
Department of Internal Medicine
Charles and Jane Pak Center for Mineral Metabolism
 and Clinical Research
University of Texas Southwestern Medical Center
Dallas, Texas
 Chapter 40, Urolithiasis

Vinay Sakhuja, MD, DM
Department of Nephrology
Post Graduate Institute of Medical Education and Research
Chandigarh, India
Chapter 80, Indian Subcontinent

Alan D. Salama, MBBS, PhD, FRCP
Professor of Nephrology
University College London Centre for Nephrology
Royal Free Hospital
London, United Kingdom
Chapter 29, The Kidney Biopsy

Jeff M. Sands, MD
Professor, Renal Division
Department of Medicine and Department of Physiology
Emory University School of Medicine
Atlanta, Georgia
Chapter 10, Urine Concentration and Dilution

Fernando Santos, MD
Professor of Pediatrics
Chair, Department of Medicine
University of Oviedo
Chairman of Pediatrics
Hospital Universitario Central de Asturias
Oviedo, Asturias, Spain
Chapter 75, Fluid, Electrolyte, and Acid-Base Disorders in Children

Anjali Saxena, MD
Clinical Assistant Professor of Medicine
Internal Medicine
Stanford University
Stanford, California;
Director of Peritoneal Dialysis
Internal Medicine
Santa Clara Valley Medical Center
San Jose, California
Chapter 66, Peritoneal Dialysis

Mohamed H. Sayegh, MD
Senior Lecturer, Harvard Medical School
Schuster Family Transplantation Research Center
Brigham and Women's Hospital
Boston, Massachusetts;
Dean and Vice President of Medical Affairs
Professor of Medicine and Immunology
Faculty of Medicine
American University of Beirut
Beirut, Lebanon
Chapter 71, Transplantation Immunobiology

Franz Schaefer, MD
Professor of Pediatrics
Head, Division of Pediatric Nephrology and KFH Children's Kidney Center
Heidelberg University Medical Center
Heidelberg, Germany
Chapter 74, Diseases of the Kidney and Urinary Tract in Children

John C. Schwartz, MD
Nephrology Division
Department of Internal Medicine
Baylor University Medical Center
Dallas, Texas
Chapter 25, Approach to the Patient with Kidney Disease

Rizaldy P. Scott, MS, PhD
Division of Nephrology and Hypertension
Department of Medicine
Feinberg School of Medicine
Northwestern University
Chicago, Illinois
Chapter 1, Embryology of the Kidney

Stuart J. Shankland, MD, MBA, FRCPC, FASN, FAHA, FACP
Professor of Medicine
Belding H. Scribner Endowed Chair in Medicine
Head, Division of Nephrology
University of Washington
Seattle, Washington
Chapter 4, The Podocyte

Asif A. Sharfuddin, MD
Associate Professor of Clinical Medicine
Division of Nephrology, Department of Medicine
Indiana University School of Medicine
Indianapolis, Indiana
Chapter 31, Acute Kidney Injury

Prabhleen Singh, MD
Assistant Professor of Medicine
Division of Nephrology and Hypertension
University of California, San Diego
VA San Diego Healthcare System
San Diego, California
Chapter 5, Metabolic Basis of Solute Transport

Karl L. Skorecki, MD, FRCP(C), FASN
Annie Chutick Professor and Chair in Medicine (Nephrology)
Technion—Israel Institute of Technology
Director of Medicine and Research Development
Rambam Health Care Campus
Haifa, Israel
Chapter 15, Disorders of Sodium Balance

Itzchak N. Slotki, MD
Associate Professor of Medicine
Hadassah Hebrew University of Jerusalem
Director, Division of Adult Nephrology
Shaare Zedek Medical Center
Jerusalem, Israel
Chapter 15, Disorders of Sodium Balance

Miroslaw J. Smogorzewski, MD, PhD
Associate Professor of Medicine
Division of Nephrology, Department of Medicine
University of Southern California, Keck School
 of Medicine
Los Angeles, California
 *Chapter 19, Disorders of Calcium, Magnesium, and
 Phosphate Balance*

Sandeep S. Soman, MD
Division of Nephrology and Hypertension
Henry Ford Hospital
Detroit, Michigan
 Chapter 87, Quality Improvement Initiatives in Kidney Disease

Stuart M. Sprague, DO
Chief, Division of Nephrology and Hypertension
Department of Medicine
NorthShore University HealthSystem
Evanston, Illinois;
Professor of Medicine
University of Chicago Pritzker School of Medicine
Chicago, Illinois
 Chapter 55, Chronic Kidney Disease–Mineral Bone Disorder

Peter Stenvinkel, MD, PhD, FENA
Professor of Renal Medicine
Karolinska Institutet
Stockholm, Sweden
 Chapter 58, Endocrine Aspects of Chronic Kidney Disease

Jason R. Stubbs, MD
Associate Professor of Medicine
Division of Nephrology and Hypertension
The Kidney Institute
University of Kansas Medical Center
Kansas City, Kansas
 *Chapter 19, Disorders of Calcium, Magnesium, and
 Phosphate Balance*

**Maarten W. Taal, MBChB, MMed, MD,
FCP(SA), FRCP**
Professor of Medicine
Division of Medical Sciences and Graduate
 Entry Medicine
University of Nottingham
Honorary Consultant Nephrologist
Department of Renal Medicine
Royal Derby Hospital
Derby, United Kingdom
 Chapter 22, Risk Factors and Chronic Kidney Disease
 *Chapter 52, Adaptation to Nephron Loss and Mechanisms of
 Progression in Chronic Kidney Disease*
 *Chapter 62, A Stepped Care Approach to the Management of
 Chronic Kidney Disease*

Manjula Kurella Tamura, MD, MPH
Associate Professor of Medicine/Nephrology
Division of Nephrology, Stanford University School
 of Medicine
VA Palo Alto Health Care System Geriatrics Research
 Education and Clinical Center
Palo Alto, California
 Chapter 59, Neurologic Aspects of Kidney Disease

Jane C. Tan, MD, PhD
Associate Professor of Medicine
Division of Nephrology
Stanford University
Stanford, California
 *Chapter 72, Clinical Management of the Adult Kidney
 Transplant Recipient*

Stephen C. Textor, MD
Professor of Medicine
Division of Hypertension and Nephrology
Mayo Clinic College of Medicine
Mayo Clinic
Rochester, Minnesota
 *Chapter 48, Renovascular Hypertension and Ischemic
 Nephropathy*

Ravi Thadhani, MD, MPH
Professor of Medicine
Harvard Medical School
Chief, Nephrology Section
Massachsetts General Hospital
Boston, Massachusetts
 Chapter 49, Hypertension and Kidney Disease in Pregnancy

James R. Thompson, PhD
Department of Physiology, Biophysics, and Bioengineering
Department of Biochemistry and Molecular Biology
Mayo Clinic College of Medicine
Mayo Clinic
Rochester, Minnesota
 *Chapter 7, The Regulation of Calcium, Magnesium, and
 Phosphate Excretion by the Kidney*

Scott C. Thomson, MD
Professor of Medicine
University of California, San Diego
Chief of Nephrology Section
Department of Medicine
VA San Diego Healthcare System
San Diego, California
 Chapter 5, Metabolic Basis of Solute Transport

Vicente E. Torres, MD, PhD
Professor of Medicine
Nephrology and Hypertension
Mayo Clinic
Rochester, Minnesota
 Chapter 46, Cystic Diseases of the Kidney

Karl Tryggvason, MD, PhD
Professor of Medical Chemistry
Department of Medical Biochemistry and Biophysics
Karolinska Institutet
Stockholm, Sweden
  Chapter 44, Inherited Disorders of the Glomerulus

Joseph G. Verbalis, MD
Professor of Medicine
Georgetown University
Chief, Endocrinology and Metabolism
Georgetown University Hospital
Washington, DC
  Chapter 16, Disorders of Water Balance

Jill W. Verlander, DVM
Scientist
Director of College of Medicine Core Electron
  Microscopy Lab
Division of Nephrology, Hypertension, and
  Transplantation
University of Florida College of Medicine
Gainesville, Florida
  Chapter 9, Renal Acidification Mechanisms

Ron Wald, MDCM, MPH
Associate Professor of Medicine
University of Toronto
Staff Nephrologist
Department of Medicine
St. Michael's Hospital
Toronto, Ontario, Canada
  Chapter 67, Critical Care Nephrology

Walter G. Wasser, MD
Attending Physician, Division of Nephrology
Mayanei HaYeshua Medical Center
Bnei Brak, Israel;
Rambam Health Care Campus
Haifa, Israel
  Chapter 50, Antihypertensive Therapy
  Chapter 81, The Far East

I. David Weiner, MD
Professor of Medicine
Division of Nephrology, Hypertension, and
  Transplantation
University of Florida College of Medicine
Nephrology and Hypertension Section
North Florida/South Georgia Veterans Health System
Gainesville, Florida
  Chapter 9, Renal Acidification Mechanisms

Matthew R. Weir, MD
Professor and Director
Division of Nephrology, Department of Medicine
University of Maryland School of Medicine
Baltimore, Maryland
  Chapter 50, Antihypertensive Therapy

Steven D. Weisbord, MD, MSc
Staff Physician, Renal Section and Center for Health
  Equity Research and Promotion
VA Pittsburgh Healthcare System
Associate Professor of Medicine and Clinical and
  Translational Science
Renal-Electrolyte Division, Department of Medicine
University of Pittsburgh School of Medicine
Pittsburgh, Pennsylvania
  Chapter 31, Acute Kidney Injury

David C. Wheeler, MD
Professor of Kidney Medicine
Centre for Nephrology
Division of Medicine
University College London
London, United Kingdom
  Chapter 56, Cardiovascular Aspects of Kidney Disease

Christopher S. Wilcox, MD, PhD
Division Chief, Professor of Medicine
George E. Schreiner Chair of Nephrology
Director of the Hypertension, Kidney, and Vascular
  Research Center
Georgetown University
Washington, DC
  Chapter 51, Diuretics

F. Perry Wilson, MD, MSCE
Assistant Professor of Medicine (Nephrology)
Yale School of Medicine
New Haven, Connecticut
  Chapter 21, Demographics of Kidney Disease

Christopher G. Wood, MD
Professor and Deputy Chairman
Douglas E. Johnson, MD Endowed Professorship
  in Urology
Department of Urology
The University of Texas MD Anderson Cancer Center
Houston, Texas
  Chapter 41, Kidney Cancer

Stephen H. Wright, PhD
Professor, Department of Physiology
University of Arizona
Tucson, Arizona
  Chapter 8, Renal Handling of Organic Solutes

Jerry Yee, MD
Division Head
Division of Nephrology and Hypertension
Henry Ford Hospital
Detroit, Michigan
  Chapter 87, Quality Improvement Initiatives in Kidney Disease

Jane Y. Yeun, MD
Clinical Professor of Medicine
Department of Internal Medicine, Division of Nephrology
University of California Davis Health System
Sacramento, California;
Staff Nephrologist
Medical Service
Sacramento Veterans Administration Medical Center
Mather, California
 Chapter 65, Hemodialysis

Alan S.L. Yu, MB, BChir
Harry Statland and Solon Summerfield Professor
 of Medicine
Director, Division of Nephrology and Hypertension
 and The Kidney Institute
University of Kansas Medical Center
Kansas City, Kansas
 *Chapter 19, Disorders of Calcium, Magnesium, and
 Phosphate Balance*

Ming-Zhi Zhang, MD
Assistant Professor of Medicine
Vanderbilt University
Nashville, Tennessee
 Chapter 14, Arachidonic Acid Metabolites and the Kidney

Foreword

Ten quadrennial editions and counting! This latest edition of Brenner and Rector's *The Kidney*, which comes 40 years after the first, is also the first in which I have had no formal role. The work of editing is now in the very capable hands of five exceptionally gifted and internationally dispersed former colleagues. It is perhaps fitting then to leave behind something of the history of how this textbook came into being. The year was 1972, the setting the Veterans Administration Medical Center at Fort Miley, perched on a high bluff overlooking the Golden Gate Bridge at the entrance to San Francisco Bay. I was then in my third year beyond renal physiology fellowship training, holding the position as Chief, Nephrology Section, overseeing a faculty of four and a single laboratory devoted to basic kidney research. Exploiting surface glomeruli in a unique strain of Wistar rats, using specially designed micropuncture techniques, our now classical studies of glomerular hemodynamics and permselectivity propelled me up the academic ladder such that a full professorship in the University of California system was soon earned. I was so self-confident and ambitious that new challenges and adventures were eagerly sought and considered.

But the one that presented itself on a Saturday morning in late 1972 could hardly have been imagined. After reviewing the week's laboratory data with my research team, I wandered, as I often did, into the nearby office of the Chair of Medicine, Marvin H. Sleisenger, whose warm and supportive words were always a treasured source of guidance and encouragement. On this particular morning's visit, I saw on his desk before him reams of long vertical galley proof of what was soon to become the first edition of a new textbook on gastroenterology, co-edited with John Fordtran. How wonderful it must feel, I remarked, to be in the position to oversee the organization and synthesis of a major field of internal medicine. He indeed expressed great pride and satisfaction in dealing with this challenge and, to my complete amazement, gazed up at me and suggested that this might be the appropriate time in my career to undertake a similar responsibility for a large-scale academic work in nephrology.

Flattered, of course, I left his office with little belief that I had the knowledge or capability to take on so formidable a challenge at this relatively early stage in my career. Not more than a week later, however, Albert Meier, Senior Editor at W.B. Saunders Publishing Company, was in my office urging me to set aside my reservations and undertake the responsibility for putting together a comprehensive compendium of nephrology, from basic science to clinical diagnosis and treatment of kidney disease. Weeks passed without decision into early 1973, when I learned that Floyd C. Rector, Jr., a world-renowned academic nephrologist, was moving to San Francisco to direct the Renal Division at the University of California, San Francisco. Imagine my excitement at the prospect of collaborating with this brilliant physician-scientist on a project of this magnitude and importance. Upon my sharing the notion with him, Dr. Rector was quick to agree that a two-volume textbook of nephrology based on fundamental physiologic principles was indeed needed, and we soon informed Saunders that a detailed outline of the scope and organization that reflected our combined personal insights and imagination would soon be forthcoming. All this was achieved in an informal 4-hour session in the living room of my Mill Valley home, where, over a lovely bottle of Napa Valley cabernet sauvignon and delicious, warm canapés prepared by my wife, Jane, we sketched out the five-section structure of a book that would remain unaltered over seven editions, namely, "Elements of Normal Renal Function," "Disturbances in Control of Body Fluid Volume and Composition," "Pathogenesis of Renal Disease," "Pathophysiology of Renal Disease," and "Management of the Patient with Renal Failure." Over the next few weeks, we added the filigree of specific chapter titles, prospective authors, timelines, and our shared editorial responsibilities and submitted the operational plan to Saunders for their executive consideration. Enthusiastic approval and contracts soon followed, and we were then busy with formal letters of invitation to authors (no e-mail in those days) for 49 chapters in nearly 2000 printed pages, with not a single turndown.

The first edition of *The Kidney* debuted at the ninth annual meeting of the American Society of Nephrology in November 1975, bearing the publication date of 1976. Acceptance was instantaneous and robust. Three subsequent editions with Dr. Rector appeared in 1980, 1984, and 1988, each extensively revised and expanded to reflect the remarkable progress in the field. I then served as sole editor for four editions, including an extensive structural redesign for the eighth edition, which consisted of 70 chapters in 12 sections. Among the newly crafted sections were the timely themes of "Epidemiology and Risk Factors in Kidney Disease," "Genetic Basis of Kidney Disease," and "Frontiers in Nephrology." The eighth edition also displayed cover art, tables, and figures redrawn in house in multicolor format and a fully functional electronic edition. In the preface to this eighth edition, which appeared in 2008, I wrote, "Just as blazing embers eventually grow dimmer, I recognize that now is the appropriate time to begin the orderly transition of responsibility for future editions…to a new generation of editors." An international team consisting of Glenn M. Chertow, Philip A. Marsden, Karl L. Skorecki, Maarten W. Taal, and Alan S. L. Yu joined me in crafting the ninth edition, to which two major new sections were added, "Pediatric Nephrology" and "Global Considerations in Kidney Disease." And for this tenth edition, which you are now reading, these five editors have operated fully independently in producing this extensively updated and further expanded latest edition, featuring several novel new chapters, by far the best ever!

In addition to the refinements mentioned, what has come to be known as the "Brenner and Rector" project has grown into a very well received library of nephrology, consisting of discrete companion volumes designed to delve more deeply into specific areas of readership interest, including *Therapy in Nephrology and Hypertension*; *Chronic Kidney Disease, Dialysis, and Transplantation*; *Hypertension*; *Acute Renal Failure*; *Acid-Base and Electrolyte Disorders*; *Diagnostic Atlas of Renal Pathology*; *Molecular and Genetic Basis of Renal Disease*, and *Pocket Companion to Brenner and Rector's The Kidney*.

Nephrology has evolved dramatically over these past 40 years and will surely continue at an ever-quickening pace in the future. This will necessitate a full thrust into multimedia electronic formats such that updating new developments will appear more and more as a continuum. This will surely require new tools and editorial flexibility not yet tested. But therein may lie the project's greatest challenge.

Looking back, I could hardly have imagined the enormous success and respect this textbook project has enjoyed. Of course, full credit rests entirely with the authors of the chapters in each edition, whose enormous commitments of time and effort provided the outstanding scholarship and synthesis their respective areas demanded, along with invaluable comprehensive bibliographies, all of which served our devoted readership so well. My gratitude to them, our editorial staff, and the readers for their generous feedback over the years is unbounded. Playing a part in documenting the ever-more complex and expanding disciplines of renal science and medicine is among my life's greatest pleasures and challenges. If only I could again be a young student and have this magnificent new edition introduce me to the kidney's many wonders and enigmas.

Barry M. Brenner, MD

Preface

The tenth edition of *The Kidney* represents a turning point in the more than 40-year history of what has rightfully become a classic in nephrology. Barry Morton Brenner, co–founding editor with his distinguished colleague, Floyd Rector, and sole editor for the fourth through eighth editions, has shepherded an orderly transition of editorial stewardship to five of his fortunate trainees. We served as co-editors with Dr. Brenner on the ninth edition, for which Maarten W. Taal was a lead editor, and have now been fully entrusted with this precious legacy, buoyed by the mentorship and training that we have each received from Dr. Brenner.

The same sense of honor, mixed with trepidation, responsibility, and pride, that accompanied each of us as we entered the vaunted nephrology clinical and research program in Dr. Brenner's division at Brigham and Women's Hospital now accompanies us as we accept into our hands this "labor of love." Although this is the first edition for which Dr. Brenner is not an editor, his presence is palpable throughout the book. A fascinating history of *The Kidney* is described in the foreword by Dr. Brenner, and the narrative very much follows the exciting history of scientific discovery and clinical advances in the rather young clinical specialty of nephrology and our emerging knowledge of kidney biology. Dr. Brenner's imprint is also evident in so many of his own scientific discoveries and insights that have transformed our understanding of all aspects of the kidney in health and disease, as described by the authors throughout all the sections of the book. *The Kidney* continues to combine authoritative coverage of the most important topics of relevance to readers worldwide with the excitement of "a work in progress" presenting novel and transformative insights based on basic and clinical research and clinical paradigms that inform and improve medical care to patients with kidney disease in every corner of the world.

The more than 200 authors with whom we have had the great privilege of working have succeeded in transmitting not only a wealth of information, but also a sense of passion for the topics at hand. We hope that the reader will readily identify for each author the specific attraction that draws the author closer to the subject. These are myriad and diverse, ranging from the sheer and exquisite beauty of the architecture, structure, and substructure of the renal system, to the intricacies of cellular and molecular function, alongside advances in our understanding of disease pathogenesis at the most fundamental level, coupled with the opportunity to offer lifesaving clinical management with a global health perspective. Indeed, the authors reflect an international fellowship of dedicated researchers, scientists, and health professionals who find their expression in narrative text, images, illustrations, Web links, review questions, and references that constitute this tenth edition of *The Kidney*.

Most of all, the book is imbued with the inspiration of Dr. Brenner. We feel that it is this ingredient that guarantees the continued success of *The Kidney* in an era when other textbooks in all specialties are supplanted by a morass of other information sources. We, the editors and publishers, together with our authors, believe in the cardinal importance of a coherent and updated source of empowering information for students and devotees of the kidney, whether in the professional, teaching, or research domain.

To this end, the ninth edition of *The Kidney*, with Maarten W. Taal as lead editor, introduced several major changes that have proven enormously successful. Therefore we have retained and extended these innovations in the tenth edition. As befitting a living textbook, all chapters have been extensively updated or entirely rewritten. All of the authors are authorities in their respective fields, and many have accompanied *The Kidney* for several editions. However, new authors have been invited to provide refreshing perspectives on existing topics or to introduce brand-new areas relevant to kidney biology and health. One of the many examples is thorough consideration of our completely transformed understanding of sodium balance, resulting from the discovery of sodium stores whose very existence had been unknown and whose fluxes are under complex hormonal and growth factor regulation. By combining the classical and authoritative with transformative discovery and perspectives, *The Kidney* has positioned itself as the "go-to" reference and also the leading learning resource for kidney health and disease throughout the world. For example, a section on pediatric kidney disease was included in the ninth edition, and the positive feedback we received resulted in greater emphasis in the tenth edition. The extension of *The Kidney* into pediatric kidney disease will allow individuals and institutions throughout the world, sometimes with limited resources, to access information from a learning resource that covers kidney health and disease from pre-conception, through fetal and infant health, childhood, adulthood, and into old age. Similarly, the section on global perspectives has been expanded, and the chapter on ethical challenges has been deepened.

A number of practical considerations were also taken into account in the production of the tenth edition. Positive feedback and reviews have reinforced the overall organization into 14 sections and 87 chapters that take the reader from normal structure and function through to current and future challenges in the concluding section.

The authors have been asked to choose 50 key references for their respective chapters, whose citations will appear in the print edition. The online edition will in turn offer access to the full repertoire of references for each chapter, allowing scholarly primary assessment of each subject. As a new resource, we have included a set of board review–style questions for those using *The Kidney* in preparation for certification and other examination purposes. As an educational resource, readers will be able to download figures for PowerPoint teaching purposes. We have also made an effort to adopt uniform terminology and nomenclature, in line with emerging consensus in the world kidney community. Thus, wherever possible, we have preferred terms such as *chronic kidney disease* and *acute kidney injury*, replacing the diverse and sometimes confusing terms that have peppered the literature in the past. Through Expert Consult, individuals who wish access to a physiology or disease topic at the most authoritative level will also be able to acquire separate chapters of interest, as might be the case for scientists and professionals outside of nephrology. Thus, through acquisition of *The Kidney*, individuals or institutions acquire a companion to accompany them on their journey in study, research, or patient care related to kidney health and disease.

Production of *The Kidney* is very much a team effort. The editors are indebted to the publication production team. Joan Ryan has served as our guide and lamppost beaconing the numerous contributors and providing expert input and support as Senior Content Development Specialist now for the ninth and tenth editions. Kate Dimock, Helene Caprari, and now Dolores Meloni have successfully assumed successive positions as Content Strategists, and Mary Pohlman as Senior Project Manager. These are but a few of the many members of the highly professional team at Elsevier, from whose wealth of experience the editors have benefited greatly.

None of this is possible without our authors, whose imprimatur, loyalty, and commitment to the highest standards continue to place *The Kidney* in its well-deserved position of international recognition. Through interactions with authors, we have also been able to strengthen long-standing bonds and to cultivate friendships. Most importantly, we owe a debt of gratitude to our readers, whose loyalty to and enthusiastic participation in each new edition energizes us as editors and reinforces our belief that the guiding spirit of Brenner and Rector for the subject matter and respect for the tradition initiated by the veritable "father" of *The Kidney*—Barry Morton Brenner—will continue to enliven this labor of love through many future editions.

On behalf of my co-editors, Maarten Taal, Glenn Chertow, Alan Yu, and Philip Marsden, I express tremendous gratification with the work that has become a major part of our lives and those of our families and friends and hope that the reader will also share this gratification upon partaking of *The Kidney*.

Karl Skorecki
Haifa, Israel

Contents

Volume 1

SECTION I NORMAL STRUCTURE AND FUNCTION, 1

1. Embryology of the Kidney, 2
   Rizaldy P. Scott | Yoshiro Maezawa | Jordan Kreidberg | Susan E. Quaggin

2. Anatomy of the Kidney, 42
   Robert A. Fenton | Jeppe Praetorius

3. The Renal Circulations and Glomerular Ultrafiltration, 83
   Karen A. Munger | David A. Maddox | Barry M. Brenner | Curtis K. Kost, Jr.

4. The Podocyte, 112
   Stuart J. Shankland | Peter W. Mathieson

5. Metabolic Basis of Solute Transport, 122
   Prabhleen Singh | Alicia A. McDonough | Scott C. Thomson

6. Transport of Sodium, Chloride, and Potassium, 144
   David B. Mount

7. The Regulation of Calcium, Magnesium, and Phosphate Excretion by the Kidney, 185
   Theresa J. Berndt | James R. Thompson | Rajiv Kumar

8. Renal Handling of Organic Solutes, 204
   Orson W. Moe | Stephen H. Wright | Manuel Palacín

9. Renal Acidification Mechanisms, 234
   I. David Weiner | Jill W. Verlander

10. Urine Concentration and Dilution, 258
    Jeff M. Sands | Harold E. Layton | Robert A. Fenton

11. The Cell Biology of Vasopressin Action, 281
    Dennis Brown | Robert A. Fenton

12. Aldosterone and Mineralocorticoid Receptors: Renal and Extrarenal Roles, 303
    David Pearce | Vivek Bhalla | John W. Funder

13. Vasoactive Molecules and the Kidney, 325
    Richard E. Gilbert | Andrew Advani

14. Arachidonic Acid Metabolites and the Kidney, 354
    Raymond C. Harris | Ming-Zhi Zhang | Richard M. Breyer

SECTION II DISORDERS OF BODY FLUID VOLUME AND COMPOSITION, 389

15. Disorders of Sodium Balance, 390
    Itzchak N. Slotki | Karl L. Skorecki

16. Disorders of Water Balance, 460
    Joseph G. Verbalis

17. Disorders of Acid-Base Balance, 511
    Thomas D. DuBose, Jr.

18. Disorders of Potassium Balance, 559
    David B. Mount

19. Disorders of Calcium, Magnesium, and Phosphate Balance, 601
    Miroslaw J. Smogorzewski | Jason R. Stubbs | Alan S.L. Yu

SECTION III EPIDEMIOLOGY AND RISK FACTORS IN KIDNEY DISEASE, 637

20. Epidemiology of Kidney Disease, 638
    Raymond K. Hsu | Chi-yuan Hsu

21. Demographics of Kidney Disease, 655
    Amanda Hyre Anderson | Jeffrey S. Berns | F. Perry Wilson | Harold I. Feldman

22. Risk Factors and Chronic Kidney Disease, 669
    Maarten W. Taal

23. Nephron Endowment and Developmental Programming of Blood Pressure and Renal Function, 693
    Valerie A. Luyckx | Paul Goodyer | John F. Bertram

24. Aging and Kidney Disease, 727
    Devasmita Choudhury | Moshe Levi

SECTION IV EVALUATION OF THE PATIENT WITH KIDNEY DISEASE, 753

25. Approach to the Patient with Kidney Disease, 754
    Michael Emmett | Andrew Z. Fenves | John C. Schwartz

26. Laboratory Assessment of Kidney Disease: Glomerular Filtration Rate, Urinalysis, and Proteinuria, 780
    Katrina Chau | Holly Hutton | Adeera Levin

27 Interpretation of Electrolyte and Acid-Base Parameters in Blood and Urine, 804
Kamel S. Kamel | Mogamet R. Davids | Shih-Hua Lin | Mitchell L. Halperin

28 Diagnostic Kidney Imaging, 846
Vinay A. Duddalwar | Hossein Jadvar | Suzanne L. Palmer | William D. Boswell, Jr.

29 The Kidney Biopsy, 915
Alan D. Salama | H. Terence Cook

30 Biomarkers in Acute and Chronic Kidney Diseases, 926
Chirag R. Parikh | Jay L. Koyner

SECTION V DISORDERS OF KIDNEY STRUCTURE AND FUNCTION, 957

31 Acute Kidney Injury, 958
Asif A. Sharfuddin | Steven D. Weisbord | Paul M. Palevsky | Bruce A. Molitoris

32 Primary Glomerular Disease, 1012
William F. Pendergraft, III | Patrick H. Nachman | J. Charles Jennette | Ronald J. Falk

33 Secondary Glomerular Disease, 1091
Gerald B. Appel | Jai Radhakrishnan | Vivette D'Agati

34 Overview of Therapy for Glomerular Disease, 1161
Daniel Cattran | Heather N. Reich | Michelle A. Hladunewich

35 Microvascular and Macrovascular Diseases of the Kidney, 1175
Piero Ruggenenti | Paolo Cravedi | Giuseppe Remuzzi

36 Tubulointerstitial Diseases, 1209
Carolyn J. Kelly | Eric G. Neilson

37 Urinary Tract Infection in Adults, 1231
Lindsay E. Nicolle

38 Urinary Tract Obstruction, 1257
Jørgen Frøkiaer

39 Diabetic Nephropathy, 1283
Peter Rossing | Paola Fioretto | Bo Feldt-Rasmussen | Hans-Henrik Parving

Volume 2

40 Urolithiasis, 1322
Khashayar Sakhaee | Orson W. Moe

41 Kidney Cancer, 1368
Kara N. Babaian | Scott E. Delacroix, Jr. | Christopher G. Wood | Eric Jonasch

42 Onco-Nephrology: Kidney Disease in Patients with Cancer, 1389
Kevin W. Finkel

SECTION VI GENETICS OF KIDNEY DISEASE, 1409

43 Genetic Basis of Kidney Disease, 1410
Friedhelm Hildebrandt

44 Inherited Disorders of the Glomerulus, 1421
Karl Tryggvason | Jaako Patrakka

45 Inherited Disorders of the Renal Tubule, 1434
Alain Bonnardeaux | Daniel G. Bichet

46 Cystic Diseases of the Kidney, 1475
Vicente E. Torres | Peter C. Harris

SECTION VII HYPERTENSION AND THE KIDNEY, 1521

47 Primary and Secondary Hypertension, 1522
William J. Elliott | Aldo J. Peixoto | George L. Bakris

48 Renovascular Hypertension and Ischemic Nephropathy, 1567
Stephen C. Textor

49 Hypertension and Kidney Disease in Pregnancy, 1610
Sharon E. Maynard | S. Ananth Karumanchi | Ravi Thadhani

50 Antihypertensive Therapy, 1640
Matthew R. Weir | Donna S. Hanes | David K. Klassen | Walter G. Wasser

51 Diuretics, 1702
Ewout J. Hoorn | Christopher S. Wilcox | David H. Ellison

SECTION VIII THE CONSEQUENCES OF ADVANCED KIDNEY DISEASE, 1735

52 Adaptation to Nephron Loss and Mechanisms of Progression in Chronic Kidney Disease, 1736
Maarten W. Taal

53 Mechanisms and Consequences of Proteinuria, 1780
Norberto Perico | Andrea Remuzzi | Giuseppe Remuzzi

54 The Pathophysiology of Uremia, 1807
Timothy W. Meyer | Thomas H. Hostetter

55 Chronic Kidney Disease–Mineral Bone Disorder, 1822
Sharon M. Moe | Stuart M. Sprague

56 Cardiovascular Aspects of Kidney Disease, 1854
Richard Haynes | David C. Wheeler | Martin J. Landray | Colin Baigent

57 Hematologic Aspects of Kidney Disease, 1875
Carlo Brugnara | Kai-Uwe Eckardt

58 Endocrine Aspects of Chronic Kidney Disease, 1912
Juan Jesús Carrero | Peter Stenvinkel | Bengt Lindholm

59 Neurologic Aspects of Kidney Disease, 1926
Manjula Kurella Tamura

60 Dermatologic Conditions in Kidney Disease, 1942
Christine J. Ko | Shawn E. Cowper

SECTION IX CONSERVATIVE MANAGEMENT OF KIDNEY DISEASE, 1955

61 Dietary Approaches to Kidney Diseases, 1956
Denis Fouque | William E. Mitch

62 A Stepped Care Approach to the Management of Chronic Kidney Disease, 1987
Damian G. Fogarty | Maarten W. Taal

63 Therapeutic Approach to Chronic Kidney Disease–Mineral Bone Disorder, 2019
L. Darryl Quarles

64 Drug Dosing Considerations in Patients with Acute Kidney Injury and Chronic Kidney Disease, 2034
Gary R. Matzke | Frieder Keller

SECTION X DIALYSIS AND EXTRACORPOREAL THERAPIES, 2057

65 Hemodialysis, 2058
Jane Y. Yeun | Daniel B. Ornt | Thomas A. Depner

66 Peritoneal Dialysis, 2111
Ricardo Correa-Rotter | Rajnish Mehrotra | Anjali Saxena

67 Critical Care Nephrology, 2137
Ron Wald | Kathleen Liu

68 Plasmapheresis, 2148
Ernesto Sabath | Bradley M. Denker

69 Elimination Enhancement of Poisons, 2166
Marc Ghannoum | Karine Mardini | Paul Ayoub

70 Interventional Nephrology, 2191
Timmy Lee | Ivan D. Maya | Michael Allon

SECTION XI KIDNEY TRANSPLANTATION, 2227

71 Transplantation Immunobiology, 2228
Mohamed H. Sayegh | Leonardo V. Riella | Anil Chandraker

72 Clinical Management of the Adult Kidney Transplant Recipient, 2251
Colin R. Lenihan | Stéphan Busque | Jane C. Tan

SECTION XII PEDIATRIC NEPHROLOGY, 2293

73 Malformation of the Kidney: Structural and Functional Consequences, 2294
Norman D. Rosenblum

74 Diseases of the Kidney and Urinary Tract in Children, 2308
Sevcan A. Bakkaloglu | Franz Schaefer

75 Fluid, Electrolyte, and Acid-Base Disorders in Children, 2365
James C.M. Chan | Fernando Santos

76 Renal Replacement Therapy (Dialysis and Transplantation) in Pediatric End-Stage Kidney Disease, 2402
Yaacov Frishberg | Choni Rinat | Rachel Becker-Cohen

SECTION XIII GLOBAL CONSIDERATIONS IN KIDNEY DISEASE, 2439

77 Latin America, 2440
Leonardo V. Riella | Miquel C. Riella

78 Africa, 2454
Saraladevi Naicker | Sagren Naidoo

79 Near and Middle East, 2468
Suheir Assady | Rawi Ramadan | Dvora Rubinger

80 Indian Subcontinent, 2494
Vinay Sakhuja | Harbir Singh Kohli

81 The Far East, 2510
Chuan-Ming Hao | Fan-Fan Hou | Walter G. Wasser

82 Oceania Region, 2538
Gavin J. Becker | John F. Collins | David C.H. Harris

SECTION XIV CHALLENGES IN NEPHROLOGY, 2557

83 Ethical Dilemmas Facing Nephrology: Past, Present, and Future, 2558
Alvin H. Moss

84 Health Disparities in Nephrology, 2574
Yoshio N. Hall | Glenn M. Chertow

85 Care of the Older Adult with Chronic Kidney Disease, 2586
Meghan J. Elliott | Ann M. O'Hare | Brenda R. Hemmelgarn

86 Tissue Engineering, Stem Cells, and Cell Therapy in Nephrology, 2602
L. Spencer Krane | Anthony Atala

87 Quality Improvement Initiatives in Kidney Disease, 2620
Sandeep S. Soman | Jerry Yee | Kevin Ho

40 Urolithiasis

Khashayar Sakhaee | Orson W. Moe

CHAPTER OUTLINE

EPIDEMIOLOGY, 1322
General Points, 1322
Calcium Stones, 1323
Uric Acid Stones, 1324
Data on Stone Incidence, 1324
HISTOPATHOLOGY, 1325
Idiopathic Calcium Oxalate Stones, 1325
Calcium Phosphate Stones, 1325
Stones in Enteric Hyperoxaluria, 1325
PATHOPHYSIOLOGY, 1325
Physical Chemistry of Urinary Saturation, 1325
Kidney Stone Inhibitors, 1329
Calcium Stones, 1331
Uric Acid Stones, 1341
Cystine Stones, 1345
Infection Stones, 1346
Uncommon Stones, 1347
GENETICS, 1348
Human Genetics, 1348

UROLITHIASIS AS A SYSTEMIC DISORDER, 1350
Obesity, Weight Gain, Diabetes Mellitus, and Risk for Urolithiasis, 1350
Urolithiasis and Risk for Cardiovascular Disease, 1351
Urolithiasis and Hypertension, 1351
Kidney Stone Disease and Chronic Kidney Disease, 1352
Urinary Tract Cancers and Kidney Stones, 1352
Calcium Stones and Bone Disease, 1352
CLINICAL EVALUATION, 1355
Presentation, 1355
LABORATORY EVALUATION, 1356
Serum Chemistry, 1356
Urine Chemistry, 1356
Stone Analysis, 1359
Imaging Studies, 1359
MANAGEMENT OF STONES, 1360
Acute Management, 1360
Chronic Management, 1361

Urolithiasis is the abnormal formation and retention of solid phase inorganic and organic concretions in the urinary tract. Kidney stone disease is not a diagnosis per se but the manifestation of a variety of underlying causative and pathophysiologic factors. Although the stones appear to be localized to the urinary tract, urolithiasis is truly a systemic disease. While the surgical treatment of urolithiasis has greatly advanced over the years, the need to understand how stones form is still of critical importance because they can be prevented from recurring. Overall, the metabolic evaluation of urolithiasis is still not performed often enough, in our opinion. In addition to the potential of uncovering treatable underlying diagnoses, the pathophysiologic definition of kidneys can also guide selection and help monitor therapy.

EPIDEMIOLOGY

GENERAL POINTS

KIDNEY STONES IN ADULT POPULATION: 1976-1994

The prevalence of kidney stones has increased steadily over the past 4 decades,[1,2] which is associated with a rise in direct and indirect expenditures for this condition in the United States.[3] In 1994, data from the U.S. National Health and Nutrition Examination Survey (NHANES) III showed a rise in the prevalence of self-reported history of kidney stones compared to the period from 1976 to 1980 (from 3.8% to 5.2%). The increase was greater in females than males and higher in the aging population.[1] African Americans had a lower risk of the disease compared to whites and Mexican Americans. Age-adjusted prevalence was shown to be higher in southern parts of the United States.[1] This is consistent with several cross-sectional studies showing a higher prevalence of kidney stones in southeastern parts of the United States.[3,4]

Previous studies explored the model that environmental factors and systemic conditions, including quality of the water supply,[5] climate,[6] intake of animal protein, and association with hypertension,[7] were important in increasing the risk of kidney stone disease, in addition to geographic distribution. The contribution of mineral content and quality of the water to the prevalence of kidney stones and its geographic distribution was questioned by a study in three Midwest U.S. regions, which showed no correlation between water calcium content and prevalence of kidney stone disease[8]; the role of other minerals were not addressed. Prevalence data from 1988 to 1994 was not able to use dietary factors to explain geographic variation in the prevalence of kidney stone diseases.[1] The lack of association between diet and the prevalence of kidney stones may be due to the cross-sectional nature of the studies and lack of temporal association between stone disease and time of the data collection.

KIDNEY STONES IN THE ADULT POPULATION: 2007-2010

A more recent NHANES cross-sectional study, from 2007-2010, involving 12,110 subjects with self-reported history of kidney stone disease[2] demonstrated a marked increase in the prevalence at 8.8%, compared to the 1994 survey showing the prevalence of stones to be 5.2%. According to the latest estimate, 1 in 11 individuals in the United States had a history of kidney stones, in contrast to a previous estimate of 1 in 20 U.S. citizens.[1] Furthermore, the overall prevalence was 10.6% in male subjects and 7.1% in females compared with the previous study,[1] which showed 6.3% in men and 4.1% in women[2] (Figure 40.1).

Aside from gender, race, age, ethnicity, and socioeconomic class, conditions associated with metabolic syndrome were shown to be predictive of kidney stone disease.[2] Again, the likelihood of kidney stones was lower among black and Hispanic than white populations. Furthermore, obesity, diabetes, gout, and low household income (≤$19,999) were more likely to be associated with kidney stone disease. The association between features of the metabolic syndrome, including obesity and diabetes, and the prevalence of kidney stone disease is consistent with a previous prospective study, which indicated that the risk of kidney stone disease increased with obesity and weight gain.[9,10]

Using pooled published data from 1965 to 2005 from seven countries, Romero and colleagues showed a continuous increase in prevalence, although the gender and age distribution profile was similar within each time period.[11] As discussed above, factors such as the rise in prevalence in metabolic syndrome and dietary changes have been suggested to underlie this rise. Brikowski and associates[12] took a different (and interesting approach) using global warming trends; they modeled the northward expansion of the U.S. stone belt in the coming decades, which predicts a dramatic increase in stone prevalence in the northern United States.

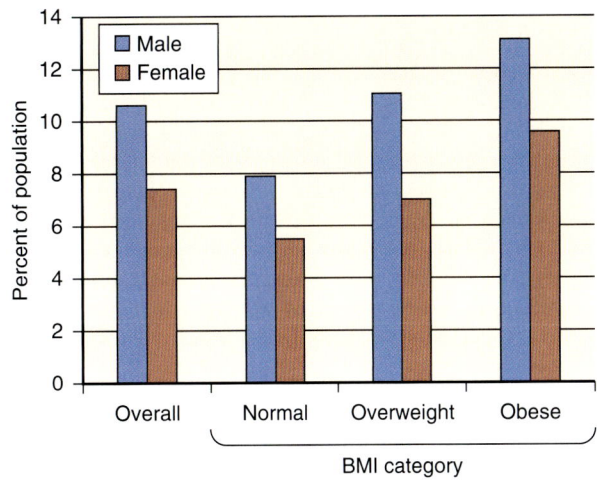

Figure 40.1 Prevalence of urolithiasis plotted as function of gender and body mass index (BMI). (Modified from Scales CD, Jr, Smith AC, Hanley JM, Saigal CS: Urologic Diseases in America Project: Prevalence of kidney stones in the United States. *Eur Urol* 62:160-165, 2012.)

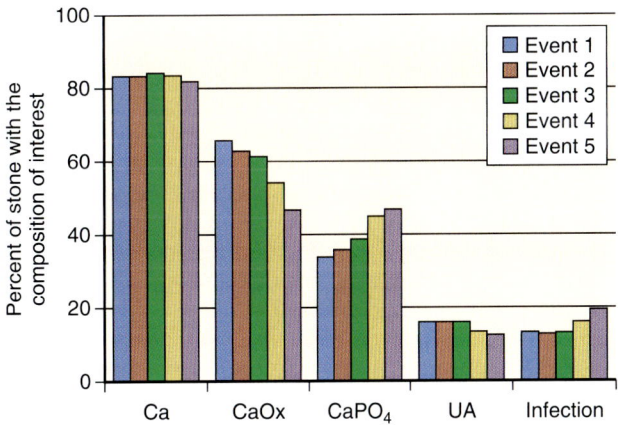

Figure 40.2 Occurrence of stone types (%). Calcium (Ca), calcium oxalate (CaOx), calcium phosphate (CaPO$_4$), uric acid (UA), and infection stones are shown as a function of the event—that is, ranging from the first to the fifth event. (From Mandel N, Mandel I, Fryjoff K, et al: Conversion of calcium oxalate to calcium phosphate with recurrent stone episodes. *J Urol* 169:2026-2029, 2003.)

CALCIUM STONES

PREVALENCE OF CALCIUM STONES

An evaluation of kidney stone composition was made using the National Veteran Administration Crystal Identification Center.[13] A comparison with a previous study showed an increased occurrence (%) of calcium oxalate and brushite stones between 1996 and 2003. Furthermore, with each recurrent stone event, there was an increased occurrence of calcium phosphate stones (%) accompanied by a decrease in occurrence of calcium oxalate stones (Figure 40.2).[13] The underlying factors for the change in stone composition are not known. A retrospective evaluation of 1201 stone formers in the past 3 decades has shown that over time, increased incidence of calcium phosphate stones coincides with increased urinary pH and the number of shock wave lithotripsy treatments.[14] Causality between lithotripsy and urinary pH and stone risk still remains to be determined.

CALCIUM INTAKE

There are several large studies that have explored the association between dietary factors and risk of kidney stone disease. The role of dietary calcium as a risk factor was assessed in a few prospective observational studies showing that low dietary calcium intake is associated with a higher risk of kidney stones in women as well as young men.[15-18] On the contrary, calcium supplementation was associated with a higher risk of kidney stones solely in older women.[17,19] The epidemiologic association of low dietary calcium with urolithiasis is consistent with the findings of a randomized controlled study in hypercalciuric men with calcium urolithiasis.[20] This study will be discussed below in more detail.

OXALATE INTAKE

One epidemiologic study using a food frequency questionnaire in men, older women, and younger women showed that oxalate intake did not correlate with kidney stone disease.[21] One has to exercise caution in drawing conclusions about such negative studies by consideration of the limitations of the questionnaire, heterogeneity of causality among the stone formers, and magnitude of the effect of dietary oxalate.

PROTEIN CONSUMPTION

Epidemiologic studies have demonstrated a positive relationship between animal protein consumption and kidney stone formation in men, but not so much in women.[15,17,19] However, in a randomized controlled trial, consumption of a low animal protein and high-fiber diet was not shown to reduce the relative risk of recurrent kidney stones in calcium oxalate stone formers compared to those instructed on a high fluid intake.[22] Nonetheless, the pathophysiologic basis and metabolic studies supporting the relationship between dietary protein and stone risk is solid; one interventional study in which multiple variables, including dietary protein, were manipulated showed benefits from protein restriction.[20]

URIC ACID STONES

PREVALENCE OF URIC ACID STONES

There are regional differences in uric acid stone prevalence, with the highest reported in the Middle East and a few European countries,[23-25] but only comprising 8% to 10% of all kidney stones in the United States.[26] In the United States, uric acid stones among Chinese and Japanese descendants have been reported to be slightly higher than the general U.S. population, at approximately 15% to 16%.[27] The highest prevalence of uric acid stones and gouty arthritis has been demonstrated in the Hmong population of Asian heritage but living in Minnesota.[27,28] The factors underlying these differences are not known.

GENETIC AND DIETARY FACTORS

The underlying causes for the global differences in uric acid stone prevalence remain unknown. However, a high prevalence of obesity, diabetes, and hypertension is commonly associated with uric acid urolithiasis in Western societies[29-31] and has also been shown to be present in Hmong populations born in the United States. Therefore, it is likely that

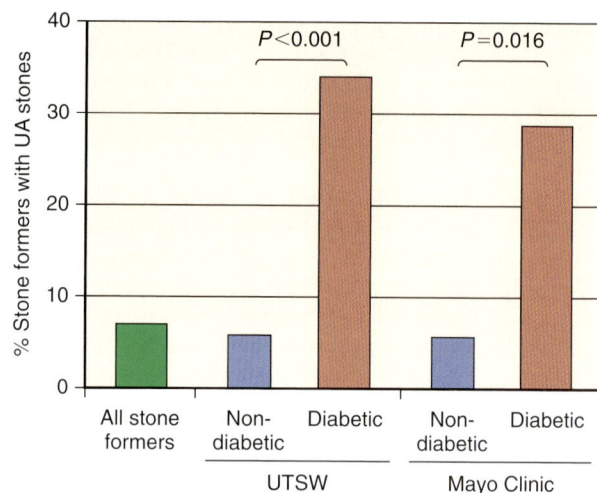

Figure 40.3 Prevalence of uric acid (UA) urolithiasis in the kidney stone population. UTSW, University of Texas Southwestern Medical Center. (From Lieske JC, de la Vega LS, Gettman MT, et al: Diabetes mellitus and the risk of urinary tract stones: a population-based case-control study. *Am J Kidney Dis* 48:897-904, 2006.)

interplay between genetic factors and diet affect the high incidence of uric acid stones. Among stone formers in the United States and Europe, uric acid stones occur more frequently in subjects with type 2 diabetes mellitus (T2DM) and obesity than in nonobese, nondiabetic stone formers (Figure 40.3).[30,32-33]

DATA ON STONE INCIDENCE

Precise information of kidney stone incidence among adult and pediatric populations is limited compared to prevalence. In adult populations, one small study from Minnesota showed an incidence rate of 101.8/100,000 patients/year.[35] Moreover, two studies using a questionnaire found an overall incidence rate among adult males and females of 306 and 95/100,000 person-years, respectively.[15,19]

One study from South Carolina used data from pediatric emergency visits and deduced that the incidence of urolithiasis in children (≤18 years of age) increased from 7.9 to 18.5/100,000 children in a little over a decade.[36] The cause is not known, but it has been suggested that childhood obesity plays a key role in the rising kidney stone incidence of children in recent years. However, larger U.S. epidemiologic studies have not supported this notion.[37]

Dietary factors, including increased sodium consumption[38] and decreased calcium intake[39] from milk, which has been substituted with sugar drinks,[40,41] have also been implicated to have a pathophysiologic role in the development of more kidney stones in the pediatric population. It has also been reported that children are currently consuming less water than in the past.[42] Data from Asia and Europe also showed incidence rates consistent with those of pediatric populations in South Carolina.[43,44] Much like adults, calcium-containing stones are the most predominant kidney stones in pediatric populations.[45,46] On the contrary, uric acid stones are less common, comprising only 2% to 3% of stones in this population.[47]

HISTOPATHOLOGY

While many urinary biochemical stone risk factors can be studied in rodents, urolithiasis that genuinely resembles human disease involving urinary and epithelial factors is actually rather unusual in rodents. The main source of histopathologic data has been derived from clinical surgical samples and will continue to be so. In addition to luminal factors, such as chemical components of stone, inhibitors, and promoters, there are also epithelial factors that initiate and promote crystal adhesion, growth, and agglomeration. This field was advanced significantly by the work of Evan, Lingeman, Coe, Worcester, and colleagues,[49-53] using human kidney samples from intraoperative biopsies, which provided histologic descriptions enabling the formulation of pathogenic models of stone formation.

In the 1930s, Randall examined the papilla of over 1000 pairs of cadaveric kidneys and observed what appeared to be seemingly benign cream-colored areas near the papillary in one of five kidneys. These areas consisted of interstitial rather than luminal plaques associated with interstitial collagen material and tubular basement membranes and were composed of calcium, nitrogen, carbon dioxide, and phosphorus.[48] More advanced lesions intruded into tubular lumens. These plaques were not normal variants according to the findings of small stones attached to some of the plaques, projecting into the lumen of the renal pelvis in more than 60 kidneys. Randall concluded that the attached stones were growing from the interstitial calcium plaque rather than directly from the epithelium.[48] These observations were confirmed by many surgeons in the decades to follow, but it was the Indiana-Chicago group of investigators who shed light on the importance of Randall plaques.

IDIOPATHIC CALCIUM OXALATE STONES

There was no clinical information on Randall's subjects but it is likely that they were calcium oxalate stone formers with idiopathic hypercalciuria. In these patients, plaques are now known to form in the papillary tip in the basement membrane of the thin loop of Henle,[49] with mineral and organic layers alternating in a concentric configuration (Figure 40.4). In the absence of longitudinal biopsies, cross-sectional data indicated that the particles move from the basement membrane into the surrounding interstitium. Individual particles are orderly, associated with type 1 collagen. Evan and coworkers[49] proposed that this is the final form of plaque composed of fused particles in close association with collagen, with the mineral phase covered by organic matrix.

En bloc examination of stones with attached tissue[50] showed that there is loss of epithelial cells, and the plaque is exposed at the attachment site. After exposure, the plaque is overlaid with new matrix, and crystals form in the new matrix, in successive waves. Immunohistochemistry reveals that osteoprotegerin is present in the stone and plaque, and Tamm-Horsfall protein (THP), known to be restricted to the urine and thick ascending limb of the loop of Henle, is present only on the urine space side of the interface and extends to the interface surface.[50] Coe and colleagues proposed that the organic material forming the overlaying of the exposed plaque comes from urine molecules adsorbed initially onto the matrix of plaque. As new crystals nucleate in this urine matrix, the crystals themselves can attract molecules that have affinities for them, thereby creating the new stone.[51]

CALCIUM PHOSPHATE STONES

Although Randall plaques are seen in calcium phosphate stone formers, they are fewer in number. In contrast to calcium oxalate, calcium phosphate stone formers[52] have apatite deposits in the lumen of ducts of Bellini and inner medullary collecting ducts, associated with massive ductal dilation (Figure 40.5). The dilated ducts seem to have lost their epithelial cell layer and are surrounded by interstitial fibrosis. The abundance of calcium phosphate (CaP) crystals is associated with higher urinary CaP supersaturation,[14] driven mostly by high urine pH and to a lesser extent by hypercalciuria. Parks and associates postulated that shock wave lithotripsy injures the epithelium and impairs local luminal acidification.[53] Interestingly, a similar pattern is observed in patients with CaP stones from primary hyperparathyroidism.[54] Luminal plugging and plaque can coexist. A scenario of persistently high pH is typical in CaP stone formers with distal renal tubular acidosis from congenital or acquired causes. Papillae show multiple dilated ducts of Bellini, with intraluminal calcium phosphate deposits. Distortion, flattening, and fibrosis are common. Atrophic remnants of nephron structures lie within fibrotic fields of interstitium.

STONES IN ENTERIC HYPEROXALURIA

In patients with enteric hyperoxaluria, crystallization is mainly driven by a high urinary luminal oxalate concentration. In patients with postgastric bypass, the epithelium appeared rather normal, with calcium oxalate crystals lodged in the lumen.[55] In hyperoxaluric calcium oxalate stone formers from small bowel resection (e.g., Crohn's disease), the inner medullary collecting ducts (IMCDs) contained crystal deposits associated with cell injury, interstitial inflammation, and structural deformity of the papillae, accompanied by tubular atrophy and interstitial fibrosis. Interestingly, Randall plaques were observed similar to those seen in idiopathic calcium oxalate stone formers. The IMCD deposits contained apatite, with calcium oxalate in some instances.[56] The birefringent thin crystalline material scattered on the IMCD cell membranes was the initial crystal lesion.

PATHOPHYSIOLOGY

PHYSICAL CHEMISTRY OF URINARY SATURATION
GENERAL CONCEPTS

Lithogenesis involves the formation of solid phase solutes in urine. Using calcium oxalate as an example, equilibrium is said to be attained when the calcium and oxalate concentrations in solution and amount of calcium oxalate crystals bathed by that solution is unchanged. The product of the free ionized calcium and oxalate concentrations in such a

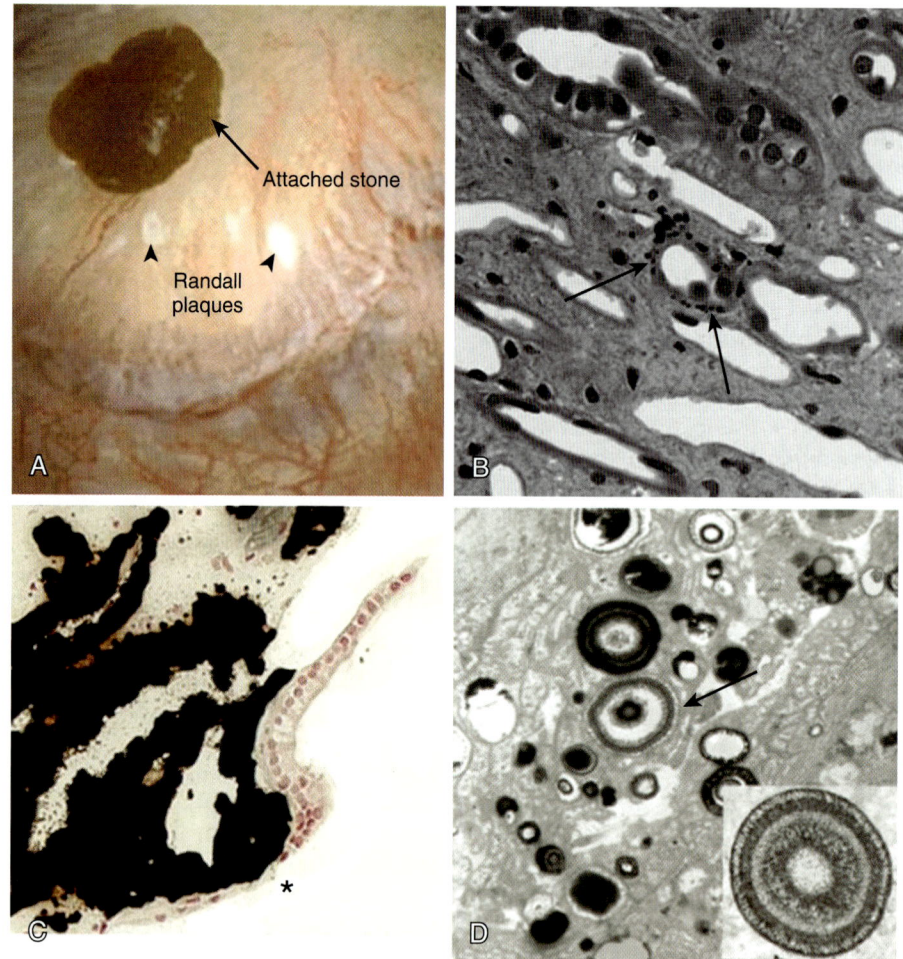

Figure 40.4 Histopathology of Randall plaques in calcium oxalate stone formers. **A,** View during endoscopic surgery. One plaque (not visible) has an overlying attached calcium oxalate stone (*arrow*). Two Randall plaques without stones are below (*arrowheads*). **B,** Light microscopic image of the locale of the initial crystal deposits in the basement membrane of the thin loops of Henle (*arrows*). **C,** Calcium phosphate stained *black* showing a more advanced lesion filling the interstitial space and extending (*), eventually protruding into the urinary space and corresponding to the cream-colored plaques in **A. D,** The individual deposits (*arrow*) assume the morphology of multilaminated spheres of alternating layers of electron-lucent inorganic crystal and electron-dense matrix (*inset*). (From Evan AP, Lingeman JE, Coe FL, et al: Randall's plaque of patients with nephrolithiasis begins in basement membranes of thin loops of Henle. *J Clin Invest* 111:607-616, 2003.)

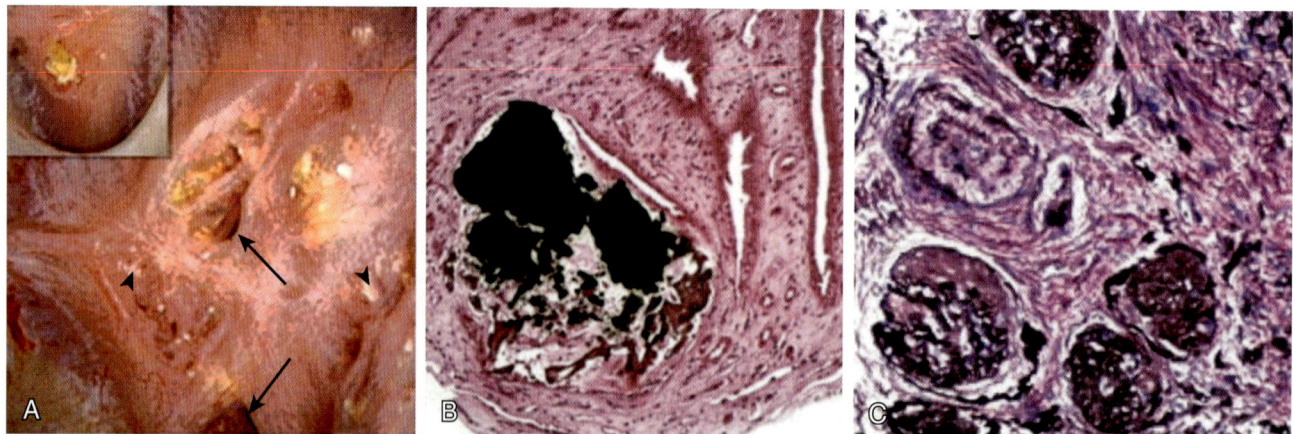

Figure 40.5 Histopathology of calcium phosphate stone formers. **A,** View during endoscopic surgery. Depressions near the papillary tips (*arrows*) are unique to calcium phosphate stone formers, which coexist with Randall plaques. The papillae show yellow crystalline deposits (*arrowheads*) coming out of the ducts of Bellini (*inset*). **B,** Micrograph of luminal deposits in inner medullary collecting duct. The crystal deposits greatly expanded the lumen, and cell injury and necrosis were found. Interstitial inflammation and fibrosis surround the intraluminal crystal deposition. **C,** Renal biopsy from a patient with calcium phosphate stones shows advanced glomerulosclerosis, tubular atrophy, and interstitial fibrosis. This is rarely seen in calcium oxalate stone formers. (From Coe FL, Evan A, Worcester E: Kidney stone disease. *J Clin Invest* 115:2598-2608, 2005.)

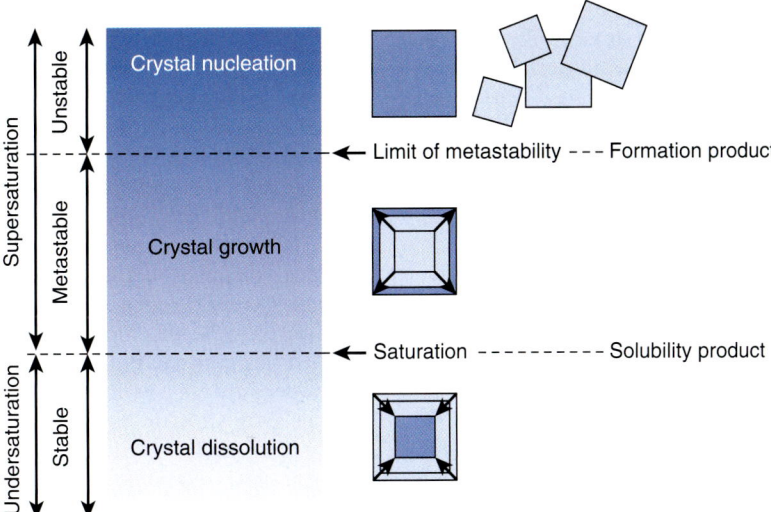

Figure 40.6 Physicochemical parameters used in assessment of kidney stone risk. These are shown in relation to the three states of crystal of dissolution, growth, and nucleation.

solution in equilibrium is termed the *equilibrium solubility product*. The solubility is the concentration of calcium oxalate complex in solution, which is about 6.2 μmol/L. Solubility for CaP (brushite; initial phase of complex formation) is about 0.35 μmol/L and is about 520 μmol/L for uric acid. When free ion activity product falls below the solubility product, the crystals will dissolve; this solution is undersaturated. A free ion activity product higher than the solubility product will lead to a supersaturated state and cause the crystals to grow (Figure 40.6).

When the crystals are removed from a saturated solution at equilibrium, and calcium and oxalate are added to raise the ion activity product beyond the equilibrium solubility product, the elevated activity product would have caused growth of preformed crystals, if these were present. However, in the absence of a preexisting solid phase, no new crystals appear. A solution that causes the growth of preformed crystals but not the appearance of a new solid phase is supersaturated and metastable. If one raises the activity product yet higher with further calcium and oxalate addition, new crystals will appear at some point (see Figure 40.6). The product of the activities of the ions has reached the formation product, also called the upper limit of metastability. Above the formation product, a solution changes from metastable to unstable, and crystallization is inevitable. Urine is undersaturated, metastable, or unstable with respect to calcium oxalate or CaP crystals (see Figure 40.6).

FACTORS INFLUENCING SATURATION

The rate of excretion of the component species of the activity products (e.g., calcium oxalate, CaP, calcium urate) and water (denominator) are primary determinants of saturation. Complexation of calcium and oxalate, and changes in urine pH, can all influence the free ion concentrations and are important in regulating saturation. Therefore, total concentration measurements provide few clues about the actual activity product. For example, citrate readily complexes calcium, reducing the ionized calcium levels[57]; a similar relationship exists for magnesium and oxalate.[58] Changes in urine pH can drastically affect the monovalent or divalent phosphate and urate/uric acid ratio. For this reason, hypercalciuria, hyperoxaluria, hypocitraturia, unusually alkaline urine, and chronic dehydration all increase the risk of calcium stones, but by themselves are not sufficient. Thus, interpretation based solely on chemical concentration can be misleading. An excellent example is when a patient with idiopathic hypercalciuria is treated with thiazide, and the urinary calcium excretion decreases. However, a state of potassium deficiency develops, which causes secondary hypocitraturia. It is not easy for a practitioner to glance at the urinary calcium and citrate excretion rates and determine whether the stone risk is reduced. Another scenario is when a patient with CaP stones from distal renal tubular acidosis and profound hypocitraturia is treated with alkali. The urinary citrate increases, but the urine pH increases concomitantly as well. Is the risk of CaP precipitation reduced or increased? We will discuss methods to address these types of questions.

URINE SATURATION MEASUREMENTS

Upper Limit of Metastability and Formation Product

The upper limit of metastability (ULM) is an empirical entity determined by raising the activity product, adding ligands, and noting the activity product at which a solid phase begins to appear spontaneously (see Figure 40.6). It takes the concentration of the lithogenic solutes and all the inhibitors and promoters into consideration.

Activity Product Ratio

Crystals of interest are seeded to urine and incubated at 37° C, with stirring at constant pH, for 2 days. After reaching equilibrium, the crystal mass has stabilized. If the crystals have grown, the equilibrium activity product is lower than the original sample, so it is less than 1. If the crystals partially dissolved, the equilibrium activity product is higher than the original sample, so it is more than 1. Thus, this describes whether preexistent crystals, once formed, will grow or shrink while suspended, but gives incomplete information about the ability of that urine to produce new crystals. In simple salt solutions, the ULM for calcium oxalate has been found to occur at an APR of 8.5 by Pak and Holt.[59] The small difference is mainly methodologic in origin.

Concentration Product Ratio

Pak and associates used an empirical method to measure urine saturation by comparing urine chemistries to their equilibrium concentration for a given crystal.[61,62] In the original assay, crystals of interest are seeded to an aliquot of urine and incubated at 37° C, with stirring at a constant pH, for 2 days. By the time equilibrium is attained, the crystal mass has stabilized. If the activity coefficients for calcium, oxalate, and phosphate—essentially the fractions of each that are free to react—remain stable throughout the incubation, the ratio of the concentration product at the start of incubation to the concentration product after incubation (equilibrium) must equal the APR, even though the concentration products themselves do not equal the activity products. Pak and coworkers have shown that the assumption of stable activity coefficients is valid, so the empirical concentration product ratio (CPR) is a valid estimation of the APR, provided the calcium concentration is below 5.0 mmol/L and oxalate is below 0.5 mmol/L.[62] This assay has been simplified technically and was used to analyze the propensity of calcium oxalate and calcium phosphate stone formation.[63-65]

Use of Software

One can use computer programs to calculate urine free ion activities for calcium, oxalate, and phosphate from their measured chemical concentration and their known tendency (association constant, K_a) to form soluble complexes with each other and with other ligands.[60,62,66] Using knowledge of the K_a of the complexes, one can calculate the free ion activity product. If one divides this by the corresponding equilibrium solubility product, the resulting ratio is the relative supersaturation ratio (RSR), which estimates the degree of saturation. A ratio above 1 connotes oversaturation; below 1 it is undersaturation. The validity of this approach has been confirmed by studies showing a correlation between the type of stone a patient forms and the prevailing supersaturation in two or three 24-hour urine samples, as estimated by the computer program known as EQUIL2.[67,68] Another computer-based program was developed called the Joint Expert Speciation System (JESS), which differs from EQUIL2 in that many more thermodynamic constants are used to calculate mixed ligand speciation.[69,70] One critical factor that distinguishes it from EQUIL2 is the calcium phosphocitrate complex, a soluble complex whose formation is pH-dependent. Pak and colleagues compared the two computer-based predictive programs to empirical physicochemical methods and found closer approximation of JESS than EQUIL2 to physicochemical methods.[63-65] While EQUIL2 provides relative supersaturation (RS) as a readout, JESS expresses the data as a solubility index (SI), calculated based on the same physicochemical principles as RS values generated by EQUIL, but the two programs use different speciation concentrations.

Urine Saturation in Stone Formers

Robertson, Pak, and Weber and colleagues independently provided evidence that urine from stone formers is more supersaturated than urine from non–stone formers.[59,71-73] Absolute values differ for the three investigative groups, likely due to different methods used. Stone formers have higher average values of urine saturation than normal subjects, whether saturation was measured with respect to calcium oxalate, brushite, octacalcium phosphate, or hydroxyapatite. Weber and coworkers showed supersaturation for calcium oxalate was higher in hypercalciuric than in normocalciuric patients.[73] In all studies, the normal urine was supersaturated with respect to calcium oxalate. Added crystals grow in urine from most normal persons.[59,73] In an important study, Hautmann and colleagues measured calcium and oxalate concentrations in tissue from the cortex, medulla, and papilla of seven human kidneys.[74] The calcium oxalate concentration product in the papillae (1×10^{-4} mol/L^2) exceeded that of urine (5×10^{-7} mol/L^2) and those of the medulla and cortex (8×10^{-7} and 6×10^{-7} mol/L^2, respectively). In addition, high calcium phosphate supersaturation is common in the tip of Henle's loop because tubular fluid pH and Ca^{2+} concentration are high due to water extraction in the descending limb.[75]

The actual ULM for calcium oxalate and brushite in human urine samples from normal subjects and from hypercalciuric, normocalciuric, and hyperparathyroid stone formers are surprisingly variable.[59] The ULMs of calcium oxalate and brushite were measured in urine from calcium stone formers and gender- and age-matched control subjects[76,77]; the gap between prevailing supersaturation of the urine and the ULM was reduced in stone formers, rendering it more likely for crystallization and stone formation to occur. The reduced ULM likely represents deranged crystallization inhibition. Urine is abnormally saturated in stone formers. Values lie close enough to the ULM for calcium oxalate and CaP that new crystal formation could be expected. Most urine, even from normal persons, is metastable with respect to calcium oxalate, so growth of crystal nuclei into a significant mass is predictable.

ASSESSMENT OF NUCLEATION

Nucleation refers to the initial formation of a crystal nidus. This is followed by crystal growth, epitaxial growth, and aggregation. Homogeneous nucleation, the spontaneous formation of new crystal nuclei in a supersaturated metastable solution, is uncommon. Usually, particles of debris in solution, irregularities on the surface of the container, or other existing crystals furnish a surface on which crystal nuclei begin to form at a lower APR than is required for homogeneous nucleation. The existence of the metastable zone reflects the greater free energy required to create new nuclei than that needed simply to enlarge preformed nuclei. Any surface that can serve as a substrate on which ions in solution can organize acts as a heterogeneous nucleus, bypassing the energetically more unfavorable costly process of creating a solid phase de novo. In other words, such a surface can lower the apparent ULM for heterogeneous nucleation.

The efficiency of heterogeneous nucleation depends on the similarity between the spacing of charged sites on the preformed surface and in the lattice of the crystal that is to grow on that surface. This matching is termed *epitaxis,* and its extent is usually referred to as a good or poor epitaxial relationship.[78]

A number of urine crystals have good epitaxial matching and behave toward one another as heterogeneous nuclei. Monosodium urate and uric acid are excellent heterogeneous nuclei for calcium oxalate,[79,80] so uric acid or urate could, by crystallizing, lower the ULM for calcium oxalate. Heterogeneous nucleation is the mechanism linking hyperuricosuria to calcium oxalate stones.[81,82] Epitaxial overgrowth of calcium oxalate on a surface of uric acid has been experimentally documented.[83] Both brushite and hydroxyapatite can also nucleate calcium oxalate,[84,85] which is the basis for Randall plaque as initiators of calcium oxalate stones.

Randall plaque is formed in the interstitium of the papilla but can erode through the papillary epithelium to be exposed to the urine, thus furnishing a preferred nucleating site for crystallization of calcium oxalate. The plaque also provides an anchoring site that allows retained new crystals to have sufficient time to grow to a clinically significant size. Apatite is frequently found at the core of calcium oxalate stones,[86] and there is increased prevalence and severity of Randall plaques in stone formers as compared to non–stone formers.[87] Randall plaque formation in patients with various types of urolithiasis[49,52,88-91] has been extensively studied and will be discussed in the relevant sections below.

ASSESSMENT OF CRYSTAL GROWTH AND AGGREGATION

Once formed, crystals will grow if bathed in urine with an APR higher than 1. Growth and aggregation are pathogenic because microscopic nuclei are too small to cause disease. Crystals are regular lattices, composed of repeating subunits, and grow by incorporation of calcium and oxalate or phosphate into new subunits on their surfaces. In metastable solutions, at 37° C, growth rates of calcium oxalate and the stone-forming CaP crystal show appreciable changes in macroscopic dimensions over hours. Growth rate increases with the extent of supersaturation and is most rapid in urine with the highest APR. Small crystals aggregate into larger crystalline masses by electrostatic attraction from the charged surface of the crystals. This process can rapidly increase particle size, producing a crystal that can lodge in the urinary tract. Stone former's urine contains larger crystal aggregates compared to that of non–stone formers.[92]

Inhibition of crystal agglomeration (ICA) can be measured[93] by adding a fixed amount of solid calcium oxalate (CaOx) to a synthetic solution metastably supersaturated with CaOx or to a similar solution spiked with the test subject's urine. ICA is expressed as the time to reach half of the maximum decline in [Ca], the half-life ($t_{1/2}$) in synthetic solution. A higher $t_{1/2}$ indicates greater ICA.

CELL-CRYSTAL INTERACTIONS

An important concept was introduced by Finlayson and Reid—crystals cannot grow or aggregate fast enough to anchor in the urinary tract during the normal transit time through the nephron.[94] This is analogous to throwing a handful of sand into a sink with the faucet wide open. All the sand will simply wash into the drain. Crystals must anchor to the renal tubule epithelium to delay its passage so they can grow large enough to be of clinical significance. Although Randall plaques[95] offer anchoring and nucleating sites, it is also clear that some stones form in the absence of Randall plaques,[87] so an alternative mechanism has been proposed. CaOx crystals can adhere to cultured collecting duct epithelial cells.[96] The in vitro adherence and uptake of crystals appear to be greater for CaOx than CaP.[97] The crystals bind to anionic sites on the cell membrane[98] and can be inhibited by a variety of anionic compounds normally found in urine.[99] Phosphatidylserine appears to be a preferred binding site, and enrichment of cell membranes with phosphatidylserine increases CaOx crystal binding by renal epithelial cells in culture.[100] The evidence is mostly from cell culture experiments, and the importance of the cell-crystal interaction in the pathogenesis of human kidney stone disease is not clear at this time.

KIDNEY STONE INHIBITORS

The common stone constituents, such as CaOx, CaP, sodium urate, and uric acid, are often supersaturated in normal urine, yet precipitation rarely occurs.[59,71-73] This implies that there are inhibitors of stone formation present in normal urine.[101,102] In terms of relevance to stone disease, the ULM is lower in patients who form stones compared to matched controls, indicating a deficiency in inhibitors in stone formers.[91] Despite this phenomenologic finding, the exact role of inhibitors is far from fully understood. One can arbitrarily classify inhibitors into four classes—multivalent metallic cations such as magnesium, small organic anions such as citrate, small inorganic anions such as pyrophosphate, or macromolecules such as osteopontin and THP (Table 40.1).

MAGNESIUM

Magnesium has been touted as a kidney stone inhibitor for many years.[103] It is present in urine in millimolar concentrations, and it readily binds to oxalate. Some have proposed that magnesium is efficacious in preventing stone formation by binding or complexing oxalate in the bowel and urine,[104-106] by inhibiting CaOx crystal formation,[105,107,108] and

Table 40.1 Natural Inhibitors of Stone Formation

Inorganic	Magnesium pyrophosphate
Small organic anion	Citrate
Macromolecules	Bikunin
	Calgranulin
	FK-binding protein 12
	Glycosaminoglycans
	Lithistathine
	Matrix-Gla protein
	Nephrocalcin
	Osteopontin
	Tamm-Horsfall protein
	Urinary prothrombin fragment F1
	Urinary trefoil factor 1

by increasing urinary citrate when given as alkali salt.[109] In vitro studies have shown that magnesium is an inhibitor of CaOx crystal growth in artificial, rodent, and human urine, but at supraphysiologic concentrations.[110-115] Magnesium inhibits nucleation and growth of CaOx crystals.[116] In a seeded crystal growth system of constant composition, magnesium was a weak inhibitor.[117] The results of clinical trials of magnesium have not been uniform. In one study, 55 stone formers were given 500 mg of magnesium daily as $Mg(OH)_2$ and experienced a decrease in stone rate from 0.8 to 0.08 stone/year.[103] The stone recurrence-free rate was 85% in treated patients compared to 59% in untreated control patients. However, more recent controlled clinical studies have suggested that magnesium does not alter the recurrence rates for CaOx stone formation, perhaps due to its poor absorption.[118] Another possibility is that the beneficial inhibitory effect of magnesium is offset by its hypercalciuric effects because luminal magnesium and low pH inhibit the calcium channel TRPV5.[119]

CITRATE

Citrate is the best studied, understood, and tested inhibitor. In addition to its chelating action on calcium, which reduces calcium's availability to bind oxalate and phosphate, citrate inhibits the nucleation, growth, and aggregation of CaOx crystals.[120,121] Citrate directly inhibits crystallization[109,122] and increases the ULM by increasing urine citrate and pH.[123] Potassium citrate has been shown, in most clinical studies, to reduce recurrent calcium urolithiasis in patients with idiopathic hypercalciuria, distal renal tubular acidosis, and even in kidney stone formers with normal urinary citrate.[124-130] The most important regulator of urinary citrate levels is the acid-base status of the organism, particularly proximal tubule cell pH. Since urinary citrate serves dual roles as a calcium chelator and the principal urinary base, this presents a conflict when base conservation is required, thus putting the urine at risk of calcium crystallization.[131] During systemic or proximal tubular acidosis, there is an increase in proximal citrate reabsorption and metabolism of citrate, reducing the amount of citrate excreted in the urine.[132] A reduction of urinary citrate, due to increase of the acid load generated from dietary protein ingestion, can promote formation of CaOx stones.[128,133]

PYROPHOSPHATE

The inhibitory role of pyrophosphate on calcium crystallization has been known for years[134] and plays an important role outside the kidney.[135] Pyrophosphate binds to the surface of basic CaP crystals, including hydroxyapatite, and arrests or at least retards the crystal growth of CaP and CaOx crystals.[136-138] The average urine pyrophosphate concentration is sufficient to inhibit crystal growth significantly.[138] There is a reduced pyrophosphate/creatinine ratio in 50% of stone formers, suggesting that a lack of pyrophosphate predisposes to urolithiasis.[137]

MACROMOLECULES

Macromolecules are potent inhibitions of CaOx crystallization.[139] Some of the macromolecules in Table 40.1 will be highlighted. These molecules are generally highly anionic and contain large amounts of acidic amino acid, which undergo posttranslational modification, with negatively charged side chains. Bergsland and associates compared the inhibitory proteins in urine from 50 stone-forming and 50 non–stone-forming matched first-degree relatives of calcium stone–forming patients.[140] They found that the profiles of inhibitory proteins were more effective in discriminating relatives of stone formers from non–stone formers than conventional measurements of supersaturation. Clinical use of inhibitor profiles is hampered by the difficulty and thus the expense of these measurements.

Osteopontin

Osteopontin (previously termed *uropontin*) is an acidic phosphoglycoprotein that was initially isolated from bone[141-144] but is excreted in urine at a rate of about 4 mg/day.[142,143] In bone, osteopontin inhibits hydroxyapatite formation during osteogenesis.[145-147] It is expressed in cells of the thick ascending limb of Henle (TAL) and distal convoluted tubules and secreted into the tubules. Osteopontin inhibits nucleation, growth, and aggregation of CaOx stones in vitro.[141,142,148] Osteopontin knockout mice develop CaOx kidney stones when given ethylene glycol, a nephrotoxin that leads to hyperoxaluria, at doses that do not induce stone formation in wild-type mice.[141,149] Osteopontin is upregulated at sites of stone formation in genetic hypercalciuric stone–forming rats.[150]

Tamm-Horsfall Protein

This is the most abundant protein found in human urine, with approximately 100 mg excreted each day. It is synthesized in the TAL and, due to self-aggregation, is the principal component of urinary casts.[151] Also known as uromodulin, THP is implicated and involved in a multitude of functions and pathobiologic mechanisms, including ion transport, innate immunity, and acute and chronic kidney injury.[152,153,154] THP inhibits CaOx crystal aggregation but does not alter growth or nucleation.[155,156] THP-deleted mice spontaneously form calcium crystals in the lumen of tubules in the papilla and medulla.[157] When these mice are given ethylene glycol to induce CaOx stone formation, there is a marked induction of renal osteopontin at sites of crystal formation.[157]

Urinary Prothrombin Fragment 1

Urinary prothrombin fragment 1 (UPTF1, crystal matrix protein) is a fragment of prothrombin made in the kidney.[158] It is a potent inhibitor of CaOx growth, aggregation, and nucleation[159] and is present in kidney stones.[160] There is evidence for differences in UPTF1 between stone formers and non–stone formers.[161]

Bikunin

This is the light chain of the inter-alpha-trypsin inhibitor (IαI), which inhibits CaOx growth and nucleation.[162] It is found in the proximal tubule and in the thin descending segment near the TAL.[163] Bikunin, along with the heavy chains of the IαI, have been isolated from kidney stones, suggesting that multiple fragments of this inhibitor are active in preventing stone formation.[164] Bikunin was present only in the collecting duct apical membranes and loop cell cytoplasm of stone formers colocalizing with osteopontin and IαI heavy chain 3, and extensive heavy chain 3 was only present in stone formers and not in controls.[165] One study has demonstrated differences in the electrophoretic mobility pattern between stone formers and non–stone formers.[166]

Glycosaminoglycans

Glycosaminoglycans (GAGs) occurring in the urine of normal individuals typically consist of about 50% chondroitin sulfate, 25% heparin sulfate, 10% low sulfated chondroitin sulfate, and 5% to 10% hyaluronic acid (HA).[167] Chondroitin sulfate retards nucleation, while dermatan sulfate inhibits nucleation.[168] In rodents induced to precipitate calcium oxalate, there is increased expression of heparin sulfate in the tubules.[169] HA, which is in the extracellular matrices, is proposed to bind at cell surfaces.[170] Human tubular cells in primary culture bind crystals when damaged, dependent on the expression of HA.[171] Canine tubular cells increase the synthesis of GAGs to protect from toxic insults of CaOx crystals and oxalate ions in vitro.[172] Human studies have shown decreased urinary GAG levels in stone formers,[173,174] but this finding has not been universal.[175,176]

Matrix-Gla Protein

This is a 14-kDa glycoprotein that was the first urinary protein found to have crystal inhibitory properties.[155,177,178] Matrix-Gla protein (MGP) contains five γ-carboxyglutamic acid (Gla) residues, which have a high affinity for calcium and phosphate ions and hydroxyapatite crystals,[179] and inhibits crystal growth, nucleation, and aggregation. It is clear that MGP protects the vasculature from calcification,[180,181] and it serves a similar role in the kidney. MGP messenger RNA (mRNA) expression is increased in renal tubular epithelial cells following exposure to CaOx crystals.[182,183] Interestingly, multilaminated crystals were formed in the injured tubules, with lack of MGP expression,[184] but no crystal formations were seen in tubules with MGP expression. Genetic MGP single-nucleotide polymorphism was associated with the individual susceptibility of urolithiasis.[185] MGP from some stone-forming patients lacks Gla and has a diminished ability to inhibit nucleation and growth of calcium oxalate crystals.[155,156,186]

Urinary Trefoil Factor 1

Urinary trefoil factor (TFF1) has potent inhibitory activity against CaOx crystal growth, similar to that of nephrocalcin.[187] Concentrations of TFF1 have been shown to be greater in stone formers compared to controls. Calgranulin has been isolated from urine and from CaOx kidney stones and is a potent inhibitor of growth and aggregation.[188]

CALCIUM STONES

CaOx is the most prevalent component of kidney stones worldwide, accounting for approximately 70% to 80% of kidney stones, while CaP stones contribute to a smaller percentage (15%).[189-193] However, the percentage of CaP stones appears to increase with each new stone event.[13] The pathogenesis of CaOx stone formation includes hypercalciuria, hyperuricosuria, hypocitraturia, hyperoxaluria, and altered urinary pH.[189,190] CaP stones share some common mechanisms with CaOx stones, including hypercalciuria and hypocitraturia, but in contrast to CaOx, unusually alkaline urine is characteristic among CaP stone formers. An ambulatory evaluation in over 1270 patients with recurrent calcium urolithiasis demonstrated hypercalciuria in 60% of patients, while hyperuricosuria was found in 35.8%, hypocitraturia in 31.3%, hyperoxaluria in 8.1%, abnormal urinary pH in 10%, and low urinary volume in 16.3%, and no metabolic abnormality was noted in 4% of patients.[191] Note that these percentages are approximate because all the variables in question are continuous in their distribution. A study of 82 brushite stone formers demonstrated hypercalciuria in about 80%, alkaline urinary pH in about 60%, and hypocitraturia in about 50% of patients. Hyperuricosuria and hyperoxaluria were uncommon, found in 18% and 10% of patients, respectively; a low urine volume was found in nearly 60%.[192]

HYPERCALCIURIA

Hypercalciuria is the most prevalent metabolic abnormality in patients with calcium urolithiasis, occurring in 60% of adults with calcium stones.[192-197] The pathophysiologic mechanisms for hypercalciuria are protean and involve increased intestinal absorption (absorptive hypercalciuria), diminished renal tubular calcium reabsorption (renal leak hypercalciuria), and enhanced calcium mobilization from the bone (resorptive hypercalciuria).[190,198-201] Intestinal hyperabsorption of calcium has been shown to be the most common abnormality in this population.[202] Nevertheless, all the physiologic derangements noted earlier coexist in individual patients.

Intestinal Hyperabsorption of Calcium

Flocks initially showed a link between hypercalciuria and urolithiasis.[203] Subsequently, Albright and colleagues used the term *idiopathic hypercalciuria* to highlight the unknown origins of hypercalciuria in this population.[204,205] The metabolic basis and its link to intestinal hyperabsorption of calcium were first alluded to by Nordin and Pak, and the term *absorptive hypercalciuria* (AH) was introduced.[206] Balance studies showed a negative calcium balance in patients with hypercalciuria compared to non–stone-forming control subjects.[207,208] Compatible with the balance data was information from dietary recall that also demonstrated that patients with hypercalciuria consumed less calcium than they excreted.[209]

Further balance studies showed a low fecal calcium content[210] and correction of hypercalciuria using an intestinal calcium binder with sodium cellulose phosphate.[211,212] Typically, the characteristic features of AH are hypercalciuria with normocalcemia, normal or suppressed serum parathyroid hormone (PTH), and/or urinary cyclic adenosine monophosphate (cAMP), a surrogate marker of PTH bioactivity in the kidney. Hyperabsorption has been recognized to be one of the most prevalent characteristic features in many patients with idiopathic hypercalciuria; furthermore, it has been proposed that AH is a heterogeneous disorder, consisting of two subtypes, calcitriol-dependent and calcitriol-independent.[202,210,213-220]

1,25-Dihydroxyvitamin D Dependence. Increased 1,25(OH)$_2$D concentration was reported in four different studies in hypercalciuric urolithiasis patients.[213-216] The diagnosis of AH was established by direct measurement of intestinal calcium absorption[219,221] or indirectly[215] by showing a lower serum PTH concentration. The underlying pathophysiologic

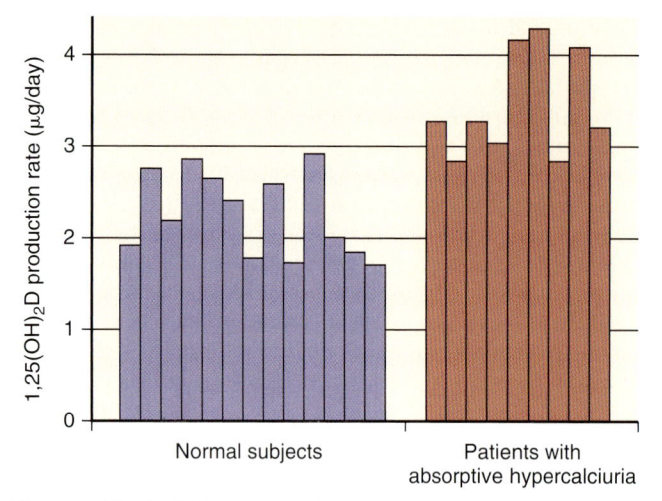

Figure 40.7 Individual values for 1,25(OH)$_2$D production rates in normal subjects and those with absorptive hypercalciuria. The mean 1,25-dihydroxyvitamin D production rate was significantly higher in patients with absorptive hypercalciuria than in the normal subjects (3.4 ± 0.5 vs. 2.2 ± 0.5 μg/day; $P < 0.001$). (From Insogna KL, Broadus AE, Dreyer BE, et al: Elevated production rate of 1,25-dihydroxyvitamin D in patients with absorptive hypercalciuria. *J Clin Endocrinol Metab* 61:490-495, 1985.)

mechanism responsible for increased serum 1,25(OH)$_2$D was likely a result of increased production rather than decreased metabolic clearance (Figure 40.7).[214]

The infusion equilibrium technique was performed in nine patients with AH (>4 mg/kg/day and/or >300 mg/day) on a defined calcium intake. A high calciuric response after an oral calcium load in association with a fasting normal or decreased PTH level or nephrogenic cAMP was compared with 13 normal subjects.[214] Further support for the role of 1,25(OH)$_2$D in enhancing urinary calcium excretion came from a study in normal subjects who became hypercalciuric after receiving high-dose 1,25(OH)$_2$D.[213] Another calcium balance study was performed in eight healthy males four on a low-calcium diet, and four on a comparable low-calcium diet while receiving large doses of oral calcitriol (0.75 μg) every 6 hours for 4 days.[222] Net intestinal calcium absorption significantly increased during calcitriol treatment in all subjects and urinary calcium excretion in stone formers exceeded that of controls, demonstrating a negative calcium balance during calcitriol administration. This was associated with an increase in urinary hydroxyproline, a surrogate marker of bone resorption, suggesting that elevated 1,25(OH)$_2$D levels in healthy men during a low-calcium diet enhances bone resorption. However, other investigators showed a direct correlation between serum 1,25(OH)$_2$D, calcium excretion and calciuric responses, suggesting the pathogenetic role of excess 1,25(OH)$_2$D in increased intestinal absorption.[213] It is still controversial whether hypercalciuria originates from the bone[222] or intestine.[213]

The reason for elevated 1,25(OH)$_2$D production in an AH population is unclear. The main regulators of 1,25(OH)$_2$D synthesis, including PTH and/or its bioactivity (urinary cAMP), were never found to be increased in this population.[191,193,202,215,219,220,223-225] However, there were no frank reductions in serum phosphorus concentration, maximal tubular reabsorption rate of phosphate (TmP), and glomerular filtration rate (GFR), the other main regulators of 1,25(OH)$_2$D production.[213-215,226]

Despite studies precluding the role of phosphorus in the increased production of 1,25(OH)$_2$D, some have suggested that some patients with absorptive hypercalciuria have a primary defect in renal tubular reabsorption of phosphorus (renal phosphorus wasting), which consequently stimulates 1,25(OH)$_2$D synthesis and enhances intestinal calcium absorption.[215,227,228] Serum phosphorus concentrations do not differ in hyperabsorptive and normal subjects when studied under the same dietary regimen[225,229]; hypophosphatemia and low TmP-GFR were found only in a minority of the patients with absorptive hypercalciuria.[225] However, it is still possible to have phosphate wasting and depletion without frank hypophosphatemia because serum phosphate is a practical but imperfect surrogate for phosphate stores.[230]

A study described two patients with an elevated serum 1,25(OH)$_2$D$_3$, urolithiasis, and nephrocalcinosis associated with hypercalciuria due to undetectable activity of 1,25(OH)$_2$D$_3$ 24-hydroxylase (CYP24A1), an enzyme that inactivates 1,25(OH)$_2$D$_3$.[231] This loss-of-function mendelian disease was ascribed to biallelic inactivating mutations of CYP24A1. The frequency of the CYP24A1 variant, based on a National Center for Biotechnology Information (NCBI) database, was estimated to be 4% to 20%. This report constitutes a proof of principle for the role of the 24-hydroxylase in D-dependent calcium stones but it is difficult to determine whether these alleles predispose to urolithiasis in the general population.

An epidemiologic analysis of men in the Health Professionals Follow-Up Study over 12 years found that within the normal range of serum 1,25(OH)$_2$D, the odds ratio of incident symptomatic kidney stones in the highest compared with the lowest quartiles was 1.73 after adjusting for body mass index (BMI), diet, plasma factors, and other covariates.[232]

1,25-Dihydroxyvitamin D–Independent Absorptive Hypercalciuria. In humans, two thirds of absorptive hypercalciuria patients exhibit increased intestinal calcium absorption with normal levels of 1,25(OH)$_2$D.[202,210,218-220,233] Moreover, a triple-lumen intestinal perfusion study supported 1,25(OH)$_2$D-independent selective jejunal hyperabsorption of calcium in this population, which differs from the less selective gastrointestinal (GI) effects of 1,25(OH)$_2$D in normal subjects.[234]

To explore this further, pharmacologic probes were used to alter serum 1,25(OH)$_2$D concentrations and assess intestinal calcium absorption in hypercalciuric subjects.[220,223-225] Ketoconazole reduced serum 1,25(OH)$_2$D in normal subjects and patients with primary hyperparathyroidism.[235-237] Nineteen patients with absorptive hypercalciuria were treated with ketoconazole (600 mg/day × 2 weeks; Figure 40.8).[223] In 12 of these patients, ketoconazole lowered 1,25(OH)$_2$D concentration, intestinal calcium absorption, and 24-hour urinary calcium. Moreover, intestinal calcium absorption assessed directly by ^{47}Ca absorption correlated with serum 1,25(OH)$_2$D and 24-hour urinary calcium excretion. Importantly, in 7 patients, despite the significant reduction of 1,25(OH)$_2$D, there was no change in calcium

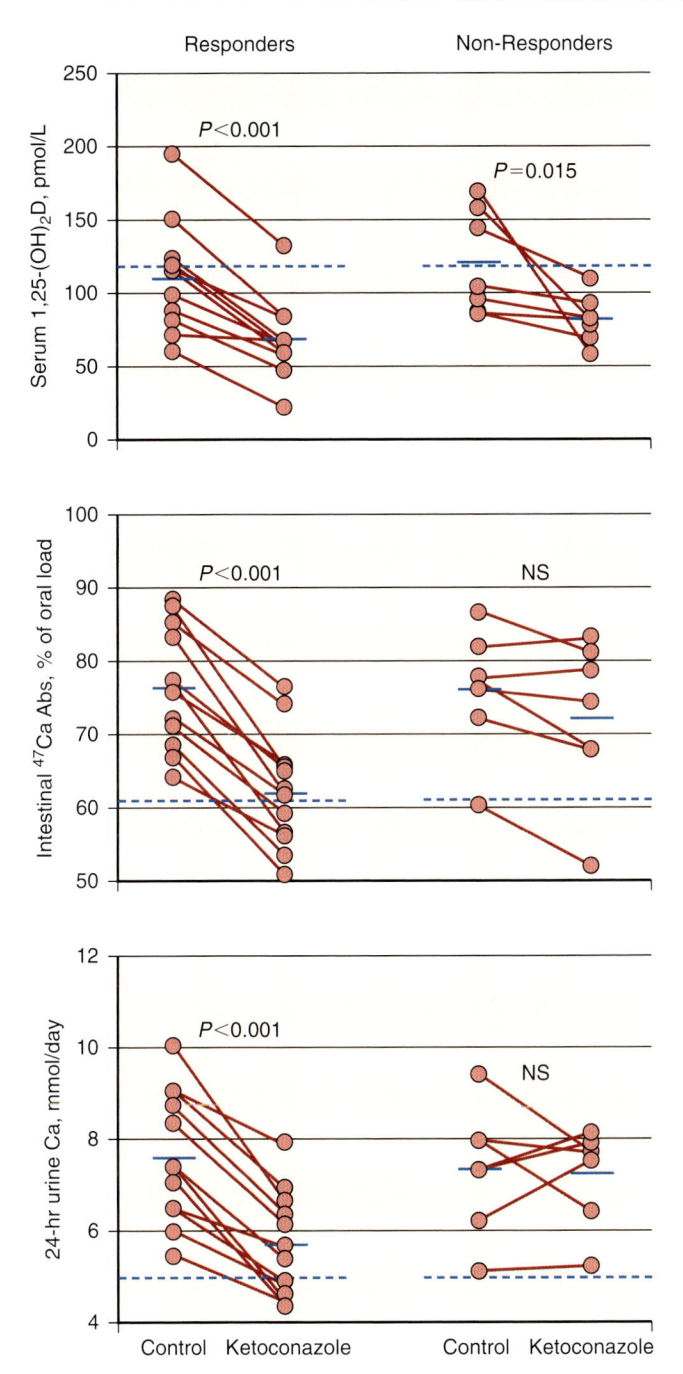

Figure 40.8 Heterogeneity of absorptive hypercalciuria. Shown are the responses of patients with hypercalciuria to a 2-week course of ketoconazole (600 mg/day). Abs, Absorption. (From Breslau NA, Preminger GM, Adams BV, et al: Use of ketoconazole to probe the pathogenetic importance of 1,25-dihydroxyvitamin D in absorptive hypercalciuria. J Clin Endocrinol Metab 75:1446-1452, 1992.)

independent mechanism in the development of hypercalciuria in this population.

Increased Abundance of Vitamin D Receptor. Expression and activation of the vitamin D receptor (VDR) are necessary for vitamin D action.[238] A genetic association of intestinal hyperabsorption of calcium and calcium stone formation with the VDR locus has been described.[239,240] Two common single-nucleotide polymorphisms (SNPs) were linked to altered expression and/or function of VDR protein,[241-244] but these results were not confirmed by others.[245,246] Since intestinal calcium absorption in hyperabsorptive kidney stone formers mainly occurs with normal serum 1,25(OH)$_2$D,[202,218-220] there might be an alteration in the amount of VDRs or sensitivity to 1,25(OH)$_2$D. VDRs are expressed in peripheral monocytes and in T and B lymphocytes.[247,248-251]

In 10 male hypercalciuric calcium oxalate stone formers compared to age- and gender-matched controls without a history of stone disease, the abundance of VDR was twofold higher in peripheral blood mononuclear cells (PBMCs) in stone formers.[252] In another study of absorptive hypercalciuric patients, a Scatchard plot showed an increase in VDR abundance in a subset of patients with normal serum 1,25(OH)$_2$D. These results suggest heterogeneous patterns with respect to VDR abundance.[247]

Genetic Hypercalciuric Rat Model of Hypercalciuria

Genetic hypercalciuric stone-forming (GHS) rats are a polygenic model for hypercalciuria.[253-256] Breeding of Sprague-Dawley rats with high physiologic calcium excretion has yielded robust, constant hypercalciuria after 60 generations.[257,258] These animals have normal serum calcium and calcitriol levels, increased intestinal calcium absorption, formation of calcium stones, excessive bone resorption, and decreased renal tubular calcium reabsorption, making this a feasible model for studying the 1,25(OH)$_2$D-VDR axis.[259-263] On a low-calcium diet, there was an increase in serum 1,25(OH)$_2$D in control and GHS rats. The increase was lower in GHS compared to controls, but there was greater net increase in intestinal calcium absorption in GHS rats, suggesting amplified bioactivity of 1,25(OH)$_2$D.[259,264] This is analogous to patients with absorptive hypercalciuria, in whom elevated intestinal calcium absorption and urinary calcium excretion are associated with normal 1,25(OH)$_2$D levels.[202,218-220] The increased abundance of duodenal and kidney VDRs[262,265,266] accounts for the heightened biologic effect of 1,25(OH)$_2$D in GHS rats.[202,218-220] The high tissue VDR levels were due to an increase in VDR gene expression, protein synthesis, and half-life of the VDR protein,[266-268] with no change in the VDR DNA sequence.[267] However, the transcription factor Snail, a negative regulator of VDR gene expression, seemed to be lower in GHS rats.[268]

Transcellular intestinal calcium transport involves initial calcium entry across the apical membrane, which is facilitated across the cells by the 9-kDa calbindin, followed by extrusion through the plasma basolateral membrane.[269] The biologic action of VDR in GHS rats was supported by increased expression of vitamin D–dependent genes, such as increased expression of calbindin-9 in the duodenum.[266] The 28-kDa calbindin is the principal calcium-binding protein in the renal distal convoluted tubule and plays a role

absorption or urinary calcium excretion.[223] In these patients, intestinal calcium absorption and urinary calcium excretion were not correlated with serum 1,25(OH)$_2$D levels. Studies using thiazide,[220] glucocorticoids,[224] and orthophosphates[225] in hyperabsorptive patients have also shown that lowering 1,25(OH)$_2$D concentration is not associated with changes in intestinal calcium absorption, indicative of a calcitriol-

in renal calcium transport.[270-274] Baseline calbindin-28k levels were higher in GHS rat kidneys and, after a single dose of 1,25(OH)$_2$D, calbindin-28k increased much more in GHS rats compared to control rats.[266] One may conclude that an abundance of tissue VDR in GHS rats and in humans with AH amplifies the biologic effect of normal serum 1,25(OH)$_2$D levels and consequently increases the expression of vitamin D–dependent genes and their protein products to regulate intestinal, renal, and bone calcium transport.

Renal Leak Hypercalciuria

Renal leak of calcium is presumed to be due to diminished renal tubular calcium reabsorption and is associated with secondary increases in serum PTH and 1,25(OH)$_2$D and a compensatory increase in intestinal calcium absorption.[275] The underlying mechanisms for impaired renal tubular calcium reabsorption have not yet been fully explored. However, several potential mechanisms have been purported to affect renal tubular calcium reabsorption, including primary proximal defect, hyperinsulinemia, calcium-sensing receptor (CaSR) gene expression and its interaction with calcitriol, and claudin-14 expression.

Seminal human metabolic studies performed by Worcester and associates have demonstrated an exaggerated fractional excretion of calcium (FE_{Ca}) in hypercalciuric patients in a postprandial state compared to normal subjects.[276] Furthermore, increased FE_{Ca} was not a consequence of differences in filtered calcium load, urinary sodium excretion, or serum PTH levels (Figure 40.9). It was proposed that the postprandial inhibition of renal tubular calcium reabsorption is due to differences in insulin levels in hypercalciuric stone formers.[277,278] This was based on previous findings showing an exaggerated calciuric response to an oral

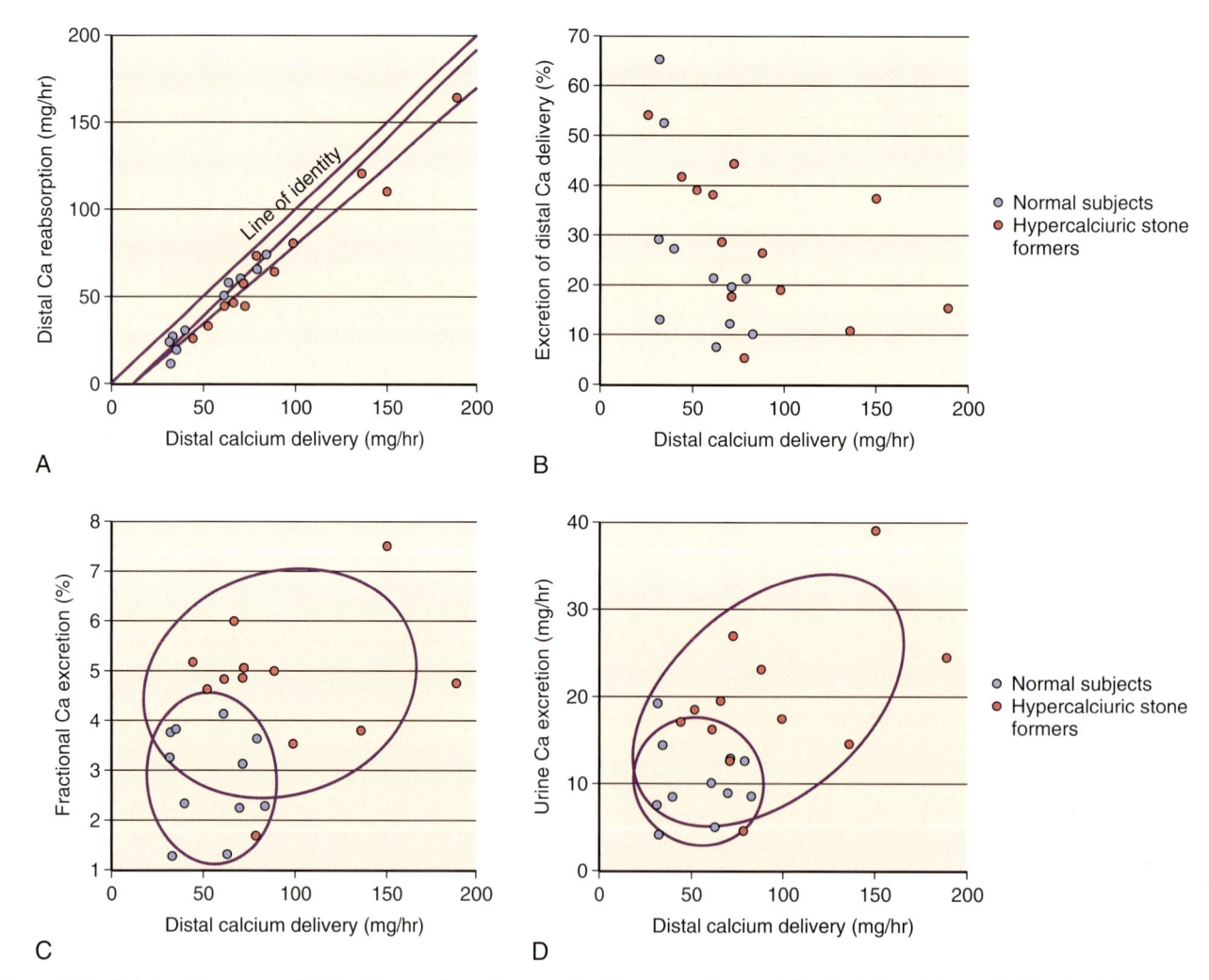

Figure 40.9 Relationship among distal calcium reabsorption, renal calcium excretion, and distal calcium delivery. **A,** Distal calcium reabsorption rises similarly with calcium delivery in normal subjects and hypercalciuric stone formers. Both lines are positioned slightly beneath the line of identity. This suggests normal distal calcium handling but higher distal calcium delivery. **B,** The actual fraction (%) of distally delivered calcium that was excreted decreased with increasing distal delivery, and stone formers lie above normal subjects at a comparable distal delivery. **C,** Fractional and total **(D)** calcium excretions were high in many stone formers versus normal subjects at comparable deliveries. (From Worcester EM, Coe FL, Evan AP, et al: Evidence for increased postprandial distal nephron calcium delivery in hypercalciuric stone-forming patients. *Am J Physiol Renal Physiol* 295(5):F1286-1294, 2008.)

carbohydrate load in hypercalciuric stone formers.[279-281] These studies did not segregate the effects of hyperinsulinemia from those of the serum glucose concentration. A study using euglycemic hyperinsulinemic clamp demonstrated that the rise in insulin-induced calciuria was small and was no different between hypercalciuric stone formers and non–stone-forming control subjects, suggesting that insulin is unlikely to play a significant pathogenic role in hypercalciuric stone formers.[282] Insulin resistance and hyperinsulinemia are features of obesity associated with hypercalciuria and risk of kidney stone formation,[9,283-285] but FE_{Ca} was comparable in the hypercalciuric stone formers, overweight and obese non–stone formers, and lean controls and independent of peripheral insulin sensitivity measured as glucose disposal rates. This study is at variance with a previous report that used insulin extracted from islets rather than recombinant insulin and that showed significant insulin-induced hypercalciuria.[286]

The CaSR is expressed in the parathyroid glands, kidney, and GI tract.[287] In the parathyroid glands, the CaSR responds to calcium and suppresses PTH release. In the kidney, the CaSR responds to increased circulating ionized calcium and reduces renal tubular calcium reabsorption in the TAL and distal convoluted tubal (DCT).[288] An Italian cohort linked hypercalciuria in stone formers to polymorphism in the CaSR gene. Serum calcitriol levels were not defined in these subjects. Vitamin D responsive elements (VDREs) have been identified in the CaSR gene, which suggests that calcitriol can upregulate kidney CaSR expression and reduce renal tubular calcium reabsorption.[289]

Tight junction proteins of the claudin family that are expressed in the TAL are critical for paracellular Ca^{2+} reabsorption in the kidney.[290] A large genomewide association study conducted in Iceland and the Netherlands found an association between sequence variations of the *CLDN14* gene and kidney stones and reduced bone mineral density at the hip.[291] One study has suggested that CaSR regulates claudin-14 expression via two microRNAs, miR-9 and miR-374, and that dysregulation of the renal CaSR–claudin-14 pathway might be a possible cause of hypercalciuria.[292] This model has proposed that CaSR increases claudin-14, which inhibits the complex of claudin-16 and claudin-19 that regulates paracellular Ca^{2+} reabsorption in the TAL.[290]

Resorptive Hypercalciuria

Resorptive hypercalciuria refers to hypercalciuria that is caused by enhanced calcium mobilization from bone.

Parathyroid Hormone–Dependent Resorptive Hypercalciuria. Primary hyperparathyroidism (PHPT) is the most common cause of resorptive hypercalciuria and is associated with calcium stones in 2% to 8% of patients.[189] Due to the much earlier diagnosis of primary hyperparathyroidism, asymptomatic cases are common, and renal complications have significantly decreased.[293] A retrospective study of 271 renal ultrasounds from asymptomatic cases with surgically proven hyperparathyroidism showed a 7% prevalence of stones compared with 1.6% in 500 age-matched subjects who underwent sonography examinations for other reasons.[294] Although hypercalciuria has been perceived as a cause of kidney stones in this population, the exact relationship between hypercalciuria and the risk of urolithiasis in patients with primary hyperparathyroidism has been debated.[295,296] The relative contribution from enhanced skeletal calcium mobilization versus enhanced intestinal calcium absorption is unclear.[295,297,298] Serum $1,25(OH)_2D$ is higher, and there is increased calciuric response to oral calcium load in patients with primary hyperparathyroidism with renal stones.[297-300] One study has shown that kidney stones are more frequently seen in younger patients due to higher synthetic capacity of $1,25(OH)_2D$ than older patients, with subsequent higher intestinal calcium absorption.[297]

Parathyroid Hormone–Independent Resorptive Hypercalciuria. Elevated serum $1,25(OH)_2D$ or amplified sensitivity to $1,25(OH)_2D$ at the target organ lead to enhanced bone resorption and diminished bone collagen synthesis in hypercalciuric stone-forming subjects.[252,301] A similar phenotype has been shown in GHS rats, in which their bones were more sensitive to exogenous $1,25(OH)_2D$ compared with bones from normal control rats.[265] Other mechanisms proposed are diminished bone expression of transforming growth factor-β (TGF-β), which stimulates bone formation and mineralization and/or perturbation in the RANK/RANK-L/OPG system, which increases bone resorption, in association with other cytokines and growth factors to act synergistically with high $1,25(OH)_2D$ to affect bone remodeling.[198,302,303]

HYPERURICOSURIA

Hyperuricosuria as a single abnormality is detected in much lower frequency than in combination with other metabolic abnormalities among calcium stone formers.[190,304] Several investigators have shown a high frequency of CaOx stones in patients with gout and kidney stone disease.[305,306] A structural similarity was described between crystals of uric acid (UA), sodium hydrogen urate, and CaOx, attributed to growth of one crystal on another.[307]

Pathophysiologic Mechanism of Hyperuricosuria

UA production has three sources—de novo synthesis, tissue catabolism, and dietary purine load. Of the typical daily UA load, 50% is provided by de novo synthesis and tissue catabolism, with the remainder from dietary sources.[308] Increased dietary purine intake has been implicated in most hyperuricosuric calcium urolithiasis (HUCU) patients. A metabolic study comparing HUCU stone formers with age- and weight-matched normal subjects showed that stone-forming patients ingest a higher intake of purine-rich foods, such as meat, fish, and poultry.[309] With kinetic studies, endogenous overproduction of UA has been suggested in approximately one third of HUCU stone formers consuming purine-free diets.[309] About one third of synthesized UA is excreted through the intestinal tract, followed by intestinal uricolysis, and the remainder by the kidney.[310] However, defective renal tubular reabsorption of UA has not been shown to be responsible for hyperuricosuria in this population.[311] In most mammals, ingested purines are converted to UA and then further converted to allantoin via a series of enzymatic reactions that occur primarily in the peroxisomes of hepatic cells.[312] However, humans and higher primates lack functional uricase, the enzyme that converts UA to allantoin, thereby making UA the final by-product of purine metabolism in these species.[313,314]

Physicochemical Mechanism of Hyperuricosuria-Induced Calcium Stones

The physicochemical basis for hyperuricosuria-induced CaOx stones has been postulated but has not yet been proven. In two studies, the underlying mechanism linking UA to CaOx crystallization was attributed to heterogeneous nucleation[79,80] (Figure 40.10). However, the in vivo role of heterogeneous nucleation is uncertain. Another study has shown that colloidal monosodium urate from supersaturated urine in these patients attenuates inhibitor activity against CaOx crystallization[315,316] but, when GAGs were specifically examined, UA did not affect its inhibitor activity.[317] Another study showed that monosodium urate diminishes the solubility of CaOx in solution, a process referred to as salting out.[318,319] Salting out is also known as antisolvent crystallization, which was classically used to precipitate a nonelectrolyte multicharged macromolecule (usually protein) at high electrolyte concentrations (usually ammonium sulfate). The mechanisms whereby sodium urate salts out CaOx still needs to be defined. Despite this controversy, clinical studies in HUCU patients have shown a significant decline in the rate of recurrent kidney stone formation in those treated with xanthine oxidase inhibition by allopurinol.[320] Increasing urinary supersaturation with monosodium urate in conjunction with the decreased limit of metastability of CaOx due to adsorption of macromolecular inhibitors of CaOx crystallization by monosodium urate in HUCU patients increases the risk of CaOx stone formation.[321] Contrary to clinical evidence, a retrospective population-based study in a large number of patients did not show a relationship between urinary UA and CaOx stone formation.[322]

HYPOCITRATURIA

Hypocitraturia as an isolated abnormality occurs in about one third of patients with calcium urolithiasis.[128] The presence of citrate in human urine was described in 1917.[323] A decade later, it was shown that acid-base homeostasis plays a key role in determining urinary citrate excretion in that higher urinary citrate excretion was observed in alkalotic patients and was very low in those with metabolic acidosis.[324] In 1954, a combination of oral sodium citrate, potassium citrate, and citric acid was used to alkalinize the urine of patients with UA and cystine stones.[325] Citrate is a prominent organic anion found in urine and is an important inhibitor of calcium stone formation via its effects on calcium chelation, prevention of crystallization, and aggregation independent of reducing ionized calcium and, some have postulated, its ability to promote detachment from cells (Figure 40.11).[128,131,326,327] Citrate has pK_a values of 2.9, 4.3, and 5.6 and so is found mostly as a trivalent anion (citrate^{3-}) in blood. Citrate is freely filtered, and approximately 10% to 35% of filtered citrate is excreted in urine; however, this varies tremendously, depending mainly on acid-base status. The reabsorption of citrate predominantly occurs from the proximal convoluted tubule and, to a lesser extent, the proximal straight tubule.[132,328,329] Apical membrane transport occurs through a coupled sodium dicarboxylate cotransporter (NaDC-1).[330,331] In contrast, basolateral citrate reabsorption occurs via a tricarboxylate transporter.[332]

Role of Acid-Base Status

It is well known that alteration of acid-base status plays a key role in renal tubular citrate reabsorption by multiple mechanisms (see Figure 8.11 and additional discussion in Chapter 8). Since the highest pK_a of citric acid is 5.6, the concentration of citrate^{2-}, the transported ionic species, increases at a lower luminal pH.[333] There is also a direct gating effect of pH on NaDC-1 activity, independent of the substrate concentration.[331] Furthermore, cytosolic adenosine triphosphate (ATP) citrate lyase and mitochondrial

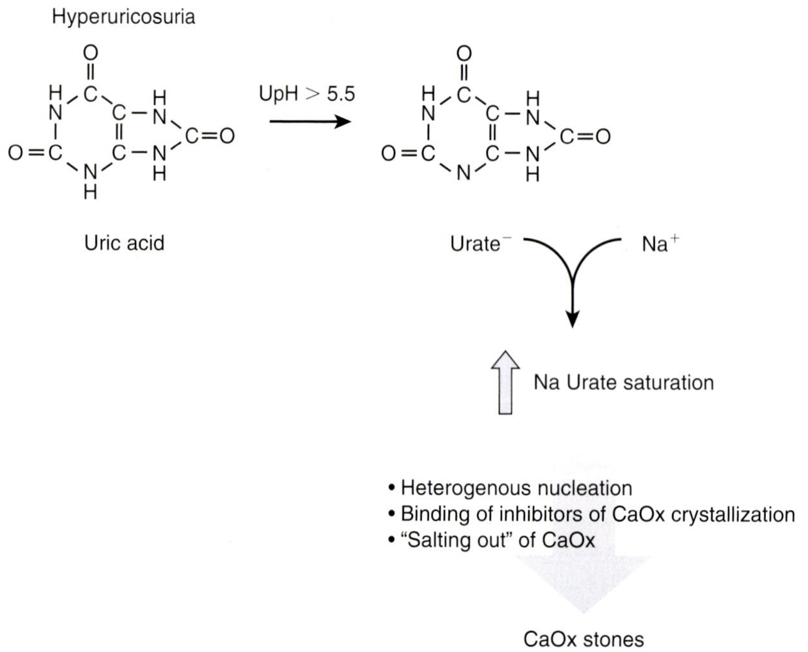

Figure 40.10 Physicochemical scheme for urate-induced CaOx stones. Hyperuricosuria in the absence of acidic urine renders high free oxalate activity levels in the urine. Sodium activity is perpetually higher than oxalate by two orders of magnitude. The higher sodium oxalate promotes CaOx crystallization by three nonexclusive mechanisms. UpH, Urinary pH.

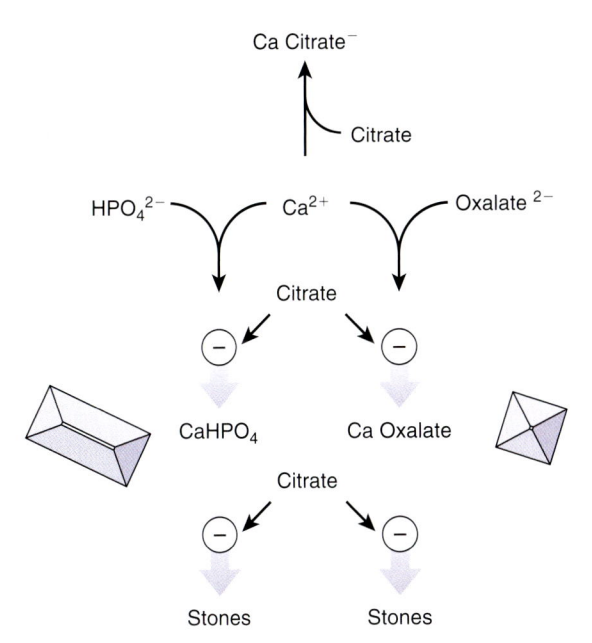

Figure 40.11 Protective effects of citrate against urolithiasis. Citrate binds calcium with high affinity to form soluble calcium citrate complexes and lowers the ionized calcium and calcium activity. Citrate also directly inhibits calcium oxalate and calcium phosphate crystallization and aggregation.

Table 40.2	Clinical Conditions Associated with Hypocitraturia
Low Extracellular Fluid pH	**Normal or High Extracellular Fluid pH**
Overproduction acidosis	Potassium deficiency
• Chronic diarrhea	
• Exercise-induced lactic acidosis	
Underexcretion acidosis	Angiotensin II–related
• Congenital or acquired distal renal tubular acidosis	• ACE inhibitors
	• Salt excess
• Acetazolamide, topiramate	Excess dietary protein

ACE, Angiotensin-converting enzyme.

aconitase activity increases in acidosis, which lowers the intracellular concentration of citrate and promotes its reabsorption.[334,335] Finally, the abundance of NaDC-1 cotransporter increases in the apical membrane of the proximal renal tubule during acidosis.[336]

Other Factors

The contribution of factors other than acid-base status to renal tubular citrate handling has not been extensively studied. However, it has been suggested that vitamin D, PTH, calcitonin, lithium, calcium, sodium,[337] magnesium, and a variety of organic anions alter urinary citrate excretion.[338] The effect of organic acid has been attributed to its competition with renal citrate for reabsorption via NaDC-1 transporters.[338] The effects of increasing apical calcium and magnesium were noted in cultured proximal tubular cells that showed decreased citrate uptake via NaDC-1 that involved a transporter other than NaDC-1.[339]

Clinical Conditions

Clinical conditions associated with significant hypocitraturia can be divided into those with systemic extracellular acidosis and those without (Table 40.2). Distal renal tubular acidosis (dRTA) is the most prominent cause of hypocitraturia and is frequently found in patients with recurrent urolithiasis.[340-344] Other conditions associated with systemic acidosis include carbonic anhydrase inhibitor treatment,[345,346] strenuous physical exercise,[347] and chronic diarrheal states.[348-350]

Hypocitraturia can also be found in normobicarbonatemic states, including incomplete dRTA, chronic renal insufficiency, mild chronic metabolic acidosis, high protein consumption and thiazide treatment with hypokalemia, primary aldosteronism, excessive salt intake, and angiotensin-converting enzyme (ACE) inhibitor treatment.[130,337,351-355]

Among these conditions, it has been demonstrated in experimental animals and, to a certain extent, in humans that ACE inhibitors lower intracellular pH or reduce hydrogen secretion by the proximal tubule.[355] Furthermore, experimental evidence in rats has shown that potassium depletion upregulates renal citrate reabsorption in the proximal tubule apical membrane from an abundance of transporters.[356]

Actions of Citrate

The physicochemical basis for the inhibitory role of citrate involves the formation of soluble complexes from the reduction of ionic calcium concentration in the urine.[357] Also, direct inhibition of crystallization of CaOx and CaP is facilitated by the inhibition of spontaneous precipitation of CaOx and the accumulation of preformed calcium oxalate crystals.[93,109]

HYPEROXALURIA

Hyperoxaluria is present in isolation or in combination with other risk factors in 8% to 50% of kidney stone formers.[191,358-360] In CaOx stone formers, urinary oxalate and calcium are responsible for driving CaOx supersaturation, although the activity of calcium is one order higher than that of oxalate (Figure 40.12).[361] Under normal circumstances, the physiologic concentrations of urinary calcium and oxalate predict the concentration of a CaOx complex in the urine, which far exceeds its solubility constant.[361,362] The mechanisms underlying hyperoxaluria can stem from multiple factors, summarized in Figure 40.13.[363-367]

Increased Hepatic Production

Monogenic disorders of oxalate metabolism are rare but serious causes of kidney stones. Oxalate is a dicarboxylic acid and, in mammals, is an end product of hepatic metabolism.[190,363,368] Primary hyperoxaluria (PH) is an autosomal recessive disorder of inborn enzymatic defects resulting in massive hepatic overproduction of oxalate. The three main forms of PH are classified as types I, II, and III. Type I PH (Online Mendelian Inheritance in Man [OMIM] 259900) is the consequence of a deficiency or mistargeting of hepatic alanine-glyoxylate transferase (AGT), which is a pyridoxal 5′-phosphate–dependent enzyme that transaminates glyoxylate to glycine.[369] It accounts for about 80% of PH cases. Type II (OMIM 260000) is due to a deficiency in the

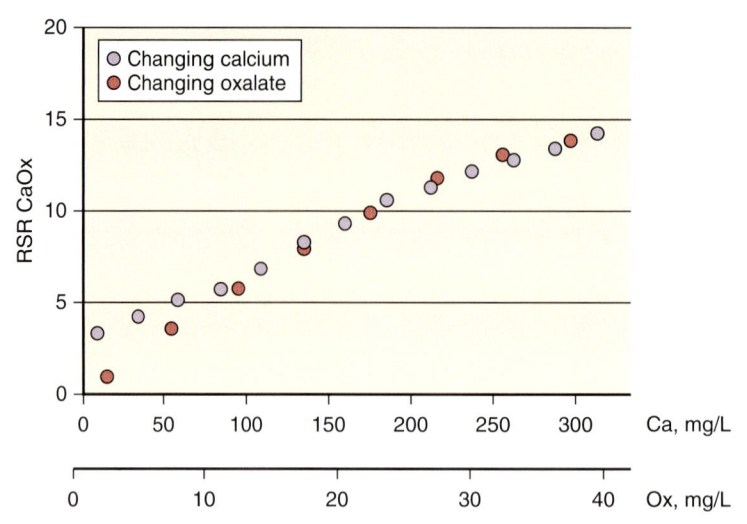

Figure 40.12 Relationship between calcium oxalate saturation and calcium or oxalate concentration. Calcium or oxalate was varied individually while the other was kept constant. RSR, Relative supersaturation ratio. (Modified from Pak CY, Adams-Huet B, Poindexter JR, et al: Rapid communication: relative effect of urinary calcium and oxalate on saturation of calcium oxalate. *Kidney Int* 66:2032-2037, 2004.)

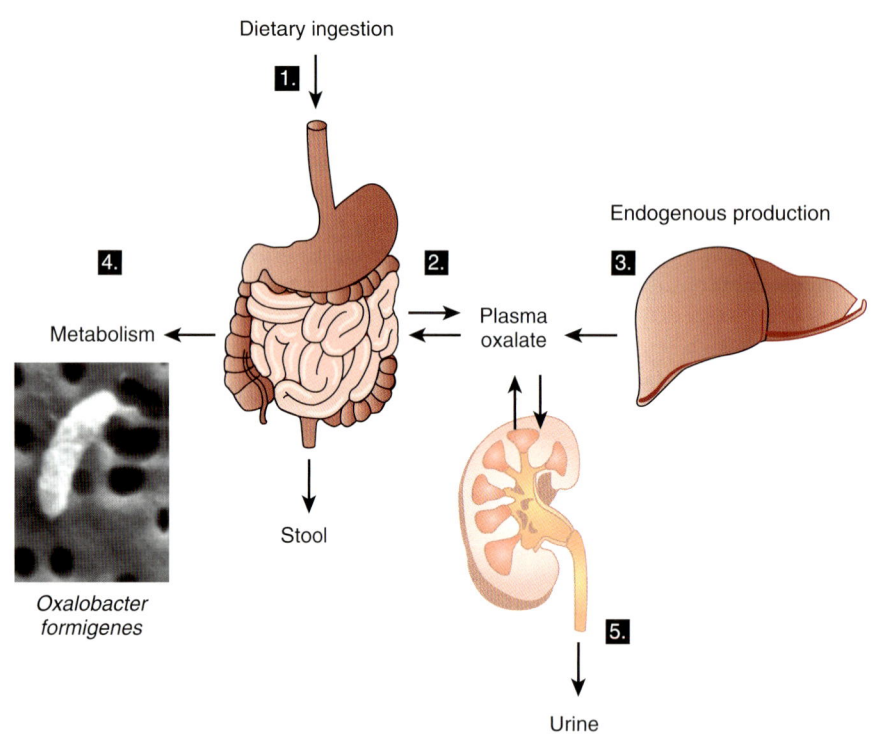

Figure 40.13 Pathophysiologic mechanisms of hyperoxaluria. Oxalate balance consists of ingestion and endogenous production versus intestinal and urinary excretion. Intestinal handling can be bidirectional, and luminal degradation is facilitated by microbial degradation. Urinary excretion is the net of filtration minus tubular reabsorption of oxalate. Hyperoxaluria can be caused by the following: (1) increased dietary ingestion; (2) increased gut absorption or decreased secretion; (3) endogenous hepatic production; (4) decreased intestinal bacterial metabolism; or (5) renal hyperexcretion.

cytosolic enzyme glyoxalate reductase–hydroxypyruvate reductase (GRHPR), which reduces glyoxalate to glycolate.[370] It accounts for about 10% of cases. The least common variety is type III (OMIM 613616), which is due to activating mutations in the mitochondrial 4-hydroxy-2-oxoglutarate aldolase (HOGA) enzyme, which converts hydroxyproline to glyoxylate.[371-374] Unlike types I and II, heterozygotes can have CaOx stones.[373,374] PH type III accounts for about 5% of cases, with another 5% of PH cases having no known genetic lesions.

A number of other metabolic precursors of oxalate metabolism, including by-products of the breakdown of ascorbic acid, fructose, xylose, and hydroxyproline, potentially contribute to oxalate production. However, their contribution under normal physiologic circumstances has not yet been fully elucidated.[375,376]

Dietary Intake and Bioavailability

Dietary oxalate plays an important role in urinary oxalate excretion. There is a wide variation in estimated intake of oxalate, ranging from 50 to 1000 mg/day.[191,360] Dietary oxalate and its bioavailability contribute to approximately 45% of the urinary oxalate excretion.[377] The main source of most bioavailable oxalate-rich food includes seeds, such as chocolate derived from tropical cocoa trees, leafy vegetables, including spinach and rhubarb, and tea. The relationship between oxalate absorption and dietary oxalate intake has been demonstrated to be nonlinear.[377]

Intestinal Absorption

Despite seminal advances in rodent intestinal physiology of oxalate handling,[378] the specific intestinal segments in humans involved in oxalate absorption is not fully known. It was proposed that the main fraction of oxalate is absorbed in the small intestine, since most oxalate is absorbed during the first 4 to 8 hours after the consumption of oxalate-rich foods,[358,366,379,380] and 5 hours of intestinal transit time is required for nutrients to move from the stomach to the colon. Nevertheless, it has also been suggested that the colon also participates, but to a lesser extent, in oxalate absorption.[380]

Oxalate is absorbed and secreted in the GI tract through paracellular and transcellular pathways. Paracellular oxalate absorption has not yet been confirmed in intact organisms. However, it has been proposed that at a low gastric pH, part of the dietary oxalate is converted into small hydrophobic molecules that could possibly diffuse through the lipid bilayer,[381-384] thereby increasing urinary oxalate excretion.

Role of Anion Exchanger Slc26a6

The anion exchange transporter Slc26a6 has been shown to be involved in intestinal oxalate transport.[385,386] This transporter is expressed in the apical membrane of the duodenum, jejunum, and ileum and, to a lesser extent, the large intestine.[387] In vitro studies have demonstrated defective net oxalate secretion in mice with targeted inactivation of Slc26a6[385] (Figure 40.14). Furthermore, in vivo studies in *Slc26a6* null mice on a controlled oxalate diet showed increased plasma oxalate concentration, decreased fecal oxalate excretion concentration, and high urinary oxalate excretion.[385] The differences in these levels were attenuated following stabilization on an oxalate-free diet. These results suggest that diminished net oxalate secretion in the gut is responsible for net oxalate absorption; this results in a rise in plasma oxalate concentration, elevated urinary oxalate excretion and bladder stones, and Yasue-positive crystals in the kidney. However, the influence of this putative anion exchange transporter on intestinal oxalate absorption—specifically, its role in kidney stone formation in humans—has not yet been demonstrated. Studies with exogenous radiolabelled oxalate in normal humans have shown that renal excretion accounts for most of the disposal of oxalate.[388] In contrast, report of a case of enteric hyperoxaluria has shown drastically diminished expression of SLC26A6 protein in the intestine.[389]

Role of *Oxalobacter formigenes*

Many gut bacteria, including *Oxalobacter formigenes* (OF), have been reported to degrade oxalate in the intestinal

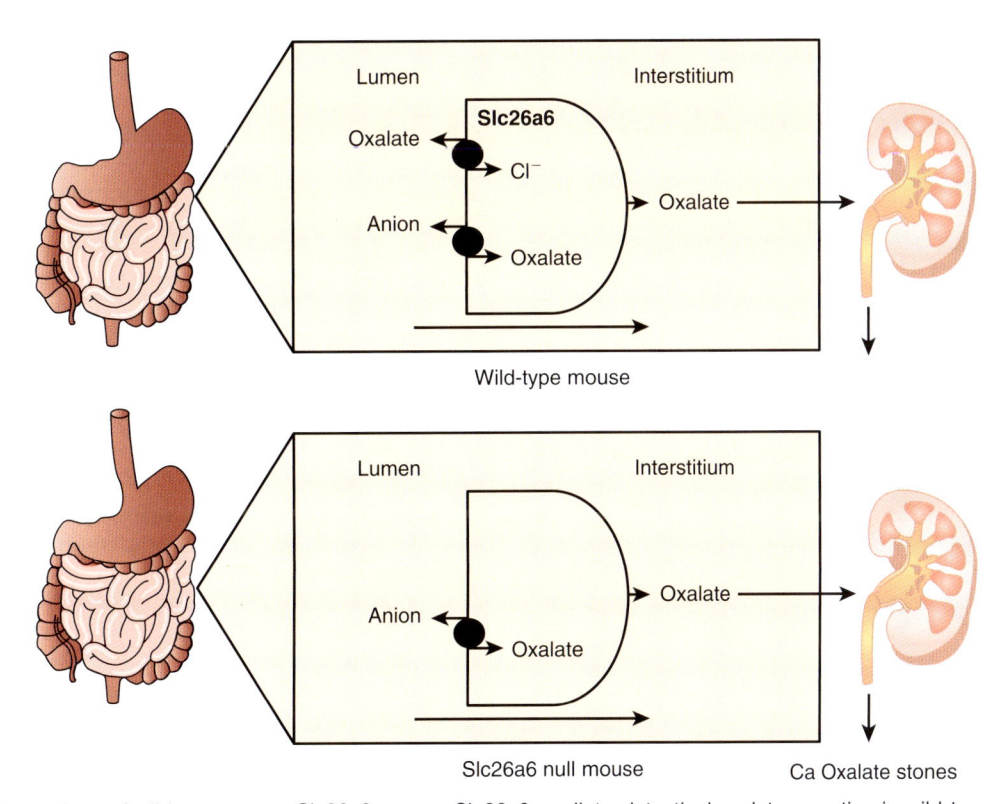

Figure 40.14 Comparison of wild-type versus Slc26a6 mouse. Slc26a6 mediates intestinal oxalate secretion in wild-type mice, so that only 10% of ingested oxalate is normally absorbed and excreted into the urine. Targeted deletion of the *Slc26a6* gene in mice unmasks a large intestinal absorptive flux of oxalate and leads to increased plasma oxalate levels, hyperoxaluria, and calcium oxalate stones.

lumen.[390] Although OF was initially found in ruminants, they have been shown to be present in other species and in humans.[391,392] Colonization of the bowels with OF begins at some point during childhood and is found in the feces of 60% to 80% of adults.[393] Dietary oxalate intake influences the colonization of OF in the intestinal tract. In animal studies, significant declines in urinary oxalate follow administration of or an increase in OF colonization.[394,395] An ex vivo Ussing chamber study demonstrated microbe-host interaction in that OF not only degrades intestinal luminal oxalate, but has the capability to stimulate net intestinal oxalate secretion.[396] The result of this pathophysiologic mechanism from animal experiments has been confirmed in patients with type I PH, in subjects with normal renal function, and in patients with chronic renal insufficiency showing a transient reduction of urinary oxalate following the oral administration of OF.[397]

Renal Excretion

The kidney plays a major role in oxalate homeostasis. Oxalate is not significantly protein-bound and is freely filtered at the glomerulus. With impaired kidney function, plasma oxalate concentration steadily increases, exceeds its saturation in the blood, and therefore enhances the risk of systemic tissue oxalate deposition, including kidney damage. Renal oxalate clearance studies in human subjects have been controversial. Radiolabeled oxalate studies[398,399] have demonstrated oxalate secretion, while endogenous renal oxalate clearance assessments using direct measurements of serum and urine oxalate have demonstrated net reabsorption.[400,401] However, renal secretion of oxalate with high fractional excretion has been reported in patients with primary or enteric hyperoxaluria.[399-401]

Reabsorption and secretion of oxalate have been shown in the renal proximal tubule.[402,403] It has been shown that Slc26a6 is expressed in the apical membrane of the proximal renal tubule and affects the activity of a number of other apical anion exchangers.[404,405] However, the physiologic role of this anion exchanger in renal oxalate handling has not yet been fully demonstrated. In *slc26a6* null mice, the high serum oxalate appears to be driven mostly by hyperoxalemia rather than by renal leak of oxalate.[385]

Clinical Hyperoxaluria

PH typically presents during early childhood with CaOx stones and nephrocalcinosis. This disease is severe and is associated with frequent stone recurrence and impaired kidney function.[406] From 1985 to 1992, the estimated prevalence of PH was reported to be 1 to 3 cases/million population, a calculated incidence rate of 1/120,000/year.[407,408] Furthermore, end-stage kidney disease (ESKD) as a result of PH has been demonstrated to occur in 1% to 10% of children.[409,410] Occasionally, milder forms of PH are found in adult subjects.

Enteric hyperoxaluria due to inflammatory bowel disease, jejunoileal bypass, and modern bariatric surgeries for morbid obesity are the most common causes of hyperoxaluria in clinical practice.[411-416] Roux-en-Y gastric bypass (RYGB) is a weight reduction procedure theoretically combining restrictive and malabsorptive mechanisms for the treatment of obesity. Urolithiasis is a well-known complication of those who have undergone RYGB. A comparison of 4690 patients following RYGB with an obese control group found 7.5% of kidney stones in RYGB patients compared with 4.63% in obese controls. Another retrospective cohort of 972 RYGB patients showed an 8.8% stone prevalence prior to surgery, while 3.2% developed new stones postoperatively.[417] The pathophysiologic mechanisms for lithogenesis are complex and can be due to hyperoxaluria, hypocitraturia, aciduria, and low urinary volume[349,350,418-426] (Table 40.3). A national private insurance claim database from 2002 to 2006 supported the notion that gastric banding is not associated with increased kidney stone risk. After gastric banding, 1.49% of subjects formed stones compared to 5.97% of obese controls.[427]

The underlying mechanisms for hyperoxaluria following inflammatory bowel disease and bariatric procedures have not yet been elucidated. Purported mechanisms have linked hyperoxaluria to intestinal fat malabsorption.[423,428] In this scheme, unabsorbed fatty acids sequester calcium that would otherwise bind oxalate in the intestinal lumen, thereby increasing the free luminal concentration of oxalate and enhancing its availability for absorption. An additional mechanism was suggested to be increased permeability of the colon from exposure to unconjugated bile acids and long-chain fatty acids following inflammatory bowel disease and bariatric procedures[367,429] (Figure 40.15). Finally, it has been proposed that changes in intestinal microbiota occur in patients with recurrent calcium oxalate urolithiasis,[394,430,431] enteric hyperoxaluria,[432,433] and cystic fibrosis,[434,435] all of which can potentially modify the colonization of lower intestinal flora with respect to OF.[434,435]

Physicochemical Effects of Hyperoxaluria

Oxalate and calcium are both important in raising CaOx supersaturation in urine.[361] In human serum, oxalate concentration is 1-5 μmol/L but its concentration in the urine is 100 times higher than in serum.[436] At physiologic pH, oxalate will form an insoluble salt with calcium. Normal urine is often supersaturated with CaOx because the solubility of CaOx in an aqueous solution is limited to approximately 5 mg/L at a pH of 7. Considering that normal urine volume ranges from 1 to 2 L/day, normal urinary excretion is more than 40 mg. In most cases, one can surmise that normal urine is supersaturated with CaOx salt. However, under normal conditions, the blood is undersaturated with respect to CaOx. Nevertheless, in patients with PH and renal insufficiency, when the serum oxalate concentration rises above 30 μmol/L, the blood becomes supersaturated with CaOx.[437]

ALTERATIONS OF URINARY pH

Both highly acidic (≤5.5) and highly alkaline (≥6.7) urine increase the propensity for calcium kidney stone formation. With unusually acidic urinary pH, urine becomes supersaturated with undissociated UA, which can contribute to CaOx crystallization.[79,438] Highly alkaline urine increases the abundance of monohydrogen phosphate (dissociation constant $pK_a \cong 6.7$), which, in combination with calcium, transforms to thermodynamically unstable brushite ($CaHPO_4 \cdot 2H_2O$) and finally to hydroxyapatite—$Ca_{10}(PO_4)_6(OH)_2$. Over the past 4 decades, the average CaP content of stones has progressively increased.[53]

The rise in the prevalence of CaP stones has been attributed to, but not proven to be, due to extracorporeal shock

Table 40.3 Kidney Stone Risk Profiles and Roux-en-Y Gastric Bypass Surgery (RYGB)

Reference	Pathophysiologic Mechanisms for Lithogenesis	Before RYGB	Following RYGB
Nelson et al[418]	Urinary oxalate (mg/day)	N/A	79
Sinha et al[349]		31 ± 16	65 ± 39*
Asplin and Coe[350]		N/A	85 ± 44*
Duffey et al[420]		31 ± 10	41 ± 18*
Penniston et al[424]		N/A	48 ± 4
Park et al[419]		32 (median)	40 (median)*
Maalouf et al[365]		N/A	45 ± 21*
Patel et al[422]		N/A	61 ± 4*
Kumar et al[423]		26 ± 13	32 ± 11 (NS)
Froeder et al[425]		N/A	26 (median; NS)
Sinha et al[349]	Urinary citrate (mg/day)	660 ± 297	444 ± 376 (NS)
Asplin and Coe[350]		N/A	477 ± 330*
Penniston et al[424]		N/A	441 ± 71*
Park et al[419]		675 (median)	456 (median)*
Maalouf et al[365]		N/A	358 ± 357*
Patel et al[422]		N/A	621 ± 40*
Froeder et al[425]		N/A	472 (median; NS)
Asplin and Coe[350]	Urinary pH	N/A	5.72 ± 0.31*
Sinha et al[349]		5.96 ± 0.38	5.78 ± 0.59 (NS)
Duffey et al[420]		5.82 ± 0.54	5.66 ± 0.43 (NS)
Park et al[419]		6.03 (median)	5.75 (median; NS)
Froeder et al[425]		N/A	5.78 (median; NS)
Duffey et al[420]	Urinary volume (mL/day)	1380 ± 400	900 ± 430*
Park et al[419]		1800 (median)	1440*
Maalouf et al[365]		N/A	1900 ± 900 (NS)
Kumar et al[423]		2091 ± 768	1316 ± 540*
Froeder et al[425]		N/A	1140*
Sinha et al[349]	Urinary calcium (mg/day)	206 ± 111	112 ± 92*
Asplin and Coe[350]		N/A	141 ± 61*
Duffey et al[420]		206 ± 111	112 ± 92*
Fleischer et al[426]		161 ± 22	92 ± 15*
Penniston et al[424]		N/A	100 ± 12*
Park et al[419]		176 (median)	135* (median)
Maalouf et al[365]		N/A	115 ± 93*
Froeder et al[425]		N/A	89* (median)

*Significant compared to control.
N/A, Not available; NS, statistically nonsignificant.

wave lithotripsy (ESWL), increasing use of medications, including topiramate, and alkali therapy.[14,192,439,440] The three main risk factors for the development of brushite stones are alkaline urine, hypercalciuria, and hypocitruria (Figure 40.16). It has been suggested that urinary pH elevation plays the most important role in the transformation of CaOx to CaP. A retrospective study of 62 patients found that high urinary pH was the primary physiologic abnormality in those in whom CaOx transformed to CaP.[53] The defective renal acidification was proposed to be related to renal tissue damage from ESWL.[14] Patients with CaP stones usually carry a greater stone burden, are less likely to be stone-free after urologic procedures, and also experience resistance to ESWL and ultrasonic lithotripsy.[441-443]

URIC ACID STONES

Higher primates have higher serum and urinary UA levels due to the lack of the enzyme uricase, which transforms uric acid into the more soluble allantoin[313,314,444] and are thus end products of metabolism. Uricase deficiency is partially compensated by repression of xanthine oxidase[445] but the high serum UA is also due to low renal fractional excretion of UA.[314] The principal sources of UA production are de novo synthesis, tissue catabolism, and dietary purine load.[308] Generally, 50% of the typical daily urate load is provided by de novo synthesis and tissue catabolism, with the remainder originating from dietary sources.[308] About 25% to 30% of synthesized UA is excreted through the intestinal tract and the remainder by the kidney.[310]

The cause of uric acid urolithiasis can be genetic[313,446,447] or acquired,[347,352,448] with the metabolic syndrome being the principal acquired cause (Table 40.4). The primary pathophysiologic mechanisms accounting for UA urolithiasis include hyperuricosuria and low urinary volume; the most important contributing factor is unusually low urinary pH.

PHYSICOCHEMISTRY OF URIC ACID

Given that UA solubility in a urinary environment is limited to about 96 mg/L, and UA excretion in humans typically exceeds 600 mg/day, the risk of UA precipitation is constant.[190,358] Uric acid has a pK_a of 5.35 at 37° C.[449,450]

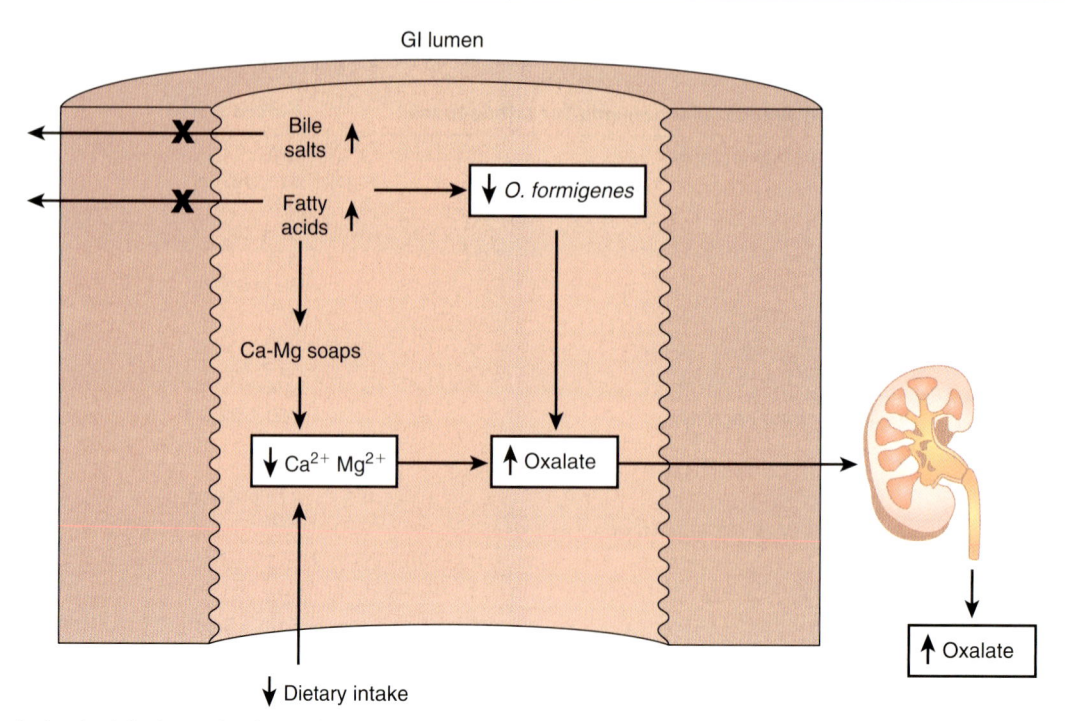

Figure 40.15 Pathophysiologic mechanisms of hyperoxaluria in inflammatory bowel disease or following bariatric surgery. Fatty acids and bile salts precipitate luminal calcium, which can be compounded by low dietary intake. Low luminal calcium frees up and increases unbound oxalate. Lack of *Oxalobacter formigenes* due to excess bile salts also contributes to high luminal oxalate.

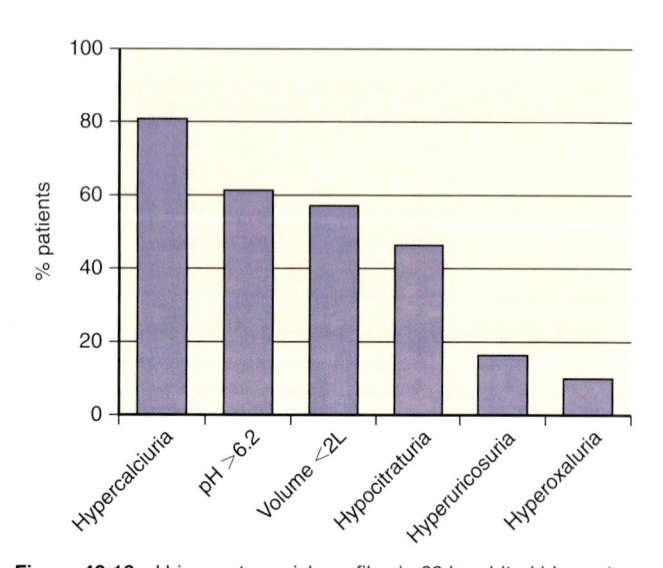

Figure 40.16 Urinary stone risk profiles in 82 brushite kidney stone formers. (Modified from Krambeck AE, Handa SE, Evan AP, Lingeman JE: Brushite stone disease as a consequence of lithotripsy? *Urol Res* 38:293-299, 2010.)

Table 40.4 Causes of Uric Acid Urolithiasis

Cause	Low Urine Volume	Low Urinary pH	Hyperuricosuria
Acquired			
Diarrhea	+	+	+
Myeloproliferative			+
High animal protein		+	+
Uricosuric drugs			+
Primary gout		+	
Metabolic syndrome		+	
Congenital			
Enzyme disorders of purine metabolism			+
Mutations in uric acid transporters			+

Consequently, urinary pH plays a principal role in that acidic urine (pH ≤ 5.5) titrates urate to UA, which is sparingly soluble and hence precipitates.[358,451,452] This also indirectly induces mixed UA-CaOx urolithiasis, which is mediated through heterogeneous nucleation and epitaxial crystal growth.[81,453,454] Generally, urine is metastably supersaturated with respect to UA. This suggests that the absence of an inhibitor influences the propensity for UA urolithiasis. This has been supported by experimental evidence demonstrating the presence of macromolecules that attenuate UA crystal adherence to the renal tubular epithelium.[455]

PATHOPHYSIOLOGY OF URIC ACID STONES

Hyperuricosuria

Hyperuricosuria can be due to genetic, metabolic, or dietary factors.[26] Hyperuricosuria is seen in rare hereditary disorders, with mutations in enzymatic pathways responsible for UA production. These conditions include X-linked phosphoribosyl synthetase overactivity, autosomal recessive glucose-6-phosphatase deficiency, and glycogenesis types III, V, and VII.[26,313,447] The clinical presentations of these disorders are unique and can be accompanied with a significant risk for gouty arthritis, kidney stone formation, and even renal failure. Biochemical abnormalities include highly elevated serum UA concentration (10 mg/dL) and urinary UA excretion of 1000 mg/day or higher. The disease manifestations commonly present during childhood; however, they remain silent until puberty.

Renal handling of UA is complex and involves secretion and reabsorption.[314] An inactivating mutation of the urate transporter, URAT1, causes renal uric acid wasting, which results in hyperuricosuria, hypouricemia, UA kidney stones, and exercise-induced acute renal failure.[456,457] In addition, specifically in the Sardinian population, a putative gene locus localized on chromosome 10q122 has been linked to UA urolithiasis. The putative culprit gene codes for a hypothetical protein with zinc finger motifs, ZNF365, of unknown function.[458]

Hyperuricosuria also occurs with excessive tissue breakdown with malignancy and chemotherapy.[459,460] Certain uricosuric drugs such as high-dose salicylates, probenecid, radiocontrast agents and losartan have been shown to increase UA excretion, which increases the risk of UA stone formation.[450,461] In the large majority of cases, however, there are no identifiable congenital or acquired causes of hyperuricosuria.

Low Urinary Volume

Low urinary volume increases the urinary supersaturation of all stone-forming constituents.[462] Volume depletion from chronic diarrhea from inflammatory bowel disease has a major impact on uric acid stone formation. It has been shown that one third of the stones are composed of uric acid, an incidence is higher than the incidence of 8% to 10% reported in the general population.[463-465] In addition, uric acid stones comprise two thirds of all stones in patients following ileostomy.[463] In this population, low urinary volume, in addition to the aciduria from alkali loss, is common.[466-468]

Low Urinary pH

In the large majority of cases, hyperuricosuria or low urine volume is not the culprit. The lithogenesis is driven by low urinary pH. Collectively, these patients are experiencing, by default, idiopathic UA urolithiasis (IUAU). This condition is caused by unusually acidic urine, which is the single invariant feature in all patients with IUAU[29,358,469] (Figure 40.17).

Origin of Low Urinary pH. IUAU is the stone type that shares numerous common characteristics with the metabolic syndrome.[31,446,470,471] Several cross-sectional studies have supported the association between UA stones, diabetes, and obesity[30,32,33,472-475] (Figure 40.18). Since 2000, two major causative factors—increased acid load to the kidneys and impaired ammonium (NH_4^+) excretion—have been shown to result in unusually acidic urine.[29,358]

Increased Acid Load to Kidneys. In a steady state, net acid excretion (NAE) equals net acid production. Higher NAE can occur as a consequence of increased endogenous production, increased dietary ingestion (high dietary acid consumption or low alkali intake), or alkali loss.[476] Several

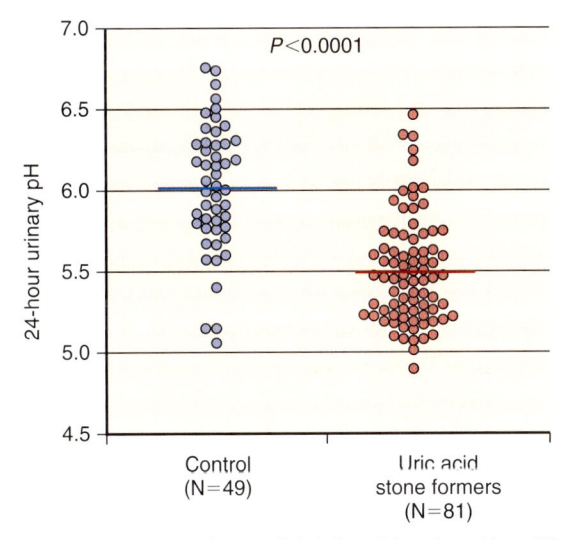

Figure 40.17 24-hour urinary pH in idiopathic uric acid urolithiasis versus control subject. Urine was collected under a fixed metabolic diet. The comparison was made by an unpaired T-test.

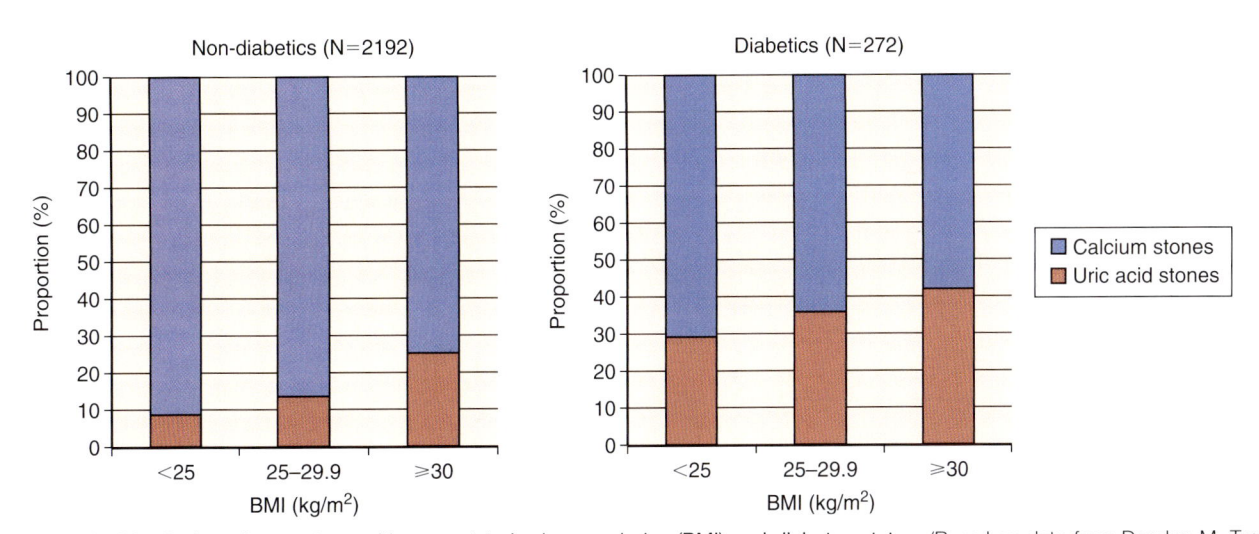

Figure 40.18 Distribution of stone type with respect to body mass index (BMI) and diabetes status. (Based on data from Daudon M, Traxer O, Conort P, et al: Type 2 diabetes increases the risk for uric acid stones. *J Am Soc Nephrol* 17:2026-2033, 2006.)

metabolic studies of a constant, controlled metabolic diet have shown that NAE is higher in IUAU patients and type 2 diabetics without stones compared to control subjects,[29,470,471,477] suggesting that endogenous acid production is elevated (Figure 40.19). The nature and source of these putative organic acids is unknown at present but likely has an enterohepatic origin.[478] Adults with type 2 diabetes without kidney stones have similar features to those with UA stones and similar differences in gut microbiota compared to nondiabetic adults.[479]

Impaired NH_4^+ Excretion. Under normal physiologic circumstances, NH_4^+ excretion plays a key role in the regulation of acid-base balance due to its high pK_a of 9.3 (NH_3/NH_4^+ system). NH_4^+ can effectively buffer a major portion of secreted H^+ due to its high capacity and high pK_a.[480,481]

The alternative source of buffering is by many H^+ acceptors, which are collectively referred to as titratable acid (TA).[480] In IUAU, there is defective NH_4^+ production and excretion (see Figure 40.19). More H^+ is buffered by TA (including urate) to maintain acid-base homeostasis.[29,358,471] The trade-off is the propensity for UA precipitation.[29,469] The defective NH_4^+ excretion in IUAU occurs at a steady state while the patient is on a fixed metabolic diet, as well as after acute acid loads.[29] Defective NH_4^+ excretion is not unique to UA stone formers but remains a shared feature between metabolic syndrome patients and type 2 diabetic non–stone formers (Figure 40.20).[31,446,471,475]

Role of Renal Lipotoxicity

Most urinary NH_4^+ is produced and secreted by the renal proximal tubular cell.[482,483] NH_4^+ is directly transported by the Na^+-H^+-exchanger (NHE3), either as Na^+-NH_4^+ into the proximal tubular lumen or by nonionic diffusion of NH_3 into the renal proximal tubular lumen, trapped as NH_4^+ by luminal H^+ secretion by NHE3.[482-488] When energy intake exceeds utilization, as occurs in patients with IUAU, obesity, diabetes, or multiple sclerosis (MS), fat accumulates; this can occur in nonadipose tissues[489] (Figure 40.21). Ectopic fat is termed *steatosis*, and the ill effects of steatosis are termed *lipotoxicity*,[489-494] which is the consequence of the accumulation of toxic metabolites such as acyl coenzyme A (acyl CoA), diacylglycerol, and ceramide.[495-497] In a rodent model of the metabolic syndrome, the Zucker diabetic fatty (ZDF) rat,[498] as well as in cultured proximal tubular cells, steatosis led to deranged ammoniagenesis and transport.[499] ZDF rats have higher renal cortical triglyceride content commensurate with lower urinary NH_4^+ and pH values[499] (see Figure 40.21). Similar findings were also seen in humans with a high BMI.[500] Kidney cell lines incubated with a mixture of long-chain fatty acids have a decrease in NH_4^+ production.[499] Treatment of ZDF rats with thiazolidinediones or removal of fatty acids from cultured cells reduced renal steatosis, and restored acid-base parameters toward normal, demonstrating causality (see Figure 40.21).[501]

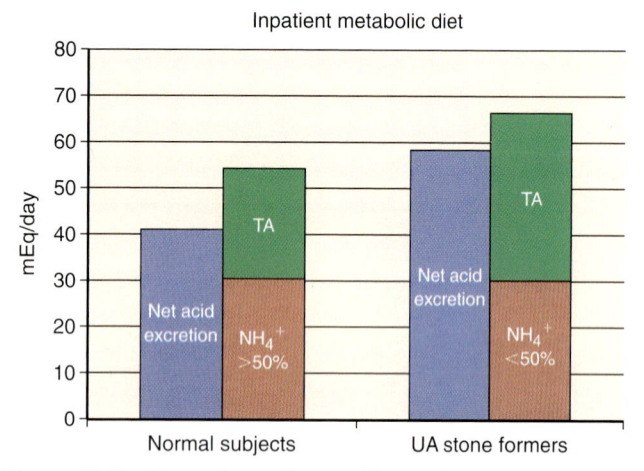

Figure 40.19 Comparison of net acid excretion between normal subjects and uric acid (UA) stone formers. Studies were performed with a controlled metabolic diet. Despite equivalent amounts of exogenous acid intake (same urinary sulfate excretion, not shown), uric acid stone formers had higher net acid excretion, and a lower fraction of the net acid was carried by ammonium. TA, Titratable acid. (Adapted from 471, 887, 888.)

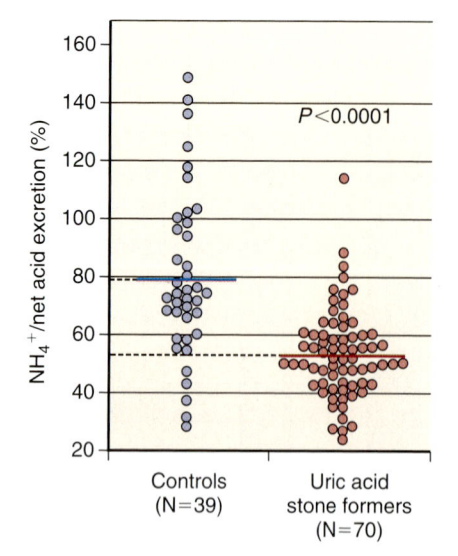

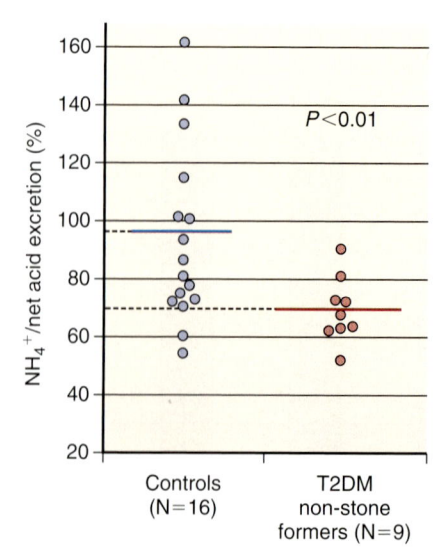

Figure 40.20 Decreased ammonium excretion as a fraction of net acid excretion in idiopathic uric acid stone formers and subjects with type 2 diabetics (T2DM). Individuals were studied under a controlled metabolic diet so all differences were intrinsic to the subjects. (From Maalouf NM, Cameron MA, Moe OW, Sakhaee K: Metabolic basis for low urine pH in type 2 diabetes. *Clin J Am Soc Nephrol* 5:1277-1281, 2010.)

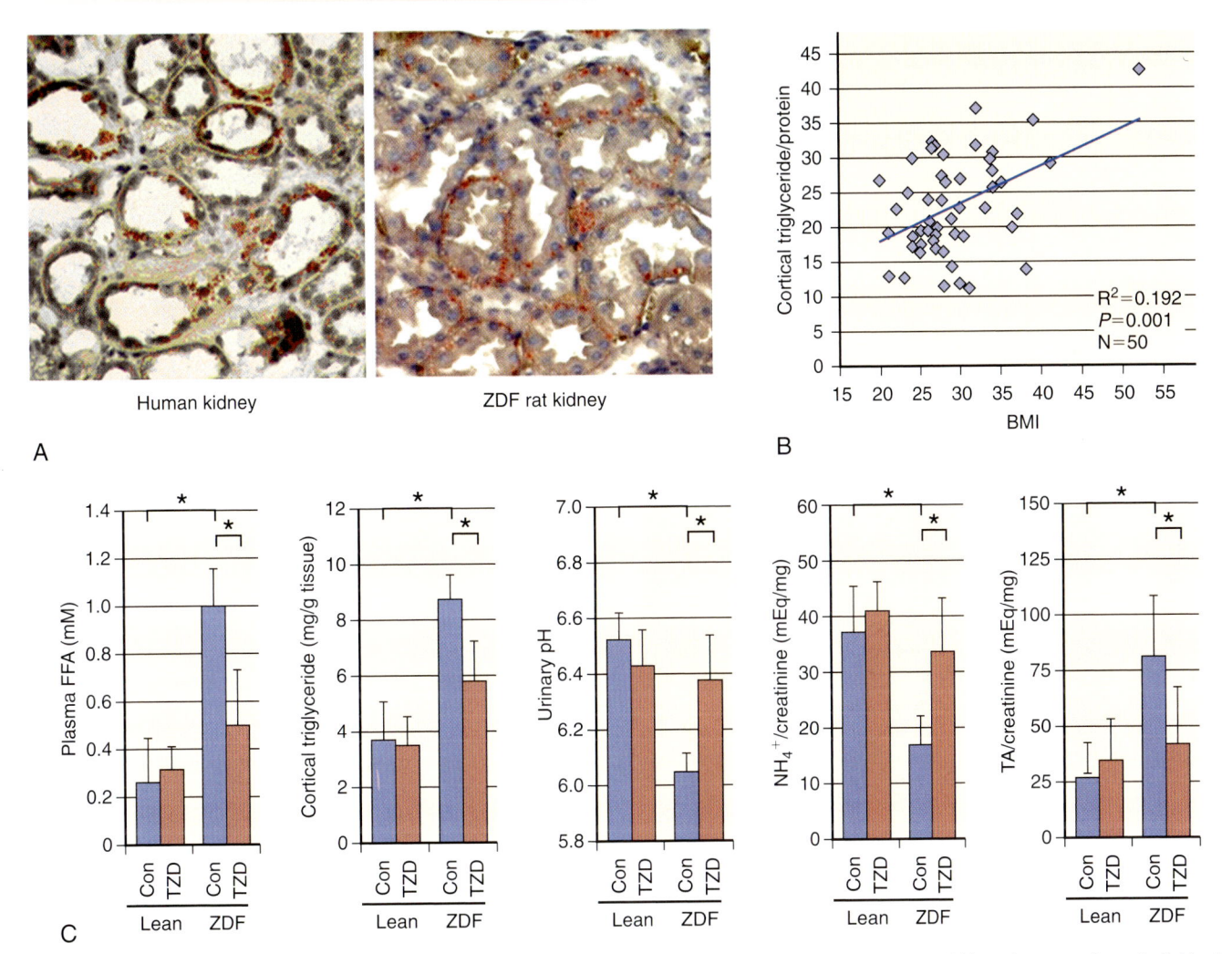

Figure 40.21 Renal steatosis and lipotoxicity in humans and rats. **A,** Oil red O stain of triglyceride in human kidney from an obese individual and Zucker diabetic fatty (ZDF) rats (×). **B,** Cortical triglyceride content in human biopsy samples showing the relationship between triglyceride and body mass index (BMI). **C,** Lean rats or ZDF rats were treated with vehicle or rosiglitazone thiazolidinedione (TZD). A number of parameters were compared among the four groups. The amelioration of plasma free fatty acid (FFA) and renal cortical triglyceride was accompanied by increase in urine pH and ammonium excretion, whereas titratable acid (TA) excretion was decreased. Con, Control. (Adapted from Bobulescu IA, Dubree M, Zhang J, et al: Effect of renal lipid accumulation on proximal tubule Na+/H+ exchange and ammonium secretion. *Am J Physiol Renal Physiol* 294:F1315-F1322, 2008; Bobulescu IA, Lotan Y, Zhang J, et al: Triglycerides in the human kidney cortex: relationship with body size. *PLoS One* 9:e101285, 2014; and Bobulescu IA, Dubree M, Zhang J, et al: Reduction of renal triglyceride accumulation: effects on proximal tubule Na+/H+ exchange and urinary acidification. *Am J Physiol Renal Physiol* 297:F1419-F1426, 2009.)

Another potential mechanism in UA stone formers and/or in ZDF rats is defective NH_4^+ synthesis due to substrate competition—namely, fatty acid instead of glutamine as a source of energy—thus removing the source of nitrogen for ammoniagenesis.[502]

CYSTINE STONES

OVERVIEW

Cystine stones are exclusively seen in cystinuria, which is a mendelian disorder caused by inactivating mutations of the subunits of a dibasic amino acid transporter in the proximal tubule, rBAT/b$^{0,+}$AT (SLC3A1/SLC7A9; heavy-light chain), which is equivalent to the system b$^{0,+}$ of amino transport (Figure 40.22; see Chapter 8). This is the most common primary inherited aminoaciduria (OMIM 220100), causing 1% to 2% of renal stones in adults and 6% to 8% in pediatric patients.[503] Normally, reabsorption of amino acids from the urine is near completion with a fractional excretion close to zero. Inactivation of rBAT/b$^{0,+}$AT leads to urinary wasting of many cationic amino acids, but only cystine has a low enough solubility to precipitate. Since rBAT/b$^{0,+}$AT is also present in the gut, there is malabsorption of cationic amino acids but no clinically discernible intestinal phenotype.

MOLECULAR BIOLOGY AND GENETICS

The rBAT and b$^{0,+}$AT subunits are linked by a disulfide bridge in the heterodimer, which is characteristic of the heteromeric amino acid transporters.[504] It mediates obligatory exchange of cationic amino acids (e.g., cystine–two cysteines bound by a disulfide bridge) and neutral amino acids with a 1:1 stoichiometry (see Chapter 8). In addition to human disease, the causal link of rBAT/b$^{0,+}$AT to cationic aminoaciduria has been corroborated by mouse models

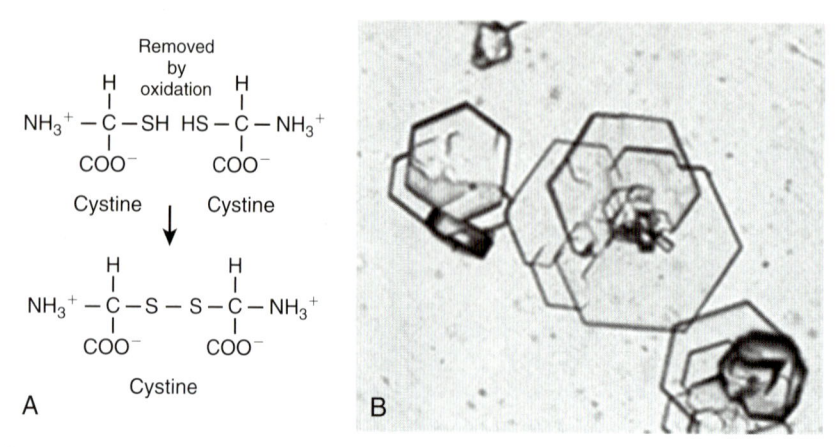

Figure 40.22 **A,** Cystine is a dimer of cysteine formed by disulfide bonding under oxidizing conditions. **B,** Appearance of cystine crystals in the urine of a patient with cystinuria.

with defective rBAT (D140G mutation)[505] or b[0,+]AT (knockout)[506] and Newfoundland dogs with defective rBAT (natural nonsense mutation),[507] which all have cystinuria similar to that in humans.

To date, a total of 133 mutations in rBAT (SLC3A1; cystinuria type A) and 95 mutations in b[0,+]AT (*SLC7A9;* cystinuria type B) have been identified in humans, including missense, nonsense, splice site, frameshift, and large chromosomal rearrangements[503] in about 90% of the subjects studied. In most cases, the disease is inherited in an autosomal recessive manner. In about 3% of patients with clinical cystinuria, there are no mutations in the two candidate loci. These can be due to mutations in promoter, regulatory, or intronic regions. The current belief is that all cases of classic and isolated cystinuria are due to mutations in system b[0,+].

Interestingly, haplotypes with b[0,+]AT polymorphisms have been reported to lead to cystinuria. This has been reported in cystine stone formers who are heterozygous for a known b[0,+]AT disease mutation.[508,509] Isolated cystinuria (cystine wasting without cationic aminoaciduria) can be caused by heterozygous b[0,+]AT mutation.[510,511,509] The molecular biology is in accordance with metabolic data. Cystine clearance approximates the GFR in classic cystinuria.[512] System b[0,+] (rBAT/b[0,+]AT) is the principal transport system for cystine reabsorption in the proximal tubule apical membrane. In contrast, clearance of cationic amino acids is only partly affected (40 to 60 mL/min/1.73 m^2) in cystinuria,[513] suggesting that other apical transport systems participate in the renal reabsorption of these amino acids.

CLINICAL PRESENTATION

Cystine was discovered in the urine of a patient with urolithiasis by Wollaston in 1810[514] and was likely the first case in medical history. The prevalence is reported to be highest in individuals of Libyan Jewish descent (1:2500). A history of parental consanguinity may or may not be present because compound heterozygotes can come from apparently unrelated marriage partners. Patients present similarly to subjects with other stones with hematuria, renal colic, and urinary obstruction, although their symptoms tend to be more severe and they are more likely to have staghorn calculi, need surgery, and progress to chronic kidney disease (CKD).[515] The age of onset varies widely, but approximately half of patients present to pediatricians.[516] The historical type I versus II classification has now been replaced by type A (mutations in both alleles, SLC3A1, genotype AA) and type B (mutations in both alleles, *SLC7A9*, genotype BB).[517] Cases of uncommon digenic inheritance (type AB) have also been described, but individuals with this pattern likely do not suffer from kidney stones.

Urinary cystine quantification is not routinely performed in all stone formers. The features that raise suspicion are family history of cystinuria, staghorn calculi, positive nonquantitative screening test with sodium nitroprusside (>75 mg/L, 0.325 mmol/L), and presence of pathognomonic hexagonal cystine crystals on urinalysis (see Figure 40.22).

Quantitation of urinary cystine excretion (normal < 30 mg/day [0.13 mmol/day]) is mandatory to diagnose cystinuria. Patients with cystinuria often excrete more than 400 mg/day (1.7 mmol/day). Poor cystine solubility and precipitation can sometimes lead to misleadingly low results, so alkalinization of collected urine is often required.[518] One caveat is the inability of current assays to distinguish cystine from soluble, adducted drug-cysteine complexes. Ex vivo disintegrated thiol cysteine can self-recombine to form dimeric cystine. These problems led to the development of a solid-phase assay, which is reliable in the presence of thiol drugs.[519] A physicochemical method similar to that for calcium stones has been tested to measure the propensity for cystine stone formation empirically.[519]

INFECTION STONES

PATHOPHYSIOLOGY

This category of stones does not form because of intrinsic host defects but because of an infected urinary environment. Struvite ($MgNH_4PO_4 \cdot 6H_2O$) stones account for a small percentage of all kidney stones and often also contain carbonate apatite, $Ca_{10}(PO_4)_6 \cdot CO_3$. These stones are rapidly growing, branch and enlarge, and fill the renal collecting system to form staghorns. The key culprits are urea-splitting bacteria. These stones are difficult to treat medically. Even with surgical removal, any remaining fragments containing the infecting bacteria furnish a nidus for further rapid stone growth. The nature of these stones to grow rapidly, recur, and cause morbidity and mortality has led to the term *stone cancer*.

Struvite stones occur more frequently in women than in men, largely because of the higher incidence of urinary tract infection. Chronic urinary stasis or infections predispose to struvite stones so that older age, neurogenic bladder, indwelling urinary catheters, and urinary tract anatomic abnormalities are all predisposing factors. The presence of large stones in infected alkaline urine should alert the clinician to the potential presence of struvite. Given their potential for rapid growth and substantial morbidity, early detection and eradication are essential.[520,521]

The urease of urea splitting organisms hydrolyzes the following reactions:

$$(H_2N)_2\text{-C=O} + H_2O \rightarrow 2NH_4^+ + HCO_3^- + OH^- \quad (1)$$

$$(H_2N)_2\text{-C=O} + H_2O + CO_2 \rightarrow 2NH_4^+ + 2HCO_3^- \quad (2)$$

Urea contains two nitrogens and one carbon. On the product side of the equation (right side), $2NH_4^+$ represents two acid equivalents, and either HCO_3^- plus OH^- or $2HCO_3^-$ represents two base equivalents. The phosphate and magnesium combine with the NH_4 to form struvite, and the calcium and phosphate combine with the carbonate to form carbonate apatite. Ammonium can bind to the sulfates on the glycosaminoglycans on the urothelium,[522] impair the hydrophilic activity of the GAGs, and increase crystal adhesion. During infections with urease-producing organisms, there is a simultaneous elevation in urine NH_4^+, pH, and carbonate concentration. With successful antimicrobial treatment of the underlying infection, the struvite can actually dissolve because the urine is generally undersaturated with respect to struvite.[523,524] However, urine is not undersaturated with respect to carbonate apatite,[524] so successful antimicrobial therapy is not expected to dissolve this component of the stone. Whether a stone will dissolve with prolonged antibiotic is dependent on the amount of carbonate apatite.

While many bacteria (gram-negative and gram-positive), *Mycoplasma*, and yeast species can produce urease, most urease-producing infections are caused by *Proteus mirabilis*. In addition, *Haemophilus*, *Corynebacterium*, and *Ureaplasma* spp. have been identified to cause struvite stones. All these bacteria use urease to split urea and supply their need for nitrogen (in the form of NH_3). Colony counts may be low so the laboratory should be instructed to identify any bacteria and determine sensitivities, no matter how low the number of colony-forming units. If routine urinary cultures are negative but a urease producer is suspected, the laboratory should be specifically instructed to culture for *Mycobacterium* or *Ureaplasma urealyticum*, which are also urease-positive.[522]

UNCOMMON STONES

Rare kidney stone disease can be genetic or acquired. Among the genetic diseases, the most common types are xanthine stones and 2,8-dihydroxyadenine (DHA) stones. Acquired causes may be iatrogenic with the use of medications or may be caused by toxins or other diseases.

GENETIC CAUSES

DHA stone formation is characterized by excessive production and urinary excretion of DHA as a consequence of adenine phosphoribosyl transferase (APRT) deficiency, which is inherited as an autosomal recessive disorder (OMIM 102600). In subjects with impaired APRT, adenine is converted to 8-hydroxyadenine, which is further metabolized to DHA by xanthine dehydrogenase.[525] Consequently, APRT deficiency results in high urinary levels of DHA, which is insoluble and forms crystals that aggregate, grow, and form kidney stones.[526,527] This disorder can present at any age but, in approximately 50% of subjects, symptoms do not occur until adulthood.[528] The diagnosis is made by the microscopic appearance of DHA crystals in the urine, which are pathognomonic for this disease. Typically, DHA crystals as seen by polarized microscopy are round and reddish-brown, with a characteristic central Maltese cross pattern.[525] However, the diagnosis is established by the absence of APRT enzyme activity in red cell lysates or identification of functionally significant mutations in *APRT*.

Xanthine stones are present in about one third of subjects with classic xanthinuria, which is an inborn error in metabolism inherited as an autosomal recessive trait.[529,530] Hereditary xanthinuria is caused by mutations in xanthine dehydrogenase (XDH),[525] leading to the overproduction of xanthine and minimal production of uric acid. Patients have very low serum urate levels but suffer from elevated levels of xanthine in the urine, leading to xanthine stones, hematuria, and sometimes occult kidney failure.[531] Urinary excretion of xanthine and hypoxanthine are significantly increased. Xanthine stones occur more often than hypoxanthine because of the lower solubility of xanthine in urine. Xanthinuria should be suspected if a patient has significant hypouricemia and hypouricosuria in the presence of radiolucent stones.

Xanthine stones may also be acquired following allopurinol treatment in patients with significant hyperuricemia such as Lesch-Nyhan syndrome and in those undergoing chemotherapy for myeloproliferative disorders.[532,533]

ACQUIRED CAUSES

Rare acquired kidney stones arise from disease and also after ingesting toxins or use of certain drugs with poor solubility in a urinary environment.[534] Ammonium urate stones are radiolucent stones that occur in patients with chronic diarrhea, inflammatory bowel disease, ileostomy, and laxative abuse; all are associated with intestinal alkali loss and compensatory renal hyperexcretion of ammonium.[535-539] This occurs due to the relative abundance of urinary ammonium accompanied by decreased urinary sodium and potassium, thereby making the urine supersaturated with respect to poorly soluble ammonium urate. The catabolic state of these patients also cause hyperuricosuria.

Consumption of over-the-counter (OTC) drugs such as guaifenesin as an expectorant and ephedrine as a stimulant and for weight reduction accounts for approximately one third of the U.S. drug-induced kidney stone incidence.[540,541] After the introduction of protease inhibitors for the treatment of HIV patients, indinavir-treated patients began to show a high incidence of indinavir-associated stones.[542,543] In later years, it was shown that other antiproteases, such as nelfinavir, tenofovir, atazanavir, and antinucleosidic drugs, including efavirenz, also cause kidney stone formation.[544-547]

Other drugs such as triamterene, various antimicrobial agents, including sulfamides, penicillin, cephalosporin, quinolones, and nitrofurantoin, and agents such as silicium derivatives (e.g., magnesium trisilicate) have been shown to be associated with drug-induced stones.[534]

Environmental factors play a role in kidney stone formation. Melamine is an organic nitrogenous compound used in the industrial productions of plastics, dyes, fertilizers, and fabrics.[548] In 2008, kidney stone cases were reported in infants and children in China who had consumed melamine-contaminated milk.[549] A study in Taiwan screened 1129 children with potential exposure to contaminated milk formula. The results showed that those with high exposure had an increased incidence of urolithiasis. The group of children with kidney stones was reported to be significantly younger than those without. Metabolic workups did not disclose any evidence of hypercalciuria, and the stones were radiolucent, indicating that these stones were related to melamine ingestion.[550,551]

GENETICS

HUMAN GENETICS

FAMILIAL CLUSTERING

It is well accepted that in humans, a significant portion of the risk of kidney stones, including their major risk factor, hypercalciuria, is hereditary in origin.[552-555] The familial clustering of kidney stones and hypercalciuria has been documented for decades.[253] Despite the fact that family members share similar lifestyles, a number of studies have corrected for confounding factors and have still shown an increased risk of kidney stones. This has certainly been the anecdotal experience of practitioners. In a large epidemiologic study of more than 300,000 patient-years, and after adjusting for dietary factors, age, and BMI, there was a 2.6-fold higher risk of kidney stones when there was a positive family history.[556] Case-control studies, with a combined number of cases and control each exceeding 1000, have shown that the relative risk is twofold to fourfold higher and hereditary contributions (defined as the ratio of genetic variance to the total phenotypic variance) are 40% to 60%.[557-560] In a segregation analysis of more than 200 stone-forming families, hypercalciuria was found to have a hereditability of 60% and was transmitted in a polygenic fashion.[561] However, the complexity of polygenic traits renders a discussion of the genetics of hypercalciuria and kidney stones a formidable task. The challenges include phenocopy, multiple loci, locus heterogeneity, and lack of an intermediate phenotype in clinical databases.

ETHNICITY

African Americans have a lower prevalence of kidney stones than whites, which cannot be accounted for by diet.[3] A longitudinal study has also shown a persistently lower stone incidence in African Americans in the 1970s through the 1990s, suggesting that the difference is inherent.[1] A similar difference has been noted in urinary calcium excretion, with much lower rates in blacks.[562] Hispanics and Asians have values intermediate between those of U.S. whites and blacks. In a cross-sectional, population-based study, immigrants of various ethnic backgrounds maintained their relative risk of stones in their native country, despite considerable assumption and homogenization of a Western lifestyle.[563]

HUMAN GENETIC STUDIES

Twin Studies

Comparison of monozygotic to dizygotic twins and/or full siblings reared in almost identical environments are informative.[564,565] Goldfarb and coworkers sampled dizygotic and monozygotic twins from the Vietnam Era Twin Registry and found a concordance rate of 32% in monozygotic twins compared to 17% in dizygotic twins, an effect that cannot be explained by the documentable dietary information.[566] Other twin studies obtained urinary chemistries and found the heritability of the urinary calcium excretion rate to be about 50%.[564,565]

Candidate Genes

This approach is based on educated guesses of suspected loci. Studies have demonstrated an association of polymorphisms of genes along the vitamin D axis with one form of phenotypic parameter or another,[567-570] but corresponding phenotype studies were negative.[245,246] Sib-pair studies in French Canadians have yielded positive results with several candidate genes, including the vitamin D receptor, 1-α-hydroxylase, CaSR, and crystallization modifiers such as osteopontin, THP, and osteocalcin-related gene, but thus far no conclusions have been reached.[240,571-573] Association studies in an Italian cohort have suggested that a CaSR functional polymorphism (R990G) mutation[574-576] is a possible locus. In a Swiss cohort, three nonsynonymous polymorphisms in the intestinal calcium channel TRPPV6 were found with higher frequency in calcium stone formers; interestingly, the contemporaneous presence of all three polymorphisms led to increased channel activity.[577]

A seminal paper by Halbritter and colleagues has exemplified the power of the candidate gene approach in a complex polygenic disease.[578] These investigators determined the percentage of cases that could be accounted for by mutations in any one of 30 known kidney stone genes using a high-throughput mutation analysis. The sample, which was drawn from multiple kidney stone clinics, consisted of 272 genetically unresolved individuals (106 children and 166 adults) from 268 families with urolithiasis or isolated nephrocalcinosis. Fifty putative disease mutations (unlikely to be polymorphisms) in 14 of 30 analyzed genes were detected, resulting in a genetic diagnosis in 15% of all cases, 40% of which had novel mutations (Figure 40.23). The frequency of monogenic cases was remarkably high in the adult (11.4%) and pediatric (20.8%) cohorts. Recessive causes were more frequent among children, and dominant disease occurred more in adults. This paper indicated that monogenic causes of urolithiasis are much more frequent than expected and illustrates the principle of "one who does not look will not find."

Genomewide Association Studies

To date, success using genomewide association studies (GWAS) has been modest in regard to identification of loci. A small-scale, whole-genome linkage analysis of absorptive hypercalciuria and low bone mineral density has found

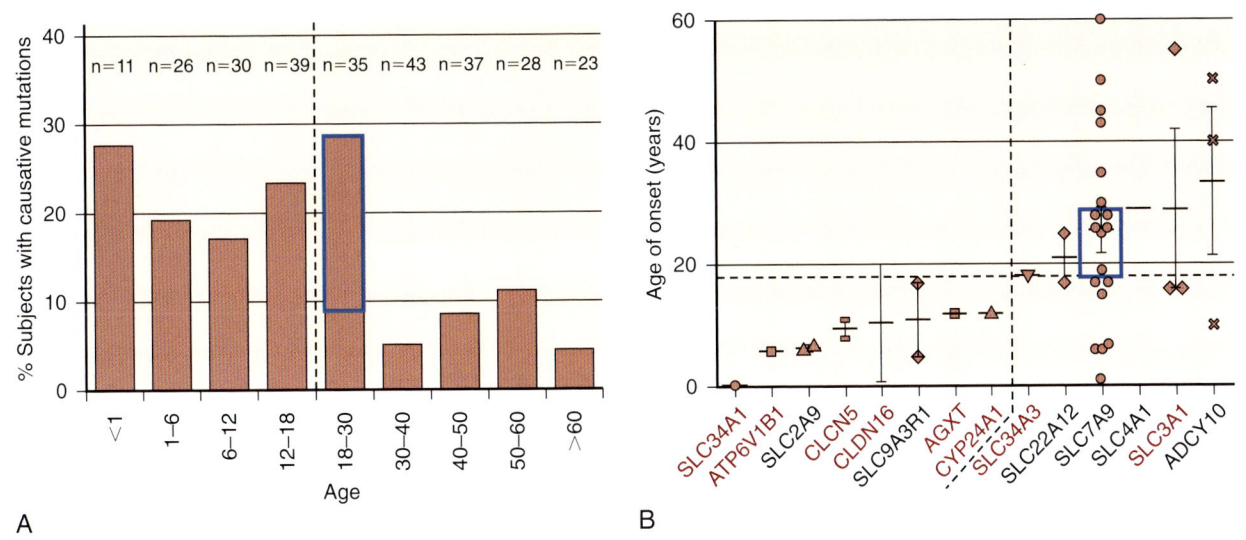

Figure 40.23 Distribution of genetic causes of urolithiasis and nephrocalcinosis. **A,** Percentage of subjects with identified genetic diagnoses grouped by age of onset. The frequency in the entire pediatric cohort (age of onset < 18 years) was 20.8% compared with 11.4% in the adult cohort (age of onset ≥ 18 years); $P \leq 0.05$). The *green rectangle* represents six subjects with heterozygous SLC7A9 mutations enriched within the age group 18 to 30 years or older. **B,** Distribution of age of onset across mutated causative genes. Inheritance mode: dominant, *black*; recessive, *red*. For SLC2A9, SLC22A12, and SLC7A9, mutations were primarily dominant, but both modes of inheritance have been reported. Mutations in four of six genes that had a median onset at 18 years or older are dominantly inherited (*upper right quadrant*), whereas mutations in six of eight genes that had a median onset in those younger than 18 years are recessive (*lower left quadrant*). Genes with identified mutations: SLC34A1 (sodium phosphate cotransporter member 1); ATP6V1B1 (H+-ATPase, V₁ subunit B1); SLC2A9 (solute carrier family 2; facilitated glucose transporter, GLUT9); CLCN5 (voltage-sensitive chloride channel 5); CLDN16 (claudin-16); SLC9A3R1 (Na-H exchange regulatory cofactor, NHERF1); AGXT (alanine-glyoxylate aminotransferase); CYP24A1 (1,25-dihydroxyvitamin D₃ 24-hydroxylase); SLC34A3 (solute carrier family 34; sodium phosphate cotransporter, NaPi-IIc); SLC22A12 (organic anion–urate transporter, URAT1); SLC7A9 (glycoprotein-associated amino acid transporter light chain, b⁰,+AT); SLC4A1 (anion exchanger, AE1); SLC3A1 (cystine, dibasic, and neutral amino acid transporter heavy chain, rBAT); ADCY10/SAC (adenylate cyclase 10). (From Halbritter J, Baum M, Hynes AM, et al: Fourteen monogenic genes account for 15% of nephrolithiasis/nephrocalcinosis. *J Am Soc Nephrol* 26:543-551, 2015.)

soluble adenylyl cyclase (sAC) as a possible locus.[82-84] Polymorphisms in this gene are also associated with bone mineral density (BMD) variations in healthy premenopausal women and men. There are many functions for the sAC protein but one appears to be a mediator of low bicarbonate-induced bone resorption.[579] A GWAS conducted in more than 3700 cases and more than 42,500 controls from Iceland and the Netherlands found synonymous variants in the claudin-14 gene that associate with kidney stones.[291] Carriers were estimated to have 1.64 times greater risk. Claudin-14 is a paracellular protein that regulates calcium transport in the renal TAL. The same variants were also found to be associated with reduced BMD.[291] From a similar Icelandic and Dutch database, another GWAS found a variant positioned next to the *UMOD* gene, which encodes uromodulin (THP), and this variant seems to protect against kidney stones.[580] Uromodulin confers protection from kidney stones through yet unknown mechanisms.[157,581]

There is no doubt that there is a prominent genetic component to hypercalciuria and kidney stones. However, the genes remain elusive after decades of study, a situation not unlike that for hypertension, dyslipidemia, and diabetes mellitus. Unraveling the origins of this complex polygenic trait will be a formidable challenge. Correlation of the candidate gene with gene product function and whole-organism physiology and pathophysiology will be a critical part of this venture. The knowledge gained from studies of monogenic diseases in humans, animals, and polygenic animal models are valuable in unraveling this mystery because the function and dysfunction of the gene products can be linked to physiology and pathophysiology, respectively.

MONOGENIC CAUSES OF UROLITHIASIS

Using intermediate or endophenotypes, one can appreciate clear mendelian conditions in humans that cause hypercalciuria and a predisposition to stones. An even larger number of candidate loci have been identified in animal gene deletion that results in hypercalciuria. The rodent models of hypercalciuria are summarized in Table 40.5. One powerful feature of monogenic diseases is that they have lesions in one gene product that allow a single point of origin to be traced to a discrete phenotypic end point. Examination of these gene products reveals that the pathophysiologic mechanisms of hypercalciuria and/or kidney stones in these conditions are extremely diverse. This underscores the point that defects in many organs can all converge on hypercalciuria as a phenotype. The question is whether some of the loci involved in these monogenic disorders also have alleles that contribute to the risk in the general hypercalciuric stone-forming population.

POLYGENIC ANIMAL MODEL

There are many animal models of monogenic stone formation. However, human urolithiasis is a polygenic disorder, and most people with calcium-containing kidney stones are hypercalciuric.[565,582] One of the most successful and powerful animal models of polygenic hypercalciuria in the GHS rat was developed by Bushinsky and associates.[150,260,261,263,265,267,583-589]

Table 40.5 Rodent Models of Monogenic Hypercalciuria

Reference	Gene/Gene Product	Phenotype
Luyckx et al[872]; Piwon et al[873]; Silva et al[874]	CLC5/chloride channel	Hypercalciuria Hyperphosphaturia Proteinuria Increased gut calcium absorption Spinal deformities
Beck et al[875]	NPT2/renal-I specific Na-coupled phosphate cotransporter	Hypercalciuria Hyperphosphaturia Renal calcifications Retarded secondary ossification
Shenolikar et al[876]	NHERF-1/Na-H-exchanger regulatory factor; docking protein	Hypercalciuria Hyperphosphaturia Hypermagnesuria Female—reduced bone mineral density and fractures
Hoenderop et al[877]	TRPV5l/epithelial calcium channel	Hypercalciuria Hyperphosphaturia Increased intestinal calcium absorption Reduced trabecular and cortical thickness of bones
Li et al[878]; Yoshizawa et al[879]; Zheng et al[880]	VDR/vitamin D receptor	Hypercalciuria on high-calcium and lactose diet Rickets
Zheng et al[880]; Airaksinen et al[881]; Lee et al[882]; Sooy et al[883]	CalB/calbindin-D28k intracellular calcium buffer	Normocalcemia Hypercalciuria Normocalciuria
Takahashi et al[884]	NKCC2/Na-K-Cl cotransporter	Hypercalciuria Polyuria, hydronephrosis Proteinuria
Cao et al[885]	CAV1/caveolin-1 scaffolding protein	Hypercalciuria in males Bladder stones
Aida et al[886]	AKR1B1/aldoketoreductase	Hypercalciuria Hypercalcemia Hypermagnesemia

As described above, GHS rats have hypercalciuria due to intestinal hyperabsorption, renal leak, and increased bone mineral resorption. Regions of five chromosomes—1, 4, 7, 10, and 14—have been linked to the hypercalciuria,[586] with no identification of specific genes as of yet. When normocalciuric Wistar-Kyoto rats were bred with GHS rats to yield congenic rats with the chromosome 1 locus on the Wistar-Kyoto background, the congenic rats were also hypercalciuric but to a lesser extent than the parenteral GHS rats,[590] supporting the importance of this locus and the polygenic nature of the hypercalciuria in the GHS rats.

UROLITHIASIS AS A SYSTEMIC DISORDER

Classically, kidney stone disease has been recognized as an isolated, benign, painful local condition of the urinary tract. However, the association of urolithiasis with gout and degenerative vascular disease in postmortem examinations was noted in the 1760s.[591] The prevalence of kidney stones has been increasing, along with the ever-expanding epidemic of obesity, type 2 diabetes, and metabolic syndrome.[9,10,592-596] Concern about metabolic syndrome and the risk for urolithiasis has not been limited to adults because this link has been reported in obese adolescents as well as in the pediatric kidney stone population.[47,597] It is presently unknown whether the link between kidney stone disease and metabolic syndrome reflects the same underlying pathophysiologic mechanisms in both disorders or is simply an association.

OBESITY, WEIGHT GAIN, DIABETES MELLITUS, AND RISK FOR UROLITHIASIS

A prospective epidemiologic study involving over 200,000 subjects demonstrated that obesity and weight gain increased the risk of kidney stone formation[9] (Figure 40.24). The relative risk for stone formation in men with a body weight of 100 kg (220 lb) or more was significantly higher than men with a body weight of 68 kg (150 lb) or less.[9]

Similarly, the relationship between T2DM and the risk of kidney stone formation was seen in three large cohorts—the Nurses' Health Study I (NHS I) comprised of older women, the Nurses' Health Study II (NHS II) consisting of younger women, and the Health Professionals Follow-up Study (HPFS) in men. These studies showed that the relative risk of prevalent kidney stones in subjects with T2DM compared to those without was 1.38 in older women, 1.60 in younger women, and 1.31 in men.[10]

ASSOCIATION BETWEEN METABOLIC SYNDROME AND NEPHROLITHIASIS

Metabolic syndrome is characterized by a cluster of features, including dyslipidemia, hyperglycemia, hypertension, obesity, and insulin resistance.[598,599] In addition to its relationship to T2DM and cardiovascular risks, metabolic

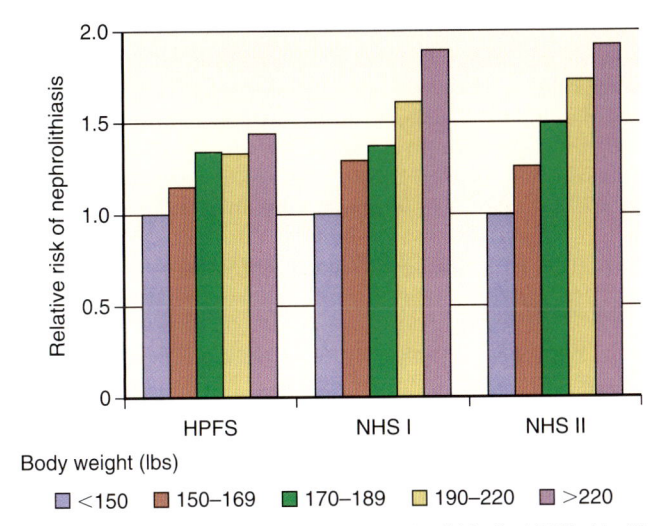

Figure 40.24 Obesity and the risk of nephrolithiasis. HPFS, Health Professionals Follow-up Study; NHS I, Nurses' Health Study I; NHS II, Nurses' Health Study II. (Data pooled from three databases; modified from Taylor EN, Stampfer MJ, Curhan GC: Obesity, weight gain, and the risk of kidney stones. *JAMA* 293:455-462, 2005.)

Figure 40.25 Increased risk for myocardial infarction in stone formers. Data were collected from Olmsted County, Minnesota residents. (Modified from Rule AD, Roger VL, Melton LJ, 3rd, et al: Kidney stones associate with increased risk for myocardial infarction. *J Am Soc Nephrol* 21:1641-1644, 2010.)

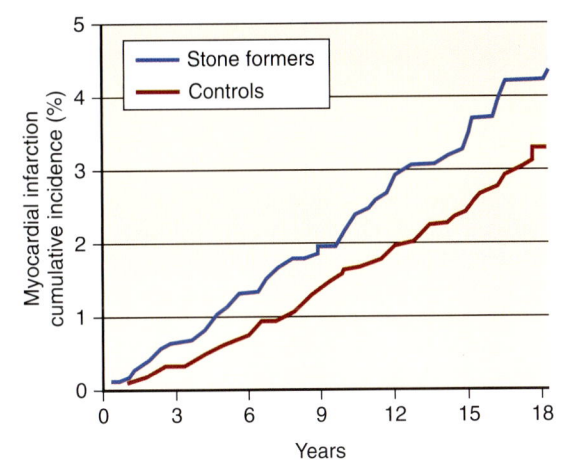

Incidence (no. at risk)				
Control	0 (10,860)	0.8 (6,689)	2 (3,184)	4.2 (1,010)
Stone formers	0 (4,564)	1.3 (2,686)	3 (1,276)	5.2 (404)

syndrome has been associated with urolithiasis and chronic renal disease.[9,10,47,592-603] Despite this strong association between metabolic syndrome and kidney stone disease, one limitation has been the lack of documentation of kidney stone composition in these studies. The link between obesity and documented CaOx urolithiasis has been in part explained by dietary factors, such as higher consumption of salt and animal protein.[283,284]

Documented uric acid stones occur more prevalently in patients with T2DM than in nondiabetic stone formers and more in obese than in nonobese stone formers.[29,30,32,33,472,474] Moreover, higher BMI and T2DM are shown to be independent risk factors for UA urolithiasis[473] (see Figure 40.24). Furthermore, cross-sectional studies in healthy, non–stone formers and in kidney stone formers have shown an inverse relationship among urinary pH, body weight, and increasing features of metabolic syndrome.[446,475] The relationship among low urinary pH, supersaturation index of UA, and adiposity has been specifically shown to be related to fat distribution, with a significant relationship between total body fat and trunk fat associated with increased risk factors for UA stone formation.[604] Further studies in ZDF rats have demonstrated the causative role of renal steatosis in the pathogenesis of urinary acidification defects in this animal model.[499] Furthermore, treatment with thiazolidinediones (TZDs) to improve insulin resistance by redistributing fat to adipocytes was shown to restore urinary biochemical profiles in this animal model compared to control animals. These changes were associated with reduced renal triglyceride accumulation.[499]

UROLITHIASIS AND RISK FOR CARDIOVASCULAR DISEASE

Risk factors for coronary artery disease include hypertension, diabetes mellitus, hyperlipidemia, and smoking.[605-608] Some of these risk factors (e.g., atherosclerosis, hypertension, diabetes, metabolic syndrome) are also seen in patients with kidney stones.[7,10,592,609-612] Cross-sectional studies linking coronary artery disease to kidney stones have been inconsistent,[613-615] with one study showing a positive association[613] and others demonstrating a lack of such association.[614,615] A cross-sectional study in a large number of Portuguese subjects showed a significant correlation between self-reported history of kidney stones and myocardial infarction solely in females, following multivariable adjustments.[616]

One 9-year longitudinal study in a population from Minnesota showed a multivariable adjusted hazard ratio (HR) for developing myocardial infarction to be significantly higher in patients with kidney stones compared to non–stone-forming control participants[617] (Figure 40.25). Although the study was adjusted for multiple variables, risk factors such as dietary calcium and use of thiazide diuretics were not accounted for. In a large number of patients in the two female cohorts in NHS I and NHS II, a positive history of kidney stones was associated with an elevated risk of coronary artery disease but such a link was not detected in a separate cohort of men in HPFS.[618] The causal relationship among kidney stones, coronary artery disease, and gender specificity has not been proven.

UROLITHIASIS AND HYPERTENSION

Multiple cross-sectional studies have demonstrated a link between urolithiasis and blood pressure.[619-623] In 895 Swedish men in whom blood pressure was measured once, the prevalence of urolithiasis increased from 1.1% in those with the lowest blood pressure to 13.3% in those with the highest blood pressure.[619] Another cross-sectional study in Italian adults detected a higher prevalence of urolithiasis in subjects in the highest quintile of diastolic blood pressure compared to those in the lowest quintile (5.22% vs. 3.36%; $P = 0.009$).[621] In a large cross-sectional study of U.S. men and women, the prevalence of urolithiasis was higher in hypertensive subjects compared with normotensive participants, adjusted for age and race.[623]

The results of these cross-sectional studies have been supported by a longitudinal study conducted over an 8-year period. This study demonstrated that 17.4% of subjects with a history of urolithiasis versus 13.1% without a history of kidney stones received a new diagnosis of hypertension when adjusted for age, BMI, dietary sodium, potassium, magnesium, and alcohol consumption.[624] Although the causal relationship among these events has not yet been fully elucidated, some have suggested that alterations in calcium metabolism potentially link the development of kidney stone disease and hypertension.[625,626] Hypercalciuria, which is prevalent in subjects with calcium urolithiasis and essential hypertension, has been proposed by some as a major underlying mechanism, but the role of calcium in human hypertension has never been established.[625-629] A model of hypercalciuria and blood pressure elevation was proposed in spontaneously hypertensive rats.[630,631] NHS I and II showed an association among alterations in acid-base balance, hypocitraturia, and hypertension.[632] Similar associations were found in spontaneously hypertensive rats demonstrating evidence of metabolic acidosis.[633,634]

KIDNEY STONE DISEASE AND CHRONIC KIDNEY DISEASE

Until rather recently, the association between kidney stones and progressive impairment of kidney function and consequently ESKD had not been explored. Such an association was attributed to infectious, stone-causing staghorn calculi.[635-637] In one epidemiologic study, the prevalence of ESKD due to urolithiasis in the general population was estimated to be approximately 3.1/million/year.[638] The results of this study are comparable with the U.S. Renal Data System study involving over 200,000 white subjects who started dialysis between 1993 and 1997, which found approximately 1.2% with urolithiasis as the cause of ESKD.[639] Data from NHANES III, which compared the GFR in 876 subjects with a history of kidney stone disease and 14,129 subjects without a history of stones, showed a link among stone history, estimated GFR (eGFR), and BMI.[640] After adjustment for confounders, the eGFR in stone formers with a BMI of 27 kg/m² or higher was significantly lower than in non–stone formers. However, no difference in eGFR was found in subjects with a BMI of 27 kg/m² or less. In a more recent study, the association between kidney stones and CKD was shown to be gender-specific, with a significantly higher risk in women with a history of kidney stones than in men for ESKD development, doubling of serum creatinine levels, and CKD (stages 3b to 5).[641]

URINARY TRACT CANCERS AND KIDNEY STONES

The association of renal pelvis cancer to kidney stones has been reported in several case-control studies.[642-644] However, the association of renal parenchymal cancer was only reported in case reports.[645] In one large population-based cohort study from a Swedish national inpatient registry and a cancer registry of 61,144 patients who were hospitalized for kidney or ureter stones from 1965 to 1983, there was an increased risk of developing renal pelvic, ureter, or bladder cancer beyond 10 years of follow-up. However, it was proposed that chronic infection or irritation play a pathogenetic role in the development of cancer.[646] In this large population-based cohort study, no association was found between kidney or ureteral stones and renal cell cancer. This result is contrary to the high risk reported in the case-control studies.[647-650] There was a possibility of selection bias.

CALCIUM STONES AND BONE DISEASE

EPIDEMIOLOGY

Bone disease is an underemphasized condition in urolithiasis. Several epidemiologic studies have established an increased association between a history of kidney stones and higher prevalence of fractures.[651-653] In a population-based study in Rochester, Minnesota, the incidence of first vertebral fracture in patients with symptomatic kidney stone disease followed for 19 years was fourfold higher than in the general population[651] (Figure 40.26).[198] The NHANES III study, which included 14,000 men and women, demonstrated an association among a history of kidney stone, low BMD, and higher incidence of fracture.[652] This risk of fracture was found to be higher in males than females. In the most comprehensive population-based study of almost 6000 men, the Osteoporotic Fractures in Men Study (Mr. OS), showed an association of kidney stones with lowered BMD at the spine and hip.[653]

PATHOPHYSIOLOGIC MECHANISMS LINKING OSTEOPOROSIS AND KIDNEY STONES

Osteoporosis is a heterogeneous disorder characterized by disordered bone remodeling resulting in reduced BMD, impairment of microarchitectural integrity, reduced bone strength, and increased fracture risk.[654] Numerous studies in calcium stone-forming subjects have shown reduced BMD in this population[227,655-683] (Table 40.6).[198]

The loss of BMD was shown to be generalized at all skeletal sites, with 40% of patients showing diminished BMD at the

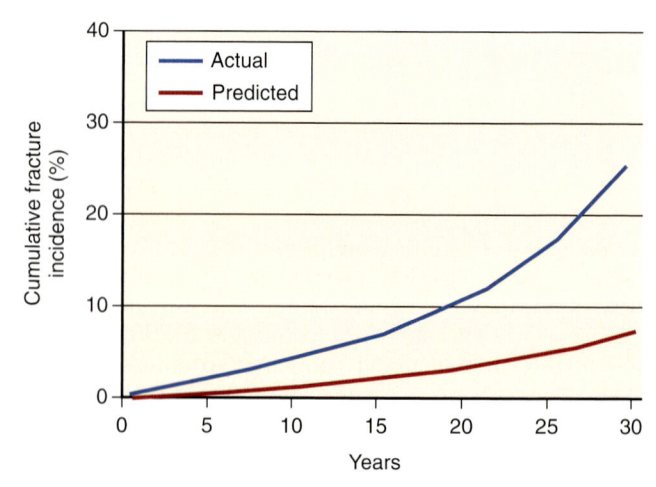

Figure 40.26 Cumulative incidence of vertebral fracture in stone formers. The elevated fracture risk was vertebral and was present in both genders. Data were obtained from Rochester, Minnesota, residents following an initial episode of symptomatic urolithiasis. (Adapted from Melton LJ, 3rd, Crowson CS, Khosla S, et al: Fracture risk among patients with urolithiasis: a population-based cohort study. *Kidney Int* 53:459-464, 1998.)

Table 40.6 Changes in Bone Mineral Density (BMD) in Calcium Kidney Stone Formers

Reference	Study Subjects	No. of Subjects			BMD Site			Measurement Technique
		Male	Female	Control	Spine	Hip	Radius	
Alhava et al[655]	Single or recurrent urolithiasis	54	21	21			↓	Americium-241 gamma ray attenuation
Lawoyin et al[656]	Absorptive hypercalciuria	94	23	Not reported			↔	Single-photon absorptiometry
	Renal hypercalciuria	28	16				↓	
	Primary hyperparathyroidism	22	31				↓	
	Osteoporosis	14	55				↓	
Fuss et al[657]	Absorptive hypercalciuria	24	19	Not reported			↓	Single-photon absorptiometry
	Renal or resorptive hypercalciuria	7	18				↓	
	Normocalciuric	35	6				↓	
Barkin et al[658]	Idiopathic hypercalciuria	86	23	84	↓ Calcium binding index			Neutron activation analysis
Fuss et al[659]	Free diet	63	0	16			↔	Single-photon absorptiometry
	Low-calcium diet	60	0				↓	
Pacifici et al[660]	Absorptive hypercalciuria	29	18	28 (24 male, 4 female)	↓			Quantitative computed tomography
	Fasting hypercalciuria	16	7		↓			
Bataille et al[661]	Dietary hypercalciuria	12	6	61 (41 male, 20 female)	↔			Quantitative computed tomography
	Dietary-independent hypercalciuria	17	7		↓			
Borghi et al[662]	Dietary hypercalciuria	13	7	0	↔			Dual-photon absorptiometry
	Dietary-independent hypercalciuria	14	7		↓			
Pietschmann et al[663]	Absorptive hypercalciuria	42	20	0	↓			Dual-energy x-ray absorptiometry, dual photon absorptiometry, and single-photon absorptiometry
	Fasting hypercalciuria	24	3		↓			
	Normocalciuric	25	6		↔			
Jaeger et al[664]	Hypercalciuric	49	0	234	↓	↓		Dual-energy x-ray absorptiometry
	Normocalciuric	61	0		↓	↓		
Zanchetta et al[665]	Fasting hypercalciuria	15	23	50 (20 male, 30 female)	↓			Dual-photon absorptiometry
	Absorptive hypercalciuria	5	7		↓ Female ↔ Male			
Weisinger et al[666]	Hypercalciuric	4	13	12 (4 male, 8 female)	↓			Dual-energy x-ray absorptiometry
	Normocalciuric	4	8		↔			
Ghazali et al[667]	Idiopathic hypercalciuria	15	1	10 (8 male, 2 female)	↓			Quantitative computerized tomography
	Dietary hypercalciuria	9	1		↔			
Giannini et al[668]	Fasting hypercalciuria	8	23	13 (10 male, 3 female)	↓	↓		Dual-energy x-ray absorptiometry
	Absorptive hypercalciuria	13	5		↓	↔		
Trinchieri et al[669]	Hypercalciuria	10		0	↔	↔		Dual-energy x-ray absorptiometry
	Normocalciuria	34			↔	↔		
Tasca et al[670]	Fasting hypercalciuria	27	12	15	↓			Dual-energy x-ray absorptiometry
	Absorptive hypercalciuria	20	11		Not reported			
Misael da Silva et al[671]	Idiopathic hypercalciuria	11	11	10 (5 male, 5 female)	↓	↓		Dual-energy x-ray absorptiometry
	Normocalciuria	8	10		↔	↔		
Asplin et al[672]	Stone formers	15	7	37 (14 male, 23 female)	↓	↓		Dual-energy x-ray absorptiometry
Vezzoli et al[673]	Hypercalciuria	29	35	0	↓	↓		Dual-energy x-ray absorptiometry
	Normocalciuria	15	27		↓	↓		
Caudarella et al[674]	Stone formers (27% with hypercalciuria)	102	94	196 (102 male, 94 female)			↓	Dual-energy x-ray absorptiometry, Quantitative Ultrasonography

↔, No change in BMD; ↓, lower BMD

Adapted from Sakhaee K, Maalouf NM, Kumar R, et al: Nephrolithiasis-associated bone disease: pathogenesis and treatment options. Kidney Int 79:393-403, 2011.

Table 40.7 Bone Histomorphometric Characteristics in Kidney Stone Formers

Reference	Study Subjects	No. of Subjects	Bone Histomorphometric Profiles
Bordier et al[227]	Dietary hypercalciuria	20	None
	Renal hypercalciuria	19	Increased osteoclastic and osteoblastic surfaces
	Hypophosphatemia	21	Increased osteoclastic and eroded surface (within normal range), decreased osteoblastic surfaces, decreased osteoid parameters
	Controls	12	
Malluche et al[676]	Absorptive hypercalciuria	15	Low-normal osteoclastic bone resorption, low osteoblastic activity, decreased fraction of mineralizing osteoid seams, decreased mineralization apposition rate
	Controls	22	
de Vernejoul et al[677]	Idiopathic hypercalciuria	30 (20 M, 10 F)	Decreased trabecular volume, decreased active osteoblastic surface, decreased active bone resorption surface,
	Controls	187	
Steiniche et al[678]	Idiopathic hypercalciuria	33 (22 M, 11 F)	Increased bone resorption surfaces (decreased refilling of lacunae with low bone formation), decreased bone formation rate, increased mineralization lag times
	Controls	30 (19 M, 11 F)	
Heilberg et al[679]	Fasting hypercalciuria	6 male	Increased eroded surface, decreased osteoid surface, decreased bone formation rate with a complete lack of tetracycline double labeling
	Controls	No information	
Bataille et al[680]	Idiopathic hypercalciuria	24 (20 M, 4 F)	Low eroded surface; low bone volume; low osteoid surface, thickness, mineral apposition rate, adjusted apposition rate, and bone formation rate
	Controls	18 (9 M, 9 F)	
Misael da Silva et al[671]	Idiopathic hypercalciuria	22	High eroded surface, increased osteoblastic bone surface, no change in trabecular thickness
	Controls	94	
Heller et al[681]	Absorptive hypercalciuria	9 (6 M, 3 F)	Relatively high bone resorption (osteoclastic surface, bone surface; mean value within normal limit), lower indices of bone formation (osteoblastic surface, bone surface), decreased wall thickness
	Controls	9 (6 M, 3 F)	

vertebral spine, 30% at the proximal hip, and 65% at the radius.[198] Although low BMD is present in hypercalciuric and normocalciuric stone formers, it is most prominent in those with hypercalciuria.[657,660,664,669,675] However, diminished BMD was not universally detected in normocalciuric kidney stone formers.[663,666,669,671] Given that BMD may be one of the important surrogates of bone strength, it is reasonable to suggest that hypercalciuric stone-forming subjects carry the highest risk of bone fracture. Altered bone remodeling is a significant finding in hypercalciuric stone formers.[227,671,676,678,679,681,684] Most histomorphometric studies have agreed unanimously that defective bone formation rather than excessive bone resorption plays a key role in the development of bone disease in this population[227,676-679,681,685] (Table 40.7).

The pathophysiologic mechanism(s) of bone disease in stone formers is not known, although it may be related to an interplay among environmental, genetic, and hormonal influences and perturbations in the formation of local cytokines.[198] A major emphasis has been placed on the link of idiopathic hypercalciuria and development of bone disease. However, the presence of negative calcium balance,[682] osteopenia, and osteoporosis has been demonstrated primarily in patients with dRTA, as well as medullary sponge kidney (MSK),[686] in whom there is a high prevalence of acidosis,[687,688] which can be the true cause of bone loss.

Dietary Factors
Salt and protein intake has been recognized to be associated with increased risk of kidney stones[198] and bone disease.[663,664] Multiple pathophysiologic mechanisms play a role in increased urinary calcium excretion because of high salt and protein consumption, including diminished renal tubular calcium reabsorption, hyperfiltration, imposition of acid load, and increased urinary prostaglandin excretion.[353,689-694] The presence of subtle metabolic acidosis is a common link between protein and salt-induced hypercalciuria.[692] Metabolic acidosis inhibits osteoblastic matrix protein synthesis and alkaline phosphatase activity by stimulating prostaglandin E_2 (PGE_2) production.[695-697] Increased PGE_2 production enhances the osteoblastic expression of receptor activator for nuclear κB ligand (RANKL), a major downstream cytokine that stimulates osteoblastic production by binding to its receptor RANK.[698] Low bicarbonate in vitro alters osteoblastic extracellular matrix proteins, including type I collagen,[695,697] osteopontin, matrix Gla protein,[696,699] and expression of cyclo-oxygenase-2[700] and RANKL.[698,701] The effect of protein is only partially mediated by its acid content[702] because in humans, the total neutralization of the acid of dietary protein does not reverse the hypercalciuria.[703]

Genetic Factors
The genetic link of vertebral bone loss in kidney stone patients with absorptive hypercalciuria was identified in a genomewide linkage approach study showing polymorphism in the soluble adenylyl cyclase gene (*ADCY10*) on chromosome 1q234-1q24.[704,705] Another genomewide screening study associated sequence variants in the claudin-14 gene (*CLDN14*) with kidney stone and reduced BMD at the hip in

a large population of kidney stone formers from Iceland and the Netherlands.[291] Although soluble *ADCY10* has been shown to regulate osteoclastic function by ambient bicarbonate concentration,[579] and claudin-14 is recognized as paracellular protein mediating renal tubular calcium reabsorption, it is unclear in both cases how these putative genes influence bone remodeling. Others have shown association between CaSR gene polymorphism and increased urinary calcium excretion in hypercalciuric patients,[574] as well as reduced forearm BMD in healthy subjects and postmenopausal women.[706,707] An initial report claimed that mutation in the sodium phosphate transporter NaPi2a is linked to kidney stones and defective bone mineralization,[708] but additional studies did not confirm this association.[709,710]

Numerous genetically heterogeneous disorders that present in childhood or early adulthood are associated with hypercalciuria, nephrocalcinosis, urolithiasis, and rachitic bone disease, including Dent's disease (mutation of the chloride proton transporter CLC-5) and Lowe's syndrome (mutation of the phosphatydylinositol 4,5-bisphosphonate 5-phosphatase, OCRL1).[711-713] However, the role of these genes in bone disease in the general kidney stone–forming population has not yet been defined.

Hormones and Local Cytokines

Elevated serum $1,25(OH)_2D$ levels occur in one third of hypercalciuric stone formers.[209,214,219,221] Moreover, peripheral blood monocyte VDR levels are increased in most of these patients, which amplifies the target organ action of circulating $1,25(OH)_2D$ on bone, kidney, and intestine.[252] High doses of $1,25(OH)_2D$ in vitro enhance bone resorption and decrease bone collagen synthesis.[301] Low expression of TGF-β, which is known to enhance bone formation and bone mineralization,[301,303] were demonstrated by immunohistochemistry in bones of hypercalciuric stone formers.[302] Increased production of bone resorptive lymphokines was shown in idiopathic hypercalciuric stone formers.[660,666,667] One study using undecalcified bone in idiopathic hypercalciuric patients found elevated bone expression of RANKL.[302] Therefore, it is plausible that an interplay of cytokines and RANK/RANKL/OPG (osteoprotegrin) stimulates bone resorption, while lowered TGF-β, high $1,25(OH)_2D$, and/or amplified vitamin D activity impair osteoblastic bone formation in this population.

CLINICAL EVALUATION

PRESENTATION

SYMPTOMS AND SIGNS

Kidney stones may be asymptomatic and incidentally present in patients during an imaging procedure. Renal colic, pain localized to the back and flank, is a common clinical manifestation of kidney stones. The pain occurs as the kidney stone is propelled through the ureter and is a consequence of increased intraluminal pressure, causing stimulation of nerve endings in the ureteral mucosa. Pain and discomfort are usually intense and intermittent, originating in the back or flank, radiating around the torso to the groin, and ending up in the testicles or labia for male or female subjects, respectively. Stones in the midportion of the ureter imitate appendicitis on the right side or diverticulitis on the left side. Renal colic can be associated with systemic symptoms such as nausea and vomiting since the GI tract shares common innervation with the genitourinary system. When the kidney stone approaches the urinary bladder, it frequently presents with bladder symptoms such as urinary frequency, dysuria, suprapubic pain, and urinary incontinence.[714]

The most important physical finding is costovertebral angle tenderness. Its presence and severity are not as consistent and intense as in pyelonephritis. The abdominal examination is usually negative. Hypertension and tachycardia may be present and are most likely due to severe, relentless pain. A presentation with fever and muscle spasm is infrequent and represents underlying diseases or complications. A toxic-appearing patient during stone passage indicates obstruction, infection, and urosepsis.

ENVIRONMENT, LIFESTYLE, AND MEDICAL HISTORY

It is important to elicit a history of any systemic disorders. These include disorders of calcium homeostasis such as primary hyperparathyroidism, conditions accompanied by extrarenal calcitriol production such as granulomatous disease, obesity, type 2 diabetes, gout, recurrent urinary tract infections, inflammatory bowel disease, bowel resection, pancreatic disease, bariatric surgery, distal renal tubular acidosis, and MSK.[190,715,716]

Patients should be asked about climate exposure, work environment, and exercise frequency and intensity because these have been shown to affect the risk of development of kidney stones. Higher temperatures and a prolonged summer season in equatorial regions increases the prevalence of kidney stones. Daily exposure to hot conditions, such as by those in the military who train in a high-temperature environment and by those who engage in physical exercise during the summer months, also plays a role in stone development.[12,716,717]

Dietary history should include the average amount of daily fluid intake (from water and beverages), intake of calcium and sodium, amount and type of protein intake, intake of food containing oxalate, and intake of alkali-rich foods, including fruits and vegetables. The history also should detail the use of OTC medications and/or supplements, including calcium, vitamin D, multivitamins, and ascorbic acid.

A careful drug history must be taken, because prescription and OTC drugs have been demonstrated to increase the risk of kidney stones.[715] In some cases, the increased risk is due to metabolic alterations in the urinary environment—for example, by calcium, vitamin D, and vitamin C supplements, carbonic anhydrase inhibitors (e.g., acetazolamide, topiramate, zonisamide), laxatives,[535,536] probenecid, ascorbic acid, lipase inhibitors,[718,719] excessive alkali treatment, and chemotherapeutic agents.[715] However, in other cases, there is a risk of crystallization of the drug in urine due to its poor solubility. This class includes triamterene, protease inhibitors (e.g., indinavir, atazanavir nelfinavir), guaifenesin, ephedrine, antacids (magnesium trisilicate), and antimicrobials (e.g., sulfonamides, quinolones).[346,440,715,716,720]

FAMILY HISTORY

It is very common to obtain a positive family history in a stone former. The pattern may or may not be mendelian in nature but nonetheless needs to be documented. The interpretation of whether a certain pedigree has a mendelian trait is often difficult due to phenocopy, incomplete penetrance, and loci heterogeneity. Certain monogenic diseases present with kidney stones that have specific phenotypic characteristics. Hypercalciuric urolithiasis among male subjects associated with renal impairment and low-molecular-weight proteinuria that is X-linked recessive is found in patients with Dent's disease.[721] The familial occurrence of kidney stones and nephrocalcinosis in male subjects with early cataracts or glaucoma is suggestive of Lowe's syndrome.[722] Aggressive urolithiasis, nephrocalcinosis, retarded growth, and deafness can be seen in patients with dRTA, presenting with autosomal dominance and recessive inheritance.[722,723] Presentation with nephrocalcinosis and impaired kidney function with hyperoxaluria should suggest the diagnosis of PH.[724]

LABORATORY EVALUATION

Laboratory diagnosis includes blood and urinary metabolic profiles, stone analysis, and imaging studies (Tables 40.8 to 40.10).[190,714]

SERUM CHEMISTRY

All kidney stone formers require the determination of full fasting serum chemistries (electrolytes, including calcium and phosphorus, renal function, UA) and PTH levels. Fasting glucose levels and a full lipid panel are also justified, considering the increased prevalence of diabetes and the metabolic syndrome in stone formers. Increased serum total calcium concentrations and low serum phosphorus levels, in association with high PTH concentrations, are indicative of primary hyperparathyroidism, although this full triad is often not present. The finding of a low serum phosphorus level with a normal serum PTH level is suggestive of a renal phosphorus leak. In the latter condition, hypercalciuria ensues due to increased intestinal calcium absorption from an elevated serum calcitriol level as a result of hypophosphatemia. The measurement of serum $1,25(OH)_2D$ concentrations is optional and may be considered for specific situations or for research purposes. A serum $25(OH)D$ measurement is helpful in patients with high or high normal PTH levels and mild hypercalcemia to exclude vitamin D deficiency as a cause of the high PTH level. The finding of a low serum potassium level and low serum total CO_2 content is suggestive of dRTA or a chronic diarrheal state. Hyperuricemia suggests the diagnosis of UA urolithiasis.[190,582,714,716]

URINE CHEMISTRY

SPOT URINALYSIS

A spot urine collection is of some value due to its simplicity. The urinary pH obtained from the colorimetric reaction of the dipstick is notoriously inaccurate, and only extreme values are informative. A very low dipstick pH (<5.5) suggests UA stones, whereas a high pH (>6.5) suggests dRTA, and a very high pH (>7.4) should raise suspicion for infection. Urine culture must be obtained in patients suspected of having a urinary tract infection (UTI) and in patients with established struvite stones. Crystalluria per se is not abnormal as it is found in normal urine, except that cystine crystals are never present in normal urine (see Figure 40.22B).

All patients, irrespective of the severity of their kidney stone disease, should have a metabolic evaluation. It has been suggested that a simplified metabolic evaluation be considered for single stone formers. An extensive evaluation is needed for recurrent kidney stone formers and individuals at a high risk for recurrent stone formation (e.g., those with primary hyperparathyroidism, dRTA, chronic diarrhea, or UA stones; obese subjects; and pediatric populations with kidney stones).

SIMPLIFIED METABOLIC EVALUATION

Although it is not perfect, studies have shown a correlation between kidney stone composition and urinary biochemical profiles.[67,68] A simple evaluation includes a single, random, 24-hour urinary profile, including total volume, pH, and creatinine, calcium, oxalate, citrate, uric acid, sulfate, chloride, and ammonium levels (see Table 40.8). There is some controversy regarding the recommended number of random 24-hour urine collections required to determine kidney stone risk.[725-727]

Regardless of the number of samples collected, physicians should take into account dietary intake of known risk factors, such as salt and protein, because these are outpatient collections on a random diet. The patient should be instructed to adhere to his or her usual daily activities and diet before and during the collection. If two collections are contemplated, restriction of dietary sodium and protein should be considered prior to a second collection to evaluate the contribution from dietary aberrations without embarking on a fully executed dietary control (see below).

EXTENSIVE METABOLIC EVALUATION

An extensive evaluation includes a 24-hour urinary sample following a 1-week instructed, fixed, metabolic diet consisting of 400 mg calcium/day, 100 mEq sodium/day, and avoidance of oxalate-rich food[728] (see Table 40.10). Generally, high-risk and recurrent stone formers benefit from an extensive metabolic evaluation. These include those with a systemic illness, such as primary hyperparathyroidism, dRTA, gout, or type 2 diabetes, patients with a family history of stone disease, and those with a solitary kidney. The 24-hour urine profile should be complemented by two additional tests, which can be performed at the completion of the restricted 24-hour urine collection—(1) a 2-hour urinary fasting calcium/creatinine ratio to assess renal leak and/or excessive skeletal calcium mobilization and urinary fractional phosphorus excretion to monitor renal phosphorus leak (TmP/GFR); and (2) a 4-hour urinary calcium/creatinine ratio following a 1-g oral calcium load to determine intestinal calcium absorption. However, these tests are usually performed only as a research tool or in a specialized stone clinic.

In those with established cystine stones, a positive family history of cystine stones or those suspected of having the condition, urinary cystine measurement must be considered. In those with urinary oxalate exceeding 100 mg/day, a diagnosis of PH should be suspected. In those cases, 24-hour urine must be tested for glycolate and L-glycerate to confirm the diagnosis of PH types I and II, respectively. Increased urinary glycolate levels are detected in approximately two thirds of hyperoxaluric type I subjects, so a normal urinary glycolate level does not exclude this diagnosis.[729,730] With renal impairment, there is a decrease in the

Table 40.8 Simplified Ambulatory Metabolic Evaluation and Interpretation of Urinary Parameters

Random 24-Hour Urinary Profile	Expected Values* (per day)	Interpretation
Total volume	≥2.5 L	Indicative of minimal daily fluid intake (minus insensible losses); diminishes with low fluid intake, sweating, and diarrhea
pH	5.9-6.2	<5.5 increases risk of uric acid precipitation; commonly found in idiopathic uric acid stone patients, subjects with intestinal disease and diarrhea, and those with intestinal bypass surgery >6.7 increases risk of calcium phosphate precipitation; commonly found in patients with dRTA, primary hyperparathyroidism, alkali, carbonic anhydrase treatment >7.0-7.5 indicates urinary tract infection from urease-producing bacteria
Creatinine	15-25 mg/kg body weight (BW); (0.13-0.22 mmol/kg BW)	Assessment of completeness of collection 15-20 mg/kg BW (0.13-0.15 mmol/kg BW) in females; 20-25 mg/kg BW (0.15-0.22 mmol/kg BW) in males; valid only in steady state of constant serum creatinine concentration with time
Sodium	100 mEq (100 mmol)	Reflects dietary sodium intake (minus extrarenal loss); much lower than dietary intake in diarrhea and excessive sweating; high sodium intake is major cause of hypercalciuria
Potassium	40-60 mEq (100 mmol)	Reflects dietary potassium intake (minus extrarenal loss); much lower than dietary intake in diarrhea states; gauge of dietary alkali intake since most dietary potassium accompanied by organic anions
Calcium	≤250-300 mg (≤6.24-7.49 mmol)	Higher value is expected in males; in states of zero balance, urinary calcium excretion is net gut absorption minus net bone deposition; secondary causes can be ruled out before definitive diagnosis of idiopathic hypercalciuria.
Magnesium	30-120 mg (1.23-4.94 mmol)	Low urinary magnesium detected with low magnesium intake, intestinal malabsorption (small bowel disease), following bariatric surgery; low magnesium increases risk of calcium stones
Oxalate	≤45 mg (≤0.51 mmol)	Commonly encountered with intestinal disease with fat malabsorption (e.g., inflammatory bowel disease, following bariatric surgery); values > 100 mg/day (1.14 mmol/day) suggest primary hyperoxaluria (PH); diagnosis of PH I and PH II further established by high urinary glycolate and L-glycerate
Phosphorus	≤1100 mg (35.5 mmol)	Indicative of dietary organic and inorganic phosphorus intake and absorption; higher excretion increases risk of calcium phosphate stone formation
Uric Acid	600-800 mg (3.57-4.76 mmol)	Hyperuricosuria encountered with overproduction of endogenous uric acid or overindulgence of purine-rich foods (e.g., red meat, poultry, fish); mainly a risk factor for calcium oxalate stones when urinary pH > 5.5 but is risk factor for uric acid stones when urinary pH < 5.5
Sulfate	≤20 mmol	Sulfate is marker of a dietary acid intake (oxidation of sulfur-containing amino acids)
Citrate	≤320 mg (≤1.67 mmol)	Inhibitor of calcium stone formation; hypocitraturia commonly encountered in metabolic acidosis, dRTA, chronic diarrhea, excessive protein ingestion, strenuous physical exercise, hypokalemia, intracellular acidosis, with carbonic anhydrase inhibitor drugs (e.g., acetazolamide, topiramate, and zonisimide), rarely with ACE inhibitors
Ammonium	30-40 mEq (30-40 mmol)	Ammonium is major carrier of H⁺ in urine; its excretion corresponds with urinary sulfate (acid load); higher ammonium/sulfate ratio indicates GI alkali loss
Chloride	100 mEq (100 mmol)	Chloride varies with sodium intake
Cystine	<30-60 mg (<0.12-0.25 mmol)	Cystine has a limited urinary solubility—250 mg/L

These limits are mean + 2 standard deviations (for calcium, oxalate, uric acid, pH, sodium, sulfate, and phosphorus) or mean − 2 standard deviations (for citrate, pH, and magnesium) from normal.
*Expected values should be cross-checked with reference laboratory recommendations since these values differ.
ACE, Angiotensin-converting enzyme; dRTA, distal renal tubular acidosis.

urinary oxalate level, so its urinary measurement will not be accurate. In these cases, the plasma oxalate level should be assessed to confirm the diagnosis of PH. It is typically elevated at 80 μmol/L compared to non-PH hyperoxaluric patients in whom plasma oxalate levels may vary from 30 to 80 μmol/L.[731-733] The most definitive diagnosis is by genetic analysis.[734-737] In cases in which clinical suspicion of PH is considered to be high but DNA screening is nondiagnostic, a liver biopsy is indicated to established the diagnosis.[730]

URINARY SUPERSATURATION ESTIMATION

The clinical utility of urinary supersaturation measurement has not been widely accepted. However, it can be used in

Table 40.9 Simplified Ambulatory Metabolic Evaluation and Interpretation of Other Parameters

Simplified Fasting Blood Chemistries	Values	Interpretation
Complete metabolic panel	Variable*	Low serum potassium, high serum chloride, low serum total CO_2 content suggestive of diarrheal state or distal renal tubular acidosis
PTH	10-65 pg/mL (1.06-6.90 pmol/L)	High serum calcium, low serum phosphorus, high PTH suggestive of primary hyperparathyroidism
1,25-dihydroxyvitamin D	Variable*	Normal serum calcium, normal PTH, elevated 1,25-dihydroxyvitamin D suggestive of absorptive hypercalciuria; normal serum calcium, normal PTH, low serum phosphorus, elevated 1,25-dihydroxyvitamin D suggestive of renal phosphorus leak
Bone mineral density measurements (DXA)	z score > –2 T-score > –2.5	z score < –2 or T-score < –2.5 indicates bone loss; this finding may be more prevalent in hypercalciuric kidney stone formers

*Expected values should be cross-checked with reference laboratory recommendations since these values differ.
PTH, Parathyroid hormone.

Table 40.10 Extensive Ambulatory Metabolic Evaluation and Interpretation*

Restricted 24-Hour Urinary Profile	Expected Values/day†	Interpretation
Calcium	<200 mg (<4.99 mmol)	A restricted diet urinary Ca below 200 mg/day (4.99 mmol/d) accompanied by a random diet urinary Ca greater than 200-250 mg/day (6.24-7.49 mmol/day) is reflective of dietary Ca indiscretion. Persistent high urinary Ca on a restricted diet is reflective of intestinal hyperabsorption of Ca.
Sodium	100 meq (100 mmol)	Urinary Na greater than 100 meq/day (100 mmol/day) reflects high dietary salt intake. An increment of 100 meq/day (100 mmol/day) of Na increases urinary calcium of approximately 40 mg/day (1 mmol/day).
Oxalate	<40 mg (<0.45 mmol)	Urinary oxalate greater than 40 mg/day (0.45 mmol/day), in absence of chronic diarrheal state, is indicative of high dietary oxalate intake.
Sulfate	<20 mmol	Urinary sulfate greater than 20 mmol/day indicates overindulgence of high acid-ash diet found in animal proteins.
2-hour fasting calcium:creatinine ratio (Ca/Cr)	<0.11 mg/100 ml GF (<2.7 umol/100 mg GF)	Elevated fasting Ca/Cr, high serum calcium, and elevated PTH is suggestive of primary hyperparathyroidism. Elevated fasting Ca/Cr, normal serum calcium, and normal or suppressed PTH suggestive of resorptive hypercalciuria; elevated fasting Ca/Cr, normal serum calcium, elevated PTH suggestive of renal hypercalciuria.
4-hour Ca/Cr ratio following 1-g oral calcium load	≤0.20 mg/mg Cr (≤0.56 mmol/mmol Cr)	Elevated Ca/Cr following 1-g oral calcium load suggestive of absorptive hypercalciuria.

These limits are mean + 2 standard deviations (for calcium oxalate, uric acid, pH, sodium, sulfate, and phosphorus) or mean – 2 standard deviations (for citrate, pH, and magnesium) from normal.
*After 1 week of dietary restrictions.
†Expected values should be cross-checked with reference laboratory recommendations since these values differ.
Ca/Cr, Calcium/creatinine.

clinical and research settings to estimate risks and monitor response to treatment.[67,68,738] Urinary supersaturation in stone research has been calculated using the EQUIL2 software program (now offered commercially).[60,739,740] Other programs, including the Joint Expert Speciation System (JESS), have also been used to calculate urinary supersaturation.[69] Furthermore, urinary supersaturation ratios are reported by commercial clinical laboratories and are available to practitioners. The relative supersaturation ratio (RSR) is defined as the ratio of calculated activity product in a given urine sample to that of the respective thermodynamic solubility product.[60] Values higher than 1 indicate supersaturation, and values less than 1 indicate undersaturation. Another method, urinary relative supersaturation (RS), is calculated as the ratio of activity product (for UA, it is the concentration of undissociated uric acid) in a particular urine specimen and corresponding mean activity product (for UA, it is the undissociated uric acid) from normal subjects. The upper limit of normal for RS of calcium oxalate, brushite, monosodium urate, and uric acid is defined as 2.[462]

Despite the lack of hard evidence correlating urinary biochemical abnormalities and urinary supersaturation of stone-forming salt following dietary and pharmacologic treatment with clinical stone occurrence, several observational and case-control studies have shown a correlation between the calculated parameter and clinical outcome.[741-743] For example, one study performed at a specialized kidney stone center has shown that a reduction of calcium oxalate supersaturation is accompanied by a reduction in the number of formed kidney stones.[744]

There is no hard rule regarding structured longitudinal monitoring of urinary parameters following initiation of a pharmacologic and/or dietary regimen. However, it is advisable to perform a 24-hour urinalysis annually, depending on the activity of stone disease.[745,746]

STONE ANALYSIS

The analysis of a stone provides valuable information that clarifies the differential diagnosis and assists in directing the management plan.[747,748] The stone crystallographic finding also helps identify the occurrence of infrequently encountered kidney stones, such as cystine and infection-induced stones, which completely change the treatment plan. Stone analysis also assists in the diagnosis of extremely rare stones, such as 2,8-hydroxyadenine or drug-induced stones.[715,716] Generally, the presence of ammonium urate stones is encountered in patients with HIV/AIDS as a consequence of laxative abuse[539] due to protracted diarrhea.[714] In addition, the presence of calcium phosphate stones suggests conditions such as dRTA, primary hyperparathyroidism, MSK, and carbonic anhydrase inhibitor treatment.[749] Although it is opinion-based, one may follow/reassess stone analysis in the management of recurrent stone formers who are unresponsive to specific medical treatment.

IMAGING STUDIES

Imaging studies could be considered in patients suspected of kidney stones as well as in the follow-up of treated stone formers to monitor the stone activity. Various recognized imaging methods include plain abdominal radiography for the kidneys, ureters and bladder (KUB), ultrasound examination, and non-contrast computerized tomography (NCCT).

KIDNEYS, URETERS, AND BLADDER X-RAY

Kidney, ureters, and bladder (KUB) radiography is a plain x-ray of the abdomen that will detect opaque calcareous or cystine stones. It has wide availability, minimal radiation exposure, and low cost. The drawback is limited sensitivity (45% to 58%) and specificity (60% to 77%)[750] due to body habitus, overlying bowel gas, and extragenitourinary calcifications. It does provide adequate information for following the stone load during therapy in patients with radiopaque stones. For stable patients, annual imaging is adequate; however, additional imaging must be considered according to the clinical activity of the patient.[751] During passage of a calcareous stone, KUB can also follow the movement of the stone.

ULTRASOUND

Although ultrasound is reliable, noninvasive, and fast and does not involve ionizing radiation, its major limitation is its low sensitivity. The lack of radiation and contrast renders it safe, particularly for children and pregnant women.[752,753] It is also inexpensive and widely available. It is excellent in detecting hydronephrosis and hydroureter.[754] Renal ultrasound is suitable for most patients with radiolucent stones (e.g., UA). However, ultrasound misses a significant fraction of ureteral stones[754] and gives a false-positive diagnosis of obstruction in patients with pyelonephritis, vesicoureteric reflux, and residual dilation following relief of obstruction. Finally, sonography tends to overestimate the size of a stone due to inaccurate determination of the boundary of the stone and tissue.

COMPUTED TOMOGRAPHY

Noncontrast computed tomography (NCCT, synonymous with unenhanced helical CT) screening has the highest sensitivity (94% to 100%) and specificity (92% to 99%)[755,756] and can be considered to be the current gold standard for kidney stone diagnosis.[757] Stones as small as 1 mm can be diagnosed by NCCT. The disadvantages of this technique include radiation exposure, limited ability to evaluate degree of obstruction, and high cost. Newer techniques have been adapted to offer lower exposure to radiation (from a former 8 to 16 millisieverts [mSv] down to 0.5 to 2 mSv).[758] If NCCT imaging can be performed effectively with lower dose radiation, it will remove the only concern with this test, which is increased risk of malignancy with long-term usage in repeated stone formers.[759-761]

Another advantage of the NCCT scan is its ability to determine stone density using the Hounsfield unit (HU), which has prognostic value in terms of success in shock wave therapy.[762] Similar to a preoperative test (e.g., prior to percutaneous urolithotomy), NCCT can detect possible altered anatomy and accurately assess stone size and location; both of these have an impact on the selection of optimal surgical intervention.

INTRAVENOUS PYELOGRAPHY

Intravenous pyelography (IVP) has been the traditional gold standard imaging approach to diagnose urolithiasis. It provides excellent anatomic detail of the minor and major calyces, infundibula, renal pelvis, and ureters, and a calculus is visualized as a discrete filling defect. The disadvantage is the use of nephrotoxic contrast agents. The sensitivity and specificity of KUB for detecting renal calculi have been reported as 59% and 71%, respectively.[763] The use of NCCT has largely supplanted IVP.[764-766] IVP is still occasionally used following NCCT in some patients to help guide percutaneous or endoureteral surgical procedures. It is also used in diabetic patients with renal colic mimicking kidney stones caused by papillary necrosis.[750]

MAGNETIC RESONANCE IMAGING

Magnetic resonance imaging (MRI) is a potential alternative to NCCT for the diagnosis of urolithiasis and urinary tract obstruction. The obvious advantage is that it does not use ionizing radiation. Akin to sonography, it is useful in pregnant women and in children and adolescents. A related technique, magnetic resonance urography, has been reported as a novel tool in the diagnosis of urinary tract obstruction, specifically in pregnant women.[767] The disadvantage of MRI is its high cost.

In general, patients with a known history of previous renal colic due to stone disease may be initially evaluated by KUB or ultrasound. NCCT can be used in patients who have not been previously diagnosed and in those with an atypical clinical presentation. Ultrasound is considered the method of choice for pregnant patients and children with kidney stone disease. IVP should be considered following NCCT if no stone was diagnosed or when planning an endoscopic evaluation or open intervention to assist the urologist in mapping the urinary tract. In situations in which NCCT is not available, one may start with KUB and ultrasound evaluations and only consider the use of IVP if these two techniques fail to diagnose kidney stones. In the follow-up of patients, due to the high risk of cumulative radiation, it is advisable to select KUB and ultrasound until newer, low-radiation NCCT can be used.

MANAGEMENT OF STONES

ACUTE MANAGEMENT

As an acute illness, urolithiasis is associated with significant pain, disability, and loss of productivity.[768] Approximately 50% of patients experiencing acute upper urinary tract stones require surgical intervention.[769,770] Medical treatment has been shown to facilitate spontaneous passage of ureteral stones. Stone size and location within the urinary tract are the major determinants of the likelihood of spontaneous stone passage. Spontaneous passage rates are higher for distal ureteral calculi compared with proximal and middle locations. Rates are also higher for smaller (<4 mm in diameter) compared to larger stones (between 4 and 6 mm) and those more than 6 mm in diameter.[771,772] Overall, spontaneous passage rates are 12%, 22%, and 45% for proximal, middle, and distal ureteral calculi, respectively, and 55%, 35%, and 8% for stones smaller than 4 mm, 4 to 6 mm, and more than 6 mm, respectively.[771] Since acute renal colic is associated with severe pain over an unpredictable time interval, adjunctive treatment to promote spontaneous stone passage and reduce the symptoms is crucially important.

RENAL COLIC

The management of renal colic is necessary until spontaneous passage of a stone, which usually occurs in patients with smaller (<4 mm) and more distal ureteral stones within 48 hours after the onset of acute renal colic.[773] During that period, patients will require supportive treatment with pain medications, including nonsteroidal antiinflammatory drugs (NSAIDs) and opioids, hydration, and antiemetics.[774] Patients with resolving colic can be discharged from the emergency room but hospitalization is indicated in cases of persistent relentless pain and intractable vomiting, established infection, and obstruction. Nephrostomy must be considered urgently to relieve the obstruction, which can be followed by ESWL, percutaneous lithotripsy, ureteroscopy with laser lithotripsy, retrograde basket extraction of the stone or, in rare cases, open surgical removal.[775,776]

Medical Expulsive Therapy

Medical expulsive therapy plays an important role in the acute management of stones because it significantly decreases the costs and complications of ESWL and ureteroscopy.[768,777] Also, it immensely improves the patient's quality of life by reducing episodes of pain,[778,779] lowers analgesic use,[780] and diminishes stone transit time.[780,781] Agents include glucocorticoids, hormones, NSAIDs, calcium channel blockers, and α-adrenergic blocker agents as medical expulsive therapy (MET).[782-785] We will focus mainly on calcium channel blockers, which suppress smooth muscle contraction and reduce ureteral spasm, and α₁-adrenergic receptor antagonists, which decrease ureteral smooth muscle tone and the frequency and force of peristalsis.[4,5] A meta-analysis of all published studies (up to 2005) that used calcium channel blockers or α-blockers has demonstrated that medical treatment with these agents, with or without steroid treatment and regardless of stone size, enhances the percentage of ureteral stone passage[782] (Figure 40.27). One small randomized controlled trial (RCT) has shown that an α-blocker (tamsulosin) in combination with corticosteroids had an advantage over tamsulosin alone in passing the stones a few days earlier.[786] Additionally, a meta-analysis of 11 RCTs of 911 patients demonstrated a significantly higher rate of spontaneous stone passage with α-blockers compared with no treatment.[783] The American Urological Association/European Urological Association's 2007 Ureteral Stones Guidelines Panel studied all available MET trials and demonstrated that α-blockers are superior to calcium channel blockers in absolute stone passage at 29% versus 9%.[77] The reader can obtain a more detailed summary of the literature on MET in a recent review.[772]

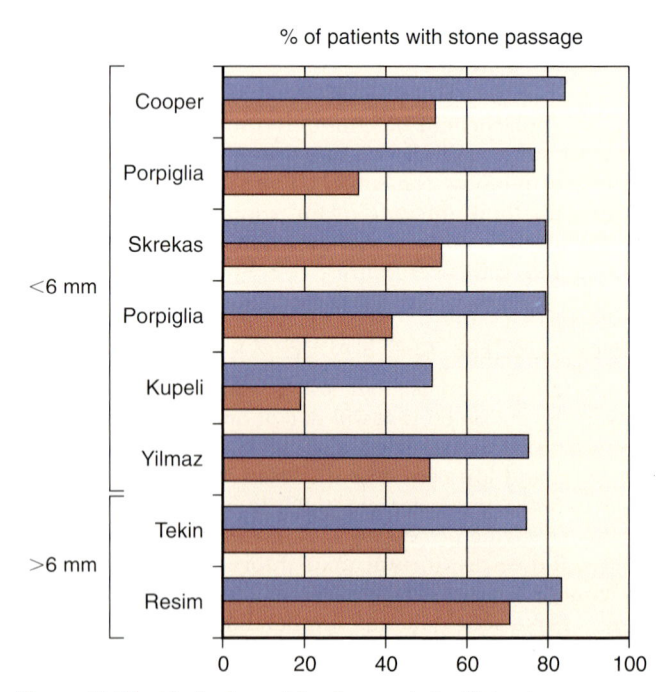

Figure 40.27 Medical expulsive therapy to facilitate stone passage. A meta-analysis was performed of nine randomized controlled trials in which calcium channel blockers or α-adrenergic blockers were used to treat ureteral stones. The figure shows the percentage of patients who passed stones stratified by study group and mean stone size. Control group, *white bars*; treatment group, *black bars*. (From Hollingsworth JM, Rogers MA, Kaufman SR, et al: Medical therapy to facilitate urinary stone passage: a meta-analysis. *Lancet* 368:1171-1179, 2006.)

CHRONIC MANAGEMENT

LIFESTYLE AND DIETARY TREATMENT

One major limitation in the field has been the scarcity of RCTs to compare the effects of specific dietary and fluid measures in recurrent kidney stone formers.

Fluid Intake

Fluid management should be considered in all patients with kidney stones, regardless of stone composition. Dilution of lithogenic elements in the urine should be the panacea of kidney stone therapy. The effect of fluid intake was first examined in 108 idiopathic stone formers over approximately 5 years, with significant declines in new stone formation. One limitation of this study was lack of a control group.[787] However, in an RCT in men with recurrent CaOx stones over 5 years, high fluid intake to ensure a urinary volume of approximately 2.5 L/day reduced stone recurrence by approximately 44% compared with a control group with no dietary restrictions.[788] In a 3-year RCT, 1009 kidney stone formers were randomized to a control group that continued drinking soft drinks and an intervention group that avoided consumption of soft drinks. This study showed a marginal benefit of avoiding soft drinks. Another study suggested that fluid intake of fruit juices, specifically orange juice, is also effective in reducing urinary CaOx saturation.[789] The same effectiveness is not seen with apple juice, grapefruit juice, cola, or some sport drinks due to their elevated oxalate and fructose concentrations.[789-791]

Fluid therapy is also recommended for cystinuria. Cystine has a limited solubility of 243 mg/L in urine.[792] Reduction of urine cystine supersaturation to less than 1.0 or of concentration to less than 243 mg/L (1 mmol/L) would require drinking about 4 L/day, including nocturnal intake.[793] Off-label use of a vasopressin receptor antagonist has been proposed to induce pharmacologic diabetes insipidus,[794] but the long-term effects of this drug have not been evaluated. In conjunction with the exorbitant cost and safe and easily available water, it is unclear whether there is an advantage to this therapy.

Dietary Adjustment

Calcium Intake. In general, high dietary calcium intake appears to be protective against CaOx stones. In one study of Italian men with recurrent CaOx stones, a traditional prescription of a low-calcium diet was compared with liberal calcium diet (1200 mg/day) but low dietary sodium (<100 mEq/day) and animal protein consumption (50 to 60 g/day).[20] Despite only partial adherence, the low-sodium and low-protein diets resulted in less recurrence of stones. In another study in first-time CaOx stone formers, those given a high-fluid, high-fiber, and low-protein diet did not show decreased stone recurrence compared to high-fluid alone.[22] A limitation of this study was that the control group had a higher urine volume. However, in another RCT, CaOx stone formers were divided into three groups (low animal protein diet, high-fiber diet, and control group without dietary instructions for 4 years), there was no statistical significance in stone recurrence.[795]

Three large epidemiologic studies using food frequency questionnaires and history of kidney stone passage have suggested that low calcium intake, low fluid intake, sugar-containing beverages, and high animal protein intake are risk factors for the development of first-time kidney stones in women and younger men.[15,17-19,796] Unlike dietary calcium, supplemental calcium increases the risk of stone formation. This association was shown in an observational study of older women treated with calcium supplements compared to those who did not take supplements.[19] However, this association was not seen in younger men and women.[17] In a large epidemiologic study (Women's Health Initiative), calcium supplementation increased the risk of CaOx stone formation; one should exercise some caution because the total calcium intake was very high in those using supplements.[797]

Dietary Oxalate. Since high urinary oxalate is associated with the risk of urolithiasis,[798] dietary oxalate restriction has generally been recommended. In epidemiologic studies, it is difficult to demonstrate the relationship between dietary oxalate and urinary oxalate.[799] While there is no doubt that dietary oxalate is absorbed, the huge variation in intestinal absorption, bacterial degradation, and superimposed endogenous synthesis renders it difficult to discern a clear relationship between dietary and urinary oxalate. The Dietary Approaches to Stop Hypertension (DASH) diet, which was not restricted in oxalate content, significantly reduced the risk of kidney stones.[800] However, the protective effect of the DASH diet may have been due to the ingestion of high fruit and vegetable content (alkali) in conjunction with low animal protein intake.

In general, urinary oxalate excretion is affected by calcium intake, which determines intestinal bioavailability of oxalate and consequently its absorption. With the recommended daily dietary calcium, CaOx stone risk has been shown not to be significantly influenced, even with relatively high dietary oxalate.[21] Therefore, it is prudent to recommend that patients with hyperoxaluria and CaOx stone consume a total calcium of 1000 to 1200 mg/day, taken with meals to complex intestinal luminal oxalate. The restriction of dietary oxalate in subjects with idiopathic hyperoxaluria may not be efficacious but likely will not increase stone risk. In contrast, in patients with inflammatory bowel disease or those who have undergone bariatric surgery, dietary oxalate restriction should be imposed, in addition to higher total calcium intake from the diet and supplements at mealtime.[104,801,802]

Ascorbic Acid. Vitamin C above the physiologic dose increases urinary oxalate. In a metabolic study, 2 g of ascorbic acid elevated 24-hour urinary oxalate (29 to 35 mg in non–stone formers; 31 to 41 mg in stone formers). Therefore, patients with hyperoxaluria should be cautious about OTC vitamin C supplements.[803,804] Fortunately, most preparations are less than 1 g/day.

Dietary Intervention in Cystinuria. Cystine excretion has been shown to be reduced by decreasing dietary sodium, although no clinical outcome studies have been performed.[793,805-808] The mechanism for this is unknown but salt regulation of the $b^{0,+}$ system for the purpose of L-dopa uptake and synthesis of nephrogenic dopamine is a possibility.[809] On a high-salt diet, we suggest that the $b^{0,+}$ system be occupied with dopamine synthesis and hence unavailable for cystine reabsorption. In the absence of ill effects of salt restriction, it is reasonable therefore to recommend restricting salt intake to about 2 g/day.

Reduction of animal protein intake has also been proposed to be beneficial because it would reduce dietary intake of cystine and its precursor methionine, which reduces cystine excretion,[810] and would also increase the solubility of urinary cystine by increasing the urinary pH. One study has shown that urinary cystine excretion decreases in cystinuric patients on a low-protein diet, in which 9% of caloric intake is from protein compared to higher protein intake.[810] Restriction of protein must be used cautiously in children because the restriction of essential amino acids compromises growth in children.

Other Dietary Interventions. It has been suggested that lowering urinary phosphorus magnesium and ammonium via dietary manipulation would lower the risk of struvite stones. There are limited data in humans exploring the efficacy of dietary modification in this population. Low phosphorus and calcium combined with aluminum hydroxide gel and estrogen have been proposed,[811] supposedly to lower urinary phosphorus excretion by limiting the intake and absorption of phosphorus. Treatment with estrogen over 3.5 years was proposed to diminish urinary calcium excretion mediated by decreasing bone resorption.[812] However, these interventions were also associated with side effects, including GI distress, lethargy, bone pain, and hypercalciuria.

PHARMACOLOGIC TREATMENT

Pharmacologic treatment is essential for most patients with UA-, cystine-, recurrent calcium-, and infection-induced stones, principally due to the lack of availability and/or consensus regarding the effectiveness of nonpharmacologic interventions. One major limitation with respect to pharmacologic treatment is the paucity of randomized control data with stone episodes as hard evidence of treatment results.[772] This is largely because stone events are rare, and these studies must be carried out in a large number of patients over a long period of time. There is also no consensus as to whether pharmacologic treatment should be targeted at specific metabolic abnormalities or should be given empirically, irrespective of underlying biochemical abnormalities.[125,813-816] Although the benefit of directed medical treatment has not been decisively proven, some observational studies have suggested the beneficial effects of directed management of kidney stones.[817,818]

Thiazide Diuretics

Thiazide diuretics and their analogs are used commonly for lowering calcium excretion in hypercalciuric, recurrent calcium stone formers.[772] To date, six RCTs have studied thiazides in recurrent calcium stone formers. One study has shown a similar decrease in stone formation among thiazide-treated versus untreated patients.[819] Another study has shown diminished hypercalciuria without any change in stone events in patients treated with hydrochlorothiazide compared to placebo.[820] The remaining four RCTs, which evaluated 408 patients over periods of 26 to 36 months, demonstrated significant reductions in recurrent kidney stones with thiazides and the thiazide analog, indapamide (Table 40.11).[815,816,821-823] The results of these RCTs are consistent with uncontrolled studies totaling over 6600 patient-years of thiazide treatment for calcium urolithiasis patients.[320,453,823-828]

Two critical but often ignored facts about thiazide therapy deserve note. First, the optimal effect of thiazide diuretics is attained with a low-salt diet. While there is likely some direct effect of thiazides on the DCT, most of its effect is to induce slight extracellular volume contraction and increase proximal calcium reabsorption; thus, simultaneous ingestion of a high-salt diet will nullify the efficacy of thiazides.[829,830] Second, the successful reduction in urinary calcium can be offset by hypocitraturia due to potassium depletion and proximal tubule intracellular acidosis. One must be vigilant in detecting potassium deficiency, and potassium supplements should be prescribed to avoid hypocitraturia if dietary potassium intake is not sufficient.[354] Potassium citrate provides an advantage over potassium chloride in these cases.[831]

Thiazide administration along with dietary sodium restriction to maximize the hypocalciuric effect of thiazide is the treatment of choice in hypercalciuric, calcium stone-forming subjects. The incidence of side effects on thiazide diuretic approach 30%,[823] but side effects requiring discontinuation of the drug are rare. To date, long-term side effects of thiazide treatment in the kidney stone population have not yet been documented. A meta-analysis of clinical trials in hypertensive subjects has demonstrated a relationship between changes in serum glucose and potassium concentrations.[832] This was also confirmed in a large cohort, the Antihypertensive and Lipid-Lowering Treatment to Prevent Heart Attack Trial (ALLHAT), in which the incidence of diabetes mellitus was higher with chlorthalidone compared with amlodipine or lisinopril over 4 years. The exact pathophysiologic mechanism has not yet been fully delineated.[833-835] One potential mechanism is the relationship between potassium deficiency and defective insulin secretion and action.[836,837] Commonly used drugs and recommended dosages in the treatment of hypercalciuric calcium urolithiasis with potential side effects are summarized in Table 40.12.

Alkali Treatment

Alkali treatment can be used alone or in combination with thiazides for recurrent calcium or UA stone formers. In four RCTs,[124,125,838] three nonrandomized, nonplacebo control studies, one retrospective study, and one non-RCT, potassium citrate reduced the risk of clinical stone events (see Table 40.11).

One study has shown no difference in stone formation.[126] This study included 50 hypocitraturic calcium urolithiasis patients treated with potassium alkali, 90 mEq/day, over 3 years. One possibility for the lack of efficacy might have been because of the small size of the study.

In three nonrandomized, non–placebo-controlled studies, alkali treatment showed a significant decrease in new stone events.[129,130,839] One retrospective study compared three groups of patients with MSK who received potassium citrate or no treatment. The results showed that treatment with potassium citrate was effective in reducing renal stones compared to nontreated groups.[840] In one nonrandomized, placebo-controlled study, 503 subjects were treated with a mixture of potassium citrate, thiazide, and allopurinol. Compared with no treatment after

Table 40.11 Major Clinical Pharmacotherapeutic Trials in Calcium and Noncalcium Urolithiasis

Trial	Reference	Treatment	No. of Patients	Design	Outcome
Thiazide diuretics	Laerum et al[816]	Hydrochlorothiazide vs. placebo	50	RCT	Decreased new stone formation, prolonged stone-free interval
	Ettinger et al[815]	Chlorthalidone vs. magnesium hydroxide vs. placebo	124	RCT	Chlorthalidone more effective than magnesium hydroxide or placebo in reducing stone events
	Ohkawa et al[821]	Trichlormethiazide vs. no treatment	175	RCT	Decreased calciuria and stone formation rate
	Borghi et al[822]	Diet vs. diet + indapamide vs. diet + indapamide + allopurinol	75	RCT	Diet + pharmacotherapy better than diet alone
	Yendt et al[823]	Hydrodiuril	33	NNT	Decreased number of stone events or invasive and noninvasive procedures
	Coe and Kavalach[453]	Trichlormethiazide	37	NNT	Decreased new stone formation
	Coe[320]	Trichlormethiazide vs. allopurinol vs. both	222	NNT	Decreased new stone formation
	Yendt and Cohanim[828]	Hydrochlorothiazide	139	NNT	Decreased new stone formation or stone growth
	Backman et al[827]	Bendroflumethiazide	44	NNT	Decreased new stone formation
	Maschio et al[825]	Hydrochlorothiazide + amiloride vs. both + allopurinol	519	NNT	Decreased new stone formation
	Pak et al[826]	Hydrochlorothiazide	37	NNT	Decreased new stone formation
Alkali treatment	Pak et al[129]	Potassium citrate vs. pretreatment in calcium and uric acid stone formers	89	NNT	Decreased stone events
	Preminger et al[130]	Potassium citrate	9	NNT	Decreased new stone formation
	Pak et al[839]	Potassium citrate	18	NNT	Decreased stone events
	Fabris et al[840]	Potassium citrate vs. no treatment	65	NNT	Decreased stone rate in those treated with potassium citrate
	Barcelo et al[124]	Potassium citrate vs. placebo	57	RCT	Decreased new stone formation and increased urinary citrate
	Hofbauer et al[126]	Diet + sodium potassium citrate vs. diet	50	RCT	No difference in stone formation
	Ettinger et al[125]	Potassium magnesium citrate vs. placebo	64	RCT	Decreased new stone formation
	Soygur et al[838]	Potassium citrate vs. no treatment after shock wave lithotripsy	110	RCT	Decreased stone recurrence
	Kang et al[818]	Mix of potassium citrate, thiazide, allopurinol vs. no treatment after percutaneous nephrolithotomy	226	NCT	Decreased stone recurrence
Allopurinol treatment	Ettinger et al[845]	Allopurinol vs. placebo	60	RCT	Decreased stone events
	Coe[320]	Thiazide vs. allopurinol vs. both	202	RCT	Decreased stone events vs. pretreatment
Febuxostat	Goldfarb et al[793]	Febuxostat vs. allopurinol or placebo	99	RCT	Febuxostat decreased 24-hour urinary uric acid excretion more significantly than allopurinol; no change in stone size or number
Other treatment	Dahlberg et al[852]	D-Penicillamine	89	R	Decreased stone event and dissolution of stones
	Pak et al[792]	D-Penicillamine or α-mercaptopropionylglycine vs. conservative therapy	66	R	Both drugs equally effective in reducing stone events
	Chow and Streem[853]	D-Penicillamine or α-mercaptopropionylglycine vs. conservative therapy	16	NNT	Decreased stone event
	Barbey et al[854]	D-Penicillamine or α-mercaptopropionylglycine vs. conservative therapy	27	R	Decreased stone events
	Williams et al[864]	Acetohydroxamic acid vs. placebo	18	RCT	Decreased stone size
	Griffith et al[863]	Acetohydroxamic acid vs. placebo	210	RCT	Decreased stone growth
	Griffith et al[862]	Acetohydroxamic acid vs. placebo	94	RCT	Decreased stone growth

NCT, Nonrandomized controlled trial; NNT, nonrandomized, non–placebo-controlled trial; R, retrospective; RCT, randomized controlled trial.
Adapted from Sakhaee K, Maalouf NM, Sinnott B: Clinical review. Kidney stones 2012: pathogenesis, diagnosis, and management. *J Clin Endocrinol Metab* 97:1847-1860, 2012.

Table 40.12 Commonly Used Drugs in Treatment of Hypercalciuric Calcium Nephrolithiasis

Drug	Recommended Dosage(s)	Comments
Hydrochlorothiazide	50 mg/day; 25 mg twice daily	A single dosage is preferred since twice-daily dosage causes nocturia, discomfort, and noncompliance.
Chlorthalidone	25 mg/day, 50 mg/day	Both dosages lower urinary calcium by the same degree, both are long-acting and cause hypokalemia and secondary hypocitraturia.
Indapamide	1.25 mg/day, 2.5 mg/day	This agent has fewer side effects than hydrochlorothiazide, including lower incidence of hypokalemia and hypotension.
Amiloride	5 mg/day	Potassium sparing and lowers urinary calcium but to a lesser degree than hydrochlorothiazide.
Amiloride, hydrochlorothiazide	5 mg, 50 mg/day	Maintains the hypocalciuric effect of thiazide while averting the development of severe hypokalemia.
Trichlormethiazide	2 mg/day; 4 mg/day	Not marketed in the United States.

percutaneous urolithotomy, for a mean duration of 41 months, there was a decreased stone formation rate, from 1.89 to 0.46 stones/year.[818] One caveat in these studies was that alkali treatment was given to patients with urinary citrate excretion ranging from normal to low normal and low urinary citrate.[124-126]

Alkali treatment is relatively safe, with minor GI side effects, although certain susceptible individuals can have considerable gastric distress. The side effects have to be weighed against its efficacy against recurrent CaOx stones[124-126] and uric acid stones[452,839] and in patients with residual stones after shock wave lithotripsy.[838] One primary potential side effect that is attracting attention is the risk of CaP stone formation. A rise of urinary pH above 6.7 favors the generation of monohydrogen phosphate. Despite this concern, in two nonrandomized, non–placebo-controlled trials[130,840] in patients with distal dRTA and MSK with preexisting high urinary pH, alkali therapy was shown to be effective in reducing recurrent calcium stone formation. Larger scale prospective RCTs are still necessary to determine the effects of alkali treatment on the incidence of CaP stone formation.

Although sodium bicarbonate offers the same degree of urinary alkalinization when used in equivalent dosages to those of potassium alkali, it increases the risk of calcium stone formation due to sodium-induced hypercalciuria and promotion of monosodium urate–induced CaOx crystallization.[452,839] The initial recommended dosage for alkali is 30 to 40 mEq/day. In practice, 24-hour urine will be measured to follow the increase in citraturia, titrate the alkali dose, and maintain urinary pH between 6.1 and 7 to avoid potential complication of calcium stone formation. The 24-hour urinary pH, however, does not reflect diurnal variation in urinary pH during the period of high urinary acidity.[841] Therefore, higher doses of alkali administered at night ameliorate abnormally acidic urine in those with recurrent UA kidney stones.[841] Since unusually acidic urine is the predominant feature of patients with UA urolithiasis, alkali therapy with potassium citrate is first-line treatment in these patients.[29] Treatment with allopurinol can be considered when there is very high urinary UA level; alkali treatment is unsuccessful in patients with inflammatory bowel disease, bowel resection, and recurrent UA stones despite adequate urinary alkalinization.

Alkalinization is also helpful in cystinuria, as cystine solubility increases with increasing pH. Generally, it is recommended that alkalinization should be conducted conservatively so as not to exceed a pH of more than 6.5 to 6.7 because highly alkaline urine increases the risk of CaP stone formation. Defective acidification and high urinary pH has been described in patients with mixed cystine and calcium stones.[842] It is often difficult to determine the optimal dose of alkali to be administered to each individual patient.[518,843] Therefore, it is advisable to monitor patient responses with direct measurements of urinary supersaturation with respect to cystine.[793] Both potassium citrate and sodium bicarbonate have been shown to be equally effective in alkalinizing urine in this population.[844] Sodium alkali can be used in patients with renal insufficiency to avoid hyperkalemia. The dosage of alkali is typically divided equally three to four times daily.

Xanthine Oxidase Inhibitors

Allopurinol is used for the treatment of hyperuricosuric calcium stone formers rather than UA stone formers. One RCT in hyperuricosuric calcium stone formers, which compared allopurinol versus placebo,[845] demonstrated significantly decreased stone events with allopurinol treatment. Another RCT, in recurrent hyperuricosuric calcium stone formers, compared thiazide versus allopurinol, and both showed significantly reduced stone events with the combination treatment[320] (see Table 40.11). The efficacy of allopurinol alone in the treatment of hyperuricosuric CaOx stone-forming patients with multiple metabolic abnormalities is less evident.[846] The effective dose of allopurinol is 300 mg/day, which can be administered as a single dose or divided into three equal doses throughout the day. Side effects of allopurinol are reported as uncommon, but include a skin rash in 2% of treated patients and more severe, but even rarer, life-threatening hypersensitivity reactions, including acute interstitial nephritis and Steven-Johnson syndrome.[847] Adjustments are needed for patients with impaired kidney function since allopurinol is primarily excreted by the kidney.

A nonpurine xanthine oxidase inhibitor analog, febuxostat, has recently been approved for the treatment of hyperuricemia associated with gouty arthritis. In a retrospective study, the use of febuxostat in patients with gout who had allergies to allopurinol was shown to be a safe alternative.[848] In a 6-month, double-blinded RCT, hyperuricosuric calcium stone formers with one or more calcium stones detected by CT were treated with 80 mg/day of febuxostat, 300 mg/day of allopurinol, or placebo. Febuxostat reduced 24-hour urinary UA levels significantly more than allopurinol, but there was no change in stone size or number over this period.[849] Therefore, no conclusion comparing the drugs can be drawn until a longer study is conducted to determine the incidence of stone events (see Table 40.11). One advantage of febuxostat is that it is principally metabolized by the liver, thereby rendering dose adjustments in those with impaired kidney function unnecessary.[850]

Cystine Chelation Therapy

The treatment of cystine stones can be challenging. Conservative management with hydration and urinary alkalinization are the first steps in the management of a cystinuric patient, but they usually do not suffice. Thiol derivatives that act as chelating agents are commonly used in patients with severe cystinuria (>1000 mg/day). These drugs reduce a single cystine molecule into two cysteines and form a highly soluble disulfide compound of the drug with the cysteine molecules.[851] The effect of a disulfide compound (D-penicillamine) on stone events was first described by Dahlberg and coworkers.[852] Subsequently, α-mercaptopropionylglycine (tiopronin) was marketed for use in cystinuric patients. In two studies, pharmacologic treatment with D-penicillamine or tiopronin was shown to be superior to hydration and alkalinization alone for reducing stone events[853,854] (see Table 40.11). However, to date, no RCTs have demonstrated the superiority of pharmacologic treatment over placebo in cystinuric patients.

A few studies have suggested that captopril, which is also a thiol derivative, might also be effective in reducing urinary cystine excretion,[855,856] but its efficacy has not been confirmed by others.[854,857] Most recently, the potential role of inhibitors of cystine crystal growth has been explored. The most effective inhibitors tested were L-cystine dimethyl ester (L-CDME) and L-cystine methyl ester (L-CME). However, their effectiveness has only been tested in experimental models and not yet in cystinuric populations.[858]

Tiopronin has a lower incidence of side effects compared to D-penicillamine, and it is therefore used most often.[792] The side effects include GI irritation, abnormalities in hepatic enzymes, pancytopenias, skin irritation and disorders, and proteinuria.[792] Effective therapy should be aimed at maintaining the urinary cystine concentration at 250 mg/L, although there is variability among individual patients. Therefore, assessment of urinary supersaturation with respect to cystine solubility is important. However, to date, there is no clinical study exploring whether such measurements will avert the complications of cystine stone formation.[518,793,843] One important caveat is that urinary cystine measurement does not differentiate between a drug-cysteine complex and unbound cystine. Furthermore, urinary measurement of cystine does not decrease with drug treatment, which can lead to the misguided attempts to increase the dose of thiol drugs to lower urinary cystine levels. Therefore it is advisable to monitor the patient's response to treatment via urinary supersaturation, which is a better guide for dosing of chelating agents.

Pharmacotherapy of Infection-Related Stones

According to the guidelines of the American Urological Association (AUA), surgical treatment is still the best management for those with infectious stones (see below). However, medical treatment can be used for those with significant comorbidities who are not amenable to surgery and also to prevent stone recurrence after successful stone removal. These treatments include antibiotics, dissolution therapy, urease inhibitors, urinary acidification, dietary modification, and other supportive measures.

Antibiotics. Antibiotics are important during the preoperative and perioperative periods to prevent urinary sepsis from surgical procedures. Antibiotics should be directed against specific microorganisms established by positive urine cultures.

Dissolution Therapy. Boric acid, permanganate, and other solutions have been instilled into kidneys to dissolve infectious stones.[859] However, dissolution treatment has fallen out of favor due to its cost, duration of hospitalization and, most importantly, significant associated risks. The increased mortality following internal irrigation led to a ban by the U.S. Food and Drug Administration (FDA) on the use of this treatment approach.

Urease Inhibitors. Urease-producing microorganisms play a key role in the supersaturation of urine with respect to ammonium magnesium phosphate (struvite) by converting urea to ammonia, which usually coexists with calcium carbonate apatite stones because both stone types are favored in an alkaline environment.[860] While inhibition of bacterial urease has been shown to retard stone growth and to prevent new stone formation, it cannot eradicate existing stones nor the underlying infection. However, when combined with antimicrobial therapy, urease inhibition provides palliation for patients who cannot undergo definitive surgical management.[522,861]

The urease inhibitor, acetohydroxamic acid (AHA), is the only FDA-approved urease inhibitor to be used orally to inhibit urease enzyme activity.[862,863] This drug is cleared by the kidney and can penetrate bacterial cell walls. It also functions synergistically with antibiotics. Three RCTs have shown significant reductions in stone growth with AHA compared with placebo.[862-864] AHA can confer serious GI, neurologic, hematologic, and dermatologic side effects in 20% of patients, but these tend to resolve on discontinuation.[862-864] The starting dose of AHA is 250 mg by mouth twice daily. AHA is also contraindicated in patients with CKD and serum creatinine concentrations more than 2.5 mg/dL, which increase the risk of toxicity and poor urinary concentration.[862,863]

Urinary Acidification. Since urine alkalinity (pH > 7.2) promotes the formation of struvite and carbonate apatite stones, urinary acidification has been used to control stone burden in this population. L-Methionine, which imposes an acid load (H_2SO_4), can lower urinary pH. An in vitro simulation of decreasing urinary pH from 6.5 to 5.7 increased the dissolution rate of struvite stones.[865] It was suggested that oral intake of L-methionine, 1500 to 3000 mg/day, can be used for the dissolution of infectious stones, although no trials have proven this to date.[865]

SURGICAL MANAGEMENT OF INFECTION-RELATED STONES

Struvite staghorn calculi generally require surgical removal and, if not properly treated, require nephrectomy.[866] The goal is eradication of stone burden and prevention of stone regrowth, renal damage, and persistent infection. A significant number of patients treated with open surgical stone removal have recurrence following surgery due to recurrent urinary tract infections. Rather than open surgical stone removal, percutaneous urolithotomy can completely remove struvite stones 90% of the time,[867,868] with a recurrence rate approaching only 10% in kidneys rendered stone free.[869] A retrospective analysis of 43 patients with pure or mixed struvite stones from Duke University Medical Center from 2005 to 2012 has shown stone recurrence in 23% of patients, with stable renal function over a median follow-up of 22 months (range, 6 to 67 months). ESWL with ureteral stenting alone will result in stone-free rates of 50% to 75%.[870] Retrograde ureteroscopy with holmium:YAG laser stone disruption can fragment almost all minor staghorn stones, with a recurrence rate of 60% at 6 months.[871] The AUA has suggested a combined approach of percutaneous urolithotomy and shock wave lithotripsy.

ACKNOWLEDGMENTS

Our work has been supported by the National Institutes of Health (R01-DK081423, R01DK091392, R01-DK092461, and U01-HL111146), O'Brien Kidney Research Center (P30 DK-079328), American Society of Nephrology, Simmons Family Foundation, and Charles and Jane Pak Foundation. We wish to acknowledge Ms. Ashlei L. Johnson and Ms. Valeria Rodela for their assistance in the preparation of the manuscript.

Complete reference list available at ExpertConsult.com.

KEY REFERENCES

2. Scales CD, Jr, Smith AC, Hanley JM, et al: Urologic Diseases in America Project: Prevalence of kidney stones in the United States. *Eur Urol* 62:160–165, 2012.
4. Curhan GC, Rimm EB, Willett WC, et al: Regional variation in nephrolithiasis incidence and prevalence among United States men. *J Urol* 151:838–841, 1994.
20. Borghi L, Schianchi T, Meschi T, et al: Comparison of two diets for the prevention of recurrent stones in idiopathic hypercalciuria. *N Engl J Med* 346:77–84, 2002.
29. Sakhaee K, Adams-Huet B, Moe OW, et al: Pathophysiologic basis for normouricosuric uric acid nephrolithiasis. *Kidney Int* 62:971–979, 2002.
49. Evan AP, Lingeman JE, Coe FL, et al: Randall's plaque of patients with nephrolithiasis begins in basement membranes of thin loops of Henle. *J Clin Invest* 111:607–616, 2003.
59. Pak CY, Holt K: Nucleation and growth of brushite and calcium oxalate in urine of stone-formers. *Metabolism* 25:665–673, 1976.
93. Kok DJ, Papapoulos SE, Bijvoet OL: Excessive crystal agglomeration with low citrate excretion in recurrent stone-formers. *Lancet* 1:1056–1058, 1986.
101. Daudon M, Hennequin C, Bader C, et al: Inhibitors of crystallization. *Adv Nephrol Necker Hosp* 24:167–216, 1995.
124. Barcelo P, Wuhl O, Servitge E, et al: Randomized double-blind study of potassium citrate in idiopathic hypocitraturic calcium nephrolithiasis. *J Urol* 150:1761–1764, 1993.
128. Pak CY: Citrate and renal calculi: an update. *Miner Electrolyte Metab* 20:371–377, 1994.
132. Hamm LL: Renal handling of citrate. *Kidney Int* 38:728–735, 1990.
191. Levy FL, Adams-Huet B, Pak CY: Ambulatory evaluation of nephrolithiasis: an update of a 1980 protocol. *Am J Med* 98:50–59, 1995.
198. Sakhaee K, Maalouf NM, Kumar R, et al: Nephrolithiasis-associated bone disease: pathogenesis and treatment options. *Kidney Int* 79:393–403, 2011.
202. Pak CY, Oata M, Lawrence EC, et al: The hypercalciurias. Causes, parathyroid functions, and diagnostic criteria. *J Clin Invest* 54:387–400, 1974.
214. Insogna KL, Broadus AE, Dreyer BE, et al: Elevated production rate of 1,25-dihydroxyvitamin D in patients with absorptive hypercalciuria. *J Clin Endocrinol Metab* 61:490–495, 1985.
223. Breslau NA, Preminger GM, Adams BV, et al: Use of ketoconazole to probe the pathogenetic importance of 1,25-dihydroxyvitamin D in absorptive hypercalciuria. *J Clin Endocrinol Metab* 75:1446–1452, 1992.
232. Taylor EN, Hoofnagle AN, Curhan GC: Calcium and phosphorus regulatory hormones and risk of incident symptomatic kidney stones. *Clin J Am Soc Nephrol* 26:2015.
233. Pak CY, Kaplan R, Bone H, et al: A simple test for the diagnosis of absorptive, resorptive and renal hypercalciurias. *N Engl J Med* 292:497–500, 1975.
245. Zerwekh JE, Hughes MR, Reed BY, et al: Evidence for normal vitamin D receptor messenger ribonucleic acid and genotype in absorptive hypercalciuria. *J Clin Endocrinol Metab* 80:2960–2965, 1995.
252. Favus MJ, Karnauskas AJ, Parks JH, et al: Peripheral blood monocyte vitamin D receptor levels are elevated in patients with idiopathic hypercalciuria. *J Clin Endocrinol Metab* 89:4937–4943, 2004.
267. Yao J, Kathpalia P, Bushinsky DA, et al: Hyperresponsiveness of vitamin D receptor gene expression to 1,25-dihydroxyvitamin D3. A new characteristic of genetic hypercalciuric stone-forming rats. *J Clin Invest* 101:2223–2232, 1998.
283. Sakhaee K, Capolongo G, Maalouf NM, et al: Metabolic syndrome and the risk of calcium stones. *Nephrol Dial Transplant* 27:3201–3209, 2012.
289. Canaff L, Hendy GN: Human calcium-sensing receptor gene. Vitamin D response elements in promoters P1 and P2 confer transcriptional responsiveness to 1,25-dihydroxyvitamin D. *J Biol Chem* 277:30337–30350, 2002.
291. Thorleifsson G, Holm H, Edvardsson V, et al: Sequence variants in the CLDN14 gene associate with kidney stones and bone mineral density. *Nat Genet* 41:926–930, 2009.
335. Melnick JZ, Preisig PA, Moe OW, et al: Renal cortical mitochondrial aconitase is regulated in hypo- and hypercitraturia. *Kidney Int* 54:160–165, 1998.
346. Welch BJ, Graybeal D, Moe OW, et al: Biochemical and stone-risk profiles with topiramate treatment. *Am J Kidney Dis* 48:555–563, 2006.
349. Sinha MK, Collazo-Clavell ML, Rule A, et al: Hyperoxaluric nephrolithiasis is a complication of Roux-en-Y gastric bypass surgery. *Kidney Int* 72:100–107, 2007.
358. Sakhaee K: Recent advances in the pathophysiology of nephrolithiasis. *Kidney Int* 75:585–595, 2009.
371. Danpure CJ, Jennings PR: Peroxisomal alanine:glyoxylate aminotransferase deficiency in primary hyperoxaluria type I. *FEBS Lett* 201:20–24, 1986.
374. Monico CG, Rossetti S, Belostotsky R, et al: Primary hyperoxaluria type III gene HOGA1 (formerly DHDPSL) as a possible risk factor for idiopathic calcium oxalate urolithiasis. *Clin J Am Soc Nephrol* 6:2289–2295, 2011.
385. Jiang Z, Asplin JR, Evan AP, et al: Calcium oxalate urolithiasis in mice lacking anion transporter Slc26a6. *Nat Genet* 38:474–478, 2006.
446. Maalouf NM, Sakhaee K, Parks JH, et al: Association of urinary pH with body weight in nephrolithiasis. *Kidney Int* 65:1422–1425, 2004.
452. Sakhaee K, Nicar M, Hill K, et al: Contrasting effects of potassium citrate and sodium citrate therapies on urinary chemistries and crystallization of stone-forming salts. *Kidney Int* 24:348–352, 1983.
473. Daudon M, Traxer O, Conort P, et al: Type 2 diabetes increases the risk for uric acid stones. *J Am Soc Nephrol* 17:2026–2033, 2006.

481. Curthoys NP, Moe OW: Proximal tubule function and response to acidosis. *Clin J Am Soc Nephrol* 9:1627–1638, 2014.
483. Nagami GT: Renal ammonium production and excretion. In Seldin DW, Giebisch GH, editors: *The kidney: physiology and pathophysiology*, Philadelphia, 2000, Lippincott Williams & Wilkins, pp 1995–2014.
501. Bobulescu IA, Dubree M, Zhang J, et al: Reduction of renal triglyceride accumulation: effects on proximal tubule Na+/H+ exchange and urinary acidification. *Am J Physiol Renal Physiol* 297:F1419–F1426, 2009.
503. Chillaron J, Font-Llitjos M, Fort J, et al: Pathophysiology and treatment of cystinuria. *Nat Rev Nephrol* 6:424–434, 2010.
553. Moe OW, Bonny O: Genetic hypercalciuria. *J Am Soc Nephrol* 16:729–745, 2005.
566. Goldfarb DS, Fischer ME, Keich Y, et al: A twin study of genetic and dietary influences on nephrolithiasis: a report from the Vietnam Era Twin (VET) Registry. *Kidney Int* 67:1053–1061, 2005.
575. Vezzoli G, Terranegra A, Arcidiacono T, et al: R990G polymorphism of calcium-sensing receptor does produce a gain-of-function and predispose to primary hypercalciuria. *Kidney Int* 71:1155–1162, 2007.
577. Suzuki Y, Pasch A, Bonny O, et al: Gain-of-function haplotype in the epithelial calcium channel TRPV6 is a risk factor for renal calcium stone formation. *Hum Mol Genet* 17:1613–1618, 2008.
604. Pigna F, Sakhaee K, Adams-Huet B, et al: Body fat content and distribution and urinary risk factors for nephrolithiasis. *Clin J Am Soc Nephrol* 9:159–165, 2014.
609. Reiner AP, Kahn A, Eisner BH, et al: Kidney stones and subclinical atherosclerosis in young adults: the CARDIA study. *J Urol* 185:920–925, 2011.
618. Ferraro PM, Taylor EN, Eisner BH, et al: History of kidney stones and the risk of coronary heart disease. *JAMA* 310:408–415, 2013.
651. Melton LJ, 3rd, Crowson CS, Khosla S, et al: Fracture risk among patients with urolithiasis: a population-based cohort study. *Kidney Int* 53:459–464, 1998.
702. Amanzadeh J, Gitomer WL, Zerwekh JE, et al: Effect of high protein diet on stone-forming propensity and bone loss in rats. *Kidney Int* 64:2142–2149, 2003.
712. Hoopes RR, Jr, Shrimpton AE, Knohl SJ, et al: Dent disease with mutations in OCRL1. *Am J Hum Genet* 76:260–267, 2005.
725. Pak CY, Peterson R, Poindexter JR: Adequacy of a single stone risk analysis in the medical evaluation of urolithiasis. *J Urol* 165:378–381, 2001.
793. Goldfarb DS, Coe FL, Asplin JR: Urinary cystine excretion and capacity in patients with cystinuria. *Kidney Int* 69:1041–1047, 2006.

41 Kidney Cancer

Kara N. Babaian | Scott E. Delacroix, Jr. | Christopher G. Wood | Eric Jonasch

CHAPTER OUTLINE

BENIGN NEOPLASMS OF THE KIDNEY, 1368
Benign Epithelial Tumors, 1368
Benign Mesenchymal Tumors, 1368
Benign Cystic Neoplasms, 1369

MALIGNANT NEOPLASMS OF THE KIDNEY, 1370
Renal Cell Carcinoma, 1370
Renal Pelvic Tumors, 1385
Other Kidney Tumors, 1386

BENIGN NEOPLASMS OF THE KIDNEY

Benign tumors of the kidney lack both the chromosomal abnormalities associated with malignant tumors and the ability to metastasize. They are infrequent, but it is challenging to estimate their true incidence because most benign lesions are asymptomatic and difficult to detect. Benign tumors can arise from any cell type within the kidney, and most are of epithelial or mesenchymal origin. Other benign tumors are cystic masses or are composed of both epithelial and mesenchymal elements.

BENIGN EPITHELIAL TUMORS

RENAL CORTICAL ADENOMA

Small benign renal cortical tumors, measuring less than 5 mm, with tubulopapillary histology of low nuclear grade are called *renal cortical adenomas*.[1] Most are asymptomatic and undetectable radiographically because of their small size. Renal adenomas are usually found incidentally during surgery or at autopsy, with an incidence of 7.2% to 22%.[2,3]

ONCOCYTOMA

Renal oncocytomas are uncommon but increasingly recognized benign tumors.[4-6] Oncocytomas are composed of a pure population of oncocytes—large, well-differentiated neoplastic cells with intensely eosinophilic granular cytoplasm. The cytoplasm of these cells is packed with mitochondria, leading to their histologic appearance. Immunohistochemical studies suggest that oncocytomas probably also arise from the intercalated cells of the distal collecting tubules.[5] Peak incidence of these tumors is in the seventh decade of life with a male-to-female predominance of 2:1 to 3:1.[7] The tumors are usually asymptomatic and discovered incidentally by imaging studies. Larger oncocytomas can have a stellate central fibrous scar, which is visible on preoperative radiologic studies in 6.7% to 50% of cases.[7] Grossly, oncocytomas are generally well encapsulated and are only rarely invasive. Pathologic differentiation of a typical renal oncocytoma from an oncocytic renal cell carcinoma (RCC) can be difficult. Some series suggest that 3% to 7% of solid renocortical tumors previously classified as RCCs are in fact oncocytomas.[4] Renal oncocytomas almost invariably have a benign clinical behavior and are rarely associated with metastases, even when the primary tumor is very large. Nephrectomy is usually the treatment of choice for large renal masses regardless of type, but the possibility of oncocytoma should be considered with incidentally discovered small renal masses or tumors in a solitary kidney.

METANEPHRIC ADENOMA

Metanephric adenoma (MA) is a rare benign tumor that is usually a solitary lesion. The peak incidence of this tumor is in the fifth and sixth decades of life[8] with a female predominance of 2.5:1.[7] It also occurs in children. Most cases are asymptomatic and are diagnosed incidentally. Reported symptoms include abdominal or flank pain, palpable mass, fever, and hematuria. Metanephric adenoma has been associated with polycythemia in 12% of cases.[8] Mean tumor size at diagnosis is 5 cm.[8] On computed tomography (CT) these tumors show mild enhancement and, therefore, can be mistaken for papillary RCC.[9] Metanephric adenomas are well circumscribed and can contain areas of necrosis, hemorrhage, calcifications, and cysts.[10,11] Although these tumors are considered benign, two cases with metastatic disease have been reported in the literature.[12,13] Surgical resection is required to rule out malignancy.

BENIGN MESENCHYMAL TUMORS

ANGIOMYOLIPOMA

Angiomyolipoma (AML) is a neoplasm consisting of blood vessels, smooth muscle, and mature adipose tissue. Most affected patients present in the fifth or sixth decade, and there is a female predominance. Eighty percent of AMLs are sporadic and the rest are associated with genetic syndromes such as tuberous sclerosis complex (TSC) and lymphangioleiomyomatosis (LAM).[14] Sporadic cases tend to be solitary, whereas patients with TSC can have multiple and bilateral AMLs. Histologically, there are two types of AMLs, classic type and epithelioid variant (eAML). The classic type contains variable amounts of vascular, smooth muscle, and adipose elements, whereas in the epithelioid variant, epithelioid cells predominate and vascular and adipose elements are usually absent.[15] Epithelioid AMLs can be locally aggressive, have the ability to metastasize, and tend to recur. There have been reports of eAMLs involving the renal vein, inferior vena cava, lymph nodes, per-renal fat, adjacent organs, lungs, and liver.[16,17] About 75% of AMLs are asymptomatic and are diagnosed by cross-sectional imaging. Symptoms include abdominal or flank pain, hematuria, palpable mass, and hemorrhagic shock from a spontaneous retroperitoneal bleed (called Wunderlich's syndrome). The mean tumor size at diagnosis is 3.5 cm.[18] The presence of fat with value of less than 20 Hounsfield units (HU) on CT is diagnostic of AML. On magnetic resonance imaging (MRI), AMLs appear hyperintense on T1- and T2-weighted images and hypointense on T1-weighted images with fat suppression.[19,20] AMLs larger than 4 cm require intervention owing to the risk of hemorrhage. Treatment options include angioembolization, partial nephrectomy, and radical nephrectomy.

LEIOMYOMA

Renal leiomyomas are benign neoplasms that arise from smooth muscle cells and usually originate from the renal capsule, but they can also originate from the muscularis of the renal pelvis or cortical vascular smooth muscle.[21] Because most renal leiomyomas are small, they are usually asymptomatic and discovered incidentally. The patient with a large leiomyoma may present with pain or a palpable mass. The estimated incidence, based on autopsy studies, is 5%.[22] Renal leiomyomas arise from the renal capsule, so they are peripherally located, in contact with only the outer surface of the kidney, and do not appear to arise from the renal parenchyma.[21] On contrast-enhanced CT, these lesions appear well-circumscribed and demonstrate homogeneous enhancement.[21] Because renal leiomyomas are indistinguishable from RCC on the basis of imaging characteristics, they require surgical excision to obtain a pathologic diagnosis.

JUXTAGLOMERULAR CELL TUMOR

A reninoma or renal juxtaglomerular cell tumor secretes renin, resulting in secondary hyperaldosteronism. This excess aldosterone leads to hypertension and hypokalemia. The peak incidence of this tumor is in the second or third decade, with a 2:1 female-to-male predominance. Most often, affected patients present with poorly controlled hypertension, polyuria, polydipsia, muscle aches, and headaches. Laboratory abnormalities include elevated plasma renin activity (PRA), elevated plasma aldosterone concentration, and hypokalemia. Surgical resection provides definitive treatment and results in reversal of hypertension and hypokalemia.

RENOMEDULLARY INTERSTITIAL CELL TUMOR

Also known as medullary fibromas, renomedullary interstitial cell tumors are small benign lesions, usually measuring less than 5 mm, that arise from interstitial cells of the medulla.[23,24] Up to 50% of adults have evidence of these tumors at autopsy.[23] On CT, this lesion appears as a small, nonenhancing, noncalcified, hypoattenuating solid mass within the renal medulla.[24]

HEMANGIOMA

Hemangiomas in the kidney are extremely rare, with an incidence of 1 in 2000 to 1 in 30,000 in autopsy studies,[25] and are associated with tuberous sclerosis, Sturge-Weber syndrome, and Klippel-Trenaunay-Weber syndrome.[21] Most cases are asymptomatic and incidentally diagnosed but can manifest as hematuria and pain. Hemangiomas are small, usually less than 2 cm,[26] and located in the tip of the papilla and the renal pelvis.[27] On unenhanced CT, renal hemangioma may appear as a lobulated hypo- to isoattenuating soft tissue mass in the region of the medulla or pelvis, and on enhanced CT, they demonstrate intense arterial enhancement.[28,29]

OTHER RARE BENIGN MESENCHYMAL TUMORS

Other rare benign mesenchymal tumors include hemangiopericytoma, lymphangioma, lipoma, and solitary fibrous tumor. Hemangiopericytomas of the kidney are rare, with less than 40 cases reported in the literature. Most patients with this tumor present in the fourth decade of life and can have hematuria or hypoglycemia due to glucose hypermetabolism within the mass.[30] Renal lymphangioma is a rare benign developmental malformation in which the developing lymphatic tissue fails to establish communication with the remainder of the lymphatic system.[31] Abnormal lymphatic channels dilate to form cystic masses in the perinephric or renal sinus region.[31] Only 50 cases have been reported in the literature. If intervention is required, therapeutic options include percutaneous[32] or laparoscopic aspiration,[33] cyst marsupialization,[34] and nephrectomy.[35] Renal lipomas are rare neoplasms, with only 20 cases reported in the literature.[27,36,37] Lipomas develop from lipomatous differentiation of primitive mesenchymal cells or from embryonic rests of adipose tissue in the kidney.[23,24] The presence of macroscopic fat is evident on imaging studies. Lastly, solitary fibrous tumors (SFTs) are rare neoplasms composed of fibrous tissue and collagen and can arise anywhere in the body, the most common site being the pleura. Within the kidney, SFTs can arise from the renal capsule, cortex, pelvis, or peripelvic connective tissue. Most patients are older than 40 years, with a slight female predominance. Clinical symptoms include flank pain, hematuria, and palpable mass.[27]

BENIGN CYSTIC NEOPLASMS

MULTILOCULAR CYSTIC NEPHROMA AND MIXED EPITHELIAL STROMAL TUMOR

Multilocular cystic nephromas have a bimodal age distribution, occurring in male children younger than 4 years and in adult women between 40 and 60 years.[38,39] Children usually present with an abdominal mass, whereas adults present with hematuria or abdominal/flank pain. On CT, cystic nephromas appear well-circumscribed and multiseptated with enhancement within the septations.[23] They also tend to herniate into the renal pelvis or proximal ureter.[23] The differential diagnosis includes cystic RCC and mixed epithelial stromal tumor (MEST). Some pathologists believe that cystic nephromas and MESTs are not separate entities but instead are part of the same spectrum of stromal epithelial tumors.[40] MESTs are composed of stromal elements that resemble ovarian stroma and an epithelial component, consisting of epithelium-lined cysts. Ninety percent of these tumors occur in women and may be associated with estrogen therapy.[41] On CT, MESTs are well-circumscribed cystic masses with multiple enhancing septations and solid components.[23]

MALIGNANT NEOPLASMS OF THE KIDNEY

Renal cell carcinomas arise within the renal cortex and account for about 80% to 85% of all primary renal neoplasms. Transitional carcinomas arising from the renal pelvis are the next most common, accounting for 7% to 8% of primary renal neoplasms. Other parenchymal epithelial tumors, such as oncocytomas, collecting duct tumors, and renal sarcomas, are uncommon but are becoming more frequently recognized pathologically. Nephroblastoma (Wilms' tumor) is common in children and accounts for 5% to 6% of all primary renal tumors.

Metastatic lesions to the kidney (secondary neoplasms) occur in 7% to 20% of patients with cancer at autopsy.[42-44] These secondary lesions are very rare in the absence of progression of the primary neoplasm.[45]

This section focuses on the epidemiology, pathology, genetics, clinical, and radiographic presentation, staging methods, and surgical and systemic management of primary renal neoplasms. A brief description of the biology and management of the less common tumors as well as evaluation of suspected metastatic disease is also presented.

RENAL CELL CARCINOMA

EPIDEMIOLOGY

In 2013, it was estimated that renal cell and renal pelvic cancer would be newly diagnosed in 65,150 people in the United States and that almost 13,680 people would die of the disease.[46] RCC represents 3.9% of all U.S. cancers and 2% of all cancer deaths. Worldwide, the mortality from RCC is estimated to exceed 100,000 per year.[47]

The incidence varies widely from country to country, with the highest rates seen in Northern Europe and North America.[48] Although the incidence is reported to be lower in individuals living in African countries,[48] the incidences are equivalent among whites and African Americans living in the United States.[49] Chronic kidney failure was more strongly associated with RCC among blacks (odds ratio [OR], 8.7; 95% confidence interval [CI], 3.3 to 22.9) than among whites (OR, 2.0; 95% CI, 0.7 to 5.6, P [interaction] = 0.03).[50] Historically, RCC was twice as common in men as in women, but later data suggest that this gap is beginning to narrow. The incidence in Asian Americans and Pacific Islanders is half that of their white and African American counterparts.[46] RCC occurs predominantly in the sixth to eighth decades; it is uncommon in patients younger than 40 years and rare in children.[51-53]

The incidence of RCC has steadily risen over time. Between 1975 and 1995 in the United States the incidence rates per 100,000 person-years increased by 2.3%, 3.1%, 3.9%, and 4.3% annually for white men, white women, African American men, and African American women, respectively.[11] Mortality rates are equivalent for whites (5.9 males and 2.7 females per 100,000 persons) and African Americans (6.0 and 2.6, respectively), whereas Asian American and Pacific Islanders have the lowest mortality rates (2.9 and 1.3, respectively).[46] American Indians and Alaskan Natives have an increased incidence of cancer of the kidney and an alarmingly high mortality rate (8.8 males and 4.1 females per 100,000 persons).[46,54]

The overall incidence of RCC in the United States for all population ancestry groups has risen at a rate that is threefold higher than the mortality rate. Since 1950, there has been a 126% increase in the incidence, accompanied by a 37% increase in annual mortality.[55,56] The 5-year survival rate of patients with a diagnosis of kidney cancer has improved from 50% for those receiving this diagnosis in 1975 to 72% for those receiving this diagnosis in 2008.[46] The proportion of RCCs discovered incidentally increased from approximately 10% in the 1970s to 60% in 1998.[56] In addition, at one major institution, the percentage of organ-confined tumors increased from 47% in 1989 to 78% in 1998.[57] Stage of disease at diagnosis has changed over this time, with incidence of stage 1 disease increasing from 43% to 57% between 1993 and 2004, and stage 2 and 3 disease showed a statistically significant decline. The incidence of stage 4 disease has remained stable over this same period.[58]

Numerous environmental and clinical factors have been implicated in the etiology of RCC.[59] They include tobacco use; occupational exposure to toxic compounds such as cadmium, asbestos, and petroleum by-products; obesity; acquired cystic kidney disease (typically associated with dialysis); and analgesic abuse nephropathy. Cigarette smoking doubles the likelihood of RCC and contributes to as many as one third of all cases.[60-62] The risk for development of kidney cancer in patients with acquired cystic kidney disease has been estimated to be 30 times greater than that in the general population.[63] In particular, it is estimated that acquired cystic kidney disease develops in 20% to 90% of patients receiving long-term dialysis, depending on the duration of dialysis,[64] and that RCC develops in between 3.8% and 4.2% of these patients.[65] Patients with large cysts appear to be an increased risk for malignant transformation. The carcinomas are multiple and bilateral in approximately half the cases, a finding consistent with the diffuse nature of the underlying disease.[35] The prolonged ingestion of analgesic combinations, particularly compounds containing phenacetin and aspirin, can lead to end-stage kidney disease. Patients with this diagnosis are at increased risk for renal pelvic tumors and possibly kidney cancer, although the latter association remains controversial.[66-68] Because of its carcinogenic properties, phenacetin was removed from the U.S. marketplace by the U.S. Food and Drug Administration (FDA) in 1983 and later from European markets.

An enhanced risk for RCC has been observed in patients with certain inherited disorders, implicating various genetic abnormalities in the etiology of this disease. The disorders include von Hippel–Lindau syndrome, hereditary papillary renal cancer, hereditary leiomyoma renal cancer syndrome, and Birt-Hogg-Dube syndrome. In addition, patients with tuberous sclerosis and autosomal dominant polycystic kidney disease, although they do not have a dramatically increased incidence of kidney cancer, can have cancers with unique features.

Hereditary polycystic kidney disease (autosomal dominant polycystic kidney disease [ADPKD]) has a long-debated association with kidney cancer; however, when kidney cancer does occur in patients with this disorder, it typically displays a number of distinct clinical characteristics.[69] The tumors are more often bilateral at presentation, multicentric, and with sarcomatoid features when symptomatic or advanced. A 2009 analysis of 89 nephrectomy specimens from patients with ADPKD who underwent extirpation for nononcologic indications reported an increased risk of kidney cancer.[70] Specifically, overall incidence rose to 8.3%. The tumors were bilateral in 10% and multifocal in 27.3% of cases, and the histologic subtypes were divided between clear cell RCCs (60%) and papillary RCCs (40%). These cancers were all staged as T1 disease, and none of the tumors were seen on preoperative imaging. An increased incidence of sarcomatoid features was not seen in this group, possibly because of the benign indications for extirpation.

Although most RCCs are sporadic, factors suggesting a hereditary cause include the occurrence of the disease in first-degree relatives,[71-74] onset before the age of 40, and bilateral or multifocal disease.[4] Several kindreds with familial clear cell carcinoma have been identified that have consistent abnormalities on the short arm of chromosome 3.[5,6,75,76] Other kindreds with papillary tumors have been identified with different genetic abnormalities,[77] suggesting that these tumors represent distinct disease entities. Although the true prevalence of hereditary RCC is unknown, it is estimated that hereditary carcinomas make up 3% to 5% of all RCCs.[78] A more detailed discussion of the molecular biology of RCC is provided in a later section.

PATHOLOGY AND CYTOGENETICS

RCC was first reported by Konig in 1826. In 1883, Grawitz hypothesized on histologic grounds that RCCs arose from rests of adrenal tissue within the kidney.[79] Although immunohistologic and ultrastructural analyses currently point toward the proximal renal tubule as the true cell of origin,[80] the term *hypernephroma* continues to be incorrectly applied to these cancers.

Renal cell tumors occur with equal frequency in right and left kidneys and are distributed equally throughout the kidney.[81] The average diameter is about 7 cm, but tumors have ranged from less than 2 cm to more than 25 cm in diameter. Previously, renal lesions smaller than 2 to 3 cm were incorrectly considered to be benign adenomas. Such distinctions between benign and malignant tumors are made no longer on the basis of size but rather according to fundamental histologic criteria. Therefore, from a practical standpoint, all solid renal masses require resection or biopsy for accurate histologic diagnosis. Improved percutaneous biopsy techniques have a role in the management of renal masses but are definitively less accurate than extirpation in providing pathologic and histologic information.

Renal cell carcinomas have historically been classified according to cell type (clear, granular, spindle, or oncocytic) and growth pattern (acinar, papillary, or sarcomatoid).[81] This classification has undergone a transformation to more accurately reflect the morphologic, histochemical, and molecular features of different types of adenocarcinomas (Table 41.1).[82-84] On the basis of research studies, the following five distinct subtypes have been identified: clear cell (conventional), chromophilic (papillary), chromophobic, oncocytic, and collecting duct (Bellini duct). Each of these tumors has a unique growth pattern, cell of origin, and cytogenetic characteristics. Table 41.1 summarizes this classification, which more accurately reflects the greater knowledge of the molecular and genetic abnormalities of these lesions than did the earlier classification.[83] Sarcomatoid variants of almost all of the aforementioned histologic subtypes have been described and represent a dedifferentiation (poor differentiation) of the individual subtype.[85]

Clear cell or conventional RCCs make up 75% to 85% of tumors and are characterized by a deletion or functional inactivation in one or both copies of chromosome arm 3p.[86] A higher nuclear grade (Fuhrman classification) or the presence of a sarcomatoid pattern correlates with a poorer prognosis.[87,88]

Chromophilic or papillary carcinomas (synonymous) make up 10% to 15% of kidney cancers. In hereditary disease papillary carcinomas are multifocal and bilateral, and they commonly manifest as small tumors.[89] These tumors also

Table 41.1 Pathologic Classification of Renal Cell Carcinoma

Carcinoma Type	Growth Pattern (Incidence, %)	Cell of Origin	Cytogenetic Characteristics	
			Major	Minor
Clear cell	Acinar or sarcomatoid (75-85)	Proximal tubule	−3p	+5, +7, +12, −6p, −8p −9, −14q, −Y
Chromophilic*	Papillary or sarcomatoid (12-14)	Proximal tubule	+7, +17, −Y	+12, +16, +20, −14
Chromophobic	Solid, tubular, or sarcomatoid (4-6)	Intercalated cell of cortical collecting duct	Hypodiploidy	—
Oncocytic	Typified by tumor nests (2-4)	Intercalated cell of cortical collecting duct	Undetermined†	—
Collecting duct	Papillary or sarcomatoid (1)	Medullary collecting duct	Undetermined†	—

*These tumors were previously classified as papillary tumors.
†This classification is based on the work of Storkel S, van den Berg E: Morphological classification of renal cancer. *World J Urol* 13:153-158, 1995.

appear to arise from the proximal tubule but are both morphologically and genetically distinct from clear cell carcinomas. These tumors often have a low stage at presentation and are thus attributed a more favorable prognosis,[89,90] but in advanced stages, they can be as aggressive as clear cell lesions.[91] The class of papillary RCC has now been subdivided into papillary type 1 and type 2.[92] This differentiation has been based on histologic appearance[92] and has been validated through microarray analysis of molecular markers.[93] Subtyping permits identification of an independent prognostic factor, because patients with type 2 papillary RCC have a worse outcome even when stratified by TNM stage.[92,93]

Chromophobe carcinomas make up about 4% of all RCCs. Histologically, they are composed of sheets of cells that are uniformly darker than those of the usual clear cell carcinoma, with a peripheral eosinophilic granularity. These cells lack the abundant lipid and glycogen characteristics of the clear cell RCC and are believed to arise from the intercalated cells of the renal collecting ducts.[94-96] They have a hypodiploid number of chromosomes, but also no 3p loss.[97-99] These tumors are usually well circumscribed and generally have an excellent prognosis. As a group, chromophobe RCCs tend to manifest at lower stages and grades, yet once metastatic, chromophobe carcinomas are highly refractory to therapy and have a prognosis equivalent to or worse than that of clear cell carcinomas.[100]

Collecting duct (Bellini duct) tumors are also very rare but are frequently very aggressive in behavior.[101] They are located in the renal medulla and pelvis and thus usually manifest as gross hematuria. In contrast to clear cell carcinomas, collecting duct tumors produce mucin and react with antibodies to both high-molecular-weight and low-molecular-weight keratins.[102] Sarcomatoid variants have also been noted. Neither oncocytomas nor collecting duct tumors have been associated with a consistent pattern of genetic abnormalities.

Medullary RCC is a rare aggressive variant usually seen in individuals with sickle cell trait.[103] Davis and colleagues designated this entity the "seventh sickle cell nephropathy."[103] Histologically, a variety of growth patterns have been described for medullary RCC, including reticular, solid, tubular, trabecular, cribriform, sarcomatoid, and micropapillary.[104] Little is known about the cytogenetics of this tumor. Gene expression profiling has shown clustering more closely associated with urothelial carcinoma than with RCC.[105,106] Classification and further characterization of this rare but lethal entity will require further molecular and pathologic research with a larger collection of specimens.

The Xp11.2 translocation carcinoma was first described in 1991 by Tomlinson and colleagues.[107] This translocation results in the fusion of a novel gene, designated *RCC17*, at chromosome band 17q25 to the gene for transcription factor for immunoglobulin heavy-chain enhancer 3 *(TFE3)* located on chromosome band Xp11.[108] These tumors usually occur in children and young adults, appearing at a median age of 20 years, and account for at least one third of carcinomas seen in childhood and adolescence.[105] Tumor cells are described as having voluminous clear cytoplasm and bulging distinct cell borders, an appearance reminiscent of soap bubbles. The architecture is predominantly solid, tubular, acinar, or alveolar, with areas with a pseudopapillary appearance.[109] Transcription factor 3 is a sensitive and specific marker for translocation carcinomas, with a sensitivity ranging from 82% to 97.5%.[105] Although relatively indolent, these tumors are refractory to systemic therapy and respond only to aggressive surgical resection.

MOLECULAR BIOLOGY AND HEREDITARY DISORDERS

Much of the late success in developing therapies for RCC has arisen out of an improved understanding of the molecular biology of clear cell kidney carcinoma and its highly prevalent mutation in *VHL*, the von Hippel–Lindau gene. Only 4% of cases of RCC are familial, yet elucidation of the genetic mutations involved in hereditary RCC has led to targeted therapies that benefit the majority of sporadic cases (Figure 41.1).[110] Cloning of the VHL gene in 1993,[111] and the subsequent functional and structural characterization of the gene product,[112] has contributed greatly to our

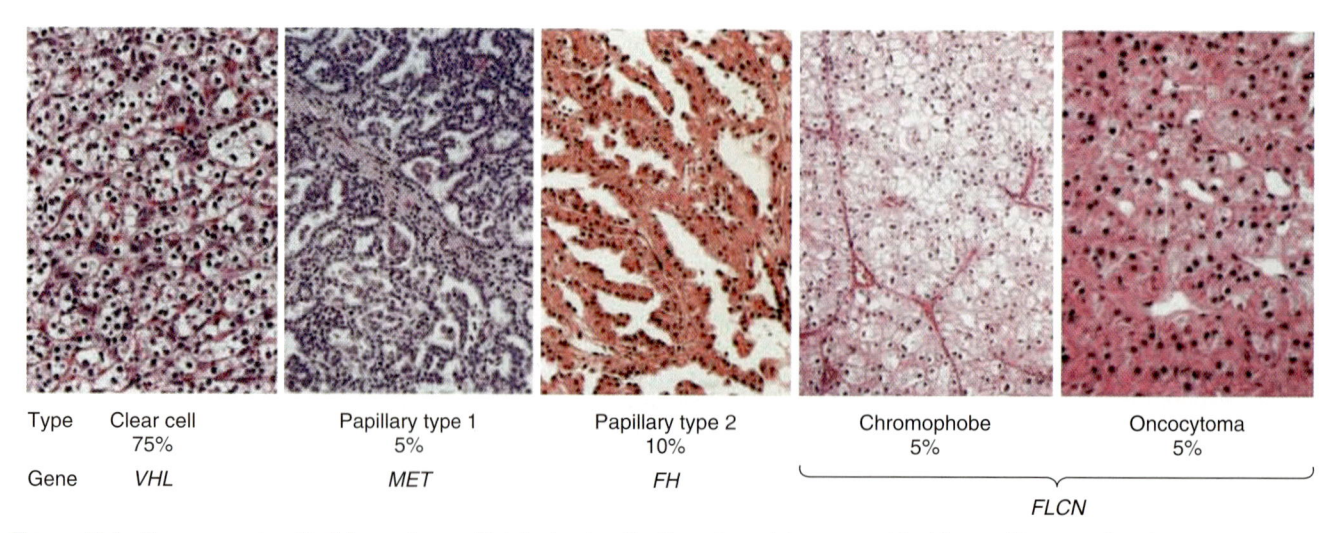

Figure 41.1 Human renal epithelial neoplasms. Histologic classification of renal tumors and incidence. The associated gene for inherited neoplasms is listed, although these genes can also be mutated in sporadic cases (especially the von Hippel–Lindau [VHL] gene in clear cell carcinomas). FH, fumarate hydratase; FLCN, folliculin; MET, Met proto-oncogene. (From Linehan WM, Walther MM, Zbar B: The genetic basis of cancer of the kidney. *J Urol* 170:2163, 2003.)

Type	Clear cell 75%	Papillary type 1 5%	Papillary type 2 10%	Chromophobe 5%	Oncocytoma 5%
Gene	VHL	MET	FH	FLCN	FLCN

understanding of the genetics of this disease and of RCC in general.

VHL syndrome is transmitted in an autosomal dominant fashion and is characterized by a predisposition to various neoplasms, including RCC (with clear cell histology), renal cysts, retinal angiomas, spinocerebellar hemangioblastomas, pheochromocytomas, and pancreatic carcinomas and cysts.[113] Renal cysts are frequently multiple and bilateral.

RCC develops in about a third of all patients with VHL syndrome and is a major cause of death in patients with the disease. Tumor development in this setting is linked to somatic inactivation of the remaining wild-type allele. Moreover, biallelic *VHL* inactivation due to somatic mutations and/or hypermethylation is observed in more than 50% of sporadic clear cell carcinomas. Restoration of VHL protein function in $VHL^{-/-}$ RCC cell lines suppresses their ability to form tumors in nude mice xenograft assays, a finding that supports the role of the *VHL* gene as a renal cancer tumor suppressor gene.[114]

Tumors associated with *VHL* mutations (including the hereditary tumors in VHL syndrome and a majority of the sporadic cases of clear cell RCC[115]) are typically hypervascular and occasionally lead to the overproduction of red blood cells (polycythemia).[116] These developments are due to overproduction of vascular endothelial growth factor (VEGF) and erythropoietin, respectively. Working from the knowledge that the two genes encoding these proteins are hypoxia inducible, several groups went on to show that cells lacking the protein encoded by *VHL* are unable to suppress the accumulation of hypoxia-inducible factors, including VEGF, under well-oxygenated conditions.[117-119] The hypoxia-inducible factor (HIF) family of transcription factors is at the center of maintaining oxygen homeostasis and regulates a variety of hypoxia-inducible genes. HIF is a heterodimer composed of HIF-α and HIF-β subunits.[120] Although the HIF-β subunit is constitutively expressed, HIF-α is normally degraded in the presence of oxygen and accumulates only under hypoxic conditions.[121,122] A 200–amino acid oxygen-dependent degradation domain lies within the central region of HIF1-α.[123,124] This region is sufficient to target HIF for degradation by the ubiquitin-proteasome pathway in the presence of oxygen[124-126] (Figure 41.2). At present, several dozen HIF target genes have been identified, including the genes for VEGF, platelet-derived growth factor (PDGF), and transforming growth factor-α. Their protein products play critical roles in cellular and systemic physiologic responses to hypoxia, including glycolysis, erythropoiesis, angiogenesis, and vascular remodeling.[120]

Papillary RCC possesses unique genetic features. In hereditary cases, it is characterized by the formation of multiple bilateral tumors with trisomy of chromosomes 7 and 17.[127] The hereditary papillary RCC gene was identified on chromosome bands 7q31.1-34, and germline missense mutations in the tyrosine kinase domain of the *c-Met* proto-oncogene were detected in several families with hereditary papillary RCC.[128] In sporadic papillary RCC, mutations of the *c-Met* proto-oncogene have been detected in 13% of patients with papillary RCC and no family history of kidney cancers.[129] These mutations are oncogenic and create a constitutively active, ligand-independent autophosphorylation of *c-Met*. These data may underestimate the significance of alterations in *c-Met*, because other mutations, chromosomal duplications (e.g., trisomy 7), and epigenetic events likely increase the frequency of *c-Met* activation.

The disorder that results from autosomal dominant mutations in the fumarate hydratase *(FH)* gene is known as

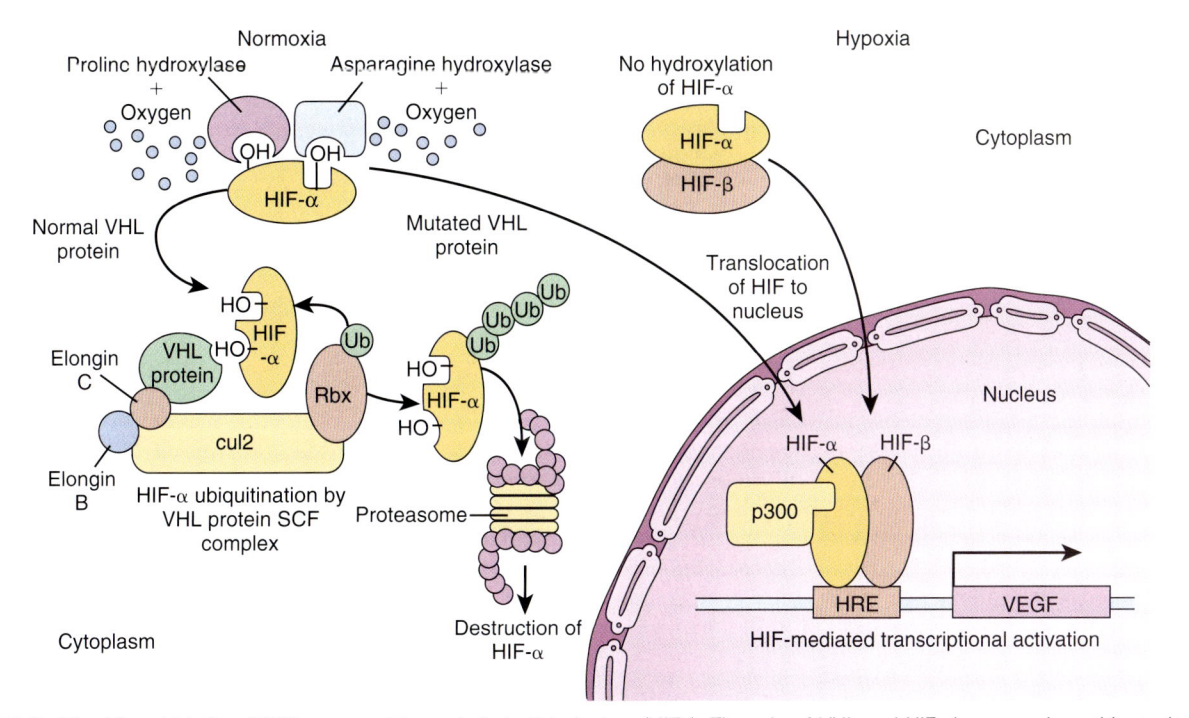

Figure 41.2 Von Hippel–Lindau *(VHL)* gene and hypoxia-inducible factors (HIFs). The role of *VHL* and HIFs in normoxic and hypoxic conditions in the *normal* cell (VHL$^{+/-}$ or VHL$^{+/+}$). Mutations in the VHL protein cause constitutive expression of HIFs and thus lead to unregulated expression of HIF-inducible pathways, which produces the effects on the *left* under all conditions. cul2, an elongin; HRE, HIF response element; OH, hydroxyl group; p, phosphorylation; Pro, proline; SCF, Skp, Cullin, F-box containing complex; Ub, ubiquitination; VEGF, vascular endothelial growth factor. (From Cohen HT, McGovern FJ: Renal-cell carcinoma. *N Engl J Med* 353:2477, 2005.)

multiple cutaneous and uterine leiomyomas (MCUL). Overlapping with this syndrome is another autosomal dominant condition, hereditary leiomyomatosis and renal cell cancer (HLRCC) syndrome. This syndrome also results from mutations in the *FH* gene. Autosomal recessive *FH* gene mutations also underlie the disorder fumarate deficiency. This condition is associated with progressive encephalopathy, cerebral atrophy, seizures, hypotonia, and renal developmental delay. Heterozygous carriers of *FH* deficiency occasionally (but only rarely) exhibit leiomyomas.[130] HLRCC syndrome is characterized by cutaneous leiomyomas, uterine fibroids, and RCCs, which are predominantly single, although multiple and bilateral tumors have been reported.[131,132] The renal tumors are aggressive, and they may metastasize and lead to death in patients in their thirties. Although HLRCC syndrome was originally classified as hereditary papillary RCC type 2, the unique cytomorphologic features of the renal tumors, as well as the finding of mutations in the *FH* gene in affected families, suggest that it may be a distinct entity.[133,134]

Birt-Hogg-Dube syndrome is characterized by prominent cutaneous manifestations, the development of spontaneous pneumothorax in association with lung cysts, and a predisposition to kidney neoplasms, which may be chromophobe renal cancers, oncocytomas, or tumors with features of both (termed *mixed oncocytic*).[135-137] The characteristic skin lesions, fibrofolliculomas (hamartomas of the hair follicle), consist of multiple painless dome-shaped papules, 2 to 3 mm in diameter, that develop on the skin of the head and neck of patients with the syndrome after age 30. The affected gene, *folliculin*, was described in 2002.[138] The identification of loss-of-function mutations in the *folliculin* gene (localized to chromosome arm 17p) suggests that it functions as a tumor suppressor gene.[138] A high frequency of somatic mutations has been detected in renal tumors from patients with germline mutations in the *BHD* gene, suggesting that malignancy results from the inactivation of both copies of the gene.[139] Mutations in the *folliculin* gene do not appear to play a role in sporadic RCC.[140,141] *Folliculin* is thought to regulate the activity of mammalian target of rapamycin (mTOR) through complex mechanisms that are yet to be delineated.[142,143] mTOR has an integral role in pathways relating to the response to hypoxia (HIF), autophagy, and independent gene expression regulation.[144]

Tuberous sclerosis is an autosomal dominant condition associated with mutations in the tuberous sclerosis complex genes (*TSC1* and *TSC2*).[145,146] The TSC1/TSC2 complex mediates multiple inputs (growth factor signals, amino acids, and adenosine triphosphate) that regulate mTOR activity and thus cell growth.[142] Affected individuals typically manifest facial angiofibromas, show cognitive impairment, and have renal angiomyolipomas.[147] Although the incidence of kidney cancer is only slightly increased, such cancers have been associated with biallelic loss of the *TSC2* gene, implicating this pathway in the pathogenesis of kidney cancer.

CLINICAL AND LABORATORY FEATURES

The propensity of RCC to manifest with diverse and often obscure signs and symptoms has led to its being labeled the *internist's tumor*. The clinical presentation of RCC can be extremely variable. Many tumors are clinically occult, leading to delayed diagnosis, when a more advanced and symptomatic stage is common. Indeed, 25% of individuals have distant metastases or locally advanced disease at the time of presentation.[84] By contrast, other patients with RCC experience a wide array of symptoms or have a variety of abnormalities on laboratory tests, even in the absence of metastatic disease. The current clinical paradigm of RCC is the ever-increasing incidental detection of kidney cancer through the use of abdominal imaging. Incidentally discovered renal tumors are estimated to represent from 40% to 60% of all pathologically diagnosed RCCs. This situation has led to the recharacterization of the disease as the *radiologist's tumor*. On the basis of an analysis of the Surveillance, Epidemiology, and End Results (SEER) database for the period 1998 through 2002, renal tumor size at presentation decreased from 6.7 cm to 5.8 cm with a concordant increase in the age-adjusted incidence in RCC.[148]

The presence or absence of local or systemic symptoms of RCC has been shown to correlate with TNM stage and grade, and, most importantly, is an independent variable (on multivariate analysis) predicting overall prognosis.[149,150] Although the presence of symptoms strongly correlates with prognosis, a significant portion of incidentally discovered (asymptomatic) tumors can cause death. In a study of 3912 patients who had been surgically treated for incidentally discovered renal masses, 3650 patients (90%) were diagnosed with a primary renal malignancy, of whom 28.3% had locally advanced tumors, 27.6% had high-grade tumors, 5.7% had nodal metastases, and 13% had distant metastases. Cancer-specific mortality in this group of patients with incidentally discovered kidney cancers was 14.4% (525 patients). This is the largest series of incidentally discovered renal tumors.[149,151]

Currently, most patients diagnosed with RCC are asymptomatic. In early reports of patients undergoing nephrectomy for RCC, the most common presenting symptom was hematuria (which occurred in up to 59% of patients), followed by abdominal mass, pain, and weight loss.[152,153] In contemporary series these symptoms are less common at presentation, and up to 60% of patients are asymptomatic.

The classic triad for RCC—flank pain, hematuria, and palpable abdominal renal mass—occurs in fewer than 10% of patients, and when present, it strongly suggests advanced disease.[149,150,152] Hematuria, gross or microscopic, is usually observed only if the tumor has invaded the collecting system. Gibbons and associates reported the absence of gross or microscopic hematuria in 63% of their patients with proven RCC.[153] Scrotal varicocele was reported in up to 11% of patients.[154] Most varicoceles due to an obstructing retroperitoneal mass are left-sided and typically fail to empty in the recumbent position (grade 3 varicocele). Varicoceles typically result from obstruction by tumor thrombus of the gonadal vein at its entry point into the left renal vein. Varicocele development in an adult should always raise the possibility of an associated neoplasm within the kidney. In addition, inferior vena cava involvement by tumor thrombus can produce a variety of clinical manifestations, including ascites, hepatic dysfunction possibly related to Budd-Chiari syndrome, pulmonary emboli, and bilateral lower extremity edema.

Often, symptoms or signs related to metastases prompt medical evaluation.[155] Most patients (75%) presenting with metastatic disease have lung involvement (most common site of metastasis). Other common sites, from most to least common, are lymph nodes, bone, liver, adrenal gland, contralateral kidney, and brain. Patients may present with pathologic fractures, cough, hemoptysis, dyspnea related to pleural effusions, or palpable nodal masses. Clear cell pathologic features in the metastatic lesion and/or the finding of a renal mass on staging CT usually lead to the proper diagnosis.

A number of patients with RCC experience systemic symptoms or paraneoplastic syndromes.[156-158] Fever is one of the more common manifestations of the disease, occurring in up to 20% of patients.[159] It is usually intermittent and is often accompanied by night sweats, anorexia, weight loss, and fatigue. Secondary amyloidosis has been reported in as many as 3% to 5% of patients.[156] Anemia is also common in patients with RCC and frequently precedes the diagnosis by several months.[154,158,160,161] Hepatic dysfunction in the absence of metastatic disease was noted and labeled *Stauffer's syndrome*.[162] This syndrome, manifested as abnormal results on liver function tests (particularly elevations of alkaline phosphatase, α_2-globulin, and transaminases) and prolonged prothrombin time, has been reported to occur in up to 7% of patients with RCC. Hepatic dysfunction frequently occurs in association with fever, weight loss, and fatigue. The syndrome likely results from the overproduction of cytokines, such as granulocyte-macrophage colony-stimulating factor or possibly interleukin-6 (IL-6), by the tumor.[163,164] Even though the laboratory abnormalities and other symptoms often revert to normal after nephrectomy, this syndrome is associated with an elevated risk of recurrence and an overall poor 5-year survival.

Hormones produced by RCCs include parathyroid-like hormone, gonadotropins, placental lactogen, adrenocorticotropic hormone–like substance, renin, erythropoietin, glucagon, and insulin.[165] Several of these hormones have been associated with specific paraneoplastic phenomena. Erythrocytosis, defined as a hematocrit value greater than 55 mL/dL, occurs in 1% to 5% of patients with RCC and appears to be due to constitutive erythropoietin production by kidney cancer cells.

Hypercalcemia occurs in up to 15% of all patients with RCC. The presence of hypercalcemia has been defined as an independent negative prognostic factor in patients with metastatic RCC and can be associated with lytic bone metastases.[166] Hypercalcemia can occur in the absence of osseous metastases, and the ectopic production of parathyroid hormone–related peptide by the primary tumor has been documented in these cases.[167] In other patients, elevated prostaglandin values have been implicated in the development of hypercalcemia, which may respond to indomethacin treatment.[168] Long-acting bisphosphonates such as pamidronate and zoledronic acid are the treatment of choice in patients with metastatic RCC and hypercalcemia.[169] These agents may be especially beneficial in patients with lytic bone metastases, in whom such therapy might also reduce the incidence of pathologic fractures.[169,170] The concurrent use of antiangiogenic therapies and bisphosphonates has been found to be associated with a higher risk for osteonecrosis of the jaw than bisphosphonate therapy alone.[171,172] This finding will prompt further investigation into the risks of concurrent usage of these agents.

RADIOLOGIC DIAGNOSIS

The prognosis for patients whose tumors were diagnosed incidentally is more favorable than that for patients whose tumors caused symptoms, partly because the former group consists of patients with smaller tumors that tend to be confined to the kidney.[151,173] For patients with symptoms suggestive of RCC, numerous radiologic approaches are available for the evaluation of the kidney. With the advent of CT, MRI, and sophisticated ultrasonography, many of the more invasive procedures of the past are largely of historical interest and are rarely used in clinical practice. Although intravenous pyelography remains useful in the evaluation of hematuria, CT and ultrasonography are the mainstays of evaluation of a suspected renal mass. As seen on CT, the typical RCC has a heterogeneous density and enhances with use of a contrast agent (Figure 41.3).[174,175]

Cystic renal masses are graded on the basis of a long-standing classification system first introduced by Bosniak in 1986 and since updated and validated in numerous studies with surgical pathologic assessment.[176] The Bosniak renal cyst classification has been classically applied in evaluation of cystic masses using contrast-enhanced CT. Ultrasonography, although less sensitive than CT in detecting renal masses,[177] can be of use (albeit limited) in characterizing simple or minimally complex renal cysts—those containing one or two hairline-thin septa.[178]

Cystic renal masses are characterized according to wall thickness; presence or absence, number, and thickness of septa; enhancement of septa and/or thickened wall; and presence or absence of solid enhancing components (Table 41.2).[179] Presence of malignancy correlates with the Bosniak classification: in category I and II lesions, malignancy is very rare; in category IIF lesions the malignancy rate is approximately 5% to 15%; in category III lesions it is 30% to 60%; and in category IV lesions it is more than 90%. Use of MRI in conjunction with a modified Bosniak system for evaluating cystic masses has been studied and is an acceptable alternative when the patient cannot undergo CT with a contrast agent.[180] In some patients unable to undergo contrast-enhanced CT because of moderate to severe chronic kidney disease, the risk of nephrogenic systemic fibrosis may outweigh the potential benefits of imaging.[181] Currently used gadolinium-based MRI contrast agents have an FDA-required "black box warning" owing to the risk of inducing nephrogenic systemic fibrosis.

Renal arteriography is rarely employed in current practice, having been supplanted by magnetic resonance angiography and CT with three-dimensional reconstruction (Figure 41.4) to delineate vascular anatomy and assist in surgical planning.[182] MRI with gadolinium enhancement is superior to CT for evaluating the inferior vena cava if tumor extension into this vessel is suspected.[183] MRI is also a useful adjunct to ultrasonography in the evaluation of renal masses if a radiographic contrast agent cannot be administered because of allergy or inadequate renal function.

Although most solid renal masses are RCCs, some benign lesions complicate the diagnosis. The most common of these rare tumors are angiomyolipomas (renal hamartomas). Unless very small, angiomyolipomas are readily distinguishable from RCCs by the finding of a distinctive fat density on CT.[184] However, given that several reports have

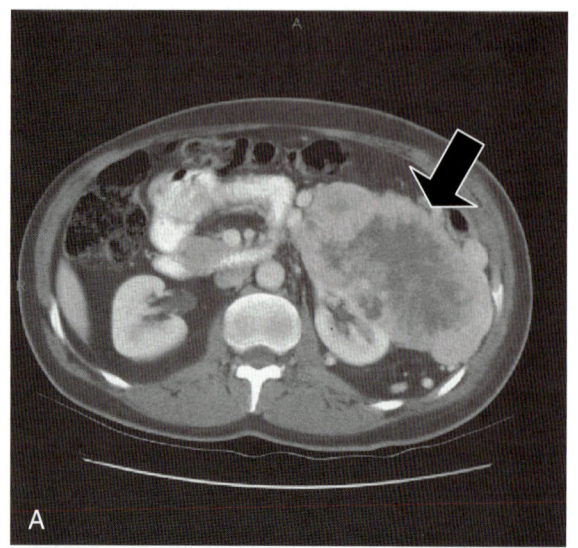

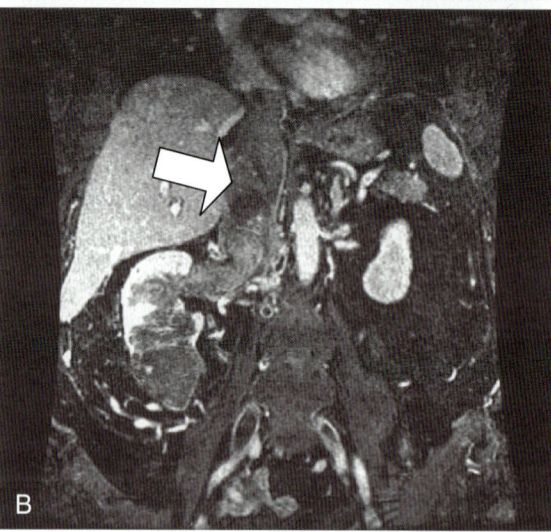

Figure 41.3 **A,** Computed tomography (CT) scan revealing massive renal cell carcinoma arising from the right kidney *(arrow)* and pushing the kidney anteriorly. Note the distortion of the collecting system. **B,** CT scan for the same patient demonstrates tumor thrombus *(arrow)* in the center of the inferior vena cava. (From Richie JP, Garnick MB: Primary renal and ureteral cancer, in Rieselbach RE, Garnick MB, editors: *Cancer and the kidney,* Philadelphia, 1982, Lea & Febiger, p 662.)

Table 41.2	Bosniak Classification of Renal Cysts
Category	**Description**
I	A benign simple cyst with a hairline-thin wall that does not contain septa, calcifications, or solid components. It measures water density and does not enhance.
II	A benign cyst that may contain a few hairline-thin septa in which "perceived" enhancement may be present. Fine calcification or a short segment of slightly thickened calcification may be present in the wall or septa. Uniformly high attenuation lesions < 3 cm (so-called high-density cysts) that are well marginated and do not enhance are included in this group. Cysts in this category do not require further evaluation.
IIF (F for follow-up)	Cysts that may contain multiple hairline-thin septa or minimal smooth thickening of their wall or septa. Perceived enhancement of their septa or wall may be present. Their wall or septa may contain calcification that may be thick and nodular, but no measurable contrast enhancement is present. These lesions are generally well marginated. Totally intrarenal nonenhancing high-attenuation renal lesions > 3 cm are also included in this category. These lesions require follow-up studies to prove benignity.
III	"Indeterminate" cystic masses that have thickened irregular or smooth walls or septa in which measurable enhancement is present. These are surgical lesions, although some will prove to be benign (e.g., hemorrhagic cysts, chronic infected cysts, multiloculated cystic nephroma), and some will be malignant (e.g., cystic renal cell carcinoma and multiloculated cystic renal cell carcinoma).
IV	These are clearly malignant cystic masses that can have all the criteria of category III but also contain enhancing soft tissue components adjacent to, but independent of, the wall of septum. These lesions include cystic carcinomas and require surgical removal.

From Israel GM, Bosniak MA: An update of the Bosniak renal cyst classification system. Urology *66:484, 2005.*

shown that macroscopic fat can be detected within RCCs, it may no longer be possible to dismiss all fat-containing lesions identified on CT as benign.[185] Fat-poor angiomyolipomas have also been described that are very difficult to distinguish from RCCs on preoperative imaging and thus frequently must be resected to rule out a malignant neoplasm.[186] As mentioned previously, renal oncocytoma has been described to appear on CT as a central stellate scar within a homogeneous, well-circumscribed solid mass.[187] This finding is nonspecific, however, and cannot be used to clinically exclude the diagnosis of clear cell carcinoma.

The role of radionuclide bone scanning in the initial diagnosis and preoperative staging of RCC is unclear. Although bone scanning demonstrates high sensitivity in the detection of osteoblastic metastases, RCC usually produces osteolytic lesions that may be missed by bone scan.

Atlas and colleagues suggested that a combination of bone pain on presentation plus an elevated serum alkaline phosphatase value were comparable to bone scan results in evaluating patients with RCC.[188] Koga and colleagues demonstrated bone scan to have a sensitivity of 94% and specificity of 86%,

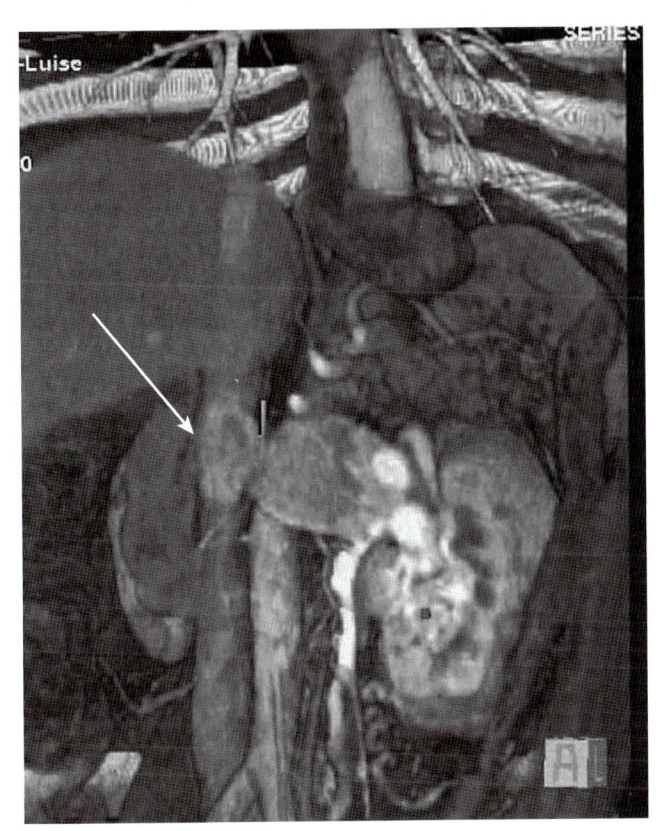

Figure 41.4 Three-dimensional reconstruction of 2-mm computed tomography slices for a patient with a venous tumor thrombus from renal cell carcinoma. Arrow points to tumor thrombus. (From Hallscheidt PJ, Fink C, Haferkamp A, et al: Preoperative staging of renal cell carcinoma with inferior vena cava thrombus using multidetector CT and MRI: prospective study with histopathological correlation. *J Comput Assist Tomogr* 29:64, 2005.)

Table 41.3 Sites and Frequencies of Metastases in Renal Cell Carcinoma

Site	Incidence (%)
Lung	50-60
Lymph node	30-40
Bone	30-40
Liver	30-40
Adrenal	20
Opposite kidney	10
Brain	5

From McDougal WS, Garnick M: Clinical signs and symptoms of kidney cancer. In Vogelzang NJ, Scardino PT, Shipley WU, et al (editors): Comprehensive textbook of genitourinary oncology, Baltimore, 1996, Williams & Wilkins.

with a low yield in patients with earlier-stage primary tumors. They recommended omitting bone scanning in patients with T1 to T3a tumors and no bone pain.[189]

A number of studies have been published evaluating the role of fluorine F 18 2-fluoro-2-deoxy-D-glucose positron emission tomography (FDG-PET) for the detection and management of RCC primary and metastatic lesions. Kang and colleagues studied 66 patients with primary RCC and reported 60% sensitivity of FDG-PET for the primary renal mass compared with 91.7% for CT, whereas the specificities for both were 100%.[190] Other studies have shown sensitivity rates as low as 31%.[191,192] FDG-PET is unlikely to be used as a stand-alone study in the evaluation of a patient with a solid renal mass.

In the restaging and follow-up of RCC, FDG-PET scanning provides information that is complementary to that of conventional imaging and can alter management decisions. The sensitivity and specificity of FDG-PET in detecting recurrent or metastatic disease are better than the sensitivity and specificity when it is used for the evaluation of primary lesions.[191] In this disease process, sensitivity of this imaging method is significantly lower when metastatic lesions smaller than 1 cm are evaluated. False-negative and false-positive readings are significant, and FDG-PET is not a substitute for contrast-enhanced CT in the detection and follow-up of metastatic RCC.

An additional application of PET involves the use of antibodies such as the chimeric monoclonal antibody chimeric G250 to carbonic anhydrase IX.[192] Carbonic anhydrase IX is expressed in more than 90% of RCCs.[193,194] In the first immune PET study, iodine 124–labeled antibody chimeric G250 (^{124}I-cG250) PET had a sensitivity of 94% in correctly identifying clear cell (cc) RCCs. G250-PET also correctly predicted all non–clear cell histologic types. A multicenter phase III clinical trial corroborated these results; ^{124}I-cG250 PET/CT was compared with contrast-enhanced CT (CECT) for the detection of ccRCC. The average sensitivity and specificity were higher for ^{124}I-cG250 PET/CT than for CECT (86.2% vs. 75.5% and 85.9% vs. 46.8%, respectively).[195] Despite the encouraging result for ^{124}I-cG250 PET in assessing primary tumors, its performance in evaluating metastatic lesions has been shown to be significantly inferior to that of FDG-PET.[196]

Although morphologic or functional imaging modalities such as CT, MRI, and PET have been used to evaluate renal masses, Doppler ultrasonography with contrast agent injection has been shown to provide both morphologic and functional information about renal lesions. The size of tumors can be accurately measured and the percentage of contrast agent uptake (which provides an approximation of tumor vascularity) can be evaluated with this technique. In the era of new antiangiogenic treatment modalities, assessment of tumor neovascularization is of major importance, and this parameter could be a potential biomarker for treatment evaluation.

STAGING AND PROGNOSIS

After the presumptive diagnosis of RCC has been made, attention must be turned to the delineation of the extent of involvement of regional and distant metastatic sites. RCCs can grow locally into very large masses and invade through surrounding fascia into adjacent organs. The most common sites of metastases are the regional lymphatics, lungs, bone, liver, brain, ipsilateral adrenal gland, and contralateral kidney. The rates of metastasis to these sites are listed in Table 41.3.[197,198] Metastases to unusual sites, such as the thyroid gland, pancreas, mucosal surfaces, skin, and soft tissue, are not uncommon in this disease. CT of the abdomen is the principal radiologic tool for defining the local and regional extent of an RCC. The accuracy of CT in staging RCC is close to 90%.[199] In clinically advanced disease, staging evaluation should also include CT of the chest and bone scanning. At initial presentation approximately 2% of patients have bilateral tumors and 25% to 30% have overt metastases.[197] If metastatic disease is suspected on the basis of staging studies, pathologic confirmation is required before therapy is contemplated. It is often more useful to perform a biopsy of a metastatic site rather than the primary tumor because of the presence of necrosis in the primary lesion. CT or ultrasound-guided percutaneous needle biopsy of a suspected lung, liver, lymph node, adrenal, or sometimes even skeletal metastasis frequently yields diagnostic material.

The TNM staging system for RCC (Table 41.4) has largely supplanted the previously used Robson system. The TNM system was modified in 2002 with the division of T1 tumors into T1a for tumors 4 cm or less in diameter and T1b for tumors larger than 4 cm. It also included renal sinus invasion in the T3a classification and renal vein invasion in the T3b subset.[200] The seventh edition of the American Joint Committee on Cancer (AJCC) staging system, released in 2010, includes relevant changes to the T3 and T4 definitions; it also defines node-positive disease as N1 regardless of number of positive nodes. This updated system accurately characterizes the disease with respect to prognosis. Pathologic stage remains the most consistent single prognostic variable that influences survival. Survival based on stage is shown in Table 41.5.

The Fuhrman grading system for RCC is based on nuclear characteristics (size, contour, and nucleoli) and uses a scale from 1 to 4, in which 4 represents the highest degree of nucleolar irregularity and indicates a poorer prognosis.[92] Mitotic activity is not considered in the grading system. Although the Fuhrman grading system as a prognostic tool has been validated for clear cell kidney carcinoma, its use for the other histologic subtypes (especially papillary and chromophobe) is a topic of debate.[92,201]

Identification of novel clinicopathologic prognosticators in RCC has resulted in a gradual transition from classifications that use clinical factors, such as the TNM staging system and Fuhrman grade, to systems that integrate multiple validated prognostic factors. Motzer and colleagues examined features predictive of survival in 670 patients with stage IV disease enrolled in clinical trials at Memorial Sloan-Kettering Cancer Center (MSKCC).[166] Significant factors predictive of poor outcome in a multivariate analysis included Karnofsky performance status score less than 80%, hemoglobin level less than 10 mg/dL, serum lactate dehydrogenase level more than 1.5 times the upper limit of normal, corrected serum calcium level more than 10 mg/dL, and lack of prior nephrectomy. A risk model was created using these five factors to assign patients to one of three groups: those with zero risk factors (favorable risk), those with one or two risk factors (intermediate risk), and those with three or more risk factors (poor risk). Median survival for the group as a whole was 10 months but ranged from 15 months for patients in the favorable-risk group to 4 months for patients in the poor-risk group (Figure 41.5).[166] These prognostic factors have been validated in cohorts heavily treated with multiple non-antiangiogenic and noncytokine

Table 41.4 TNM Staging for Renal Cell Carcinoma

Category	Code	Description
Primary tumor (T)	TX	Primary tumor cannot be assessed
	T0	No evidence of primary tumor
	T1a	Tumor 4 cm in greatest dimension, limited to the kidney
	T1b	Tumor > 4 cm but ≤ 7 cm in greatest dimension, limited to the kidney
	T2a	Tumor > 7 cm but ≤ 10 cm in greatest dimension, limited to the kidney
	T2b	Tumor >10 cm, limited to the kidney
	T3a	Tumor grossly extends into the renal vein or its segmental (muscle-containing) branches, or tumor invades perirenal and/or renal sinus fat, but not beyond Gerota's fascia
	T3b	Tumor grossly extends into the vena cava below the diaphragm
	T3c	Tumor grossly extends into the vena cava above the diaphragm or invades the wall of the vena cava
	T4	Tumor invades beyond Gerota's fascia (including contiguous extension into the ipsilateral adrenal gland)
Regional lymph nodes (N)	NX	Regional lymph nodes cannot be assessed
	N0	No regional lymph node metastases
	N1	Regional lymph node metastases
Distant metastasis (M)	M0	No distant metastases
	M1	Distant metastases

Adapted from Edge SB, et al; American Joint Committee on Cancer: AJCC cancer staging manual, 7th ed, New York, 2010, Springer, xiv.

Table 41.5 Correlation of Stage Grouping with Survival in Patients with Renal Cell Cancer

Stage	Grouping			5-Year Survival (%)
I	T1	N0	M0	90-95
II	T2	N0	M0	70-85
III	T3a	N0	M0	50-65
	T3b	N0	M0	50-65
	T3c	N0	M0	45-50
	T1	N1	M0	25-30
	T2	N1	M0	25-30
	T3	N1	M0	15-20
IV	T4	Any N	M0	10
	Any T	N2	M0	10
	Any T	Any N	M1	<5

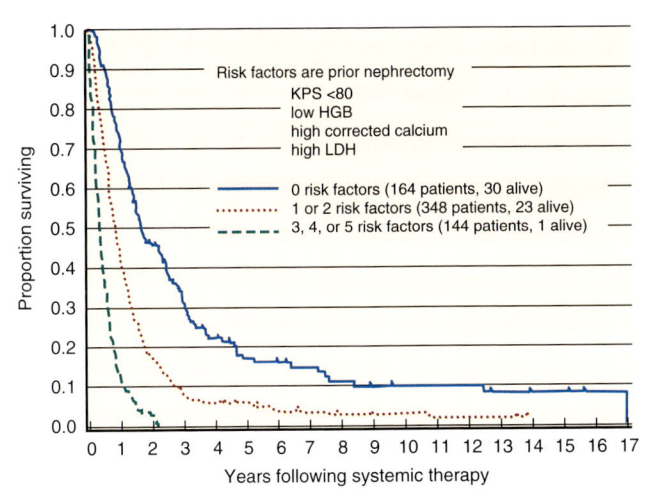

Figure 41.5 Survival and prognostic stratification for renal cell carcinoma. Survival rates in a series of 86 patients with metastatic renal cell carcinoma treated by various modalities are compared with the survival of patients treated with adjunctive nephrectomy. HGB, hemoglobin; KPS, Karnofsky performance status; LDH, lactate dehydrogenase. (From Motzer RJ, Mazumdar M, Bacik J, et al: Survival and prognostic stratification of 670 patients with advanced renal cell carcinoma. *J Clin Oncol* 17:2530, 1999.)

therapies.[202] The MSKCC criteria have been validated across multiple institutions, and adding the number of metastatic sites to this model even better defines outcomes for patients with favorable, intermediate, and poor risk.[166-168,203-205] Currently, the Memorial Sloan-Kettering Prognostic Factors Model is the most commonly used nomogram for prognostication in clinical and experimental settings.

Investigators at the University of California at Los Angeles (UCLA) have developed the UCLA Integrated Staging System (UISS), a system based on TNM stage, grade, and Eastern Cooperative Oncology Group (ECOG) performance status.[206] Patients are stratified into three risk groups according to the probability of tumor recurrence and survival, and risk group–specific surveillance guidelines are offered. On the basis of data from a large sample of patients, investigators at the Mayo Clinic devised the stage, size, grade, and necrosis (SSIGN) scoring system, in which patients with clear cell kidney carcinoma were assigned a score based on tumor stage, tumor size, nuclear grade, and the presence of necrosis.[207] With use of the SSIGN score, cancer-specific survival at 1 to 10 years after treatment can be estimated for an individual patient. Investigators at MSKCC combined tumor stage, tumor size, histologic subtype, and symptoms at presentation into a nomogram that predicted the probability of freedom from recurrence at 5 years after treatment.[206] This nomogram has been updated for the clear cell variant of RCC and includes tumor stage, tumor size, nuclear grade, necrosis, vascular invasion, and symptoms at presentation as prognostic factors.[208] For clear cell carcinomas, clinical factors that influence survival include performance status grade and the presence of paraneoplastic signs or symptoms such as anemia, hypercalcemia, hepatopathy, fever, and weight loss.[172-174,209-211] Various microscopic features, such as Fuhrman nuclear grade and sarcomatoid histologic features, as well as biologic features like IL-6 and VEGF production may be useful in predicting survival.[73,210,212-214]

SURGICAL TREATMENT

Nephrectomy

The mainstay of treatment of primary RCC is surgical excision or nephrectomy. Nephrectomy represents the only proven curative modality. Radical nephrectomy, which involves the early ligation of the renal artery and renal vein and excision en bloc of the kidney with surrounding Gerota's fascia and ipsilateral adrenal gland, became the procedure of choice in the 1960s. Various surgical approaches (open and minimally invasive) are available for the effective performance of this procedure. Minimally invasive approaches have been shown to have equivalent oncologic outcomes to those of open approaches. Laparoscopic partial nephrectomy is a viable alternative to an open procedure, with equivalent surgical efficacy and safety and substantially reduced postoperative recovery time.[215]

With better understanding of tumor biology and changing patterns of presentation, the value of radical nephrectomy is being reassessed. Involvement of the ipsilateral adrenal gland occurs only 4% of the time, and in most instances, it is associated with direct extension from a large upper-pole lesion or with the presence of nodal or distant metastases.[216-218] As a consequence, adrenalectomy is often reserved for patients with large upper-pole lesions or those in whom solitary ipsilateral adrenal metastases have been identified on preoperative staging studies.

Nephron-Sparing Surgery

The American Urological Association released guidelines for nephron-sparing surgery or partial nephrectomy.[219] This release has expanded the role of nephron-sparing surgery from an elective option to the standard of care for patients with clinical stage T1a (cT1a) tumors (tumors < 4 cm) amenable to partial nephrectomy, and as an option in patients with tumors from 4 to 7 cm in whom preservation of renal function is a priority. The generally accepted criteria for consideration of nephron-sparing or partial nephrectomy are listed in Table 41.6. These include bilateral tumors, tumor in a solitary kidney, and compromised renal function.[220,221] Overall survival of patients undergoing partial nephrectomy is equivalent to that of patients with disease of a comparable stage who underwent radical nephrectomy.[221-223] A retrospective review of data for 648 patients who underwent either radical or partial nephrectomy for cT1a renal masses suggested a survival advantage with partial nephrectomy.[224] This advantage may be explained by the increased rate of future development of renal insufficiency in patients who undergo radical nephrectomy.[225,226]

In patients with small, solitary tumors, the rate of local recurrences is 0% to 7%,[227] with a number of series reporting no local recurrences. Several retrospective series[57,228-231] and one prospective study[232] have demonstrated equivalent survivals for patients who undergo partial nephrectomy and those who undergo radical nephrectomy.

Minimally invasive techniques (including laparoscopic and robotic partial nephrectomies) are being used in the setting of nephron-sparing surgery.[233-235] Laparoscopic partial nephrectomy has been associated with a higher

Table 41.6	Indications for Partial Nephrectomy
Absolute	All renal masses < 4 cm amenable to partial nephrectomy (clinical T1a) Bilateral tumors Tumor in solitary kidney Tumor in functionally solitary kidney Compromised renal function Multiple recurrent tumors (von Hippel–Lindau syndrome)
Relative	Localized tumor with progressive disorder that may impair renal function History of familial renal cell carcinoma Oncocytoma (preoperative pathologic diagnosis)
Elective	Tumors 4-7 cm (clinical T1b) amenable to partial nephrectomy
Controversial	Large (>5 cm) tumors in patients with normal contralateral kidney Centrally located tumors in patients with normal contralateral kidney

complication rate (from 1.5 to 2.0 times greater) than open surgery and with a warm ischemia time that is approximately 1.5 times longer. Postoperative nadir creatinine levels have not been significantly different in multiple series comparing open partial nephrectomy with laparoscopic partial nephrectomy.[236] Oncologic outcomes for the laparoscopic procedure have been equivalent to those for open partial nephrectomy at large experienced centers.[237] Robotic partial nephrectomy is currently being evaluated at multiple sites, and after short follow-up, outcomes seem to duplicate those of laparoscopic partial nephrectomy.[238] In several retrospective series, robotic partial nephrectomy has been associated with decreased overall blood loss and shorter warm ischemia time than that associated with laparoscopic partial nephrectomy.[239-243] The proposed benefit of robotic in comparison with laparoscopic partial nephrectomy is in reconstruction of the renal unit after extirpation (especially of more complex masses), but this claim awaits validation in larger series with adequate follow-up.

Impact of Surgical Treatment for Renal Cell Carcinoma on Kidney Function

Partial nephrectomy is the treatment of choice for cT1a renal masses in order to preserve renal function, especially in patients with already existing chronic kidney disease (CKD). An analysis of renal function outcomes from the European Organization for Research and Treatment of Cancer (EORTC) randomized trial 30904 (partial nephrectomy versus radical nephrectomy for renal masses ≤ 5 cm) revealed that partial nephrectomy was associated with less moderate renal dysfunction (estimated glomerular filtration rate [eGFR] < 60 mL/min/1.73 m^2 in comparison with radical nephrectomy (eGFR < 45 mL/min/1.73 m^2) at a median follow-up of 6.7 years.[244] This benefit in renal function did not result in improved survival, because overall survival favored the radical nephrectomy arm ($P = 0.032$).[245] However, there was no difference in advanced kidney disease (eGFR < 30 mL/min/1.73 m^2) and kidney failure (eGFR < 15 mL/min/1.73 m^2) between the two treatment arms. In a retrospective review of more than 4000 partial and radical nephrectomies, Lane and coworkers found that patients with preexisting CKD had worse overall survival than patients with surgically induced renal dysfunction.[246] In addition, postoperative eGFR predicted survival only for patients with preexisting CKD, not for patients with normal preoperative kidney function.[246] These findings suggest that patients with preexisting CKD are most likely to benefit from nephron-sparing surgery.

Energy-Based Tissue Ablation

Over the past decade, cryoablation and radiofrequency ablation have emerged as treatment alternatives for a select group of patients with localized renal tumors. Although long-term follow-up has not been achieved, oncologic effectiveness in the intermediate term is comparable to that of the current gold standard treatment modalities.[247,248] Ablative techniques are hindered by their association with a substantially higher risk of *local* tumor recurrence than with extirpative procedures and the need for retreatment. Identification of residual disease also seems to be more problematic with radiofrequency ablation than with cryoablation. There are no randomized trials comparing radiofrequency ablation with cryoablation. A meta-analysis comparing the two modalities favored cryoablation with regard to need for repeat ablation (1.3% for cryoablation vs. 8.5% for radiofrequency ablation) and local tumor progression (5.2% for cryoablation vs. 12.9% for radiofrequency ablation), but a comparison trial needs to be performed because of the many inherent flaws in a comparative analysis of this type.[240,249]

Surveillance

Surveillance is an option for the patient with a small renal mass (<4 cm) and for the patient with multiple and/or bilateral tumors, for example, patients with von Hippel–Lindau syndrome. Some writers have advocated waiting until the largest lesion is more than 3 cm in diameter before performing a partial nephrectomy.[250] For tumors smaller than 4 cm, the rate of progression to metastatic disease has been very low (<2%) in all retrospective series. Active surveillance is a reasonable option for patients with limited life expectancy or for those unfit for intervention.[219] Patients should be counseled about the risk, albeit small, of progression to metastatic disease. Increased use of renal mass biopsy may help better select patients for active surveillance by identifying benign or indolent cancers.[243]

Lymph Node Dissection

The benefit of performing a regional lymph node dissection in conjunction with the radical nephrectomy is controversial.[251] With improved preoperative CT staging, the incidence of unsuspected nodal metastases in patients with low-stage tumors is less than 1%. Multiple preoperative and intraoperative evaluative nomograms exist and can aid the surgeon in determining the benefit of lymph node dissection in conjunction with nephrectomy.[252,253] The only randomized trial to evaluate lymph node dissection in patients with RCC showed no improvement in survival with such dissection.[254] The results of this study are tempered by the fact that the majority of patients enrolled had low-stage (T1 and T2) tumors, and thus, the higher-risk patients most likely to derive a therapeutic benefit from lymph node dissection were not adequately studied. A therapeutic benefit of lymph node dissection in patients with metastatic disease undergoing cytoreductive nephrectomy was supported (level 2 evidence) by the findings of several series.[255-257] A therapeutic benefit of extended lymphadenectomy in patients with clinically evident lymphadenopathy but with no evidence of distant metastasis has been suggested.[258,259] In locally advanced disease, regional lymph node dissection should be performed when technically feasible.[251]

Vena Caval Involvement

Inferior vena caval involvement with tumor thrombus is found in about 5% of patients undergoing radical nephrectomy.[260] It occurs more frequently with right-sided tumors and is commonly associated with metastases. The anatomic location of the tumor thrombus is prognostically relevant. Although 5-year survival in patients with subdiaphragmatic lesions approaches 50%, patients with supradiaphragmatic thrombi do considerably less well.[261,262] Even at experienced centers, the operative mortality may be as high as 5% to 10%.[263,264] Five-year survival in patients with coexisting nodal or systemic metastases is extremely low,[260] yet a distinct subset of patients may benefit from resection and subsequent systemic therapy.[265]

Cytoreductive Nephrectomy

In 2001, results of two randomized studies were published demonstrating a significant survival advantage in patients with metastatic disease who underwent nephrectomy prior to embarking on a course of cytokine therapy.[266,267] UCLA investigators reported a median survival of 16.7 months and a 19.6% 5-year survival rate in patients treated with IL-2–containing therapy after debulking nephrectomy.[268] In addition, the Cytokine Working Group reported a 21% to 24% response rate in patients who received cytokine therapy following recent nephrectomy.[269] These two analyses suggested that IL-2–based therapy should be considered after nephrectomy in patients who have metastatic kidney cancer.

Several other reports indicated that anywhere from 13% to 77% of patients treated in this way never progressed to immunotherapy because of complications of treatment or rapid, symptomatic disease progression, further emphasizing the need for proper patient selection if debulking nephrectomy is to be entertained.[270-273] Recognizing this need, Fallick and associates developed strict criteria for determining which patients should undergo debulking nephrectomy before receiving systemic IL-2 therapy.[274] These criteria included removal of more than 75% of the tumor burden, no central nervous system (CNS), bone, or liver metastases, adequate pulmonary and cardiac function, no significant comorbid conditions, and ECOG performance status of 0.[274]

Cytoreductive nephrectomy in the era of molecular targeted agents has not been prospectively evaluated but is generally accepted on the basis of the earlier studies with cytokine-based therapy.[275,276] Newer targeted therapies are better than immunotherapy at downsizing the primary tumor, but reductions are generally less than 20% by volume. The largest series of metastatic patients undergoing cytoreductive nephrectomy after pretreatment with targeted agents confirmed an increased risk for specific wound-related complications, but overall and severe complications (Clavien-Dindo grade > 3) were not significantly different from those in patients undergoing immediate cytoreductive surgery.[277] These data, combined with those from small case series, have generated hypotheses that should be further evaluated in larger prospective trials.[278,279]

Resection of Metastatic Disease

Surgical resection of metastatic disease has been actively pursued in certain clinical situations. Patients who have a synchronous solitary metastasis at presentation have lower survival than patients in whom metastasis develops after the primary tumor is removed (metachronous metastasis).[280] Nonetheless, it is common to resect solitary or oligometastatic disease, often in the ipsilateral lung or adrenal gland, in conjunction with nephrectomy, and occasionally patients remain disease free long term.[281-283] On the other hand, 5-year survival rates as high as 50% have been reported for patients undergoing resection of isolated metachronous metastases.[284-286] Time to presentation of metastatic disease (after initial nephrectomy) is a significant prognostic indicator for those undergoing metastasectomy.

SYSTEMIC THERAPY

Although surgical resection of localized disease can be curative, 25% to 30% of patients have metastatic disease at presentation, and as many as 30% to 40% of patients with a surgical "cure" later experience a recurrence. The current median survival for patients with metastatic RCC can vary greatly, depending on multiple prognostic factors.[202] The MSKCC-defined risk categories "favorable," "intermediate," and "poor" are associated with median overall survival rates of 26 months, 14.4 months, and 7.3 months, respectively.[202,204] Patient selection greatly influences response rate and survival, and this factor must be kept in mind when one evaluates the results of any phase II or III study. Treatment options over the years have included hormonal therapy, chemotherapy, and immunotherapy; however, attention has lately been given to targeted therapy approaches.

Adjuvant Therapy

Because a substantial number of patients with high-risk features experience recurrence after primary nephrectomy, an adjuvant therapy could be useful in their treatment. The risk of recurrence after nephrectomy for an individual patient can be calculated with one of the validated models discussed in the staging and prognosis section of this chapter.[287] The ECOG completed a trial comparing adjuvant interferon alfa therapy with observation after resection of high-risk RCC. At a minimum follow-up of 36 months and a mean of 68 months overall, no statistically significant difference in disease-free survival was observed between the two study arms.[288]

A smaller study performed by the EORTC also showed no benefit for the adjuvant administration of interferon alfa. Although the results were disappointing, the study was useful in providing information on the natural history of stage III RCC. Specifically, it identified a high-risk group, those with T3c, T4, and/or N2 or N3 disease, who had only a 20% to 25% chance of remaining disease free at 2 years.[288] This population was believed to be at sufficient risk of relapse to justify exploration of more aggressive therapy, such as high-dose IL-2, in an effort to prevent or delay relapse. Consequently, the Cytokine Working Group performed a trial randomly assigning patients who met these high-risk staging criteria to either a single cycle of high-dose IL-2 or observation. Unfortunately, this trial showed no survival benefit.[289] There is no evidence to support the use of interferon or IL-2 in the adjuvant setting in patients with high-risk kidney cancer. Two trials that have investigated vaccine-based treatment in the adjuvant setting are discussed later in this chapter; one has shown promising results.[290-292]

Several adjuvant studies have been performed. ECOG trial No. 2805, the Adjuvant Sorafenib or Sunitinib for Unfavorable Renal Carcinoma (ASSURE) study, is a double-blinded phase III trial randomly assigning 1923 patients to receive no treatment, 1 year of sunitinib treatment, or 1 year of sorafenib treatment.[293] The major endpoint being assessed is disease-free survival. Five other phase III trials are currently accruing patients for adjuvant therapy or have completed accrual: Sunitinib Treatment of Renal Adjuvant Cancer (S-TRAC), SORCE (A phase III randomized double-blind study comparing SOrafenib with placebo in patients with Resected primary renal CEll carcinoma at high or intermediate risk of relapse), ATLAS (Adjuvant Axitinib Therapy of Renal Cell Cancer in High Risk Patients), PROTECT (A Study to Evaluate Pazopanib as an Adjuvant Treatment for Localized Renal Cell Carcinoma), and SWOG (Southwest Oncology Group)S0931, which are evaluating sunitinib, sorafenib, axitinib, pazopanib, and everolimus, respectively.

Neoadjuvant Therapy

The use of targeted agents as neoadjuvant therapy is on the verge of being explored in a large prospective trial. Their use could be initiated through a clinical trial in two subsets of patients: (1) patients with metastatic disease, to provide a test of the benefits of cytoreductive nephrectomy, and (2) patients with locally advanced or marginally resectable disease, in hopes of reducing severity of disease or at least maintaining stability of disease and determining which patients have early presentation of nonresponsive metastases. Several studies have shown variable mean primary tumor shrinkage with neoadjuvant targeted therapy ranging from 9.6% to 21.1%.[294-299] In addition, studies have shown contradictory results regarding the effect on vena caval tumor thrombus. A 2013 abstract reported results of a phase II trial investigating the effect of axitinib on tumor downsizing in 19 patients. All patients had locally advanced, biopsy-proven ccRCC and were treated with 12 weeks of axitinib prior to undergoing radical nephrectomy. Nine patients (47%) demonstrated a partial response and none progressed.[300]

Targeted Agents

Given the frequency of biallelic loss of the *VHL* gene and associated dysregulation of hypoxia-inducible genes, including those for the proangiogenic growth factors VEGF and PDGF, RCC has been a particularly promising target for antiangiogenic therapy. The use of the term *targeted agents* is a misnomer, however, because most of these drugs act on multiple systems within the cell and so have multiple targets (Figure 41.6).[301,302] The monoclonal antibodies are an exception to this statement. Currently seven drugs have shown to improve progression-free survival or overall survival in large phase III randomized trials, with several more awaiting data maturity. Response rates and tolerability of these agents are better than those of cytokines, but there are only sporadic cases of durable complete responses. Despite the advances brought by targeted agents, there is still a role for cytokine therapy in selected patients. With the influx of so many new targeted agents and a second generation of agents currently being tested, questions that remain to be answered are "What is the appropriate sequencing of the agents?" and "Is combination therapy safe and is it more effective than single-agent therapy?" The development of novel clinical trial designs with multi-institutional and multinational cooperation will be crucial in answering these questions.

Sunitinib. Sunitinib is a small-molecule multitargeted kinase inhibitor of VEGF receptor (VEGFR), PDGF receptor (PDGFR), the proto-oncogene *c-Kit*, and the receptor FLT3 (FMS-like tyrosine kinase 3). Two phase II studies were performed in patients with metastatic RCC refractory to cytokine therapy. The first trial enrolled 63 patients, the majority of whom had tumors with clear cell histologic features and had undergone nephrectomy. The response rate was 40% with no patients showing a complete response, and the progression-free survival was 8.1 months.[303] A subsequent 106-patient study, in which all individuals had clear cell carcinoma, had undergone nephrectomy, and had shown no response to cytokine therapy, demonstrated a 25% response rate after independent review. On the basis of these phase II data, sunitinib was approved by the FDA in January 2006.

A phase III trial randomly assigning 750 patients to receive either sunitinib or interferon alfa was completed in July 2005.[304] Progression-free and overall survival rates were significantly different between the two groups, in favor of sunitinib (11 months vs. 5 months, $P = 0.001$ and 26.4 months vs. 21.8 months, $P = 0.049$, respectively). Objective response rate as measured by Response Evaluation Criteria in Solid Tumors (RECIST) was 47% for sunitinib and 12% for interferon alfa. The most commonly reported sunitinib-related grade 3 adverse events were hypertension (12%), fatigue (11%), diarrhea (9%), and hand-foot syndrome (9%). Thyroid abnormalities can be found in more than 80% of patients and warrant monitoring.[305] The development of grade 3 systemic hypertension during receipt of treatment may be predictive of efficacy.[306]

Sorafenib. Sorafenib is a bis-aryl urea originally developed as a potent inhibitor of both wild-type and mutant (V599E) B-Raf and c-Raf kinase isoforms. It was also found to possess inhibitory activity against VEGFR, PDGFR, c-KIT, and FLT3. A phase III trial (Treatment Approaches in Renal Cancer Global Evaluation Trial [TARGET]) was completed in early 2005.[307] Patients with metastatic RCC for whom one prior therapy had failed were randomly assigned to receive either sorafenib or placebo. Median progression-free survival was 5.5 months in the treatment arm and 2.8 months in the placebo arm, which were highly statistically significant ($P = 0.000001$). Sorafenib was FDA approved in December 2005 for use in the treatment of advanced RCC. Results of a study comparing sorafenib with interferon as first-line therapy were published in 2009.[308] Progression-free survival was 5.7

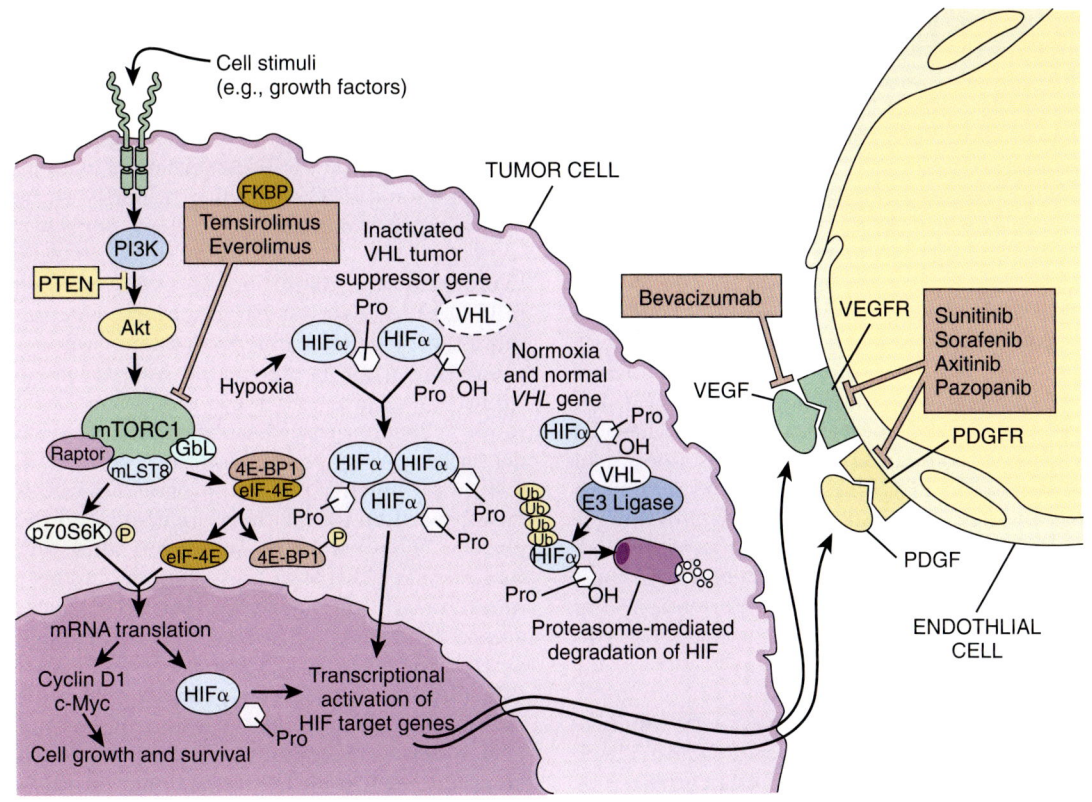

Figure 41.6 Therapeutically relevant biologic pathways in renal cell carcinoma. In conditions of normoxia and normal von Hippel–Lindau (VHL) gene function, VHL protein is the substrate recognition component of an E3 ubiquitin ligase complex that targets hypoxia-inducible factor-α (HIF-α) for proteolysis. In cellular hypoxia or with an inactivated VHL gene, the VHL protein–HIF interaction is disrupted, leading to stabilization or accumulation of HIF transcription factors. HIF accumulation can also result from activation of mammalian target of rapamycin (mTOR) downstream of cellular stimuli and the phosphatidylinositol-3-kinase/protein kinase B (PI3K/Akt) pathway. mTOR phosphorylates and activates p70S6 kinase (p70S6K), resulting in enhanced translation of certain proteins, including HIF. Activated mTOR also phosphorylates 4E binding protein 1 (4E-BP1), promoting dissociation of this complex and allowing a eukaryotic translation initiation factor 4E (eIF-4E) to stimulate an increase in the translation of messenger RNAs (mRNAs) that encode cell cycle regulators, such as c-Myc and cyclin D1. Activated HIF translocates into the nucleus and causes transcription of a large repertoire of hypoxia-inducible genes, including vascular endothelial growth factor (VEGF) and platelet-derived growth factor (PDGF). These ligands bind to their cognate receptors present on the surfaces of endothelial cells, leading to cell migration, proliferation, and permeability. Sites of action of targeted therapies are illustrated. Temsirolimus and everolimus bind to FK506-binding protein (FKBP), and the resultant protein-drug complex inhibits the kinase activity of mTOR complex 1 (mTORC1). Bevacizumab is a VEGF ligand–binding antibody. Sunitinib, sorafenib, axitinib, and pazopanib are small-molecule inhibitors of multiple tyrosine kinase receptors, including the receptors for VEGF (VEGFR) and PDGF (PDGFR). GbL, G protein beta subunit-like; OH, hydroxyl; P, phosphorylation; Pro, proline; Ub, ubiquitin. (From Rini BI: Metastatic renal cell carcinoma: many treatment options, one patient. *J Clin Oncol* 27:3225, 2009; and Rini BI, Campbell SC, Escudier B: Renal cell carcinoma. *Lancet* 373:1119, 2009.)

months for sorafenib-treated patients, and 5.6 months for interferon-treated patients. Owing to the relatively disappointing progression-free survival data in this study, sorafenib has fallen out of favor as an agent of first choice.

Pazopanib. Pazopanib is an oral second-generation multi-targeted kinase inhibitor of VEGFR types 1, 2, and 3, PDGFR-α, PDGFR-β, and c-Kit.[309] In a phase II clinical trial, the tolerability profile was different from that of other multitargeted kinase inhibitors, with hypertension in 8%, grade 4 myelosuppression in 7%, fatigue in 4%, and diarrhea in 3% of patients. An international phase III trial in patients with RCC was reported in 2009.[310] Patients were randomly assigned in a 2:1 ratio to receive 800 mg pazopanib orally per day or placebo. The primary end point was progression-free survival. Median progression-free survival was 9.2 months in the pazopanib-treated group and 4.2 months in the placebo arm (hazard ratio [HR], 0.42; 95% CI, 0.34 to 0.62, $P < 0.0000001$). In a phase III trial comparing pazopanib with sunitinib as first-line therapy, pazopanib was not inferior to sunitinib with respect to progression-free and overall survival. However, there was a difference in the side-effect profile between the two drugs. Patients in the sunitinib group had a significantly higher risk of hand-foot syndrome, stomatitis, hypothyroidism, fatigue, and thrombocytopenia, whereas patients in the pazopanib group had a significantly higher risk of weight loss, alopecia, and increased alanine transferase (ALT) level.[311]

Axitinib. Axitinib is an oral second-generation multitargeted kinase inhibitor against VEGFR types 1, 2, and 3. A phase II clinical trial involving 52 patients in whom cytokines had been ineffective recorded an overall response rate (complete plus partial responses by RECIST criteria) of

44.2%.[312] At a median follow-up of 20 months, median progression-free survival was 15.7 months and median overall survival was 31.1 months. Dosage reduction was required in 29% of patients because of serious adverse events. Unlike with pazopanib, there were no cases of grade 3 or 4 myelosuppression.

Another phase II study enrolled 62 patients who showed no response to sorafenib and 72% had received prior systemic therapy. Axitinib dosages were titrated up and down from 5 mg/day. Overall response rate was 22.6%. Median progression-free and overall survival were 7.4 and 13.6 months, respectively. Serious adverse events (grade 3 or 4) were hand-foot syndrome (16.1%), fatigue (16.1%), hypertension (16.1%), dyspnea (14.5%), diarrhea (14.5%), and hypotension (6.5%).[312] A prospective randomized phase III trial of 723 patients comparing axitinib to sorafenib in patients with metastatic RCC that did not respond to a prior first-line therapy demonstrated significantly longer progression-free survival for axitinib than for sorafenib (6.7 months vs. 4.7 months, respectively, $P < 0.0001$). The most common adverse events were diarrhea, hypertension, and fatigue in the axitinib group, and diarrhea, hand-foot syndrome, and alopecia in the sorafenib group.[313]

Bevacizumab. Bevacizumab is an intravenously administered human monoclonal antibody directed against VEGF. All circulating VEGF isoforms are bound and neutralized by this antibody, thus prohibiting ligand binding to the VEGF receptor and consequently inhibiting signal transduction in the endothelial cell. Bevacizumab in combination with interferon alfa was approved by the FDA in July 2009 as a first-line therapy for treatment-naive patients with metastatic RCC. A phase III trial enrolling 723 treatment-naive patients showed a median progression-free survival of 8.5 months in patients receiving bevacizumab plus interferon alfa versus 5.2 months in patients receiving interferon alfa monotherapy ($P < 0.001$). Overall toxicity was greater in the bevacizumab plus interferon group, including significantly more grade 3 hypertension (95% vs. 0%), anorexia (17% vs. 8%), fatigue (35% vs. 28%), and proteinuria (13% vs. 0%). No overall survival difference was reported in this study.[314,315]

Temsirolimus. A rapamycin analog, temsirolimus inhibits mTOR downstream of the serine-threonine protein kinase Akt. It is administered intravenously. A randomized phase III three-arm study, in which one group received 25 mg of intravenous temsirolimus weekly, one group received 9 million U of interferon alfa three times weekly, and one group received 15 mg of intravenous temsirolimus weekly plus 6 million U of interferon alfa three times weekly, showed significant differences among treatment groups.[316] Patient inclusion criteria showed significant differences from criteria in contemporary phase III trials: 35% of patients had not undergone cytoreductive nephrectomy; 80% of patients had a Karnofsky performance status score less than 80; and 20% of patients had tumors with non–clear cell histologic features. The median survival of patients in the temsirolimus-only arm was significantly longer than that of patients receiving interferon alfa monotherapy (10.9 months vs. 7.1 months, respectively, $P = 0.0069$). The objective response rates as measured by RECIST criteria did not differ among the three arms. The median survival of patients receiving the combination therapy was 8.4 months and was not significantly different from that in the temsirolimus-only arm. The most common serious adverse events in the temsirolimus-only arm were anemia (20%), asthenia (11%), and hyperglycemia (11%). Temsirolimus is currently first-line monotherapy for treatment-naive patients with poor-risk metastatic RCC (including tumors with non–clear cell histologic characteristics).

Everolimus. Everolimus is an orally bioavailable mTOR inhibitor. A phase III clinical trial evaluating everolimus randomly assigned subjects—patients whose cancer had progressed while being treated with at least one targeted agent—to receive either everolimus or placebo in a 2:1 ratio.[317] Patients receiving everolimus demonstrated both decreased risk of progression (HR, 0.30; 95% CI, 0.22 to 0.40) and longer median progression-free survival (4.0 months vs. 1.9 months) in comparison with those receiving placebo. There were no significant differences in overall survival, likely because most patients in the placebo arm were crossed over to receive everolimus once disease progression was documented. Serious adverse events (grade 3 or 4) in the everolimus and placebo groups were stomatitis (3% and 0%, respectively), fatigue (3% and 1%, respectively), and pneumonitis (3% and 0%, respectively). The FDA approved everolimus for the treatment of patients with metastatic RCC after failure of treatment with sunitinib or sorafenib.

Vaccines

The goal of tumor vaccines is to stimulate the host immune system to recognize and attack existing tumor cells. There are four types of tumor vaccines: autologous tumor cells, genetically modified tumor cells, antigen-loaded dendritic cells, and peptides derived from tumor-associated antigens. Only three randomized phase III studies have investigated the use of vaccines in the treatment of RCC. Two of these vaccines were tested in the adjuvant setting and one was tested in the metastatic setting.[290-292,318] An autologous tumor vaccine (Reniale) was evaluated in a phase III trial and found to improve progression-free survival in patients with high-risk nonmetastatic RCC ($P = 0.0476$).[290,291] In the subgroup with T3 tumors (staged according to AJCC edition 4), the 5-year progression-free survival was 67.5%, versus 49.7% in the untreated control group. A subset analysis of patients with T3 disease also showed a benefit in overall survival ($P = 0.024$). The vaccine is not commercially available in Europe or the United States at this time. A multinational clinical trial that integrates the current staging system could provide more insight into patient selection and the role of this vaccine in adjuvant treatment of high-risk disease.

In a phase III multinational open-label clinical trial, more than 800 patients with high-risk tumors were randomly assigned to receive a heat shock protein complex derived from autologous tumors (vitespen) or to observation alone. No difference in recurrence-free survival was seen between the groups.[292] The third phase III trial used the attenuated virus, modified vaccinia Ankara (MVA), to deliver the tumor antigen 5T4 (TroVax) to immune cells. 5T4 is a transmembrane glycoprotein that is rarely expressed in normal tissue but has high expression in most tumors and is retained in the metastatic tissues.[318] Patients were randomly assigned to receive placebo or TroVax along with IL-2, interferon alfa, or sunitinib. Although significant survival advantage was seen in good-prognosis patients treated with IL-2 plus TroVax than in those treated with IL-2 alone, there was no difference in overall survival between the TroVax and placebo groups (20.1 months and 19.2 months, respectively, $P = 0.55$).[318]

CHEMOTHERAPY

Many studies of single-agent chemotherapy for RCC have been performed, with most agents showing minimal or no activity.[319] In a review of the chemotherapy literature in the mid-1990s, Yagoda and colleagues[320] reported a 4% overall response rate in 3635 patients with RCC treated with various chemotherapy approaches. Later studies evaluated gemcitabine chemotherapy for RCC. When gemcitabine was used as a single agent, response rates between 6% and 30% were reported.[321-323] A combination of gemcitabine and 5-fluorouracil demonstrated a response rate of 17% in 41 patients with metastatic RCC.[324] Median progression-free survival in this pretreated group of patients was 28.7 weeks. Follow-up studies using gemcitabine and capecitabine, the oral prodrug form of 5-fluorouracil, demonstrated response rates of 11% and overall survival of 14 months.[325] Another study demonstrated median progression-free survival and overall survival of 4.6 and 17.9 months, respectively.[326] A case series involving 18 patients with sarcomatoid RCC and other aggressive RCCs treated with doxorubicin (50 mg/m^2) and gemcitabine (1500 or 2000 mg/m^2) every 2 to 3 weeks along with granulocyte colony–stimulating factor support was reported in 2004. Two patients had a complete response, five had a partial response, three had a mixed response, and one had stable disease. The median duration of response was 5 months (range 2-21+ months).[327] Prospective studies need to be performed to validate this observation.

IMMUNOTHERAPY

Immunotherapeutic strategies for treatment of RCC have included therapy with nonspecific stimulators of the immune system, specific antitumor immunotherapy, and adoptive immunotherapy. The most consistent results have been reported with interferon alfa and IL-2. Although the mechanism of action of these cytokines is incompletely understood, the induction of antitumor responses in mice by interferon alfa and IL-2 has been linked to the direct killing of tumor cells by activated T and natural killer cells as well as to the antiangiogenic effects of these agents.

Interferon alfa

Interferon alfa (denoted hereforth as interferon) underwent extensive clinical evaluation as treatment for metastatic RCC. Results of these investigations are thoroughly described in several reviews.[328-330] Although no clear dose-response relationship exists, daily doses in the 5 million to 10 million U range appear to have the highest therapeutic index.[331] Toxic effects of interferon include flu-like symptoms such as fever, chills, myalgias, and fatigue, as well as weight loss, altered taste, depression, anemia, leukopenia, and elevated liver function values. Most adverse effects, especially the flu-like symptoms, tend to diminish with time during long-term therapy.

Later studies have suggested that the antitumor effects of interferon are quite limited. For example, a French Immunotherapy Group phase III trial comparing interferon alone with both IL-2 and IL-2 plus interferon reported a response rate of only 7.5% for the interferon arm with a 1-year event-free survival rate of only 12%.[332] Efforts to improve upon the clinical activity of interferon have included combining it with 5-fluorouracil, 13-*cis*-retinoic acid, interferon-γ, thalidomide, and IL-2. For the most part these efforts have met with limited success, with occasionally promising phase II findings failing to be confirmed in phase III trials.[333,334]

Interleukin-2

In 1992, high-dose bolus IL-2 therapy received FDA approval for treatment of metastatic RCC on the basis of data from 255 patients treated in seven clinical trials at 21 institutions. In these studies, recombinant IL-2 (Proleukin) at a dose of 600,000 to 720,000 IU/kg was administered by 15-minute intravenous infusion every 8 hours on days 1 to 5 and 15 to 19 (maximum, 28 doses). Treatment was repeated at approximately 12-week intervals for a maximum of three cycles in patients showing a tumor response. There were 12 complete responses (5% of patients) and 24 partial responses (9% of patients). Follow-up data on the study patients were accumulated through late 1998 (median follow-up, 8 years). The clinical results appear to have steadily improved over time. At last report, 17 patients (7%) were classified as having complete responses and 20 (8%) as having partial responses. The median survival for the group as a whole was 16.3 months, with 10% to 15% of patients estimated to remain alive 5 to 10 years after treatment with high-dose IL-2. A large percentage of patients showing a response—particularly those remaining free from progression for longer than 2 years and those who underwent resection that achieved disease-free status after their tumors responded to high-dose IL-2—appear unlikely to experience progression and may actually be "cured."[335]

Attempts to improve the efficacy of IL-2 have included the addition of interferon alfa and 5-fluorouracil. Despite publication of promising data by several groups, follow-up trials conducted by the Cytokine Working Group did not confirm the promise of cytokine combination therapy.[336,337] IL-2 and interferon alfa administered subcutaneously with or without weekly 5-fluorouracil produced response rates and median survival similar to those observed with high-dose IL-2 alone or high-dose IL-2 and interferon alfa; however, the quality and durability of the responses appeared to be considerably less than those observed with high-dose IL-2 alone.[338]

RENAL PELVIC TUMORS

The cellular lining of the urinary collecting system, originating in the proximal renal pelvis, traversing the ureter and urinary bladder, and ending in the distal urethra, is composed of transitional epithelium or urothelium. This entire surface may be affected by carcinogenic influences, a characteristic that may help explain the multiplicity in time and place of "urothelial" tumors, which some have termed *polychronotropism*. Renal pelvic tumors account for approximately 10% of all primary kidney cancers.

Tumors of the upper tract are twice as common in men, generally occur in patients older than 65 years, and are usually unilateral. The disease is more common in the

Balkan region (Bulgaria, Greece, Romania, Yugoslavia) and in regions of China, where it is often bilateral, and is associated with exposure to aristolochic acid.[339,340] As with urothelial tumors of the urinary bladder, exposure to cigarette smoke, certain chemicals, plastics, coal, tar, and asphalt may also increase the incidence of the disease. Long-term exposure to the analgesic phenacetin has been associated with the development of renal pelvic tumors.

Although most tumors of the upper tract are transitional cell carcinomas, which account for more than 90% of lesions, squamous carcinomas also occur, usually in the setting of chronic infections with kidney stones.

Adenocarcinomas and other miscellaneous subtypes are rare.

CLINICAL FEATURES AND DIAGNOSTIC EVALUATION

The most common presenting feature of a renal pelvic tumor is gross hematuria, which occurs in 75% of patients, followed by flank pain, which is seen in 30%. Evaluation may reveal either a nonfunctioning kidney and nonvisualization of the collecting system or, more commonly, a filling defect of the calyceal system, renal pelvis, or ureter on CT urogram. Exfoliative cytologic analysis commonly has positive findings, as in bladder cancers. A positive cytologic result in the presence of a filling defect of the renal pelvis or ureter confirms the diagnosis. Results of retrograde pyelography with brush biopsy of suspicious lesions may also yield the diagnosis of cancer. If there is still uncertainty about the diagnosis after pyelography, including a retrograde evaluation, ureteroscopy may be performed to further evaluate the filling defect or obstruction.

STAGING AND GRADING OF RENAL PELVIC TUMORS

Upper tract urothelial carcinomas (UTUCs) are graded on a scale from grade I, representing a well-differentiated lesion, to grade IV, representing an anaplastic and undifferentiated lesion. Because of the difficult access to some tumors of the upper tract, clinical staging is problematic. Histologic grade of biopsy specimens can be used to predict pathologic stage of disease.[341] In a staging system similar to that used for urinary bladder cancer, stage 0 is disease limited to the mucosa; stage A is invasion into the lamina propria without muscularis invasion; stage B is invasion into the muscularis; stage C is invasion into the serosa; and stage D is metastatic disease. Lymphatic metastases usually indicate that more widespread metastatic disease is or will be present. The AJCC TNM classification of renal pelvic tumors is also similar to the staging for bladder carcinoma.[342]

TREATMENT

For low-grade, low-stage transitional cancers, the general approach to treatment is conservative, consisting of local excision and preservation of the kidney parenchyma. For high-stage and high-grade lesions that have infiltrated into the renal parenchyma, the surgical treatment of choice is nephroureterectomy and removal of a cuff of bladder that encompasses the ipsilateral ureteral orifice. This approach is generally required because of the high likelihood of local recurrence in the bladder at the ureterovesical junction or in the distal ureter. Five-year recurrence-free and cancer-specific survival rates for patients with UTUC who undergo radical nephroureterectomy are 69% and 73%, respectively.[343] In patients with regionally advanced or metastatic renal pelvic tumors, systemic chemotherapy, identical to that administered for bladder cancer, is often employed.

Adjuvant therapy has not been adequately assessed, but one study identified 415 patients with T3N0 and T4N0 UTUCs, of whom 16% and 25%, respectively, received adjuvant chemotherapy. Chemotherapy status was not associated with any significant cancer-specific or overall survival differences.[344] Another problem when reviewing the literature on adjuvant chemotherapy for high-risk disease is the paucity of descriptions of lymph node dissection in the initial surgical procedure. Nevertheless, definitions of regional templates for lymphadenectomy in this disease have been developed.[112] For patients with pathologically determined T3 disease, the extent of lymph node dissection is a significant prognostic indicator and correlates with cancer-specific survival.[112] Standard first-line regimens for patients with locally advanced or metastatic transitional cell carcinoma mirror those used in bladder cancer and include methotrexate, vinblastine, doxorubicin (Adriamycin), and cisplatin (MVAC) as well as gemcitabine with cisplatin (GC). Initial response rates may vary depending on prognostic factors, but long-term survival is poor.

Another consideration is neoadjuvant chemotherapy in high-risk/locally advanced disease because of the risk to the patient of renal insufficiency after nephroureterectomy and the resultant inability to receive optimal adjuvant chemotherapy.[345] This is a difficult argument to make considering the clear lack of data regarding the overall effectiveness of adjuvant treatment in UTUC, but management practice has been extrapolated from the literature on bladder transitional cell carcinoma. Data reported for a large cohort of patients who underwent nephroureterectomy for UTUC provided some insight into operative decisions.[346] According to the criterion of a GFR of 60 mL/min or above, only 48% of patients were eligible for chemotherapy preoperatively, and that number decreased to 22% postoperatively.[346] After nephroureterectomy the opportunity for treatment with optimal chemotherapy was lost in 61% of patients able to receive it preoperatively.[346] In a patient at risk for postoperative renal insufficiency and a significant risk for advanced UTUC, strong consideration should be given to the neoadjuvant administration of chemotherapy.

OTHER KIDNEY TUMORS

RENAL SARCOMAS

Renal sarcomas account for approximately 1% to 2% of primary kidney cancers. Fibrosarcomas are the most common and have a poor prognosis as a result of typically late presentation and the presence of locally advanced involvement into the renal vein or metastatic disease at presentation. Five-year survival rates are less than 20%. Other, rarer sarcoma variants that may occur are leiomyosarcoma, rhabdomyosarcoma, osteogenic sarcoma, and liposarcoma.

WILMS' TUMOR

In children, Wilms' tumor (nephroblastoma) is the most common cancer of the kidney, accounting for approximately 400 new cases per year in the United States. The development of a successful treatment regimen for the disease in the 1990s was due to the coordinated efforts of a multidisciplinary team of oncologists, radiation therapists, and surgeons. The disease tends to occur more frequently in African American children. A variety of etiologic factors have been suggested to increase the risk of Wilms' tumor, but for none has a definitive link been established.

Genetics

Several well-described genetic abnormalities are associated with Wilms' tumor. Patients with Wilms' tumor may also manifest other abnormalities, which include aniridia, WAGR syndrome (Wilms' tumor, aniridia, other genitourinary abnormalities, mental retardation), Denys-Drash syndrome (Wilms' tumor, glomerulitis, pseudohermaphrodism), hemihypertrophy, trisomy, other rare physical abnormalities such as macroglossia, and developmental sexual disorders.

Abnormalities of the genes *WT1* (chromosome arm 11p13) and *WT2* (11p15), and mutations at 16q have all been implicated in the molecular genetics of Wilms' tumor. Loss of heterozygosity in *WT1* and at 16q occur in 20% of patients; inactivation of *WT2* has also been described. Other genetic abnormalities have suggested the presence of other abnormal chromosomal locations. Patients with trisomy[347] and XX/XY mosaicisms have been reported to have an increased incidence of Wilms' tumor.

Pathology and Staging

Microscopically, Wilms' tumors consist of blastemic, epithelial, and stromal cells, often arranged in patterns that resemble tubular or glomeruloid features. The multipotential aspects of Wilms' tumors may be characterized by the presence of teratomatous or teratoid features, including components of mesenchymal structures such as muscle, cartilage, and lipoid tissues. In contrast to these differentiated structures, undifferentiated or sarcomatoid lesions can also occur and are associated with a worse prognosis. The presence of nephrogenic rests in the setting of Wilms' tumors is common; they are thought to be precursor lesions. According to Wilimas and associates,[348] such a rest is "defined as a focus of persistent nephrogenic cells, some of which can be induced to form a Wilms' tumor."

Clinical Features

The most common presentation of Wilms' tumor is as an asymptomatic abdominal mass in a young patient (median age, 3.5 years). Hematuria, anemia, hypertension, and/or acute severe abdominal pain may also be present. Abdominal ultrasonography is an important diagnostic test to further evaluate the mass and its anatomic extension, which may include inferior or superior extension into the vena cava. Intravenous pyelography and CT are also warranted. Assessment for metastases to liver, chest, and bone complement the evaluation. The lungs are the most common site of metastasis. The diagnosis is usually established by surgery. If the diagnostic tests and clinical features suggest the presence of a Wilms' tumor, preoperative needle biopsy should be avoided because of the attendant risks of tumor spillage and subsequent "upstaging" of the patient's disease.

Multimodality Treatment

High cure rates have been achieved with the concerted effort of multimodality teams performing surgery, radiation therapy, and chemotherapy. Surgical removal of the affected kidney along with examination of the regional lymph nodes and detailed abdominal exploration is the goal. Removal of all gross tumors should be attempted and justifies the radical resection that is often required. Tumors are classified as favorable or unfavorable in histologic features. All patients receive at least two-drug chemotherapy with dactinomycin and vincristine; those with more advanced disease receive additional doxorubicin, cyclophosphamide, and etoposide with abdominal radiation (1080 Gy) and possibly radiation to the chest (1200 Gy). Specific recommendations regarding the exact protocols to be used are determined by the operative findings, the histologic subtype of the tumor, and whether there was evidence of tumor spillage during the resection.

Chemotherapy is an important component of treatment for Wilms' tumors. Not only is chemotherapy administered after surgery, but neoadjuvant chemotherapy can diminish the size of the primary tumor and cause regression of metastatic lesions as well as reduce tumors in patients with stage 5 disease (bilateral disease). Before the extensive use of chemotherapy, the survival rate for patients with stage 2 or 3 tumors was less than 45%. Now, cure rates approaching 80% to 90% are routinely achieved; survival rates of 92% to 97% are obtainable in earlier stages of disease. Chemotherapy administration in the adjuvant and neoadjuvant settings varies greatly between Europe (studies of the International Society of Paediatric Oncology [SIOP]) and the United States (Wilms' Tumor Study Group [WTSG]).

As these excellent results continue to accumulate, treatment programs aimed at lessening treatment duration and minimizing long-term consequences, such as induction of second tumors, continue to be evaluated. Such programs include the more selective use of radiation therapy and a decrease in the duration of chemotherapy.

Complete reference list available at ExpertConsult.com.

KEY REFERENCES

4. Ligato S, Ro JY, Tamboli P, et al: Benign tumors and tumor-like lesions of the adult kidney. Part I: Benign renal epithelial neoplasms. *Adv Anat Pathol* 6:1, 1999.
21. Katabathina VS, Vikram R, Nagar AM, et al: Mesenchymal neoplasms of the kidney in adults: imaging spectrum with radiologic-pathologic correlation. *Radiographics* 30:1525, 2010.
23. Raman SP, Hruban RH, Fishman EK: Beyond renal cell carcinoma: rare and unusual renal masses. *Abdom Imaging* 37:873, 2012.
27. Tamboli P, Ro JY, Amin MB, et al: Benign tumors and tumor-like lesions of the adult kidney. Part II: Benign mesenchymal and mixed neoplasms, and tumor-like lesions. *Adv Anat Pathol* 7:47, 2000.
40. Jevremovic D, Lager DJ, Lewin M: Cystic nephroma (multilocular cyst) and mixed epithelial and stromal tumor of the kidney: a spectrum of the same entity? *Ann Diagn Pathol* 10:77, 2006.
45. Sanchez-Ortiz RF, Madsen LT, Bermejo CE, et al: A renal mass in the setting of a nonrenal malignancy: When is a renal tumor biopsy appropriate? *Cancer* 101:2195, 2004.
46. Siegel R, Naishadham D, Jemal A: Cancer statistics, 2013. *CA Cancer J Clin* 63:11, 2013.
58. Kane CJ, Mallin K, Ritchey J, et al: Renal cell cancer stage migration: analysis of the National Cancer Data Base. *Cancer* 113:78, 2008.
76. Zbar B, Brauch H, Talmadge C, et al: Loss of alleles of loci on the short arm of chromosome 3 in renal cell carcinoma. *Nature* 327:721, 1987.
78. Coleman JA, Russo P: Hereditary and familial kidney cancer. *Curr Opin Urol* 19:478, 2009.
92. Delahunt B: Advances and controversies in grading and staging of renal cell carcinoma. *Mod Pathol* 22(Suppl 2):S24, 2009.
105. Srigley JR, Delahunt B: Uncommon and recently described renal carcinomas. *Mod Pathol* 22(Suppl 2):S2, 2009.

110. Linehan WM, Walther MM, Zbar B: The genetic basis of cancer of the kidney. *J Urol* 170:2163, 2003.
112. Kondo T, Nakazawa H, Ito F, et al: Impact of the extent of regional lymphadenectomy on the survival of patients with urothelial carcinoma of the upper urinary tract. *J Urol* 178:1212, 2007.
115. Kim WY, Kaelin WG: Role of VHL gene mutation in human cancer. *J Clin Oncol* 22:4991, 2004.
144. Brugarolas J: Renal-cell carcinoma–molecular pathways and therapies. *N Engl J Med* 356:185, 2007.
149. Patard JJ, Leray E, Cindolo L, et al: Multi-institutional validation of a symptom based classification for renal cell carcinoma. *J Urol* 172:858, 2004.
166. Motzer RJ, Mazumdar M, Bacik J, et al: Survival and prognostic stratification of 670 patients with advanced renal cell carcinoma. *J Clin Oncol* 17:2530, 1999.
179. Israel GM, Bosniak MA: An update of the Bosniak renal cyst classification system. *Urology* 66:484, 2005.
195. Divgi CR, Uzzo RG, Gatsonis C, et al: Positron emission tomography/computed tomography identification of clear cell renal cell carcinoma: results from the REDECT trial. *J Clin Oncol* 31:187, 2013.
202. Motzer RJ, Bacik J, Schwartz LH, et al: Prognostic factors for survival in previously treated patients with metastatic renal cell carcinoma. *J Clin Oncol* 22:454, 2004.
207. Frank I, Blute ML, Cheville JC, et al: An outcome prediction model for patients with clear cell renal cell carcinoma treated with radical nephrectomy based on tumor stage, size, grade and necrosis: the SSIGN score. *J Urol* 168:2395, 2002.
239. Kural AR, Atug F, Tufek I, et al: Robot-assisted partial nephrectomy versus laparoscopic partial nephrectomy: comparison of outcomes. *J Endourol* 23:1491, 2009.
240. Benway BM, Bhayani SB, Rogers CG, et al: Robot assisted partial nephrectomy versus laparoscopic partial nephrectomy for renal tumors: a multi-institutional analysis of perioperative outcomes. *J Urol* 182:866, 2009.
241. Ellison JS, Montgomery JS, Wolf JS, Jr, et al: A matched comparison of perioperative outcomes of a single laparoscopic surgeon versus a multisurgeon robot-assisted cohort for partial nephrectomy. *J Urol* 188:45, 2012.
243. Tsivian M, Rampersaud EN, Jr, Laguna Pes MD, et al: Small renal mass biopsy—how, what and when: report from an international consensus panel. *BJU Int* 113:854, 2013.
245. Van Poppel H, Da Pozzo L, Albrecht W, et al: A prospective, randomised EORTC intergroup phase 3 study comparing the oncologic outcome of elective nephron-sparing surgery and radical nephrectomy for low-stage renal cell carcinoma. *Eur Urol* 59:543, 2011.
246. Lane BR, Campbell SC, Demirjian S, et al: Surgically induced chronic kidney disease may be associated with a lower risk of progression and mortality than medical chronic kidney disease. *J Urol* 189:1649, 2013.
249. Kunkle DA, Uzzo RG: Cryoablation or radiofrequency ablation of the small renal mass: a meta-analysis. *Cancer* 113:2671, 2008.
252. Blute ML, Leibovich BC, Cheville JC, et al: A protocol for performing extended lymph node dissection using primary tumor pathological features for patients treated with radical nephrectomy for clear cell renal cell carcinoma. *J Urol* 172:465, 2004.
253. Hutterer GC, Patard JJ, Perrotte P, et al: Patients with renal cell carcinoma nodal metastases can be accurately identified: external validation of a new nomogram. *Int J Cancer* 121:2556, 2007.
254. Blom JH, van Poppel H, Marechal JM, et al: Radical nephrectomy with and without lymph-node dissection: final results of European Organization for Research and Treatment of Cancer (EORTC) randomized phase 3 trial 30881. *Eur Urol* 55:28, 2009.
256. Pantuck AJ, Zisman A, Dorey F, et al: Renal cell carcinoma with retroperitoneal lymph nodes. Impact on survival and benefits of immunotherapy. *Cancer* 97:2995, 2003.
259. Delacroix SE, Jr, Chapin BF, Chen JJ, et al: Can a durable disease-free survival be achieved with surgical resection in patients with pathological node positive renal cell carcinoma? *J Urol* 186:1236, 2011.
266. Mickisch GH, Garin A, van Poppel H, et al: Radical nephrectomy plus interferon-alfa-based immunotherapy compared with interferon-alfa alone in metastatic renal-cell carcinoma: a randomised trial. *Lancet* 358:966, 2001.
267. Flanigan RC, Salmon SE, Blumenstein BA, et al: Nephrectomy followed by interferon alfa-2b compared with interferon alfa-2b alone for metastatic renal-cell cancer. *N Engl J Med* 345:1655, 2001.
277. Chapin BF, Delacroix SE, Jr, Culp SH, et al: Safety of presurgical targeted therapy in the setting of metastatic renal cell carcinoma. *Eur Urol* 60:964, 2011.
290. Jocham D, Richter A, Hoffmann L, et al: Adjuvant autologous renal tumour cell vaccine and risk of tumour progression in patients with renal-cell carcinoma after radical nephrectomy: phase III, randomised controlled trial. *Lancet* 363:594, 2004.
291. May M, Kendel F, Hoschke B, et al: Adjuvant autologous tumour cell vaccination in patients with renal cell carcinoma. Overall survival analysis with a follow-up period in excess of more than 10 years. *Urologe A* 48:1075, 2009.
292. Wood C, Srivastava P, Bukowski R, et al: An adjuvant autologous therapeutic vaccine (HSPPC-96; Vitespen) versus observation alone for patients at high risk of recurrence after nephrectomy for renal cell carcinoma: a multicentre, open-label, randomised phase III trial. *Lancet* 372:145, 2008.
295. Abel EJ, Culp SH, Tannir NM, et al: Primary tumor response to targeted agents in patients with metastatic renal cell carcinoma. *Eur Urol* 59:10, 2011.
304. Motzer RJ, Hutson TE, Tomczak P, et al: Overall survival and updated results for sunitinib compared with interferon alfa in patients with metastatic renal cell carcinoma. *J Clin Oncol* 27:3584, 2009.
306. Rixe O, Billemont B, Izzedine H: Hypertension as a predictive factor of Sunitinib activity. *Ann Oncol* 18:1117, 2007.
312. Rixe O, Bukowski RM, Michaelson MD, et al: Axitinib treatment in patients with cytokine-refractory metastatic renal-cell cancer: a phase II study. *Lancet Oncol* 8:975, 2007.
317. Motzer RJ, Escudier B, Oudard S, et al: Efficacy of everolimus in advanced renal cell carcinoma: a double-blind, randomised, placebo-controlled phase III trial. *Lancet* 372:449, 2008.
318. Amato RJ, Hawkins RE, Kaufman HL, et al: Vaccination of metastatic renal cancer patients with MVA-5T4: a randomized, double-blind, placebo-controlled phase III study. *Clin Cancer Res* 16:5539, 2010.
335. Fisher RI, Rosenberg SA, Fyfe G: Long-term survival update for high-dose recombinant interleukin-2 in patients with renal cell carcinoma. *Cancer J Sci Am* 6(Suppl 1):S55, 2000.
343. Margulis V, Shariat SF, Matin SF, et al: Outcomes of radical nephroureterectomy: a series from the Upper Tract Urothelial Carcinoma Collaboration. *Cancer* 115:1224, 2009.
344. Hellenthal NJ, Shariat SF, Margulis V, et al: Adjuvant chemotherapy for high risk upper tract urothelial carcinoma: results from the Upper Tract Urothelial Carcinoma Collaboration. *J Urol* 182:900, 2009.
346. Lane BR, Smith AK, Larson BT, et al: Chronic kidney disease after nephroureterectomy for upper tract urothelial carcinoma and implications for the administration of perioperative chemotherapy. *Cancer* 116:2967, 2010.

Onco-Nephrology: Kidney Disease in Patients with Cancer

Kevin W. Finkel

CHAPTER OUTLINE

ACUTE KIDNEY INJURY, 1390
MULTIPLE MYELOMA, 1390
Pathogenesis, 1390
Kidney Involvement and Pathology, 1391
Light-Chain Deposition Disease, 1391
HEMATOPOIETIC STEM CELL TRANSPLANTATION, 1393
Acute Kidney Injury, 1394
Chronic Kidney Disease, 1394
Specific Kidney Diseases after Hematopoietic Stem Cell Transplantation, 1394
TUMOR LYSIS SYNDROME, 1395
Definitions, 1396
Pathophysiology, 1396
Treatment, 1396
CHEMOTHERAPEUTIC AGENTS, 1397
Cisplatin, 1397
Ifosfamide, 1397
Cyclophosphamide, 1397
Methotrexate, 1398
Biologic Agents, 1398
Anti-Angiogenic Agents, 1398
Cetuximab, 1398
MISCELLANEOUS AGENTS, 1398
Calcineurin Inhibitors, 1398
Bisphosphonates, 1399

HYPERCALCEMIA OF MALIGNANCY, 1399
RADIATION-ASSOCIATED KIDNEY INJURY, 1400
Pathogenesis, 1400
Epidemiology, 1400
Total-Body Irradiation and Transplantation, 1400
Clinical Presentation, 1401
Diagnosis, 1401
Treatment, 1401
Prognosis, 1401
LEUKEMIA AND LYMPHOMA, 1401
Lymphoma, 1402
Cytotoxic Nephropathy/Hemophagocytic Syndrome, 1402
Leukemia, 1403
PARANEOPLASTIC GLOMERULAR DISEASES, 1403
RENAL INFECTIONS, 1404
Renal Candidiasis, 1404
Adenovirus Infections, 1404
Epstein-Barr Virus Infection, 1404
Polyomavirus (BK-Type) Infection, 1404
Zygomatosis, 1405
Disseminated Histoplasmosis, 1405
THROMBOTIC MICROANGIOPATHY, 1405

The care of patients with kidney disease has become increasingly complex and requires even further subspecialization. In the past general nephrologists provided care to recipients of kidney transplantation, but because of the extensively observed patient comorbid conditions after transplantation and the growing armamentarium of immunosuppressive medications utilized for it, care is increasingly delegated to transplant nephrologists. For similar reasons, Onco-Nephrology is emerging as a new subspecialty dedicated to the management of kidney disease in patients with cancer.

There are several reasons for this development. First is the recognition that both acute kidney injury (AKI) and chronic kidney disease (CKD) increase the morbidity and mortality in all patients, including those with cancer. Because many oncology practices are associated with a comprehensive care center, nephrologists have become an integral part of the treatment team. Second, patients with cancer, in addition to presenting with kidney diseases seen in the general population, can experience unique disorders related to the malignancy itself or its treatment. This possibility requires nephrologists to develop a specialized knowledge related to these specific clinical entities. Third, because the prevalences of both cancer and CKD are high, a growing number of patients require the expertise of onco-nephrologists, who must be knowledgeable about the array of new chemotherapeutic agents and their potential effects on kidney function as well as the effects of various dialytic modalities on drug clearance. Finally, as patients with cancer survive longer, there is a need for long-term management of patients in whom CKD develops from cancer treatment.

ACUTE KIDNEY INJURY

AKI is characterized by an abrupt decline in glomerular filtration rate (GFR) over hours or days. Mortality rates of patients with AKI in the intensive care unit (ICU) approach 50% to 70%.[1,2] Cancer patients are a group particularly at risk for the development of AKI secondary to exposure to chemotherapeutic and other nephrotoxic agents, infections and sepsis, tumor lysis syndrome, hematopoietic stem cell transplantation, and direct effects of malignancy (Table 42.1). In a large cohort of Danish patients with cancer, the highest incidence of AKI occurred in renal cancers (44%), multiple myeloma (33%), liver cancer (32%), and acute myelogenous leukemia (28%).[3] In critically ill patients with cancer the incidence of AKI is as high as 49% with up to 32% of patients requiring dialysis.[4-7] These rates are higher than in patients without cancer with similar illness severity of kidney disease.[4,8,9]

In addition to the morbidity and mortality associated with AKI, reduced renal function adversely affects cancer treatment. In the presence of AKI, therapy may be delayed, chemotherapeutic dose may be reduced (thus decreasing the "killing effect"), and certain agents may be precluded altogether.

In patients with severe AKI, the use of dialysis can lead to unpredictable chemotherapeutic and antibiotic concentrations, resulting in either toxicity or inadequate treatment. Finally, patients who survive an initial episode of AKI are at increased risk for development of CKD, which could adversely affect future cancer therapy while also reducing quality of life and survival.

As in other patient cohorts, the utility of consensus definitions of AKI (risk, injury, failure, loss of kidney function, and end-stage kidney disease [RIFLE] and AKI Network [AKIN] criteria) in patients with cancer has been substantiated. In a retrospective cohort study of 3795 critically ill patients with cancer, increases in serum creatinine concentrations as small as 10% were associated with significantly prolonged ICU length of stay and a twofold increase in mortality; likewise, the RIFLE criteria were shown to be accurate predictors of increased mortality.[1] In another study of 537 patients with acute myelogenous leukemia, the RIFLE criteria had prognostic utility in mortality prediction.[10] Risk factors for the development of AKI included advanced age, mechanical ventilation, use of vasopressors, diuretics, amphotericin B or vancomycin, leukopenia, and hypoalbuminemia. Finally, in a cross-sectional analysis of 3558 hospitalized patients with cancer over a 3-month period, AKI developed in 12% of patients on the basis of RIFLE criteria; 4% required dialysis.[11] Length of stay, hospital costs, and mortality were significantly increased in patients with AKI. Risk factors associated with AKI were presence of diabetes mellitus, use of chemotherapy, antibiotics, or intravenous radiocontrast agent, and presence of hyponatremia.

Table 42.1 Causes of Acute Kidney Injury in Cancer Patients

Prerenal	Sepsis
	Volume depletion (vomiting, diarrhea, mucositis)
	Hepatorenal syndrome (venoocclusive disease of the liver)
	Capillary leak syndrome (interleukin-2 administration)
	Hypercalcemia
Intrinsic	Acute tubular necrosis:
	Ischemia (sepsis/shock)
	Nephrotoxic (aminoglycosides, amphotericin B, chemotherapy)
	Tubulointerstitial nephritis:
	Tumor lysis syndrome (urate and phosphate nephropathy)
	Allergic reaction
	Pyelonephritis
	Opportunistic infections
	Infiltration (lymphoma/leukemia)
	Vascular:
	Thrombotic microangiopathy
	Cancer treated
	Drug induced
	Bone marrow transplantation
	Radiation injury
	Amyloidosis
	Light-chain deposition disease
	Paraneoplastic syndromes (membranous, antineutrophil cytoplasmic antibody associated, focal segmental glomerulosclerosis)
Postrenal	Intrarenal (urate, acyclovir, methotrexate)
	Extrarenal (retroperitoneal fibrosis, lymphadenopathy, direct invasion)

MULTIPLE MYELOMA

PATHOGENESIS

Multiple myeloma (MM) is a hematologic malignancy involving the pathologic proliferation of terminally differentiated plasma cells. It is the second most common hematologic malignancy, behind non-Hodgkin's lymphoma, with an annual incidence of 4 to 7 cases per 100,000 in the United States. Men are more commonly affected than women and the median age at diagnosis is 62 years. Less than 2% of patients are younger than 40 years. African Americans are affected more often than Caucasians, with Asians having the lowest incidence of disease. Clinical symptoms are due to osteolysis of the bone marrow, suppression of normal hematopoiesis, and the overproduction of monoclonal immunoglobulins that deposit in organ tissues.

Clinical symptoms include bone pain and fractures, anemia, infections, hypercalcemia, edema, heart failure, and renal disease.

KIDNEY INVOLVEMENT AND PATHOLOGY

More than half of patients with MM initially present with varying degrees of AKI. Nearly 20% of patients present with a serum creatinine greater than 2.0 mg/dL, and 10% of patients require dialysis on presentation.[12] The presence of AKI is associated with higher mortality, but this association may be reflective of patients with more advanced disease.[13]

The kidneys are particularly vulnerable to injury from circulating free light chains (FLCs) secondary to high plasma flow and glomerular filtration. Normally, the kidneys filter less than 1 g per day of FLCs, which are reabsorbed through the megalin-cubilin receptor system and digested by lysozymes within the proximal tubule. In MM, the kidneys may filter more than 80 g per day of FLCs, which overwhelm the absorptive capacity of the proximal tubule. Given that not all patients with MM have AKI, it is apparent that only certain light chains have a predilection for depositing within the glomeruli, tubules, interstitium, or vasculature of the kidney. Glomerular deposition leads to proteinuria, whereas tubulointerstitial deposition manifests as AKI. Rarely, proximal tubule damage may present as Fanconi's syndrome.[14] Unless markedly advanced, vascular deposition of FLCs is generally not clinically apparent. Light chains isolated from human urine have been shown to replicate patterns of renal injury in animal models, supporting the theory of the inherent pathogenicity of certain FLCs.[15]

The major diseases in the spectrum of myeloma-related kidney disease include cast nephropathy, light-chain deposition disease (LCDD), and amyloid light-chain (AL) amyloidosis. Renal biopsy demonstrates the presence of monotypic light chains on immunofluorescence examination as well as characteristic ultrastructural features of deposits on electron microscopy. Renal injury from cryoglobulinemia, proliferative glomerulonephritis, heavy-chain deposition disease, and immunotactoid glomerulonephritis has also been described.[16]

CAST NEPHROPATHY

Cast nephropathy has been diagnosed in 41% of patients with MM and renal disease.[17] Excess light chains precipitate with Tamm-Horsfall protein (THP) secreted by the thick ascending limb of the loop of Henle and produce casts in the distal tubule. Reduced GFR may increase the concentration of light chains in the distal tubule and enhance the formation of casts. Therefore, hypercalcemia, volume depletion, diuretics, and nonsteroidal antiinflammatory drugs have traditionally been avoided in patients with this disease.

In some cases of AKI associated with MM, cast formation is a rare finding on renal biopsy. Instead, renal injury is attributed to the direct toxic effects of urinary FLCs on proximal tubule cells.[18,19] After reabsorption, lysosomal degradation of FLCs can activate the nuclear factor kappaB (NFκ-B) pathway, leading to oxidative stress with an inflammatory response, apoptosis, and fibrosis. This lesion is characterized histologically by loss of brush border and cell vacuolization and necrosis; it can be caused by either κ or λ light chains.[20]

The classic presentation consists of unexplained AKI, anemia, and bone pain or fractures in an elderly patient. Proteinuria, which is generally subnephrotic, is primarily composed of monoclonal light chains (Bence Jones proteins). The qualitative measurement for protein on dipstick urinalysis, which mainly detects albuminuria, is generally minimally reactive. The kidneys may appear normal or enlarged on imaging studies.

Most patients with myeloma cast nephropathy are diagnosed without kidney biopsies, serum and urine immunofixation and serum FLC analysis being used instead. When biopsy is performed, casts in the specimen are eosin positive, fractured, and waxy in appearance on light microscopy. Multinucleated giant cells may surround casts, and an interstitial inflammatory infiltrate composed of lymphocytes and monocytes may also be present. Widespread tubular atrophy and interstitial fibrosis eventually develops. Immunofluorescence staining generally demonstrates light-chain restriction within the casts, although patterns may be mixed or nondiagnostic. Casts have a lattice-like appearance and may contain needle-shaped crystals on electron microscopy. The glomeruli and vessels appear normal, unless LCDD is concurrently present.

On the basis of foregoing, recommendations for diagnostic investigation and follow-up suggest that patients with or without a known diagnosis of MM who are being evaluated for unexplained kidney injury for less than 6 months in duration should have the following tests to exclude cast nephropathy: serum FLC measurement, serum protein electrophoresis and immunofixation, 24-hour quantitation of urinary total protein excretion, and electrophoresis. Only selected patients with enigmatic presentations might require kidney biopsy for a definitive diagnosis. In patients who have a known diagnosis of myeloma and who present with unexplained kidney injury that occurs over less than 6 months, serum FLC concentrations of 1500 mg/L or higher can be considered suspicious for cast nephropathy. Among patients with known diagnosis of myeloma, unexplained kidney injury, and a serum FLC concentration lower than 1500 mg/L, other myeloma-related causes (LCDD, amyloidosis, membranoproliferative glomerulonephritis) and nonmyeloma causes of kidney injury should be considered. After prerenal and postrenal causes have been ruled out (usually by administration of fluids and renal ultrasonography), a kidney biopsy can be considered (see also Chapter 29).

LIGHT-CHAIN DEPOSITION DISEASE

LCDD has been diagnosed at autopsy in 19% of patients with MM and renal disease.[17] The renal manifestations are most apparent clinically, whereas light-chain deposits within the heart, liver, spleen, and peripheral nervous system may remain asymptomatic. The hallmark of the disease is the development of mesangial nodules secondary to the upregulation of platelet-derived growth factor-β and transforming growth factor-β.

Clinically, patients present with proteinuria, renal insufficiency, and a nodular sclerosing glomerulopathy. Several retrospective reviews have reported on the clinical characteristics of these patients.[21,22] The mean age was 58 years with no significant preference with respect to gender. Marked reduction in GFR was common on presentation, with a median serum creatinine concentration greater than 4 mg/dL, and renal function rapidly declined thereafter. Nephrotic-range proteinuria was detected in 26% to 40% of patients and correlated with the extent of glomerular involvement. Hypertension and microscopic hematuria were also present in the majority of patients.

Light-chain deposition stimulates mesangial and matrix expansion, leading to nodule formation. On light microscopy, mesangial nodules are more uniform in distribution and size in LCDD than in diabetic nephropathy. Irregular thickening and double contours of the glomerular basement membrane may also be present. Eosin-positive deposits may be seen diffusely throughout the tubular basement membranes. Immunofluorescence demonstrates a characteristic linear staining of basement membranes with monotypic light chains, which are most commonly restricted to κ type. On electron microscopy, granular-powdery deposits are distributed within the mesangium and midportion of the glomerular, tubular, and vessel wall basement membranes.

AMYLOID LIGHT-CHAIN AMYLOIDOSIS

AL amyloidosis occurs when pathogenic light chains unfold and deposit as insoluble fibrils extracellularly within tissues. This disorder occurs in 30% of patients with underlying MM and renal involvement.[17] Amyloid fibrils may deposit within any organ but most commonly affect the kidneys, heart, liver, and peripheral nervous system.

Patients often present with fatigue, weight loss, and nephrotic syndrome. The clinical characteristics of patients with biopsy-proven renal amyloidosis were described in a retrospective review of 84 patients at the Mayo Clinic.[23] The median age at diagnosis was 61 years, and 62% of patients were men. The median serum creatinine level on presentation was 1.1 mg/dL. The majority of patients had nephrotic syndrome (86%) with a median 24-hour protein loss of 7 g/day. Renal replacement therapy was eventually required in 42% of patients, and median survival after the start of dialysis was less than 1 year. In general, cardiac involvement occurs in nearly a third of patients and portends a poor prognosis.

AL amyloid manifests as an amorphous hyaline substance within the mesangium, glomerular basement membranes, and vessel walls. Mesangial involvement may be diffuse or nodular. Amyloid stains positive for Congo red and reveals a characteristic apple-green birefringence under polarized light. Immunofluorescence staining reveals the underlying monotypic light chain, which has a λ:κ ratio of 6:1. Electron microscopy demonstrates nonbranching, randomly oriented 8- to 10-nm fibrils. Amyloid deposits may appear as subepithelial spikes along the basement membrane similar to those seen in membranous nephropathy.

OTHER DISORDERS IN MULTIPLE MYELOMA

Patients with MM are more susceptible to infections, and AKI may develop secondary to sepsis or nephrotoxic antiinfective drugs. Osteoclast-mediated bone destruction may result in hypercalcemia, which may manifest as AKI, interstitial nephritis, nephrogenic diabetes insipidus, or nephrolithiasis. Tubular damage from the light-chain deposits may also cause nephrogenic diabetes insipidus. Rarely, malignant plasma cells may directly invade the kidney and cause AKI.[24]

TREATMENT OF CAST NEPHROPATHY
General Measures

Volume resuscitation (100 to 150 mL/hr of normal or half-normal saline) to ensure optimum hemodynamic support and adequate urine output (≈3 L/day) are of critical importance in the initial management. On the basis of experimental evidence that furosemide promotes intratubular cast formation by increasing sodium delivery to the distal tubule, the use of loop diuretics should be avoided. Hypercalcemia should be aggressively treated because it can lead to renal vasoconstriction, volume depletion, and enhanced cast formation. It has been suggested that urinary alkalinization decreases cast formation by reducing the net positive charge of FLCs and the interaction with THP.[25] However, there is no clinical data supporting this approach. Given the risk of causing renal calcium precipitation in the setting of hypercalcemia, urinary alkalinization cannot be recommended. Colchicine was shown to reduce cast formation through decreasing THP secretion and binding in rats, but human studies of this approach have been disappointing.[26,27]

Chemotherapy and Stem Cell Transplantation

The key to treating myeloma cast nephropathy is rapid reduction in FLC concentrations. An early decrease in FLC levels is associated with the highest rate of renal recovery. In severe AKI due to cast nephropathy, a 60% reduction in FLC levels by day 21 after diagnosis is associated with renal recovery in 80% of cases.[28] Previous studies with conventional chemotherapy protocols demonstrated that high-dose dexamethasone rapidly reduced FLCs. Newer agents such as thalidomide and the proteasome inhibitor bortezomib also rapidly lower FLC concentrations; this approach has been referred to as "renoprotective chemotherapy."

Significant improvement in renal dysfunction has been reported for patients with MM treated with bortezomib-based regimens.[29-31] Reversal of renal dysfunction with bortezomib may be more frequent and rapid than with other agents, on the basis of observational analysis. No dose adjustment for renal function is necessary for bortezomib.

Thalidomide and lenalidomide are two related chemotherapeutic agents commonly used in the treatment of MM. Lenalidomide dose must be adjusted for renal dysfunction.[32] Thalidomide does not depend on glomerular filtration for clearance so a dose adjustment is not required for renal function status; however its use may predispose to hyperkalemia in the setting of renal failure.[33,34] Regimens with thalidomide or lenalidomide have shown superior effectiveness to traditional therapy with alkylating agents in terms of reversing renal failure in MM; these agents may be nearly as effective as bortezomib regimens.[35] Their effects are likely due to rapid lowering of serum FLC levels.

Hematopoietic stem cell transplantation (HCT) is an important and potentially curative therapy in MM; however, patient selection criteria are stringent, and significant kidney disease has traditionally excluded patients from transplantation. Studies have shown that HCT may be safe and effective in highly selected patients with renal failure.[36]

Extracorporeal Removal of Free Light Chains

Light chains are small molecular weight proteins. κ-Light chains usually circulate as monomers with a molecular weight of 22.5 kDa, whereas λ-light chains are typically dimeric with a molecular weight of 45 kDa.[37] Because of their size, there has been a keen interest in the use of extracorporeal therapy as a means of FLC removal.

Therapeutic Plasma Exchange. Several small trials initially suggested that therapeutic plasma exchange (TPE) was effective in rapidly lowering FLC concentrations and improving renal function. However, these studies were small, conducted in single centers, and therefore statistically underpowered. The largest randomized controlled trial of TPE did not demonstrate any benefit in patients with cast nephropathy.[38] This study assessed the benefit of five to seven TPE sessions in 104 patients (30% requiring dialysis) with presumed cast nephropathy (not all patients had biopsy confirmation). There was no difference in the two groups with respect to the composite outcome of death, dialysis, or reduced renal function at 6 months. This lack of benefit may be related to the volume of distribution of FLCs. On the basis of their molecular weights, 85% of light chains are confined to the extravascular space.[39] Therefore, a traditional 2-hour TPE session would be ineffective in removing significant amounts of FLCs because of the excessive rebound effect. Most of the previous trials were performed prior to the availability of bortezomib-containing regimens. In a study of 14 patients with presumed myeloma kidney treated with bortezomib and TPE, 12 had complete or partial renal response by 6 months; however there were no control patients.[40] Although there is still interest in TPE as a therapy for cast nephropathy, its routine use cannot be recommended on the basis of current evidence.

High-Cutoff Hemodialysis. Interest has developed in another method of extracorporeal removal of FLCs, high-cutoff hemodialysis (HCO-HD). In this technique, a hemofilter with a large pore size (45 kDa) and a surface area of 1.1 m² is used for extended periods in order to remove FLCs.

In a pilot trial, 5 patients with biopsy-proven cast nephropathy requiring dialysis were treated with dexamethasone, thalidomide, cyclophosphamide, and extended HCO-HD for 4 to 10 hours per day.[39] Three of the patients became dialysis independent after a mean of 16 dialysis treatments; all 3 patients received daily extended HCO-HD and showed response to chemotherapy. In the 2 "nonresponder" patients, chemotherapy had to be suspended because of complications, and rapid rebounds in the FLC concentrations occurred after dialysis. Therefore, response to chemotherapy is an essential component in treating cast nephropathy. There was no control group for comparison.

In an open-label study of 19 patients with biopsy-proven cast nephropathy and dialysis requiring AKI, treatment with HCO-HD with two filters in series was added to treatment with cyclophosphamide, thalidomide, doxorubicin, and dexamethasone.[41] Patients with relapsing disease received bortezomib. A total of 13 patients had response to chemotherapy, all of whom recovered renal function at a median of 4 weeks. Of the 6 patients in whom chemotherapy was interrupted, only 1 recovered renal function. The absence of a control group precludes determining that addition of HCO-HD is more beneficial in cast nephropathy than current renoprotective chemotherapy.

In the largest study of dialysis-dependent renal failure secondary to MM, 67 patients were treated with HCO-HD and chemotherapy.[42] Only 57% of patients had undergone renal biopsy, of which 87% were found to have cast nephropathy. Most patients (85%) received combination chemotherapy with dexamethasone and either bortezomib or thalidomide. The median number of HCO-HD sessions was 11, and all patients had extended (> 4-hour) treatments. Overall, 63% of the patients became dialysis independent. The factors that predicted renal recovery were the degree of FLC reduction at days 12 and 21, and the time to initiation of HCO-HD. Unfortunately, this trial also did not have a control group to allow assessment of the benefit of HCO-HD in comparison with renoprotective chemotherapy alone.

It is not known whether HCO-HD offers any *additional* benefit over current chemotherapeutic regimens. Randomized controlled trials proving the benefit of adding HCO-HD to current chemotherapy in patients with cast nephropathy will be necessary before its routine use can be recommended.

HEMATOPOIETIC STEM CELL TRANSPLANTATION

Acute kidney injury and CKD are common complications of HCT and their etiologies are often multifactorial (Table 42.2). Patients undergoing HCT are at risk for kidney injury from preexisting kidney disease, conditioning chemotherapy, irradiation, antimicrobials, infections, sinusoidal obstruction syndrome (SOS), transplantation-associated thrombotic microangiopathy (TA-TMA), and graft-versus-host disease (GVHD).[43,44] Both AKI and CKD can increase short- and long-term morbidity and mortality.[45] Further complications of HCT, such as fluid imbalances, electrolyte abnormalities, glomerular disease, and hypertension, may occur independent of, or concomitant with, reductions in the GFR.

The purpose of HCT is to allow otherwise lethal doses of chemoradiotherapy followed by engraftment of stem or progenitor cells for bone marrow recovery. Stem and progenitor cells can be harvested from bone marrow, peripheral blood, or umbilical cord blood. Cells can be obtained either from the patient (autologous) or from related or unrelated donors (allogeneic). In conventional myeloablative HCT,

Table 42.2 Renal Syndromes Associated with Hematopoietic Cell Transplantation

Immediate	Tumor lysis syndrome
	Marrow infusion syndrome
Early	Sinusoidal obstruction syndrome
	Acute tubular necrosis (ischemic/nephrotoxic)
	Sepsis/shock
	Tubulointerstitial nephritis
	Graft-versus-host disease
Late	Transplantation-associated microangiopathy
	Calcineurin toxicity
	Radiation-associated kidney injury
	Graft-versus-host disease

high-dose chemotherapy and radiotherapy are given to eradicate the disease and the bone marrow, followed by reconstitution of the marrow with infusion of stem or progenitor cells. Myeloablative HCT is quite toxic, so sicker and older patients are often excluded from transplant candidacy. Therefore, nonmyeloablative regimens have been devised that are less toxic and depend on a "graft-versus-tumor" effect for therapeutic efficacy.

ACUTE KIDNEY INJURY

The incidence and clinical course of AKI has been described best in allogeneic HCT. In one study, AKI occurred in 53% of patients, of which half required dialysis, with a mortality rate of 84% at 2 months.[46] In later studies in patients undergoing allogeneic HCT, the incidence of moderate to severe AKI (defined as a doubling of the baseline serum creatinine value) ranged from 36% to 78%, with dialysis required in 21% to 33%.[47-49] The mortality in patients receiving dialysis was 78% to 90%.

The incidence of AKI with autologous HCT is less common.[47] In a series of patients with breast cancer, autologous HCT was associated with the development of moderate to severe AKI in 21% of patients and a mortality rate of 18%. One reason given for the lower incidence of AKI with autologous HCT is the avoidance of calcineurin inhibitors for prevention of the GVHD seen with allogeneic HCT.[50]

Nonmyeloablative HCT is also associated with a lower incidence of AKI.[51] In a study of patients undergoing nonablative HCT, the cumulative incidence of AKI at 4 months (defined as a doubling of the baseline creatinine value) was 40.4%, and dialysis was necessary in only 4.4% of patients. In contrast to myeloablative HCT, AKI in these patients was more commonly associated with the use of calcineurin inhibitors, whereas SOS was uncommon. The timing of AKI was also different. In contrast to myeloablative HCT, during which AKI typically develops in the first 3 weeks, development of AKI during nonmyeloablative HCT was distributed over the first 3 months. This difference is attributed to the milder conditioning regimen used with nonmyeloablative HCT.

The reported risk of needing acute dialysis after HCT-associated AKI varies widely. Later literature cites a risk of dialysis ranging from 0% to 30%,[51-57] and the risk is higher with myeloablative therapy than with reduced-intensity therapy.[58] However, there is less uncertainty about the outcome of patients who require acute renal replacement therapy, because almost all studies report that acute dialysis in this population is associated with an extremely high mortality rate, often from 80% to approaching 100%.[44,51-54,57,59,60]

CHRONIC KIDNEY DISEASE

As in the AKI literature, studies reporting the risk of CKD after HCT are difficult to compare because the definitions of CKD are not consistent, the populations studied are often heterogeneous, and follow-up times vary.[61] Although several disease processes, such as TA-TMA, radiation nephritis, nephrotic syndrome, chronic GVHD, and BK virus nephropathy, have been associated with CKD after HCT, much of the long-term kidney injury in patients undergoing HCT remains unexplained.[62] GVHD may lead to CKD via direct T-cell damage, via cytokine-induced inflammation, or through concomitant calcineurin therapy.[63]

A meta-analysis reviewed the published data on CKD after HCT through 2006.[61] Patients in the studies had survived to at least 100 days; only 18% of the identified studies were prospective. Kidney function was assessed with creatinine-based, radioisotope, or inulin measurements of GFR. The overall prevalence of CKD was 16.6% (range, 3.6% to 89%) and prevalences were similar in those receiving autologous and allogeneic transplants, although the allogeneic transplant recipients had a greater decrease in kidney function. The risk of CKD was noted to be higher in adults than children. At 2 years, overall estimated GFR decreased from a mean of 102 mL/min/1.73 m^2 before transplantation to 77 mL/min/1.73 m^2. Risk factors for CKD included a history of AKI, chronic GVHD, long-term cyclosporine use, and total-body irradiation (TBI). In comparison with the community population, GFR decreased more rapidly in the HCT recipients (0.75 mL/min/1.73 m^2 per year vs. 12-25 mL/min/1.73 m^2 per year after HCT) and the risk of CKD after HCT was almost double that reported in the age-matched Framingham Study cohort (9.4% vs. 16.6%).

SPECIFIC KIDNEY DISEASES AFTER HEMATOPOIETIC STEM CELL TRANSPLANTATION

MARROW INFUSION SYNDROME

Within the first few days of transplantation, AKI may develop from hemoglobinuria caused by infusion of hemolyzed red blood cells. Preservation of stem cells with dimethyl sulfoxide (DMSO) will cause hemolysis of red blood cells present in the stored specimen, and subsequent infusion will result in hemoglobinuria. Three mechanisms are involved in the pathogenesis of hemoglobinuric AKI: renal vasoconstriction, direct cytotoxicity of hemoglobin, and intratubular cast formation. By scavenging nitric oxide and stimulating the release of endothelin and thromboxane, hemoglobin causes renal vasoconstriction. Hemoglobin is also toxic to renal tubular epithelial cells either directly or through release of iron and by generation of reactive oxygen species.[64] Intratubular cast formation occludes urinary flow, thereby decreasing GFR, and prolongs cellular exposure to the harmful effects of hemoglobin.

SINUSOIDAL OCCLUSION SYNDROME

Another renal syndrome typically occurs between 10 and 21 days after transplantation and is associated with the development of SOS (formerly referred to as *venoocclusive disease of the liver*).[65] It is characterized by tender hepatomegaly, fluid retention with ascites formation, and jaundice. It is the result of fibrous narrowing of small hepatic venules and sinusoids triggered by the pretransplantation cytoreductive regimen and is more common after allogeneic than autologous HCT. The development of SOS is most commonly associated with pretreatment with cyclophosphamide, busulfan, and/or TBI.[66] The AKI is similar in appearance to hepatorenal syndrome. Patients have hyperdynamic vital signs along with hyponatremia, oliguria, and low urinary sodium concentration. The urinalysis shows minimal proteinuria and muddy brown granular casts as a result of bile salts and bilirubin in the urine. The fluid retention is usually resistant to diuretics, and spontaneous recovery is rare. Risk factors for the development of AKI include weight gain, hyperbilirubinemia, use of amphotericin B, vancomycin, or acyclovir, and a baseline serum creatinine level greater than 0.7 mg/dL. The development of AKI adversely affects survival. In patients who require dialysis, the mortality rate approaches 80%. Although SOS can be diagnosed by either direct measurement of sinusoidal pressures or liver biopsy, these procedures are difficult or hazardous in patients who have undergone HCT. Therefore the diagnosis of SOS is usually made on clinical criteria. However, studies have shown that clinical criteria alone may not be sufficient to recognize or exclude a diagnosis of SOS.[67] Results of small trials using infusions of prostaglandin E, pentoxifylline, low-dose heparin, and defibrotide (an antithrombotic and fibrinolytic agent) have shown promise in the prevention and treatment of SOS.[68-70] Smaller trials with defibrotide, an antithrombotic and fibrinolytic agent, have shown benefit in patients with SOS.[71,72] However, their use is not commonplace because of the associated risk of bleeding.

TRANSPLANTATION-ASSOCIATED THROMBOTIC MICROANGIOPATHY

TA-TMA is a pathologically defined entity characterized as endothelial damage leading to thickened glomerular and arteriolar vessels, the presence of fragmented red blood cells, thrombosis, and endothelial cell swelling.[73,74] It can lead to subclinical disease, AKI, or CKD after HCT.[62,75,76] Given the challenges of obtaining kidney tissue in the HCT population, two consensus guidelines have been published outlining clinical criteria for the diagnosis of TA-TMA.[77,78] Both guidelines require the presence of schistocytes on peripheral smear and an elevated lactate dehydrogenase concentration. The Blood and Marrow Transplant (BMT) Clinical Trials Network also includes AKI (doubling of serum creatinine level), unexplained central nervous system dysfunction, and a negative Coombs test result.[77] The International Guidelines from the European Group for Blood and Marrow Transplantation include thrombocytopenia, anemia, and a decreased haptoglobin level.[78] Diagnosing TA-TMA remains challenging and often requires a high index of suspicion, as supported by validation studies[79] and autopsy studies in which clinical criteria often do not correlate with histologic findings.

Whether TA-TMA is a distinct disease after HCT or merely a manifestation of other post-HCT complications, such as GVHD and infection, is a matter of ongoing debate.[80-83] However, the distinct histologic findings support the importance of endothelial cell damage, primarily in the renal vasculature, in the pathogenesis of TA-TMA. Although histologically similar, TA-TMA appears to be distinct from thrombotic thrombocytopenic purpura (TTP), in that patients with TA-TMA do not have markedly low levels of von Willebrand factor–cleaving protease ADAMTS13.[84-88] In some patients, HCT may unmask a previously undiagnosed genetic mutation in the alternate complement pathway, resulting in atypical hemolytic-uremic syndrome (HUS).[89] In that case, treatment with a monoclonal antibody that binds C5 complement protein and inhibits formation of the terminal attack complex (eculizumab) may be appropriate.[90]

Transplantation-associated thrombotic microangiopathy in the kidney may reflect direct injury to endothelial cells of the kidney by GVHD. Studies of patients with TA-TMA suggest that GVHD is a potential trigger for its development. The risk of TA-TMA diagnosed on renal pathology at autopsy was increased fourfold in patients with acute GVHD after transplantation. Endothelial injury in the kidney may be secondary to circulating inflammatory cytokines or may reflect direct injury to endothelial cells of the kidney by GVHD. Plasma markers of endothelial injury and coagulation activation are elevated in patients with acute GVHD after HCT, suggesting an association among endothelial injury, acute GVHD, and the subsequent development of TA-TMA.[91,92]

Treatment for TA-TMA remains challenging, and current studies have been limited by retrospective study designs and the inclusion of heterogeneous patient populations. Current options include adjustment of GVHD prophylaxis (especially either stopping or reducing dosage of calcineurin inhibitors), TPE, rituximab, and defibrotide.[77,79,93-95] Response rates for TPE are reported between 27% and 80% in uncontrolled studies,[96-102] but the procedure is not without risks.[103,104] In a prospective study of 112 patients who had undergone HCT, TA-TMA developed in 11. There was a 64% response rate in patients treated with both TPE and cyclosporine withdrawal.[98] In case reports, rituximab has been shown to have benefit.[86,92,105-109]

GRAFT-VERSUS-HOST DISEASE–RELATED CHRONIC KIDNEY DISEASE

CKD develops in many patients after HCT without evidence of TA-TMA or viral infection and has been labeled idiopathic CKD. Later data, however, suggest that CKD is due to acute or chronic GVHD, particularly in patients whose pre-HCT conditioning regimen did not include TBI.[63,110]

In a large retrospective study of 1635 HCT recipients, neither TBI nor cyclosporine use was associated with the development of CKD (defined as a GFR <60 mL/min/1.73 m^2) at 1 year after transplantation. A subgroup analysis of all patients receiving cyclosporine further supported the theory that GVHD, independent of calcineurin inhibitor therapy, raised the risk of CKD.[63]

TUMOR LYSIS SYNDROME

TLS is often a dramatic presentation of AKI in patients with malignancy.[111] It is characterized by the development of hyperphosphatemia, hypocalcemia, hyperuricemia, and hyperkalemia. TLS can occur spontaneously during the rapid growth phase of malignancies, such as bulky lymphoblastomas and Burkitt's and non-Burkitt's lymphomas, that have extremely rapid cell turnover rates.[112] More commonly it is seen when cytotoxic chemotherapy induces lysis of malignant cells in patients with large tumor burdens. The syndrome has developed in patients with non-Hodgkin's lymphoma, acute lymphoblastic leukemia, chronic myelogenous leukemia in blast crises, small cell lung cancer, and metastatic breast cancer.[113] Because of more potent chemotherapeutic agents, however, the frequency of TLS is rising among patients whose tumors were once rarely associated with the complication. In most patients the AKI is reversible after aggressive supportive therapy, including dialysis. Risk factors for the development of TLS are listed in Table 42.3.

Table 42.3	Risk Factors for Tumor Lysis Syndrome	
Tumor Histology	**Disease Features**	**Renal Function**
Burkitt's lymphoma	Bulky tumor	Chronic kidney disease
Lymphoblastic lymphoma/acute lymphocytic leukemia;	Elevated lactate dehydrogenase	Hypovolemia
Diffuse large cell lymphoma	Rapid turnover	Hyperuricemia
Acute leukemia	Elevated white blood cell count	Acute kidney injury pretreatment
	High sensitivity to therapy	Concomitant nephrotoxins

Table 42.4	Cairo-Bishop Classification of Tumor Lysis Syndrome (TLS)
Laboratory TLS Requires ≥2 of 4	Uric acid ≥8.0 mg/dL
	Potassium ≥6.0 mEq/L
	Phosphorus ≥4.6 mg/dL
	Calcium ≤7.0 mg/dL
Clinical TLS Laboratory TLS plus ≥1 of the following	Acute kidney injury (creatinine 1.5 × upper limit of normal)
	Cardiac arrhythmia
	Seizure, tetany, or other symptoms

From Cairo M, Bishop M. Tumor lysis syndrome: new therapeutic stategies and classification, Br J Haematol 127:3-11, 2004.

DEFINITIONS

Tumor lysis syndrome is classified as either a laboratory or a clinical entity (Table 42.4). Laboratory TLS requires the presence of two or more metabolic abnormalities (hyperuricemia, hyperkalemia, hyperphosphatemia, and hypocalcemia) and clinical disease is present when laboratory TLS is accompanied by AKI, seizures, cardiac arrhythmias, or death due to hyperkalemia or hypocalcemia.[114] For a diagnosis of TLS to be established, metabolic abnormalities should occur within 3 days before or up to 7 days after initiation of treatment.

PATHOPHYSIOLOGY

The pathophysiology of AKI associated with TLS is classically attributed to two main factors, preexisting volume depletion prior to the onset of kidney injury and the precipitation of uric acid and calcium phosphate complexes in the renal tubules and tissue.[115] Patients may be volume depleted either from anorexia or nausea and vomiting associated with the malignancy or from increased insensible losses due to fever or tachypnea.

Hyperuricemia either is present before treatment with chemotherapy or develops after therapy despite prophylaxis with allopurinol.[116] Uric acid is nearly completely ionized at physiologic pH but becomes progressively insoluble in the acidic environment of the renal tubules. Precipitation of uric acid causes intratubular obstruction, leading to increased renal vascular resistance and decreased GFR. Moreover, a granulomatous reaction to intraluminal uric acid crystals and necrosis of tubular epithelium can be found in biopsy specimens.

Keen interest has developed in the potential noncrystalline effects of uric acid in precipitating renal injury.[117,118] Mild elevations in serum uric acid have been found to predict AKI in patients receiving cisplatin. In addition, retrospective analysis of two large randomized studies of patients undergoing cardiac bypass surgery demonstrated that a preoperative or postoperative serum uric acid level greater than 7.5 mg/dL was associated with a twofold to fourfold increase in rate of AKI after adjustment for age, gender, and baseline creatinine. Proposed mechanisms of renal injury include vasoconstriction due to reduced nitric oxide production and stimulation of the renin angiotensin aldosterone axis as well as increased oxidative stress and inflammation via activation of nuclear factor-kappaB (NF-κB) and P38 mitogen–activated protein kinases (p38MAPKs).

Hyperphosphatemia and hypocalcemia also occur in TLS. In patients in whom hyperuricemia does not develop, AKI has been attributed to metastatic intrarenal calcification or acute nephrocalcinosis.[119] Tumor lysis with release of inorganic phosphate results in acute hypocalcemia and metastatic calcification, leading to AKI.

Therefore, AKI associated with TLS is the result of the combination of volume depletion in the presence of varying degrees of vasoconstriction, inflammation, urinary precipitation of uric acid in the renal tubules and parenchyma, and acute nephrocalcinosis from severe hyperphosphatemia. Because patients at risk for TLS often have intraabdominal lymphoma, urinary tract obstruction can be a contributing factor in the development of AKI.

TREATMENT

The optimal management of TLS reduces the risk of AKI and prevents development of symptomatic electrolyte abnormalities. Key components to management are ensuring a high urine output, reducing uric acid levels, and controlling serum phosphate levels. It is recommended that urine output be maintained at a rate of 2 mL/kg/hr by infusion of isotonic crystalloid solutions. The use of loop diuretics should be avoided because they acidify the urine and can lead to volume depletion. A consensus statement on the treatment of TLS was published by the American Society of Clinical Oncology in 2008.[120]

The treatment algorithm to prevent TLS is now based on risk stratification into low-risk versus medium/high-risk groups on the basis of tumor and clinical characteristics.[121] In patients at low risk of TLS, allopurinol is administered to inhibit uric acid formation. Through its metabolite oxypurinol, allopurinol inhibits xanthine oxidase and thereby blocks the conversion of hypoxanthine and xanthine to uric acid. During massive tumor lysis, uric acid excretion can still increase despite the administration of allopurinol, so intravenous hydration is still necessary to prevent AKI. Allopurinol and its metabolites are excreted in the urine, so the dose should be reduced in the patient with impaired renal function. Other limitations to allopurinol use include hypersensitivity reaction, drug interactions, and slow lowering of uric acid levels.

In the past, because uric acid is very soluble at physiologic pH, sodium bicarbonate was added to the intravenous fluid to achieve a urinary pH greater than 6.5. However, this therapy is associated with several potential side effects, and its use can no longer be recommended. The systemic alkalosis from alkali administration can aggravate hypocalcemia, resulting in tetany and seizures. An alkaline pH markedly decreases the urinary solubility of calcium phosphate and can precipitate phosphate nephropathy.

In medium- and high-risk patients, rasburicase (recombinant urate oxidase) should be started if evidence of TLS is present. This agent converts uric acid to water-soluble allantoin, thereby decreasing both serum uric acid levels and urinary uric acid excretion.[122] The use of rasburicase obviates the need for urinary alkalinization, but good urine flow with hydration should be maintained, given the probability of preexisting volume depletion. Its use reduced the area under the serial plasma uric acid concentration curve of 96-hour uric acid exposure in comparison with allopurinol.[123] In another study of 100 adult patients with aggressive non-Hodgkin's lymphoma, prophylactic rasburicase given 24 hours before chemotherapy lowered uric acid levels within 4 hours.[124] No patient had an increase in serum creatinine level or required dialysis. Rasburicase treatment should be avoided in patients with glucose-6-phosphate dehydrogenase deficiency because hydrogen peroxide, a breakdown product of uric acid, can cause methemoglobinemia and, in severe cases, hemolytic anemia.[125,126] Rasburicase is recommended as first-line treatment for patients at high risk for TLS. Because of cost considerations, there is no consensus on the use of rasburicase in low- to medium-risk patients.

CHEMOTHERAPEUTIC AGENTS

As various new agents to treat malignancy become available, the potential for an expanding list of substances causing nephrotoxic injury increases. Many chemotherapeutic agents have been reported to induce renal injury in case reports thus far.[127,128] In addition, several chemotherapy agents need dose adjustment for kidney dysfunction. Because serum creatinine levels are an unreliable marker of GFR, it is recommended that the estimated GFR (MDRD [Modification of Diet in Renal Disease Study] and Epi-CKD [Chronic Kidney Disease Epidemiology Collaboration] formulas) be used when drug doses are being adjusted (see Chapter 26). Agents associated with more established forms of nephrotoxicity are described here.

CISPLATIN

Nephrotoxicity is the most common dose-limiting side effect of cisplatin administration. The primary site for clearance of cisplatin is the kidney. The most common clinical scenario is the gradual onset of nonoliguric AKI; however, electrolyte wasting is seen, especially with high doses of cisplatin.[129] Apoptosis of renal proximal tubular cells is induced, resulting in wasting of electrolytes such as potassium, magnesium, calcium, and bicarbonate. A common electrolyte abnormality is hypomagnesemia, which often occurs with prolonged exposure to the drug.[130] The direct tubular toxicity associated with cisplatin is exacerbated in a low-chloride environment. In the intracellular compartment, chloride molecules are replaced with water molecules in the *cis*- position of cisplatin, forming hydroxyl radicals that injure the neutrophilic binding sites on DNA.[131,132] The decline in glomerular filtration associated with cisplatin toxicity usually occurs 3 to 5 days after the exposure. Doses of cisplatin higher than $50\ mg/m^2$ are sufficient to cause renal injury. The renal injury is typically reversible, but repeated doses of cisplatin in excess of $100\ mg/m^2$ may cause irreversible renal damage. Hydration with isotonic saline and avoidance of concomitant nephrotoxins are the most effective way to prevent cisplatin-induced nephrotoxicity. Amifostine has been shown to reduce cisplatin nephrotoxicity through promotion of better DNA repair and elimination of free radicals.[133,134] With the cessation of cisplatin therapy the majority of patients recover renal function. However, it has been reported that GFR is reduced on average 15% in patients followed long term for resolved AKI from cisplatin nephrotoxicity.[135]

Newer platinum agents such as carboplatin and oxaliplatin are less nephrotoxic than cisplatin and are alternate agents in patients with underlying kidney disease.[136,137] However, AKI and electrolyte disorders still occur with these agents.

IFOSFAMIDE

Ifosfamide is an alkylating drug that causes renal toxicity either directly or through a metabolite, chloroacetaldehyde, which directly damages tubular epithelial cells.[138] The renal injury occurs throughout the kidney, including the glomerulus, proximal and distal tubule, and interstitium. The proximal tubule is most seriously affected, causing wasting of electrolytes as with cisplatin. The degree of hypokalemia, hypophosphatemia, hypomagnesemia, and hyperchloremic acidosis experienced with ifosfamide toxicity can be severe. Patients can experience Fanconi's syndrome with hypophosphatemic rickets and osteomalacia, as well as nephrogenic diabetes insipidus.[139] A potential marker for ifosfamide nephrotoxicity is increased urinary β_2-microglobulin excretion.[140] Risk factors for ifosfamide nephrotoxicity include previous exposure to cisplatin, CKD, and a cumulative dose more than $84\ g/m^2$.[141,142] Data suggest that amifostine may have a protective role against ifosfamide as well as cisplatin nephrotoxicity.[143] Mesna is a synthetic sulfhydryl compound that detoxifies metabolites in the urine and is efficacious in preventing hemorrhagic cystitis, but it is ineffective in preventing tubular injury.[139,144] The majority of patients recover from ifosfamide-induced tubular injury; however, there are reports of long-term complications. Ifosfamide has been linked to chronic renal fibrosis with a decline in the GFR over time and in one case leading to end-stage kidney disease.[145,146] In pediatric literature the chronic and progressive nature of ifosfamide-induced renal toxicity is well documented.[147]

CYCLOPHOSPHAMIDE

Cyclophosphamide has been associated with hemorrhagic cystitis but not tubular injury. Hyponatremia resulting from increased antidiuretic hormone activity is the primary clinical abnormality associated with cyclophosphamide.[148] As with ifosfamide, the metabolites of cyclophosphamide can cause hemorrhagic cystitis and occasional AKI due to bladder outlet obstruction.

METHOTREXATE

Methotrexate (MTX)–induced AKI is caused by the precipitation of the drug and its more insoluble metabolite, 7-hydroxymethotrexate, in the tubular lumen.[149] At a pH lower than 5.5, MTX and its metabolite precipitate when their concentration exceeds 2×10^{-3} molar, whereas solubility increases with a urine pH of 7.[150] AKI occurs from intrarenal obstruction, direct tubular toxicity, and prerenal azotemia due to afferent arteriolar vasoconstriction. AKI is reported in 30% to 50% of patients treated with high-dose MTX ($>1g/m^2$). For the prevention of renal toxicity, hydration and high urine output are essential. Isotonic saline infusion and furosemide may be necessary to keep the urine output more than 1 mL/kg/hr. An increase in the clearance rate of MTX is seen when the urine pH is increased from 5.5 to 8.4, which can be accomplished with an isotonic solution containing bicarbonate.[151] Once AKI develops, the excretion of MTX is reduced, the systemic toxicity of MTX is increased, and treatment is mainly supportive. It may be necessary to remove the drug with dialysis. Hemodialysis, using high blood flow rates with a high-flux dialyzer, is an effective method of removing MTX.[152] High-dose leucovorin therapy can reduce the systemic toxicity associated with MTX and AKI.[153,154] In the majority of cases MTX-induced AKI resolves. Often the plasma creatinine peaks within 1 week and returns to baseline at 3 weeks.

BIOLOGIC AGENTS

Acute kidney injury is well described with the administration of interferon alfa and interleukin-2 (IL-2).[155,156] The AKI secondary to interferon alfa therapy is uncommon and is sometimes associated with massive proteinuria.[157] Renal biopsy in interferon alfa–associated AKI has revealed glomerular lesions including focal segmental glomerulosclerosis, minimal change disease, acute interstitial nephritis, and acute tubular necrosis.[158-161] The AKI can be reversed with cessation of the drug, although some patients may have CKD or require long-term dialysis. After recovery of the AKI proteinuria may persist, and patients with this condition should be monitored for progression of renal disease.

With IL-2–induced renal dysfunction a systemic capillary leak syndrome occurs, resulting in volume depletion, hypotension, and oliguric prerenal AKI.[162,163] Unlike interferon alfa, IL-2 decreases GFR in the majority of patients who receive the drug, and the incidence of AKI is high.[164] Proteinuria and pyuria reported in some cases of IL-2–induced AKI suggest that IL-2 might have a direct injurious effect on the kidneys.[162] The onset of IL-2–induced AKI usually occurs at 24 to 48 hours and is dose related. Antihypertensive agents should be withdrawn, and fluid resuscitation initiated. Administration of low-dose dopamine (2 μg/kg/min) may prevent the renal toxicity of IL-2, reversing oliguria and improving renal recovery time.[165]

ANTI-ANGIOGENIC AGENTS

Over the last several years a variety of chemotherapy agents have been developed to prevent angiogenesis as an antitumor effect (bevacizumab, sorafenib, sunitinib, vatalanib, and axitinib).

Bevacizumab is a monoclonal antibody against vascular endothelial growth factor (VEGF) that is associated with hypertension and proteinuria.[166,167] The mechanism of hypertension and proteinuria is thought to be the result of inhibition of VEGF-related micro-angiogenesis, and nitric oxide synthesis, leading to increased peripheral resistance and endothelial cell dysfunction.[168,169] The effects of anti-VEGF therapy on the development of hypertension were reviewed in a meta-analysis of seven trials. The relative risk for development of hypertension was threefold to sevenfold higher, depending on dose.[167] Proteinuria was also more common. Proteinuria is usually mild and reversible upon drug discontinuation. Nephrotic-range proteinuria is rare (1%-2%). Limited biopsies in these cases have revealed a variety of lesions, including immune-mediated focal proliferative glomerulonephritis, cryoglobulinemic glomerulonephritis, and collapsing glomerulopathy.[170,171]

Because the mechanism of hypertension may be related to the drug's antitumor effect, the development of hypertension may be used as a biomarker of responsiveness. Two retrospective studies showed that the development of hypertension was associated with improved cancer outcomes.[172,173] An expert panel from the National Institute of Cancer has proposed guidelines on the therapy of anti-VEGF therapy–induced hypertension.[174] These guidelines recommend treatment for sustained hypertension exceeding 140 mm Hg systolic/90 mm Hg diastolic. The panel did not recommend any specific agent, but if there is concurrent proteinuria, the use of an angiotensin-converting enzyme (ACE) inhibitor or an angiotensin receptor blocker (ARB) would be prudent.

CETUXIMAB

Cetuximab, a monoclonal antibody against the epidermal growth factor (EGF) receptor, is approved for use in metastatic colon cancer.[175] The primary renal abnormality associated with EGF receptor antagonists is renal magnesium wasting. EGF normally activates the renal magnesium channel in the apical membrane of the distal convoluted tubule to stimulate magnesium absorption.[176] The incidence of severe hypomagnesemia is 10% to 15%.[177]

MISCELLANEOUS AGENTS

CALCINEURIN INHIBITORS

The calcineurin inhibitors cyclosporin A (CsA) and tacrolimus are widely used as immunosuppressants in HCT to prevent GVHD. Both CsA and tacrolimus cause AKI. Nephrotoxicity is the result of direct afferent arteriolar vasoconstriction leading to a decrease in the glomerular filtration pressure and GFR. The vascular effect associated with CsA or tacrolimus is reversible with discontinuation of the drug. A dose reduction is sometimes enough to reverse the prerenal effect. Chronic nephrotoxicity is a potential complication with more prolonged use of the calcineurin inhibitors. Proteinuria, tubular dysfunction, arterial hypertension, and rising creatinine concentration are clinical findings consistent with long-term CsA or tacrolimus nephrotoxicity. It typically takes more than 6 months of therapy for the chronic changes to occur. Arteriolar damage, interstitial fibrosis, tubular atrophy, and glomerulosclerosis are found in renal biopsy specimens. The pathologic changes of the chronic nephrotoxicity are irreversible.[178-180] A rare complication of CsA and tacrolimus therapy is TMA. The mechanism of CsA- or tacrolimus-induced TMA is direct damage to the vascular endothelium in a dose-dependent fashion. With discontinuation of the drug, patients may have partial recovery.[181-183] Calcineurin inhibitors have also been associated with hyperkalemia, thought to be secondary to tubular resistance to aldosterone.[184]

BISPHOSPHONATES

Bisphosphonates are commonly used to manage hypercalcemia of malignancy and to reduce skeletal complications in patients with bone metastases and multiple myeloma. Bisphosphonates are excreted unchanged by the kidneys, and AKI has been reported in both animals and humans.

All three generations of bisphosphonates have been shown to cause kidney injury although it is more common with older agents. The most common pathologic finding on renal biopsy is acute tubular necrosis (ATN). One study reported biopsy-proven toxic ATN in six patients treated with zoledronate (Zometa), a potent bisphosphonate; renal function did improve with cessation of the drug but did not return to baseline levels.[185] Pamidronate has been shown to cause AKI as well as the nephrotic syndrome from a collapsing variant of focal segmental glomerulosclerosis.[186,187] The exact mechanism of bisphosphonate induced kidney injury is not known, but direct toxicity to the tubular epithelial cells is suspected. A newer agent, ibandronate, is highly protein-bound, a feature that reduces the risk of rapid influx of the drug into the tubular cells, thereby reducing the risk of renal toxicity. This property makes ibandronate useful in patients with renal failure in multiple myeloma.[188]

In 2007 the American Society of Clinical Oncology updated the guidelines for the use of bisphosphonates in patients with reduced GFR.[189] The guidelines recommend reduction of zoledronate dose in patients with mild to moderate CKD (estimated GFR [eGFR] 30 to 60 mL/min) and avoiding it in those whose eGFR is less than 30 mL/min. Pamidronate 90 mg is administered over 4 to 6 hours (rather than over 2 hours) in patients with advanced CKD (eGFR < 30 mL/min). A decrease in the initial dose is also recommended. Recently, the treatment of osteoporosis has been advanced even in patients with stage 4 CKD (eGFR 15-30 mL/min) with the use of denosumab, a monoclonal antibody antiresorptive agent that is not cleared by the kidney and that may be preferred to the use of oral bisphosphonates at reduced doses. Use of these drugs has been advocated for women at severe risk for fractures and mortality without evidence of hyperparathyroidism and metabolic bone disease (specifically adynamic bone disease). Experience with the use of drugs for these indications is currently still limited and should be considered only by experts in appropriate at-risk patients after thoughtful discussions of the risks and benefits.[190]

HYPERCALCEMIA OF MALIGNANCY

Malignancy is the most common cause of hypercalcemia in hospitalized patients. In general, hypercalcemia is a late finding when the cancer is very advanced and is associated with a poor prognosis. The major mechanisms involved in malignancy-associated hypercalcemia are (1) secretion of parathyroid hormone–related protein (PTHrP), which is the major mechanism for most cases of the condition known as humoral hypercalcemia of malignancy; (2) direct osteolytic metastases with release of local cytokines; and (3) secretion of 1,25-dihydroxy vitamin D (Table 42.5). Rarely do tumors secrete intact parathyroid hormone (PTH).[191]

Secretion of PTHrP by malignant tumors is the main cause of hypercalcemia in patients with nonmetastatic solid tumors (especially squamous cell carcinoma of the lung, and head and neck cancer) and some non-Hodgkin's lymphomas. It is rare in multiple myeloma.[192,193] PTHrP has a 13–amino acid N-terminal sequence homology with intact PTH, which enables it to bind to PTH receptors, stimulate cyclic adenosine monophosphate (cAMP) production, and mimic the actions of intact PTH. Both PTH and PTHrP stimulate bone turnover through the receptor of NF-κB (RANK) ligand (RANKL) signaling pathway. Binding to the PTH receptor present on osteoblasts increases cell activity and RANKL signaling, resulting in osteoclast proliferation and differentiation into mature, multinucleated cells.[194]

When tumor cells metastasize to bone, direct local osteolysis can occur, resulting in local bone destruction and hypercalcemia.[195] Local osteolysis contributes to hypercalcemia in multiple myeloma, breast, and prostate cancer as well as non–small cell carcinoma of the lung. Cancers metastatic to bone stimulate the production of a number of soluble osteoclast-activating factors, leading to bone resorption, including IL-1, IL-6, and tumor necrosis factor-α (TNF-α).

Some malignancies secrete an active form of vitamin D, resulting in hypercalcemia. This occurs in multiple myeloma,

Table 42.5 Hypercalcemia of Malignancy

Cancer	Frequency (%)	Mechanism
Lung	35	PTHrP
		Local osteolysis
Breast	25	PTHrP
		Local osteolysis
Head and neck	6	PTHrP
Renal	3	PTHrP
		Local osteolysis
Multiple myeloma	15	PTHrP (rare)
		Local osteolysis
		1,25-Dihydroxyvitamin D
Prostate	7	Local osteolysis
Lymphoma	15	1,25-Dihydroxyvitamin D
		PTHrP

PTHrP, Parathyroid hormone related protein.

Hodgkin's and non-Hodgkin's lymphoma, and, rarely, solid tumors.[196,197] Active vitamin D causes increased gastrointestinal absorption of calcium and is associated with decreased urinary excretion of calcium as well as increased renal phosphate reabsorption.

Hypercalcemia induces prerenal azotemia by causing nephrogenic diabetes insipidus, renal vasoconstriction, and intratubular calcium deposition.[198] When the serum calcium level exceeds 13 mg/dL, most patients have some degree of volume depletion. Volume repletion and a saline diuresis are essential to the therapy. Isotonic saline should be infused intravenously in large volumes to increase calcium excretion. Furosemide may be used to increase the calciuresis once volume depletion is corrected. However, the effectiveness of loop diuretics in reducing serum calcium levels has been questioned.[199] Thiazide diuretics should be avoided because they decrease urinary calcium excretion.

Bisphosphonates, pyrophosphate analogs with a high affinity for hydroxyapatite, may be necessary to control the serum calcium in severe cases.[200,201] Pamidronate and clodronate, two second-generation bisphosphonates, are commonly used preparations.[202] Pamidronate can be given as a single intravenous dose of 30 to 90 mg and may normalize the calcium for several weeks. However, its onset is somewhat delayed with a mean time to achieve normocalcemia of 4 days. Therefore, other means of lowering the calcium level must be implemented in the immediate period.

Calcitonin, derived from the thyroid C cell, inhibits osteoclast activity. The onset of action of calcitonin is rapid but with a short half-life and is usually not given as a sole therapy, often being combined with pamidronate.[203] Tachyphylaxis to calcitonin is frequently seen at 48 hours as a result of downregulation of the calcitonin receptor. Concomitant administration of glucocorticoids can prolong calcitonin's effective duration of action.[204]

Plicamycin (mithramycin), an inhibitor of RNA synthesis, impairs osteoclast activity. It is an effective means to acutely lower serum calcium. However, the multiple toxicities associated with plicamycin have made its use uncommon.

Glucocorticoids are also effective in the therapy of hypercalcemia in patients with hematologic malignancies or multiple myeloma. In these cases, glucocorticoids inhibit osteoclastic bone resorption by decreasing tumor production of locally active cytokines.

A later addition to agents used to treat hypercalcemia of malignancy is denosumab. It is a humanized monoclonal antibody directed against RANKL that thereby decreases osteoclast differentiation and proliferation.[205] Denosumab has been effective in lowering calcium levels in breast and prostate cancer as well as multiple myeloma.

Hemodialysis with a low-calcium bath is the preferred method of reducing serum calcium levels in the patient with a severely depressed GFR.

RADIATION-ASSOCIATED KIDNEY INJURY

Ionizing radiation was first used to treat breast cancer in 1896, a year after the discovery of x-rays. Since that time, it has become an increasingly utilized modality in the treatment of malignant and benign conditions alike. For almost as long, it has been known that irradiation of normal tissue can have toxic effects. Modern-day radiation therapy seeks to balance the curative potential of ionizing radiation with the potentially serious adverse effects on normal tissue.

Previously, the kidneys were believed to be very radiation-resistant organs and the true renal sensitivity to ionizing radiation was not fully appreciated.[206] Today, however, the kidney is often regarded as the dose-limiting organ for TBI in many gynecologic cancers, gastrointestinal cancers, sarcomas, and lymphomas.

PATHOGENESIS

The pathogenesis of radiation-associated kidney injury is poorly understood in humans. Much of the published research focuses on long-term clinical outcomes of patients with CKD who have received irradiation in the past. Few studies focus on the actual mechanism of injury to the kidney, and those that do have primarily been conducted in animals.

Radiation causes cellular damage through direct and indirect mechanisms. One third of cellular radiation damage is caused by direct ionization of DNA, leading to double-strand breaks. Two thirds of damage is indirect, being caused by a combination of free electrons released when ionizing radiation strikes an intracellular molecule and intracellular free radicals interacting with DNA. The result of both direct and indirect damage is aberrations in cellular DNA. The pattern of injury in the kidney is a combination of both tubular and glomerular lesions.[207-209] The tubulointerstitium develops fibrosis and atrophy. Radiation-damaged glomeruli exhibit basement membrane duplication and vascular changes, including capillary loop thickening with subendothelial expansion.[208] Glomerulosclerosis tends to increase in severity from the cortex to the medulla and is accelerated with increased dose.

In addition to the early changes, characteristic late findings include loss of renal mass and volume, sclerosed intralobular and arcuate arteries, and associated interstitial fibrosis. Late endothelial damage in the small blood vessels results in fibrin deposition, platelet aggregation, and red blood cell injury.[210]

EPIDEMIOLOGY

Radiation-associated kidney injury is uncommon even in patients receiving large doses of radiation to one or both kidneys. In a large cohort of patients who received more than 25 Gray (Gy) to both kidneys, only 20% of the subjects experienced renal adverse effects.[211] Other series report a wide range of kidney injury, depending on patient and treatment-related factors.[212-217] Rates of kidney injury can be as high as 71% to 76% in patients with ovarian cancer receiving abdominal irradiation and cisplatin but can be significantly lower for patients receiving no chemotherapy and/or a low dose of radiation.

TOTAL-BODY IRRADIATION AND TRANSPLANTATION

TBI has been used to prepare both pediatric and adult patients for HCT. Radiation-associated injury can occur at a much lower dose during TBI than bilateral whole-kidney irradiation.[218-227] This observation is attributed to the fact that radiation for HCT is given in higher dose per fraction, which does not allow the normal tissue to undergo appropriate DNA repair. Published case series report rates of renal toxicity to be anywhere from 0 to 46.7% in children and adults, depending on dose and dose rate.[228,229] When studies with patients of all ages were included, dose rate, dose, and use of fludarabine chemotherapy were significant factors in the incidence of renal adverse effects.[230]

Several writers describe radiation nephropathy following irradiation for HCT as a separate and distinct clinical syndrome. It tends to occur in a shorter time course than chronic forms of radiation-associated kidney injury and can occur at much lower doses of radiation. Severe cases can mimic the presentation of hemolytic-uremic syndrome, and hypertension is more consistently present than with radiation nephropathy from other causes.[231]

CLINICAL PRESENTATION

Luxton and Kunkler first characterized the four clinical syndromes produced by radiation damage to the kidneys in the 1950s while studying the effects of abdominal irradiation for seminomas.[232]

HISTORY

Radiation-associated kidney injury has a long latency period. With the exception of patients who undergo a HCT, there is no acute form that manifests during or shortly after radiation therapy. Patients do not experience signs of kidney dysfunction until at least 6 months after irradiation, and for many patients it may take several years to progress to overt renal dysfunction.[233,234]

Common symptoms of radiation-associated kidney injury include edema, fluid retention, increased weight, and malaise. Additionally, symptoms can overlap with those of other renal diseases such as malignant hypertension (headaches, vomiting, and blurry vision) and other end-organ damage (dyspnea, confusion, and coma). It is important to recognize that these symptoms in themselves do not differentiate radiation nephropathy from many other causes of renal failure.

LABORATORY FINDINGS

The complete blood count may reveal a microangiopathic hemolytic anemia with schistocytes on the peripheral smear. Thrombocytopenia is also present.[235]

Urinalysis typically demonstrates proteinuria, granular casts, and microscopic hematuria. Although present, proteinuria usually does not reach nephrotic-range levels. These findings are not typically present until 6 months or more after irradiation and may increase in severity as time progresses and symptoms begin to become more clinically evident.

There are no specific radiographic findings for radiation-associated kidney injury. Computed tomography (CT) and magnetic resonance imaging may show progressive kidney atrophy beginning 6 months to 1 year after irradiation with the possibility of asymmetric contrast uptake if only one kidney was in the target field. Technetium Tc 99m-labeled diethylenetriaminepentaacetic acid (^{99m}Tc-DTPA) renography demonstrates decreased glomerular function and Tc 99m-labeled dimercaptosuccinic acid (^{99m}Tc-DMSA) renography shows decreased tubular function. Iodohippurate sodium iodine-131 scintigraphy will likely show a perfusion defect.

DIAGNOSIS

The diagnosis of radiation nephropathy is made clinically through identification of a syndrome of progressive CKD in a patient with cancer who received irradiation to the total body, spine, abdomen, or pelvis. A thorough history and physical examination should be performed, and the clinician should have a strong index of suspicion in patients with a history of radiation therapy. It is important to contact the radiation oncologist who delivered the radiation to determine what dose of radiation the kidneys received. A kidney biopsy does not necessarily need to be performed. Many of the histopathologic findings in radiation nephropathy are nonspecific and common to a large host of other causes of CKD; however, kidney biopsy may demonstrate thrombotic microangiopathy. Unless a biopsy needs to be performed for another indication, the added diagnostic information is often not worth the cost and the potential risk to the patient.

TREATMENT

Patients who receive drugs inhibiting the renin angiotensin aldosterone system (RAAS) after exposure to radiation have a lower incidence of radiation-associated kidney injury.[236,237] This protective effect was first shown with the ACE inhibitor captopril but has now been shown with other ACE inhibitors and ARBs.[238-244] One small randomized trial suggested that a protective effect in patients who receive HCT, though this effect was not statistically significant (15% incidence of nephropathy or HUS for placebo vs. 3.7% for captopril; $P = 0.1$).

Blockade of the RAAS is also useful once radiation-induced injury has developed. Various studies have shown ACE inhibitors to have beneficial effects on the course of the disease. As opposed to treatment prior to the development of clinical disease, the use of ARBs does not appear to be effective. It is unclear why this discrepancy between ACE inhibitors and ARBs exists, although it may be related to the extent of blood pressure control.

PROGNOSIS

The prognosis for patients in whom radiation-associated kidney injury develops is generally poor. Once kidney injury caused by radiation therapy becomes clinically evident it usually continues to progress. The time course of progression is somewhat variable, and many patients can remain stable for years but others show rapid decompensation. A case-control study of patients who had end-stage kidney disease after irradiation for HCT showed that they had poorer survival than controls with no history of irradiation.[245]

LEUKEMIA AND LYMPHOMA

The development of kidney disease is common in patients with lymphoma and leukemia. As with all hospitalized patients, those with lymphoma and leukemia are at risk for development of AKI due to hypotension, sepsis, or administration of radiocontrast, antifungal, or antibacterial agents. With the presence of cancer, renal injury can also result from chemotherapy, immunosuppressive drugs, HCT, or TLS. Furthermore, patients are at risk for renal syndromes specific to the presence of lymphoma or leukemia. Various types of paraneoplastic glomerulonephritides are associated with lymphoma and leukemia and are described elsewhere in the chapter. This section focuses on infiltrative diseases of the kidney.

LYMPHOMA
BACKGROUND

Although a variety of cancers can metastasize to the kidneys and invade the parenchyma, the most common malignancies that do so are lymphomas and leukemia. The true incidence of renal involvement is unknown because it is usually a silent disease and only occasionally causes renal failure. Autopsy studies suggest that renal involvement occurs in 90% of patients with lymphoma whereas radiographic evidence sets the figure significantly lower.[246]

CLINICAL FEATURES

Renal involvement in lymphoma is often clinically silent so patients can present with slowly progressive CKD attributed to other etiologies. Therefore a high index of suspicion is needed to make a diagnosis. Patients may present with AKI but this presentation is rare and is most commonly seen in highly malignant and disseminated disease.[247-250] Other presentations include proteinuria in both the nephrotic and nonnephrotic range, as well as a variety of glomerular lesions, such as pauci-immune crescentic glomerulonephritis.[251] Patients may also present with flank pain and hematuria.

The cause of impaired renal function from lymphomatous infiltration is poorly understood. On the basis of biopsy series, patients who present with AKI have predominantly bilateral interstitial infiltration of the kidneys with lymphoma cells and uniformly are found to have increased renal size on radiographic imaging.[252] These findings suggest that increased interstitial pressure results in reduced intrarenal blood flow with subsequent renal tubular injury. Patients who present with proteinuria, on the other hand, often have intraglomerular infiltration with lymphoma.[252] It is not known how proteinuria develops in these cases, but the local release of permeability factors and cytokines has been suggested.[253,254]

DIAGNOSIS

The diagnosis of kidney disease resulting from lymphomatous infiltration is necessarily one of exclusion because more common explanations are often present. The diagnosis may be suspected from clinical features and imaging studies. Renal ultrasonography may reveal diffusely enlarged kidneys, sometimes with multiple focal lesions. However, most times radiology is unrevealing. In a study of 668 consecutive patients with lymphoproliferative disease who underwent diagnostic CT, only 3% with non-Hodgkin's lymphoma were found to have kidney abnormalities.[255] Both diffuse enlargement and solitary lesions were detected. This discrepancy between radiologic and autopsy/histopathologic results may be due to the fact that renal involvement is often indolent and detectable only on histopathologic examination. Owing to increased metabolic activity within lymphomatous deposits, positron emission tomography may be a more sensitive imaging technique.[256,257] Although definitive diagnosis depends on renal biopsy, this procedure often is impossible because of the presence of contraindications. In such cases the following criteria support the diagnosis of kidney disease due to lymphomatous infiltration: (1) renal enlargement without obstruction, (2) absence of other causes of kidney disease, and (3) rapid improvement of kidney function after radiotherapy or systemic chemotherapy.

TREATMENT

The treatment of lymphomatous involvement of the kidney is directed at the underlying malignancy. There are numerous case reports of improvement in renal function after initiation of antitumor therapy. In indolent malignant disease that is usually treated by observation alone, kidney involvement is an indication for starting systemic therapy.

CYTOTOXIC NEPHROPATHY/ HEMOPHAGOCYTIC SYNDROME
BACKGROUND

Hemophagocytic syndrome (HPS) is a reactive disorder that results from intense macrophage activation and cytokine release.[258,259] It is characterized by histiocytic proliferation, hemophagocytosis, fever, hypotension, hepatosplenomegaly, generalized lymphadenopathy, and hypofibrinogenemia. It is the result of an intense cytokine storm similar to the systemic inflammatory response syndrome seen in patients with severe sepsis. HPS was first described as a familial disorder of immune dysfunction in children. It is inherited in an autosomal recessive pattern with an estimated incidence of 1 per 50,000 live births.[260,261] Familial HPS is a fatal disease if untreated with a mean survival rate of 2 months. It typically manifests in infancy or early adolescence and can be triggered by infection.

It is now recognized that there are numerous forms of secondary HPS that can develop in a variety of diseases, including malignant lymphoma, juvenile rheumatoid arthritis, and severe bacterial and viral infections, and in patients receiving prolonged parenteral nutrition with soluble lipids.[262]

CLINICAL FEATURES

The clinical presentation of HPS is nonspecific and can be confused with sepsis, given their overlapping features. The most common symptoms are fever, hepatosplenomegaly, and cytopenias.[263] Other findings include liver dysfunction (50%-90%), coagulopathy with hypofibrinogenemia, and neurologic dysfunction (33%). Less commonly patients can have diffuse lymphadenopathy, jaundice, rash, respiratory failure, and AKI (16%). Histopathologic examination of tissue reveals diffuse accumulation of lymphocytes and macrophages with occasional hemophagocytosis. There have been reports of HPS in association with occult peripheral T-cell lymphomas causing severe AKI.[264,264a] Renal biopsy specimens are characterized by an unusually severe degree of interstitial edema with limited interstitial cellular infiltrate. Natural killer (NK) cells tend to be low, whereas a number of cytokines, including interferon-α, soluble interleukin-2 receptor, TNF-α, interleukin-6, and macrophage colony-stimulating factor are upregulated.

DIAGNOSIS

Diagnosis should be suspected in any patient with malignant lymphoma in whom unexplained multiple-organ dysfunction including AKI develops. Diagnostic criteria for diagnosis of familial HPS were first developed in 1991 and later modified in 2004.[263] However, many of the criteria have poor specificity for differentiating HPS from malignant lymphoma. Fever, splenomegaly, anemia, thrombocytopenia, and hypofibrinogenemia are common to both. Therefore, bone marrow aspiration may be required for definitive diagnosis.

TREATMENT

In the past, treatment of familial HPS included cytotoxic agents, intravenous immunoglobulin (IVIG), TPE, and HCT. It is not clear whether such regimens are effective in secondary cases of HPS due to lymphoma. Current standard of care consists of a course of dexamethasone and etoposide in diminishing dosages.[259] Therapy should be started even in the presence of organ dysfunction or infection. Etoposide dose should be adjusted for impaired kidney or liver function.

LEUKEMIA

BACKGROUND

Leukemia cells can infiltrate any organ, and the kidneys are the most frequent extramedullary site of infiltration. Autopsy studies reveal that 60% to 90% of patients have renal involvement.[265] On biopsy cells are usually found to be located in the renal interstitium, although occasional glomerular lesions are noted.[266] Increased interstitial pressure leads to vascular and tubular compression and subsequent tubular injury. Occasional nodular lesions are found but they are more common with lymphoma.

CLINICAL FEATURES

Leukemic infiltration of the kidneys is often an indolent and clinically silent disease. Most often it is incidentally noted after autopsy or by detection of renal enlargement on ultrasound or CT scan. Although leukemic infiltration is uncommon, many cases of AKI attributable to it have been described.[267-269] Patients may also experience hematuria or proteinuria. Occasionally renal enlargement is accompanied by flank pain or fullness. AKI can develop from leukostasis in patients with significantly elevated white blood cell counts. Leukemic cells occlude the peritubular and glomerular capillaries, thereby decreasing GFR. Patients may be oliguric but their renal function often improves with therapeutic leukapheresis or chemotherapy. Leukostasis has been described in both acute and chronic leukemia. There are also reports of patients with chronic lymphocytic leukemia in whom AKI develops from leukemic infiltration and who are infected with polyomavirus (BK).[270] Urine from patients demonstrates viral inclusions in tubule cells ("decoy" cells) and blood is positive for BK viral DNA. Therefore, in patients with leukemia and AKI considered due to leukemic infiltration, evidence for coexisting BK virus infection should be sought.

DIAGNOSIS

The diagnosis of leukemic infiltration as a cause of AKI requires a high level of vigilance because it is often clinically silent and leukemic patients usually have multiple alternative explanations for renal injury. A presumptive diagnosis can be made if there is no other obvious cause of AKI, bilateral renal enlargement is demonstrated radiographically, and there is prompt improvement in renal function after chemotherapy. Screening for leukemic infiltration with radiographic imaging is not appropriate. In a study of 668 consecutive patients with lymphoproliferative disease who underwent diagnostic CT, only 5% with leukemia were found to have kidney abnormalities.[256] As with lymphoma, this discrepancy between radiologic and autopsy/histopathologic results may be due to the fact that renal involvement is often indolent and detectable only on histopathologic examination.

TREATMENT

Treatment is directed by the type of leukemia. Although some patients do not recover, renal function does improve in the majority of cases as the leukemia responds to systemic treatment.

PARANEOPLASTIC GLOMERULAR DISEASES

Glomerulonephritis, usually manifesting as nephrotic syndrome, is associated with the presence of various types of cancer and GVHD (Table 42.6). The strongest association is with membranous nephropathy and solid tumors (lung, colon, breast, and prostate).[271] In a cohort study of 240 patients with membranous nephropathy, 24 had cancer at the time of renal biopsy or within 1 year.[272] In comparison with the incidence in the general population, the incidence of cancer was significantly higher in this cohort (standardized incidence ratios of 9.8 and 12.3 for men and women, respectively). At the time of diagnosis, clinical presentations

Table 42.6 Glomerulonephritis Associated with Malignancy

Membranous glomerulonephritis:
    Breast cancer
    Lung cancer
    Colon cancer
    Prostate cancer
    Graft-versus-host disease
Minimal change disease:
    Hodgkin's lymphoma
    Non-Hodgkin's lymphoma
    Graft-versus-host disease
Case reports
    Immunoglobulin A nephritis
    Antineutrophil cytoplasmic antibody vasculitis
    Focal segmental glomerulosclerosis

did not differ between patients with cancer-associated and those with idiopathic membranous nephropathies. Given this association, it is recommended that any patient older than 40 years with idiopathic membranous glomerulonephritis undergo cancer screening as recommended by the American Cancer Society guidelines. The mechanism of the paraneoplastic syndrome is unknown, although it may involve in situ immune complex formation and complement activation.[273,274]

There also appears to be a strong association between Hodgkin's lymphoma and minimal change disease.[275-277] The nephrotic syndrome occurs early, often preceding the diagnosis of lymphoma by several months. It also rapidly disappears after effective treatment of the lymphoma.

A variety of other glomerular diseases, such as focal sclerosis, membranoproliferative glomerulonephritis, IgA nephropathy, and antineutrophil cytoplasmic antibody (ANCA)–associated vasculitis, have been described in patients with cancer.[271,278] In a retrospective case-control study of 200 consecutive patients with ANCA-associated vasculitis, the patients with ANCA disease had a higher risk of malignancy than age- and gender-matched controls (relative risk, 6.02).[279] However, most of these associations form the basis of case reports or case series. Given the high prevalence of cancer in the general population and the low incidence of glomerulonephritis, it is difficult to prove any true cause-and-effect relationship.

GVHD has also been associated with glomerulonephritis manifesting as the nephrotic syndrome. Membranous nephropathy is the most common glomerular lesion reported and often occurs after withdrawal of cyclosporine. Minimal change disease and IgA nephropathy have also been reported. In most cases there was favorable response to immunosuppressive therapy with improvement in the nephrotic-range proteinuria.[280-283]

RENAL INFECTIONS

Patients with cancer are at increased risk for infection because of either direct effects of the malignancy or adverse effects of therapy. Several infections associated with cancer may specifically involve the kidneys.

RENAL CANDIDIASIS

Mucosal ulceration and long-dwelling intravascular catheters are major risk factors for invasion of the bloodstream by *Candida* species. Other important risk factors are prolonged hospitalization, prior exposure to antimicrobial agents, corticosteroid therapy, the postoperative state, surgical wounds, long-term indwelling urinary catheters, and underlying malignancy. The kidneys are particularly vulnerable to candidal invasion. The presence of hyphae in the urine does not have diagnostic significance, although the absence of pyuria does not rule out a diagnosis of renal candidiasis, especially in the severely neutropenic patient. Therefore, identification of *Candida* on urine culture in the septicemic patient is considered proof of renal candidiasis.[284] The *Candida* organisms progressively penetrate the renal parenchyma, forming hyphae and microabscesses especially in the cortical regions. Involvement of renal vasculature may result in renal infarction and papillary necrosis. Penetration of the organisms into the renal tubules may cause multiple sites of tubular obstruction or the formation of large aggregates of fungi within the collecting system in the form of fungal balls or bezoars.[285] Obstruction should be suspected in the presence of flank pain and microscopic hematuria. *Candida* species differ in virulence capacity to involve the kidneys. *Candida albicans* and *Candida tropicalis* have the greatest propensity to cause widespread metastatic disease and renal invasion.

The patient with renal candidiasis usually presents with fever, candiduria, and unexplained progressive renal failure.[286] There usually are no symptoms referable to the kidneys, although there may be symptoms arising from involvement of other organs including skin, mucosa, muscle, and eyes. Contrary to the case with bacterial urinary tract infections, there is no consensus as to the critical concentration of candiduria required for a diagnosis of renal candidiasis. High colony count may be a reflection of colonization rather than infection in the patient with an indwelling bladder catheter or nephrostomy tube. Diagnosis is further complicated by the lack of any tests to localize infection to the kidneys. *Candida* casts are highly suggestive of renal infection but are an unusual finding. The presence of fungal bezoars in the upper urinary tract can be excluded with renal ultrasonography or another suitable imaging procedure. A useful diagnostic test in the catheterized patient with candiduria, bladder washings with amphotericin B, will clear the urine of colonization but not renal candidosis.[287] The routine use of prophylactic fluconazole in patients undergoing HCT has reduced the incidence of invasive candidiasis, but the rate of fluconazole resistance has increased.[288]

ADENOVIRUS INFECTIONS

Opportunistic infections secondary to systemic adenovirus infection occur in immunocompromised patients. Adenovirus type II appears to have a predilection for urothelial membrane surfaces, and infections of the urothelium are frequent. As a result, adenovirus type II has been associated with urinary tract obstruction and hemorrhagic cystitis in this patient population. There are several reports of acute tubulointerstitial nephritis (TIN) with oliguric AKI in the setting of severe pneumonitis, hepatitis, meningoencephalitis, myocarditis, and hemorrhagic cystitis.[289,290] Although there is no standard treatment, cidofovir appears to be a safe and effective choice.[291]

EPSTEIN-BARR VIRUS INFECTION

Epstein-Barr virus (EBV) is associated with acute TIN and renal failure in both immunocompetent and immunocompromised patients.[292] Other renal lesions associated with EBV and infectious mononucleosis include acute glomerulonephritis, HUS, and rhabdomyolysis-induced AKI.[293] Reduction in immunosuppression is recommended in these circumstances.

POLYOMAVIRUS (BK-TYPE) INFECTION

BK virus is a double-stranded DNA virus in the polyomavirus family. Infection with the virus is almost ubiquitous by early adulthood, in that seroprevalence rates of 80% have been reported in healthy blood donors.[294] The virus then remains dormant in the urothelial cells without clinical effects in immunocompetent individuals. In the immunosuppressed population, BK virus has most commonly been associated with nephropathy after kidney transplantation and with hemorrhagic cystitis (>1 week after stem cell infusion) after HCT.[295] In transplant recipients, primary BK virus infection may be acquired from the environment, blood transfusions, or donor and has been associated with renal dysfunction and urinary tract obstruction from ureteral ulcerations and strictures.[296] An acute TIN (BK nephropathy) has been reported in patients who undergo renal transplantation or HCT.[297] The diagnosis of BK nephropathy is suggested by the presence of inclusion-bearing cells in the urine ("decoy" cells) and the detection by polymerase chain reaction analysis of BK-virus DNA in the serum.

Current treatment options for hemorrhagic cystitis include pain control, bladder irrigation, and urologic intervention for clot removal or obstruction. Pharmacologic interventions include cidofovir, leflunomide, and fluoroquinolones.[298-300] Ciprofloxacin has been reported to decrease BK urinary viral loads, but not the risk of hemorrhagic cystitis, when given as prophylaxis during the first 2 months after HCT.[301] CMX100, an oral formulation of cidofovir with activity against double-stranded DNA viruses, may have less renal toxicity, and clinical trials are currently ongoing.[302] Given the nephrotoxicity of cidofovir, its use should be restricted to patients with biopsy evidence of BK nephropathy.

ZYGOMATOSIS

Invasive zygomycosis (mucormycosis) occurs predominantly in immunocompromised patients. Patients present with bilateral flank pain, fever, hematuria, pyuria, and renal failure.[303] Radiographic assessment demonstrates bilaterally enlarged, nonfunctioning kidneys. Oral antifungal prophylaxis with triazoles and nystatin is ineffective. Treatment consists of amphotericin B, reduction of immunosuppression, and surgical debridement.

DISSEMINATED HISTOPLASMOSIS

Multiple organ failure can develop from disseminated histoplasmosis in immunocompromised patients. The disease usually follows a rapidly progressive course with a high mortality rate. Although uncommon, AKI does occur.[304,305] Biopsy specimens show aggregates of phagocytosed macrophages in the glomerular capillaries and the tubular interstitium. Treatment consists of reduction of immunosuppression and administration of amphotericin B.

THROMBOTIC MICROANGIOPATHY

TMA in the form of HUS and TTP is a disease of multiple etiologies manifesting as nonimmune hemolytic anemia, thrombocytopenia, varying degrees of encephalopathy, and renal failure due to platelet thrombi in the microcirculation of the kidneys. Laboratory findings include elevated indirect bilirubin and lactate dehydrogenase (LDH) values, depressed serum haptoglobin values, and the finding of schistocytes on peripheral blood smear. The characteristic renal lesion consists of vessel wall thickening in capillaries and arterioles, with swelling and detachment of endothelial cells from the basement membranes and accumulation of subendothelial fluffy material.[306] These vascular lesions are indistinguishable from those seen in malignant hypertension and scleroderma renal crisis.

Typically, HUS develops in children with hemorrhagic colitis from verotoxin-producing *Escherichia coli* infection associated with ingestion of undercooked meat.[307] Renal failure is pronounced, and altered sensorium is not consistently present. In contrast, idiopathic TTP is usually seen in adult women in whom encephalopathy is the predominant clinical feature and renal involvement is less severe. However, because of similar laboratory findings and the great overlap in clinical features, these syndromes likely have the same pathogenesis, endothelial cell dysfunction.[308]

In patients with cancer, malignancy, chemotherapy, irradiation, immunosuppressive agents, and HCT can induce endothelial dysfunction leading to TMA and renal failure (Table 42.7). TMA has been most commonly associated with carcinomas. Gastric carcinoma accounts for more than half of the cases, followed by breast and lung cancer.[309]

Chemotherapy agents are likewise associated with the development of TMA. Mitomycin C is the classic drug, with an incidence of TMA during its use as high as 10%.[310,311] Bleomycin, cisplatin, and 5-fluorouracil are less frequently reported in association with the syndrome's development. Gemcitabine, a nucleoside analog, has been reported to cause TMA with an incidence of 0.31%.[312]

Treatment of renal failure and TMA in patients with cancer is mainly supportive, with initiation of dialysis as necessary. Stopping any causative medications is advised. However, the role of TPE remains controversial. Although all forms of TMA share the underlying pathogenesis of endothelial cell injury and dysfunction, the actual inciting event may be different in each case and not amenable to TPE. As an example, TPE has not been found to be an effective therapy for HUS in children despite its clear benefit in the treatment of idiopathic TTP.[313] In TTP, an autoantibody to the von Willebrand factor–cleaving protease ADAMTS13

Table 42.7 Causes of Thrombotic Microangiopathy in Patients with Cancer

Chemotherapy	Mitomycin C
	Cisplatin
	Bleomycin
	Gemcitabine
Immunosuppressive agents	Cyclosporine
	Tacrolimus
	Rapamycin
Malignancy	Gastric carcinoma
	Breast carcinoma
	Lung carcinoma
Hematopoietic cell transplantation	Transplantation-associated microangiopathy
	Radiation-associated kidney injury

has been described.[314] Inhibition of the cleaving enzyme leads to unusually large von Willebrand factor multimers that may agglutinate circulating platelets at sites with high levels of intravascular shear stress, triggering TMA. Plasma infusion may provide an exogenous source of cleaving protease to compete with the autoantibody, whereas plasmapheresis removes the pathogenic antibody. In HUS, the autoantibody is rarely found, potentially explaining the ineffectiveness of TPE in this disorder.[315] Reports on the use of TPE in patients with cancer are confined to those with TMA after bone marrow transplantation. Most studies are small case series that are unable to clearly demonstrate true benefit. Nevertheless, for a patient with the clinical characteristics of severe TTP after HCT, a trial of TPE is probably warranted.

Complete reference list available at ExpertConsult.com.

KEY REFERENCES

1. Samuels J, Ng CS, Nates J, et al: Small increases in serum creatinine are associated with prolonged ICU stay and increased hospital mortality in critically ill patients with cancer. *Support Care Cancer* 19:1527–1532, 2011.
2. Uchino S, Kellum JA, Bellomo R, et al: Acute renal failure in critically ill patients: a multinational, multicenter study. *JAMA* 294:813–818, 2005.
3. Christiansen CF, Johansen MB, Langeberg WJ, et al: Incidence of acute kidney injury in cancer patients: a Danish population-based cohort study. *Eur J Intern Med* 22:399–406, 2011.
4. Darmon M, Ciroldi M, Thiery G, et al: Clinical review: specific aspects of acute renal failure in cancer patients. *Critical Care* 10:211, 2006.
12. Kyle RA, Gertz MA, Witzig TE, et al: Review of 1027 patients with newly diagnosed multiple myeloma. *Mayo Clin Proc* 78:21–33, 2003.
13. Eleutherakis-Papaiakovou V, Bamias A, Gika D, et al: Renal failure in multiple myeloma: incidence, correlations, and prognostic significance. *Leuk Lymphoma* 48:337–341, 2007.
15. Solomon A, Weiss DT, Kattine AA: Nephrotoxic potential of Bence Jones proteins. *N Engl J Med* 324:1845–1851, 1991.
18. Sanders PW: Mechanisms of light chain injury along the tubular nephron. *J Am Soc Nephrol* 23:1777–1781, 2012.
22. Pozzi C, D'Amico M, Fogazzi GB, et al: Light chain deposition disease with renal involvement: clinical characteristics and prognostic factors. *Am J Kidney Dis* 42:1154–1163, 2003.
23. Kyle RA, Gertz MA: Primary systemic amyloidosis: clinical and laboratory features in 474 cases. *Semin Hematol* 32:45–59, 1995.
28. Hutchison CA, Cockwell P, Stringer S, et al: Early reduction of serum-free light chains associates with renal recovery in myeloma kidney. *J Am Soc Nephrol* 22:1129–1136, 2011.
31. Dimopoulos MA, Roussou M, Gkotzamanidou M, et al: The role of novel agents on the reversibility of renal impairment in newly diagnosed symptomatic patients with multiple myeloma. *Leukemia* 27:423–429, 2013.
35. Roussou M, Kastritis E, Christoulas D, et al: Reversibility of renal failure in newly diagnosed patients with multiple myeloma and the role of novel agents. *Leuk Res* 34:1395–1397, 2010.
42. Hutchison CA, Heyne N, Airia P, et al: Immunoglobulin free light chain levels and recovery from myeloma kidney on treatment with chemotherapy and high cut-off haemodialysis. *Nephrol Dial Transplant* 27:3823–3828, 2012.
43. Hingorani SR, Guthrie K, Batchelder A, et al: Acute renal failure after myeloablative hematopoietic cell transplant: incidence and risk factors. *Kidney Int* 67:272–277, 2005.
46. Zager RA, O'Quigley J, Zager BK, et al: Acute renal failure following bone marrow transplantation: a retrospective study of 272 patients. *Am J Kidney Dis* 13:210–216, 1989.
53. Kersting S, Koomans HA, Hene RJ, et al: Acute renal failure after allogeneic myeloablative stem cell transplantation: retrospective analysis of incidence, risk factors and survival. *Bone Marrow Transplant* 39:359–365, 2007.
62. Hingorani S: Chronic kidney disease in long-term survivors of hematopoietic cell transplantation: epidemiology, pathogenesis, and treatment. *J Am Soc Nephrol* 17:1995–2005, 2006.
65. Zager RA: Acute renal failure in the setting of bone marrow transplantation. *Kidney Int* 46:1443–1458, 1994.
77. Ho VT, Cutler C, Carter S, et al: Blood and marrow transplant clinical trials network toxicity committee consensus summary: thrombotic microangiopathy after hematopoietic stem cell transplantation. *Biol Blood Marrow Transplant* 11:571–575, 2005.
78. Ruutu T, Barosi G, Benjamin RJ, et al: Diagnostic criteria for hematopoietic stem cell transplant-associated microangiopathy: results of a consensus process by an International Working Group. *Haematologica* 92:95–100, 2007.
82. Kojouri K, George JN: Thrombotic microangiopathy following allogeneic hematopoietic stem cell transplantation. *Curr Opin Oncol* 19:148–154, 2007.
90. Zuber J, Fakhouri F, Roumenina L, et al: Use of eculizumab for atypical haemolytic uraemic syndrome and C3 glomerulopathies. *Nat Rev Nephrol* 8:643–659, 2012.
104. Shemin D, Briggs D, Greenan M: Complications of therapeutic plasma exchange: a prospective study of 1,727 procedures. *J Clin Apher* 22:270–276, 2007.
111. Howard SC, Jones DP, Pui CH: The tumor lysis syndrome. *N Engl J Med* 364:1844–1854, 2011.
114. Cairo M, Bishop M: Tumor lysis syndrome: New therapeutic stategies and classification. *Brit J Haematol* 127:3–11, 2004.
118. Ejaz AA, Mu W, Kang DH, et al: Could uric acid have a role in acute renal failure? *Clin J Am Soc Nephrol* 2:16–21, 2007.
121. Wilson F, Berns J: Onco-Nephrology: Tumor lysis syndrome. *Clin J Am Soc Nephrol* 7:1730–1739, 2012.
124. Coiffier B, Mounier N, Bologna S, et al: Efficacy and safety of rasburicase (recombinant urate oxidase) for the prevention and treatment of hyperuricemia during induction chemotherapy of aggressive non-Hodgkin's lymphoma: results of the GRAAL1 (Groupe d'Etude des Lymphomes de l'Adulte Trial on Rasburicase Activity in Adult Lymphoma) study. *J Clin Oncol* 21:4402–4406, 2003.
126. Jeha S, Pui CH: Recombinant urate oxidase (rasburicase) in the prophylaxis and treatment of tumor lysis syndrome. *Contrib Nephrol* 147:69–79, 2005.
129. Arany I, Safirstein RL: Cisplatin nephrotoxicity. *Semin Nephrol* 23:460–464, 2003.
132. Ries F, Klastersky J: Nephrotoxicity induced by cancer chemotherapy with special emphasis on cisplatin toxicity. *Am J Kidney Dis* 8:368–379, 1986.
163. Memoli B, De Nicola L, Libetta C, et al: Interleukin-2-induced renal dysfunction in cancer patients is reversed by low-dose dopamine infusion. *Am J Kidney Dis* 26:27–33, 1995.
166. Izzedine H, Rixe O, Billemont B, et al: Angiogenesis inhibitor therapies: focus on kidney toxicity and hypertension. *Am J Kidney Dis* 50:203–218, 2007.
174. Maitland ML, Bakris GL, Black HR, et al: Initial assessment, surveillance, and management of blood pressure in patients receiving vascular endothelial growth factor signaling pathway inhibitors. *J Natl Cancer Inst* 102:596–604, 2010.
189. Kyle RA, Yee GC, Somerfield MR, et al: American Society of Clinical Oncology 2007 clinical practice guideline update on the role of bisphosphonates in multiple myeloma. *J Clin Oncol* 25:2464–2472, 2007.
194. Rosner M, Dalkin A: Onco-Nephrology: The pathophysiology and treatment of malignancy associated hypercalcemia. *Clin J Am Soc Nephrol* 7:1722–1729, 2012.
199. LeGrand S, Leskuski D, Zam I: Narrative review: furosemide for hypercalcemia: an unproven yet common practice. *Ann Intern Med* 149:259–263, 2008.
205. Castellano D, Sepulveda J, Garcia-Escobar I, et al: The role of RANK-ligand inhibition in cancer: the story of denosumab. *Oncologist* 16:136–145, 2011.
208. Cohen EP, Robbins ME: Radiation nephropathy. *Semin Nephrol* 23:486–499, 2003.
239. Cohen EP, Hussain S, Moulder JE: Successful treatment of radiation nephropathy with angiotensin II blockade. *Int J Radiat Oncol Biol Phys* 55:190–193, 2003.

252. Tornroth T, Heiro M, Marcussen N, et al: Lymphomas diagnosed by percutaneous kidney biopsy. *Am J Kidney Dis* 42:960–971, 2003.
259. Jordan M, Allen C, Weitzman S, et al: How I treat hemophagocytic lymphohistiocytosis. *Blood* 118:4041–4052, 2011.
272. Lefaucheur C, Stengel B, Nochy D, et al: Membranous nephropathy and cancer: Epidemiologic evidence and determinants of high-risk cancer association. *Kidney Int* 70:1510–1517, 2006.
277. Dabbs DJ, Striker LM, Mignon F, et al: Glomerular lesions in lymphomas and leukemias. *Am J Med* 80:63–70, 1986.
288. Maschmeyer G, Haas A: The epidemiology and treatment of infections in cancer patients. *Int J Antimicrob Agents* 31:193–197, 2008.
295. Dropulic LK, Jones RJ, Polyomavirus BK: infection in blood and marrow transplant recipients. *Bone Marrow Transplant* 41:11–18, 2008.
296. O'Donnell PH, Swanson K, Josephson MA, et al: BK virus infection is associated with hematuria and renal impairment in recipients of allogeneic hematopoetic stem cell transplants. *Biol Blood Marrow Transplant* 15:1038–1048 e1, 2009.
299. Ramos E, Drachenberg CB, Wali R, et al: The decade of polyomavirus BK-associated nephropathy: state of affairs. *Transplantation* 87:621–630, 2009.
315. Furlan M, Robles R, Galbusera M, et al: von Willebrand factor-cleaving protease in thrombotic thrombocytopenic purpura and the hemolytic-uremic syndrome. *N Engl J Med* 339:1578–1584, 1998.

SECTION VI
GENETICS OF KIDNEY DISEASE

43 Genetic Basis of Kidney Disease

Friedhelm Hildebrandt

CHAPTER OUTLINE

DEGREES OF GENETIC DISEASE CAUSALITY AND PREDICTIVE POWER OF GENETIC ANALYSIS, 1411
SINGLE-GENE KIDNEY DISEASES, 1412
Mutation Analysis, 1412
CRITERIA TO ASSESS GENETIC "CAUSATION", 1412
INDICATION-DRIVEN DIAGNOSTIC MUTATION ANALYSIS PANELS, 1412
STEROID-RESISTANT NEPHROTIC SYNDROME, 1413
Monogenic Causation of Steroid-Resistant Nephrotic Syndrome, 1413
Genotype-Phenotype Correlations, 1414
Genotype-Treatment Correlations, 1415
Insights into Disease Pathways, 1415
Animal Models, 1415
CONGENITAL ANOMALIES OF THE KIDNEYS AND URINARY TRACT, 1415
Monogenic Causation, 1415
Genotype-Phenotype Correlations, 1416

Pathogenesis, 1416
RENAL CYSTIC CILIOPATHIES, 1416
Polycystic Kidney Disease, 1416
Nephronophthisis-Related Ciliopathies, 1416
Genotype-Phenotype Correlation, 1417
Pathogenesis, 1417
NEPHROLITHIASIS/NEPHROCALCINOSIS, 1417
INHERITED RENAL TUBULOPATHIES, 1417
ATYPICAL HEMOLYTIC UREMIC SYNDROMES, 1418
IDENTIFICATION OF NOVEL SINGLE-GENE KIDNEY DISORDERS, 1418
Whole-Exome Sequencing, 1418
FUTURE DIRECTIONS IN SINGLE-GENE DISORDERS, 1418
COMMON AND POLYGENIC RENAL DISORDERS, 1419
Polygenic Diseases, 1419
The Territory between Monogenic and Polygenic Disease, 1419

Knowledge of the primary cause of a disease is essential to understanding its pathomechanism, assessing its prognosis, and instituting adequate treatment. For most kidney diseases the primary causes are still unknown. This situation is rapidly changing, due to the advances in molecular genetics that started with the Human Genome Project. Insights into kidney diseases have mainly come from two complementary genetic approaches:

1. In rare single-gene (monogenic) kidney diseases, hundreds of novel disease-causing genes have been discovered, using genetic mapping and whole-exome sequencing (WES) techniques, and they follow mendelian inheritance patterns in families and pedigrees. Rare kidney diseases, such as autosomal dominant polycystic kidney disease (ADPKD), are caused by single monogenic mutations with strong pathogenic effects that are alone sufficient to cause disease.
2. In common polygenic kidney diseases, dozens of risk alleles have been detected using genomewide association studies (GWAS). Polygenic kidney diseases, such as diabetic nephropathy, are caused by genetic variants that act together to increase disease risk in adult-onset disease, where each genetic variant contributes only a small fraction to the phenotypic variance of a disease.

There has been a surge in the discovery of hundreds of novel single-gene causes of kidney disease. This was followed by the surprising realization that seemingly similar disorders that lead to early-onset chronic kidney disease (CKD), such as focal segmental glomerulosclerosis, are caused by single-gene mutations in one of dozens of different single genes, a different gene being mutated in each individual. Knowledge of the disease-causing mutation in a single-gene disorder represents one of the most robust diagnostic measures available to clinical medicine, because the mutation conveys an almost 100% risk for developing the disease by a defined age. Since each mutation may convey a specific pathogenic process, knowledge of the causative single-gene mutation of an individual with kidney disease

Table 43.1 Degrees of Genetic Causality and Power of Molecular Genetic Diagnostics in Recessive, Dominant, and Polygenic Diseases

	Monogenic		Polygenic
	Recessive	**Dominant**	
Genetic causality	Strong	Intermediate	Weak
Penetrance	Full	Can be incomplete	Weak
Predictive power of mutation analysis	Almost 100%	Strong*	Weak
Age of onset	Fetus, child, young adult	Adult	Adult
Molecular genetic approaches	Detection of causative mutations by direct exon sequencing	Detection of causative mutations by direct exon sequencing	Only assignment of relative risk possible
Frequency	<1:40,000 (rare)	<1:1000 (rare)	<1:5 (common)
Source from which data are usually derived	Gene mapping and whole-exome sequencing	Gene mapping and whole-exome sequencing	Genomewide association studies
Confirmation by animal model	Very feasible	Feasible	Difficult

*Except for incomplete penetrance and variable expressivity.

will likely enable approaches of personalized medicine in the near future.

This chapter will discuss prominent renal single-gene disorders, as well as polygenic risk alleles of common renal disorders. It will delineate how emerging techniques of WES assist molecular genetic diagnosis, prognosis, and specific treatment and lead to an improved elucidation of disease mechanisms, thus enabling the development of new targeted drugs.

DEGREES OF GENETIC DISEASE CAUSALITY AND PREDICTIVE POWER OF GENETIC ANALYSIS

Single-gene disorders are also known as "monogenic diseases" or "mendelian diseases." They are characterized by the fact that a mutation in a single gene (of the ≈20,000 genes that are contained within our genome) is sufficient to cause disease in an individual. In contrast to single-gene disorders, polygenic disorders are caused by genetic variants in several different genes that work together to increase disease risk.[1]

Mutations in single-gene disorders may display recessive or dominant inheritance patterns. For each autosomal gene we possess two copies, one from each parent. In a recessive disease gene, both parental copies have to be mutated to cause disease. If the mutation inherited from each parent is identical, the mutations are termed "homozygous." If each parent contributed a different mutation in the same gene, the mutations are termed "compound heterozygous." The parents will be healthy heterozygous carriers. And, as a rule, no one in the ancestry will ever have had this disease, because only heterozygous mutations are expected to be present in the ancestors of the parents. (The term "heterozygosity" indicates that only one parental allele is mutated.) An example of a recessive disease is autosomal recessive PKD, in which the *PKHD1* gene is mutated. In monogenic disease with dominant inheritance, a mutation in one parental copy is sufficient to cause disease. Therefore one of the parents will also express the dominant disorder, and the disease will have been transmitted through the ancestry in an autosomal dominant mendelian inheritance pattern. The term "monogenic" does not preclude, however, that in different individuals different genes may cause a similar disease. This situation is known as "gene locus heterogeneity." For instance, steroid-resistant nephrotic syndrome may be caused by recessive mutations in the *NPHS1* or the *NPHS2* gene, as well as other genetic loci.

The degree of genetic causality is determined by the mode of inheritance (Table 43.1). Recessive diseases reside at one extreme of this spectrum and show a very tight genotype-phenotype correlation. In recessive diseases the disease phenotype is almost exclusively determined by the single-gene causative mutation, so that virtually all individuals who carry two mutations in a recessive-disease gene (one mutation on the paternal and one on the maternal allele) will develop disease by a certain age. This situation is referred to as "full penetrance" and generally reflects loss of function attributable to mutations in both parental copies. It lends a very high predictive power to mutation analysis (see Table 43.1). Diseases with recessive mendelian inheritance usually manifest prenatally, in childhood, or in young adults (e.g., autosomal recessive PKD), whereas those caused by genes with dominant inheritance typically manifest in adulthood (e.g., autosomal dominant PKD1) (see Table 43.1). Recessive diseases are usually rare (e.g., 1 in ≈40,000 individuals). However, the related heterozygous mutations are found once in hundreds of individuals (see Table 43.1), which allows identification of parents who are at risk for having a child with a recessive disease.[2] Recessive mutations are usually identified by exon sequencing or WES (see Table 43.1). The effect of recessive mutations is easily amenable to functional studies in animal models of gene knockdown or knockout (e.g., in mice or zebrafish) (see Table 43.1).

In diseases with dominant inheritance, the tightness of genotype-phenotype correlation may be reduced in comparison to recessive inheritance diseases, because the corresponding dominant inheritance genes may show incomplete penetrance (i.e., skipping of the disease phenotype in a generation). They may also show variable expressivity, even within a family carrying the same mutation (i.e., different degrees of organ involvement or disease severity) (see Table 43.1). Dominant diseases as a rule manifest in adulthood. They often exhibit the phenomenon of age-related penetrance. For instance, the age of onset and progression of CKD in the most frequent dominant lethal disease in humans (ADPKD) is distributed over the fourth to seventh decades of life.

At the other extreme of the range of causality are polygenic diseases, in which genotype-phenotype correlation is weak (see Table 43.1). In contrast to autosomal recessive diseases, where there is often 100% penetrance, in polygenic diseases usually only a relative disease risk can be attributed to a genetic variant, as for instance in an association between the markers of the *APOL1* locus and focal segmental glomerulosclerosis.[3,4] Polygenic disease variants are mostly identified by GWAS (see Table 43.1). Specific disease-associated alleles of many different genes often explain only very small percentages of the phenotypic variance (missing heritability).[5] Polygenic diseases usually manifest in adulthood and are much more frequent than monogenic diseases. Since the penetrance of pathogenic disease alleles is weak, these diseases are more susceptible to environmental influences on the disease phenotype. It is very difficult to test the pathogenic effects of polygenic disease variants in animal models due to the small effect that each genetic variant contributes to the disease phenotype.

SINGLE-GENE KIDNEY DISEASES

MUTATION ANALYSIS

In single-gene disorders identification of the causative mutation has the following important clinical consequences: (1) it provides the patient with an unequivocal molecular genetic diagnosis; (2) it makes prenatal diagnostic testing possible; (3) for individuals participating in clinical studies, it permits a causation-based classification of disease; (4) detection of specific mutations may allow specific therapeutic approaches in way of "personalized medicine"; (4) it allows the development of relevant animal models; and (5) it permits screening for therapeutic molecules in high-throughput cell-based or animal-based disease model systems. Therefore, due to the high penetrance of mutations in monogenic disorders, mutation analysis has a very high diagnostic and prognostic value (see Table 43.1).

Diagnostic mutation analysis in single-gene disorders is usually performed by sequencing all exons (the protein-encoding sequences) of a gene and the adjacent intronic splice sites. (Splice sites are used to splice exons together following gene transcription, to generate a continuous protein-encoding messenger RNA.) Even though exonic sequence represents only 1% of the human genome, for reasons of practicality it is sufficient to concentrate on exonic sequence and adjacent splice sites (whole-exome sequence), because it is thought that these DNA segments contain 85% of all disease-causing mutations in single-gene disorders.

CRITERIA TO ASSESS GENETIC "CAUSATION"

Molecular genetic diagnostics by exon sequencing is initiated following written consent of the patient whose DNA is examined. It is performed by diagnostic laboratories that are licensed for clinical genetic testing (i.e., Clinical Laboratories Improvement Amendments [CLIA] certification). Genomic DNA for molecular genetic diagnostics is extracted usually either from a 4-mL ethylenediaminetetraacetic acid (EDTA) sample of whole blood or from a saliva sample. Exon sequencing is performed by classical Sanger sequencing, by high-throughput sequencing using diagnostic panels of disease-causing genes, or by WES. The DNA sequence data that result from diagnostic exome sequencing of a patient's DNA is aligned with the sequence of normal reference individuals. Differences in exon or splice-site sequence between patient and reference individual are termed "genetic variants." If genetic variants are considered disease causing, they are termed "mutations."[6-12] A genetic variant has to fulfill a graded set of multiple criteria to qualify as a mutation. These include (1) whether the mutation truncates the encoded protein ("truncating mutation") or only leads to an exchange of an amino acid residue (missense mutation), (2) the degree of evolutionary conservation of an amino acid residue affecting a missense mutation, (3) whether inheritance of the genetic variant within the pedigree travels together with the disease phenotype ("cosegregation"), and (4) experimental data showing that the mutation conveys loss of biologic function in cell-based or animal models (Table 43.2).

INDICATION-DRIVEN DIAGNOSTIC MUTATION ANALYSIS PANELS

Over last 2 years it has become apparent that a surprisingly high proportion (≈20%) of CKD that manifests before 25 years of age is caused by a single-gene (monogenic) mutation. These mutations can be identified by mutation analysis using high-throughput exon-sequencing techniques.[13-16] The most frequent diagnostic groups of CKD that manifests before 25 years of age are listed in Table 43.3 as determined in approximately 9000 persons from North American Pediatric Renal Trials and Collaborative Studies (NAPRTCS) data.[17] CKD is caused by congenital anomalies of the kidneys and urinary tract (CAKUT) in 50% of cases, by steroid-resistant nephrotic syndrome (SRNS) in 15%, by glomerulonephritis in 14%, and by cystic kidney diseases in 6%. Genetic mapping techniques and the acceleration of next-generation sequencing techniques have permitted identification of dozens of monogenic disease genes for each of these diagnostic groups of early-onset CKD (see Table 43.3). The number of newly discovered monogenic causes of CKD is rapidly increasing.

Furthermore, it was shown that in a high fraction of early-onset CKD a causative single-gene mutation can be identified in one of the dozens of these disease genes. These fractions are 15% for CAKUT,[18-20] 30% for SRNS,[15] 50% to 70% for cystic kidney diseases,[14,21] 20% for renal tubulopathies,[22] and 15% for nephrolithiasis[16] (see Table 43.3). The

Table 43.2 DNA Variant Criteria for Mutation Analysis in Single-Gene Disorders

Disease-causing variants in *recessive genes* are considered if two alleles were found in the same individual that fulfilled at least one of the following criteria:

1. At least one of the two alleles is protein truncating (stop, abrogation of start or stop, obligatory splice site, or frameshift); OR
2. At least one of the two alleles was reported in the Human Gene Mutation Database (http://www.hgmd.org/) as disease-causing; AND

for those individuals the second allele needs to meet at least one of the following criteria:

3. Missense mutation exhibiting high evolutionary conservation; OR
4. Two out of three prediction scores classify the allele as disease causing: PolyPhen-2 prediction HumVar of greater than 0.9 (http://genetics.bwh.harvard.edu/pph2), SIFT (http://sift.jcvi.org), Mutation Taster (http://www.mutationtaster.org); OR
5. Loss of function of the identified allele is supported by functional data.
6. For recessive genes the two variants have to be present "in trans" (i.e., each on different parental chromosomes).

Exclusion criteria: Minor allelic frequency (MAF) needs to be less than 1% in genotyping data of the NHLBI GO Exome Sequencing Project Exome Variant Server (EVS; http://evs.gs.washington.edu/EVS/). Variants are excluded if they do not segregate in a recessive way with the affected status in family members.

Disease-causing variants in *dominant genes* are considered if one allele fulfills at least one of the following criteria:

1. Truncating mutation (stop, abrogation of start or stop, obligatory splice site, and frameshift); OR
2. Variant was reported in the Human Gene Mutation Database (http://www.hgmd.org/) as disease causing; OR
3. Missense mutation, if at least conserved in vertebrates; OR
4. Two out of three prediction scores classify the allele as disease causing: PolyPhen-2 prediction HumVar of greater than 0.9 (http://genetics.bwh.harvard.edu/pph2), SIFT (http://sift.jcvi.org), Mutation Taster (http://www.mutationtaster.org); OR
5. Loss of function or dominant-negative effect of the identified allele is supported by functional data; OR
6. Full segregation exists in the affected status for seven or more affected family members.

Exclusion criteria: Variants are excluded if the allele occurred at least once heterozygously or homozygously in the EVS server (http://evs.gs.washington.edu/EVS/), or if the allele does not segregate with the affected status in the family.

NHLBI, National Heart, Lung, and Blood Institute.

---

fraction of individuals with CKD in whom a causative mutation can be detected will keep rising, as more monogenic disease genes are discovered and as "mild" mutations will be incriminated in adult-onset disease.[23,24]

The reason why this high proportion of single-gene causation in CKD was recognized only recently is likely twofold. (1) First, high-throughput WES techniques have become available and affordable only very recently. Second, (when assuming monogenic causation, familial occurrence is often expected. However, familial occurrence is atypical for recessive diseases, because parents and ancestors are usually healthy heterozygous carriers of any causative mutation, and only one in four children of heterozygous carrier parents will carry mutations on both parental alleles and thereby be affected with disease. Therefore most individuals with recessive disease-causing mutations will appear as "sporadic cases" with no positive family history.

As a consequence of the high proportion of monogenic causation of early-onset CKD, **gene panels** have been developed to identify the causative mutation in these subgroups of CKD (see Table 43.3). Studies that demonstrated the high proportion of detectable single-gene mutations in CKD that manifests before age 25 years used simple and reproducible clinical indications to decide if mutation analysis was warranted.[13-16] These indication-driven diagnostic panels (Table 43.4) allow one to expect similar likelihoods of detecting a causative mutation when applying identical indications to run a diagnostic panel. Clinical indications (for individuals developing CKD before 25 years of age) were as follows (see Table 43.4): (1) in SRNS, proteinuria (>150 mg/dL) for at least 3 consecutive days[15]; (2) in cystic kidney diseases, demonstration of two or more cysts, increased echogenicity, or reduced corticomedullary differentiation upon renal ultrasonographic examination[13,14]; (3) in CAKUT, demonstration of renal or urinary tract malformation by imaging; (4) in nephrolithiasis, the presence of at least one stone in the urinary tract or the presence of nephrocalcinosis demonstrated by ultrasonography[16]; and (5) in renal tubulopathies, a suspected diagnosis of a defect of renal tubular transport (see Table 43.4).

Overall these indication-driven monogenic diagnostic panels currently interrogate the exons of approximately 215 kidney disease genes and have a likelihood of detecting a monogenic cause of CKD in greater than 20% of individuals with CKD manifesting before 25 years of age (see Table 43.4). For many of these disease groups, the likelihood of detecting the causative mutations is inversely related to age of onset.[15] However, as less severe mutations will be called disease-causing on the basis of functional studies of these mutations (see Table 43.1), the proportion of monogenic causation in CKD will rise also in late-onset CKD.[25]

STEROID-RESISTANT NEPHROTIC SYNDROME (See Chapter 44)

SRNS, which mostly manifests histologically as focal segmental glomerulosclerosis, remains one of the most intractable kidney diseases. Genetic mapping and next-generation sequencing have permitted identification of more than 30 monogenic causative genes, and this number is rapidly increasing (Figure 43.1).[26] Twenty-one genes follow an autosomal recessive mode of inheritance, and seven genes are autosomal dominant (see Figure 43.1).

MONOGENIC CAUSATION OF STEROID-RESISTANT NEPHROTIC SYNDROME

Using a high-throughput exon-sequencing technique,[13,27] it was shown in a worldwide cohort of individuals from 1780

Table 43.3 Single-Gene Causes of Chronic Kidney Disease Manifesting by 25 Years of Age

Diagnostic Group of Chronic Kidney Disease[17]	Chronic Kidney Disease (%)	Genes (No.)	Monogenic (%)
CAKUT	50	30	≈15
Steroid-resistant nephrotic syndrome	15	30	30
Chronic glomerulonephritis	14	—	—
(MPGN, SLE, IgA, granulomatosis with polyangiitis [formerly designated as Wegener's granulomatosis])			
Cystic kidney disease	6	95	≈70
(ARPKD, ADPKD, nephronophthisis, MCKD)			
Tubulopathies	3	45	≈20
Other	12	—	—
Total (n = 8990)	100	200	≈20

ADPKD, Autosomal dominant polycystic kidney disease; ARPKD, autosomal recessive polycystic kidney disease; CAKUT, congenital anomalies of the kidneys and urinary tract; IgA, immunoglobulin A; MCKD, medullary cystic kidney disease; MPGN, membranoproliferative glomerulonephritis; SLE, systemic lupus erythematosus.

Table 43.4 Indication-Driven Mutation Analysis Panels for Single-Gene Causes of Chronic Kidney Disease Manifesting by 25 Years of Age

CKD Disease Group (Indication to Perform Mutation Analysis)	Genes (No.)	Causative Mutation Detected (%)	Reference
Steroid-resistant nephrotic syndrome (proteinuria)	30	30	Sadowski et al, 2015[15]
Cystic kidney disease (ultrasonographic cysts or echogenicity)	95	>70	Halbritter et al, 2015[107]
CAKUT (imaging showing malformation)	30	>15	Kohl et al, 2014[19]
Kidney stones (stone or nephrocalcinosis)	60	>21	Halbritter et al, 2015[16]
All monogenic causes of CKD < 25 yr	≈215	>20	—

CAKUT, Congenital anomalies of kidney and urinary tract; CKD, chronic kidney disease.

different families in whom SRNS manifested before 25 years of age, that in 29.5% of these families a causative mutation can be detected in 1 of 27 genes.[15] Mutations were called disease causing based on strict genetic criteria (see Table 43.4). We found causative *NPHS2* (podocin) mutations in 10%, *NPHS1* (nephrin) mutations in approximately 7%, *WT1* (Wilms' tumor 1 gene) mutations in 5%, and *PLCE1* (phospholipase Cε_1)[28,29] mutations in 2% (Table 43.5). Another 22 rare genes shared 6% of the causative mutations. The earlier the age of onset, the more likely SRNS was of monogenic origin.[15] The fraction of single-gene causation of SRNS depends on the age of manifestation, being 60% in infants, 25% in schoolchildren, and approximately 15% in young adults. A similar proportion of detectable single-gene causes in 23% to 30% of SRNS that manifests by 25 years was confirmed by two other groups.[30,31]

GENOTYPE-PHENOTYPE CORRELATIONS

NPHS1 mutations are most frequent in congenital nephrotic syndrome (onset by 90 days of life).[15,32] Mutations in *NPHS2*, *LAMB2*, or *PLCE1* cause childhood-onset SRNS, whereas mutations in dominant genes, including *ACTN4* (α-actinin-4),[33] and *TRPC6*[34,35] lead to onset in young adults with few exceptions.[36,37] These data are consistent with the previous findings that 85% of all cases that manifest with

Table 43.5 Steroid-Resistant Nephrotic Syndrome

Causative Gene	Families (No.)	Families (%)
NPHS2 (podocin)	170	10
NPHS1 (nephrin)	125	7
WT1	85	5
PLCE1	35	2
Other genes (22)	105	6
Total	520	30

SRNS in the first 3 months of life and 66% of all those that manifest in the first year of life are caused by mutations in **one of only four genes** (*NPHS1*, *NPHS2*, *LAMB2*, or *WT1*).[32] Age of onset of SRNS is governed not only by the type of gene mutated, but also by specific **combinations of the two recessive causative mutations**. For instance, in *NPHS2* mutations the presence of at least one protein-truncating mutation or the mutation R138Q leads to very early onset of SRNS at a median age of 1.7 years rather than a median onset of 4.7 years.[38] Compound heterozygosity for the R229Q variant of podocin and one of several specific other podocin mutations was shown to cause adult-onset syndrome in up to 15% of cases.[25]

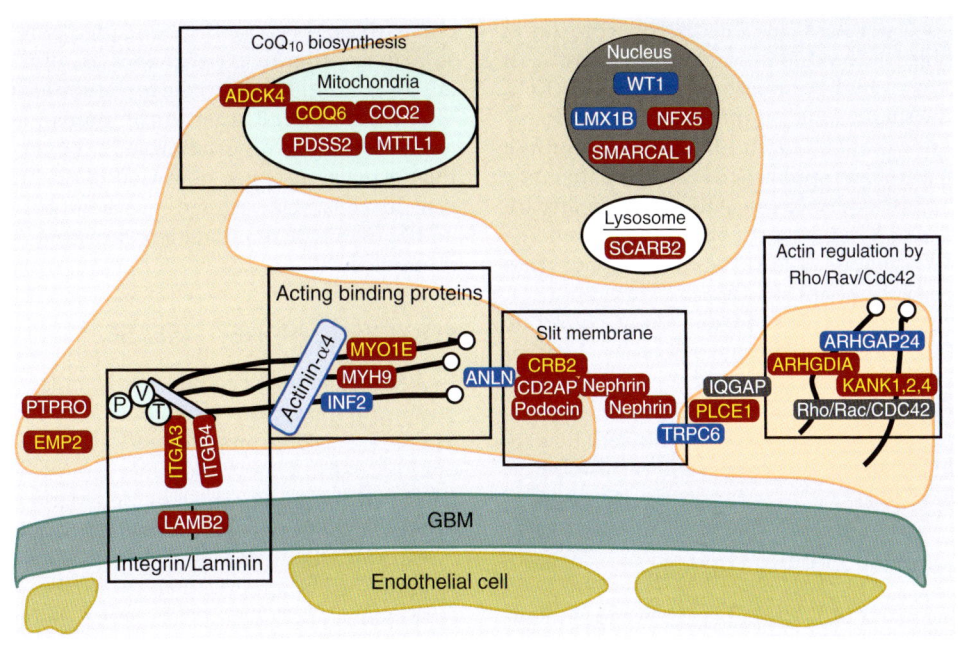

Figure 43.1 Identification of single-gene causes of steroid-resistant nephrotic syndrome (SRNS) moved the glomerular podocyte to the center of the pathogenesis of SRNS. Podocyte cell body and foot processes are shown in *manila*. Foot processes attach to the glomerular basement membrane (GBM, *green*). Identification of 27 single-gene (monogenic) causes of SRNS revealed the function *(in black boxes)* of the encoded proteins as central to the pathogenesis of SRNS. The gene products of these monogenic SRNS genes converge onto distinct protein complexes and signaling pathways depicted in *boxes*. Products of dominant genes are shown in *blue*, products of recessive genes in *red*.

GENOTYPE-TREATMENT CORRELATIONS

Identification of single-gene causes of nephrotic syndrome has revealed that mutations often define treatment response. For instance, in virtually all patients in whom a single-gene cause is detected in one of the 30 SRNS genes (see Figure 43.1), there is no response to standard steroid treatment.[39-41] Conversely, single-gene mutations have almost never been detected in individuals with typical steroid-sensitive nephrotic syndrome[39] with the exception of mutations in the *EMP2* gene.[39a] Childhood SRNS is generally associated with a 30% risk for recurrence in a kidney transplant. However, patients with two recessive mutations of the podocin gene have a **substantially reduced likelihood of recurrence** of focal segmental glomerulosclerosis in a kidney transplant (35% versus 8%).[39] Interestingly, individuals with mutations in the genes *COQ6* or *ADCK4*, which encode components of the coenzyme Q_{10} (CoQ_{10}) biosynthesis pathway, may respond to treatment with CoQ_{10}.[42,43] It will therefore be important to identify these individuals by mutation analysis using a proteinuria gene panel (see Table 43.4), as they may represent treatable cases of SRNS for which no effective treatment exists.

INSIGHTS INTO DISEASE PATHWAYS

Identification of single-gene causes of SRNS has moved the glomerular podocyte to the center of the pathogenesis of SRNS.[44] In this way disease gene identification has furthered the conceptual assembly of protein components necessary for glomerular function. Increasingly, data are generated showing that the proteins encoded by the approximately 30 monogenic SRNS genes known so far coalesce around distinct structural protein complexes and signaling pathways that reveal functional aspects essential for glomerular function (see Figure 43.1). These functional complexes include actin-binding proteins, laminin/integrin-signaling components, the actin-regulating small GTPases Rho/Rac/CDC42, lysosomal proteins, transcription factors, and proteins of CoQ_{10} biosynthesis (see Figure 43.1). For the study of pathogenic aspects of SRNS the so-called "podocyte migration assay" has been a useful cell-based platform for pathogenic and therapeutic studies.[42,45]

ANIMAL MODELS

Mouse models have been used extensively to study pathogenic aspects of SRNS. It was found that the study of the zebrafish pronephric kidney also provides a useful model for the pathogenesis of nephrotic syndrome[46] by generating transgenic models of nephrotic syndrome.[47] Some of these models have permitted studying the effect of potential treatment modalities for SRNS (e.g., Rac inhibitors).[45,48] Certain animal models might hold the promise of allowing high-throughput screening for small molecules that may mitigate the pathogenesis of SRNS.

CONGENITAL ANOMALIES OF THE KIDNEYS AND URINARY TRACT
(See Chapter 73)

MONOGENIC CAUSATION

Almost 50% of CKD that manifests before age 25 years is caused by CAKUT (see Table 43.3). CAKUT is present in approximately 3 to 6 per 1000 live births and constitutes 20% to 30% of all birth defects identified in neonates.[20,49] It was hypothesized that a high number of cases with CAKUT may be caused by single-gene (monogenic) mutations[23] based on the evidence that (1) dozens of monogenic mouse models of CAKUT have been published, (2) more than two dozen monogenic causes of isolated CAKUT in humans are known (for review see Vivante and colleagues[20]), and (3) there are over 100 genetic syndromes in humans that contain CAKUT as a subphenotype. Currently mutations in approximately 30 genes are known to cause nonsyndromic CAKUT, cumulatively explaining approximately 15% of case (see Table 43.3).[18-20,50] An indication-driven panel allows identification of disease-causing mutations in these genes (see Table 43.4). As CAKUT is likely genetically very heterogeneous, many additional causative genes will be discovered in the near future.

GENOTYPE-PHENOTYPE CORRELATIONS

The phenotypic spectrum of CAKUT is very broad, including renal agenesis,[51,52] renal hypodysplasia,[53] multicystic dysplastic kidneys,[54] hydronephrosis, ureteropelvic junction obstruction, megaureter, ureter duplex or fissus, prevesical stenosis, and vesicoureteral reflux.[55-58] These congenital abnormalities may present as an isolated feature or as part of a clinical syndrome[59-61] in association with extrarenal manifestations, such as in branchio-oto-renal syndrome,[62-64] or Kallmann's syndrome.[65] In some instances different classes of mutations may determine whether syndromic or isolated CAKUT develops. For instance, two recessive protein-truncating mutations in any one of the genes *FRAS1*, *FREM2*, *GRIP1*, *FREM1*, and *GREM1* cause Fraser's syndrome, whereas two recessive hypomorphic (mild) mutations in any of these genes only cause isolated CAKUT.[19,66]

PATHOGENESIS

The pathologic basis of CAKUT is the disturbance of normal nephrogenesis[67] as a result of mutations in genes that govern this process.[50] Many of these genes encode transcription factors.[20] Because different mutations in transcription factor genes may cause stochastic effects of genetic dosing, mutations in transcription factors may partly account for the variable expressivity (i.e., different severity of bilateral malformations) seen in CAKUT. In the future many forms of CAKUT will likely be recognized as single-gene defects, which will allow important advances in preventive diagnostic tests.

RENAL CYSTIC CILIOPATHIES
(See Chapter 46)

Cystic kidney diseases are almost exclusively of monogenic origin. Currently over 90 genes have been identified as causing cystic kidney diseases, if mutated (see Table 43.3). Virtually all of these genes are recessive genes, with the exception of *PKD1* and *PKD2*, which if mutated cause ADPKD, and the two genes *UMOD* and *MUC1* mutated in medullary cystic kidney disease (MCKD). Cystic kidney diseases have been summarized under the term "renal cystic ciliopathies," because their encoded gene products localize to primary cilia or basal bodies, from which primary cilia are assembled. Primary cilia are antenna-like cellular organelles that most cell types in the human body may generate and that play an important role in the reception of extracellular signals. It seems, however, that centrosomes and their role in cell cycle regulation are more important for the pathogenesis of renal cystic ciliopathies than primary cilia themselves.[68-70]

POLYCYSTIC KIDNEY DISEASE

In PKD, kidneys become grossly enlarged, and cysts are uniformly spread out over the entire kidney parenchyma. There are two dominant genes (*PKD1* and *PKD2*) and one recessive gene (*PKHD1*). In MCKD, on the other hand, kidneys may or may not be enlarged, and distribution of renal cysts is very inhomogeneous. There are two genes causing MCKD (*UMOD* and *MUC1*).[71] In the nephronophthisis-related ciliopathies (NPHP-RCs), for which over 90 causative genes are known (see later), kidneys usually retain their normal size or are diminished in size.

ADPKD is the most frequent lethal dominant disease in the United States and Europe, afflicting approximately 1 in 1000 individuals.[72] CKD develops by 60 to 70 years of age. The two genes mutated in ADPKD, *PKD1* and *PKD2*, encode polycystin 1 and polycystin 2, respectively, transmembrane proteins that are important for maintenance of renal tubular cell differentiation.[73] Although these mutations segregate in families in an autosomal dominant way, the cellular defect leading to renal cysts most likely involves a "loss-of-function" mechanism, with the cumulative stochastic occurrence of second-hit mutations that arise spontaneously throughout life in distinct renal tubular cells, thereby inducing growth of cysts.[72] Because of the presence of four PKD1-related pseudogenes, development of molecular genetic diagnostics was difficult to develop for ADPKD. However, up to 90% of cases of ADPKD can now be diagnosed by mutation testing. This may aid clinical decision making, especially if living related donor transplantation is planned within PKD families.[74,75]

Autosomal recessive PKD (ARPKD is characterized by bilateral renal cystic enlargement that may start in utero.[69] CKD develops postnatally, in childhood or adolescence, depending on the severity of the two recessive mutations in the *PKHD1* gene. Specifically, the presence of truncating mutations in *PKHD1* is associated with perinatal onset of ARPKD. Intrahepatic bile duct dysplasia causes chronic liver fibrosis with abnormal bile duct structure (Caroli's disease) as an extrarenal manifestation of ARPKD.

Renal cysts may also be caused by genes that if mutated cause benign and malignant tumors of the kidney, including mutations in *TSC1*, *TSC2*, *VHL*, and *WT1*. Molecular genetic diagnostic tests play an important role in the diagnosis and prevention of such tumors in families with mutations in these genes.[76]

NEPHRONOPHTHISIS-RELATED CILIOPATHIES

In NPHP-RC over 90 causative recessive genes are known (see Table 43.3).[77-80] CKD develops by a median age of 13 years.[81,82] Unlike in PKD, cysts are mostly restricted to the corticomedullary border of the kidneys. Upon renal ultrasonography, cortical medullary differentiation is lost and kidney size is normal or reduced. NPHP-RCs are often associated with extrarenal manifestations, including retinal degeneration (Senior-Loken syndrome), liver fibrosis, or cerebellar vermis aplasia (Joubert's syndrome). Bardet-Biedl syndrome is a form of NPHP-RC that is characterized by the cardinal features of retinitis pigmentosa, polydactyly, mental retardation, hypogenitalism, and obesity together with NPHP-RC.[83,84] For molecular genetic diagnostics the high number of NPHP-RC genes is best examined using WES (see later), interrogating the exome data for mutations in the approximately 90 known NPHP-RC genes.

GENOTYPE-PHENOTYPE CORRELATION

For both ADPKD and ARPKD it was noted that protein-truncating mutations have a higher likelihood of leading to earlier onset of CKD than missense mutations.[85-87] Also in NPHP-RC the nature of the two recessive mutations determines disease severity and extent of organ involvement, leading to seemingly different disorders. Within this genotype-phenotype association, protein-truncating mutations cause severe, early-onset, dysplastic, multiorgan disease in the disease phenotype of Meckel-Gruber syndrome, whereas hypomorphic (missense) mutations cause mild, late-onset, degenerative disease with less extrarenal organ involvement.[80,88] The extent and severity of extrarenal organ involvement in NPHP-RC is determined by three genetic mechanisms: (1) mutations in different genes cause phenotypes of different severities; (2) whereas two truncating mutations of NPHP3, CEP290, or RPGRIP1L cause Meckel-Gruber syndrome, the presence of at least one missense mutation leads to the milder phenotype of Joubert's syndrome with degenerative disease of kidney, eye, and cerebellum; and (3) in homozygous NPHP1 deletions, the presence of an additional heterozygous mutation in CEP290, or RPGRIP1L may cause additional eye or cerebellar involvement.[89,90] So-called oligogenicity has been postulated in Bardet-Biedl syndrome.[91] The concept of oligogenicity assumes that under certain circumstances the presence of two or more heterozygous mutations of different recessive genes may cause disease.[91,92] However, so far there is no direct proof of this concept. This concept will have to be established on the basis of studies in mouse models before conclusions about its clinical effect can be drawn in humans. The validity of zebrafish models of morpholino oligonucleotide knockdown to model the pathogenesis of NPHP-RC within the concept of oligogenicity has been questioned.[93]

PATHOGENESIS

The pathogenesis of renal cystic diseases is still obscure. A unifying pathogenic theory for cystic kidney diseases was developed following the discovery that all gene products defective in cystic kidney diseases localize to the primary cilia–centrosome complex.[80,94] Centrosomes, which convert into the spindle poles during mitosis, play an important part in cell-cycle regulation and in the assembly of primary cilia. Therefore PKD, NPHP-RC, Meckel-Gruber syndrome, and Bardet-Biedl syndrome have been summarized under the term "renal cystic ciliopathies."[80,94] Multiple cellular signaling pathways have been implicated in the pathogenesis of renal cystic ciliopathies, including Wnt,[95,96] Sonic hedgehog,[97,98] Hippo,[99] and DNA damage response signaling.[68-70,80,100-102] Many mouse models have been generated to study the pathogenesis of renal cystic ciliopathies, which has partially led to therapeutic approaches toward these mouse models.[103-105] Finally, identification of monogenic disease genes has allowed initial insights into the pathogenesis of renal cystic ciliopathies that have been the basis of therapeutic trials in patients with ADPKD.[106]

NEPHROLITHIASIS/NEPHROCALCINOSIS
(See Chapter 40)

Nephrolithiasis is a prevalent condition with a high morbidity. Several single-gene defects have been identified, many of them representing rare abnormalities of specific renal tubular transport channel and renal transporter genes. Highly parallel exon sequencing of 30 candidate genes was performed in 268 families with nephrolithiasis (n = 256) or nephrocalcinosis (n = 16).[107] Fifty causative mutations have been detected in 14 of 30 analyzed genes, leading to a molecular diagnosis in 15% of all cases.[107] The cystinuria gene SLC7A9 (n = 19) was most frequently mutated. The detection rate of monogenic causes of nephrolithiasis was notably high in both the adult (11.4%) and pediatric cohorts (20.8%). Mutations in recessive genes were more frequent among children, whereas dominant disease occurred more frequently in adults. In some individuals mutation detection had consequences for clinical management.[107] In conclusion, in families or single individuals with at least one episode of nephrolithiasis, molecular genetic exon sequencing using a nephrolithiasis/nephrocalcinosis panel (see Table 43.4) is warranted to determine the molecular genetic cause of nephrolithiasis and nephrocalcinosis. The findings may guide personalized treatment of nephrolithiasis.

INHERITED RENAL TUBULOPATHIES
(See Chapter 45)

Due to early advances in renal physiology, combined with expression cloning, genes that if mutated cause renal tubulopathies were among the first monogenic kidney disease genes to be identified. Renal tubular function governs reabsorption of water and solutes from the glomerular filtrate. In renal tubulopathies the primary genetic defect causes loss of function of a specific renal transport protein or signaling molecule. For some diseases, such as Bartter's syndrome, similar phenotypes may be caused by mutations in different genes (SLC12A1, CLCNKB, KCNJ1, or BSND), whose encoded proteins act in concert regarding well-defined tasks of sodium reabsorption in the thick ascending limb of Henle's loop.[108-112]

Functional disturbances of some tubule segments lead to segment-specific defects in tubular reabsorption: **Proximal tubule defects** cause glucosuria, phosphaturia, aminoaciduria, or proximal renal tubular acidosis. This combination of features is known as renal Fanconi's syndrome. Dysfunction of sodium reabsorption in the **thick ascending limb of Henle's loop** causes Bartter's syndrome, renal salt loss, and secondary hypokalemic metabolic alkalosis. Defects of the distal convoluted tubule cause Gitelman's syndrome[113] and other forms of hypomagnesemia.[114-117] Finally, tubulopathies of the collecting duct impair reabsorption of water, sodium, potassium, and protons, resulting in polyuria, salt loss, hyperkalemia, and acidosis, respectively. Mutations in the aquaporin-2 water channel cause recessive nephrogenic diabetes insipidus,[117] and mutations in the vasopressin V_2 receptor cause X-linked nephrogenic diabetes insipidus.[118,119] In secondary tubulopathies the genetic defect does not directly affect a tubular transport or transport signaling proteins but rather nonspecifically leads to damage of renal tubular cells and thereby impairs renal tubular function. Gene identification has rendered the often-enigmatic disease group of tubulopathies accessible to unequivocal diagnostic tests that use a panel of 30 genes that cause renal tubulopathies if mutated.

ATYPICAL HEMOLYTIC UREMIC SYNDROMES (See Chapter 35)

In atypical hemolytic uremic syndrome (aHUS) multiple monogenic causes of disease have been described. They involve regulators of the complement system that modulate complement activation and protect host cells against complement damage. Monogenic causes of aHUS include the genes for complement factor I *(CFI)*[120] and complement factor B *(CFB)*,[121] mutations of which are inherited in an autosomal dominant fashion. Autosomal recessive variants of aHUS are caused by mutations in the gene for diacylglycerol kinase ε*(DGKE)*,[122] complement factor H *(CFH)*,[123] complement factor H-related 1, 3, or 4 *(CFHR1, CFHR3, or CFHR4)*.[124] Mutations in the genes for complement component 3 *(C3)*[124] or for complement regulatory protein *(CD46*, alias *MCP)*[125] may be inherited in either a recessive or dominant fashion. Monogenic forms of aHUS often feature renal histologic characteristics of membranoproliferative glomerulonephritis.

Mutation analysis to identify the causative mutation is particularly important in the autosomal dominant versions of aHUS, because dominant diseases occur throughout multiple generations. In autosomal dominant inheritance there can be age-related penetrance and incomplete penetrance (i.e., a generation may be skipped by the disease altogether). Therefore mutation analysis will be helpful for identifying who in a family is at risk for a potential treatment approach (e.g., the likelihood of responding to eculizumab) before an episode of the disease occurs.

IDENTIFICATION OF NOVEL SINGLE-GENE KIDNEY DISORDERS

WHOLE-EXOME SEQUENCING

The development of WES has greatly facilitated identification of novel disease-causing genes in single-gene disorders. When WES is performed, DNA of an individual is broken into random fragments using an air jet. The fragments are then hybridized to an array of oligonucleotides that represent the entire human "exome" (i.e., all ≈330,000 exons that encode proteins in the human genome). Non–exon-containing fragments are discarded (99% of the genome), and the exon-containing fragments are eluted, followed by one next-generation sequencing run. Because approximately 85% of all disease-causing mutations in mendelian disorders reside within coding exons,[126] exome capture with consecutive large-scale sequencing currently has a high likelihood of identifying a disease-causing mutation. However, modern techniques of WES and large-scale sequencing will produce a high number of sequence variants when the exome sequence of a patient under study is compared to a normal reference sequence. This renders identification of a mutation in the single disease-causing gene difficult. This problem can be overcome by evaluating WES data a priori only for the candidate genes from the indication-driven diagnostic panels that are suggested by the patient's clinical "indication criteria." The use of WES has greatly furthered the success rate of molecular genetic diagnostics.[6-12,127,128]

Of approximately 7200 mendelian disorders, the disease-causing gene is still unknown in roughly 3200 disorders (http://www.omim.org/statistics/entry). Specifically in single-gene renal disorders, many causative genes are still unknown. The application of WES, particularly when combined with genetic mapping, has greatly helped the identification of novel disease genes.[117,118,129] The identification of single-gene causes of renal disease offers the unique advantage that it leads to the discovery of components of renal function, each of which *alone* is necessary to maintain renal function (i.e., to avoid development of the respective disease). In this way discovery of monogenic disease genes has helped our understanding of many mechanisms of renal disease. This effect is currently strongly enhanced by the finding that many proteins encoded by monogenic disease genes are part of functional protein complexes, thereby elucidating signaling pathways and other complex functional components of renal function.

FUTURE DIRECTIONS IN SINGLE-GENE DISORDERS

For individuals who develop CKD before 25 years of age the likelihood is approximately 20% that a causative mutation can be detected by WES (see Table 43.4). Given this opportunity, molecular genetic diagnostics should be offered if indicated (e.g., by the indication clinical criteria listed in Table 43.3). Molecular genetic diagnostics are initiated following informed consent. And often, especially in the setting of familial disease, genetic counseling is advisable.

An important feature of monogenic diseases is the fact that the disease-causing mutation represents the primary cause of the disease. The identification of single-gene causes of renal disease will have a major impact on the understanding of disease mechanisms, diagnostics, prophylaxis, and treatment for the following reasons:

1. Single-gene disorders allow unequivocal molecular genetic diagnostics with a very high sensitivity, specificity, and positive predictive value. For instance, recessive disease gene mutations represent "biomarkers" that have virtually 100% specificity, because virtually all individuals who carry a mutation on both gene copies will inescapably develop disease.

2. Unequivocal molecular genetic diagnostic tests can be offered to avoid invasive diagnostic procedures such as renal biopsy.
3. Molecular genetic diagnostics also permit prenatal diagnosis (e.g. for the diagnosis of the perinatal lethal Meckel-Gruber syndrome).
4. Specific prognostic outcomes can be delineated for specific mutations (e.g., the risk for developing gonadoblastoma in specific *WT1* mutations.[130]
5. Subgroups of diseases can be classified on an etiologic basis (e.g., for therapeutic trials).
6. In rare instances identification of the causative mutation reveals that a personalized treatment option is available, as exemplified by CoQ_{10} treatment in SRNS caused by CoQ_{10} biosynthesis defects.
7. Single-gene (monogenic) causes of disease provide deep mechanistic insights, because they constitute one of the strongest cause-effect relationships known to medicine (e.g., in a *recessive* disease there is virtually 100% disease penetrance).
8. Because of this strong cause-effect relationship, single-gene disorders permit powerful mechanistic studies that commence at the primary cause of the defect (i.e., the gene mutation).
9. Recessive single-gene defects can easily be recapitulated in animal models of gene knockout or knockdown to perform detailed pathophysiologic studies.
10. New treatment modalities can be developed by screening for small molecules, using high-throughput cell-based assays or animal models (e.g., in SRNS, for which currently no curative treatment exists).

COMMON AND POLYGENIC RENAL DISORDERS

POLYGENIC DISEASES

Disease-causing mutations of **single-gene disorders** are rare, strongly affect the disease phenotype with (almost) full penetrance, manifest early in life, are seldom influenced by environmental effects, and are usually detected by linkage mapping and WES (see Table 43.1). By contrast, **polygenic disorders**, in which several mutated alleles in different genes have to act in concert to cause disease, are more common, exert weak causality on the disease phenotype, manifest later in life, and are more commonly subject to gene-by-environment influences (see Table 43.1). Polygenic diseases usually represent common diseases, whereas single-gene disorders are rare diseases (as defined by a prevalence of less than 200,000 affected individual in the United States at any given time). The pathogenic effect of a polygenic disease gene can usually not be assigned as causative, but rather as conveying a relative risk for developing disease. The respective genetic variant is then considered as "associated" with disease and is usually discovered by GWAS.[1] An up-to-date consideration of models that describe the contribution of allelic variants at multiple loci to polygenic disease shows patterns ranging from the cumulative effect of very many rare variants to stronger effects of higher-frequency risk variants at a limited number of loci.[131]

An example of successful identification of disease risk alleles in kidney diseases is that of specific haplotypes in the *APOL1* locus that were associated with an increased risk for focal segmental glomerulosclerosis and CKD in African American patients.[3,132-134] Approximately 60% of African Americans in the United States (compared with 4% of European Americans) carry this risk allele, and the risk for developing focal segmental glomerulosclerosis is increased fivefold.[3,4,132,133,135]

Other examples of the discovery of risk alleles in renal diseases are variants of the *ELMO1* gene that have been associated with nephropathy in type 2 diabetes.[136,137] Furthermore, Köttgen and colleagues identified a polymorphic single-nucleotide polymorphism (rs12917707) near the *UMOD* gene (in which dominant monogenic mutations cause autosomal dominant MCKD type 2) that was strongly associated with CKD.[138,139] In addition, risk allele associations have been described for hypertension (Online Mendelian Inheritance in Man [OMIM] #145500), aHUS (OMIM #235400), and ureteropelvic junction obstruction (OMIM *300034) (OMIM website: http://www.omim.org).

A limitation of GWAS is that GWAS results often account for only a small proportion of the variance of the disease phenotype (usually ≈1%) and that any assignment of an associated genetic marker to a disease mechanism or loss of gene function of a specific gene is difficult.[1] This limits the utility for genetic counseling for an individual regarding the genetic risk alleles. Another limitation rests with the fact that a risk marker allele identified by GWAS is only considered "associated" with disease, because it is positioned in a chromosomal location that is significantly more frequently found in cases versus controls. Due to this associative rather than causative relation between risk markers and disease, it is possible that the true disease-relevant genetic variant may be missed. This was the case when on the basis of GWAS data initially a polymorphic allele in the *MYH9* gene was attributed to conveying increased risk for developing focal segmental glomerulosclerosis in African American individuals.[140,141] Later this finding was revised to instead implicate the *APOL1* gene as associated with this disease risk.[3,4]

THE TERRITORY BETWEEN MONOGENIC AND POLYGENIC DISEASE

The clear-cut border between single-gene and polygenic diseases has become blurred: For example, most patients with complete absence of *NPHP1* function based on a homozygous deletion in this gene develop isolated nephronophthisis only. However, in these patients the presence of a heterozygous mutation in *NPHP6* causes the additional disease phenotypes of retinal degeneration or ataxia.[89,142,143] In this context the heterozygous mutation in *NPHP6* is thought to exert a **modifier gene effect** on *NPHP1*, because a heterozygous mutation alone in the recessive gene *NPHP6* does not elicit any disease phenotype.

Complete reference list available at ExpertConsult.com.

KEY REFERENCES

1. Altshuler D, Daly MJ, Lander ES: Genetic mapping in human disease. *Science* 322:881–888, 2008.

3. Genovese G, Friedman DJ, Ross MD, et al: Association of trypanolytic ApoL1 variants with kidney disease in African Americans. *Science* 329:841–845, 2010.
7. MacArthur DG, Manolio TA, Dimmock DP, et al: Guidelines for investigating causality of sequence variants in human disease. *Nature* 508:469–676, 2014.
14. Halbritter J, Porath JD, Diaz KA, et al: Identification of 99 novel mutations in a worldwide cohort of 1,056 patients with a nephronophthisis-related ciliopathy. *Hum Genet* 132:865–884, 2013.
18. Hwang DY, Dworschak GC, Kohl S, et al: Mutations in 12 known dominant disease-causing genes clarify many congenital anomalies of the kidney and urinary tract. *Kidney Int* 85:1429–1433, 2014.
19. Kohl S, Hwang DY, Dworschak GC, et al: Mild recessive mutations in six Fraser syndrome-related genes cause isolated congenital anomalies of the kidney and urinary tract. *J Am Soc Nephrol* 25:1917–1922, 2014.
20. Vivante A, Kohl S, Hwang DY, et al: Single-gene causes of congenital anomalies of the kidney and urinary tract (CAKUT) in humans. *Pediatr Nephrol* 29:695–704, 2014.
23. Hildebrandt F: Genetic kidney diseases. *Lancet* 375:1287–1295, 2010.
26. Antignac C: Molecular basis of steroid-resistant nephrotic syndrome. *Nefrologia* 25:25–28, 2005.
32. Hinkes BG, Mucha B, Vlangos CN, et al: Nephrotic syndrome in the first year of life: two thirds of cases are caused by mutations in 4 genes (*NPHS1*, *NPHS2*, *WT1*, and *LAMB2*). *Pediatrics* 119:e907–e919, 2007.
33. Kaplan JM, Kim SH, North KN, et al: Mutations in ACTN4, encoding alpha-actinin-4, cause familial focal segmental glomerulosclerosis. *Nat Genet* 24:251–256, 2000.
34. Reiser J, Polu KR, Moller CC, et al: TRPC6 is a glomerular slit diaphragm-associated channel required for normal renal function. *Nat Genet* 37:739–744, 2005.
36. Hildebrandt F, Heeringa SF: Specific podocin mutations determine age of onset of nephrotic syndrome all the way into adult life. *Kidney Int* 75:669–671, 2009.
38. Hinkes B, Vlangos C, Heeringa S, et al: Specific podocin mutations correlate with age of onset in steroid-resistant nephrotic syndrome. *J Am Soc Nephrol* 19:365–371, 2008.
42. Ashraf S, Gee HY, Woerner S, et al: ADCK4 mutations promote steroid-resistant nephrotic syndrome through CoQ10 biosynthesis disruption. *J Clin Invest* 123:5179–5189, 2013.
43. Heeringa SF, Chernin G, Chaki M, et al: COQ6 mutations in human patients produce nephrotic syndrome with sensorineural deafness. *J Clin Invest* 121:2013–2024, 2011.
44. Wiggins RC: The spectrum of podocytopathies: a unifying view of glomerular diseases. *Kidney Int* 71:1205–1214, 2007.
45. Gee HY, Saisawat P, Ashraf S, et al: ARHGDIA mutations cause nephrotic syndrome via defective RHO GTPase signaling. *J Clin Invest* 123:3243–3253, 2013.
47. Zhou W, Hildebrandt F: Inducible podocyte injury and proteinuria in transgenic zebrafish. *J Am Soc Nephrol* 23:1039–1047, 2012.
50. Chen F: Genetic and developmental basis for urinary tract obstruction. *Pediatr Nephrol* 24:1621–1632, 2009.
55. Lu W, van Eerde AM, Fan X, et al: Disruption of ROBO2 is associated with urinary tract anomalies and confers risk of vesicoureteral reflux. *Am J Hum Genet* 80:616–632, 2007.
63. Ruf RG, Xu PX, Silvius D, et al: SIX1 mutations cause branchio-oto-renal syndrome by disruption of EYA1-SIX1-DNA complexes. *Proc Natl Acad Sci U S A* 101:8090–8095, 2004.
68. Chaki M, Airik R, Ghosh AK, et al: Exome capture reveals *ZNF423* and *CEP164* mutations, linking renal ciliopathies to DNA damage response signaling. *Cell* 150:533–548, 2012.
69. Lans H, Hoeijmakers JH: Genome stability, progressive kidney failure and aging. *Nat Genet* 44:836–838, 2012.
70. Zhou W, Otto EA, Cluckey A, et al: FAN1 mutations cause karyomegalic interstitial nephritis, linking chronic kidney failure to defective DNA damage repair. *Nat Genet* 44:910–915, 2012.
72. Torres VE, Harris PC: Autosomal dominant polycystic kidney disease: the last 3 years. *Kidney Int* 76:149–168, 2009.
73. Kim E, Walz G: Sensitive cilia set up the kidney. *Nat Med* 13:1409–1411, 2007.
76. Henske EP: The genetic basis of kidney cancer: why is tuberous sclerosis complex often overlooked? *Curr Mol Med* 4:825–831, 2004.
80. Hildebrandt F, Benzing T, Katsanis N: Ciliopathies. *N Engl J Med* 364:1533–1543, 2011.
88. Chaki M, Hoefele J, Allen SJ, et al: Genotype-phenotype correlation in 440 patients with NPHP-related ciliopathies. *Kidney Int* 80:1239–1245, 2011.
91. Katsanis N, Ansley SJ, Badano JL, et al: Triallelic inheritance in Bardet-Biedl syndrome, a mendelian recessive disorder. *Science* 293:2256–2259, 2001.
94. Hildebrandt F, Otto E: Cilia and centrosomes: a unifying pathogenic concept for cystic kidney disease? *Nat Rev Genet* 6:928–940, 2005.
95. Otto EA, Schermer B, Obara T, et al: Mutations in INVS encoding inversin cause nephronophthisis type 2, linking renal cystic disease to the function of primary cilia and left-right axis determination. *Nat Genet* 34:413–420, 2003.
96. Watnick T, Germino G: From cilia to cyst. *Nat Genet* 34:355–356, 2003.
98. Attanasio M, Uhlenhaut NH, Sousa VH, et al: Loss of GLIS2 causes nephronophthisis in humans and mice by increased apoptosis and fibrosis. *Nat Genet* 39:1018–1024, 2007.
106. Torres VE: Treatment strategies and clinical trial design in ADPKD. *Adv Chronic Kidney Dis* 17:190–204, 2010.
107. Halbritter J, Baum M, Hynes AM, et al: Fourteen monogenic genes account for 15% of nephrolithiasis/nephrocalcinosis. *J Am Soc Nephrol* 26:543–551, 2015.
108. Simon DB, Karet FE, Hamdan JM, et al: Bartter's syndrome, hypokalaemic alkalosis with hypercalciuria, is caused by mutations in the Na-K-2Cl cotransporter NKCC2. *Nat Genet* 13:183–188, 1996.
111. Birkenhager R, Otto E, Schurmann MJ, et al: Mutation of BSND causes Bartter syndrome with sensorineural deafness and kidney failure. *Nat Genet* 29:310–314, 2001.
113. Simon DB, Nelson-Williams C, Bia MJ, et al: Gitelman's variant of Bartter's syndrome, inherited hypokalaemic alkalosis, is caused by mutations in the thiazide-sensitive Na-Cl cotransporter. *Nat Genet* 12:24–30, 1996.
117. Deen PM, Verdijk MA, Knoers NV, et al: Requirement of human renal water channel aquaporin-2 for vasopressin-dependent concentration of urine. *Science* 264:92–95, 1994.
126. Lifton RP: Individual genomes on the horizon. *N Engl J Med* 362:1235–1236, 2010.
127. Otto EA, Hurd TW, Airik R, et al: Candidate exome capture identifies mutation of SDCCAG8 as the cause of a retinal-renal ciliopathy. *Nat Genet* 42:840–850, 2010.
128. Gee HY, Otto EA, Hurd TW, et al: Whole-exome resequencing distinguishes cystic kidney diseases from phenocopies in renal ciliopathies. *Kidney Int* 85:880–887, 2014.
129. Hildebrandt F, Heeringa SF, Ruschendorf F, et al: A systematic approach to mapping recessive disease genes in individuals from outbred populations. *PLoS Genet* 5:e1000353, 2009.
132. Freedman BI, Kopp JB, Langefeld CD, et al: The apolipoprotein L1 (APOL1) gene and nondiabetic nephropathy in African Americans. *J Am Soc Nephrol* 21:1422–1426, 2010.
136. Divers J, Freedman BI: Susceptibility genes in common complex kidney disease. *Curr Opin Nephrol Hypertens* 19:79–84, 2010.
138. Köttgen A, Glazer NL, Dehghan A, et al: Multiple loci associated with indices of renal function and chronic kidney disease. *Nat Genet* 41:712–717, 2009.
141. Kopp JB, Smith MW, Nelson GW, et al: MYH9 is a major-effect risk gene for focal segmental glomerulosclerosis. *Nat Genet* 40:1175–1184, 2008.
142. Sayer JA, Otto EA, O'Toole JF, et al: The centrosomal protein nephrocystin-6 is mutated in Joubert syndrome and activates transcription factor ATF4. *Nat Genet* 38:674–681, 2006.

Inherited Disorders of the Glomerulus

44

Karl Tryggvason | Jaako Patrakka

CHAPTER OUTLINE

INHERITED DISORDERS PRIMARILY AFFECTING THE GLOMERULAR BASEMENT MEMBRANE, 1421
Type IV Collagen Disease, 1421
Laminin Disease: Pierson's Syndrome, 1426
INHERITED DISORDERS PRIMARILY AFFECTING THE PODOCYTE, 1426
Nephrin Disease: Congenital Nephrotic Syndrome of the Finnish Type, 1426
Podocin Disease: Steroid-Resistant Nephrotic Syndrome, 1428
INF2 Disease: Focal Segmental Glomerulosclerosis and Charcot-Marie Tooth Neuropathy–Associated Glomerulopathy, 1429
APOL1 Gene: Susceptibility to Focal Segmental Glomerulosclerosis, 1429

PLCE1 Disease: Familial Diffuse Mesangial Sclerosis, 1429
Focal Segmental Glomerulosclerosis, 1430
Glepp1 Disease: Steroid-Resistant Nephrotic Syndrome, 1431
INHERITED PRIMARY GLOMERULAR DISORDERS OF UNKNOWN CAUSE, 1431
Galloway-Mowat Syndrome, 1431
Immunoglobulin A Nephropathy, 1431
INHERITED SYSTEMIC SYNDROMES AFFECTING THE GLOMERULUS, 1431
Nail-Patella Syndrome, 1431
Denys-Drash and Frasier's Syndromes, 1431
Mitochondrial Disorders, 1432
Schimke's Immuno-Osseous Dysplasia, 1432
Scarb2 Disease, 1432

Most kidney disease cases that progress to end-stage kidney disease (ESKD) originate in glomerular insults. However, the causes and pathomechanisms of this large group of kidney diseases are still poorly understood. Since 1990, the underlying cause of several rare glomerular diseases has been elucidated at the gene level. This new information has revealed the existence of a large number of proteins that are crucial for different parts of the filtration barrier, such as the glomerular basement membrane (GBM), slit diaphragm, and podocyte cells. Identification of mutations in genes for these proteins has provided new insight into the molecular nature of the filtration barrier, protein function, and functionally important parts of the proteins and how some of these proteins normally interact. Although the causes of most of the glomerular diseases still remain to be clarified, new information that has accumulated at an increasingly rapid pace has yielded new diagnostic possibilities for many glomerular diseases.

INHERITED DISORDERS PRIMARILY AFFECTING THE GLOMERULAR BASEMENT MEMBRANE

The GBM is a specialized type of basement membrane that forms a central part of the glomerular filtration barrier. In adults, this sheetlike extracellular structure, which is about 300 to 350 nm thick, is composed of basement membrane proteins, such as type IV collagen, laminin, proteoglycans (perlecan and agrin), and nidogens. Triple-helical type IV collagen molecules composed of three α-chains assemble extracellularly to form the structural framework of the GBM (Figure 44.1). There are three types of type IV collagen trimers with chain compositions α1:α1:α2, α3:α4:α5, and α5:α5:α6. The genes for these chains are located in pairs head to head on three different chromosomes (see Figure 44.1). Mutations in any of the genes can lead to defects in the GBM and, in some cases, defects in the basement membranes of other tissues; these defects, in turn, result in diseases such as Alport's syndrome, thin basement membrane nephropathy (TBMN), and the syndrome of hereditary angiopathy, nephropathy, aneurysms, and muscle cramps (HANAC syndrome). Laminins are also trimeric proteins consisting of α-, β-, and γ-chains that exist in five, four, and three genetically distinct forms, respectively.[1] These chains can form at least 15 different isoforms in vivo. Mutations in the gene for the β2-chain present in laminin-521 (α5:β2:γ1) lead to Pierson's syndrome, a distinct type of nephrotic syndrome.

TYPE IV COLLAGEN DISEASE

ALPORT'S SYNDROME (HEREDITARY NEPHRITIS)

Alport's syndrome is an inherited disorder of type IV (basement membrane) collagen. It affects primarily renal

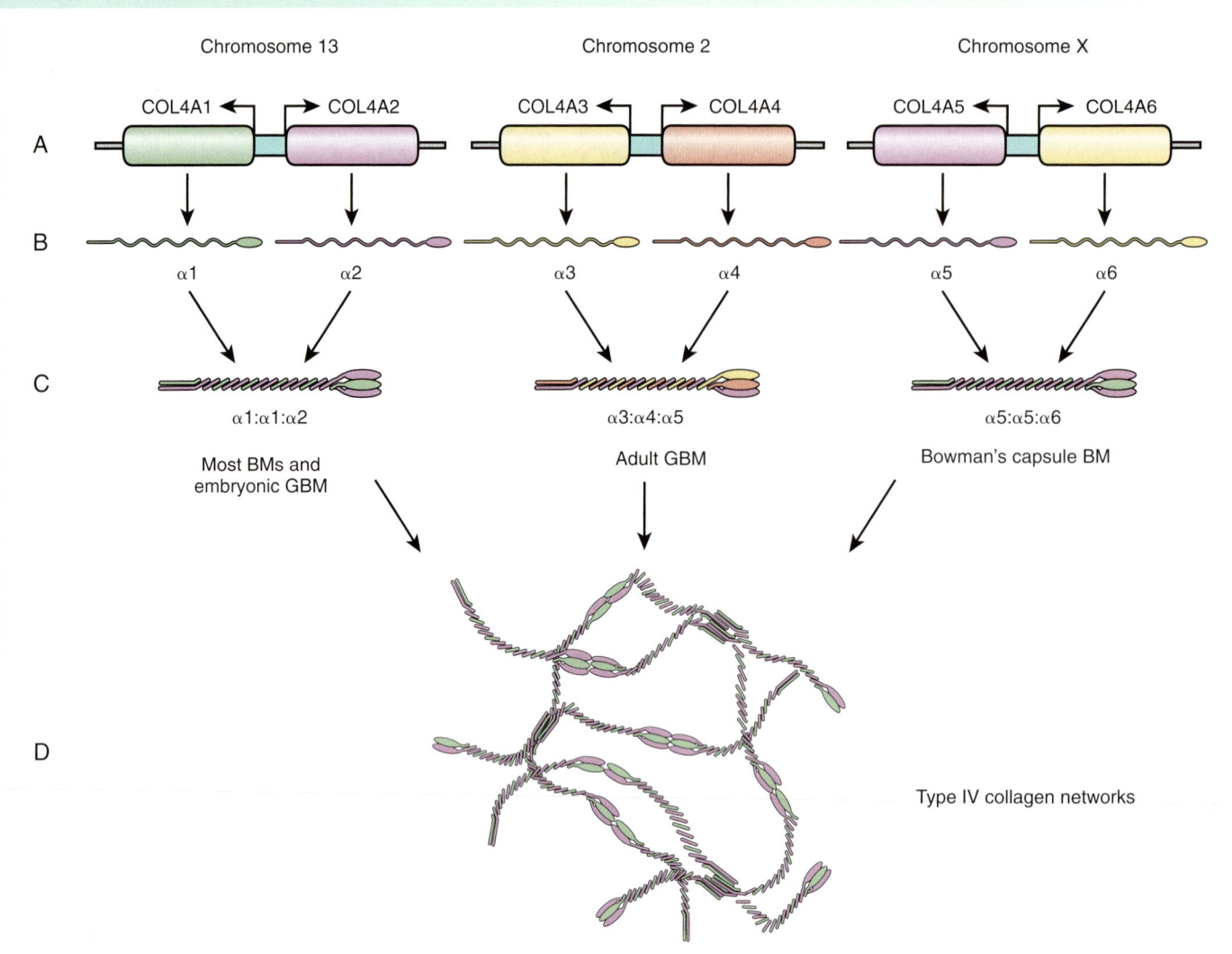

Figure 44.1 Type IV collagen genes, α-chains, and glomerular isoforms. **A,** The six collagen IV genes (*COL4A1* to *COL4A6*) are located pairwise in a head to head manner on three different chromosomes. **B,** The *COL4A* genes generate six different α-chains that have a globular noncollagenous domain at their C-terminus. **C,** Three chains form three combinations of triple-helical molecules. **D,** Extracellularly, the triple-helical type IV collagen molecules form a network by associating with each other at their ends so that two molecules are cross-linked through their C-terminal globular domain (NC1) and four trimers associate with each other at the N-termini. In the embryonic glomerular basement membrane (GBM), the ubiquitous α1:α1:α2 trimer is the only isoform. After birth, this isoform is gradually replaced by an α3:α4:α5 isoform, which is more cross-linked through disulfide bonds within the collagenous regions (*black spots*) and more resistant to extracellular proteolysis. Defects in the α3:α4:α5 trimers lead to thin basement membrane nephropathy (TBMN) or Alport's syndrome, depending on the extensiveness of alleles involved (see text). A single-allele mutation in *COL4A1* has been shown to cause the syndrome of hereditary angiopathy, nephropathy, aneurysms, and muscle cramps (HANAC syndrome).

glomeruli but is also associated with sensorineural hearing loss and ocular lesions.[2-4] About 85% of the cases are X-linked; the rest are mainly autosomal recessive. Thus, most patients with Alport's syndrome are males. The disease was first described by Alport in 1927 as hematuria-associated deafness and uremia in affected male patients.[2] The disease usually manifests in childhood with persistent hematuria and mild proteinuria. The pathomechanism of the disease began to be elucidated in the early 1990s with the identification of three novel type IV collagen genes.[5-7] Clinical variability within kindreds with Alport's syndrome reflects the complexity of collagen genetics involving three gene loci and variability with regard to the site and nature of gene mutations. Absence of a functionally specific type IV collagen isoform that is essential for the integrity of adult GBM leads to breakdown and disintegration of this specialized basement membrane. The disease is usually identified through the identification of hematuria in association with hearing loss in children or young adults.

Genetics and Pathogenesis

Alport's syndrome is caused by mutations in genes encoding α-chains of type IV collagen that forms the structural skeleton of basement membranes. Type IV collagen molecules are large triple-helical proteins containing three α-chains (see Figure 44.1). Six genetically distinct α-chains are present in vivo in three trimeric isoforms—α1:α1:α2, α3:α4:α5, and α5:α5:α6.[8] The α1:α1:α2 trimer, a ubiquitous isoform present in basement membranes of most tissues, is expressed in the GBM during embryogenesis, but after birth it is replaced by an adult isoform, α3:α4:α5, which is a more stable protein containing more cross-links and is more resistant to proteinases.[3] The α3-, α4-, and α5-chains are encoded by the *COL4A3*, *COL4A4*, and *COL4A5* genes, respectively. *COL4A5* is located head to head with *COL4A6* on the X chromosome, and *COL4A3* and *COL4A4* are located head to head on chromosome 2 (see Figure 44.1).[3] As a consequence of structurally abnormal α3:α4:α5 collagen molecules or their absence, the GBM structural framework becomes distorted and regionally broken down, which, in turn, allows for limited passage of red blood corpuscles into the urine.

Male patients with X-linked Alport's syndrome are hemizygous for mutations in a single allele of the *COL4A5* gene.[5] Several hundred mutations, including missense and nonsense (frameshift) mutations, splice mutations, deletions, insertions, and inversions have been described, and new mutations are continuously identified.[9-11] On occasion, concomitant mutations in the adjacent COL4A6 gene can also result in leiomyomatosis.[12]

Autosomal recessive Alport's syndrome is caused by compound heterozygous or homozygous mutations in the *COL4A3* and *COL4A4* genes that are located on chromosome 2q.[7,13-16] Single-allele mutations do not result in actual Alport's syndrome, but are associated with TBMN (see later discussion).

Data are strongly suggestive about the pathomechanisms of GBM distortion in Alport's syndrome. As is the case for other genetic collagen diseases, a large body of data suggests that an abnormal collagen chain does not usually incorporate intracellularly into a functional triple-helical molecule; instead, it is degraded intracellularly.[17] It is also evident that α3:α4:α5 trimers can be formed only if all chains are present intracellularly. Thus, if one chain is abnormal or absent and a trimer cannot be formed, then the other two chains are degraded. In response to the absence of α3:α4:α5 form trimers, the embryonic α1:α1:α2 form replaces them. However, this isoform is not capable of forming a structurally functional adult GBM. A similar lack of a developmental switch has been described in the cochlear basement membrane in patients with Alport's syndrome who have hearing loss.[18]

In patients with X-linked Alport's syndrome, the α3-, α4-, and α5-chains are usually completely undetectable in immunostained kidney sections. However, in autosomal recessive Alport's syndrome, in which the defects are in the *COL4A3* or *COL4A4* gene, the α5-chain is expressed in Bowman's capsule, where it is incorporated into an α5:α5:α6 trimer.[19]

Clinical Manifestations

Alport's syndrome is usually identified as persistent hematuria in children or young adults, particularly boys, often accompanied by reduced hearing.[20,21] Proteinuria is usually mild but becomes more severe with age.[4,22,23] In some cases, episodes of gross hematuria occur in connection with upper respiratory infections. As the disease progresses, hypertension may occur, particularly in male patients. The disease course is usually milder in female patients with persistent hematuria.

In a large study on 401 affected male patients in 195 kindreds with X-linked Alport's syndrome, hearing loss was present in about 82% of patients and ocular lesions developed in more than 44%.[4] The ocular lesions included mainly lenticonus, maculopathy, or both. Congenital or early-onset cataract formation was also found in some patients.[4] About 22% of patients did not have a family history, which suggests that de novo mutations are common. Moderate hypertension had variable occurrences, most often as a later manifestation. Leiomyomatosis, which is associated with defects in the *COL4A6* gene, is sometimes associated with X-linked inheritance.[12,24] Progression to ESKD occurs in about 80% of male patients.[4] An analysis of female patients in the same 195 kindreds revealed that about 95% of the female carriers for the disease have hematuria and proteinuria, and hearing loss and ocular defects developed with time in 75%, 30%, and 15% of patients, respectively.[4] However, the probability of developing ESKD by the age of 40 years was only about 10% in the female patients, as opposed to 90% in male hemizygotes.

Pathologic Findings and Diagnosis

The diagnosis of Alport's syndrome is based on findings from electron microscopic studies, immunofluorescence analysis and, more recently, DNA analysis. Normal light microscopy reveals no pathognomonic changes. At early stages (before age 5 years), kidney biopsy findings are usually normal. Once the presence of persistent microscopic hematuria and possibly signs of hearing loss have been established, kidney biopsies often reveal glomerular and tubular lesions. In children between 5 and 10 years of age, mesangial and capillary lesions, such as segmental to diffuse mesangial cell proliferation, matrix accumulation, and thickening of the capillary wall may be evident.[25] Tubulointerstitial damage may also be present, characterized by interstitial fibrosis, tubular atrophy, focal basement membrane thickening, and interstitial foamy cells.[26,27] With time, these changes progress from segmental to widely diffuse when the condition progresses to ESKD.

Immunofluorescence studies can be diagnostic. In X-linked and autosomal disease, glomeruli of male patients usually lack the type IV collagen α3-, α4-, and α5-chains.[19] However, in occasional cases, staining for these chains yields positive results; therefore, positive immunostaining results do not completely rule out Alport's syndrome. These cases may represent mutations that do not prevent the intracellular formation of triple-helical α3:α4:α5 molecules, although the secreted protein is not fully functional. About two thirds of female carriers of X-chromosomal *COL4A5* mutations exhibit a segmental absence of GBM staining for α3-, α4-, and α5-chains.[28]

On electron microscopy, the earliest visible changes are thinning of the GBM, which is similar to findings in thin basement membrane disease (see later discussion). However, with progression of the disease, the hallmark findings of Alport's syndrome become evident—irregular thinning and thickening of the GBM, with lamellation and a woven basket pattern (Figure 44.2). The endothelial cells usually appear normal, and the slit diaphragms can also look normal, with occasional effacement of the foot processes on the distorted GBM. These findings, although typical for Alport's syndrome, are not totally specific for the disease, inasmuch as foci and lamellation have been observed in 6% to 10% of unselected renal biopsy samples from patients with focal segmental glomerulosclerosis (FSGS), immunoglobulin A (IgA) nephropathy, postinfectious glomerulonephritis, and mesangioproliferative disease.[29] However, a combination of

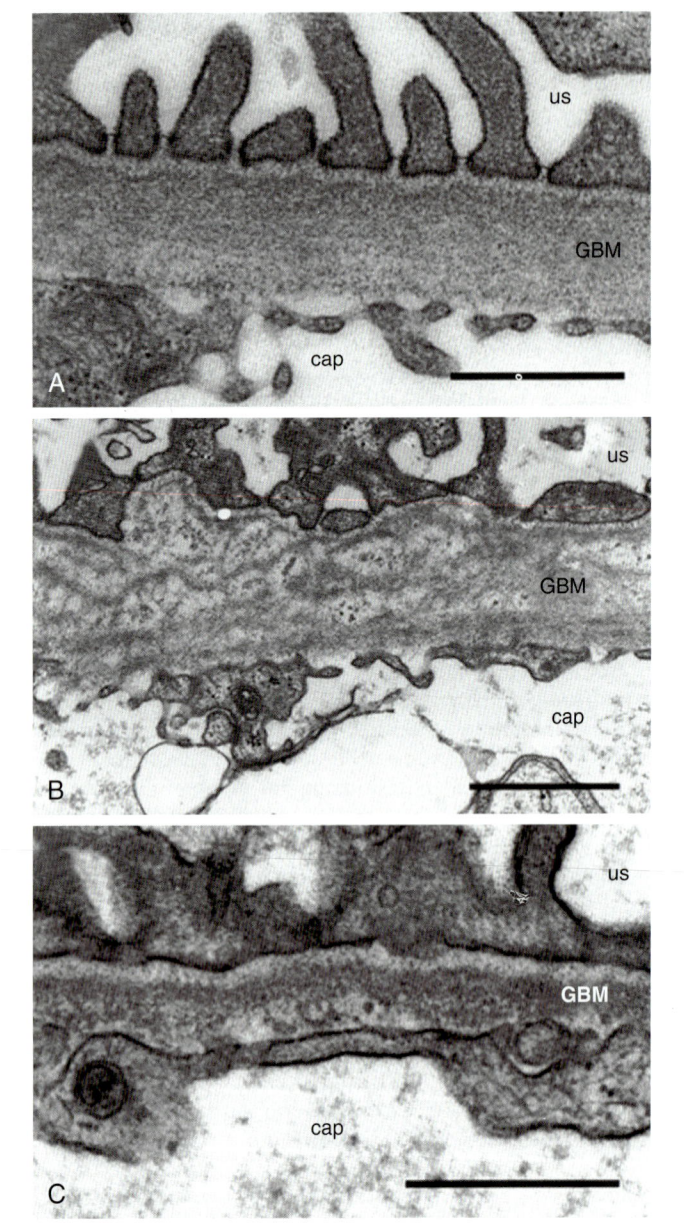

Figure 44.2 Morphologic nature of the glomerular basement membrane (GBM) in normal conditions, Alport's syndrome, and thin basement membrane nephropathy (TBMN). **A,** In the normal glomerulus, the width of the GBM is uniformly between 300 and 350 nm. **B,** In Alport's syndrome, electron microscopy reveals focal thickening and thinning of the GBM. On occasion, lamination of the GBM is observed. **C,** In TBMN, the GBM is characteristically thinned; its thickness is only about half that of a normal kidney. *Bars* represent 500 nm; cap, capillary lumen; us, urinary space. (**A** courtesy Dr. Finn P. Reinholt, Karolinska University Hospital, Huddinge, Sweden; **B** courtesy Dr. Kjell Hultenby, Karolinska University Hospital, Huddinge, Sweden.)

Alport's syndrome–specific immunostaining results with typical electron microscopy findings is strongly suggestive of the diagnosis of Alport's syndrome.

To date, the most accurate method for diagnosing Alport's syndrome is DNA analysis revealing mutations in any of the COL4A5, COL4A4, or COL4A5 genes. Tests for mutation analysis of the COL4A3, COL4A4, and COL4A5 genes are commercially available and can reveal larger gene rearrangements or small mutations by sequencing of the promoter and exon regions. At present, sequencing can reveal more than 90% of the mutations. In some cases, the mutations can be difficult or impossible to identify if they are small and located within large introns or at sites distant from the actual structural gene. This problem may be alleviated with the rapid development of high-throughput sequencing technologies. However, the combination of immunofluorescence and electron microscopy findings, together with DNA analysis, almost guarantees an accurate diagnosis of Alport's syndrome.

Course and Treatment

Recurrent hematuria with mild proteinuria may be present for years before it progresses to renal insufficiency and ESKD. ESKD develops in almost all male patients with X-linked disease and in male and female patients who are homozygotes or compound heterozygotes for mutations in the COL4A3 and COL4A4 genes on chromosome 2q. The rate of progression varies significantly, depending on the nature of mutations, but intrakindred variation may be considerable; the cause is not understood.

There is currently no proven treatment for Alport's syndrome. Because weakening of the GBM is considered to contribute to the disease, reduction of intraglomerular pressure by hypertension therapy and angiotensin-converting enzyme (ACE) inhibitors may slow down the rate of progression.[30] In some cases, long-term cyclosporine treatment has been reported to stabilize the disease.

Dialysis and kidney transplantation are common treatments for ESKD. However, transplantation is not totally free of risk; many patients who do not express $\alpha 3{:}\alpha 4{:}\alpha 5$ molecules in the GBM may react to those molecules as foreign antigens.

THIN BASEMENT MEMBRANE NEPHROPATHY

TBMN is the most common cause of persistent hematuria in children and adults, occurring in as much as 1% of the population.[31-33] TBMN is associated with mutations in type IV collagen genes (see Figure 44.1), but the course of this disorder is usually not progressive. Although TBMN is not a true disease that necessitates treatment, it is still a major clinical problem because clinical findings are similar to those of early stages of Alport's syndrome, and affected individuals have a mutation in one type IV collagen gene allele.

Genetics

TBMN has been reported in all population ancestry groups and has been diagnosed at all ages. It manifests mainly as an inherited disorder with dominant transmission, affecting 50% of successive generations.[34-36] About two thirds of patients with TBMN have at least one relative with hematuria.[34]

It has become apparent that the disorder is associated with heterozygous mutations in genes for any of the $\alpha 3$-, $\alpha 4$-, or $\alpha 5$-chains of type IV collagen, the same genes that are mutated in Alport's syndrome (see Figure 44.1). Lemmink and associates first reported that some carriers for autosomal forms of Alport's syndrome had TBMN; they identified a heterozygous mutation in the COL4A4 gene.[14] Since then, numerous reports have described heterozygous mutations in *COL4A3* or *COL4A4* genes in individuals with TBMN.[13,15,34,37] Thus, TBMN-affected individuals may have a similar type of carrier status for autosomal Alport's syndrome, as do female relatives of male patients with X-linked Alport's syndrome. To date, researchers in only a few studies have attempted to correlate type IV collagen gene mutations with the clinical phenotype; however, interestingly, the same mutation can result in clinical symptoms of differing severity.[38]

Most current evidence suggests that TBMN is a disorder of the α3:α4:α5 isoform of type IV collagen, although some TBMN-affected families do not show linkage with any of the *COL4A3*, *COL4A4*, or *COL4A5* genes.[39] This might be explained by a high rate of de novo mutations, as has been shown to be the case in X-linked Alport's syndrome (22%), but the presence of mutations in other genes cannot as yet be ruled out.[4]

Pathogenesis

The development of autosomal nonprogressive TBMN involves heterozygous mutations in the *COL4A3* or *COL4A4* genes, whereas homozygous or compound heterozygous mutations in the same genes result in progressive autosomal Alport's syndrome. A similar TBMN phenotype is usually the case in female individuals with heterozygosity for mutations in the X-chromosomal *COL4A5* gene. The differences in clinical effects may be explained by a so-called dose effect, whereby absence of a single allele leads to lower production of the α3:α4:α5 trimer and loss of two alleles leads to a total loss or malfunction of the α3:α4:α5 trimer and development of Alport's syndrome.[40]

Clinical Manifestations

The characteristic clinical manifestation of TBMN is persistent microscopic hematuria.[31-33] Most individuals present with only hematuria and no additional symptoms, such as proteinuria. The disorder is usually detected incidentally during preventive medicine screening of asymptomatic healthy individuals or of healthy controls in clinical research studies or in certain population screening settings (e.g., recruitment for military service). The onset of TBMN can occur at any age.[36] At least a single episode of macroscopic hematuria occurs in 5% to 22% of affected individuals, but occurrence of macroscopic hematuria is more common in patients with Alport's syndrome or IgA nephropathy.[41,42] On occasion, the hematuria disappears over time.[32] Renal function in children with TBMN is normal, but affected adults have been reported to have a low prevalence of renal insufficiency.[32,43-47] In general, the prognosis for patients with nephropathy in true TBMN is excellent.

Pathologic Findings

Light microscopic study of kidney biopsy samples usually reveals normal histologic features, with only occasional mild mesangial cellular proliferation and matrix expansion.[48] In about 5% to 25% of cases, FSGS and tubular fibrosis may be observed with aging.[46,48]

Electron microscopic study reveals the typical TBMN finding (i.e., thinning of the GBM), but it does not distinguish between pure TBMN and thin GBM in the early stages of Alport's syndrome (see Figure 44.2).

Diagnosis

TBMN is the major cause of persistent hematuria; therefore, it is important to differentiate it from other causes of hematuria, such as Alport's syndrome, IgA nephropathy, mesangiocapillary glomerulonephritis, and lupus nephritis. The major early clinical challenge is to distinguish benign TBMN from early-stage Alport's syndrome because the two conditions have completely different outcomes (one very mild and the other very severe, respectively), despite very similar clinical findings. Because the family history does not help distinguish between the two conditions, kidney biopsy may be indicated in some cases in which the benefits outweigh the risks. Immunostaining for the α3-, α4-, and α5-chains normally reveals the presence of all the three chains, whereas in Alport's syndrome, they are usually absent. However, such analysis can in rare cases yield false-negative results, inasmuch as low levels of the protein are expressed in 20% of patients with autosomal Alport's syndrome and in 30% of female carriers for X-linked Alport's syndrome.[49,50] Electron microscopy is not diagnostic because it does not differentiate between TBMN and thin GBM findings in early-stage Alport's syndrome.

Genetic analyses can verify diagnosis by identification of mutations in the *COL4A3* or *COL4A4* gene in autosomal form and by identifying carriers for X-linked Alport's syndrome (see Figure 44.1). Thus, a combination of immunofluorescence analysis and DNA sequencing of the two genes can almost guarantee an exact diagnosis.

Treatment

TBMN is a benign GBM disorder that does not necessitate treatment if a correct diagnosis can be made.

HEREDITARY ANGIOPATHY, NEPHROPATHY, ANEURYSMS, AND MUSCLE CRAMPS

Heterozygous mutations have been identified in the type IV collagen α1-chain gene *(COL4A1)* in a rare complex familial disease referred to as HANAC syndrome (**h**ereditary **a**ngiopathy, **n**ephropathy, **a**neurysms, and **m**uscle **c**ramps).[51] The disease is characterized by autosomal dominant hematuria and cystic kidney disease, accompanied by intracranial aneurysms and muscle cramps. Mutations in the *COL4A1* gene have also been reported to cause cerebral hemorrhage and porencephaly in humans and mice.[52] Kidney biopsy samples exhibit no abnormalities, and immunofluorescence studies reveal normal expression of the α1-chain and other type IV collagen chains in renal vascular and epithelial basement membranes. Expression of the α3-, α4-, and α5-chains is normal in the GBM. Electron microscopy reveals normal appearance of the GBM but irregular thickening and lamellation of basement membranes in interstitial capillaries, with numerous focal interruptions. Typically, patients have intracranial aneurysms, tortuous retinal arteries, and development of muscle cramps. The pathogenesis of the disease is not clear, but it may be related to low expression of the α1-chain that is the major component of the ubiquitous α1:α1:α2 type IV collagen present in almost all basement membranes. Thus far, it is not known whether a heterozygous mutation in the α2-chain gene causes a disease in humans.

LAMININ DISEASE: PIERSON'S SYNDROME

Pierson's syndrome is a rare, lethal, autosomal recessive form of congenital nephrotic syndrome manifested by proteinuria, diffuse mesangial sclerosis, and distinctive ocular anomalies characterized by microcoria (fixed narrowing of the pupil).[53,54] The disease is caused by mutations in the *LAMB2* gene encoding the β2-chain of laminin. In a mutation analysis study of 89 children from 80 families with nephrotic syndrome occurring in the first year of life, Hinkes and colleagues showed that 2.5% of cases were caused by mutations in the *LAMB2* gene.[55] At birth, most affected patients exhibit massive proteinuria, with rapid progression to renal failure that leads to death before age 2 months. However, a number of milder variants have been identified which are diagnosed in early childhood.

As noted earlier, laminins are trimeric basement membrane proteins containing α-, β-, and γ-chains, which exist in five, four, and three genetically distinct forms, respectively.[1,56] These chains can form at least 16 different isoforms in vivo.[57] In the embryonic GBM, the laminin-511 (α5:β1:γ1) isoform is expressed, but after birth it is replaced by laminin-521 (α5:β2:γ1) in a developmental switch analogous to that of embryonic GBM type IV collagen (α1:α1:α2) to adult type IV collagen (α3:α4:α5).[56] The actual role of laminin-521 in the GBM is not known, but it must be essential for maintaining a functional glomerular filter structure and function. This is highlighted by the fact that knockout mice for laminin α5 and laminin β2 exhibit disorganization of the GBM and proteinuria.

INHERITED DISORDERS PRIMARILY AFFECTING THE PODOCYTE

Discoveries during the last 15 years have revealed that defects in genes encoding protein components of the podocyte slit diaphragm and foot processes are the underlying causes of a number of rare glomerular disorders that lead to proteinuria, nephrotic syndrome, and ESKD. Although the causes of most glomerular diseases are unknown, the new information has shed light on the molecular nature and function of the renal filter (Figure 44.3).

NEPHRIN DISEASE: CONGENITAL NEPHROTIC SYNDROME OF THE FINNISH TYPE

Congenital nephrotic syndrome of the Finnish type (CNF) is a rare disease; however, it is particularly common in Finland and has also been described in other countries.[58] Affected individuals have defects in the gene for nephrin that is a major structural and functional component of the slit diaphragm located between podocyte foot processes.

GENETICS

CNF is inherited as an autosomal recessive trait. Although cases of this disease have been described worldwide, most of them have been identified in Finland, where the incidence has been reported to be 1/8200 births.[59] The mutated nephrotic syndrome 1 gene *(NPHS1)*, which was identified by positional cloning, is located on chromosome 19 and was shown to encode a novel protein termed *nephrin*.[60] The gene has a size of 26 kb and contains 29 exons. More than 100 mutations have been identified in the *NPHS1* gene.

In Finns, two main nonsense mutations account for more than 90% of cases of CNF.[60,61] The Fin-major mutation is a two-base pair deletion in exon 2 that results in a frameshift and a stop codon in the same exon. This mutation leads to formation of only a 90-residue truncated protein. The Fin-minor mutation is a nonsense mutation in exon 26 and leads to a truncated 1109-residue protein. The homogeneous pattern of *NPHS1* mutations in Finnish patients can be explained by the founder effect. A few missense mutations have also been identified in Finnish patients.

In other populations, the mutations vary extensively among families, with most mutations being missense mutations, but nonsense and splice-site mutations, deletions, and insertions have also been described.[62,63] Enrichment of some mutations has been detected in a few isolated populations; for example, in Mennonites, a common 1481delC mutation leading to a truncated 547-residue protein has been described and, in Maltese patients, a homozygous nonsense mutation R1160X in exon 27 is highly enriched.[63] Hinkes and colleagues have shown, in a worldwide case study, that 22.5% of 89 cases of nephrotic syndrome occurring in the first year of life are caused by mutations in the *NPHS1* gene.[55]

Some *NPHS1* mutations do not lead to typical CNF but rather to a later onset nephrotic syndrome that resembles that caused by podocin gene mutations.[64] Homozygous or compound heterozygous nephrin mutations have been found even in a few adult-onset cases, but their incidence is low.

NEPHRIN AND PATHOGENESIS OF CNF

In the kidney, nephrin is expressed specifically in podocytes.[65] It is a 1241-residue transmembrane protein with an approximately 35-nm-long extracellular domain that reaches out from the foot process membrane into the 40-nm-wide slit (see Figure 44.3). In the middle of the slit, nephrin molecules from two neighboring foot processes are believed to interact to form a zipper-like structure with pores on both sides.[66,67] Nephrin has been reported to interact with NEPH1 and NEPH2 in the slit diaphragm.[68] Intracellularly, nephrin molecules normally bond with podocin, which is mutated in steroid-resistant nephrotic syndrome.[69]

In CNF, mutations in the *NPHS1* gene lead to loss or a malfunctioning nephrin so that the slit diaphragm cannot form or function normally. The size-selective filter is lost, and the slit collapses.[70] The foot processes do not form, and because the slit diaphragm and filter structure are absent, massive proteinuria occurs. Nephrin knockout mice have similarly massive proteinuria present at birth, and they also lack the slit diaphragm.[71] Absence of nephrin apparently results in distortion of the slit diaphragm and consequent massive leakage of albumin through the slit. Several missense mutations detected in non-Finnish patients have been shown to result in defective intracellular trafficking of nephrin and in absence of nephrin from the slit diaphragm.[72] Thus, even these missense mutations that appear to be "mild" can result in severe clinical phenotypes, similar to those caused by truncating mutations.

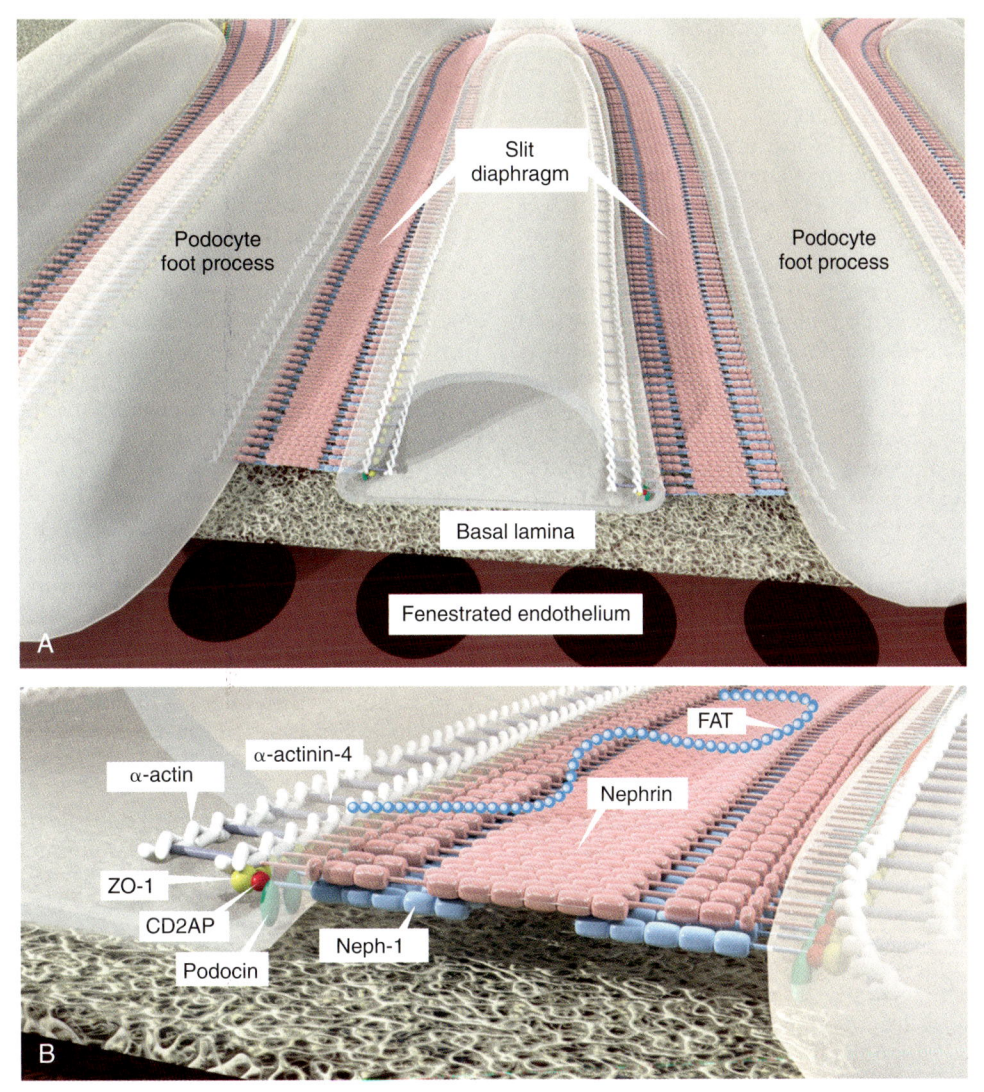

Figure 44.3 Schematic depiction of the three layers of the glomerular filtration barrier and molecular composition of the slit diaphragm and foot processes. **A,** The renal ultrafiltration barrier is made up of fenestrated endothelial cells, basal lamina (basement membrane), and podocyte foot processes interconnected by slit diaphragms. **B,** Molecular components of the slit diaphragm complex include nephrin, Neph1, fat, and podocin. The cytoplasmic components of the slit diaphragms include Cd2ap and ZO-1. α-Actin and α-actinin-4 are components of the foot process cytoskeleton.

CLINICAL MANIFESTATIONS

CNF usually develops already in utero, which is observed in the form of leakage of alpha-fetoprotein into the amniotic fluid and maternal blood.[58] Premature birth and a placenta weighing more than 25% of the birth weight are typical findings. Massive proteinuria and nephrotic syndrome develop soon after birth. Typically, hypoalbuminemia, hyperlipidemia, abdominal distension, and edema develop in affected neonates.[58,73] The protein loss in these patients usually leads to severe hypoalbuminemia, and the serum albumin concentration is typically less than 10 g/L. In light microscopy, cystic dilations of proximal tubules are a typical but not pathognomonic finding. In some cases, the pathologic findings are similar to those observed in FSGS, minimal-change nephrosis, or diffuse mesangial sclerosis.[59,74] Electron microscopy and electron tomography reveal effacement of podocytes, a narrow slit, and absence of the slit diaphragm.[70] Before effective treatment was developed, the disease was always lethal. Affected patients had marked growth and mental retardation, bacterial infections, and poor psychomotor development.

POSTTRANSPLANTATION RECURRENCE OF PROTEINURIA

After kidney transplantation, patients with nephrin mutations are at risk for recurrence of proteinuria and nephrotic syndrome.[75] This may lead to graft loss. In Finnish patients with recurrence, approximately 50% of patients have circulating anti-nephrin antibodies, which may react against the glomerular filter and induce proteinuria.[75] Similarly, injection of anti-nephrin antibodies in a rat model has been shown to cause massive proteinuria.[76] Thus far, all Finnish patients with recurrence have been homozygous for the Fin-major mutation.[75] In these patients, antibodies are produced against a novel antigen, inasmuch as no nephrin (or only 90 amino acids) has been present during maturation of the immunologic system. Patients with recurrence are treated with steroids, cyclophosphamide, and plasmapheresis.

TREATMENT

CNF is a potentially lethal disease that cannot be cured by immunosuppressive therapy. Therefore, all treatment should be aimed toward kidney transplantation, which is curative and carries an excellent prognosis.[77,78] Today, among patients with CNF, the rate of survival 5 years after renal transplantation is more than 90%.[79] Before transplantation, the treatment was albumin substitution, intravenous nutrition, and nephrectomy. Patients with mutations leading to seriously malfunctioning nephrin or its absence do not usually respond to ACE inhibitors or immunosuppressive therapy, but those with some milder mutations may respond to such therapies.[61,64] At least 50% of transplant recipients have circulating nephrin antibodies that may have a pathogenic influence on recurrence of the disease.[75]

PODOCIN DISEASE: STEROID-RESISTANT NEPHROTIC SYNDROME

Mutations in the *NPHS2* gene, which encodes the slit diaphragm protein podocin, were originally identified in a familial form of FSGS.[69] This disease is characterized by childhood onset, steroid resistance, and rapid progression to ESKD. Since the initial description, mutations in *NPHS2* have been found to be a common cause of congenital and childhood-onset, steroid-resistant nephrotic syndrome.[55,80-82]

GENETICS

Podocin disease is inherited as an autosomal recessive trait.[69] It is a relatively common cause of neonatal nephrotic syndrome. Hinkes and colleagues showed in a worldwide study that podocin mutations underlay 37.5% of cases in 89 children in whom nephrotic syndrome appeared during the first year of life.[55] The gene for podocin, termed *NPHS2* (for nephrotic syndrome 2), contains eight exons and is located on chromosome 1q25. Podocin has 383 amino acid residues and belongs to the stomatin protein family. The protein has a hairpin structure and is located in the foot process membrane; its N- and C-terminal ends extend into the intracellular space. In the kidney, podocin is located specifically at the slit diaphragm of the glomerulus.[83]

Over 100 different *NPHS2* mutations have been identified worldwide so far. These include missense, nonsense, and deletion mutations scattered along the whole *NPHS2* gene. The mutation of arginine-138 to glutamine is a so-called founder mutation and is detected commonly in the central European population.[69] It results in retention of the mutant podocin in the endoplasmic reticulum and failure of the podocin protein to reach the slit diaphragm.[84] Therefore, this mutation can be considered a severe mutation. Several other missense mutations seem to result in a similar mistargeting of podocin mutants.[85]

Another mutation, from arginine-229 to glutamine, is of special interest. It is common especially in the European population, in which the observed allele frequency ranges from 0.03 to 0.13.[86-90] The pathogenic effect has been shown, on the basis of in vitro findings, to decrease binding of the protein to nephrin.[89] Also, arginine-229 in podocin is conserved in podocin orthologs, which suggests that this residue is crucial for normal functional podocin. Machuca and associates assessed the pathogenic effect of this mutation in 546 patients with steroid-resistant nephrotic syndrome and noted that the frequency of the mutation was significantly higher in patients with steroid-resistant nephritic syndrome than among controls.[91] Homozygosity for this mutation does not seem to cause renal disease but, in combination with the pathogenic podocin mutation from arginine-229 to glutamine, it leads to nephrotic syndrome. Of importance is that patients with compound heterozygosity for this mutation and one pathogenic podocin mutation have a significantly later onset of nephrotic syndrome than patients with two pathogenic mutations. A total of 18 patients in whom nephrotic syndrome was diagnosed after the age of 18 years had this podocin genotype. Similar results were reported by Tsukaguchi and colleagues.[89] However, results of three studies of three large cohorts have not supported this finding: *NPHS2* mutations were found to be rare among patients with adult-onset nephrotic syndrome.[20,54,101] Thus, the podocin mutation from arginine-229 to glutamate, in combination with a pathogenic podocin mutation, may explain some cases with adult-onset nephrotic syndrome; how common this podocin genotype is among affected patients is, however, still unclear.

PATHOGENESIS

As a molecular component of the slit diaphragm (Figure 44.3), podocin has been shown to interact directly with nephrin, CD2-associated protein (CD2AP), and NEPH1.[83,92] Podocin can form oligomers in lipid rafts, and it seems to be needed for the recruitment of nephrin and CD2AP in these microdomains.[84] Therefore, the presence of podocin is essential for the formation of the slit diaphragm, inasmuch as no slit diaphragm is formed in the absence of nephrin.[61] This conclusion has been confirmed in podocin-deficient mice, which exhibit massive proteinuria at birth, and no nephrin is detected in foot processes.[93] Thus, truncating mutations, as well as many missense mutations that have been shown to result in entrapment of misfolded protein to endoplasmic reticulum, probably result in the absence of podocin and nephrin from the slit diaphragm and therefore result in massive protein leakage through the glomerular filtration barrier. A mouse model for the missense mutation from arginine-138 to glutamate has confirmed the occurrence of this phenomenon. The milder phenotype observed in some missense podocin mutants is probably attributable to the fact that these mutants can reach the slit diaphragm, but their functional properties within the slit are compromised because of amino acid alterations. The podocin protein, with the mutation from arginine-229 to glutamate, has been shown to have weaker interaction with nephrin, which may explain the milder phenotype in these patients.[89]

CLINICAL MANIFESTATIONS

In contrast to nephrin disease, the clinical manifestations of podocin disease vary considerably. Truncating mutations and severe missense mutations (see earlier discussion) can lead to congenital nephrotic syndrome or steroid-resistant nephrotic syndrome, both of which manifest at a very early age. Hinkes and colleagues identified *NPHS2* mutations in

39% of patients with congenital nephrotic syndrome and in 35% of those with infantile nephrotic syndrome.[55] In older children, podocin mutations are responsible for 10% to 30% of cases of steroid-resistant nephrotic syndrome.[94] Of importance is that patients with podocin mutations do not seem to respond to steroids; furthermore, podocin disease seems to be resistant to cyclosporine and to cyclophosphamide therapy.[82] Thus, podocin mutations seem to result in a nephrotic syndrome that is resistant to immunosuppressive therapy. However, He and associates reported an interesting exception to this rule—patients with the mutation from arginine-229 to glutamate in one allele and a pathogenic mutation in the other allele achieved complete remission after steroid treatment.[95]

Podocin mutations have also been identified in patients who develop nephrotic syndrome in early adulthood.[91] These patients often carry one disease-causing mutation in the compound heterozygous state, together with the mutation from arginine-229 to glutamine.[89] After kidney transplantation, patients with podocin mutation have a decreased risk for recurrence of the disease.[82] In fact, only a few patients with podocin mutations have been reported to develop recurrence of the disease in the graft.[96] NPHS2 variants detected in these patients were originally considered to be disease-causing mutations, but this has since been questioned.[97] Obviously, patients with a primary nephropathy caused by podocin mutations should not have any (or only minimal) risk for recurrence of the disease in the graft.

TREATMENT

Proteinuria in patients with podocin disease–related nephropathy should be treated according to standard protocol, including treatment with ACE inhibitors or angiotensin receptor blockers. The indications for immunosuppressive therapy should be carefully evaluated on an individual basis. In general, patients with podocin mutations do not respond to any immunosuppressive therapy.[82] However, one exception to this rule has been reported—patients with the mutation from arginine-229 to glutamine in one allele and a pathogenic mutation in the other allele.[95] In some cases, it may be difficult to detect a real pathogenic mutation from a polymorphism, and population genetic or functional studies may be needed to sort this out.

INF2 DISEASE: FOCAL SEGMENTAL GLOMERULOSCLEROSIS AND CHARCOT-MARIE TOOTH NEUROPATHY–ASSOCIATED GLOMERULOPATHY

Heterozygous mutations in inverted formin, FH2, and WH2 domains containing INF2 seem to be the most common genetic cause of autosomal dominant FSGS.[98,99] In one large cohort, INF2 mutations were found to be the cause of dominant FSGS in 17% of familial cases, whereas in sporadic cases the INF2 mutations were rare.[98]

The INF2 protein is a member of the diaphanous-related formin family, which participates in regulating actin and microtubule cytoskeletons. The protein is composed of an N-terminal diaphanous-inhibitory domain (DID), the forming homology domains FH1 and FH2, and a C-terminal diaphanous-autoregulatory domain (DAD). The mutations associated with FSGS are clustered to the DID.[98,99] INF2 interacts with diaphanous-related formins (mDia) and inhibits mDia-mediated actin polymerization.[100] Mutations in FSGS patients may compromise the interplay between INF2 and the foot process actin cytoskeleton, and thus result in progressive proteinuric disease.

Interestingly, mutations in INF2 have been found to be the cause of Charcot-Marie-Tooth neuropathy (CMT)–associated nephropathy.[101] CMT is a heterogenous group of hereditary disorders affecting peripheral neurons that is typified by progressive muscle weakness and atrophy distally in limbs, reduced tendon reflexes, and deformities in the feet and hands. INF2 is expressed in Schwann cell cytoplasm, in which it interacts with myelin and lymphocyte protein (MAL), which has an essential role in myelination. This can explain why some INF2 mutations lead to demyelinization.

APOL1 GENE: SUSCEPTIBILITY TO FOCAL SEGMENTAL GLOMERULOSCLEROSIS

In African Americans, variants in the APOL1 gene (encoding apolipoprotein L-1) have been found to underlie the susceptibility to develop renal disease.[102,103] The variants of APOL1 lyse the parasite *Trypanosoma brucei rhodesiense,* which is why they have become so common through natural selection.

APOL1 is expressed in podocytes, and this expression can be induced in podocytes in culture in response to cytokine triggers.[104] In FSGS patients, APOL1 expression is decreased.[105] In vitro studies in cell culture systems have suggested that APOL1 sequesters phosphatidic acid and cardiolipin and promotes autophagocytic cell death, although more recent studies in human podocytes in culture have suggested possible pyroptotic and lysosomal-mediated injury pathways.[103] Because autophagy plays a key role in the maintenance of normal podocyte function, APOL1 may be contributing to podocyte homeostasis and survival. APOL1 variants may compromise these functions and lead to podocyte death and the development of FSGS. The fact that kidney transplants obtained from donors carrying APOL1 risk variants have a poorer prognosis supports the idea that the intrinsic defect in the kidney is behind APOL1-related susceptibility, although a role for secreted APOL1 has not been entirely ruled out.[106]

PLCE1 DISEASE: FAMILIAL DIFFUSE MESANGIAL SCLEROSIS

Phospholipase C, epsilon 1 (PLCE1), is encoded by the PLCE1 gene. Nephropathy caused by PLCE1 mutations is inherited as an autosomal recessive trait.[107] In the original description of PLCE1 disease–related nephropathy, all patients with PLCE1 mutations developed glomerular disease by the age of 4 years. The histologic picture was dependent on the type of mutation; all truncating mutations led to diffuse mesangial sclerosis, whereas missense mutations in two patients (from one family) resulted in FSGS. Gbadegesin and associates have investigated the incidence of PLCE1 mutations in isolated (nonsyndromic) diffuse mesangial sclerosis (IDMS).[108] They examined 40 children from 35 families with IDMS in a worldwide cohort.

Truncating mutations in *PLCE1* were detected in 10 families (28.6%). Thus, mutations in *PLCE1* seem to be a common cause of IDMS. Ismaili and colleagues detected *PLCE1* mutations in 3 of 10 Belgian families with congenital nephrotic syndrome.[81] Thus, PLCE1 disease also seems to explain some cases of congenital nephrotic syndrome. To determine whether mutations in *PLCE1* are a common cause of FSGS, the gene was analyzed in a total of 69 families with 231 affected individuals with FSGS.[81] No known disease-causing mutations were identified in the families screened, and *PLCE1* mutations therefore seem to be a rare cause of FSGS.

It is not clear how mutations in the PLCE1 enzyme lead to glomerular disease. PLCE1 belongs to the phospholipase family of proteins that catalyze the formation of secondary messengers, such as inositol 1,4,5-trisphosphate and diacylglycerol in cells. These signals launch cascades that mediate several cellular responses, including cell growth and differentiation. PLCE1 is expressed widely, but in the kidneys it is enriched in podocytes, in which PLCE1 localizes to the cytoplasm of the podocyte cell body and major processes.[107] PLCE1 is highly expressed, particularly during development of the glomerulus. Because glomeruli of patients with *PLCE1* mutations display developmental abnormalities, it has been proposed that the morphologic phenotype of diffuse mesangial sclerosis is a result of a cessation in glomerular development.[107] However, because nephropathy in some patients with *PLCE1* mutations can be reversible, as well as having a late onset, PLCE1 may also have a role in the maintenance of the podocytes and glomerulus filtration barrier. Of note, *Plce1*-knockout mice do not have any obvious renal phenotype; therefore, the pathomechanisms behind PLCE1 disease–related nephropathy remain to be poorly understood.

FOCAL SEGMENTAL GLOMERULOSCLEROSIS

α-ACTININ-4 DISEASE

FSGS caused by mutations in the α-actinin-4 gene *(ACTN4)* is inherited as an autosomal dominant trait.[109] The disease is very rare, and most patients with *ACTN4* mutations exhibit proteinuria first during adolescence or later and develop slowly advancing renal dysfunction. In some patients, this dysfunction progresses to renal failure. The disease is not fully penetrant: Individuals with *ACTN4* mutations but without any obvious renal disease have been identified.[109] To date, all disease-causing mutations identified are missense mutations located in the actin-binding domain of α-actinin-4. This suggests that they are gain-of-function mutations. In fact, mutated α-actinin-4 proteins bind more strongly to filamentous actin than the wild-type protein.[109,110] Therefore, it is reasonable to believe that the pathomechanism behind the renal disease in patients with *ACTN4* mutations involves dysregulation of the actin cytoskeleton in podocyte foot processes. The pathogenic nature of the mutated α-actinin-4 has been confirmed in a mouse model that expresses the mutated protein specifically in podocytes; these mice developed proteinuria and FSGS.[111] In podocyte cell culture, the mutated protein also impairs cytoskeletal dynamics.[112] Of note, even mice lacking α-actinin-4 develop a proteinuric glomerular disease, and studies performed on a podocyte cell line lacking α-actinin-4 have shown that α-actinin-4 is involved in the adhesion of podocytes to the GBM.[113,114] Thus, α-actinin-4 has a role in actin dynamics and cell matrix adhesion in podocytes and, in patients with *ACTN4* mutations, the former seems to be impaired.

TRPC6 DISEASE

Mutations in the gene that encodes the transient receptor potential cation channel, subfamily C, member 6 *(TRPC6)* were originally identified by two independent groups in six families with autosomal dominant FSGS.[115,116] These families had missense mutations in the *TRPC6* gene, and the disease was characterized by adult onset and incomplete penetrance. Since these reports, only a few studies have found *TRPC6* mutations in patients with FSGS. A Chinese study of 31 pedigrees with late-onset familial FSGS identified one patient with a new missense mutation, and another study of 130 Spanish patients from 115 families with FSGS revealed three additional missense substitutions in three unrelated patients.[117,118] In the latter study, one patient had unusual clinical features for TRPC6 disease–related nephropathy—mesangial proliferative FSGS in childhood (onset at age 7 years). So far, other patients identified with TRPC6 disease have had late-onset nephrotic syndrome with histologic features of FSGS.

TRPC6 is a member of a family of nonselective cation channels that are involved in the regulation of the intracellular calcium concentration in response to the activation of G protein–coupled receptors and receptor tyrosine kinases. In podocytes, the TRPC6 protein localizes to the slit diaphragm.[115] Many *TRPC6* mutations found in patients result in increased amplitude and duration of calcium influx after stimulation.[115,116] In addition, transient overexpression of TRPC6 through in vivo gene delivery results in proteinuria, whereas TRPC6-deficient mice do not exhibit any obvious renal phenotype.[119,120] Together, these data suggest that TRPC6 disease–related nephropathy is caused by gain-of-function mutations that might interfere with slit diaphragm signaling.

CD2AP DISEASE

Mutations in the *CD2AP* gene seem to be a rare cause of FSGS.[121] The mode of inheritance is unclear because dominant and recessive cases have been reported.[121,122] The importance of CD2AP for the glomerular filtration barrier has been demonstrated in CD2AP-deficient mice; they die within a few weeks after birth from massive proteinuria and renal failure.[123] Similarly, mice with CD2AP haploinsufficiency develop proteinuria.[121] These mice show defects in the formation of multivesicular bodies in podocytes, which suggests that an impairment of the intracellular degradation pathway may be involved in the pathogenesis of proteinuria in these mice. CD2AP interacts directly with the intracellular tail of nephrin (see Figure 44.3); therefore, impaired interaction with the slit diaphragm and actin cytoskeleton may also be involved in the pathogenesis of CD2AP disease–related nephropathy.[124]

MYO1E DISEASE

Mutations in *MYO1E* encoding nonmuscle myosin 1e has been identified as a cause of childhood-onset, steroid-resistant FSGS in a consanguineous Italian pedigree.[125] Myosin 1e is a member of class 1 myosins, whose C-terminus interacts with cell membranes and their N-terminal motor domain with actin filaments Myosin 1e is found in podocyte foot processes, and *MYO1E* knockout mice develop foot process effacement and proteinuria.[125] It is plausible to speculate that myosin 1e contributes to the function of actin cytoskeleton in podocyte foot processes and that mutated *MYO1E* results in impairment of this contractile apparatus.

GLEPP1 DISEASE: STEROID-RESISTANT NEPHROTIC SYNDROME

Mutations in the *PTPRO* gene encoding Glepp1 have been identified in two Turkish families with steroid-resistant nephrotic syndrome (SRNS).[126] Glepp1 is a tyrosine phosphatase receptor present on the apical cell surface of the glomerular podocyte. Two distinct mutations identified are loss-of-function mutations, and the Glepp1-associated disease seems to follow a recessive inheritance. In contrast to this, knockout mice for GLEPP-1 exhibit widened foot processes with clinical findings of hypertension and reduction in the glomerular filtration rate but no proteinuria.[127] Why the mouse model and humans behave so differently is not known, and the role of Glepp1 in podocytes and the kidney filter is still unsolved.

INHERITED PRIMARY GLOMERULAR DISORDERS OF UNKNOWN CAUSE

GALLOWAY-MOWAT SYNDROME

In 1968, Galloway and Mowat described a clinical constellation of an early nephrotic syndrome, congenital microcephaly, and hiatal hernia.[128] Since then, over 50 patients have been reported to have Galloway-Mowat syndrome.[129] In this condition, nephrotic syndrome is usually diagnosed within the first 4 months of life. It is steroid-resistant and soon progresses to ESKD. However, milder variants of Galloway-Mowat syndrome have been described, in which the nephropathy first manifests after the age of 10 years.[130,131] Renal histopathologic findings are also highly variable, although FSGS is included in most cases. The manifestation of extrarenal symptoms can also vary considerably in affected patients. For example, hiatal hernia is not observed in all cases of Galloway-Mowat syndrome. The variation in clinical features of this syndrome probably results from genetic heterogeneity of the disease. No disease gene(s) underlying Galloway-Mowat syndrome have been identified so far.

IMMUNOGLOBULIN A NEPHROPATHY

IgA nephropathy is the most common primary form of glomerulonephritis worldwide. Although the pathogenesis of IgA nephropathy remains unclear, there is strong evidence that it is an immune complex disease. IgA nephropathy is described in more detail elsewhere in this text. A familial form of IgA nephropathy was first described in 1973 by de Werra and associates.[132] Several studies in families with IgA nephropathy have since confirmed that at least in some cases, genetic factors play a role in the pathogenesis.[133] It has been estimated that 15% to 20% of the pedigrees of IgA nephropathy have an inherited form of the disease.[133]

Genomewide association studies (GWASs) of IgA nephropathy have identified multiple loci, but no underlying causal variants have yet been found.[134-137] Future genomewide sequencing studies will probably result in the discovery of genetic variants behind the hereditary factors that cause IgA nephropathy and lead to a better understanding of the disease process.

INHERITED SYSTEMIC SYNDROMES AFFECTING THE GLOMERULUS

NAIL-PATELLA SYNDROME

Nail-patella syndrome is an autosomal dominant disease manifesting with symmetric nail, skeletal, ocular, and renal abnormalities.[138] The incidence of this disease is about 1/50,000 live births. The onset and outcome of the renal disease vary significantly. Some patients develop renal failure in early childhood, whereas a few patients show no signs of clinical nephropathy. However, characteristic pathologic features of the GBM thickening and splitting and fibrillar collagen deposits are observed in most cases. The disease is caused by loss-of-function mutations in the gene that encodes the LIM homeobox transcription factor 1β (LMX1B).[139-141] LMX1B is expressed in the kidney mainly by podocytes, and it regulates the expression of many crucial podocyte proteins, including nephrin, podocin, CD2AP, and α3 and α4 type IV collagen chains.[142-144] Dysregulation of these podocyte genes probably plays a role in the development of nail-patella syndrome–associated nephropathy.

DENYS-DRASH AND FRASIER'S SYNDROMES

Denys-Drash and Frasier's syndromes are characterized by male pseudohermaphroditism and progressive glomerulopathy.[145-147] In addition, patients with Denys-Drash syndrome have a predisposition for Wilms' tumor, whereas gonadoblastomas are associated with Frasier's syndrome. In Denys-Drash syndrome, nephropathy develops in infancy and progresses to ESKD by the age of 3 years. The typical glomerular lesion is diffuse mesangial sclerosis. In contrast, nephropathy in Frasier's syndrome usually manifests at a later stage, with a histologic picture of FSGS. However, clinical signs of the two syndromes can overlap.[148] Of importance is that the nephropathies in Denys-Drash and Frasier's syndromes are resistant to drug treatment, and kidney transplantation remains the only therapeutic alternative. Of note, mutations in WT1 have also been identified in patients without any obvious extrarenal abnormalities.[149]

Denys-Drash and Frasier's syndromes are caused by dominant mutations in the Wilms' tumor oncogene, *WT1*.[150-153] Denys-Drash syndrome is caused by several different mutations distributed along the *WT1* gene, whereas patients with Frasier's syndrome have mutations in the donor splice site of intron 9 in the gene. The *WT1* gene encodes a transcription factor that controls the expression of many key podocyte genes, and nephropathy may be caused by a failure in the regulation of these genes.[154] However, the phenotype of chimeric *WT1* mutant mice suggests that glomerulopathy may be mediated by the systemic effects of *WT1* mutations.[155]

MITOCHONDRIAL DISORDERS

Mitochondrial diseases are a heterogeneous group of syndromes affecting basically all organs dependent on mitochondrial energy supply.[156] These diseases are caused by mutations in genes coding for mitochondrial enzyme complexes that are important for oxidative phosphorylation and energy production. Mitochondrial diseases are primarily neuromuscular syndromes, but renal manifestations have also been reported in several cases.[156] The clinical course of the mitochondrial disease–related nephropathy varies significantly. Some patients exhibit proteinuria in early childhood, whereas others develop the first renal symptoms in adulthood. The rate of progression to end-stage renal disease is variable. Renal pathologic studies have not revealed any alterations specific for mitochondrial disorders, although FSGS is a common histologic finding.

SCHIMKE'S IMMUNO-OSSEOUS DYSPLASIA

Schimke's immuno-osseous dysplasia (SIOD) is an autosomal recessive syndrome manifesting with disproportional growth failure, impaired cellular immune function, cerebrovascular complications, and steroid-resistant nephrotic syndrome. Patients with severe SIOD develop nephrotic syndrome and renal insufficiency by preschool age.[157] A typical histopathologic finding is FSGS, although cases with minimal changes have also been reported. Disproportional growth failure manifests typically as a more prominent reduction of trunk length than of leg length. Cerebrovascular complications include life-threatening neurologic events, such as transient ischemic attacks and cerebral infarctions. However, patients with milder disease may not develop cerebrovascular complications, and other typical manifestations of SIOD can also be missing.

SIOD is caused by mutations in *SMARCAL1*, a gene encoding a putative chromatin remodeling protein of unknown function.[157,158] A number of different mutations have been identified in this gene, and missense mutations apparently often lead to a mild form of the disease. Mutations associated with SIOD seem to affect SMARCAL1 protein expression, stability, subcellular location, chromatin binding, and enzymatic activity. How these altered properties lead to SIOD is, however, not understood.

SCARB2 DISEASE

Action myoclonus–renal failure syndrome is a rare autosomal recessive disorder manifesting, typically at age 15 to 25 years, as a combination of FSGS (sometimes with glomerular collapse) and progressive myoclonus epilepsy in association with storage material in the brain.[159,160] Two independent studies have identified mutations in the gene that encodes scavenger receptor B2 (Scarb2), a lysosomal-membrane protein; this gene is thought to be responsible for this syndrome.[161,162]

Mutations in a lysosomal protein are suggestive of a previously unknown pathogenic mechanism for the genesis of proteinuria and FSGS. Scarb2 is expressed in podocytes.[162] Mutations in *SCARB2* result in a lack of the gene product.[159,162] Lack of Scarb2 probably leads, on the other hand, to abnormal lysosomal function, podocyte dysfunction, and proteinuria. The exact mechanism is unknown, but altered recycling or degradation of critical podocyte proteins may contribute to cellular damage. The role of Scarb2 in renal function has been confirmed by studies on *Scarb2*-knockout mice that exhibit subtle glomerular changes. Of note, tubular dysfunction has also been observed in *Scarb2*-knockout mice.

Complete reference list available at ExpertConsult.com.

KEY REFERENCES

2. Alport AC: Hereditary familial congenital haemorrhagic nephritis. *BMJ* 1:504–506, 1927.
3. Hudson BG, Tryggvason K, Sundaramoorthy M, et al: Alport's syndrome, Goodpasture's syndrome, and type IV collagen. *N Engl J Med* 348:2543–2556, 2003.
5. Barker DF, Hostikka SL, Zhou J, et al: Identification of mutations in the COL4A5 collagen gene in Alport syndrome. *Science* 248:1224–1227, 1990.
6. Hostikka SL, Eddy RL, Byers MG, et al: Identification of a distinct type IV collagen alpha chain with restricted kidney distribution and assignment of its gene to the locus of X chromosome–linked Alport syndrome. *Proc Natl Acad Sci U S A* 87:1606–1610, 1990.
7. Mochizuki T, Lemmink HH, Mariyama M, et al: Identification of mutations in the alpha 3(IV) and alpha 4(IV) collagen genes in autosomal recessive Alport syndrome. *Nat Genet* 8:77–81, 1994.
9. Martin P, Heiskari N, Pajari H, et al: Spectrum of COL4A5 mutations in Finnish Alport syndrome patients. *Hum Mutat* 15:579, 2000.
14. Lemmink HH, Nillesen WN, Mochizuki T, et al: Benign familial hematuria due to mutation of the type IV collagen alpha4 gene. *J Clin Invest* 98:1114–1118, 1996.
32. Savige J, Rana K, Tonna S, et al: Thin basement membrane nephropathy. *Kidney Int* 64:1169–1178, 2003.
37. Buzza M, Dagher H, Wang YY, et al: Mutations in the COL4A4 gene in thin basement membrane disease. *Kidney Int* 63:447–453, 2003.
40. Gregory MC: Alport syndrome and thin basement membrane nephropathy: unraveling the tangled strands of type IV collagen. *Kidney Int* 65:1109–1110, 2004.
43. Blumenthal SS, Fritsche C, Jr, Lemann J: Establishing the diagnosis of benign familial hematuria. The importance of examining the urine sediment of family members. *JAMA* 259:2263–2266, 1988.
51. Plaisier E, Gribouval O, Alamowitch S, et al: COL4A1 mutations and hereditary angiopathy, nephropathy, aneurysms, and muscle cramps. *N Engl J Med* 357:2687–2695, 2007.
52. Gould DB, Phalan FC, Breedveld GJ, et al: Mutations in Col4a1 cause perinatal cerebral hemorrhage and porencephaly. *Science* 308:1167–1171, 2005.
60. Kestila M, Lenkkeri U, Mannikko M, et al: Positionally cloned gene for a novel glomerular protein—nephrin—is mutated in congenital nephrotic syndrome. *Mol Cell* 1:575–582, 1998.
65. Ruotsalainen V, Ljungberg P, Wartiovaara J, et al: Nephrin is specifically located at the slit diaphragm of glomerular podocytes. *Proc Natl Acad Sci U S A* 96:7962–7967, 1999.
67. Tryggvason K, Patrakka J, Wartiovaara J: Hereditary proteinuria syndromes and mechanisms of proteinuria. *N Engl J Med* 354:1387–1401, 2006.
69. Boute N, Gribouval O, Roselli S, et al: NPHS2, encoding the glomerular protein podocin, is mutated in autosomal recessive steroid-resistant nephrotic syndrome. *Nat Genet* 24:349–354, 2000.
70. Wartiovaara J, Ofverstedt LG, Khoshnoodi J, et al: Nephrin strands contribute to a porous slit diaphragm scaffold as revealed by electron tomography. *J Clin Invest* 114:1475–1483, 2004.
83. Schwarz K, Simons M, Reiser J, et al: Podocin, a raft-associated component of the glomerular slit diaphragm, interacts with CD2AP and nephrin. *J Clin Invest* 108:1621–1629, 2001.
89. Tsukaguchi H, Sudhakar A, Le TC, et al: NPHS2 mutations in late-onset focal segmental glomerulosclerosis: R229Q is a common disease-associated allele. *J Clin Invest* 110:1659–1666, 2002.

92. Sellin L, Huber TB, Gerke P, et al: NEPH1 defines a novel family of podocin interacting proteins. *FASEB J* 17:115–117, 2003.
99. Brown EJ, Schlondorff JS, Becker DJ, et al: Mutations in the formin gene INF2 cause focal segmental glomerulosclerosis. *Nat Genet* 42:72–76, 2010.
101. Boyer O, Nevo F, Plaisier E, et al: INF2 mutations in Charcot-Marie-Tooth disease with glomerulopathy. *N Engl J Med* 365(25):2377–2388, 2011.
102. Genovese G, Friedman DJ, Ross MD, et al: Association of trypanolytic ApoL1 variants with kidney disease in African Americans. *Science* 329:841–845, 2010.
103. Tzur S, Rosset S, Skorecki K, et al: APOL1 allelic variants are associated with lower age of dialysis initiation, and thereby increased dialysis vintage in African and Hispanic Americans with non-diabetic end-stage kidney disease. *Nephrol Dial Transplant* 27:1498–1505, 2012.
107. Hinkes B, Wiggins RC, Gbadegesin R, et al: Positional cloning uncovers mutations in PLCE1 responsible for a nephrotic syndrome variant that may be reversible. *Nat Genet* 38:1397–1405, 2006.
109. Kaplan JM, Kim SH, North KN, et al: Mutations in ACTN4, encoding alpha-actinin-4, cause familial focal segmental glomerulosclerosis. *Nat Genet* 24:251–256, 2000.
110. Weins A, Kenlan P, Herbert S, et al: Mutational and biological analysis of alpha-actinin-4 in focal segmental glomerulosclerosis. *J Am Soc Nephrol* 16(12):3694–3701, 2005.
113. Kos CH, Le TC, Sinha S, et al: Mice deficient in alpha-actinin-4 have severe glomerular disease. *J Clin Invest* 111:1683–1690, 2003.
115. Reiser J, Polu KR, Moller CC, et al: TRPC6 is a glomerular slit diaphragm-associated channel required for normal renal function. *Nat Genet* 37:739–744, 2005.
116. Winn MP, Conlon PJ, Lynn KL, et al: A mutation in the TRPC6 cation channel causes familial focal segmental glomerulosclerosis. *Science* 308:1801–1804, 2005.
121. Kim JM, Wu H, Green G, et al: CD2-associated protein haploinsufficiency is linked to glomerular disease susceptibility. *Science* 300:1298–1300, 2003.
123. Shih NY, Li J, Karpitskii V, et al: Congenital nephrotic syndrome in mice lacking CD2-associated protein. *Science* 286:312–315, 1999.
125. Mele C, Iatropoulos P, Donadelli R, et al: MYO1E mutations and childhood familial focal segmental glomerulosclerosis. *N Engl J Med* 365:295–306, 2011.
126. Ozaltin F, Ibsirlioglu T, Taskiran EZ, et al: Disruption of PTPRO causes childhood-onset nephrotic syndrome. *Am J Hum Genet* 89:139–147, 2011.
127. Wharram BL, Goyal M, Gillespie PJ, et al: Altered podocyte structure in GLEPP1 (Ptpro)-deficient mice associated with hypertension and low glomerular filtration rate. *J Clin Invest* 106:1281–1290, 2000.
135. Gharavi AG, Yan Y, Scolari F, et al: IgA nephropathy, the most common cause of glomerulonephritis, is linked to 6q22-23. *Nat Genet* 26:354–357, 2000.
136. Paterson AD, Liu XQ, Wang K, et al: Genomewide linkage scan of a large family with IgA nephropathy localizes a novel susceptibility locus to chromosome 2q36. *J Am Soc Nephrol* 18:2408–2415, 2007.
139. Dreyer SD, Zhou G, Baldini A, et al: Mutations in LMX1B cause abnormal skeletal patterning and renal dysplasia in nail patella syndrome. *Nat Genet* 19:47–50, 1998.
140. McIntosh I, Dreyer SD, Clough MV, et al: Mutation analysis of LMX1B gene in nail-patella syndrome patients. *Am J Hum Genet* 63:1651–1658, 1998.
142. Miner JH, Morello R, Andrews KL, et al: Transcriptional induction of slit diaphragm genes by Lmx1b is required in podocyte differentiation. *J Clin Invest* 109:1065–1072, 2002.
143. Morello R, Zhou G, Dreyer SD, et al: Regulation of glomerular basement membrane collagen expression by LMX1B contributes to renal disease in nail patella syndrome. *Nat Genet* 27:205–208, 2001.
144. Rohr C, Prestel J, Heidet L, et al: The LIM-homeodomain transcription factor Lmx1b plays a crucial role in podocytes. *J Clin Invest* 109:1073–1082, 2002.
149. Guaragna MS, Lutaif AC, Piveta CS, et al: Two distinct WT1 mutations identified in patients and relatives with isolated nephrotic proteinuria. *Biochem Biophys Res Commun* 441:371–376, 2013.
150. Barbaux S, Niaudet P, Gubler MC, et al: Donor splice-site mutations in WT1 are responsible for Frasier syndrome. *Nat Genet* 17:467–470, 1997.
151. Haber DA, Buckler AJ, Glaser T, et al: An internal deletion within an 11p13 zinc finger gene contributes to the development of Wilms' tumor. *Cell* 61:1257–1269, 1990.
153. Pelletier J, Bruening W, Kashtan CE, et al: Germline mutations in the Wilms' tumor suppressor gene are associated with abnormal urogenital development in Denys-Drash syndrome. *Cell* 67:437–447, 1991.
154. Guo JK, Menke AL, Gubler MC, et al: WT1 is a key regulator of podocyte function: reduced expression levels cause crescentic glomerulonephritis and mesangial sclerosis. *Hum Mol Genet* 11:651–659, 2002.
155. Patek CE, Fleming S, Miles CG, et al: Murine Denys-Drash syndrome: evidence of podocyte de-differentiation and systemic mediation of glomerulosclerosis. *Hum Mol Genet* 12:2379–2394, 2003.
157. Zivicnjak M, Franke D, Zenker M, et al: SMARCAL1 mutations: a cause of prepubertal idiopathic steroid-resistant nephrotic syndrome. *Pediatr Res* 65:564–568, 2009.

45 Inherited Disorders of the Renal Tubule

Alain Bonnardeaux | Daniel G. Bichet

CHAPTER OUTLINE

INHERITED DISORDERS ASSOCIATED WITH GENERALIZED DYSFUNCTION OF THE PROXIMAL TUBULE (RENAL FANCONI'S SYNDROME), 1435
Pathogenesis, 1435
Clinical Presentation of Renal Fanconi's Syndrome, 1436
Dent's Disease, 1437
Oculocerebrorenal Dystrophy (Lowe's Syndrome), 1438
Mistargeting to Mitochondria of Peroxisomal EHHADH, an Enzyme Involved in Peroxisomal Oxidation of Fatty Acids, 1439
Idiopathic Causes of Renal Fanconi's Syndrome, 1439
Cystinosis, 1439
Glycogenosis (von Gierke's Disease), 1442
Tyrosinemia, 1443
Galactosemia, 1444
Wilson's Disease, 1444
Hereditary Fructose Intolerance, 1445
INHERITED DISORDERS OF RENAL AMINO ACID TRANSPORT, 1445
Cystinuria, 1445
Lysinuric Protein Intolerance, 1449
Hartnup's Disorder, 1449
Iminoglycinuria, 1450
Dicarboxylic Aminoaciduria, 1450
INHERITED DISORDERS OF RENAL PHOSPHATE TRANSPORT, 1450
Renal Phosphate Excretion, 1450
X-Linked Hypophosphatemic Rickets, 1451
Autosomal Dominant Hypophosphatemic Rickets, 1452
Autosomal Recessive Hypophosphatemic Rickets, 1452
Hereditary Hypophosphatemic Rickets with Hypercalciuria, 1453
Familial Tumoral Calcinosis, 1453
Hereditary Selective Deficiency of $1\alpha,25(OH)_2D_3$, 1453

Hereditary Generalized Resistance to $1\alpha,25(OH)_2D_3$, 1453
Resistance to Parathormone Action, 1453
INHERITED DISORDER OF URATE TRANSPORT, 1453
Familial Renal Hypouricemia, 1453
INHERITED DISORDERS OF RENAL GLUCOSE TRANSPORT, 1453
Renal Glucosuria, 1454
Glucose-Galactose Malabsorption, 1454
INHERITED DISORDERS OF ACID-BASE TRANSPORTERS, 1454
Proximal Renal Tubular Acidosis, 1455
Distal Renal Tubular Acidosis, 1457
BARTTER'S AND GITELMAN'S SYNDROMES, 1457
Bartter's Syndrome, 1457
Gitelman's Syndrome, 1459
INHERITED DISORDERS WITH HYPERTENSION AND HYPOKALEMIA, 1459
Congenital Adrenal Hyperplasia, 1461
Liddle's Syndrome, 1462
Apparent Mineralocorticoid Excess, 1463
Autosomal Dominant Early-Onset Hypertension with Severe Exacerbation during Pregnancy, 1463
Glucocorticoid-Remediable Hyperaldosteronism, 1463
Familial Hyperaldosteronism Type II, 1464
PSEUDOHYPOALDOSTERONISM, 1464
Pseudohypoaldosteronism Type I, 1464
Pseudohypoaldosteronism Type II, 1464
INHERITED DISORDERS OF RENAL MAGNESIUM PROCESSING, 1465
Familial Hypomagnesemia with Hypercalciuria and Nephrocalcinosis, 1466
Familial Hypomagnesemia with Secondary Hypocalcemia, 1466
Isolated Dominant Hypomagnesemia with Hypocalciuria, 1466

Ca²⁺/Mg²⁺-Sensing Receptor–Associated Disorders, 1466
Isolated Recessive Hypomagnesemia with Normocalciuria, 1466
Dominant and Recessive Hypomagnesemia, 1467
DIABETES INSIPIDUS, 1467
Pathogenesis, 1467
Clinical Presentation and History of X-Linked Nephrogenic Diabetes Insipidus, 1470
Polyuria, Polydipsia, Electrolyte Imbalance, and Dehydration in Cystinosis, 1473
Polyuria in Hereditary Hypokalemic Salt-Losing Tubulopathies, 1473
Carrier Detection, Perinatal Testing, and Treatment, 1473

Considerable progress has been made in understanding the molecular basis of several inherited renal tubule disorders. These advances have allowed the identification of genes expressed in the renal tubule (Table 45.1), increasing our knowledge of basic renal physiology and pathobiology. Other benefits include potential prenatal and postnatal screening and better phenotype characterization and knowledge. Although most diseases described in this section are relatively rare (1:2000 or less; affecting fewer than 200,000 persons in the United States) and previously restricted to pediatric nephrology, advances in therapy have increased longevity for many patients, thus confronting the adult nephrologist with new challenges.

INHERITED DISORDERS ASSOCIATED WITH GENERALIZED DYSFUNCTION OF THE PROXIMAL TUBULE (RENAL FANCONI'S SYNDROME)

Renal Fanconi's syndrome is a generalized dysfunction of the proximal tubule with no primary glomerular involvement. It is characterized by variable degrees of phosphate, glucose, amino acid, and bicarbonate wasting. Isolated or partial defects are described in other sections of this chapter. The clinical presentation of Fanconi's syndrome in children consists of rickets and impaired growth. In adults, bone disease manifests as osteomalacia and osteoporosis. Polyuria, renal sodium and potassium wasting, metabolic acidosis, hypercalciuria, and low-molecular-weight proteinuria may be part of the clinical spectrum.

There are hereditary and acquired variants of Fanconi's syndrome. Acquired forms in adults are usually associated with abnormal proteinurias such as paraproteinemias or the nephrotic syndrome, with residual cases being secondary to tubular damage caused by toxic or immunologic factors.[1] Hereditary Fanconi's syndrome occurs principally by one of two mechanisms: primary proximal tubule transport defects or accumulation of toxic metabolic products in the kidneys (Table 45.2).

PATHOGENESIS

The proximal tubule is responsible for reclaiming most of the filtered load of bicarbonate, glucose, urate, amino acids and low-molecular-weight proteins as well as an important fraction of the filtered load of sodium, chloride, phosphate, and water. It exhibits a very extensive apical endocytic apparatus consisting of an elaborate network of coated

Table 45.1 Impact of DNA Variation on Protein Function

Loss of function	A mutation that reduces or abolishes a normal physiologic function (likely to be recessive)
Gain of function	A mutation that increases the function of a protein (likely to be dominant)
Dominant negative	A mutation that dominantly affects the phenotype by means of a defective protein or RNA molecule that interferes with the function of the normal gene product in the same cell (likely to be dominant)

Table 45.2 Inherited and Acquired Causes of Fanconi's Syndrome

Inherited	Idiopathic (AD)
	Dent's disease (XL)
	"Sporadic"
	Cystinosis (AR)
	Tyrosinomia type I (AR)
	Galactosemia (AR)
	Glycogen storage disease type I (AR)
	Wilson's disease (AR)
	Mitochondrial diseases (cytochrome-c oxidase deficiency)
	Oculocerebrorenal syndrome of Lowe (XL)
	Hereditary fructose intolerance (AR)
	Mistargeting to mitochondria of peroxisomal EHHADH
Acquired	Paraproteinemias (multiple myeloma)
	Nephrotic syndrome
	Chronic tubulointerstitial nephritis
	Renal transplantation
	Malignancy
Exogenous factors	Heavy metals (cadmium, mercury, lead, uranium, platinum)
	Drugs (cisplatin, aminoglycosides, 6-mercaptopurine, valproate, outdated tetracyclines, methyl-3-chrome, ifosfamide)
	Chemical compounds (toluene, maleate, paraquat, Lysol)

AD, Autosomal dominant; AR, autosomal recessive; EHHADH, enoyl–coenzyme A (CoA), hydratase/3-hydroxyacyl CoA dehydrogenase; XL, X-linked.

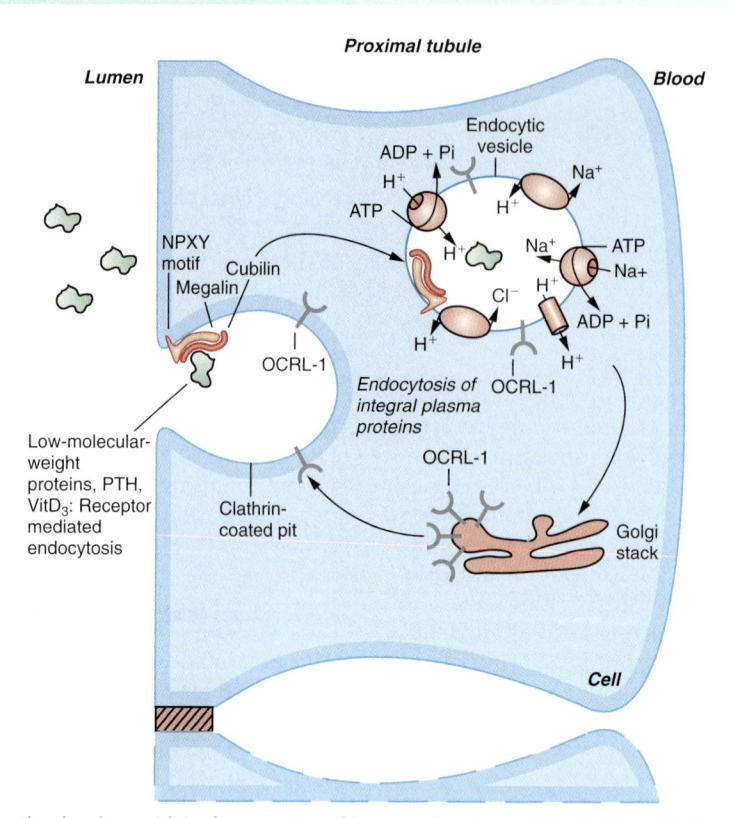

Figure 45.1 The glomerular filtration barrier restricts the passage of large molecules, particular those that are negatively charged molecules. The proteins appearing in the proximal tubule are reabsorbed by endocytosis (see luminal part of the schematic representation). Vitamins and iron that are complexed to carrier proteins bind to megalin and/or cubilin followed by endocytosis. The ligands are released from the receptors by the low pH in the endosomes, and receptors recycle through the membrane recycling compartment. The protein component is degraded, whereas the vitamin, as well as iron, is transported across the epithelial cell (not represented). 1,25-dihydroxyvitamin D_3 is activated by mitochondrial 1α-hydroxylase, implying that the vitamin is transported to the cytoplasm, possibly by diffusion, before its release to the basolateral membrane. The regulation and maintenance of an endocytic vesicle pH are represented here according to Weisz,[376] whereby protons are pumped into the organelle by vacuolar H^+-ATPase and can leave by the chloride proton exchanger ClC-5. The *ClC5* gene is mutated in patients with type 1 Dent's disease, and the *OCRL1* gene is mutated in patients with type 2 Dent's disease. OCRL1 encodes a phosphatase that is present on the trans-Golgi network and is important for regulating the traffic between the network, early endosomes, and clathrin-coated intermediate particles. ADP, Adenosine diphosphate; ATP, adenosine triphosphate; NPXY, asn-pro-any amino acid-tyrosine motif; OCRL-1, phosphatidylinositol 4,5-bisphosphate 5-phosphatase encoded by *OCRL1* gene; P_i, inorganic phosphate; PTH, parathyroid hormone; Vit, vitamin.

pits and small, coated and noncoated endosomes. In addition, the cells contain a large number of late endosomes, prelysosomes, lysosomes, and so-called dense apical tubules involved in receptor recycling from the endosomes to the apical plasma membrane. This endocytic apparatus is involved in the reabsorption of molecules filtered by the glomeruli (Figure 45.1). The process is very effective, as demonstrated by the fact that although several grams of proteins are filtered daily, the urine is virtually devoid of protein under physiologic conditions. Reabsorption of solutes by proximal tubule cells is achieved by transport systems at the brush border membrane that are directly or indirectly coupled to sodium movement, by energy production and transport from the mitochondria, and by the Na^+-K^+-adenosine triphosphatase (ATPase) at the basolateral membrane. The Na^+-K^+-ATPase lowers intracellular Na^+ concentration and provides the electrochemical gradient that allows Na^+-coupled solute to enter the cell. A second route, the paracellular pathway, is responsible for reclaiming up to half of the sodium and most of the water through tight junctions.

Because multiple transport anomalies characterize renal Fanconi's syndrome, the defects responsible must lead to the functional disruption of the proximal tubule cell itself. Storage diseases leading to Fanconi's syndrome are potentially reversible. For example, the defect is reversed after dietary restriction of tyrosine and phenylalanine in tyrosinemia,[2] fructose in hereditary fructose intolerance,[3] and galactose in galactosemia.[4] The duration of the exposure is also important for the disorder to be expressed and is protracted in cadmium intoxication[5] or shortened in fructose intolerance following a fructose load.[6]

CLINICAL PRESENTATION OF RENAL FANCONI'S SYNDROME

AMINOACIDURIA

Amino acids are filtered by the glomerulus with more than 98% subsequently reabsorbed by multiple proximal tubule transporters. In Fanconi's syndrome, all amino acids are excreted in excess. The pattern of excretion of amino acids parallels that in physiologic conditions, so those excreted at the highest levels are histidine, serine, cystine, lysine, and glycine. Aminoaciduria is usually quantified by one of several chromatographic methods in specialized centers. Clinically, losses are relatively modest and do not lead to specific deficiencies. There is no need to give amino acid supplements to affected subjects.

PHOSPHATURIA AND BONE DISEASE

Phosphate wasting is a cardinal manifestation but bone features are variable. Serum phosphate levels are usually decreased, and tubular reabsorption of phosphate (TRP) and maximal capacity—calculated by dividing maximum tubular reabsorption of phosphate (Tm_P) by glomerular filtration rate (GFR) or Tm_P/GFR—are systematically reduced. Rickets and osteomalacia, which are caused by increased urinary losses of phosphate as well as by impaired 1α-hydroxylation of 1,25-dihydroxyvitamin D_3, can compose the dominant clinical picture. Rickets manifests as the bowing deformity of the lower limbs with metaphyseal widening of the proximal and distal tibia, distal femur, ulna, and radius. Bone manifestations in subjects with adult-onset renal Fanconi's syndrome are severe bone pain and spontaneous fractures.

RENAL TUBULAR ACIDOSIS

Hyperchloremic metabolic acidosis is a frequent finding and is caused by defective bicarbonate reabsorption. Hence, renal acidification by the distal tubule is normal, as demonstrated by the ability to acidify urine at a pH below 5.5 when plasma bicarbonate is below the threshold. Because the more distal segments have substantial bicarbonate reabsorptive capacity, the plasma bicarbonate concentration is usually maintained between 12 and 20 mmol/L. The diagnosis can be established by raising the plasma bicarbonate concentration with an intravenous sodium bicarbonate infusion (0.5 to 1 mmol/kg per hour) to 18 to 20 mmol/L. The fractional excretion of bicarbonate will usually rise to 15% to 20% in proximal RTA but will remain lower (3%) in distal RTA. Treatment with large doses of alkali may be necessary to correct the acidosis.

GLUCOSURIA

Glucosuria is a common manifestation although the serum glucose level is normal, and the amount of glucose lost in the urine varies from 0.5 to 10 g per day. Glucosuria (and hypoglycemia) may be massive in glycogenosis type I.[7]

POLYURIA, SODIUM, AND POTASSIUM WASTING

Polyuria, polydipsia, and dehydration may be prominent features. The decreased concentrating ability of the kidney may also be related to abnormal tubule function of the distal tubule and collecting duct, caused by hypokalemia. Renal sodium losses may be significant and may lead to hypotension, hyponatremia, and metabolic alkalosis. Supplementation with sodium chloride is indicated and achieves clinical improvement. Potassium losses are secondary to increased delivery of sodium to the distal tubule and activation of the renin angiotensin aldosterone system from hypovolemia. Supplementation is indicated to correct low serum potassium levels.

PROTEINURIA

Low-molecular-weight proteinuria is almost always present in low to moderate amounts. Endosomal machinery proteins, including the vacuolar type H^+-ATPase (V-ATPase), ClC-5 chloride/proton exchanger channels, and the endocytotic receptors megalin and cubilin,[8] are important in protein reabsorption. The urine dipstick test result is frequently positive because of the presence of albuminuria, typically at levels of 1 g/day. Rates of $β_2$-microglobulin excretion are also elevated.

HYPERCALCIURIA

Hypercalciuria is a frequent manifestation in patients with renal Fanconi's syndrome. The pathogenesis is not known but could be related to abnormal recycling of proteins involved in calcium reabsorption by the proximal tubule, natriuresis, and increased vitamin D synthesis from hypophosphatemia. Hypercalciuria is only occasionally associated with nephrolithiasis, possibly because of the presence of polyuria.

DENT'S DISEASE

PATHOGENESIS

Dent's disease, X-linked recessive hypophosphatemic rickets, and X-linked recessive nephrolithiasis (Online Mendelian Inheritance in Man [OMIM] entry #300009)[9] are clinical manifestations of the same disease. Clinical features include primary Fanconi's syndrome, low-molecular-weight proteinuria, hypercalciuria with calcium nephrolithiasis, nephrocalcinosis, rickets, and progressive renal failure. Dent's disease is caused by mutations in the *CLCN5* gene located on chromosome Xp11.22 encoding a lysosomal transport protein, ClC-5, a 2 chloride/1 proton antiporter.[10] Defects in the *OCRL1* gene (oculocerebrorenal syndrome of Lowe), encoding a phosphatidylinositol 4,5-bisphosphate 5-phosphatase (Ocrl) and usually found mutated in patients with Lowe's syndrome, also can induce a Dent-like phenotype (type 2 Dent's disease [OMIM #300555]; see later)[11,12] (see Figure 45.1) Of the 32 families with the clinical diagnosis of Dent's disease reported by Hoopes and colleagues,[13] 19 (60%) had mutations in *CLCN5* and 5 families (16%) had mutations in *OCRL1* (for whom the diagnosis of Lowe's syndrome had been excluded because of absence of cataracts). Because these two genes do not account for all patients with the phenotype of Dent's disease, it is likely that other genes involved in proximal tubular function will be found in such patients.[13]

ClC-5 mutations expressed in vitro lead to a disorder manifesting as defects in receptor-mediated endocytosis and/or endosomal acidification.[14] ClC-5 co-localizes with the proton pump and internalized proteins early after uptake and is also expressed in type A intercalated cells. ClC-5 forms a dimer of two identical subunits, each of which contains a complete ion conduction pathway and is composed of 18 α-helices. It is thought to provide an electrical shunt for the acidification of vesicles of the endocytotic pathway required for receptor-ligand interactions and cell sorting events.[15] Inhibition of the acidification interferes with cell-surface receptor recycling, reducing endocytosis of albumin and resulting in mistargeting of megalin, cubilin, Na^+-H^+-exchanger isoform 3 (NHE3), and the sodium/phosphate transporter NPT2a.

CLINICAL PRESENTATION

The clinical presentation is explained by the predominant expression of ClC-5 in the proximal tubule. Patients have varying degrees of low-molecular-weight proteinuria, hypercalciuria with calcium nephrolithiasis, rickets, nephrocalcinosis, and renal failure.[16] There is considerable intrafamilial variability,[17] probably because of genetic and/or environmental modifiers. The disease affects male patients predominantly, and female patients have an attenuated phenotype. However, renal failure develops only in male patients.

The excretion of low-molecular-weight proteins in the urine such as albumin, $β_2$-microglobulin, and $α_1$-microglobulin is thought to be the most reliable marker for the disease. Affected male patients usually excrete $β_2$-microglobulin in amounts that are more than 100-fold the upper limit of normal. Female carriers can also have low-molecular-weight proteinuria, but it is usually less pronounced than in male patients and sometimes absent. Low-molecular-weight proteinuria is not a specific finding because it can be seen in tubulointerstitial diseases as well. The degree of proteinuria is relatively constant and amounts to 0.5 to 2 g/day in adults and up to 1 g/day in children.[18-20] The nephrotic syndrome does not occur, and albumin excretion represents less than half of the proteins excreted. An attenuated form of the disease with low-molecular-weight proteinuria as the only or predominant feature appears to be prevalent in Japan.[21]

Hypercalciuria is also a common finding in this disorder and is present in most cases, beginning in childhood. It is usually overt and predominant in male patients (exceeding 7.5 mmol/day). Female patients are also frequently hypercalciuric, but their values are usually closer to the upper limit of the normal range. Nephrolithiasis is frequent, with 50% of male patients affected. Stones are composed of calcium phosphate or a mixture of calcium phosphate and oxalate.[20] Multiple episodes starting during the teenage years are common. Radiologic nephrocalcinosis of the medullary type is seen in most affected male patients and occasionally in female patients. Serum phosphate levels are usually below normal values or at the lower limit of the normal range. Tm_P/GFR is decreased, indicating defective reabsorption by the proximal tubule. Rickets may be present in children and is cured by the administration of pharmacologic doses of vitamin D. Osteomalacia occurs in adults and is also corrected after administration of vitamin D. Serum levels of 1,25-dihydroxyvitamin D_3 are normal or slightly raised, whereas 25-hydroxyvitamin D levels are normal. The cause of hypercalciuria and renal stones is not known, but one possible explanation is that renal phosphate leak and reduced degradation of luminal parathyroid hormone (PTH) results in increased 1α-hydroxylase activity and 1,25-dihydroxycholecalciferol (1,25[OH]$_2$D$_3$) production. Other explanations are abnormal trafficking (recycling) of transporters or channels necessary for calcium transport to the apical membrane, and decreased reabsorption of a regulatory protein by the proximal tubule.[22]

Systemic acidosis is typically not seen before renal function deteriorates significantly. Male patients usually have urinary acidification defects detectable by an ammonium chloride load, but these are not consistent features of the phenotype. Spontaneous hypokalemia is common in male patients, and there is inability to concentrate urine maximally. Aminoaciduria and glucosuria are also frequent. Half the male patients have raised serum creatinine with progressive renal failure. End-stage kidney disease occurs at age 47 ± 13 years. Renal biopsy specimens show a pattern of a chronic interstitial nephritis with scattered calcium deposits.[18,20] The glomeruli are normal or hyalinized. There is prominent tubular atrophy with diffuse inflammatory infiltrate composed of lymphocytes, and foci of calcification around and within epithelial cells. Molecular genetic testing is available and confirms the diagnosis.

TREATMENT

Renal stones and hypercalciuria are treated with supportive measures (and in particular, increasing fluid intake). Dietary restriction of calcium reduces calcium excretion but is not recommended because it might contribute to the bone disease.[23] Thiazide diuretics can be given in small doses and may decrease calciuria,[24] but in patients with Dent's disease, who have a tendency for salt wasting, response to these agents seems to consist of excessive diuresis, kaliuresis, and blood pressure reduction.[20] Rickets are treated with small doses of vitamin D, but this treatment should be given with caution as it might increase urine calcium excretion and the risk of nephrolithiasis. Verifying urine calcium excretion before and after vitamin D therapy might be appropriate.[23] There is no specific treatment for preventing progression of renal failure, although citrate has been shown to delay progression in a *Clc-5* knockout mouse model.[25] This goal has to be balanced against the possibility of increasing calcium phosphate supersaturation and stone formation by urine alkalinization.

OCULOCEREBRORENAL DYSTROPHY (LOWE'S SYNDROME)

The oculocerebrorenal syndrome (OCRL) of Lowe (OMIM #309000) is an X-linked recessive multisystem disorder characterized by congenital cataracts, mental retardation, and renal Fanconi's syndrome.[26]

PATHOGENESIS

Mutations in the *OCRL1* gene are responsible for OCRL.[27,28] *OCRL1* encodes a 105-kDa Golgi protein with phosphatidylinositol 4,5-bisphosphate (PIP$_2$) 5-phosphatase activity. Therefore, OCRL1 is mainly a lipid phosphatase that may control cellular levels of a critical metabolite, PIP$_2$,[29] and is involved in the inositol phosphate signaling pathway. OCRL1 is likely to regulate cellular trafficking. It is present in the trans-Golgi network, in early endosomes, and in clathrin-coated intermediates that move between these compartments.[29] Phosphorylation of phosphatidylinositol at the 3, 4, or 5 position of the inositol ring generates seven phosphoinositides (PIs) that play key regulatory functions in cell physiology (reviewed by Pirruccello and De Camilli[30]). The related soluble inositol polyphosphates and pyrophosphates, generated from inositol 1,4,5-trisphosphate (IP$_3$)—a product of PI(4,5)P$_2$ cleavage by phospholipases—are also important signaling molecules. PIs function in diverse processes, including signal transduction, transport of ions and metabolites across membranes, exocytosis and endocytosis, regulation of the actin cytoskeleton, transcriptional regulation, and membrane trafficking. Their phosphorylated headgroups, which are localized on the cytosolic leaflets of membranes and help define membrane identity, interact with a variety of amino acid motifs or protein domains, and thus regulate protein-bilayer interactions. Thus, OCRL1 deficiency may result in reductions in recycling of receptors and delivery of cargo to the plasma membrane. This possibility is consistent with the apparent loss of megalin from the apical membrane and protein absorption defects seen in patients (see Figure 45.1). It is not clear why the loss of OCRL1, a ubiquitously expressed protein, should result in defects to only the eyes, brain, and kidney proximal tubule. Compensation by another enzyme with overlapping specificity in the unaffected tissues is a possible explanation.

CLINICAL PRESENTATION

OCRL is a multisystem disorder characterized by ocular, neurologic, and renal defects. Renal dysfunction (Fanconi's syndrome) is a major feature and occurs in the first year of life, but the severity and age of onset vary. It is characterized by proteinuria (0.5 to 2 g of daily urinary protein per square meter of body surface area), generalized aminoaciduria (100 to 1000 mmol of daily urinary amino acid per kg of body weight), carnitine wasting (mean fractional excretion, 0.05 to 0.15), phosphaturia, and bicarbonaturia.[26] Glucosuria is variably present. Linear growth decreases after 1 year of age. Glomerular function also decreases with age, with end-stage kidney failure predicted between the second and fourth decade of life.

Neurologic findings include infantile hypotonia, mental retardation, and areflexia. Prenatal development of cataracts is universal, and other ocular anomalies are glaucoma, microphthalmos, and corneal keloid formation. Visual acuity is frequently decreased. Mental retardation is very common. Cranial magnetic resonance imaging (MRI) shows mild ventriculomegaly and cysts in the periventricular regions. Status epilepticus is also frequent. Death usually occurs in the second or third decade from renal failure or infection.

Some patients with a phenotype indistinguishable from Dent's disease (see previous discussion in "Dent's Disease" section) carry mutations in the *OCRL1* gene and have an attenuated form of OCRL.[11]

The diagnosis is established in affected individuals by the demonstration of reduced (<10% of normal) activity of inositol polyphosphate 5-phosphatase OCRL-1 in cultured skin fibroblasts. Molecular genetic testing of *OCRL* detects mutations in approximately 95% of affected males and a similar proportion of carrier females.[31] Carrier detection by slit-lamp examination has high but not absolute sensitivity. Concentrations of the muscle enzymes creatine kinase, aspartate aminotransferase, and lactate dehydrogenase, as well as of total serum protein, serum α_2-globulin, and high-density lipoprotein cholesterol, are elevated.

TREATMENT

Treatment of OCRL is supportive and includes taking care of ocular (cataract extraction, treatment of glaucoma), neurologic (anticonvulsants, speech therapy), and renal complications. Nasogastric tube feedings or feeding gastrostomy and antipsychotic therapy may be required. Bicarbonate therapy is usually given at a dose of 2 to 3 mmol/kg/day every 6 to 8 hours but may vary from 1 to 8 mmol/kg/day to maintain a serum bicarbonate concentration of 20 mmol/L. Sodium or potassium phosphate can be given in amounts 1 to 4 g/day for phosphate depletion, and vitamin D may be added if that approach is unsuccessful.

MISTARGETING TO MITOCHONDRIA OF PEROXISOMAL EHHADH, AN ENZYME INVOLVED IN PEROXISOMAL OXIDATION OF FATTY ACIDS

Peroxisomes were first identified by Christian de Duve, and it was originally thought that the primary function of these organelles was the metabolism of hydrogen peroxide. One of their main metabolic functions is β-oxidation of very long-chain fatty acids (for review see Lodhi and Semenkovich[32]). An EHHADH (enoyl-CoA, hydratase/3-hydroxyacyl CoA dehydrogenase) dominant mutant has been shown to mistarget to mitochondria and not to perixosomes, impaired mitochondrial oxydative phosphorylation and caused renal Fanconi's syndrome (Figure 45.2).[33]

IDIOPATHIC CAUSES OF RENAL FANCONI'S SYNDROME

Renal Fanconi's syndrome occurs in the absence of both known inborn errors of metabolism and acquired causes. Sporadic and familial cases unlinked to *CLCN5* (Dent's disease), *OCRL1* (Lowe's syndrome), or *EHHADH*[33] have been described,[13] with variable progressive renal failure.[26,34,35]

CYSTINOSIS

PATHOGENESIS

Cystinosis (OMIM #219800) is a rare autosomal recessive disease of lysosomal transport of the disulfide amino acid cystine.[36-38] Lysosomes are intracellular organelles containing enzymes responsible for the digestion of macromolecules. Lysosomal hydrolases are optimally active at low pH. The by-products of the hydrolytic digestion exit the lysosome through specific transporters. A defect in one of the lysosomal hydrolases results in the accumulation of macromolecules or by-products that lead to lysosomal, cellular, and eventually organ dysfunction. Cystine accumulation and crystallization destroy tissues, causing renal failure.[39] Inactivating mutations in the *CTNS* (cystinosis) gene on chromosome 17p13, encoding an integral lysosomal membrane protein termed *cystinosin*,[40] cause cystinosis. Approximately half of patients who have cystinosis and are of northern European descent carry at least one allele that bears a specific 57-kb deletion that encompasses the *CTNS* gene. This lysosomal cystine transporter has seven transmembrane domains and at least two lysosomal targeting signals (GYDQL in the C-terminus and YFPQA in the fifth intertransmembrane loop).

CLINICAL PRESENTATION

Cystinosis, which affects 1 in 100,000 to 1 in 200,000 newborns, is the most frequent cause of the inherited forms of renal Fanconi's syndrome. The clinical presentation is variable[41,42] and encompasses classic nephropathic cystinosis, a rare "adolescent" form, and also a mild adult-onset variant (Table 45.3). The most severe form manifests in the first year of life as failure to thrive, increased thirst, polyuria, and poor feeding. White patients with the disease frequently have blond hair and blue eyes and are more

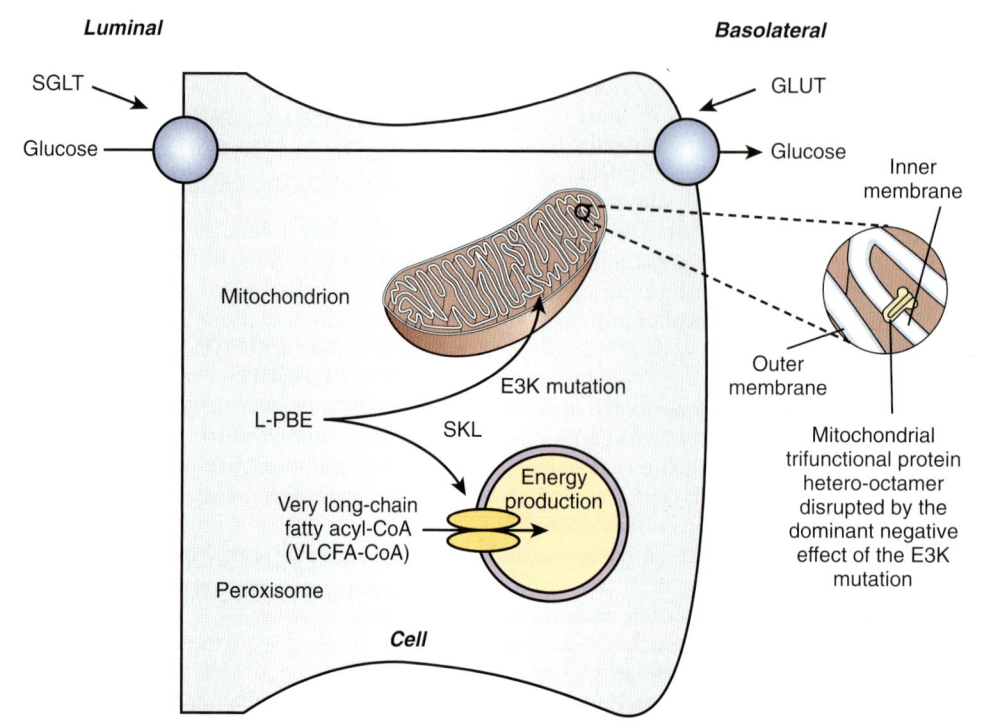

Figure 45.2 **Proposed model of a dominant negative effect of mutant peroxisomal L-bifunctional enzyme disrupting the mitochondrial trifunctional protein hetero-octamer in the renal proximal tubule.** Glucose is reabsorbed from the luminal (urine-side) membranes to the basolateral (blood-side) membranes and is not used for energy production. Most of the basolateral fatty acid uptake is used for mitochondrial energy production by means of trifunctional protein. A small fraction of the fatty acid uptake is used for peroxisomal energy production by means of bifunctional protein (D-bifunctional enzyme [D-PBE]). The physiologic targeting motif, SKL (serine-lysine-leucine), normally directs L-bifunctional enzyme (L-PBE) to the peroxisome. The E3K mutation instead creates a targeting motif that directs L-PBE to the mitochondrion, where its homology causes it to interfere with the assembly and function of trifunctional protein. GLUT, Glucose transporter; SGLT, sodium-glucose linked transporter. (Redrawn from Klootwijk ED, Reichold M, Helip-Wooley A, et al: Mistargeting of peroxisomal EHHADH and inherited renal Fanconi's syndrome. *N Engl J Med* 370:129-138, 2014.)

Table 45.3 Age-Related Clinical Characteristics of Untreated Nephropathic Cystinosis

Age (yr)	Symptom or Sign	Prevalence of Affected Patients (%)
6-12 mo	Renal Fanconi's syndrome (polyuria, polydipsia, electrolyte imbalance, dehydration, rickets, growth failure)	95
5-10	Hypothyroidism	50
8-12	Photophobia	50
8-12	Chronic renal failure	95
12-40	Myopathy, difficulty swallowing	20
13-40	Retinal blindness	10-15
18-40	Diabetes mellitus	5
18-40	Male hypogonadism	70
21-40	Pulmonary dysfunction	100
21-40	Central nervous system calcifications	15
21-40	Central nervous system symptomatic deterioration	2

From Gahl WA, Thoene JG, Schneider JA: Cystinosis. *N Engl J Med* 347:111-121, 2002.

lightly pigmented. Additional clinical findings include phosphaturia, aminoaciduria, glucosuria, and bicarbonaturia. Rickets occurs frequently. Renal wasting of sodium, calcium, and magnesium and tubular proteinuria are usually present. If the cystinosis is not treated, progressive renal damage culminates in end-stage kidney failure by the end of the first decade of life.

Damage in multiple organ systems, including ocular, endocrine, hepatic, muscular, and central nervous, has been reported. Cystinosis can affect most of the structures of the eye, with variable rates of progression. In the cornea, crystal deposits are absent at birth and appear by the end of the first year of life. Those can be seen by slit-lamp examination as fusiform crystals involving the anterior third of the central cornea and the full thickness of the peripheral cornea. Eventually, these deposits progress to develop a characteristic haziness. They can also be found in the iridis and conjunctiva as well as the retina, with consequent development of a characteristic peripheral retinopathy.

Other features include hypothyroidism from cystine crystallization in the follicular cells of the thyroid gland. It is present in more than 70% of patients older than 10 years. Insulin-dependent diabetes mellitus develops from long-standing cystine crystal accumulation in the pancreas, particularly after renal transplantation.[43] Hepatomegaly and splenomegaly with little clinical impact also occur in more than 40% of subjects older than 10 years.[41] A distal vacuolar myopathy is a late finding in 25% of cystinotic patients, with wasting in the small muscles of the hand. Facial weakness and dysphagia are often seen. In a previous study, muscle biopsies revealed marked fiber size variability, prominent acid phosphatase–positive vacuoles, and an absence of fiber-type grouping or inflammatory cells. Crystals of cystine were detected in perimysial cells but not within the muscle cell vacuoles. The muscle cystine content of clinically affected muscles is markedly elevated.[44] Central nervous system involvement has been described in the late stages of the disease,[37] and cystine crystal accumulation has been reported. The accumulation of intracellular cystine itself may also be a risk factor for vascular calcifications.[45]

The diagnosis is usually established by measuring the cystine content in peripheral leukocytes. Patients usually have values higher than 2 nmol of half-cystine per milligram of protein (normal < 0.2 nmol). Alternatively, the diagnosis can be made through recognition of the characteristic corneal crystals on slit-lamp examination. Molecular analysis of the cystinosin gene allows early diagnosis and can be used for prenatal diagnosis as well. Prenatal diagnosis of cystinosis can also be made by measuring S-labeled cystine accumulation in cultured amniocytes or chorionic villi samples[35]; and by a direct measurement of cystine in uncultured chorionic villi samples. Over 90 mutations have been reported, with a detection ratio close to 100%.[46]

TREATMENT

Patients with cystinosis who are treated at an early age are now expected to live a nearly normal life, but a limited access to cysteamine still exists in developing nations.[48] Prior to development of the cystine-depleting drug cysteamine, dialysis had to be initiated on average in patients reaching age 10. Cysteamine enters the lysosome by a specific transporter for aminothiols or aminosulfides and cleaves cystine into cysteine and a cysteine-cysteamine mixed disulfide (Figure 45.3). Oral cysteamine is given at doses of 60 to 90 mg/kg/day every 6 hours and generally achieves approximately 90% depletion of cellular cystine, as measured in circulating leukocytes.[49] A long-acting form appears to have similar efficacy.[50] It slows the rate of progression of renal failure and increases growth in affected subjects.[51-53] Kidney function stabilizes on initiation of therapy, and even some recovery can be seen if therapy is begun in the first year or two of life.[52] The growth rate becomes normal, but there is no "catching up." Topical cysteamine eye drops[54] and a new gel formulation[55] are used to treat ocular complications of cystinosis; they cause dissolution of corneal crystals.

Symptomatic treatment also involves rehydration, particularly during episodes of gastroenteritis. Replacement of bicarbonate losses with citrate- or bicarbonate-containing salts is frequently necessary. Phosphate losses are replaced with phosphate salts and oral vitamin D therapy. Indomethacin has been used to decrease renal salt and water wasting. Recombinant human growth hormone increases growth but not the rate of progression of renal failure.[53] Kidney transplantation is routinely performed, and most recipients do well.[56] Kidneys from heterozygous family donors are widely accepted because there is no evidence of cystine accumulation in kidney transplants.

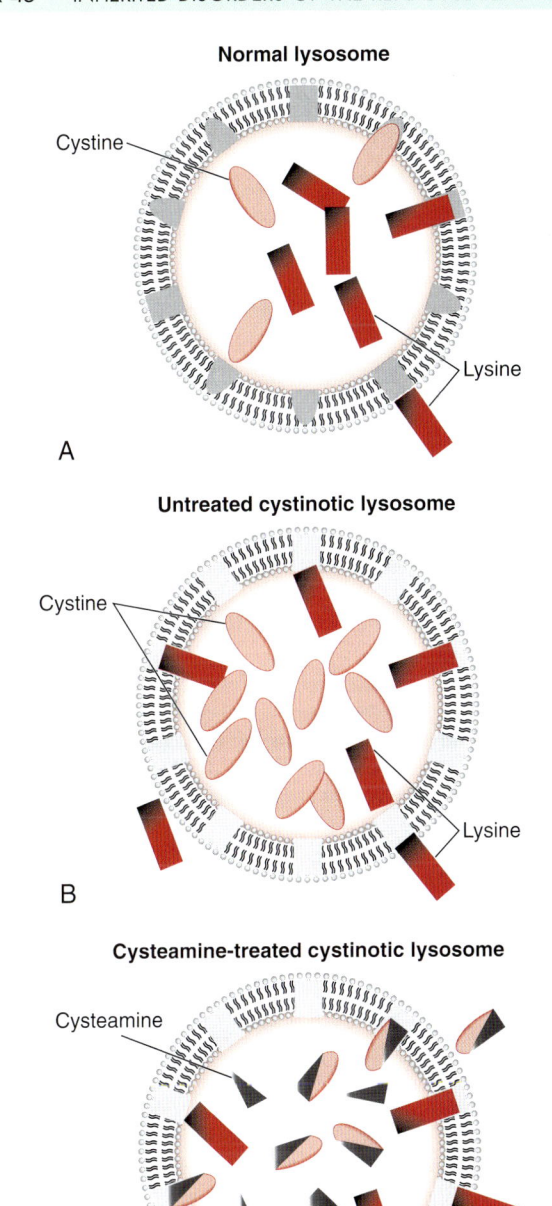

Figure 45.3 Mechanism of cystine depletion by cysteamine. **A,** In normal lysosomes, cystine and lysine freely traverse the lysosomal membrane through specific transporters (*rectangles* for the lysine transporter; *ovals* for the cystine transporter). **B,** In cystinotic lysosomes (note the absence of specific cystine transporters), lysine can freely traverse through specific transporters in the lysosomal membrane, but cystine cannot and therefore accumulates inside the lysosome. **C,** In cysteamine-treated lysosomes, cysteamine combines with half-cystine (i.e., cysteine) to form the mixed disulfide cysteine-cysteamine, which uses the lysine transporter to exit the lysosome. (Modified with permission from Gahl WA, Thoene JG, Schneider JA: Cystinosis. *N Engl J Med* 347:111-121, 2002. Copyright © 2002 Massachusetts Medical Society. All rights reserved.)

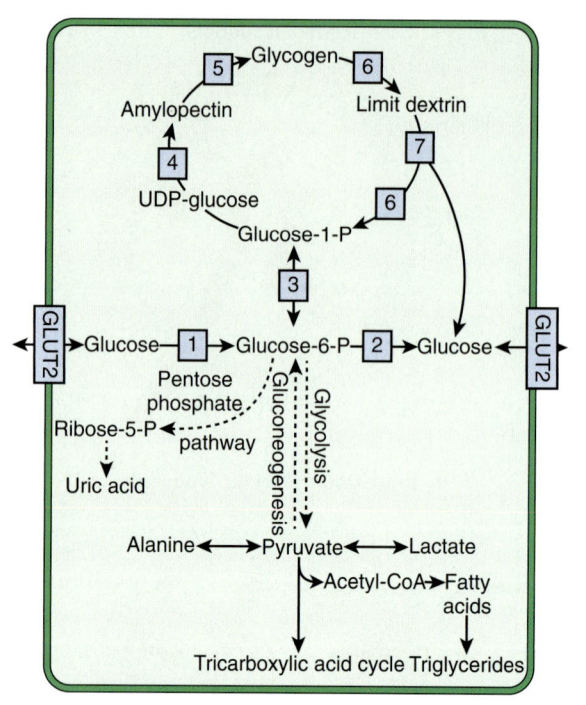

Figure 45.4 Simplified scheme of glycogen synthesis and breakdown. 1, Hexokinase/glucokinase; 2, glucose-6-phosphatase (G6Pase); 3, phosphoglucomutase; 4, glycogen synthase; 5, branching enzyme; 6, glycogen phosphorylase; 7, debranching enzyme. CoA, Coenzyme A; GLUT2, glucose transporter 2; P, phosphate; UDP-glucose, uridine diphosphoglucose. (From Wolfsdorf JI, Weinstein DA: Glycogen storage diseases. *Rev Endocr Metab Disord* 4:95-102, 2003.)

GLYCOGENOSIS (VON GIERKE'S DISEASE)

Glycogen storage diseases are inherited disorders that affect glycogen metabolism (Figure 45.4).[57] Both the liver and muscle store physiologically important quantities of glycogen. These organs are primarily affected, with the symptoms usually including hepatomegaly, hypoglycemia, muscle cramps and weakness, exercise intolerance, and fatigue. This section discusses type I glycogen storage disease because it is the only form associated with primary renal involvement. Type V glycogen storage disease (McArdle's disease) as well as other rare glycogenoses associated with rhabdomyolysis, myoglobinuria, and acute tubular necrosis are not discussed further.

PATHOGENESIS

Glycogen storage disease type I (GSD-I), also known as von Gierke's disease, is a group of autosomal recessive metabolic disorders caused by deficiencies in the activity of the glucose-6-phosphatase system that consists of at least two membrane proteins, glucose-6-phosphate transporter (G6PT) and glucose-6-phosphatase (G6Pase).[57] G6PT and G6Pase work in concert to maintain glucose homeostasis. G6Pase catalyzes the hydrolysis of glucose-6-phosphate (G6P) to produce glucose and phosphate. GSD-Ia (G6Pase deficiency),[58,59] the most frequent form, is caused by deficiency in enzymatic activity. GSD-Ib is caused by mutations in G6PT, which translocates G6P from the cytoplasm to the lumen of the endoplasmic reticulum (ER). Other variants include GSD-Ic (defect in microsomal phosphate or pyrophosphate transport) and GSD-Id (defect in microsomal glucose transport). The molecular basis of these variants remains to be determined.

CLINICAL PRESENTATION

GSD-I manifests as functional G6Pase deficiency, characterized by growth retardation, hypoglycemia, hepatomegaly, kidney enlargement, hyperlipidemia, hyperuricemia, and lactic acidemia. Patients with type Ib disease also suffer from chronic neutropenia and functional deficiencies of neutrophils and monocytes, resulting in recurrent bacterial infections as well as ulceration of the oral and intestinal mucosae. GSD-Ia manifests in the first year of life with hepatomegaly and/or hypoglycemic seizures with lactic acidosis. Hypoglycemia occurs because of impaired gluconeogenesis, glycogenolysis, and recycling of glucose through G6P to the glucose system. Adults usually present with hypoglycemic symptoms that are exacerbated by exercise and relieved by food. However, 48-hour fasting blood glucose levels are frequently normal.[60] The accumulation of G6P leads to an increase in glycolysis and lactic acidosis. Hyperuricemia and gout are caused by increased activity of hepatic adenosine monophosphate (AMP)–deaminase and adenine nucleotide production, thus increasing uric acid production. Hyperuricemia also results from decreased renal excretion because urate competes with lactate for secretion in the proximal tubule. Gout occurs in adults but is rarely seen in children. An enlarged abdomen from hepatomegaly, short stature from impaired growth, and skin manifestations from dyslipidemia (xanthomas) are frequent findings. Dyslipidemia is a result of increased synthesis of very low-density lipoprotein (VLDL), and low-density lipoprotein (LDL), and decreased lipolysis. Impairment of platelet adhesion and aggregation with prolonged bleeding time lead to easy bruising and epistaxis.

A renal Fanconi's syndrome occurs in GSD-I, with aminoaciduria, low-molecular-weight proteinuria, phosphaturia, and bicarbonaturia.[61,62] Renal disease is common in adult patients[63] with untreated GSD-I. It evolves slowly and is a late finding. In children, increased kidney size, hyperfiltration, and moderate proteinuria are common.[64] Distal renal tubular acidosis, hypocitraturia, hypercalciuria, nephrocalcinosis, and calcium nephrolithiasis can be variably associated,[65] but virtually all patients have impaired distal tubular acidification. The most common finding is focal and segmental glomerulosclerosis with tubulointerstitial atrophy. Glomerular changes include thickening, lamellation, and glycogen deposition in the glomerular basement membrane.[66]

The diagnosis of GSD-I is established by DNA testing or liver biopsy.[67] A 1-mg intramuscular glucagon test can be used and the result is frequently abnormal (an increase in blood glucose level < 4 mmol/L, usually at 30 minutes). Liver histology reveals prominent storage of glycogen and fat, large lipid vacuoles with hepatocyte distension, and steatosis with little fibrosis. Abnormally high glycogen levels are noted in liver biopsy samples. Electron microscopy shows moderate to large excesses of glycogen in the cytoplasm, often displacing the organelles in the hepatocyte. Enzyme analysis of fresh and frozen samples can distinguish type Ia from type Ib GSD.

TREATMENT

Life expectancy for patients with GSD-I has improved considerably. The treatment goal is to maintain normoglycemia to avoid the metabolic complications that are secondary to hypoglycemia and lactic acidosis. This can be accomplished at night with nasogastric feeding of glucose[68] or with orally administered uncooked cornstarch. A single dose of cornstarch (1.75 to 2.5 g/kg) at bedtime will maintain serum glucose concentrations above 3.9 mmol/L for 7 hours or longer in most young adults.[69] Because hypoglycemia and lactic acidosis occur in adults as well, treatment might also be indicated after childhood.[70] Guidelines for the management of GSD-I published by the European Study on Glycogen Storage Disease Type I[71] include a preprandial blood glucose level higher than 3.5 to 4.0 mmol/L (60 to 70 mg/dL), a urine lactate/creatinine ratio lower than 0.06 mmol/mmol, a serum uric acid concentration in the high normal range for age, a venous blood bicarbonate level above 20 mmol/L (20 mEq/L), a serum triglyceride concentration below 6.0 mmol/L (531 mg/dL), normal fecal alpha$_1$-antitrypsin concentration for GSD-Ib, and a body mass index within two standard deviations of normal. Enzyme replacement therapy is not currently available for GSD-I. Kidney transplantation has been successfully performed but does not correct the hypoglycemia.

TYROSINEMIA

Hepatorenal tyrosinemia (tyrosinemia type I) is a rare autosomal recessive disorder caused by deficiency of fumarylacetoacetate hydrolase (FAH).[72] Worldwide, the incidence is 1 in 100,000. The disorder is characterized by severe liver disease, which either causes liver failure in infancy or may take a more protracted course, with death often occurring during childhood or adolescence because of hepatocarcinoma.[73] The accumulation of tyrosine in body fluids and tissues affects principally the liver, kidneys, and peripheral nerves. The disorder is particularly prevalent in a genetic isolate in Canada (Saguenay-Lac-Saint-Jean), in which the carrier rate is 1 in 20 and the incidence is 1 in 2000, and in which nearly 80% of the gene pool comes from founders who settled in the seventeenth century.[74]

PATHOGNESIS

Mutations in the gene encoding FAH on chromosome 15q23-q25 are responsible for tyrosinemia type I.[75-79] The hepatic toxicity is caused by accumulation of fumarylacetoacetate, which apparently induces the release of cytochrome c, which in turn triggers the activation of the caspase cascade in hepatocytes as seen in affected animal models.[80] It is unlikely that tyrosine accumulation leads to the hepatic and renal manifestations of the disease, because hypertyrosinemia has been described in other settings without renal and liver involvement.

CLINICAL PRESENTATION

Most patients present clinically in regions without a specific newborn screening program for tyrosinemia type 1, although a few may be identified because of affected siblings or abnormalities of plasma or urine amino acids. Renal involvement is almost always present in tyrosinemic subjects and is probably caused by succinylacetone toxicity.[81,82] It ranges from mild tubular dysfunction to renal failure. Hypophosphatemic rickets is the principal sign of tubular dysfunction, and acute decompensation can exacerbate the dysfunction. Generalized aminoaciduria is frequent. Nephrocalcinosis and nephromegaly can often be seen on renal ultrasonography.[83] Glucosuria and proteinuria are usually mild. Glomerular filtration rate is frequently decreased. Tubular defects respond to diet but may be irreversible in chronic cases.

The liver is the main organ affected in tyrosinemia type I. Initially, liver dysfunction often affects coagulation factors, even before other signs of liver failure appear. In fact, jaundice and liver enzyme elevations are rare in the early stages of tyrosinemia. A common presentation mode is the "acute hepatic crisis," in which ascites, jaundice, and gastrointestinal bleeding are precipitated by an acute event such as an infection. Acute hepatic crises usually resolve spontaneously but on occasion progress to complete liver failure and encephalopathy. Cirrhosis eventually develops in most patients with the disease, and hepatocellular carcinoma is frequent in tyrosinemic subjects with chronic liver disease.[84] It is believed that toxic metabolites that accumulate in tyrosinemia, such as fumarylacetoacetate, are mutagenic and contribute to the elevated rate of liver carcinoma.[85] Serial liver imaging (ultrasonography and/or MRI) is indicated. Neurologic crises are acute episodes of peripheral neuropathy with painful paresthesias and, eventually, autonomic dysfunction.[86]

The diagnosis of tyrosinemia type I is made with the detection of excess succinylacetone in urine or plasma. Succinylacetone can be detected in the biologic fluid of all untreated patients with the disorder. The increase in succinylacetone is typically detected by gas chromatography/mass spectroscopy of extracted organic acids. Confirmatory testing can be performed with the measurement of FAH in cultured skin fibroblasts or the documentation of pathogenic mutations from DNA. Enzymatic analysis of FAH is not readily available as a common clinical assay, and only a few laboratories perform DNA mutation analysis of the *FAH* gene. Molecular genetic studies may be needed for counselling, prenatal diagnosis, and family screening. One splice mutation is prevalent in French-Canadians, and more than 40 mutations are now known (reviewed by de Laet et el[73]).

TREATMENT

Since 1992, nitisinone has been used in tyrosinemia.[87] It is an effective inhibitor of *p*-hydroxyphenylpyruvic acid oxidase that blocks an enzyme proximal in the catabolic pathway of tyrosine and prevents substrate from reaching the FAH enzyme. Thus, the intracellular accumulation of the toxic fumarylacetoacetate (FAA) and its eventual extracellular conversion to succinylacetone are prevented. A nutritionist skilled in metabolic disorders is essential to assist with the use of special formulas for infants and low-protein diet for older patients. At least 90% of patients with the acute form of tyrosinemia type I show response to nitisinone therapy. It is the unusual child in whom liver damage is so severe that insufficient hepatocytes exist to allow clinical recovery. Such a child requires liver transplantation. Orthotopic liver transplantation has been used for several years in tyrosinemia type I but carries a significant mortality rate (10% to 20%).

The decision to perform liver transplantation depends on the patient's liver status and neurologic symptoms.[73] The renal dysfunction may persist following transplantation because the renal enzyme is still defective.[88]

GALACTOSEMIA

Galactosemia is an inherited metabolic disorder in which the individual is unable to metabolize lactose.[89,90] Three inherited disorders of galactose metabolism resulting in galactosemia have been described and are transmitted by an autosomal recessive mode. Clinical manifestations appear after exposure to galactose and can produce failure to thrive, vomiting, inanition, liver disease, cataracts, and developmental delays.

PATHOGNESIS

The genetic defect responsible for galactosemia may be a defect in galactose-1-phosphate uridyltransferase, galactokinase, or uridine diphosphate galactose-4-epimerase. All of these enzymes catalyze the reactions in the unique pathway converting galactose to glucose. *Classic galactosemia* (OMIM #230400), which affects approximately 1 in 30,000 to 60,000 live births, is the most frequent form. The underlying basis of most pathophysiology in galactosemia remains poorly understood. Untreated and treated patients with galactosemia experience abnormal accumulation and/or depletion of specific metabolites. Specific abnormalities of glycosylation can also be demonstrated, suggesting that aberrant biosynthesis of glycoproteins and/or glycolipids may contribute not only to the acute but also to some of the long-term complications experienced by galactosemic patients.[90,91]

CLINICAL PRESENTATION

The clinical manifestations of galactosemia range from cataracts caused by galactokinase deficiency to important toxicity syndromes resulting from galactose exposure in deficiencies of galactose-1-phosphate uridyltransferase and uridine diphosphate galactose-4-epimerase. Vomiting, diarrhea, jaundice, hepatomegaly, and ascites occur in transferase deficiency. Tubular proteinuria, generalized aminoaciduria, and bicarbonaturia occur but may quickly disappear following withdrawal of galactose.

The diagnosis is suggested by elevation of galactose or galactose-1-phosphate in serum or of galactose in the urine. The definitive diagnosis is made by the demonstration of the enzyme deficiency in erythrocytes.[92,93] Prenatal diagnosis can be offered to parents with a family history of the disease.[94]

In the United States and many other industrialized nations, inclusion of galactosemia in the mandated panel of conditions tested during newborn screening has all but eliminated the acute presentation.

TREATMENT

With early diagnosis and simple dietary intervention, galactosemia is no longer a lethal condition. The only therapy for patients with classical galactosemia is a galactose-restricted diet, and initially all galactose must be removed from the diet as soon as the diagnosis is suspected.[93,95] A newborn with a positive screening result should immediately be started on a soy-based infant formula. In spite of the strict diet, long-term complications such as retarded mental development, verbal dyspraxia, motor abnormalities, and hypergonadotrophic hypogonadism are frequently seen in patients with classic galactosemia.

WILSON'S DISEASE

Wilson's disease (OMIM #277900) is an autosomal recessive disorder in which biliary excretion of copper and its incorporation into ceruloplasmin are impaired, leading to liver, kidney, and corneal damage from accumulation of copper.[96] The frequency of the disease is approximately 1 to 3 per 100,000 live births.

PATHOGNESIS

ATP7B, the gene responsible for Wilson's disease, encodes a P-type ATPase, and is located on chromosome 13q14.3. This copper-transporting P-type ATPase (the WND protein) has a crucial role in copper excretion into the bile[97-99] and is targeted to the mitochondria. These findings suggest that WND protein plays its role in copper-dependent processes in this organelle.[100] More than 380 mutations in this gene have been identified in patients with Wilson's disease worldwide.

CLINICAL PRESENTATION

The primary consequence is liver disease for approximately 40% of patients with Wilson's disease. Affected adults often show most features of Fanconi's syndrome, with aminoaciduria, bicarbonaturia, phosphaturia, glucosuria, and low-molecular-weight proteinuria,[101] probably from copper accumulation. Children do not frequently have renal manifestations. Hypercalciuria is frequent, and kidney stones and nephrocalcinosis have been described in several cases.[102-104] Ultrastructural findings on renal biopsies include electron-dense deposits in the tubular cytoplasm.[105]

Most patients with Wilson's disease present with liver dysfunction, neurologic symptoms, or a combination of the two. Liver symptoms can take multiple forms, that is, chronic and acute liver failure. Copper accumulates in the liver, with progressive damage, and overflow to the brain. This causes central nervous system anomalies such as dysarthria and coordination defects of voluntary movements. Pseudobulbar palsy is frequent and is a common cause of death in undiagnosed cases. Psychiatric symptoms can encompass a spectrum of personality changes, depression, bipolar disorder, schizophrenia, and dementia.[106] Wilson's disease should be suspected in all subjects with acute or chronic liver dysfunction. The most useful laboratory tests for diagnostic purposes are those measuring 24-hour urinary copper excretion, hepatic copper concentration, serum-free copper concentration, and ceruloplasmin concentration. Increased liver copper level (>300 mg/g dry weight) is a reliable finding. The Kayser-Fleischer ring is an important clinical sign for making the diagnosis; it is seen in 50% of patients with liver dysfunction and in 90% of those with neurologic disease.[107] This ring is a yellow-brown (dull copper colored) granular deposit on Descemet's membrane at the limbus of the cornea, usually seen earliest at the upper and lower poles. Given the variability of the biochemical and clinical features of Wilson's disease, mutation analysis is becoming more and more essential to confirm a suspicion of the disorder.[96] Molecular genetic diagnosis is available.[108] The lack of genotype-phenotype correlation remains unexplained, the causes of fulminant liver failure are not known, and the treatment of neurologic symptoms is only partially successful.[109]

TREATMENT

D-Penicillamine, which mobilizes copper and forms copper-penicillamine complexes that are excreted in the urine, is very effective.[110] Adults usually require 1 g/day divided in two doses, but it is best to start with small doses (125 mg/day) to avoid hypersensitivity reactions. Twenty-four hour urinary excretion of copper should be monitored to achieve copper losses of 2 mg/day. Doses of D-penicillamine can be decreased after 1 or 2 years to achieve urinary losses of 1 mg/day. Alternative treatments include trientine, a copper chelator, and zinc salts, which block intestinal copper absorption by inducing metallothionein synthesis in the mucosal intestinal cells. Tetrathiomolybdate, a copper chelator, appears to be an excellent form of initial treatment in patients with neurologic symptoms and signs. In contrast to penicillamine therapy, initial treatment with tetrathiomolybdate can often be effective in preventing further neurologic deterioration.[111]

Patients should be considered for liver transplantation when suitable medical therapy has failed or for the development of acute liver failure, when there is no time for other therapies to take effect. Patients with a combination of hepatic and neuropsychiatric conditions warrant careful neurologic assessment, but liver transplantation is contraindicated only in cases of severe neurologic impairment.[96]

HEREDITARY FRUCTOSE INTOLERANCE

There are several disorders of fructose metabolism, secondary to deficiencies in aldolase B (OMIM #229600), fructose 1-phosphate aldolase, and fructokinase, respectively.[112] Hereditary fructose intolerance due to fructose 1-phosphate aldolase deficiency (fructose 1,6-bisphosphate aldolase [EC 4.1.2.13]) is an autosomal recessive disorder characterized by vomiting shortly after the intake of fructose. The disease can be associated with proximal tubule dysfunction and lactic acidosis. Kidney biopsies show discrete findings. Liver dysfunction, hepatomegaly, cirrhosis, and jaundice appear from prolonged exposure. Unfortunately, hypoglycemia is frequently absent. Continued ingestion of noxious sugars leads to hepatic and renal injury and growth retardation. The most common mutation has a prevalence of 1.3%, suggesting a frequency of 1 in 23,000 homozygotes.[113] Because of the difficulty in making the diagnosis, genetic analysis is useful.[114]

The pathophysiology of renal Fanconi's syndrome is not clear but could be related to vacuolar proton pump dysfunction in the proximal tubule, because a direct binding interaction between V-ATPase and aldolase was demonstrated for the regulation of the V-ATPase. This study showed that aldolase B was abundant in endocytosis zones of the proximal tubule, a subcellular domain also abundant in V-ATPase.[115] V-ATPases are essential for acidification of intracellular compartments and for proton secretion from the plasma membrane in kidney epithelial cells and osteoclasts. Perhaps the release of nonfunctional aldolase B in response to fructose ingestion impairs the coupling of the V-ATPase to glycolysis. For these reasons, mechanistic similarities in organelle dysfunction between Dent's disease and hereditary fructose intolerance are apparent.

The management of hereditary fructose intolerance involves withdrawal of sucrose, fructose, and sorbitol from the diet.

INHERITED DISORDERS OF RENAL AMINO ACID TRANSPORT

Proteins ingested in the regular diet and degraded in the intestine are absorbed by the mucosa as amino acids and small oligopeptides. Intestinal apical and basolateral transporters carry the amino acids into the blood, where they are used for metabolic needs, but are also freely filtered by the kidneys as they are not significantly bound to proteins in the plasma (except for tryptophan, which is 60% to 90% bound). However, the proximal tubule reabsorbs 95% to 99.9% of the filtered load. Thus the excretion of more than 5% of the filtered load of an amino acid is abnormal. Renal amino acid reabsorption occurs in the proximal tubule through a variety of transporters. Most amino acids are reabsorbed by more than one transporter and almost completely reclaimed, except for histidine, which has a fractional excretion of 5%.[116] Amino acids can share transporters with low affinity but high transport capacity, and have a specific transporter for one amino acid that has a high affinity and low maximal transport capacity. Because most amino acid carriers have not been extensively studied, a more detailed discussion is not possible at this stage. Common carriers have been divided into five groups, which transport neutral and cyclic amino acids, glycine and imino acids, cystine and dibasic amino acids, dicarboxylic amino acids, and β-amino acids.[116] The transport of amino acids is coupled to the sodium gradient established by the basolateral Na^+-K^+-ATPase.

Aminoaciduria occurs when a renal transport defect of the proximal tubule decreases the reabsorptive capacity for one or several amino acids or when the threshold for reabsorbing an amino acid is exceeded when its plasma concentration is elevated as a result of a metabolic defect ("overflow aminoaciduria").[117] This latter category is not discussed in this section. Theoretically, renal aminoacidurias can be secondary to defects in brush border or basolateral transporters and intracellular trafficking of amino acids. They are usually detected by newborn urine screening programs, and the most frequent abnormalities identified (apart from phenylketonuria, now normally detected by blood screening) are cystinuria, histidinemia, Hartnup's disease, and iminoglycinuria (Figure 45.5).[118] Clinically, the most significant renal aminoaciduria is cystinuria (Table 45.4). In the past 10 years, all major apical neutral amino acid transporters have been identified on a molecular level.[119] This has considerably improved our understanding of rare inherited aminoacidurias and helped explain some of the features of Fanconi's syndrome.

CYSTINURIA

Cystinuria (OMIM #220200) is the most frequent and best known of the aminoacidurias.[120] The existence of cystinuria

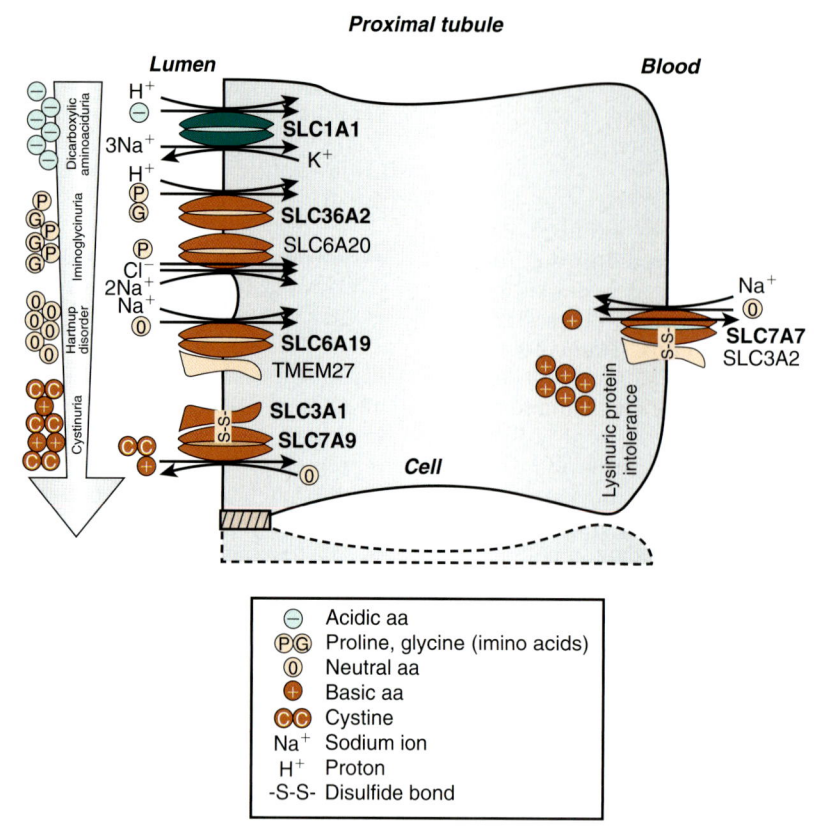

Figure 45.5 A model of the renal proximal tubule, illustrating the principal epithelial transporters involved in amino acid reabsorption, which are mutated in human aminoacidurias. A crosssection of the proximal convoluted tubule is represented. Four of the aminoacidurias—dicarboxylic aminoaciduria (DA), iminoglycinuria, Hartnup disorder, and cystinuria—manifest at the apical surface of the renal tubule, whereas lysinuric protein intolerance manifests at the basolateral surface. Mutations in the high-affinity glutamate and aspartate transporter SLC1A1 are responsible for DA.[166] Iminoglycinuria results from complete inactivation of SLC36A2, a proline and glycine transporter, or from additional modifying mutations in the high-affinity proline transporter SLC6A20 when SLC36A2 is not completely inactivated.[182] Mutations in the neutral amino acid transporter SLC6A19 are responsible for Hartnup disorder.[163,377] The neutral amino acid transport defect can also be exacerbated by a kidney-specific loss of heterodimerization of mutant SLC6A19 with TMEM27.[378] Cystinuria has a heterogeneous phenotype and arises from mutations in individual or both subunits of the disulfide bridge–linked heterodimer comprising the type II membrane protein SLC3A1[379] and the cystine and basic amino acid transporter SLC7A9.[380] Lysinuric protein intolerance[151,154] results from mutations in the basolaterally expressed basic amino acid transporter SLC7A7, which forms a disulfide bridge–linked heterodimer with type II membrane protein SLC3A2. aa, Amino acid. (Adapted from Bailey CG, Ryan RM, Thoeng AD, et al: Loss-of-function mutations in the glutamate transporter SLC1A1 cause human dicarboxylic aminoaciduria. J Clin Invest 121:446-453, 2011.)

has been recognized since 1810,[121,122] first suspected in two patients with bladder stones, hence the name—cystic oxide and cystine to characterize the chemical composition of the stones. It is an autosomal recessive disorder associated with defective transport of cystine and of the dibasic amino acids ornithine, lysine, and arginine. It involves the epithelial cells of the renal tubule and gastrointestinal tract (see Figure 45.5). The formation of cystine calculi in the urinary tract, potentially leading to infection and renal failure, is the hallmark of the disorder. Cystine is the least soluble of the naturally occurring amino acids, particularly at low pH. Worldwide, the prevalence of cystinuria is approximately 1 in 7000 and varies according to geographic location, being 1 in 15,000 in the United States,[123] 1 in 2000 in England,[124] 1 in 4000 in Australia,[125] and 1 in 2500 in Jews of Libyan origin.[126] Thus, it is one of the most common mendelian disorders. Newborn screening programs worldwide now help identify cases.

PATHOGNESIS

Cystinuria is caused by mutations in the genes that encode the two subunits—neutral and basic amino acid transport protein rBAT and $b^{(0,+)}$-type amino acid transporter 1—of the amino acid transport system $b^{(0,+)}$.[120] By itself, the subunit $b^{0,+}$AT is sufficient to catalyze transmembrane amino acid exchange (i.e., the exchange of dibasic amino acids for neutral amino acids).[127] A model for the reabsorption of cystine and dibasic amino acids is shown in Figure 45.6. Cystinuria also manifests as defective intestinal absorption of dibasic amino acids, implying that there is a transporter defect in the gut similar to that in the renal proximal tubule cells.[120] Why defective intestinal amino acid transport does not lead to more serious metabolic problems is not known, but the reason could be either the ability of the intestine to absorb small (di- and tri-) peptides or the presence of other transporters of dibasic amino acids in the gut.

Table 45.4 Classification of the Aminoacidurias

Aminoaciduria	Gene	Gene Name	Protein	Chromosome	Hallmark (Amino Acid[s] Elevated in Urine)
Cystinuria A	SLC3A1	Solute carrier family 3 (cystine, dibasic, and neutral amino acid transporters, activator of cystine, dibasic, and neutral amino acid transport), member 1	rBAT	2p21	Cystine, lysine, arginine, ornithine
Cystinuria B	SLC7A9	Solute carrier family 7 (cationic amino acid transporter, y$^+$ system), member 9	b$^{0,+}$AT	19q13.11	Cystine, lysine, arginine, ornithine
Cystinuria AB	SLC3A1/SLC7A9				Cystine, lysine, arginine, ornithine
Lysinuric protein intolerance	SLC7A7	Solute carrier family 7 (cationic amino acid transporter, y$^+$ system), member 7	y$^+$LAT1	14q11.2	Lysine, arginine, ornithine
Hartnup's disorder	SLC6A19	Solute carrier family 6 (neutral amino acid transporter), member 19	B^{0}AT1	5p15.33	Neutral amino acids
Iminoglycinuria	SLC36A2	Solute carrier family 36 (imino and glycine transporter), member 2	PAT2	5q33.1	Proline, hydroxyproline, glycine
Dicarboxylic aminoaciduria	SLC1A1	Solute carrier family 1	EAAT$_3$	9p24	Aspartate, glutamate

Adapted from Tanzi RE, Petrukhin K, Chernov I, et al: The Wilson disease gene is a copper transporting ATPase with homology to the Menkes disease gene. Nat Genet 5:344-350, 1993.

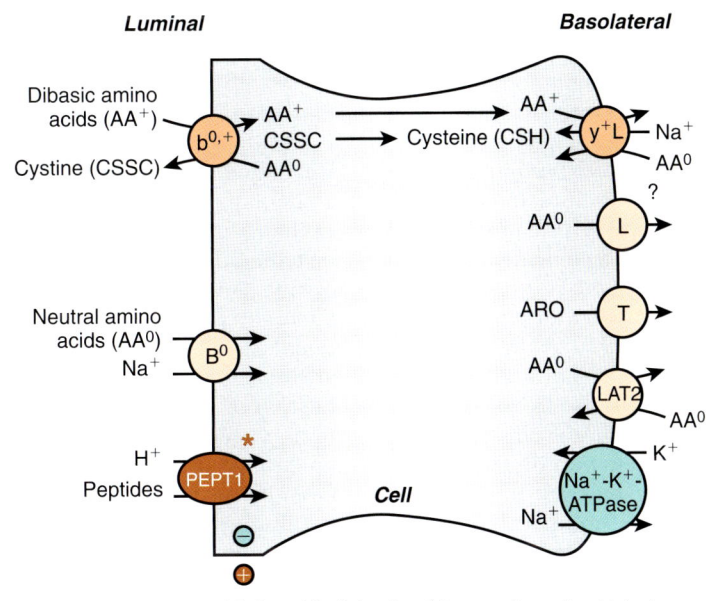

Figure 45.6 Trafficking of cystine and dibasic amino acids in epithelial cells of the renal proximal tubule or small intestine. The apical transport system b$^{0,+}$ mediates influx of AA$^+$ and CSSC in exchange for AA^0. The Na$^+$-dependent transporter B^0 is believed to be the major apical contributor to the high intracellular content of AA^0 exploited by b$^{0,+}$. In the small intestine (but not in kidney), uptake of dipeptides and tripeptides through apical H$^+$-dependent solute carrier family 15 member 1 (PEPT1) compensates the defective absorption of AA$^+$ and CSSC. AA$^+$ exit the basolateral membrane through system y$^+$L, mutations in which cause lysinuric protein intolerance. The basolateral efflux of CSH and AA^0 are not well understood. The general AA^0 exchanger LAT2 and the aromatic transporter T have been suggested to participate in the excretion of CSH and aromatic amino acids (ARO). In addition, an unidentified transporter L for unidirectional efflux of AA^0 is believed to have a role in AA^0 reabsorption. *Only in intestinal cells. (Redrawn from Chillaron J, Font-Llitjos M, Fort J, et al: Pathophysiology and treatment of cystinuria. Nat Rev Nephrol. 6:424-434, 2010.)

CLINICAL PRESENTATION

Cystinuria is classified according to the gene responsible, but this classification currently has no clinical utility. It may prove to be important if gene or pharmacologic therapy becomes more targeted. Type A cystinuria (also called type I; OMIM #220100) is caused by mutations in the *SLC3A1* gene (chromosome 2). It is a completely recessive disease because both parents excrete normal amounts of cystine (0 to 100 mmol per g creatinine). Jejunal uptake of cystine and dibasic amino acids is absent, and there is no plasma response to an oral cystine load. The risk of nephrolithiasis is very high. The *SLC3A1* gene encodes the renal proximal tubule S3 segment and intestinal dibasic rBAT amino acid transporter (see Figure 45.6).[128] More than 100 different mutations have been reported to date.[120] The most common point mutation, the M467T and its relative M467K, result in retention of the transporter in the ER with impaired maturation and export to the plasma membrane.[129]

Type B cystinuria (also called non–type I cystinuria; OMIM #600918) is an incompletely recessive form caused by mutations in the *SLC7A9* gene encoding BAT1 and located on chromosome 19q13. Both parents excrete intermediate amounts of cystine (100 to 600 mmol per g creatinine) but may also have a normal pattern. More than 90 mutations have been identified.[120] BAT1 is a subunit linked to the rBAT through a disulfide bond. It belongs to a family of light subunits of amino acid transporters, expressed in the kidney, liver, small intestine, and placenta. Cotransfection of $b^{0,+}AT$ and rBAT brings the latter to the plasma membrane, and results in the uptake of L-arginine in vitro.

Type AB cystinuria is caused by one mutation in *SLC3A1* and one mutation in *SLC7A9*, but this digenic inheritance is exceptional. The observed prevalence of patients with AB cystinuria is much lower than anticipated, because they may present with a mild phenotype and therefore, in most cases, escape detection or, alternatively, carry two mutations in *SLC7A9* (which was not detected) and a coincidental carrier state for an *SLC3A1* mutation.[130]

The only known manifestation of cystinuria is nephrolithiasis. Cystine stones account for 1% to 2% of all kidney stones, and cystinuria should be suspected in all staghorn calculi.[131] Clinical expression of the disease frequently starts during the first to third decade of life but may occur any time from the first year of life up to the ninth decade. The disease occurs equally in both sexes, but male patients tend to be more severely affected. Cystine stones are made of a yellow-brown substance, are very hard, and appear radiopaque on radiographs because of their sulfur molecules. Stones are frequently multiple and staghorn, and they tend to be smoother than calcium stones. Magnesium ammonium phosphate and calcium stones can also form as a result of infection.

Diagnosis can be made through the analysis of a simple urine sample in which typical hexagonal crystals appear. Acidification of concentrated urine with acetic acid can also precipitate crystals not initially visible. Diagnosis is ultimately made from the measurement of cystine excretion in the urine. This measurement is usually performed in specialized centers using a variety of methods. Molecular diagnosis is not necessary.

TREATMENT

Unfortunately, there have been few advances in the treatment of cystinuria. A regularly followed medical program based on high diuresis and alkalinization with a second-line addition of thiols slows down stone formation and precludes the need for urologic procedures in more than half of patients.[132] Patients who are poorly compliant with hyperdiuresis remain at risk for recurrence.

Diet

Cystine production arises from the metabolism of methionine. Previous attempts at reducing methionine in the diet have been both uncomfortable and of limited usefulness.[133,134] Reducing sodium in the diet results in lower urine cystine.[135-137]

Decreasing Urine Cystine Saturation

A combination of increasing both fluid intake and urine pH usually decreases urine cystine saturation. Fluid intake should ideally reach 4 L/day, because many cystinuric patients excrete 1 g/day or more of cystine. A daily urine output of at least 3 L seems necessary.[132] It is also important for patients to drink at bedtime and during sleep (using an alarm clock helps) to prevent supersaturation during periods of reduced urine output.[138] Cystine solubility can be increased by alkalinization of the urine with potassium citrate or bicarbonate, but the solubility of cystine does not increase until the pH reaches 7.0 to 7.5. Use of citrate is the preferred method because alkalinization lasts longer. The requirements for alkali often reach 3 to 4 mmol/kg/day.

Penicillamine

Patients who are unable to comply with a regimen of high fluid intake and urine alkalinization or in whom adequate treatment fails may be given D-penicillamine in doses of 30 mg/kg/day up to a maximum of 2 g. Through a disulfide exchange reaction, D-penicillamine can form the disulfide cysteine-penicillamine, which is much more soluble than cystine. Several studies have reported that D-penicillamine is generally well tolerated in cystinuric patients,[139,140] but frequent side effects such as rash, fever, and, more rarely, arthralgias and medullary aplasia have led a significant proportion of patients to discontinue therapy.[141,142] Other reactions include proteinuria and membranous nephropathy, epidermolysis, and loss of taste. Inhibition of pyridoxine by D-penicillamine is also a potential side effect.[143]

Another drug that may be useful in cystinuria is mercaptopropionylglycine, with recommended dosing ranges of 400-1200mg per day in 3 divided doses.[144,145] Identical in mechanism of action to D-penicillamine, mercaptopropionylglycine is as effective in reducing urine cystine excretion. Side effects are similar and include skin rash, fever, nausea, proteinuria, and membranous nephropathy. Finally, captopril has been advocated as a potential treatment for cystinuria, but its efficacy is controversial.

Surgical Management

Patients with cystinuria frequently require stone-removing procedures.[146] It is important to achieve a stone-free state because recurrent stone activity has been demonstrated to be higher in those with residual calculi.[147] The type of procedure does not impact recurrence rates. The introduction of extracorporeal shock wave lithotripsy has not been of great benefit to cystinuric patients. Cystine stones are hard and have proved difficult to pulverize. Consequently, percutaneous lithotripsy is more effective and is the preferred approach. Progress in urologic treatment of kidney stones has decreased the need for open surgery.[148] Urinary alkalinization, as well as direct irrigation of the urinary tract with D-penicillamine, N-acetylpenicillamine, or tromethamine to form disulfide compounds, has resulted in the dissolution of stones, but this approach requires irrigation for several weeks with a risk for potential complications of catheterization and has been largely abandoned.

Transplantation is sometimes necessary for patients with terminal renal failure from chronic obstruction or infection (or both). A kidney from an unaffected donor will not form cystine stones once transplanted.

LYSINURIC PROTEIN INTOLERANCE

PATHOGNESIS

Lysinuric protein intolerance (LPI) (OMIM #222700) is a very rare recessively inherited dibasic amino acid transport disorder, mostly reported in Finland[149,150] but also present in Japan and Italy. It is caused by defective basolateral membrane efflux of the cationic amino acids lysine, arginine, and ornithine in intestinal, hepatic, and renal tubular epithelia. Inactivating mutations in *SLC7A7* have been found in several families with LPI.[151-153] *SLC7A7* encodes a 511–amino acid protein, y$^+$LAT-1, predicted to harbor 12 membrane-spanning domains, with both amino and carboxy termini located intracellularly. This protein is thought to be part of the y$^+$L multimeric unit. Cationic amino acid transport occurs through five different systems: y$^+$, y$^+$L, b$^+$, b^{0+}, and B^{0+}. Defective system y$^+$L transport explains the abnormality in cationic amino acid transport as it mediates sodium-independent high-affinity transport of cationic amino acids and the transport of zwitterionic amino acids with low affinity. It is responsible for renal reabsorption and intestinal absorption of dibasic amino acids at the basolateral membranes. y$^+$L transport is induced by a cell surface glycoprotein heavy chain (4F2hc) that represents the heavy-chain subunit of a disulfide-linked heterodimer.[149] The amino acid deficiency in LPI leads to impaired urea cycle and postprandial hyperammonemia.

CLINICAL PRESENTATION

Infants with LPI are usually asymptomatic while breast feeding. After weaning, they show protein aversion, a delay in bone growth, and prominent osteoporosis, hepatosplenomegaly, muscle hypotonia, and sparse hair. Jaundice, hyperammonemia, coma, and metabolic acidosis occur. Micronodular cirrhosis occurs from protein malnutrition, and pulmonary alveolar proteinosis is an occasional finding.[154] Various renal disorders, including immunoglobulin A (IgA) nephropathy have been described.[155] Several immunologic abnormalities have also been described[156] and are possibly secondary to low levels of arginine, the substrate for nitric oxide synthase and nitric oxide production.[157] The urinary excretion of lysine and all cationic amino acids is increased, and the plasma levels are decreased. The biochemical diagnosis can be uncertain, requiring confirmation by DNA testing. So far, approximately 50 different mutations have been identified in the *SLC7A7* gene.[158]

TREATMENT

The current treatment of lysinuric protein intolerance involves moderate protein restriction as well as supplementation with 3 to 8 g of citrulline daily during meals and lysine.[159] Citrulline is transported by a different pathway from that of dibasic amino acids and can be converted to ornithine and arginine in the liver. Lysine cannot be made from citrulline.

HARTNUP'S DISORDER

PATHOGNESIS

Described initially in 1956 in the Hartnup family, Hartnup's disorder (OMIM #234500) is an autosomal recessive and usually benign condition, consisting of excessive urinary excretion of the monoamino, monocarboxylic (neutral) amino acids alanine, asparagine, glutamine, histidine, isoleucine, leucine, methionine, phenylalanine, serine, threonine, tryptophan, tyrosine, and valine.[160] Its incidence has been estimated at 1 in 26,000 in newborn screening programs.[161] Hartnup's disorder is caused by mutations in the neutral amino acid transporter B^{0}AT1 (*SLC6A19*).[162] The transporter is found in the kidney and intestine, where it is involved in the resorption of all neutral amino acids.[119]

CLINICAL PRESENTATION

Most newborns identified prospectively by genetic screening programs as having Hartnup's disorder have been completely asymptomatic. In affected individuals there is also a decreased intestinal absorption of neutral amino acids, particularly tryptophan. The clinical features of this disorder, if any, are caused by deficiency of nicotinamide, which is partly derived from tryptophan. They include a photosensitive erythematous rash (pellagra-like) clinically identical with that seen in niacin deficiency, intermittent cerebellar ataxia, and, rarely, mental retardation. Emotional instability, psychosis, and depression have been rarely noted, particularly during episodes of ataxia. Although in the Hartnup family there were several cases with mental retardation, most affected subjects described subsequently have not had mental retardation. Hartnup's disorder should be suspected in all subjects with pellagra and unexplained intermittent ataxia. Siblings of affected patients should be screened as well. Clinical manifestations can be triggered by periods of inadequate dietary intake or increased metabolic needs. For example, a young woman presenting with pellagra precipitated by prolonged lactation and increased activity was diagnosed with Hartnup's disorder.[163]

The diagnosis is easily made with a urinary aminogram, which shows increased excretion of neutral amino acids but not of glycine, cystine, or dibasic, dicarboxylic, or imino amino acids. Thus, any confusion with renal Fanconi's syndrome is avoided through a complete evaluation of amino acids in the urine using one of several chromatographic methods. The pattern of amino acid excretion, rather than the total amount, is the determining factor. The reabsorption defect involves 12 amino acids, and most patients with Hartnup's disorder have the same pattern of aminoaciduria.

The levels of amino acids in the monoamino, dicarboxylic group (such as glutamic acid and aspartic acid), and basic group (lysine, ornithine, arginine) are normal or slightly increased. The excretion of proline, hydroxyproline, and cystine is also normal. In spite of the defect, substantial reabsorption of the involved amino acids occurs through other transporters.

TREATMENT

Treatment of symptomatic cases involves the administration of nicotinamide in doses of 50 to 300 mg/day. The value of treating asymptomatic cases is not known, but given the harmlessness of the treatment, this might be a rational choice.

IMINOGLYCINURIA

Familial iminoglycinuria (OMIM #242600) is a benign autosomal recessive disorder with no clinical symptoms, in which our main interest is that it suggests the presence of a common carrier for the imino acids, proline and hydroxyproline, as well as glycine.[164] Iminoglycinuria was discovered after the application of chromatographic methods to the investigation of disorders of amino acid metabolism. *SLC36A2*, the gene encoding proton amino acid transporter 2 (PAT2) has been identified as the major gene responsible for iminoglycinuria.[165] Mutations in *SLC36A2* that retain residual transport activity result in the iminoglycinuria phenotype when combined with mutations in the gene encoding the imino acid transporter *SLC6A20*. Additional mutations have been identified in the genes encoding the putative glycine transporter SLC6A18 (XT2) and the neutral amino acid transporter SLC6A19 (B⁰AT1) in families with either iminoglycinuria or hyperglycinuria, suggesting that mutations in the genes encoding these transporters may also contribute to these phenotypes.

The diagnosis is usually suggested by increased urinary excretion of imino acids and glycine. Newborns and infants usually excrete detectable amounts of imino acids and glycine for up to 3 months. Thus, the presence of increased urinary excretion of imino acids and glycine in infants older than 6 months can be considered abnormal.

DICARBOXYLIC AMINOACIDURIA

Dicarboxylic aminoaciduria (OMIM #222730) is an autosomal recessive disorder with, in a limited number of cases, an association with mental retardation. It is secondary to loss-of-function mutations in the glutamate transporter SLC1A1, a high-affinity anionic amino acid transporter expressed in the kidney and a wide variety of epithelial tissues, the brain, and the eye.[166]

INHERITED DISORDERS OF RENAL PHOSPHATE TRANSPORT

Inherited disorders of renal phosphate transport are hypophosphatemic conditions caused by a reduction in renal tubule reabsorption of phosphate[167] with frequent metabolic bone disease manifesting as rickets in childhood and osteomalacia in adults.

RENAL PHOSPHATE EXCRETION

Determinants of inorganic phosphate (Pi) homeostasis are ingestion, intestinal absorption, and renal excretion. In a steady state, urine Pi excretion reflects dietary intake. Normal phosphate intake in adults varies from 800 to 1600 mg/day, and average serum phosphate levels remain normal over a wide range of intake. Unlike dietary calcium, ingested phosphate is generally efficiently absorbed (65% to 90% in children) from the gastrointestinal tract, although complex plant phosphate (phytate) is almost totally excreted. Most dietary phosphate is absorbed by passive concentration-dependent processes, but the active metabolite of vitamin D increases intestinal Pi absorption marginally. Contrary to active calcium absorption, which is greatest in the duodenum with a lower rate in the jejunum, ileum, and colon, active Pi absorption is highest in the jejunum and ileum with a lower rate in the duodenum and colon.[168]

Inorganic phosphate is filtered by the glomerulus and reabsorbed in the proximal tubule. The difference between the amounts of Pi filtered and reabsorbed determines the net appearance of Pi in the urine. Phosphate reabsorption by the proximal tubule occurs by a Tm-limited active process. The fractional reabsorption of filtered phosphate is usually estimated by the tubular reabsorption of Pi (TRP). There is a simple equation to assess the renal tubular phosphate transport, as follows:

$$TRP = \frac{(1 - U_P \times P_{Cr})}{U_{Cr} \times P_P}$$

where P_{Cr} is plasma creatinine concentration, P_P is plasma phosphate concentration, U_{Cr} is urine creatinine concentration, and U_P is urine phosphate concentration. Given normal renal function and normal diet, the TRP is usually above 85%. A more precise way of estimating the tubular reabsorption of Pi is to calculate the theoretical threshold, as follows:

$$\frac{Tm_P}{GFR} = P_P - \frac{(U_P \times P_{Cr})}{U_{Cr}}$$

RENAL PHOSPHATE TRANSPORTERS

Inorganic phosphate is reabsorbed almost exclusively in the renal proximal tubule through a transcellular pathway.[169] The limiting step of this transepithelial transport system is the entry of phosphate at the apical domain of proximal tubular cells. This process requires sodium-phosphate cotransporters that use the inward sodium gradient established and maintained by the activity of Na⁺-K⁺-ATPase (Figure 45.7). There are three types of sodium-phosphate cotransporters (members of the SLC34 and SLC20 families) at the apical (brush border) renal proximal tubular cells.[169] The putative proteins responsible for basolateral P_i flux have not been identified. The transport mechanism of the two kidney-specific SLC34 proteins (NaPi-IIa and NaPi-IIc) and of the ubiquitously expressed SLC20 protein (PiT-2) has been studied by heterologous expression to reveal important differences in kinetics, stoichiometry, and substrate specificity. NaPi-IIa is central to renal phosphate reabsorption and phosphate balance. It is found almost

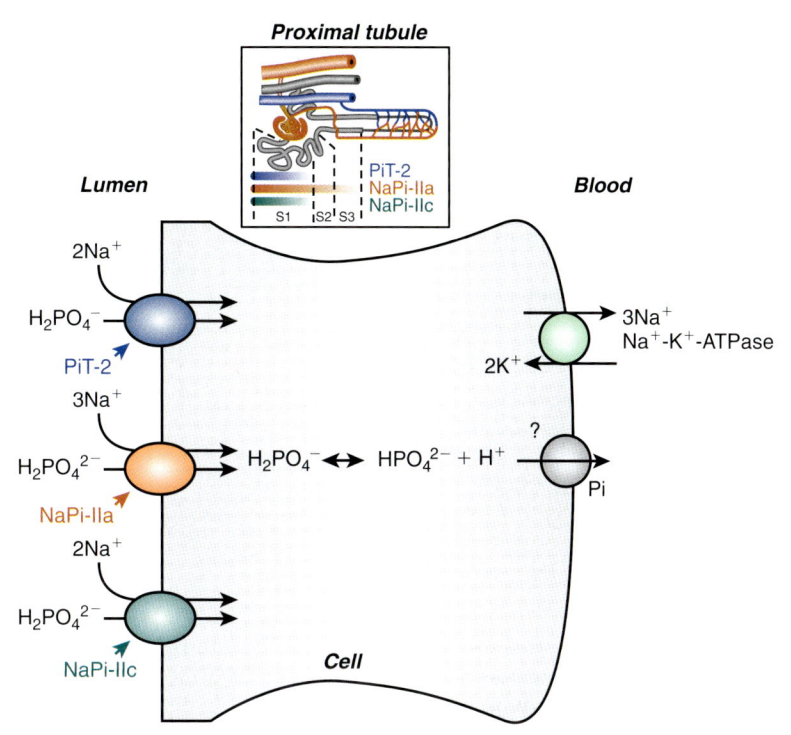

Figure 45.7 Crosssection of mammalian kidney and schematic representation of renal tubular phosphate reabsorption in segments of the proximal tubule (S1, S2, and S3) through sodium-phosphate cotransporters. This task is accomplished by two distinct families of sodium-dependent phosphate transporters, one being NaPiII-a/NaPiII-c and the other PiT-2, which are expressed in the luminal membrane of proximal tubular cells. The number of sodium-phosphate cotransporter units of NPT2a/c expressed at the membrane is regulated by parathyroid hormone (PTH) and fibroblast growth factor-23 (FGF-23). NaPi-IIa and NaPi-IIc transport divalent P_i (HPO_4^{2-}), whereas PiT-2 prefers monovalent P_i ($H_2PO_4^-$). The basolateral exit pathway remains unknown. The basolaterally localized Na^+-K^+-ATPase maintains an inwardly directed Na^+ gradient to drive cotransport. (Redrawn from Biber J, Hernando N, Forster I: Phosphate transporters and their function. *Annu Rev Physiol* 75:535-550, 2013.)

exclusively in the apical membrane of renal proximal tubular cells. The amount of NaPi-IIa protein at the brush border membrane determines the capacity of the proximal tubule to reabsorb phosphate; this finding explains why NaPi-IIa/SLC34A1-deficient mice have increased urinary phosphate excretion and marked hypophosphatemia.[170] NaPi-IIa is the target of the two main hormones that control renal phosphate reabsorption, PTH and fibroblast growth factor 23 (FGF-23), both of which decrease the amount of NaPi-IIa at the brush border membrane. The contribution of NaPi-IIa to renal phosphate balance was established by Magen and coworkers when they reported autosomal recessive hypophosphatemic rickets with renal Fanconi's syndrome secondary to a loss-of-function mutation in NaPi-IIa.[171]

Membrane sorting of NaPi-IIa requires sodium-hydrogen exchanger regulatory factor 1 (NHERF-1), a multifunctional intracellular protein with two structural domains, the PSD95, Discs-large, ZO-1 (PDZ1) domain and the PSD95, Discs-large, ZO-2 (PDZ2) domain. These domains can interact with specific sequences of the carboxy terminus of various membrane proteins, among them NaPi-IIa[172,173] and the PTH type 1 receptor (PTH1R).[174,175] Disruption of *NHERF1* in mice results in a phenotype that is very similar to that of *NaPi-IIa* knockout mice, including increased urinary phosphate excretion and hypophosphatemia due to decreased NPT2a in brush border membranes.[176]

Two other bone-specific proteins, PHEX (see discussion of XLH) and dentin matrix protein 1 (DMP1), appear to be necessary for limiting the expression of FGF-23, thereby allowing sufficient renal conservation of phosphate.[177] A reduction in serum phosphate levels also leads to increased $1,25(OH)_2D_3$ levels from greater activity of the 1α-hydroxylase. The decrease in serum phosphate levels also inhibits bone deposition, and the rise in serum $1,25(OH)_2D_3$ increases bone resorption, thus favoring a net shift of phosphate from bone. Higher serum levels of $1,25(OH)_2D_3$ also increase intestinal phosphate and calcium absorption. As a consequence, serum calcium levels rise and inhibit PTH secretion. The reduction in PTH levels does not lead to a further increase in phosphate reabsorption by the kidney because the proximal tubule is insensitive to the action of PTH in states of phosphate deprivation. As a result, one should predict that a renal phosphate leak will lead to raised serum $1,25(OH)_2D_3$ levels, decreased PTH, and induction of hypercalciuria.

X-LINKED HYPOPHOSPHATEMIC RICKETS

PATHOGNESIS

X-linked hypophosphatemic rickets (XLH; OMIM #307800) is the most common inherited hypophosphatemic disorder, accounting for more than 50% of cases of familial phosphate wasting (see Table 45.5). It is characterized by

Table 45.5 Inherited Hypophosphatemias—Mutated Proteins and Laboratory Findings

Disease	Protein	Laboratory Values			
		Serum Ca^{2+}	$1,25(OH)_2D$	FGF-23	PTH
Hypophosphatemic rickets, X-linked dominant (XLH)	PHEX	Normal	Low/Normal	High/Normal	Normal
Hypophosphatemic rickets, autosomal recessive (ARHP)	DMP1	Normal	Normal	Normal	High/Normal
Hypophosphatemic rickets, autosomal dominant (ADHR)	FGF-23	Normal	Normal	High	Normal
Nephrolithiasis/osteoporosis, hypophosphatemic 2	NHERF-1	Normal	High	Normal	Normal
Hypophosphatemic rickets and hyperparathyroidism	KLOTHO	High	High	High	High
Nephrolithiasis/osteoporosis, hypophosphatemic 1	SLC34A1 (?)	High	n.d.	High	n.d.
Hypophosphatemic rickets with hypercalciuria (HHRH)	SLC34A3	High	Low	High	Low

DMP1, Dentin matrix protein 1; FGF-23, fibroblast growth factor-23; n.d., not determined; NHERF-1, sodium-hydrogen exchanger regulatory factor 1; PHEX, M13 zinc metalloprotease encoded by *PHEX*; PTH, parathyroid hormone; SLC, solute carrier.
Adapted from Amatschek S, Haller M, Oberbauer R: Renal phosphate handling in human—what can we learn from hereditary hypophosphataemias? Eur J Clin Invest 40:552-560, 2010.

hypophosphatemia, phosphaturia, normal serum calcium and PTH levels, and inappropriately normal to low serum $1,25$-$(OH)_2D_3$ levels. XLH is caused by mutations in the *PHEX* gene (phosphate-regulating gene with homologies to endopeptidases on the X chromosome). *PHEX* encodes an M13 zinc metalloprotease expressed in osteoblasts and odontoblasts but not in the kidney. Although it is not immediately apparent how loss of PHEX function leads to a decrease in renal Pi reabsorption, it has been suggested that PHEX is involved in the inactivation of a phosphaturic hormone or the activation of a Pi-conserving hormone.[178,179] FGF-23 synthesis and secretion appear reduced through yet unknown mechanisms that involve PHEX.[180]

CLINICAL PRESENTATION

Early in life, patients with XLH demonstrate short stature (growth retardation), femoral and/or tibial bowing, and histomorphometric evidence of rickets and osteomalacia. Male patients are usually more severely affected than female patients, with variable penetrance. Serum phosphate levels are usually lower than 0.8 mmol/L (2.5 mg/dL) and the Tm_P/GFR is lower than 0.56 mmol/L (1.8 mg/dL). The $1,25(OH)_2D_3$ levels are normal or near normal. There is apparently no correlation between the serum levels of phosphate and the severity of the disease. Affected children tend to have higher serum phosphate and Tm_P/GFR values than affected adults, as is the case with normal subjects. The earliest sign of the disease in children can be increased serum alkaline phosphatase levels.[180]

TREATMENT

Early therapy with $1,25(OH)_2D_3$ (1.0 to 3.0 mcg/day) and phosphate (1 to 2 g/day in divided doses) has a beneficial effect on growth, bone density, and deformations.[181] Nephrocalcinosis caused by vitamin D and phosphate therapy can lead to deterioration of renal function.

AUTOSOMAL DOMINANT HYPOPHOSPHATEMIC RICKETS

Autosomal dominant hypophosphatemic rickets (ADHR; OMIM #193100) is a very rare cause of rickets (see Table 45.5) characterized by hypophosphatemia, phosphaturia, inappropriately low or normal $1,25(OH)_2D$ levels, and bone mineralization defects that can result in bone pain, fracture, rickets, osteomalacia, lower extremity deformities, and muscle weakness.[182] These features are similar to those of XLH. However, ADHR is far less common than XLH and has incomplete penetrance with a variable age of onset. The gene responsible for ADHR encodes a member of the FGF family, FGF-23, a 251–amino acid peptide that is secreted and processed to amino- and carboxy-terminal peptides at a consensus pro-protein convertase (furin) site, RHTR (ArgHisThrArg),[183] by a subtilisin-like pro-protein convertase. Missense mutations in FGF-23 identified in all families with ADHR abrogate peptide processing.[184] The mutant FGF-23 is predicted to have a longer circulating half-life than the wild type and to be associated with higher serum concentrations. Iron deficiency may trigger late-onset ADHR (in pregnancy and adolescence, for example) by increasing FGF-23 production.[185]

AUTOSOMAL RECESSIVE HYPOPHOSPHATEMIC RICKETS

Autosomal recessive hypophosphatemic rickets (ARHR1; OMIM #241520) is a very rare form of hypophosphatemic rickets caused by inactivating mutations of the DMP-1 gene *(DMP1)* that result in secondary elevation of FGF-23 concentrations.[186] The *DMP1* gene is located at chromosome 4q21 and is one of a cluster of genes encoding a class of tooth and bone noncollagenous matrix proteins known as SIBLINGs (small *i*ntegrin-*b*inding *li*gand, *N*-linked *g*lycoproteins). ARHR2 (OMIM #613312) is caused by mutations in ENPP1 (ectonucleotide pyrophosphatase/phosphodiesterase family member 1), a regulator of extracellular pyrophosphate, and has previously been linked to the development of generalized arterial calcification of infancy (*GACI*; OMIM #208000).[187] The biochemical features are similar to those of XLH—hypophosphatemia, phosphaturia, and inappropriately low $1,25(OH)_2D_3$. The clinical presentation is usually found not at birth but later, during childhood and even in adulthood.

HEREDITARY HYPOPHOSPHATEMIC RICKETS WITH HYPERCALCIURIA

Hereditary hypophosphatemic rickets (OMIM #241530) associated with hypercalciuria is a rare autosomal disease caused by mutations in *SLC34A3*, the gene encoding the renal sodium-phosphate cotransporter NaPi-IIc.[188,189] Affected subjects appear to have a chronic renal phosphate leak with an appropriate response to hypophosphatemia, because serum levels of calcitriol are increased. Consequently, intestinal calcium absorption is enhanced, resulting in hypercalciuria. Serum calcium levels are normal, and other features include rickets, short stature, and suppressed PTH. The condition responds to administration of daily oral phosphate (1 to 2.5 g/day), which leads to an increase in serum phosphate and decreases in serum $1,25(OH)_2D_3$, calcium, and alkaline phosphatase. Growth rate can be restored, and the clinical manifestations of rickets and osteomalacia (e.g., bone pain, muscle weakness) disappear.

FAMILIAL TUMORAL CALCINOSIS

Familial tumoral calcinosis (FTC; OMIM #211900) is a severe autosomal recessive metabolic disorder that manifests as hyperphosphatemia and massive calcium deposits in the skin and subcutaneous tissues.[190] Loss-of-function mutations in *FGF23*,[191] as well as *GALNT3*[192] and *KL*,[193] cause familial tumoral calcinosis because of inadequate concentrations or action of intact FGF-23. Affected individuals report recurrent painful, calcified subcutaneous masses of up to 1 kg, often resulting in secondary infection and incapacitating mutilation. The *GALNT3* gene encodes a glycosyltransferase responsible for initiating mucin-type O-glycosylation, whereas Klotho (encoded by *KL*) functions as a cofactor essential for interactions between FGF-23 and FGF receptors.[194]

HEREDITARY SELECTIVE DEFICIENCY OF $1\alpha,25(OH)_2D_3$

A rare form of autosomal recessive vitamin D responsive rickets, hereditary selective deficiency of $1\alpha,25(OH)_2D_3$ (OMIM #264700) is not a disease of tubule transport per se, but a 1α-hydroxylation deficiency. It is described in this chapter because the enzyme is specifically expressed in the proximal tubule. It results from inactivating mutations in the *CYP27B1* gene.[195,196] Vitamin D is metabolized by sequential hydroxylations in the liver (25-hydroxylation) and the kidney (1α-hydroxylation). Hydroxylation of 25-hydroxyvitamin D_3 is mediated by $25(OH)D_3$ 1α-hydroxylase in the kidney. Patients usually appear normal at birth, but muscle weakness, tetany, convulsions, and rickets start to develop at 2 months of age. Serum calcium levels are low; PTH levels are high with low to undetectable $1,25(OH)_2D_3$. Serum levels of $25(OH)D_3$ are normal or slightly increased. Once recognized, this rare disorder is easily treated with physiologic doses of calcitriol, which leads to healing of rickets and restoration of the plasma calcium, phosphate, and PTH levels.

HEREDITARY GENERALIZED RESISTANCE TO $1\alpha,25(OH)_2D_3$

Hereditary vitamin D–resistant rickets (HVDRR) is a rare monogenic autosomal recessive disorder caused by mutations in the vitamin D receptor (VDR) and is similar to selective deficiency of $1\alpha,25(OH)_2D_3$. Its salient features are increased serum levels of $25(OH)D_3$ and $1\alpha,25(OH)_2D_3$, and the disease does not respond to doses of $1\alpha,25(OH)_2D_3$ and $1\alpha,(OH)D_3$. In addition, approximately half of the patients described with the disease have alopecia. In a subset of affected kindreds, premature stop codons in the vitamin D receptor gene lead to the absence of the ligand-binding domain.[197]

RESISTANCE TO PARATHORMONE ACTION

Pseudohypoparathyroidism (PHP) is associated with biochemical hypoparathyroidism (i.e., hypocalcemia, hyperphosphatemia) caused by resistance to, rather than deficiency of PTH. Patients with PHP type 1a have a generalized form of, hormone resistance plus a constellation of, developmental defects termed *Albright's hereditary osteodystrophy*. Within PHP type 1a families, some individuals show osteodystrophy but have normal hormone responsiveness, a variant phenotype termed *pseudo-PHP*. By contrast, patients with PHP type 1b manifest only PTH resistance and lack features of osteodystrophy. These various forms of PHP are caused by defects in the *GNAS1* gene that lead to decreased expression or activity of the α subunit of the stimulatory G protein ($G_{\alpha s}$). Tissue-specific genomic imprinting of *GNAS1* accounts for the variable phenotypes of patients with *GNAS1* defects.[198]

INHERITED DISORDER OF URATE TRANSPORT

FAMILIAL RENAL HYPOURICEMIA

Renal hypouricemia is an autosomal recessive disorder characterized by impaired urate handling in the renal tubules.[199] Type 1 (more than 90% of cases) is caused by a loss-of-function mutation in the *SLC22A12* gene (OMIM #220150) encoding the apical urate/anion exchanger URAT1,[200] whereas type 2 is caused by defects in the *SLC2A9* gene (OMIM #612076) encoding glucose transporter 9 (GLUT9), a high-capacity basolateral urate transporter belonging to the facilitated glucose transporter family.[201,202] The disorder is associated with exercise-induced acute renal failure and nephrolithiasis. Hyperuricosuria, combined with dehydration or exercise, results in acute uric acid nephropathy and causes an obstructive acute renal failure. This can be prevented by forced hydration with bicarbonate or saline solutions. Affected subjects typically have very high urate fractional excretion (50% or higher) and their parents have intermediate levels.[203] In addition, polymorphisms in *SLC2A9* explain 1.7% to 5.3% of the variance in serum uric acid concentrations.[204]

INHERITED DISORDERS OF RENAL GLUCOSE TRANSPORT

Under normal conditions, glucose is almost completely reabsorbed by the proximal tubule. Thus, very small amounts of glucose are present in the urine. The appearance

Table 45.6 Causes of Glucosuria
Hyperglycemia
Diabetes mellitus
Iatrogenic:
Glucocorticoids
Catecholamines
Angiotensin I–converting enzyme inhibitors
Dextrose intravenous solutions
Total parenteral nutrition
Renal Glucosuria
Idiopathic
Glucose-galactose malabsorption
Fanconi's syndrome
Pregnancy

of glucose in the urine (500 mg or 2.75 mmol/day in adults) is caused most often by hyperglycemia (overload glucosuria) and rarely by abnormal handling of glucose by the kidney (Table 45.6). Renal glucosuria may be part of a generalized defect of the proximal tubule (Fanconi's syndrome) or may manifest as an isolated defect.

RENAL GLUCOSURIA

Familial renal glucosuria (FRG; OMIM #233100) is an inherited renal tubular disorder characterized by persistent isolated glucosuria in the absence of hyperglycemia. It is usually a benign clinical condition. FRG is transmitted as a codominant trait with incomplete penetrance. Homozygotes can show glucosuria of more than 60 g/day, evidence of renal sodium wasting, mild volume depletion, and raised basal plasma renin and serum aldosterone levels.[205]

The definition of *glucosuria* is arbitrary, and different investigators have proposed different guidelines to distinguish abnormal from normal glucosuria. A currently accepted stringent definition of glucosuria proposes the following criteria:

- The oral glucose tolerance test result and the levels of plasma insulin and free fatty acids and of glycosylated hemoglobin should all be normal.
- The amount of glucose in the urine (10 to 100 g/day) should be relatively stable except during pregnancy, when it may increase.
- The degree of glucosuria should be largely independent of diet but may fluctuate according to the amount of carbohydrates ingested. All specimens of urine should contain glucose.
- The carbohydrate excreted should be glucose. Other sugars are not found (fructose, pentoses, galactose, lactose, sucrose, maltose, and heptulose).

Subjects with renal glucosuria should be able to store and use carbohydrates normally. Mutations in the sodium-glucose cotransporter SGLT2 and the coding gene, *SLC5A2*, are responsible for the disorder.[206] Some Japanese patients might have mutations in GLUT2.[207] SGLT2 and SGLT1 mediate apical glucose uptake in the S1 and S3 segments of the proximal tubule, respectively. SGLT2 inhibitors could help diabetic patients control hyperglycemia by augmenting urinary glucose excretion.[208] These drugs have been shown to lower weight and blood pressure as well as the hyperfiltration seen in diabetic kidney disease and are being evaluated in humans to determine whether they prevent progression of nephropathy.[209,210]

GLUCOSE-GALACTOSE MALABSORPTION

Glucose-galactose malabsorption (OMIM #606824) is a rare autosomal recessive congenital disease resulting from a selective defect in the intestinal transport of glucose and galactose. It is characterized by the neonatal onset of severe watery and acidic diarrhea that results in death unless these sugars are removed from the patient's diet.[211] Significant weight loss from hyperosmolar dehydration and metabolic acidosis is frequent. The disease occurs occasionally in adults. Mutations in SGLT1—which couples transport of sugar to sodium gradients across the intestinal brush border[212]—cause absence of the transporter in the intestine and the kidney plasma membranes, leading to glucose-galactose malabsorption. The acidic diarrhea results from bacterial metabolism of sugar in the stools. Normally, lactose in milk is broken down into glucose and galactose by lactase, an ectoenzyme on the brush border, and the hexoses are transported into the cell by SGLT1.

The disease is usually suspected from the clinical history and the presence of glucosuria despite normal serum glucose levels. Dramatic improvement occurs after withdrawal of glucose and galactose from the patient's diet. The acidic diarrhea can be improved with antibacterial treatment.

INHERITED DISORDERS OF ACID-BASE TRANSPORTERS

A typical Western diet generates an acid load of approximately 1 mmol of mineral acid per kg of body weight, which must be excreted by the kidney. In addition, the kidney filters approximately 4000 mmol of bicarbonate daily and must reclaim most of the filtered load to maintain acid-base balance. Excretion of the ingested acid load and reabsorption of filtered bicarbonate are accomplished by complex processes requiring coordinated actions of transport and enzymatic activities in the apical and basolateral membranes (Figure 45.8).

In the proximal tubule, filtered bicarbonate (HCO_3^-) is almost completely reabsorbed by an indirect mechanism. H^+ and HCO_3^- are generated by intracellular hydration of CO_2 by carbonic anhydrase II (CA II). H^+ secretion occurs across the apical membrane via NHE3, the Na^+-H^+ exchanger, and an H^+-ATPase, and HCO_3^- is transferred via a basolateral Na^+-HCO_3^- cotransporter. The secreted hydrogen ions react with filtered HCO_3^- to form H_2CO_3, which is rapidly converted to CO_2 and H_2O by carbonic anhydrase IV (CA IV) present in the apical membrane. The CO_2 and H_2O then diffuse into the cell. The result is the removal of a filtered HCO_3^- and its replacement by another in the plasma, but the process is neutral for net urinary H^+ excretion because the secreted hydrogen ions are used to reabsorb filtered

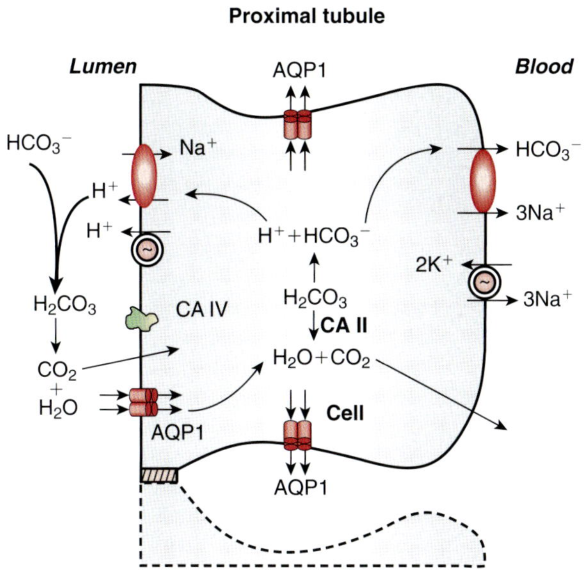

Figure 45.8 Mechanisms of renal acidification. AQP1, Aquaporin-1; CA II/IV, carbonic anhydrase II/IV.

HCO_3^-. Carbonic anhydrases are zinc metalloenzymes that catalyze the reversible hydration of CO_2 to form HCO_3^- and protons, according to the following reaction:

$$CO_2 + H_2O \leftrightarrow H_2CO_3 \leftrightarrow H^+ + HCO_3^-$$

The first reaction is catalyzed by carbonic anhydrase, and the second reaction occurs instantaneously. Net urinary elimination of H^+ depends on its buffering and excretion as titratable acid (mainly phosphate: $HPO_4^{2-} + H^+ \leftrightarrow H_2PO_4^-$), and excretion as NH_4^+. The production of NH_4^+ from glutamine by the proximal tubule and its secretion generate new plasma HCO_3^-. This process is stimulated in metabolic acidosis.

In the distal and collecting tubule, the connecting segment and type A intercalated cells secrete H^+ into the lumen via a vacuolar Mg^{2+}-dependent H^++ATPase and possibly an exchanger, H^+-K^+-ATPase (Figure 45.9). The generation of H^+ is catalyzed by carbonic anhydrase II and HCO_3^- is transported across the basolateral membrane through the anion exchanger 1 (AE1), or Cl^-/HCO_3^- exchanger. Luminal H^+ is trapped by urinary buffers, including ammonium secreted by the proximal tubule, and phosphate.

Renal tubular acidosis (RTA) is a clinical syndrome characterized by hyperchloremic (normal anion gap) metabolic acidosis secondary to abnormal urine acidification.[213] It can be identified from inappropriately high urine pH, bicarbonaturia, and reduced net acid excretion. Clinical and functional studies allow classification into four types, historically numbered in the order of discovery: proximal (type 2), classical distal (type 1), hyperkalemic distal (type 4), and combined proximal and distal (type 3). Rare forms of hereditary proximal and distal renal tubular acidosis have been identified[213-215] and are discussed here (Table 45.7).

PROXIMAL RENAL TUBULAR ACIDOSIS

Proximal renal tubular acidosis (PRTA) usually occurs as part of the spectrum of Fanconi's syndrome, in which the excretion of glucose, amino acids, and phosphate is also increased. Primary, isolated hereditary PRTA is an extremely rare disorder that may be inherited as an autosomal recessive or dominant trait.[216] The diagnosis of PRTA rests on an appropriately acid urine pH (pH < 5.5) in patients with acidosis and a high fractional excretion of bicarbonate (>10% to 15%) during intravenous loading with sodium bicarbonate ($NaHCO_3$). The underlying defect is a failure of proximal bicarbonate reabsorption. It results in an abnormally low threshold for renal bicarbonate reabsorption because the distal nephron is unable to compensate and reabsorb the large bicarbonate load presented to it. However, distal acidification mechanisms are intact, and acid urine can be produced. The metabolic acidosis is generally mild and associated with hypokalemia, and although metabolic bone disease is common, nephrocalcinosis and nephrolithiasis are rare. Because of a lowering of the tubular threshold for bicarbonate reabsorption, once the plasma bicarbonate is reduced, the threshold can be reached and a steady state maintained at a serum concentration of approximately 15 mM. In contrast, levels can fall to less than 10 mM in DRTA. Administration of large amounts of alkali (10 to 20 mmol/kg/day) may be required to normalize serum bicarbonate in the patient with PRTA.

SODIUM-BICARBONATE SYMPORTER MUTATIONS

Inactivating mutations in *SLC4A4*, the gene coding for the Na^+-HCO_3^- (NBC1) symporter, cause autosomal recessive PRTA with various ocular abnormalities such as band keratopathy, glaucoma, and cataracts (OMIM #604278).[217] The Na^+-HCO_3^- symporter is expressed in multiple ocular tissues,[218] thus explaining the abnormalities. Pancreatitis can be associated with mutations in NBC1, which is expressed in the pancreas.[219]

CARBONIC ANHYDRASE II DEFICIENCY

Recessive mixed proximal-distal (type 3) RTA accompanied by osteopetrosis and mental retardation (OMIM #259730) is caused by inactivating mutations in the cytoplasmic carbonic anhydrase II gene.[220] The pathogenesis of the mental subnormality and cerebral calcification is poorly understood. More than 50 cases have been described, predominantly from the Middle East and Mediterranean regions. The disorder is discovered late in infancy or early in childhood because of developmental delay, short stature, fracture, weakness, cranial nerve compression, dental malocclusion, and/or mental subnormality. Typical radiographic features of osteopetrosis are present, and histopathologic study of the iliac crest reveals unresorbed calcified primary spongiosa. The radiographic findings are unusual, however, in that cerebral calcification appears by early childhood and the osteosclerosis and skeletal modeling defects may gradually resolve by adulthood. Patients are usually not anemic. A hyperchloremic metabolic acidosis, sometimes with hypokalemia, is caused by RTA, which may be a proximal, distal, or combined type.[221] Bilateral recurrent renal stones, hypercalciuria, and medullary nephrocalcinosis have been described.[222] There is no established medical therapy, and the long-term outcome remains to be characterized. Treatment involves alkali supplementation for the acidosis and, potentially, bone marrow transplantation for osteopetrosis.[223]

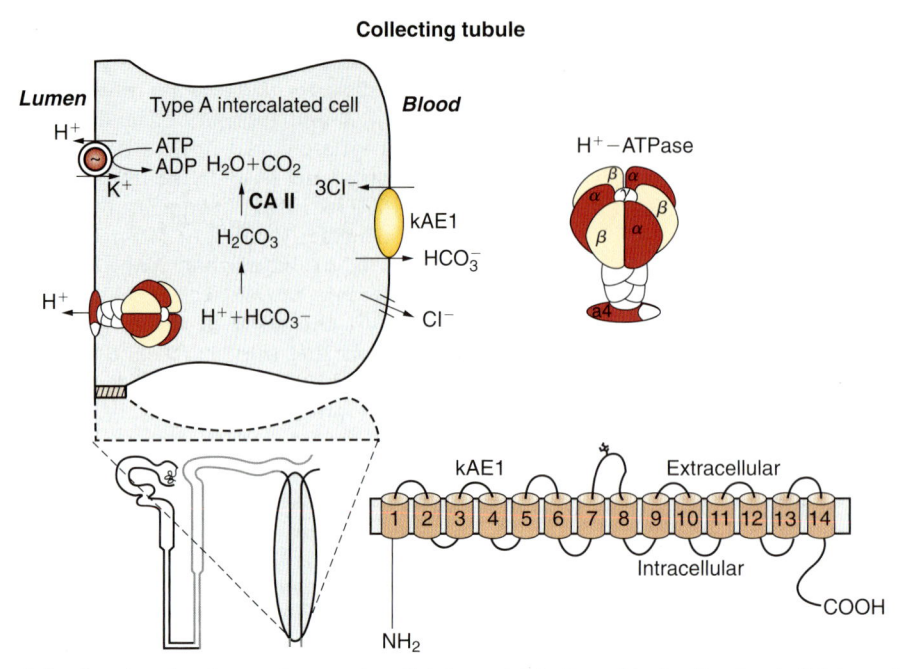

Figure 45.9 Autosomal dominant and autosomal recessive distal renal tubular acidosis. Dominant distal renal tubular acidosis (RTA) is caused by mutations in the gene *SLC4A1* encoding the chloride-bicarbonate exchanger AE1.[225,381] The *AE1* gene (chromosome 17) encodes both the erythroid (eAE1) and the kidney (kAE1) isoforms of the band 3 protein.[382] Mutations in the gene encoding the β_1-subunit of H⁺-ATPase (*ATP6V1B1*; chromosome 2p13) cause recessive distal renal tubular acidosis with sensorineural deafness.[228] Distal RTA with preserved hearing is secondary to mutations in *AIP6V0A4*, which encodes the α_4 subunit of the proton pump.[383] Both H⁺ and H⁺-K⁺-ATPases are represented. The H⁺-ATPase is schematically represented according to the proposed structure of the F-type F₁-ATPase of the inner mitochondrial membrane.[384] F₁ is represented as a flattened sphere 80 Å high and 100 Å across. The three α- and three β-subunits are arranged alternately like the segments of an orange around a central α-helix 90 Å long. Mutations in the β-subunit cause autosomal recessive distal RTA. Autosomal recessive distal RTA has also been found, in small kindred, for the *SLC4A1* mutation G701D.[227] ADP, Adenosine diphosphate; ATP, adenosine triphosphate.

Table 45.7 Classifications, Features, and Underlying Molecular Transport Defect(s) in Inherited Renal Tubular Acidoses

	Clinical Features	Protein	Gene
Proximal RTA			
Autosomal recessive PRTA with ocular abnormalities	Band keratopathy, glaucoma, cataracts, short stature, mental retardation, dental enamel defects, pancreatitis, basal ganglia calcification	NBC1	SLC4A4
Autosomal recessive PRTA with osteopetrosis and cerebral calcification (inherited carbonic anhydrase II deficiency)	Mental retardation, osteopetrosis, cerebral calcification	CA II	CA2
Autosomal dominant PRTA	Short stature, osteomalacia	Unknown	Unknown
Distal RTA			
Autosomal dominant DRTA	Complete or incomplete DRTA, hypercalciuria, nephrocalcinosis, nephrolithiasis, hypokalemia, short stature, osteomalacia, rickets	AE1	SLC4A1
Autosomal recessive DRTA	Complete or incomplete DRTA Other features as above Reported in Asian populations	H⁺-ATPase (A4 subunit) AE1	ATP6V0A4 SLC4A1
Autosomal recessive DRTA with progressive nerve deafness	Complete or incomplete DRTA (B1 subunit) As above but with late-onset nerve deafness	H⁺-ATPase H⁺-ATPase (A4 subunit)	ATP6V1B1 ATP6V0A4

AE1, Ion exchanger 1; CA II, cytosolic carbonic anhydrase; D, distal; NBC1, Na⁺-HCO₃⁻ cotransporter; P, proximal; RTA, renal tubular acidosis.
Adapted from Laing CM, Toye AM, Capasso G, et al: Renal tubular acidosis: developments in our understanding of the molecular basis. Int J Biochem Cell Biol 37:1151-1161, 2005.

DISTAL RENAL TUBULAR ACIDOSIS

Hereditary DRTA is a genetically heterogeneous disorder with dominant and recessive forms caused by dysfunction of type A intercalated cells[213,214,224] (see Figure 45.9). Implicated transporters include the AE1 (Cl^-/HCO_3^-) exchanger of the basolateral membrane and at least two subunits of the apical membrane V-ATPase, the V_1 (head) subunit B1 (associated with deafness) and the V_0 (stalk) subunit A4. Clinical features include inability to acidify urine, variable hyperchloremic hypokalemic metabolic acidosis, hypercalciuria, nephrocalcinosis, and nephrolithiasis. Patients with recessive DRTA present with either acute illness or growth failure at a young age, sometimes accompanied by deafness. Dominant DRTA is usually a milder disease and involves no hearing loss.

CHLORIDE-BICARBONATE EXCHANGER MUTATIONS

Mutations in the *SLC4A1* gene encoding AE1 can lead to dominant (OMIM #179800) or recessive DRTA.[225] AE1 is the basolateral Cl^-/HCO_3^- exchanger located in alpha intercalated cells of the collecting duct.[226] The renal AE1 contributes to urinary acidification by providing the major exit route for HCO_3^- across the basolateral membrane. DRTA results from aberrant targeting of AE1.

The dominant form is usually a mild disorder that can be discovered incidentally after a kidney stone episode. Serum bicarbonate concentrations are usually between 14 and 25 mmol/L, and serum potassium levels between 2.1 and 4.2 mmol/L. Minimum urine pH following an acid load varies from 5.95 to 6.8 (normal < 5.30). Nephrocalcinosis and kidney stones are present in approximately 50% of subjects. Deafness is usually absent.

The recessive form of DRTA (OMIM #109270) is diagnosed at a younger age, often before 1 year. It is found in Southeast Asia (Thailand, Papua–New Guinea, and Malaysia), where it is associated with ovalocytosis.[227] Affected subjects present with vomiting, dehydration, failure to thrive, or delayed growth. Nephrocalcinosis, kidney stones, or both are frequent, and rickets can be present. Severe metabolic acidosis with serum pH less than 7.30 and serum bicarbonate less than 15 mmol/L is common. Serum potassium levels are also lower than in autosomal dominant DRTA.

PROTON ATPASE SUBUNIT MUTATIONS

Mutations in ATP6V1B1, the B_1-subunit of the apical proton pump ATP6B1 that mediates distal nephron acid secretion (OMIM #267300), cause DRTA with sensorineural deafness in a significant proportion of families.[228,229] In type A intercalated cells, the H^+-ATPase pumps protons against an electrochemical gradient. Active proton secretion is also necessary to maintain proper endolymph pH. These findings implicate ATP6B1 in endolymph pH homeostasis and in normal auditory function, because nearly all patients with ATP6V1B1 mutations also have sensorineural hearing loss.

Mutations in the *ATP6V0A4* gene on chromosome 7 (OMIM #602722) also give rise to recessive DRTA,[230] but hearing is preserved. ATP6V0A4 encodes a kidney-specific A4 isoform of the proton pump's 116-kDs accessory a subunit. The treatment of DRTA involves the correction of dehydration, electrolyte, and bicarbonate anomalies, which will improve symptoms. In adults, administration of alkali 1 to 3 mmol kg/day usually corrects the metabolic abnormality. In children, up to 5 mmol/kg/day may be required. Potassium supplementation may be needed even after correction of the acidosis.

BARTTER'S AND GITELMAN'S SYNDROMES

In 1962, Bartter and coworkers described two patients with hypokalemic metabolic alkalosis, hyperreninemic hyperaldosteronism, normal blood pressure, as well as hyperplasia and hypertrophy of the juxtaglomerular apparatus.[231] Since then, familial hypokalemic, hypochloremic metabolic alkalosis has been recognized as not a single entity but, rather, a set of closely related disorders.[232] Although Bartter's syndrome and Bartter mutations are used commonly as diagnoses, it is likely, as explained by Jeck and colleagues, that the two patients with a mild phenotype originally described by Bartter had Gitelman's syndrome, a thiazide-like salt-losing tubulopathy with a defect in the distal convoluted tubule.[232] As a consequence, salt-losing tubulopathy of the furosemide type is a more physiologically appropriate definition for Bartter's syndrome. Bartter's syndrome is a genetically heterogeneous disorder affecting the loop of Henle, where 30% of the filtered sodium chloride is reabsorbed, that typically manifests during the neonatal period and is associated with hypercalciuria and nephrocalcinosis (Figure 45.10). In contrast, Gitelman's syndrome is a disorder affecting the distal tubule[233] that is usually diagnosed at a later stage and is associated with hypocalciuria and hypomagnesemia, with predominant muscular signs and symptoms (Figure 45.11).[234]

BARTTER'S SYNDROME

PATHOGNESIS

Bartter's syndrome (OMIM #601678, #241200, #607364, and #602522) is an autosomal recessive disorder affecting the function of the thick ascending limb (TAL) of the loop of Henle, giving a clinical picture of salt wasting and hypokalemic metabolic alkalosis. It is caused by inactivating mutations in one of at least four genes encoding membrane proteins (Bartter's syndrome types 1 through 4)[235-239]: type 1, the Na^+-K-$2Cl^-$ cotransporter (*SLC12A1* encoding NKCC2); type 2, the apical inward-rectifying potassium channel (*KCNJ1* encoding ROMK); type 3, a basolateral chloride channel (*CLCNK* encoding ClC-Kb), and type 4, *BSND*, encoding Barttin, a protein that acts as an essential activator β-subunit for ClC-Ka and ClC-Kb chloride channels (see Figure 45.10). Gain-of-function mutations in the extracellular calcium-sensing receptor (CaSR) cause a variant of Bartter's syndrome[240,241] with hypocalcemia. In this regard, it is of interest that a Bartter-like syndrome has been described in patients treated with aminoglycosides such as gentamicin and amikacin, characterized by transient hypokalemia, metabolic alkalosis, hypomagnesemia with urinary magnesium wasting, and hypercalciuria, which resolve weeks after drug termination. Drugs in this class are polycations acting as calcimimetics and stimulating the CaSR. This disorder can be thought of as an acquired form of type 5 Bartter's syndrome. Alternatively, direct drug-induced tubular damage may be the etiologic mechanism.[242]

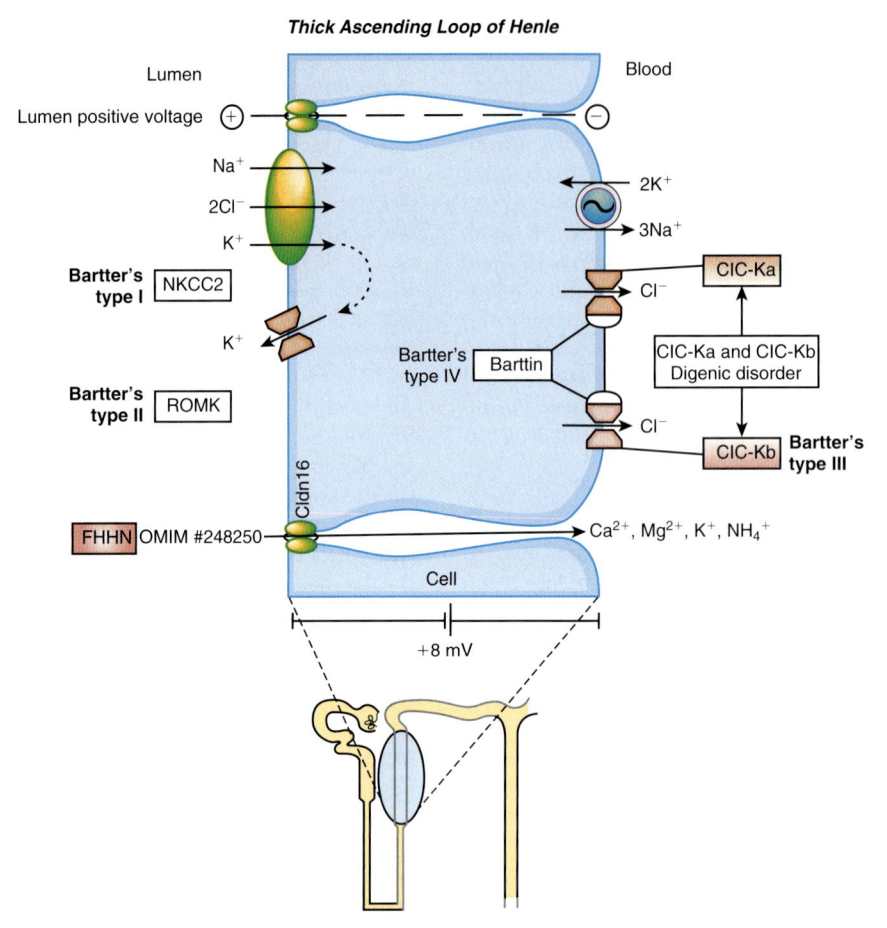

Figure 45.10 Schematic representation of transepithelial salt reabsorption in a cell of the thick ascending limb of the loop of Henle. Thirty percent of the filtered sodium chloride is reabsorbed in the thick ascending limb (TAL). Most of the energy for concentrating and diluting the urine is used on active NaCl transport in the TAL. Filtered NaCl is reabsorbed through Na^+-K^+-$2Cl^-$ cotransporter type 2 (NKCC2), which uses the sodium gradient across the membrane to transport chloride and potassium into the cell. The potassium ions are recycled (100%) through the apical membrane by the potassium channel ROMK. Sodium leaves the cell actively through the basolateral Na^+-K^+-ATPase. Chloride diffuses passively through two basolateral channels, ClC-Ka and ClC-Kb. Both of these chloride channels must bind to the β-subunit of Barttin to be transported to the cell surface. Four types of Bartter's syndrome (types I, II, III, and IV) are attributable to recessive mutations in the genes that encode NKCC2, ROMK, ClC-Kb, and Barttin, respectively. A fifth type of Bartter's syndrome has also been shown to be a digenic disorder that is attributable to loss-of-function mutations in the genes that encode the chloride channels ClC-Ka and ClC-Kb.[222] As a result of these different molecular alterations, sodium chloride is lost into the urine, positive lumen voltage is abolished, and calcium (Ca^{2+}), magnesium (Mg^{2+}), potassium (K^+), and ammonium (NH_4^-) cannot be reabsorbed in the paracellular space. In the absence of mutations, the recycling of potassium maintains a lumen-positive gradient (+8 mV). Claudin-16 (CLDN16) is necessary for the paracellular transport of calcium and magnesium. FHHN, Familial hypomagnesemia with hypercalciuria and nephrocalcinosis. (Modified with permission from Bichet DG, Fujiwara TM: Reabsorption of sodium chloride—lessons from the chloride channels. *N Engl J Med* 350:1281-1283, 2004.)

An additional type of Bartter's syndrome has been shown to be a digenic disorder that is attributable to loss-of-function mutations in the genes that encode the chloride channels ClC-Ka and ClC-Kb.[238]

CLINICAL PRESENTATION

Most cases of Bartter's syndrome present antenatally or in neonates. Polyhydramnios and premature labor are common findings. Postnatal findings include polyuria, polydipsia, failure to thrive, growth retardation, dehydration, low blood pressure, muscle weakness, seizures, tetany, paresthesias, and joint pain from chondrocalcinosis.[243] In contrast to patients with Gitelman's syndrome, those with Bartter's syndrome are virtually always hypercalciuric and normomagnesemic.

Nephrocalcinosis occurs in almost all patients with Bartter's syndrome with NKCC2 (type 1) and ROMK (type 2) mutations but in only 20% of those with CLC-Kb mutations. This finding could be attributable to lower urine calcium excretion. Patients with ROMK mutations may show hyperkalemia at birth, which converts to hypokalemia within the first weeks of life.[244] Thus, they can be misdiagnosed with pseudohypoaldosteronism type I (see earlier discussion of pseudohypoaldosteronism). This pattern could be explained by the fact that ROMK, in addition to being required for sodium reabsorption in the TAL, is also expressed in the collecting duct. Patients do not need important K^+ supplementation, contrary to other patients with Bartter's syndrome, but still demonstrate hypokalemia due to reduced reabsorption in the TAL and possibly to K secretion by maxi-K channels in the late distal tubule.[245] The type 3 Bartter's syndrome (CLC-Kb) phenotype is highly variable and may manifest as either a typical antenatal variant or a

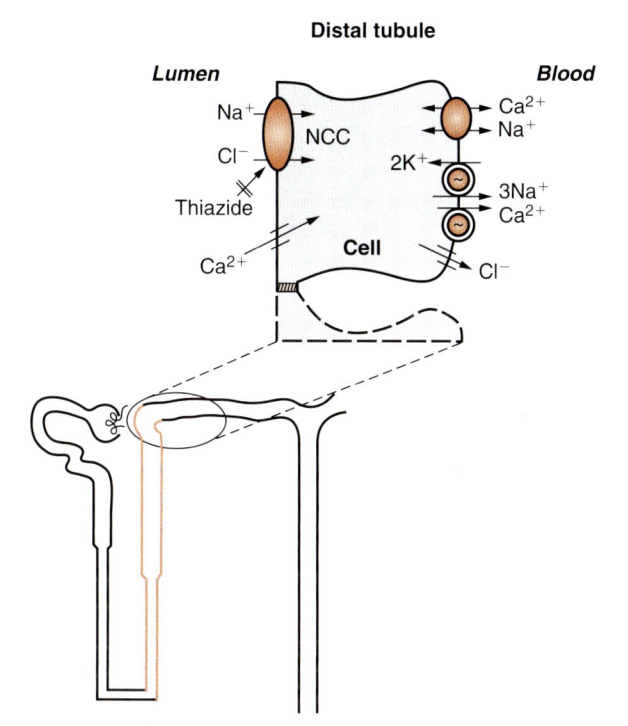

Figure 45.11 Gitelman's syndrome: loss-of-function mutations of the thiazide-sensitive Na-Cl cotransporter (NCC).

"classic" Bartter's variant characterized by an onset in early childhood and lower severity or absence of hypercalciuria and nephrocalcinosis. BSND mutations (type 4 Bartter's syndrome) are usually associated with an extremely severe phenotype with intrauterine onset, profound renal salt and water wasting, renal failure, sensorineural deafness, and motor retardation.[246] Sensorineural deafness is specific for Barttin (type 4) because it is an essential subunit of chloride channels in the inner ear, necessary for generating the endocochlear potential.[247] The severity of type 4 Bartter's syndrome would be consistent with contributions of both ClC-Ka and ClC-Kb to basolateral chloride exit in the TAL.

TREATMENT

Treatment of Bartter's syndrome usually involves potassium and magnesium supplements, spironolactone, and nonsteroidal antiinflammatory drugs. Indomethacin has been widely used, for which elevations of urinary prostaglandin E_2 have provided a rationale.[232] Angiotensin I–converting enzyme inhibitors have been used successfully in conjunction with potassium supplements.[248,249] Therapy should lead to catch-up growth in infants.[250]

GITELMAN'S SYNDROME

PATHOGNESIS

Gitelman's syndrome (OMIM #263800), a milder disorder than Bartter's syndrome,[251] is usually diagnosed in adolescents and adults.[252] It is an autosomal recessive trait caused by inactivating mutations in the SLC12A3 gene encoding the thiazide-sensitive Na^+-Cl^- cotransporter (NCC).[233] Rare cases are caused by mutations in the CLCNKB gene, which encodes the renal chloride channel CLC-Kb, located in basolateral membrane of cells of the TAL and the distal tubules. These patients appear to have a Gitelman's and not the expected Bartter's phenotype.[237] Gitelman's syndrome results in a thiazide-like effect, consisting of sodium and chloride wasting with secondary hypovolemia and metabolic alkalosis. Activation of the renin angiotensin aldosterone system from volume depletion, plus increased sodium load to the cortical collecting duct, leads to increased sodium reabsorption by the epithelial sodium channel, which is counterbalanced by potassium and hydrogen excretion, resulting in hypokalemia and metabolic alkalosis. Enhanced passive Ca^{2+} transport in the proximal tubule rather than active Ca^{2+} transport in the distal convoluted tubule explains the hypocalciuria. Downregulation of TRPM6 (epithelial Mg^{2+} channel transient receptor potential channel subfamily M, member 6) explains the hypomagnesemia.[253]

CLINICAL PRESENTATION

The carrier state of SLC12A3 mutations occurs in 1% of the general population, suggesting a prevalence of Gitelman's syndrome of 25 per million population and making it the most common inherited renal tubule disorder.[254,255] Contrary to patients with Bartter's syndrome, those with Gitelman's syndrome are usually asymptomatic in the neonatal period and often discovered incidentally (Figure 45.12).[232] Subjects have hypokalemic metabolic alkalosis, but unlike those with Bartter's syndrome, they are hypocalciuric and hypomagnesemic and do not have signs of overt volume depletion.[256] Polyuria and polydipsia are not features of Gitelman's syndrome either. Patients suffer from arthritis due to chondrocalcinosis in several joints,[257] possibly secondary to hypomagnesemia. Urinary prostaglandin E_2 levels are normal,[258] a finding compatible with the poor response observed to prostanoid synthetase inhibition. The major conditions in the differential diagnosis of Gitelman's syndrome are diuretic abuse, laxative abuse, and chronic vomiting. A careful history, as well as measurement of urinary chloride and detection of diuretics, should help differentiate among these conditions.

TREATMENT

The treatment of Gitelman's syndrome includes potassium supplementation and spironolactone.[259] Nonsteroidal antiinflammatory drugs are usually not helpful because prostaglandin levels are normal.

INHERITED DISORDERS WITH HYPERTENSION AND HYPOKALEMIA

Most patients with hypokalemia and hypertension have essential hypertension associated with the use of diuretics, secondary aldosteronism from renal artery stenosis, or primary hyperaldosteronism.[260] Hereditary causes of hypertension and hypokalemia include excess secretion of aldosterone or other mineralocorticoids and abnormal sensitivity to mineralocorticoids. They are primarily characterized by low or low-normal plasma renin concentration and salt-sensitive hypokalemic hypertension, suggesting enhanced mineralocorticoid activity.[261] The molecular basis for several of these traits has been elucidated.

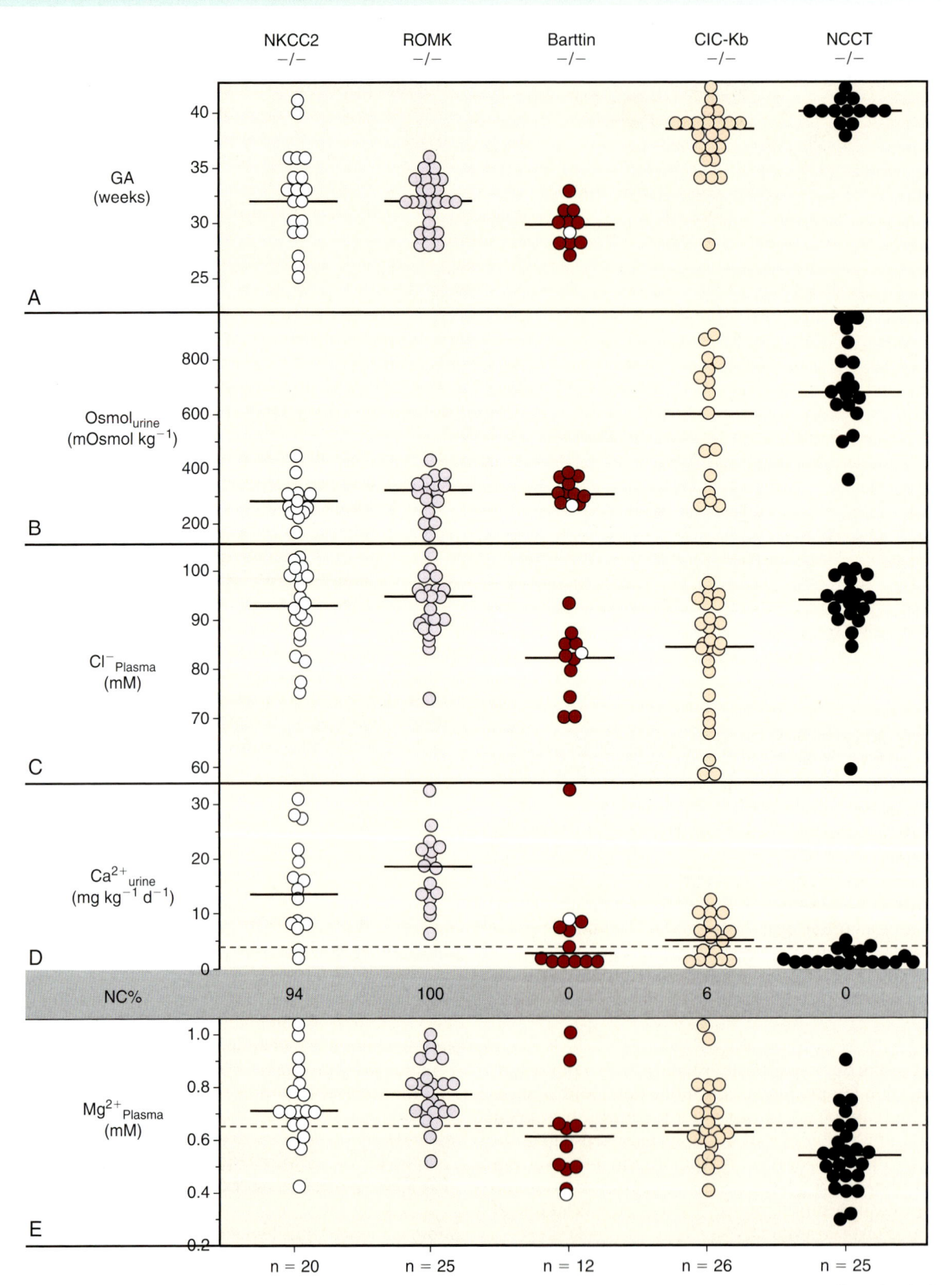

Figure 45.12 Genotype-phenotype correlation in untreated salt-losing tubulopathies. **A,** Age of gestation at birth (GA). **B,** Maximal urine osmolality in random morning urine samples. **C,** Minimal plasma Cl⁻ concentration. **D,** Maximal urinary Ca^{2+} excretion (*dashed line* indicates the upper normal limit, about 4 mg·kg^{-1}× day^{-1}) and percentage of medullary nephrocalcinosis (NC%). **E,** Minimal plasma Mg^{2+} concentration (*dashed line* indicates the lower normal limit, 0.65 mM). *Horizontal lines* indicate the median; the *open symbol* in the Barttin group indicates the digenic ClC-Ka/ClC-Kb disorder. ClC-Kb, Basolateral chloride channel b; NCCT, Na-Cl transporter; NKCC2, Na^+-K^+-$2Cl^-$ cotransporter 2; ROMK, potassium channel. (With permission from Jeck N, Schlingmann KP, Reinalter SC, et al: Salt handling in the distal nephron: lessons learned from inherited human disorders. *Am J Physiol Regul Integr Comp Physiol* 288:R782-R795, 2005.)

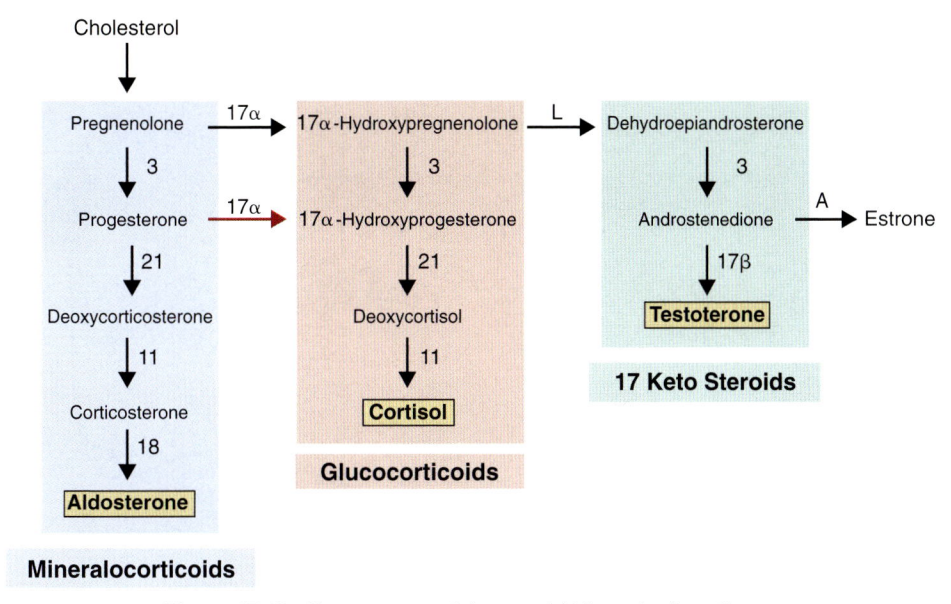

Figure 45.13 Key enzymes of the steroid biosynthesis pathway.

CONGENITAL ADRENAL HYPERPLASIA

Inherited abnormalities in steroid biosynthesis cause hypertension in some cases of congenital adrenal hyperplasia. These autosomal recessive disorders arise from deficiencies of key enzymes of the steroid biosynthesis pathway (Figure 45.13).[262,263] The decrease in cortisol production causes an increase in adrenocorticotropic hormone (ACTH) secretion and subsequent hyperplasia of the adrenal glands. The phenotypes are determined by deficiencies as well as by overproduction of steroids unaffected by the enzymatic defect. Hypertension is observed in only two of the three major subtypes of congenital adrenal hyperplasia (11β-hydroxylase and 17α-hydroxylase deficiencies), because metabolic blockade distal to 21α-hydroxylase allows the formation of 21-hydroxyl groups necessary for mineralocorticoid precursor biosynthesis. Other clinical manifestations depend on the consequences of the enzymatic defect on androgen biosynthesis with either an increase (11β-hydroxylase) or a decrease (17α-hydroxylase) in production. In both deficiencies, overproduction of cortisol precursors that are metabolized to mineralocorticoid agonists or that have intrinsic mineralocorticoid activity induce volume and salt-dependent forms of hypertension. The elevated zona fasciculata deoxycorticosterone (DOC) produces mineralocorticoid hypertension with suppressed renin and reduced potassium concentrations. Aldosterone, the most important mineralocorticoid, regulates electrolyte excretion and intravascular volume mainly through its effects on renal distal convoluted tubules and cortical collecting ducts.

11β-HYDROXYLASE DEFICIENCY

Inactivating mutations in the gene encoding 11β-hydroxylase[264,265] cause the second most common form of congenital adrenal hyperplasia (OMIM #202010), representing 5% of cases (90% are caused by 21-hydroxylase deficiency). This disorder is associated with excess production of DOC, 18-deoxycortisol, and androgens. By virtue of the significant intrinsic mineralocorticoid activity of DOC, subjects with mutations in both alleles of the gene exhibit hypokalemic hypertension. Because the androgen pathway is unaffected, prenatal masculinization occurs in female patients and postnatal virilization in both sexes. The diagnosis of 11β-hydroxylase deficiency is established by means of an ACTH test showing elevation of deoxycorticosterone and 11-deoxycortisol and marked suppression of plasma renin activity.[263] The treatment consists of exogenous corticoids that inhibit ACTH secretion.

17α-HYDROXYLASE DEFICIENCY

17α-Hydroxylase deficiency (OMIM #202110) results in reduced conversion of pregnenolone to progesterone and androgens and absence of sex hormone production.[262,266] The absence of sex hormone formation in both the adrenal glands and the gonads, which causes hypogonadism and male pseudohermaphroditism, is usually detected at adolescence because of failure to undergo puberty. Patients have a decreased ability to synthesize cortisol, leading to elevated ACTH, which increases serum levels of deoxycorticosterone and, especially, corticosterone, resulting in low-renin hypertension, hypokalemia, and metabolic alkalosis. The clinical features vary depending on the enzymatic activity affected. In severe 17α-hydroxylase deficiency, both the 17α-hydroxylase and 17,20-lyase activities are reduced or absent. This deficiency results in high mineralocorticoid activity and hypertension, and produces a female phenotype in all subjects due to the absence of sex steroid production in both the adrenal and gonads. Partial 17α-hydroxylase deficiency leads to sexual ambiguity in male patients without hypertension. Corticosteroid replacement corrects ACTH levels and hypertension. Women usually require hormonal therapy. Genetic male patients reared as female patients also require estrogen replacement. Genetic male patients reared as male patients require surgical correction of their external genitalia and androgen replacement therapy.

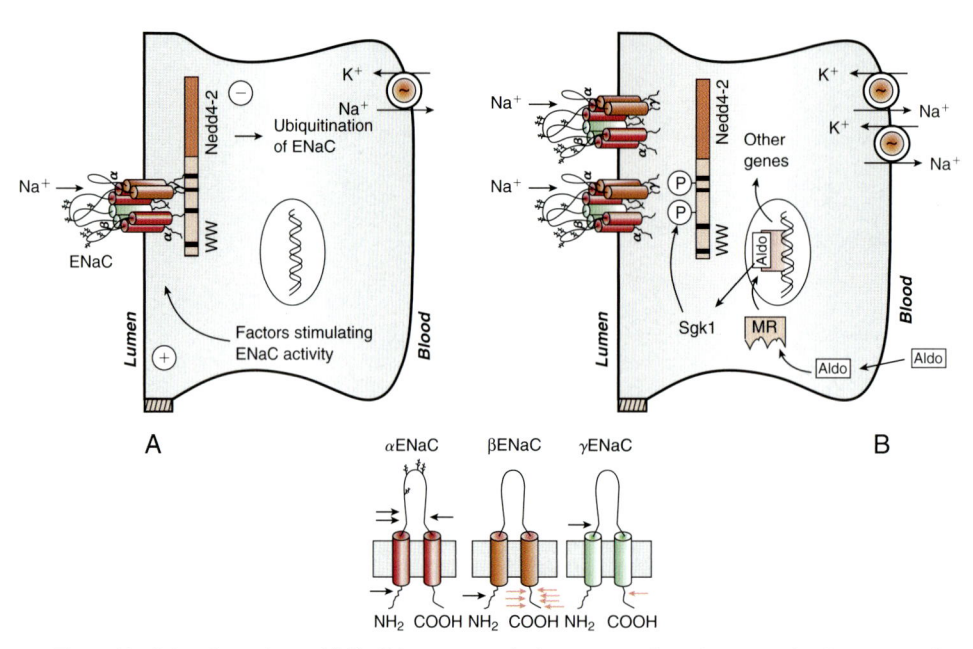

Figure 45.14 Bottom, The epithelial sodium channel (ENaC) is composed of two α, one β, and one γ-subunits surrounding the channel pore.[361] Each subunit has two transmembrane domains with short cytoplasmic amino and carboxy termini and a large ectocytoplasmic loop. Mutations in subunits of ENaC cause either Liddle's syndrome (pink arrows) (β- or γ-subunits) or the autosomal recessive form of pseudohypoaldosteronism type I (PHA I [black arrows]) (α-, β-, or γ-subunits).[251] The autosomal dominant form of PHA I is secondary to mutations in the mineralocorticoid receptor (MR) gene.[272] These ENaC and mineralocorticoid receptor mutations recapitulate the main pathway for sodium reabsorption and potassium secretion across the principal cell of the cortical and medullary collecting duct. Sodium transport in tight epithelia of the distal nephron is mediated by the ENaC and the Na$^+$-K$^+$-ATPase. The ENaC is located at the apical membrane and constitutes the rate-limiting step for electrogenic sodium transport, whereas the Na$^+$-K$^+$-ATPase, located at the basolateral membrane, creates the driving force for this process. Note that only the α-subunit is glycosylated. **Top,** The mechanism of ENaC expression in an aldosterone-sensitive epithelial cell is represented. **A,** In a resting state, few ENaCs, which facilitate sodium reabsorption in a rate-limiting fashion, are resident in the apical membrane. Factors known to enhance ENaC surface expression and activity are counterbalanced by retrieval of these channels from the membrane through the ubiquitin pathway mediated by ubiquitin-protein ligase Nedd4-2. **B,** Shortly after aldosterone exposure and binding to the mineralocorticoid receptor (MR), transcriptional stimulation of serum and glucocorticoid-regulated kinase 1 (Sgk1) leads to phosphorylation of Nedd4-2, which subsequently disrupts ENaC/Nedd4-2 interactions. In this situation, ubiquitination of ENaCs is reduced, thus favoring both their residence in the apical membrane and enhanced sodium reabsorption. Black arrows in the **lower panel** refer to the location of inactivating mutations (pseudohypoaldosteronism type I), while *pink arrows* refer to location of activating mutations (Liddle syndrome).

LIDDLE'S SYNDROME

PATHOGNESIS

Liddle's syndrome (OMIM #177200) is an autosomal dominant form of hypertension characterized by hypokalemia and low levels of plasma renin and aldosterone, resulting from either premature termination or frameshift mutations in the carboxy-terminal tail of the epithelial sodium channel (ENaC) β- or γ-subunits.[267] The amiloride-sensitive epithelial Na$^+$ channel is a tetramer formed by the assembly of three homologous subunits, α, β, and γ, with the α subunit being present in two copies (Figure 45.14).[268] The NH$_2$ and carboxy-terminal terminal segments are cytoplasmic and contain potential regulatory segments that are able to modulate the activity of the channel. Mutations in the β- and γ-subunits of ENaC lead to channel hyperactivity by deleting or altering a conserved proline-rich amino acid sequence referred to as the PY-motif. *SCNN1B* β-subunit or *SCNN1G* γ-subunit mutations could lead to an increase in the number of channels in the membrane or in their "openness." The identification of specific binding domains for Nedd4 (for all subunits) and α-spectrin (for the α-subunit only) within the cytosolic carboxy-terminal region of the ENaC subunits suggests that interactions with cytoskeletal elements control the expression of ENaC at the apical membrane.[269] Therefore, Nedd4 (neural precursor cell expressed developmentally downregulated protein 4) and α-spectrin appear to play a role in the assembly, insertion, and/or retrieval of the ENaC subunits in the plasma membrane.[270]

CLINICAL PRESENTATION

Liddle's syndrome is characterized by inappropriate renal sodium reabsorption, blunted sodium excretion, and low-renin hypertension.[268] The features of this syndrome were described by Liddle and colleagues in 1963 in a large pedigree.[271] Affected subjects are at increased risk of cerebrovascular and cardiovascular events. Liddle's syndrome can be differentiated from other rare mendelian forms of low-renin hypertension with the use of urinary/plasma hormonal profiles. Glucocorticoid-remediable aldosteronism is associated with increased production of 18-hydroxycortisol and aldosterone metabolites. Apparent mineralocorticoid excess is associated with an elevated ratio of urinary

Table 45.8 Urinary Steroid Profiles in Mendelian Forms of Low-Renin Hypertension

	Liddle's Syndrome	GRA	AME
Aldosterone	⇓⇓	⇑	⇓
TH-Aldo	⇓⇓	⇑	⇓
18-OH-TH-Aldo	⇓⇓	⇑	⇓
18-OH F	—	⇑⇑⇑	—
TH-F	nl	nl	⇑
TH-E	nl	nl	⇓
TH-F/TH-E ratio	nl	nl	⇑⇑⇑

Aldo, Aldosterone; AME, apparent mineralocorticoid excess; E, cortisone; F, cortisol; GRA, glucocorticoid-remediable aldosteronism; nl, normal; TH- tetrahydro-; —, not usually detected.
Adapted from Warnock DG: Liddle syndrome: an autosomal dominant form of human hypertension. Kidney Int 53:18-24, 1998.

cortisol (tetrahydrocortisol) to cortisone (tetrahydrocortisone) metabolites (Table 45.8).

TREATMENT

Hypertension is *not* improved by spironolactone but can be corrected by a low-salt diet and an ENaC antagonist (amiloride or triamterene).

APPARENT MINERALOCORTICOID EXCESS

PATHOGNESIS

The syndrome of apparent mineralocorticoid excess (AME; OMIM #207765) is a rare autosomal recessive disorder that results in hypokalemic hypertension with low serum levels of renin and aldosterone.[272,273] AME is caused by a deficiency in 11β-hydroxysteroid dehydrogenase type 2 enzymatic activity (11β-HSD2), which is responsible for the conversion of cortisol to the inactive metabolite cortisone, therefore protecting the mineralocorticoid receptors from cortisol intoxication. In AME, cortisol acts as a potent mineralocorticoid and causes salt retention, hypertension, and hypokalemia with a suppression of the renin angiotensin aldosterone system. A milder phenotype, or type 2 variant, also results from abnormal activity of the enzyme.[274] Cushing's syndrome and extremely high cortisol levels can overcome the ability of 11β-HSD2 to convert cortisol to cortisone.

CLINICAL PRESENTATION

AME is associated with severe juvenile low-renin hypertension, hypokalemic alkalosis, low birth weight, failure to thrive, poor growth, nephrocalcinosis, and variable degrees of polyuria.[276] The urinary metabolites of cortisol demonstrate an abnormal ratio, with predominance of cortisol metabolites (i.e., tetrahydrocortisol plus 5α-tetrahydrocortisol/tetrahydrocortisone in the range 6.7 to 33, the normal ratio being 1.0).[277] The milder form of AME (type 2) lacks the typical urinary steroid profile (i.e., biochemical analysis reveals a moderately elevated ratio of cortisol to cortisone metabolites).[274] The heterozygote state is phenotypically normal but is associated with subtle defects in cortisol metabolism.

TREATMENT

The treatment of AME is sodium restriction and either triamterene or amiloride. Spironolactone is *not* effective. Additional antihypertensive agents may be used as needed.

AUTOSOMAL DOMINANT EARLY-ONSET HYPERTENSION WITH SEVERE EXACERBATION DURING PREGNANCY

Autosomal dominant early-onset hypertension with severe exacerbation during pregnancy is a rare autosomal dominant disorder (OMIM #605115) described in a family that is associated with activating mutations in the mineralocorticoid receptor. By screening the mineralocorticoid receptor in 75 patients with early onset of severe hypertension, Geller and colleagues identified a 15-year-old boy with severe hypertension, suppressed plasma renin activity, low aldosterone, and no other underlying cause of hypertension, who had a heterozygous missense mutation (S810L) in the mineralocorticoid receptor gene.[278] Of 23 relatives evaluated, 11 had been diagnosed with severe hypertension before age 20, whereas the remaining 12 had unremarkable blood pressures. Two L810 carriers had undergone five pregnancies, all of which had been complicated by marked exacerbation of hypertension with suppressed aldosterone levels. The S810L mutation alters a conserved amino acid, resulting in a constitutively active and altered mineralocorticoid receptor. In addition, progesterone and other steroids lacking 21-hydroxyl groups, normally mineralocorticoid receptor antagonists, become potent agonists. Spironolactone is also a potent agonist of L810, so its use is contraindicated in L810 carriers.

GLUCOCORTICOID-REMEDIABLE HYPERALDOSTERONISM

PATHOGNESIS

Glucocorticoid-remediable hyperaldosteronism (GRA) is also known as familial hyperaldosteronism type I (OMIM #103900), aldosteronism sensitive to dexamethasone, glucocorticoid-suppressible hyperaldosteronism, and syndrome of ACTH-dependent hyperaldosteronism. It is an autosomal dominant hypertensive disorder caused by a chimeric gene duplication arising from unequal crossover between genes encoding aldosterone synthase and 11β-hydroxylase,[279] two highly similar genes with the same transcriptional orientation lying 45,000 base pairs apart on chromosome 8. Humans have two isozymes with 11β-hydroxylase activity that are required for synthesis of cortisol and aldosterone, respectively. CYP11B1 (11β-hydroxylase) is expressed at high levels and is regulated by ACTH, whereas CYP11B2 (aldosterone synthase) is normally expressed at low levels and is regulated by angiotensin II. In addition to 11β-hydroxylase activity, the latter enzyme has 18-hydroxylase and 18-oxidase activities and can synthesize aldosterone from deoxycorticosterone.[280] Thus, with the unequal crossover between the two genes, the aldosterone synthase gene is under the control of regulatory promoter sequences of the 11β-hydroxylase. The chimeric gene product is expressed at high levels in both the zona glomerulosa and zona fasciculata and is controlled by ACTH, leading to increased production of 18-hydroxycortisol and aldosterone metabolites.

CLINICAL PRESENTATION

The phenotype of GRA is highly variable.[281] Affected individuals may have mild hypertension and normal biochemistry and may be clinically indistinguishable from patients with essential hypertension. However, some subjects have early-onset severe hypertension, hypokalemia, and metabolic alkalosis. In a study of 376 patients from 27 genetically proven GRA pedigrees, 48% of all GRA families and 18% of all patients with GRA had cerebrovascular complications, findings similar to the frequency of aneurysm in adult polycystic kidney disease.[282] The diagnosis is usually established by measuring 18-hydroxycortisol or 18-oxocortisol metabolites in the urine or with the dexamethasone suppression test.[283] In addition, because patients with GRA secrete aldosterone in response to ACTH, glucocorticoid administration can suppress excessive aldosterone secretion.[284] The dexamethasone suppression test is a variably reliable method for establishing the diagnosis. Patients without the disease (i.e., subjects with an aldosterone-producing adenoma or with idiopathic hyperaldosteronism) can suppress aldosterone secretion.[285] The diagnosis of GRA can be definitively established by demonstration of the chimeric gene by molecular techniques.

TREATMENT

Simple glucocorticoid replacement is the treatment for GRA. Salt restriction combined with either spironolactone or ENaC inhibition is also effective.

FAMILIAL HYPERALDOSTERONISM TYPE II

Familial hyperaldosteronism type II (FH-II; OMIM #605635) is characterized by hypersecretion of aldosterone due to adrenocortical hyperplasia, an aldosterone-producing adenoma, or both. In contrast to familial hyperaldosteronism type I, FH-II is not suppressible by dexamethasone. Stowasser and colleagues reported five families with this phenotype with a segregation pattern supporting dominant inheritance.[283] Analysis of an extended kindred has revealed linkage between FH-II and markers on chromosome 7p22, but the gene implicated has not been clearly identified.[286]

PSEUDOHYPOALDOSTERONISM

PSEUDOHYPOALDOSTERONISM TYPE I

PATHOGNESIS

Pseudohypoaldosteronism type I (PHA I) is a rare disorder characterized by salt wasting, hypotension, hyperkalemia, metabolic acidosis, and failure to thrive in infants. There are two subtypes of PHA I.[287] The autosomal recessive form (OMIM #264350 and #177735) leads to severe manifestations that persist in adulthood and is caused by inactivating mutations in any of the three subunits (α, β, γ) of ENaC. The autosomal dominant form (OMIM #177735) is associated with milder manifestations that remit with age and is caused by mutations in the mineralocorticoid receptor (MR) gene[288] that result in haploinsufficiency or in dominant negative actions. Homozygous MR mutations are probably lethal in humans, because knockout mice show a severe salt wasting syndrome and die a few days after birth.[289]

CLINICAL PRESENTATION

The clinical contrast between PHA I due to ENaC and that due to MR mutations is striking.[287] Autosomal recessive PHA I manifests neonatally or in childhood as renal salt wasting, hypotension, hyperkalemia, metabolic acidosis, and, on occasion, failure to thrive. Other biologic features include hyponatremia, high plasma and urinary aldosterone levels despite hyperkalemia, and elevated plasma renin activity. Autosomal dominant PHA I is associated with milder manifestations and remits with age. PHA I must be differentiated from aldosterone synthase deficiency, salt-wasting forms of congenital adrenal hyperplasia, and adrenal hypoplasia congenita, all of which cause aldosterone deficiency and are associated with hyponatremia, hyperkalemia, hypovolemia, elevated plasma renin activity, and occasionally shock and death.[290] Bartter's syndrome type 2 (ROMK gene mutations) can also manifest in the neonatal period with a similar (transient) clinical picture.

TREATMENT

Treatment of PHA I consists of salt supplementation, which can greatly improve hyponatremia, hyperkalemia, and growth. Administration of aldosterone, fludrocortisone, or deoxycorticosterone is not helpful. Patients with the recessive form usually need lifelong treatment for salt wasting and hyperkalemia, whereas for those with the dominant form, treatment can usually be withdrawn in adulthood.

PSEUDOHYPOALDOSTERONISM TYPE II

PATHOGNESIS

Pseudohypoaldosteronism type II (PHA II; OMIM #145260), also known as familial hyperkalemia and hypertension or Gordon syndrome, is a volume-dependent, low-renin hypertension characterized by persistent hyperkalemia despite a normal renal GFR. Variants within at least four genes—the with-no-lysine-(K) kinases, WNK1 and WNK4, Cullin3, and KLHL3 (encoding the Kelch-like 3 protein)—can cause the phenotype.[291,292] Details are still emerging for some of these genes, but it is likely that they all cause a gain of function in thiazide-sensitive NCC and, hence, salt retention. Hypertension is attributable to increased renal salt reabsorption, and hyperkalemia to reduced renal K^+ excretion. Reduced renal H^+ secretion is also commonly seen, resulting in metabolic acidosis. The features of PHA II are chloride dependent, because they are corrected when infusion of sodium sulfate or sodium bicarbonate is substituted for sodium chloride.[293]

WNK1 and WNK4 function as molecular switches, eliciting coordinated effects on diverse ion transport pathways to maintain homeostasis during physiologic perturbation. In PHA II, mutations that appear to activate WNK1 and inactivate WNK4 have been proposed to result in increased thiazide-sensitive cotransporter (TSC) activity and decreased ROMK activity (Figure 45.15).[294] Kelch-like 3 and Cullin 3

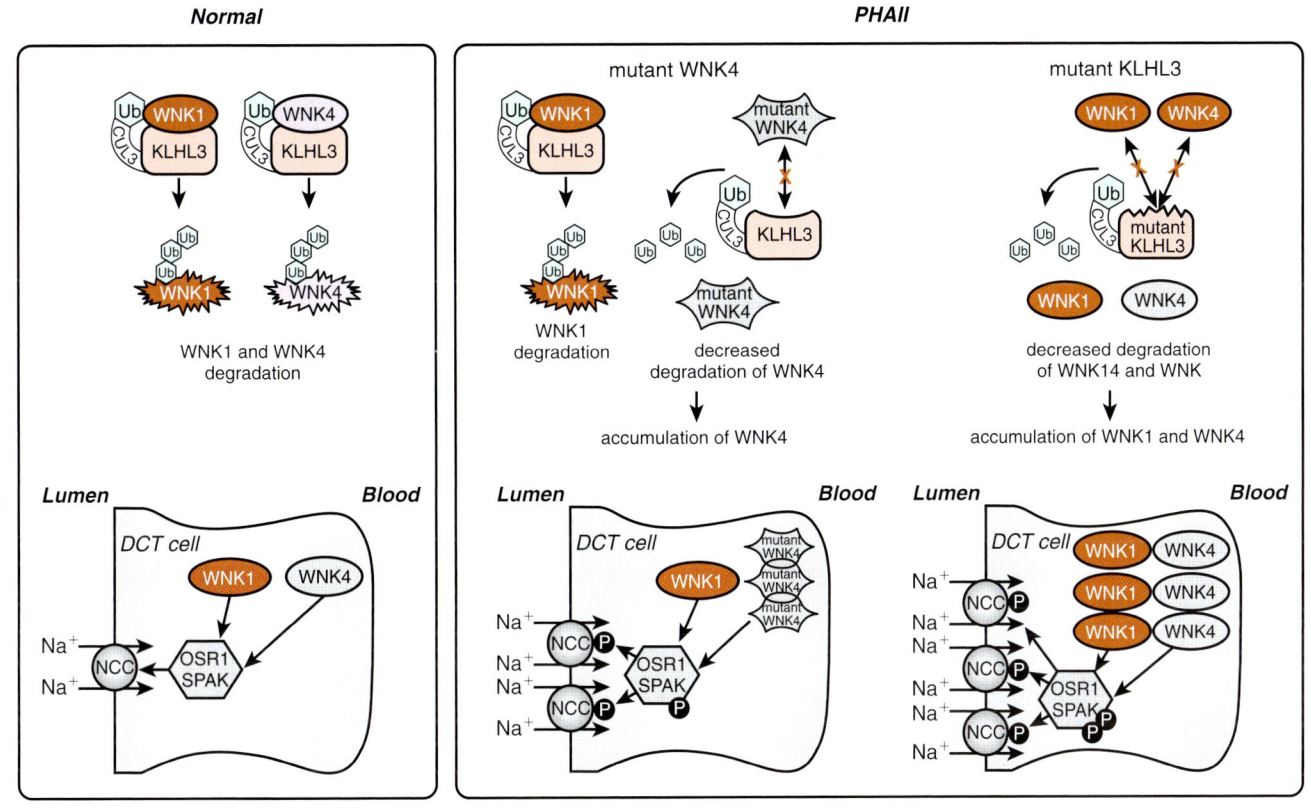

Figure 45.15 Molecular mechanism of pseudohypoaldosteronism type II in the distal convoluted tubule. Left, Normally kinases WNK1 and WNK4 can stimulate Na-Cl cotransporter (NCC) trafficking to the plasma membrane and phosphorylation of NCC by Ste20-related proline alanine-rich kinase (SPAK) and oxidative stress–responsive kinase (OSR1). This is the WNK-OSR1/SPAK-NCC phosphorylation signaling cascade, recognized now as the major pathogenic mechanism of pseudohypoaldosteronism type II (PHA II) (shown at right). WNK1 and WNK4 are substrates of KLH$_3$ (Kelch-like 3)–Cullin3 E3 ligase–mediated ubiquitination. Not represented here are (1) the downregulation of ROMK by increased WNK activity, resulting in decreased K$^+$ excretion, and (2) increase in sodium reabsorption and decrease in potassium secretion leading to urinary hydrogen excretion, which causes metabolic acidosis. DCT, Distal convoluted tubule; Ub, ubiquitin. (From Susa K, Sohara E, Rai T, et al: Impaired degradation of WNK1 and WNK4 kinases causes PHAII in mutant KLHL3 knock-in mice. *Hum Mol Genet* 23:5052-5060, 2014; and Pathare G, Hoenderop JG, Bindels RJ, et al: A molecular update on pseudohypoaldosteronism type II. *Am J Physiol Renal Physiol* 305:F1513-F1520, 2013.)

regulate electrolyte homeostasis via ubiquitination and degradation of WNK1 and WNK4.[295,296] On one hand is the overactivity of TSC and on the other is the increased paracellular reabsorption of Cl$^-$, also known as the *chloride shunt* hypothesis. The action of these kinases may serve to increase salt reabsorption and intravascular volume in volume-depleted states and decrease potassium secretion in K depletion, by enabling the distal nephron to allow either maximal NaCl reabsorption or maximal K$^+$ secretion in response to hypovolemia or hyperkalemia, respectively.

CLINICAL PRESENTATION

PHA II is usually diagnosed in adults but can also be seen neonatally.[297] Unexplained hyperkalemia is the usual presenting feature and occurs prior to the onset of hypertension. The severity of hyperkalemia varies greatly and is influenced by prior intake of diuretics and salt.[298] Causes of spurious elevation of potassium should be ruled out before this diagnosis is made. In its most severe form, PHA II is associated with muscle weakness (from hyperkalemia), short stature, and intellectual impairment. Mild hyperchloremia, metabolic acidosis, and suppressed plasma renin activity are findings variably associated with the trait. Aldosterone levels vary from low to high depending on the level of hyperkalemia. Urinary concentrating ability, acid excretion, and proximal tubular function are all normal.

TREATMENT

Thiazides reverse all biochemical abnormalities. Lower than average doses can be given if overcorrection occurs. Loop diuretics may also be used.

INHERITED DISORDERS OF RENAL MAGNESIUM PROCESSING

Magnesium, the second most abundant intracellular cation, plays an important role as a cofactor in energy metabolism, nucleotide and protein synthesis, neuromuscular excitability, and oxidative phosphorylation and as a regulator of sodium, potassium, and calcium channels. Under normal conditions, extracellular magnesium concentration is maintained at nearly constant values (0.70 to 1.1 mmol/L). Hypomagnesemia results from decreased dietary intake but more commonly is caused by intestinal malabsorption, renal losses, or use of drugs including cyclosporine, omeprazole, cetuximab, and cisplatin.[299]

Primary hypomagnesemia is composed of a heterogeneous group of disorders characterized by renal and intestinal Mg wasting often associated with hypercalciuria (Table 45.9).[299-303] The genetic basis and cellular defects of a number of primary hypomagnesemias have been elucidated. These inherited conditions affect different nephron segments and different cell types, leading to variable but increasingly distinguishable phenotypic presentations.

FAMILIAL HYPOMAGNESEMIA WITH HYPERCALCIURIA AND NEPHROCALCINOSIS

The syndrome of renal hypomagnesemia with hypercalciuria and nephrocalcinosis (OMIM #248250), or familial hypomagnesemia with hypercalciuria and nephrocalcinosis (FHHNC), is a rare autosomal recessive trait characterized by profound Mg wasting that results in severe hypomagnesemia not correctable by oral or intravenous magnesium supplementation. The disorder is caused by mutations in claudin-16 (CLDN16), previously known as paracellin-1,[304] a protein located in tight junctions of the TAL and related to the claudin family of tight junction proteins (see Figure 45.10). A study of nine additional families with severe hypomagnesemia identified mutations in CLDN19 (OMIM #24190) that share the same renal phenotype as FHHNC. CLDN19 encodes claudin-19, a tight junction protein expressed in renal tubules and the eye.[305]

Every patient with FHHNC has hypomagnesemia with inappropriately high urinary Mg excretion (Mg^+ fractional excretions above 10%). Renal calcium wasting is present in every case initially and leads to parenchymal calcification (nephrocalcinosis) and renal failure, often requiring dialysis. The progression rate of renal insufficiency correlates with the severity of nephrocalcinosis. Other clinical findings are polyuria, polydipsia, ocular abnormalities, recurrent urinary tract infections, and renal colic with stone passage. Serum PTH levels are abnormally high. Serum levels of calcium, phosphorus, and potassium and urinary excretion of uric acid and oxalate are normal. In contrast to patients with a CLDN16 defect, affected individuals with a CLDN19 mutation have ocular symptoms that include severe visual impairment, macular colobomata, horizontal nystagmus, and marked myopia.[305] Long-term oral Mg administration does not normalize serum Mg^{2+} levels. Thiazides are effective to reduce urinary Ca excretion.[306] After kidney graft, tubular handling of Mg^{2+} and Ca is normal.

FAMILIAL HYPOMAGNESEMIA WITH SECONDARY HYPOCALCEMIA

Familial hypomagnesemia with secondary hypocalcemia (OMIM #602014) is an autosomal recessive disease that results in electrolyte abnormalities shortly after birth and is caused by mutations in TRPM6 (Figure 45.16). TRPM6 holds 39 exons that code for a protein of 2022 amino acids. Affected individuals show extremely low serum Mg^{2+} levels (0.1 to 0.3 mmol/L) and hypocalcemia, causing muscular and neurologic complications including seizures in early infancy that can lead to neurologic damage or cardiac arrest if left untreated. The disorder is caused by impaired intestinal uptake and renal Mg^{2+} wasting.[307] Restoring the concentrations of serum magnesium to normal values with high-dose magnesium supplementation can overcome the apparent defect in magnesium absorption and in serum concentrations of calcium. Life-long magnesium supplementation is required to overcome the defect in the seizures and magnesium handling in these individuals.

ISOLATED DOMINANT HYPOMAGNESEMIA WITH HYPOCALCIURIA

A rare autosomal dominant disorder, isolated dominant hypomagnesemia with hypocalciuria (OMIM #154020) is caused by a dominant negative mutation of the FXYD2 gene resulting in a trafficking defect of the γ-subunit of the Na^+-K^+-ATPase at the basolateral membrane of the distal convoluted tubule,[308] the main sites of active renal Mg^{2+} reabsorption. The hypomagnesemia in patients with the disorder can be as low as 0.40 mmol/L, resulting in convulsions. Mutation of FXYD2 leads to misrouting of the Na^+/K^+-ATPase γ-subunit, so Mg^{2+} reabsorption is abnormal. Hypomagnesemic patients have lower urinary excretion of calcium, presumably as a consequence of increased reabsorption in the loop of Henle.[309]

The transcription factor hepatocyte nuclear factor 1 homeobox B (HNF1B) has been linked to the regulation of the FXYD2 gene, and hypomagnesemia, hypermagnesuria, and hypocalciuria have been observed in 44% of HNF1B mutation carriers (OMIM #137920). Mutations have also been described in PCBD1, which encodes hepatocyte nuclear factor 1 homeobox A (PCBD1) (see Figure 45.16).[310]

Ca^{2+}/Mg^{2+}-SENSING RECEPTOR–ASSOCIATED DISORDERS

An important regulator of magnesium homeostasis is the Ca^{2+}/Mg^{2+}(calcium)–sensing receptor (CaSR). CaSR senses ionized serum calcium and magnesium concentrations and is involved in renal calcium and magnesium reabsorption as well as in PTH secretion.[311] Activating mutations of the CaSR gene were first described in families affected with autosomal dominant hypocalcemia.[240,312] Affected individuals present with hypocalcemia, hypercalciuria, and polyuria, and approximately 50% of them have hypomagnesemia.[302] Clinically, autosomal dominant hypocalcemia may be mistaken for primary hypoparathyroidism, because of the decreased PTH secretion in the setting of mild to moderate hypocalcemia. Most affected individuals have hypomagnesemia and renal magnesium wasting.

ISOLATED RECESSIVE HYPOMAGNESEMIA WITH NORMOCALCIURIA

Isolated recessive hypomagnesemia (IRH; OMIM #131530) is a rare hereditary disease that was originally described in a consanguineous family.[313] The affected individuals presented with symptoms of hypomagnesemia during early infancy. IRH is caused by a mutation of the epidermal growth factor (EGF) precursor protein pro-EGF, which is expressed in the gastrointestinal tract, the respiratory tract, and the basolateral membrane of the distal convoluted

Table 45.9 Inherited Disorders of Magnesium Transport

Disease/OMIM* Entry	Gene/Inheritance	Protein	Key Clinical/Biochemical Symptoms
Gitelman's syndrome/#263800	SLC12A3/AR	NCC	Muscle weakness/tetany Fatigue Chondrocalcinoisis Hypomagnesemia Hypocalciuria
Familial hypomagnesemia with hypercalciuria and nephrocalcinosis/#248250/#248190	CLDN16/AR CLDN19/AR	Claudin-16 Claudin-19	Polyuria Renal stones/nephrocalcinosis Ocular abnormalities Severe hypomagnesemia Hypercalciuria
Autosomal dominant isolated renal Mg loss/#154020	FXYD2/AD	γ-Subunit sodium-potassium ATPase	Seizures Chondrocalcinosis Hypomagnesemia Hypocalciuria
Autosomal dominant hypomagnesemia, hypermagnesemia, and hypocalcinuria/#137920	HNF1B/AD	Transcription factor hepatocyte nuclear factor 1 homeobox B (HNF1B) is linked to the regulation of FXYD2	
Maturity-onset diabetes of the young (MODY) with hypomagnesemia and renal Mg^{2+} loss/#126090	PCBD1/AR	Hepatocyte nuclear factor 1 homeobox A (PCBD1)	
Familial hypomagnesemia with secondary hypocalcemia/#602014	TRPM6/AR	Epithelial magnesium channel TRPM6	Tetany/seizures Hypomagnesemia Hypocalcemia
Autosomal recessive isolated Mg loss/#611718	EGF/AR	Epidermal growth factor	Tetany/seizures Hypomagnesemia Normocalciuria
Autosomal dominant hypomagnesemia/#176260	KCNA1/AD	Voltage-gated potassium channel Kv1.1	Muscle cramps Tetany Tremor Muscle weakness Cerebral atrophy Myokymia
Epilepsy, ataxia, sensorineural deafness and tubulopathy (EAST)/#612780	KCNJ10/AR	K^+ channel Kir4.1	Polyuria Hypokalemic metabolic alkalosis Hypomagnesemia Hypocalciuria
Dominant and recessive hypomagnesemia with impaired brain development and seizures/#607803	CNNM2/AD/AR	CNNM2 Mg-ATP	Mental retardation Seizures

AD, Autosomal dominant; AR, autosomal recessive; ATP, adenosine triphosphate; CLDN, claudin; CNNM2, cyclin M2; EGF, epidermal growth factor; FXYD2, FXYD domain–containing ion transport regulator 2; NCC, Na-Cl cotransporter; OMIM, Online Mendelian Inheritance in Man; SLC, solute carrier; TRPM6, transient receptor potential channel 6.
*OMIM numbers. Available at http://www.ncbi.nlm.gov/omim/OMIM.

tubule. On membrane insertion, pro-EGF is processed by unknown proteases into a functional EGF peptide hormone, which activates EGF receptors (EGFRs) on the basolateral membrane (see Figure 45.16). As a result, EGF stimulates the trafficking of TRPM6 channels to the luminal membrane, increasing the reabsorption of Mg^{2+} through TRPM6.[299]

DOMINANT AND RECESSIVE HYPOMAGNESEMIA

Dominant and recessive hypomagnesemia with impaired brain development (recessive) and seizures secondary to CNNM2 mutations (OMIM #607803). Mutations in the gene encoding cyclin M2 (CNNM2) have been found in two unrelated families with dominant isolated hypomagnesemia, mental retardation, and seizures.[314] Recessive forms have also been identified.[315]

DIABETES INSIPIDUS

PATHOGENESIS

The conservation of water by the human kidney is regulated by the action of the neurohypophyseal antidiuretic hormone arginine vasopressin (AVP) on renal medulla cells of the collecting tubules.[316] AVP has multiple cellular actions, including the inhibition of diuresis, contraction of smooth

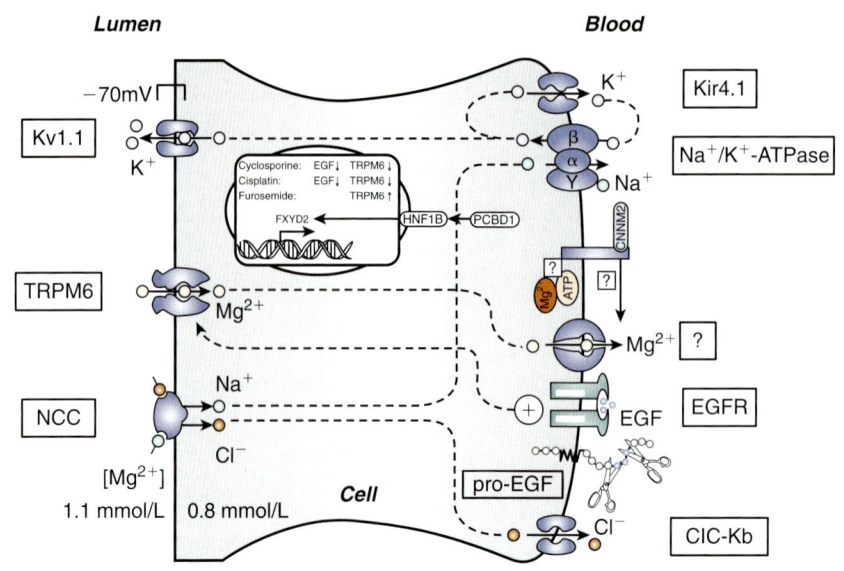

Figure 45.16 Magnesium reabsorption in the distal convoluted tubule. Transient receptor potential 6 (TRPM6) channels, located in the luminal membrane, facilitate transport of Mg^{2+} from the pro-urine into the cell, which is driven primarily by the luminal membrane potential established by the voltage-gated K^+ channel Kv1.1. Epidermal growth factor (EGF) and insulin function as magnesiotropic hormones, stimulating TRPM6 activity through activation of the PI3K-Akt pathway. Insulin can also act on TRPM6 via phosphorylation of cyclin-dependent kinase 5 (CDK5). The expression of TRPM6 in the distal convoluted tubule (DCT) is affected by treatment with furosemide, cyclosporine A, and cisplatin; the last two have been shown to also downregulate EGF levels. The Mg^{2+} buffering and extrusion systems are not yet known. CNNM2, the gene encoding cyclin M2, is suggested as playing a role in the Mg^{2+} extrusion and can bind Mg–adenosine triphosphate (ATP), which might play a role in this process. Transcription factor HNF1B, together with its regulator PCBD1, is proposed to regulate the expression of FXYD2, which encodes the γ-subunit of the Na^+/K^+-ATPase. ClC-Kb, Basolateral chloride channel b; EGFR, EGF receptor; NCC, Na-Cl Cotransporter. (Redrawn from van der Wijst J, Bindels RJ, Hoenderop JG: Mg^{2+} homeostasis: the balancing act of TRPM6. *Current Opinion Nephrol Hypertens* 23:361-369, 2014; and Glaudemans B, Knoers NV, Hoenderop JG, et al: New molecular players facilitating Mg(2+) reabsorption in the distal convoluted tubule. *Kidney Int* 77:17-22, 2010.)

muscle, aggregation of platelets, stimulation of liver glycogenolysis, and modulation of ACTH release from the pituitary, as well as central regulation of somatic functions (thermoregulation and blood pressure) and modulation of social and reproductive behavior.[317] In the kidney, the important function of AVP is to promote urinary concentration by allowing water to be transported passively down an osmotic gradient between the tubular fluid and the surrounding interstitium.

THE AVP-AVPR2-AQP SHUTTLE PATHWAY

Water homeostasis in the kidney is regulated by three key proteins. AVP, secreted from the posterior pituitary, activates the process of water excretion by binding to the vasopressin V_2 receptor (AVPR2; see Figure 45.17) located on the basolateral membrane of collecting duct cells. This step activates the stimulatory G protein (G_s) and adenylyl cyclase, resulting in the production of cyclic AMP (cAMP) and stimulation of protein kinase A (PKA). The final step in the antidiuretic action of AVP is the exocytic insertion of a specific water channel, aquaporin-2 (AQP2), into the luminal membrane, thereby increasing the water permeability of that membrane. These water channels are members of a superfamily of integral membrane proteins that facilitate water transport.[318,319] Six aquaporins are expressed in the kidney, AQP1, AQP2, AQP3, AQP6, AQP7, and AQP11.[319] Aquaporin-1 (AQP1), also known as CHIP (channel-forming integral protein) was the first protein shown to function as a molecular water channel and is constitutively expressed in mammalian red blood cells, renal proximal tubules, thin descending limbs of the loop of Henle, and other water-permeable epithelia.[320]

Murata and colleagues described an atomic model of AQP1 at 3.8 Å resolution,[321] and "real-time" molecular dynamic simulations of water permeation through human AQP1 were conducted by de Groot and Grubmüller.[322] The latter proposed that conserved fingerprint (asparagine-proline-alanine [NPA]) motifs form a selectivity-determining region, and that a second (aromatic/arginine) region functions as a proton filter. These data have solved a long-standing physiologic puzzle—how membranes can be freely permeable to water but impermeable to protons. AQP2 is the vasopressin-regulated water channel in renal collecting ducts. It is exclusively present in principal cells of inner medullary collecting duct cells and is diffusely distributed in the cytoplasm in the euhydrated condition, whereas apical staining of AQP2 is intensified in the dehydrated condition or after vasopressin administration. These observations are thought to represent the exocytic insertion of preformed water channels from intracellular vesicles into the apical plasma membrane (the shuttle hypothesis) (see Figure 45.17).

The short-term regulation of AQP2 by AVP involves the movement of AQP2 from the intracellular vesicles to the luminal membrane; in the long-term regulation, which requires a sustained elevation of circulating AVP for 24

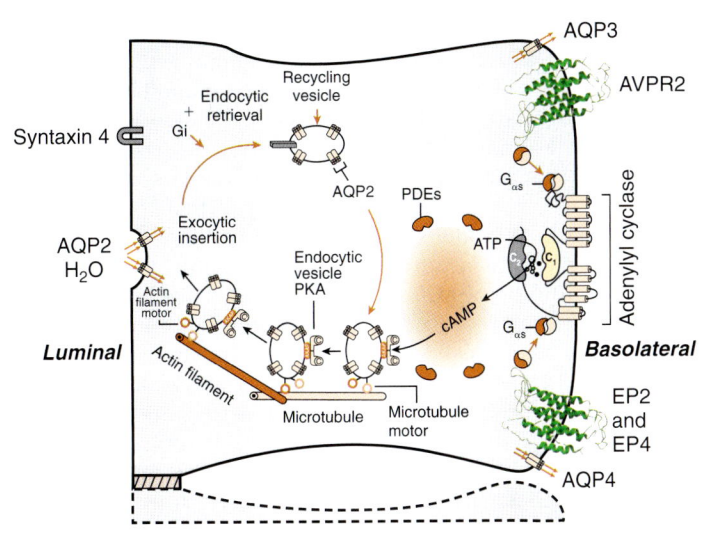

Figure 45.17 Schematic representation of the effect of vasopressin to increase water permeability in the principal cells of the collecting duct. Vasopressin (AVP) is bound to the V₂ receptor (AVPR2, a G protein–coupled receptor) on the basolateral membrane. The basic process of G protein–coupled receptor signaling consists of three steps: (1) a hepta-helical receptor detects a ligand (in this case, AVP) in the extracellular milieu; (2) a G protein ($G_{\alpha s}$) dissociates into a subunit bound to guanosine triphosphate (GTP) and G$\beta\gamma$ subunits after interaction with the ligand-bound receptor; and (3) an effector (in this case, adenylyl cyclase) interacts with dissociated G protein subunits to generate small-molecule second messengers. AVP activates adenylyl cyclase, increasing the intracellular concentration of cyclic adenosine monophosphate (cAMP). The topology of adenylyl cyclase is characterized by two tandem repeats of six hydrophobic transmembrane domains separated by a large cytoplasmic loop and terminates in a large intracellular tail. The dimeric structure (C_1 and C_2) of the catalytic domains is represented. Conversion of ATP to cAMP takes place at the dimer interface. Two aspartate residues (in C_1) coordinate two metal co-factors (Mg^{2+} or Mn^{2+}, represented here as two *small black circles*), which enable the catalytic function of the enzyme. Adenosine is shown as a *large open circle* and the three phosphate groups (ATP) as *small open circles*. Protein kinase A (PKA) is the target of the generated cAMP. The binding of cAMP to the regulatory subunits of PKA induces a conformational change, causing these subunits to dissociate from the catalytic subunits. These activated subunits as shown here are anchored to an aquaporin-2 (AQP2)–containing endocytic vesicle via an A-kinase anchoring protein. The local concentration and distribution of the cAMP gradient is limited by phosphodiesterases (PDEs). Cytoplasmic vesicles carrying the water channels (represented as homotetrameric complexes) are fused to the luminal membrane in response to AVP, thereby increasing the water permeability of this membrane. The dissociation of the A-kinase anchoring protein from the endocytic vesicle is not represented. Microtubules and actin filaments are necessary for vesicle movement toward the membrane. When AVP is not available, AQP2 water channels are retrieved by an endocytic process, and water permeability returns to its original low rate. Aquaporin-3 (AQP3) and aquaporin-4 (AQP4) water channels are expressed constitutively at the basolateral membrane. Other G protein–coupled receptors, such as prostaglandin receptors EP2 and EP4, and the secretin receptor, may also contribute to an increase in intracellular cAMP. Gi, Inhibitory guanine nucleotide-binding protein.

hours or more, AVP increases the abundance of water channels. This increase is thought to be a consequence of increased transcription of the *AQP2* gene.[323] AQP3 and AQP4 are the water channels in basolateral membranes of renal medullary collecting ducts. In addition, vasopressin increases the water reabsorptive capacity of the kidney by regulating the urea transporter UT-A1, which is expressed in the inner medullary collecting duct, predominantly in its terminal part.[324] AVP also increases the permeability of principal collecting duct cells to sodium.[325] In summary, in the absence of AVP stimulation, collecting duct epithelia exhibit very low permeabilities to sodium, urea, and water. These specialized permeability properties permit the excretion of large volumes of hypotonic urine formed during intervals of water diuresis. In contrast, AVP stimulation of the principal cells of the collecting ducts leads to selective increases in the permeabilities of the apical membrane to water (P_f), urea (P_{Urea}), and sodium (P_{Na}).

In neurohypophyseal diabetes insipidus, termed *familial neurohypophyseal diabetes insipidus* (FNDI), levels of AVP are insufficient, and patients show a positive response to treatment with desmopressin (DDAVP). Growth retardation might be observed in untreated children with autosomal dominant FNDI (adFNDI).[326] More than 50 mutations in the prepro-arginine-vasopressin-neurophysin II *AVP* gene located on chromosome 20p13 have been reported in adFNDI. Knock-in mice heterozygous for a nonsense mutation in the AVP carrier protein neurophysin II showed progressive loss of AVP-producing neurons over several months that correlated with increased water intake, increased urine output, and decreased urine osmolality. The data suggest that vasopressin mutants accumulate as fibrillar aggregates in the ER and cause cumulative toxicity to magnocellular neurons, explaining the later age of onset.[327,328]

To date, recessive FNDI has been described in only two studies.[329,330] A study by Christensen and colleagues examining the differences in cellular trafficking between dominant and recessive AVP mutants found that dominant forms were concentrated in the cytoplasm whereas recessive forms were localized to the tips of neurites.[331] The expression of regulated secretory proteins such as granins and prohormones, including pro-vasopressin, generates granule-like structures in a variety of neuroendocrine cell lines because of aggregation in the trans-Golgi network.[332] Co-staining experiments unambiguously distinguished between these granule-like structures and the accumulations by pathogenic dominant mutants formed in the ER, because the latter, but not the trans-Golgi granules, co-localized with specific ER markers.[327]

As studies concerning both dominant and recessive FNDI accumulate, it is becoming evident that FNDI exhibits a variable age of onset, which may be related to the cellular handling of the mutant AVP. This progressive toxicity, sometimes called a *toxic gain of function*, shares mechanistic pathways with other neurodegenerative diseases such as Huntington's and Parkinson's.

In nephrogenic diabetes insipidus (NDI), AVP values are normal or elevated, but the kidney is unable to concentrate urine. The clinical manifestations of polyuria and polydipsia can be present at birth and must be immediately recognized to avoid severe episodes of dehydration. Most (>90%) of patients with congenital NDI have X-linked mutations in the *AVPR2* gene, the Xq28 gene coding for the vasopressin V_2 (antidiuretic) receptor. In less than 10% of the families studied, congenital NDI has an autosomal recessive inheritance, and approximately 42 mutations have been identified in the AQP2 gene *(AQP2)*, located in chromosome region 12q13.[333] For the *AVPR2* gene, 211 putative disease-causing mutations in 326 unrelated families with X-linked NDI have now been published. When studied in vitro, most *AVPR2* mutations lead to receptors that are trapped intracellularly and are unable to reach the plasma membrane.[334] A minority of the mutant receptors reach the cell surface but are unable to bind AVP or to trigger an intracellular cAMP signal. Similarly, AQP2 mutant proteins are trapped intracellularly and cannot be expressed at the luminal membrane. This AQP2 trafficking defect is correctable, at least in vitro, by chemical chaperones. Other inherited disorders with mild, moderate, or severe inability to concentrate urine include Bartter's syndrome (MIM 601678),[243] cystinosis, autosomal dominant hypocalcemia,[36,302] nephronophthisis, and apparent mineralocorticoid excess.[276]

CLINICAL PRESENTATION AND HISTORY OF X-LINKED NEPHROGENIC DIABETES INSIPIDUS

X-linked NDI (OMIM #304800) is secondary to *AVPR2* mutations, which result in a loss of function or dysregulation of the V_2 receptor.[335] Male patients who have an *AVPR2* mutation have a phenotype characterized by early dehydration episodes, hypernatremia, and hyperthermia as early as the first week of life. Dehydration episodes can be so severe that they lower arterial blood pressure to a degree that is not sufficient to sustain adequate oxygenation to the brain, kidneys, and other organs. Mental and physical retardation and renal failure are the classic "historical" consequences of a late diagnosis and lack of treatment. Heterozygous female patients may exhibit variable degrees of polyuria and polydipsia because of skewed X chromosome inactivation.[336]

The "historical" clinical characteristics include hypernatremia, hyperthermia, mental retardation, and repeated episodes of dehydration in early infancy.[337] Mental retardation, a consequence of repeated episodes of dehydration, was prevalent in the Crawford and Bode study, which found that only 9 of 82 patients (11%) had normal intelligence.[337] Early recognition and treatment of X-linked NDI with an abundant intake of water allows a normal life span with normal physical and mental development.[338] Two characteristics suggestive of X-linked NDI are the familial occurrence and the confinement of mental retardation to male patients. It is then tempting to assume that the family described in 1892 by McIlraith and discussed by Reeves and Andreoli was a family with X-linked NDI.[339,340] Lacombe and Weil described a familial form of diabetes insipidus with autosomal transmission and without any associated mental retardation.[341,342] The descendants of the family originally described by Weil were later found to have neurohypophyseal adFNDI (OMIM #192340).[343] Patients with adFNDI retain some limited capacity to secrete AVP during severe dehydration, and the polyuropolydipsic symptoms usually appear after the first year of life, when the infant's demand for water is more likely to be understood by adults.

The severity in infancy of NDI was clearly described by Crawford and Bode.[337] The first manifestations of the disease can be recognized during the first week of life. The infants are irritable, cry almost constantly, and although eager to suck, will vomit milk soon after ingestion unless prefed with water. The history given by the mothers often includes persistent constipation, erratic unexplained fever, and failure to gain weight. Even though the patients characteristically show no visible evidence of perspiration, increased water loss during fever or in warm weather exaggerates the symptoms. Unless the condition is recognized early, children experience frequent bouts of hypertonic dehydration, sometimes complicated by convulsions or death. Mental retardation is a common consequence of these episodes. The intake of large quantities of water, combined with the patient's voluntary restriction of dietary salt and protein intake, lead to hypocaloric dwarfism beginning in infancy. Affected children frequently have lower urinary tract dilation and obstruction, probably secondary to the large volume of urine produced. Dilation of the lower urinary tract is also seen in patients with primary polydipsia and in patients with neurogenic diabetes insipidus.[344,345] Chronic renal insufficiency may occur by the end of the first decade of life and could be the result of episodes of dehydration with thrombosis of the glomerular tufts.[337] More than 20 years ago the authors' group observed that the administration of desmopressin, a V_2 receptor agonist, caused an increase in plasma cAMP concentrations in normal subjects but had no effect in 14 male patients with X-linked NDI.[346] Intermediate responses were observed in obligate carriers of the disease, possibly corresponding to half of the normal receptor response. On the basis of these results, our group predicted that the defective gene in these patients with X-linked NDI was likely to code for a defective V_2 receptor (Figure 45.18).[346]

X-linked NDI is a rare disease, with an estimated prevalence of approximately 8.8 per million male live births in the province of Quebec (Canada).[336] In defined regions of North America, the prevalence is much higher. Our group estimated the incidence in Nova Scotia and New Brunswick (Canada) to be 58 per million male live births because of shared ancestry.[336] An additional example has been identified in a Mormon pedigree whose members reside in Utah (Utah families). This pedigree was originally described by Cannon.[347] The "Utah mutation" is a nonsense mutation (L312X) predictive of a receptor that lacks transmembrane domain 7 and the intracellular COOH-terminus.[348] The largest known kindred with X-linked NDI is the Hopewell family, named after the Irish ship *Hopewell*, which arrived in Halifax, Nova Scotia, in 1761.[349] Aboard the ship were members of the Ulster Scot clan, descendants of Scottish

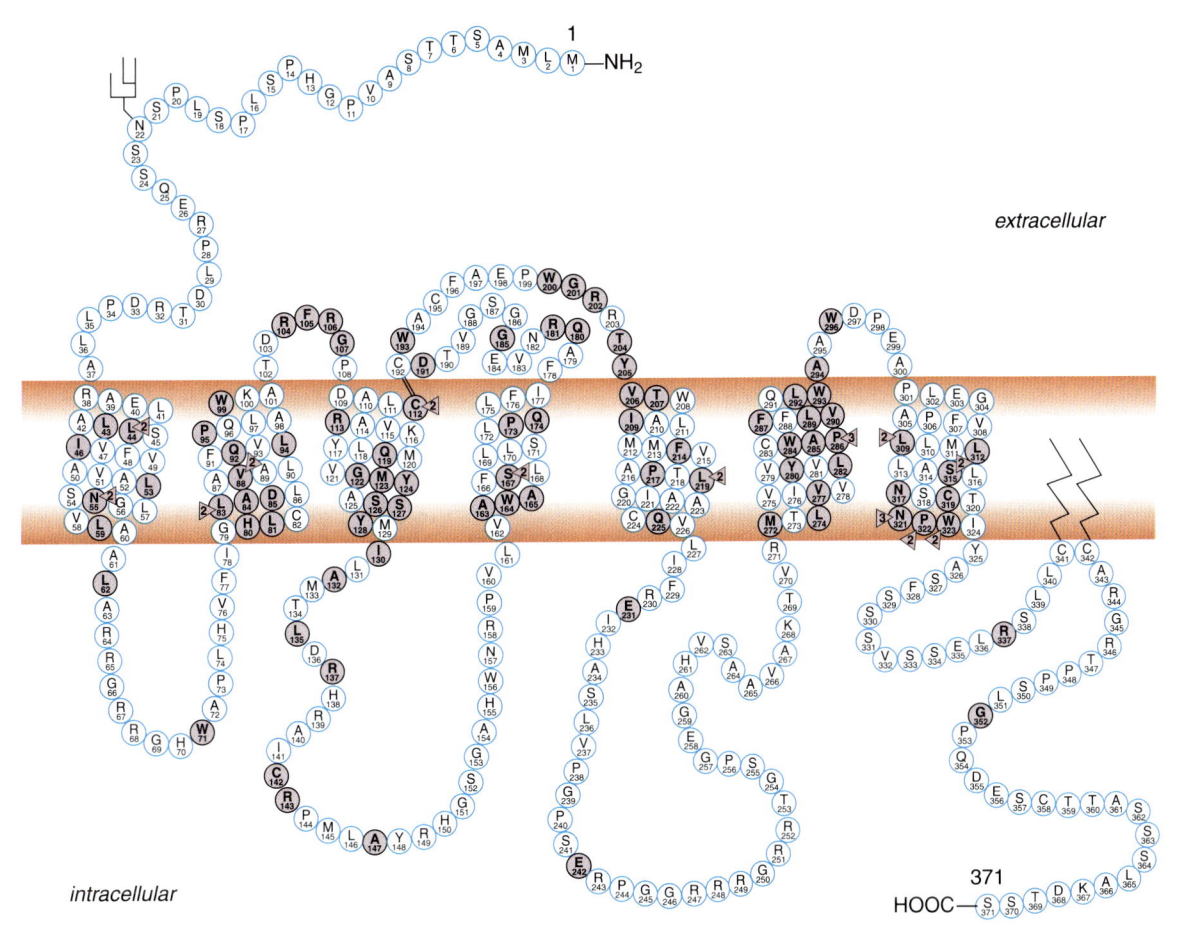

Figure 45.18 Schematic representation of the V_2 receptor (AVPR2) and identification of 193 putative disease-causing AVPR2 mutations. Predicted amino acids are shown as their one-letter amino acid codes. A **solid symbol** indicates a codon with a missense or nonsense mutation; a **number** (within a triangle) indicates more than one mutation in the same codon; other types of mutations are not indicated on the figure. There are 95 missense, 18 nonsense, 46 frameshift deletion or in-sertion, 7 in-frame deletion or insertion, 4 splice-site, and 22 large deletion mutations, and one complex mutation.

Presbyterians who migrated to Ulster province in Ireland in the seventeenth century and left Ireland for the New World in the eighteenth century. Although families arriving with the first emigration wave settled in northern Massachusetts in 1718, the members of a second emigration wave, passengers of the *Hopewell*, settled in Colchester County, Nova Scotia. According to the "Hopewell hypothesis,"[349] most patients with NDI in North America are progeny of female carriers of the second emigration wave. This assumption is based mainly on the high prevalence of NDI among descendants of the Ulster Scots residing in Nova Scotia. In two villages with a total of 2500 inhabitants, 30 patients have been diagnosed, and the carrier frequency has been estimated at 6%.

Given the numerous mutations found in North American X-linked NDI families, the Hopewell hypothesis cannot be upheld in its originally proposed form. However, among X-linked NDI patients in North America, the W71X mutation (the Hopewell mutation) is more common than the other *AVPR2* mutation. It is a null mutation (W71X), predictive of an extremely truncated receptor consisting of the extracellular NH_2-terminus, the first transmembrane domain, and the NH_2-terminal half of the first intracellular loop.[348,350] Because the original carrier cannot be identified, it is not clear whether the Hopewell mutation was brought to North America by *Hopewell* passengers or by other Ulster Scot immigrants. The diversity of *AVPR2* mutations found in many ethnic groups (whites, Japanese, African Americans, and Africans), and the low frequency of the disease are consistent with an X-linked recessive disease that in the past was lethal for male patients and was balanced by recurrent mutations. In X-linked NDI, loss of mutant alleles from the population occurs because of the higher mortality of affected male patients compared with healthy male patients, whereas gain of mutant alleles occurs by mutation. If affected male patients with a rare X-linked recessive disease do not reproduce and if mutation rates are equal in mothers and fathers, then, at genetic equilibrium, one third of new cases in affected male patients will be caused by new mutations. Our group has described ancestral mutations, de novo mutations, and potential mechanisms of mutagenesis.[336] These data are reminiscent of those obtained from patients with late-onset autosomal dominant retinitis pigmentosa. In one fourth of patients, the disease is caused by mutations in the light receptor rhodopsin. Here, too, many different mutations (approximately 100) spread throughout the coding region of the rhodopsin gene have been found.[351]

The basis of loss of function or dysregulation of 28 different mutant V_2 receptors (including nonsense, frameshift, deletion, and missense mutations) has been studied with the use of in vitro expression systems. Most of the mutant V$_2$ receptors tested were not transported to the cell membrane and were retained within the intracellular compartment. Our group also demonstrated that misfolded *AVPR2* mutants could be rescued in vitro but also in vivo by nonpeptide vasopressin antagonists acting as pharmacologic chaperones.[352,353] This new therapeutic approach could be applied to the treatment of several hereditary diseases resulting from errors in protein folding and kinesis.[354]

Only four *AVPR2* mutations (D85N, V88M, G201D, and P322S) have been associated with a mild phenotype.[355-357] In general, the male infants bearing these mutations are identified later in life and the "classic" episodes of dehydration are less severe. This mild phenotype is also found in expression studies. The mutant proteins are expressed on the plasma membranes of cells transfected with these mutants and demonstrate a stimulation of cAMP for higher concentrations of agonists.[355,357,358]

LOSS-OF-FUNCTION MUTATIONS OF *AQP2* (OMIM #107777)

The *AQP2* gene is located on chromosome region 12q12-q13. Approximately 10% of NDI cases are caused by autosomal mutations in *AQP2*. Forty-six mutations have been reported, which are either autosomal recessive (32 mutations reported) or autosomal dominant (8 mutations reported).[319] Bot male and female patients who are affected with congenital NDI have been described as homozygous for a mutation in the *AQP2* gene or carry two different mutations (Figure 45.19).[356,359] Autosomal recessive mutations give rise to misfolded proteins that are retained in the ER and are eventually degraded.[333] Autosomal dominant mutations are believed to be restricted to the carboxy-terminal end of the AQP2 protein and to operate through a dominant negative effect whereby the mutant protein associates with functional AQP2 proteins within intracellular stores, thus preventing normal targeting and function.[319,360]

Oocytes of the African clawed frog (*Xenopus laevis*) have provided a useful system for studying the behavior of various AQP2 mutants on membrane water permeability. Functional expression studies showed that *Xenopus* oocytes injected with mutant chromosomal RNA (cRNA) had abnormal coefficient of water permeability, whereas *Xenopus* oocytes injected with both normal cRNA and mutant cRNA had coefficient of water permeability similar to that of normal constructs alone. These findings provide conclusive evidence that NDI can be caused by homozygosity for mutations in the *AQP2* gene. A patient with a partial phenotype has also been described to be a compound heterozygote for the L22V and C181W mutations.[361] In the same study,

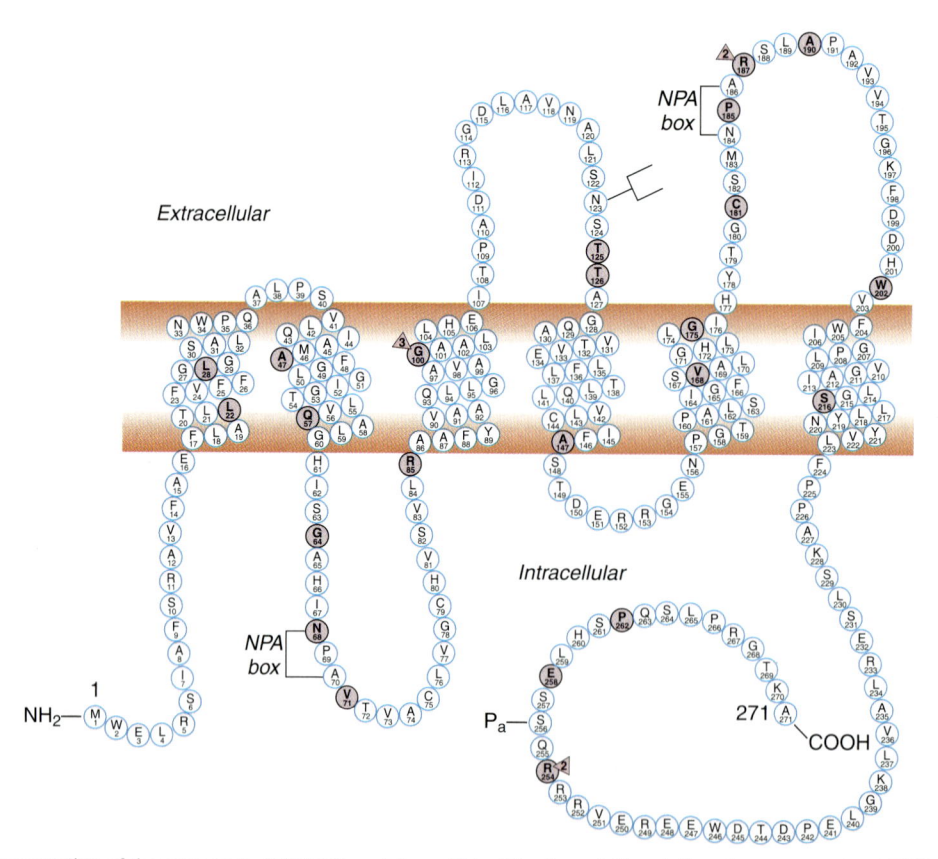

Figure 45.19 A representation of the aquaporin-2 (AQP2) protein and identification of 46 putative disease-causing AQP2 mutations. Predicted amino acids are shown as their one-letter amino acid codes. A monomer is represented with six transmembrane helices. The location of the protein kinase A (PKA) phosphorylation site (P$_a$) is indicated. The extracellular, transmembrane, and cytoplasmic domains are defined according to Deen et al, 1994.[359] **Triangles** are indicating aminoacids with more than one mutation in the same codon. **Solid symbols** indicate locations of the mutations: *M1I; L22V; V24A; L28P; G29S; A47V; Q57P; G64R, N68S, A70D; V71M; R85X; G100X; G100V; G100R; I107D; 369delC; T125M; T126M; A147T; D150E; V168M; G175R; G180S; C181W; P185A; R187C; R187H; A190T; G196D; W202C; G215C; S216P; S216F; K228E; R254Q; R254L; E258K;* and *P262L*. GenBank accession numbers—AQP2: AF147092, exon 1; AF147093, exons 2 through 4. NPA (asparagine-proline-alanine) motifs and the *N*-glycosylation site are also indicated by the fork like symbol on aminoacid N123.

immunolocalization of AQP2-transfected Chinese hamster ovary cells showed that the C181W mutant had an ER-like intracellular distribution, whereas L22V and wild-type AQP2 showed endosome and plasma membrane staining. The investigators suggested that the L22V mutation is the cause of the patient's unique response to desmopressin. The leucine 22 residue might be necessary for proper conformation or for binding of another protein important for normal targeting and trafficking of the molecule.[361]

In later studies, our group obtained evidence suggesting that both autosomal dominant and autosomal recessive NDI phenotypes could be secondary to novel mutations in the *AQP2* gene.[360,362-366] Reminiscent of expression studies done with AVPR2 proteins, Mulders and coworkers demonstrated that the major cause underlying autosomal recessive NDI is the misrouting of AQP2 mutant proteins.[367-372] To determine whether the severe AQP2 trafficking defect observed with the naturally occurring mutations T126M, R187C, and A147T is correctable, cells were incubated with the chemical chaperone glycerol for 48 hours. Redistribution of AQP2 from the ER to the membrane-endosome fractions was observed through immunofluorescence. This redistribution was correlated to improved water permeability measurements.[370] Our group also studied the ability of myoinositol to stimulate water permeability in oocytes expressing six different mutant AQP2s. Only two mutants (D150E and S256L) were sensitive to the effect of myoinositol, whereas no changes were seen with mutants A70D, V71M, and G196D.[373]

POLYURIA, POLYDIPSIA, ELECTROLYTE IMBALANCE, AND DEHYDRATION IN CYSTINOSIS

Polyuria may be as mild as persistent enuresis or so severe as to contribute to death from dehydration and electrolyte abnormalities in infants with cystinosis who have acute gastroenteritis.[36]

POLYURIA IN HEREDITARY HYPOKALEMIC SALT-LOSING TUBULOPATHIES

Patients with polyhydramnios, hypercalciuria, and hyposthenuria or isosthenuria have been found to bear *KCNJ1* (ROMK) and *SLC12A1* (NKCC2) mutations.[234,243] Patients with polyhydramnios, profound polyuria, hyponatremia, hypochloremia, metabolic alkalosis, and sensorineural deafness have been found to bear *BSND* mutations.[239,246,374,375] These studies demonstrate the critical importance of the proteins ROMK, NKCC2, and Barttin in transferring NaCl to the medullary interstitium and thereby generating, together with urea, a hypertonic milieu (see Figure 45.10).

CARRIER DETECTION, PERINATAL TESTING, AND TREATMENT

We encourage physicians who observe families with X-linked and autosomal recessive diabetes insipidus to recommend mutation analysis before the birth of an infant because early diagnosis and treatment can avert the physical and mental retardation associated with episodes of dehydration. Diagnosis of X-linked NDI was accomplished by mutation testing of cultured amniotic cells or chorionic villus samples (N = 17), or cord blood obtained at birth (N = 65) in 82 of our patients from 69 families. Thirty-six male patients were found to bear mutant sequences, and 26 had normal sequences. Diagnosis of AQP2 autosomal recessive mutants was made in 4 families for a total of 6 subjects, of whom 3 were found to be homozygous for the previously identified mutation, 2 were heterozygous, and 1 had a normal sequence on both alleles. The affected patients were immediately treated with abundant water intake, a low-sodium diet, and hydrochlorothiazide. They never experienced episodes of dehydration, and their physical and mental development is normal. Gene analysis is also important for the identification of nonobligatory female carriers in families with X-linked NDI. Most female patients heterozygous for a mutation in the V_2 receptor do not present with clinical symptoms, and a few are severely affected,[336] (Bichet, unpublished observations). Mutational analysis of polyuric patients with cystinosis, hypokalemic salt-losing tubulopathy, nephronophthisis, and apparent mineralocorticoid excess is also of importance for definitive molecular diagnosis.

All complications of congenital NDI can be prevented by an adequate water intake. Thus, patients should be provided with unrestricted amounts of water from birth to ensure normal development. In addition to a low-sodium diet, the use of diuretics (thiazides) or indomethacin may reduce urinary output. This advantageous effect must be weighed against the side effects of these drugs (thiazides: electrolyte disturbances; indomethacin: reduction of the GFR and gastrointestinal symptoms). Many affected infants frequently vomit because of an exacerbation of physiologic gastroesophageal reflux. These young patients often improve with the absorption of a histamine H_2 blocker and with metoclopramide, which could induce extrapyramidal symptoms, or domperidone, which seems to be efficacious and better tolerated.

Complete reference list available at ExpertConsult.com.

KEY REFERENCES

8. Christensen EI, Birn H, Storm T, et al: Endocytic receptors in the renal proximal tubule. *Physiology (Bethesda)* 27:223–236, 2012.
9. McKusick VA: Mendelian Inheritance in Man and its online version, OMIM. *Am J Hum Genet* 80:588–604, 2007.
10. Lloyd SE, Pearce SH, Fisher SE, et al: A common molecular basis for three inherited kidney stone diseases. *Nature* 379:445–449, 1996.
14. Gorvin CM, Wilmer MJ, Piret SE, et al: Receptor-mediated endocytosis and endosomal acidification is impaired in proximal tubule epithelial cells of Dent disease patients. *Proc Natl Acad Sci U S A* 110:7014–7019, 2013.
16. Devuyst O, Thakker RV: Dent's disease. *Orphanet J Rare Dis* 5:28, 2010.
26. Charnas LR, Bernardini I, Rader D, et al: Clinical and laboratory findings in the oculocerebrorenal syndrome of Lowe, with special reference to growth and renal function. *N Engl J Med* 324:1318–1325, 1991.
30. Pirruccello M, De Camilli P: Inositol 5-phosphatases: insights from the Lowe syndrome protein OCRL. *Trends Biochem Sci* 37:134–143, 2012.
33. Klootwijk ED, Reichold M, Helip-Wooley A, et al: Mistargeting of peroxisomal EHHADH and inherited renal Fanconi's syndrome. *N Engl J Med* 370:129–138, 2014.
36. Gahl WA, Thoene JG, Schneider JA: Cystinosis. *N Engl J Med* 347:111–121, 2002.

50. Dohil R, Cabrera BL: Treatment of cystinosis with delayed-release cysteamine: 6-year follow-up. *Pediatr Nephrol* 28:507–510, 2013.
55. Labbe A, Baudouin C, Deschenes G, et al: A new gel formulation of topical cysteamine for the treatment of corneal cystine crystals in cystinosis: the Cystadrops OCT-1 study. *Mol Genet Metab* 111:314–320, 2014.
117. Camargo SM, Bockenhauer D, Kleta R: Aminoacidurias: clinical and molecular aspects. *Kidney Int* 73:918–925, 2008.
120. Chillaron J, Font-Llitjos M, Fort J, et al: Pathophysiology and treatment of cystinuria. *Nat Rev Nephrol* 6:424–434, 2010.
149. Palacin M, Bertran J, Chillaron J, et al: Lysinuric protein intolerance: mechanisms of pathophysiology. *Mol Genet Metab* (Suppl 1):S27–S37, 2004.
169. Biber J, Hernando N, Forster I: Phosphate transporters and their function. *Annu Rev Physiol* 75:535–550, 2013.
171. Magen D, Berger L, Coady MJ, et al: A loss-of-function mutation in NaPi-IIa and renal Fanconi's syndrome. *N Engl J Med* 362:1102–1109, 2010.
204. Vitart V, Rudan I, Hayward C, et al: SLC2A9 is a newly identified urate transporter influencing serum urate concentration, urate excretion and gout. *Nat Genet* 40:437–442, 2008.
208. Chao EC, Henry RR: SGLT2 inhibition—a novel strategy for diabetes treatment. *Nat Rev Drug Discov* 9:551–559, 2010.
213. Fry AC, Karet FE: Inherited renal acidoses. *Physiology (Bethesda)* 22:202–211, 2007.
231. Bartter FC, Pronove P, Gill JRJ, et al: Hyperplasia of the juxtaglomerular complex with hyperaldosteronism and hypokalemic alkalosis: a new syndrome. *Am J Med* 33:811–828, 1962.
232. Jeck N, Schlingmann KP, Reinalter SC, et al: Salt handling in the distal nephron: lessons learned from inherited human disorders. *Am J Physiol Regul Integr Comp Physiol* 288:R782–R795, 2005.
243. Peters M, Jeck N, Reinalter S, et al: Clinical presentation of genetically defined patients with hypokalemic salt-losing tubulopathies. *Am J Med* 112:183–190, 2002.
261. Lifton RP, Gharavi AG, Geller DS: Molecular mechanisms of human hypertension. *Cell* 104:545–556, 2001.
271. Liddle G, Bledsoe T, Coppage W: A familial renal disorder simulating primary aldosteronism but with negligible aldosterone secretion. *Trans Am Assoc Phys* 76:199–213, 1963.
276. Bockenhauer D, van't Hoff W, Dattani M, et al: Secondary nephrogenic diabetes insipidus as a complication of inherited renal diseases. *Nephron Physiol* 116:p23–p29, 2010.
279. Lifton RP, Dluhy RG, Powers M, et al: A chimaeric 11 beta-hydroxylase/aldosterone synthase gene causes glucocorticoid-remediable aldosteronism and human hypertension. *Nature* 355:262–265, 1992.
291. Glover M, O'Shaughnessy KM: Molecular insights from dysregulation of the thiazide-sensitive WNK/SPAK/NCC pathway in the kidney: Gordon syndrome and thiazide-induced hyponatraemia. *Clin Exp Pharmacol Physiol* 40:876–884, 2013.
292. Boyden LM, Choi M, Choate KA, et al: Mutations in kelch-like 3 and cullin 3 cause hypertension and electrolyte abnormalities. *Nature* 482(7383):98–102, 2012.
296. Shibata S, Zhang J, Puthumana J, et al: Kelch-like 3 and Cullin 3 regulate electrolyte homeostasis via ubiquitination and degradation of WNK4. *Proc Natl Acad Sci U S A* 110:7838–7843, 2013.
298. Hadchouel J, Delaloy C, Faure S, et al: Familial hyperkalemic hypertension. *J Am Soc Nephrol* 17:208–217, 2006.
300. Knoers NV: Inherited forms of renal hypomagnesemia: an update. *Pediatr Nephrol* 24:697–705, 2009.
307. van der Wijst J, Bindels RJ, Hoenderop JG: Mg2+ homeostasis: the balancing act of TRPM6. *Curr Opin Nephrol Hypertens* 23:361–369, 2014.
311. Brown EM, Pollak M, Seidman CE, et al: Calcium-ion-sensing cell-surface receptors. *N Engl J Med* 333:234–240, 1995.
315. Arjona FJ, de Baaij JH, Schlingmann KP, et al: CNNM2 mutations cause impaired brain development and seizures in patients with hypomagnesemia. *PLoS Genet* 10:e1004267, 2014.
316. Moeller HB, Rittig S, Fenton RA: Nephrogenic diabetes insipidus: essential insights into the molecular background and potential therapies for treatment. *Endocr Rev* 34:278–301, 2013.
317. Bichet DG: Central vasopressin: dendritic and axonal secretion and renal actions. *Clin Kidney J* 7:242–247, 2014.
320. Agre P, Preston GM, Smith BL, et al: Aquaporin CHIP: the archetypal molecular water channel. *Am J Physiol* 34:F463–F476, 1993.
321. Murata K, Mitsuoka K, Hirai T, et al: Structural determinants of water permeation through aquaporin-1. *Nature* 407:599–605, 2000.
327. Birk J, Friberg MA, Prescianotto-Baschong C, et al: Dominant pro-vasopressin mutants that cause diabetes insipidus form disulfide-linked fibrillar aggregates in the endoplasmic reticulum. *J Cell Sci* 122:3994–4002, 2009.
335. Fujiwara TM, Bichet DG: Molecular biology of hereditary diabetes insipidus. *J Am Soc Nephrol* 16:2836–2846, 2005.
336. Arthus M-F, Lonergan M, Crumley MJ, et al: Report of 33 novel AVPR2 mutations and analysis of 117 families with X-linked nephrogenic diabetes insipidus. *J Am Soc Nephrol* 11:1044–1054, 2000.
344. Ulinski T, Grapin C, Forin V, et al: Severe bladder dysfunction in a family with ADH receptor gene mutation responsible for X-linked nephrogenic diabetes insipidus. *Nephrol Dial Transplant* 19:2928–2929, 2004.
348. Bichet DG, Arthus M-F, Lonergan M, et al: X-linked nephrogenic diabetes insipidus mutations in North America and the Hopewell hypothesis. *J Clin Invest* 92:1262–1268, 1993.
349. Bode HH, Crawford JD: Nephrogenic diabetes insipidus in North America: The Hopewell hypothesis. *N Engl J Med* 280:750–754, 1969.
352. Morello JP, Salahpour A, Laperrière A, et al: Pharmacological chaperones rescue cell-surface expression and function of misfolded V2 vasopressin receptor mutants. *J Clin Invest* 105:887–895, 2000.
353. Bernier V, Morello JP, Zarruk A, et al: Pharmacologic chaperones as a potential treatment for X-linked nephrogenic diabetes insipidus. *J Am Soc Nephrol* 17:232–243, 2006.
359. Deen PMT, Verdijk MAJ, Knoers NVAM, et al: Requirement of human renal water channel aquaporin-2 for vasopressin-dependent concentration of urine. *Science* 264:92–95, 1994.
365. Kuwahara M, Iwai K, Ooeda T, et al: Three families with autosomal dominant nephrogenic diabetes insipidus caused by aquaporin-2 mutations in the C-terminus. *Am J Hum Genet* 69:738–748, 2001.
368. Marr N, Bichet DG, Hoefs S, et al: Cell-biologic and functional analyses of five new aquaporin-2 missense mutations that cause recessive nephrogenic diabetes insipidus. *J Am Soc Nephrol* 13:2267–2277, 2002.
370. Tamarappoo BK, Verkman AS: Defective aquaporin-2 trafficking in nephrogenic diabetes insipidus and correction by chemical chaperones. *J Clin Invest* 101:2257–2267, 1998.

Cystic Diseases of the Kidney

46

Vicente E. Torres | Peter C. Harris

CHAPTER OUTLINE

CLASSIFICATION OF RENAL CYSTIC DISEASES, 1475
DEVELOPMENT OF RENAL EPITHELIAL CYSTS, 1475
HEREDITARY CYSTIC KIDNEY DISORDERS, 1479
Autosomal Dominant Polycystic Kidney Disease, 1479
Autosomal Recessive Polycystic Kidney Disease, 1496
Tuberous Sclerosis Complex, 1500
Von Hippel–Lindau Syndrome, 1502
Familial Renal Hamartomas Associated with Hyperparathyroidism–Jaw Tumor Syndrome, 1503
Hepatocyte Nuclear Factor-1β–Associated Nephropathy, 1503
Oro-Facial-Digital Syndrome Type 1, 1504
Medullary Cystic Kidney Disease (Autosomal Dominant Tubulointerstitial Kidney Disease), 1504
AUTOSOMAL RECESSIVE CILIOPATHIES WITH INTERSTITIAL NEPHRITIS AND RENAL CYSTIC DISEASE, 1505
Nephronophthisis, 1508
Joubert Syndrome, 1508
Meckel Syndrome, 1509

Bardet-Biedl Syndrome, 1509
Alström Syndrome, 1509
Nephronophthisis Variants Associated with Skeletal Defects (Skeletal Ciliopathies), 1509
RENAL CYSTIC DYSPLASIAS, 1510
Multicystic Dysplastic Kidneys, 1510
OTHER CYSTIC KIDNEY DISORDERS, 1511
Simple Cysts, 1511
Localized or Unilateral Renal Cystic Disease, 1512
Medullary Sponge Kidney, 1513
Acquired Cystic Kidney Disease, 1514
RENAL CYSTIC NEOPLASMS, 1516
Cystic Renal Cell Carcinoma, 1516
Multilocular Cystic Nephroma, 1517
Cystic Partially Differentiated Nephroblastoma, 1517
Mixed Epithelial and Stromal Tumor, 1517
RENAL CYSTS OF NONTUBULAR ORIGIN, 1517
Cystic Disease of the Renal Sinus, 1517
Perirenal Lymphangiomas, 1517
Subcapsular and Perirenal Urinomas (Uriniferous Pseudocysts), 1517
Pyelocalyceal Cysts, 1518

CLASSIFICATION OF RENAL CYSTIC DISEASES

Renal cystic diseases encompass a large number of sporadic and genetically determined congenital, developmental, and acquired conditions that have in common the presence of cysts in one or both kidneys. *Renal cysts* are cavities lined by epithelium and filled with fluid or semisolid matter. Cysts are derived primarily from tubules. Whereas cystic kidneys of different etiologies may appear morphologically similar, the same etiologic entity may cause a wide spectrum of renal abnormalities. Classifications of renal cystic diseases are based on morphologic, clinical, and genetic information (Table 46.1) and change as the understanding of the underlying etiologies and pathogeneses continues to expand.

DEVELOPMENT OF RENAL EPITHELIAL CYSTS

Epithelial cysts develop from preexisting renal tubule segments and are composed of a layer of partially dedifferentiated epithelial cells enclosing a cavity filled with either a urinelike liquid or semisolid material. They may develop in any tubular segment between Bowman's capsule and the tip

Table 46.1	Classification of Cystic Kidney Disorders

Autosomal dominant polycystic kidney disease (ADPKD)
Autosomal recessive polycystic kidney disease (ARPKD):
    Tuberous sclerosis complex
    von Hippel–Lindau syndrome
    Familial renal hamartomas associated with hyperparathyroidism–jaw tumor syndrome
    Hepatocyte nuclear factor-1–associated nephropathy
    Oro-facial-digital syndrome
Autosomal dominant medullary cystic kidney disease (autosomal dominant tubulointerstitial kidney disease)
Hereditary recessive ciliopathies with interstitial nephritis, cysts, or both:
    Nephronophthisis
    Joubert syndrome
    Meckel syndrome
    Bardet-Biedl syndrome
    Alström syndrome
    Nephronophthisis variants associated with skeletal defects (skeletal ciliopathies)
Renal cystic dysplasias:
    Multicystic kidney dysplasia
Other cystic kidney disorders:
    Simple cysts
    Localized or unilateral renal cystic disease
    Medullary sponge kidney
    Acquired cystic kidney disease
Renal cystic neoplasms:
    Cystic renal cell carcinoma
    Multilocular cystic nephroma
    Cystic partially differentiated nephroblastoma
    Mixed epithelial and stromal tumor
Cysts of nontubular origin:
    Cystic disease of the renal sinus
    Perirenal lymphangiomas
    Subcapsular and perirenal urinomas
Pyelocalyceal cysts

of the renal papilla, depending on the nature of the underlying disorder. After achieving a size of perhaps a few millimeters, most cysts lose their attachments to their parent tubule segment.

Pathophysiologic processes that contribute to the development of cysts include disruption of programs responsible for the establishment and maintenance of normal tubular diameter (i.e., convergent extension, or the process of cell intercalation by which cells elongate along an axis perpendicular to the proximal-distal axis of the tubule and actively crawl among one another to produce a narrower, longer tubule; and oriented cell division or alignment of the mitotic spindle axis and cell division with the proximal-distal axis of the tubule),[1,2] excessive cell proliferation, active solute and fluid transport into the expanding cysts, cross talk between epithelial cells and interstitial macrophages, and interactions between epithelial cells and extracellular matrix[3,4] (Figure 46.1).

Renal cysts have been regarded as benign neoplasms that arise from individual cells or restricted segments of the renal tubule. Transgenic insertions of activated proto-oncogenes and growth factor genes into rodents results in the formation of renal cysts. Therefore, processes that stimulate renal cell proliferation along with the inability to maintain planar cell polarity have the potential to generate the cystic phenotype.

Conditional knockouts of *Pkd1* or of ciliogenesis (*Ift88* and *Kif3a*) at various time points have shown that the timing of their inactivation determines the rate of development of cystic disease.[5-8] Inactivation in newborn mice leads to rapid cyst development. Inactivation after about 13 days leads to slowly progressive disease evident only in the adult kidneys, but progression can be hastened by maneuvers such as ischemic or reperfusion injury to stimulate cell proliferation.[9] The underlying rate of epithelial cell proliferation may account for increased susceptibility to cyst development during nephrogenesis as well as for the migration of cysts as the kidney matures in humans and in animal models of PKD from being located predominantly proximal to appearing predominantly distal and in the collecting duct.[10] Immature early tubules (S-shaped bodies) exhibit very high rates of proliferation. Later, when the epithelium differentiates into nephron segments recognizable on light microscopy, proliferative indices become very low in proximal tubules but remain elevated in the distal nephrons and collecting ducts. In pediatric and adult kidneys, proliferative indices are very low in all tubular segments but remain higher in collecting ducts than in proximal tubules.[11,12]

The finding of fluid secretion in renal epithelial cysts led to a re-investigation of fluid secretion mechanisms in otherwise normal renal tubules. Beyond the loop of Henle, tubule cells have the capacity to secrete solutes and fluid upon stimulation with cyclic adenosine monophosphate (cAMP).[13] This secretory flux operates in competition with the more powerful mechanism by which Na^+ is absorbed through apical epithelial Na^+ channels (ENaCs). Under conditions in which Na^+ absorption is diminished, the net secretion of NaCl and fluid can be observed at rates that could have a significant impact on the net economy of body salt and water content. Thus, renal cystic disease has led to a heightened appreciation of an "ancient" solute and water secretory mechanism that has been largely overlooked in modern studies of renal physiology.[14]

Three decades ago it was noted that a germ-free environment inhibits cyst development in CFW mice and in a model of polycystic kidney disease (PKD) induced by nordihydroguaiaretic acid; the administration of endotoxin rescued the cystic phenotype.[15,16] Chemokines and cytokines were found at high concentrations in cyst fluid and produced by epithelial cells of the cyst lining.[17] In later studies, alternatively activated macrophages aligned along cyst walls were detected in polycystic kidneys from conditional *Pkd1* knock-out and the *Pkd2*[WS25/−] model.[18,19] Macrophage depletion inhibited epithelial cell proliferation and cyst growth and improved renal function. These observations led to the hypothesis that alternatively activated M2 macrophages contribute to cell proliferation in PKD, as has been described during development, during recovery from acute kidney injury, and in cancer.

Evidence indicates that alterations in focal adhesion complexes, basement membranes, and extracellular matrix (ECM) contribute to the pathogenesis of PKD.[20] Focal adhesion complexes contain integrin αβ heterodimer receptors and multiple structural and signaling molecules, including polycystin 1. The integrin receptors link the actin

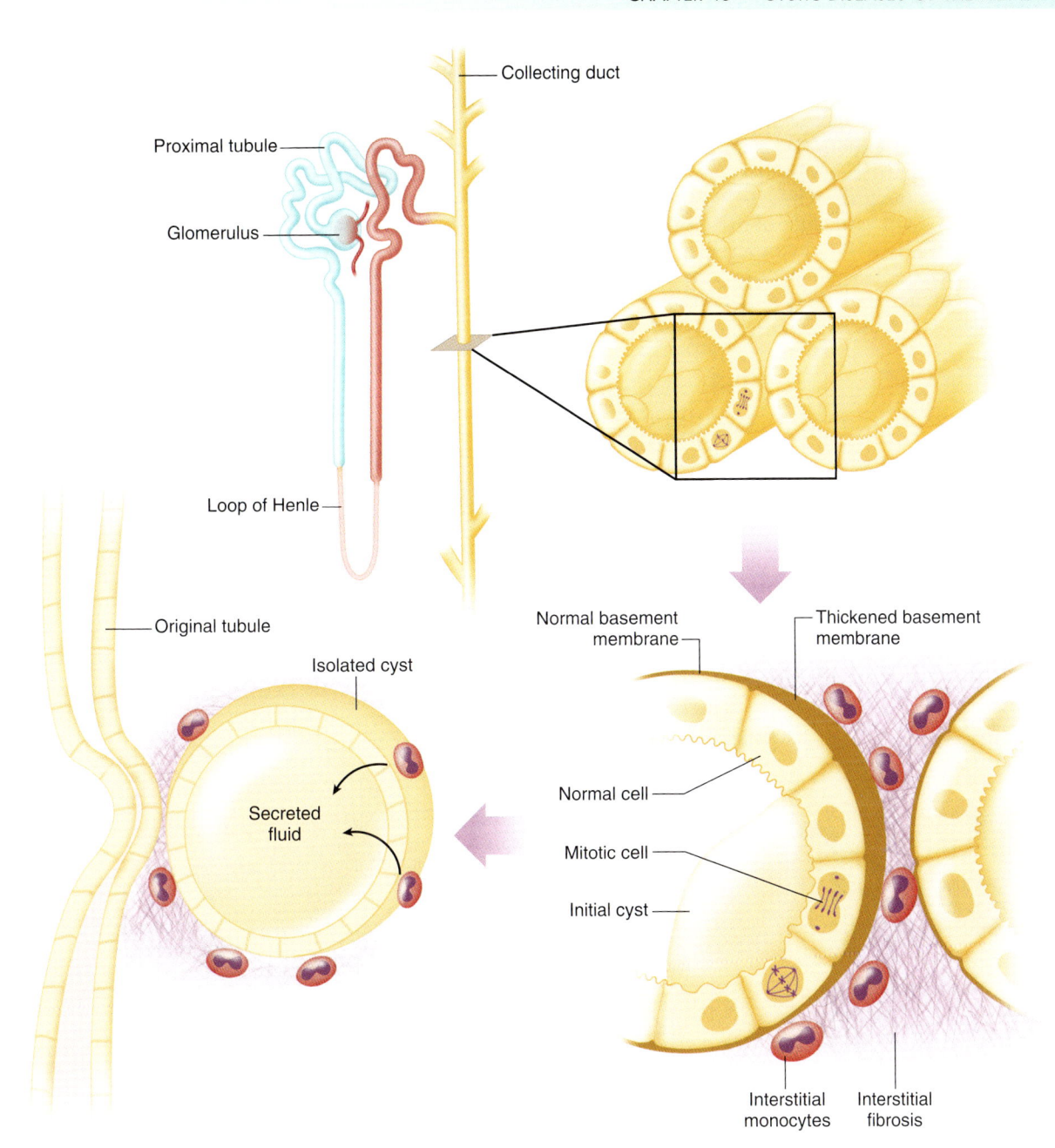

Figure 46.1 Evolution of cysts from renal tubules. Abnormal proliferation of tubule epithelium begins in a single cell after a "second-hit" process disables the function of the normal allele or if the level of functional polycystin falls below a specific threshold. Repeated cycles of cell proliferation lead to expansion of the tubule wall into a cyst. The cystic epithelium is associated with thickening of the adjacent tubule basement membrane and with an influx of inflammatory cells into the interstitium. The cystic segment eventually separates from the original tubule, and net epithelial fluid secretion contributes to the accumulation of liquid within the cyst cavity.

cytoskeleton laminin αβγ heterotrimers and collagens in the basement membrane. Integrins $β_4$ and $β_1$ may mediate the increased adhesion of cyst-lining epithelial cells to laminin-322 and collagen and are all overexpressed in cystic tissues.[21,22] Periostin, an ECM protein, and its receptor $α_v$ integrin as well as $α_1$ and $α_2$ integrins are also overexpressed.[23,24] Laminin-322 and periostin stimulate, whereas antibodies to laminin-332 and $α_v$ integrin inhibit cyst formation in three-dimensional gel culture.[23,25] Renal cystic disease develops in $β_1$ integrin knockout and laminin $α_5$ hypomorphic mutant mice, the latter associated with overexpression of laminin-322.[26,27] Mutations in exons 24 and 25 of the gene *COL4A1*, which encodes procollagen type IV, have been found in patients with autosomal dominant (*h*ereditary) *a*ngiopathy with *n*ephropathy (consisting of hematuria and bilateral large renal cysts), *a*neurysms, and muscle *c*ramps (HANAC syndrome).

Evidence accumulated during the last roughly 15 years strongly suggests that the primary cilium is essential to maintain epithelial cell differentiation and that structural and functional defects in the primary cilium of tubular epithelia have a central role in various forms of human and rodent cystic diseases. The *primary cilium* is a single hairlike organelle that projects from the surface of most mammalian cells, including epithelial and endothelial cells, neurons, fibroblasts, chondrocytes, and osteocytes. It is involved in left–right embryonic patterning as well as in mechanosensing (renal tubular and biliary epithelia), photosensing (retinal pigmented epithelia), and chemosensing (olfactory neurons).[28-32] In renal tubule epithelial cells, the cilium projects into the lumen and is thought to have a sensory role (Figure 46.2). The cilium arises from the mother centriole in the centrosome. The centrosome comprises a mother centriole and a daughter centriole plus a "cloud" of pericentriolar material.[33] The centrosome serves as the microtubule-organizing center for interphase cells, and the mother and daughter centrioles form the poles of the spindle during cell division.

The first clue connecting PKD and cilia was that polycystin 1 (PC1) and polycystin 2 (PC2) homologs in *Caenorhabditis elegans* are located in cilia of male sensory neurons; loss of these proteins is associated with mating behavior defects.[34] Next, a known intraflagellar transport (IFT) protein, polaris, was found to be defective in a hypomorphic mouse mutant, *orpk*, in which PKD, left–right patterning defects, and a variety of other abnormalities develop and that has

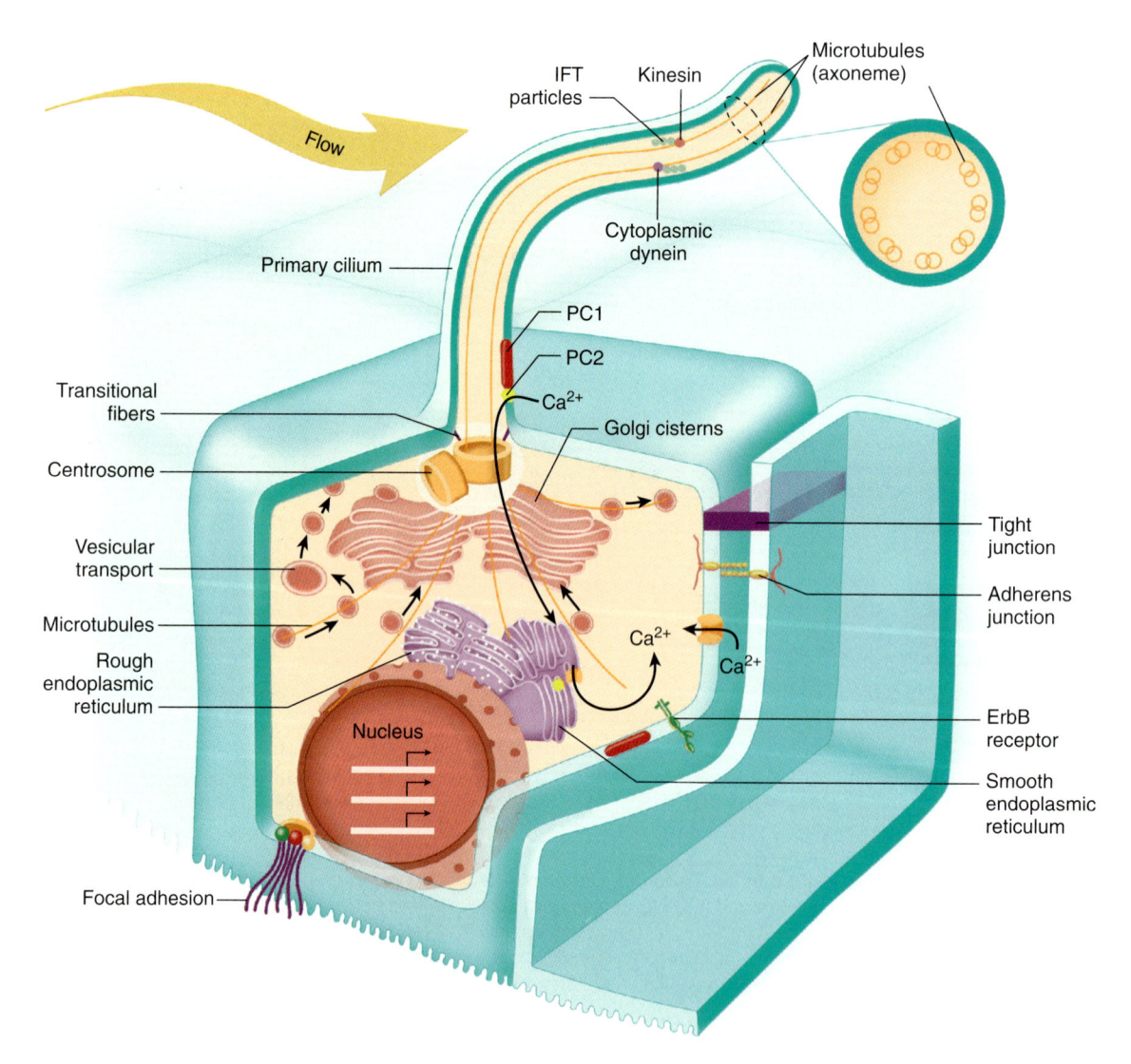

Figure 46.2 Diagram depicting the primary cilium and hypothetical functions of the polycystins. Polycystin 1 (PC1) and polycystin 2 (PC2) are found on the primary cilium, a single hairlike structure that projects from the apical surface of the cell into the lumen. It consists of a membrane continuous with the cell membrane and a central axoneme composed of nine peripheral microtubule doublets. It arises from the mother centriole in the centrosome, the microtubule-organizing center of the cell. The centrosome comprises a mother centriole and a daughter centriole plus a "cloud" of pericentriolar material. In response to mechanical stimulation of the primary cilium by flow, the PC1 and PC2 complex mediates Ca^{2+} entry into the cell. This triggers Ca^{2+}-induced release of Ca^{2+} from the smooth endoplasmic reticulum (ER) through ryanodine receptors. The function of the polycystins extends beyond the cilium because PC1 is also found in the plasma membrane and PC2 is predominantly expressed in the ER. PC2 is an intracellular Ca^{2+} channel that is required for the normal pattern of $[Ca^{2+}]_i$ responses involving ryanodine receptors and inositol 1,4,5-trisphosphate (IP3) receptors and may also affect the activity of store-operated Ca^{2+} channels. ErbB, Epidermal growth factor receptor; IFT, intraflagellar transport. (Reproduced from Torres VE, Harris PC, Pirson Y: Autosomal dominant polycystic kidney disease. *Lancet* 369:1287-1301, 2007.)

shortened cilia in the kidney.[35] Subsequently, the proteins mutated in other rodent models of PKD—such as the *cpk* (centrin) and *inv* (inversin) mice, autosomal dominant PKD (ADPKD; PC1 and PC2), autosomal recessive PKD (ARPKD; fibrocystin), autosomal recessive ciliopathies (see later in the chapter), and possibly tuberous sclerosis complex (TSC) and von Hippel–Lindau disease—have been localized to the ciliary axoneme, the basal body, or centrosomal structures.[30,36,37] Conditional inactivation of the ciliary motor protein KIF3A (kinesin family member 3A) in collecting duct epithelial cells reproduced all of the clinical and biologic features of PKD.[38]

The polycystin complex on cilia seems to detect changes in flow and transduce it into a Ca^{2+} influx through the PC2 channel, thus functioning as a mechanosensor,[38a] although a chemosensory role has not been excluded. The Ca^{2+} influx may in turn induce release of Ca^{2+} from intracellular stores. The increased Ca^{2+} concentration in intracellular microenvironments may then modulate specific signaling pathways that regulate cellular differentiation, proliferation, and apoptosis, such as cAMP, receptor-tyrosine kinase, extracellular signal–regulated kinase (ERK), and mTOR (mammalian target of rapamycin) signaling.[4]

The ciliocentric model of cystogenesis is attractive but may be too reductionist. Several cyst-associated proteins have other functions, including participation in cell–cell and cell–matrix interactions at adherens junctions and focal adhesions. Dysfunction of these subcellular domains most likely contributes to the aberrant epithelial growth and tubular architecture that are common to virtually all forms of renal cystic disease. Although ciliary dysfunction may be the initiating event in cystogenesis, defects in other cellular mechanisms may modulate the final cystic disease phenotype.

HEREDITARY CYSTIC KIDNEY DISORDERS

AUTOSOMAL DOMINANT POLYCYSTIC KIDNEY DISEASE

EPIDEMIOLOGY

ADPKD occurs worldwide and in all races, with a prevalence estimated to be between 1 in 400 and 1 in 1000.[39] The yearly incidence rates for end-stage kidney disease (ESKD) due to ADPKD are 8.7 and 6.9 per million (1998-2001, United States),[40] 7.8 and 6.0 per million (1998-1999, Europe),[41] and 5.6 and 4.0 (1999-2000, Japan)[42] in men and women, respectively. Age-adjusted gender ratios greater than unity (1.2-1.3) suggest a more progressive disease in men than in women. Approximately 30,000 patients have ESKD due to ADPKD in the United States (1:3500 individuals aged 65-69 years).[43] The proceedings of a 2014 Kidney Disease: Improving Global Outcomes (KDIGO) Controversies Conference to assess the current state of knowledge related to the evaluation, management and treatment of ADPKD have now been published.[44]

GENETICS AND GENETIC MECHANISMS

ADPKD is inherited as an autosomal dominant trait with complete penetrance in terms of cyst development. Therefore, each child of an affected parent has a 50% chance of inheriting the abnormal gene. Most patients with ADPKD have an affected parent but at least 10% of families can be traced to an apparent de novo mutation.[45] ADPKD is genetically heterogeneous with two genes identified, *PKD1* (chromosome region 16p13.3) and *PKD2* (4q21).[46-49] Current data do not support theories about a third gene accounting for a small number of unlinked families.[50]

In groups identified through renal clinics, *PKD1* accounts for about 78% of pedigrees and *PKD2* for about 13%, and no mutation is detected (NMD) in about 9%.[51,52] *PKD2* may account for up to approximately 25% of mutation-characterized cases in population-based studies.[53] In the latest version of the ADPKD Mutation Database (PKDB), 1272 *PKD1* mutations are described accounting for 1874 families, with 202 mutations to *PKD2* causing disease in 438 pedigrees.[54] For *PKD1*, about 65% of mutations are predicted to truncate the protein, leaving about 35% nontruncating.[51,52] Corresponding levels for *PKD2* are about 87% truncating and 13% nontruncating; about 3% of ADPKD mutations are larger rearrangements involving deletion or duplication of at least one exon.[51,52,55] A next-generation sequencing method for ADPKD screening based on sequencing the locus-specific LR-PCR (long-range polymerase chain reaction) products has been described.[56] Such methods can identify unusual mutations, such as gene conversions with one of the pseudogenes.

Inheritance of two *PKD1* or two *PKD2* alleles with inactivating mutations is lethal in utero.[57] Individuals heterozygous for both a *PKD1* and *PKD2* mutation live to adulthood but have more severe renal disease than those heterozygous for only one mutation.[58] Patients with a *PKD1* mutation have more severe disease than those with a *PKD2* mutation, the average ages at ESKD being 58.1 years and 79.7 years, respectively.[59] Viable ADPKD cases homozygous/compound heterozygous for *PKD1* pathogenic variants suggests the presence of hypomorphic alleles.[60] Up to 50% of nontruncating *PKD1* changes have been suggested to be hypomorphic alleles, resulting in ESKD at 55 years in patients with truncating *PKD1* mutations and 67 years in those with nontruncating changes.[59,61] Patients with mutations in the 5′ region of *PKD1* may be more likely to have intracranial aneurysms (ICAs) and aneurysm ruptures than patients with 3′ mutations.[62] No clear correlations with mutation type or position have been found in *PKD2* mutations.[63]

A small number (<1%) of patients with ADPKD exhibit early-onset disease, with a diagnosis made in utero or infancy from the presence of enlarged echogenic kidneys that may resemble those seen in ARPKD.[64,65] Most early-onset cases have been linked to *PKD1*, but a family with *PKD2* mutation and perinatal death in two severely affected infants has been described.[66] Some cases of early-onset ADPKD, or cases mimicking ARPKD, are due to an *in trans* combination of two *PKD1* mutations, at least one of which is hypomorphic.[60,67] Studies of a *Pkd1* mouse model with a missense change, p.R3277C, confirmed the hypomorphic nature of this allele and its role in causing early-onset disease.[10,60] Unilateral parental disomy involving a hypomorphic *PKD2* allele can also cause early-onset ADPKD.[68] Mutations in other cystogenes, such as *HNF1B* (associated with the renal cysts and diabetes [RCAD] syndrome) and *PKHD1* (the ARPKD gene), in combination with a ADPKD mutant allele have also been suggested to be associated with early-onset PKD.[69]

The contiguous deletion of the adjacent *PKD1* and *TSC2* (see later discussion of tuberous sclerosis complex) genes is characterized by childhood PKD with additional clinical signs of TSC.[69a]

Significant intrafamilial variability in the severity of renal and extrarenal manifestations points to genetic and environmental modifying factors. Analysis of the variability in renal function between monozygotic twins and siblings supports a role for genetic modifiers.[70,71] Parental hypertension, particularly in the nonaffected parent, increases the risk for hypertension and ESKD.[72] Parents are as likely to show more severe disease as children.[73] Mosaicism can also modulate disease presentation and result in marked intrafamilial variability.[55,74]

Cysts in ADPKD kidneys appear to be derived through clonal proliferation of single epithelial cells in fewer than 1% of the tubules. A two-hit model of cystogenesis has been proposed to explain the focal nature of the cysts. In this model, a mutated *PKD1* (or *PKD2*) gene is inherited from one parent, and a wild-type gene is inherited from the unaffected parent. During the lifetime of the individual, the wild-type gene undergoes a somatic mutation and becomes inactivated. Loss of heterozygosity owing to somatic mutations of the *PKD1* and *PKD2* genes has been identified in the cells lining the cysts in both the kidney and the liver.[75,76] Support for this model of cystogenesis is provided by the embryonic lethality and severe PKD of homozygous *Pkd1* or *Pkd2* knockout mice, the late development of cysts in the kidney or liver in heterozygous mutant mice, and the increased severity of the disease in $Pkd2^{WS25/-}$ mice carrying a *Pkd2* allele (WS25) prone to genomic rearrangement.[77]

Evidence suggests, however, that other genetic mechanisms may also be involved. Most cysts in ADPKD kidneys overexpress PC1 or PC2. Transgenic overexpression of *PKD1* or *PKD2* induces renal cystic disease.[78-80] The presence of somatic transheterozygous mutations in human polycystic kidneys (somatic mutation of the PKD gene not involved by the germline mutation) and the greater severity of cystic disease in mice with transheterozygous mutations of *Pkd1* and *Pkd2* than could be predicted by a simple additive effect suggest that haploinsufficiency may play a role in cyst formation.[58] Comparative genomic hybridization and loss of heterozygosity analysis have shown multiple molecular cytogenetic aberrations in epithelial cells from individual cysts in polycystic kidneys, suggesting the involvement of additional genes in the initiation and progression of the cystic disease.[81] Mice that are homozygous for *Pkd1* hypomorphic alleles indicate that complete inactivation of both *Pkd1* alleles is not required for cystogenesis in ADPKD.[10,82,83] *Pkd2* haploinsufficiency has been associated with a higher rate of cell proliferation in noncystic tubules of $Pkd2^{+/-}$ mice.[84] These observations suggest that diminished expression of native polycystins below a certain threshold is sufficient to induce renal cystic disease and may also be relevant for the extrarenal manifestations of the disease. Reduction of PC2 levels to 50% of normal in the vascular smooth muscle of $Pkd2^{+/-}$ mice causes significant alterations in $[Ca^{2+}]_i$ (intracellular calcium concentration) and cAMP; moreover, it results in higher rates of cell proliferation and apoptosis, contractility, and vasculature susceptibility to hemodynamic stress.[85] Reduction of PC1 levels to 50% of normal causes significant alterations in $[Ca^{2+}]_i$ homeostasis and increased vascular reactivity with compensatory changes in the transport proteins involved in calcium signaling in the aorta of $Pkd1^{+/-}$ mice.[86]

PATHOGENESIS

PC1 (4303 aa; ≈600 kDa, uncleaved and glycosylated) is a receptor-like protein with a large ectodomain (3074 aa) that comprises a number of domains involved in protein-protein and protein-carbohydrate interactions and 16 PKD repeats with an immunoglobulin (Ig) domain–like fold (Figure 46.3).[47,48] PC1 also has 11 transmembrane domains and a cytoplasmic tail. PC2 (968 aa; ≈110 kDa) is a six-transmembrane, Ca^{2+}-responsive cation channel of the transient receptor potential (TRP) family (also known as TRPP2).[49] PC1 and PC2 interact via their C-terminal tails with the resulting polycystin complex thought to play a role in intracellular Ca^{2+} regulation. Data also indicate an interdependence of the proteins for maturation and localization.[87,88]

Like many other proteins implicated in renal cystic diseases, the polycystins are located in the plasma membrane overlying primary cilia.[88a,88b] The polycystins are required for induction of calcium transients in response to ciliary bending.[38a] PC1 is also found in plasma membranes at focal adhesion, desmosomes, and adherens junction sites,[89-92] whereas PC2 is found in the endoplasmic reticulum,[93-95] and both proteins are abundant in exosomes.[96,97] The PC1 protein in the plasma membrane may interact with PC2 in the adjacent endoplasmic reticulum. PC2 interacts with the inositol 1,4,5-trisphosphate receptor (IP3R), ryanodine receptor 2 (RyR2), and TRP channels TRPC1, TRPC4, and TRPV4.[98-100]

Precisely how intracellular calcium homeostasis is altered in ADPKD remains uncertain.[101] Cells overexpressing PC2 exhibit an amplified Ca^{2+} release from intracellular stores after agonist stimulation.[102] A 50% reduction in PC2 lowers capacitative calcium entry, sarcoplasmic reticulum Ca^{2+} stores, and $[Ca^{2+}]_i$ in vascular smooth muscle cells (VSMCs).[85] Increases in $[Ca^{2+}]_i$ levels evoked by platelet-activating factor are reduced in unciliated B-lymphoblastoid cells from patients with *PKD1* or *PKD2* mutations.[103] Loss of PC2 localization to the mitotic spindles by knockdown of the interacting cytoskeletal protein, mDia1, blunts agonist-evoked $[Ca^{2+}]_i$ increases in dividing cells that lack primary cilia.[104] The majority of studies that have measured resting intracellular calcium, endoplasmic reticulum calcium stores, and store-operated calcium entry in primary cell cultures or microdissected samples from human and rodent polycystic tissues have found them to be reduced.[85,86,98,105-111]

Tissue levels of cAMP are increased in numerous animal models of PKD, not only in the kidney[10,112-115] but also in cholangiocytes,[116] vascular smooth muscle cells,[117] and choroid plexus (Figure 46.4).[118] Levels of cAMP are determined by the activities of membrane-bound (under the positive or negative control of G protein–coupled receptors [GPCRs] and extracellular ligands) and soluble adenylyl cyclases (ACs), and of cAMP phosphodiesterases (PDEs), themselves subject to complex regulatory mechanisms. The increased levels in cystic tissues may be directly related to changes in $[Ca^{2+}]_i$ homeostasis. Reduced calcium activates calcium inhibitable AC-6, directly inhibits calcium/calmodulin–dependent PDE_1 (also increasing the levels of cyclic guanosine monophosphate [cGMP]), and indirectly

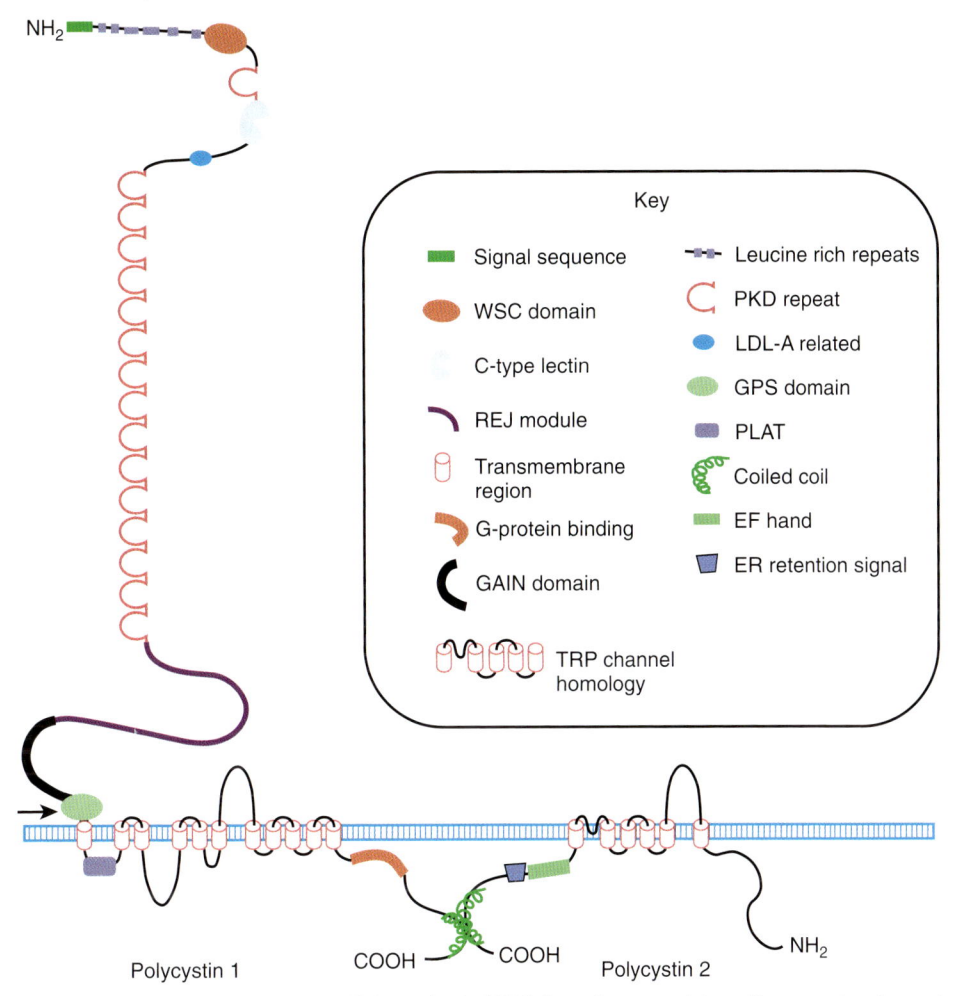

Figure 46.3 Structure of the polycystin proteins. Polycystin 1 (PC1) is a large protein with an extensive extracellular region, an 11-transmembrane area, and a short cytoplasmic tail. The protein contains a number of recognized domains and motifs (see **Key**). The protein is cleaved at the GPS (G protein–coupled receptor proteolytic site) domain (*arrow*). Polycystin 2 (PC2) is a 6-transmembrane, transient receptor potential (TRP)–like channel with cytoplasmic N and C termini. The proteins are thought to interact through coiled-coil domains. ER, Endoplasmic reticulum; GAIN, G protein-coupled receptor-Autoproteolysis INducing; LDL-A, low-density lipoprotein A module; PKD, polycystic kidney disease; PLAT, Polycystin-1, Lipoxygenase, Alpha-Toxin; REJ, receptor of egg jelly protein.

inhibits cGMP-inhibitable PDE$_3$[113,119] (see Figure 46.4). Additional mechanisms include the following:

1. Dysfunction of a ciliary protein complex (comprising A-kinase anchoring protein 150, AC-5/6, PC2, PDE$_{4C}$, and protein kinase A [PKA]) that normally restrains cAMP signaling via inhibition of AC-5/6 activity by PC2–mediated calcium entry and degradation of cAMP by PDE$_{4C}$ transcriptionally controlled by hepatocyte nuclear factor-1β (HNF-1β).[120]
2. Depletion of the endoplasmic reticulum calcium stores, which triggers oligomerization and translocation of stromal interaction molecule 1 (STIM1) to the plasma membrane, where it recruits and activates AC-6.[110]
3. Other contributory factors, such as disruption of PC1 binding to heterotrimeric G proteins, upregulation of the vasopressin V$_2$ receptor, and increased levels of circulating vasopressin or accumulation of forskolin, lysophosphatidic acid, adenosine triphosphate (ATP), or other adenylyl cyclase agonists in the cyst fluid.[121-124]

The marked amelioration of the cystic disease in collecting duct–specific *Pkd1* knockout mice by a concomitant *Ac6* knockout provides strong support for the central role of calcium-inhibitable AC-6.[125] PDEs are likely important in PKD because maximal rates of degradation by PDEs exceed by an order of magnitude those of synthesis by ACs and hence control compartmentalized pools of cAMP, which are likely more crucial than total intracellular cAMP. PDE$_1$ and PDE$_3$ may be particularly important. PDE$_1$ accounts for most PDE activity in renal tubules, it is the only PDE activated by calcium (which is reduced in PKD cells), and its activity is reduced in cystic kidneys.[119] The knockdown of *pde1a* using morpholinos induces or aggravates the cystic phenotype of wild-type or *pkd2* morphant zebrafish embryos, respectively, whereas PDE$_{1a}$ RNA partially rescues the phenotype of *pkd2* morphants.[126] PDE$_3$ controls a compartmentalized cAMP pool that stimulates mitogenesis in MDCK cells[127] as well as cystic fibrosis transmembrane conductance regulator (CFTR)–driven chloride secretion in pig trachea submucosal and shark rectal glands.[128,129] A small-molecule,

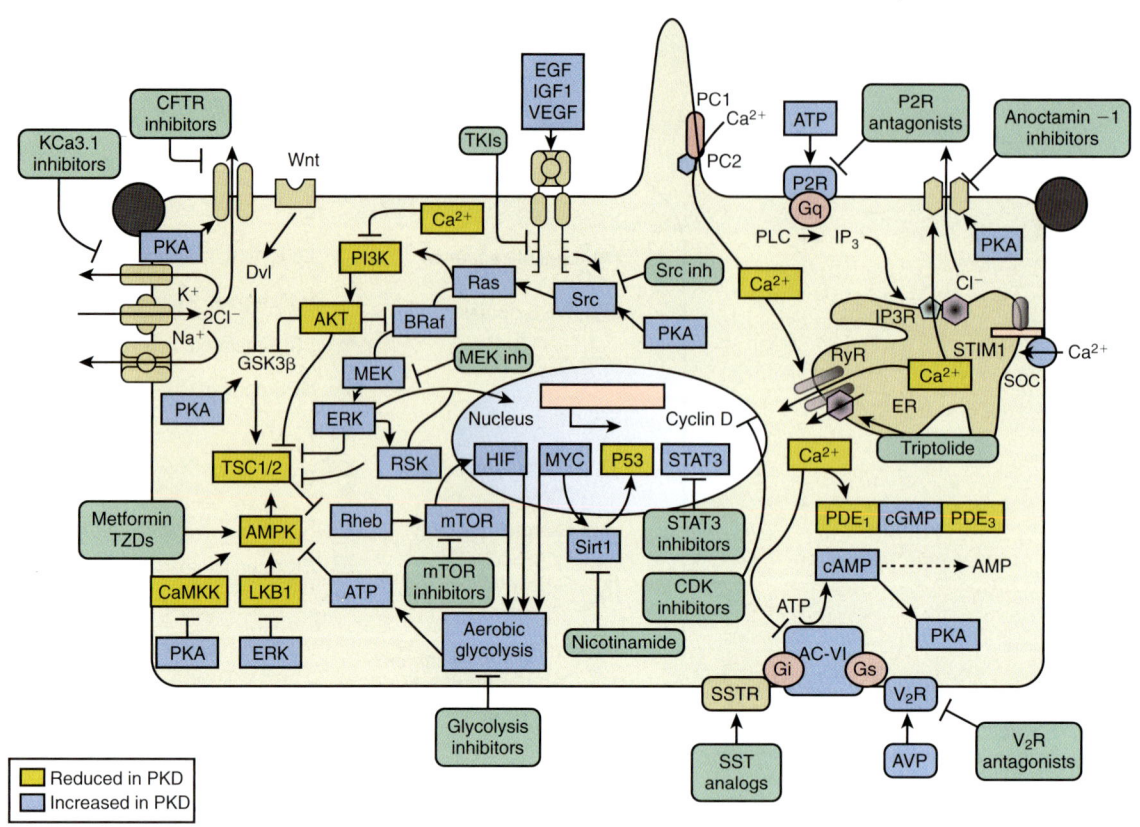

Figure 46.4 Diagram depicting hypothetical pathways upregulated or downregulated in polycystic kidney disease and rationale for treatments targeting these pathways (*green boxes*). Aberrant crosstalk between intracellular calcium (Ca^{2+}) and cyclic adenosine monophosphate (cAMP) signaling may be one of the first consequences of polycystic kidney disease (PKD) mutations. Disrupted calcium may enhance cAMP and protein kinase A (PKA) signaling through activation of calcium-inhibitable adenylyl cyclases and inhibition of calcium-dependent phosphodiesterases (PDE_1 and, indirectly, cyclic guanosine monophosphate [cGMP]–inhibited PDE_3). Enhanced PKA activity may in turn disrupt intracellular calcium homeostasis through phosphorylation of calcium-cycling proteins in the endoplasmic reticulum. PKA-induced phosphorylation of the cystic fibrosis transmembrane conductance regulator (CFTR) allows chloride and fluid secretion into the cysts; anoctamin-1 may synergistically interact with CFTR, further enhancing fluid secretion. PKA activation inhibits cell proliferation in wild-type cells but has a stimulatory effect in PKD cells. Calcium deprivation in wild-type cells and delivery of calcium in PKD cells reverse these effects. A proposed mechanism for the proliferative response in PKD and calcium-deprived wild-type cells is inhibition of phosphoinositide 3-kinase (PI3K) and protein kinase B (AKT), which releases protein BRaf from AKT inhibition. This in turn leads to dysregulation of signaling pathways (BRaf/MEK/ERK; AMPK/mTOR) and transcription factors (HIF1, MYC, P53, STAT3) that control cell cycle progression and energy metabolism. Mislocalization of ErbB (epidermal growth factor receptor) receptors and overexpression of growth factors, cytokines, chemokines, and their receptors further contribute to disease progression. AC-VI, Adenylate cyclase 6; AMPK, AMP-activated kinase; ATP, adenosine triphosphate; AVP, vasopressin; CaMKK, calcium/calmodulin-dependent protein kinase kinase; CDK, cyclin-dependent kinase; EGF, epidermal growth factor; ER, endoplasmic reticulum; ERK, extracellular signal–regulated kinase; Gi, inhibitory G protein; Gq, a G protein subunit; Gs, stimulatory G protein; GSK3β, glycogen synthase kinase 3β; HIF, hypoxia-inducible factor; IGF1, insulin-like growth factor 1; inh, inhibition/inhibitor; IP3R, inositol 1,4,5-trisphosphate (IP3) receptor; KCa3.1, a calcium channel; LKB1, liver kinase B1; MEK, mitogen-activated protein kinase kinase; mTOR, mammalian target of rapamycin; PC1, polycystin 1; P2R, purinergic 2 receptor; PC2, polycystin 2; PLC, phospholipase C; Rheb, Ras homolog enriched in brain; RSK, ribosomal s6 kinase; RYR, ryanodine receptor; Sirt1, sirtuin 1; SOC, store operated channel; STAT3, signal transducer and activator of transcription 3; STIM1, stromal interaction molecule 1; SSTR, somatostatin receptor; TKIs, tyrosine-kinase inhibitors; TSC, tuberous sclerosis proteins tuberin (TSC2) and hamartin (TSC1); TZDs, thiazolidinediones; V_2R, vasopressin V_2 receptor.

nonselective PDE activator lowers cAMP and inhibits the growth of MDCK cysts.[130]

The reduction in $[Ca^{2+}]_i$ and the increase in cAMP may play a central role in the pathogenesis of PKD (see Figure 46.4). Cyclic AMP stimulates mitogen-activated protein kinase/extracellularly regulated kinase (MAPK/ERK) signaling and cell proliferation in PKD renal epithelial cells in a manner dependent on PKA, the proto-oncogene tyrosine protein kinase Src, and the protein Ras. On the other hand, cAMP has an inhibitory effect in wild-type cells.[131,132] The abnormal proliferative response to cAMP is directly linked to the alterations in $[Ca^{2+}]_i$ because it can be reproduced in wild-type cells by lowering of $[Ca^{2+}]_i$.[133] Conversely, calcium ionophores or channel activators can rescue the abnormal response of cyst-derived cells.[105] Activation of mTOR signaling also occurs downstream from PKA, through ERK-mediated phosphorylation of tuberin in cystic tissues.[134,135] Activation of mTOR has in turn been linked to transcriptional activation of aerobic glycolysis and increased levels of ATP, which together with ERK-dependent inhibition of liver kinase B1 (LKB1) and inhibition of AMP kinase (AMPK)[136-138] further enhance mTOR signaling.[139] Phosphorylation and inhibition of glycogen synthase kinase type 3β (GSK3β)[140] and direct phosphorylation and stabilization

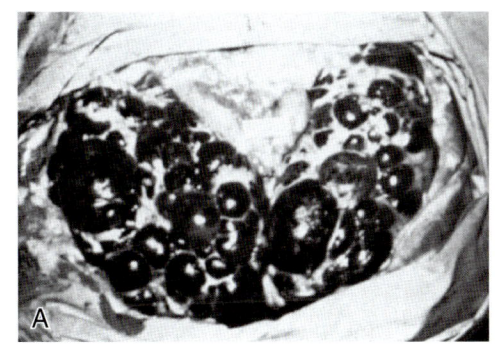

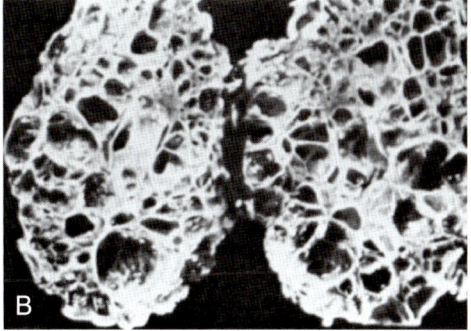

Figure 46.5 Autosomal dominant polycystic kidney disease in situ (**A**) and on cut section (**B**). Note diffuse, bilateral distribution of cysts. (Courtesy FE Cuppage, Kansas City, KS.)

of β-catenin by PKA[141] enhance Wnt/β-catenin signaling. PKA-dependent upregulation of CREB (cAMP response element-binding transcription factor),[142] Pax-2 (paired box gene 2),[103,143] and STAT3 (signal transducer and activator of transcription 3)[144-147] also contribute to the proliferative phenotype of the cystic epithelium. Cyst-derived epithelial cells also exhibit increased expression and apical localization of the epidermal growth factor (EGF) receptors ErbB1 and ErbB2.[148,149] Activation of these receptors by EGF-related compounds, which are present in cyst fluid, is likely to contribute to the stimulation of MAPK/ERK signaling and cell proliferation.

Upregulation of PKA signaling promotes cystogenesis via phosphorylation of CFTR in the apical membrane, stimulation of chloride-driven fluid secretion,[148-155] and possibly other mechanisms such as disruption of tubulogenesis[156] and effects on cell-ECM and epithelial cell–macrophage interactions.[3]

Additional ways that extracellular cues detected by the polycystin complex may be transmitted to the nucleus include canonical and noncanonical Wnt, JAK/STAT (Janus kinase–signal transducer and activator of transcription), and NFAT (nuclear factor of activated T cells) pathways.[154,155] A cleavage event in the G protein–coupled receptor proteolytic site (GPS) domain, separating the extracellular region from the transmembrane part of the protein, may be important for activation of PC1.[157] It has also been proposed that PC1 may activate transcription directly by cleaving at additional sites and through the translocation of the resulting C-terminal fragments to the nucleus, a process that may be regulated by flow.[158,159]

PATHOLOGY

Cystic kidneys usually maintain their reniform shape (Figure 46.5). Their size ranges from minimally or moderately enlarged in early disease to more than 20 times normal size in advanced disease. Although unusual, striking asymmetry of cyst development may be seen. Both the outer and the cut surfaces show numerous cysts ranging in size from barely visible to several centimeters in diameter. They are distributed evenly throughout both the cortical and medullary parenchyma. The papillae and pyramids are distinguishable in early cases but are difficult or impossible to identify in advanced examples, and the calyces and pelves are often greatly distorted.

Nephron reconstruction and microdissection studies revealed that cysts begin as outpouchings from preexisting renal tubules. With enlargement beyond a few millimeters in diameter, most cysts become detached from the tubule of origin. In the early stages of the disease, the noncystic parenchymal elements appear relatively normal because fewer than 1% of the tubules appear to become cystic. The cells in the vast majority of the cysts are not typical of fully differentiated, mature renal tubular epithelium and are thought to be partially dedifferentiated or relatively immature. A minority of the cysts continue to function, as evidenced by their capacity to generate transepithelial electrical gradients and to secrete NaCl and fluid in vitro. The majority of cysts (75%) with Na^+ levels approximating the level in plasma and relatively leaky apical junctions probably represent cysts with epithelium that is less well differentiated than cysts with low Na concentrations.

ADPKD cysts have been thought to arise from all segments of the nephron and collecting ducts. Microdissection studies of ADPKD kidneys in the 1960s and 1970s suggested that collecting ducts are diffusely enlarged and that collecting duct cysts are more numerous and larger than those derived from other tubular segments. Most cysts of at least 1 mm in diameter stain positively for collecting duct markers.[160,161] Studies of *Pkd1* or *Pkd2* rodent models with postnatal development of cystic disease have shown that most cysts originate from the collecting ducts and distal nephron[77,82,83,162] but that proximal tubule cysts may be common at early stages.[10] Cultured epithelial cells from human ADPKD cysts exhibit a larger cAMP response to 1-deamino-8-D-arginine vasopressin (DDAVP) and vasopressin than to the parathyroid hormone, a reaction consistent with a collecting duct origin.[163] These observations indicate that the majority of cysts in adults with ADPKD are derived from the distal nephron and the collecting duct (Figure 46.6).

At the end stage of the disease, the kidneys are usually several times larger than normal and exhibit innumerable fluid-filled cysts that make up almost all of the total renal mass. In these far-advanced cases, only scant normal-appearing parenchyma may be found in isolated patches. Abundant fibrous tissue is plastered along the surface of the kidney beneath the capsule, and on the cut surfaces of transected kidneys, cysts may be found encapsulated by fibrous bands. Tubulointerstitial fibrosis and arteriolar sclerosis are cardinal features of end-stage polycystic kidney. The disappearance of noncystic parenchyma implicates apoptosis as a primary mechanism in progressive renal dysfunction in ADPKD.

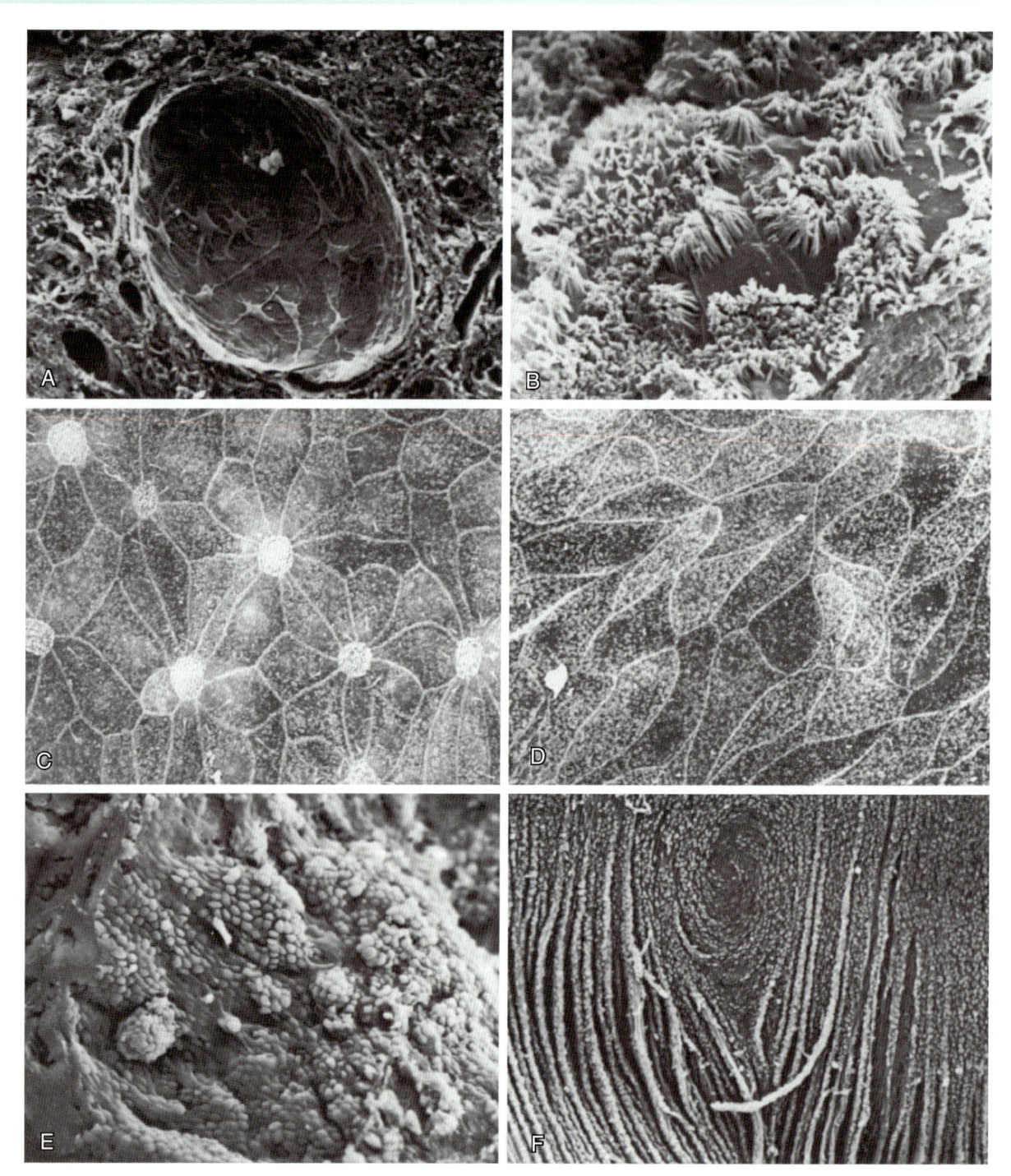

Figure 46.6 Scanning electron micrographs of epithelium lining a cyst in autosomal dominant polycystic kidney disease. **A,** Epithelium typical of glomerular visceral layer (×250). **B,** Epithelium typical of proximal tubule (×3000). **C,** Epithelium typical of cortical collecting duct (×1000). **D,** Epithelium not typical of any normal tubule segment (×1000). **E,** Micropolyps (×250). **F,** Cordlike hyperplasia (×80). (From Grantham JJ, Geiser JL, Evan AP: Cyst formation and growth in autosomal dominant polycystic kidney disease. *Kidney Int* 31:1145-1152, 1987, with permission.)

Up to 90% of adults with ADPKD have cysts in the liver.[164] These cysts are lined by a single layer of epithelium resembling that of the biliary tract and contain fluid that resembles the bile salt–independent fraction of the bile. The electrolyte composition and osmolality are similar to those in the serum; the concentrations of phosphorus, cholesterol, and glucose are lower.[165] The cysts are derived by progressive proliferation and dilatation of the biliary ductules (biliary microhamartomas or von Meyenburg complexes) and peribiliary glands.[166,167] Like kidney cysts, liver cysts become detached as they grow, so macroscopic cysts usually do not communicate with the biliary system. Minimal to moderate dilation of the extrahepatic bile ducts is common. In rare kindreds, hepatic changes indistinguishable from those seen in congenital hepatic fibrosis (CHF) can be seen.

DIAGNOSIS

The diagnosis of ADPKD in an individual with a positive family history relies on imaging. Counseling should be performed before testing. Benefits of testing include certainty regarding diagnosis that may influence family planning, early detection and treatment of disease complications, and selection of genetically unaffected family members for living related donor renal transplantation. Potential discrimination in terms of insurability and employment associated with a positive diagnosis should be discussed. Renal ultrasonography is commonly used because of its lower cost and safety (Figure 46.7).

Revised criteria have been proposed to improve the diagnostic performance of ultrasonography in ADPKD (Table 46.2). The presence of at least three (unilateral or bilateral) renal cysts and of two cysts in each kidney has a positive predictive value (PPV) of 100% in 15- to 39- and 40- to 59-year-old at-risk individuals, respectively.[168] For at-risk individuals ages 60 years and older, four or more cysts in each kidney are required. Although the positive predictive values of these criteria are very high, their sensitivity and negative predictive value are low, particularly when applied to 15- to 59-year-old patients with PKD2. This is a problem in the evaluation of potential kidney donors, in which exclusion of the diagnosis is important. Information on the age at ESKD in other affected family members may be helpful in this setting.[169] A history of at least one affected family member who had ESKD secondary to ADPKD by age 55 years has 100% positive predictive value for PKD1. Conversely, a history of at least one affected family member without ESKD by age 70 or older is predictive of PKD2 or a hypomorphic *PKD1* allele. Different criteria have therefore been proposed to exclude a diagnosis of ADPKD in an individual at risk from a family with an unknown genotype (see Table 46.2). An ultrasonographic finding of normal kidneys or one renal cyst in an individual age 40 years or older has a negative predictive value of 100%. The absence of any renal cyst provides near certainty that ADPKD is absent in at-risk individuals ages 30 to 39 years with a negative predictive value (NPV) of 98.3%. A negative or indeterminate ultrasonography scan result does not exclude ADPKD with certainty in an at-risk individual younger than 30 years. In this setting, the results of magnetic resonance imaging (MRI) or contrast-enhanced computed tomography (CT) provide further assurance, and one study has shown that the finding of a total of fewer than five renal cysts on MRI is sufficient for disease exclusion.[170]

In the absence of a family history of ADPKD, the finding of bilateral renal enlargement and cysts with or without hepatic cysts as well as absence of other manifestations suggesting a different renal cystic disease provides presumptive evidence for the diagnosis. Contrast-enhanced CT and MRI provide better anatomic definition than ultrasonography

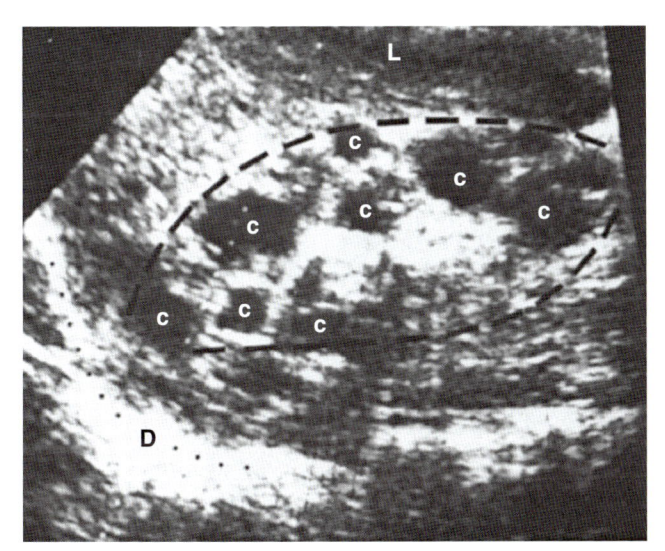

Figure 46.7 Autosomal dominant polycystic kidney disease seen in a parasagittal or longitudinal sonogram. This view of the right kidney was obtained with the patient in the right anterior oblique position. The approximate outline of the kidney is indicated by the *broken line*. Some of the larger renal cysts are indicated by Cs. The liver (L) is at the top of the figure. The right dome of the diaphragm (D) is at the lower left.

Table 46.2 Sonographic Criteria for Diagnosis or Exclusion of Autosomal Dominant Polycystic Kidney Disease

		Family Genotype					
		Unknown		PKD1		PKD2	
Age (yr)	Criteria for Positive Diagnosis	PPV (%)	Sensitivity (%)	PPV (%)	Sensitivity (%)	PPV (%)	Sensitivity (%)
15-29	≥3 cysts, unilateral or bilateral	100	81.7	100	94.3	100	69.5
30-39	≥3 cysts, unilateral or bilateral	100	95.5	100	96.6	100	94.9
40-59	≥2 cysts in each kidney	100	90.0	100	92.6	100	88.8
≥60	≥4 cysts in each kidney	100	100	100	100	100	100
	Revised Criteria For Diagnosis Exclusion	NPV (%)	Specificity (%)	NPV (%)	Specificity (%)	NPV (%)	Specificity (%)
15-29	≥1 cyst	90.8	97.1	99.1	97.6	83.5	96.6
30-39	≥1 cyst	98.3	94.8	100	96.0	96.8	93.8
40-59	≥2 cysts	100	98.2	100	98.4	100	97.8

NPV, Negative predictive value; PPV, positive predictive value.

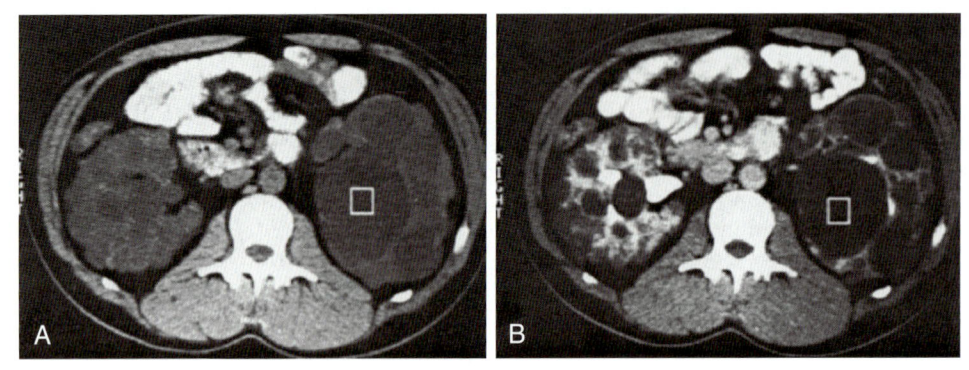

Figure 46.8 Computed tomography (CT) scans of polycystic kidneys. This male patient has autosomal dominant polycystic kidney disease, and his serum creatinine level is within the normal range. An oral contrast agent was given to highlight the intestine. **A,** CT scan without contrast. **B,** CT scan at the same level as **A** but after intravenous infusion of iodinated radiocontrast material. The cursor *(box)* is used to determine the relative density of cyst fluid, which in this case is equal to that of water. Contrast enhancement highlights functioning parenchyma, which here is concentrated primarily in the right kidney. The renal collecting system also is highlighted by contrast material in both kidneys.

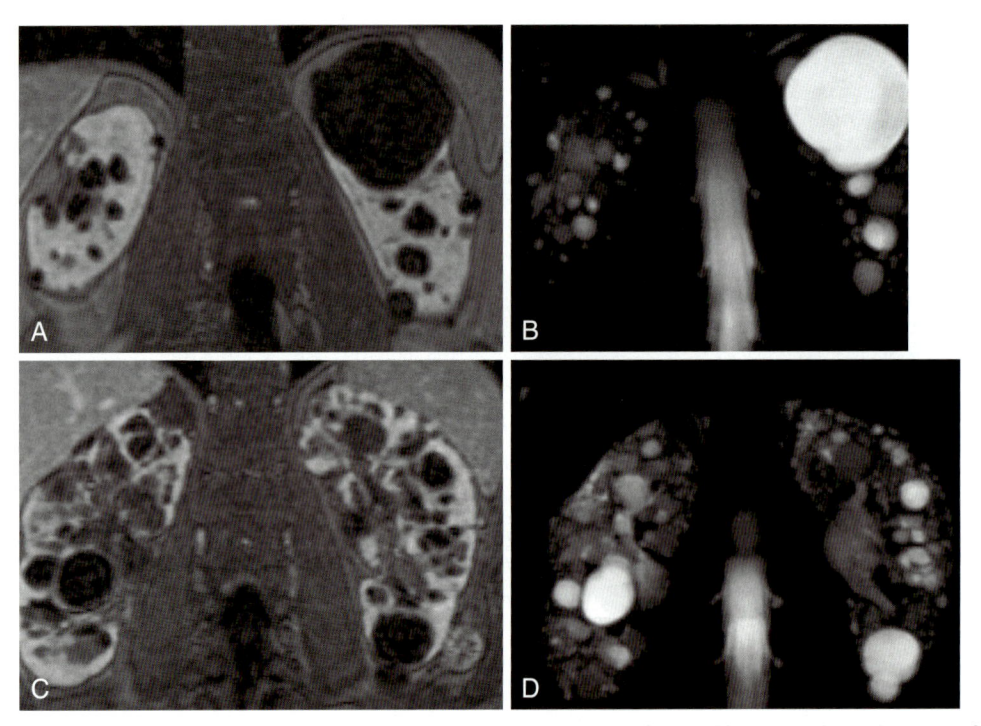

Figure 46.9 Magnetic resonance imaging studies of two female patients with mild (A and B) and moderately severe (C and D) disease. In neither subject was the serum creatinine value higher than 1.1 mg/dL. For the images in **A** and **C**, gadolinium was infused intravenously a few minutes previously. The residual, normal parenchyma between cysts is highlighted by gadolinium. In **B** and **D**, heavy T2-weighted images are shown at the same kidney level as in **A** and **C**. The cysts are emphasized, illustrating that cysts smaller than 3 mm can be detected.

and are more helpful to ascertain the severity and prognosis of the disease (Figures 46.8 and 46.9).

Genetic testing can be used when the imaging results are equivocal and when a definite diagnosis is required in a younger individual, such as a potential living related kidney donor. It may also be helpful in patients with a negative family history, atypical radiologic presentations, and unusually severe or mild disease.[171] Prenatal testing is rarely considered for ADPKD.[172,173] Preimplantation genetic diagnosis, which is most commonly used in severe genetic diseases with early manifestations, such as cystic fibrosis and ARPKD, may become more frequently used in ADPKD, but it is available only in certain countries and the acceptance of this technique is influenced by personal values as well as the severity of the disease.[172,174]

Genetic testing can be performed by linkage or sequence analysis. Linkage analysis uses highly informative microsatellite markers flanking *PKD1* and *PKD2* and requires an accurate diagnosis, availability, and willingness of a sufficient number of affected family members to be tested. Moreover, the test results are indirect and can be confounded by de novo mutations, mosaicism, and bilineal disease. Because of these constraints, linkage analysis for the diagnosis of ADPKD is now rarely used. The large size and complexity of *PKD1* and marked allelic heterogeneity are obstacles to molecular testing by direct DNA analysis. Mutation scanning by direct sequencing of *PKD1* and *PKD2* now yields detection rates higher than 90%.[52,175] However, because most mutations are unique and up to one third of *PKD1* changes are missense, the pathogenicity of some changes is difficult to prove. Advances in resequencing (i.e., next-generation sequencing [NGS]) technologies have enabled high-throughput mutation screening of both *PKD1* and *PKD2* with a recent "proof-of-principle" study showing promising results.[56] The adaptation of this new technology to molecular diagnostics in ADPKD is expected to facilitate mutation screening while reducing costs.[176]

RENAL MANIFESTATIONS

Cyst Development and Growth

Many manifestations of ADPKD are directly related to renal cyst development and enlargement. A study of 241 nonazotemic patients followed prospectively with yearly MRI examinations by the Consortium for Radiologic Imaging Studies of Polycystic Kidney Disease (CRISP) has provided invaluable information to the understanding of how the cysts develop and grow.[177,178] Total kidney volume (TKV) and cyst volumes increased exponentially (Figure 46.10). At baseline, TKV was 1060 ± 642 mL, and the mean increase over 3 years was 204 mL or 5.3% per year. The rates of change of total kidney and total cyst volumes and of right and left kidney volumes were strongly correlated. Baseline TKV predicted the subsequent rate of increase in renal volume and decline in renal function.[179] Furthermore, TKV, particularly when used together with age and kidney function, identifies individuals who are at risk for progression to ESKD and may be useful to select patients whose disease characteristics are most likely to be informative in clinical trials and who are most likely to benefit from treatment as they become available.[180] Higher urine sodium excretion and lower serum high-density lipoprotein (HDL) cholesterol at baseline were also associated with greater kidney growth.[181]

Renal Function Abnormalities

Impaired urinary concentrating capacity is common even at early stages of ADPKD.[182] Sixty percent of children cannot maximally concentrate their urine. Plasma vasopressin levels are increased. The vasopressin-resistant concentrating defect is not explained by reduced cAMP or expression of concentration-associated genes, which are consistently increased in animal models. It has not been determined whether the defect is attributable to disruption of the medullary architecture by the cysts or to a cellular defect directly linked to the disruption of the polycystin function. Newer studies suggest that the urinary concentrating defect and elevated vasopressin values may contribute to cystogenesis. They may also contribute to the glomerular hyperfiltration seen in children and young adults[183] and to the development of hypertension and the progression of chronic kidney disease (CKD). Defective medullary trapping of ammonia and transfer to the urine caused by the concentrating defect may contribute to the low urine pH values, hypocitric aciduria, and predisposition to stone formation.

Reduced renal blood flow is another early functional defect.[184] It may be caused by the changes in intrarenal pressures, neurohumoral or local mediators, and/or intrinsic vascular abnormalities. Mild to moderate persistent proteinuria (150-1500 mg/day) may be found in a significant number of patients in the middle to late stages of the disease. It is an indicator of a more progressive disease.[185] Patients with proteinuria may also excrete doubly refractile lipid bodies (oval fat bodies).[186]

Hypertension

Hypertension (blood pressure ≥ 140 mm Hg systolic /90 mm Hg diastolic), found in approximately 50% of 20- to 34 year-old patients with ADPKD and normal renal function, is present in nearly 100% of patients with ESKD.[187] Development of hypertension is accompanied by a reduction in renal blood flow, an increase in filtration fraction, abnormal renal handling of sodium, and extensive remodeling of the renal vasculature.

The association between renal size and the prevalence of hypertension supports the hypothesis that stretching and compression of the vascular tree by cyst expansion causes ischemia and activation of the renin angiotensin aldosterone system (RAAS).[188] The expression of PC1 and PC2 in vascular smooth muscle[189-191] and endothelium,[192] along with enhanced vascular smooth muscle contractility[193] and impaired endothelium-dependent vasorelaxation,[194] suggests that a primary disruption of polycystin function in the vasculature may also play a role in the early development of hypertension and renal vascular remodeling.

Whether circulating angiotensin is instrumental in causing hypertension is controversial.[195,196] Plasma renin activity and aldosterone values are normal in most studies. Because blood pressures are higher than those of control participants, it has been argued that the renin and aldosterone levels are not appropriately suppressed. A 1990 study showed higher levels after short- or long-term administration of an angiotensin-converting enzyme (ACE) inhibitor in normotensive and hypertensive patients with ADPKD and normal renal function than in both normal subjects and patients with essential hypertension.[195] Another study found no differences in hormonal or blood pressure responses between patients with ADPKD and patients with essential hypertension matched in terms of renal function and blood pressure under conditions of high- and low-sodium intake and after the administration of an ACE inhibitor.[196] Sodium intake was not controlled in the former study, and differences in selection and ethnic composition of the control groups have been offered as possible explanations for the different results.

There is stronger evidence for the local activation of the intrarenal RAAS. It includes (1) partial reversal of the reduced renal blood flow, increased renal vascular resistance, and increased filtration fraction by short- or long-term administration of an ACE inhibitor,[195,197,198] (2) shift of immunoreactive renin from the juxtaglomerular apparatus to the walls of the arterioles and small arteries,[199,200] (3) ectopic synthesis of renin in the epithelium of dilated tubules and cysts,[201,202] and (4) ACE-independent generation of angiotensin II by a chymase-like enzyme.[202]

Nitric oxide associated endothelium–dependent vasorelaxation has been shown to be impaired in small subcutaneous resistance vessels from patients with normal renal function before the development of hypertension.[203-205] Other factors proposed to contribute to hypertension in

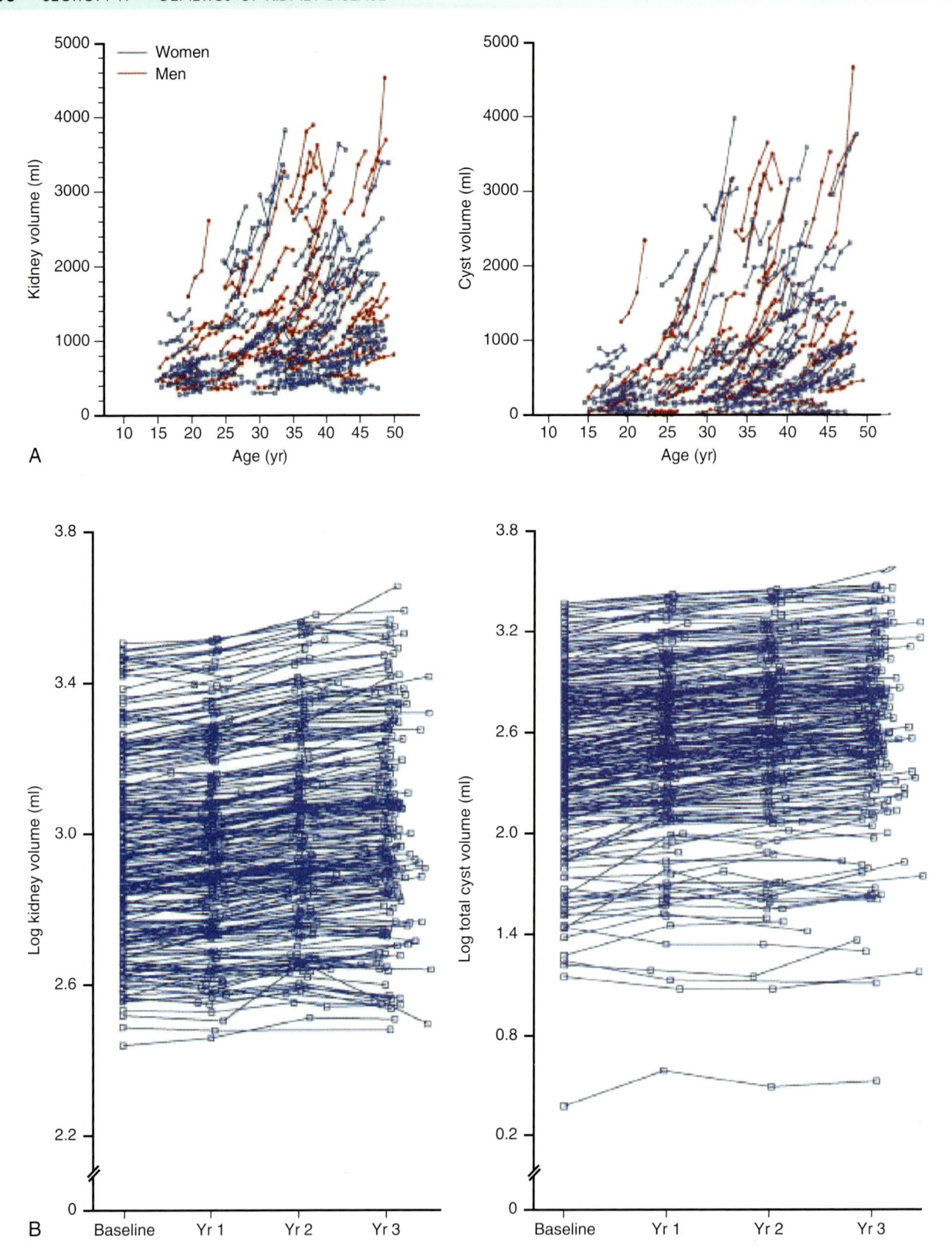

Figure 46.10 Progression of autosomal dominant polycystic kidney disease. **A,** Combined left and right total kidney (TKV) and cyst (TCV) volumes in relation to age in women *(blue)* and men *(red)*. The lines connecting the four measurements for each patient in the 3 years of follow-up exhibit a concave upward sweep suggestive of an exponential growth process. **B,** Log_{10} combined total kidney (TKV) and cyst (TCV) volumes in relation to time. The linearity of the four measurements for each patient in the 3 years of follow-up is consistent with an exponential growth process. (Reproduced from Grantham JJ, Torres VE, Chapman AB, et al: Volume progression in polycystic kidney disease. *N Engl J Med* 354:2122-2130, 2006.)

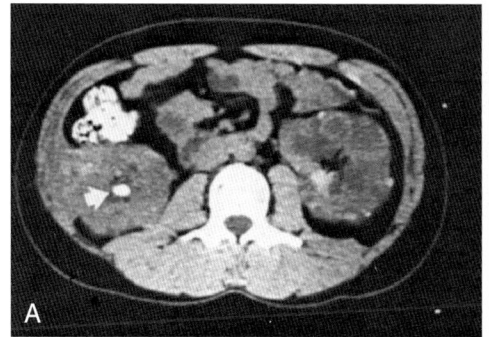

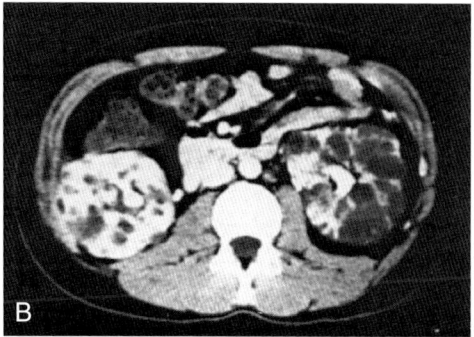

Figure 46.11 Computed tomography (CT) of polycystic kidneys in a male patient whose serum creatinine level is within the normal range. **A,** CT scan without contrast shows a radiopaque stone in the pelvis of the right kidney *(arrow)*. **B,** CT scan after intravenous administration of an iodinated radiocontrast agent. The stone now is obscured by contrast medium in the renal pelvis.

ADPKD include increases in sympathetic nerve activity and plasma endothelin 1 levels as well as insulin resistance.[206]

The diagnosis of hypertension in ADPKD is often made late. Twenty-four-hour ambulatory blood pressure monitoring of children or young adults without hypertension may reveal blood pressure elevations, attenuated nocturnal blood pressure dipping, and exaggerated blood pressure response during exercise, which may be accompanied by left ventricular hypertrophy and diastolic dysfunction. Early detection and treatment of hypertension are important because cardiovascular disease is the main cause of death in patients with ADPKD.[39,207] Uncontrolled blood pressure increases the morbidity and mortality from valvular heart disease and aneurysms as well as the risk of proteinuria, hematuria, and a faster decline of renal function. The presence of hypertension also increases the risk of fetal and maternal complications during pregnancy. Normotensive women with ADPKD usually have uncomplicated pregnancies.[208]

Pain

Pain is the most frequent symptom (60%) reported by adult patients with ADPKD.[209,210] Acute pain may be associated with renal hemorrhage, passage of stones, and urinary tract infections. Some patients have chronic flank pain without an identifiable etiology other than the cysts.

Vascular endothelial growth factor (VEGF) produced by the cystic epithelium[211] may promote angiogenesis, hemorrhage into cysts, and gross hematuria. Symptomatic episodes likely underestimate the frequency of cyst hemorrhage because more than 90% of patients with ADPKD have hyperdense (CT) or high-signal (MRI) cysts, reflecting blood or high protein content. Most hemorrhages resolve within 2 to 7 days. If symptoms last longer than 1 week or if the initial episode occurs after the age of 50 years, investigation to exclude neoplasm should be undertaken.

Approximately 20% of patients with ADPKD have kidney stones, usually composed of uric acid and calcium oxalate.[212,213] Metabolic factors include decreased ammonia excretion, low urinary pH, and low urinary citrate concentration. Urinary stasis secondary to the distorted renal anatomy may also play a role. CT of the abdomen before and after contrast enhancement is the best imaging technique to detect small uric acid stones that may be very faint on plain films with tomograms and to differentiate stones from cyst wall and parenchymal calcifications. Stones may be missed if only a contrast-enhanced CT is obtained (Figure 46.11). Dual-energy CT can be used to distinguish between calcium and uric acid stones.[214,215]

As in the general population, urinary tract infections affect women more frequently than men. Most are caused by Enterobacteriaceae.[216] CT and MRI are useful to detect complicated cysts and provide anatomic definition, but the findings are not specific for infection (Figure 46.12). Nuclear imaging (^{67}Ga or ^{111}In-labeled leukocyte scans) may be helpful, but false-negative and false-positive results are possible. Fluorine 18 2-fluoro-2-deoxy-D-glucose (FDG) positron emission tomography (PET) has become a promising agent for detection of infected cysts, but its use to diagnose kidney infections may be difficult because FDG is filtered by the kidneys, is not reabsorbed by the tubules, and appears in the collecting system.[217-219] Cyst aspiration should be considered when the clinical setting and imaging are suggestive and blood and urine cultures are negative.

Renal cell carcinoma (RCC) is a rare cause of pain in ADPKD. Although it does not occur more frequently than in the patients with other renal diseases,[220] it may manifest at an earlier age in patients with ADPKD, with frequent constitutional symptoms and a higher proportion of sarcomatoid, bilateral, multicentric, and metastatic tumors.[221] A solid mass on ultrasonography, speckled calcifications on CT and contrast enhancement, and tumor thrombus and regional lymphadenopathies on CT or MRI should raise the suspicion of a carcinoma.

Renal Failure

The development of renal failure in ADPKD is highly variable. In most patients, renal function is maintained within the normal range because of compensatory adaptation, despite relentless growth of cysts, until the fourth to sixth decade of life (Figure 46.13). By the time renal function starts declining, the kidneys usually are markedly enlarged and distorted with little recognizable parenchyma on imaging studies. At this stage, the average rate of decline in glomerular filtration rate (GFR) is approximately 4.4 to 5.9 mL/min/yr.[222] The mutated gene (*PKD1* vs. *PKD2*), type of mutation in *PKD1* (truncating versus nontruncating), and modifier genes determine to a significant extent the clinical course of ADPKD (see earlier discussion). Other risk factors are male gender, diagnosis before the age of 30 years, a first episode of hematuria before age 30 years, onset of hypertension before age 35 years, hyperlipidemia, low

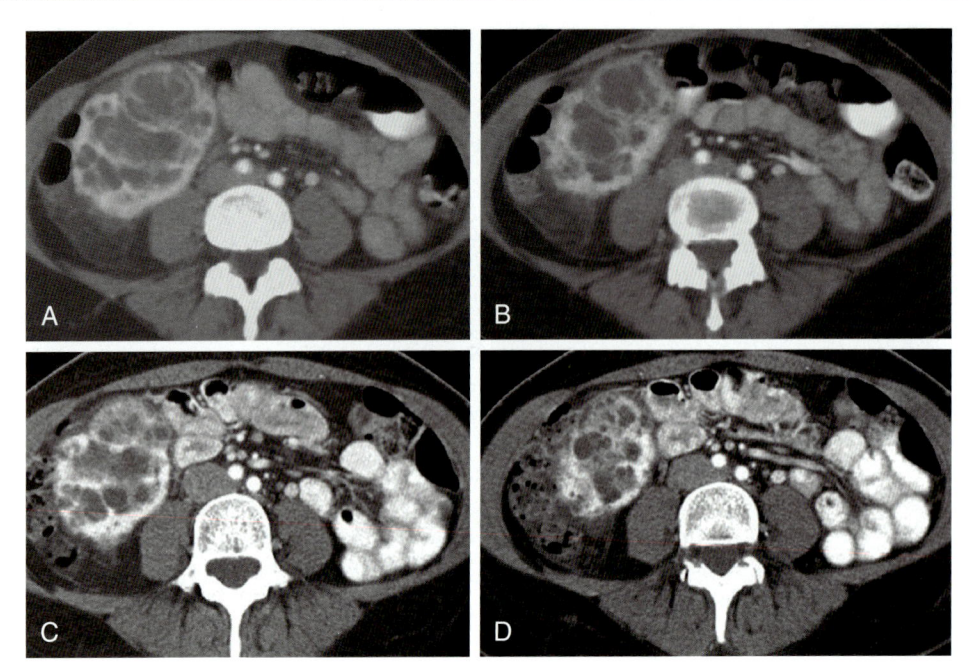

Figure 46.12 Cyst infection. A and **B,** Contrast-enhanced computed tomography (CT) scans demonstrate a 4-cm infected cyst in the anterior portion of the lower pole of the right kidney and inflammatory stranding in the perirenal fat. **C** and **D,** CT scans obtained after 3 weeks of antibiotic therapy show a decrease in the size of the cyst and improved enhancement of the renal parenchyma.

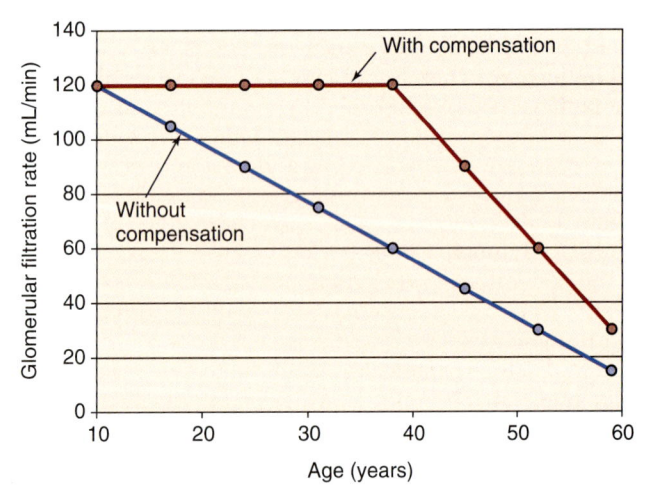

Figure 46.13 Effects of compensatory maintenance of glomerular filtration rate (GFR) on the pattern of progression in autosomal dominant polycystic kidney disease. It was assumed that, beginning at the age of 10 years, the patient loses an amount of parenchyma each year that normally contributes 2 mL/min of GFR. It was further assumed that each residual normal glomerulus can double the single-nephron GFR by compensatory mechanisms (as seen in normal individuals by the maintenance of total GFR after uninephrectomy for kidney donation). As seen in the model, total GFR is maintained until parenchymal loss precludes complete compensation; at that point, total GFR begins to fall at a rate that appears more "precipitous" than what had actually occurred. This model illustrates that GFR is a poor indicator of ADPKD progression and that more sensitive markers of parenchymal loss are needed to facilitate earlier monitoring.

level of high-density lipoprotein cholesterol, and sickle cell trait.[223,224] Whether blacks or individuals with specific *ACE* or *ENOS* genotypes are at an increased risk for disease progression is uncertain. Smoking raises the risk for ESKD, at least in some patient subsets, such as male smokers with no history of ACE inhibitor treatment.[225]

Several factors contribute to renal function decline. A strong relationship with renal enlargement has been noted. CRISP has confirmed this relationship and has shown that kidney and cyst volumes are the strongest predictors of renal functional decline.[226] After a mean follow-up of 7.9 years, 30.7% of CRISP enrollees reached stage 3 CKD. Correlations of height-adjusted TKV at baseline with GFR at different time points increased from −0.22 (GFR at baseline) to −0.65 (GFR at year 8).[179] A height-adjusted TKV of 600 mL/m or higher at baseline most accurately defined the risk for development of stage 3 CKD within 8 years (area under the curve of 0.84 in a receiver operator characteristic analysis, 95% confidence interval [CI], 0.79 to 0.90). Kidney volume was a better predictor of GFR decline than baseline age, serum creatinine, blood urea nitrogen (BUN), urinary albumin, and monocyte chemotactic protein-1 (MCP-1) excretion.

CRISP has also shown that reduced renal blood flow (or increased vascular resistance) is an additional independent predictor of GFR decline.[184] This factor points to the importance of vascular remodeling in the progression of the disease and may account for cases in which the decline of renal function seems to be out of proportion to the severity of the cystic disease. Angiotensin II, transforming growth factor-β, and reactive oxygen species may contribute to the vascular lesions and interstitial inflammation and fibrosis by stimulating the synthesis of chemokines, ECM, and metalloproteinase inhibitors. The expression of MCP-1 and osteopontin is increased in cyst epithelial cells. MCP-1 is found in cyst fluids in high concentrations, and the urinary excretion is increased.[227] Other factors such as heavy use of analgesics may contribute to CKD progression in some patients.

Patients with ADPKD and advanced CKD have less anemia than patients with other renal diseases because of enhanced production of erythropoietin by the polycystic kidneys.

EXTRARENAL MANIFESTATIONS
Polycystic Liver Disease

Polycystic liver disease (PLD) is the most common extrarenal manifestation of ADPKD. It is associated with both *PKD1* and non-*PKD1* genotypes. PLD also occurs as a genetically distinct disease in the absence of renal cysts. Similar to ADPKD, autosomal dominant PLD (ADPLD) is genetically heterogeneous, with three genes identified. *PRKCSH* (chromosome 19) and *SEC63* (chromosome 6) account for approximately one third of isolated ADPLD cases.[228-230] Whole-exome sequencing has now shown that *LRP5* mutations (chromosome 11) are associated with hepatic cystogenesis.[231]

Although hepatic cysts are rare in children, the frequency increases with age and may have been underestimated by ultrasonography and CT studies. Their prevalences according to MRI in the CRISP study were 58%, 85%, and 94% in 15- to 24-year-old, 25- to 34-year-old, and 35- to 46-year-old participants, respectively.[164] Hepatic cysts are more prevalent and hepatic cyst volume is larger in women than in men. Women who have multiple pregnancies or who have used oral contraceptive agents or estrogen replacement therapy have more severe disease, suggesting an estrogen effect on hepatic cyst growth.[188,232] Estrogen receptors are expressed in the epithelium lining the hepatic cysts, and estrogens stimulate proliferation of hepatic cyst–derived cells.

Typically PLD is asymptomatic, but symptoms have become more frequent as the life span of patients with ADPKD has lengthened because of dialysis and transplantation. Symptoms may result from the mass effect or from complicating infection and hemorrhage (Figure 46.14). Symptoms typically caused by massive enlargement of the liver or by mass effect from a single or a limited number of dominant cysts include dyspnea, early satiety, gastroesophageal reflux, and mechanical lower back pain. Other complications caused by mass effect include hepatic venous outflow obstruction, inferior vena cava compression, portal vein compression, and bile duct compression manifesting as obstructive jaundice.[233]

Symptomatic complications of hepatic cysts include cyst hemorrhage, infection, and, rarely, torsion or rupture. The typical manifestation of cyst infection consists of localized pain, fever, leukocytosis, elevated erythrocyte sedimentation rate, and, often, elevated alkaline phosphatase. It is usually monomicrobial and caused by Enterobacteriaceae.[234-236] MRI sensitively differentiates between complicated and uncomplicated hepatic cyst. On CT, fluid-debris levels within cysts, cyst wall thickening, intracystic gas bubbles, and heterogeneous or increased density have been associated with infection. Radionuclide imaging and FDG-PET scanning have been used for diagnosis.[237]

Mild dilation of the common bile duct has been observed in 40% of patients with PLD studied by CT and may rarely be associated with episodes of cholangitis.[238] Rare associations of PLD include CHF, adenomas of the ampulla of Vater, and cholangiocarcinoma.

Cysts in Other Organs

Cysts are found in the pancreas in approximately 5%, arachnoid in approximately 8%, and seminal vesicles in approximately 40% of patients with ADPKD.[239-244] Seminal vesicle cysts rarely result in infertility.[245] Defective sperm motility is another cause of male infertility in ADPKD.[246] Pancreatic cysts are almost always asymptomatic, with very rare occurrences of recurrent pancreatitis. It is uncertain whether the reported association of carcinoma of the pancreas represents more than chance. Arachnoid membrane cysts are asymptomatic but may increase the risk for subdural hematomas.[244,247] Spinal meningeal diverticula may occur with increased frequency and rarely manifest as intracranial hypotension due to a cerebrospinal fluid leak.[248] Ovarian cysts are not associated with ADPKD.

Vascular Manifestations

Vascular manifestations of ADPKD include intracranial aneurysms and dolichoectasias, thoracic aortic and cervicocephalic artery dissections, and coronary artery aneurysms.

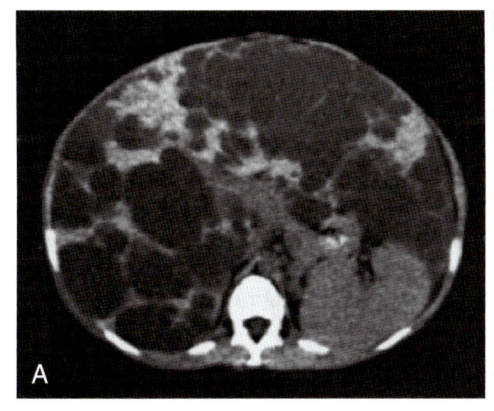

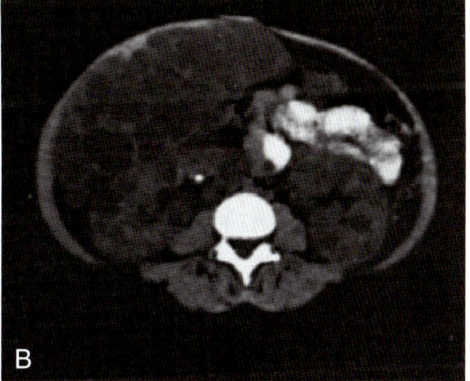

Figure 46.14 Computed tomography (CT) scan of polycystic liver and kidneys in female patient with autosomal dominant polycystic kidney disease. The serum creatinine level and liver function test results were within the normal range. An oral contrast agent was given to highlight the intestine, but no intravenous contrast was used. **A,** Massive enlargement of the liver caused by intraparenchymal cysts. **B,** CT scan at a lower level in the abdomen shows cystic kidneys and the lower portion of the cystic liver.

They are caused by alterations in the vasculature directly linked to mutations in *PKD1* or *PKD2*. PC1 and PC2 are expressed in VSMCs.[189-191] *Pkd2*[+/−] VSMCs exhibit increased rates of proliferation and apoptosis, and *Pkd2*[+/−] mice have a greater susceptibility to vascular injury and premature death when hypertension is induced to develop.[85,117]

ICAs occur in approximately 6% of patients with a negative family history and in 16% of those with a positive family history of aneurysms.[249] They are most often asymptomatic. Focal findings such as cranial nerve palsy and seizure result from compression of local structures. The risk of rupture depends on many factors (see later discussion). Rupture carries a 35% to 55% risk of combined severe morbidity and mortality.[250] The mean age at rupture is lower than in the general population (39 years vs. 51 years, respectively). Most patients have normal renal function, and up to 29% have normal blood pressure, at the time of rupture.

Cardiac Manifestations

Mitral valve prolapse observed by echocardiography is the most common valvular abnormality, found in up to 25% of patients with ADPKD.[251,252] Aortic insufficiency may occur in association with dilation of the aortic root.[253] Although these lesions may progress with time, they rarely require valve replacement. Screening echocardiography is not indicated unless a murmur is detected on physical examination.

Diverticular Disease

Colonic diverticulosis and diverticulitis are more common in patients with ADPKD and ESKD than in those with other renal diseases. Whether this increased risk extends to patients before the onset of ESKD is uncertain.[254] There have been reports of extracolonic diverticular disease.[255] It may become clinically significant in a minority of patients. Subtle alterations in polycystin function may enhance the smooth muscle dysfunction from aging, which is thought to underlie the development of diverticula.

Bronchiectasias

PC1 is expressed in the motile cilia of airway epithelial cells. Bronchiectasis occurs three times more frequently in patients with ADPKD than in control individuals (37% vs. 13%, respectively; $P < 0.002$), as detected by CT.[256]

TREATMENT

Current therapy of ADPKD is directed toward limiting the morbidity and mortality from the complications of the disease.

Hypertension

There is no proven antihypertensive agent of choice in ADPKD. ACE inhibitors or angiotensin receptor blockers (ARBs) increase renal blood flow, have a low side effect profile, and may have renoprotective properties beyond blood pressure control. Some studies have shown better preservation of renal function or reduction in proteinuria and left ventricular hypertrophy with ACE inhibitors or ARBs than with diuretics or calcium channel blockers,[257-259] but other studies have been unable to detect the superiority of these drugs.[260] A meta-analysis of 142 patients with ADPKD in eight randomized clinical trials showed that ACE inhibitors were more effective in lowering urine protein excretion and slowing kidney disease progression in patients with higher levels of proteinuria, but the overall kidney disease progression was not significantly different (29% in the inhibitor group vs. 41% in the control group).[261] Most studies have been limited by inadequate power, short follow-ups, wide ranges of renal function, and the use of doses with inadequate pharmacologic effects.

Equally controversial has been the optimal blood pressure target. In the Modification of Diet in Renal Disease (MDRD) study, patients with ADPKD and a baseline GFR between 13 and 24 mL/min/1.73 m^2 assigned to a low blood pressure target (≤92 mm Hg) had faster declines in GFR than those assigned to a standard blood pressure goal (≤107 mm Hg). The reason may be the inability to autoregulate renal blood flow.[222] The rate of decline in participants with a baseline GFR between 25 and 55 mL/min/1.73 m^2 was not affected by the blood pressure target over a mean intervention period of 2.2 years. However, an extended follow-up of these patients showed a delayed onset of kidney failure and a reduced composite outcome of kidney failure and all-cause mortality in the low blood pressure target group (51% of them taking ACE inhibitors) in comparison with those in the standard blood pressure target group (32% of them taking ACE inhibitors).[262] The magnitude of this beneficial effect was similar to that observed in patients with other renal diseases.

The results of the HALT Progression of Polycystic Kidney Disease (HALT-PKD) clinical trials have been published.[263,264] In study A, 558 hypertensive patients with ADPKD (15 to 49 years of age, with estimated GFRs [eGFRs] greater than 60 mL/min/1.73 m^2 of body surface area) were randomly assigned to either a standard blood pressure target (120/70 to 130/80 mm Hg) or a low blood pressure target (95/60 to 110/75 mm Hg) and to either lisinopril plus telmisartan or lisinopril plus placebo.[263] In study B, 486 hypertensive patients with ADPKD (18 to 64 years of age, with eGFRs 25 to 60 mL/min/1.73 m^2) were randomly assigned to receive lisinopril plus telmisartan or lisinopril plus placebo, with the doses adjusted to achieve a blood pressure of 110/70 to 130/80 mm Hg.[264] Both studies showed that an ACE inhibitor alone adequately controlled hypertension in most patients, justifying its use as first-line treatment for hypertension in this disease. Study A showed that lowering blood pressure to levels below those recommended by current guidelines in young patients with good kidney function reduced the rate of increase in kidney volume by 14%, the increase in renal vascular resistance, urine albumin excretion (all identified in CRISP as predictors of renal function decline), left ventricular mass index, and, marginally (after the first 4 months of treatment), the rate of decline in eGFR.[263] The overall effect of low blood pressure on eGFR, however, was not statistically significant, possibly because the reduction of blood pressure to low levels was associated with an acute reduction in eGFR within the first 4 months of treatment. Although these results may not be viewed universally as positive, they do underline the importance of early detection and treatment of hypertension in ADPKD. The addition of an ARB to an ACE inhibitor did not show additional benefit.

Several studies suggest that improved blood pressure control in patients with ADPKD over the last two decades has been associated with reduced cardiovascular morbidity and mortality. A small prospective study from the University of Colorado showed that rigorous blood pressure control caused a greater decrease in left ventricular mass without a detectable effect on renal function.[265] A population-based study using the U.K. General Practice Research Database found that increased use of antihypertensive drugs over the period from 1991 to 2008 in patients with ADPKD, particularly of agents blocking the RAAS, was accompanied by reduced mortality.[266] The low prevalence of left ventricular hypertrophy (LVH) assessed by MRI in 543 hypertensive patients with ADPKD (mean age 36 years) who had normal renal function and were enrolled in the HALT-PKD study at entry into the study—3.9% by nonindexed left ventricular mass (LVM) and 0.9% by LVM index (LVMI), much lower than that observed in earlier studies[267]—likely reflects the excellent blood pressure control (mean approximately 124/82 mm Hg) and the high utilization of RAAS blockers (61%).[268] In Danish patients with ADPKD and ESKD, cardiovascular and cerebrovascular deaths decreased from 1993 to 2008, possibly owing to a greater effectiveness of antihypertensive treatment.[269]

There is less evidence that the better control of hypertension over the last two decades has delayed the progression to ESKD. Two observational studies have suggested that in patients with ADPKD, the average age at start of renal replacement therapy (RRT) has increased considerably during the last two decades.[270,271] A study of European Renal Association–European Dialysis and Transplant Association (ERA-EDTA) Registry data on patients starting RRT between 1991 and 2010, spanning 12 European countries with 208 million inhabitants, also showed that mean age at onset of RRT among patients with ADPKD (n = 20,596) has risen, albeit considerably less than in the two aforementioned studies, from 56.6 to 58.0 years.[272] Although the RRT incidence did not change among patients with ADPKD younger than 50 years, it increased among older patients (> 70 years). These data suggest that the greater age of patients with ADPKD at the start of RRT may be explained by increased access of the elderly to RRT or by the lower competing risk of mortality prior to the start of RRT, rather than the consequence of effective renoprotective therapies.[273,274]

Pain

Causes of pain in ADPKD that may require intervention, such as infections, stones, and tumors, should be excluded. Long-term administration of nephrotoxic agents should be avoided. Narcotic analgesics should be reserved for acute episodes. Psychological evaluation and an understanding and supportive attitude on the part of the physician are essential to minimize the risk for narcotic and analgesic dependence in patients with chronic pain. Reassurance, lifestyle modification, avoidance of aggravating activities, tricyclic antidepressants, and pain clinic interventions such as splanchnic nerve blockade with local anesthesia or steroids may be helpful.[209,210]

When conservative measures fail, surgical interventions can be considered. Aspiration of large cysts under ultrasonographic or CT guidance is a simple procedure and may help identify the cause of the pain. Sclerosing agents may be used to prevent the reaccumulation of fluid. When multiple cysts contribute to pain, laparoscopic or surgical cyst fenestration through lumbotomy or flank incisions may be of benefit.[275] Laparoscopy is as effective as open surgical fenestration for patients with limited disease and has a shorter, less complicated recovery period.[276,277] Surgical interventions do not accelerate the decline in renal function as was once thought, but they do not preserve declining renal function either. Laparoscopic renal denervation or thoracoscopic sympathosplanchnicectomy can be considered, particularly in polycystic kidneys without large cysts.[278,279] Percutaneous transluminal renal denervation has been proposed as a potential treatment option for PKD-related pain but has not yet been adequately tested.[280,281] Laparoscopic or retroperitoneoscopic nephrectomy is indicated for symptomatic patients with ESKD. Arterial embolization is an alternative when the surgical risk is high, but its role has not been fully defined.

Cyst Hemorrhage

Cyst hemorrhages are usually self-limiting and respond to conservative management with bed rest, analgesics, and hydration. When a subcapsular or retroperitoneal hematoma is causing significant decrease in hematocrit and hemodynamic instability, hospitalization, transfusion, and investigation by CT or angiography become necessary. In cases of unusually severe or persistent hemorrhage, segmental arterial embolization can be successful. If not, surgery may be required to control bleeding. Segmental arterial embolization or surgery may be required in some cases. The antfibrinolytic agent tranexamic acid has been successfully used in some cases, but no controlled studies of its use have been performed[282] and the dose needs to be reduced in the presence of renal insufficiency. Potential adverse effects of this treatment include glomerular thrombosis and ureteral obstructions due to clots.

Cyst Infection

Cyst infections are often difficult to treat.[216] Treatment failure may occur because of poor antibiotic penetration into the cysts. Lipophilic agents penetrate the cysts consistently. If fever persists after 1 to 2 weeks of appropriate antimicrobial therapy, percutaneous or surgical drainage of infected cysts or, in the case of end-stage polycystic kidneys, nephrectomy should be undertaken. If fever recurs after antibiotic therapy is stopped, a complicating feature such as obstruction, perinephric abscess, or a stone should be excluded. If none is identified, several months of antibiotic therapy may be required to eradicate the infection.

Nephrolithiasis

Treatment is similar to that in patients without ADPKD. Potassium citrate is indicated for the three causes of stones associated with ADPKD, that is, uric acid lithiasis, hypocitraturic calcium oxalate nephrolithiasis, and distal acidification defects. Extracorporeal shock wave lithotripsy and percutaneous nephrostolithotomy have been performed successfully without undue complications.

End-Stage Kidney Disease

Patients with ADPKD do better on dialysis than patients with other causes of ESKD, perhaps because of higher levels of erythropoietin and hemoglobin or lower comorbidity.[283] Despite renal size and increased risk for hernias, peritoneal dialysis is usually possible.

Transplantation is the treatment of choice for ESKD in ADPKD. There is no difference in patient or graft survival between patients with ADPKD and other ESKD populations. Graft survival after living donor transplants is also no different in patients with and without ADPKD. However, data are more limited for those with ADPKD, in whom living related donor transplantation was not widely practiced in the past. In 1999, for instance, 30% of kidney transplants for ADPKD patients were from living donors, compared with 12% in 1990.

Complications after transplantation are no greater in the ADPKD population than in the general population, and specific complications directly related to ADPKD are rare. Cyst infection is not increased after transplantation, and there is no significant increase in the incidence of symptomatic mitral valve prolapse or hepatic cyst infection. One study showed a higher rate of diverticulosis and bowel perforation in ADPKD. Whether ADPKD increases the risk for development of new-onset diabetes mellitus after transplantation is controversial.

Pretransplantation nephrectomy, commonly used in the past, has fallen out of favor. By 1 and 3 years following renal transplantation, kidney volumes decrease by 37.7% and 40.6%, and liver volumes increase by 8.6% and 21.4%, respectively.[284] Indications for nephrectomy include a history of infected cysts, frequent bleeding, severe hypertension, and massive renal enlargement with extension into the pelvis. There is no evidence for an increased risk for development of renal cell carcinoma in native ADPKD kidneys after transplantation. When nephrectomy is indicated, hand-assisted laparoscopic nephrectomy is associated with less intraoperative blood loss, less postoperative pain, and faster recovery than open nephrectomy and is increasingly being used.[277]

Polycystic Liver Disease

PLD is usually asymptomatic and requires no treatment. When it is symptomatic, therapy is directed toward reducing cyst volume and hepatic size. Noninvasive measures include avoiding ethanol, other hepatotoxins, and possibly cAMP agonists (e.g., caffeine), which have been shown to stimulate cyst fluid secretion in vitro. Estrogens are likely to contribute to cyst growth, but the use of oral contraceptive agents and postmenopausal estrogen replacement therapy are contraindicated only if the liver is significantly enlarged and the risk for further hepatic cyst growth outweighs the benefits of estrogen therapy. Rarely, symptomatic PLD may require invasive measures to reduce cyst volume and hepatic size. Options include percutaneous cyst aspiration and sclerosis, laparoscopic fenestration, open surgical hepatic resection/cyst fenestration, selective hepatic artery embolization, and liver transplantation.[285,286] Cyst aspiration is the procedure of choice if symptoms are caused by one or a few dominant cysts or by cysts that are easily accessible to percutaneous intervention. To prevent the reaccumulation of cyst fluid, sclerosis with minocycline or 95% ethanol is often successful. Laparoscopic fenestration can be considered for large cysts that are more likely to recur after ethanol sclerosis or if several cysts are present that would require multiple percutaneous passes to be treated adequately. Partial hepatectomy with cyst fenestration is an option because PLD often spares a part of the liver with adequate preservation of hepatic parenchyma and liver function.[287] In cases in which no segments are spared, liver transplantation may be necessary.

When a hepatic cyst infection is suspected, any cyst with unusual appearance on an imaging study should be aspirated for diagnostic purposes. The best management is percutaneous cyst drainage in combination with antibiotic therapy. Long-term oral antibiotic suppression or prophylaxis should be reserved for relapsing or recurrent cases. Antibiotics of choice are trimethoprim-sulfamethoxazole and the fluoroquinolones, which are effective against the typical infecting organisms and concentrate in the biliary tree and cysts.

Intracranial Aneurysm

Widespread presymptomatic screening is not indicated because it yields mostly small aneurysms in the anterior circulation with a low risk of rupture. Indications for screening in patients with good life expectancy include a family history of aneurysm or subarachnoid hemorrhage, previous aneurysm rupture, preparation for major elective surgery, high-risk occupations (e.g., airline pilots), and patient anxiety despite adequate information.[249] MR angiography does not require intravenous contrast material. CT angiography is a satisfactory alternative when there is no contraindication to intravenous contrast agents.

When an asymptomatic aneurysm is found, a recommendation on whether to intervene depends on its size, site, and morphology; prior history of subarachnoid hemorrhage from another aneurysm; patient age and general health; and whether the aneurysm is coilable or clippable. The prospective arm of the International Study of Unruptured Intracranial Aneurysms (ISUIA) has provided invaluable information to assist in the decision.[288] The 5-year cumulative rupture rates for patients without a previous history of subarachnoid hemorrhage with aneurysms located in the internal carotid artery, anterior communicating or anterior cerebral artery, or middle cerebral artery were 0%, 2.6%, 14.5%, and 44.0% for aneurysms less than 7 mm, 7 to 12 mm, 13 to 24 mm, and 25 mm or greater, respectively, compared with rates of 2.5%, 14.5%, 18.4%, and 50%, respectively, for the same size categories involving the posterior circulation and posterior communicating artery. Among unruptured noncavernous segment aneurysms less than 7 mm in diameter, the rupture risks were higher among patients who had a previous subarachnoid hemorrhage from another aneurysm. These risks need to be balanced with those associated with surgical or endovascular surgery also reported by the ISUIA. The 1-year mortality and combined morbidity (Rankin score 3 to 5 or impaired cognitive status) and mortality rates were 2.7% and 12.6%, respectively, for open surgery and 3.4% and 9.8%, respectively, for endovascular repair.

The risk for development of new aneurysms or enlargement of an existing one in patients with ADPKD is very low in those with small (<7 mm) aneurysms detected by presymptomatic screening and moderate in those with a previous rupture from a different site.[289-291] On the basis of these and the ISUIA data, conservative management is usually recommended for patients with ADPKD who have small (<7 mm) aneurysms detected by presymptomatic screening, particularly in the anterior circulation. Semiannual or annual imaging studies of an aneurysm are appropriate initially, but reevaluation at less frequent intervals may be sufficient after the stability of the aneurysm has been documented. Elimination of tobacco use and aggressive treatment of hypertension and hyperlipidemia should be recommended.

The risk for development of a new aneurysm after an initial negative study result is small, about 3% at 10 years in patients with a family history of ICAs.[292] Therefore, rescreening of patients with a family history of after an interval of 5 to 10 years seems reasonable.

Novel Therapies

A better understanding of the pathophysiology and the availability of animal models has facilitated the development of preclinical trials and identification of promising candidate drugs for clinical trials (http://www.clinicaltrials.gov).

Vasopressin V_2 Receptor Antagonists. The effect of vasopressin, via V_2 receptors, on cAMP levels in the collecting duct, the major site of cyst development in ADPKD, and the role of cAMP in cystogenesis provided the rationale for preclinical trials that showed effectiveness of vasopressin V_2 receptor (V_2R) antagonists in animal models of ARPKD, ADPKD, and nephronophthisis (NPHP).[113,162,306] Preliminary dosing studies showed that twice daily administration of the V_2R antagonist tolvaptan was necessary to maintain urine hypotonicity (a surrogate for V_2R blockade) throughout a 24-hour period.[293-295] Two small phase II, open-label, uncontrolled, 3-year clinical trials provided preliminary support for its long-term safety and tolerability.[296] Two additional short-term studies showed that the aquaretic effect of tolvaptan was accompanied by a small, rapidly reversible reduction in GFR, uric acid clearance, and kidney and cyst volumes.[297,298]

The results of a phase III, global, multicenter, randomized, double-blind, placebo-controlled, parallel-arm trial of tolvaptan in ADPKD (TEMPO [Tolvaptan Efficacy and Safety in Management of ADPKD and its Outcomes], 3:4; NCT00428948) have been published.[299,300] Subjects with ADPKD (n = 1445) and rapid disease progression reflected by kidney volumes of at least 750 mL at a relatively young age (between 18 and 50 years), but still with preserved renal function (estimated creatinine clearance [eCrCl] > 60 mL/min), were randomly assigned at a rate of 2:1 to tolvaptan or placebo. Morning and afternoon split 45/15-mg doses were titrated at weekly intervals to 60/30 and 90/30 mg. The maximally tolerated dose was maintained for 3 years. Participants were instructed to drink enough water to prevent thirst. Serum creatinine and laboratory parameters were measured every 4 months, and renal MRI was obtained yearly. Twenty-three percent of tolvaptan-treated subjects withdrew from the trial, 15% because of adverse events, including aquaresis-related symptoms in 8%, in comparison with 14%, 5%, and 0.4%, respectively, in the placebo group. Of the subjects assigned to tolvaptan therapy and completing 3 years of treatment, 24%, 21%, and 55% were tolerating doses of 45/15, 60/30, and 90/30 mg, respectively, at the end of the study. Seventeen percent of subjects receiving placebo were unable to tolerate the 90/30 mg dose.

Tolvaptan reduced the rate of kidney growth by 50%, from 5.5% to 2.8% per year. The treatment effect was greatest from baseline to year 1, but also significant from year 1 to year 2, and from year 2 to year 3. The analysis of time to development or progression of multiple clinical events (worsening kidney function, severe kidney pain, hypertension, and albuminuria) showed fewer clinical events for tolvaptan than for placebo, with a hazard ratio of 0.87. This result was driven by a 61% lower risk of 25% reductions in reciprocal serum creatinine value and a 36% lower risk of kidney pain events. Tolvaptan also reduced the rate of decline of reciprocal serum creatinine value, from −3.81 to −2.61 mg/mL per year.

Frequencies of adverse events were similar in the two groups; those related to aquaresis were more common in the tolvaptan group, whereas those related to ADPKD, such as kidney pain, hematuria, and urinary tract infection, were more common in the placebo group. Increases in serum sodium and uric acid were more frequently seen in tolvaptan-treated subjects. Tolvaptan-treated subjects also had more frequent, clinically significant elevations of liver enzymes, leading to discontinuation of tolvaptan in 1.8%.

Tolvaptan was approved in March 2014 by the regulatory authorities in Japan for the suppression of progression of ADPKD in patients with rapid rate of increase in kidney volume.[301] In the United States, the U.S. Food and Drug Administration (FDA) requested the manufacturer of tolvaptan to provide additional data to further evaluate the efficacy and safety of this drug in patients with ADPKD.[302] Concerns raised during the review process included: (1) not accepting TKV as an established surrogate; (2) uncertainty introduced by missing data and a post-treatment baseline for the key secondary end point; (3) potential risk for hepatotoxicity; and (4) the "small" 1 mL/min/1.73 m^2 per year (26%) improvement in renal function decline. Applications for approval of tolvaptan for the treatment of ADPKD have recently been approved by the European Medicines Agency (EMA) and Health Canada.

Somatostatin Analogs. Binding of somatostatin to its receptors, (SSTR1 through SSTR5) inhibits adenylyl cyclase and MAPK, cell proliferation, and secretion of several hormones (growth hormone, insulin, glucagon, gastrin, cholecystokinin, vasoactive intestinal peptide and secretin, thyroid-stimulating hormone [TSH], and adrenocorticotropic hormone [ACTH]) and growth factors (insulin-like growth factor 1 [IGF-I] and VEGF).[303,304] All five SSTRs are expressed in renal tubular epithelial cells and cholangiocytes. Because somatostatin has a half-life of approximately 3 minutes, more stable synthetic peptides (octreotide, lanreotide, and pasireotide) have been developed for clinical use. They differ in stability and in affinity for the different SSTRs. Half-lives in the circulation are 2 hours for octreotide and lanreotide and 12 hours for pasireotide. Octreotide and lanreotide bind with high affinity to SSTR2 and SSTR3, with moderate affinity to SSTR5, and have no affinity to SSTR1 and SSTR4. Pasireotide binds with high affinity to SSTR1, SSTR2, SSTR3, and SSTR5. In preclinical studies, octreotide and pasireotide reduced cAMP levels and proliferation of cholangiocytes in vitro, expansion of liver cysts in three-dimensional (3D) collagen culture, and development of kidney and liver cysts and fibrosis in PCK rats and $Pkd2^{WS25/-}$ mice.[116,305] In agreement with the longer half-life and higher affinity to a broader range of SSTRs, the effects of pasireotide are more potent than those of octreotide. Pasireotide and tolvaptan have been shown to have an additive beneficial effect in the $Pkd1^{RC/RC}$ mouse model of ADPKD.[306]

Several small randomized, placebo-controlled studies of octreotide or lanreotide have been completed.[307-310] Most of these studies have been of short duration, but two of them have been extended as open-label, uncontrolled studies.[311,312] The recent ALADIN study randomly assigned 79 patients ADPKD with and eGFR values of 40 mL/min/1.73m² or higher to intramuscular injections of a long-acting form of octreotide or placebo and monitored them for 3 years.[313] The primary outcome variable, a mean increase in TKV at 3 years of follow-up, showed numerically smaller growth in the octreotide group than in the placebo group (220 mL versus 454 mL). The difference, however, was not statistically significant. A favorable effect was noted on the secondary outcome of kidney function, but this end point also did not reach statistical significance. These findings provide support for larger randomized controlled trials to test the protective effect of somatostatin analogs against renal function loss. An ongoing clinical trial involves 300 patients with ADPKD and CKD stages 3a and 3b.[314] Until the results of larger trials become available, somatostatin analogs should not be prescribed for renoprotection outside of a research study.

The somatostatin analogs have also shown a potential beneficial effect on the progression of polycystic liver disease. Liver volume decreased by 4% to 6% during the first year of treatment, and this reduction was sustained during the second year. Young female patients appear to have the greatest benefit from this treatment.[315] The addition of everolimus to treatment with octreotide does not provide added benefit.

Octreotide and lanreotide are overall well tolerated. Self-resolving abdominal cramps and loose stools are common in the first few days following the injections. Other adverse effects include injection site granuloma and pain, cholelithiasis, steatorrhea, weight loss, and, rarely, hair loss. The adverse event profile of pasireotide in patients with ADPKD may include hyperglycemia because pasireotide inhibits insulin more potently than glucagon secretion, whereas the contrary is true for octreotide and pasireotide.[316]

Rapalogs. There is overwhelming evidence for enhanced mTOR complex 1 (mTORC1) signaling in PKD cystic tissues, and results of preclinical trials of mTOR-inhibiting rapalogs (sirolimus and everolimus) in rodent models were mostly encouraging. At doses and blood levels achievable in humans, sirolimus and everolimus were effective in a rat model of PKD affecting proximal tubules,[317,318] but not in an ARPKD model affecting the distal nephron and collecting duct.[319] Mice tolerate much higher doses and blood levels than rats and humans, and at these high levels rapalogs were consistently effective in orthologous and nonorthologous mouse models.[320,321] However, the results of clinical trials have been mostly discouraging,[322-324] likely because blood levels capable of inhibiting mTOR in peripheral blood mononuclear cells do not inhibit mTOR in the kidney.[325]

Several strategies may overcome the systemic toxicity and limited renal bioavailability of rapalogs. One is to target the drug specifically to the kidney by conjugating it to folate, and treatment of *bpk* mice was effective in reducing renal cyst growth and preserving kidney function without toxicity.[326] Another approach takes advantage of the mechanism of action of sirolimus, which forms a complex with the binding protein FKBP12 that competes with phosphatidic acid for binding to mTOR. Phosphatidic acid, a phospholipase D product generated by the hydrolysis of phosphatidylcholine, is required for the association of mTOR with component Raptor in mTORC1 and with component Rictor in mTORC2. One study showed that PKD cells have a slightly higher phospholipase D activity and that blockade of its activity by either specific inhibitors or "alcohol trap" treatment retrains mTORC1 and decreases cell viability and proliferation.[327] A third approach is the use of mTOR-catalytic inhibitors that cause a more potent and durable inhibition of mTORC1 than rapalogs, which are currently being tested in rodent PKD models.[328]

Other Agents. Many other drugs have been shown to be effective in preclinical trials and of potential value for the treatment of human PKD. Some act on tyrosine kinase receptors, downstream signaling pathways such as MAPK and Wnt/β-catenin signaling, effectors and inhibitors of cell cycling, or energy metabolism to inhibit cell proliferation.[148,149,329,330] Other potential therapies target fluid secretion (cystic fibrosis transmembrane conductance regulator [CFTR] and KCa3.1 inhibitors) or important pathogenic interactions between epithelial cells and ECM and the interstitial inflammatory microenvironment. Of particular interest are drugs that have shown effectiveness in animal models and that are currently used for other indications with relatively little toxicity, such as metformin, the thiazolidinediones, and nicotinamide.[139,331-335]

Clinical Trials and Renal Function

In planning for clinical trials for ADPKD, the use of renal function as the primary outcome becomes an issue. This is because decades of normal renal function remain despite progressive enlargement and cystic transformation of the kidneys. By the time the GFR starts declining, the kidneys are markedly enlarged, distorted, and unlikely to benefit from treatment. On the other hand, early interventional trials would require unrealistic periods of follow-up if renal function were to be used as the primary outcome. The results of CRISP have shown that the rate of renal growth is a good predictor of functional decline and justify the use of kidney volume as a marker of disease progression in clinical trials for ADPKD.[178,179]

AUTOSOMAL RECESSIVE POLYCYSTIC KIDNEY DISEASE

EPIDEMIOLOGY

ARPKD is generally characterized by relatively rapid, symmetric, bilateral renal enlargement in infants due to collecting duct cysts in association with CHF.[336-338] Nonobstructive intrahepatic bile duct dilatation (Caroli's disease) is variably seen. A minority of cases may occur in older children, teenagers, or young adults, usually with manifestations of portal hypertension or cholangitis. In rare cases, the presentation may be in older adults, mostly with complications of the liver disease but sometimes with renal manifestations such as proteinuria, nephrolithiasis, and renal insufficiency.[339,340]

Prevalence and carrier frequencies are thought to be 1 in 20,000 and 1 in 70, respectively.[341] Molecular data indicate that ARPKD is likely to be found in all racial groups.[342,343]

GENETICS

ARPKD is inherited as an autosomal recessive trait and therefore may occur in siblings but not in the parents. The disease is observed in one fourth of the offspring of carrier parents. All cases of typical ARPKD are caused by mutations in a gene on chromosome 6p21.1-p12 (*PKHD1*).[344-346] Studies have shown that *PKHD1* mutations are also responsible for nonsyndromic CHF and Caroli's disease.[339]

PKHD1 is among the largest genes in the human genome, extending approximately 470 kb and including 67 exons.[347,348] Mutations are scattered throughout the gene without "hot spots."[342,343] Most have been described in just a single family, but some are more frequent in particular populations (e.g., R496X in Finland and 9689delA in Spain).[349,350] One missense substitution, T36M, has been found on approximately 16% of mutant alleles and seems to be an ancestral mutation that arose in Europe more than a 1000 years ago.[351] There is evidence of genotype-phenotype correlations. The presence of two truncating mutations results in a lethal phenotype by the neonatal period. Surviving patients with severe or milder renal disease have at least one nontruncation mutation, indicating that many nontruncating mutations are hypomorphic.[349,350,352] Despite the importance of the germline mutations, affected sibling pairs may exhibit phenotypes of markedly discordant severity, most likely because of the effect of modifier genes.

PATHOGENESIS

The ARPKD protein, fibrocystin (460 kDa), has a single-transmembrane pass, a large extracellular region containing IPT/TIG (immunoglobulin-like fold shared by plexins and transcription factors) and PbH1 (parallel beta-helix 1) repeats, and an intracellular carboxyl tail with potential phosphorylation sites.[347,348] Cleavage of the protein in the extracellular region at the proprotein convertase site is likely important to form a functional protein.[97,353] This possibility suggests that fibrocystin may be a cell surface receptor implicated in protein-protein interactions. Like the polycystins, fibrocystin is localized in primary cilia. Fibrocystin, PC2, and the kinesin-2 motor subunit KIF3B (kinesin family member 3B) form a protein complex in which KIF3B acts as a linker between fibrocystin and PC2.[354] The physical interaction between fibrocystin and the motor protein KIF3B may explain the structural abnormalities described in the primary cilia of PCK rat cholangiocytes.[355] Within the fibrocystin-KIF3B-PC2 complex, fibrocystin is capable of enhancing the channel function of PC2. Fibrocystin has also been shown to interact with calcium-modulating cyclophilin ligand, a protein that participates in the regulation of cytosolic calcium pools.[356] These observations suggest that an alteration of the intracellular calcium homeostasis plays an important role in ARPKD, as also seems to be the case in ADPKD. Aberrant activation of mTOR has been shown in ARPKD kidneys as it has in ADPKD kidneys.[357] The expression of fibrocystin in ureteric bud branches, intrahepatic and extrahepatic biliary ducts, and pancreatic ducts during embryogenesis is consistent with the histologic features of ARPKD.[358]

PATHOLOGY

ARPKD affects both the kidneys and the liver in approximately inverse proportions. That is, the disease may be viewed as a spectrum ranging from severe renal damage and mild liver damage at one end to mild renal damage and severe liver damage at the other. The form with severe renal damage is the more common and is the form that manifests at or near the time of birth. The form with less severe renal damage and more severe liver damage is less common and usually manifests in infancy, childhood, or later.

The kidneys in the perinatal and neonatal forms of ARPKD are symmetrically and bilaterally enlarged up to more than 20 times normal (Figure 46.15) and may be the cause of dystocia because of their size. Average combined weight of the kidneys in one series was about 300 g (range,

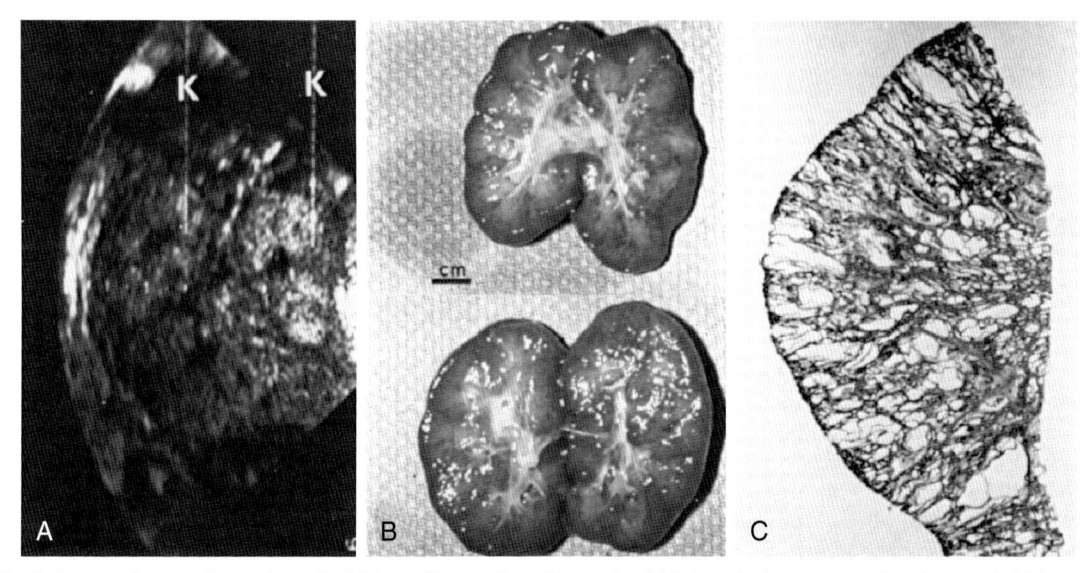

Figure 46.15 Autosomal recessive polycystic kidney disease in a 32-week-old fetus. **A,** A sonogram showing cystic kidneys (K) of a fetus in utero. Gross (**B**) and microscopic (**C**) sections show radially oriented cysts of collecting ducts.

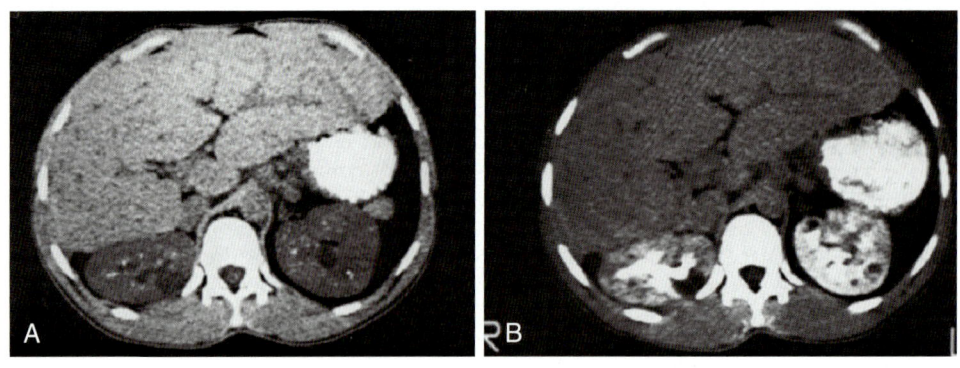

Figure 46.16 Computed tomography (CT) scan of autosomal recessive polycystic kidney disease in an 18-year-old man whose serum creatinine and liver function test results were within normal ranges. The patient had clinical evidence of portal hypertension (gastric varices, enlarged spleen). An oral contrast agent was given to highlight the intestines. **A,** CT scan without contrast enhancement. The liver is enlarged but not cystic. The kidneys are slightly enlarged and contain focal radiodense areas (nephrolithiasis). **B,** CT scan after intravenous administration of iodinated radiocontrast agent showing cystic areas in both kidneys. The renal calcifications are now obscured by contrast medium in the collecting systems.

240 to 563 g), a normal combined weight being about 25 g. The renal enlargement is caused by fusiform dilation of collecting ducts to 1 to 2 mm in the cortex and medulla. Almost 100% of collecting ducts are affected in the most severe cases. Dilation of the collecting ducts occurs in the fetal period, and the glomeruli and more proximal tubular elements of the nephron appear normal. However, there is evidence in early human fetuses (14-24 weeks) that proximal tubule cysts occur, as in some rodent models of recessive PKD,[359-361] but these are no longer evident after 34 weeks of gestation.[362] The dilated collecting ducts are lined by typical cuboidal cells.[363,364] In many cases of neonatal ARPKD, an overall reduction in size may occur as the children age, and macroscopic cysts may develop. Renal calcifications are common in children with the disease.

In later presentations of ARPKD, mainly with complications of portal hypertension caused by CHF or episodes of cholangitis caused by Caroli's disease, the renal involvement may be much less prominent, consisting of medullary ductal ectasia with minimal or no renal enlargement. The picture resembles and may be confused with medullary sponge kidney (MSK), a distinct disease with a far different prognosis (see later discussion).

The hepatic lesion is diffuse but limited to the portal areas. CHF is characterized by enlarged and fibrotic portal areas with apparent proliferation of bile ducts, absence of central bile ducts, hypoplasia of the portal vein branches, and sometimes prominent fibrosis around the central veins. Bulbar protrusions from the walls of dilated ducts also occur, and bridges sometimes form. This malformation has been found to occur occasionally as an isolated event (Caroli's disease), but most often it is associated with ARPKD.

DIAGNOSIS

The diagnosis is often made by sonography in utero or shortly after birth. The typical sonogram (see Figure 46.15) shows enlarged kidneys with increased echogenicity in the cortex and medulla, with poor definition of the collecting system and fuzzy delineation of the kidneys from surrounding tissues. Although the appearance of the kidneys on sonography, CT, and MRI may be very suggestive of ARPKD, a definite diagnosis based on renal imaging alone is not possible, particularly in utero and the neonatal period, when the appearance of the kidney may be indistinguishable from ADPKD and other recessive renal cystic diseases. The family history, ultrasonographic or histologic evaluation of the liver for the presence of hepatic fibrosis, and absence of extrarenal malformations associated with multiple malformation syndromes and with renal dysplasia help in the diagnosis.

Older children and adolescents may present with symptoms and signs referable to the hepatic fibrosis and portal hypertension, including gastrointestinal bleeding from varices, hepatosplenomegaly, and hypersplenism, with or without associated renal manifestations such as a urinary concentrating defect, nephrolithiasis, hypertension, and renal insufficiency. Collecting duct ectasia and macrocystic changes may be observed in the kidneys of these patients (Figure 46.16). Combined use of conventional and high-resolution ultrasonography with MR cholangiography in patients with ARPKD and CHF allows detailed definition of the extent of kidney and hepatobiliary manifestations without requiring ionizing radiation and contrast agents.[365]

Owing to the severity of disease in ARPKD, there is significant demand for prenatal diagnostics. This interest largely comes from couples with a previously affected pregnancy, detected either in utero (which may have resulted in termination) or with the birth of an affected child (who may have died in the neonatal period).[366] Preimplantation genetic diagnosis (PGD), which avoids the trauma of a termination of pregnancy in the case of an affected fetus, has been performed in only a few cases.[367] There is also demand for molecular diagnostics in older patients with less severe disease to differentiate ARPKD from other causes of childhood PKD. Molecular diagnostics have been offered since *PKHD1* was localized using a linkage-based approach with flanking markers. This method requires material from an affected individual with a firm diagnosis of ARPKD and can be complicated by crossovers between flanking markers. With the gene discovery, mutation-based diagnostics have become possible.[368] This method has the advantages that DNA from a previously affected family member is not required and that patients with an uncertain diagnosis can be tested. However, it is complicated by the marked allelic heterogeneity and prevalence of novel missense mutations of uncertain pathogenicity. If two clearly pathogenic mutations are identified, the diagnosis is highly reliable. When only one mutation is identified, diagnosis is often possible in combination with a focused linkage approach.[351] In one study, a definitive prenatal diagnosis (presence or absence of two identified mutations) was feasible in 72% of the cases, and an improved risk assignment (presence or absence of one identified mutation) was possible in an additional 25% of the studied families.[342]

The phenotype of greatly enlarged and echogenic kidneys in neonates is not pathognomonic for ARPKD, and other possible cystic disorders should also be considered. Rarely (<1% cases), ADPKD manifests in utero or in the neonatal period as clinical symptoms very similar to those of ARPKD.[64,369] In approximately 50% of these cases, an affected parent is recognized only after the diagnosis of a severely affected child.[370] In addition, rare de novo, early-onset ADPKD may occur. Most early-onset cases have been linked to *PKD1*, although a *PKD2* family with perinatal death in two severely affected infants has been described.[66] CHF is not normally part of the ADPKD phenotype, but rare reports of an association have been described.

The high risk of recurrence of early-onset ADPKD in affected families suggested a common familial modifying background for early and severe disease expression (e.g., mutations or variants in genes encoding other cystoproteins).[64] Emerging family data suggested that *in trans* inheritance of a null and an incompletely penetrant *PKD1* allele could result in early-onset ADPKD with an ARPKD-like phenotype.[60,67,68,372] This hypothesis has been confirmed by a knockin mouse model mimicking the naturally occurring *PKD1* variant p.R3277C highlighted by later family studies.[60,67] Mirroring observation in the human studies, gradual cystic disease developed in $Pkd1^{RC/RC}$ animals over 1 year, whereas early-onset, rapidly progressive disease occurred in $Pkd1^{RC/null}$ mice.[10] Early-onset severe ADPKD has been linked to contiguous deletion of *PKD1* and *TSC2*[373,374] as well as co-inheritance of an ADPKD and a *HNF1B* or *PKHD1* allele.[69]

Glomerulocystic kidney disease can rarely manifest in the neonatal period with an ARPKD-like phenotype.[375] Rare families with ARPKD-like disease and skeletal and facial anomalies[376,377] or recessively inherited renal and hepatic cystic diseases with hypoglycemia[351,378] that are not linked to *PKHD1* have been described. Infantile NPHP may also be confused with ARPKD. A number of syndromic congenital hepatorenal disorders that are lethal in infancy can be associated with renal abnormalities resembling those in ARPKD and with CHF. These include Joubert, Meckel, Elejalde (acrocephalopolysyndactyly), and Ivemark (renal-hepatic-pancreatic dysplasia) syndromes and glutaric aciduria type II. Mutations to *ANKS6* have also been shown to sometimes result in an ARPKD-like phenotype but usually also with cardiovascular abnormalities.[379]

MANIFESTATIONS

Children with ARPKD are typically identified in utero from the finding of enlarged, echogenic kidneys. In the most severe cases, poor urine output may result in oligohydramnios and the Potter sequence, characterized by typical facies, wrinkled skin, compression deformities of the limbs, and pulmonary hypoplasia. The presentation of ARPKD at birth may be dominated by respiratory difficulties from pulmonary hypoplasia or from restrictive disease caused by massive kidney enlargement. The need for neonatal ventilation predicts the development of CKD and death. Approximately 30% of affected neonates die shortly after birth.[380-383]

Most patients who survive the neonatal period live to adulthood. Hypertension, electrolyte abnormalities, and renal insufficiency are the major disease complications in surviving infants, with liver disease becoming more important in older patients. Hypertension developed in between 55% and 86% of patients reported in two studies, with blood pressure elevations often seen at birth or at diagnosis.[380,381] The pathogenesis of hypertension remains undefined. The ectopic expression of components of the RAAS in cystic-dilated tubules suggests that increased intrarenal angiotensin II production contributes to its development.[384] However, the circulating plasma renin level is usually low,[382] and the intravascular volume expanded, particularly in patients with concomitant hyponatremia.[381] Increased sodium reabsorption in the ectatic collecting ducts may contribute to the hypertension,[385,386] but conflicting data have been reported.[387] The inability to concentrate and dilute urine can cause major electrolyte abnormalities. During the first year or two of life, renal function can improve, and renal size relative to body mass often decreases.[363,388,389] Renal function may remain stable for many years or may slowly progress to renal failure. The consequences of chronic renal insufficiency, growth failure, anemia, and osteodystrophy become apparent during childhood. Because complications of liver disease become more important as these children age, careful examination for splenomegaly and blood counts for cytopenias should be regularly performed.

Adolescents and adults present most often with complications of portal hypertension (variceal esophageal bleeding, splenomegaly and hypersplenism with leukopenia, thrombocytopenia, or anemia).[339] Up to 50% of patients with CHF may exhibit segmental dilation of intrahepatic bile ducts (Caroli's disease), sometimes with episodes of cholangitis or sepsis and complications of biliary sludge or lithiasis. Hepatocellular function is rarely deranged, and enzyme values are only occasionally mildly elevated. Increased bilirubin or enzyme values suggest the possibility of cholangitis. The kidneys in these patients may be normal or may exhibit various degrees of medullary collecting duct ectasia or macrocystic disease without marked renal enlargement.

Three reports have described cases of ARPKD with ICAs.[390-392] It is not clear whether the prevalence of ICAs is increased in ARPKD or whether these cases are coincidental findings.

Heterozygote carriers of *PKHD1* mutations have usually been considered to be entirely normal. However, an ultrasonographic study of 110 obligate carriers of ARPKD showed increased medullary echogenicity in 6 (5.5%), multiple small liver cysts in 10 (9.1%), a moderately increased liver echo pattern suggestive of CHF in 4 (3.6%), and mild splenomegaly in 9 (8.2%) patients.[393]

TREATMENT

Later studies suggest that the prognosis of ARPKD for children who survive the first month of life is far less bleak than was initially thought.[336,380-382] In patients with respiratory insufficiency, the cause (pulmonary hypoplasia, abdominal mass, pneumothorax, pneumomediastinum, atelectasis, pneumonia, heart failure) should be assessed fully, and artificial ventilation and aggressive resuscitative measures are indicated. Severely affected neonates may require unilateral or bilateral nephrectomies because of respiratory and nutritional compromise. An aggressive nutritional program and correction of acidosis and other electrolyte disorders are needed to optimize linear growth. The hypertension generally responds to salt restriction and antihypertensive drugs. Like patients with other renal cystic disorders, patients with ARPKD are susceptible to urinary tract infections, so urinary tract instrumentation is best avoided.

For infants with ESKD, peritoneal dialysis is preferable, but peritoneal dialysis and hemodialysis are options for children with renal failure. Kidney transplantation is limited by body size, but in experienced centers, it can be performed even in small children with a minimal weight of 7 kg.[394] Pretransplantation splenectomy may be indicated for patients with marked leukopenia or thrombocytopenia due to hypersplenism. These patients should receive pneumococcal vaccinations. Rejection rates and survival beyond 3 years for such patients are not different from those in patients with other renal diseases who undergo transplant surgery. Biliary sepsis is a frequent contributor to the mortality in patients with ARPKD who undergo transplant surgery.[395]

Surviving patients and those whose disease manifests during adolescence are likely to require portosystemic shunting to prevent life-threatening hemorrhages from esophageal varices. The renal disease may progress to renal failure years later even after successful shunting. Patients with associated nonobstructive intrahepatic biliary dilation (Caroli's disease) may have recurrent episodes of cholangitis and may require antimicrobial therapy or segmental hepatic resection. Combined kidney and liver transplantation has been advocated for selected patients with ESKD who have significant bile duct dilation and episodes of cholangitis.[396-398]

TUBEROUS SCLEROSIS COMPLEX

Epidemiology

TSC is an autosomal dominant disease that affects up to 1 in 6000 individuals.

Genetics

It is caused by mutations in one of two genes, *TSC1* and *TSC2*. *TSC1* is located on chromosome 9q34, which encodes for hamartin. *TSC2* is located on chromosome 16p13 and encodes for tuberin. The disease tends to be less severe in patients with *TSC1* mutations than in those with *TSC2* mutations.[399-401]

Pathogenesis

Hamartin and tuberin physically interact, and this interaction is important for their function. The hamartin-tuberin complex antagonizes an insulin-signaling pathway that plays an important role in the regulation of cell size, cell number, and organ size.[402,403] In the absence of growth factor stimulation, tuberin-hamartin complexes maintain Rheb (Ras homolog enriched in the brain) in an inactive guanosine diphosphate (GDP)–bound state by stimulating its intrinsic guanosine triphosphatase (GTPase) activity and inhibit downstream signaling from Rheb via mTOR. Growth factor stimulation of phosphoinositide 3-kinase (PI3K) signaling leads to Akt-dependent phosphorylation of tuberin, dissociation of the tuberin-hamartin complex, and activation of Rheb and mTOR. Tuberin or hamartin mutations prevent the formation of tuberin-hamartin complexes and lead to constitutive activation of mTOR.

Diagnosis

A definite diagnosis of TSC requires one of the following conditions:

- Two major features from the following list: renal angiomyolipoma, facial angiofibromas or forehead plaques, nontraumatic ungual or periungual fibroma, three or more hypomelanotic macules, shagreen patch, multiple retinal nodular hamartomas, cortical tuber, subependymal nodule, subependymal giant cell astrocytoma, cardiac rhabdomyoma, lymphangioleiomyomatosis
- One major feature from previous list plus two minor features from the following list: multiple renal cysts, nonrenal hamartoma, hamartomatous rectal polyps, retinal achromic patch, cerebral white matter radial migration tracts, bone cysts, gingival fibromas, "confetti" skin lesions, multiple enamel pits

Manifestations

Renal involvement is second only to the involvement of the central nervous system (CNS) as a cause of death in patients with TSC. The main renal manifestations are angiomyolipomas (including rare epithelioid angiomyolipomas), cysts, oncocytomas, clear cell RCC, lymphangiomatous cysts, and (rarely) focal segmental glomerulosclerosis.[404-407]

Angiomyolipomas (AMLs) are benign tumors consisting of abnormal blood vessels, smooth muscle, and fat cells. They are derived from perivascular epithelioid cells (PEComas) and exhibit immunoreactivity for both melanocytic markers (as detected by the antibodies HMB-45 and melan-A) and smooth muscle markers (actin and desmin). The diagnosis of renal AML relies on the demonstration of fat in the tumor by imaging studies. The fat appears hyperechogenic on ultrasonography, has a low attenuation value on CT, and on MRI appears bright on T1-weighted images, dark on T2-weighted images with fat saturation, and intermediate on T2-weighted images.[7,38,41,407a] Approximately 5% of renal AMLs contain minimal amounts of fat and are called minimal-fat or fat-poor lesions. The differential diagnosis can be challenging and includes classic AMLs (predominantly composed of smooth muscle cells), epithelioid AMLs, RCC, and oncocytoma. When the distinction between minimal-fat renal AMLs and renal cell carcinoma cannot be reliably established by imaging techniques, imaging-guided percutaneous needle biopsy and staining for melanocyte markers should be considered as an alternative to surgical exploration.[408] The risk of bleeding after needle biopsy of a minimal-fat AML does not appear to be higher than that of a biopsy for other renal tumors, particularly when fine needles are used.

In patients with TSC, AMLs are extremely common, are usually multiple and bilateral, and affect both genders, in contrast to the general population, in which they are uncommon, usually single, and mainly found in middle-aged women. They develop after the first year of age, and by the third decade, 60% of patients with TSC have renal AMLs. The lesions express receptors for estrogen and progesterone, and women have more and larger angiomyolipomas than men. The early small lesions have a characteristic radial, striated, or wedge-shaped pattern with the base of the wedge facing the surface of the kidney. As the lesions increase in size, they penetrate deeper into the renal parenchyma or become exophytic, extending into the perirenal fat. The main manifestations relate to their potential for hemorrhage (hematuria, intratumoral, or retroperitoneal) and mass effect (abdominal or flank mass and tenderness, hypertension, or renal insufficiency). Because of the potential for renal AML development and growth, it is recommended that renal surveillance in patients with TSC be performed with ultrasonography at diagnosis and thereafter every 1 to 2 years (3 years in those in whom no AMLs are identified and at least yearly in patients with known AMLs).[409] In patients with known renal lesions, the serum creatinine concentration should be measured at least once a year.

The epithelioid AML variant is differentiated from the classic variant by the presence of an epithelioid cell component with abundant eosinophilic and granular cytoplasm.[410] There is no consensus on the percentage of epithelioid cells that is required to make a diagnosis of the epithelioid variant, with values ranging from 10% to 100% in published studies.[411,412]

In contrast to the uniformly benign prognosis of classic renal AMLs, as described in the preceding section, epithelioid variants infrequently undergo malignant transformation that manifests as local recurrence and/or distal metastases.

Unlike angiomyolipomas, renal cysts may be present in the first year of life, and cystic disease may be the presenting manifestation of TSC. *TSC2* and *PKD1* lie adjacent to each other in a tail-to-tail orientation on chromosome 16 at 16p13.3. Deletions inactivating both genes are associated with polycystic kidneys diagnosed during the first year of life or early childhood (*TSC2/PKD1* contiguous gene syndrome).[373,374] Therefore, TSC should be considered in children with renal cysts and no family history of PKD. Rarely, *TSC2/PKD1* contiguous gene syndrome can be diagnosed in adults.[413] Patients with the contiguous gene syndrome usually reach ESKD at an earlier age than patients with ADPKD alone, but the disease severity in patients who have mosaicism is more variable.[374] Patients with *TSC1* or *TSC2* mutations without the contiguous gene syndrome also can have renal cysts. The renal cysts in TSC are often lined by a very distinct, perhaps unique, epithelium of markedly hypertrophic and hyperplastic cells with prominent eosinophilic cytoplasm. The combination of cystic kidneys and angiomyolipomas has been said to be virtually pathognomonic for TSC.

Oncocytomas—benign tumors derived from intercalated cells in the collecting ducts—and clear cell RCCs occur with increased frequency in TSC. RCCs in TSC have a female predominance and an earlier age of presentation as well as increased bilaterality. Early detection is essential. They should be suspected in cases of enlarging lesions without demonstrable fat and in the presence of intratumoral calcifications.

Treatment

Angiomyolipomas are benign lesions and often require no treatment. Because of their increased frequency and size in women and reports of hemorrhagic complications during pregnancy, patients with multiple AMLs should be cautioned about the potential risks of pregnancy and estrogen administration. Annual reevaluations with ultrasonography or CT are necessary to assess for growth and development of complications. Renal-sparing surgery is indicated for symptoms such as pain and hemorrhage, growth with compromise of functioning renal parenchyma, and inability to exclude an associated RCC. Because angiomyolipomas larger than 4 cm are more likely to grow, develop microaneurysms and macroaneurysms, and cause symptoms, some writers suggest that prophylactic intervention should be considered in these cases. Some lesions, because of their size or central location, may be more amenable to selective arterial embolization. Radiofrequency ablation and cryoablation have also been successful in the treatment of renal AMLs less than 4 cm in diameter without bleeding complications.[414-416]

Elucidation of the TSC protein function at a molecular level and preclinical studies have identified mTOR as a target for intervention in TSC.[417,418] The efficacy of mTOR inhibitors has also been demonstrated in patients with TSC who have subependymal giant cell astrocytomas or pulmonary lymphangioleiomyomatosis. Multiple open-label, nonrandomized studies have shown that sirolimus produces a reduction in the volume of renal AMLs, mostly achieved in the first few months of treatment,[419-422] but the effect is not maintained after discontinuation of treatment. The best data on the efficacy of mTOR inhibitors come from the double-blind EXIST-2 study (Efficacy and safety of everolimus for subependymal giant cell astrocytomas associated with tuberous sclerosis complex or sporadic lymphangioleiomyomatosis, which included 118 patients, 18 years or older, who had a definite diagnosis of TSC (n = 113) or sporadic lymphangioleiomyomatosis (LAM) (n = 5) and at least one renal AML 3 cm or more in its largest diameter. The patients were randomly assigned in a 2 : 1 ratio to everolimus 10 mg/day or placebo, and treated for a median duration of 38 or 34 weeks, respectively.[423] At the data cutoff, therapy had been discontinued in 20 patients, because of disease progression in 9 receiving placebo and because of adverse effects in 1 receiving everolimus and 4 receiving placebo. The primary end point, at least a 50% reduction in the total volume of all target AMLs identified at baseline, was achieved in 42% of the patients treated with everolimus and in none of the patients treated with placebo ($P < 0.001$). The median time to response to everolimus was 2.9 months. Progression of AMLs was significantly more common in the placebo group (21% vs. 4%). The response rate of skin lesions was significantly more common with everolimus (26% vs. 0%). The patients treated with everolimus had significantly higher rates of stomatitis (48% vs. 8%) and acne-like skin lesions (22% vs. 5%). On the basis of these findings, the FDA approved everolimus tablets for the treatment of adults with renal AMLs and TSC who do not require immediate surgery. At present, the place of everolimus or other mTOR inhibitors for the treatment of renal AMLs needs to be further defined. Benefits and risks need to be balanced, because the administration of mTOR inhibitors can be associated with significant adverse events, the reduction in renal AML volume is reversible after discontinuation of treatment, and long-term outcome results are not available.

Case reports have suggested efficacy of mTOR inhibitors in patients with unresectable or metastatic malignant epithelioid AMLs.

The main clinical problems associated with cystic disease in TSC are hypertension and renal failure. The treatment consists of strict control of hypertension. Bilateral nephrectomy should be considered before transplantation surgery because of the risk of life-threatening hemorrhage and the development of RCC

VON HIPPEL–LINDAU SYNDROME

Epidemiology

von Hippel–Lindau (VHL) syndrome is a rare autosomal dominant disease with a prevalence of 1 in 36,000. It is characterized by retinal hemangiomas, clear cell RCCs, cerebellar and spinal hemangioblastomas, pheochromocytomas, and, less frequently, pancreatic cysts and neuroendocrine tumors, endolymphatic sac tumors of the inner ear, and epididymal cystadenomas.[424,425] In approximately 20% of patients with VHL syndrome have a de novo mutation, they do not have a family history of VHL syndrome.

Genetics

The VHL protein (pVHL) is encoded by a highly conserved tumor suppressor gene in chromosome 3p25-p26. Genotype-phenotype correlations in VHL syndrome have classified four VHL subtypes.[281] Patients with VHL type 1 have no pheochromocytomas. Mutations in patients with VHL type 1 are mostly loss-of-function type, leading to a truncated pVHL or no pVHL at all. Patients with complete germline deletions have a lower rate of RCC than patients with partial deletions (22.6% vs. 49%, respectively).[225a] Mutations in patients with VHL type 2 are mostly missense mutations with some residual function. Whereas type 2 families have pheochromocytomas and are divided into subtypes with a low (type 2A) or high (type 2B) risk of RCC, type 2C families present with pheochromocytoma only. Dysregulation of VHL-dependent degradation of the α-subunit of hypoxia-inducible factor (HIF-α) is observed in subtypes 1, 2A, and 2B. By contrast, VHL-dependent HIF-α degradation is not observed in type 2C VHL mutants.

Pathogenesis

VHL encodes two proteins with relative molecular masses of approximately 30 kDa and 19 kDa. Although these isoforms may have different functions, both are capable of suppressing RCC growth in vivo. However, the best-characterized function of pVHL is to act as an essential component in the degradation of HIF-α subunits. pVHL is the substrate-binding subunit of an E3 ubiquitin ligase that ubiquitinates HIF-α.[425b] The HIF transcription factors consist of an oxygen-sensitive α-subunit and a constitutively expressed β-subunit, also known as the aryl hydrocarbon receptor nuclear translocator (ARNT). There are three isoforms of the α-subunit, HIF-1α, HIF-2α and HIF-3α, and one β subunit, HIF-1β. In normoxic conditions, HIF-1α and HIF-2α are hydroxylated by prolyl hydroxylases, recognized by pVHL, and targeted for proteasomal degradation. In conditions of low oxygen tension, HIF-1α and HIF-2α are stable and bind to HIF-1β. HIF-α/HIF-β dimers are translocated to the nucleus, bind to R-C-G-T-G DNA sequences called *hypoxia response elements*, and induce expression of numerous proteins, including proteins controlling angiogenesis (e.g., VEGF), erythropoiesis (e.g., erythropoietin), glucose uptake and metabolism (e.g., the Glut1 glucose transporter and various glycolytic enzymes), extracellular pH (e.g., carbonic anhydrases IX and XII), and mitogenesis (e.g., transforming growth factor-α (TGF-α), and platelet-derived growth factor [PDGF]).[425c]

Upregulation of HIF is not sufficient but is necessary to induce the RCC and CNS tumors associated with *VHL* mutations. A homozygous *VHL* missense mutation (p.R200W) causes Chuvash polycythemia. This condition is endemic to the Chuvash population of Russia, but it occurs worldwide.[426] VHL p.R200W homozygosity causes elevations of HIF, VEGF, erythropoietin, and hemoglobin, vertebral hemangiomas, varicose veins, low blood pressure, and premature mortality (42 years; range, 26 to 70 years) related to cerebral vascular events and peripheral thrombosis. The absence of RCCs, spinocerebellar hemangioblastomas, and pheochromocytomas typical of classic VHL syndrome, however, suggest that overexpression of HIF and VEGF is not sufficient for tumorigenesis. On the other hand, HIF upregulation is required for the development of VHL-associated RCC, and short hairpin HIF RNAs suppress tumor formation by VHL-defective renal carcinoma cells.

The demonstration that HIF upregulation is not sufficient to induce RCC suggests that pVHL has other cellular functions in addition to controlling HIF levels.[427,428] These include its ability to regulate apoptosis and senescence as well as its role in the maintenance of primary cilia and orchestration of the deposition of ECM.

Loss of heterozygosity at the *VHL* locus in microscopic renal cysts from patients with inherited VHL syndrome established cyst formation as an early step in the pathogenesis of RCC.[428a] Renal cysts and RCCs from patients with VHL syndrome show increased concentrations of both HIF-1α and HIF-2α. Renal cysts in patients with VHL syndrome and in renal clear cell carcinoma cell lines lacking pVHL have either no cilia or sparse, rudimentary cilia.[36,37,429] Importantly, ectopic expression of the VHL gene in renal clear cell carcinoma cell lines restores cilia formation, suggesting that pVHL directly supports ciliogenesis.

Diagnosis

The diagnosis of VHL syndrome should be made in a person with multiple CNS or retinal hemangioblastomas or a single hemangioblastoma plus one of the other characteristic physical abnormalities, or in families with a history of VHL syndrome. In some cases, the diagnosis may be warranted in a patient with a positive family history but without CNS or retinal lesions who has one or more of the less specific findings, with the exception of epididymal cysts, which are too nonspecific.

The molecular genetic diagnosis of VHL syndrome has greatly facilitated the evaluation and management of families whose members have the disease. Using a variety of techniques, the current detection rate of mutations is nearly 100%. Candidates for mutation analysis are patients with classic VHL syndrome (meeting clinical diagnostic criteria) and their first-degree family members and members of a family in which a germline *VHL* gene mutation has been identified (presymptomatic test). Genetic testing should also be considered for patients with findings suggestive but not diagnostic for VHL syndrome (i.e., multicentric tumors in one organ, bilateral tumors, two organ systems affected, one hemangioblastoma or pheochromocytoma in a patient younger than 50 years, or one RCC in a patient younger than 30 years) and for family members who have hemangioblastomas, RCCs, or pheochromocytomas only.

Manifestations

Renal cysts usually, but not always, precede the development of renal tumors. VHL syndrome–associated RCC manifests early in life, with a mean age at diagnosis of 35 years. The histology is uniformly clear cell. The cumulative probability of development of RCCs rises progressively beginning at age 20 years, reaching 70% by age 60 years. In contrast to RCCs in the general population, RCCs in individuals with VHL syndrome are more often multicentric and bilateral. Metastatic RCC is the leading cause of death from the syndrome.

Treatment

Patients with VHL syndrome need annual physical and ophthalmologic examinations; annual measurements of blood or urinary catecholamines and metanephrines; yearly ultrasonography, MRI, or CT of the abdomen; and yearly or biannual MRI or CT of the head and upper spine.[430] Positron emission tomography (PET) or iodine 131 (^{131}I)–metaiodobenzylguanidine scanning may be indicated for further evaluation of biochemical or imaging abnormalities. Early detection of complications, especially RCC and CNS lesions, followed by appropriate treatment is essential to reduce mortality from VHL syndrome. Because it tends to be recurrent, bilateral, and multifocal, strategies have been developed to preserve renal parenchyma and minimize the number of invasive procedures. The National Cancer Institute developed the 3-cm rule for surgical intervention on the basis of absence of documented metastasis from tumors smaller than 3 cm. Renal-sparing surgery provides effective initial treatment, with 5- and 10-year cancer-specific survival rates similar to those obtained with radical nephrectomy. Minimally invasive techniques that include percutaneous or laparoscopically guided cryotherapy or radiofrequency ablation represent suitable treatment options for selected patients with VHL syndrome that have high technical success rates and cause minor changes in renal function.[431,432]

The demonstration that HIF is required for VHL-associated carcinogenesis provides a rationale for therapies targeting this transcription factor.[433,434] HIF can be downregulated by mTOR inhibitors, heat shock protein 90 inhibitors such as geldanamycin and 17-(allylamino)-17-demethoxygeldanamycin, histone deacetylase (HDAC) inhibitors, topoisomerase I inhibitors, thioredoxin-1 inhibitors, and microtubule disrupters. Two mTOR inhibitors, temsirolimus and everolimus, have shown efficacy in the treatment of sporadic RCC.[435] Treatments can be directed against HIF-responsive gene products, such as VEGF, or against receptors for VEGF, PDGF, or TGF-β. Sunitinib, a VEGF and PDGF tyrosine kinase inhibitor, is currently used in patients with VHL-associated advanced RCC, pancreatic neuroendocrine tumors, and malignant pheochromocytomas.[436]

FAMILIAL RENAL HAMARTOMAS ASSOCIATED WITH HYPERPARATHYROIDISM–JAW TUMOR SYNDROME

The autosomal dominant disease familial renal hamartomas associated with hyperparathyroidism–jaw tumor syndrome is characterized by primary hyperparathyroidism (parathyroid adenoma or carcinoma) and ossifying fibroma of the jaw. Kidney lesions may also occur as bilateral cysts, renal hamartomas, or Wilms' tumors.[437] Renal cysts are a common finding, and in some cases, they have been clinically diagnosed as PKD. The gene mutated in this disease (*HRPT2*) is ubiquitously expressed and evolutionarily conserved and encodes a protein of 531 amino acids (parafibromin) with moderate identity and similarity to a protein of *Saccharomyces cerevisiae* (cdc73p) that is important in transcriptional initiation and elongation.[438]

HEPATOCYTE NUCLEAR FACTOR-1β–ASSOCIATED NEPHROPATHY

Hepatocyte nuclear factor-1β (HNF-1β) is a transcription factor encoded by the gene *HNF1B* (*TCF2*), which is expressed in polarized epithelia of the pancreas, liver, renal, and genital tracts. HNF-1β is expressed in the wolffian duct, the developing mesonephros and metanephros, and the müllerian ducts from the earliest stages of differentiation. In adults, it is expressed in kidney tubules and collecting ducts, oviducts, uterus, epididymis, vas deferens, seminal vesicles, prostate, and testes. HNF-1β regulates the transcription of a number of genes involved in tubulogenesis, nephron maturation, and tubular transport, including genes mutated in polycystic kidney disease (*PKHD1* and *PKD2*) and medullary cystic kidney disease (*UMOD*) and in autosomal dominant renal hypomagnesemia with hypocalciuria (*FXYD2*).[438a]

Heterozygous mutations of *HNF1B* are responsible for a dominantly inherited disease with renal and extrarenal phenotypes, HNF-1β–associated nephropathy.[439,440] Thirty percent to 50% of patients have de novo mutations. Whole-gene deletions occur in approximately 40% of the patients diagnosed in adulthood and in a higher percentage of the patients diagnosed in utero or infancy.[441-443] The disease is characterized by high phenotypic heterogeneity even within the same family.

The renal manifestations include structural and tubular transport abnormalities.[439-441] The structural abnormalities, often detected in utero, include bilateral hyperechogenic kidneys,[293] unilateral or bilateral agenesis or hypoplasia, multicystic dysplasia, abnormal calyces and papillae, and renal cysts. Histologic evaluation may reveal glomerular cysts and oligomeganephronia. Eight percent of congenital solitary kidneys are due to *HNF1B* mutations.

During childhood, the disease is characterized by defective kidney growth and impairment of renal function in approximately 50% of cases with evolution to ESKD in approximately 5% to 10%.[444]

The renal phenotype in adults is that of a chronic tubulointerstitial nephropathy with bland urinalysis, absence of hematuria, absence of or low-grade proteinuria, low prevalence of hypertension, and slowly progressive kidney failure (yearly eGFR decline of 2 to 2.5 mL/min/1.73 m^2). Renal cysts are present in 60% to 80% of the patients but usually are few in number, and unlike in ADPKD, the course of the cystic disease is not characterized by a progressive increase in the number of cysts or in kidney size.

Hypomagnesemia is present in approximately 50% of patients, likely because of the control of the expression of *FXYD2* by HNF-1β.[445] Hypokalemia is also present in 40% of adult patients but has not been observed in children; the underlying mechanism is uncertain. Hyperuricemia and gout have also been associated with the disease with variable frequency. Rarely a generalized dysfunction of proximal tubular function results in renal Fanconi's syndrome. Chromophobe RCCs have been described in a few patients.

The extrarenal manifestations include maturity-onset diabetes of the young type 5 (MODY5), exocrine pancreatic failure, fluctuating liver test abnormalities, and genital tract abnormalities.[439-441] Pancreatic atrophy is found in approximately one third and diabetes mellitus in approximately half of the patients. For reasons not understood, diabetic nephropathy is extremely rare in these patients. Liver function abnormalities, mainly fluctuating levels of serum alkaline phosphatase and γ-glutamyl transpeptidase, may occur in 40% to 80% of the patients, but liver biopsy findings are usually normal. The genital tract malformations may include absence of fallopian tubes or uterus, vaginal atresia, fusion abnormality such as bicornuate uterus or biseptate vagina, and male genital tract abnormalities. *HNF1B* mutations are found in approximately 18% of women with both renal and uterine malformations, but not in patients with isolated uterine malformations. Cognitive defects, autistic features, and epilepsy have also been associated with *HNF1B* mutations.

Patients with HNF-1β–associated nephropathy are good candidates for kidney transplantation, but they are at risk for early development of new-onset diabetes after transplantation. The immunosuppressive regimen should avoid tacrolimus and reduce corticosteroid dosage to minimize the risk of development of diabetes mellitus in nondiabetic transplant recipients.[446] In diabetic patients with HNF-1β–associated nephropathy and ESKD, simultaneous pancreatic and kidney transplantation should be considered.

ORO-FACIAL-DIGITAL SYNDROME TYPE 1

Oro-facial-digital syndrome type 1 is a rare X-linked dominant disorder with prenatal lethality in boys.[447] Affected girls may have kidneys indistinguishable from those in ADPKD. The correct diagnosis should be suggested by the extrarenal manifestations, which may include oral (hyperplastic frenula, cleft tongue, cleft palate or lip, malposed teeth), facial (broad nasal root with hypoplasia of nasal alae and malar bone), and digital (brachydactyly, syndactyly, clinodactyly, camptodactyly, polydactyly) anomalies.

Some patients have structural CNS anomalies such as agenesis of the corpus callosum, cerebellar agenesis, or the Dandy-Walker malformation. Renal cystic disease is present in 60% of cases after 18 years of age.[448] These individuals may also have liver and pancreatic cysts.[449] Mental retardation and tremor can be present in up to 50% of patients. The *OFD1* gene has been mapped to chromosome Xp22 and identified.[449a] A combination of direct DNA sequencing and gene dosage methods, to detect deletions, yield an 85% mutation detection rate.[450] Most mutations are private and predicted to result in a prematurely truncated protein. The 120-kDa OFD1 protein contains an N-terminal LisH motif, which is important in microtubule dynamics. This protein is a core component of the human centrosome throughout the cell cycle.[451] Most reported *OFD1* mutations are predicted to cause protein truncation with loss of coiled-coil domains necessary for centrosomal localization. A novel X-linked mental retardation syndrome associated with recurrent respiratory tract infections and macrocephaly caused by ciliary dyskinesia, but no renal phenotype, has been associated with an *OFD1* mutation.[452]

MEDULLARY CYSTIC KIDNEY DISEASE (AUTOSOMAL DOMINANT TUBULOINTERSTITIAL KIDNEY DISEASE)

MCKD is an autosomal dominant disorder characterized by the pathologic appearance of the kidneys (small to normal size with cysts at the corticomedullary junction, irregular thickening of the tubular basement membrane, and marked tubular atrophy and interstitial fibrosis; see Figure 46.17) and clinical manifestations (polydipsia and polyuria followed by development of renal insufficiency with low-grade proteinuria and a benign urine sediment) similar to those seen in NPHP (see later). The distinguishing features are the pattern of inheritance, distinct pathogenesis, later age at diagnosis and ESKD, and absence of extrarenal organ involvement except for gout.[453,454]

Because the development of medullary cysts is neither an early nor a typical feature of the disease, many now consider the term medullary cystic kidney disease to be a misnomer

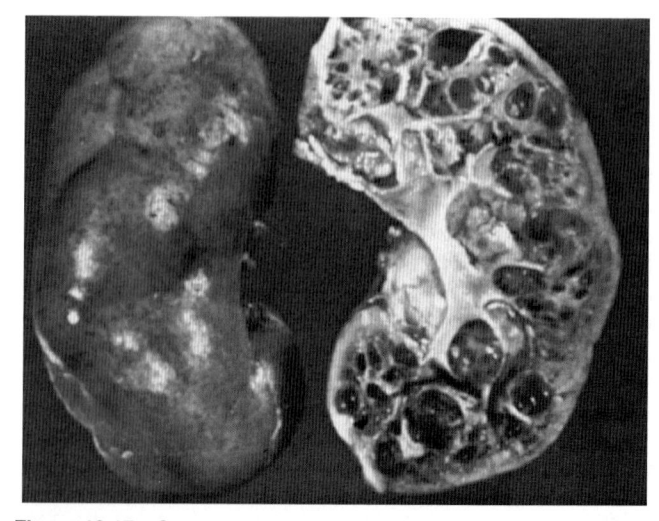

Figure 46.17 Outer and cut surface of kidney with severe medullary cystic disease.

and have proposed the term *autosomal dominant tubulointerstitial kidney disease* (ADTKD)[455,455a] to refer to a group of diseases caused by at least four genes: *MUC1* encoding the mucoprotein mucin-1 (MUC-1) (chromosomal location 1q22)[456]; *UMOD* encoding uromodulin, also known as Tamm-Horsfall protein (chromosome 16p12.3)[457,458]; *HNF1B* encoding hepatocyte nuclear factor-1β (chromosome 17q12); and *REN* encoding renin (chromosome 1q32.1). Mucin-1 and uromodulin, which are found in the thick ascending limb of loop of Henle, protect against infection. Although HNF-1β–associated extrarenal features may accompany the nephropathy, they are not obligatory, and these four entities can be reliably identified only through genetic analysis.

ADTKD-*MUC1* (or MCKD type 1) is caused by a heterozygous mutation in the variable-number tandem repeat (VNTR) region of *MUC1*.[456] All identified mutations add one cytosine to a tract of seven cytosine nucleotides, resulting in a frameshift mutation causing truncation of the VNTR and the creation of a new amino acid sequence on the terminal end of the MUC-1 protein. This new protein appears to be improperly processed in the cytoplasm, leading to apoptosis of tubular cells and slowly progressive tubular cell death and nephron dropout, resulting in chronic kidney disease.[456]

ADTKD-*UMOD* (or MCKD type 2) is caused by a heterozygous mutation, usually a missense mutation in exon 3, 4, 5, 6, 7, or 8, that results in an amino acid change that either creates or replaces a cysteine residue.[459,460] The correct protein folding is disrupted, leading to intracellular accumulation of mutant uromodulin, retention in the endoplasmic reticulum, and increased apoptosis.[461,462] This process explains the fact that $Umod^{-/-}$ mice do not have a MCKD phenotype, although they are more susceptible to urinary tract infections and stone formation.[463-465] A consanguineous family with multiple heterozygous cases and three more severely affected but viable homozygous cases for the same mutation has been described.[466] The association of a *UMOD* mutation and glomerulocystic kidney disease has been described in one family.[467] Furthermore, single nucleotide polymorphisms in *UMOD* have been associated with an increased risk of CKD.[468] Polydipsia, polyuria, and a tendency to waste sodium are common manifestations of the disease. MCKD2 is frequently but not always associated with hyperuricemia and gout at an early age. It is thought that the accumulation of abnormal uromodulin in the epithelial cells of the thick ascending limb of loop of Henle prevents the proper function of ion channels, results in mild natriuresis, and increases proximal tubular reabsorption of urate. Hyperuricemia and gout also occur in MCKD1, but usually at advanced stages of the disease. Patients with MCKD1 and MCKD2 reach ESKD at median ages of 62 and 32 years, respectively, with large patient-to-patient variability.

A diagnosis of MCKD should be considered in patients with a family history of chronic kidney disease, bland urinary sediment, and segregation suggesting autosomal dominant inheritance.[469] If there is a history of gout at an early age or a strong family history of gout, molecular genetic testing for *UMOD* mutations should be performed.[453] If there is a history of anemia in childhood and mildly elevated serum potassium concentrations, familial juvenile hyperuricemic nephropathy 2 should be considered, and genetic testing for *REN* (renin gene) mutations performed.[470] If none of the preceding clinical characteristics is present or if molecular genetic testing has not revealed a disease-causing mutation, *MUC1* molecular genetic testing should be considered.[454]

The treatment of choice for ESKD secondary to MCKD is kidney transplantation.[471] If a kidney from a living related donor is considered for transplantation, precautions should be taken to obtain it only from an older relative, who should be subjected to meticulous diagnostic evaluation.

AUTOSOMAL RECESSIVE CILIOPATHIES WITH INTERSTITIAL NEPHRITIS AND RENAL CYSTIC DISEASE

Autosomal recessive ciliopathies with interstitial nephritis and renal cystic disease are large group of diseases caused by mutations in genes encoding ciliary or basal body proteins.[472,473] The primary cilium is a single hairlike organelle that projects from the surface of most mammalian cells, including epithelial and endothelial cells, neurons, fibroblasts, chondrocytes, and osteocytes.[473a] It arises from the mother centriole, or basal body, in the centrosome. In addition to the basal body, the cilium comprises a transition zone, which anchors it to the cell membrane and regulates protein traffic in and out of the cilium, and the axoneme, which contains a ring of microtubule bundles connecting the ciliary base to the tip (Figure 46.18). There is a distinctive proximal segment of the ciliary axoneme known as the inversin compartment, but its function is uncertain. A specific process of intraflagellar transport (IFT) involving anterograde transport of cargo toward the tip of the cilium (using the kinesin II motor in association with the IFT complex B [IFT-B] proteins) and retrograde movement (employing the cytoplasmic dynein motor 2 in association with the IFT complex A [IFT-A] proteins) is required for ciliary formation and function.

Primary cilia are important for cell migration or fate determination and tissue patterning during development and for maintenance of cell differentiation thereafter.[473a] The ciliopathies exhibit marked genetic heterogeneity and multiple organ involvement (pleiotropy). Nephronophthisis (NPHP), Joubert syndrome (JBTS), and Meckel (MKS) syndrome are autosomal recessive ciliopathies manifesting with cystic kidneys/interstitial nephritis, retinal degeneration, cerebellar/neural tube malformation, and hepatic fibrosis. The impact of the gene involved, the combination of mutations, and likely other genetic and nongenetic factors determine whether the resulting phenotype is mainly of a developmental (e.g., vermis aplasia, encephalocele, severe renal cystic disease) or degenerative (e.g., retinitis pigmentosa, interstitial nephritis, hepatic fibrosis) nature.[473] Mutations in the same gene can result in different phenotypes. For example, in the case of MKS3, two *TMEM67* truncating mutations can cause MKS. However, *TMEM67* mutations can also cause JBTS and NPHP with liver fibrosis (COACH [*c*erebellar vermis hypoplasia/aplasia, *o*ligophrenia, *a*taxia, *c*oloboma, and *h*epatic fibrosis] syndrome. In this case although there is higher frequency of missense changes in these disorders, a complete genotype/phenotype

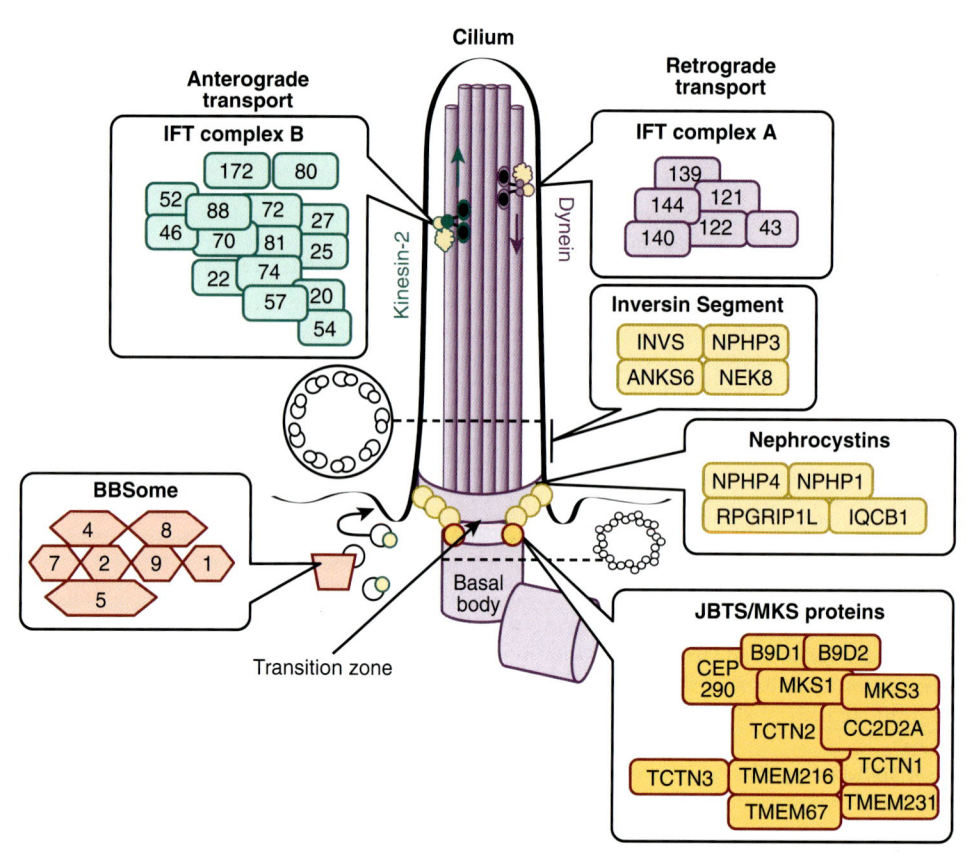

Figure 46.18 Structure of the primary cilium showing localization of groups of cilioproteins. Primary cilia are sensory organelles that have been implicated in the pathogenesis of polycystic kidney disease, and a large group of the proteins that cause ciliopathies have now been identified. Intraflagellar transport (IFT) moves proteins along the cilium and is involved in cilia formation. Two specific complexes of IFT proteins are involved in anterograde (IFT complex B; kinesin 2 motor) and retrograde (IFT complex A, dynein motor) movements within the cilium. (Numbers inside each complex signify specific IFT proteins.) Many of the proteins involved in Meckel syndrome (MKS) and Joubert syndrome (JBTS) and some of the nephronophthisis (NPHP) proteins form a complex at the transition zone and are thought to regulate the protein composition of the cilium. Another group of proteins, including inversin (INVS), are localized to the proximal region of the ciliary axoneme (inversin segment), but their function is less clear. Many of the Bardet–Biedl syndrome (BBS) proteins form the BBSome and regulate trafficking of membrane proteins to the cilium. (Numbers inside BBSome signify various BBS proteins.) Mutations in these ciliopathy proteins alter the normal composition, sensory functions, and signaling of the cilium and are associated with the pleiotropic phenotypes typical of these diseases. ANKS6, Ankyrin repeat and SAM (sterile alpha motif) domain–containing protein 6; B9D1/2, B9 domain containing proteins 1/2; CC2D2A, coiled-coil and C2-domain containing 2A protein; CEP290, centrosomal protein of 290 kDa; $IQCB_1$, IQ motif containing B_1; NEK8, serine/threonine-protein kinase 8; RPGRIP1L, RPGR (retinitis pigmentosa guanosine triphosphatase regulator)–interacting protein 1–like protein; TCTN, tectonic family member; TMEM, transmembrane protein.

correlation has not been defined. Therefore, NPHP, JBTS, and MKS can be considered to be allelic disorders.[474] There is also substantial phenotypic and some genetic overlap between these diseases and other disorders such as Bardet-Biedl syndrome (BBS) and Alström syndrome (ALMS). A remarkable feature of these ciliopathies is their large and overlapping genetic heterogeneity, with a total of 55 genes now implicated: NPHP (18), JBTS (21), MKS (11), BBS (19), and ALMS (1) (see Table 46.3 for details).[475]

Proteomics and assays of ciliogenesis and epithelial morphogenesis have suggested that the NPHP/JBTS/MKS proteins are organized into a network of functionally connected modules.[476,477] The role of these complexes seems to be to regulate protein trafficking into the cilium. In most cases, mutation leads not to ciliary loss but to an impaired functionality of the cilium. The NPHP1, NPHP4, and RPGRIP1L module localizes to the ciliary transition zone and to cell-cell contacts. It is not essential for ciliogenesis, but it is important for the organization of specialized structures at the apical surface of polarized cells and for epithelial morphogenesis. The IQCB1 and CEP290 module is localized to centrosomes and transition fibers and is indispensable for ciliogenesis in terminal inner medullary collecting duct (IMCD3) cells and for tissue organization. The module consisting of MKS proteins is localized to the transition zone and functionally connected to hedgehog signal transduction. INVS, NPHP3, and NEK8 interact in the inversin compartment but their function is unknown. The NPHP-JBTS-MKS network does not overlap with the module integrated by the proteins mutated in BBS (BBSome),[478] despite significant phenotypic overlap, nor with the components of the IFT-A or IFT-B complex proteins despite the fact that defects in IFT may lead to cystic kidney disease and retinal degeneration.

The convergence of proteins mutated in these related ciliopathies at cilia and centrosomes is starting to reveal the

Table 46.3 Genes Mutated in Autosomal Recessive Ciliopathies with Interstitial Nephritis, Cysts, or Both

OFFICAL GENE NAME	NPHP	Disease Designations						
		LCA	SLS	JBTS*	MKS	BBS	ALMS	OFDS
NPHP1	NPHP1		SLS1	JBTS4				
INVS	NPHP2							
NPHP3	NPHP3				MKS7			
NPHP4	NPHP4		SLS4					
IQCB1	NPHP5		SLS5					
CEP290	NPHP6	LCA10†	SLS6	JBTS5	MKS4	BBS14		
GLIS2	NPHP7							
RPGRIP1L	NPHP8			JBTS7	MKS5			
NEK8	NPHP9							
SDCCAG8	NPHP10		SLS7					
TMEM67	NPHP11			JBTS6	MKS3	BBS16		
TTC21B	NPHP12							
WDR19	NPHP13							
ZNF423	NPHP14			JBTS19				
CEP164	NEPH15							
ANKS6	NPHP16							
IFT172	NPHP17							
CEP63	NPHP18							
INPP5E				JBTS1				
TMEM216				JBTS2	MKS2			
AHI1				JBTS3				
ARL13B				JBTS8				
CC2D2A				JBTS9	MKS6			
OFD1				JBTS10				OFDS1
KIF7				JBTS12				
TCTN1				JBTS13				
TMEM237				JBTS14				
CEP41				JBTS15				
TMEM138				JBTS16				
C5ORF42				JBTS17				OFDSVI
TCTN3				JBTS18				OFDSIV
TMEM231				JBTS20	MKS11			
CSPP1				JBTS21				
PDE6D				JBT322				
MKS1					MKS1	BBS13		
TCTN2					MKS8			
B9D1					MKS9			
B9D2					MKS10			
BBS1						BBS1		
BBS2						BBS2		
ARL6						BBS3		
BBS4						BBS4		
BBS5						BBS5		
MKKS						BBS6		
BBS7						BBS7		
TTC8						BBS8		
PTHB1						BBS9		
BBS10						BBS10		
TRIM32						BBS11		
BBS12						BBS12		
C2orf86						BBS15		
LZTFL1						BBS17		
BBIP1						BBS18		
IFT127						BBS19		
ALMS1							ALMS1	

*Includes CORS (cerebellooculorenal syndrome) and COACH (cerebellar vermis hypoplasia or aplasia, oligophrenia, congenital ataxia, coloboma, and congenital hepatic fibrosis) syndrome.
†Hypomorphic mutations.
ALMS, Alström syndrome; BBS, Bardet-Biedl syndrome; JBTS, Joubert syndrome; LCA, Leber congenital amaurosis; MKS, Meckel syndrome; NPHP, nephronophthisis; OFDS, oral-facial-digital syndrome; SLS, Senior-Loken syndrome.

pathogenesis of these diseases, which are likely associated with abnormal regulation of protein entry into cilia.[479] Multiple signaling pathways require cilia for proper functioning and have been implicated in ciliopathies, including Wnt and sonic hedgehog signaling.[473] The pleiotropic features seen in ciliopathies are likely a combination of defects of cilia sensor/mechanosensory functions and cilia-associated signaling that are disrupted by an abnormal cilia-gating process. The observation that proteins that cause NPHP and related ciliopathies when mutated exhibit dual localization at centrosomes and at nuclear foci and play a role in in DNA damage response has led to the hypothesis that defects in DNA damage response participate in the pathogenesis of these diseases.[480]

NEPHRONOPHTHISIS

NPHP is an autosomal recessive disorder with an estimated prevalence of 1 in 50,000 live births. It accounts for approximately 5% of ESKD in North American children.[481] It is genetically heterogeneous, with 18 genes identified (see Table 46.3).[482-488] Homozygous deletions in *NPHP1* account for approximately 21% of all cases of NPHP; the other genes contribute less than 3% each. No mutations in any of the known genes are found in approximately 60% of patients, indicating that many other genes remain to be discovered.[489]

Mutations in *INVS* and less frequently *NPHP3* lead to renal failure between birth and age 3 years (infantile NPHP). Mutations in the other genes, including *NPHP3*, cause renal failure in the first three decades of life (juvenile NPHP).[484] Severe retinitis pigmentosa (Senior-Loken syndrome) is frequently associated with *IQCB1*, *CEP290*, and *RPGRIP1L* mutations, but it is less severe and more rarely associated with mutations in other *NPHP* genes. Oculomotor apraxia (Cogan's syndrome) is occasionally observed with *NPHP1* and *NPHP4* mutations. *CEP290* and *RPGRIPL1* mutations are frequently associated with cerebellar aplasia or hypoplasia and mental retardation (overlap with JBTS; see later). *INVS* and, more rarely, *NPHP3* mutations can be associated with situs inversus, cardiac ventricular septal defect, hepatic fibrosis, and retinitis pigmentosa. Hypomorphic mutations of *TMEM67* cause NPHP associated with hepatic fibrosis.

The nephrocystins form a multifunctional complex localized in primary cilia, centrosomes, and actin- and microtubule-based structures involved in cell-cell and cell-matrix adhesion signaling as well as in cell division.[483,485,486,488,490-492] In the kidney, these functional roles could be particularly important for establishing and maintaining the differentiated state of tubular epithelial cells. Localization of nephrocystins to the cilia explains the association with renal cystic disease and hepatic fibrosis (primary cilia in tubular epithelial cells and cholangiocytes; see earlier discussions of ADPKD and ARPKD), retinitis pigmentosa (rods and cones are modified cilia), and situs inversus and ventricular septal defect (primary cilia in the embryonic node are essential for left-right axis determination).

In the juvenile form, the kidneys are small with a granular capsular surface. On cut sections, the cortex and medulla are thinned, and the corticomedullary margin is indistinct with a variable number of small, thin-walled cysts of distal convoluted and collecting tubule origin. Similar cysts may also be present in the medulla. Grossly visible cysts are often absent. The tubular basement membranes are thickened, even fairly early in the course of the disease, and tubule segments of a single nephron may be encompassed by very dense sclerotic interstitium with sparse chronic inflammatory cell infiltrates. The histologic features of the infantile form are different. The kidneys are often enlarged and cystic, and thickening of the tubular basement membranes is less prominent.

Excretory urography and ultrasonography frequently fail to detect cysts because they are small.[493] Excretory urography may show inhomogeneous streaking in the medulla caused by accumulation of contrast material in the collecting ducts. Contrast-enhanced CT and MRI are more sensitive to detect small corticomedullary and medullary cysts, but failure to detect cysts does not exclude the diagnosis.

The onset of the disease is insidious. Polyuria and polydipsia are the presenting symptoms. Hypertension is common in the infantile form, but whether absent or present, it is not a prominent feature in the juvenile form. Sodium wasting is common. The urine sediment is characteristically benign. Proteinuria is absent or low grade. There is no microhematuria. Progression to ESKD occurs within the first 3 years in the infantile form and within the first 2 to 3 decades in the juvenile form.

The treatment of NPHP is supportive. Because of the tendency for sodium wasting, volume contraction, and renal azotemia, unnecessary sodium restriction or use of diuretics should be avoided. If kidneys from siblings are considered for transplant surgery, precautions should be taken to obtain them only from unaffected, older relatives, who should be subjected to meticulous diagnostic evaluation.[495]

JOUBERT SYNDROME

JBTS is an autosomal recessive neurologic disease characterized by cerebellar vermis aplasia or hypoplasia with abnormal superior cerebellar peduncles (the "molar tooth sign"), mental retardation, hypotonia, an irregular breathing pattern, and eye movement abnormalities.[496] In addition to these core features, patients may exhibit retinal defects (ranging in severity from Leber congenital amaurosis to slowly progressive retinopathies with partially preserved vision), renal defects (nephronophthisis or cystic dysplastic kidneys), and CHF. Rarer features include chorioretinal or optic nerve colobomas, congenital heart malformations, situs inversus, severe scoliosis, skeletal dysplasia, Hirschsprung's disease, and midline oral and facial defects, such as cleft lip, cleft palate, or both, notched upper lip, lobulated tongue with multiple frenula, and lingual or oral soft tumors. The association of JBTS with polydactyly and midline orofacial defects defines the so-called orofacial-digital type VI syndrome. A distinct subgroup of JBTS defined by *c*erebellar vermis hypoplasia or aplasia, *o*ligophrenia, congenital *a*taxia, *c*oloboma, and *h*epatic fibrosis is known by the acronym COACH, which is usually associated with *TMEM67*, *CC2D2A*, or *RPGRIP1L* mutations. Gentile syndrome applies to patients who present with JBTS and CHF in the absence of other clinical features.

Like NPHP and MKS, JBTS exhibits marked genetic heterogeneity. The genetic bases of JBTS are extremely complex and only partly understood, despite the tremendous acceleration in gene discovery enabled by next-generation sequencing techniques. So far, 21 causative genes have been identified, with autosomal or X-linked recessive inheritance (see Table 46.3).[496]

MECKEL SYNDROME

MKS is characterized by bilateral renal cystic dysplasia or polycystic kidney disease, CNS defects (typically occipital encephalocele, but can include the Dandy-Walker malformation or hydrocephalus), postaxial polydactyly, and biliary dysgenesis/CHF. It is a lethal disorder, and most affected infants are stillborn or die within few hours or days after birth.

MKS is genetically heterogeneous, and 11 genes have been associated with it (see Table 46.3).[497-501] The MKS proteins have been localized to the centrosome, the pericentriolar region, or the cilium itself, and their function is likely involved in forming the barrier between the cell and the cilium at the transition zone.[479]

BARDET-BIEDL SYNDROME

BBS is characterized by retinitis pigmentosa, obesity, postaxial polydactyly, learning disabilities, hypogenitalism, and renal abnormalities. Four of these six cardinal features are required for the diagnosis. Other manifestations are diabetes, hypertension, congenital heart disease, ataxia, spasticity, deafness, hepatic fibrosis, and Hirschsprung's disease. The manifestations may appear after several years of development.[502]

Although rare (1 in 120,000 live births), its prevalence in certain geographically isolated communities, such as the Canadian province of Newfoundland and in Kuwait, is more common (1 in 13,500 to 1 in 17,500).[366]

BBS is genetically heterogeneous. Nineteen known BBS genes account for approximately 80% of patients clinically diagnosed with the syndrome.[502-505] The majority of pathogenic mutations are found in BBS1 and BBS10, accounting for 23.2% and 20%, respectively. The disease is primarily inherited in an autosomal recessive manner but with some evidence of a more complex, oligogenic form of inheritance (triallelism and digenic).[506,507] The localization of the BBS proteins at a subcellular level points to a role in the function of the cilium–centrosome axis. BBS4, BBS6, and BBS8 interact with the *pericentriolar material protein 1*, a protein important for centriolar duplication. BBS6, BBS10, and BBS12 are chaperone-like proteins. BBS proteins 1, 2, 4, 5, 7, 8, and 9 constitute the BBSome, implicated in vesicular transport toward the cilium. BBS7 and BBS8 play a role in IFT. BBS11 is an ubiquitin ligase.[478,508]

The diagnosis of BBS is often missed in childhood and made only later in life. Targeted fetal sonography in the second trimester of pregnancy to detect digital and renal abnormalities has been proposed for the prenatal diagnosis of the disease. The prenatal appearance of enlarged hyperechoic kidneys without corticomedullary differentiation should prompt the diagnosis in a family with BBS, especially when polydactyly is present.[509,510] In nonaffected families, BBS should be included in the differential diagnosis whenever such an appearance is discovered in utero. The postnatal evolution of the renal ultrasonographic findings is variable, and normalization generally occurs by the age of 2 years.

Renal abnormalities are very common in BBS.[511] Calyceal clubbing, diverticula, or cysts can be detected in up to 96% of cases. The most common and earliest functional abnormality is a reduced ability to concentrate the urine, resulting in polyuria and polydipsia. Hypertension develops in approximately 50% of patients, and chronic renal insufficiency in 25% to 50%. Despite mental retardation, obesity, and severe visual problems, patients tolerate hemodialysis well. Renal transplantation can be performed, but special attention must be given to controlling hyperphagia and obesity.

ALSTRÖM SYNDROME

Alström syndrome is an autosomal recessive disease that has some phenotypic overlap with BBS. It is characterized by obesity, type 2 diabetes mellitus, retinitis pigmentosa, nerve deafness, CHF, cardiomyopathy, chronic respiratory tract infections, and, frequently, slowly progressive chronic tubulointerstitial nephropathy.[512,513] The Alström syndrome protein (ALMS1) is of unknown function, is widely expressed in human and mouse tissues, and localizes to centrosomes and the base of cilia.

NEPHRONOPHTHISIS VARIANTS ASSOCIATED WITH SKELETAL DEFECTS (SKELETAL CILIOPATHIES)

The association of NPHP with cone-shaped epiphyses of the phalanges, known as Mainzer-Saldino syndrome, occurs in patients who also have retinal degeneration and cerebellar ataxia. Mutations in *IFT80*, a component of IFT-B complex, cause Jeune syndrome (asphyxiating thoracic dysplasia), a genetically heterogeneous disorder characterized by a severely constricted thoracic cage and respiratory insufficiency, retinal degeneration, cystic renal disease, and polydactyly.[514] Sensenbrenner syndrome, or cranioectodermal dysplasia, is characterized by skeletal abnormalities (e.g., craniosynostosis, narrow rib cage, short limbs, brachydactyly), ectodermal defects, NPHP leading to progressive renal failure, hepatic fibrosis, heart defects and retinitis pigmentosa. Other syndromic forms of NPHP with skeletal disorders include Ellis–van Creveld syndrome (short stature, short ribs, postaxial polydactyly, nail dystrophy, oral and cardiac defects) and RHYNS syndrome (*r*etinitis pigmentosa, *h*ypopituitarism, *n*ephronophthisis, and *s*keletal dysplasia).

Whereas proteins associated with NPHP, JBTS, and MKS mainly function at the ciliary transition zone, most proteins associated with skeletal ciliopathies have been shown to participate in intraflagellar transport. Ciliary proteins found to be defective in skeletal disorders currently encompass the following four main subgroups: (1) IFT-A subunits and its motor protein, DYNC2H1, whose defects disrupt retrograde transport and cause IFT protein accumulation at the ciliary tip; (2) IFT80 and IFT172, two of 14 subunits of IFT-B; (3) NEK1, a serine-threonine kinase involved in cell-cycle control and ciliogenesis; and (4) EVC- and EVC2-positive regulators of sonic hedgehog signaling located at the basal body.[515-525]

RENAL CYSTIC DYSPLASIAS

Renal cystic dysplasias result from an interference with a normal ampullary activity that leads to abnormal metanephric differentiation. When the inhibition of the ampullary activity occurs very early, few collecting ducts are formed and few nephrons develop. The kidney becomes a cluster of cysts with little or no residual parenchyma, and the ureter is absent or atretic. These kidneys may be normal size, larger than normal (multicystic dysplastic kidney [MCDK]), or markedly shrunken (hypodysplastic kidney). These variations probably represent different stages of the same pathologic process because renal cysts can involute and disappear completely during intrauterine life. When the interference with the ampullary activity occurs later (e.g., as the result of urethral or ureteral obstruction), there may be mild irregularities in branching with a mild generalized dilation of the collecting tubules in the medulla. Most nephrons, however, except the last to be formed, are normal. The cysts are found under the capsule and generally derive from Bowman's spaces (glomerular cysts), the loop of Henle, or terminal ends of collecting tubules. A variety of renal abnormalities in the contralateral kidney can be found in association with cystic dysplastic kidneys. These include renal agenesis, ectopy or fusion, and ureteral duplication or obstruction that may result from injury to the ureteric bud during various stages of development. When the injury to the ureteric bud occurs before a communication with the metanephric blastema has been established, secondary atrophy of the metanephric blastema and renal agenesis ensue. On the other hand, if the injury of the bud or ureteral obstruction occurs after renal development is completed, dysplasia does not occur. Thus, a spectrum of renal abnormalities ranging from agenesis and severe dysplasia to mild cystic dysplasia with glomerular cysts and a variety of related renal and ureteral abnormalities may result from interferences with normal ampullary activity and metanephric differentiation.

Renal cystic dysplasias may be the consequence of an intrinsic (malformation) or extrinsic (disruption) defect in organogenesis. An intrinsic defect may be caused by a single gene mutation, a chromosomal aberration, or a combination of genetic and environmental factors (multifactorial determination). Extrinsic causes include teratogenic chemicals, metabolic abnormalities, and infections. Evidence for intrinsic or extrinsic defects should be sought by careful review of the pregnancy, family history, and physical examination (pattern of associated abnormalities) as well as by the study of the karyotype. Renal cystic dysplasias frequently occur as sporadic events, but they can also occur in the context of many multiorgan malformation syndromes, several of which have defined genetic bases.[526]

Although most dysplastic kidneys are grossly deformed in a fairly characteristic way, most writers accept only two absolute criteria for dysplasia, both of which require histologic confirmation (Figure 46.19). Of greater importance is the finding of primitive ducts encompassed by mantles of variably differentiated mesenchyma and lined by cuboidal to columnar, sometimes ciliated, epithelium unlike that in any normally developing or mature ducts. Somewhat less important, because of its variable presence, is the finding of metaplastic cartilage (see Figure 46.19). Cysts of glomerular, tubule, and ductal origin may also be present, but because they might represent either a maldevelopment or a histologically similar degenerative change in previously normal but immature structures, they do not provide absolute evidence of parenchymal maldevelopment.

MULTICYSTIC DYSPLASTIC KIDNEY

MCDK is the most common cause of an abdominal mass in infancy and the most common type of bilateral cystic disease in newborns (Figure 46.20). With the widespread use of fetal sonography, MCDK is now most often diagnosed in utero, usually during the third trimester. MCDK is more often unilateral than bilateral, and boys are more frequently affected than girls. Because affected kidneys tend to involute over weeks or months prenatally and postnatally, the prevalence of unilateral MCDK is higher on fetal screening (1 in 2000) than on neonatal screening (1 in 4000).

Differentiation of MCDK from hydronephrosis in fetuses and newborns is essential because the therapeutic approaches to these conditions differ. The most useful sonographic criteria for identifying a MCDK include the presence of interphases between cysts, a nonmedial location of the larger cysts, absence of an identifiable renal sinus in 100% of the cases, and the absence of parenchymal tissue. The

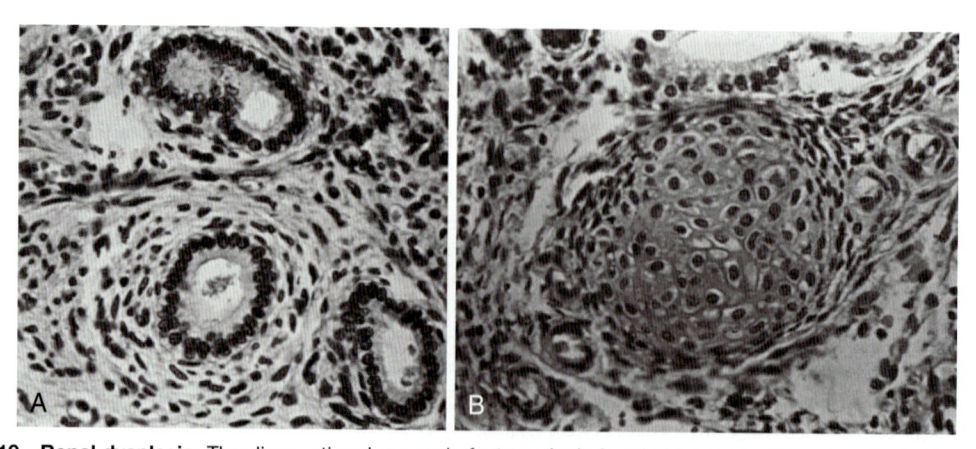

Figure 46.19 Renal dysplasia. The diagnostic microscopic features include primitive ducts (**A**) and metaplastic cartilage (**B**).

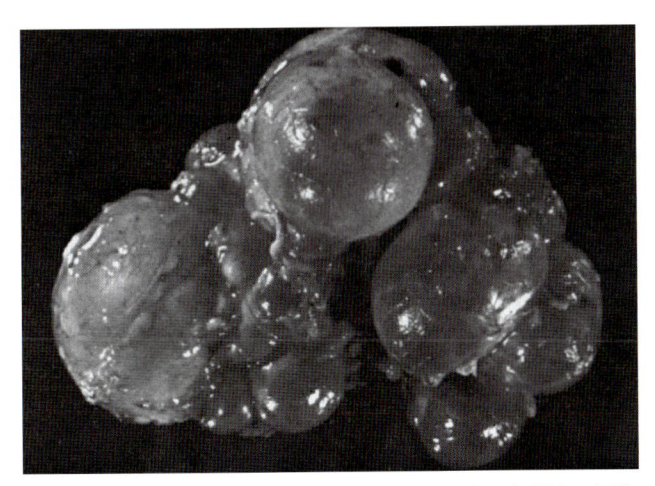

Figure 46.20 Severe renal cystic dysplasia (multicystic kidney). The renal architecture is markedly distorted.

diagnosis can be confirmed by retrograde pyelography, which shows an absence or atresia of proximal ureter, and by angiography, which demonstrates absence or hypoplasia of the renal artery. Cyst walls often calcify in older patients and may appear as ringlike densities in the region of the kidney.

The manifestations of MCDK depend on whether it is bilateral or unilateral. Bilateral MCDK results in oligohydramnios and the Potter sequence and is incompatible with life. Unilateral MCDK may be diagnosed in a newborn during an evaluation of a renal mass or may go unnoticed until later in life, during evaluation for abdominal or flank discomfort caused by the mass effect of the lesion.[527] Serial ultrasonography shows that 33% of the MCDKs have completely involuted at 2 years of age, 47% at 5 years, and 59% at 10 years. The development of hypertension or malignant degeneration is very rare.[528] Because of its low risk and tendency to involute, MCDK in children is usually managed conservatively.[529] When indicated, laparoscopic nephrectomy is preferable to open nephrectomy. Attention should be paid to an increased risk for associated urinary tract malformations of the contralateral kidney (e.g., pelviureteric junction obstruction and vesicoureteric reflux), but voiding cystography is indicated only when the ultrasonographic findings in the contralateral kidney or ureter are abnormal.[530]

OTHER CYSTIC KIDNEY DISORDERS

SIMPLE CYSTS

PREVALENCE

Simple cysts are the most common cystic abnormality encountered in human kidneys.[531] They may be solitary or multiple and are filled with a fluid that is chemically similar to an ultrafiltrate of plasma. The cysts are very rare in children, but the frequency increases with age.[532] In autopsy studies and as incidental CT findings, they are found in approximately 25% and 50% in patients 40 and 50 years of age, respectively. Ultrasonography is less sensitive than CT or MRI and turns up lower percentages. A CT angiographic study of 1948 potential kidney donors (42% men; mean age, 43 years) showed that 39%, 22%, 7.9%, and 1.6% of 19- to 49-year-old individuals and 63%, 43%, 22%, and 7.8% of 50- to 75-year-old individuals had at least one cortical or medullary cyst at least 2, 5, 10, and 20 mm in diameter, respectively. The 97.5th percentile for number of cortical and medullary cysts 5 mm or larger increased with age (1 cyst in men and 1 in women 18-29 years old, 2 in men and 2 in women 30-39 years old, 3 in men and 2 in women 40-49 years old, 5 in men and 3 in women 50-59 years old, and 10 in men and 4 in women 60-69 years old).[533]

PATHOGENESIS

Simple renal cysts are acquired, although the contribution of genetic factors has not been studied. Several hypotheses have been proposed to explain their pathogenesis. Tubular obstruction and ischemia might play a role. Microdissection studies revealed that diverticula of distal convoluted and collecting tubules are common after age 20 years and increase in number with age. Cysts are thought to derive from progressive dilation and detachment of these diverticula. The cyst walls also appear to be relatively impermeable to low-molecular-weight solutes and to antibiotics. Nonetheless, the turnover of cyst fluid may be as great as 20 times per day, as measured by tritiated water diffusion. Another study has shown a positive association between the plasma levels of copeptin, a surrogate for vasopressin, and the presence of renal cysts, suggesting the possibility that vasopressin may favor the development of simple renal cysts.[534]

PATHOLOGY

Simple renal cysts are usually lined by a single layer of epithelial cells and filled with a clear, serous fluid. They grow slowly, but huge cysts, up to 30 cm in diameter, have been described. The inner surface of these cysts is glistening and usually smooth, but some cysts may be trabeculated by partial septa that divide the cavity into broadly interconnecting locules. These septated simple cysts should not be confused with multilocular cysts. The cysts are often cortical and distort the renal contour, but they may be deep cortical or apparently medullary in origin. They do not communicate with the renal pelvis. The walls typically are thin and transparent but may become thickened, fibrotic, and even calcified, possibly from earlier hemorrhage or infection.

DIAGNOSIS

Most simple cysts are found on routine imaging studies (Figure 46.21). Differentiation of simple cysts from RCC is a common problem. Because the appearance of a renal mass on the excretory urogram alone never excludes a malignancy, ultrasonography, CT, or MRI is commonly required to characterize the lesion. Acceptance of definite criteria for the diagnosis of a simple cyst by these imaging techniques has eliminated the use of renal angiography and percutaneous cyst aspiration to characterize renal masses. Calcium deposits are found in 2% of simple cysts and 10% of RCCs. Whereas calcifications appear to be peripheral in simple cysts, they are more central in tumors. Improvements in the imaging techniques have also reduced the indications for surgery in the management of patients with benign simple cysts. When the cysts are numerous and bilateral, differentiation from ADPKD may be difficult if liver cysts are

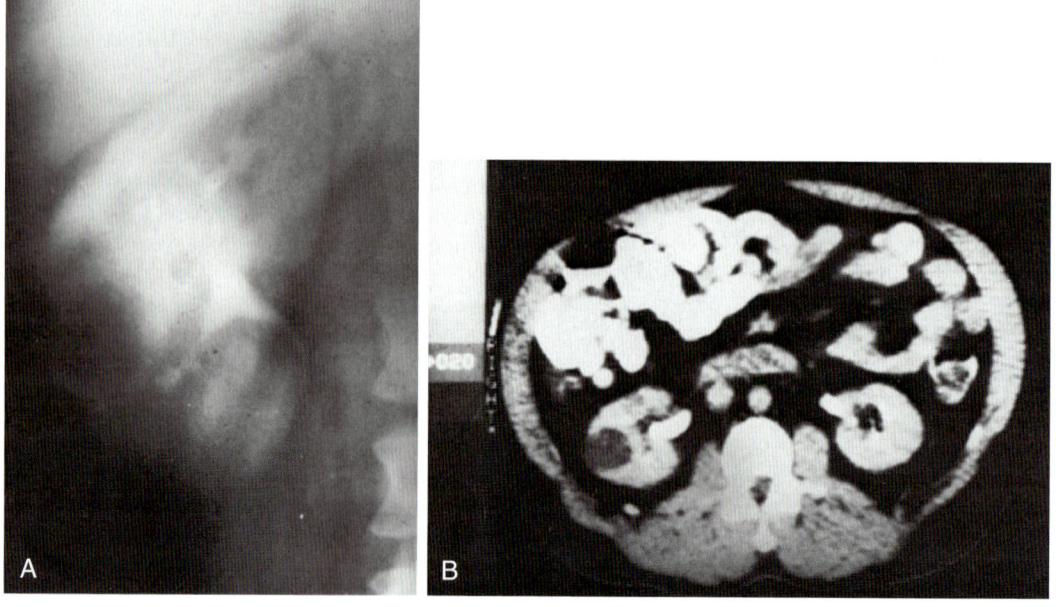

Figure 46.21 Simple renal cysts. **A,** Solitary cortical cyst of the right kidney seen on intravenous urography. **B,** Solitary cyst of right renal cortex seen on computed tomography with intravenous contrast enhancement. Oral contrast material was given to highlight the intestine.

not also found. Because of the obvious implications, it is important to avoid a diagnosis of ADPKD in questionable cases unless a familial history consistent with autosomal dominant transmission can be documented or the diagnosis can be confirmed by genetic testing.

MANIFESTATIONS

The cysts are usually asymptomatic, being discovered at the time of a nephro-urologic evaluation for some unrelated problem. They should not distract from the diagnosis of more important intrarenal or extrarenal lesions. Large renal cysts may cause abdominal or flank discomfort, often described as a sensation of weight or a dull ache. Frequently, however, this pain can be explained by a coexisting abnormality such as nephrolithiasis. Rare cases of gross hematuria due to vascular erosion by an enlarging cyst have been documented. However, hematuria is usually attributable to another cause. When the simple cysts lie at or near the hilus, a urographic pattern of calyceal obstruction or hydronephrosis is frequently found. In most but not all cases, these apparent obstructive changes are of no functional significance. A dynamic Hippuran/diethylenetriaminepentaacetic acid (DTPA) radioactive renal scan before and after administration of furosemide can help assess the degree of obstruction. Rare cases of renin-dependent hypertension caused by solitary intrarenal simple cysts have been described. The proposed mechanism is arterial compression by the cyst that causes segmental renal ischemia. Infection is a rare but dramatic complication of a renal cyst. Simple cysts are not thought to impair renal function, but the presence of simple cysts has been associated with reduced renal function in hospitalized patients younger than 60 years.[535] A CT angiographic study of 1948 potential kidney donors showed an association of cortical and medullary cysts 5 mm or larger with higher 24-hour urine albumin excretion as well as with increased body surface area, hypertension, and higher GFR in some analyses, after adjustment for patient age and sex.[533] Renal cysts are common, particularly in older men, and may be a marker of early kidney injury because they associate with albuminuria, hypertension, and hyperfiltration. Simple cysts infrequently become infected; affected patients present with high fever, flank pain and tenderness, and, frequently, a sympathetic pleural effusion. Most patients are women, and the most common pathogen is *Escherichia coli*. Urine culture results can be negative. Carcinomas do not arise from benign simple cysts. For asymptomatic patients with unequivocal simple cysts, periodic follow-up with ultrasonography is reasonable.

TREATMENT

Treatment of simple renal cyst is indicated only if it is symptomatic or causing obstruction. Intermediate-sized cysts can be aspirated percutaneously, and a sclerosing agent can be instilled into the cavity in an attempt to prevent recurrence. Cysts more than 500 mL in volume are usually drained surgically. Laparoscopic methods are now used routinely. Hypertension has sometimes disappeared after successful aspiration of the cyst fluid or surgical removal of the cyst. Renal vein plasma renin activity is usually elevated in such cases, and the mechanism is thought to be compression of adjacent vessels by cysts with selective renal ischemia and increased renin production. A surgical approach is usually taken to infected renal cysts, but percutaneous aspiration and drainage of infected cysts have also been used.

LOCALIZED OR UNILATERAL RENAL CYSTIC DISEASE

Localized or unilateral renal cystic disease is a rare condition that involves part or, more rarely, the whole of one kidney with cysts that are indistinguishable from those in ADPKD.[536] The absence of a family history and the fact that the remaining renal tissue and the liver appear intact help differentiate this condition from asymmetric forms of ADPKD. Its etiology and pathogenesis are not understood. The clinical presentation includes a palpable mass, flank pain, gross or microscopic hematuria, and hypertension with well-preserved renal function.

MEDULLARY SPONGE KIDNEY

EPIDEMIOLOGY

Medullary sponge kidney, or precalyceal canalicular ectasia, is a common disorder characterized by tubular dilation of the collecting ducts and cyst formation strictly confined to the medullary pyramids, especially to their inner, papillary portions.[537] In studies using strict criteria for the quality of acceptable intravenous urograms, the incidence of MSK has been about 13% in patients with calcium urolithiasis but only about 2% in otherwise normal patients. In particular, MSK is associated with a 60% lifetime risk for renal stones, and the prevalence of MSK in patients with renal stones is significantly higher (8.5%; $P < 0.01$) than in the control population[538] (1.5%). Among all patients with calcium stones, women have a greater incidence of MSK than men.

PATHOGENESIS

MSK has been usually regarded as a nonhereditary disease, but autosomal dominant inheritance has been suggested in several families. In five MSK families, *GDNF* (glial cell–derived neurotrophic factor) gene variants were found to cosegregate with the disease.[539] A study of family members of 50 patients with MSK identified 59 first- and second-degree relatives of 27 probands in all generations who also had MSK.[540] There were progressively lower values for urine volume, pH, and excretion of sodium and calcium, and progressively higher levels of serum phosphate noted in probands compared to relatives with bilateral MSK, those with unilateral MSK, and those unaffected by MSK. The investigators interpreted these observations as indicative of a milder form of MSK in the affected relatives. These findings suggest that familial clustering of MSK is common and that the disease has an autosomal dominant inheritance, reduced penetrance, and variable expressivity.

There have been several reports of MSK in patients with Ehlers-Danlos syndrome and in patients with hemihypertrophy. Precalyceal canalicular ectasia can be observed frequently in patients with ADPKD. MSK has been associated with primary hyperparathyroidism. The rarity of reported cases of this disorder among children favors the interpretation that this is an acquired rather than a congenital disease. Progression of the tubular ectasia and development of tubule dilation and medullary cysts have been documented in some patients.

PATHOLOGY

Despite the name of this disorder, the affected kidney does not closely resemble a sponge. It is usually normal in size or slightly enlarged. The precalyceal canalicular ectasia may involve one or more renal papillae in one or both kidneys, and the lesions are bilateral in 70% of cases. The dilated ducts communicate proximally with collecting tubules of normal size and often show a relative constriction to approximately normal diameter at the point of their

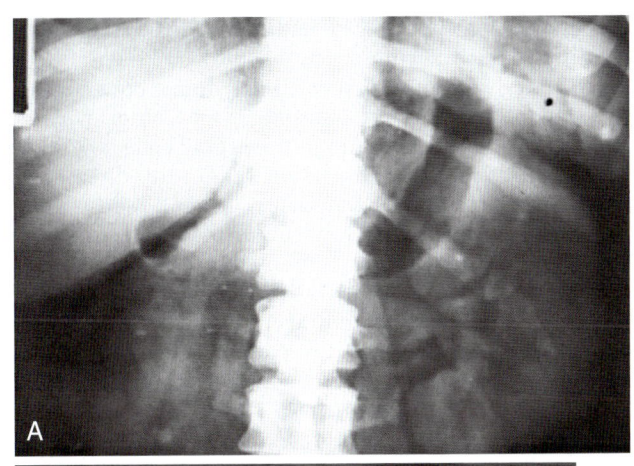

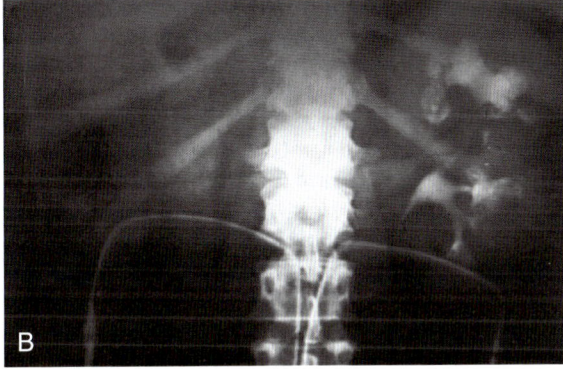

Figure 46.22 Medullary sponge kidney. **A,** Plain radiograph of a large solitary left kidney containing several calcific densities. **B,** Urogram showing the pronounced tubular ectasia of all papillae that is typical of medullary sponge kidney.

communication with the calyx. Their diameter is often 1 to 3 mm, occasionally 5 mm, and rarely up to 7.5 mm. They often contain small calculi and may be surrounded by normal-looking medullary interstitium or, in cases of more prominent cystic disease, inflammatory cell infiltration or interstitial fibrosis.

DIAGNOSIS

A definitive diagnosis of MSK can be made by excretory urography when the dilated collecting ducts are visualized on early and later radiographs without the use of compression and in the absence of ureteral obstruction (Figure 46.22). Deposition of calcium salts within these dilated tubules occurs as renal calculi or nephrocalcinosis. The distribution of the renal calculi in MSK patients is characteristically found in clusters fanning away from the calyx. Because conventional CT has almost completely replaced excretory urography, the diagnosis of MSK may now be made less often. The finding of medullary nephrocalcinosis on CT or medullary hyperechogenicity on ultrasonography may be suggestive, but is not diagnostic, of MSK. Diagnosis of MSK by CT requires multidetector-row CT using high-resolution three-dimensional displays and late urographic images.

MANIFESTATIONS

MSK is usually a benign disorder that may remain asymptomatic and undetected for life. The disease is associated with gross and microscopic hematuria that may be recurrent and with urinary tract infections that often are the first signs of an underlying abnormality. Renal stones consisting of calcium oxalate, calcium phosphate, and other types of calcium salts commonly form in the ectatic collecting ducts and are the most common presentation of this disease.

Impairment of tubular functions, such as a mild concentration defect, a reduced capacity to lower the urine pH after administration of ammonium chloride in comparison with controls, and, possibly, a low maximal excretion of potassium after short-term intravenous potassium chloride loading, may be documented in patients with MSK. Incomplete distal renal tubular acidosis may be found in as many as 30% to 40% of patients.

Whether patients with MSK exhibit specific metabolic abnormalities that predispose them to stone formation different from abnormalities in other patients with stone-forming disorders has been a controversial issue.[541] Hypercalciuria and hypocitraturia, a marker of renal tubular acidosis, have been the metabolic risk factors for stone formation more frequently identified in patients with ADPKD. Many, but not all, studies find hypocitraturia to be more common in patients with MSK with stones than in patients with other stone-forming disorders, and the same can be said for hypercalciuria. Some small studies have shown that the hypercalciuria is due to increased intestinal absorption but others have demonstrated a calcium leak. The calcium leak hypothesis could explain reported associations with parathyroid hyperplasia or adenomas and with osteopenia and osteoporosis. An alternative hypothesis is that hypercalciuria in patients with MSK reflects an abnormally high bone turnover as a result of the incomplete renal tubular acidosis seen in many patients with the disease.

Several studies have emphasized the association of hypocitraturia, distal renal tubular acidosis,[542,543] and hypercalciuria[541] with MSK. However, other studies have not found hypocitraturia to occur more frequently in patients with MSK than in other patients with renal stones. It has also been suggested that hypercalciuria from a calcium leak may lead to the development of parathyroid adenomas.[544] However, a critical examination of calcium excretion in patients with MSK and other stone-forming disorders showed that absorptive hypercalciuria was the most common abnormality in MSK, occurring in 59% of patients, whereas only 18% had hypercalciuria resulting from a renal calcium leak.[545] MSK seldom progresses to ESKD, although reduced GFRs have been observed, and a few patients have a relatively poor prognosis because of recurring urolithiasis, bacteriuria, and pyelonephritis.

TREATMENT

There is no specific treatment for MSK. Most patients discovered incidentally to have MSK can be advised that the disorder is benign and that they can anticipate no serious morbidity and that it is not life-threatening. The treatment of nephrolithiasis and urinary tract infection, when present, is the same as it would be for any patient with these problems. As a general rule, patients with nephrolithiasis should excrete about 2.5 L of urine each day to reduce the risk of stone formation. Potassium citrate and thiazides have been found to be effective in preventing stones in these patients. Fabris and colleagues recommend using potassium citrate as the first step in patients with MSK and a metabolic risk factor regardless of whether this is hypercalciuria, hypocitraturia, hyperuricosuria, or hyperoxaluria.[546] They recommend starting with 20 mEq of citrate per day in two divided doses, increasing the administration gradually by 10 mEq at a time, if tolerated, for patients in whom a citraturia level above 450 mg/24 hr is not achieved initially, until the desired citrate level is reached, provided that the urine pH in a 24-hour collection is less than 7.5. Careful monitoring of the urine pH is necessary to ensure that pH stays below 7.5 in a 24-hour urine collection so as to prevent further formation of calcium phosphate stones in the ectatic tubules. With this regimen, these investigators have achieved not only an increase in urine citrate but also a significant reduction in urine calcium excretion (presumably as a result of the activation of the epithelial calcium channel TRPV5 in the distal nephron by the higher luminal pH) and, most importantly, a marked reduction in the stone event rate, from 0.58 to 0.10 stones per year per patient. They also observed an improvement in bone densitometry, with a total vertebral T-score increasing from −2.82 to −1.98 and a total hip T-score increasing from −2.03 to −1.86 after an average follow-up of 6.5 years.[547] These investigators reserve the use of thiazides for patients who continue to pass stones or have hypercalciuria despite receiving an optimal dose of citrate.

Patients with MSK appear to be more susceptible to urinary tract infections, and routine preventive measures seem warranted, especially in female patients. Repeated unnecessary investigations for hematuria should be avoided. Relapsing urinary tract infections may be due to infected renal stones and may require long-term antimicrobial suppression when the source of the infections cannot be eliminated.

ACQUIRED CYSTIC KIDNEY DISEASE

EPIDEMIOLOGY

Acquired cystic kidney disease (ACKD) is characterized by small cysts distributed throughout the renal cortex and medulla of patients with ESKD and is unrelated to inherited renal cystic disease. There is no agreement on the extent of cystic change required for the diagnosis, ranging from one to five cysts per kidney in radiologic studies to cystic changes in 25% to 40% of renal volume for tissue-based studies. Its prevalence and severity are higher in men than in women and increase with the duration of azotemia. Acquired cysts are found in 7% to 22% of patients with renal failure and serum creatinine values exceeding 3 mg/dL before dialysis, in 35% who have undergone dialysis for less than 2 years, in 58% for 2 to 4 years, in 75% for 4 to 8 years, and in 92% for longer than 8 years.[547a] ACKD is unrelated to age, dialysis methods, race, and the causes of renal failure. In one study, no reduction in the frequency or severity of this disease was observed in 43 patients treated with hemodiafiltration in comparison with 43 patients treated with conventional hemodialysis after a mean follow-up of 63 months despite significantly lower levels of serum parathyroid hormone and alkaline phosphatase with hemodiafiltration. Multiple logistic regression analysis indicated that the duration of renal replacement therapy (RRT) was the only risk factor for the presence of ACKD.[548] Cysts can regress after successful renal transplant surgery but conversely can develop in transplanted kidneys affected by long-term rejection. Cyclosporine has been incriminated as predisposing native kidneys to cyst formation.

A very important feature in ACKD is the occurrence of renal tumors. The overall prevalence of RCC in patients undergoing hemodialysis evaluated radiologically or at autopsy is approximately 1% to 4%.[549] Carcinoma in dialysis recipients is three times more common in the presence than in the absence of acquired renal cysts, and six times more common in large than in small cystic kidneys. Overall, the incidence of renal malignancy in patients undergoing dialysis has been estimated to be 50 to 100 times greater than in the general population. The RCCs associated with ACKD have a lower risk for metastasis and a better prognosis than RCCs not associated ACKD.

The risk for RCC remains high after renal transplantation in patients with ACKD. A study of 961 patients who received a kidney transplant between 1970 and 1998, included 561 patients who underwent prospective ultrasound screening of the native kidneys between 1997 and 2003.[550] Twenty-three percent of them were found to have ACKD. Including 19 patients with formerly diagnosed RCC, the study found that the prevalence of RCC was 4.8% among all patients, 19.4% among the patients with ACKD, and 0.5% in those without ACKD. RCC was bilateral in 26% of cases. Tumor histology was clear cell RCC in 58% and papillary RCC in 42% of cases. Only one patient had a lung metastasis, and no patient died. Another study conducted ultrasound examination of the native kidneys every 6 months after renal transplantation between 1991 and 2007.[551] Renal cell carcinomas were diagnosed in 10 patients after a mean follow-up of 61.8 months. Two lesions were solid and eight were cystic, with the average size 2.1 cm. Four were clear cell type, and six papillary carcinomas. None of the patients had metastatic disease.

PATHOGENESIS

The development of the cysts and tumors seems to be tied to the pronounced epithelial hyperplasia observed microscopically. The hyperplasia, in turn, seems to be a result of the uremic state even though there appears to be no relation between the occurrence of acquired cysts and the efficacy of dialysis. If ACKD is present at the time of successful transplantation, that process seems to regress or at least not to increase in severity. Conceivably, the loss of renal mass causes the production of renotropic factors that stimulate hyperplasia.

PATHOLOGY

ACKD is usually bilateral and equal, with even severely affected kidneys weighing less than 100 g (30% less than 50 g), although about 25% weigh more than 150 g, including a few exceptional specimens of more than 1000 g (Figure 46.23). In nephrectomy and autopsy specimens, the cysts vary in number and type from a few subcapsular cysts up to 2 to 3 cm in diameter to numerous smaller cysts that are diffusely distributed. The cysts are generally smaller than those in ADPKD. Microdissection studies have demonstrated the continuity of the cysts with both proximal and distal tubules and have suggested their origin both in the fusiform dilation of tubule segments and in multiple small tubule diverticula. Some, but not all, immunohistochemical studies have shown that the cysts in ACKD are mostly derived from proximal tubules.[552]

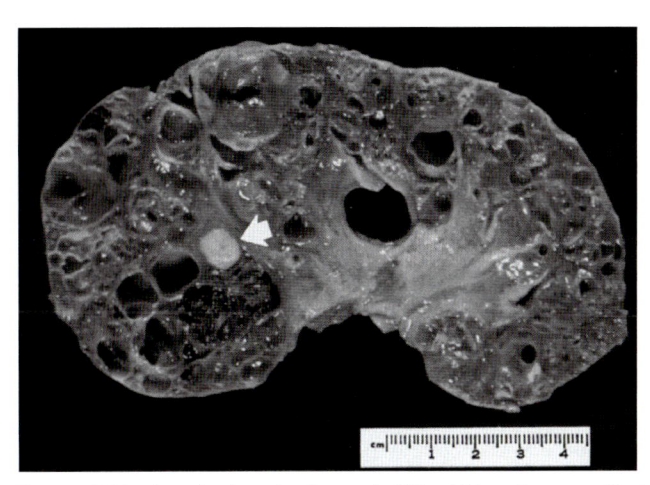

Figure 46.23 Acquired cystic disease in 320-g kidney from a patient with a 10-year history of hemodialysis. There were bilateral, multifocal renal cell carcinomas *(arrow)* with multiple systemic metastases.

In a significant fraction of reported cases, the cysts contain single or, more often, multiple papillary, tubular, or solid neoplasms arising from the cyst lining and consistent with renal cell "adenomas" or adenocarcinomas. The genetic changes underlying the development of most of these tumors are different from those occurring in sporadic clear cell RCCs. Compared with sporadic RCC, ACKD-associated RCC tends to display lower Fuhrman nuclear grade, less proliferative activity, and diploidy in most cases, reflecting less aggressive behavior. The predominant type is clear cell, but papillary renal cell carcinomas are over-represented in comparison with the sporadic RCC in the general population.[549,550] In addition, RCC with distinctive histologic features has been associated with ACKD. These tumors are characterized by abundant eosinophilic cytoplasm; a variably solid, cribriform, tubulocystic, and papillary architecture; and deposits of calcium oxalate crystals.[553-555]

DIAGNOSIS

Ultrasonography is a sensitive method to detect renal cysts and ACKD. However, complex cysts with intracystic septations, intracystic hemorrhage, mural nodules, and peripheral calcifications are sometimes difficult to distinguish from RCC with this method. CT with contrast enhancement is superior to ultrasonography in the evaluation of complex cysts (see Figure 46.23), but contrast enhancement is required to differentiate between benign and potentially malignant cystic lesions, and the intravenous administration of iodinated contrast media carries a risk of worsening the renal function in patients who are not yet undergoing dialysis or who have impaired renal function after transplantation. MRI, on the other hand, provides high-resolution images with excellent tissue contrast even without the administration of gadolinium, which is contraindicated in patients with impaired renal function.[556] T1- and T2-weighted turbo spin-echo MRI sequences provide very good contrast among different tissues, and modern techniques such as diffusion-weighted sequences help improve diagnostic accuracy.

Because RCC is an important complication of ACKD, screening with ultrasonography has been recommended after 3 years of dialysis, followed by screening for neoplasm at 1- or 2-year intervals thereafter. However, because RCC is a relatively rare cause of death among dialysis recipients, a more aggressive renal imaging program, including annual screening, would be unlikely to significantly reduce mortality and therefore would not be cost effective.[557] In the end, the clinical decision must be based on the individual patient, with consideration given both to the known risk factors for carcinoma—including prolonged dialysis, the presence of ACKD, large kidneys, and male sex—and the patient's age and general fitness. Screening with ultrasonography or MRI at 1- to 2-year intervals may be beneficial in selected populations such as young dialysis recipients or in transplant recipients with ACKD.

MANIFESTATIONS

ACKD develops insidiously. Most patients have no symptoms. When symptoms occur, gross hematuria, flank pain, renal colic, fever, palpable renal mass, and rising hematocrit are most common. Retroperitoneal hemorrhage may manifest as acute pain, hypotension, and shock. Rarely, the presentation consists of symptoms from metastatic RCC. Approximately 20% of ACKD-associated RCCs metastasize (vs. 50% for sporadic RCCs).

TREATMENT

Bleeding episodes in ACKD, either intrarenal or perirenal, are often treated conservatively with bed rest and analgesics. Persistent hemorrhage, however, may require nephrectomy or therapeutic renal embolization and infarction. Because the risk of undetected RCC is high in patients with retroperitoneal hemorrhage, nephrectomy is recommended in those in whom carcinoma cannot be ruled out. If a few larger cysts are associated with flank pain, percutaneous aspiration (with cytologic examination) is a reasonable temporizing measure. ACKD may regress after successful renal transplantation (Figure 46.24).

Renal masses larger than 3 cm detected in patients with ACKD are treated by excision. For tumors smaller than 3 cm, the options are nephrectomy for those who can undergo surgery or annual CT follow-up with resection if the lesions enlarge. Although metastases are less likely to occur from small than from large tumors, small tumor size is not a guarantee against metastasis. Resection even of small neoplasms seems prudent in preparation for transplantation. Because carcinoma in the setting of ACKD is often multicentric and bilateral, some writers recommend bilateral nephrectomy in these cases. If this procedure is not performed, frequent monitoring of the contralateral kidney is advised. Laparoscopic bilateral radical nephrectomy in patients with ESKD, ACKD, and suspicious tumors has been proposed as a more desirable alternative to traditional open surgery.[558]

RENAL CYSTIC NEOPLASMS

Renal cystic neoplasms encompass a number of entities that cannot be reliably distinguished from one another on preoperative imaging studies. These entities include cystic RCC, multilocular cystic nephromas, cystic partially differentiated nephroblastomas, and mixed epithelial and stromal tumors.[559]

CYSTIC RENAL CELL CARCINOMA

Multilocular and unilocular RCCs account for about 5% of RCCs and are characterized by their cystic nature—less than 25% of solid component—and by the absence of necrosis. They are usually clear cell type and of low grade and virtually never metastasize or cause death.[560] They should be distinguished from RCCs with a large cystic component due to extensive necrosis (pseudocystic necrotic carcinoma), which have an aggressive behavior, often leading to metastasis and death. Surgical excision is usually needed for diagnosis because fine-needle aspiration is not sufficiently accurate.

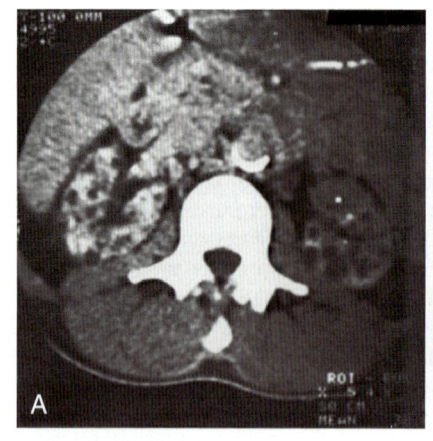

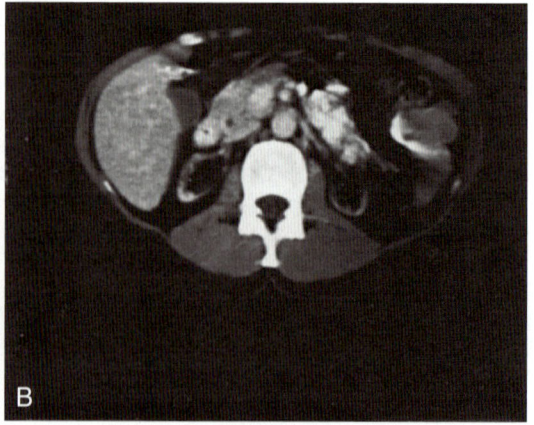

Figure 46.24 Acquired renal cystic disease. **A,** Computed tomography (CT) scan with intravenous contrast. This man had renal failure caused by diabetic nephropathy and had received hemodialysis for 6 years before this examination. There is bilateral renal enlargement with diffuse cysts in the cortex and medulla. A solid tissue tumor *(white dot)* is seen in the anterior part of the left kidney. **B,** CT scan of the original kidneys in a patient with a functioning renal allograft. Note the marked atrophy of the renal parenchyma in contrast to the cystic changes seen in **A.**

MULTILOCULAR CYSTIC NEPHROMA

Cystic nephroma is a rare benign cystic neoplasm encountered in children and adults, with a bimodal distribution of age and gender (65% in patients younger than 4 years with a male/female ratio of 2:1 and the remainder in patients older than 30 years of age with a male/female ratio of 1:8). Cystic nephroma appears as an encapsulated multilocular mass, the locules of which are not connected to each other or to the pyelocalyceal system. They are lined by a single layer of nondescript, flattened or cuboidal cells and "hobnail" cells with abundant eosinophilic cytoplasm and large apical nuclei. The septa are composed of connective tissue and may contain scattered atrophic renal tubules. Multilocular cystic nephroma is a benign lesion, but malignant transformation can occur in rare cases.

CYSTIC PARTIALLY DIFFERENTIATED NEPHROBLASTOMA

Cystic partially differentiated nephroblastoma is a rare benign cystic renal neoplasm that is histologically identical to cystic nephroma except for Wilms' tumor elements within the septa. It mostly occurs in children younger than 2 years, with rare adult occurrences. It is cured by complete excision.

MIXED EPITHELIAL AND STROMAL TUMOR

Mixed epithelial and stromal tumor is a rare type of cystic renal neoplasm, with about 50 cases reported. Contrary to cystic nephroma and cystic partially differentiated nephroblastoma, which are purely cystic and have thin septa, the mixed epithelial and stromal tumor is partly cystic and has thicker wall-forming solid areas. All affected patients but one have been female, with a mean age of 46 years. The role of female hormone in the pathogenesis of this tumor is supported by a female predominance, a history of long-term estrogen treatment in many patients, and the expression of estrogen and progesterone receptors by tumor stromal cells. Mixed epithelial and stromal tumors are benign, and resection is curative.

RENAL CYSTS OF NONTUBULAR ORIGIN

CYSTIC DISEASE OF THE RENAL SINUS

The cystic disorders of the renal sinus are benign conditions that with modern imaging techniques can be clearly distinguished from more serious mass-occupying lesions of the renal pelvis or renal parenchyma. Two types of cystic lesions have been described in this area: hilus cysts and parapelvic cysts.

Hilus cysts, which have been identified only at autopsy, are thought to be caused by regressive changes in the fat tissue of the renal sinus, especially in kidneys with abundant fat in the renal sinus associated with renal atrophy. The cysts result from fluid replacement of adipose tissue that undergoes regressive changes owing to localized vascular disease and atrophy because of recent wasting. A single layer of flattened mesenchymal cells lines the wall of such a cyst, and the cystic fluid is clear and contains abundant lipid droplets.

Parapelvic cysts are of lymphatic origin and are much more common. The walls of the cysts are very thin and are lined by flat endothelial cells. The composition of the cystic fluid resembles that of lymph. The mechanism responsible for the dilation of the lymphatics is not known. Parapelvic cysts may be multiple and bilateral. They are in direct contact with the extrarenal pelvic surface and extend into the renal sinus, distorting the infundibula and calyces. The kidneys may appear slightly enlarged, but the enlargement is exclusively caused by the expansion of the renal sinus, and the area of the renal parenchyma remains normal. Bilateral parapelvic cysts (cystic disease of the renal sinus) can be confused with ADPKD on excretory urography, but the distinction between the two entities is straightforward on CT or MRI.

Parapelvic cysts are most frequently diagnosed after the fourth decade of life. They are usually discovered in the course of evaluations for conditions such as urinary tract infections, nephrolithiasis, hypertension, and prostatism. Despite considerable calyceal distortion, the pressure in these lymphatic cysts is low and not likely to result in significant functional obstruction. Indeed, renal function in patients with bilateral multiple parapelvic cysts is usually normal. Occasionally, parapelvic cysts are the only finding in the course of evaluation for otherwise unexplained lumbar or flank pain. The therapeutic approach to parapelvic cysts should be conservative.

PERIRENAL LYMPHANGIOMAS

Perirenal lymphangiomas are characterized by dilation of the lymphatic channels around the kidneys that leads to the development of unilocular or multilocular cystic masses.[561] Lymphatic obstruction may play a role in its pathogenesis, and rare familial cases suggest a genetic component. Perirenal lymphangiomas have also been observed in patients with TSC.[562] Pregnancy is reported to exacerbate the condition, possibly because the renal lymphatics play a role in handling an enhanced interstitial fluid flow during this condition.[563] Mild renal functional impairment and hypertension can occur transiently and revert to normal in the postpartum period.

SUBCAPSULAR AND PERIRENAL URINOMAS (URINIFEROUS PSEUDOCYSTS)

Subcapsular and perirenal urinomas are encapsulated collections of extravasated urine in the subcapsular and perirenal spaces. They are usually secondary to obstructive uropathies, such as posterior urethral valve, pelviureteric junction, or vesicoureteric junction obstruction, ureteric calculus, or trauma. They are caused by pyelosinus backflow, which can occur when the intrapelvic pressure rises to 35 cm H_2O or greater, leading to rupture of calyceal fornices. Whereas subcapsular urinomas are situated between the renal parenchyma and renal capsule, perirenal urinomas are located between the renal capsule and Gerota's fascia. Treatment includes temporary decompression by placement of a pigtail catheter in the most dependent point of the urinoma and correction of the underlying disorder.

PYELOCALYCEAL CYSTS

Also termed *pyelocalyceal diverticula* or *calyceal* or *pyelorenal cysts* or *diverticula*, pyelocalyceal cysts represent congenital, probably developmental, saccular diverticula from a minor calyx (type I) or from the pelvis or adjacent major calyx (type II). Type I is more common, is usually located in the poles (especially the upper), and tends to be smaller and less often symptomatic than the centrally located type II. Both types are usually less than 1 cm in diameter but occasionally may be quite large. The cysts are encompassed by a muscularis, are lined by a usually chronically inflamed transitional epithelium, and usually contain urine or cloudy fluid.

Pyelocalyceal cysts occur sporadically, affect all age groups, and usually are unilateral. They may be detected in as many as 0.5% of excretory urograms but normally are asymptomatic unless they are complicated by nephrolithiasis or infection. The frequency of stone formation in calyceal diverticula has been reported to be between 10% and 40%. Transitional cell carcinoma arising in a pyelocalyceal cyst has been seldom reported. Surgical intervention is indicated only when conservative management of this complication fails.

Complete reference list available at ExpertConsult.com.

KEY REFERENCES

3. Torres VE, Harris PC: Strategies targeting cAMP signaling in the treatment of polycystic kidney disease. *J Am Soc Nephrol* 25:18–32, 2014.
10. Hopp K, Ward CJ, Hommerding CJ, et al: Functional polycystin-1 dosage governs autosomal dominant polycystic kidney disease severity. *J Clin Invest* 122:4257–4273, 2012.
59. Cornec-Le Gall E, Audrezet MP, Chen JM, et al: Type of PKD1 mutation influences renal outcome in ADPKD. *J Am Soc Nephrol* 24:1006–1013, 2013.
61. Harris PC, Hopp K: The mutation, a key determinant of phenotype in ADPKD. *J Am Soc Nephrol* 24:868–870, 2013.
69. Bergmann C, von Bothmer J, Ortiz Bruchle N, et al: Mutations in multiple PKD genes may explain early and severe polycystic kidney disease. *J Am Soc Nephrol* 22:2047–2056, 2011.
101. Chebib FT, Sussman CR, Wang X, et al: Vasopressin and disruption of calcium signaling in polycystic kidney disease. *Nat Clin Nephrol* Epub April 14, 2015.
105. Yamaguchi T, Hempson SJ, Reif GA, et al: Calcium restores a normal proliferation phenotype in human polycystic kidney disease epithelial cells. *J Am Soc Nephrol* 17:178–187, 2006.
168. Pei Y, Obaji J, Dupuis A, et al: Unified criteria for ultrasonographic diagnosis of ADPKD. *J Am Soc Nephrol* 20:205–212, 2009.
169. Barua M, Cil O, Paterson AD, et al: Family history of renal disease severity predicts the mutated gene in ADPKD. *J Am Soc Nephrol* 20:1833–1838, 2009.
170. Pei Y, Hwang YH, Conklin J, et al: Imaging-based diagnosis of autosomal dominant polycystic kidney disease. *J Am Soc Nephrol* 26:746–753, 2014.
175. Harris PC, Bae KT, Rossetti S, et al: Cyst number but not the rate of cystic growth is associated with the mutated gene in autosomal dominant polycystic kidney disease. *J Am Soc Nephrol* 17:3013–3019, 2006.
179. Chapman AB, Bost JE, Torres VE, et al: Kidney volume and functional outcomes in autosomal dominant polycystic kidney disease. *Clin J Am Soc Nephrol* 7(3):479–486, 2012.
180. Irazabal MV, Rangel LJ, Bergstralh EJ, et al: Imaging classification of autosomal dominant polycystic kidney disease: a simple model for selecting patients for clinical trials. *J Am Soc Nephrol* 26:160–172, 2015.
181. Torres VE, Grantham JJ, Chapman AB, et al: Potentially modifiable factors affecting the progression of autosomal dominant polycystic kidney disease. *Clin J Am Soc Nephrol* 6:640–647, 2011.
219. Jouret F, Lhommel R, Beguin C, et al: Positron-emission computed tomography in cyst infection diagnosis in patients with autosomal dominant polycystic kidney disease. *Clin J Am Soc Nephrol* 6:1644–1650, 2011.
220. Wetmore JB, Calvet JP, Yu AS, et al: Polycystic kidney disease and cancer after renal transplantation. *J Am Soc Nephrol* 25:2335–2341, 2014.
234. Lantinga MA, Drenth JP, Gevers TJ: Diagnostic criteria in renal and hepatic cyst infection. *Nephrol Dial Transplant* Epub June 20, 2014.
235. Suwabe T, Ubara Y, Sumida K, et al: Clinical features of cyst infection and hemorrhage in ADPKD: new diagnostic criteria. *Clin Exp Nephrol* 16:892–902, 2012.
263. Schrier RS, Abebe KZ, Perrone RD, et al: Angiotensin blockade, blood pressure and autosomal dominant polycystic kidney disease. *N Engl J Med* 371:2255–2266, 2014.
264. Torres VE, Abebe KZ, Chapman AB, et al: Angiotensin blockade in late autosomal dominant polycystic kidney disease. *N Engl J Med* 371:2267–2276, 2014.
266. Patch C, Charlton J, Roderick PJ, et al: Use of antihypertensive medications and mortality of patients with autosomal dominant polycystic kidney disease: a population-based study. *Am J Kidney Dis* 57:856–862, 2011.
269. Orskov B, Sorensen VR, Feldt-Rasmussen B, et al: Changes in causes of death and risk of cancer in Danish patients with autosomal dominant polycystic kidney disease and end-stage renal disease. *Nephrol Dial Transplant* 27:1607–1613, 2012.
272. Spithoven E, Kramer A, Meijer E, et al: Renal replacement therapy for autosomal dominant polycystic kidney disease (ADPKD) in Europe: prevalence and survival—an analysis of data from the ERA-EDTA Registry. *Nephrol Dial Transplant* 29(Suppl 4):iv15–iv25, 2014.
284. Yamamoto T, Watarai Y, Kobayashi T, et al: Kidney volume changes in patients with autosomal dominant polycystic kidney disease after renal transplantation. *Transplantation* 93:794–798, 2012.
285. Abu-Wasel B, Walsh C, Keough V, et al: Pathophysiology, epidemiology, classification and treatment options for polycystic liver diseases. *World J Gastroenterol* 19:5775–5786, 2013.
286. Drenth JP, Chrispijn M, Nagorney DM, et al: Medical and surgical treatment options for polycystic liver disease. *Hepatology* 52:2223–2230, 2010.
291. Irazabal MV, Huston J, 3rd, Kubly V, et al: Extended follow-up of unruptured intracranial aneurysms detected by presymptomatic screening in patients with autosomal dominant polycystic kidney disease. *Clin J Am Soc Nephrol* 6:1274–1285, 2011.
300. Torres VE, Chapman AB, Devuyst O, et al: Tolvaptan in patients with autosomal dominant polycystic kidney disease. *N Engl J Med* 367:2407–2418, 2012.
306. Hopp K, Hommerding CJ, Wang X: Tolvaptan plus pasireotide shows enhanced efficacy in a PKD1 model. *J Am Soc Nephrol* 26(1):39–47, 2015.
312. Hogan MC, Masyuk TV, Page L, et al: Somatostatin analog therapy for severe polycystic liver disease: results after 2 years. *Nephrol Dial Transplant* 27:3532–3539, 2012.
313. Caroli A, Perico N, Perna A, et al: Effect of long acting somatostatin analogue on kidney and cyst growth in autosomal dominant polycystic kidney disease (ALADIN): a randomised, placebo-controlled, multicentre trial. *Lancet* 382:1485–1495, 2013.
315. Gevers TJ, Inthout J, Caroli A, et al: Young women with polycystic liver disease respond best to somatostatin analogues: a pooled analysis of individual patient data. *Gastroenterology* 145:357–365.e1–2, 2013.
322. Serra AL, Poster D, Kistler AD, et al: Sirolimus and kidney growth in autosomal dominant polycystic kidney disease. *N Engl J Med* 363:820–829, 2010.
324. Walz G, Budde K, Mannaa M, et al: Everolimus in patients with autosomal dominant polycystic kidney disease. *N Engl J Med* 363:830–840, 2010.
393. Gunay-Aygun M, Turkbey BI, Bryant J, et al: Hepatorenal findings in obligate heterozygotes for autosomal recessive polycystic kidney disease. *Mol Genet Metab* 104:677–681, 2011.
397. Telega G, Cronin D, Avner ED: New approaches to the autosomal recessive polycystic kidney disease patient with dual kidney-liver complications. *Pediatr Transplant* 17:328–335, 2013.
423. Bissler JJ, Kingswood JC, Radzikowska E, et al: Everolimus for angiomyolipoma associated with tuberous sclerosis complex or

sporadic lymphangioleiomyomatosis (EXIST-2): a multicentre, randomised, double-blind, placebo-controlled trial. *Lancet* 381:817–824, 2013.

425. Maher ER, Neumann HP, Richard S: von Hippel-Lindau disease: a clinical and scientific review. *Eur J Hum Genet* 19:617–623, 2011.

439. Faguer S, Decramer S, Chassaing N, et al: Diagnosis, management, and prognosis of HNF1B nephropathy in adulthood. *Kidney Int* 80:768–776, 2011.

455. Ekici AB, Hackenbeck T, Morinière V, et al: Renal fibrosis is the common feature of autosomal dominant tubulointerstitial kidney diseases caused by mutations in mucin 1 or uromodulin. *Kidney Int* 86:589–599, 2014.

459. Moskowitz JL, Piret SE, Lhotta K, et al: Association between genotype and phenotype in uromodulin-associated kidney disease. *Clin J Am Soc Nephrol* 8:1349–1357, 2013.

468. Trudu M, Janas S, Lanzani C, et al: Common noncoding UMOD gene variants induce salt-sensitive hypertension and kidney damage by increasing uromodulin expression. *Nat Med* 19:1655–1660, 2013.

469. Bleyer AJ, Kmoch S, Antignac C, et al: Variable clinical presentation of an MUC1 mutation causing medullary cystic kidney disease type 1. *Clin J Am Soc Nephrol* 9:527–535, 2014.

473. Hildebrandt F, Benzing T, Katsanis N: Ciliopathies. *N Engl J Med* 364:1533–1543, 2011.

502. Forsythe E, Beales PL: Bardet-Biedl syndrome. *Eur J Hum Genet* 21:8–13, 2013.

511. Putoux A, Attie-Bitach T, Martinovic J, et al: Phenotypic variability of Bardet-Biedl syndrome: focusing on the kidney. *Pediatr Nephrol* 27:7–15, 2012.

533. Rule AD, Sasiwimonphan K, Lieske JC, et al: Characteristics of renal cystic and solid lesions based on contrast-enhanced computed tomography of potential kidney donors. *Am J Kidney Dis* 59:611–618, 2012.

534. Ponte B, Pruijm M, Ackermann D, et al: Copeptin is associated with kidney length, renal function, and prevalence of simple cysts in a population-based study. *J Am Soc Nephrol* Epub September 30, 2014.

541. Fabris A, Anglani F, Lupo A, et al: Medullary sponge kidney: state of the art. *Nephrol Dial Transplant* 28:1111–1119, 2013.

HYPERTENSION AND THE KIDNEY

SECTION VII

47 Primary and Secondary Hypertension

William J. Elliott | Aldo J. Peixoto | George L. Bakris

CHAPTER OUTLINE

HYPERTENSION DEFINITIONS, 1524
Evolution of Blood Pressure Goals, 1524
EPIDEMIOLOGY, 1524
Age and Hypertension, 1525
Gender and Hypertension, 1525
Race/Ethnicity and Hypertension, 1526
BLOOD PRESSURE CONTROL RATES, 1527
ECONOMICS OF HYPERTENSION, 1528
PATHOPHYSIOLOGY, 1528
Pressure Natriuresis and Salt Sensitivity, 1528
Genetics of Hypertension, 1529
Nonosmotic Sodium Storage, 1530
Renin Angiotensin Aldosterone System, 1530
Sympathetic Nervous System, 1532
Obesity, 1533
Natriuretic Peptides, 1534
The Endothelium, 1534
Arterial Stiffness in Hypertension, 1535
Role of the Immune System in Hypertension, 1535
Novel Metabolic Peptides and Hypertension, 1536
CLINICAL EVALUATION, 1536

History and Physical Examination, 1536
Blood Pressure Measurement, 1538
Laboratory and Other Complementary Tests, 1542
SECONDARY HYPERTENSION, 1543
Risk Factors and Epidemiology, 1544
HYPERTENSIVE URGENCY AND EMERGENCY, 1550
CLINICAL OUTCOME TRIALS, 1552
Blood Pressure Control and Chronic Kidney Disease Progression, 1552
Trials in Nondiabetic Chronic Kidney Disease That Contributed to Blood Pressure Goal, 1553
Diabetes, 1553
Albuminuria, Blood Pressure, and Diabetic Nephropathy, 1556
Clinical Trials in Older Adults, 1557
Blood Pressure Management in Patients Undergoing Dialysis, 1561
MANAGEMENT OF PRIMARY HYPERTENSION IN CHRONIC KIDNEY DISEASE, 1562
Antihypertensive Medications, 1563
RESISTANT HYPERTENSION, 1565

Hypertension has consistently been one of the major contributors to premature morbidity and mortality in the United States.[1] Hypertension is ranked first worldwide in an analysis of all risk factors for global disease burden in 2010[2] (Figure 47.1). By the year 2025, hypertension is expected to increase in prevalence worldwide by 60% and will affect 1.56 billion people.[3] Developing nations will experience an 80% increase (from 639 million to 1.15 billion afflicted persons). As emerging countries have improved sanitation and other basic public health measures, cardiovascular (CV) disease has or soon will become the most common cause of death, and hypertension will be its most common reversible risk factor, as it already is in the United States.

The major public health importance of hypertension can be amply demonstrated using data from the United States, but similar conclusions are emerging as other industrialized countries analyze national health care databases.[4] Hypertension was listed as either the principal or a contributing cause of death in nearly 15% of the death certificates filed in the United States in 2010.[1]

Hypertension is the most important modifiable risk factor for stroke.[1] It fell from the second most common cause of death in the United States in 1958, to third between 1959 and 2007, to fourth between 2008 and 2012, to fifth in 2013.[5] Current estimates are that 77% of those who have a first stroke have had a blood pressure (BP) above 140/90 mm Hg.

High BP is the leading antecedent condition for either the systolic or diastolic type of heart failure and the most common reason for acute care hospitalization among

1990

Mean rank (95% UI)	Risk factor
1.1 (1–2)	1 Childhood underweight
2.1 (1–4)	2 Household air pollution
2.9 (2–4)	3 Smoking (excluding SHS)
4.0 (3–5)	4 High blood pressure
5.4 (3–8)	5 Suboptimal breastfeeding
5.6 (5–6)	6 Alcohol use
7.4 (6–8)	7 Ambient PM pollution
7.4 (6–8)	8 Low fruit
9.7 (9–12)	9 High fasting plasma glucose
10.9 (9–14)	10 High body mass index
11.1 (9–15)	11 Iron deficiency
12.3 (9–17)	12 High sodium
13.9 (10–19)	13 Low nuts and seeds
14.1 (11–17)	14 High total cholesterol
16.2 (9–38)	15 Sanitation
16.7 (13–21)	16 Low vegetables
17.1 (10–23)	17 Vitamin A deficiency
17.3 (15–20)	18 Low whole grains
20.0 (13–29)	19 Zinc deficiency
20.6 (17–25)	20 Low omega-3
20.8 (18–24)	21 Occupational injury
21.7 (14–34)	22 Unimproved water
22.6 (19–26)	23 Occupational low back pain
23.2 (19–29)	24 High processed meat
24.2 (21–26)	25 Drug use
	26 Low fiber
	30 Lead

2010

Risk factor	Mean rank (95% UI)	% change (95% UI)
1 High blood pressure	1.1 (1–2)	27% (19 to 34)
2 Smoking (excluding SHS)	1.9 (1–2)	3% (−5 to 11)
3 Alcohol use	3.0 (2–4)	28% (17 to 39)
4 Household air pollution	4.7 (3–7)	−37% (−44 to −29)
5 Low fruit	5.0 (4–8)	29% (25 to 34)
6 High body mass index	6.1 (4–8)	82% (71 to 95)
7 High fasting plasma glucose	6.6 (5–8)	58% (43 to 73)
8 Childhood underweight	8.5 (6–11)	−61% (−66 to −55)
9 Ambient PM pollution	8.9 (7–11)	−7% (−13 to −1)
10 Physical inactivity	9.9 (8–12)	0% (0 to 0)
11 High sodium	11.2 (8–15)	33% (27 to 39)
12 Low nuts and seeds	12.9 (11–17)	27% (18 to 32)
13 Iron deficiency	13.5 (11–17)	−7% (−11 to −4)
14 Suboptimal breastfeeding	13.8 (10–18)	−57% (−63 to −51)
15 High total cholesterol	15.2 (12–17)	3% (−13 to 19)
16 Low whole grains	15.3 (13–17)	39% (32 to 45)
17 Low vegetables	15.8 (12–19)	22% (16 to 28)
18 Low omega-3	18.7 (17–23)	30% (21 to 35)
19 Drug use	20.2 (18–23)	57% (42 to 72)
20 Occupational injury	20.4 (18–23)	12% (−22 to 58)
21 Occupational low back pain	21.2 (18–25)	22% (11 to 35)
22 High processed meat	22.0 (17–31)	22% (2 to 44)
23 Intimate partner violence	23.8 (20–28)	0% (0 to 0)
24 Low fiber	24.4 (19–32)	23% (13 to 33)
25 Lead	25.5 (25–29)	160% (143 to 176)
26 Sanitation		
29 Vitamin A deficiency		
31 Zinc deficiency		
33 Unimproved water		

——— Ascending order in rank
- - - - Descending order in rank

Figure 47.1 Global risk factor ranks with 95% uncertainty interval (UI) for all ages and sexes combined in 1990 and 2010 and percentage change. PM, Particulate matter; SHS, secondhand smoke. (From Lim SS, Vos T, Flaxman AD, et al: A comparative risk assessment of burden of disease and injury attributable to 67 risk factors and risk factor clusters in 21 regions, 1990-2010: a systematic analysis for the Global Burden of Disease Study 2010. *Lancet* 380:2224-2260, 2012.)

Medicare beneficiaries (approximately 1.023 million in 2010); approximately 74% of people experiencing an initial hospitalization for heart failure either had or have BP of 140/90 mm Hg or higher.[1]

Currently, end-stage kidney disease has the highest per-patient annualized cost to Medicare,[6] and hypertension is the second most common cause of end-stage kidney disease. After tobacco and diabetes, hypertension is the most important risk factor for peripheral vascular disease (the second leading cause of loss of limbs in the United States).[1] Hypertension is likely the most important treatable cause of vascular dementia, which ranked eighth among causes of death in the United States in 2010, and is the third leading cause of admission to nursing homes. Hypertension ranks first among the chronic conditions for which Americans visit a health care provider. This may be secondary to its high age-adjusted prevalence (29.1% of adults age 18 years and over between 2011 and 2012) and the fact that treatment clearly improves prognosis.

All health care providers routinely encounter people who are likely to benefit from lowered BP levels. In the future more people will likely become candidates for antihypertensive therapy, as the prevalence of hypertension is increasing secondary to the increasing prevalence of obesity and increased longevity of the general population.[7]

HYPERTENSION DEFINITIONS

High blood pressure is defined traditionally as a persistent BP elevation in the office above 140/90 mm Hg.[8] Blood pressure is the phenotypic expression of the genetically predisposed disease hypertension. Blood pressure is a continuous variable. The "threshold BP value" to secure a diagnosis of hypertension comes from large epidemiologic studies demonstrating a higher mortality at levels above 140/90 mm Hg.[9] In the United States, the national guidelines promulgated by the Seventh Report of the Joint National Committee on Prevention, Detection, Evaluation, and Treatment of High Blood Pressure (JNC 7) in 2003 simplified the classification of hypertension and related conditions (Table 47.1).[8] This classification is endorsed by later guidelines as well.[7] The four categories of BP (normal, prehypertension, stage 1 hypertension, and stage 2 hypertension) are associated with progressively increasing CV risk and are independent of any other risk factor (including age).[2,8] JNC 8 provided once again evidence-based guidelines and did not redefine high BP. The expert panel concluded that the 140/90 mm Hg definition from JNC 7 remains reasonable.

The diagnosis of hypertension is based on properly measured office BP readings (Table 47.2).[8,10] Not following this procedure usually leads to inaccurate BP readings.

EVOLUTION OF BLOOD PRESSURE GOALS

As more data became available, the traditional definition of hypertension in guidelines has evolved over the last 35 years (Figure 47.2). The change of the diastolic cutoff from 95 to 90 mm Hg occurred concomitantly with the recommendation to use Korotkoff phase V disappearance of sound, rather than phase IV ("muffling" of sounds) in diagnosis.

Table 47.1 "Traditional" Cut Points of Blood Pressure for Hypertension and Its Related Diagnoses in the United States*

Condition	Systolic Blood Pressure (mm Hg)		Diastolic Blood Pressure (mm Hg)
Normal	≤120	and	<80
Prehypertension	120-139	or	80-89
Stage 1 hypertension	140-159	or	90-99
Stage 2 hypertension	≥160	or	≥100

*If the systolic and diastolic blood pressure levels fall into two different diagnostic categories, the higher category is used (e.g., 162/92 mm Hg is stage 2 hypertension; 122/72 mm Hg is prehypertension). These definitions are those of the Seventh Report of the Joint National Committee on Prevention, Detection, Evaluation, and Treatment of High Blood Pressure (JNC 7).[1] Different classification schemes are used outside the United States.

The inclusion of systolic BP in the definition of hypertension has been much more gradual (see Figure 47.2).

In JNC I and II (1977-1982), the diagnosis of hypertension was made **solely** on diastolic BP values. In JNC III and IV, "isolated systolic hypertension" (systolic BP ≥ 160 mm Hg, but diastolic BP < 90 mm Hg) was defined, but no recommendations about therapy were made (see Figure 47.2).

Since 1993 both the JNC and the European guidelines recognize isolated systolic hypertension as worthy of treatment.[11] BP-lowering therapy in this subgroup of older adults has morbidity and mortality benefits.[12,13] Hypertension is diagnosed in adults if either systolic **or** diastolic BP is elevated. A pooling of data from over 1 million patients from 61 long-term epidemiologic studies concluded that systolic BP predicts approximately 89% of age-stratified stroke deaths and 93% of coronary heart disease deaths, whereas diastolic BP is much less predictive (83% and 73%, respectively).[9]

The importance of systolic BP, especially in people over age 55 years, was validated and extended by linking electronic medical records from 1.25 million English subjects with 5.2 years' median follow-up enrolled in the National Health Service from 1997 to 2010.[4] Moreover, 11 clinical trials, comparing active antihypertensive drugs to either placebo or no treatment in 28,436 patients, demonstrate morbidity and mortality benefits of treatment tied to reductions in systolic but not diastolic BP.[13]

EPIDEMIOLOGY

Hypertension is widely treated because of its increased risk for long-term morbidity and mortality and the fact that antihypertensive treatment prevents some of these events. The risks attributable to elevated BP levels are documented in numerous epidemiologic studies, beginning in 1948 with

Table 47.2 Essential Elements of Proper Blood Pressure Measurement in the Office

Allow patient to rest in the seated position for at least 3 to 5 minutes prior to measuring BP.
Neither patient nor examiner should talk during measurements.
The patient should have the legs uncrossed and should be seated comfortably on a chair with arm and back support.
Use the arm as the preferred site of measurement.
Make sure the measuring device is adequately maintained and calibrated.
Use a cuff that fits the arm circumference properly. The bladder length should cover at least 80% of the arm circumference. Recommended cuff sizes for adults are as follows:
- "Small adult" (12 × 22 cm): for arm circumferences between 22 and 26 cm
- "Adult" (16 × 30 cm): for arm circumferences between 27 and 34 cm
- "Large adult" (16 × 36 cm): for arm circumferences between 35 and 44 cm
- "Adult thigh" (16 × 42 cm): for arm circumferences between 45 and 52 cm

Place the lower end of the cuff approximately 2-3 cm above the antecubital fossa.
Have the arm positioned at the level of the heart.
Take at least 2 BP measurements and average them. Obtain more measurements if there is disparity between the first 2 values.
Measure BP in both arms to identify interarm differences (approximately 20% of individuals may have a difference >10 mm Hg). If different, report the values obtained on the arm with higher BP.
If using the auscultatory method with a stethoscope, use Korotkoff phase I (appearance) and V (disappearance) to define systolic and diastolic BP, respectively.
If using an aneroid or mercury manometer, use a deflation rate of 2-3 mm Hg/sec. (Deflation rates with automated oscillometric devices vary substantially and are defined based on proprietary algorithms.)

BP, Blood pressure.
Data from reference 10.

the Framingham Heart Study and extending to the present.[14,15] Meta-analyses of pooled data confirm the robust, continuous relationship between BP level and cerebrovascular disease and coronary heart disease in both Western and Eastern populations.[9] In addition, BP is linked directly in epidemiologic studies to incident left ventricular hypertrophy (LVH), heart failure, peripheral vascular disease, carotid atherosclerosis, end-stage kidney disease, and "subclinical CV disease." A natural history study that involved almost 12,000 veterans, studied over 15 years, noted that the level of BP corresponds to the risk for end-stage kidney disease (Figure 47.3).[16] Note that the highest risk is at levels above the autoregulatory range of the kidney (i.e., a systolic BP > 180 mm Hg).

CV risk factors tend to cluster; thus hypertensive individuals are much more likely than normotensive people to have type 2 diabetes mellitus or dyslipidemia, especially elevated triglyceride levels and low high-density lipoprotein cholesterol levels. The common denominator may be insulin resistance, perhaps because of the frequent coexistence of hypertension and obesity.

AGE AND HYPERTENSION

Increasing age is a major risk factor for developing hypertension (Figure 47.4), as well as a very strong confounder of its independent influence on CV and renal events. In the analysis of nearly a million individuals in 61 epidemiologic studies followed for an average of 13.3 years, those with BP levels in the highest decile had roughly the same risk for death from either ischemic heart disease or stroke as people who were 20 years older but had BP levels in the lowest decile.[9] In the Framingham study the lifetime risk of 55- to 65-year-old men or women for developing hypertension was above 90%.[17] In this study, of those who survived to ages 65 to 89 years, systolic BP elevations were found in 87% of the hypertensive men and 93% of the hypertensive women. In an analysis of the Framingham data set, classification of people with hypertension over age 60 years into the appropriate BP stages was done correctly in 99% of the cases using systolic rather than diastolic BP.[18]

These data highlight the great public health importance of systolic BP, particularly among those older than 50 years. In such individuals, systolic BP is a much better predictor of hypertensive target-organ damage and future CV and renal events than is diastolic BP.[9,19,20] Overall, each 20–mm Hg increase in systolic BP doubled the risk for CV death.[9] Systolic BP was less likely to be controlled to less than 140 mm Hg than diastolic to less than 90 mm Hg in the general U.S. population, according to every National Health and Nutrition Examination Survey (NHANES) data set from 1974 to 2012. Nearly 71% of those with treated but uncontrolled hypertension in the United States in 2012 were 60 years of age and older.[21] Yet antihypertensive drug therapy reduces the risk for CV events across the full age spectrum and has its greatest absolute benefit in older people, including individuals older than 80 years of age.[22,23]

The diagnosis of hypertension in children and adolescents is becoming more important, due to the epidemic of obesity in young Americans.[24] Current U.S. guidelines recommend BP measurement in children at least annually, but "normative values" depend on gender, age, and height of the child.[25] As a result, interpretation of BP levels in children and adolescents usually involves comparison of a child's average BP (from three visits) to a complex table that provides threshold values for "prehypertension" (traditionally, BP between the 90th and 95th percentiles), "hypertension" (BP between the 95th and 99th percentiles), and "severe hypertension" (99th percentile or higher).

GENDER AND HYPERTENSION

Hypertension is a major problem for both men and women, but men tend to develop it at an earlier age (Figure 47.5), which is also true of the adverse clinical consequences of hypertension. Among individuals older than 70 years, women are more likely to have hypertension[1,21] and to have a CV event compared to men. Age and body mass index have been much stronger predictors of incident hypertension than gender in epidemiologic studies. Drug treatment of hypertension has roughly the same benefits for women and men.[26,27]

Figure 47.2 The evolution of the Joint National Committee (JNC) reports. **A,** Systolic blood pressure (SBP). **B,** Diastolic blood pressure (DBP). ISH, Isolated systolic hypertension.

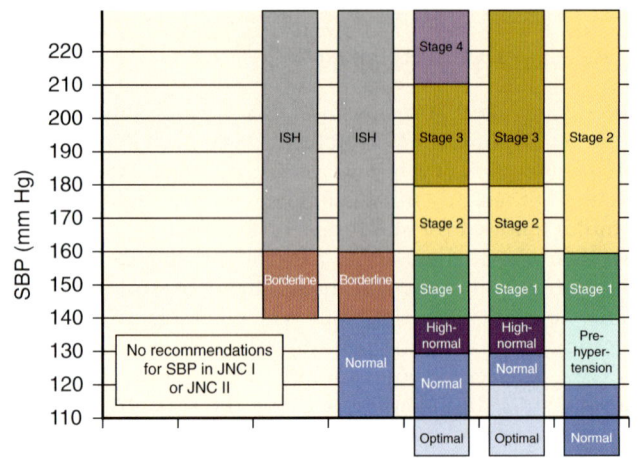

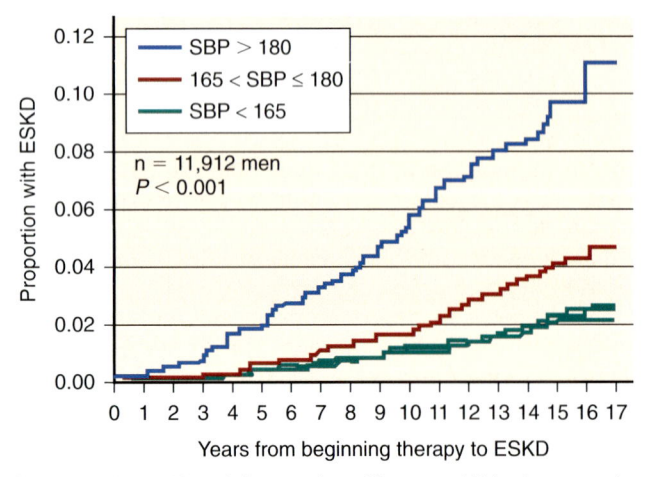

JNC I. *JAMA.* 237:255-261, 1977.
JNC II. *Arch InternMed.* 40:1280-1285, 1980.
JNC III. *Arch InternMed.* 144:1047-1057, 1984.
JNC IV. *Arch InternMed.* 148:1023-1038, 1988.
JNC V. *Arch InternMed.* 153:154-183, 1993.
JNC VI. *Arch InternMed.* 157:2413-2446, 1997.
JNC 7. *JAMA.* 289:2660-2672, 2003.

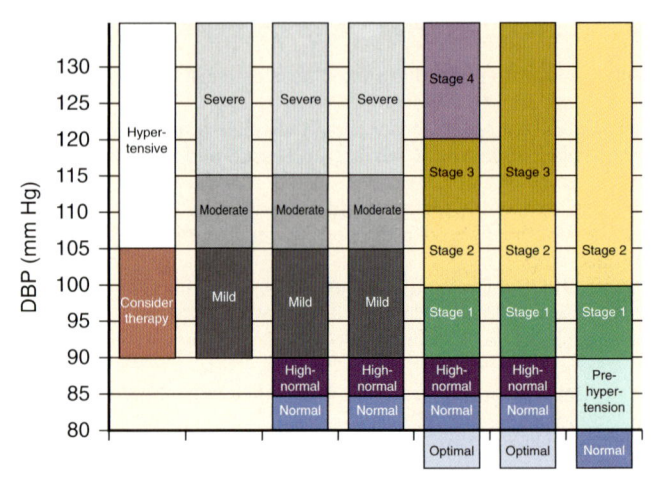

Figure 47.3 17-Year follow-up from Veterans Affairs hypertension clinics on end-stage kidney disease (ESKD). SBP, Systolic blood pressure.

RACE/ETHNICITY AND HYPERTENSION

Similar to previous surveys, NHANES 2011-2012 concluded that non-Hispanic blacks had approximately a 50% higher prevalence of hypertension than non-Hispanic whites, even after age adjustment (42.1% vs. 28.0%).[21] The prevalence of hypertension in either non-Hispanic Asians or Hispanics was slightly but not significantly lower (at 24.7% and 26.0%, respectively) than non-Hispanic whites. The prevalence of hypertension is geographically heterogeneous, with the highest prevalence in both blacks and whites in the southeastern United States ("the Stroke Belt"). Perhaps because of persistent public health initiatives, non-Hispanic blacks had the highest awareness (at 85.7%) and treatment (at 77.4%) of hypertension, but their control rate lagged that of non-Hispanic whites (49.5% to 53.9%, age–adjusted). This pattern has been consistent over the last decade.

Although the prevalence of hypertension has increased between NHANES 1988-1991 and 2011-2012, the increase is greatest for non-Hispanic blacks, compared to either Mexican Americans or non-Hispanic whites. In contrast to non-Hispanic whites and Mexican Americans, a higher prevalence of hypertension was observed in NHANES 2007-2010 for non-Hispanic black women, compared to men (47.0% vs. 42.6%). In all three racial/ethnic groups, women had higher rates of awareness, treatment, and control of BP in NHANES 2005-2010.

Perhaps because of the persistent historical difference in BP control rates, the adverse long-term consequences of hypertension are still more common in blacks than whites, but disparities have decreased in the last decade.[1] In 2010, the age-adjusted death rate from heart disease was 20% higher in blacks, as was stroke (by approximately 40%) and hypertension or hypertensive renal disease (by 140%).[28] Incident end-stage kidney disease was 3.4 or 1.6 times more common in 2011 in blacks or Native Americans, compared to whites.[29] Although diuretics or calcium channel blockers (CCBs) may have an advantage as initial therapy for reducing CV events in blacks, an angiotensin-converting enzyme (ACE) inhibitor (ACEI) was better than either a CCB or a β-blocker in preventing the decline of renal function in African Americans with hypertensive nephrosclerosis.[12,30] Most current guidelines therefore recommend controlling hypertension with multidrug regimens in all racial/ethnic groups.[8,11,31]

Although the prevalence of hypertension in Hispanics is lower than in non-Hispanic blacks and whites, hypertension is a concern. Mexican Americans continue to have the

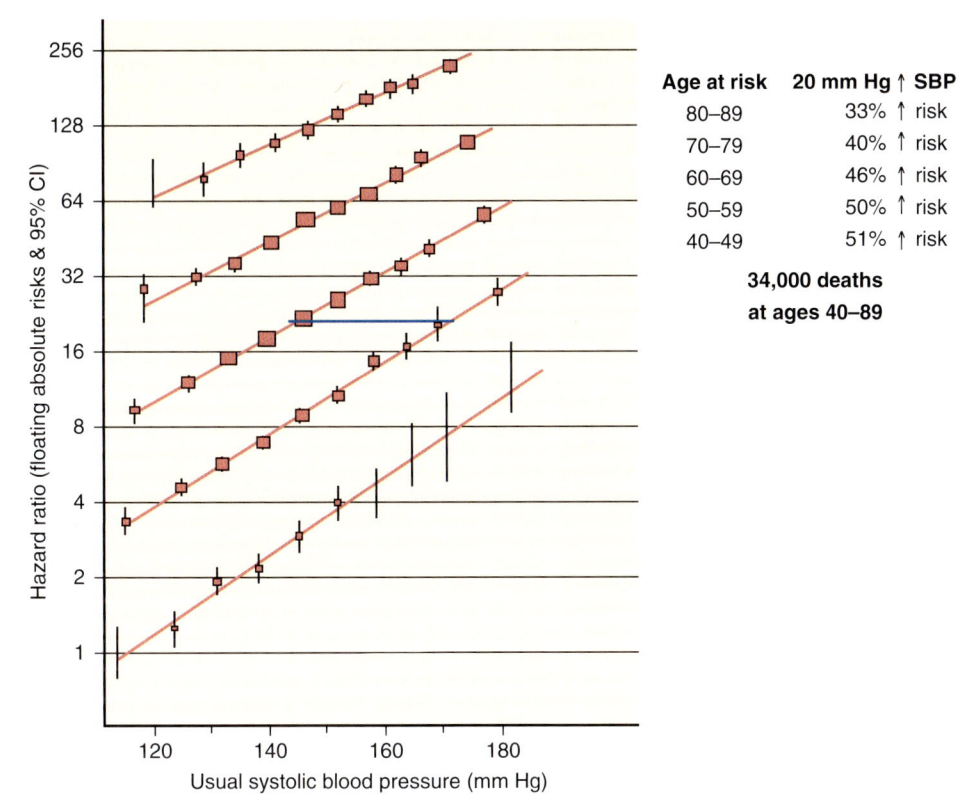

Figure 47.4 Coronary heart disease mortality in each decade of age versus systolic blood pressure (SBP) at the start of that decade. CI, Confidence interval.

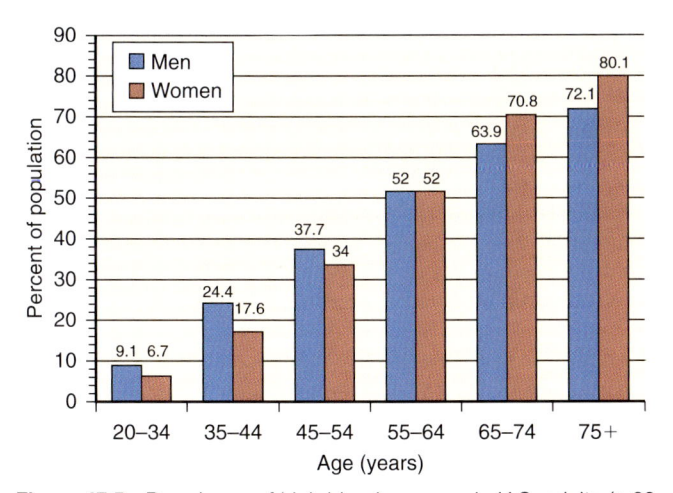

Figure 47.5 Prevalence of high blood pressure in U.S. adults (≥ 20 years of age) by age and gender, according to the National Health and Nutrition Examination Surveys 2007-2010.

lowest prevalence of controlled hypertension in both men and women (23.3% and 29.6%, respectively, in NHANES 1999-2004, compared to 35.1% and 41.6% in NHANES 2011-2012).[1]

BLOOD PRESSURE CONTROL RATES

Despite major progress in identifying the risks associated with elevated BP and demonstration that reducing BP to within a certain range reduces risk for death from CV disease and stroke as well as kidney disease progression, control rates are poor in the world. There are over 125 different medications encompassing eight different antihypertensive drug classes to help lower BP, as well as more than 20 single-pill combination agents for BP control. In spite of this, BP control remains suboptimal in many parts of the world.[8,21,32]

BP control rates (to < 140/90 mm Hg) have improved substantially in the United States since 1974 (Figure 47.6) and have stabilized at just over 50% in the last three biennial NHANES reports.[1] Successful national efforts to increase hypertension treatment and control rates have been associated with significant reductions in CV hospitalizations or death in both Canada[33] and the United Kingdom.[34]

The prevalence of uncontrolled hypertension is greater for undiagnosed, untreated, or older individuals and for systolic (rather than diastolic) BP. Some health care delivery organizations have reported BP control rates in excess of 60% to 80%.[35] They attribute their improvement in BP control to systems improvements that routinely call the health care provider's attention to the uncontrolled BP at every clinical encounter, development of a hypertension registry, increasing convenience for BP measurements, and widespread use of single-pill combination therapy.[35]

The wisdom of controlling BP over a relatively short time course after its discovery, rather than taking months to do so, was most clearly demonstrated in the Valsartan Antihypertensive Long-term Use Evaluation (VALUE) trial.[36] Although the randomized comparison was between high-risk patients with hypertension who received either valsartan or amlodipine initially, prevention of CV events

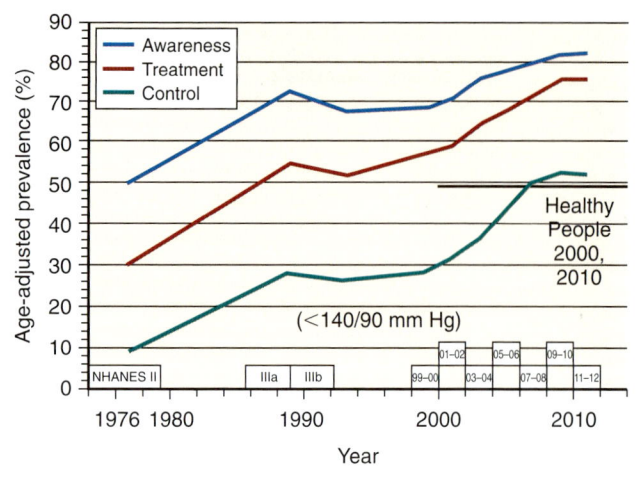

Figure 47.6 Awareness, treatment, and control of hypertension (to < 140/90 mm Hg) in U.S. National Health and Nutrition Examination Surveys (NHANES), from 1973 to 2012. The horizontal line at 50%, starting at the year 2000, corresponds to the national target for hypertension control promulgated by Healthy People 2000 and 2010, which has been increased to 61.2% by Healthy People 2020. The small numbers (e.g., "IIIa, IIIb, 99-00") in *boxes* just above the *x*-axis of the figure reflect the nomenclature of the NHANES data collection period.

was clearly better among individuals who achieved their goal BP during the *first 6 months* of treatment, regardless of initial randomized therapy. Similar long-term benefits of "early" control of BP have been seen for stroke or CV events in the Systolic Hypertension in Europe trial[37] and for death in the Systolic Hypertension in the Elderly Program (SHEP).[38]

ECONOMICS OF HYPERTENSION

Cost considerations are now increasingly important in the pharmacologic management of hypertension in the United States, and they have always been a major consideration in the rest of the world. No regimen, no matter how carefully and appropriately selected, will be effective if the patient cannot afford it. Moreover, if an antihypertensive agent does not appear on the national formulary or the formulary of the insurance company from which a patient receives medication, the cost will not be covered. Generic preparations tend to be the least expensive options for initial therapy and are available for every class of antihypertensive agent except the renin inhibitor. In general, brand-name CCBs are the most expensive, with brand-name angiotensin receptor blockers (ARBs) and ACEIs the next most expensive drugs.

For many of the single-pill combinations, generic medications are now available. Thus the cost is less than what would be paid for the individual components if they were purchased separately. It has also become common for single-pill combinations that include a thiazide diuretic to cost no more than the nondiuretic component alone.

A proper analysis of the economics of hypertension and its treatment should include more than what is spent on drugs, patient visits, and/or laboratory tests.[39] For many high-risk patients the expensive complications of untreated hypertension far outweigh the inconvenience and costs associated with effective treatment. For the United States in 2011, hypertension was expected to cost approximately $46.4 billion (related to CV disease),[1] and roughly another $32 billion related to chronic kidney disease (CKD). Approximately $19 billion (or 24% of the expenditures for hypertension) will pay for antihypertensive drugs. This proportion of expenditures has decreased steadily over the last decade due to the approval of generic formulations. Generic formulations recently constituted about 90% of the dispensed antihypertensive medications in the United States.

PATHOPHYSIOLOGY

The physiology that generates BP involves the integration of cardiac output (CO) and systemic vascular resistance (SVR) (BP = CO × SVR), with each of these having its own determinants ([CO = heart rate × stroke volume]; [SVR = 80 × (mean arterial pressure − central venous pressure)/CO]). This view is simplified, but it provides a framework to define the relevant factors in BP regulation. Changes in CO typically produce short-lived BP changes (hours to days), as adaptive mechanisms adjust SVR to normalize BP. However, changes in SVR are able to produce sustained increases in BP. The following sections summarize relevant mechanisms leading to BP regulation.

PRESSURE NATRIURESIS AND SALT SENSITIVITY

A key factor in the regulation of BP as a factor of CO and SVR is the phenomenon of pressure natriuresis. Pressure natriuresis is defined as the increase in renal sodium excretion because of mild increases in BP, allowing BP to remain in the normal range.[40,41] This occurs over hours to days and is modulated by both biophysical and humoral factors.

In the normal state, increased sodium intake causes an increase in extracellular volume and BP. Because of the steep relationship between volume and pressure, small increases in BP produce natriuresis that restores sodium balance and returns BP to normal (Figure 47.7). The ability of the kidneys to adjust to sodium loading is remarkable, adapting to fluctuations in sodium intake as high as 50-fold.[41]

However, this response becomes abnormal whenever there is abnormal sodium handling, leading to states of sodium-sensitive hypertension, such as in conditions of reduced glomerular filtration rate (GFR) or high levels of angiotensin II (see Figure 47.7). In such situations the change in extracellular fluid volume is relatively small (3% to 5%), but a state of chronic high BP develops resulting from increased SVR. The mechanisms responsible for this vascular effect are not completely understood but likely involve increased activity of the renin angiotensin aldosterone system (RAAS) (high angiotensin II level) and several other vasoconstricting substances, as will be discussed later in this section.

The pressure natriuresis process is also mediated by biophysical factors. Increased renal interstitial hydrostatic pressure is an important factor. Sodium loading results in increased pressure in the vasa recta, which have noticeably poor autoregulation, while pressure in cortical peritubular capillaries remains normal.[42,43] Vasa recta blood flow approximates 10% of total renal blood flow. This

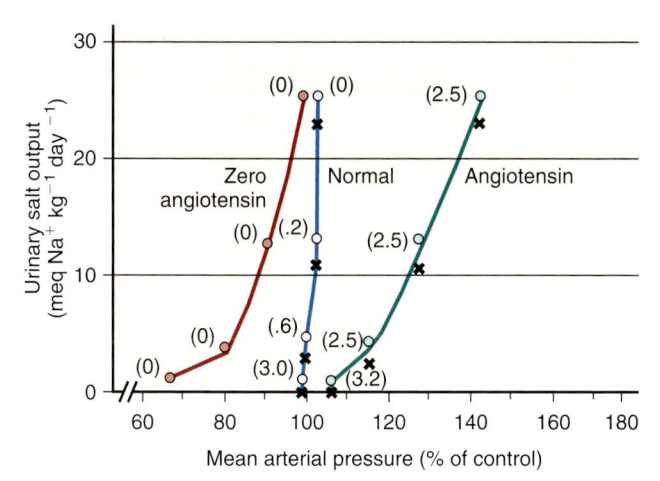

Figure 47.7 Pressure natriuresis curves in dogs at different levels of sodium intake (reflected in urinary salt output, y-axis). In the normal state, massive fluctuations in sodium intake produce minimal changes in blood pressure (BP). In states of high angiotensin II levels (angiotensin II infusion in this model), BP increases significantly even with modest increases in sodium intake. Conversely, in states where angiotensin II is absent or low (administration of captopril in this model), the increased sodium results in increased BP only at low BP levels; once BP becomes normal, the relationship is similar to that of normal kidneys. Values in parentheses are the relative estimated concentrations of angiotensin II (1 being the reference). *(From reference 41.)*

increase in interstitial pressure inhibits sodium transport largely by increasing 20-hydroxyeicosatetraenoic acid, an inhibitor of sodium-potassium adenosine triphosphatase (Na^+-K^+-ATPase), whose inhibition causes decreased activity of the Na^+-H^+-exchanger isoform 3 (NHE3).[42] In addition, increased interstitial pressure limits proximal tubular paracellular pathways, thus maximizing natriuresis.

Because abnormalities in pressure-sodium relationships are essential to maintaining chronic elevations in BP, they represent a fundamental step in the pathogenesis of any type of hypertension, not only primary, but also in the maintenance phase of most secondary causes, such as renal and renovascular hypertension, hyperaldosteronism, glucocorticoid excess, coarctation of the aorta, and pheochromocytoma.

The interplay between renal sodium retention and hypertension involves changes in sodium handling throughout the nephron. A theory with substantial experimental support proposes that increased renal vasoconstriction due to a variety of possible mechanisms (e.g., increased levels of angiotensin II, catecholamines, or uric acid, progressive aging) induces a preglomerular (afferent) arteriolopathy that results in impaired sodium filtration.[44,45] In addition, renal vasoconstriction results in tubular ischemia, another mediator of increased sodium avidity.

GENETICS OF HYPERTENSION

Hypertension clusters in families; an individual with a family history of hypertension has a fourfold greater chance of developing hypertension,[46] and it is estimated that the heritability of hypertension ranges from 31% to 68%. Genome-wide association studies (GWAS) in several multinational cohorts have identified a large number of single-nucleotide polymorphisms (SNPs) associated with hypertension. However, these individual SNPs are responsible for only minor BP effects (0.5 to 1 mm Hg), and the overall impact of these identified SNPs on the overall BP variance is only approximately 1% to 2%.[46] The shortcomings of the use of GWAS and other large population approaches are multiple.[47] The SNP platforms used for testing are not hypothesis driven; they simply include common genetic variants for exploratory analyses that might provide clues for molecular pathways leading to better understanding of disease or new targets for therapy. In addition, BP measurement is not uniform, and large numbers of patients are receiving treatment at the time of testing, thus limiting the strength of any associations. Finally, hypertensive phenotypes are not well defined, so patients with very different phenotypes (e.g., isolated diastolic hypertension, isolated systolic hypertension of the young, isolated systolic hypertension of older adults) are all lumped together.[48]

We now understand that each of these phenotypes likely has different underlying pathophysiologic mechanisms, and that even within each group there is substantial variability in hemodynamic profile.[49,50] With the improvement in techniques that allow expeditious, cheaper whole-exome or whole-genome analyses, it is probable that phenotype-driven studies will become obsolete and greater mechanistic insights on the genetics of hypertension will become available, but this is not true as of the writing of this book.

Whereas the attempts at using current genetic approaches to understand essential hypertension in general have not been fruitful, the study of monogenic hypertension has. Monogenic causes of hypertension, although rare, have provided substantial insight into the pathogenesis of hypertension. Of the monogenic forms of hypertension with well-described molecular mechanisms, all have one thing in common: a defect in renal sodium handling. This commonality points to the primacy of the kidney in regulating BP by way of sodium balance.

In Liddle's syndrome, mutations in the epithelial sodium channel (ENaC) lead to increased ENaC expression and decreased removal from the luminal membrane, both of which contribute to persistent channel activation leading to sodium avidity, volume expansion, hypertension, hypokalemia, and metabolic alkalosis with suppressed aldosterone levels.[51] In Gordon's syndrome (pseudohypoaldosteronism type 2), a variety of mutations have been described leading to changes in the function of the thiazide-sensitive sodium-chloride cotransporter (NCC).[51] These mutations were initially mapped to the with-no-lysine (WNK) kinases 1 and 4, which regulate NCC phosphorylation and activity. Mutations in two E3 ubiquitin ligase complex proteins (kelch-like 3 and cullin 3) were discovered later.[52] These mutations are responsible for the majority of cases of the syndrome.

The presumed mechanism is related to decreased channel ubiquitination and therefore persistent presence in the luminal membrane leading to the clinical phenotype of hypertension, hyperkalemia, and metabolic acidosis. Mutations in the mineralocorticoid receptor can also produce hypertensive syndromes, such as hypertension exacerbated by pregnancy (Geller's syndrome), in which there is constitutive activity of the receptor in addition to marked sensitivity to progesterone, leading to hypertension during pregnancy in addition to chronic, severe hypertension with hypokalemia.[53] Likewise, increases in aldosterone level due to a chimeric gene duplication involving the 11β-hydroxylase and the aldosterone synthase genes result in control of aldosterone synthase by adrenocorticotropic hormone (ACTH), independently of sodium balance or angiotensin II or serum potassium levels. Such patients have hyperaldosteronism that is only blunted by ACTH suppression, thus the term *glucocorticoid-remediable hyperaldosteronism*.[54]

Other patients may have "apparent mineralocorticoid excess" due to mutations in the 11β-hydroxysteroid dehydrogenase type 2 gene. This enzyme is responsible for the conversion of cortisol to the inactive cortisone in target epithelia, including the kidneys. As a result, excess cortisol is available to activate the mineralocorticoid receptor leading to a state of apparent mineralocorticoid excess (salt-sensitive hypertension, hypokalemia, metabolic alkalosis) in the absence of aldosterone.

Similarly, patients with congenital adrenal hyperplasia due to 11β-hydroxylase or 17α-hydroxylase deficiency have an excess production of 21-hydroxylated steroids such as deoxycorticosterone and corticosterone, which are potent activators of the mineralocorticoid receptor, thus also producing the syndrome of apparent mineralocorticoid excess in addition to the well-known sexual developmental abnormalities of the syndromes.[55] Taken together, this is strong evidence of the importance of renal sodium handling in the genesis of hypertension.

NONOSMOTIC SODIUM STORAGE

The paradigm of sodium balance described earlier assumes that sodium and its accompanying anion are osmotically active and therefore retained isosmotically with water. However, this paradigm cannot explain the observation that acute sodium loading in humans and animals results in positive sodium balance without the expected water (weight) gain. Consequently, sodium may accumulate without water, most prominently in the skin,[56] where negatively charged glycosaminoglycans bind sodium.[57] This system of interstitial sodium buffering adds to the classical Guytonian approach wherein nonosmotic accumulation occurs acutely and is presumably followed by increased removal from skin (via an enhanced lymphatic network) for ultimate renal excretion.

The mechanisms explaining isosmotic sodium storage are under intense investigation. Mice and rats receiving a high-salt diet develop hypertonicity of the skin interstitium, which triggers a series of mechanisms to keep interstitial volume constant.[58] The hypertonic sodium content activates the tonicity-responsive enhancer–binding protein (TonEBP) present in mononuclear cells infiltrating the skin. Consequently, these skin macrophages secrete vascular endothelial growth factor type C, resulting in increased density and hyperplasia of the skin lymphocapillary network and increased endothelial nitric oxide synthase (eNOS). If these responses are blocked, salt-sensitive hypertension develops.[58,59] These findings link the mononuclear phagocyte system to extracellular fluid volume control.

The translation of these findings into clinical implications was addressed in a study evaluating sodium balance in cosmonauts undergoing prolonged training (up to 205 days) in a facility simulating life in space.[60] By carefully monitoring water and electrolyte intake and excretion, as well as factors regulating sodium balance, individuals exhibited a large variability in sodium excretion on a day-to-day basis despite relatively stable diets. In the long term, approximately 95% (70% to 103%) of ingested sodium was recovered, but daily sodium excretion during stable sodium intake varied considerably and was independent of BP and sodium intake. Instead, urine sodium excretion varied as a function of circaseptan fluctuations (6 to 9 days in this case) in levels of aldosterone and cortisol/cortisone Moreover, total body sodium stores had even longer infradian variations (averaging several weeks).

The factors regulating these intriguing changes are still unknown. These observations have clinical implications for the use of urine sodium excretion to assess sodium intake because they suggest wide day-to-day variations that cannot[60] be captured in a single 24-hour urine collection.

RENIN ANGIOTENSIN ALDOSTERONE SYSTEM

The RAAS has wide-ranging effects on BP regulation. Figure 47.8 summarizes the most relevant elements of the RAAS and its role in the pathogenesis of hypertension and its complications. The different elements of the RAAS have key roles in mediating sodium retention, pressure natriuresis, salt sensitivity, vasoconstriction, endothelium dysfunction, and vascular injury. Taken together, the RAAS has an important role in the pathogenesis of hypertension. However, in a very large GWAS of 2.5 million genotyped or imputed SNPs in 69,395 individuals of European ancestry from 29 studies,[61] the meta-analysis showed that the majority of SNPs involved issues with natriuretic peptide abnormalities. Thus these hormones play a prominent role in the pathogenesis of hypertension and may be more important than the RAAS system, which did not have prominent SNPs associated with this analysis.[61]

Renin and prorenin are synthesized and stored in the juxtaglomerular cell apparatus and released in response to decreased renal afferent perfusion pressure, decreased sodium delivery to the macula densa, activation of renal nerves (via $β_1$-adrenergic receptor stimulation), and a variety of metabolic products, including prostaglandin E_2 and several others. Renin's main function is to cleave angiotensinogen into angiotensin I. Prorenin, previously viewed as an inactive substrate for renin production, is now known to also stimulate the (pro)renin receptor (PRR). This receptor leads to more efficient cleavage of angiotensinogen and activates downstream intracellular signaling through the mitogen-activated protein (MAP) kinases extracellular signal–regulated kinases 1 and 2 (ERK1/2) pathways that have been associated with profibrotic effects in some, but not all, experimental models.[62,63] At this point, it is uncertain that the PRR is involved in the genesis or complications of hypertension in a manner that is independent of the effects of angiotensin II.

Angiotensin II, formed by the cleavage of angiotensin I by the ACE, is at the center of the pathogenetic role of the RAAS in hypertension. Primarily through its actions mediated by the angiotensin II type 1 receptor (AT_1R), angiotensin II is a potent vasoconstrictor of vascular smooth muscle, causing systemic vasoconstriction as well as increased

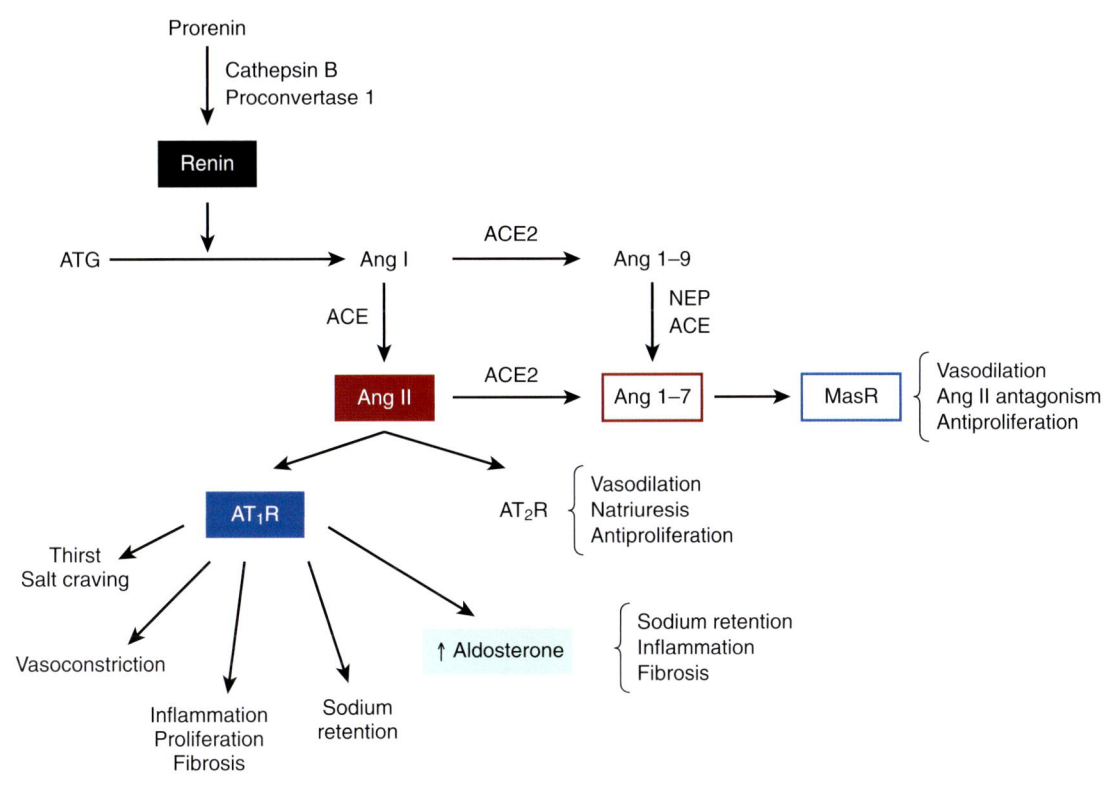

Figure 47.8 Key elements of the renin angiotensin aldosterone system. ACE, Angiotensin-converting enzyme; Ang, angiotensin; ATG, angiotensinogen; AT_1R, angiotensin II type 1 receptor; AT_2R, angiotensin II type 2 receptor; MasR, Mas receptor; NEP, neutral endopeptidase.

renovascular resistance and decreased medullary flow, which is a mediator of salt sensitivity. It produces increased sodium reabsorption in the proximal tubule by increasing the activity of NHE3, the sodium-bicarbonate exchanger, and Na^+-K^+-ATPase and by inducing aldosterone synthesis and release from the adrenal zona glomerulosa. In addition, it is associated with endothelial cell dysfunction and produces extensive profibrotic and proinflammatory changes, largely mediated by increased oxidative stress, resulting in renal, cardiac, and vascular injury, thus giving angiotensin II a tight link to target-organ injury in hypertension.[64] Conversely, stimulation of the angiotensin II type 2 receptor (AT_2R) is associated with opposite effects, resulting in vasodilation, natriuresis, and antiproliferative effects.

The relative importance of the renal and vascular effects of angiotensin II was evaluated in classical cross-transplantation studies using both wild-type mice and mice lacking the AT_1R.[65,66] By cross transplanting the kidneys of wild-type mice into AT_1R knockout mice and vice versa, investigators were able to generate animals that were selective renal AT_1R knockouts or selective systemic (nonrenal) AT_1R knockouts. In physiologic conditions, renal, systemic, and total knockout animals had lower BP than wild-type animals, indicating a role of both renal and extrarenal AT_1R in BP regulation.[66] The systemic AT_1R absence was associated with approximately 50% lower aldosterone levels, but the lower BP observed in this group was independent of this lower aldosterone production, as BP remained low despite aldosterone infusions to supraphysiologic levels following adrenalectomy in the systemic knockout animals. In addition, the BP reduction in kidney knockout animals occurred despite normal aldosterone excretion, again confirming the independence of renal angiotensin II effects from aldosterone.

In the hypertensive environment, it is the presence of renal AT_1R that mediates both hypertension and organ injury[66] (Figure 47.9). When animals were infused with angiotensin II for 4 weeks, animals lacking renal AT_1R did not develop sustained hypertension, whereas wild-type and systemic knockout mice had a significant increase in BP. Additionally, only animals with elevated BP developed cardiac hypertrophy and fibrosis. This indicates that cardiac injury is largely dependent on hypertension and not on the presence of AT_1R in the heart, as the (hypertensive) systemic knockout animals developed significant cardiac abnormalities despite the absence of AT_1R in the heart.[65] In summary, these experiments indicate that both systemic and renal actions of angiotensin II are relevant to physiologic BP regulation, but in hypertension, the detrimental effects of angiotensin II are mediated via its renal effects.

Aldosterone, the adrenocortical hormone synthesized in the zona glomerulosa, plays a critical role in hypertension through its well-known effects on sodium reabsorption that are largely mediated by genomic effects through the mineralocorticoid receptor leading to increased expression of ENaC. An extensive body of literature has identified other genomic and nongenomic effects of aldosterone with relevance to hypertension. Extensive nonepithelial effects include vascular smooth muscle cell proliferation, vascular extracellular matrix deposition, vascular remodeling and fibrosis, and increased oxidative stress leading to endothelial dysfunction and vasoconstriction.[64,67]

Several other elements of the RAAS have been identified as having potentially important roles in hypertension. The

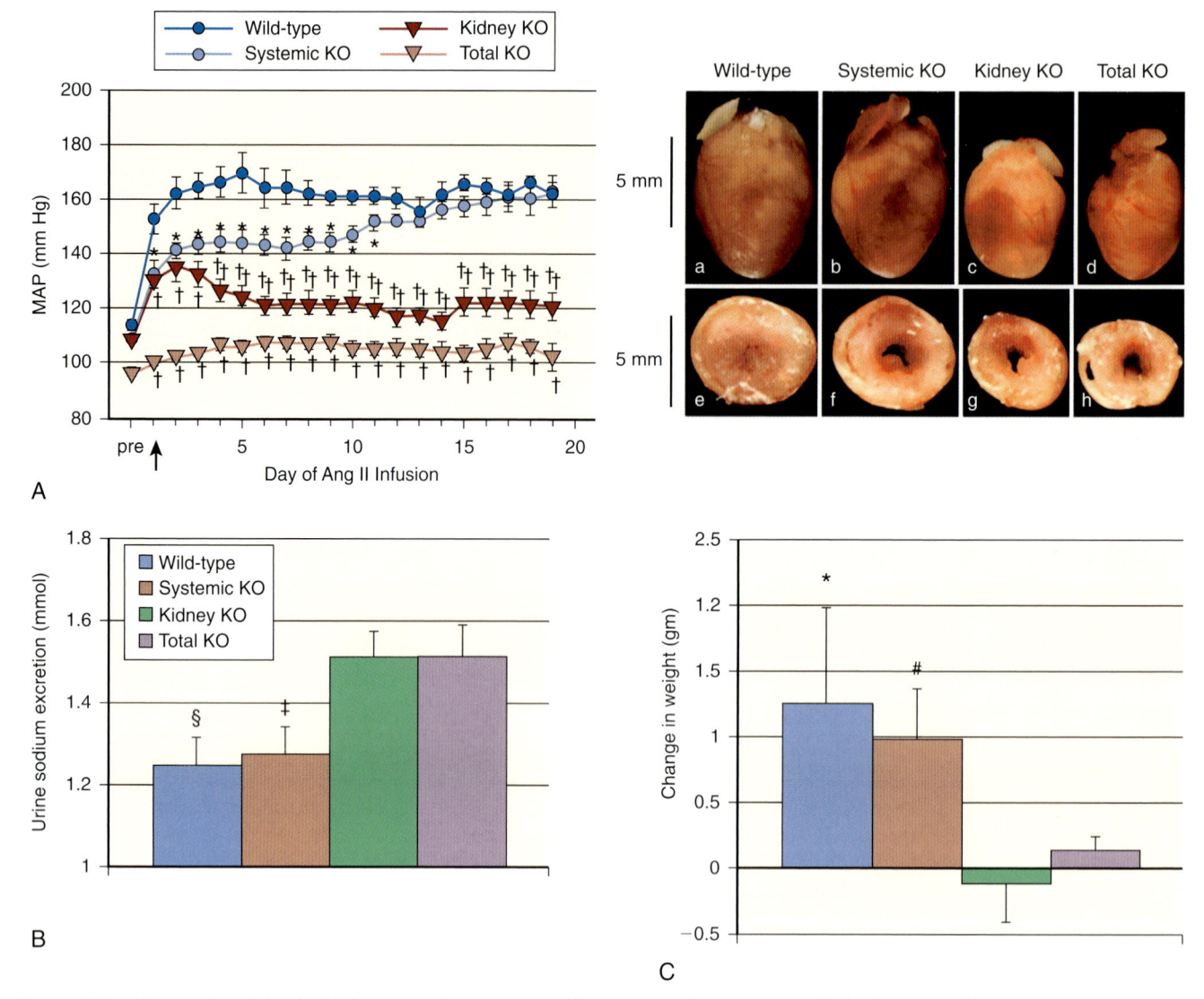

Figure 47.9 Effects of angiotensin II infusion on blood pressure (**A**), urinary sodium excretion (**B**), body weight (**C**), and cardiac hypertrophy (photos) according to renal and extrarenal presence of angiotensin II type 1 receptor. See text for details. KO, Knockout; MAP, mean arterial pressure. (From Crowley SD, Gurley SB, Herrera MJ, et al: Angiotensin II causes hypertension and cardiac hypertrophy through its receptors in the kidney. *Proc Natl Acad Sci U S A* 103:17985-17990, 2006.)

importance of ACE2 and angiotensin-(1-7) to BP regulation and angiotensin II–associated target-organ injury has become apparent. ACE2 is expressed largely in heart, kidney, and endothelium; it has partial homology to ACE and is unaffected directly by ACEIs.[68] It has a variety of substrates, but its most important action is the conversion of angiotensin II to angiotensin-(1-7). Angiotensin-(1-7) is formed primarily though the hydrolysis of angiotensin II by ACE2, and its actions are opposite to those of angiotensin II, including vasodilatory and antiproliferative properties that are mediated by the Mas receptor, a G protein–coupled receptor that, upon activation, forms complexes with the AT_1R, thus antagonizing the effects of angiotensin II. The vasodilatory effects are mediated by increased cyclic guanosine monophosphate, decreased norepinephrine release, and amplification of bradykinin effects. Studies have identified ACE2 and angiotensin-(1-7) as protective factors in the development of atherosclerosis and cardiac and renal injury,[68,69] and administration of recombinant ACE2 or its activator, xanthenone, has resulted in improved endothelial function, decreased BP, and improved renal, cardiac, and perivascular fibrosis in hypertensive animals.[70-72]

SYMPATHETIC NERVOUS SYSTEM

The sympathetic nervous system (SNS) is activated consistently in patients with hypertension compared with normotensive individuals, particularly in the obese (Figure 47.10). Many patients with hypertension are in a state of autonomic imbalance that encompasses increased sympathetic and decreased parasympathetic activity.[73,74] SNS hyperactivity is relevant to both the generation and maintenance of hypertension and is observed in human hypertension from very early stages. For example, studies in humans have identified markers of sympathetic overactivity in normotensive individuals with a family history of hypertension.[73] Among

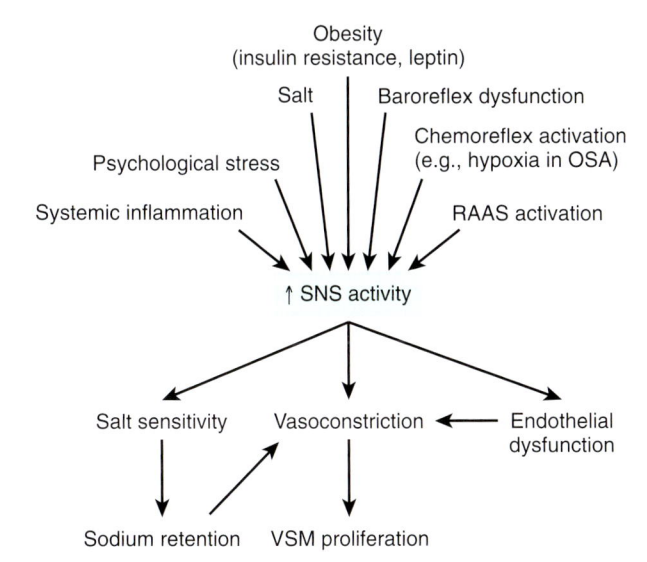

Figure 47.10 Causes and consequences of sympathetic nervous system (SNS) activation in the pathogenesis of hypertension. OSA, Obstructive sleep apnea; RAAS, renin angiotensin aldosterone system; VSM, vascular smooth muscle.

patients with hypertension, increasing severity of hypertension is associated with increasing levels of sympathetic activity measured by microneurography.[75,76] In human hypertension, plasma catecholamine levels, microneurographic recordings, and systemic catecholamine spillover studies have shown consistent elevation of these markers in obesity, the metabolic syndrome, and hypertension complicated by heart failure or kidney disease.[73] In addition, SNS hyperactivity is observed in most hypertensive subgroups, though it appears more pronounced in men than in women, and in younger than in older patients.

Several experimental models have outlined the importance of the SNS in generating hypertension. Different models of obesity-related hypertension indicate that the SNS is activated early in the development of increased adiposity,[74] and the key factor in the maintenance of sustained hypertension is increased renal sympathetic nerve activity and its attendant sodium avidity.[74]

SNS-mediated induction of salt sensitivity is a key element to sustaining high BP in other models of hypertension as well. For instance, rats receiving daily infusions of phenylephrine for 8 weeks developed hypertension during the infusions, but BP normalized under a low-salt diet after discontinuation of phenylephrine.[77] However, once exposed to a high-salt diet, the animals again became hypertensive. The degree of BP elevation on a high-salt diet was directly related to the degree of renal tubulointerstitial fibrosis and decrement of GFR. These findings can be interpreted within the paradigm that catecholamine-induced hypertension causes renal interstitial injury that associates with a salt-sensitive phenotype even after sympathetic overactivity is no longer present.[77] In addition, enhanced SNS activity results in α_1-receptor–mediated endothelial dysfunction, vasoconstriction, vascular smooth muscle proliferation, and arterial stiffness, all of which contribute to the development of hypertension. Finally, evidence indicates that sympathetic overactivity results in salt sensitivity due to a reduction in the activity of WNK4. This results in increased sodium avidity through the thiazide-sensitive NCC.[78] Figure 47.10 summarizes the causes and consequences of SNS activation in the genesis of hypertension.

Renalase is a flavoprotein highly expressed in kidney and heart that metabolizes catecholamines and catecholamine-like substances to aminochrome.[79] Tissue and plasma renalase is decreased in experimental models with renal mass reduction, and renalase knockout mice have increased BP and elevated circulating catecholamine levels. A normal phenotype is restored by administration of recombinant renalase. Also of relevance to catecholamine metabolism is catestatin, a product of the proteolysis of the neuroendocrine peptide chromogranin A.[80] Catestatin acts at nicotinic cholinergic receptors in adrenal chromaffin cells as an inhibitor of catecholamine release. Chromogranin A knockout mice are hypertensive and have elevated catecholamine levels, both of which are normalized by administration of catestatin. Moreover, serum catestatin levels are decreased in patients with hypertension and their normotensive offspring, raising the possibility of a regulatory role in the development of hypertension. The role of renalase and catestatin in the modulation of SNS-mediated hypertension, as well as their possible value in the treatment of hypertension in humans, remains uncertain.

Because increased SNS activity is associated with vascular smooth muscle proliferation, LVH, large artery stiffness, myocardial ischemia, and arrhythmogenesis, there is also a mechanistic role for the SNS in the complications of hypertension. In support of this concept, there are several cohort studies reporting an association between physiologic or biochemical markers of SNS activation and adverse outcomes in heart failure, stroke, and end-stage kidney disease.[73,81] However, there are no such studies among patients with hypertension, and the indirect evaluation of the impact of treatment-induced heart rate reduction in hypertension has yielded "paradoxical" results.

In a meta-analysis of hypertension trials, heart rate reduction during treatment with β-blockers was associated with increased risk for death and CV events in patients with hypertension.[82] In contrast, in a very large (n = 10,000) patient outcome trial, a post hoc analysis of heart rate at baseline demonstrated that those with a resting heart rate above 80 beats per minute even with a BP below 140/90 mm Hg had a higher mortality rate.[83] Therefore, while apparent that SNS activation is deleterious to patients with CV disease, and presumably with hypertension, a cause for the overactivity should be sought and an attempt made to affect that mechanism.

OBESITY

Obesity-related hypertension is characterized primarily by impaired sodium excretion and endothelial dysfunction, both of which are dependent on SNS overactivity, activation of the RAAS, and increased oxidative stress.[73,84] Fat tissue in obesity is hypertrophied and marked by increased macrophage infiltration.[85] As it is now well described, adipose tissue is not inert and secretes a wide range of cytokines and chemokines whose profile is abnormal in obesity, marked by increased levels of leptin, resistin, interleukin-6, and tumor necrosis factor-α secretion, elevated free fatty acid release, and reduced adiponectin level. Decreased adiponectin level results in insulin resistance, decreased induction of eNOS, and possibly increased sympathetic activity. Resistin impairs nitric oxide (NO) synthesis (eNOS inhibition) and enhances endothelin-1 (ET-1) production, shifting the vasodilation/vasoconstriction balance toward vasoconstriction. Hyperleptinemia directly stimulates the SNS through complex mechanisms that involve central leptin receptors as well as activation of the pro-opiomelanocortin system (via the melanocortin 4 receptor).[84] Lastly, visceral adipocyte mass is directly correlated with aldosterone secretion by the zona glomerulosa, a process mediated by angiotensinogen production by adipocytes as well as increased secretion of Wnt signaling molecules that modulate steroidogenesis.[86-88] All of these factors compound the tendency toward sodium retention and shifting the pressure-natriuresis curve to the right. Activation of these same systems leads to a proinflammatory state related to increased reactive oxygen species, factors directly associated with endothelial dysfunction and vascular proliferation. Therefore, multiple mechanisms contribute to the development and maintenance of hypertension in obese individuals.

NATRIURETIC PEPTIDES

Natriuretic peptides (atrial [ANP], brain [BNP], and urodilatin) also play a role in salt sensitivity and hypertension. These peptides have important natriuretic and vasodilatory properties that allow maintenance of sodium balance and BP during sodium loading. Upon administration of a sodium load, atrial and ventricular stretch lead to release of ANP and BNP, respectively, which result in immediate BP lowering due to systemic vasodilation and decreased plasma volume, the latter caused by fluid shifts from the intravascular to the interstitial compartment.[89] Finally, all natriuretic peptides increase GFR, which in volume-expanded states is mediated by an increase in efferent arteriolar tone. They also inhibit renal sodium reabsorption through both direct and indirect effects. Direct effects include decreased activity of Na^+-ATPase and the sodium-glucose co-transporter in the proximal tubule and inhibition of the ENaC in the distal nephron. The inhibitory effects of natriuretic peptides on renin and aldosterone release mediate indirect effects. Unfortunately, understanding the contribution of natriuretic peptides to the development of hypertension in humans is complicated by the elevation of their levels in association with increased BP (due to increased afterload) and hypertensive heart disease.

Some studies have tested whether polymorphisms in ANP or BNP genes resulting in higher levels of these peptides would associate with lower BP; results of these studies have been inconsistent, and effects have been small.[90-92] There are no published studies evaluating sequential changes in natriuretic peptides and risk for incident hypertension.

Attention has been given to corin, the serine protease that is largely expressed in the heart and converts pro-ANP and pro-BNP to their active forms. Experiments suggest that states of corin deficiency are associated with sodium overload, heart failure, and salt-sensitive hypertension,[93] and clinical studies have observed an association between certain corin gene polymorphisms and risk for preeclampsia and increased BP levels and hypertension risk, particularly among African Americans but not Chinese populations.[94]

THE ENDOTHELIUM

The endothelium is a major regulator of vascular tone and thus plays a key role in BP regulation. Endothelial cells produce a host of vasoactive substances, of which NO is the most important to BP regulation. NO is continuously released by endothelial cells in response to flow-induced shear stress, leading to vascular smooth muscle relaxation through activation of guanylate cyclase and generation of intracellular cyclic guanosine monophosphate.[95] Interruption of its production via inhibition of the constitutively expressed eNOS causes BP elevation and development of hypertension in both animals and humans. Using brachial artery flow-mediated vasodilation and measurement of urinary excretion of NO metabolites as methods to evaluate NO activity in humans, several studies have demonstrated decreased whole-body production of NO in patients with hypertension compared with normotensive controls.

Several elements are responsible for endothelial dysfunction in hypertension. Normotensive offspring of patients with hypertension have impaired endothelium-dependent vasodilation despite normal endothelium-independent responses, thus suggesting a genetic component to the development of endothelial dysfunction. Besides direct pressure-induced injury in the setting of chronically elevated BP, a mechanism of major importance is increased oxidative stress. Reactive oxygen species are generated from enhanced activity of several enzyme systems, reduced nicotinamide adenine dinucleotide phosphate-oxidase (NADPH-oxidase), xanthine oxidase, and cyclo-oxygenase in particular, and decreased activity of the detoxifying enzyme superoxide dismutase.[95,96] Excess availability of superoxide anions leads to their binding to NO, leading to decreased NO bioavailability, in addition to generating the oxidant, proinflammatory peroxynitrite. It is the decreased NO bioavailability that links oxidative stress to endothelial dysfunction and hypertension.[97] Angiotensin II is a major enhancer of NADPH-oxidase activity and plays a central role in the generation of oxidative stress in hypertension, although several other factors are also involved, including cyclic vascular stretch, ET-1, uric acid, systemic inflammation, norepinephrine, free fatty acids, and tobacco smoking.[98]

ET-1 is the endothelial cell product that counteracts NO to maintain balance between vasodilation and vasoconstriction. ET-1 expression is increased by shear stress, catecholamines, angiotensin II, hypoxia, and several proinflammatory cytokines such as tumor necrosis factor-α, interleukins 1 and 2, and transforming growth factor-β.[95] ET-1 is a potent vasoconstrictor through stimulation of ET-A receptors in vascular smooth muscle.[99] In hypertension, increased ET-1 levels are not consistently found. However, there is a trend of increased sensitivity to the vasoconstrictor effects of ET-1. ET-1 therefore is considered a relevant mediator of BP elevation, as ET-A and ET-B receptor antagonists attenuate or abolish hypertension in several experimental models of hypertension (angiotensin II–mediated models, deoxycorticosterone acetate–salt hypertension, and Dahl salt-sensitive rats) and are effective in lowering BP in humans.[100]

Endothelial cells also secrete a variety of other vasoregulatory substances. These include the vasodilating prostaglandin prostacyclin and several vasodilating endothelium-derived hyperpolarizing factors, the identity of which remains uncertain. There are also endothelium-derived contracting factors besides ET-1, such as locally generated angiotensin II and vasoconstricting prostanoids such as thromboxane A_2 and prostaglandin A_2. The balance of these factors, along with NO and ET-1, determine the final impact of the endothelium on vascular tone.

Other non–endothelium-derived factors may be of relevance to the genesis of hypertension via endothelium dysfunction. Much attention is given to uric acid, which can induce endothelial dysfunction and produce salt-sensitive hypertension through mechanisms that involve renal microvascular injury.[101,102] These changes can be abrogated by therapies that lower uric acid in animals and may be of value in lowering BP and limiting renal injury in humans with hyperuricemia. Also of relevance is the possible role of high dietary fructose consumption in intracellular adenosine triphosphate depletion, increased oxidative stress, increased uric acid production, and endothelial dysfunction.[103]

The net result observed in patients with hypertension is one of endothelial dysfunction. In cross-sectional analyses, the lower the degree of forearm flow-mediated vasodilation, the greater the prevalence of hypertension.[96,104] Prospective cohort studies have used flow-mediated vasodilation as a measure of endothelial dysfunction (regardless of specific mechanism) to evaluate its relationship with hypertension and test whether endothelial dysfunction is cause or consequence of hypertension, or both.[105] These studies have shown conflicting results, but the larger of them was unable to demonstrate an association between endothelial dysfunction and incident hypertension among 3500 patients followed for 4.8 years,[105] so as it stands, the evidence is stronger for endothelial dysfunction as a consequence, not a cause, of hypertension.[104]

ARTERIAL STIFFNESS IN HYPERTENSION

Arterial stiffness is an important factor in the pathogenesis of hypertension, particularly the syndrome of isolated systolic hypertension, as it is a common accompaniment of elevated systolic BP and pulse pressure. Arterial stiffness develops as a result of structural changes in large arteries, particularly elastic arteries.[106] These include loss of elastic fibers and substitution with less distensible collagen fibers. Factors strongly associated with arterial stiffening include aging, hypertension, diabetes mellitus, CKD, smoking, and high-sodium intake.[107]

The most commonly used measure to assess arterial stiffness in humans is carotid-femoral pulse wave velocity (cf-PWV). The traditional view linking arterial stiffness (measured as increased cf-PWV) to hypertension invoked that faster PWV produced faster reflection of the incident pulse wave, which resulted in an earlier reflected wave that returned to the central circulation before the end of systole, resulting in increased systolic BP.[108] While these mechanisms still hold true, later data have brought forth the importance of two other factors: increased amplitude of the forward wave and increased characteristic impedance of the proximal aorta.[108] When these specific factors are taken into account, the relative contribution of wave reflection to the observed age-dependent change in pulse pressure is only 4% to 11%.

Arterial stiffness was previously thought to be a consequence of hypertension. Cyclical pulsatile load is associated with fracture of elastin fibers and wall stiffening, and increased distending pressure demands recruitment of the less distensible collagen fibers, thus making vessels stiffer.[106] Evidence from several studies, however, indicates that arterial stiffness may precede and predispose to hypertension.[108] For example, in the Framingham Heart Study, markers of arterial stiffness (cf-PWV and amplitude of the forward pressure wave) were associated with a 30% to 60% increased risk for incident hypertension (per standard deviation of each variable) during 7 years of follow-up.[109] Conversely, baseline BP levels did not associate with future changes in arterial stiffness. Other studies corroborate these findings, but other studies also suggest a bidirectional relationship such that arterial stiffness is also a consequence of chronic hypertension.[108]

Arterial stiffening is relevant to target-organ damage in hypertension. Increased PWV is associated with increased mortality and CV events[110] as well as with a variety of subclinical CV injury markers, such as coronary calcification, cerebral white matter lesions, ankle-brachial index, and albuminuria. The relationship with cardiac complications is easily grasped: increased impedance to left ventricular ejection results in LVH, diastolic dysfunction, and subendocardial myocardial ischemia.

The relationship to brain and renal complications is more complex. It is now apparent that the mechanism of damage of these organs, which are characterized by vasculatures with high flow and low impedance, is mediated by increased transmission of increased pulsatile pressure to the brain and renal parenchyma. The reason for this is related to the abnormal process of "impedance matching." For individuals with normal vessels, the elastic arteries are much less stiff than muscular arteries, thus creating an impedance mismatch. This mismatch provokes wave reflection, thus protecting the tissue located distally to this reflection point from injury from the traveling pulse wave. In states of increased arterial stiffness, the stiffening of elastic arteries approximates the stiffness of muscular arteries, thus eliminating the protective impedance mismatch. Once impedances become "matched," there is less reflection and greater tissue injury, as supported by a growing body of clinical and experimental literature.[108]

ROLE OF THE IMMUNE SYSTEM IN HYPERTENSION

Immune responses, both innate and adaptive, participate in several of the mechanisms discussed earlier, including the generation of reactive oxygen species, mediation of the afferent arteriolopathy thought important to maintain salt sensitivity, and participation in the inflammatory changes noted in the kidneys, vessels, and brain in hypertension.[111,112] Innate responses, especially those mediated by macrophages, have been linked to hypertension induced by angiotensin II, aldosterone, and NO antagonism. Reductions in macrophage infiltration of the kidney or the periadventitial space of the aorta and medium-sized vessels lead to improvements in BP and salt sensitivity in several experimental models.[112,113] Adaptive responses via T cells have been linked to the genesis and complications of hypertension. T cells express AT_1R and mediate angiotensin II–dependent hypertension, as demonstrated by the observations that adoptive transfer of T cells restored the hypertensive phenotype in response to angiotensin II infusion that was absent in mice without lymphocytes.[113] Abnormalities in both proinflammatory T cells and regulatory T cells alike are implicated in complications of hypertension, as they appear to regulate vascular and renal inflammation that underlies target-organ injury.

Suppression of these inflammatory responses can improve BP control.[111,114] B lymphocytes may also play a causative role in hypertension as suggested by reports of several autoantibodies, including agonistic antibodies against adrenergic receptors, vascular calcium channels, and AT_1R, and antibodies against endothelial cells causing endothelial dysfunction, or heat shock proteins (hsp70) causing salt-sensitive hypertension.[115] Further research will determine if manipulation of immune targets is of value in the prevention and treatment of hypertension.

NOVEL METABOLIC PEPTIDES AND HYPERTENSION

Several vasodilating substances act as compensatory vasodilators to balance the heavily provasoconstrictive milieu in hypertension. Some of these vasodilators act primarily through an increase in NO release from endothelial cells, such as calcitonin gene–related peptide, adrenomedullin, and substance P. The glucose-regulating, gut hormone glucagon-like peptide-1 (GLP-1) has vasodilating properties, and its administration to Dahl salt-sensitive rats improves endothelial function, induces natriuresis, and lowers BP.[116] Additionally, the use of recombinant GLP-1 to treat diabetes in humans (exenatide) results in significant BP reduction, especially in those with high BP at baseline.[117]

CLINICAL EVALUATION

The evaluation of patients with hypertension focuses on six key components: (1) the confirmation that the patient is indeed hypertensive through a careful measurement of BP levels; (2) an assessment of clinical features that suggest specific causes of hypertension; (3) the identification of comorbid conditions that confer additional CV risk or that may impact treatment decisions; (4) the discussion of patient-related lifestyle practices and preferences that will affect management; (5) the systematic evaluation of hypertensive target-organ damage; and (6) shared decision making about the treatment plan. In order to accomplish this, the clinician often needs multiple visits and judicious use of the clinical examination and a variety of laboratory and imaging tests.

HISTORY AND PHYSICAL EXAMINATION

The medical history and physical examination are essential to uncovering possible secondary causes of hypertension and to identifying symptoms suggestive of hypertensive target-organ damage and comorbid conditions that may affect treatment decisions. While there is a focus on the CV, neurologic, and renal systems, a complete review of systems is indicated when the patient is first evaluated. This is because some patients will present with hypertension because of sleep apnea (snoring, witnessed apneas/gasping), hyperthyroidism or hypothyroidism (each with their litany of possible symptoms), hyperparathyroidism (symptoms of hypercalcemia), Cushing's syndrome (symptoms of cortisol excess), pheochromocytoma or paraganglioma (symptoms of catecholamine excess), or acromegaly with its distinctive features. These conditions are discussed in detail later in this chapter.

High BP is typically asymptomatic, but some symptoms are common among patients with very high BP levels, such as headaches, epistaxis, dyspnea, chest pain, and faintness, all of which were present in more than 10% of patients presenting with diastolic BP levels above 120 mm Hg.[118] Other common symptoms are nocturia and unsteady gait, whereas treated patients often complain of fatigue in addition to symptoms of overtreatment and those related to specific side effects of medications. In patients with lower BP levels, the occurrence of symptoms is often difficult to tie to observed BP, as demonstrated in a study evaluating the relationship between headaches and BP levels, where the frequently observed headaches in patients with hypertension did not correlate well with office or ambulatory BP levels.

When searching for target-organ damage, one looks for symptoms to suggest a previous stroke or transient ischemic attack, previous or ongoing coronary ischemia, heart failure, peripheral arterial disease, or a past history of kidney disease or current symptoms such as hematuria or flank pain.

Obtaining a detailed family history as it pertains to hypertension is essential. Focus should be on the development of hypertension at a young age or clustering of endocrine (pheochromocytoma, multiple endocrine neoplasia, primary aldosteronism) or renal problems (polycystic kidney disease or any inherited form of kidney disease). The young patient with hypertension and a family history of hypertension poses a particular challenge and should be evaluated in detail. Table 47.3 provides a guide to possible causes to be entertained.[119]

Knowledge of several conditions with potential relevance to treatment is important. For example, issues related to CV risk management such as diabetes mellitus, hypercholesterolemia, and tobacco smoking need to be evaluated. Patients with established CV disease will need some treatments for both their hypertension and their underlying disorder (e.g., β-blockers for angina pectoris), so knowledge of specific CV diagnoses is essential. Lastly, some non-CV conditions may have an impact on treatment options. For example, patients with reactive airways disease (asthma) probably should not receive β-blockers, patients with prostatic hyperplasia may benefit from a regimen that includes an α-blocker, and patients with attention-deficit/hyperactivity disorder or anxiety may benefit from a central sympatholytic (e.g., guanfacine), whereas those with major depression should probably not be treated with this drug class.

It is also important to recognize that it is during the history that the clinician has the opportunity to explore issues related to lifestyle, cultural beliefs, and patient preferences that will be essential in designing an effective treatment plan. It is important to define eating and physical activity patterns and, when problems are identified, to determine if the patient is willing and/or able to modify them. Cultural beliefs related to the treatment of hypertension,

Table 47.3 Clinical Clues to Guide the Investigation in Young Patients with Hypertension with a Potential Hereditary Cause

Specific Conditions	Possible Causes of Familial Hypertension	Clinical Clues
Catecholamine-Producing Tumors		
Pheochromocytoma/paraganglioma	Familial cases are responsible for <30% of cases, including MEN2A and MEN2B, von Hippel–Lindau disease, neurofibromatosis, and familial paraganglioma syndromes (SDH complex mutations)	Paroxysmal palpitations, headaches, diaphoresis, pale flushing; syndromic features of any of the associated disorders
Neuroblastomas (adrenal)	1%-2% of neuroblastomas are familial	
Aortic or renovascular lesions		
Coarctation of the aorta	Overrepresented in families but no familial distribution	Asymmetry between upper- and lower-extremity BP, radial-formal pulse delay; associated with Turner's syndrome, Williams' syndrome, and bicuspid aortic valve
Renal artery stenosis caused by fibromuscular dysplasia or inherited arterial wall lesions	<10% familial with AD pattern	Abnormal renal vascular imaging results; vascular disease in the carotid territory at an early age; common in neurofibromatosis and Williams' syndrome; also present in tuberous sclerosis, Ehlers-Danlos syndrome, and Marfan's syndrome
Parenchymal kidney disease GN	Alport disease (X-linked, AR, or AD), familial IgA nephropathy (AD with incomplete penetrance)	Proteinuria, hematuria, low eGFR
PKD	ADPKD type 1 or 2, ARPKD	Multiple renal cysts (as few as 3 in patients under 30 yr)
Adrenocortical disease		
Glucocorticoid-remediable aldosteronism (familial hyperaldosteronism type I)	AD chimeric fusion of the 11β-hydroxylase and aldosterone synthase genes	Cerebral hemorrhages at young age, cerebral aneurysms; mild hypokalemia; high plasma aldosterone, low renin
Familial hyperaldosteronism	AD; unknown defect	Severe type 2 hypertension in early adulthood; high plasma aldosterone, low renin; no response to glucocorticoid treatment
Familial hyperaldosteronism type III	AD; unknown defect	Severe hypertension in childhood with extensive target-organ damage; high plasma aldosterone, low renin; marked bilateral adrenal enlargement
Congenital adrenal hyperplasia	AR mutations in 11β-hydroxylase or 21-hydroxylase	Hirsutism, virilization; hypokalemia and metabolic alkalosis, low plasma aldosterone and renin
Monogenic Primary Renal Tubular Defects		
Gordon's syndrome	AD mutations of *KLHL3*, *CUL3*, *WNK1*, and *WNK4*; AR mutations of *KLHL3*	Hyperkalemia and metabolic acidosis with normal renal function
Liddle's syndrome	AD mutations of the epithelial sodium channel	Hypokalemia and metabolic alkalosis; low plasma aldosterone and renin
Apparent mineralocorticoid excess	AD mutation in 11β-hydroxysteroid dehydrogenase type 2	Hypokalemia and metabolic alkalosis; low plasma aldosterone and renin
Geller's syndrome	AD mutation in the mineralocorticoid receptor	Hypokalemia and metabolic alkalosis; low plasma aldosterone and renin; increased BP during pregnancy or exposure to spironolactone
Hypertension-Brachydactily syndrome	AD mutations in the phosphodiesterase E3A enzyme	
Unknown Mechanisms		
Hypertension-brachydactyly syndrome	AD	Short fingers (small phalanges) and short stature; brainstem compression from vascular tortuosity in the posterior fossa
Essential Hypertension		
	Polygenic	When obesity or metabolic syndrome is present, the likelihood of essential hypertension is higher

AD, Autosomal dominant; ADPKD, autosomal dominant polycystic kidney disease; AR, autosomal recessive; ARPKD, autosomal recessive polycystic kidney disease; BP, blood pressure; eGFR, estimated glomerular filtration rate; GN, glomerulonephritis; IgA, immunoglobulin A; MEN, multiple endocrine neoplasia; PKD, polycystic kidney disease; SDH, succinate dehydrogenase.

health illiteracy, and mistrust in physicians and the pharmaceutical industry are several of the items that can affect the relationship with the patient and that should be openly raised. It is only then that patients will be able to participate in shared decision making about their treatment, an essential tenet of patient-centered care.

The physical examination is designed to complement the items discussed in the history. One should pay attention to syndromic features of cortisol excess (moon face, central obesity, frontal balding, cervical and supraclavicular fat deposits, skin thinning, abdominal striae), hyperthyroidism (tachycardia, anxiety, lid lag/proptosis, hypertelorism, pretibial myxedema), hypothyroidism (bradycardia, coarse facial features, macroglossia, myxedema, hyporeflexia), acromegaly (frontal bossing, widened nose, enlarged jaw, dental separation, acral enlargement), neurofibromatosis (neurofibromas, café au lait spots, as neurofibromatosis is associated with pheochromocytoma and renal artery stenosis), or tuberous sclerosis (hypopigmented ash leaf patches, facial angiofibromas, as tuberous sclerosis is associated with renal hypertension, usually related to angiomyolipomas). Many other even rarer associations exist but fall beyond the scope of this chapter.

In younger patients or in patients with unexplained, difficult-to-treat hypertension, it is worth exploring the possibility of coarctation of the aorta by measurement of BP in both arms and in one thigh. If present, there will be a significantly lower BP in the thigh (typically by more than 30 mm Hg). Sometimes, in case of a lesion proximal to the left subclavian, there may be a significant interarm difference, lower on the left. In addition, there is significant decrease in intensity of the femoral pulses and a palpable radial-femoral pulse delay.

All patients should have a funduscopic examination to evaluate vascular changes associated with hypertension. The retinal changes are associated with severity of both acute and chronic BP elevation. Acute changes can happen quite abruptly (hours to days) and range from arteriolar spasm in most patients with uncontrolled BP to retinal infarcts (exudates) and microvascular rupture (flame hemorrhages), to papilledema once the protection afforded by vasoconstriction is overcome. Chronic changes take much longer to develop and include vascular tortuosity (arteriovenous nicking) due to perivascular fibrosis, followed by progressive arteriolar wall thickening that prevents visualization of the blood column, thus leading to the appearance of copper wiring, then silver wiring. Several studies have demonstrated a relationship between severity of hypertensive retinopathy and risk for LVH and stroke.

The CV examination focuses on the identification of volume overload (jugular venous distension, lung crackles, edema), cardiac enlargement (deviated cardiac impulse), and the presence of a third or fourth heart sound as markers of impaired left ventricular compliance. We also routinely look for bruits over the carotid arteries, as the prevalence of carotid atherosclerosis is increased in patients with hypertension, as well in the abdomen, primarily looking for renal arterial bruits heard over the epigastrium and/or flanks. These bruits are of greater significance if occurring on both systole and diastole. Finally, detailed palpation of the peripheral pulses of the arms and legs is important to look for signs of peripheral arterial disease.

To wrap up the examination, a focused neurologic examination looks for obvious cranial nerve abnormalities, motor deficits, or speech or gait abnormalities. Any further testing is based on specific symptoms or on focal findings on the screening examination.

BLOOD PRESSURE MEASUREMENT

Because treatment decisions are based largely on BP levels, accurate BP measurement is essential. Cuff-based brachial BP is the most used method to measure BP, typically in the office setting. However, a rapidly growing body of evidence points to the value of out-of-office BP methods, such as 24-hour ambulatory BP monitoring (ABPM) and home BP monitoring, as superior methods to evaluate BP burden and evaluate BP-related risk in patients with hypertension.[8,10]

OFFICE BLOOD PRESSURE MEASUREMENT

Office BP measurement is the time-honored method for the diagnosis and management of hypertension. It is strongly associated with hypertension-related outcomes based on more than 50 years of observational and clinical trial data. Accordingly, guidance provided to clinicians for the diagnosis and treatment of hypertension by most major guidelines is based on office BP values (see Table 47.2).[10] The British National Institute for Health and Care Excellence (NICE) guidelines recommend ABPM or home BP monitoring as preferred methods for the initial diagnosis of hypertension but still recommend office BP for monitoring treatment. The rationale for and controversy associated with these recommendations is discussed later.

Attention to measurement technique is essential. Table 47.2 summarizes essential elements of proper BP measurement technique. Most patients should have their BP measured in the arm in the seated position. In selected situations, such as the malformations, injuries, or extensive vascular disease of the upper extremities, or when comparing BP levels in the upper and lower extremities, it may be necessary to use thigh measurements with an appropriately sized thigh cuff, which should be obtained in the supine position to allow the cuff to be at the level of the heart. Mercury sphygmomanometers are now seldom available in clinical practice because of environmental concerns. Aneroid and electronic oscillometric manometers are accurate but should have periodic maintenance (every 12 months) to ensure that they are properly calibrated, as well as any time poor function is suspected.

A development in office BP measurement is the use of an electronic oscillometric device for multiple measurements by both staff and patient while in the office but with the patient alone in the room for five self-measured readings. Using this method, the "white coat effect" is largely eliminated (Figure 47.11).[120] In addition, this automated approach results in better correlations with ambulatory BP averages and with left ventricular mass than routine office BP.[121]

ORTHOSTATIC BLOOD PRESSURE MEASUREMENT

Orthostatic hypotension is a common accompaniment of uncontrolled hypertension, especially among older patients, where it occurs in 8% to 34% of patients.[122] Some guidelines now provide specific recommendations for measurement of

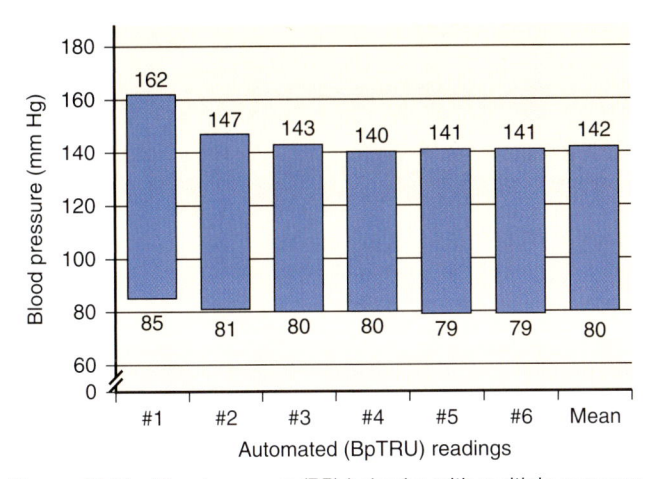

Figure 47.11 Blood pressure (BP) behavior with multiple measurements in the office in 50 patients with hypertension. The first BP reading was taken by the physician. The following five readings were taken by the patient with only the patient in the examination room. (From Myers MG: The great myth of office blood pressure measurement. *J Hypertens* 30:1894-1898, 2012.)

standing BP to screen for orthostatic hypotension in older patients with hypertension, as well as in patients at increased risk for autonomic dysfunction, such as those with diabetes and kidney disease.[123]

The frequency of orthostatic hypotension is influenced by increasing age, the presence of hypertension, and the number of antihypertensive drugs, while it is unclear that the type of antihypertensive drug has any specific impact on its development. The development of orthostatic hypotension is significant because it is a risk factor for syncope and falls. Therefore, it is important to evaluate for the presence of orthostatic hypotension as part of the assessment of risks and benefits of drug treatment for BP control in patients with hypertension.

Orthostatic vital signs (heart rate and BP) are best obtained after at least 5 minutes in the supine position followed by immediate assumption of the standing position, when sequential measurements are taken for up to 3 minutes. The difficulties of following this protocol in a busy clinical practice are recognized, so it is acceptable to compare values in the seated position with those after standing for 1 minute; this approach results in decreased sensitivity for the detection of orthostatic hypotension but is better than no measurement at all.[124] The generally accepted definition of orthostatic hypotension is a drop in BP of more than 20/10 mm Hg that occurs after 3 minutes of standing. Among patients with supine hypertension, it has been proposed that the definition of systolic fall in BP for the diagnosis is a drop of more than 30 mm Hg as the level of baseline BP is directly proportional to the orthostatic BP fall.

Integration of the heart rate response to changes in BP during orthostasis is important to guide the differential diagnosis and further evaluation of orthostatic hypotension. In the absence of medications with a negative chronotropic effect, the lack of a tachycardic response to orthostatic hypotension is indicative of baroreflex or sympathetic autonomic dysfunction. Patients with an appropriate tachycardic response, on the other hand, likely have volume depletion or excessive vasodilation.

Management of orthostasis is dependent on the pathophysiology of the cause. If baroreceptor abnormalities or autonomic dysfunction are a cause, a general approach requiring nocturnal β-blockers with compression stocking and increased morning sodium intake has been shown to be beneficial to reducing the symptoms and closing the pressure gap.[125]

OFFICE VERSUS OUT-OF-OFFICE BLOOD PRESSURE

Figure 47.12 summarizes the most relevant differences between office and out-of-office BP measurements (home BP and ABPM). Office BP measurement is the time-honored method to evaluate hypertension. It is easy to perform and is widely available at low cost. Home BP is also widely available, though accessibility to low-income patients is still a problem despite the availability of low-cost devices. ABPM, on the other hand, is less widely available due to costs and limited reimbursement by third-party payers in the United States. Both home BP monitoring protocols and ABPM include larger numbers of readings, thus decreasing variability and improving reproducibility.[126]

Office brachial BP values, generally obtained under standardized conditions in the seated position, are strongly associated with CV outcomes and mortality in the general population and in patients with hypertension. In the last 30 years, however, ABPM and home BP have become accepted as better markers of hypertensive target-organ damage and adverse clinical outcomes. ABPM has stronger associations with several measures of LVH, albuminuria, kidney dysfunction, retinal damage, carotid atherosclerosis, and aortic stiffness than office BP, although this is not consistent among studies.[127] Likewise, home BP is a better marker than office BP for LVH and proteinuria, though it is not consistently superior for other measures of target-organ damage.

In the assessment of hard CV end points, a systematic review by the NICE clinical guidelines group in the United Kingdom identified nine cohort studies comparing ABPM with office BP; ABPM was superior in eight and equal to office BP in one.[128] For home BP, they identified three studies comparing it with office BP; home BP was superior in two and equal in one. Lastly, two studies compared ABPM, home BP, and office BP; of these, one showed superiority of both ABPM and home BP while the other study did not show differences among any of the three methods.

In a meta-analysis of studies that evaluated both office and ABPM on outcomes, only ABPM values retained significance.[129] Likewise, in the largest home BP cohort study that included simultaneous use of office and home BP to predict CV events and mortality, only home BP remained significantly associated with these adverse outcomes.[130] Similar observations of the superior prognostic performance of out-of-office methods exist for patients with resistant hypertension, CKD, hemodialysis, and the general population.

In summary, evidence from prospective cohort studies convincingly demonstrates the superiority of out-of-office BP measurements as predictors of hypertension outcomes.

There are several possible explanations for the superiority of out-of-office measurements in outcomes assessment:

1. There is lower variability and better reproducibility afforded by the larger number of readings across a longer

White coat hypertension vs. normotension

Study name	Hazard ratio	Lower limit	Upper limit	Z value	P value
Verdecchia 1994	1.170	0.253	5.402	0.201	0.841
Kario 2001	0.760	0.164	3.529	−0.350	0.726
Fagard 2005	1.000	0.372	2.686	0.000	1.000
Ohkubo 2005	0.950	0.389	2.322	−0.112	0.910
Hansen 2006	0.960	0.500	1.842	−0.123	0.902
Pierdomenico 2008	0.970	0.381	2.468	−0.064	0.949
Summary	0.964	0.654	1.421	−0.186	0.852

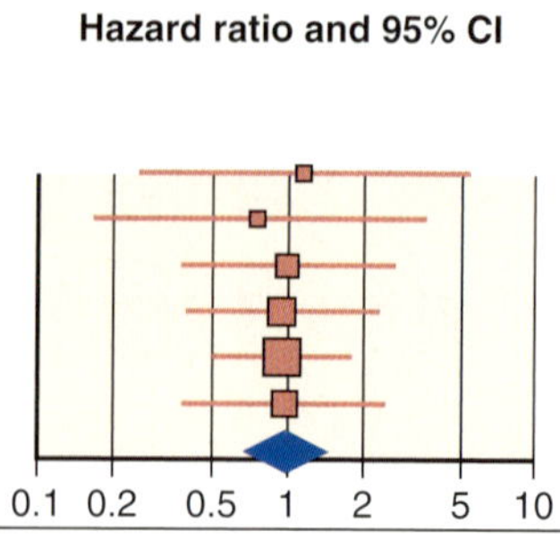

Masked hypertension vs. normotension

Study name	Hazard ratio	Lower limit	Upper limit	Z value	P value
Bjorklund 2003	2.770	1.149	6.676	2.270	0.023
Fagard 2005	1.650	0.526	5.172	0.859	0.390
Ohkubo 2005	2.560	1.410	4.649	3.088	0.002
Hansen 2006	1.660	1.056	2.610	2.195	0.028
Pierdomenico 2008	2.650	1.177	5.966	2.354	0.019
Summary	2.088	1.550	2.812	4.844	0.000

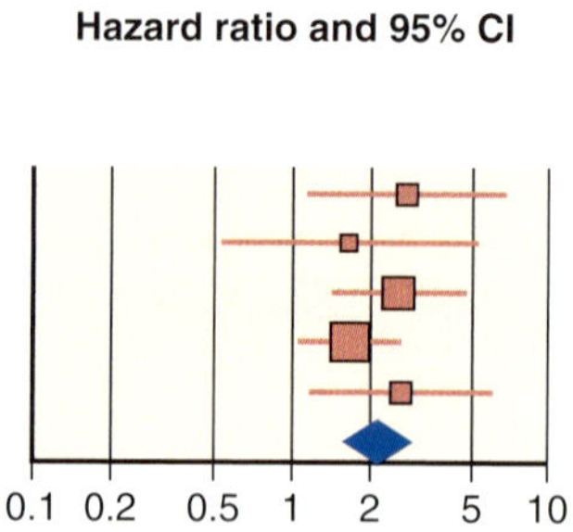

Figure 47.12 Results of a meta-analysis of the effects of white coat hypertension (*top*) and masked hypertension (*bottom*) on the occurrence of fatal and nonfatal cardiovascular events. There is no statistical difference between white coat hypertension and normotension (hazard ratio, 0.96; $P = 0.85$), whereas masked hypertension is associated with a 2.09-fold increase in risk ($P < 0.0001$). (From Pierdomenico SD, Cuccurullo F: Prognostic value of white-coat and masked hypertension diagnosed by ambulatory monitoring in initially untreated subjects: an updated meta analysis. *Am J Hypertens* 24:52-58, 2011.)

period of observation, thus making ABPM/home BP better reflections of "BP burden."

2. Home BP and ABPM can detect "white coat" and "masked" hypertension (see Figure 47.12).

   White coat hypertension (WCH), or isolated office hypertension, is the occurrence of high BP in the office and normal BP values in the out-of-office environment. It occurs in 20% to 30% of patients with a diagnosis of office hypertension.[131] It has generally been noted that patients with WCH have similar CV outcomes as normotensive individuals.[132] However, data from the large International Database of Home Blood Pressure in Relation to Cardiovascular Outcome have shown a significant increase in fatal and nonfatal CV events among untreated WCH patients diagnosed based on home BP compared with untreated normotensive persons (hazard ratio [HR], 1.42; $P = 0.02$).[133] Interestingly, treated patients with hypertension who retained a white coat effect had the same overall risk as treated patients whose BP was controlled both in the office and at home (HR, 1.16; $P = 0.45$).

   Moreover, WCH has been associated with an "intermediate phenotype" between normotension and hypertension as it pertains to left ventricular mass, carotid intima-media thickness, aortic pulse wave velocity, and albuminuria.[133] However, there are no data available to demonstrate that patients with WCH benefit from drug therapy. Therefore, it appears that WCH may not be as benign as previously considered, and patients should be advised on general lifestyle changes to improve BP levels and overall vascular risk, especially as their risk for progressing to sustained hypertension is approximately 40% after 10 years of follow-up.[134]

   Masked hypertension, conversely, consists of normal BP in the office but high BP in the ambulatory setting, with an estimated prevalence of 10% to 15% in population studies. It has been consistently and strongly associated with increased risk for adverse CV end points and mortality, to a level that is indistinguishable from that associated with sustained hypertension.[132] The very existence of masked hypertension is troublesome, as its identification is only possible with BP measurement in the out-of-office environment. This finding has important public policy implications related to screening that remain unresolved at this time.

   Because WCH and masked hypertension afflict such a substantial number of patients and have diametrically different impact on outcomes, their identification improves outcome prediction in patients with hypertension.

3. The ability to evaluate BP during sleep was a characteristic until now restricted to ABPM, though newer home BP monitors can be programmed for activation during sleep. In some, but not all, studies nighttime BP is a better marker of CV disease than daytime or 24-hour-average BP.[129,135,136] The importance of nighttime BP (compared with daytime levels) appears greater among treated patients, perhaps because antihypertensive treatment, often taken in the morning, might result in better BP control during the day than during the night.[136]

   The pattern of BP fluctuation between day and night also associates with prognosis. The normal circadian BP pattern includes a fall in BP of approximately 15% to

20% during sleep. Patients who lack this normal BP dip during sleep are called "nondippers" (arbitrarily defined as a sleep BP that falls by less than 10% compared with awake levels) and have increased target-organ damage and overall CV risk. In large observational studies, patients whose systolic BP falls by 20% or more during the night have lower fatal and nonfatal CV event rates than those whose BP decreases by less than 20%, while those whose BP does not fall at all during the night have significantly worse CV outcomes than all other patients.[137]

4. ABPM also provides information on BP variability throughout the day, which may add further prognostic information. Increased BP variability (measured as the standard deviation of BP) has been associated with increased event rates, though these findings are of small magnitude when taken independently from BP values.[138]

Despite these observations, objective evidence demonstrating that outcomes are better when patients are managed using an out-of-office method is lacking. Three randomized clinical trials have compared management of hypertension with office or out-of-office BP, one using 24-hour ABPM[139] and two using home BP.[37,140] All of these studies showed that more patients managed with out-of-office methods could have treatment stopped or de-escalated, thus resulting in marginal cost savings. However, none of them could demonstrate the superiority of ABPM or home BP in achieving better BP control (the primary outcome of all three trials) or less LVH (evaluated in all studies as a secondary outcome).

CLINICAL USE OF AMBULATORY AND HOME BLOOD PRESSURE MONITORING

ABPM has been in clinical use for almost 50 years. In the United States, problems related to limited reimbursement have significantly limited its expansion compared with other parts of the world. Despite this limitation, there is general agreement on its value in several clinical circumstances, as outlined in Table 47.4.

ABPM is performed, typically, over a period of 24 hours, although it can be extended for longer periods (e.g., 48 hours) in order to provide information covering more than one wake/sleep cycle, or to cover a specific period in detail, such as a 2-day interdialytic period for a patient undergoing hemodialysis. Clinicians should use an independently validated monitor (for a list, refer to www.dableducational.org). A typical measurement interval is every 20 minutes during the daytime (7 AM to 11 PM) and every 30 minutes at night (11 PM to 7 AM), though the frequency and time windows can be adjusted based on clinical needs, such as the need to identify frequent BP swings, atypical sleep patterns, etc. Patients should keep a log of activities during the day, the time of retiring to bed and waking up, and time of taking vasoactive medications (if applicable). It is preferred that the periods designated as "night" and "day" reflect the actual periods of sleep and wakefulness obtained from the patient's diary. Most patients tolerate the procedure well, although sometimes sleep is compromised (<10% of cases), and, rarely, patients have excessive bruising or discomfort from the frequent cuff inflations. Up-to-date instructions on how to perform and interpret ABPM studies are available in guideline format from the European Society of Hypertension.

Home BP is performed by the patient in the home (or sometimes work) environment. It is used commonly in clinical practice and is associated with improved adherence to therapy. It has also been used successfully for treatment self-titration of BP medications and is amenable to telemedicine approaches, in which the patient can upload BP values via telephone or direct entry to a Web server so that clinicians can inspect the BP logs and make treatment decisions remotely.

Just as with office BP, it is important that the equipment fits the patient well and that measurements are obtained using the same technique as outlined earlier for office BP. Independently validated devices are listed at www.dableducational.org; unfortunately, many of the marketed devices have not been independently validated. The preferred devices use arm cuffs. Finger cuffs are inaccurate, and wrist cuffs often provide incorrect readings because of inappropriate technique. As a result, only arm devices are recommended by current guidelines.[10,141]

In order to allow management decisions, home BP monitoring is best performed using specific periods of monitoring. For most patients, a BP log obtained over 7 days before each office visit suffices, as it retains excellent

Table 47.4 Indications for 24-Hour Ambulatory and Home Blood Pressure Monitoring

Indication	Home BP Monitoring	ABPM	Comment
Identify white coat hypertension	++	+++	ABPM still the gold-standard when patients have home BP values that are "borderline" (125-135/80-85 mm Hg)
Identify masked hypertension	++	+++	
Identify true resistant hypertension	++	+++	
Evaluate borderline office BP values without target-organ damage	++	+++	
Evaluate nocturnal hypertension	—	+++	
Evaluate labile hypertension	++	++	Home BP better for infrequent symptoms or paroxysms; ABPM better if frequent within a 24-hr period
Evaluate hypotensive symptoms	+++	++	
Evaluate autonomic dysfunction	+	++	Home BP useful to monitor orthostatic hypotension; ABPM useful to quantify supine hypertension and determine overall (average) BP levels
Clinical research (treatment, prognosis)	++	+++	

ABPM, Ambulatory blood pressure monitoring; BP, blood pressure.

Table 47.5	Normative Values for ABPM and Home Blood Pressure Monitoring	
	Blood Pressure Equivalent to Office Blood Pressure of	
	120/80 mm Hg	140/90 mm Hg
24-Hour Ambulatory BP Monitoring		
24-hour BP	117/74 mm Hg	131/79 mm Hg
Awake BP	122/79 mm Hg	138/86 mm Hg
Sleep BP	101/65 mm Hg	120/71 mm Hg
Home BP Monitoring		
Average BP*	121/78 mm Hg	133/82 mm Hg

*Average of all values during the monitoring period, usually 7 days.
Normative data based on equivalent of cardiovascular event rates observed at each level of office BP.
ABPM, Ambulatory blood pressure monitoring; BP, blood pressure.
Data from reference 142 and Kikuya M et al: Diagnostic thresholds for ambulatory blood pressure monitoring based on 10-year cardiovascular risk. Circulation 115;2145-2152, 2007.

reproducibility.[141] We recommended that the patient obtain readings in duplicate (approximately 1 minute apart), twice daily (in the morning before taking medications and in the evening before dinner). In selected situations, more frequent or more prolonged monitoring may be needed. For example, patients with hypotensive symptoms may benefit from BP measurements during peak action of medications, such as in the mid to late morning or late evening, depending on the time when medications are taken. Likewise, patients with labile BP can be monitored more often in order to capture the overall BP variability better, though we prefer to use ABPM in such patients. As for ABPM, detailed home BP guidelines are available from the European Society of Hypertension[141] and the American Heart Association.[10]

Normative values for the interpretation of ABPM and home BP results are available based on observed outcomes in longitudinal studies[142] (Table 47.5). For ease of use, these thresholds were matched to specific office BP levels at which the observed rate of CV events was the same, thus allowing clinicians to relate to office values that have historically driven clinical decisions. For ABPM, other measures such as the nocturnal dip, early morning surge (magnitude of BP rise during the first hours post awakening), BP load (percentage of time BP remains above a certain threshold, such as 140/90 mm Hg during the day and 120/80 mm Hg during the night), and overall BP variability (standard deviation of the 24-hour BP or awake BP), were not studied in relationship to hard outcomes for precise normative results.

LABORATORY AND OTHER COMPLEMENTARY TESTS

Similar to the history and physical examination, laboratory tests, imaging, and other complementary tests also focus on the evaluation of comorbid conditions, established target-organ damage, and possible secondary causes. In the absence of worrisome signs or symptoms during the initial evaluation, the clinician should obtain a basic set of tests, including renal function; levels of electrolytes, calcium, glucose, and hemoglobin; lipid profile, urinalysis, and electrocardiogram (Table 47.6).

Further testing may be required in case any of these initial test results are abnormal or in case there are specific symptoms or physical findings suggesting a diagnosis (see "Secondary Hypertension" section). Likewise, patients who are resistant to treatment during follow-up have higher rates of secondary causes of hypertension, in particular sleep apnea, hyperaldosteronism, and renovascular disease, thus deserving a more dedicated search for secondary causes in their evaluation.

ECHOCARDIOGRAPHY

LVH is the most common target-organ damage in hypertension and is independently associated with worse prognosis, marked by increased risk for CV events (coronary, cerebrovascular), heart failure, and death.[143] The electrocardiogram is very specific but insensitive for the detection of LVH. Not surprisingly, the prevalence of LVH among patients with hypertension is only approximately 18% based on electrocardiographic criteria, whereas this number increases to approximately 40% when more sensitive echocardiographic criteria are used. The echocardiogram also provides information on left ventricular diastolic function, which is often impaired early in the course of hypertensive heart disease and does not require the presence of LVH. Finally, it allows assessment of left ventricular systolic dysfunction, which is uncommonly present in hypertension (approximately 4%) but is associated with worse prognosis. Even though echocardiography is not recommended as a routine test in patients with hypertension, it often provides important information to help guide treatment, such as defining the need to initiate or escalate treatment in patients with borderline office or ambulatory BP levels.

EVALUATION OF SODIUM AND POTASSIUM INTAKE

Because of the importance of sodium and potassium as dietary interventions in hypertension, it is often useful to quantify intake objectively. Diary recall is the most often used method in clinical practice; however, it is often problematic because many patients have difficulty defining portions. In situations where detailed knowledge of sodium and potassium intake is important to management, our practice is to obtain a 24-hour urine collection to evaluate sodium and potassium on a stable diet. These ions are measured in milliequivalents per day, then converted to dietary target in milligrams per day (1 mEq of sodium = 23 mg of sodium or 58 mg of "salt" as NaCl, and 1 mEq of potassium = 39 mg of potassium). A diuretic can be maintained as long as the dose has been stable over time. One must recognize that sodium excretion may follow a circaseptan rhythm[60] and may therefore be imprecise on a single 24-hour collection, but it is still valuable as a general guide to allow more precise dietary advice to patients.

RENIN PROFILING

The evaluation of plasma renin activity has been proposed by Laragh as an empiric method for the evaluation and

Table 47.6 Initial Laboratory Evaluation of the Hypertensive Patient to Investigate the Presence of Comorbid Conditions, Secondary Causes, or Established Target-Organ Damage

Test	Clinical Usefulness
Serum creatinine (and estimated glomerular filtration rate)	Assessment of renal function. Identifies parenchymal kidney disease as a possible secondary cause as well as established TOD.
Serum potassium	Low potassium (of renal origin) suggests mineralocorticoid excess (primary or secondary), glucocorticoid excess, Liddle's syndrome. High potassium with normal renal function suggests Gordon's syndrome. Low levels raise caution about the use of thiazides and loop diuretics. High levels preclude the use of ACEIs, ARBs, renin inhibitors, and potassium-sparing diuretics.
Serum sodium	If high, suggests primary aldosteronism. If low, alerts to the need to avoid thiazide diuretics.
Serum bicarbonate	If high, suggests aldosterone excess (primary or secondary). If low with normal renal function, suggests Gordon's syndrome (with high potassium) or primary hyperparathyroidism (with high calcium).
Serum calcium	If high, suggests primary hyperparathyroidism.
Serum glucose	Identifies prediabetes or diabetes. In the appropriate setting, suggests glucocorticoid excess, pheochromocytoma, or acromegaly.
Lipid profile	Identifies hyperlipidemia.
Hemoglobin/hematocrit	If high, in the absence of other hematologic abnormalities or underlying lung disease, suggests sleep apnea.
Urinalysis*	Proteinuria and hematuria identify a possible secondary cause (glomerulonephritis). Proteinuria can also be a marker of TOD.
Electrocardiogram	Identifies left ventricular hypertrophy, old myocardial infarction, or other ischemic changes. Identifies conduction abnormalities that may preclude the use of β-blockers or nondihydropyridine CCBs.

*Some organizations recommend screening microalbuminuria as a more sensitive tool to identify early renal injury.
The most recent guidelines do not recommend BUN measurement alone.
ACEI, Angiotensin-converting enzyme inhibitor; ARB, angiotensin receptor blocker. CCB, calcium channel blocker; TOD, target-organ damage.

treatment of hypertension.[144] The premise for this approach is mechanistic: patients with high renin levels (>0.65 ng/mL/hr, and particularly >6.5 ng/mL/hr) have vasoconstriction mediated by the RAAS as the primary operative mechanism of hypertension, whereas those with suppressed renin levels (<0.65 ng/mL/hr) are volume overloaded. Accordingly, patients with high levels of renin are treated with blockers of the RAAS (ACEIs, angiotensin receptor antagonists, renin inhibitors, β-blockers), and those with low levels of renin are treated with diuretics (including aldosterone antagonists), CCBs, or α-blockers. The approach not only includes using drugs that directly address the underlying pathophysiology but also proposes removal of drugs from the opposite group as there are reports of paradoxical BP elevations in such cases.[145] A case series reported streamlined drug regimens and improved BP control in patients with resistant hypertension, and a small randomized trial of renin-guided therapy versus conventional therapy yielded greater systolic BP lowering with the renin-guided system (−29 vs. −19 mm Hg, $P = 0.03$).[146] It is reasonable to entertain renin profiling, especially in patients who do not respond to initial therapy. In such cases, renin measurement, along with plasma aldosterone measurement, will also be useful to rule out primary hyperaldosteronism.

SYSTEMIC HEMODYNAMICS AND EXTRACELLULAR FLUID VOLUME

An alternative to the renin-profiling approach is to measure systemic hemodynamics and extracellular fluid volume, noninvasively. Such measurements can be achieved with several methodologies, but impedance cardiography has the advantage of simultaneously obtaining both volume (thoracic fluid content) and hemodynamic (CO, SVR) data. This approach has been used in patients with resistant hypertension with some success in two randomized trials.[147,148] In one study, patients managed using the hemodynamic approach achieved better BP control while receiving more diuretics, while in the other, control was also better but not associated with the specific extra use of any particular drug class. Direct measurement of volume excess and hemodynamics and availability of the information at the point of care make this methodology more attractive than renin profiling. However, high costs associated with the technology make the wide use of this method out of reach for most physicians and their patients.

SECONDARY HYPERTENSION

Secondary (or remediable) hypertension is elevated BP due to a specific cause.[7,8] It is worth consideration in every newly diagnosed or referred patient with hypertension, for several reasons. The proportion of patients with secondary hypertension who can eventually be cured is far greater than those with primary hypertension. This is particularly important in young hypertensive people (especially in children and adolescents),[149] who are more likely to harbor nearly all types of secondary hypertension with the important exception of atherosclerotic renovascular hypertension. For such people, and those with an otherwise long life expectancy, the cost of diagnosis and treatment (and even "cure") of secondary hypertension may be less than the cost of chronic medical therapy (including drugs, office visits, and laboratory monitoring). Lastly, it is intellectually appealing to consider the possibility of "cure" for patients with hypertension, which not only keeps the health care provider mentally awake, but also may help to avoid "failure to diagnose" torts in patients who actually harbor a secondary cause, but its presence is never contemplated or formally evaluated.

RISK FACTORS AND EPIDEMIOLOGY

In general clinical practice, there is a higher probability of secondary hypertension in patients: (1) with higher levels of untreated blood pressure (except primary hyperaldosteronism), (2) with characteristic physical signs (for details, see later), (3) with refractory hypertension (now more commonly called *resistant hypertension*, and defined as a patient who, despite proper doses of three appropriately chosen antihypertensive drugs, one of which is a diuretic, has a persistent office blood pressure ≥ 140/90 mm Hg[5]), or (4) seen in tertiary referral centers (largely due to "referral bias"). Because of these factors, the prevalence of secondary hypertension varies widely.

The largest prospective study reported from a primary care setting evaluated 1020 consecutive patients with hypertension in Yokohama, Japan. The authors found 9.1% of patients had a secondary cause, which was primary hyperaldosteronism in 6%, Cushing's syndrome (full-blown in 1% and preclinical in 1%), pheochromocytoma (0.6%), and renovascular hypertension (0.5%).[150]

The largest series of consecutive patients evaluated by a whole-day protocol from 1976 to 1994 in a tertiary referral center came from Syracuse, New York. In this study, 10.1% of 4429 patients with hypertension had secondary hypertension: 3.1% with renovascular hypertension, 1.4% with primary hyperaldosteronism, 0.5% with Cushing's syndrome, 0.3% with pheochromocytoma, 3% with primary hypothyroidism, and 1.8% with hypertension attributed to CKD.[151] Later series from all over the globe have suggested that primary hyperaldosteronism (especially due to sleep-disordered breathing and obstructive sleep apnea) is far more common than it was before the year 2000, with an average prevalence of approximately 10% to 11.2% in population-based studies[152]; its prevalence is approximately twice that in resistant hypertension. These estimates have been based largely on a single determination of the plasma aldosterone/renin ratio (discussed later) and probably represent an overestimate of the prevalence.

EVALUATION OF SECONDARY HYPERTENSION

Hypertension guidelines and a great deal of clinical experience suggest a more detailed evaluation for secondary causes in patients with hypertension younger than 30 years who have no family history of hypertension. Additionally, those older than 55 years with new-onset hypertension, sudden worsening of BP control (despite years of previously controlled BP levels), recurrent flash pulmonary edema, an abdominal bruit (especially with a louder diastolic component), and sudden increases of serum creatinine level by 30% or more after a blocker of the RAAS should prompt evaluation for secondary causes of hypertension. Such patients have a higher pretest probability of renovascular hypertension.

The initial set of laboratory tests recommended for newly diagnosed patients with hypertension includes serum levels of blood urea nitrogen and creatinine and a urinalysis, which is generally sufficient for identifying patients with underlying intrinsic renal disease, even if the 3-month criterion for CKD is not yet met (see Table 47.6).

Either hyperthyroidism or hypothyroidism can be a cause of hypertension, but the presence of either is detected commonly with a serum ultrasensitive thyroid-stimulating hormone (thyrotropin) level.

Sometimes the demographic and clinical features of the patient help direct the search for a secondary cause: Fibromuscular dysplasia is much more common in young white women, whereas atherosclerotic renovascular disease is more common in older smokers (both current and former). Some symptoms, when elicited by a careful history, are also quite suggestive (although incompletely sensitive and not very specific).

Classically, paroxysmal "spells" occur in approximately 25% to 30% of patients with pheochromocytoma; the associated symptoms are variable across patients but commonly experienced repetitively in a given patient. Sadly, the specificity of these paroxysms, even when they include headache, sweating, and elevated BP levels, is less than 5% in most large series. Similarly, the classical symptoms of large muscle weakness (particularly when rising from a chair or climbing stairs) reported with Cushing's syndrome, or lower extremity weakness and leg cramps reported in primary hyperaldosteronism and attributed to hypokalemia, are uncommon in today's literature and patients. Given the relatively low prevalence of secondary hypertension, the decision to undertake a formal evaluation for specific causes can (and should) be individualized.

EXACERBATION OF PREEXISTING HYPERTENSION DUE TO LIFESTYLE FACTORS

Although generally not considered in most discussions of secondary (or remediable) hypertension, BP can be influenced by prescription or nonprescription medications or both,[153] excessive dietary sodium intake,[154] body weight/obesity, and excessive alcohol intake.[8] The health care provider or the patient may not immediately appreciate some of these factors. Appropriate attention to these issues can result in improved BP profiles and a better prognosis.[155]

Modification of these factors is the cornerstone of therapy for primary hypertension and can mimic secondary hypertension. Of these factors, the most common issues relate to excessive sodium intake, poor sleep hygiene (i.e., getting less than 6 hours of uninterrupted sleep a night),[156] and excessive caffeine or other stimulants, as well as use of nonsteroidal antiinflammatory drugs (NSAIDs).

INTRINSIC KIDNEY DISEASE

Hypertension can be both a cause and a consequence of CKD (i.e., estimated GFR [eGFR] < 60 mL/min/1.73 m^2). It is often difficult to discern which occurred first when a patient presents initially with both, but the screening and diagnostic processes are identical to those used for each individually. The diagnosis of hypertension requires repeated, correctly taken measurements in adults showing BP of 140/90 mm Hg or higher (amended to ≥ 150/90 mm Hg for those over age 60 years by the 2014 expert panel).¹² CKD is currently diagnosed using the 2012 Kidney Disease: Improving Global Outcomes (KDIGO) criteria from the National Kidney Foundation: persistent (≥3 months) evidence of kidney damage (e.g., proteinuria, abnormal urinary sediment, abnormal blood or urine chemistry levels, imaging studies, or biopsy), but primarily based on the eGFR.[157] Although it is possible to have CKD with eGFR above 60 mL/min/1.73 m², most authorities recommend this threshold for common use. Management strategies for hypertension due to CKD are also identical to those used in primary hypertension except that doses and frequency of antihypertensive (and other) medications normally cleared by the kidney are decreased inversely to the eGFR. While most antihypertensive drugs do not need dose adjustments in stage 3b or higher CKD, some agents that affect the RAAS mechanistically need reduction. Specifically, the β-blockers, atenolol, bisoprolol, nadolol, and acebutolol need dose reductions to avoid toxicity. Additionally, all ACEIs except for fosinopril and trandolapril need dose reductions since they are all renally excreted. However, no serious adverse effects other than possibly hyperkalemia have occurred with not adjusting ACEI dosing.

Restriction of dietary protein intake was recommended in the distant past, based on several small trials (primarily in Australia), but had marginal success in the Modification of Diet in Renal Disease trial,[158] and is usually challenging to carry out effectively, even in tertiary centers with a dedicated renal nutritionist. Dietary sodium restriction, although somewhat a lesser challenge, has benefits in patients with CKD and hypertension, not only to lower BP, but also to reduce urinary protein (and albumin) excretion.[31]

PRIMARY HYPERALDOSTERONISM

This form of secondary hypertension has been increasing in prevalence worldwide over the last 25 years[152] and is generally due to one of six subtypes: (1) an aldosterone-producing ("Conn's") adenoma, nearly always in one adrenal gland (approximately 35% of cases); (2) bilateral adrenal hyperplasia (also known as "idiopathic primary hyperaldosteronism," approximately 60% of cases); (3) primary (or unilateral) adrenal hyperplasia (approximately 2% of cases); (4) aldosterone-producing adrenal carcinoma (approximately 35 cases in the world's literature); (5) familial hyperaldosteronism, which takes one of two forms: glucocorticoid-suppressible hyperaldosteronism, due to a chimeric chromosome 8, in which the 5′-regulatory sequence for corticotropin responsiveness of 11β-hydroxylase is fused to the enzyme coding sequence for aldosterone synthase (<1% of cases), or familial occurrences of either an aldosterone-producing adenoma or bilateral adrenal hyperplasia (<2% of cases); or (6) ectopic production of aldosterone by an adenoma or carcinoma outside the adrenal gland (< 0.1% of cases). In addition, obstructive sleep apnea and sleep-disordered breathing often cause hyperaldosteronism. This is classically described as secondary hyperaldosteronism, but its evaluation and medical treatment are often quite similar to that of bilateral adrenal hyperplasia.

The prevalence of primary hyperaldosteronism depends on where and how one looks and is controversial. Some referral centers report a prevalence of hyperaldosteronism related to sleep apnea at approximately 20%, similar to the original prevalence of aldosterone-secreting adenomas estimated by Conn in the 1950s. In large population-based studies the prevalence of primary hyperaldosteronism has been estimated at approximately 10% to 11.2% of hypertensives. The condition appears to be more common in people with higher levels of BP (2% for BP levels 140-159/90-99 mm Hg, 8% for BP levels 160-179/100-109 mm Hg, and 13% for BP levels > 180/110 mm Hg), treatment-resistant hypertension (17% to 23% in several series), patients with hypertension with either spontaneous or diuretic-associated hypokalemia, and hypertension and a serendipitously discovered adrenal mass (1% to 10%).

In the last millennium, hypokalemia was thought to be very common (if not nearly universal) among patients with primary hyperaldosteronism, particularly if provoked by diuretic therapy. Today, however, more afflicted patients have eukalemia than hypokalemia, although sometimes more severe cases have weakness, muscle cramps, and even periodic paralysis. Patients with primary hyperaldosteronism experience higher CV morbidity and mortality than age-, gender-, and BP-matched patients with primary hypertension.[43]

Screening for primary hyperaldosteronism is most efficiently performed in potassium-repleted patients using the ratio of plasma aldosterone concentration to plasma renin activity (ARR). The ARR can be affected by many factors, including antihypertensive drug therapy, dietary sodium restriction, posture, time of day, and sample handling (Table 47.7). Most authorities recommend sustained-release verapamil, hydralazine, and peripheral α₁-adrenoceptor antagonists as medications that have little, if any, effect on the ARR. The likelihood of a false-positive ARR is increased by a low plasma renin activity (e.g., <0.5 ng of angiotensin II per milliliter per hour), so some investigators require the plasma aldosterone concentration to be above a given threshold (e.g., >15 ng/dL), for the screening to be considered positive. The most common cutoff value for an ARR that usually leads to further investigation is 30 (when aldosterone level is measured in nanograms per deciliter and plasma renin activity in nanograms of angiotensin II per milliliter per hour), but higher thresholds lead to more falsely negative tests.

Clinical practice guidelines from the Endocrine Society recommend one of four confirmatory tests before proceeding to an imaging study, because of the expense and radiation involved in the latter. There are only a few comparative studies of these four tests; they seem to have similar performance characteristics (75% to 90% sensitivity, 80% to 100% specificity). Cost, patient preference, local experience, local laboratory methods, and insurance reimbursement all factor into which confirmatory test is chosen.

The traditional "saline-loading test" (2 L infused over 4 hours) is confirmatory if the postinfusion plasma aldosterone concentration is greater than 10 ng/mL, but intravenous saline is not often recommended for patients with heart failure, CKD, or uncontrolled hypertension.

Many centers have reported success with an oral sodium-loading protocol, which involves liberalizing sodium intake to approximately 6 gm/day for 3 to 5 days and then assaying 24-hour urine collections for sodium (to ensure loading) and aldosterone content. The test is considered positive if the urinary aldosterone excretion is greater than 12 to

Table 47.7 Factors That May Cause False-Positive or False-Negative Results of the Aldosterone/Renin Ratio

	False Positives	False Negatives
Aldosterone relatively high Renin relatively low	Potassium loading β-Blockers Central antiadrenergics Direct renin inhibitors Nonsteroidal antiinflammatory drugs Chronic kidney disease Sodium loading	
Aldosterone relatively low Renin relatively high		Hypokalemia Diuretics ACE inhibitors, angiotensin receptor blockers Calcium channel blockers (dihydropyridines) Acute sodium depletion

ACE, Angiotensin-converting enzyme.

14 μg/day, but oral sodium loading can be as problematic in some patients as intravenous saline.

The fludrocortisone suppression test involves giving 0.1 mg of fludrocortisone every 6 hours for 4 days, and then assaying the plasma aldosterone concentration when the patient is standing upright. It is considered confirmatory if the concentration is greater than 6 ng/dL and plasma renin activity and serum cortisol levels are low. Execution of the test may be difficult for patients who have a long journey to the office or who are nonadherent.

Lastly, the captopril challenge test is performed by assaying the plasma aldosterone concentration before and 1 and 2 hours after administration of 25 to 50 mg of oral captopril. It is considered confirmatory if the plasma aldosterone concentration remains elevated (and unchanged from baseline); many false-negative and equivocal captopril challenge test results have been reported, although several Japanese series show excellent results with this method.

After the diagnosis of primary aldosteronism is confirmed, a computed tomographic scan of the adrenals is undertaken, which is quite useful in detecting large masses that might be adrenal carcinomas. Adrenal carcinomas typically have larger size (>4 cm diameter), an inhomogeneous character (often with internal hemorrhage), internal calcifications (in approximately 40%), and irregular borders (often due to micrometastases) and show enhancement after intravenous contrast medium is administered. Aldosterone-producing adenomas are most commonly small (<2 cm diameter), hypodense, unilateral nodules. Idiopathic hyperaldosteronism usually has normal-appearing adrenal glands, but sometimes nodular changes or general enlargement are visible in one or both adrenals. Magnetic resonance imaging is no better at detecting these abnormalities than computed tomography, which is usually less expensive. Both techniques often detect nonfunctioning nodules, especially in older patients. At some centers, patients with hypertension with proven primary hyperaldosteronism younger than 40 years of age with a single typical hypodense nodule in one adrenal gland are directly offered an adrenalectomy.

Because computed tomographic scans identify unilateral adrenal disease with a sensitivity of only 78% and specificity of only 75%, the Endocrine Society recommends adrenal venous sampling for most surgical candidates. Despite being invasive, expensive, technically challenging, and potentially dangerous and requiring an experienced and well-coordinated team, it has sensitivity and specificity of 95% and 100% for detecting unilateral aldosterone production. It is most often performed at 8 AM, with continuous cosyntropin administration, and simultaneous adrenal vein cortisol level measurement. Most centers use a 4:1 cutoff value of the cortisol-corrected aldosterone ratio to define a positive lateralization.

Several older (some would prefer "classical") tests remain available for the presumably rare circumstance in which adrenal venous sampling was technically unsuccessful or nondiagnostic; these are usually much less expensive and therefore can sometimes be preauthorized when financial and other roadblocks are erected to adrenal venous sampling. The postural stimulation test, developed in the 1970s, depends on the propensity of patients with an aldosterone-producing adenoma to retain diurnal variation in the plasma aldosterone concentration, whereas those with idiopathic hyperaldosteronism often show an increased sensitivity to small increases in angiotensin II levels (e.g., after standing). In some centers, this test is performed by drawing two additional blood samples (before and after standing) at the conclusion of the intravenous saline infusion test. In a review of the Mayo Clinic experience from the last millennium in 246 patients with surgically proven adenomas, the test was only 85% accurate.

Iodocholesterol scintigraphy was developed at the University of Michigan in the 1970s; its sensitivity correlates directly with tumor size, so it is not very helpful in discerning microadenomas from bilateral hyperplasia. Serum 18-hydroxycorticosterone levels, typically measured in the recumbent position at 08:00 are often higher than 100 ng/dL in patients with an adenoma, but the opposite is true in patients with bilateral hyperplasia, so blood was traditionally taken for this analyte before the 2-L saline infusion test. However, the accuracy of this test was even lower than the postural stimulation test.

Testing for familial forms of primary hyperaldosteronism is recommended for those who are younger than 20 years of age at diagnosis and in those with a family history of primary aldosteronism or stroke at an early age (typically <30 years of age). This strategy was successful in approximately half of large, qualifying, unrelated cohorts. Genetic testing by either Southern blot or long polymerase chain reaction techniques is both sensitive and specific for glucocorticoid-remediable hyperaldosteronism (familial hyperaldosteronism, type I, the most common monogenetic cause of hypertension). Such testing is expensive; so many managed care organizations will not pay for the test unless an appropriate response (in both BP and plasma aldosterone concentration) is seen after weeks of empirical glucocorticoid administration. Familial hyperaldosteronism type II is genetically heterogeneous, despite being autosomal dominant in most affected cases. Genetic testing is not yet available for this more common type of familial hyperaldosteronism, so the diagnosis is primarily clinical, based on the biochemical findings and the pedigree.

Laparoscopic procedures for unilateral adrenalectomy have improved to the point that most patients with adrenal venous sampling–proven hyperaldosteronism have shorter hospital stays, fewer complications, and lower costs than open procedures. Although nearly all return to eukalemia, hypertension is "cured" (i.e., follow-up BP levels of <140/90 mm Hg without antihypertensive drug therapy) in only approximately 50%. This is more likely in younger people, those with a short duration of hypertension, prior BP control with only one or two agents, and a family history of hypertension that includes no first-degree relatives or only one. Typically, plasma aldosterone concentration and plasma renin activity are measured shortly after successful surgery, and potassium supplementation and aldosterone antagonists are discontinued. Intravenous saline is often required, as the remaining adrenal gland recovers its normal function (which may take a few weeks). The nonsurgical option for patients with idiopathic hyperaldosteronism is spironolactone, which had significantly better efficacy than its successor, eplerenone, in an international randomized clinical trial in hypertensive subjects with primary aldosteronism. Most physicians use dexamethasone or prednisone at bedtime (over twice-daily hydrocortisone) for glucocorticoid-remediable hyperaldosteronism, but the doses are kept low to avoid iatrogenic Cushing's syndrome (see later).

HYPERALDOSTERONISM ASSOCIATED WITH SLEEP-DISORDERED BREATHING

Several publications have highlighted this association, which is thought to account for approximately 20% of resistant hypertension and typically responds very nicely to selective aldosterone antagonists. The ratio of serum aldosterone to plasma renin activity is most often used to diagnose the condition, and (if the Berlin questionnaire or a sleep study is sufficiently suggestive) is often followed by a therapeutic trial of spironolactone.

MINERALOCORTICOID EXCESS STATES

Several unusual diagnoses manifest with a similar set of signs and symptoms (especially hypokalemia and often other cushingoid features) that result from an apparent mineralocorticoid excess. These are most easily distinguished from the several types of hyperaldosteronism by the suppressed plasma aldosterone level.

The most common type, classical congenital adrenal hyperplasia, is due to one of several autosomal recessive genetic deficiencies in enzymes involved in adrenal steroidogenesis, most often resulting in mineralocorticoid and androgen excess. Although most common in infants and children, some patients (especially those with milder loss-of-function mutations) go undiagnosed until adulthood. The most common deficiency, 21-hydroxylase, accounts for approximately 95% of cases and is often discovered by universal screening programs, particularly for female newborns with ambiguous genitalia. If left untreated, approximately 75% of such babies suffer salt wasting, failure to thrive, hyponatremia, hypovolemia, shock, and death.

Hypertension occurs in approximately two thirds of patients with congenital adrenal hyperplasia due to either 11β-hydroxylase deficiency (approximately 5% of cases of congenital adrenal hyperplasia, and a prevalence of approximately 1:100,000 in whites) or 17α-hydroxylase deficiency (which is rare). More than 40 mutations have been identified that lead to 11β-hydroxylase deficiency, which results in high circulating levels of deoxycorticosterone and 11-deoxycortisol, with increased production of adrenal androgens. Thus girls present in infancy or childhood with hypertension, hypokalemia, acne, hirsutism, and virilization; whereas boys present with pseudoprecocious puberty. Because 17α-hydroxylase is required for production of both cortisol and sex steroids, its deficiency can delay puberty and present as pseudohermaphroditism or phenotypic female features (in genetic 45, XY boys), or as primary amenorrhea in girls. After appropriate diagnosis (typically by determination of levels of steroid precursors in serum), patients with congenital adrenal hyperplasia receive supplementation with glucocorticoids, which suppress corticotropin secretion, and reduction of the signs and symptoms of mineralocorticoid excess. Long-term care of adults with congenital adrenal hyperplasia is challenging.

Very rare causes of mineralocorticoid excess include deoxycorticosterone-producing tumors (which are usually quite large and often malignant), primary cortisol resistance, or 11β-hydroxysteroid dehydrogenase deficiency (of which approximately 50 cases worldwide are congenital; most are acquired and associated with imported licorice or licorice-flavored chewing tobacco). Some would also include Liddle's syndrome (hypertension, hypokalemia, and inappropriate kaliuresis, associated with low plasma aldosterone and renin activity), due to an autosomal dominant condition that results in mutations in the β- or γ-subunits of the renal amiloride-sensitive ENaC.

RENOVASCULAR HYPERTENSION

Hypertension due to renal artery stenosis (fibromuscular dysplasia or atherosclerotic disease) has been heavily studied since the pioneering work of Harry Goldblatt. The probability of renovascular hypertension can be calculated, based on clinical characteristics in a given patient, which eliminates the need for a screening test in most cases. The choice among the several screening tests for renovascular hypertension is usually based on patient and physician preference, local expertise, and a favorable decision about prior authorization for the test from insurance companies, which has become less common since the publication of several outcome studies that showed no significant benefit to renal angioplasty (usually with stenting) over medical management in atherosclerotic renal artery disease.[159]

PHEOCHROMOCYTOMA

Although chromaffin tumors (pheochromocytomas and paragangliomas) that secrete catecholamines are rare (estimated incidence: 2 to 8 cases per million per year), their diagnosis and management are important because they can possibly cause fatal hypertensive crises (despite otherwise appropriate treatment), probably more than 10% are metastatic at diagnosis, specific therapy can be curative, and a much higher proportion of cases are heredofamilial than once thought.

Catecholamine-secreting tumors are found in 0.2% to 0.6% of patients with hypertension, may be more common in hypertensive children (1.7%), and are too often found incidentally, or worse, only at autopsy. The clinical presentation of patients with these tumors is quite variable, as symptoms may occur constantly or in paroxysms. The classical triad of headache, sweating attacks, and hypertension was said to be present in 95% of patients in one large French series, but most centers report having to see more than 100 such patients on referral before one is positively diagnosed.

The differential diagnosis includes many disorders, some of which are functional or factitious, so a high index of suspicion is required, even when faced with common admitting conditions (e.g., heart failure, which can be precipitated, if not exacerbated, by a functioning tumor). Some heredofamilial conditions that include pheochromocytoma have characteristic physical signs (e.g., café au lait spots and neurofibromas, retinal hemangiomas, port-wine stains, subungual fibromas, ash leaf or shagreen patches, adenoma sebaceum, marfanoid body habitus) that provide clues to the underlying syndromes.

There seem to be more "exceptions" to pheochromocytoma than with many other conditions: approximately 10% of such tumors are extraadrenal, multiple or bilateral, recurrent (after surgical extirpation), discovered as "incidentalomas," or in children; more than 10% are likely heredofamilial or metastatic at presentation (and both of these have increased in the last 30 years). Although approximately 90% of pheochromocytomas are found in or in close proximity to an adrenal gland, paragangliomas can occur anywhere along the sympathetic ganglia, but most commonly in or near the organ of Zuckerkandl (at the aortic bifurcation) or near the bladder (which gives rise to rather unusual symptoms of "micturition headache," syncope, or the like).

Pheochromocytomas play important parts in the multiple endocrine neoplasia (MEN) syndromes, especially MEN2A (pheochromocytoma in approximately 50%—usually bilateral, medullary carcinoma of the thyroid, parathyroid adenomas, and cutaneous lichen amyloidosis, associated with the *RET* proto-oncogene), and MEN2B (usually bilateral pheochromocytomas, medullary carcinoma of the thyroid, submucosal neuromas, hyperplastic corneal nerves, joint laxity, Hirschsprung's disease, and sometimes marfanoid body habitus). Pheochromocytomas are also found in patients with phakomatoses.

Approximately 20% of patients with von Hippel–Lindau disease type 2 (retinal and/or cerebellar hemangioblastomas, occasionally with clear cell renal carcinoma, pancreatic neuroendocrine tumors, retinal angiomas or hemangioblastomas, mediated by the *VHL* tumor suppressor gene, located on chromosome 3p25-26) will have pheochromocytomas or paragangliomas. Approximately 2% of patients with neurofibromatosis type 1 (autosomal dominant von Recklinghausen's disease: neurofibromas, with café au lait spots, axillary and/or inguinal freckling, hamartomas of the iris—Lisch nodules, bony abnormalities, central nervous system gliomas, and sometimes macrocephaly, or cognitive deficits, mediated by the *NF1* tumor-suppressor gene on chromosome 17q11.2) will develop a catecholamine-secreting tumor, usually an adrenal pheochromocytoma. Both of these conditions can be diagnosed using genetic screening, although this is often more fruitful for screening family members after an index case has been identified.

Neither the prevalence nor the genetics of pheochromocytoma in Sturge-Weber syndrome (choroidal and leptomeningeal angiomas, port-wine stain in the trigeminal distribution) or tuberous sclerosis (sometimes called Bourneville's or Pringle's disease: adenoma sebaceum, subungual fibromas, and occasionally mental retardation) are as well understood. Familial paraganglioma is an autosomal dominant syndrome with paragangliomas in the skull base and neck, thorax, abdomen, pelvis, or urinary bladder wall; much work in the last 2 decades has characterized mutations in one of several genes that code for components of the mitochondrial succinate dehydrogenase complex: *SDHD*, located on chromosome 11q23, or *SDHB*, located on chromosome 1p35-36. Availability of genetic testing for these mutations has made disease surveillance for those who carry these genes (typically relatives of index cases) much simpler.

The process of case finding for catecholamine-secreting tumors typically begins with biochemical testing for catecholamine metabolites. Measurements of plasma-free or urinary fractionated metanephrines are most commonly recommended, but a wide variety of factors are known to produce both false-positive and false-negative results. In some centers, plasma-free metanephrines (which provide a very brief "snapshot" of catecholamine production and metabolism) can be assayed quickly and accurately; in others, integration of catecholamine production and metabolism over a longer time period is less expensively performed using urinary collections. False-negative urinary collections are common in patients with pheochromocytomas that are familial, normotensive, dopamine β-hydroxylase deficient, or intermittently secreting. Pharmacologic testing for pheochromocytoma is occasionally used in equivocal cases; clonidine suppression testing is usually preferred over glucagon stimulation testing, although most managed care organizations recommend a repeat plasma or urinary collection 6 or more months after the initial evaluation.

To improve cost-effectiveness and reduce radiation exposure, imaging studies for pheochromocytoma and related tumors are generally not obtained until after biochemical evidence of catecholamine overproduction is obtained. In this setting the higher resolution available from computed tomographic scans (with thin cuts of the adrenals) outweighs the more specific finding of a T2-weighted "bright spot" on magnetic resonance imaging. For some patients (e.g., those with metastatic disease, intraabdominal surgical clips, allergies to radiocontrast media, pregnancy) magnetic resonance imaging may be a more suitable option. Positron emission tomographic scans using fluorine 18–labeled fludeoxyglucose or nuclear medicine scans using iodine 123–labeled *m*-iodobenzylguanidine (^{123}I-MIBG) can localize and define the extent of metastatic disease, especially if delivery of a ^{131}I-MIBG scan is a viable therapeutic option. Prior to performing this scan a number of antihypertensive medications must be discontinued.

The role of genetic testing in routine care of patients with pheochromocytoma is evolving; current guidelines recommend a shared decision-making process, often involving more family members than just the index patient. Eight studies have shown a high prevalence of germline mutations in patients with presumed sporadic pheochromocytoma/ganglioma, so some authorities recommend genetic screening for all afflicted patients; others base the decision on the pedigree, syndromic features, or extent of disease (multifocal, bilateral, or metastatic tumors at diagnosis).

Proper pharmacologic preparation of the patient with pheochromocytoma is critical for successful extirpation of the tumor: α-blockers (e.g., phentolamine intravenously or phenoxybenzamine orally) are given first, followed by β-blockers (if needed to control tachycardia). Most experts use a calcium antagonist before adding a β-blocker and recommend delaying the operation for 7 to 14 days after localization of the tumor, to normalize BP, heart rate, and intravascular volume, which helps minimize hypotension after removal of the tumor.

Many surgeons favor laparoscopic procedures for small adrenal pheochromocytomas or paragangliomas in accessible locations. Postoperatively, vigilant monitoring may reduce the risk for severe hypotension, hypoglycemia, or adrenal insufficiency. The diagnostic technique that originally demonstrated the overproduction of catecholamines in a given patient is usually repeated 4 to 6 weeks postoperatively to document successful tumor removal, and occasionally (often annually) during long-term follow-up. The specific frequency is best individualized, based on the pedigree, results of genetic testing, and risk factors that predict recurrence.

HYPERCORTISOLISM

Most cases of Cushing's syndrome today are iatrogenic (due to prescribed oral corticosteroids), but occasional sporadic cases are still seen and were found in 0.5% to 1.0% of hypertensive subjects in two large series. The pathophysiology of hypertension in Cushing's syndrome overlaps somewhat with mineralocorticoid excess states, since excess cortisol often overwhelms the capacity of 11β-hydroxysteroid dehydrogenase type 2 and can increase circulating levels of deoxycorticosterone, which has only mineralocorticoid activity.

The full-blown syndrome of hypertension, truncal obesity with striae, diabetes, hirsutism, acne, hyperglycemia, hypokalemia, and muscular weakness is less common today than in Cushing's era, and the recommended diagnostic sequence is much shorter as well. After an appropriate screening test (urinary free cortisol, late night salivary cortisol, or overnight dexamethasone suppression test) has positive results, an endocrine referral for a second test is recommended, before imaging studies are ordered. In some centers, plasma corticotropin levels are used to discriminate between corticotropin-dependent Cushing's syndrome (>15 pg/mL, probably 85% to 90% of cases) and corticotropin-independent Cushing's syndrome (<5 pg/mL). In the majority of the cases, dynamic testing of the hypothalamic-pituitary-adrenal axis is performed next, with either a corticotropin-releasing hormone test (which assays plasma cortisol and corticotropin levels before and after intravenous releasing hormone) or a high-dose dexamethasone (2 mg every 6 hours) suppression test (which assays serum cortisol level).

Most expert centers report that this localizes the tumor to the pituitary in 60% to 75% of the cases, a single adrenal gland in approximately 20% (split approximately 60:40 between adenomas and carcinomas), or ectopic production of corticotropin (10% to 12%, most often by small cell lung cancers), with less than 1% due to ectopic production of corticotropin-releasing hormone (typically by bronchial carcinoid tumors). Petrosal venous sinus sampling is not needed very often today. The anatomic site of hormonal overproduction is then usually approached surgically, although other modalities (e.g., radiation of the sella turcica) can be used in special circumstances. Medical therapy is also possible in some cases, especially those in which surgery is not feasible.

THYROID DYSFUNCTION

The literature about thyroid dysfunction being associated with hypertension is inconsistent.[160] Many patients with hyperthyroidism have wide pulse pressures (and therefore elevated systolic BP levels) and high pulse rates, but this is seldom missed, especially in younger patients. The ultrasensitive serum thyroid-stimulating hormone (TSH) level is widely available, and most commonly used for screening. After diagnosis, a nonselective β-blocker such as propranolol may be specifically useful, as it treats the tachycardia and hypertension and allegedly inhibits peripheral conversion of thyroxine to triiodothyronine (although some now question this "classical" clinical pharmacologic literature).

The role of hypothyroidism as a potential cause of hypertension (especially isolated diastolic) is less clear, despite the experience in upstate New York, in which 3% of patients with hypertension reverted to normotension after treatment of hypothyroidism.[151] The hypertension in hypothyroidism is predominantly diastolic and usually in the range of stage 1 (i.e., diastolic BP <99 mm Hg). In children and adolescents, especially in areas of iodide deficiency, a positive association between serum TSH and BP has been seen. A pooling of seven population-based European data sets showed similar findings in adults, but there was no consistent relationship with either a 5-year change in BP or incident hypertension. It is likely that targeted screening of patients with hypertension for hypothyroidism with determination of serum TSH level may be useful, but routine screening for all newly diagnosed patients with hypertension is not currently recommended by any set of national or international guidelines.

HYPERPARATHYROIDISM, CALCIUM INTAKE, VITAMIN D, AND HYPERTENSION

Although hypercalcemia and hypertension associated with hyperparathyroidism often improve after appropriate treatment, causal relationships between calcium and vitamin D intake, serum parathyroid hormone levels, and BP have not been consistently seen in large populations.[161] As a result, most current guidelines recommend a serum calcium (and not parathyroid hormone) determination during blood testing for patients with an initial diagnosis of hypertension.

COARCTATION OF THE AORTA

Although most discrete isthmic constrictions of the aorta occur in or near the ductus arteriosus, there is growing awareness that this fifth most common form of congenital CV disorders constitutes a spectrum of aortic and vasculopathic disorders and is not always "cured" by surgical procedures that relieve the obstruction. Most patients with the condition are hypertensive[162] and are diagnosed in infancy or childhood, but some escape detection until adulthood. Many cases are identified by suggestive physical findings (e.g., murmur, BP lower in the legs than the arms, radial-femoral pulse delay), some after imaging studies done for other reasons (e.g., rib notching or a "3" sign on chest radiograph, the latter of which results from indentation of the aorta, with prestenotic and poststenotic dilation), and others during investigation of associated abnormalities (e.g., bicuspid aortic valve).

Echocardiography is highly recommended for diagnosis and localization of the coarctation, although some patients (especially adults and those with associated anomalies) may require cardiac catheterization. Most pediatric patients undergo percutaneous catheter balloon dilation with stent placement; this can be followed by definitive surgical correction later, if needed. In a systematic review, 25% to 68% of patients with a coarctation had persistent hypertension despite satisfactory procedure results, with age at the time of surgery, age at follow-up, and the type of intervention being strong predictors of persistent hypertension.[163] A β-blocker can lower BP, and is often used in patients with coarctation, but this is not an indication approved by the U.S. Food and Drug Administration.

ACROMEGALY

Hypertension occurs in more than 40% of patients with excessive growth hormone release causing acromegaly, and it can be exacerbated by concomitant sleep apnea.[164] Most such patients are easily identified by symptoms or signs of acral bony overgrowth, particularly in children or adolescents before epiphyseal closure, although some patients ignore or tolerate these changes for a decade or more. The vast majority (98%) of cases are caused by a pituitary adenoma; serum insulin-like growth factor-1 is the most useful initial laboratory screening test, although other tests (including the response of plasma growth hormone levels to an oral 75-g glucose load and prolactin levels) are often performed.

As with coarctation, successful treatment of acromegaly usually lowers BP, but hypertension often persists, especially in older and overweight patients.[165] No specific antihypertensive drug therapy seems to be more effective than others, but because acromegaly is a very unusual cause of resistant hypertension, antihypertensive drug therapy is usually effective.

HYPERTENSIVE URGENCY AND EMERGENCY

A hypertensive emergency is the combination of elevated BP levels (with no specific diagnostic BP level) and signs or symptoms of acute, ongoing target-organ damage. Such patients are traditionally admitted to an intensive care unit and given parenteral infusions of short-acting antihypertensive agents to restore autoregulation in vascular beds. This is done because historical data from the 1920-1940 era (antedating effective antihypertensive drug therapy) showed a prognosis similar to that of many cancers. Patients who present with very elevated BP levels, but no acute, ongoing target-organ damage, were traditionally diagnosed with a "hypertensive urgency." They were observed for a few hours after treatment with one or more oral antihypertensive agents and then discharged to a site of ongoing care for their hypertension.[166] This practice is currently undertaken for medicolegal reasons, rather than prospective data showing that such treatment improves prognosis.[167]

The initial evaluation of a severely hypertensive patient includes a thorough inspection of the optic fundi (looking for acute hemorrhages, exudates, or papilledema); a mental status assessment; a careful cardiac, pulmonary, and neurologic examination; a quick search for clues that might indicate secondary hypertension (e.g., abdominal bruit, striae, radial-femoral delay); and laboratory studies to assess renal function (dipstick and microscopic urinalysis, determination of serum creatinine level).

Several options for intravenous drug treatment exist, but nitroprusside is the least expensive and most widely available. It must be kept in the dark and is metabolized to cyanide and/or thiocyanate, particularly during long-term infusions. Fenoldopam mesylate, a dopamine-1 agonist, is very effective and acutely improves several parameters of renal function. Clevidipine is a dihydropyridine (DHP) calcium antagonist that is hydrolyzed within minutes by ubiquitous serum esterases; it is administered in an emulsion containing soy and egg proteins (either of which can cause immunologic reactions in allergic patients). Clevidipine and its older, longer-acting cousin, nicardipine, are often used for patients with coronary disease, because the reflex tachycardia is usually offset by coronary vasodilation. Nimodipine is typically used only for subarachnoid hemorrhage.

The quickest therapeutic response to a hypertensive emergency is required with an acute aortic dissection. In this condition the BP should be lowered **within 20 minutes** to a systolic BP below 120 mm Hg, typically with a β-blocker (to reduce shear stress on the dissection) and a vasodilator. Controversy exists about, if, and when BP lowering is recommended in the setting of an acute ischemic stroke. If the patient is a candidate for acute thrombolytic therapy and the BP is higher than 180/110 mm Hg, acute BP lowering is recommended.

Most U.S. authorities suggested attempting slow and gradual BP lowering only if the BP is "very high" (e.g., ≥180/110 mm Hg) with a short-acting, rapidly titratable drug. However, two large, randomized trials done outside the United States suggested that BP lowering is safe but does not produce significant outcome benefits in either ischemic[168] or hemorrhagic stroke.[169]

All other types of hypertensive emergency can be handled with a gradual lowering of BP (typically 10% to 15% during the first hour and a further 10% to 20% during the next hour, for a total of approximately 25%) (Table 47.8).

Frequent monitoring of the patient's clinical status is important, because not all patients can reestablish the

Table 47.8 Various Types of Hypertensive Emergencies, Therapies, and Target Blood Pressures

Type of Emergency	Drug of Choice	Blood Pressure Target
Aortic dissection	β-Blocker plus nitroprusside*	120 mm Hg systolic in 20 min (if possible)
Cardiac		
Ischemia/infarction	Nitroglycerin, nitroprusside* nicardipine, or clevidipine	Cessation of ischemia
Heart failure (or pulmonary edema)	Nitroprusside* and/or nitroglycerin	Improvement in failure (typically only a 10%-15% decrease is required)
Hemorrhagic		
Epistaxis, gross hematuria, or threatened suture lines	Any (perhaps with anxiolytic agent)	To decrease bleeding rate (typically only 10%-15% reduction over 1-2 hr is required)
Obstetric		
Eclampsia or preeclampsia	$MgSO_4$, hydralazine, methyldopa	Typically <90 mm Hg diastolic, but often lower
Catecholamine Excess States		
Pheochromocytoma	Phentolamine	To control paroxysms
Drug withdrawal	Drug withdrawn	Typically only one dose necessary
Cocaine (and similar drugs)	Phentolamine	Typically only 10%-15% reduction over 1-2 hr
Renal		
Major hematuria or acute kidney injury	Nitroprusside,* Fenoldopam	0%-25% reduction in mean arterial pressure over 1-12 hr
Neurologic		
Hypertensive encephalopathy	Nitroprusside*	25% reduction over 2-3 hr
Acute head injury/trauma	Nitroprusside*	0%-25% reduction over 2-3 hr (controversial)

*Many physicians prefer an intravenous infusion of either clevidipine, fenoldopam, or nicardipine, none of which has potentially toxic metabolites, over nitroprusside, especially if a long duration of treatment is planned. Acute improvements in renal function occur during therapy with fenoldopam, but not with nitroprusside.

normal autoregulatory capacity of the circulation in important vascular beds during the same short time period. Because hypertensive encephalopathy is a diagnosis of exclusion, it is often very rewarding to monitor these patients closely, since their mental status improves markedly (and usually rather quickly) as the BP is carefully lowered.

Patients who present with hypertensive crises involving cardiac ischemia/infarction or pulmonary edema can be managed with nitroglycerin, clevidipine, nicardipine, or nitroprusside, although typically a combination of drugs (including an ACEI for heart failure or left ventricular systolic dysfunction) is used in these settings. Efforts to preserve myocardium and open the obstructed coronary artery (by thrombolysis, angioplasty, or surgery) also are indicated.

Hypertensive emergency involving the kidney commonly is followed by a further deterioration in renal function even when BP is lowered properly. The most important predictor of the need for acute dialysis is not the BP level, but instead the degree of renal dysfunction (both eGFR and degree of albuminuria). Some physicians prefer fenoldopam to nicardipine or nitroprusside in this setting because of its lack of toxic metabolites and specific renal vasodilating effects.[170] The need for acute dialysis often is precipitated by BP reduction in patients with preexisting stage 3 to 5 CKD, but many patients are able to avoid dialysis (and a remarkable few even discontinue it) in the long term if BP is carefully and well controlled during follow-up.

Hypertensive crises resulting from catecholamine excess states (e.g., pheochromocytoma, monoamine oxidase inhibitor crisis, cocaine intoxication) are most appropriately managed with an intravenous α-blocker (e.g., phentolamine), with a β-blocker added later, if needed. Many patients with severe hypertension caused by sudden withdrawal of antihypertensive agents (e.g., clonidine) are easily managed by giving one acute dose of the missed drug.

Hypertensive crises during pregnancy must be managed in a more careful and conservative manner because of the presence of the fetus. Magnesium sulfate, methyldopa, and hydralazine are the drugs of choice, with oral labetalol and nifedipine being drugs of second choice in the United States; nitroprusside, ACEIs, and ARBs are contraindicated.[22] Delivery of the infant is often hastened by the obstetrician to assist in management of hypertension in pregnancy.

Whether hypertensive urgencies (elevated BP, but without acute ongoing target-organ damage) require acute treatment is controversial, as there is no evidence that such treatment improves prognosis. The BP in many such patients spontaneously falls during a 30-minute period of quiet rest.

Conversely, immediate-release nifedipine capsules can cause precipitous hypotension, stroke, myocardial infarction, and death. According to the U.S. Food and Drug Administration, they "should be used with great caution, if at all." In such instances, true "hypotension" (e.g., systolic BP < 90 mm Hg) may not be observed, yet the BP may fall below the autoregulatory threshold (which is likely different for every patient, and unknown to the treating physician until it is surpassed), precipitating ischemia.

Clonidine, captopril, labetalol, several other short-acting antihypertensive drugs, and even amlodipine, have been used in this setting, but none has a clear advantage over the others, and each is usually effective in most patients. The most important aspect of managing a hypertensive urgency is to refer the patient to a good source of ongoing care for hypertension, where adherence to antihypertensive therapy during long-term follow-up will be more likely.

In short, patients presenting with a hypertensive emergency should be diagnosed quickly and started promptly on effective parenteral therapy (often nitroprusside 0.5 μg/kg/min) in an intensive care unit. BP should be reduced approximately 25% gradually over 2 to 3 hours. Oral antihypertensive therapy should be instituted, usually after approximately 8 to 24 hours of parenteral therapy; evaluation for secondary causes of hypertension may be considered after transfer from the intensive care unit. Because of advances in antihypertensive therapy and management, "malignant hypertension" is a term that should be relegated to the dustbin of history (and used only by billers and coders), as the prognosis of patients with this condition has improved greatly since the term was introduced in 1927.

CLINICAL OUTCOME TRIALS

There are hundreds of clinical studies that have evaluated the efficacy and safety of the eight different classes of antihypertensive medications. All BP-lowering agents need to have at least two appropriately powered, placebo-controlled studies to meet specific U.S. Food and Drug Administration criteria for approval as antihypertensive agents. This chapter will not focus on the details of these studies but rather on data supporting BP reductions with certain BP-lowering classes and the impact of CKD progression as well as trials evaluating CV outcomes in patients with kidney disease. This section will not be an exhaustive evaluation of all CV end point trials but rather focus on trials associated with renal outcomes or CV outcome trials with substudies in patients with kidney disease.

Meta-analyses of all commonly used antihypertensive drug classes demonstrate that, regardless of the agent used, reduction in BP corresponds to reduction in CV events if BP reduction is achieved.[171,172] This reduction in CV risk, however, is predominantly seen in people with stage 2 hypertension with much less outcome data to support risk reduction in stage 1 hypertension.

Events that drive the risk reduction are derived predominantly from reduced incidence of stroke, myocardial infarction, and heart failure. In all trials to date it is the group with the best overall BP control that has the best outcomes.[173] An exception to this generalization is Avoiding Cardiovascular Events Through Combination Therapy in Patients Living with Systolic Hypertension (ACCOMPLISH), a CV outcome trial in over 11,000 people. In this trial both groups had similar BP control, and both randomized to the same ACEI (benazepril), yet the group initially randomized to a single-pill combination of benazepril with a calcium antagonist had a 20% CV risk reduction compared to the ACEI plus diuretic group.[174] This benefit by the benazepril-amlodipine combination was extended to slowing CKD progression as well.[175]

Almost all people with an eGFR of less than 60 mL/min/1.73 m² and hypertension will require two or more medications to achieve a BP goal of less than 140/90 mm Hg. Single-pill combinations, including the matching of an RAAS blocker with either a calcium antagonist or diuretic, are preferred agents.[176] These combinations when given, generally in an additive fashion, reduce CV events and CKD progression.[7] Other combinations that are efficacious for reducing BP but not tested in clinical trials include β-blockers with DHP calcium antagonist and DHP calcium antagonists with diuretics.[176]

There have been a number of trials assessing both CV outcome and changes in CKD progression. All these trials assume adherence with antihypertensive medications. However, according to one report, only 71% of subjects with hypertension in the United States are on treatment, and only 48% have their BP under adequate (<140/90 mm Hg) control. Moreover, two separate studies, one in the United Kingdom and the other in Germany, evaluating medication adherence, showed that only approximately 45% of patients who claimed to be taking BP-lowering medication actually were, as assessed by urine analysis of drug metabolites.[177,178] Although there has been significant reduction in the age-adjusted death rate for stroke and coronary artery disease since the early 1980s as a result of better BP control (and better treatment of other risk factors such as hyperlipidemia), heart disease and stroke remain the first and third leading causes of death in Western countries. This emphasizes the importance of identifying and treating patients with hypertension. This section will discuss outcome trials focused on BP reduction that evaluated CKD progression as well as CV outcomes in people with CKD.

BLOOD PRESSURE CONTROL AND CHRONIC KIDNEY DISEASE PROGRESSION

There is clear evidence that partial blockade of the RAAS slows nephropathy progression among those with stage 3 or higher proteinuric kidney disease. While there is no evidence as to whether an ACEI or ARB yields a better CKD outcome, it is clear that both classes have similar benefits between trials.

It is also clear that a lower level of BP does not slow nephropathy progression. Three prospective randomized long-term CKD outcome trials in nondiabetic kidney disease failed to show a benefit on slowing nephropathy progression among the groups with the lower BP.[158,179,180] Hence, the updated KDIGO BP guidelines recommend a BP goal of less than 140/90 mm Hg in those with CKD and is backed by the highest level of evidence. The previous goal of less than 130/80 mm Hg has a much lower level of evidence and is endorsed in the presence of a very high urine albumin level (>300 mg/day), and even then the evidence level is low.

TRIALS IN NONDIABETIC CHRONIC KIDNEY DISEASE THAT CONTRIBUTED TO BLOOD PRESSURE GOAL

MODIFICATION OF DIET IN RENAL DISEASE STUDY

This was the first appropriately powered study to test whether a lower BP goal was associated with a slower progression of CKD. A low BP goal (target mean arterial pressure ≤92 mm Hg for patients ≤60 years old or 98 mm Hg for patients ≥61 years old) was associated with a significant reduction in proteinuria and to a slower subsequent decline in GFR, albeit not significant compared to the higher pressure group with a mean arterial pressure of 102 to 107 mm Hg.

THE AFRICAN AMERICAN STUDY OF KIDNEY DISEASE AND HYPERTENSION

The effect of antihypertensive therapy on the progression of CKD secondary to hypertension is more controversial. In the Multiple Risk Factor Intervention Trial (MRFIT), where thiazide diuretics and β-blockers were primarily used to control BP, slowing or stabilization of kidney function was not seen in African American men but was seen in all other racial groups studied.[181]

In the African American Study of Kidney Disease and Hypertension (AASK), the use of an ACEI (ramipril) was found to be more effective at slowing CKD progression compared to either the dihydropyridine CCB (DCCB), amlodipine, or metoprolol[30] (Figure 47.13). This trial in over 1000 African Americans failed to show superior protection with BP reduced to levels below 130/80 mm Hg compared to conventional BP targets of 140/90 mm Hg in subjects with hypertensive nephrosclerosis. Masked hypertension may be a confounder to these outcomes. A subanalysis of over 50% of the AASK participants who had 24-hour ABPM showed inadequate 24-hour BP control in approximately 36% of the cohort.[182] Masked hypertension and failure of nocturnal dipping were the two most common reasons for poor out-of-office BP control.

Further studies were performed to assess whether change in antihypertensive dose timing corrected the failure of nocturnal dipping, and the results were negative.[183] In contrast, studies performed in Spain in white patients with CKD stages 2 to 3b demonstrate an improvement in dipping status when dosing BP medications at night.[184]

RAMIPRIL EFFICACY IN NEPHROPATHY TRIAL

This multicenter, randomized controlled trial was conducted in Italy among patients with proteinuria associated with immunoglobulin A nephropathy who were receiving background treatment with the ACEI ramipril (2.5 to 5 mg/day). The aim was to assess the effect of intensified versus conventional BP control on progression to end-stage kidney disease. Subjects were randomly assigned to either conventional (diastolic < 90 mm Hg; n = 169) or intensified (systolic/diastolic < 130/80 mm Hg; n = 169) BP control. To achieve the intensified BP level, patients received add-on therapy with the DCCB, felodipine (5 to 10 mg/day). The primary outcome measure was time to end-stage kidney disease over 36 months' follow-up. The authors found that over a median follow-up of 19 months 38 out of 167 (23%) patients assigned to intensified BP control and 34 out of 168 (20%) allocated conventional control progressed to end-stage kidney disease (HR, 1.00; 95% confidence interval [CI], 0.61 to 1.64; $P = 0.99$). Hence, there was no benefit of aggressive BP lowering in slowing this nondiabetic nephropathy.

DIABETES

There are no randomized trials of BP level and CKD outcome among patients with diabetes. The lower-goal BP in diabetes resulted from post hoc analyses of trials that evaluated CV outcomes in subjects with diabetic kidney disease. All these studies showed a benefit on CV risk reduction and some in slowing CKD progression in the group randomized to the lower pressures.

A key study that many have used to argue for a lower BP in diabetes is the Hypertension Optimal Treatment (HOT) trial. This was the first CV outcome trial that evaluated different levels of diastolic BP (80 mm Hg, 85 mm Hg, and 90 mm Hg) in 18,790 patients with hypertension, from 26 countries, mean age 61.5 years. Felodipine was given as baseline therapy with the addition of other agents, according to a five-step regimen. In the subgroup of patients with diabetes mellitus there was a 51% reduction in major CV events in the target group of 80 mm Hg or less compared with the target group of 90 mm Hg or less (P for trend = 0.005). Nevertheless, if the primary end point of the trial fails to reach statistical significance on CV outcome at the lowest randomized BP level, the diabetes subgroup cannot be considered positive even if significant as the hypothesis tested did not specifically apply to this subgroup.

The Ongoing Telmisartan Alone and in combination with Ramipril Global Endpoint Trial (ONTARGET) and the International Verapamil-Trandolapril Study (INVEST), like the Action to Control Cardiovascular Risk in Diabetes (ACCORD) trial, failed to show a benefit on CV outcomes.[185-187] Taken together, these three studies demonstrate

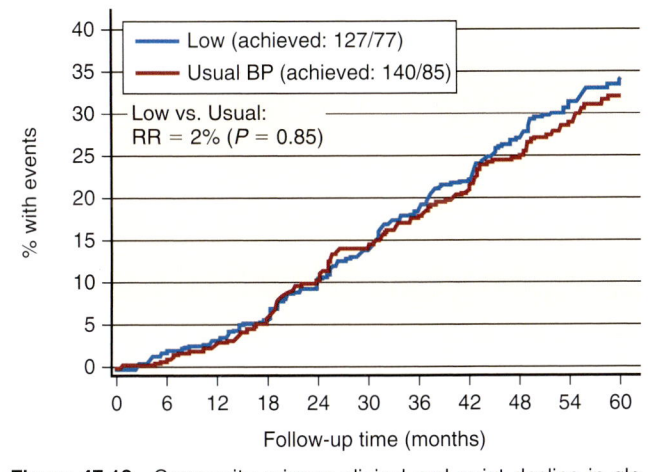

Figure 47.13 Composite primary clinical end point decline in glomerular filtration rate, end-stage kidney disease, or death in the African American Study of Kidney Disease. BP, Blood pressure; RR, relative risk.

no additional benefit of BP lowering below 130/80 mm Hg on CV risk reduction compared to being 130-139/80-85 mm Hg (Table 47.9).

INVEST also demonstrated an increase in CV events at systolic BP levels below 115 mm Hg, although 100% of these patients had coronary artery disease. The exception, however, is stroke reduction, which in ACCORD demonstrated a linear benefit between level of BP and risk reduction; this was not seen in the INVEST analysis but was seen in the ACCOMPLISH analysis[188] (Figure 47.14).

The only prospective outcome trials that randomized groups to different BP levels and were powered statistically for CV outcomes were United Kingdom Prospective Diabetes Study (UKPDS) and ACCORD. However, only the intensive treatment group in the ACCORD study attained a BP of less than 130/80 mm Hg.[187,189]

In ACCORD there was no significant difference in the primary end point, all-cause and CV mortality, between the standard and intensive BP groups. Moreover, there was a significantly higher side-effect profile in the intensive treatment group. A post hoc analysis evaluated CV outcomes in patients with and without CKD (eGFR < 60 mL/min/1.73 m^2).

Renal function data were available on 10,136 patients of the original ACCORD cohort. Of those, 6506 were free of CKD at baseline and 3636 met the criteria for CKD. Risk for the primary outcome was 87% higher in patients with CKD

Table 47.9 Achieved Blood Pressure Levels in Diabetes Outcome Clinical Trials

Clinical Outcome Trial	Achieved Level of Systolic Blood Pressure (mm Hg)
ACCORD (primary)	119 (intensive); 133 (conventional)
UKPDS (primary)	144 (intensive); 154 (conventional)
ACCOMPLISH (secondary)	Overall mean 133
INVEST (secondary)	144 (tight control); 149 (conventional)
ONTARGET (secondary)	Averaging approximately 140
VADT (secondary)	127 (intensive); 125 (conventional)
ADVANCE (secondary)	145 (in both intensive and conventional glucose control)

ACCOMPLISH, Avoiding Cardiovascular Events Through Combination Therapy in Patients Living with Systolic Hypertension; ACCORD, Action to Control Cardiovascular Risk in Diabetes; ADVADT, Veterans Affairs Diabetes Trial; ADVANCE, Action in Diabetes and Vascular Disease: Preterax and Diamicron Modified Release Controlled Evaluation; INVEST, International Verapamil-Trandolapril Study; ONTARGET, Ongoing Telmisartan Alone and in combination with Ramipril Global EndpoinT trial; UKPDS, United Kingdom Prospective Diabetes Study.

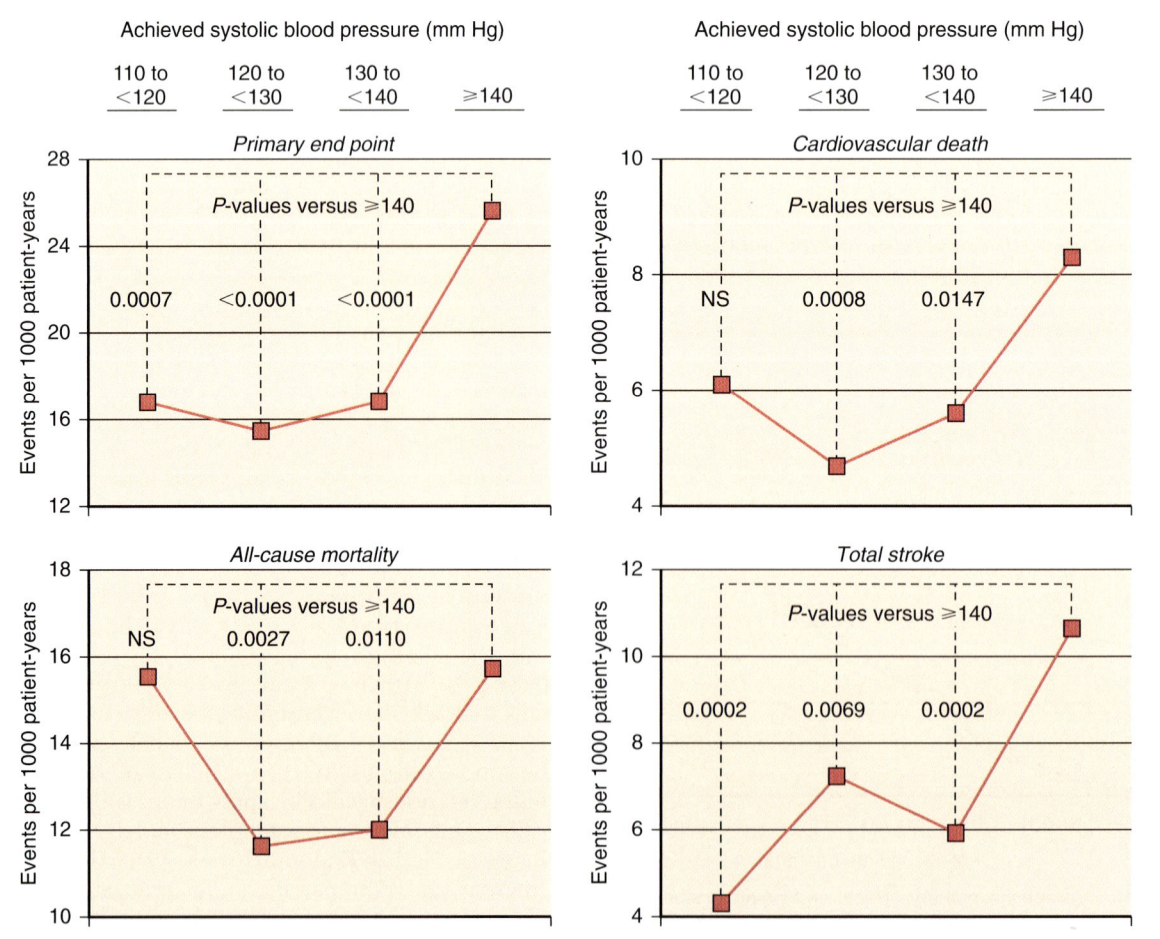

Figure 47.14 Event rates (per 1000 patient-years) for major clinical outcomes in the Avoiding Cardiovascular Events Through Combination Therapy in Patients Living with Systolic Hypertension (ACCOMPLISH) trial categorized by systolic pressure. NS, Not significant.

(HR, 1.866; 95% CI, 1.651 to 2.110).[190] In patients with CKD, compared with standard therapy, intensive lowering of glucose level was significantly associated with both 31% higher all-cause mortality (HR, 1.306; CI, 1.065 to 1.600) and 41% higher CV mortality (HR, 1.412; CI, 1.052 to 1.892). This study confirms a higher CV risk in patients with CKD and that intensive glycemic control increases risk for CV and all-cause mortality in diabetes.

The UKPDS did not show a benefit from the lower BP group, which averaged above 140/90 mm Hg (see Table 47.9). Additional findings from post hoc analyses of diabetes subgroups of other trials also fail to show benefit of BP levels below 130/80 mm Hg, demonstrating additional CV outcome benefit except for stroke in most cases.

A number of studies demonstrate that some classes of antihypertensive drugs should be used preferentially in patients with diabetes who have nephropathy (i.e., blockers of the RAAS system). However, this class of agents does not possess any specific advantages over other antihypertensive classes in people with diabetes who do not have nephropathy. Moreover, there is no evidence that blockers of the RAAS system benefit people with normotension with or without microalbuminuria from developing declines in kidney function.[191-193]

Many post hoc analyses demonstrate that diuretics and β-blockers both worsen blood glucose control among those with diabetes and increase the development of new-onset diabetes in those with impaired fasting glucose. Thiazide diuretics worsen glycemic status through hypokalemia and other mechanisms related to increased visceral adiposity. β-Blockers that result in vasoconstriction, such as metoprolol and atenolol, worsen insulin sensitivity. The vasodilating β-blockers, such as carvedilol and nebivolol, have neutral effects on glycemic control and increase insulin sensitivity.

Post hoc analyses of two different CV outcome trials note that CV event rates were not higher in the diuretic group in spite of a higher incidence of new-onset diabetes. An analysis of the Antihypertensive and Lipid-Lowering Treatment to Prevent Heart Attack Trial (ALLHAT) subgroup with diabetes failed to show a higher CV event rate in the diuretic group even though they had the greatest worsening of glycemic control.[27] Note that blood glucose level was managed in this trial. In a 12-year follow-up of the ALLHAT, participants on chlorthalidone with incident diabetes had consistently lower, nonsignificant risk for CV disease mortality versus no diabetes or participants on amlodipine or lisinopril with incident diabetes.[194] Moreover, participants with incident diabetes had elevated coronary heart disease risk compared with those with no diabetes, but those on chlorthalidone had significantly lower risk for events compared to those on lisinopril. Thus, thiazide-related incident diabetes has less adverse long-term CV disease impact than incident diabetes that develops while on other antihypertensive medications.

CHRONIC KIDNEY DISEASE HARD END POINT TRIALS IN DIABETES

While there are many studies that evaluate changes in albuminuria and changes in eGFR, there are four CKD outcome trials statistically powered for meaningful outcomes on CKD progression; those trials are discussed in this section.

The Captopril Trial

The first clinical outcome trial to put RAAS blocking agents on the map for slowing CKD progression was this trial in 1993. It was a randomized, controlled trial comparing captopril with placebo in 472 patients with hypertension and type 1 diabetes in whom urinary protein excretion was greater than 500 mg/day and the serum creatinine concentration less than 2.5 mg/dL.[195] The primary end point was a doubling of the baseline serum creatinine concentration. Captopril reduced doubling of serum creatinine concentration by 48% over placebo (25 patients, captopril group, vs. 43 patients, placebo group; $P = 0.007$). The benefit was even higher in those with a serum creatinine concentration above 2 mg/dL. The mean rate of decline in creatinine clearance was 11% ± 21% per year in the captopril group and 17% ± 20% per year in the placebo group ($P = 0.03$). Captopril treatment was associated with a 50% reduction in the risk for the combined end points of death, dialysis, and transplantation. There was a 4–mm Hg significantly lower systolic BP in the captopril group; however, the benefit was independent of this lower BP. To date, this is the only outcome trial with an ACEI in advanced nephropathy to be done.

Reduction of Endpoints in Non–Insulin Dependent Diabetes Mellitus with the Angiotensin II Antagonist Losartan (RENAAL)

The RENAAL study was a randomized, double-blind study in 1513 patients comparing losartan (50 to 100 mg once daily) with placebo, both taken in addition to conventional antihypertensive treatment for a mean of 3.4 years.[196] The primary outcome was the composite of a doubling of the baseline serum creatinine concentration, end-stage kidney disease, or death. Secondary end points included a composite of morbidity and mortality from CV causes, proteinuria, and the rate of progression of renal disease. Losartan reduced the incidence of a doubling of the serum creatinine concentration (risk reduction, 25%; $P = 0.006$) and end-stage kidney disease (risk reduction, 28%; $P = 0.002$) but had no effect on the rate of death. The benefit exceeded that attributable to changes in BP. The composite of morbidity and mortality from CV causes was similar in the two groups, although the rate of first hospitalization for heart failure was significantly lower with losartan (risk reduction, 32%; $P = 0.005$). Proteinuria declined by 35% percent with losartan compared to placebo ($P < 0.001$).

Irbesartan Diabetic Nephropathy Trial

In this study, 1715 patients with hypertension with nephropathy due to type 2 diabetes were randomized to treatment with irbesartan (300 mg daily), amlodipine (10 mg daily), or placebo.[197] The target BP was 135/85 mm Hg or less in all groups. The primary composite end point was a doubling of the baseline serum creatinine level, development of end-stage kidney disease, or death from any cause. We also compared them with regard to the time to a secondary, CV composite end point. Treatment with irbesartan had a 20% risk reduction of the primary composite end point compared to placebo ($P = 0.02$) and a 23% lower risk than the amlodipine group ($P = 0.006$) at 2.6 years. The risk for a doubling of the serum creatinine level was 33% lower in the irbesartan group compared to placebo ($P = 0.003$), and 37%

lower in the irbesartan group than in the amlodipine group ($P < 0.001$). Like the RENAAL trial, there were no significant differences in the rates of death from any cause or in the CV composite end point. Thus, irbesartan, like losartan, is effective in protecting against the progression of nephropathy due to type 2 diabetes.

The next trials examined whether the *combination* of an ACEI and ARB would further slow nephropathy progression associated with type 2 diabetes.

Veterans Affairs Nephropathy in Diabetes Trial

The Veterans Affairs Nephropathy in Diabetes (VA NEPHRON D) trial studied 1448 male veterans with type 2 diabetes, hypertension, and nephropathy. They were randomly assigned to either losartan 100 mg per day and then randomized to receive either lisinopril (at a dose of 10 to 40 mg per day) or placebo.[198] The primary end point was the first occurrence of a change in the eGFR (a decline of ≥30 mL/min/1.73 m² if the initial eGFR was ≥ 60 mL/min/1.73 m² or a decline of ≥50% if the initial eGFR was < 60 mL/min/1.73 m²), end-stage kidney disease, or death. Safety outcomes included mortality, hyperkalemia, and acute kidney injury. The study was stopped early secondary to safety concerns with a median follow-up of 2.2 years. There was no difference in the primary end points between groups ($P = 0.30$). There was no benefit with respect to mortality or CV events. Combination therapy increased the risk for hyperkalemia (6.3 events per 100 person-years vs. 2.6 events per 100 person-years with monotherapy; $P < 0.001$) and acute kidney injury (12.2 vs. 6.7 events per 100 person-years; $P < 0.001$). Thus, combining an ACEI and an ARB is associated with far more risk than benefit in diabetic nephropathy irrespective of albuminuria or BP level.

A second study in persons with diabetic nephropathy to examine combination therapy was the Aliskiren Trial in Type 2 Diabetes Using Cardio-Renal Endpoints (ALTITUDE), although this had as a primary end point a CV outcome rather than CKD progression,[199] although CKD was part of the primary composite outcome.

This was a double-blind randomized trial of 8561 patients allocated to aliskiren (300 mg daily) or placebo as an adjunct to background ACEI or an ARB. The primary end point was a composite of the time to CV death or a first occurrence of cardiac arrest with resuscitation; nonfatal myocardial infarction; nonfatal stroke; unplanned hospitalization for heart failure; end-stage kidney disease, death attributable to kidney failure, or the need for renal replacement therapy with no dialysis or transplantation available or initiated; or doubling of the baseline serum creatinine level.

Like the VA NEPHRON D trial, this trial was also stopped prematurely after the second interim efficacy analysis, at a median of 32.9 months. The primary reasons for stopping were hyperkalemia and hypotension in the combined aliskiren group. Moreover, at the time of stopping there was no difference in the primary end point between groups ($P = 0.12$), nor was there a difference in the secondary renal end points. Systolic and diastolic BP levels were lower with aliskiren (between-group differences, 1.3 and 0.6 mm Hg, respectively), and the mean reduction in the urine albumin to creatinine ratio was greater in the aliskiren group. Thus, this is the second study that precludes the use of combined RAAS blockade in patients with advanced CKD.

ALBUMINURIA, BLOOD PRESSURE, AND DIABETIC NEPHROPATHY

We will not discuss trials of microalbuminuria and BP as it is well documented that BP reduction with all antihypertensive drug classes reduces microalbuminuria.[191] The exception for antihypertensive agents on very high albuminuria reduction are summarized in Table 47.10. These findings hold predominantly for those with more than 500 mg/day of albumin.

An analysis performed in 2014 of all studies that used microalbuminuria as either synonymous with diabetic nephropathy or as an end point implying slowed nephropathy progression are misleading, since the premise that microalbuminuria is indicative of kidney disease is highly controversial.[191,192,200] The rationale for this analysis was to review the data on microalbuminuria, an amount of albumin in the urine of 30 to 299 mg/day, in patients with diabetes in the context of CV risk and development of kidney disease. The objective was to review the pathophysiology of microalbuminuria in patients with diabetes and review the data from trials regarding microalbuminuria in the context of risk for CV events or kidney disease progression.

The data suggest that microalbuminuria is a risk marker for CV events and possibly for kidney disease development. Its presence alone, however, does not indicate established kidney disease, especially if the eGFR is greater than 60 mL/min/1.73 m².[191] An increase in microalbuminuria, when BP and other risk factors are controlled, portends a poor prognosis for kidney outcomes over time. Early in the course of diabetes, aggressive risk factor management focused on glycemic and BP goals is important to delay kidney disease development and reduce CV risk. Thus, microalbuminuria

Table 47.10 Changes in Proteinuria at Six Months to a Year Following Treatment Predict Long-Term Renal Outcomes

Increased Time to Dialysis	No Change in Time to Dialysis
(30%–35% proteinuria reduction) • AASK Trial (nondiabetic) • RENAAL (diabetes) • IDNT (diabetes)	(NO proteinuria reduction) • DCCB arm-IDNT (diabetes) • DCCB arm-AASK (nondiabetic)

>30% reduction in proteinuria at 6 months to a year following antihypertensive therapy. Effect independent of magnitude of blood pressure reduction.
AASK, African American Study of Kidney Disease and Hypertension; DCCB, dihydropyridine calcium channel blocker; IDNT, Irbesartan Diabetic Nephropathy Trial; RENAAL, Reduction of Endpoints in Non–Insulin Dependent Diabetes Mellitus with the Angiotensin II Antagonist Losartan.
From Hart P, Bakris GL: Managing hypertension in the diabetic patient. In Egan BM, Basile JN, Lackland DT, editors: Hot topics in hypertension, *Philadelphia, 2004, Hanley and Belfus, pp 249–252.*

is a marker of CV disease risk and should be monitored per guidelines once or twice a year for progression to very high albuminuria and kidney disease development, especially if levels of plasma glucose, lipids, and BP are at guideline goals.

There are two statistically powered studies in patients with hypertension who have a very high urine albumin level that demonstrated nice reductions in the level.[201,202] Both these studies had greater than 300 mg/day baseline levels of albuminuria.

A TRIAL TO COMPARE TELMISARTAN VERSUS LOSARTAN IN PATIENTS WITH HYPERTENSION WITH TYPE 2 DIABETES WITH OVERT NEPHROPATHY

Two different ARBs were compared in a double-blind, prospective trial of 860 patients with type 2 diabetes whose BP levels were over 130/80 mm Hg or who were receiving antihypertensive medication and had a morning spot urine albumin to creatinine ratio of 700 or more. Patients were randomized to telmisartan or losartan.[202] The primary end point was the difference in the urine albumin to creatinine ratio between the groups at 52 weeks. The geometric coefficient of variation and the mean of the urine albumin to creatinine ratio fell in both groups at 52 weeks, but both were significantly greater for the telmisartan compared to losartan. Mean systolic BP reductions were not significantly different between groups at the end of the trial. This trial suggests that longer-acting telmisartan is superior to losartan in reducing albuminuria in patients with hypertension with diabetic nephropathy, despite a similar reduction in BP. Keep in mind that there are no renal outcome studies powered with telmisartan. However, there is a renal substudy of the ONTARGET study that shows a similar effect in albuminuria reduction between ramipril and telmisartan with the combined group having the greatest reduction but the worst outcome.[203]

A second trial that compared the effects of BP lowering albuminuria reduction in diabetic nephropathy was the Gauging Albuminuria Reduction with Lotrel in Diabetic Patients with Hypertension (GUARD) trial.[201] This double-blind, randomized controlled trial of 322 patients with hypertension, albuminuria, and type 2 diabetes tested the hypothesis that combining an ACEI with either a thiazide diuretic or a CCB will result in similar reductions in BP and albuminuria. Groups were randomized to either benazepril plus amlodipine or benazepril plus hydrochlorothiazide for 1 year. The trial employed a noninferiority design. Both combinations significantly reduced the urine albumin to creatinine ratio and sitting BP of the entire cohort. The percentage of patients progressing to overt proteinuria was similar for both groups. When only patients with microalbuminuria and hypertension were examined, a larger percentage of patients receiving the diuretic and ACEI normalized their albuminuria. In contrast, BP reduction, particularly the diastolic component, favored the combination with amlodipine. This finding was also seen in the large CV outcome trial ACCOMPLISH. Hence, reductions in albuminuria are NOT a surrogate for CV or CKD outcomes, as discussed earlier.

ONTARGET and Telmisartan Randomized Assessment Study in ACE Intolerant Subjects with Cardiovascular Disease (TRANSCEND) also studied many patients with diabetes and high CV risk. ONTARGET involved 25,620 patients extending in a follow-up of more than 5 years. It compared the effects of ACEI treatment (ramipril, 10 mg), ARB treatment (telmisartan, 80 mg), and treatment with the combination of both (an ACEI plus ARB together: ramipril 10 mg plus telmisartan 80 mg), in patients at high risk for CV disease (population with established coronary artery disease, stroke, peripheral vascular disease, or diabetes with end-organ damage). The primary end point of the trial was a composite of CV death, myocardial infarction, stroke, and hospitalization for heart failure.[204] Secondary end points included reduction in the development of diabetes mellitus, nephropathy, dementia, and atrial fibrillation. This trial and the parallel study TRANSCEND (evaluating 5776 patients unable to tolerate an ACEI who have been randomized to receive telmisartan or placebo, with the same primary and secondary end points) are expected to provide new insights into the optimal treatment of patients at high risk for complications from atherosclerosis.[205] These are the largest ARB clinical trials ever conducted.

ADVANCE TRIAL

In the Action in Diabetes and Vascular Disease: Preterax and Diamicron Modified Release Controlled Evaluation (ADVANCE) factorial trial, the combination of perindopril and indapamide reduced mortality among patients with type 2 diabetes.[206] While this trial did not randomize to different levels of BP control, it did maintain systolic BP control to levels below 140 mm Hg. After a 6-year posttrial follow-up, surviving participants were invited for reassessment. The primary end points were death from any cause and major macrovascular events. The authors found the baseline characteristics similar among the 11,140 patients who originally underwent randomization and the 8494 patients who participated in the posttrial follow-up for a median of 5.9 years (blood pressure–lowering comparison) or 5.4 years (glucose control comparison). Between-group differences in BP and glycated hemoglobin levels during the trial were no longer evident by the first posttrial visit. The reductions in the risk for death from any cause and of death from CV causes that had been observed in the group receiving active blood pressure–lowering treatment during the trial were attenuated but significant at the end of the posttrial follow-up period ($P = 0.04$). Thus, in this long-term diabetes trial the mortality benefits originally observed among patients assigned to blood pressure–lowering therapy were attenuated but still evident.

CLINICAL TRIALS IN OLDER ADULTS

According to the latest NHANES,[207] 67% of adults aged 60 years and older were found to be hypertensive, and with increasing age, not only is it more likely that someone will develop hypertension, but the person's risk for dying from CV disease is increased, even during the prehypertensive range[9,208] (see Figure 47.4). Despite the relative high incidence of hypertension, older adults are not represented in clinical trials as the trials have upper age limits or do not present age-specific results.

All major clinical trials involving persons older than 65 years are summarized in Table 47.11. Most patients recruited

Table 47.11 Clinical Trials in Older Adults

Clinical Trials	Mean Age	N	Drugs Used	Achieved BP (Control)	Achieved BP (Rx)	Outcome
EWHPE, 1985	72	840	HCTZ + triamterene, ± methyldopa	159/85	155/84	+ CV risk reduction
Coope and Warrender trial, 1986	68	884	Atenolol ± bendrofluazide	180/89	178/87	Stroke reduction
SHEP, 1991	72	4736	Chlorthalidone ± atenolol or reserpine	155/72	143/68	Stroke reduction
STOP, 1991	72	1627	Atenolol ± HCTZ or amiloride	161/97	159/81	Stroke and MI reduction
MRC, 1992	70	3496	HCTZ ± amiloride vs. atenolol	≈169/79	≈150/80	Stroke, MI, and CHD reduction
CASTEL, 1994	83	665	Clonidine, nifedipine and atenolol + chlorthalidone	181/97	165.2/85.6	Reduced mortality
STONE, 1996	67	1632	Nifedipine	155/87	147/85	Stroke and CV event reduction
Syst-Eur, 1997	70	4695	Nitrendipine + enalapril or HCTZ	161/94	151/79	Stroke and CVD reduction
Syst-China, 2000	67	2394	Nitrendipine + captopril or HCTZ	178/93	151/76	Stroke, CVD, and HF reduction
HYVET, 2008	84	3845	Indapamide + perindopril	158.5/84	143/78	Stroke and HF reduction
JATOS, 2008	75	4418	Efonidipine hydrochloride	145.6/78.1	136/74	No difference between aggressive BP on renal and CV events

BP, Blood pressure; CASTEL, Cardiovascular Study in the Elderly; CHD, coronary heart disease; CV, cardiovascular; CVD, cardiovascular disease; EWHPE, European Working Party on High Blood Pressure in the Elderly; HCTZ, hydrochlorothiazide; HF, heart failure; HYVET, Hypertension in the Very Elderly Trial; JATOS, Japanese Trial to Assess Optimal Systolic Blood Pressure in Elderly Hypertensive Patients; MI, myocardial infarction; MRC, Medical Research Council; Rx, medication; SHEP, Systolic Hypertension in the Elderly Program; STONE, Shanghai Trial of Nifedipine in the Elderly; STOP, Hypertension, Swedish Trail in Old Patients with Hypertension; Syst-China, Systolic Hypertension in China; Syst-Eur, Systolic Hypertension in Europe.

in these trials prior to Hypertension in the Very Elderly Trial (HYVET) were less than 80 years of age, limiting information about octogenarians.[23] Results in these trials showed reduction in the incidence of both stroke and CV morbidity, but a trend toward an increase in all-cause mortality. Previous clinical trials showed that lowering BP in older adults has no effect on overall mortality or on the incidence of fatal or nonfatal myocardial infarction.[209,210] However, there was a benefit in stroke outcomes. Thus, clinical practice guidelines prior to HYVET and subsequently the American College of Cardiology (ACC)/AHA recommended that in subjects aged 80 years and above "evidence for benefits of anti-hypertensive treatment is as yet inconclusive."[8]

The release of the HYVET,[23] and the subsequent publication of the "ACCF/AHA 2011 Expert Consensus Document on Hypertension in the Elderly,"[211] changed the management of hypertension particularly in patients more than 80 years old. The 2014 expert panel recommended that older adults, aged 60 or greater, have a BP goal of less than 150/90 mm Hg. This was based on a review of five trials, only two of which randomized to different BP levels that were below a systolic of 140 mm Hg. The trials were SHEP, Systolic Hypertension in Europe (Syst-Eur), HYVET, Japanese Trial to Assess Optimal Systolic Blood Pressure in Elderly Hypertensive Patients (JATOS), and Valsartan in Elderly Isolated Systolic Hypertension (VALISH)[212] (see Table 47.11). Both randomized BP trials with the lower BP levels were carried out in Japan. The results from these two studies showed no additional benefit of achieving a BP of less than 140/90 mm Hg compared to less than 150/90 mm Hg.

A concern in patients with isolated systolic hypertension is the reduction of diastolic BP after initiation of antihypertensive therapy. A diastolic BP that is too low may interfere with coronary perfusion and possibly increase CV risk. The relationship between diastolic BP and CV death, particularly myocardial infarction, is like a J-shaped curve; thus, excessive reduction in diastolic pressures should be avoided in patients with coronary artery disease who are being treated for hypertension. A BP of 119/84 mm Hg was identified as a nadir when treating patients with coronary artery disease[213]; however, among patients with CKD, a nadir of 131/71 mm Hg was identified as a level below which higher CV mortality was present[214] (Figure 47.15).

When treating patients with isolated systolic hypertension, the JNC 7 suggests a minimum posttreatment diastolic BP of 60 mm Hg overall or perhaps 65 mm Hg in patients with known coronary artery disease,[8] unless symptoms that could be attributed to hypoperfusion occur at higher pressures. This was seen in the findings of the SHEP trial,[215] where older patients with lower diastolic BP have higher CV event rates.

Additionally, in some trials involving older individuals, there is concern about thiazide diuretic use, hyponatremia, and worsening of kidney function in subjects with hypertension. In the European Working Party on High Blood

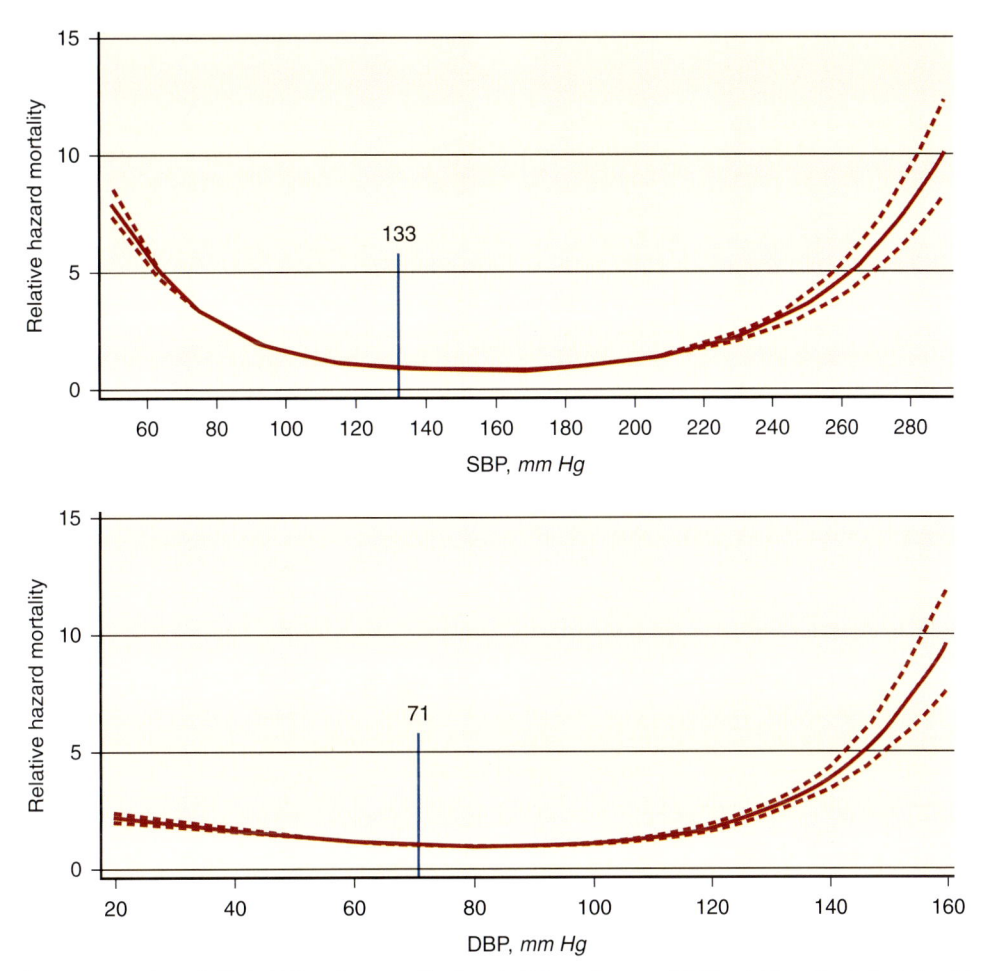

Figure 47.15 Blood pressure and mortality in U.S. veterans with chronic kidney disease. (Multivariable-adjusted relative hazards [hazard ratios (95% confidence intervals)] of all-cause mortality associated with systolic blood pressure (SBP) and diastolic blood pressure (DBP) relative to a hypothetical patient with the mean time-varying SBP (133 mm Hg) and DBP (71 mm Hg).

Pressure in the Elderly trial, a significantly higher incidence of impaired kidney function was found in those receiving diuretics compared with placebo.[216] In the SHEP trial, serum creatinine level increased significantly in the subjects treated with thiazide diuretics compared to placebo.[217] In ALLHAT the chlorthalidone-treated group showed worse kidney function than either the amlodipine- or lisinopril-treated groups at both the 2- and 4-year end points.[187] While this could likely be accounted for by volume depletion in many cases, diuretics have been shown to induce mild renal injury in various animal models, possibly because of hypokalemia, hyperuricemia, and stimulation of the RAAS related to the reduction in renal perfusion pressure.

The HYVET trial in 2008 changed how hypertension in older adults is managed. It randomly assigned almost 4000 patients who were 80 years old and above and had systolic BP above 160 mm Hg to either indapamide or placebo. Results of HYVET provided clear evidence that BP lowering with treatment using antihypertensive medications is associated with definite CV benefits. The use of indapamide supplemented by perindopril showed reductions in the incidence of stroke, congestive heart failure, and CV fatal events.[23]

Stricter BP goals showed no benefit in CV morbidity and mortality in older populations. The JATOS study showed that systolic BP goals of less than 140 mm Hg did not have any statistical significance in the CV mortality of patients older than 65 years.[218]

There are no specific trials powered to assess CKD progression in older people. There are prespecified and post hoc analyses of trials where the mean age is above 65 examining changes in CKD progression. A notable example is the prespecified analysis of the ACCOMPLISH trial, where more than 40% of the people with CKD were age 70 or greater. This trial showed a benefit of the RAAS blocker–CCB combination over the RAAS blocker–diuretic for slowing progression and time to dialysis (see Table 47.11).[175] A post hoc analysis of the ALLHAT study in people over 65 years also showed that BP control slowed progression.[219] In this trial we have no information about albuminuria, however.

MANAGEMENT OF HYPERTENSION IN OLDER ADULTS WITH CHRONIC KIDNEY DISEASE

Nonpharmacologic Intervention

In the Trial of Nonpharmacologic Interventions in the Elderly (TONE),[220] the combination of weight loss and sodium restriction showed a drop of 5.3 ± 1.2 mm Hg in the systolic BP and 3.4 ± 0.8 mm Hg diastolic BP in obese, older patients with hypertension. The goal of sodium restriction was 1.8 g/24 hr, and the goal for weight reduction was 10 lb. Other lifestyle changes recommended in the older patient include watching potassium intake to keep the level of serum potassium in a safe range. Patient education about high-potassium foods is important. Intake of NSAIDs should also be decreased to a minimum, as these patients are more likely to take NSAIDs for arthritis and pain. These drugs are known to cause elevations in BP by inhibiting the production of vasodilatory prostaglandins and may increase BP by as much as 6 mm Hg.[221,222] Their BP-raising effects can be blunted by both calcium antagonists and, to a lesser extent, diuretics.[223]

Pharmacologic Intervention

According to the 2011 ACCF/AHA consensus guidelines, the initial antihypertensive drug should be started at the lowest dose and gradually increased depending on the BP response up to the maximum tolerated dose.[211] If the response to initial therapy is inadequate after reaching full dose (not necessarily the maximum recommended dose), a second drug from another class should be added. The full dose of the drug is the highest pharmacologic dose of drug available, while the maximum dose is the highest dose that the person can tolerate without side effects. If the person is having no therapeutic response or had significant side effects, a drug from another class should be substituted. In fact, most older patients require two or more drugs to achieve the recommended goals in clinical trials.

Either a diuretic or calcium antagonist may be an initial drug, or a diuretic should be one of the first two agents when starting combination drugs.[12] When the BP is more than 20/10 mm Hg above goal, the recommendation is to initiate with two antihypertensive medications, with one of the choices being a diuretic. Single-pill combinations that incorporate logical doses of two agents may enhance convenience and compliance in older patients.[211] However, there is still a need for individualization of treatment; thus, treatment options should be carefully considered in older adults. The benefits of lowering BP must be weighed against the risks of side effects and the concomitant morbidity of the patient.

Thiazide diuretics such as hydrochlorothiazide, chlorthalidone, indapamide, and bendrofluazide, as well as calcium antagonists, are recommended for initiating therapy.[8,12] Diuretics cause an initial reduction of intravascular volume, peripheral vascular resistance, and BP in more than 50% of patients and are well tolerated and inexpensive.[224,225] However, they can cause hypokalemia, hypomagnesemia, and hyponatremia and are therefore not recommended in patients with baseline electrolyte abnormalities or those with a history of hyponatremia. Serum potassium level should be monitored, and supplementation should be given if needed.[211]

Calcium antagonists are well suited for older patients whose hypertensive profile is based on increasing arterial dysfunction secondary to decreased atrial and ventricular compliance. This class of drugs dilates coronary and peripheral arteries in doses that do not severely affect myocardial contractility.[226,227] Most adverse effects relate to vasodilation like ankle edema, headache, and postural hypotension. Ankle edema is not secondary to sodium retention, as calcium antagonists are natriuretic when given initially, but the profound vasodilation with poor venous return in older people is the major contributor.

First-generation drugs, such as nifedipine, verapamil, and diltiazem should be avoided in patients with left ventricular dysfunction. Nondihydropyridines can precipitate heart blocks in older adults with underlying conduction defects.[228]

RAAS blockers, such as ACEIs, ARBs, and direct renin inhibitors, may be used in older adults.[229,230] Theoretically, as aging occurs, there is a reduction in angiotensin levels; thus, ACEIs may not be an effective medication for hypertension in older adults. However, several clinical trials have shown otherwise. The use of ACEIs is beneficial in the reduction of morbidity and mortality in patients with myocardial infarction, reduced systolic function, heart failure, and reduction in the progression of diabetic renal disease and hypertensive nephrosclerosis.[231,232] In older patients with hypertension and diabetes, ARBs are considered first-line treatment, and as an alternative to ACEIs in patients who cannot tolerate the latter.[233]

Lastly, it appears that use of a blocker of the RAAS may provide greater benefit for CV and renal risk reduction than use of a diuretic, based on data from ACCOMPLISH, a large outcome trial of 11,506 persons with a mean age of 68 years. While there are very few data on kidney disease in older adults, ACCOMPLISH[234] did provide some evidence worthy of being tested in a prospective trial (i.e., that a calcium antagonist–ACEI combination led to fewer people going on dialysis than a diuretic–ACEI combination) (Table 47.12). Note that this outcome could not be explained by differences in BP of 1.2 mm Hg systolic. It must be noted that those over 70 years of age tend to drink small amounts of fluid, and hence this makes them more vulnerable to decline in kidney function by RAAS blockade, as already discussed. Thus it is recommended that they increase their fluid intake to prevent volume depletion.

The clinical benefits of β-blockers as monotherapy in uncomplicated older patients are poorly documented. They may have a role in combination therapy, especially with diuretics. β-Blockers have established roles in patients with hypertension complicated by certain arrhythmias, migraine headaches, senile tremors, coronary artery disease, or heart failure.[235] Nebivolol, a selective $β_1$-blocker with NO properties, does not show any associated symptoms of depression, sexual dysfunction, dyslipidemia, and hyperglycemia in older adults, unlike earlier generations of β-blockers.[236,237]

Potassium-sparing diuretics are useful when combined with other agents. Aldosterone-blocking agents like spironolactone and eplerenone reduce vascular stiffness and systolic BP.[238,239] They are also useful for patients with hypertension with heart failure or primary hyperaldosteronism. Gynecomastia and sexual dysfunction are the limiting adverse events, reactions that occur in men using spironolactone but are less frequent with eplerenone. The epithelial sodium transport antagonists (amiloride, triamterene) are most useful when combined with another diuretic.

Other agents, such as α-blockers, centrally acting drugs (e.g., clonidine), and nonspecific vasodilators (e.g., minoxidil) should not be used as first- or second-line agents in an older adult with hypertension. Instead, they are reserved as part of a combination regimen to maximize BP control after other agents have been deployed.[211]

Table 47.12 Outcomes in the Intention-to-Treat Population and in Patients Aged 65 Years or Older in the ACCOMPLISH Renal Study

	Benazepril Plus Amlodipine	Benazepril Plus Hydrochlorothiazide	Hazard Ratio (95% CI)	P Value
Intention-to-Treat Population (N = 11,506)				
Main end point of progression of chronic kidney disease	113 (1.97%)	215 (3.73%)	0.52 (0.41-0.65)	<0.0001
Doubling of serum creatinine concentration	105 (1.83%)	208 (3.61%)	0.51 (0.39-0.63)	<0.0001
Dialysis	7 (0.12%)	13 (0.23%)	0.53 (0.21-1.35)	0.180
eGFR < 15 mL/min/1.73 m^2	18 (0.31%)	17 (0.30%)	1.06 (0.54-2.05)	0.868
Progression of chronic kidney disease and cardiovascular death	220 (3.83%)	345 (5.99%)	0.63 (0.53-0.74)	<0.0001
Progression of chronic kidney disease and all-cause mortality	346 (6.02%)	465 (8.07%)	0.73 (0.64-0.84)	<0.0001
Patients Aged ≥ 65 Years (n = 7640)				
Main end point of progression of chronic kidney disease	70 (1.83%)	138 (3.62%)	0.50 (0.37-0.67)	<0.0001
Doubling of serum creatinine concentration	66 (1.73%)	132 (3.46%)	0.49 (0.37-0.67)	<0.0001
Dialysis	3 (0.08%)	10 (0.26%)	0.30 (0.08-1.09)	0.053
eGFR < 15 mL/min/173 m^2	11 (0.29%)	11 (0.29%)	1.00 (0.43-2.31)	0.99
Progression of chronic kidney disease and cardiovascular death	160 (4.18%)	234 (6.13%)	0.68 (0.55-0.83)	0.0002
Progression of chronic kidney disease and all-cause mortality	266 (6.96%)	327 (8.57%)	0.81 (0.68-0.95)	0.010

ACCOMPLISH, Avoiding Cardiovascular Events Through Combination Therapy in Patients Living with Systolic Hypertension; CI, confidence interval; eGFR, estimated glomerular filtration rate.

BLOOD PRESSURE MANAGEMENT IN PATIENTS UNDERGOING DIALYSIS

Elevations in BP in dialysis patients are almost exclusively due to excessive volume. Hence hypertension control is much more a problem in hemodialysis than in peritoneal dialysis. There are no large multicenter randomized trials in patients undergoing dialysis to evaluate different levels of BP on CV outcomes. However, there is a prospective, randomized trial that evaluated the effects of an ACEI versus a β-blocker on LVH and as a secondary end point CV mortality in patients undergoing dialysis.[240]

The purpose of the study was to determine in 200 hypertensive patients undergoing hemodialysis with echocardiographic LVH whether a β-blocker or an ACEI used for BP lowering results in a greater regression of LVH. Subjects were randomly assigned to either open-label lisinopril (n = 100) or atenolol (n = 100), each administered three times per week after dialysis. Monthly monitored home BP was controlled to less than 140/90 mm Hg with medications, dry weight adjustment, and sodium restriction. The primary outcome was the change in left ventricular mass index from baseline to 12 months. The results demonstrated that there was no between-group difference in 44-hour ambulatory BP. However, monthly measured home BP was consistently higher in the lisinopril group despite the need for both a greater number of antihypertensive agents and a greater reduction in dry weight. An independent data safety monitoring board recommended termination because of CV safety. Serious CV events were more prominent in the lisinopril group (20 events, atenolol versus 43 events, lisinopril; $P = 0.001$). Combined serious adverse events of myocardial infarction, stroke, and hospitalization for heart failure or CV death were much lower in the atenolol group ($P = 0.021$). Thus it appears that β-blocker therapy is superior to RAAS blockade in patients undergoing hemodialysis to reduce CV morbidity and all-cause hospitalizations.

Retrospective analysis of patients on hemodialysis support other β-blockers such as carvedilol for also lowering CV events in patients who were undergoing hemodialysis and hypertensive. Japanese investigators further corroborate the results supporting β-blocker use in patients undergoing dialysis. The effect of β-blocker use on mortality among a cohort of patients undergoing hemodialysis was evaluated in a database analysis from the Dialysis Outcomes and Practice Patterns Study phase II of 2286 randomly selected patients on hemodialysis in Japan.[241] The main outcome measure was all-cause mortality. The authors found β-blocker use was low (i.e., only 247 patients [10.8%] were administered β-blockers, and 1828 patients [80%] were not). A Kaplan-Meier analysis revealed that all-cause mortality rates were significantly ($P < 0.007$) decreased in patients treated with β-blockers compared to the group not on β-blockers. In multivariable, fully adjusted models, treatment with β-blockers was also independently associated with reduced all-cause mortality (HR, 0.48; $P = 0.02$).[241]

Data from the United States Renal Data System demonstrates a U-shaped relationship between systolic BP goals in patients undergoing dialysis and CV outcomes, suggesting that BP should be consistently above 120 mm Hg and below 150 mm Hg.[242] A meta-analysis by Agarwal and Sinha of antihypertensive medications in patients undergoing dialysis demonstrates that regardless of class, reducing BP reduces CV events.[243] Data from epidemiologic studies consistently show that in patients undergoing maintenance dialysis, low BP values are associated with higher death rates when compared with normal to moderately high values.

Based on the available data, no generalizable approach can be suggested for all patients undergoing dialysis other than to ensure that euvolemia exists by both clinical examination and perhaps newer techniques of bioimpedance and, based on this data, to consider altering antihypertensive medications.

MANAGEMENT OF PRIMARY HYPERTENSION IN CHRONIC KIDNEY DISEASE

There are many guidelines written on the management of hypertension in the general population, and those have been summarized at the beginning of this chapter. Both the Kidney Disease Outcomes Quality Initiative (KDOQI) and the KDIGO guidelines focus on the evidence for certain BP levels and classes of medication in patients with CKD. These guidelines have also been discussed in this chapter. To summarize the key findings, the strongest level of evidence supports a BP goal below 140/90 mm Hg and the use of RAAS-blocking agents in people with stage 3 or higher CKD who have very high albuminuria. Nevertheless, there is weaker evidence to support RAAS-blocker use in people with CKD in general, as well as very weak evidence supporting a BP of less than 130/80 mm Hg for those who have a urine albumin level of 1 g or more and an eGFR of less than 60 mL/min/1.73 m^2.[123,244,245] These BP levels and recommendations for RAAS blockers are focused on the primary outcome of slowing CKD progression. A summary of all trials and changes in eGFR decline are in Figure 47.16.

Nuances in the management of BP in the patient with CKD are necessary as these patients have problems not seen in the general population. First, risk for hyperkalemia is a problem especially in certain subgroups of patients. A review of clinical trials where hyperkalemia developed when managing hypertension in CKD found three risk predictors. If a patient was already receiving an appropriate diuretic for level of kidney function, then these were reliable risk predictors for hyperkalemia (i.e., [K$^+$]$_s$ > 5.5 mEq/L): (1) eGFR of less than 45 mL/min/1.73 m^2, (2) serum potassium level above 4.5 mEq/L, (c) body mass index of less than 25.[246] Hyperkalemia has limited our ability to assess whether RAAS blockers are effective in slowing CKD progression in stage 3b and higher CKD. Newer agents to manage hyperkalemia will open the door to safer management and expanded research.[247,248]

Another nuance in BP management in the patient with CKD is the critical importance of sodium restriction to less than 2400 mg/day and reduced alcohol consumption, as well as aerobic NOT isometric exercise.[8,249] Studies evaluating the effect of sodium intake on BP control in people with stage 4 CKD show that approximately every 400 mg above a sodium intake base of 3000 mg/day requires an additional BP medication to maintain BP control.[250] Moreover, failure to reduce sodium intake suppresses the RAAS system and hence reduces efficacy of RAAS blockers. Thus failure to reduce sodium intake is a cause of resistant hypertension as noted earlier in the chapter. Additionally, BP targets need to be clearly defined and finally, the appropriate antihypertensive agents indicated as initial therapy by evidence based guidelines should be used.

The role of initial combination therapy in patients with CKD is clear since the guidelines recommend that all people with a BP that is 20/10 mm Hg above the goal be initiated on single-pill combination therapy to enhance adherence and efficacy.[7,8,176] Studies evaluating initial monotherapy versus single-pill combination on achieving BP goal have uniformly shown an advantage to achieving BP goal more quickly and with better tolerability.[36,251]

These new guidelines and concepts have been integrated into an algorithm that was in the original National Kidney Foundation consensus report. It is meant to provide an approach to pharmacologically meaningful agents that when combined actually further reduce BP. Table 47.13

Nondiabetes

MDRD. *N Engl J Med.* 1993
AIPRI. *N Engl J Med.* 1996
REIN. *Lancet.* 1997
AASK. *JAMA.* 2002
Hou FF et al. *N Engl J Med.* 2006
Parsa A et al. *N Engl J Med.* 2013

Diabetes

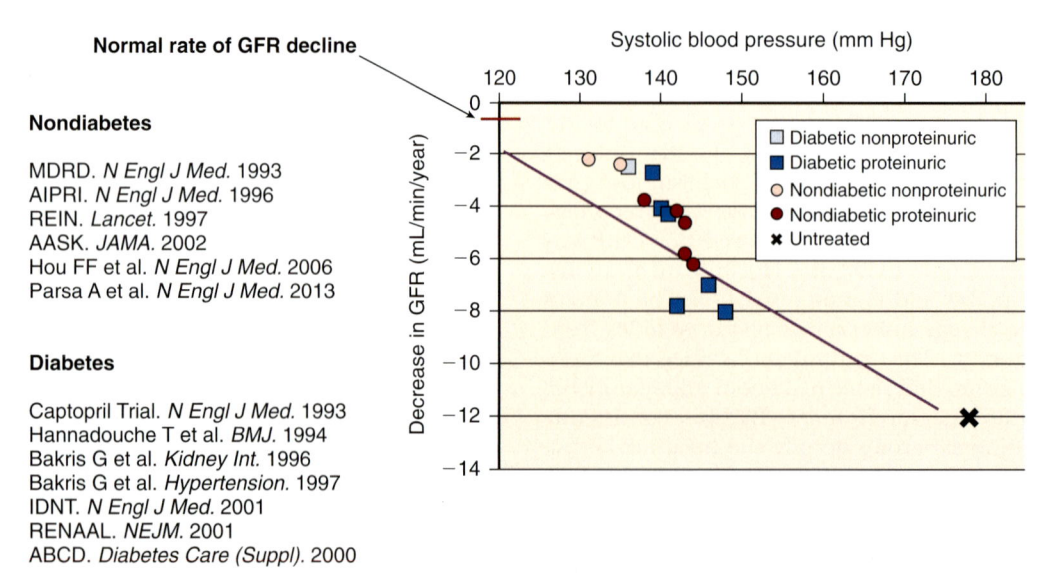

Captopril Trial. *N Engl J Med.* 1993
Hannadouche T et al. *BMJ.* 1994
Bakris G et al. *Kidney Int.* 1996
Bakris G et al. *Hypertension.* 1997
IDNT. *N Engl J Med.* 2001
RENAAL. *NEJM.* 2001
ABCD. *Diabetes Care (Suppl).* 2000

Figure 47.16 Relationship between achieved blood pressure and decline in kidney function from primary renal end point trials.

Table 47.13 American Society of Hypertension Evidence-Based Fixed Dose Antihypertensive Combinations

Preferred
- ACE inhibitor/diuretic*
- ARB/diuretic*
- ACE inhibitor/CCB*
- ARB/CCB*

Acceptable
- β-blocker/diuretic*
- CCB (dihydropyridine)/β-blocker
- CCB/diuretic
- Renin inhibitor/diuretic*
- Renin inhibitor/ARB*
- Thiazide diuretics/K+-sparing diuretics*

Less Effective
- ACE inhibitor/ARB
- ACE inhibitor/β-blocker
- ARB/β-blocker
- CCB (nondihydropyridine)/β-blocker
- Centrally acting agent/β-blocker

*Single-pill combination available in United States.
ACE, Angiotensin-converting enzyme; ARB, angiotensin receptor blocker; CCB, calcium channel blocker.
From Gradman A et al: Combination therapy in hypertension. J Am Soc Hypertens 4:42-50, 2010.

provides an approved list of combination agents noting which are meaningful for optimal BP reduction and which are not. Figure 47.17 presents an evidence-based algorithm to help achieve BP control in the patient with advanced CKD.

ANTIHYPERTENSIVE MEDICATIONS

All information about antihypertensive medications used for general management of hypertension may be found in a compendium of these medications published by the American Society of Hypertension.[252] This section will focus on antihypertensive medications in patients with CKD, dosage adjustments, and other related issues.

ANGIOTENSIN-CONVERTING ENZYME INHIBITORS

The most compelling indication to use this class of agents comes from the AASK trial, where ramipril was superior to either amlodipine or metoprolol for slowing CKD progression.[30] However, no other ACEIs have been tested in hypertensive nephropathy (HN), and a systematic review and meta-analysis by the Cochrane group found that there are not enough data to make claims that ACEIs prevent or delay any nephropathy in the early stages 1 or 2.[253]

ANGIOTENSIN RECEPTOR BLOCKERS

The data on ARBs are exclusively in diabetic nephropathy with no outcome data in hypertension. Given the mechanism of action and the benefit seen in diabetic nephropathy, discussed elsewhere in this book, there is no reason to think

---

If Blood Pressure >140/90 mm Hg in CKD

(if systolic BP <20 mm Hg above goal) Start ARB or ACEI titrate upwards

(if systolic BP ≥20 mm Hg above goal) Start with ACEI or ARB + thiazide-like diuretic* or CCB

If BP still not at goal (140/90 mm Hg)

Add thiazide-like diuretic* or CCB

Add CCB or thiazide-like diuretic*

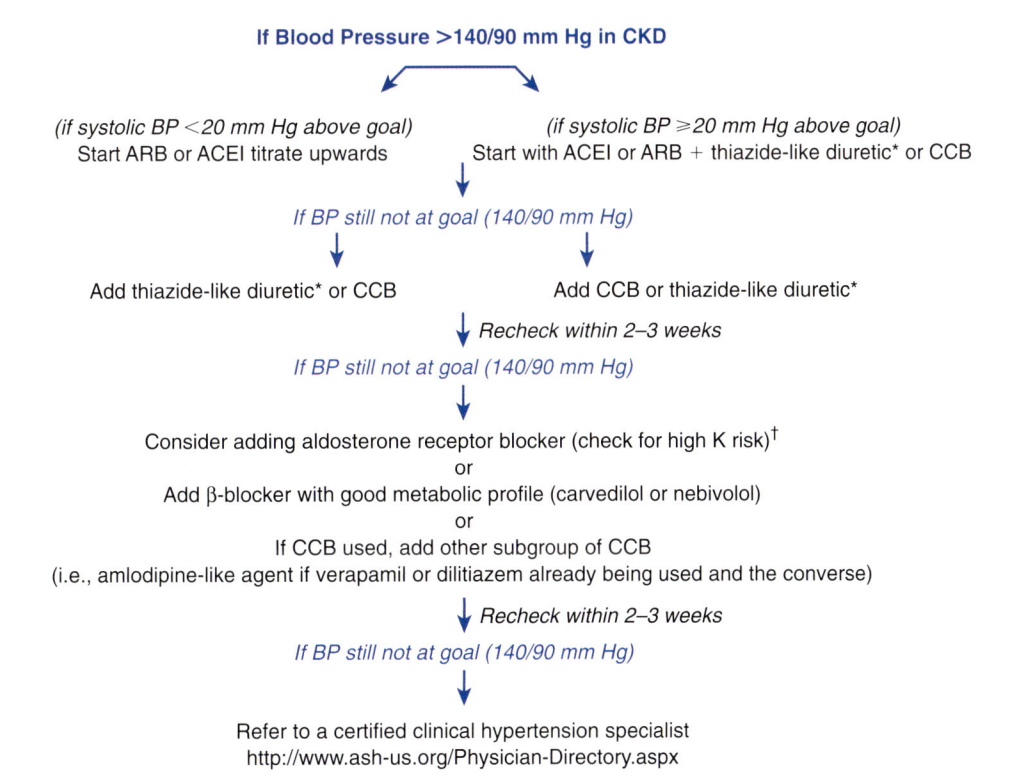

Recheck within 2–3 weeks

If BP still not at goal (140/90 mm Hg)

Consider adding aldosterone receptor blocker (check for high K risk)†
or
Add β-blocker with good metabolic profile (carvedilol or nebivolol)
or
If CCB used, add other subgroup of CCB
(i.e., amlodipine-like agent if verapamil or dilitiazem already being used and the converse)

Recheck within 2–3 weeks

If BP still not at goal (140/90 mm Hg)

Refer to a certified clinical hypertension specialist
http://www.ash-us.org/Physician-Directory.aspx

Figure 47.17 An evidence-based approach to blood pressure (BP) management in stage 3 or higher chronic kidney disease (CKD) updated from the National Kidney Foundation consensus report. *Chlorthalidone or indapamide are preferred diuretics as they work to estimated glomerular filtration rate (eGFR) 30 mL/min. Below this GFR torsemide, the long-acting loop diuretic, is preferred. †Risk for hyperkalemia—if on diuretic, eGFR < 45 mL/min/1.73 m² or $[K^+]_s$ > 4.5 mEq/L. ACE, Angiotensin-converting enzyme; ACEI, angiotensin-converting enzyme inhibitor; ARB, angiotensin receptor blocker; CCB, calcium channel blocker.

these agents would not be as effective in hypertension; however, there are no outcome data. Moreover, there are no adequately powered trials that directly compare progression of CKD between ARBs and ACEIs. In general, one major difference between ACEIs and ARBs is that ARBs are better tolerated than ACEIs due to lower incidence of cough, angioedema, taste disturbances, and hyperkalemia.[153,249]

It is important to understand that in patients with advanced nephropathy, increases in serum creatinine level of up to 30% are commonly seen within 1 to 2 weeks of starting ACEIs or ARBs.[254-256] This increase in serum creatinine level is especially true if BP was previously not controlled and now is within goal. However, in patients under age 66 years with baseline serum creatinine values of more than 3.5 mg/dL, a rise in serum creatinine level of up to 30% within the first 4 months of starting ACEIs or ARBs correlated with slowed long-term decline in kidney function over a mean follow-up period of 3 or more years.[254] For acute, sustained increases in serum creatinine level of more than 35%, patients should be evaluated for (1) volume depletion *(the most common cause)*, (2) decompensated congestive heart failure, or (3) bilateral renal artery stenosis. Hyperkalemia should be managed with avoidance of high-potassium foods, appropriately dosing diuretics, and stopping agents known to increase potassium levels, such as NSAIDs.[254]

DIRECT RENIN INHIBITORS

Aliskiren is currently the first and only approved oral direct renin inhibitor for reduction of BP. There are no direct outcome data available describing the use of aliskiren in patients with HN. However, there are data from 24-hour ABPM studies evaluating the effect of this agent alone and in combination on BP control. Aliskiren was tested alone and in combination with valsartan in people with stage 2 CKD from hypertension to evaluate BP control. The 24-hour ABPM showed additive BP reduction with the combination and improvement in nocturnal dipping in people with stage 2 nephropathy. Moreover, there were no problems with elevated potassium level or reduced kidney function that emerged in the combination group.[257]

ALDOSTERONE ANTAGONISTS

Aldosterone antagonists such as spironolactone are recommended for treating hypertension in patients with advanced heart failure and post myocardial infarction,[8] but their role in kidney disease is unclear. As there are no outcome data in HN, this class will not be discussed in this chapter. It should be noted, however, that obesity is common in HN and aldosterone antagonists are most efficacious for lowering BP in patients with sleep apnea and obesity and do not work well in thin people.[258,259] This is due to the contribution of the adipocyte to aldosterone production.[260]

DIURETICS

Thiazide-like diuretics (chlorthalidone and indapamide) have a strong evidence base for reducing CV risk even in patients with stage 3 CKD. However, their role in renal outcome studies is unclear. Post hoc analyses of ALLHAT demonstrated that chlorthalidone was as good as ACEIs for slowing CKD progression in stage 3 nephropathy.[219] This post hoc analysis of ALLHAT included both those with HN and diabetic nephropathy, so the data should be considered as less than definitive.

Data from the updated international guidelines clearly have thiazide-type diuretics in a supportive role following RAAS blockade and calcium antagonists in people with high CV risk and hypertension.[11,38] There are major differences between chlorthalidone, indapamide, and hydrochlorothiazide. Chlorthalidone has a much longer half-life compared to hydrochlorothiazide at the same milligram dose.[261] This difference in duration of action by chlorthalidone translated into an additional 7–mm Hg reduction in systolic BP when substituted for hydrochlorothiazide.[261,262]

CALCIUM CHANNEL BLOCKERS

When used in patients with HN, both dihydropyridine CCBs (DCCBs) and nondihydropyridine CCBs (NDCCBs) are effective in lowering BP and CV events in high-risk populations.[173,263] These agents are particularly efficacious for CV risk reduction when combined with an ACEI as shown by the results of ACCOMPLISH.[174,175] In this trial, patients at high risk for a CV event and CKD progression treated with a single-pill combination of an ACEI with amlodipine had a 20% relative risk reduction in CV events and slower CKD progression when compared to an ACEI plus hydrochlorothiazide.

Also, a prespecified post hoc analysis of ACCOMPLISH evaluated CKD outcomes showing that the DCCB plus ACEI inhibitor decreased CKD progression to a greater extent than the ACEI and diuretic (HR, 0.52; $P < 0.001$).[175] Note that approximately 60% of the patients in this substudy were thought to have HN.

As an antihypertensive class, DCCBs do not reduce albuminuria to the same degree as NDCCBs.[263] The mechanism of this difference is due to changes in glomerular permeability that occur in patients with advanced nephropathy[264] and has translated into worse CKD outcomes when compared with those treated with RAAS blockers.[265] Note that when used with a RAAS blocker DCCB does not have adverse effects.[175,266]

In summary, both DCCBs and NDCCBs are effective BP-reducing agents in patients without albuminuric kidney disease. However, in those with advanced albuminuric nephropathy, NDCCBs are preferred, but DCCBs must be used in combination with a RAAS blocker to maximally slow progression of nephropathy.

β-ADRENERGIC BLOCKERS

β-Blockers on the most updated guidelines are no longer a first-line option to lower BP.[11,38] Some patients with HN have an increase in sympathetic activity and a high CV event rate and should benefit from β-blockers, however.[267] Despite being quite effective at lowering BP, physicians have been reluctant to use β-blockers because of significant adverse metabolic profiles and marked bradycardia.[268]

The vasodilating and metabolically neutral β-blockers have expanded the role for these agents, especially in patients with diabetes and hypertensive nephropathy. The combined α- and β-blocker, carvedilol, and the $β_1$-vasodilating agent nebivolol have neutral glycemic and lipid parameters.[269,270] There are major pharmacologic and outcome differences between labetalol and carvedilol. Specifically, the ratio of β- to α-blockade is 7:1 for labetalol and 3:1 for carvedilol; hence, oral labetalol behaves like a typical β-blocker.[271] Moreover, it has a short half-life and ideally should be given three to four times daily. Lastly, labetalol has no outcome data, whereas carvedilol reduces CV morbidity and reduces mortality in those with CKD, hypertension, and diabetes.[272] Thus, in patients with HN, vasodilating β-blockers can be used and are excellent add-on agents to reduce CV risk and achieve BP goal.

Other classes of BP-lowering medications such as α-adrenergic antagonists, vasodilators such as hydralazine and minoxidil, as well as central α-agonists will not be discussed, as there are no CV or CKD outcome data on their usefulness in HN.

DIRECT-ACTING VASODILATORS

Hydralazine and minoxidil are direct-acting vasodilators that have different mechanisms of action but the same clinical consequences. They both increase sodium reabsorption dramatically by the proximal tubule, increase sympathetic tone, and as a result should never be used long term without concomitant use of loop diuretics and beta blockers.[273-277] Moreover, hydralazine is well known to increase genesis of peroxynitrite, which damages cells and reduces NO. Thus, nitrates need to be given with hydralazine to reduce this risk.

RESISTANT HYPERTENSION

Resistant hypertension is currently defined as the failure to achieve a goal BP of less than 140/90 mm Hg in patients who are adherent with maximal tolerated doses of a minimum of three antihypertensive drugs, one of which must be a diuretic appropriate for kidney function.[152] The increasing prevalence of obesity and hypertension in the general population has resulted in this disorder's gaining attention in the past decade. Large-scale population-based studies such as the NHANES have specifically examined the prevalence and incidence of resistant hypertension and associated risk factors. The findings suggest the prevalence of resistant hypertension is approximately 8% to 12% of adult patients with hypertension (6 to 9 million people).[278] The increasing prevalence of resistant hypertension contrasts with the improvement in BP control rates during the same period. Studies also show that patients with resistant hypertension who are older than 55 years, of black ethnicity, with high body mass index, diabetes, or CKD have an increased risk for CV events compared to patients with nonresistant hypertension. The effects of WCH and pseudoresistant hypertension have not been factored into many of the prevalence studies, and hence the true prevalence is not known. The white coat effect contributes greatly to the high perceived incidence of resistant hypertension, as was evidenced by the over 60% screen failure in the Renal Denervation in Patients with Uncontrolled Hypertension (SYMPLICITY HTN-3) trial of renal denervation due to WCH.[279,280]

Thus this is a diagnosis frequently seen by nephrologists and is most commonly due to nonadherence with medication as well as volume overload secondary to poor kidney function and nonadherence with a low-sodium diet. Once a diagnosis of resistant hypertension is made using a 24-hour ABPM and a fourth drug is needed after use of a calcium antagonist, diuretic, and RAAS blocker, a mineralocorticoid inhibitor has demonstrated significant benefit in controlling BP in newer studies.[281-283] A detailed discussion of this topic is beyond the scope of this chapter, but the reader is referred to two good reviews by Kwok and associates and Achelrod and colleagues.[284,285]

Complete reference list available at ExpertConsult.com.

KEY REFERENCES

1. Mozaffarian D, Benjamin EJ, Go AS, et al: Executive summary: heart disease and stroke statistics-2015 update: a report from the American Heart Association. *Circulation* 131:434–441, 2015.
9. Lewington S, Clarke R, Qizilbash N, et al: Age-specific relevance of usual blood pressure to vascular mortality: a meta-analysis of individual data for one million adults in 61 prospective studies. *Lancet* 360:1903–1913, 2002.
10. Pickering TG, Hall JE, Appel LJ, et al: Recommendations for blood pressure measurement in humans and experimental animals: part 1: blood pressure measurement in humans: a statement for professionals from the Subcommittee of Professional and Public Education of the American Heart Association Council on High Blood Pressure Research. *Hypertension* 45:142–161, 2005.
11. Mancia G, Fagard R, Narkiewicz K, et al: 2013 ESH/ESC guidelines for the management of arterial hypertension: the Task Force for the Management of Arterial Hypertension of the European Society of Hypertension (ESH) and of the European Society of Cardiology (ESC). *J Hypertens* 31:1281–1357, 2013.
12. James PA, Oparil S, Carter BL, et al: 2014 Evidence-based guideline for the management of high blood pressure in adults: report from the panel members appointed to the Eighth Joint National Committee (JNC 8). *JAMA* 311:507–520, 2014.
14. Franklin SS, Jacobs MJ, Wong ND, et al: Predominance of isolated systolic hypertension among middle-aged and elderly US hypertensives: analysis based on National Health and Nutrition Examination Survey (NHANES) III. *Hypertension* 37:869–874, 2001.
23. Beckett NS, Peters R, Fletcher AE, et al: Treatment of hypertension in patients 80 years of age or older. *N Engl J Med* 358:1887–1898, 2008.
24. Skinner AC, Skelton JA: Prevalence and trends in obesity and severe obesity among children in the United States, 1999-2012. *JAMA Pediatr* 168:561–566, 2014.
31. Flack JM, Sica DA, Bakris G, et al: Management of high blood pressure in blacks: an update of the International Society on Hypertension in Blacks consensus statement. *Hypertension* 56:780–800, 2010.
35. Jaffe MG, Lee GA, Young JD, et al: Improved blood pressure control associated with a large-scale hypertension program. *JAMA* 310:699–705, 2013.
37. Staessen JA, Thijisq L, Fagard R, et al: Effects of immediate versus delayed antihypertensive therapy on outcome in the Systolic Hypertension in Europe Trial. *J Hypertens* 22:847–857, 2004.
42. O'Connor PM, Cowley AW, Jr: Modulation of pressure-natriuresis by renal medullary reactive oxygen species and nitric oxide. *Curr Hypertens Rep* 12:86–92, 2010.
51. Jain G, Ong S, Warnock DG: Genetic disorders of potassium homeostasis. *Semin Nephrol* 33:300–309, 2013.
52. Boyden LM, Choi M, Choate KA, et al: Mutations in kelch-like 3 and cullin 3 cause hypertension and electrolyte abnormalities. *Nature* 482:98–102, 2012.
55. Lifton RP, Gharavi AG, Geller DS: Molecular mechanisms of human hypertension. *Cell* 104:545–556, 2001.
59. Machnik A, Neuhofer W, Jantsch J, et al: Macrophages regulate salt-dependent volume and blood pressure by a vascular endothelial growth factor-C-dependent buffering mechanism. *Nat Med* 15:545–552, 2009.
61. Ehret GB, Munroe PB, Rice KM, et al: Genetic variants in novel pathways influence blood pressure and cardiovascular disease risk. *Nature* 478:103–109, 2011.
67. McCurley A, Jaffe IZ: Mineralocorticoid receptors in vascular function and disease. *Mol Cell Endocrinol* 350:256–265, 2012.

74. DiBona GF: Sympathetic nervous system and hypertension. *Hypertension* 61:556–560, 2013.
83. Julius S, Palatini P, Kjeldsen SE, et al: Usefulness of heart rate to predict cardiac events in treated patients with high-risk systemic hypertension. *Am J Cardiol* 109:685–692, 2012.
85. Dorresteijn JA, Visseren FL, Spiering W: Mechanisms linking obesity to hypertension. *Obes Rev* 13:17–26, 2012.
86. Flynn C: Increased aldosterone: mechanism of hypertension in obesity. *Semin Nephrol* 34:340–348, 2014.
99. Kohan DE, Barton M: Endothelin and endothelin antagonists in chronic kidney disease. *Kidney Int* 86:896–904, 2014.
108. Mitchell GF: Arterial stiffness: insights from Framingham and Iceland. *Curr Opin Nephrol Hypertens* 24:1–7, 2015.
110. Ben-Shlomo Y, Spears M, Boustred C, et al: Aortic pulse wave velocity improves cardiovascular event prediction: an individual participant meta-analysis of prospective observational data from 17,635 subjects. *J Am Coll Cardiol* 63:636–646, 2014.
112. Harrison DG: The immune system in hypertension. *Trans Am Clin Climatol Assoc* 125:130–138, 2014.
127. Bliziotis IA, Destounis A, Stergiou GS: Home versus ambulatory and office blood pressure in predicting target organ damage in hypertension: a systematic review and meta-analysis. *J Hypertens* 30:1289–1299, 2012.
142. Niiranen TJ, Asayama K, Thijs L, et al: Outcome-driven thresholds for home blood pressure measurement: international database of home blood pressure in relation to cardiovascular outcome. *Hypertension* 61:27–34, 2013.
156. Bruno RM, Palagini L, Gemignani A, et al: Poor sleep quality and resistant hypertension. *Sleep Med* 14:1157–1163, 2013.
163. Canniffe C, Ou P, Walsh K, et al: Hypertension after repair of aortic coarctation—a systematic review. *Int J Cardiol* 167:2456–2461, 2013.
171. Sundstrom J, Arima H, Woodward M, et al: Blood pressure–lowering treatment based on cardiovascular risk: a meta-analysis of individual patient data. *Lancet* 384:591–598, 2014.
172. Emdin CA, Rahimi K, Neal B, et al: Blood pressure lowering in type 2 diabetes: a systematic review and meta-analysis. *JAMA* 313:603–615, 2015.
173. Turnbull F, Neal B, Ninomiya T, et al: Effects of different regimens to lower blood pressure on major cardiovascular events in older and younger adults: meta-analysis of randomised trials. *BMJ* 336:1121–1123, 2008.
175. Bakris GL, Sarafidis PA, Weir MR, et al: Renal outcomes with different fixed-dose combination therapies in patients with hypertension at high risk for cardiovascular events (ACCOMPLISH): a prespecified secondary analysis of a randomised controlled trial. *Lancet* 375:1173–1181, 2010.
176. Gradman AH, Basile JN, Carter BL, et al: Combination therapy in hypertension. *J Clin Hypertens (Greenwich)* 13:146–154, 2011.
180. Appel LJ, Wright JT, Jr, Greene T, et al: Intensive blood-pressure control in hypertensive chronic kidney disease. *N Engl J Med* 363:918–929, 2010.
183. Rahman M, Greene T, Phillips RA, et al: A trial of 2 strategies to reduce nocturnal blood pressure in blacks with chronic kidney disease. *Hypertension* 61:82–88, 2013.
191. Bakris GL, Molitch M: Microalbuminuria as a risk predictor in diabetes: the continuing saga. *Diabetes Care* 37:867–875, 2014.
195. Lewis EJ, Hunsicker LG, Bain RP, et al: The effect of angiotensin-converting-enzyme inhibition on diabetic nephropathy. The Collaborative Study Group. *N Engl J Med* 329:1456–1462, 1993.
196. Brenner BM, Cooper ME, de Zeeuw D, et al: Effects of losartan on renal and cardiovascular outcomes in patients with type 2 diabetes and nephropathy. *N Engl J Med* 345:861–869, 2001.
197. Lewis EJ, Hunsicker LG, Clarke WR, et al: Renoprotective effect of the angiotensin-receptor antagonist irbesartan in patients with nephropathy due to type 2 diabetes. *N Engl J Med* 345:851–860, 2001.
198. Fried LF, Emanuele N, Zhang JH, et al: Combined angiotensin inhibition for the treatment of diabetic nephropathy. *N Engl J Med* 369:1892–1903, 2013.
214. Kovesdy CP, Bleyer AJ, Molnar MZ, et al: Blood pressure and mortality in U.S. veterans with chronic kidney disease: a cohort study. *Ann Intern Med* 159:233–242, 2013.
240. Agarwal R, Sinha AD, Pappas MK, et al: Hypertension in hemodialysis patients treated with atenolol or lisinopril: a randomized controlled trial. *Nephrol Dial Transplant* 29:672–681, 2014.
244. Taler SJ, Agarwal R, Bakris GL, et al: KDOQI US commentary on the 2012 KDIGO clinical practice guideline for management of blood pressure in CKD. *Am J Kidney Dis* 62:201–213, 2013.
246. Lazich I, Bakris GL: Prediction and management of hyperkalemia across the spectrum of chronic kidney disease. *Semin Nephrol* 34:333–339, 2014.
250. Boudville N, Ward S, Benaroia M, et al: Increased sodium intake correlates with greater use of antihypertensive agents by subjects with chronic kidney disease. *Am J Hypertens* 18:1300–1305, 2005.
252. Ferdinand KC: A compendium of antihypertensive therapy. *J Clin Hypertens (Greenwich)* 13:636–638, 2011.
254. Bakris GL, Weir MR: Angiotensin-converting enzyme inhibitor-associated elevations in serum creatinine: is this a cause for concern? *Arch Intern Med* 160:685–693, 2000.
261. Ernst ME, Carter BL, Goerdt CJ, et al: Comparative antihypertensive effects of hydrochlorothiazide and chlorthalidone on ambulatory and office blood pressure. *Hypertension* 47:352–358, 2006.

Renovascular Hypertension and Ischemic Nephropathy

Stephen C. Textor

CHAPTER OUTLINE

HISTORICAL PERSPECTIVE, 1568
PATHOPHYSIOLOGY OF RENOVASCULAR HYPERTENSION AND ISCHEMIC NEPHROPATHY, 1570
Renal Artery Stenosis versus Renovascular Hypertension, 1570
Role of the Renin Angiotensin System in One-Kidney and Two-Kidney Renovascular Hypertension, 1571
Mechanisms Sustaining Renovascular Hypertension, 1572
Phases of Development of Renovascular Hypertension, 1574
Mechanisms of Ischemic Nephropathy, 1574
Adaptive Mechanisms to Reduced Renal Perfusion, 1575
Mechanisms of Tissue Injury in Azotemic Renovascular Disease, 1577
Consequences of Restoring Renal Blood Flow, 1579
EPIDEMIOLOGY OF RENAL ARTERY STENOSIS AND RENOVASCULAR HYPERTENSION, 1580
CLINICAL FEATURES OF RENOVASCULAR HYPERTENSION, 1581
Fibromuscular Disease versus Atherosclerosis, 1581
CLINICAL FEATURES OF RENAL ARTERY STENOSIS, 1582
Progressive Vascular Occlusion, 1585
Role of Changing Antihypertensive Therapy, 1587

CHANGING POPULATION DEMOGRAPHICS, 1587
Role of Concurrent Diseases, 1587
DIAGNOSTIC TESTING FOR RENOVASCULAR HYPERTENSION AND ISCHEMIC NEPHROPATHY, 1588
Goals of Evaluation, 1588
Physiologic and Functional Studies of the Renin Angiotensin System, 1588
Studies of Individual Renal Function, 1589
Imaging of the Renal Vasculature, 1590
MANAGEMENT OF RENAL ARTERY STENOSIS AND ISCHEMIC NEPHROPATHY, 1594
Overview, 1594
Medical Therapy for Renovascular Disease, 1595
Endovascular Renal Angioplasty and Stenting, 1599
PROSPECTIVE TRIALS, 1602
Medical Therapy Compared to Angioplasty Plus Stents, 1602
COMPLICATIONS OF RENAL ARTERY ANGIOPLASTY AND STENTING, 1604
SURGICAL TREATMENT OF RENOVASCULAR HYPERTENSION AND ISCHEMIC NEPHROPATHY, 1604
PREDICTORS OF LIKELY BENEFIT REGARDING RENAL REVASCULARIZATION, 1607
SUMMARY, 1607

Few areas within nephrology are undergoing more dramatic paradigm shifts than occlusive renovascular disease. Aging population demographics coupled with advances in imaging technology, effective medical therapy, and clinical trials with negative results must be reconciled with an established record of clinical success and improving techniques of renal revascularization. Although trial data repeatedly fail to provide compelling evidence in favor of stenting for many patients with atherosclerotic disease, experienced clinicians recognize that renal revascularization in these disorders sometimes should be undertaken both to improve hypertension and to salvage renal function. Selecting patients and determining optimal timing for vascular intervention at reasonable risk is rarely simple.

The study and treatment of renovascular disease overlaps numerous medical disciplines and subspecialties, including nephrology, internal medicine, cardiovascular diseases, interventional radiology, and vascular surgery. These

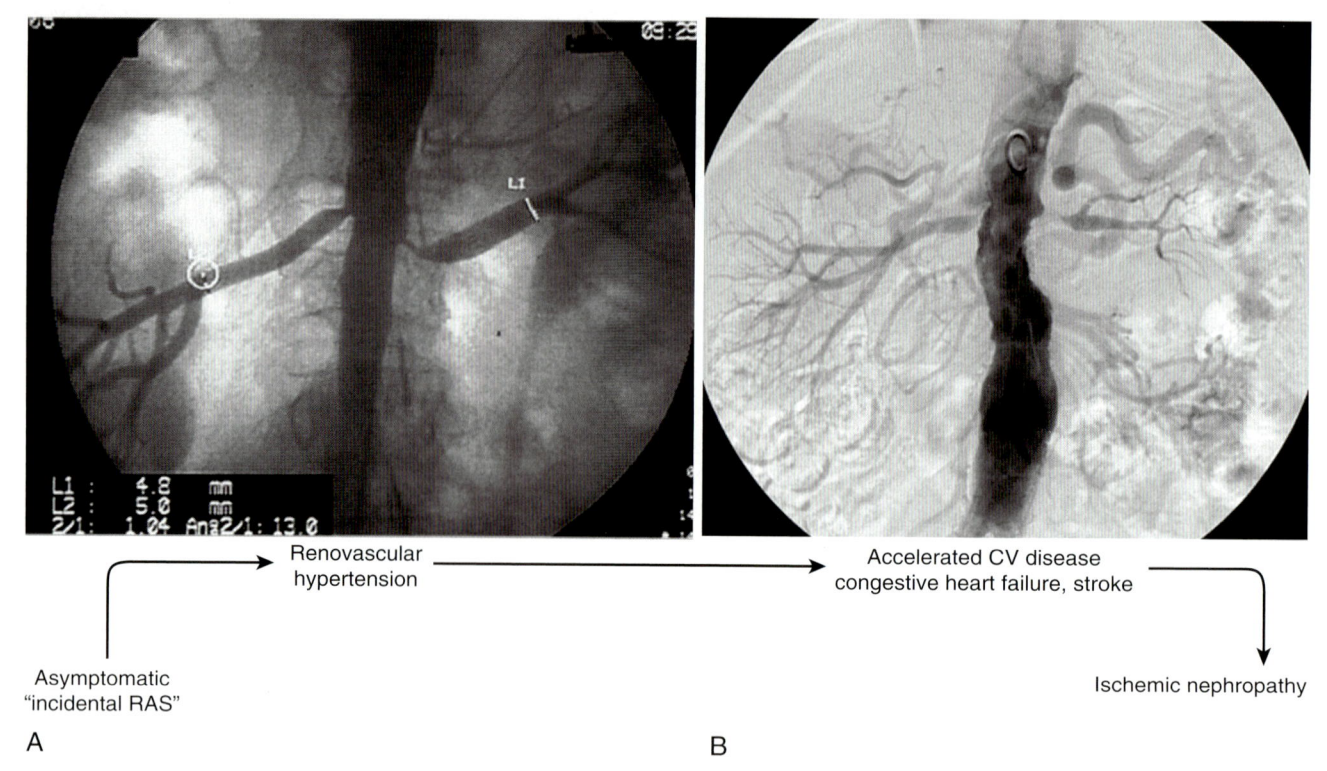

Figure 48.1 Spectrum of atherosclerotic renovascular disease (ARVD) manifestations. A, Aortogram obtained during coronary angiography demonstrating moderate "incidental" stenosis in both renal arteries in a 67-year-old man with symptomatic coronary disease. B, More severe occlusive disease observed in a 68-year-old woman presenting with severe hypertension and episodes of flash pulmonary edema. ARVD commonly develops in the setting of atherosclerotic disease elsewhere and may be associated with any of multiple clinical syndromes ranging from renovascular hypertension to accelerated cardiovascular (CV) decompensation and ischemic nephropathy. Trends favor initial management with intensive medical therapy, often including agents that block the renin angiotensin system. Clinicians face the challenge of recognizing the role of ARVD in more advanced disease and balancing the risks and benefits of renal revascularization in high-risk subsets. RAS, Renal artery stenosis. (Modified from Herrmann SM, Saad A, Textor SC: Management of atherosclerotic renovascular disease after Cardiovascular Outcomes in Renal Atherosclerotic Lesions (CORAL). *Nephrol Dial Transplant.* Epub April 9, 2014.)

subspecialty groups often deal with widely different patient subgroups and clinical issues that shape different points of view. Cardiologists, for example, more commonly manage patients with refractory congestive heart failure at risk for "flash" pulmonary edema than internists, who may deal with established patients with progressive hypertension or a rise in serum creatinine level (Figure 48.1). Nephrologists may encounter declining kidney function with high-grade stenosis to a solitary functioning kidney. All of these conditions can represent clinical manifestations of renovascular disease but present different comorbid risk and management issues. Not surprisingly, perceptions related to renovascular hypertension and ischemic nephropathy often differ even among informed clinicians. Initial results from prospective, randomized trials, such as Angioplasty and Stenting for Renal Artery Lesions (ASTRAL)[1] in the United Kingdom and Cardiovascular Outcomes in Renal Atherosclerotic Lesions (CORAL)[2] in the United States, comparing optimal medical therapy with or without endovascular stent procedures continue to provoke controversy. Some of the authors of these "negative" trials report "high-risk" subsets not enrolled in those studies that have major clinical and mortality benefits from restoring renal blood flow.[3-5] These observational studies underscore the ambiguity that clinicians encounter in practice. Ultimately, renovascular disease threatens blood flow to the kidney. The consequences of impaired blood flow not only affect blood pressure and cardiovascular risk, but also threaten the viability of the kidney. It can lead to irreversible loss of kidney function, sometimes designated "ischemic nephropathy" or "azotemic renovascular disease."[6] Restoring blood flow and perfusion by relieving vascular occlusion intuitively offers a means to halt or reverse this process. It must be recognized, however, that renal revascularization is a two-edged sword. The benefits include the potential to improve systemic arterial blood pressures and to preserve or salvage renal function. The potential risks of renal intervention are all too familiar to nephrologists. Endovascular procedures themselves may threaten the affected kidney through vascular thrombosis, dissection, restenosis, or atheroemboli. These events sometimes precipitate the need for renal replacement therapy, including dialysis or transplantation. It is therefore important that nephrologists have a solid foundation related to the implications of reduced renal perfusion and the risks and benefits of both medical management and restoration of renal artery patency.

HISTORICAL PERSPECTIVE

Renovascular disease is among the most intensely studied forms of secondary hypertension. Early observations regarding blood pressure regulation revealed important connections between fluid volume, renal arterial pressures, and vascular resistance. The sequence of these observations related to identification of the renin angiotensin system ahas been reviewed.[7] In 1898 Tigerstedt and Bergman established that extracts of the kidney had pressor effects in the whole animal and are credited with the identification of renin. Identification of each component of the renin angiotensin system represents a remarkable series of research ventures spanning a half century and investigators in many countries. Goldblatt and others provided seminal experiments, published between 1932 and 1934, with the development of an animal model in which reduced renal perfusion regularly produced hypertension. Numerous investigators thereafter identified the peptide nature of angiotensin, the role of "renin-substrate" or angiotensinogen, the role of nephrectomy in sensitizing the animal to the pressor effects of angiotensin, and the sequential "phases" of renovascular hypertension. Hence the renin-angiotensin system owes its initial discovery and nomenclature primarily to early studies related to regulation of blood pressure by the kidney. Much later, many additional actions of angiotensin became evident regarding vascular remodeling, modulation of inflammatory pathways, and interaction with fibrogenic mechanisms. Understanding that reduced renal blood flow produces sustained elevations in arterial pressure led to broad study of the mechanisms underlying many forms of hypertension. Experimental models of two-kidney and one-kidney renal clip (two-kidney and one-kidney "Goldblatt" hypertension) represent some of the most extensively studied models of blood pressure and cardiovascular regulation. Extension of these studies into clinical medicine followed soon thereafter. Some forms of hypertension were designated as malignant in character during the late 1930s and 1940s based on poor survival if patients were untreated. Few antihypertensive agents were known until the 1950s, and intervention consisted mainly of lumbar sympathectomy and/or extremely low-sodium-intake diets. Some of the major events in identification and treatment of renovascular hypertension are summarized in Figure 48.2.[8] Recognition that some forms of severe hypertension were secondary to occlusive vascular disease in the kidney led surgeons to undertake unilateral nephrectomy for small kidneys in 1937.[9] The fact that some of these were indeed "pressor" kidneys and blood pressure fell to normal levels provided "proof of concept" and led to more widespread use of nephrectomy. Unfortunately, achieving "cure" of hypertension after nephrectomy was rare, and Homer Smith reviewed the poor results overall in a 1956 paper discouraging this practice.

The 1960s marked the introduction of methods of vascular surgery to restore renal blood flow. These carried substantial morbidity but offered an opportunity to improve the renal circulation and potentially to reverse renovascular hypertension. One result of this development was a series of studies to characterize the functional role of each vascular lesion in producing hypertension, thereby allowing prediction of the outcomes of vascular surgery.[9] The large Cooperative Study of Renovascular Hypertension included major vascular centers and reported on the results of more than 500 surgical procedures. These results provided limited support for vascular repair but identified relatively high associated morbidity and mortality, particularly for patients with atherosclerotic disease.

In the 1980s and 1990s further developments led to both improved medications and the introduction of endovascular procedures, including percutaneous angioplasty and stents.[10] These both broadened the options for treating patients with vascular disease and raised new issues regarding timing and overall goals of intervention. Later developments highlight the need for intensive reduction of cardiovascular risk factors and more stringent standards of blood pressure control. Antihypertensive medications have improved dramatically, with regard to both efficacy and tolerability. As emphasized later, broad application of angiotensin-converting enzyme (ACE) inhibitors and angiotensin receptor antagonists, for reasons other than hypertension alone, changed the clinical presentation of disorders associated with renal artery stenosis. Prospective, randomized trials emphasize the limited additional benefits from restoring renal blood flow for many patients with moderate vascular disease.[3] Uncontrollable hypertension is now less commonly the reason to intervene in renovascular disease. Often the main objective is the long-term preservation of renal function. Endovascular techniques make renal

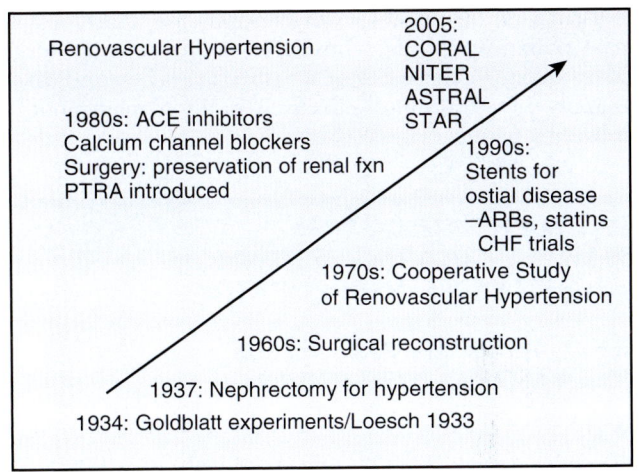

Figure 48.2 Historical timeline of major milestones in renovascular disease. Although pressor substances derived from the kidney were identified more than a century ago, recognition that renal perfusion regulates arterial blood pressure occurred only in the 1930s. Technical advances allowing surgical reconstruction, more effective arterial imaging, and endovascular revascularization gradually evolved from 1970 to the present. Important advances in antihypertensive drug therapy, particularly with agents that block the renin angiotensin system, and other advances in managing atherosclerotic disease such as statins continue to define optimal medical management of patients with renovascular disease. Results from several prospective, randomized clinical trials indicate that renal revascularization often fails to add substantial benefits to effective medical therapy in the near term for patients with moderate atherosclerotic renovascular disease, although high-risk subsets likely are an exception (see text). ACE, Angiotensin-converting enzyme; ARBs, angiotensin receptor blockers; ASTRAL, Angioplasty and Stenting for Renal Artery Lesions; CHF, congestive heart failure; CORAL, Cardiovascular Outcomes in Renal Atherosclerotic Lesions; fxn, function; NITER, Nephropathy Ischemic Therapy; PTRA, percutaneous transluminal renal angioplasty; STAR, Stent Placement and Blood Pressure and Lipid-Lowering for the Prevention of Progression of Renal Dysfunction Caused by Atherosclerotic Ostial Stenosis of the Renal Artery.

revascularization possible with relatively low morbidity in many patients previously considered as unacceptable surgical candidates. The challenge for clinicians is how and when to apply these tools most effectively in the management of individual patients[11]

PATHOPHYSIOLOGY OF RENOVASCULAR HYPERTENSION AND ISCHEMIC NEPHROPATHY

RENAL ARTERY STENOSIS VERSUS RENOVASCULAR HYPERTENSION

As with most vascular lesions, the presence of a renovascular abnormality alone does not translate directly into functional importance. Some degree of renal artery stenosis can be identified in as many as 20% to 45% of patients undergoing vascular imaging for other reasons, such as coronary angiography or lower extremity peripheral vascular disease.[12,13] Most of these incidentally detected stenoses are of minor hemodynamic significance. Failure to limit treatment trials to patients with hemodynamically important lesions has been a serious barrier to understanding the role for renal revascularization (see later). The term "renovascular hypertension" refers to a rise in arterial pressure induced by reduced renal perfusion. A variety of lesions can lead to the syndrome of renovascular hypertension, some of which are listed in Table 48.1. Studies of vascular obstruction using latex rubber casts indicate that between 70% and 80% of lumen obstruction must occur before measurable changes in blood flow or pressure across the lesion can be detected. Measurements of pressure gradients undergoing renal angiography confirm that a pressure gradient of at least 10 to 20 mm Hg between the aorta and the poststenotic renal artery is required before measurable release of renin develops.[14,15] When advanced stenosis is present, the fall in pressure and flow develops steeply as illustrated in Figure 48.3. When lesions have reached this degree of hemodynamic significance, they are deemed to have reached "critical" stenosis.

When renal artery lesions reach critical dimensions, a series of events leads to a rise in systemic arterial pressure

Table 48.1 Examples of Vascular Lesions Producing Renal Hypoperfusion and the Syndrome of Renovascular Hypertension

Unilateral Disease (Analogous to Two-Kidney–One-Clip Hypertension)

Unilateral atherosclerotic renal artery stenosis
Unilateral fibromuscular dysplasia[193]
   Medial fibroplasia
   Perimedial fibroplasia
   Intimal fibroplasia
   Medial hyperplasia
Renal artery aneurysm
Arterial embolus
Arteriovenous fistula (congenital/traumatic)
Segmental arterial occlusion (posttraumatic)
Extrinsic compression of renal artery (e.g., pheochromocytoma)
Renal compression (e.g., metastatic tumor)

Bilateral Disease or Solitary Functioning Kidney (Analogous to One-Kidney–One-Clip Model)

Stenosis to a solitary functioning kidney
Bilateral renal artery stenosis
Aortic coarctation
Systemic vasculitis (e.g., Takayasu's arteritis, polyarteritis)
Atheroembolic disease
Vascular occlusion due to endovascular aortic stent graft

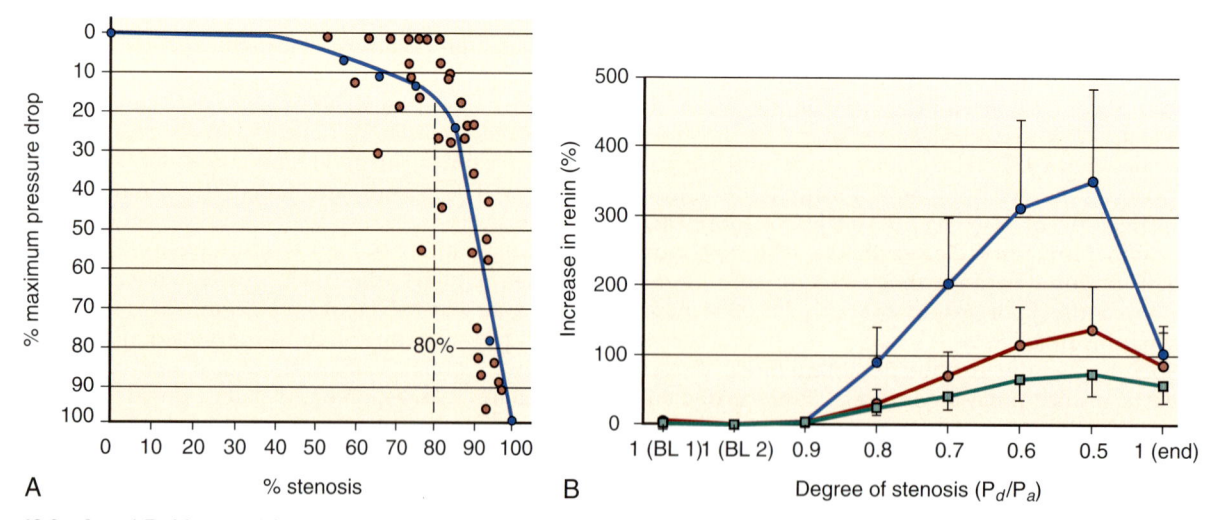

Figure 48.3 A and B, Measured fall in arterial pressure and blood flow across stenotic lesion induced in experimental animals. The degree of stenosis was determined using latex casts after completion of the experiment. These data indicate that critical lesions require 70% to 80% luminal obstruction before hemodynamic effects can be detected. Studies from human subjects with translesional pressure gradients indicate that aortic-renal pressure gradient of 10% to 20% is necessary to detect renin release (**A** from Textor SC: Renovascular hypertension and ischemic nephropathy. In Brenner BM, editor: *Brenner and Rector's: the kidney*, Philadelphia, 2008, Saunders, pp 1528-1566; **B** reprinted with permission from De Bruyne B, Manoharan G, Pijls NHJ, et al: Assessment of renal artery stenosis severity by pressure gradient measurements. *J Am Coll Cardiol* 48:1851-1855, 2006.)

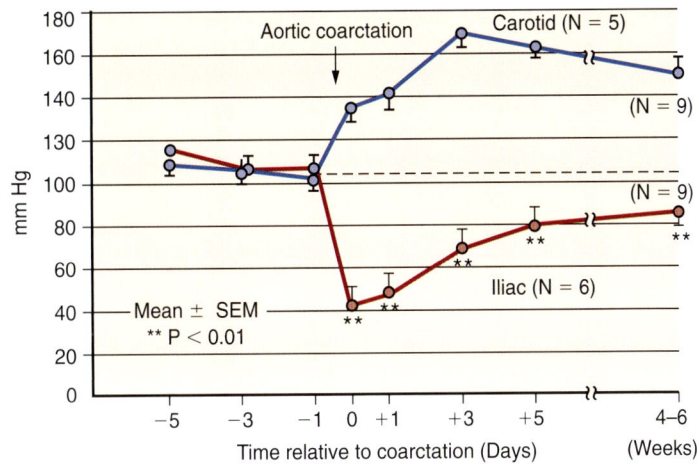

Figure 48.4 Systemic arterial pressure (carotid) and poststenotic renal perfusion pressures (iliac) in an aortic coarctation model with the clip placed between the right and left renal arteries. These measurements were obtained in conscious animals during development of renovascular hypertension. They illustrate the fact that despite a persistent gradient across the stenosis, renal perfusion pressure rises and is maintained at near normal levels at the expense of systemic hypertension. Reduction of systemic pressures thereby reduces post stenotic perfusion pressures due to the gradient across the lesion. SEM, Standard error of the mean. (Reprinted with permission from Textor SC, Smith-Powell L: Post-stenotic arterial pressure, renal haemodynamics and sodium excretion during graded pressure reduction in conscious rats with one- and two-kidney coarctation hypertension. *J Hypertens* 6:311-319, 1988.)

and restoration of renal perfusion pressure as illustrated in Figure 48.4. Hence one can view the development of rising pressures in this context as an integrated renal response to maintain renal perfusion. It is important to distinguish between experimental models of "clip" stenosis, at which time a sudden change in renal perfusion is induced, and the more common clinical situation of gradually progressive lumen obstruction. In the latter instance, hemodynamic characteristics change slowly and are likely to produce hypertension over a prolonged time interval. The rise in systemic pressure restores normal renal perfusion, often with normal-sized kidneys and no discernible hemodynamic compromise. If the renal artery lesion progresses further (or is experimentally advanced), the cycle of reduced perfusion and rising arterial pressures recurs until malignant-phase hypertension develops. Experimental swine models emphasize gradually progressing vascular lesions that mimic human renovascular disease.[16]

A corollary to critical arterial stenosis is that reduction of elevated systemic pressures to normal in renovascular hypertension reduces renal pressures beyond the stenotic lesion. Poststenotic pressures may fall below levels of autoregulation that maintain blood flow. This underperfusion of the kidney activates counterregulatory pathways and leads to a sequence of events directed toward restoring kidney perfusion.

ROLE OF THE RENIN ANGIOTENSIN SYSTEM IN ONE-KIDNEY AND TWO-KIDNEY RENOVASCULAR HYPERTENSION

Reduction in renal perfusion pressures activates the release of renin from juxtaglomerular cells within the affected kidneys. Experimental studies indicate that hypertension in two-kidney–one-clip models can be delayed indefinitely so long as agents that block this system are administered. Animals genetically modified to lack the angiotensin (AT_1) receptor fail to develop two-kidney–one-clip hypertension as illustrated in Figure 48.5.[17] Experiments using kidney transplantation from AT_1 receptor knockout mice indicate that both systemic and renal angiotensin receptors participate in additive fashion to blood pressure regulation.[18]

Demonstration of the role of the renin angiotensin axis in renovascular hypertension depends in part upon whether or not a contralateral, nonstenotic kidney is present. Classically, human renovascular hypertension is considered analogous to two-kidney–one-clip experimental (Goldblatt) hypertension. The contralateral, nonstenotic kidney is subjected to elevated systemic perfusion pressures. Effects of rising perfusion pressure are to force natriuresis from the nonstenotic kidney and to suppress renin release. Hence the nonstenotic kidney tends to prevent the rise in systemic pressures, thereby perpetuating reduced perfusion to the stenotic side and fostering continued renin release from the stenotic kidney. Blood pressure in these models is demonstrably angiotensin dependent and associated with elevated circulating levels of plasma renin activity, as illustrated in Figure 48.6. The two-kidney–one-clip model of renovascular hypertension provides the basis for many of the early functional studies of surgically curable hypertension in which side-to-side function was compared (e.g., glomerular filtration, sodium excretion). This paradigm is also the basis for comparing kidneys side-to-side using radionuclide studies, such as captopril renograms, and renal vein renin determinations. Unilateral renal ischemia represents a classical model for the study of angiotensin-dependent hypertension and target organ injury.

When no such contralateral kidney is present or able to respond to pressure natriuresis, mechanisms sustaining hypertension differ. This model corresponds to the one-kidney–one-clip (one-kidney Goldblatt) hypertensive animal. Although renin release occurs initially, elevated systemic pressures develop with sodium and volume retention, because there is limited sodium excretion by the contralateral kidney. Rising pressures eventually restore renin levels to normal. Hypertension in this model is not demonstrably

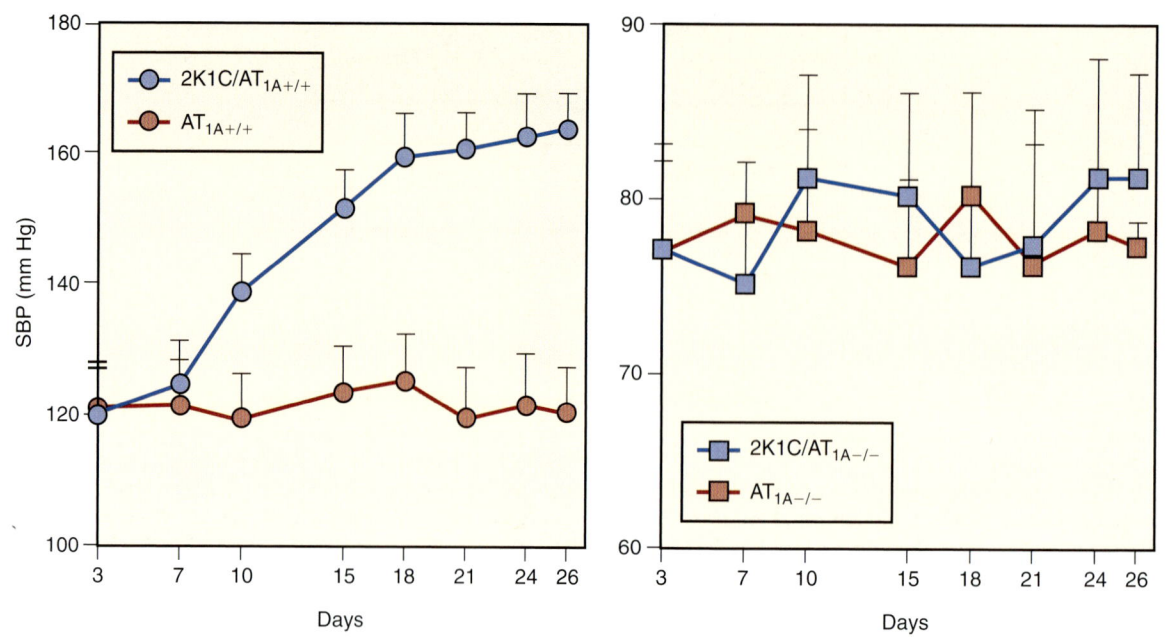

Figure 48.5 Systolic blood pressure (SBP) measurements in mice before and after placement of a renal artery clip in experimental two-kidney–one-clip renovascular hypertension (2K1C). The rise in SBP after clip placement develops rapidly only in mice with an intact angiotensin 1A receptor (AT_{1A+}, blue circles, left). This rise is blocked by administration of an angiotensin receptor blocker (red circles, left). A genetic knockout mouse strain with no AT_{1A} receptor ($AT_{1A-/-}$) has lower SBP and has no change after renal artery clipping (blue squares, right). No additional effect is noted with an angiotensin receptor blocker (red squares, right). These data reinforce the essential role of the renin angiotensin system and an intact angiotensin 1 receptor for development of renovascular hypertension. (Modified with permission from Cervenka L, Horacek V, Vaneckova I, et al: Essential role of AT1-A receptor in the development of 2K1C hypertension. Hypertension 40:735-741, 2002.)

dependent upon angiotensin II unless prior sodium depletion is achieved. Clinical examples of this situation are those of bilateral renal artery stenoses or stenosis to a solitary functioning kidney in which the entire renal mass is affected. In such cases diagnostic comparison of side-to-side renin release is not possible or has little meaning.

MECHANISMS SUSTAINING RENOVASCULAR HYPERTENSION

For more than a century the kidney has been recognized as a source of multiple pressor materials. Recruitment of numerous pathways that raise arterial pressure increases the complexity of managing hypertension in this setting. Identification of components of the renin angiotensin system provides a crucial link to understanding several of these systems. Circulating renin is derived primarily from the kidney in response to a reduction of renal perfusion pressure detected by loss of afferent arteriolar stretch.[19] Renin itself has biologic activity directed mainly to the enzymatic release of angiotensin I from its circulating substrate, angiotensinogen, in plasma and possibly other sites. Two further peptides are cleaved from angiotensin I through the action of ACE to produce angiotensin II. Generation of angiotensin II in plasma occurs mainly during passage through the lung. Hence the signal of reduced kidney pressures is amplified and transmitted to a major circulating vasopressor system that acts throughout the body, accounting for one major mechanism by which renovascular hypertension develops.

Following its discovery, the renin angiotensin system has been found to have widespread effects beyond its vasoconstrictor action in renovascular hypertension. Some actions of the angiotensin II are illustrated in Figure 48.7. Activation of this system increases vascular resistance, sodium retention, and aldosterone stimulation. Further studies indicate that complex interactions between angiotensin II and tissue and cellular systems occur, leading to vascular remodeling, left ventricular hypertrophy, and activation of inflammatory and fibrogenic mechanisms.

Hypertension and peripheral vasoconstriction reflect further complex interactions between angiotensin and other vasoactive systems. Renovascular disease leads to disturbances in sympathetic nerve traffic, which may differ between one-kidney and two-kidney models. Muscle sympathetic nerve activity is increased in humans with renovascular hypertension, and blood pressure responses to adrenergic inhibition are magnified.[20]

A major transition occurs with recruitment of altered oxidative stress within the systemic vasculature, leading to increased oxygen free radicals.[21] Experimental models of two-kidney–one-clip hypertension develop a rise in oxidative stress (reflected by F_2-isoprostanes) that can be reversed, in part, with angiotensin blockade and/or antioxidants.[22] Vascular injury itself produces disturbances in endothelium-derived mechanisms, such as endothelin production and vasodilator systems, including prostacyclin.[23] The roles for endothelial dysfunction and increased oxidative stress in human renovascular disease and their reversal after revascularization have been supported by clinical studies in patients with both atherosclerotic and fibromuscular renal artery stenosis.[24] Studies in a swine model of renovascular disease demonstrate an important interaction between "atherosclerosis" induced by cholesterol feeding and

UNILATERAL RENAL ARTERY STENOSIS

Reduced renal perfusion → ↑ Renin angiotensin system (RAS), ↑ Renin, ↑ Angiotensin II, ↑ Aldosterone → Angiotensin II–dependent hypertension

Increased renal perfusion → Suppressed RAS, Increased Na⁺ excretion (pressure natriuresis)

Effect of blockade of RAS
Reduced arterial pressure
Enhanced lateralization of diagnostic tests
Glomerular filtration rate (GFR) in stenotic kidney may fall

Diagnostic tests
Plasma renin activity elevated
Lateralized features, e.g., renin levels in renal veins, captopril-enhanced renography

A

BILATERAL RENAL ARTERY STENOSIS

Bilateral / Stenosis of solitary kidney → Reduced renal perfusion

↑ Renin angiotensin system (RAS), ↑ Renin, ↑ Angiotensin II, ↑ Aldosterone → Normal or low angiotensin II

Impaired Na⁺ and water excretion → Volume expansion → Increased arterial pressure

Inhibit RAS

Effect of blockade of RAS
Reduced arterial pressure only after volume depletion
May lower GFR

Diagnostic tests
Plasma renin activity normal or low
Lateralized features: none

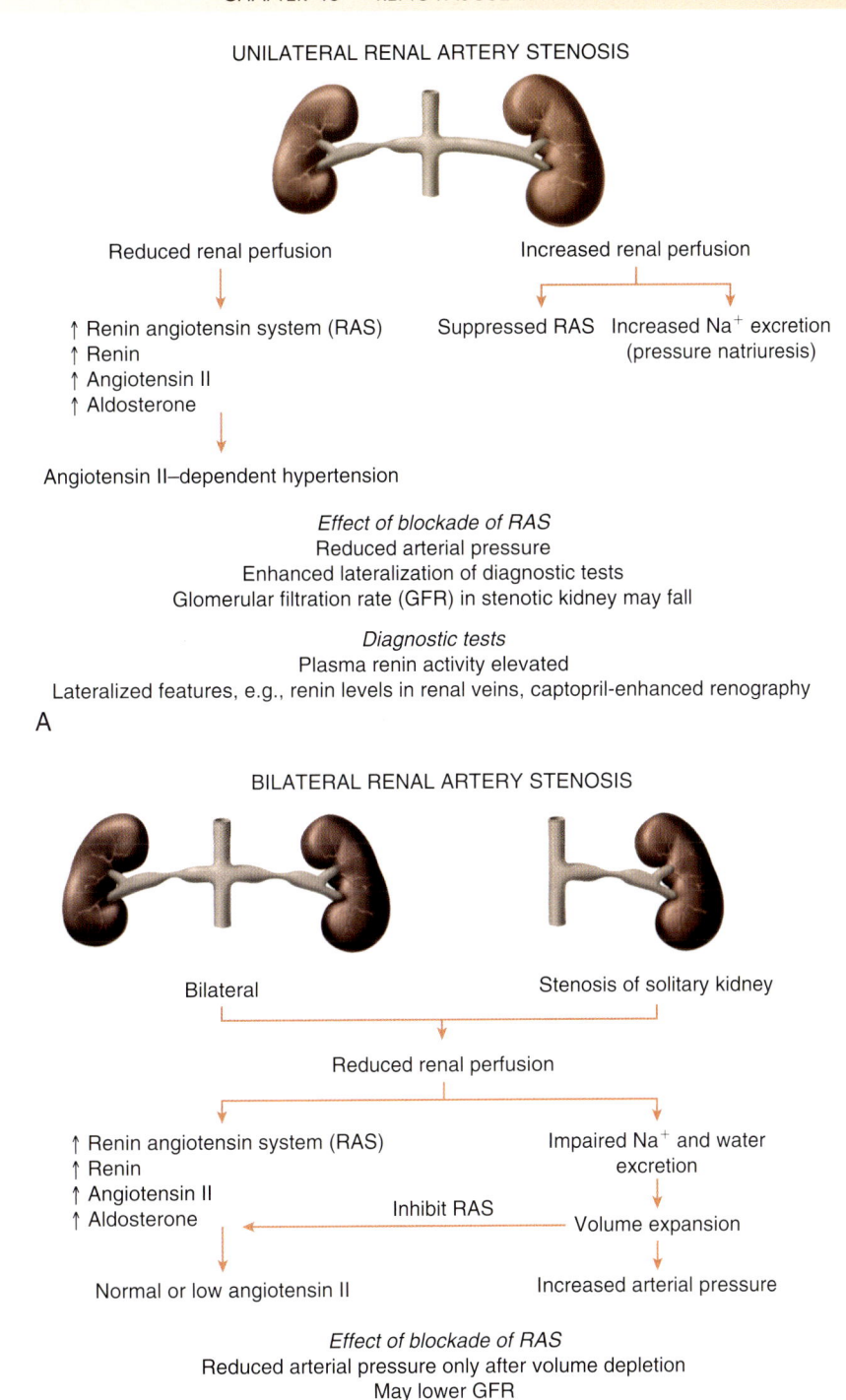

B

Figure 48.6 Schematic view of two-kidney (A) and one-kidney (B) renovascular hypertension. These models differ by the presence of a contralateral kidney exposed to elevated perfusion pressures in two-kidney hypertension. The nonstenotic kidney tends to allow pressure natriuresis to ensue and produces ongoing stimulation of renin release from the stenotic kidney. The one-kidney model eventually produces sodium retention and a fall in renin level with minimal evidence of angiotensin dependence unless sodium depletion is achieved.

renovascular disease. Measures of endothelial dysfunction in the kidney and tissue fibrosis are magnified by the atherosclerotic process. Some of these changes can be abrogated experimentally by intensive therapy with statins and antioxidants.[25,26] These data have been reinforced in atherosclerotic renovascular disease demonstrating a rise in nitric oxide level and reduction in malondialdehyde level within 24 hours of endovascular revascularization.[27] These studies indicate that oxidative stress can be reversed both by infusion of antioxidants and by successful revascularization.

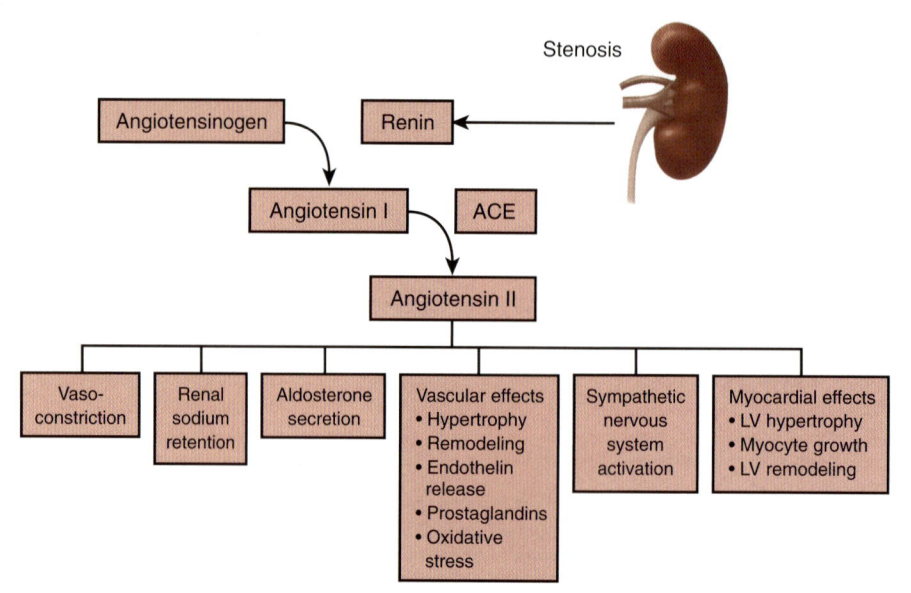

Figure 48.7 Schematic view of activation of the renin angiotensin system beyond a renal artery stenotic lesion. Generation of circulating and local angiotensin II leads to widespread effects, including sodium retention, efferent arteriolar vasoconstriction, and elevated systemic vascular resistance. Studies implicate angiotensin II in many other pathways of vascular and cardiac smooth muscle remodeling, activation of inflammatory and fibrogenic cytokines, coagulation factors, and induction of other vasoactive systems. ACE, Angiotensin-converting enzyme; LV, left ventricular.

Experimental infusion of agents capable of protecting mitochondria from reactive oxygen species by inhibiting the opening of the mitochondrial transition pore is associated with improved recovery of microvascular structures and renal function after revascularization.[28]

PHASES OF DEVELOPMENT OF RENOVASCULAR HYPERTENSION

Experimental models of renovascular hypertension indicate that mechanisms sustaining hypertension change over time (Figure 48.8). Even before occlusive lesions are evident, the renal vascular wall accumulates inflammatory monocytes, and levels of circulating cytokines are elevated.[29] An early pressor phase is characterized by elevated circulating indices of renin activity and hypertension, both of which return to normal after removing the vascular lesion. A second phase has been described with a return of circulating renin activity to normal or low levels, during which hypertension persists and blood pressure can still respond to clip removal. A third phase has been proposed, during which removal of the clip no longer leads to reduction in arterial pressure. These observations have been interpreted to underscore the transition between differing mechanisms of vascular control, some of which no longer depend upon reduced renal perfusion. Some data indicate that microvascular injury to the contralateral kidney sustains hypertension in this latter phase. Studies in a swine model indicate that the fall in renin activity follows a transition to mechanisms related to oxidative stress with persistent elevation of levels of oxidative metabolites such as isoprostanes.[21] Whether these phases translate directly to human renovascular disease is not well known.

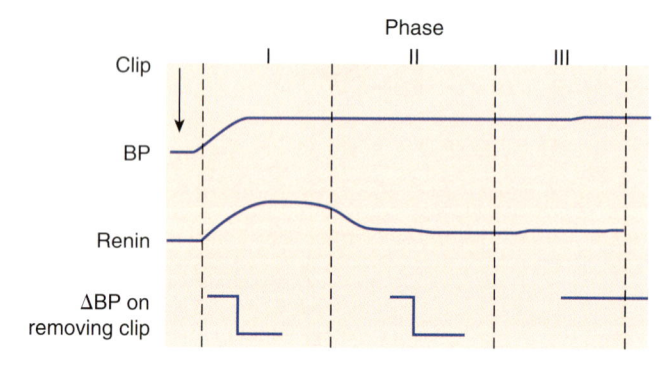

Figure 48.8 Schematic depiction of phases observed in experimental renovascular hypertension. Initially high levels of renin activity fall in the chronic phase, although removal of the renal artery clip corrects hypertension. These observations support the concept of renal artery stenosis leading to recruitment of additional structural and pressor mechanisms after initial activation of the renin angiotensin system (see text). Whether human renovascular hypertension follows these patterns is not well known. (Reprinted with permission from Textor SC: Renovascular hypertension and ischemic nephropathy. In Taal MW, Brenner BM, editors: *Brenner and Rector's the kidney*, Philadelphia, 2012, Elsevier Saunders, pp 1752-1791.)

MECHANISMS OF ISCHEMIC NEPHROPATHY

Reduced renal perfusion beyond critical stenosis ultimately leads to loss of viable kidney function, as illustrated in Figure 48.9. Patients with stenosis affecting the entire renal mass develop reduced blood flow and glomerular filtration when poststenotic pressures fall below the range of autoregulation. This process can be reversible if pressure is restored and/or the vascular lesion is removed. The

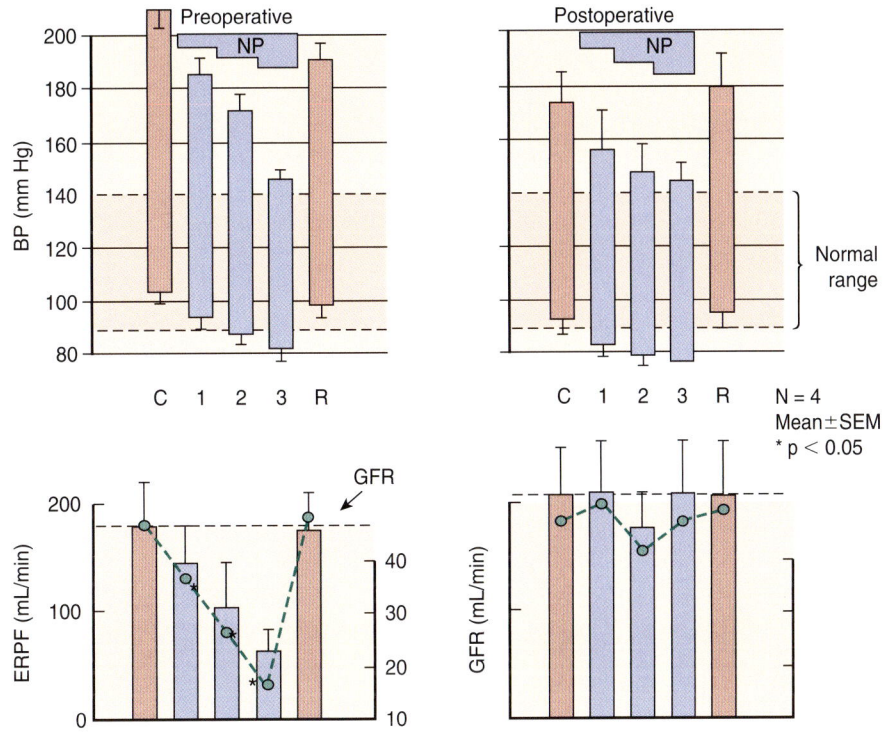

Figure 48.9 Effective renal plasma flow (ERPF) and glomerular filtration rate (GFR) in patients with critical bilateral renal artery stenosis (RAS) during pressure reduction with sodium nitroprusside (NP). Reducing systemic blood pressure (BP) to normal levels produced a reversible fall in both plasma flow and GFR. Repeat studies in the same patients (**right**) after unilateral surgical revascularization demonstrate that the sensitivity of blood flow and GFR to pressure reduction can be reversed. SEM, Standard error of the mean. (Reprinted with permission from Textor SC. Renovascular hypertension and ischemic nephropathy. In Taal MW, Brenner BM, editors: *Brenner and Rector's the kidney*, Philadelphia, 2012, Elsevier Saunders, pp 1752-1791.)

mechanisms by which this occurs differ from those that govern the development of hypertension. The term "ischemic" nephropathy may itself be a misnomer, as we have discussed previously.[15,30]

ADAPTIVE MECHANISMS TO REDUCED RENAL PERFUSION

Unlike brain or cardiac tissue, the kidney is vastly oversupplied with oxygenated blood, consistent with its function as a filtering organ. Measurements of both renal vein oxygen saturation and erythropoietin level in patients with high-grade renovascular lesions indicate that whole-organ ischemia is rarely present. It has long been postulated that local areas of reduced oxygen delivery within the kidney predispose to injury. Imaging using blood oxygen level–dependent (BOLD) magnetic resonance imaging (MRI) demonstrates markedly reduced oxygenation in deeper medullary regions despite preserved cortical oxygenation in both normal kidneys and in patients with renal artery stenosis.[30] Much of the oxygen consumption within the kidney is a result of energy consumed in solute transport. Studies using BOLD MRI of patients with renal artery stenosis sufficient to reduce blood flow, kidney volume, and glomerular filtration rate (GFR) indicate remarkable preservation of tissue oxygenation (Figure 48.10). This protection of oxygen gradients is due partly to the surplus of oxygenated blood to the cortex and to reduced oxygen consumption as a result of reduced solute filtration and thereby reduced reabsorptive work of the affected kidney. When more severe vascular occlusion produces cortical hypoxia, these adaptive measures are overwhelmed and tissue injury ensues.

The kidney maintains autoregulation of blood flow in the face of reduced arterial diameters of up to 75%. Under basal conditions, renal blood flow is among the highest of all organs, reflecting its filtration function. Less than 10% of delivered oxygen is sufficient to maintain overall renal metabolic needs. Under conditions of impaired renal perfusion, oxygen delivery is sometimes maintained by development of collateral vessels, associated with intrarenal redistribution of blood flow. The kidney medulla normally functions at levels closer to hypoxia and is sensitive to acute changes in perfusion.[31] During chronic reduction of blood flow, the medulla is partially protected by adaptive maintenance of tissue perfusion at the expense of cortical blood flow, which parallels whole-kidney renal blood flow.[32] Hence gradual reduction of renal perfusion pressures allows recruitment of protective mechanisms, which remain incompletely understood, leading to different functional and morphologic changes from those observed after acute ischemic injury.

A fall in renal blood flow is accompanied by decreased oxygen consumption, in part due to reduced metabolic

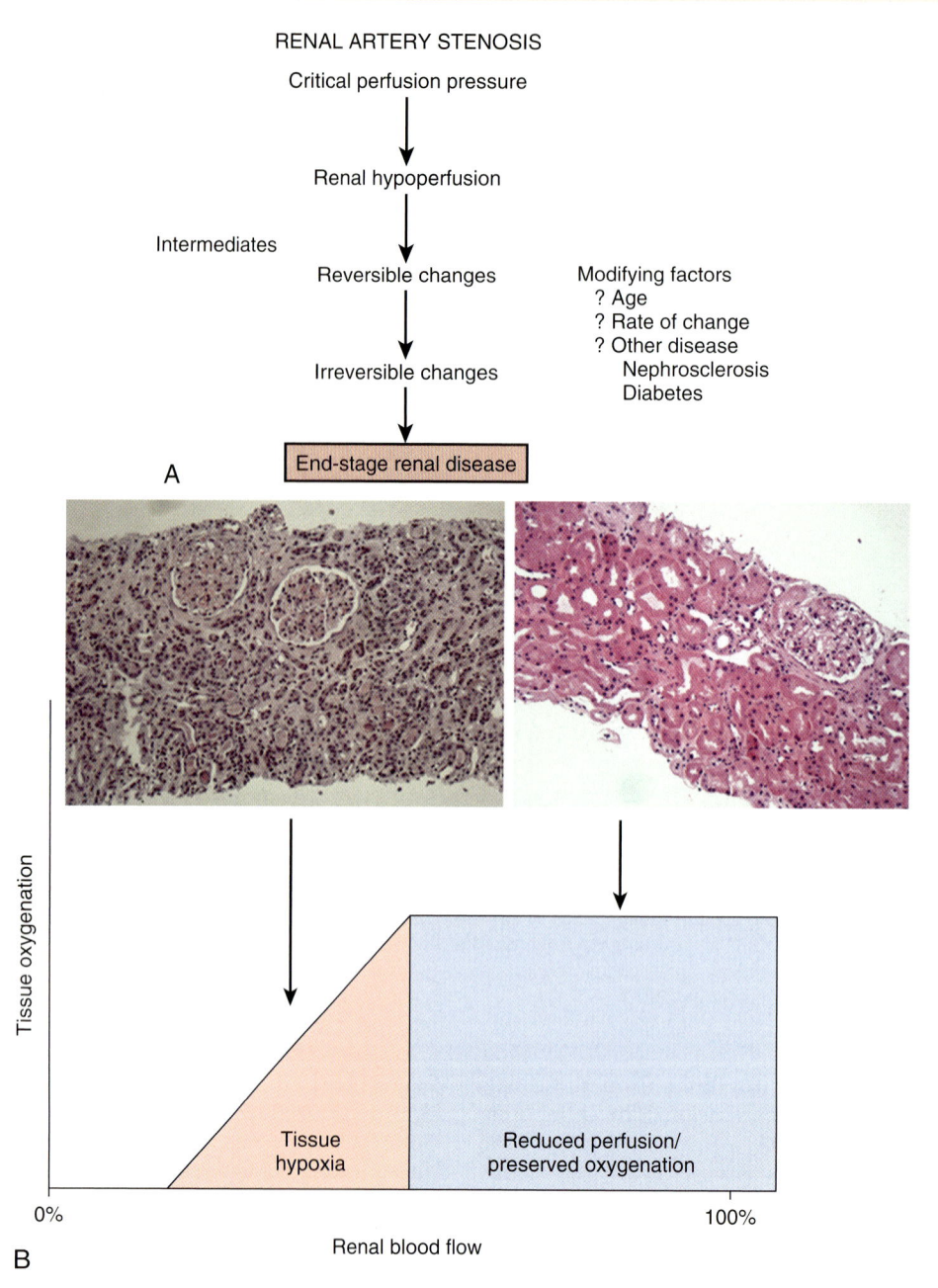

Figure 48.10 **A,** Schematic depiction of the "adaptation" of tissue oxygenation within the kidney to moderate reduction in blood flow, whereby both oxygen gradients and tissue histologic characteristics can be preserved. The fact that such adaptation occurs may partly explain the stability of kidney function during antihypertensive drug therapy that lowers systemic pressure and renal blood flow in patients with atherosclerotic renal artery stenosis. Eventually, more severe reductions of blood flow overwhelm adaptation, leading to overt tissue hypoxia. Transjugular biopsy samples from patients with cortical hypoxia demonstrate loss of tubular structures and accumulation of inflammatory T cells and macrophages with diffuse activation of transforming growth factor-β. **B,** General clinical paradigm that reversible reduction in glomerular filtration rate related to hypoperfusion of the kidney undergoes a transition to irreversible injury at some point that no longer responds to restoration of blood flow alone. (Modified from Gloviczki ML, Keddis MT, Garovic VD, et al: TGF expression and macrophage accumulation in atherosclerotic renal artery stenosis. *Clin J Am Soc Nephrol* 8:546-553, 2013.)

demands of filtration and tubular solute reabsorption.[31,33] When severe, reduced blood flow leads to accumulation of deoxygenated molecular hemoglobin (Figure 48.11A and D).[34,35] Eventually, structural atrophy of the renal tubules occurs, partly due to necrosis and apoptosis.[36] The latter is an active, programmed form of cellular death that appears to be closely regulated and differs from tissue necrosis. Tubular atrophy is potentially reversible, and the kidney maintains the capacity for tubular cell regeneration under many conditions, features that support the concept that underperfused kidney tissue sometimes can achieve a "hibernating" state capable of restoring function if blood flow is restored.[37] Eventually, pathologic examination demonstrates reduced glomerular volume, loss of tubular structures near underperfused glomeruli, and areas of local inflammatory reaction as illustrated in Figure 48.10B.

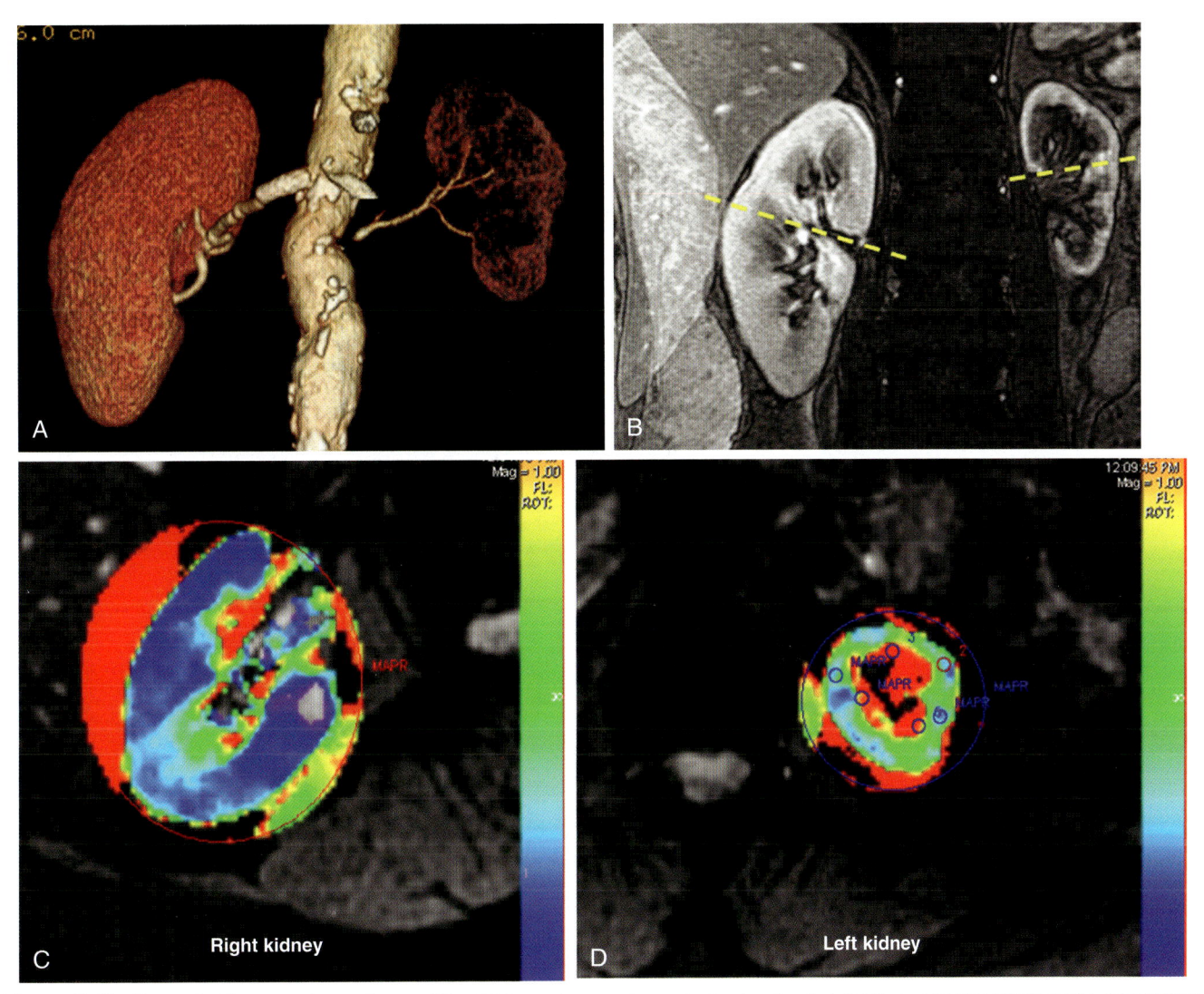

Figure 48.11 Computed tomography angiogram (**A**) of high-grade vascular occlusion leading to left kidney atrophy, whereas the right kidney is well perfused beyond an endovascular stent. T2 signals from magnetic resonance imaging (**B**) illustrate a gradient of perfusion from cortex to lower levels in the deeper medullary sections, especially in the left kidney. Mapping of the blood oxygen level–dependent (BOLD) magnetic resonance R2* levels (a function of deoxyhemoglobin) (**C** and **D**) illustrates the normal gradient in the right kidney from cortex (low R2*, *blue*) to deeper medullary segments that have progressively higher levels of R2* (*green* to *red*). The R2* map of the left kidney (**D**) illustrates overt cortical hypoxia evident beyond critical vascular occlusion associated with a larger fraction of the slice having high R2* values (*red*) and fractional hypoxia.

MECHANISMS OF TISSUE INJURY IN AZOTEMIC RENOVASCULAR DISEASE

Reduction of blood flow to the kidney activates numerous pathways of vascular and tissue injury, including increased angiotensin II, endothelin release, and oxidative stress, as noted earlier. Experimental studies demonstrate complex interactions with renal microvessels, leading to vascular rarefaction (Figure 48.12) and stimulation of inflammatory signaling and cellular infiltration to injured renal tubules.[38] Under the right conditions, these factors trigger ongoing release of inflammatory cytokines that eventually activate fibrogenic mechanisms and tissue fibrosis.

The role of angiotensin II during renal hypoperfusion is complex. The generation of angiotensin II acts to raise perfusion pressure and to protect glomerular filtration by efferent arteriolar constriction, as noted earlier. Angiotensin II induces cellular hypertrophy and hyperplasia in several cell types, in addition to direct stimulation of local hormone production and ion transport. Experimental infusion of angiotensin II leads to parenchymal renal injury with focal and segmental glomerulosclerosis.[39] ACE inhibition and angiotensin II receptor blockade in several experimental models diminish renal cell proliferation and suppress infiltration of mononuclear cells that trigger expression of extracellular matrix proteins and progressive nephrosclerosis. Angiotensin II may participate in vascular smooth muscle cell growth, platelet aggregation, generation of superoxide radicals, activation of adhesion molecules and macrophages, induction of gene transcription for proto-oncogenes, and oxidation of low-density lipoproteins.[40] These observations underscore the multiple roles of angiotensin II, both for adaptation and maintenance of kidney function and for

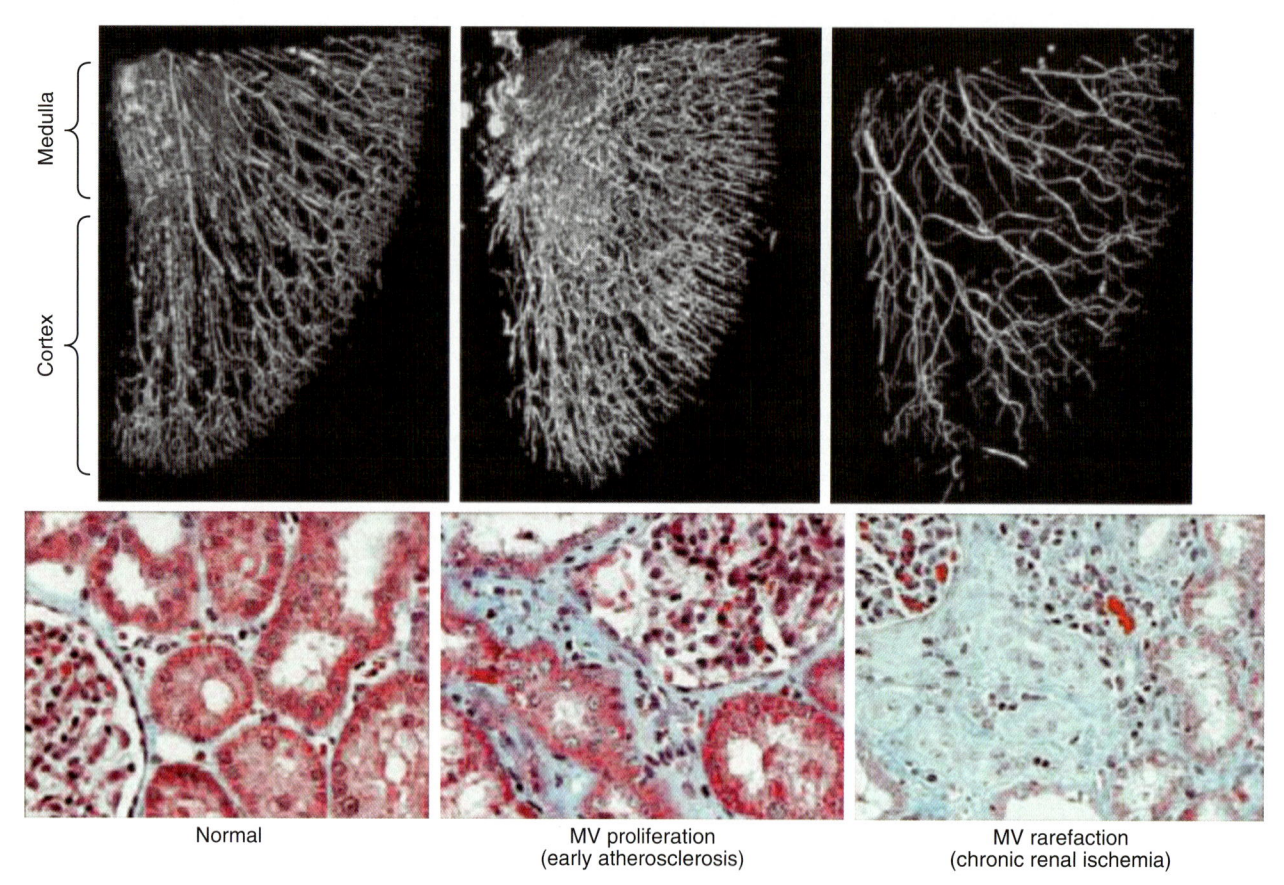

Figure 48.12 **Illustrations of micro–computed tomography reconstructions of vessels in experimental atherosclerosis and superimposed large vessel renovascular disease.** Studies demonstrate complex microvascular dysfunction and rarefaction that develop in poststenotic kidneys. These are accelerated and/or modified by angiogenic stimuli, oxidative stress pathways, and a variety of cytokines leading eventually to interstitial fibrosis. Studies in experimental animals suggest that angiogenic stimuli such as intrarenal infusion of endothelial progenitor cells or mesenchymal stem cells may offer the potential to repair microvascular injury (see text). Microvascular rarefaction in particular is accompanied by severe renal fibrosis **(bottom)**. MV, Microvascular. (Reprinted with permission from Lerman LO, Chade AR: Angiogenesis in the kidney: a new therapeutic target? *Curr Opin Nephrol Hypertens* 18:160-165, 2009.)

modulating many steps in the pathologic cascade underlying progressive renal injury.

Experimental studies indicate an independent effect of hypercholesterolemia in modifying parenchymal renal injury in ischemic nephropathy. Cholesterol feeding is used as a model of "early atherosclerosis" and itself alters renal vascular reactivity to acetylcholine and changes renal tubular functional characteristics.[41] Levels of oxidized low-density lipoprotein rise in this model, associated with markers of oxidative stress and activation of tissue nuclear factor-kappaB, transforming growth factor-β (TGF-β), and inducible nitric oxide synthase. The effect of these changes in producing kidney fibrosis is magnified in the presence of renal artery stenosis. Many of these effects can be reduced experimentally by endothelin blockade, antioxidants, or statins.[42]

The vascular endothelium is a source of multiple vasoactive factors, the most widely recognized of which are nitric oxide and endothelin. Endothelial *nitric oxide* is synthesized from L-arginine by a family of nitric oxide synthases and participates in the regulation of kidney function by counteracting the vasoconstrictor effects of angiotensin II. In addition to its effects on blood flow and tubular reabsorption of sodium, nitric oxide inhibits growth of vascular smooth muscle cells, mesangial cell hypertrophy and hyperplasia, and synthesis of extracellular matrix.

A reduction in renal perfusion leads to diminished "shear stress" distal to the stenosis. This condition reduces production of nitric oxide and accelerates release of renin and generation of angiotensin II in the stenotic kidney. Hence the effects of nitric oxide are diminished in the poststenotic kidney, allowing predominance of intrarenal vasoconstrictors, including angiotensin II and vasoconstrictor prostaglandins, such as thromboxane.[43] The decrease in nitric oxide removes its antithrombotic effects and the inhibition of responses to tissue injury. A direct consequence of reduced perfusion within the poststenotic kidney is progressive rarefaction of small vessels in both cortex and medulla, eventually producing tubular collapse (see Figure 48.12). Glomerular sclerosis is a late event and usually accompanies severe loss of GFR. Experimental studies infusing autologous endothelial progenitor cells into the renal artery demonstrate that functional recovery of GFR and restoration of vascular function can sometimes be achieved, suggesting that angiogenesis may be an achievable goal in this vascular bed.[44]

The *endothelin* (ET) peptides are potent and long-lasting vasoconstrictor peptides produced and released from endothelial cells. ET itself is released from renal epithelial cells after simulation with a variety of substances such as thrombin and local cytokines, including TGF-β), interleukin-1, and tumor necrosis factor. It must be emphasized that renal ischemia is a potent stimulus for expression of the endothelin-1 gene in the kidney, which persists for days after resolution of the ischemic injury. Sustained vascular effects of ET may participate in the hypoperfusion that lasts long beyond the vascular insult to postischemic kidneys.

The kidney is a rich site for production of *prostaglandins*, which are cyclo-oxygenase derivatives of arachidonic acid. These mediators are produced in arteries, arterioles, and glomeruli in the cortex, where they have important actions to maintain renal blood flow and filtration, particularly under conditions of elevated angiotensin II levels. Enhanced synthesis of prostacyclin and prostaglandin E_2 occurs during tissue hypoperfusion and ischemia, which may protect against some forms of hypoxic injury. Conversely, thromboxane A_2 (TXA_2) is a vasoconstrictor prostaglandin that lowers GFR by reducing renal plasma flow and can accelerate structural renal damage. It is stimulated by production of angiotensin II and reactive oxygen species and may in turn modify the hemodynamic properties of angiotensin II. TXA_2 modulates vascular permeability, which may contribute to interstitial matrix composition and target organ damage. Blockade of TXA_2 receptors in some models can reduce severity of experimental tissue damage, including acute ischemic injury.

Oxidative stress refers to an imbalance between tissue oxygen radical generating systems and radical scavenging systems toward "pro-oxidant" species. This process increases the presence and toxicity of reactive oxygen species, which in turn can promote the formation of vasoactive mediators, including endothelin-1, leukotrienes, and prostaglandin $F_{2\alpha}$ and isoprostanes, which are products of lipid peroxidation. As noted earlier, these mediators affect renal function and hemodynamics, both by inducing renal vasoconstriction and by changing glomerular capillary ultrafiltration characteristics. Reactive oxygen species themselves can magnify ischemic renal injury by causing lipid peroxidation of cell and organelle membranes. These disrupt structural integrity and capacity for cell transport and energy production, particularly within the proximal tubule. Other cytokine pathways, including activation of nuclear factor-kappaB and growth factors may play a role.

The role of TGF-β merits emphasis. It belongs to a family of polypeptides that regulate normal cell growth, development, and tissue remodeling after injury.[45] TGF-β is an important and ubiquitous fibrogenic factor, which modifies extracellular matrix synthesis by both glomerular and extraglomerular mesenchymal cells. These actions modify both tissue healing and progression to advanced renal failure. TGF-β is essential for tissue repair after many forms of injury, including ischemic conditions, during which it participates in restoring extracellular matrix in proximal tubular basement membranes. Activation of the AT_1 receptor stimulates generation of TGF-β, which plays a major role in tissue fibrosis through increases in type IV collagen deposition. TGF-β acts synergistically with endothelin and has interactions with platelet-derived growth factor, interleukin-1, and basic fibroblast growth factor in progressive interstitial fibrosis. Some investigators propose that many forms of renal scarring represent an overabundance of TGF-β activity due to failure to suppress its activity after repair of an original injury.[46] Activation of TGF-β develops in experimental models of renal artery stenosis and is magnified by hypercholesterolemia.[41] Conversely, animals lacking downstream effector pathways for TGF-β (e.g., Smad3 knockout mice) are protected from parenchymal injury in renovascular disease models.[47]

Although whole-kidney oxygen saturation and delivery remains preserved in the poststenotic kidney, it is inescapable that local areas within the kidney are exposed to at least *intermittent, recurrent ischemia*. The potential for repetitive acute renal injury to induce long-term irreversible fibrosis is evident from studies of acute heme protein exposure.[48] The hallmark of acute ischemia is a rapid decline in cellular adenosine triphosphate, which in turn allows accumulation of intracellular calcium, activation of phospholipases, and generation of oxygen free radicals.

Tissue ischemia appears to be a common denominator in many forms of progressive tubulointerstitial injury.[49] Such injury is associated commonly with interstitial inflammatory reactions and activation of fibroblasts and heat shock proteins. Disruption of the tubular epithelium alters the antigenic profile of these cells, initiating a cell-mediated immune response, sometimes associated with infiltration of B lymphocytes, T lymphocytes, and macrophages. As noted earlier, sustained tubulointerstitial injury leads to increased TGF-β production, enhanced expression of plasminogen activator inhibitor-1, tissue inhibitor of metalloprotease 1, collagen α_1 IV, and fibronectin-EIIA, and thus to increased synthesis of extracellular matrix.

Many of the mechanisms mentioned earlier interact with each other. Taken together, the kidney is subject to a wide variety of vasoactive and inflammatory mediators, which can be disturbed by loss of blood flow and perfusion pressure. These disturbances appear to activate a variety of fibrogenic and local destructive mechanisms, which can lead to irreversible parenchymal damage within the kidney.

CONSEQUENCES OF RESTORING RENAL BLOOD FLOW

As illustrated in Figure 48.9, restoring renal perfusion can allow recovery of renal function when these changes remain reversible. At some point, both inflammatory and fibrogenic mechanisms appear to no longer respond with recovery of renal function.

RENAL REPERFUSION INJURY

The course of recovery after restoration of blood supply to an underperfused kidney depends upon the extent and duration of the perfusion injury, in addition to the adequacy of reperfusion.[50] Paradoxically, some tissues subjected to ischemia undergo morphologic and functional changes that worsen during the reperfusion phase. This is thought to reflect vascular endothelial damage and activated leukocytes, which may be "primed" to obstruct distal capillaries after restoring perfusion pressure contributing to a so-called no-reflow phenomenon. Under experimental conditions, reperfusion injury appears to require major degrees of pro-oxidant stress with excess prostaglandin $F_{2\alpha}$ isoprostanes and free oxygen radicals, particularly with a deficit of nitric oxide. Hence antioxidants and reactive oxygen metabolite scavengers improve outcomes following experimental reperfusion. Within the kidney, ischemia-reperfusion models are most pronounced in the proximal tubules, with local necrosis and tubular obstruction as observed in acute tubular necrosis. Studies in experimental renovascular disease suggest that pretreatment with a mitochondrial transition pore inhibiting agent allows improved recovery of blood flow, microvascular integrity, and function in a swine model consistent with ischemia-reperfusion injury prevention.[28]

Angiotensin II may participate in some of these changes because activation of AT_1 receptors impairs glomerular filtration in the postischemic kidney.[51] Local imbalance of nitric oxide production is particularly prominent within the kidney; it has a dual action with the potential drawback of accelerating reoxygenation injury and initiating lipid peroxidation. However, systemic treatment with nitric oxide donors improves renal function and blunts local inflammation before reperfusion in some conditions.[52]

EPIDEMIOLOGY OF RENAL ARTERY STENOSIS AND RENOVASCULAR HYPERTENSION

The syndrome of renovascular hypertension can be produced by a wide variety of lesions affecting renal blood flow. In unselected mild to moderate hypertensive populations, the frequency appears to be between 0.6% and 3%, whereas in a referral clinic of patients with "treatment-resistant" hypertension, the prevalence may exceed 20%.[53] Some specific examples of lesions producing renal ischemia are listed in Table 48.1. A rapidly developing form of this disorder can be seen after spontaneous or traumatic renal artery dissection or iatrogenic occlusion, sometimes produced by endovascular aortic stent grafts.[10] The majority of stenotic lesions are either "fibromuscular diseases" or atherosclerotic renal artery stenosis (ARAS). The reported prevalence depends heavily upon differences between patient groups studied. As noted later, the prevalence of anatomic renal artery stenosis far exceeds that of renovascular hypertension.

Fibromuscular dysplasia (FMD) commonly refers to one of several conditions affecting the intimal, medial, or fibrous layers of the vessel wall. In some cases multiple layers of the vessel wall may be affected. Reports from arteriograms obtained in "normal" renal organ donors indicate that 3% to 5% of persons may have one of these lesions, many of which are present at an early age and do not affect either renal blood flow or arterial pressure.[54] Such lesions can lead to renovascular hypertension, sometimes associated with dissection or progression. Smoking is a risk factor for disease progression. Medial fibroplasia is the most common subtype, often associated with a "string-of-beads" appearance as illustrated in Figure 48.13A. These lesions consist primarily of intravascular "webs," each of which may have only moderate hemodynamic effect. The combination of multiple webs in series, however, can impede blood flow characteristics and activate responses within the kidney to reduced perfusion. FMD appears in the renal arteries in 65% to 70% of cases and in cerebral arteries in 25%. Both renal and cerebral vessels may be abnormal in 10% to 25%. The

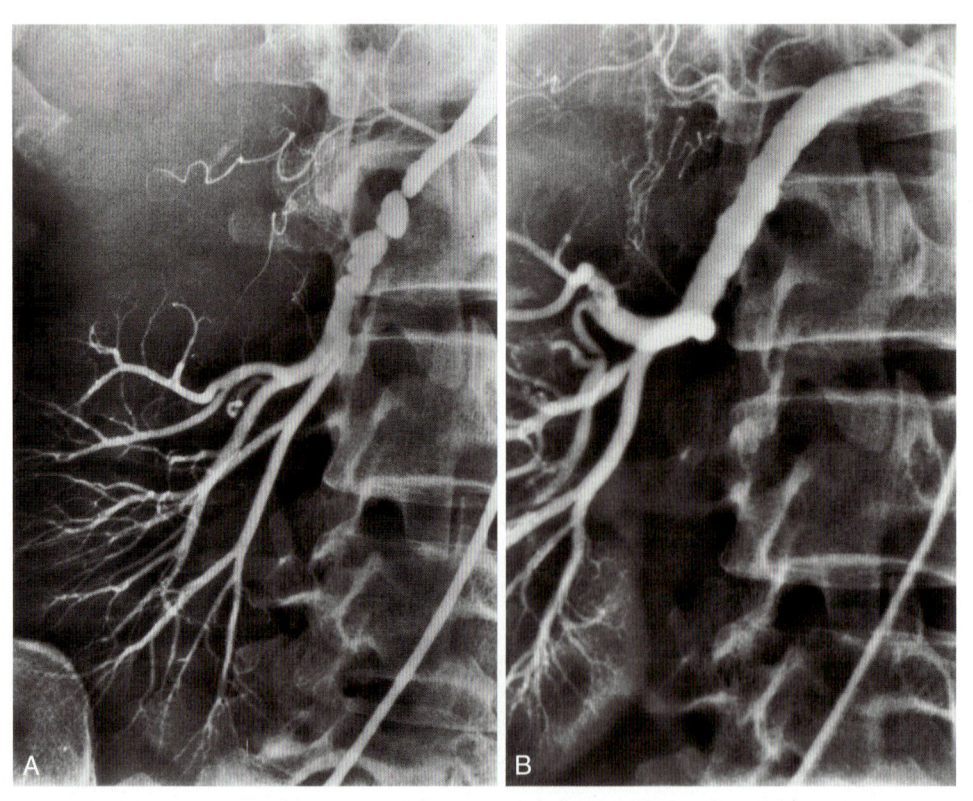

Figure 48.13 **A,** Angiographic appearance of medial fibroplasia with serial intravascular webs with small aneurysmal dilatations between them. These lesions appear in the midportion of the vessel and have a strong predilection for the right renal artery and are most commonly found in women. As shown in **B,** these lesions can often be improved substantially by balloon angioplasty.

preponderance of hypertensive cases coming to vascular intervention occur in women with a bias toward the right renal artery.[55] FMD lesions are classically located away from the origin of the renal artery, often in the midportion of the vessel or at the first arterial bifurcation. Some of these expand to develop small vascular aneurysms. Although less common, other dysplastic lesions, particularly intimal hyperplasia, can progress and lead to renal ischemia and atrophy. Although loss of renal function is unusual with FMD, quantitative imaging of cortical and medullary kidney volumes indicates parenchymal "thinning" occurs both in the stenotic and contralateral kidneys beyond FMD.[56] Interventional studies suggest that among patients referred for renal revascularization for hypertension FMD accounts for 16% or less.[57]

Atherosclerosis affecting the renal arteries is the most common renovascular lesion in the United States. ARAS can be identified commonly in patients with disease affecting other vascular beds and may be magnified by inflammatory vascular injury.[29] Population-based surveys identify incidental renal artery stenosis (more than 60% occlusion by Doppler criteria) in 6.8% of individuals older than 65 years in the United States.[58] A systematic review of imaging studies for other vascular conditions confirms that the prevalence of lesions with more than 50% luminal occlusion rises progressively with the extent of overall atherosclerotic burden.[13] Hence patients undergoing coronary angiography have identifiable ARAS in 14% to 20% of cases.[12,59,60] Aortograms obtained in patients with peripheral vascular disease demonstrate that 30% to 50% of such patients have renal artery lesions of some degree. Table 48.2 summarizes multiple reports related to the coexistence of atherosclerotic lesions in various vascular territories. The prevalence of ARAS increases with age and with the presence of atherosclerotic risk factors such as elevated cholesterol levels, smoking, and hypertension. The probability of identifying high-grade renal artery stenosis in hypertensive patients with azotemia rises from 3.2% in the sixth decade to above 25% in the eighth decade.[61] Population-based studies in the United States confirm that more than 70% of older patients with renal artery stenosis above 60% occlusion have clinical manifestations of cardiovascular disease.[62] The prevalence of ARAS may be rising as a result of more individuals surviving to older ages. These figures confirm previous postmortem observations indicating that many patients dying of cardiovascular disease have renal artery lesions at autopsy. They underscore the fact that some renal artery lesions remain undetected on clinical grounds for many years (see later).

The location of atherosclerotic disease is most often near the origin of the artery (Figure 48.14A), although it can be observed anywhere. Many such lesions represent a direct extension of an aortic plaque into the renal arterial segment. It should be emphasized that ARAS is strongly associated with preexisting hypertension, cardiovascular lipid risk, diabetes, smoking, and abnormal renal function.[12,59]

CLINICAL FEATURES OF RENOVASCULAR HYPERTENSION

FIBROMUSCULAR DISEASE VERSUS ATHEROSCLEROSIS

As noted earlier, renovascular hypertension may develop as a result of many lesions (see Table 48.1). The two most common are the FMDs and atherosclerosis. FMD represents several types of intimal or medial disorders of the vessel wall, commonly affecting midportions of the renal artery in younger individuals. These lesions rarely lead to major renal functional loss, although some progression may be seen, particularly in smokers. FMD lesions appear most often as hypertension of early onset (between 30 and 50 years of age) and unusual severity. Occasionally FMD presents as hypertension during pregnancy. Many lesions respond well to percutaneous angioplasty (see Figure 48.13B).[63]

By contrast, atherosclerotic lesions more commonly arise near the origin of the renal artery and amplify the risks of systemic atherosclerosis elsewhere. ARAS is commonly associated with reduced glomerular filtration rates.[11] Clinical manifestations may fall across a wide spectrum (see Figure 48.1), although they are not related simply to the anatomic severity of the lesion.[64] Ambulatory blood pressure recordings indicate exaggerated systolic pressure variability and frequent loss of the circadian pressure rhythm,[65] commonly associated with left ventricular hypertrophy. Sympathetic nerve traffic recordings indicate heightened adrenergic outflow. A population-based study of 870 subjects older than 65 years indicated that those with renal artery stenosis had a 2- to 3-fold increased risk for adverse cardiovascular events during the subsequent 2 years.[62] These data are supported by a review of Medicare claims data between 1999 and 2001 for a random sample of Medicare recipients above 67 years of age.[66] The authors indicate that the incidence of newly treated atherosclerotic renovascular disease was 3.7 per 1000 patient-years and was associated with preexisting

Table 48.2 Prevalence Rates of Atherosclerotic Renal Artery Stenosis in Patients with Vascular Disease Affecting Other Regional Beds Identified by Angiography

"Suspected renovascular HTN"	14.1%
Coronary angiography	10.5%
With HTN	17.8%
Peripheral vascular disease	25.3%
AAA	33.1%
ESKD	40.8%?
Congestive heart failure	54.1%?

N = 40 studies: 15,879 patients. Prevalence of patients with "50% luminal" narrowing: pooled prevalence rates.
Pooled prevalence rates for various imaging modalities indicating identified atherosclerotic RAS associated with vascular disease in other vascular beds.
(?) marks refer to limited data suggesting high prevalence in unexplained advanced chronic kidney disease (CKD) in older subjects and patients with congestive heart failure.
AAA, Abdominal aortic aneurysm; ESKD, end-stage kidney disease; HTN, hypertension; RAS, renal artery stenosis.
de Mast Q, Beutler JJ: The prevalence of atherosclerotic renal artery stenosis in risk groups: a systematic literature review. J Hypertens 27:1333-1340, 2009.

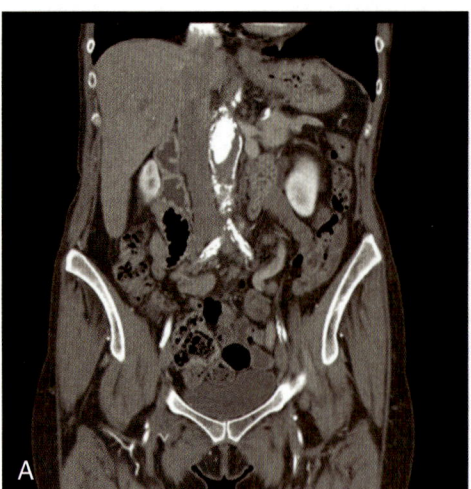

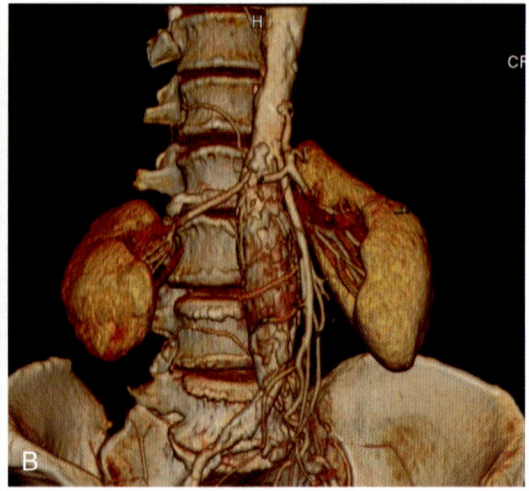

Figure 48.14 Atherosclerotic disease commonly affects both the renal arteries and abdominal aorta. **A** and **B,** Images from a computed tomography angiogram with high-grade stenosis to a small right kidney arising from diffuse aortic disease. The coronal section (**A**) demonstrates extensive thrombotic debris along the aortic wall. A reconstructed view of the aorta (**B**) demonstrates diffuse calcification and early aneurysm formation. The mean age of series presenting for renal revascularization for atherosclerotic disease has risen to more than 70 years. The decision about endovascular or surgical intervention in such cases must balance the hazards of aortic manipulation and the potential benefits regarding blood pressure control and/or renal function (see text).

peripheral and coronary disease. After detection, subsequent development of claims for heart disease, transient ischemic attack, renal replacement therapy, and congestive heart failure was 3- to 20-fold higher in such patients as compared to contemporaries without renovascular disease. Adverse cardiovascular events were more than 10-fold more common than the need for renal replacement therapy. As a result, one of the major current controversies in cardiovascular disease is how to identify and manage clinically significant renal artery stenosis as a modifying factor for cardiovascular outcomes. The major U.S. trial of renal revascularization (CORAL) specifically targeted overall cardiovascular outcomes in treating this disorder (see later).[2,3] This controversy is compounded by changes produced by (1) evolving medical therapy and (2) changing population characteristics.

CLINICAL FEATURES OF RENAL ARTERY STENOSIS

Manifestations of renal artery disease vary widely across a spectrum illustrated in Figure 48.1 and Table 48.3. This spectrum may range from an *incidental finding noted during imaging* for other indications to advancing renal failure leading to the need for dialytic support. As described earlier, multiple mechanisms raise systemic arterial pressure and tend to restore renal perfusion pressures to levels close to baseline. Clinical features of patients with essential hypertension were compared to those in patients subjected to revascularization for renovascular hypertension in the Cooperative Study of Renovascular Hypertension in the 1960s and are summarized in Table 48.3. Many features, including short duration of hypertension, early age of onset, funduscopic findings, and hypokalemia, were more common in those with renovascular hypertension but had limited discriminating or predictive value.

If renal artery lesions progress to critical stenosis, they can produce a *rapidly developing form of hypertension*, which may be severe and associated with polydipsia, hyponatremia, and central nervous system findings.[67] These cases are most often seen with acute renovascular events, such as sudden occlusion of a renal artery or branch vessel.

More commonly, renal artery stenosis presents as a progressive *worsening of preexisting hypertension*, often with a modest rise in serum creatinine levels. Because the prevalence of both hypertension and atherosclerosis increases with age, this disorder must be considered particularly in older subjects with progressive hypertension. Some of the most striking examples of renovascular hypertension are older individuals whose previously well-controlled hypertension deteriorates to an accelerated rise in systolic blood pressure and target injury, such as stroke. Studies from hypertension referral centers in the Netherlands are typical in this regard. Of 477 patients undergoing detailed evaluation for renal artery stenosis because of "treatment resistance," 107 (22.4%) were identified with renovascular disease (>50% stenosis by angiography). Clinical features predictive of renal artery stenosis included older age, recent progression, other vascular disease (e.g., claudication), an abdominal bruit, and elevated serum creatinine level. The authors derived a multivariate regression equation of predictive features for the presence of angiographic renal artery stenosis. They presented a clinical scoring system to determine the pretest probability of identifying renal artery disease (Figure 48.15).[57] The strongest predictors included age and serum creatinine level. Clinical features alone could provide pretest predictive value nearly as accurate as radionuclide scans.[57]

Declining renal function during antihypertensive therapy is a common manifestation of progressive renal arterial disease. Not surprisingly, blood flow and perfusion pressures to the kidney fall beyond a critical renal artery stenosis. This can be magnified by reduction in systemic arterial pressure by

> **Table 48.3 Clinical Features of Patients with Renovascular Hypertension**
>
> **A. Syndromes Associated with Renovascular Hypertension**
> 1. Early- or late-onset hypertension (<30 years, >50 years)
> 2. Acceleration of treated essential hypertension
> 3. Deterioration of renal function in treated essential hypertension
> 4. Acute renal failure during treatment of hypertension
> 5. Flash pulmonary edema
> 6. Progressive renal failure
> 7. Refractory congestive cardiac failure
>
> These syndromes should alert the clinician to the possible contribution of renovascular disease in a given patient. The bottom three are most common in patients with bilateral disease, many of whom are treated for essential hypertension until these characteristics appear (see text).
>
> **B. Clinical Features of Patients with Renovascular Hypertension**
>
> | Clinical Feature | Essential HTN (%) | Renovascular HTN (%) |
> |---|---|---|
> | Duration < 1 yr | 12 | 24 |
> | Age of onset > 50 yr | 9 | 15 |
> | Family history of HTN | 71 | 46 |
> | Grade 3 or 4 fundi | 7 | 15 |
> | Abdominal bruit | 9 | 46 |
> | Blood urea nitrogen > 20 mg/dL | 8 | 16 |
> | Potassium < 3.4 mEq/L | 8 | 16 |
> | Urinary casts | 9 | 20 |
> | Proteinuria | 32 | 46 |
>
> Clinical features that differed ($P < 0.05$) between closely matched groups of 131 patients with essential and renovascular hypertension taken from the Cooperative Study of Renovascular Hypertension in the 1960s. These observations underscore the potential severity of hypertension in candidates for surgery, but none of these features allows clinical discrimination with confidence (see text).
> HTN, Hypertension.

any antihypertensive regimen. Reduced GFR during antihypertensive therapy has become particularly common since the introduction of ACE inhibitors, and later with angiotensin receptor blockers (ARBs). A precipitous rise in serum creatinine level soon after starting these agents may occur because of a loss of transcapillary filtration pressure produced by removing the efferent arteriolar vasoconstriction from angiotensin II. This particular "functional" loss of GFR is reversible if detected promptly and should lead the clinician to consider large vessel renovascular disease when it occurs.[68] Clinically important changes in serum creatinine level develop mainly when the entire renal mass is affected, such as with bilateral renal artery stenosis or stenosis to a solitary functioning kidney. Most such patients tolerate reintroduction of renin angiotensin blockade when challenged after successful revascularization.[69]

Other syndromes heralding occult renal artery stenosis are becoming more commonly recognized. Among the most important are rapidly developing episodes of circulatory congestion (so-called flash pulmonary edema).[70] This usually arises in patients with hypertension and with left-ventricular systolic function, which may be well preserved. Underlying arterial compromise may favor volume retention and resistance to diuretics in such cases. A sudden rise in arterial pressure impairs cardiac function because of rapidly developing diastolic dysfunction. Such episodes tend to be rapid both in onset and in resolution. Patients with treatment-resistant congestive cardiac failure, often with reduced arterial pressures, may harbor unsuspected renovascular disease. Restoration of renal blood flow in such patients can improve volume control and sensitivity to diuretics with lower risk for azotemia during therapy.[71] A similar sequence of events may produce symptoms of "crescendo" angina from otherwise stable coronary disease.[72] Registry data indicate that patients with episodic pulmonary edema with renal artery stenosis have substantially increased hospitalization and mortality that can be reduced with successful revascularization.[5]

Another clinical presentation of renal artery stenosis is *advanced renal failure*, occasionally at end stage requiring renal replacement therapy. This manifestation has been controversial in the past, particularly because it raises the possibility of an undetected, potentially reversible, form of chronic renal failure. As discussed earlier, this is designated by some as ischemic nephropathy or azotemic renovascular disease[73] and is defined as loss of renal function beyond an arterial stenosis because of impaired renal blood flow. Studies in patients with bilateral renal artery stenosis indicate that reduction of systemic pressures to normal levels using sodium nitroprusside can abruptly reduce both renal plasma flow and GFR, indicating that the poststenotic pressures are at critical levels beyond autoregulation (see Figure 48.9). Some estimates suggest that as many as 12% to 14% of patients reaching end-stage kidney disease (ESKD) with no other identifiable primary renal disease may have occult, bilateral renal artery stenosis.[74] A survey using spiral computed tomography (CT) angiography examined 49 of 80 patients starting dialysis therapy and identified ARAS (estimated more than 50% lumen occlusion) in 20 of them (41%), and in 8 (16%) it was bilateral. Assuming correctly that these lesions were the primary cause of ESKD, the authors proposed that up to 27% of patients with new ESKD may have lost kidney function on this basis.[75] A more conservative review of United States Renal Data System data for patients older than 67 years in the United States starting dialysis suggests that identified renovascular disease may be present in 7.1% to 11.1% of patients, although clinicians caring for such patients attributed their renal failure to renal artery stenosis in only 5.0%.[76] Multivariate analysis indicates that male gender and advancing age correlated positively with this disorder, whereas being African American, Asian-American, or Native American correlated negatively.[77] Patients with rapidly progressive dysfunction and accelerated hypertension have a mortality benefit from revascularization and were rarely included in prospective, randomized trials (see later).[4,5,78]

Only patients with vascular lesions affecting the entire renal mass are at risk for large loss of kidney function on this basis. The role of vascular impairment in producing renal dysfunction is established most firmly when renal revascularization leads to recovery of renal function. Unfortunately, this does not occur commonly, as has been

Predictor	Score	
	Persons who never smoked	Former or current smokers
Age (yr)		
20	0	3
30	1	4
40	2	4
50	3	5
60	4	5
70	5	6
Female	2	2
Signs and symptoms of atherosclerosis	1	1
Onset of HTN within 2 yr	1	1
BMI <25 kg/m²	2	2
Abdominal bruit	3	3
Serum creatinine concentration (µmol/L)		
40	0	0
60	1	1
80	2	2
100	3	3
150	6	6
200	9	9
Serum cholesterol level >6.5 mmol/L or cholesterol-lowering therapy	1	1

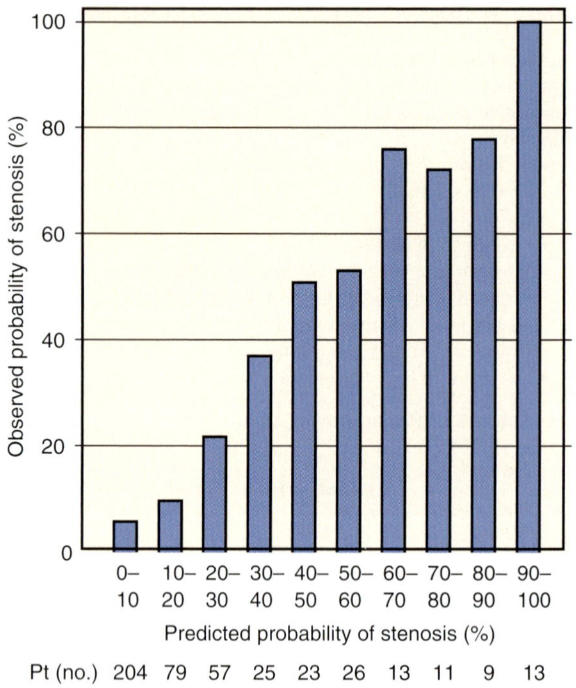

Figure 48.15 **Probability of identifying renal artery stenosis based upon clinical features.** These data were obtained from 477 patients in referral centers for treatment-resistant hypertension in the Netherlands. Overall prevalence was 22.4%, illustrating that even in "enriched" patient populations, renovascular disease is not present in the majority. Clinical features allowed selection of patients for testing with relatively high pretest probability of disease, which affects the validity of testing schemes. BMI, Body mass index; HTN, hypertension. (Reprinted with permission from Krijnen P, van Jaarsveld BC, Steyerberg EW, et al: A clinical prediction rule for renal artery stenosis. *Ann Intern Med* 129:705-711, 1998.)

reviewed.[6] Studies over the last decade have produced a shift in the paradigm related to hemodynamically induced renal dysfunction. Measurements of tissue oxygenation in human subjects using BOLD MRI with ARAS sufficiently severe to reduce GFR and kidney volume most often demonstrate preserved oxygenation gradients between cortex and medulla. This is explained in part by the surfeit of blood flow to the kidney and by reduced oxygen consumption from reduced solute filtration.[79] Hence many subjects can be treated with antihypertensive drug therapy without evident further loss of GFR, sometimes for many years, as demonstrated by prospective, randomized controlled trials (RCTs) such as ASTRAL and CORAL. A subset of patients with more severe or long-standing vascular occlusion (usually defined as peak systolic velocities above 385 cm/sec on duplex ultrasonography) manifest overt cortical hypoxia using BOLD MRI. Such patients demonstrate more advanced tissue histologic injury with loss of tubular structures on biopsy and interstitial cellular infiltrates consistent with inflammatory injury[80,38] (see Figures 48.10B and 48.11). These observations underscore the gradual transition from a primarily "hemodynamic" reduction in kidney function (potentially improved by restoring blood flow) to an inflammatory injury that no longer predictably recovers function after restoring vessel patency. Patients with advanced renal dysfunction have high comorbidity associated with cardiovascular disease and commonly have interstitial renal injury on biopsy.[81,82] Prospective treatment trials specifically directed at slowing the loss of kidney function by renal revascularization have failed to identify much benefit in the intermediate term.[1,83] Those with declining renal function have a poor survival rate regardless of intervention, the strongest predictor of which is low baseline GFR.

The potential benefit of revascularization regarding salvage, or at least stabilization, of renal function is greatest when the serum creatinine level is less than 3 mg/dL, so the diagnosis of ischemic nephropathy is best considered early in its course. Remarkably, renal artery stenosis can be associated with *proteinuria*, occasionally to nephrotic levels.[84-86] Proteinuria can diminish or resolve entirely following renal revascularization,[87] suggesting that intrarenal hemodynamic changes and/or stimulation of local hormonal or cytokine activity alter glomerular membrane permeability in a reversible fashion. Although other glomerular diseases can develop in patients with renal artery disease, including diabetic nephropathy and focal sclerosing glomerulonephritis, the presence of proteinuria alone does not establish a second disorder.

Clinical manifestations and prognosis differ when renovascular disease affects one of two kidneys or affects the entire functioning renal mass. Although blood pressure levels may be similar, the fall in blood pressure after renal revascularization is greater in bilateral disease.[88] Most patients with episodic pulmonary edema have bilateral disease or a solitary kidney. Long-term mortality during

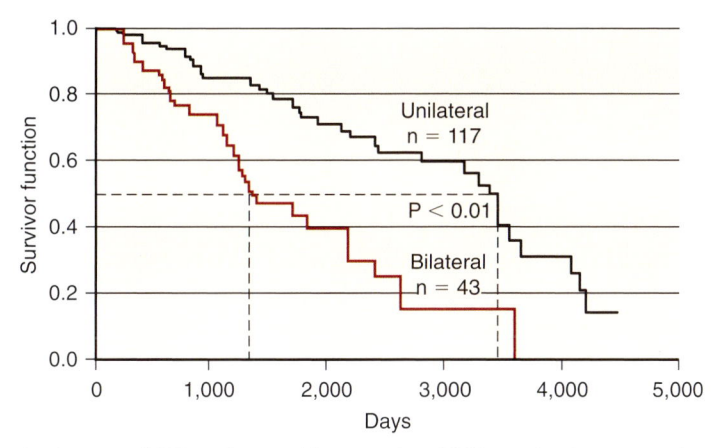

Figure 48.16 Kaplan-Meier survival curve of 160 patients with more than 70% renal artery stenosis managed without revascularization. Those with bilateral disease had lower survival, primarily due to cardiovascular disease. The mean age of death was 79 years. These data underscore the close relationship between extent of vascular disease and mortality. Less than 10% of these subjects developed advanced kidney disease during follow-up, although long-term survival even in treated patients is related to levels of kidney function at the time of intervention.[10] Prospective randomized clinical trials indicate that between 16% and 22% of medically treated patients with atherosclerotic renal artery stenosis progress to more advanced renal dysfunction over 3 to 5 years.[3] (Reprinted with permission from Textor SC: Renovascular hypertension and ischemic nephropathy. In Taal MW, Brenner BM, editors: *Brenner and Rector's the kidney*, Philadelphia, 2012, Elsevier Saunders, pp 1752-1791.)

follow-up is higher when bilateral disease is present, regardless of whether renal revascularization is undertaken.[64,89,90] These data suggest that the extent and severity of renovascular disease reflects the overall atherosclerotic burden of the individual. Patients with incidental renal artery stenosis (>70%) managed without revascularization have reduced survival with bilateral disease, despite reasonable blood pressure control, as illustrated in Figure 48.16. The causes of death are mainly related to cardiovascular disease, including stroke and congestive heart failure.

PROGRESSIVE VASCULAR OCCLUSION

Atherosclerosis is a progressive disorder, although individual rates of progression vary widely. The clinical manifestations from renal artery stenosis depend partly upon the severity and extent of vascular occlusion. The most ominous of these manifestations (e.g., renal failure or pulmonary edema) are related to bilateral disease or stenosis to a solitary functioning kidney and pose the greatest hazard when total arterial occlusion develops. Hence the impetus to intervene in renal artery stenosis depends upon predicting, or establishing, the "natural history" of vascular stenosis within an individual. Retrospective studies of serial angiograms obtained in the 1970s and early 1980s indicated that atherosclerotic lesions progressed to more severe levels in 44% to 63% of patients followed from 2 to 5 years. Up to 16% of renal arteries developed total occlusion. Later prospective studies in patients undergoing cardiac catheterization or serial Doppler ultrasound measurements suggest that current rates of progression may be lower. Zierler and colleagues reported a 20% rate of disease progression overall with 7% advancing to total occlusion over 3 years.[91] A later report from the same group using different Doppler velocity criteria suggested higher rates of progressive stenosis. Overall progression was detectable in 31%, but primarily those with the most severe baseline stenosis (>60%) and severe hypertension were more likely to progress (51%) (Figure 48.17). The occurrence of total occlusion was rare (9 of 295, or 3%).[92] Data from medical treatment trials suggest that progressive occlusion can develop silently in up to 16% of treated subjects.[93] These observations are supported by development of renal end points (defined as progressive renal deterioration) ranging between 16% and 22% in prospective RCTs.[3]

Importantly, clinical events such as detectable changes in renal function or accelerating hypertension bear only a limited relationship to anatomic vascular progression. The occurrence of renal "atrophy" (loss in renal size by 1 cm or more by ultrasonography) developed in 20.8% of the most severe lesions in the prospective series.[94] Most series of medically treated patients indicate that despite evident progression of vascular disease, changes in kidney function are modest and uncommon. Results reported during medical follow-up of 41 patients managed medically before the introduction of ACE inhibitors for an average of 36 months identified a loss of renal length in 35%, whereas a significant rise in serum creatinine level developed in 8 out of 41 (19.5%) patients. Results of 160 patients with high-grade (>70%) stenosis identified incidentally and managed without revascularization are summarized in Table 48.4. Patients were followed for many years and divided into cohorts spanning the introduction of ACE inhibitors into clinical practice. Blood pressure control improved during these intervals. Medical management was associated with increased requirements for antihypertensive agents. The number developing clinical progression with refractory hypertension or progressive renal insufficiency fell from 21% in the earliest period to less than 10% in the later cohort after introduction of ACE inhibitors. This conclusion is consistent with long-term studies from Europe in which incidental renal artery lesions were rarely associated with progressive renal failure over more than 9 years of follow-up.[95] These data support the observation that many renal artery lesions remain stable in some patients over many years without adverse clinical effects or evident

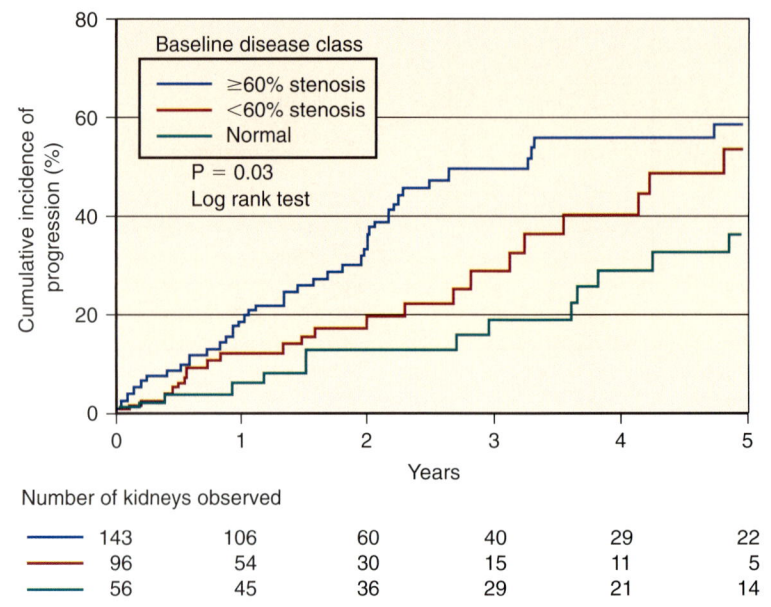

Figure 48.17 Cumulative rates of anatomic disease progression in atherosclerotic renal artery stenosis, as measured by renal artery Doppler ultrasonography. During a follow-up period of 5 years, overall progression was 31%, but those with the most severe baseline lesion progressed in 50% of cases. The progression of vascular disease was not closely related to changes in serum creatinine level or renal atrophy (see text). (Modified from Caps MT, Perissinotto C, Zierler RE, et al: Prospective study of atherosclerotic disease progression in the renal artery. *Circulation* 98:2866-2872, 1998.)

Table 48.4 Incidental Renal Artery Stenosis: Medical Management between 1980 and 1993 during Introduction of ACE Inhibition

	1980-1984	1985-1989	1990-1993
Number	34	57	69
Age	69.3	70.3	71.5
Mean follow-up (months)	58	54	35
Blood pressure (mm Hg)			
Initial	172/91	163/88	155/81*
Last follow-up	163/83†	160/84	154/79
Creatinine level			
Initial	1.6	1.6	1.4
Last follow-up	2.0†	2.1†	2.0†
Renal failure‡	2.9%	5.3%	7.2%
BP medications at follow-up (no.)	2.5	2.0	2.1
ACE inhibitors (%) (initial)		21	41*§
Subsequent revascularization	20.6	14.0	5.7*

*$P < 0.05$ versus 1980-1984.
†$P < 0.01$ at last follow-up versus initial.
‡Creatinine rise ≥ 50%.
§$P < 0.05$ versus 1985-1989.

Management of renal artery stenosis without revascularization in patients with incidentally identified disease between 1980 and 1993 during introduction of blockade of the renin angiotensin system. These cohorts bridged the period of the first ACE inhibitors, during which the use rose from 0% to 40.6% of patients. Achieved blood pressures improved during this interval, and the number of patients referred for revascularization because of refractory hypertension or progressive renal insufficiency fell from 20.6% to less than 10% during several years of follow-up. Such observations underscore the fact that some patients can be managed medically without adverse effects for many years, although a residual group does face progressive loss of glomerular filtration rate in clinical use.

ACE, Angiotensin-converting enzyme; BP, blood pressure.

Reprinted from Textor SC: Renovascular hypertension and ischemic nephropathy. In Taal MW, Brenner BM, editors: Brenner and Rector's the kidney, Philadelphia, 2012, Elsevier Saunders, pp 1752-1791.

progression,[96] as observed in prospective treatment trials, including ASTRAL and CORAL.[3] It is likely that overall rates of atherosclerotic disease progression are falling due to more widespread use of statin-class drugs, aspirin, diminishing tobacco use, and more intense antihypertensive therapy. Hence worsening vascular occlusion is an important clinical risk but does not occur in all patients.

ROLE OF CHANGING ANTIHYPERTENSIVE THERAPY

Before the 1980s the literature of renovascular disease concerned primarily identification of functionally important lesions in patients with severe hypertension. Drug therapy was limited in scope and often produced intolerable side effects. Most importantly, the available drugs did not yet include agents capable of interrupting the renin angiotensin system (see Figure 48.2). As a result, patients commonly appeared with accelerated or malignant hypertension, a large fraction of which was related to renal artery stenosis. Among 123 patients whose average age was 44 years presenting with accelerated hypertension, more than 30% of whites were identified as having renovascular hypertension. Some patients could not be effectively controlled with available medications and were subjected to "urgent" bilateral nephrectomy as a life-saving measure. The evaluation for renal artery stenosis centered upon identifying those patients whose blood pressures could be improved, perhaps "cured," by renal revascularization.

Since the 1980s several new classes of antihypertensive agents have become available and widely used. These include calcium channel blockers and, most importantly, drugs that functionally block the renin angiotensin system, such as ACE inhibitors and ARBs. Later orally active direct renin inhibitors were added (e.g., aliskiren). The impact of these agents has been enormous. Reviews of medical therapy for renovascular hypertension indicate that regimens using these agents increased the likelihood of achieving good blood pressure control from 46% to more than 90%.[11] The concept of emergency bilateral nephrectomy for control of hypertension has almost disappeared. Most importantly, it is likely that many patients with renovascular disease and hypertension now go undetected because blood pressure and renal function are well controlled and stable.[60] This may be happening even more commonly than before with the expanded use of ACE inhibitors for congestive cardiac failure, proteinuric renal disease, and other constellations of cardiovascular risk factors, particularly since the publication of the Heart Outcomes Prevention Evaluation (HOPE) trial[97] and others. This raises the interesting hypothesis that the use of ACE inhibitors and/or ARBs may delay the onset of renovascular hypertension in humans, as it does in experimental animals. To date this hypothesis has not been adequately addressed.

CHANGING POPULATION DEMOGRAPHICS

The last several decades have been characterized by longer life spans in many Western countries. These likely result from several factors, including major declines in mortality related to stroke and cardiovascular disease. Population groups above age 65 years are now among the most rapidly growing segments in the United States. One consequence of lower mortality from coronary and cerebrovascular events is the delayed appearance of vascular disease affecting other beds, such as the aorta and kidneys. As a result, clinical manifestations of renal artery stenosis are appearing in older individuals, often combined with other conditions. These features change the clinical presentation and affect the risk/benefit considerations inherent in undertaking renal revascularization. Series with renal artery intervention now routinely include average age values between 68 and 71 years, whereas a decade ago the mean age was between 61 and 63 years.[98,99] These mean values are more than 15 years older than those from the 1960s and 1970s. As might be expected, the prevalence of advanced coronary disease, congestive heart failure, previous stroke/transient ischemic attack and aortic disease, as well as impaired renal function, is rising in patients with atherosclerotic renal artery disease.

ROLE OF CONCURRENT DISEASES

ARAS rarely occurs as an isolated entity. It is a manifestation of atherosclerotic disease, which often affects multiple other sites. Follow-up studies related to survival of "incidentally" identified renal arterial disease suggest that the presence of renal artery stenosis independently predicts mortality, particularly in the presence of elevated levels of serum creatinine. It bears emphasis that the mortality risk of a patient with serum creatinine level above 1.4 mg/dL (but less than 2.3 mg/dL) for any reason is higher than the risk for those with normal creatinine levels.[97] The major causes of death are cardiovascular events, including congestive cardiac failure, stroke, and myocardial infarction. It is essential to consider the role of these competing risks in planning management of patients with all forms of vascular disease, especially older adults.[100] These disorders often dominate the clinical outcomes of patients with renal arterial disease, independent of the level of renal function. As one result, it has been difficult to establish improved survival in prospective trials of patients treated either with medical therapy or renal revascularization. Although many patients experience blood pressure more easily controlled and some recover renal function, current methods of revascularization are not free of risks. Even after successful renovascular procedures, other comorbid events may obscure long-term benefit, challenging the cost-effectiveness of renal revascularization. Reviews of Medicare claims in the United States for 2 years after identification of ARAS indicate that cardiovascular events, many of which are fatal, are more than 10-fold more likely than progression to advanced renal failure.[66] Conversely, others argue that renal artery stenosis accelerates these cardiovascular risks by increasing arterial pressures and activating adverse neurohumoral pathways, predisposing to both congestive heart failure and renal dysfunction.[101] These divergent views form the basis for several prospective RCTs related to renal revascularization over the past decade (see later) that partly address these issues.

DIAGNOSTIC TESTING FOR RENOVASCULAR HYPERTENSION AND ISCHEMIC NEPHROPATHY

GOALS OF EVALUATION

The literature related to diagnosis and evaluation of renovascular hypertension is complex and inconsistent. Some of the confusion likely reflects the widely different patient groups being considered for evaluation and divergent goals for intervention. It behooves the clinician to identify the objectives of initiating expensive and sometimes ambiguous studies beforehand. As with all tests, the reliability and value of diagnostic studies depend heavily on the pretest probability of disease[102] (Table 48.5). Furthermore, it is essential to consider from the outset exactly what is to be achieved. Is the major goal to exclude high-grade renal artery disease? Is it to exclude bilateral (as opposed to unilateral) disease? Is it to identify stenosis and estimate the potential for clinical benefit from renal revascularization? Is it to evaluate the role of renovascular disease in explaining deteriorating renal function? The specific approach to diagnosis will differ depending upon which of these is the predominant clinical objective.

Noninvasive diagnostic tests for renovascular hypertension and ischemic nephropathy remain imperfect. For the purposes of this discussion, diagnostic tests fall into the following general categories (Table 48.6): (1) physiologic and functional studies to evaluate the role of stenotic lesions particularly related to activation of the renin angiotensin system, (2) perfusion and imaging studies to identify the presence and degree of vascular stenosis, and (3) studies to predict the likelihood of benefit from invasive maneuvers, including renal revascularization.

PHYSIOLOGIC AND FUNCTIONAL STUDIES OF THE RENIN ANGIOTENSIN SYSTEM

Efforts have been made for years to link measurement of activation of the renin angiotensin system as a marker of underlying renovascular hypertension. Although these studies are promising when performed in patients with known renovascular hypertension, they have lower performance as diagnostic tests when applied to wider populations, as has been reviewed.[103] Plasma renin activity is sensitive to changes in sodium intake, volume status, renal function, and many medications. The sensitivity and specificity of such maneuvers are heavily dependent upon the a priori probability of renovascular hypertension. In practice the major utility of these studies depends upon their negative predictive value, specifically the certainty with which one can exclude significant renovascular disease if the test results are negative. Because negative predictive value rarely exceeds 60% to 70%, these tests offer limited value in clinical decision making.

Measurement of renal vein renin levels has been widely applied in planning surgical revascularization for hypertension. These measurements are obtained by sampling renal vein and inferior vena cava blood individually. The level of the vena cava is taken as comparable to the arterial levels into each kidney and allows estimation of the contribution of each kidney to total circulating levels of plasma renin activity. Lateralization is defined usually as a ratio exceeding 1.5 between the renin activity of the stenotic kidney and the nonstenotic kidney. Some authors propose detailed examination not only of the relative ratio between kidneys but the degree of suppression of renin release from the nonstenotic or contralateral kidney. In general, the greater the degree of lateralization, the more probable that clinical blood pressure benefit will accrue from surgical or other revascularization. Results from many studies support the observation that large differences between kidneys identify high-grade renal artery stenosis. These observations have been reinforced by studies of renal vein measurements before considering nephrectomy for refractory hypertension and advanced renovascular occlusive disease.[104] As with many tests of hormonal activation, study conditions are crucial. A number of measures to enhance renin release and magnify differences between kidneys have been proposed, including sodium depletion with diuretic administration, hydralazine, tilt-table stimulation, or captopril. Strong and colleagues demonstrated that nonlateralization can be changed to strongly lateralizing measurements by administration of diuretics between sequential studies.[104a] A review of more than 50 studies of renal vein renin measurements indicated that when lateralization could be demonstrated, clinical benefit regarding blood pressure control could be expected in more than 90% of cases. Failure to demonstrate lateralization, however, still was associated with significant benefit in more than 50% of cases.[89] Later series reached similar conclusions, indicating that overall sensitivity of renal vein

Table 48.5 Renovascular Disease and Ischemic Nephropathy

Goals of Diagnostic Evaluation

1. Establish presence of renal artery stenosis: location and type of lesion
2. Establish whether unilateral or bilateral stenosis (or stenosis to a solitary kidney) is present
3. Establish presence and function of stenotic and nonstenotic kidneys
4. Establish hemodynamic severity of renal arterial disease
5. Plan vascular intervention: degree and location of atherosclerotic disease

Goals of Therapy

1. Improved blood pressure control
   a. Prevent morbidity and mortality of high blood pressure
   b. Improve blood pressure control and reduce medication requirement
2. Preservation of renal function
   a. Reduce risk for renal adverse perfusion from use of antihypertensive agents
   b. Reduce episodes of circulatory congestion (flash pulmonary edema)
   c. Reduce risk for progressive vascular occlusion causing loss of renal function: preservation of renal function
   d. Salvage renal function (i.e., recover glomerular filtration rate)
3. Recovery of volume regulation and fluid excretion
   a. Reduce circulatory overload and diuretic resistance
   b. Reduce episodes of flash pulmonary edema

Table 48.6 Noninvasive Assessment of Renal Artery Stenosis

Study	Rationale	Strengths	Limitations
Physiologic Studies to Assess the Renin Angiotensin System			
Measurement of peripheral plasma renin activity	Reflects the level of sodium excretion	Measures the level of activation of the renin angiotensin system	Low predictive accuracy for renovascular hypertension; results influenced by medications and many other conditions
Measurement of captopril-stimulated renin activity	Produces a fall in pressure distal to the stenosis	Enhances the release of renin from the stenotic kidney	Low predictive accuracy for renovascular hypertension; results influenced by many other conditions
Measurement of renal-vein renin activity	Compares renin release from the two kidneys	Lateralization predictive of improvement in blood pressure with revascularization	Nonlateralization has limited predictive power of the failure of blood pressure to improve after revascularization; results influenced by medications and many other conditions
Perfusion Studies to Assess Differential Renal Blood Flow			
Captopril renography with technetium ^{99m}Tc mercaptoacetyltriglycine (^{99m}Tc-MAG3)	Captopril-mediated fall in filtration pressure amplifies differences in renal perfusion	Normal study excludes renovascular hypertension	Multiple limitations in patients with advanced atherosclerosis or creatinine >2.0 mg/dL (177 µmol/L)
Nuclear imaging with technetium mercaptoacetyltriglycine or diethylenetriaminepentaacetic acid (DTPA) to estimate fractional flow to each kidney	Estimates fractional flow to each kidney	Allows calculation of single-kidney glomerular filtration rate	Results may be influenced by other conditions, e.g. obstructive uropathy
Vascular Studies to Evaluate the Renal Arteries			
Duplex ultrasonography	Shows the renal arteries and measures flow velocity as a means of assessing the severity of stenosis	Inexpensive; widely available; suitable for sequential measurement to follow disease progression and/or restenosis	Heavily dependent on operator's experience; less useful than invasive angiography for the diagnosis of fibromuscular dysplasia and abnormalities in accessory renal arteries
Magnetic resonance angiography	Shows the renal arteries and perirenal aorta	Not nephrotoxic, but concerns for gadolinium toxicity exclude use in GFR < 30 mL/min/1.73 m^2; provides excellent images	Expensive; gadolinium excluded in renal failure; unable to visualize stented vessels
Computed tomographic angiography	Shows the renal arteries and perirenal aorta	Provides excellent images; stents do not cause artifacts	Expensive; moderate volume of contrast required, potentially nephrotoxic

GFR, Glomerular filtration rate.
Modified with permission from Safian RD, Textor SC: Medical progress: renal artery stenosis. N Engl J Med 344:431-442, 2001.

renin measurements was no better than 65% and that positive predictive value was 18.5%.[105] For these and other reasons, renal vein assays are performed less commonly than before. A major factor is that the goals of renal revascularization have shifted substantially and are often directed toward "preservation of renal function," rather than for blood pressure control per se. In cases for which it is important to establish the degree of pressor effect of a specific kidney or site, such as before considering nephrectomy of a pressor kidney, measurement of renal vein renin levels can provide strong supportive evidence.

STUDIES OF INDIVIDUAL RENAL FUNCTION

Serum creatinine level, iothalamate clearance, and other estimates of total GFR are measures of overall renal excretory function and do not address changes within each kidney. A large body of literature addresses the potential for individual "split" renal function studies to establish the functional importance of each kidney in renovascular disease.

Split renal function studies classically use separate ureteral catheters to allow individual urine collection for measurement of separate GFR, renal blood flow, sodium excretion, concentrating ability, and the response to blockade of angiotensin II. These studies demonstrate that hemodynamic effects of renal artery lesions translate directly into functional changes, such as avid sodium retention, before major changes in blood flow occur. They emphasize that autoregulation of blood flow and GFR can occur over a wide range of pressures in humans and may be affected in both stenotic and contralateral kidneys by the effects of angiotensin II. These studies require urinary tract instrumentation and provide only indirect information regarding the probability of benefit from revascularization. They are now rarely performed.

Separate renal functional measurements can be obtained less invasively with radionuclide techniques. These methods use a variety of radioisotopes (e.g., technetium 99m–labeled mercaptoacetyltriglycine [^{99m}Tc-MAG3] or technetium 99m–labeled diethylenetriaminepentaacetic acid [^{99m}Tc-DTPA]) to estimate fractional blood flow and filtration to each kidney. Administration of captopril beforehand magnifies differences between kidneys, primarily by delaying excretion of the filtered isotope due to removal of the efferent arteriolar effects of angiotensin II. Some authors advocate such measurements to follow progressive renal artery disease and its effect on unilateral kidney function as a guide to consider revascularization.[106] Serial measurements of individual renal function by radionuclide studies allow more precise identification of progressive ischemic injury to the affected kidney in unilateral renal artery disease than can be determined from overall GFR. Studies indicate that single-kidney GFR measurements by this method accurately reflect changes in three-dimensional volume parameters measured by MRI.[107] These authors argue that demonstrating well-preserved parenchymal volume with disproportionate reduction in single-kidney GFR supports the concept of "hibernating" kidney parenchyma and might provide a predictive parameter for recovery of kidney function after revascularization.[107]

IMAGING OF THE RENAL VASCULATURE

Advances in Doppler ultrasonography, radionuclide imaging, magnetic resonance (MR) angiography, and CT angiography continue to introduce major changes in the field of renovascular imaging. The details of these methods are beyond the scope of this discussion. They are addressed more fully elsewhere. What follows is a discussion of some of the specific merits and limitations of each modality as they apply to application in renovascular hypertension and ischemic nephropathy.[102]

Current practice favors limiting invasive arteriography to the occasion of endovascular intervention (e.g., stenting and/or angioplasty). Although angiography remains for many the gold standard for evaluation of the renal vasculature, its invasive nature, potential hazards, and cost make it most suitable for those in whom intervention is planned, often during the same procedure. As a result, most clinicians favor preliminary noninvasive studies. When noninvasive studies are equivocal, arterial angiography may be warranted to establish the presence of transstenotic pressure gradients, as recommended for treatment trials.[108,109]

NONINVASIVE IMAGING

Doppler Ultrasonography of the Renal Arteries

Duplex interrogation of the renal arteries provides measurements of localized velocities of blood flow and characteristics of renal tissue. In many institutions this provides an inexpensive means for measuring vascular occlusive disease at sequential time points, both to establish the diagnosis of renal artery stenosis and to monitor its progression. After renal revascularization, Doppler studies are commonly used to monitor restenosis and target vessel patency[110,111] (Figure 48.18). Its main drawbacks relate to the difficulties of obtaining adequate studies in obese patients. The utility and reliability of Doppler ultrasonography depend partly upon the specific operator and the time allotted for optimal studies. These factors vary considerably between institutions.

The primary criteria for renal artery studies are a peak systolic velocity above 180 cm/sec and/or a relative velocity above 3.5 as compared to the adjacent aortic flow.[112] Using these criteria, sensitivity and specificity with angiographic estimates of lesions exceeding 60% can surpass 90% and 96%, respectively,[113] although not universally.[114] Increasing the threshold for peak systolic velocities reduces the rate of false-positive estimates of stenosis. When main vessel velocities cannot be determined reliably, segmental waveforms within the arcuate vessels in the renal hilum can provide additional information. Damping of these waveforms, labeled "parvus" and "tardus," have been proposed as indirect signs of upstream vascular occlusive phenomena.[115] Some authors challenge the use of angiographic estimates of stenosis as representing a gold standard altogether.[116] These authors argue that Doppler velocities correlate highly ($r = 0.97$) with a truer estimate of vascular occlusion, specifically stenosis determined by intravascular ultrasonography.

In the author's own experience, Doppler study of the renal arteries is highly reliable when adequate imaging of the renal arteries can be obtained. Positive Doppler velocities in an artery clearly identified as the renal artery are rarely proven to be negative later. False-negative studies are more common. In subjects with accessible vessels, Doppler ultrasonography provides the most practical means of following vessel characteristics sequentially over time. A drawback of renal artery Doppler studies includes frequent failure to identify accessory vessels. Because the correlation between velocity and degree of stenosis is only approximate, clinical trials such as CORAL have raised the peak velocity threshold to 300 cm/sec. This seems warranted, particularly when the risk for overdiagnosis of renal arterial lesions is high, as in the Stent Placement and Blood Pressure and Lipid-Lowering for the Prevention of Progression of Renal Dysfunction Caused by Atherosclerotic Ostial Stenosis of the Renal Artery (STAR) trial, in which 18 out of 64 patients assigned to stenting were found not to have significant renovascular disease at the time of angiography despite noninvasive estimates to the contrary.[83]

Additional studies emphasize the potential for Doppler ultrasonography to characterize small vessel flow characteristics within the kidney. The resistive index provides an estimate of the relative flow velocities in diastole and systole. In a study of 138 patients with renal artery stenosis, a resistive index above 80 provided a predictive tool for identification of parenchymal renal disease that did not respond to renal

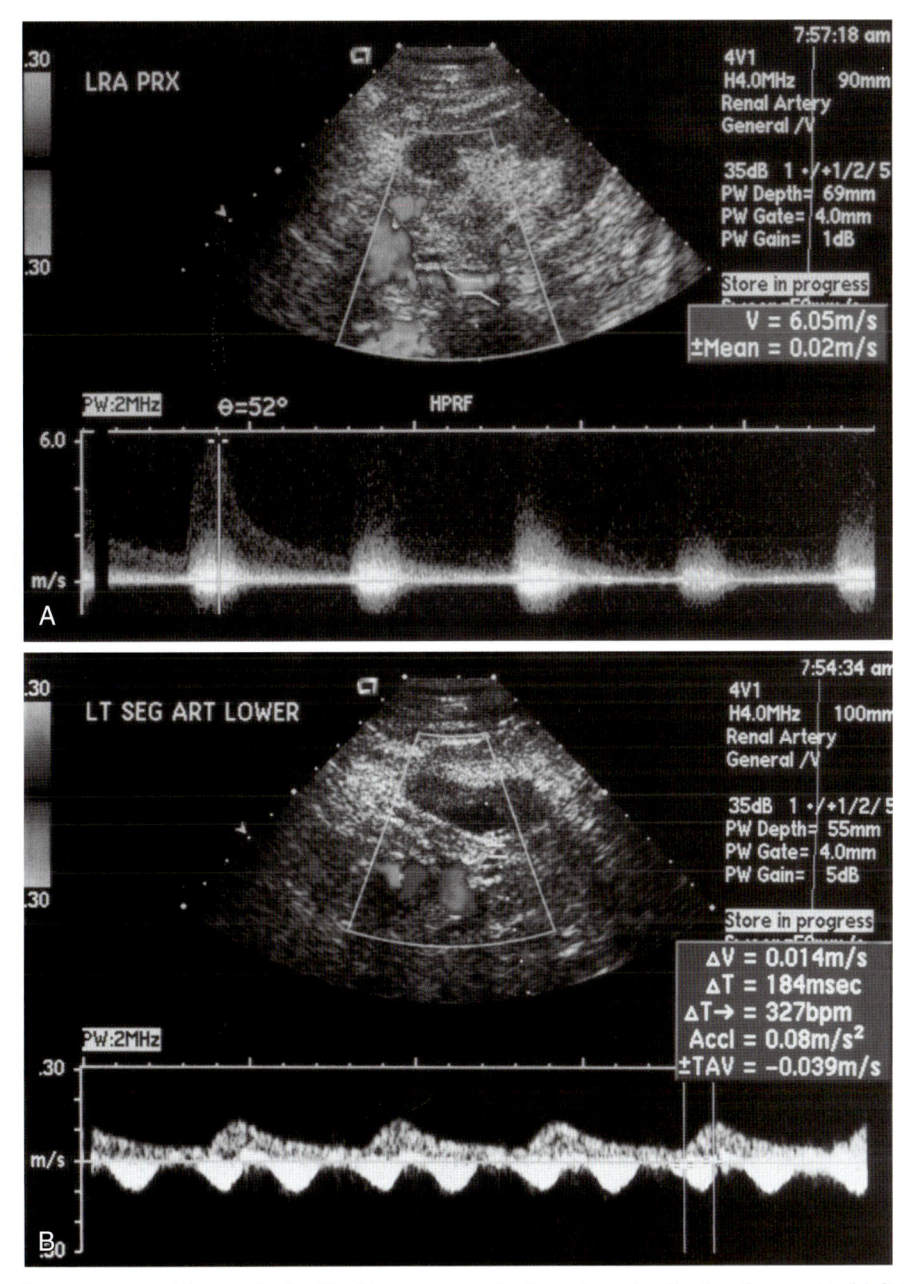

Figure 48.18 **A,** Velocity measurement in a patient with high-grade renal artery stenosis affecting the proximal left renal artery (LRA PRX). Velocities reach 605 cm/sec, well above the normal upper limit of 180 cm/sec. **B,** Segmental branch ultrasonography in the distal segmental renal arteries demonstrates parvus and tardus dampening of the signal characteristic of poststenotic waveforms. The utility of these measurements depends upon the ability to obtain reliable identification of vessel segments and the skills of the operator. Once the location of a vascular lesion is known, subsequent studies can be performed more easily to track progression of vascular occlusion, restenosis, and/or the results of endovascular intervention (see text).

revascularization[117] (Figure 48.19). A sizable portion of this group eventually progressed to renal failure. Resistive index is measured in the segmental arteries, usually the first two vessels that branch off the main renal artery, and is an index of the peak velocity of blood in systole relative to the minimum diastolic velocity $\{100 \times [1 - (V_{min}/V_{max})]\}$. A higher number would reflect important falls in flow during diastole versus systole. When diastolic flow is 20% of systolic flow, the resistive index is 80, a reflection of augmented resistance in the downstream vascular bed.

A resistive index less than 80 was associated with more than 90% favorable blood pressure response and stable or improved renal function. The authors emphasize that accurate predictive power depended upon using the highest resistive index observed, even when present in the nonstenotic kidney. A subsequent study of 215 subjects with mean preintervention serum creatinine levels of 1.51 mg/dL failed to confirm the predictive value of resistive index measurements. Of 99 subjects with "improved" renal function after 1 year, 18% had a resistive index above 80 before intervention, whereas 15% of 92 subjects with no improvement had an index above 80 (not significant). In this series, preintervention level of serum creatinine itself was the strongest predictor of improved renal function.[118] Most

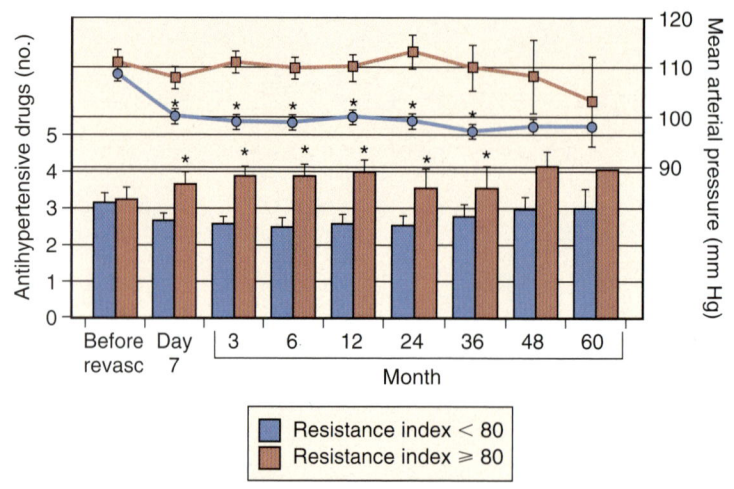

Figure 48.19 Outcome of revascularization as measured by mean arterial blood pressure and number of antihypertensive agents in 138 patients with renal artery stenosis. These patients were divided into groups with an ultrasound-determined resistive index of 80 or higher and those below 80 in the most severely affected kidney. The authors indicate that a high resistive index reflects intrinsic parenchymal and small vessel disease in the kidney that does not improve after revascularization. Those with lower indices had both lower blood pressures during follow-up and lower antihypertensive medication requirements. (Reprinted with permission from Radermacher J, Chavan A, Bleck J, et al: Use of Doppler ultrasonography to predict the outcome of therapy for renal-artery stenosis. N Engl J Med 344:410-417, 2001.)

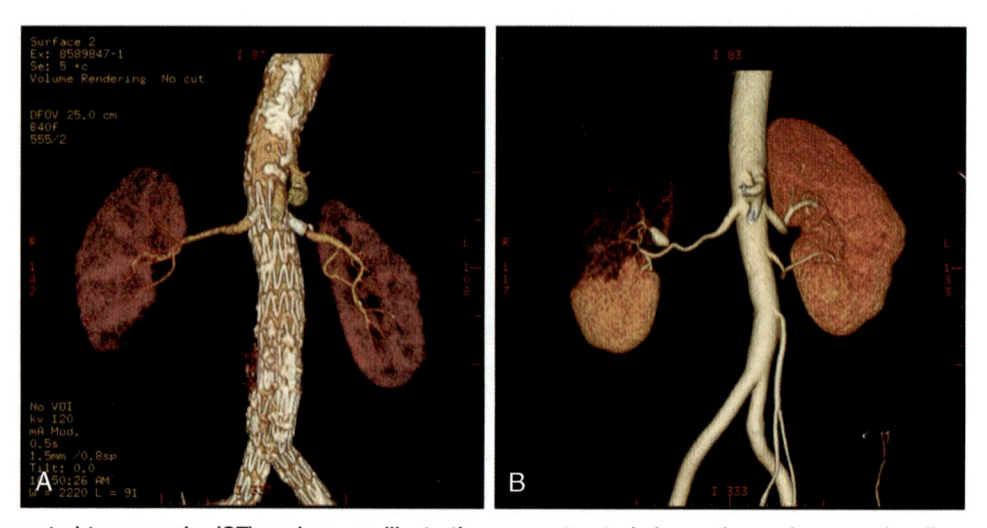

Figure 48.20 Computed tomography (CT) angiograms illustrating reconstructed views of complex vascular disease. A, Aortic endovascular stent extending beyond the origins of the renal arteries. Renal artery stents have been placed through the aortic graft to restore blood flow, although the nephrograms demonstrate patchy defects consistent with small vessel occlusion and/or atheroembolic events. B, CT angiogram with a small aneurysm of the right renal artery that has produced segmental infarction, leading to accelerated hypertension. Although CT angiography requires contrast, current multidetector CT studies allow excellent image resolution at rapid acquisition and less contrast exposure than ever before.

clinicians agree that detecting a low resistive index indicates a well-preserved vasculature within the kidney with improved likelihood of recovering or stabilizing after vascular intervention.[119,120]

Computed Tomography Angiography

CT angiography using helical and/or multiple detector scanners and intravenous contrast can provide excellent images of both kidneys and the vascular tree. Resolution and reconstruction techniques render this modality capable of identifying smaller vessels, vascular lesions, and parenchymal characteristics, including malignancy and stones[121] (Figure 48.20). When used for detection of renal artery stenosis, CT angiography agrees well with conventional arteriography (correlation 95%), and sensitivity may reach 98% and specificity 94%.[122] Studies indicate that CT provides excellent accuracy regarding evaluation of in-stent restenosis,[123] and evolving quantitative three-dimensional image analysis may improve on intraarterial methods.[122] Although this technique offers excellent noninvasive examination of the vascular tree, it does require iodinated contrast. As a result, it raises concerns for evaluation of renovascular hypertension and/or ischemic nephropathy for older patients with impaired renal function and/or diabetes. Concerns regarding toxicity associated with MR angiographic contrast nonetheless encourage wider use of multidetector

CT as a diagnostic imaging test for patients suspected of renovascular disease. Limitations include reduced visibility of vessel lumens in the presence of substantial calcium deposition. A single study comparing both CT angiography and MR angiography with intraarterial studies in 402 subjects indicated substantially worse performance for detection of lesions with greater than 50% stenosis.[124] In this particular study, CT angiography had sensitivity of 64% and specificity of 92%, whereas MR angiography had sensitivity of 62% and specificity of 84%. This was an unusual population with only 20% of the screened population having stenotic lesions, nearly half of which were FMD. The results of such studies reinforce the importance of careful patient selection for study and establishing in advance exactly what questions the imaging is addressing.[125]

Magnetic Resonance Angiography

Gadolinium-enhanced images of the abdominal and renal vasculature had been a mainstay of evaluating renovascular disease in many institutions.[121,126] Comparative studies indicate that sensitivity ranges from 83% to 100% and specificity from 92% to 97% in renal artery stenosis.[127,128] Meta-analyses of published literature including 998 subjects support more than 97% sensitivity using gadolinium-enhanced imaging.[129] The nephrogram obtained from gadolinium filtration provides an estimate of relative function and filtration, as well as parenchymal volume. Quantitative measurement of parenchymal volume determined by MRI appears to correlate closely with isotopically determined single-kidney GFR in some institutions.[107] Since 2006, concerns about the potential for gadolinium-based contrast to produce nephrogenic systemic fibrosis effectively have eliminated contrast-enhanced MRI for patients with impaired kidney function in the United States.[130]

Technologic advances are allowing high-resolution vascular MRI without contrast in many patients. An example of MR angiography without contrast is shown in Figure 48.21. Drawbacks include expense and the tendency to overestimate the severity of lesions, which in fact appear as a signal void.[121,131] The limits of resolution with current instrumentation make detection of small accessory vessels limited, and quantitating fibromuscular lesions is difficult with current technology. Both of these are improving with newer generations of scanners. High-spatial-resolution three-dimensional contrast-enhanced MR scanners provide up to 97% sensitivity and 92% specificity for renal artery stenotic lesions.[132] Importantly, signal degradation due to metallic stents renders MR angiography unsuitable for follow-up studies after endovascular procedures in which stents are used.

Captopril Renography

Imaging the kidneys before and after administration of an ACE inhibitor (e.g., captopril) traditionally provided a functional assessment of the change in blood flow and GFR to the kidney related to both changes in arterial pressure and removal of the efferent arteriolar effects of angiotensin II. Because hypertension is not commonly the primary motivation for evaluating renovascular disease, these tests are less frequently applied now. The most commonly used radiopharmaceuticals are ^{99m}Tc-DTPA and ^{99m}Tc-MAG3. The latter agent has clearance characteristics similar to hippuran and is often taken as reflecting renal plasma flow. Both can be used, although specific interpretive criteria differ.[133] Both provide information regarding size and filtration of both kidneys and the change in these characteristics after inhibition of ACE allows inferences regarding the dependence of glomerular filtration upon angiotensin II. Patient groups with prevalence of renovascular disease rates between 35% and 64% of subjects suggest that sensitivity and specificity range between 65% and 96% and 62% and 100%, respectively.[133] Because of its high specificity, captopril renography can be applied to populations at low pretest probability with an expectation that normal study results will exclude significant renovascular hypertension in more than 96% of cases.[134] Some series report 100% accurate negative predictive values.[135]

Renographic imaging studies are less sensitive and specific for renovascular disease in the presence of renal insufficiency (usually defined as creatinine level higher than 2.0 mg/dL). These performance characteristics also deteriorate for patients who cannot be prepared carefully, (i.e., withdrawal of diuretics and ACE inhibitors for 4 to 14 days before the study).[133] It should be emphasized that renography provides functional information but no direct anatomic information (e.g., the location of renal arterial disease, the number of renal arteries, or associated aortic and/or ostial disease) (Figure 48.22). Some authors argue that renographic screening of patients using this technique is among the most cost-effective methods of identifying candidates for further diagnostic studies and superior to functional studies of the renin angiotensin system. On the other hand, prospective studies of renovascular disease from the Netherlands did observe changes in the renogram during follow-up but did not find captopril renography predictive of angiographic findings or outcomes.[93] A prospective study of 74 patients undergoing both renography and Doppler ultrasonography evaluation before renal revascularization could identify only limited predictive value of scintigraphy (sensitivity of 58% and specificity of 57%) regarding blood pressure outcomes.[136]

Some authors argue that under carefully controlled conditions changes in renographic appearance correlate with changes in blood pressure after revascularization. Changes in split renal function indicate that stenotic kidneys regain

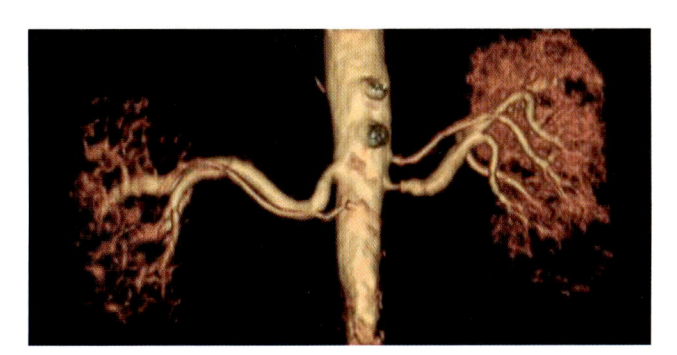

Figure 48.21 Magnetic resonance (MR) angiogram reconstructed without gadolinium contrast. After warnings about the association of gadolinium with nephrogenic systemic fibrosis, contrast MR is less commonly used for atherosclerotic renovascular imaging than before. Newer techniques can allow excellent vascular imaging without contrast as shown here.

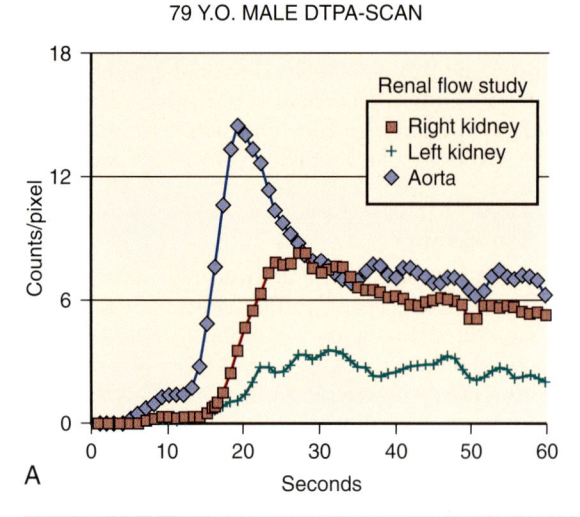

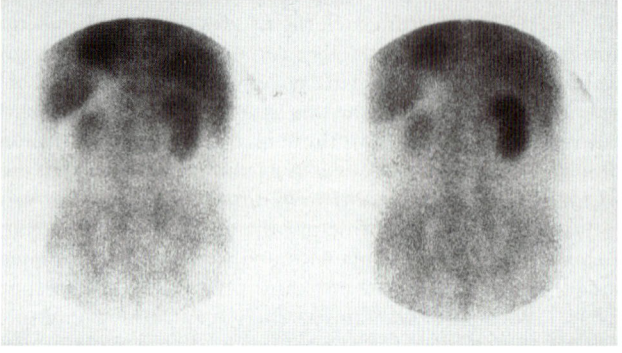

Figure 48.22 Isotope renography in a patient with unilateral renal artery stenosis. A, Technetium 99m–labeled diethylenetriaminepentaacetic acid (^{99m}Tc-DTPA) scan demonstrates delayed circulation and excretion of isotope on the left. **B,** Hippuran scan (now replaced with technetium 99m–labeled mercaptoacetyltriglycine) provides a renogram demonstrating a small kidney with impaired renal function on the affected side. Radionuclide scans provide a comparative estimate of function from each kidney that may facilitate selection of intervention, including the potential effect of nephrectomy (see text).

GFR after revascularization, sometimes with a decrement in contralateral GFR, thereby leaving overall kidney function unchanged.[137]

INVASIVE IMAGING

Intraarterial angiography currently remains the gold standard for definition of vascular anatomy and stenotic lesions in the kidney. Often it is completed at the time of a planned intervention, such as endovascular angioplasty and/or stenting. What is the current role of including angiography of the renal arteries during imaging of other vascular beds such as "drive-by" angiography during coronary artery imaging? Several studies confirm that the prevalence of renal artery lesions exceeding 50% lumen occlusion in patients with hypertension and coronary artery disease is high, usually between 18% and 24%.[101] Some individuals (7% to 10%) will have high-grade stenoses above 70% occlusion, and some will be bilateral. Accepting the fact that an arterial puncture and catheterization of the aorta and coronary vessels produces some risk, the *added* risk from including aortography of the renal vessels is small, almost negligible. Follow-up studies of individuals with identified incidental renal artery lesions suggest that the presence of these lesions does provide additive predictive risk for mortality.[62,138] Screening angiography is less commonly performed since the publication of prospective RCTs suggesting little benefit for stable patients with atherosclerotic renovascular disease from renal revascularization (see later). Hence endovascular procedures for such lesions should be confined to individuals with strong indications for renal revascularization, as even ardent advocates of catheter-based intervention have suggested.[101]

Contrast toxicity remains an issue with conventional iodinated agents.[139] Intravascular ultrasound procedures have been undertaken using papaverine to evaluate "flow reserve" beyond stenotic lesions.[140] Various reports indicate that either a reduced or preserved flow reserve may identify a poststenotic kidney that may improve after successful revascularization.[140,141] Previous studies of pressure gradients measured across stenotic lesions failed to predict the clinical response to renal revascularization. Measurements using currently available low-profile wire probes do, however, indicate a relationship between pressure gradients and activation of the renin angiotensin system.[14] Outcomes of patients with translesional pressure gradients measured after vasodilation suggest that measurement of hyperemic systolic gradient above 21 mm Hg most accurately predicts high-grade stenosis (average 78% by intravascular ultrasonography) and a beneficial response of blood pressure after stenting.[142] The latter observation and increasing reliability of technical measurements underscore the value of measuring gradients to establish a hemodynamic role for vascular lesions of marginal severity.

MANAGEMENT OF RENAL ARTERY STENOSIS AND ISCHEMIC NEPHROPATHY

OVERVIEW

Few areas in medicine have seen a greater pendulum swing than the shift from renal revascularization for cure of renovascular hypertension to primary reliance on medical antihypertensive therapy for atherosclerotic renovascular disease. This pendulum swing may be excessive in some cases, however, requiring nephrologists to deal with advanced renal failure that might be prevented. Considering the array of potential interventions and the complexity of these patients, clinicians need to formulate a clear set of therapeutic goals for each patient. Because each treatment—ranging from medical therapy alone to surgical revascularization—carries with it both benefits and risks, the clinician's task is to weigh the role of each of these within the context of the individual's comorbid conditions. In most cases, long-term management of the patient with renovascular disease represents integrated pharmacologic management of blood pressure and cardiovascular risk and optimal timing of renal revascularization for those with high-risk manifestations and/or disease progression. The objective of this section is to provide a framework by which to plan a balanced approach to the patient with unilateral or bilateral renal artery stenosis. It should be emphasized that consideration of renal artery disease takes place in the broad context of managing other cardiovascular risk factors, including withdrawal of tobacco use, reduction of cholesterol levels, and treatment of diabetes and obesity.

MEDICAL THERAPY FOR RENOVASCULAR DISEASE

The overall goals of therapy are summarized in Table 48.5. Foremost among these is the objective identified from multiple reports from the Joint National Committee of the National High Blood Pressure Education Program: "The goal of treating patients with hypertension is to prevent morbidity and mortality associated with high blood pressure."[143] This task may include the effort to simplify or potentially to eliminate long-term antihypertensive drug therapy, particularly in younger individuals with fibromuscular disease. A further goal is to preserve kidney function and to prevent loss of kidney function related to impaired renal blood flow. In some instances, renal revascularization is undertaken to allow improved management of salt and water balance in the process of managing patients with congestive cardiac failure. This may allow safer use of diuretic agents and ACE inhibitor and ARB classes of medication in patients with critical renal artery lesions to the entire renal mass. Because prospective clinical trial data are limited to relatively low-risk patients included for randomization, each patient must be considered individually. Several prospective RCTs have been undertaken over the last decade and are now published. Although each has limitations, results of medical therapy over time periods ranging from 2 to 5 years have been equivalent to those observed with medical therapy plus renal revascularization with relatively limited treatment crossovers (Tables 48.7 to 48.9). Taken together, these data underscore the importance of optimizing medical antihypertensive therapy as part of the decision-making process.

If blood pressure can be well controlled with a tolerable regimen and kidney function remains stable, it is difficult to justify moving forward with costly and potentially hazardous imaging and/or vascular intervention procedures. As a practical matter, these measures must be considered within the entire context of patient management over time.

UNILATERAL VERSUS BILATERAL RENAL ARTERY STENOSIS

Consideration of these disorders differs in some respects. "Bilateral" in this context refers to the circumstances when the entire functional renal mass is affected by vascular occlusion. This may be caused either by bilateral stenoses or stenosis to a solitary functioning kidney. Not only are the putative mechanisms related to blood pressure and volume control different in the presence of a nonstenosed, functioning contralateral kidney with unilateral disease (as outlined under the earlier discussion of pathophysiology), but the potential hazards of intervention and/or medical therapy differ. Patient survival is reduced in patients with bilateral disease or stenosis to a solitary functioning kidney. Progressive arterial disease in this group also poses the most immediate hazard of declining renal function. Patient survival depends upon the extent of vascular involvement[90] regardless of whether renal revascularization is undertaken.

MANAGEMENT OF UNILATERAL RENAL ARTERY STENOSIS

Most patients with atherosclerotic renal artery disease have preexisting hypertension. As a result, most are exposed to antihypertensive therapy before identification of the lesion and may be well controlled with only moderate medication use.[60] As noted earlier, such patients commonly come to clinical attention when recognizable clinical progression occurs. Occasionally, clinical decision making is influenced strongly by concerns about the hazards of medical therapy

Table 48.7 Outcomes of Endovascular Renal Artery Revascularization

Hypertension: Effect on Blood Pressure

	Cured	Improved	No Change
14 series N = 678 patients 98% technical success	Weighted mean: 17% Range: 3-68%	Weighted mean: 47% Range: 5-61%	Weighted mean: 36% Range: 0-61%
Renovascular hypertension N = 472	12%	73%	15%

Ischemic Nephropathy: Effect on Renal Function in Patients with Azotemia

	Improved	Stabilized	Worse
14 series Reporting impaired renal function N = 496 patients	Weighted mean: 30% Range: 10-41%	Weighted mean: 42% Range: 32-71%	Weighted mean: 29% Range: 19-34%
Ischemic nephropathy N = 469	41%	37% no change	22%

Several early series targeting hypertension reported results with angioplasty alone, whereas later series for both hypertension and ischemic nephropathy included primary angioplasty plus stents for atherosclerotic RVD (see text).
Modified and summarized from Textor SC: Renovascular hypertension and ischemic nephropathy. In Taal MW, Brenner BM, editors: Brenner and Rector's the kidney, Philadelphia, 2012, Elsevier Saunders, pp 1752-1791.

Table 48.8 Prospective, Randomized Trials of Medical versus Interventional Therapy for Hypertension in Patients with Atherosclerotic Renal Artery Stenosis

Author/No. Patients	Inclusion/BP Measurement	BP Outcome (mm Hg)	Renal Outcome	Comments
SNRAS: Webster et al, 1998 N = 55 (unilateral = 27) N = 135 eligible RAS > 50%	DBP ≥95 mm Hg, 2 drugs Exclusion: CVA, MI within 3 months: Creatinine > 500 µmol/L BP: random zero device No ACEI allowed	Unilateral: PTRA: 173/95 Med Rx: 161/88 Bilateral: PTRA: 152/83 Med Rx: 171/91 ($P < 0.01$)	Creatinine (µmol/L) Bilateral PTRA: 188 Med Rx: 157 Unilateral PTRA: 144 Med Rx: 168	"... unable to demonstrate any benefit in respect of renal function or event free survival" (follow-up 40 mo).
EMMA: Plouin et al, 1998 N = 49 (unilateral RAS only) RAS > 75% or > 60%, lateralizing study	<75 years Normal contralateral kidney Exclusion: malignant HTN, CVA, CHF, MI within 6 mo BP: automated sphygmomanometer, ABPM at 6 mo	PTRA: 140/81 Med Rx: 141/84 No. drugs (DDD): PTRA 1.0 Med Rx: 1.78 ($P < 0.01$) Crossover to PTRA: 7/26 (27%)	Creatinine clearance (mL/min) (6 mo): PTRA: 77 Med Rx: 74 Renal artery occlusion: PTRA: 0 Med Rx: 0	"BP levels and the proportion of patients given antihypertensive treatment were similar one year after randomization in the control and angioplasty groups, confirming that the BP-lowering effect of angioplasty in the short and medium terms is limited in atherosclerotic RAS."
DRASTIC: van Jaarsveld et al, 2000 N = 106 ASO RAS > 50%	Resistant: 2 drugs DBP > 95 mm Hg or creatinine rise with ACEI Exclusion: creatinine ≥ 2.3 Solitary kidney/total occlusion Kidney < 8 cm BP: automated oscillometric	BP outcomes at 3 mo: PTRA: 169/89 Med Rx: 163/88 At 12 mo: PTRA: 152/84 Med Rx: 162/88 No. drugs: 1.9 vs. 2.4 ($P < 0.01$)	Creatinine clearance (mL/min) (3 mo): PTRA: 70 Med Rx: 59 ($P = 0.03$) Abnormal renograms PTRA: 36% Med Rx: 70% ($P = 0.002$) Renal artery occlusion PTRA: 0 Med Rx: 8	"In the treatment of patients with hypertension and renal artery stenosis, angioplasty has little advantage over antihypertensive drug therapy"

The table is a summary of prospective, randomized trials for renovascular hypertension comparing medical therapy to percutaneous transluminal renal angioplasty (PTRA) with and without stenting. These studies contained selected patient populations with well-preserved kidney function and variable clinical parameters (e.g., unilateral vs. bilateral disease). Importantly, they sought to standardize blood pressure outcome measurement and to randomize patients prospectively. Each study differed from the others, but all found less major benefits accrued in interventional groups than reported by observational studies alone. Crossover rates from medical to angioplasty arms were significant in the early trials, however, and emphasize the importance of restoring blood supply in selected patients, particularly those with bilateral disease.

ABPM, Overnight ambulatory readings; ACEI, angiotensin-converting enzyme inhibitor; ASO, atherosclerotic occlusive disease; BP, blood pressure; CHF, congestive heart failure; CVA, cerebrovascular accident; DBP, diastolic blood pressure; DDD, defined daily doses; DRASTIC, Dutch Renal Artery Stenosis Intervention Cooperative; EMMA, Essai Multicentrique Medicaments vs. Angioplastie; MI, myocardial infarction; N, number of patients; RAS, renal artery stenosis; SNRAS, Scottish and Newcastle Renal Artery Stenosis Collaborative Group; Tx, therapy.

Modified from Textor SC: Renovascular hypertension and ischemic nephropathy. In Taal MW, Brenner BM, editors: Brenner and Rector's the kidney, Philadelphia, 2012, Elsevier Saunders, pp 1752-1791; Webster J, Marshall F, Abdalla M, et al: Randomised comparison of percutaneous angioplasty vs continued medical therapy for hypertensive patients with atheromatous renal artery stenosis. J Hum Hypertens 12:329-335, 1998; Plouin PF, Chatellier G, Darne B, et al: Blood pressure outcome of angioplasty in atherosclerotic renal artery stenosis: a randomized trial. Hypertension 31:822-829, 1998; and van Jaarsveld BC, Krijnen P, Pieterman H, et al: The effect of balloon angioplasty on hypertension in atherosclerotic renal-artery stenosis. N Engl J Med 342:1007-1014, 2000.

and failing to achieve restored blood flow soon enough. Examination of the results of medical therapy alone is important before evaluating the role of vascular reconstruction or dilation.

Since the introduction of agents blocking the renin angiotensin system have been introduced, most patients (86% to 92%) with unilateral renal artery disease can achieve blood pressure levels below 140/90 mm Hg with medical regimens based upon these agents. Treatment trials confirm that target blood pressure levels can regularly be achieved.[1,2] It should be understood that widespread application of these agents to patients with many forms of cardiovascular disease ensures that subcritical cases of renovascular disease are treated without being identified.

Table 48.9 Prospective, Randomized Clinical Trials for Renal Function and/or Cardiovascular Outcomes Comparing Medical Therapy versus Renal Artery Stenting

Trials	N	Population	Inclusion Criteria	Exclusion Criteria	Outcomes
STAR (2009) 10 centers Follow-up 2 yr	Med Tx: 76 PTRA: 64	Patients with impaired renal function, ostial ARVD detected by various imaging studies and stable blood pressure on statin and aspirin	ARVD > 50% Creatinine clearance < 80 mL/min/1.73 m^2 Controlled blood pressure 1 mo before inclusion	Kidney <8 cm and renal artery diameter <4 mm Estimated creatinine clearance < 15 mL/min/1.73 m^2 DM with proteinuria (>3 g/day), malignant hypertension	No difference in GFR decline (primary end point ≥20% change in clearance), but many did not undergo PTRA due to ARVD <50% on angiography Serious complication in the PTRA group Study was underpowered
ASTRAL (2009) 57 centers Follow-up 5 yr	Med Tx: 403 PTRA: 403	Patients with uncontrolled or refractory hypertension or unexplained renal dysfunction with unilateral or bilateral ARVD on statin and aspirin	ARVD substantial disease suitable for endovascular and patient's physician uncertainty of clinical benefit from revascularization	High likelihood of PTRA in < 6 mo Without ARVD, previous ARVD, PTRA FMD	No difference in BP, renal function, mortality, CV events (Primary end point: 20% reduction in the mean slope of the reciprocal of the serum creatinine level) Substantial risk in the PTRA group
CORAL (2013) 109 centers Follow-up 5 yr	Med Tx: 480 PTRA: 467	Hypertension on 2 or more antihypertensives or CKD stage ≥3 with ARVD with unilateral or bilateral disease on statin	SBP >155 mm Hg, at least 2 drugs ARVD >60% Subsequent changes included that the SBP > 155 mm Hg for defining systolic hypertension was no longer specified as long as patient had CKD stage 3	FMD Creatinine > 4.0 mg/dL Kidney length < 7 cm and use of > 1 stent	No difference of death from CV or renal causes Modest improvement of SBP in the stented group Total 26 complications (5.5%)

ARVD, Atherosclerotic renovascular disease; ASTRAL, Angioplasty and Stenting for Renal Artery Lesions; BP, blood pressure; CKD, chronic kidney disease; CORAL, Cardiovascular Outcomes in Renal Artery Lesions; CV, cardiovascular; DM, diabetes mellitus; FMD, fibromuscular dysplasia; GFR, glomerular filtration rate; N, number of patients; PTRA, percutaneous transluminal renal angioplasty; SBP, systolic blood pressure; STAR, Stent Placement and Blood Pressure; and Lipi-Lowering for the Prevention of Progression of Renal Dysfunction Caused by Atherosclerotic Ostial Stenosis of the Renal Artery; Tx, therapy.

Do the risks of treating unidentified renal artery stenoses with antihypertensive drug therapy pose a long-term hazard to kidney function? This issue is at the crux of clinical debates regarding management of patients with renovascular hypertension. Early studies with experimental clip hypertension emphasized renal fibrosis and scarring that occurred in the stenotic kidney in animals treated with ACE inhibitors. It is well recognized that removal of the efferent arteriolar effects of angiotensin II pose the possibility of loss of glomerular filtration in a kidney with reduced renal perfusion (Figure 48.23). Experimental studies in two-kidney–one-clip rats indicate that the loss of kidney function is sometimes irreversible, although survival is improved in ACE inhibitor–treated animals as compared to minoxidil treatment.[144] The unique role of ACE inhibitors and ARBs must be understood in this regard. Any drug capable of reducing systemic arterial pressure has the potential to lower renal pressures beyond a critical stenosis. As a result, successful antihypertensive therapy in renovascular disease has the theoretical result of reducing blood flow to the poststenotic kidney sufficient to induce vascular thrombosis. The unique feature of agents that block the renin angiotensin system is the reduction of efferent arteriolar resistance sufficient to lower transcapillary filtration pressures, despite preserved blood flow to the glomerulus (see Figure 48.23B). This property is central to the benefits of this class of agent in "hyperfiltration" states thought to accelerate renal damage in other settings. In the presence of renovascular disease, the fall in glomerular filtration beyond a stenotic lesion can be observed despite relatively preserved plasma flows. The fall in GFR heralds an approaching degree of critical vascular compromise before blood flow itself is reduced.[145] Studies in a porcine renovascular model suggest that angiotensin receptor blockade may have protective effects within the kidney as compared to drug therapy without renin angiotensin system blockade.[146] Earlier studies in renovascular hypertensive animals confirm that despite a reduction in filtration, renal structural integrity can be

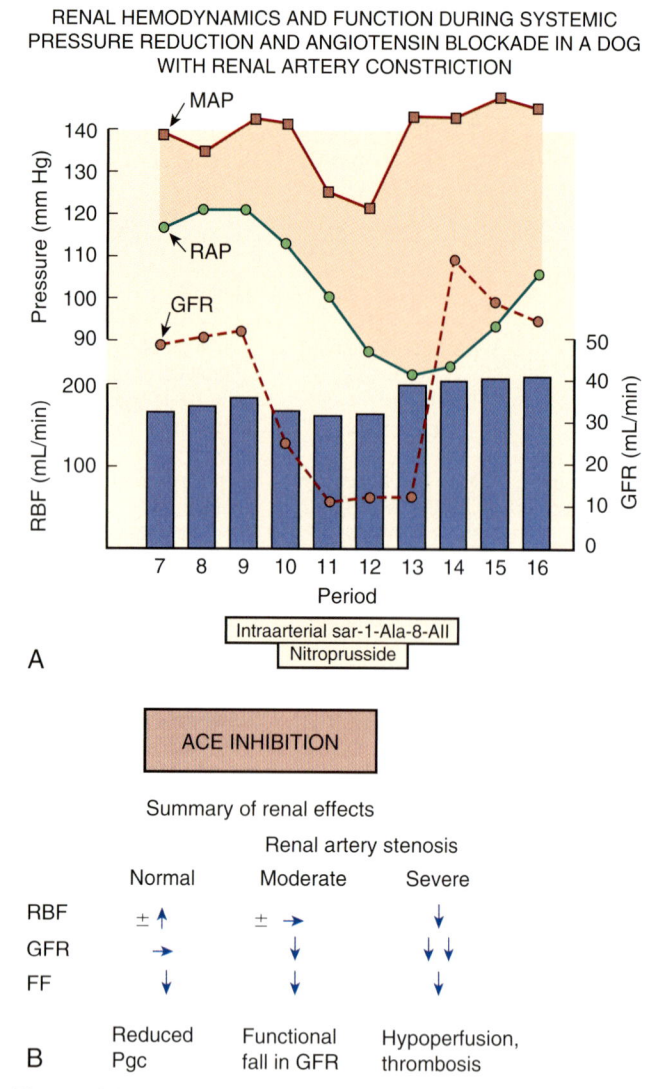

Figure 48.23 **A,** Glomerular filtration rate (GFR) falls beyond a renal artery stenotic lesion during blockade of angiotensin II (produced by intrarenal infusion of sar-1-ala-8-angiotensin II) and pressure reduction induced by sodium nitroprusside. The fall in GFR occurs despite preserved renal blood flow (RBF, measured by electromagnetic flow probe). These observations illustrate the specific role of angiotensin II in maintaining GFR in the poststenotic kidney at reduced perfusion pressures. **B,** Summary of the effects of angiotensin-converting enzyme (ACE) inhibition and/or angiotensin receptor blockade on RBF, GFR, and filtration fraction (FF) in normal, moderate, and severe levels of renal artery stenosis. As compared to other antihypertensive agents, ACE inhibitors and angiotensin receptor blockers lead to a fall in GFR and FF due to removal of the efferent arteriolar effects of angiotensin II. When stenosis is sufficiently severe that pressure reduction compromises RBF, the potential for complete occlusion is present, as with other effective antihypertensive agents as well. MAP, Mean arterial pressure; Pgc, glomerular capillary pressure; RAP, renal artery pressure. (Reprinted with permission from Textor SC: Renal failure related to ACE inhibitors. *Semin Nephrol* 17:67-76, 1997.)

preserved and recovered[147] after removal of the clip and/or removal of the ACE inhibitor. Hence it is unlikely that ACE inhibitors or ARBs themselves pose a unique hazard beyond that attributable to reduction in renal blood flow.

It is important to recognize that the contralateral kidney usually supports total glomerular filtration despite reduced filtration in the stenotic kidney. Changes in overall GFR may be undetectable. This may be interpreted in several ways. Some authors argue in favor of using split renal function measurements, such as radionuclide renal scans, to detect loss of individual kidney function as a means of timing revascularization.[103] Depending upon the circumstances, loss of one kidney may be an acceptable price if one can assure the patient that the remaining kidney has adequate function and blood supply. The fall in GFR from a loss of one kidney represents a loss of GFR similar to that of donating a kidney for renal transplantation or nephrectomy for malignancy. In such instances the long-term hazard to the remaining kidney is small, although not negligible.[148,149] As the age and comorbidity burden of the population at risk rises, the loss of one kidney may pose little additional hazard if overall glomerular filtration is adequate. The experience with ACE inhibition in trials of congestive cardiac failure is reassuring in this regard. Thousands of patients with marginal arterial pressures and clinical heart failure have been treated over many years with a variety of ACE inhibitors, and later ARBs. These patients are at high risk for undetected renal artery lesions as part of the atherosclerotic burden associated with coronary disease. Although a minor change in creatinine level is observed in 8% to 10% of these patients, a rise sufficient to lead to withdrawal of these agents under trial monitoring conditions occurs in only 1% to 2%.[145] Data from patients with high cardiovascular disease risk treated with ramipril included patients with creatinine levels up to 2.3 mg/dL. Those with creatinine levels between 1.4 and 2.3 mg/dL were at higher risk for cardiovascular mortality and had a major survival benefit from ACE inhibition. Close follow-up of kidney function indicated that withdrawal of ACE inhibition due to deterioration of renal function was less than 5% and no greater than placebo.[97] Registry data from the United Kingdom further support the tolerability of renin angiotensin system blockade in more than 90% of patients with atherosclerotic renovascular disease, including more than 75% of patients with bilateral disease.[69] Importantly, there appeared to be a mortality benefit in patients treated with these agents.

PROGRESSIVE RENAL ARTERY STENOSIS IN MEDICALLY TREATED PATIENTS

The potential for vascular occlusive disease to worsen is central to long-term management of patients with renovascular disease. It may be argued that failure to revascularize the kidneys exposes the individual to the hazard of undetected, progressive occlusion, potentially leading to total blood flow cessation and/or irreversible loss of renal function. Because the treatment trials have been relatively brief, this issue remains an important consideration for long-term treatment of atherosclerotic renovascular disease. A firm understanding of the data regarding progressive atherosclerotic disease of the kidney is important for planning both endovascular and surgical revascularization.

Atherosclerosis is a variably progressive disorder. Management of disorders of the carotid, coronary, aortic, and peripheral vasculatures all recognize the potential for progression, which occurs at widely different rates between individuals. Medical therapy for all of these disorders should incorporate measures aimed at intensive reduction of risk factors, of which smoking cessation, blood pressure control, and correction of dyslipidemias are paramount. Treatment of these risk factors reduces mortality rates related to cardiovascular disease.[150]

How does progressive renal artery occlusive disease affect management of renovascular hypertension? Moderate *anatomic progression* alone does not reliably predict functional changes in terms of deteriorating blood pressure control or renal function. Results from Doppler ultrasound studies from Seattle indicate that a decrement in measured renal size by 1 cm (renal atrophy) developed in 5.5% of those with normal initial vessels and 20.8% of those with baseline stenosis greater than 60% during a follow-up interval of 33 months.[94] Changes in serum creatinine levels were infrequent but did occur in a subset of patients, particularly those with bilateral renal artery stenosis. These findings are in general agreement with early studies during medical therapy for renovascular hypertension in which 35% of patients had a detectable fall in measured renal length, but only 8 out of 41 (20%) had a significant rise in creatinine level during a follow-up of 33 months. Follow-up of the medical treatment arms during short-term studies fails to show major changes in kidney function, although occasional loss of renal perfusion by radionuclide scan is observed.[93]

How often does management of renal artery stenosis without revascularization lead to *clinical progression*, either in terms of refractory hypertension or advancing renal insufficiency? Follow-up of patients with incidentally identified renal artery stenosis is helpful in this regard. Review of peripheral aortograms identified 69 patients with high-grade renal arterial stenoses (>70%) followed without revascularization for more than 6 months. Their long-term follow-up identified generally satisfactory blood pressure control, although some required more intensive antihypertensive therapy during an average of 36 months of follow-up.[96] Four of these eventually underwent renal revascularization for refractory hypertension and/or renal dysfunction. Five developed ESKD, of which only one was thought related to renal artery stenosis directly. Overall, serum creatinine levels rose from 1.4 mg/dL to 2.0 mg/dL. These data indicate that many such patients can be managed without revascularization for years and that clinical progression leading to urgent revascularization develops in between 10% and 14% of such individuals. Expansion of this data set to 160 patients allowed comparison of different antihypertensive regimens. The rates of progression did not appear related to the introduction of ACE inhibitors, although the level of blood pressure control improved in later years (see Table 48.4).[151] These observations are supported by a report of 126 patients with incidental renal artery stenosis compared to 397 patients matched for age. Measured serum creatinine level was higher and calculated (Cockcroft-Gault) GFR was lower in patients with renal artery stenosis followed 8 to 10 years. However, none of the patients progressed to ESKD. These observations are consistent with results of prospective trials of medical versus surgical intervention started in the 1980s and extended into the 1990s.[152] Remarkably similar data are evident from the later RCTs in which both the medical therapy and revascularization arms developed progression to renal end points in 16% to 22% of cases in CORAL and ASTRAL (see Table 48.9). No differences in patient survival or renal function could be identified. Taken together, these studies indicate that rates of progression of renovascular disease are moderate and occur at widely varying rates. Many such patients can be managed well without revascularization for many years.

Although these reports are informative, they leave many questions unanswered. How often does suboptimal blood pressure control in renovascular hypertension accelerate cardiovascular morbidity and mortality? Does one lose the opportunity to reverse hypertension effectively by delaying renal revascularization? These issues will depend upon further prospective studies. It is equally clear that for a subset of high-risk patients with progressive disease and advancing clinical manifestations of pulmonary edema, accelerating hypertension, and rapidly falling GFR, optimal long-term stability of kidney function and blood pressure control can be achieved by successful surgical or endovascular restoration of the renal blood supply.

ENDOVASCULAR RENAL ANGIOPLASTY AND STENTING

The ability to restore renal perfusion in high-risk patients with renovascular hypertension and ischemic nephropathy using endovascular methods represents a major advance in this disorder. Restoration of blood flow to the kidney beyond a stenotic lesion seems to provide an obvious means of improving renovascular hypertension and halting progressive vascular occlusive injury. In the 1990s a major shift from surgical reconstruction ensued toward preferential application of endovascular procedures.[10] The total volume of renal revascularization procedures registered for the U.S. Medicare population above 65 years of age rose 61% from 13,380 to 21,600 between 1996 and 2000. This change reflected an increase in endovascular procedures by 2.4-fold, whereas surgical renovascular procedures fell by 45%. The trend continued with an estimate of 35,000 endovascular procedures in 2005.[8,153] Since the publication of the ASTRAL trial, this trend has reversed dramatically, leading to few revascularization procedures in the United Kingdom.

Revascularizing the kidney has both benefits and risks. With older patients developing renal artery stenosis in the context of preexisting hypertension, the likelihood of a cure for hypertension is small, particularly in atherosclerotic disease. Although complications are not common, they can be catastrophic, including atheroembolic disease and aortic dissection. Knowing when to pursue renal revascularization is central to the dilemma of managing renovascular disease.

ANGIOPLASTY FOR FIBROMUSCULAR DISEASE

Most lesions of medial fibroplasia are located at a distance away from the renal artery ostium. Many of these have multiple webs within the vessel, which can be successfully traversed and opened by balloon angioplasty. Experience in the 1980s indicated more than 94% technical success rates.[154] Some of these lesions (approximately 10%) develop restenosis for which repeat procedures have been used.[63] Clinical benefit regarding blood pressure control has been reported in observational outcome studies in 65% to 75% of patients, although the rates of cure are less secure.[55] Cure of hypertension, defined as sustained blood pressure levels less than 140/90 mm Hg with no antihypertensive medications, may be obtained in 35% to 50% of patients. Predictors of cure (normal arterial pressures without medication at 6 months and beyond after angioplasty) include lower systolic blood pressures, younger age, and shorter duration of hypertension.[155]

A large majority of patients with FMD are female. The age at which hypertension is detected is usually younger than in the series of patients with atherosclerotic disease.[55] In general, such patients have relatively less aortic disease and are at less risk for major complications of angioplasty. Because the risk for major procedural complications is low, most clinicians favor early intervention for hypertensive patients with FMD with the hope of reduced antihypertensive medication requirements after successful angioplasty.

ANGIOPLASTY AND STENTING FOR ATHEROSCLEROTIC RENAL ARTERY STENOSIS

During the introduction of percutaneous transluminal renal angioplasty (PTRA) it was soon evident that ostial lesions commonly failed to respond, in part because of extensive recoil of the plaque, which extended into the main portion of the aorta.[156] These lesions develop restenosis rapidly even after early success. Endovascular stents were introduced for ostial lesions in the late 1980s and early 1990s.[157]

The technical advantage of stents is indisputable. An example of successful renal artery stenting is shown in Figure 48.24. Prospective comparison between angioplasty

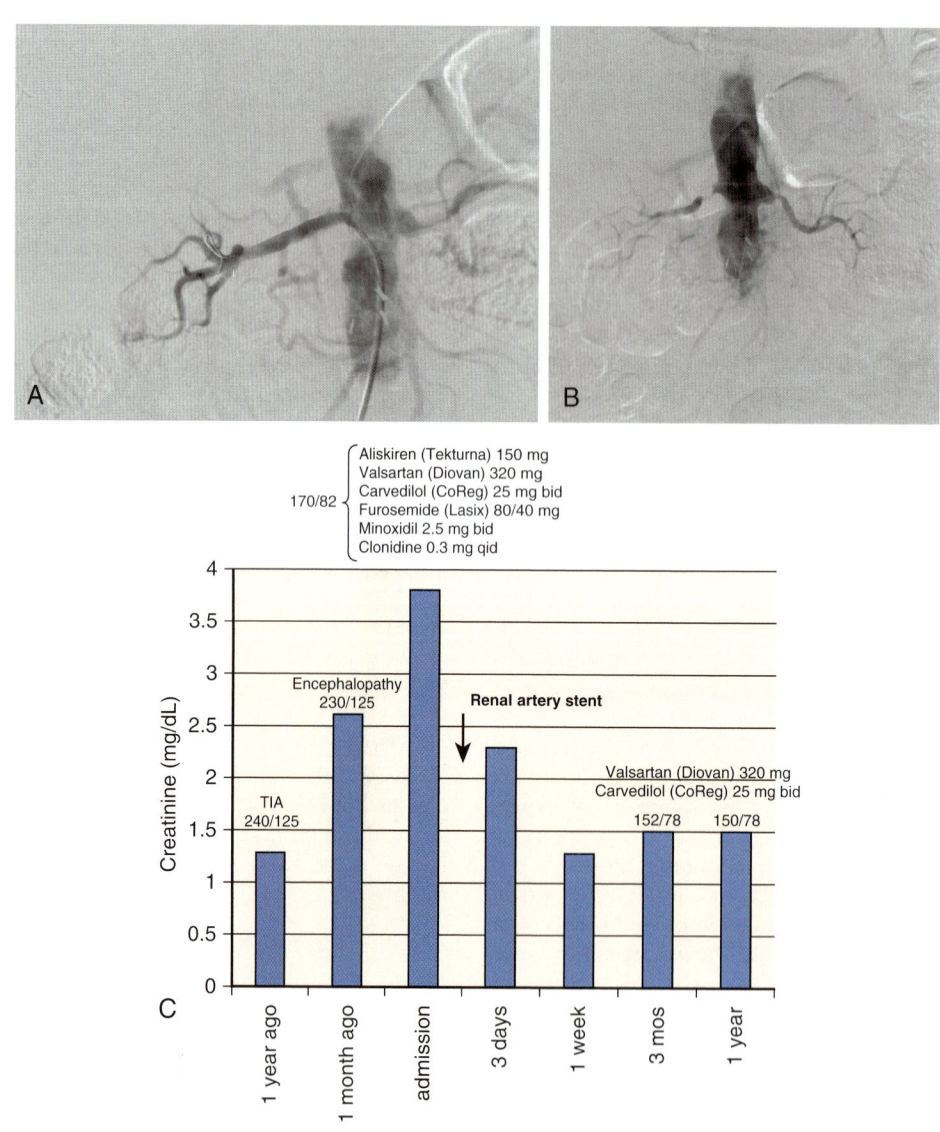

Figure 48.24 **A,** Renal aortogram illustrating high-grade, bilateral renal arterial lesions in a 73-year-old male who developed accelerated hypertension a few months before. **B,** Aortogram after placement of endovascular stents, illustrating excellent vessel patency and early technical success. This was followed by resolution of his hypertension. **C,** Serum creatinine levels, blood pressure levels, and antihypertensive drug regimen in an individual with high-grade bilateral renal artery stenosis. Rapidly developing hypertension and loss of glomerular filtration rate were associated with transient neurologic deficits. Successful renal artery stenting led to sustained reduction in serum creatinine levels, improved blood pressure levels, and reduced drug requirements. Such cases reflect high-risk subsets that were not well represented in the prospective randomized controlled trials (see text). TIA, transient ischemic attack. (Reprinted with permission from Textor SC: Attending rounds: a patient with accelerated hypertension and an atrophic kidney. *Clin J Am Soc Nephrol* 9:1117-1123, 2014.)

alone versus angioplasty with stents indicates intermediate (6 to 12 months) vessel patency was 29% and 75%, respectively. Restenosis fell from 48% to 14% in stented patients.[156] As technical success continues to improve, many reports suggest nearly 100% technical success in early vessel patency, although rates of restenosis continue to reach 14% to 25%.[10,101]

The introduction of endovascular stents has expanded renal revascularization, in part because of improved technical patency possible with ostial atherosclerotic lesions as compared to angioplasty alone. It should be emphasized that much of the shift to endovascular procedures relates to their applicability in older patients and widespread availability of interventional radiology.

What are the outcomes of patients undergoing renal artery stenting? These are commonly considered in terms of (1) *blood pressure control* and (2) preservation or salvage of *renal function* in ischemic nephropathy. Results from observational cohort blood pressure studies after stenting face the same limitations as observed with angioplasty alone. Results during follow-up from 1 to 4 years are summarized for representative series in Tables 48.7 to 48.9. These have been reviewed elsewhere.[158] Typical fall in blood pressure levels is in the range of 25 to 30 mm Hg systolic, the best predictor of which was the initial systolic blood pressure.[159] Some authors report 42% improvement in blood pressure with fewer medications needed, although cures were rare and renal function was unchanged.[160] Careful attention to degree of residual patency led to more than 91% patency at 1 year and 79% at 5 years in 210 patients with stents.[111] Blood pressures were "cured" or "improved" in more than 80% of patients. In some cases, angina and recurrent congestive cardiac failure subsides.[161,162] As noted under the trials summarized later, prospective RCTs have been less impressive regarding the benefits of angioplasty (Figure 48.25). The ambiguity of blood pressure responses in these studies produced widely different recommendations. These range from "we are left with whether renal angioplasty should be considered at all"[163] to a general conviction expressed within the interventional cardiology community that "open renal arteries are better than closed renal arteries" and that nearly all renal artery lesions should be opened (and probably stented).[101]

What results regarding *recovery of renal function* can be expected after endovascular revascularization? Tables 48.7 to 48.9 summarize some of the series. In general, changes in renal function for ARAS, as reflected by serum creatinine levels, have been small.[73] Remarkably, the changes in renal function in patients with azotemia after surgical reconstruction are similar.[164,165] As has been observed, overall group changes in kidney function can be misleading. Careful evaluation of the literature indicates that three distinctly

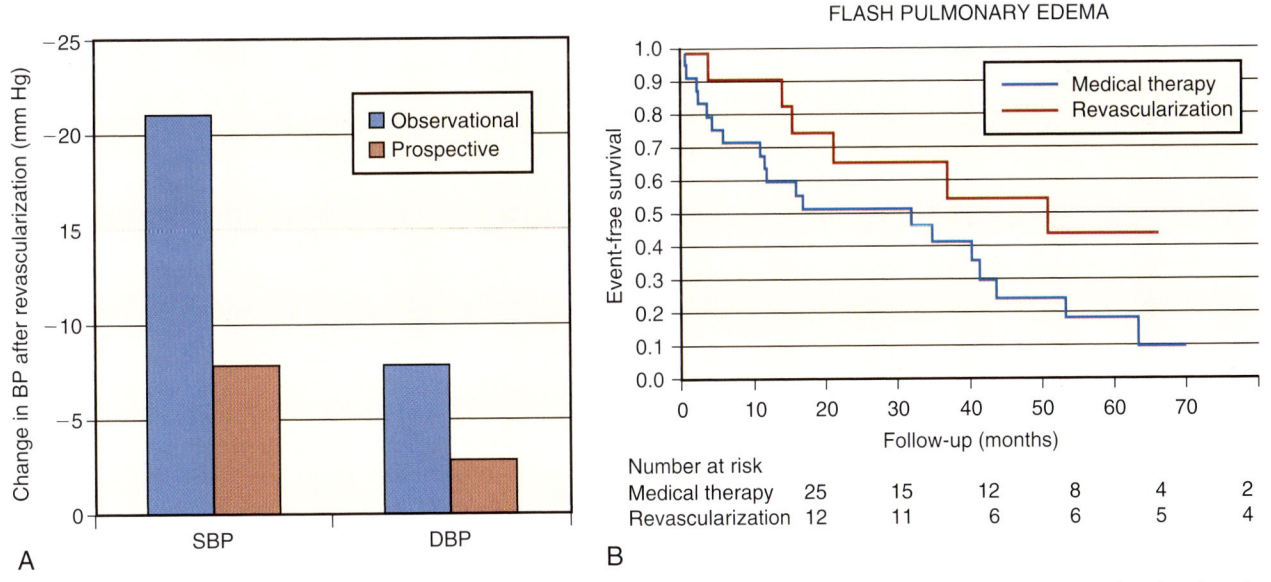

Figure 48.25 **A,** Comparison of blood pressure (BP) changes reported after renal revascularization from a large, observational registry (more than 1000 patients) and from a meta-analysis of three prospective randomized trials (210 patients). The large difference between these BP effects is reflected in variable enthusiasm for intervention between clinicians. Initial results from prospective trials (ASTRAL and CORAL, see text) identified only minor differences in achieved BP levels. Although results from observational series may overstate treatment benefits, results from prospective trials likely underestimate changes, in part due to limitations in patient recruitment and crossover between treatment arms, ranging from 27% to 44% in early series (see text). **B,** Follow-up data from a registry in the United Kingdom; most of these patients were not considered candidates for ASTRAL. This report identified a major mortality risk for patients with renal artery stenosis and episodes of pulmonary edema that was reduced for patients submitted for renal revascularization. A similar mortality benefit was identified for patients with rapidly progressive renal failure (see text). DBP, Diastolic blood pressure; SBP, systolic blood pressure. (**A** data from Dorros G, Jaff M, Mathiak L, et al: Multicenter Palmaz stent renal artery stenosis revascularization registry report: four-year follow-up of 1,058 successful patients. *Catheter Cardiovasc Interv* 55:182-188, 2002; and Nordmann AJ, Woo K, Parkes R, et al: Balloon angioplasty or medical therapy for hypertensive patients with atherosclerotic renal artery stenosis? A meta-analysis of randomized controlled trials. *Am J Med* 114:44-50, 2003; **B** reprinted with permission from Ritchie J, Green D, Chrysochou C, et al: High-risk clinical presentations in atherosclerotic renovascular disease: prognosis and response to renal artery revascularization. *Am J Kidney Dis* 63:186-197, 2014.)

different clinical outcomes are routinely observed. In some instances (approximately 27%), revascularization produces meaningful improvements in kidney function. For this group the mean serum creatinine level may fall from a mean value of 4.5 mg/dL to an average of 2.2 mg/dL. There can be no doubt that such patients benefit from the procedure and can avoid major morbidity (and probably mortality) associated with advanced renal failure. The bulk of patients, however, have no measurable change in renal function (approximately 52%). Whether such patients benefit much depends upon the true clinical likelihood of progressive renal injury if the stenotic lesion were managed without revascularization, as discussed earlier. Those without much risk for progression gain little. The most significant concern, however, is the group of patients whose renal function deteriorates further after a revascularization procedure. In most reports this ranges from 19% to 25%.[73,166] In some instances this represents atheroembolic disease or a variety of complications, including vessel dissection with thrombosis.[167] Hence nearly 20% of patients with azotemia face a relatively rapid progression of renal insufficiency and the potential for requiring renal replacement therapy, including dialysis and/or renal transplantation.[165,168,169] Possible mechanisms for deterioration include atheroembolic injury, which may be nearly universal after any vascular intervention,[170] and acceleration of oxidative stress producing interstitial fibrosis.[171] Whether improving techniques, including the application of distal "protection" devices for endovascular catheters, will reduce these complications is not yet certain.

Several studies suggest that progression of renal failure attributed to ischemic nephropathy may be reduced by endovascular procedures.[166,172] Harden and associates presented reciprocal creatinine plots in 23 (of 32) patients suggesting that the slope of loss of GFR could be favorably changed after renal artery stenting.[166] It should be emphasized that 69% of patients "improved or stabilized," indicating that 31% worsened, consistent with results from other series. These reports and a guideline document from the American Heart Association promote the use of break-point analysis to analyze and report the results of renovascular procedures. Caution must be applied regarding the use of break points using reciprocal creatinine plots in this disorder, however. Vascular disease does not affect both kidneys symmetrically, nor is it likely to follow a constant course of progression, in contrast to diabetic nephropathy, for example. As a result, a gradual loss of renal function with subsequent stabilization can be observed equally with unilateral disease leading to total occlusion as well as successful revascularization. Perhaps the most convincing group data in this regard derives from serial renal functional measurement in 33 patients with high-grade (>70%) stenosis to the entire affected renal mass (bilateral disease or stenosis to a solitary functioning kidney) with creatinine levels between 1.5 and 4.0 mg/dL. Follow-up over a mean of 20 months indicates that the slope of GFR loss converted from negative (−0.0079 dL/mg per month) to positive (0.0043 dL/mg per month).[172] These studies agree with other observations that long-term survival is reduced in bilateral disease and that the potential for renal dysfunction and accelerated cardiovascular disease risk is highest in such patients (see earlier).

PROSPECTIVE TRIALS

MEDICAL THERAPY COMPARED TO ANGIOPLASTY PLUS STENTS

RENOVASCULAR HYPERTENSION

As noted earlier, many patients with unilateral renal artery stenosis are managed without restoration of blood flow for a long period, sometimes indefinitely. The judgment about endovascular intervention in a specific case revolves about the anticipated outcome as summarized later. There are now several prospective, randomized trials comparing medical therapy with revascularization using PTRA with or without stents upon which to draw. Familiarity with the available trials and their limitations is important for nephrologists. The major features of these trials are summarized in Tables 48.8 and 48.9.

Three early trials in renovascular hypertension from the 1990s address the relative value of endovascular repair, specifically PTRA as compared to medical therapy for ARAS. To the credit of these investigators, care was taken to standardize blood pressure measurement before and after endovascular repair and to select antihypertensive regimens carefully. All of these trials have limitations, but they are instructive. Webster and associates randomized 55 patients with ARAS to either medical therapy or PTRA. Follow-up blood pressure measurements were obtained using a random-zero sphygmomanometer after a run-in period. The run-in period produced considerable reduction in blood pressures in all patients. Those with unilateral disease had no difference between medical therapy and PTRA[88] after 6 months. There was greater blood pressure benefit after PTRA in those with bilateral renal artery stenosis. The authors indicated they were "unable to demonstrate any benefit in respect of renal function or event free survival" during follow-up, which was presented up to 40 months. Plouin and colleagues randomized 49 patients with unilateral ARAS greater than 75% or greater than 60% with lateralizing functional studies. Blood pressure measurements were based upon overnight ambulatory readings, which are thought to yield more reproducible trial data and to be relatively free from placebo or office effects. Seven of 26 assigned to medical therapy eventually crossed over to the PTRA group (27%) for refractory hypertension. There were six procedural complications in the PTRA group, including branch dissection and segmental infarction. Final blood pressures were not different between groups, but slightly fewer medications were required in the PTRA group. Taken together, this trial suggested that PTRA produced more complications in the near term, was useful in some medical treatment failures, and required slightly fewer medications after 6 months. Medical therapy for this study specifically excluded agents that block the renin angiotensin system (such as ACE inhibitors).[173] A third prospective trial included 106 patients enrolled in the Dutch Renal Artery Stenosis Intervention Cooperative (DRASTIC) study.[93] These patients were selected for resistance to therapy including two drugs and were required to have serum creatinine values below 2.3 mg/dL. Blood pressures were evaluated using automated oscillometric devices at 3 and 12 months after entry. Patients were evaluated on an intention-to-treat basis. Blood pressures did not differ between groups overall at either 3 or 12 months, although the PTRA group was taking fewer medications (2.1 ± 1.3 vs. 3.2 ± 1.5 defined daily doses, $P < 0.001$). The authors concluded that in the treatment of hypertension and renal artery stenosis, "angioplasty has little advantage over antihypertensive drug therapy."[93] Many critics emphasize, however, that 22 of 50 (44%) patients assigned to medical therapy were considered treatment failures and referred for PTRA after 3 months. There were eight instances of total arterial occlusion in the medical group, as compared to none in the angioplasty group. Many clinicians interpret these data to support an important role for PTRA in management of patients with refractory hypertension and renal artery stenosis. Regardless, the results of these trials indicate that benefits of endovascular procedures, even in the short term, are moderate compared to effective antihypertensive therapy. Patients failing to respond to medical therapy often improve after revascularization. Some authors have combined these prospective studies into meta-analyses, indicating that taken together, renal revascularization produced modest but definite reductions in blood pressures, averaging −7/−3 mm Hg.[174,175]

STENTS FOR PROGRESSION OF RENAL INSUFFICIENCY AND CARDIOVASCULAR OUTCOMES

Several prospective RCTs sought to compare medical therapy with endovascular stenting targeted primarily to progression of chronic kidney disease (CKD) and/or adverse cardiovascular outcomes such as stroke and coronary disease events. Among these, the largest are the United States–based CORAL trial and the U.K.-based ASTRAL trial (see Table 48.9). Although these have been published and add important information, they have substantial limitations of which nephrologists should be aware.

CORAL was designed to test whether renal artery stenting, when added to optimal (standardized) medical therapy, including blockade of the renin angiotensin system, improves cardiovascular outcomes for individuals with ARAS. The authors list more than 110 participating centers with a total of 947 participants enrolled over a 5-year period to stenting plus medical therapy (467 patients) or to medical therapy alone (480 patients). Average entry estimated GFR (eGFR) values were 58 mL/min/1.73 m². This trial attempted to standardize evaluation of stenosis by requiring translesional gradient measurement and review by an angiographic core laboratory. After a mean of 43 months of follow-up, no differences were apparent for any or all of the composite end point (death from cardiovascular or renal causes, myocardial infarction, stroke, hospitalization for congestive heart failure, progressive renal insufficiency, or the need for renal replacement therapy) between the stent group and the medical therapy only group (35.1% and 35.8%, respectively; hazard ratio, 0.94; 95% confidence interval, 0.76 to 1.17; $P = 0.58$).[2] Systolic blood pressure was slightly lower in the revascularization arm (−2.3 mm Hg). Importantly, procedural complications per vessel treated were only 5.2% in the stent group (Table 48.10). CORAL has several important limitations, as has been discussed elsewhere.[3,78] The authors acknowledge that recruitment for CORAL was difficult and took longer than anticipated. Most centers enrolled fewer than 10 subjects over the 4- to 5-year period. Several criteria for enrollment and intervention changed during the trial. The original intention had been to include patients with severe renal artery stenosis and systolic blood pressure above 155 mm Hg while receiving two or more antihypertensive medications. Severe renal artery stenosis was defined as more than 80% stenosis in isolation or 60% to 80% with a gradient of at least 20 mm Hg. As the protocols evolved, patients could be enrolled with or without hypertension if the eGFR was less than 60 mL/min/1.73 m². Requirements for translesional gradients were dropped, and patients could be enrolled using duplex ultrasonography, MR angiography, or CT angiographic criteria. Ultimately, the average level of stenosis (67%) measured in the core laboratory was lower than estimates by the investigators on site (73%). As with other RCTs it is likely that many of these lesions were below the threshold of 75% to 80% usually required to produce a reduction in blood flow in experimental studies. Twenty-five percent

Table 48.10 Complications after PTRA and Stenting of the Renal Arteries

Minor (Most Frequently Reported)
Groin hematoma
Puncture site trauma
Major (Reported in 71/799 treated arteries [9%])[179]
Hemorrhage requiring transfusion
Femoral artery pseudoaneurysm needing repair
Brachial artery traumatic injury needing repair
Renal artery perforation leading to surgical intervention
Stent thrombosis: surgical or antithrombotic intervention
Distal renal artery embolus
Iliac artery dissection
Segmental renal infarction
Cholesterol embolism: renal
Peripheral atheroemboli
Aortic dissection[167]
Restenosis
16% (range: 0-39%)
Deterioration of Renal Function
26% (range: 0-45%) combined complication rate over 24 mo
Stenting after failed PTRA: 24%[194]
Mortality Attributed to Procedure: 0.5%
Procedure-Related Complications
51/379 patients in 10 series (13.5%)[168]
Procedure Complications Reported from CORAL Angiographic Core Laboratory (2014)[2]
Dissection: 11/495 (2.2%)
Branch occlusion: 6/495 (1.2%)
Distal embolization: 6/495 (1.2%)
Single events: wire perforation, vessel rupture, pseudoaneurysm
Total events: 26/495 (5.3%)

CORAL, Cardiovascular Outcomes in Renal Atherosclerotic Lesions; PTRA, percutaneous transluminal renal angioplasty.

of patients had reached goal blood pressures before entry. Specific high-risk groups, including those with congestive heart failure within 30 days, were excluded. Based on Medicare claims data indicating more than 20,000 renal artery stent procedures annually (estimates from 2000), it is clear that screening and enrollment for CORAL included only a small fraction of treatment candidates, for which no contemporaneous U.S. registry comparison is available. Based on difficult enrollment and relaxed criteria, it appears that the CORAL cohort represented a relatively low-risk atherosclerotic population. This is based on the preserved levels of eGFR at baseline, easily controlled blood pressures, and exclusion of recent congestive heart failure and low 5-year cardiovascular mortality. Remarkably, fewer than 5% of enrolled patients died of cardiovascular causes during CORAL, substantially less than the registry population reported by Ritchie and coworkers, and less even than the ASTRAL cohort, which specifically excluded patients that clinicians thought would "definitely benefit" from revascularization.[1,5]

Results from the ASTRAL trial from the United Kingdom were published for 806 subjects followed for several years. The mean serum creatinine level was above 2.0 mg/dL, and the severity of vascular occlusion was estimated by a variety of imaging methods above 70%. Patients were considered eligible for the trial if clinicians were uncertain about optimal management. No differences were apparent regarding changes in kidney function, blood pressure, hospitalizations, mortality, or episodes of circulatory congestion.[1] Rates of progression to renal end point were 16% to 22% in both medically treated and revascularized groups. A smaller trial, STAR, enrolled 140 subjects and aimed to evaluate progression of CKD based upon initial creatinine clearance level of less than 80 mL/min and atherosclerotic stenosis of more than 50% luminal narrowing. No differences for the change in creatinine clearance were detected during follow-up of 2 years, although some substantial complications occurred in the stent-treated group.[83] This study in particular highlights the drawbacks of including trivial vascular lesions in a treatment trial. Only 46 of 64 patients assigned to stent therapy underwent stenting, mainly because lesions were often not hemodynamically significant.

These modest benefits present a striking contrast between the present and the situation a few decades ago. Reports from the 1970s underscore the fact that some patients experienced recurrent episodes of malignant-phase hypertension with encephalopathy, fluid retention, and progressive renal insufficiency. Over the years since then, malignant hypertension is becoming less prevalent in most Western countries, although not universally. Introduction of ACE inhibitors and calcium channel blockers in the 1980s coincided with reduced occurrence of severe hypertension and improved medical management of patients with high-renin states, including renovascular hypertension. Reported results from the prospective trials of angioplasty are less favorable than those reported from retrospective series. A representative report of more than 1000 successfully stented patients followed in a registry suggests that average blood pressure levels fell during follow-up −21/−8 mm Hg[98] (see Figure 48.25A). The differences between prospective trials and registry values sometimes reflect an element of outcome reporting bias. An important alternative possibility, however, is that enrollment in prospective trials itself reflects recruitment bias in favor of more "stable" patients in less urgent clinical need of restoring renal circulation. Hence the randomized trials almost certainly underestimate the benefits of renal revascularization for the patients at the greatest risk for both accelerated hypertension and/or renal failure. Taken together, however, results of the trials underscore the efficacy of medical therapy for many patients and weaken the argument for revascularization for moderate ARAS.

COMPLICATIONS OF RENAL ARTERY ANGIOPLASTY AND STENTING

Atherosclerotic plaque is commonly composed of multiple layers with calcified, fibrotic, and inflammatory components. Physical expansion of such a lesion applies considerable force to the wall and may lead to cracking and release of small particulate debris into the bloodstream. Effective balloon angioplasty and stenting requires applying optimal techniques for limiting the damage to blood vessels during the procedure. A review of 10 published series with 416 stented vessels indicates that significant complications arise in 13% of cases, not counting those that led to the need for dialysis. These include several of the events listed in Table 48.10, including hematomas and retroperitoneal bleeding requiring transfusion. Renal function deteriorated in these series on average 26% of the time, and 50% (7 of 14) subjects with preprocedure creatinine levels above 400 μmol progressed to advanced renal failure requiring dialysis.[168] Most complications are minor, including local hematomas and false aneurysms at the insertion site. Occasional severe complications develop, including aortic dissection,[167] stent migration, and vessel occlusion with thrombosis.[176] Local renal dissections can be managed by judicious application of additional stents. Mortality related directly to this procedure is small but has been reported in 0.5% to 1.5% of patients.[168,177]

Restenosis remains a significant clinical limitation. Rates vary widely between 13% and 30%, most often developing within the first 6 to 12 months.[99,168,178,179] Most later series report 13% to 16% restenosis, sometimes leading to repeat procedures.

SURGICAL TREATMENT OF RENOVASCULAR HYPERTENSION AND ISCHEMIC NEPHROPATHY

Early experience with vascular disease of the kidney was based entirely upon surgical intervention, either nephrectomy or vascular reconstruction, with the objective of "surgical curability."[9] For that reason, much of the original data regarding split renal function measurement was geared toward identifying "functionally" significant lesions as a guide by which patients should be selected for a major surgical procedure. Surgical intervention is less commonly performed now and is most often reserved for complex vascular reconstruction and/or failed endovascular procedures. Generally speaking, age and comorbid risks of patients with atherosclerotic disease favor endovascular procedures when feasible.

Methods of surgical intervention have changed over the decades. A review in 1982 emphasized the role for ablative techniques, including partial nephrectomy. Use of ablative operative means was guided by the difficulty of controlling blood pressure during this period. They are less common since the expansion of tolerable medication regimens, as noted earlier. Introduction of laparoscopic techniques, including hand-assisted nephrectomy, may return attention to nephrectomy as a means to reduce medication requirements with low morbidity in high-risk patients.

Surgical series from the 1960s and early 1970s indicated that cure of hypertension was present only in 30% to 40% of subjects, despite attempts at preselection. Survival of groups chosen for surgery appeared to be better than those chosen for medical management. This likely reflected the heavy disease burden and preoperative risks identified in those for whom surgery was excluded. The Cooperative Study of Renovascular Hypertension in the 1960s and 1970s examined many of the clinical characteristics of renovascular hypertension. These studies identified some of the limitations and hazards of surgical intervention and reported mortality rates of 6.8%, even in excellent institutions. The mean age in this series was 50.5 years. Definitions of operative mortality included events as late as 375 days after the procedure and may overestimate the hazard. Had the authors considered only deaths within the first week, for example, the immediate perioperative mortality was 1.7%.[89]

Subsequent development of improved techniques for patient selection, including screening for coronary and carotid disease, for renal artery bypass and endarterectomy, and for combined aortic and renal artery repair, represents a major element in the history of vascular surgery.[9] Several of the options developed for renal artery reconstruction are listed in Table 48.11. Most of these methods focus upon reconstruction of the vascular supply for preservation of nephron mass. Transaortic endarterectomy can effectively restore circulation to both kidneys. It requires aortic cross-clamping and may be undertaken as part of a combined procedure with aortic replacement. Identification and treatment of carotid and coronary disease led to reductions in surgical morbidity and mortality. By addressing associated cardiovascular risk before surgery, early surgical mortality falls below 2% for patients without other major diseases.

Surgical reconstruction of the renal blood supply usually requires access to the aorta. A variety of alternative surgical procedures have been designed to avoid manipulation of the badly diseased aorta, including those for which previous surgical procedures make access difficult. These include extraanatomic repair of the renal artery using hepatorenal or splenorenal conduits that avoid the requirement of manipulation of a badly diseased aorta.[180] An example of contemporary surgical reconstruction to protect renal function is illustrated in Figure 48.26. It should be emphasized that success with extrarenal conduits depends upon the integrity of the alternative blood supply. Hence careful preoperative assessment of stenotic orifices of the celiac axis is undertaken before using either the hepatic or splenic arteries. The results of these procedures have been good, both in the short term and during long-term follow-up studies.[181] Analysis of 222 patients treated more than 10 years earlier

Table 48.11 Surgical Procedures Applied to Reconstruction of the Renal Artery and/or Reversal of Renovascular Hypertension*

Ablative surgery: removal of a pressor kidney
  Nephrectomy: direct or laparoscopic
  Partial nephrectomy
Renal artery reconstruction (require aortic approach)
  Renal endarterectomy
  Transaortic endarterectomy
  Resection and reanastomosis: suitable for focal lesions
  Aortorenal bypass graft
Extraanatomic procedures (may avoid direct manipulation of the aorta)—require adequate alternate circulation without stenosis at celiac origin
  Splenorenal bypass graft
  Hepatorenal bypass graft
  Gastroduodenal, superior mesenteric, iliac-to-renal bypass grafts
Autotransplantation with ex vivo reconstruction

*See text.
Modified from Libertino JA, Zinman L: Surgery for renovascular hypertension. In Breslin DL, Swinton NW, Libertino JA, et al, editors: Renovascular hypertension, Baltimore, 1982, Williams and Wilkins, pp 166-212.

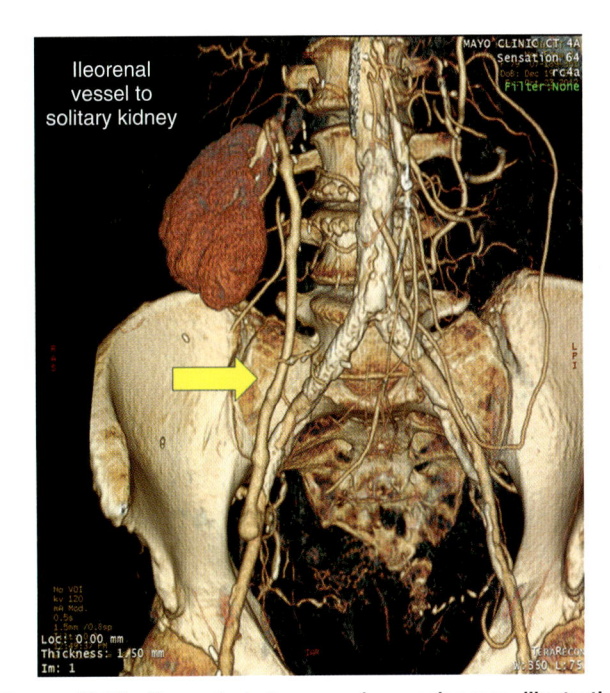

Figure 48.26 Computed tomography angiogram illustrating complex surgical repair of aortic and vascular perfusion to a solitary functioning kidney. Although surgical reconstruction of the renal vessels is less commonly performed since the introduction of endovascular techniques, it provides an essential alternative for complex occlusive disease and failed endovascular stenting in selected patients. *Arrow* identifies ileorenal bypass vessel providing blood flow to a solitary kidney.

indicates that these procedures were performed with 2.2% mortality and low rates of restenosis (7.3%) and good long-term survival. The predictors of late mortality were age above 60 years, coronary disease, and previous vascular surgery.

The durability of surgical vascular reconstruction is well established. Follow-up studies after 5 and 10 years for all forms of renal artery bypass procedures indicate excellent long-term patency (above 90%) both for renal artery procedures alone and when combined with aortic reconstruction.[182] Results of surgery have been good despite increasing age in the reported series. Patient selection has been important in all of these reports. Whereas long-term outcome data are established for surgery, limited information is available for endovascular stent procedures, which are more prone to restenosis and technical failure. This proven record of surgical reconstruction leads some clinicians to favor this approach for younger individuals with longer life expectancy.

Some studies have compared endovascular intervention (PTRA without stents) and surgical repair. A single study of nonostial, unilateral atherosclerotic disease in which patients were randomly assigned to surgery or PTRA indicates that although surgical success rates were higher and PTRA was needed on a repeat basis in several cases, the 2-year patency rates were 90% for PTRA and 97% for surgery.[183] A prospective comparison of endovascular stents compared to open surgical renal revascularization argues that patency over 4 years was better with open surgical repair, but that otherwise the outcome of the two procedures did not differ.[184]

In many institutions, surgical reconstruction of the renal arteries is most often undertaken as part of aortic surgery.[185] Those with impaired renal function at the Mayo Clinic (creatinine level ≥ 2.0 mg/dL) underwent simultaneous aortic and renal procedures in 75% of cases.[164] Experience indicates that combining renal revascularization with aortic repair does not increase the risk of the aortic operation. As with endovascular techniques, the results regarding changes in renal function include improvement in 22% to 26%, no change (some consider this stabilization) in 46% to 52%, and progressive deterioration in 18% to 22% (Figure 48.27). Using intraoperative color flow Doppler ultrasonography allows immediate correction of suboptimal results and improved long-term patency.[186] Results from several contemporary surgical series are summarized in Table 48.12. Despite good results, open operations for renal artery revascularization continue to decline. A review of the National Inpatient Sample indicates relatively high mortality rates (approximately 10%) overall, leading the authors to support lower-risk endovascular methods where possible or referral to high-volume surgical centers.[187] For experienced centers using current techniques, operative risk is below 4% in good-risk candidates.[188,189] Risk factors for higher risk include advanced age, elevated creatinine level (above 2.7 to 3.0 mg/dL), and associated aortic or other vascular disease. In some cases, nephrectomy of a totally infarcted kidney provides major improvement in blood pressure control at low operative risk. The introduction of laparoscopic surgical techniques makes nephrectomy technically easier in some patients for whom vascular reconstruction is not an option. These series reflect widely variable methods of determining blood pressure benefit as discussed later.

Studies in patients with bilateral renal artery lesions or vascular occlusion to the entire renal mass indicate that restoration of blood flow can lead to preservation of renal function in some cases.[190] Most often this has been undertaken when a clue of preserved blood supply, sometimes from capsular vessels, is evident by renography. Occasionally

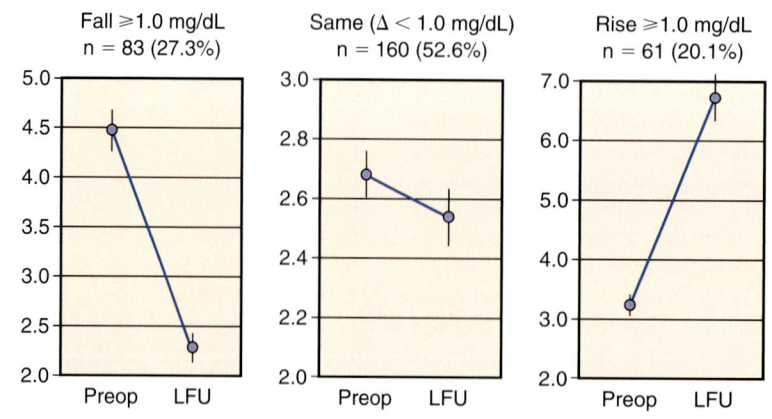

Figure 48.27 Renal functional outcomes after renal revascularization in 304 patients with azotemia (creatinine ≥ 2.0 mg/dL) with atherosclerotic renal artery stenosis (RAS). On average, mean serum creatinine level does not change during a follow-up period exceeding 36 months, as observed with most reported series (see text). Group mean values obscure major differences in clinical outcomes as shown here. Some patients experience major clinical benefit (defined as a fall in serum creatinine level of ≥1.0 mg/dL) (**left**). The largest group (**middle**) has minor changes (<1.0 mg/dL), which might be considered stabilization of renal function. The degree of benefit in these patients depends upon whether renal function is deteriorating before intervention. The data for the group on the **right** emphasize the failure to observe consistent overall improvement in function, because 18% to 22% of patients develop worsening renal function. The exact causes of this deterioration are not clear, although atherosclerotic disease is responsible for a portion. This potential hazard of revascularization must be considered when offering these procedures. LFU, Latest follow-up. (From Textor SC, Wilcox CS: Renal artery stenosis: a common, treatable cause of renal failure? *Annu Rev Med* 52:421-442, 2001).

Table 48.12 Selected Series of Surgical Renal Artery Revascularization: 2000-2005

Author	Pts.	Bil. Repair (%)	Preop RI	Renal Function Response (%)		Hypertension Response (%)		Perioperative Outcome (%)	
				Improved	Unchanged	Cured	Improved or Stable	Death	Morbidity
Hansen	232	64	100	58	35	11	76	7.3	30
Paty*	414	NR	4	26	68	NR		5.5	11.4
Cherr	500	59	49	43	47	73	12	4.6	16
Marone	96	27	100	42	41	NR		4.1	NR
Mozes	198	65	57	28	67	2	59	2.5	19

*Pts. operated for either hypertension or renal salvage. Improvement was noted in 26, 68% remained stable, and 6% worsened. Specific renal function decline occurred in 3%.
Bil., Bilateral; NR, not reported; preop RI, preoperative renal insufficiency.
With permission of Mayo Foundation for Medical Education and Research. All rights reserved. From Bower TC, Oderich GS: Surgical revascularization. In Lerman LO, Textor SC, editors: *Renal vascular disease*, London, 2014, Springer, pp 325-340.

revascularization can lead to functional recovery sufficient to eliminate the need for dialysis.

PREDICTORS OF LIKELY BENEFIT REGARDING RENAL REVASCULARIZATION

Identification of patients most likely to experience improved blood pressure and/or renal function after renal revascularization remains an elusive task. As noted earlier, functional tests of renin release, such as measurement of renal vein renin levels, have not performed universally well. Many of these studies are most useful when their results are positive (e.g., the likelihood of benefit improves with more evident lateralization) but have relatively poor negative predictive value, that is, when results of such studies are negative, outcomes of vessel repair may still be beneficial. As a clinical matter, recent progression of hypertension, deterioration of renal function, and/or pulmonary edema remain among the most consistent predictors of improved blood pressure after intervention.

Predicting favorable renal functional outcomes is also difficult. Either surgical or endovascular procedures are least likely to benefit those with advanced renal insufficiency, usually characterized by serum creatinine levels above 3.0 mg/dL. Nonetheless, occasional patients with recent progression to far-advanced renal dysfunction can recover GFR with durable improvement over many years (see Figure 48.26). Small kidneys, as identified by length less than 8 cm, are less likely to recover function, particularly when little function can be identified on radionuclide renography.[191] Reports of renal resistance index measured by Doppler ultrasonography in 5950 patients indicate that identification of lower resistance was a favorable marker for improvement in both GFR and blood pressure, whereas elevated resistance index was an independent marker of poor outcomes[117] (see Figure 48.19). None of these is absolute, and some studies identify favorable outcomes in some patients with adverse predictors.[177] Some authors suggest that detecting abnormalities in "fractional flow reserve" measured by translesional flows and gradients after dilation with papaverine may predict benefits of revascularization.[142,192] Recent deterioration of kidney function or hypertension portends more likely improvement with revascularization.

SUMMARY

Renovascular disease is common, particularly in older subjects with other atherosclerotic disease. It can produce a wide array of clinical effects, ranging from asymptomatic incidentally discovered disease to accelerated hypertension and progressive renal failure. With improved imaging and older patients, significant renal artery disease is detected more often than ever before. It is incumbent upon the clinician to evaluate both the role of renal artery disease in the individual patient and the potential risk/benefit ratio for renal revascularization. An algorithm to guide treatment and reevaluation of patients with ARAS is presented in Figure 48.28. Application of this strategy relies heavily upon considering comorbid risks and the evolution of both blood pressure control and kidney function over a period of time. Management of cardiovascular risk and hypertension is the primary objective of medical therapy. For most patients the realistic goals of renal revascularization are to reduce medication requirements and to stabilize renal function over time. Patients with bilateral disease or stenosis to a solitary functioning kidney may have lower risk for circulatory congestion (flash pulmonary edema or its equivalent) and lower risk for advancing renal failure after revascularizing the kidney. It is essential to appreciate the risks inherent in either surgical or endovascular manipulation of the diseased aorta. These include a hazard of atheroembolic complications and potential deterioration of renal function related to the procedure itself (estimated at 20% for patients with preexisting kidney dysfunction). Hence the decision to undertake these procedures should include consideration of whether the potential gain warrants such risks. In many cases, improved blood pressure and recovery of renal function justify the costs and hazards completely. Follow-up of both blood pressure and renal function is important,

MANAGEMENT OF RENOVASCULAR HYPERTENSION AND ISCHEMIC NEPHROPATHY

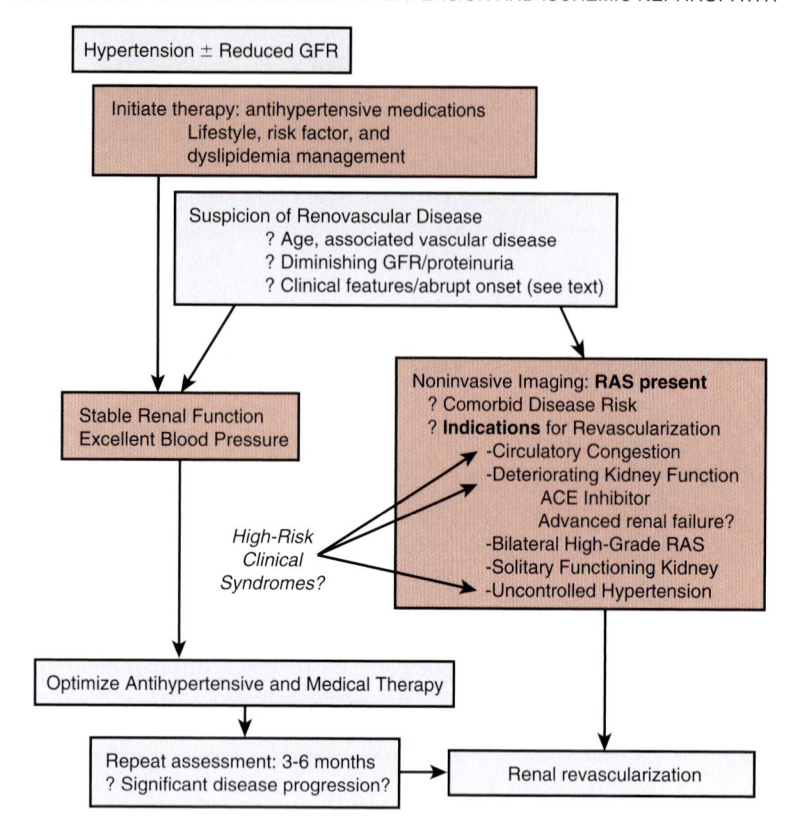

Figure 48.28 Algorithm summarizing a management scheme for patients with renovascular hypertension and/or ischemic nephropathy. Optimizing antihypertensive and medical therapy for comorbid conditions, including dyslipidemia and smoking, is paramount to reducing cardiovascular morbidity and mortality in atherosclerotic disease. Decisions regarding timing of renal revascularization procedures depend both upon the clinical manifestations (see text) and whether blood pressures and kidney function remain stable. *ACE,* Angiotensin-converting enzyme; *GFR,* glomerular filtration rate; *PTRA,* percutaneous transluminal renal angioplasty; *RAS,* renal artery stenosis.

particularly because of the potential for restenosis and/or recurrent disease. Optimal selection and timing for medical management and revascularization depend largely upon the comorbid conditions for each patient.

Complete reference list available at ExpertConsult.com.

KEY REFERENCES

1. The ASTRAL Investigators: Revascularization versus medical therapy for renal-artery stenosis. *N Engl J Med* 361:1953–1962, 2009.
2. Cooper CJ, Murphy TP, Cutlip DE, et al: Stenting and medical therapy for atherosclerotic renal artery stenosis. *N Engl J Med* 370:13–22, 2014.
3. Herrmann SM, Saad A, Textor SC: Management of atherosclerotic renovascular disease after Cardiovascular Outcomes in Renal Atherosclerotic Lesions (CORAL). *Nephrol Dial Transplant* 30:366–375, 2015.
4. Kalra PA, Chrysochou C, Green D, et al: The benefit of renal artery stenting in patients with atheromatous renovascular disease and advanced chronic kidney disease. *Catheter Cardiovasc Interv* 75:1–10, 2010.
5. Ritchie J, Green D, Chrysochou C, et al: High-risk clinical presentations in atherosclerotic renovascular disease: prognosis and response to renal artery revascularization. *Am J Kidney Dis* 63:186–197, 2014.
10. Textor SC, Misra S, Oderich G: Percutaneous revascularization for ischemic nephropathy: the past, present and future. *Kidney Int* 83(1):28–40, 2013.
13. de Mast Q, Beutler JJ: The prevalence of atherosclerotic renal artery stenosis in risk groups: a systematic literature review. *J Hypertens* 27:1333–1340, 2009.
14. De Bruyne B, Manoharan G, Pijls NHJ, et al: Assessment of renal artery stenosis severity by pressure gradient measurements. *J Am Coll Cardiol* 48:1851–1855, 2006.
21. Lerman LO, Nath KA, Rodriguez-Porcel M, et al: Increased oxidative stress in experimental renovascular hypertension. *Hypertension* 37(2 Pt 2):541–546, 2001.
28. Eirin A, Li Z, Xhang X, et al: A mitochondrial permeability transition pore inhibitor improves renal outcomes after revascularization in experimental atherosclerotic renal artery stenosis. *Hypertension* 60:1242–1249, 2012.
29. Kotliar C, Juncos L, Inserra F, et al: Local and systemic cellular immunity in early renal artery atherosclerosis. *Clin J Am Soc Nephrol* 7:224–230, 2012.
30. Textor SC, Glockner JF, Lerman LO, et al: The use of magnetic resonance to evaluate tissue oxygenation in renal artery stenosis. *J Am Soc Nephrol* 19:780–788, 2008.
34. Warner L, Gomez SI, Bolterman R, et al: Regional decrease in renal oxygenation during graded acute renal arterial stenosis: a case for renal ischemia. *Am J Physiol Regul Integr Comp Physiol* 296(1):R67–R71, 2009.
36. Cheng J, Zhou W, Warner GM, et al: Temporal analysis of signaling pathways activated in a murine model of 2-kidney,1-clip hypertension. *Am J Physiol Renal Physiol* 297:F1055–F1068, 2009.
38. Gloviczki ML, Keddis MT, Garovic VD, et al: TGF expression and macrophage accumulation in atherosclerotic renal artery stenosis. *Clin J Am Soc Nephrol* 8(4):546–553, 2013.
44. Chade AR, Zhu X, Lavi R, et al: Endothelial progenitor cells restore renal function in chronic experimental renovascular disease. *Circulation* 119:547–557, 2009.
47. Warner GM, Cheng J, Knudsen BE, et al: Genetic deficiency of Smad3 protects the kidneys from atrophy and interstitial fibrosis in 2K1C hypertension. *Am J Physiol Renal Physiol* 302(11):F1455–F1464, 2012.
54. Slovut DP, Olin JW: Current concepts: fibromuscular dysplasia. *N Engl J Med* 350:1862–1871, 2004.
56. Mounier-Vehier C, Lions C, Jaboureck O, et al: Parenchymal consequences of fibromuscular dysplasia in renal artery stenosis. *Am J Kidney Dis* 40:1138–1145, 2002.
58. Hansen KJ, Edwards MS, Craven TE, et al: Prevalence of renovascular disease in the elderly: a population based study. *J Vasc Surg* 36:443–451, 2002.

62. Edwards MS, Hansen KJ, Craven TE, et al: Associations between renovascular disease and prevalent cardiovascular disease in the elderly: a population-based study. *Vasc Endovascular Surg* 38:25–35, 2004.
65. Iantorno M, Pola R, Schinzari F, et al: Association between altered circadian blood pressure profile and cardiac end-organ damage in patients with renovascular hypertension. *Cardiology* 100:114–119, 2003.
66. Kalra PA, Guo H, Kausz AT, et al: Atherosclerotic renovascular disease in United States patients aged 67 years or older: risk factors, revascularization and prognosis. *Kidney Int* 68:293–301, 2005.
69. Chrysochou C, Foley RN, Young JF, et al: Dispelling the myth: the use of renin-angiotensin blockade in atheromatous renovascular disease. *Nephrol Dial Transplant* 27(4):1403–1409, 2012.
70. Messerli FH, Bangalore S, Makani H, et al: Flash pulmonary oedema and bilateral renal artery stenosis: the Pickering syndrome. *Eur Heart J* 32(18):2231–2237, 2011.
76. Guo H, Kalra PA, Gilbertson DT, et al: Atherosclerotic renovascular disease in older US patients starting dialysis, 1996-2001. *Circulation* 115:50–58, 2007.
78. Textor SC, Lerman LO: Reality and renovascular disease: when does renal artery stenosis warrant revascularization. *Am J Kidney Dis* 63(2):175–177, 2014.
80. Gloviczki ML, Glockner JF, Crane JA, et al: Blood oxygen level-dependent magnetic resonance imaging identifies cortical hypoxia in severe renovascular disease. *Hypertension* 58:1066–1072, 2011.
88. Webster J, Marshall F, Abdalla M, et al: Randomised comparsion of percutaneous angioplasty vs continued medical therapy for hypertensive patients with atheromatous renal artery stenosis. *J Hum Hypertens* 12:329–335, 1998.
92. Caps MT, Perissinotto C, Zierler RE, et al: Prospective study of atherosclerotic disease progression in the renal artery. *Circulation* 98:2866–2872, 1998.
93. van Jaarsveld BC, Krijnen P, Pieterman H, et al: The effect of balloon angioplasty on hypertension in atherosclerotic renal-artery stenosis. *N Engl J Med* 342:1007–1014, 2000.
100. Welch HG, Albertsen PC, Nease RF, et al: Estimating treatment benefits for the elderly: the effect of competing risks. *Ann Intern Med* 124:577–584, 1996.
102. Boudewijn G, Vasbinder C, Nelemans PJ, et al: Diagnostic tests for renal artery stenosis in patients suspected of having renovascular hypertension: a meta-analysis. *Ann Intern Med* 135:401–411, 2001.
103. Safian RD, Textor SC: Medical progress: renal artery stenosis. *N Engl J Med* 344:431–442, 2001.
113. Weinberg I, Jaff MR: Renal artery duplex ultrasonography. In Lerman LO, Textor SC, editors: *Renal vascular disease*, London, 2014, Springer, pp 211–229.
115. Stavros AT, Parker SH, Yakes WF, et al: Segmental stenosis of the renal artery: pattern recognition of tardus and parvus abnormalities with duplex sonography. *Radiology* 184:487–492, 1992.
117. Radermacher J, Chavan A, Bleck J, et al: Use of Doppler ultrasonography to predict the outcome of therapy for renal-artery stenosis. *N Engl J Med* 344:410–417, 2001.
119. Herrmann SMS, Textor SC: Diagnostic criteria for renovascular disease: where are we now? *Nephrol Dial Transplant* 27(7):2657–2663, 2012.
138. Levin A, Linas SL, Luft FC, et al: Controversies in renal artery stenosis: a review by the American Society of Nephrology Advisory Group on Hypertension. *Am J Nephrol* 27:212–220, 2007.
142. Leesar MA, Varma J, Shapria A, et al: Prediction of hypertension improvement after stenting of renal artery stenosis: comparative accuracy of translesional pressure gradients, intravascular ultrasound, and angiography. *J Am Coll Cardiol* 53:2363–2371, 2009.
153. Murphy TP, Soares G, Kim M: Increase in utilization of percutaneous renal artery interventions by Medicare beneficiaries, 1996-2000. *Am J Roentgenol* 183:561–568, 2004.
156. van de Ven PJ, Kaatee R, Beutler JJ, et al: Arterial stenting and balloon angioplasty in ostial atherosclerotic renovascular disease: a randomised trial. *Lancet* 353:282–286, 1999.
167. Bloch MJ, Trost DW, Sos TA: Type B aortic dissection complicating renal artery angioplasty and stent placement. *J Vasc Interv Radiol* 12:517–520, 2001.
172. Watson PS, Hadjipetrou P, Cox SV, et al: Effect of renal artery stenting on renal function and size in patients with atherosclerotic renovascular disease. *Circulation* 102:1671–1677, 2001.
173. Plouin PF, Chatellier G, Darne B, et al: Blood pressure outcome of angioplasty in atherosclerotic renal artery stenosis: a randomized trial. *Hypertension* 31:822–829, 1998.
183. Weibull H, Bergqvist D, Bergentz SE, et al: Percutaneous transluminal renal angioplasty versus surgical reconstruction of atherosclerotic renal artery stenosis: a prospective randomized study. *J Vasc Surg* 18:841–850, 1993.
185. Bower TC, Oderich GS: Surgical revascularization. In Lerman LO, Textor SC, editors: *Renal vascula disease*, London, 2014, Springer, pp 325–340.
187. Modrall JG, Rosero EB, Smith ST, et al: Operative mortality for renal artery bypass in the United States: results from the National Inpatient Sample. *J Vasc Surg* 48:317–322, 2008.

49 Hypertension and Kidney Disease in Pregnancy

Sharon E. Maynard | S. Ananth Karumanchi | Ravi Thadhani

CHAPTER OUTLINE

PHYSIOLOGIC CHANGES OF PREGNANCY, 1610
Hemodynamic and Vascular Changes of Normal Pregnancy, 1610
Renal Adaptation to Pregnancy, 1611
Respiratory Alkalosis of Pregnancy, 1612
Diabetes Insipidus of Pregnancy, 1612
Mechanism of Vasodilation in Pregnancy, 1612
PREECLAMPSIA AND HELLP SYNDROME, 1613
Epidemiology and Risk Factors, 1613
Diagnosis and Clinical Features, 1615
Pathogenesis of Preeclampsia, 1618
Screening for Preeclampsia, 1624
Prevention of Preeclampsia, 1625
Management and Treatment of Preeclampsia, 1626
CHRONIC HYPERTENSION AND GESTATIONAL HYPERTENSION, 1627
Secondary Hypertension in Pregnancy, 1628
Approach to Management of Chronic Hypertension in Pregnancy, 1628
Gestational Hypertension, 1629
Management of Hypertension in Pregnancy, 1629
ACUTE KIDNEY INJURY IN PREGNANCY, 1631
Acute Tubular Necrosis and Bilateral Cortical Necrosis, 1631
Acute Kidney Injury and Thrombotic Microangiopathy, 1632
Obstructive Uropathy and Nephrolithiasis, 1632
Urinary Tract Infection and Acute Pyelonephritis, 1633
CHRONIC KIDNEY DISEASE AND PREGNANCY, 1633
Diabetic Nephropathy and Pregnancy, 1634
Lupus Nephritis and Pregnancy, 1634
Pregnancy During Long-Term Dialysis, 1635
Pregnancy in the Kidney Transplant Recipient, 1636

Pregnancy is characterized by a myriad of physiologic changes, of which the emergence of a placenta and growing fetus are the most dramatic. Hypertension and/or renal disease occurring in the setting of pregnancy presents a unique set of clinical challenges. This chapter includes a detailed discussion of preeclampsia, a syndrome specific to pregnancy that remains one of the most enigmatic human disorders and continues to claim the lives of thousands of mothers and neonates yearly. Other causes of acute renal failure in pregnancy are also discussed. The chapter reviews current data on epidemiology and management issues regarding chronic hypertension, chronic renal disease, and pregnancy in the setting of kidney transplantation as well. Our hope is that this chapter will offer the reader insights into our emerging understanding of the pathogenesis of preeclampsia and provide a sound basis for the management of pregnancy from a nephrologist's perspective.

PHYSIOLOGIC CHANGES OF PREGNANCY

HEMODYNAMIC AND VASCULAR CHANGES OF NORMAL PREGNANCY

Normal pregnancy is characterized by profound vascular and hemodynamic changes that reach far beyond the fetus and placenta (Table 49.1). Early in pregnancy, systemic vascular resistance decreases and arterial compliance increases.[1] These changes are evident by 6 weeks of gestation, prior to the establishment of the uteroplacental circulation.[2] This decrease in systemic vascular resistance leads directly to several other cardiovascular changes. Mean arterial blood pressure falls by an average of 10 mm Hg below nonpregnant levels by the second trimester (Figure 49.1). Sympathetic activity is increased, reflected in a 15% to 20% increase in heart rate.[3] The combination of increased heart rate and

Table 49.1 Physiologic Changes in Pregnancy

Physiologic Variable	Change In Pregnancy
Hemodynamic Parameters	
Plasma volume	Increases 30%-50% above baseline
Blood pressure	Decreases by approximately 10 mm Hg below prepregnancy level, with nadir in second trimester; gradual increase toward prepregnancy levels by term
Cardiac output	Increases 30%-50%
Heart rate	Increases by 15-20 beats/min
Renal blood flow	Increases to 80% above baseline
Glomerular filtration rate	150-200 mL/min (increases to 40%-50% above baseline)
Serum Chemistry and Hematologic Changes	
Hemoglobin	Decreases by an average of 2 g/L (from 13 g/L to 11 g/L) owing to plasma volume expansion out of proportion to the increase in red blood cell mass
Creatinine	Decreases to 0.4-0.5 mg/dL
Uric acid	Decreases to a nadir of 2.0-3.0 mg/dL by 22-24 wk, then increases back to nonpregnant levels toward term
pH	Increases slightly to 7.44
PCO_2	Decreases by approximately 10 mm Hg to an average of 27-32 mm Hg
Calcium	Increased calcitriol stimulates increases both intestinal calcium reabsorption and urinary calcium excretion
Sodium	Decreases by 4-5 mEq/L below nonpregnancy levels
Osmolality	Decreases to a new osmotic set point of approximately 270 mOsm/kg

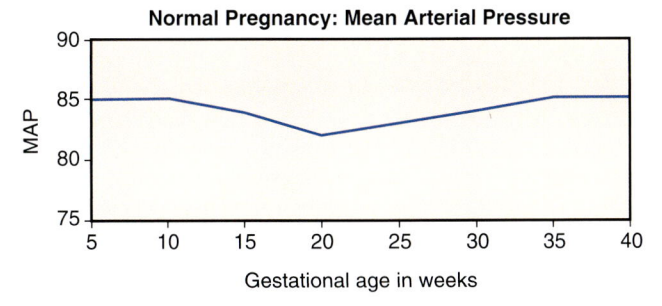

Figure 49.1 Changes in mean arterial pressure in normal pregnancy. Mean arterial blood pressure (MAP) according to gestational age in weeks in a large representative cohort of pregnant women followed longitudinally. (Adapted from Thadhani R, Ecker JL, Kettyle E, et al: Pulse pressure and risk of preeclampsia: a prospective study. *Obstet Gynecol* 97:515-520, 2001.)

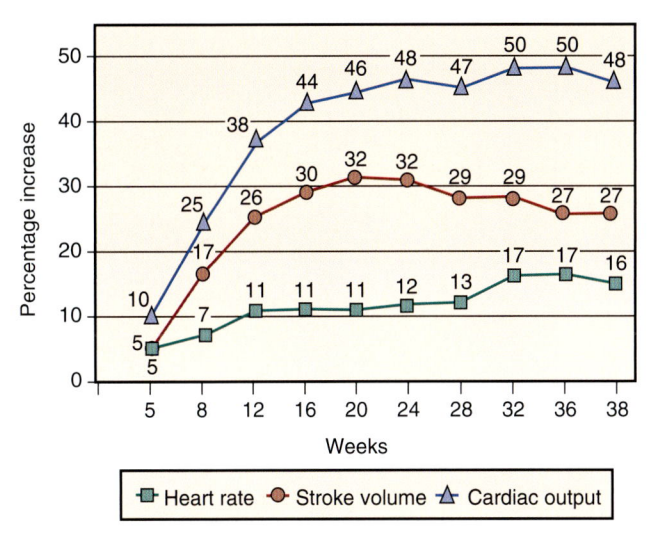

Figure 49.2 Hemodynamic changes in pregnancy. Shown are the percentage changes from prepregnancy values in heart rate, stroke volume, and cardiac output measured throughout pregnancy. (Modified from Robson SC, Hunter S, Boys RJ, et al: Serial study of factors influencing changes in cardiac output during human pregnancy. *Am J Physiol* 256:H1060-H1065, 1989.)

decreased afterload leads to a large increase in cardiac output in the early first trimester, which peaks at 50% above prepregnancy levels by the middle of the third trimester (Figure 49.2).

The renin aldosterone angiotensin system is activated in pregnancy,[4] leading to renal salt and water retention. Increased renal interstitial compliance may also contribute to volume retention via an attenuation of the renal pressure natriuretic response.[5] Total body water increases by 6 to 8 liters, leading to expansion of both plasma volume and interstitial volume. Thus, most women have demonstrable clinical edema at some point during pregnancy. There is also cumulative retention of about 950 mmol of sodium distributed between the maternal extracellular compartments and the fetus.[6] The plasma volume increases out of proportion to the red blood cell mass, leading to mild physiologic anemia.[7] Plasma volume expansion is followed by increased secretion of atrial natriuretic peptide (ANP) late in the first trimester.[2]

RENAL ADAPTATION TO PREGNANCY

In pregnancy, the kidney length increases by 1 to 1.5 cm and kidney volume increases by up to 30%.[8] There is physiologic dilation of the urinary collecting system with hydronephrosis in up to 80% of women, usually more prominent on the right than the left. These changes are likely due to mechanical compression of the ureters between the gravid uterus and the linea terminalis.[9] Estrogen, progesterone, and prostaglandins may also affect ureteral structure and peristalsis. Hydronephrosis of pregnancy is usually asymptomatic, but abdominal pain, and rarely obstruction, can occur (see "Obstructive Uropathy" section).

Glomerular filtration rate (GFR) rises by 40% to 65% as a result of an even larger increase in renal blood flow (RBF) (Figure 49.3).[10] This increase is observed within weeks of conception and is maintained until the middle of the third trimester, when RBF begins to decline toward prepregnancy levels. The increase in GFR results in a physiologic decrease in levels of circulating creatinine, urea, and uric acid. Normal creatinine clearance in pregnancy rises to 150 to 200 mL/min, and average serum creatinine falls from 0.8 mg/dL to approximately 0.5 to 0.6 mg/dL. Hence, a serum creatinine of 1.0 mg/dl, which would be considered

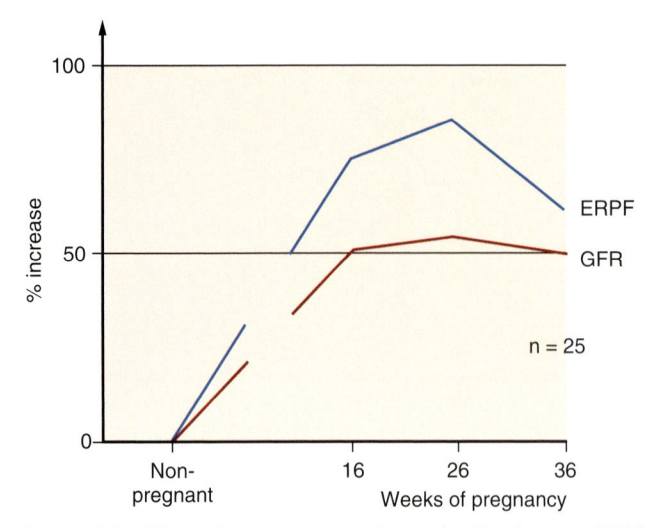

Figure 49.3 Effect of pregnancy on glomerular filtration rate (GFR) and effective renal plasma flow (ERPF). Renal plasma flow rises out of proportion to the GFR, leading to a decrease in filtration fraction. Both GFR and ERPF peak at midgestation, at approximately 50% and 80% above prepregnancy levels, respectively, and decrease slightly toward term. (From Davison JM: Overview: kidney function in pregnant women. *Am J Kidney Dis* 9:248, 1987.)

normal in a nonpregnant individual, reflects renal impairment in a pregnant woman. Similarly, urea (measured as blood urea nitrogen [BUN]) falls from an average of 13 mg/dL in the nonpregnant state to approximately 8 to 10 mg/dl. Although proteinuria is not a feature of normal pregnancy, women with preexisting proteinuric renal disease have an exacerbation of proteinuria in the second and third trimesters that is more exaggerated than that which would be expected from the increased GFR alone[11] (see "Chronic Kidney Disease and Pregnancy" section).

Serum uric acid declines in early pregnancy because of the rise in GFR, reaching a nadir of 2.0 to 3.0 mg/dL by 22 to 24 weeks.[12] Thereafter, the uric acid level begins to rise, reaching nonpregnant levels by term. The late gestational rise in uric acid levels is attributed to increased renal tubular absorption of urate.

Pregnancy is characterized by several changes in renal tubular function. Owing to the large increase in GFR, glomerular tubular balance requires a concomitant increase in tubular solute reabsorption in order to avoid excessive renal losses. The kidney achieves this balance flawlessly, and sodium balance is maintained normally: Pregnant women have normal excretion of an exogenous solute load and appropriately conserve sodium when intake is restricted.[13]

The ability to excrete a water load is also normally maintained, albeit at a lower osmotic set point. The osmotic threshold for stimulation of both antidiuretic hormone (ADH) release and thirst is decreased, by a mechanism that appears to be mediated by human chorionic gonadotropin (hCG)[14] and relaxin.[15] This change results in mild hyponatremia: The serum sodium typically falls by 4 to 5 mmol/L below nonpregnancy levels. Animal studies suggest that increased aquaporin-2 expression in the collecting tubule may contribute to this effect.[16]

Mild glucosuria and aminoaciduria can occur in normal pregnancy. They occur in the absence of hyperglycemia and renal disease. These conditions are thought to be due to a combination of the increased filtered load of glucose and amino acids and less efficient tubular reabsorption.

RESPIRATORY ALKALOSIS OF PREGNANCY

Minute ventilation begins to rise by the end of the first trimester and continues to increase until term. Progesterone mediates this response by directly stimulating respiratory drive and increasing sensitivity of the respiratory center to CO_2.[17] The result is a mild respiratory alkalosis—PCO_2 falls to approximately 27 to 32 mm Hg—and a compensatory increase in renal excretion of bicarbonate. This large increase in minute ventilation allows maintenance of high-normal PO_2 despite the 20% to 33% increase in oxygen consumption in pregnancy.

DIABETES INSIPIDUS OF PREGNANCY

For reasons that are obscure, circulating levels of vasopressinase, an enzyme that hydrolyzes arginine vasopressin, are increased during normal pregnancy. The gene product mediating placental vasopressinase activity has been characterized as a novel placental leucine aminopeptidase.[18] Occasionally, this increase is so pronounced that circulating antidiuretic hormone (arginine vasopressin) disappears, resulting in the polyuria and polydipsia of diabetes insipidus. This syndrome of transient diabetes insipidus manifests during the second trimester and disappears after delivery.[19] It is important to recognize this entity because affected women may become dangerously hypernatremic, especially if they undergo cesarean section using general anesthesia and/or water restriction in the delivery room. The polyuria can be controlled by the administration of desamino-8-D-arginine vasopressin (DDAVP), which is not destroyed by vasopressinase.[20]

MECHANISM OF VASODILATION IN PREGNANCY

The mechanisms mediating the widespread pregnancy-induced decrease in vascular tone are not fully understood. The drop in systemic vascular resistance is only partially attributable to the presence of the low-resistance circulation in the pregnant uterus, as blood pressure and systemic vascular resistance (SVR) are noted to fall before this system is well developed. Reduced vascular responsiveness to vasopressors such as angiotensin II (Ang II), norepinephrine, and vasopressin in pregnancy is well documented (Figure 49.4).[21] The mechanism of this primary systemic vasodilatory response likely reflects effects of several hormones and signaling pathways, including estrogen, progesterone, prostaglandins, and relaxin.

Pregnancy differs fundamentally from other conditions of peripheral vasodilation, such as sepsis, cirrhosis, and high-output congestive heart failure (CHF), all of which are characterized by increased, rather than decreased, renal vascular resistance. This difference suggests that in pregnancy there is a specific renal vasodilating effect that overrides vasoconstricting factors such as renin angiotensin aldosterone activation. A review—mostly of studies of pregnant rats—suggested that the hormone relaxin is central to

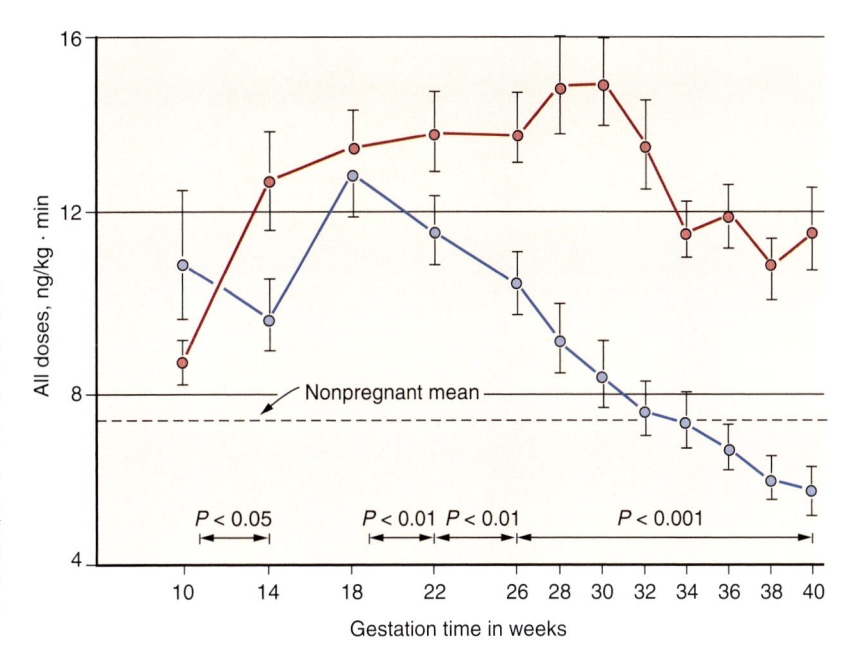

Figure 49.4 Effect of pregnancy on sensitivity to the pressor effects of angiotensin II. The ordinate displays the dose of angiotensin II needed to raise diastolic blood pressure 20 mm Hg. In normal pregnancy (red circles; N = 120), a higher dose was required than for nonpregnant women (dashed line). In women in whom preeclampsia ultimately developed (blue circles; N = 72), insensitivity to angiotensin II was lost beginning in mid–second trimester. (From Gant NF, Daley GL, Chand S, et al: A study of angiotensin II pressor response throughout primigravid pregnancy. *J Clin Invest* 52:2682-2689, 1973, by copyright permission of the American Society for Clinical Investigation.)

this global vasodilatory response, and specifically to the increase in GFR and RBF.[22] Relaxin is a 6-kDa peptide hormone first isolated from pregnant serum in the 1920s and noted to produce relaxation of the pelvic ligaments.[23] Relaxin is released predominantly from the corpus luteum and its level rises early in gestation in response to hCG. Gestational renal hyperfiltration and vasodilation were completely abolished in pregnant rats either administered relaxin-neutralizing antibodies or lacking a functional corpus luteum, suggesting a critical role for relaxin in mediating the renal circulatory changes during pregnancy.[24] Relaxin acts by upregulating endothelin and nitric oxide production in the renal circulation, leading to generalized renal vasodilation, decreased renal afferent and efferent arteriolar resistance, and a subsequent increase in RBF and GFR.[22]

The low-resistance, high-flow circulation of the fetoplacental unit also contributes to the low SVR characteristic of the second and third trimesters of pregnancy. During placental development, the high-resistance uterine arteries are transformed into larger-caliber capacitance vessels (Figure 49.5). This transformation appears to be driven by invasion of the maternal spiral arteries by fetal-derived cytotrophoblasts, which transform from an epithelial to an endothelial phenotype as they replace the endothelium of the maternal spiral arteries.[25] The mechanisms governing this process, termed *pseudovasculogenesis*, are still being elucidated. Angiogenic factors, such as vascular endothelial growth factor (VEGF) and angiopoietins, have a complex spatial and temporal expression in developing placenta, and these factors may be involved in placental vascular development.[26-28] Increased skin capillary density in pregnancy[29] suggests that angiogenic factors may be acting systemically as well as locally in the placenta. Dysregulation of these angiogenic factors may contribute to disorders of placental vasculogenesis, such as preeclampsia (discussed more fully in the "Pathogenesis of Preeclampsia" section).

PREECLAMPSIA AND HELLP SYNDROME

Preeclampsia is systemic syndrome that is specific to pregnancy, characterized by the new onset of hypertension and proteinuria after 20 weeks of gestation. Preeclampsia affects approximately 5% of pregnancies worldwide.[30] Despite many advances in our understanding of the pathophysiology of preeclampsia, delivery of the neonate remains the only definitive treatment. Hence, preeclampsia is still a leading cause of preterm birth and consequent neonatal morbidity and mortality in the developed world as well as the most common cause of maternal death in the United States.[31] In developing countries, where access to safe emergency delivery is less readily available, preeclampsia continues to claim the lives of more than 60,000 mothers every year.[32]

EPIDEMIOLOGY AND RISK FACTORS

The incidence of preeclampsia varies among populations. Most cases of preeclampsia occur in healthy nulliparous women, in whom the incidence of preeclampsia has been reported as high as 7.5%.[33] Although preeclampsia is classically a disorder of first pregnancies, multiparous women who are pregnant with new partners appear to have an elevated preeclampsia risk similar to that of nulliparous women.[34] This effect may be due to longer interpregnancy interval rather than the change in partner per se.[35]

Although most cases of preeclampsia occur in the absence of a family history, the presence of preeclampsia in a first-degree relative increases a woman's risk of severe preeclampsia twofold to fourfold,[36] suggesting a genetic contribution to the disease. Results of several large genome-wide scans seeking a specific linkage to preeclampsia have been fairly discordant and disappointing, with significant LOD (logarithm [base 10] of odds) scores in isolated

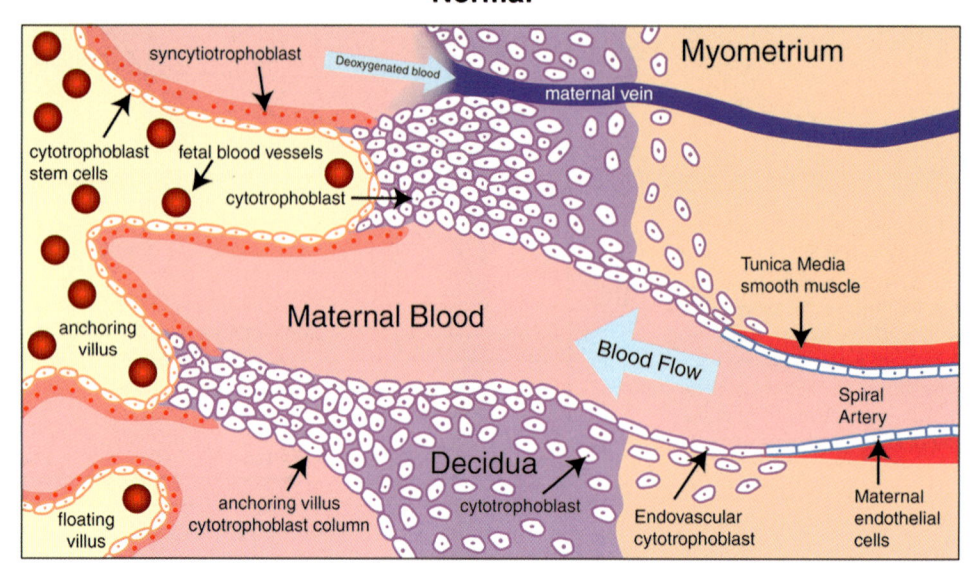

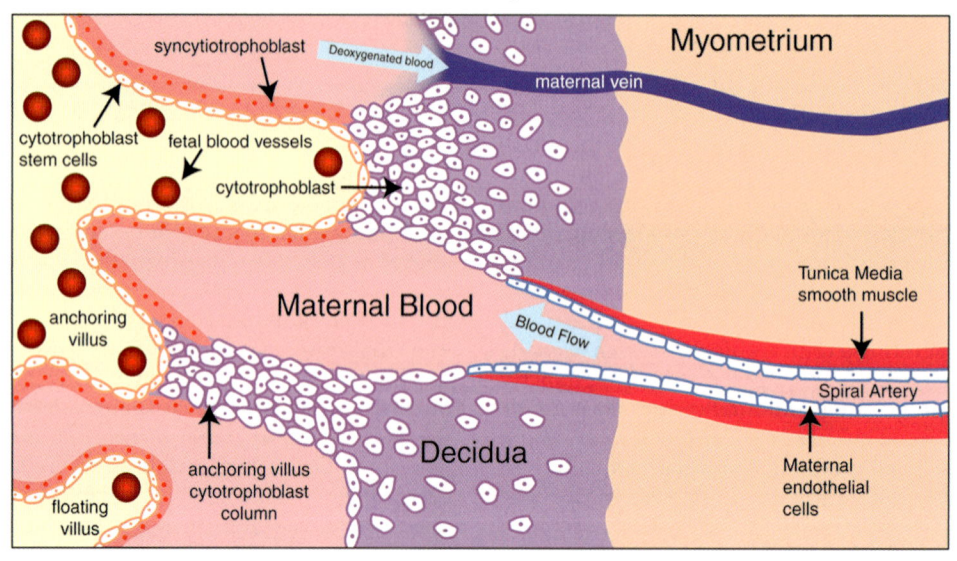

Figure 49.5 Placentation in normal and preeclamptic pregnancies. In normal placental development **(upper panel)**, invasive cytotrophoblasts of fetal origin invade the maternal spiral arteries, transforming them from small-caliber resistance vessels to high-caliber capacitance vessels capable of providing placental perfusion adequate to sustain the growing fetus. During the process of vascular invasion, the cytotrophoblasts differentiate from an epithelial phenotype to an endothelial phenotype, a process referred to as *pseudovasculogenesis* or *vascular mimicry*. In preeclampsia **(lower panel)**, cytotrophoblasts fail to adopt an invasive endothelial phenotype. Instead, invasion of the spiral arteries is shallow, and they remain small-caliber resistance vessels. (From Lam C, Kim KH, Karumanchi SA: Circulating angiogenic factors in the pathogenesis and prediction of preeclampsia. *Hypertension* 46:1077-1085, 2005.)

Finnish (2p25, 9p13)[37] and Icelandic (2p12)[38] populations. Specific genetic mutations consistent with these loci have remained elusive.

Several medical conditions are associated with increased preeclampsia risk, including chronic hypertension, diabetes mellitus, renal disease, obesity, and antiphospholipid antibody syndrome (Table 49.2). Women who had preeclampsia in a prior pregnancy have a high risk of preeclampsia in subsequent pregnancies. Conditions associated with increased placental mass, such as multifetal gestations and hydatidiform mole, are also associated with increased preeclampsia risk. Trisomy 13 is associated with a high risk of preeclampsia.[39] In vitro fertilization has also emerged as an important risk factor for preeclampsia.[40] Although none of these risk factors is fully understood, they have provided insights into the pathogenesis of the disorder.

Several putative risk factors remain controversial. Teen pregnancy has been identified as a risk factor in some studies,[41] but this finding was not confirmed in a meta-analysis and systematic review.[42] Congenital or acquired thrombophilia is associated with preeclampsia in some[43,44] but not all[45,46] studies. Racial differences in the incidence and severity of preeclampsia have been difficult to assess because of confounding socioeconomic and cultural factors.

Table 49.2 Major Risk Factors for Preeclampsia	
Risk Factor	OR or RR (95% CI)
Antiphospholipid antibody syndrome	9.7 (4.3-21.7)[42]
Renal disease	7.8 (2.2-28.2)[398]
Prior preeclampsia	7.2 (5.8-8.8)[42]
Nulliparity	5.4 (2.8-10.3)[48]
Chronic hypertension	3.8 (3.4-4.3)[399]
Diabetes mellitus	3.6 (2.5-5.0)[42]
High altitude	3.6 (1.1-11.9)[400]
Multiple gestations	3.5 (3.0-4.2)[401]
Strong family history of cardiovascular disease (heart disease/stroke in ≥2 first-degree relatives)	3.2 (1.4-7.7)[402]
Systemic lupus erythematosus	3.0 (2.7-3.3)[403]
Obesity	2.5 (1.7-3.7)[404]
Family history of preeclampsia	2.3-2.6 (1.8-3.6)[36]
Advanced maternal age (>40 yr)	1.68 (1.23-2.29) nulliparas 1.96 (1.34-2.87) multiparas[41,42]
Excessive gestational weight gain (>35 lb)	1.88 (1.74-2.04)[251,405]
In vitro fertilization	1.78 (1.05-3.06)[40]

CI, Confidence interval; OR, odds ratio; RR, relative risk.
Superscript numbers indicate chapter references.

Table 49.3 Diagnostic Criteria for Preeclampsia	
Diagnostic Criteria for Preeclampsia	
Hypertension	≥140 mm Hg systolic or ≥ 90 mm Hg diastolic after 20 weeks of gestation on two occasions at least 4 hours apart in a woman with a previously normal blood pressure OR With blood pressures ≥ 160 mm Hg systolic or ≥ 105 mm Hg diastolic, hypertension can be confirmed within a short interval (minutes) to facilitate timely antihypertensive therapy
AND	
Proteinuria	≥ 300 mg/24 hr (or this amount extrapolated from a timed collection) OR Protein-to-creatinine ratio ≥ 0.3 mg protein/mg creatinine OR Dipstick 1+ (used only if other quantitative methods not available)
OR in the absence of proteinuria, new-onset hypertension with the new onset of any of the following:	
Thrombocytopenia	≤100,000 platelets/mL
Renal insufficiency	Serum creatinine concentrations > 1.1 mg/dL or a doubling of the serum creatinine concentration in the absence of other renal disease
Impaired liver function	Elevated blood concentrations of liver transaminases to twice normal
Pulmonary edema	
Cerebral or visual symptoms	
Diagnostic Criteria for Superimposed Preeclampsia	
Hypertension	A sudden increase in blood pressure in a woman with chronic hypertension that was previously well controlled or escalation of antihypertensive medications to control blood pressure
OR	
Proteinuria	New onset of proteinuria in a woman with chronic hypertension or a sudden increase in proteinuria in a woman with known proteinuria before or in early pregnancy

Adapted from American College of Obstetricians and Gynecologists; Task Force on Hypertension in Pregnancy: Hypertension in pregnancy. Report of the American College of Obstetricians and Gynecologists' Task Force on Hypertension in Pregnancy. Obstet Gynecol 122:1122-1131, 2013.

Although population-based studies have reported a higher rate of preeclampsia among black women,[47,48] these findings have not been confirmed in studies confined to healthy, nulliparous women.[49,50] This situation suggests that the increased preeclampsia incidence noted in some studies may be attributable to the higher rate of chronic hypertension in African Americans, because chronic hypertension is itself a strong risk factor for preeclampsia (see Table 49.2).[51] Black women with preeclampsia also have a higher case-mortality rate,[52] which may be due to more severe disease or to deficiencies in prenatal care. In Hispanic women, the incidence of preeclampsia appears to be increased, with a concomitant decrease in risk for gestational hypertension.[53]

The possibility that infectious agents contribute to preeclampsia risk has continued to have sporadic support. A systematic review and meta-analysis of 49 studies reported small but significant associations between preeclampsia and urinary tract infections (odds ratio [OR], 1.57) and periodontal disease (OR, 1.76), but no association with other infections, including human immunodeficiency virus (HIV), cytomegalovirus, *Chlamydia*, and malaria.[54]

DIAGNOSIS AND CLINICAL FEATURES

The American College of Obstetrics and Gynecologists' Task Force on Hypertension in Pregnancy published updated criteria for the diagnosis of preeclampsia in 2013 that is summarized in Table 49.3.[55] These guidelines help distinguish preeclampsia from other hypertensive disorders of pregnancy, such as chronic and gestational hypertension. The diagnosis of preeclampsia in women with chronic hypertension and/or underlying proteinuric renal disease on clinical criteria alone remains challenging.

HYPERTENSION

For the diagnosis of preeclampsia, *hypertension* is defined as a systolic blood pressure of 140 mm Hg or higher or a diastolic blood pressure of 90 mm Hg or higher after 20 weeks of gestation in a woman with previously normal blood pressure.[55] Hypertension should be confirmed by two separate measurements made at least 4 hours apart. The severity of hypertension in preeclampsia can vary widely, from mild blood pressure elevations easily managed with antihypertensive medication to severe hypertension associated with headache and visual changes resistant to multiple medications. The latter situation can often herald seizures (eclampsia) and is an indication for urgent delivery. Medical management of hypertension in preeclampsia is discussed in the next section.

PROTEINURIA

Proteinuria is a hallmark of preeclampsia. For a diagnosis of preeclampsia, proteinuria greater than 300 mg protein in a 24-hour urine collection or a urine protein-to-creatinine (P:C) ratio higher than 0.3 is sufficient. However, preeclampsia can be diagnosed even in the absence of proteinuria if a patient presents with evidence of thrombocytopenia or elevated liver enzymes in the setting of hypertension (see Table 49.3). Routine obstetric care includes dipstick protein testing of a random voided urine sample at each prenatal visit—a screening method that has been shown to have a high rate of false-positive and false-negative results in comparison with 24-hour urine protein measurement.[56] However, the 24-hour urine collection for proteinuria is cumbersome for the patient and often inaccurate because of undercollection,[57] and results are not available for at least 24 hours, while the collection is being completed. The urinary P:C ratio has become the preferred method for quantification of proteinuria in the nonpregnant population. A meta-analysis showed a pooled sensitivity of 84% and specificity of 76% using a P:C ratio cutoff value of greater than 0.3, in comparison with the gold standard of 24-hour urine protein excretion greater than 300 mg/day.[58] Hence, it is reasonable to use the urine P:C ratio for the diagnosis of preeclampsia, with 24-hour collection undertaken when the ratio result is equivocal.

The degree of proteinuria in preeclampsia can range widely, from minimal to nephrotic range. However, the degree of proteinuria is a poor predictor of adverse maternal and fetal outcomes,[59] so heavy proteinuria alone is not an indication for urgent delivery. New-onset proteinuria is particularly useful among women with chronic hypertension to diagnose superimposed preeclampsia (see Table 49.3). However, among women with underlying proteinuria, other signs of preeclampsia, such as elevated transaminases, thrombocytopenia, and cerebral signs and symptoms, are more useful to diagnose superimposed preeclampsia.[55]

EDEMA

Although edema was historically part of the diagnostic triad for preeclampsia, it is also recognized to be a feature of normal pregnancy, diminishing its usefulness as a specific pathologic sign. Still, the sudden onset of severe edema, especially in the hands and face, can be an important presenting symptom in this otherwise insidious disease and should prompt evaluation.

URIC ACID

Serum uric acid is elevated in most women with preeclampsia primarily as a result of enhanced tubular urate reabsorption. It has been suggested that hyperuricemia may contribute to the pathogenesis of preeclampsia by inducing endothelial dysfunction[60] or by impairing trophoblast invasiveness, a key element in placental vascular remodeling.[61] Serum uric acid levels are correlated with the presence and severity of preeclampsia and with adverse pregnancy outcomes,[62] even in gestational hypertension without proteinuria.[63] Unfortunately, uric acid measurement is of limited clinical utility either in distinguishing preeclampsia from other hypertensive disorders of pregnancy or as a clinical predictor of adverse outcomes.[64-66] One clinical scenario in which serum uric acid measurement may be useful is in the diagnosis of preeclampsia in women with chronic kidney disease, in whom the usual diagnostic criteria of new-onset hypertension and proteinuria are often impossible to apply. In such patients, a serum uric acid level greater than 5.5 mg/dL in the presence of stable renal function might suggest superimposed preeclampsia.

CLINICAL FEATURES OF SEVERE PREECLAMPSIA

Several clinical and laboratory findings suggest severe or progressive disease and should prompt consideration of immediate delivery.[55] Oliguria (<500 mL urine in 24 hours) is usually transient; acute kidney injury, though uncommon, can occur. Persistent headache or visual disturbances can be a prodrome to seizures. Pulmonary edema complicates 2% to 3% of severe preeclampsia[34] and can lead to respiratory failure. Epigastric or right upper quadrant pain may be associated with liver injury. Elevated liver enzymes and thrombocytopenia can occur alone or as part of the HELLP (hemolytic anemia, elevated liver enzymes, and low platelets) syndrome (see later).

ECLAMPSIA

Seizures complicate approximately 2% of cases of preeclampsia in the United States.[67] Although eclampsia most often occurs in the setting of hypertension and proteinuria, it can occur without these warning signs. Up to a third of eclampsia cases occur postpartum, sometimes days to weeks after delivery.[68] Late postpartum preeclampsia in particular is often a difficult and potentially missed diagnosis, often seen by non-obstetricians in the emergency department. Radiologic imaging of the head using computed tomography (CT) or magnetic resonance imaging (MRI) is usually not indicated when the diagnosis is apparent but typically shows vasogenic edema, predominantly in the subcortical white matter of the parieto-occipital lobes (see Pathogenesis of preeclampsia: Cerebral changes). Women who have had eclampsia may have subtle long-term impairment of cognitive function.[69]

HELLP SYNDROME

There remains considerable confusion and variability regarding the precise diagnostic criteria for the HELLP syndrome in the medical literature (Table 49.4). The HELLP syndrome is generally considered to be a severe variant of preeclampsia, although it can occur in the absence of proteinuria. The HELLP syndrome is associated with higher rates of maternal and neonatal adverse outcomes than preeclampsia alone, including eclampsia (affecting 6% of cases), placental abruption (10%), acute renal failure (5%), disseminated intravascular coagulation (8%), pulmonary edema (10%),[70] and (rarely) hepatic hemorrhage and rupture.[71]

Table 49.4 Comparison of Clinical and Laboratory Characteristics, Effect on Delivery, and Management of HELLP, HUS/TTP, and AFLP

	HUS/TTP	HELLP	AFLP
Clinical characteristic:			
Hemolytic anemia	+++	++	±
Thrombocytopenia	+++	++	±
Coagulopathy	−	±	+
CNS symptoms	++	±	±
Renal failure	+++	+	++
Hypertension	±	+++	±
Proteinuria	±	++	±
Elevated AST	±	++	+++
Elevated bilirubin	++	+	+++
Anemia	++	+	±
Ammonia	Normal	Normal	High
Effect of delivery on disease	None	Recovery	Recovery
Management	Plasma exchange	Supportive care, delivery	Supportive care, delivery

AFLP, Acute fatty liver of pregnancy; AST, aspartate aminotransferase; CNS, central nervous system; HELLP, hemolytic anemia, elevated liver enzymes, and low platelets; HUS/TTP, hemolytic-uremic syndrome/thrombotic thrombocytopenic purpura; − absent; ± present or absent; + mild; ++ moderate; +++ severe.

Data derived from Allford SL, Hunt BJ, Rose P, et al: Guidelines on the diagnosis and management of the thrombotic microangiopathic haemolytic anaemias. Br J Haematol 120:556-573, 2003; Egerman RS, Sibai BM: Imitators of preeclampsia and eclampsia. Clin Obstet Gynecol 42:551-562, 1999; Stella CL, Dacus J, Guzman E, et al: The diagnostic dilemma of thrombotic thrombocytopenic purpura/hemolytic uremic syndrome in the obstetric triage and emergency department: lessons from 4 tertiary hospitals. Am J Obstet Gynecol 200:381-386, 2009.

MATERNAL AND NEONATAL MORTALITY

Approximately 500,000 women die in childbirth each year worldwide,[72] and preeclampsia and eclampsia are estimated to account for 10% to 15% of these deaths.[73] In the United States, the rate of severe preeclampsia has been rising since the 1980s,[41] and preeclampsia and eclampsia account for 16% to 20% of all pregnancy-related maternal mortality.[31,52] Maternal death is most often due to eclampsia, cerebral hemorrhage, renal failure, hepatic failure, pulmonary edema, and the HELLP syndrome. Most preventable errors in preeclampsia management leading to maternal death involve inattention to blood pressure control and signs of pulmonary edema.[31] Risk of death in preeclampsia is increased for women with little or no prenatal care, those of black race, those older than 35 years, and those with early-onset preeclampsia.[52] Adverse maternal outcomes can often be avoided with timely delivery; hence in the developed world the burden of morbidity and mortality falls on the neonate.

Worldwide, preeclampsia is associated with a perinatal and neonatal mortality rate of 10%[74]; as with maternal mortality, the risk of neonatal mortality increases substantially for preeclampsia presenting earlier in gestation. Neonatal death is most commonly due to iatrogenic premature delivery undertaken to preserve the health of the mother. In addition, fetal growth restriction can occur, likely as a result of impaired uteroplacental blood flow or placental infarction. Oligohydramnios and placental abruption are less common complications.

POSTPARTUM RECOVERY

Generally, preeclampsia begins to remit soon after delivery of the fetus and placenta, and complete recovery is the rule. However, normalization of blood pressure and proteinuria often takes days to weeks.[75] Postpartum monitoring is important because, as discussed, eclampsia can occur after delivery.

LONG-TERM CARDIOVASCULAR AND RENAL OUTCOMES

Previously, women with preeclampsia were reassured that the syndrome remits completely after delivery, with no long-term consequences aside from increased preeclampsia risk in future pregnancies. Epidemiologic studies have refuted this claim.[76,77] Fifty percent of women with preeclampsia experience hypertension later in life. As early as 1 year after the affected pregnancy, women with preeclampsia have a dramatically (OR, 13.9) higher risk of hypertension than control women who have not had preeclampsia[78] and the risk of new-onset diabetes mellitus is doubled.[79] Relative risks for subsequent ischemic heart disease, stroke, and cardiovascular death are more than doubled in women who have had preeclampsia (Figure 49.6).[76,77] Women who have had preeclampsia have alterations in physical and biochemical markers of cardiovascular risk (obesity, hypercholesterolemia, hypertension, microalbuminuria) 1 year after their affected pregnancies.[80] In particular, severe preeclampsia, recurrent preeclampsia, preeclampsia with preterm birth, and preeclampsia with intrauterine growth restriction are most strongly associated with adverse cardiovascular outcomes. The American Heart Association guidelines include a history of preeclampsia as a risk factor for cardiovascular disease in women.[81]

Preeclampsia, especially in association with low neonatal birth weight, also carries an increased risk of later maternal kidney disease requiring a kidney biopsy.[82] A large Norwegian study using birth and renal registry data on more than 570,000 women showed that preeclampsia increases the risk

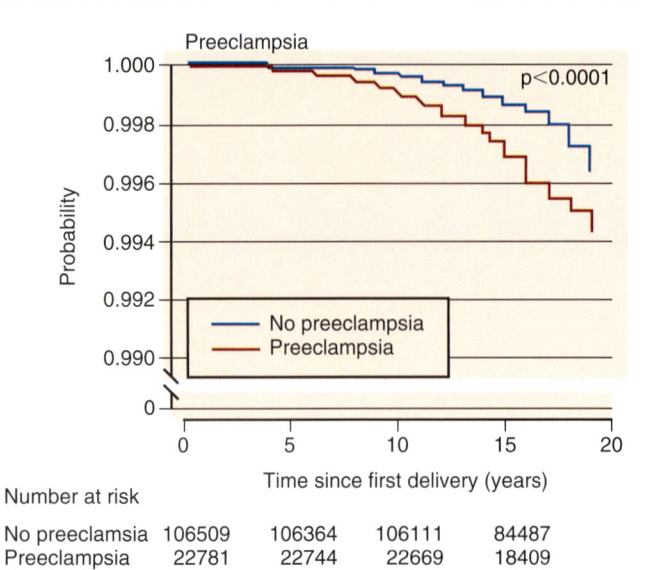

Figure 49.6 Preeclampsia increases the risk for cardiovascular disease later in life. Kaplan-Meier plot of the cumulative probability of survival without admission to the hospital for ischemic heart disease or death from ischemic heart disease in women with and without a history of preeclampsia. (From Smith GC, Pell JP, Walsh D: Pregnancy complications and maternal risk of ischaemic heart disease: a retrospective cohort study of 129,290 births. *Lancet* 357:2002-2006, 2001.)

of subsequent end-stage kidney disease (ESKD) by almost fivefold.[83] A later study suggested that familial aggregation of risk factors does not seem to explain increased ESKD risk after preeclampsia.[84] Although it appears that preeclampsia is associated with increased risk of subsequent ESKD, the absolute risk is low.

Preeclampsia and cardiovascular disease share many risk factors, such as chronic hypertension, diabetes, obesity, renal disease, and the metabolic syndrome. Still, the increase in long-term cardiovascular mortality holds even for women in whom preeclampsia develops in the absence of any overt vascular risk factors. Whether these observations result from vascular damage or persistent endothelial dysfunction caused by preeclampsia, or simply reflect the common risk factors for preeclampsia and cardiovascular disease, remains speculative. Regardless of etiology, it is recommended that women who experience preeclampsia, especially with preterm birth or intrauterine growth restriction, receive screening for potentially modifiable cardiovascular and kidney disease risk factors (hypertension, diabetes mellitus, hyperlipidemia, obesity) at the postpartum obstetrician visit and yearly thereafter.[55,85]

Epidemiologic evidence suggests that low birth weight (with or without preeclampsia) is associated with the development of hypertension, diabetes, cardiovascular disease, and chronic kidney disease in the offspring of affected pregnancies.[86] It has been hypothesized that this association may be due to low nephron number.

PATHOGENESIS OF PREECLAMPSIA

THE ROLE OF THE PLACENTA

Observational evidence suggests the placenta has a central role in preeclampsia. Preeclampsia occurs only in the presence of a placenta—though not necessarily a fetus, as in the case of hydatidiform mole—and almost always remits after its delivery. In a case of preeclampsia with extrauterine pregnancy, removal of the fetus alone was not sufficient; symptoms persisted until the placenta was delivered.[87] Severe preeclampsia is associated with pathologic evidence of placental hypoperfusion and ischemia. Findings include acute atherosis, a lesion of diffuse vascular obstruction that includes fibrin deposition, intimal thickening, necrosis, atherosclerosis, and endothelial damage.[88] Infarcts, likely due to occlusion of maternal spiral arteries, are also common. Although these findings are not universal, they appear to be correlated with severity of clinical disease.[89]

Several clinical and laboratory observations strongly support the role of placental ischemia in the pathophysiology of preeclampsia. Abnormal uterine artery Doppler ultrasound findings, consistent with decreased uteroplacental perfusion, are observed before the clinical onset of preeclampsia.[90] The incidence of preeclampsia is increased twofold to fourfold in women residing at high altitude, implying that hypoxia may be a contributing factor.[91] Indeed, global gene expression profiles are similar for hypoxia-treated placental explants, high-altitude placentas, and placentas from preeclamptic pregnancies.[92] Pregnant subjects with sickle cell disease, who often have pathologic evidence of placental ischemia and infarction, have an increased risk for preeclampsia.[93-95] Hypertension and proteinuria can be induced by constriction of uterine blood flow in pregnant primates and other mammals.[96] These observations suggest that placental ischemia may be an important trigger for the maternal syndrome.

However, evidence for a causative role for placental ischemia alone remains circumstantial, and several observations call the hypothesis into question. For example, the animal models based on uterine hypoperfusion fail to induce several of the multiorgan features of preeclampsia, including seizures, elevated liver enzyme values, and thrombocytopenia. In most cases of preeclampsia, there is no evidence of growth restriction or fetal intolerance of labor, both of which are expected consequences of placental ischemia. It may be that the placental ischemic damage that accompanies late-stage preeclampsia is a secondary event.

PLACENTAL VASCULAR REMODELING

Early in normal placental development, extravillous cytotrophoblasts invade the uterine spiral arteries of the decidua and myometrium (see Figure 49.5). These invasive fetal cells replace the endothelial layer of the uterine vessels, transforming them from small-caliber resistance vessels to flaccid, high-caliber capacitance vessels.[97] This vascular transformation, which is most dramatic in the myometrial vessels, allows the increase in uterine blood flow needed to sustain the fetus through the pregnancy.[98] In preeclampsia, this transformation is incomplete.[99] Cytotrophoblast invasion of the arteries is limited to the superficial decidua, and the myometrial segments remain narrow and undilated.[100] Zhou and colleagues have shown that in normal placental development, invasive cytotrophoblasts downregulate the expression of adhesion molecules characteristic of their epithelial cell origin and adopt an endothelial cell-surface adhesion phenotype (pseudovasculogenesis).[101] In preeclampsia, cytotrophoblasts do not undergo this switching of cell-surface integrins and adhesion molecules and fail to adequately invade the myometrial spiral arteries.

The factors that regulate this process are just beginning to be elucidated. Hypoxia-inducible factor-1 (HIF-1) activity is increased in preeclampsia, and HIF-1 target genes such as transforming growth factor-β_3 may block cytotrophoblast invasion.[102] Invasive cytotrophoblasts express several angiogenic factors and receptors, also regulated by HIF, including vascular endothelial growth factor (VEGF), placental growth factor (PlGF), and vascular endothelial growth factor receptor 1 (VEGFR-1 or soluble fms-like tyrosine kinase-1 [sFlt1]); expression of these proteins by immunolocalization is altered in preeclampsia.[103] A genetic study identified polymorphisms in STOX1, a paternally imprinted gene and member of the winged helix gene family, in a Dutch preeclampsia cohort.[104] The investigators hypothesized that loss-of-function mutations in this gene could result in defective polyploidization of extravillous trophoblast, leading to loss of cytotrophoblast invasion. However, a subsequent cohort study failed to confirm an association between preeclampsia and STOX polymorphisms.[105] More work is needed to uncover the molecular signals governing cytotrophoblast invasion early in placentation, defects in which may underlie the early stages of preeclampsia.

MATERNAL ENDOTHELIAL DYSFUNCTION

Although the origins of the preeclampsia syndrome appear to be placental, the target organ is the maternal endothelium. The clinical manifestations of preeclampsia reflect widespread endothelial dysfunction resulting in vasoconstriction and end-organ ischemia.[106,107] Incubation of endothelial cells with serum from women with preeclampsia results in endothelial dysfunction; hence, it has been hypothesized that factors present in maternal syndrome, likely originating in the placenta, are responsible for the manifestations of the disease (Figure 49.7).

Dozens of serum markers of endothelial activation are deranged in women with preeclampsia, including von Willebrand antigen, cellular fibronectin, soluble tissue factor, soluble E-selectin, platelet-derived growth factor, and endothelin.[107] C-reactive protein[108] and leptin[109] are increased early in gestation. There is evidence for oxidative stress and platelet activation.[110] Decreased production of prostaglandin I_2, an endothelium-derived prostaglandin, occurs well before the onset of clinical symptoms.[111] Inflammation is often present; for example, there is neutrophil infiltration in the vascular smooth muscle of subcutaneous fat, with increased vascular smooth muscle expression of interleukin-8 and intercellular adhesion molecule-1.[112] Several of these aberrations occur well before the onset of symptoms, supporting the central role of endothelial dysfunction in the pathogenesis of preeclampsia.

HEMODYNAMIC CHANGES

The decreases in peripheral vascular resistance and arterial blood pressure that occur during normal pregnancy are absent or reversed in preeclampsia. Systemic vascular resistance is higher and cardiac output is lower than in normal pregnancies.[113] These changes are due to widespread vasoconstriction resulting from endothelial dysfunction. This hypothesis is supported by both in vivo and in vitro evidence. Women with preeclampsia have impaired endothelium-dependent vasorelaxation, which has been noted prospectively prior to the onset of hypertension and proteinuria[114] and persists for years after the preeclampsia episode.[115] There is exaggerated sensitivity to vasopressors such as Ang II and norepinephrine (see Figure 49.4).[107] Subtle increases in blood pressure and pulse pressure are present prior to the onset of overt hypertension and proteinuria, suggesting that arterial compliance is decreased early in the course of the disease.[42,116] Mechanisms underlying endothelial dysfunction are discussed in the next section.

RENAL CHANGES

The pathologic swelling of glomerular endothelial cells in preeclampsia was first described in 1924.[117] Thirty years later, Spargo and associates coined the term "glomerular endotheliosis" and characterized the ultrastructural changes, including generalized swelling and vacuolization of the endothelial cells and loss of the capillary space (Figure 49.8).[118] There are deposits of fibrinogen and fibrin within and under the endothelial cells, and electron microscopy shows loss of glomerular endothelial fenestrae.[119] The primary injury is specific to endothelial cells: The podocyte foot processes are intact early in disease, a finding atypical of other nephrotic diseases. However, podocyte injury as evidenced by podocyturia has been observed in preeclampsia.[120] Changes in the afferent arteriole, including atrophy of the macula densa and hyperplasia of the juxtaglomerular apparatus, have also been described.[121] Although mild glomerular endotheliosis was once considered pathognomonic for preeclampsia, later studies have shown that it also occurs in pregnancy without preeclampsia, especially in gestational hypertension.[122] This finding suggests the endothelial dysfunction of preeclampsia may in fact be an exaggeration of a process present toward term in all pregnancies.

Both RBF and GFR are lower in preeclampsia than in normal pregnancy. RBF falls as a result of high renal vascular resistance, primarily due to increased afferent arteriolar resistance. GFR decreases as a result of both the fall in RBF and a decrease in the ultrafiltration coefficient (Kf), which is attributed to endotheliosis in the glomerular capillary.[123] Although acute kidney injury can occur in preeclampsia, proteinuria (with a bland urinary sediment) and renal sodium and water retention are typically the only renal manifestations of disease.

CEREBRAL CHANGES

Cerebral edema and intracerebral parenchymal hemorrhage are common autopsy findings in women who die from eclampsia. The presence of cerebral edema in eclampsia correlates with markers of endothelial damage but not the severity of hypertension,[124] suggesting that the edema is secondary to endothelial dysfunction rather than a direct result of blood pressure elevation. Findings on head CT and MRI are similar to those seen in hypertensive encephalopathy, with vasogenic cerebral edema and infarctions in the subcortical white matter and adjacent gray matter, predominantly in the parieto-occipital lobes.[68] A syndrome that includes these characteristic MRI changes, together with headache, seizures, altered mental status, and hypertension, has been described in patients with acute hypertensive encephalopathy in the setting of renal disease, eclampsia, or immunosuppression.[125] This syndrome, termed *reversible*

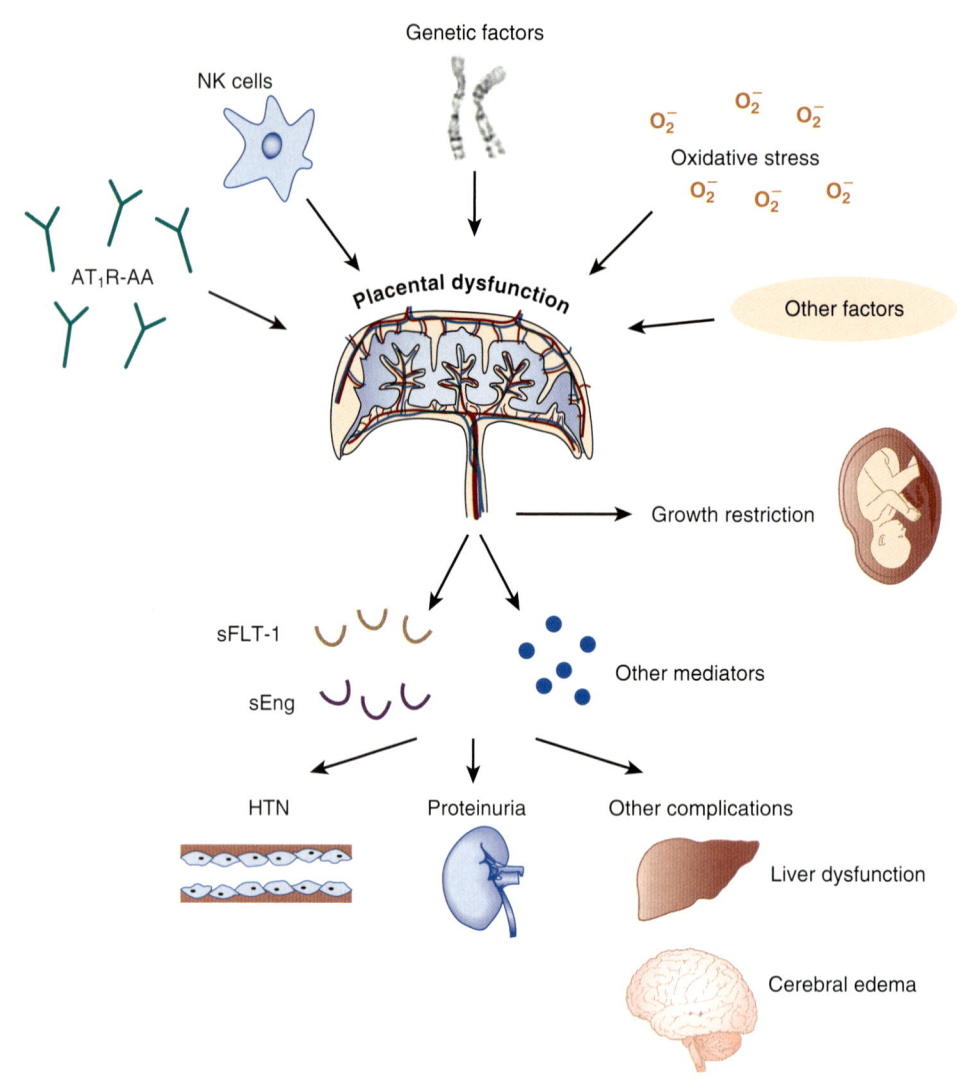

Figure 49.7 Placental dysfunction and endothelial dysfunction in the pathogenesis of preeclampsia. Placental dysfunction triggered by genetic, immunologic (natural killer [NK] cells and angiotensin receptor autoantibodies [AT₁R-AAs]), and other factors (altered heme oxygenase expression, oxidative stress) plays an early and primary role in the pathogenesis of preeclampsia. The diseased placenta in turn secretes anti-angiogenic factors (soluble fms-like tyrosine kinase-1 [sFlt-1], soluble endoglin [sEng]) and other toxic mediators into the systemic circulation, causing maternal endothelial dysfunction. Nearly all the manifestations of preeclampsia, including hypertension, proteinuria (glomerular endotheliosis), seizures (cerebral edema), and HELLP (hemolysis, elevated liver enzymes, and low platelets) syndrome, can be attributable to vascular endothelial damage secondary to excess circulating anti-angiogenic factors. (Adapted from Powe CE, Levine RJ, Karumanchi SA: Preeclampsia, a disease of the maternal endothelium: the role of antiangiogenic factors and implications for later cardiovascular disease. *Circulation* 123:2856-2869, 2011).

posterior leukoencephalopathy, has subsequently been associated with the use of calcineurin inhibitors or anti-angiogenic agents for cancer therapy.[126] This latter observation supports the possible role for innate anti-angiogenic factors in the pathophysiology of preeclampsia/eclampsia, as detailed later in this section.

OXIDATIVE STRESS AND INFLAMMATION

Oxidative stress, the presence of reactive oxygen species in excess of antioxidant buffering capacity, is a prominent feature of preeclampsia. Oxidative stress is known to damage proteins, cell membranes, and DNA and is a potential mediator of endothelial dysfunction. It has been hypothesized that in preeclampsia, placental oxidative stress is transferred to the systemic circulation, resulting in oxidative damage to the maternal vascular endothelium.[110] However, the absence of any clinical benefit of antioxidant supplementation in the prevention of preeclampsia suggests that oxidative stress is likely to be a secondary phenomenon in preeclampsia and not a promising therapeutic target.[127] Circulating placental cytotrophoblast debris with the accompanying inflammation has also been proposed as a pathogenic mechanism to explain the maternal endothelial dysfunction, but causal evidence for this hypothesis is still lacking.[128]

IMMUNOLOGIC INTOLERANCE

The possibility of immune maladaptation remains an intriguing but unproven theory of the pathogenesis of preeclampsia. Normal placentation requires the development of immune tolerance between the fetus and the mother. The fact that preeclampsia occurs more often in first pregnancies or after a change in partners suggests an etiologic

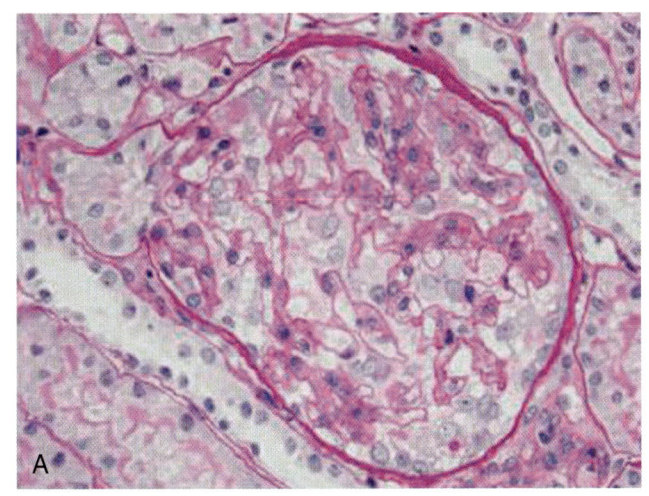

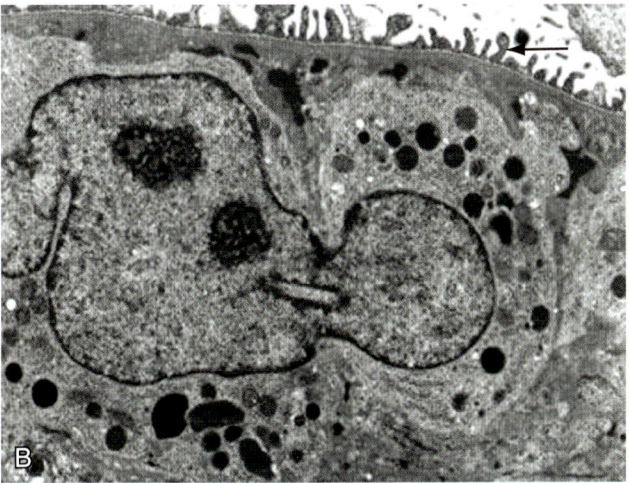

Figure 49.8 Glomerular endotheliosis. **A,** Human preeclamptic glomerulus on light microscopy (periodic acid–Schiff [PAS] stain). Renal biopsy findings from a 29-year-old woman with twin gestation and severe preeclampsia are shown. Patient's blood pressure was 170/112 mm Hg, and random urine protein-to-creatinine ratio was 9.8. Note the "bloodless" appearance of the glomeruli and absence of the capillary lumen. (Original magnification, ×40.) **B,** Electron microscopy of biopsy specimen of the glomerulus from the same patient. Note occlusion of capillary lumen cytoplasm and expansion of the subendothelial space with some electron-dense material. Podocyte cytoplasm shows protein resorption droplets and relatively intact foot processes. (Original magnification, ×1500.) (Courtesy IE Stillman.)

role for abnormal maternal immune response to paternally derived fetal antigens. This response could result in failure of fetal cells to successfully invade the maternal vessels during placental vascular development.

Observational studies suggest that preeclampsia risk increases in cases of exposure to novel paternal antigens, not only in first pregnancies but also in pregnancies with new partners[129] and with long interpregnancy interval.[35] Women using contraceptive methods that reduce exposure to sperm have higher preeclampsia incidence.[130] Women impregnated by intracytoplasmic sperm injection (ICSI) with sperm that were surgically obtained (i.e., the woman was never exposed to the partner's sperm in intercourse) had a threefold higher risk of preeclampsia than women undergoing ICSI with sperm that were obtained by ejaculation.[131] Conversely, prior exposure to paternal antigens appears to be protective. The risk of preeclampsia is inversely proportional to the length of cohabitation,[132] and oral tolerance to paternal antigens through oral sex and swallowing is associated with decreased risk.[133] None of these clinical observations has yet provided insights into immunologic triggers of or pathogenic links to the paternal syndrome.

On a molecular level, HLA-G expression appears to be abnormal in preeclampsia. HLA-G is normally expressed by invasive extravillous cytotrophoblasts and may play a role in inducing immune tolerance at the maternal-fetal interface. In preeclampsia, HLA-G expression by cytotrophoblasts is reduced or absent,[134] and HLA-G protein concentrations are reduced in maternal serum[135] and in placental tissue.[136] These alterations in HLA-G expression could contribute to the ineffective trophoblast invasion seen in preeclampsia. Decidual natural killer (NK) cells, which promote angiogenesis and are involved in trophoblast invasion, has also been hypothesized to contribute to the abnormal placental development seen in the disease.[137,138] Genetic studies have noted that the susceptibility to preeclampsia may be influenced by polymorphisms in killer immunoglobulin receptors (KIRs, present on NK cells) and HLA-C (KIR ligands present on trophoblasts).[139]

ANGIOGENIC IMBALANCE

Overwhelming evidence from epidemiologic studies and experimental studies in animals suggests that excess placental production of soluble VEGF receptor 1, referred to as soluble fms-like tyrosine kinase-1 (sFlt1, or sVEGFR-1), plays a causal role in mediating the signs and symptoms of preeclampsia.[140] A truncated splice variant of the VEGF receptor Flt1, sFlt1 antagonizes VEGF and PlGF by binding them in the circulation and preventing interaction with their endogenous receptors in the vasculature (Figure 49.9). sFlt1 inhibits VEGF- and PlGF-mediated angiogenesis and is upregulated in the placentas of women with preeclampsia, resulting in elevated circulating sFlt1 values.[141] The increase in maternal circulating sFlt1 precedes the onset of clinical disease (Figure 49.10)[142-144] and is correlated with disease severity.[144,145] Increased circulating sFlt1 is accompanied by decreased circulating free PlGF in serum (Figure 49.11). In vitro effects of sFlt1 include vasoconstriction and endothelial dysfunction. Exogenous sFlt1 administered to pregnant rats produces a syndrome resembling preeclampsia, including hypertension, proteinuria, and glomerular endotheliosis.[141] The preeclampsia-like syndrome induced by sFlt1 in animals can be rescued by exogenous VEGF or PlGF administration.[146-148] In summary, this work has suggested that sFlt1 is a key pathogenic circulating toxin that mediates the signs and symptoms of preeclampsia (see Figure 49.7). Several novel isoforms of sFlt1 have been described, but the exact role of the various forms in human disease is still being investigated.[149,150]

Derangements in other angiogenic molecules have also been observed. Endostatin, another anti-angiogenic factor, is elevated in preeclampsia.[151] Expression of $VEGF_{165b}$, an anti-angiogenic isoform of VEGF, is reduced in the first trimester in women in whom preeclampsia later develops.[152] Circulating values of soluble endoglin (sEng), a truncated form of the transforming growth factor-β (TGF-β) receptor, are elevated in preeclampsia. Soluble endoglin amplifies the vascular damage mediated by sFlt1 in pregnant rats, inducing a severe preeclampsia-like syndrome with features of the HELLP syndrome.[153] Maternal serum levels of sEng rise prior to preeclampsia onset,[154-156] in a pattern similar to that of sFlt1.[157] Because TGF-β regulates podocyte VEGF-A expression,[158] soluble endoglin may result in impaired local VEGF signaling in the glomerulus. Semaphorin 3B, a novel trophoblastic secreted anti-angiogenic protein, has also been found to be upregulated in preeclamptic placentas to inhibit trophoblast migration and invasion by downregulating VEGF signaling.[159] The precise role of these novel anti-angiogenic proteins and their relationship with sFlt1 in the systemic vasculature continues to be explored.

There is circumstantial evidence suggesting that interference with VEGF signaling may lead to preeclampsia.[140] VEGF appears to be important in the stabilization of endothelial cells in mature blood vessels. VEGF is particularly important in the health of the fenestrated and sinusoidal endothelium found in the renal glomerulus, brain, and liver[160,161]—organs disproportionally affected in preeclampsia. VEGF is highly expressed by glomerular podocytes, and VEGF receptors are present on glomerular endothelial cells.[162] In experimental glomerulonephritis, VEGF is necessary for glomerular capillary repair.[163] In a podocyte-specific VEGF knockout mouse, heterozygosity for VEGF-A resulted in renal disease characterized by proteinuria and glomerular endotheliosis.[164] In anti-angiogenesis cancer trials, VEGF antagonists produce proteinuria and hypertension in human subjects.[165-168] This evidence suggests that VEGF deficiency induced by excess sFtl1 has the capacity to produce the characteristic renal lesion of preeclampsia.

Although the glomerular capillary endothelial cell appears to be the primary glomerular target in preeclampsia, the podocyte is clearly affected in severe disease, as evidenced by podocyturia during clinical disease and even before overt proteinuria.[120,169] However, podocyturia is also noted in other proteinuric disorders and is not specific for preeclampsia. Renal autopsy examination in women who died of preeclampsia demonstrates markedly reduced podocyte expression of nephrin,[170] and serum from preeclamptic women reduces nephrin expression by cultured podocytes.[171] In a study using a mouse model of preeclampsia induced by administration of anti-VEGF antibodies, it was noted that nephrin expression is reduced in podocytes.[172] The effect of sFlt1 on podocyte nephrin expression appears to be via increased release of endothelin-1 by endothelial cells,[171] another finding implicating the glomerular endothelial cell as the primary site of injury in preeclampsia.

Alterations in circulating sFlt1 have been noted in certain preeclampsia risk groups. Higher sFlt1 levels have been noted in first than in second pregnancies,[173] in twin than in singleton pregnancies,[174,175] in women with prior preeclampsia,[176] and in women carrying fetuses affected by trisomy

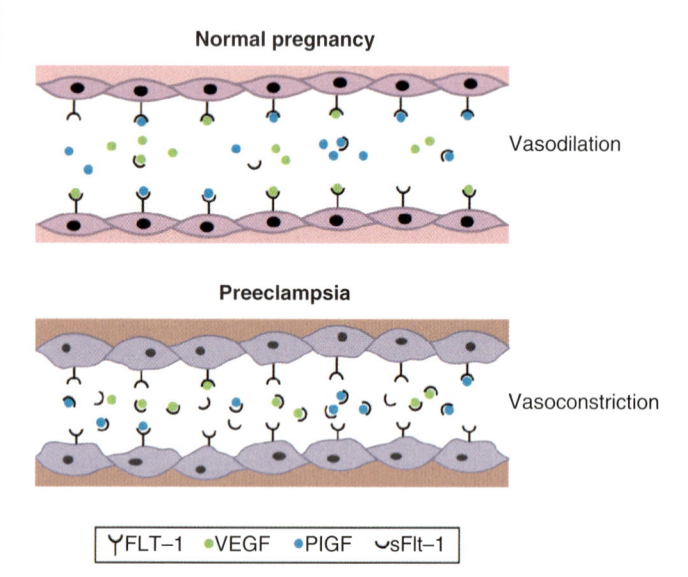

Figure 49.9 Proposed mechanism of soluble fms-like tyrosine kinase-1 (sFlt1)–induced endothelial dysfunction. sFlt1 protein, derived from alternative splicing of Flt1, lacks the transmembrane and cytoplasmic domains but still has the intact vascular endothelial growth factor (VEGF) and placental growth factor (PlGF) binding extracellular domain. During normal pregnancy, VEGF and PlGF signal through the VEGF receptors (Flt1) and maintain endothelial health. In preeclampsia, excess sFlt1 binds to circulating VEGF and PlGF, thus impairing normal signaling of both VEGF and PlGF through their cell surface receptors. Thus, excess sFlt1 leads to maternal endothelial dysfunction. (From Bdolah Y, Sukhatme VP, Karumanchi SA: Angiogenic imbalance in the pathophysiology of preeclampsia: newer insights. *Semin Nephrol* 24:548-556, 2004.)

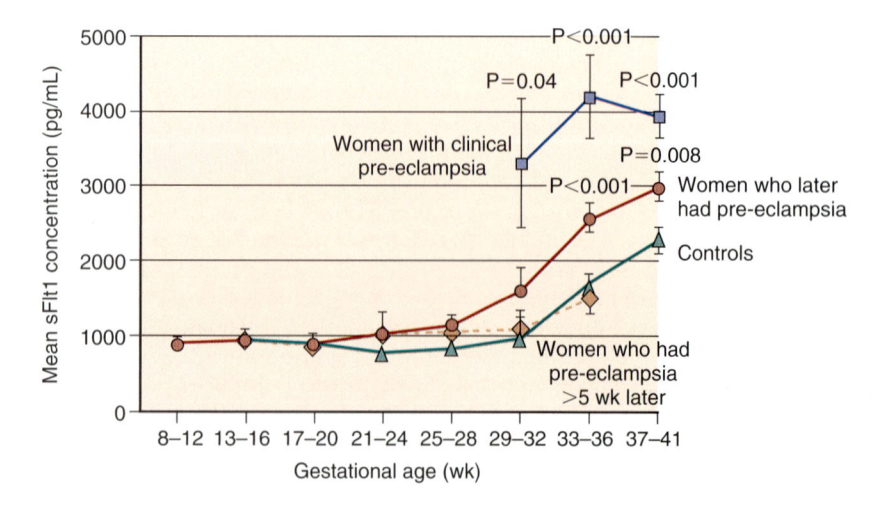

Figure 49.10 Concentrations of sFlt1 in preeclampsia and normal pregnancy. Shown are the mean serum sFlt1 concentrations (± standard error of mean [SEM]) before and after onset of clinical preeclampsia according to the gestational age of the fetus. The *P* values given are for comparisons, after logarithmic transformation, with specimens from controls obtained during the same gestational-age interval. All specimens were obtained before labor and delivery. (From Levine RJ, Maynard SE, Qian C, et al: Circulating angiogenic factors and the risk of preeclampsia. *N Engl J Med* 350:672-683, 2004.)

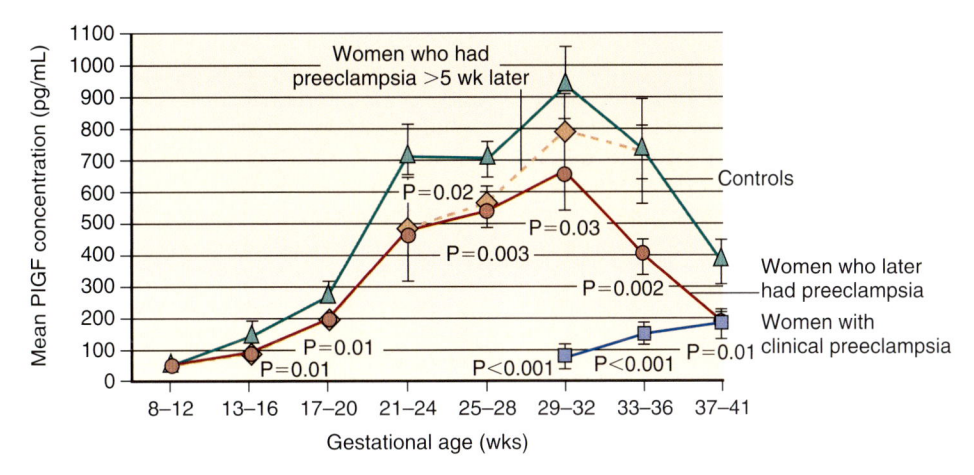

Figure 49.11 Concentrations of placental growth factor (PlGF) in preeclampsia and normal pregnancy. Shown are the mean serum PlGF concentrations (± SEM) before and after onset of clinical preeclampsia according to the gestational age of the fetus. The *P* values given are for comparisons, after logarithmic transformation, with specimens from controls obtained during the same gestational-age interval. All specimens were obtained before labor and delivery. (From Levine RJ, Maynard SE, Qian C, et al: Circulating angiogenic factors and the risk of preeclampsia. *N Engl J Med* 350:672-683, 2004.)

13,[177,178] potentially accounting for the increased preeclampsia risk in these groups. In the case of twin pregnancies, the increased sFlt1 production appears to be due to greater placental mass rather than placental ischemia.[175] Conversely, lower levels of sFlt1 in pregnant smokers[157,179] may explain the protective effect of smoking in preeclampsia.[180,181]

Angiogenic factors are likely to be important in the regulation of placental vasculogenesis. VEGF ligands and receptors are highly expressed by placental tissue in the first trimester.[182] sFlt1 decreases cytotrophoblast invasiveness in vitro.[103] Circulating sFlt1 levels are relatively low early in pregnancy and begin to rise in the third trimester. This pattern may reflect a physiologic anti-angiogenic shift in the placental milieu toward the end of pregnancy, corresponding to completion of the vasculogenic phase of placental growth. It is intuitive to hypothesize that placental vascular development might be regulated by a local balance between proangiogenic and anti-angiogenic factors and that excess antiangiogenic sFlt1 in early gestation could contribute to inadequate cytotrophoblast invasion in preeclampsia. By the third trimester, excess placental sFlt1 is detectable in the maternal circulation, producing end-organ effects. In this case, placental ischemia, rather than causative, may reflect that the placenta is the earliest organ affected by this derangement of angiogenic balance.

The pathways regulating placental angiogenic factor expression, and the reasons for their dysregulation in preeclampsia, are yet unknown (see Figure 49.7). Pieces of the puzzle may be starting to emerge, however. Animal models of preeclampsia based on induction of uteroplacental ischemia are characterized by increased endogenous sFlt1[96,183] and sEng.[184] Agonistic Ang II type 1 (AT$_1$) receptor autoantibodies produce a preeclampsia-like syndrome in mice (see later), in association with increased circulating sFlt1 levels.[185] Elaboration of the upstream pathways involved in placental angiogenic factor expression remains an area of intense research. Heme oxygenase 1 and its downstream metabolite, carbon monoxide, act as a vascular protective factor by inhibiting the production of sFlt1.[186] Animal studies suggest that enzyme cystathionine lyase (which regulates hydrogen sulfide) may also contribute to preeclampsia by disrupting placental angiogenesis.[187] However, human studies demonstrating alterations in heme oxygenase or cystathionine γ-lyase expression prior to alterations in anti-angiogenic factor are still lacking.

In addition to angiogenic alterations, women in whom preeclampsia develops also have evidence of insulin resistance.[188] Moreover, women with pregestational or gestational diabetes mellitus have an increased risk for development of preeclampsia.[42] In accordance with this finding, in vitro models suggest that insulin signaling and angiogenesis are intimately related at a molecular level,[189] and epidemiologic data show that altered angiogenesis and excess insulin resistance may be additive insults that lead to preeclampsia.[190] Furthermore, altered levels of biomarkers linked with angiogenesis and insulin resistance persist in the postpartum state,[191] possibly explaining the long-term cardiovascular risk in affected women.

ANGIOTENSIN II TYPE 1 RECEPTOR AUTOANTIBODIES

In preeclampsia, plasma renin levels are suppressed in relation to normal pregnancy as a secondary response to systemic vasoconstriction and hypertension. As noted in the previous section, preeclampsia is characterized by increased vascular responsiveness to Ang II and other vasoconstrictive agents. Wallukat and colleagues identified agonistic AT$_1$ receptor autoantibodies in women with preeclampsia.[192] They hypothesized that these antibodies, which activate the AT$_1$ receptor, may account for the increased Ang II sensitivity observed in preeclampsia. The same investigators later showed that these AT$_1$ autoantibodies, like Ang II itself, stimulate endothelial cells to produce tissue factor, an early marker of endothelial dysfunction. Xia and associates found that AT$_1$ autoantibodies decreased invasiveness of immortalized human trophoblasts in an in vitro invasion assay, suggesting that these autoantibodies might contribute to defective placental pseudovasculogenesis as well.[193] The same group showed that AT$_1$ autoantibodies isolated from the serum of women with preeclampsia produce a preeclampsia-like syndrome in pregnant rats, with increased endogenous sFlt1 production,[185] suggesting that AT_1 autoantibodies and sFlt1 may be part of the same pathophysiologic pathway leading to preeclampsia. Increased endogenous sFlt1 and the phenotype of proteinuria and glomerular endotheliosis in the pregnant dams but not in nonpregnant animals provided further evidence that placental sFlt1 specifically mediates the proteinuria secondary to AT_1 autoantibodies.

AT_1 autoantibodies are not limited to pregnancy; they also appear to be increased in malignant renovascular hypertension in nonpregnancy.[194] In addition, these antibodies have been identified in women with abnormal second-trimester uterine artery Doppler study findings in whom preeclampsia did not develop, suggesting that AT_1 antibodies may be a nonspecific response to placental hypoperfusion.[195]

The angiotensinogen T235 polymorphism, a common molecular variant associated with essential hypertension and microvascular disease, has also been associated with preeclampsia in several studies in different populations, though with significant ethnic heterogeneity.[196] Functional implications of this polymorphism remain unclear. Work by Abdalla and colleagues has suggested that heterodimerization of AT_1 receptors with bradykinin-2 receptors may contribute to Ang II hypersensitivity in preeclampsia.[197] This work remains to be validated in other studies.

SCREENING FOR PREECLAMPSIA

Although there is not yet any definitive therapeutic or preventive strategy for preeclampsia, clinical experience seems to show that early detection, monitoring, and supportive care are beneficial to the patient and the fetus. For example, lack of adequate antenatal care is strongly associated with poor outcomes, including eclampsia and fetal death.[198] Risk assessment early in pregnancy is important to identify those who require close monitoring after 20 weeks. Women with first pregnancies or other preeclampsia risk factors (see Table 49.2) should be assessed frequently after 20 weeks of gestation for the development of hypertension, proteinuria, headache, visual disturbances, and epigastric pain.

Higher blood pressure in the first or second trimester, even in the absence of overt hypertension, is associated with elevated risk for preeclampsia in healthy nulliparous women.[199] Unfortunately, these small elevations in midtrimester blood pressure are subtle and their positive predictive value as a screening test is low (especially given the relatively low prevalence), limiting routine clinical utility.

Presumably as a result of failed placental vascular remodeling, preeclampsia is associated with increased placental vascular resistance and uterine artery waveform abnormalities in the second trimester, as measured by uterine artery Doppler ultrasonography.[200] Dozens of studies have investigated the use of uterine artery Doppler ultrasonography for prediction of preeclampsia. Test performance varies widely among studies because of differences in populations studied, gestational age at the time of measurement, definition of an abnormal result, and severity and timing of preeclampsia detected: Sensitivities and specificities range from 65% to 85%. Even meta-analyses have differed in their conclusions, with some reporting limited diagnostic accuracy for uterine artery Doppler ultrasonography in predicting preeclampsia[200,201] and others suggesting that it is accurate enough to be recommended for preeclampsia screening in routine clinical practice.[202] Thus, there is wide regional variability in the use of this examination for routine screening, and it remains uncommon in the United States. Some data suggest that there may be promise in combining uterine artery Doppler ultrasonography with measurement of serum biomarkers in screening for preeclampsia.[203,204]

Of dozens of putative serum markers for preeclampsia, only a handful have been shown to be elevated prior to the onset of clinical disease, and none has yet proved to be an effective and useful screening tool for preeclampsia. Placental protein 13 and angiogenic biomarkers (sFlt1, PlGF, and sEng) hold promise for screening and/or early diagnosis of preeclampsia.

Placental protein 13 (PP13) is thought to be involved in normal placentation and maternal vascular remodeling. A low level of PP13 could identify a woman at high risk for preeclampsia as early as the first trimester,[205,206] although it appears to be a robust biomarker only for early-onset disease and may be less useful for preeclampsia close to term.[207] Polymorphisms in *LGALS13*, the gene encoding PP13, have been detected in cases of preeclampsia.[208] This polymorphism may result in production of a shorter splice variant of PP13 that is not detected by conventional assays, contributing to low circulating levels and decreased local activity of PP13.

Alterations in circulating levels of the angiogenic factors sFlt1 and sEng occur weeks prior to the onset of preeclampsia and may be useful for screening and/or diagnosis.[209,210] Significant elevations in maternal sFlt1 and sEng are observed from midgestation onwards[142,154-157,211,212] and appear to rise 5 to 8 weeks prior to preeclampsia onset (see Figure 49.10).[144] Maternal sFlt1 levels are particularly high in severe preeclampsia, early-onset preeclampsia, and preeclampsia complicated by a small-for-gestational-age (SGA) infant.[144,213] Serum levels of PlGF are lower during the first[214] or early second[144,215-217] trimester in women who eventually have preeclampsia (see Figure 49.11). Because PlGF passes into the urine, low urinary PlGF has been identified as a potential marker for preeclampsia. Urinary levels of PlGF are significantly lower in women in whom preeclampsia develops from the late second trimester[218] and may prove to be useful in screening and diagnosis of preeclampsia, especially in early-onset and severe preeclampsia. Prospective studies are ongoing to evaluate the clinical utility of these biomarkers for preeclampsia screening and risk assessment.

Later studies have suggested that circulating angiogenic factors in plasma or serum can be used to differentiate preeclampsia from other diseases that mimic preeclampsia, such as chronic hypertension, gestational hypertension, lupus nephritis, and chronic kidney disease.[219-223] Several groups have also demonstrated a role for angiogenic biomarkers in the prediction of preeclampsia-related adverse outcomes among women evaluated for suspected preeclampsia.[224-228] Measurements of circulating angiogenic factors (sFlt1, PlGF, sEng) robustly predicted adverse maternal and perinatal outcomes in women presenting with signs or symptoms of preeclampsia, and these biomarkers outperformed the standard battery of clinical diagnostic measures, including blood pressure, proteinuria, uric acid, and other laboratory assays. Importantly, sFlt1 and/or PlGF levels at presentation were strongly associated with the remaining duration of pregnancy.[224,227] By providing more accurate identification of women at high risk for adverse pregnancy outcomes, use of angiogenic biomarkers may reduce costs and unnecessary resource use in women with possible preeclampsia.[229]

PREVENTION OF PREECLAMPSIA

Strategies to prevent preeclampsia have been extensively studied, but no intervention to date has yet proved unequivocally effective.[55]

ANTIPLATELET AGENTS

Because of prominent alterations in prostacyclin-thromboxane balance in preeclampsia,[230] aspirin has been posited as a preventive strategy. Aspirin and other antiplatelet agents have been evaluated in dozens of trials for the prevention of preeclampsia, both in high-risk groups and in healthy nulliparous women. Among women at high risk for preeclampsia, results of several small, early trials suggested that daily aspirin had a significant protective effect.[231] Unfortunately, these initially promising findings were not confirmed in three large randomized controlled trials with a cumulative enrollment of 12,000 high-risk women.[232-234] All three studies found a small, nonsignificant trend toward a lower incidence of preeclampsia in the aspirin-treated groups. A subsequent comprehensive meta-analysis of antiplatelet agents to prevent preeclampsia, which included more than 32,000 women of varying risk status from 31 trials, found that antiplatelet agents have a modest benefit, with a relative risk of preeclampsia of 0.90 (95% confidence interval [CI], 0.84 to 0.97) for aspirin-treated patients (Figure 49.12).[235] The magnitude of the protective effect did not appear to differ among risk groups, although the reduction in absolute risk was greatest in women at highest baseline risk. Nevertheless, low-dose aspirin clearly appears to be safe: Early concerns about an increased risk of postpartum hemorrhage have clearly been assuaged. Given the small but significant protective effect, aspirin prophylaxis should be considered as primary prevention for preeclampsia only in women at high baseline risk, in whom the absolute risk reduction will be greatest.

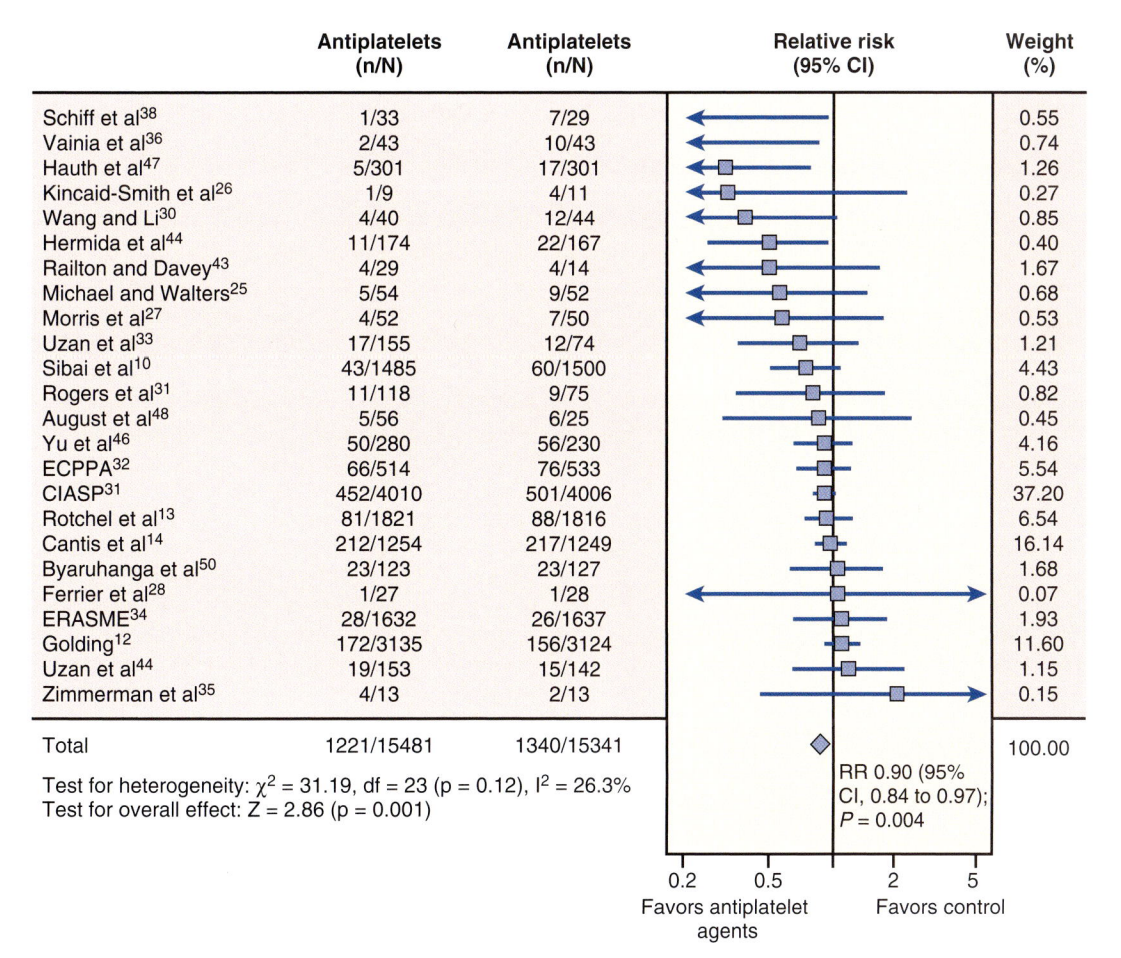

Study	Antiplatelets (n/N)	Antiplatelets (n/N)	Relative risk (95% CI)	Weight (%)
Schiff et al[38]	1/33	7/29		0.55
Vainia et al[36]	2/43	10/43		0.74
Hauth et al[47]	5/301	17/301		1.26
Kincaid-Smith et al[26]	1/9	4/11		0.27
Wang and Li[30]	4/40	12/44		0.85
Hermida et al[44]	11/174	22/167		0.40
Railton and Davey[43]	4/29	4/14		1.67
Michael and Walters[25]	5/54	9/52		0.68
Morris et al[27]	4/52	7/50		0.53
Uzan et al[33]	17/155	12/74		1.21
Sibai et al[10]	43/1485	60/1500		4.43
Rogers et al[31]	11/118	9/75		0.82
August et al[48]	5/56	6/25		0.45
Yu et al[46]	50/280	56/230		4.16
ECPPA[32]	66/514	76/533		5.54
CIASP[31]	452/4010	501/4006		37.20
Rotchel et al[13]	81/1821	88/1816		6.54
Cantis et al[14]	212/1254	217/1249		16.14
Byaruhanga et al[50]	23/123	23/127		1.68
Ferrier et al[28]	1/27	1/28		0.07
ERASME[34]	28/1632	26/1637		1.93
Golding[12]	172/3135	156/3124		11.60
Uzan et al[44]	19/153	15/142		1.15
Zimmerman et al[35]	4/13	2/13		0.15
Total	1221/15481	1340/15341	RR 0.90 (95% CI, 0.84 to 0.97); P = 0.004	100.00

Test for heterogeneity: $\chi^2 = 31.19$, df = 23 (p = 0.12), $I^2 = 26.3\%$
Test for overall effect: Z = 2.86 (p = 0.001)

0.2 0.5 ← Favors antiplatelet agents | 2 5 Favors control →

Figure 49.12 Effect of antiplatelet drugs on preeclampsia in moderate-risk and high-risk women. Summary of studies of the effect of antiplatelet drugs on preeclampsia incidence. "Subtotal" indicates the results of a meta-analysis of all studies, suggesting a small but significant benefit. For both risk groups, the largest studies (N > 1000 for moderate-risk and N > 100 for high-risk women) did not show a statistically significant protective effect. CI, Confidence interval. (From Askie LM, Duley L, Henderson-Smart DJ, et al: Antiplatelet agents for prevention of pre-eclampsia: a meta-analysis of individual patient data. *Lancet* 369:1791-1798, 2007.)

CALCIUM FOR THE PREVENTION OF PREECLAMPSIA

Several studies have examined the effectiveness of calcium supplementation to prevent preeclampsia. Among low-risk primiparous North American women, calcium supplementation did not reduce incidence of preeclampsia.[50] A meta-analysis of 12 trials, involving 15,528 women, reported a significant reduction in preeclampsia risk with calcium supplementation, with the greatest effect among women with low baseline calcium intake and at high preeclampsia risk.[236] This finding was tested directly in a large randomized, placebo-controlled trial of calcium supplementation in more than 8000 women with low baseline calcium intake (<600 mg/day).[237] Although there was no difference in incidence of preeclampsia, the calcium group had lower rates of eclampsia, gestational hypertension, preeclampsia complications, and neonatal mortality. Thus, calcium supplementation may be useful in women with low baseline calcium intake.

ANTIOXIDANTS AND NUTRITIONAL INTERVENTIONS

On the basis of the hypothesis that oxidative stress may contribute to pathogenesis, it has been suggested that antioxidants may prevent preeclampsia.[238] However, four large randomized, controlled trials have failed to show a benefit of vitamin C and vitamin E supplementation for the prevention of preeclampsia in various populations,[239-243] even in women at high risk for preeclampsia who were recruited from communities at risk for poor nutritional status.[239] Vitamin D deficiency has also been suggested as an important factor contributing to preeclampsia,[244-246] but none of the studies adjusted for vitamin D–binding proteins, which are upregulated during pregnancy. More work is needed to evaluate whether true deficiency of vitamin D is associated with preeclampsia.

Nutritional interventions have generally not been effective in decreasing preeclampsia risk. Protein and calorie restriction for obese pregnant women effects no reduction in the risk for preeclampsia or gestational hypertension and may increase risk for intrauterine growth restriction (IUGR), so should be avoided.[247] Women who have had bariatric surgery for severe obesity have had a lower incidence of preeclampsia than obese controls in some[248] but not all[249] studies. Obese women with lower gestational weight gain (<15 kg) have a reduced incidence of preeclampsia.[250,251]

MANAGEMENT AND TREATMENT OF PREECLAMPSIA

TIMING OF DELIVERY

The timing of delivery in severe preeclampsia has been contentiously debated. In women presenting prior to 24 weeks of gestation with severe preeclampsia, perinatal and neonatal mortality rates are extremely high (>80%) even with attempts to postpone delivery, and maternal complications are common.[252] For this reason, pregnancy termination is usually recommended in women with severe preeclampsia prior to 24 weeks of gestation. In addition, the presence of nonreassuring fetal test results, suspected abruptio placentae, thrombocytopenia, worsening liver and/or kidney function, and symptoms such as unremitting headache, visual changes, nausea, vomiting, and epigastric pain are generally considered indications for expedient delivery.

In preeclampsia manifesting between 24 and 34 weeks of gestation without the severe signs and symptoms just described, postponing delivery may improve neonatal outcome. The potential neonatal benefit needs to be balanced against the possibility of increased maternal morbidity as a result of delaying delivery. Two small randomized controlled trials demonstrated that in women presenting with severe preeclampsia between 28 and 32 weeks of gestation, expectant management (with delivery postponed 1 to 2 weeks after presentation) resulted in decreases in rate of neonatal complications rates and duration of neonatal intensive care unit stay, with no significant increase in rate of maternal complications.[253,254] Most subsequent observational studies have confirmed that delivery can be safely and effectively postponed in women with severe preeclampsia with careful and intensive fetal and maternal monitoring.[252] In addition, expectant management of preeclampsia in the mother appears to decrease the rate of childhood respiratory disorders in the infant.[255]

There are no randomized controlled trials to evaluate optimal mode of delivery in severe preeclampsia. Retrospective studies suggest that maternal and neonatal outcomes are similar among women undergoing induction of labor and those undergoing cesarean section.[256]

BLOOD PRESSURE MANAGEMENT

Management of blood pressure in women with preeclampsia is substantially different from that in the nonpregnant population. Rather than seeking to minimize long-term cerebrovascular and cardiovascular complications, the goal of care is to maximize the likelihood of successful delivery of a healthy infant while minimizing the chance of acute complications in the mother. Aggressive treatment of hypertension in pregnancy can compromise placental blood flow and fetal growth. Treatment of mild to moderate hypertension in pregnancy has not been shown to improve outcomes[257] and has been associated with increased risk of SGA infants (Figure 49.13).[258] Acute aggressive lowering of blood pressure can lead to fetal distress or demise, especially if placental perfusion is already compromised. For this reason, antihypertensive therapy for preeclampsia is usually withheld unless the blood pressure rises above 150 to 160 mm Hg systolic or 100 to 110 mm Hg diastolic, above which the risk of cerebral hemorrhage becomes significant.[55] The next section reviews details regarding the use of specific antihypertensive agents for blood pressure management in pregnancy.

MAGNESIUM AND SEIZURE PROPHYLAXIS

Magnesium has been widely used for the management and prevention of eclampsia for decades. Prior to the mid-1990s, evidence for its use was largely derived from clinical experience and from small uncontrolled studies. Over the last 20 years, magnesium has been proved to be superior to other agents for the prevention and treatment of seizures in preeclampsia, although not for the prevention of preeclampsia per se. In 1995, two randomized controlled trials in an international population and a U.S. population showed magnesium sulfate superior to diazepam and phenytoin in reducing risk of seizures in women in preeclampsia/

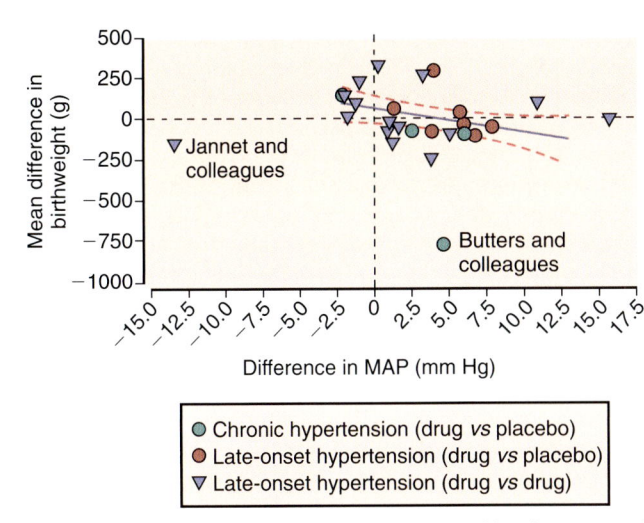

Figure 49.13 Treatment-induced decrease in blood pressure is associated with lower mean birth weight. Results from a meta-analysis of 25 trials of antihypertensive therapy in pregnancy. MAP, Mean arterial pressure. (From von Dadelszen P, Ornstein MP, Bull SB, et al: Fall in mean arterial pressure and fetal growth restriction in pregnancy hypertension: a meta-analysis. *Lancet* 355:87-92, 2000.)

eclampsia.[259,260] Subsequently, the Magpie study confirmed this benefit with a randomized, controlled trial comparing magnesium and placebo for seizure prevention in more than 10,000 women with preeclampsia from 33 countries, finding that magnesium decreased the incidence of eclamptic seizure by 50% (0.8% with magnesium vs. 1.9% with placebo).[74] A global public health effort over the past 10 to 15 years has led to improved access to magnesium in developing countries, where the rate of use of magnesium in preeclampsia/eclampsia has now reached 75% to 90%.[261]

Magnesium is now categorized as a pregnancy category D agent by the U.S. Food and Drug Administration (FDA), primarily because of adverse fetal effects with long-term (>5-7 days) use as a tocolytic in preterm labor.[261a] Despite this labeling change, short-term (<48 hours) intravenous magnesium is still recommended by the American College of Obstetricians and Gynecologists for the prevention and treatment of seizures in women with preeclampsia and eclampsia.[262] Magnesium is generally given intravenously as a bolus, followed by a continuous infusion. In the therapeutic range (5 to 9 mg/dL), magnesium sulfate slows neuromuscular conduction and depresses central nervous system irritability. Women receiving continuous infusions of magnesium should be monitored carefully for signs of toxicity, including loss of deep tendon reflexes, flushing, somnolence, muscle weakness, and decreased respiratory rate. Such monitoring is especially important in women with impaired renal function, who also have impaired urinary magnesium excretion.

MANAGEMENT OF THE HELLP SYNDROME

The clinical course of the HELLP syndrome usually involves inexorable and often sudden and unpredictable deterioration. Given the high incidence of maternal complications, some writers recommend immediate delivery in all cases of confirmed HELLP syndrome. Among women in the 24- to 34-week gestational window whose clinical status appears relatively stable and with reassuring fetal status, expectant management is often a viable alternative. For many years intravenous steroids have been suggested as an adjunct to usual management, on the basis of retrospective and uncontrolled studies. A randomized controlled trial, however, showed no benefit to high-dose dexamethasone treatment in HELLP syndrome.[263] Post-hoc analysis suggested that the subgroup with severe preeclampsia (platelet count < 50,000/mm³) may have a shorter average platelet count recovery and shorter hospitalization when given steroids, so further studies are required to evaluate the benefit in this population.

On the basis of pathophysiologic similarities of HELLP syndrome to thrombotic thrombocytopenic purpura, there are reports of using plasmapheresis in the management of HELLP syndrome. Data for the antepartum period are limited to a few cases series with mixed results and no clear benefit.[264] Potential drawbacks include fetal compromise due to diminishment of already compromised placental blood flow.

NOVEL THERAPIES FOR PREECLAMPSIA

Advances in our understanding of the pathophysiology of preeclampsia have revealed new potential therapeutic targets. Interfering with the production or signaling of sFlt1 may ameliorate the endothelial dysfunction of preeclampsia, allowing delivery to be more safely postponed. In a pilot study limited to three women with severe early preeclampsia (24-32 weeks of gestation), Thadhani and colleagues lowered sFlt1 levels using dextran sulfate apheresis and prolonged pregnancy by 2 to 4 weeks; importantly, this therapy promoted fetal growth with no adverse effects on the fetus or the mother.[265] If confirmed this approach could lead to targeted therapy for patients with preterm preeclampsia who present with an abnormal angiogenic profile.[265] Statins have also been proposed as potential therapeutic agents for preeclampsia on the basis of their promotion of heme oxygenase activity and improvement of angiogenic imbalance in animal models of preeclampsia.[186,266] However, statins are currently categorized as pregnancy category X agents by the FDA because of potential teratogenic effects. Pilot human trials to test the safety and efficacy of pravastatin during the third trimester in patients with severe preeclampsia are ongoing.[267] Other investigators are exploring the safety and efficacy of relaxin (a vasodilator) in the treatment of preeclampsia.[268] Dietary choline, which acts by decreasing placental sFlt1 expression, has also been suggested as novel strategy to prevent preeclampsia.[269] Results from these and other prospective therapeutic trials are eagerly awaited.

CHRONIC HYPERTENSION AND GESTATIONAL HYPERTENSION

The diagnosis of chronic hypertension in pregnancy is usually based on a documented history of hypertension prior to pregnancy or a blood pressure higher than 140/90 mm Hg prior to 20 weeks of gestation. Gestational hypertension, in contrast, is usually first noted after 20 weeks of gestation and, by definition, resolves after delivery. These diagnoses, based on the timing of the first recorded blood pressure elevation, can be subject to pitfalls, however. The physiologic dip in blood pressure in the second trimester, which reaches a nadir at about 20 weeks of gestation (see Figure 49.1), occurs in women with chronic hypertension and can mask the presence of underlying chronic hypertension early in pregnancy. In such cases, a woman with chronic hypertension may be inappropriately labeled as having gestational hypertension when her blood pressure rises in the third trimester. On the other hand, preeclampsia can occasionally manifest prior to 20 weeks of gestation; hence, preeclampsia should always be suspected in women presenting with new hypertension and proteinuria close to midgestation.

Chronic hypertension is present in 3% to 5% of pregnancies[270] and is more common with advanced maternal age, obesity, and black race.[271] Pregnant women with chronic hypertension have an increased risk of preeclampsia (21%-25%), premature delivery (33%-35%), intrauterine growth restriction (10%-15%), placental abruption (1%-3%), and perinatal mortality (4.5%).[272,273] However, most adverse outcomes occur in women with severe hypertension (diastolic blood pressure > 110 mm Hg) and those with preexisting cardiovascular and renal disease. Women with mild, uncomplicated chronic hypertension usually have obstetric outcomes comparable to those in the general obstetric population.[271] Both the duration and the severity of hypertension are correlated with perinatal morbidity and preeclampsia risk.[274,275] The presence of baseline proteinuria increases the risk of preterm delivery and IUGR but not that of preeclampsia per se.[273]

The diagnosis of preeclampsia superimposed on chronic hypertension can be difficult. In the absence of underlying kidney disease, the new onset of proteinuria (>300 mg/day), usually with worsening hypertension, is the most reliable sign of superimposed preeclampsia.[55] When proteinuria is present at baseline, preeclampsia is likely when a sudden increase in blood pressure is observed in a woman whose blood pressure was previously well-controlled. Other signs and symptoms of preeclampsia, such as headache, visual changes, epigastric pain, and pulmonary edema, and laboratory derangements, such as thrombocytopenia, new or worsening renal insufficiency, and elevated liver enzymes, also should prompt consideration of preeclampsia and, when present, are an indication of preeclampsia severity.[55]

SECONDARY HYPERTENSION IN PREGNANCY

Prepregnancy evaluation of women with chronic hypertension should include consideration of secondary causes of hypertension such as renal artery stenosis, primary hyperaldosteronism, and pheochromocytoma. Renal artery stenosis due to fibromuscular dysplasia or, less often, atherosclerotic vascular disease occasionally manifests in pregnancy and should be suspected when hypertension is severe and resistant to medical therapy. Diagnosis with magnetic resonance (MR) angiography followed by successful angioplasty and stent placement in the second or third trimester of pregnancy has been described.[276]

Although rare, pheochromocytoma can be devastating when it first manifests during pregnancy. This syndrome is occasionally unmasked during labor and delivery, when fatal hypertensive crisis can be triggered by vaginal delivery, uterine contractions, and anesthesia.[277] Maternal and neonatal morbidity and mortality are much better when the diagnosis is made antepartum, with attentive and aggressive medical management. Surgical intervention is typically postponed until after delivery whenever possible.

Hypertension and hypokalemia from primary hyperaldosteronism might be expected to improve during pregnancy, because progesterone antagonizes the effect of aldosterone on the renal tubule. However, such remission is not universal and many women with primary hyperaldosteronism have a pregnancy-induced exacerbation of hypertension.[278] In the case of a functional adrenal adenoma, there is little data to favor either immediate surgical adrenalectomy or medical management until after delivery, although case reports have suggested success with both approaches. Although the use of spironolactone has been reported during pregnancy, theoretical risks to the fetus are significant, and aldosterone antagonists should be avoided if possible.

A rare cause of early-onset hypertension is due to a mutation in the mineralocorticoid receptor. The mutation results in inappropriate receptor activation by progesterone, and affected women demonstrate a marked exacerbation of hypertension and hypokalemia in pregnancy, but without proteinuria or other features of preeclampsia.[279]

APPROACH TO MANAGEMENT OF CHRONIC HYPERTENSION IN PREGNANCY

Blood pressure control should be optimized prior to conception whenever possible, and the woman with chronic hypertension should be counseled regarding the risks of adverse pregnancy outcomes, including preeclampsia. Once she is pregnant, changes in antihypertensive agents may be appropriate (see later), and the woman should be followed closely as pregnancy progresses for signs of superimposed preeclampsia.

GOALS OF THERAPY

When hypertension is severe (diastolic blood pressure > 100 mm Hg), antihypertensive therapy is clearly indicated for the prevention of stroke and cardiovascular complications.[55] However, there is little evidence that treatment of mild to moderate hypertension has a clear benefit for either mother or fetus. Several clinical trials have evaluated the impact of antihypertensive therapy in comparison with no treatment in women with mild to moderate hypertension, and their results have been evaluated in three meta-analyses.[257,270,280] Although antihypertensive therapy lowered the risk for development of severe hypertension, there was no beneficial effect on the development of preeclampsia, neonatal death, preterm birth, SGA babies, or other adverse outcomes (Figure 49.14). In addition, aggressive treatment of mild to moderate hypertension in pregnancy may impair fetal growth. Treatment-induced drops in mean arterial pressure are associated with decreased birth weight and fetal growth restriction, presumably as a result of decreased uteroplacental perfusion (see Figure 49.13).[258] For this reason, the American College of Obstetricians and Gynecologi (ACOG) Task Force on Hypertension in Pregnancy recommends against use of antihypertensive medication in pregnant women with chronic hypertension and blood pressure less than 160/105 mm Hg in the absence of evidence

Comparison or outcome	Peto odds ratio (95% CI)	No. of trials
Maternal		
Severe hypertension	0.27 (0.14 to 0.53)	3
Additional antihypertensives	0.36 (0.23 to 0.57)	5
Admission before delivery	0.23 (0.07 to 0.70)	1
Proteinuria	0.70 (0.45 to 1.08)	6
Cesarean section	1.22 (0.81 to 1.82)	4
Abruption	0.42 (0.15 to 1.22)	3
Changed drugs owing to side effects	2.79 (0.39 to 20.04)	2
Perinatal		
Perinatal mortality	0.40 (0.12 to 1.32)	7
Prematurity	1.47 (0.75 to 2.88)	3
Small for gestational age infants	1.28 (0.69 to 2.36)	6
Neonatal hypoglycemia	2.06 (0.41 to 10.29)	2
Low Apgar score (5 minutes <7)	0.90 (0.32 to 2.53)	3

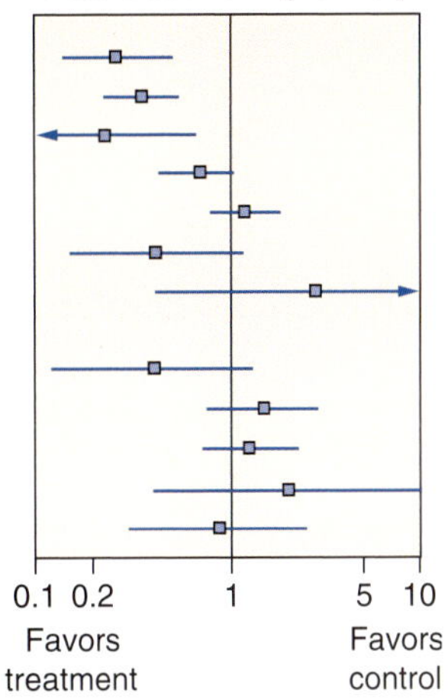

Figure 49.14 Effect of antihypertensive treatment versus no treatment for mild chronic hypertension in pregnancy. Results from a meta-analysis of seven trials of the effect of antihypertensive treatment on maternal and perinatal outcomes. (From Magee LA, Ornstein MP, von Dadelszen P: Fortnightly review: management of hypertension in pregnancy. *BMJ* 318:1332-1336, 1999.)

of end-organ damage.[55] Similarly, in women already receiving long-term antihypertensive therapy prior to pregnancy, consideration could be given to tapering or discontinuing treatment unless blood pressures exceed these levels.

GESTATIONAL HYPERTENSION

Gestational hypertension is defined as the new onset of hypertension without proteinuria after 20 weeks of gestation that resolves postpartum. Gestational hypertension likely represents a mix of several underlying etiologies. A subset of women with gestational hypertension have previously existing essential hypertension that is undiagnosed. In such cases, if the woman presents for medical care during the second-trimester nadir in blood pressure, she may be inappropriately presumed to be previously normotensive. In such a circumstance the diagnosis of chronic hypertension is established postpartum, when blood pressure fails to return to normal.

Gestational hypertension progresses to overt preeclampsia in about 10% to 25% of cases.[281] When gestational hypertension is severe, it carries similar risks for adverse outcomes to those of preeclampsia, even in the absence of proteinuria.[282] A renal biopsy study suggests that a significant proportion of women with gestational hypertension have renal glomerular endothelial damage.[122] Hence, gestational hypertension may have the same pathophysiologic underpinnings as preeclampsia and should be monitored and treated as such. In recognition of the syndromic nature of preeclampsia, new ACOG guidelines have eliminated the dependence on proteinuria for the diagnosis of preeclampsia (see Table 49.3). In a subset of women with gestational hypertension, the disorder may represent a temporary unmasking of an underlying predisposition to chronic hypertension. Such women often present with a strong family history of chronic hypertension and experience hypertension in the third trimester with low uric acid values and no proteinuria. Although the hypertension often resolves after delivery, these women are at risk for the development of hypertension and cardiovascular disease later in life.[283,284]

MANAGEMENT OF HYPERTENSION IN PREGNANCY

CHOICE OF AGENTS

Recommendations for the use of antihypertensive agents in pregnancy are summarized in Table 49.5. Methyldopa continues to be the first-line oral agent for the management of hypertension in pregnancy. Methyldopa is a centrally acting α_2-adrenergic agonist now seldom used outside pregnancy. Of all antihypertensive agents, it has the most extensive safety data and appears to have no adverse fetal effects. Drawbacks include a short half-life, sedation, and rare adverse effects such as elevated liver enzymes and hemolytic anemia. Clonidine appears to be comparable to methyldopa in terms of mechanism and safety, but data on its use in pregnancy are fewer.

β-Adrenergic antagonists have been used extensively in pregnancy and are effective without known teratogenicity or known adverse fetal effects. One possible exception is atenolol, which has been associated with fetal growth restriction.[285] Labetalol, which may result in better preservation of uteroplacental blood flow because of to its α-adrenergic–blocking action, has found widespread use and acceptance both as an oral and an intravenous agent.[286]

Calcium channel blockers appear to be safe in pregnancy, and clinical experience with them is growing. Long-acting nifedipine, the most well studied, appears to be safe and effective.[286,287] Non-dihydropyridine calcium channel blockers such as verapamil have also been used without apparent adverse effects. However, experience with these agents is more limited than that with some other classes.

Although diuretics are often avoided in preeclampsia, with the reasoning that circulating volume is already low, there is no evidence that diuretics are associated with adverse fetal or maternal outcomes. Similarly, diuretics are not considered first line in the management of chronic

Table 49.5 Safety of Antihypertensive Medications in Pregnancy

Drug*	Advantage(s)	Disadvantage(s)
First-Line Agents		
Oral		
Methyldopa (B)	First-line; extensive safety data	Short duration of action/bid or tid dosing
Labetalol (C)	Appears to be safe Labetalol is preferred over other β-blockers owing to theoretical beneficial effect of α-blockade on uteroplacental blood flow	Short duration of action/tid dosing
Long-acting nifedipine (C)	Appears to be safe Available in a slow-release preparation, allowing once-daily dosing	
Intravenous		
Labetalol (C)	Good safety data	
Nicardipine (C)	Extensive safety data on use as a tocolytic during labor; effective	
Second-Line Agents		
Hydralazine (PO or IV) (C)	Extensive clinical experience	Increased risk of maternal hypotension and placental abruption when used acutely
Metoprolol (C)	Potential for once-daily dosing using long-acting formulation	Safety data less extensive than for labetalol
Verapamil (C), diltiazem (C)	No evidence of adverse fetal effects	Limited data
Generally Avoided		
Diuretics	No clear evidence of adverse fetal effects	Theoretically may impair pregnancy-associated expansion in plasma volume
Atenolol		May impair fetal growth
Nitroprusside		Risk of fetal cyanide poisoning if used for more than 4 hr
Contraindicated		
ACE inhibitors		Multiple fetal anomalies; see text
Angiotensin receptor antagonists		Similar risks to those of ACE inhibitors

ACE, angiotensin-converting enzyme; bid, twice daily; IV, intravenous; PO, by mouth; tid, thrice daily.
*U.S. Food and Drug Administration (FDA) pregnancy-use category designations for the individual drugs are shown in parentheses.

hypertension in pregnancy because of their theoretical impact on the normal plasma volume expansion of pregnancy. When hypertension in pregnancy is complicated by pulmonary edema, diuretics are appropriate and effective.

Angiotensin-converting enzyme inhibitors (ACEIs) and angiotensin receptor blockers (ARBs) are contraindicated in the second and third trimesters of pregnancy. Exposure during this time leads to major fetal malformations, including renal dysgenesis, perinatal renal failure, oligohydramnios, pulmonary hypoplasia, hypocalvaria, and IUGR.[288] Evidence for teratogenicity with first-trimester exposure is less compelling. In a large population-based study, Cooper and associates reported that congenital malformations of the central nervous and cardiovascular systems were higher among women with first-trimester exposure to ACEIs.[289] However, this study has been criticized for the presence of potential confounding factors and ascertainment bias. Women with a compelling indication for ACEI/ARB therapy (such as diabetic nephropathy) can probably continue on these agents while attempting conception, with discontinuation as soon as pregnancy is diagnosed. However, risks and benefits of this strategy should be discussed with the patient, with shared and individualized decision making. Women inadvertently exposed in early pregnancy can be reassured by normal midtrimester ultrasound findings. Fewer data are available on the effects of ARBs, but a case series strongly suggests that the fetal effects are similar to those of ACEIs,[290] as would be expected on a theoretical basis.

INTRAVENOUS AGENTS FOR URGENT BLOOD PRESSURE CONTROL

Severe hypertension in pregnancy occasionally requires inpatient management with intravenous agents. All intravenous medications commonly used for urgent control of severe hypertension are classified as pregnancy class C (lack of controlled studies in humans). Nevertheless, there is extensive clinical experience with several agents, which are widely used with no evidence of adverse effects. Options for intravenous use include labetalol, calcium channel blockers such as nicardipine, and hydralazine.

Intravenous labetalol, like oral labetalol, is safe and effective, with the major drawback being its short duration of action. Intravenous nicardipine has been used safely for tocolysis during premature labor, and reports suggest that it is safe for the treatment of hypertension as well.[291] The use of short-acting nifedipine is controversial owing to well-documented adverse effects in the nonpregnant population. However, one trial suggests that oral short-acting nifedipine can be safely used for hypertensive emergencies during pregnancy,[292] and it may be a good option in areas where intravenous agents are unavailable.

Hydralazine has been widely used as a first-line agent for severe hypertension in pregnancy. However, a meta-analysis of 21 trials comparing intravenous (IV) hydralazine with either labetalol or nifedipine for acute management of hypertension in pregnancy found an increased risk of maternal hypotension, maternal oliguria, placental abruption, and low Apgar scores with hydralazine.[293] Hence, hydralazine should probably be considered a second-line agent, and its use limited when possible. Nitroprusside carries risk of fetal cyanide poisoning if used for more than 4 hours and is generally avoided.

ANTIHYPERTENSIVE DRUGS DURING BREASTFEEDING

There are few well-designed studies of the safety of antihypertensive medications in breastfeeding women. In general, the agents that are considered safe during pregnancy remain so for breastfeeding. Methyldopa, if effective and well-tolerated, should be considered the first-line agent. β-Blockers with high protein binding, such as labetalol and propranolol, are preferred over atenolol and metoprolol, which are concentrated in breast milk.[286] Diuretics may decrease milk production and should be avoided.[286] ACEIs are poorly excreted in breast milk and generally considered safe in lactating women.[294] Enalapril and captopril have been best studied and are preferred in lactating women. Hence, in women with proteinuric renal disease, re-initiation of ACEIs should be considered immediately after delivery. Finally, specific data on the pharmacokinetics of each medication should be used to guide mothers to time breastfeeding to occur before or well after peak breast milk excretion to avoid significant exposure of the baby to the medication.

ACUTE KIDNEY INJURY IN PREGNANCY

The incidence of acute kidney injury (AKI) in pregnancy in the developed world has fallen dramatically over the past 40 years.[295] This trend is due to a variety of factors, including improved availability of safe and legal abortion and more widespread and aggressive use of antibiotics (both of which have decreased the incidence of septic abortion) as well as improvement in overall prenatal care.

The most common cause of AKI during pregnancy is prerenal azotemia due to hyperemesis gravidarum or vomiting from acute pyelonephritis. Occasionally pregnancy-specific conditions such as preeclampsia, HELLP syndrome, and acute fatty liver of pregnancy (AFLP) are complicated by AKI. Obstetric complications such as septic abortion and placental abruption are associated with severe acute tubular necrosis (ATN) and bilateral cortical necrosis. Obstructive uropathy is a rare cause of renal failure in pregnancy.

ACUTE TUBULAR NECROSIS AND BILATERAL CORTICAL NECROSIS

ATN in pregnancy can be precipitated by a variety of factors. Volume depletion complicating hyperemesis gravidarum or uterine hemorrhage (due to placental abruption, placenta previa, failure of the postpartum uterus to contract, or uterine lacerations and perforations) can lead to renal ischemia and subsequent ATN. AKI may also occur following intraamniotic saline administration, amniotic fluid embolism, and diseases or accidents unrelated to pregnancy.

Bilateral cortical necrosis is a severe and often irreversible form of ATN that is associated with septic abortion and placental abruption. Septic abortion is an infection of the uterus and the surrounding tissues following any abortion, most commonly nonsterile illicit abortion. Septic abortion is now rare where safe therapeutic abortion is available but remains a serious clinical problem in countries where induced abortion is illegal and/or inaccessible. Women with septic abortion usually present with vaginal bleeding, lower abdominal pain, and fever hours to days after the attempted abortion. If the condition is untreated, progression to shock may be rapid, and patients can manifest a peculiar bronze color from hemolytic jaundice with cutaneous vasodilatation, cyanosis, and pallor. Renal failure, which complicates up to 73% of cases,[296] is often characterized by gross hematuria, flank pain, and oligoanuria. Other complications include acute respiratory distress syndrome, severe anemia, leukocytosis, severe thrombocytopenia, and disseminated intravascular coagulopathy. An abdominal radiograph may demonstrate air in the uterus or abdomen secondary to gas-forming organisms and/or perforation.

The bacteria associated with septic abortion are usually polymicrobial and derived from the normal flora of the vagina and endocervix, in addition to sexually transmitted pathogens. *Clostridium welchii*, *Clostridium perfringens*, *Streptococcus pyogenes*, and gram-negative organisms such as *Escherichia coli* and *Pseudomonas aeruginosa* are all known pathogens. Fatal toxic shock syndrome with *Clostridium sordellii* has also been reported following medical termination of pregnancy using mifepristone (RU-486) and intravaginal misoprostol.[297] Pregnancy has long been known to confer a peculiar susceptibility to the vascular effects of gram-negative endotoxin (Shwartzman reaction [or phenomenon]). Perhaps because of the physiologic increase in procoagulant factors that occurs in normal pregnancy, the thrombotic microangiopathy and renal cortical necrosis that characterize septic shock—notably with gram-negative organisms—are particularly pronounced during pregnancy.

AKI with bilateral cortical necrosis in the last trimester of pregnancy can also be precipitated by placental abruption. Cortical necrosis can involve the entire renal cortex, often leading to irreversible renal failure, but more commonly involvement is incomplete or patchy. In such cases, a protracted period of oligoanuria is followed by a variable return of renal function. The diagnosis of renal cortical necrosis can be usually be established by CT scan, which characteristically demonstrates hypodense areas in the renal cortex.

The treatment of AKI in pregnancy is supportive with prompt restoration of fluid volume deficits and, in later pregnancy, expedient delivery. No specific therapy is effective in acute cortical necrosis except for dialysis when needed. Both peritoneal dialysis and hemodialysis have been used during pregnancy, although peritoneal dialysis carries the risk of impairing uteroplacental blood flow.[298] In patients with septicemia, death occurs rapidly in a small percentage, but most respond to antibiotics and volume resuscitation. Survival is intimately linked with the management of and recovery from the AKI.[299]

ACUTE KIDNEY INJURY AND THROMBOTIC MICROANGIOPATHY

The presence of thrombotic microangiopathy and acute renal failure in pregnancy is one of the most challenging differential diagnoses to face the nephrologist caring for pregnant patients. Five pregnancy syndromes share many clinical, laboratory, and pathologic features: preeclampsia/HELLP syndrome, thrombotic thrombocytopenic purpura/hemolytic-uremic syndrome (HUS/TTP), acute fatty liver of pregnancy, systemic lupus erythematosus (SLE) with the antiphospholipid antibody syndrome, and disseminated intravascular coagulation (usually complicating sepsis). Although it is difficult to establish clinical distinctions between these entities with certainty, the confluence of clinical clues can often establish a likely diagnosis (see Table 49.4).

SEVERE PREECLAMPSIA

AKI is a rare complication of preeclampsia and is most frequently seen in the setting of coagulopathy, hepatic rupture, liver failure, or preexisting renal disease. When acute renal failure occurs in the patient with preeclampsia, urgent delivery is indicated.

ACUTE FATTY LIVER OF PREGNANCY

AFLP is a rare but potentially fatal complication of pregnancy, affecting about 1 in 10,000 pregnancies, with a 10% case-fatality rate.[300] The clinical picture is dominated by liver failure, with elevated serum aminotransferase values and hyperbilirubinemia. Severely affected patients have elevations in blood ammonia values and hypoglycemia. Preeclampsia can also be present in up to half of cases. Hemolysis and thrombocytopenia are not prominent features, and the presence of these findings should suggest the diagnosis of HELLP syndrome or HUS/TTP (see Table 49.4). Acute renal failure in association with acute fatty liver is seen mainly near term but can occur any time after midgestation.[301] The kidney lesion is mild and nonspecific, and the cause of renal failure is obscure. It may be due to hemodynamic changes akin to those seen in the hepatorenal syndrome or to a thrombotic microangiopathy.

Although liver biopsy is rarely undertaken clinically, AFLP is a pathologic diagnosis: Histologic changes include swollen hepatocytes filled with microvesicular fat and minimal hepatocellular necrosis. This histologic picture resembles that seen in Reye's syndrome and Jamaican vomiting sickness. A defect in mitochondrial fatty acid oxidation due to mutations in the long-chain 3-hydroxyacyl coenzyme A dehydrogenase gene was hypothesized as a risk factor for the development of AFLP.[302]

Management of AFLP includes supportive care, including aggressive management of the coagulopathy, and prompt termination of the pregnancy. The syndrome typically remits postpartum with no residual hepatic or renal impairment, although it can recur in subsequent pregnancies.

HEMOLYTIC-UREMIC SYNDROME/THROMBOTIC THROMBOCYTOPENIC PURPURA

HUS/TTP is characterized by hemolysis, thrombocytopenia, and variable organ dysfunction including acute renal failure.[303] Patients are thought to have TTP when neurologic symptoms dominate and HUS when renal failure is the dominant presenting feature.[304] Pregnancy appears to be associated with an increased risk of both TTP (usually manifesting prior to 24 weeks) and HUS (typically occurring near term or postpartum),[305] and pregnancy can precipitate relapse in women with a history of TTP.[306] Deficiency in the von Willebrand factor–cleaving protease (ADAMTS13) has been linked to the pathogenesis of TTP in nonpregnant states, but this relationship has not been well-studied in pregnancy. ADAMTS13 levels fall during the second and third trimesters, potentially contributing to the increased incidence of TTP in the latter half of pregnancy.[307]

The often challenging clinical distinction between HUS/TTP and preeclampsia/HELLP is important for patient management, because plasma exchange is beneficial in HUS/TTP but not in the HELLP syndrome. A history of preceding proteinuria, hypertension, and severe liver injury is more suggestive of HELLP syndrome, whereas the presence of renal failure and severe nonimmune hemolytic anemia is more typical of HUS/TTP (see Table 49.4). Although plasmapheresis for HUS/TTP in pregnancy and postpartum has not been evaluated in controlled studies, case series suggest that it is safe and effective.[306] Termination of pregnancy does not appear to alter the course of HUS/TTP, so thus is not generally recommended unless the fetus is compromised.

OBSTRUCTIVE UROPATHY AND NEPHROLITHIASIS

AKI due to bilateral ureteral obstruction is a rare complication of pregnancy. Because of the physiologic hydronephrosis of pregnancy (see "Physiologic Changes of Pregnancy" section), the diagnosis of frank urinary obstruction can be challenging. If clinical suspicion is high (e.g., marked hydronephrosis, abdominal pain, elevated serum creatinine), a percutaneous nephrostomy may be needed as a diagnostic and therapeutic trial to confirm the diagnosis of obstructive uropathy. If present, obstruction can be managed with ureteral stenting.[308] Massive hematuria from the right ureter in the postpartum period, subsiding spontaneously following decompression of the partially obstructed right collecting system, has been reported.[309]

Circulating levels of 1,25-dihydroxyvitamin D_3 are increased during normal pregnancy, resulting in increased intestinal calcium absorption. Urinary excretion of calcium is also increased, leading to a tendency in some women to form kidney stones. Excessive intake of calcium supplements can lead to hypercalcemia and hypercalciuria.

Although intestinal absorption and urinary excretion of calcium are increased, there is no evidence that the risk of nephrolithiasis is increased, possibly because of a concomitant increase in urine flow and physiologic dilation of the urinary tract.

Calcium oxalate and calcium phosphate constitute the majority of the stones produced during pregnancy. As in nonpregnant patients, ureteral calculi in pregnant women produce flank pain and lower abdominal pain with hematuria. Premature labor is sometimes induced by the intense pain, and the risk of infection is increased. Ultrasound examination is the preferred method to visualize obstruction and stones. The management of renal calculi is conservative with adequate hydration, analgesics, and antiemetics. Thiazide diuretics and allopurinol are contraindicated during pregnancy. Twenty-four–hour urine collection to quantify urinary calcium and uric acid excretion is recommended after delivery. Nephrolithiasis complicated by urinary tract infection should be treated with antibiotics for 3 to 5 weeks, followed by suppressive treatment after delivery, because the calculus may serve as a nidus of infection. Most stones pass spontaneously, but ureteral catheterization and placement of a ureteral stent may be required. Lithotripsy is relatively contraindicated during pregnancy because of adverse effects on the fetus. However, extracorporeal shock wave lithotripsy has been used during the first 4 to 8 weeks of pregnancy without known adverse consequences to the fetus.[310]

URINARY TRACT INFECTION AND ACUTE PYELONEPHRITIS (see also Chapter 37)

Infection of the urinary tract is the most common renal problem encountered during gestation.[311] Although the prevalence of asymptomatic bacteriuria in pregnant women—which ranges between 2% and 10%—is similar to that in nonpregnant populations, it needs to be managed more aggressively for several reasons. Physiologic hydronephrosis predisposes pregnant women to ascending pyelonephritis in the setting of cystitis. Hence, although asymptomatic bacteriuria in the nonpregnant state is usually benign, untreated asymptomatic bacteriuria in pregnancy can progress to overt cystitis or acute pyelonephritis in up to 40% of patients.[312] Acute pyelonephritis is a serious complication during pregnancy, usually manifesting between 20 and 28 weeks of gestation with fevers, loin pain, and dysuria. Sepsis resulting from pyelonephritis can progress to endotoxic shock, disseminated intravascular coagulation, and acute renal failure. Asymptomatic bacteriuria has also been associated with an increased risk of premature delivery and low birth weight.[313] Treatment of asymptomatic bacteriuria during pregnancy has been shown to reduce these complications and improve perinatal morbidity and mortality.[314] Thus, early detection and treatment of asymptomatic bacteriuria are warranted.

The usual signs and symptoms of urinary tract infection can be unreliable in pregnancy. Dysuria and urinary frequency are common during the latter half of pregnancy in the absence of infection, owing to pressure on the bladder from the gravid uterus. Low-grade pyuria is often present because of contamination by vaginal secretions. The use of the urinary dipstick to screen for bacteriuria is associated with a high false-negative rate, so quantitative urine culture is preferred for screening. More than 10^5 bacteria/mL of a single species indicates significant bacteriuria. Screening for asymptomatic bacteriuria is recommended during the first prenatal visit and is repeated only in high-risk women such as those with a history of recurrent urinary infections or urinary tract anomalies.

If asymptomatic bacteriuria is found, prompt treatment is warranted (usually with a cephalosporin) for at least 3 to 7 days.[315] Treatment with a single dose of fosfomycin has also been used successfully. Trimethoprim-sulfamethoxazole and tetracycline are contraindicated in early pregnancy because of their association with birth defects. A follow-up culture 2 weeks after treatment is necessary to ensure eradication of bacteriuria. Suppressive therapy with nitrofurantoin or cephalexin is recommended for patients with bacteriuria that persists after two courses of therapy.[316] Longer-term suppressive treatment of bacteriuria has been shown to reduce the incidence of pyelonephritis.[317] Because of the high maternal morbidity and mortality associated with pyelonephritis, it is usually treated aggressively with hospitalization, intravenous antibiotics, and hydration.

CHRONIC KIDNEY DISEASE AND PREGNANCY

Women who enter pregnancy with chronic kidney disease are at increased risk for adverse maternal and fetal outcomes, including rapid decline of renal function and perinatal mortality. Although the frequency of live births now exceeds 90% in such women, the risks for preterm delivery, IUGR, perinatal mortality, and preeclampsia are significantly elevated.[318,319] Preterm delivery results in both immediate and long-term morbidity for the offspring, with an increased risk of cardiovascular and renal diseases later in life.[320] The goals for pregnancy in women with chronic kidney disease are to preserve maternal renal function during and after pregnancy and to maximize the likelihood of successful term or near-term delivery for the fetus.

The physiologic increase in RBF and GFR characteristic of normal pregnancy is attenuated in chronic renal insufficiency.[319] The stress of greater RBF during pregnancy may exacerbate renal damage in the setting of preexisting renal disease, as in nonpregnancy states in which the impaired kidney is more sensitive to such insults. Indeed, worsening of hypertension and proteinuria are common during pregnancy if these conditions exist prior to pregnancy,[321] and in concert with these observations, overall maternal and fetal prognosis correlates with the severity of hypertension, proteinuria, and renal insufficiency prior to conception.

Fortunately, there is good evidence to suggest that women with underlying kidney disease but only mild renal impairment, normal blood pressure, and no proteinuria have good maternal and fetal outcomes, with little risk for accelerated progression toward ESKD.[319,322] However, even women with stage 1 chronic kidney disease are at increased risk for cesarean section, preterm delivery, and the need for neonatal intensive care in comparison with low-risk control pregnancies.[323] Although debate exists whether specific renal diseases are more commonly associated with an accelerated decline in renal function, data suggest that the degree of renal insufficiency, presence and severity of hypertension, and severity of proteinuria, rather than the underlying renal diagnosis, are the primary determinants of outcome.[323] Women who become pregnant with a serum creatinine value above 1.4 to 1.5 mg/dL are more likely to experience a decline in renal function than women with a comparable degree of renal dysfunction who do not become pregnant.[319] Initiating pregnancy with a serum creatinine value in excess of 2.0 mg/dL carries a high risk (>30%) for accelerated decline in renal function both during and after pregnancy.[318] Furthermore, of women with serum creatinine values higher than 2.5 mg/dL, more than 70% experience preterm delivery and more than 40% experience preeclampsia.[318,321] Measures to predict which women will experience rapid decline postpartum do not exist, and terminating pregnancy does not reliably reverse the decline in renal function. Data from women with autosomal dominant polycystic kidney disease and normal renal function suggest that there is high rate of successful uncomplicated pregnancies.[324] Other specific conditions, including diabetic nephropathy and lupus nephritis, are discussed later; however, regardless of the cause of renal disease, the tenet that a serum creatinine level above 1.4 to 1.5 mg/dL puts a woman at increased risk for renal decline holds true.

DIABETIC NEPHROPATHY AND PREGNANCY

The incidence and prevalence of diabetes throughout the world are rising, leading to an increase in the incidence and prevalence of diabetic nephropathy. Currently, more than 50% of patients with ESKD have diabetes.[325] Although diabetes is less common among women of childbearing age, the number of women entering pregnancy with diabetes is rising.[326] Women with pregestational diabetes, with or without nephropathy, have a higher risk of adverse fetal and maternal outcomes during pregnancy than nondiabetic women.[327-329] For example, the risk of preeclampsia in women with pregestational diabetes is more than double that seen in the general population.[328] The presence of albuminuria confers an additional risk: women with pre-pregnancy microalbuminuria are at increased risk for preeclampsia and preterm delivery.[330] Poor glycemic control before and during pregnancy has also been linked to preeclampsia and serious adverse fetal outcomes; hence endocrinologic consultation before pregnancy is strongly advised.[331,332]

Although it has been suggested that pregnancy negatively affects renal function in women with pregestational diabetes, pregnancy itself does not appear to adversely affect the progression of kidney disease if kidney function is normal or near normal at the start of pregnancy.[333] The prognosis changes, however, if renal function is impaired at that time. In comparison with preconception value, creatinine clearance is notably lower even within the first few months postpartum in women initiating pregnancy with impaired renal function.[334] In a study of 11 patients with diabetic nephropathy and serum creatinine values higher than 1.4 mg/dL at pregnancy onset, more than 40% progressed to end-stage kidney failure within 5 to 6 years after pregnancy.[335] Aggressive blood pressure control before and after pregnancy may attenuate the postpartum decline in renal function.[333] Nevertheless, inexorable decline in renal function following pregnancy is the rule rather than the exception in women initiating pregnancy with diabetic nephropathy and impaired renal function. For this reason, women with diabetic nephropathy are strongly advised to postpone pregnancy until after renal transplantation, which improves fertility status and fetal outcomes and does not lead to impaired renal function if allograft function is normal.

ACEIs and ARBs are contraindicated during pregnancy, and the inability to use these medications may contribute to the more rapid progression to renal failure in pregnant women with diabetic nephropathy and impaired renal function. Notably, these medications are toxic to the fetus if exposure occurs during the second or third trimester, leading to adverse outcomes, including hypocalvaria (hypoplasia of the membrane bones of the skull), renal tubular dysplasia, and IUGR.[286] Although surveillance studies find little to no adverse fetal consequences among women taking ACEIs in the first trimester,[286,336] exencephaly and unilateral renal agenesis were found in the fetus of a mother who was taking an ARB at conception.[337] Therefore, although preconception and postpartum (e.g., during breastfeeding) use of these medications appears to be safe, exposure during pregnancy, especially in the second or third trimester, is contraindicated.

The diabetic milieu during pregnancy may also subsequently affect metabolism and renal function in the offspring.[338,339] For example, in a cross-sectional study of 503 Pima Indians with type 2 diabetes, the prevalence of albuminuria was significantly higher in the offspring of mothers with diabetes during pregnancy (58%) than in the offspring of mothers without evidence of diabetes during pregnancy (40%).[339] It is speculated that abnormal in utero exposure in the offspring of diabetic mothers leads to impaired nephrogenesis and reduced nephron mass, and putting the offspring at higher risk for development of renal disease and hypertension in later life.

LUPUS NEPHRITIS AND PREGNANCY

SLE is one of the most common autoimmune diseases in women of childbearing age. During pregnancy, women with SLE are at increased risk for preterm birth, IUGR, spontaneous abortion, and preeclampsia.[340] The presence of superimposed renal disease increases the risk of these complications even further.[341,342] Over the last 20 years, improvements in disease management and perinatal monitoring have led to a decrease in pregnancy loss and preterm deliveries.[343] Outcomes, however, still appear to be poor in developing countries.[344] With careful planning, monitoring, and management, the majority of patients with SLE—especially those with normal baseline renal function—can complete pregnancy without serious maternal or fetal complications.[345]

Although there remains a long-standing debate about whether pregnancy itself induces a lupus flare, it is clear that active disease, compromised renal function, hypertension, or proteinuria at conception is associated with an increased risk of adverse fetal (e.g., fetal loss and preterm delivery) and maternal (e.g., preeclampsia, renal deterioration) outcomes.[346-348] Specific subsets of women with SLE are at especially high risk. For example, women with SLE and antiphospholipid antibodies have an increased risk of thrombosis, fetal loss, and preeclampsia.[349] Proliferative (World Health Organization [WHO] class III or IV) lupus nephritis is associated with a higher risk of preeclampsia and lower birth weights than mesangial (WHO class II) or membranous (WHO class V) lupus nephritis.[350] Women with lupus should postpone pregnancy until lupus activity is quiescent for approximately 6 months and doses of immunosuppressive agents are minimized.[351,352] Mycophenolate mofetil is teratogenic and should be replaced by azathioprine prior to conception; this approach is associated with a low risk of renal flares.[353] Importantly, prophylactic therapy with steroids does not appear to prevent a lupus flare during pregnancy[354]; however, immunosuppressives (e.g., steroids, azathioprine) have been used to manage lupus flares during pregnancy in hopes of extending pregnancy duration.

Pregnant women with a history of lupus nephritis are at risk both for a flare of the underlying renal disease and for preeclampsia. Unfortunately, both syndromes share the common presenting symptoms of hypertension and proteinuria, so distinguishing the two can be a clinical challenge.[355] In addition, women with proteinuric renal disease of any etiology usually have an increase in proteinuria as pregnancy continues owing to increased GFR (see "Renal Adaptation to Pregnancy" section), further clouding the differential diagnosis. The distinction between preeclampsia and lupus flare is critical, however, especially in women presenting prior to 37 weeks of gestation, because the treatments differ. For a lupus nephritis flare, steroids and azathioprine may quell the disease, allowing pregnancy to continue, whereas for preeclampsia, induction of delivery is the definitive treatment. Even in the medical literature reports of preeclampsia in the setting of lupus renal disease are prone to misclassification, because the diagnosis of preeclampsia is often based on blood pressure elevation and development of proteinuria[62] and not on results of renal biopsy or specific serologic testing. Alterations in components of the complement cascade (e.g., reductions in C_3, C_4, CH_{50}) have been used to identify pregnant women with a lupus flare and to distinguish lupus flare from preeclampsia.[356] Unfortunately, low complement levels and the presence of hematuria are neither sensitive nor specific for diagnosis of a lupus nephritis flare.[355,357] An "active" urinary sediment is common in lupus nephritis, whereas the sediment in preeclampsia is typically "bland." Nonetheless, distinguishing lupus flare from preeclampsia remains a challenge and requires frequent clinical assessment by a multidisciplinary team. Often a kidney biopsy is required. Although data on the safety of kidney biopsy during pregnancy are limited, clinical experience suggests that it is safe if undertaken prior to about 30 weeks of gestation.[358] Later in gestation, kidney biopsy is technically difficult because the gravid uterus makes the requisite prone position difficult. On the horizon, novel serologic tests for preeclampsia based on angiogenic factors may aid clinical decision making, especially during the critical period before term[62,355] (see "Screening for Preeclampsia" section).

Treatment of severe proliferative lupus nephritis in pregnancy is challenging, because conventional induction therapies are contraindicated owing to risk of congenital malformations with mycophenolate[359] and fetal loss associated with cyclophosphamide.[360] Prednisone is safe and commonly used in both patients with lupus nephritis and those with kidney transplants, though the risk of gestational diabetes is increased.[351] Calcineurin inhibitors are nonteratogenic and can be used to treat lupus nephritis in pregnancy, with some data to support their efficacy in the nonpregnant population.[351] Rituximab lacks safety data in pregnancy and is not recommended for use in pregnancy. Azathioprine, despite assignment to category D (evidence for human fetal risk based on human studies) by the FDA, is considered relatively safe in pregnancy and can be used as adjunctive or maintenance therapy in pregnant patients with lupus nephritis.

PREGNANCY DURING LONG-TERM DIALYSIS

End-stage kidney disease is characterized by severe hypothalamic-pituitary-gonadal dysfunction that is reversed by transplantation but not by conventional dialysis. Women of childbearing age undergoing dialysis have menstrual disturbances, anovulation, and infertility.[361] Animal studies suggest that uremia impairs fertility via aberrant neuroendocrine regulation of hypothalamic gonadotropin-releasing hormone (GnRH) secretion.[362] Gonadal function is impaired in men as well, who can experience testicular atrophy, hypospermatogenesis, infertility, and impotence.

Conception during dialysis is unusual but not impossible. Hence, adequate contraception remains important in women of childbearing age undergoing dialysis who do not wish to become pregnant. Although in a recent report U.S. Renal Data System investigators (USRDS) found that pregnancy and live birth rates over the past decade have increased in young women (<30 years of age) undergoing dialysis,[363] the literature on pregnancy in patients on dialysis remains dominated by case reports and small, single-center case series. Two surveys provide some insight into epidemiology. A 1994 survey of 206 U.S. dialysis units reported that 1.5% of 1281 women of childbearing age became pregnant over a 2-year period while on hemodialysis.[364] This finding was confirmed in a 1998 survey of 930 dialysis units, which reported that 2% of 6230 women of childbearing age became pregnant over a 4-year period.[365] In both studies, approximately half of pregnancies resulted in successful delivery of live infants, although the majority (84% in the 1994 study) were premature. Later reports of pregnancies in the setting of long-term hemodialysis have reported somewhat higher neonatal survival (70%-75%).[366-368] Adverse fetal outcomes are most often due to preterm labor, premature rupture of membranes, polyhydramnios, and IUGR. Likelihood of successful pregnancy is higher for women who conceive prior to initiation of dialysis than for women who conceive after initiation.[368]

When pregnancy does occur in a woman undergoing long-term hemodialysis, significant changes in management are required. Current guidelines recommend increasing the weekly dialysis dose to 20 or more hours per week, because this approach has been associated with improved neonatal outcomes and longer gestations.[365,369] Later data support this suggestion.[370] Increase in dialysis dose is often most realistically attained by daily nocturnal dialysis. Management of volume status is challenging because the dry weight increases throughout pregnancy, and hypovolemia needs to be vigilantly avoided. Medications must be carefully reviewed so as to avoid drugs toxic to the fetus, such as ACEIs. Erythropoietin dosing should be adjusted to approximate the physiologic anemia of pregnancy (10-11 g/dL), because high hematocrit has been associated with adverse fetal outcomes. Exacerbation of hypertension is common, although the incidence of preeclampsia is difficult to ascertain because of the inability to apply standard diagnostic criteria. Close monitoring of fetal well-being, in collaboration with an obstetrician, is essential after 24 weeks of gestation because early fetal distress is common. Data on pregnancy outcomes in peritoneal dialysis are even more limited but appear to be similar to those seen in patients undergoing hemodialysis.[365,371]

PREGNANCY IN THE KIDNEY TRANSPLANT RECIPIENT

Although women with ESKD who are undergoing dialysis are typically infertile, successful kidney transplantation results in a return to normal hormonal function and fertility within 6 months in approximately 90% of women of childbearing age.[372] More than 14,000 pregnancies in renal allograft recipients have been documented since 1958 (Figure 49.15).[373] Although the majority of pregnancies following kidney transplantation have excellent outcomes for both mother and fetus, such pregnancies are not without risk and require close monitoring and collaboration between the nephrologist and the obstetrician.[374,375] The goals of care in these patients are to optimize maternal health, including graft function and detection and management of hypertensive disorders of pregnancy, and to maximize the possibility of a healthy newborn.

FETAL AND NEONATAL OUTCOMES

Most data on pregnancy outcomes in transplant patients are derived from voluntary registries, case reports, and single-center retrospective studies. Four major registries, the U.S. National Pregnancy Transplantation Registry (NPTR),[376] the European Dialysis and Transplant Association Registry,[377] the UK Transplant Pregnancy Registry,[378] and the Australia New Zealand Dialysis and Transplant Registry,[379] have documented pregnancy outcomes on more than 2600 pregnancies in women with solid organ transplants. Statistics on the major complications of pregnancy are remarkably consistent. Approximately 22% of pregnancies among renal transplant recipients end in the first trimester, 13% because of miscarriage and the remainder because of elective termination.[376] Of pregnancies that continue, more than 90% result in a successful outcome for both mother and fetus; however, there is a substantial risk of low birth weight (25%-50%) and/or preterm delivery (30%-50%).[376,380] Ectopic pregnancy appears to be slightly increased, especially in pregnancies that occur soon after transplantation, but the rate remains below 1%. The rate of structural birth defects is no higher than the general population. Vaginal delivery is safe, and cesarean section should be performed only for obstetric indications.

TIMING OF PREGNANCY AFTER TRANSPLANTATION

Several factors need to be considered in the decision on how long to wait after transplantation before pregnancy can be attempted. Pregnancy within the first 6 to 12 months after transplantation is undesirable for several reasons. The risk of acute rejection is relatively high, immunosuppressant medications are at higher dosages, and risk of infection is greatest.[373] Traditionally it has been recommended that women wait about 2 years after transplantation before attempting conception.[381] However, many women who have undergone renal transplantation are of advanced maternal age, so delaying pregnancy may lead to age-related decreases in fertility. The American Society of Transplantation currently suggests that for women taking stable, low doses of immunosuppressive agents who have normal renal function and have had no prior rejection episodes, conception could be safely considered as early as 1 year after transplantation.[373]

EFFECT OF PREGNANCY ON RENAL ALLOGRAFT FUNCTION

Pregnancy itself does not appear to adversely affect graft function in transplant recipients, provided that baseline graft function is normal and significant hypertension is not present.[381] In general, when pregnancy occurs 1 to 2 years after transplantation, the rejection rate is similar to that seen in nonpregnant controls (3%-4%).[376] When moderate renal insufficiency is present (serum creatinine > 1.5-1.7 mg/dL), pregnancy does carry a risk of progressive renal dysfunction[382] as well as an increased risk of an SGA infant and of preeclampsia.[383]

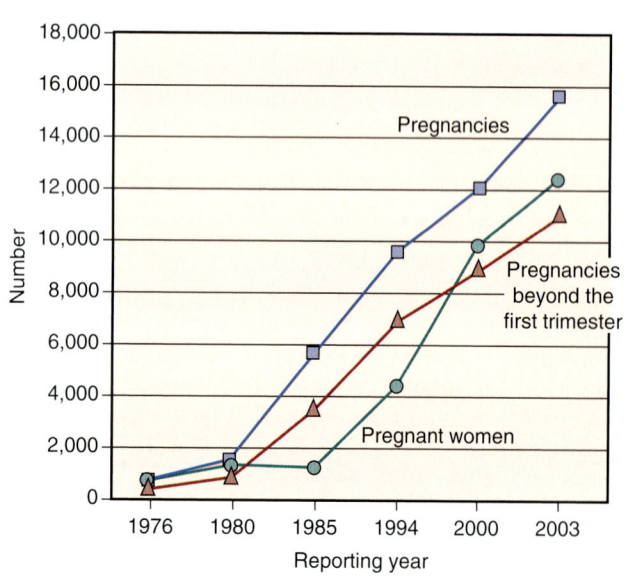

Figure 49.15 Pregnancies in kidney transplant recipients worldwide. The *circles* represent the numbers of pregnancies reported worldwide in kidney transplant recipients during the indicated year. The *numbers* include therapeutic terminations, spontaneous abortions, ectopic pregnancies, and stillbirths. The *squares* represent the numbers of transplant recipients reported to have been pregnant during that year, again including all outcomes. The *triangles* represent the numbers of pregnancies beyond the first trimester reported in the literature during the indicated year. The data are from the U.S. National Transplantation Pregnancy Registry, the European Dialysis and Transplant Association Registry, and the U.K. Transplant Pregnancy Registry. (From McKay DB, Josephson MA: Pregnancy in recipients of solid organs—effects on mother and child. *N Engl J Med* 354:1281-1293, 2006.)

Only two small case-control studies have reported long-term (>10-year) graft function after pregnancy. One study found that 10-year graft survival may be diminished in transplant recipients who became pregnant than in controls who did not become pregnant.[384] A second study reported no significant difference.[385] Further studies reporting long-term outcomes in the era of calcineurin inhibitors are needed.

Because of ongoing immunosuppression, transplant recipients are at risk for infections that have implications for the fetus, including cytomegalovirus, herpes simplex, and toxoplasmosis. The rate of bacterial urinary tract infections is increased (≈13%-40%),[382] but they are usually treatable and uncomplicated.

The most common complication of pregnancy in transplant recipients is hypertension, which affects between 30% and 75% of pregnancies among transplant recipients.[376,386] Hypertension is likely due to a combination of underlying medical conditions and the use of calcineurin inhibitors. Preeclampsia complicates 25% to 30% of pregnancies in kidney transplant recipients,[376,380,382] and diagnosis is often challenging because of the frequent presence of hypertension and/or proteinuria at baseline. The American Society of Transplantation recommends that hypertension in pregnant renal transplant recipients should be managed aggressively, with target blood pressure close to normal—a goal that differs from somewhat higher blood pressure goals in women with hypertension during pregnancy who have not undergone transplantation.[286,373] Agents of choice (see Table 49.5) include methyldopa, nonselective β-adrenergic antagonists (e.g. labetalol), and calcium channel blockers. ACEIs are contraindicated at every point in pregnancy except the early first trimester and even then should be avoided. Details about the use of these agents in pregnancy are discussed in greater detail in the section on chronic hypertension and gestational hypertension.

MANAGEMENT OF IMMUNOSUPPRESSIVE THERAPY IN PREGNANCY

The FDA classifies drugs as pregnancy categories A (no risk in controlled studies), B (no evidence of risk in humans), C (risk cannot be ruled out), D (positive evidence of risk), and X (contraindicated). Because controlled studies on developmental toxicity due to immunosuppressive agents cannot be performed for ethical reasons, most immunosuppressive agents fall into category C. Nevertheless, there is a significant amount of published data that can inform decisions to use some of these agents safely in pregnancy (Table 49.6).

Cyclosporine (or tacrolimus) and steroids, with or without azathioprine, form the basis of immunosuppression during pregnancy. Corticosteroids at low to moderate doses (5-10 mg/day) are safe and prednisone is classified as pregnancy category B.[387] Stress-dose steroids are needed at the time of delivery and for 24 to 48 hours after delivery. Azathioprine is generally considered safe at doses less than 2 mg/kg/day, although higher doses are associated with congenital anomalies, immunosuppression, and IUGR and thus should be avoided if possible.[381]

Although high doses of both cyclosporine and tacrolimus are associated with fetal resorption in animal studies, both animal and human data suggest that lower doses of calcineurin inhibitors are safe in pregnancy.[387,388] Experience with tacrolimus is more limited than that for cyclosporine, but growing.[388,389] Clinical data have not demonstrated an increased incidence of congenital malformations with the possible exception of low birth weight.[387] Owing to decreased gastrointestinal absorption, increased volume of distribution, and increased GFR, levels of cyclosporine and tacrolimus can fluctuate significantly in pregnancy, with concomitant risk of acute rejection. Hence, close monitoring of blood levels with dosing adjustment are required to maintain optimal levels.[388]

Sirolimus is contraindicated in pregnancy as it is teratogenic in rats at doses used clinically.[387] The risk of fetal malformations is highest at 30 to 71 days of gestation, so there is a window during which sirolimus should be stopped if pregnancy is detected early. Nevertheless, sirolimus should be discontinued preemptively in women of childbearing age who are not using contraception.

Mycophenolate mofetil is associated with developmental toxicity, malformations, and intrauterine death in animal

Table 49.6 Immunosuppressive Medications in Pregnancy

Drug*	Recommendations
Prednisone (B)	Safe when used long term at low to moderate doses (5-10 mg/day) Safe when given acutely at high doses
Cyclosporine (C)	Extensive clinical data suggest safe at low to moderate clinical doses Changes in absorption and metabolism require close monitoring of levels and frequent dose adjustments in pregnancy
Tacrolimus (C)	Similar to those for cyclosporine, although somewhat less data available
Sirolimus (C)	Embryo/fetal toxicity in rodents was manifested as mortality and reduced fetal weights (with associated delays in skeletal ossification); human studies are lacking
Azathioprine (D)	Considered safe at dosages less than 2 mg/kg per day, but at higher doses associated with fetal growth restriction
Mycophenolate mofetil (D)	Contraindicated in pregnancy (teratogenic in animal and human studies)
Muromonab-CD3 (OKT-3) (C)	Case reports of successful use for induction in unsuspected pregnancy and for acute rejection, but data are limited
Antithymocyte globulin (C)	Animal studies have not been reported, and there are no controlled data from use in human pregnancy

*U.S. Food and Drug Administration (FDA) pregnancy-use category designations for the individual drugs are shown in parentheses.
(Adapted from McKay DB, Josephson MA: Pregnancy after kidney transplantation. Clin J Am Soc Nephrol 3(Suppl 2):S117-S125, 2008.)

studies at therapeutic dosages. Human data are limited to isolated case reports but suggest that mycophenolate mofetil may be associated with spontaneous abortion and with major fetal malformations,[390] especially when used in combination with cyclosporine.[387] Hence mycophenolate mofetil, like sirolimus, should be avoided in pregnancy. For a more detailed discussion of data on the effects of these agents on neonatal immunologic function and long-term outcomes, the reader is referred to reviews by Josephson and McKay.[375,391]

MANAGEMENT OF ACUTE REJECTION IN PREGNANCY

The incidence of acute kidney transplant rejection during pregnancy is similar to that of the nonpregnant transplant population[376,381]; however, the diagnosis of acute rejection during pregnancy can be difficult. Acute rejection should be suspected if fever, oliguria, graft tenderness, or deterioration in renal function is noted. Biopsy of the renal graft should be performed to confirm the diagnosis prior to initiation of treatment. Although high-dose steroid therapy has been associated with fetal malformations and maternal infections, it remains a mainstay of treatment of acute rejection during pregnancy.[381,392] Little data are available on the safety of agents such as OKT-3, antithymocyte globulin, daclizumab, and basiliximab in pregnancy (see Table 49.6).[387] The National Transplantation Pregnancy Registry reported five cases of OKT-3 use during pregnancy, with four surviving infants.[376] Polyclonal and monoclonal antibodies would be expected to cross the placenta, but their fetal effects are largely unknown.

BREASTFEEDING AND IMMUNOSUPPRESSIVE AGENTS

Studies on the transfer of calcineurin inhibitors to the babies of breastfeeding mothers are inconsistent, with some studies reporting undetectable levels[387,393] and others reporting high neonatal blood concentrations.[394] There are no reports on adverse neonatal effects with use of cyclosporine or tacrolimus in breastfeeding. Limited data suggest that tacrolimus levels are very low in breast milk. Investigators from the National Transplantation Pregnancy Registry recommend that breastfeeding should not be discouraged in women taking tacrolimus.[395] When cyclosporine or tacrolimus is used in a lactating mother, consideration should be given to monitoring neonatal blood concentrations for potential toxicity. Theoretically, mycophenolate mofetil should be safe in breastfeeding because the active metabolite secreted in breast milk, mycophenolic acid, is not gastrointestinally available; however, human evidence of safety is lacking. Nevertheless, breastfeeding among transplant recipients remains controversial.[375]

PREGNANCY OUTCOME FOLLOWING KIDNEY DONATION

Data on pregnancy outcomes after kidney donation in young women of childbearing age suggest that such women have a lower risk for full-term deliveries and higher risks for fetal loss and for development of gestational diabetes, gestational hypertension, and preeclampsia during pregnancy.[396] If these data are corroborated (some were derived from questionnaire responses and hence subject to recall and response bias), eligibility criteria for future donors may be changed.[397]

Complete reference list available at ExpertConsult.com.

KEY REFERENCES

1. Poppas A, Shroff SG, Korcarz CE, et al: Serial assessment of the cardiovascular system in normal pregnancy. Role of arterial compliance and pulsatile arterial load. *Circulation* 95:2407–2415, 1997.
2. Chapman AB, Abraham WT, Zamudio S, et al: Temporal relationships between hormonal and hemodynamic changes in early human pregnancy. *Kidney Int* 54:2056–2063, 1998.
24. Novak J, Danielson LA, Kerchner LJ, et al: Relaxin is essential for renal vasodilation during pregnancy in conscious rats. *J Clin Invest* 107:1469–1475, 2001.
32. Duley L: The global impact of pre-eclampsia and eclampsia. *Semin Perinatol* 33:130–137, 2009.
41. Ananth CV, Keyes KM, Wapner RJ: Pre-eclampsia rates in the United States, 1980-2010: age-period-cohort analysis. *BMJ* 347:f6564, 2013.
55. American College of Obstetricians and Gynecologists; Task Force on Hypertension in Pregnancy: Hypertension in pregnancy. Report of the American College of Obstetricians and Gynecologists' Task Force on Hypertension in Pregnancy. *Obstet Gynecol* 122:1122–1131, 2013.
58. Cote AM, Brown MA, Lam E, et al: Diagnostic accuracy of urinary spot protein:creatinine ratio for proteinuria in hypertensive pregnant women: systematic review. *BMJ* 336:1003–1006, 2008.
70. Haddad B, Barton JR, Livingston JC, et al: Risk factors for adverse maternal outcomes among women with HELLP (hemolysis, elevated liver enzymes, and low platelet count) syndrome. *Am J Obstet Gynecol* 183:444–448, 2000.
77. Bellamy L, Casas JP, Hingorani AD, et al: Pre-eclampsia and risk of cardiovascular disease and cancer in later life: systematic review and meta-analysis. *BMJ* 335:974, 2007.
81. Mosca L, Benjamin EJ, Berra K, et al: Effectiveness-based guidelines for the prevention of cardiovascular disease in women—2011 update: a guideline from the American Heart Association. *Circulation* 123:1243–1262, 2011.
83. Vikse BE, Irgens LM, Leivestad T, et al: Preeclampsia and the risk of end-stage renal disease. *N Engl J Med* 359:800–809, 2008.
92. Soleymanlou N, Jurisica I, Nevo O, et al: Molecular evidence of placental hypoxia in preeclampsia. *J Clin Endocrinol Metab* 90:4299–4308, 2005.
98. Lyall F, Robson SC, Bulmer JN: Spiral artery remodeling and trophoblast invasion in preeclampsia and fetal growth restriction: relationship to clinical outcome. *Hypertension* 62:1046–1054, 2013.
101. Zhou Y, Fisher SJ, Janatpour M, et al: Human cytotrophoblasts adopt a vascular phenotype as they differentiate. A strategy for successful endovascular invasion? *J Clin Invest* 99:2139–2151, 1997.
111. Mills JL, DerSimonian R, Raymond E, et al: Prostacyclin and thromboxane changes predating clinical onset of preeclampsia: a multicenter prospective study. *JAMA* 282:356–362, 1999.
114. Khan F, Belch JJ, MacLeod M, et al: Changes in endothelial function precede the clinical disease in women in whom preeclampsia develops. *Hypertension* 46:1123–1128, 2005.
119. Lafayette RA, Malik T, Druzin M, et al: The dynamics of glomerular filtration after caesarean section. *J Am Soc Nephrol* 10:1561–1565, 1999.
127. Roberts JM, Myatt L, Spong CY, et al: Vitamins C and E to prevent complications of pregnancy-associated hypertension. *N Engl J Med* 362:1282–1291, 2010.
140. Powe CE, Levine RJ, Karumanchi SA: Preeclampsia, a disease of the maternal endothelium: the role of antiangiogenic factors and implications for later cardiovascular disease. *Circulation* 123:2856–2869, 2011.
141. Maynard SE, Min JY, Merchan J, et al: Excess placental soluble fms-like tyrosine kinase 1 (sFlt1) may contribute to endothelial dysfunction, hypertension, and proteinuria in preeclampsia. *J Clin Invest* 111:649–658, 2003.
144. Levine RJ, Maynard SE, Qian C, et al: Circulating angiogenic factors and the risk of preeclampsia. *N Engl J Med* 350:672–683, 2004.

148. Bergmann A, Ahmad S, Cudmore M, et al: Reduction of circulating soluble Flt-1 alleviates preeclampsia-like symptoms in a mouse model. *J Cell Mol Med* 14:1857–1867, 2010.
150. Sela S, Itin A, Natanson-Yaron S, et al: A novel human-specific soluble vascular endothelial growth factor receptor 1: cell type-specific splicing and implications to vascular endothelial growth factor homeostasis and preeclampsia. *Circ Res* 102:1566–1574, 2008.
153. Venkatesha S, Toporsian M, Lam C, et al: Soluble endoglin contributes to the pathogenesis of preeclampsia. *Nat Med* 12:642–649, 2006.
157. Levine RJ, Lam C, Qian C, et al: Soluble endoglin and other circulating antiangiogenic factors in preeclampsia. *N Engl J Med* 355:992–1005, 2006.
164. Eremina V, Sood M, Haigh J, et al: Glomerular-specific alterations of VEGF-A expression lead to distinct congenital and acquired renal diseases. *J Clin Invest* 111:707–716, 2003.
167. Eremina V, Jefferson JA, Kowalewska J, et al: VEGF inhibition and renal thrombotic microangiopathy. *N Engl J Med* 358:1129–1136, 2008.
168. Patel TV, Morgan JA, Demetri GD, et al: A preeclampsia-like syndrome characterized by reversible hypertension and proteinuria induced by the multitargeted kinase inhibitors sunitinib and sorafenib. *J Natl Cancer Inst* 100:282–284, 2008.
169. Garovic VD, Wagner SJ, Turner ST, et al: Urinary podocyte excretion as a marker for preeclampsia. *Am J Obstet Gynecol* 196:320.e1–320.e7, 2007.
185. Zhou CC, Zhang Y, Irani RA, et al: Angiotensin receptor agonistic autoantibodies induce pre-eclampsia in pregnant mice. *Nat Med* 14:855–862, 2008.
204. Poon LC, Kametas NA, Maiz N, et al: First-trimester prediction of hypertensive disorders in pregnancy. *Hypertension* 53:812–818, 2009.
210. Noori M, Donald AE, Angelakopoulou A, et al: Prospective study of placental angiogenic factors and maternal vascular function before and after preeclampsia and gestational hypertension. *Circulation* 122:478–487, 2010.
222. Rolfo A, Attini R, Nuzzo AM, et al: Chronic kidney disease may be differentially diagnosed from preeclampsia by serum biomarkers. *Kidney Int* 83:177–181, 2013.
223. Perni U, Sison C, Sharma V, et al: Angiogenic factors in superimposed preeclampsia: a longitudinal study of women with chronic hypertension during pregnancy. *Hypertension* 59:740–746, 2012.
224. Rana S, Powe CE, Salahuddin S, et al: Angiogenic factors and the risk of adverse outcomes in women with suspected preeclampsia. *Circulation* 125:911–919, 2012.
235. Askie LM, Duley L, Henderson-Smart DJ, et al: Antiplatelet agents for prevention of pre-eclampsia: a meta-analysis of individual patient data. *Lancet* 369:1791–1798, 2007.
239. Villar J, Purwar M, Merialdi M, et al: World Health Organisation multicentre randomised trial of supplementation with vitamins C and E among pregnant women at high risk for pre-eclampsia in populations of low nutritional status from developing countries. *BJOG* 116:780–788, 2009.
254. Sibai BM, Mercer BM, Schiff E, et al: Aggressive versus expectant management of severe preeclampsia at 28 to 32 weeks' gestation: a randomized controlled trial. *Am J Obstet Gynecol* 171:818–822, 1994.
258. von Dadelszen P, Ornstein M, Bull S, et al: Fall in mean arterial pressure and fetal growth restriction in pregnancy hypertension: a meta-analysis. *Lancet* 355:87–92, 2000.
260. Lucas MJ, Leveno KJ, Cunningham FG: A comparison of magnesium sulfate with phenytoin for the prevention of eclampsia. *N Engl J Med* 333:201–206, 1995.
265. Thadhani R, Kisner T, Hagmann H, et al: Pilot study of extracorporeal removal of soluble fms-like tyrosine kinase 1 in preeclampsia. *Circulation* 124:940–950, 2011.
286. Podymow T, August P, Umans JG: Antihypertensive therapy in pregnancy. *Semin Nephrol* 24:616–625, 2004.
289. Cooper WO, Hernandez-Diaz S, Arbogast PG, et al: Major congenital malformations after first-trimester exposure to ACE inhibitors. *N Engl J Med* 354:2443–2451, 2006.
302. Ibdah JA, Bennett MJ, Rinaldo P, et al: A fetal fatty-acid oxidation disorder as a cause of liver disease in pregnant women. *N Engl J Med* 340:1723–1731, 1999.
312. Hill JB, Sheffield JS, McIntire DD, et al: Acute pyelonephritis in pregnancy. *Obstet Gynecol* 105:18–23, 2005.
323. Piccoli GB, Attini R, Vasario E, et al: Pregnancy and chronic kidney disease: a challenge in all CKD stages. *Clin J Am Soc Nephrol* 5:844–855, 2010.
340. Wagner SJ, Craici I, Reed D, et al: Maternal and foetal outcomes in pregnant patients with active lupus nephritis. *Lupus* 18:342–347, 2009.
353. Fischer-Betz R, Specker C, Brinks R, et al: Low risk of renal flares and negative outcomes in women with lupus nephritis conceiving after switching from mycophenolate mofetil to azathioprine. *Rheumatology (Oxford)* 52:1070–1076, 2013.
370. Asamiya Y, Otsubo S, Matsuda Y, et al: The importance of low blood urea nitrogen levels in pregnant patients undergoing hemodialysis to optimize birth weight and gestational age. *Kidney Int* 75:1217–1222, 2009.
391. Josephson MA, McKay DB: Pregnancy and kidney transplantation. *Semin Nephrol* 31:100–110, 2011.

50 Antihypertensive Therapy

Matthew R. Weir | Donna S. Hanes | David K. Klassen | Walter G. Wasser

CHAPTER OUTLINE

PHARMACOLOGY OF THE NONDIURETIC ANTIHYPERTENSIVE DRUGS, 1640
Angiotensin-Converting Enzyme Inhibitors, 1640
Angiotensin II Type 1 Receptor Antagonists, 1651
β-Adrenergic Antagonists, 1656
Calcium Channel Blockers, 1662
Central Adrenergic Agonists, 1671
Central and Peripheral Adrenergic Neuronal Blocking Agent, 1673
Direct-Acting Vasodilators, 1673
Endothelin Receptor Antagonists, 1675
Moderately Selective Peripheral α_1-Adrenergic Antagonists, 1675
Peripheral α_1-Adrenergic Antagonists, 1676
Renin Inhibitors, 1677
Selective Aldosterone Receptor Antagonists, 1678
Tyrosine Hydroxylase Inhibitor, 1679

SELECTION OF ANTIHYPERTENSIVE DRUG THERAPY, 1680
Determination of Blood Pressure Goal, 1680
Single-Pill Combination Therapy, 1681
Choice of Appropriate Agents, 1682
Strategies for Selecting the Optimal Combination Antihypertensive Therapy, 1689
Specific Drug Combinations, 1690
Bedtime Antihypertensive Dosing Versus Morning Dosing, 1692
Resistant Hypertension, 1693
DRUG TREATMENT OF HYPERTENSIVE URGENCIES AND EMERGENCIES, 1695
Parenteral Drugs and Direct-Acting Vasodilators, 1696
Rapid-Acting Oral Drugs, 1699
Clinical Considerations in the Rapid Reduction of Blood Pressure, 1699

This chapter is divided into three major sections. The first section reviews the pharmacology of nondiuretic antihypertensive drugs to provide clinicians with a complete overview of how to use these therapies safely in practice (Table 50.1; see Chapter 51 for a review of diuretic drugs). The first section also discusses individual drug classes and highlights the class mechanisms of action, members, renal effects, and efficacy and safety. Individual similarities and differences within and between classes are then addressed. The second section reviews clinical decision making with regard to the selection of antihypertensive therapy, blood pressure (BP) goals, and considerations in choosing the first agent or using fixed-dose combination therapy, as well as methods of dealing with refractory hypertension. The third section reviews the pharmacology of the parenteral and oral drugs available for the management of hypertensive urgencies and emergencies and discusses clinical considerations in seeking to achieve rapid reduction of BP. The history of the development of modern antihypertensive drug therapy is shown in Figure 50.1.

PHARMACOLOGY OF THE NONDIURETIC ANTIHYPERTENSIVE DRUGS

ANGIOTENSIN-CONVERTING ENZYME INHIBITORS

CLASS MECHANISMS OF ACTION

Angiotensin-converting enzyme (ACE) inhibitors inhibit the activity of ACE, which converts the inactive decapeptide angiotensin I (Ang I) into the potent hormone angiotensin II (Ang II) (Figure 50.2). Because Ang II plays a crucial role in maintaining and regulating BP levels by promoting vasoconstriction and renal sodium and water retention, ACE inhibitors are powerful tools for targeting multiple pathways that contribute to hypertension. ACE inhibitors directly reduce the circulating and tissue levels of Ang II, thus blocking the potent vasoconstriction induced by the hormone (see Table 50.2).[1] The resulting decrease in peripheral vascular resistance is not accompanied by cardiac output or

Table 50.1	Pharmacologic Classification of Nondiuretic Antihypertensive Drugs

Angiotensin-converting enzyme inhibitors
    Sulfhydryl
    Carboxyl
    Phosphinyl
Angiotensin II type 1 receptor antagonists
    Biphenyl tetrazoles
    Nonbiphenyl tetrazoles
    Nonheterocyclics
β-Adrenergic antagonists and α1- and β-adrenergic antagonists
    Nonselective β-adrenergic antagonists
    Nonselective β-adrenergic antagonists with partial agonist activity
    β1-Selective adrenergic antagonists
    β1-Selective adrenergic antagonists with partial agonist activity
    Nonselective β-adrenergic and α1-adrenergic antagonists
Calcium antagonists
    Benzothiazepines
    Dihydropyridines
    Diphenylalkylamines
    Tetralines
Central α2-adrenergic agonists
Central and peripheral adrenergic-neuronal blocking agents
Direct-acting vasodilators
Moderately selective peripheral α1-adrenergic antagonists
Peripheral α1-adrenergic antagonists
Peripheral adrenergic-neuronal blocking agents
Renin inhibitors
Selective aldosterone receptor antagonists
Tyrosine hydroxylase inhibitors
Vasopeptidase inhibitors*

*Not approved for the treatment of hypertension.

Table 50.2	Antihypertensive Mechanisms of Action of Angiotensin-Converting Enzyme Inhibitors

Lower peripheral vascular resistance.
Inhibit the breakdown of vasodilatory bradykinins.
Enhance vasodilatory prostaglandin synthesis.
Improve nitric oxide–mediated endothelial function.
Reverse vascular hypertrophy.
Decrease aldosterone secretion.
Induce natriuresis.
Augment renal blood flow.
Blunt sympathetic nervous system activity and pressor responses.
Inhibit norepinephrine and arginine vasopressin release.
Inhibit baroreceptor reflexes.
Reduce endothelin-1 levels.
Inhibit thirst.
Inhibit oxidation of cholesterol.
Inhibit collagen deposition in target organs.

glomerular filtration rate (GFR) changes; the heart rate is unchanged or may be reduced in patients with baseline heart rates higher than 85 beats/min.[2]

A reduction in systemic and local levels of Ang II leads to effects beyond vasodilation that contribute to the antihypertensive efficacy of ACE inhibitors (Table 50.2).[3] Additional mechanisms include the following: (1) inhibition of the breakdown of vasodilatory bradykinins catalyzed by ACE or kininase II (the hypotensive action of ACE inhibitors is blocked, in part, by bradykinin antagonists)[4]; (2) enhancement of vasodilatory prostaglandin synthesis; (3) improvement of nitric oxide–mediated endothelial function[5,6] and upregulation of endothelial progenitor cells[7]; (4) reversal of vascular hypertrophy[8]; (5) decrease in aldosterone secretion; (6) augmentation of renal blood flow to induce natriuresis[9]; (7) blunting of sympathetic nervous system activity[10-12] through presynaptic modulation of norepinephrine release; (8) inhibition of postjunctional pressor responses to norepinephrine or Ang II[11,13]; (9) inhibition of central Ang II–mediated sympathoexcitation, norepinephrine synthesis, and arginine vasopressin release; (10) inhibition of centrally controlled baroreceptor reflexes, which results in increased baroreceptor sensitivity[13]; (11) decrease in vasoconstrictor endothelin-1 levels[14]; (12) inhibition of thirst; (13) inhibition of cholesterol oxidation[15]; and (14) inhibition of collagen deposition in target organs.[16]

CLASS MEMBERS

Currently, there are more than 15 ACE inhibitors in clinical use. Each drug has a unique structure that determines its potency, tissue receptor binding affinity, metabolism, and prodrug compound, but they have remarkably similar clinical effects (Tables 50.3 and 50.4).[3] The drugs are classified into sulfhydryl, carboxyl, or phosphinyl categories on the basis of the ligand that binds to the ACE-zinc moiety.

Sulfhydryl Angiotensin-Converting Enzyme Inhibitors

Captopril is a sulfhydryl-containing ACE inhibitor that is available in tablets of 12.5, 25, and 50 mg (see Tables 50-3 and 50-4).[12,17,18] The usual starting dosage for hypertension treatment is 25 mg two or three times daily (see Table 50.2), and the dosage can be titrated at 1- to 2-week intervals.[12] Captopril has 75% bioavailability, with peak onset within 1 hour. The half-life is 2 hours; with long-term administration, the hemodynamic effects are maintained for 3 to 8 hours.[12] Food may decrease captopril absorption by up to 54%, but this decrease is clinically insignificant.[19] Captopril is partially metabolized in the liver into an inactive compound; 95% of the parent compound and metabolites are eliminated in the urine within 24 hours. The elimination half-life increases markedly in patients with creatinine clearances of less than 20 mL/min/1.73 m^2. In such patients, the initial dosages should be reduced, and smaller increments should be used for titration. Hemodialysis removes approximately 35% of the dose.[12,20]

Carboxyl Angiotensin-Converting Enzyme Inhibitors

Benazepril hydrochloride is a long-acting, non–sulfhydryl-containing, carboxyl ACE inhibitor that is available as 10- or 20-mg tablets alone or in combination with amlodipine.[18] The usual initial dosage is 10 mg daily, with maintenance dosages of 20 to 40 mg daily. Some patients respond better

THE HISTORY OF ANTIHYPERTENSIVES
Reserpine, Pentolinium, Guanethidine, Methyl dopa (1950–1960), Clonidine (1980)

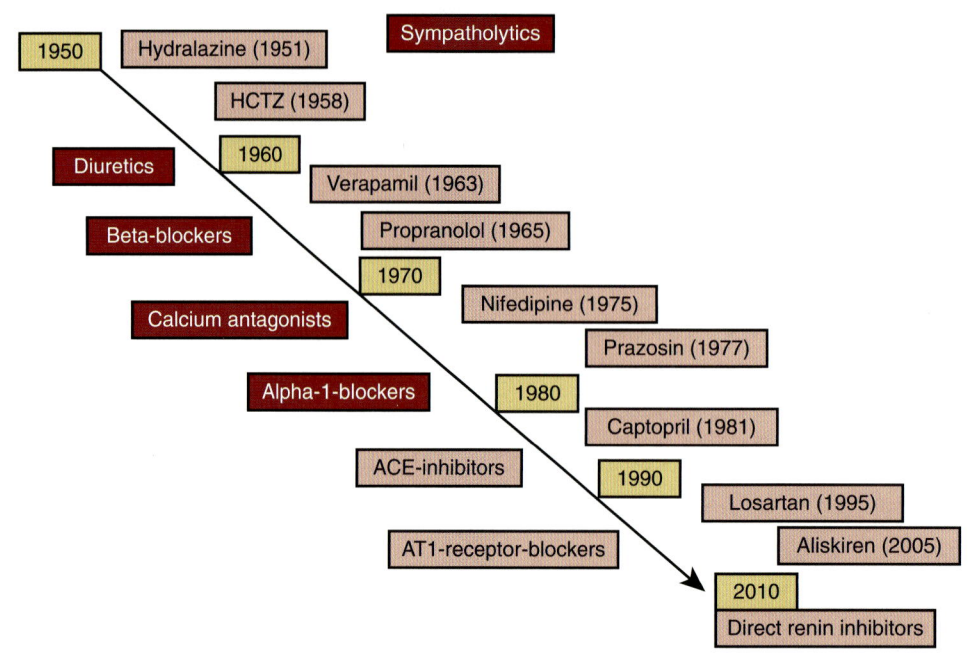

Figure 50.1 History of modern antihypertensive drug therapy. The first antihypertensive drug, hydralazine, was a nonspecific vasodilator discovered in the 1950s. This was followed by blockade of calcium channels on vascular smooth muscle cells, the calcium channel blockers in the 1960s, and blockade of postsynaptic α-adrenoceptors on peripheral sympathetic neurons, the alpha blockers in the late 1970s. Blockade by the renin angiotensin aldosterone system (RAAS) by angiotensin-converting enzyme inhibitors was discovered in the 1980s, angiotensin receptor blockers in the 1990s, and direct renin inhibitors just 10 years ago. HCTZ, Hydrochlorothiazide. (From Sever PS, Messerli FH: Hypertension management 2011: optimal combination therapy. *Eur Heart J* 32:2499-2506, 2011.)

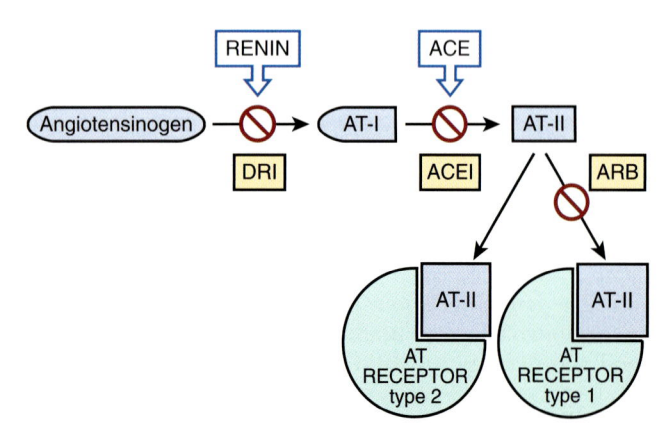

Figure 50.2 Renin angiotensin aldosterone system (RAAS)—effect site for each type of RAAS blocking drugs. The two major classes of drugs that target the RAAS are the angiotensin-converting enzyme inhibitors (ACEIs) and the selective AT_1 receptor blockers (ARBs). Both these drug classes target angiotensin II, but the differences in their mechanisms of action have implications for their effects on other pathways and receptors. Both ACEIs and ARBs are effective antihypertensive agents that have been shown to reduce the risk of cardiovascular and renal events. Direct inhibition of renin—the most proximal aspect of the RAAS—became clinically feasible in 2007 with the introduction of aliskiren. AT, Angiotensin. (From Robles NR, Cerezo I, Hernandez-Gallego R: Renin-angiotensin system blocking drugs. *J Cardiovasc Pharmacol Ther* 19:14-33, 2014.)

to twice-daily dosing (see Tables 50-3 and 50-4).[21] The onset of action occurs in 2 to 6 hours; maximal antihypertensive responsiveness occurs in 2 weeks. Benazepril is a prodrug that is rapidly bioactivated in the liver into the active benazeprilat compound, which is 200 times more potent than benazepril. The elimination half-life of benazeprilat is 22 hours. Benazeprilat is excreted primarily in the urine. Dialysis does not remove benazepril, but the initial dose should be no more than 10 mg in patients with a creatinine clearance of less than 60 mL/min/1.73 m², and the dose should be reduced to 5 mg in patients with a creatinine clearance of less than 30 mL/min/1.73 m².[22]

Cilazapril is a nonsulfhydryl prodrug of the long-acting ACE inhibitor cilazaprilat.[12,18] The usual dosage is 2.5 to 10 mg daily or in divided doses. After absorption, cilazapril is rapidly de-esterified in the liver to its active metabolite, cilazaprilat. The initial antihypertensive response occurs in 1 to 2 hours, peaks at 6 hours, and lasts for 8 to 12 hours.[23] Dosages should be reduced by 25% in renal failure patients.[22,24]

Enalapril maleate is a nonsulfhydryl prodrug of the long-acting ACE inhibitor enalaprilat.[18,25] The oral preparations are available in tablets of 2.5, 5, 10, and 20 mg. The initial dosage of enalapril is 5 mg once daily (see Table 50.3). The usual daily dose is 10 to 40 mg, singly or in divided doses. Initial responses occur in 1 hour, and peak serum levels of enalaprilat are achieved in 3 to 4 hours. Enalapril undergoes biotransformation in the liver into the active compound, enalaprilat (see Table 50.4). Enalapril is excreted

Table 50.3 Pharmacodynamic Properties of Angiotensin-Converting Enzyme Inhibitors

Generic Name (Trade Name)	Initial Dose (mg)	Usual Dose (mg)	Maximum Dose (mg)	Interval	Peak Response (hr)	Duration of Response (hr)
Alacepril (Cetapril)	12.5	12.5-100	100	qd	3	24
Captopril (Capoten)	25	12.5-50	150	tid	1-2	3-8
Benazepril (Lotensin)	10	20-40	40	qd	2-6	24
Enalapril (Vasotec)	5	10-40	40	qd, bid	3-4	12-24
Moexipril (Univasc)	7.5	7.5-30	30	qd, bid	3-6	24
Quinapril (Accupril)	10	20-80	80	qd	2	24
Ramipril (Altace)	2.5	2.5-20	40	qd, bid	2	24
Trandolapril (Mavik)	1	2-4	8	qd	2-12	24
Fosinopril (Monopril)	5	5-40	40	qd, bid	2-7	24
Cilazapril (Dynorm)	2.5	2.5-10	10	qd, bid	6	8-12
Perindopril (Aceon)	4	4-8	8	qd	3-7	24
Spirapril (SCH 33844)	6	6	6	qd	3-6	24
Zofenopril (SQ 26991)	30	30-60	60	qd	—	—
Lisinopril (Zestril, Prinivil)	10	20-40	40	qd	6	24
Imidapril (TA 6366)	10	10-40	40	qd	5-6	24

Table 50.4 Pharmacokinetic Properties of Angiotensin Converting Enzyme Inhibitors

Drug	Absorption (%)	Bioavailability (%)	Affected by Food	Peak Blood Level (hr)	Elimination Half-Life (hr)	Metabolism	Excretion	Active Metabolites
Alacepril	—	70	—	1	1.9	L	U (70%)	Captopril
Captopril	60-75	75	Yes	1	2	L	U	Inactive
Benazepril	35	>37	No	2-6	22	L, K	F, U	Benazeprilat
Enalapril	55-75	73	—	3-4	11-35	L	F, U	Enalaprilat
Lisinopril	25	6-60	—	1	12	K	U	Enalaprilat
Moexipril	>20	13-22	Yes	1.5	2-10	L	F (50%), U	Moexiprilat
Quinapril	60	50	Yes	1	25	L	U (50%)	Quinaprilat
Ramipril	50-60	60	—	1-2	13-17	L	F, U	Ramiprilat
Trandolapril	70	10	No	2-12	16-24	L	F (66%), U	Trandalaprilat
Fosinopril	36	36	—	1	12	L, K, I	F, U	Fosinoprilat
Cilazapril	—	57-76	No	1-2	30-50	L	U (52%)	Cilazaprilat
Spirapril	—	50	Yes	1	33-41	L	F (60%), U (40%)	Spiraprilat
Perindopril	—	75	Yes	1.5	3-10	L	F, U (75%)	Perindoprilat
Imidapril	—	40	—	3-10	10-19	L	U	Imidaprilat
Zofenopril	>80	96	Yes	5	5	K	F (26%), U (69%)	Zofenoprilat

F, Feces; I, intestine; K, kidney; L, liver; U, urine.

primarily in the urine. Dosages should be reduced by 25% to 50% in patients with end-stage kidney disease (ESKD).[22]

Imidapril is the nonsulfhydryl prodrug of the long-acting ACE inhibitor imidaprilat.[18,26] The usual daily dose is 10 to 40 mg (see Table 50.3). The peak response occurs in 5 to 6 hours and lasts for 24 hours. Imidapril is metabolized in the liver (see Table 50.4). The elimination half-life of the metabolites is 10 to 19 hours. No dosage adjustments are necessary in patients with renal failure. Imidapril has a unique advantage over other ACE inhibitors in that it is less likely to cause cough.[27]

Lisinopril is a nonsulfhydryl analogue of enalaprilat.[18,28] The initial dosage is 10 mg/day, and the usual daily dose is 20 to 40 mg (see Table 50.3). The initial antihypertensive response occurs in 1 hour, peaks at 6 hours, and lasts for 24 hours (see Table 50.4). The maximal effect may not be observed for 24 hours. The elimination half-life is 12 hours. Lisinopril is not metabolized, and it is exclusively eliminated in the urine unchanged. Lisinopril is dialyzable, and patients undergoing dialysis may require supplemental doses. The initial dosage should be reduced to 2.5 to 7.5 mg/day in patients with moderate to advanced renal failure.[22]

Moexipril hydrochloride is the nonsulfhydryl prodrug of the ACE inhibitor moexiprilat.[18,29] The usual daily dose is 7.5 to 30 mg in single or divided doses (see Table 50.3).[12] The oral bioavailability of moexipril is approximately 20%, and its absorption is impaired by high-fat meals. The peak response occurs at 3 to 6 hours and lasts for 24 hours (see Table 50.4). Moexipril is rapidly converted in the liver to moexiprilat, which is 1000 times more potent than the parent compound. The dosage should be reduced by 50% in patients with renal failure.[22,30]

Perindopril is a nonsulfhydryl prodrug of the long-acting ACE inhibitor perindoprilat.[12,30] The usual daily dose is 4 to 8 mg (see Table 50.3). The response peaks at 3 to 7 hours. A single dose has a duration of action of 24 hours.

Perindopril undergoes extensive first-pass hepatic metabolism into the active metabolite, perindoprilat (see Table 50.4). Renal excretion accounts for 75% of the clearance. The dosage should be reduced by 75% and 50% in patients with creatinine clearances of less than 50 and less than 10 mL/min/1.73 m^2, respectively.[22,30]

Quinapril hydrochloride is a nonsulfhydryl prodrug of the ACE inhibitor quinaprilat.[18,30,31] The initial dose is 10 mg, and the usual daily dose is 20 to 80 mg, which should be adjusted at 2-week intervals (see Table 50.3). Twice-daily therapy may provide a more sustained BP reduction. The onset of action occurs in 1 hour, and the peak response occurs in 2 hours and lasts for 24 hours. Quinapril is extensively metabolized in the liver into the active metabolite, quinaprilat (see Table 50.4). Renal excretion by way of filtration and active tubular secretion accounts for 50% of the clearance. Quinapril is not dialyzable. The dosage should be reduced by 25% to 50% in patients with renal failure.[22]

Ramipril is a potent, nonsulfhydryl prodrug of the ACE inhibitor ramiprilat.[12,18] Ramipril capsules are available in 1.25, 2.5, or 5 mg. The initial daily dose is 2.5 mg (see Table 50.3). The usual daily dose is 2.5 to 20 mg, and it can be titrated by doubling the current dose at 2- to 4-week intervals. Ramipril is well absorbed from the gastrointestinal tract; peak concentrations are achieved in 1 to 2 hours (see Table 50.4). The peak response occurs in 2 hours and lasts for 24 hours. Ramipril is extensively metabolized in the liver into the active metabolite, ramiprilat. The elimination half-life of the active compound is 13 to 17 hours, and it is prolonged in renal failure patients to approximately 50 hours. The dosage should be reduced by 50% to 75% in patients with a creatinine clearance of less than 50 mL/min/1.73 m^2.[18,22]

Trandolapril is a nonsulfhydryl ethyl ester prodrug of the ACE inhibitor trandolaprilat.[12,18] It is available in tablets of 1, 2, and 4 mg or in combination with verapamil. The usual starting dosage is 1 mg/day (see Table 50.3). Trandolapril is only 10% bioavailable, and its absorption is not affected by food (see Table 50.4).[32] Trandolapril undergoes extensive first-pass hepatic metabolism into trandolaprilat. The peak serum concentrations of trandolaprilat occur within 2 to 12 hours; the duration of action is 24 hours, but it may be as long as 6 weeks. The recommended starting dose in patients with a creatinine clearance of less than 30 mL/min/1.73 m^2 is 0.5 mg.

Phosphinyl Angiotensin-Converting Enzyme Inhibitor

Fosinopril sodium is a nonsulfhydryl prodrug of fosinoprilat, a long-acting ACE inhibitor.[18,33] The usual daily dose is 5 to 40 mg (see Table 50.3). Its maximal effects may not occur until 4 weeks. The initial response occurs in 1 hour, the peak response occurs in 2 to 7 hours, and the duration of response is 24 hours, which is prolonged in patients with ESKD (see Tables 50-3 and 50-4). The elimination half-life of fosinoprilat is 12 hours. All metabolites are excreted in the urine and feces. Hepatic biliary clearance increases significantly as renal function declines. Thus, the dosage must be reduced by 25% in patients with ESKD.[22]

CLASS RENAL EFFECTS

There has been considerable interest in the ability of ACE inhibitors to protect the kidney from the unrelenting deterioration that occurs with hypertension and renal insufficiency. ACE inhibitors have extensive hemodynamic and nonhemodynamic effects that afford such protection (Table 50.5). In hypertensive patients, ACE inhibitors can restore the pressure-natriuresis relationship to normal, thereby maintaining sodium balance at a lower arterial BP.[34] The response is exaggerated in a restricted sodium intake setting. The mechanism responsible for this effect is the direct inhibition of proximal, and possibly distal, tubule sodium reabsorption.[35] The increased renal excretory capacity plays a major role in the long-term antihypertensive activity of the drugs. Clinically, the increase in sodium excretion is transitory because the reduced arterial pressure allows the sodium excretion to return to normal. However, the maintenance of normal sodium excretion at lower arterial pressures correlates with increased excretion in the setting of hypertension.[34] After several days, inhibition of Ang II and aldosterone contributes to the natriuresis.[36] The long-term effects on water excretion are less certain. ACE inhibitors initially induce an increase in free water clearance, but there are no long-term changes in total body weight, plasma, or extracellular fluid volume. The decreased aldosterone level caused by ACE inhibition also correlates with decreased potassium excretion,[36] particularly in patients with impaired renal function. The antikaliuretic effect appears to be transient, but it can be exacerbated by concomitant administration of potassium-sparing diuretics, supplements, and nonsteroidal antiinflammatory drugs (NSAIDs); it should be monitored rigorously.

The effects of ACE inhibitors on angiotensin peptide levels depend on the responsiveness of renin secretion.[37,38] All ACE inhibitors decrease the level of Ang II and increase the levels of angiotensin-(1-7) (a potential vasodilator) and plasma renin. When renin levels show little increase in response to ACE inhibition, the levels of Ang II and its metabolites decrease markedly, with little change in the levels of Ang I. Large increases in renin levels in response to ACE inhibition increase the levels of Ang I and its metabolites. The increased levels of angiotensin I can produce higher levels of Ang II through uninhibited ACE and other pathways, thereby blunting the effect of reduced Ang II. This phenomenon is termed *ACE escape* and may contribute to reduced ACE inhibitor efficacy when used over a long term.[39]

Table 50.5 Renal Protective Mechanisms of Angiotensin-Converting Enzyme Inhibitors

Restore pressure-natriuresis relationship to normal.
Inhibit tubule sodium resorption.
Decrease arterial pressure.
Decrease aldosterone production.
Decrease proteinuria.
Improve altered lipid profiles.
Decrease renal blood flow.
Decrease filtration fraction.
Decrease renal vascular resistance.
Reduce scarring and fibrosis.
Attenuate oxidative stress and reduce free radicals.

Recent experimental reports have highlighted the potential importance of the tissue specificity of ACE inhibitors,[40] as well as disagreement about the role played by systemic generation of Ang II versus the local generation of Ang II within the kidneys and its relative importance in terms of hypertension. An important role for intrarenal ACE has been demonstrated in murine hypertension models, as mice lacking only renal ACE are protected against hypertension.[40] The intrarenal Ang II production and local regulation of renal sodium transport represents a new mechanistic understanding of the underlying inappropriate regulation of salt and water balance. However, what remains unclear is the role that intrarenal renin angiotensin aldosterone system (RAAS) plays in human disease. It is clear that local inhibition of ACE in the vascular wall and renal vessels contributes to the antihypertensive activity of hypertension drugs. ACE inhibitor–induced changes in BP correlate with the degree of inhibition of RAAS in plasma and tissues.[41] The ACE inhibitors with the greatest tissue specificity, however, are associated with prolonged activity at the tissue level, even after serum ACE levels have returned to normal.[41] Consequently, they are more efficacious with once-daily dosing.[41] Other potential renoprotective effects that have been noted in experimental models include attenuation of oxidative stress,[42] scavenging of free radicals, and attenuation of lipid peroxidation.[43] The clinical importance of these effects is under investigation.

Because the degree of proteinuria correlates best with the rate of declining renal function, and a decrease in proteinuria correlates better with renal protection than with decreased BP, the reduction of proteinuria can have a substantial impact.[44] All ACE inhibitors decrease urinary protein excretion[45-47] in normotensive and hypertensive patients with renal disease of various origins. Individual response rates vary from an increase of 31% to a decrease of 100%, and they are strongly influenced by drug dosage and dietary sodium changes.[46,48] There is a clear dose-response relationship between increased doses and reduced proteinuria, and this relationship is not dependent on changes in BP, renal plasma flow, or GFR. Furthermore, the effect of ACE inhibitors on the reduction of proteinuria is eliminated with high salt intake.

Studies have demonstrated that in normotensive diabetic patients, ACE inhibitors can normalize GFR, markedly reduce the progression of renal disease, and normalize microalbuminuria.[49,50] These findings are discussed in depth in Chapter 39. The effect is noted in the first month of therapy and is maximal at 14 months. Several mechanisms account for the reduction in urinary protein excretion, including the following: a decrease in glomerular capillary hydrostatic pressure; a decrease in mesangial uptake and clearance of macromolecules; and improved glomerular basement membrane perm-selectivity.[3,51] The ACE inhibitors have better antiproteinuric efficacy than other classes of antihypertensive agents, with the exception of angiotensin receptor blockers (ARBs). In the treatment of proteinuria, the noninferiority of ARBs to ACE inhibition was recently confirmed in a meta-analysis of 24 studies.[47] Furthermore, the antiproteinuric effect is additive with the ARBs and does not depend on changes in creatinine clearance, GFR, or BP, but it does not necessarily portend a better outcome.[52,53] The beneficial effect of ACE inhibition may not be enhanced by combined nondihydropyridine calcium channel antagonist therapy beyond BP lowering.[54,55] A suggested goal of ACE inhibition or ARB therapy is to reduce proteinuria to less than 1000 mg/day or reduce proteinuria to more than 50% from baseline, in addition to protein excretion at less than 3.5 g/day.[56] Blood pressure should be reduced to less than 140/90 mm Hg in all hypertensive patients and to less than 130/80 mm Hg in patients with protein excretion more than 500 mg/day.[57]

Up to 0.7% of patients treated with captopril develop proteinuria, with total urinary protein excretion exceeding 1 g/day.[58-60] In most cases, proteinuria subsides within 6 months, regardless of whether captopril is continued, with no residual change in GFR. Renal biopsy specimens reveal a membranous nephropathy. The sulfhydryl group of captopril is thought to invoke an immune complex–mediated nephropathy similar to that which occurs with penicillamine administration.[61]

Most of the vasoconstrictor action of Ang II is confined to the efferent arteriole. ACE inhibitors preferentially dilate the efferent arteriole by reducing the systemic and intrarenal levels of Ang II. The effect is a reduction in intraglomerular capillary pressure. In patients with hypertension, ACE inhibitors uniformly increase renal blood flow, decrease filtration fraction, decrease renal vascular resistance, reduce urinary protein excretion, impair microvascular autoregulation, and restore normal circadian BP patterns,[62-64] with variable to no effect on GFR. In patients with nondiabetic glomerular renal damage, short-term ACE inhibitor administration causes a decrease in renal perfusion, glomerular filtration, and pressure and an increase in afferent resistances.[65] Long-term administration is associated with a decrease in renal perfusion, as well as a tendency to a higher filtration fraction and lower afferent resistances. Marked improvement in GFR occurs and is sustained for up to 3 years.[36,66] However, many patients with impaired renal function exhibit a reversible fall in GFR with ACE inhibitor therapy that is not detrimental. The GFR declines initially because of the hemodynamic changes, but the long-term reduction in perfusion pressure is renoprotective. Even in patients receiving hemodialysis, ACE inhibitor therapy significantly preserves residual renal function and helps maintain urine output.[67] Patients with type 1 diabetes who have the greatest initial decline in GFR have the slowest rate of loss of renal function over time.[68] It should be emphasized that ACE inhibitors should not be withdrawn immediately if an increase in serum creatinine level is noted; a 20% to 30% decline in GFR can be expected, and close monitoring is warranted.

An inherited trait of disordered regulation of the RAAS contributes to the pathogenesis of hypertension in approximately 45% of patients.[69] Such patients have sodium-sensitive hypertension, abnormalities in renal vascular responses to changes in sodium intake and Ang II, blunted decrements of renin release in response to saline or Ang II, and accentuated vasodilator responses to ACE inhibition; they have been termed *nonmodulators*.[69] In these patients, ACE inhibition not only increases renal blood flow substantially more than it does in normal subjects, but also restores the renal vascular and adrenal responses to Ang II, renin release, renal sodium handling, and BP.[69,70]

Treatment with ACE inhibitors is frequently associated with an initial decrease in kidney function.[71] The significance of this increase in the serum creatinine level after the initiation of RAAS inhibitor therapy is uncertain because it is due in part to a reduction in intraglomerular pressure, which might be expected to contribute to the slowing of disease progression. An initial elevation in the serum creatinine level of up to 30% above baseline, which stabilizes within the first 2 months of therapy, has been considered acceptable, and it is no reason to discontinue therapy in the absence of hypotension.[72,73] Rather than being an adverse effect, a review of 12 randomized trials has shown that in patients receiving ACE inhibitors, a stable rise in the serum creatinine level of less than 30% was associated with long-term preservation of kidney function.[72,73]

In patients with an activated RAAS, however, ACE inhibitors can decrease GFR and perhaps even precipitate acute kidney injury (AKI). Patients with severe bilateral renal artery stenosis,[74] unilateral renal artery stenosis of a solitary kidney, severe hypertensive nephrosclerosis, volume depletion, congestive heart failure, cirrhosis, or a transplanted kidney[75] are at higher risk for deterioration in kidney function with ACE inhibitor therapy.[76,77] These patients typically have a precipitous drop in BP and deterioration of renal function when treated with ACE inhibitors. In these states of reduced renal perfusion related to low effective arterial circulating volume or flow reduced by an obstructed artery, the maintenance of renal blood flow and GFR is highly dependent on increased efferent arteriolar vasoconstriction mediated by Ang II. Interruption of the increased tone causes a critical reduction in perfusion pressure and can lead to dramatic reductions in GFR and urinary flow, worsening of renal ischemia and, in selected cases, anuria. The hemodynamic effect is often reversible with cessation of therapy.[78] Even paradoxic severe hypertension has been described in rare patients with renal artery stenosis treated with ACE inhibitors.[79] In a recent prospective study, reports of 26 older patients with hemodynamically significant renal artery stenosis who received renin angiotensin blockers and developed more than 25% worsening of kidney function, 19% (5 of 26) developed ESKD, and 73% (19 of 26) showed estimated GFR (eGFR) improvement.[80]

These mostly reversible azotemic events described in 1983 stigmatized the use of renin angiotensin blockade of patients with significant renovascular disease.[81] However, multiple randomized controlled trials have shown that RAAS blockade effectively decreases the progression of kidney disease,[82-84] and observational studies have demonstrated the benefit of RAAS blockade in BP control, adverse cardiovascular outcomes, and all-cause mortality. Recent studies of atherosclerotic renovascular disease demonstrating the efficacy of medical therapy, including use of ACE inhibitors and ARBs over renal artery stenting, have indicated that perhaps many of the risks of renin angiotensin therapy (e.g., azotemia, hyperkalemia, angioedema) can be balanced by their benefits when patients are carefully monitored.[81,85,86]

CLASS EFFICACY AND SAFETY

ACE inhibitors are recommended for initial monotherapy in patients with mild, moderate, and severe hypertension, regardless of age, ancestry, or gender.[87] They are effective in diabetic patients, obese patients, and patients with renal transplants,[88] and they are safe to use in patients with mild, moderate, and severe renal insufficiency. In general, patients with high-renin hypertension and chronic renal parenchymal disease respond particularly well, presumably because they have inappropriately high intrarenal renin and Ang II levels. African Americans with hypertension have been found to respond less well to lower dosages than whites, but higher dosages are equally effective.[89-91] In most studies, ACE inhibitors elicit an adequate response in 40% to 60% of patients.[92] An immediate fall in BP occurs in 70% of patients. The enhanced efficacy of ACE inhibitors in the presence of salt restriction is paralleled by the additive effects of diuretic therapy.[93] The addition of low-dose hydrochlorothiazide enhances the efficacy more than 80%, normalizing BP in another 20% to 25% of patients.[94] Adding a diuretic is more effective than increasing the dosage of the ACE inhibitor.[94,95] Recent clinical trials have examined the use of the combination of an ACE inhibitor and ARB to prevent target-organ damage.[96] The Renal Outcomes with Telmisartan, Ramipril, or Both, in People at High Vascular Risk (ONTARGET) trial compared the ACE inhibitor ramipril with the ARB telmisartan, alone and in combination, in patients at high risk for vascular disease.[97,98] Although the achieved mean BP was lower in the patients who received telmisartan or both agents than in those who received ramipril alone, there was no difference in the primary outcomes between any of the groups, and more adverse outcomes were noted in the combination group. Importantly, this trial did not evaluate ARB and ACE inhibitor therapy in patients with advanced proteinuric renal disease. The VA NEPHRON-D study, a trial using combination therapy (ACE inhibitor and ARB therapy vs. ARB monotherapy) in proteinuric diabetic nephropathy was stopped due to increased adverse events of hyperkalemia and AKI.[99] The Aliskiren Trial in Type 2 Diabetes Using Cardiorenal Endpoints (ALTITUDE) randomly assigned 8561 patients to aliskiren (300 mg daily) or placebo as an adjunct to ACE or ARB monotherapy as an angiotensin receptor blocker. The trial was stopped prematurely due to adverse events (hyperkalemia and hypotension).[100] Therefore, ACE inhibitors should not be used concomitantly with ARBs and renin inhibitors due to an increased risk of hypotension, hyperkalemia, and renal dysfunction.[101]

Many studies have attempted to achieve further benefit from ACE inhibitors and other RAAS blocking agents by increasing the doses of these drugs. This reasoning is based on the original observation that the optimal antiproteinuric dose does not necessarily equal the optimal antihypertensive dose. Many of these study results have shown further proteinuria reduction,[102-106] whereas others have not.[107-109] However, similar to the initial studies of the combination therapy with RAAS blocking agents, many of these high-dosage studies were also short-term studies that used BP and albuminuria as outcome variables. These studies have not been sufficiently powered, or they lacked duration to detect safety signals and side effects rates that may emerge with end point trials.[101] Therefore, before ultrahigh-RAAS blocking agent dosing as renoprotective therapy can be recommended, more studies with hard kidney and cardiovascular event points are warranted.[101]

Neither the duration nor the degree of BP lowering is predicted by the effect on blood ACE or Ang II levels, and all ACE inhibitors appear to have comparable efficacy. The response may be due in part to interindividual variability of the ACE genotype.[91,110] The activity of ACE is partially dependent on the presence or absence of a 287–base pair element in intron 16, and this insertion-deletion (I/D) polymorphism of a human Al repetitive DNA element accounts for 47% of the total phenotypic variation in plasma ACE. Deletion-deletion (D/D) subjects have the highest ACE concentrations, I/D subjects have intermediate ACE concentrations, and insertion-insertion (I/I) subjects have the lowest. Genotype also influences tissue ACE activity, but the clinical implications are under investigation.

ACE inhibitors are indicated as first-line therapy in hypertensive patients with heart failure and systolic dysfunction,[111] type 1 diabetes and proteinuria,[68] reduced systolic function after myocardial infarction,[112] coronary artery disease or new atrial fibrillation,[113,114] and left ventricular dysfunction,[87,114,115] as well as patients undergoing dialysis.[116] ACE inhibitors reduce ventricular hypertrophy independent of the BP decrease.[117] All patients with diabetes, even those without evidence of nephropathy, should be given ACE inhibitors for cardiovascular risk reduction.[118-122] Primary and secondary prevention trials[118,123,124] have shown that ACE inhibitors improve endothelial dysfunction and cardiac and vascular remodeling, retard the progression of atherosclerosis, improve arterial distensibility, and reduce the risk of myocardial ischemia and infarction, stroke, and cardiovascular death. Some but not all studies have shown a small decrease in the risk of new and recurrent atrial fibrillation due to the beneficial structural and electrical effects on the atria.[125,126] The use of ACE inhibitors is also associated with improved exercise performance in patients with hypertension and intermittent claudication,[127] reduced pain perception,[128] and reduced perioperative myocardial ischemia,[112] as well as the retardation of the progression of aortic stenosis,[129] protection against cognitive decline and dementia,[130,131] promotion of atrial structural remodeling,[132] prolongation of the survival of arteriovenous polytetrafluoroethylene grafts,[133] and possible reduced risk of pneumonia[134] and prevention of osteoporosis.[135] Long-term use of these agents has been associated with a lower risk for breast cancer, but the importance of this finding has yet to be substantiated.[136]

ACE inhibitors may cause fetal or neonatal injury or death when used during the second and third trimesters of pregnancy[137] because angiotensin appears to be required for normal fetal growth and development.[138] Concern has been expressed regarding first-trimester use of ACE inhibitors since their use during this period might be associated with congenital malformations, but these malformations may also be related to maternal factors.[139] A recent study has found that maternal use of ACE inhibitors in the first trimester shows a risk profile similar to that of other antihypertensives.[140]

A systemic review of published case reports and case series dealing with intrauterine exposure to ACE inhibitors or ARBs has shown 118 cases of ACE inhibitor exposure and 68 cases of ARB exposure. Among 118 cases of ACE inhibitor exposure, 27% were taken only in the first trimester; in 68 cases of ARB exposure, 38% were taken throughout the entire pregnancy. Neonatal complications were more frequent following exposure to ARBs; 52% of the newborns exposed to ACE inhibitors did not exhibit any complications, whereas only 13% of the newborns exposed to ARBs did not ($P < 0.0001$); however, many of the patients exposed to ARBs received therapy throughout the pregnancy.[141] In 26 children, 23% developed kidney failure, 8% required dialysis, 15% demonstrated hypertension, 8% developed acidosis, 12% developed polyuria, 15% showed small or echogenic kidneys on ultrasound, 8% had polycythemia, 15% had growth retardation, and 12% experienced neurodevelopmental delay. The outcome was normal in 50% of cases, mild in 42%, and bad in 8%. Complications were similar whether the children were exposed to ACE inhibitors or ARBs. The authors commented that the congenital malformations that occurred following in utero RAAS exposure might have resulted from the drug as well as the underlying maternal illness, usually hypertension or diabetes.

A prospective, observational, controlled cohort study of ACE inhibitors and ARB exposure during the first trimester was recently reported.[142] The subjects were enrolled from women contacting a teratogen information service. There were two comparison groups, women with hypertension treated with other antihypertensives (including methyldopa or calcium channel blockers) and healthy controls. In the ACE-ARB and disease-matched groups, the offspring exhibited significantly lower birth weights and gestational ages than those of the healthy controls ($P < 0.001$ for both variables). A significantly higher rate of miscarriage was noted in the ACE-ARB group ($P < 0.001$). These results suggest that ACE inhibitors and ARBs are not major human teratogens during the first trimester. There was, however, a higher rate of spontaneous abortions in the ACE-ARB group.

When a patient becomes pregnant during treatment with an ACE inhibitor or ARB, the drug should be discontinued immediately, and alternative antihypertensive therapy should be started. Pregnancy termination is at the discretion of the patient and treatment team, but physicians and patients can derive some reassurance from the small studies quoted above if the drug is discontinued during the first trimester. Many caregivers may try to avoid ACE inhibitors and ARBs in women planning to conceive, given the fact that 50% of pregnancies are unplanned, the clear contraindication of ACE inhibitors in the second and third trimesters, and the often late presentation for prenatal care. Responsible patients can plan to stop the drugs with the first missed menstrual cycle, obtain a pregnancy blood test, and substitute an antihypertensive, such as methyldopa, labetalol, or a nondihydropyridine calcium channel blocker (CCB)[143] if proteinuria is being treated for diabetic or nondiabetic chronic kidney disease (CKD).[144] (See Chapter 49 and Figure 50.7.)

ACE inhibitors are transferred into breast milk, but the drug levels in milk are low. Captopril and enalapril have been reviewed by the American Academy of Pediatrics[145] and the NICE guidelines for the management of hypertension in pregnancy from the United Kingdom,[146] and they are compatible with lactation. However, newborns may be more susceptible to the hemodynamic effects of these drugs (e.g., hypotension) and sequelae (e.g., oliguria, seizures).

Overall, ACE inhibitors are well tolerated and have relatively neutral or beneficial metabolic effects. ACE inhibitors are associated with 8% to 11% reductions in levels of low-density lipoprotein (LDL) cholesterol and triglycerides and 5% increases in levels of high-density lipoprotein (HDL) cholesterol.[147] They do not cause perturbations of serum sodium or uric acid levels. ACE inhibitors reduce the levels of plasminogen activator inhibitor-1 and may improve fibrinolysis.[148]

The effects of ACE inhibitors on glucose metabolism are favorable.[149] They may improve glucose tolerance by augmenting the insulin secretory response to glucose[149] and may also help ameliorate obesity and hyperinsulinemia.[150] The use of ACE inhibitors has been clinically associated with a 25% to 30% reduction in the risk of developing diabetes.[151] Several large clinical trials are have been evaluating the clinical relevance of this finding.[152] Many of the ACE inhibitors require dosage adjustment in the presence of renal dysfunction[22] (Table 50.6).

There are few adverse effects of this class of drugs, and they may occur with all ACE inhibitors. The newer agents appear to have a lower incidence of adverse effects, possibly because of lack of the sulfhydryl moiety found in captopril. The most common adverse effect of ACE inhibitors is a dry, hacking, nonproductive, and often intolerable cough, which has been reported in up to 20% of patients.[153] In the ONTARGET trial, cough sufficiently severe to permanently discontinue the drug was described in 4.2% of patients treated with ramipril[154]; cough is much less common with ARBs. The cough is thought to be secondary to hypersensitivity to bradykinins, which are increased by ACE,[155] increased levels of prostaglandins,[156] accumulation of substance P,[153] a potent bronchoconstrictor,[157] or polymorphisms in the neurokinin-2 receptor gene.[158] The cough can begin initially or many months after the start of therapy.[159] It is more common in women, African Americans,[160] and Asians in Hong Kong[161] and Korea,[162] and it may spontaneously disappear.[159] It may be more common in patients with bronchial hyperreactivity, but ACE inhibitors are safe to use in asthmatic patients.[163] NSAIDs, oral iron supplements, and sodium cromoglycate have been reported to improve the cough,[164] but cessation of ACE therapy is the only absolute cure. In a dosage of 600 mg twice daily, picotamide (a thromboxane antagonist) was effective in treating ACE inhibitor–induced cough.[165] Patients may be effectively switched to ARBs if an antihypertensive effect is observed with ACE inhibitors.

Angioedema is a rare but potentially life-threatening complication of ACE inhibitor therapy. It occurs in 0.1% to 0.7% of patients within hours of the first dose of ACE inhibitor or after prolonged use.[166-168] In the ONTARGET Trial, the occurrence of angioedema, although potentially life-threatening, was reported and was listed as a reason to discontinue from the study permanently in just 0.3% of more than 8500 individuals given ramipril.[154]

This absolute risk of ACE inhibitor–induced angioedema is low, but with large numbers of prescriptions written annually, many patients are at risk for this disorder.[169] ACE inhibitor–induced angioedema accounts for one third of all cases of angioedema seen in emergency departments.

Our understanding of the mechanism of ACE inhibitor–induced angioedema is evolving. The side effect occurs five times more frequently in individuals of African ancestry. ACE inhibitors act by inhibiting bradykinin breakdown in addition to blocking the conversion of Ang I to Ang II. ACE inhibitor–induced angioedema involves several components, including tissue accumulation of bradykinin and inhibition of C1 esterase activity.[166,170] Susceptible individuals typically have defects in non-ACE, non–kininase I vasoactive pathways of bradykinin degradation, possess the XPNPEP2 gene variant,[171,172] have elevated des-Arg9-BK,[173] or are taking dipeptidyl peptidase inhibitors (e.g., sitagliptin, saxagliptin, linagliptin) to treat diabetes.[166,174-176] Some patients also have defective degradation of substance P, thereby increasing vascular permeability.[177]

Clinical features, including asymmetric swelling confined to the face, subcutaneous or submucous membranes, and lips, usually resolves with discontinuation of the therapy, but obstructive sleep apnea may be exacerbated.[178] If the ACE inhibitor is not discontinued, the episode usually resolves, but the frequency and severity of future episodes will escalate.[179,180] Angioedema of the small intestine and acute appendicitis have also been reported.[181-184]

Involvement of the glottis and larynx requiring airway management occurs in 10% of all cases and may result in laryngeal obstruction and death.[185] Administration of epinephrine, histamine-2 blockers, glucocorticoids, and/or fresh-frozen plasma is indicated.[186] Recently, icatibant, a selective bradykinin B2 receptor antagonist approved for the treatment of hereditary angioedema, has also been shown to be effective for the treatment of ACE inhibitor–induced angioedema in a multicenter, double-blind, phase 2 study. In 27 patients, the median time to resolution was 8 hours with icatibant (interquartile range, 3.0 to 16.0 hours) compared to 27.1 hours with standard therapy (interquartile range, 20.3 to 48.0 hours) with a glucocorticoid and an antihistamine. Patients experiencing an episode of angioedema associated with ACE inhibitor usage should be switched to ARBs or other agents.[187] ACE inhibitors are contraindicated in patients with a known hypersensitivity to ACE inhibitors.

First-dose hypotension, with a reduction in BP of up to 30%, has been reported with all ACE inhibitors in up to 2.5% of patients. In the Studies of Left Ventricular Dysfunction (SOLVD trial), hypotension was observed in 14.8% of patients versus 7.1% of individuals who received a placebo ($P < 0.0001$).[188] In the ONTARGET Trial, of the 8579 patients who received ramipril, only 1.7% and 0.2% permanently stopped therapy due to hypotension and syncope, respectively.[154]

Hypotension occurs more commonly in patients with effective arterial volume depletion, patients with high-renin hypertension, and those with systolic heart failure.[188,189] Hypotension is usually well tolerated, although occasionally it is associated with syncope. In older patients, ACE inhibitor therapy more frequently causes nocturnal hypotension.[190] The accompanying increase in the plasma norepinephrine level may explain the low incidence of orthostatic symptoms.[190] In patients at high risk of orthostatic symptoms, therapy should be initiated at lower dosages, preferably after discontinuing diuretics. Rebound hypertension has not been reported with discontinuation of ACE inhibitors.

Adverse effects related to the chemical structure are more frequently seen with the sulfhydryl-containing captopril than with the other agents. Dysgeusia appears to be related to the binding of zinc by the ACE inhibitors.[191] Approximately 2% to 4% of patients experience a diminution or loss of taste sensation that is associated with a metallic taste. It is usually self-limited and resolves in 2 to 3 months, even with continued therapy. However, it may be severe enough to interfere with nutrition and cause weight loss.[192]

Table 50.6 Dose Modifications of Antihypertensive Drugs Required for Renal Insufficiency*

Drug	Estimated Glomerular Filtration Rate (Creatinine Clearance; mL/min/1.73 m^2)			Dialysis†
	>50	10-15	<10	
Angiotensin-Converting Enzyme Inhibitors				
Benazepril	No change	50%	25%	Negligible
Captopril	No change	50%	25%	H: 50%
Cilazapril	No change	50%	25%	H: 50%
Enalapril	No change	50%	25%	H: 50%
Fosinopril	No change	No change	75%	—
Imidapril	No change	No change	—	—
Lisinopril	No change	50%	25%	H: 50%
Moexipril	No change	50%	25%	—
Perindopril	No change	75%	50%	—
Quinapril	No change	50%	25%	—
Ramipril	No change	50%	25%	—
Trandolapril	No change	50%	25%	—
Zofenopril	No change	—	—	—
Angiotensin Receptor Blockers				
Candesartan	No change	No change	No change	Negligible
Eprosartan	No change	No change	50%	Negligible
Irbesartan	No change	No change	—	Negligible
Losartan	No change	No change	No change	Negligible
Olmesartan	No change	—	—	—
Telmisartan	No change	No change	No change	Negligible
Valsartan	No change	No change	No change	—
Adrenergic Antagonists				
Nadolol	No change	50%	25%	H: 50%
Carteolol	No change	50%	25%	—
Penbutolol	No change	No change	50%	Negligible
Pindolol	No change	No change	50%	Negligible
Atenolol	No change	50%	25%	H: 50%
Betaxolol	No change	No change	50%	H: 50%
Bisoprolol	No change	50%	25%	Negligible
Acebutolol	No change	50%	30%-50%	H: 50%
Celiprolol	No change	50%	Avoid	—
Nebivolol	No change	50%	—	—
Calcium Channel Blockers				
Diltiazem	No change	No change	No change	Negligible
Verapamil	No change	No change	No change	Negligible
Nifedipine	No change	No change	No change	Negligible
Amlodipine	No change	No change	No change	Negligible
Felodipine	No change	No change	No change	Negligible
Isradipine	No change	No change	No change	Negligible
Manidipine	No change	No change	No change	Negligible
Nicardipine	No change	No change	No change	Negligible
Nisoldipine	No change	No change	No change	Negligible
Lacidipine	No change	No change	No change	Negligible
Lercanidipine	Dosage adjustment in renal failure unknown			
Central α$_2$-Adrenergic or I$_1$ Imidazole Receptor Agonists				
Methyldopa	No change	No change	50%	H: 50%
Clonidine	No change	50%	25%	Negligible
Moxonidine	No change	50%	—	—
Rilmenidine	No change	50%	25%	—
Direct-Acting Vasodilators				
Hydralazine	No change	No change	75%‡	Negligible
Minoxidil	No change	50%	50%	H and P: 50%

Continued on following page

Table 50.6 Dose Modifications of Antihypertensive Drugs Required for Renal Insufficiency* (Continued)

Drug	Estimated Glomerular Filtration Rate (Creatinine Clearance; mL/min/1.73 m^2)			
	>50	10-15	<10	Dialysis[†]
Peripheral Adrenergic Neuronal Blocking Agents				
Guanethidine	No change	No change	—	—
Guanadrel	No change	50%	25% (avoid)	—
Renin Inhibitor				
Aliskiren	No change	No change	Not studied	Not studied
Tyrosine Hydroxylase Inhibitor				
Metyrosine	No change	50%	25%	—
Selective Aldosterone Receptor Antagonist				
Eplerenone	Dosage adjustment in renal failure unknown Caution in regard to hyperkalemia			

*Percentage of usual dose given.
[†]Replacement dose at end of dialysis as percentage of dose prescribed for patient with glomerular filtration rate < 10 mL/min.
[‡]Slow acetylators.
H, Hemodialysis; P, peritoneal dialysis; —, not applicable.

Cutaneous reactions manifest as a nonallergic, pruritic, maculopapular eruption that appears during the first few weeks of therapy. These reactions may be associated with a fever or arthralgias and may disappear, even with continuation of the ACE inhibitor.[193]

Leukopenia and anemia have been reported with ACE inhibitor therapy. Among patients with normal renal function, ACE inhibitors may reduce hemoglobin levels in a dose-dependent manner.[194] ACE inhibitors have been demonstrated to interfere with the response to erythropoietin. Hemodialysis and renal transplant patients receiving erythropoietin frequently require higher dosages to maintain hemoglobin levels.[195] Consequently, ACE inhibitors can be used effectively to reduce posttransplantation erythrocytosis,[196] but appear to have little effect on erythropoiesis in hemodialysis patients.[197] Neutropenia (<1000 neutrophils/mm^3) with myeloid hypoplasia occurs almost exclusively in patients with renal insufficiency, immunosuppression, collagen vascular disease, or autoimmune disease.[12] It is associated with systemic and oral cavity infections common with agranulocytosis. Neutropenia occurs within 3 months of initiation of therapy and generally resolves 2 weeks after therapy is discontinued.[12,193] Although it is usually reversible, it may be fatal.

Anaphylactoid reactions ranging from mild pruritus to bronchospasm and cardiopulmonary collapse have been reported in patients treated with ACE inhibitors who undergo dialysis with equipment that uses high-flux polyacrylonitrile, cellulose acetate, or cuprophane membranes or who undergo apheresis with equipment that uses dextran sulfate membranes.[198] The frequency of reactions is unknown, but they occur within the first few minutes of treatment. Such membranes should be avoided when patients are receiving ACE inhibitors. The use of ACE inhibitors in patients on plasmapheresis or an exchange protocol is safe as long as effective arterial volume is managed appropriately.

Few significant drug interactions occur with ACE inhibitors. Studies have shown that aspirin dosages of 100 mg/day or less do not negate the effects of ACE inhibitors.[199] Ang II stimulates the production of vasodilatory prostaglandins. Aspirin inhibits the production of vasodilator and antithrombotic prostaglandins. Theoretically, either agent may antagonize the effectiveness of the other. Concomitant use of ACE inhibitors and cyclosporine may exacerbate renal hypoperfusion.[12] Use of the mammalian target of rapamycin (mTOR) inhibitors sirolimus or everolimus in transplant recipients decreases the metabolism of bradykinins and predisposes them to angioedema with ACE inhibitors.[200]

Hyperkalemia of more than 5.5 mmol/L was observed in 3.3% of patients taking ramipril in the ONTARGET study.[154] Production of Ang II systemically and locally in the zona glomerulosa of the adrenal gland, which is blocked by ACE inhibitors, will reduce subsequent aldosterone synthesis and urinary potassium excretion. In a Veterans Administration Medical Center case-control study of 1818 patients using ACE inhibitors, 194 (11%) developed hyperkalemia.[201] The results of laboratory studies indicated that a serum urea nitrogen level higher than 6.4 mmol/L and a creatinine level higher than 136 μmol/L, as well as congestive heart failure and long-acting ACE inhibitors, were independently associated with hyperkalemia; concurrent use of a loop or thiazide diuretic agent was associated with reduced risk. After 1 year of follow-up, 15 (10%) of 146 patients who remained on a regimen of an ACE inhibitor developed severe hyperkalemia (potassium level > 6.0 mmol/L). A serum urea nitrogen level higher than 8.9 mmol/L, and age older than 70 years were independently associated with subsequent severe hyperkalemia.

Hyperkalemia has been effectively and safely treated with patiromer and sodium zirconium cyclosilicate recently in an outpatient setting.[202,203] These two new drugs add to the outpatient pharmacopoeia that until now has been limited to sodium and calcium polystyrene sulfonate, with its gastrointestinal adverse effects.

ACE inhibitors have no effect on C-reactive protein levels.[204]

ANGIOTENSIN II TYPE 1 RECEPTOR ANTAGONISTS

CLASS MECHANISMS OF ACTION

The Ang II receptor blockers (ARBs) allow more specific and complete blockade of the RAAS than the ACE inhibitors because they circumvent all pathways that lead to the formation of Ang II (see Figure 50.2). For example, Ang I is metabolized not only by ACE to form Ang II but also by chymase, cathepsin G, tissue plasminogen activator, and other enzymes.[205] Ang II can be formed at sites other than those in the systemic circulation, such as the brain, kidney, and heart. Furthermore, long-term ACE inhibitor therapy is associated with a return of Ang II levels to baseline, which possibly contributes to reduced efficacy. The ARBs selectively antagonize Ang II directly at the Ang II type 1 (AT_1) receptor, regardless of the source of production. Because Ang II plays a crucial multifactorial role in maintaining and regulating BP, blockade of the AT_1 receptor with ARBs is a powerful tool for targeting multiple pathways that contribute to hypertension.

Like ACE inhibitors, ARBs directly block the vasoconstrictive action of Ang II and cause a decrease in peripheral vascular resistance.[206] The hypotensive effect is not accompanied by changes in cardiac output, heart rate, or GFR. Interruption of the binding of Ang II at the tissue level also leads to other effects (beyond vasodilation) that contribute to the antihypertensive effect. Additional mechanisms include the following: (1) augmentation of renal blood flow and reduction of aldosterone release to induce natriuresis and attenuate the compensatory increase in sodium retention that accompanies a fall in BP; (2) direct depression of tubular sodium reabsorption[207,208]; (3) improvement of nitric oxide–mediated endothelial function[209]; (4) reversal of vascular hypertrophy[209]; (5) blunting of sympathetic nervous system activity and presynaptic noradrenaline release; (6) inhibition of postjunctional pressor responses to norepinephrine or Ang II; (7) inhibition of central Ang II–mediated sympathoexcitation and vasopressin release[210-212]; (8) inhibition of centrally controlled baroreceptor reflexes[213]; (9) inhibition of central nervous system (CNS) norepinephrine synthesis; (10) inhibition of thirst[214]; and (11) possible inhibition of RAAS-mediated action on endothelin-1.[215] The antihypertensive action of ARBs is dependent on activation of the RAAS and is associated with clinically insignificant increases in circulating levels of Ang II.[206] ARBs also increase bradykinin levels by antagonizing angiotensin II at its type 1 receptor and diverting Ang II to its counterregulatory type 2 receptor, which potentiates vasodilation.[216] ARBs also increase the level of other angiotensin peptides, including angiotensin-(1-7), Ang II, and angiotensin IV, which can act on their respective receptors to modulate vasoconstriction, renal blood flow, and vascular hypertrophy.[217-222]

CLASS MEMBERS

The ARB class is composed of peptide and nonpeptide analogues that vary in structure, mechanism of receptor inhibition, metabolism, and potency. There are currently eight drugs in clinical use. Many of the newer drugs were developed by modifying losartan, the first biologically active ARB oral agent. These drugs are categorized according to the substitution of carboxylic and other moieties into several groups—the biphenyl tetrazoles (derivatives of losartan), nonbiphenyl tetrazoles, and nonheterocyclic compounds. They are also classified according to their ability to antagonize Ang II.[223] The competitive (surmountable) antagonists shift the dose-response curve for Ang II–mediated contraction to the right without depressing the maximal response to Ang II. The noncompetitive (insurmountable) antagonists also depress the maximal response to Ang II. The variable effects of ARBs are mediated by differences in the interaction with allosteric binding sites on the receptor, dissociation of the drug-receptor complex, removal of the agonists from tissues or by the ability to modulate the amount of internalized receptors[223] (see Tables 50.7 to 50.9).

Biphenyl Tetrazole and Oxadiazole Derivatives

Azilsartan medoxomil (Edarbi), the most recently approved selective AT_1 receptor blocker, has demonstrated a potent 24-hour sustained antihypertensive effect. At the approved dosage, it reduces systolic BP by 12 to 15 mm Hg and diastolic BP by 7 to 8 mm Hg,[224-226] which is a decrease in BP compared with other ARBs, without any significant side effects.[227] Azilsartan medoxomil is a prodrug that is hydrolyzed to azilsartan in the gastrointestinal tract during absorption. It possesses a unique moiety (5-oxo-1,2,4-oxadiazole) in place of the tetrazole ring that offers a very strong inverse antagonism at the AT_1 receptor.[228,229] This bond is chemically stronger than that of its predecessors, which may explain its superior potency when compared to other members of its class or ACE inhibitors.[228] The estimated oral bioavailability is about 60%; peak plasma concentration is reached after 1.5 to 3 hours following ingestion.[227] Food does not affect the bioavailability of the drug. More than 99% of azilsartan is bound to albumin The initial starting dose is 20 mg once daily, and it is available in 20-, 40-, and 80-mg tablets. The terminal half-life is 9 hours, and approximately 55% of the parent compound is excreted by the kidney.[227] In a recent study to assess the pharmacokinetics of kidney disease of azilsartan, no dosage adjustment was advised for kidney disease or hemodialysis.[230] In a recent report, 17 hemodialysis patients who switched to azilsartan showed a decrease in systolic BP from 150.9 ± 16.2 to 131.3 ± 21.7 mm Hg ($P < 0.008$) and a decrease in diastolic BP from 84.1 ± 6.3 to 74.9 ± 8.3 mm Hg.[231]

Candesartan cilexetil is an esterified prodrug imidazole that is rapidly and completely converted into the active 7–carboxylic acid candesartan (CV-11974) in the intestinal wall.[12] Candesartan is a selective, nonpeptide, noncompetitive (insurmountable) ARB with the second highest receptor binding affinity and a slow detachment rate from the receptor (Table 50.7). Consequently, the effects are long-lasting and unlikely to be overcome by the upregulation of Ang II that commonly accompanies AT_1 receptor blockade. The initial dose is 16 mg daily, and the usual daily dose is 8 to 32 mg in one or two divided doses. The antihypertensive response occurs initially in 2 to 4 hours, peaks at 6 to 8 hours, and lasts for 24 hours (Tables 50.8 and 50.9).[223,232] Radioreceptor assays demonstrate the presence of candesartan at the receptor site for longer than predicted periods (from plasma half-life analysis), which correlates with the clinical observation of a sustained effect beyond 24 hours.[232,233] Maximal response is achieved in 4 weeks. The terminal half-life of candesartan is approximately 9 hours, and it is not affected by renal failure. No unchanged parent compound is detected in the serum or urine. Candesartan is not dialyzable.

Eprosartan is a nonpeptide selective ARB that was modified to more closely resemble Ang II.[234] It is a noncompetitive antagonist, with a high affinity for the AT_1 receptor (see Table 50.7).[12] The initial daily dose is 200 mg (see Table 50.8), and the usual daily dose is 200 to 400 mg. Eprosartan is rapidly absorbed, but its absorption is delayed by food (see Table 50.9). The initial response occurs in 4 hours and lasts for 24 hours. The elimination half-life is 6 hours. Dosages should be reduced by 50% in patients with renal failure.

Irbesartan is a nonpeptide-specific imidazolinone derivative of losartan that acts as a noncompetitive AT_1 receptor blocker with a very high receptor binding affinity[235] (see Table 50.7).[12] The initial dose is 150 mg daily, and the usual daily dose is 150 to 300 mg. The initial response occurs in 2 hours. The peak response is bimodal; in hypertensive patients, peak responses occur in 4 to 6 hours and 14 hours, corresponding to the peak increases in plasma renin activity and Ang II levels, respectively.[235] With continuous dosing, the maximal effect may not be seen for up to 6 weeks. The duration of action is 24 hours. Irbesartan is not dialyzable.

Losartan potassium is the prototype ARB. The tetrazole moiety on the biphenyl ring accounts for its activity in oral form and its duration of action. It was the first oral active agent, and it is a nonpeptide competitive, selective AT_1 receptor inhibitor, with moderate receptor binding affinity (see Table 50.7).[12,236] The usual starting dosage is 50 mg once daily (see Table 50.8). Dosage adjustments should be made at weekly intervals. The antihypertensive efficacy may be improved with divided doses. The usual daily dose is 50 to 100 mg. The potassium content of the 25-, 50-, and 100-mg tablets is 0.054, 0.108, and 0.216 mEq, respectively. The oral bioavailability of losartan is 25%, and it is unaffected by food (see Table 50.9). The initial response occurs in 1 hour, and the response peaks at 6 hours and lasts for 24 hours. Only 5% of losartan is recovered unchanged in

Table 50.7 Pharmacokinetic Interactions between Angiotensin II Type 1 (AT_1) Receptor Blockers and Receptor

Agent	AT_1 Receptor–Receptor Antagonist Dissociation Rate	Affinity (Kd)	Type of AT_1 Antagonism
Candesartan cilexetil (candesartan)	Slow	280	Noncompetitive
Irbesartan	Slow	5	Noncompetitive
Valsartan	Slow	10	Noncompetitive
Telmisartan	Slow	10	Noncompetitive
Losartan	Fast	50	Competitive
Eprosartan	Fast	100	Competitive

Table 50.8 Pharmacodynamic Properties of Angiotensin Receptor Blockers

Generic Name (Trade Name)	Initial Dose (mg)	Usual Dose (mg)	Maximum Dose (mg)	Interval	Peak Response (hr)	Duration of Response (hr)
Eprosartan (Teveten)	200	200-400	400	qd, bid	4	24
Irbesartan (Avapro)	150	150-300	300	qd	4-6, 14	24
Losartan (Cozaar)	50	50-100	100	qd/bid	6	12-24
Valsartan (Diovan)	80	80-160	300	qd	4-6	24
Candesartan (Atacand)	16	8-32	32	qd	6-8	24
Telmisartan (Micardis)	40	40-80	80	qd	3	24
Azilsartan (Edarbi)	20	40-80	80	qd	1.5 to 3 hours peak response	24+
Olmesartan (Benicar) Azilsartan	20	20-40	40	qd	1-2	24

Table 50.9 Pharmacokinetic Properties of Angiotensin Receptor Blockers

Drug	Absorption (%)	Bioavailability (%)	Affected by Food	Peak Blood Level (hr)	Elimination Half-Life (hr)	Metabolism	Excretion	Active Metabolites
Eprosartan	>80	13	Yes	4	6	L	F (70%), U (7%)	Inactive
Irbesartan	>80	60-80	No	1.5-2	10-14	L, K	F (65%), U (20%)	Inactive
Losartan	>80	25	No	1	4-9	L, K	F (60%), U (40%)	Active
Valsartan	>80	25	Yes	2-4	6-9	L, K	F (83%), U (13%)	Inactive
Candesartan	—	15	No	2-4	9	I, L, K	F (67%), U (33%)	None
Telmisartan	—	42	Yes	0.5-1	24	L	F	Inactive
Olmesartan	—	26	No	1	13	I	F (50%), U (50%)	Active

F, Feces; I, intestine; K, kidney; L, liver; U, urine.

the urine, which supports extensive metabolism and biliary secretion. Neither the parent drug nor metabolites are removed by dialysis.[22]

Olmesartan medoxomil is a nonpeptide selective ARB prodrug that is rapidly and completely bioactivated by hydrolysis to olmesartan during absorption from the gastrointestinal tract.[237] The initial dosage is 20 mg daily, and the usual dosage is 20 to 40 mg daily (see Table 50.8). The peak plasma concentration is reached in 1 hour (see Table 50.9). The BP-lowering effect lasts for 24 hours and peaks at 2 weeks. Olmesartan is eliminated in a biphasic manner, with a terminal half-life of 13 hours. Dosing and pharmacokinetics have not been studied in dialysis patients.

Nonbiphenyl Tetrazole Derivatives

Telmisartan incorporates a carboxylic acid as the biphenyl acidic group. Telmisartan is a nonpeptide, noncompetitive ARB, with high specificity and receptor affinity.[12,238] The usual starting dosage is 40 mg daily, and the usual daily dose is 40 to 80 mg. The initial response occurs in 3 hours, and it is dose-dependent (see Table 50.9). The duration of action is 24 hours but may last up to 7 days after discontinuing the drug. Women typically achieve plasma levels two to three times higher than those of men, but this result is not associated with differences in BP response. Less than 3% of the drug is metabolized in the liver into inactive compounds. The elimination half-life is 24 hours. Telmisartan is not dialyzable, and dosage adjustment is not necessary in patients with renal disease.

Nonheterocyclic Derivatives

Valsartan is a nonheterocyclic ARB in which the imidazole of losartan is replaced by an acetylated amino acid.[12] Valsartan is a noncompetitive antagonist with high specificity and receptor binding affinity (see Table 50.7). The initial starting dosage is 80 mg once daily (see Table 50.8), and the usual dosage is 80 to 160 mg daily. The maximal BP response is achieved after 4 weeks of therapy. The initial response occurs in 2 hours, peaks at 4 to 6 hours, and lasts 24 hours. Valsartan does not undergo significant metabolism. The elimination half-life is 6 to 9 hours, and it is not affected by renal failure (see Table 50.9).

CLASS RENAL EFFECTS

Intrarenal Ang II receptors are widely distributed in the afferent and efferent arterioles, glomerular mesangial cells, inner stripe of the outer medulla, and medullary interstitial cells,[239] as well as on the luminal and basolateral membranes of the proximal and distal tubule cells, collecting ducts, podocytes, and macula densa cells.[240] Most receptors are of the AT_1 subclass. Circulating and predominantly locally produced Ang II interacts with the receptors; the complex is internalized and Ang II is released into the intracellular compartment, where it exerts its effects. Studies have suggested that most renal interstitial Ang II is formed at sites not readily accessible to ACE inhibition or is formed by non-ACE pathways.

ARBs antagonize the binding of Ang II and cause a number of intrarenal changes. The overall renal hemodynamic responses of AT_1 receptor blockade are variable, depending on the counteracting influences of the decrease in arterial pressure.[207,241] Decreases in systemic arterial pressure by ARBs may be associated with compensatory activation of the intrarenal sympathetic nervous system, resulting in decreased renal function. This effect is more pronounced in sodium-depleted states because activation of the RAS helps maintain arterial and renal pressure. By contrast, direct intrarenal infusions of ARBs cause an increase in sodium excretion.[242] The enhanced sodium excretion has been shown to be due to direct inhibition of sodium reabsorption by the proximal tubules, but it may also be due to hemodynamic changes in medullary blood flow and tubule absorption in distal nephron segments. Because Ang II blockade enhances the ability of the kidneys to excrete sodium, sodium balance can be maintained at lower arterial pressures. Ang II blockade also reduces tubuloglomerular feedback sensitivity by decreasing macula densa transport of sodium chloride to the afferent arteriole.[243] This leads to increased delivery of sodium chloride to the distal segments for excretion, without compensatory changes in GFR.

In addition to the natriuretic and diuretic actions, short-term administration of some ARBs has been observed to induce reversible kaliuresis in salt-depleted normotensive subjects in the absence of changes in GFR.[244] However, long-term Ang II receptor blockade does not cause appreciable changes in urinary electrolyte excretion or volume. The kaliuretic effect may be due to specific intrinsic pharmacologic effects of the losartan molecule.

Another property unique to the losartan molecule is induction of uricosuria.[245] This effect is not observed with ACE inhibitors or other ARBs, including the active metabolite of losartan, and does not appear to be related to inhibition of the RAAS.[245] Losartan has a greater affinity for the urate-anion exchanger than other antagonists, and it inhibits urate reabsorption in the proximal tubule.[246] The uricosuria is associated with a concomitant decrease in serum uric acid levels in normal subjects, hypertensive subjects, and patients with renal disease and kidney transplants.[246] The effect occurs within 4 hours of drug administration and is dose-dependent. Long-term administration reduces uric acid levels by approximately 0.4 mmol/L.[247] The clinical implications of this effect are unknown. Concerns that increased uric acid supersaturation might perpetuate renal uric acid deposition have not been borne out clinically because losartan simultaneously increases urinary pH, which protects against crystal nucleation.[248] However, the decrease in the serum uric acid level might be beneficial because it has been suggested that hyperuricemia is a risk factor for renal disease progression[249] and coronary artery disease.[250]

Hypertensive patients treated with ARBs—both those with normal and those with impaired renal function—exhibit renal responses similar to or slightly greater than the responses of patients treated with ACE inhibitors.[251] In addition to decreases in systolic and diastolic BPs, patients demonstrate increases in renal blood flow and decreases in filtration fraction and renal vascular resistance, with no substantial changes in GFR.[252] These effects are probably a result of combined decreases in preglomerular and postglomerular resistances. It has been suggested that elevated intrarenal Ang II levels in the presence of AT_1 receptor blockade stimulates AT_2 receptors, which can increase the preglomerular vasodilator actions of bradykinin, cyclic guanosine monophosphate, and nitric oxide.[253] ACE inhibitors can potentiate this effect, but the clinical importance of this finding has not been established. Ang II blockade may significantly reduce GFR in underperfused kidneys. Patients with low perfusion pressures, dehydration, or renal artery stenosis may experience severe decreases in GFR but less severe decreases than with ACE inhibitors.[254] Under conditions of overperfusion, such as in hypertension associated with glomerulosclerosis and nephron loss or diabetes, Ang II blockade is protective. Such patients often have a suboptimal suppression of the RAAS. The lowering of efferent arteriole resistance reduces intraglomerular hydrostatic pressure, which attenuates the progression of renal injury, and increases renal sodium excretory capacity. In concert with the reduction in systemic arterial pressure, these actions may provide more renal protection than other classes of antihypertensive agents, despite equivalent reductions in BP.[82,255,256]

In healthy and hypertensive patients, ARBs produce dose-dependent increases in circulating Ang II levels and plasma renin activity.[257] The increases occur at the peak plasma drug levels and persist for up to 24 hours; they remain elevated with long-term administration. Decreases in plasma levels of aldosterone have been reported, but they are variable.[258] In normal individuals, the decreases coincide with the peak interval of ARB activity; in hypertensive patients consuming a fixed-sodium diet, there are no significant changes in aldosterone level from baseline.[244] ARBs suppress the Ang II–mediated adrenal cortical release of aldosterone, but these effects appear to be quantitatively less important than the intrarenal suppression of Ang II action. Long-term AT_1 receptor blockade does not appear to induce aldosterone escape.[259]

Urinary protein excretion is significantly decreased with administration of ARBs and parallels findings with ACE inhibitor therapy.[47] Antiproteinuric effects have been described in diabetic and nondiabetic patients, as well as renal transplantation patients.[47,260] The antiproteinuric effect has a slow onset, and the dose-response curves differ from those of the antihypertensive effects, in which the maximal effect occurs at 3 to 4 weeks. Currently, the peak of the dose-response curve has not been determined. Whether the antiproteinuric effects are equivalent to or better than those of ACE inhibitors remains to be determined, but it is evident that the suppression of albuminuria is equivalent at all stages of CKD.[261] ARBs and ACE inhibitors do appear to have additive and similar hemodynamic and antiproteinuric effects.[47] In a number of trials, ACE inhibitor therapy or ARB therapy reduced proteinuria by up to 40%. Combined therapy resulted in a 70% reduction of proteinuria, with no further changes in BP.[262,263] However, combination therapy appears to reduce intrarenal Ang II and transforming growth factor-β (TGF-β) levels more than high doses of either agent alone.[30] Combining ACE inhibitors and ARBs for renoprotection and proteinuria reduction is no longer recommended owing to the significant development of hyperkalemia, hypotension, and renal hypoperfusion, particularly in patients with underlying CKD.[101,154,264,265] Like ACE inhibitors, ARBs have nonhemodynamic effects that may contribute to renoprotection, including antiproliferative actions on the vasculature and mesangium, inhibition of TGF-β,[30,266] inhibition of atherogenesis[267] and vascular deterioration,[268] improved superoxide production and nitric oxide bioavailability,[269] reduction of collagen formation, reduction of mesangial matrix production, improved vascular wall remodeling, decreased vasoconstrictor effects of endothelin-1, improved endothelial function,[268] reduction of oxidative stress and inflammation,[270] modulation of peroxisome proliferator–activated receptor γ (PPARγ) activity, and protection from calcineurin inhibitor injury. ARBs also reduce salt sensitivity by restoring renal nitric oxide synthesis.[271] The clinical importance of these effects remains under investigation.

CLASS EFFICACY AND SAFETY

All AT_1 receptor blockers have been demonstrated to lower BP effectively and safely in patients with mild, moderate, and severe hypertension, regardless of age, gender, or ancestry.[272-274] The Trial of Preventing Hypertension (TROPHY) study evaluated the feasibility of treating patients with prehypertension (defined as a systolic BP of 130 to 139 mm Hg and a diastolic pressure of 85 to 89 mm Hg) with the ARB candesartan. After 4 years, patients randomly assigned to the ARB arm were significantly less likely to develop incident hypertension than those treated with placebo.[275] Prehypertension is a predictor of cardiovascular risk, but whether these data will change clinical practice remains speculative.

ARBs are indicated as first-line monotherapy or add-on therapy for hypertension and are comparable in efficacy to other agents.[276-278] They are safe and effective in patients with CKD (even when used at high dosages), diabetes, heart failure, renal transplants, coronary artery disease, arrhythmias, and left ventricular hypertrophy (LVH)[279-282] and have been shown to protect against hypertensive end-organ damage,[154,283,284] such as LVH, stroke, ESKD,[47,285] retinopathy,[286] exercise-induced inflammatory and prothrombotic stress, and possibly diabetes and dementia.[282,287-290a] Some but not all studies have shown a weak lowering of the risk for new and recurrent atrial fibrillation due to the beneficial structural and electrical effects on the atria.[125,126] ARBs have been shown to diminish the rate of persistent atrial fibrillation in patients with preexisting recurrent atrial fibrillation.[291] The Prevention Regimen for Effectively Avoiding Second Strokes (PRoFESS) study did not show any significant benefit of ARBs for the prevention of recurrent stroke but may have been underpowered to show an effect in its well-treated patient population.[292]

Although ARBs may not be the most efficacious agents in terms of BP reduction in African Americans, they are equally or more efficacious in providing target-organ protection and arresting disease progression compared to other antihypertensive agents that do not inhibit the RAAS.[293] Moreover, their antihypertensive activity is not attenuated by high-salt diets in African Americans.[277,293,294] In most patients, ARBs offer BP lowering comparable to that of all other antihypertensive drug classes, with an improved tolerability profile.[295]

ARBs provide effective control over a 24-hour period and are suitable for once-daily dosing.[296,297] Response rates vary from 40% to 60%. ARBs do not affect the normal circadian BP variation.[298] The long onset of action (4 to 6 weeks) avoids the first-dose hypotension and rebound hypertension that are commonly observed with other drugs. There is a dose-dependent response with newer agents, but losartan and valsartan have a relatively flat dose-response curve.[299]

Azilsartan, candesartan, irbesartan, and olmesartan may have the greatest efficacy, with a longer duration of action because of their noncompetitive binding, and telmisartan may have an added advantage by the inhibition of sympathetic nervous system (SNS) activation through an antioxidant effect in experimental models.[300,301]

The addition of thiazide diuretics to ARBs potentiates the therapeutic effect, increases response rates to 70% to 80%, and is more effective than increasing the ARB dosage. ARBs may also abrogate the adverse metabolic effects of thiazides.[302] Combining ARBs with ACE inhibitors is additive in reducing BP and effectively suppressing sympathetic activity, but this therapy has been shown to be associated with more adverse outcomes in high-risk patients, as previously discussed, and therefore is not recommended.[101,154,303]

An enhanced BP-lowering efficacy after 16 weeks of olmesartan-based treatment ($P = 0.0005$) may be observed in hypertensive patients with CKD-associated sympathetic hyperactivity, as evidenced by a baseline morning home systolic BP of 165 mm Hg or higher and patients with a morning home pulse rate of 70 beats/min or more in the Home BP Measurement With Olmesartan-Naive Patients to Establish Standard Target Blood Pressure (HONEST) study.[304] Similarly, the addition of mineralocorticoid receptor antagonists to ARBs provides added benefits for BP control and reduction of proteinuria in diabetic patients over the long term but has not been found to be protective from the decline in eGFR.[305] Combination therapy with ARBs plus dihydropyridines has additive effects in reducing BP and is well tolerated.[306]

ARBs may decrease kidney function and elevate serum potassium levels; serum chemistries should be checked after initiation or increase in dosage of these drugs. The overall incidence of hyperkalemia from ARBs is 3.3%, similar to that of ACE inhibitors.[154] Participants in the CHARM (Candesartan in Heart Failure-Assessment of Reduction in Mortality and Morbidity; $N = 7599$) program were randomized to standard heart failure therapy plus candesartan or placebo, with recommended monitoring of serum potassium and creatinine levels.[307] The authors assessed the incidence and predictors of hyperkalemia over the median 3.2 years of follow-up. Candesartan increased the risk of incident hyperkalemia compared to placebo from 5.2% from 1.8% (difference, 3.4%; $P < 0.0001$). The risk of hyperkalemia is increased in symptomatic heart failure patients with advanced age, male gender, baseline hyperkalemia, renal failure, diabetes, or combined RAAS blockade. Hyperkalemia has been treated with patiromer and sodium zirconium cyclosilicate in addition to sodium and calcium polystyrene sulfonate.[202,203] Judicious and careful use of ARBs is indicated, especially in patients with known renovascular hypertension and with especially careful attention to kidney function and serum potassium levels.[81]

ARBs should be stopped immediately at the onset of pregnancy with the first missed menstrual period in the first trimester, as discussed previously, as these drugs may cause fetal or neonatal death and congenital abnormalities when used during the second and third trimesters of pregnancy.[142] Breast feeding is not contraindicated, as per Kidney Disease: Improving Global Outcomes (KDIGO) and National Institute for Health and Care Excellence (NICE) guidelines; however, low drug levels are detected in breast milk.[145,146]

Overall, ARBs have neutral metabolic effects and are superior to other hypertensive classes with respect to tolerability. ARBs do not cause hypernatremia or hyponatremia, and hyperkalemia is relatively uncommon. In the ONTARGET study, a potassium level higher than 5.5 mmol/L was observed in 3.3% of patients who resigned from the study and is comparable to that observed with ACE inhibitor therapy[154]; it is amenable to treatment with new antihyperkalemia therapy.[202,203] Hyperkalemia is more likely to develop in patients with renal insufficiency or diabetes or in those taking potassium-sparing drugs. ARBs tend to lower levels of brain natriuretic peptide, which may explain their benefit in heart failure.[308] ARBs have no effect on serum lipid levels in hypertensive patients but may improve the abnormal lipoprotein profile of patients with proteinuric renal disease and reduce obesity-related morbidity.[309,310] ARBs have favorable effects on serum glucose levels and insulin sensitivity.[311-313] Clinical trials comparing ARB-based therapy with treatment with other antihypertensives in patients with hypertension with and without LVH demonstrated a 25% reduced risk of the development of diabetes in the ARB-treated group.[314,315] The mechanism for this effect has not been defined.[287,316] Increased levels of liver transaminases are occasionally reported, but the effects are usually transient, even with continued therapy.[12]

Clinically relevant adverse effects are not observed more frequently than in placebo-treated patients. Because ARBs do not interfere with kinin metabolism, cough is rare, which is a major clinical advantage.[154] The incidence of cough in patients with a history of ACE inhibitor–induced cough is no greater than in those receiving placebo.[317] Similarly, the incidence of angioedema and facial swelling is no greater than that with placebo, but such swelling can occur.[318] ARBs are typically associated with a more potent antiinflammatory response than ACE inhibitors.[319] The most frequent adverse effects are headache (14%), dizziness (2.4%), and fatigue (2%), which occur at rates lower than those with placebo.[320] ARB therapy not only does not worsen sexual activity, but may improve it.[321] Like ACE inhibitors, ARBs may cause minor decreases in the serum hemoglobin level; they may also lower the hemoglobin effectively in posttransplantation erythrocytosis.[322] There have been rare associated cutaneous eruptions.

A spruelike enteropathy associated with olmesartan therapy has been reported.[323,324] In a recent systematic review of 54 patients,[324] the clinical presentation was diarrhea (95%) and weight loss (89%). Less common symptoms were fatigue, nausea, vomiting, and abdominal pain. The patients had been taking olmesartan for 6 months to 7 years. A laboratory examination showed a normochromic, normocytic anemia (45%) and hypoalbuminemia (39%). HLA-DQ2 or HLA-DQ8 was observed in more than 70%. Antibody testing for celiac disease was negative. Duodenal villous atrophy in varying degrees was described in all the reported patients, and they all showed resolution of diarrhea. The FDA issued a drug safety communication on July 13, 2013 (http://www.fda.gov/Drugs/DrugSafety/ucm359477.htm).

ARBs have not been shown to have an increased cancer risk. An initial trial showed a slightly increased risk of cancer (relative risk [RR], 1.08; 95% confidence interval [CI], 1.01 to 1.15) in a meta-analysis of various antihypertensive drugs.[325] The methodology of this trial had been criticized

Table 50.10 Pharmacologic Properties of β-Adrenergic Antagonists

Generic Name (Trade Name)	β₁ Selectivity	Partial Agonist Activity	Membrane-Stabilizing Activity	α-Adrenergic Antagonist Activity
Nadolol (Corgard)				
Propranolol (Inderal)			+	
Carteolol (multiple)		+		
Penbutolol (Levatol)		+		
Pindolol (Visken)		+	+	
Labetalol (Trandate)		+		+
Carvedilol (Coreg)			+	+
Atenolol (Tenormin)	+			
Metoprolol (Lopresser)	+			
Betaxolol (Kerlone)	+		+	
Acebutolol (Sectral)	+	+	+	
Celiprolol (none in United States)	+			+
Bisoprolol (Zebeta)	+			
Nebivolol (Bystolic)	+			

because some randomized controlled trials were not included; had they been, the cancer signal would have disappeared. Subsequent meta-analyses[326-329] and cohort studies[330-334] were performed. The conclusion was that there was no evidence that ARBs are associated with cancers of any type in large populations, and one study indicated that ARBs may actually lower the incidence.[330] A subsequent systematic review of observational and interventional studies suggested that the use of ACE inhibitors and ARBs may improve cancer outcomes.[335]

Drug interactions with ARBs are uncommon but, as with ACE inhibitors, NSAIDs may blunt the natriuretic effect of ARBs.[336] ARBs have an increased incidence of hypotension and kidney impairment compared to ACE inhibitors.[154] Acute reversible renal failure has been reported with Ang II receptor blockade therapy in salt-depleted patients.[337] Thus, therapy should not be instituted in hypovolemic patients or in the setting of active diuresis. Concomitant use with ACE and renin inhibitors should be avoided in patients with a GFR lower than 60 mL/min and is contraindicated in patients with diabetes due to an increased risk of hypotension, hyperkalemia, and renal dysfunction.[101,265,338]

β-ADRENERGIC ANTAGONISTS

CLASS MECHANISMS OF ACTION

β-Adrenergic antagonists exert their antihypertensive effects by the attenuation of sympathetic stimulation through the competitive antagonism of catecholamines at the β-adrenergic receptor.[339] In addition to β-blockade properties, certain drugs have antihypertensive effects that are mediated through different mechanisms (Table 50.10), including α₁-adrenergic blocking activity, β₂-adrenergic agonist activity, and perhaps effects on nitric oxide–dependent vasodilator action. Partial agonist activity is a property of certain β-adrenergic blockers that results from a small degree of direct stimulation of the receptor by the drug, which occurs at the same time that receptor occupancy blocks the access of strongly stimulating catecholamines.[340-342] Whether the presence of partial agonist activity is advantageous or disadvantageous remains unclear. Drugs with partial agonist activity slow the resting heart rate less than drugs that lack this pharmacologic effect.[343] The exercise-induced increase in heart rate is similarly blocked by both groups of drugs.[343] However, β-adrenergic blockers with nonselective partial agonist activity may reduce peripheral vascular resistance and cause less atrioventricular (AV) conduction depression than drugs without partial agonist activity. The specificity of partial agonist activity for β₁- or β₂-receptors may also have a role in the antihypertensive response to a given drug.

β-Adrenergic receptor blockers may be nonspecific and block β₁- and β₂-adrenergic receptors, or they may be relatively specific for β₁-adrenergic receptors. β₁-Receptors are found predominantly in heart, adipose, and brain tissue, whereas β₂-receptors predominate in the lung, liver, smooth muscle, and skeletal muscle. Many tissues, however, have both β₁- and β₂-receptors, including the heart, and it is important to realize that the concept of a cardioselective drug is only relative.

β-Adrenergic blockers differ significantly in gastrointestinal absorption, first-pass hepatic metabolism, protein binding, lipid solubility, penetration into the CNS, and hepatic or renal clearance. β-Blockers that are eliminated primarily by hepatic metabolism have a relatively short plasma half-life; however, the duration of the clinical pharmacologic effect does not correlate well with the plasma half-life in many of these drugs. Water-soluble drugs that are eliminated by the kidney may have longer half-lives. Bioavailability varies greatly.

Overall, the precise mechanism of the antihypertensive effect of β-adrenergic blockers remains incompletely understood. β₁-Adrenergic receptor blockade has generally been considered responsible for the BP-lowering effect; however, β₂-receptor blockade has an independent antihypertensive effect.[344] Inhibition of β₁-adrenergic receptors in the juxtaglomerular cells in the kidney may inhibit renin release. A direct action on the CNS, with a reduction in CNS sympathetic outflow, may also be involved. Attenuation of cardiac pressor stimuli related to β-blockade may result in baroreceptor resetting. In addition, adrenergic neuron output may be blocked because of the inhibition of β₂-adrenergic receptors at the vascular wall.

Table 50.11 Pharmacokinetic Properties of β-Adrenergic Antagonists

Drug	Bioavailability (%)	Affected by Food	Peak Blood Level (hr)	Elimination Half-Life (hr)	Metabolism	Excretion	Active Metabolites
Nadolol	20-40	No	2-4	20-24	—	U, F	—
Propranolol	16-60	Yes	—	3-4	L	—	—
Timolol	50-90	—	—	2-4	L	U (20%)	—
Carteolol	84	Yes	—	5-8.5	L	—	—
Penbutolol	100	No	—	17-24	L	U	—
Pindolol	95	No	2	3-11	L	U (40%)	—
Atenolol	40-60	Yes	—	14-16	—	U, F	—
Metoprolol	50	—	1.5-2	3-7	L	U	—
Betaxolol	78-90	No	2-6	12-22	L	U	—
Bisoprolol	90	—	2.3	9.6	L	U	—
Acebutolol	90	No	2-3	3-8	L	U	—

F, Feces; L, liver; U, urine.

Table 50.12 Pharmacodynamic Properties of β-Adrenergic Antagonists

Drug	Initial Dose (mg)	Usual Dose (mg)	Maximum Dose (mg)	Interval	Peak Response (hr)	Duration of Response (hr)
Nadolol	40	40-80	320	qd	—	—
Propranolol	40	80-320	640	bid	—	—
Timolol	10	20-40	60	bid	—	—
Carteolol	2.5	2.5-10	60	qd	6	24
Penbutolol	20	20-40	80	qd, bid	2	20-24
Pindolol	5	10-40	60	qd, bid	—	24
Atenolol	25	50-100	200	qd	3	24
Metoprolol	12.5-50	100-200	450	qd, bid	1	3-6
Betaxolol	10	10-40	40	qd	3	23-25
Bisoprolol	2.5	2.5-20	40	qd	2-4	24
Acebutolol	400	400-800	1200	qd	3	24

Nonselective β-Adrenergic Antagonists

Nadolol is a nonselective β-adrenergic blocking agent without partial agonist activity (Table 50.11). The average adult dosage is 40 to 80 mg given once daily, with a maximum daily dose of 320 mg (Table 50.12). Nadolol is not appreciably metabolized, and elimination occurs predominantly in the urine and feces. Dosage adjustment is indicated in patients with renal failure. Dosage intervals should be increased to 24 to 36 hours, 24 to 48 hours, and 40 to 60 hours in patients with creatinine clearances of 30 to 50, 10 to 30, and less than 10 mL/min/1.73 m^2, respectively.[22] Dosage adjustment is not necessary in patients with hepatic insufficiency. Hemodialysis reduces the serum concentration of nadolol, but specific recommendations for dosage during dialysis are not available.

Propranolol is a noncardioselective β-adrenergic blocker (see Tables 50-11 and 50-12) that has no partial adrenergic activity. The usual daily dosage range is 80 to 320 mg. The drug may be administered in a single daily dose if a long-acting preparation is used. The drug is metabolized by the liver. The major metabolite, 4-hydroxypropranolol, has β-adrenergic blocking activity. Renal excretion is less than 1%. Dosage adjustment in patients with renal failure is not necessary.[22] Patients with liver disease may require variable dosage adjustments and more frequent monitoring.

Timolol is a nonselective β-adrenergic blocking agent without partial adrenergic activity (see Tables 50.11 and 50.12). The recommended initial dosage of timolol in the management of hypertension is 10 mg twice daily. The maintenance dosage generally ranges from 20 to 40 mg daily. No dosage adjustment is necessary in patients with renal failure.[22] Because timolol undergoes extensive hepatic metabolism, patients with liver disease may require a dosage adjustment and frequent monitoring. Timolol is not removed by dialysis.

Carteolol is a long-acting nonselective β-adrenergic blocker (see Tables 50-11 and 50-12).[345,346] It has moderate partial agonist activity,[347,348] and its recommended dosing is 2.5 to 10 mg daily. Doses of up to 60 mg/day have been used. Carteolol is eliminated primarily by the kidney. Dosage adjustment should be made for decreased renal function. The recommended dosing interval is 72 hours for a creatinine clearance less than 20 mL/min/1.73 m^2 and 48 hours for a creatinine clearance between 20 and 60 mL/min/1.73 m^2.[22]

Penbutolol is a nonselective, β-adrenergic blocking agent (see Tables 50-11 and 50-12).[345] This drug has low partial agonist activity. Usually, dosages are 20 to 40 mg given as a single dose or divided twice daily. Hepatic metabolism to inactive metabolites occurs with subsequent renal

Table 50.13 Pharmacokinetic Properties of β-Adrenergic Antagonists with Vasodilatory Properties

Drug	Bioavailability (%)	Affected by Food	Peak Blood Level (hr)	Elimination Half-Life (hr)	Metabolism	Excretion	Active Metabolites
Labetalol	25-40	Yes	1-2	5-8	L	U (50%-60%)	—
Carvedilol	25-35	No	1-1.5	6-8	L	F	—
Celiprolol	30-70	Yes	—	5-6	—	F, U	—
Nebivolol	12-96	No	2.4-3.1	8-27	L	—	—

F, Feces; L, liver; U, urine.

elimination. The optimal antihypertensive effect is observed at an average of 14 days after initiation of therapy. Dosage adjustments for patients with renal insufficiency are not recommended, but adjustment may be required for patients with hepatic insufficiency.[22]

Pindolol is a nonselective, β-adrenergic blocking agent with high partial agonist activity (see Tables 50-11 and 50-12). The usual adult oral dosage is 5 mg twice daily, with incremental 10- mg increases every 3 to 4 weeks. The maximum daily recommended dose is 60 mg. Approximately 40% of a dose of pindolol is excreted unchanged in the urine; 60% is metabolized in the liver. The drug half-life increases modestly in patients with renal impairment. Dosage adjustments do not appear be necessary.[22] Dosage adjustments may be necessary in patients with severely impaired hepatic function and in patients with concomitant cirrhosis and renal failure.

$β_1$-Selective Adrenergic Antagonists

Atenolol is a long-acting, $β_1$-selective, adrenergic blocking agent, with no partial agonist activity. The usual dosage is 50 to 100 mg once daily. Approximately 50% of the drug is eliminated by the kidneys, and 50% is excreted in the feces. Dosages of more than 100 mg/day are unlikely to produce additional benefits. The time required to achieve the optimal antihypertensive effect is 1 to 2 weeks. In patients with moderate renal insufficiency, the dosing interval should be increased to 48 hours, and in patients with advanced renal disease, dosing intervals should be increased to 96 hours.[22] Atenolol is not significantly metabolized by the liver, and no dosage adjustment is necessary in patients with hepatic disease. The drug is removed by dialysis, and a maintenance dose should be given after a dialysis treatment.

Metoprolol is a $β_1$-selective adrenergic blocker with no partial agonist activity. Extensive hepatic metabolism occurs primarily by the cytochrome P450 (CYP) 2D6 system (CYP2D6), and 3% to 10% of the drug is excreted unchanged in the urine. Metoprolol pharmacokinetics is heavily influenced by the CYP2D6 genotype and metabolizer phenotype, with up to a 15-fold difference in clearance between ultrarapid and poor metabolizers.[349] The initial oral dosage is 12.5 to 50 mg once or twice daily, increasing to 100 to 200 mg twice daily. Sustained-release (SR) preparations may be substituted as a once-daily dose.

Betaxolol is a long-acting, $β_1$-selective, adrenergic blocking agent,[350] with no partial agonist activity. The usual oral dosage for hypertension is 10 to 40 mg once daily. Therapy is typically started at a dosage of 10 mg once daily. Most patients respond to 20 mg once daily. The time to achieve the optimal antihypertensive effect is approximately 1 to 2 weeks. Renal dysfunction results in a decrease in betaxolol clearance. Titration should begin at 5 mg once daily in those with severe renal impairment. Betaxolol is metabolized predominantly in the liver, with metabolites excreted by the kidney. Approximately 15% of the dose is recovered unchanged in the urine.

Bisoprolol is a long-acting, $β_1$-selective, adrenergic blocking agent,[351] with no partial agonist activity. The usual oral dosage is 2.5 to 20 mg given once daily. Hepatic metabolism occurs with the renal excretion of metabolites; however, 50% of the drug is excreted by the kidney unchanged. In patients with renal failure, the initial oral dosage should be 2.5 mg once daily, with careful monitoring of dose titration. The maximum recommended dosage of bisoprolol in patients with renal failure is 10 mg/day. Similar dosage reduction is also required for patients with hepatic insufficiency.

Acebutolol is a $β_1$-selective, adrenergic blocking agent, with low partial agonist activity. Dosages of 400 to 1200 mg/day are effective in treating hypertension. The drug is metabolized to diacetolol, an active metabolite, with the parent compound being excreted renally and in bile. Diacetolol is excreted mainly by the kidneys. Dosage reduction of 50% to 75% is recommended for patients with advanced renal insufficiency.[22]

Nonselective β-Adrenergic Antagonists with α-Adrenergic Antagonism or other Mechanisms of Antihypertensive Action

Labetalol is a nonselective β-adrenergic blocking agent[352] that also possesses selective α-adrenergic blocking activity (Tables 50-13 and 50-14). It has weak partial agonist activity. The blocking of $β_1$- and $β_2$-adrenergic receptors is approximately equivalent. In addition, labetalol is highly selective for postsynaptic $α_1$-adrenergic receptors. After an oral dose, the ratio of $α_1$- to β-blocking potency is approximately 1:3. With intravenous administration, the β-blocking potency seems more prominent. The usual initial dosages for treatment of hypertension are 100 mg orally twice daily, increasing gradually to a maintenance dosage of 200 to 400 mg twice daily. The drug is metabolized in the liver, with 50% to 60% of a dose excreted in the urine and the remainder in the bile. Dosing adjustment is not required for any degree of renal failure.[22] Chronic liver disease has been demonstrated to decrease the first-pass metabolism of labetalol. Dosage reduction is required in these patients to avoid excessive decreases in heart rate and supine BP.

Table 50.14 Pharmacodynamic Properties of β-Adrenergic Antagonists with Vasodilatory Properties

Drug	Initial Dose (mg)	Usual Dose (mg)	Maximum Dose (mg)	Interval	Peak Response (hr)	Duration Of Response (hr)
Labetalol	100	200-800	1200-2400	bid	3	8-12
Carvedilol	6.25	12.5-25	50	bid	4-7	24
Celiprolol	200	200-600	—	qd	—	—
Nebivolol	5	5	—	qd	6	24

Carvedilol is a nonselective, β-adrenergic blocking agent with peripheral $α_1$-blocking activity (see Tables 50-13 and 50-14)[353,354] and no partial agonist activity. The drug is approximately equipotent in blocking $β_1$- and $β_2$-adrenergic receptors. Carvedilol is highly selective for postsynaptic $α_1$-adrenergic receptors. The ratio of $α_1$- to $β_1$-blocking activity is estimated to be 1:7.6. There is evidence that the therapeutic actions of carvedilol may depend in part on the endogenous production of nitric oxide, which may improve endothelial dysfunction in hypertensive patients. For the management of hypertension, an initial oral dosage of 6.25 mg twice daily is recommended and may be increased to 12.5 to 25 mg twice daily, if needed. Dosing adjustments are not required for patients with renal insufficiency. Carvedilol is extensively metabolized in the liver, and dosage reductions are suggested for patients with hepatic insufficiency.

Celiprolol is a β-blocker with several unique properties.[355,356] It is a $β_1$-adrenergic blocking agent with $α_2$-receptor blocking activity (see Tables 50-13 and 50-14). Celiprolol also causes vasodilation through $β_2$-receptor stimulation and possibly nitric oxide, with a subsequent decrease in systemic vascular resistance. In contrast to other β-blockers, celiprolol does not appear to induce bronchospasm or have negative inotropic effects. It does have moderate partial agonist activity. The initial dosage of celiprolol is 200 mg once daily and can be increased to 400 to 600 mg once daily. Renal excretion is 35% to 42%. A 50% dosage reduction is suggested in patients with a creatinine clearance of 15 to 40 mL/min/1.73 m^2. Celiprolol is not recommended for patients with a creatinine clearance less than 15 mL/min/1.73 m^2.

Nebivolol is a long-acting, $β_1$-selective adrenergic antagonist (see Tables 50-13 and 50-14).[357-361] The compound is a 1:1 racemic mixture of two enantiomers, D-nebivolol and L-nebivolol. The actions of nebivolol, which are unique and unlike those of other β-blocking agents, are attributable to the individual effects of the isomers. The $β_1$-adrenergic blocking effects are related to the D-isomer, whereas the L-isomer is essentially devoid of β-blocking properties at therapeutic doses. When administered alone, the L-isomer does not produce significant effects on BP; however, the antihypertensive effects of the D-isomer are enhanced by the presence of the L-isomer. The hypotensive effects of the racemic mixture are associated with a decrease in peripheral vascular resistance.[362] The mechanism whereby the L-isomer enhances the hypotensive effects of the D-isomer is unclear. It has been suggested that L-nebivolol may potentiate the effects of endothelium-derived nitric oxide and induce decreases in BP and peripheral vascular resistance. These effects may improve endothelial dysfunction and potentially influence cardiovascular risks.[363,364] It has also been suggested that the L-isomer may inhibit norepinephrine actions at the presynaptic β-receptors. The initial oral dosage is 5 mg once daily. The drug is metabolized in the liver; rapid and slow metabolizers have been identified. The half-life of nebivolol is 8 hours in rapid metabolizers and 27 hours in slow metabolizers. Reduced initial dosages are recommended for patients with renal insufficiency.

CLASS RENAL EFFECTS

Both α- and β-adrenergic receptors in the kidney mediate vasoconstriction and vasodilation as well as renin secretion. β-Adrenergic blockers may influence renal blood flow and GFR through their effects on cardiac output and BP in addition to direct effects on intrarenal adrenergic receptors. β-Adrenergic receptors have been localized to the juxtaglomerular apparatus in autoradiographic studies.[365] $β_2$-Receptors predominate in the kidney. The degree of specificity of β-adrenergic blockers for $β_1$- and $β_2$-receptors might be expected to influence the effect on renal function, as might the degree of intrinsic partial agonist activity. In general, the short-term administration of a β-adrenergic blocker usually results in a reduction of GFR and effective renal plasma flow.[366] This effect is independent of whether the drug has $β_1$-selectivity or intrinsic partial agonist activity. Nebivolol, carvedilol, and celiprolol, however, have vasodilatory properties and have been shown to increase GFR and renal plasma flow.[367] Nebivolol dilates glomerular afferent and efferent arterioles by a nitric oxide–dependent mechanism, in contrast to metoprolol, which had no similar effect.[368] This effect may be mediated by the increased synthesis of vasodilatory nitric oxide. Nadolol has been shown in some studies to increase renal plasma flow and glomerular filtration with intravenous administration; however, oral administration may result in decreased blood flow and GFR. $β_1$-Selective drugs, when administered orally, tend to produce smaller reductions in GFR and renal plasma flow. The long-term use of propranolol has been characterized by a 10% to 20% decrease in renal plasma flow and GFR. The degree of reduction in GFR and renal plasma flow is modest and probably not of great clinical significance in most cases.

The fractional excretion of sodium has been observed to decrease by up to 20% to 40% in some studies of the acute renal effects of β-blockade.[369] A combined α- and β-blockade with labetalol has shown little effect on renal hemodynamics.

β-Adrenergic antagonist therapy is usually associated with suppression of plasma renin activity.[370] Long-term effects, however, are less well defined. The degree of partial agonist activity may have a direct effect on renin secretion, regardless of the degree of $β_1$-selectivity of the adrenergic blocking agent, although not all studies have yielded consistent results. The exercise-induced increase in plasma renin activity has been shown to be suppressed by β-blockade.[371]

CLASS EFFICACY AND SAFETY

β-Adrenergic antagonists provide effective therapy for the management of mild to moderate hypertension; however, their use as first-line therapy has become controversial.[372-374] Based largely on data from the Antihypertensive and Lipid-Lowering Treatment to Prevent Heart Attack Trial (ALLHAT), the Seventh Report of the Joint National Committee on Prevention, Detection, Evaluation, and Treatment of High Blood Pressure (JNC 7) has strongly recommended a thiazide-type diuretic as appropriate initial therapy for most patients with hypertension.[87,375] The use of β-adrenergic antagonists is suggested mainly as secondary therapy for patients with specific comorbid conditions for which β-adrenergic antagonists have been shown to be of specific value, such as heart failure or angina, or after myocardial infarction.[339,376-378] Meta-analyses have suggested that compared with therapy with other agents, the reduction in major cardiovascular events associated with β-adrenergic antagonist therapy is not seen in older patients. In patients older than 60 years, β-blockers did not lower rates of myocardial infarction, heart failure, or death and were associated with higher rates of stroke compared to other therapies.[373,376,379] β-Blockers should not be considered first-line therapy for older patients without specific indications for their use.[326,380] In younger patients (<60 years), primary β-blocker therapy is associated with protection from major cardiovascular events equivalent to that associated with diuretic therapy. These recommendations are based on the results of numerous randomized clinical trials comparing therapy with β-blockers to treatment with other agents. A Cochrane review by Wiysonge and colleagues has concluded that the available evidence does not support the use of β-blockers as first-line drugs for the treatment of hypertension based on the relatively weak effect of β-blockers in reducing stroke and a trend toward worse outcomes compared with CCBs, RAAS inhibitors, and thiazide diuretics.[381] Wright and Musini obtained similar findings.[382] Messerli and associates examined the results of 10 trials involving more than 16,000 older patients randomly assigned to treatment with diuretics, β-blockers, or both.[383] Diuretic therapy was associated with a greater reduction in cerebrovascular events, fatal stroke, cardiovascular mortality, and all-cause mortality. In this analysis in older patients, β-blockers were effective in reducing cerebrovascular events and heart failure. This meta-analysis was complicated by the concurrent use of diuretics and β-blockers in 52% to 60% of patients. In another large meta-analysis, however, Law and coworkers concluded that all classes of BP-lowering drugs have a similar effect in reducing coronary heart disease events and stroke for a given reduction in BP.[384] Fretheim and colleagues found little or no difference among commonly used antihypertensive medications for the primary prevention of cardiovascular disease.[385]

Recent studies have suggested that β_1-selective blockers may have a slightly greater antihypertensive effect than nonselective agents. This effect may be in the range of 2 to 3 mm Hg. It may be that β_2-blockade in some fashion blunts the antihypertensive effects of β_1-blockade.[386] The β_2 partial agonist activity may mediate peripheral vasodilator effects that could contribute to the antihypertensive action. A β_1-selective antagonist with partial agonist activity at the β_1-receptor may result in less hypotensive effect. The magnitude and clinical significance of these differences are unclear.

β-Adrenergic antagonists provide useful therapy for patients in all ethnic groups.[387-389] Data reported by the Department of Veterans Affairs Cooperative Study Group on Antihypertensive Agents have suggested that the antihypertensive response to β-blocker therapy is lower in older African American patients.[388] Other studies have also suggested that β-adrenergic blockers may be less efficacious in African Americans than in white patients compared with therapy with CCBs and diuretics.[387,388,390] As a group, these drugs remain useful in African American patients, leading to significant reductions in BP, particularly when the more highly β_1-selective agents are used. β-Adrenergic blockers have been used to treat women with hypertension in the third trimester of pregnancy, although the birth weights of their infants have been observed to be lower. β-Adrenergic blockers are generally avoided in early pregnancy.[144,391-393] Labetalol with α- and β-adrenergic blocking characteristics is, however, commonly used in pregnancy.

β-Adrenergic antagonists have been shown to have important effects on outcome in patients with coronary artery disease.[394,395] The use of a β-blocker after an acute myocardial infarction (MI) has been shown to reduce morbidity and mortality.[396] Despite the clear benefit, β-blockers have been underused in this setting. When prescribed, they are often used in dosages considerably lower than those proved to be effective in the clinical trials. A survey of postinfarction β-blockade usage involving more than 200,000 patients found that a survival benefit from β-blockade was apparent, regardless of systolic BP, age, or ejection fraction.[395] Different subtypes of β-blockers did not differ with regard to survival post-MI because the effects of atenolol, metoprolol, and propranolol were similar in a retrospective study of more than 200,000 patients, although these drugs differ in β_1-selectivity.[397] β-Blockers with intrinsic sympathetic activity were associated with reduced clinical benefits post-MI.[398] Patients with chronic obstructive pulmonary disease, which is commonly regarded as a contraindication to β-blockade, also had a significant decrease in the risk of death when treated with a β-blocker.[395] Other studies have shown a 20% reduction in total mortality and a 32% to 50% reduction in sudden death with β-blocker therapy in patients who have experienced an MI.[394] In a study of stable outpatients with coronary artery disease, β-blocker use was associated with cardiovascular end points only in those with an MI in the last year and not in those with coronary artery disease.[396] For hypertensive patients with a previous MI (at least in the last year), β-adrenergic antagonists may be the drugs of choice for antihypertensive therapy.[87,395,399]

Patients with coexisting heart failure and hypertension are an appropriate population for treatment with β-adrenergic antagonists.[400-402] The Cardiac Insufficiency Bisoprolol Study II demonstrated a 20% reduction in mortality in patients with moderate heart failure randomly assigned to therapy with a β-blocker.[403] Hospitalizations for heart failure were reduced, and sudden death was reduced by 44%. Similar results were observed in a large randomized intervention trial using metoprolol in patients with congestive heart failure. Over the long term, treatment with β-adrenergic blockers improves exercise tolerance, left ventricular geometry, and left ventricular structure and reduces myocardial oxygen demand. The magnitude of heart rate reduction with β-blockers, but not the dose, is significantly associated with the survival benefit in heart failure.[404] β-Blockers may differ in effects on cardiovascular outcomes. A meta-analysis has suggested that the vasodilatory β-blocker carvedilol has a greater effect on all-cause mortality in systolic heart failure compared to $β_1$-selective β-blockers, although this has not been observed in all studies.[379,404,405] Genetic polymorphisms affecting the $β_1$-adrenergic receptor, the $α_{2C}$-adrenergic receptor and the G protein–coupled receptor kinase have been suggested to modify heart failure risk and the response to β-blocker therapy.[406] Whether β-adrenergic blockers have a role in the primary prevention of cardiac disease in hypertensive patients is less clear than their role in patients with preexisting cardiac disease, for whom the benefits are quite apparent.[407-409] A meta-analysis has shown β-blockade to be significantly associated with a reduced risk of stroke and congestive heart failure.[407]

Agents with $β_1$-selectivity or intrinsic sympathetic activity have a therapeutic advantage over nonselective β-adrenergic antagonists in the treatment of patients with bronchospastic airway disease, chronic obstructive pulmonary disease, peripheral vascular disease, and diabetes mellitus.[340,410,411] Bronchoconstriction is mediated in part by $β_2$-adrenergic receptors in the airways. β-Blockade with nonselective agents can lead to increased airway resistance. This increase is less likely to occur with $β_1$-selective agents. $β_1$-Selectivity is relative, however, and may be less apparent at higher dosages. Patients with severe bronchospastic airway disease should not receive β-blockers. In patients with mild to moderate disease, $β_1$-selective agents may be used cautiously; it has been proposed that they have beneficial effects on airway hyperresponsiveness.[412] Symptoms of peripheral vascular disease may be exacerbated by β-blocker therapy.[413] Cold extremities and absent pulses have been described in patients with severe disease. Reynaud's phenomenon has been reported with nonselective β-blockade.[414] Blockade of $β_2$-receptor–mediated skeletal muscle vasodilation as well as decreased cardiac output may contribute to vascular insufficiency.[415] A meta-analysis has shown that treatment with β-adrenergic blockers does not worsen intermittent claudication or walking capacity in patients with mild to moderate peripheral vascular disease.[416]

The CNS symptoms of sedation, sleep disturbance, depression, and visual hallucinations have been reported with β-adrenergic blockade. These symptoms may be more common with lipid-soluble β-blockers and less common with nebivolol.[417] Sexual dysfunction has been reported but is less of a problem with $β_1$-selective, non–lipid-soluble agents.[418] In a review of 15 randomized trials involving more than 35,000 subjects, β-blocker therapy was not associated with a significant annual increase in the risk of reported depressive symptoms (6/1,000 patients; 95% CI, −7 to 19). β-Blockers were associated with a small but significant annual increase of reported fatigue (18/1,000 patients; 95% CI, 5 to 30). β-Blockers were associated with a small but significant annual increase in reported sexual dysfunction (5/1,000 patients; 95% CI, 2 to 8). None of the adverse effects differed by lipid solubility.[419] Changes in cognitive function—both improvement and worsening—have been reported; however, there is no clear mechanism whereby such symptoms may arise. Constipation, diarrhea, nausea, and indigestion may occasionally occur with β-blockers. These symptoms are probably less common with $β_1$-selective agents.

β-Adrenergic receptors have important effects on glucose metabolism, mediating increases in glycogenolysis and gluconeogenesis from amino acids and glycerol, and inhibit glucose uptake in the periphery. These effects may result in impaired glucose tolerance and an increased blood glucose level in some diabetic patients. β-Blockers differ in terms of their effects on glucose metabolism. Nonvasodilating β-blockers, such as metoprolol, are associated with a worsening of glycemic control. Metoprolol has been shown to decrease insulin sensitivity significantly, whereas nebivolol does not.[420] Numerous studies have shown that vasodilating β-blockers are associated with more favorable effects on glucose metabolism.[421] β-Blockers are associated with weight gain and an increased risk of new-onset diabetes mellitus.[422,423] β-Blockade can result in the blunting of the effects of epinephrine secretion resulting from hypoglycemia and lead to hypoglycemia unawareness.[424,425] Nonselective β-adrenergic blockers and, to a lesser degree, $β_1$-selective agents, have been associated with a rise in the serum potassium level.[426] Suppression of aldosterone and inhibition of $β_2$-linked, sodium-potassium membrane transport in skeletal muscle have been proposed as possible mechanisms.[427,428] This effect is of limited clinical importance in patients who have normal renal function and are not taking other medications that might affect serum potassium levels. Acceleration of the development of antinuclear antibodies (ANAs) was reported with the β-blockers atenolol (10.9%), labetalol (13.8%), and acebutolol (33%) compared to other β-blockers, with which the fraction of patients developing ANAs was less than 10%.[429]

β-Adrenergic blocking agents can affect lipid levels.[430] Long-term use of β-adrenergic blockers has been associated with an increase in triglyceride levels and a decrease in the level of HDL cholesterol. β-Blockers with increased $β_1$-selectivity or with partial agonist activity appear to have less effect on the lipid profile. Nonselective β-blockers without partial agonist activity may decrease the HDL cholesterol level by up to 20%; an increase in triglyceride levels of up to 50% has been reported. The effects of β-blockade on lipid metabolism are due primarily to the modulation of lipoprotein lipase activity. Very-low-density lipoprotein (VLDL) cholesterol and triglyceride metabolism is reduced in the setting of unopposed β-adrenergic stimulation of lipoprotein lipase activity. Decreased VLDL metabolism results in decreases in HDL cholesterol levels.

Abrupt withdrawal of β-adrenergic blockers may be associated with overshoot hypertension and worsening angina in patients with coronary artery disease.[431] Myocardial infarction has been reported. These withdrawal symptoms may be due to increased sympathetic activity, which is a reflection of possible adrenergic receptor upregulation during long-term sympathetic blockade. Gradual tapering of β-blockers decreases the risk of withdrawal. Withdrawal symptoms have been reported more commonly with abrupt discontinuation of relatively short-acting drugs. Withdrawal symptoms are relatively unusual with longer acting agents.[432]

CALCIUM CHANNEL BLOCKERS

CLASS MECHANISMS OF ACTION

CCBs remain an important therapeutic class of medications for a variety of cardiovascular disorders.[433-436] Initially introduced in the 1960s as antianginal agents, CCBs are now widely advocated as first-line therapy for hypertension.[87,437] The pharmacologic effects of these drugs are related to their ability to attenuate cellular calcium uptake.[438-442] CCBs do not directly antagonize the effects of calcium; rather, they inhibit the entry of calcium or its mobilization from intracellular stores.

Calcium channels have binding sites for activators and antagonists. The voltage-dependent, L-type calcium channel is a multimeric complex composed of α_1-, α_2-, ω-, β-, and γ-subunits.[433] These channels have different binding sites for the various CCBs and are regulated by voltage-dependent and receptor-dependent events involving protein phosphorylation and G protein coupling resulting from, for example, β-adrenergic stimulation.[443] Each class of CCB is quantitatively and qualitatively unique; the CCB classes possess different sensitivities and selectivities for binding pharmacologic receptors and the slow calcium channel in various vascular tissues. Even within the dihydropyridine class, there is considerable pharmacologic variability.[444] This differential selectivity of action has important clinical implications for the use of these drugs and explains why the CCBs vary considerably in their effects on regional circulatory beds, sinus and AV nodal function, and myocardial contractility. The selectivity further explains the diversity of indications for clinical use, ancillary effects, and side effects.[445]

CCBs represent ideal antihypertensive agents because they uniformly lower peripheral vascular resistance in patients, regardless of ancestry, salt sensitivity, age, or comorbid conditions. There are at least three mechanisms through which CCBs lower BP. First, CCBs reduce peripheral vascular resistance by attenuating the calcium-dependent contractions of vascular smooth muscle. Contraction of vascular smooth muscle depends on the total cytosolic calcium concentration, which in turn is regulated by two distinct mechanisms. Depolarization of vascular smooth muscle tissue depends on the inward flux of calcium through voltage-sensitive L-type and T-type calcium channels. Hypertensive patients have an abnormal influx of calcium, which promotes increased peripheral vascular resistance.[438] Calcium is released from the sarcoplasmic reticulum in response to extracellular calcium influx via a non–voltage-dependent pathway. Cytosolic calcium binds to calmodulin, initiating a sequence of cellular events that promotes the interaction between actin and myosin and results in smooth muscle contraction. Therefore, the importance of the calcium channels lies in their pivotal role in linking cell membrane electrical activity to biologic responses. Calcium influxes through L-type channels from extracellular sources and intracellular sources are both attenuated by CCBs.[435,439]

Second, CCBs decrease vascular responsiveness to Ang II and the synthesis and secretion of aldosterone.[441] CCBs also interfere with α_2-adrenergic receptor–mediated vasoconstriction and possibly α_1-adrenergic receptor–mediated vasoconstriction.[440,446] The maximal vasodilatory response, as measured by forearm blood flow, appears to be inversely related to the patient's plasma renin activity and Ang II concentration. Thus, it is possible that there is a greater influence of the calcium influx–dependent vasoconstriction in patients with low-renin hypertension, such as African Americans, which explains the clinical observation that CCBs are often more potent than other agents in such groups.

Finally, the CCBs may induce a mild diuresis. It is well known that the dihydropyridines, in particular, reduce preglomerular resistance and maintain or increase the GFR because of their preferential vasodilatory action on the renal afferent arteriole.[442] Subsequently, decreased tubular sodium reabsorption and improved renal blood flow and natriuresis are observed. The sodium excretion rate tends to correlate with the reduction in BP.

Antihypertensive activity has not uniformly been demonstrated to be secondary to changes in nitric oxide release. The vasorelaxant properties of nifedipine and verapamil appear to be nitric oxide–independent, whereas those of amlodipine are partly nitric oxide–dependent.[447,448] This effect of amlodipine is thought to be mediated by the inhibition of local ACEs and increases in vasodilatory bradykinins.

CLASS MEMBERS

Despite their shared mechanism of action, the CCBs are a very heterogeneous group of compounds. They differ with respect to pharmacologic profile, chemical structure, pharmacokinetic profile, tissue specificity, receptor binding, clinical indications, and side effect profile (Tables 50.15 and 50-16). Two primary subtypes are distinguished on the basis of their behavior, dihydropyridines and nondihydropyridines. The nondihydropyridines are further divided into two classes—benzothiazepines (diltiazem) and diphenylalkylamines (verapamil). Their distinctly different pharmacologic effects are summarized in Tables 50-15 and 50-16.

Although all CCBs vasodilate coronary and peripheral arteries, the dihydropyridines are the most potent. Because those in this subclass of CCBs are membrane-active drugs, they exert a greater effect on the peripheral vessels than on myocardial cells, which depend less heavily on the external calcium influx than on vessels.[439] Their potent vasodilatory action prompts a rapid compensatory increase in sympathetic nervous activity, as mediated by baroreceptor reflexes creating a neutral or positive inotropic stimulus.[449] Longer acting dihydropyridines, however, do not appear to activate the SNS.[450] By contrast, the nondihydropyridines are moderately potent arterial vasodilators but directly decrease AV nodal conduction and have negative inotropic and chronotropic effects, which are not abrogated by the reflex increase in sympathetic tone. Because of their negative inotropic action, their use is contraindicated in patients with systolic heart failure. As expected, these drugs are more effective at reducing stress-induced cardiovascular responses than dihydropyridines.[451]

A clinically useful classification system for CCBs categorizes them by their duration of action into short-acting and long-acting agents (to be given once daily; see Tables 50-15 and 50-16). This schema is helpful because the short-acting agents are no longer recommended for the management of hypertension due to their stimulation of the SNS, which may predispose patients to angina, myocardial infarction, and stroke.[452] The long-acting drugs are commonly divided into three generations. First-generation agents, such

Table 50.15 Pharmacodynamic Properties of Calcium Channel Blockers

Generic Name (Trade Name)	First Dose (mg)	Usual Daily Dosage (mg)	Maximum Daily Dose (mg)	Peak Response (hr)	Duration of Response (hr)
Diltiazem (Cardizem)	60	60-120 tid, qid	480	2.5-4	8
Diltiazem SR (Cardizem SR)	180	120-240 bid	480	6	12
Diltiazem CD (Cardizem CD)	180	240-280 qd	480	—	24
Diltiazem XR (Dilacor XR)	180	180-480 qd	480	3-6	24
Diltiazem ER (Tiazac)	180	180-480 qd	480	4-6	24
Amlodipine (Norvasc)	5	5-10 qd	10	30-50	24
Felodipine (Plendil ER)	5	2.5 qd	20	2-5	24
Isradipine (DynaCirc)	2.5	2.5-5 bid	20	2-3	12
Isradipine CR (DynaCirc CR)	5	5-20 qid	20	2	7-18
Nicardipine (Cardene)	20	20-40 tid	120	0.5-2	8
Nicardipine SR (Cardene SR)	30	30-60 bid	120	1.4	12
Nifedipine (Procardia, Adalat)	10	10-30 tid, qid	120	0.1	4-6
Nifedipine GITS (Procardia XL)	30	30-90 qd	120	4-6	24
Nifedipine ER (Adalat CC)	30	30-90 qd	120	2-6	24
Nisoldipine (Sular)	20	20-40 qd	60	—	24
Verapamil (Calan, Isoptin)	80	80-120 tid	480	6-8	8
Verapamil SR (Calan SR, Isoptin SR)	120	120-240 bid	480	—	12-24
Verapamil SR Pellet (Verelan)	120	240-480 qd	480	—	24
Verapamil COER-24 (Covera-HS)	180	180-480 qhs	480	>4-5	24
Mibefradil (Posicor)	50	50-100 qd	100	2-4	17-25

CD, Controlled-diffusion; CODAS, chronotherapeutic oral drug absorption system; COER, controlled-onset extended release; CR, controlled release; ER, extended release; F, feces; GITS, gastrointestinal therapeutic system; L, liver; SR, sustained release; U, urine; XR, extended release.

Table 50.16 Pharmacokinetic Properties of Calcium Channel Blockers

Drug	Oral Absorption (%)	First-Pass Effect	Bioavailability (%)	Peak Blood Level	Elimination Half-Life (hr)	Metabolism and Excretion	Protein Binding (%)	Active Metabolites
Diltiazem	98	50%	40	2-3 hr	4-6	L, F, U	77-93	Yes
Diltiazem SR	>80	50%	35	6-11 hr	5-7	L, F, U	77-93	Yes
Diltiazem CD	95	E	35	12 hr	5-8	L, F, U	77-93	Yes
Diltiazem XR	95	E	41	4-6 hr	5-10	L, F, U	95	Yes
Diltiazem ER	93	E	40-60	4-6 hr	10	L, F, U	95	Yes
Amlodipine	>90	M	88	6-12 hr	30-50	L/U	>95	Yes
Felodipine	>90	E	13-18	2.5-5 hr	11-16	L/U	>95	No
Isradipine	>90	E	15-25	2-3 hr	8	L, F, U	>95	No
Isradipine CR	>90	E	15-25	7-18 hr	—	L, F, U	>95	No
Nicardipine	>90	E	35	0.5-2 hr	8.6	L, F, U	>95	No
Nicardipine SR	>90	E	35	1-4 hr	—	L, F, U	>95	No
Nifedipine	>90	20%-30%	60	<30 min	2	L, U	98	Yes
Nifedipine GITS	>90	25%-35%	86	6 hr	—	L, U	98	Yes
Nifedipine ER	>90	25%-35%	86	2.5-5 hr	7	L, U	98	Yes
Nisoldipine	>85	E	4-8	6-12 hr	10-22	L, F, U	99	No
Verapamil	>90	70%-80%	20-35	1-2 hr	2.8-7.4	L, F, U	85-95	Yes
Verapamil SR	>90	70%-80%	20-35	5-6 hr	4-12	L, F, U	85-95	Yes
Verapamil SR pellet	>90	70%-80%	20-35	7-9 hr	12	L, F, U	85-95	Yes
CODAS Verapamil	>90	70%-80%	20-35	11 hr	—	L, F, U	85-95	Yes

CD, Controlled-diffusion; CODAS, chronotherapeutic oral drug absorption system; CR, controlled release; E, extensive; ER, extensive release; F, feces; GITS, gastrointestinal therapeutic system; L, liver; M, minimal; SR, sustained release; U, urine; XR, extended release.

as nifedipine, have shorter half-lives and require multiple daily doses. Second-generation agents have been modified into SR formulations, requiring once-daily dosing. The third-generation agents have intrinsically longer plasma or receptor half-lives, possibly related to their greater lipophilicity.[453]

Benzothiazepines

Diltiazem hydrochloride is the prototype of the benzothiazepine CCBs. Diltiazem is 98% absorbed from the gastrointestinal tract, but because of extensive first-pass hepatic metabolism, its bioavailability is only 40% compared with intravenous dosing[12] (see Tables 50-15 and 50-16). In vivo, the competitively inhibited liver CYP2D6 isoenzyme is the most important metabolic pathway and probably accounts for the substantial proportion of drug interactions that occur with diltiazem.[454] The rates of elimination are lower in older persons and those with chronic liver disease but unchanged in patients with renal insufficiency.

Oral forms of diltiazem have been modified to improve delivery and currently include tablets, SR capsules, controlled-diffusion (CD) capsules, Geomatrix extended-release (XR) capsules, extended-release (ER) capsules, and buccoadhesive formulations.[455-457] The usual starting dosage for the drug in tablet form is 180 mg/day in three divided doses, and the drug may be titrated to a total dosage of 480 mg/day (see Table 50.15).

The SR tablet release rate varies with the size of the matrix.[458] Therefore, the long-acting preparations should not be divided. The usual daily dose is 120 to 240 mg, and the peak response usually occurs within 6 hours. The CD capsules are composed of two types of diltiazem beads; 40% of the beads release the drug within 12 hours, and the remaining 60% release the drug over the next 12 hours.[12] The usual daily dose is 240 to 480 mg. Approximately 95% of the drug is absorbed, peak plasma levels occur in 10 to 14 hours, and the plasma half-life is 5 to 8 hours but increases with increasing dose. The XR capsules contain a degradable "swellable" controlled-release (CR) matrix that slowly releases the drug over 24 hours. The usual daily dose is 180 to 480 mg; 95% of the drug is absorbed. The onset of action is within 3 to 6 hours, and the half-life ranges from 5 to 10 hours. ER capsules contain microgranules that dissolve at a constant prolonged rate. Peak blood levels are achieved after 4 to 6 hours, and bioavailability is 93%. The usual daily dose is 180 to 480 mg, with an elimination half-life of up to 10 hours. A buccoadhesive formulation has been developed to avoid the effects of hepatic first-pass metabolism and improve bioavailability.[457] The dissolution and diffusion of the buccoadhesive hydrophilic matrices of diltiazem polymers provide reliable delivery for up to 10 hours. The optimal use of this vehicle is still under investigation.[459]

Diphenylalkylamine

Verapamil hydrochloride, the oldest CCB, is the prototype diphenylalkylamine derivative. Verapamil inhibits membrane transport of calcium in myocardial cells, particularly the AV node, and smooth muscle cells, which renders it antiarrhythmic, antihypertensive, and a negative inotrope. The drug is available for oral administration as film-coated tablets containing 40, 80, or 120 mg of racemic verapamil hydrochloride.[12] The usual daily dose is 80 to 120 mg three times daily (see Table 50.15). The elimination half-life increases with long-term administration and in older patients with renal insufficiency (see Table 50.16).

The SR caplets are available in scored 120-, 180-, and 240-mg forms. The usual antihypertensive dose is equivalent to the total daily dose of immediate-release tablets and can be given as 240 to 480 mg/day. An adequate antihypertensive response may be improved by divided twice-daily dosing.

The SR pellet–filled verapamil capsules are gel-coated capsules with an onset of action of 7 to 9 hours that is not affected by food. The peak concentrations are approximately 65% of those of immediate-release tablets, but the trough concentrations are 30% higher. The usual daily dose is 240 to 480 mg.

The controlled-onset, extended-release (COER) and chronotherapeutic oral drug absorption system (CODAS) tablets have unique pharmacologic properties and deliver verapamil 4 to 5 hours after ingestion. A delay coating is inserted between the outer semipermeable membrane and active inner drug core. As the delay coating expands in the gastrointestinal tract, the pressure causes drug from the inner core to be released through laser-drilled holes in the outer membrane, making this formulation ideal for nighttime dosing by providing maximal plasma levels in the early morning hours, from 6 AM to noon, and minimizing nighttime diurnal BP variations.[460] A buccal gel formulation of verapamil that provides sustained release of the drug up to 6 hours has recently been reported.[461]

Of the 13 known metabolites of verapamil, norverapamil is the only one with cardiovascular activity; it has 20% of the potency of the parent compound. Renal excretion accounts for 70% of clearance and occurs within 5 days. The remainder is excreted in the feces. Clearance decreases with increasing age and decreasing weight.[462] With long-term administration, there is a significant increase in bioavailability, possibly as a result of saturation of hepatic enzymes. Dosage adjustment is necessary in patients with hepatic but not renal failure; however, verapamil should be used with caution in patients who ingest large amounts of grapefruit juice or those with renal insufficiency who are taking concurrent AV nodal blocking agents.[463]

Dihydropyridines

Nifedipine is a dihydropyridine CCB that causes decreased peripheral resistance, with no clinically significant depression of myocardial function. Because of the reflex sympathetic stimulation triggered by vasodilation, nifedipine has no tendency to prolong AV conduction or sinus node recovery or slow the sinus rate. Clinically, there is usually a small increase in heart rate and cardiac index. The labeling for immediate-release nifedipine capsules has been revised to recommend against using this dosage form for the management of chronic hypertension.[12,464] In older persons, use of the immediate-release form has been associated with a greater than threefold increase in mortality compared with the use of other antihypertensive agents, including other CCBs.[465] In most patients, immediate-release nifedipine causes a modest hypotensive effect that is well tolerated. However, in occasional patients, the hypotensive effect is profound and has resulted in myocardial infarction, stroke, and death.[464] This effect appears to be more pronounced in patients also taking β-blockers.[466] Consequently, its use should be reserved for short periods, but not in the setting of acute syndromes. The usual adult dosage is 10 to 30 mg three times daily, and the dose can be titrated weekly (see Table 50.15). Nifedipine is rapidly and fully absorbed, and drug levels are detectable within 10 minutes of ingestion. Peak levels are achieved within 30 minutes, and the half-life is 2 hours. There is no clinical advantage to ingestion using the technique of bite and swallow or bite and hold sublingually.

Nifedipine is extensively metabolized in the liver and then excreted in the urine. Most of the population is reported to metabolize the drug rapidly. Because nifedipine is 98% protein-bound, the dosage should be adjusted in patients with hepatic insufficiency or severe malnutrition.

The ER tablets of nifedipine are available in 30-, 60-, and 90-mg doses. These tablets consist of an outer semipermeable membrane surrounding an active drug core.[467] The core is composed of an inner active drug layer surrounded by an osmotically active, inert layer that forces the dissolution of the drug core as it swells from gastrointestinal juice absorption. The drug is then slowly and steadily released over 16 to 18 hours. This method of delivery is termed the *gastrointestinal therapeutic system*, or GITS, formulation. The ER form should not be bitten or divided. The time to peak concentration is 6 hours, and plasma levels remain steady for 24 hours. The bioavailability of the ER tablet is 86% compared with that of immediate-release forms, and tolerance does not develop.[467] Of the metabolites, 80% are excreted in the urine. The remainder is excreted in the feces, along with the outer semipermeable membrane shell. The usual adult maintenance dosage is 30 to 90 mg/day. Conversion from the immediate-release form to ER tablets can be done on an equal-milligram basis.

A similar ER formulation is composed of a coat and core.[468] The outer layer contains a slow-release form of nifedipine; the inner core is a fast-release preparation. Peak concentrations are reached within 2.5 to 5 hours, and there is a second peak after 6 to 12 hours as the inner core is released. When the drug is administered in this way, the half-life is extended from 2 to 7 hours. The usual daily dose is 30 to 90 mg, and the dose should be titrated by 30-mg increments in 7 to 14 days for maximal effect. Because of the unique delivery system, which provides a rapid-release core, peak plasma concentrations are not always reliable. Ingestion of three 30-mg tablets simultaneously, but not two, results in a 29% higher peak plasma concentration than the ingestion of a single 90-mg tablet. Consequently, two tablets may be substituted for 60 mg, but the substitution of three 30-mg tablets to make 90 mg is not recommended.[12]

Amlodipine besylate is unique among the dihydropyridine CCBs. It appears to bind to dihydropyridine and nondihydropyridine sites to produce peripheral arterial vasodilation without significant activation of the SNS.[22] The parent compound has substantially slower but more complete absorption than others in the class (see Table 50.16). After ingestion, amlodipine is almost completely absorbed, peak concentrations are achieved in 6 to 12 hours, and the clinical response can be detected at 24 hours. The mean peak serum levels are linear, age- independent, and achieved after 7 to 8 days of continuous dosing.[469] The elimination half-life is long, ranging from 30 to 50 hours, and is prolonged in older adults. The long half-life permits once-daily dosing, the hypotensive response may last up to 5 days,[470] 90% of amlodipine is metabolized in the liver, and 10% is excreted unchanged. The metabolites are excreted primarily in the urine, but no dosage adjustment is necessary with renal impairment. The minimum effective dose is 2.5 mg, particularly in older patients. Most patients require a dosage of 5 to 10 mg/day.

Benidipine is a long-acting dihydropyridine CCB that is available for the management of mild to moderate hypertension. It has several unique mechanisms of action[471]: it has a high vascular selectivity and inhibits L-, N-, and T-type calcium channels. This drug is widely available in Japan and has a proven safety record for use as an antihypertensive agent and renoprotective drug. The usual dosage is 2 to 4 mg once daily, but the dosage can be increased to 4 mg twice daily for those with angina pectoris.

Clevidipine is a novel ultra–short-acting dihydropyridine CCB administered intravenously for the treatment of hypertensive emergencies or acute increases in BP in the perioperative setting.[472] It has a high degree of vascular selectivity and an ultrafast onset and offset for immediate titratability. Clevidipine has a high clearance (0.05 L/min/kg) and is rapidly hydrolyzed to inactive metabolites by arterial esterases.[472]

Felodipine is a dihydropyridine CCB that is administered in ER tablets of 2.5, 5, and 10 mg (see Table 50.15).[12] Felodipine is almost completely absorbed from the gastrointestinal tract, with a time to peak concentration of 2 to 5 hours (see Table 50.16).

There is extensive first-pass hepatic metabolism. Bioavailability is influenced by food. Large meals and the flavonoids in grapefruit juice increase the bioavailability by approximately 50%.[473] The overall half-life is 11 to 16 hours. Felodipine is metabolized in the liver to inactive metabolites, most of which are excreted in the urine. The usual daily dose is 2.5 to 10 mg, and titration can be instituted at 2-week intervals. The dosage should be adjusted for hepatic, but not renal, insufficiency.

Isradipine is a dihydropyridine CCB that is effective alone or in combination with other antihypertensive agents for the management of mild to moderate hypertension[12] (see Tables 50-15 and 50-16). Isradipine is rapidly and almost completely absorbed after oral administration. Extensive first-pass hepatic metabolism reduces bioavailability to less than 25%. The hypotensive effect peaks at 2 to 3 hours for the regular release form. The drug is active for 12 hours; however, the full antihypertensive response does not occur until 14 days. The usual dosage is 2.5 to 5 mg two to three times daily. The onset of action of the SR formulation is achieved in 2 hours and lasts for 7 to 18 hours. The usual daily dose of the CR tablet is 5 to 20 mg. Isradipine is extensively protein-bound. The elimination half-life is biphasic, with a terminal half-life of 8 hours. Dosage adjustment is unnecessary for those in renal or liver failure.

Manidipine is a third-generation dihydropyridine CCB that is structurally related to nifedipine.[474,475] The usual adult dosage is 10 to 20 mg once daily. Dosage should be adjusted at 2-week intervals. Manidipine is highly protein-bound and extensively metabolized in the liver. Metabolism is impaired by grapefruit juice[476]; 63% of the drug is excreted in the feces. The peak plasma concentration occurs after 2 to 3.5 hours, with an elimination half-life of 5 to 8 hours. Dosage adjustment is not necessary in renal failure.

Nicardipine hydrochloride is a dihydropyridine CCB that is available as 20- and 40-mg immediate-release gelatin capsules or 30-, 45-, and 60-mg SR capsules.[12] The usual dosage is 20 to 40 mg three times daily for the immediate-release form and 30 to 60 mg twice daily for the SR preparation. When conversion is made to the SR form, the previous daily total of immediate-release drug should be administered on a twice-daily regimen. Titration should be instituted at least 3 days after administration. Nicardipine is well absorbed orally but has only 35% systemic bioavailability because of its extensive first-pass hepatic metabolism. The time to peak concentration is 30 minutes to 2 hours for immediate-release capsules and 1 to 4 hours for SR forms. The elimination half-life is 8.6 hours. Nicardipine is 100% oxidized in

Table 50.17 Renal Effects of Calcium Channel Blockers						
Class	Sodium Excretion	Glomerular Filtration Rate	Filtration Fraction	Renal Blood Flow	Renal Vascular Resistance	Proteinuria
Dihydropyridines	↑	↑ to ↔	↔	↑ to ↔	↓	↑
Diltiazem	↑	↑ to ↔	↔	↑ to ↔	↓	↓
Verapamil	↑	↑ to ↔	↔	↑ to ↔	↓	↑

the liver to inactive pyridine metabolites. There is no evidence of microsomal enzyme induction. Metabolites are excreted primarily in the urine and feces. The parent compound is not dialyzable. Dosage adjustments are necessary with hepatic, but not renal, insufficiency.

Nisoldipine is a dihydropyridine CCB that is formulated as ER tablets of 10, 20, 30, and 40 mg (see Tables 50-15 and 50-16).[12] The initial starting dose is 20 mg, and the usual maintenance dose is 20 to 40 mg given once daily, which can be titrated at weekly intervals. The bioavailability of nisoldipine is low and variable (4% to 8%). The coat core design affords a full 24-hour effect after oral administration. The drug reaches therapeutic concentrations in 6 to 12 hours, and absorption is slowed by high-fat meals. The elimination half-life ranges from 10 to 22 hours. Nisoldipine is metabolized in the liver and intestine. Variable hepatic blood flow induced by the drug probably contributes to its pharmacokinetic variability. Most of the metabolites are excreted in the urine and the remainder in the feces. Dosage adjustments are necessary with hepatic, but not renal, impairment.

Lacidipine is a second-generation dihydropyridine CCB that is available in tablet form. It is reported to be unusually potent and long acting, possibly because it diffuses deeper into lipid bilayer membranes. A unique attribute of this drug is its apparently greater vascular selectivity, but the clinical relevance of this remains unclear.[477] The usual dosage is 4 to 6 mg once daily, and the dose should be titrated at 2- to 4-week intervals.[478] The duration of action is 12 to 24 hours. The elimination half-life is 12 to 19 hours. The parent compound is converted 100% by the liver into inactive fragments that are excreted primarily in the feces (70%) and kidney. Dosage adjustment is necessary in older persons and in patients with hepatic, but not renal, impairment.

Lercanidipine is a novel dihydropyridine CCB whose molecular design imparts greater solubility within the arterial cellular membrane bilayer, conferring a 10-fold higher vascular selectivity than that of amlodipine.[478] In contrast to amlodipine, lercanidipine has a relatively short half-life but a long-lasting effect at the receptor and membrane levels and is associated with significantly less peripheral edema.[478] The drug is administered at a starting dose of 10 mg and increased to 20 mg daily as needed. It has a gradual onset of action, and its effects last for 24 hours.[479] Lercanidipine is unique among the dihydropyridines in that it also appears to dilate the efferent renal arteriole.[480]

CLASS RENAL EFFECTS

The potential benefits of CCBs in acute and chronic kidney disease have been well described. There are multiple mechanisms whereby CCBs alter or protect renal function, notably as natriuretics, vasodilators, and antiproteinuric agents (Table 50.17). All CCBs exert natriuretic and diuretic effects.[481,482] Experimental studies and studies in humans with hypertension have indicated that the increase in sodium excretion is, in part, independent of vasodilatory action or changes in GFR, renal blood flow, or filtration fraction. This effect is probably the result of changes in renal sodium handling that can potentiate the antihypertensive vascular effect. In normal individuals, CCBs acutely increase sodium excretion, frequently in the absence of changes in BP. In hypertensive individuals, the short-term administration of CCBs uniformly increases sodium excretion 1.1- to 3.4-fold; the magnitude of the increase is not related to the decrease in BP.[481]

The natriuretic effect appears to persist in the long term. Long-term administration of CCBs to hypertensive patients results in a cumulative sodium deficit that is abruptly reversed with the discontinuation of the drug. Natriuresis frequently occurs 3 to 6 hours after the morning dose.[482] The net negative sodium balance levels off after the first 2 to 3 days of administration but persists for the duration of therapy.[483] There are no significant changes in long-term body weight, levels of potassium, urea nitrogen, or catecholamines, or GFR. Moreover, stimulation of renin release and aldosterone does not occur to an appreciable degree. It has been postulated that the natriuresis induced by CCBs increases distal sodium delivery to the macula densa, suppressing renin release. Because Ang II mediates aldosterone synthesis by way of cytosolic calcium messengers, CCBs blunt this response as well.[484]

The mechanism whereby CCBs induce natriuresis appears to be direct inhibition of renal tubular sodium and water absorption. Dihydropyridines increase urinary flow rate and sodium excretion without changing the filtered water and sodium load. Studies have suggested that CCBs may diminish sodium uptake at the amiloride-sensitive sodium channels.[485] Inhibition of water reabsorption occurs distally to the late distal tubule. Proximal tubular sodium reabsorption may be inhibited by higher dosages. One possible mediator of this effect is atrial natriuretic peptide. In human studies, CCBs augment atrial natriuretic peptide release and potentiate its action at the level of the kidney. Other potential mediators are under investigation. How much the natriuretic effects contribute to the antihypertensive response is unknown, but unlike with other vasodilators, the changes attenuate the expected adaptive changes in sodium handling.

The renal hemodynamic effects of CCBs are variable and depend primarily on which vasoconstrictors modulate the renal vascular tone.[486] Experimentally, CCBs improve GFR in the presence of the vasoconstrictors norepinephrine and Ang II, as well as others, by preferentially attenuating afferent arteriolar resistance.[487] The efferent arteriole appears to be refractory to these vasodilatory effects. Patients with primary hypertension appear to be more sensitive to the renal hemodynamic effects of CCBs than normotensive subjects, and this effect is more pronounced with advancing kidney disease.[488] Short-term administration of CCBs results in little change in or augmentation of the GFR and renal plasma flow, no change in the filtration fraction, and reduction of renal vascular resistance. Long-term administration is not associated with significant changes in renal hemodynamics. The response is maximal in the presence of Ang II, which selectively causes postglomerular vasoconstriction. Clinically significant changes are counteracted by the reduction in renal perfusion pressure coincident with a reduction of BP.

The long-term effects of CCBs on renal function are variable.[489,490] In hypertensive patients, the effects on renal hemodynamics vary. Some patients exhibit no change in GFR, whereas others have an exaggerated increase in GFR and renal plasma flow.[486] Even normotensive patients with a family history of hypertension have an exaggerated hemodynamic response.[491]

The antiproteinuric effects of CCBs also vary with respect to the type of drug and level of BP reduction achieved.[492] Some dihydropyridines increase protein excretion by up to 40%. It is not clear whether this increase is a result of hemodynamic vasodilation at the afferent arteriole, resulting in increased glomerular capillary pressure (because CCBs directly impair renal autoregulation), changes in glomerular basement membrane permeability, or increased intrarenal Ang II. By contrast, felodipine, diltiazem, verapamil, and others do not appear to have this effect and may lower protein excretion, possibly by also decreasing the efferent arteriolar tone and glomerular pressure.[143] The clinical implications remain to be determined.

Large clinical trials underscore this controversy. In African Americans with hypertension and mild to moderate renal insufficiency with proteinuria of more than 1 g of protein/day, renoprotection with an ACE inhibitor far exceeded any effect of the dihydropyridine CCB amlodipine. In the latter group of patients, renal function deteriorated.[493] This effect was independent of BP reduction and was more evident in proteinuric patients; it was also suggestive in patients with a baseline proteinuria of less than 300 mg of protein/day. Hypertensive patients with diabetic nephropathy also fared considerably worse with amlodipine therapy than with ARB therapy.[255] Patients experienced higher rates of progression of renal disease and all-cause mortality in the amlodipine- and placebo-treated groups. This effect was also independent of the BP levels achieved. However, it should be emphasized that coadministration of a dihydropyridine and an ARB does not abrogate the ARB's protective effect on kidney function.[82] It has been postulated that the selective dilation of the afferent arteriole favors an increase in glomerular capillary pressure that perpetuates renal disease progression.

CCBs have many nonhemodynamic effects that may also afford renoprotection (Table 50.18).[494] In addition to lowering BP, CCBs act as free-radical scavengers, retard renal growth and increase kidney weight,[495,496] reduce the entrapment of macromolecules in the mesangium, attenuate the mitogenic actions of platelet-derived growth factor and platelet-activating factor,[496] block the mitochondrial overload of calcium,[497] decrease lipid peroxidation, decrease glomerular basement membrane thickness, augment the antioxidant activities of superoxide dismutase, catalase, and glutathione peroxidase,[498] inhibit metalloproteinase 1 and collagenolytic activity, suppress the expression of angiogenic growth factors and suppress selectins (which are important for leukocyte adhesion to the vascular endothelium),[499] vascular endothelial growth factor, fibroblast growth factor, TGF-β, and endothelial nitric oxide synthase,[500,501] prevent renal cortical remodeling and scarring and improve fibrinolysis, and improve endothelial dysfunction and inhibit mesangial cell damage, as elicited by advanced glycation end products (see Table 50.18).[486,502-505]

Because of their renal hemodynamic effects and the inhibition of calcium-mediated injury, CCBs have the ability to attenuate various types of kidney damage, including radiocontrast-induced nephropathy and hypoperfusion ischemic injury, such as that occurring during cardiac surgery.[506,507] In experimental models, pretreatment with a CCB variably preserved GFR and renal blood flow.[508] The clinical effectiveness of this class of drugs in these settings requires further evaluation.

CCBs represent an important treatment option for renal transplant recipients.[342,509,510] Administration of CCBs in the renal allograft perfusate and to renal allograft recipients reduces initial graft nonfunction by attenuating ischemic and reperfusion injury and preserves long-term renal function by protecting against cyclosporine nephrotoxicity and by contributing to immunomodulation. Cyclosporine causes direct tubular injury and induces intrarenal vasoconstriction. The thromboxane- and endothelin-induced vasoconstriction of the afferent arteriole, as stimulated by cyclosporine, is reversed by CCBs.[511]

Table 50.18 Renal Protective Mechanisms of Calcium Channel Blockers

Lower blood pressure.
Decrease proteinuria.
Scavenge free radicals.
Retard kidney growth.
Reduce mesangial molecule entrapment.
Attenuate antigenic platelet-derived growth factor and platelet-activating factor.
Block mitochondrial calcium overload.
Decrease lipid peroxidation.
Reduce glomerular basement membrane thickness.
Augment antioxidant effects of superoxide dismutase-catalase and glutathione peroxidase.
Inhibit collagenic activity.
Suppress angiogenic growth factors—vascular endothelial growth factor, basic fibroblast growth factor, transforming growth factor-β, and endothelial nitric oxide synthase.
Prevent renal cortical remodeling.
Ameliorate cyclosporine toxicity.
Block thromboxane- and endothelin cyclosporine–induced vasoconstriction.
Inhibit advanced glycation end product–elicited mesangial cell damage.

CLASS EFFICACY AND SAFETY

All CCBs are considered initial antihypertensive agents and appear to be equally efficacious and safe.[434,437] Approximately 70% to 80% of patients with stage 1 or, 2 hypertension respond to monotherapy. Up to 50% of unselected patients respond to monotherapy.[388] In contrast to other vasodilators, CCBs attenuate the reflex increase of neurohormonal activity that accompanies a reduction in BP and in the long term, they inhibit or do not change the sympathetic activity.[512,513] The long-acting agents produce sustained BP reductions of 16 to 28 mm Hg systolic and 14 to 17 mm Hg diastolic, with no appreciable development of tolerance.

The CCBs are effective in young, middle-aged, and older patients with white coat hypertension and mild, moderate, or severe hypertension.[514-517] Their efficacy may be determined by genetic polymorphisms.[518] CCBs are equally efficacious in men and women, in patients with a high or low plasma renin activity regardless of dietary salt intake, and in African American, white, and Hispanic patients.[519] The effects of CCBs are diminished in smokers.[520] CCBs are effective and safe in patients with hypertension and coronary artery disease,[521] as well as in those with ESKD.[522] CCBs also reduce adverse cardiovascular events and slow the progression of atherosclerosis in normotensive patients with coronary artery disease.[523]

Among the different categories, dihydropyridines appear to be the most powerful for reducing BP but may also be associated with greater activation of baroreceptor reflexes.[524] Dihydropyridines induce a greater shift in the sympathovagal balance that favors sympathetic predominance compared to nondihydropyridines.[451] In general, however, compared with other vasodilators, CCBs attenuate the reflex increase in sympathetic activity—increased heart rate, cardiac index, and plasma norepinephrine levels and renin activity.

Verapamil and, to a lesser extent, diltiazem exert greater effects on the heart and have less vasoselectivity. These drugs typically reduce the heart rate, slow AV conduction, and depress contractility (Table 50.19). The second- and third-generation CCBs consist of pharmacologically manipulated formulations, whose half-lives are progressively longer.[453]

The use of CCBs is contraindicated in patients with severely depressed left ventricular function (except, perhaps, amlodipine or felodipine), hypotension, sick sinus syndrome (unless a pacemaker is in place), second- or third-degree heart block, and atrial arrhythmias associated with an accessory pathway.[439] The nondihydropyridines have been associated with heart block in hyperkalemic patients.[525] These drugs should not be used as first-line antihypertensive agents in patients with heart failure, those who have experienced myocardial infarction, those with unstable angina, or African Americans with proteinuria of more than 300 mg protein/day.[493] By contrast, CCBs are indicated and may be preferred in patients with metabolic disorders, such as diabetes, peripheral vascular disease, and stable ischemic heart disease. CCBs may also be ideal agents for older hypertensive patients because they tend to lower the risk of stroke more than other hypertensive drug classes.[526] Because CCBs are particularly effective in stroke prevention, they may also retard cognitive decline in older adults.[380,527-529]

CCBs are generally well tolerated and are not associated with significant impairments in glycemic control or sexual dysfunction.[434] The rapid antihypertensive action of CCBs may encourage patient adherence. Orthostatic changes do not occur because venoconstriction remains intact. Adverse effects are usually transient and are the direct result of vasodilation. Hypotension is most common with intravenous administration. The most common adverse effect of the dihydropyridines is peripheral edema[530]; it is dose-related and thought to be the result of uncompensated precapillary vasodilation, which causes increased intracapillary hydrostatic pressure. The edema is not responsive to diuretics but improves or resolves with the addition of an ACE inhibitor or ARB, which preferentially vasodilates postcapillary beds and reduces intracapillary hydrostatic pressure.[510] Other adverse effects related to vasodilation include headache, nausea, dizziness, and flushing and occur more commonly in women. The nondihydropyridines verapamil and isradipine more commonly cause constipation and nausea. The gastrointestinal effects are directly related to the inhibition of calcium-dependent smooth muscle contraction—reduced peristalsis and relaxation of the lower esophageal sphincter. Another common adverse effect of the dihydropyridines is gingival hyperplasia, which is exacerbated in patients who are also taking cyclosporine. Dihydropyridines lead to the accumulation of gingival inflammatory B cell infiltrates as stimulated by bacterial plaque, immunoglobulins, and folic acid, which causes the growth of the gingiva.[531] This growth can be controlled with regular periodontal treatment and reversed with discontinuation of the drug.[532]

CCBs are notable among antihypertensive agents because of their metabolic neutrality. Because the calcium influx across β cell membranes helps regulate insulin release,[533] CCBs might predispose to low insulin levels. At typical therapeutic levels, CCBs have no effect on the serum glucose level, insulin secretion, or insulin sensitivity in nondiabetic

Table 50.19	Hemodynamic Effects of Calcium Channel Blockers									
Class	Arteriolar Dilation	Coronary Dilation	Cardiac Afterload	Cardiac Contractility	Myocardial O$_2$ Demand	Cardiac Output	AV Conduction	SA Automaticity	Heart Rate: Short Term/Long Term	Activation of Baroreceptor Reflexes
Dihydropyridines	↑↑↑	↑↑↑	↓↓	↔	↓	↓ or ↔	↔	↔	↑/↑	↑ or ↔
Diltiazem	↑↑	↑↑↑	↓	↓	↓	↔	↓	↓↓	↓/↓ or ↔	↔
Verapamil	↑↑	↑↑	↓	↓↓	↓	↔	↓↓	↓	↓/↓ or ↔	↔

AV, Atrioventricular; SA, sinoatrial.

and diabetic individuals. The use of CCBs was not significantly associated with incident diabetes compared to other antihypertensive agents in a meta-analysis of randomized controlled trials.[534] The association with diabetes was lowest for ACE inhibitors and ARBs, followed by CCBs, β-blockers, and diuretics.[534] Furthermore, it was recently demonstrated that CCBs can even prevent diabetes and increase β-cell survival in vitro. The mechanism behind the β-cell mass destruction is the human islet cell protein TXNIP (thioredoxin-interacting protein), which is upregulated by hyperglycemia. Orally administered verapamil resulted in a reduction of TXNIP expression and β-cell apoptosis, enhanced endogenous insulin levels, and rescued mice from streptozotocin (STZ)-induced diabetes. Verapamil also promoted β cell survival and improved glucose homeostasis and insulin sensitivity in ob/ob mice.[535]

CCBs do not increase triglyceride or cholesterol levels and do not reduce HDL cholesterol levels. CCBs do not precipitate hyponatremia, hyperkalemia, hypokalemia, or hyperuricemia. Therefore, they are ideal agents for patients with dysmetabolic syndromes or diabetes. Initial trials have indicated that CCBs are more efficacious in African Americans and older persons or those with low-renin hypertension. However, CCBs are equally efficacious in young and old, African American, white, diabetic, and obese patients. In older patients with hypertension or coronary artery disease, verapamil may cause more bradycardia than other agents, but second- or third-degree heart block is not seen.[521] In older patients receiving long-term treatment with ACE inhibitors, the addition of verapamil can reverse ACE inhibitor–induced increases in creatinine levels safely without further lowering BP.[536] The hypothesis is that the ACE inhibition causes excess bradykinin and increases glomerular pressure to vasoconstriction in afferent and efferent arterioles with endothelial damage and mesangial contraction. The addition of verapamil to an ACE inhibitor dilates afferent and efferent arterioles and reduces the mesangial contraction produced by endothelin-1. In addition, verapamil reduces consumption and may reduce glomerular injury by decreasing oxygen radicals.[536] CCBs are safe and effective in older patients with stage 1 isolated systolic hypertension and can reduce progression to higher stages of hypertension.[537] The latter may be a result of their ability to correct altered arteriole resistance vessels and endothelial function.[538]

Properties beyond their antihypertensive actions make the CCBs particularly useful in certain clinical situations. CCBs not only lower arterial pressure but also have variable effects on cardiac function. All CCBs are vasodilators and increase coronary blood flow. With the exception of the short-acting dihydropyridines, most CCBs reduce heart rate, improve myocardial oxygen demand, improve ventricular filling, diminish ventricular arrhythmias, reduce myocardial ischemia, and conserve contractility,[539,540] making them ideal for patients with angina or diastolic dysfunction.[521] In short-term use, CCBs improve diastolic relaxation; when administered over a long term, they reduce left ventricular wall thickness,[541] may prevent the development of hypertrophy, and may improve arterial compliance.[542-544] This may be crucial in hypertensive patients because LVH is one of the strongest risk predictors for cardiovascular morbidity and mortality.[545] Verapamil may also be used for secondary cardioprotection to reduce reinfarction rates in patients who are intolerant of β-blockers (unless they have concomitant heart failure)[546] and in patients with chronic headaches.[547] The BP-independent inhibition of atherogenesis by CCBs may be another indication to use a CCB, particularly in high-risk patients, such as those with diabetes and ESKD.[548,549] Furthermore, dihydropyridine CCBs are useful in the expulsion of ureteral stones[550] in patients with asthmatic bronchospasm[551] for the treatment of primary pulmonary hypertension.[552,553]

Ongoing trials are evaluating the use of CCBs in preventing or slowing the decline of dementia. A randomized trial that has confirmed a protective effect of antihypertensive treatment on the incidence of dementia has been the systolic hypertension in Europe (SYST-EUR) trial.[528] In the SYST-EUR trial, subjects using nitrendipine were at a 55% lower risk of dementia compared to those receiving a placebo. Moreover, the specific effects of CCBs were supported by observational studies.[554,555]

In general, the antihypertensive effects of CCBs are enhanced more in combination with β-blockers or ACE inhibitors than in combination with diuretics.[556-559] Perhaps this reflects the fact that CCBs themselves have intrinsic diuretic activity. In combination with ACE inhibitors, response rates approach 70% in patients with stage 1 to 3 hypertension.[558] It has been theorized that this particular combination (a dihydropyridine and ACE inhibitor) maximizes precapillary and postcapillary vasodilation to lower peripheral vascular resistance.

The combination of dihydropyridine CCBs with β-blockers is efficacious and even desirable in selected patients. CCBs have the potential to blunt the adverse effects associated with β-blockade, such as vasoconstriction, and β-blockers have the ability to attenuate the increased sympathetic stimulation induced by CCBs. Concomitant therapy with β-blockers and nondihydropyridine CCBs is potentially more dangerous because they may have additive effects in suppressing heart rate, AV node conduction, and cardiac contractility (Table 50.20). This combination may be particularly dangerous in patients with ESKD due to the effects of hyperkalemia on cardiac conduction.

Drug interactions are not uncommon (see Table 50.20). Concurrent use of a CCB and amiodarone exacerbates sick sinus syndrome and AV block. Diltiazem, verapamil, and nicardipine have been shown to increase the levels of cyclosporine (including the microemulsion formulation), tacrolimus, and sirolimus by 25% to 100%.[560] This interaction may be clinically useful for reducing the dosage and cost associated with immunosuppressive therapy. Frequent monitoring of calcineurin inhibitor levels is recommended. By contrast, nifedipine and isradipine have no effect on these concentrations and can be used safely. Diltiazem is a potent inhibitor of CYP3A4, which is responsible for the metabolism of methylprednisolone. Coadministration of diltiazem and methylprednisolone resulted in a more than a 2.5-fold increase in the steroid blood level and enhanced adrenal suppressive responses.[561] Coadministration of diltiazem also increased nifedipine levels by 100% to 200%.[562] This combination has additive antihypertensive efficacy and appears to be safe.[563] Concomitant administration of CCBs with the digitalis glycosides resulted in up to a 50% increase in serum digoxin concentrations due to reduced

Table 50.20 Drug-Drug Interactions with Calcium Channel Blockers

Calcium Channel Blocker	Interacting Drug	Result
Verapamil	Digoxin	Digoxin level ↑ by 50%-90%
Diltiazem	Digoxin	Digoxin level ↑ by 40%
Verapamil	β-Blockers	AV nodal blockade, hypotension, bradycardia, asystole
Verapamil, diltiazem	Cyclosporine-tacrolimus and sirolimus	Cyclosporine level ↑ by 25%-100%
Verapamil, diltiazem	Cimetidine	Verapamil and diltiazem levels ↑ by decreased metabolism
Verapamil	Rifampin-phenytoin	Verapamil level ↓ by enzyme induction
Dihydropyridines	Amiodarone	Exacerbation of sick sinus syndrome and AV nodal blockade
Dihydropyridines	α-Blockers	Excessive hypotension
Dihydropyridines	Propranolol	Increases propranolol level
Dihydropyridines	Cimetidine	Increased area under the curve and plasma level of calcium channel blocker
Nicardipine	Cyclosporine	Cyclosporine level ↑ by 40%-50%
Amlodipine	Cyclosporine	Cyclosporine level ↑ by 10%
Felodipine	Flavonoids	Bioavailability ↑ by 50%
Diltiazem	Methylprednisone	Methylprednisone ↑ 2.5-fold
Nifedipine	Diltiazem	Nifedipine level ↑ 100%-200%

AV, Atrioventricular.

renal clearance of digoxin, an effect that appears to be dose-dependent.[564] Insofar as dihydropyridine CCBs partially suppress aldosterone synthesis, they provide an attractive alternative for patients who cannot tolerate a blockade of the RAAS.[565]

Several issues regarding the inherent safety of CCBs have come under scrutiny. CCBs may be associated with an increased risk of gastrointestinal hemorrhage, particularly in older persons.[566] Diltiazem inhibits platelet aggregation in vitro,[567] but the clinical relevance of this finding has not been substantiated. Nonetheless, it is prudent to use caution when coadministering CCBs with NSAIDs because NSAIDs may exacerbate the risk of bleeding and may antagonize the antihypertensive effects of CCBs.[568,569]

Concern regarding a possible relationship between the long-term use of CCBs and breast cancer has recently been re-introduced.[136,570] In view of previous small studies showing a breast cancer risk with CCBs, a meta-analysis has shown breast cancer risk in CCB users for longer than 10 years. This meta-analysis consisted of 17 observational studies, 9 cohort studies, and 8 case-control studies.[571] The studies included 149,607 subjects, of whom 53,812 were CCB users who were followed for 2 to 16 years. The relative risk for breast cancer in CCB users for more than 10 years was 1.71 (95% CI, 1.01 to 2.42)—nifedipine 1.10 (95% CI, 0.87 to 1.33) and diltiazem 0.75 (95% CI, 0.4 to 1.1).[571]

A recent population case-control study of breast cancer in the three-county Seattle–Puget Sound metropolitan area Cancer Surveillance System has shown that the use of CCBs for more than 10 years is associated with a more than twofold increase in the risk of invasive ductal and invasive lobular breast cancer.[570] Participants were postmenopausal women aged 55 to 74 years; 880 had invasive ductal breast cancer, 1027 had invasive lobular breast cancer, and 856 individuals who had no cancer served as controls. The use of CCBs for more than 10 years was associated with ductal breast cancer (odds ratio [OR], 2.4; 95% CI, 1.2 to 4/9; $P = 0.04$) and lobular breast cancer (OR, 2.6; 95% CI, 1.3 to 5.3; $P = 0.01$), respectively. This association was consistent for short-acting and long-acting dihydropyridines and nondihydropyridines. Diuretics, β-blockers, ACE inhibitors and ARBs, by contrast, were not associated with breast cancer.

The Seattle–Puget Sound Breast Cancer Study is a large, carefully performed, case-control study that attempted to exclude potential sources of bias (e.g., confounding by indication—hypertension, recall bias [as the medication was ascertained by self-report], and unknown confounders inherent in all nonrandomized studies).[572] If true, the conclusion has major public health implications because CCBs are the ninth most commonly prescribed drug in the United States, with more than 90 million prescriptions filled. The two- to threefold fold increase in breast cancer, if confirmed, would represent a major modifiable risk factor for breast cancer. As such, efforts are presently underway to replicate these findings in general practice research database cohorts that link prescription information and cancer. Larger numbers would estimate the effect more precisely. Should the use of CCB be discontinued in individuals taking the drug for more than 10 years? At this point, probably not in most cases. The above results need to be confirmed as they emerge from an observational study; thus, they cannot prove causality. These results should not by themselves cause a change in clinical practice.[572] These new findings need to be interpreted with caution but warrant additional investigation, especially in the context of prior studies that have had mixed results,.

The safety of CCBs in treating hypertension and cardiovascular disease is no longer controversial. There is clear evidence that CCBs reduce cardiovascular mortality and morbidity, particularly stroke; however, short-acting agents, such as nifedipine, have been associated with a small increased risk of MI in meta-analyses[407,464] when compared with other agents. It has been speculated that the disadvantageous activation of the RAAS and SNS induced by the short-acting agents may predispose to myocardial ischemia. Currently, there is no evidence to prove the existence of additional beneficial or detrimental effects of CCBs on coronary disease events, including fatal or nonfatal MIs and other deaths from coronary heart disease. Because of a potential risk, however, as well as for simplicity and improved patient adherence, longer acting agents should be considered over short-acting CCBs for the management of hypertension.

CENTRAL ADRENERGIC AGONISTS

CLASS MECHANISMS OF ACTION

Central adrenergic agonists act by crossing the blood-brain barrier and have a direct agonist effect on α_2-adrenergic receptors located in the midbrain and brainstem.[559,573,574] Binding to the more recently described I_1 imidazoline receptors in the brain may also play a role in the inhibition of central sympathetic output.[575-580,5] Drugs in this class bind to the α-adrenergic or I_1 imidazoline receptors with some degree of specificity (Table 50.21). Moxonidine and rilmenidine have a 30-fold greater specificity for the I_1 imidazoline receptor than the α_2-receptor. Clonidine, by contrast, exhibits a fourfold greater specificity for the I_1 imidazoline receptor than for the α_2-receptor. The central adverse effects are thought to be largely related to α_2-receptor binding. Moxonidine and rilmenidine have reduced central side effects because of the lower activity at the α_2-receptor relative to other agents.[580,581] In addition to decreasing the total sympathetic outflow, binding to these receptors results in increased vagal activity. A reduction in catecholamine release and turnover, as evidenced by decreased biochemical markers of noradrenergic activity, such as plasma norepinephrine levels, correlated with the magnitude of BP decreases.

Stimulation of both receptor types is probably mediated through the same neuronal pathways.[581] The classic α_2-receptor agonists, such as clonidine and α-methyldopa (acting through its active metabolite, α-methylnoradrenaline), result in vasodilation in the resistance vessels and thus a reduction in peripheral vascular resistance. As a result, BP is reduced. Despite vasodilator action, reflex tachycardia generally does not occur, probably as a result of peripheral sympathetic inhibition.

The selective I_1 receptor agonists moxonidine and rilmenidine are predominantly arterial vasodilators that lead to a reduction in peripheral vascular resistance.[576] Moxonidine is associated with a reduction in plasma renin activity. The central α_2-adrenergic agonists may also stimulate peripheral α_2-adrenergic receptors. This effect predominates at high drug concentrations. These receptors mediate vasoconstriction, which may result in a paradoxic increase in BP.[573] Overall, these drugs generally result in a decrease in peripheral vascular resistance, slowing of the heart rate, and either no change or a mild decrease in cardiac output.[581,582] Orthostatic hypotension is generally not a feature of these drugs. The pharmacokinetic and pharmacodynamic properties of these drugs are shown in Tables 50.22 and 50.23.

CLASS MEMBERS

Methyldopa is a methyl-substituted amino acid that is active after conversion to an active metabolite. This active metabolite, α-methylnorepinephrine, accumulates in the CNS and is selective for α_2-adrenergic receptors. The initial dosage of methyldopa in hypertension is 250 mg two to three times daily. This dose may be increased at intervals of not less than 2 days until a therapeutic response is achieved. The usual maintenance dosage is 500 mg to 2 g daily in two to four doses. The maximum recommended daily dose is 3 g. An initial response occurs within 3 to 6 hours after dosing. The peak response occurs at 6 to 9 hours. The drug is approximately 50% metabolized by the liver. The drug half-life is increased in patients with renal failure. Excretion in the urine is largely in the form of an inactive metabolite. The dosing interval should be increased to every 12 to 24 hours

Table 50.21 Receptor Binding of Centrally Acting Antihypertensives

Drug	Receptor
Clonidine	α_2, I_1
α-Methyldopa	α_2
Guanabenz	α_2
Guanfacine	α_2
Rilmenidine	$I_1 > \alpha_2$
Moxonidine	$I_1 > \alpha_2$

α_2, α_2-Adrenergic receptor; I_1, imidazole receptor.

Table 50.22 Pharmacokinetic Properties of Central Adrenergic Agonists

Drug	Bioavailability (%)	Affected by Food	Peak Blood Level (hr)	Elimination Half-Life (hr)	Metabolism	Excretion	Active Metabolites
Clonidine (Catapres)	50	—	—	6-23	L	F (30%-50%) U (24%)	Methyldopa-o-sulfite
α-Methyldopa (Aldomet)	65-96	—	1.5-5	6-23	L	F (22%) U (65%)	—
Guanabenz (Wytensin)	75	—	2-5	7-10	L	F (16%)	—
Guanfacine (Tonex)	80	—	1-4	17	L	U (40%-75%)	—
Rilmenidine (Hyperium)	80-90	No	2	2-3	L	U (90%)	—
Moxonidine (Physiotens)	100	No	0.5-3	2	L	U (90%)	—

F, Feces; L, liver; U, urine.

Table 50.23	Pharmacodynamic Properties of Central Adrenergic Agonists					
Drug	Initial Dose (mg)	Usual Dose (mg)	Maximum Dose (mg)	Interval	Peak Response (hr)	Duration of Response (hr)
Clonidine	0.1	0.1-0.6	1.2	bid	2-4	6-10
α-Methyldopa	250	250-500	3000	bid, qid	6-9	24-48
Guanabenz	4	16-32	96	bid	2-4	10-12
Guanfacine	1	1-3	6	qd, bid	6	24
Moxonidine	0.1-0.2	0.2-0.3	0.6	bid	1.5-4	48-72
Rilmenidine	1	1-2	—	qd, bid	1-2	10-12

in patients with severe renal failure. Approximately 60% of methyldopa is removed with hemodialysis. A supplemental dose is recommended after dialysis treatment.

Clonidine is a central-acting α-adrenergic agonist.[157,577,583] The usual oral dosage is 0.1 mg twice daily, adjusted as necessary in 0.1- to 0.2-mg increments. The usual maintenance dosage is 0.2 to 0.6 mg once daily in two divided doses. Total doses more than 1.2 mg daily are usually not associated with a greater effect. The onset of activity is 30 to 60 minutes after an oral dose. The peak antihypertensive activity occurs within 2 to 4 hours. The duration of the antihypertensive effect is 6 to 10 hours. The half-life of the absorbed drug is 6 to 23 hours. Hepatic metabolism to inactive metabolites is followed by renal excretion. Transdermal patches are available and may be applied on a once-weekly basis. The drug half-life with the transdermal patch is approximately 20 hours after removal of the patch. With a transdermal patch, steady-state drug levels are reached within approximately 3 days. Dosage adjustment is not needed for patients with any degree of renal dysfunction, including severe renal failure. Approximately 5% of clonidine body stores are removed after a 5-hour dialysis treatment.

Guanabenz is an orally active, central α$_2$-adrenergic agonist.[573] The usual starting dosage for the management of hypertension is 4 mg twice daily. Dosages may be increased to 4 to 8 mg/day at 1- to 2-week intervals. Dosages as high as 96 mg/day have been used. The onset of antihypertensive activity usually occurs within 60 minutes, and the activity lasts approximately 10 to 12 hours. The drug is highly protein-bound and extensively metabolized. Less than 1% of the unchanged drug is excreted in the urine. The half-life of the drug is 7 to 10 hours. Dosage adjustment in patients with renal failure is not necessary. It appears that dosage reductions may be necessary in patients with severe hepatic insufficiency. Because of extensive protein binding, drug removal by dialysis or peritoneal dialysis is minimal.

Guanfacine is a centrally acting antihypertensive drug with actions similar to those of clonidine.[573] Effective dosages are 1 to 3 mg daily. Peak levels are noted between 1 and 4 hours. The drug half-life is approximately 17 hours. The drug is 70% protein-bound. It is metabolized in the liver, with a renal excretion of 40% to 75% as an unchanged drug. Limited data are available on dosing in renal failure; however, dosage adjustments do not appear warranted.

Moxonidine is a central I$_1$ imidazole and α$_2$-receptor agonist.[157,584,585] Serum concentration peaks are reached within 30 to 180 minutes; 90% of the dose is excreted through the urine within 24 hours, and 50% of this is as unchanged drug. The average half-life is 2 hours. For the management of hypertension, the starting dosage is 0.2 to 0.4 mg/day. The dosage may be increased after several weeks to 0.2 to 0.3 mg twice daily. The maximum daily dose is 0.6 mg. Selectivity for the I$_1$ imidazoline receptor results in fewer central adverse effects, such as dry mouth and sedation, compared with those of clonidine. Drug clearance is delayed in those with renal impairment. Single doses of 0.2 mg and a maximum daily dosage of 0.4 mg should not be exceeded in patients with renal failure.

Rilmenidine is a centrally acting imidazole receptor and α$_2$-adrenergic receptor agonist.[157,579,586-590] Rilmenidine binds preferentially to central I$_1$ imidazoline receptors in the brainstem. At higher doses, rilmenidine can bind and activate central α$_2$-adrenergic receptors. Antihypertensive effects occur within 1 hour after a single 1-mg dose. The duration of action is 10 to 12 hours. The concentration after oral dosing peaks at approximately 2 hours. Steady-state plasma levels are reached by day 3. Rilmenidine is eliminated primarily unchanged in the urine. In chronic renal failure, clearance of the drug is decreased. The usual oral dosage is 1 mg once or twice daily. Dosage reductions are required for patients with renal dysfunction. In patients with advanced renal disease, the dosage should be decreased to 1 mg every other day.

CLASS RENAL EFFECTS

Central α$_2$- and I$_1$ imidazoline receptor agonists have little if any clinically important effect on renal plasma flow, GFR, or the RAAS. The fractional excretion of sodium is unchanged. Body fluid composition and weight are not altered. A water diuresis may be associated with the use of guanabenz through inhibition of the central release of vasopressin or altered renal responsiveness to vasopressin. These agents may result in decreased renal vascular resistance, as mediated by a decrease in preglomerular capillary resistance related to decreased levels of circulating catecholamines.

CLASS EFFICACY AND SAFETY

The antihypertensive efficacy of this class of drugs has been confirmed in large numbers of patients. These agents provide effective monotherapy for hypertension.[573] Combination with a diuretic is associated with additive effects. Drugs in this class are effective for young and old patients, and the effects do not differ in different racial or ethnic groups. Moxonidine and rilmenidine have been associated with decreased plasma glucose levels and may improve insulin sensitivity. These drugs may also decrease total cholesterol, LDL, and triglyceride levels[575,591,592] and may play a role in the management of metabolic syndrome. They may also be of benefit in patients with congestive heart failure. Treatment with rilmenidine and moxonidine reverses LVH and improves arterial compliance. This effect was associated with a reduction in plasma levels of atrial natriuretic peptide.

Stimulation of α_2-adrenergic receptors in the CNS induces several adverse effects of these drugs, including sedation and drowsiness. The most common adverse effect related to α_2-adrenergic activation is dry mouth caused by a decrease in salivary flow. This decrease is due to centrally mediated inhibition of cholinergic transmission. Clonidine in high doses may precipitate a paradoxic hypertensive response related to the stimulation of postsynaptic vascular α_2-adrenergic receptors.[573] Methyldopa use has been associated with a positive result on the direct Coombs test in patients with and without hemolytic anemia.[573] Because of a long history of safe use during pregnancy, methyldopa remains a common therapeutic agent for hypertensive disorders of pregnancy and for essential hypertension during pregnancy.[559,574] The α_2-adrenergic agonists are associated with sexual dysfunction and may produce gynecomastia in men and galactorrhea in men and women.

Abrupt cessation of α_2-adrenergic blockers may result in rebound hypertension, which occurs 18 to 36 hours after the cessation of short-acting agents.[593] Patients may experience tachycardia, tremor, anxiety, headache, nausea, and vomiting. This syndrome may be related to downregulation of the α_2-adrenergic receptors in the CNS as associated with long-term therapy. These agents have a higher specificity for the I_1 receptor and appear to produce significantly fewer CNS effects, such as dry mouth and drowsiness. Rebound hypertension secondary to abrupt withdrawal has not been associated with moxonidine or rilmenidine.

CENTRAL AND PERIPHERAL ADRENERGIC NEURONAL BLOCKING AGENT

MECHANISMS OF ACTION AND CLASS MEMBER

Reserpine, a *Rauwolfia* alkaloid, reduces BP by decreasing the activity of central and peripheral noradrenergic neurons. Reserpine blocks noradrenaline and dopamine uptake into the storage granules of noradrenergic neurons. The result is noradrenaline depletion. A similar effect is seen in central dopaminergic and serotoninergic neurons. At the dosages currently used to treat hypertension, the major effect of the use of reserpine is in the CNS. Reserpine results in a rapid reduction in cardiac output, heart rate, and peripheral vascular resistance. Enhanced vagal activity may also be involved. Tolerance to the antihypertensive effects of reserpine does not occur.

Reserpine is used at initial dosages of 0.1 to 0.25 mg daily.[594] Approximately 40% of an oral dose is absorbed. The half-life is 50 to 100 hours. Extensive hepatic metabolism occurs; 1% is recovered as unchanged compound in the urine. The maximal clinical effect is observed 2 to 3 weeks after initiation of therapy. No dosage adjustment is necessary for patients with renal insufficiency. Dosage supplementation is not required after hemodialysis.

RENAL EFFECTS

The GFR and renal plasma flow are not affected by reserpine therapy. Renal vascular resistance may be reduced, perhaps mediated by decreased sympathetic stimulation of vascular α-adrenergic receptors. Significant effects on the RAAS have not been observed. Renal handling of sodium and potassium is unchanged.

EFFICACY AND SAFETY

Reserpine provides effective therapy as a single agent or in combination with hydrochlorothiazide.[594,595] This has been observed in numerous large and small trials, including the Veterans Administration Cooperative Study on Antihypertensive Agents, Hypertension Detection and Follow-up Program, and the Multiple Risk Factor Intervention Trial. Reserpine used in combination with a diuretic has shown comparable efficacy to combinations of β-blockers and diuretics. In these studies, the dosage of reserpine was between 0.1 and 0.3 mg daily, which is many times lower than the dosages used in the 1960s that led to reserpine's reputation as having a poor side effect profile. The most common adverse effect of reserpine is nasal congestion, which is reported in 6% to 20% of patients. Unlike other adverse effects, nasal congestion does not appear to decrease at lower drug dosages and is thought to be related to the cholinergic effects of the drug. Increased gastric motility and gastric acid secretion can occur; however, the incidence of dyspepsia or peptic ulcer disease with reserpine therapy is not greater than that with other antihypertensive drug treatments. Inability to concentrate, sedation, sleep disturbance, and depression have been reported. Other adverse effects include weight gain, increased appetite, and sexual dysfunction. Early suggestions that reserpine causes breast cancer in women were not confirmed.

DIRECT-ACTING VASODILATORS

CLASS MECHANISMS OF ACTION

The direct-acting vasodilators reduce systolic and diastolic BPs by decreasing peripheral vascular resistance. These drugs act directly on vascular smooth muscle with the selective vasodilation of the arteriolar resistance vessels and have little or no effect on the venous capacitance vessels.[596] There is no effect on the functioning of carotid or aortic baroreceptors. The vasodilating effects are thought to involve inhibition of calcium uptake into the cells. Decreases in arterial pressure are associated with a decrease in peripheral resistance and a reflex increase in cardiac output. Sodium and water retention are promoted secondary to the stimulation of renin release and possibly by direct effects on renal tubules. The arteriolar dilation produced by these drugs causes a decrease in cardiac afterload,[596] and the absence of venodilation leads to an increase in venous return to the heart, which produces an elevated preload. These combined effects result in increased cardiac output.[596] The pharmacokinetic and pharmacodynamic properties of these drugs are shown in Tables 50-24 and 50-25.

CLASS MEMBERS

The initial oral dosages of hydralazine for hypertension should be 10 mg four times daily, increasing to 50 mg four times daily over several weeks. Patients may require dosages of up to 300 mg/day. Dosing can be changed to twice daily for maintenance. The drug may also be used as an intravenous bolus injection or as a continuous infusion. The

Table 50.24	Pharmacokinetic Properties of Direct-Acting Vasodilators						
Drug	Bioavailability (%)	Affected by Food	Peak Blood Level (hr)	Elimination Half-Life (hr)	Metabolism	Excretion	Active Metabolites
Hydralazine (Apresoline)	20-50	No	1-2	1.5-8	L	U (3%-14%) F (3%-12%)	—
Minoxidil (Loniten)	90-100	—	1	4.2	L	U (90%) F (3%)	Glucuronide

F, Feces; L, liver; U, urine.

Table 50.25	Pharmacodynamic Properties of Direct-Acting Vasodilators					
Drug	Initial Dose (mg)	Usual Dose (mg)	Maximum Dose (mg)	Interval	Peak Response (hr)	Duration of Response (hr)
Hydralazine	10	200-400	400	bid, qid	1	3-8
Minoxidil	2.5	10-20	40	qd, qid	4-8	10-12

elimination half-life is 1.5 to 8 hours and varies with the acetylation rate in the liver. Slow and fast acetylators have been described. The onset of action is approximately 1 hour. In patients with mild to moderate renal insufficiency, the dosing interval should be increased to every 8 hours. In patients with severe renal failure, the dosing interval should be increased to every 8 to 24 hours. No dosage supplement is required after hemodialysis or peritoneal dialysis (see Table 50.6).

Minoxidil is more potent than hydralazine. For severe hypertension, the initial recommended dosage is 2.5 mg as a single daily dose, increasing to 10 to 20 or 40 mg in single or divided doses. Minoxidil is usually used in conjunction with salt restriction and diuretics to prevent fluid retention. Concomitant therapy with a β-adrenergic blocking agent is often required to control tachycardia related to minoxidil use. The onset of the antihypertensive effect is within 30 to 60 minutes. The peak response occurs at 4 to 8 hours. The drug is 90% metabolized by the liver. The glucuronide metabolite has reduced pharmacologic effects but accumulates in patients with ESKD. Renal excretion is 90%. Dosage adjustments may be required for patients with renal failure, although the mean daily doses required to control BP are similar in patients with normal renal function and in those with renal failure (see Table 50.6).

The effectiveness of minoxidil in patients with resistant hypertension has been well established.[597,598] Minoxidil is frequently a therapy of last resort in patients with CKD unresponsive to other therapies. It must generally be used in combination with a β-blocker and a loop diuretic to prevent tachycardia and fluid retention.

CLASS RENAL EFFECTS

Hydralazine and minoxidil both increase the juxtaglomerular cell secretion of renin, which is associated with increased Ang II and aldosterone levels. Long-term use is associated with the return of plasma aldosterone levels to baseline. Retention of salt and water may be due to direct drug effects on the proximal convoluted tubule. Renal vascular resistance is decreased in association with a relaxation of resistance vessels.[596] GFR and renal plasma flow are preserved.

Hydralazine may reduce BP compared to placebo in patients with primary hypertension; however, these results are based on before and after studies, not on randomized controlled trials. Furthermore, the effect of this drug on cardiovascular outcomes remains unstudied.

CLASS EFFICACY AND SAFETY

Although minoxidil has been used to treat mild to moderate hypertension, it is commonly reserved for severe or intractable hypertension. When added to a diuretic and β-blocker, minoxidil is generally well tolerated. Hypertrichosis is, unfortunately, a common adverse effect and is not tolerated well by many patients. Pericarditis and pericardial effusions have been described.[599] An increase in left ventricular mass has been reported, which may be due to adrenergic hyperactivity.

Similar findings have been observed with hydralazine. In addition to adrenergic activation and fluid retention, long-term treatment with hydralazine has been associated with the development of systemic lupus erythematosus. Generally, this syndrome occurs early in therapy, but can develop after many years of treatment. A positive result in the antinuclear antibody titer is used to confirm a clinical diagnosis of lupus. It has been estimated that between 6% and 10% of patients receiving high doses of hydralazine for longer than 6 months develop hydralazine-induced lupus.[600] It is seen most frequently in women and rarely in African Americans. This syndrome occurs primarily in slow acetylators and is reversible when hydralazine is discontinued, but months may be required for complete clearing of symptoms. Hydralazine has been frequently used to treat pregnancy-associated hypertension in view of its relatively low teratogenicity.

ENDOTHELIN RECEPTOR ANTAGONISTS

Endothelin receptor antagonists may have a future role in the management of hypertension.[601] Endothelin is among the most potent endogenous vasoconstrictors known.[602] It also enhances mitogenesis and induces extracellular matrix formation. The drug is thought to be involved in vascular remodeling and end-organ damage under several different cardiovascular conditions.[603] As a result of the understanding of these actions, endothelin receptors are attractive targets for the development of blocking agents.

CLASS MECHANISM OF ACTION AND CLASS MEMBERS

An effort to explore the usefulness of endothelin receptor antagonists in the management of hypertension is logical, given the fact that endothelin is such a powerful vasoconstrictor. The two primary receptor sites, endothelin type A (ET-A) and endothelin type B (ET-B), can be selectively blocked with different chemicals, or both sites can be blocked simultaneously. These compounds function as specific vasodilators.

Originally, these compounds were studied in patients with heart failure or pulmonary hypertension.[604-608] The results of the studies in pulmonary hypertension have been encouraging. Bosentan, a mixed ET-A/ET-B receptor antagonist, has shown strong promise. Its use has led to improvement in exercise capacity, hemodynamic parameters, and World Health Organization functional class over 1 year. It has been hypothesized that selective ET-A receptor antagonists might offer greater benefits in patients with systolic heart failure than nonselective agents, such as bosentan. It is thought that stimulation of ET-B receptors by the endothelin-induced release of nitric oxide and prostaglandins may lead to vasorelaxation. ET-B receptors may also regulate the clearance of endothelin from the circulation.[609] Thus, some consider the use of selective ET-A receptor blockers to be a better therapeutic strategy.[610] Other studies of the use of endothelin blockers to treat heart failure have not been encouraging, particularly when the drugs were used in conjunction with other approved therapies[604,605]

Bosentan has been studied in the management of hypertension. A large placebo-controlled trial lasting 4 weeks demonstrated a dose-dependent reduction in BP compared with placebo when bosentan was dosed from 100 mg once daily up to 1000 mg twice daily.[611] The mean reduction in diastolic BP of 5.8 mm Hg across all dosages at or above 5 mg/day was almost identical to that seen with 20 mg of enalapril. The most common adverse effects were peripheral edema, flushing, headache, and some alterations in liver enzyme levels.

Darusentan, a selective ET-A receptor antagonist, has also been studied in a large placebo-controlled trial comparing dosages of 10 to 100 mg/day over a 6-week period.[612] Placebo-subtracted reductions in BP were best with the 100-mg dose and approximated 11.3 mm Hg. This dosage was associated with adverse side effects more than lower dosages, with reports of headache, flushing, and peripheral edema. There was no evidence of alteration in hepatic enzyme levels. Subsequent studies have demonstrated that darusentan has important BP-lowering effects in patients with resistant hypertension.

CLASS RENAL EFFECTS

Endothelin receptor antagonists have been used to study the role of endothelin in the development of acute and chronic renal failure in different experimental models.[613] Clinical studies using endothelin receptor blockers have shown improvement in proteinuria. This effect is independent of the antiproteinuric effects of inhibition of the RAAS and may help relieve renal injury.[614] What is unknown is whether the selective blockage of the ET-A receptor over the ET-B receptor will provide a greater opportunity for using endothelin receptor antagonists, not only to control BP but also to mitigate renal ischemia and reduce proteinuria.

CLASS EFFICACY AND SAFETY

Despite the BP reduction evident with these drugs, clinical progress in defining the therapeutic index of bosentan and darusentan or other similar compounds is not yet evident. Whether this is related to concerns about tolerability, development of competing products with a better tolerability profile, or teratogenic potential of endothelin receptor blockade, as shown in experimental models, is unknown. These drugs may ultimately have a benefit for patients with resistant hypertension.

MODERATELY SELECTIVE PERIPHERAL α_1-ADRENERGIC ANTAGONISTS

CLASS MECHANISMS OF ACTION

The nonselective agents phentolamine and phenoxybenzamine have an occasional role in hypertension management. Phentolamine is administered parenterally, and the longer acting agent phenoxybenzamine has been used orally for the management of hypertension associated with pheochromocytoma.[615] Phenoxybenzamine is a moderately selective, peripheral α_1-adrenergic antagonist. Its specificity for the α_1-adrenergic receptor is 100 times greater than that for the α_2-adrenergic receptor.

CLASS MEMBERS

Phenoxybenzamine is a long-acting α-adrenergic blocking agent. This agent irreversibly and covalently binds to α-receptors only. β-Receptors and the parasympathetic system are not affected by phenoxybenzamine. The total peripheral resistance is decreased, and cardiac output increases with phenoxybenzamine. Phenoxybenzamine is also believed to inhibit the uptake of catecholamines into adrenergic nerve terminals and extraneural tissues. The usual oral dosage of phenoxybenzamine for the treatment of pheochromocytoma is initially 10 mg twice daily, with the dosage gradually increased every other day to dosages ranging between 20 and 40 mg two or three times daily. The final dosage should be determined by the BP response. Phenoxybenzamine may be administered with a β-blocking agent if tachycardia becomes excessive during therapy. The pressor effects of a pheochromocytoma must be controlled by α-blockade before β-blockers are initiated. With oral use, the pheochromocytoma symptoms decrease after several days. The oral bioavailability is 20% to 30%. The drug is extensively metabolized by the liver. Phenoxybenzamine should be administered cautiously to patients with renal impairment. Specific dosage recommendations are not available.

Table 50.26 Pharmacokinetic Properties of Peripheral α_1-Adrenergic Antagonists

Drug	Bioavailability (%)	Affected by Food	Peak Blood Level (hr)	Elimination Half-Life (hr)	Metabolism	Excretion	Active Metabolites
Doxazosin (Cardura)	62-69	No	2-5	9-22	L	F (63%-65%) U (1%-9%)	—
Prazosin (Minipress)	—	No	1-3	2-4	L	F	—
Terazosin (Hytrin)	90	Yes	1	12	L	F (45%-60%) U (10%)	—

F, Feces; L, liver; U, urine.

Table 50.27 Pharmacodynamic Properties of Peripheral α_1-Adrenergic Antagonists

Drug	Initial Dose (mg)	Usual Dose (mg)	Maximum Dose (mg)	Interval	Peak Response (hr)	Duration of Response (hr)
Doxazosin	1	8	16	qd, qid	4-8	24
Prazosin	1	3-20	20	bid, qid	0.5-1.5	10
Terazosin	1	5	20	qd, bid	3	24

Phentolamine is an α-adrenergic blocking agent that produces peripheral vasodilation and cardiac stimulation, with a resulting decrease in BP in most patients. The drug is used parenterally. The usual dose is 5 mg, repeated as needed. The onset of activity with intravenous dosing is immediate. The drug is not absorbed well orally; its half-life is 19 minutes. It is metabolized by the liver, with 10% excreted in the urine as unchanged drug.

CLASS RENAL EFFECTS

Phenoxybenzamine has no clear effect on the RAAS. Blood volume and body weight are not altered. Salt and water retention do not occur. GFR and effective renal plasma flow would be expected to increase. Renal vascular resistance probably decreases in proportion to the degree of blockade of α-adrenergic receptors.

CLASS EFFICACY AND SAFETY

Phenoxybenzamine is used primarily as an agent to counteract the excessive α-adrenergic tone associated with pheochromocytoma. Tachycardia may result from an α-adrenergic blockade, which unmasks β-adrenergic effects with epinephrine-secreting tumors. This may be controlled with concurrent use of a β-adrenergic antagonist. α-Adrenergic blockade must be initiated before β-adrenergic blockade to avoid paradoxic hypertension. Adverse effects of phenoxybenzamine are sedation, weakness, nasal congestion, hypertension, and tachycardia.

PERIPHERAL α_1-ADRENERGIC ANTAGONISTS

CLASS MECHANISMS OF ACTION

Drugs of the peripheral α_1-adrenergic antagonist class, including doxazosin, prazosin, and terazosin, are selective antagonists of the postsynaptic α_1-adrenergic receptor. These drugs, which blunt the increases in arteriolar and venous tone mediated by norepinephrine released from sympathetic nerve terminals, act at the α_1-adrenergic receptor located postjunctionally in the blood vessel wall. The affinity of these drugs for the α_2-receptor is very low. Because of the selective α_1 action, there is no interference with the negative feedback control mechanisms that are mediated by the prejunctional α_2-receptors. As a result, the reflex tachycardia associated with the blockade of the presynaptic α_2-receptor decreases substantially. The pharmacokinetic and pharmacodynamic properties of these drugs are shown in Tables 50-26 and 50-27.

CLASS MEMBERS

Doxazosin is a selective long-acting α_1-adrenergic antagonist. The initial antihypertensive dosage is 1 mg daily. This dose can be titrated up to a maximum of 16 mg daily. The maximal antihypertensive effect is seen 4 to 8 hours after a single dose. The drug is highly plasma protein-bound and extensively metabolized. Most of the administered dose is excreted in the feces. The estimated half-life ranges from 9 to 22 hours. Doxazosin pharmacokinetics are not altered in patients with renal impairment. The drug should be used with caution in patients with advanced liver dysfunction.

The availability of extended-release formulations of these drugs has improved tolerability. The use of doxazosin has declined after the Data Safety Monitoring Board for the ALLHAT study decided to discontinue the doxazosin-treatment arm of the study based on the finding that a significantly higher percentage of patients on doxazosin developed stroke and congestive heart failure.[616] The ASCOT study conducted a nonrandomized, non–placebo-controlled study that showed doxazosin to be an effective and safe third-line antihypertensive agent.[617] The ASCOT trial conducted an observational analysis of blood among 10,069 participants as a third-line drug. A doxazosin GITS was given to 10,069 participants in dosages ranging from 4 to 7 mg. The BP fell by an average of almost 12/7 mm Hg and modest reductions were seen in total and LDL cholesterol levels but only a small increase in fasting plasma glucose concentrations. There was no excess of heart failure seen.

Prazosin is a selective α_1-adrenergic antagonist that is structurally related to doxazosin and terazosin. Oral dosing is 3 to 20 mg/day. A first-dose phenomenon with postural hypotension resulting in palpitations, tachycardia, and potentially syncope has been associated with prazosin. This can be minimized by limiting the initial dose to 1 mg at bedtime. Full therapeutic effects are seen within 4 to 8 weeks after initiation of therapy. Peak serum levels are reached 1 to 3 hours after an oral dose. The drug is highly protein-bound. The elimination half-life is 2 to 4 hours. There is extensive hepatic metabolism followed by renal excretion of a very small amount of unchanged drug. Dosage adjustment is not required for patients with renal failure. Patients with significant liver disease may require a dosage adjustment and more frequent monitoring.

Terazosin is a selective, long-acting α_1-adrenergic antagonist that has structural similarities to prazosin and doxazosin. The initial dosage is 1 mg orally at bedtime, with titration to 5 mg daily. Doses of 10 to 20 mg orally have been given. Peak serum levels after oral administration occur within 1 hour. The half-life is approximately 12 hours. Terazosin is extensively metabolized in the liver and eliminated primarily through the biliary tract. Renal insufficiency does not affect the pharmacokinetics of terazosin, and dosage adjustment is not required. Patients with severe hepatic insufficiency may require dosage adjustments.

CLASS RENAL EFFECTS

GFR and renal blood flow are maintained during long-term treatment with prazosin. In some studies, there was a slight increase in renal blood flow. Renal vascular resistance may be reduced, perhaps mediated by a reduction in preglomerular capillary resistance related to inhibition of α_1-mediated vasoconstriction. Urinary protein excretion has been reported to be reduced. The RAAS is not significantly affected by specific α_1-adrenergic antagonists. Extracellular fluid volume has been reported to be increased, and fractional excretion may be decreased.

CLASS EFFICACY AND SAFETY

Comparative clinical studies of the efficacy of α_1-adrenergic blockers have shown that the antihypertensive responses are similar to those elicited by other antihypertensive drugs.[92] This conventional viewpoint has come under criticism with the results of ALLHAT, in which patients receiving doxazosin as their initial antihypertensive drug were found to have poorer BP control than those receiving a chlorthalidone-based treatment.[616] In this study, no difference was seen in the primary outcomes of fatal coronary heart disease or nonfatal MI in patients receiving doxazosin, but these patients had higher rates of stroke and congestive heart failure.[618] The data from ALLHAT have prompted a reassessment of the appropriateness of using doxazosin or other peripheral α_1-adrenergic antagonists as primary hypertensive therapeutic agents. These drugs can be considered as secondary agents in the management of resistant hypertension.

These drugs have been shown to increase insulin sensitivity.[619] There are potentially beneficial effects of α_1-blockers on lipid metabolism.[92,262,620-622] They have been consistently shown to result in a modest reduction in levels of total and LDL cholesterol and a small increase in HDL cholesterol levels. This metabolic benefit may be linked to the beneficial effect on insulin responsiveness, leading to increased peripheral glucose uptake.

The most important adverse effect of α_1-adrenergic receptor blockers is the first-dose orthostatic hypotension effect, resulting in lightheadedness, palpitations, and occasionally syncope. This is related to the drug effect on the venous capacitance vessels, which results in venous dilation and inadequate venous return. It may occur when peak drug levels are reached 30 to 90 minutes after the first dose; it can be minimized by initiating therapy with a small dose taken at bedtime.[623] This effect can be exacerbated in patients with underlying autonomic insufficiency.

α_1-Adrenergic antagonists are also used for the symptomatic management of prostatic hypertrophy. Prostatic smooth muscle has significant α_1-adrenal receptor expression. Blockade of these receptors results in smooth muscle relaxation within the prostate.[624,625] Terazosin has been marketed in combination with amlodipine for male patients with hypertension and lower urinary tract symptoms.[626]

RENIN INHIBITORS

The earliest renin-inhibiting compounds in development included aliskiren, zankiren, and remikiren. However, due to problems with oral bioavailability, only aliskiren has been approved for the treatment of hypertension.

CLASS MECHANISM OF ACTION AND CLASS MEMBER

Aliskiren was designed through a combination of molecular modeling techniques and crystal structure elucidation.[627] It is a potent and specific inhibitor of human renin in vitro (the concentration that inhibits 50% = 0.6 nmol/L). Aliskiren was the first in a new class of orally effective, nonpeptide, low-molecular-weight renin inhibitors used for the management of hypertension (see Figure 50.2).[628,629] Renin inhibition interferes with the first and rate-limiting step in the renin enzyme cascade, the interaction of renin with its substrate angiotensinogen. The renin blockade step is an attractive target for hypertension therapeutics, in large part due to the remarkable specificity of renin for its substrate.[630] This specificity reduces the likelihood of unwanted interactions and possible adverse effects. In addition, unlike ACE inhibitors or ARBs, which lead to a reactive increase in renin and associated angiotensin peptides, only renin inhibition renders the RAAS quiescent. Although aliskiren has low inherent bioavailability (2.6%), it is potent in reducing BP and has an effective half-life of 40 hours.[631] The drug is not actively metabolized by the liver and is primarily excreted in the urine, with most of it as unchanged drug. CYP enzymes are not involved in the metabolism of aliskiren. Thus, clinically significant CYP inhibition by aliskiren is unlikely.[632]

CLASS RENAL EFFECTS

Renin inhibitors offer substantial promise for renal protection in that they provide not only BP reduction, but also an opportunity to attenuate the activity of the RAAS without a reactive increase in renin or other angiotensin peptides. Experimental studies have demonstrated the usefulness of aliskiren in providing renal protection in hypertensive diabetic nephropathy in double-transgenic (Ren-2) rats.[633] These rats provide a model of activated tissue RAAS. After the animals were made diabetic with streptozotocin, the rats were treated with vehicle or aliskiren by osmotic minipumps. Aliskiren not only lowered the systolic BP, but also prevented the development of albuminuria and reduced the urinary excretion of TGF-β. The gene expression of TGF-β was significantly suppressed.[634] In another study, these investigators compared aliskiren and enalapril in the same model of Ren-2 double-transgenic rats without diabetes.[635] Both therapeutic strategies significantly reduced BP and urinary albumin excretion for the duration of therapy. However, even after therapy was stopped, the reduction of urinary TGF-β excretion and albuminuria was maintained in the rats that had received both the renin inhibitor and ACE inhibitor.

In another experimental study, aliskiren was compared with the ARB valsartan in the same model of the Ren-2 double-transgenic rat, which, because of its overexpression of human renin and angiotensinogen genes, rapidly develops cardiovascular and renal disease. Aliskiren and valsartan demonstrated an important ability to lower BP, reverse LVH and albuminuria, and delay the onset of death.[635] On the basis of these studies, it was suggested by the investigators that the renin inhibitor provides renal protection comparable to that of an ACE inhibitor or an ARB that extends beyond the dosing interval of the drug.

Clinical trial data in humans have indicated that aliskiren reduces proteinuria in conjunction with decreasing BP.[630] In a study involving 600 patients with hypertension, diabetes, and nephropathy, the administration of aliskiren, 300 mg/day, facilitated a 20% incremental reduction in proteinuria compared with placebo in patients being treated concurrently with losartan, 100 mg/day. The baseline BP was 135 mm Hg with losartan treatment before random assignment to aliskiren therapy and did not change with the addition of aliskiren.[338] Renal vascular response curves for ACE inhibition or renin inhibition at the top of the dose-response curve indicated greater improvement in renal blood flow with the renin inhibitor, despite similar changes in BP.[630] However, despite these encouraging clinical observations, a subsequent clinical trial, ALTITUDE, did not demonstrate an incremental benefit of aliskiren when used with an ACE inhibitor or ARB in patients with diabetic kidney disease on cardiovascular or renal end points.[265] From a safety standpoint, there were more adverse events in the patients receiving both classes of RAAS-blocking drugs.

CLASS EFFICACY AND SAFETY

Clinical trials of aliskiren have demonstrated a dose-dependent efficacy in reducing systolic and diastolic BP. In an 8-week, double-blind, placebo-controlled trial, aliskiren was studied in dosages from 150 to 600 mg/day.[636] The placebo-corrected reduction in sitting systolic BP was approximately 10 to 11 mm Hg for both the 300- and 600-mg doses. Also evaluated in the same study was irbesartan, an ARB, at a dosage of 150 mg/day. This dosage provided BP reduction comparable to that of aliskiren at a dosage of 150 mg/day. Other clinical studies have confirmed the antihypertensive efficacy of aliskiren compared with placebo or with other active therapies, such as the ARB losartan. As expected, BP reduction was comparable with that produced by the active agents. The only observed difference was suppression of plasma renin activity and Ang I and Ang II levels with aliskiren but increased levels of Ang I and Ang II with ARB therapy.

The tolerability of aliskiren is comparable to that of placebo, with a relatively low incidence of adverse events at all dosages tested in the 150- to 600-mg range.[636] Aliskiren treatment was comparable in tolerability to treatment with an ARB or placebo, with a low discontinuation rate and no statistical difference in the incidence of different types of adverse events, except for some diarrhea at the 600-mg dose.

Aliskiren has also been studied in combination with hydrochlorothiazide, CCBs, ARBs, and ACE inhibitors in the management of hypertension.[637-640] In one small clinical trial, all patients received aliskiren 150 mg once daily for 3 weeks. Patients who had a daytime BP above 130/80 mm Hg, as measured by ambulatory BP monitoring, were given hydrochlorothiazide, 25 mg daily, for an additional 3 weeks. Adding 25 mg of hydrochlorothiazide resulted in an additional 10 mm Hg of systolic BP reduction. Not surprisingly, there was no difference in plasma renin activity between the patients receiving aliskiren with hydrochlorothiazide and those receiving aliskiren alone. Adding aliskiren to amlodipine, valsartan, or ramipril provides incremental and statistically significant improvements in BP reduction. However, the ALTITUDE study did raise safety concerns about using aliskiren with RAAS blocking drugs with regard to changes in renal function and hyperkalemia.[265] Therefore, this combination is not currently recommended and should be avoided. The additional BP reduction may or may not be related to the neutralization of plasma renin activity that occurs with the addition of the renin inhibitor.

SELECTIVE ALDOSTERONE RECEPTOR ANTAGONISTS

CLASS MECHANISM AND CLASS MEMBER

Potassium-sparing diuretics, including spironolactone, a nonselective aldosterone receptor antagonist, are discussed below. However, eplerenone is a selective aldosterone receptor antagonist that is the first in its class to be evaluated for its antihypertensive and cytoprotective properties. It may have antihypertensive effects distinct from its diuretic properties.

Eplerenone is a 9α,11α-epoxy derivative of spironolactone that is approximately 24 times less potent in blocking mineralocorticoid receptors than spironolactone. However, this drug is substantially more selective than spironolactone and has little agonist activity at estrogen and progesterone receptors.[641] Therefore, eplerenone is associated with a lower incidence of gynecomastia, breast pain, and impotence in men and diminished libido and menstrual irregularities in women. The time to peak concentration is 1 to 2 hours. No significant accumulation occurs with multiple-dose administration, but up to 4 weeks may be required for the full antihypertensive effects to be evident. It appears to be well absorbed, but absolute (oral vs. intravenous) data are unavailable; specific data on protein binding and metabolism are also unavailable. The elimination half-life of eplerenone is 4 to 6 hours. Bioavailability is 69%, with approximately 50% protein binding. It is metabolized primarily by the hepatic CYP3A4 system to inactive metabolites excreted two thirds in the urine and one third in the feces.

The mineralocorticoid receptor forms part of the steroid–thyroid–retinoid–orphan receptor family of nuclear transactivating factors.[642] When unbound, these receptors are in an inactive multiprotein complex of chaperones. On binding of aldosterone, the chaperones are released, and the receptor hormone complex is translocated into the nucleus, where it binds to hormone response elements on DNA and interacts with transcription initiation complexes, which ultimately modulate gene expression.[643] In the kidney, mineralocorticoid receptors are located primarily in the epithelial cells of the distal nephron. These receptors bind physiologic glucocorticoids and mineralocorticoids with a similar affinity. Activation of mineralocorticoid receptors by aldosterone results in the activation of epithelial sodium channels, which leads to a rapid increase in sodium and water reabsorption and promotes the tubular secretion of potassium.[644,645] A persistent increase in sodium balance does not occur, even with continued stimulation of mineralocorticoid receptors by aldosterone. The mechanism of this escape phenomenon has not been fully elucidated. Studies have suggested that eplerenone and spironolactone lower BP by a mechanism that is independent of distal tubular effects on vascular smooth muscle cells.[646]

There is evidence indicating the presence of biologic activity of mineralocorticoid receptors in nonepithelial tissues.[647] These receptors have been identified in blood vessels of the heart and brain and may be involved in vascular injury and repair responses.[648,649] Aldosterone mediates fibrosis and collagen formation through the upregulation of Ang II receptor responsiveness.[583,647] Aldosterone increases sodium influx in vascular smooth muscle and inhibits norepinephrine uptake in vascular smooth muscle and myocardial cells.[650] Aldosterone also directly participates in vascular smooth muscle cell hypertrophy. Clinical trials are underway to validate the hypothesis that aldosterone receptor antagonism may inhibit vascular, myocardial, and renal injury. A meta-analysis of randomized controlled trials has shown a positive impact on changes in the cardiac structure and left ventricular function in patients with heart failure.[651]

Recently, the role of aldosterone antagonists in treating hypertensive obese patients with sleep apnea has been reported, representing approximately 20% of all individuals with sleep apnea. The aldosterone production relates directly to the adipocyte.[652-655]

CLASS RENAL EFFECTS

Selective aldosterone receptor antagonism may have benefits for the kidney, independently of its effects on BP. Experimental and clinical studies have demonstrated that Ang II may be the primary mediator of the RAAS associated with the progression of renal disease.[656,657] The relative importance of aldosterone in this cascade has been the subject of experimental and clinical studies. Hyperaldosteronism and adrenal hypertrophy are common observations in remnant kidney models and correlate with progressive loss of renal function.[656] Investigators have demonstrated that hypertension, proteinuria, and structural injury are less prevalent in subtotally nephrectomized rats that have undergone adrenalectomy, even when given large doses of replacement glucocorticoids.[658] Other investigators have demonstrated that aldosterone infusion can reverse the renal protective effects of an ACE inhibitor in stroke-prone, spontaneously hypertensive rats.[659] Interestingly, in this model, the renal injury induced by aldosterone was independent of BP increases, suggesting a toxic tissue effect of aldosterone. Other experimental studies have indicated that aldosterone receptor antagonism can prevent the development of proteinuria.[659]

Even though selective aldosterone receptor antagonists have no observable effects on glomerular hemodynamics, therapy with these drugs may provide an incremental effect in protecting the kidney when added to ACE inhibitors or ARBs by inhibiting the effects of aldosterone that persist, despite treatment with the latter drugs. Studies in patients with diabetic nephropathy or other glomerular diseases have demonstrated that the addition of spironolactone for ACE inhibition markedly reduces albuminuria.[660,661]

CLASS EFFICACY AND SAFETY

Eplerenone lowers BP in a dose-dependent fashion when administered at dosages of 25, 50, or 200 mg twice daily.[662] Changes in BP were found to be greater with twice-daily dosing (50 mg twice daily yielded a 11.7-mm Hg reduction in systolic pressure) than with a single daily dose (100 mg daily produced a 7.9-mm Hg systolic BP reduction), as measured by 24-hour ambulatory BP monitoring.[662]

Clinical trials have also demonstrated that eplerenone has antihypertensive activity that is additive to that of an ACE inhibitor or ARB. Additional reductions in BP were 5.9 mm Hg systolic with the ACE inhibitor and 6.8 mm Hg systolic with the ARB.[662a] Another clinical trial has demonstrated that in diabetic hypertensive patients with microalbuminuria, adding eplerenone to ACE inhibitor therapy was capable of reducing proteinuria more than the ACE inhibitor alone, independently of BP reduction.[663]

The advantage of eplerenone over spironolactone in clinical practice is relates to its fewer antiandrogenic adverse effects because of its more selective aldosterone receptor antagonism. Eplerenone is less potent and has a shorter half-life (3 to 4 hours), leading to reduced antihypertensive efficacy and a requirement for twice-daily dosing.[664]

TYROSINE HYDROXYLASE INHIBITOR

MECHANISMS OF ACTION

Metyrosine, the only drug in the tyrosine hydroxylase inhibitor class, blocks the rate-limiting step in the biosynthetic pathway of catecholamines. Metyrosine inhibits tyrosine hydroxylase, the enzyme responsible for the conversion of tyrosine to dihydroxyphenylalanine. This inhibition results in decreased levels of endogenous catecholamines. In patients with pheochromocytomas, metyrosine reduces catecholamine biosynthesis by up to 80%, resulting in a decrease in total peripheral vascular resistance. The heart rate and cardiac output increase because of the vasodilation.

CLASS MEMBER

The recommended initial dosage of metyrosine is 250 mg four times a day orally. The dose may be increased by 250 to 500 mg every day until a maximum of 4 g/day is given. Following oral absorption, metyrosine is eliminated primarily unchanged in the urine. The half-life is 7.2 hours. Dosage reduction is appropriate in patients with renal failure.

RENAL EFFECTS

Little information is available on the renal effects of metyrosine. On the basis of its mechanism of action, which would counteract the renal effects of excessive circulating catecholamines, renal plasma flow and glomerular filtration would probably increase. Renal vascular resistance would be expected to decrease.

EFFICACY AND SAFETY

Metyrosine is used in the preoperative or intraoperative management of pheochromocytoma. Hypertension and reflex tachycardia may result from vasodilation. These effects can be minimized by volume expansion. Adverse effects include sedation, changes in sleep patterns, and extrapyramidal signs. Metyrosine crystals have been noted in the urine in patients receiving high dosages. Patients taking metyrosine should maintain a generous fluid intake; some patients have occasionally experienced diarrhea.

SELECTION OF ANTIHYPERTENSIVE DRUG THERAPY

DETERMINATION OF BLOOD PRESSURE GOAL

Numerous factors confound the management of high BP, which is a lifelong, progressive, asymptomatic disease process. The treatment is often delayed many years. Worldwide surveys of BP recommended targets consistently reveal that the goal of less than 140/90 mm Hg is reached only by a minority of people.[665] Consequently, it is not uncommon for the patient to have subclinical or even clinically evident target-organ damage at the initiation of treatment. Moreover, the mechanistic underpinnings of high BP have not been well elucidated, and pharmacotherapy is frequently based simply on what "brings the numbers down" and not necessarily on what may be well tolerated or what may be best for preventing the development of cardiovascular disease or renal disease.

The whole purpose of treating BP elevation is to prevent the development of cardiovascular events. From this perspective, BP is nothing more than one of many surrogate markers of risk contributing to cardiovascular disease. Consequently, the word *hypertension* is a nebulous concept. A factual definition of hypertension would be the level of BP at which there is a greater net attributable risk of cardiovascular disease. Thus, the optimal BP goal for different patients may be somewhat different, depending on coexistent cardiovascular risk factors. The management of high BP is much more complex than it was once assumed to be, and the determination of the BP goal must be carefully individualized for each patient.

Clinicians must ask themselves three major questions:

- How low should the BP go?
- What drugs should be used?
- What are the best strategies for facilitating the attainment of the target BP?

The question of how low BP should go is not easy to answer because there are so many different aspects of patient care that require consideration. Observational data indicate the advantages of lower systolic and diastolic BPs, preferably below 120/80 mm Hg.[666,667] However, treated BPs of the same levels as observed BPs may not provide the same cardiovascular risk reduction. Most recent guidelines have based their recommendations for goal BP on clinical trial evidence.[437,668-670] Despite the enthusiasm for lower BP treatment goals of 130/80 mm Hg or less for people with heart disease, kidney disease, or diabetes, there are insufficient clinical trial data to support these lower BP goals. Consequently, guidelines have refocused BP targets at below 140/90 mm Hg for patients younger than age 60 and below 150/90 mm Hg for those older than 60 years. The only demonstrable benefit for lower BP goals has been based on secondary analyses of clinical trials, such as the ACCORD study,[671] which suggested that lower BP goals in patients with type 2 diabetes may reduce the incidence of stroke, or on clinical trials in patients with type 2 diabetes and nephropathy, which suggested that patients with more than 1 g of protein in their urine/day had a slower progression of renal disease if their BP was below 130/80 mm Hg than if their BP was 140/90 mm Hg. The ongoing SPRINT trial may help answer some important questions concerning optimum target BP; the authors of this study have randomized more than 9250 patients to compare a systolic pressure of 140 versus 120 mm Hg in a large cohort of older patients and in patients with CKD. Once this study is completed, there will be more opportunity to determine the usefulness of lower BP goals on cardiovascular and renal outcomes.

A recent systematic review and meta-analysis was performed to investigate the effects of BP lowering in persons with grade 1 hypertension (systolic BP of 149 to 159 mm Hg and/or diastolic BP of 90 to 99 mm Hg) and no overt cardiovascular disease. The patients were randomly assigned to an active antihypertensive drug or control (placebo) regimen and had substantial benefit, especially patients at risk for cardiovascular disease.[672] There were 8905 patients identified from trials included in the BPLTTC (Blood Pressure Lowering Treatment Trialists' Collaboration). The difference in mean BP reduction was 3.6 mm Hg/2.4 mm Hg between actively treated and control groups. Over the 5 years of the study, the ORs were 0.86 for total cardiovascular events (95% CI, 0.74 to 1.01), 0.72 for strokes (CI, 0.55 to 0.94), 0.91 for coronary events (CI, 0.74 to 1.12), 0.80 for heart failure (CI, 0.57 to 1.12), 0.75 for cardiovascular deaths (CI, 0.57 to 0.98), and 0.78 for total deaths (CI, 0.67 to 0.92). These findings are in line with reductions in risk from large-scale trials of BP reduction conducted among patients with high BP and preexisting cardiovascular disease.[673] A previous review failed to show benefit for this population of patients with grade 1 hypertension.[674] The more recent study differed from the previous study in that persons with diabetes were included, and the number of patients studied was nearly double that of the previous study. Consequently, more information from randomized controlled trials are needed before the present BP goals of 150/90 mm Hg for people older than 60 years and 140/90 mm Hg for people younger than 60 years can be changed.[437]

Whether one should treat the systolic, diastolic, or pulse pressure is another important consideration. This is particularly true when one considers the vast number of patients with isolated systolic hypertension, who have traditionally been assumed to have normal BP because their diastolic pressure was below 90 mm Hg. Interventional trials have demonstrated the advantage of lowering systolic BP.[675-677] Evidence from three large clinical trials on the management of isolated systolic hypertension has indicated a consistent benefit related to a reduction in the incidence of congestive heart failure, MI, and stroke with the control of systolic BP to an intermediate goal of less than 160 mm Hg and preferably to a final goal of less than 150 mm Hg.

Epidemiologic data have also demonstrated the importance of pulse pressure (systolic pressure minus diastolic BP) in predicting cardiovascular events.[678-680] Pulse pressure correlates directly with the risk of MI and the development of LVH. Because the measurement of diastolic BP is frequently difficult in older patients with vascular disease, the exact assessment of pulse pressure may not always be possible. Consequently, relying on the systolic BP may give the clinician a more realistic opportunity to gauge the adequacy of antihypertensive therapy. It is important to realize that the management of systolic BP may provide one of the most important opportunities to achieve cardiovascular risk reduction, particularly in patients with lower diastolic pressures who have a wider pulse pressure.

The promptness of achieving BP control has long been thought to be an important strategy for the clinical care for patients with hypertension. Clinical trials and observational studies have indicated that initiating treatment with a two-drug combination of medications results in a more rapid achievement of target BP goals compared to monotherapy. A retrospective analysis of the Valsartan Antihypertensive Long-term Use Evaluation (VALUE) trial has indicated that earlier BP control results in a significant reduction in the 5-year risk of cardiovascular events, regardless of the type of medication used.[681] More recently, a matched cohort study has demonstrated that initial combination therapy reduces the risk of cardiovascular events in hypertensive patients.[399] This reduction was thought to be related to an earlier achievement of target BP as the main contributor of risk reduction.

Decisions about which drug(s) should be used for a given patient require careful consideration and individualization. As discussed later, the appropriate pharmacotherapy may depend on age, gender, race, obesity, and associated cardiovascular or renal disease. Clinical trials in patients with vascular disease, heart disease, or kidney disease have demonstrated the important therapeutic advantage of drugs that block the RAAS—ACE inhibitors or ARBs[82,255,256,682-687]—to prevent progression of cardiac or renal disease as part of a multidrug regimen to lower BP. In the aggregate, RAAS are blocking drugs that provide an approximately 20% relative risk reduction benefit compared to other therapies. These drugs should be part of every antihypertensive regimen in patients with heart disease or kidney disease unless there are specific contraindications.[684] RAAS-blocking drugs are also some of the best-tolerated therapies available for treating hypertension. Although these drugs provide important risk reduction opportunities, they are not a substitute for achieving BP control.

SINGLE-PILL COMBINATION THERAPY

With the shift in emphasis on treatment from diastolic BP to systolic and diastolic BPs,[87] later stage treatment in the disease process, greater salt intake, and more patients who are overweight or obese, there has been a substantial increase in the complexity of medical regimens to treat hypertension. Most available antihypertensive drugs, when appropriately dosed, reduce systolic BP by approximately 8 to 10 mm Hg (Figure 50.3). Therefore, the number of drugs needed to reach the BP goal can generally be predicted by dividing the number 10 into the difference between the current and target systolic BPs. For many patients, three or four drugs may be required. Ideally, medications that are long-acting, can be taken once daily, are well tolerated, and preferably work well with other medications to facilitate BP control should be used. In addition, there has been a marked increase in the number of single-pill, fixed-dose combination antihypertensive drugs that are available in the marketplace, developed in large part to facilitate adherence by reducing the complexity of the antihypertensive regimen (Table 50.28).

Drugs that block the RAAS system, such as ACE inhibitors, ARBs, renin inhibitors, or β-blockers, can be prescribed with a low dose of chlorthalidone (half of a 25-mg tablet) or hydrochlorothiazide (6.25 or 12.5 mg). The advantage of the low-dose thiazide or thiazide-like drug is that it nearly doubles the antihypertensive effects of the parent drug without adding any toxicity to the regimen (Figure 50.4).[688] Single-pill combinations of an ACE inhibitor or ARB and CCB are also available. Clinical studies have demonstrated that these drugs are also additive in their ability to lower diastolic and systolic BPs.[689-693] Moreover, there is good clinical evidence that the ACE inhibitor or ARB in such combinations antagonizes the development of pedal edema, which is not uncommonly observed with CCBs.[694] Two triple single-pill combinations (ARB, CCB, hydrochlorothiazide) have been approved for the treatment of hypertension.[695] An ARB has also been formulated with the thiazide-like diuretic chlorthalidone. Some single-pill combinations are now approved by the U.S. Food and Drug Administration (FDA) for initial treatment in patients with moderate to severe hypertension.

Given that the efficacy of drugs that block the RAAS is enhanced with thiazide, thiazide-like diuretics, or CCBs, a clinical trial was conducted to examine whether long-term cardiovascular outcomes would be improved if a thiazide diuretic or CCB was paired with the full dose of an ACE inhibitor. In the Avoiding Cardiovascular Events through Combination Therapy in Patients Living with Systolic Hypertension (ACCOMPLISH) study, approximately 11,000 hypertensive patients at high risk for a cardiovascular event were randomized to receive an ACE inhibitor with a CCB or an ACE inhibitor with a thiazide diuretic.[696] The trial was stopped prematurely because there was a 20% relative risk reduction benefit of cardiovascular events in those patients receiving a CCB with an ACE inhibitor (Figure 50.5). This observation was notable, given that there was no difference in the achievement in goal levels of BP between the

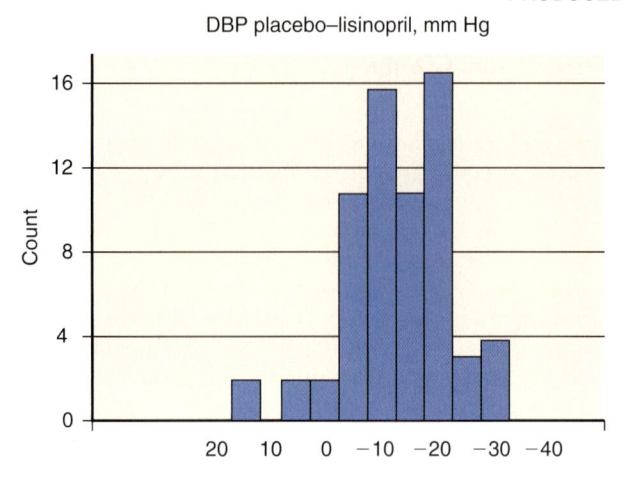

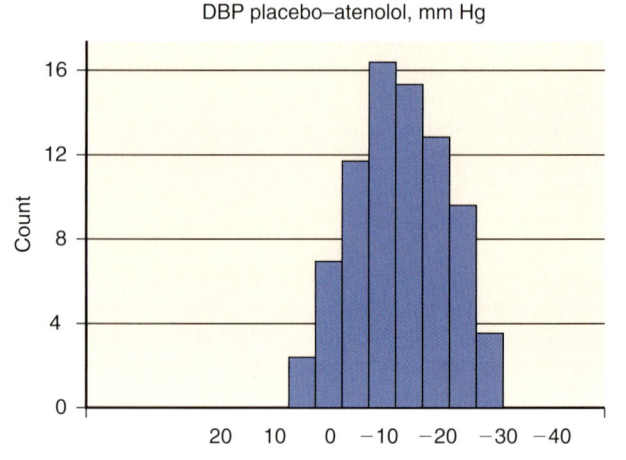

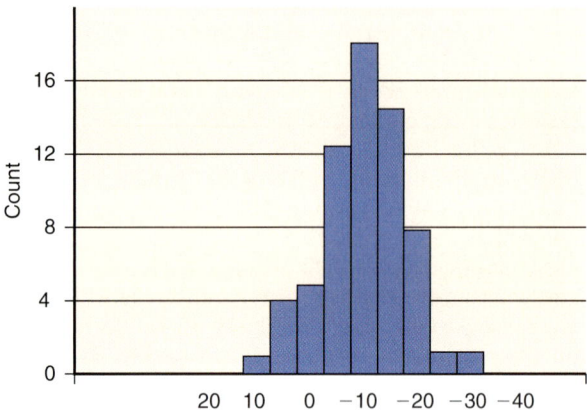

Figure 50.3 Frequency distribution of changes in diastolic blood pressure (DBP) produced by three different antihypertensive drugs. Negative values represent placebo-corrected reductions in diastolic pressure. A meta-analysis of placebo-controlled trials of monotherapy in unselected hypertensives reports averaged placebo-corrected blood pressure responses to single agents of 9.1 mm Hg systolic and 5.5 mm Hg diastolic pressures. These average values disguise the extremely wide-ranging responses in individuals across a fall of 20 to 30 mm Hg systolic pressure at one extreme, to no effect at all, or even a small rise in blood pressure at the other. (Modified from Attwood S, Bird R, Burch K, et al: Within-patient correlation between the antihypertensive effects of atenolol, lisinopril and nifedepin. *J Hypertens* 12:1053-1060, 1994.)

treatment regimens. The benefit of the ACE inhibitor–CCB combination in reducing cardiovascular and renal end points was evident, regardless of age, gender, ethnicity, or presence of diabetes. The explanation for this improvement in outcome is unknown.

Considerations for physicians about how to consolidate and simplify pharmacotherapy to control BP are of great interest, given the complexity of the current multidrug regimens that many patients require. Administering four drugs in two pills or three drugs in a single pill is possible with available fixed-dose combinations. This goal is important because many patients require eight to ten medications to control their various medical problems, including diabetes, dyslipidemia, and angina. High BP is a disease that is largely asymptomatic and, consequently, the therapeutic approach should be simple, effective, and well tolerated.

CHOICE OF APPROPRIATE AGENTS

This section of the chapter considers the initial therapy for various types of patients depending on factors such as age, gender, ancestry, obesity, and coexistent cardiovascular or renal disease. These suggestions are primarily generalizations based on clinical experience and should not be viewed as rigorous guidelines. Because each patient is different, variation in the approach is frequently necessary (Figure 50.6).

TREATMENT OF OLDER PATIENTS

The major considerations for initial therapy in older patients (Table 50.29) relate to the primary pathophysiologic problem, which is an increase in peripheral vascular resistance. With associated proximal aortic stiffening, there is frequently an increase in systolic BP, decrease in diastolic pressure, and wider pulse pressure.[679] There is also an associated reduction in cardiovascular baroreceptor reflex function, greater BP lability, and consequent propensity for orthostasis.[697] Older patients also tend to have hypertrophic cardiomyopathy with impaired diastolic function, which may impair cardiac output.[698]

An ideal therapeutic strategy for these patients is the use of a vasodilator, such as a thiazide or thiazide-like diuretic. Thiazide diuretics function primarily as vasodilators and have minimal long-term effects on blood volume. At lower dosages (hydrochlorothiazide, 12.5 to 25 mg, or chlorthalidone, 12.5 mg), these drugs are well tolerated and effective when used with ACE inhibitors and ARBs and cause minimal problems related to glycemia control, potassium homeostasis, and cholesterol metabolism.[699,700] They are more effective in controlling systolic BP when used in higher doses

Table 50.28 Single-Pill Combinations Available for the Treatment of Hypertension

Type of Combination	First Drug (Doses)	Second Drug (Doses)	Third Drug (Doses)
Dual Combinations			
Thiazide/K sparing diuretic	HCTZ (25/50)	Triamterene (37.5/75)	
	HCTZ (25/50)	Spironolactone (25/50)	
	HCTZ (25/50)	Amiloride (2.5/5)	
	Furosemide (20)	Spironolactone (50)	
ACE inhibitor/diuretic	Captopril (25/50)	HCTZ (15/25)	
	Enalapril (10/20)	HCTZ (12.5/25)	
	Lisinopril (10/20)	HCTZ (12.5/25)	
	Cilazapril (5)	HCTZ (12.5)	
	Fosinopril (10/20)	HCTZ (12.5)	
	Quinapril (10/20)	HCTZ (12.5)	
	Benazepril (5/10/20)	HCTZ (6.25/12.5/25)	
	Moexipril (7.5/15)	HCTZ (12.5/25)	
	Ramipril (2/5)	HCTZ (12.5/25)	
	Ramipril (5)	Piretanide (6)	
	Zofenopril (30)	HCTZ (12.5)	
	Perindopril (2.5/5/10)	Indapamide (0.625/1.25, 2.5)	
ACE inhibitor/CCB	Perindopril (5/10)	Amlodipine (5/10)	
	Benazepril (10/20/40)	Amlodipine (2.5/5/10)	
	Enalapril (5)	Diltiazem (180)	
	Enalapril (10)	Nitrendipine (20)	
	Enalapril (10/20)	Lercanidipine (10)	
	Ramipril (2.5/5)	Felodipine ER (2.5/5)	
	Trandolapril (1/2/4)	Verapamil (180, 240)	
	Delapril (10)	Manidipine (30)	
ARB/diuretic	Losartan (50/100)	HCTZ (12.5/25)	
	Valsartan (80/160)	HCTZ (12.5/25)	
	Irbesartan (150/300)	HCTZ (12.5/25)	
	Candesartan (8/16/32)	HCTZ (12.5/25)	
	Telmisartan (40/80)	HCTZ (12.5)	
	Eprosartan (600)	HCTZ (12.5/25)	
	Olmesartan (20/40)	HCTZ (12.5/25)	
	Azilsartan (40)	Chlorthalidone (12.5/25)	
ARB/CCB	Valsartan (80/160)	Amlodipine (5/10)	
	Telmisartan (40/80)	Amlodipine (5/10)	
	Olmesartan (20/40)	Amlodipine (5/10)	
	Candesartan (8)	Amlodipine (5)*	
	Irbesartan (100/150)	Amlodipine (5/10)*	
Renin inhibitor/diuretic	Aliskiren (150/300)	HCTZ (12.5/25)	
Renin inhibitor/CCB	Aliskiren (150/300)	Amlodipine (5/10)	
Beta-blocker/diuretic	Atenolol (50/100)	Chlorthalidone (25)	
	Atenolol (50)	HCTZ (25)	
	Metoprolol (50/100)	HCTZ (25/50)	
	Bisoprolol (2.5/5/10)	HCTZ (6.25)	
	Bisoprolol (1)	Chlorthalidone (25)	
	Nadolol (40/80)	Bendroflumethiazide (5)	
	Oxprenolol (120)	Chlorthalidone (20)	
	Pindolol (10)	Clopamide (5)	
	Propranolol (40/80)	HCTZ (25)	
	Propranolol LA (80/160)	HCTZ (50)	
	Timolol (10)	HCTZ (25)	
Beta-blocker/CCB	Atenolol (25/50)	Nifedipine (10/20)	
	Metoprolol (50/100)	Felodipine (5/10)	
Alpha-blocker/diuretic	Methyldopa (250)	HCTZ (15)	
	Clonidine (0.1/0.2/0.3)	Chlorthalidone (15)	
	Reserpine (0.1)	HCTZ (10)	
Triple Combinations			
ARB/CCB/diuretic	Valsartan (160/320)	Amlodipine (5/10)	HCTZ (12.5/25)
	Olmesartan (20/40)	Amlodipine (5/10)	HCTZ (12.5/25)
	Telmisartan (40/80)	Amlodipine (5/10)	HCTZ (12.5/25)
ACE inhibitor/CCB/diuretic	Perindopril (5/10)	Amlodipine (5/10)	Indapamide (1.25/2.5)
Renin inhibitor/CCB/diuretic	Aliskiren (150/300)	Amlodipine (5/10)	HCTZ (12.5/25)

ACE, Angiotensin converting enzyme, ARB, angiotensin receptor blocker, CCB, calcium channel blocker, HCTZ, hydrochlorothiazide; K, potassium; LA, long acting.
*Some dosages may be available only in certain countries. The list is not exhaustive.
From Burnier M: Antihypertensive combination treatment: state of the art. Curr Hyperten Rep 17:51, 2015.

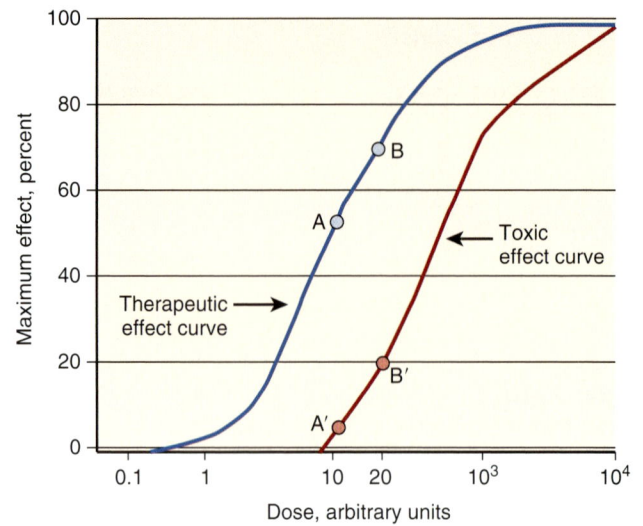

Figure 50.4 Dose relationship between therapeutic effect and toxicity with antihypertensive drugs. For the initial therapy of hypertension, a strategy to reduce side effects and enhance the tolerability of multiple antihypertensive drugs in combination has been identified using low doses of more than one antihypertensive agent with different combined modes of action to minimize side effects. With a low dose of drug A, a partial therapeutic effect is obtained, and adverse effects (A′) are minimal. If the dose is raised to B, a greater therapeutic effect will be accompanied by more adverse effects (B′). If a low dose of a second drug is added with its own minimal side effects, an extra effect will be obtained without more adverse effects, which will remain at A′. (Modified from Epstein M, Bakris G: Newer approaches to antihypertensive therapy. Use of fixed-dose combination therapy. *Arch Intern Med* 156:1969-1978, 1996.)

Table 50.29	Considerations for Initial Therapy in Older Patients
Clinical Observation	**Pharmacologic Considerations**
Decreased vascular compliance and peripheral vascular resistance	Use vasodilator (e.g., HCTZ, ACEI, ARB, CCB, α-blocker).
Isolated systolic hypertension and wide pulse pressure	Use vasodilator (e.g., HCTZ, CCB).
Reduction of cardiovascular baroreflex function with blood pressure lability	Avoid sympatholytics and volume depletion. Use β-blockers cautiously.
Orthostatic hypertension during recumbency	Consider using short-acting medications (<8-hr duration) at bedtime.
Reduced metabolic capability	Adjust all medications for renal and hepatic function; start at half-dose.
Prostatic hypertrophy	Use α-blocker.
More than 20 mm Hg from systolic goal	Use fixed-dose combination therapy (ACEI/CCB, ARB/CCB, ACEI/HCTZ, ARB/HCTZ, β-blocker/HCTZ).

ACEI, Angiotensin-converting enzyme inhibitor; ARB, angiotensin II receptor blocker; CCB, calcium channel blocker; HCTZ, thiazide diuretic.

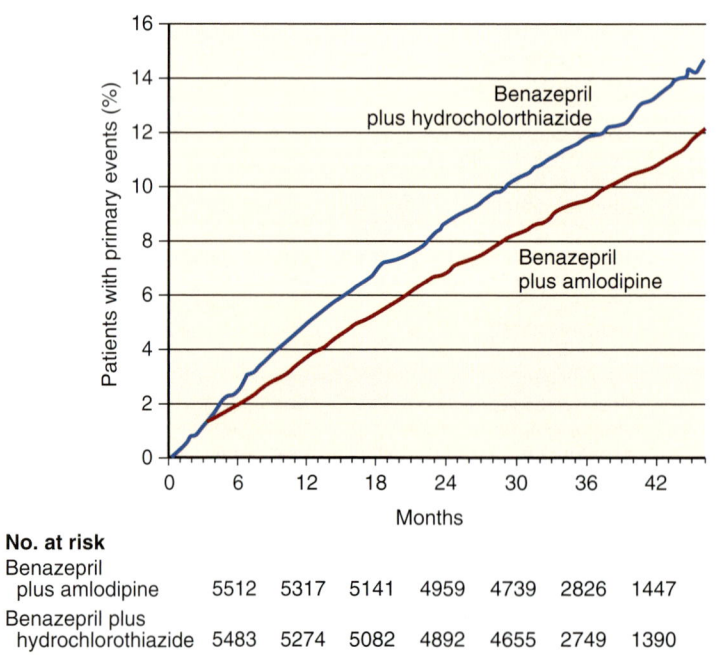

Figure 50.5 Comparison of combined therapies for patients at high risk for a cardiovascular event. In this study, 11,506 patients with hypertension at high risk for cardiovascular events received treatment with benazepril plus amlodipine or benazepril plus hydrochlorothiazide, the benazepril-amlodipine combination was superior to the benazepril-hydrochlorothiazide combination in reducing cardiovascular events (9.6 vs. 11.8%; HR, 0.8; 95% CI, 0.72 to 0.90), and chronic kidney disease (CKD) occurred less often (2% vs. 3.7%). The direct implication for practice is that an ARB plus a dihydropyridine calcium channel blocker (CCB) is preferred in individuals with systolic/diastolic blood pressures more than 20/10 mm Hg above the 140/90 mm Hg blood pressure goal. (From Jamerson K, Michael A. Weber MA, et al; ACCOMPLISH Trial Investigators: Benazepril plus amlodipine or hydrochlorothiazide for hypertension in high-risk patients. Benazepril plus amlodipine or hydrochlorothiazide for hypertension in high-risk patients. *N Engl J Med* 359:2417-2428, 2008.)

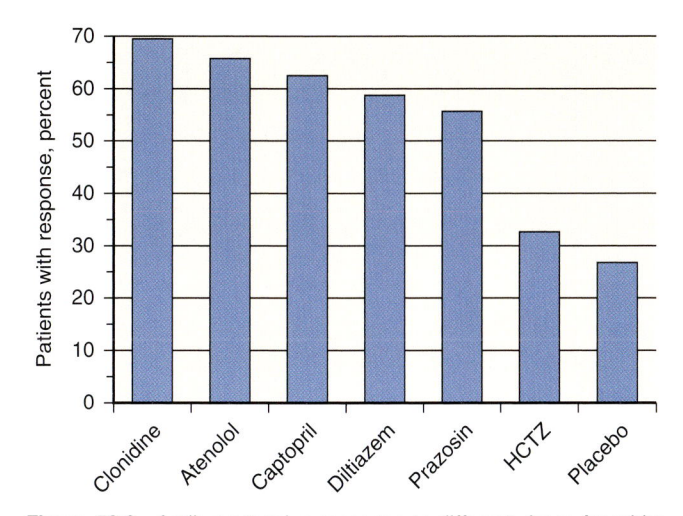

Figure 50.6 Antihypertensive response to different drugs for white individuals younger than 60 years. Hydrochlorothiazide (HCTZ) appears to be the least effective as a single agent. (From Materson BJ, Reda DJ, Cushman WC, et al: Single-drug therapy for hypertension in men. A comparison of six antihypertensive agents with placebo. The Department of Veterans Affairs Cooperative Study Group on Antihypertensive Agents. N Engl J Med 328:914-921, 1993.)

(e.g., hydrochlorothiazide, 50 to 100 mg; chlorthalidone, 25 to 50 mg).[701] Their biologic half-life extends well beyond their pharmacologic half-life.

Thiazide and thiazide-like diuretics also facilitate vasodilation in combination with other therapeutic classes, particularly those that block the RAAS.[688] These drugs can be used together in fixed-dose combinations.

Thiazide-like diuretics are not commonly prescribed for the treatment of hypertension, despite the fact that chlorthalidone has been studied extensively in large-scale clinical trials and has been demonstrated to reduce cardiovascular mortality.[686] A meta-analysis of diuretic trials has demonstrated that the equivalent dose of chlorthalidone to reduce systolic BP is 8.6 mg, compared to 26.4 mg for hydrochlorothiazide.[687] Many clinicians and authors have debated about the preferred diuretic for the treatment of hypertension. Although chlorthalidone is more potent than hydrochlorothiazide, there is presently no convincing evidence of the superiority of one over the other in large-scale clinical trials.[701a]

CCBs are also useful vasodilators in older patients. They are much better tolerated in the lower half of their dosing range and are quite effective even in the presence of a high-salt diet, perhaps owing to their natriuretic effects[702] or intrinsic vasodilatory effects.[703,704] α-Blockers may be useful in older men with benign prostatic hypertrophy because they facilitate prostatic urethral relaxation and improve urinary stream. ACE inhibitors and ARBs are also effective vasodilators in older patients. They are well tolerated, and their efficacy is enhanced when they are combined with low-dose thiazide diuretic therapy of chlorthalidone (half of a 25-mg tablet) or hydrochlorothiazide (6.25 or 12.5 mg).[688] Concerns about β-blocker use in older patients have raised questions about their safety.[705] Although β-blockers remain a cornerstone therapy in the management of patients with a previous MI or with heart failure, there is evidence to suggest that the reduction of heart rate with these drugs paradoxically increases the risk of cardiovascular events and stroke in hypertensive patients. Thus, individualization of their use and heart rate response needs to be carefully considered in older patients.[705] β-Blockers may also impair baroreceptor responses in older patients and worsen orthostasis.

Older patients have a higher likelihood of orthostasis than younger patients. As many as 18% of untreated older patients with hypertension have a decrease in systolic BP of more than 20 mm Hg after standing for 1 to 3 minutes.[706] Older patients may also have pseudohypertension, which may interfere with a true determination of BP.[707] Consequently, three-position BP measurements should always be used during the initiation and titration of medications. If recumbent BPs remain elevated, short-acting medications taken before bedtime, such as clonidine or captopril, may be useful in controlling BP overnight.

Management of isolated systolic hypertension in older patients frequently requires multiple drugs. Regardless of the agents used, an approach of slow, careful titration is recommended, preferably with dosage increments no more frequently than every 3 months. A careful assessment of the metabolic and excretory routes of the drugs, as well as possible drug-drug interactions, is recommended because older patients frequently have impaired metabolic function.

TREATMENT BASED ON GENDER

Differences in gender may be important regarding the selection of antihypertensive therapy (Table 50.30).[708] Men and women benefit equally from a more intensive control of BP, which results in a reduction in the risk of cardiovascular events.[709] In general, men have a lower resting heart rate, longer left ventricular ejection fraction time, and higher pulse pressure when stressed than women.[708] Women tend to have lower peripheral vascular resistance and a greater blood volume than men[708]; they also have a lower likelihood of coronary disease before menopause. However, when menopause occurs, or in the presence of diabetes, women have the same risk of coronary disease as men.[708] Vasodilation is always a good choice for treatment because elevated peripheral vascular resistance is almost always involved in BP elevation, regardless of gender. Thiazide diuretics, ACE inhibitors, ARBs, and CCBs are all effective treatments. Many patients require two or more of these drugs, and fixed-dose combinations can be used.

Women should avoid the use of ACE inhibitors and ARBs in pregnancy because of their possible teratogenic effects. CCBs may delay labor. Optimal therapy in a pregnant woman remains α-methyldopa, hydralazine, or β-blockers because they have a safety record with a minimal risk of teratogenic effects on the fetus (Figure 50.7).

In women with osteoporosis, thiazide and thiazide-like diuretics are ideal agents because they antagonize calciuria and facilitate bone mineralization.[710]

Women experience more cough with ACE inhibitors and more pedal edema with CCBs than men.[711] These differences in adverse effects may require adjustment in the dose or switching of medications. Interestingly, despite differences in the underlying pathophysiologic mechanisms of high BP between genders, there does not appear to be a substantial difference in the response rate to similar dosages of commonly used antihypertensive drugs.

Table 50.30 Considerations for Initial Therapy Based on Gender

Clinical Observation	Pharmacologic Considerations
Men have lower resting heart rate, longer left ventricular ejection time, and higher stressed pulse pressure compared with women.	Use vasodilator (e.g., HCTZ, ACEI, ARB, CCB).
Women have lower total peripheral resistance and greater blood volume compared with men.	Use drugs that provide vasodilation, heart rate reduction; may need diuresis (e.g., HCTZ, ACE inhibitor, ARB, β-blocker, CCB).
Postmenopausal women more frequently have coronary artery disease with atypical chest pain.	Use drugs that counter angina and reduce heart rate (β-blocker, CCB).
Osteoporosis	Antagonize calciuria (HCTZ).
Pregnancy	Avoid teratogenic drugs (ACEI, ARB). Avoid drugs that may cause ureteroplacental insufficiency (loop diuretics). Optimal choices are α-methyldopa, hydralazine, and β-blockers.
Women report more pedal edema with CCBs and cough with ACEIs than men.	Adjust dosage or discontinue drug.
More than 20 mm Hg from systolic goal	Use fixed-dose combination therapy (ACEI/CCB, ARB/CCB, ACEI/HCTZ, β-blocker/HCTZ, ARB/HCTZ).

ACEI, Angiotensin-converting enzyme inhibitor; ARB, angiotensin II receptor blocker; CCB, calcium channel blocker; HCTZ, thiazide diuretic.

Table 50.31 Considerations for Initial Therapy in African American Patients

Clinical Observation	Pharmacologic Considerations
High peripheral vascular resistance and increased salt sensitivity	Use vasodilator (e.g., HCTZ, ACEI, CCB, ARB). Use natriuretic (HCTZ, ACEI, ARB, CCB). Have patient reduce salt intake.
Tendency to increase blood volume relative to the peripheral vascular resistance	Use natriuretic, diuretic (HCTZ; if creatinine level > 2.0 mmol/L, loop diuretic).
More than 20 mm Hg from systolic goal	Use fixed-dose combination therapy (ACEI/CCB, ARB/CCB, ACEI/HCTZ, β-blocker/HCTZ, ARB/HCTZ).

ACEI, Angiotensin-converting enzyme inhibitor; ARB, angiotensin II receptor blocker; CCB, calcium channel blocker; HCTZ, thiazide diuretic.

ETHNIC AND RACIAL FACTORS

Ethnicity may play a role in the choice of antihypertensive agents (Table 50.31). African Americans frequently present with high BP at an earlier age and have more substantial elevations in BP, as well as earlier development of target-organ damage, than similar, demographically matched white counterparts.[390,712,713] Ethnic differences in the response to antihypertensive medications have been demonstrated in numerous clinical trials.[390,703] The mechanisms for these differences are not yet elucidated but appear to be independent of dietary salt or potassium intake. Some investigators have suggested possible genetic differences in renal sodium handling, but this has not been conclusively demonstrated in clinical trials. Despite this observation, African Americans frequently display BP salt sensitivity.[714,715] A careful assessment of the dose response for different medication classes, with adjustment for differences in dietary sodium consumption and body mass index among races and ethnic groups, has not been performed.

In general, thiazide diuretics and CCBs have more robust antihypertensive properties at lower dosages in African Americans than other commonly used therapeutic classes.[703,704,716] Drugs that block the RAAS are effective in African Americans, but higher dosages are frequently required to achieve the same level of BP as observed in non–African Americans.[293] As in most population groups, elevated peripheral vascular resistance contributes to BP elevation. Some investigators have suggested that African Americans have a modest volume component contributing to BP elevation that may also contribute to antihypertensive drug resistance.[714] It is not uncommon for multiple drugs to be required to reach the target BP, given the greater degree of BP elevation and somewhat different patterns in responses to antihypertensive agents. Consequently, fixed-dose combinations may be most useful in this population group as part of a strategy to simplify the approach.

Hispanics and Asians do not appear to have different hypertensive responses to commonly used drugs from those of whites.[390] However, Caribbean Hispanics who have a higher proportion of African ancestry may respond to commonly prescribed antihypertensive agents in a way that is characteristic of non-Hispanic black hypertensives.[715]

TREATMENT OF OBESE PATIENTS

Obese patients with hypertension frequently have other medical problems that complicate the management of their hypertension (Table 50.32).[90] These patients tend to have a hyperdynamic circulation, increased peripheral vascular resistance, expanded plasma volume and, like African Americans, a greater sensitivity to the influence of dietary salt in increasing BP.

In the previously mentioned ACCOMPLISH trial, when calcium channel blockade was compared with thiazide diuretic treatment in ACE inhibitor–treated patients at high cardiovascular risk, thiazide-based treatment was associated with less cardiovascular protection in normal weight than in

A

Antihypertensive Therapies Commonly Used in Pregnancy*					
Agent	Indication	Dose range	FDA classification	Potential side effects	Comments
α–Methyldopa	Often used as first line	250 mg – 1.5 g orally twice a day	B	Lethargy	Data on offspring up to 7.5 y of age demonstrating long-term safety
Labetalol	Often used as first line	100 – 1200 mg orally twice a day	C	Exacerbation of asthma	Widely used in pregnancy
Calcium channel blockers	Second line or alternative first line (nifedipine)	Varies according to drug used	C	Concern for synergy with magnesium sulfate for neuromuscular depression	
β-blockers	Second line	Varies according to drug used	C	Exacerbation of asthma	Same recommend avoiding atenolol during pregnancy and lactation
Thiazide diuretics	Second line	12.5 – 50 mg orally once a day	C	Volume depletion and hypokalemia	

- FDA indicates Food and Drug Administration.
- –* Angiotensin-converting enzyme inhibitors and angiotensin receptor blockers are contraindicated in the second and third trimesters of pregnancy and are class D. Safety in the first trimester is controversial; in this trimester, they are class C.

B

FDA Classification of Drugs in Pregnancy
Category A: controlled studies in pregnant women have demonstrated no risk of fetal abnormalities.
Category B: reproduction studies in animal indicate no fetal risk, but there are no adequate and well-controlled studies in pregnant women; or animal reproduction studies have shown an adverse effect of the drug but not in well-controlled studies in pregnant women.
Category C: animal reproduction studies have shown an adverse effect of the fetus but no adequate human or animal studies; or animal reproduction studies have not been conducted and it is not known whether the drug can cause fetal harm when administered to a pregnant woman.
Category D: evidence of human fetal risk, but benefits outweigh risks. Women taking this drug during pregnancy should be informed of potential fetal risk.
Category X: evidence of human fetal risk. Drug is contraindicated in women who are pregnant or who may become pregnant. If this drug is used during pregnancy or if the patient becomes pregnant while taking this drug, the patient should be apprised of the potential hazard to a fetus.

- FDA indicates Food and Drug Administration.

Figure 50.7 Antihypertensive therapies used in pregnancy. **A,** Therapies commonly used in pregnancy. **B,** FDA classification of drugs in pregnancy. ACE, Angiotensin-converting enzyme; ARB, angiotensin receptor blocker; CCB, calcium channel blocker; RAAS, renin angiotensin aldosterone system. (From Seely EW, Ecker J: Cardiovascular management in pregnancy: chronic hypertension in pregnancy. *Circulation* 129:1254-1261, 2014.)

Table 50.32 Considerations for Initial Therapy in Obese Patients with Hypertension

Clinical Observation	Pharmacologic Considerations
Hyperdynamic circulation	Reduce heart rate and sympathoadrenal outflow (β-blocker).
Increased peripheral vascular resistance	Use vasodilator (e.g., HCTZ, ACEI, ARB, CCB).
Salt sensitivity	Use natriuretic (HCTZ, ACEI, ARB, CCB). Have patient reduce salt intake.
Expanded plasma volume	Use diuretic (HCTZ). Have patient reduce salt intake.
Hypoventilation	Order sleep study to evaluate need for positive pressure ventilation at night.
More than 20 mm Hg from systolic goal	Use fixed-dose combination therapy (ACEI/CCB, ARB/CCB, ACEI/HCTZ, β-blocker/HCTZ, ARB/HCTZ).

ACEI, Angiotensin-converting enzyme inhibitor; ARB, angiotensin II receptor blocker; CCB, calcium channel blocker; HCTZ, thiazide diuretic.

Table 50.33 Considerations for Initial Therapy in Patients with Heart Disease

Clinical Observation	Pharmacologic Considerations
Angina	Reduce heart rate and induce coronary vasodilation (reduce heart rate 20% or to 60-65 beats/min; β-blocker, nitrates, CCB).
Left ventricular hypertrophy	Reduce systolic blood pressure (HCTZ, ACEI, CCB, ARB). Avoid nonspecific vasodilator or therapies that result in reflex increase in heart rate.
Systolic dysfunction	Reduce afterload and preload; promote natriuresis (ACEI, HCTZ, ARB; antineurohormonal agents, β-blocker, spironolactone).
Diastolic dysfunction	Improve myocardial compliance, reduce heart rate, and avoid volume depletion (β-blocker, CCB, ACEI, ARB; avoid loop diuretics).
Myocardial infarction	Reduce heart rate (β-blocker, ACEI).
More than 20 mm Hg from systolic goal	Use fixed-dose combination therapy (ACEI/CCB, ARB/CCB, ACEI/HCTZ, β-blocker /HCTZ, ARB/HCTZ).

ACEI, Angiotensin-converting enzyme inhibitor; ARB, angiotensin II receptor blocker; CCB, calcium channel blocker; HCTZ, thiazide diuretic.

obese patients.[717] However, amlodipine-based therapy was equally effective across body mass index subgroups and offered superior cardiovascular protection in nonobese patients with hypertension.[696]

β-Blockers may be helpful in diminishing sympathoadrenal drive. Vasodilators such as hydrochlorothiazide and ACE inhibitors, ARBs, and CCBs are useful for reducing peripheral vascular resistance. Combinations of these drugs may also be helpful. Because of the tendency toward expanded plasma volume, thiazide or thiazide-like diuretics can be helpful because they provide an opportunity to produce vasodilation and mild volume reduction. Frequently, obese patients require multiple drugs to achieve BP goals, and simplification strategies are important. Given the increased frequency of cardiovascular risk clustering phenomena in these patients, metabolically neutral drug therapies are ideal. One also should use β-blockers carefully because they could increase the likelihood of weight gain and may compromise glucose tolerance.[703,718] Recently the role of aldosterone antagonism has been reported in obese, hypertensive individuals requiring treatment with multiple medications due to adipocyte production of aldosterone.[652-655]

TREATMENT OF PATIENTS WITH CARDIOVASCULAR OR KIDNEY DISEASE

Cardiovascular Disease

Patients with hypertension and cardiac disease require tailored approaches because the medications used to control BP are all quite different with regard to their effects on the heart (Table 50.33). In patients with coronary artery disease, it is important to remember that most coronary artery perfusion occurs during diastole. Hence, pharmacotherapy should be targeted toward slowing the heart rate to enhance perfusion during diastole. β-Blockers and heart rate–lowering CCBs, such as the nondihydropyridines, would be ideal in this respect. However, as previously discussed, there is a theoretical concern about reducing heart rate excessively (<60 to 65 beats/min) in older patients; therefore, caution should be used for each individual in regard to the goal heart rate, and patients should be carefully monitored.

LVH provides evidence of the duration and magnitude of BP elevation. All the drugs that lower BP, except for direct-acting vasodilators, effectively cause the LVH to regress.[719] Thus, most antihypertensives can be useful in this regard. Some trials have indicated that drugs that block the RAAS may be more effective than other drugs in reducing LVH. A large-scale clinical trial has demonstrated that the ARB losartan is more effective in reducing overall cardiovascular morbidity and mortality (primarily related to the reduction in the incidence of stroke) in patients with hypertension and LVH than a β-blocker–based antihypertensive regimen.[684]

The lack of ability of a β-blocker to reduce LVH may be related to heart rate slowing and associated aortic pulse wave augmentation. If patients have dyspnea, it is important to use echocardiography to distinguish between diastolic and systolic dysfunction. The management of diastolic dysfunction should include therapies that facilitate ventricular relaxation and modest reduction of heart rate (β-blockers and CCBs). With systolic dysfunction, drugs that block the RAAS are more suitable for providing both preload and afterload reduction and diminishing the sympathoadrenal response.[720] β-Blockers and mineralocorticoid receptor antagonists in addition to ACE inhibitor therapy are also

Table 50.34 Considerations for Initial Therapy in Patients with Renal Disease*	
Clinical Observation	**Pharmacologic Considerations**
Increased blood volume (common in glomerular diseases)	Reduce blood volume (HCTZ, loop diuretic if creatinine level >2.0 mmol/L).
Decreased blood volume (common in tubular diseases)	Salt supplementation may be needed.
Increased peripheral vascular resistance	Use vasodilator (ACEI, CCB, ARB).
Proteinuria	Reduce proteinuria (ACEI, ARB, NDCCB) (recommended target systolic blood pressure ≤ 130 mm Hg).
Diabetes with proteinuria	Control blood pressure and glycemia (ACEI if type 1 diabetes, ARB if type 2; recommended target systolic blood pressure < 130 mm Hg).
More than 20 mm Hg from systolic goal	Use fixed-dose combination therapy (ACEI/CCB, ARB/CCB, ACEI/HCTZ, β-blocker/HCTZ, ACEI/CCB). Use of HCTZ depends on renal function.

*All medications adjusted according to renal function.
ACEI, Angiotensin-converting enzyme inhibitor; ARB, angiotensin II receptor blocker; CCB, calcium channel blocker; HCTZ, thiazide diuretic; NDCCB, nondihydropyridine calcium channel blocker.

helpful in these patients. Diuretic therapy should be used to adjust the blood volume, as necessary.

Kidney Disease

In patients with kidney disease (Table 50.34), BP control is more complex to achieve because such patients not only have increased vascular resistance but also frequently have increased blood volume, contributing to the hypertensive process.[721] The understanding of renal autoregulation provides some insight into the appropriate levels of BP control and the relative importance of different types of antihypertensive drugs in preserving renal function.

Glomerular circulation operates optimally at one half to two thirds of the systemic BP.[722] Preglomerular vasoconstriction is necessary to decrease the systemic pressure to glomerular capillary pressure levels that are optimal for filtration yet low enough to avoid mechanical injury to the filtering apparatus.[722,723] The efferent glomerular arteriole also serves an important purpose—it vasoconstricts during situations of diminished effective arterial blood volume to maintain adequate pressure for glomerular filtration. With the development of vascular disease, the afferent glomerular arteriole does not vasoconstrict properly, which permits the transmission of systemic BP into the glomerulus. A clinical clue that could indicate the failure of autoregulation is the presence of microalbuminuria or protein in the urine. Under these circumstances, systemic BP should be reduced more substantially to minimize the risk of mechanical injury

to the glomerulus. Current recommendations suggest a target BP below 140/90 mm Hg based on patients with kidney disease in clinical trial evidence.[437] It is possible that even lower pressures may be necessary to optimally delay the progression of renal disease, particularly in patients with proteinuria and diabetes.

Drugs that block the RAAS, such as ACE inhibitors[682,683] and ARBs,[686,689] provide a more consistent opportunity to reduce the progression of renal disease as part of an intensive BP–lowering strategy than other commonly used antihypertensive drugs. The benefit of these drugs resides, in part, on their ability to facilitate efferent glomerular arteriolar dilation by antagonizing the effects of Ang II as they lower blood pressure.[724] Renin inhibitors have similar clinical effects on reducing both BP and proteinuria to those of ACE inhibitors and ARBs, but have not been studied alone in renal protection trials.[725] Overall, there is a more consistent reduction in systemic and glomerular capillary pressures with RAAS-blocking drugs. Additional medications can be added to these drugs to achieve better BP control and help reduce glomerular capillary pressure and proteinuria. Sufficient dosages of diuretics to control the blood volume should also be used. When the serum creatinine level reaches 2 mmol/L, volume reduction is more amenable to the use of loop diuretics as opposed to thiazides, which are more effective as peripheral vasodilators.

Some investigators have questioned the safety of using CCBs in patients with kidney disease, given their preferential effects on dilating the afferent glomerular arteriole.[54] Some studies have demonstrated that CCBs can increase proteinuria, despite lowering BP.[726] However, there is no clinical evidence that these drugs are detrimental and worsen the progression of renal disease if they are given with ACE inhibitors or ARBs, which dilate the efferent glomerular arteriole. If anything, the lower BP achieved using these drugs in combination may provide better protection against the loss of kidney function, as was observed in the ACCOMPLISH study.[717]

Antiproteinuric strategies should be considered in patients with kidney disease because a reduction in proteinuria by specific antihypertensive drugs, such as ACE inhibitors or ARBs, correlates with slowing the progression of renal disease.[727,728] However, dual RAAS blockade, despite reducing proteinuria, has not provided incremental benefit on renal disease progression and is associated with a greater risk for increased serum creatinine and potassium levels.[99,265] For further discussion of drugs for the treatment of hypertension associated with renal disease, see Chapter 62.

STRATEGIES FOR SELECTING THE OPTIMAL COMBINATION ANTIHYPERTENSIVE THERAPY

A meta-analysis involving 40,000 treated patients evaluated the usefulness of low-dose combination treatments separately and in combination.[729] The average BP reduction achieved with low-dose therapy was only 20% in 354 randomized, double-blind, placebo-controlled trials of thiazides, β-blockers, ACE inhibitors, ARBs, and CCBs. Thiazides and CCBs cause side effects infrequently at a half-standard dose (2% and 1.6%, respectively), whereas side effects occur commonly at standard doses (9.9% and 8.3%, respectively).

β-Blockers, however, cause an equivalently high number of side effects at both dosage levels (5.5% vs. 7.5%; $P = 0.04$). The only side effect observed with ACE inhibitors was cough (3.9%), which did not vary with dosage. ARBs were not associated with an excess of side effects at a standard dose. The reduction in BP was additive; however, the prevalence of adverse effects was not additive. Therefore, combinations of two or three drugs at low doses are preferable to one or two drugs at standard doses. In the absence of cough, ACE inhibitors and ARBs can be used at higher doses due to the lack of adverse effects associated with these drugs. In a subsequent meta-analysis, the authors quantified the effect of a combination of drugs from the four drug classes on BP reduction. The extra BP reduction achieved by combining two drugs from different classes is approximately five times greater than that achieved when the dosage of one drug is doubled.[730] This confirms what might be expected based on knowledge of the dose-effect relationship between the therapeutic effects of antihypertensive drugs and their toxicity (see Figure 50.4).

The rationale for fixed-dose combination therapy is as follows[731]:

- To combine drugs acting on different systems, thus initiating a pharmacologic attack on two systems with greatly enhanced impact compared with monotherapy
- To combat counterregulatory responses that interfere with BP reduction

For example, CCBs activate the sympathetic nervous system and RAAS, which can attenuate BP-lowering effects.[732,733] This action can be buffered by RAAS blockers. The antihypertensive effect of an RAAS blocker can be enhanced by the negative sodium balance created by the diuretic and natriuretic properties of a CCB.[734]

- To decrease the pill burden and enhance adherence to prescribed therapy

Many individuals with BP s that are 20 mm Hg (systolic) and 10 mm Hg (diastolic) above the target pressure will require more than one drug. Clinical trials have documented that achieving BP targets necessitates the use of multiple drugs. In the ALLHAT study, for example, only one third of patients achieved their target BP with monotherapy after 5 years.[735]

- To decrease BP variability

Blood pressure has been shown to be less variable with combination therapy versus monotherapy.[736] Variability in visit to visit systolic BPs was shown to be a strong predictor of stoke and myocardial infarction.[737] CCBs and diuretics were found to be the most useful agents for reducing this variability, whereas β-blockers increased the variability.[737]

- To decrease adverse effects

Combining two antihypertensive drugs at lower doses may actually reduce adverse effects compared with higher doses of both drugs. Studies have shown that the combination of an ACE inhibitor and ARB with a CCB reduces the

Preferred
- ACE-inhibitor/CCB
- ARB/CCB
- ACE-inhibitor/thiazide-like diuretic
- ARB/thiazide-like diuretic

Acceptable
- Beta-blocker/thiazide-like diuretic
- CCB (dihydropyridine)/beta-blocker
- CCB/thiazide-like diuretic
- Renin inhibitor/thiazide-like diuretic
- Renin inhibitor/CCB
- Dihydropyridine CCB/non-dihydropyridine CCB

Unacceptable
- ACE-inhibitor/ARB
- Renin inhibitor/ARB
- Renin inhibitor/ACE-Inhibitor
- RAS inhibitor/beta-blocker
- CCB (non-dihydropyridine)/beta-blocker
- Centrally acting agent/beta-blocker

Figure 50.8 Recommendations for specific hypertensive drug combinations. (From Sever PS, Messerli FH: Hypertension management 2011: optimal combination therapy. *Eur Heart J* 32:2499-2506, 2011.)

incidence of CCB-related peripheral edema by as much as 38%.[738] Combining an RAAS blocker with a thiazide reduces the occurrence of diuretic-induced hypokalemia.

Dual therapy and sequential monotherapy are currently being compared in ongoing trials. JNC 8 was unable to recommend administration of multiple antihypertensive drugs over uptitration, use of a combination of drugs at low doses, and initiation of two drugs at the same time due to the lack of available randomized controlled trials available on combination drug therapy.[437] It is presently not known whether one of these strategies will improve mortality or cardiovascular, cerebrovascular, and kidney outcomes. Limitations have been identified with the single pill combination approach, however, and are listed in Table 50.35.

SPECIFIC DRUG COMBINATIONS

See Figure 50.8.[731,739,740]

PREFERRED COMBINATIONS

Renin Angiotensin Aldosterone System Inhibitors and Calcium Channel Blockers

The ACCOMPLISH trial demonstrated the superiority of an ACE inhibitor and CCB in single-pill form versus an ACE inhibitor plus hydrochlorothiazide. The ACCOMPLISH trial compared BP reduction and cardiovascular outcomes achieved with two combination therapies, benazepril-amlodipine and benazepril-hydrochlorothiazide

> **Table 50.35 Advantages and Limits of the Use of Single-Pill Combinations in Hypertension**
>
> **Advantages**
> - Reduction of the pill burden
> - Simplification of the treatment schedule
> - Increased adherence to therapy (better long-term persistence)
> - Improved efficacy with reduced incidence of side effects
> - Better prevention of cardiovascular events (to be demonstrated prospectively)
>
> **Limits**
> - Reduction of the prescription flexibility
> - Difficulty to identify the precise cause of an unexpected side effect
> - Difficulty to memorize the exact content of the single-pill combinations
> - Risk of a more pronounced rebound hypertension in case of repeated omissions
> - Risk of acute hypotension when restarting a triple combination after interruptions
> - Increased cost versus free combinations of generics
>
> *From Burnier M: Antihypertensive combination treatment: state of the art. Curr Hyperten Rep 17:51, 2015.*

in a single tablet. The trial included more than 11,000 individuals, and the mean BP was nearly equivalent between the benazepril-amlodipine and benazepril-hydrochlorothiazide groups (131.6 and 73.3 vs. 132.5 and 74.3, respectively). The outcome in this study was time to reach a primary end point—a composite of cardiovascular events or death. The trial was terminated early (after a mean of 36 months) because the benazepril-amlodipine group had reached a lower event rate (9.6%) than the benazepril- hydrochlorothiazide group (11.8%; RR, 19.6%; hazard ratio [HR], 0.80; $P > 0.001$).

Renin Angiotensin Aldosterone System Inhibitors and Thiazide-like Diuretics

By depleting intravascular volume, diuretics activate the RAAS system, which causes vasoconstriction as well as salt and water retention. The RAAS blockade attenuates the counterregulatory response and causes additional BP reduction. This combination has several advantages—the RAAS mitigates diuretic-induced hypokalemia and glucose intolerance. In a recent report on individuals older than 80 years, the Hypertension in the Very Elderly (HYVET) trial, indapamide, a thiazide-like diuretic, combined with the ACE inhibitor perindopril reduced the incidence of stroke (30%) and heart failure (64%).

ACCEPTABLE COMBINATIONS

β-Blockers and Thiazide-like Diuretics

β-Blockers and diuretics have been shown to reduce cardiovascular end points in randomized controlled trials; however, meta-analyses have suggested that they are less effective than other agents.[372,741] The addition of diuretics increases the effectiveness of β-blockers in individuals of African ancestry and in others with low-renin hypertension. Both these drug classes have similar adverse effects, including the development of glucose intolerance, new-onset diabetes, fatigue, and sexual dysfunction. However, in 2007, the European Society of Hypertension warned against the use of this combination for patients with metabolic syndrome or for those at high risk of diabetes.[742] A meta-analysis has demonstrated a 35% risk of new-onset diabetes with diuretics compared to non–β-blocker antihypertensives and a 31% risk of new-onset diabetes with diuretics compared to nondiuretic antihypertensives.[743] Given the possibility of adverse metabolic consequences, it seems reasonable to avoid the use of this combination for initial therapy without other compelling indications.[739]

Calcium Channel Blockers and Thiazide-like Diuretics

The combination of a CCB and diuretic provides a partially additive antihypertensive effect.[744] CCBs increase kidney sodium excretion, albeit not to the same extent as diuretics. This combination performed well in the VALUE trial, in which hydrochlorothiazide was administered to participants randomized to amlodipine as a second step compared to the valsartan arm.[745] Adverse effects included peripheral edema and hypokalemia as well as a slight increase in the incidence of new-onset diabetes.

Calcium Channel Blockers and β-Blockers

Additive BP reduction can be achieved with the combination of a β-blocker and a dihydropyridine CCB. In one study, the antihypertensive effects of combination ER metoprolol succinate and ER felodipine produced dose-related BP-lowering effects over a wide dose range; moreover, the incidence of edema and adverse effects was low. Nondihydropyridine CCBs such as verapamil and diltiazem should not be given together with β-blockers due to dual negative chronotropic effects, which may result in heart block or severe bradycardia.

Dual Calcium Channel Blockade

In a meta-analysis of six studies consisting of 153 patients, dual CCB therapy (dihydropyridine CCB with verapamil or diltiazem) was shown to have additive antihypertensive effects without an increase in adverse events.[746] Long-term prospective clinical trials are required to assess the long-term safety of this combination and to obtain cardiovascular outcome data. Dual CCB therapy should not be used as an alternative treatment for resistant hypertension until outcome data are available.

UNACCEPTABLE OR INEFFECTIVE COMBINATIONS

Dual Renin Angiotensin Aldosterone System Blockade

A dual RAAS blockade is not recommended. Two recent negative trials and a retracted earlier study have lessened the enthusiasm for RAAS blockade combinations. In the ALTITUDE trial, aliskiren or placebo was added to ACE inhibitors or ARBs, which inhibit RAAS, in diabetics with CKD.[100] The trial was halted early due to an increased incidence of hypotension, AKI, hyperkalemia and stroke. In the

ONTARGET trial, there were more adverse events, including worsening kidney function, with a combination of telmisartan and ramipril than with the individual drugs, and the combination did not improve cardiovascular outcomes.[154] Additionally, the COOPERATE study, which claimed that 263 patients with nondiabetic renal disease were randomly allocated to treatment with an ACE inhibitor, ARB, or combination of both medications at equivalent doses,[747] concluded in 2003 that the combination therapy was superior to monotherapy with an ACE inhibitor or ARB. However, the study was eventually retracted in 2009.[748]

Renin Angiotensin Aldosterone System Blockers and β-Blockers

These two drug classes are often combined after an MI or in those with heart failure. However, the combination achieves minimal additional antihypertensive effects compared with either drug as a monotherapy.

β-Blockers and Central Adrenergic Agonists

β-Blockers and central adrenergic agents (e.g., clonidine, α-methyldopa) both interfere with the SNS. No studies have explored the potential additive antihypertensive effects of these agents. However, it is known that additive adverse effects, including bradycardia, heart block, and rebound hypertension, occur when the drugs are abruptly discontinued.

OTHER DRUG CLASSES IN COMBINATION THERAPY

Peripheral α₁-Adrenergic Antagonists

Peripheral α₁-adrenergic antagonists (e.g., doxazosin, prazosin, terazosin) are often used in combination regimens to achieve BP targets. These drugs are reported to lower BP effectively while reducing plasma lipid levels, ameliorating insulin sensitivity and enhancing glucose metabolism.[622] The availability of ER formulations of these drugs has improved tolerability. The use of doxazosin has declined after the Data Safety Monitoring Board for the ALLHAT Study decided to discontinue the doxazosin treatment arm of the study based on the finding that a significantly higher percentage of patients on doxazosin developed stroke and congestive heart failure.[616] The ASCOT was a nonrandomized, non–placebo-controlled study showing that doxazosin is an effective and safe third-line antihypertensive agent.[617] In this study, an observational analysis of BP from 10,069 participants was performed to determine the efficacy of doxazosin as a third-line drug. A doxazosin GITS was given to all participants in doses ranging from 4 to 7 mg. The BP of the participants decreased by an average of almost 12/7 mm Hg, and modest reductions were noted in total and LDL cholesterol. However, there was a small increase in fasting plasma glucose concentrations. No excess of heart failure was observed.

Aldosterone Antagonists and Epithelial Sodium Channel Inhibitors

The aldosterone antagonists spironolactone and eplerenone, and the mineralocorticoid receptor antagonists and potassium-sparing diuretics amiloride and triamterene, block the action of aldosterone on the epithelial sodium channel located in the distal collecting tubule and collecting duct.[749] Spironolactone, eplerenone, amiloride and triamterene can provide enhanced antihypertensive therapy in patients with resistant hypertension and those who have elevated aldosterone levels,[750] as well as those with normal urinary aldosterone levels.[749] Spironolactone has been extensively studied for its role in treating resistant hypertension.

In the ASCOT study, the antihypertensive effect of spironolactone was evaluated among 1411 participants who received the drug as a fourth-line antihypertensive agent at a dosage beginning at 12.5 mg and increasing up to 50 mg daily. During spironolactone therapy, the participants' BP decreased by 21.9/9.5 mm Hg (95% CI, 20.8 to 23.0 and 9.0 to 10.1 mm Hg; $P < 0.001$). The drug was generally well tolerated; the most frequent adverse event was gynecomastia or breast discomfort in male participants (6%) and hyperkalemia (>5.5 mmol/L [4%] and >6.0 mmol/L [2%]). Collectively, these data suggest that spironolactone at 12.5 to 50 mg/day is an effective treatment option for individuals with resistant hypertension (uncontrolled on three or more medicines including a diuretic).

A smaller study of 52 patients has demonstrated the efficacy of the selective aldosterone blocker eplerenone at a dose of 50 to 100 mg daily in patients with resistant hypertension. After eplerenone treatment, the clinical BP was reduced by 18/8 mm Hg compared with baseline ($P < 0.0001$ for systolic and diastolic BPs).[751] Individuals treated with aldosterone antagonists require careful monitoring for hyperkalemia.

Direct-Acting Vasodilators

Direct-acting vasodilator drugs such as minoxidil and hydralazine are held in reserve for patients with advanced stage 2 hypertension who have not responded to conventional multidrug antihypertensive regimens.[597,598] The rationale is that the direct vasodilatory mode of action is different and complementary to the modes of action of other drug classes. Minoxidil is effective in patients with resistant hypertension; it is frequently a drug of last resort in patients with CKD and must be administered together with a β-blocker and loop diuretic. The initial dosage is 2.5 mg, with a maintenance dose generally ranging from 10 to 40 mg/day.

BEDTIME ANTIHYPERTENSIVE DOSING VERSUS MORNING DOSING

Shifting one nondiuretic antihypertensive medicine from morning to evening can reduce the total 24-hour mean BP and restore the normal nocturnal BP decrease (generally, ≈15%, failure of the BP to decrease at night is termed *nondipping*). Nondipping is a cardiovascular disease risk factor.[752] After a median follow-up of 5.4 years, patients who took at least one BP-lowering medication at bedtime had an adjusted risk for total cardiovascular events (a composite of death, myocardial infarction, angina pectoris, revascularization, heart failure, arterial occlusion of lower extremities, occlusion of the retinal artery, and stroke) that was approximately one third that of patients who took all medications on awakening (adjusted HR, 0.31; 95% CI, 0.21 to 0.46; $P \leq 0.001$).)[753] Similar results were demonstrated in patients with CKD.[754]

RESISTANT HYPERTENSION

Resistant hypertension is a term used to characterize high BP that fails to respond to what the clinician thinks is an adequate antihypertensive regimen (Table 50.36).[755,756] Resistant hypertension has also been defined as the inability to reach a desired BP goal, despite the use of three optimally dosed drugs, one of which is a diuretic, or the need for four or more medications to reach the desired BP goal.[757] A variety of factors can interfere with the ability of what is deemed to be appropriate antihypertensive therapy to normalize BP. Perhaps most important is nonadherence to the therapy regimen. Nonadherence is common and is one of the most serious problems that interfere with attaining the BP goal. This problem has many sources, including inadequate education, poor clinician-patient relationship, lack of understanding of side effects, and complexity of multidrug regimens. The health care provider should make every effort to determine whether adherence to therapy is part of the problem before pursuing other potential explanations for resistant hypertension. If nonadherence is eliminated, a methodologic approach can be used to help diagnose the cause of resistant hypertension and then correct it.

Pseudohypertension is another cause of resistant hypertension. It is usually observed in older hypertensive patients who have hardened atherosclerotic arteries, which are not easily compressible. This condition interferes with auscultatory measurements of BP. It is also known as Osler's phenomenon.[758] Because of the conformational changes of the vessels, greater apparent pressure is required to compress the sclerotic vessel than the intraarterial BP requires.

Another common cause of pseudohypertension is improper measurement, which occurs when the BP is taken with an inappropriately small cuff in a person with a large arm circumference. Because of the substantial proportion of hypertensive patients who are obese, it is critical to have a cuff of the appropriate size to determine the auscultatory pressure. The bladder within the cuff should encircle at least 80% of the arm to provide an accurate determination.

Ambulatory BP monitoring can assist in phenotyping patients with hypertension. This may be particularly important in patients with chronic kidney disease, for whom out of office BP and both cardiovascular and renal outcomes are more strongly related than office BP measures.[707] These important observations have been noted in several clinical trials. Moreover, these studies have also demonstrated that masked hypertension and nocturnal hypertension (nondipping) are also usually associated with cardiovascular events and renal disease progression[759] A comparison of national recommendations for normative threshold values of ambulatory BP monitoring matched to an office BP of 140/90 mm Hg is presented in Figure 50.9.

Volume overload is an important and common cause of resistant hypertension. It may be related to excessive salt intake or to the inability of the kidney to excrete an appropriate salt and water load because of endocrine abnormalities or intrinsic renal disease.

Increasing the dietary salt intake offsets the antihypertensive activities of all antihypertensive medications.[703] Some patients are more salt-sensitive than others. Salt sensitivity is common in patients of African ancestry.[715] This sensitivity is also a more common problem in patients with renal disease and congestive heart failure. A careful clinical examination coupled with the judicious use of a thiazide-like or loop diuretic (depending on the level of renal function) is critical in achieving an ideal blood volume to restore the antihypertensive efficacy of most classes of drugs. It is also appropriate to consider educating the patient about avoiding foods that are high in salt content, such as processed foods.

Drug-related causes of resistant hypertension are common and need to be carefully assessed in each patient. Perhaps the most common drugs that cause resistant hypertension are over the counter (OTC) preparations of sympathomimetics, such as nasal decongestants, appetite suppressants, and NSAIDs.[760] In addition, oral contraceptives, immunosuppressants (e.g., cyclosporine), and even some antidepressants can increase BP. Caffeine, licorice, and even erythropoiesis-stimulating agents (ESAs) erythropoietin may also increase BP. Unfortunately, patients may not always recognize OTC preparations as medications. Therefore, careful questioning specifically focusing on these types of medications should be routine during the

---

Table 50.36 Causes of Resistant Hypertension

Pseudoresistance
    White coat hypertension or office elevations
    Pseudohypertension in older patients
    Use of small cuff on very obese arm
Nonadherence to therapeutic regimen
Volume overload
Drug-related causes
    Antihypertensive drug dosage too low
    Wrong type of diuretic
    Inappropriate combinations of antihypertensive drugs
    Drug actions and interactions
        Sympathomimetics
        Nasal decongestants
        Appetite suppressants
        Cocaine
        Caffeine
        Oral contraceptives
        Adrenal steroids
        Licorice (may be found in chewing tobacco)
        Cyclosporine, tacrolimus
        Erythropoiesis-stimulating agents (ESAs) and Erythropoietin
        Antidepressants
        Nonsteroidal antiinflammatory drugs
Concomitant conditions
    Obesity
    Sleep apnea
    Ethanol intake > 1 oz (30 mL)/day
    Anxiety, hyperventilation
Secondary causes of hypertension
    Renovascular hypertension
    Primary aldosteronism
    Pheochromocytoma
    Hypothyroidism
    Hyperthyroidism
    Hyperparathyroidism
    Aortic coarctation
    Renal disease

National Guideline	Clinic BP	ABP Equivalents, mm Hg		
		24 h	Night	Day
Seventh joint National Committee (USA, 2003)	140/90	Not stated	120/75	135/85
European Society of Hypertension (2013)	140/90	130/80	120/70	135/85
Japanese Circulation Society (2012)	140/90	130/80	120/70	135/85
Canadian Hypertension Society (1999)	140/90	130/80	120/75	135/85
Australian National Heart High BP Research Council Consensus (2012)	140/90	130/80	120/75	135/85
National Institute for Health and Clinical Excellence (UK, 2011)	140/90	Not stated	Not stated	135/85

- All values in mm Hg. Note that the only discrepancy is for nighttime diastolic BP.
- ABP indicates ambulatory blood pressure and BP, blood pressure.

Figure 50.9 Comparison of national recommendations for ABP equivalents of hypertension clinic values of 140/90 mm Hg. (From Head GA, McGrath BP, Mihailidou AS, et al: Ambulatory blood pressure monitoring is ready to replace clinic blood pressure in the diagnosis of hypertension: pro side of the argument. Hypertension 64:1175-1181, 2014.)

evaluation for refractory hypertension. In addition, alcohol use, smoking, and cocaine use can be complicating factors that interfere with the ability of medications to lower BP.

Some medications may interfere with the antihypertensive activity of other drugs. For example, NSAIDs interfere with the antihypertensive activity of diuretics and ACE inhibitors.[755] Interestingly, only the antihypertensive activity of CCBs appears to be immune to the effects of NSAIDs.[761] Drug-drug interactions that can interfere with drug absorption, drug metabolism, or the pharmacodynamics of the concomitantly administered drugs can also interfere with antihypertensive activity.

Secondary causes of hypertension might also be considered a cause of resistant hypertension. These causes can be divided into two groups, renal parenchymal and renal vascular and endocrine. Renal parenchymal and renal vascular diseases are not uncommon (90% of the total causes of secondary hypertension). A chemistry profile and urinalysis facilitate the diagnosis of renal disease, whereas renal vascular assessment with Doppler ultrasonography or a direct imaging technique determines whether renal vascular hypertension is present. Associated endocrine abnormalities include hyperaldosteronism, pheochromocytoma, hypothyroidism or hyperthyroidism, and hyperparathyroidism. Rarely, aortic coarctation can be a cause of resistant hypertension. With the realization that hyperaldosteronism may explain 15% to 20% of resistant hypertension, all patients should be screened for occult hyperaldosteronism by measuring the ratio of plasma aldosterone level to plasma renin activity. In a retrospective study, more widespread use of the plasma aldosterone concentration/plasma renin activity ratio in hypertensive patients resulted in a 1.3- to 6.3-fold increase in the annual detection rate for primary aldosteronism (1% to 2% before screening and 5% to 10% after screening). Although these results are complicated by selection bias, they indicate that this type of screening should be considered for patients with resistant hypertension, despite the fact that it is unusual to find an adenoma.[762] Often, patients with subtle hyperaldosteronism respond to the addition of a selective aldosterone receptor blocker to their antihypertensive regimen.

Coexisting medical conditions can also interfere with the ability of medications to control BP. Obesity is a cause of resistant hypertension that is often overlooked because it is commonly associated with the obesity hypoventilation syndrome of obstructive sleep apnea.[652] It is thought that the accumulation of dependent edema in overweight patients, when it redistributes in a cephalad direction during recumbency at night, may enhance airway closure and facilitate obstruction.[763]

Nighttime ventilation techniques, such as continuous positive airway pressure, enhance the control of BP.[652] Visceral adipose tissue increases the production of aldosterone and causes hyperaldosteronism by the zona glomerulosa in obese patients.[653-655,764] This process is mediated by the adipocyte production of angiotensinogen and WNT signaling molecules that cause steroidogenesis. These factors contribute to sodium retention, a shift to the right of the pressure-natriuresis curve, endothelial dysfunction, and vascular proliferation. Resistant hypertension in this setting can be evaluated for hyperaldosteronism and treated with a therapeutic trial of a selective aldosterone receptor antagonist, such as eplerenone.[653-655,764]

Strategies to control BP in patients with refractory hypertension should first address issues related to adherence, simplification of the medical regimen, and determination of whether side effects play a role. Subsequently, one can evaluate the medications and try to choose those that work well with one another to facilitate a almost additive antihypertensive response. As previously noted, most drugs reduce systolic BP by approximately 8 to 10 mm Hg. Consequently, it is not unusual for patients who are 40 or 50 mm Hg from their target systolic BP to require four or five medications, or possibly even more.

One should also be careful to ensure that volume excess is controlled and that there are no drug-drug interactions or clinical situations that would promote diuretic resistance, such as excessive salt intake, impaired drug bioavailability, impaired diuretic secretion by the proximal tubule, increased protein binding in the tubule lumen, or reduced GFR. Both pseudohypertension and secondary causes of hypertension should be eliminated as possibilities. True resistant hypertension is unusual, and a methodologic approach should be taken to help facilitate BP control in these patients because a lack of control puts these patients at a greater risk of cardiovascular complications.

Refractory hypertension refers to patients whose BP cannot be controlled with maximal medical therapy (more than four drugs with complementary mechanisms, given at maximal tolerable doses) under the care of a specialist.[765] It is an important clinical phenotype that is commonly associated with those of African heritage, patients with diabetes, and/or those with albuminuria.[765] Recent large observational studies have noted that 0.5% of patients receiving antihypertensive treatment and 3.6% of individuals with resistant hypertension have refractory hypertension, and that these individuals have much higher 10-year Framingham coronary heart disease and stroke risk scores. Strategies for improving treatment in these types of patients are unknown but may require higher doses of mineralocorticoid receptor antagonists.

Many hypertensive patients are not controlled due to nonadherence or lack of tolerance to available antihypertensive therapy. In one study, as many as 35% of these individuals, who may be prescribed as many as three to five antihypertensive medications, blood and urine samples revealed no trace of medication.[766,767] Thus, there is a need for novel new drug therapies and devices to lower BP in individuals with refractory hypertension. Fortunately, there are many new drugs in preclinical and clinical trials.[768] A recent large, blinded clinical trial evaluating catheter-based renal denervation did not show a significant reduction of systolic BP 6 months after the procedure compared to that of sham controls.[769] However, it has become clear that results are difficult to interpret due to the procedural and technical shortcomings of the renal denervation procedure itself as only a few participants (9 of 253) received a complete four-quadrant ablation (covering 360 degrees of the renal artery), and systolic BP was significantly higher in participants who underwent incomplete renal denervation compared to those with complete renal denervation.[768,770]

Hopefully, one may be optimistic that these shortcomings will be resolved in the near-future to allow renal denervation procedures to reach clinical applicability.[768] The drugs in development, and innovative novel interventional approaches, should provide physicians with the tools to provide better care for their patients with hypertension that is not yet controlled Novel antihypertensive drug and device treatments are the subject of a recent review[768] (Figure 50.10).

DRUG TREATMENT OF HYPERTENSIVE URGENCIES AND EMERGENCIES

It is important to distinguish between hypertensive urgency and hypertensive emergency (Table 50.37). These terms are used loosely in clinical practice, with a great deal of overlap. The distinction between the two is important because the management approach is substantially different.

A hypertensive emergency is a clinical syndrome in which marked elevation in BP results in ongoing target-organ damage in the body. The syndrome can be manifested by encephalopathy, retinal hemorrhage, papilledema, acute MI, stroke, or acute renal dysfunction. Any delay in the control of BP may lead to irreversible sequelae, including death. This syndrome is unusual but requires immediate hospitalization in an intensive care unit (ICU), with careful and judicious use of intravenous vasodilators to lower systolic and diastolic BPs cautiously to approximately 140/90 mm Hg.

Hypertensive urgency is a clinical situation in which a patient may have a marked elevation in BP (>200/130 mm Hg) but no evidence of ongoing target-organ damage. Such a patient can be treated with rapid-onset drugs, such as captopril or clonidine, and be observed cautiously, with the administration of long-acting medications on an outpatient basis as progressive restoration of a more appropriate BP level is attained.

Thus, the history and physical examination findings are the critical factors in delineating the difference between these two syndromes. The decision about whether to hospitalize the patient in an ICU and use intravenous medication or to observe the patient carefully and use oral medications to facilitate better BP control depends in a large part on the presence or absence of ongoing target-organ injury.

A variety of different antihypertensive therapeutic drug classes are effective in the treatment of hypertensive emergencies. These drugs can be given parenterally and include the following: direct-acting vasodilators—diazoxide, hydralazine, nitroprusside, and nitroglycerin; β_1-selective adrenergic antagonist esmolol; α- and β-adrenergic antagonist

Table 50.37 Hypertensive Emergencies

Hypertensive encephalopathy*
Acute aortic dissection*
  Central nervous system bleeding*
  Intracranial hemorrhage
  Thrombotic cerebrovascular accident
  Subarachnoid hemorrhage
Acute left ventricular failure refractory to conventional medical therapy*
Myocardial ischemia or infarction associated with persistent chest pain*
Accelerated or malignant hypertension†
Toxemia of pregnancy—eclampsia*
Renal failure or insufficiency†
Hypertension associated with hyperadrenergic states*
  Pheochromocytoma
  Interaction between monoamine oxidase inhibitors and tyramine-containing foods
  Interaction between an α-adrenergic agonist and nonselective β-adrenergic antagonist
  After abrupt withdrawal of clonidine or guanabenz
  After severe body burns
  Neurogenic hypertension
Hypertension in the surgical patient†
  Associated with postoperative bleeding
  After open heart or vascular surgery
  Preceding emergency surgery
  After kidney transplantation
  Hypertension in a diabetic patient with retinal hemorrhage*

*Considered by some authors to be a true hypertensive emergency.
†Considered by some authors to be a hypertensive urgency.

Drug	Mechanism of Action	Status
BAY 94-8862 (finerenone)	Mineralocorticoid receptor antagonist	Phase IIb
LCI699	Aldosterone synthase inhibitor	Phase II trials*
C21	AT2 receptor agonist	Preclinical
XNT	ACE2 activator	Preclinical*
DIZE	ACE2 activator	Preclinical*
rhACE2	ACE2 activator	Phase I
HP-β-CD/Ang 1-7	Ang1-7 analogue	Preclinical
AVE0991	Nonpeptide agonist of MAS	Preclinical
CGEN-856S	Peptide agonist of MAS	Preclinical
Alamandine/HPβCD	Mas-related-G-protein coupled receptor, member D agonist	Preclinical
PC18	Aminopeptidase N inhibitor	Preclinical
RB150 (OGC001)	Aminopeptidase A inhibitor	Phase I
LCZ696	Dual-acting angiotensin receptor-neprilysin inhibitor	Phase III
SLV-306 (Daglutril)	Dual-acting endothelin-converting enzymes-neprilysin inhibitor	Phase II
PL-3994	Natriuretic peptide A agonist	Phase II
C-ANP$_{4-23}$	ANP analog, selective for NPR-C	Preclinical
AR9281	Soluble epoxide hydrolase inhibitors	Phase II*
Vasomera (PB1046)	Vasoactive intestinal peptide receptor 2 (VPAC2) agonist	Phase II
AZD1722 (Tenapanor)	Intestinal Na$^+$/H$^+$ exchanger 3 inhibitor	Phase I
Etamicastat	Dopamine β-hydroxylase inhibitor	Phase I
Vaccines		
CYT006-Ang0β	Vaccine against angiotensin II	Phase II
Angil-KLH	Vaccine against angiotensin II	Preclinical
pHAV-4Anglis	Vaccine against angiotensin II	Preclinical
ATR0β-001	Vaccine against angiotensin II type 1 receptor	Preclinical
ATR12181	Vaccine against angiotensin II type 1 receptor	Preclinical
Preeclampsia drugs		
DIF	Anti-digoxin antibody tragment	Phase II expedited
ATryn	Recombinant antithrombin	Phase III

ANP indicates atrial natriuretic peptide; ATR, angiotensin II type 1 receptors; DIF, digoxin-immune Fab; KLH, keyhole limpet hemocyanin; and rhACE2, recombinant human ACE2.

*Stopped.

Figure 50.10 New drugs for hypertension. (From Oparil S, Schmieder RE. New approaches in the treatment of hypertension. *Circ Res* 116:1074-1095, 2015.)

labetalol; central adrenergic agent methyldopate; ganglionic blocking agent trimethaphan; ACE inhibitor enalaprilat; peripheral α-adrenergic blocker phentolamine; CCBs (nicardipine or clevidipine); and dopamine D$_1$–like receptor agonist fenoldopam mesylate.

PARENTERAL DRUGS AND DIRECT-ACTING VASODILATORS

Diazoxide is a benzothiadiazine drug used primarily in the treatment of acute hypertensive emergencies.[771,772] It is a pure arterial dilator. The so-called minibolus (1 mg/kg administered at intervals of 5 to 15 minutes) and continuous infusion of diazoxide have become the preferred methods of administration to avoid excessive reduction in BP. Diazoxide acts rapidly, and the BP effect persists for up to 12 hours. It has a plasma half-life of 17 to 31 hours. In the urine, 20% is eliminated unchanged, and the remainder undergoes hepatic metabolism to inactive metabolites. In renal disease, the plasma half-life is prolonged, and dosage reduction is required.

Because diazoxide relaxes smooth muscle at peripheral arterioles, a reduction in BP is accompanied by an increase in the cardiac output and heart rate, which in susceptible

Table 50.38 Parenteral Drugs Used in the Treatment of Hypertensive Emergencies

Drug	Dosage	Onset of Action	Peak Effect	Duration of Action
Diazoxide	7.5-30–mg/min infusion or 1-mg/kg bolus q5-15min (300 mg maximum)	1-5 min	30 min	4-12 hr
Hydralazine	0.5-1.0–mg/min infusion or 10-50 mg intramuscularly	1-5 min	10-80 min	3-6 hr
Nitroglycerine	5-100-µg/min infusion	1-2 min	2-5 min	3-5 min
Nitroprusside	0.25-10–µg/kg/min infusion	Immediate	1-2 min	2-5 min
Esmolol	250-500 µg/kg/min × 1 (loading dose), then 50-100 µg/kg/min × 4 (maintenance); maintenance dosage may be increased to maximum of 300 µg/kg/min	1-2 min	5 min	0-30 min
Labetalol	2-mg/min infusion or 0.25 mg/kg	5 min	10 min	3-6 hr
Methyldopa	250-500–mg bolus every 6 hr (2 g maximum)	2-3 hr	3-5 hr	6-12 hr
Trimethaphan	0.5-10–mg/min infusion bolus over 2 min (300 mg maximum)	Immediate	1-2 min	5-10 min
Enalaprilat	0.625-5.0–mg bolus over 5 min q6h	5-15 min	1-4 hr	6 hr
Phentolamine	0.5-1.0–mg/min infusion or 2.5-5.0 mg bolus	Immediate	3-5 min	10-15 min
Nicardipine	5-15 mg/hr	5-10 min	45 min	50 hr
Clevidipine	16 mg/hr	1-2 min	5-6 min	15 min
Fenoldopam	0.01-1.6–µg/min constant infusion	5-15 min	30 min	5-10 min

patients can provoke cardiac ischemia. Concurrent administration of a β-adrenergic antagonist controls these reflex vasodilatory responses. Transient hyperuricemia and hyperglycemia occur in most patients. Consequently, the blood glucose level should be monitored. Salt and water retention also occur, and concurrent diuretic administration is often required. Diazoxide and its metabolites are removed by hemodialysis and peritoneal dialysis, but clearance is relatively low because of extensive protein binding.

Hydralazine is a direct-acting vasodilator and may be given intramuscularly or as a rapid intravenous bolus injection (Table 50.38). It acts rapidly, and the BP effect persists for up to 6 hours.[771,772] Hydralazine is less potent than diazoxide, and the BP response is less predictable. It may also cause a reflex increase in heart rate and sodium and water retention.

Sodium nitroprusside is the most potent of the parenteral vasodilators.[771,772] Nitroprusside acts on the excitation-contraction coupling of vascular smooth muscle by interfering with the intracellular activation of calcium. Unlike diazoxide and hydralazine, nitroprusside dilates arteriolar resistance and venous capacitance vessels. It has the advantages of being immediately effective when given as an infusion and of having an extremely short duration of action, which permits minute to minute adjustments in BP control (see Table 50.38). Disadvantages of nitroprusside therapy include the following: (1) need for intraarterial BP monitoring; (2) need for the drug to be prepared fresh every 4 hours; (3) need to protect the solution from light during infusion; and (4) potential for toxic effects from metabolic side products. Nitroprusside is not excreted intact; it is rapidly metabolized to cyanide and thiocyanate through a reaction with hemoglobin, which yields methemoglobin and an unstable intermediate that dissociates to release cyanide. The major elimination pathway of cyanide is conversion in the liver and kidney to thiocyanate. Back conversion of thiocyanate to cyanide may occur. Thiocyanate is largely excreted in the urine; it has a plasma half-life of 1 week in normal individuals and accumulates in those with renal insufficiency.

Toxic concentrations of cyanide or thiocyanate may occur if nitroprusside infusions are given for longer than 48 hours or at infusion rates higher than 2 mg/kg/min; the drug should not be administered at the maximal dose of 10 mg/kg/min for longer than 10 minutes.[773] Toxic manifestations include air hunger, hyperreflexia, confusion, and seizures. Lactic acidosis and venous hyperoxemia are laboratory indicators of cyanide intoxication. The appearance of drug unresponsiveness may reflect an increase in the concentration of free cyanide. In such cases, the drug should be promptly discontinued and the levels of cyanide measured. Nitroprusside is hemodialyzable.

Intravenous nitroglycerin produces dilation of arterial and venous beds in a dose-related manner. At lower dosages, the primary effect is on preload; at higher infusion rates, afterload is reduced. Nitroglycerin may also dilate epicardial coronary vessels and their collaterals, increasing the blood supply to ischemic regions. Effective coronary perfusion is maintained, provided that the BP does not fall excessively or that the heart rate does not increase significantly. Nitroglycerin has an immediate onset of action but is rapidly metabolized to dinitrates and mononitrates (see Table 50.38). Because nitroglycerin is absorbed by many plastics, dilution should be performed only in glass parenteral solution bottles. Nitroglycerin is also absorbed by polyvinyl chloride (PVC) tubing; non-PVC intravenous administration sets should be used.

Patients with normal or low left ventricular filling pressure or pulmonary wedge pressure may be hypersensitive to the effects of nitroglycerin. Therefore, continuous monitoring of BP, heart rate, and pulmonary capillary wedge pressure must be performed to assess the correct dose. Intravenous nitroglycerin may be the drug of choice in the treatment of patients with moderate hypertension associated with coronary ischemia because it provides collateral coronary vasodilation, a property that is not seen with the other direct-acting arteriolar vasodilators. The principal adverse effects are headache, nausea, and vomiting. Tolerance may develop with prolonged use.

β_1-SELECTIVE ADRENERGIC ANTAGONIST

Esmolol hydrochloride is a short-acting, β_1-selective adrenergic antagonist. Esmolol hydrochloride concentrate for injection must be diluted to a final concentration of 10 mg/mL.[771,772] Extravasation of esmolol hydrochloride may cause serious local irritation and skin necrosis. Esmolol shares all the toxic potential of the β_1-adrenergic antagonists, as previously discussed.

After intravenous injection of a loading dose of 250 to 500 mg/kg and then infusion of a maintenance dose ranging from 50 to 100 mg/kg/min, steady-state blood concentrations are achieved within 5 minutes (see Table 50.38). Efficacy should be assessed after the 1-minute loading dose and 4 minutes of maintenance infusion. If an adequate therapeutic effect is observed, as assessed by BP and heart rate response, then the maintenance infusion should be maintained. If an adequate therapeutic effect is not observed, the same loading dose can be repeated for 1 minute, followed by maintenance infusion at an increased rate.

Esmolol has pharmacologic actions similar to those of other β_1-selective adrenergic antagonists; it produces negative chronotropic and inotropic activity. It has been used to prevent or treat hemodynamic changes induced by surgical events, including increases in systolic and diastolic BPs and doubling of the product of heart rate multiplied by systolic BP. Esmolol may be particularly useful for the treatment of postoperative hypertension and hypertension associated with coronary insufficiency.[771,772] Esmolol is hydrolyzed rapidly in the blood, and negligible concentrations are present 30 minutes after discontinuance. Because the kidneys eliminate the de-esterified metabolite of esmolol, the drug should be used cautiously in patients with renal insufficiency.

α_1- AND β-ADRENERGIC ANTAGONISTS

The α_1- and β-adrenergic antagonist labetalol may be given by repeated intravenous injection or slow continuous infusion[771,772] (see Table 50.38). The maximal BP-lowering effect occurs within 5 minutes of the first injection. The drug should be administered to patients in the supine position to avoid symptomatic postural hypotension. The adverse effects of labetalol have been previously discussed. This drug has been proven safe and useful in hypertensive urgencies and emergencies in pregnant women.

CENTRAL α_2-ADRENERGIC AGONIST

Methyldopate hydrochloride is a central α_2-adrenergic agonist that may be administered intravenously as a bolus infusion[771,772] (see Table 50.38). It has a delayed onset of action and peak effect, and its effect on BP is unpredictable. The adverse effects of methyldopa were discussed previously.

GANGLIONIC BLOCKING AGENT

Trimethaphan camsylate is a ganglionic blocking agent. It blocks transmission of impulses at sympathetic and parasympathetic ganglia by occupying receptor sites and by stabilizing the postsynaptic membranes against the action of acetylcholine liberated from presynaptic nerve endings. Peripheral vascular resistance is decreased, the heart rate is usually increased, and cardiac output is decreased because of venous dilation and peripheral pooling of blood. Trimethaphan is used exclusively for the treatment of hypertensive emergencies.[771,772] Trimethaphan has been shown to be useful for immediate BP reduction in patients with acute aortic dissection. It has an immediate onset of action when administered as a continuous infusion (see Table 50.38). The resulting dramatic reduction in BP requires intraarterial monitoring. The main disadvantage is that the drug must be administered with the patient supine to avoid profound postural hypotension. Other disadvantages include the following: (1) potential for tachyphylaxis after sustained infusion (48 hours); (2) appearance of adverse effects associated with parasympathetic and sympathetic blockade; and (3) histamine release.

ANGIOTENSIN-CONVERTING ENZYME INHIBITOR

Enalaprilat, the active metabolite of the oral ACE inhibitor enalapril, is administered as a slow intravenous infusion for 5 minutes (see Table 50.38) in an intravenous dose that is approximately 25% of the oral dose. The onset of action occurs within 15 minutes, and the maximal effect is observed within 1 to 4 hours.[774] The duration of action is approximately 6 hours. Adverse effects of enalapril were previously discussed. In patients with renal insufficiency, the initial dose should be no more than 0.625 mg.

α-ADRENERGIC ANTAGONIST

Phentolamine mesylate is a nonselective, α-adrenergic antagonist used primarily in the treatment of hypertension associated with pheochromocytoma.[771,772] It has a rapid onset of action when administered intravenously as a bolus or continuous infusion (see Table 50.38). The duration of action is 10 to 15 minutes. The drug has a plasma half-life of 19 minutes. Approximately 13% of a single dose appears in the urine as unchanged drug. Adverse effects include those associated with nonselective α-adrenergic blockade, as previously discussed.

CALCIUM CHANNEL BLOCKERS

Nicardipine hydrochloride, a dihydropyridine CCB, is administered by slow continuous infusion at a concentration of 0.1 mg/mL; each 1-mL ampule (25 mg) should be diluted with 240 mL of a compatible intravenous fluid (not including sodium bicarbonate or lactated Ringer's solution) to produce 250 mL of solution at a concentration of 0.1 mg/mL.[775] There is a dose-dependent decrease in BP. The onset of action is within minutes; 50% of the ultimate decrease in BP occurs within 45 minutes, but a final steady state is not reached for approximately 50 hours (see Table 50.38). The discontinuation of infusion is followed by a 50% offset of action within 30 minutes, but gradually decreasing antihypertensive effects exist for approximately 50 hours. Adverse effects of nicardipine have been previously discussed. This drug has been shown to be safe and effective in the treatment of pediatric hypertensive emergencies.[775,776]

Clevidipine is a dihydropyridine CCB that is available in a lipid emulsion for intravenous infusion for the treatment of hypertensive emergencies.[777] Steady-state concentrations of clevidipine in arterial or venous blood are attained within

Table 50.39 Rapid-Acting Oral Drugs Used in the Treatment of Hypertensive Emergencies

Drug	Dosage	Onset of Action	Peak Effect	Duration of Action
α_1- and β-Adrenergic Antagonist				
Labetalol	100-400 mg q12h (2400 mg maximum)	1-2 hr	2-4 hr	8-12 hr
α_1-Adrenergic Antagonist				
Prazosin	1-5 mg q2h (20 mg maximum)	<60 min	2-4 hr	6-12 hr
Central α_2-Agonist				
Clonidine	0.2 mg initially, then 0.1 mg/hr (0.8 mg maximum)	30-60 min	2-4 hr	6-8 hr
Calcium Channel Blockers				
Diltiazem	30-120 mg q8h (480 mg maximum)	<15 min	2-3 hr	8 hr
Verapamil	80-120 mg q8h (480 mg maximum)	<60 min	2-3 hr	8 hr
Angiotensin-Converting Enzyme Inhibitors				
Captopril	12.5-25 mg qh (150 mg maximum)	<15 min	1 hr	6-12 hr
Enalapril	2.5-10 mg q6h (40 mg maximum)	<60 min	4-8 hr	12-24 hr

2 and 10 minutes in healthy volunteers receiving 0.91 and 3.2 µg/kg/min, respectively. The relationship between the intravenous infusion dose and steady-state blood concentrations is linear in patients with mild to moderate hypertension and in healthy volunteers. Clevidipine is highly protein-bound and rapidly distributed. This drug is rapidly hydrolyzed by esterases in the blood and extravascular tissues. Blood concentrations decrease rapidly after termination of the infusion. The initial phase is rapid (half-life of ≈1 minute) and accounts for 85% to 90% of elimination. The terminal elimination half-life is 15 minutes. Clevidipine treatment results in a prompt reduction in BP (≥15% from baseline) in less than 6 minutes.[778] Clevidipine has a safety profile comparable to that of nitroglycerin, sodium nitroprusside, and nicardipine. The most common adverse events are sinus tachycardia, headache, nausea, and chest discomfort.[779]

DOPAMINE D_1–LIKE RECEPTOR AGONIST

Fenoldopam mesylate, a dopamine D_1–like receptor agonist, is formulated as a solution to be diluted for intravenous infusion for the treatment of acute hypertension.[777,780] It is a rapid-acting agent that produces vasodilation by functioning as an agonist for dopamine D_1–like receptors and has moderate affinity for α_2-adrenoreceptors.

Fenoldopam is a racemic mixture in which the R isomers are responsible for its biologic activity. It has vasodilatory effects on coronary, renal, mesenteric, and peripheral arteries in experimental studies; however, not all vascular beds respond uniformly. In humans, the drug increases renal blood flow in hypertensive and normotensive subjects.

Fenoldopam comes in 1-mL ampules that contain 10 mg of fenoldopam and is diluted for administration as a constant infusion at a rate of 0.01 to 1.6 mg/kg/min (see Table 50.38). It produces steady-state plasma concentrations in proportion to its infusion rate, its elimination half-life is 5 minutes, and steady-state concentrations are reached within 20 minutes.

Clearance of the active compound is not altered by ESKD or hepatic disease. Approximately 90% of infused fenoldopam is eliminated in urine and 10% in feces. Elimination occurs largely by conjugation that does not involve CYP enzymes. There are no data on drug-drug interactions.

Adverse effects include reflex increase in heart rate, increase in intraocular pressure, headache, flushing, nausea, and hypotension.

RAPID-ACTING ORAL DRUGS

A more gradual, progressive reduction in systemic BP may be achieved after the oral administration of drugs with rapid absorption.[781] These drugs include the following: (1) α_1- and β-adrenergic antagonist labetalol; (2) central α_2-adrenergic agonist clonidine; (3) CCBs diltiazem and verapamil; (4) ACE inhibitors captopril and enalapril; (5) postsynaptic α_1-adrenergic antagonist prazosin; and (6) a combination of oral therapies. The dosages and pharmacodynamic effects of rapid-acting oral drugs that are commonly used in the treatment of hypertensive emergencies are given in Table 50.39. Note that rapid-acting oral dihydropyridine CCBs, such as sublingual nifedipine, are no longer recommended because they may cause large and unpredictable reductions in BP, with resultant ischemic events.[782]

CLINICAL CONSIDERATIONS IN THE RAPID REDUCTION OF BLOOD PRESSURE

The rapid reduction of BP carries the risk of impairing blood supply to vital structures, such as the brain and heart. Consequently, every effort should be made to avoid an excessive reduction of BP. The risk of overreduction of BP in a rapid fashion is linked to the use of sublingual nifedipine capsules with stroke and heart attack in hypertensive subjects.[782] Because this approach is variable and rapid, clinicians are unable to set a lower limit of BP that is achieved with therapy.

Cerebral blood flow is normally carefully autoregulated so that perfusion is maintained at a sufficient level when BP is low but is diminished during states of chronic hypertension to avoid cerebral edema. With chronic hypertension, the short-term, rapid reduction of BP may decrease cerebral blood flow sufficiently to precipitate ischemia and infarction. This decrease may be particularly important in patients with atherosclerotic disease of the cerebral blood vessels in whom there may be areas of uneven cerebral perfusion. Although drugs that do penetrate the blood-brain barrier, such as hydralazine, sodium nitroprusside, and nicardipine, dilate cerebral vessels, which may lessen the likelihood of ischemia, intrinsic vascular disease may render some areas more ischemic than others with BP reduction. In addition, potent cerebral vasodilators can conceivably cause an increase in intracranial pressure, creating the potential for cerebral edema and possible herniation.

Sudden drops in BP can also interfere with coronary perfusion during diastole and result in myocardial ischemia, infarction, or arrhythmia. In addition, rapid reduction of BP may result in a reflex increase in heart rate, which would also interfere with coronary perfusion during diastole. For these reasons, careful, cautious, and controlled reduction in BP is necessary for these patients. For most hypertensive emergencies, a parenteral drug, such as sodium nitroprusside, is ideal. However, if the patient has coronary disease, the use of intravenous nitroglycerin, esmolol, or both is a useful approach because these drugs can induce coronary dilation and slow heart rate, respectively. Intravenous nicardipine can also be used because it facilitates coronary vasodilation. Patients with acute aortic dissection are best treated with a β-adrenergic antagonist plus nitroprusside or a ganglionic blocker, such as trimethaphan. Patients with hypertensive encephalopathy or CNS hemorrhage are best treated with drugs that do not cause cerebral vasodilation, such as hydralazine, nitroprusside, nicardipine, or fenoldopam. Fenoldopam may be helpful for patients with kidney disease because it maintains renal blood flow.

Complete reference list available at ExpertConsult.com.

KEY REFERENCES

40. Gonzalez-Villalobos RA, et al: The absence of intrarenal ACE protects against hypertension. *J Clin Invest* 123:2011–2023, 2013.
45. Gansevoort RT, de Zeeuw D, de Jong PE: Dissociation between the course of the hemodynamic and antiproteinuric effects of angiotensin I converting enzyme inhibition. *Kidney Int* 44:579–584, 1993.
47. Kunz R, et al: Meta-analysis: effect of monotherapy and combination therapy with inhibitors of the renin angiotensin system on proteinuria in renal disease. *Ann Intern Med* 148:30–48, 2008.
50. Mercier K, Smith H, Biederman J: Renin-angiotensin-aldosterone system inhibition: overview of the therapeutic use of angiotensin-converting enzyme inhibitors, angiotensin receptor blockers, mineralocorticoid receptor antagonists, and direct renin inhibitors. *Prim Care* 41:765–778, 2014.
55. Remuzzi G, Macia M, Ruggenenti P: Prevention and treatment of diabetic renal disease in type 2 diabetes: the BENEDICT study. *J Am Soc Nephrol* 17(Suppl 2):S90–S97, 2006.
74. Hricik DE, et al: Captopril-induced functional renal insufficiency in patients with bilateral renal-artery stenoses or renal-artery stenosis in a solitary kidney. *N Engl J Med* 308:373–376, 1983.
80. Onuigbo MA, Onuigbo NT: Worsening renal failure in older chronic kidney disease patients with renal artery stenosis concurrently on renin angiotensin aldosterone system blockade: a prospective 50-month Mayo-Health-System clinic analysis. *QJM* 101:519–527, 2008.
81. Cohen JB, Townsend RR: Use of renin-angiotensin system blockade in patients with renal artery stenosis. *Clin J Am Soc Nephrol* 9:1149–1152, 2014.
98. Investigators O, et al: Telmisartan, ramipril, or both in patients at high risk for vascular events. *N Engl J Med* 358:1547–1559, 2008.
100. Parving HH, et al: Cardiorenal end points in a trial of aliskiren for type 2 diabetes. *N Engl J Med* 367:2204–2213, 2012.
139. Cooper WO, et al: Major congenital malformations after first-trimester exposure to ACE inhibitors. *N Engl J Med* 354:2443–2451, 2006.
140. Li DK, et al: Maternal exposure to angiotensin converting enzyme inhibitors in the first trimester and risk of malformations in offspring: a retrospective cohort study. *BMJ* 343:d5931, 2011.
244. Burnier M, Brunner HR: Angiotensin II receptor antagonists and the kidney. *Curr Opin Nephrol Hypertens* 3:537–545, 1994.
245. Puig JG, et al: Effect of eprosartan and losartan on uric acid metabolism in patients with essential hypertension. *J Hypertens* 17:1033–1039, 1999.
256. Parving HH, et al: The effect of irbesartan on the development of diabetic nephropathy in patients with type 2 diabetes. *N Engl J Med* 345:870–878, 2001.
261. Ogawa S, et al: Identification of the stages of diabetic nephropathy at which angiotensin II receptor blockers most effectively suppress albuminuria. *Am J Hypertens* 26:1064–1069, 2013.
302. Sowers JR, et al: Angiotensin receptor blocker/diuretic combination preserves insulin responses in obese hypertensives. *J Hypertens* 28:1761–1769, 2010.
303. Rossing K, et al: Dual blockade of the renin-angiotensin system in diabetic nephropathy: a randomized double-blind crossover study. *Diabetes Care* 25:95–100, 2002.
326. Bangalore S, et al: Antihypertensive drugs and risk of cancer: network meta-analyses and trial sequential analyses of 324,168 participants from randomised trials. *Lancet Oncol* 12:65–82, 2011.
373. Poirier L, Lacourcière Y: The evolving role of β-adrenergic receptor blockers in managing hypertension. *Can J Cardiol* 28:334–340, 2012.
373. Kizer JR, et al: Stroke reduction in hypertensive adults with cardiac hypertrophy randomized to losartan versus atenolol: the Losartan Intervention For Endpoint reduction in hypertension study. *Hypertension* 45:46–52, 2005.
381. Wiysonge CS, et al: Beta-blockers for hypertension. *Cochrane Database Syst Rev* (11):CD002003, 2012.
382. Wright JM, Musini VM: First-line drugs for hypertension. *Cochrane Database Syst Rev* CD001841, 2009.
399. Gradman AH, et al: Initial combination therapy reduces the risk of cardiovascular events in hypertensive patients: a matched cohort study. *Hypertension* 61:309–318, 2013.
433. Triggle DJ: L-type calcium channels. *Curr Pharm Des* 12:443–457, 2006.
434. Abernethy DR, Schwartz JB: Calcium-antagonist drugs. *N Engl J Med* 341:1447–1457, 1999.
136. Li CI, et al: Use of antihypertensive medications and breast cancer risk among women aged 55 to 74 years. *JAMA Intern Med* 173:1629–1637, 2013.
572. Coogan PF: Calcium-channel blockers and breast cancer: a hypothesis revived. *JAMA Intern Med* 173:1637–1638, 2013.
601. Kaoukis A, et al: The role of endothelin system in cardiovascular disease and the potential therapeutic perspectives of its inhibition. *Curr Top Med Chem* 13:95–114, 2013.
614. Barton M: Endothelin antagonism and reversal of proteinuric renal disease in humans. *Contrib Nephrol* 172:210–222, 2011.
633. Rakusan D, et al: Persistent antihypertensive effect of aliskiren is accompanied by reduced proteinuria and normalization of glomerular area in Ren-2 transgenic rats. *Am J Physiol Renal Physiol* 299:F758–F766, 2010.
641. Delyani JA: Mineralocorticoid receptor antagonists: the evolution of utility and pharmacology. *Kidney Int* 57:1408–1411, 2000.
646. Sowers JR, Whaley-Connell A, Epstein M: Narrative review: the emerging clinical implications of the role of aldosterone in the metabolic syndrome and resistant hypertension. *Ann Intern Med* 150:776–783, 2009.

654. Flynn C, Bakris GL: Interaction between adiponectin and aldosterone. *Cardiorenal Med* 1:96–101, 2011.
660. Bomback AS, et al: Change in proteinuria after adding aldosterone blockers to ACE inhibitors or angiotensin receptor blockers in CKD: a systematic review. *Am J Kidney Dis* 51:199–211, 2008.
668. Daskalopoulou SS, et al: The 2012 Canadian hypertension education program recommendations for the management of hypertension: blood pressure measurement, diagnosis, assessment of risk, and therapy. *Can J Cardiol* 28:270–287, 2012.
669. Krause T, et al: Management of hypertension: summary of NICE guidance. *BMJ* 343:d4891, 2011.
670. American Diabetes, A.: Standards of medical care in diabetes–2013. *Diabetes Care* 36(Suppl 1):S11–S66, 2013.
675. SHEP Cooperative Research Group: Prevention of stroke by antihypertensive drug treatment in older persons with isolated systolic hypertension. Final results of the Systolic Hypertension in the Elderly Program (SHEP). *JAMA* 265:3255–3264, 1991.
695. Calhoun DA, et al: Triple antihypertensive therapy with amlodipine, valsartan, and hydrochlorothiazide: a randomized clinical trial. *Hypertension* 54:32–39, 2009.
696. Weber MA, et al: Effects of body size and hypertension treatments on cardiovascular event rates: subanalysis of the ACCOMPLISH randomised controlled trial. *Lancet* 381:537–545, 2013.
699. Neutel JM: Metabolic manifestations of low-dose diuretics. *Am J Med* 101:71S–82S, 1996.
717. Jamerson K, et al: Benazepril plus amlodipine or hydrochlorothiazide for hypertension in high-risk patients. *N Engl J Med* 359:2417–2428, 2008.
724. Weir MR, Dworkin LD: Antihypertensive drugs, dietary salt, and renal protection: how low should you go and with which therapy? *Am J Kidney Dis* 32:1–22, 1998.
728. de Remuzzi G, Parving HH, Zeeuw D: Proteinuria, a target for renoprotection in patients with type 2 diabetic nephropathy: Lessons from RENAAL. *Kidney Int* 65:2004.
757. Calhoun DA, et al: Resistant hypertension: diagnosis, evaluation, and treatment. A scientific statement from the American Heart Association Professional Education Committee of the Council for High Blood Pressure Research. *Hypertension* 51:1403–1419, 2008.
758. Messerli FH, Ventura HO, Amodeo C: Osler's maneuver and pseudohypertension. The New England journal of medicine. *N Engl J Med* 312:1548–1551, 1985.
759. Agarwal R, Andersen MJ: Prognostic importance of ambulatory blood pressure recordings in patients with chronic kidney disease. *Kidney Int* 69:1175–1180, 2006.
764. Dudenbostel T, Calhoun DA: Resistant hypertension, obstructive sleep apnoea and aldosterone. *J Hum Hypertens* 26:281–287, 2012.
771. Elliot WJ: Hypertensive emergencies. *Crit Care Clin* 17:435–451, 2001.

51 Diuretics

Ewout J. Hoorn | Christopher S. Wilcox | David H. Ellison

CHAPTER OUTLINE

INDIVIDUAL CLASSES OF DIURETICS, 1702
Carbonic Anhydrase Inhibitors, 1702
Osmotic Diuretics, 1704
Loop Diuretics, 1705
Thiazides and Thiazide-like Diuretics
(Distal Convoluted Tubule Diuretics), 1710
Distal Potassium-Sparing Diuretic
Agents, 1712
Miscellaneous Agents, 1713
ADAPTATION TO DIURETIC THERAPY, 1714
Diuretic Braking Phenomenon, 1714

Humoral and Neuronal Modulators of the
Response to Diuretics, 1716
Diuretic Resistance, 1717
Diuretic Combinations, 1719
CLINICAL USES OF DIURETICS, 1719
Edematous Conditions, 1719
Nonedematous Conditions, 1725
ADVERSE EFFECTS OF DIURETICS, 1727
Fluid and Electrolyte Abnormalities, 1727
Metabolic Abnormalities, 1730
Other Adverse Effects, 1731

This chapter reviews the mechanisms of action of, physiologic adaptations to, clinical uses of, and adverse effects of diuretics. The major transport targets for diuretic drugs have been defined and their genes cloned. The effects of disease on diuretic kinetics are discussed because they predict the required dosage modifications. Loop diuretics and thiazides are the most widely used diuretics, and the physiologic adaptations to their prolonged use are described. Diuretic resistance, its management, and the major adverse effects of therapy are discussed. This discussion provides a framework for the design of strategies to maximize the desired actions while minimizing the unwanted effects. The chapter also includes a discussion of the practical use of diuretics in the treatment of specific clinical conditions.

Other chapters discuss the treatment of hypertension by diuretic drugs (Chapter 50), diuretic-induced changes in potassium excretion (Chapter 18), acid-base disturbances (Chapter 17), divalent cation excretion and nephrolithiasis (Chapters 19 and 40), the syndrome of inappropriate antidiuretic hormone (SIADH) secretion (Chapter 16), and acute kidney injury (AKI) (Chapter 31). Diuretics have been reviewed extensively.[1-4] More extensive and historical references appeared in previous editions of this chapter; the interested reader is referred to editions 7, 8, and 9 of *Brenner and Rector's The Kidney* for more detailed references.

INDIVIDUAL CLASSES OF DIURETICS

The major sites of action of diuretics and the fractions of filtered Na^+ reabsorbed at the corresponding nephron segments are summarized in Figure 51.1.

CARBONIC ANHYDRASE INHIBITORS

SITES AND MECHANISMS OF ACTION

In the kidney, carbonic anhydrase inhibitors (CAIs) act primarily on proximal tubule cells to inhibit bicarbonate absorption (Figure 51.2). An additional, more modest, effect along the distal nephron, however, is also observed.[5] Carbonic anhydrase (CA), a metalloenzyme containing one zinc atom per molecule, is important in sodium bicarbonate reabsorption and hydrogen ion secretion by renal epithelial cells. The biochemical, morphologic, and functional properties of carbonic anhydrase have been reviewed.[6,7]

CA is expressed by many tissues, including erythrocytes, kidney, gut, ciliary body, choroid plexus, and glial cells. Although at least 14 isoforms of CA have been identified, two play predominant roles in renal acid-base homeostasis, CA II and CA IV. CA II is widely expressed, comprising the enzyme expressed by red blood cells and a variety of secretory and absorptive epithelia. In the kidney, CA II is expressed in the cytoplasm and accounts for 95% of renal CA.[7] It is present in proximal tubule cells and intercalated cells of the aldosterone-sensitive distal nephron (ASDN).[7] Carbonic anhydrase IV is expressed at the luminal border of the cells of the proximal, thick ascending limb (TAL) of the loop of Henle, and α-intercalated cells of the ASDN.[8]

CAIs block the catalytic dehydration of luminal carbonic acid at the brush border of the proximal tubule, decrease the intracellular generation of H^+ required for countertransport with Na^+, and decrease the peritubular capillary fluid uptake.[9] CAIs also are also weak inhibitors of reabsorption in TAL,[10] but the natriuretic efficacy of CAIs and

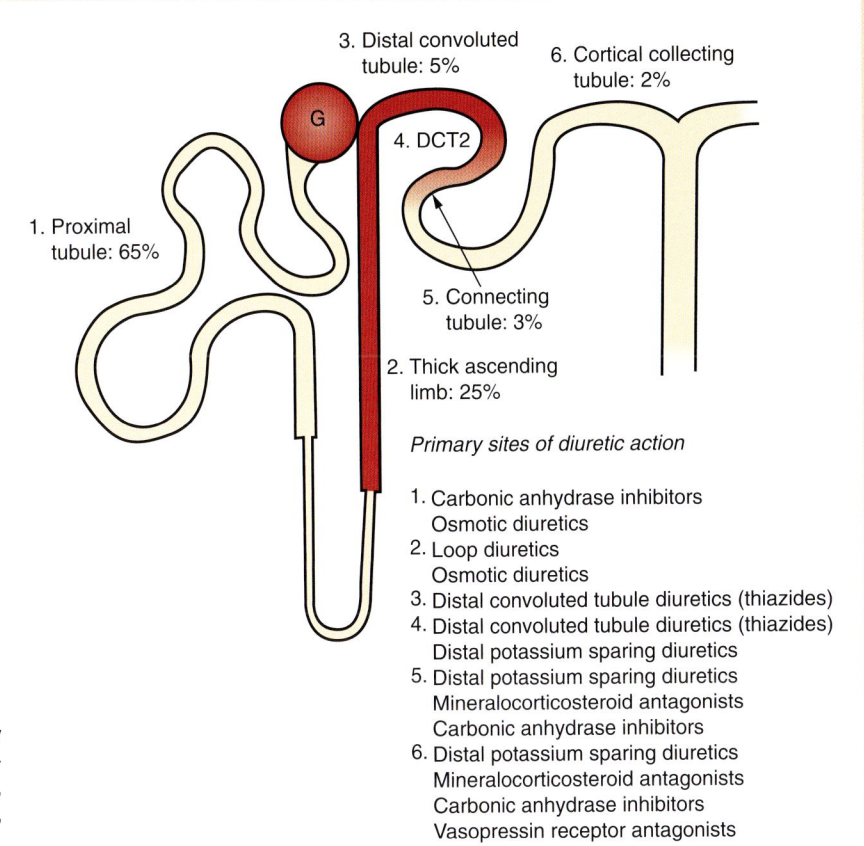

Figure 51.1 Nephron diagram showing the primary sites of diuretic action and the approximate percentage of filtered sodium reabsorbed at each. DCT2, Late segment of distal convoluted tubule; G, glomerulus.

1. Proximal tubule: 65%
2. Thick ascending limb: 25%
3. Distal convoluted tubule: 5%
4. DCT2
5. Connecting tubule: 3%
6. Cortical collecting tubule: 2%

Primary sites of diuretic action

1. Carbonic anhydrase inhibitors
   Osmotic diuretics
2. Loop diuretics
   Osmotic diuretics
3. Distal convoluted tubule diuretics (thiazides)
4. Distal convoluted tubule diuretics (thiazides)
   Distal potassium sparing diuretics
5. Distal potassium sparing diuretics
   Mineralocorticosteroid antagonists
   Carbonic anhydrase inhibitors
6. Distal potassium sparing diuretics
   Mineralocorticosteroid antagonists
   Carbonic anhydrase inhibitors
   Vasopressin receptor antagonists

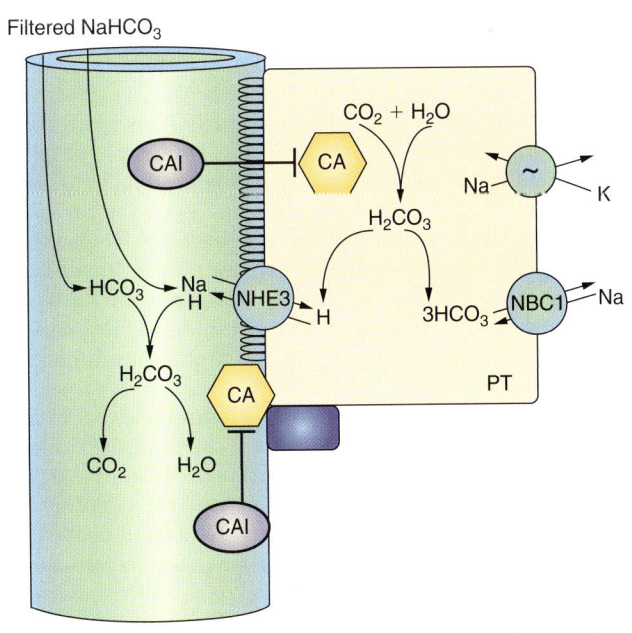

Figure 51.2 Mechanisms of diuretic action in the proximal tubule. The figure shows a functional model of proximal tubule cells; many transport proteins are omitted from the model for clarity. Inside the cell carbonic anhydrase (CA) catalyzes the formation of HCO_3^- from OH^- and CO_2. Bicarbonate leaves the cell via the sodium-bicarbonate transporter (NHE3). A second pool of carbonic anhydrase is located in the brush border. This participates in disposing of carbonic acid formed from filtered bicarbonate and secreted H^+. Both pools of carbonic anhydrase are inhibited by acetazolamide and other carbonic anhydrase inhibitors (CAIs; see text for details). NBC1, Sodium-bicarbonate cotransporter 1.

loop diuretics (see later) is additive, confirming their independent mechanisms of action.[11] CAIs also inhibit bicarbonate reabsorption along the distal tubule, presumably by interfering with the action of α-intercalated cells.[7] The first administration of a CAI causes a brisk alkaline diuresis. The excretion of Na^+, K^+, HCO_3^-, and PO_4^{2-} increases, whereas titratable acid and NH_4^+ decrease sharply. Excretion of Ca^{2+} remains essentially unchanged. There is substantial kaliuresis, owing to the presence of nonreabsorbable HCO_3^- and high flow rates in the distal nephron. However, hypokalemia is uncommon, because acidosis partitions K^+ out of cells.

Long-term CAI administration causes only a modest natriuresis, despite the magnitude of carbonic anhydrase–dependent proximal Na^+ reabsorption. Several factors account for this fact. First, carbonic anhydrase is required for reabsorption of HCO_3^-, whereas about two thirds of the proximal Na^+ reabsorption is accompanied by Cl^-. Second, some proximal HCO_3^- reabsorption persists even after apparently full inhibition of carbonic anhydrase.[12] Third, some of the HCO_3^- that is delivered out of the proximal tubule can be reabsorbed at more distal sites.[12] Fourth, the metabolic acidosis that develops limits the filtered load to HCO_3^- and thereby curtails the natriuresis. Fifth, the increased delivery of filtered Na^+ to the macula densa elicits a tubuloglomerular feedback (TGF)–induced reduction in the glomerular filtration rate (GFR).[13] Micropuncture studies of mice with deletion of the proximal Na^+-H^+ exchanger, NHE3, show that inhibition of proximal Na reabsorption is largely balanced by reduced GFR,[14] supporting this mechanism. One experimental study, however, has shown that the combined use of a thiazide and the CAI acetazolamide resulted in a brisk natriuresis.[15]

Most diuretics have some CAI action.[16] This characteristic contributes to the weak inhibition of proximal reabsorption by furosemide and chlorothiazide and to the relaxation of vascular smooth muscle cells by high-dose furosemide.[16]

PHARMACOKINETICS

Acetazolamide (Diamox) is readily absorbed. It is eliminated with a half-life ($t_{1/2}$) of 13 hours by tubular secretion, which is diminished during hypoalbuminemia.[17] Methazolamide (Neptazane) has less plasma protein binding, a longer $t_{1/2}$, and greater lipid solubility, all of which favor penetration into aqueous humor and cerebrospinal fluid. This agent has less renal effect and therefore is preferred for treatment of glaucoma.

CLINICAL INDICATIONS

The use of CAIs as diuretics is limited by their transient action, the development of metabolic acidosis, and a spectrum of adverse effects. They can be used with $NaHCO_3$ infusion to initiate an alkaline diuresis that increases the excretion of weakly acidic drugs (e.g., salicylates and phenobarbital) or acidic metabolites (urate). Chloride-responsive metabolic alkalosis is best treated by administration of Cl^- with K^+ or Na^+. However, if it produces unacceptable extracellular volume (ECV) expansion, acetazolamide (250-500 mg/day) and KCl can be used to increase HCO_3^- excretion.

Metabolic alkalosis due to loop diuretics or thiazides can depress respiration in patients with chronic respiratory acidosis, for example, due to chronic obstructive pulmonary disease. This effect provides the rationale for use of a CAI. Indeed, the administration of acetazolamide to such subjects can reduce the arterial partial pressure of arterial carbon dioxide ($Paco_2$) and improve the partial pressure of oxygen (Pao_2). Because both $Paco_2$ and plasma bicarbonate concentration (P_{HCO3}) decrease, there is little change in blood pH.[18] However, a reduction in P_{HCO3} limits the buffer capacity of blood. CAIs can increase the $Paco_2$ during metabolic acidosis or exercise, perhaps by depressing hypoxic ventilatory drive[19] and hypoxic pulmonary vasoconstriction,[20] and can cause ventilation-perfusion imbalance.[21] Nevertheless, acetazolamide (250 mg twice a day) can improve blood gas parameters in patients with chronic obstructive pulmonary disease.[22] Careful surveillance is required when CAIs are administered to such patients.

When used to treat glaucoma, CAIs diminish the transport of HCO_3^- and Na^+ by the ciliary process, thereby reducing the intraocular pressure.[23] CAIs also limit formation of cerebrospinal fluid[24] and endolymph.[25]

Acute mountain sickness is characterized by headache, nausea, drowsiness, insomnia, shortness of breath, dizziness, and malaise after an abrupt ascent. Acetazolamide is useful in a dose of 250 mg daily as prophylaxis against mountain sickness, probably through stimulating respiration and diminishing cerebral blood flow and cerebrospinal fluid formation.[26,27] Used in established mountain sickness, acetazolamide improves oxygenation and pulmonary gas exchange.[28] It can stimulate ventilation in patients with central sleep apnea.[29] In patients with idiopathic intracranial hypertension, acetazolamide administration along with a low-sodium weight-reduction diet modestly improved visual field function.[30]

CAIs are effective in prophylaxis of hypokalemic periodic paralysis because they diminish the influx of K^+ into cells.[31] Paradoxically, they are also useful in the treatment of hyperkalemic periodic paralysis.[32]

Other indications for CAIs that are experimental but emerging include possible application in diseases as diverse as obesity, cancer, and infection.[33]

ADVERSE EFFECTS

Patients taking CAIs may complain of weakness, lethargy, abnormal taste, paresthesia, gastrointestinal distress, malaise, and decreased libido. These symptoms can be diminished by $NaHCO_3$ but this agent increases the risk of nephrocalcinosis and nephrolithiasis.[34] Overall, symptomatic metabolic acidosis develops in half of patients with glaucoma treated with CAIs.[35]

Elderly patients or those with diabetes mellitus or chronic kidney disease (CKD) can experience a serious metabolic acidosis if given a CAI.[35] An alkaline urine favors partitioning of renal ammonia into blood rather than its elimination in urine. An increase in blood ammonia may precipitate encephalopathy in patients with liver failure.[35]

Acetazolamide increases the risk of nephrolithiasis by more than 10-fold.[36] CAIs occasionally cause allergic reactions, hepatitis, and blood dyscrasias.[37] They can cause osteomalacia when used with phenytoin or phenobarbital.[38]

OSMOTIC DIURETICS

SITES AND MECHANISMS OF ACTION

Osmotic diuretics are substances that are freely filtered but poorly reabsorbed.[39] Mannitol is the prototypic osmotic diuretic, although sorbitol and glycerol have similar actions. In the water-permeable nephron segments of the proximal nephron and the thin limbs of the loop of Henle, fluid reabsorption concentrates filtered mannitol sufficiently to diminish tubular fluid reabsorption. Ongoing Na^+ reabsorption lowers the tubular fluid $[Na^+]$ and creates a gradient for back flux of reabsorbed Na^+ into the tubule. Increased distal flow stimulates K^+ secretion.

Mannitol is a hypertonic solute that abstracts water from cells. The increase in total renal blood flow (RBF) relates in part to hemodilution and a decrease in blood hematocrit and viscosity. Mannitol increases the medullary blood flow and decreases the medullary solute gradient, thereby preventing urinary concentration. The rise in renal plasma flow and drop in plasma colloid osmotic pressure can increase the GFR.[40]

PHARMACOKINETICS AND DOSAGE

Mannitol is distributed in extracellular fluid. It is filtered freely at the glomerulus. Consequently, the $t_{1/2}$ for plasma clearance of mannitol depends on the GFR and is prolonged from 1 to 36 hours in advanced renal failure.[41] It can be infused intravenously in daily doses of 50 to 200 g as a 15% or 20% solution or 1.5 to 2.0 g/kg of 20% mannitol over 30 to 60 minutes to treat raised intraocular or intracranial pressure.[39]

CLINICAL INDICATIONS

Mannitol has been evaluated for the prophylaxis of AKI, but controlled trials of its use in patients at risk for AKI have not had positive results.[42,43] The rationale for such trials includes mannitol's ability to expand the ECV, block TGF, maintain GFR, increase RBF and tubule fluid flow, prevent tubule obstruction from shed cell constituents or crystals, reduce renal edema, redistribute blood flow from the outer cortex to the relatively hypoxic inner cortex and outer medulla, and scavenge oxygen radicals.[39,40] It can protect against AKI in cadaveric kidney transplant recipients.[39] The use of diuretics to convert oliguric to nonoliguric AKI is discussed later (see under "Clinical Uses of Diuretics").

A trial of mannitol therapy for cerebral edema complicating hepatic failure demonstrated a markedly better survival of 47%, compared with only 6% in the control group.[44] Mannitol is recommended for management of severe head injury.[45,46] It is more effective than loop diuretics or hypertonic saline in reducing brain water content.[47] Mannitol can reverse the dialysis disequilibrium syndrome.[48]

ADVERSE EFFECTS

The effects of mannitol on plasma electrolyte concentrations are complex. The osmotic abstraction of cell water initially causes hypertonic hyponatremia and hypochloremia. Later, when the excess extracellular fluid (ECF) is excreted, the decrease in cell water concentrates K^+ and H^+ within cells, thereby increasing the gradient for their diffusion into the ECF, leading to hyperkalemic acidosis. Normally these electrolyte changes are rapidly corrected by the kidney, provided that renal function is adequate. Later, hypernatremic dehydration may develop if free water is not provided, because urinary concentrating ability is inhibited. In fact, when mannitol-induced hypernatremia exceeds serum sodium levels of 150 mmol/L, its positive effects are outweighed by untoward effects, including renal failure, and higher mortality.[49]

Expansion of ECV, hemodilution, and hyperkalemic metabolic acidosis occur in patients with renal failure whose bodies cannot eliminate the drug. Circulatory overload, pulmonary edema, central nervous system depression, and severe hyponatremia require urgent hemodialysis.[50] Doses of more than 200 g/day can cause renal vasoconstriction and AKI.[39]

LOOP DIURETICS

SITES AND MECHANISMS OF ACTION

The primary action of loop diuretics occurs from the luminal aspect of the TAL (Figure 51.3). An electroneutral Na-K-2Cl cotransporter, termed NKCC2, is located at the luminal membrane.[51,52] This cotransporter, a member of the solute carrier family 12 (SLC12A1), mediates Na^+ and Cl^- movement across the cell. A high luminal K^+ conductance, via the renal outer medullary K^+ (ROMK) channel, allows the majority of K^+ to recycle across the luminal membrane.[53] Coupled with electrogenic exit of Cl^- across the basolateral membrane, the activity of the NKCC2 generates a transepithelial voltage, oriented with the lumen positive relative to interstitial fluid. The primary energy for transport across TAL cells is provided via the basolateral sodium pump, Na^+-K^+–adenosine triphosphatase (ATPase), which maintains a low intracellular $[Na^+]$. Additional details concerning mechanisms of solute reabsorption by TAL cells can be found in Chapter 6. Loop diuretics are organic anions that bind to the NKCC2 from the luminal surface. Early studies showed that $[^3H]$ bumetanide binds to membranes that express the NKCC proteins and that Cl^- competes for the same binding site on the transport protein.[54] Studies using chimeric NKCC molecules have investigated sites of bumetanide binding and interactions with ions by determining effects on ion transport of heterologously expressed NKCC proteins; they have found that changes in amino acids that affect bumetanide binding are not the same as patterns of changes affecting the kinetics of ion translocation.[55,56] Nevertheless, the second membrane-spanning segment of NKCC2 does appear to participate in both anion affinity and bumetanide affinity.[55,56] A clearer picture of the details of diuretic and ion interaction with the NKCC protein must await achievement and study of its crystal structure.

NKCC2 is expressed on the apical membranes of medullary and cortical TALs and macula densa segments.[57,58] Its abundance is increased by prolonged infusion of saline or furosemide.[57] A closely related gene, NKCC1, encodes a protein that is widely expressed in transporting epithelia.[51] In contrast to NKCC2, NKCC1 is implicated in uptake and secretion of Cl^- and NH_4^+ at the basolateral membrane of the medullary CDs.[59]

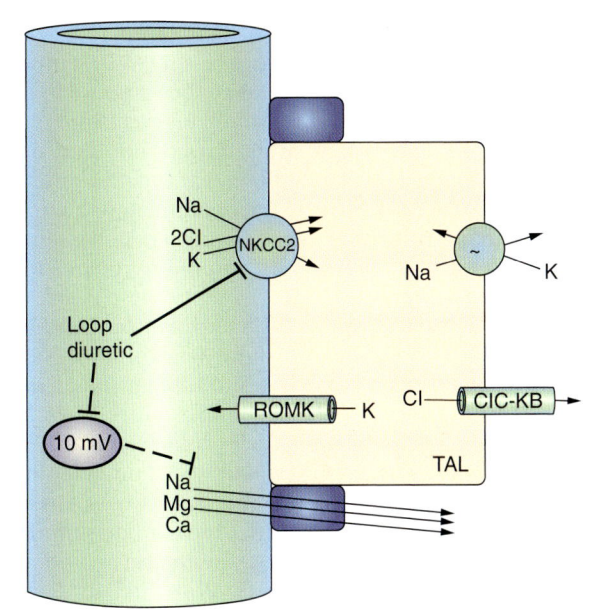

Figure 51.3 Mechanisms of diuretic action along the loop of Henle. The figure shows a model of thick ascending limb cells. Na^+ and Cl^- are reabsorbed across the apical membrane via the loop diuretic–sensitive Na-K-2Cl cotransporter 2 (NKCC2). Loop diuretics bind to and block this pathway directly. Note that the transepithelial voltage along the thick ascending limb is oriented with the lumen positive relative to blood (circled value, given in millivolts [mV]). This transepithelial voltage drives a component of Na^+ (and calcium and magnesium; see Figure 51.4) reabsorption via the paracellular pathway. This component of Na^+ absorption is also reduced by loop diuretics because they reduce the transepithelial voltage. ClC-KB, A chloride channel protein; ROMK, renal outer medullary K^+ channel.

Hormones that stimulate cyclic adenosine monophosphate (cAMP), such as arginine vasopressin (AVP), enhance TAL reabsorption and should enhance the response to loop diuretics. In contrast, those that stimulate cyclic guanosine monophosphate (cGMP), such as nitric oxide and atrial natriuretic peptide (ANP), or those that increase intracellular [Ca^{2+}], such as 20-hydroxyeicosatetraenoic acid (20-HETE), or that activate the Ca^{2+} (polyvalent cation)–sensing protein[60] inhibit TAL reabsorption and reduce the response to loop diuretics.[61]

The rat TAL also transports NH_4^+,[62] which can substitute for K^+ on NKCC2. In the rat, there is a luminal Na^+-H^+ countertransporter that contributes to tubular fluid acidification. Loop diuretics block the luminal entry of Na^+ via NKCC2, but not the peritubular exit via the Na^+-K^+-ATPase, and thereby reduce the intracellular [Na^+] sufficiently to promote luminal Na^+ uptake via the Na^+-H^+ countertransport process. This is one reason that furosemide stimulates acid excretion in the rat.[63] In some studies, furosemide has not affected net acid excretion or urine pH in normal human subjects.[64]

Loop diuretics reduce proximal fluid reabsorption modestly. This effect has been ascribed to a weak CAI action. However, furosemide depresses proximal reabsorption in tubules perfused with HCO_3^--free solutions.[65] Moreover, bumetanide, which is a much less potent inhibitor of carbonic anhydrase, also impairs proximal fluid reabsorption.[66]

Furosemide exerts two contrasting effects on reabsorption in the superficial distal tubule. Increased delivery to the unsaturated distal tubule reabsorption process increases Na^+ reabsorption.[63] However, Velazquez and Wright perfused rat distal tubules in vivo to obviate the confounding effects of altered delivery.[67] They concluded that furosemide, but not bumetanide, was a weak inhibitor of the thiazide-sensitive Na-Cl cotransporter (NCC). Loop diuretics also inhibit NaCl transport in short descending limbs of the loop of Henle[68] and collecting ducts (CDs).[69] Although the TAL is clearly the major site of action of loop diuretics, actions at other nephron segments contribute to the natriuresis by blunting the expected increase in reabsorption in the proximal tubule (in response to volume depletion) and the distal nephron (in response to increased load). Reabsorption of solute from the water-impermeable TAL segments dilutes the tubular fluid and concentrates the interstitium. Its inhibition by loop diuretics impairs both free water excretion during water loading and free water reabsorption during dehydration.[70] Loop diuretics increase the fractional excretion of Ca^{2+} by up to 30%.[71] The predominant mechanism is a decrease in the magnitude of the lumen-positive transepithelial potential (see Figures 51.3 and 51.4). A large fraction of transepithelial Ca^{2+} transport along the TAL traverses a paracellular pathway involving claudins 16 and 19 and is driven by the lumen-positive transepithelial potential.[72] By reducing its magnitude, loop diuretics lower passive calcium absorption along this segment. A second mechanism has been observed in some experiments, involving active Ca^{2+} transport, but this pathway is not affected by loop diuretics.[73]

The loop of Henle is the major nephron segment for reabsorption of Mg^{2+}.[71] Mg^{2+} transport along the TAL, like Ca^{2+} transport, traverses a paracellular pathway that involves claudins and is driven by the transepithelial potential difference. Loop diuretics can increase fractional Mg^{2+} excretion by more than 60%[74] by diminishing voltage-dependent paracellular transport[71] (see Figures 51.3 and 51.4) (see later discussion of adverse effects). Loop diuretics initially increase urate excretion by inhibiting proximal urate transport.[75] However, there is a succeeding reduction in urate clearance that is largely secondary to volume depletion.[76] The total RBF is maintained or increased and the GFR is little changed during administration of loop diuretics to normal subjects.[77] However, there is a marked redistribution of blood flow from the inner to the outer cortex.[78] The fall in papillary plasma flow depends on angiotensin II.[79] Furosemide increases the renal generation of prostaglandins.[80] Blockade of cyclo-oxygenase prevents furosemide-induced renal vasodilation.[81]

The macula densa participates importantly both in renin secretion and in TGF-mediated control of GFR. NaCl entry into macula densa cells regulates both processes; thus, loop diuretics affect both TGF and renin secretion. When the luminal NaCl concentration at the macula densa rises, as during ECV expansion, NaCl entry into macula densa cells leads to the production of adenosine, which interacts with adenosine 1 receptors on vascular smooth muscle and/or extraglomerular mesangial cells, activating phospholipase C. This activation leads to depolarization and activation of voltage-dependent Ca^{2+} channels, which contract afferent arterioles and reduce GFR (the TGF response).[82] NaCl transport across the luminal membrane of macula densa cells traverses the NKCC2.[58] Loop diuretics, by blocking NaCl entry into macula densa cells, block TGF completely.[83] This is one reason that loop diuretics tend to preserve GFR despite ECV depletion.

Loop diuretics also stimulate renin secretion, both short term and long term. Although this effect results, in part, from ECV depletion, a major component is from direct effects of loop diuretics on the macula densa. NaCl uptake into macula densa cells inhibits renin secretion acutely and inhibits renin synthesis chronically.[84] Macula densa cells were shown to express cyclo-oxygenase-2 (COX-2). Schnermann and colleagues showed that lowering NaCl concentration bathing a macula densa cell line acutely increased the release of PGE_2, followed by a delayed induction of COX-2 expression. A similar stimulation of COX-2 expression was also caused by furosemide and bumetanide. A lowering of medium Cl concentration was followed by rapid phosphorylation of p44/42 and p38 MAP kinases, and the presence of p44/42 and p38 inhibitors prevented the stimulation of COX-2 expression by low chloride. In summary, a decrease in luminal NaCl concentration activates and transcriptionally induces COX-2, causing release of prostaglandin E_2 (PGE_2) release, and prostaglandin E_2 receptor type 4 (EP4)–mediated stimulation of renin secretion and renin synthesis. Nitric oxide synthase inhibition with L-NAME has been found to completely block the increase in renin messenger RNA (mRNA) after administration of furosemide for 4 days by minipump infusion.[85] Similarly, the increase in renin content in renal microvessels caused by a 5-day furosemide treatment was completely prevented by the nitric oxide inhibitor L-NAME (N^G-nitro-L-arginine methyl ester).[86] Yet mice made deficient in both the neuronal and endothelial forms of nitric oxide synthase display relatively normal renin

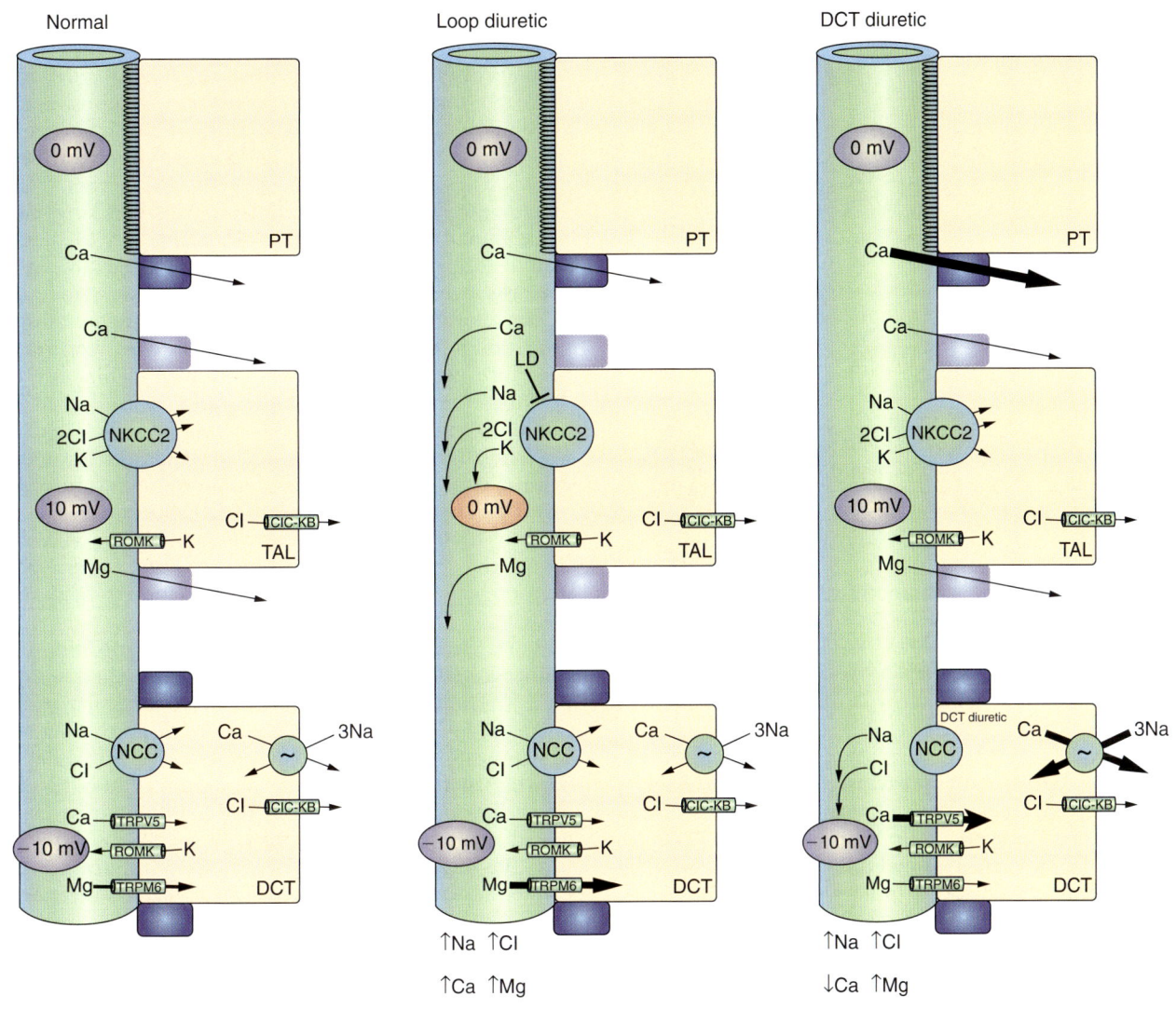

Figure 51.4 Possible mechanisms of diuretic effects on calcium and magnesium excretion. Typical cells from the proximal tubule (PT), thick ascending limb (TAL), and distal convoluted tubule (DCT) are shown. Calcium reabsorption occurs along the distal convoluted tubule largely via a transient receptor potential channel (TRPV5). Magnesium reabsorption occurs along the distal convoluted tubule largely via a transient receptor potential channel (TRPM6). Transepithelial voltages (representative but arbitrary values, given in millivolts [mV]) are shown. Net effects on electrolyte excretion are shown at the *bottom*. Normal conditions are at the *left*. Treatment with loop diuretics (LD) is shown in the *middle*; treatment with DCT diuretics is shown on the *right*. Loop diuretics reduce the magnitude of the lumen-positive transepithelial voltage, thereby retarding passive calcium and magnesium reabsorption. Passive calcium and magnesium reabsorption appears to traverse the paracellular pathway. Long-term treatment, especially with DCT diuretics, increases proximal Na^+ and Ca^{2+} reabsorption; thus, less calcium is delivered distally. Enhanced distal calcium absorption, driven by DCT diuretics, also occurs. Effects of DCT diuretics to increase magnesium excretion remain incompletely understood. ClC-KB, A chloride channel protein; NCC, Na-Cl transporter; NKCC2, Na-K-2Cl cotransporter 2; ROMK, renal outer medullary K^+ channel; ↑, increase(d); ↓, decrease(d).

responses to loop diuretics.[87] These data have been interpreted to suggest that nitric oxide synthesis plays a permissive role in macula densa–mediated renin secretion.

PHARMACOKINETICS AND DIFFERENCES BETWEEN DRUGS

Loop diuretics are absorbed promptly after ingestion, but their bioavailabilities vary. Because bumetanide and torsemide are more completely absorbed than furosemide, changing from intravenous to oral dosing requires a doubling of the furosemide dose but does not require changing the bumetanide or torsemide dose. Moreover, there is considerable variation in furosemide absorption, both between patients and over time,[88] that is accentuated by food intake.[89,90]

Once absorbed, loop diuretics circulate largely bound to albumin (91% to 99%), greatly limiting their clearance by glomerular filtration. The diuretic volume of distribution varies inversely with the serum albumin concentration,[91] but this is not usually a major determinant of diuretic responsiveness (see later).[92] The metabolism of loop diuretics comprises both hepatic and renal mechanisms; the relative fractions that are cleared by each mechanism differ among agents. Loop diuretics, thiazides, and CAIs are all secreted avidly by a probenecid-sensitive organic anion transporter in proximal tubule cells (Figure 51.5).[93,94] Diuretics gain

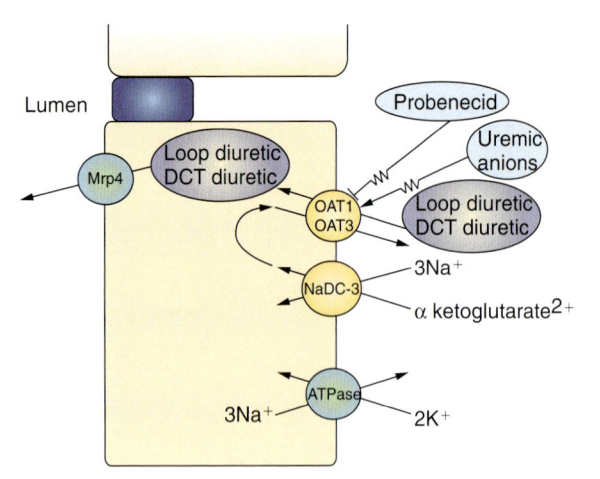

Figure 51.5 Mechanisms of diuretic secretion by proximal tubule cells. Cell diagram of the S2 segment of the proximal tubule showing secretion of anionic diuretics, including loop diuretics and distal convoluted tubule (DCT) diuretics. Peritubular uptake by an organic anion transporter (primarily OAT1, although OAT3 may play a smaller role) occurs in exchange for α-ketoglutarate, which is brought into the cell by the Na⁺-dependent cation transporter NaDC-3. Luminal secretion can occur via a voltage-dependent pathway or in exchange for luminal hydroxyl (OH⁻) or urate. A portion of the luminal transport traverses multidrug resistance–associated protein 4 (Mrp4). ATPase, adenosine triphosphatase.

access to tubular fluid almost exclusively by proximal secretion. Studies have characterized this weak organic anion (OA^-) transport process. Four isoforms of an OA transporter (OAT) have been cloned and are expressed in the kidney.[94,95] Peritubular uptake by an OAT is a tertiary active process (see Figure 51.5). Energy derives from the basolateral Na^+-K^+-ATPase that provides a low intracellular [Na^+] that drives an uptake of Na^+ coupled to α-ketoglutarate (α-KG) to maintain a high intracellular level of α-KG. This in turn drives a basolateral OA-α-KG countertransporter. OAT1 is expressed on the basolateral membrane of the S2 segment of the proximal tubule.[96] A mouse colony deficient in OAT1 was generated and shown to exhibit dramatically impaired renal OA secretion and furosemide resistance.[97] A similar effect was observed in OAT3-deficient mice, suggesting that both OAT1 and OAT3 mediate secretion of loop diuretic by proximal cells, and that a lack of either is not fully compensated by the other.[98]

OATs translocate diuretics into the proximal tubule cell, where they can be sequestered in intracellular vesicles. They are secreted across the luminal membrane by a voltage-driven OA transporter[99] and by a countertransporter in exchange for urate or OH^-.[95] The orphan transporter hNPT4 (human sodium phosphate transporter 4; SLC17A3) has been identified as an organic anion efflux transporter that likely also secretes furosemide and bumetanide.[100] In addition, the multidrug resistance–associated protein 4 (MRP4) has been identified as the third type of transporter involved in the urinary excretion of diuretics; mice lacking Mrp4 exhibited an almost two-fold lower excretion of furosemide and hydrochlorothiazide.[101] Approximately 50% of furosemide is eliminated by metabolism to the inactive glucuronide. Only the unmetabolized and secreted fraction is available to inhibit NaCl reabsorption. In contrast, bumetanide and torsemide are metabolized in the liver.[102,103] Slow-release furosemide is more effective in reducing blood pressure and treating edema, highlighting the importance of pharmacokinetics in diuretic responsiveness.[104] Torsemide's action is approximately twice as long as furosemide's,[105] and bumetanide's action is shorter than furosemide's. These differences may be clinically relevant,[106,107] but large controlled trials studying this issue are lacking. Unlike the elimination of bumetanide or torsemide,[105] the elimination of furosemide in patients with CKD is greatly reduced because its metabolism to the inactive glucuronide occurs in the kidney; in contrast, metabolic inactivation of bumetanide and torsemide occurs mainly in the liver and therefore they are unaffected by uremia.[4] This difference prolongs the $t_{1/2}$ of furosemide in CKD, leading to drug accumulation. However, the fraction of a dose excreted unchanged in patients with CKD is greater for furosemide, leading to an enhanced natriuretic response (Figure 51.6). There is therefore a tradeoff in the selection of a loop diuretic in CKD: Furosemide can accumulate and cause ototoxicity at high doses, whereas bumetanide retains its metabolic inactivation but is therefore somewhat less potent.

Renal clearance of the active form of loop diuretics is reduced in CKD in proportion to the creatinine clearance.[108] There is competition both for peritubular uptake[94] and for luminal secretion[99] with other OAs, including urate, which accumulates in uremia. Metabolic acidosis depolarizes the membrane potential of proximal tubule cells,[109] which decreases OA secretion,[99] an effect that may explain why diuretic secretion is enhanced by alkalosis.[110] Therefore, the increased plasma levels of OAs and urate and the metabolic acidosis of CKD impair proximal tubule secretion of diuretics and, hence, impair their delivery to their active sites in the nephron.

Proximal secretion of active furosemide is potentiated by albumin.[111] In the rabbit, an equal fraction of administered furosemide is taken up by probenecid-sensitive mechanisms in the S2 (secretory) or the S1 segment of the proximal tubule, where it is conjugated and excreted as the inactive glucuronide (Figure 51.7).[112] Unlike the uptake and secretion of active furosemide by the S2 segment, uptake and metabolism by the S1 segment is enhanced by a drop in albumin concentration. Therefore, a low serum albumin concentration enhances furosemide metabolism[113] yet decreases tubular secretion of active diuretic.[111] The consequences of this process are described later (see "Nephrotic Syndrome").

The relationship between fractional sodium excretion and the log of the serum diuretic concentration is sigmoidal. There is a similar sigmoidal relation between fractional sodium excretion and the log of the urinary diuretic concentration (Figure 51.8). Inhibition of proximal secretion with probenecid shifts the curve of the plasma dose-response to the right but does not perturb the relationship between natriuresis and diuretic excretion.[114] Thus, natriuresis is related to the urinary concentration, but not the plasma concentration, of diuretic. The administration of indomethacin or other nonsteroidal anti-inflammatory drugs (NSAIDs) reduces the responsiveness of the tubule to furosemide.[115] This reduction is due predominantly to reduced generation of PGE_2, because a natriuretic response to

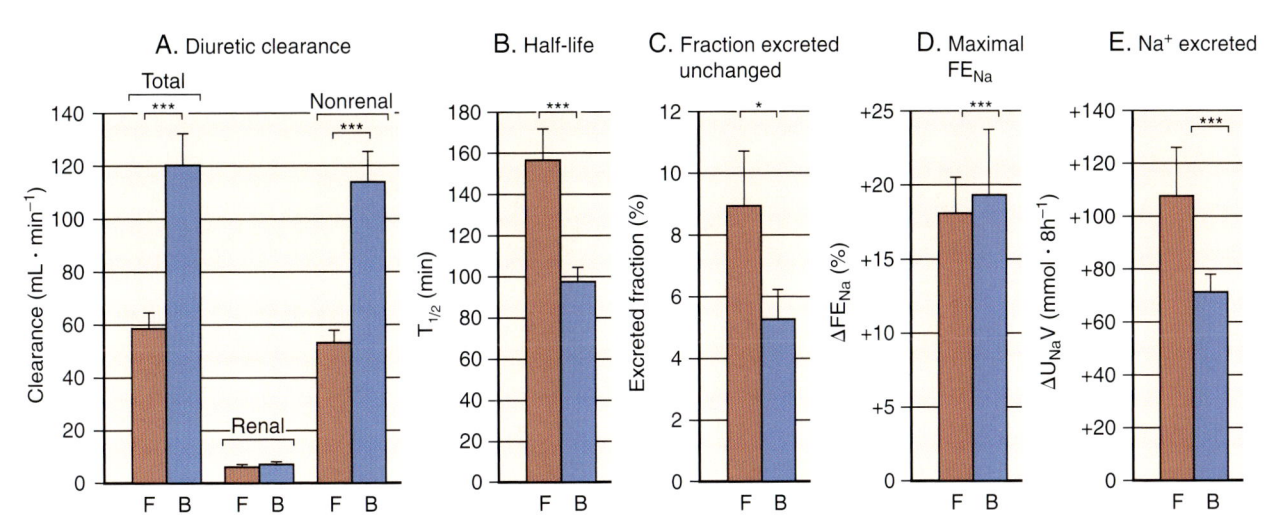

Figure 51.6 Comparison of the pharmacokinetics and dynamics of furosemide (F, 160 mg; metabolically inactivated in the kidney) and bumetanide (B, 4 mg; metabolically inactivated in the liver) in 10 subjects with chronic kidney disease (mean creatinine clearance 12 ± 2 mL/min). Significance of difference: *, $P < .05$; ***, $P < .005$. FE_{Na}, fractional excretion of sodium; $T_{1/2}$, half-life; U_{Na}, urinary sodium. (Redrawn from data in Voelker JR, Cartwright-Brown D, Anderson S, et al: Comparison of loop diuretics in patients with chronic renal insufficiency. *Kidney Int* 32:572-578, 1987.)

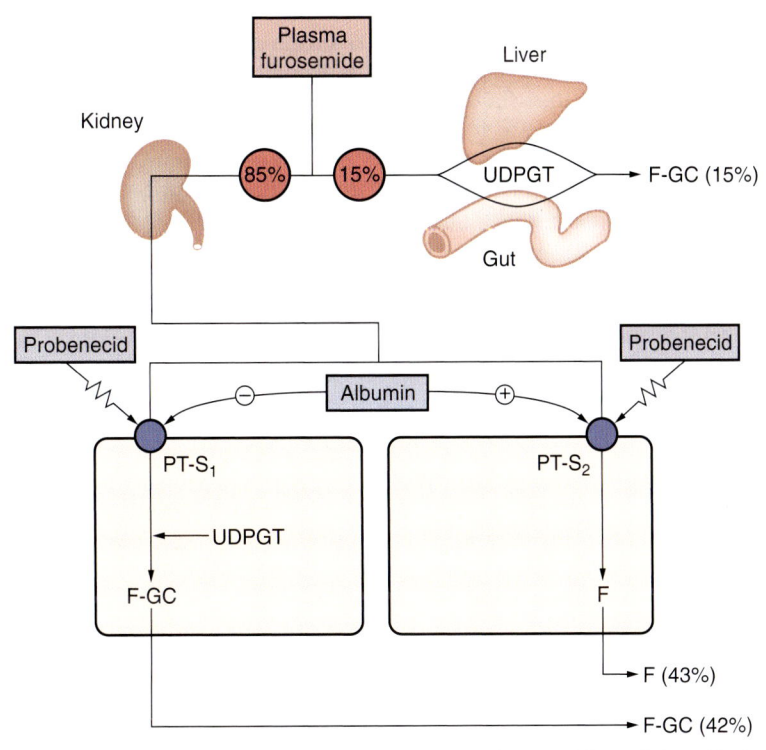

Figure 51.7 Diagrammatic representation of the disposition of intravenous furosemide and the effects of hypoalbuminemia or probenecid in normal or hypoalbuminemic rabbits. After intravenous administration of furosemide, 15% is metabolized by uridine diphosphate glucuronyl transferase (UDPGT) in the liver and gut to the inactive furosemide gluconide (F-GC). Of the remainder, 85% is transported by the kidney. Some 42% is taken up in the S1 segment of the proximal tubule ($PT-S_1$) and metabolized to the inactive gluconide, and the remainder is taken up by the S2 segment ($PT-S_2$) and secreted in active form into the lumen. Both uptake processes are inhibited by probenecid. Plasma albumin concentration facilitates uptake and secretion by $PT-S_2$ but inhibits uptake and metabolism by $PT-S_1$. (Drawn from data in Pichette V, Geadah D, du Souich P: The influence of moderate hypoalbuminemia on the renal metabolism and dynamics of furosemide in the rabbit. *Br J Pharmacol* 119:885-890, 1996.)

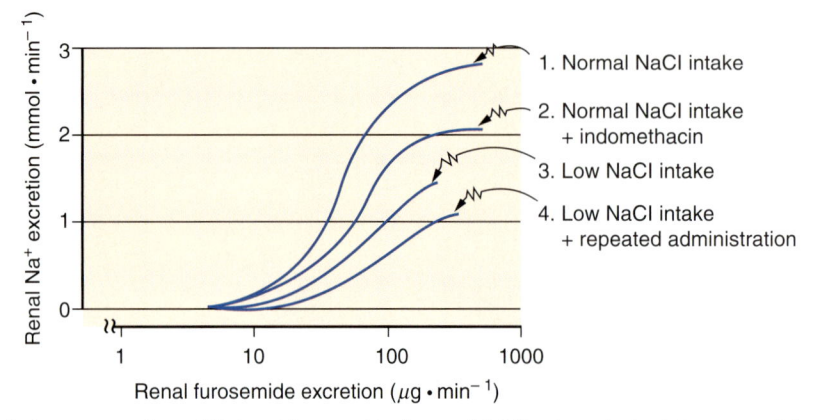

Figure 51.8 Relationship between excretion of Na⁺ and furosemide (log scale) following a bolus intravenous injection of 40 mg furosemide in normal subjects with a normal NaCl intake (1), with a normal NaCl intake after indomethacin (2), with a low Na⁺ intake (20 mmol/24 hours) (3), and for the third day of furosemide administration with a low Na⁺ intake (4). (Redrawn from data in Wilcox CS, Mitch WE, Kelly RA, et al: Response of the kidney to furosemide. *J Lab Clin Med* 102:450, 1983; and Chennavasin P, Seiwell R, Brater DC: Pharmacokinetic-dynamic analysis of the indomethacin-furosemide interaction in man. *J Pharmacol Exp Ther* 215:77, 1980.)

furosemide can be restored in indomethacin-treated rats by infusion of PGE_2.[116] A reduced dietary salt intake and repeated administration of furosemide during salt restriction[117] both diminish the renal tubular response to furosemide (see Figure 51.8).

Although knowledge of the pharmacogenetics of diuretics is still rudimentary, a number of studies have demonstrated that certain polymorphisms contribute to individual differences in the response to loop diuretics. For example, in 97 healthy whites, one study reported that the acute effects of loop diuretics were greater in subjects with polymorphisms in the genes encoding NCC and the β-subunit of ENaC, but smaller in those with a polymorphism in the gene encoding the γ-subunit of ENaC.[118] This finding suggests that individual variations in loop diuretic response may, in part, be attributed to lower or higher activities of transporters located distal to NKCC2. Another pharmacokinetic study identified female gender and polymorphisms in the gene encoding the organic anion transporter OATP1B1 as predictors for slower elimination of torsemide.[119]

CLINICAL INDICATIONS

Clinical indications for the use of loop diuretics are discussed later (see "Clinical Uses of Diuretics").

ADVERSE EFFECTS

Adverse effects of loop diuretics are discussed later (see "Adverse Effects of Diuretics").

THIAZIDES AND THIAZIDE-LIKE DIURETICS (DISTAL CONVOLUTED TUBULE DIURETICS)

SITES AND MECHANISMS OF ACTION

Thiazides and thiazide-like diuretics are moderately active drugs that increase excretion of sodium, chloride, and potassium while reducing excretion of calcium. The major site of action of thiazide and thiazide-like diuretics is the distal convoluted tubule (DCT), where they block coupled reabsorption of Na⁺ and Cl⁻ (Figure 51.9).[67,90,120] The true thiazides (benzothiadiazines) are chlorothiazide, hydrochlorothiazide, bendroflumethiazide, and others. Subsequent to their development, non-thiazide drugs with similar activities were developed. Substitution of the ring sulfone in the thiazides with a carbonyl group provides a group of quinazolinones with diuretic activity that is similar to the thiazides (cf. metolazone). Chlorthalidone, a substituted benzophenone that does not contain the benzothiadiazine molecular structure, exhibits strong carbonic anhydrase activity and a prolonged half-life and has seen widespread use as an antihypertensive.

The predominant effect of the thiazide diuretics is to inhibit the thiazide-sensitive Na-Cl cotransporter (NCC; SLC12A3). This protein is expressed in the DCT[121,122] and is inhibited directly by thiazides (see later). Several thiazides and thiazide-like drugs (e.g., chlorothiazide, hydrochlorothiazide, and chlorthalidone) also inhibit carbonic anhydrase, contributing to their natriuretic efficacy.[123] Yet patients with Gitelman's syndrome, who have a loss-of-function mutation in the NCC, demonstrate a dramatically impaired natriuretic response to thiazides,[124] confirming that the principal effect of these drugs is to inhibit NCC. Further, Na⁺ reabsorption by the proximal tubule is enhanced during long-term treatment with thiazides, even when the drug has significant CA-inhibiting capacity.[125] Finally, a sodium-dependent chloride-bicarbonate exchanger has been shown to mediate electroneutral sodium transport in the collecting duct and to also be inhibited by thiazides.[126]

Like loop diuretics, diuretics that are active in the DCT, including the thiazides, are organic anions that bind to the transport protein from the luminal surface. The mechanism(s) of NCC inhibition have been studied using two approaches. First, Beaumont and colleagues showed that [³H]metolazone binds avidly to kidney membrane proteins; its binding is inhibited competitively by Cl⁻, suggesting that Cl⁻ and diuretic compete for the same binding site.[127,128] These results are reminiscent of those of studies that utilized [³H]bumetanide to study properties of the NKCC proteins and were used to develop a kinetic model for the NCC.[129]

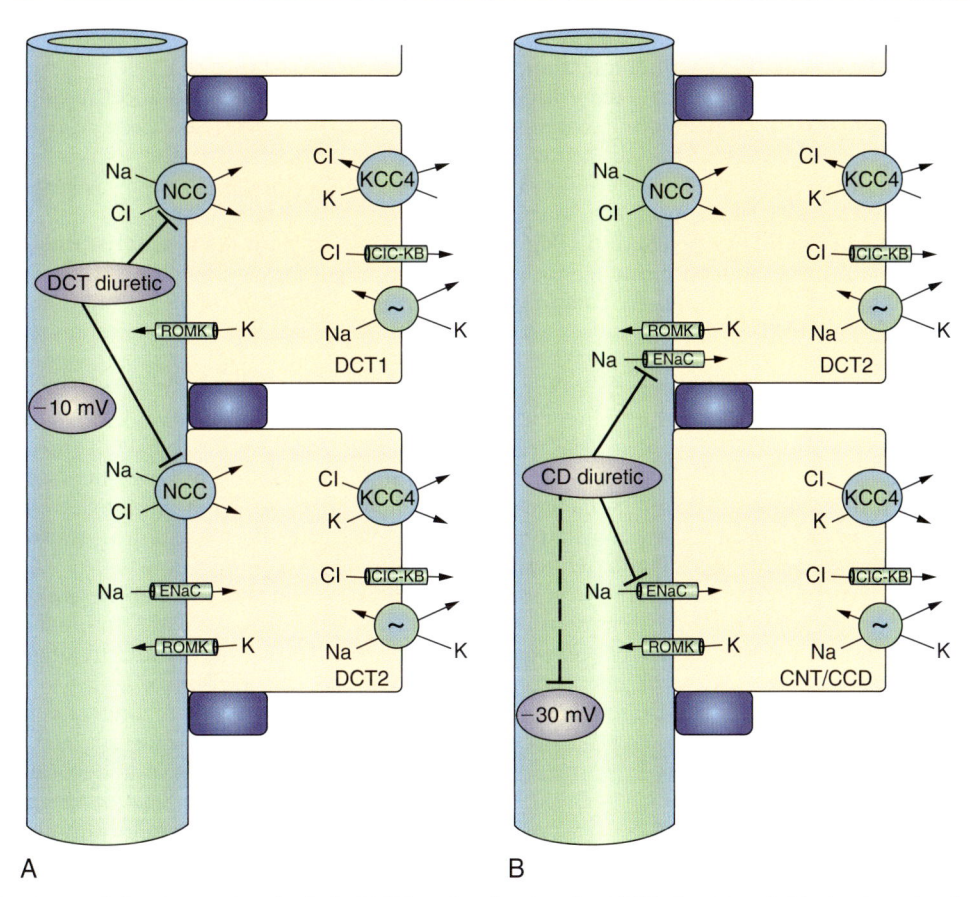

Figure 51.9 Mechanisms of distal convoluted tubule (DCT) and collecting duct (CD) diuretics. **A,** Mechanism of action of DCT diuretics. In rat, mouse, and human, two types of DCT cells have been identified, referred to here as DCT1 and DCT2. Na^+ and Cl^- are reabsorbed across the apical membrane of DCT1 cells only via the thiazide-sensitive Na^+-Cl^- cotransporter (NCC). This transport protein is also expressed by DCT2 cells where Na^+ can also cross through the epithelial Na^+ channel (ENaC; see text for details). Thus, the transepithelial voltage along the DCT1 is near to 0 mV, whereas it is finite and lumen-negative along the DCT2. **B,** Mechanism of action of CD diuretics. The late distal convoluted tubule cells (DCT2 cells) and connecting tubule (CNT) or cortical collecting duct (CCD) cells are shown. Na^+ is reabsorbed via ENaC, which lies in parallel with a renal outer medullary K^+ channel (ROMK). The transepithelial voltage is oriented with the lumen negative, relative to the interstitium (shown in the *circled value*), generating a favorable gradient for transepithelial K^+ secretion. Drugs that block the epithelial Na^+ value reduce the voltage toward 0 mV (effect indicated by *dashed line*), thereby inhibiting K^+ secretion. ClC-KB, A chloride channel protein.

Gamba and colleagues have expressed chimeras of the NCC in *Xenopus* oocytes and defined thiazide affinity on the basis of transport inhibition. The results suggest a more complicated picture. They conclude that thiazide diuretic affinity is conferred by transmembrane segments 8 through 12, whereas transmembrane segments 1 through 7 affect chloride affinity. Both domains are involved in determining Na^+ affinity.[130] These data suggest that the affinity of thiazide diuretics for binding to the transport protein is in a region distinct from the region that participates in Cl^- transport.

Thiazides increase potassium excretion, but they do not augment DCT secretion of K^+ directly.[90,131] Instead, their effects result from their tendency to stimulate aldosterone secretion, to increase distal flow, and to increase calcium reabsorption.[132] Mineralocorticoids, glucocorticoids,[133] and estrogens[134] enhance thiazide binding and tubular actions. Thiazides reduce Ca^{2+} excretion. Three potential and nonredundant mechanisms have been postulated (see Figure 51.4).[135,136] First, blockade of luminal NaCl entry reduces the tubule cell intracellular $[Na^+]$ sufficiently to enhance basolateral Na^+-Ca^{2+} exchange.[137] Second, thiazide-induced blockade of luminal NaCl entry reduces cell $[Cl^-]$ concentration, thereby hyperpolarizing the membrane voltage (making the interior of the cell more negative, electrically). Hyperpolarization increases calcium entry via the transient receptor potential channel subfamily V, member 5 (TRPV5) channel, which is expressed at the apical membrane of DCT and connecting tubule cells.[138,139] Third, thiazides stimulate proximal reabsorption of Ca^{2+} owing to ECV depletion.[140] The importance of this proximal effect has been highlighted because thiazides reduce Ca^{2+} excretion even when the TRPV5 channel has been knocked out and the major distal calcium reabsorptive pathway is absent.[141] However, other mechanisms in the DCT must also play a role, because a study in mice deficient for the DCT-specific protein parvalbumin showed that hydrochlorothiazide did not increase natriuresis but did increase hypocalciuria.[142] Similarly, a study in humans showed that hypovolemia is not the sole cause of hypocalciuria in patients with Gitelman's syndrome, who have a genetic inactivation of NCC.[143] Thiazides produce a sustained reduction in renal Ca^{2+} excretion that is accompanied by a small rise in serum Ca^{2+} concentration. Mg^{2+} excretion is enhanced by thiazide diuretics, at least during prolonged therapy[144] (see Figure 51.4). It has also been shown that transient receptor potential channel melastatin 6 (TRPM6) is a magnesium channel of the distal nephron.[145,146] Long-term thiazide treatment of mice diminishes TRPM6 mRNA expression modestly and reduces TRPM6 protein abundance by approximately 80%. Such changes would be expected to reduce magnesium reabsorption along the distal nephron, leading to Mg^{2+} wasting. Mg^{2+} depletion that can occur during chronic thiazide administration may be augmented by K^+ depletion.[144] Thiazides reduce urate clearance secondary to ECV depletion[76] and competition for tubular uptake.[93]

Expression of the water channel aquaporin-2 (AQP2) begins at the junction between the DCT and the connecting tubule. Thus, the NCC-expressing DCT comprises the terminal diluting segment of the kidney. Thiazides impair maximal urinary dilution but not maximal urinary concentration.[147] Thiazides also enhance water absorption from inner medullary collecting ducts in an AVP-independent manner.[148] This effect is correlated with an increase in AQP2 expression during long-term thiazide treatment.[149] These effects may contribute to the tendency of thiazide diuretics to produce hyponatremia. Central effects on thirst, however, may also contribute (see later discussion of adverse effects).

PHARMACOKINETICS OF AND DIFFERENCES AMONG THIAZIDES

Thiazides are readily absorbed. They are extensively bound to plasma proteins. They are eliminated largely through secretion by the S2 segment of the proximal tubule, mostly via OAT1 and OAT3.[94,98] The $t_{1/2}$ is prolonged in renal failure and in the elderly, reducing natriuretic efficacy.[150] The more lipid-soluble drugs (e.g., bendroflumethiazide and polythiazide) are more potent, have a more prolonged action, and are more extensively metabolized.[151] Chlorthalidone has a particularly prolonged action.[151] Indapamide is sufficiently metabolized to limit accumulation in renal failure.[151] Extrarenal effects of thiazide diuretics, including effects on platelet aggregation and vascular permeability, vary among the types of thiazide diuretics, possibly explaining differences in their cardiovascular effects.[152]

As stated previously, little is known about the pharmacogenetics of diuretics, but the available studies suggest that differences in individual responses are important. In one study, diuretic therapy in carriers of a variant of α-adducin, a cytoskeleton protein important for the function of renal Na^+-K^+-ATPase, was found to be associated with a lower risk of combined myocardial infarction and stroke than other antihypertensive therapies.[153] In another study, polymorphisms in with-no-lysine kinase 1 (WNK1), a kinase involved in the regulation of NCC, also affected the response to a thiazide diuretic.[154] Finally, polymorphisms in Nedd4-2, a ubiquitin ligase that regulates the sodium chloride cotransporter,[155] predicts the blood pressure response to hydrochlorothiazide in white subjects and cardiovascular outcome with hydrochlorothiazide in black subjects.[156]

CLINICAL INDICATIONS

The clinical indications for the use of thiazides and thiazide-like drugs are discussed later (see "Clinical Uses of Diuretics").

ADVERSE EFFECTS

Adverse effects of thiazides and thiazide-like drugs are discussed later (see "Adverse Effects of Diuretics").

DISTAL POTASSIUM-SPARING DIURETIC AGENTS

Distal K^+-sparing diuretics comprise those that directly block the epithelial Na^+ channel ENaC (amiloride and triamterene) and antagonists of the mineralocorticoid receptor (MRA) (spironolactone and eplerenone).

SITES AND MECHANISMS OF ACTION

Distal K^+-sparing diuretics act on the cells in the late DCT, connecting tubule, and cortical CD (the ASDN), where they inhibit luminal Na^+ entry via ENaC (see Figure 51.9).[120,157] They depolarize the lumen-negative transepithelial voltage, diminishing the electrochemical gradient for K^+ and H^+ secretion.[120,158]

Both amiloride and triamterene are organic cations that block ENaC directly from the luminal surface. Amiloride also inhibits NHE3, but the affinity of amiloride for NHE3 is low enough that the distal effects predominate in clinical use. In experimental work, congers of amiloride that are more selective for either ENaC or NHE3 have been developed, although they have not been employed clinically. Amiloride appears to bind ENaC in its conducting pore and is thus a pore blocker.[159] Amiloride binding is sensitive to the electric field, and the agent appears to compete with Na^+ for binding to the pore of the channel.[160] Amiloride may interact with several regions on the ENaC protein, but one amiloride-binding region comprises a short amino acid stretch within the extracellular loop.[161]

Spironolactone and eplerenone are competitive antagonists of the mineralocorticoid receptor. MRAs were developed when it was discovered that aldosterone is an 18-aldehyde derivative of corticosterone and that progesterone increases Na^+ excretion by blocking exogenously administered mineralocorticoid. Eventually, spironolactone was developed. It was found not to have any effect on urinary Na^+ or K^+ directly, but instead to competitively block the mineralocorticoid receptor. Structurally, spirolactone strongly resembles aldosterone. Eplerenone was developed as an attempt to find an MRA with fewer estrogenic side effects.

These drugs were employed for many years primarily to reduce the excretion of K^+ and net acid, especially when used in combination with other diuretics.[162] Amiloride and triamterene reduce the excretion of Ca^{2+} and Mg^{2+},[144,163] because these drugs cause a very modest natriuresis. Under certain circumstances, however, their natriuretic efficacy can be significant.

For example, spironolactone is more effective than furosemide in reducing cirrhotic ascites.[164] Furthermore, spironolactone is often an effective adjunct in the treatment of resistant hypertension.[165] This agent has achieved an important role in the treatment of congestive heart failure caused by systolic dysfunction,[166] although the mechanisms by which it achieves protection continue to be debated.

PHARMACOKINETICS

Triamterene is well absorbed. It is rapidly hydroxylated to active metabolites.[167] The drug and its metabolites are secreted by the organic cation pathway in the proximal tubule,[3] with half-lives of 3 to 5 hours. Triamterene and its active metabolites accumulate in patients with cirrhosis because of decreased biliary secretion,[168] and in the elderly,[169,170] and in patients with CKD[150] because of decreased renal excretion.

Amiloride is incompletely absorbed. Its duration of action is approximately 18 hours. It is secreted into the tubular fluid by the organic cation transport pathway.[171] Other organic cations, such as cimetidine, inhibit its secretion and prolong its half-life.[171] It accumulates in renal failure[172] and may worsen renal function.[173] Spironolactone is readily absorbed and circulates bound to plasma proteins. Its intrinsic half-life is short, but it is metabolized to active compounds with considerably prolonged actions. Spironolactone is metabolized to canrenones ($t_{1/2}$ = 16 hr) and to sulfur-containing metabolites, predominantly 7 alpha-thiomethylspirolactone ($t_{1/2}$ = 13 hr).[174] Canrenones are metabolized by the cytochrome P-4503A system.[175] Clinically, spironolactone has a $t_{1/2}$ of approximately 20 hours. It takes 10 to 48 hours to become maximally effective.[176] It is lipid soluble and enters distal renal tubules from the plasma.[177] Eplerenone has fewer antiandrogenic and proestrogenic effects.[178,179] However, it is metabolized with a half-life of 3 hours and therefore should be given twice daily.[180]

CLINICAL INDICATIONS

Distal K^+-sparing agents are used to prevent or treat hypokalemic alkalosis, especially in combination with a thiazide diuretic.[181] Amiloride can prevent amphotericin-induced hypokalemia and hypomagnesemia.[182] Spironolactone is indicated as a first-line agent for ECV expansion in the setting of cirrhotic ascites, in which it is more effective than daily furosemide.[183-185] It is indicated for heart failure associated with systolic dysfunction, in which its effects may include renal and extrarenal mineralocorticoid receptor blockade[186] and recommended doses are limited to 25 and 50 mg/day, respectively. Spironolactone is also used commonly to treat hypertension associated with hyperaldosteronism and for resistant hypertension,[165,187,188] and it may reduce proteinuria and progressive loss of kidney function in CKD[189,190] (however, see the following discussion of adverse effects). Eplerenone is indicated to prevent cardiac remodeling and systolic dysfunction in the setting of recent myocardial infarction.[191,192] Preliminary experimental data suggest that spironolactone may help prevent the development of CKD after ischemic AKI ("AKI-induced CKD").[193]

ADVERSE EFFECTS AND DRUG INTERACTIONS

Hyperkalemia is the most common complication of the distal K^+-sparing diuretics. The risk is dose dependent and increases considerably in patients with CKD or in those receiving K^+ supplements, angiotensin-converting enzyme (ACE) inhibitors, angiotensin receptor blockers (ARBs), NSAIDs, β-blockers, heparin, or ketoconazole.[194] The incidence of hyperkalemia-associated morbidity and mortality in Canada rose sharply after the publication of the Randomized Aldactone Evaluation Study (RALES), which demonstrated the efficacy of spironolactone in improving outcome in heart failure, and may relate to the consequent widespread use of this agent in patients with congestive heart failure and impaired renal function.[195] It is important to note that the original RALES study specifically excluded patients with several of these comorbidities. Renal failure appears to be another complication in this group.[196]

Gynecomastia may occur in men, especially as the dose is increased,[197] but even at low doses[198]; decreased libido and impotence have also been reported. Women may experience menstrual irregularities, hirsutism, or swelling and tenderness of the breast. Impaired net acid excretion can cause metabolic acidosis,[199] which worsens hyperkalemia.

Amiloride and triamterene accumulate in renal failure,[170,200] and triamterene accumulates in cirrhosis.[168] Therefore, these drugs should be avoided in patients with these conditions. Triamterene occasionally precipitates in the urinary collecting system and causes obstruction.[201] It can cause acute kidney injury when given with indomethacin.[202]

MISCELLANEOUS AGENTS

DOPAMINERGIC AGENTS

When given to normal subjects in low doses (1-3 μg/kg/minute), dopamine causes a modest increase in the GFR, reduces proximal reabsorption via a cAMP-induced inhibition of the Na^+-H^+ antiporter and increases Na^+ excretion.[203] Fenoldopam is a selective dopamine type 1 receptor agonist with little cardiac stimulation.[203] Unfortunately, these beneficial effects are reduced in patients who are critically ill and/or receiving vasopressors.[204] A comprehensive review of the literature has concluded that in controlled trials low-dose dopamine universally failed to improve renal outcomes in patients at high risk for AKI and that in the largest trials it had no effect on renal function, need for dialysis, or mortality in critically ill patients with early renal dysfunction.[204] Thus, there is currently no justification for the use of low-dose dopamine for renal protection. Dopamine infusion at higher rates has a role as a pressor agent in septic shock or refractory heart failure, but the benefits can be offset by arrhythmias.[204]

VASOPRESSIN RECEPTOR ANTAGONISTS

Vasopressin receptor antagonists are nonpeptide molecules that competitively inhibit one or more of the human vasopressin receptors, $V_{1a}R$, $V_{1b}R$, and V_2R.[205] Conivaptan is a combined $V_{1a}R/V_2R$ antagonist for intravenous use, whereas tolvaptan, mozavaptan, and lixivaptan are orally active V_2R-selective antagonists. All of these agents cause a free water diuresis without appreciable natriuresis or kaliuresis and they are therefore sometimes referred to as "aquaretics."[206] This effect is mainly attributed to inhibition of V_2R in the collecting duct, which prevents vasopressin from recruiting AQP2 water channels to increase water reabsorption. Therefore, vasopressin receptor antagonists can be used to treat hypervolemic or euvolemic hyponatremia, in which increased vasopressin is considered "inappropriate." Co-inhibition of $V_{1a}R$, which is located in vascular smooth muscle, could be beneficial to reduce coronary vasoconstriction, myocyte hypertrophy, and vascular resistance in patients with heart failure,[207] but definitive studies on this effect are lacking. At present, some 20 clinical trials have tested these agents against placebo or conventional therapy in patients with liver cirrhosis, heart failure, or hyponatremia secondary to SIADH.[208] In all trials, vasopressin receptor antagonists effectively raised serum sodium and helped correct hyponatremia. In addition, a positive effect on some secondary end points was observed in patients with heart failure, including improved mental condition and reductions in body weight, dyspnea, and ascites.[209–211] However, the Efficacy of Vasopressin Antagonist in Heart Failure Outcome Study with Tolvaptan (EVEREST), which involved 4133 patients hospitalized for heart failure (with or without hyponatremia), did not show a beneficial effect of tolvaptan on the primary outcome of death and rehospitalization for heart failure.[210] Thus, vasopressin receptor antagonists appear effective in the correction of hyponatremia but have not yet shown an effect on primary outcomes.

ADENOSINE TYPE I RECEPTOR ANTAGONISTS

Aminophylline is an adenosine receptor antagonist that inhibits NaCl reabsorption in the proximal tubule and diluting segments and causes a modest increase in GFR.[212] Highly selective adenosine I (A_1) receptor antagonists are natriuretic[213] and antihypertensive, and they potentiate furosemide-induced natriuresis in normal humans[214] and in patients with diuretic-resistant heart failure. A_1 antagonists disrupt glomerulotubular balance and TGF, thereby decreasing proximal reabsorption and increasing GFR.[213] Several A_1 receptor antagonists have been tested in patients with acute heart failure, but a large trial with the drug rolofylline did not show improvement in survival, heart failure status, or kidney function.[215]

UREA CHANNEL INHIBITORS

Urea channel inhibitors are a new class of diuretics that induce an osmotic diuresis by inhibiting urea reabsorption in the renal medulla. They are currently undergoing preclinical testing. An inhibitor of the urea channel UT-B (SLC14A1), increased urine output in rats without commensurate urinary sodium and potassium loss.[216] A small molecule screen recently also identified selective inhibitors of UT-A1 (SLC14A2).[217]

NESIRITIDE

Nesiritide is the recombinant form of B-type natriuretic peptide, which can be administered intravenously in acute decompensated congestive heart failure (see later discussion of clinical uses of diuretics in congestive heart failure). By stimulating cyclic guanosine monophosphate, this agent causes both a natriuresis and relaxation of smooth muscle.

NEPRILYSIN INHIBITORS

Neprilysin inhibitors prevent the breakdown of natriuretic peptides, and therefore contribute to natriuresis. The combined use of an ARB and neprilysin inhibitor (LCZ696) has been shown to reduce rates of cardiovascular death and hospitalization for heart failure in patients with class II, III, or IV heart failure.[218]

ADAPTATION TO DIURETIC THERAPY

Diuretics entrain a set of homeostatic mechanisms that limit their fluid-depleting actions and contribute to both resistance to these agents and their adverse effects.

DIURETIC BRAKING PHENOMENON

The first dose of a diuretic normally produces a reassuring diuresis. However, in normal subjects a new equilibrium is attained within 1 day, when body weight stabilizes and daily fluid and electrolyte excretion no longer exceeds intake.[117] This reaction is called the "diuretic braking phenomenon." The effects of dietary salt intake on the diuretic braking phenomenon during 3 days of loop diuretic administration to normal human subjects are shown in Figure 51.10.[117,219-221] During high Na^+ intake (270 mmol/24 hours), the first dose of furosemide (F_1) causes a large negative Na^+ balance over the ensuing 6 hours (*blue bars* in Figure 51.10A) followed by 18 hours during which Na^+ excretion is reduced well below intake (postdiuresis salt retention), which results in positive Na^+ balance (*light green areas* in Figure 51.10A) that offsets the preceding negative Na^+ balance. The natriuresis caused by the third daily dose of furosemide (F_3) is comparable to that caused by the first dose and also is followed by a restoration of Na^+ balance. Consequently, at high levels of Na^+ intake, subjects regain neutral Na^+ balance within 24 hours of each dose of furosemide and maintain their original body weight. A similar diuretic braking phenomenon occurs during established furosemide therapy.[77] During severe dietary Na^+ restriction (20 mmol/24 hours; Figure 51.10C), the first dose of furosemide produces a blunted natriuresis. However, Na^+ balance cannot be restored because of the low level of dietary Na^+ intake. Consequently, virtually all the Na^+ lost during the diuretic phase is represented as negative Na^+ balance for the day. Unlike in the high-salt protocol, tolerance manifests as a 40% reduction in the natriuretic response to the drug over 3 days. However, despite a blunted initial response and the development of tolerance, all subjects lose Na^+ and body weight. A loop diuretic given during a Na^+ intake of 120 mmol/24 hours (equivalent to a salt-restricted diet) causes Na^+ loss, but the loss is curtailed by a combination of postdiuretic renal salt retention and diuretic tolerance (Figure 51.10B).[221]

Furosemide kinetics and GFR are unchanged over 3 days of furosemide administration. What, then, mediates diuretic tolerance? During a low NaCl intake, the curve representing the relationship between natriuresis and furosemide excretion on a graph is shifted to the right by the third day of diuretic administration (see Figure 51.8), indicating a blunting of diuretic responsiveness.

One month of furosemide therapy for hypertension reduces the natriuretic response to a test dose of furosemide by 18%.[77] This tolerance cannot be ascribed to aldosterone, nor to a fall in plasma or ECV, because tolerance to furosemide is not prevented by spironolactone and does not develop during thiazide therapy, which causes similar reductions in body fluids. In fact, the natriuretic response to a test dose of a thiazide is augmented during furosemide therapy. Thus, tolerance to furosemide is class specific and depends on increased NaCl reabsorption at a downstream, thiazide-sensitive nephron site.

Furosemide activates the r RAAS and the sympathetic nervous system (SNS). However, postdiuretic Na^+ retention is not blunted by doses of an ACE inhibitor, which prevents any changes in plasma angiotensin II or aldosterone concentrations,[219,222,223] or by prazosin, which blocks adrenergic receptors even when an ace inhibitor and prazosin are given in combination.[220]

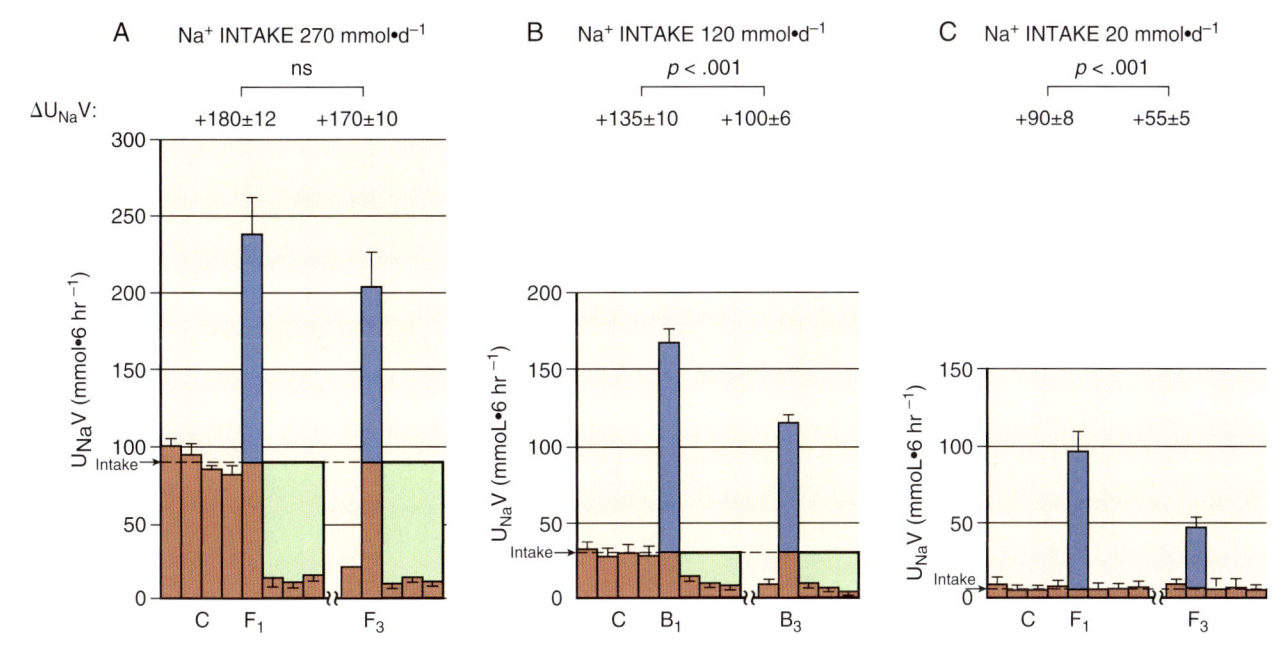

Figure 51.10 Effects of dietary salt intake on diuretic braking phenomenon. Renal Na$^+$ excretion (mmol/6 hours) for 24 hours before and after the first (F_1) and third (F_3) daily doses of (**A** and **C**) furosemide (40 mg intravenously) and (**B**) bumetanide (B_1, B_3, 1 mg intravenously) in groups of 8 to 10 normal subjects equilibrated to fixed daily Na$^+$ intakes. The average level of Na$^+$ intake (mmol/6 hours) is shown by *broken horizontal lines*. Negative Na$^+$ balance is indicated by *blue bars* and positive Na$^+$ balance by *light green areas*. The mean ± standard error of the mean (SEM) values for diuretic-induced increases in Na$^+$ excretion above baseline values ($\Delta U_{Na}V$) for 6 hours after the administration of the diuretic are shown at the *top*. (Redrawn from data in Wilcox CS, Mitch WE, Kelly RA, et al: Response of the kidney to furosemide. *J Lab Clin Med* 102:450, 1983.)

Micropuncture studies have shown that the blunted natriuretic response to furosemide during repeated administration can be attributed to three factors: (1) reduced NaCl delivery to the site of furosemide action; (2) limited inhibition of NaCl reabsorption by furosemide in the loop of Henle; and (3) enhanced ability of the distal tubule to reabsorb the extra NaCl load delivered during furosemide's upstream action.[224]

Rats receiving prolonged infusions of loop diuretics have considerable structural hypertrophy of the DCT, connecting tubule, and intercalated cells of the CD[225] that is partially dependent on angiotensin II.[226] The DCT and CD have a large increase in mRNA for insulin-like growth factor–binding protein-1[227] and increases in both Na$^+$-K$^+$-ATPase[228] and H$^+$-ATPase.[229] The Na$^+$-K$^+$-ATPase activity of rat cortical CD segments increases abruptly following an increase in cellular [Na$^+$], owing to mobilization of a latent pool of enzyme.[230] There is doubling of NCC expression in the distal tubules of rats adapted to diuretics.[231] Microperfusion studies of rats adapted to prolonged diuretic infusion have shown enhanced, aldosterone-independent distal Na$^+$ and Cl$^-$ absorption and K$^+$ secretion.[232] Therefore, diuretics induce structural and functional adaptations of downstream nephron segments, apparently in response to increased rates of NaCl delivery and to some extent to RAAS activation. Nephronal adaptation could underlie the inappropriate renal Na$^+$ retention that can persist for up to 2 weeks after abrupt cessation of diuretic therapy.[233]

Normal subjects fully eliminate a modest (100 mmol) NaCl load over 2 days.[234] However, when these subjects are challenged with the same NaCl load delivered after administration of bumetanide during simultaneous infusion of sufficient fluid, Na$^+$, K$^+$, and Cl$^-$ to prevent any losses, elimination of the load is prevented.[234] Thus, diuretics can entrain an ECV-independent NaCl retention; this is apparent when distal delivery is enhanced, as during high NaCl intake. Even a single dose of loop diuretic can cause a Cl$^-$ depletion "contraction" alkalosis, which may contribute to diuretic tolerance and the braking phenomenon.[64] In a study of normal subjects in whom mild metabolic alkalosis was produced by equimolar substitution of NaHCO$_3$ for NaCl, bumetanide-induced natriuresis was reduced during alkalosis despite enhanced delivery of bumetanide to the urine (Figure 51.11).[110] This finding implies a profound defect in tubular responsiveness to the diuretic. Several mechanisms may contribute. First, the Na-K-2Cl cotransporter has affinities for Na$^+$, K$^+$, and Cl$^-$ of 7.0, 1.3, and 67 mM, respectively. Thus, the [Cl$^-$] of tubular fluid may be low enough during Cl$^-$ depletion alkalosis to limit reabsorption by this transporter and thereby to limit the responsiveness to loop diuretics. Second, alkalosis causes glycosylation of the bumetanide-sensitive cotransporter, which could alter its transport function.[57] Third, thiazide-sensitive cotransporters in the rat DCT are increased by 40% during NaHCO$_3$ administration.[235]

Findings of these studies have several clinical implications (Table 51.1). First, dietary salt intake must be restricted, even in subjects receiving powerful loop diuretics, to obviate postdiuretic salt retention and to ensure the development of a negative NaCl balance. Second, during prolonged diuretic administration, subjects may be particularly responsive to another class of diuretic. Third, diuretic therapy should not be stopped abruptly unless dietary salt intake is curtailed, because the adaptive mechanisms limiting salt

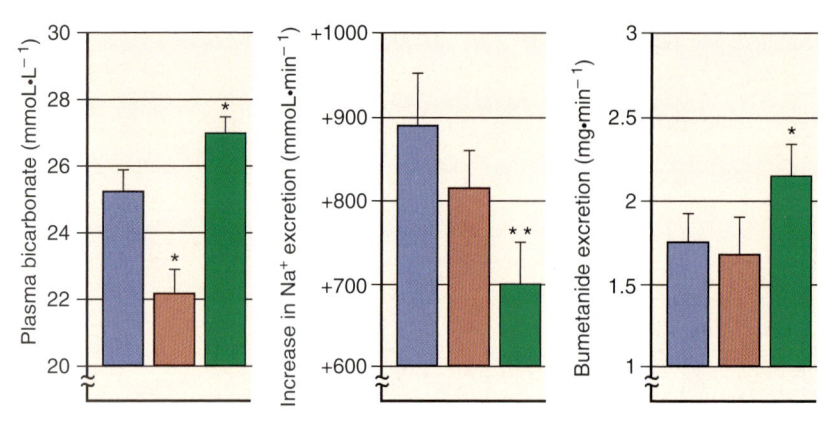

Figure 51.11 Mean ± standard error of the mean (SEM) values for plasma bicarbonate concentration, increase in Na⁺ excretion with bumetanide (1 mg intravenously), and rate of bumetanide excretion in normal subjects (n = 8) after equilibration to equivalent diets containing 100 mmol/24 hours of NaCl (control, *blue bars*), NH_4Cl (mild metabolic acidosis, *pink bars*), or $NaHCO_3$ (mild metabolic alkalosis, *green bars*). Compared with control: *P <.05; **P <.01. (Redrawn from Loon NR, Wilcox CS: Mild metabolic alkalosis impairs the natriuretic response to bumetanide in normal human subjects. *Clin Sci [Colch]* 94:287, 1998.)

Table 51.1 Strategies to Overcome Diuretic Braking

1. Restrict dietary salt to prevent postdiuretic salt retention.
2. Consider adding another class of diuretic.
3. Consider multiple daily dosing or a diuretic with prolonged action.
4. Do not stop diuretic therapy abruptly.
5. Prevent or reverse diuretic-induced metabolic alkalosis.

---

excretion persist for days after diuretic use. Fourth, selection of a diuretic with a prolonged action, or more frequent administration of the diuretic, will enhance NaCl loss by limiting the time available for postdiuretic salt retention. Indeed, a continuous infusion of a loop diuretic is somewhat more effective than the same dose given as a bolus injection in volunteers[236] and in patients with chronic kidney disease[237] despite a similar delivery of diuretic to the urine. Although a previous study showed that a continuous infusion is also more effective in cardiac disease,[238] a later study showed similar efficacy.[239] Fifth, prevention or reversal of diuretic-induced metabolic alkalosis may enhance diuretic efficacy.

There are similar patterns of furosemide-induced K⁺ loss followed by renal K⁺ retention[240] associated with an increase in the transtubular K⁺ gradient.[241] In contrast, loop diuretics induce ongoing renal K⁺ losses during severe salt restriction due to hyperaldosteronism[240] that can be countered by distal, K⁺-sparing diuretics.[241]

HUMORAL AND NEURONAL MODULATORS OF THE RESPONSE TO DIURETICS

RENIN ANGIOTENSIN ALDOSTERONE SYSTEM

Diuretic therapy increases plasma renin activity and serum aldosterone concentrations, as described previously. The initial rise in plasma renin activity with loop diuretics is independent of volume depletion or the sympathetic nervous system (SNS) and is related to inhibition of NaCl reabsorption at the macula densa.[242] Loop diuretics also stimulate renal prostacyclin release, which promotes renin secretion.[243] Later, renin secretion depends on ECV depletion and the SNS.

Activation of the RAAS in patients treated with diuretics and salt restriction for edema limits the natriuresis.[244] In a study of patients with heart failure (HF), ACE inhibition potentiated the diuretic and natriuretic responses to furosemide despite a drop in blood pressure.[245] However, severe volume depletion and azotemia can complicate overzealous therapy with ACE inhibitors, particularly in patients with HF who are receiving high doses of diuretics or in those with stenosis of both renal arteries or the artery to a single or dominant kidney.[246] Thus, the combination of diuretics and ACE inhibitors can be highly effective but requires careful surveillance.

During stimulation of the RAAS by severe dietary salt restriction, further diuretic-induced increases in serum aldosterone concentration promote renal K⁺ losses.[247] ACE inhibitors counter diuretic-induced increases in serum aldosterone concentration and blunt diuretic-induced hypokalemia.[240]

EICOSANOIDS

Prostaglandin E_2, acting on luminal prostaglandin receptor type 4 (EP_4), inhibits NaCl reabsorption via the NKCC2[248] and inhibits free water and Na⁺ reabsorption in the CDs via changes in cAMP (Figure 51.12).[249] Loop diuretics, thiazides, triamterene, and spironolactone increase prostaglandins substantially.[250] Inhibition of PG synthesis by NSAIDs can diminish the natriuresis and diuresis induced by furosemide,[251] hydrochlorothiazide,[252] spironolactone,[250] or triamterene (see Figure 51.12).[253] Microperfusion of the loop segment with PGE_2[116] restores the response to furosemide in indomethacin-treated rats. Indomethacin also blunts furosemide-induced renal[254] and capacitance vessel vasodilation[255] and stimulation of renin.[256] The blunting of furosemide-induced natriuresis by NSAIDs is potentiated by salt depletion[257] and is prominent in edematous patients.[251] The NSAIDs ibuprofen, naproxen, and sulindac blunt

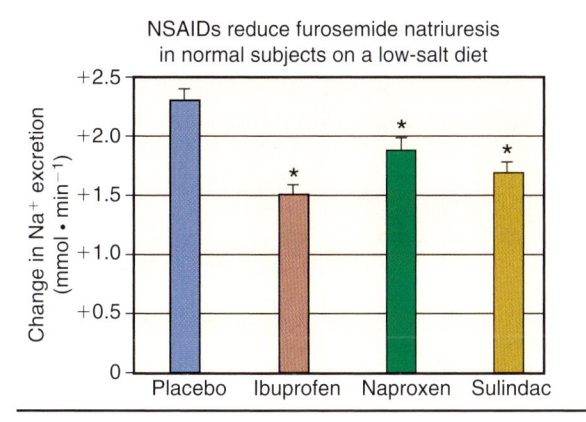

Figure 51.12 Mean ± standard error of the mean (SEM) values for change in Na⁺ excretion for 11 normal subjects given 40 mg of furosemide intravenously after placebo or after each of three nonsteroidal anti-inflammatory drugs: ibuprofen, 600 mg/6 hr for 3 doses; naproxen, 375 mg/12 hr for 2 doses; or sulindac, 200 mg/12 hr for 2 doses. (Drawn from data from Brater DC, Anderson S, Baird B, et al: Effects of ibuprofen, naproxen, and sulindac on prostaglandins in men. *Kidney Int* 27:66-73, 1985. Printed with permission.)

Table 51.2 Common Causes of Diuretic Resistance

Incorrect diagnosis (e.g., venous or lymphatic edema)
Inappropriate NaCL or fluid intake
Inadequate drug reaching tubule lumen in active form because of:
  Noncompliance
  Dose inadequate or too infrequent
  Poor absorption (e.g., due to uncompensated HF)
  Decreased renal blood flow (e.g., due to HF or cirrhosis of liver, or in elderly patient)
  Decreased functional renal mass (e.g., due to AKI or CKD, or in elderly patient)
  Proteinuria (e.g., due to nephrotic syndrome)
Inadequate renal response because of:
  Low glomerular filtration rate (e.g., due to AKI, CKD)
  Decreased effective extracellular fluid volume (e.g., due to edematous conditions)
  Activation of renin angiotensin aldosterone system (e.g., due to edematous conditions)
  Nephron adaptation (e.g., due to prolonged diuretic therapy)
  Nonsteroidal antiinflammatory drugs (e.g., indomethacin, aspirin)

AKI, Acute renal failure; HF, heart failure; CKD, chronic kidney disease.

furosemide-induced natriuresis similarly. A COX-2 inhibitor blocks furosemide-induced renin secretion but not natriuresis, although other studies show an effect of COX-2 inhibition on Na⁺ reabsorption.[258] It is COX-1 that facilitates natriuresis in the distal nephron.[259] Salt-sensitive hypertensive subjects have a blunted natriuretic response to furosemide that may be related to a paradoxical reduction in renal excretion of 20-HETE. Thus, COX-1 products mediate a part of furosemide-induced natriuresis, whereas COX-2 products mediate renin secretion. 20-HETE may be an important positive modulator of salt excretion.

Loop diuretics also increase the excretion of the thromboxane A_2 (TxA_2) metabolite TxB_2. Inhibition of TxA_2 synthesis or receptors in the rat increases furosemide diuresis[260] and diminishes the renal vasodilation.[261] Thus, TxA_2 may antagonize the actions of loop diuretics.

ARGININE VASOPRESSIN

AVP increases after administration of furosemide.[262] This may be a response to a reduced blood volume. Plasma AVP is increased in many edematous states, such as HF and liver cirrhosis,[263] especially in those who demonstrate hyponatremia during thiazide treatment.[264] AVP stimulates K⁺ secretion in the rat distal tubule.[265] Diuretic-induced AVP release contributes to hypokalemia, because the kaliuretic response to furosemide is reduced by 40% in subjects whose AVP release is suppressed by a water load.[247] In addition, despite its classic role as a water balance hormone, AVP has been shown to increase the activity of both NCC and ENaC, possibly compounding sodium retention in edematous states.[266,267]

CATECHOLAMINES AND SYMPATHETIC NERVOUS SYSTEM

The first dose of furosemide raises the heart rate and plasma catecholamine concentrations.[110,220] Blockade of α_2-adrenergic receptors with prazosin does not modify the ensuing renal salt retention[220] but blockade of these receptors blunts the renin release.[242] Short-term, furosemide-induced ECV depletion in the conscious rat activates sympathetic nerve activity that stabilizes the blood pressure.[268]

ATRIAL NATRIURETIC PEPTIDE

Diuretics are often used to treat patients who have an expanded blood volume and elevated levels of ANP. Administration of furosemide to dogs with congestive heart failure (CHF) reduces ANP levels.[269] Infusion of ANP in this dog model promotes furosemide-induced natriuresis and blunts both activation of the RAAS and the fall in GFR. Thus, a drop in ANP contributes to postdiuretic renal NaCl retention.[269]

DIURETIC RESISTANCE

Diuretic resistance implies an inadequate clearance of edema despite a full dose of diuretic. The principal causes are summarized in Table 51.2. The first step is to select the appropriate target response (e.g., a specific body weight) and to ensure that the edema is due to inappropriate renal NaCl and fluid retention rather than to lymphatic or venous obstruction or redistribution (Figure 51.13). Diuretics do not prevent edema caused by dihydropyridine calcium

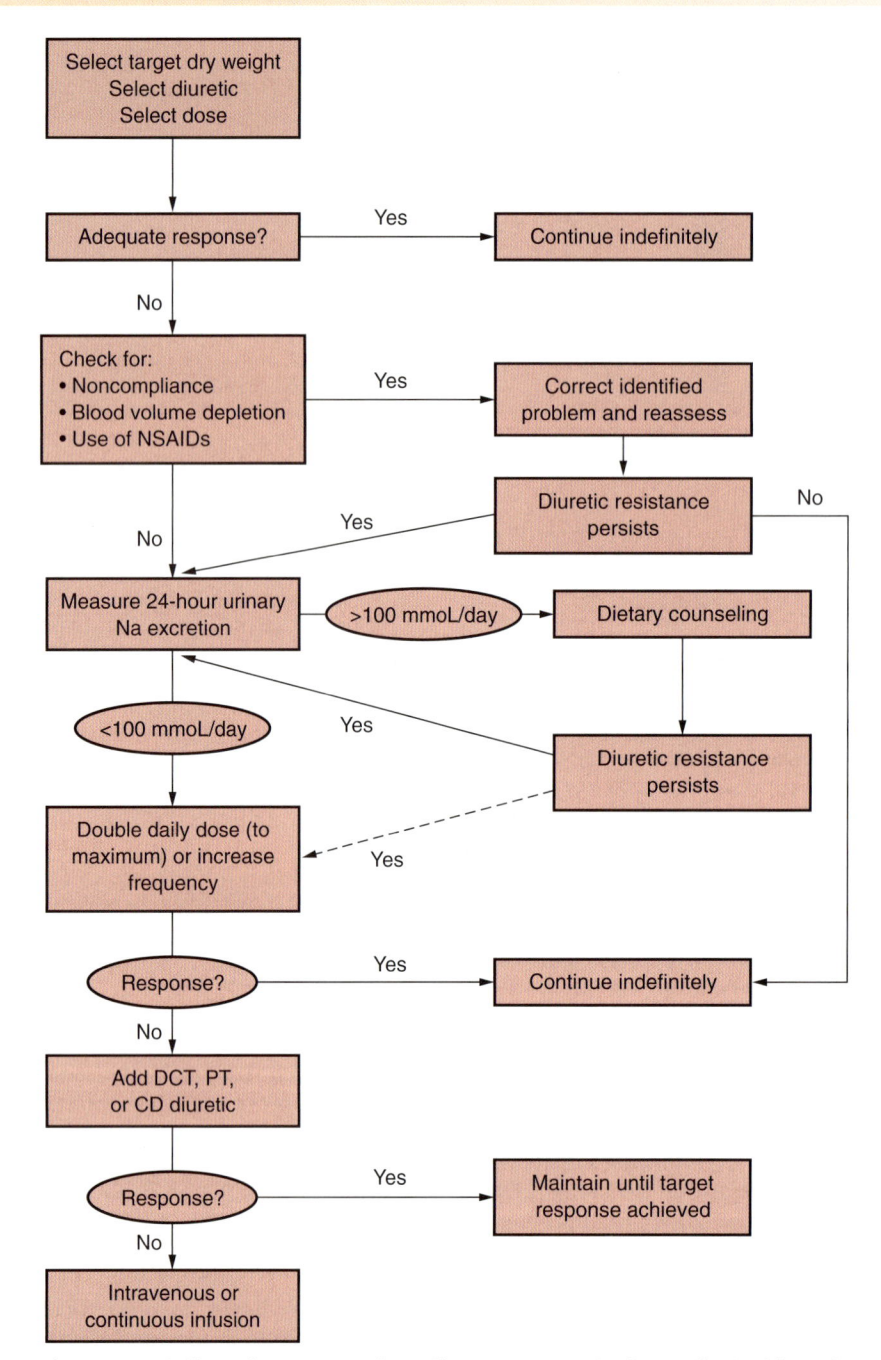

Figure 51.13 Diagrammatic representation of an approach to the management of a patient with resistance to a loop diuretic. CD, Collecting duct diuretic (e.g., amiloride, triamterene, or spironolactone); DCT, distal convoluted tubule diuretic (e.g., thiazide); NSAIDs, nonsteroidal antiinflammatory drugs; PT, proximal tubule diuretic (e.g., acetazolamide). (From Ellison DH, Wilcox CS: Diuretics: use in edema and the problem of resistance. In Brady HR, Wilcox CS, editors: *Therapy in nephrology and hypertension,* 2nd ed, London, 2003, Elsevier Science.)

channel blockers.[270] The next step is to exclude noncompliance, severe blood volume depletion, and concurrent NSAID use. Thereafter, dietary NaCl intake should be quantitated. In the steady state, this can be assessed from measurements of 24-hour Na^+ excretion. For patients with mild edema or hypertension, a daily Na^+ intake of 100 to 120 mmol may be sufficient. For patients with diuretic resistance, the help of a dietitian is usually necessary to reduce daily Na^+ intake to 80 to 100 mmol. In patients who are not in steady state (e.g., patients with worsening heart failure), urine sodium will decrease, a step that may be used as an indication to intensify diuretic therapy.[271] The diuretic dose must be above the natriuretic threshold (the steep part of the dose-response curve in Figure 51.8). Outpatients should be able to detect an increase in urinary volume within 4 hours of an administered dose; urine volume can be measured directly in patients who are hospitalized. If a diuresis does not occur, the next step is to double the dose until an effective dose or the maximum safe dose is reached. The next step is to give two daily doses of the diuretic. Furosemide and bumetanide act for only 3 to 6 hours. Two daily half-doses, by interrupting postdiuretic salt retention, produce a greater response than the same total dose given once daily, as long as both are above the diuretic threshold. Concurrent disease may impair absorption of the diuretic. Thus, a more bioavailable diuretic, such as torsemide, may be preferable to furosemide.[106] Diuretic resistance is often accompanied by a pronounced metabolic alkalosis,[110] which may be reversed by administration of KCl or addition of a distal K^+-sparing diuretic.

A progressive increase in diuretic dosage may produce an inadequate reduction in body fluids because of activation of NaCl-retaining mechanisms. ACE inhibitors can sometimes restore a diuresis in resistant patients with HF,[244] but a fall in blood pressure often limits the response. Adaptive changes in downstream nephron segments during prolonged diuretic therapy[77,225] provide a rational basis for combining diuretics (see the following section). Highly resistant patients can be admitted for a trial of intravenous infusion of loop diuretic or ultrafiltration.[272]

DIURETIC COMBINATIONS

Full doses of more than one diuretic acting on the same transport mechanism are less than additive, whereas use of several diuretics acting on a separate mechanism may be synergistic.[5,273]

LOOP DIURETICS AND THIAZIDES

A loop diuretic and a thiazide or thiazide-like drug (e.g., hydrochlorothiazide or metolazone) are synergistic in normal subjects and in subjects with edema or renal insufficiency.[273-277] Metolazone is equivalent to bendrofluazide in enhancing NaCl and fluid losses in furosemide-resistant subjects with heart failure or the nephrotic syndrome.[278] During prolonged furosemide therapy, the responsiveness to a thiazide is augmented.[77] Patients with advanced CKD (GFR < 30 mL/min) that is unresponsive to thiazide alone show a marked natriuresis when a thiazide is added to loop diuretic therapy,[276] probably by blockade of enhanced distal tubular Na^+ reabsorption.[279] However, such combination therapy should be initiated under close surveillance because of a high associated incidence of hypokalemia, excessive ECV depletion, and azotemia.[280]

LOOP DIURETICS OR THIAZIDES AND DISTAL POTASSIUM-SPARING DIURETICS

Amiloride or triamterene increases furosemide natriuresis only modestly but curtails the excretion of K^+ and net acid[63] and preserves total body K^+.[281] Distal K^+-sparing agents are generally contraindicated in renal failure because they may cause severe hyperkalemia and acidosis.

CLINICAL USES OF DIURETICS

A general algorithm for diuretic therapy in the treatment of renal insufficiency, nephrotic syndrome, liver cirrhosis, and heart failure is shown in Figure 51.14.[282]

EDEMATOUS CONDITIONS

The first aim in the treatment of edema is to reverse the primary cause by restoring hemodynamics and cardiac output in patients with heart failure (e.g., use of vasodilators or elimination of cardiac depressant drugs), by improving hepatic function in patients with cirrhosis and ascites (e.g., stopping alcohol intake), or by diminishing proteinuria in patients with the nephrotic syndrome (e.g., administration of ACE inhibitors or ARBs). Although the GFR is not reduced by low-dose diuretic therapy in normal subjects, it can be reduced in those with CKD or if there is an abrupt fall in BP, especially if this is complicated by orthostatic hypotension. Moreover, overzealous diuresis decreases the cardiac output, BP, and renal function, and stimulates the RAAS, the SNS, prostaglandins, and AVP, all of which may compromise the desired hemodynamic and renal responses.[283] Therefore, diuretic therapy for edema should be initiated with the lowest effective dose. Additional drugs can be used to counteract unwanted actions. For example, ACE inhibitors, ARBs, or MRAs can prevent the expression of an activated RAAS and enhance fluid losses, yet diminish K^+ depletion (see Figure 51.20). The use of a second diuretic can have a synergistic action, whereas the use of a distal K^+-sparing agent may counteract unwanted hypokalemia, alkalosis, or Mg^{2+} depletion (see "Adaptation to Diuretic Therapy").

Dietary Na^+ intake should be restricted to 2.5 to 3 g daily (corresponding to 107 to 129 mmol/24 hours) in patients with mild edema. Increasingly severe Na^+ restrictions to 2 grams daily (86 mmol/24 hours) are required for patients with refractory edema.

Some resistance to diuretic therapy should be anticipated in all patients with CKD and those with more than mild edema (Figure 51.15).

CONGESTIVE HEART FAILURE

Congestive heart failure is classified as systolic and diastolic heart failure (i.e., symptomatic heart failure with preserved ejection fraction). The therapeutic approach to cardiac failure depends on the cause and whether there is acute decompensation or a compensated chronic state.[284,285] This section first reviews the role of diuretics in acute decompensated heart failure in general and as secondary to acute coronary syndrome, then discusses the role of diuretics as maintenance therapy in systolic and diastolic heart failure. The reader is referred to the joint guidelines published by the American College of Cardiology and American Heart Association for more detailed recommendations and an overview of the level of evidence for each treatment.[286]

Acute Decompensated Heart Failure

In the absence of obvious causes such as acute coronary syndrome and valve abnormalities, acute decompensated heart failure (ADHF) often results from an imbalance in the neurohumoral systems that regulate cardiac and renal function.[287] Therefore, it is rational to target these mechanisms with selective therapy. After initial stabilization, the mainstay of treatment is vasodilator and diuretic therapy. Intravenous vasodilators such as nitroglycerine, nitroprusside, and nesiritide counteract the effects of baroreceptor-dependent increases in sympathetic tone, angiotensin II and aldosterone, endothelin, and AVP. Vasodilators are usually combined with intravenous loop diuretics (e.g., furosemide 40 mg, bumetanide 1 mg, torsemide 10-20 mg). For example, a study in patients with severe heart failure showed

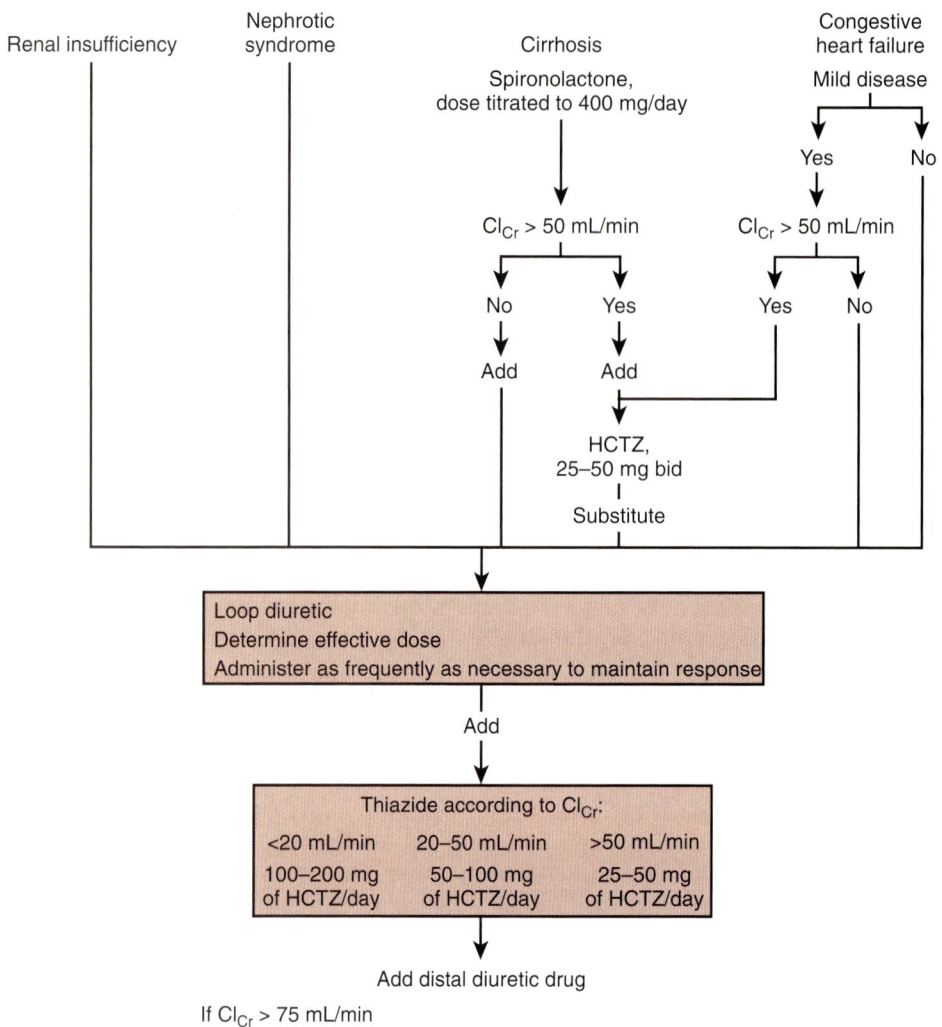

Figure 51.14 Algorithm for diuretic therapy in patients with edema due to renal, hepatic, or cardiac disease. bid, Twice a day; Cl$_{Cr}$, creatinine clearance; HCTZ, hydrochlorothiazide. (From Brater DC: Diuretic therapy. *N Engl J Med* 339:387-395, 1989, with permission.)

that therapy with vasodilators and diuretics aimed at improving overall hemodynamic status led to rapid neurohumoral improvement when central filling pressure declined.[288] Another study found that although "aggressive decongestion" during ADHF was associated with worsening renal function, survival was actually improved.[289] In a carefully performed randomized trial, no differences between continuous dosing and bolus dosing of furosemide were observed; furthermore, no differences in global symptom improvement were observed between a low dose (equivalent of oral dose) and a high dose (2.5 times the oral dose).[239] It should be noted, however, that this trial did not study patients shown to be diuretic resistant. Longer-acting loop diuretics, such as torsemide[290] and azosemide,[291] produce less neurohumoral activation and may be preferable.

Diuretic kinetics are impaired in decompensated HF.[292,293] The bioavailability of furosemide, unlike that of bumetanide or torsemide, is erratic in HF.[294] This feature, and a longer duration of action, may account for the finding of a 50% reduction in the requirement for readmission to hospital in patients with HF randomly assigned to receive torsemide rather than furosemide.[106] There is decreased plasma clearance in decompensated HF because of a decreased RBF.[292] Together, these effects can limit the peak diuretic concentration in the tubular fluid to the foot of the dose-response curve and thereby diminish the response (see Figure 51.15).

Nesiritide is a recombinant human B-type natriuretic peptide (BNP) that was approved by the U.S. Food and Drug Administration (FDA) for the treatment of acute decompensated heart failure.[295] Studies of mice deficient in natriuretic peptide receptor A mice implicate this system in the natriuretic response to blood volume expansion[296] and provide a rationale for BNP in the treatment of ADHF. Nesiritide given short term to patients with decompensated HF can reduce pulmonary capillary wedge pressure.[297] However, some subsequent studies have shown that nesiritide is not a diuretic in patients with heart failure and, in comparison with placebo, may be associated with higher risks of death and worsening renal function.[298-300] Conversely, other studies indicate a potential role for nesiritide

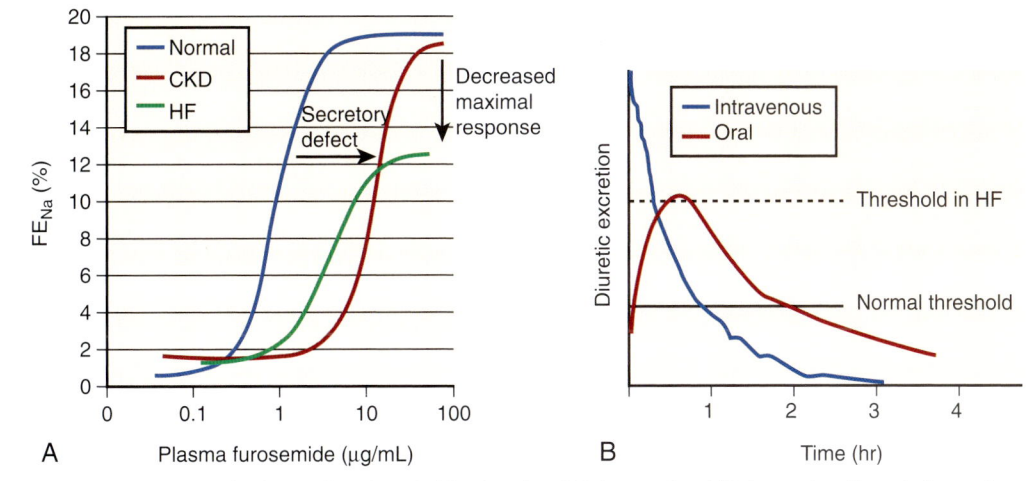

Figure 51.15 Dose-response curve for loop diuretics. **A,** The fractional Na⁺ excretion (FE$_{Na}$) as a function of plasma loop diuretic concentration. Compared with normal subjects, patients with chronic kidney disease (CKD) show a rightward shift in the curve owing to impaired diuretic secretion. The maximal response is preserved when expressed as FE$_{Na}$, but not when expressed as absolute Na⁺ excretion. Patients with congestive heart failure (HF) demonstrate a rightward and downward shift, even when expressed as FE$_{Na}$, and thus are relatively diuretic resistant. **B,** Comparison of the response to intravenous and oral doses of loop diuretics. In a normal individual, an oral dose may be as effective as an intravenous dose because the time during which this individual is above the natriuretic threshold (indicated by the *Normal threshold* line) are approximately equal. If the natriuretic threshold increases (as indicated by the *Threshold in HF* line), then the oral dose may not provide a high enough plasma level to elicit natriuresis.

in the perioperative treatment of patients with left ventricular dysfunction who are undergoing cardiac surgery. In this context, these agents may improve renal function and possibly even survival.[301,302] Current guidelines recommend nesiritide for alternative vasodilator therapy in patients with ADHF without hypotension and with volume overload who remain dyspneic despite receiving intravenous loop diuretics.[286,303]

In the past few years, there has been substantial interest in venovenous ultrafiltration as treatment for ADHF. Nevertheless, a randomized trial conducted by the Heart Failure Clinical Research Network, comparing diuretic therapy with ultrafiltration, found that creatinine rose more in the ultrafiltration group than in the diuretic group, despite similar volume losses.[304] It should be emphasized, however, that this trial specifically excluded individuals in whom dialysis, in addition to volume removal, was indicated. Thus a role for pure ultrafiltration in treating HF remains to be established. The supplementary material in this publication[304] also provides protocols that have been widely promulgated by the Heart Failure Clinical Research Network for volume reduction in decompensated CHF.

Finally, the intravenous inotropes dobutamine and milrinone are reserved for situations in which ADHF is complicated by unresponsiveness to standard therapies, diminished peripheral perfusion, end-organ dysfunction, and/or hypotension ("low-output syndrome"). One trial has shown no added benefit of low-dose dopamine or nesiritide in either decongestion or kidney function.[305]

ACUTE DECOMPENSATED HEART FAILURE IN ACUTE CORONARY SYNDROME

Patients with acute myocardial infarction (AMI) require the rapid establishment of coronary reperfusion (e.g., by thrombolysis and percutaneous coronary intervention) and treatment of arrhythmias. The aim of concomitant treatment is to counter the increase in left ventricular end-diastolic pressure, which enhances wall tension and O$_2$ usage, and the accumulation of pulmonary edema without further curtailing the cardiac output. Judicious use of diuretics may meet these requirements. In one study, intravenous furosemide for left ventricular failure (LVF) complicating acute AMI reduced the left ventricular filling pressure from 20 to 15 mm Hg within 5 to 15 minutes and increased the venous capacitance by 50%.[306] This rapid venodilation is blocked by NSAIDs[255] and ACE inhibitors.[307] The ensuing diuresis reduces left ventricular end-diastolic pressure further.

A study of first-line therapy for 48 patients with acute LVF following AMI compared the responses to intravenous furosemide, a venodilator (isosorbide dinitrate), an arteriolar dilator (hydralazine), and a positive inotrope (prenalterol).[308] The venodilator and furosemide both reduced left ventricular filling pressure while maintaining the cardiac index and heart rate. The investigators concluded that these were the best first-line agents but that they should be combined with an arteriolar vasodilator. In contrast, a study randomly assigned 110 patients with acute LVF to receive either high-dose isosorbide dinitrate (3 mg intravenously every 5 minutes) or high-dose furosemide (80 mg intravenously every 15 minutes).[309] An adverse end point occurred more frequently in those receiving furosemide (46%) than in those receiving nitrate (25%). The investigators cautioned against the use of high-dose furosemide in acute LVF. Although intravenous furosemide decreases left ventricular filling pressure in patients with LVF, the shape of the Frank-Starling ventricular function curve predicts little change in cardiac output at elevated filling pressures. Nevertheless, most investigators recommend a trial of loop diuretics after ECV depletion and preload-dependent right heart failure have been ruled out by targeted volume boluses.[310]

Furosemide can be given as an IV bolus of up to 100 mg or as a short-term infusion to limit the risk of ototoxicity.

Although controversial, an intermittent infusion produces a slightly greater natriuresis in most comparative studies.[311] Ideally, lower doses are used initially and titrated up to a good effect, for instance, a pulmonary capillary wedge pressure of 16 mm Hg.[311] Hemodynamic and biochemical parameters should be monitored frequently during loop diuretic therapy, especially because patients with AMI are usually also treated with β-blockers, ACE inhibitors, or vasodilators.

Chronic Heart Failure

Diuretics are extremely useful in the long-term management of chronic, systolic HF. Avid renal NaCl and fluid retention leads to pulmonary edema that limits ventilation. Cardiac dilation limits cardiac function and increases wall tension and O_2 usage. This combination can create a spiral of decreasing oxygenation and cardiac output. In a study of 13 patients with severe edema due to HF, furosemide therapy increased stroke volume by 15% and decreased peripheral vascular resistance despite reducing body weight by an average of 10 kg.[312] In another study, combined therapy using a diuretic and a vasodilator reduced left and right atrial volumes, corrected atrioventricular valvular regurgitation, and improved stroke volume by 64%.[308] A meta-analysis of trials for HF concluded that odds ratios were reduced to 0.25 for mortality and 0.31 for hospitalization for subjects randomly selected to receive diuretics.[313] These remarkable data strongly support the use of diuretics in HF.

On the other hand, the failing heart has a decreased capacity to regulate its contractility in response to changes in venous return, so if diuretic therapy is too abrupt or severe, the patient suffers from a decreased effective blood volume (orthostatic hypotension, weakness, fatigue, decreased exercise ability, and prerenal azotemia). This is especially true for patients with diastolic dysfunction, an increasingly recognized form of symptomatic heart failure with preserved ejection fraction.[314] Therefore, salt-depleting therapy requires continual reassessment and judicious use of other measures (e.g., vasodilators, ACE inhibitors, ARBs, or MRAs). Mild HF often responds to dietary Na^+ restriction (100-120 mmol/day) and low doses of a thiazide diuretic. As cardiac failure progresses, larger, more frequent doses of loop diuretics and tighter control of dietary salt (80-100 mmol/day) are required. It is important to emphasize that diuretic responsiveness is impaired in patients with advanced HF, as shown by a shift to the right in the natriuresis/excretion relationship of diuretics (see Figure 51.15).[293] For the refractory patient, the addition of a second diuretic acting at the proximal tubule (e.g., acetazolamide) or a downstream site (e.g., a thiazide) can produce a dramatic diuresis, even in individuals with impaired renal function.[315,316] For example, additional therapy with metolazone[317] or hydrochlorothiazide[318] can increase fluid losses by an average of 7 to 8 kg. Although drug therapy for chronic heart failure should be individualized, a suggested step-up algorithm consists of diuretics and ACE inhibitors or ARBs as the first agents, β-blockers second, and MRAs or hydralazine-isosorbide dinitrate (in blacks) third, with digoxin, cardioverter-defibrillator, and resynchronization devices being saved as final resorts.[319] The lesson from the excess morbidity from hyperkalemia observed during trials of spironolactone therapy is to use MRAs within guidelines.[195] The guidelines exclude men with creatinine concentrations higher than 2.5 mg/dL (221 μmol/L) and women with creatinine concentrations higher than 2.0 mg/dL (177 μmol/L).[320] However, within guidelines, both MRAs and loop diuretics are important because they can improve ventricular remodeling.[321,322] In patients with preserved ejection fraction, spironolactone may improve left ventricular diastolic dysfunction but it has been found not to improve symptoms and outcome.[323,324]

Despite these options, heart failure often progresses and introduces a vicious circle. Decompensated HF stimulates the RAAS and AVP,[325] predisposing to hypokalemia, hypomagnesemia, hyponatremia, and arrhythmias. Hypokalemia potentiates the binding of digitalis to cardiac myocytes,[326] decreases its renal elimination,[327] and enhances its cardiac toxicity.[328] Although this circle can be curtailed by higher doses of diuretics or continuous intravenous infusion of a loop diuretic,[329] the risks of volume depletion, azotemia, and electrolyte abnormalities increase sharply.[330] Continuous infusion should be tried in patients known to show response to maximum bolus doses of diuretics, because bolus therapy results in higher initial serum concentrations and therefore higher initial rates of urinary diuretic excretion than continuous infusion. If the patient has received one or more intravenous boluses within the previous few hours, then an infusion can be started without a loading dose.

Infusion rates of up to 240 mg/hour are reported in the literature. The risk of ototoxicity and other side effects associated with these infusion rates must be weighed against alternative strategies, such as the addition of a thiazide-type diuretic or fluid removal via ultrafiltration.

Therefore, new therapies are required, because a decrement in renal function predicts a bad outcome in patients treated for HF.[331] Renal dysfunction can be ameliorated by an ARB, provided that blood pressure is maintained. The combination of an ARB with a neprilysin inhibitor, which prevents the breakdown of natriuretic peptides, may be especially advantageous in terms of cardiovascular and renal outcomes, according to one study.[218] In the scenario in which deteriorating heart failure worsens kidney function, often referred to as the cardiorenal syndrome, therapy must be aimed at improving cardiac function (if possible) and treating congestion with diuretics, β-blockers, ACE inhibitors, or ARBs and MRAs.[332]

Right Ventricular Failure

The requirement for diuretic therapy in patients with pure right heart failure or cor pulmonale is not compelling. A decrease in venous return induced by vigorous diuresis may worsen right heart function. Furosemide administration increases angiotensin II–induced hypoxic pulmonary vascular resistance.[328] Therefore, the emphasis should be on reversal of chronic hypoxemia.

CIRRHOSIS OF THE LIVER

Most patients with cirrhotic ascites and peripheral edema have expansion of the ECV owing to arteriolar underfilling, caused by peripheral vasodilation and impaired cardiac function.[333-335] Studies in patients with cirrhosis also demonstrate increases in proximal reabsorption in response to a diminished effective arterial blood volume.[336] Finally, patients with liver cirrhosis have increases in both the natriuretic response to a thiazide and serum aldosterone concentrations.[337] Thus, diuretics acting on the distal nephron and MRAs are rational for cirrhosis and are usually well tolerated.[164] The American Association for the Study of Liver Disease practice guidelines suggest that first-line treatment of patients with cirrhosis and ascites should consist of sodium restriction (2000 mg or 88 mmol daily) and diuretics (oral spironolactone with or without oral furosemide).[338] The guideline suggests an initial regimen of 40 mg furosemide and 100 mg spironolactone, with titration upwards maintaining the same diuretic ratio.[338] Maximally recommended doses are 400 mg of spironolactone and 160 mg of furosemide.

Patients with cirrhosis and ascites cannot normally tolerate ACE inhibitors or ARBs because of a fall in blood pressure.[339] Mild edema without ascites can be treated with dietary restriction of Na+ (100 mmol/day). Dietary fluid restriction is not necessary in most patients with cirrhotic ascites. The guideline does not recommend fluid restriction in patients with cirrhosis and ascites, unless serum sodium falls below 125 mmol/L.[338] Although it has never been shown that treating hyponatremia in liver disease improves prognosis, hyponatremia by itself has been a consistent predictor of poor prognosis.[340] Ascitic fluid is largely cleared by the lymphatics. Diuretics increase thoracic duct lymph flow.[341] Thus, diuretics decrease ascites formation by decreasing venous and portal hydraulic pressures, concentrating the plasma proteins,[342] and increasing ascites absorption.[341,343]

The maximal daily ascites drainage into the systemic circulation is limited to 300 to 900 ml.[344] Therefore the maximum daily weight loss in *nonedematous* patients should not exceed 0.3 to 0.5 kg. In patients with ascites and edema, daily diuretic-induced weight losses of 1 to 3 kg do not perturb the plasma volume or renal function.[345] The same diuretic regimen maintained after the peripheral edema has cleared, however, or given to nonedematous patients reduces plasma volume by as much as 24% and raises the risks of hyponatremia, alkalosis, and azotemia. Furthermore, the reduced serum albumin and an increased portal venous pressure coupled with preexisting diuretic use can lead to true "underfill edema." Diuretic therapy for patients with these findings is complicated by hypotension, azotemia, and electrolyte dysfunction. Thus a diuretic prescription that is initially safe must be reviewed continuously. In addition, patients with ascites but without peripheral edema seem more prone to development of the side effects of diuretics.[345]

The most common problems with furosemide in cirrhosis are electrolyte disturbances and volume depletion. Hypokalemia, which is related to preexisting K+ depletion and hyperaldosteronism, can be countered with the use of spironolactone, eplerenone, or a distal K+-sparing agent, as noted previously. However, hyperkalemic metabolic acidosis can develop in patients with cirrhosis who are given spironolactone.[346] More severe diuretic resistance requires paracentesis. It is important, however, to differentiate diuretic resistance from noncompliance with NaCl restriction. This can be done by determining 24-hour NaCl excretion or by using a spot urine Na/K ratio (higher ratios suggest noncompliance, lower ratios diuretic resistance; the optimal cutoff varies among studies, between 1 and 2.5[347]).

Controlled trials in patients with refractory ascites have shown that large-volume paracentesis is more effective than diuretic therapy in reducing hospital stay and electrolyte complications but does not influence mortality.[348] Even repeated, large-volume paracenteses (4-6 L/day) are safe if intravenous albumin (40 g with each procedure) is administered.[348] Most investigators, however, recommend paracentesis only for cases that are relatively resistant to diuretics and dietary Na+ restriction (Figure 51.16).[349]

Patients with mild cirrhosis of the liver have a normal or reduced natriuretic response to furosemide with little change in diuretic kinetics.[2] However, in those with advanced disease, furosemide absorption is slowed,[350] its volume of distribution is increased because of hypoalbuminemia and an expanded ECV, and its elimination is delayed because of hypoalbuminemia, which limits proximal tubule diuretic secretion, and a low RBF, which limits renal clearance.[2] Resistance to loop diuretics in early cirrhosis is largely due

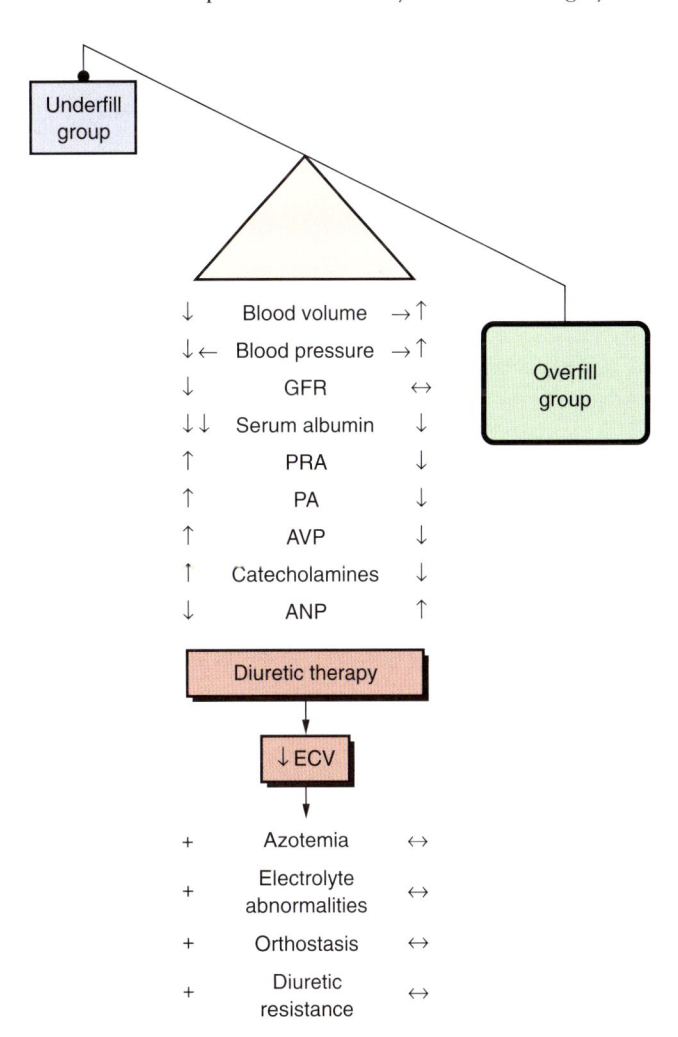

Figure 51.16 Comparison of clinical and biochemical characteristics and responses in patients with nephrotic syndrome and underfill edema versus overfill edema. ANP, Atrial natriuretic peptide; AVP, arginine vasopressin; ↓ECV, decrease in extracellular fluid volume; GFR, glomerular filtration rate; PA, plasma aldosterone; PRA, plasma renin activity. ↑, increase; ↓, decrease; ↔, no effect; +, potential side-effect (Based on Schrier RW, Fassett RG: A critique of the overfill hypothesis of sodium and water retention in the nephrotic syndrome. *Kidney Int* 53:1111, 1998.)

to decreased responsiveness to the drug, which correlates with elevated serum aldosterone.[164] With the development of ascites, a further decrease in natriuretic response correlates with decreased delivery of furosemide to the urine[351] and with further stimulation of the RAAS.[164]

Diuretic resistance is common in advanced cirrhosis. In addition to the usual causes (see Table 51.2), it may herald the development of infection, bleeding, or a critical drop in cardiac output. Patients whose disease is refractory and who are disabled by recurrent paracentesis may show response to body compression[352] or a transjugular intrahepatic portosystemic shunt.[353] Intravenous loop diuretics are generally discouraged, because they may precipitate the hepatorenal syndrome.

NEPHROTIC SYNDROME

Renal albumin losses and reduced hepatic synthesis in the nephrotic syndrome eventually lead to hypoalbuminemia. The ensuing fall in plasma oncotic pressure increases the flux of fluid into the interstitial spaces, leading to underfill edema.[354,355] Additionally, a primary renal salt retention can lead to overfill edema (Figure 51.17). Patients with minimal change disease often have contracted plasma volume and stimulated RAAS, whereas those with diabetes and hypertension usually have expanded plasma volume and suppressed RAAS.[356] Micropuncture studies of sodium-retaining animal models of the nephrotic syndrome demonstrate pronounced NaCl reabsorption in the distal

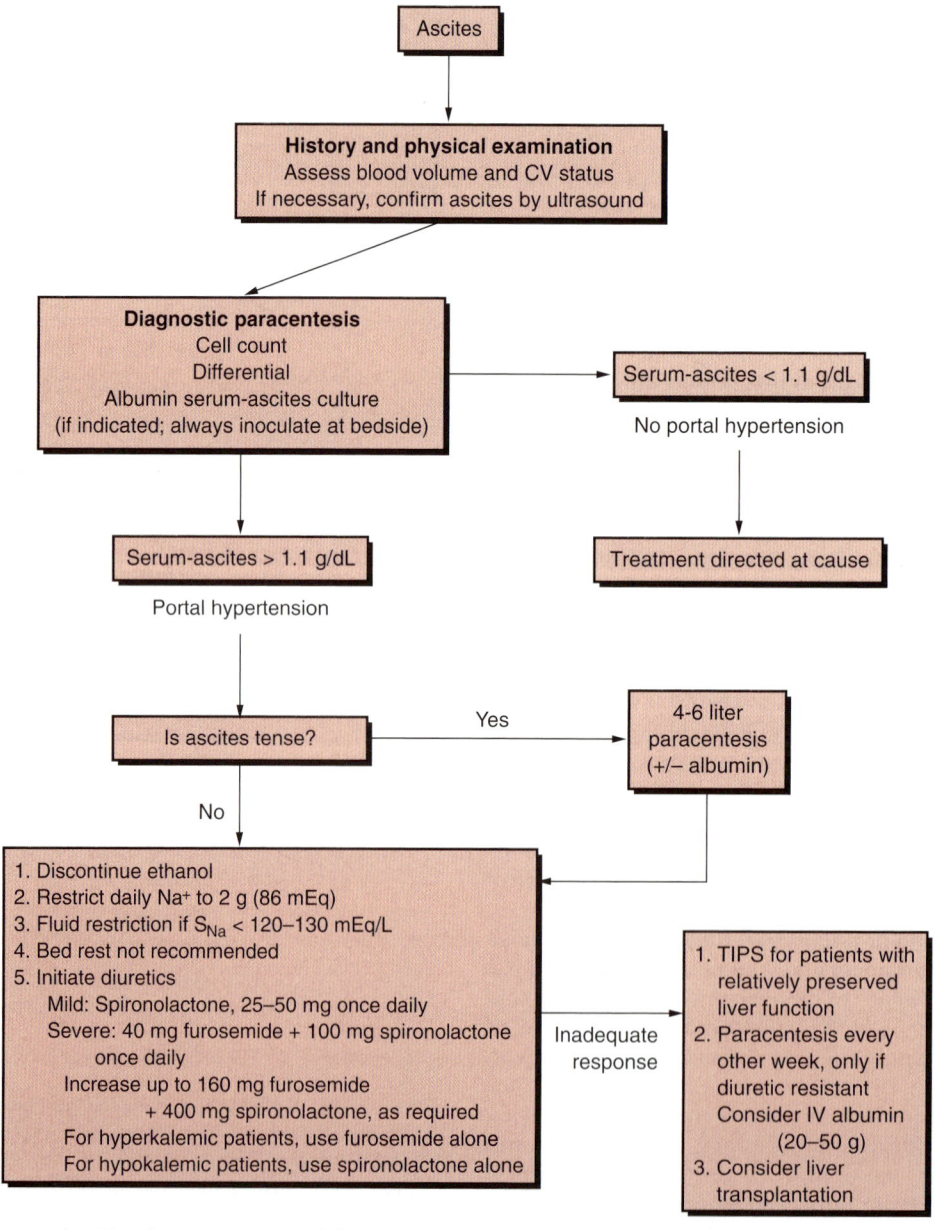

Figure 51.17 Treatment algorithm for management of fluid retention in patients with hepatic cirrhosis and ascites. CV, Cardiovascular; IV, intravenous; S_{Na}, serum Na+ concentration; TIPS, transjugular intrahepatic portosystemic shunt. (From Ellison DH, Wilcox CS: Diuretics: use in edema and the problem of resistance. In Brady HR, Wilcox CS, editors: *Therapy in nephrology and hypertension*, 2nd ed. London, 2003, Elsevier Science.)

nephron and TAL.[357,358] The proteinuric kidney of a rat model of unilateral nephrotic syndrome has an enhanced Na⁺ reabsorption in the CDs[359] and a diminished response to ANP.[360] Hyperaldosteronism reinforces NaCl reabsorption at these sites. Renin and aldosterone levels are highly variable in patients with the nephrotic syndrome.[361] Hypoalbuminemia reduces the binding of furosemide to plasma proteins and thereby enlarges its volume of distribution.[362] Whereas one study reported that premixing furosemide with albumin in the syringe prior to intravenous injection enhanced the diuresis of patients with the nephrotic syndrome,[91] this finding has not been confirmed.[92,363,364] Indeed, two studies have shown that patients with a serum albumin level of 2 g/dL can deliver normal quantities of furosemide into the urine.[362,365] Iso-oncotic plasma volume expansion with albumin in patients with the nephrotic syndrome fails to induce negative NaCl balance[366] or to enhance the response to furosemide[363] and so is not generally recommended for treatment of resistant nephrotic syndrome.[363,367] One study found that a fractional sodium excretion of 0.2% differentiated volume-contracted from volume-expanded nephrotic syndrome in children; treatment with diuretics alone proved effective and safe for the volume-expanded group.[368]

A more logical approach to diuretic resistance is to limit albuminuria with an ACE inhibitor or ARB or both, which also may combat the associated coagulopathy, dyslipidemia, edema, and progressive loss of renal function. The addition of a loop diuretic to an ACE inhibitor or an ARB reduces proteinuria further but increases the serum creatinine concentration.[369]

The secretion of CAIs[17] and loop diuretics[112] by the S2 segment of the proximal tubule depends on albumin. However, in the rabbit, the uptake of loop diuretics into the S1 portion of the proximal tubule, where furosemide is inactivated by glucuronidation, is inhibited by albumin (see Figure 51.7).[113,370] Albumin infusion into nephrotic patients does indeed increase renal furosemide excretion, whereas hypoalbuminemia enhances its metabolic clearance.[371]

The interaction of furosemide with its receptor in the lumen of the TAL is restricted by binding to filtered albumin.[372] Addition of albumin to the tubular perfusate of the loop of Henle attenuates the response to perfused furosemide because of binding to albumin and is reversed by coperfusion with warfarin, which displaces it from its albumin-binding site.[373] However, Agarwal and colleagues found that displacing furosemide from albumin via coadministration of sulfisoxazole did not affect natriuresis in patients with the nephrotic syndrome.[374] This study's results are not definitive, however, because subjects did not have diuretic resistance.

Animal studies demonstrate five mechanisms that could impair the responsiveness to loop diuretics in patients with the nephrotic syndrome: decreased delivery and/or decreased tubular secretion of the diuretic, increased renal metabolism, decreased blockade by the diuretic, and increased NaCl reabsorption by other nephron segments. Clinical studies confirm that nephrotic patients have an impaired tubular response to loop diuretics.

Nephrotic edema is best managed with dietary salt and fluid restriction. Most patients show initial response to a loop diuretic when it is required. Spironolactone or eplerenone is effective in some patients.[355] Decreasing renal function[262] or administration of indomethacin[251] causes marked resistance to loop diuretics in these patients. The combination of a thiazide diuretic with furosemide dissipates edema but at the expense of marked kaliuresis.[375] Data suggest that primary sodium retention in nephrotic syndrome is related to the presence of plasma proteinases in nephrotic urine, such as plasmin, which can activate the epithelial sodium channel.[376] Although this suggestion would provide a rationale for treatment with amiloride or triamterene, clinical studies are lacking.

IDIOPATHIC EDEMA

Idiopathic edema affects women predominantly. It causes fluctuating salt retention and edema, exacerbated by orthostasis.[377] The effects of diuretic withdrawal during controlled salt intake were studied in 10 such patients.[378] Although their body weight increased by 0.5 to 5.0 kg within 2 to 8 days, 7 returned to their original weight by 3 weeks without reinstitution of diuretic therapy. The investigators concluded that diuretic abuse could cause idiopathic edema. However, this conclusion has been challenged.[379] Remarkably, 83% of habitual furosemide abusers who consume high doses over prolonged periods demonstrate medullary nephrocalcinosis and tubulointerstitial fibrosis.[380] Patients with idiopathic edema are best treated with salt restriction.

NONEDEMATOUS CONDITIONS

HYPERTENSION

Hypertension is discussed in Chapters 47 to 50.

ACUTE KIDNEY INJURY

A review of 11 randomized trials of loop diuretics or mannitol for prophylaxis or treatment of established AKI found no benefit.[381] Diuretics can be used to convert oliguric to nonoliguric AKI. One study involving 58 patients found that sustained diuresis can be provoked in most patients given 1 g furosemide orally three times daily, but this very large dose produced deafness in 2 patients, which was permanent in 1,[382] and therefore cannot be recommended. Older observational and randomized studies have indicated that furosemide does not improve the prognosis of AKI,[383-385] and some have suggested that diuretics worsen the prognosis.[386] Evidence of adverse effects of ECF volume overload in critically ill patients has been growing. The Fluid and Catheter Treatment Trial was a randomized trial comparing treatment strategies in patients with respiratory distress syndrome. A post hoc analysis of patients within this trial in whom AKI developed suggested that patients randomly assigned to lower central venous pressure (CVP) targets exhibited lower mortality. These patients received substantially higher diuretic doses than those randomly assigned to higher CVP targets. Because this approach eliminated the confounding by indication that has complicated other studies, it provides substantial evidence that loop diuretics can be used safely in this population.[387] Furosemide can reduce the need for dialysis by diminishing hyperkalemia, acidosis, or fluid overload.[381] One protocol is to give 40 mg of furosemide, 1 mg of bumetanide, or 25 mg of torsemide intravenously and to double the dose every 60 minutes if there is no response, up to a total daily dose of 1 g of

Table 51.3 Ceiling Doses (in mL) of Loop Diuretics

Condition	Furosemide IV	Furosemide PO	Bumetanide, IV or PO	Torsemide, IV or PO
Chronic renal insufficiency:				
Moderate (GFR 20-50 mL·min^{-1})	80-160	160	6	50
Severe (GFR < 20 mL·min^{-1})	200	240	10	100
Nephrotic syndrome with normal GFR	120	240	3	50
Cirrhosis with normal GFR	40-80	80-160	1	20
Heart failure with normal GFR	40-80	80-160	1	20

GFR, Glomerular filtration rate; IV, intravenous; PO, oral.
Data from references 5, 7, and 8.

furosemide or the equivalent.[381] Bumetanide and torsemide are metabolized by the liver and so may be preferred to furosemide, which is metabolized by the kidney and therefore accumulates to a greater degree in patients with renal insufficiency (see Figure 51.6).

CHRONIC KIDNEY DISEASE

In subjects who are in balance, the fractional reabsorption of NaCl and fluid by the renal tubules is reduced in proportion to the fall in GFR. The renal clearance of loop diuretics falls in parallel with the GFR because of a decreased renal mass and the accumulation of organic acids that compete for proximal secretion.[388] Thus, although the maximal increase in fractional excretion of Na$^+$ produced by furosemide is maintained quite well in CKD,[5,389,390] the absolute response to diuretics is limited by reductions in absolute rate of NaCl reabsorption and in delivery of the diuretic to its target (see Figure 51.15). Although CKD decreases proximal reabsorption, there is enhanced fractional reabsorption in the loop segment, distal tubule, and CDs[391] with a relative increase of threefold to fourfold per residual nephron in the expression of the NKCC2 in the TAL and the NCC in the DCT.[392] Torsemide has the greatest oral bioavailability in CKD.[103] For refractory cases, a loop diuretic infusion (e.g., bumetanide, 1 mg/hour for 12 hours) produces a greater natriuresis and less myalgia than two bolus injections.[238] Thiazides when used alone become relatively ineffective in patients with creatinine clearance below 35 mL/min. When used in combination with a loop diuretic that increases NaCl delivery and reabsorption at the distal tubule, larger doses of thiazides are effective in patients with moderate azotemia, although at the cost of a sharp further rise in the serum creatinine and blood urea concentrations and a high incidence of hypokalemia and electrolyte disorders.[280] Moreover, high plasma levels of furosemide can cause ototoxicity.[393] Therefore, care should be taken not to exceed the ceiling dose (Table 51.3).[389,390] Epidemiologic studies have correlated diuretic use with end-stage CKD,[394] but this may be an epiphenomenon.[395] In fact, continuing diuretics in patients undergoing dialysis who have residual renal function was associated with lower interdialytic weight gain, less hyperkalemia, and lower cardiac-specific mortality.[396] References 4 and 397 are recommended for further reading on diuretics in CKD.

RENAL TUBULAR ACIDOSIS

Furosemide increases the distal delivery of NaCl and fluid and stimulates aldosterone secretion and phosphate elimination, which enhance acid elimination.[398] In addition, a direct effect of both furosemide and thiazide on distal acidification with increased abundance of the H$^+$-ATPase B1 subunit has been demonstrated.[399] Hence, furosemide can be used in patients with hyperkalemic (type IV) renal tubular acidosis to increase renal acid excretion.[400,401] Because hyperkalemic renal tubular acidosis is usually due to hypoaldosteronism, mineralocorticoid therapy is also often indicated.[402]

HYPERCALCEMIA

Ca^{2+} excretion is increased by osmotic or loop diuretics but decreased by thiazides and distal agents. Hypercalcemia activates the Ca^{2+}-sensing receptor[403,404] that inhibits fluid and NaCl reabsorption in the TAL and impairs renal concentration. The ensuing ECV depletion further limits Ca^{2+} excretion by reducing the GFR and enhancing proximal fluid and Ca^{2+} reabsorption. Therefore, the initial therapy for hypercalcemia is volume expansion with saline with or without bisphosphonates or steroids, depending on the cause. Loop diuretics may help prevent or treat fluid overload, but there is little evidence to support a role in the treatment of hypercalcemia.[405]

NEPHROLITHIASIS

Thiazides reduce stone formation in hypercalciuric and even normocalciuric patients by reducing excretion of Ca^{2+} and oxalate.[406] Some patients continue to form stones and require additional citrate therapy.[407] Ca^{2+} excretion can be enhanced by the addition of amiloride[408] or a low-salt diet. KHCO$_3$ produces a greater reduction in Ca^{2+} excretion than KCl when given with hydrochlorothiazide.[409]

OSTEOPOROSIS

Bone cells express an Na$^+$-Cl$^-$ cotransporter[410] that, when blocked by a thiazide, enhances bone Ca^{2+} uptake.[411] Thiazides inhibit osteocalcin, an osteoblast-specific protein that retards bone formation,[412] and directly stimulate the production of the osteoblast differentiation markers runt-related transcription factor 2 (runx2) and osteopontin.[413]

They inhibit bone reabsorption[414] and augment bone mineralization, independent of parathyroid hormone.[415] Thus, thiazides may promote bone mineralization both by reducing renal Ca^{2+} excretion and through direct effects on bone. These biologic effects are supported by epidemiologic studies. Thiazide therapy is associated with an increase in bone mineral density and a reduction in hip fractures in elderly persons.[416,417] In a placebo-controlled trial in postmenopausal women,[418] hydrochlorothiazide (50 mg/day) slowed cortical bone loss significantly. Surprisingly, despite having opposite effects on Ca^{2+} excretion, a thiazide and a loop diuretic both enhance bone formation in postmenopausal women, at least in the short term.[419] However, loop diuretics alone have been associated with hip bone loss in older men, increased risk of fractures in postmenopausal women, and increased risk of revision following primary total hip arthroplasty in men and women.[420-422]

GITELMAN'S SYNDROME

In addition to potassium supplementation, potassium-sparing diuretics may be used in Gitelman's syndrome to treat hypokalemia. Spironolactone (200 to 300 mg/day) was shown to be more effective than amiloride (10 to 30 mg/day).[423] In a later study, the efficacy of indomethacin (75 mg/day), amiloride (30 mg/day), and eplerenone (150 mg/day) in correcting hypokalemia was compared in a crossover trial.[424] Although all three drugs significantly increased plasma potassium, indomethacin was most effective but also was associated with the most adverse effects.

DIABETES INSIPIDUS

Thiazides can reduce urine flow by up to 50% in patients with central or nephrogenic diabetes insipidus.[425] This paradoxic effect is related to decreased GFR, enhanced water reabsorption in the proximal and distal nephron,[426,427] and an increase in papillary osmolarity leading to distal water reabsorption. A small placebo-controlled crossover trial and an animal study have shown that amiloride prevents lithium-induced polyuria.[428,429] This effect is attributed to blockage by amiloride of the entry of lithium via ENaC in the principal cell, where it can downregulate the water channel AQP2 via glycogen synthase kinase 3.[430]

ADVERSE EFFECTS OF DIURETICS

Although diuretic therapy is generally well tolerated, a Medical Research Council trial showed that the following adverse effects occurred more frequently with thiazide than with placebo: impaired glucose tolerance, gout, impotence, lethargy, nausea, dizziness, headache, and constipation.[431] However, the withdrawal rate of those receiving a thiazide was similar to that for a β-blocker, and the dose of thiazide was higher than that used currently.

FLUID AND ELECTROLYTE ABNORMALITIES

EXTRACELLULAR VOLUME DEPLETION AND AZOTEMIA

Diuretics normally do not decrease the GFR.[77,432] However, renal failure can be precipitated by vigorous diuresis in patients with impaired renal function, severe edema, or cirrhosis and ascites. A rise in the ratio of blood urea nitrogen to creatinine suggests ECV depletion. This change can be ascribed to decreased renal urea clearance because of greater urea reabsorption in the distal nephron[433] and to increased urea appearance due to greater arginine uptake by the liver with metabolism by arginase.[434-436] In addition, combining diuretics with ACE inhibitors and NSAIDs raises the risk of AKI.[437]

HYPONATREMIA

Several mechanisms may play a role. One, illustrated in a self-experiment by McCance (Figure 51.18) of severe salt depletion by a salt-free diet and forced perspiration, shows that the loss of the first 2 L of body fluid occurs isotonically.[138] However, further obligated NaCl losses are not accompanied by corresponding fluid losses, leading to progressive hyponatremia, likely a consequence of AVP release

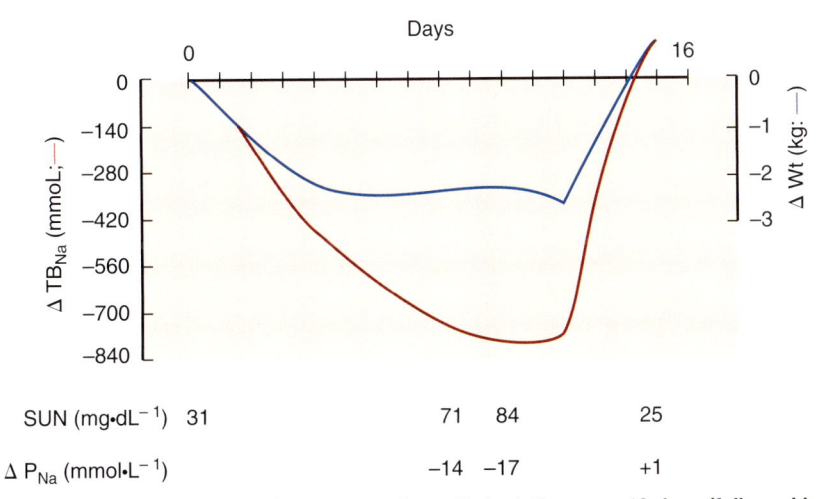

Figure 51.18 Data from normal volunteers subjected to progressive salt depletion over 12 days (followed by 3 days of salt repletion) caused by a zero salt intake and forced perspiration. Results shown are for changes in total body Na^+ (Δ TB_{Na}), body weight (Δ Wt), and plasma sodium concentration (Δ P_{NA}), and serum urea nitrogen (SUN). (Drawn from data in McCance RA: Experimental sodium chloride deficiency in man. *Proc R Soc Lond B Biol Sci* 119:245-268, 1936.)

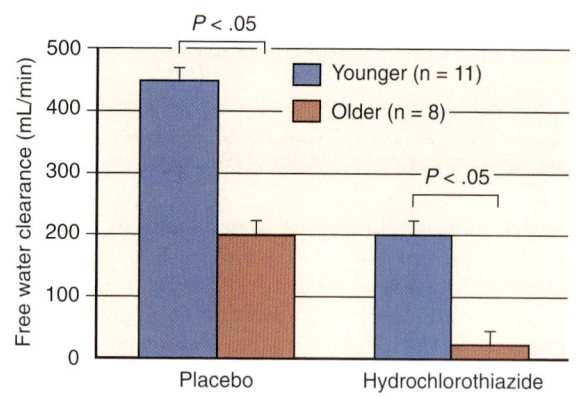

Figure 51.19 Mean ± standard error of the mean (SEM) values for positive free water clearance during water loading. Data shown compare values in younger and older normal volunteers given placebo or hydrochlorothiazide. Note that both older age and thiazide diuretics impair free water excretion. (Redrawn from Clark BA, Shannon RP, Rosa RM, Epstein FH: Increased susceptibility to thiazide-induced hyponatremia in the elderly. *J Am Soc Nephrol* 5:1106, 1994.)

in response to severe plasma volume depletion. Despite salt depletion, the hyponatremia is mild.

A second mechanism is illustrated in the study of Clark and colleagues.[439] They showed that older age and thiazide diuretics are additive in impairing maximal free water excretion following a water load (Figure 51.19). This effect is relatively specific for thiazides, which inhibit urinary dilution, whereas loop diuretics inhibit urinary concentration and dilution.[440] Indeed, thiazides are 12-fold more likely than loop diuretics to cause hyponatremia.[441] Thiazide-induced hyponatremia usually entails inappropriate fluid intake and expanded total body water.[441,442] Estradiol enhances the expression of the thiazide-sensitive cotransporters in the DCT.[443] Eighty percent of thiazide-induced hyponatremia occurs in females,[444] most of whom are elderly.[445] As noted previously, thiazide diuretics also increase both AVP-independent water reabsorption along the medullary collecting duct and AQP2 expression when administered long term.[148,149] Hyponatremia can develop during rechallenge with a thiazide.[442,446] It often develops within the first 2 weeks of thiazide therapy.[441,446] Mild hyponatremia can be treated by withdrawal of diuretics, restriction of the daily intake of free water to 1.0 to 1.5 liter, restoration of any K$^+$ and Mg^{2+} losses, and replenishment of NaCl if the patient is clearly volume-depleted.[441,447]

It is becoming increasingly clear that even mild hyponatremia can produce symptoms. Renneboog and associates showed that patients in whom hyponatremia had been classified as chronic and asymptomatic actually had various neurologic deficits when analyzed more closely.[448] These deficits included attention deficits and gait disturbances leading to more frequent falls. Therefore, the development of diuretic-induced hyponatremia should probably be regarded as a contraindication to continue using the agent responsible. Severe, symptomatic hyponatremia complicated by seizures or coma is an emergency requiring intensive treatment.[449] Conversely, osmotic demyelination has been related to overcorrection of hyponatremia or to a rapid correction of serum sodium by more than 12 and more than 18 mmol/L in the first 24 and 48 hours, respectively.[444,447,450] Patients with concurrent hypokalemia, liver disease, or malnutrition may be more susceptible to osmotic demyelination.[451]

Despite the importance of diuretic-induced hyponatremia (and hypokalemia, see later) for individual cases, these side effects are relatively mild on a population basis and should therefore not discourage prescription of these effective drugs. For example, a study among 3000 patients starting antihypertensive monotherapy, serum sodium and potassium values were only marginally lower in thiazide users, with more than 90% of patients maintaining normal levels.[452]

HYPOKALEMIA

Four mechanisms have been identified that increase renal K$^+$ elimination during therapy with thiazides or loop diuretics (Figure 51.20): increased tubular flow, secretion of AVP and aldosterone, and alkalosis. Flow-dependent K$^+$ secretion by the distal nephron provides a universal mechanism for increased K$^+$ secretion in response to diuretics that act more proximally.[157] The basal and flow-dependent components of K$^+$ secretion have been shown to be largely mediated by distinct channels. Whereas basal secretion traverses ROMK (see previous discussion) channels, flow-dependent K$^+$ secretion is mediated by calcium-activated maxi or big K$^+$ (BK) channels.[453,454] Normally, a flow-dependent rise in K$^+$ secretion during increased water intake is offset by a drop in AVP concentration that diminishes distal K$^+$ secretion. Diuretic therapy, however, is unusual because it combines increased distal tubule flow with maintained or increased AVP release due to nonosmotic stimulation, the second mechanism contributing to kaliuresis. Indeed, inhibition of AVP release in normal human subjects undergoing a furosemide diuresis inhibits the kaliuresis.[247] Nonosmotic AVP release is common in edematous subjects.[447] Therefore, enhanced release of AVP and increased distal tubule fluid delivery combine to promote ongoing K$^+$ losses during diuretic therapy for edema. Diuretic-induced aldosterone secretion also promotes distal K$^+$ secretion and provides a further mechanism for K$^+$ secretion.[157,265,455] The effects of flow and aldosterone on distal K$^+$ secretion are normally counterbalanced during changes in salt intake, just as are the effects of flow and AVP induced by changes in water intake (see Figure 51.20). Diuretic treatment, however, uncouples the two because it enhances the secretion of aldosterone and AVP but increases distal flow, thereby accounting for the particular importance of aldosterone and AVP in promoting K$^+$ loss with diuretics.[247] Finally, diuretic-induced alkalosis enhances distal secretion of K$^+$.[157]

The serum potassium concentration in patients not receiving KCl supplements falls by an average of 0.3 mmol/L with furosemide and by 0.6 mmol/L with thiazides.[456] This 20% fall in serum potassium is accompanied by a fall in total body K$^+$ that averages less than 5%.[456] Moreover, in normal subjects receiving daily doses of loop diuretics, there is no detectable change in K$^+$ balance despite a reproducible fall in serum potassium of about 0.5 mmol/L.[247] This finding implies that the primary cause of hypokalemia during diuretic administration is a redistribution of K$^+$ into cells, likely related to the accompanying metabolic alkalosis.[64,110]

Mild diuretic-induced hypokalemia (serum potassium 3.0-3.5 mmol/L) increases the frequency of ventricular ectopy.[457] Some writers have shown that thiazide-induced

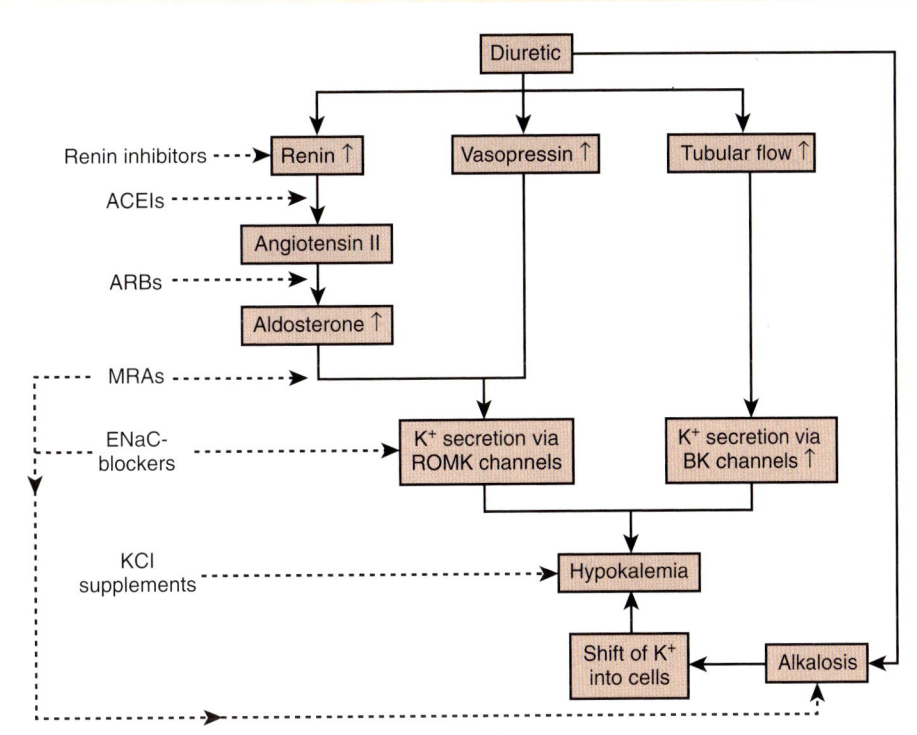

Figure 51.20 Diagrammatic representation of mechanisms that increase (↑) K⁺ excretion by the collecting ducts or partition K⁺ into cells during therapy with a thiazide or loop diuretic, and strategies for prevention or treatment (*dashed lines*) with direct renin inhibitors, angiotensin-converting enzyme inhibitors (ACEIs), angiotensin receptor blockers (ARBs), mineralocorticoid receptor antagonists (MRAs; e.g., spironolactone), epithelial Na⁺ channel (ENaC) blockers (amiloride or triamterene), or KCl supplements. Diuretics stimulate the renin angiotensin aldosterone system (RAAS), increase distal tubule flow and release of arginine vasopressin, and generate a metabolic alkalosis, all of which enhance K⁺ secretion in the collecting ducts. Two distinct mechanisms are responsible for K⁺ secretion in the collecting ducts, one mediated by the renal outer medulla K⁺ (ROMK) channels, and the other by big K⁺ (BK) channels.

hypokalemia does not pose a risk of clinically significant cardiac dysrhythmia even in large populations of hypertensive patients.[343,458] In contrast, others report a dose-dependent risk of cardiac arrest in patients receiving thiazides that is prevented by therapy with a K⁺-sparing diuretic such as amiloride.[459] In one study in rats, thiazide-induced hypokalemia was associated with hypomagnesemia, hypertriglyceridemia, insulin resistance, hyperaldosteronism, and renal injury, all of which were absent in rats with a similar degree of hypokalemia due to a dietary potassium depletion.[460] Although of concern, these data may be species specific and may also be ascribed to the dose given (10 mg/kg).[461] In a large population-based study of older adults, chlorthalidone was shown to be as effective in reducing cardiovascular outcomes as hydrochlorothiazide but more often resulted in hospitalization for hypokalemia or hyponatremia.[462]

Adverse effects of hypokalemia are clearly important in certain circumstances. First, severe hypokalemia (serum potassium < 3.0 mmol/L) requires treatment because it is associated with a doubling of serious ventricular dysrhythmias, muscular weakness, and rhabdomyolysis.[463] Second, mild hypokalemia can precipitate dangerous dysrhythmias in patients with cardiac dysfunction due to left ventricular hypertrophy, coronary ischemia, HF, prolonged QT interval, anoxia, or ischemia as well as in patients with known dysrhythmias. Third, hypokalemia enhances the toxicity of cardiac glycosides by diminishing the renal tubule secretion of digoxin and by enhancing its binding to cardiac Na⁺-K⁺-ATPase, thereby exaggerating its actions on the heart. Fourth, hypokalemia stimulates renal ammoniagenesis. This effect is dangerous for patients with cirrhosis and ascites who are prone to development of hepatic encephalopathy due to hyperammonemia. Moreover, the accompanying diuretic-induced alkalosis partitions ammonia into the brain. Fifth, catecholamines partition K⁺ into cells and lower serum potassium. Myocardial infarction provokes sufficient catecholamine release to lower serum potassium by approximately 0.5 mmol/L, which is potentiated in patients who have received prior thiazide therapy.[464] Sixth, hypokalemia impairs insulin release and predisposes to hyperglycemia.[465] Seventh, hypokalemia limits the antihypertensive action of thiazides.[466] In a placebo-controlled study of hypokalemic subjects receiving thiazide diuretics, coadministration of KCl that restored serum potassium also reduced blood pressure significantly.[466]

Diuretic-induced hypokalemia can be easily prevented, and the adverse consequences can be clinically significant. Therefore, it is prudent to prevent even mild degrees of hypokalemia. Hypokalemia can be prevented by increasing intake of K⁺ with Cl⁻ (see Figure 51.20) but doing so often requires 40 to 80 mmol daily. Moreover, in the presence of alkalosis, hyperaldosteronism, or Mg²⁺ depletion, hypokalemia is quite unresponsive to dietary KCl. A more effective, convenient, and predictable strategy is to prescribe a combined therapy with a distal K⁺-sparing agent such as amiloride or triamterene, which maintains serum potassium during short- or long-term hydrochlorothiazide therapy (see Figure

51.20).[467] It also prevents diuretic-induced alkalosis and provides further natriuresis and antihypertensive efficacy. An alternative strategy is to administer an ACE inhibitor, ARB, or MRA to counter angiotensin II–induced hyperaldosteronism, which would promote distal K^+ secretion. The fall in blood pressure and the beneficial cardiovascular actions of these agents are clearly a further advantage. Finally, a small study showed that combining torsemide with hydrochlorothiazide led as expected to a synergistic increase in sodium excretion but surprisingly reduced urinary potassium and magnesium losses in comparison with hydrochlorothiazide alone,[468] possibly owing to the antialdosteronic effects of torsemide.[469]

HYPERKALEMIA

Diuretics acting in the ASDN decrease K^+ secretion and predispose to hyperkalemia.[455,470] As noted previously, this complication was observed more frequently after increased use of distal K^+-sparing diuretics in Canada,[195] although a later report from Scotland was not able to reproduce these findings.[471] The risk of hyperkalemia may rise, especially when spironolactone is combined with other drugs that interfere with renal potassium secretion, such as trimethoprim-sulfamethoxazole.[472]

HYPOMAGNESEMIA

Loop diuretics inhibit Mg^{2+} reabsorption in the TAL[71,74] by reducing the transepithelial voltage that drives Mg^{2+} and Ca^{2+} paracellularly (see Figure 51.4).[473] Thiazides first enhance Mg^{2+} uptake in the DCT, but during prolonged therapy, there is enhanced renal Mg^{2+} excretion.[144] Although this greater excretion has been attributed to a fall in cellular $[Na^+]$ that stimulates basolateral Na^+-Mg^{2+} exchange,[473] later molecular data suggest that long-term thiazide use leads to downregulation of TRPM6, the predominant apical Mg^{2+} channel of the distal nephron.[141] Distal K^+-sparing agents and spironolactone diminish Mg^{2+} excretion. During prolonged therapy with thiazides and loop diuretics, serum Mg^{2+} concentration falls by 5% to 10%. Diuretic-induced hyponatremia and hypokalemia cannot be reversed fully until any Mg^{2+} deficit is replaced.[474] Mg^{2+}-depleted rats secrete K^+ inappropriately into the distal tubule and independent of aldosterone,[475] possibly because a decrease in intracellular magnesium releases the magnesium-mediated inhibition of ROMK channels.[476]

HYPERCALCEMIA

Thiazides increase the serum concentrations of total and ionized calcium but rarely result in frank hypercalcemia. During established thiazide treatment, parathyroid hormone concentrations are inversely related to ionized serum calcium.[477] The increased serum calcium can be ascribed primarily to enhanced Ca^{2+} reabsorption (the mechanism is discussed previously). Persistent hypercalcemia should prompt a search for a specific cause, for example, an adenoma of the parathyroid glands.[477,478]

ACID-BASE CHANGES

Metabolic alkalosis induced by thiazides or loop diuretics is an important adverse factor in patients with hepatic cirrhosis and ascites, in whom the alkalosis may provoke hepatic coma by partitioning ammonia into the brain, and in those with underlying pulmonary insufficiency, in whom the alkalosis diminishes ventilation.[479] The generation of metabolic alkalosis with loop diuretics results from contraction of the extracellular HCO_3^- space by the excretion of a relatively HCO_3^--free urine.[64,480] The maintenance of metabolic alkalosis involves increased net acid excretion in response to hypokalemia-induced ammoniagenesis and mineralocorticoid excess during continued Na^+ delivery and reabsorption at the distal nephron sites of H^+ secretion.[481] Diuretic-induced metabolic alkalosis is best managed with administration of KCl, but a distal K^+-sparing diuretic[482] or, occasionally, a CA inhibitor should be considered.[18] Metabolic alkalosis impairs the natriuretic response to loop diuretics[110] (see Figure 51.11) and may thereby contribute to diuretic resistance.

CA inhibitors produce metabolic acidosis. Spironolactone, eplerenone, amiloride, and triamterene can cause hyperkalemic metabolic acidosis, especially in elderly patients, patients with renal impairment, and those receiving KCl supplements.

METABOLIC ABNORMALITIES

HYPERGLYCEMIA

Diuretic therapy, especially with thiazides, impairs carbohydrate tolerance and occasionally precipitates diabetes mellitus.[431,483,484] The increase in blood glucose concentration is greatest during initiation of therapy. In one study, hydrochlorothiazide given to patients with non–insulin-dependent diabetes mellitus increased the fasting serum glucose concentration by 31% at 3 weeks. This increase was attributed to decreased hepatic utilization of glucose.[485] Hyperglycemia persists[486] but is reversed rapidly after diuretic discontinuation, even after 14 years of thiazide therapy.[487] The increase in blood glucose provoked by thiazides is worsened by concurrent β-adrenergic-receptor blockade.[485]

Thiazides impair glucose uptake into muscle[488,489] and liver.[485] This effect is more pronounced during initiation of therapy. It has been ascribed to a diuretic-induced reduction in cardiac output with reflex activation of the SNS and catecholamine secretion, which lead to reductions in hepatic glucose uptake, muscle blood flow, and muscle glucose uptake (Figure 51.21). During sustained thiazide therapy, there is decreased insulin release, which can be corrected by reversal of hypokalemia with KCl,[490] hypomagnesemia with magnesium oxide,[491] or administration of spironolactone. Experimental K^+ deficiency causes glucose intolerance and impairs insulin secretion in the absence of diuretics.[492] Hydrochlorothiazide and ACE inhibitors have opposite effects on glucose disposal, which are attributed to their opposing effects on serum potassium.[489] The increase in serum glucose levels that occurs with thiazide therapy is more pronounced in obese patients and correlates with a fall in intracellular $[K^+]$ or $[Mg^{2+}]$.[493] It can be prevented by reducing the thiazide dosage[465] or by KCl replacement.[490] Therefore, care should be taken to monitor blood glucose during thiazide therapy, particularly in obese or diabetic patients, and to prevent hypokalemia.

Thiazide-induced hyperglycemia should be anticipated and prevented. Measures include coadministration of a distal K^+-sparing diuretic, MRA, ACE inhibitor, or ARB, prescribing extra KCl, or reducing the thiazide dosage.[494]

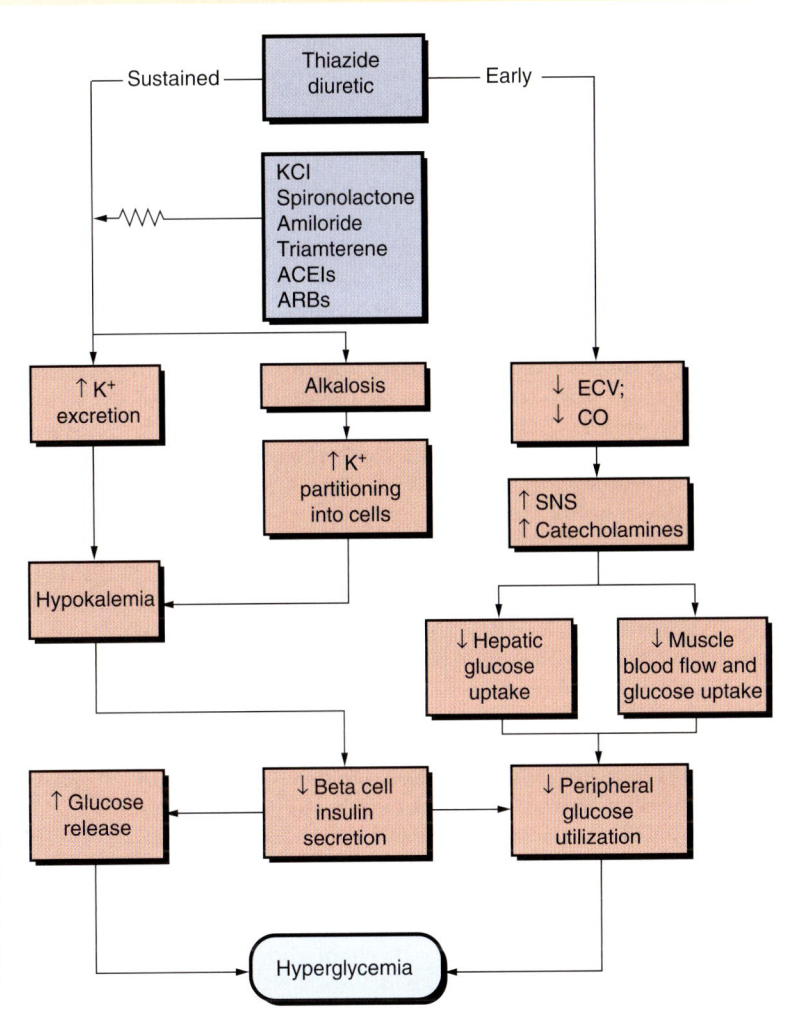

Figure 51.21 Hypothesis for the hyperglycemic actions of thiazide diuretics. ACEI, Angiotensin-converting enzyme inhibitor; ARB, angiotensin receptor blocker; ECV, extracellular fluid volume; SNS, sympathetic nervous system; ↑, increase(d); ↓, decrease(d). (From Wilcox CS: Metabolic and adverse effects of diuretics. *Semin Nephrol* 19:557-568, 1999.)

Thiazide diuretics are not contraindicated in patients with diabetes mellitus. Indeed, diuretics produce an even greater reduction in the absolute risk for cardiovascular events in hypertensive patients who are diabetic.[495] Therefore, diabetes mellitus is an indication for close surveillance and attention to coadministration of agents designed to prevent hypokalemia (see Figure 51.21).

HYPERLIPIDEMIA

Administration of loop diuretics or thiazides raises the plasma concentrations of total cholesterol, triglycerides, and low-density lipoprotein cholesterol, but reduces the concentration of high-density lipoprotein cholesterol. These adverse changes average 5% to 20% during initiation of therapy.[496] The mechanism is uncertain; it may relate to ECV depletion, because severe dietary NaCl restriction has similar metabolic effects[497] whereas increasing NaCl intake lowers serum cholesterol. Alternatively, it may relate to hypokalemia, which impairs insulin secretion.[490,493] Importantly, most studies have shown that serum cholesterol returns to baseline over 3 to 12 months of thiazide therapy.[496,498] In fact, when combined with lifestyle management, 4 years of thiazide therapy for hypertension is associated with a modest improvement in lipid profile.[499,500]

HYPERURICEMIA

Prolonged thiazide therapy for hypertension increases the serum urate concentration by approximately 35%. Renal urate clearance falls because of competition for secretion between urate and the diuretic,[75] and ECV depletion–induced urate reabsorption (see Figure 51.5).[76] Hyperuricemia is dose-related and can lead to gout. A very long-term outcome analysis of 3693 patients detected no adverse effects of diuretic-induced hyperuricemia in hypertensive subjects who did not have gout.[501] However, later studies have correlated raised serum urate with higher cardiovascular death rate.[502] One possibility is to combine diuretic treatment with ARB losartan, which has weak uricosuric properties.[503]

OTHER ADVERSE EFFECTS

IMPOTENCE

In the Medical Research Council trial involving 15,000 hypertensive subjects, impotence was much higher in those receiving a thiazide.[431] In the Treatment of Mild Hypertension Study, erection problems were twice as high in subjects receiving a thiazide as in those who were not.[504] A controlled trial demonstrated the efficacy of sildenafil in reversing impotence in hypertensive patients receiving multiple antihypertensive agents including diuretics.[505]

OTOTOXICITY

Loop diuretics can cause deafness that may occasionally be permanent.[506] The risk is greater with ethacrynic acid than with other loop diuretics and is also greater when a loop diuretic is combined with another ototoxic drug (e.g., an aminoglycoside).[507] It is especially common during high-dose bolus intravenous therapy in patients with renal failure, in whom plasma levels are increased, and in hypoalbuminemic subjects.[508] In a crossover trial, no ototoxicity was noted in patients with severe HF when they were given an infusion of 250 to 2000 mg of furosemide over 8 hours, whereas reversible deafness occurred in 25% when the same dose was given as a bolus.[318]

HAZARDS IN PREGNANCY AND NEWBORNS

Diuretics do not prevent preeclampsia. They have little effect on perinatal mortality.[509] Thiazide therapy can be continued during pregnancy in patients whose hypertension has been controlled by these agents or used to treat pulmonary edema.[510]

Intensive therapy with loop diuretics for neonates with respiratory distress syndrome increases the prevalence of patent ductus arteriosus because of increased generation of prostaglandins,[511] cholelithiasis, secondary hyperparathyroidism, bone disease, and drug fever.[512] Prolonged furosemide therapy in preterm infants can cause renal calcification.[513] Diuretics can be transferred from the mother to the infant in breast milk,[513] in whom they can cause serious fluid and electrolyte abnormalities.[514]

B VITAMIN DEFICIENCY

Diuretics increase the excretion of water-soluble vitamins.[515] Long-term diuretic therapy for HF reduces folate and vitamin B1 (thiamine) levels[516] and increases plasma homocysteine. Thiamine can improve left ventricular function in some patients with HF being treated with furosemide.[517]

DRUG ALLERGY

A reversible photosensitivity dermatitis occurs rarely during thiazide or furosemide therapy.[518] High-dose furosemide in renal failure can cause bullous dermatitis.[519] Diuretics may cause a more generalized dermatitis, sometimes with eosinophilia, purpura, or blood dyscrasia. Occasionally, they cause a necrotizing vasculitis or anaphylaxis.[520] Acute allergic reactions to sulfonamides are mediated via immunoglobulin E, whereas delayed-onset hypersensitivities are mediated by antibodies to specific protein epitopes.[521] Severe necrotizing pancreatitis is a rare complication.[522] Acute interstitial nephritis with fever, rash, and eosinophilia may develop abruptly some months after initiation of therapy with a thiazide or, less often, furosemide.[523,524] Ethacrynic acid is chemically dissimilar from other loop diuretics and can be a substitute.

MALIGNANCY

Although previous epidemiologic studies suggested associations between diuretic use and cancer (renal cell carcinoma and colon carcinoma), a 2011 meta-analysis has refuted the suggestion of a higher risk of cancer or cancer-related death with use of any antihypertensive drugs.[525]

ADVERSE DRUG INTERACTIONS

Hyperkalemia in patients receiving distal K^+-sparing diuretics, spironolactone, or eplerenone can be precipitated by concurrent therapy with KCl, ACE inhibitors, ARBs, heparin, ketoconazole, trimethoprim, or pentamidine. Therefore, these drugs should not normally be prescribed in combination, especially in patients with impaired renal function or diabetes. ACE inhibitors increase the risk of severe hyperkalemia in patients with decompensated HF receiving spironolactone.[526,527] Loop diuretics and aminoglycosides potentiate ototoxicity and nephrotoxicity.[508,528] Diuretic-induced hypokalemia increases digitalis toxicity fourfold.[529] Plasma lithium concentrations rise during loop diuretic therapy[530] because of increased proximal lithium reabsorption.[531] NSAIDs may impair the diuretic, natriuretic, antihypertensive, and venodilating responses to diuretics and predispose to renal vasoconstriction and a drop in GFR (see earlier discussion "Adaptation to Diuretic Therapy"). Used together, indomethacin and triamterene may precipitate renal failure.[532]

Complete reference list available at ExpertConsult.com.

KEY REFERENCES

1. Bleich M, Greger R: Mechanism of action of diuretics. *Kidney Int Suppl* 59:S11–S15, 1997.
2. Brater DC: Use of diuretics in cirrhosis and nephrotic syndrome. *Semin Nephrol* 19:575–580, 1999.
3. Brater DC: Pharmacology of diuretics. *Am J Med Sci* 319:38–50, 2000.
4. Wilcox CS: New insights into diuretic use in patients with chronic renal disease. *J Am Soc Nephrol* 13:798–805, 2002.
77. Loon NR, Wilcox CS, Unwin RJ: Mechanism of impaired natriuretic response to furosemide during prolonged therapy. *Kidney Int* 36:682–689, 1989.
82. Schnermann J, Homer W: Smith Award lecture: the juxtaglomerular apparatus: from anatomical peculiarity to physiological relevance. *J Am Soc Nephrol* 14:1681–1694, 2003.
90. Ellison DH, Velazquez H, Wright FS: Thiazide-sensitive sodium chloride cotransport in early distal tubule. *Am J Physiol* 253:F546–F554, 1987.
98. Vallon V, Rieg T, Ahn SY, et al: Overlapping in vitro and in vivo specificities of the organic anion transporters OAT1 and OAT3 for loop and thiazide diuretics. *Am J Physiol Renal Physiol* 294:F867–F873, 2008.
110. Loon NR, Wilcox CS: Mild metabolic alkalosis impairs the natriuretic response to bumetanide in normal human subjects. *Clin Sci* 94:287–292, 1998.
112. Pichette V, Geadah D, du Souich P: The influence of moderate hypoalbuminaemia on the renal metabolism and dynamics of furosemide in the rabbit. *Br J Pharmacol* 119:885–890, 1996.
115. Chennavasin P, Seiwell R, Brater DC: Pharmacokinetic-dynamic analysis of the indomethacin-furosemide interaction in man. *J Pharmacol Exp Ther* 215:77–81, 1980.
117. Wilcox CS, Mitch WE, Kelly RA, et al: Response of the kidney to furosemide: I: effects of salt intake and renal compensation. *J Lab Clin Med* 102:450–458, 1983.
141. Nijenhuis T, Vallon V, van der Kemp AW, et al: Enhanced passive Ca^{2+} reabsorption and reduced Mg^{2+} channel abundance explains thiazide-induced hypocalciuria and hypomagnesemia. *J Clin Invest* 115:1651–1658, 2005.
186. Pitt B, Zannad F, Remme WJ, et al: The effect of spironolactone on morbidity and mortality in patients with severe heart failure. *N Engl J Med* 341:709–717, 1999.
195. Juurlink DN, Mamdani MM, Lee DS, et al: Rates of hyperkalemia after publication of the randomized aldactone evaluation study. *N Eng J Med* 351:543–551, 2004.

225. Kaissling B, Bachmann S, Kriz W: Structural adaptation of the distal convoluted tubule to prolonged furosemide treatment. *Am J Physiol* 248:F374–F381, 1985.
234. Almeshari K, Ahlstrom NG, Capraro FE, et al: A volume-independent component to post-diuretic sodium retention in man. *J Am Soc Nephrol* 3:1878–1883, 1993.
273. Ellison DH: The physiologic basis of diuretic synergism: its role in treating diuretic resistance [see comments]. *Ann Intern Med* 114:886–894, 1991.
282. Brater DC: Diuretic therapy. *N Engl J Med* 339:387–395, 1998.
286. Jessup M, Abraham WT, Casey DE, et al: 2009 focused update: ACCF/AHA guidelines for the diagnosis and management of heart failure in adults: a report of the American College of Cardiology Foundation/American Heart Association Task Force on Practice Guidelines: developed in collaboration with the International Society for Heart and Lung Transplantation. *Circulation* 119:1977–2016, 2009.
316. Jentzer JC, DeWald TA, Hernandez AF: Combination of loop diuretics with thiazide-type diuretics in heart failure. *J Am Coll Cardiol* 56:1527–1534, 2010.
332. Sarnak MJ: A patient with heart failure and worsening kidney function. *Clin J Am Soc Nephrol* 9:1790–1798, 2014.
334. Gines P, Cardenas A, Arroyo V, et al: Management of cirrhosis and ascites. *N Engl J Med* 350:1646–1654, 2004.
338. Runyon BA: AASLD. Introduction to the revised American Association for the Study of Liver Diseases Practice Guideline management of adult patients with ascites due to cirrhosis 2012. *Hepatology* 57:1651–1653, 2013.
355. Schrier RW, Fassett RG: A critique of the overfill hypothesis of sodium and water retention in the nephrotic syndrome. *Kidney Int* 53:1111–1117, 1998.
387. Stewart RM, Park PK, Hunt JP, et al: Less is more: improved outcomes in surgical patients with conservative fluid administration and central venous catheter monitoring. *J Am Coll Surg* 208:725–735, discussion 735–727, 2009.
390. Voelker JR, Cartwright Brown D, Anderson S, et al: Comparison of loop diuretics in patients with chronic renal insufficiency. *Kidney Int* 32:572–578, 1987.
397. Sica DA, Gehr TW: Diuretic use in stage 5 chronic kidney disease and end-stage renal disease. *Curr Opin Nephrol Hypertens* 12:483–490, 2003.
424. Blanchard A, Vargas-Poussou R, Vallet M, et al: Indomethacin, amiloride, or eplerenone for treating hypokalemia in Gitelman syndrome. *J Am Soc Nephrol* 26:468–475, 2015.
428. Bedford JJ, Weggery S, Ellis G, et al: Lithium-induced nephrogenic diabetes insipidus: renal effects of amiloride. *Clin J Am Soc Nephrol* 3:1324–1331, 2008.
438. McCance RA: Experimental sodium chloride deficiency in man. *Proc R Soc Lond B Biol Sci* 119:245–268, 1936.
439. Clark BA, Shannon RP, Rosa RM, et al: Increased susceptibility to thiazide-induced hyponatremia in the elderly. *J Am Soc Nephrol* 5:1106–1111, 1994.
442. Friedman E, Shadel M, Halkin H, et al: Thiazide-induced hyponatremia: reproducibility by single dose rechallenge and an analysis of pathogenesis. *Ann Intern Med* 110:24–30, 1989.
449. Spasovski G, Vanholder R, Allolio B, et al: Clinical practice guideline on diagnosis and treatment of hyponatraemia. *Nephrol Dial Transplant* 29(Suppl 2):i1–i39, 2014.
461. Ellison DH, Loffing J: Thiazide effects and adverse effects: insights from molecular genetics. *Hypertension* 54:196–202, 2009.

THE CONSEQUENCES OF ADVANCED KIDNEY DISEASE

SECTION VIII

52 Adaptation to Nephron Loss and Mechanisms of Progression in Chronic Kidney Disease

Maarten W. Taal

CHAPTER OUTLINE

STRUCTURAL AND FUNCTIONAL ADAPTATION OF THE KIDNEY TO NEPHRON LOSS, 1737
Alterations in Glomerular Physiology, 1737
Mediators of the Glomerular Hemodynamic Responses to Nephron Loss, 1738
Renal Hypertrophic Responses to Nephron Loss, 1741
Mechanisms of Renal Hypertrophy, 1743
ADAPTATION OF SPECIFIC TUBULE FUNCTIONS IN RESPONSE TO NEPHRON LOSS, 1745
Adaptation in Proximal Tubule Solute Handling, 1745
Loop of Henle and Distal Nephron, 1746
Glomerulotubular Balance, 1746
Sodium Excretion and Extracellular Fluid Volume Regulation, 1747
Urinary Concentration and Dilution, 1748
Potassium Excretion, 1748
Acid-Base Regulation, 1749
Calcium and Phosphate, 1749
LONG-TERM ADVERSE CONSEQUENCES OF ADAPTATIONS TO NEPHRON LOSS, 1750
Hemodynamic Factors, 1750

Mechanisms of Hemodynamically Induced Injury, 1752
Nonhemodynamic Factors in the Development of Nephron Injury Following Extensive Renal Mass Ablation, 1755
A Unified Hypothesis of Chronic Kidney Disease Progression, 1763
INSIGHTS FROM MODIFIERS OF CHRONIC KIDNEY DISEASE PROGRESSION, 1764
Pharmacologic Inhibition of the Renin Angiotensin Aldosterone System, 1764
Arterial Hypertension, 1765
Dietary Protein Intake, 1767
Gender, 1768
Nephron Endowment, 1769
Ethnicity, 1769
Obesity and Metabolic Syndrome, 1770
Sympathetic Nervous System, 1771
Dyslipidemia, 1772
Calcium and Phosphate Metabolism, 1774
Anemia, 1776
Tobacco Smoking, 1776
Acute Kidney Injury, 1777
FUTURE DIRECTIONS, 1778

The introduction of a classification system for chronic kidney disease (CKD) by the National Kidney Foundation Kidney Disease Outcomes Quality Initiative (KDOQI) and its adoption worldwide have made a valuable contribution to raising awareness of the problem of CKD.[1] Importantly, the division of the spectrum of CKD into stages has emphasized the progressive nature of CKD and facilitated the development of stage-specific strategies for slowing the progression of CKD, as well as treating the complications of CKD. These developments highlight the importance of understanding the mechanisms that contribute to CKD progression in order to inform strategies for slowing such progression. Central to these mechanisms are the adaptations observed in the kidney when nephrons are lost.

The kidney's primary function of maintaining constancy of the extracellular fluid (ECF) volume and composition is remarkably well preserved until late in the course of CKD. When nephrons are lost through disease or surgical ablation, those remaining or least affected undergo remarkable physiologic responses resulting in hypertrophy and hyperfunction that combine to compensate for the acquired loss of renal function. Effective kidney function requires close integration of glomerular and tubular functions. Indeed, the preservation of *glomerulotubular balance* seen until the terminal stages of CKD is fundamental to the *intact nephron hypothesis* of Bricker, which essentially states that as CKD advances, kidney function is supported by a diminishing pool of functioning (or hyperfunctioning) nephrons, rather than relatively constant numbers of nephrons, each with diminishing function. This concept has important implications for the mechanisms of disease progression in CKD.

Several decades ago, clinical studies of patients with CKD established that once GFR fell below a critical level, a relentless progression to end-stage kidney disease (ESKD) inevitably ensued, even when the initial disease activity had abated. The rate of decline of GFR in a given individual followed a near-constant linear relationship with time, enabling remarkably accurate predictions of the date at which ESKD would be reached and renal replacement therapy required. Among patients with diverse kidney diseases, the slope of the GFR/time relationship was found to be a characteristic of individual patients rather than typical of their specific kidney disease. This observation suggested that the progressive nature of kidney disease could be attributed to a final "common pathway" of mechanisms, independent of the primary cause of nephropathy.[2] Within this framework, Brenner and colleagues formulated a unifying hypothesis for kidney disease progression based on the physiologic adaptations observed in experimental models of CKD.[3] The central tenets of the common pathway theory state that CKD progression occurs, in general, through focal nephron loss and that the adaptive responses of surviving nephrons, although initially serving to increase single nephron GFR (SNGFR) and offset the overall loss in clearance, ultimately prove detrimental to the kidney. Over time, glomerulosclerosis and tubular atrophy further reduce nephron number, fueling a self-perpetuating cycle of nephron destruction culminating in uremia.

In this chapter we describe in detail the functional and structural adaptations observed in remaining nephrons following substantial reductions in functioning renal mass and the mechanisms thought to be responsible for them. We then consider how these changes may in time prove maladaptive and contribute to the progressive renal injury described earlier. Given the growing worldwide burden of CKD that causes substantial morbidity and mortality in individuals and threatens to overburden health care systems, it could be argued that the further elucidation of the mechanisms of CKD progression resulting in more effective interventions to slow its advance should remain among the highest priorities for nephrologists and health care systems today.

STRUCTURAL AND FUNCTIONAL ADAPTATION OF THE KIDNEY TO NEPHRON LOSS

ALTERATIONS IN GLOMERULAR PHYSIOLOGY

Glomerular hemodynamic responses to nephron loss have been studied largely in animals subjected to surgical ablation of renal mass. It was recognized several decades ago that unilateral nephrectomy in rats resulted in a rapid

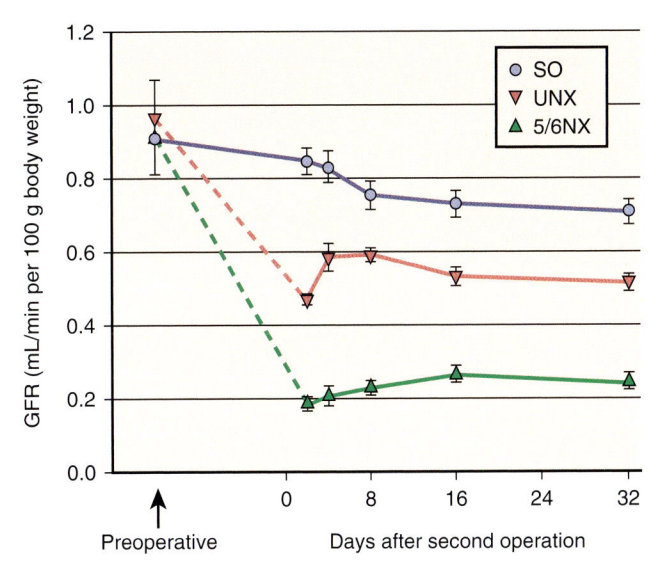

Figure 52.1 Glomerular filtration rate (GFR) in conscious rats before and after sham operation (SO), uninephrectomy (UNX), or 5/6 nephrectomy (5/6NX). Values are means ± standard error of means (SEM). (Used with permission from Chamberlain RM, Shirley DG: Time course of the renal functional response to partial nephrectomy: measurements in conscious rats. *Exp Physiol* 92:251-262, 2007.)

increase in function of the remaining kidney, detectable 3 days after nephrectomy, such that the GFR achieved a maximum of 70% to 85% of the previous two-kidney value after 2 to 3 weeks. Observations in conscious rats have reported a maximal increase of approximately 50% in GFR of a single kidney at 8 days after uninephrectomy and a 300% increase in GFR of the remnant kidney at 16 days after 5/6 nephrectomy (Figure 52.1).[4] As no new nephrons are formed in mature rodents, the observed rise in GFR represents an increase in the filtration rate of remaining nephrons.

Detailed study of glomerular hemodynamics was facilitated by the identification of a rat strain, Munich-Wistar, which is unique in regularly bearing glomeruli on the kidney surface. This allowed micropuncture of the glomerulus and direct measurement of intraglomerular pressures as well as sampling of blood from afferent and efferent arterioles. These techniques made possible the study of mechanisms underlying the compensatory rise in GFR after renal mass ablation. Increases in whole-kidney GFR at 2 to 4 weeks after unilateral nephrectomy were attributable to an increase in SNGFR averaging 83%, achieved in large part by a rise in glomerular plasma flow rate (Q_A), which in turn resulted from dilation of afferent and, to a lesser extent, efferent arterioles. Although systemic blood pressure was not elevated, glomerular capillary hydraulic pressure (P_{GC}) and the glomerular transcapillary pressure difference (ΔP) were increased significantly post uninephrectomy, accounting for an estimated 25% of the rise in SNGFR.[5] The glomerular ultrafiltration coefficient, K_f (the product of glomerular hydraulic permeability and surface area available for filtration) was unaltered at this stage but may become elevated later.[6]

With more extensive nephron loss, even greater compensatory increases in SNGFR were observed. In Munich-Wistar rats studied 7 days after unilateral nephrectomy and infarction of 5/6 of the contralateral kidney, SNGFR in the remnant was more than double that of two-kidney controls. This increment was again attributable to large increases in Q_A, and a substantial rise in P_{GC}. Efferent and afferent arteriolar resistances were reduced, but the decrease in afferent arteriolar resistance was again proportionately greater, accounting for the observed rise in P_{GC}.[7] Comparison of renal infarction versus surgical excision models of 5/6 nephrectomy subsequently found that changes in arteriolar resistance were similar but that P_{GC} was significantly more elevated in the infarction model, indicating that glomerular transmission of elevated systemic blood pressure (absent in the surgical excision model) also contributes to the increase in P_{GC}.[8] Changes in K_f after extensive renal mass ablation appear to be time dependent, with a decrease reported at 2 weeks after surgery,[9] and an increase at 4 weeks.[10] Further studies indicated that glomerular hemodynamic responses to nephron loss seem to be similar between the superficial cortical and juxtamedullary nephrons.[11] The rise in SNGFR associated with renal mass ablation is often referred to as *glomerular hyperfiltration*, and the elevated P_{GC} is termed *glomerular hypertension*. Together these terms encompass the central concepts underlying the hemodynamic adaptations in the remnant kidney.

Glomerular hemodynamic adaptations to nephron loss may show interspecies variation. In dogs, increases in SNGFR observed 4 weeks after 3/4 or 7/8 nephrectomy were attributable largely to increases in Q_A and K_f. In contrast to the findings in rodents, ΔP was only modestly elevated. After ablation of 7/8 of their renal mass, dogs developed a significant rise in P_{GC} independent of arterial pressure, again as a result of relatively greater relaxation of afferent versus efferent arterioles.[12]

In humans, the effects of nephron loss on the physiology of the remnant kidney have been studied mainly in healthy individuals undergoing donor nephrectomy for kidney transplantation. Inulin clearance studies of the earliest kidney donors revealed that total GFR in the donor's remaining kidney had increased to 65% to 70% of the previous two-kidney value by 1 week post nephrectomy. A meta-analysis of data from 48 studies that included 2988 living kidney donors estimated that GFR decreased, on average, by only 17 mL/min after uninephrectomy.[13] These observations imply that single-kidney GFR (and therefore also the average SNGFR) increases by 30% to 40% after uninephrectomy in humans. There is currently no method for measuring SNGFR or P_{GC} in humans, but detailed studies in 21 healthy kidney donors have reported that the observed increase in single-kidney GFR could be accounted for by the observed increase in renal plasma flow (RPF) and a rise in K_f resulting from glomerular hypertrophy without need for an increase in P_{GC}.[14]

MEDIATORS OF THE GLOMERULAR HEMODYNAMIC RESPONSES TO NEPHRON LOSS

The factors that are sensed after renal mass ablation and serve as signals to initiate the adjustments in glomerular hemodynamics responsible for the increase in remnant kidney GFR remain to be identified. However, the effector mechanisms have been studied extensively, and the hemodynamic changes can be attributed to the net effects of complex interactions of several factors, each having specific, and sometimes opposing actions on the various determinants of glomerular ultrafiltration. Several vasoactive substances, including angiotensin II (Ang II), aldosterone, natriuretic peptides (NPs), endothelins (ETs), eicosanoids, and bradykinin, have been implicated. Moreover, sustained increases in SNGFR also require resetting of the autoregulatory mechanisms that normally govern GFR and RPF. For a detailed discussion of vasoactive peptides in the kidney, see Chapter 13.

RENIN ANGIOTENSIN ALDOSTERONE SYSTEM

Ang II appears to play a critical role in the development of glomerular capillary hypertension following renal mass ablation and may also contribute to changes in K_f. Acute infusion of Ang II in normal rats results in a rise in P_{GC}, due to a greater increase in efferent than afferent resistance, and reductions in Q_A and K_f.[15,16] Chronic administration of Ang II for 8 weeks resulted in systemic hypertension and lowered single-kidney GFR and, with the exception of K_f, elicited similar glomerular hemodynamic changes to those observed after acute infusion in both normal and uninephrectomized rats.[6] The importance of the influence of endogenous Ang II on glomerular hemodynamics in remnant kidneys was revealed by studies with pharmacologic inhibitors of the renin angiotensin aldosterone system (RAAS). Chronic treatment of 5/6 nephrectomized rats with either an angiotensin-converting enzyme inhibitor (ACEI)[17,18] or Ang II subtype 1 receptor blocker (ARB$_1$)[19,20] results in normalization of P_{GC} through reduction in systemic blood pressure and dilation of both afferent and efferent arterioles. SNGFR, however, remains elevated due to an increase in K_f. Furthermore, acute infusion of an ACEI or saralasin, a peptide analogue receptor antagonist of Ang II, was found to normalize P_{GC} in 5/6 nephrectomized rats through efferent arteriolar dilation, without affecting mean arterial pressure (MAP).[9,21] It is unclear why these findings could not be confirmed with the ARB$_1$, losartan.[22]

These effects of RAAS inhibition imply that there is increased local activity of endogenous Ang II, yet plasma renin levels show only a transient increase following 5/6 nephrectomy.[8,23] This suggests differential regulation of the systemic versus intrarenal RAAS and that Ang II is formed locally. Detailed studies have identified that all components of the RAAS are expressed in the kidney.[24] Renin messenger RNA (mRNA) and protein levels are both increased in glomeruli adjacent to the infarction scar in 5/6 nephrectomized rats.[25-27] Furthermore, renal renin mRNA levels are increased at day 3 and 7 after renal mass ablation by infarction but not when renal mass is excised surgically, suggesting that renal infarction activates the RAAS by creating a margin of ischemic tissue around the organizing infarct and explaining the greater severity of hypertension as well as glomerulosclerosis associated with the infarction model.[8] Detailed studies of intrarenal Ang II levels following 5/6 nephrectomy achieved by infarction have confirmed these findings by showing higher Ang II levels in the periinfarct portion of the kidney than the intact portion at all time points.[23] On the other hand, the studies also showed that the rise in intrarenal Ang II following 5/6 nephrectomy was transient. Whereas Ang II levels in the periinfarct portion were elevated compared to sham-operated controls at 2 weeks after surgery, they were not statistically different at 5 or 7 weeks. In the intact portion of the remnant kidney, Ang II levels were similar to controls at 2 and 5 weeks and were lower at 7 weeks.[23] Sustained increases in intrarenal Ang II levels are therefore not required to maintain the hypertension and progressive renal injury characteristic of this model. Nevertheless, subsequent studies have shown that the renoprotective effects of ACEI and ARB_1 treatment are associated with a reduction in intrarenal Ang II levels in both the periinfarct and intact portions of the remnant kidney.[28] In contrast, treatment with the dihydropyridine calcium antagonist, nifedipine, did not reduce proteinuria despite lowering blood pressure to the same levels as the RAAS antagonist, and was associated with an increase in intrarenal Ang II.[28] Thus intrarenal Ang II appears to play a central role in the pathogenesis of hypertension and renal injury in this model even in the absence of sustained increases in Ang II levels. Further research is required to fully explain these findings. It could be argued that apparently normal intrarenal Ang II levels are inappropriately high in the context of the hypertension and ECF volume expansion seen in these animals or that the average intrarenal Ang II levels measured may have failed to detect important local elevations of Ang II.

Later attention focused on the potential role of aldosterone in progressive renal injury. In addition to evidence that aldosterone may exert profibrotic effects in the kidney (see later), observations suggest that it may also have important glomerular hemodynamic effects. Previous observations that the deoxycorticosterone-salt model of hypertension is associated with glomerular capillary hypertension prompted detailed studies of microperfused rabbit afferent and efferent arterioles that found dose-dependent constriction of both arterioles in response to nanomolar concentrations of aldosterone, with greater sensitivity observed in efferent arterioles.[29] These effects were not inhibited by spironolactone and were still present with albumin-bound aldosterone, indicating that they may be mediated by specific membrane receptors rather than the intracellular receptors responsible for most of the actions of aldosterone. Interestingly, aldosterone may also counteract rabbit afferent arteriolar vasoconstriction via a nitric oxide (NO)-dependent pathway, an action that would also be expected to increase P_{GC}.[30,31]

ENDOTHELINS

ETs are potent vasoconstrictor peptides that act via at least two receptor subtypes, ET type A (ET-A) and ET type B (ET-B). ET receptors have been identified throughout the body and are most abundant in the lungs and kidneys. ET-A receptors are primarily located on vascular smooth muscle cells and mediate vasoconstriction as well as cellular proliferation. ET-B receptors are expressed on vascular endothelial and renal epithelial cells and appear to play a role as clearance receptors as well as mediating endothelium-dependent vasodilation via NO.[32-34] Renal production of ETs is increased after 5/6 nephrectomy, raising the possibility that they may also contribute to the observed glomerular hemodynamic adaptations.[35,36] Acute and chronic infusion of ET elicits dose-dependent reductions in RPF and GFR in normal rats.[37-40] Observations regarding the relative effects of ET on afferent and efferent arterioles are to some extent contradictory, possibly reflecting different experimental conditions. Despite some differences, most studies in intact animals reported greater increases in efferent than afferent arteriolar resistance resulting in an increase in P_{GC}. The ultrafiltration coefficient (K_f) was significantly reduced, and thus, SNGFR was unchanged or was decreased.[41-44] On the other hand, observations in microperfused arterioles found that ET caused greater constriction of the afferent than efferent arteriole. Studies with selective ET-A and ET-B receptor antagonists and ET-B receptor knockout mice were somewhat contradictory, suggesting a complex interaction between ET-A and ET-B receptors in determining the response.[45,46] In short-term studies of human subjects with CKD, ET receptor antagonists increased renal blood flow but had little effect on GFR due to a decrease in filtration fraction, observations consistent with a greater vasodilatory effect on the efferent arteriole.[47,48] Interestingly, these observations were made in subjects already receiving treatment with an ACEI or ARB_1. The potential interaction between ETs and other vasoactive molecules is further illustrated by observations that chronic infusion of Ang II results in increased production of ET[49] and that endothelin-1 (ET-1) transgenic mice are not hypertensive but evidence induction of inducible nitric oxide synthase (iNOS) resulting in increased NO production as a probable counterregulatory mechanism to maintain normal blood pressure.[50] Furthermore, some of the glomerular hemodynamic effects of ET appear to be modulated by prostaglandins.[44] Detailed micropuncture studies to elucidate the role of ETs in remnant kidney hemodynamics have not yet been published. These studies should be facilitated by the ongoing development of specific ET-A and ET-B receptor antagonists.

NATRIURETIC PEPTIDES

Atrial natriuretic peptide (ANPs) and other structurally related NPs mediate, in large part, the functional adaptations in tubular sodium reabsorption that maintain sodium excretion in 5/6 nephrectomized rats[51] but also exert important hemodynamic effects. Circulating ANP levels are elevated in 5/6 nephrectomized rats, and acute administration of an NP antagonist elicited profound decreases in GFR and RPF in 5/6 nephrectomized rats on high-salt (but not low-salt) diet, indicating that NPs play an important role in the observed hemodynamic responses to 5/6 nephrectomy.[52] In another study brain natriuretic peptide (BNP) levels were found to be elevated after 3/4 nephrectomy in the absence of cardiac dysfunction or upregulation of myocardial BNP gene expression.[53] Further insights into the renal hemodynamic effects of NP were gained from observations in normal rats infused with a synthetic ANP. Whole-kidney GFR and SNGFR increased by approximately 20% due entirely to a rise in P_{GC}, resulting from significant afferent arteriolar dilation and efferent arteriolar constriction.[54] In these experiments some residual elevation in remnant kidney GFR appeared to persist even after the NP system was suppressed by sodium restriction or an NP receptor antagonist, suggesting that factors other than NP make contributions to glomerular hyperfiltration following renal mass ablation. The potential interaction between NP and other vasoactive molecules is illustrated by the observation that ANP infusion in normal rats induced an increase in renal nitric oxide synthase (NOS) activity.[55]

EICOSANOIDS

Eicosanoids, another family of potent vasoactive molecules present in abundance in the kidney, may also play a role in mediating glomerular hyperfiltration. Urinary excretion per nephron of both vasodilator and vasoconstrictor prostaglandins is increased in rats and rabbits after renal mass ablation.[56-58] Infusion of prostaglandin E_2 (PGE_2), prostacyclin (PGI_2), or 6-keto-PGE_1 into the renal artery elicits significant renal vasodilation.[59] Whereas acute inhibition of prostaglandin synthesis by infusion of the cyclo-oxygenase (COX) inhibitor, indomethacin, had no effect on GFR or glomerular hemodynamics in normal rats, indomethacin lowered both SNGFR and Q_A after 3/4 or 5/6 nephrectomy.[56,57] On the other hand, chronic treatment with a selective COX-2 inhibitor attenuated the systemic and glomerular hypertension observed in 5/6 nephrectomized rats but had no effect on GFR.[60] The relative effects of prostaglandin synthesis inhibitors on afferent and efferent arterioles may vary with time post nephrectomy. Afferent arteriolar constriction was the predominant finding reported at 24 hours post surgery, whereas constriction of both afferent and efferent arterioles was observed at 3 to 4 weeks.[56,57] Some contribution of thromboxanes to glomerular hemodynamic adjustments after 5/6 nephrectomy in rats is suggested by the increase in GFR seen after acute infusion of a selective thromboxane synthesis inhibitor.[58] Thus, different eicosanoids appear to exert opposite effects, but the general impression is that the combined effects of vasodilator prostaglandins outweigh those of the vasoconstrictors. This interaction is illustrated by the observation that perfusion of isolated glomeruli with bradykinin resulted in vasodilation of the efferent arteriole that was completely blocked by indomethacin but that this blockade was reversed by a specific antagonist of 20-hydroxyeicosatetraenoic acid (20-HETE), a vasoconstrictor eicosanoid, indicating that the glomerulus produced both vasodilator and vasoconstrictor eicosanoids.[61]

NITRIC OXIDE

The extremely short half-life of NO precludes direct measurement of NO levels or administration of exogenous NO in experimental models. The actions of NO have thus been inferred from experiments with inhibitors of NOS. Intravenous infusion of NOS inhibitors results in systemic and renal vasoconstriction as well as a reduction in GFR in normal rats.[62,63] Thus NO appears to exert a tonic effect on the physiologic maintenance of systemic blood pressure and renal perfusion under resting conditions. It is unclear, however, whether NO plays a specific role in the adaptive hemodynamic changes that follow renal mass ablation. Indeed, renal expression of NOS and renal NO generation are reduced in 5/6 nephrectomized rats, whereas systemic production of NO is increased.[64,65] MAP and renal vascular resistance increased, whereas renal blood flow (RBF) and GFR decreased to a similar extent after acute infusion of an endothelial NOS (eNOS) inhibitor, N^G-monomethyl-L-arginine (L-NMMA), irrespective of whether given to normal rats or 3 to 4 weeks after unilateral or 5/6 nephrectomy.[63] Chronic NOS inhibition with N^G-nitro-L-arginine methyl ester (L-NAME) produced elevations in systemic blood pressure and P_{GC} in 5/6 nephrectomized rats without affecting GFR,[66] whereas chronic treatment with aminoguanidine, an inhibitor of iNOS, had no effect on GFR, RPF, or P_{GC}.[65] Similarly, greater increases in blood pressure and proteinuria were observed after 5/6 nephrectomy in eNOS knockout versus wild-type mice.[67] On the other hand, renal NOS expression and activity are increased early after unilateral nephrectomy, and pretreatment of rats with a subpressor dose of L-NAME prevents the early increase in RBF and decrease in renal vascular resistance usually observed after unilateral nephrectomy.[68,69] It therefore appears that NO plays a role in early hemodynamic adaptations to nephron loss resulting in an increase in RBF, but in the longer term NO retains a tonic influence on systemic and renal hemodynamics without being a specific determinant of the adaptive changes in glomerular hemodynamics.

BRADYKININ

Bradykinin is a potent vasodilatory peptide that is elevated in the remnant kidney[23] and may therefore contribute to hemodynamic adaptations after nephron loss. Acute and chronic infusion of bradykinin results in increased RPF but has no effect on GFR.[70,71] Micropuncture studies in intact animals are lacking, but studies of isolated perfused afferent arterioles have shown that bradykinin induces a biphasic response with vasodilation at low concentrations and vasoconstriction at higher concentrations. Both effects appear to be mediated by products of COX.[72] Similar experiments with efferent arterioles found dose-dependent vasodilation (no biphasic response) that was dependent on cytochrome P450 metabolites but independent of COX products or NO.[73] When glomeruli were perfused with bradykinin, vasodilation of efferent arterioles was again observed but was inhibited by a COX inhibitor, indicating that bradykinin induces glomerular production of COX metabolites (prostaglandins) that also contribute to efferent arteriolar dilation.[61] Further studies are required to elucidate the role of bradykinin after nephron loss.

UROTENSIN II

Urotensin II (U-II) is the most potent vasoconstrictor identified to date, but its actions appear to vary in different vascular territories, and in some vessels it may even produce vasodilation. Infusion of exogenous U-II has been reported to increase or decrease GFR in normal rodents in different experiments (see Chapter 13). U-II is produced in the kidney, and urotensin receptors have been localized on glomerular arterioles.[74] Increased renal expression of mRNA for urotensin-related protein (which also binds to the urotensin receptor) and urotensin receptor has been reported in rats after 5/6 nephrectomy,[75] but the potential role of U-II in the hemodynamic adaptations that follow nephron loss has yet to be investigated.

ADJUSTMENTS IN RENAL AUTOREGULATORY MECHANISMS

After extensive renal mass ablation, there is a marked readjustment of the autoregulatory mechanisms that control RPF and GFR.[76-78] The role of myogenic mechanisms is uncertain, but detailed studies of afferent arteriolar myogenic responses suggest that their primary role is to protect the glomerulus from elevations in systolic blood pressure (SBP).[79] The tubuloglomerular feedback system is reset

Table 52.1 Hemodynamic Effects of Vasoactive Molecules Mediating Glomerular Hemodynamic Adaptations After Partial Renal Mass Ablation

	R_A	R_E	P_{GC}	Q_A	K_f	SNGFR	RPF	GFR
Angiotensin II	↑	↑↑	↑	↓	↓↔	↓↔	↓	↔
Aldosterone	↑	↑↑	↑	?	?	?	?	?
Endothelins	↑↔	↑	↑↔	↓	↓↔	↓↔	↓	↓↔
Natriuretic peptides	↓	↑ (?)	↑	↔	↔	↑	↑↔	↑
Prostaglandins	↓	↓	↔	↑	↑	↑	↑	↑
Bradykinin	↓↑	↓	?	?	?	?	↑	↔
Observed changes after partial renal ablation	↓↓	↓	↑	↑	↑↓	↑	—	↓

GFR, Glomerular filtration rate; K_f, glomerular ultrafiltration coefficient; P_{GC}, glomerular capillary hydraulic pressure; Q_A, glomerular plasma flow rate; R_A, afferent arteriolar resistance; R_E, efferent arteriolar resistance; RPF, renal plasma flow; SNGFR, single nephron GFR.

---

after renal mass ablation to permit and sustain the elevations in SNGFR and P_{GC} described earlier.[80,81] Resetting appears to occur as early as 20 minutes after unilateral nephrectomy,[82] in proportion to the extent of renal ablation. The adjustments observed after uninephrectomy are of lesser magnitudes than those seen after 5/6 nephrectomy.[80]

INTERACTION OF MULTIPLE FACTORS

As is readily appreciated from the earlier discussion, the adjustments in glomerular hemodynamics seen after renal mass ablation represent the net effect of several endogenous vasoactive factors. NPs and vasodilator prostaglandins dilate the preglomerular vessels, whereas bradykinin dilates both afferent and efferent arterioles. On the other hand, Ang II, vasoconstrictor prostaglandins, and possibly ETs constrict both afferent and efferent arterioles with a greater effect on the latter. A net fall in preglomerular vascular resistance is observed, whereas efferent arteriolar resistance decreases to a lesser extent. Together with greater transmission of the raised systemic blood pressure to the glomerular capillary network, these alterations in microvascular resistances result in the observed elevations in Q_A, P_{GC}, ΔP, and SNGFR (Table 52.1). The importance of multiple vasoactive factors is illustrated by the observation that treatment of 5/6 nephrectomized rats with omapatrilat, an inhibitor of both angiotensin-converting enzyme (ACE) and neutral endopeptidase that results in reduced Ang II production as well as increased NP and bradykinin levels, lowered P_{GC} more than ACE inhibition alone.[83] The complexity of factors involved is further illustrated by observations that other molecules involved in the modulation of progressive renal injury may exert hemodynamic effects by influencing the mediators discussed earlier. Acute infusion of hepatocyte growth factor (HGF) has been shown to induce a decline in blood pressure and GFR, an effect that is mediated by a short-term increase in ET-1 production.[84] In isolated perfused preparations, platelet-activating factor (PAF) at picomolar concentrations has been shown to induce glomerular production of NO, resulting in dilation of preconstricted efferent arterioles, whereas at nanomolar concentrations, PAF constricts efferent arterioles through local release of COX metabolites.[85] The potential role of other identified vasoactive molecules such as U-II remains to be elucidated.

RENAL HYPERTROPHIC RESPONSES TO NEPHRON LOSS

The notion that a single kidney enlarges to compensate for the loss of its partner has been entertained since antiquity. Aristotle (384-322 BC) noted that a single kidney was able to sustain life in animals, and that such kidneys were enlarged. In preparation for the first human nephrectomy in 1869 a German surgeon, Gustav Simon uninephrectomized dogs and noted a 1.5-fold increase in the size of the remaining kidney at 20 days.[86] Compensatory renal hypertrophy has been studied in a variety of species, including toads, mice, rats, guinea pigs, rabbits, cats, dogs, pigs, and baboons. The majority of experimental work has been conducted in rodents subjected to uninephrectomy, but hypertrophic responses have also been studied in response to unilateral ureteric obstruction (UUO) or after nephrotoxin administration.[87]

WHOLE-KIDNEY HYPERTROPHIC RESPONSES

Among the earliest responses to unilateral nephrectomy are biochemical changes that precede cell growth. Increased incorporation of choline, a precursor of cell membrane phospholipid, has been detected as early as 5 minutes and increased choline kinase activity at 2 hours after nephrectomy. Activity of ornithine decarboxylase, the enzyme catalyzing the first step of polyamine synthesis, is elevated at 45 to 120 minutes, and polyamine levels peak at 1 to 2 days post nephrectomy. Early alterations in mRNA metabolism have also been observed. Although there is no change in the half-life or cytoplasmic distribution of mRNA, a near 25% increase in the fraction of newly synthesized poly(adenylic acid)–deficient mRNA occurs within 1 hour of uninephrectomy, and total RNA synthesis in the kidney increases by 25% to 100% relative to that in the liver. Ribosomal RNA synthesis is increased by 40% to 50% at 6 hours. The rate of protein synthesis is increased at 2 hours and is nearly doubled at 3 hours. Data on cyclic nucleotide levels, which are thought to affect cell growth and proliferation, are conflicting. Some studies report elevated levels of cyclic guanosine monophosphate (cGMP) in the remaining kidney as early as 10 minutes after surgery, whereas others have found no consistent changes in cyclic adenosine monophosphate (cAMP) or cGMP levels.[87] Genomewide analysis of gene expression using cDNA microarrays in remaining

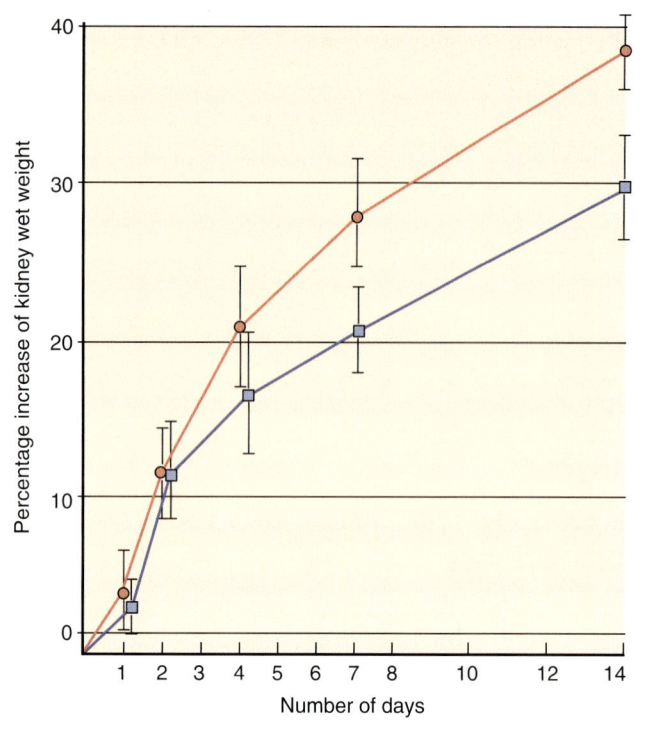

Figure 52.2 Rate of compensatory renal growth after unilateral nephrectomy (*circles*) and ureter ligation (*squares*). (Reproduced with permission from Dicker SE, Shirley DG: Compensatory hypertrophy of the contralateral kidney after unilateral ureteral ligation. *J Physiol [Lond]* 220:199-210, 1972.)

rat kidneys up to 72 hours after uninephrectomy has revealed the dominant response to be suppression of genes responsible for inhibition of growth and apoptosis.[88]

Early biochemical changes are followed by a period of rapid growth. DNA synthesis is increased at 24 hours, and increased numbers of mitotic figures are evident at 28 to 36 hours. Both reach a maximum increase of 5- to 10-fold at 40 to 72 hours. In rats, kidney weight is increased at 48 to 72 hours after uninephrectomy and achieves a 30% to 40% gain at 2 to 3 weeks (Figure 52.2).[69,87] As nephron number is fixed shortly before birth in most species, this gain in kidney weight is attributable to increased nephron size. Growth is thought to occur largely through cell hypertrophy, accounting for 80% of the increase in renal mass seen in adult rats and, to a lesser extent, through hyperplasia. Renal mass continues to rise for 1 to 2 months until a 40% to 50% increase is achieved. The degree of compensatory growth is a function of the extent of renal ablation. Uninephrectomy has been shown to provoke an 81% increase of residual renal mass at 4 weeks compared to an increase of 168% after 70% renal ablation. Normal controls gained 31% in kidney weight over the same period. Age diminishes renal hypertrophic responses: after uninephrectomy, greater increases in kidney weight and more extensive hyperplasia were observed in 5-day-old versus 55-day-old rats, and aging rats exhibited gains in kidney weight of only one third to three quarters of those seen in younger controls.[87]

In humans, assessment of renal hypertrophy after nephrectomy is dependent on radiologic studies. Ultrasonographic studies have reported increases of 19% to 100% in kidney volume,[89] and in computed tomography (CT) studies, an increase of 30% to 53% in renal cross-sectional area.[90,91] Contrast-enhanced CT has been used to measure renal parenchymal volume post unilateral nephrectomy. One study reported increases of 12.1% and 8.9% at 1 week and 6 months, respectively. The degree of hypertrophy correlated positively with the function of the kidney removed and negatively with patient age.[92] One relatively large study of living kidney donors observed a 27.6 ± 9.7% increase in the remaining kidney volume at 6 months post donor nephrectomy,[93] and a detailed study reported an increase in renal cortical volume of 27% at a median of 0.8 years post nephrectomy that increased to 35% after a median of 6.1 years.[14] The relatively small number of subjects included, wide variation in the time intervals between nephrectomy and assessment of renal size, and differing indications for nephrectomy make interpretation of these results difficult.

GLOMERULAR ENLARGEMENT

The principal morphometric change observed in glomeruli after uninephrectomy is an increase in volume. Glomerular enlargement appears to parallel whole-kidney growth and has been detected as early as 4 days after surgery.[94] The degree of enlargement of superficial and juxtamedullary glomeruli is similar. Proportionally similar increases in number and size of all cell types occur, with preservation of the relative volumes of different glomerular cells.[87] There is consensus that glomerular capillaries increase in length and number (i.e., more branching), but most studies show that diameter or cross-sectional surface area of the glomerular capillaries remains constant or increases only minimally.[95,96] Transplantation of hypertrophied kidneys into uninephrectomized recipients has demonstrated regression of glomerular hypertrophy within 3 weeks, yet the increase in capillary length was maintained.[96]

Glomerular hypertrophy, as evidenced by elevated RNA/DNA and protein/DNA ratios, as well as by increased glomerular volume (V_G) on electron microscopy, has been detected at 2 days after 5/6 nephrectomy.[97] The initial increase in V_G was due, almost entirely, to increases in visceral epithelial cell volume, whereas at 14 days the increase in V_G was largely accounted for by mesangial matrix expansion. Although several studies report glomerular capillary lengthening after 5/6 nephrectomy, few have detected any increase in cross-sectional area or diameter of the glomerular capillaries.[98-101] These observations should, however, be considered in the light of important technical considerations. In vitro perfusion of isolated glomeruli demonstrates that V_G increases as perfusion pressure is raised through physiologic and pathophysiologic ranges. Moreover, glomerular capillary "compliance" in these studies was a function of the baseline V_G, and glomeruli obtained from remnant kidneys post 5/6 nephrectomy had a higher compliance than those from control animals.[102] These findings have two important implications. First, although glomerular pressures are only minimally elevated after uninephrectomy, the glomerular capillary hypertension associated with more extensive renal ablation is likely to contribute significantly to the increase in V_G. Second, estimates of V_G in tissues that have not been perfusion fixed at the appropriate blood pressure should be interpreted with caution. Direct comparison of V_G in perfusion-fixed versus immersion-fixed kidney from the same rats yielded estimates of V_G in immersion-fixed samples that were 61% lower than those from perfusion-fixed kidneys.[103]

MECHANISMS OF RENAL HYPERTROPHY

Despite more than a century of research that identified a large number of mediators or modulators of renal hypertrophy, the identities of the specific factors that regulate hypertrophy and the stimuli to which these factors respond remained elusive. Renal innervation does not appear to play a role as kidneys transplanted into bilaterally nephrectomized rats exhibit the same degree of hypertrophy after 3 weeks as kidneys remaining after uninephrectomy.[104] The absence of any reduction in renal hypertrophy when rats are treated with an ACEI after uninephrectomy indicates that the RAAS also does not play a major role.[105] Several hypotheses were advanced to account for the observed changes associated with renal hypertrophy and have been discussed in detail in other publications[86,87]; they are summarized next.

SOLUTE LOAD

The notion that hypertrophy after uninephrectomy is stimulated by the need for the remaining kidney to excrete larger amounts of metabolic waste products, necessitating more excretory "work," was proposed by Sacerdotti in 1896. Subsequently, it became apparent that urea excretion is largely a function of glomerular filtration, whereas the main energy-requiring function of the renal tubules is reabsorption of filtered electrolytes (principally sodium) and water. The hypothesis was therefore modified to view hypertrophy as a response to the increased demand for water and solute reclamation imposed by increased SNGFR ("solute load hypothesis"). Several lines of evidence supported the concepts underlying the solute load hypothesis. After uninephrectomy RBF increased by 8% in the remaining kidney and preceded hypertrophy, but treatment with a subpressor dose of the NOS inhibitor L-NAME prevented the rise in RBF and substantially attenuated increases in renal weight as well as glomerular and proximal tubule area at 7 days post nephrectomy.[69] In the remnant kidney, proximal tubule sodium absorption increased in parallel with GFR (glomerulotubular balance), and tubules continued to display enhanced fluid reabsorption in vitro, implying that the adaptive changes were intrinsic to the tubular epithelial cells. In chronic glomerulonephritis, a lesion characterized by marked heterogeneity in SNGFR, there is preservation of the SNGFR to proximal fluid reabsorption ratio and a close correlation between glomerular and proximal tubule hypertrophy. Moreover, sustained increases in GFR in the absence of renal mass ablation result in renal hypertrophy in some conditions, including pregnancy (in some but not all studies) and diabetes mellitus.[86]

On the other hand, experimental maneuvers dissociating renal solute load from hypertrophy appear to contradict the solute load hypothesis. Total diversion of urine from one kidney into the peritoneum by ureteroperitoneostomy is associated with an increase in GFR in the contralateral kidney of similar magnitude to that seen after uninephrectomy, but no increase in renal mass or mitotic activity. In another example, potassium depletion results in renal hypertrophy without any increase in GFR. Moreover, the findings that some of the early biochemical changes associated with hypertrophy precede increases in glomerular filtration or sodium reabsorption argue against a causal association of hypertrophy and increased solute load. It is, however, possible to offer alternative explanations for each of the earlier observations. Despite these conflicting data, there is nevertheless considerable evidence of an association between GFR and proximal tubule hypertrophy that may play a role in stimulating renal growth in the remnant kidney.[86]

RENOTROPIC FACTORS

Failure of the solute load hypothesis to explain all of the experimental data led others to propose instead that the primary stimulus for renal hypertrophy was a change in renal mass and that renal growth was under the control of specific growth and/or inhibitory factors. Evidence in support of this theory was derived from three types of experiment. In the first, a stable connection was established between the extracellular space and microcirculation of two animals (parabiosis), and the effects of renal mass ablation in one animal were assessed in the intact kidneys of its partner. Despite some inconsistencies due to variations in methodology, these experiments generally found that uninephrectomy in one animal resulted in hypertrophy of the contralateral kidney and, to a lesser extent, of both kidneys of the parabiotic partner. Bilateral nephrectomy in one partner or triple nephrectomy produced incremental degrees of hypertrophy in the remaining kidney(s). Furthermore, the hypertrophy was rapidly reversed following cessation of cross circulation.[86]

A second strategy was to inject serum or plasma from uninephrectomized animals into intact subjects and then assess renal hypertrophy by radiolabeled thymidine uptake or mitotic count. Although results of studies using single small intraperitoneal or subcutaneous doses were negative, the administration of repeated, large doses by intraperitoneal or intravenous routes elicited renal hypertrophy in most subjects studied.[86]

The data that most consistently supported the existence of a renotropic factor were derived from in vitro experiments in which renal tissues were incubated in the presence or absence of plasma or serum from rats subjected to renal mass ablation. Evidence for hypertrophy was generally assessed by incorporation of radiolabeled thymidine or uridine into DNA or RNA, respectively. In general these experiments showed increased uptake of radiolabeled nucleotides after incubation with serum from uninephrectomized animals. This effect appeared to be organ but not species specific. That a tissue factor produced by kidneys and upregulated after nephrectomy may be required for the activity of a circulating "renotropin," was suggested by experiments in which kidney extract from rats taken 20 hours after uninephrectomy, in the presence of normal rat serum, was found to stimulate tritiated thymidine (^{3}H thymidine) incorporation in normal renal cortex, but addition of the same extract in the absence of the serum tended to depress ^{3}H thymidine uptake. Serum taken from bilaterally nephrectomized animals lacked renotropic effects, but these were restored after dialysis of the serum, suggesting the presence of renotropin inhibitory factors that accumulated in the absence of renal function. Although the specific identity of renotropin remained elusive, several lines of evidence suggested that it was a small protein. Retention of activity after ultrafiltration, dialysis, and removal of albumin from serum implied that renotropin was a molecule of 12 to 25 kDa with no significant binding to albumin.[86,87]

Several hypotheses were advanced to reconcile the earlier observed effects and operation of a putative renotropic system. It was variously proposed that (1) renotropin was a circulating substance normally catabolized or excreted by the kidneys; (2) renal growth was regulated by a specific renotropin-producing tissue that was inhibited by a factor produced by normal kidneys; or (3) renal growth was tonically inhibited by a substance produced by normal kidneys, a decrease in the levels of which induced an enzyme in the renal cortex that cleaved a circulating precursor of renotropin to produce the active molecule.[86,87]

ENDOCRINE EFFECTS

Several of the major endocrine systems influence renal growth, but each lacks selective effects on the kidney. There is little evidence that any of these systems represent the specific mediators of compensatory renal hypertrophy. Whereas early experiments suggested that hypophysectomy inhibits compensatory hypertrophy after uninephrectomy, later studies that controlled for the reduction in renal mass that usually accompanies hypopituitarism found a degree of hypertrophy comparable to that seen in normal rats. Nevertheless, specific renotropic activity has been identified in a subfraction of ovine pituitary extract associated with a lutropin-like substance.[86,87] Uninephrectomy is accompanied by a transient increase in the pulsatile release of growth hormone (GH) in male but not female rats, suggesting a role for this hormone in the early phase of hypertrophy in males.[106] When the increase in GH was prevented by administration of an antagonist to GH-releasing factor or the effects of GH are blocked by a GH-receptor blocker, renal hypertrophy is significantly attenuated.[107,108] Adrenal hormones appear to play little role in renal hypertrophy. Adrenalectomy does not inhibit compensatory growth after uninephrectomy. Whereas renal weight relative to body weight is reduced in hypothyroidism and increased by excess thyroid hormone, compensatory hypertrophy still occurs in thyroidectomized rats. Progesterone and estradiol in excess or ovariectomy have little effect on renal weight, but testosterone appears to play a role, as evidenced by a fall in kidney/body weight after orchidectomy and an increase in kidney weight with excess testosterone. Whereas orchidectomy does not inhibit hypertrophy after uninephrectomy, exogenous testosterone did increase the degree of hypertrophy observed, in some, but not all studies.[86,87]

GROWTH FACTORS

Of the numerous growth factors and their receptors that have been localized in the kidney, at least four are associated with renal hypertrophy.[109,110] Several lines of evidence suggest a role for insulin-like growth factor-1 (IGF-1). Renal IGF-1 levels were elevated at 1 to 5 days after uninephrectomy and started to decline within days in some[111,112] but not all studies.[113] In one study the level of renal IGF-1 expression was significantly correlated with the extent of renal mass ablation.[114] On the other hand, Shohat and colleagues found an increase in serum IGF-1 levels only at 10 days post nephrectomy, which was still present on day 60.[111] That IGF-1 may be induced independent of GH in the setting of renal hypertrophy is illustrated by preservation of the increase in renal IGF-1 in hypophysectomized[115] and GH-deficient rats.[116] Other molecules related to IGF function are also upregulated: renal IGF-1 receptor gene expression was increased 2- to 4-fold in female rats after uninephrectomy,[106] IGF-1 binding protein mRNA was upregulated in the remnant kidney at 2 weeks after 5/6 nephrectomy,[117] and analysis of the genomewide transcriptional response to unilateral nephrectomy identified insulin-like growth factor-2 (IGF-2)-binding protein as one of the few activated genes.[88] Further evidence suggests that IGF-1 may in turn promote production of vascular endothelial growth factor (VEGF), implying that VEGF may be a downstream mediator of IGF-1 effects, at least in the pathogenesis of diabetic retinopathy.[118] That VEGF is important for compensatory renal hypertrophy is confirmed by the observation that treatment of mice with VEGF antibodies after uninephrectomy completely prevented glomerular hypertrophy and inhibited renal growth at 7 days.[112] Epidermal growth factor (EGF) in the remaining kidney is increased on day 1 in mice[119] and by day 5 in rats.[120] In addition, EGF has been shown to induce IGF-I mRNA production in collecting duct cells in vitro, suggesting the existence of a local paracrine system.[121] Increased mRNA levels for both HGF and its receptor, c-Met, have been demonstrated in the remaining kidney as early as 6 hours after uninephrectomy.[122,123] In another study the rise in HGF message was found to be nonspecific, occurring in both liver and kidney and also in sham-operated rats, whereas the increase in mRNA for c-Met was specific for the outer renal medulla.[124] Despite these associations, the timing of the changes in growth factor levels remains unclear. Whereas some investigators report early increases,[119,125] several others report changes only at time points when significant hypertrophy is already present, thus failing to provide convincing evidence that they represent the proximal effectors in a renotropic system.[111,120]

MESANGIAL CELL RESPONSES: A UNIFYING HYPOTHESIS

Mesangial cells play a central role in glomerular function, modulating glomerular capillary blood flow and ultrafiltration surface area. In addition, mesangial cells are both a source of and target for vasoactive molecules, growth factors, cytokines, and extracellular matrix (ECM) proteins. Evidence suggests that they also play a major role in compensatory renal hypertrophy. In vitro experiments found that when mesangial cells from a remaining kidney after uninephrectomy were cultured with serum obtained from rats after uninephrectomy, they induced hypertrophy in tubular cells.[126] Uninephrectomy induces significant transient proliferation of mesangial cells, reaching a peak at 24 hours and ceasing within 72 hours. This proliferation occurs in an environment of increased circulating as well as renal growth factors and cytokines such as GH, IGF-1, and interleukin-10 (IL-10), as well as reduced levels of antiproliferative factors such as transforming growth factor-β (TGF-β) and ANP. The reduction in mesangial cell proliferation occurs in parallel with the onset of tubular cell hypertrophy. IL-10 and TGF-β have been identified as the major mediators of the mesangial regulation of tubular cell hypertrophy. Mesangial cells are the main source of IL-10 in the kidney, where it acts as an autocrine growth factor and induces expression of TGF-β.[127] Mesangial cells are the only resident renal cells known to produce and activate TGF-β, a process that is regulated by multiple factors, including Ang II, IGF-1, HGF, basic fibroblast growth factor, tumor necrosis factor-α (TNF-α), EGF, and platelet-derived growth factor (PDGF), all of which are produced by mesangial cells. IL-10 expression starts to increase in the remaining kidney within hours of uninephrectomy, peaks at 24 hours, and returns to normal within several days. In contrast, circulating and renal TGF-β levels fall in the first 24 hours after nephrectomy and start to rise from 72 hours, reaching a peak at 1 week.[127] The importance of IL-10 was confirmed by experiments in which inhibition of IL-10 production resulted in lower TGF-β levels and reduced tubular hypertrophy, resulting in a 20% to 25% reduction in the weight of the remaining kidney.[127] IL-10 has no direct effect on tubular cells, whereas TGF-β has been identified as an important mediator of tubular cell hypertrophy.[128] The data presented are therefore consistent with the hypothesis that hyperfiltration after unilateral nephrectomy induces mesangial cell proliferation, as well as production of IL-10 and other growth factors that induce expression and activation of TGF-β in mesangial cells. TGF-β in turn stimulates tubular cell hypertrophy[129] (Figure 52.3). This hypothesis goes a long way to unifying the components of the solute load and renotropin hypotheses into a single paradigm to explain the mechanisms of compensatory renal hypertrophy.

TUBULAR CELL RESPONSES

Detailed investigation of cellular responses to renal mass reduction has begun to elucidate some of the mechanisms involved in compensatory hypertrophy at the cellular level. Renal hypertrophy is achieved by modulation of the cell cycle, which becomes arrested in the late G1 phase and therefore does not progress to the S phase, resulting in cell hypertrophy instead of hyperplasia. This is achieved through activation of cyclin-dependent kinase (CDK) 4/cyclin D without subsequent engagement of CDK 2/cyclin E, a process thought to be regulated by TGF-β and CDK inhibitor proteins $p21^{Waf1}$, $p27^{kip1}$, and $p57^{kip2}$. Activity of CDK 4/cyclin D complexes increases at 4, 7, and 10 days post nephrectomy, and CDK 2/cyclin E increases at days 2, 4, and 7 to 14, implying that $p21^{Waf1}$, $p27^{kip1}$, and $p57^{kip2}$ may play an important role in regulating tubular cell hypertrophy.[130-132] The required increase in RNA and protein synthesis appears to be mediated by mammalian target of rapamycin (mTOR), a protein kinase that controls protein synthesis as well as cell growth and metabolism. In cells, mTOR exists in two distinct multiprotein complexes, mTORC1 and mTORC2. mTORC1 acts through multiple mediators to regulate protein synthesis and cell size. Two important downstream effectors of mTORC1 are 4E-binding protein 1 and ribosomal protein S6 kinase 1 (S6K1). The importance of mTORC1 is confirmed by the observation that pretreatment of rats with rapamycin, an inhibitor of mTORC1, inhibited renal hypertrophy after uninephrectomy.[133] Furthermore, experiments in S6K1 knockout mice found inhibition of 60% to 70% of the hypertrophy observed after uninephrectomy, indicating that S6K1 plays a major role in compensatory hypertrophy.[134]

ADAPTATION OF SPECIFIC TUBULE FUNCTIONS IN RESPONSE TO NEPHRON LOSS

As noted earlier, the bulk of the increase in renal mass following uninephrectomy is due to hypertrophy of the proximal nephron. The more distal nephron segments also enlarge, but to a lesser extent. In uninephrectomized rats the proximal convoluted tubule is increased on average by 17% in luminal diameter and 35% in length, yielding a 96% increase in total volume; the distal convoluted tubule is enlarged by 12% in luminal diameter and 17% in length, yielding a 25% increase in total volume.[135] Maintenance of homeostasis for various solutes in the face of a declining GFR requires highly integrated responses from each tubule segment. Whereas some solutes, including creatinine and urea, are chiefly cleared by glomerular filtration and therefore rise gradually in plasma with declining GFR, for others, the tubule solute handling adapts so that plasma levels remain constant, virtually until ESKD is reached (Figure 52.4).

ADAPTATION IN PROXIMAL TUBULE SOLUTE HANDLING

In renal ablation models, as with the increase in remnant kidney SNGFR, the extent to which the proximal tubule enlarges is inversely proportional to the remnant kidney mass. Proximal tubule enlargement is associated with an increase in proximal fluid reabsorption. In studies of both animals and humans with reduced renal mass, the increase

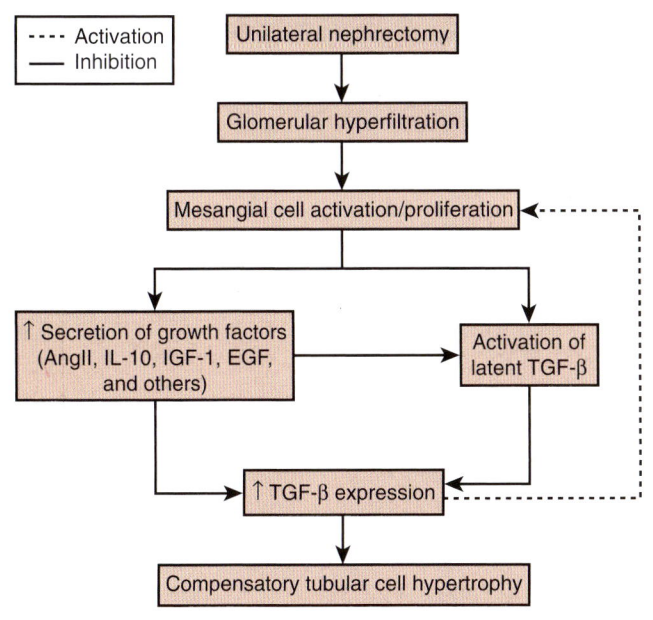

Figure 52.3 Possible mechanisms involved in compensatory renal growth after unilateral nephrectomy. AngII, Angiotensin II; EGF, epidermal growth factor; IGF-1, insulin-like growth factor-1; IL-10, interleukin-10. (Used with permission from Sinuani I, Beberashvili I, Averbukh Z, et al: Mesangial cells initiate compensatory tubular cell hypertrophy. *Am J Nephrol* 31:326-331, 2010.)

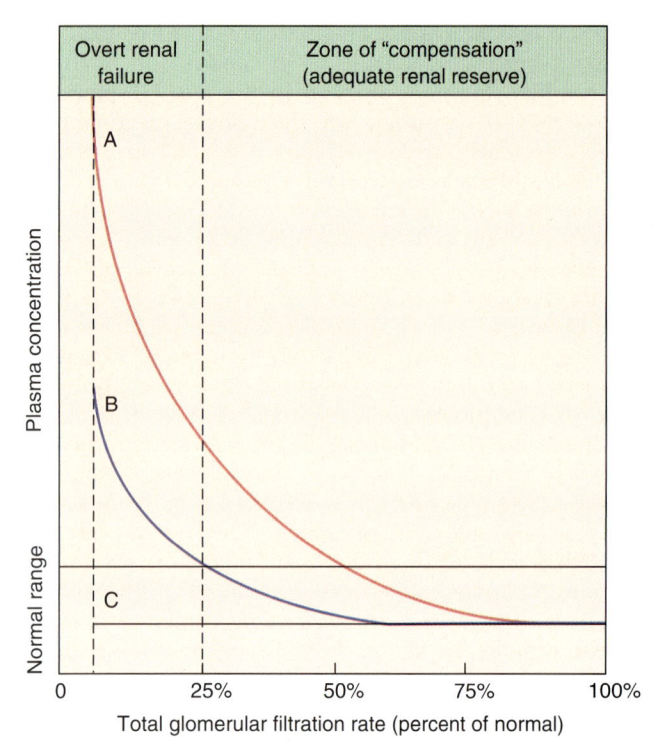

Figure 52.4 Representative patterns of adaptation for different types of solutes in body fluids in chronic kidney disease. Pattern A, rise in serum concentration with each permanent reduction in GFR (e.g., creatinine); pattern B, rise in serum concentration only after GFR falls below a critical value due to adaptive increases in tubular secretion (e.g., phosphate); pattern C, serum concentration remains normal through almost entire period of progression of renal failure (e.g., sodium). GFR, Glomerular filtration rate. (Modified from Bricker NS, et al: In Brenner BM, Rector FC, editors: *The kidney*, ed 2, Philadelphia, 1981, WB Saunders.)

in proximal fluid reabsorption observed was found to be proportional to both the increase in remnant kidney GFR and the increase in tubular volume.[136] Similarly, in proximal tubules isolated from remnant kidneys, the observed increase in transtubular fluid flux was proportional to the increases in size and protein content of the tubular epithelial cells.[137,138] Folding of the basolateral membrane of the proximal tubule epithelium was also found to increase, resulting in augmentation of the basolateral surface area, in proportion to the increase in cell volume.[139] This increase in surface area was accompanied by an increase in activity of sodium-potassium adenosine triphosphatase (Na^+-K^+-ATPase), the membrane pump that generates the main driving force for proximal tubule solute and water transport.[139]

Increases in proximal tubule size and surface area are not, however, the only determinants of increased transport activity in this nephron segment. Fluid reabsorption in isolated proximal tubule segments increases within 24 hours of nephrectomy (i.e., when GFR is already increasing, but well before significant hypertrophy occurs), implying an intrinsic tubular epithelial cell adaptation to nephron loss.[140] This observation also raises the possibility that the increases in proximal fluid reabsorption occurring in response to nephron loss are driven by the increase in SNGFR.[86,87] As solute reclamation is an energy-requiring process, it is not surprising that in uninephrectomized rabbits the increase in proximal tubule volume was accompanied by a proportional increase in mitochondrial volume.[141] The observation that the increase in renal mass is outstripped by the rise in GFR in models of progressive nephron loss implies that renal energy consumption per unit of remnant renal mass increases as renal function declines.[135]

The rise in SNGFR that occurs in the remnant kidney presents increased loads of glucose, amino acids, and other solutes that would normally be reabsorbed entirely in the proximal tubule, provided that the maximal transport capacity was not exceeded. Maximal proximal tubular reabsorptive capacities for glucose and amino acids have been shown to increase in proportion to tubule mass after partial renal ablation.[142] Some metabolic functions of proximal tubules are also augmented in the remnant kidney, so as to maintain adequate plasma levels of important metabolites, including citrulline, arginine, and serine.[143] Other proximal tubule functions, however, are not adjusted in proportion to proximal tubule mass: fractional phosphate reabsorption is decreased, whereas ammoniagenesis increases.[142,144,145] These adaptations are appropriate homeostatic responses that permit continued excretion of daily phosphate and acid loads, respectively, as the number of functioning nephrons declines.

LOOP OF HENLE AND DISTAL NEPHRON

Although there is little change in cross-sectional area in the thick ascending limb of the loop of Henle, fluid reabsorption in this segment also increases in proportion to SNGFR.[135] In contrast, both the distal tubule and the cortical collecting duct enlarge in response to nephron loss.[135] Unlike the proximal tubule, however, where the increased reabsorptive capacity is chiefly due to increased tubule dimensions, the increased reabsorptive capacity observed in the distal segments is far greater than would be expected for the corresponding increase in tubule volume, implying a major adaptive increase in active solute transport.[135] Levels of mRNA for the Na^+/myo-inositol cotransporter (SMIT) and Na^+/Cl^-/betaine-γ-amino-N-butyric acid transporter (BGT-1) are increased in the cortex and outer medulla of remnant kidneys from 5/6 nephrectomized rats.[146] Likewise, potassium secretion by the distal nephron increases in compensation for nephron loss, facilitated by an increased basolateral surface area of cortical collecting duct principal cells and an increase in Na^+-K^+-ATPase activity.[147,148]

GLOMERULOTUBULAR BALANCE

Micropuncture studies have confirmed that proximal fluid reabsorption remains proportional to glomerular filtration over a wide range of SNGFR in both glomerular and tubulointerstitial diseases.[149,150] This glomerulotubular balance is critical to the physiologic integrity of remnant nephron function and hence ECF homeostasis. Compensatory increases in SNGFR in surviving nephrons must be accompanied by similar increases in proximal tubule solute and water reabsorption, so as to avoid overwhelming the distal nephron transport capacity and disrupting its regulation of the volume and composition of the final urine. Conversely, reductions in SNGFR in damaged nephrons must be matched by similar reductions in proximal fluid reabsorption so as to maintain adequate solute and water delivery to the distal tubule, again permitting excretion of urine of appropriate volume and composition.

Glomerulotubular balance is maintained as follows. The degree of single-nephron hyperfiltration occurring as a consequence of nephron loss determines the passive Starling forces operating in the postglomerular microcirculation, which in turn govern net transtubular solute reabsorption.[151] Increases in SNGFR associated with an increased filtration fraction result in elevated postglomerular capillary protein concentrations, which determine nonlinear increases in oncotic pressure, Π_E, the major determinant of peritubular capillary reabsorptive force (P_r). Reductions in SNGFR, in contrast, result in a lowered peritubular oncotic pressure, thereby reducing P_r. Thus SNGFR and proximal fluid reabsorption remain in direct proportion to one another. Prevention of hyperfiltration by dietary protein restriction has been shown to abrogate the increase in proximal fluid reabsorption in the remnant kidney, underscoring the dependence of proximal tubular function on the level of glomerular filtration.[151] In the remnant kidney of rats subjected to extensive renal mass ablation, absolute fluid reabsorption was found to be markedly increased in proximal portions of both superficial and juxtamedullary nephrons, yet fluid delivery to the more distal segments of the nephron was also somewhat increased.[152] In the setting of nephron loss, sodium reabsorption by the loop of Henle has been shown to remain proportional to sodium delivery to that segment, indicating preservation of tubulotubular balance, a mechanism that maintains appropriate distal solute and water delivery in the face of progressive nephron loss. Until the adaptive capacities of these mechanisms are finally exhausted, the operation of glomerulotubular balance and tubulotubular balance ensures that the distal tubule mechanisms that determine final urine volume and composition are not overwhelmed by unregulated distal delivery of water and solute.[153] In keeping with these physiologic observations, morphologic studies have shown that within the same kidney, nephrons associated with damaged glomeruli are usually atrophic and presumably hypofunctioning or nonfunctioning, whereas those associated with healthier glomeruli are usually hypertrophic and hyperfunctioning.[154]

In order to maintain homeostasis in the face of continued food and water intake, specific mechanisms that enhance single-nephron water and solute excretion must come into play, in addition to the adjustments in SNGFR and tubular reabsorption that occur in response to nephron loss. These mechanisms are not unique to the setting of renal insufficiency, however, and are also engaged when the normal kidney is challenged to excrete extraordinary loads of solute and water. In general, the adaptive physiology of the chronically injured kidney is adequate to preserve homeostasis for many solutes under baseline conditions, but the adaptive capacity may easily become overwhelmed by fluctuations in fluid intake and especially by increases in electrolyte and acid loads. Patients with CKD are therefore susceptible to developing volume overload, volume loss, hyperkalemia, and acidosis when the excretory capacity of the kidney is challenged by relatively modest increases in excretory demands.

SODIUM EXCRETION AND EXTRACELLULAR FLUID VOLUME REGULATION

In CKD, ECF volume is often maintained very close to normal until end-stage failure is reached.[155] This remarkable feat is accomplished by an increase in fractional sodium excretion (FE_{Na}) in inverse proportion to the decline in GFR.[156] Many studies have been carried out in an attempt to identify which nephron segments are responsible for the decrease in sodium reabsorption: micropuncture studies in uninephrectomized rats have shown that tubule fluid transit times, as well as the half-time for reabsorption of a stationary saline droplet in the proximal tubule lumen, were not different from controls[135]; in remnant kidneys of rats receiving high-, normal-, or low-sodium diets, *absolute* sodium reabsorption was found to increase, but *fractional* sodium and fluid reabsorption were found to decrease in all groups[157]; micropuncture studies in dogs and rats have failed to detect significant reductions in fractional proximal tubule fluid and sodium reabsorption[158]; distal sodium delivery was found to be markedly increased in the rat remnant kidney[157]; increased solute transport activity has been demonstrated in the distal tubule of uninephrectomized rats[135]; and under conditions of hydropenia and salt loading, sodium reabsorption by the medullary collecting duct of the rat remnant kidney was markedly reduced.[159] Taken together, these data suggest that proximal fractional reabsorption remains largely unchanged, and that in the setting of renal insufficiency, adjustments in sodium excretion occur predominantly in the loop and distal nephron segments.[160] These physiologic observations were supported by studies investigating changes in sodium transporters after 5/6 nephrectomy. At 4 weeks after surgery a substantial increase in abundance of the Na^+-K^+-$2Cl^-$ and Na^+-Cl^- cotransporters (expressed chiefly in the loop of Henle and distal tubule, respectively) was observed, whereas marked decrease was observed in both at 12 weeks. Expression of epithelial sodium channel-α increased throughout the observation period.[161]

In addition to load-dependent tubular adaptations in sodium handling, sodium excretion is also modulated by hormonal influences. Levels of NPs are elevated in CKD as a result of reduced clearance and in response to alterations in sodium and volume status.[52,162] In rats with extensive renal mass ablation, plasma ANP levels may be restored toward normal levels by dietary sodium restriction, but, in response to increases in sodium intake, they rise progressively along with sodium excretion.[163] The notion that ANP plays an important role in mediating adaptive changes in sodium excretion in the setting of renal ablation is confirmed by observations that administration of an NP receptor antagonist reduced both FE_{Na} and GFR in 5/6 nephrectomized rats receiving either normal or high-salt diets but did not alter these variables in rats fed low-salt diets.[164] Significantly, NPs not only modulate sodium excretion but may also contribute to the attendant glomerular hyperfiltration and thereby further exacerbate renal injury (see earlier).

Systemic hypertension has also been proposed by Guyton and associates as a contributor to the increase in FE_{Na} observed with renal insufficiency.[165] Their hypothesis states that a constant sodium intake in the face of a reduced number of functioning nephrons leads to positive sodium balance as a result of reduced excretory capacity. Positive sodium balance leads to an increase in ECF volume and a rise in systemic blood pressure that in turn leads to an increase in FE_{Na} and reestablishes the steady state. In support of this hypothesis, salt intake has been shown to be critical to the development of hypertension in subtotally nephrectomized dogs,[166] and uremic patients have been found to exhibit marked sodium retention when treated with vasodilating antihypertensive agents.[167] On the other hand, a lowered salt intake in 5/6 nephrectomized rats does not prevent the development of systemic hypertension,[100] suggesting that sodium excretion and hypertension are not always interdependent in the setting of extensive renal mass ablation. Sodium conservation, on the other hand, is also impaired with renal insufficiency, and, in response to an acute reduction in sodium intake, most patients were unable to reduce sodium excretion below 20 to 30 mEq/day.[168] The "salt-losing" tendency associated with CKD appears to be dependent upon the salt load per nephron and may therefore be reversible with adequate dietary sodium restriction. Other factors modulating FE_{Na} in the setting of renal insufficiency include changes in sympathetic nervous system activity, aldosterone, prostaglandins, and parathyroid hormone (PTH) levels.[160,169] Sodium homeostasis and volume regulation are discussed in further detail in Chapters 6 and 10.

URINARY CONCENTRATION AND DILUTION

ECF homeostasis is usually well maintained until renal insufficiency is far advanced, when the ability of the kidney to excrete a volume load becomes significantly reduced.[160] Normal generation of solute-free water is approximately 12 mL per 100 mL of GFR and is dependent on dilution of tubule fluid in the thick ascending limb, maintenance of low water permeability in the distal nephron segments in the absence of antidiuretic hormone (arginine vasopressin [AVP]), and decreased hypertonicity of the medullary interstitium during water diuresis. Although the single nephron capacity to excrete free water per milliliter of GFR is not reduced in patients with advanced kidney disease,[170] the absolute reduction in GFR reduces the overall capacity of the kidney to excrete a water load. Patients with CKD therefore cannot adequately dilute their urine and are prone to water intoxication and hyponatremia. Hypothetically, in addition to excretion of the equivalent of 2 L of "isotonic urine" per day (obligatory excretion of 600 mOsm/day), normal kidneys, with a GFR of 150 L/day, can excrete up to 18 L of free water, whereas failing kidneys, with a GFR of 15 L/day, can excrete only approximately 1.8 L of free water per day. The minimum urinary osmolality achievable by normal kidneys would therefore approach 30 mOsm/L (600 mOsm/20 L), whereas that of diseased kidneys would be 160 mOsm/L (600 mOsm/3.8 L).

Urinary concentration is also impaired in renal insufficiency. Normal urinary concentration requires preservation of the countercurrent mechanism to maintain hypertonicity of the medullary interstitium and normal water transport across the distal nephron segments in response to AVP. Maximal urinary osmolality in normal subjects is approximately 1200 mOsm/L. As GFR decreases, however, maximal urinary osmolality falls and with a GFR of 15 mL/min is reduced to approximately 400 mOsm/L.[171] A normal individual can therefore excrete the obligatory daily 600 mOsm in as little as 0.5 L of urine, whereas the patient with a GFR of 15 mL/min can excrete the same load in a minimum of 1.5 L. Part of the defect in urinary concentration observed with renal damage may be attributed to the high solute load imposed per surviving nephron. In patients with CKD, however, the osmotic effect of urea was shown to be inadequate to account fully for the reduction in maximal urine concentration, indicating that factors other than osmotic diuresis contribute to reduction in urinary concentrating ability in these patients.[171] Furthermore, in patients with chronic glomerulonephritis, reduction in urine concentrating capacity was found to correlate significantly with the degree of medullary fibrosis on renal biopsy,[172] suggesting that disruption of the medullary architecture, with the consequent loss of medullary hypertonicity, may result in disproportionate impairment of urinary concentrating ability at any given level of GFR. Consistent with this observation, patients with primary tubulointerstitial injury (e.g., analgesic nephropathy and sickle cell disease) have markedly impaired urinary concentrating abilities, even early in the course of their illness.[171,173,174] Similarly, in animal experiments, surgical exposure of the renal papilla in intact hydropenic rats was found to lead to reduction in urinary osmolality because of the accompanying alterations in vasa recta flow and ensuing washout of medullary solutes.[175] Interestingly, similar exposure of papillae in rats with remnant kidneys did not affect urinary osmolality, presumably because medullary solute washout had already occurred due to the adaptive responses to nephron loss.

Urinary concentration also depends on water reabsorption in the distal nephron segments of the remnant nephron. Reduction in water reabsorption may be the result of several mechanisms in the failing kidney. Defective cAMP-mediated response to AVP may render the cortical collecting duct resistant to the effects of AVP, resulting in increased water delivery to the papillary collecting duct.[176] Urinary osmolality is inversely proportional to fractional water delivery to the papillary collecting duct in 5/6 nephrectomized rats, despite an increase in absolute water reabsorption per functioning collecting tubule when compared with controls.[175] Patients with renal insufficiency are therefore prone to volume depletion in the presence of water deprivation or impaired thirst mechanisms. More commonly, the inability to concentrate urine becomes manifest as nocturia, which develops as renal function deteriorates. Urinary concentrating and diluting mechanisms are discussed in further detail in Chapters 10 and 11.

POTASSIUM EXCRETION

In order to maintain potassium homeostasis in the face of continued dietary intake and a reduced number of functioning nephrons, potassium excretion per nephron must increase. In both normal and diseased kidneys, almost all of the filtered potassium is reabsorbed in the proximal tubule and loop of Henle. Potassium excretion is therefore determined predominantly by distal secretion,[160] although a reduction in potassium reabsorption by the loop of Henle has been shown to contribute to increased potassium excretion in rats with reduced renal mass.[177] In both normal and partially nephrectomized dogs, urinary potassium excretion was found to correlate directly with serum potassium concentration.[178] Similarly, in intact and uninephrectomized rats, net potassium secretion in the distal convoluted tubule occurred only during potassium infusion, whereas potassium secretion by cortical collecting tubules (CCTs) occurred under all conditions and was greater after uninephrectomy.[179] Other studies have confirmed that the CCT is an important site of potassium secretion in the remnant kidney.[147,159] Secretion of potassium by CCTs isolated from remnant kidneys of rabbits fed normal or high-potassium diets was shown to persist in vitro and to be directly related to the dietary potassium content,[147] indicating an intrinsic tubular adaptation to potassium load. This adaptation was absent in CCTs from rabbits in which dietary potassium had been reduced in proportion to the amount of renal mass lost. In addition to variation with dietary potassium load, the increase in potassium secretion by remnant CCTs was also found to correlate with plasma aldosterone levels, but not with intracellular potassium concentration or Na^+-K^+-ATPase activity.[147] In contrast, however, others have reported an increase in cortical and outer medullary Na^+-K^+-ATPase activity in homogenates from rat remnant kidneys that was abrogated when potassium intake was reduced in proportion to the reduction in GFR.[180] Finally, the frequent occurrence of hyperkalemia in patients with CKD after treatment with an aldosterone antagonist or an ACEI suggests that "normal" aldosterone levels are required to maintain adequate potassium excretion in this population.[181] In general, therefore, the increase in potassium secretion by surviving nephrons appears to be predominantly determined by the rise in plasma potassium level after potassium ingestion and by intrinsic tubular adaptation to the increased filtered potassium load.[178,179] In both dogs and patients with CKD, however, the kaliuretic response to an oral potassium load is attenuated compared to normals despite higher serum potassium levels.[178,182] The eventual, complete excretion of a potassium load therefore occurs at the expense of a sustained increase in serum potassium level. Control of potassium excretion is discussed further in Chapters 6 and 18.

ACID-BASE REGULATION

Reduction of GFR in patients with CKD is associated with the development of systemic metabolic acidosis, due to a reduction in serum bicarbonate concentration. Normal acid-base balance requires reabsorption of filtered bicarbonate, excretion of titratable acid, ammonia generation, and acidification of tubular luminal fluid by the distal nephron.[160] In CKD, acidosis develops as a result of varying degrees of impairment in each of these processes.[183]

Reduction in renal ammonia synthesis is the greatest limitation to acid excretion in CKD. Low serum bicarbonate levels result in maintenance of acid urine, which stimulates proximal tubule ammoniagenesis and also protonates ammonia, resulting in its entrapment as ammonium in the tubule lumen. Net ammonia production per hypertrophied proximal tubule has been shown to increase in response to nephron loss.[176] With decreasing GFR, however, this increase becomes inadequate to compensate for further nephron loss, and absolute ammonia excretion falls.[145] In addition, disruption of the tubulomedullary ammonium concentration gradient as a result of structural injury may impair ammonia trapping and therefore reduce ammonium excretion.[145] Bicarbonate reabsorption by the nephron occurs predominantly in association with sodium reclamation in the proximal tubule and is dependent upon generation of a proton gradient in the distal nephron. Conflicting data with respect to bicarbonate reabsorption in remnant kidneys may reflect species differences. In dogs with remnant kidneys, bicarbonate reabsorption was increased at both proximal and distal micropuncture sampling sites compared to intact controls.[184] In contrast, bicarbonate reabsorption per unit GFR is reduced in both humans and rats with CKD,[160] and some patients with renal failure demonstrate bicarbonate wasting until serum bicarbonate drops below 20 mEq/L.[185] Bicarbonate reabsorption is also reduced in the setting of hyperkalemia, increased ECF volume, and hyperparathyroidism, all of which may be present in patients with CKD.[186-188] Distal urinary acidification tends to be relatively well preserved in patients with CKD, and urinary pH, although higher than in normal individuals with experimental acidosis, is usually approximately 5.[189] Urinary excretion of titratable acid is also generally well preserved in the setting of nephron loss, as a consequence of increased fractional phosphate excretion.[142,145] As renal failure progresses, acid excretion becomes more dependent on excretion of titratable acid. Renal acidification mechanisms are discussed more comprehensively in Chapters 9 and 17.

CALCIUM AND PHOSPHATE

Derangements of calcium and phosphate metabolism occurring with renal insufficiency are not only the result of impaired urinary excretion of these solutes, but also of associated abnormalities in vitamin D metabolism and PTH secretion. With progressive renal dysfunction, 1-hydroxylation of vitamin D by the kidney decreases, calcium absorption from the gut decreases, serum calcium level tends to decrease, serum phosphate level tends to increase, and PTH secretion increases. In response to increased PTH, calcium is mobilized from bone, renal phosphate excretion is enhanced, and the steady state becomes reestablished, with secondary hyperparathyroidism as the "trade-off."[190] In CKD, serum phosphate level does not increase until GFR falls below 20 mL/min, and phosphate balance is maintained predominantly by an increase in fractional phosphate excretion.[191] With moderate renal failure, therefore, filtered phosphate is not greatly increased, and the increase in phosphate excretion must be achieved by a reduction in phosphate reabsorption per nephron.[192] With more severe reductions in GFR, however, phosphate excretion is maintained by an increase in serum phosphate level as well as reduced reabsorption per nephron. Sodium-dependent phosphate transport measured in proximal tubular brush border membrane vesicles prepared from the remnant kidneys of dogs was shown to be decreased when compared to that in vesicles derived from normal dogs.[142] Interestingly, however, this decrease was abolished if the partially nephrectomized dog had also undergone parathyroidectomy, indicating that PTH plays an important role in proximal tubular adaptation to phosphate excretion. Studies of isolated proximal tubules from euparathyroid uremic rabbits showed a reduction in net phosphate flux per unit of reabsorptive surface area and an increase in sensitivity to PTH.[144] The authors postulated that the number of PTH receptors per tubule must increase in the remnant kidney, concomitant with tubular hypertrophy. The levels of mRNA encoding the sodium-coupled phosphate transporter, Na^+-PO_4^{3-}-exchanger type 2 (NaPi-2), are reduced by approximately 50% in remnant kidneys from 5/6 nephrectomized rats.[193] In contrast, tubules from hyperparathyroid uremic rabbits demonstrated reduced PTH sensitivity, consistent with downregulation or persistent occupancy of the PTH receptors. On the other hand, studies in animals with reduced renal mass subjected to parathyroidectomy have shown that fractional excretion of phosphate remains inversely proportional to the reduction in GFR,[194] indicating that phosphate excretion is not entirely dependent on the presence of PTH. Fibroblast growth factor 23 (FGF-23) has been identified as a major mediator of increased phosphaturia after nephron loss.[195] First identified as the primary mediator of autosomal dominant hypophosphatemia, increased FGF-23 expression has been shown in transgenic models to increase urinary phosphate excretion through downregulation of NaPi-2a expression in proximal tubules.[196] Further experiments utilizing gene deletion models found that decreased expression of NaPi-2a and NaPi-2c by exogenous FGF-23 was mediated predominantly by FGF receptor 1.[197] Activation of FGF receptors by FGF-23 is critically dependent on binding with its coreceptor, Klotho.[195] Circulating levels of FGF-23 become elevated early in the course of CKD, with levels rising once GFR falls below 70 mL/min in humans.[195] That FGF-23 is important in mediating increased phosphaturia after nephron loss has been demonstrated by experiments in which administration of neutralizing anti–FGF-23 antibodies after renal mass reduction resulted in decreased fractional excretion of phosphate and increased serum phosphate level.[198] Whereas most of the reduction in phosphate reabsorption is achieved in the proximal tubule, there is also some evidence of increased fractional phosphate excretion by the distal tubule in uremic dogs and rats.[199] As renal failure advances, renal 1-hydroxylation of vitamin D decreases, and as a result, calcium absorption from the gut is reduced.[200] In addition to its effects on renal phosphate excretion, FGF-23 inhibits renal 1α-hydroxylase activity, thereby reducing levels of 1,25-dihydroxyvitamin D $(1,25[OH]_2D)$.[196,198] In renal failure, fractional intestinal calcium absorption is inversely proportional to blood urea nitrogen level.[200] Calcium excretion, on the other hand, varies widely in patients with kidney disease, probably due to differences in diet, heterogeneity of vitamin D production, and predominance of glomerular versus tubulointerstitial injury.[201] In normal individuals, calcium excretion is mediated by suppression of PTH-induced reabsorption in the distal nephron and by suppression of PTH-independent mechanisms in the thick ascending limb. In patients with CKD, fractional calcium excretion remains unchanged until GFR falls below 25 mL/min, when fractional excretion increases due to the obligatory solute diuresis.[160] Absolute calcium excretion, however, remains low. Hypocalciuria in patients with CKD has been shown to be due in part to the attendant hyperparathyroidism.[202] Similar findings were obtained in rats with reduced renal mass, in which parathyroidectomy resulted in increased calcium excretion compared to nonparathyroidectomized controls.[203] Renal calcium clearance is increased in patients with tubulointerstitial disease and in rats with surgical papillectomy, suggesting that regulation of calcium reabsorption depends on intact medullary structures, and that regulation of calcium excretion may be largely modulated by the distal nephron segments.[160] The potential contribution of calcium and phosphate to kidney disease progression is discussed later. Calcium and phosphate metabolism are also discussed in greater detail in Chapters 7 and 19.

LONG-TERM ADVERSE CONSEQUENCES OF ADAPTATIONS TO NEPHRON LOSS

The functional and structural adaptations to nephron loss described earlier may be regarded as a beneficial response that minimizes the resultant loss of total GFR. It has been appreciated for several decades, however, that rats subjected to partial nephrectomy subsequently develop hypertension, albuminuria, and progressive renal failure. Detailed histopathologic studies in rat remnant kidneys after 5/6 nephrectomy revealed mesangial accumulation of hyaline material that progressively encroached on capillary lumina, obliterating Bowman's space and finally resulting in global sclerosis of the glomerulus. These findings, together with the observation that sclerosed glomeruli are a common finding in human CKD of diverse causes, led to the hypothesis that glomerular hyperfiltration ultimately results in damage to remaining glomeruli and contributes to a vicious cycle of progressive nephron loss. The 5/6 nephrectomy model has been extensively studied, and considerable progress has been made in elucidating how the physiologic adaptations of remaining nephrons that initially permit greatly augmented function per nephron ultimately produce a complex series of adverse effects that eventuate in progressive renal injury and an inexorable decline in function.[7]

HEMODYNAMIC FACTORS

As early as 1 week after extensive renal mass ablation, glomerular hyperfiltration and glomerular capillary hypertension were associated with morphologic changes, including visceral epithelial cell cytoplasmic attenuation, protein reabsorption droplets and foot process fusion, mesangial expansion, and focal lifting of endothelial cells from the basement membrane (Figures 52.5 and 52.6).[7] Evidence that these morphologic changes were a consequence of the glomerular hemodynamic alterations was provided by studies in rats fed a low-protein diet after 5/6 nephrectomy. This intervention prevented the hemodynamic changes, effectively normalizing Q_A, P_{GC}, and SNGFR, and abrogated the structural lesions observed in rats on standard diet.[7] Similar findings were subsequently described in a variety of animal models of CKD, including diabetic nephropathy[204,205] and deoxycorticosterone acetate (DOCA)-salt hypertension.[206] Together, these observations led Brenner and colleagues to propose that the hemodynamic adaptations following renal mass ablation ultimately prove injurious to glomeruli and initiate processes that eventuate in glomerulosclerosis. The resulting obliteration of further glomeruli would induce hyperfiltration in remaining, less affected glomeruli, thereby establishing a vicious cycle of progressive nephron loss. These mechanisms constituted a "common pathway" for renal damage that could account for the inexorable progression of CKD, regardless of the cause of the initial renal injury.[3] The hypothesis also explained the finding of both atrophic and hypertrophic nephrons typically encountered in chronically diseased kidneys. Further evidence supportive of the "hyperfiltration hypothesis" was gleaned from the study of experimental diabetic nephropathy in which glomerular hyperfiltration was also found to be a forerunner of glomerular pathologic processes.[7,205] Maneuvers such as unilateral nephrectomy, which exacerbates hyperfiltration in the remaining kidney, were also found to exacerbate diabetic renal injury.[207] Furthermore, when the kidney was shielded from elevated perfusion pressure and from glomerular capillary hypertension by creating unilateral renal artery stenosis, the ipsilateral kidney was protected against the development of diabetic injury, which progressed unabated in the contralateral kidney.[208] In addition, when glomerular hyperfiltration was reversed in 5/6 nephrectomized rats by transplantation of an isogeneic kidney, hypertension and proteinuria were ameliorated, and glomerular injury was limited.[209] Similarly, augmenting renal mass in the Fisher-to-Lewis rat transplant model normalized P_{GC} and greatly reduced the development of chronic renal allograft injury.[210,211] Direct evidence that similar mechanisms may operate in human kidneys is derived from a study of 14 patients with solitary kidneys who had undergone varying degrees of partial nephrectomy of the remaining kidney for malignancy.[212] Before renal-sparing surgery, proteinuria was absent in all patients. Although serum creatinine level remained stable after an initial rise of 50% in 12 patients, the 2 patients subjected to the most extensive nephrectomy (75% and 67%, respectively) developed progressive renal failure and required long-term dialysis. Moreover, among the remaining patients, 7 developed proteinuria, the levels of which were inversely related to the amount of renal tissue preserved. Renal biopsy specimens in 4 patients with moderate-to-severe proteinuria showed focal segmental glomerulosclerosis (FSGS),[212] which later morphometric analysis revealed to involve virtually all glomeruli examined.[213] The importance of renal mass in humans is further

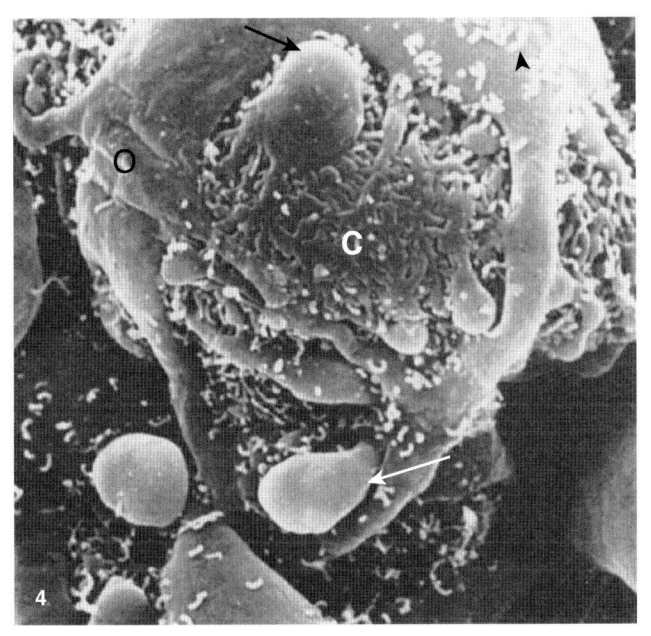

Figure 52.5 Scanning electron micrograph of a glomerulus from a rat following 5/6 nephrectomy. View from urinary space. Cytoplasmic blebs (*arrows*), numerous microvilli (*arrowhead*), focal obliteration (O) and coarsening (C) of foot processes are seen (×3600). (Reproduced with permission from Hostetter TH, Olson JL, Rennke HG, et al: Hyperfiltration in remnant nephrons: a potentially adverse response to renal ablation. *Am J Physiol* 241:F85-F93, 1981.)

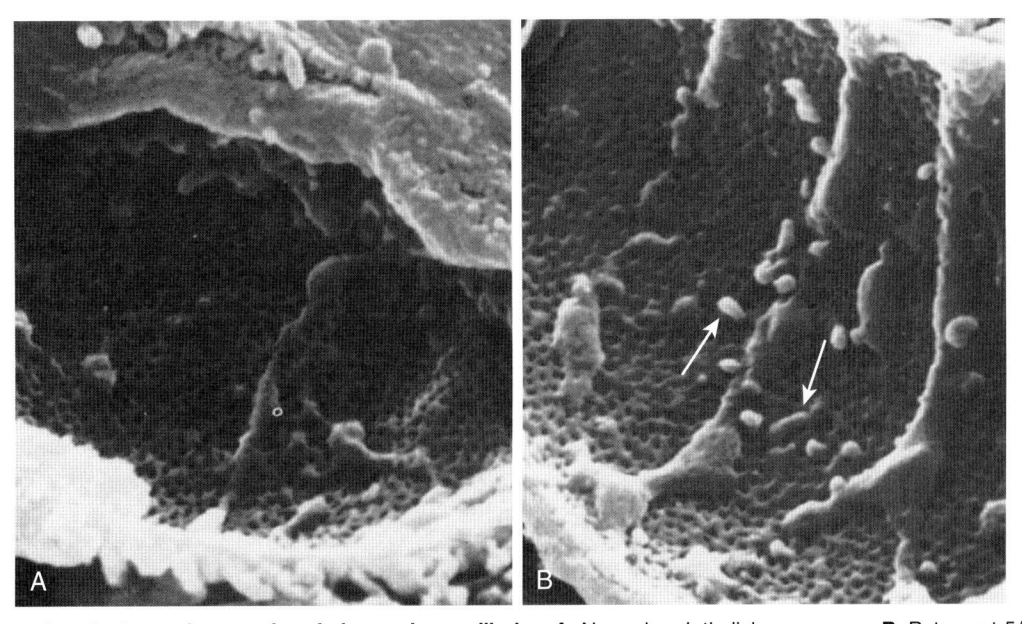

Figure 52.6 Scanning electron micrographs of glomerular capillaries. **A,** Normal endothelial appearance. **B,** Rats post 5/6 nephrectomy. Scattered endothelial blebs (*arrows*) are often present in this group (×18,000.). (Reproduced with permission from Hostetter TH, Olson JL, Rennke HG, et al: Hyperfiltration in remnant nephrons: a potentially adverse response to renal ablation. *Am J Physiol* 241: F85-F93, 1981.)

illustrated by an observational study of 749 patients who underwent either radical nephrectomy or nephron-sparing surgery for removal of a renal mass. Those who had nephron-sparing surgery evidenced a significantly lower incidence of reduced GFR (16.0% versus 44.7%) and proteinuria (13.2% versus 22.2%).[214] Similarly, a large meta-analysis that included data from 31,729 people who had a radical nephrectomy and 9281 people who had a partial nephrectomy for cancer found a 61% reduction in risk for developing CKD stages 3 to 5 after partial nephrectomy.[215] Finally, whereas unilateral donor nephrectomy is associated with an excellent prognosis in the majority, two case-controlled studies have reported a small absolute increase in long-term risk for ESKD.[216,217] One detailed study in 51 living donors has reported that hypertension in kidney donors older than 50 years was associated with a lower estimated number of functioning nephrons per kidney, and it is therefore possible that donors with low nephron number are at increased risk for subsequent kidney damage.[218]

The importance of glomerular hemodynamic factors in the development of progressive renal injury was further illustrated by studies that reported dramatic protective effects against the development of glomerulosclerosis after chronic inhibition of the RAAS with either ACEI or ARB treatment in 5/6 nephrectomized rats.[17-20] Micropuncture studies showed that like the low-protein diet, the renoprotective effects of RAAS inhibition were associated with near normalization of the P_{GC}, yet, in contrast to the effects of dietary protein restriction, SNGFR remained elevated.[219] This suggested that glomerular capillary hypertension, rather than hyperfiltration per se, was the key factor in the initiation and progression of glomerular injury. Confirmation of this view came from an experiment in which rats were treated with a combination of reserpine, hydralazine, and hydrochlorothiazide ("triple therapy") to lower arterial pressure to levels similar to those obtained with an ACEI. In contrast to the glomerular hemodynamic effects of the ACEI, however, triple therapy did not alleviate glomerular hypertension or proteinuria, and glomerular injury progressed unabated[18,19] (Figure 52.7). Interestingly, within the context of pharmacologic inhibition of the RAAS, the level to which systemic blood pressure is reduced remains a critical determinant of the extent of the renal protection conferred.[220] The effectiveness of both ACEI and ARB in lowering glomerular pressure and ameliorating glomerular injury has since been observed in several other animal models of CKD, including diabetic nephropathy,[204,221,222] hypertensive kidney disease,[223,224] experimental chronic renal allograft failure (a model that lacks systemic hypertension but exhibits glomerular capillary hypertension),[225-227] age-related glomerulosclerosis,[228,229] and obesity-related glomerulosclerosis.[230] It is noteworthy that the phase of transition from an acute, nonhypertensive experimental injury induced by puromycin aminonucleoside (PAN) administration to a chronic nephropathy characterized by proteinuria and glomerulosclerosis is also associated with the development of glomerular capillary hypertension.[231] That similar mechanisms are relevant in human CKD progression has been strongly suggested by the results of clinical trials showing substantial renoprotective effects with ACEI and ARB treatment.[232-236] The importance of glomerular capillary hypertension has been further illustrated by studies of

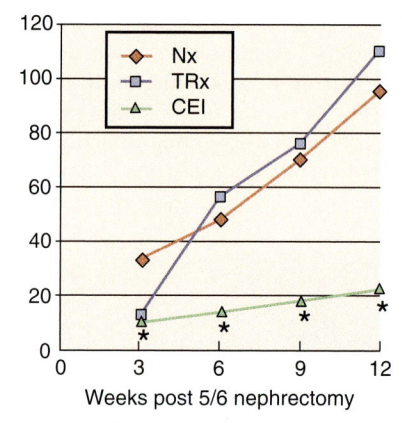

Figure 52.7 Proteinuria levels following 5/6 nephrectomy in untreated rats (NX) versus treatment with triple therapy (reserpine, hydralazine, and hydrochlorothiazide [TRx]), (NX + TRX) or enalapril (NX + CEI). Despite equivalent levels of blood pressure control, enalapril therapy almost completely prevented proteinuria and glomerulosclerosis, whereas triple therapy afforded no renoprotection. *P <0.05 versus Nx. (Reproduced with permission from Anderson S, Rennke HG, Brenner BM: Therapeutic advantage of converting enzyme inhibitors in arresting progressive renal disease associated with systemic hypertension in the rat. J Clin Invest 77:1993-2000, 1986.)

the effects of omapatrilat, a vasopeptidase inhibitor. Micropuncture studies after 5/6 nephrectomy showed even greater lowering of P_{GC} with omapatrilat than with ACEI treatment, despite equivalent effects on systemic blood pressure. In subsequent chronic studies, omapatrilat produced more effective renoprotection than the ACEI.[83] Thus, among the determinants of glomerular hyperfiltration, glomerular capillary hypertension has been identified as a critical factor in the initiation and progression of glomerular injury.

MECHANISMS OF HEMODYNAMICALLY INDUCED INJURY

MECHANICAL STRESS

Several mechanisms have been proposed whereby elevated P_{GC} may result in glomerular cell injury. Experiments in isolated perfused rat glomeruli have reported significant increases in V_G with increases in perfusion pressure over the normal and relevant abnormal range.[102] These increases in wall tension and V_G can be predicted to result in stretching of glomerular cells. Experimental evidence suggests that such stretching may have adverse consequences for all three major cell types in the glomerulus. Furthermore, advances in the study of cellular responses to mechanical stress raise the possibility that glomerular hyperperfusion may also promote the development of glomerulosclerosis through more subtle and complex pathways that induce profibrotic phenotypic alterations in glomerular cells.[237]

ENDOTHELIAL CELLS

The vascular endothelium serves multiple complex functions, including acting as a dynamic barrier to leukocytes and plasma proteins, secretion of vasoactive factors (PGI_2, NO, and ET), conversion of Ang I to Ang II, and expression of cell adhesion molecules. It is also the first cellular structure in the kidney that encounters the mechanical forces imparted by glomerular hyperperfusion. After 5/6 nephrectomy, endothelial cells are activated or injured, resulting in detachment and exposure of the basement membrane. This in turn may induce platelet aggregation, deposition of fibrin, and intracapillary microthrombus formation.[7,238] It has been recognized for some time that segmental glomerulosclerosis is associated with focal obliteration of capillary loops[239] and that interstitial fibrosis is associated with loss of peritubular capillaries.[240] Furthermore, it has been shown that this loss of capillaries in the remnant kidney is associated with a decrease in endothelial cell proliferation and reduced constitutive expression of VEGF by podocytes and renal tubular cells, as well as increased expression of the antiangiogenic factor, thrombospondin-1, by the renal interstitium.[241] Since VEGF is an important endothelial cell angiogenic, survival, and trophic factor, these findings suggest that capillary loss may be due in part to failure of recovery from hemodynamically mediated endothelial cell injury. Indeed, inhibition of endothelial and mesangial cell proliferation by treatment with everolimus after 5/6 nephrectomy resulted in increased proteinuria, glomerulosclerosis, and interstitial fibrosis associated with reduced glomerular expression of VEGF.[242] Furthermore, short-term treatment of rats with VEGF ameliorated both glomerular and peritubular capillary loss after 5/6 nephrectomy.[243] This preservation of capillaries was associated with a trend toward less glomerulosclerosis and significantly less interstitial deposition of collagen III, as well as better preservation of renal function. Further evidence of the importance of endothelial cells in the preservation of function after nephron loss is provided by experiments in which bone marrow–derived endothelial progenitor cells (EPCs) were administered to mice after 5/6 nephrectomy. EPC-treated mice evidenced better preservation of renal function, less proteinuria, and relatively preserved renal structure, as well as decreased expression of proinflammatory molecules and restored levels of the angiogenic molecules VEGF, VEGF receptor 2, and thrombospondin-1.[244] Long-term studies are required to evaluate further the potential benefit of improving renal angiogenesis in the setting of progressive renal injury.

Endothelial cells bear numerous receptors that allow them to detect and respond to changes in mechanical forces. Thus exposure of endothelial cells to changes in shear stress, cyclic stretch, or pulsatile barostress that result from glomerular hyperperfusion may induce changes in expression of genes involved in inflammation, cell cycle control, apoptosis, thrombosis, and oxidative stress.[245] The in vitro responses of endothelial cells to mechanical forces have largely been studied in the context of vascular remodeling and atherosclerosis, but it can readily be appreciated that similar responses may impact the development of inflammation and fibrosis within the remnant kidney. Of particular interest are observations that shear stress can stimulate endothelial expression of adhesion molecules[246] and proinflammatory cytokines.[247] It is clear from this discussion why biomechanical activation has emerged as an important paradigm in endothelial cell biology,[248] but further studies focusing on glomerular endothelial responses to mechanical stress are required to elucidate the role of such mechanisms in progressive renal injury.

MESANGIAL CELLS

Mesangial cells are closely associated with the capillaries in the glomerulus and are therefore also exposed to mechanical forces. Evidence from in vitro studies indicates that mesangial cells respond to changes in these mechanical forces in ways that may promote inflammation and fibrosis. Subjecting mesangial cells to cyclical stretch or strain has been shown to induce proliferation[249] and synthesis of ECM constituents.[250,251] Cyclical stretch also activates the transcription factor nuclear factor κ light-chain enhancer of activated B cells (NF-κB),[252] stimulates synthesis of intercellular cell adhesion molecule-1 (ICAM-1),[253] monocyte chemoattractant protein-1 (MCP-1),[253] TGF-β[254] and its receptor,[255] as well as connective tissue growth factor (CTGF).[256] Cyclical stretch also activates the RAAS in cultured mesangial cells,[257] and Ang II in turn may induce TGF-β synthesis.[258] In vitro studies have identified several signaling pathways responsible for stretch-induced signal transduction in mesangial cells. Cyclical stretch activates the serine/threonine kinase Akt through a mechanism requiring phosphatidylinositol-3-kinase and transactivation of EGF receptor and is necessary for the increased synthesis of collagen $α_1I$ observed in the mesangial cells. Furthermore, Akt activation was observed in remnant kidney glomeruli, indicating that these mechanisms are also present in vivo.[259] The actin cytoskeleton is an important transmitter of mechanical signals, and the GTPase RhoA, a central regulator of the cytoskeleton, is activated by cyclical stretch. Stretch-induced activation of the mitogen-activated protein kinase ERK, linked to increased matrix production, is dependent on activation of RhoA.[260] Mesangial cells cultured at ambient pressures of 50 to 60 mm Hg (i.e., levels corresponding to glomerular capillary hypertension) also show enhanced synthesis and secretion of ECM when compared with cells grown at "normal" pressures of 40 to 50 mm Hg.[261] Exposure of mesangial cells to barostress, achieved by culture under increased barometric pressure, stimulates expression of cytokines, including platelet-derived growth factor-B (PDGF-B)[262] and MCP-1.[263] Transduction of mechanical forces by mesangial cells has been associated with tyrosine phosphorylation[264] and protein kinase C–induced increases in S6 kinase activity.[265]

PODOCYTES

A growing body of evidence attests to the importance of podocyte injury in a variety of kidney diseases and in CKD progression.[266] Podocytes display morphologic evidence of injury as early as 1 week after 5/6 nephrectomy[7] and 6 months after uninephrectomy.[267] Increased numbers of podocytes have been observed in the urine from rats after 5/6 nephrectomy and in human CKD.[266] In 5/6 nephrectomized rats the number of podocytes correlated with the severity of proteinuria as well as mean arterial blood pressure, suggesting that podocyte loss may contribute to CKD progression.[268] The importance of podocyte injury in CKD progression is further supported by the observation that amelioration of glomerular damage in 5/6 nephrectomized rats treated with $1,25(OH)_2D_3$ is associated with preservation of podocyte number as well as prevention of podocyte hypertrophy and injury.[269] Detailed in vitro studies have shown that early podocyte injury is associated with dysregulation of calcium homeostasis and disruption of the actomyosin contractile apparatus. The Rho family of small guanosine triphosphatases plays a key role in this process. Calcium influx via transient receptor potential cation channel (TRPC) type 5 results in activation of Ras-related C3 botulinum toxin substrate 1 (Rac1) and is associated with increased podocyte migration and proteinuria, whereas calcium influx via TRPC type 6 activates RhoA, resulting in preservation of stress fibers, prevention of podocyte migration, and maintenance of the filtration barrier.[270] As podocytes are attached to the outer aspect of the glomerular basement membrane, it is reasonable to expect that they would be exposed to increased mechanical forces resulting from glomerular hypertension. Confirmation that podocytes respond to such physical forces is derived from several in vitro experiments that examined podocyte responses to stretching. Activation of voltage-sensitive potassium channels was observed in response to stretching of the podocyte cell membrane,[271] and culture of podocytes under constant stretch induced activation of the protein kinases ERK1/2 and c-Jun N-terminal kinase (JNK) via the EGF receptor as well as other changes in cell signaling.[272] Mechanical stretch inhibited podocyte proliferation[273] and (in common with TGF-β) reduced $α_3β_1$-integrin expression and podocyte adhesion in vitro.[274] Exposure to cyclical stretching that mimics pulsatile strain within the glomerulus has been shown to cause reorganization of the actin cytoskeleton,[275] upregulation of COX-2, and E-prostanoid 4 (EP4) receptor expression[276] as well as podocyte hypertrophy.[277] Subsequent experiments utilizing mice with podocyte-specific depletion or overexpression of EP4 receptors found that PGE_2 acting via EP4 receptors contributes to the development of proteinuria after 5/6 nephrectomy and therefore probably contributes to podocyte injury.[278] In another experiment, cyclical stretching of podocytes was associated with increased production of Ang II and TGF-β, as well as upregulation of angiotensin subtype 1 receptors (AT_1Rs), resulting in increased Ang II–dependent apoptosis.[279] Cyclical stretch of podocytes also resulted in a 50% reduction of nephrin (a key component of the slit diaphragm) mRNA and protein levels via an Ang II–dependent mechanism that was inhibited by the peroxisome proliferator–activated receptor γ (PPARγ) agonist, rosiglitazone, which prevented AT_1R upregulation.[280] Taken together, these data suggest that stretch-induced podocyte injury is a further mechanism whereby glomerular hypertension contributes to glomerular injury.

Detailed studies of podocyte hypertrophy have found that impaired podocyte hypertrophy in response to glomerular enlargement is a further mechanism that may contribute to the development of proteinuria and FSGS. Using a transgenic rat model (dominant negative AA-4E-BP1 transgene) that resulted in impaired podocyte hypertrophy, the investigators observed a remarkable linear relationship between gain in body weight, proteinuria, and glomerulosclerosis that was accelerated after uninephrectomy. Dietary caloric restriction that prevented weight gain and glomerular enlargement also prevented the proteinuria. Analysis of the kidneys from rats with proteinuria demonstrated a mismatch between glomerular tuft volume and total podocyte volume, and electron microscopy revealed pulling apart of podocyte foot process, resulting in exposed areas of glomerular basement membrane and adhesions to Bowman's capsule.[281] Further studies are required to identify whether impaired podocyte hypertrophy contributes to proteinuria and glomerulosclerosis in human kidney diseases associated with glomerular enlargement such as diabetic nephropathy, obesity-related glomerulopathy, and oligomeganephronia.

CELLULAR INFILTRATION IN REMNANT KIDNEYS

Despite the lack of an obvious immune stimulus, an inflammatory cell infiltrate composed predominantly of macrophages and smaller numbers of lymphocytes is observed in remnant kidneys after 5/6 nephrectomy.[282] Interestingly, similar observations have been reported in a rat model of spontaneous renal agenesis associated with a 60.2% reduction in nephron endowment.[283] As discussed earlier, it is possible that the glomerular hemodynamic adaptations to nephron loss may provoke an inflammatory cell response through the effects of mechanical forces on endothelial and mesangial cells. Thus upregulation of renal endothelial adhesion molecules may facilitate egress of leukocytes from the circulation into the mesangium, where they may participate in further renal injury. The recruited cellular infiltrate may constitute an abundant source of potent pleiotropic cytokine products that in turn influence other infiltrating leukocytes, dendritic cells, and kidney cells, stimulating cell proliferation, elaboration of ECM components, and increased endothelial adhesiveness.[284] Evidence is now emerging that these proposed mechanisms, based largely on in vitro observations, are indeed relevant in vivo. In the two-kidney–one-clip model of renovascular hypertension, upregulated expression of adhesion molecules and TGF-β, as well as cell infiltration, is observed only in the nonclipped kidney that is exposed to the hypertensive perfusion pressure.[285,286] In the 5/6 nephrectomy model, coordinated upregulation of a variety of cell adhesion molecules, cytokines, and growth factors in association with macrophage infiltration has been observed at time points that precede the development of severe glomerulosclerosis.[287,288] Furthermore, the renoprotection afforded by ACEI or ARB treatment in this model was associated with inhibition of cytokine upregulation and prevention of renal infiltration by macrophages.[288,289]

Infiltrating macrophages, although present in the glomeruli of remnant kidneys, are chiefly distributed in the tubulointerstitial regions,[282,288] suggesting that they play a role in the development of the tubulointerstitial fibrosis (TIF) that accompanies glomerulosclerosis. Further analysis of the cellular infiltrate has also identified mast cells in close proximity to areas of TIF.[290] It is possible that interstitial infiltrates are recruited as the result of tubulointerstitial cell activation by the downstream effects of cytokines released in the glomeruli. Alternatively it has been proposed that excessive uptake of filtered proteins by tubular epithelial cells stimulates expression of cell adhesion and chemoattractant molecules that recruit macrophages and other monocytic cells to tubulointerstitial areas[291] (see later for further discussion). The chemokine C-C motif receptor 1 (CCR1) has been shown to be important in interstitial but not glomerular recruitment of leukocytes. Treatment with a nonpeptide CCR1 antagonist has been shown to reduce interstitial macrophage infiltration and ameliorate interstitial fibrosis in the UUO model but data are still lacking in the 5/6 nephrectomy model.[292] Furthermore, antagonism of MCP-1 signaling through gene therapy–induced production of a mutant form of MCP-1 by skeletal muscle resulted in reduced interstitial macrophage infiltration and amelioration of interstitial fibrosis in mice after UUO.[293] The identification of renal tubular cells expressing α-smooth muscle actin after 5/6 nephrectomy raised the possibility that tubular cells may undergo transdifferentiation to a myofibroblast phenotype that contributes to interstitial fibrosis.[294] Furthermore, the renoprotection observed with mycophenolate treatment in 5/6 nephrectomized rats is associated with reductions in interstitial myofibroblast infiltration and collagen III deposition.[295] There is, however, ongoing debate regarding the origin of interstitial myofibroblasts in CKD. Fate mapping studies have indicated that mesenchymal cells called pericytes are the predominant source of myofibroblasts and that epithelial to mesenchymal transdifferentiation is not a source of myofibroblasts or accounts for only a small minority.[296] Other cells that may give rise to interstitial myofibroblasts include resident fibroblasts, endothelial cells, and bone marrow–derived cells.[297,298]

Several lines of evidence suggest that this cellular infiltrate contributes to renal injury and is not merely a consequence of it.[299] In one study, multiple linear regression analysis identified glomerular macrophage infiltration in the remnant kidney as a major determinant of mesangial matrix expansion and adhesion formation between Bowman's capsule and glomerular tufts.[282] Furthermore, depletion of leukocytes in rats by irradiation delayed the onset of glomerular injury after renal ablative surgery.[300] Several studies have reported amelioration of the cellular infiltrate and renal injury in the 5/6 nephrectomy model following treatment with the immunosuppressive agent mycophenolate mofetil.[301-304] One study found that mycophenolate also lowers P_{GC}, which may account for some of its renoprotective effects.[305] Several other antiinflammatory interventions have been shown to ameliorate renal injury after 5/6 nephrectomy: treatment with the antiinflammatory agent nitroflurbiprofen, also an NO donor, was associated with moderate renoprotection.[306] Rats treated with a PPARγ agonist evidenced significant attenuation of the proteinuria and glomerulosclerosis observed in untreated rats, despite the failure of treatment to lower blood pressure. This renoprotection was observed in association with marked reductions in glomerular cell proliferation, glomerular macrophage infiltration, and renal expression of plasminogen activator inhibitor-1 (PAI-1) as well as TGF-β.[307] The authors speculate that some of these effects may have resulted from the known actions of PPARγ activation to antagonize the activities of the transcription factors activating protein-1 (AP-1) and NF-κB. Administration of a sphingosine-1 phosphate receptor (S1PR) agonist, a novel immunosuppressant that inhibits egress of T cells and B cells from lymph nodes, attenuated the increase in chemokine receptor expression observed in untreated rats, and tended to normalize RANTES (regulated on activation, normal T expressed, and secreted) and MCP-1 gene expression. Glomerular and interstitial inflammation and fibrosis were also reduced.[308] Overexpression of the antiinflammatory cytokine IL-10 in rats was associated with reduced interstitial inflammation and lower levels of MCP-1, RANTES, interferon-γ, and IL-2 expression, as well as attenuation of proteinuria, glomerulosclerosis, and TIF.[309] Finally, overexpression of the gene for angiostatin, an anti-angiogenic factor that also inhibits leukocyte recruitment as well as neutrophil and macrophage migration, was associated with inhibition of macrophage and T cell infiltrates in glomeruli as well as the interstitium, reduced MCP-1 expression and attenuation of glomerulosclerosis as well as interstitial fibrosis.[310] Taken together, these findings strongly support the hypothesis that in addition to direct glomerular cell injury, glomerular hemodynamic adaptations to nephron loss provoke a complex series of proinflammatory and profibrotic responses that further contribute to renal damage. Treatments that antagonize the mediators of these responses may therefore be of benefit in slowing the rate of CKD progression.

NONHEMODYNAMIC FACTORS IN THE DEVELOPMENT OF NEPHRON INJURY FOLLOWING EXTENSIVE RENAL MASS ABLATION

The weight of evidence in support of the hypothesis that glomerular hemodynamic adaptations are central to progressive renal injury does not exclude the possibility that the kidney may also be affected by a variety of factors not directly attributable to hemodynamic changes. These nonhemodynamic factors have been extensively studied and may offer new therapeutic targets for future renoprotective interventions.

TRANSFORMING GROWTH FACTOR-β

TGF-β is associated with chronic fibrotic states throughout the body, including CKD.[311] In vitro TGF-β elicits overproduction of ECM constituents by mesangial cells, and its expression is increased in several experimental models of kidney disease, including diabetic nephropathy,[312] anti–Thy-1 glomerulonephritis,[313] doxorubicin (Adriamycin)-induced nephropathy,[314] and chronic allograft nephropathy,[315] as well as in human glomerulonephritis,[316,317] human immunodeficiency virus (HIV) nephropathy,[318] diabetic nephropathy,[319] and chronic allograft nephropathy.[320] The role of TGF-β in renal fibrosis is further illustrated by experiments in which transfection of the gene for TGF-β into one renal artery produced ipsilateral renal fibrosis.[321] In 5/6 nephrectomized rats a 2- to 3-fold increase in remnant kidney mRNA levels for TGF-β was observed, and in situ hybridization revealed elevations in TGF-β mRNA throughout glomeruli, tubules, and interstitium. Treatment with an ACEI or an ARB resulted in substantial renal protection and prevented upregulation of TGF-β.[288,289] Furthermore, in rats treated with an ACEI or an ARB the extent of glomerulosclerosis correlated closely with remnant kidney TGF-β mRNA levels.[220] Several interventions that inhibit the effects of TGF-β have been shown to afford renoprotection in animal models of kidney disease: Transfection of the gene for decorin, a naturally occurring inhibitor of TGF-β, into skeletal muscle limited the progression of renal injury in anti–Thy-1 glomerulonephritis[322]; administration of anti–TGF-β antibodies to salt-loaded Dahl–salt sensitive rats ameliorated the hypertension, proteinuria, glomerulosclerosis, and interstitial fibrosis typical of this model[323]; treatment with tranilast (N-[3,4-dimethoxycinnamoyl] anthranilic acid), an inhibitor of TGF-β–induced ECM production, significantly reduced albuminuria, macrophage infiltration, glomerulosclerosis, and interstitial fibrosis in 5/6 nephrectomized

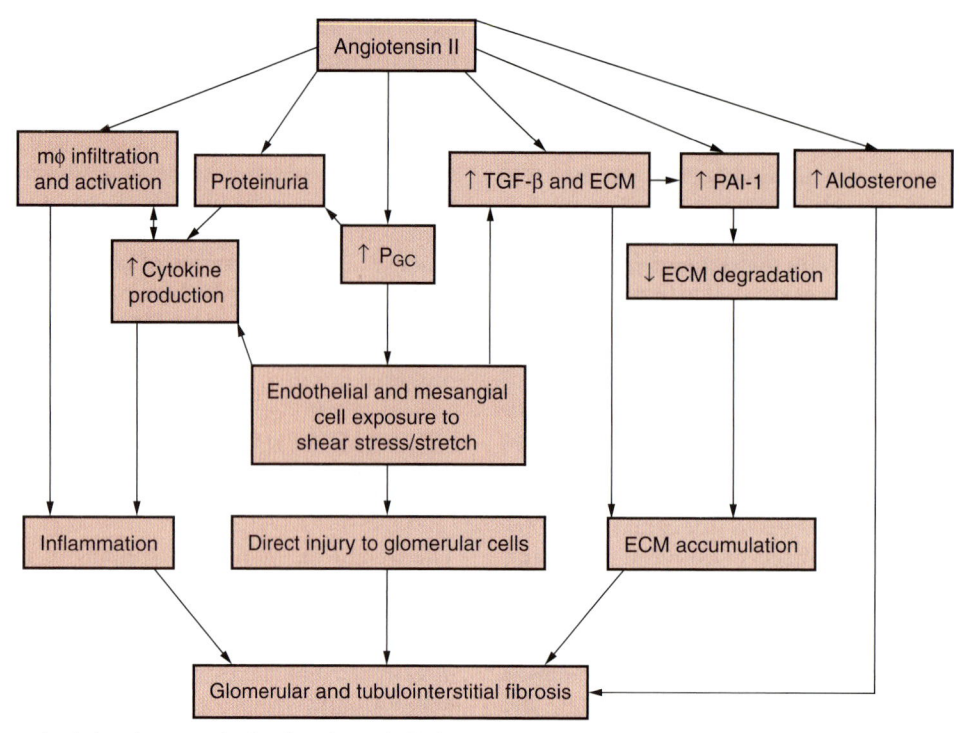

Figure 52.8 Scheme depicting the central role of angiotensin II, through hemodynamic and nonhemodynamic effects, in the pathogenesis of progressive renal injury and fibrosis following nephron loss. ECM, Extracellular matrix; mφ, macrophage; PAI-1, plasminogen activator inhibitor-1; P_{GC}, glomerular capillary hydraulic pressure; TGF-β, transforming growth factor-β. (Reproduced with permission from Taal MW, Brenner, BM: Renoprotective benefits of RAS inhibition: from ACEI to angiotensin II antagonists. *Kidney Int* 57:1803-1817, 2000.)

rats[324]; transfer of an inducible gene for Smad 7, which blocks TGF-β signaling by inhibiting Smad 2/3 activation, inhibited proteinuria, fibrosis, and myofibroblast accumulation after 5/6 nephrectomy[325]; and 2 weeks of treatment with a polyamide compound designed to suppress transcription of the TGF-β gene, significantly reduced proteinuria and prevented upregulation of TGF-β, CTGF, collagen I α1, and fibronectin mRNA in the renal cortex, as well as suppressing urinary TGF-β excretion and staining for TGF-β by immunofluorescence in salt-loaded Dhal–salt sensitive rats.[326] Another fibrogenic molecule, CTGF, has also been observed to be overexpressed in kidney biopsy specimens from patients with a variety of kidney diseases.[327] The specific induction of CTGF expression by exogenous TGF-β in mesangial cells[256,328] and fibroblasts,[329] together with the finding that blocking antibodies to TGF-β inhibited increased CTGF expression in mesangial cells exposed to high-glucose concentrations,[328] suggests that CTGF may serve as a downstream mediator of the profibrotic effects of TGF-β.[330] Further experiments have shown that the fibrotic effects of TGF-β in the remnant kidney are mediated at least in part by induction of the microRNA miR-192 via Smad 3. In vitro overexpression of miR-192 promotes but inhibition of miR-192 attenuates TGF-β–induced production of collagen I in rat tubular cells.[331]

ANGIOTENSIN II

As discussed earlier, Ang II plays a central role in the glomerular hemodynamic adaptations observed after renal mass ablation. AT_1Rs are, however, distributed on many cell types within the kidney, including mesangial, glomerular epithelial, endothelial, tubular epithelial, and vascular smooth muscle cells, suggesting multiple potential actions of Ang II within the kidney.[332] Experimental studies have revealed several nonhemodynamic effects of Ang II that may be important in CKD progression (Figure 52.8). In isolated, perfused kidneys, infusion of Ang II results in loss of glomerular size permselectivity and proteinuria, an effect that has been attributed to both hemodynamic effects of Ang II resulting in elevations in P_{GC} and a direct effect of Ang II on glomerular permselectivity.[333] Furthermore, overexpression of AT_1Rs on podocytes resulted in albuminuria and FSGS in the absence of hypertension in transgenic rats.[334] In vitro Ang II has been shown to stimulate mesangial cell proliferation and induce expression of TGF-β, resulting in increased synthesis of ECM.[258] In vivo transfection of rat kidneys with human genes for renin and angiotensinogen resulted in glomerular ECM expansion within 7 days.[335] Ang II also stimulates production of PAI-1 by endothelial cells and vascular smooth muscle cells[336-338] and may therefore further increase accumulation of ECM through inhibition of ECM breakdown by matrix metalloproteinases (MMPs) that require conversion to an active form by plasmin. Other reports indicate that Ang II may directly induce the transcription of a variety of cell adhesion molecules and cytokines, as well as activating the transcription factor NF-κB[339-341] and directly stimulating monocyte activation.[342] Ang II infusion provoked upregulation of COX-2 expression in rats that was not dependent on blood pressure elevation,[343] and 5/6 nephrectomized rats evidenced Ang II–dependent upregulation of interstitial COX-2 expression.[344] In other experiments Ang II infusion has been shown to induce interstitial macrophage infiltration and increased expression of MCP-1 and TGF-β that were sustained for up to 6 days after cessation of the infusion.[345] Finally, Ang II may have fibrogenic effects via mineralocorticoids (see later). Interestingly, Ang II may also have antifibrotic effects via the angiotensin subtype 2 receptor (AT_2R). Ang II appears to upregulate AT_2R expression via an AT_2R-dependent mechanism after 5/6 nephrectomy, and treatment with an AT_2R antagonist exacerbated renal damage[346] and increased renal PAI-1 expression.[347] Furthermore, overexpression of AT_2R in transgenic mice was associated with reduced albuminuria as well as decreased glomerular expression of PDGF-BB chain and TGF-β after 5/6 nephrectomy.[348]

ALDOSTERONE

Observations that aldosterone stimulates collagen synthesis in the myocardium and that spironolactone treatment affords survival benefit in addition to that achieved with ACEI alone in heart failure patients[349] gave impetus to studies investigating the potential role of aldosterone in renal fibrosis. In the remnant kidney model, adrenal hypertrophy and markedly elevated plasma aldosterone levels have been reported. Furthermore, administration of exogenous aldosterone during inhibition of the RAAS with combination ACEI and ARB therapy in the 5/6 nephrectomy model negates the renal protective effects of the latter.[350] Further evidence of the role of aldosterone was provided by experiments in which rats subjected to adrenalectomy after 5/6 nephrectomy received replacement glucocorticoid but not mineralocorticoid therapy, resulting in less severe renal injury than in rats with intact adrenal glands.[351] Mechanisms whereby aldosterone may contribute to renal damage include the following: hemodynamic effects (see earlier); mesangial cell proliferation,[352] apoptosis,[353] hypertrophy, and transdifferentiation[354]; podocyte injury and apoptosis associated with reduced expression of nephrin and podocin, resulting in proteinuria[355-357]; proximal tubular cell transdifferentiation and increased production of collagen III and IV[358]; and increased renal production of reactive oxygen species (ROS),[355,357] PAI-1,[359,360] TGF-β,[361] and CTGF.[362,363] Early experimental use of aldosterone receptor blockers in 5/6 nephrectomized rats yielded only modest renoprotective effects,[350,364] but other studies have found significant amelioration of glomerulosclerosis in 5/6 nephrectomized rats treated with spironolactone, alone or in combination with triple antihypertensive therapy or an ARB.[359,365,366] In some rats spironolactone was associated with apparent regression of glomerulosclerosis. Furthermore, the observed renoprotection was associated with inhibition of PAI-1 mRNA expression in the renal cortex.[359] In another experiment renoprotection achieved with combination ACEI and spironolactone treatment was associated with abrogation of increase in mesangial cells and decrease in podocytes observed in untreated rats. Combination treatment also attenuated the increase in expression of collagen IV, TGF-β, and desmin.[365] Spironolactone has also been shown to ameliorate renal damage in other experimental models, including diabetic nephropathy,[362,367] Ren2 transgenic rats,[368] radiation nephritis,[369] and stroke-prone hypertension.[370] Several small clinical trials have reported additional reduction of proteinuria by 15% to 54%, blood pressure by approximately 40%, and GFR by approximately 25% when aldosterone receptor blockers were added to ACEI or ARB treatment,[371] but large randomized trials are required to fully assess the potential benefits of these treatments in CKD, and their use in CKD is currently limited by the associated risk for hyperkalemia.[372]

HEPATOCYTE GROWTH FACTOR

Investigations have shed light on the role of HGF as a potential antifibrotic factor in CKD. Initial studies focused on the property of HGF to ameliorate tubular cell injury in models of renal ischemia,[373,374] but studies in models of CKD suggest that HGF may also ameliorate CKD through its mitogenic, motogenic, morphogenic, and antiapoptotic actions.[375] As discussed earlier, HGF is upregulated in the remaining kidney after uninephrectomy and may play a role in compensatory renal hypertrophy.[122] Further studies have confirmed that HGF and its receptor, c-Met, are also upregulated in the remnant kidney after 5/6 nephrectomy.[376] Furthermore, blockade of HGF action with anti-HGF antibodies resulted in a more rapid decline in GFR and more severe renal fibrosis that was associated with increased ECM accumulation and a greater number of myofibroblasts in the interstitium and tubules. Other studies have identified multiple mechanisms whereby HGF may contribute to renoprotection, including the following: amelioration of podocyte injury and apoptosis as well as proteinuria[377]; increased apoptosis of myofibroblasts[378]; decreased ECM accumulation associated with increased expression of MMP-9 and decreased expression of endogenous inhibitors of MMPs, tissue inhibitor of metalloproteinase (TIMP)-1 and TIMP-2 in proximal tubular cell cultues[376]; disruption of NF-κB signaling in tubular cells[379,380] and suppression of TGF-β–induced CTGF expression in tubular cells.[381] Multiple experiments have confirmed the renoprotective effects of HGF. The renoprotective effects of ACEI and ARB treatment were associated with increased renal expression on HGF mRNA.[382] Treatment with anti-HGF antibodies resulted in increased TGF-β levels in a mouse model of chronic glomerulonephritis.[383] HGF treatment ameliorated the progression of chronic allograft nephropathy in a renal transplant model.[384] HGF blocked the TGF-β–induced transdifferentiation of tubular epithelial cells to myofibroblasts.[385] Exogenous HGF administration[385] or HGF overexpression[386] blocked myofibroblast activation and prevented interstitial fibrosis in the UUO model. HGF gene transfer into skeletal muscle ameliorated glomerulosclerosis and interstitial fibrosis after 5/6 nephrectomy.[387] HGF treatment suppressed CTGF expression and attenuated renal fibrosis after 5/6 nephrectomy.[388] In contrast, other studies have reported adverse renal effects associated with excess HGF exposure. Transgenic mice that overexpressed HGF developed progressive kidney disease characterized by tubular hypertrophy, glomerulosclerosis, and cyst formation,[389] and HGF administration resulted in more rapid deterioration of creatinine clearance as well as increased albuminuria in obese db diabetic mice.[390] Available evidence thus suggests that HGF may play a role in ameliorating CKD, but inappropriate or excessive exposure to HGF may have adverse renal effects.

BONE MORPHOGENETIC PROTEIN-7

Bone morphogenetic protein 7 (BMP-7), also termed osteogenic protein-1, is a bone morphogen involved in embryonic development and tissue repair. Preliminary evidence suggests that BMP-7 may also play a role in renal repair.

BMP-7 is downregulated after acute renal ischemia,[391] early in the course of experimental diabetes,[392] and after 5/6 nephrectomy.[393] Furthermore, administration of exogenous BMP-7 increased tubular regeneration after 5/6 nephrectomy,[393] attenuated interstitial inflammation and fibrosis after UUO,[394] and ameliorated glomerulosclerosis in rats with diabetic nephropathy.[395] In one model of diabetic nephropathy BMP-7 was noted to be most effective at inhibiting tubular inflammation and TIF.[396] In vitro experiments have identified several potential renoprotective effects attributable to BMP-7, including inhibition of proinflammatory cytokine as well as ET expression in tubular cells exposed to TNF-α,[397] reversal of renal tubular epithelial to mesenchymal cell transdifferentiation,[398] antagonism of the fibrogenic effects of TGF-β in mesangial cells,[399] and protection from injury in podocytes exposed to high levels of glucose.[400] The renoprotective effect is further illustrated by the observation that expression of a transgene for BMP-7 in podocytes and proximal renal tubular cells was associated with prevention of podocyte dropout as well as amelioration of albuminuria, glomerulosclerosis, and interstitial fibrosis after induction of diabetes.[401] Further studies evaluating the effects of chronic treatment with BMP-7 or small molecule BMP-7 agonists are still awaited.

MicroRNAs

Attention has focused on the potential role of microRNAs (miRNAs) in promoting renal fibrosis. These are small, noncoding RNAs that have been shown to have important post-transcriptional gene regulatory function. MiRNAs miR-21 and miR-214 have been shown to be upregulated in several experimental models of CKD,[402,403] and miR-21 has been reported to be upregulated in human transplant kidneys with nephropathy.[402] Deletion of miR-21 or treatment with anti–miR-21 oligonucleotides were each associated with amelioration of interstitial fibrosis in animal models.[402] Similarly, deletion of miR-214 and treatment with anti–miR-214 were each associated with attenuation of interstitial fibrosis in the UUO model. Importantly, the effects of miR-214 appear to be independent of TGF-β signaling, and TGF-β blockade had additive antifibrotic effects with miR-214 deletion.[404]

OXIDATIVE STRESS

CKD is associated with increased oxidative stress that likely contributes to the progression of renal damage as well as the pathogenesis of the associated cardiovascular disease.[405] Superoxide is the primary ROS that accounts for oxidative stress. Its major source is production by nicotinamide adenine dinucleotide phosphate-oxidase (NADPH-oxidase), and it is removed (by conversion to hydrogen peroxide) by superoxide dismutase (SOD). Following 5/6 nephrectomy, significant upregulation of NADPH-oxidase and downregulation of SOD were observed in the liver and kidneys, indicating that the increase in superoxide is due to a combination of increased production and decreased removal.[406] Blood pressure was elevated, and nitrotyrosine levels were increased, whereas urine NO metabolites were decreased, observations consistent with increased NO inactivation by superoxide. The effects of increased levels of ROS are further compounded by reduced abundance and activity of antioxidant enzymes (catalase, glutathione peroxidase, glutathione),[407] as well as reduced levels of high-density lipoprotein, apolipoprotein A-I, and thiols.[408] Adverse consequences of oxidative stress that may contribute to CKD progression include hypertension (due to inactivation of NO and oxidation of arachidonic acid to generate vasoconstrictive isoprostanes),[409] inflammation (due to activation of NF-κB),[407] fibrosis, and apoptosis,[408] as well as glomerular filtration barrier damage.[410] Inflammation may in turn increase oxidative stress due to generation of ROS by activated leukocytes, thus establishing a vicious cycle of oxidative stress and inflammation.[405] Other factors that may contribute to increased ROS production in CKD include Ang II,[411] reduced production of NO,[67] and hypertension.[412] The importance of ROS in the progression of CKD has been shown by experiments in which antioxidant therapies, including melatonin,[413] niacin,[414] and ω-3 fatty acids,[415] have reduced oxidative stress and ameliorated renal damage in the 5/6 nephrectomy model. On the other hand, treatment with tempol, a SOD-mimetic, reduced plasma malondialdehyde levels and the number of superoxide-positive cells but did not reduce overall renal oxidative stress, inflammation, or renal damage.[416]

ACIDOSIS

As GFR declines, the ability of kidneys to excrete hydrogen ions becomes impaired, and a new steady state is achieved that allows excretion of acid at the cost of a persistent metabolic acidosis (see "Acid-Base Regulation" section). Acidosis is present in the majority of patients when GFR falls below 20% to 25% of normal.[417] Chronic metabolic acidosis has multiple adverse consequences, including increased protein catabolism, increased bone turnover, induction of inflammatory mediators, insulin resistance, and increased production of corticosteroids as well as PTH.[417,418] These observations make it reasonable to consider whether acidosis may also contribute to progressive renal damage in CKD. Early experiments found no persisting renal damage after dietary acid loading in rats with normal renal function and no renoprotection associated with sodium bicarbonate treatment in the 5/6 nephrectomy model, suggesting that acidosis did not initiate or exacerbate renal damage.[419] Later experiments, however, found that an acid-generating diet of casein protein induced tubulointerstitial injury in rats with normal renal function, whereas a non–acid-inducing diet of soy protein did not. Furthermore, dietary acid supplementation with ammonium sulfate ($[NH_4]_2SO_4$) in soy protein–fed rats was associated with tubulointerstitial injury.[420] Similarly in the 5/6 nephrectomy model, a casein-rich diet was associated with metabolic acidosis and a progressive decline in GFR and increasing albuminuria, whereas a soy protein diet was not. Dietary acid supplementation with $(NH_4)_2SO_4$ in soy protein–fed rats provoked a decline in GFR and albuminuria. Treatment with sodium bicarbonate or calcium bicarbonate ($Ca[HCO_3]_2$) but not sodium chloride was renoprotective in the casein-fed rats but only if the resultant hypertension (in sodium bicarbonate- but not $Ca[HCO_3]_2$-treated rats) was adequately treated.[421] Furthermore, when rats were subject to 2/3 rather than 5/6 nephrectomy, a level of renal mass reduction not associated with metabolic acidosis, microdialysis identified tissue acid accumulation in muscle and kidney that correlated with subsequent GFR decline. Amelioration of tissue acid accumulation by low acid–generating diet or alkali supplementation was associated with abrogation of GFR decline, whereas dietary acid supplementation was associated with exacerbation of GFR decline.[422] Treatment with calcium citrate has also been shown to improve acidosis and reduce glomerular as well as interstitial injury in the 5/6 nephrectomy model.[423] Mechanisms whereby acidosis may contribute to renal damage after nephron loss include activation of the alternative complement pathway by increased ammoniagenesis,[424] increased plasma and kidney Ang II,[425] and induction of ET as well as aldosterone production.[426] Observational clinical studies have identified acidosis as an independent risk factor for CKD progression,[427,428] but to date only small studies have investigated the renoprotective potential of alkali supplementation in human subjects. In the first randomized study in adults with creatinine clearance of 15 to 30 mL/min/1.73 m^2, randomization to treatment of acidosis (serum bicarbonate 16 to 20 mmol/L) with sodium bicarbonate was associated with less decline in creatinine clearance (1.88 versus 5.93 mL/min/1.73 m^2) and lower incidence of ESKD (6.5% versus 33%). The authors concede, however, that the study was not blinded or placebo controlled.[429] In a second nonrandomized study, treatment of 30 subjects with sodium citrate was associated with reduced urinary excretion of ET-1 and N-acetyl- β-D-glucosaminidase (a marker of tubulointerstitial injury), as well as a lower rate of estimated GFR decline, than observed in 29 untreated controls who were unwilling or unable to take sodium citrate.[430] One study has reported renoprotective effects following sodium bicarbonate treatment in early CKD. In a randomized, placebo-controlled trial in subjects with a mean estimated GFR of 75 mL/min/1.73 m^2, treatment with sodium bicarbonate for 5 years was associated with a slower reduction in estimated GFR (derived from plasma cystatin C measurements) than placebo or treatment with sodium chloride.[431] Further studies have reported that correction of acidosis with a diet rich in fruits and vegetables was as effective in ameliorating kidney damage in early (CKD stage 1 to 2)[432] and more advanced (CKD stage 4) disease.[433] In one trial, people with CKD stage 3 and serum bicarbonate level of 22 to 24 mmol/L were randomized to oral bicarbonate supplementation, diet rich in fruits and vegetables, or "usual care." All participants received treatment with RAAS inhibitor (RAASi), and SBP was controlled to less than 130 mm Hg. Both interventions achieved an increase in serum bicarbonate level and were associated with a decrease in urinary angiotensinogen level. After 3 years, both interventions were associated with less albuminuria and GFR decline than the "usual care" group.[434] Bicarbonate supplementation is already recommended for patients with levels below 22 mEq/L, but further studies are required to further investigate whether it is beneficial in the setting of less severe acidosis.[435]

HYPERTROPHY

The consistent observation of renal and in particular glomerular hypertrophy after renal mass reduction has prompted investigators to propose that processes involved in or resulting from hypertrophy may contribute to progressive renal injury in CKD.[436] The well-documented observation that renal and glomerular hypertrophy precede the development of diabetic nephropathy and the finding of a positive association between glomerular size and early sclerosis in rats subjected to renal mass ablation[437] further suggests that hypertrophy may play a direct role in pathogenesis of glomerulosclerosis. Several clinical observations also support an association between glomerular hypertrophy and renal injury. Oligomeganephronia, a rare congenital condition with a nephron number 25% of normal or less, is characterized by marked hypertrophy of the remaining glomeruli and development of proteinuria and renal failure in adolescence, with FSGS as the typical renal biopsy finding.[438] In children with minimal change disease, a glomerulopathy generally associated with spontaneous remission and lack of progression to renal failure, investigators noted an association between glomerular size and the risk for developing FSGS and renal failure.[439]

Several interventions have been employed in experiments to interrupt the development of glomerular hypertrophy after renal mass reduction and thereby assess its role in kidney disease progression but have produced contradictory results. Rats subjected to 5/6 nephrectomy were compared to rats in which two thirds of the left kidney was infarcted and the right ureter drained into the peritoneal cavity (an intervention that apparently results in decreased renal clearance without compensatory renal hypertrophy). Micropuncture studies confirmed similar degrees of elevation of P_{GC} and SNGFR in both models. At 4 weeks, however, the maximal planar area of the glomerulus was significantly less and glomerular injury, as assessed by sclerosis index, significantly reduced in ureteroperitoneostomized rats versus 5/6 nephrectomized controls. Accordingly, the authors concluded that glomerular hypertrophy was more important than glomerular capillary hypertension in the progression of glomerular injury in this model.[436] Dietary sodium restriction has also been utilized to inhibit renal hypertrophy after 5/6 nephrectomy. Although sodium restriction had no effect on glomerular hemodynamics, V_G was significantly reduced in 5/6 nephrectomized rats fed low- versus normal-sodium diets. Moreover, urinary protein excretion was lower and glomerulosclerosis was less severe in rats on restricted sodium intake.[100] These findings were extended by another study in which the effect of sodium restriction in preventing glomerular hypertrophy and ameliorating glomerular injury was confirmed, but which also found that these benefits were overcome by administration of an androgen that stimulated glomerular hypertrophy despite sodium restriction. Glomerular hemodynamics were similar among the groups.[440] On the other hand, treatment with seliciclib, a cyclin-dependent kinase inhibitor, reduced renal hypertrophy by 45% after 5/6 nephrectomy but had no effect on kidney damage.[441]

Glomerular hypertrophy may contribute to glomerulosclerosis through a number of different mechanisms. According to Laplace's law, the increase in V_G could result in an increase in capillary wall tension only if the capillary wall diameter was also increased (Figure 52.9). Cyclic stretch would then exert stress capable of damaging epithelial, mesangial, and endothelial cells as described earlier. Alternatively, glomerulosclerosis may be viewed as a maladaptive growth response following loss of renal mass and resulting in excessive mesangial proliferation and ECM production.[436] The identification of TGF-β as a key mediator of renal hypertrophy as well as an important promoter of renal fibrosis provides an obvious link between renal hypertrophy and fibrosis.[129]

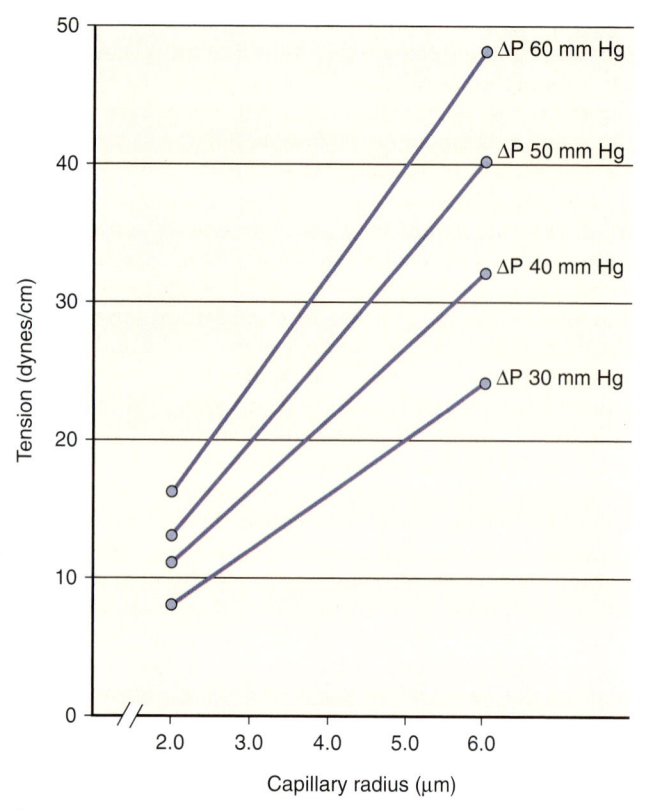

Figure 52.9 Illustration of the synergistic effects of changes in transcapillary hydrostatic pressure difference (ΔP; mm Hg) and mean glomerular capillary radius (μm) on the calculated capillary wall tension (dynes/cm). (Reproduced with permission from Bidani AK et al. Absence of progressive glomerular injury in a normotensive rat remnant kidney model. *Kidney Int* 38:28-38, 1990.)

PROTEINURIA

Abnormal excretion of protein in the urine is the hallmark of experimental and clinical glomerular disease. Whereas immune complex deposition and resulting inflammation account for abnormal permeability of the glomerular filtration barrier to proteins in glomerulonephritis, studies in rats subjected to extensive renal ablation have shown loss of glomerular barrier function to proteins of similar molecular size, yet in the apparent absence of primary immune-mediated renal injury or inflammatory response. Sieving studies using dextrans and other macromolecules in rats 7 or 14 days after 5/6 nephrectomy revealed loss of both size- and charge-selectivity of the glomerular filtration barrier. Ultrastructural examination of the remnant kidneys revealed detachment of glomerular endothelial cells and visceral epithelial cells from the glomerular basement membrane. In addition, protein reabsorption droplets and attenuation of cytoplasm resulting in bleb formation was observed in podocytes. The authors concluded that the altered permselectivity may be due in part to separation of endothelial cells from the glomerular basement membrane, allowing access of macromolecules, and in part to loss of anionic sites in the lamina rara externa, resulting in both loss of charge selectivity and detachment of podocytes.[442] Studies have identified decreased nephrin expression in podocytes as a further mechanism contributing to proteinuria after 5/6 nephrectomy,[443] and in vitro studies have reported a 50% reduction in nephrin expression when podocytes were exposed to cyclical stretching.[280] A direct role for Ang II in modulating glomerular capillary permselectivity is suggested by the observation of marked increases in urinary protein excretion during infusion of Ang II in normal rats. While some investigators have attributed this to a direct effect of Ang II on the cellular components of the glomerular filtration barrier, resulting in opening of interendothelial junctions and epithelial cell disruption, others have shown that the increase in proteinuria may be accounted for almost completely by the associated hemodynamic changes, principally a reduction in Q_A and an increase in filtration fraction.[444] On the other hand, the notion that Ang II may mediate changes in glomerular permselectivity independent of its effects on glomerular hemodynamics is supported by studies in an isolated perfused rat kidney preparation in which infusion of Ang II augmented urinary protein excretion and enhanced the clearance of tracer macromolecules independent of any change in filtration fraction.[333] Furthermore, Ang II and aldosterone have been shown to reduce nephrin expression in podocytes and may therefore directly affect glomerular permselectivity.[280,357,445]

Proteinuria, long considered simply a marker of glomerular injury, has also been implicated as an effector of injury processes involved in kidney disease progression, especially those resulting in TIF.[446] In rats with aminonucleoside-induced nephrotic syndrome, the proteinuric phase of the disease was associated with an acute interstitial nephritis, the intensity of which correlated closely with the severity of the proteinuria.[291] Furthermore, in an overload proteinuria model induced by daily intraperitoneal administration of bovine serum albumin to uninephrectomized rats, proximal tubular cell injury and interstitial infiltration of macrophages and lymphocytes were evident after 1 week.[447] The severity of the proteinuria showed a positive correlation with the intensity of the infiltrate. At 4 weeks, focal areas of chronic interstitial inflammation were noted.[447] Other experiments have identified mast cells as a component of the inflammatory infiltrate observed after protein overload. The number of mast cells correlated with the severity of interstitial inflammation as well as with levels of stem cell factor and TGF-β.[448] A causative association between excessive proteinuria and interstitial inflammation has been suggested by in vitro studies of proximal tubule epithelial cells cultured in media supplemented with high concentrations of albumin, immunoglobulin (Ig) G, or transferrin. Cellular uptake of these proteins by endocytosis was observed to increase secretion of ET-1,[449] MCP-1,[450] RANTES,[451] IL-8,[452] and fractaline.[453] Electrophoretic mobility shift assay of cell nucleus extracts revealed intense activation of the transcription factor NF-κB that was dependent on the concentration of protein in the medium.[451] Furthermore, the liberation of these molecules was noted to be predominantly from the basolateral aspect of the cells. This would be in keeping with secretion into the renal interstitium in vivo, thereby contributing to the development of tubulointerstitial inflammation and fibrosis. On the other hand, secretion of TGF-β by tubular cells in response to albumin was not inhibited by inhibitors of endocytosis, implying that a different mechanism must be responsible.[454] Exposure of tubular cells to albumin has also been shown to result in increased levels of intracellular ROS and activation of the signal transducer and activator of transcription (STAT) signaling pathway.[455] The STAT pathway in turn mediates a variety of cellular responses, including proliferation and induction of cytokines as well as growth factors. Preliminary evidence suggests that exposure of tubular cells to albumin may also induce apoptosis.[456] Other experiments have found apoptosis in tubular cells exposed to high-molecular-weight plasma proteins but not smaller proteins.[457] Albumin and transferrin exposure also induced complement activation in tubular cells and reduced binding of factor H, a natural inhibitor of the alternative complement pathway.[458] The involvement of immune cells in the processing of absorbed proteins has been shown in studies in which tubular cells were found to cleave albumin into an N-terminal 24–amino acid peptide that was further processed by dendritic cells into antigenic peptides with binding sites for major histocompatibility complex (MHC) class I molecules that were capable of activating $CD8^+$ T cells. After 5/6 nephrectomy dendritic cells were found in the interstitium, peaking at 1 week and decreasing at 4 weeks, coinciding with their appearance in renal lymph nodes. Dendritic cells from the lymph nodes were able to activate $CD8^+$ T cells in culture.[459]

Despite this evidence, other investigators have raised concerns regarding the interpretation of these observations.[460] They point out that the concentrations of plasma proteins used in vitro were nonphysiologic and far exceeded those observed in proximal tubule fluid from experimental models of nephrotic syndrome. Furthermore, many of the experiments were performed in cells that were routinely cultured in the presence of high concentrations of protein (serum) that may significantly alter their phenotype. Not all investigators have been able to confirm the observations described earlier. In particular, some have found proliferative or profibrotic responses when proximal tubular cells are exposed to serum or serum fractions, but no response after exposure to purified forms of albumin or transferrin, suggesting that factors other than albumin or transferrin may be involved.[461,462] Furthermore, experiments in mice with tubules deficient in megalin, the key molecule responsible for the endocytosis of filtered proteins by tubular cells, have reported that tubulointerstitial inflammation was not inhibited in the absence of megalin, implying that it was not dependent on endocytosis.[463] They propose instead that tubulointerstitial inflammation is provoked by misdirection of protein-rich glomerular filtrate into the interstitium due to formation of adhesions between the glomerular tuft and Bowman's capsule or, in the case of crescentic glomerulonephritis, encroachment of the crescent onto the proximal tubule, resulting in occlusion and tubule degeneration.[464] Moreover, they propose that the increase in cytokine and adhesion molecule production observed in tubular cells that have endocytosed excess protein may in fact be a protective response.[463]

Several lines of evidence suggest that filtered molecules other than albumin or immunoglobulin may play a role in the progression of chronic nephropathies. It has been proposed that free fatty acids (FFAs) bound to albumin may play an important role provoking a proinflammatory response in tubular cells. In one experiment albumin-bound fatty acids stimulated macrophage chemotactic activity whereas delipidated albumin did not.[465] Albumin-bound FFA has also been shown to activate PPARγ and induce apoptosis in proximal tubular cells.[466] High-density lipoprotein (HDL) and low-density lipoprotein (LDL) have been identified in the urine, renal interstitium, and tubular cells in renal biopsies of patients with nephrotic syndrome. In vitro, cultured human proximal tubule epithelial cells take up LDL and HDL.[467] Oxidized LDL may cause tubular cell injury and exposure of tubular epithelial cells to HDL is associated with increased synthesis of ET-1.[467,468] A role has also been proposed for other compounds bound to filtered proteins such as IGF-1, which has been detected in increased amounts in the proximal tubule fluid of rats with doxorubicin (Adriamycin) nephrosis. Proximal tubular cells cultured in the presence of proximal tubule fluid from nephrotic rats exhibit enhanced cell proliferation and increased secretion of collagen I and IV. Both effects were inhibited by neutralizing IGF-1 receptor antibodies.[469] Other growth factors in plasma, including HGF and TGF-β, may also appear in glomerular ultrafiltrate with proteinuria and exert effects on tubular cells.[470] Furthermore, cytokines produced in injured glomeruli may have downstream proinflammatory effects. Whereas complement components are normally absent from tubule fluid, C3 and C5b-9 neoantigen were observed along the luminal border of tubular epithelial cells in the protein-overload proteinuria model. To examine the role of filtered complement in renal injury, rats with puromycin aminonucleoside nephrosis were subjected to complement depletion with cobra venom factor or inhibition of complement activation by administration of soluble recombinant human complement receptor type 1, before the onset of proteinuria. In control rats, proximal tubular degeneration, interstitial leukocyte infiltrate, and renal impairment (as assessed by inulin and p-aminohippurate clearances) occurred at 7 days, together with positive staining for C3 and C5b-9 along the proximal tubule brush border. Both interventions were associated with significantly less tubulointerstitial pathologic processes and greater clearance of p-aminohippurate but not inulin, whereas the severity of the proteinuria was unaffected, suggesting that filtered complement plays a significant role in the tubulointerstitial injury associated with proteinuria.[471] A more selective approach, using recombinant complement inhibitory molecules targeted to proximal tubular cells with carrier antibodies to brush border antigen resulted in significant reduction of interstitial fibrosis in the same model.[472] Similarly, mice with C3 deficiency were protected against interstitial inflammation after protein overload, and wild-type kidneys transplanted into C3-deficient mice were protected, whereas kidneys from C3-deficient mice were not protected when transplanted into wild-type mice, implying that filtered rather than locally synthesized C3 is important in the pathogenesis of interstitial inflammation associated with proteinuria.[473]

In experimental models of proteinuric renal disease, filtered proteins have also been found to accumulate in the glomerular mesangium[442] and may therefore contribute to glomerular as well as tubulointerstitial injury. Further support for this notion is derived from a meta-analysis of 57 studies of experimental CKD that found a consistent positive correlation between the severity of proteinuria and the extent of glomerulosclerosis.[474] Lipoproteins, in particular, accumulate in the glomeruli of patients with glomerulonephritis.[475,476] Furthermore, LDL stimulates mesangial cells to proliferate in vitro[477,478] and enhances mesangial cell synthesis of the ECM protein fibronectin.[479] LDL exposure is also associated with increased mesangial cell mRNA levels for MCP-1[479] and PDGF.[478] Oxidation of LDL by mesangial cells or macrophages may enhance its toxicity.[477] Thus accumulation of proteins in the mesangium may stimulate a number of different mechanisms that contribute to glomerulosclerosis.

The relevance of these findings to the processes occurring in vivo has been borne out by studies in rats. In the protein-overload model the development of proteinuria at 1 week was associated with significant increases in TGF-β at both protein and mRNA levels, in interstitial as well as proximal tubular cells.[447] Similarly, renal cortical mRNA levels encoding the macrophage chemoattractant, osteopontin, were increased on day 4, and immunofluorescence localized increased osteopontin staining to cortical tubules at day 7. MCP-1 and osteopontin mRNA and protein levels were elevated at 2 and 3 weeks. Furthermore, a significant effect of proteinuria on molecules involved in ECM protein turnover was observed. Although mRNA levels for various renal matrix proteins were variable, staining for the proteins in the cortical interstitium increased progressively. Levels of mRNA for the protease inhibitors PAI-1 and TIMP-1 were elevated at 2 weeks, at which time significant renal fibrosis was present.[447] Gene expression profiling has identified over 100 genes that are upregulated in the proximal tubular cells of mice exposed to overload proteinuria.[480] Consistent with the hypothesis that protein-bound FFAs are important, rats receiving FFA-replete bovine serum albumin developed more severe tubulointerstitial injury and more extensive macrophage infiltration than those receiving FFA-depleted bovine serum albumin.[481,482] In other models of proteinuric renal disease, including 5/6 nephrectomy and passive Heymann's nephritis, accumulation of albumin and IgG by proximal tubular cells occurred before infiltration of the interstitium by macrophages and MHC-II positive mononuclear cells. The infiltrates localized to areas where proximal tubular cells stained positive for intracellular IgG, or where luminal casts were present. Furthermore, proximal tubular cells that stained positive for IgG also showed evidence of increased osteopontin production.[483] The IgG staining in proximal tubular cells was subsequently associated with peritubular accumulation of macrophages and α-smooth muscle actin–positive cells as well as upregulation of TGF-β mRNA in the tubular and infiltrating cells.[484] The importance of inflammatory factors in the development of interstitial fibrosis is illustrated by the observation that treatment of rats with experimental membranous nephropathy with rapamycin was associated with reduced expression of profibrotic and proinflammatory genes as well as amelioration of interstitial inflammation and fibrosis.[485] Further studies in the 5/6 nephrectomy model have suggested that tubulointerstitial injury may play an important role in the decline of GFR, especially in the late stages of progressive renal injury.[486] By examining serial sections of remnant kidneys, the investigators were able to show that in association with a doubling in serum creatinine level, there was a substantial increase in the proportion of glomeruli no longer connected to glomeruli (atubular glomeruli) or connected to atrophic tubules. The majority of these glomeruli were not globally sclerosed, implying that the tubular injury was responsible for the final loss of function in these nephrons. The authors speculate that the absorption of excess filtered protein may play an important role in this tubular injury.[486] Finally, evidence is accumulating for the role of proteinuria in the development of interstitial damage in human CKD. Among 215 patients with CKD, urine albumin to creatinine ratio (ACR) correlated with urinary MCP-1 levels and interstitial macrophage numbers. Furthermore, urine ACR and interstitial macrophage number independently predicted renal survival.[487]

Establishing a cause-and-effect relationship between proteinuria and kidney damage in humans is difficult, but several clinical studies provide evidence in support of this notion. A meta-analysis of 17 clinical studies of CKD revealed a positive correlation between the severity of proteinuria and the extent of biopsy-proven glomerulosclerosis,[474] and data from a meta-analysis that included over 1 million participants identified albuminuria as a strong independent risk factor of progression to ESKD.[488] Observations from the Modification of Diet in Renal Disease (MDRD) trial also suggest that proteinuria is an independent determinant of CKD progression. Greater levels of baseline proteinuria were strongly associated with more rapid declines in GFR; reduction of proteinuria, independent of reduction in blood pressure, was associated with lesser rates of decline in GFR. Furthermore, the degree of benefit achieved by lowering blood pressure below usual target levels was highly dependent on the level of baseline proteinuria.[489] The severity of proteinuria at baseline has been shown to be the most important independent predictor of renal outcomes in randomized trials of ACEI or ARB treatment in diabetic nephropathy[490] and nondiabetic CKD.[233] Furthermore, the percentage reduction in proteinuria over the first 3 to 6 months and the absolute level of proteinuria at 3 or 6 months are strong independent predictors of the subsequent rate of decline in GFR among patients with diabetic nephropathy[490] and nondiabetic CKD.[491] A meta-analysis that included data from 1860 patients with nondiabetic CKD confirmed these findings and showed that during antihypertensive treatment the current level of proteinuria was a powerful predictor of the combined end point of doubling of baseline serum creatinine level or onset of ESKD (relative risk [RR], 5.56 for each 1.0 g/day protein level).[492] Similarly a meta-analysis of 21 randomized trials of drug treatment in CKD that included 78,342 participants found that for each 30% initial reduction in albuminuria on treatment, the risk for ESKD decreased by 23.7% (95% confidence interval [CI], 11.4% to 34.2%), independent of the class of drug used for treatment.[493] The Renoprotection of Optimal Antiproteinuric Doses (ROAD) study has provided the most direct evidence of the clinical benefit of proteinuria reduction to date. Subjects with proteinuric CKD were randomized to standard therapy with an ACEI or ARB (separate groups) or to ACEI or ARB therapy titrated to the maximum antiproteinuric dose (two further groups). Despite comparable blood pressure control, subjects in the groups randomized to maximum antiproteinuric doses evidenced 51% and 53% relative risk reductions in the combined primary end point of creatinine level doubling, ESKD, or death.[494] Taken together, the evidence from experimental and clinical studies provides support for the hypothesis that impaired glomerular permselectivity results in excessive filtration of proteins and/or protein-bound molecules that contribute to kidney damage, but many questions regarding the tubulotoxic potential of filtered plasma proteins and the identity of the specific molecules involved remain unanswered. Despite these uncertainties, the close association between the severity of proteinuria and renal prognosis implies that reduction of proteinuria should be regarded as an important independent therapeutic goal in clinical strategies seeking to slow the rate of progression of CKD. The mechanisms and consequences of proteinuria are discussed further in Chapter 53.

TUBULOINTERSTITIAL FIBROSIS

Together with secondary FSGS, TIF constitutes a major component of the progressive renal injury observed in CKD. Several of the mechanisms that are proposed to initiate TIF have been discussed earlier, but here we review briefly the downstream mechanisms of fibrosis. TIF is characterized by inflammatory cell and fibroblast infiltration, accumulation of ECM, tubular cell loss, and rarefaction of peritubular capillaries. Fibrogenesis starts at small sites of inflammation and then expands if a profibrotic milieu persists. The inflammatory infiltrate is composed of lymphocytes, macrophages, dendritic cells, and mast cells.[495] Lymphocytes are recruited early in the process, and their importance is highlighted by the protection from fibrosis observed in *Rag2* null mice, which lack B and T lymphocytes.[496] Monocytes are recruited and transdifferentiate into macrophages. The profibrotic role of macrophages is illustrated by observations that the extent of macrophage accumulation correlates closely with the severity of fibrosis,[497] and macrophage depletion attenuates fibrosis.[498] Nevertheless it has been proposed that alternatively activated M2 macrophages exert antiinflammatory actions, and infusion of cells enriched for M2 macrophages has been shown to reduce renal fibrosis in mice.[499] Myofibroblasts are the chief source of ECM production, and the accumulation of interstitial myofibroblasts is central to the pathogenesis of TIF. There is considerable ongoing controversy regarding the cellular origins of interstitial myofibroblasts in TIF. Different investigators have identified resident fibroblasts,[500] transdifferentiation from tubular epithelial cells and endothelial cells,[501,502] bone marrow–derived fibrocytes,[503] and pericytes[296] as possible sources.[298] Fate mapping studies have indicated that pericytes are the predominant source of myofibroblasts and that epithelial to mesenchymal transdifferentiation is not a source of myofibroblasts or accounts for only a small minority.[296] The excessive ECM is composed largely of collagen I and II as well as fibronectin. Matrix accumulation is proposed to commence with the appearance of collagen nucleators in the interstitial fluid that act as a scaffold for the deposition of fibrillar collagens. Fibroblasts use collagen fibrils as a scaffold to move through damaged tissue along chemoattractant gradients. Fibrogenesis is promoted by the expression of key growth factors, principally TGF-β.[504] The role of tissue proteases in TIF is complex and has not been fully characterized. Whereas MMP-2 and MMP-9 degrade collagen IV (and possibly collagen I and III) in vitro, they do not consistently abrogate TIF in vivo.[505,506] Indeed, in some models MMPs appear to exert profibrotic effects.[506] Rarefaction of peritubular capillaries is a hallmark of TIF. In the early stages, capillaries may be damaged by transient ischemia that promotes apoptosis.[507] Further capillary loss is attributable to an imbalance between proangiogenic and antiangiogenic factors[508,509] or loss of peritubular endothelial cells through endothelial-mesenchymal transdifferentiation.[501] Tissue hypoxia results from rarefaction of peritubular capillaries, as well as accumulation of ECM, requiring oxygen to diffuse over greater distances to reach cells. Hypoxia contributes to TIF by promoting EMT and apoptosis of tubular cells as well as fibroblast activation and ECM production.[510,511] The importance of hypoxia in provoking interstitial (and glomerular) injury has been demonstrated by studies in which induction of hypoxia-inducible factor, a key mediator of protective responses to hypoxia, was associated with amelioration of proteinuria, glomerulosclerosis, and TIF as well as decreased macrophage infiltration, expression of collagen IV, and osteopontin.[512,513] Tubulointerstitial inflammation and fibrosis are discussed in more detail in Chapter 36.

A UNIFIED HYPOTHESIS OF CHRONIC KIDNEY DISEASE PROGRESSION

In the past there has tended to be a dichotomy of viewpoints regarding the relative importance of hemodynamic and nonhemodynamic factors in the pathogenesis of glomerulosclerosis and TIF after nephron loss.[436,514] Proponents of the "hypertrophy hypothesis" pointed out that in some experiments a disassociation between glomerular hemodynamic changes and glomerulosclerosis has been observed and that in one study, antihypertensive therapy was renoprotective without lowering P_{GC}.[436] On the other hand, those favoring the "hemodynamic hypothesis" noted that treatment with an ACEI[18] or ARB[20] in 5/6 nephrectomized rats resulted in renoprotection without preventing renal or glomerular hypertrophy and that many of the studies purporting to show a positive association between glomerular hypertrophy and sclerosis failed to report glomerular hemodynamic data. Furthermore, rats subjected to ureteroperitoneostomy developed significantly more glomerulosclerosis than sham-operated controls despite a lack of increase in glomerular size.[514] Several other observations suggest that hemodynamic factors override the potential role of hypertrophy in progressive renal damage. The renoprotection achieved after 5/6 nephrectomy by a low-protein diet (associated with prevention of glomerular hypertrophy) can be reversed by treatment with calcium channel blockers that inhibit renal autoregulation but have no effect on glomerular size.[515] Comparison of rats subjected to 5/6 nephrectomy by excision versus infarction of two-thirds of the remaining kidney shows similar increases in V_G, but the infarction model is associated with more severe glomerular hypertension and glomerulosclerosis.[8] Despite these apparently conflicting views, it is clear from the earlier discussion that hemodynamic and nonhemodynamic mechanisms often overlap. For example, Ang II, a key mediator of glomerular hemodynamic adaptations after nephron loss, also exerts multiple nonhemodynamic deleterious effects. Furthermore, the inflammatory and profibrotic mechanisms that eventuate in glomerulosclerosis and TIF may be provoked by both hemodynamic and nonhemodynamic stimuli. A growing appreciation of the complexity of the multiple adaptations that follow nephron loss has facilitated the

Figure 52.10 Schema illustrating the hypothesized interaction of multiple hemodynamic and nonhemodynamic factors in the pathogenesis of progressive nephron injury in chronic kidney disease. Ang II, Angiotensin II.

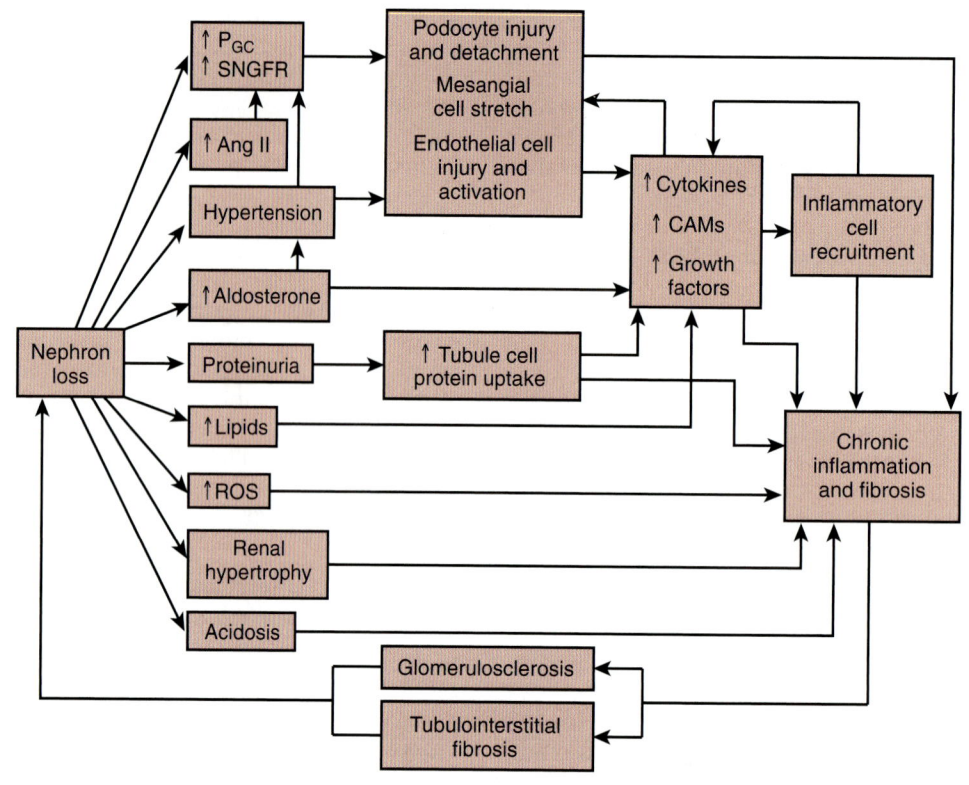

P_{GC} – glomerular capillary hydraulic pressure
SNGFR – single nephron GFR
CAMs – cell adhesion molecules
ROS – reactive oxygen species

development of a consensus view that continues to regard raised glomerular capillary pressure as a central factor in initiating glomerulosclerosis but also acknowledges that other nonhemodynamic pathogenetic mechanisms may act in concert with hemodynamic factors in a complex interplay that eventuates in a vicious cycle of progressive renal damage (Figure 52.10).

INSIGHTS FROM MODIFIERS OF CHRONIC KIDNEY DISEASE PROGRESSION

PHARMACOLOGIC INHIBITION OF THE RENIN ANGIOTENSIN ALDOSTERONE SYSTEM

Experimental evidence showing a central role for Ang II in mechanisms of CKD progression through hemodynamic and nonhemodynamic effects has been borne out in randomized clinical trials of ACEI and ARB treatment in patients with all forms of CKD. ACEI treatment has been shown to be renoprotective in patients with microalbuminuria and type 2 diabetes mellitus,[516] type 1 diabetes and overt nephropathy,[232] and nondiabetic CKD.[233,236,517,518] Treatment with an ARB affords renoprotection in patients with type 2 diabetes and microalbuminuria[519] or overt nephropathy.[234,235] Evidence is also accumulating that ARB treatment at doses higher than the maximum antihypertensive dose may afford additional renoprotection.[520,521] More complete inhibition of the RAAS with combination ACEI and ARB treatment was associated with additional lowering of proteinuria in several small clinical studies.[522] However, the largest randomized study of combination ACEI and ARB treatment versus monotherapy in CKD was unfortunately withdrawn due to serious concerns regarding the integrity of the data.[523] A large trial of combination therapy in patients with hypertension and increased cardiovascular risk reported no additional benefit with respect to cardiovascular outcomes, but combination therapy was associated with greater reductions in proteinuria than monotherapy. However, the trial reported an increase in the combined end point of creatinine level doubling, ESKD, or death with combination therapy, indicating that combination ACEI and ARB therapy may be associated with adverse outcomes in some patient groups.[524] It should be noted, however, that subjects were selected on the basis of cardiovascular risk profile and that the majority did not have reduced GFR or proteinuria. A similar study in 1448 people with type 2 diabetes and urine ACR of 300 mg/g or higher also found no benefit with respect to the primary outcome of CKD progression, ESKD, or death in participants randomized to combination ACEI and ARB therapy versus monotherapy, but those receiving combination therapy evidenced a significantly higher incidence of acute kidney injury (AKI) and hyperkalemia.[525] Thus in two large randomized trials, combination ACEI and ARB therapy did not confer additional benefit and was associated with increased risk for adverse effects. Combination therapy should therefore not be used in the patient groups included in these studies. Further studies are required to assess the risks versus benefits of combination therapy in people with proteinuric, nondiabetic CKD. The development of direct renin inhibitors (DRIs) made it possible to inhibit the RAAS at its rate-limiting step (the conversion of angiotensinogen to angiotensin I) and thereby to achieve more complete blockade. DRIs were effective as antihypertensive agents and reduced proteinuria in animal models.[526,527] Two early randomized trials reported additional lowering of albuminuria in subjects with diabetic nephropathy receiving combination DRI and ARB therapy versus ARB therapy alone.[528,529] However, a large randomized trial that included 8561 people with type 2 diabetes and albuminuria or cardiovascular disease was stopped prematurely after the second interim efficacy analysis. Despite greater lowering of blood pressure and albuminuria with combination DRI and ARB therapy, no benefit was observed with respect to the composite primary end point of cardiovascular event, CKD progression, ESKD, or death versus ARB monotherapy, but combination therapy was associated with a higher incidence of hyperkalemia and hypotension.[530] Taken together, published data from large randomized trials have to date failed to show additional renoprotective benefit with combination RAASi therapy, and all have reported increased adverse effects. This implies that near-complete blockade of the RAAS may be undesirable in many patient groups, but this does not exclude the possibility that it may be beneficial in selected patients who are at high risk for CKD progression, resistant to monotherapy, and at low risk for the reported adverse effects. Further studies are required to investigate this possibility before combination RAASi therapy can be recommended in clinical practice.

One meta-analysis has called into question the importance of RAAS inhibition,[531] but it should be noted that this study was dominated by data from the Antihypertensive and Lipid-Lowering Treatment to Prevent Heart Attack Trial (ALLHAT), which found no difference in fatal coronary heart disease or nonfatal myocardial infarction among hypertensive patients with at least one cardiovascular risk factor randomized to treatment with a thiazide diuretic, a calcium channel blocker, or an ACEI.[532] In a post hoc analysis there was also no difference in the secondary outcome of ESKD or greater than 50% decrement in GFR, but patients with serum creatinine level above 2 mg/dL were specifically excluded, resulting in only a minority of patients (5662 of 33,357) having kidney disease (estimated GFR < 60 mL/min/1.73 m^2). Furthermore, there was no assessment of proteinuria.[533] Thus inclusion of the ALLHAT data was inappropriate and significantly affected the results of the meta-analysis.[534] Other meta-analyses that did not include ALLHAT data have shown significant renoprotective benefit in patients receiving ACEI treatment.[535,536] In summary, there is now evidence from multiple randomized trials showing significant renoprotection associated with pharmacologic inhibition of the RAAS in a wide variety of forms of CKD, confirming that Ang II is a critical mediator of mechanisms of CKD progression in humans and providing support for the consensus that RAAS inhibition should be central to treatment strategies for slowing CKD progression.[537] The role of RAASi treatment in achieving optimal renoprotection is discussed further in Chapter 62.

ARTERIAL HYPERTENSION

Malignant hypertension frequently leads to renal injury, but whether or not less severe forms of hypertension cause "hypertensive nephrosclerosis" remains a subject of debate.[538,539] An increased risk for developing progressive renal failure with higher levels of blood pressure has been observed in several population-based studies[540-543] and is exemplified by findings from the Multiple Risk Factor Intervention Trial (MRFIT).[544] In a population of 332,544 men there was a strong, graded relationship between blood pressure and the risk for developing or dying with ESKD over a 15- to 17-year follow-up period. Renal function was not assessed at screening or during follow-up, however, so it is not possible to establish with any certainty whether higher blood pressure initiated kidney disease or accelerated a nephropathy that was already present. In one study the importance of hypertension as a risk factor for ESKD was further illustrated by the observation that lowering SBP by 20 mm Hg reduced the risk for ESKD by two thirds.[541] Even small increases in blood pressure, below the threshold usually used to define hypertension, are associated with an increased risk for ESKD.[540,542,545] Hypertension has also been identified as a risk factor for developing albuminuria or renal impairment among patients with type 2 diabetes mellitus.[546]

Whereas the role of hypertension in initiating kidney disease requires further clarification, there is clear evidence that hypertension accelerates the rate of progression of preexisting kidney disease, most likely through transmission of raised hydraulic blood pressure to the glomerulus resulting in exacerbation of glomerular capillary hypertension associated with nephron loss.[2] Among patients with diabetic nephropathy and nondiabetic CKD, the initiation of antihypertensive therapy results in significant reductions in rates of GFR decline, implying that hypertension, an almost universal consequence of impaired renal function, also contributes to the progression of CKD.[547] The potential impact of hypertension on the kidney is exemplified by case reports of patients with unilateral renal artery stenosis who manifested diabetic nephropathy or FSGS only in the nonstenotic kidney, and not in the stenotic side that was shielded from the hypertension.[548,549] Analysis of data from the Chronic Renal Insufficiency Cohort (CRIC) study has emphasized the importance of blood pressure control over time. Time-updated SBP above 130 mm Hg was more strongly associated with increased risk for CKD progression than a single baseline measurement.[550]

Uncertainty remains, however, as to what level of blood pressure lowering is required to achieve optimal renoprotection. Several randomized trials have sought to resolve this issue. In the MDRD study patients with predominantly nondiabetic CKD were randomized to a target MAP of less than 92 mm Hg (equivalent to < 125/75 mm Hg) versus a target MAP of less than 107 mm Hg (equivalent to 140/90 mm Hg). Whereas there was no difference between the overall rate of change in GFR during a mean of 2.2 years follow-up, patients randomized to the low blood pressure target evidenced an early rapid decrease in GFR, likely due to associated renal hemodynamic effects, that obscured a later significantly slower rate of GFR decline. Furthermore, the effect of blood pressure control was strongly modulated by the severity of proteinuria. Among patients with a urine protein level above 3 g/day at baseline, randomization to the low blood pressure target was associated with a significantly slower rate of GFR decline.[551] Secondary analysis also revealed significant correlations between the rate of GFR decline and *achieved* blood pressure, an effect that was more marked among those with greater baseline proteinuria.[552] In study 1 (patients with GFR of 25 to 55 mL/min/1.73 m²), rates of GFR decline increased above a MAP of 98 mm Hg among patients with baseline urine protein level of 0.25 to 3.0 g/day, and above 92 mm Hg in those with baseline urine protein level higher than 3.0 g/day. In study 2 (patients with GFR of 13 to 24 mL/min/m²), higher achieved blood pressure was associated with greater rates of GFR decline at all levels among patients with baseline urine protein level above 1 g/day (Figure 52.11). That the benefits of lower blood pressure may become evident only over a longer period is illustrated by the observation that further follow-up (mean 6.6 years) of patients from the MDRD study revealed a significant reduction in the risk for ESKD (adjusted hazard ratio [HR], 0.68; 95% CI, 0.57 to 0.82) or a combined end point of ESKD or death (adjusted HR, 0.77; 95% CI, 0.65 to 0.91) among patients randomized to the low blood pressure target even though treatment and blood pressure data were not available beyond the 2.2 years of the original trial.[553] In contrast, in the African American Study of Kidney Disease and Hypertension (AASK) no significant difference in the rate of GFR decline was observed between patients randomized to MAP goals of 92 mm Hg or less versus 102 to 107 mm Hg. Even after prolonged follow-up of the randomized groups, no difference in the combined end point of creatinine level doubling, ESKD, or death was observed.[554] It should be noted, however, that patients in AASK generally had low levels of baseline proteinuria (mean urine protein level 0.38 to 0.63 g/day),[518] and after prolonged follow-up, some reduction in the risk for the primary end point was observed among those with baseline urine protein to creatinine ratio above 0.22 mg/mg.[554] Thus the MDRD and AASK study results support the notion that lower blood pressure targets afford additional renoprotection in patients with more severe proteinuria. Since not all the patients in the MDRD study received ACEI treatment, it remained unclear to what extent the level of blood pressure attained is important in CKD patients receiving ACEI or ARB treatment. Experimental studies have found SBP to be a major determinant of glomerular injury in rats receiving either ACEI or ARB treatment.[220,555] Moreover, among patients with type 1 diabetes and established nephropathy receiving ACEI treatment, randomization to a low (MAP < 92 mm Hg) versus "usual" (MAP of 100 to 107 mm Hg) blood pressure target was associated with significantly lower levels of proteinuria after 2 years, although there was no significant difference in GFR decline.[556] Furthermore, secondary analysis of data from the Irbesartan in Diabetic Nephropathy Trial (IDNT) did show greater renoprotection among patients who achieved lower blood pressure targets such that achieved SBP above 149 mm Hg was associated with a 2.2-fold increased risk for developing ESKD or a doubling of serum creatinine level versus achieved SBP of less than 134 mm Hg.[557] Importantly, the relationship between improved outcomes and lower achieved SBP persisted among those patients treated with irbesartan. Similarly, in a meta-analysis of data from 1860 patients without diabetes with CKD the lowest risk for CKD progression was observed in patients with SBP of 110 to 129 mm Hg.[558] The Effect of Strict Blood Pressure Control and ACE Inhibition on the Progression of CRF in Pediatric Patients (ESCAPE) trial investigated the optimal level of blood pressure control for renoprotection in the setting of ACEI treatment. The study found that among children with CKD receiving treatment with an ACEI, those randomized to a lower blood pressure target evidenced a significantly reduced risk for reaching ESKD or doubling of serum creatinine level.[559] Another trial

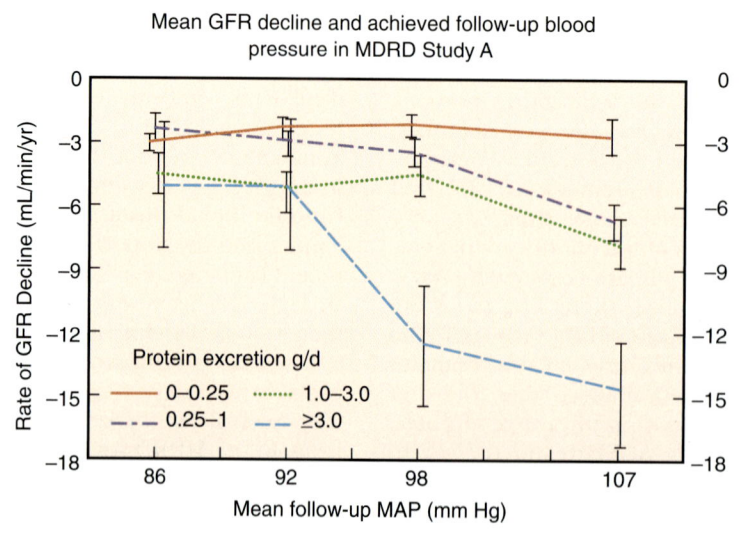

Figure 52.11 The interaction of blood pressure reduction and proteinuria at baseline on the rate of decline in glomerular filtration rate (GFR). MAP, Mean arterial pressure; MDRD, Modification of Diet in Renal Disease. (Reproduced with permission from Peterson JC, Adler S, Burkart JM, et al: Blood pressure control, proteinuria, and the progression of renal disease. The Modification of Diet in Renal Disease Study. *Ann Intern Med* 123:754-762,1995.)

has reported significant benefit associated with a lower blood pressure target in young (age < 50 years) people with autosomal dominant polycystic kidney disease and GFR above 60 mL/min/1.73 m². Participants randomized to a low blood pressure target (110/75 to 95/60 mm Hg) in addition to RAASi treatment evidenced a slower rate of increase in kidney volume as well as a greater decrease in albuminuria and left ventricular mass index than those randomized to usual blood pressure control (120/70 to 130/80 mm Hg),[560] but these findings cannot be applied to patients who do not meet the inclusion criteria for this study. On the other hand, additional blood pressure reduction with a calcium channel blocker in patients with nondiabetic CKD on ACEI treatment failed to produce additional renoprotection, but the degree of additional blood pressure reduction was modest (4.1/2.8 mm Hg) and may have been insufficient to improve outcomes in patients already receiving optimal ACEI therapy.[561] Several lines of evidence have drawn attention to the possibility that aggressive lowering of blood pressure may be associated with adverse effects in some patients. In the IDNT study achieved SBP of less than 120 mm Hg was associated with increased all-cause mortality and no further improvement in renal outcomes,[557] and in the meta-analysis described earlier, achieved SBP of less than 110 mm Hg was associated with a higher risk for CKD progression.[558] Furthermore, secondary analysis of data from the Ongoing Telmisartan Alone and in combination with Ramipril Global EndpoinT (ONTARGET) trial found that subjects who achieved a SBP of less than 120 mm Hg had a significantly higher cardiovascular mortality than those who achieved a SBP of 120 to 129 mm Hg.[562] Similarly, the ACCORD study reported no additional benefit with respect to cardiovascular end points among patients with diabetes randomized to achieve a SBP below 120 mm Hg (versus conventional control to < 130/80 mm Hg), but the lower blood pressure target was associated with more treatment-related adverse events and a greater decline in GFR.[563] Whereas the results of randomized trials comparing "low" and "usual" blood pressure targets among CKD patients have not yielded unequivocal results, the overall picture is one of lower blood pressure targets being associated with more effective renoprotection among those with more severe proteinuria. These observations have led to a consensus that blood pressure should be lowered to less than 130/80 mm Hg in all patients with diabetic or proteinuric CKD and less than 140/90 mm Hg in patients without these risk factors,[564] though the strength of the evidence supporting these specific recommendations has been called into question.[565] It is hoped that the ongoing Systolic Blood Pressure Intervention Trial (SPRINT; NCT01206062 at www.clinicaltrials.gov), which randomized more than 9000 subjects, including approximately one third with nondiabetic CKD, to SBP targets of less than 140 mm Hg or 120 mm Hg, will yield new data to guide future recommendations.[566]

DIETARY PROTEIN INTAKE

Increased dietary protein intake and intravenous protein loading in animals or humans with intact kidneys are associated with increases in renal mass, renal blood flow, and GFR, as well as a decrease in renal vascular resistance. The magnitude of the increases in GFR and renal blood flow in response to a protein load is a function of renal reserve. In patients with renal insufficiency some studies have shown that the percentage increase in GFR in response to a protein meal is reduced in those with a lower baseline GFR.[567] In contrast, a study comparing the renal response to an oral protein load in patients with moderate and advanced renal failure found a similar percent increase in GFR over baseline in both groups, demonstrating that even with advanced kidney disease, some renal reserve is still present and that elevated intake of dietary protein may have undesirable effects on glomerular hemodynamics at all levels of renal function.[568]

To understand the mechanisms whereby protein loading acutely augments renal function, various components of protein diets have been examined individually. Administration of equivalent quantities of urea, sulfate, acid, and vegetable protein to dogs or humans all failed to reproduce a meat protein–induced rise in GFR.[569-571] In contrast, feeding or infusion of mixed or individual amino acids (e.g., glycine, L-arginine) was shown to effect increases in GFR of similar magnitude to those seen with meat ingestion.[572,573] Micropuncture experiments demonstrated that amino acid infusion resulted in increases in glomerular plasma flow and transcapillary hydraulic pressure difference, thereby raising SNGFR without affecting the ultrafiltration coefficient.[572] Interestingly, however, perfusion of the isolated kidney with an amino acid mixture resulted in only a modest increase in GFR.[574] Taken together, these observations suggest that amino acids themselves do not have a major direct effect on renal hemodynamics, but their effects appear to be mediated by an intermediate compound generated only in the intact organism. Glucagon, the secretion of which is stimulated by protein feeding, has been proposed as such a mediator. GFR and renal blood flow increase in response to glucagon infusion in dogs.[573] Furthermore, administration of the glucagon antagonist, somatostatin, consistently blocks amino acid–induced augmentation in renal function both in humans and rats.[572,575] Large protein meals are also rich in minerals, potassium, phosphate, and acids. Indeed, after feeding a protein meal to dogs, the excretions of sodium, potassium, phosphorus, and urea were found to increase in parallel to the increase in GFR.[569] On the other hand, sodium chloride reabsorption in the proximal tubule and loop of Henle was found to be increased in rats maintained on a high-protein diet.[576] As result, less sodium and chloride would be delivered to the macula densa, thereby inhibiting tubuloglomerular feedback and adding a further stimulus to renal hyperemia. Since dietary protein does not affect systemic blood pressure,[572] other factors have been suggested to contribute to the renal hemodynamic changes following a protein load. Administration of the NO inhibitor L-NMMA or nonsteroidal antiinflammatory agents has been shown to blunt the renal hyperemic response to an oral protein load in both rats and humans, invoking a role for NO and prostaglandins.[576,577] In addition, Ang II and ET have been proposed as mediators of protein-induced renal injury as low-protein diets have been shown to reduce renal ET-1, ET receptors A and B, and AT_1R mRNA expression in PAN-injected and normal rats.[578,579]

It has been proposed that the augmented renal function induced by dietary protein may be an evolutionary adaptation of the kidney to the intermittent heavy protein intake of the hunter-gatherer.[3] Renal hyperfunction following a protein load would serve to facilitate excretion of the waste products of protein catabolism and other dietary components, thereby achieving homeostasis in the face of an abrupt increase in consumption in times of nutritional plenty; the subsequent decline of GFR to baseline during the intervals between meals would then favor mechanisms suited to conservation of fluid and electrolytes in times of scarcity. Persistent renal hyperfunction due to continuous excessive protein intake, however, leads to renal injury in experimental models. Laboratory animals with intact kidneys and ingesting food ad libitum become proteinuric and develop glomerulosclerosis with age.[3,151,580] This progression was significantly attenuated by feeding animals on alternate days only.[151] Furthermore, aging rats fed a high-protein diet ad libitum showed marked acceleration and increased severity of renal injury compared to rats receiving a normal-protein diet, whereas rats fed a low-protein diet were protected from renal injury.[580] Similarly, in diabetic rats, progression of nephropathy was markedly accelerated in the setting of a high-protein diet and substantially attenuated by a low-protein diet.[205] In this study, kidney weight in high protein–fed diabetic rats was significantly greater than in diabetic rats receiving normal-protein diets, suggesting that protein-induced renal hypertrophy may itself contribute to acceleration of renal functional deterioration. As discussed earlier, the renoprotective effects of dietary protein restriction in experimental animals are associated with virtual normalization of P_{GC} and SNGFR.[7]

Despite unambiguous evidence from experimental studies, confirmation of a beneficial effect of protein restriction in clinical trials has proved elusive. Following the publication of several smaller studies that generally suggested a beneficial effect from protein restriction but that suffered from deficiencies in design or patient compliance, a large, multicenter, randomized study, the MDRD study, was conducted to resolve the issue.[551] In this study, 585 patients with moderate CKD (GFR of 25 to 55 mL/min/1.73 m^2) were randomized to "usual" (1.3 g/kg/day) or "low" (0.58 g/kg/day) protein diet (study 1), and 255 patients with severe CKD (GFR of 13 to 24 mL/min/1.73 m^2) to "low" (0.58 g/kg/day) or "very low" (0.28 g/kg/day) protein diet. All causes of CKD were included, but patients with diabetes mellitus requiring insulin therapy were excluded. Patients were also assigned to different levels of blood pressure control. After a mean of 2.2 years' follow-up, the primary analysis revealed no difference in the mean rate of GFR decline in study 1 and only a trend toward a slower rate of decline in the very low protein group in study 2. Secondary analyses of the MDRD data, however, revealed that dietary protein restriction probably did achieve beneficial effects. In study 1 low-protein diet was associated with an initial reduction in GFR that likely resulted from the functional effects of decreased protein intake and not from loss of nephrons. This initial reduction in GFR obscured a later reduction in the rate of GFR decline that was evident after 4 months in the low-protein group and that may have resulted in more robust evidence of renoprotection had follow-up been continued for a longer period.[581] Disappointingly, long-term follow-up of 255 participants in study 2 of the MDRD trial found no renoprotective benefit associated with randomization to very low-protein diet in the original study but did report a higher risk for death in this group (HR, 1.92; CI, 1.15 to 3.20).[582] Despite inconclusive findings in several of the individual studies, three meta-analyses have each concluded that dietary protein restriction is associated with a reduced risk for ESKD (odds ratio of 0.62 and 0.67, respectively),[583,584] as well as a modest reduction in the rate of estimated GFR decline (0.53 mL/min/yr).[585] Whereas the renoprotective benefit of dietary protein restriction in humans appears modest, such dietary restriction is associated with other benefits, including improvement in acidosis as well as reduction in phosphorus and potassium load. Thus comprehensive dietary intervention with a moderate restriction in dietary protein intake should remain an important part of the management of patients with CKD.[586] The interaction of diet and kidney disease is discussed further in Chapter 61.

GENDER

Laboratory studies indicate that male animals appear to be at greater risk for developing kidney disease and for disease progression than females. Age-associated glomerulosclerosis is much more pronounced in male than in female rats, and it is notable that the male propensity for age-related glomerulosclerosis can be prevented by castration.[587] This gender difference was found to be independent of P_{GC} or glomerular hypertrophy, suggesting a role for the sex hormones as modulators of renal injury. Ovariectomy, on the other hand, had no effect on the development of glomerular injury seen in nonovariectomized female rats, implying that the presence of androgens, and not the lack of estrogens promotes renal injury.[587,588] In contrast, in the hypercholesterolemic Imai rat the development of spontaneous glomerulosclerosis in males can be significantly reduced by castration or by administration of exogenous estrogens.[589,590] These data again suggest an important role for androgens in the development of renal injury and raise the possibility that estrogens may to some extent counteract the adverse effects of androgens. In an apparently conflicting observation, female Nagase analbuminemic rats (NARs) develop renal injury of greater severity than males, a characteristic that is ameliorated by ovariectomy.[591] These rats may be unique, however, in that triglyceride levels, which are higher in females, may have an independent and overriding effect on kidney disease propensity. Glomerulosclerosis also develops to a significantly greater extent in male versus female rats subjected to extensive renal ablation.[592] This difference was independent of blood pressure and glomerular hypertrophy, but the degree of glomerulosclerosis and the extent of mesangial expansion each were found to correlate significantly with an increased expression of glomerular procollagen α_1(IV) mRNA in males. Similarly, in aging Munich-Wistar rats, glomerular metalloproteinase activity was found to decrease with age in males but not in females or castrated rats, suggesting that suppression of metalloproteinase activity by androgens could account for the gender difference in disease susceptibility.[593] Finally, estrogens, but not androgens, possess antioxidant activity and have been shown to inhibit mesangial cell LDL oxidation,[594] a property that may contribute to renoprotection.

Clinical studies suggest that humans also evidence a gender difference with respect to CKD progression. Data from the United States Renal Data System show a substantially higher incidence of ESKD among males (413 per million population in 2003) versus females (280 per million population),[595] and several studies have reported worse renal outcomes in males. In a Japanese community-based mass screening program the risk for developing ESKD (if baseline serum creatinine level was greater than 1.2 mg/dL for males or 1 mg/dL for females) was almost 50% higher in men than in women.[596] In a large population-based study in the United States, male gender was associated with a significantly increased risk for ESKD or death associated with CKD.[542] Similarly, in France, studies of factors influencing development of ESKD in patients with moderate and severe kidney disease found that disease progression was accelerated in males versus females, especially in those with chronic glomerulonephritis or autosomal dominant polycystic kidney disease (ADPKD). Furthermore, the effect of hypertension as a risk factor for CKD progression appeared to be greater in males.[597,598] Other studies of patients with CKD have reported a lower risk for ESKD among female patients with CKD stage 3[599] and a shorter time to renal replacement therapy among male patients with CKD stages 4 and 5.[600] One meta-analysis of 68 studies that included 11,345 patients with CKD reported a higher rate of decline in renal function in men,[601] but another meta-analysis of individual patient data from 11 randomized trials evaluating the efficacy of ACEI treatment in CKD did not show an increased risk for doubling of serum creatinine level or ESKD, or ESKD alone among men.[602] On the contrary, after adjustment for baseline variables, including blood pressure and urinary protein excretion, women evidenced a significantly higher risk for these end points than men.[602] One limitation of these studies is that the menopausal status of the women was often not documented. In general, the prevalence of hypertension and uncontrolled hypertension is higher among men, men tend to consume more protein than women, and the prevalence of dyslipidemias is greater in men than in premenopausal women. All of these factors may contribute to the increased severity of kidney disease observed in men, but they do not explain all of the differences.[603,604] The role of gender in kidney disease is reviewed in more detail in Chapters 20 and 21.

NEPHRON ENDOWMENT

Experimental and clinical studies have shown that the number of nephrons per kidney is variable and may be influenced by several factors during development in utero. Furthermore, low nephron endowment predisposes individuals to hypertension and CKD. This has been confirmed in studies using a rat model of spontaneous renal agenesis. Rats born with a single kidney had 19% fewer nephrons per kidney than their two-kidney littermates, resulting in a 60.2% reduction in nephron endowment that was associated with subsequent renal and glomerular hypertrophy, proteinuria, glomerular sclerosis, and TIF.[283] It has been proposed that reduced nephron endowment results in an increase in SNGFR and therefore a reduction in renal reserve.[605] Whereas the glomerular hemodynamic changes associated with mild-to-moderate congenital nephron deficiencies may not in themselves be sufficient to provoke renal injury, they could be predicted to compound the effects of an acquired nephron loss and predispose the individual to progressive renal damage. Thus CKD should be viewed as a "multi-hit" process in which the first "hit" may be reduced nephron endowment.[606] Nephron endowment is discussed in detail in Chapter 23.

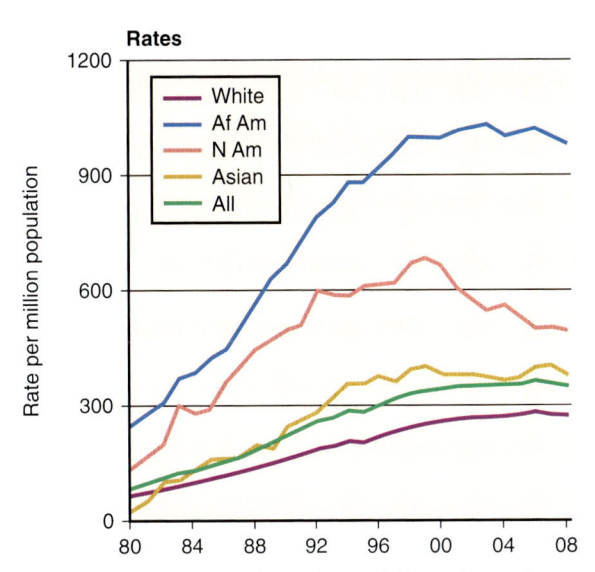

Figure 52.12 Incident rates for end-stage kidney disease by race in the U.S. population, adjusted for age and gender. The standard population was the U.S. population in 2011. Af Am, African American; N Am, Native American. (Reproduced with permission from United States Renal Data System: *2014 Annual data report: epidemiology of kidney disease in the United States*, Bethesda, Md, 2014, National Institutes of Health, National Institute of Diabetes and Digestive and Kidney Diseases.)

ETHNICITY

Data from the United States Renal Data System show a consistent and substantially higher incidence of ESKD among African Americans, Hispanics, and Native Americans versus whites. In 2012 the incidence rate was 3.3 times higher in African Americans and 1.8 times higher in Native Americans than in whites. In Hispanics the incidence rate was 1.5 times that in non-Hispanics (Figure 52.12).[607] Similarly, the prevalence of ESKD in 2008 was higher among minority groups: African Americans, 5671 per million population (pmp); Native Americans, 2600 pmp; Hispanics, 2932 pmp; Asians, 2272 pmp; whites, 1432 pmp.[607] The reasons for this obvious discrepancy are complex and include both social and biologic factors.[608,609] Interestingly, data from the Reasons for Geographic and Racial Differences in Stroke (REGARDS) cohort study show a lower prevalence of estimated GFR of 50 to 59 mL/min/1.73 m^2 among African American versus white subjects but a higher prevalence of estimated GFR of 10 to 19 mL/min/1.73 m^2, suggesting that African Americans have a lower risk for developing CKD but a higher risk for progression of CKD to ESKD.[610]

African Americans appear to be more susceptible to FSGS. One retrospective analysis of 340 routine kidney biopsies detected a significantly higher prevalence of FSGS and a significantly lower prevalence of membranous glomerulonephritis, IgA, and immunotactoid nephropathies among black versus white patients.[611] Similarly, among pediatric transplant recipients a higher proportion of African

American and Hispanic children had FSGS as a primary diagnosis versus whites.[612] The same investigators found that despite similar treatment modalities and similar durations of nephrotic syndrome, black children with FSGS reached ESKD almost twice as frequently as white children.[612]

More significant in terms of patient numbers and morbidity, however, are the racial discrepancies in the incidence of ESKD due to hypertensive and diabetic nephropathies. One longitudinal study that examined data from 1,306,825 Medicare beneficiaries reported substantially increased risks for developing ESKD in black versus white subjects in all categories: among diabetic subjects 2.4- to 2.7-fold increased, among hypertensive subjects 2.5- to 2.9-fold increased, and among subjects with neither hypertension nor diabetes 3.5-fold increased.[613] MDRD study data showed the prevalence of hypertension to be higher in blacks versus whites among patients with CKD, despite a higher mean GFR in the black patients.[604] Hypertensive patients were found to have had more rapid progression of kidney disease before entry into the study, suggesting that the higher prevalence of hypertension in black patients is likely to be a significant contributor to accelerated progression of CKD. On the other hand, both higher MAP and black race were independent predictors of a faster decline in GFR in the MDRD study.[614] In a large community-based epidemiologic study, black patients were found to have a 5.6 times higher unadjusted incidence of hypertensive ESKD with respect to the entire study population.[615] This increased incidence was directly related to the prevalence of hypertension, severe hypertension, and diabetes in the study population and inversely related to age at diagnosis of hypertension and socioeconomic status. After adjustment for these factors the risk for hypertensive ESKD remained 4.5 times greater among blacks compared to whites, providing further evidence that black patients have an increased susceptibility to kidney disease beyond that attributable to their increased prevalence of hypertension and diabetes. Salt-sensitive hypertension, in particular, is more prevalent in the black population than in the white population.[616] Comparing renal responses to a high sodium intake in salt-sensitive versus salt-resistant patients, renal blood flow was found to decrease in the face of an increased filtration fraction (implying an increased P_{GC}) in salt-sensitive patients, whereas the converse occurred in salt-resistant patients.[538] These observations are consistent with the notion that salt loading injures the glomerulus through glomerular capillary hypertension and that salt-sensitive individuals, and blacks in particular, are at added risk for this form of injury. The incidence of ESKD due to diabetic nephropathy is fourfold higher among African Americans than among white Americans.[617] It is notable that after controlling for the higher prevalence of diabetes and hypertension, as well as age, socioeconomic status, and access to health care, the excess incidence of ESKD due to diabetes in blacks versus whites was confined to patients with type 2 diabetes.[618] Among patients with type 1 diabetes, blacks were not found to be at higher risk than whites. Indeed, the majority of blacks with diabetic ESKD (77%) had type 2 diabetes, whereas the majority of whites with diabetic ESKD (58%) had type 1 diabetes.[619] Black race was also found to be associated with a threefold higher risk for early renal function decline (increase in serum creatinine level of 0.4 mg/dL or higher) among adults with diabetes.[620]

Several potential factors contributing to the different prevalence and severity of kidney disease among population groups have been analyzed. Adjustment for socioeconomic factors reduces, but does not eliminate, the increased risk for African Americans to develop ESKD.[609,617,620] African Americans have lower birth weights than their white counterparts and may therefore have programmed or genetically determined deficits in nephron number, rendering them more susceptible to hypertension and subsequent ESKD.[621,622] Finally, 40% of African American patients with hypertensive ESKD and 35% with type 2 diabetes–associated ESKD have a first-, second-, or third-degree relative with ESKD, implying a strong familial susceptibility to ESKD and therefore a genetic predisposition.[623] Evidence of a genetic explanation for the high incidence of ESKD observed in African Americans was provided by research that identified a strong association between ESKD and two coding variants of the gene for apolipoprotein L1 (*APOL1*).[624] These gene variants confer resistance to infection with *Trypanosoma brucei rhodesiense*, which causes sleeping sickness, providing an explanation for how selection likely resulted in a high prevalence of these variants in the population.[625] Subsequent studies have identified associations between *APOL1* risk variants and several renal pathologic processes, including FSGS, HIV-associated nephropathy, sickle cell kidney disease, and severe lupus nephritis. *APOL1* risk variants have also been associated with HIV nephropathy in black South Africans.[626] Moreover, cohort studies have reported associations between *APOL1* risk variants and risk for progression to ESKD. Risk for progression was the lowest in European Americans (with no risk variants), intermediate in African Americans with no or one risk variant, and highest in African Americans with two risk variants.[627] It is estimated that *APOL1* variants account for 40% of disease burden due to CKD in African Americans. The biologic role of APOL1 in the progression of CKD remains to be elucidated. The APOL1 protein is expressed in the kidney but is also secreted and is bound to circulating HDL particles. Current evidence suggests that it is the locally expressed form of APOL1 that is involved in CKD pathogenesis.[628] Despite the strong association between inheritance of two *APOL1* risk variants and ESKD, only the minority of people with this genotype actually develop kidney disease, suggesting that the action of a second factor is required to cause disease in genetically susceptible individuals. HIV is one example of such a "second hit," but it has been proposed that other viruses and other gene variants may also be important.[625] Other ethnic groups, including Asians,[546,629] Hispanics,[630] Native Americans,[631] Mexican Americans,[632] and Aboriginal Australians,[633] have also been found to be at increased risk for developing CKD and ESKD. See Chapters 20 and 21 for further discussion of ethnicity and the epidemiology of CKD and Chapter 43 for a detailed discussion of genetic factors in the pathogenesis of CKD.

OBESITY AND METABOLIC SYNDROME

Obesity may directly cause a glomerulopathy characterized by proteinuria and histologic features of FSGS,[634] but it is likely that it also exacerbates progression of other forms of CKD. Micropuncture studies have confirmed that obesity is another cause of glomerular hypertension and hyperfiltration that may contribute to the progression of CKD.[635,636]

Griffin and associates have pointed out that whereas obesity is widespread, only a minority of obese individuals develop obesity-related glomerulopathy. They propose that low nephron endowment (associated with an increased risk for later life obesity in low-birth-weight babies) or acquired nephron loss constitute a necessary additional factor that increases glomerular hypertrophy as well as preglomerular vasodilation and transmission of elevated systemic blood pressure to the glomerulus, eventuating in glomerulosclerosis.[637] Detailed investigation of adipocyte function has revealed that adipocytes are not merely storage cells but produce a variety of hormones and proinflammatory molecules that may contribute to progressive renal damage.[638,639] In addition, adiponectin, an adipokine produced by adipocytes, may exert a protective effect on podocyte function. Adiponectin levels are reduced in obesity and are inversely correlated with the magnitude of albuminuria.[640] Moreover, adiponectin knockout mice develop albuminuria associated with podocyte foot process effacement that is corrected by administration of exogenous adiponectin.[641] Obesity is also associated with increased production of aldosterone and expanded extracellular volume, both of which may contribute to progressive renal damage.[642]

In humans, severe obesity is associated with increased RPF, glomerular hyperfiltration, and albuminuria, abnormalities that are reversed by weight loss.[643] Several large population-based studies have identified obesity as an independent risk factor for developing CKD,[543,644] and one study has found a progressive increase in relative risk for developing ESKD associated with increasing body mass index (BMI) (relative risk [RR], 3.57; CI, 3.05 to 4.18 for BMI 30.0 to 34.9 kg/m² versus BMI 18.5 to 24.9 kg/m²) among 320,252 subjects with no evidence of CKD at initial screening.[645] On the other hand, analysis of data from the Framingham Heart Study confirmed an increased risk for developing CKD stage 3 associated with obesity but found that this was no longer significant after adjustment for known cardiovascular risk factors. Nevertheless the increased risk for incident proteinuria persisted in multivariable models.[646] Change in body weight has also been identified as a risk factor for incident CKD. In one study of 8792 previously healthy men, an increase in body weight of 0.75 kg/yr or more (and a decrease of less than 0.75 kg/yr) was associated with an increased risk for developing CKD in previously obese and nonobese subjects.[647] The metabolic syndrome (insulin resistance), defined by the presence of abdominal obesity, dyslipidemia, hypertension, and fasting hyperglycemia, is also associated with an increased risk for developing CKD. Analysis of the Third National Health and Nutrition Examination Survey (NHANES) data revealed a significantly increased risk for CKD and microalbuminuria in subjects with the metabolic syndrome as well as a progressive increase in risk associated with the number of components of the metabolic syndrome present.[648] Furthermore, a longitudinal study of 10,096 patients without diabetes or CKD at baseline identified metabolic syndrome as an independent risk factor for the development of CKD over 9 years (adjusted odds ratio [OR], 1.43; 95% CI, 1.18 to 1.73). Again there was a progressive increase in risk associated with the number of traits of the metabolic syndrome present (OR, 1.13; 95% CI, 0.89 to 1.45 for one trait versus OR, 2.45; 95% CI, 1.32 to 4.54 for five traits).[649] The metabolic syndrome has also been identified as a risk factor for incident CKD among Native Americans[650] and in Taiwan.[651] Patient waist-to-hip ratio (WHR), a marker of central fat distribution and insulin resistance, was independently associated with impaired renal function even in lean individuals (BMI < 25 kg/m²) among a population-based cohort of 7676 subjects.[652] Furthermore, analysis of data from the Atherosclerosis Risk in Communities (ARIC) study found that WHR but not BMI was associated with an increased risk for incident CKD and mortality,[653] suggesting that accumulation of visceral fat is more important as a risk factor than obesity per se. The effect of obesity on progression in cohorts of patients with established CKD is less well documented. In one study, increased BMI was an independent predictor of CKD progression among 162 patients with IgA nephropathy,[654] and BMI was independently associated with more rapid CKD progression in a cohort of CKD subjects (predominantly CKD stage 3).[655] On the other hand, obesity may be less relevant to progression in more advanced stages of CKD as evidenced by the observation that BMI was unrelated to the risk for ESKD among a cohort of patients with CKD stage 4 and 5.[600] The association of obesity with CKD and increased risk for CKD progression suggests that weight loss may represent an important intervention for achieving renoprotection. Sustained weight loss is notoriously difficult to achieve, but a meta-analysis of several small, short-duration studies found that weight loss achieved through diet or medication was associated with a reduction in proteinuria and blood pressure. Surgical procedures to achieve weight loss in the morbidly obese were associated with normalization of glomerular hyperfiltration and reductions in microalbuminuria and blood pressure.[656] A systematic review analyzed the effects of weight loss achieved by bariatric surgery, medication, or diet in 31 studies and found that in the majority of studies weight loss was associated with reductions in proteinuria. In people with glomerular hyperfiltration, GFR tended to decrease with weight loss, and in those with reduced GFR it tended to increase.[657]

SYMPATHETIC NERVOUS SYSTEM

Overactivity of the sympathetic nervous system has been observed in patients with CKD, and several lines of evidence suggest that this may be another factor that contributes to progressive renal injury.[658] The kidneys are richly supplied with afferent sensory and efferent sympathetic innervation and may therefore act as both a source and target of sympathetic activation. That the former is true is suggested by a study that compared postganglionic sympathetic nerve activity (SNA) measured via microelectrodes in the peroneal nerve in normal individuals and patients undergoing hemodialysis subdivided into those who retained their native kidneys and those who had undergone bilateral nephrectomy.[659] SNA was 2.5 times higher in nonnephrectomized patients undergoing dialysis compared to both normals and nephrectomized patients, in whom SNA was similar. Furthermore, increased SNA was associated with increased vascular tone and MAP in nonnephrectomized patients. SNA did not vary as a function of age, blood pressure, antihypertensive agents, or body fluid status. The authors speculated that intrarenal accumulation of uremic compounds stimulates renal afferent nerves via chemoreceptors, leading to reflex activation of efferent sympathetic nerves and increased SNA. Other studies, however, have observed increased SNA in the absence of uremia in patients with renovascular disease,[660] hypertensive ADPKD,[661] and nondiabetic CKD[662] or increased noradrenaline secretion in patients with nephrotic syndrome[663] and ADPKD.[661,664] Furthermore, correction of uremia by renal transplantation does not abrogate the increased SNA.[665] Interestingly, investigation of eight living kidney donors found no increase in SNA after donor nephrectomy, suggesting that the rise in SNA is related to renal damage rather than nephron loss.[662] Together, these findings suggest that a variety of forms of renal injury may provoke increased SNA and that uremia is not required for this response.

Evidence from experimental studies indicates that sympathetic overactivity resulting from kidney disease may also accelerate renal injury. Ablation of afferent sensory signals from the kidneys by bilateral dorsal rhizotomy in 5/6 nephrectomized rats prevented the expected rise in systemic blood pressure, attenuated the rise in serum creatinine level, and reduced the severity of glomerulosclerosis in the remnant kidneys when compared with sham-rhizotomized controls.[666] Moreover, the renoprotective effects of rhizotomy were found to be additive to that of ACEI treatment.[667] To further investigate whether the benefits of rhizotomy were solely attributable to the prevention of hypertension, 5/6 nephrectomized rats were treated with nonhypotensive doses of the sympatholytic drug moxonidine.[668] Despite the lack of effect on blood pressure, moxonidine treatment was associated with lower levels of proteinuria and less severe glomerulosclerosis than untreated rats. In a similar study, 5/6 nephrectomized rats were treated with the α-blocker phenoxybenzamine, the β-blocker metoprolol, or a combination.[669] As in the previous study, the doses used did not lower blood pressure, but all three treatments significantly lowered albuminuria and almost normalized the reductions in capillary length density (an index of glomerular capillary obliteration) and podocyte number. Metoprolol and combination therapy significantly lowered the glomerulosclerosis index versus untreated controls. Taken together, these results indicate that increased SNA accelerates renal injury independent of its effect on blood pressure, and that the adverse effects are not mediated by sympathetic cotransmitters but by catecholamines. Furthermore, sympathetic nerve overactivity has been proposed to contribute to the development of tubulointerstitial injury by reducing peritubular capillary perfusion to the extent that tubular and interstitial ischemia result.[670]

Preliminary evidence suggests that sympathetic overactivity may also be important in the progression of human CKD. Among patients with type 1 diabetes mellitus and proteinuria, evidence of parasympathetic dysfunction (which permits unopposed sympathetic tone) was associated with an increase in serum creatinine level over the next 12 months.[671] Analysis of data from the ARIC study found that higher resting heart rate and reduced heart rate variability, markers of autonomic dysfunction, were each independently associated with an increased risk for developing ESKD or a CKD-related hospital admission during 16 years of follow-up.[672] Several drug treatments may improve sympathetic overactivity in CKD patients. Among 15 normotensive patients with type 1 diabetes, 3 weeks' treatment with moxonidine significantly lowered albumin excretion rates without affecting blood pressure.[673] In other studies, chronic treatment with an ACEI or ARB, of proven benefit in renoprotection, was associated with reduction but not normalization of sympathetic overactivity.[674-676] In contrast, treatment with amlodipine was associated with increased SNA. Since ACEIs and ARBs do not readily enter the central nervous system, it is possible that RAAS inhibition modulates neurotransmitter release in the kidney and reduces afferent signaling. Several questions remain to be answered regarding the role of increased SNA in CKD progression. Whereas the renoprotective effects of sympatholytic drugs appear to be independent of effects on systemic blood pressure, it is as yet unknown what effect they have on glomerular hemodynamics. Further studies are also required to determine the extent to which chronic inhibition of sympathetic overactivity may be beneficial in a variety of forms of human CKD and whether or not this benefit is additive to that derived from inhibition of the RAAS.

DYSLIPIDEMIA

Moorhead and colleagues advanced the hypothesis that abnormalities in lipid metabolism may contribute to the progression of CKD.[677] Glomerular injury, accompanied by an alteration in basement membrane permeability, was envisaged as the initiator of a vicious cycle of hyperlipidemia and progressive glomerular injury. They proposed that urinary losses of albumin and lipoprotein lipase activators result in an increase in circulating LDLs, which in turn bind to the glomerular basement membrane, further impairing its permselectivity; filtered lipoproteins accumulate in the mesangium, stimulating ECM synthesis and mesangial cell proliferation; and filtered LDL is taken up and metabolized by the tubules, leading to cell injury and interstitial disease. Notably, this hypothesis did not propose hyperlipidemia as an initiating factor in renal injury, but rather as a participant in a self-sustaining mechanism of disease progression.

Several lines of experimental evidence confirm the association between dyslipidemia and renal injury. Both intact and uninephrectomized rats with dietary-induced hypercholesterolemia developed more extensive glomerulosclerosis than their normocholesterolemic controls, and the severity of glomerulosclerosis correlated with serum cholesterol levels[678]; aging female NARs have endogenous hypertriglyceridemia and hypercholesterolemia and develop proteinuria and glomerulosclerosis by 9 and 18 months of age, respectively, whereas male NARs have lower lipid levels and have no glomerulosclerosis by 22 months of age.[591] Interestingly, ovariectomy in female NARs lowers triglyceride levels and reduces their renal injury. In seeming contradiction, however, young and aging male Sprague-Dawley rats developed more extensive glomerulosclerosis than age- and sex-matched NAR, despite increased cholesterol levels in the NAR.[679] Triglyceride levels, however, were lower in the NARs, again suggesting an independent role for triglycerides in lipid-mediated renal injury. Whereas data regarding the role of lipids in initiating kidney disease are conflicting, several studies support the notion that dyslipidemia may promote renal damage. Cholesterol feeding has been shown to exacerbate glomerulosclerosis in uninephrectomized rats, prediabetic rabbits, rats with PAN nephropathy, and in the unclipped kidney of rats with two kidney–one clip hypertension. When hypertension and dyslipidemia are superimposed, a synergistic effect that dramatically accelerates renal functional deterioration is observed.[680,681] In the 5/6 nephrectomy model, progressive renal damage is associated with renal tissue accumulation of lipids, as well as upregulation of pathways involved in tubular reabsorption of protein-bound lipids and downregulation of pathways involved in lipid catabolism.[682]

In humans the role of lipids in initiation and progression of kidney disease remains unclear. At autopsy a highly significant correlation was found between the presence of systemic atherosclerosis and the percentage of sclerotic glomeruli in normal individuals, fostering speculation that the development of glomerulosclerosis may be analogous to that of atherosclerosis.[683] A study designed to identify the clinical correlates of hypertensive ESKD found a strong association between atherosclerosis and hypertensive ESKD among older white patients.[684] Furthermore, dyslipidemia has been identified in several large studies as a risk factor for subsequent development of CKD in apparently healthy individuals.[543,685,686] The common forms of primary hypercholesterolemia are not associated with an increased incidence of kidney disease in the general population, but renal injury has been described in association with rare inherited disorders of lipoprotein metabolism.[687,688]

Whereas primary lipid-mediated renal injury is rare among patients with CKD, the latter is frequently accompanied by elevations in serum lipid levels, as a result of urinary loss of albumin and lipoprotein lipase activators, defective clearance of triglycerides, modification of LDL by advanced glycation end products, reduced plasma oncotic pressure, adverse effects of medication, and underlying systemic diseases.[689,690] Among a cohort of adult patients with CKD, the most frequent lipid abnormalities noted were hypertriglyceridemia, low HDL levels, and increased apolipoprotein levels.[691] Furthermore, in a study of 631 routine renal biopsies, lipid deposits were detected in nonsclerotic glomeruli in 8.4% of kidneys, and staining for apolipoprotein B was positive in approximately one quarter of biopsies, suggesting that lipid deposition is not infrequent in diverse kidney diseases.[475] Several epidemiologic studies have found a strong association between CKD progression and dyslipidemia. In the MDRD study, low serum HDL cholesterol level was found to be an independent predictor of more rapid rates of decline in GFR.[692] Elevated total cholesterol, LDL cholesterol, and apolipoprotein B levels have been found to correlate strongly with GFR decline in CKD patients.[693] Hypercholesterolemia was shown to be a predictor of loss of renal function in patients with type 1 and type 2 diabetes.[694,695] Among patients without diabetes, CKD advanced more rapidly in patients with hypercholesterolemia and hypertriglyceridemia, independent of blood pressure control.[696] Among patients with IgA nephropathy, hypertriglyceridemia was independently predictive of progression.[697] However, not all studies confirm these findings. In MRFIT, dyslipidemias were not associated with a decline in renal function.[698] After 10 years of follow-up in the MDRD study, measures of dyslipidemia were not predictive of cardiovascular events or ESKD.[699] In a retrospective analysis of patients with nephrotic syndrome, hypercholesterolemia at diagnosis was not found to be a predictor of kidney disease progression.[700] In the CRIC study, no association was observed between levels of total or LDL cholesterol and the risk for ESKD or 50% reduction in estimated GFR (eGFR).[701] Interpretation of these data is complicated by the fact that in patients with renal insufficiency, dyslipidemias do not occur in isolation and are associated with other factors that also affect kidney disease progression, including hypertension, hyperglycemia, and proteinuria. Levels of serum cholesterol and triglycerides have been found to correlate with blood pressure and circulating Ang II levels in patients with type 1 and type 2 diabetes with kidney disease and to rise with increasing proteinuria in patients with nephrotic syndrome.[688]

The possible mechanisms whereby hyperlipidemia may contribute to renal injury have not been fully elucidated. Cholesterol feeding has been associated with an increase in mesangial lipid content,[678] glomerular macrophages, and TGF-β as well as fibronectin mRNA levels.[702,703] Furthermore, reduction of glomerular macrophages by whole-body x-irradiation in the setting of nephrotic syndrome significantly reduced albuminuria without affecting serum lipid levels, indicating that macrophages play a central role in hyperlipidemic glomerular injury.[703] Mesangial cells express receptors for LDL, and uptake is stimulated by vasoconstrictor and mitogenic peptides such as ET-1 and PDGF.[478] Metabolism of LDL by mesangial cells leads to increased synthesis of fibronectin and MCP-1, which may contribute to mesangial matrix expansion and recruitment of circulating macrophage/monocytes into the glomerulus.[479] Moreover, triglyceride-rich lipoproteins (very low-density lipoprotein [VLDL] and intermediate-density lipoprotein) induce mesangial cell proliferation and elaboration of IL-6, PDGF, and TGF-β in vitro.[704] Mesangial cells, macrophages, and renal tubular cells all have the capacity to oxidize LDL via formation of ROS, a step that may be inhibited by antioxidants and HDL.[467,705,706] Oxidized LDL may induce dose-dependent mesangial cell proliferation or mesangial cell death as well as production of TNF-α, eicosanoids, monocyte chemotaxins, and glomerular vasoconstriction. These pathways, together with free radicals generated during LDL oxidation, may each contribute to renal inflammation and injury.[704,705] Hyperlipidemia is also associated with elevated P_{GC}, raising the possibility of a further pathway to glomerulosclerosis via hemodynamic injury.[678] The elevated P_{GC} appears to be mediated, in part, by an increase in renal vascular resistance that occurs in the context of increased plasma viscosity. In patients with diabetes, circulating Ang II levels have been found to correlate with serum cholesterol levels,[707] and both oxidized LDL and lipoprotein (a) have been shown to stimulate renin production by juxtaglomerular cells in vitro.[706] Moreover, oxidized LDL has been found to reduce NO synthesis by endothelial cells[706] raising the possibility that alterations in activity of the RAAS and NO metabolism could also contribute to the increase in P_{GC} observed with hyperlipidemia.

It would follow that if hyperlipidemia exacerbates renal injury, interventions designed to lower serum lipid levels should ameliorate disease progression. Treatment with a 3-hydroxy-3-methylglutaryl–coenzyme A (HMG-CoA) reductase inhibitor (statin) or clofibric acid in the obese Zucker rat (a strain with endogenous hyperlipidemia and spontaneous glomerulosclerosis) and 5/6 nephrectomized rats (which develop hyperlipidemia secondary to renal insufficiency) resulted in lowering of serum lipid levels, reduction in albuminuria, reduction in mesangial cell DNA synthesis, and attenuation of glomerulosclerosis, despite a lack of effect on either systemic blood pressure or P_{GC}.[10,708] Indeed, statin treatment resulted in additional lowering of proteinuria, regression of glomerulosclerosis, normalization of podocyte number, and abrogation of tubulointerstitial injury when added to combination ACEI and ARB treatment.[709] In rats in the nephrotic phase of PAN nephropathy, statin treatment resulted in reduction of albuminuria and serum cholesterol levels, reduction of MCP-1 mRNA expression, and a 77% reduction in glomerular macrophage accumulation.[710] The statins may therefore exert beneficial effects on kidney disease progression, not only by reducing serum lipid levels, but also by inhibiting mesangial cell proliferation and mechanisms for the recruitment of macrophages due to decreased expression of chemotactic factors and cell adhesion molecules.[711] Cholesterol-fed rats with PAN nephropathy treated with the antioxidants probucol or vitamin E showed significant reductions in proteinuria and glomerulosclerosis compared to untreated controls.[712] Furthermore, plasma VLDL and LDL from the treated animals were less susceptible to in vitro oxidation, and less renal lipid peroxidation was evident, implying that lipid peroxidation plays an important role in renal injury associated with hyperlipidemia. Niacin treatment after 5/6 nephrectomy resulted in lower blood pressure, less proteinuria, less renal tissue accumulation of lipids, and attenuation of tubulointerstitial injury, indicating that lipid lowering through strategies other than statins may also be renoprotective.[713]

In some clinical studies, dietary or pharmacologic lowering of serum lipid levels has also been associated with a reduction in proteinuria and lower rates of decline in renal function, but other studies have failed to demonstrate significant beneficial effects of lipid-lowering therapy on proteinuria or decline of renal function, despite adequate therapeutic reductions in serum lipid levels. A meta-analysis of 13 small studies that included both diabetic and nondiabetic kidney disease found that lipid-lowering therapy significantly reduced the rate of decline in GFR (mean reduction of 1.9 mL/min/yr).[714] Several secondary analyses of data from clinical trials suggest that lipid-lowering therapy may slow progression in human CKD, but these data should be interpreted with caution. Secondary analysis of data from a randomized trial of pravastatin treatment for patients with a history of myocardial infarction found that pravastatin slowed the rate of GFR decline in patients with eGFR of less than 40 mL/min/1.73 m^2, an effect that was also more pronounced in those with proteinuria.[715] Similarly, patients with previous cardiovascular disease or diabetes randomized to simvastatin treatment in the Heart Protection Study evidenced a smaller increase in serum creatinine level than those who received placebo.[716] In a placebo-controlled open-label study, atorvastatin treatment in patients with CKD, proteinuria, and hypercholesterolemia was associated with preservation of creatinine clearance, whereas those receiving placebo evidenced a significant decline.[717] In a meta-analysis of studies in which patients with CKD before dialysis were randomized to therapy with a statin, analysis of data from a relatively small subgroup in which renal end points were available found that statin therapy was associated with a reduction in proteinuria but no improvement in creatinine clearance.[718] Whereas these renoprotective effects were associated with cholesterol lowering, it is possible that they may also be due to the direct pleiotropic effects of HMG-CoA reductase inhibitors. This notion is further supported by the observation that lipid lowering with fibrates was not associated with preservation of renal function,[719,720] although one study did show reduced progression to microalbuminuria among patients with type 2 diabetes receiving fenofibrate.[721] The Study of Heart and Renal Protection (SHARP) investigated the cardiovascular and renoprotective effects of lipid lowering with simvastatin and ezetimibe in 9438 subjects with CKD and ESKD. Whereas the treatment arm evidenced a mean reduction of 43 mg/dL in LDL cholesterol and a 17% reduction in major atherosclerotic events, no significant effect was observed on the incidence of the renal end points ESKD (risk ratio [RR], 0.97; 95% CI, 0.89 to 1.05) and ESKD or creatinine doubling (RR, 0.93; 95% CI, 0.86 to 1.01).[722] It should be noted, however, that the subjects with CKD had relatively advanced disease (mean eGFR 27 ± 13 mL/min/1.73 m^2), and these observations therefore do not exclude the possibility that lipid lowering may have renoprotective effects in less advanced CKD. However, a meta-analysis of 38 studies that included 37,274 participants with CKD found that statin therapy was associated with a reduction in mortality and cardiovascular events but no clear effect on CKD progression.[723]

CALCIUM AND PHOSPHATE METABOLISM

As is the case with many of the adaptations that follow nephron loss, evidence is accumulating that alterations in calcium and phosphate metabolism may also contribute to progressive renal damage. A retrospective analysis of 15 patients with nonprogressing CKD (GFR 27 to 70 mL/min, followed for up to 17 years) revealed that the single feature common to all these patients was an enhanced capacity to excrete phosphate when compared to patients with similar GFR but progressive kidney disease.[724] In all of the nonprogressors, serum phosphate and calcium levels remained within normal limits without use of phosphate binders, calcium supplementation, or vitamin D. It is not yet clear which factors are most important, but evidence suggests that hyperphosphatemia, renal calcium deposition, hyperparathyroidism, and activated vitamin D deficiency may each play a role. FGF-23 has been identified as a key mediator of bone mineral and vitamin D metabolism in CKD and may emerge as the dominant factor.

HYPERPHOSPHATEMIA

Uninephrectomized rats receiving a high-phosphate diet (1%) developed renal calcium and phosphate deposition and tubulointerstitial injury within 5 weeks of nephrectomy.[192] Similar changes were observed in a proportion of intact rats fed a 2% phosphate diet. Phosphate excess, therefore, does appear to have some intrinsic nephrotoxicity that is enhanced in the setting of reduced nephron number. A high-phosphate diet has also been associated with the development of parathyroid hyperplasia and hyperparathyroidism in remnant kidney rats.[725] Conversely, in both animals and humans with renal insufficiency, dietary phosphate restriction or treatment with oral phosphate binders has been associated with reductions in proteinuria and glomerulosclerosis and attenuation of disease progression as well as prevention of hyperparathyroidism.[726-729] A further mechanism whereby hyperphosphatemia may contribute to kidney damage is suggested by the observation that high-phosphate diet increased and phosphate binder therapy decreased renal expression of ACE after 5/6 nephrectomy.[730] Dietary phosphate restriction, however, almost inevitably also imposes dietary protein restriction. It is therefore not clear whether the benefit was derived directly from reduced phosphate intake or indirectly from protein restriction. One study in humans has reported additional renoprotection when phosphate restriction was superimposed on protein restriction.[731]

RENAL CALCIUM DEPOSITION

Calcium-phosphate deposition is a frequent histologic finding in end-stage kidney biopsies, irrespective of the underlying cause of renal failure.[200,732] Calcium levels in end-stage kidneys have been found to be approximately nine times greater than levels in control kidneys.[732] Histologically, deposits were seen in cortical tubular cells, basement membranes, and the interstitium.[732,733] Furthermore, the severity of renal parenchymal calcification has been found to correlate with the degree of renal dysfunction, implicating calcium-phosphate deposition in disease progression.[726,734] To determine whether the calcium deposits observed in end-stage kidneys precede or follow renal parenchymal fibrosis, investigators maintained rats with reduced renal mass on a high-phosphate diet, thus ensuring a high calcium-phosphate product. A subgroup was treated with 3-phosphocitrate, an inhibitor of calcium-phosphate deposition.[734] Treatment with 3-phosphocitrate led to a significant reduction in renal injury compared to controls, indicating that calcium-phosphate deposition within the kidney occurs during the evolution of renal injury and may exacerbate nephron loss. Calcium deposition in the renal parenchyma is associated with ultrastructural evidence of mitochondrial disorganization and calcium accumulation[733] and may therefore contribute to renal injury via uncoupling of mitochondrial respiration and generation of ROS.[735] Mitochondrial calcium deposition was reduced by dietary protein restriction or calcium channel blocker therapy.[733,735] Other potential roles for cellular calcium in kidney disease progression include effects on vascular smooth muscle tone, mesangial cell contractility, cell growth and proliferation, ECM synthesis and immune cell modulation.[736]

HYPERPARATHYROIDISM

Podocytes express a unique transcript of PTH receptor, and PTH has been shown to have several effects on the kidney, including decreasing SNGFR (without change in Q_A, P_{GC}, or ΔP), lowering K_f, and stimulating renin production.[729] Furthermore, increased PTH levels may exacerbate renal damage through effects on blood pressure,[737] glucose intolerance, and lipid metabolism.[738,739] Two experimental studies have provided evidence that PTH may contribute to CKD progression. In the first, parathyroidectomy was shown to improve survival, reduce the increase in renal mass as well as renal calcium content, and attenuate the rise in serum creatinine level observed in 5/6 nephrectomized rats fed a high-protein diet.[740] In the other, calcimimetic treatment and parathyroidectomy after 5/6 nephrectomy each abrogated TIF and glomerulosclerosis.[741] Interpretation of these data are, however, complicated by the observation in the latter study that both interventions also lowered blood pressure.

ACTIVATED VITAMIN D DEFICIENCY

It is perhaps not surprising that vitamin D, normally 1-hydroxylated in the kidney and therefore reduced in CKD, has several potentially beneficial effects on the kidney. Several experiments have reported amelioration of renal damage in rats treated with $1,25(OH)_2D_3$ or vitamin D analogue after 5/6 nephrectomy.[742-744] Interestingly, a further study found that $1,25(OH)_2D_3$ treatment also preserved podocyte number, volume, and structure after 5/6 nephrectomy.[269] In other experimental models, vitamin D or vitamin D analogues have been shown to abrogate interstitial inflammation by promoting sequestration of NF-κB signaling,[745] inhibit renal hypertrophy after uninephrectomy,[746] reduce renin[729,747] as well as TGF-β expression,[744] and restore glomerular filtration barrier structure as well as slit diaphragm protein expression.[747] Several small trials have reported reductions in proteinuria among patients with diabetic[748] and nondiabetic CKD[749,750] randomized to treatment with the vitamin D analogue paricalcitol, but larger long-term studies are required to further evaluate the potential renoprotective effects of vitamin D replacement.

FIBROBLAST GROWTH FACTOR 23

FGF-23 has been identified as a key regulator of the bone mineral and vitamin D changes observed in CKD and may also mediate some of the adverse cardiovascular consequences, as well as contributing to CKD progression. It is produced by osteoblasts and osteocytes, and levels rise early in the course of CKD. FGF-23 is stimulated chiefly by $1,25(OH)_2D_3$ and dietary phosphate intake.[751] Its chief actions are to reduce phosphate reabsorption in the proximal tubule by downregulating sodium-phosphate cotransporters and to reduce $1,25(OH)_2D_3$ levels by inhibiting renal $25(OH)D_3$ 1α-hydroxylase as well as stimulating the catabolic $25(OH)D_3$ 24-hydroxylase.[751] Thus decreased phosphate excretion early in the course of CKD stimulates FGF-23 production, which increases phosphate excretion to prevent hyperphosphatemia until late in the course of CKD. This response is achieved at the expense of low $1,25(OH)_2D_3$ levels, which in turn facilitate the development of secondary hyperparathyroidism.[198,752] In addition to the role of FGF-23 in bone mineral metabolism, longitudinal studies have identified FGF-23 as an independent risk factor for mortality in patients undergoing hemodialysis[753,754] and an independent risk factor for progression of CKD in patients with diabetes[755] as well as those without diabetes,[756] including African Americans.[757] Whether FGF-23 contributes directly to CKD progression or is simply a risk marker remains to be elucidated. Indeed, overexpression of mutant FGF-23 in the Thy-1 model of glomerulonephritis resulted in lowering of serum phosphate levels and amelioration of glomerulosclerosis.[758] Possible mechanisms whereby FGF-23 may contribute to CKD progression include aggravation of $1,25(OH)_2D_3$ deficiency and secondary hyperparathyroidism (Figure 52.13; see earlier sections).

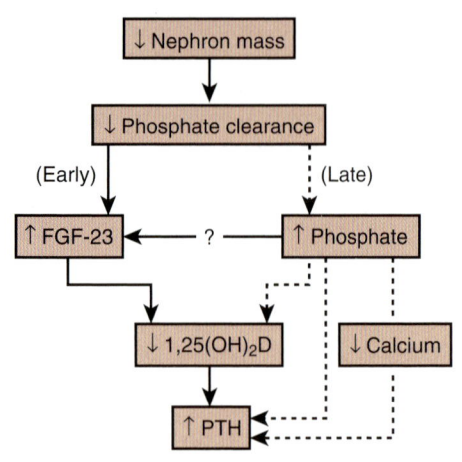

Figure 52.13 Schema to explain the possible interactions between phosphate, vitamin D (1,25[OH]$_2$D), fibroblast growth factor 23 (FGF-23), and parathyroid hormone (PTH) in regulating serum phosphate and calcium after nephron loss. (Reproduced with permission from Gutierrez OM: Fibroblast growth factor 23 and disordered vitamin D metabolism in chronic kidney disease: updating the "trade-off" hypothesis. Clin J Am Soc Nephrol 5:1710-1716, 2010.)

ANEMIA

Anemia is a frequent consequence of CKD but may also influence its progression. Both acute and chronic anemia are associated with reversible increases in renal vascular resistance and a normal or reduced filtration fraction in animals and humans. Conversely, an increase in hematocrit is associated with an increase in filtration fraction. Thus hematocrit may influence renal hemodynamics and thereby affect the rate of progression of CKD. The effects of anemia on glomerular hemodynamics have been studied in rats subjected to 5/6 nephrectomy, DOCA-salt hypertension, and diabetes.[759-761] Irrespective of the model, anemia was associated with significant amelioration of glomerulosclerosis and a reduction in P$_{GC}$. Reduced P$_{GC}$ resulted predominantly from reductions in efferent arteriolar resistance in rats with renal ablation, lowered SBP in DOCA-salt rats, and increased afferent arteriolar resistance in diabetic rats. Similarly, in the Munich-Wistar-Frömter/Ztm rat, which develops spontaneous glomerulosclerosis with age, anemia induced by dietary iron deficiency was associated with lower blood pressure, reduced urinary protein excretion, and less extensive glomerulosclerosis compared with controls fed a diet of normal iron content.[762] In contrast, prevention of anemia by administration of erythropoietin to remnant kidney rats to maintain a normal hematocrit resulted in increased systemic and glomerular blood pressures as well as markedly increased glomerulosclerosis.[759] In another apparently contradictory study, treatment with epoetin delta after 5/6 nephrectomy was associated with slower rates of decline in renal function, decreased renal fibrosis, and less interstitial macrophage accumulation. Interestingly, these effects were observed at subhemopoietic doses, indicating that they may have resulted from direct actions of the epoetin, rather than anemia correction.[763]

Despite the apparently favorable hemodynamic effects of anemia in experimental models of CKD, human studies suggest that anemia may in fact accelerate CKD progression. In patients with inherited hemoglobinopathies, chronic anemia is associated with glomerular hyperfiltration that eventuates in proteinuria, hypertension, and ESKD.[764,765] Furthermore, reduced hemoglobin level was an independent predictor of increased risk for developing ESKD among patients with diabetic nephropathy in the Reduction of Endpoints in NIDDM with the Angiotensin II Antagonist Losartan (RENAAL) trial.[766] Several longitudinal studies of patients with other forms of CKD have identified lower hemoglobin level as a risk factor for progression.[767,768] Further confirmation that anemia has an adverse effect on CKD progression is derived from two small randomized studies that have reported renoprotective benefit when anemia is corrected with erythropoietin. Among patients without diabetes with serum creatinine level of 2 to 6 mg/dL, early treatment (started when hemoglobin level < 11.6 g/dL) with erythropoietin alpha was associated with a 60% reduction in the risk for doubling serum creatinine level, ESKD, or death versus delayed treatment (started when hemoglobin level < 9.0 g/dL),[769] and in patients with serum creatinine level of 2 to 4 mg/dL and hematocrit below 30%, erythropoietin treatment was associated with significantly improved renal survival.[770] On the other hand, two other studies that had effect on left ventricular mass as their primary end point,[771,772] as well as the Trial to Reduce Cardiovascular Events with Aranesp Therapy (TREAT),[773] found no effect of high versus low hemoglobin target on rate of decline in GFR, and in the Cardiovascular Risk Reduction by Early Anemia Treatment with Epoetin Beta (CREATE) study, randomization to a higher hemoglobin target (13 to 15 mg/dL) was associated with a shorter time to initiation of dialysis than the lower target (10.5 to 11.5 mg/dL).[774]

The reasons for the apparent contradiction between the beneficial hemodynamic effects of anemia in experimental models and the identification of anemia as a risk factor for CKD progression in clinical studies are unknown. It is possible that the benefit of the hemodynamic effects is outweighed by other factors such as increased renal hypoxia and ROS formation that may contribute to progressive renal damage.[775] Nevertheless, several studies indicate that normalization of hemoglobin level in CKD may be associated with several serious adverse effects, including increased risk for stroke[773] and death.[776] Issues related to the treatment of anemia in CKD are discussed further in Chapter 57.

TOBACCO SMOKING

Smoking produces acute sympathetic nervous system activation resulting in tachycardia and an increase in SBP of up to 21 mm Hg.[777] Vasoconstriction occurs in several vascular beds, including the kidneys. Among healthy, nonsmoking volunteers, acute exposure to cigarette smoke caused an 11% increase in renovascular resistance accompanied by a 15% reduction in GFR and an 18% decrease in filtration fraction. These effects appear to be mediated, at least in part, by nicotine, since similar responses were observed after chewing nicotine gum.[778] The renal hemodynamic effects of smoking can be blocked by pretreatment with a β-blocker, indicating that β-adrenergic stimulation is also involved.[779] The effects of chronic smoking on the normal kidney are less well defined. RPF but not GFR is reduced in chronic smokers, and plasma ET levels are elevated. In one population-based study, chronic smoking was associated with a small increase in creatinine clearance, implying that smoking may cause glomerular hyperfiltration.[780] That these functional abnormalities may result in structural changes to blood vessels is suggested by the observation of abnormal intrarenal vasculature in smokers.[781,782] Moreover, epidemiologic studies have found smoking to be an important predictor of albuminuria in the general population.[780,783] In one study, heavy smoking (>20 cigarettes per day) was associated with a relative risk for albuminuria of 1.92.[783] Furthermore, in other epidemiologic studies, smoking has been identified as a significant risk factor for CKD[543,784,785] and the development of ESKD.[542] On the other hand, smoking was associated with an increased risk for developing glomerular hyperfiltration (eGFR ≥ 117 mL/min/1.73 m^2; OR, 1.32 versus nonsmokers) as well as proteinuria (OR, 1.51 versus nonsmokers) in one longitudinal study of 10,118 middle-aged Japanese workers.[786] Two other similar longitudinal studies from Japan confirmed that smoking is associated with an increased risk for developing proteinuria but with a higher mean eGFR than in nonsmokers.[787,788] In one of the studies, smoking was associated with a reduced risk for developing CKD stage 3.[788]

Whereas more studies are required to elucidate the effects of smoking on healthy kidneys, a growing body of evidence attests to the role of smoking as an important risk factor for disease progression in a variety of forms of CKD. The first published studies focused on diabetic nephropathy. Among patients with type 1 diabetes, smoking has been found to be a significant risk factor for the development of microalbuminuria and overt nephropathy.[789,790] Furthermore, smoking was associated with more rapid progression from microalbuminuria to overt nephropathy[791] and with almost double the rate of decline in GFR in nonsmokers.[792] Similar observations have been made among patients with type 2 diabetes,[793-795] and smoking cessation was associated with less progression to macroalbuminuria and a slower rate of GFR decline than continued smoking.[796] Several studies have also reported associations between smoking and accelerated CKD progression among nondiabetic forms of CKD. Among men with ADPKD or IgA nephropathy, a dose-dependent association between smoking and ESKD was observed, with an odds ratio of 5.8 for those with more than 15 pack years versus those with less than 5 pack years.[797] The median time to ESKD was almost halved in smokers versus nonsmokers in patients with lupus nephritis.[798] Among 295 patients with a primary glomerulonephritis, those with a serum creatinine level above 1.7 mg/dL were significantly more likely to be smokers than those with a normal creatinine level.[799] Similarly, among 73 patients with primary renal disease, the rate of decline in GFR was doubled in heavy smokers versus nonsmokers.[800] Smoking was the most powerful predictor of a rise in serum creatinine level among patients with severe essential hypertension.[801] In the CRIC study, nonsmoking was associated with a reduced risk for CKD progression (HR, 0.68; 95% CI, 0.55 to 0.84), atherosclerotic cardiovascular events (HR, 0.55; 95% CI, 0.40 to 0.75), and mortality (HR, 0.45; 95% CI, 0.34 to 0.60).[802]

Mechanisms whereby cigarette smoking may result in renal injury are the subject of ongoing research but are thought to include sympathetic nervous system activation, glomerular capillary hypertension, endothelial cell injury, and direct tubulotoxocity.[803] Furthermore, nicotine administration in Thy-1 rats increased mesangial cell accumulation, and in vitro nicotine increased COX-2 expression and mesangial cell proliferation.[804] Similarly, in a mouse model of diabetic nephropathy, nicotine increased proteinuria, glomerular hypertrophy, and mesangial area. NADPH-oxidase 4, nitrotyrosine, and Akt were also increased. In vitro nicotine and high glucose levels were found to have additive effects in stimulating generation of ROS and Akt phosphorylation in mesangial cells.[805] Nicotine administration after 5/6 nephrectomy in rats was associated with a small increase in blood pressure as well as increased proteinuria (but not albuminuria). Glomerular injury score at 12 weeks was exacerbated by nicotine in association with increased expression of fibronectin, NADPH-oxidase, and TGF-β.[806] Among patients with CKD the hemodynamic effects of smoking were variable, but smoking was associated with a consistent increase in urine ACR.[778] Analysis of urine from smokers and nonsmokers has revealed significantly higher excretions of thromboxane- and PGI$_2$-derived products in smokers.[807] The authors suggest that increased synthesis of thromboxanes and PGI$_2$ may have pathologic importance for vascular injury given the biologic effects of these compounds on platelets and smooth muscle cells. An important role for sympathetic nervous system activation was suggested by an experimental study in which sympathetic denervation abrogated renal injury induced by exposure to cigarette smoke condensate.[808] A growing body of evidence thus supports the notion that the kidney is yet another organ that is adversely affected by smoking and that smoking cessation may contribute to slowing the rate of progression of CKD.[809,796]

ACUTE KIDNEY INJURY

A growing body of evidence indicates that recovery from AKI is associated with a substantially increased risk for CKD, and AKI superimposed on CKD has been proposed as a previously underappreciated mechanism for CKD progression. Following publication of several individual cohort studies, a meta-analysis of 13 studies reported a significantly increased risk for developing CKD and ESKD in patients who had survived an episode of AKI versus participants without AKI (pooled adjusted HR for CKD, 8.8; 95% CI, 3.1 to 25.5) (pooled HR for ESKD, 3.1; 95% CI, 1.9 to 5.0).[810] Studies in animal models of AKI have identified failure of dedifferentiation of tubular cells as a key mechanism associated with progressive TIF after AKI. After acute tubular necrosis, regeneration of tubules is achieved by dedifferentiation of remaining tubular cells followed by proliferation to replace lost cells and redifferentiation. If this process fails, tubule cells become arrested in the dedifferentiated state and continue to produce proinflammatory and profibrotic cytokines that drive progressive interstitial fibrosis. Activation of pericytes results in differentiation into myofibroblasts that contribute to fibrosis. The loss of pericytes contributes to loss of endothelial integrity and capillary rarefaction that exacerbates tissue hypoxia and fibrosis.[811] The specific factors that provoke progressive kidney damage after AKI remain to be elucidated. It is proposed that a single episode of AKI normally heals without progressive kidney damage but that repeated episodes of AKI, a single

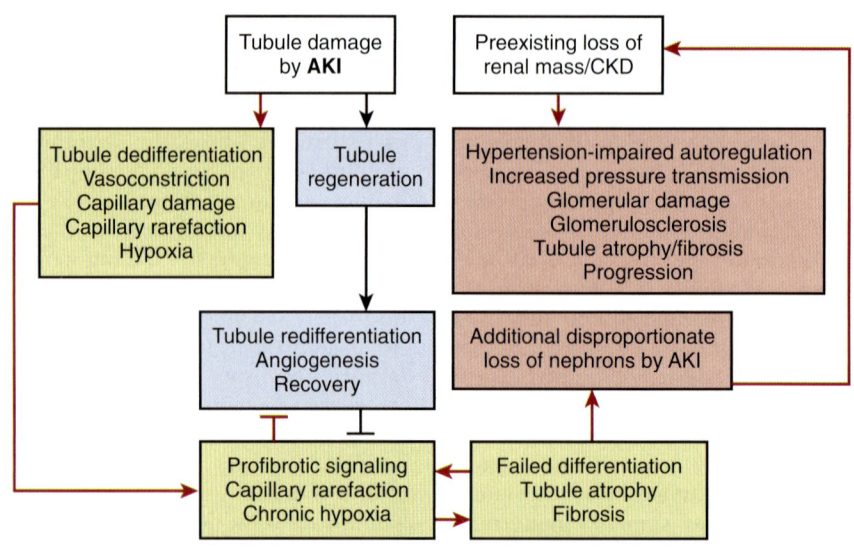

Figure 52.14 Failed tubule differentiation and loss of renal mass after acute kidney injury (AKI) lead to hemodynamic abnormalities that cause chronic kidney disease (CKD) progression. Schematic diagram illustrating the effects of AKI that lead to tubulointerstitial fibrosis, the renal mass reduction that retards recovery of tubules regenerating after AKI, and the resulting disproportionate further reduction of renal mass that triggers hemodynamic mechanisms of renal disease progression. (Reproduced with permission from Venkatachalam MA, et al: Failed tubule recovery, AKI-CKD transition, and kidney disease progression. *J Am Soc Nephrol* pii:ASN.2015010006. Epub Mar 25, 2015.)

very severe episode of AKI, or AKI superimposed on preexisting CKD may provoke these mechanisms.[812] The interaction between AKI and CKD progression is demonstrated by a study of 39,805 patients with eGFR of less than 45 mL/min/1.73 m² before hospitalization. Those who survived an episode of AKI that required dialysis had a very high risk for developing ESKD within 30 days of hospital discharge (i.e., nonrecovery of AKI) that was related to preadmission eGFR. For eGFR of 30-44 mL/min/1.73 m² the incidence of ESKD was 42%, and for eGFR of 15 to 29 mL/min/1.73 m² it was as high as 63%, whereas the incidence of ESKD was only 1.5% among those who did not have AKI that required dialysis. Among patients who survived longer than 30 days after hospital discharge without ESKD, the incidence of ESKD and death at 6 months were 12.7% and 19.7%, respectively, versus 1.7% and 7.4% in the comparator group with CKD but no AKI. After adjustment for multiple risk factors, AKI was associated with a 30% increase in long-term risk for death or ESKD (adjusted HR, 1.30; 95% CI, 1.04 to 1.64).[813] The interaction between AKI and CKD has been explored further in rats subjected to renal ischemia 2 weeks after 3/4 nephrectomy, uninephrectomy, or sham operation. Despite comparable acute injury, ischemia after 3/4 nephrectomy was associated with a sustained increase in serum creatinine level and more tubules that failed to redifferentiate associated with more severe capillary rarefaction and TIF. Furthermore, rats that were initially normotensive after 3/4 nephrectomy developed hypertension and proteinuria at 2 to 4 weeks after ischemia.[814] The investigators propose that loss of autoregulation results in greater transmission of elevated systemic blood pressure to the glomerulus that exacerbates glomerular damage and contributes to CKD progression.[812] Proposed interactions between mechanisms of kidney injury post AKI and mechanisms of CKD progression are illustrated in Figure 52.14.

FUTURE DIRECTIONS

The development of pharmacologic inhibitors of the RAAS provided powerful and incisive tools to explore renal hemodynamic and other associated adaptations in the setting of progressive renal injury. These insights paved the way for clinical studies that have now provided clear evidence for the use of ACEI and ARB treatment as the mainstay of renoprotective strategies. Nevertheless, these studies have shown at best a halving of the rate of CKD progression. Ongoing research involving cell biology and molecular cloning, as well as genomics and proteomics, continues to yield novel insights into the mechanisms of progressive renal injury that promise to direct researchers to potential new molecular targets for renoprotective interventions. The development of the means to specifically inhibit molecular targets may provide new forms of therapy for those with CKD and enable physicians to realize the ultimate goal of achieving remission of progressive renal injury in the majority of patients and even regression of renal damage in some.

Complete reference list available at ExpertConsult.com.

KEY REFERENCES

7. Hostetter TH, Olson JL, Rennke HG, et al: Hyperfiltration in remnant nephrons: a potentially adverse response to renal ablation. *J Am Soc Nephrol* 12:1315–1325, 2001.
14. Lenihan CR, Busque S, Derby G, et al: Longitudinal study of living kidney donor glomerular dynamics after nephrectomy. *J Clin Invest* 125:1311–1318, 2015.
78. Carlstrom M, Wilcox CS, Arendshorst WJ: Renal autoregulation in health and disease. *Physiol Rev* 95:405–511, 2015.
83. Taal MW, Nenov VD, Wong W, et al: Vasopeptidase inhibition affords greater renoprotection than angiotensin-converting enzyme inhibition alone. *J Am Soc Nephrol* 12:2051–2059, 2001.

215. Kim SP, Murad MH, Thompson RH, et al: Comparative effectiveness for survival and renal function of partial and radical nephrectomy for localized renal tumors: a systematic review and meta-analysis. *J Urol* 2012. doi: 10.1016/j.juro.2012.10.026. pii: S0022-5347(12)05254-8. [Epub Oct 18, 2012].
216. Mjoen G, Hallan S, Hartmann A, et al: Long-term risks for kidney donors. *Kidney Int* 86:162–167, 2014.
217. Muzaale AD, Massie AB, Wang MC, et al: Risk of end-stage renal disease following live kidney donation. *JAMA* 311:579–586, 2014.
218. Lenihan CR, Busque S, Derby G, et al: The association of predonation hypertension with glomerular function and number in older living kidney donors. *J Am Soc Nephrol* 26:1261–1267, 2015.
281. Fukuda A, Chowdhury MA, Venkatareddy MP, et al: Growth-dependent podocyte failure causes glomerulosclerosis. *J Am Soc Nephrol* 23:1351–1363, 2012.
283. Wang X, Johnson AC, Williams JM, et al: Nephron deficiency and predisposition to renal injury in a novel one-kidney genetic model. *J Am Soc Nephrol* 2014. pii: ASN.2014040328. [Epub Oct 27, 2014].
291. Remuzzi G, Bertani T: Pathophysiology of progressive nephropathies. *N Engl J Med* 339:1448–1456, 1998.
297. Duffield JS: Cellular and molecular mechanisms in kidney fibrosis. *J Clin Invest* 124:2299–2306, 2014.
298. Falke LL, Gholizadeh S, Goldschmeding R, et al: Diverse origins of the myofibroblast-implications for kidney fibrosis. *Nat Rev Nephrol* 11:233–244, 2015.
299. Meng XM, Nikolic-Paterson DJ, Lan HY: Inflammatory processes in renal fibrosis. *Nat Rev Nephrol* 10:493–503, 2014.
402. Chau BN, Xin C, Hartner J, et al: MicroRNA-21 promotes fibrosis of the kidney by silencing metabolic pathways. *Sci Transl Med* 4:121ra18, 2012.
403. Denby L, Ramdas V, McBride MW, et al: miR-21 and miR-214 are consistently modulated during renal injury in rodent models. *Am J Pathol* 179:661–672, 2011.
404. Denby L, Ramdas V, Lu R, et al: MicroRNA-214 antagonism protects against renal fibrosis. *J Am Soc Nephrol* 25:65–80, 2014.
425. Wesson DE, Jo CH, Simoni J: Angiotensin II-mediated GFR decline in subtotal nephrectomy is due to acid retention associated with reduced GFR. *Nephrol Dial Transplant* 30:762–770, 2015.
432. Goraya N, Simoni J, Jo C, et al: Dietary acid reduction with fruits and vegetables or bicarbonate attenuates kidney injury in patients with a moderately reduced glomerular filtration rate due to hypertensive nephropathy. *Kidney Int* 81:86–93, 2012.
433. Goraya N, Simoni J, Jo CH, et al: A comparison of treating metabolic acidosis in CKD stage 4 hypertensive kidney disease with fruits and vegetables or sodium bicarbonate. *Clin J Am Soc Nephrol* 8:371–381, 2013.
434. Goraya N, Simoni J, Jo CH, et al: Treatment of metabolic acidosis in patients with stage 3 chronic kidney disease with fruits and vegetables or oral bicarbonate reduces urine angiotensinogen and preserves glomerular filtration rate. *Kidney Int* 86:1031–1038, 2014.
435. Dobre M, Rahman M, Hostetter TH: Current status of bicarbonate in CKD. *J Am Soc Nephrol* 26:515–523, 2015.
488. Gansevoort RT, Matsushita K, van der Velde M, et al: Lower estimated GFR and higher albuminuria are associated with adverse kidney outcomes in both general and high-risk populations: a collaborative meta-analysis of general and high-risk population cohorts. *Kidney Int* 80:93–104, 2011.
493. Lambers Heerspink HJ, Kropelin TF, Hoekman J, et al: Drug-induced reduction in albuminuria is associated with subsequent renoprotection: a meta-analysis. *J Am Soc Nephrol* 2014. pii: ASN.2014070688. [Epub Nov 24, 2014].
525. Fried LF, Emanuele N, Zhang JH, et al: Combined angiotensin inhibition for the treatment of diabetic nephropathy. *N Engl J Med* 369:1892–1903, 2013.
530. Parving HH, Brenner BM, McMurray JJ, et al: Cardiorenal end points in a trial of aliskiren for type 2 diabetes. *N Engl J Med* 367:2204–2213, 2012.
550. Anderson AH, Yang W, Townsend RR, et al: Time-updated systolic blood pressure and the progression of chronic kidney disease: a cohort study. *Ann Intern Med* 162:258–265, 2015.
560. Schrier RW, Abebe KZ, Perrone RD, et al: Blood pressure in early autosomal dominant polycystic kidney disease. *N Engl J Med* 371:2255–2266, 2014.
564. Stevens PE, Levin A: Evaluation and management of chronic kidney disease: synopsis of the Kidney Disease: Improving Global Outcomes 2012 clinical practice guideline. *Ann Intern Med* 158:825–830, 2013.
566. Ambrosius WT, Sink KM, Foy CG, et al: The design and rationale of a multicenter clinical trial comparing two strategies for control of systolic blood pressure: the Systolic Blood Pressure Intervention Trial (SPRINT). *Clin Trials* 11:532–546, 2014.
606. Nenov VD, Taal MW, Sakharova OV, et al: Multi-hit nature of chronic renal disease. *Curr Opin Nephrol Hypertens* 9:85–97, 2000.
625. Freedman BI, Skorecki K: Gene-gene and gene-environment interactions in apolipoprotein L1 gene-associated nephropathy. *Clin J Am Soc Nephrol* 9:2006–2013, 2014.
626. Kasembeli AN, Duarte R, Ramsay M, et al: APOL1 risk variants are strongly associated with HIV-associated nephropathy in black South Africans. *J Am Soc Nephrol* 2015. pii:ASN.2014050469. [Epub Mar 18, 2015].
627. Parsa A, Kao WH, Xie D, et al: APOL1 risk variants, race, and progression of chronic kidney disease. *N Engl J Med* 369:2183–2196, 2013.
628. Kruzel-Davila E, Wasser WG, Aviram S, et al: APOL1 nephropathy: from gene to mechanisms of kidney injury. *Nephrol Dial Transplant* 2015. pii:gfu391. [Epub Jan 5, 2015].
657. Bolignano D, Zoccali C: Effects of weight loss on renal function in obese CKD patients: a systematic review. *Nephrol Dial Transplant* 28(Suppl 4):iv82–iv98, 2013.
701. Rahman M, Yang W, Akkina S, et al: Relation of serum lipids and lipoproteins with progression of CKD: the CRIC study. *Clin J Am Soc Nephrol* 9:1190–1198, 2014.
722. Haynes R, Lewis D, Emberson J, et al: Effects of lowering LDL cholesterol on progression of kidney disease. *J Am Soc Nephrol* 25:1825–1833, 2014.
723. Palmer SC, Navaneethan SD, Craig JC, et al: HMG CoA reductase inhibitors (statins) for people with chronic kidney disease not requiring dialysis. *Cochrane Database Syst Rev* (5):CD007784, 2014.
730. Eraranta A, Riutta A, Fan M, et al: Dietary phosphate binding and loading alter kidney angiotensin-converting enzyme mRNA and protein content in 5/6 nephrectomized rats. *Am J Nephrol* 35:401–408, 2012.
757. Scialla JJ, Astor BC, Isakova T, et al: Mineral metabolites and CKD progression in African Americans. *J Am Soc Nephrol* 24:125–135, 2013.
786. Maeda I, Hayashi T, Sato KK, et al: Cigarette smoking and the association with glomerular hyperfiltration and proteinuria in healthy middle-aged men. *Clin J Am Soc Nephrol* 6:2462–2469, 2011.
787. Noborisaka Y, Ishizaki M, Nakata M, et al: Cigarette smoking, proteinuria, and renal function in middle-aged Japanese men from an occupational population. *Environ Health Prev Med* 17:147–156, 2012.
788. Noborisaka Y, Ishizaki M, Yamada Y, et al: The effects of continuing and discontinuing smoking on the development of chronic kidney disease (CKD) in the healthy middle-aged working population in Japan. *Environ Health Prev Med* 18:24–32, 2013.
802. Ricardo AC, Anderson CA, Yang W, et al: Healthy lifestyle and risk of kidney disease progression, atherosclerotic events, and death in CKD: findings from the Chronic Renal Insufficiency Cohort (CRIC) study. *Am J Kidney Dis* 65:412–424, 2015.
806. Rezonzew G, Chumley P, Feng W, et al: Nicotine exposure and the progression of chronic kidney disease: role of the alpha7-nicotinic acetylcholine receptor. *Am J Physiol Renal Physiol* 303:F304–F312, 2012.
810. Coca SG, Singanamala S, Parikh CR: Chronic kidney disease after acute kidney injury: a systematic review and meta-analysis. *Kidney Int* 81:442–448, 2012.
812. Venkatachalam MA, Weinberg JM, Kriz W, et al: Failed tubule recovery, AKI-CKD transition, and kidney disease progression. *J Am Soc Nephrol* 2015. pii:ASN.2015010006. [Epub Mar 25, 2015].
814. Polichnowski AJ, Lan R, Geng H, et al: Severe renal mass reduction impairs recovery and promotes fibrosis after AKI. *J Am Soc Nephrol* 25:1496–1507, 2014.

53 Mechanisms and Consequences of Proteinuria

Norberto Perico | Andrea Remuzzi | Giuseppe Remuzzi

CHAPTER OUTLINE

MECHANISMS OF PROTEINURIA, 1780
Structure and Function of the Glomerular Capillary Wall, 1780
Protein Reabsorption by the Proximal Tubule, 1784
Proteinuria of Glomerular Origin, 1785
Tubular Handling of Excessive Filtered Proteins, 1786
RENAL CONSEQUENCES OF PROTEINURIA, 1786
Glomerular Damage, 1786

Tubular Damage, 1790
Interstitial Inflammation and Injury, 1792
Endogenous Systems of Tissue Repair, 1794
SYSTEMIC CONSEQUENCES OF NEPHROTIC-RANGE PROTEINURIA, 1796
Hypoalbuminemia, 1796
Edema Formation, 1798
Hyperlipidemia, 1801
Hypercoagulability, 1803
Susceptibility to Infection, 1805

MECHANISMS OF PROTEINURIA

One of the most common features of glomerular diseases is an abnormal excretion of plasma proteins in the urine. Proteinuria is the cause and effect of several complications not only at the kidney but also at the systemic level. Complex changes in the structure and function of the glomerular capillary, as well as the entire nephron, are responsible for the final elevation in urine protein concentration in several kidney disorders. In this chapter, before the consequences of proteinuria are described, the pathophysiology of protein excretion is reviewed.

Functional properties of the glomerular filtration barrier, tubular interaction with filtered proteins, and the mechanisms of proteinuria have been reviewed in detail,[1] and characterization of structural molecules relevant to the filtration barrier in glomerular endothelial cells and in particular on podocytes has been reported.[2,3] There are in principle two distinct phenomena that can result in proteinuria. The first is elevation of glomerular filtration of circulating plasma proteins that are almost completely retained in the circulating plasma in physiologic conditions; the second is a defective or incomplete reabsorption of proteins by the proximal tubule. The two phenomena are interrelated, and likely are both present in so-called glomerular proteinuria, in which proteins in the urine are the size of albumin and larger. Despite several experimental and clinical observations investigating the structural and molecular alterations involved in kidney diseases that result in proteinuria,[4] the precise nature of the functional changes responsible and their quantification remain the subject of numerous ongoing investigations.[5]

STRUCTURE AND FUNCTION OF THE GLOMERULAR CAPILLARY WALL

The function of the glomerular capillary is to allow a large amount of water and small solute filtration while efficiently restricting glomerular passage of protein macromolecules within the blood circulation. This selective function is specific to the glomerular capillary membrane, which is far more permeable to water than any other capillary membrane in the body. With the development of glomerular diseases the capillary membrane structure at molecular and/or cellular level may be altered, resulting in loss of hydraulic permeability, reduction in surface area available for filtration, and consequent reduction in glomerular filtration rate (GFR). Despite the reduction in permeability to water, the capillary membrane often becomes more permeable to circulating macromolecules. Experimental research has elucidated a number of glomerular structural and molecular alterations that are responsible for these functional changes.

GLOMERULAR CAPILLARY WALL ORGANIZATION

Morphologic studies available in the literature describe in detail the complex organization of the glomerular capillary and the capillary membrane (see Chapter 2); however, the interpretation of filtration barrier function has been largely based on major simplifications. Thus, although the glomerular capillary comprises numerous branching segments, the glomerular capillary organization has usually been considered a simple capillary segment or a set of several uniform segments in parallel. Similarly, the capillary membrane has been considered a uniform three-layer structure. As described later, investigations now allow a better understanding of the functional effects of geometric and spatial organization of the glomerular capillary as well as of specific features of cell organization and interactions at the capillary membrane level. These aspects have revealed some new insights into the mechanisms responsible for glomerular capillary dysfunction.

Glomerular Capillary Network

According to classic optical microscopy observations of kidney tissue sections, the capillary network is composed of a number of capillary segments connecting afferent and efferent arterioles within a tuft that, in humans, has a mean diameter of 120 to 150 μm. More realistic and direct visualizations of the capillary organization are usually derived from scanning electron microscopy, but this technique allows predominantly views only from the outer surface of the capillary. Specific investigations with reconstructions from serial sections[6] or confocal microscopy[7] allow investigation of capillary segment organization and, in particular, calculation of blood flow distribution and water filtration along the network.[8] Owing to the large number of capillary segments, around 200 in the rat, and their apparent uniform size, the blood flow is expected to be uniformly distributed along the network with lower blood velocity than that in afferent arterioles. This hemodynamic arrangement allows the blood to remain in close contact with the filtration membrane. However, more detailed geometric reconstructions of the glomerular capillary show that the network has some heterogeneity. The size of some capillary segments (with a diameter less than 3-4 μm)[6] would suggest that they are perfused only by plasma, excluding red blood cell transit, and may represent a sort of shunt in the network to decrease overall network pressure. This finely organized geometry is the result of cellular organization and remodeling and seems to be importantly affected by disease processes, which result in simplification of the capillary network and changes in local pressure and flow distribution, ultimately leading to capillary obliteration in areas of segmental sclerosis.[9] These local hemodynamic changes affect the filtration function of the capillary network, because elevation of blood flow and hydraulic pressure is expected to occur in some capillary segments, leading to abnormal filtration of circulating proteins.[10]

Glomerular Capillary Wall

On a smaller scale the organization of the glomerular capillary membrane is rather heterogeneous. The arrangement that is generally described usually refers to the portion of the capillary wall that is considered the filtering surface, characterized by the three-layer composition consisting of endothelial cells, glomerular basement membrane (GBM), and epithelial cells. The structure and function of this highly differentiated arrangement of cells and matrix are presented in Chapter 2. Mechanisms whereby structural and functional changes may result in abnormal protein filtration and ultimately to proteinuria are reviewed later.

According to the classic concept, hydraulic resistance and macromolecule retention are functions of the so-called filtering surface of the glomerular capillary membrane, but newer evidence indicates that the entire structure of the epithelial cells and the relative position of capillary membrane within the tuft may also affect water and macromolecule filtration. As reported by Neal and coworkers, a large fraction of the filtration membrane is actually covered by epithelial cell bodies or by the presence of adjacent epithelial cells.[11] The three-dimensional spaces created by these structures have been called subpodocyte space (SPS) and interpodocyte space (IPS), respectively. Theoretical analysis of the transport of both water and macromolecules through the SPS indicates that structural organization of this compartment induces significant resistance to water flow from the filtration membrane to the urinary space.[12] This resistance appears to be not insignificant in comparison with that of the three-layer membrane structure. Macromolecule transport may also be influenced by the SPS.[13]

Specific evaluations of the structural changes that characterize SPS and IPS, and their functional consequence in experimental models of kidney disease or in patients with renal dysfunction, are not yet available. The difficulties in obtaining such quantitative evaluations derive from the heterogeneous nature of these three-dimensional structures. In addition, they can be visualized only with use of electron microscopy, both transmission electron microscopy (TEM) and scanning electron microscopy (SEM), but their quantification is not easy because they are located in the inner portion of the glomerular capillary tuft.[14]

ULTRASTRUCTURE OF THE GLOMERULAR CAPILLARY MEMBRANE

Endothelial Cell Layer

Glomerular endothelial cells are the most fenestrated in the circulation, with a pore area in the peripheral zone that occupies from 20% to 50% of the cell surface.[15] The surface of endothelial cells has been considered to have negative electric charge because of the presence of the electrical charges of glycoproteins, glycosaminoglycans, and membrane-associated proteoglycans (glycocalyx).[16] These negative charges are expected to act as a barrier to the interaction of anionic circulating proteins such as albumin. Thus, even if endothelial fenestrae are much larger than albumin (about 60 nm in diameter, in comparison with a diameter of 7.2 nm for albumin), negatively charged circulating macromolecules stay away from the endothelial surface because of electrical repulsion and remain within the circulation. It is now evident that the first restriction to albumin filtration across glomerular membrane consists in the endothelial surface layer and that its role is to substantially decrease protein concentration in the fluid that enters the GBM layer.[1] Endothelial cell glycocalyx expression is significantly affected by fluid shear stress.[17] Increased shear stress is associated with glycocalyx formation and reorganization on the cell surface in contact with fluid flow, with lower expression in static conditions. Thus, pathologic conditions in which changes in glomerular capillary flow may occur are expected to decrease glycocalyx formation and consequently reduce the retention of anionic proteins within the bloodstream.

It has been demonstrated that disruption of the endothelial glycocalyx increases glomerular albumin filtration even in the presence of only minor changes in both the GBM and glomerular epithelial cells.[18] The role of the glomerular polysaccharide-rich endothelial surface layer (ESL) to act as a filtration barrier for large molecules such as albumin has been confirmed in C57BL/6 mice given long-term infusions of hyaluronidase, a hyaluronan-degrading enzyme that disrupts the endothelial glycocalyx proteoglycans.[19,20] An electron microscopy technique that allows visualization of the ESL and albumin transport within the entire glomerular section at nanometer resolution was used in this set of experiments.[21] The study showed that glomerular fenestrae are filled with dense negatively charged polysaccharide structures that are largely removed in the presence of circulating hyaluronidase, leaving the polysaccharide surfaces of other glomerular cells intact.[19] Both retention of cationic ferritin in the GBM and systemic blood pressure were unaltered. In hyaluronidase-treated animals, however, albumin passed across the endothelium in 90% of glomeruli, whereas this process could not be observed in untreated control animals. Nevertheless, there was no net albuminuria because of binding and uptake of filtered albumin by the podocytes and parietal epithelium. The ESL structure and function completely recovered after cessation of hyaluronidase infusion. Thus the polyanionic ESL component hyaluronan is a key component of the glomerular endothelial permeability barrier whose reduction facilitates albumin passage across the endothelial layer and the GBM toward the epithelial compartment.

Organization of the Glomerular Basement Membrane

The basement membrane layer that characterizes the capillary wall (see Chapter 2) has been shown to make an important contribution to protein retention by the capillary wall. The molecular composition and organization of this basement membrane suggest a sieving function based on both size and charge.[22] Structural proteins such as collagen type IV and laminin, as well as heparan sulfate proteoglycans, represent not only a steric hindrance but also exert a charge effect on the filtration of circulating molecules. In vivo and in vitro studies indicate that small neutral and charged solutes are freely filtered across this extracellular matrix layer but an important restriction is observed for macromolecules the size of albumin or larger.[23] Thus, changes in composition and/or organization of GBM molecules are expected to reduce water filtration and retention of circulating macromolecules.[24] The role of the GBM in glomerular permselectivity is highlighted by the discovery of mutations affecting genes encoding GBM components in humans and mouse models.[25] Mutations in the *COL4A3*, *COL4A4*, or *COL4A5* genes that encode collagen type IV α3, α4, and α5 chains, respectively, cause Alport's syndrome, a hereditary glomerular, auditory, and ocular disease.[26] Mutations in the gene encoding laminin β2 (*LAMB2*) cause Pierson's syndrome, a congenital nephrotic syndrome with associated extrarenal manifestations.[27] Studies using knockout mouse models of Alport's and Pierson's syndromes have documented that GBM lacking these specific components is more permeable to ferritin or albumin than the normal GBM, indicating it has a role in glomerular permselectivity.[28,29]

Epithelial Filtration Slits

A large amount of experimental and clinical research has been generated in the last few decades on the molecular and structural composition of the epithelial junctional complex, known as *filtration slits*. The characterization of several molecular components of this structure has allowed detailed definition of the proteins that compose the filtration slits (Figure 53.1)[30]; however, detailed information on the ultrastructure of this intracellular junction is still under investigation.[5] The original observations by Rodewald and Karnowsky[31] suggested a zipper-like structure of the epithelial filtration slit, with 4-nm by 14-nm rectangular openings. These dimensions are in contrast with the observation that a limited amount of albumin can traverse the filtration barrier in physiologic conditions,[1] because the mean molecular radius of albumin is 3.6 nm. Observations with high-resolution SEM and three-dimensional (3D) electron microscopy reconstruction suggest that the filtration slits are perforated by larger openings of the size of albumin, with more complex geometry.[32] The morphology of the filtration slit has been further imaged with high-resolution SEM, providing evidence of a new ultrastructure composed of circular pores of different sizes with an average radius of 12 nm (Figure 53.2).[33] Despite the small size of filtration slit openings, a large amount of plasma water is filtered because of the high filtration slit length per unit surface area. As

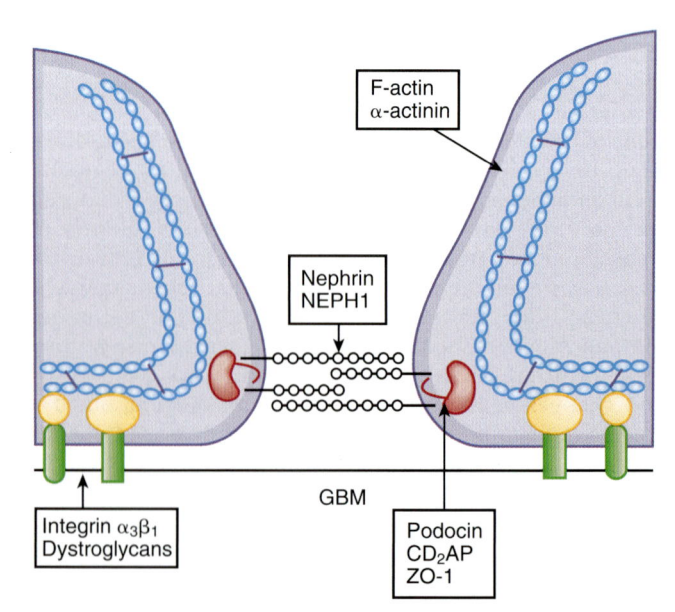

Figure 53.1 Hypothetical model of the podocyte slit diaphragm. See text for discussion. CD₂AP, CD (cluster of differentiation 2)–associated protein; GBM, glomerular basement membrane; NEPH1, a nephrin-like protein; ZO-1, tight junction protein-1. (From Jalanko H: Pathogenesis of proteinuria: lessons learned from nephrin and podocin, *Pediatr Nephrol* 18:487-491, 2003.)

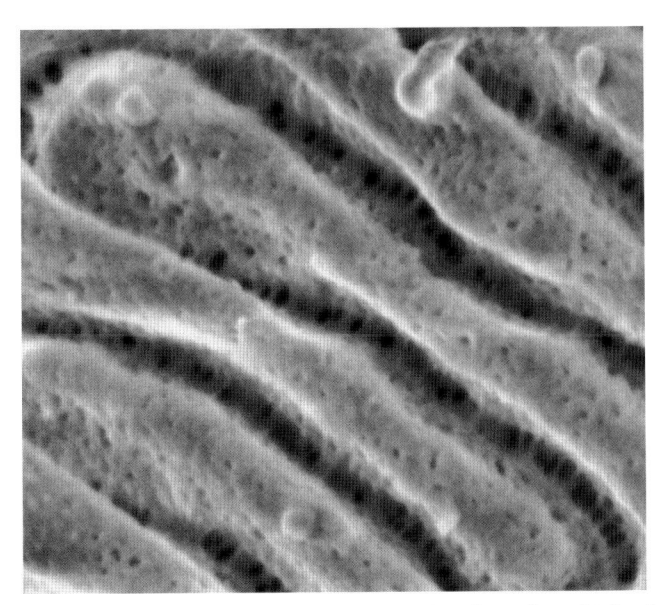

CHAPTER 53 — MECHANISMS AND CONSEQUENCES OF PROTEINURIA

Figure 53.2 Visualization of epithelial filtration slits obtained using scanning electron microscopy and an in-lens detector to enhance electron detection. The sample was obtained from a Wistar rat and dehydrated with a critical point dryer. The ultrastructure of the filtration slit appears different from the model conventionally proposed in the literature (see Rodewald and Karnovsky[31]). The radius of the circular pores averages 12 nm. (From Gagliardini E, Conti S, Benigni A, et al: . Imaging of the porous ultrastructure of the glomerular epithelial filtration slit, *J Am Soc Nephrol* 21: 2081-2089, 2010).

mentioned earlier, under physiologic conditions about 20% of peripheral capillary filtering surface is directly in communication with Bowman's space, and the epithelial slits are the last resistance encountered by water and filtered solutes.[11] In the remaining portion of the glomerular membrane water and solutes, after passing through the filtration slits, must traverse the SPS and the IPS before arriving in Bowman's capsule.[11]

THEORETICAL MODELS OF GLOMERULAR PERMSELECTIVITY

In addition to structural investigation, functional evaluations of the glomerular capillary wall have been extensively used to characterize physiologic conditions and to quantify the effect of pathologic changes. These studies are based on the estimation of filtration of endogenous plasma molecules, such as albumin, immunoglobulin G (IgG) and other proteins, or on the use of test macromolecules of different size, either neutral or electrically charged. Macromolecule filtration depends on convective and diffusive transport, which is influenced by glomerular hemodynamic conditions (flow and pressure) and water filtration. As described later, several investigators developed theoretical models to derive intrinsic sieving properties of the capillary wall from estimation of macromolecule filtration in both experimental and human studies.

Heteroporous Models of Glomerular Size-Selectivity

The most widely used theoretical models of glomerular size-selective function are based on the assumption that water-filled pores of different sizes are functional equivalents of the glomerular membrane. The passage of water is calculated along the network by taking into account the balance between hydraulic pressure and oncotic pressure as well as membrane hydraulic permeability.[9,34] For the calculation of solute filtration, convective and diffusive transport are taken into account, whereas pore resistance to solute filtration is based on steric and hydrodynamic hindrance.[10,34] The use of these models indicated that glomerular hypothetical pores have mean radius of 4.5 to 5.0 nm in humans, and a statistical distribution of pore size log normally distributed around the mean. However, the best simulation of experimental measurements has been obtained on the assumption that in parallel to restrictive pores, there is a nonselective shunt pathway.[35]

Application of these theoretical models clearly showed that in several proteinuric conditions the increased glomerular filtration of neutral test macromolecules was associated not with important change in the size of restrictive pores but rather with changes in the nonselective shunt pathway.[36] This finding suggests that in normal conditions the small amount of albumin present in the urine may be the result of a small amount of protein filtration that takes place in some focal area of the epithelial junction, while most of the filtration slits retain the protein.

Fiber Models of Glomerular Size-Selectivity

Fiber models of solute filtration across the glomerular membrane have also been developed and used.[1] Similar to porous models, the fiber models allow separation of the effect of glomerular hemodynamic changes from those related to intrinsic changes of glomerular membrane selective properties. The advantage of the fiber model is that, in addition to steric hindrance, the effect of membrane and protein electrical charge can be embedded in the model, allowing estimation of changes in membrane properties in terms of both molecular structural organization and electrical charge.[37] This modeling approach indicates that filtration of albumin is significantly affected by electrical charge, whereas on the basis of size-selectivity alone the molecule could easily escape the capillary membrane.

Multilayer Membrane Models

The structural complexity of the glomerular capillary wall suggested a need to develop more complex theoretical models to more reliably simulate the resistance to water and solute movement across the membrane. These models have been developed and tested by Edwards and colleagues[22] with the aim of estimating the role of individual layers on the filtration of water and solutes. In these models the resistance of endothelial cells, GBM, and epithelial cells is assumed to act in series. In normal conditions hydraulic resistance of endothelial layer is negligible, and GBM and epithelial resistances are comparable. The contribution of the three layers to solute hindrance has been considered and the major contribution to membrane selectivity is exerted by the filtration slit.[38] Although these models describe in detail the physical interaction of water and macromolecules with the membrane structure, their application is difficult because they require extensive measurement of structural parameters.

Models of Glomerular Charge-Selectivity

As mentioned previously, the fact that negative electrical charges are present in the glomerular membrane (in the glycocalyx of endothelial cells, the negatively charged heparan sulfate of the GBM, and the glycoproteins of the cell membrane of podocytes) strongly suggests that circulating proteins that are negatively charged, like albumin, are restricted within the circulation not only for their size but also for electrical charges. The use of theoretical models for the simulation of the charge-selective function of the glomerular membrane allowed estimation of the amount of electrical charge present within the membrane.[10] These studies indicated that electrical charge is an important component of glomerular permselective function and that changes in membrane electrical charge can explain abnormal albumin filtration even without changes in membrane structural parameters such as pore size, fiber size, and length per unit volume. However, the use of these models to investigate glomerular membrane charge is limited by the difficulties in measuring glomerular filtration of charged test solutes that interfere with circulating macromolecules and are not filtered simply on the basis of their molecular shape and electric charge alone.[39]

PROTEIN REABSORPTION BY THE PROXIMAL TUBULE

PROXIMAL TUBULE STRUCTURE AND FUNCTION

The glomerular ultrafiltrate, once flowing inside the proximal tubule, undergoes important changes in composition owing to processes of water and solute reabsorption. In addition to small solutes and electrolytes, proteins such as albumin are reabsorbed.[39] Thus, final urinary excretion of proteins depends largely on the interaction of proteins with proximal tubular epithelial cells. These cells form a compact epithelial layer with a basal side in contact with tubular basement membrane, an intercellular junction, and a luminal surface in contact with tubular fluid. They are characterized by large number of mitochondria, an index of important metabolic activity, and a prominent layer of microvilli (Figure 53.3) that results in the extension of the luminal cell surface area.

The microvillar membrane is the site for receptor-mediated endocytosis of low-density lipoprotein and negatively charged proteins. Albumin in the proximal tubule undergoes specific binding to the extracellular domain of a membrane receptor complex, megalin-cubilin receptor[40] (Figure 53.4), and following that, internalization of the protein by membrane vesicles. These vesicles are then processed for protein degradation, amino acid transport to basal membrane of tubular cells, and release into the interstitial space and ultimately into the peritubular capillaries. Receptors are recycled to luminal cell membrane by dense apical tubules.

The amount of filtered albumin at glomerular level and that reabsorbed by proximal tubular cells are not easy to quantify. Ideally one would have to sample the early proximal tubule and quantify albumin concentration in the microsamples. Despite technical difficulties, micropuncture techniques have been used to avoid sample contamination with plasma present very near the puncture site (in interstitial space and peritubular capillaries). The protein concentration in the urinary space was estimated to range from 10 to 25 µg/mL.[41,42] In a later study, direct in vivo imaging of fluorescent albumin by two-photon microscopy has been used to directly estimate albumin concentration in Bowman's capsule fluid.[43] It has also been demonstrated that reliable measurements of albumin fractional clearance, the ratio between urinary space and plasma albumin concentration, allow estimation of an albumin concentration of about 60 µg/mL in Bowman's capsule under normal conditions in the rat,[44] corresponding to a fractional clearance of 0.002. Once filtered at glomerular level, albumin and smaller proteins are almost entirely reabsorbed at the proximal tubular level. In pathologic conditions, when the filtered load overwhelms the reabsorptive capacity, proteins are detected in the urine.

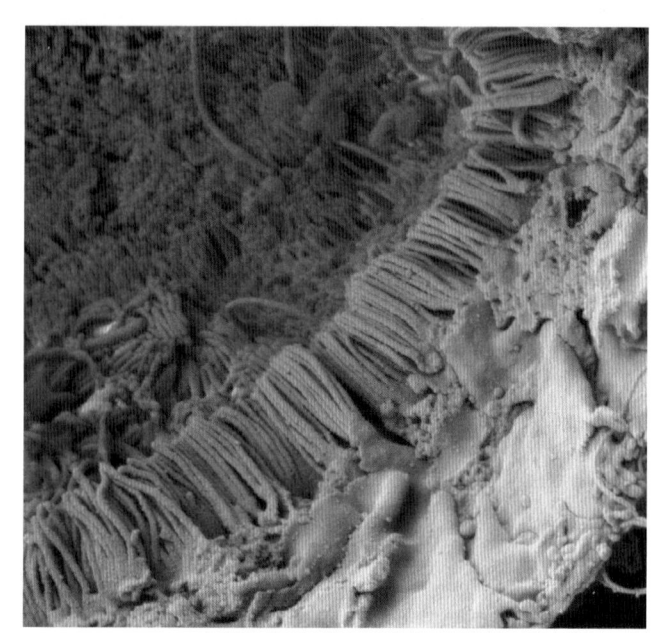

Figure 53.3 Scanning electron microscopy of proximal tubular cells. The inner cell membrane is covered by microvilli of the brush border. In order to be taken up by cell receptors, albumin must diffuse through the dense layer of microvilli.

THEORETICAL MODELS OF TUBULAR REABSORPTION

The process of albumin reabsorption by proximal tubular cells has been modeled to allow a quantitative assessment of the relationship between albumin ultrafiltration at glomerular level, proximal tubular uptake, and final excretion in the urine.[45] In this model the process of diffusion of albumin across the microvillar space and the uptake of the protein by tubular cell receptors are taken into consideration. The amount of albumin that is reabsorbed during proximal tubule passage is simulated, with the presence of a high-affinity site for binding and internalization of albumin at the base of tubular cell microvilli assumed. According to in vitro and ex vivo data, these receptors are assumed to be half-saturated at concentrations similar to those mentioned for albumin in Bowman's capsule (20-30 µg/mL). The effect of the assumption of different values for the maximum absorptive capacity (V_{max}) on the albumin concentration along the proximal tubule is reported in Figure 53.5. This modeling approach showed that the transport of albumin

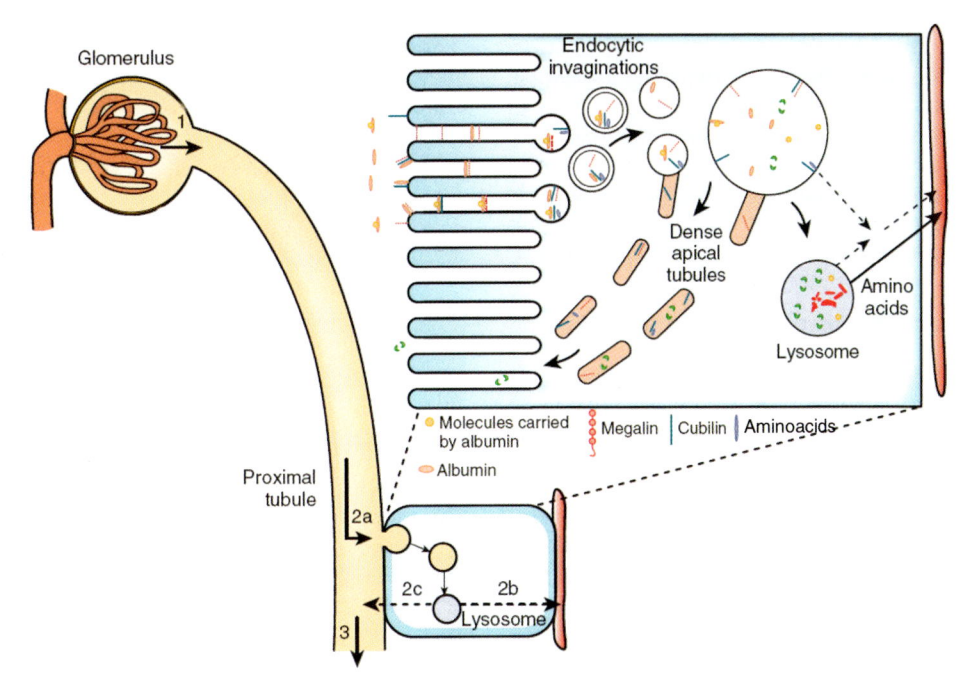

Figure 53.4 Pathways of albumin degradation in the proximal tubule. Albumin is filtered in the glomeruli (1) and reabsorbed by the proximal tubular cells by receptor-mediated endocytosis (2a). Internalization by endocytosis is followed by transport into lysosomes for degradation. Some intact albumin may escape tubular reabsorption (3), the amount being greater as the glomerular filtration fraction of albumin increases or tubular function is compromised. The upper right shows a schematic representation of the intracellular pathways following endocytic uptake of albumin and possible associated substances. After binding to the receptors, cubilin or megalin, the receptor-albumin complex is directed into coated pits for endocytosis. The complex dissociates following vesicular acidification, most likely also leading to the release of any bound substances. Albumin is transferred to the lysosomal compartment for degradation (2b). Some albumin may be degraded within a late endocytic compartment and recycled as fragments to be released at the luminal surface (2c). Alternatively, albumin fragments may be recycled from the lysosomal compartment by a yet unknown route. Receptors recycle through dense apical tubules, whereas released substances carried by albumin may be released into the cytosol or transported across the tubular cell. (From Birn H, Christensen EI: Renal albumin absorption in physiology and pathology, *Kidney Int* 69:440-449, 2006.)

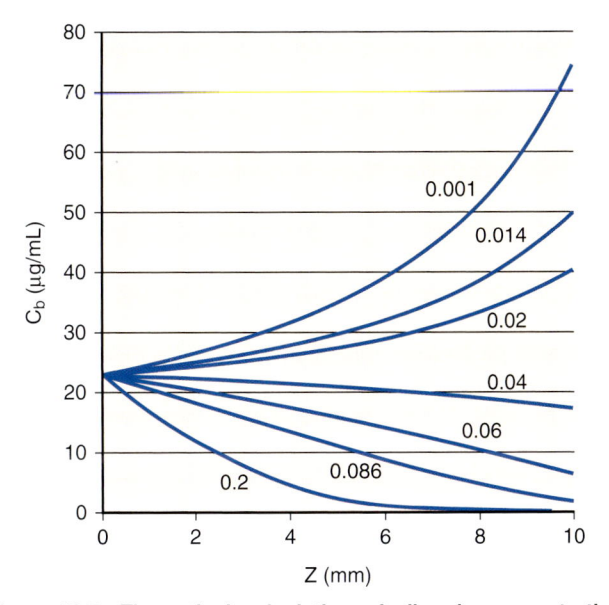

Figure 53.5 Theoretical calculation of albumin concentration along the proximal tubule. Predictions of bulk albumin concentration (C_b) vs. axial position (z) in rats for maximum uptake rate at receptor saturation (V_{max}) ranging from 0.001 to 0.2 ng/sec/mm². The curve that most closely corresponds to normal rats is that for V_{max} = 0.086 ng/sec/mm². (From Lazzara MJ, Deen WM: Model of albumin reabsorption in the proximal tubule, *Am J Physiol Renal Physiol* 292:430-439, 2007.)

across the microvillar space has a modest effect on the value of V_{max} needed to fit micropuncture data.

The two most important parameters that determine the fraction of reabsorption of albumin are the single-nephron GFR (SNGFR) and the bulk albumin concentration in the filtrate fluid (C_b). A 50% increase in SNGFR is predicted to cause a fourfold to fivefold increase in albumin excretion in the rats and humans. For large increases in C_b, such as those measured by micropuncture,[46] there is a threshold above which the reabsorption of albumin is overwhelmed, and the protein appears in the urine. According to theoretical analysis, this value corresponds to an albumin fractional clearance of approximately 0.001.[45] The combination of increased SNGFR and elevation in filtrate albumin concentration is shown to have important additive effects.

PROTEINURIA OF GLOMERULAR ORIGIN

Changes in glomerular protein filtration and/or defects in tubular reabsorption cause the appearance of proteins in the urine. At values exceeding 300 mg per day, or 200 mg/L, the condition is termed *proteinuria*. Smaller amounts of protein may appear in the urine in the early stages of progressive diseases, such as diabetic nephropathy. Albumin excretion between 30 and 300 mg/day (20-200 mg/L) was previously termed *microalbuminuria*.[47] Proteinuria is considered severe or in the "nephrotic range" when protein excretion is greater than 3.5 g/day.[1] When proteins in the urine have high molecular weight, they are considered to have glomerular origin. For proteins with low molecular weight, there is evidence that the defect causing proteinuria is likely related to abnormal proximal tubular reabsorption, often related to toxic damage of tubular cells.[48] Proteinuria associated with progressive kidney disease is predominantly of glomerular origin and mainly composed of plasma albumin. Mechanisms responsible for glomerular proteinuria are discussed in the next section.

GLOMERULAR PERMSELECTIVE DYSFUNCTION

As mentioned previously, abnormal plasma protein filtration at the glomerular level may be caused by a defect in both size-selectivity and charge-selectivity. Glomerular size-selective dysfunction has been extensively investigated in several kidney diseases with the use of neutral test macromolecules, usually neutral dextrans.[36,49] These studies demonstrated that in most cases there are statistically significant changes in fractional clearance of the largest test macromolecules while the fractional clearance (sieving coefficient) of molecules the size of albumin is unaltered. These data consistently indicate that permselectivity defects that are responsible for albumin filtration must be focal and probably due to changes in glomerular cell components, most likely the podocytes. These proteinuric conditions are frequently associated with podocyte foot process effacement and simplification, and likely with defective intercellular junctions.[50]

Quantification of the contribution of defects in charge-selectivity to proteinuria is more difficult. A few experimental and clinical investigations clearly indicate that proteinuria is indeed associated with abnormal filtration of charged macromolecules,[51,52] but these data have been questioned because electrically charged test or endogenous macromolecules in the circulation are expected to interfere with other circulating charged solutes and cell membranes.[1] This interference would result in the failure of measured fractional clearance to represent effective transport of probe macromolecules. However, even without direct evidence that glomerular membrane charge distribution is altered in proteinuric conditions, the evidence that glomerular albumin filtration is increased without important changes in the fractional clearance of test macromolecules of the same size strongly suggests a role for a charge-selectivity defect in proteinuria of glomerular origin.[36,52]

Experimental and clinical research has allowed identification of molecular defects underlying some genetic disorders associated with nephrotic syndrome. In Finnish-type nephropathy a defect in the nephrin gene *NPHS1* is responsible for glomerular dysfunction, proteinuria, and end-stage renal disease.[3,53] Similarly defects in other genes (*NPHS2, LMX1B*, and several others) have been shown to result in defective structure and function of filtration slit proteins or glomerular epithelial cells.[54]

Another condition in which proteinuria is manifest is ischemia-reperfusion injury.[55] Studies in kidney transplantation and in experimental settings suggest that abnormal elevation of proteins in the urine in this condition occurs without major changes in glomerular capillary membrane structure. The evidence indicates that ischemia is per se responsible for loss of glomerular endothelial glycocalyx, and the previously mentioned effect of fluid shear stress on endothelial cell glycocalyx would reinforce this evidence.[56] Thus, abnormal elevation of glomerular protein filtration may derive from selective changes in ultrastructure and function of membrane components.

TUBULAR HANDLING OF EXCESSIVE FILTERED PROTEINS

EFFECTS OF PROTEIN FILTRATION ON PROXIMAL TUBULAR CELLS

An excessive increase in albumin and other plasma protein filtration may result from defective glomerular capillary membrane and/or increase in SNGFR. Both conditions, and their combination, result in elevated protein concentration in the ultrafiltrate. These filtered proteins are expected not to be entirely reabsorbed by proximal tubular cells, because protein reabsorption is believed to operate near maximum under physiologic conditions.

The presence of high protein concentration within the renal tubule may influence the progression of disease processes. At least two phenomena are expected to occur. The first is related to the fact that if albumin is still present in tubular fluid at the end of the proximal tubule, its concentration increases substantially along the remaining portion of the nephron because of water reabsorption. Thus, protein concentration in distal tubule and collecting duct can reach very high values even for a small amount of protein filtered at glomerular level, with the possibility that these proteins may precipitate and form protein casts.[57] Tubular obstruction may then occur and the entire nephron function is lost, with complete loss of glomerular water filtration.

In addition, structural changes are expected to occur with tubular atrophy, disconnection of the tubule from Bowman's capsule, and structural changes in the glomerular capillary tuft. This condition is frequently observed in proteinuric kidney diseases at experimental and clinical level.[58]

Even before tubular obstruction, important functional changes are expected to occur in proximal tubular cells exposed to abnormal protein concentrations. The protein overload of these cells exposes them to increased workload, which can lead to loss of reabsorptive capacity due to loss of receptor activity.[59] In this condition the elevated protein concentration along the proximal tubule further increases owing to the lower level of absorption and the concomitant water reabsorption. Thus a vicious circle develops, inducing further damage in tubular cells and progressively higher protein concentration along the entire nephron. The consequences of this abnormal glomerular filtration of plasma proteins at both organ and systemic levels are discussed in the following sections.

RENAL CONSEQUENCES OF PROTEINURIA

GLOMERULAR DAMAGE

Data from animal models have shown that a wide variety of insults results in a common pathway of glomerular capillary hypertension, increased permeability with excess passage of proteins across the glomerular capillary wall, and progressive glomerular injury[60] (Figure 53.6). The key glomerular lesion is sclerosis, characterized by accumulation of

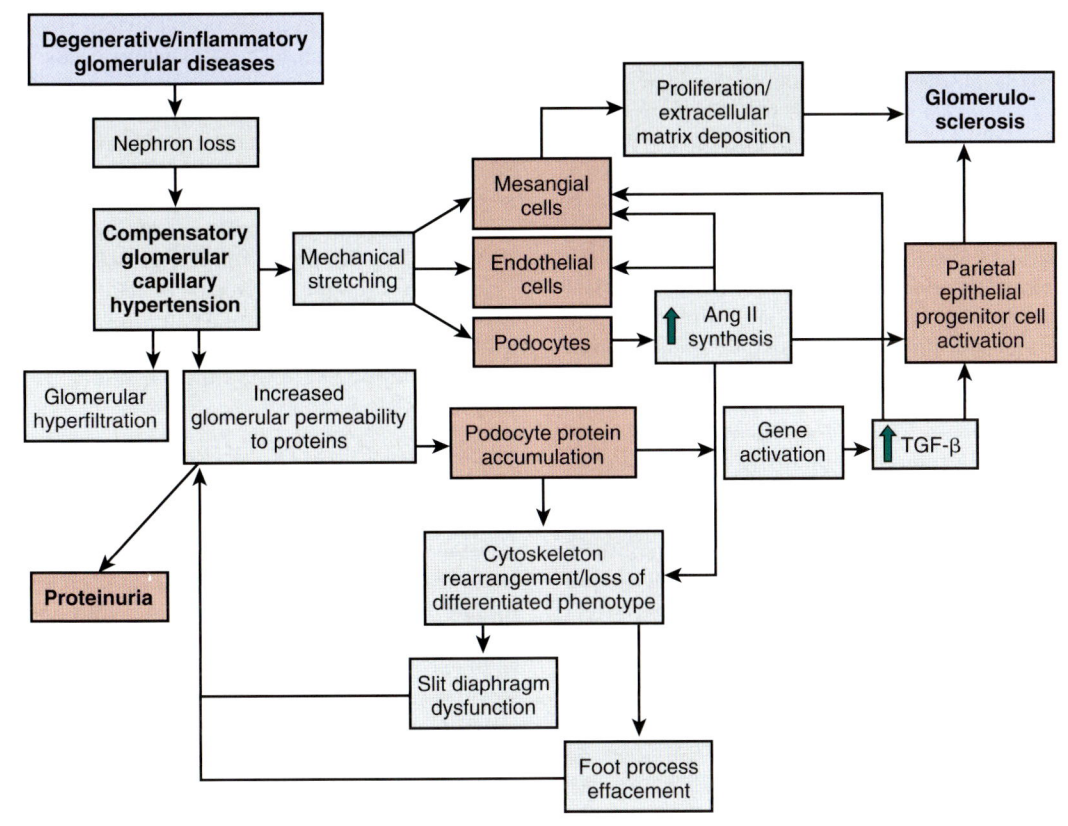

Figure 53.6 **Mechanisms of progressive glomerular injury.** A reduction in the number of nephrons as a consequence of various glomerular diseases results in compensatory glomerular hemodynamic changes that are ultimately detrimental. In particular, by mechanical stretching, the increased glomerular capillary pressure directly injures glomerular cells. Glomerular hypertension also impairs the glomerular capillary size-selective function, which causes excessive protein ultrafiltration and, eventually, podocyte injury and proteinuria. Ang II, angiotensin II; TGF-β, transforming growth factor-β; ⇧, increased.

extracellular matrix and obliteration of the capillary tuft leading to the loss of renal function.

PODOCYTES: CHANGES IN FUNCTION AND CELL NUMBER

Podocytes show a fairly uniform pattern of response to damage. The intercellular junction and cytoskeletal structure of the foot processes are altered, and the cell shows a simplified, effaced phenotype.[61,62] These alterations result in the disappearance of the typical slit diaphragm structures and the development of proteinuria. Although podocyte effacement is a hallmark of podocyte disease and nephrotic syndrome, damage to these cells may manifest as very subtle changes that are difficult to quantify.[63] Major advances in the field of live imaging have allowed the investigation of podocyte biology in unprecedented detail.[64-66] These new tools are likely to facilitate the next stage in gaining insights into podocyte responses to injury. So far there is evidence that experimental models of chronic proteinuria as well as their human counterparts (that is, minimal change glomerulopathy, focal and segmental sclerosis, diabetic nephropathy, and membranous nephropathy) have in common ultrastructural findings of severe glomerular epithelial cell damage that include vacuolization, fusion of foot processes, and focal detachment of epithelial cells from the underlying basement membrane.[67] These changes appear to be the consequence mainly of persistent abnormalities in intraglomerular capillary hemodynamics.

Increased capillary hydraulic pressure and flow, as well as activation of local tissue renin angiotensin system in podocytes,[68] eventually impairs the size-selective function of the glomerular capillary wall, allowing excess plasma protein to move into the urinary space.[69]

Besides being affected by mechanical stress, podocytes are damaged by excessive protein load resulting from alterations of glomerular permeability to macromolecules. Protein uptake by podocytes may occur through binding to megalin, a receptor for albumin and immunoglobulin light chains that is endocytosed after ligand binding, as shown in cultured murine podocytes.[70] Mice with protein overload proteinuria induced by repeated injections of bovine serum albumin demonstrated podocyte injury followed by glomerulosclerosis.[71-73] Evidence of a causal link between podocyte protein overload and podocyte damage is provided by studies showing that in rats with renal mass reduction, protein accumulation in podocytes preceded cell dedifferentiation and injury, as characterized by loss of synaptopodin and an increase in desmin expression.[74]

Podocyte abnormalities were accompanied by upregulation of transforming growth factor-β (TGF-β) messenger RNA (mRNA) and enhanced production of the related protein.[74] In vitro, albumin loading of immortalized mouse podocytes promoted actin-cytoskeleton rearrangement and upregulation of intracellular transduction signals, such as activating protein-1 (AP-1), which is a known stimulus of TGF-$β_1$ synthesis.[75]

Podocytes possess a complex contractile structure composed of F-actin microfilaments, which are most abundant in the foot process, connected with adaptor molecules that anchor the slit diaphragm proteins and $\alpha_3\beta_1$ integrins, transmembrane proteins that form focal adhesion complexes and mediate podocyte-GBM matrix interaction.[76,77] In vitro, actin filament disorganization, as occurs after albumin loading of mouse podocytes,[75] is closely associated with changes in podocyte shape that affect cell adhesion to the extracellular matrix. Podocyte detachment from the GBM likely underlies the decrease in podocyte number in proteinuric glomerular diseases that has been demonstrated in many experimental and clinical studies.[78,79]

Apoptosis is considered an additional cause of podocyte loss in proteinuric glomerulopathies. Once detached from the GBM, podocytes become extremely susceptible to apoptosis.[61] Furthermore, apoptosis may be promoted by locally produced proapoptotic factors. Studies have demonstrated that exogenous TGF-β_1–induced apoptosis in cultured podocytes via the p38 mitogen–activated protein kinase (MAPK) and classic caspase-3 pathways.[80] This effect occurred only in wild-type, not in p21-null cultured podocytes, indicating that the cyclin-dependent kinase (CDK) inhibitor p21 is required for TGF-β_1–induced apoptosis.[81] Of note, like TGF-β_1, p21 is increased in podocytes in experimental models of membranous nephropathy[82] and diabetic nephropathy.[83] In summary, protein accumulation in podocytes induces TGF-β_1 production, leading to podocyte apoptosis.

Evidence now indicates that angiotensin II (Ang II) contributes to perpetuate podocyte injury in proteinuric nephropathies, eventually promoting progression to end-stage kidney disease.[84] Mechanical strain increases Ang II production and expression of angiotensin II type 1 (AT$_1$) receptors in podocytes,[68] potentially contributing to further sustaining the glomerular hypertension–induced damage in chronic kidney disease. However, there is also evidence that, independent of its hemodynamic effect, Ang II may directly impair the glomerular barrier sieving function, possibly through inhibition of podocyte expression of nephrin, the essential protein component of the glomerular slit diaphragm.[85,86] This observation has been confirmed in studies in diabetic animals showing that blockade of Ang II synthesis/activity preserved the expression of nephrin in the glomeruli and prevented overt proteinuria.[87,88] Thus, at least in diabetes, a pathogenetic relationship between Ang II and early proteinuria via functional podocyte alteration through modulation of nephrin protein level has been suggested. Moreover, in the setting of diabetes, after the initial insult of hyperglycemia and intraglomerular hypertension, Ang II plays a relevant role in sustaining glomerular injury via persistent activation of the transmembrane receptor Notch1 and upregulation of the transcription factor Snail in podocyte, eventually resulting in persistent downregulation of nephrin expression.[89] The consistency of these findings in Zucker diabetic fatty (ZDF) rats with overt nephropathy and in patients with type 2 diabetes and established nephropathy provides robust reason to infer an important role for the Ang II Notch1/Snail axis in perpetuating podocyte damage.

A crosstalk with proximal tubular cells has been suggested to contribute to podocyte function through the release of nicotinamide mononucleotide (NMN), a suggestion that might have implications for persistent podocyte dysfunction in proteinuric diseases.[90] In a mouse model, diabetes induced downregulation of Sirtuin 1 (Sirt1), a highly conserved protein deacetylase in proximal tubules.[91] The low Sirt1 expression reduces the release of NMN by tubular cells, eventually decreasing local NMN concentrations. In vitro studies have shown that in the absence of NMN the expression of the tight junction protein claudin-1 in podocytes is no longer silenced.[90] Claudin-1 is reported to activate the intracellular β-catenin–Snail pathway[92] that eventually leads to glomerular barrier dysfunction through downregulating synaptopodin or podocin expression in podocytes.[93]

MESANGIAL CELLS: PROLIFERATION AND DEPOSITION OF EXTRACELLULAR MATRIX

Because it is close to the capillary lumen, the mesangium may be exposed to macromolecules crossing the endothelial layer, although under normal conditions they do not accumulate.[94] However, in rats having undergone unilateral nephrectomy[95] or in puromycin-aminoglycoside–induced nephrosis,[96] intravenous infusion of colloidal carbon leads to the accumulation of the macromolecular tracer in the mesangial space. To prevent accumulation of proteins, mechanisms exist for their effective removal. These include transport along the mesangial stalk in cleftlike spaces as well as phagocytosis and degradation by mesangial cells.[97]

It has been shown that IgG and IgA can be taken up by both receptor-independent and receptor-mediated processes.[98] Another important factor for clearance of immunoglobulins from the mesangium may be complement factor D, a serine protease essential for activation of the complement system through the alternative pathway, which is constitutively expressed within the glomerulus.[99] Interestingly, in mice deficient in complement factor D, a mesangial immune complex deposition disease associated with albuminuria develops spontaneously.[100] This development indicates that complement factor D is necessary to prevent mesangial accumulation of immunoglobulin deposits.

Whether abnormal local accumulation of proteins promotes mesangial cell proliferation and mesangial matrix deposition remains, however, ill-defined. Nevertheless, the significance of the protein-clearing function of the mesangial cells has been illustrated by the deleterious consequences of mesangial immune complex accumulation—complement activation and generation of mediators of inflammation, such as reactive oxygen species, prostanoids, and cytokines such as tumor necrosis factor-α (TNF-α) and interleukin-6 (IL-6).[101]

The mesangial cell is a critical part of the glomerular functional unit, interacting closely with endothelial cells and podocytes.[99] Alterations in one cell type can produce changes in the others. As such, key survival factors for mesangial cells, including platelet-derived growth factor-B (PDGF-B) are generated by endothelial cells, and mesangiolysis has been shown in knockout mice lacking endothelial PDGF-B.[99] Whether cytokines generated by podocytes also influence mesangial cells has yet to be clearly defined, but the observation that podocyte injury frequently results in mesangial cell proliferation supports the existence of such cytokine crosstalk.[99]

Growth factors besides PDGF-B shown to influence mesangial cell proliferation and mesangial matrix accumulation include PDGF-C, fibroblast growth factor, hepatocyte growth factor, epidermal growth factor (EGF), connective tissue growth factor, and TGF-β.[99] Effects of vasoactive hormones such as Ang II on mesangial cell proliferation may be mediated indirectly through the generation of growth factors such as EGF.[102] In rats with renal mass ablation, glomerular TGF-$β_1$ upregulation is associated with phenotypic transformation of mesangial cells.[74] In vitro exposure of cultured murine mesangial cells to TGF-β induced a sclerosing phenotype, as shown by α-smooth muscle actin (SMA) expression, which was blocked by anti–TGF-$β_1$ antibodies.[74] Moreover, the transfection of the TGF-$β_1$ gene into normal kidneys in rats or the transgenic TGF-β expression in mice increased extracellular matrix accumulation in the mesangial space.[103]

ENDOTHELIAL CELLS: APOPTOSIS

Glomerular endothelial injury is a common feature of many human diseases, such as diabetic nephropathy, hypertension, thrombotic microangiopathy, and preeclampsia. Evidence has been provided that there is close crosstalk of podocytes with glomerular endothelial cells, a key interaction for the normal function of the glomerular capillary barrier.[104] The final steps in glomerular endothelial cell differentiation involve the formation of fenestrae, plasma membrane–lined circular pores that perforate the flattened glomerular endothelium.[105] The fenestrated phenotype of glomerular endothelial cells is induced by vascular endothelial growth factor (VEGF), a molecule constitutively expressed and secreted by podocytes.[104,105] That VEGF regulates fenestra formation was suggested by the observation that mature fenestrated endothelium is typically located adjacent to podocytes expressing high levels of VEGF mRNA.[106] There is also in vitro evidence that VEGF types A and C regulate glycosaminoglycan synthesis, its charge, and its shedding by glomerular microvascular endothelial cell glycocalyx.[107] Moreover, deletion of the podocyte-specific transcription factor LMX1B in mice, which results in the loss of many features of podocyte differentiation, including VEGF-A expression, is associated with failure of glomerular endothelium to differentiate and develop fenestrae.[108] Thus, loss of podocytes secondary to protein-induced cell injury may lead to reduced VEGF production, influencing glomerular endothelial fenestra formation and eventually leading to endothelial cell apoptosis.[109] How VEGF reaches endothelial cells against the urine flow is not yet known, however. Conversely, in vitro evidence has shown that blockade of VEGF in glomerular endothelial cells enhanced the release of endothelin-1 (ET-1), which induced nephrin shedding from podocytes,[110] leading to further dysfunction of glomerular protein permeability.

Taken together, these studies indicate that the toxic effects of excess plasma ultrafiltered proteins on podocytes may alter podocyte-endothelial interaction, thereby further enhancing glomerular permeability to proteins through a complex interplay of molecular signaling.

PARIETAL EPITHELIAL CELLS: ACTIVATION

Glomerular injury from multiple etiologies can lead to activation and accumulation of parietal epithelial cells within Bowman's space as a common response to damage,[111] as shown in several human proliferative glomerulonephritides. Although extracapillary proliferation is a relatively straightforward pathologic change to recognize, determining its cellular components has been more controversial. The traditional concepts, largely from immunoistochemical studies, indicate that the multilayered cellular lesions are a mixture of glomerular parietal epithelial cells, macrophages, and myofibroblasts,[112-114] the proportion of such cells in the lesion being variable. In both animal models and human tissues, parietal epithelial cells predominate when Bowman's capsule is intact. A heterogeneous population of renal progenitor cells, previously identified in normal human Bowman's capsule,[115] has been documented in hyperplastic lesions of human crescentic glomerulonephritis.[116] The extracapillary lesions could therefore be the result of dysregulated proliferation of renal progenitor cells in response to the injured podocytes.[116] This possibility is supported by findings in Munich Wistar Frömter rats, which are genetically programmed to undergo renal damage characterized by excessive migration and proliferation of progenitor cells, leading to their accumulation into cellular lesions and glomerulosclerosis.[117]

Parietal epithelial cells expressing the progenitor cell marker $CD133^+CD24^+$ have also been reported to proliferate and accumulate into the multilayered cellular lesions in patients with glomerulonephritides characterized by extracapillary proliferation but not in nonproliferative nephropathies such as membranous or diabetic nephropathies.[118] Upregulation of the CXCR4 chemokine receptor on these progenitor cells was found to be accompanied by high expression of its ligand, SDF-1, in podocytes.[118] Moreover, parietal epithelial cell proliferation was associated with increased expression of the Ang II subtype 1 receptor. Renin angiotensin system blockade normalized CXCR4 and Ang II subtype 1 receptor expression on parietal progenitor cells concomitant with regression of crescentic lesions. Together these findings suggest that the glomerular hyperplastic lesions derive from the proliferation and migration of renal progenitors in response to injured podocytes, and that the Ang II/AT_1 receptor pathway may contribute, together with SDF-1/CXCR4 axis, to the dysregulated response of parietal epithelial cell precursors.

Parietal epithelial cell activation is increasingly recognized and seems to be present also in most forms of focal segmental glomerulosclerosis (FSGS), characterized by nephrotic syndrome and often leading to a progressive decline in renal function.[119] A lineage tagging approach in mice has documented that activated parietal epithelial cells invade the affected segment of the capillary tuft and initiate glomerular and epithelial basement membrane adhesion and glomerulosclerosis.[120] Notch signaling pathway has been proposed to play a role in orchestrating parietal epithelial cell phenotypic changes in FSGS.[121] This possibility rests on in vitro evidence that in cultured mouse parietal epithelial cells, TGF-β enhanced Notch mRNA expression, leading to a significant upregulation of target genes associated with mesenchymal cell phenotype, such as SMA, vimentin, and Snail.[121] Concurrent inhibition of Notch signaling with the γ-secretase inhibitor DBZ blocked both epithelial-to-mesenchymal transition gene expression changes and cell migration in response to

TGF-β, demonstrating a dependence on Notch signaling for induction of mesenchymal gene marker activation in the parietal epithelial cell line.[122] Moreover, in LMB-2 antibody–treated NEP25 transgenic mice, a model of collapsing FSGS,[123] Notch inhibition in vivo significantly decreased parietal epithelial cell lesions, pointing to the role of Notch-mediated cell activation in the formation of such lesions.[121]

LOSS OF GLOMERULAR CAPILLARIES: POSTGLOMERULAR HYPOXIA

Irrespective of the underlying process leading to glomerular endothelial damage, such as increased intracapillary pressure and/or podocyte loss, the net result is rarefaction of glomerular capillaries. Loss of glomerular capillary loops translates into diminished postglomerular blood flow from affected glomeruli and downstream injury of the peritubular capillary network. Microvascular dysfunction causes progressive scarring of renal tissue by creating a hypoxic environment, which triggers a fibrotic response in tubulointerstitial cells.[124] This, in turn, has an impact on adjacent unaffected capillaries and glomeruli, further extending the hypoxic area and leading to a vicious circle of progressive destruction of the kidney and decline of renal function to end-stage organ failure.

Indeed, in animal models of proteinuric chronic kidney disease, including anti-Thy1 glomerulonephritis, 5/6 remnant kidney, diabetic nephropathy, and Adriamycin-induced nephrosis, the immunohistochemical detection of hypoxia-dependent pimonidazole protein adducts has shown that renal tissue hypoxia is present early in the course of the disease.[125] Moreover, blood oxygen–dependent magnetic resonance imaging has shown hypoxia in diabetic nephropathy.[126] Although data from animal models provide a compelling argument for postglomerular hypoxia in proteinuric diseases as a primary mediator of progressive renal scarring, data in humans are scarce. Nevertheless, that hypoxia-related injury also applies to humans may be deduced by the finding that there is increased expression of hypoxia-inducible factor (HIF)—a key regulator of the adaptive response to hypoxia controlling expression of hundreds of genes[127]—in biopsy specimens from patients with diabetic nephropathy, IgA nephropathy, and chronic allograft nephropathy.[128]

TUBULAR DAMAGE

Glomerular ultrafiltration of excessive amounts of plasma protein–associated factors incites tubulointerstitial damage and further promotes the effects of glomerular disease on the tubular compartment. The noxious substances in the proteinuric ultrafiltrate may set off tubular epithelial injury with tubular apoptosis, secondary generation of inflammatory mediators, and peritubular inflammation.[4] The mechanisms whereby increased urinary protein concentration leads to nephrotoxic injury are multifactorial and involve complex interactions among numerous pathways of cellular damage (Figure 53.7).

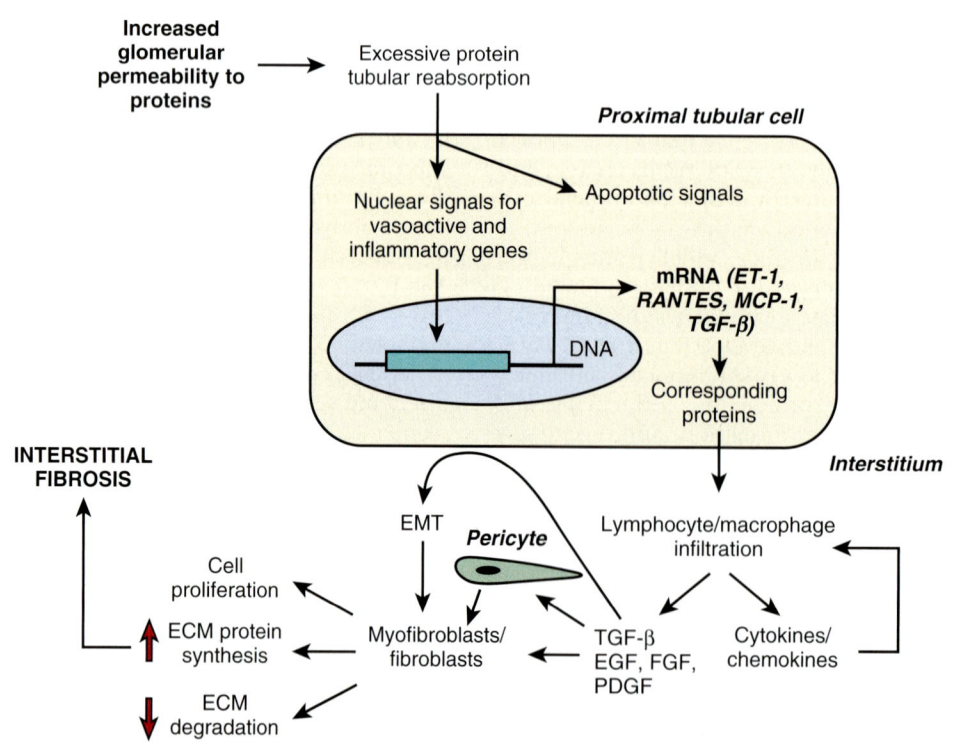

Figure 53.7 Mechanisms of tubulointerstitial damage induced by proteins. Protein overload of proximal tubular cells as a consequence of increased glomerular permeability to proteins activates intracellular signals that promote cell apoptosis or cause increased production of inflammatory and vasoactive mediators and of growth factors. These substances are released into the interstitium, inducing progressive inflammation and injury. ECM, extracellular matrix; EGF, epidermal growth factor; EMT, epithelial-to-mesenchymal transdifferentiation; ET-1, endothelin-1; FGF, fibroblast growth factor.; MCP-1, monocyte chemoattractant protein-1; PDGF, platelet-derived growth factor; RANTES, regulated upon activation, normal T cell expressed and secreted; TGF-β, transforming growth factor-β.

TUBULAR CELLS: APOPTOSIS AND TUBULOGLOMERULAR DISCONNECTION

Emerging evidence suggests that proteinuria causes tubular cell apoptosis. In cultured proximal tubular cells, de-lipidated albumin induced apoptosis in a dose- and time-dependent manner,[129] as characterized by internucleosomal DNA fragmentation, morphologic changes including cell shrinkage and nuclear condensation, and plasma membrane alterations.[129] Kidneys of rats with albumin-overload proteinuria[130] or with passive Heymann nephritis[58] showed increased numbers of terminal deoxynucleotidyl transferase (dUTP) nick-end labeling–positive apoptotic cells in the tubulointerstitial compartment. In tubules, most of the positive cells expressed Ang II subtype 2 (AT_2) receptors.[130] Findings of reduced phosphorylation of extracellular signal–regulated kinase (ERK) and Bcl-2 suggested an AT_2 receptor–mediated mechanism underlying tubular cell apoptosis.[130]

Apoptotic cells expressing both proximal and distal tubular phenotypes were detected in biopsy specimens from patients with primary FSGS.[131] A strong positive correlation was found between proteinuria and incidence of tubular cell apoptosis.[131]

Renal proximal tubular cells have a remarkable ability to reabsorb large quantities of albumin through clathrin- and megalin receptor–mediated endocytosis.[59] Megalin is the sensor that determines whether cells will be protected from or injured by albumin. It has been shown that megalin binds the serine/threonine kinase protein kinase B (PKB), which is crucial for the phosphorylation of Bad, the Bcl-2-associated death promoter.[132] Low concentrations of albumin lead to activated PKB and phosphorylation of the Bad protein, which inhibits apoptosis.[133] On the other hand, overload of albumin leads to a decrease in megalin expression on the plasma membrane of proximal tubular cells that is associated with reduction of PKB activity and Bad phosphorylation.[134] The result is albumin-induced apoptosis.

Proximal tubular cell apoptosis was found to contribute to tubuloglomerular disconnection and atrophy in response to proteinuria in animal models of proteinuric nephropathies.[58] Injured or dying cells release molecules that serve as danger signals.[135] Danger molecules trigger inflammation by engaging pattern recognition receptors such as Toll-like receptors (TLRs)[136] and nucleotide-binding domains, leucine-rich repeat-containing proteins (NLRs),[137] and are thus referred to as danger-associated molecular patterns (DAMPs).[138] Through TLRs, DAMPs signal cytokine and chemokine production and upregulate the expression of cell adhesion molecules. When DAMPs interact with NLRs, they stimulate NLRs to complex with apoptosis-associated speck-like proteins to form macromolecular complexes, the inflammasomes that cleave proinflammatory cytokines to their mature forms.[139] Thus, besides promoting tubuloglomerular disconnection, proximal tubular cell apoptosis contributes to create a local proinflammatory microenvironment.

TUBULAR CELLS: ACTIVATION

Receptor-mediated endocytosis of excessive proteins at the apical pole of the proximal tubular cells is also associated with phenotypic changes characteristic of an activated state.

Insights into specific mechanisms linking protein uptake to cell activation have come from in vitro studies using polarized proximal tubular cells to assess the effect of apical exposure to proteins. Collectively, they show that protein overload induces a proinflammatory phenotype.[140-143] Indeed upregulation of inflammatory and fibrogenic genes and production of related proteins have been reported following a challenge of proximal tubular cells with plasma proteins. They include cytokines and chemokines such as monocyte chemoattractant protein-1 (MCP-1), RANTES (regulated upon activation, normal T cell expressed and secreted), IL-8, and fractalkine.[140-143] Moreover, levels of the profibrogenic cytokine TGF-β and its type I receptor,[144] tissue inhibitors of metalloproteinase TIMP-1 and TIMP-2, as well as membrane surface expression of the $\alpha_v\beta_5$ integrin[145] were also highly increased in vitro upon stimulation by plasma proteins.

Investigations of the molecular mechanisms underlying chemokine and growth factor upregulation in proximal tubular cells on protein challenge have focused on the activation of transcription factor nuclear factor kappaB (NF-κB).[140] Other studies confirmed this pathway[146,147] and revealed reactive oxygen as a second messenger.[142,148]

Extrapolation from such in vitro data to the human situation may be difficult in light of the conflicting data observed with different proteins in different cell systems[149] as well as the reported changes in the expression of several genes of unknown function.[150] However, the in vitro observations have been confirmed through transcription analysis by complementary DNA (cDNA) microarray of renal proximal tubule epithelial cells isolated by laser capture microdissection from patients with proteinuric nephropathies.[151] More than 160 genes, including those encoding for signal transduction, transcription and translation, and apoptotic and inflammatory proteins, were identified as being regulated differently from those in proximal tubular cells from control subjects.

Evidence implicates megalin as a central element of the signaling pathway linking protein reabsorption and gene regulation in proximal tubular cells.[159] Megalin is subjected to regulated intramembrane proteolysis (RIP), an evolutionarily conserved process linking receptor function with transcriptional regulation.[153] Through RIP megalin is subjected to protein kinase C–regulated, metalloprotease-mediated ectodomain shedding, which produces a membrane-associated C-terminal fragment (MCTF).[152] The MCTF in turn forms the substrate for γ-secretase, which releases the C-terminal cytosolic domain. The latter translocates to the nucleus, where it interacts with other proteins to regulate expression of specific genes. This function may explain the phenotypic change in proximal tubules in proteinuric kidney disease.

As previously described, that megalin contributes to the early activation of proximal tubular cells in nonselective proteinuria has been documented in megalin-knockout/*NEP25* mice given immunotoxin LMB-2, a model for nephrotic syndrome, focal segmental glomerulosclerosis, and tubulointerstitial injury.[154] Megalin-deficient proximal tubular cells reabsorbed fewer proteins in vivo and expressed fewer tubular injury markers, such as MCP-1 and heme oxygenase 1.[154]

The proteinuric ultrafiltrate may also activate TLRs and promote an innate inflammatory immune response.[155] Besides being expressed by cells of the immune system, such as macrophages, dendritic cells, neutrophils, B cells, and natural killer cells, TLRs are expressed by nonimmune cells, including renal tubule epithelial cells.[155] The cellular effects of TLR include the production of proinflammatory cytokines and chemokines that contribute to local inflammation and leukocyte accumulation. It has been demonstrated that proximal tubule epithelial cells were sites of robust expression of TLR9 mRNA and protein—a receptor for CpG DNA—in (NZB × NZW)F1 lupus mice with overt nephropathy.[156] Upregulation of TLR9 expression was accompanied by the development of proteinuria and correlated with tubulointerstitial damage. Furthermore, abundant TLR-9 staining in proximal tubular cells of patients with lupus nephritis correlated with tubulointerstitial damage. Thus, tubular TLR activation may occur as a result of filtration of plasma proteins, which include immune complexes containing DNA enriched in CG motifs.[157,158]

The proximal tubule bears other receptors for ultrafiltered proteins, such as cytokines and growth factors.[4] Usually these molecules are present in high-molecular-weight precursor forms or bound to specific binding proteins that regulate their biologic activity. They can be found in nephrotic tubular fluid. In experimental proteinuria in rats there is translocation of insulin-like growth factor-1 (IGF-1) from plasma into tubular fluid (primarily as the 50-kDa complex).[159] Similarly, hepatocyte growth factor (HGF) is present in early proximal tubular fluid from rats with streptozotocin-induced diabetic nephropathy and excreted in the urine of diabetic animals.[160] Under physiologic conditions the high molecular weight of TGF-β complexes prevents glomerular ultrafiltration of this pluripotent cytokine. However, in proteinuric glomerular diseases, TGF-β is present in early proximal tubular fluid and at least a portion is bioactive.[160] IGF-1, HGF, and TGF-β are also present in the urine of patients with proteinuric diseases.[161]

Collectively the tubular response to these growth factors can be described as activation or as a moderate change toward a cell phenotype resembling cell injury, which includes a moderate increase in collagen type I and IV production in response to IGF-1[159] and upregulation of the expression of fibronectin by HGF.[162] TGF-β also increases the transcription in proximal tubular cells of the genes encoding collagen α_1III *(Col3A1)* and collagen α_2I *(Col1A2)* as well as fibronectin.

With proteinuria, a putative key factor in tubular cell activation and damage is the excess glomerular filtration of serum-derived complement C3, the central molecule in the complement system that exerts proinflammatory potential.[163] Renal tubule epithelial cells appear most susceptible to luminal attack by the C5b-9 membrane attack complex because of the relative lack of membrane-bound complement regulatory proteins, such as membrane cofactor protein (CD46), decay-accelerating factor (CD55), and CD59 on the apical surface.[164] In rats with severely reduced renal mass[165,166] or with protein overload proteinuria,[167] C3 co-localized with proximal tubular cells engaged in high protein uptake. By limiting the transglomerular passage of proteins, treatment with angiotensin-converting enzyme (ACE) inhibitors was an effective maneuver to reduce the C3 load of tubular cells in remnant kidneys.[165] C3 and other complement proteins are also found in proximal tubules in renal biopsy material from patients with nephrosis.[163,168]

Furthermore, proximal tubular cells are able to synthesize C3 and other complement factors[169] and to upregulate C3 in response to serum proteins in vitro.[170]

The injurious role of plasma-derived C3, as opposed to tubular cell–derived C3, has been documented in C3-deficient kidneys transplanted into wild-type mice.[167] Protein overload led to the development of glomerular injury, accumulation of C3 in proximal tubules, and tubulointerstitial changes. Conversely, when wild-type kidneys were transplanted into C3-deficient mice, protein overload led to a milder disease and abnormal C3 deposition was not observed. Thus, ultrafiltered C3 contributes more to tubulointerstitial damage induced by protein overload than locally synthesized C3.

INTERSTITIAL INFLAMMATION AND INJURY

In proteinuric kidney disease, progressive inflammation and injury to the renal interstitium are secondary events following glomerular or vascular injury. Tubular epithelial cells synthesize cytokines and chemokines and accumulate complement components that recruit inflammatory cells and lymphocytes into the interstitium causing progressive fibrosis.

RESIDENT MONOCYTE/DENDRITIC CELLS

The interstitium of normal kidneys contains numerous resident monocytic myelocytes, which express dendritic cell (DC) markers and can indeed present antigens.[171] DCs have been described to form an immune sentinel network through the entire kidney, where they probe the environment in search of antigens.[172] An inflammatory environment converts the tolerogenic status of resident DCs into an immunogenic one, favoring recruitment of T cells. It is known that cross-presentation by DCs is a major mechanism for the immune surveillance of tissue against foreign antigens.[173] In this process professional antigen-presenting cells, such as DCs, acquire proteins from other tissue cells through endocytic mechanisms, especially phagocytosis or macropinocytosis. The internalized antigen can then be processed and presented on major histocompatibility complex (MHC) class I molecules to the extracellular environment.[174] The outcome of cross-presentation with regard to immunity depends on the expression of immunostimulatory signals after the uptake of the antigen.[173]

In the past, the role of resident DCs that accumulate in the renal parenchyma of non–immune-mediated proteinuric nephropathies remained poorly understood. Later studies, however, provided new insights into the activation of DCs in the setting of proteinuria. Administration of ovalbumin—which is freely filtered by the glomerulus—to normal mice leads to concentration of the protein principally in proximal tubules and to its transfer to DCs in the kidney and renal lymph nodes.[175] Here, ovalbumin is presented to CD8+ T cells, thereby inducing proliferation of these cells.

The importance of kidney DC activation to renal injury has been demonstrated by the fact that in transgenic NOH mice (which selectively express the model antigens ovalbumin and hen egg lysozyme in podocytes), DC depletion resolved established periglomerular mononuclear infiltrates.[176] In vitro experiments have also shown that exposure of rat proximal tubular cells to excess autologous albumin, as in the case of proteinuric nephropathies, results in the formation of the N-terminal 24-residue fragment of albumin (ALB_{1-24}).[177] This peptide is taken up by DCs, where it is further processed by proteasomes into antigen peptides. These peptides were shown to have the binding motif for MHC class I and to be capable of activating $CD8^+$ T cells. Moreover, in vivo, in the rat 5/6 nephrectomy model, accumulation of DCs in the renal parenchyma peaked 1 week after surgery and decreased thereafter, concomitant with their appearance in the renal draining lymph nodes. DCs from renal lymph nodes loaded with the albumin peptide ALB_{1-24}–activated syngeneic $CD8^+$ T cells in primary culture.[177] Thus inflammatory stimuli released from damaged tubules after protein overload may represent danger signals that, in the presence of albumin peptides, alert DCs to promote local immunity via $CD8^+$ T cells, which are activated in regional lymph nodes and recruited in the renal interstitium.

MACROPHAGES AND LYMPHOCYTES

The interstitial infiltrate in most human chronic renal diseases consists of a number of different effector cells, including macrophages and $CD4^+$ and $CD8^+$ T cells.[178] In animal models, macrophages are the dominant infiltrating cells in both the early and later stages of chronic renal injury. More specifically, tubulointerstitial macrophage accumulation in chronic nephropathies correlates with the severity of the glomerular and interstitial lesions and the degree of renal dysfunction.[178] Direct damage to resident cells is caused by reactive oxygen species (ROS), nitric oxide (NO), complement factors, and proinflammatory cytokines generated by macrophages.[179] Macrophages can also affect the supporting matrix and vasculature through the expression of metalloproteinases and vasoactive peptides.

Macrophages are only one component of the cellular infiltrate that characterizes inflammation in the renal interstitium. Models of overload proteinuria have emphasized the importance of tubulointerstitial infiltration with mononuclear cells. Indeed, helper T cells and cytotoxic T cells as well as macrophages are observed in the tubulointerstitial infiltrate 2 weeks after protein overload.[180] T-cell depletion with intraperitoneal administration of anti–T cell monoclonal antibodies did not modify macrophage infiltration, indicating that the influx of these cells was independent of lymphocytes[180] and more likely resulted from local tubular cell expression of osteopontin, MCP-1, and the cellular adhesion molecules vascular CAM (VCAM) and intercellular CAM (ICAM).

T lymphocytes are also abundantly present in the tubulointerstitial infiltrate early after renal mass ablation in rats and remain there in significant numbers for the following weeks.[181] Although the infiltration of macrophages is part of a nonspecific inflammatory reaction, the presence of lymphocytes within lesions indicates that their recruitment and activation are mediated by an antigen-specific immune response. Their role is to maintain and amplify the inflammatory response in the renal interstitium.

Because B cells are considered to be important mostly in lymph nodes and spleen, and in humoral immune responses, little attention has been paid to their potential role as intrarenal infiltrating cells.[182] However, a prominent accumulation of $CD20^+$ B cells has been described in membranous nephropathy.[183] Furthermore, $CD20^+$ B cells formed a prominent part of the infiltrating cells in renal biopsy specimens from patients with IgA nephropathy and chronic interstitial nephritis.[184] Together with $CD3^+$ T cells, the $CD20^+$ B cells formed large nodular structures, like tertiary lymphatic organs in inflamed tissues.[185]

The level of mRNA expression of the chemokine CXCL13 was increased and correlated with $CD20^+$ mRNA in the tubulointerstitial space. The localization of enhanced CXCL13 immunoreactivity to the nodular infiltrates and that of the corresponding receptor CXCR5 to B cells in the infiltrates point to a role for CXCL13-CXCR5 in B-cell recruitment into the lymphoid follicle–like structures. In the interstitium, B cells may release proinflammatory cytokines and chemokines, present antigens, and activate T cells as well as play a role in the development of tissue fibrosis.[185]

BONE MARROW–DERIVED FIBROCYTES

In proteinuric renal disease, chemokines generated in the inflammatory milieu may contribute to the recruitment of bone marrow–derived fibrocytes to the renal interstitium.[186] Fibrocytes are circulating connective tissue cell progenitors with a high capacity for collagen I synthesis. In progressive kidney fibrosis induced by unilateral ureteral obstruction in mice, fibrocytes infiltrated the interstitium, and the number of these cells increased with the progression of fibrosis.[187] In addition, the number of infiltrating fibrocytes correlates well with the extent of interstitial fibrosis in several human kidney diseases.[186] Although fibrocytes isolated from mice and humans express chemokine receptors, including CCR2, CCR3, CCR5, CCR7, and CXCR4,[186] the specific chemokine and receptor pair involved in the recruitment of these cells in the damaged tubulointerstitium remains uncertain.

FIBROBLASTS: ACTIVATION AND DEPOSITION OF EXTRACELLULAR MATRIX

The process of tubulointerstitial fibrosis involves the loss of renal tubules and the accumulation of myofibroblasts and extracellular matrix (ECM) proteins.[188] Resident interstitial fibroblasts and myofibroblasts proliferate in response to macrophage-derived profibrogenic cytokines, and their number correlates with the subsequent formation of a scar.[189] These cells may be derived from transdifferentiated tubular epithelial cells or pericytes of peritubular capillaries, a process promoted by profibrogenic cytokines, including TGF-β expressed by macrophages.[190,191]

During the developmental stage embryonic epithelia of different organs, including the collecting duct epithelium of the kidney, may give rise to mesenchymal cells, a process known as epithelial-to-mesenchymal transition (EMT).[192] EMT has been suggested as a process that contributes to interstitial fibrosis in chronic kidney diseases through transformation of injured renal tubular cells into mesenchymal cells.[192] However, the evidence for EMT in the adult kidneys and in chronic renal disease is controversial, and there are no solid data supporting EMT as an in vivo process in kidney fibrosis. The most supportive data have come from a study in a model of unilateral ureteral obstruction.[193] With the use of genetically tagged proximal tubule epithelial cells, it has been demonstrated that up to 36% of all matrix-producing cells within the tubulointerstitial space may be of tubular origin.[193] However, the contribution of EMT to the formation of myofibroblasts is less in other models.[194,195] Moreover, using cell fate–tracing techniques in the unilateral ureteral obstruction model, other investigators did not find any evidence for a contribution of EMT to renal fibrosis.[196] This result is in line with the finding that after the onset of proteinuria in the remnant kidney model in rats, SMA, a marker of transdifferentiation to myofibroblasts, was initially expressed by nonepithelial cells in the peritubular compartment. Also, peritubular pericytes have been identified as the source of myofibroblasts in this transdifferentiation process.[196]

Activated renal fibroblasts may secrete chemokines that, in turn, may further attract macrophages and perpetuate tubulointerstitial injury.[155] Eventually activated fibroblasts produce interstitial matrix components that contribute to interstitial collagen deposition and fibrosis. Increased tubulointerstitial fibrosis is a common feature of kidney injury and results from accumulation of ECM structural proteins. It is maintained by continuous remodeling through the proteolytic action of matrix metalloproteinases (MMPs) and the synthesis of new proteins.

MMPs are inhibited by tissue inhibitors of matrix metalloproteinases (TIMPs). Therefore, the balance between TIMPS and MMPs determines the ECM integrity. Among the four members of the TIMP family, TIMP-3 is unique in that it is ECM bound and is highly expressed in the kidney.[197] TIMP-3$^{-/-}$ mice had more interstitial fibrosis, increased synthesis and deposition of type I collagen, increased activation of fibroblasts, and greater activation of MMP-2 after unilateral obstruction than wild-type mice.[198] TIMP-3 levels are upregulated in patients with diabetic and chronic allograft nephropathy.[198]

CHRONIC HYPOXIA

One of the most important contributors to the development of tubulointerstitial fibrosis is chronic ischemia.[199] Production of Ang II and inhibition of production of NO underlie chronic vasoconstriction, which may contribute to tissue ischemia and hypoxia.[200] In that regard histologic studies of biopsy specimens from animal models and human kidneys have documented that there is often a loss of peritubular capillaries in areas of tubulointerstitial fibrosis.[192] Downregulation of vascular endothelial growth factor (VEGF) may be functionally implicated in the progressive attrition of peritubular capillaries and tissue hypoxia, as shown in mouse folic acid nephropathy.[201]

Pericytes play a critical role in the stabilization and proliferation of peritubular capillaries via interaction with endothelial cells.[202-204] This process is mediated by several angioregulatory factors, including angiopoietin-1, produced by pericytes, and angiopoietin-2, produced by activated endothelial cells.[204-206] Renal ischemia, as it occurs in chronic kidney disease due to microvascular rarefaction,[207] promotes an imbalance in angiopoietins that, besides leading to proliferation of pericytes, may induce interstitial fibrosis in the long term.[208]

Moreover, given that the size of the interstitial compartment determines the diffusion distance between peritubular capillaries and tubular cells, interstitial fibrosis further impairs tubular oxygen supply. Focal reduction of capillary blood flow leading to starvation of tubules may underlie tubular atrophy and loss. Under these conditions, the remaining tubules are subjected to functional hypermetabolism with increased oxygen consumption, which in turn creates an even more severely hypoxic environment in the renal interstitium. In vitro, such hypoxia stimulates fibroblast proliferation and ECM production by tubular epithelial cells.[209]

ENDOGENOUS SYSTEMS OF TISSUE REPAIR

PROTECTIVE MACROPHAGES

Much remains to be learned about macrophages in tubulointerstitial injury. The role of interstitial macrophages was elucidated in mice with progressive Adriamycin-induced nephropathy.[210] Treatment of mice with the monoclonal antibody ED7 directed against the CD11b/CD18 integrin, which is expressed by macrophages, reduces renal cortical macrophages (ED1-positive cells) by almost 50%, whether ED7 was administered before or after Adriamycin administration.[211] However, ED7 reduced renal structural and functional injury only when treatment was started prior to Adriamycin administration.[211]

Among several possible explanations for these observations is a temporal change in the predominant macrophage phenotype. If pathogenic macrophages predominated early and protective macrophages later in the course of the disease, then only early antimacrophage treatment would be expected to protect against progression. Indeed, macrophages can exhibit distinctly different functional phenotypes and can be polarized toward proinflammatory (M1 macrophages) or tissue-reparative (M2 macrophages) phenotype.[212] In the peritubular interstitium macrophages have been shown to mediate tissue repair in response to acute kidney injury by adopting an M2 phenotype and producing a cytokine environment that supports tubular repair and proliferation rather than inflammation.[213] Colony-stimulating factor-1 (CSF-1) signaling mediated M2 macrophage–induced recovery from renal injury, because pharmacologic blockade of CSF-1 decreased M2 polarization and eventually inhibited tissue repair.[214]

Further observations also support the importance of macrophage phenotype. For example, in mice with unilateral ureteric obstruction reconstituted with bone marrow from Ang II subtype 1 receptor gene knockout or wild-type mice, infiltrating macrophages were shown to play a beneficial antifibrotic role.[215]

Other studies have demonstrated marked macrophage heterogeneity and context specificity, depending on the nature of the injury and location within the kidney.[216] Evidence is available that macrophages perform both injury-inducing and repair-promoting tasks in different models of inflammation. This feature has been shown in a reversible model of liver injury, in which the injury and recovery phases are distinct.[217] Macrophage depletion when liver fibrosis was advanced resulted in reduced scarring and fewer myofibroblasts. Macrophage depletion during recovery, by contrast, led to a failure of matrix degradation.[217] These findings provide clear evidence that functionally distinct subpopulations of macrophages exist in the same tissue.

Further studies on possible temporal variations in the phenotype, activation status, and net effect on injury of macrophages should yield a better understanding of the complex role of macrophages in tubulointerstitial injury and repair of chronic renal disease, particularly in the proteinuric setting.

REGULATORY T CELLS

CD4[+] T cells constitute a critical component of the adaptive immune system and are typified by their capacity to help both humoral and cell-mediated responses. However, there is a substantial functional diversity among CD4[+] T cells, and it is clear that certain subpopulations hinder rather than help the immune response. The best-characterized example of an inhibitory subpopulation is the CD4[+]CD25[+] cells, which appear to play an active role in downregulating pathogenic autoimmune responses.[218] CD4[+]CD25[+] T cells are potent immunoregulatory cells that suppress T-cell proliferation in vitro and have the capacity to suppress immune responses to autoantigens, alloantigens, tumor antigens, and infectious antigens in vivo.[219]

The regulatory activity of these cells in the setting of chronic renal diseases is highlighted by studies in SCID (severe combined immunodeficiency) mice reconstituted with CD4[+]CD25[+] T cells after induction of Adriamycin nephrosis.[211] Mice reconstituted with these regulatory cells had significantly reduced glomerulosclerosis, tubular injury, and interstitial expansion in comparison with unreconstituted mice with Adriamycin-induced nephrosis.

Findings of a study utilizing the green fluorescence protein (GFP)–*Foxp3* mouse suggest that *Foxp3* expression identifies the regulatory T-cell population.[220] In the murine model of Adriamycin nephropathy, the adoptive transfer of *Foxp3*-transduced T cells protected against renal injury. Urinary protein excretion and serum creatinine were reduced, and there were significant decreases in glomerulosclerosis, tubular damage, and interstitial infiltrates.[221]

KIDNEY-DERIVED PROGENITOR CELLS

In chronic proteinuric renal disease, regression of glomerular structural changes is associated with remodeling of the glomerular architecture.[222] Instrumental to this discovery were three-dimensional reconstruction studies of the glomerular capillary tuft, which allowed the quantification of sclerosis volume reduction and of capillary regeneration upon treatment.[222] The reversal of early glomerular damage in animal models and humans[223] argues for the existence of a regenerative mechanism that promotes glomerular repair. However, mature podocytes are post-mitotic cells with limited capacity to divide in situ and therefore are unable to regenerate.[223] A potential mechanism for podocyte replacement by bone marrow–derived stem cells was described in the Alport mouse model as well as in kidney transplants.[224,225] Nevertheless, most studies concluded that regeneration occurs predominantly from resident renal progenitors,[50,61] although the source of these cells remains ill-defined.

A study using a triple-transgenic mouse model that allowed permanent marking of glomerular parietal cells and their progeny upon administration of doxycycline showed that the parietal epithelial cells of Bowman's capsule possess the capability to migrate into the glomerular tuft via the vascular stalk, where they differentiate into podocytes.[226] Similarly, in the adult human kidney, cells localized between the urinary pole and vascular pole of Bowman's capsule—which expressed both progenitor and podocyte markers (CD24[+]CD133[+]PDX[+]cells)—were shown to differentiate into podocytes by losing stem cell markers and expressing markers indicative of a podocyte phenotype while progressing from the urinary pole to the surface of the glomerular tuft.[227]

Experimental evidence indicates that intravenous injection of human progenitor cells harvested from Bowman's capsule into SCID mice with Adriamycin-induced nephropathy reduced proteinuria and mitigated chronic glomerular damage.[227] Even more intriguing from the clinical perspective is the finding that ACE inhibition induces glomerular repair in the Munich Wistar Frömter (MWF) rat, a model of spontaneous glomerular injury.[228] In these proteinuric animals, besides halting age-related podocyte loss, lisinopril increased the number of glomerular podocytes above baseline, a change associated with an increased number of proliferating Wilms' tumor-1 (WT)-1 positive cells, loss of cycling-dependent kinase inhibitor p27 expression, and an increased number of parietal podocytes. This finding indicates that remodeling of Bowman's capsule epithelial cells contributes to the ACE inhibitor–induced restructuring of the damaged glomerular capillary, primarily by restoring the podocyte population.

Similarly, glomerular repair was augmented when glucocorticoid treatment was given to mice with experimental FSGS at a time when podocyte number was already decreased.[229] Prednisone increased podocyte number in correlation with reductions in proteinuria and glomerulosclerosis. This result could be the result of direct biologic effects on glomerular epithelial cells by reducing podocyte apoptosis and by enhancing podocyte regeneration through an increase in the number of parietal epithelial cell precursors.

Along with ACE inhibitors,[117,118] and prednisone,[229] Notch inhibitors,[230] blockers of chemokine stromal cell–derived factor-1[231] and retinoids[232] can be added to the list of agents that improve podocyte regeneration by augmenting the number of parietal epithelial cell progenitors. Indeed, in vitro exposure of human renal progenitor cells to human serum albumin inhibited their differentiation into podocytes by sequestering retinoic acid and preventing retinoic acid response element (RARE)–mediated transcription of podocyte-specific genes.[233] Similarly, in vivo in mice with Adriamycin-induced nephropathy, a model of human FSGS, blocking endogenous retinoic acid synthesis increased proteinuria and exacerbated glomerulosclerosis.[233] This effect was related to a reduction in podocyte number. In *RARE-lacZ* transgenic mice, albuminuria reduced retinoic acid bioavailability and impaired *RARE* activation in renal progenitors, inhibiting their differentiation into podocytes.[233] Treatment with retinoic acid restored *RARE* activity and induced the expression of podocyte markers in renal progenitors, decreasing proteinuria and increasing podocyte number, as demonstrated in serial biopsy specimens.[233]

Together these experimental studies suggest that restoring the capacity of parietal epithelial progenitor cells to differentiate into podocytes could promote the regeneration of podocytes and potentially result in the regression of glomerular disease.

SYSTEMIC CONSEQUENCES OF NEPHROTIC-RANGE PROTEINURIA

Nephrotic-range proteinuria is accompanied by a cluster of abnormalities that is known collectively as nephrotic syndrome. It is characterized by systemic complications that result from profound alterations in the composition of the body protein pool, a state of sodium retention, dyslipidemia, abnormalities of coagulation factors, and a variable degree of renal insufficiency.

HYPOALBUMINEMIA

Clinical manifestations of nephrotic syndrome become evident in patients with levels of proteinuria in excess of 3.5 g/day. Proteinuria in overtly nephrotic subjects usually exceeds this lower bound by a factor of 2 to 3, however. Immunochemical analysis shows that albumin accounts for more than 80% of the excreted proteins.[234] The second most abundantly excreted protein is immunoglobulin, which after albumin is the next most abundant protein in plasma. One of the most common systemic abnormalities associated with nephrotic proteinuria is hypoalbuminemia, which develops in most patients.

PATHOGENESIS OF HYPOALBUMINEMIA

Under normal conditions, albumin production by the liver is 12 to 14 g/day (130-200 mg/kg). Production equals the amount catabolized, predominantly in extrarenal locations.[235] However, about 10% is catabolized in the proximal tubule of the kidney after reabsorption of filtered albumin.[235] In patients with nephrotic syndrome hypoalbuminemia results from excessive urinary loss, decreased hepatic synthesis, and increased rates of albumin catabolism (Figure 53.8).

Urinary albumin loss is an important contributor to the development of hypoalbuminemia. However, it is not a sufficient cause in most patients with nephrotic syndrome, because the rate of hepatic albumin synthesis can increase by at least threefold, thereby compensating for urinary albumin loss.[235] Enhanced loss of albumin in the gastrointestinal tract has also been proposed to contribute to hypoalbuminemia, but there is little evidence for this hypothesis.[236] Therefore, for hypoalbuminemia to develop there must be either an insufficient increase in hepatic synthetic rate or an increase in albumin catabolism.

Normally the rate of hepatic albumin synthesis may increase by as much as 300%. However, studies of nephrotic syndrome in animal models and in humans with hypoalbuminemia demonstrate that the rate of albumin synthesis is at or only slightly above the upper limit of normal as long as dietary protein is adequate,[237] indicating an inadequate synthetic response to hypoalbuminemia by the liver.

Oncotic pressure of the plasma perfusing the liver is one major regulator of protein synthesis.[174] Experimental evidence in rats that are genetically deficient in circulating albumin showed a twofold higher hepatic transcription rate of the albumin gene than in normal rats.[174] However, in the deficient rats the increase in hepatic albumin synthesis was inadequate to compensate for the degree of hypoalbuminemia, indicating an impaired synthetic response.[174] Similarly, in nephrotic patients, reduced oncotic pressure is unable to enhance the liver's albumin synthesis rate enough to restore plasma albumin concentration.[237] There is also evidence in normal subjects that hepatic interstitial albumin regulates albumin synthesis.[238] Because in nephrotic syndrome the hepatic interstitial albumin pool is not depleted, the albumin synthetic response is normal or slightly increased, but it remains inadequate relative to the level of hypoalbuminemia.[238]

Dietary protein intake further contributes to the synthesis of albumin. Hepatic synthesis of albumin mRNA and albumin was not increased in nephrotic rats when fed a low-protein diet, but increased when they were given a high-protein diet.[239] However, serum albumin levels were not altered because hyperfiltration resulting from increased protein intake led to higher albuminuria.

The contribution of renal albumin catabolism to hypoalbuminemia in nephrotic syndrome is controversial. Some investigators have argued that renal tubular albumin transport capacity is already saturated at physiologic levels of filtered albumin and that any increase in filtered protein, instead of being absorbed and catabolized, is simply excreted in the urine.[240] Studies in isolated perfused proximal tubules in rabbits, however, demonstrated a dual transport system for albumin uptake.[241] In addition to a low-capacity system that became saturated when the protein load exceeded physiologic levels, a high-capacity low-affinity system was also present that allowed the tubular absorptive rate for albumin to increase as the filtered load rose. Thus, an increase in the fractional catabolic rate may occur in nephrotic syndrome.

This hypothesis is supported by the positive correlation between fractional albumin catabolism and albuminuria in rats with puromycin aminonucleoside (PAN)–induced nephrosis.[242] Nevertheless, because total body albumin stores are substantially decreased in nephrotic syndrome, absolute catabolic rates may be normal or even reduced.[236] This outcome is affected by nutritional state, as documented by the fact that absolute albumin catabolism was reduced in

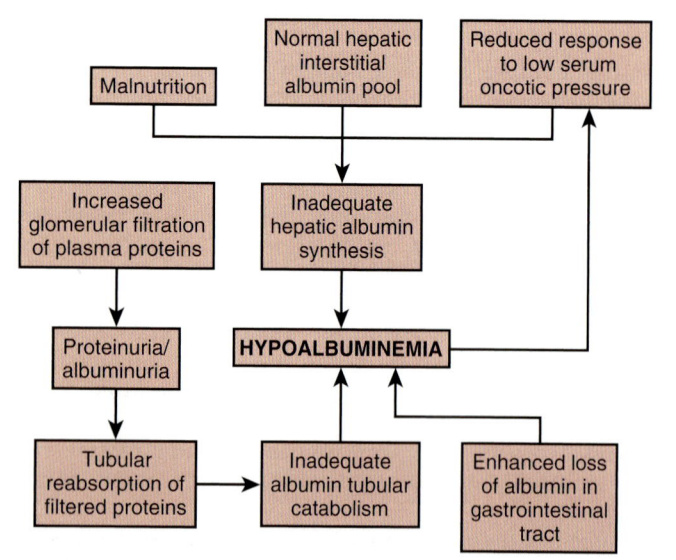

Figure 53.8 Schematic representation of mechanisms leading to nephrotic hypoalbuminemia. Compensatory mechanisms such as increases in albumin synthesis and decreases in albumin catabolism are insufficient to correct the hypoalbuminemia.

nephrotic rats nourished with a low-protein diet, but not in those with normal dietary protein intake.[243]

In summary, hypoalbuminemia in nephrotic syndrome results from multiple alterations in albumin homeostasis that are not sufficiently compensated for by hepatic albumin synthesis and by decreased renal tubular albumin catabolism.

CONSEQUENCES OF HYPOALBUMINEMIA

Impairment of kidney function is the rule in patients with nephrotic hypoalbuminemia and usually manifests in two ways. One is the inability of the kidney to maintain sodium and fluid homeostasis. The other is loss of intrinsic ultrafiltration capacity of glomerular capillary walls, a phenomenon that leads, in turn, to reduction in GFR.[244]

When viewed in physiologic terms, the GFR can be defined as the net rate of water flux across the walls of the capillaries in the glomerular tufts of the kidney. It is determined by the product of the net pressure for ultrafiltration and the ultrafiltration coefficient—Kf—a measure of intrinsic ultrafiltration capacity, derived from the product of the available filtering surface area (s) and the hydraulic permeability of the glomerular capillary wall (k). Estimating GFR and its determinants in humans has been shown that a reduced GFR in some forms of nephrotic syndrome (minimal change and membranous nephropathy) is exclusively a consequence of profoundly lowered hydraulic permeability.[245] In nephrotic syndrome associated with lupus nephritis, idiopathic focal and segmental glomerulosclerosis, and diabetic nephropathy, both reduction of the surface area available for filtration and impairment of hydraulic permeability contribute to Kf depression.[246,247]

The principal cause of impaired hydraulic permeability in nephrotic disorders is broadening and effacement of epithelial foot processes.[245] These changes lower the frequency of interpodocytic slit diaphragms through which water must pass to gain access to Bowman's space, thereby increasing the resistance to water flow. The low Kf is partially offset by an increase in net ultrafiltration pressure, which is largely due to a substantial lowering of the intraglomerular capillary oncotic pressure. As a result the drop in GFR is not proportional to the decrease in Kf. This compensatory elevation in net ultrafiltration pressure explains why reduced values of SNGFR are not consistently observed in all experimental nephrosis models.[248]

The low ultrafiltration capacity induced by glomerular disease and protein depletion makes the nephrotic patient particularly vulnerable to acute exacerbations of hypofiltration and renal insufficiency.[249] Because the prevailing level of GFR depends heavily on ultrafiltration pressure in the presence of a low Kf, any maneuver that lowers the glomerular capillary perfusion pressure can, therefore, cause a precipitous fall in the GFR. The susceptibility of nephrotic patients to episodes of acute kidney injury should thus be borne in mind when one is prescribing drugs that can compromise the ultrafiltration pressure, such as diuretics, cyclooxygenase inhibitors, and cyclosporine.

An additional consequence of hypoalbuminemia is the potential for enhanced drug toxicity.[250] Indeed, many drugs are bound to albumin. Hypoalbuminemia reduces the number of available binding sites and raises the proportion of circulating free drug, but in the steady state this process is counterbalanced by faster metabolism. Furthermore, because protein binding may enhance tubular drug secretion, diminished protein binding in nephrotic syndrome may delay renal excretion of some drugs.[251] Although the clinical consequences of altered protein binding may be difficult to predict, higher levels of free drug may be toxic, as shown with prednisolone.[252]

The case of diuretics is intriguing. Resistance to a loop diuretic, which often occurs in patients with nephrotic syndrome, may be due to reduced delivery of the diuretic to its site of action secondary to hypoalbuminemia. Anecdotal reports suggest that the administration of furosemide with small amounts of albumin (6-20 g) can enhance the response to furosemide in nephrotic patients.[253] These observations are not conclusive, because other reports did not show a difference in excretion of intravenous furosemide in urine between nephrotic patients and normal controls.[254] On the other hand, excessive amounts of filtered albumin in the tubule may bind furosemide and make it less effective.[255]

In animals, the inhibition of fractional loop Cl^- reabsorption by furosemide was blunted by the presence of albumin in the proximal tubule, and prevention of albumin-furosemide binding with warfarin and sulfisoxazole partially restored the response to the diuretic.[255] However, these findings were not confirmed in nephrotic patients given sulfisoxazole, raising doubt about the importance of excessive albumin-bound furosemide at the active tubular site in resistance to diuretics.[256] Sodium-retaining mechanisms, such as low effective arterial blood volume and activation of neurohumoral factors, may be relatively more important.

Many binding proteins are lost in the urine in nephrotic syndrome.[257] Consequently, in patients with the disease, the plasma levels of many ions (iron, copper, and zinc), vitamins (vitamin D metabolites), and hormones (thyroid and steroid hormones) are low, because the level of protein-bound ligands is reduced. Urinary loss of protein-bound ligands can theoretically cause depletion, but there is little convincing clinical evidence for such a theory, with the possible exception of vitamin D.[258] Indeed one of the proteins lost in the urine of patients with nephrotic syndrome is cholecalciferol-binding globulin (also known as vitamin D–binding protein [DBP]), which is a 59-kDa protein easily filtered by nephrotic glomeruli.[259] 25-Hydroxycholecalciferol [$25\text{-}(OH)D_3$] circulates as a complex with DBP, there also is an associated urinary loss of $25\text{-}(OH)D_3$ in nephrotic syndrome.[260] The oral administration of ^{3}H-labeled cholecalciferol indicated that the serum half-life of $25\text{-}(OH)D_3$ was reduced and urinary excretion increased in nephrotic syndrome.[261] Nevertheless, in general, nephrotic patients have normal to decreased plasma levels of 1,25-dihydroxycholecalciferol [$1,25\text{-}(OH)_2D_3$].[260]

Although the hypocalcemia of nephrotic syndrome was once attributed solely to the reduction in protein-bound calcium secondary to hypoalbuminemia, a subset of patients has been noted in whom hypocalcemia is out of proportion to the hypoalbuminemia. In these patients ionized serum calcium is decreased.[262] Secondary hyperparathyroidism is seen in some patients, even in the absence of renal failure, as are changes in bone histology consistent with mixed osteomalacia and osteitis fibrosa cystica bone disease.[263] Not all investigators, however, have observed abnormalities in calcium homeostasis in nephrotic syndrome.[264] Why only a subset of patients is predisposed to alterations in calcium, vitamin D, and parathyroid hormone homeostasis has not been determined, but it has been suggested that factors such as age, duration of disease, renal function, degree of proteinuria, serum albumin concentration, and corticosteroid therapy might be involved.[258]

Finally, hypoalbuminemia may play a role in platelet hyperaggregability.[265] Because albumin normally binds arachidonic acid, thus limiting its conversion to thromboxane A_2 by platelets, hypoalbuminemia might allow increased platelet arachidonate metabolism to take place, and platelet hyperreactivity may result.[265]

EDEMA FORMATION

The clinical manifestation that most frequently brings the nephrotic patient to medical attention is the formation of edema. This development represents an increase in the size of the interstitial fluid compartment. The interstitial fluid accumulates most readily in dependent areas, where tissue pressure is low. It thus manifests as periorbital edema upon awakening in the morning and pedal edema at the end of the day. Even when edema is generalized and massive, a condition referred to as *anasarca*, it remains most marked in the lower extremities. Not infrequently, anasarca is also accompanied by large effusions into the peritoneal, pleural, and pericardial spaces. The mechanisms responsible for extravascular fluid accumulation in nephrotic patients are complex and only partially understood.

REDUCED PLASMA ONCOTIC PRESSURE

Low oncotic pressure as a result of hypoalbuminemia favors the movement of water from the intravascular to the interstitial space. Under normal conditions, edema formation is halted by expansion and proliferation of lymphatics that increase lymphatic flow and by reduction of interstitial oncotic pressure due to accumulation of protein-free fluid. In addition the increase in hydraulic pressure in the interstitium due to fluid accumulation lowers the transcapillary pressure gradient, further reducing the transudation of plasma fluid into the interstitial space. However, there is no clear evidence of alterations in these normal defense mechanisms against edema formation in nephrotic patients.[266] For example, comparable changes in interstitial and plasma oncotic pressure have been documented during relapse and remission phases in patients with nephrotic syndrome.[266] Moreover, the capillary hydraulic conductivity is elevated in nephrotic patients,[267] possibly because of disruption of the intercellular macromolecular complex between endothelial cells, which enhances capillary filtration capacity and may lead to sustained edema formation.[268] These observations suggest that hypoalbuminemia per se may not be the primary determinant of the severity of edema formation and that intrarenal mechanisms may have a prominent contributory role.

ALTERATIONS IN BLOOD VOLUME

According to the traditional view, lowering of the plasma albumin concentration eventually induces renal sodium and fluid retention in nephrotic syndrome by causing hypovolemia, the so-called underfill mechanism (Figure 53.9). Indeed, hypovolemia as a consequence of reduced plasma

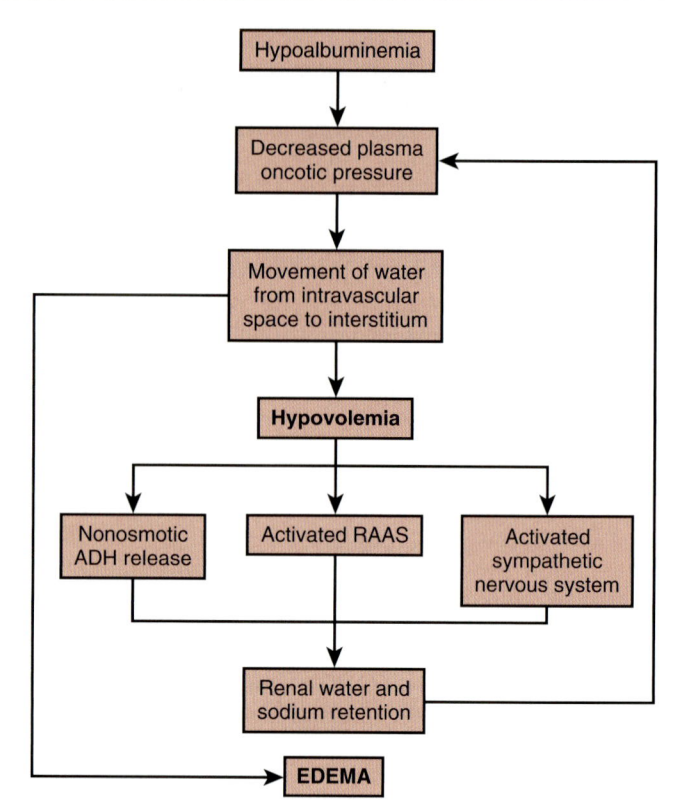

Figure 53.9 The "underfill" mechanism of edema formation. Hypovolemia, as a consequence of reduced plasma oncotic pressure, is the key event that signals the kidney to retain the filtered sodium and water. ADH, vasopressin; RAAS, renin angiotensin aldosterone system.

colloid oncotic pressure triggers a cascade of events that signal the kidney to retain the filtered sodium and water.[269] Thus hypovolemia is the afferent stimulus of a complex pathway of responses mediated by low- and high-pressure baroreceptors in the cardiac atria, carotid arteries, and aorta that activate the sympathetic nervous system and the renin angiotensin system. Moreover, hypovolemia also promotes excessive nonosmotic secretion of arginine vasopressin (AVP), which further contributes to water retention by the kidneys.[269]

The homeostatic response of renal sodium and water retention that serves to restore intravascular volume also exacerbates hypoalbuminemia, thereby sustaining transudation of plasma fluid into the interstitial space. The fact that salt retention may be the consequence of an underfilled circulation is consistent with the finding that head-out water immersion, a maneuver that raises plasma volume, is followed by a natriuretic and diuretic response in some nephrotic patients.[270]

This mechanistic scenario of edema formation in nephrotic syndrome would also imply consistently reduced plasma volume[271] as well as an elevated plasma renin activity (PRA)[272] and increased plasma and urinary levels of catecholamines.[273] However, in one study, only a minority of nephrotic patients had a low plasma volume[273]; in fact, approximately 70% of patients had normal or even high values in some studies.[274] In some cases plasma volume was lower during remission than during the acute phase of the disease.[273,274] However, methodologic issues have been raised about the measurement of plasma volume in nephrotic patients that may limit the interpretation of the findings of these studies.[275]

Measurement of vasoactive hormones, which are responsive to low plasma volume and can be taken as surrogate markers of the intravascular volume, also documented that only 50% of nephrotic patients have higher than normal PRA and plasma as well as urinary aldosterone levels.[276] Moreover, pharmacologic blockade of the renin angiotensin aldosterone system (RAAS) in nephrotic patients with high PRA values does not change sodium excretion.[277] Similarly, plasma levels of norepinephrine, AVP, and atrial natriuretic peptide (ANP) are near normal or inconsistently changed.[278] The diuretic and natriuretic responses to hyperoncotic plasma or albumin infusions[279] or to central volume expansion with head-out water immersion also vary widely from patient to patient.[279] Evidence that PRA often increases rather than decreases after steroid-induced remission of nephrotic syndrome is an additional, albeit indirect argument that argues against a key role for hypovolemia in edema formation in most nephrotic patients.[276]

INTRARENAL MECHANISMS

Alternatively, the "overfill" theory hypothesizes that there is a dominant mechanism by which the kidneys retain sodium independent of circulating plasma volume, leading to hypervolemia (Figure 53.10).[269] Examination of the edema-forming, nephrotic patient during consumption of a known amount of sodium reveals a positive sodium balance. This results in increased blood volume, which by altering Starling's forces across the capillary wall leads to plasma leakage into the interstitium and overflow edema. This mechanism has been illustrated in a unilateral model of PAN-induced nephrosis in rat.[280] In such a model, in which albumin concentration in the systemic circulation is normal, only the proteinuric kidney (not the contralateral intact one) retained excessive amounts of sodium and water. This finding indicates that abnormal sodium retention by the proteinuric kidney is brought about by intrarenal rather than circulating or systemic factors.

These findings can be partly explained by a lowered filtered sodium load, a consequence of the diminished GFR that frequently accompanies nephrotic-range proteinuria. However, because the fractional sodium excretion is low, enhanced tubular sodium reabsorption appears to be the predominant cause of sodium retention in nephrotic syndrome. Analysis of segmental sodium transport in nephrotic rats has identified the collecting duct as the major site of enhanced sodium reabsorption.[280] Refractoriness to the natriuretic action of ANP (which increases urinary sodium and water excretion) in experimental[281] and clinical[282] studies further indicates the distal segments of the nephron as the likely site of sodium retention in nephrotic syndrome. Indeed, the inner medullary segment of the collecting duct is the tubule segment most richly endowed with receptors for ANP.[283]

The crucial observation was that natriuretic and diuretic responses to intravenously infused atrial extract (from normal or nephrotic rats) or synthetic ANP were markedly lower in nephrotic than in normal rats.[284] In a rat model of unilateral glomerulopathy, the blunted natriuretic and diuretic responses to ANP were confined to the "nephrotic" kidney as opposed to the contralateral normal kidney, despite a comparable increase in GFR.[281] Moreover, both enhanced release of endogenous ANP during water

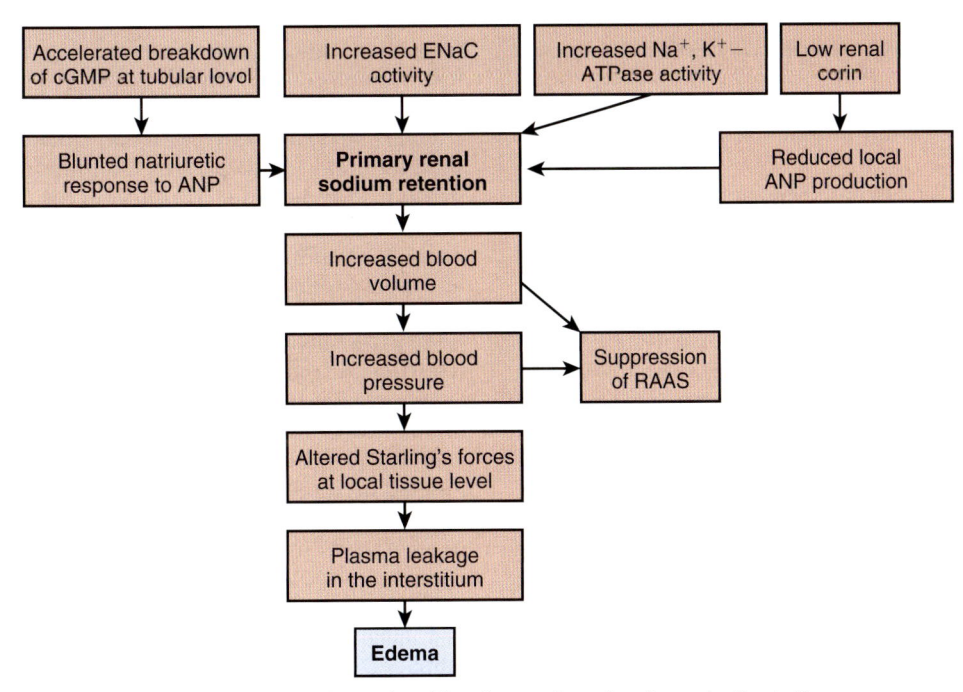

Figure 53.10 **The "overfill" mechanism of edema formation.** The abnormal renal sodium retention is the consequence of blunted natriuretic response to atrial natriuretic peptide (ANP) and increases in activity of epithelial sodium channel (ENaC) and Na+/K+-ATPase, and is the key event of the process. The resulting hypervolemia alters Starling's forces across the capillary wall at local tissue level, leading to overflow edema. cGMP, cyclic guanosine monophosphate; RAAS, renin angiotensin aldosterone system.

immersion and infusion of exogenous ANP failed to promote an appropriate natriuretic response in nephrotic patients.[282]

Taken together, these findings support a role for ANP in intrarenal sodium retention in nephrotic syndrome. In addition, it can be inferred that alterations in the intrinsic transport properties of the collecting duct render this tubule segment unresponsive to the natriuretic action of ANP.

In some studies, increased activity of efferent sympathetic nerves has been related to the blunted ANP natriuretic response.[285] More consistent evidence points to enhanced phosphodiesterase activity in collecting duct cells from nephrotic animals, leading to accelerated breakdown of normally produced cyclic guanosine monophosphate (cGMP), which is important for intracellular signaling after ANP binding to its specific receptors.[286]

With the discovery of corin, a 1042–amino acid transmembrane serine protease that converts proANP and pro–brain natriuretic peptide (proBNP) into the active forms ANP and BNP,[287,288] understanding of the pathogenesis of edema formation in nephrotic syndrome has been revised. Beside being initially localized in the heart,[287] corin has been shown to be also expressed in renal tissue.[289] Through the use of immunohistochemical analysis, co-localization of corin and ANP in renal tissue has been documented.[289] It is noteworthy that kidneys of corin$^{-/-}$ mice displayed larger amounts of renal β-epithelial Na$^+$ channel (ENaC), phosphodiesterase-5 (PDE$_5$), and protein kinase G II than wild-type mice. Induction of nephrotic syndrome by PAN or of glomerulonephritis by anti-Thy1 antibody induced concomitant increase in proANP and decrease in ANP in the kidney in association with low renal immunoreactive levels of corin.[289,290] Upregulation of PDE$_5$ and kinase G II resulted in reduced cGMP in the collecting duct and, subsequently, in increased ENaC abundance in both nephrotic syndrome and glomerulonephritis.[290] These findings suggest that corin deficiency might be involved in the primary salt retention seen in edematous glomerular diseases by lowering locally produced ANP.[291] In this regard, reduced urinary corin levels have been reported in patients with chronic kidney disease.[292]

In the kidney, the ultimate regulation of sodium reabsorption occurs in the collecting duct through the low-conductance ENaC,[293] located on the apical membrane of principal cells. Evidence is also available that the proteolytic removal of an inhibitory domain from the γ-subunit of ENaC by the serine protease plasmin can activate ENaC.[294] Plasmin, present in the urine of nephrotic rats and humans, has been shown to activate ENaC via this mechanism.[295] Additionally, urokinase-type plasminogen activator present in the rat and human kidney can convert inactive plasminogen (which is filtered by the nephrotic kidney) to the active form plasmin.[295] In the rat PAN nephrosis model, amiloride increased urine sodium excretion and reduced ascites volume. This effect was attributed to the ability of amiloride to inhibit both ENaC and urokinase-type plasminogen activator and thus to reduce the amount of active plasmin present.[295]

ENaC is also regulated by aldosterone.[293] In rat models of nephrotic syndrome, activation of ENaC together with elevated plasma aldosterone levels has been reported.[296] Nevertheless, in puromycin-induced nephrosis in rats with corticosteroid, clamped aldosterone plasma levels, sodium retention persisted even when ENaC recruitment to the apical membrane was inhibited.[297] Conversely, the transport activity of sodium-potassium-adenosine triphosphatase (Na$^+$-K$^+$-ATPase), the ubiquitous sodium pump localized exclusively on the basolateral membrane, was increased.[297] These findings indicate that increased Na$^+$-K$^+$-ATPase activity is the driving force behind enhanced sodium reabsorption in nephrotic syndrome, an observation confirmed by several studies in the cortical collecting ducts in nephrotic rats.[298]

Because the Na$^+$-K$^+$-ATPase pump in the basolateral membrane promotes secondary passive sodium entry from the lumen through the ENaC, Na retention in the collecting duct of nephrotic rats can result from the coordinated overactivity of these tubular sodium transporters. A role for the proximal tubule in the avid sodium retention of nephrotic syndrome has been proposed on the basis of the observation that in PAN-nephrotic rats, increased sodium reabsorption was associated with a shift of the apical Na$^+$-H$^+$ exchanger isoform 3 (NHE3) from an inactive to an active pool.[299] The increase in NHE3-specific activity may be a response to the increased albumin load presented to the proximal tubule, as indicated by the correlation between albumin exposure and enhanced NHE3 abundance and activity in opossum kidney (OKP) cells.[300]

An additional hypothesis concerning intrarenal mechanisms of nephrotic edema proposes that interstitial inflammation of the kidney plays a major role in the pathogenesis of primary sodium retention.[301] The generation of vasoconstrictor and the reduction of vasodilator substances in the interstitium, driven by the inflammatory cell infiltrate, can lead to a reduction in Kf and SNGFR. These glomerular hemodynamic changes that reduce filtered sodium load combine with the increased net tubular sodium reabsorption induced by mediators released from the inflammatory cell infiltrate, leading to primary sodium retention, an "overfilled" intravascular volume, and increased capillary hydrostatic pressure. The decrease in plasma oncotic pressure again promotes fluid movement out of the vascular compartment, thereby buffering the changes in blood volume induced by primary sodium retention. A renal inflammatory infiltrate is, however, minimal or absent in most children with minimal change nephrotic syndrome. Thus, the nephrotic edema may derive from a combination of primary sodium retention and relative arterial underfilling. The predominance of one or the other mechanism is perhaps in accordance with the pathogenesis of nephrotic syndrome or the stage of the disease.

Deranged renal water handling is also a cardinal feature of nephrotic syndrome. Defects in both urinary diluting ability[302] and concentrating capacity[302] have been documented in nephrotic patients. The cause of the concentrating defect has been explored in experimental models of nephrotic syndrome. The extensive downregulation of the expression of the water channels aquaporins 1, 2, and 3 in the collecting duct[303] and of the urea transporter[304] as well as a marked decrease in the abundance of thick ascending limb Na$^+$ transporters, represent an appropriate renal response to the extracellular volume expansion observed in nephrotic syndrome despite increased circulating vasopressin, but may occur at the expense of decreased urinary concentrating capacity.

HYPERLIPIDEMIA

Both quantitative and qualitative changes in lipid metabolism occur in nephrotic syndrome, with virtually all plasma lipid and lipoprotein fractions being elevated.[305] Blood levels of cholesterol are almost always increased and continue to rise as the severity of nephrotic syndrome increases.[305] Total cholesterol and cholesterol esters are all increased.[306] Levels of triglycerides are more variable and in many patients do not increase, except when the nephrotic state is very severe.[305] Plasma levels of free fatty acids are within normal limits in nephrotic syndrome, although a smaller than normal fraction is bound to plasma albumin.[305] Levels of very low-density lipoprotein (VLDL), intermediate-density lipoprotein (IDL), and low-density lipoprotein (LDL) have been found to increase early in nephrotic syndrome[305,307]; data on high-density lipoprotein (HDL) are less clear. Plasma levels of HDL are usually normal, but may decrease due to HDL excretion in the urine in severely proteinuric patients.[305]

The composition of the lipoprotein molecules is also abnormal. Greater than usual amounts of cholesterol and triglycerides are present in VLDL, IDL, and LDL. Moreover, an alteration in the specific type and quantity of various apolipoprotein moieties in the lipoprotein molecules has been described, with reduced apolipoprotein C (apo C) despite elevations in apo B, apo C-II and apo E, and an increased ratio of apo C-III to apo C-II.[308] These abnormalities return to normal fairly promptly when nephrotic syndrome remits.

PATHOGENESIS OF NEPHROTIC HYPERLIPIDEMIA

Two mechanisms contribute to nephrotic dyslipidemia: overproduction and impaired catabolism/clearance of serum lipids and lipoproteins (Figure 53.11). There is general agreement that hepatic synthesis of both lipids and apolipoproteins is increased and that the clearance of chylomicrons (CMs) and VLDL[309] is reduced in nephrotic syndrome. Cholesterol synthesis has been shown to increase both in animals and humans in response to the hypoalbuminemia associated with nephrotic syndrome.[310] Hepatic activity of hydroxymethylglutaryl CoA reductase, the rate-limiting step for hepatic synthesis of cholesterol, is elevated.[274] In general, serum cholesterol levels are inversely proportional to serum albumin levels,[274] and cholesterol levels generally normalize upon remission. Conversely, triglyceride synthesis does not appear to be increased.

It has been suggested that lipoprotein synthesis increases in parallel with albumin synthesis because they have a common secretory pathway.[311] This hypothesis was supported by studies showing that infusion of albumin partially corrected nephrotic hyperlipidemia. It has also been reported that apo B secretion by cultured hepatocytes can be reduced by a rise in the oncotic pressure of the culture medium.

Most evidence still indicates that reduced extracellular albumin concentration and/or reduced extracellular oncotic pressure in some way regulates apolipoprotein synthesis and lipogenesis by the liver. Although hepatic apolipoprotein synthesis is increased in nephrotic syndrome, not all apolipoproteins are affected to the same degree, and mechanisms causing greater synthesis of the various apolipoproteins are also different. Secretion of apo A is increased approximately sixfold,[311] whereas synthesis of apo B and E is increased by only twofold, and synthesis of the apo C is not increased.

Apo A-I mRNA is increased at the transcriptional level in the livers of nephrotic and analbuminemic rats,[312] suggesting that reduced plasma oncotic pressure or albumin concentration is responsible for the change in apo A-I gene expression. Although plasma levels of apo B and E are both increased in nephrotic and analbuminemic rats, there is little or no change in transcription rates. Thus, if greater synthesis is causing higher levels of these apolipoproteins in plasma, the mechanisms involved are most likely posttranscriptional, at the level of translational or protein processing, in contrast to the mechanism affecting apo A-I.

In addition to greater synthesis, studies in animals and humans have determined alterations in the catabolism of lipids in the syndrome. The clearance of chylomicrons and

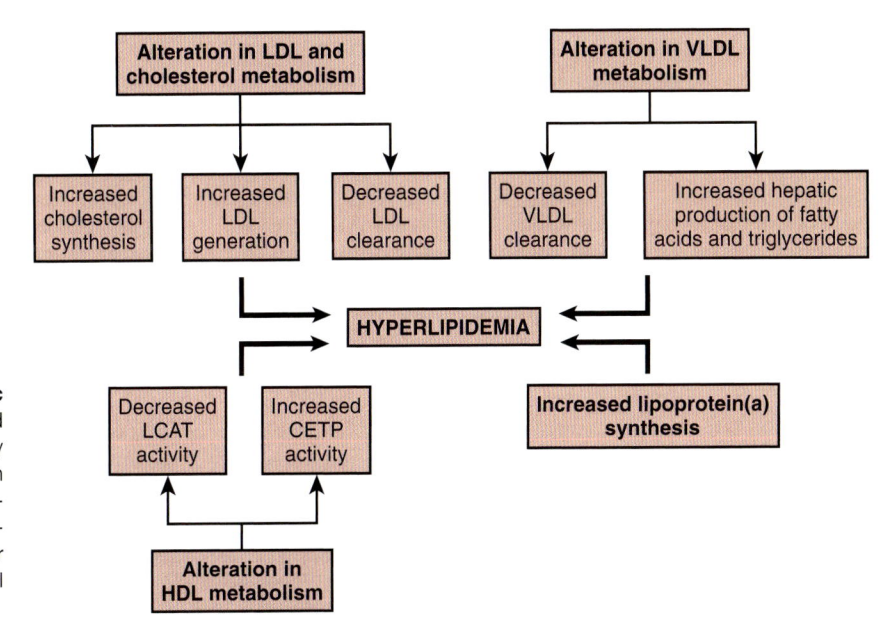

Figure 53.11 **Pathophysiology of nephrotic hyperlipidemia.** All abnormalities of lipid profile originate from alterations in low-density lipoprotein (LDL), very low-density lipoprotein (VLDL), high-density lipoprotein (HDL), and cholesterol metabolism as well as increased synthesis of lipoprotein(a). CETP, cholesterol ester transfer protein; LCAT, lecithin-cholesterol acyl transferase.

VLDL is reduced following the onset of proteinuria but is normal in rats with hereditary analbuminemia,[311,313] suggesting that urinary loss of a lipo-regulatory substance, and not reduced albumin concentration or oncotic pressure, plays a role in defective lipolysis.

One possible explanation for the defective removal of lipoproteins is a decrease in the activity of lipoprotein lipase (LPL), which hydrolyzes triglycerides in VLDL and chylomicrons, releasing free fatty acids. LPL activity is reduced in nephrotic rats, providing a potential mechanism for delayed lipolysis.[311] In one study, chylomicron catabolism in hearts isolated from nephrotic rats was decreased in vitro and the LPL pool bound to vascular endothelium was reduced by approximately 90%; LPL activity not bound to the vascular endothelium, and hence unable to interact with large lipoproteins, was normal.[313] Thus, a specific reduction in LPL attached to the vascular endothelium may be involved in the reduced catabolism of chylomicrons and VLDL in nephrotic syndrome.

The relationship between decreased endothelium-bound LPL activity and reduced catabolism of chylomicrons and VLDL is by no means clear. VLDL and chylomicron catabolism by analbuminemic rats is normal despite a marked reduction in heparin-releasable LPL activity.[314] Moreover, it has been reported that HDL isolated from normal animals corrects defective lipolysis of VLDL isolated from nephrotic rats, whereas HDL isolated from nephrotic animals may be dysfunctional. Indeed, HDL isolated from nephrotic animals has been found to be structurally abnormal.[315] Thus multiple separate defects in the peripheral catabolism of triglyceride-rich lipoproteins may be responsible for delayed lipolysis.

Studies in patients with nephrotic syndrome have not been as detailed as in the rat; however, when comparable studies are evaluated, the two groups exhibit similar disturbances in lipid metabolism. The fractional turnover rate of triglycerides is reduced in nephrotic subjects compared to controls, and the half-life of triglycerides in VLDL is prolonged from 4 to 11 hours.[316] Not only is VLDL catabolism decreased, but the concentration curve over time has an unusual shape, presumably as a result of a delay in the conversion of VLDL into LDL.[317]

It has been suggested that the delay in lipolysis in humans, as in rats, is due to a decrease in LPL activity. Support of this hypothesis comes from the finding that LPL activity is reduced in children with nephrotic syndrome and increases after remission. Furthermore, there is a strong inverse correlation between LPL activity and the concentration of triglycerides in the VLDL fraction,[318] although not all investigators report decreased LPL activity in nephrotic patients.[319]

LDL catabolism has been shown to be either normal or reduced[320] in patients with nephrotic syndrome and only marginally reduced in nephrotic rats.[321] Decreased receptor-mediated LDL clearance has been reported in some clinical studies,[322] which may account in part for elevations in LDL. A defect in LDL receptor translation or enhanced receptor protein turnover has been hypothesized, because normal LDL receptor mRNA was found in the nephrotic rat despite marked reduction in LDL receptor protein expression in the liver.[323]

Nephrotic syndrome is also associated with abnormalities in the activity of enzymes required for effective function of HDL. Cholesterol ester transfer protein (CETP) catalyzes the transfer of the cholesterol ester–rich core of HDL_2 to VLDL remnant particles, creating LDL and thereby increasing LDL cholesterol at the expense of HDL cholesterol. CETP is increased in the plasma of nephrotic patients and correlates positively with VLDL cholesterol and negatively with HDL cholesterol.[324]

The enzyme lecithin-cholesterol acyl transferase (LCAT) catalyzes the esterification of cholesterol and its incorporation into HDL particles and promotes the conversion of HDL_3 to HDL_2. The observation that HDL_3 is preserved in plasma from nephrotic patients at the apparent expense of HDL_2 suggests that the LCAT reaction is reduced in nephrotic syndrome.[325] However, increased activity of CETP could also explain this pattern of HDL distribution because it rapidly may cycle the core of HDL_2 to VLDL remnant particles, thus increasing the flux of cholesterol from the surface of nascent HDL into the core of LDL. Furthermore, mature HDL also transports a number of apolipoproteins that serve as co-factors. One of these apolipoproteins, Apo C-II, is an endogenous activator of LPL activity. Apo C-II is normally transported by HDL_2 to nascent VLDL and chylomicrons. Apo C-II may be lost in the urine of nephrotic patients, either as free protein or bound to HDL.[326] Additionally, an inhibitor of Apo C-II, Apo C-III, is increased in nephrotic syndrome; with the resulting decreased Apo C-II to Apo C-III ratio, the activity of LPL is also significantly decreased.

CLINICAL CONSEQUENCES OF HYPERLIPIDEMIA

The most important consequence of hyperlipidemia is its potential for inducing cardiovascular disease. The changes that occur in blood lipoprotein composition in nephrotic syndrome—reduced HDL_2 cholesterol, a relative increase in HDL_3 cholesterol, and a massive increase in total cholesterol, mostly found in the LDL, IDL, and VLDL fractions[307]—are likely to raise the risk of atherosclerotic disease. Nevertheless, the presence of additional risk factors for atherosclerosis in nephrotic patients, notably hypertension, hypercoagulability and chronic renal failure, makes it difficult to determine the individual contribution of hyperlipidemia to the rise in risk.

Given the natural history of atherosclerosis, one would predict that the patient with a protracted form of nephrotic syndrome has the highest risk of dying from premature cardiovascular disease.[327] Accelerated atherosclerosis has been reported in patients with proteinuria and hyperlipidemia and, in some studies, has been associated with a strongly increased incidence of cardiovascular disease and stroke.[327] One study reported an 85-fold increase in the incidence of ischemic heart disease in nephrotic patients.[328] In another retrospective analysis of 142 patients with proteinuria greater than 3.5 g/day, the relative risk of myocardial infarction was found to be 5.5, and the risk of cardiac death 2.8 in comparison with age- and sex-matched controls.[327]

A number of studies have indicated a potential role for hyperlipidemia in the progression of chronic kidney disease. It was proposed that filtered lipoproteins might accumulate in the mesangium and promote sclerosis.[329] In animals, lipogenic diets have been shown to induce focal sclerosis, and the extent of glomerular damage correlates with the serum

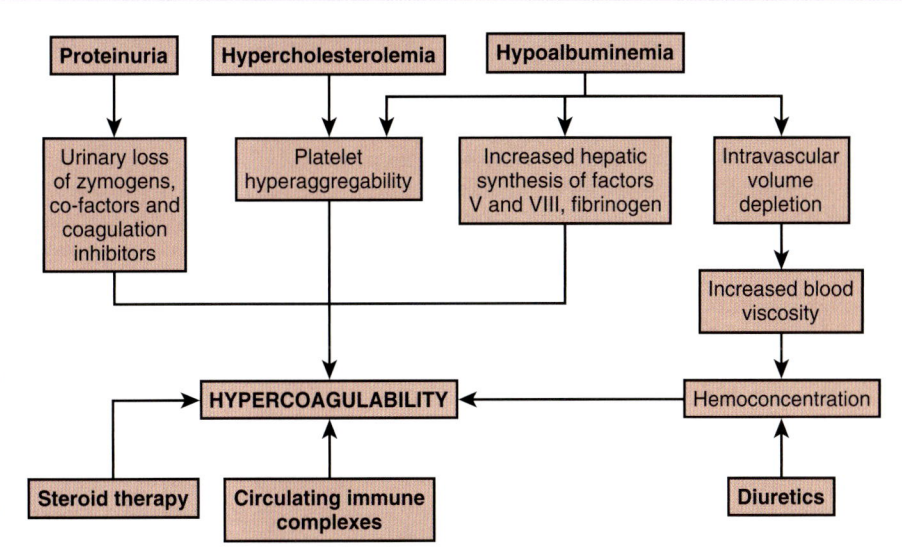

Figure 53.12 **Mechanisms in the pathophysiology of hypercoagulability in nephrotic syndrome.** Alterations in levels and activity of factors in the intrinsic and extrinsic coagulation cascades, levels of antithrombotic and fibrinolytic components of plasma, platelet count and function, and other factors, such as steroids and diuretics, are the numerous abnormalities that contribute to hypercoagulability in nephrotic syndrome.

cholesterol; in the obese Zucker rat, focal sclerosis correlates with hyperlipidemia and can be ameliorated by lipid-lowering drugs.[330] Similarly, free and esterified cholesterol was found in the glomeruli of nephrotic rats, and a close correlation was noted between plasma cholesterol levels and the number of sclerosing glomerular lesions.[331]

Whether hyperlipidemia also plays a role in the progression of chronic kidney disease in human nephrotic syndrome has yet to be determined. There is no specific indication to treat the qualitative abnormalities that characterize the lipid disorder of nephrotic syndrome, but if the duration of hyperlipidemia is anticipated to be prolonged, it is wise to initiate therapy. Treatment of nephrotic patients with ACE inhibitors[332] results in a decline in both proteinuria and blood lipid levels even if plasma albumin concentration does not increase. The decline in blood lipid levels includes decreases in total cholesterol, lipoprotein(a), and VLDL and LDL cholesterol as well as in the activities of CETP and LCAT.[333]

It is prudent to restrict dietary cholesterol and saturated lipids in patients with nephrotic syndrome. The long-term effects of dietary supplementation with fish oil (rich in omega-3 polyunsaturated fatty acids) are as yet unknown, and it cannot be recommended as standard treatment except within the context of a controlled investigative trial. If reduction of proteinuria and dietary fat restriction do not effectively reduce hyperlipidemia, a variety of lipid-lowering drugs, including the 3-hydroxy-3-methyl-glutaryl coenzyme A reductase inhibitors, antioxidants, and fibric acid derivatives, may be useful.

HYPERCOAGULABILITY

Urinary loss of some of the proteins involved in the coagulation cascade and the adaptive increased synthesis of others can induce a hypercoagulable state.[334] Although arterial thrombosis has been reported, it is venous thrombosis that occurs with a particularly high incidence in nephrotic subjects.[335]

PATHOGENESIS OF HYPERCOAGULABILITY

In nephrotic syndrome, there are widespread alterations in synthesis, turnover, and urinary losses of proteins involved in both coagulation and fibrinolysis. The numerous coagulation abnormalities that occur in nephrotic syndrome are summarized in Figure 53.12. Alterations in the concentrations of almost every coagulation factor, including zymogens (factors II, V, VII, IX, X, XI, and XII), co-factors (factors V and VIII), and fibrinogen, can occur.[335] Plasma proteins lost in the urine in patients with nephrotic syndrome include factors IX, X, and XII, which become deficient because the increase in the synthetic rates that occurs is insufficient.[335] In contrast, proteins of higher molecular weight, including factors V and VIII and fibrinogen, accumulate because of increased synthesis.[334] Levels of factor VIII typically increase as much as twofold to threefold.[334] However, because factor VIII is also an acute phase reactant, high factor VIII levels may be an epiphenomenon rather than a causal factor in the development of venous thrombosis.

There is an inverse correlation between serum albumin and fibrinogen levels in nephrotic syndrome.[336] The fibrinogen elevations in plasma likely result from increased hepatic synthesis, because catabolism is normal.[337] Hyperfibrinogenemia may contribute to the procoagulant state by providing more substrate for fibrin formation and by promoting platelet hyperaggregability, increased blood viscosity, and red blood cell aggregation. Greater fibrin deposition, however, may also occur as a result of increased thrombin formation by the higher levels of factors V and VIII.[338]

Nephrotic patients exhibit abnormalities in endogenous coagulation inhibitors, including antithrombin III, which is deficient in 40% to 80% of patients.[339] Plasma levels of antithrombin III correlate negatively with proteinuria and positively with serum albumin levels as a result of urinary losses of this factor.[339] Antithrombin III deficiency has been associated with serum albumin levels less than 2.0 g/dL[340] and correlates with deep vein thrombosis (DVT) and pulmonary embolism in some studies,[340] but not in others.[341]

Alterations in other endogenous anticoagulants may also occur in patients with nephrotic syndrome, but the findings are conflicting. Although plasma levels of total protein S are increased, the active free fraction level is reduced as a consequence of urinary loss, accounting for the decrease in activity of this coagulation inhibitor.[342] Results for protein C have been contradictory.[342] Levels of tissue factor pathway inhibitor (TFPI) were increased in patients with nephrotic syndrome in one study even though this inhibitor is of relatively low molecular weight.[343] Two additional factors that may predispose to thrombosis in nephrotic patients are elevations in serum values of thrombin-activatable fibrinolysis inhibitor (TAFI) and reductions in levels of protein Z.[344]

A number of factors may lead to a reduction in plasmin-induced fibrinolysis in nephrotic syndrome; much of the work has focused on plasminogen, the precursor for plasmin, and two major regulators of plasmin formation, plasminogen activator inhibitor (PAI-1) and tissue plasminogen activator (t-PA). Several studies noted decreased plasminogen levels in nephrotic syndrome that correlated with the magnitude of proteinuria.[345] Furthermore, hypoalbuminemia itself has been postulated to negatively affect fibrinolysis. Albumin is a co-factor for the binding of plasminogen to fibrin and their interaction with t-PA. One study demonstrated suppressed glomerular fibrinolytic activity in nephrotic syndrome, because there was a sixfold increase in PAI-1 but not t-PA levels in patients with membranous glomerulopathy compared with levels in controls.[346]

Maintenance of hemostasis also involves the formation of platelet plugs through platelet activation and aggregation. Studies examining platelet abnormalities have suggested a role for enhanced platelet-vessel wall interaction and platelet aggregation in the development of thromboembolism in nephrotic syndrome. Thrombocytosis, decreased red blood cell deformability, and increased von Willebrand factor level all favor platelet transport towards the vessel wall and increased platelet adhesion,[347] and all are observed in nephrotic syndrome.

In vitro studies have demonstrated greater platelet aggregation in nephrotic patients.[347] In addition to platelet hyperaggregability, markers of platelet activation, including plasma P-selectin levels and circulating CD62P-positive platelets, were higher in nephrotic patients than in healthy controls. Increased CD62P expression was found in pediatric patients during the nephrotic episodes but not during remission.[348]

Platelet hyperaggregability is associated with hypoalbuminemia, hypercholesterolemia, and hyperfibrinogenemia.[348] Hypoalbuminemia results in greater availability of normally albumin-bound arachidonic acid, leading to increased formation of thromboxane A_2 in platelets, which promotes platelet aggregation.[349] Elevations of LDL cholesterol may increase platelet aggregation, as suggested by the observation that lipid-lowering therapy reverses the spontaneous platelet hyperaggregability seen in such patients.[350] This effect, however, has not been conclusively shown in the general population.[351]

To date, observations suggest that platelet activation and aggregation may play a role in the increased risk of thromboembolism in patients with nephrotic syndrome. However, attempts to correlate in vitro functional tests with clinically overt thromboembolic events have had conflicting results.[341] Other clinical features of the nephrotic state, such as intravascular volume depletion and exposure to steroids, also contribute to hypercoagulability. Increased blood viscosity is associated with hemoconcentration and enhanced by the use of diuretics[352] and by hyperfibrinogenemia.[334] The nature of the underlying immunologic injury may also play a role and may account for the predilection of thrombosis for the renal vein and for the higher incidence of thrombotic complications in membranous glomerulopathy. The identification of circulating immune complexes in patients with membranous glomerulopathy with renal vein thrombosis, but not in those without thrombosis, supports this possibility.[335] The use of steroids has been also suggested to predispose patients to thromboembolic complications,[335] but other studies have reported a high incidence of thromboembolic complications in the absence of steroid therapy as well.[353]

Thus, abnormalities in any of the steps that promote coagulation—activation and termination of the coagulation cascade, fibrinolysis, and platelet activation and aggregation—may contribute to the hypercoagulable state seen in nephrotic syndrome. The specific role of each of these alterations remains ill-defined.

CLINICAL CONSEQUENCE OF HYPERCOAGULABILITY

Thromboembolic events are serious complications of nephrotic syndrome. The most common site of thrombosis is the renal vein. Retrospective and prospective studies have shown an incidence of renal vein thrombosis (RVT) in nephrotic syndrome ranging from 5% to 62%.[335] Nephrotic syndrome is associated with RVT regardless of the underlying disease. Observational studies evaluated patients who underwent renal venography.[354,355] These studies show that the prevalence of RVT is highest in patients with membranous nephropathy, on average 37%. However, the risk is still clinically important in other primary glomerular diseases, particularly in membranoproliferative glomerulonephritis and minimal change disease. Furthermore, the risk for development of RVT may have been underestimated in these largely cross-sectional studies, because the complication may have developed subsequently in patients who were initially found not to have it. In the largest prospective study, which assessed RVT in 151 patients with nephrotic syndrome, the cumulative incidence of RVT was 22%.[354]

RVT manifests clinically in two ways,[354] acute and chronic. Acute RVT is usually unilateral and characterized by acute flank pain, flank tenderness, macroscopic hematuria, and some deterioration of renal function. Chronic RVT is usually asymptomatic and occurs in the elderly. Selective renal venography is the gold standard for the diagnosis of RVT, and demonstration of venous collaterals establishes chronicity. However, renal venography is invasive and associated with complications that include pulmonary embolism due to clot dislodgement, inferior vena cava perforation, and contrast agent–induced acute kidney injury.[356] Consequently, noninvasive diagnostic tests are preferred, such as intravenous pyelography, computed tomography, and magnetic resonance imaging.[356] Nevertheless, there is need for further studies because the usefulness of these latter techniques in the diagnosis or exclusion of acute RVT remains unproven. Doppler ultrasonography appears to be inferior to renal venography in establishing the diagnosis of RVT and cannot be recommended on the basis of current data.[357]

Early data on the prognosis of nephrotic patients with RVT suggested a dismal outcome. Later it became clear that in the presence of anticoagulation therapy, symptomless chronic RVT is benign.[354] DVT of the lower extremities is also observed in nephrotic syndrome and can occur in isolation in up to 15% of patients[355] or in association with RVT.[354]

Pulmonary embolism may complicate either DVT involving the lower extremities or inferior vena cava or RVT. In a case series of 151 patients with nephrotic syndrome,[354] of whom 94 underwent ventilation-perfusion lung scanning, symptomatic pulmonary embolism was observed in 25% of patients with acute RVT and 20% of patients with chronic RVT. The incidence of asymptomatic pulmonary embolism was 12.8%. In both prospective and retrospective studies, the incidence of thromboembolic complications other than RVT ranges from 8% to 44%, with an average incidence of 20%.[335]

Many clinical studies have demonstrated an association between hypoalbuminemia and venous thromboembolism, but serum albumin levels in patients with and without thromboembolic events were not significantly different.[354] These data suggest that hypoalbuminemia is associated with, but not a prerequisite for, the development of thromboembolic complications in nephrotic patients.

The patterns of thrombosis are remarkably different between children and adults. Despite lower incidence (1.8% to 5%),[358] thromboembolic complications in children tend to be more severe, and half of the children have arterial thrombosis that may cause clinical problems, such as persistent hemiplegia, mesenteric infarction, and peripheral occlusion leading to amputation.[358] In adults, arterial thrombosis is much less common than venous thrombosis, but it is a serious complication causing important morbidity. One case series described 43 patients with nephrotic syndrome who had arterial thromboembolism at the aortic, renal, femoral, mesenteric, cerebral, or brachial sites.[353] An increased risk of coronary events in patients with nephrotic syndrome has been documented in a retrospective study.[327]

The treatment of venous thromboembolism in nephrotic patients is similar to that in the general population. First-line treatment consists of conventional anticoagulation with low-molecular-weight heparin and oral vitamin K antagonists.[335] When therapy is initiated early in the course of acute RVT, renal function and other symptoms of RVT have been shown to improve significantly.[354] Oral vitamin K antagonists are usually continued for the duration of nephrotic-range proteinuria,[359] because RVT can recur in the setting of ongoing nephrosis after withdrawal of anticoagulation therapy. Low-molecular-weight heparins have a reasonable safety profile but should be used cautiously in patients with renal insufficiency because of excessive anticoagulant activity and a higher risk of bleeding due to drug accumulation.[360]

Controversy exists regarding the use of prophylactic anticoagulation therapy in patients with nephrotic syndrome who do not have RVT. The potential benefit of prophylactic anticoagulant therapy for patients with membranous glomerulopathy has been documented with the use of decision-analysis methodology.[336] Uncontrolled series show a high mortality from pulmonary embolism among patients not receiving anticoagulant therapy and very low rates of RVT and pulmonary embolism in patients given anticoagulant therapy. Prophylactic anticoagulation is warranted as long as the patient has nephrotic proteinuria, an albumin level below 2 g/dL, or both. In patients with other underlying diseases, a more cautious approach may be indicated, and prophylactic anticoagulant therapy should be initiated only if the risk of thromboembolic events is considered high.

SUSCEPTIBILITY TO INFECTION

Loss of high filtered protein load through both urinary excretion and tubular catabolism,[361] as well as a reduced rate of synthesis,[362] may result in concurrent deficiencies of IgG and components of the alternative complement pathway, including factor B. Indeed, patients with nephrotic syndrome have low serum levels of various IgG subclasses. Also, IgA levels are decreased in nephrotic syndrome, whereas IgM level is usually increased, particularly in patients with minimal change disease and normal renal function.[363] Furthermore, defective cell-mediated immunity has been reported in nephrotic syndrome,[364,365] including reduced number of total circulating T lymphocytes and blunted blastogenic response by lymphocytes to the mitogens concanavalin A and phytohemagglutinin.

The defects in both humoral and cell-mediated immunity renders the nephrotic patient highly susceptible to infection.[366] The organisms most frequently encountered are *Streptococcus pneumoniae* and *Escherichia coli*. Although such susceptibility to infection is generalized, there seems to be a particular vulnerability to local infection at the sites of edema formation. Splits in the skin caused by edema and malnutrition may predispose nephrotic patients to cellulites.[274] Peritonitis has been reported in patients who have ascites.[366] It also occurred in approximately 6% of children with nephrotic syndrome, who suffered one or more episodes of the infection.[366]

The unusual susceptibility of children to infections with encapsulated microorganisms is associated with urinary losses of the alternative pathway complement components, particularly factor B, or C3 pro-activator, and D, which are essential for the destruction of encapsulated bacteria in the absence of specific antibody.[361] The capacity to opsonize the encapsulated bacteria can be restored to normal by addition of pure factor B to nephrotic serum.[361] Fungemia due to *Candida lusitaniae* has been also reported in low-birth-weight premature infants with congenital nephrotic syndrome.[367]

New potent antibiotics have contributed to considerably decrease the incidence of fatal infections in nephrotic syndrome. However, prophylactic measures, such as pneumococcal vaccine, are recommended in adults with severely depressed immunoglobulin levels and nephrotic children more than 2 years of age, especially when early remission of nephrotic syndrome is not anticipated.[368]

Complete reference list available at ExpertConsult.com.

KEY REFERENCES

1. Haraldsson B, Nystrom J, Deen WM: Properties of the glomerular barrier and mechanisms of proteinuria. *Physiol Rev* 88:451–487, 2008.
3. Patrakka J, Tryggvason K: New insights into the role of podocytes in proteinuria. *Nat Rev Nephrol*. 5:463–468, 2009.
5. Haraldsson B, Jeansson M: Glomerular filtration barrier. *Curr Opin Nephrol Hypertens* 18:331–335, 2009.
6. Antiga L, Ene-Iordache B, Remuzzi G, et al: Automatic generation of glomerular capillary topological organization. *Microvasc Res* 62:346–354, 2001.
10. Deen WM, Bridges CR, Brenner BM: Biophysical basis of glomerular permselectivity. *J Membr Biol* 71:1–10, 1983.
11. Neal CR, Crook H, Bell E, et al: Three-dimensional reconstruction of glomeruli by electron microscopy reveals a distinct

12. restrictive urinary subpodocyte space. *J Am Soc Nephrol* 16:1223–1235, 2005.
13. Salmon AH, Toma I, Sipos A, et al: Evidence for restriction of fluid and solute movement across the glomerular capillary wall by the subpodocyte space. *Am J Physiol Renal Physiol* 293:F1777–F1786, 2007.
19. Dane MJ, van den Berg BM, Avramut MC, et al: Glomerular endothelial surface layer acts as a barrier against albumin filtration. *Am J Pathol* 182:1532–1540, 2013.
33. Gagliardini E, Conti S, Benigni A, et al: Imaging of the porous ultrastructure of the glomerular epithelial filtration slit. *J Am Soc Nephrol* 21:2081–2089, 2010.
34. Deen WM, Bridges CR, Brenner BM, et al: Heteroporous model of glomerular size selectivity: application to normal and nephrotic humans. *Am J Physiol* 249:F374–F389, 1985.
40. Christensen EI, Nielsen R: Role of megalin and cubilin in renal physiology and pathophysiology. *Rev Physiol Biochem Pharmacol* 158:1–22, 2007.
63. Brinkkoetter PT, Ising C, Benzing T: The role of the podocyte in albumin filtration. *Nat Rev Nephrol.* 9:328–336, 2013.
66. Peti-Peterdi J, Sipos A: A high-powered view of the filtration barrier. *J Am Soc Nephrol* 21:1835–1841, 2010.
68. Durvasula RV, Petermann AT, Hiromura K, et al: Activation of a local tissue angiotensin system in podocytes by mechanical strain. *Kidney Int* 65:30–39, 2004.
69. Macconi D, Abbate M, Morigi M, et al: Permselective dysfunction of podocyte-podocyte contact upon angiotensin II unravels the molecular target for renoprotective intervention. *Am J Pathol* 168:1073–1085, 2006.
75. Morigi M, Buelli S, Angioletti S, et al: In response to protein load podocytes reorganize cytoskeleton and modulate endothelin-1 gene: implication for permselective dysfunction of chronic nephropathies. *Am J Pathol* 166:1309–1320, 2005.
78. Lemley KV, Lafayette RA, Safai M, et al: Podocytopenia and disease severity in IgA nephropathy. *Kidney Int* 61:1475–1485, 2002.
89. Gagliardini E, Perico N, Rizzo P, et al: Angiotensin II contributes to diabetic renal dysfunction in rodents and humans via Notch1/Snail pathway. *Am J Pathol* 183:119–130, 2013.
90. Hasegawa K, Wakino S, Simic P, et al: Renal tubular Sirt1 attenuates diabetic albuminuria by epigenetically suppressing claudin-1 overexpression in podocytes. *Nat Med* 19:1496–1504, 2013.
99. Schlondorff D, Banas B: The mesangial cell revisited: no cell is an island. *J Am Soc Nephrol* 20:1179–1187, 2009.
107. Foster RR, Armstrong L, Baker S, et al: Glycosaminoglycan regulation by VEGFA and VEGFC of the glomerular microvascular endothelial cell glycocalyx in vitro. *Am J Pathol* 183:604–616, 2013.
115. Sagrinati C, Netti GS, Mazzinghi B, et al: Isolation and characterization of multipotent progenitor cells from the Bowman's capsule of adult human kidneys. *J Am Soc Nephrol* 17:2443–2456, 2006.
118. Rizzo P, Perico N, Gagliardini E, et al: Nature and mediators of parietal epithelial cell activation in glomerulonephritides of human and rat. *Am J Pathol* 183:1769–1778, 2013.
121. Ueno T, Kobayashi N, Nakayama M, et al: Aberrant Notch1-dependent effects on glomerular parietal epithelial cells promotes collapsing focal segmental glomerulosclerosis with progressive podocyte loss. *Kidney Int* 83:1065–1075, 2013.
124. Fine LG, Norman JT: Chronic hypoxia as a mechanism of progression of chronic kidney diseases: from hypothesis to novel therapeutics. *Kidney Int* 74:867–872, 2008.
134. Caruso-Neves C, Pinheiro AA, Cai H, et al: PKB and megalin determine the survival or death of renal proximal tubule cells. *Proc Natl Acad Sci U S A* 103:18810–18815, 2006.
140. Zoja C, Donadelli R, Colleoni S, et al: Protein overload stimulates RANTES production by proximal tubular cells depending on NF-kappa B activation. *Kidney Int* 53:1608–1615, 1998.
142. Tang S, Leung JC, Abe K, et al: Albumin stimulates interleukin-8 expression in proximal tubular epithelial cells in vitro and in vivo. *J Clin Invest* 111:515–527, 2003.
151. Rudnicki M, Eder S, Perco P, et al: Gene expression profiles of human proximal tubular epithelial cells in proteinuric nephropathies. *Kidney Int* 71:325–335, 2007.
152. Biemesderfer D: Regulated intramembrane proteolysis of megalin: linking urinary protein and gene regulation in proximal tubule? *Kidney Int* 69:1717–1721, 2006.
162. Wang SN, Hirschberg R: Growth factor ultrafiltration in experimental diabetic nephropathy contributes to interstitial fibrosis. *Am J Physiol Renal Physiol* 278:F554–F560, 2000.
165. Abbate M, Zoja C, Rottoli D, et al: Antiproteinuric therapy while preventing the abnormal protein traffic in proximal tubule abrogates protein- and complement-dependent interstitial inflammation in experimental renal disease. *J Am Soc Nephrol* 10:804–813, 1999.
166. Nangaku M, Pippin J, Couser WG: Complement membrane attack complex (C5b-9) mediates interstitial disease in experimental nephrotic syndrome. *J Am Soc Nephrol* 10:2323–2331, 1999.
176. Heymann F, Meyer-Schwesinger C, Hamilton-Williams EE, et al: Kidney dendritic cell activation is required for progression of renal disease in a mouse model of glomerular injury. *J Clin Invest* 119:1286–1297, 2009.
177. Macconi D, Chiabrando C, Schiarea S, et al: Proteasomal processing of albumin by renal dendritic cells generates antigenic peptides. *J Am Soc Nephrol* 20:123–130, 2009.
187. Sakai N, Wada T, Yokoyama H, et al: Secondary lymphoid tissue chemokine (SLC/CCL21)/CCR7 signaling regulates fibrocytes in renal fibrosis. *Proc Natl Acad Sci U S A* 103:14098–14103, 2006.
196. Humphreys BD, Lin S-L, Kobayashi A, et al: Fate tracing reveals the stromal pericyte and not epithelial origin of myofibroblasts in the obstructive model of kidney fibrosis. *J Clin Invest* 176:85–97, 2010.
208. Khairoun M, van der Pol P, de Vries DK, et al: Renal ischemia-reperfusion induces a dysbalance of angiopoietins, accompanied by proliferation of pericytes and fibrosis. *Am J Physiol Renal Physiol* 305:F901–F910, 2013.
221. Wang YM, Zhang GY, Wang Y, et al: Foxp3-transduced polyclonal regulatory T cells protect against chronic renal injury from Adriamycin. *J Am Soc Nephrol* 17:697–706, 2006.
226. Appel D, Kershaw DB, Smeets B, et al: Recruitment of podocytes from glomerular parietal epithelial cells. *J Am Soc Nephrol* 20:333–343, 2009.
228. Macconi D, Sangalli F, Bonomelli M, et al: Podocyte repopulation contributes to regression of glomerular injury induced by ACE inhibition. *Am J Pathol* 174:797–807, 2009.
233. Peired A, Angelotti ML, Ronconi E, et al: Proteinuria impairs podocyte regeneration by sequestering retinoic acid. *J Am Soc Nephrol* 24:1756–1768, 2013.
239. Kaysen GA, Jones H, Jr, Martin V, et al: A low-protein diet restricts albumin synthesis in nephrotic rats. *J Clin Invest* 83:1623–1629, 1989.
245. Drumond MC, Kristal B, Myers BD, et al: Structural basis for reduced glomerular filtration capacity in nephrotic humans. *J Clin Invest* 94:1187–1195, 1994.
280. Ichikawa I, Rennke HG, Hoyer JR, et al: Role for intrarenal mechanisms in the impaired salt excretion of experimental nephrotic syndrome. *J Clin Invest* 71:91–103, 1983.
281. Perico N, Delaini F, Lupini C, et al: Blunted excretory response to atrial natriuretic peptide in experimental nephrosis. *Kidney Int* 36:57–64, 1989.
282. Peterson C, Madsen B, Perlman A, et al: Atrial natriuretic peptide and the renal response to hypervolemia in nephrotic humans. *Kidney Int* 34:825–831, 1988.
296. Kim SW, Wang W, Nielsen J, et al: Increased expression and apical targeting of renal ENaC subunits in puromycin aminonucleoside-induced nephrotic syndrome in rats. *Am J Physiol Renal Physiol* 286:F922–F935, 2004.
334. Kanfer A: Coagulation factors in nephrotic syndrome. *Am J Nephrol* 10(Suppl 1):63–68, 1990.

The Pathophysiology of Uremia

Timothy W. Meyer | Thomas H. Hostetter

CHAPTER OUTLINE

SOLUTES CLEARED BY THE KIDNEY AND RETAINED IN UREMIA, 1808
Individual Uremic Solutes, 1808
Solute Removal by Different Forms of Renal Replacement Therapy, 1813
Effects of Diet and Gastrointestinal Function, 1814
Solute Clearance by Organic Transport Systems, 1815
METABOLIC EFFECTS OF UREMIA, 1815
Oxidant Stress and the Modification of Protein Structure, 1815
Effects of Uremia, 1815
Overall Nutrition, 1817
SIGNS AND SYMPTOMS OF UREMIA, 1818
Well-Being and Physical Function, 1818
Neurologic Function, 1818
Appetite, Taste, and Smell, 1819
Cellular Functions, 1819
Why Is the Glomerular Filtration Rate So Large?, 1819

The word *uremic* is generally used to describe those ill effects of kidney failure that we cannot yet explain. Hypertension caused by volume overload, tetany caused by hypocalcemia, and anemia caused by erythropoietin deficiency were once considered uremic signs, but were removed from this category as their causes were discovered. Uremia may thus now be defined as the illness that would remain if the extracellular volume and inorganic ion concentrations were kept normal and the known renal synthetic products were replaced in patients without kidneys (Table 54.1).

Some features of uremia, thus defined, could reflect the lack of unidentified renal synthetic products. We presume, however, that uremia is caused largely by the accumulation of organic waste products that are normally cleared by the kidneys. In general, the study of renal organic waste removal lags far behind the study of inorganic ion excretion. A major problem is the multiplicity of waste solutes. The most comprehensive reviews to date, prepared by the European Uremic Toxin Work Group (EUTox[1,2]), list more than 80 uremic solutes, and new studies are adding to this number.[3-5] With so many substances to study, it is hard to establish which ones are toxic. Bergstom[6] has suggested criteria for identifying uremic toxins that are analogous to Koch's postulates for identifying infectious agents. According to these criteria, a uremic toxin must have a known chemical structure and the following features:

- Its plasma and/or tissue concentrations should be higher in patients with kidney failure than in normal persons.
- The high concentrations should be related to specific uremic symptoms that are ameliorated when the concentration is reduced.
- The effects observed in uremic patients should be replicated by raising the solute concentration to similar levels in normal persons, experimental animals, or in vitro systems.

No uremic solute has so far been shown to satisfy these criteria. Given the complexity of uremia, it is unlikely that the accumulation of a single solute in isolation could recapitulate uremia or that removal of the same could eliminate uremia; therefore, progress in uremia research has been relatively slow. Most solutes that accumulate with advanced chronic kidney disease (CKD) are probably not toxic. Others that are toxic may exert their ill effects only when administered in combination. The difficulty imposed by the multiplicity of solutes is compounded by the multiplicity of ill effects encountered in uremia. Investigators of uremic toxicity thus face the daunting task of matching a solute or group of solutes to an appropriate end point. Many of the effects of uremia are hard to quantify, which makes the problem even more difficult. This is particularly true of major uremic symptoms. such as fatigue, anorexia, and diminished mental acuity.

A related problem encountered in studies of uremia is distinguishing the effects of uremia from those of related conditions. Paradoxically, the widespread availability of dialysis has made uremia somewhat more difficult to study. The

Table 54.1 Metabolic Effects, Symptoms, and Signs of Uremia

Metabolic

Increased oxidant levels
Reduced resting energy expenditure
Reduced body temperature
Insulin resistance
Muscle wasting
Amenorrhea and sexual dysfunction

Neural and Muscular

Fatigue
Loss of concentration ranging to coma and seizures
Sleep disturbances
Restless legs
Peripheral neuropathy
Anorexia and nausea
Diminution in taste and smell
Itching
Cramps
Reduced muscle membrane potential

Other

Serositis (including pericarditis)
Hiccups
Granulocyte and lymphocyte dysfunction
Platelet dysfunction
Shortened erythrocyte lifespan
Albumin oxidation

Table 54.2 Uremic Abnormalities Transferable with Uremic Serum or Plasma

Inhibition of Na^+-K^+-ATPase
Inhibition of platelet function
Leukocyte dysfunction
Loss of erythrocyte membrane lipid asymmetry
Insulin resistance

ATPase, Adenosine triphosphatase.

---

severity of the classic uremic symptoms is attenuated, and patients now suffer from a new illness, which Depner[7] has aptly named the *residual syndrome*, comprised of partially treated uremia and the side effects of dialysis. In most patients, features of the residual syndrome are further combined with the effects of age and of systemic diseases responsible for kidney failure. Disturbances of inorganic ion metabolism, including acidemia and hyperphosphatemia, although excluded from our definition of uremia, undoubtedly also contribute to untoward clinical manifestations of kidney failure. Given these difficulties, it is not surprising that although we have identified many uremic solutes, we know relatively little about their toxicity. In a few cases, uremic abnormalities have been reproduced by the transfer of uremic serum or plasma to normal animals or addition of these factors to the media of cultured cells (Table 54.2). However, the role of particular solute(s) in causing the abnormalities remains uncertain.

SOLUTES CLEARED BY THE KIDNEY AND RETAINED IN UREMIA

The long list of solutes retained in uremia has been assembled in two ways. Initially, biochemists would find a substance in the urine and then look for it in the blood of uremic patients. Several dozen uremic solutes were identified in this way as the biochemical pathways of intermediary metabolism were worked out. Beginning about 1970, improved analytic techniques, including gas chromatography, mass spectroscopy, and high-performance liquid chromatography, were used to identify additional uremic solutes.[3,8] Recent technical advances, including proteomic and metabolomic screening methods, are lengthening the list of putative uremic solutes. However, the problem of determining which solutes are toxic remains. In general, the compounds that are present in the highest concentrations, and were therefore identified first, have been studied most extensively. Experiments showing that uremic signs and symptoms can be replicated by raising solute levels in normal persons or animals to equal those observed in uremic patients are lacking. When attempted, such experiments have generally shown that the solutes being studied are more toxic than urea, but that the levels required to produce toxic effects are higher than those measured in patients. Because so little is known about their toxicity, the discussion of uremic solutes is usually organized on the basis of their structure and not necessarily their contribution to disease.

INDIVIDUAL UREMIC SOLUTES

UREA

Urea is quantitatively the most abundant solute excreted by the kidney, and levels rise higher than those of any other solute when the kidney fails. Early studies indicated that urea causes only a minor part of uremic illness.[9-11] In the most often cited of these studies, Johnson and colleagues[10] dialyzed patients with kidney failure against bath solutions containing urea. They found that initiation of hemodialysis improved uremic symptoms, including weakness, fetor, and gastrointestinal upset, even when urea was added to the dialysate to maintain the blood urea nitrogen (BUN) level at approximately 90 mg/dL. In patients already on dialysis, increasing the BUN level to 140 mg/dL did not cause recurrence of uremic symptoms. Increasing the BUN level above 140 mg/dL caused nausea and headaches, and increasing the BUN level above 180 mg/dL caused weakness and lethargy. However, symptoms in dialyzed patients whose BUN values were increased to these levels were less severe than symptoms in undialyzed patients with similar BUN values. Studies in patients without kidney failure suggest that urea by itself does not cause uremia. Uremic symptoms have not been observed in patients in whom BUN levels are maintained at approximately 60 mg/dL by high protein intake or increased tubular urea absorption.[12-14] Similarly, patients on high-dose glucocorticoids or those with heart failure, conditions commonly seen in modern medical practice, do not experience uremia when kidney function, estimated by other solutes (typically serum creatinine), is not severely impaired.

The finding that uremia is not replicated by an isolated elevation of the plasma urea concentration does not mean that urea has no toxic effects.[15] The full expression of uremia may require accumulation of urea plus other solutes. Johnson and associates[10] noted that patients dialyzed against solutions of urea exhibited increased bleeding, and subsequent studies suggested that urea promotes bleeding by promoting synthesis of guanidinosuccinic acid (GSA), which in turn impairs platelet function.[16,17] Increased plasma urea concentrations may cause other ill effects by increasing isocyanate concentration and thereby promoting protein carbamylation (Figure 54.1).[18-22] Isocyanate can also combine reversibly with –OH and –SH groups of amino acids, and the various isocyanate-induced alterations in structure could impair protein function.

D-AMINO ACIDS

In comparison to urea, we know much less about most other potential uremic toxins. The D–amino acids exemplify this problem. Aggregate plasma concentrations of D–amino acids increase as kidney function declines.[23,24] However, the source, clearance, and toxicity of the D–amino acids found

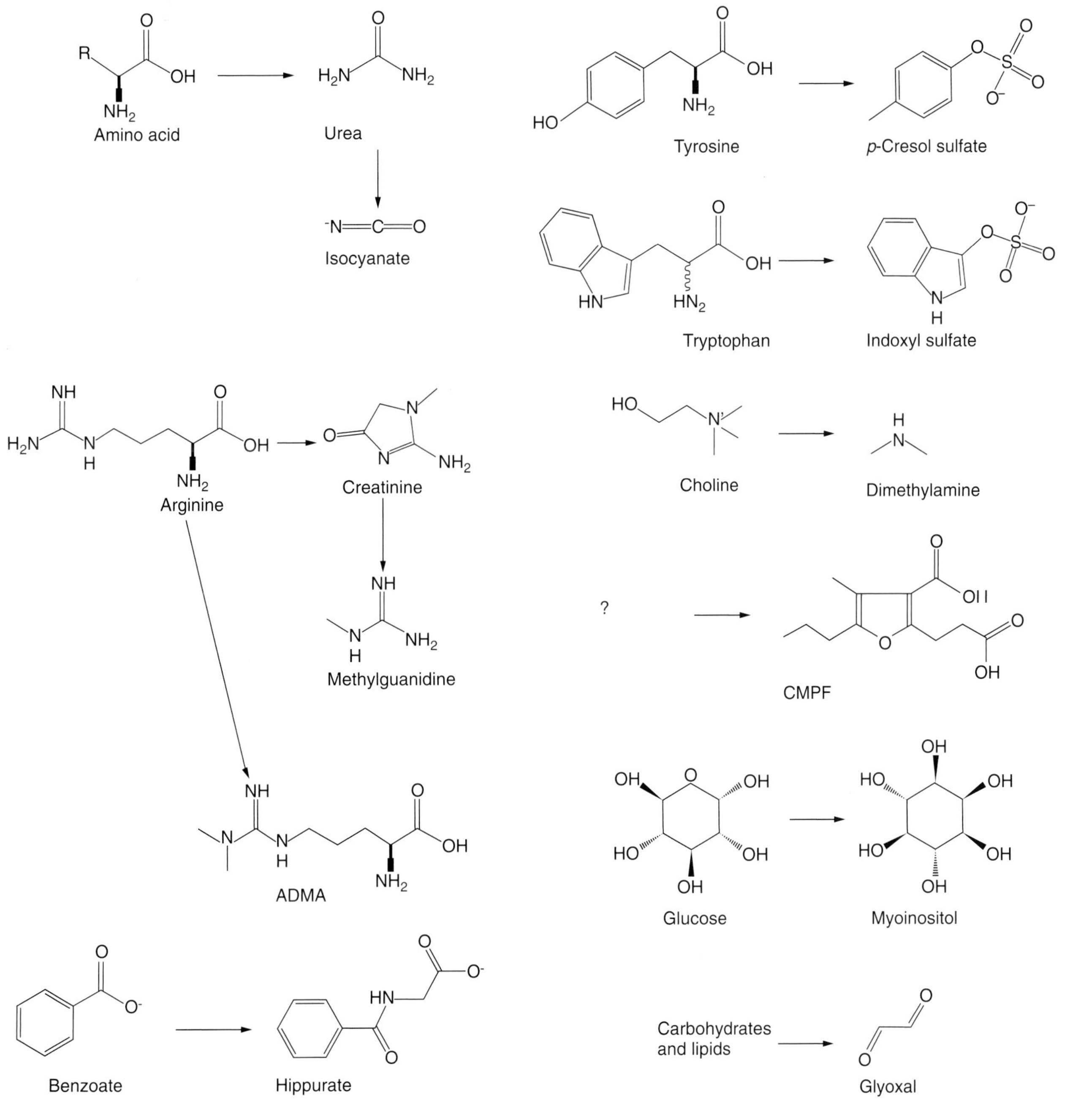

Figure 54.1 Generation of potential uremic toxins. The substances in the *right column* of each panel are metabolites that are normally excreted by the kidney and therefore accumulate in the extracellular fluid when kidney function is lost. The *left column* shows the substances from which these potential "uremic toxins" are derived. In some cases, the biochemical derivation of the potential toxins is uncertain. For example, it is not known what fraction of the dimethylamine normally excreted is derived from choline, and the source of 3-carboxy-4-methyl-5-prophy-2-furanpropanoic acid (CMPF) is obscure. See text for details. ADMA, Asymmetric dimethyl arginine.

in the plasma are not well defined. D-Amino acids can be synthesized by mammalian cells, as well as derived from food, or produced by colonic bacteria.[25] Circulating D-amino acids are filtered by the glomerulus and then, in varying proportion, reabsorbed intact, degraded by D-amino acid oxidase (DAO) or D-aspartic acid oxidase in the proximal straight tubule, or excreted unaltered in the urine.[26,27] The liver can also clear D-amino acids, but the relative importance of renal and hepatic clearance is unknown. Aggregate D-amino acid concentrations have been found to increase almost in proportion to the serum creatinine level in kidney failure, suggesting that renal clearance predominates.[23,28,29] However, concentrations of individual D-amino acids measured so far, including D-serine, increase less than the creatinine.[28,29] This discrepancy remains unexplained. It is tempting to speculate that D-amino acids are cleared rapidly from the extracellular fluid (ECF) because they have toxic effects. Also, it has long been presumed that high levels of D-amino acids could impair protein synthesis or function.[25] D-Amino acid accumulation could also interfere with the effects of endogenous D-serine and D-alanine on neuronal function,[30] but no major ill effects of D-amino acid accumulation have been observed in DAO-deficient mice, which have higher D-amino acid levels than humans with impaired kidney function.[31,32] Exogenous D-amino acids have so far been shown to be toxic only when administered in large quantities.[31,33]

PEPTIDES AND PROTEINS

The kidney clears circulating dipeptides and tripeptides, which may comprise a significant portion of the extracellular amino acid pool.[34] Filtered dipeptides and tripeptides can be broken down by brush border peptidases and reabsorbed as amino acids or reabsorbed by a brush border peptide transporter and then hydrolyzed within proximal tubule cells.[35] Peritubular uptake, again followed by hydrolysis to amino acids, makes the renal clearance of many peptides higher than the glomerular filtration rate (GFR).[34,36] Small peptides are also taken up by other organs and generally do not accumulate in kidney failure. Peptides containing altered amino acids, which are normally cleared by the kidney, may be an exception to this rule.[36]

The kidney plays a proportionally larger role in the clearance of larger peptides. Proteins with a molecular weight of 10 to 20 kDa, such as β_2-microglobulin and cystatin C, are normally filtered by the glomerulus and then endocytosed and hydrolyzed in the lysozomes of proximal tubular cells.[37,38] Their plasma concentrations therefore rise in parallel with the plasma creatinine level as kidney function declines. Indeed, the plasma concentration of cystatin C, which is released at a near-constant rate by nucleated cells, may yield a more reliable estimate of GFR than the concentration of creatinine.[39] The role of the kidney in the removal of peptides with molecular weight between 500 Da and 10 kDa is less well-defined. Peptides in this range are also filtered by the glomerulus and then hydrolyzed by brush border peptidases or endocytosed, depending on their size and structure. Biologically active peptides such as insulin may also be cleared by peritubular uptake. Studies in patients with inherited dysfunction of proximal tubular endocytosis suggest that the normal kidney clears approximately 350 mg/day of peptides with molecular weights of 5 to 10 kDa from the circulation.[40] The relative importance of renal to extrarenal clearance has not been defined for most substances in this size range. The extent to which circulating levels of such peptides are increased in kidney failure is therefore unpredictable. Even less is known about the kidneys' contribution to the clearance of peptides in the range of 500 Da to 5 kDa.

Table 54.3 Low-Molecular-Weight Proteins and Protein Fragments That Accumulate in Uremia

α_1-Microglobulin
β_2-Microglobulin
β-Trace protein
Clara cell protein
Chromogranin A
Cystatin C
Free immunoglobulin light chains
Retinol-binding protein
Transcobalamin
Leptin
Ghrelin
Resistin

Although the aggregate peptide levels in kidney failure remain ill defined, we have some knowledge of individual peptides that are retained in uremia. The best known are small proteins or fragments of large proteins for which immunoassays have been developed.[41-53] Table 54.3 provides a partial list of these substances. Retinol-binding protein, α_1-microglobulin, and β-trace protein are members of the lipocalin superfamily, and future studies may identify elevated levels of other proteins of this group. Studies using proteomic techniques have yielded a more complete picture.[54-56] These studies have shown that as expected, uremic plasma contains a vast array of protein fragments that are normally cleared by the kidney. Many of these are derived from fibrinogen and the complement cascade.[56,57] One study has identified more than 1000 peptides with molecular weights from 800 Da to 10 kDa in the plasma of patients undergoing dialysis.[58] The central question, of course, is whether any of these substances are toxic. It has been widely speculated that retained peptides can cause inappropriate activation of various hormone or cytokine receptors. For example, retained complement protein D (molecular weight [MW], 24 kDa) could contribute to the systemic inflammation and accelerated vascular disease observed in patients receiving dialysis.[59] Such hypotheses remain largely unproven, however, and β_2-microglobulin is the only retained peptide that has been convincingly shown to cause disease.

GUANIDINES

Among the compounds most frequently considered uremic toxins are guanidines, which, like urea, are derived from arginine (see Figure 55.1).[60-62] One group of guanidines that accumulate in uremia includes creatinine and its breakdown products. Creatinine is produced by nonenzymatic degradation of creatine, which in turn is made from guanidinoacetic acid (GAA).[63] Creatinine itself appears nontoxic, and levels have been increased transiently to more than 100 mg/dL in subjects undergoing clearance studies. Instead, interest has been focused on the potential toxicity of various creatinine metabolites, including creatol and methylguanidine in particular.[64,65] The production of these substances increases as plasma creatinine concentrations rise and may be stimulated by increased levels of intracellular oxidants.[61,63,64] Methylguanidine is also produced by colonic bacteria, and its production may be increased by increasing the dietary intake of protein or creatinine.[66] Another guanidine that has attracted interest is GSA, a substance formed not from creatinine but from the urea cycle intermediate, argininosuccinate.[67,68] Rising plasma urea concentrations impede the conversion of argininosuccinate to urea and increase the production of GSA. The production of GSA thus depends on dietary protein intake as well as on kidney function, and may also be stimulated by increased concentrations of intracellular oxidants.[68,69]

Creatol, methylguanidine, and GSA share the interesting property that their plasma concentrations rise out of proportion to urea and creatinine levels as the GFR declines. This is because they are cleared largely by the kidney, and their production rates increase when plasma creatinine and urea concentrations are elevated.[61,63,64] In addition, large volumes of distribution, combined with restricted intercompartmental diffusion, limit the removal of creatol, methylguanidine, and GSA by intermittent hemodialysis.[60] In patients undergoing conventional hemodialysis, these compounds therefore exhibit high concentrations relative to normal.[1] The finding that they are present in relatively high concentrations does not prove that they are toxic. However, the evidence for toxicity of various guanidines, although incomplete, is stronger than that for most other solutes. Administration of methylguanidine aggravates uremic symptoms in dogs, whereas GSA contributes to uremic platelet dysfunction, and a number of guanidines impair neutrophil function.[16,70,71] In addition, various guanidines have been shown to accumulate in the brain and cerebrospinal fluid in uremia and may contribute to central nervous system dysfunction.[72]

The methylated arginines, asymmetric dimethyl arginine (ADMA) and symmetric dimethyl arginine (SDMA) also accumulate in kidney failure (see Figure 54.1). The metabolism of methylated arginines is quite different from that of the other uremic guanidines. ADMA and SDMA are formed by the methylation of arginine residues in nuclear proteins and released when these proteins are degraded. Interest has focused largely on ADMA because it inhibits nitric oxide (a potent local vasodilator) synthesis, whereas SDMA is relatively inactive.[73,74] The urinary clearance of ADMA is similar to that of creatinine, but most plasma ADMA is taken up and degraded in various tissues, including the kidney.[73,75] The increase in plasma ADMA concentrations observed in patients with impaired kidney function has therefore generally been attributed to a reduction in extrarenal clearance, although there may also be some increase in production. The mechanism responsible for reducing the extrarenal clearance of ADMA is unknown. It is notable that ADMA levels may rise to approximately twice normal very early in the course of CKD and then do not increase much further as patients advance to end-stage renal disease (ESRD).[75,76] Increases in plasma ADMA concentration, although modest in proportion to other uremic solutes, has been associated with an increased risk for cardiovascular disease and death in patients with CKD.[74] It should be noted that differences in assay methods and reported reference ranges for ADMA greatly complicate the interpretation of these studies.

PHENOLS AND OTHER AROMATIC COMPOUNDS

Phenols are compounds that have one or more hydroxyl groups attached to a benzene ring. In discussions of uremia, phenols are usually considered together with other aromatic compounds, such as hippurates, and the term *phenols* is sometimes used loosely to include these other substances. The aromatic compounds normally found in ECF are for the most part derived from the amino acids tyrosine and phenylalanine or from aromatic compounds contained in vegetable foods. Medications provide an additional source in patients. The compounds in ECF are mostly metabolites; these are derived from their parent compounds by a combination of methylation, dehydroxylation, oxidation, reduction, and/or conjugation. Many of these reactions take place in colonic bacteria. The final step, which is usually conjugation with sulfate, glucuronic acid, or an amino acid, may take place in the liver, intestinal wall or, to a lesser extent, kidney.[77,78] In general, conjugation tends to make the aromatic compounds at once less toxic and more polar, which facilitates their excretion by various organic ion transport systems.

The metabolic processes described earlier produce a bewildering array of aromatic compounds that are normally excreted in the urine or feces. The aggregate urinary excretion of aromatics is about 1000 mg/day and varies widely with the diet. The compounds normally excreted by the kidney accumulate in uremia and contribute to elevation of the anion gap, because most aromatic conjugates are negatively charged.[79] The concentration of individual aromatic compounds in uremic patients ranges from barely detectable up to 500 μm.[1,80-82] The relatively few compounds that have been studied extensively, including the examples described later, are among those found in the highest concentration. Interest in the contribution of phenols and other aromatic compounds to uremic toxicity has been encouraged by reports that uremic symptoms are better correlated with plasma concentration of these compounds than with those of other solutes.[11,83-85] Evidence obtained so far on the toxicity of individual aromatic compound is incomplete.

The most extensively studied aromatic uremic solute is hippurate (see Figure 54.1). Because it is the aromatic waste compound normally excreted in the largest quantity, the concentration of free hippurate rises higher than those of other aromatic solutes in the plasma of patients with kidney failure. Hippurate is the glycine conjugate of benzoate, derived largely from vegetable foods, with only a small amount formed endogenously from the amino acid phenylalanine.[86,87] Diet therefore determines hippurate production, and hippurate excretion in aboriginal people eating vegetable diets may exceed hippurate excretion in people from industrialized nations by many-fold.[88] In persons with normal kidneys, active tubular secretion maintains a plasma hippurate concentration much lower than it would be if hippurate were cleared solely by glomerular filtration. Hippurate, however, is not toxic. The plasma hippurate concentration in a normal person can be increased to equal that of a uremic patient, without apparent ill effect.[89] Moreover, increasing the hippurate concentration by benzoate feeding in a patient with kidney failure does not aggravate uremic symptoms.[90]

Another extensively studied aromatic compound is *p*-cresol. In contrast to hippurate, which is derived from aromatic compounds in plants, *p*-cresol is formed by the action of colonic bacteria on tyrosine and phenylalanine. The portion of amino acids that escapes absorption in the small intestine may be increased in uremic patients, leading to increased production of *p*-cresol and other bacterial metabolites.[91,92] Studies have shown that *p*-cresol circulates almost exclusively as *p*-cresol sulfate, and reports of unconjugated *p*-cresol in the plasma of uremic patients now appear to have been the result of inadvertent hydrolysis of *p*-cresol sulfate during sample processing.[93,94] *p*-Cresol sulfate binds avidly to serum albumin, and the effect of different renal replacement therapies on albumin-bound solutes has often been tested by measuring plasma *p*-cresol sulfate concentrations.[95-97] High concentrations of *p*-cresol sulfate (often measured as *p*-cresol) have been associated with cardiovascular death in patients undergoing hemodialysis, and *p*-cresol sulfate has been related to indices of endothelial injury, including endothelial microparticle production.[98,99] These results, along with evidence that *p*-cresol sulfate can injure endothelial cells and impair neutrophil function in vivo, have increased the focus on *p*-cresol sulfate as a potential uremic toxin.[99,100]

Other aromatic uremic solutes have been identified in great numbers but studied less extensively.[6,81,82] Metabolites of tyrosine and phenylalanine, which accumulate in uremia, include phenylacetylglutamate, parahydroxyphenylacetic acid, and 3,4-dihydroxybenzoic acid, as well as *p*-cresol.[101-103] The structural relationship of these aromatic amino acid metabolites to neurotransmitters has stimulated interest in their potential role as uremic toxins. So far, 3,4-dihydroxybenzoate has been shown to cause central nervous system (CNS) dysfunction in rats, but only at levels higher than those encountered in patients with kidney failure.[102] The work of testing the toxicity of other aromatic uremic solutes is daunting, and little progress has been made.

INDOLES AND OTHER TRYPTOPHAN METABOLITES

Indoles are compounds containing a benzene ring fused to a five-membered nitrogen containing a pyrrole ring (see Figure 54.1). Many similarities are encountered when considering the indoles and phenols in uremia. As with phenols, some indoles are derived from plant foods, and others are produced endogenously. However, the endogenous indoles are derived mostly from tryptophan, whereas the phenols are derived from phenylalanine and tyrosine. As with the phenols, minor chemical modifications in various combinations yield a remarkable variety of structures, with more than 600 indoles derived from tryptophan.[104] Those with known physiologic function include the neurotransmitter 5-hydroxytryptamine (serotonin) and melatonin. Other indoles are considered to be waste products and are often conjugated prior to urinary excretion. These uremic indoles accumulate when kidney function is impaired.

The most extensively studied of the uremic indoles is indoxyl sulfate; this is produced from tryptophan in a manner reminiscent of the production of *p*-cresol sulfate from tyrosine and phenylalanine. Gut bacteria convert tryptophan to indole, which is then oxidized to indoxyl and conjugated with sulfate in the liver. There is evidence that indoxyl sulfate is toxic in vitro, but early studies of indoxyl sulfate infusion failed to replicate uremic symptoms.[11,105-107] Like *p*-cresol sulfate, indoxyl sulfate is extensively bound to plasma albumin. It has also been suggested that indoxyl sulfate is toxic to renal tubular cells, and that higher plasma indoxyl sulfate concentrations accelerate the loss of remnant nephrons in kidneys that have been damaged by disease.[108]

Other indoles that accumulate in uremia include indoleacetic acid, indoleacrylic acid, and 5-hyroxyindoleacetic acid.[1,109,110] As with the phenols, indoles are structurally related to potent neuroactive substances, including serotonin and (famously) D-lysergic acid diethylamide (D-LSD). This structural similarity has stimulated interest in the potential role of indoles as neurotoxins, but few uremic indoles have been administered to normal animals, and none have convincingly been shown to alter CNS function at the levels encountered in patients with kidney failure.

Only a minor portion of dietary tryptophan is excreted as indoles. Most is metabolized by the kynurenine pathway, which allows tryptophan to be converted to glutarate and oxidized or, when necessary, used in the synthesis of nicotinamide. Kidney failure causes members of the kynurenine pathway, including L-kynurenine and quinolinic acid, to accumulate in the plasma.[111,112] Knowledge that these substances play a physiologic role in the modulation of CNS function has stimulated interest in their possible contribution to uremic toxicity. As usual, however, evidence that they are toxic at the levels encountered in patients has not been obtained.

ALIPHATIC AMINES

The methylamines monomethylamine (MMA), dimethylamine (DMA), and trimethylamine (TMA) are among the simplest compounds that have been considered to be uremic toxins. Reported serum levels are two- to threefold higher in patients with ESRD compared to persons with normal or near-normal kidney function.[113,114] However, available data and predictions based on their chemistry suggest that the methylamines are poorly removed by dialysis, and limited data suggest that they may even be produced in excess in those with uremia.[113-115]

A large volume of distribution may contribute to poor removal of the methylamines by dialysis. These compounds are bases, with a pH ranging from 9 to 11. Thus, they exist as positively charged species at a physiologic pH. The lower intracellular pH compared to extracellular pH should lead to their preferential intracellular sequestration, with volumes of distribution exceeding total body water. Indeed, measurements in experimental animals and humans have confirmed these predictions for DMA and TMA.[114,116,117]

Because they circulate as small organic compounds that are not protein-bound, these three amines are likely freely filtered. However, because they exist as organic cations, they also have the potential to be secreted by one or another of the family of organic cation transporters and also may also travel through Rh channels.[118,119] Hence, they may achieve clearances that are in fact higher than the GFR. The chemically similar exogenous compound, tetraethyl ammonium, has long been a prototype test solute for organic cation secretion and is cleared at rates up to (and in one study higher than) the renal plasma flow.[120,121] Although formal renal clearances of DMA and TMA are not available, the total metabolic clearance of DMA and TMA by plasma disappearance of labeled compounds in rats approaches that of renal plasma flow.[116] On the other hand, the urinary clearance of MMA in normal subjects is about one third that of creatinine, indicating no net secretion for this amine.[115]

The biochemical pathways leading to MMA, DMA, and TMA are not well delineated. Both the host's mammalian tissues and resident gut flora have been thought to contribute to the net appearance of these amines. However, plasma MMA and DMA concentrations were not different among patients with ESRD with and without colons.[122] The dietary precursors for MMA, DMA, and TMA include choline and trimethylamine oxide (TMAO).[123-125] Production of these compounds may actually be increased with kidney failure, perhaps caused by overgrowth of intestinal bacteria.[115,117,126] Thus, data support the possibility that in ESRD, production of aliphatic amines may be increased in the face of impaired renal removal.

Incomplete data also implicate the amines as toxic. MMA may be the most toxic in the class, and its effects include a variety of neural toxicities, hemolysis, and inhibition of lysosomal function.[127] MMA is a potent anorectic agent when administered into the cerebrospinal fluid in mice.[128] Despite toxicities in cells and animals, however, MMA and DMA were not associated with all-cause mortality in a cohort of patients with ESRD.[129] Although of utmost importance, mortality is obviously a blunt metric of uremic toxicity. Other signs of toxicity of MMA and DMA should be explored.

The uremic fetor or fishy breath noted in uremic patients is attributable to TMA.[130] Although the malodor may be of no major consequence in itself, the potentially important and well-described diminutions in taste (dysgeusia) and smell (dysosmia) among patients with kidney failure (which may contribute to poor nutritional status) may also be related to the amines. Plasma MMA concentrations were not related to olfactory defects in ESRD.[131] TMA can be both a precursor to TMAO and, as noted, a product of dietary TMAO.[132] TMAO has been identified as a risk factor for cardiovascular disease in persons with normal renal function, and its levels are markedly elevated in patients with ESRD.[132,133] Whether the high risk for cardiovascular disease in ESRD is in some degree related to TMAO is unknown.

OTHER UREMIC SOLUTES

A wide variety of other compounds accumulate in kidney failure. One group is the polyols, of which the most extensively studied is myoinositol (see Figure 54.1).[134,135] Myoinositol is different from most other uremic solutes in that it is normally oxidized by the kidney. Its accumulation in uremia therefore reflects impaired degradation and not impaired excretion. Evidence that myoinositol causes nerve damage, although stronger than most of the evidence for the toxicity of uremic solutes, is far from conclusive.[136]

The purine metabolite uric acid is the only known organic substance with a plasma level actively regulated by variation of its renal excretion. With advanced chronic kidney disease, the capacity of the kidney to increase the fractional excretion of uric acid is exceeded, and uric acid levels increase, along with those of its precursor molecules, xanthine and hypoxanthine. Other nucleic acid metabolites excreted by the kidney are produced in much lesser quantities. Many are derived from the modified nucleosides contained in transfer RNAs (tRNAs).[137] They appear to be cleared largely by filtration and to accumulate in the plasma as the GFR falls. It has been suggested that pseudouridine, which is the most abundant of these substances, contributes to insulin resistance and altered CNS development but, as usual, the demonstration of its toxicity is not conclusive.[137,138]

Oxalate is also excreted by the kidney and accumulates in kidney failure. Oxalate is derived from catabolism of endogenous substances, including vitamin C, as well as from plant foods.[139,140] The potential for oxalate deposition in tissues may limit our ability to maintain normal plasma vitamin C concentrations in patients receiving dialysis.[141,142] Additional substances excreted by the kidney that accumulate in kidney failure include various pteridines, dicarboxylic acids, isoflavins, and furancarboxylic acids, including 3-carboxy-4-methyl-5-prophy-2-furanpropanoic acid (CMPF).[96,137,143-146] Recently completed studies continue to add new solutes to the list, and the number reported will likely soon rise above 1000, including many compounds that are at present identified only by their molecular mass and do not appear in standard databases of human metabolites as yet. The possibility of toxicity is invariably considered when new solutes are identified, but experiments to test the solute toxicity are rarely performed.

SOLUTE REMOVAL BY DIFFERENT FORMS OF RENAL REPLACEMENT THERAPY

Although investigators have not succeeded in replicating uremic illness by administering uremic solutes to normal humans or animals, reversing illness by removing solutes has become a part of everyday practice. Because renal replacement therapies remove solutes indiscriminately, the improvement they effect cannot be attributed to removal of specific compounds. However, different forms of renal replacement therapy do clear solutes at different rates based on some characteristics, including molecular size, protein binding, and sequestration within cells or other body compartments. The demonstration that different therapies have different effects on some features of uremia might therefore reveal properties of the responsible toxin(s).

ORIGINAL MIDDLE MOLECULE HYPOTHESIS

The suggestion that the nature of uremic toxins could be deduced by comparing the effects of different renal replacement methods was first advanced by Babb and colleagues.[147] In the 1960s, hemodialysis was performed with membranes that provided very limited clearance of solutes with molecular weight larger than 1000 Da. Treatment with these membranes wakened patients from coma, relieved vomiting, and partially reversed other uremic symptoms. This provided evidence, which remains convincing, that some important uremic toxins are small. Babb and coworkers were impressed that patients on peritoneal dialysis were generally healthier than patients on hemodialysis who had the same plasma urea and creatinine concentrations. They further observed that increasing the dialysis duration from 6.5 to 9 hours three times weekly prevented neuropathy.

These observations led them to conclude that important toxins were larger than 300 Da because, as compared to contemporary hemodialysis membranes, the peritoneal membrane afforded greater relative permeability in this size range and because increasing the hemodialysis session length was expected to reduce the plasma concentration of larger molecules more than the concentrations of creatinine and urea. Based on their further impression that no additional benefit was obtained using membranes that provided superior clearance for solutes larger than 2000 Da, they concluded that some important toxins were "middle molecules," with a molecular weight greater than 300 Da but less than 2000 Da.[148]

LARGE SOLUTES—CHANGING DEFINITION OF "MIDDLE MOLECULES"

Studies during the 1970s provided only equivocal evidence that increasing the clearance of solutes with a molecular weight between 350 and 2000 Da improved the health of uremic patients.[147] The proposition that no benefit could be obtained by increasing the clearance of solutes with molecular weight greater than 2000 Da was never prospectively tested. The original middle molecule hypothesis was thus never proven to be correct. And, although the phrase *middle molecules* remains in use, its meaning has gradually shifted to include larger solutes. The 2003 report of the EUTox work group[1] thus defined middle molecules as those with a size ranging from 500 Da to less than 60,000 Da, with the larger molecule nearly the size of albumin. In practice, the adoption of new membrane materials, which was in part a response to the original middle molecule hypothesis, has squelched investigation of the relative toxicity of solutes that fall into different parts of the size range less than 1000 Da. The question of whether solutes with molecular weight greater than 1000 Da exert toxic effects remains under investigation. Henderson and colleagues[149] showed that such solutes can be cleared more effectively by hemofiltration than by hemodialysis. The results of recent large trials combining hemofiltration with hemodialysis to increase the clearance of large solutes have been equivocal. One problem may be that the concentration of hypothetical high-molecular-weight toxins may not decline in proportion to the increase in clearance during treatment because they move slowly from the interstitial fluid to the extracellular fluid during treatment and because they are cleared by extrarenal mechanisms at a significant rate.[150]

PROTEIN-BOUND SOLUTES

Other solutes that are poorly removed by standard hemodialysis include those that bind to albumin.[96,151] Their dialytic clearance is low, not because they are large molecules, but because only the free, unbound solute concentration contributes to the gradient-driving solute across the dialysis membrane. In the normal kidney, the combination of protein binding and tubular secretion allows molecules to be excreted while keeping their concentrations in the extracellular fluid very low.[5] This presumably represents an evolutionary adaption to excrete toxic substances, and there is indeed suggestive evidence that some important uremic toxins are protein-bound.[152] The clearance of protein-bound solutes can be increased by raising dialysate flow and membrane size above the levels used in conventional hemodialysis or by combining a high hemofiltration rate with dialysis in hemodiafiltration treatment.[153,154] The aggregate toxicity of protein-bound solutes could thus theoretically be assessed by comparing the effects of different renal replacement prescriptions, but this has not been attempted in large-scale clinical trials or in practice. Peritoneal dialysis clears protein-bound solutes at a very low rate, and the total clearance of protein-bound solutes in patients maintained on peritoneal dialysis therefore depends heavily on the level of residual kidney function.[155,156] Surprisingly, however, plasma concentrations of the bound solutes *p*-cresol sulfate and indoxyl sulfate are not much higher in patients undergoing peritoneal dialysis patients without residual kidney function than in those with residual kidney function, suggesting that production of these solutes may diminish as residual kidney function is lost.[156]

SEQUESTERED SOLUTES

Some solutes are sequestered, or held in compartments where their concentration does not equilibrate rapidly with that of the plasma.[157] Application of a high dialytic clearance may rapidly lower the plasma concentration of such solutes while removing only a small portion of the total body content. When this happens, intermittent dialysis treatment will be followed by a rebound in the plasma solute concentration toward predialysis levels.[60,158] Theoretically, the contribution of sequestered solutes to uremic toxicity, like the contribution of large solutes or protein-bound solutes, could be assessed by comparing the efficacy of different dialysis prescriptions. When treatment is intermittent, the removal of sequestered relative to freely equilibrating solutes can be increased by lengthening the treatment while simultaneously reducing the plasma clearance. It has been suggested that this effect may be responsible in part for the exceptional results reported with slow, thrice-weekly hemodialysis.[159]

EFFECTS OF DIET AND GASTROINTESTINAL FUNCTION

It may be possible to identify uremic toxins by comparing the effect of different diets as well as by comparing the effect of different renal replacement therapies. Patients with kidney failure tend to reduce their intake of protein spontaneously.[160] Before dialysis was available, physicians found that the protein restriction could ameliorate uremic symptoms.[161] These findings suggest that important uremic toxins are derived from protein catabolism. They call into question current recommendations that patients undergoing dialysis ingest a higher protein intake than what has been recommended for the general population.[162] Uremic solutes whose production depends on protein intake include urea, methylguanidine, GSA, and the indoles and phenols produced by the action of gut bacteria on tryptophan, phenylalanine, and tyrosine.[69,80,163-165] This group overlaps with the large group of uremic solutes made by colon microbes.[122] The production of such solutes may depend not only on dietary intake but on gut function. Impaired small bowel function may increase the delivery of peptides to the colon in uremia, and the composition of the colon microbiome may also be altered.[166,167] If colonic bacteria produce uremic toxins, uremic symptoms could theoretically be relieved by altering the delivery of substrates to the colon, modifying colonic flora, or adding sorbents to the diet. Only limited studies of such maneuvers have so far been performed.[168,169] Historically, once hemodialysis became widely available, attempts to modify uremic solute production were largely abandoned. However, interest in this area may be revived by the imperfect efficacy of conventional dialysis and by the relatively disappointing results to date of trials evaluating more intensive dialysis treatment.[92]

SOLUTE CLEARANCE BY ORGANIC TRANSPORT SYSTEMS

The cloning of transporters, which move organic solutes into the lumen of the proximal tubule, has provided a potential new means to identify potential uremic toxins. To the extent that uremia is caused by accumulation of organic solutes, knocking out these transporters would be expected to recapitulate uremic symptoms. To date, knocking out individual transporters has been found not to cause detectable illness, likely because of redundancy of the transport systems.[170,171] The accumulation of uremic solutes may interfere with organic solute transport important for detoxification at other sites, most notably the liver and blood-brain barrier.[172,173]

METABOLIC EFFECTS OF UREMIA

The loss of kidney function has numerous metabolic effects. Some of the most prominent are listed in Table 54.1. A few can be related to the loss of specific renal processes, such as the hydroxylation of vitamin D. However, most have no clear cause, and can at present only be attributed to the retention of uremic solutes.

OXIDANT STRESS AND THE MODIFICATION OF PROTEIN STRUCTURE

Studies have suggested that loss of kidney function increases oxidant stress.[174] The term *oxidant stress* is acknowledged to be vague, although a wealth of evidence points to increased oxidant effects in uremia. Increased levels of primary oxidants cannot be documented because they are evanescent species, which act locally, such as superoxide anion, hydrogen peroxide, hydroxyl radical, and hypochlorous acid. The accumulation of various products of oxidant reactions is therefore taken as evidence of increased oxidant activity. Although the accumulation of these markers of oxidant activity is well documented, there is at present no explanation as to why the production of oxidants should be increased in uremia. Leukocyte activation leading to increased production of hypochlorous acid has been described in patients undergoing dialysis and may be especially prominent when uremia is accompanied by systemic inflammation.[175]

Among the most commonly measured markers of oxidant activity have been oxidized amino acids and related compounds and substances that react with thiobarbituric acid, including malondialdehyde.[176] The accumulation of these low-molecular-weight compounds could reflect reduced renal clearance as well as increased production. More convincing evidence of oxidant stress is the accumulation of intact proteins containing oxidized amino acids.[177,178] The accumulation of these larger markers of oxidation cannot be attributed to reduced renal clearance. Further potential evidence of oxidative stress in uremia is the loss of extracellular reducing substances. The extracellular compartment is normally provided with several reducing substances, of which the reduced forms of ascorbic acid and plasma albumin are considered to be the most important. In uremia, the portion of ascorbic acid and albumin circulating in the oxidized form is increased. The case of albumin, which undergoes oxidation at its single free cysteine thiol (SH) group, is particularly interesting. Plasma albumin in patients with kidney failure is rapidly restored to the reduced form during hemodialysis.[179] The shift to oxidized albumin in untreated uremia is associated with the accumulation of cystine, which is the oxidized form of the thiol amino acid cysteine, and the shift back to reduced albumin during hemodialysis is associated with a lowering of cystine levels toward normal. One explanation for these phenomena is that normal kidney function is required to accomplish the steady reduction of cystine and albumin, which must take place to offset normal oxidant production.

The major ill effect of increased oxidant activity in uremia is thought to be modification of proteins. Proteins are modified not only by direct oxidation of amino acids but by the combination of amino acid side chains with carbonyl (C=O) compounds. The terminology in this area is confusing. The first carbonyl compounds shown to react with proteins were sugars, and the modified proteins formed after several reaction steps were therefore referred to as advanced glycosylation end products, or AGEs. Elevated sugar concentrations could account for the increased concentrations of AGEs found in persons with diabetes mellitus, but not for the subsequent findings of similarly increased AGE concentrations in patients with ESRD. Studies have shown that the high levels of active nonsugar carbonyls are responsible for the increased production of these modified proteins when renal function is reduced.[180] The active carbonyls have not been fully characterized, but they include compounds such as glyoxal (see Figure 54.1), which can be produced by oxidation of sugars and lipids. It has therefore been suggested that the protein end products of carbonyl modification in uremia should be referred to not as advanced glycosylation end products but as advanced glycoxidation and lipoxidation end products. Terminology aside, interest in both directly oxidized and carbonyl-modified proteins has centered on the possibility that alterations in protein structure contribute to uremia.[181,182] The hypothesis that oxidant stress contributes to adverse health consequences in ESRD has prompted trials of various antioxidants. So far, administration of vitamin C, various forms of vitamin E, folate, and α-lipoic acid has failed to reverse plasma indices of oxidant stress in patients undergoing dialysis.[183-186]

EFFECTS OF UREMIA
ON RESTING ENERGY EXPENDITURE

Resting energy expenditure has been reported as increased, decreased, and normal in patients with kidney failure.[187-191] The choice of control populations and other methodologic issues, such as corrections for altered body composition, have probably contributed to this uncertainty. The effect of dialysis treatment, which may transiently increase energy expenditure, must also be considered. Uremia apart from dialysis likely reduces resting energy expenditure.[189,191] Lower energy expenditure accords with observations of lower body temperatures in those with uremia, although additional factors may be at play in thermoregulation.[11] However, dialysis treatment may itself speed metabolism and increase energy expenditure.[190] Effects of inflammation in patients with ESRD add further complexity to the assessment of energy requirements.[192]

Alterations in metabolic rate in uremia likely reflect the cumulative result of multiple changes. Lean body mass tends to be diminished with CKD and ESRD and is a major determinant of energy expenditure.[191] Reduced food intake and body weight may also tend to reduce basal metabolic rates.[193] The normal kidneys consume appreciable energy, given their high filtration rate and attendant transport work. Loss of this basal kidney function presumably tends to reduce total energy use with kidney failure.[189,194] Finally, early studies have suggested that retained uremic solute(s) reduce oxygen consumption.[195]

New knowledge of the physiologic control mechanisms for appetite and energy expenditure has rekindled interest in uremic energy metabolism. Recent studies have focused on the signaling molecules ghrelin, produced by the stomach, and leptin, produced by adipose tissue along with other adipose tissue–derived hormones (adipokines). Levels of these small proteins tend to rise in kidney failure because of reduced clearance by the kidney and possibly because of increased production.[51,196]

ON CARBOHYDRATE METABOLISM

Insulin resistance is the most conspicuous derangement in uremic carbohydrate metabolism.[197] The defect is clearly present in ESRD but, in cross-sectional studies, impairment can be detected when the GFR falls below 50 mL/min/1.73 m^2, with a graded relation to GFR.[198,199] There are probably several causes of this phenomenon.[200] However, some obvious possibilities do not seem to contribute. Insulin binds normally to its receptor in uremia, and the receptor density is unchanged.[201,202] Moreover, excess levels of glucagon or fatty acids do not account for the disorder.[197] As is the case with overall energy metabolism, interest has recently focused on the contribution of adipokines, including leptin, resistin, and adiponectin to insulin resistance. Adipose tissue has also been identified as a source of inflammatory cytokines that impair insulin action in various experimental systems and circulate at increased levels in many patients with advanced renal insufficiency. However, correlations among levels of individual substances with measures of insulin resistance are poor, and the extent to which adipose tissue products contribute to uremic insulin resistance remains uncertain.[52,197,203]

Because dialysis, transplantation, and low-protein diets tend to restore insulin responsiveness, it has also been suggested that unidentified nitrogenous product(s) mediate insulin resistance.[197] Acidosis has been shown to provoke insulin resistance and accumulation of acid, as well as nitrogenous wastes, may contribute to insulin resistance in uremia.[204] 11-β-Hydroxysteroid dehydrogenase type 1 provokes insulin resistance by regenerating glucocorticoids. In experimental uremia, liver and fat tissue express increased activity of this enzyme as well as insulin resistance. The insulin resistance associated with 11-β-hydroxysteroid dehydrogenase can be mitigated with an inhibitor of the enzyme, all suggesting a role for this steroid pathway in insulin resistance.[205] The cause for increased enzymatic activity is unknown. Resistin is a protein capable of inducing insulin resistance, and its levels are high when kidney function is impaired. However, the plasma concentrations of resistin are not associated with insulin resistance if the GFR is taken into account.[52] Retinol-binding protein is also associated with insulin resistance (and also rises in ESRD) but is not related to markers of glucose control.[206] Finally, physical inactivity and deconditioning may contribute to insulin resistance. Exercise programs have been shown to mitigate insulin resistance but must be relatively protracted and intensive to be effective.[207,208]

Insulin resistance may have several adverse effects. Most importantly, it has been recognized as a risk factor for cardiovascular disease.[209] The connections between insulin resistance and vascular disease are not clear. A tendency to hyperglycemia is one presumably toxic effect. Some investigators have suggested that the sodium retentive effect of insulin on the kidney remains intact, whereas other tissues become insulin-resistant in uremia. Increased plasma insulin concentrations could thus contribute to arterial hypertension in patients with impaired kidney function.[210,211] Outside of vascular disease, the loss of insulin's anabolic action may contribute to uremic muscle wasting.[197,212]

Even though insulin resistance is the rule in uremia, hypoglycemia can be a significant effect of renal insufficiency.[213] Hypoglycemia is likely to occur, despite insulin resistance, for two main reasons. First, the kidney is a major site of insulin catabolism. Patients with diabetes mellitus treated with insulin, or insulin secretagogues (e.g., sulfonylureas) frequently become hypoglycemic if doses are not adjusted downward as the GFR declines. Second, the kidney is a major site of gluconeogenesis.[213] The liver produces the bulk of glucose in postabsorptive and starvation states, but even in these situations, the kidney produces some glucose. With prolonged fasting, the kidney is responsible for approximately half of the total glucose production.[214,215] Thus, advanced CKD may predispose to hypoglycemia, both by prolonging insulin action and by reducing gluconeogenesis. These effects may become particularly apparent when other hypoglycemic factors, such as ethanol ingestion or liver disease, are also evident.

ON LIPID METABOLISM

Nephrotic syndrome and even lower-grade proteinuria are regularly associated with hyperlipidemia.[216] However, lipid abnormalities are modest when kidney function is impaired without significant proteinuria.[217] Indeed, total cholesterol falls on average as the GFR drops below about 30 mL/min/1.73 m^2.[160] Metabolite profiling in plasma of patients with ESRD using liquid chromatography and tandem mass spectrometry has revealed that lipid products deviate from normal levels far less than polar compounds. However, lower-molecular-weight triacylglycerols were generally decreased, and an increase in intermediate-weight triacylglycerols was observed.[3] The causes and consequences of these changes in lipids are uncertain. However, demonstration that uremic serum induces lipolysis in cultured adipocytes may bear on some of these findings.[218] With respect to conventionally recognized hazardous changes in plasma lipid levels, falls in high-density lipoprotein (HDL) levels, and rises in triglyceride levels have been described. Low-density lipoprotein (LDL) concentrations are usually not elevated and may be less than in normal controls.[216] The causes for these trends are unclear, although the decline in total cholesterol is taken to reflect, at least in part, progressive reduction in food intake. Numerous hypotheses have been advanced to account for the finding that atherosclerosis is accelerated but lipid levels are not markedly elevated in renal failure. Although total lipid levels are not significantly elevated, there may be an increase in oxidized forms due to oxidant stress and reduced lipoprotein clearance rates.[219] The high prevalence of cardiovascular disease patients with ESRD has prompted several randomized clinical trials of statin agents. The largest trials performed to date have identified no clear benefit of statins in patients on dialysis, in sharp contrast to persons with normal or near-normal kidney function and, in one study,[220] to patients with advanced, non–dialysis-requiring CKD.[221-223] These trials are discussed in more detail in the chapter on cardiovascular disease (Chapter 56).

ON AMINO ACID AND PROTEIN METABOLISM

The normal kidney participates in the metabolism of several amino acids.[6,224-227] For example, the kidney converts citrulline to arginine. Loss of this function likely contributes to the increasing ratio of citrulline to arginine as the GFR declines below 50 mL/min/1.73 m^2.[225,226] Similarly, reduced renal production of serine from glycine probably underlies the rise in the plasma glycine-to-serine ratio. Increased concentrations of the sulfur-containing amino acids—cystine, taurine, and homocysteine—are especially intriguing. Cystine and homocysteine accumulate in the oxidized form, consistent with the concept that uremia is a state of oxidant stress, and homocysteine levels have been associated with the progression of cardiovascular disease.[225,226,228] Administration of folate to lower homocysteine levels neither restores the plasma redox state toward normal nor reduces the frequency of cardiovascular events.[185,229] The mechanism responsible for the accumulation of oxidized cystine and homocysteine remains unclear, but this change can be detected as the GFR drops below roughly half of normal and becomes more extreme at ESRD approaches.

Tissue protein loss reflected by muscle wasting is a major concern in patients with kidney failure. Factors that predispose to protein wasting include reduced appetite, along with insulin resistance and altered amino acid metabolism, as described earlier. Dialysis also results in some protein loss, with amino acids lost in the hemodialysate and plasma proteins and amino acids lost in the peritoneal dialysate. In the absence of other complications, the effect of uremia on protein metabolism at the levels now seen clinically is usually modest, at least over the short term.[212] Patients with advanced CKD can maintain nitrogen balance on low-protein diets as long as acidosis and inflammation are absent. Several factors may combine with defects in insulin resistance and altered amino acid and adipose metabolism to produce muscle wasting. The best studied of these is acidosis, which has been shown to stimulate the ubiquitin-proteasome pathway of intracellular protein degradation. Activation of caspase-3 seems to be an important step in proteolysis, which is followed by disposal of protein cleavage fragments through the proteasome.[230] In addition to these effects, acidosis contributes to insulin resistance and thereby attenuates protein anabolic actions of insulin. Base supplements can mitigate the catabolic effects of acidosis, but a long-term study establishing the value of normalizing bicarbonate levels in patients with impaired is lacking (although several studies are ongoing).[204,231-233]

Inflammation may be an even more important contributor to protein wasting than acidosis in patients with kidney failure. Muscle loss in patients with ESRD has been linked to an inflammatory state, characterized by increased serum concentrations of C-reactive protein and various cytokines. How these inflammatory mediators trigger net protein degradation in muscle and other tissues remains to be elucidated, although their presence is regularly accompanied by muscle loss. High levels of inflammatory mediators are also associated with lower serum albumin concentrations, which have been attributed largely to reduced hepatic production of albumin. Both muscle loss and reduced albumin concentration predict early death. The exact cause(s) of inflammation remains elusive. In some cases, inflammation can be ascribed to known episodes of infection or other intercurrent illness although, in most cases, no cause can be identified. Occult inflammatory stimuli in these cases may include subclinical infection at hemodialysis catheter or arteriovenous graft sites, exposure to dialysate and various synthetic materials, and accelerated vascular injury that is common in ESRD.[234-236] Oxidant stress has also often been invoked. Attempts to reduce inflammation with free radical scavengers have been unsuccessful.[237] An interesting possibility is that organic solutes retained in kidney failure, although they do not regularly trigger inflammation over the short term, cause the late appearance of inflammation in a subset of patients with ESRD. Some evidence has suggested that accumulation of proteins modified by glycation and oxidation can trigger a self-perpetuating inflammatory loop in these cases.[238,239]

Another factor contributing to muscle wasting is dialysis inactivity. Johansen and associates have shown that self-reported physical activity in patients starting dialysis is at or below the first percentile for population reference range,[240] and lower levels of physical activity are strongly associated with mortality.[241] In these patients, inactivity may be caused by fatigue and loss of energy, which are invariable although difficult-to-measure features of uremia, and by depression and other comorbid illnesses,[242] which are common in the ESRD population.

OVERALL NUTRITION

As emphasized by Depner,[7] the condition of patients undergoing dialysis reflects a combination of residual uremia, side effects of dialysis mixed with the effects of comorbid conditions, and increasing age. Most patients starting on dialysis in Europe and the United States are overweight. This reflects population-wide overeating, which can contribute to, and accelerate the progression of, CKD. The protein wasting exhibited by a subset of patients undergoing dialysis is thus not malnutrition in the sense of limited nutrient availability. It is often accompanied by anorexia and reduced food intake, particularly when inflammation is prominent. It cannot, however, be reversed simply by increasing food intake.[243] Other measures of restoring body protein and muscle mass toward normal, including exercise, appetite stimulants, and newer anabolic and antiinflammatory agents, are under study.[244]

SIGNS AND SYMPTOMS OF UREMIA

Frequently identified signs and symptoms of uremia are listed in Table 54.1. That a fundamental metabolic disturbance such as uremia should have such a wide variety of consequences is not remarkable. The complications of untreated diabetes or hyperthyroidism are similarly extensive. However, uremia is different in that we cannot trace all its complications to dysregulation of a single key compound. And, except for renal transplantation, current therapy for uremia cannot return patients as close to normal as thyroid hormone or insulin replacement.

The level of renal function at which uremia can be said to appear is obscure. Furthermore, the diminution of functions other than solute clearance likely contributes to the symptoms and signs of uremia. In general, these other functions, such as ammoniagenesis, erythropoietin, and 1,25-dihydroxyvitamin D synthesis, urine-concentrating capacity, and tubular secretion, tend to decline in parallel with GFR, but not always. Nevertheless, defining the level of kidney function solely by GFR may be misleading. For example, certain potentially toxic solutes depend more on tubular secretion than glomerular filtration for their excretion, and renal synthetic processes are probably linked to GFR only by virtue of the loss of functioning renal tissue. However, until particular renal dysfunctions are attached to specific aspects of the uremic syndrome, GFR will remain the principal index of kidney function.

Most of the clinical and biochemical characteristics of uremia have been defined in ESRD or at a level of GFR very near to ESRD. Thus, as noted at the beginning of this chapter, uremic characteristics may be hard to dissect from complications of the dialysis procedure. Other morbidities considered separate from the uremia also commonly interact with it. For example, the cardiovascular disease suffered especially by patients with diabetes and hypertension appears to be accelerated by CKD. However, the myocardial infarctions, strokes, and peripheral vascular diseases suffered by these patients have not traditionally been considered features of the uremic syndrome. These conditions nevertheless add to patients' disabilities in ways that are often not easily distinguishable from uremia or the residual syndrome of ESRD. Similarly, the peripheral neuropathy and gastroparesis of diabetes are difficult to disentangle from uremic neuropathy and uremic anorexia, nausea, and vomiting.

WELL-BEING AND PHYSICAL FUNCTION

Given the list of signs and symptoms in Table 54.1, it is not surprising that health-related quality of life (HRQOL) tends to decline in patients with CKD. The point in the course of CKD at which quality of life begins to decline has not been dissected in great detail, but some data exist. The authors of the National Kidney Foundation Kidney Disease Outcomes Quality Initiative (NKF KDOQI) guidelines have concluded that notable reductions in well-being appear when the GFR is less than 60 mL/min. Dialysis undoubtedly imposes a burden on patients. Interestingly, however, comparisons of HRQOL in patients on dialysis and patients with advanced CKD who are not on dialysis have yielded discordant results.[245-248] Other, often neglected features of treatment, such as pill burden, may also contribute to reduction in the quality of life.[249] Patients with ESRD are on average more depressed than healthy controls. However, it is difficult to distinguish the extent to which depression is caused by uremic solutes as compared to the effects of comorbid disease and the knowledge of ill health and limited life expectancy. Not surprisingly, transplantation has rather consistently been found to improve quality of life.[250]

Physical functioning in patients treated with dialysis is decidedly below normal. The self-reported activity of people initiating dialysis is below the fifth percentile for healthy people.[240] Treatment of anemia improves this situation but does not normalize it.[251,252] The most detailed studies have identified multiple defects that are associated with fatigability.[253] These include muscle energetic failure and neural defects. The degree to which they are attributable to the uremic environment itself, deconditioning, and/or comorbid conditions such as diabetes mellitus is difficult to establish. Even highly functional patients on dialysis display notable physical limitations. Blake and O'Meara[254] have reported that middle-aged patients undergoing dialysis, with good nutrition and no significant comorbidities, exhibit a wide range of quantifiable deficiencies. For example, balance, walking, speed, and sensory function in these patients were clearly below those of matched controls.

NEUROLOGIC FUNCTION

A particularly interesting group of uremic signs and systems reflects altered nerve function. Classic descriptions emphasized that uremic patients could appear alert, despite defects in memory, planning, and attention.[11,255] As kidney function worsened, patients progressed to coma or catatonia, which could be relieved by dialysis. Today, patients maintained on dialysis exhibit more subtle cognitive defects.[256] A difficulty in identifying the effects of uremia in these patients is that the hemodialysis procedure and/or associated factors (e.g., hypotension) may transiently impair cognitive function.[257] Studies in patients with CKD have suggested that cognitive impairment can be detected when the GFR falls below 60 mL/min/1.73 m^2 and worsens as the GFR declines.[258-260] As with other signs and symptoms of uremia, the degree to which cognition is influenced by uremia, as opposed to other comorbidities, especially cerebrovascular disease, is difficult to ascertain. The population studies cited earlier have identified cognitive impairment in chronic kidney disease independent of clinically recognized vascular disease and other comorbidities. Imaging studies suggest that subclinical cerebrovascular disease is common in CKD, and its role in poor cognition needs further definition.[256,261,262] The finding that kidney transplantation improves cognitive function suggests, however, that at least some of the impairment observed in ESRD patients is due to solute accumulation.[263,264] A further reflection of altered CNS function in uremia is impaired sleep.[265,266] Sleep is fragmented by brief arousals and apneic episodes, which are often associated with bursts of repetitive leg movement. When awake, patients may feel a need to move their legs continuously, termed the *restless legs syndrome*.[267]

Sensorimotor neuropathy was a recognized component of the uremic syndrome decades ago.[11] Studies of conduction velocity and other nerve functions have since repeatedly found that most patients with uremia have peripheral neuropathy, albeit often subclinical.[255,268,269] Morphologic studies have shown that these functional changes are associated with axonal loss. The extent to which peripheral nerve function is impaired earlier in the course of chronic kidney disease is not certain. Autonomic neuropathy also develops in ESRD, but has been less extensively studied than peripheral neuropathy.[269] As with other uremic disturbances, the cause of neuropathy is unknown. Parathyroid hormone, multiple retention solutes, and more recently potassium have been associated with peripheral neuropathy, but without definitive proof of causality.[255,268]

APPETITE, TASTE, AND SMELL

Loss of appetite is a common uremic symptom and presumably contributes to malnutrition in patients with advanced renal failure. A large number of causes have been proposed. Acidosis and inflammatory cytokines, including tumor necrosis factor (TNF) and various interleukins, have been identified as contributing factors.[270] As with the uremic defects in energy metabolism, attention has been focused on the accumulation of small proteins produced by the gut and adipose tissue and act on the brain to regulate appetite in normal people.[271,272] Levels of leptin, an anorexigen produced by adipose tissue, are elevated in ESRD. Antagonism of leptin in mice with experimental CKD attenuates a number of the molecular markers of proteolysis.[273] An interesting feature of uremic anorexia that remains to be explained is a disproportionate reduction in the intake of protein.[160] Along with overall loss of appetite, erosion of taste and smell has long been recognized in the ESRD population.[274,275] As with most defects, transplantation reverses the blunted smell.[274] Some studies have reported that odor threshold declines gradually with creatinine clearance, whereas others have found that even in patients undergoing dialysis, odor detection remains normal unless malnutrition is present.[131,274] Taste acuity has been reported as lower in patients undergoing dialysis than in those with renal insufficiency, and self-reported altered taste is associated with poor nutritional status.[276,277] The factors responsible for these defects are again unknown.

CELLULAR FUNCTIONS

The most general cellular abnormality reported has been the inhibition of sodium-potassium adenosine triphosphatase (Na^+-K^+-ATPase). Decreased Na^+-K^+-ATPase activity in red cells of uremic patients was reported in 1964.[278] In general, subsequent reports have confirmed the observation, noted the same effect in other cell types, and emphasized that the inhibition was attributable to some factor in uremic serum.[279] The evidence for a circulating inhibitor includes the findings that dialysis reduces the inhibitory activity and uremic plasma can acutely suppress the pump activity.[279] However, the factor or factors have remained elusive. A number of candidates have been considered. Much attention has focused on digitalis-like substances. Several such compounds have been found in excess in humans with ESRD. These include marinobufagenin and telocinobufagin, which have a structure related to that of digitalis.

WHY IS THE GLOMERULAR FILTRATION RATE SO LARGE?

Glomerular filtration, the initial step in urine formation, is quantitatively huge, with a volume equaling that of the entire extracellular fluid filtered every 2 hours. At rest, approximately 10% of the body's energy consumption is devoted to reabsorption of valuable solutes and water necessitated by this massive filtration rate. The rate of fluid processing clearly exceeds that required to rid the body of the daily intake of water and inorganic ions. Theoretically, the large tubular flow rate provided by the GFR could supply a sink into which organic solutes are secreted more favorably than at lower tubular flows. This hypothesis accounts for the presence of a large GFR, but leaves unanswered the question of which solutes must be handled by secretion and thereby maintained at a low level in the ECF.

Homer Smith recognized that the mammalian GFR was large in proportion to the kidney's known functions. He suggested that our high GFR was an evolutionary residual of the mechanism that allowed early vertebrates living in fresh water seas to excrete large volumes of water. If this were correct, the superfluity of GFR would constitute an expensive vestige in land-dwelling mammals, and the value of tubular secretion would remain unaccounted for. An alternate explanation for the apparent superfluity of kidney function is that it provides a safety factor, similar to the capacity of bone to withstand greater than usual mechanical loads. In the case of the kidney, the ingestion of toxins could constitute an analogous increase in load. It is noteworthy, however, that the proportion of GFR and kidney size to metabolic rate appears to be nearly constant across mammalian species, including herbivores and carnivores.[280,281] This suggests that the substances with excretion that necessitate a large kidney are products of common metabolic pathways rather than specific foodstuffs. The remarkable ability of bears to reduce kidney function and net protein breakdown to near zero during winter denning further suggests that these substances are end products of protein catabolism.[282,283]

We can further suppose that kidney capacity appears excessive because our clinical criteria are too coarse to detect the consequences of mild impairment in kidney function. Fitness in an evolutionary sense may require the concentrations in body water of some excreted solutes to be maintained below the levels at which we detect disease. That is, our clinical criteria for uremic illness may be too coarse to detect the consequences of mild impairment of renal function. One might speculate that disturbances in an important but sensitive parameter, perhaps fertility, growth in children or peak physical performance, would occur with less than a twofold increase of some retained toxin. A particularly interesting finding has been the identification of similar transport systems in the kidney tubule and blood-brain barrier.[173,284] This finding suggests that the kidney, together with the liver, may be designed to keep organic waste levels in the extracellular fluid sufficiently low so that a second-stage pumping system in the blood-brain barrier can keep the brain interstitium exquisitely clean.

Complete reference list available at ExpertConsult.com.

KEY REFERENCES

1. Vanholder R, De Smet R, Glorieux G, et al: Review on uremic toxins: classification, concentration, and interindividual variability. *Kidney Int* 63:1934–1943, 2003.
2. Duranton F, Cohen G, De Smet R, et al: Normal and pathologic concentrations of uremic toxins. *J Am Soc Nephrol* 23:1258–1270, 2012.
5. Sirich TL, Aronov PA, Plummer NS, et al: Numerous protein-bound solutes are cleared by the kidney with high efficiency. *Kidney Int* 84:585–590, 2013.
6. Bergstrom J: Uremic toxicity. In Kopple JD, Massry SG, editors: *Nutritional management of renal disease*, Baltimore, 1997, Williams & Wilkins, pp 97–190.
7. Depner TA: Uremic toxicity: urea and beyond. *Semin Dial* 14:246–251, 2001.
10. Johnson WJ, Hagge WW, Wagoner RD, et al: Effects of urea loading in patients with far-advanced renal failure. *Mayo Clin Proc* 47:21–29, 1972.
11. Schreiner G, Maher J: Biochemistry of uremia. In *Uremia*, Springfield, Ill, 1960, Charles C Thomas, pp 55–85.
19. Koeth RA, Kalantar-Zadeh K, Wang Z, et al: Protein carbamylation predicts mortality in ESRD. *J Am Soc Nephrol* 24:853–861, 2013.
37. Verroust PJ, Birn H, Nielsen R, et al: The tandem endocytic receptors megalin and cubilin are important proteins in renal pathology. *Kidney Int* 62:745–756, 2002.
40. Norden AG, Sharratt P, Cutillas PR, et al: Quantitative amino acid and proteomic analysis: very low excretion of polypeptides >750 Da in normal urine. *Kidney Int* 66:1994–2003, 2004.
52. Axelsson J, Bergsten A, Qureshi AR, et al: Elevated resistin levels in chronic kidney disease are associated with decreased glomerular filtration rate and inflammation, but not with insulin resistance. *Kidney Int* 69:596–604, 2006.
54. Richter R, Schulz-Knappe P, Schrader M, et al: Composition of the peptide fraction in human blood plasma: database of circulating human peptides. *J Chromatogr B Biomed Sci Appl* 726:25–35, 1999.
60. Eloot S, Torremans A, De Smet R, et al: Kinetic behavior of urea is different from that of other water-soluble compounds: the case of the guanidino compounds. *Kidney Int* 67:1566–1575, 2005.
63. Wyss M, Kaddurah-Daouk R: Creatine and creatinine metabolism. *Physiol Rev* 80:1107–1213, 2000.
75. Ronden RA, Houben AJ, Teerlink T, et al: Reduced renal plasma clearance does not explain increased plasma asymmetric dimethylarginine in hypertensive subjects with mild to moderate renal insufficiency. *Am J Physiol Renal Physiol* 303:F149–F156, 2012.
85. Bammens B, Evenepoel P, Keuleers H, et al: Free serum concentrations of the protein-bound retention solute p-cresol predict mortality in hemodialysis patients. *Kidney Int* 69:1081–1087, 2006.
89. Cathcart-Rake W, Porter R, Whittier F, et al: Effect of diet on serum accumulation and renal excretion of aryl acids and secretory activity in normal and uremic man. *Am J Clin Nutr* 28:1110–1115, 1975.
90. Mitch WE, Brusilow S: Benzoate-induced changes in glycine and urea metabolism in patients with chronic renal failure. *J Pharmacol Exp Ther* 222:572–575, 1982.
92. Meyer TW, Hostetter TH: Uremic solutes from colon microbes. *Kidney Int* 81:949–954, 2012.
97. Sirich TL, Luo FJ, Plummer NS, et al: Selectively increasing the clearance of protein-bound uremic solutes. *Nephrol Dial Transplant* 27:1574–1579, 2012.
99. Meijers BK, Van Kerckhoven S, Verbeke K, et al: The uremic retention solute p-cresyl sulfate and markers of endothelial damage. *Am J Kidney Dis* 54:891–901, 2009.
111. Saito K, Fujigaki S, Heyes MP, et al: Mechanism of increases in L-kynurenine and quinolinic acid in renal insufficiency. *Am J Physiol Renal Physiol* 279:F565–F572, 2000.
114. Ponda MP, Quan Z, Melamed ML, et al: Methylamine clearance by haemodialysis is low. *Nephrol Dial Transplant* 25:1608–1613, 2010.
118. Wright SH, Dantzler WH: Molecular and cellular physiology of renal organic cation and anion transport. *Physiol Rev* 84:987–1049, 2004.
120. Roch-Ramel F, Besseghir K, Murer H: Renal excretion and tubular transport of organic anions and cations. In Windhager EE, editor: *Handbook of physiology: renal physiology*, Oxford, England, 1992, Oxford University Press, pp 2189–2262.
122. Aronov PA, Luo FJ, Plummer NS, et al: Colonic contribution to uremic solutes. *J Am Soc Nephrol* 22:1769–1776, 2011.
130. Simenhoff ML, Burke JF, Saukkonen JJ, et al: Biochemical profile or uremic breath. *N Engl J Med* 297:132–135, 1977.
132. Tang WH, Wang Z, Levison BS, et al: Intestinal microbial metabolism of phosphatidylcholine and cardiovascular risk. *N Engl J Med* 368:1575–1584, 2013.
149. Henderson LW, Colton CK, Ford CA, et al: Kinetics of hemodiafiltration. II. Clinical characterization of a new blood-cleansing modality. 1975. *J Am Soc Nephrol* 8:494–508, 1997.
150. Ward RA, Greene T, Hartmann B, et al: Resistance to intercompartmental mass transfer limits beta2-microglobulin removal by post-dilution hemodiafiltration. *Kidney Int* 69:1431–1437, 2006.
154. Luo FJ, Patel KP, Marquez IO, et al: Effect of increasing dialyzer mass transfer area coefficient and dialysate flow on clearance of protein-bound solutes: a pilot crossover trial. *Am J Kidney Dis* 53:1042–1049, 2009.
157. Schneditz D, Daugirdas JT: Compartment effects in hemodialysis. *Semin Dial* 14:271–277, 2001.
158. Eloot S, Torremans A, De Smet R, et al: Complex compartmental behavior of small water-soluble uremic retention solutes: evaluation by direct measurements in plasma and erythrocytes. *Am J Kidney Dis* 50:279–288, 2007.
161. Giovannetti S, Maggiore Q: A low-nitrogen diet with proteins of high biological value for severe chronic uraemia. *Lancet* 37:1000–1003, 1964.
162. Uribarri J: The obsession with high dietary protein intake in ESRD patients on dialysis: is it justified? *Nephron* 86:105–108, 2000.
171. Eraly SA, Vallon V, Vaughn DA, et al: Decreased renal organic anion secretion and plasma accumulation of endogenous organic anions in OAT1 knock-out mice. *J Biol Chem* 281:5072–5083, 2006.
172. Nolin TD: Altered nonrenal drug clearance in ESRD. *Curr Opin Nephrol Hypertens* 17:555–559, 2008.
174. Himmelfarb J: Uremic toxicity, oxidative stress, and hemodialysis as renal replacement therapy. *Semin Dial* 22:636–643, 2009.
179. Himmelfarb J, McMenamin E, McMonagle E: Plasma aminothiol oxidation in chronic hemodialysis patients. *Kidney Int* 61:705–716, 2002.
182. Thornalley PJ, Rabbani N: Highlights and hot spots of protein glycation in end-stage renal disease. *Semin Dial* 22:400–404, 2009.
184. Lu L, Erhard P, Salomon RG, et al: Serum vitamin E and oxidative protein modification in hemodialysis: a randomized clinical trial. *Am J Kidney Dis* 50:305–313, 2007.
190. Ikizler TA, Wingard RL, Sun M, et al: Increased energy expenditure in hemodialysis patients. *J Am Soc Nephrol* 7:2646–2653, 1996.
191. Avesani CM, Draibe SA, Kamimura MA, et al: Decreased resting energy expenditure in non-dialysed chronic kidney disease patients. *Nephrol Dial Transplant* 19:3091–3097, 2004.
217. Kwan BC, Kronenberg F, Beddhu S, et al: Lipoprotein metabolism and lipid management in chronic kidney disease. *J Am Soc Nephrol* 18:1246–1261, 2007.
218. Axelsson J, Astrom G, Sjolin E, et al: Uraemic sera stimulate lipolysis in human adipocytes: role of perilipin. *Nephrol Dial Transplant* 26:2485–2491, 2011.
225. Laidlaw SA, Berg RL, Kopple JD, et al: Patterns of fasting plasma amino acid levels in chronic renal insufficiency: results from the

feasibility phase of the Modification of Diet in Renal Disease Study. *Am J Kidney Dis* 23:504–513, 1994.
229. Jamison RL, Hartigan P, Kaufman JS, et al: Effect of homocysteine lowering on mortality and vascular disease in advanced chronic kidney disease and end-stage renal disease: a randomized controlled trial. *JAMA* 298:1163–1170, 2007.
230. Rajan VR, Mitch WE: Muscle wasting in chronic kidney disease: the role of the ubiquitin proteasome system and its clinical impact. *Pediatr Nephrol* 23:527–535, 2008.
237. Himmelfarb J, Ikizler TA, Ellis C, et al: Provision of antioxidant therapy in hemodialysis (PATH): a randomized clinical trial. *J Am Soc Nephrol* 25:623–633, 2014.
240. Johansen KL, Chertow GM, Kutner NG, et al: Low level of self-reported physical activity in ambulatory patients new to dialysis. *Kidney Int* 78:1164–1170, 2010.
248. Abdel-Kader K, Unruh ML, Weisbord SD: Symptom burden, depression, and quality of life in chronic and end-stage kidney disease. *Clin J Am Soc Nephrol* 4:1057–1064, 2009.
254. Blake C, O'Meara YM: Subjective and objective physical limitations in high-functioning renal dialysis patients. *Nephrol Dial Transplant* 19:3124–3129, 2004.
257. Murray AM, Pederson SL, Tupper DE, et al: Acute variation in cognitive function in hemodialysis patients: a cohort study with repeated measures. *Am J Kidney Dis* 50:270–278, 2007.
280. Singer MA, Morton AR: Mouse to elephant: biological scaling and Kt/V. *Am J Kidney Dis* 35:306–309, 2000.
284. Ohtsuki S: New aspects of the blood-brain barrier transporters; its physiological roles in the central nervous system. *Biol Pharm Bull* 27:1489–1496, 2004.

55 Chronic Kidney Disease–Mineral Bone Disorder

Sharon M. Moe | Stuart M. Sprague

CHAPTER OUTLINE

PATHOPHYSIOLOGY OF CKD-MBD, 1822
Phosphorus and Calcium Homeostasis, 1822
Hormonal Regulation of CKD-MBD, 1826
Bone Biology, 1831
Pathophysiology of Vascular Calcification, 1833
DIAGNOSIS OF CKD-MBD, 1839
Measurement of the Biochemical Abnormalities in CKD-MBD, 1839
Bone Biopsy Assessment of Bone in CKD-MBD, 1842
Noninvasive Assessment of Bone, 1846
Assessment of Vascular Calcification, 1847

CLINICAL CONSEQUENCES OF THE ABNORMALITIES IN CKD-MBD, 1847
Biochemical Abnormalities, 1847
Nutritional Vitamin D Deficiency, 1848
Fracture, 1849
Extraskeletal Calcification, 1850
CKD-MBD IN KIDNEY TRANSPLANT RECIPIENTS, 1850
Biochemical Changes After Transplantation, 1851
Bone Changes After Transplantation, 1851
Vascular Calcification Changes After Transplantation, 1852
SUMMARY, 1852

In persons with healthy kidneys, normal serum levels of phosphorus and calcium are maintained through the interaction of three hormones: parathyroid hormone (PTH), $1,25(OH)_2$ (1,25-dihydroxyvitamin D; calcitriol), which is the active metabolite of vitamin D, and fibroblast growth factor 23 (FGF-23). Circulating or soluble klotho also plays a role in mineral homeostasis. These hormones act on four primary target organs: bone, kidney, intestine, and parathyroid glands. The kidneys play a critical role in the regulation both of normal serum calcium and phosphorus concentrations and of the three hormones. Thus derangements are common in patients with chronic kidney disease (CKD). Abnormalities begin early in the course of CKD and are nearly universally observed at a glomerular filtration rate (GFR) less than 30 mL/min. With progression of CKD, the body attempts to maintain normal serum concentrations of calcium and phosphorus by altering the production of calcitriol, PTH, FGF-23, and klotho. Eventually this compensatory response becomes unable to maintain normal mineral homeostasis, resulting in (1) altered serum levels of calcium, phosphorus, PTH, calcitriol, FGF-23, and klotho, (2) disturbances in bone remodeling and mineralization (renal osteodystrophy) and/or impaired linear growth in children, and (3) extraskeletal calcification in soft tissues and arteries. In 2006, the term chronic kidney disease–mineral and bone disorder (CKD-MBD) was developed to describe this triad of abnormalities in biochemical measures, skeletal abnormalities, and extraskeletal calcification (Table 55.1).[1] These abnormalities that constitute CKD-MBD are interrelated in both the pathophysiology of the disease and the response to treatment. All three components of CKD-MBD are associated with increased risk of fractures, cardiovascular disease, and mortality in patients with CKD stages 4 through 5D. However, to enhance understanding of the complex integration of these abnormalities in CKD, each component is first discussed independently.

PATHOPHYSIOLOGY OF CKD-MBD

PHOSPHORUS AND CALCIUM HOMEOSTASIS

PHOSPHORUS BALANCE AND HOMEOSTASIS

Inorganic phosphorus is critical for numerous physiologic functions, including skeletal development, mineral metabolism, cell membrane phospholipid content and function, cell signaling, platelet aggregation, and energy transfer through mitochondrial metabolism. Because of its importance, normal homeostasis maintains serum phosphorus concentrations between 2.5 and 4.5 mg/dL (0.81 and 1.45 mmol/L). Levels are highest in infants and decrease throughout growth, reaching adult levels in the late teens. Total adult body stores of phosphorus are approximately 700 g, of which 85% is contained in bone in the form of hydroxyapatite $[(Ca)_{10}(PO_4)_6(OH)_2]$. Of the remainder, 14% is intracellular, and only 1% is extracellular. Of this

CHAPTER 55 — CHRONIC KIDNEY DISEASE–MINERAL BONE DISORDER

Table 55.1	Kidney Disease: Improving Global Outcomes (KDIGO) Classification of Chronic Kidney Disease–Mineral Bone Disease (CKD-MBD) and Renal Osteodystrophy
Definition of CKD-MBD	A systemic disorder of mineral and bone metabolism due to CKD manifested by one or a combination of the following: Abnormalities of calcium, phosphorus, parathyroid hormone, or vitamin D metabolism Abnormalities in bone turnover, mineralization, volume, linear growth, or strength Vascular or other soft tissue calcification
Definition of renal osteodystrophy	Renal osteodystrophy is an alteration of bone morphology in patients with CKD. It is one measure of the skeletal component of the systemic disorder of CKD-MBD that is quantifiable by histomorphometry of bone biopsy.

Moe S, Drüeke T, Cunningham J, et al: Definition, evaluation, and classification of renal osteodystrophy: a position statement from Kidney Disease: Improving Global Outcomes (KDIGO). Kidney Int 2006;69:1945-1953, 2006.

extracellular phosphorus, 70% is organic (phosphate) and contained within phospholipids, and 30% is inorganic. The inorganic fraction is 15% protein bound, and the remaining 85% is either complexed with sodium, magnesium, or calcium or circulates as the free monohydrogen or dihydrogen form. It is this inorganic fraction that is freely circulating and measured. At a pH of 7.4, it is in a ratio of about 4:1 HPO_4^{-2} to H_2PO^{-1}. For that reason, the phosphorus level is usually expressed in mmol/L rather than mEq/L. Thus, serum measurements reflect only a minor fraction of total body phosphorus and therefore do not accurately reflect total body stores in the setting of the abnormal homeostasis that occurs in CKD. Furthermore, there is considerable diurnal variation in serum phosphorus levels in both healthy individuals[2] and in those with advanced CKD.[3] The terms phosphorus and phosphate are often used interchangeably, but strictly speaking, *phosphate* means the inorganic freely available form (HPO_4^{-2} and H_2PO^{-1}). However, most laboratories report phosphate, the measurable inorganic component of total body phosphorus, as "phosphorus." For simplicity we use the abbreviation Pi to represent phosphate and/or phosphorus throughout this chapter.

Pi is contained in almost all foods and is generally associated with a food's protein content or the addition of additives. In most commonly ingested foods without additives, the mean Pi content ranges from 9.0 to 14.6 mg per gram of protein, with many foods having up to a 28% higher Pi content because of additives and preservatives.[4] Although the recommended daily allowance (RDA) for Pi is 800 mg/day, the average American diet contains approximately 1000 to 1400 mg Pi and that amount does not necessarily include the inorganic Pi that is added as a preservative, a common practice.[5] The source of Pi has a significant impact on bioavailability. Pi in the form of preservatives or additives is nearly 100% bioavailable, whereas Pi bound to phytate, as in legumes, is less bioavailable owing to the lack of the enzyme phytase in humans.[6] In studies, the source of Pi directly affects Pi homeostasis.[3] As a result, it is challenging to balance dietary Pi restriction against the need for adequate protein intake in patients with CKD, especially with malnutrition present in up to 50% of patients undergoing dialysis. Pi balance in earlier stages of CKD (stage 3 to 4) is generally neutral because of the phosphaturic effects of PTH and FGF-23[7]; as these compensatory mechanisms begin to fail and/or patients became anuric, however, positive Pi balance likely ensues.

Sixty percent to 70% of dietary Pi is absorbed by the gastrointestinal tract, predominantly in the small intestine, although transport can occur in all intestinal segments. Pi absorption occurs via passive sodium-independent transport and active sodium-dependent transport. Although it can vary depending on the study and experimental design, active transport is approximately 50% of total transport (Figure 55.1).[8] Passive transport occurs down electrochemical gradient through paracellular tight junctions; claudins and occludins appear to be involved and to control transport rates and ion specificity.[9] Active absorption occurs via the epithelial brush border type II (solute carrier A34 [SLCA34]) transporters, specifically the sodium-Pi cotransporter (NaPi-IIb) utilizing energy from the basolateral sodium-potassium ATPase transporter. Complete ablation of the *NaPi-IIb* gene in mice demonstrates that this transporter is responsible for 90% of sodium-dependent transport but only 50% of total intestinal Pi transport.[10] In animals with CKD induced by adenine, ablation of the *NaPi-IIb* gene lowers serum Pi, with additional lowering by the Pi binder sevelamer, suggesting that both active transport and passive transport are important in CKD.[11] The NaPi-IIb transporter is predominantly stimulated by high dietary Pi and $1,25(OH)_2D$.[8] In addition, studies suggest that the phosphatonins matrix extracellular phosphoglycoprotein (MEPE)[12] and FGF-23[13] may play a role in intestinal transport. However, dietary Pi appears the most important regulator of intestinal absorption.

The kidneys are responsible for maintaining Pi balance by excreting the net amount of Pi that is absorbed (see Chapter 7). Most inorganic Pi is freely filtered by the glomerulus with approximately 70% to 80% reabsorbed in the proximal tubule, which serves as the primary regulated site of the kidney. The remaining 20% to 30% is reabsorbed in the distal tubule. Pi transport across the apical lumen occurs via an active transport process that is driven by active sodium transport on the basolateral side by the sodium-potassium adenosine triphosphatase (Na^+-K^+-ATPase). The primary transporters on the luminal surface are NaPi-IIa (SLC34A1) and NaPi-IIc (SLC34A3), with a minor component via the type III sodium-dependent Pi cotransporter Pit-2 (SLC20A2). PTH and FGF-23 both downregulate these NaPi transporters, but through different signaling mechanisms. FGF-23 stimulates endocytosis of the transporters after signaling through the FGF receptor–klotho complex described later. PTH, after binding to PTHR1 receptor, leads to increased cyclic adenosine monophate/protein

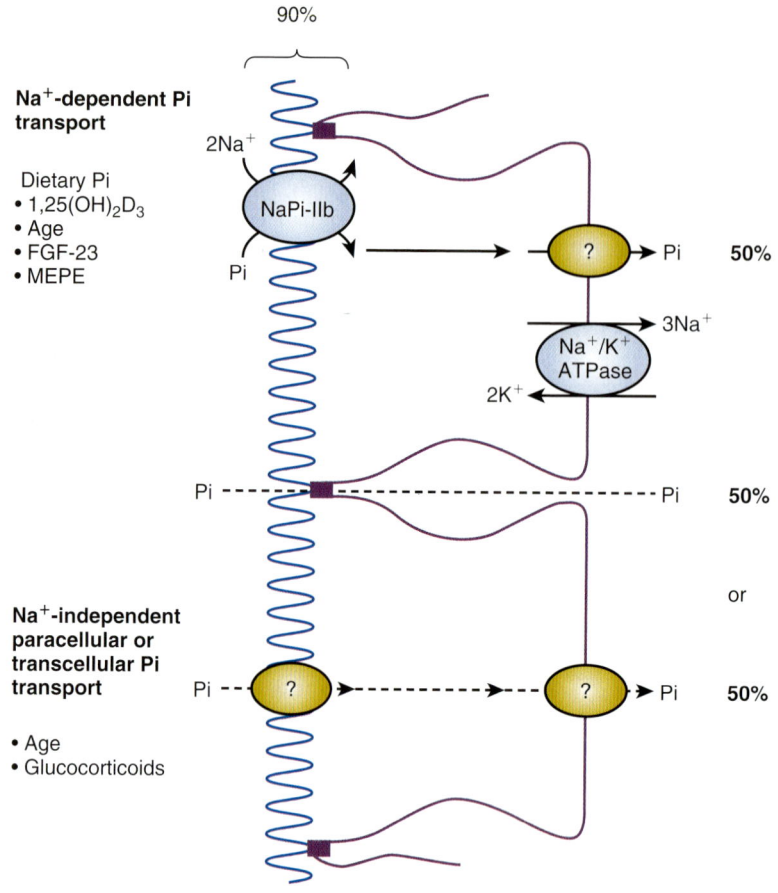

Figure 55.1 Intestinal phosphate transport. Approximately 50% of phosphate (Pi) transport is sodium (Na$^+$) dependent, due to active transport, and regulated by a number of factors. The remaining phosphate transport is sodium independent and due to paracellular or transcellular transport. FGF-23, Fibroblast growth factor 23; MEPE, matrix extracellular phosphoglycoprotein; Na$^+$/K$^+$ ATPase, sodium-potassium adenosine triphosphatase; NaPi-IIb, the sodium Pi cotransporter. (Reprinted with permission from Lee GJ, Marks J: Intestinal phosphate transport: a therapeutic target in chronic kidney disease and beyond? *Pediatr Nephrol* 30:363-371, 2015.)

kinase A (cAMP/PKA) signaling with the scaffolding protein Na$^+$-H$^+$ exchanger regulatory factors 1 and 3 (NHERF1 and NHERF3) playing an important role. FGF-23 also decreases 1,25(OH)$_2$D production by reducing the conversion of 25(OH)D to 1,25(OH)$_2$D and increasing the catabolism of 1,25(OH)$_2$D. This, in turn, further reduces intestinal phosphate absorption.

CALCIUM BALANCE AND HOMEOSTASIS

Serum calcium concentrations are normally tightly controlled within a narrow range, usually 8.5 to 10.5 mg/dL (2.1 to 2.6 mmol/L). However, the serum calcium concentration is a poor reflection of overall total body calcium, because serum levels are less than 1% of total body calcium. The remainder of total body calcium is stored in bone. Ionized calcium, generally 40% of total serum calcium, is physiologically active, whereas the non-ionized calcium is bound to albumin or anions such as citrate, bicarbonate, and Pi. In the presence of hypoalbuminemia, there is a relative increase in the ionized calcium relative to the total calcium; thus total serum calcium measurement may underestimate the physiologically active (ionized) serum calcium. A commonly utilized formula for estimating the ionized calcium from the total calcium value is to add 0.8 mg/dL for every 1-mg decrease in serum albumin below 4 mg/dL. However, in a study in patients with CKD stages 3 to 5 not undergoing dialysis, total calcium concentration and albumin-corrected total calcium values failed to correctly classify 20% of patients as either hypocalcemic or hypercalcemic whose state was documented by ionized calcium measurement.[14] The sensitivity to detect true hypocalcemia or hypercalcemia was only 40% and 21% for total calcium concentration, and 36% and 21% for albumin-corrected total calcium value, respectively.[14] The primary causes of this discordance are albumin, PTH, and pH, although the last has been questioned.[15] Thus, whenever possible, ionized calcium measurement should be utilized. Serum levels of ionized calcium are maintained in the normal range by the secretion of PTH as discussed later.

In normal individuals, the net calcium balance (intake—output) varies with age. Children and young adults are usually in a slightly positive net calcium balance to enhance linear growth; beyond ages 25 to 35 years, when bones stop growing, the calcium balance tends to be neutral. Normal individuals have protection against calcium overload by virtue of their ability to increase renal excretion of calcium and reduce intestinal absorption of calcium through the actions of PTH and 1,25(OH)$_2$D. However, in CKD the ability to maintain normal homeostasis, including a normal serum ionized calcium level and appropriate calcium balance for age, is lost. Two studies in patients with CKD stages late 3 to 4 demonstrate that 1000 mg per day of dietary or calcium supplement/binder leads to near-neutral calcium balance (reviewed in Chapter 19).[7,16]

Calcium absorption across the intestinal epithelium occurs via a vitamin D–dependent, saturable (transcellular) pathway and a vitamin D–independent, nonsaturable (paracellular) pathway. In states of adequate dietary calcium, the paracellular mechanism prevails, but the vitamin D–dependent pathways are critical in calcium-deficient states. The transcellular absorption occurs via three steps: (1) calcium enters from the lumen into the cells via transient receptor potential vanilloid (TRPV) channels, of which TRPV6 is most important in the intestine[17]; (2) the intracellular calcium associates with calbindin-D9K to be "ferried" to the basolateral membrane; and (3) calcium is removed from the enterocytes predominantly via the calcium-ATPase, with the Na^+-Ca^{2+} exchanger playing a minor role. The duodenum is the major site of calcium absorption, although the other segments of the small intestine and the colon also contribute to net calcium absorption. All of the key regulatory components of active calcium transport—TRPV, calbindin, the Ca^{2+}-ATPase (PMCA1b), and the Na^+-Ca^{2+} exchanger (NCX1)—are upregulated by $1,25(OH)_2D$.[18] However, mice with intestinal knockdown of the vitamin D receptor (VDR) are still able to maintain normal calcium levels because of increased bone resorption; in contrast, global knockdown of VDR leads to hypocalcemia. However, this state can be corrected with either a high-calcium diet (and presumed intestinal paracellular calcium transport) or the administration of $1,25(OH)_2D$.[19] Thus bone and kidney can compensate for impaired responsiveness of the intestinal VDR, and diet alone can compensate for a total lack of vitamin D. The 1α-hydroxylase enzyme (CYP27B1) is also located throughout the intestine; to date, however, conversion of $25(OH)D$ to $1,25(OH)_2D_3$ has been identified only in the colonic epithelial cells in inflammation.[20]

The renal transport of calcium is further detailed in Chapter 7. In the kidney, the majority (60% to 70%) of calcium is reabsorbed passively in the proximal tubule, a process driven by a transepithelial electrochemical gradient that is generated by sodium and water reabsorption. In the thick ascending limb, another 10% of calcium is reabsorbed via paracellular transport. Calcium-sensing receptor (CaSR) activation in this segment inhibits calcium absorption. This paracellular reabsorption also requires the specific protein paracellin-1, and genetic defects in paracellin-1 lead to a syndrome of hypercalciuria and hypomagnesemia.[21] However, the more regulated aspect of calcium reabsorption occurs via transcellular pathways in the distal convoluted tubule and connecting tubule (Figure 55.2). The mechanism is similar to intestinal transport: Calcium enters these cells via TRPV5 calcium channels down electrochemical gradients. In the cells, calcium binds with calbindin-D28k and is transported to the basolateral membrane, where calcium is actively reabsorbed by the NCX1 and/or PMCA1b. As in the intestinal epithelial cell, $1,25(OH)_2D$ upregulates all of these transport proteins.[22] Parathyroid hormone has an indirect effect on renal calcium handling via its action on $1,25(OH)_2D$ synthesis and increases TRPV5 activity.[22a] The enzymatic activity of circulating klotho has been shown to cleave the extracellular domain of TRPV5 channels, keeping these channels at the cell membrane and thereby facilitating calcium reasbsorption.[23]

CALCIUM-SENSING RECEPTOR

Physiologic studies in animals and humans in the 1980s demonstrated the rapid release of PTH in response to small reductions in blood ionized calcium, lending support to the existence of a CaSR in the parathyroid gland that was cloned in 1993.[24] The CaSR was shown to belong to the super family of G protein–coupled receptors and is a glycosylated protein with a very large extracellular domain, seven membrane–spanning segments, and a relatively large cytoplasmic domain. The primary ligand for the CaSR is Ca^{2+}, but it also senses other divalent and polyvalent cations, including Mg^{2+}, Be^{2+}, La^{3+}, Gd^{3+}, and polyarginine.[25] Extracellular calcium binds to multiple sites, leading to conformational changes that result in activation of phospholipases C, A_2, and D as well as inhibition of cAMP production.[26] Activation of the CaSR stimulates phospholipase C, leading to an increase in inositol 1,4,5-triphosphate (IP_3), which mobilizes intracellular calcium and decreases PTH secretion (Figure 55.3). In contrast, inactivation of the CaSR reduces intracellular calcium and increases PTH secretion. CaSR messenger RNA (mRNA) is widely expressed in multiple tissues, including organs responsible for CKD-MBD (parathyroid, kidney, thyroid, bone, intestine, vasculature). Studies have demonstrated a diverse role for the CaSR in disease, including in the gastrointestinal tract, where it regulates gastrin, glucagon-like peptide-1 (GLP-1), acid, and hormone secretion and is involved in taste, gastrointestinal fluid transport, and cell turnover.[27]

$CaSR^{-/-}$ mice die shortly after birth owing to hypercalcemia, hypocalciuria, and hyperparathyroidism. If the *Pth* gene is also ablated, the mice survive and most organs appear histologically normal, with healing of bone mineralization defects but no change in hypocalciuria.[29] However, these $CaSR^{-/-}/PTH^{-/-}$ mice demonstrate hypercalcemia in response to oral calcium, infusion of PTH, or administration of $1,25(OH)_2D$, whereas the $CaSR^{+/+}/PTH^{-/-}$ mice are able to decrease gastrointestinal calcium absorption and increase renal calcium excretion to maintain normal levels of serum calcium.[30,31] These data indicate that CaSR activation corrects hypocalcemia by increasing PTH, whereas in hypercalcemia, the CaSR acts independent of PTH by increasing renal calcium excretion. In uremic animals, the expression of CaSR in the parathyroid gland is downregulated by a high-Pi diet and upregulated by magnesium[32] and calcimimetics. In parathyroid glands from patients with secondary hyperparathyroidism, the expression of the CaSR is downregulated in comparison with expression in nonuremic patients[33] but can be upregulated with the administration of cinacalcet.[34]

The CaSR is expressed throughout the kidney, where it is found in diverse locations and performs multiple physiologic functions: podocyte (cytoskeleton changes), proximal tubule (phosphate reabsorption, $1,25[OH]_2D_3$ synthesis, acidification/fluid reabsorption), macula densa (renin secretion), thick ascending loop of Henle (calcium, sodium, potassium, and chloride handling), distal convoluted tubule/connecting tubule (calcium transport), and connecting duct

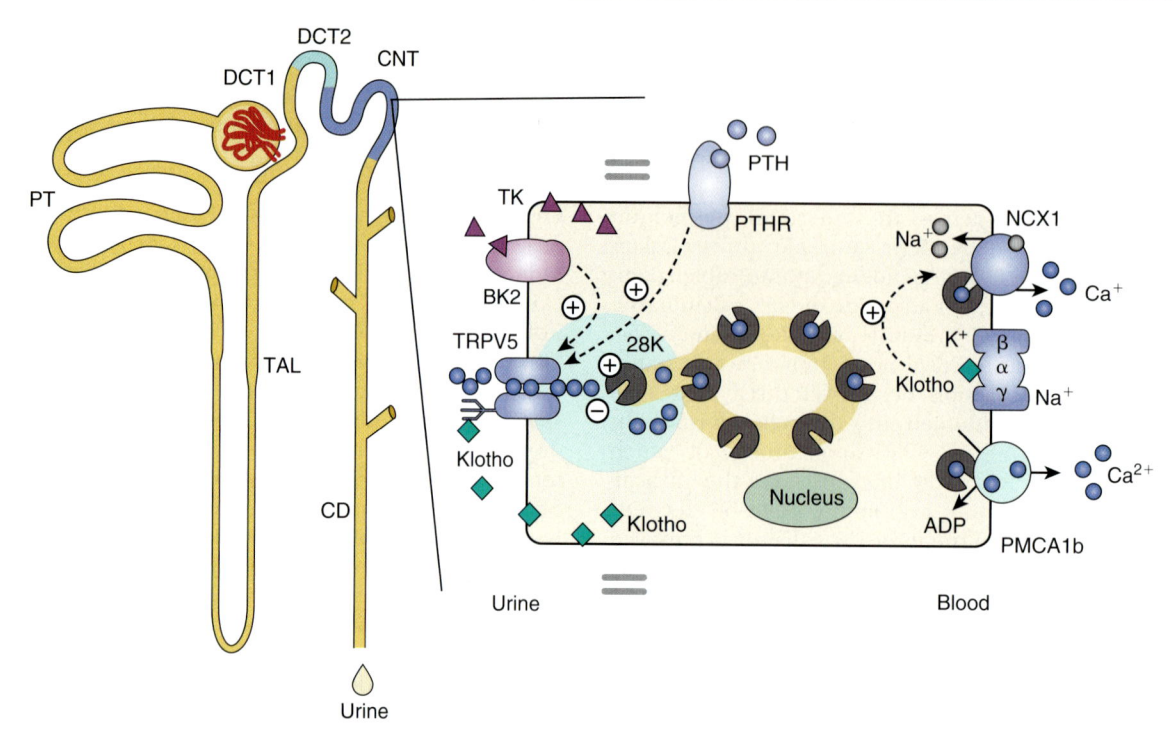

Figure 55.2 Epithelial calcium active transport. The late part of the distal convoluted tubule (DCT) and connecting tubule (CNT) play an important role in fine-tuning renal excretion of Ca^{2+}. The epithelial Ca^{2+} channel (TRPV5) is primarily expressed apically in these segments and co-localizes with calbindin-D_{28K} (28K), Na^+/Ca^{2+} exchanger (NCX1), and the plasma membrane adenosine triphosphatase (ATPase) (PMCA1b). Upon entry via TRPV5, Ca^{2+} is buffered by 28K and diffuses to the basolateral membrane, where it is released and extruded by a concerted action of NCX1 and PMCA1b. In addition, the basolateral membrane exposes a parathyroid hormone receptor (PTHR) and the Na^+/K^+-ATPase consisting of the α-, β-, and γ-subunits. PTHR activation by PTH stimulates TRPV5 activity, and entered Ca^{2+} can subsequently control the expression level of the Ca^{2+} transporters. At the apical membrane, there is a bradykinin receptor (BK2) that is activated by urinary tissue kallikrein (TK) to activate TRPV5-mediated Ca^{2+} influx. In the cell, entered Ca^{2+} acts as a negative feedback on channel activity, and 28K plays a regulatory role by association with TRPV5 under low intracellular Ca^{2+} concentrations. Extracellular urinary klotho directly stimulates TRPV5 at the apical membrane by modification of the N-glycan, whereas intracellular klotho enhances Na^+/K^+-ATPase surface expression, which in turn activates NCX1-mediated Ca^{2+} efflux. ADP, Adenosine diphosphate; DCT1, early part of distal convoluted tubule; PT, proximal tubule; TAL, thick ascending limb of Henle. (From Boros S, Bindels RJM, Hoenderop JGJ: Active Ca^{2+} reabsorption in the connecting tubule. *Pflügers Arch–Eur J Physiol.* 458:99-109, 2009.)

(acid/base, water handling).[35] The diverse functions in the kidney signify how important calcium homeostasis is to normal renal function and vice versa. Furthermore, many of these functions avoid renal calcium precipitation. Most notably, activation of the luminal CaSR in the collecting duct by elevated calcium values leads to urinary acidification and polyuria,[36] a common clinical symptom in hypercalcemia, and prevents calcium-Pi precipitation.

There is some disagreement as to the role of the CaSR in bone and whether or not this role depends on PTH. Clearly bone cells respond to calcium. The CaSR is important in fetal bone development; conditional deletion of the CaSR in early osteoblasts leads to altered bone phenotype, although the results vary depending on the construct used.[37] Studies suggest that the CaSR modulates both bone resorption and bone formation induced by PTH.[38] In vitro, mesenchymal stem cells appear to require CaSR for differentiation,[39] but in more differentiated cells, calcium channels appear more involved in calcium transport.[40] An initial report found that calcium also regulates FGF-23 synthesis in bone, although it does not appear to be mediated via the CaSR.[41] Calcimimetics, allosteric activators of the CaSR, are used to treat secondary hyperparathyroidism as discussed in Chapter 63.

Data also suggest a role for the CaSR in vascular calcification. Immunohistochemical staining demonstrates expression of CaSR on normal human arteries with downregulation in areas of calcification.[42] The CaSR is expressed on cultured vascular smooth muscle cells, and calcimimetics inhibit in vitro calcification.[42,43] The calcimimetic R-568 reverses calcitriol-induced arterial calcification[44] and inhibits proliferation of both vascular smooth muscle cells (VSMCs) and endothelial cells in the nephrectomy rat model.[45] Calcimimetics also retards uremia-enhanced vascular calcification and atherosclerosis in the ApoE$^{-/-}$ mouse[46] and prevents arterial and myocardial calcification in the Cy/+ model of slowly progressive CKD-MBD.[47] Calcimimetics also upregulate a potential local inhibitor of arterial calcification, matrix gla protein.[48] A trial in humans with end-stage kidney disease (ESKD) showed an amelioration in calcification.[49] These data support a role for the CaSR in all three components of CKD-MBD.

HORMONAL REGULATION OF CKD-MBD

PARATHYROID HORMONE

The primary function of PTH is to maintain calcium homeostasis (Figure 55.4) by (1) increasing bone mineral

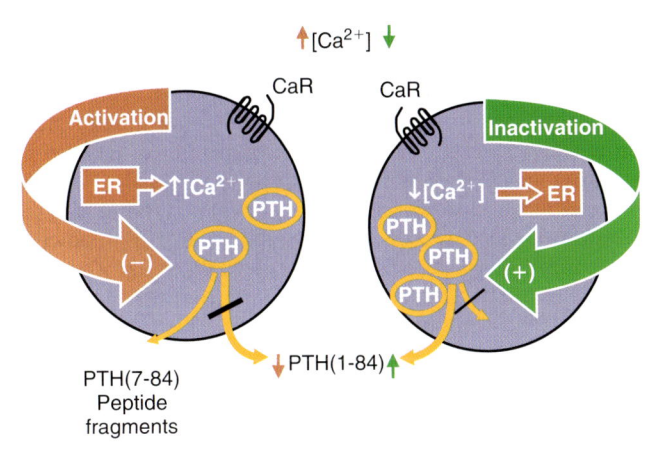

Figure 55.3 Calcium-sensing receptor (CaR). Activation of the CaR by calcium stimulates phospholipase C, leading to increased inositol 1,4,5-triphosphate (IP_3), which mobilizes intracellular calcium and inhibits parathyroid hormone (PTH) synthesis. A decrease in serum calcium (Ca^{2+}) inhibits intracellular signaling, leading to increased PTH synthesis and secretion. ER, Endoplasmic reticulum. (From Friedman PA, Goodman WG: PTH(1-84)/PTH(7-84): a balance of power. *Am J Physiol Renal Physiol.* 290:F975-F984, 2006.)

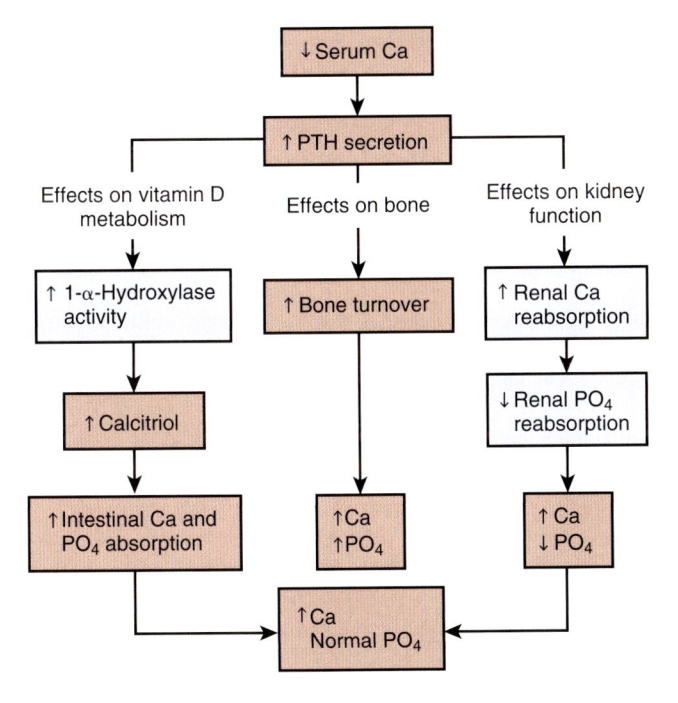

Figure 55.4 Normalization of serum calcium by multiple actions of parathyroid hormone (PTH). Serum levels of ionized calcium (Ca) are maintained in the normal range by induction of increases in the secretion of PTH. PTH acts to increase bone resorption, renal calcium reabsorption, and the conversion of 25(OH)D to $1,25(OH)_2D$ in the kidney, thereby increasing gastrointestinal calcium absorption. The *green boxes* indicate processes that are abnormal in chronic kidney disease (CKD), leading to altered calcium homeostasis. PO_4, Phosphate. (From Moe SM: Calcium, phosphorus, and vitamin D metabolism in renal disease and chronic renal failure. In Kopple JD, Massry SG, editors: *Nutritional management of renal disease,* Philadelphia, 2004, Lippincott Williams & Wilkins, pp 261-285.)

dissolution, thus releasing calcium and Pi, (2) increasing renal reabsorption of calcium and excretion of Pi, (3) increasing the activity of the renal CYP27B1 enzyme to convert 25(OH)D to $1,25(OH)_2D$, and (4) enhancing the gastrointestinal absorption of both calcium and Pi indirectly through its effects on the synthesis of $1,25(OH)_2D$. In healthy subjects, the increase in serum PTH concentration in response to hypocalcemia effectively restores serum calcium levels and maintains serum Pi levels. The kidneys are critical to this normal homeostatic response, and thus patients with more severe CKD may not be able to appropriately maintain calcium homeostasis.

PTH is cleaved to an 84–amino acid protein in the parathyroid gland, where it is stored as fragments in secretory granules for release. Once released, the circulating 1-84 amino acid protein has a half-life of 2 to 4 minutes and is further metabolized in the liver and kidney. PTH secretion occurs in response to hypocalcemia, hyperphosphatemia, elevated FGF-23 levels, and $1,25(OH)_2D$ deficiency. The extracellular concentration of ionized calcium is the most important determinant of minute-to-minute secretion of PTH from stored secretory granules. The rapid response, occurring within seconds, in response to changes in ionized calcium concentration is mediated by the CaSR. Inactivating mutations have been associated with neonatal severe hyperparathyroidism and benign familial hypocalciuric hypercalcemia. Affected patients have asymptomatic elevations of serum calcium in the presence of nonsuppressed PTH. Activating mutations have been found in patients with autosomal dominant hypocalcemia resulting in inhibition of PTH secretion at relatively lower serum calcium. PTH is released as both an intact (1-84) protein and as carboxy (C)–terminal fragments (often called PTH(7-84); see Figure 55.3). C-terminal PTH has the opposite effect on calcium release from bone in animals and cultured calvariae from that of PTH with an intact N terminus.[50] In addition, the C-terminal PTH inhibits apoptosis in osteoblasts, whereas the N-terminal PTH induces apoptosis.[50] Regulators of PTH secretion act by changing the proportion of intact 1-84 and C-terminal fragments.

PTH binds to the PTH1 receptor (PTH1R), which is a member of the G protein–linked seven membrane–spanning receptor family and is widely expressed. PTH-related peptide (PTHrp) shares homology with the first few amino acids of PTH and also binds the PTH1R. Activation of the PTH1R stimulates heterodimeric G proteins G_s (leading to stimulation of cAMP and protein kinase A signaling), and $G_{\alpha q}$ (leading to activation of IP_3 and protein kinase C), ultimately resulting in changes in intracellular calcium.[51] PTH1R activation may vary in response to time exposure, secondary conformational changes after binding, and which cell signaling mechanism is preferentially activated. In general the effects of PTH are systemic and those of PTHrp are autocrine.

The interrelationship of calcium, Pi, FGF-23, and calcitriol in the development of secondary hyperparathyroidism in CKD is complex and nearly impossible to fully evaluate in humans, because changes in one leads to rapid changes in the others. The response to a decrease in ionized calcium mediated by the CaSR is likely the most potent stimulus for PTH release. Pi increases PTH production by enhancing the stability of PTH mRNA.[52] FGF-23 directly stimulates PTH release in a klotho-independent manner.[53] $1,25(OH)_2D$ suppresses PTH release via the VDR to lead to direct suppression of the gene. Other vitamin D compounds that bind to the VDR with lower affinity still reduce PTH release if given in high enough quantities.[54] Although PTH-induced signaling predominantly affects mineral metabolism, there are also many extraskeletal manifestations of PTH excess in CKD. These include encephalopathy, anemia, extraskeletal calcification, peripheral neuropathy, cardiac dysfunction, hyperlipidemia, pain, pruritus, and impotence.[55]

In the kidney, PTH facilitates calcium reabsorption and Pi excretion, as noted earlier. In bone, PTH receptors are located on osteoblasts, with a time-dependent effect. PTH administered long term inhibits osteoblast differentiation and mineralization. In contrast, the administration of PTH to osteoblasts in a pulse rather than a continuous manner stimulates osteoblast proliferation, forming the basis for the administration of PTH as an anabolic therapy for osteoporosis. Parathyroid hormone also interacts with wnt/β-catenin signaling, as discussed later in the bone section.

VITAMIN D

Cholesterol is synthesized to 7-dehydrocholesterol, which in turn is metabolized in the skin to vitamin D_3 (Figure 55.5). This reaction is facilitated by ultraviolet light (UVB) and increased temperature, and is therefore reduced in individuals with high skin melanin content and inhibited by sunscreen containing sun protection factor (SPF) 8 or higher. In addition, there are dietary sources of vitamin D_2 (ergocalciferol) and vitamin D_3 (cholecalciferol). The difference between D_2 (plant source) and D_3 (animal source) compounds is the presence of a double bound (D_2) between carbon numbers 22 and 23 in the side chain. Once in the blood, both D_2 and D_3 bind with vitamin D–binding protein (DBP) and are carried to the liver, where they are hydroxylated by CYP27A1 (25-hydroxylase) in an essentially unregulated manner to yield $25(OH)D$, often called calcidiol. Once they are converted to calcidiol, there appears to be no difference between the biologic activities of D_2 and D_3. Calcidiol is then converted in the kidney (or other cells) to $1,25(OH)_2D$ by the action of CYP27B1. This active metabolite is also degraded by other kidney enzymes, 24,25-hydroxylase (CYP24A1), and CYP3A4, providing the primary metabolism of the active compound.

Vitamin D–binding protein is a 58-kDa protein synthesized in the liver. Its serum levels in humans are between 4 and 8 mM, and the protein has a half-life of 3 days. Both the parent vitamin D, $25(OH)D$ and $1,25(OH)_2D$ are carried

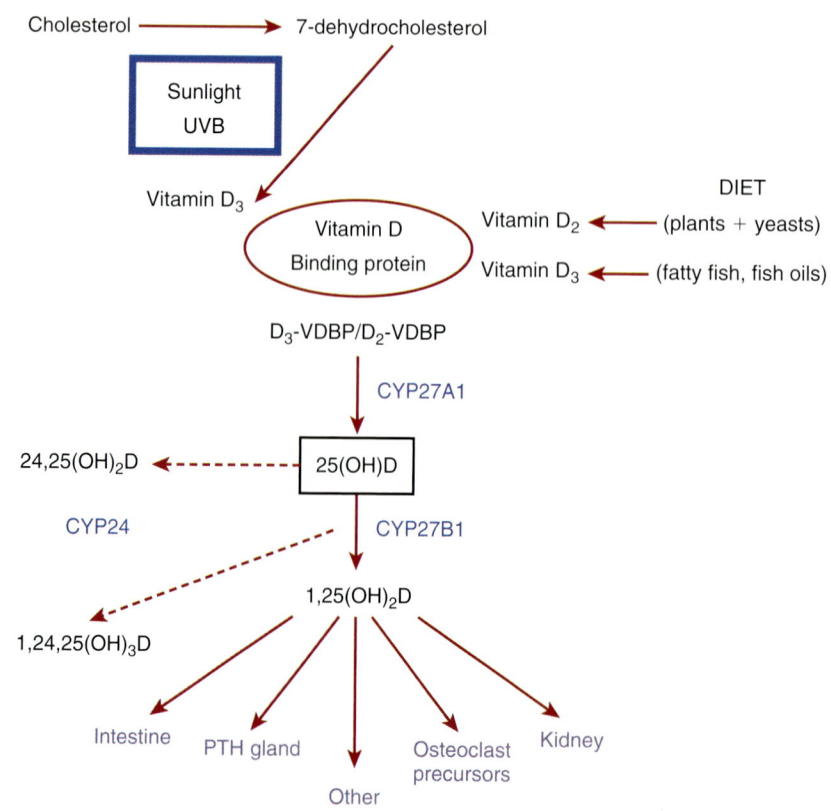

Figure 55.5 Overview of vitamin D metabolism. Vitamin D is obtained from dietary sources and is metabolized via ultraviolet light (UVB) from 7-dehydrocholesterol in the skin. Both sources (diet and skin) of vitamin D_2 and vitamin D_3 bind to vitamin D–binding protein (VDBP) and circulate to the liver. In the liver, vitamin D is hydroxylated by CYP27A1 (25-hydroxylase) to $25(OH)D$, commonly referred to as calcidiol. Calcidiol is then further metabolized to calcitriol by the 1α-hydroxylase enzyme (CYP27B1) at the level of the kidney. The active metabolite $1,25(OH)_2D$ (calcitriol) acts principally on the target organs of intestine, parathyroid (PTH) gland, bone cell precursors, and the kidney. Calcitriol is metabolized to the inert $1,24,25(OH)_3D$ through the action of the 24,25-hydroxylase enzyme (CYP24). Calcidiol is similarly hydroxylated to $24,25(OH)_2D$. (Adapted from Moe SM: Renal osteodystrophy. In Pereira BJG, Sayegh M, Blake P, editors: *Chronic kidney disease: dialysis and transplantation*, 2nd ed, Philadelphia, 2004, Elsevier Saunders.)

in the circulation by DBP, but its greater affinity is for 25(OH)D. Targeted gene disruption studies show that DBP-null mice have a marked reduction in both circulating and tissue distributions of 1,25(OH)$_2$D and yet are normocalcemic, indicating that the primary role of DBP is to maintain stable serum stores of vitamin D metabolites.[56] At the cellular level, both 25(OH)D and 1,25(OH)$_2$D are endocytosed. Inside the cell, 1,25(OH)$_2$D can be inactivated by mitochondrial 24-hydroxylase (CYP24A1) or can bind to the VDR in the cytoplasm. Once the VDR-ligand binding has occurred, the VDR translocates to the nucleus, where it heterodimerizes with the retinoid X receptor (RXR). This complex binds the vitamin D response element (VDRE) of target genes and recruits transcription factors and co-repressors/coactivators that modulate the transcription.[57] These co-repressors and coactivators appear to be specific for the ligand, and thus different forms and analogs of vitamin D may produce different effects at each tissue, forming the basis for the pharmacologic development of analogs. Degradation of calcitriol is believed to occur principally in the kidney, from side cleavage and oxidation, to form 24,25(OH)$_2$D.[57]

It is generally accepted that the major source of the circulating levels of 1,25(OH)$_2$D is the kidney, but there is also evidence that both 25(OH)D and 1,25(OH)$_2$D have local tissue effects because the VDR, CYP27B1, and CYP24A1 are found in many cells throughout the body.[58] There is also evidence for extrarenal conversion of 25(OH)D to 1,25(OH)$_2$D in multiple other organs, with evidence for CYP27B1 expression and/or activity in both normal and abnormal cells. These include osteoblasts, breast epithelial cells (normal and cancerous), prostate gland (normal and cancerous), alveolar and circulating macrophages, pancreatic islet cells, synovial cells, and arterial endothelial cells. Some of these cells may directly take up 1,25(OH)$_2$D, and others may endocytose the DBP–25(OH)D complex in a megalin-mediated manner (Figure 55.6), after which the 25(OH)D is hydroxylated by CYP27B1 to act on that specific

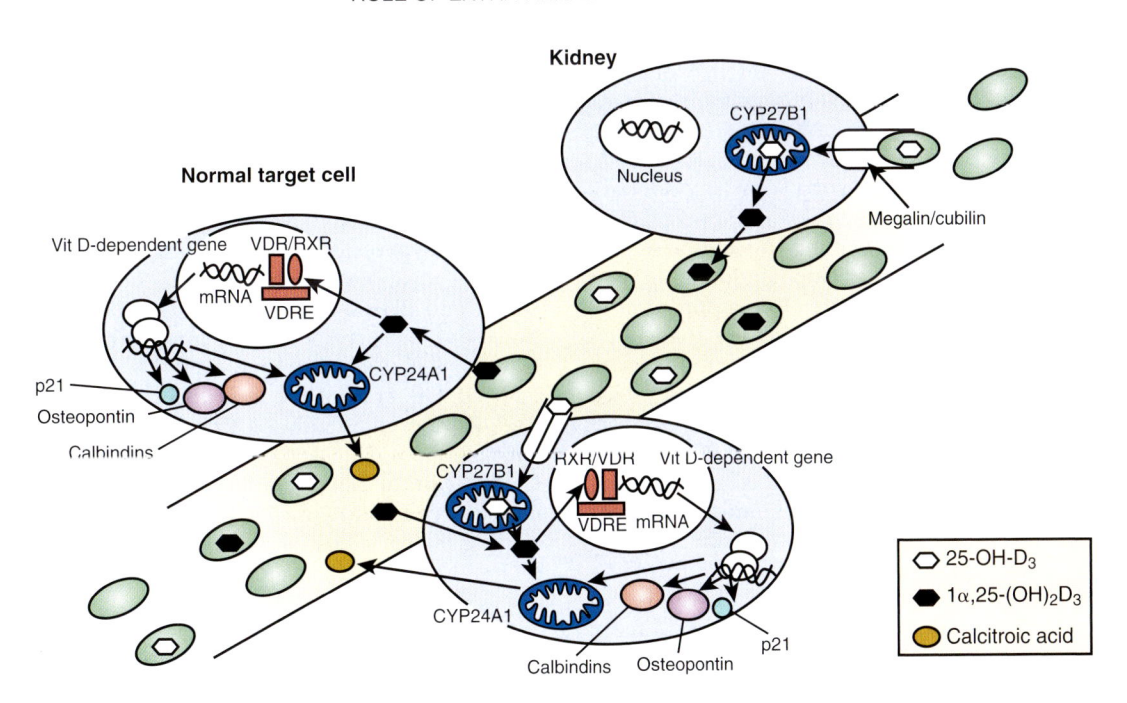

Figure 55.6 Concept of the role of the extrarenal 1α-hydroxylase. The metabolism of vitamin D in the context of the cells involved is shown. **Upper right,** Proximal tubular cell showing the key elements in the uptake of 25(OH)D$_3$ and its conversion to 1α,25(OH)$_2$D$_3$. Megalin/cubilin are cell surface receptors that execute endocytosis of the vitamin D–binding protein (DBP–25(OH)D$_3$ complex, and CYP27B1 is the main component of the 1α-hydroxylase, responsible for making 1α,25(OH)$_2$D$_3$. **Middle left,** Simple target cell that takes up 1α,25(OH)$_2$D$_3$ as the free ligand originally ferried to the target cell bound to DBP. The picture shows the key elements of the transcriptional machinery as well as some representative gene products, including the cell division protein p21, the bone matrix protein osteopontin, the calcium transport protein calbindin, and the autoregulatory protein CYP24A1. **Lower right,** Target cell expressing extrarenal 1α-hydroxylase, which possesses megalin/cubilin machinery to take up the DBP/25(OH)D$_3$ complex and also expresses CYP27B1, enabling it to make 1α,25(OH)$_2$D$_3$ intracellularly and also to respond in a likewise manner to the simple target cell because it also possesses the vitamin D receptor (VDR) and other transcriptional machinery. The expectation is that cells involved in cell differentiation or in control of cell division require higher concentrations of 1α,25(OH)$_2$D$_3$ in order to modulate a different set of genes, and that the CYP27B1 boosts local production to augment "circulating" 1α,25(OH)$_2$D$_3$ arriving from the kidney in the bloodstream. With normal physiologic processes, locally produced 1α,25(OH)$_2$D$_3$ would not enter the general circulation, although in pathologic conditions (e.g., sarcoidosis) it might. At this time, it is not clear how many cell types can be considered simple target cells and how many possess the CYP27B1 and megalin/cubilin to allow for local production of hormone. mRNA, Messenger RNA; RXR, retinoid X receptor. (Reprinted with permission from Jones G: Expanding role for vitamin D in chronic kidney disease: importance of blood 25-OH-D levels and extra-renal 1α-hydroxylase in the classical and nonclassical actions of 1α,25-dihydroxyvitamin D$_3$. Semin Dial 20:316-324, 2007.)

cell. The presence of CYP24A1 in cells also indicates that the metabolism of 1,25(OH)$_2$D may be regulated at a cellular level. The circulating levels of 25(OH)D are 1000 times greater than those of 1,25(OH)$_2$D, and thus 25(OH)D will have a local, or autocrine/paracrine effect on many cell types.[58]

Circulating 1,25(OH)$_2$D mediates its cellular function via both nongenomic and genomic mechanisms. 1,25(OH)$_2$D facilitates the uptake of calcium in intestinal and renal epithelium by increasing the activity of the voltage-dependent calcium channels TRPV5 and TRPV6. Calcitriol then enhances the transport of calcium through and out of the cells, by upregulating the calcium transport protein calbindin (calbindin-D9k in intestine, and calbindin-D28k in kidney) and the basolateral calcium-ATPase as detailed earlier in this chapter. The CYP27B1 in the kidney is the site of regulation of 1,25(OH)$_2$D synthesis by numerous other factors, including low calcium, low Pi, estrogen, prolactin, growth hormone, FGF-23, and 1,25(OH)$_2$D itself. Studies show that FGF-23 and inflammatory mediators such as interferon regulate CYP27B1 at nonrenal sites.[59] In vitamin D knockout animals, parathyroid gland hyperplasia is consistently observed despite normalization of serum calcium level. However, gland growth can be blunted by exogenous administration of calcitriol even in the absence of VDR, demonstrating a role for 1,25(OH)$_2$D in regulation of parathyroid gland growth.[60] In vivo in the rat, a single small dose of 1,25(OH)$_2$D decreases PTH secretion by nearly 100%. Studies in the 1970s demonstrated that oral 1,25(OH)$_2$D, but not the precursor hormone vitamin D$_3$, suppressed PTH in patients undergoing dialysis, leading to widespread use of calcitriol or its analogs. However, later studies in animals have demonstrated efficacy of 25(OH)D in suppression of PTH, but the levels required are much greater than levels of 1,25(OH)$_2$D. Studies in humans have shown efficacy of 25(OH)D in suppressing PTH in patients with advanced CKD, but direct comparison studies are lacking.[61]

1,25(OH)$_2$D has multiple effects on many cells that are important in bone remodeling; therefore it is not surprising that bone defects are well described in vitamin D–deficient states. However, the direct effects of the vitamin D system on bone have been difficult to differentiate from the secondary effects of hypocalcemia and hyperparathyroidism in vitamin D–deficient models. However, transgenic animals, including 1α-hydroxylase$^{-/-}$/VDR$^{-/-}$, and 1α-hydroxylase$^{-/-}$/VDR$^{-/-}$, have impaired bone mineralization. In these animals, mineralization can be corrected with normalization of serum calcium level; even exogenous calcitriol does not fully correct mineralization in the 1α-hydroxylase$^{-/-}$ animals unless calcium levels are also restored. Studies evaluating bone remodeling also demonstrate an important role for the 1,25(OH)$_2$D/VDR system. If hypocalcemia is not corrected (leading to secondary hyperparathyroidism), there is increased osteoblast activity and bone formation from the anabolic effects of PTH. The activation of osteoclasts by PTH is blunted, suggesting a synergistic effect of vitamin D and PTH. Supporting this suggestion is the finding that when calcium levels are corrected by "rescue" diets and secondary hyperparathyroidism is prevented, osteoblast numbers, mineralization activity, and bone volume are still reduced. Comparison studies of 1α-hydroxylase$^{-/-}$ and PTH$^{-/-}$ mice demonstrate a predominant role for PTH in appositional bone growth and for vitamin D in endochondral bone formation. Thus, the 1,25(OH)$_2$D/VDR system has anabolic bone effects that are necessary for bone formation and are supplemental to the effect of PTH.[62]

FGF-23 AND KLOTHO

Phosphatonins are circulating factors that regulate urinary Pi excretion. Three main phosphatonins have been described: FGF-23, secreted frizzled-related protein 4 (sFRP-4), and matrix extracellular phosphoglycoprotein (MEPE). Various forms of rickets have now all been found to be due to abnormalities in FGF-23. Autosomal dominant hypophosphatemic rickets (ADH) is rare and is associated with a mutation that limits normal degradation of FGF-23. Autosomal recessive hypophosphatemic rickets is also rare and is due to a mutation in dentin matrix protein (DMP), a locally produced inhibitor of FGF-23. X-linked hypophosphatemic rickets is the most common form of rickets due to a mutation in *PHEX* (phosphate-regulating gene with homologies to endopeptidases located on the X chromosome). Mutations in *PHEX* have been found to degrade FGF-23 in the osteocyte, leading to inappropriate levels of FGF-23.[63] Thus, what previously was thought to be disorders of different etiologies are now all linked back to FGF-23.

FGF-23 is a 251–amino acid hormone predominantly produced from bone cells (osteocytes and osteoblasts) during active bone remodeling, but its mRNA is also found in heart, liver, thyroid/parathyroid, intestine, and skeletal muscle.[64] FGF-23 production in the osteocyte is stimulated by PTH[65] and inhibited by 1,25(OH)$_2$D.[66] Elevated Pi or Pi load and hypercalcemia may also stimulate FGF-23 but this stimulation appears to be indirect. In the osteocyte, both DMP1 and PHEX protein degrade FGF-23 such that mutations in their corresponding genes lead to excess FGF-23.[63] In turn, 1,25(OH)$_2$D increases PHEX and FGF-23 inhibits 1,25(OH)$_2$D, completing a feedback loop. FGF-23 regulates NaPi-IIa independently of PTH; FGF-23 also inhibits the conversion of 25(OH)D to 1,25(OH)$_2$D by inhibition of CYP27B1 in the renal tubules[67] and at extrarenal sites,[59] and increases catabolism of 1,25(OH)$_2$D by activation of CYP24,[67] leading to hypophosphatemia and inappropriately normal or low 1,25(OH)$_2$D levels. An overview of the FGF-klotho axis is shown in Figure 55.7.

FGF-23 is a member of a diverse family of 18 FGFs that bind to one of four receptors (FGFRs) via a heparan sulfate co-factor or klotho co-receptor–dependent manner, leading to diverse biologic effects.[68] Identification of klotho as a co-receptor for FGF-23 was due to nearly identical phenotypes of the knockout mice, including hyperphosphatemia, hypercalcemia, and excess 1,25(OH)$_2$D levels associated with early mortality, growth retardation, vascular calcification, cardiac hypertrophy, and osteopenia.[69] Klotho was originally identified as an aging suppressor gene. α-Klotho is expressed in the kidney and parathyroid gland and forms complexes with FGFR1 and FGFR4 to enhance FGF-23 signaling. β-klotho is expressed in the liver and fat, forms complexes with FGFR1 and FGFR4, and supports FGF-15/19 and FGF-21 signaling. γ-klotho increases FGF-19 activity and is expressed in the eye, fat, and kidney. All three klothos are transmembrane proteins, with short intracellular domains and large extracellular domains that have β-glucosidase cleavage sites. In animals, α-klotho

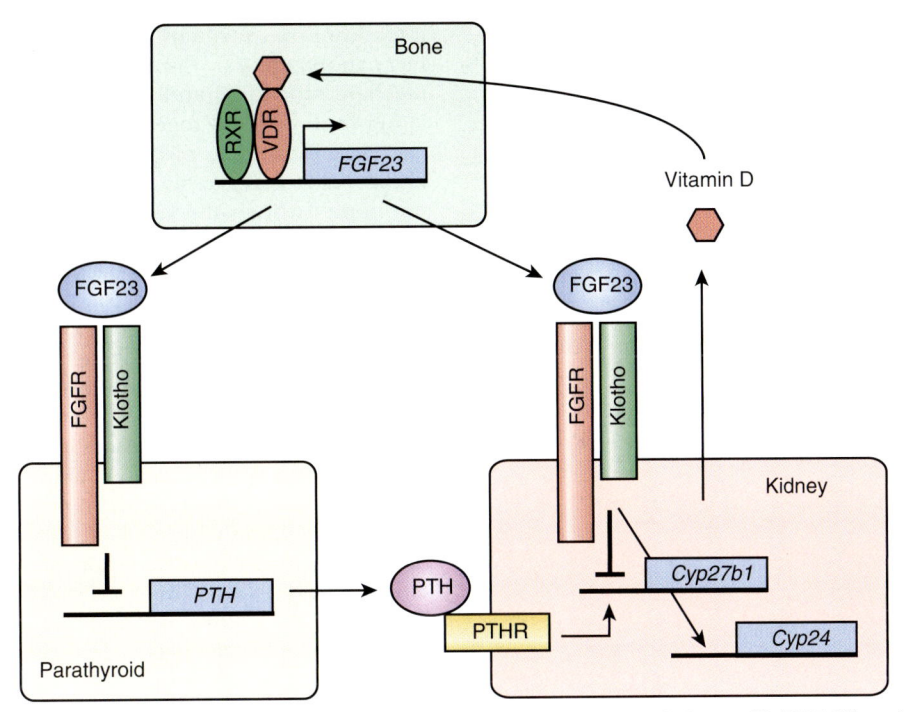

Figure 55.7 The bone-kidney-parathyroid endocrine axes mediated by fibroblast growth factor 23 (FGF-23) and klotho. Active form of vitamin D (1,25-dihydroxyvitamin D_3) binds to vitamin D receptor (VDR) in the bone (osteocytes). The ligand-bound VDR forms a heterodimer with a nuclear receptor (RXR) and transactivates expression of the FGF-23 gene. FGF-23 secreted from bone acts on the klotho-FGF receptor (FGFR) complex expressed in the kidney (the bone-kidney axis) and parathyroid gland (the bone-parathyroid axis). In the kidney, FGF-23 suppresses synthesis of active vitamin D by downregulating expression of the *Cyp27b1* gene and promotes its inactivation by upregulating expression of the *Cyp24* gene, thereby closing a negative feedback loop for vitamin D homeostasis. In the parathyroid gland, FGF-23 suppresses production and secretion of parathyroid hormone (PTH). PTH binds to the PTH receptor (PTHR) expressed on renal tubular cells, leading to upregulation of *Cyp27b1* gene expression. Thus, suppression of PTH by FGF-23 reduces expression of the *Cyp27b1* gene and serum levels of 1,25-dihydroxyvitamin D_3. This step closes another long negative feedback loop for vitamin D homeostasis. (Reprinted with permission from Kuro-o M: Overview of the FGF23-Klotho axis. *Pediatr Nephrol.* 25:583-590, 2010.)

expressed in the distal tubule can be cleaved to release the extracellular domain into the circulation. Further, alternative splicing of the α-klotho gene leads to only the extracellular domain that is released from cells and is called circulating or soluble klotho.[69] The soluble α-klotho acts as a co-receptor at nonrenal sites, and prevents FGF23 induced cardiac hypertrophy.[70] The kidney regulates both renal production of soluble klotho and renal excretion.[69]

In the kidney, tissue klotho is downregulated early in CKD[69] and FGF-23 is upregulated early in the course of CKD.[71] Klotho is shed from the distal convoluted tubule to serve as a co-receptor with FGF-23 on the proximal tubule, where it inhibits excretion of Pi that is regulated by NaPi-IIa, NaPi-IIc, and Pit-1 (similar to PTH but via different signaling mechanisms), and suppresses CYP27B1 to inhibit $1,25(OH)_2D_3$ production (opposite of PTH).[72] Klotho also increases calcium reabsorption by stimulating TRPV5,[73] decreases potassium excretion through effects on the ROMK1 (renal outer medullary potassium 1) channel,[74] protects against kidney injury and fibrosis,[75] and decreases insulin resistance.[72] Table 55.2 demonstrates the parallel changes in klotho deficiency and CKD.

In addition to klotho's role in mineral metabolism, it and FGF-23 are implicated in cardiovascular disease. FGF-23 can induce cardiac hypertrophy and increases intracellular calcium in a klotho-independent manner.[70,76,77] Klotho is localized in the heart at the sinoatrial node, and klotho deficiency may lead to arrhythmias.[78] Klotho suppresses cardiomyocyte apoptosis[79] and downregulates TRPC6 (transient receptor potential cation 6) calcium channel in the cardiomyocyte.[80] Both klotho and FGFR1 and FGFR3, but not FGF-23 and FGFR4, are expressed in human arteries.[81,82] In human arteries from patients with CKD, both klotho and FGFR1 and FGFR3 are downregulated in the presence of calcification. VDR activators upregulate klotho, leading to an anticalcific effect on FGF-23–induced calcification.[82] Decreased klotho impairs endothelial function.[83] Activation of the renin angiotensin aldosterone system (RAAS) reduces renal klotho expression.[84] The pace of discovery of the systemic effects of FGF-23 and klotho has revolutionized our understanding of CKD-MBD.

BONE BIOLOGY

The majority of the total body stores of calcium and Pi is located in bone and therefore bone plays an integral role in homeostasis. Trabecular (cancellous) bone is located predominantly in the epiphyses of the long bones, is 15% to 25% calcified, and serves a metabolic function, with a relatively short turnover time as shown by calcium[45] studies. In contrast, cortical (compact) bone is located in the shafts of long bones and is 80% to 90% calcified. This bone

Table 55.2	Comparison of Phenotypes of Klotho Deficiency and Chronic Kidney Disease (CKD)	
	Klotho Deficiency	**Chronic Kidney Disease**
Blood chemistry:		
Phosphate	↑↑↑↑	↑ or ↑↑↑*
Calcium	↑	↔ or ↓↓
Creatinine	↑	↑↑↑
1,25 vitamin D_3	↑↑↑	↓↓↓
Parathyroid hormone	↔ or ↓	↑↑
Fibroblast growth factor 23	↑↑↑	↑↑
Klotho	↓↓↓ or disappears	↓↓ at ESKD†
Gross phenotypes:		
Body weight	↓↓↓	↓↓
Growth retardation	↓↓↓↓	↓↓ in children
Physical activity	↓↓↓	↓
Fertility	↓↓↓↓	↓↓
Life span	↓↓↓↓	↓↓
Cardiovascular disease:		
Cardiac hypertrophy	↑↑	↑↑↑
Cardiac fibrosis	↑↑	↑↑↑
Vascular calcification	↑↑↑↑	↑↑
Atherosclerosis	↑↑	↑↑↑
Blood pressure	↑	↑↑↑↑
Hematocrit levels	↓	↓↓↓↓
Bone disease	↓↓↓	↓↓↓

ESKD, End-stage kidney disease; ↓, decreases; ↑, increases; ↔, unchanged.
*During early chronic kidney disease, blood phosphate level is in the normal range.
†Blood klotho may be increased in early CKD.
Modified from Hu MC, Kuro-o M, Moe OW: Renal and extrarenal actions of Klotho. Semin Nephrol. 33:118-129, 2013.

serves primarily a protective and mechanical function and has a calcium turnover time of months. Bone consists principally (90%) of highly organized cross-linked fibers of type I collagen; the remainder consists of proteoglycans and "non-collagen" proteins such as osteopontin, osteocalcin, osteonectin, and alkaline phosphatase. Hydroxyapatite—$Ca_{10}(PO_4)_6(OH)_2$—is the primary bone crystal.

The cellular components of bone are cartilage cells, which are critical to bone development; osteoblasts, which are the bone-forming cells; and osteoclasts, which are the bone-resorbing cells. Osteoblasts are derived from progenitor mesenchymal cells located in the bone marrow. They are then induced to become osteoprogenitor cells, then endosteal or periosteal progenitor cells, then mature osteoblasts. The control of this differentiation pathway is complicated and involves integration of circulating hormones, locally produced factors from the mesenchymal-hematopoietic cell niche, and transcription factors. Once bone formation is complete, osteoblasts may undergo apoptosis or may become quiescent cells trapped within the mineralized bone in the form of osteocytes.[85] The osteocytes are interconnected through a series of canaliculi and serve as mechanoreceptors. Osteocytes detect and respond to mechanical loading and initiate bone remodeling by regulating local osteoclastogenesis via paracrine signals. Osteoclasts are derived from hematopoietic precursor cells that differentiate and are signaled to arrive at a certain place in the bone through the OPG/RANKL system detailed later. Once there, they fuse to form the multinucleated cells known as osteoclasts, which become highly polarized, reabsorbing bone through the release of derivative enzymes. These cells move along a resorption surface via changes in the cytoskeleton. PTH, cytokines, and $1,25(OH)_2D$ are all important in inducing the fusion of the committed osteoclast precursors.

The control of bone remodeling is highly complex, but appears to occur in very distinct phases, as follows: (1) osteoblast activation, (2) osteoclast recruitment resorption, (3) pre-osteoblast migration and differentiation, (4) osteoblast deposition of matrix (osteoid or unmineralized bone), (5) mineralization, and (6) quiescence. At any one time, less than 15% to 20% of the bone surface is undergoing remodeling, and this process in a single bone remodeling unit can take 3 to 6 months.[86] How a certain piece of bone is chosen to undergo a remodeling cycle is not completely clear. The three main systems that interact to regulate remodeling are OPG/RANKL, sclerostin/Wnt/β-catenin, and PTH/PTHR1, which are discussed separately.

The identification of the osteoprotegerin (OPG) and RANK (receptor activator of nuclear factor κB) system in the 1980s shed new light on the control of osteoclast function and the long observed coupling of osteoblasts and osteoclasts. RANK is located on osteoclasts, and RANK ligand (RANKL) is secreted by osteoblasts. Osteoblasts also synthesize the decoy protein OPG, which can bind to OPG ligand (OPGL) on osteoblasts and inhibit the subsequent binding of OPGL to RANK on osteoclasts, thus inhibiting bone resorption (Figure 55.8). Alternatively, if OPG production is decreased, RANKL can bind with RANK on osteoclasts and induce osteoclastic bone resorption. This control system is regulated by nearly every cytokine and hormone thought important in bone remodeling, including PTH, $1,25(OH)_2D$, estrogen, glucocorticoids, interleukins, prostaglandins, and members of the transforming growth factor-β (TGF-β) superfamily of cytokines.[87] OPG has been successful in preventing bone resorption in models of osteoporosis as well as hormone- and cytokine-induced bone resorption,[87] and denosumab, an anti-RANKL antibody, is an approved anabolic drug for the treatment of osteoporosis.[88] Interestingly, abnormalities in the OPG/RANKL system have been found in kidney disease,[89] and early animal models suggest that treatment with OPG may have a protective role in hyperparathyroid bone disease.[90] Initial studies in patients undergoing dialysis have demonstrated hypocalcemia as a severe adverse effect of this agent.[91] More information is required to understand how this system regulates bone remodeling in the context of CKD.

Genetic defects in the gene SOST have been identified in rare bone disorders. Sclerostin, the protein product of this gene, binds to low-density lipoprotein (LDL) receptor–related proteins 5 and 6 (LRP5/LRP6) on the osteocyte to competitively inhibit the binding of the protein wnt (Figure

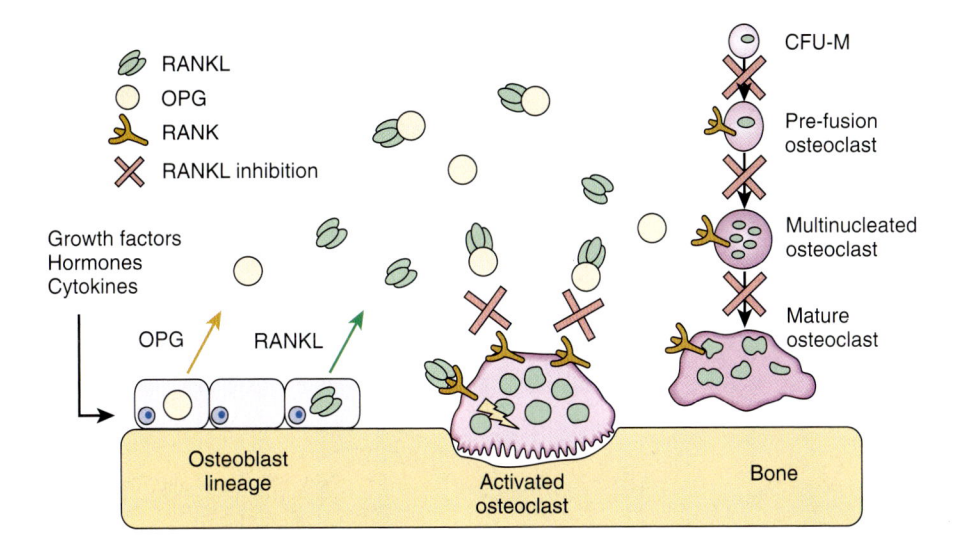

Figure 55.8 Role of OPG/RANKL in bone remodeling. Mechanisms of action for OPG (osteoprotegerin), RANKL (receptor activator of nuclear factor kappaB ligand), and RANK (receptor activator of nuclear factor kappaB) is depicted in this diagram. RANKL is produced by osteoblasts, bone marrow stromal cells, and other cells under the control of various proresorptive growth factors, hormones, and cytokines. Osteoblasts and stromal cells produce OPG, which binds to and thereby inactivates RANKL. The major binding complex is likely to be a single OPG homodimer interacting with high affinity with a single RANKL homotrimer. In the absence of OPG, RANKL activates its receptor, RANK, found on osteoclasts and preosteoclast precursors. RANK-RANKL interactions lead to preosteoclast recruitment, fusion into multinucleated osteoclasts, osteoclast activation, and osteoclast survival. Each of these RANK-mediated responses can be fully inhibited by OPG. CFU-M, Macrophage colony-forming unit. (From Kearns AE, Khosla S, Kostenuik PJ: Receptor activator of nuclear factor kappaB ligand and osteoprotegerin regulation of bone remodeling in health and disease. *Endocr Rev.* 29:155-192, 2008.)

55.9). Normally, wnt binding to LRP5/LRP6 leads to stabilization of β-catenin (canonical pathway) and regulation of normal bone accrual via osteoblast differentiation. In the presence of sclerostin, the β-catenin is degraded and mesenchymal stem cell differentiation to mature bone cells is inhibited. In animal models sclerostin deletion enhances bone accrual,[92] and in early human trials treatment with an antibody to sclerostin was found to be anabolic.[93,94] Given that sclerostin values are elevated in both blood and bone of patients with CKD[95] and bone in animals with CKD,[96] the anabolic agent anti-sclerostin antibody may be efficacious in the treatment of renal osteodystrophy. However, initial studies in animals found that anti-sclerostin antibody was not efficacious in the setting of elevated PTH, although it did improve bone volume when PTH was suppressed.[97] Dickkopf-related protein 1 (dkk-1) also inhibits wnt binding to LRP5/LRP6, and an antibody to this circulating inhibitor of wnt signaling improved bone remodeling in a model of early CKD.[98] In osteocytes, PTH directly suppresses sclerostin and dkk-1 secretion[65,99] and thus inhibits the production of circulating inhibitors of wnt signaling.

In bone, PTH binds to its receptor, PTH1R, and activates β-catenin signaling via multiple mechanisms (see Figure 55.9): (1) direct activation through cAMP signaling, (2) indirect activation via osteoclast activation, which then increases β-catenin activity in osteoblasts, and (3) by binding to LRP6 to activate LRP5/LRP6 signaling even in the absence of wnt ligands.[92] Thus, PTH can activate β-catenin through non–wnt-mediated pathways and through pathways not regulated by sclerostin or dkk-1. There are also differences in responses to continuous and intermittent PTH exposures. Mice expressing a constitutively active PTH1R or animals receiving continuous infusion of PTH(1-84) (analogous to secondary hyperparathyroidism) also have wnt-dependent remodeling with increased osteoclast bone resorption via the OPG/RANKL system, leading to osteoblast activation and β-catenin activation.[100,101] Hyperphosphatemia also activates β-catenin signaling.[102] Thus, in CKD with hyperphosphatemia and secondary hyperparathyroidism there is activation of β-catenin by PTH-mediated inhibition of circulating inhibitors of wnt signaling (sclerostin and dkk-1), PTH-mediated effects independent of wnt signaling, and phosphorus-mediated effects. They all lead to enhanced mesenchymal differentiation to osteoblasts, increased RANKL-induced osteoclast activation, and increased bone resorption.

PATHOPHYSIOLOGY OF VASCULAR CALCIFICATION

Vascular disease may be due to a variety of different pathologic processes in different arterial segments, all of which can be calcified. Atherosclerotic disease is characterized by fibro-fatty plaque formation, and on the basis of autopsy data and animal models, calcification had been thought to occur late in the disease course. These plaques can protrude into the arterial lumen, leading to a filling defect on angiography (Figure 55.10A). However, advances in imaging,

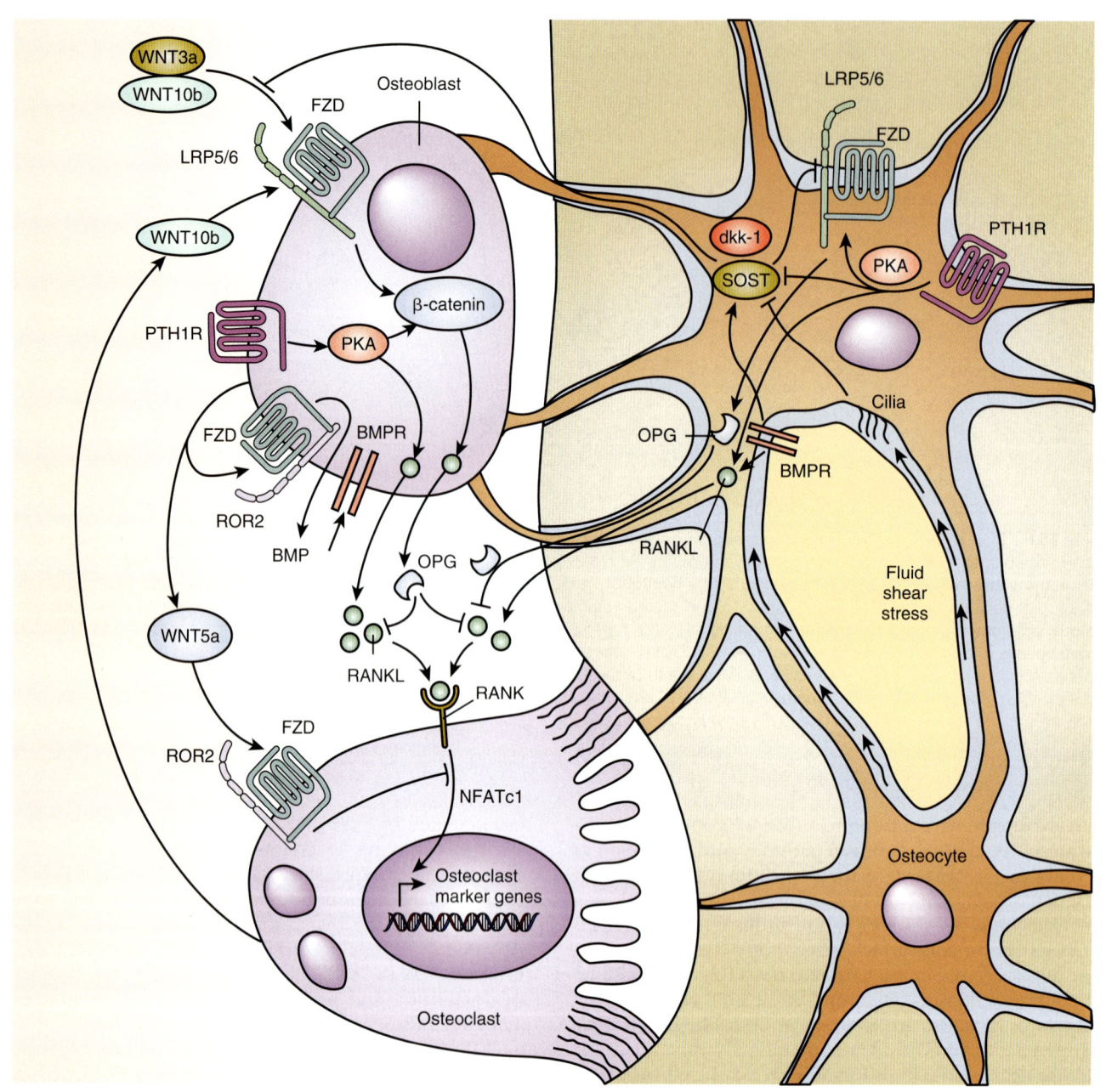

Figure 55.9 Parathyroid hormone (PTH) and β-catenin signaling in bone remodeling. Osteocytes control bone formation through the secretion of the WNT antagonists sclerostin (SOST) and Dickkopf WNT signaling pathway inhibitor 1 (dkk-1), the expression of which is regulated by mechanosignals and by signaling of PTH and bone morphogenetic protein (BMP). PTH represses expression of these antagonists, whereas BMP signaling, which is mediated by BMP receptor 1A (BMPR1A), induces their expression. Moreover, WNT signaling in osteocytes controls the production of osteoprotegerin (OPG), which is the decoy receptor for the key osteoclast differentiation factor RANKL (receptor activator of nuclear factor kappaB ligand). Osteoblast-expressed WNT5a stimulates differentiation of osteoclast precursors as a result of binding to the FZD–ROR2 (frizzled and receptor tyrosine kinase–like orphan receptor 2) receptor complex. In a feedback loop for bone remodeling, osteoclasts stimulate the local differentiation of osteoblasts at the end of the resorption phase by secreting WNT ligands. In addition, activation of parathyroid hormone 1 receptor (PTH1R)–mediated signaling in osteoblasts and osteocytes leads to stabilization of β-catenin and, thus, activation of WNT signaling. LRP5/6, Low-density lipoprotein (LDL) receptor–related proteins 5 and 6; PKA, protein kinase signaling. (Reprinted with permission from Baron R, Kneissel M: WNT signaling in bone homeostasis and disease: from human mutations to treatments. *Nat Med.* 19:179-192, 2013.)

especially intravascular ultrasonography, have demonstrated that atherosclerosis can also be a circumferential lesion (without an obstructed lumen) with calcification earlier in the course of the disease.[103] The medial layer may also be affected in arteriosclerosis, leading to thickening of the medial layer that is most commonly found in elastic arteries (Figure 55.10*B*). In addition to the larger elastic arteries, the smaller elastic arteries may be affected by medial thickening and calcification, classically described as Mönckeberg's calcification, or medial calcinosis. This disease

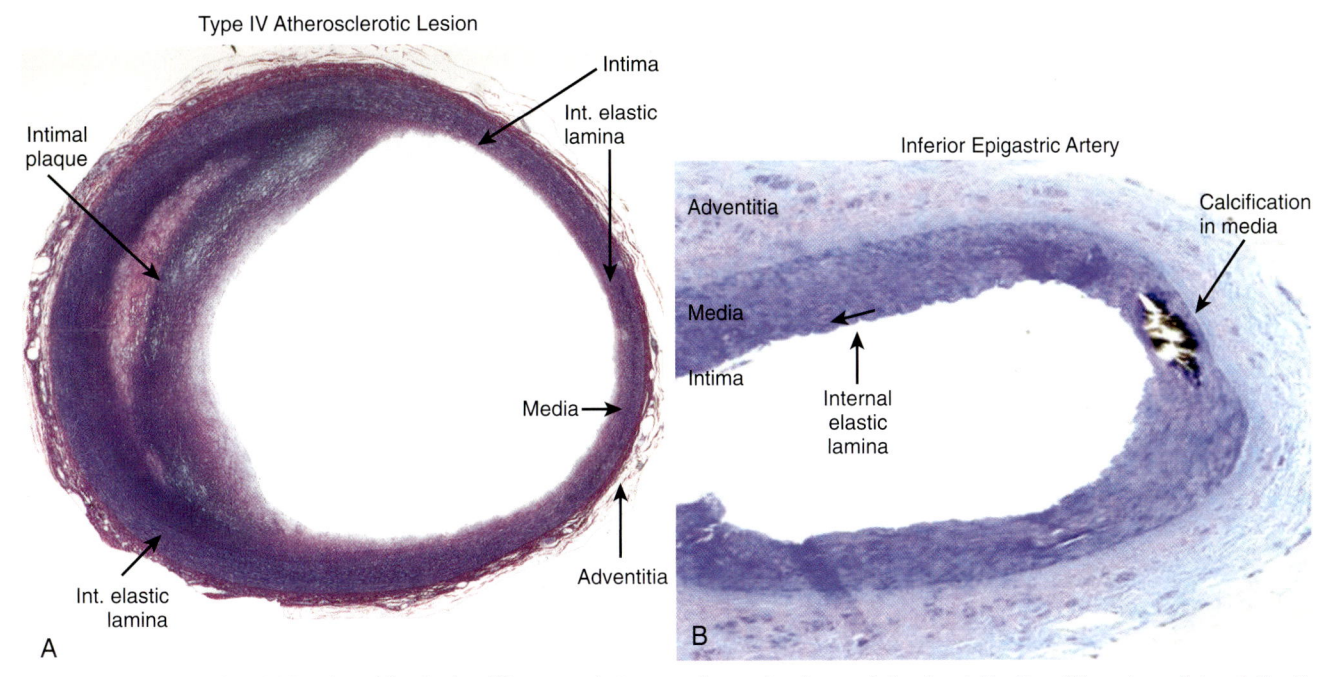

Figure 55.10 Arterial calcification. Histologic differences between atherosclerotic, or intimal calcification **(A)** and medial calcification **(B)**. Int., internal.

is more common in patients with diabetes, kidney disease, and advanced aging and is associated with increased all-cause and cardiovascular mortality in diabetic patients without CKD as well as in patients with CKD with or without diabetes.

Although initially believed to be due to spontaneous precipitation, vascular calcification is now known to be a tightly regulated process that resembles mineralization in bone, a process kept "in check" through the actions of inhibitors of calcification. The current hypothesis accepted by most investigators is that VSMCs dedifferentiate or transform to osteocyte/chondrocyte–like cells (Figure 55.11). These cells then lay down an extracellular matrix of collagen and noncollagenous proteins and make matrix vesicles that attach to the extracellular matrix to initiate and propagate mineralization. This process is regulated by the cells, the extracellular matrix proteins, and inhibitors that may act locally or systemically. In advanced CKD, there is abnormal bone remodeling and reduced renal clearance of phosphate, generating a positive calcium and Pi balance that "feeds" the mineral composition of matrix vesicles and augments the ability of existing calcification to expand. The evidence for each of these steps is discussed.

CELLULAR TRANSFORMATION

VSMCs, osteoblasts, chondrocytes, and adipocytes differentiate from mesenchymal precursors with normal differentiation and in transformation (de-differentiation), which are controlled by various transcription factors (Figure 55.12) Expression of the osteoblast differentiation factor core binding factor α-1 (Cbfα1), now called Runx-2, has been identified in the inferior epigastric artery of adults undergoing kidney transplantation[104] and in sections from the brachial arteries of children undergoing dialysis.[105] Runx-2 is critical in normal bone development, in that Runx-2

knockout mice fail to form a skeleton.[106] Genetic techniques have confirmed that VSMCs give rise to osteochondrogenic-like cells in calcified blood vessels (as opposed to circulating cells).[107] Osteoclast-like cells can also be seen, more commonly in intimal lesions, and as in bone, they appear to arise from circulating precursors.[108]

In vitro, VSMCs upregulate Runx-2 in response to elevated Pi mediated by the type III sodium-dependent Pi cotransporters Pit-1 and Pit-2.[109] In addition, VSMCs incubated with uremic serum (pooled from anuric patients undergoing dialysis), in comparison with normal serum, express Runx-2 and its downstream protein osteopontin via a non–Pi-mediated mechanism.[110] Excess calcium can also induce mineralization in vitro, and the effects of calcium are additive to those of increased Pi.[111] Lastly, FGF-23 enhances Pi-induced vascular calcification in rat aortic rings and rat aorta VSMCs by promoting osteoblastic differentiation.[112] Numerous traditional and nontraditional cardiovascular risk factors in CKD can induce the transformation of VSMCs into osteoblast-like cells, with subsequent calcification in vitro (see Figure 55.12). Given these data, it is not surprising that arterial calcification is so common in patients with CKD.

In animal models of CKD, secondary hyperparathyroidism develops spontaneously with loss of kidney function and can be associated with vascular calcification.[47,113,114] Unfortunately, it is difficult to distinguish between the effects of Pi and PTH. However, one study found that vascular calcification developed in nephrectomized animals achieving supraphysiologic PTH levels by infusion, regardless of the Pi intake.[115] In a similar study, Runx-2 was upregulated in animals in three of the four Pi/PTH intake groups—those fed normal PTH + high Pi, high PTH + high Pi, and high PTH + low Pi—indicating that both Pi and PTH may lead to Runx-2 upregulation in arteries. However, the

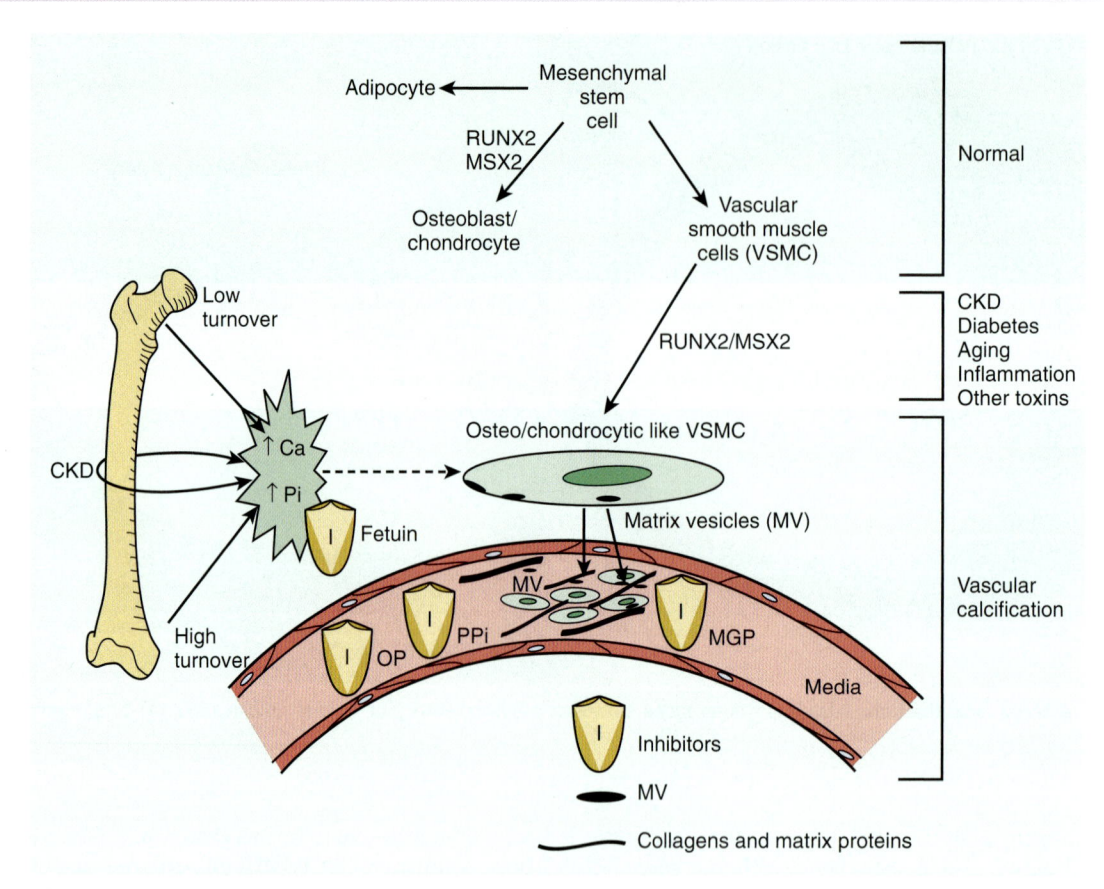

Figure 55.11 **Overview of the pathophysiology of vascular calcification.** Normally, mesenchymal stem cells differentiate to adipocytes, osteoblasts, chondrocytes, and vascular smooth muscle cells (VSMCs). In the setting of chronic kidney disease (CKD), diabetes, aging, inflammation, and the presence of multiple other toxins, these VSMCs can dedifferentiate or transform to chondrocyte/osteoblast–like cells by upregulation of transcription factors such as runt-related transcription factor 2 (RUNX-2) and homeobox protein MSX2. These transcription factors are critical for normal bone development, and thus their upregulation in VSMCs is indicative of a phenotypic switch. These osteocyte/chondrocyte–like VSMCs then become calcified in a process similar to bone formation. The cells lay down collagen and noncollagenous proteins in the intima or media *and* incorporate calcium (Ca) and phosphorus (Pi) into matrix vesicles to initiate mineralization and further grow the mineral into hydroxyapatite. The overall positive calcium and phosphorus balance of most patients undergoing dialysis feeds both the cellular transformation and the generation of matrix vesicles (MVs). In addition, the extremes of bone turnover in CKD (low and high turnover or adynamic and hyperparathyroid bone, respectively) increases the available calcium and phosphorus by altering the bone content of these minerals. Ultimately, whether an artery calcifies or not depends on the strength of the army of inhibitors (Is) standing by in the circulation (fetuin-A) and in the arteries—for example, pyrophosphate (PPI), matrix gla protein (MGP), and osteopontin (OP). (Reprinted with permission from Moe SM, Chen NX: Mechanisms of vascular calcification in chronic kidney disease. *J Am Soc Nephrol.* 19:213-216, 2008.)

animals given high PTH + low Pi did not demonstrate arterial calcification,[116] suggesting that Pi is needed to provide the substrate for calcification to progress.

There is also a relationship of bone and arterial calcification. In animal models of excessive bone resorption, treatments aimed at decreasing bone remodeling by inhibition of osteoclast activity (i.e., bisphosphonates, calcimimetics) have been found helpful in preventing vascular calcification in some[117-119] but not all studies.[120] Correction of low-turnover bone disease also appears to improve arterial calcification in animals.[121,122] The role of vitamin D has been controversial, but data now suggest that it is only when the circulating levels of calcitriol are increased (and thus induce hypercalcemia or hyperphosphatemia) that calcification is observed.[123] Treatment studies in humans are reviewed in Chapter 63.

MATRIX VESICLES AND APOPTOSIS

In chondrocytes and osteoblasts, normal mineralization is believed to be initiated when matrix vesicles are released into the extracellular space from the cell surface via polarized budding with subsequent attachment to extracellular matrix proteins. Matrix vesicles are characterized by both their appearance as small (50-200 nm), electron-dense spherical particles on electron microscopy and the biochemical presence of calcium and Pi, alkaline phosphatase, and the membrane protein annexins. Matrix vesicles have been identified in nearly all forms of mineralization/calcification in human tissues, including bone, cartilage, tendon, calciphylaxis, and atherosclerosis. Cultured VSMCs incubated with elevated concentrations of calcium and Pi release matrix vesicles into the media, and the presence of fetuin-A (AHSG or α-2-Heremans-Schmid glycoprotein), the circulating inhibitor of mineralization (see later), decreases calcium uptake of the matrix vesicles.[124] Collagenase digestion of VSMCs has been found to lead to two populations of matrix vesicles, a secreted form in the media that had high fetuin-A and low annexin II content and could not mineralize type I collagen, and cellular matrix vesicles

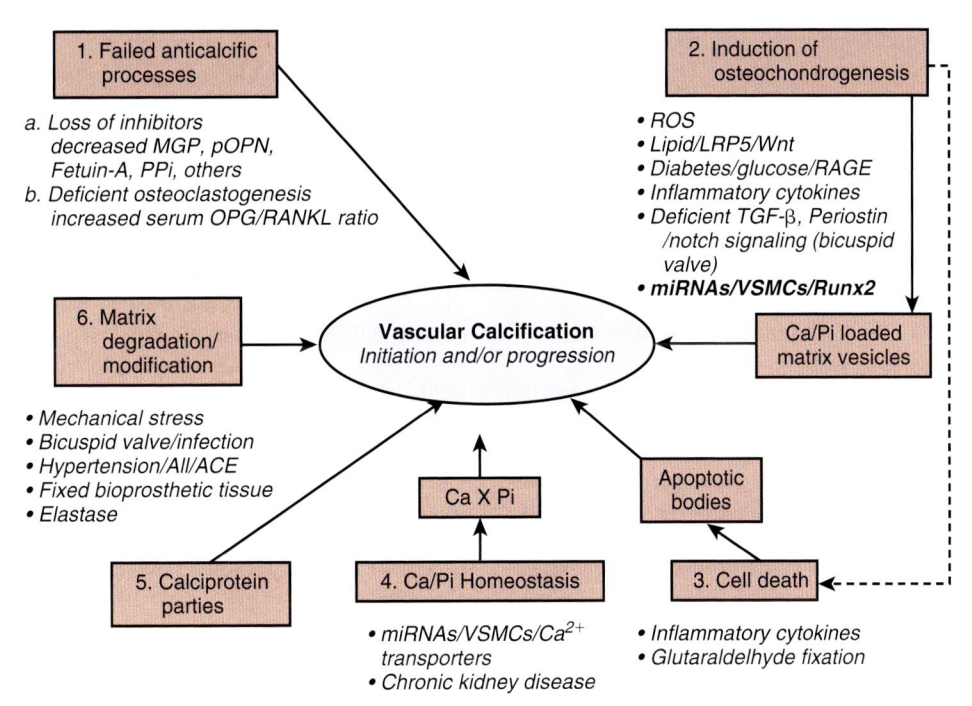

Figure 55.12 Factors that regulate pathways involved in the pathogenesis of vascular calcification. Multiple factors regulate each step of extraskeletal calcification. ACE, Angiotensin-converting enzyme; AII, Angiotensin II; Ca, calcium; LRP5, low-density lipoprotein (LDL) receptor–related protein 5; MGP, matrix gamma-carboxyglutamate (Gla) protein; miRNA, microRNA; OPG, osteoprotegerin; Pi, phosphate; PPi, pyrophosphate; RAGE, advanced glycosylation end product receptor; RANKL, receptor activator of nuclear factor kappaB ligand; ROS, reactive oxygen species; Runx2, runt-related transcription factor 2; TGF-β, transforming growth factor β; VSMCs, vascular smooth muscle cells; Wnt, wingless-type MMTV integration site family member. (Reprinted with permission from Wu M, Rementer C, Giachelli CM: Vascular calcification: an update on mechanisms and challenges in treatment. *Calcif Tissue Int.* 93:365-373, 2013.)

that had low fetuin-A and high annexin II content and could mineralize.[125] Matrix vesicles are similar to exosomes, which are known to transfer microRNAs from cell to cell and thus may play a role in calcification.[126] MicroRNAs have been found to regulate the phenotypic switch from contractile to synthetic VSMCs[127] and are involved in the regulation of arterial calcification in vitro in animal models.[126,128] These results suggest that the cellular regulation of the content of matrix vesicles may regulate the type and mineralizing capacity of the vesicle.

In addition to matrix vesicles, apoptotic bodies can induce calcification in vitro in VSMCs. Apoptotic bodies stimulated by calcium-Pi crystals of approximately 1 μm or less in diameter cause a rapid rise in intracellular calcium concentration and apoptosis, an effect triggered by lysosomal degradation.[129] Apoptosis has been identified in arterial segments with calcification obtained from children with ESKD.[105] Activation of the DNA damage response by prelamin A accelerates arterial calcification.[130] Autophagy, a regulated process of cell survival, counteracts Pi-induced calcification by reducing matrix vesicle release.[131] In contrast, atorvastatin protects against calcification by inducing autophagy via suppression of the β-catenin pathway.[132] Thus, cells appear to guard against calcification when able via a number of pathways.

INHIBITORS OF VASCULAR CALCIFICATION

Vascular calcification, although prevalent in patients with CKD and particularly in patients undergoing dialysis, is not uniform. Approximately 20% (depending on the published series) of patients undergoing dialysis have no vascular calcification and continue to have no calcification on follow-up despite risk factors similar to those in patients who do have calcification. These data support the concept of calcification inhibitors. Knockout animal models have demonstrated that selective deletion of many genes leads to vascular calcification.[133] These studies imply that mineralization (or calcification) of arteries will occur, at least in some species or individuals, unless inhibited. This concept, that the regulation of calcification in blood vessels occurs principally via inhibition rather than promotion, may also be true in bone.[134] Inhibitors can be circulating or locally produced and site specific. Three inhibitors that have been well characterized in the arterial calcification of CKD are fetuin-A, matrix gamma-carboxyglutamate (Gla) protein (MGP), and OPG.

Many other inhibitors of calcification exist. In aggregate, the data discussed in this section support the diversity and abundance of naturally occurring inhibitors of calcification. Thus, vascular calcification in CKD represents a state of increased procalcific factors and decreased calcification inhibitors.

Fetuin-A

Fetuin-A is a circulating inhibitor of calcification that is abundant in the plasma and mainly produced by the liver in adults. The transcription and synthesis of fetuin-A are downregulated during inflammation and thus it is also a reverse acute phase reactant, like serum albumin and other hepatic proteins. Fetuin-A binds to both calcium and Pi in the serum, forming small "calciparticles" that are removed through the reticuloendothelial system. Fetuin-A inhibits the de novo formation and precipitation of the apatite precursor mineral basic calcium-Pi but does not dissolve it once the basic calcium-Pi is formed.[135] Therefore, fetuin-A could be viewed as acting as a host defense to clean the blood of unwanted calcium and Pi and to prevent undesirable calcification in the circulation without causing bone demineralization. Fetuin-A has been found in matrix vesicles from VSMCs, and its presence renders the vesicles incapable of mineralization.[125,136] Fetuin-A is abundant in serum and is a major factor in the calcification propensity of serum,[137] a measure of which has been shown to reflect overall mortality in patients with CKD.[138]

Targeted disruption of fetuin-A leads to diffuse and profound soft tissue calcification and to arteriole calcification of muscle, kidney, and lung but not large arteries.[139] When Ahsg$^{-/-}$ mice were crossed with ApoE$^{-/-}$ mice, the latter known to have increased cholesterol and atherosclerosis, both aorta and coronary artery calcification developed in the double-deficient Ahsg$^{-/-}$/ApoE$^{-/-}$ mice with high-Pi diet alone and was further increased by CKD.[140] Thus, extensive and multisite arterial calcification in this animal model required genetic predisposition to atherosclerosis (Apo E$^{-/-}$), a genetic defect in an inhibitor of mineralization (Ahsg$^{-/-}$), and hyperphosphatemia that was further accelerated by CKD. These data support the redundancy of the inhibitor system, in which multiple local regulators compensate for the absence of the circulating inhibitor fetuin-A. In patients with ESKD low fetuin-A levels are associated with mortality.[141,142] Serum levels of fetuin-A in individual patients undergoing dialysis were found to be inversely correlated with coronary artery calcification assessed by spiral computed tomography (CT),[143] with carotid artery plaques,[144] and, in children undergoing dialysis, arterial stiffness.[105] Fetuin-A deficiency in CKD is likely due to chronic inflammation. However, gene polymorphisms may also play a role. It is also possible that there is inappropriate upregulation, leading to a relative deficiency of fetuin-A in the setting of elevated calcium and Pi.

MATRIX GAMMA-CARBOXYGLUTAMATE (Gla) PROTEIN

MGP is a vitamin K–dependent protein expressed in a number of tissues but highly expressed in arteries and bone, where it acts predominantly as a local regulator of vascular calcification. MGP knockout mice have excessive cartilage and growth plate mineralization and arterial medial calcification, resulting in early mortality.[145] In MGP-deficient mice, calcification depends on elastin fragmentation due to increased elastase production.[146] Warfarin use and/or nutritional vitamin K deficiency results in undercarboxylation of MGP and impaired function.[147] Warfarin use is also a known risk factor for calciphylaxis and can induce calcification in an animal model of CKD.[148] The administration of vitamin K can prevent calcification, although definitive trials are underway in CKD.[147] Serum levels of carboxylated MGP were found to be nearly undetectable in patients undergoing dialysis and in patients with atherosclerotic disease.[147] Furthermore, lower levels of carboxylated MGP were associated with increased coronary artery calcification, arterial stiffness, and high serum Pi in patients undergoing dialysis.[149] Progression of coronary calcification was greater in individuals taking warfarin.[150] Supplementation of vitamin K$_2$ in patients undergoing dialysis can restore carboxylated MGP levels,[151] and studies to determine whether such supplementation improves calcification and cardiovascular events are under way.[147]

Pyrophosphate

Another naturally occurring inhibitor of mineralization is pyrophosphate, which inhibits the formation of calcium-Pi crystals in vitro. Pyrophosphate is produced by vascular smooth muscle cells and inhibits arterial calcification. Pyrophosphate is inhibited by tissue-nonspecific alkaline phosphatase (TNAP), and TNAP activity is increased in calcified arteries from uremic animals[152] and patients with stage 5 CKD.[105] Pyrophosphate is also inhibited by another enzyme, ectonucleotide pyrophosphate/phosphodiesterase I (NPPI). Children deficient in NPPI have infantile arterial calcification.[153] Circulating levels of pyrophosphate are decreased in patients undergoing dialysis[154] and are negatively associated with arterial calcification in patients with CKD.[155] The intraperitoneal administration of pyrophosphate reduced vascular calcification in a rodent model of CKD.[156]

Osteoprotegerin

Osteopenia and arterial calcification develop in mice null for OPG, implying that OPG is an important direct inhibitor of vascular calcification, but it was not clear whether this development was due to abnormalities in bone[157] or a direct arterial effect. Studies in the low-density lipoprotein receptor null mice, a model of atherogenesis, demonstrated that the administration of OPG did not prevent atherosclerotic lesions but did prevent calcification of those lesions.[158] Both bone marrow and vessel wall OPG reduces atherosclerosis and calcification,[159] via regulation of the procalcific effects of RANKL on VSMCs.[160] Such procalcific effects appear related to inflammation[161] and may explain mechanisms of calcification in areas of macrophage-laden atherosclerotic plaques.

INTEGRATED REGULATION OF PHOSPHORUS AND CALCIUM

The four hormones PTH, FGF-23, 1,25(OH)$_2$D, and Klotho work together to maintain normal Pi and calcium homeostasis to achieve appropriate balance in the blood and urine of these ions so as to avoid extraskeletal calcification and ensure adequate availability of these ions for bone that is growing (modeling) or remodeling. A summary of the integrated physiologic response to hyperphosphatemia is depicted in Figure 55.13. This response is a very complex system of multiple integrated feedback loops and is easier to understand if broken into loops that regulate 1,25(OH)$_2$D, Pi, and calcium.

PTH–FGF-23–1,25(OH)2D Loop

PTH and FGF-23 have similar effects in stimulating Pi excretion. However, these hormones differ in their effects on the vitamin D axis. PTH stimulates CYP27B1 activity, thus increasing the production of 1,25(OH)$_2$D, which in turn negatively feeds back on the parathyroid gland to decrease PTH secretion. In contrast, FGF-23 inhibits CYP27B1 and stimulates CYP24, thereby decreasing the production of

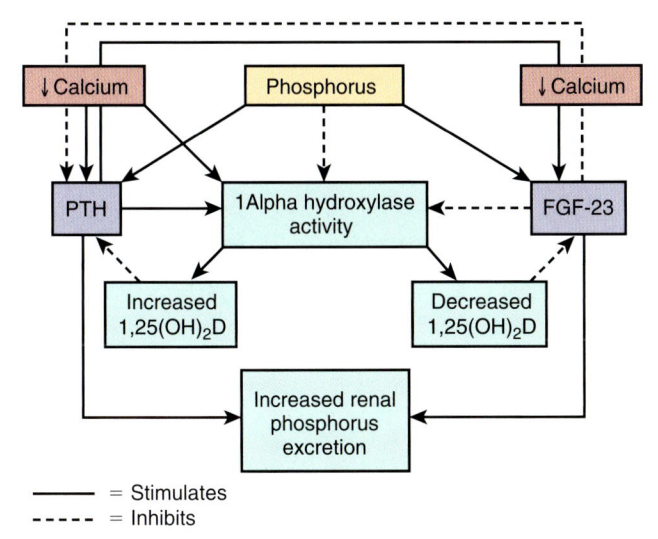

Figure 55.13 Regulation of serum phosphorus levels. As phosphorus levels increase (or there is a long-term phosphorus load), levels of both parathyroid hormone (PTH) and fibroblast growth factor 23 (FGF-23) are increased. Both of these elevations in turn increase urinary Pi excretion. The two hormones differ in respect to their effects on the vitamin D axis. PTH stimulates 1α-hydroxylase activity, thereby increasing the production of 1,25(OH)$_2$D, which in turn negatively feeds back on the parathyroid gland to decrease PTH secretion. In contrast, FGF-23 inhibits 1α-hydroxylase activity, thereby decreasing the production of 1,25(OH)$_2$D, thereby feeding back to stimulate further secretion of FGF-23. FGF-23 and PTH also regulate each other. Finally, low calcium levels stimulate PTH, whereas high calcium levels stimulate FGF-23. Lastly, there is some evidence that FGF-23 also inhibits PTH secretion.

1,25(OH)$_2$D and feeding back to limit further secretion of FGF-23—as normally 1,25(OH)$_2$D stimulates FGF-23 production.

Pi–PTH–FGF-23 Loop

As Pi levels increase (or more likely there is a long-term Pi load), both PTH and FGF-23 are increased, the latter from bone. Both the elevated PTH and FGF-23 increase urinary Pi excretion through downregulation of NaPi transporters. The effect of FGF-23 in the kidney is klotho dependent. PTH increases renal calcium reabsorption, minimizing the possibility of high calcium and Pi concentrations in urine at a time when there is a desire to increase Pi urinary excretion. PTH stimulates the secretion of FGF-23 from osteocytes, and increased FGF-23 inhibits PTH by decreasing both *PTH* gene expression and PTH secretion.[162,163]

Calcium–PTH–FGF-23 Loop

Hypocalcemia, a potent stimulator of PTH, blunts FGF-23 release.[164] The latter would therefore "remove" both the FGF-23 inhibition of PTH and the FGF-23 inhibition of 1,25(OH)$_2$D synthesis during times of hypocalcemia. This process would maximize both the PTH effects to increase renal calcium reabsorption, increase bone resorption, and enhance 1,25(OH)$_2$D stimulation of intestinal calcium absorption with the goal of normalizing calcium levels. High calcium has opposing effects: It stimulates FGF-23[165] (which reduces PTH and 1,25[OH]$_2$D synthesis) and directly inhibits 1,25(OH)$_2$D synthesis and PTH secretion. The result is decreased intestinal calcium absorption, renal reabsorption, and bone resorption.

DIAGNOSIS OF CKD-MBD

MEASUREMENT OF THE BIOCHEMICAL ABNORMALITIES IN CKD-MBD

The measurement of calcium and Pi were discussed earlier in this chapter. Table 55.3 summarizes currently measured biomarkers used for the diagnosis and management of CKD-MBD.

PARATHYROID HORMONE

PTH concentration in plasma or serum serves not only as an indicator of abnormal mineral metabolism in CKD-MBD but also as a noninvasive biochemical sign for the initial diagnosis of renal osteodystrophy, the bone component of CKD-MBD. PTH measurement also can be a useful index for monitoring the evolution of renal osteodystrophy and can serve as a surrogate measure of bone turnover in patients with CKD. Although the sensitivity and specificity of PTH as a marker of bone remodeling are not ideal, it is the best marker available at the current time.[166] However, the definitive method for establishing the specific type of renal osteodystrophy in individual patients requires bone biopsy, an invasive diagnostic procedure, and access to specialized laboratory personnel and equipment capable of providing assessments of bone histology as described later.

PTH circulates not only in the form of the intact 84–amino-acid peptide but also as multiple fragments of the hormone, particularly from the middle and C-terminal regions of the PTH molecule. These PTH fragments arise from direct secretion from the parathyroid gland as well as from metabolism of PTH(1-84) by peripheral organs, especially liver and kidney. The biologically active hormone produced (PTH[1-84]) exerts its effects through the interaction of its first 34 amino acids with PTHR1. PTH(1-84) has a plasma half-life of 2 to 4 minutes. In comparison, the half-life of C-terminal fragments, which are cleared principally by the kidney, is five to ten times longer with normal kidney function and even longer in the presence of CKD. There is also a diurnal variation in the secretion of PTH and the release is oscillatory, further complicating measurement.

The assays for PTH have undergone a number of improvements over the years (Figure 55.14). In the early 1960s radioimmunoassays were developed for measurement of PTH. However, these assays proved not to be reliable owing to different characteristics of the antisera used and are referred to as "first-generation" assays; consequently, two-site immunometric assays (IMAs) are referred to as "second- and third-generation" assays. The typical second-generation IMAs (known as intact PTH assays) measure PTH(1-84) and other large C-terminal PTH fragments because the antibodies do not bind to amino acid 1. These assays are most commonly used in clinical practice. In contrast, third-generation assays (bioactive, whole, or biointact PTH assays) use capture antibody similar to that of the intact PTH assays but also use detection antibodies directed against epitopes at the extreme N-terminal end (epitopes 1-4) of the molecule, and therefore are believed to detect exclusively the biologically

Table 55.3 Biomarkers for Chronic Kidney Disease–Mineral Bone Disease (CKD-MBD)*

	Affected by Sample Processing	Assay Validity	Renally Excreted	Diurnal Variation	Seasonal Variation	Variation with Meals	Variation with Dialysis Time
Parathyroid hormone	Yes	No; some assays pick up fragments	No	Yes	No	No	Yes
25(OH)D (calcidiol)	No	Good (uncertain importance of differentiating D_2 from D_3)	No	No	Yes	No	No
1,25(OH)$_2$D (calcitriol)	No	Good	No	Yes	No	No	?
Fibroblast growth factor 23	No	Intact vs. C-terminal	No	?	?	Yes	No
Soluble α-klotho	?	Uncertain	Yes	?	?	?	?
Sclerostin	?	Uncertain, likely valid	No	?	?	?	?
Bone alkaline phosphatase (BALP)	No	Good	No	No	No	?	No

Assay validity indicates that the measurement is of the biologically active hormone or marker, not fragments.
? indicates insufficient data.

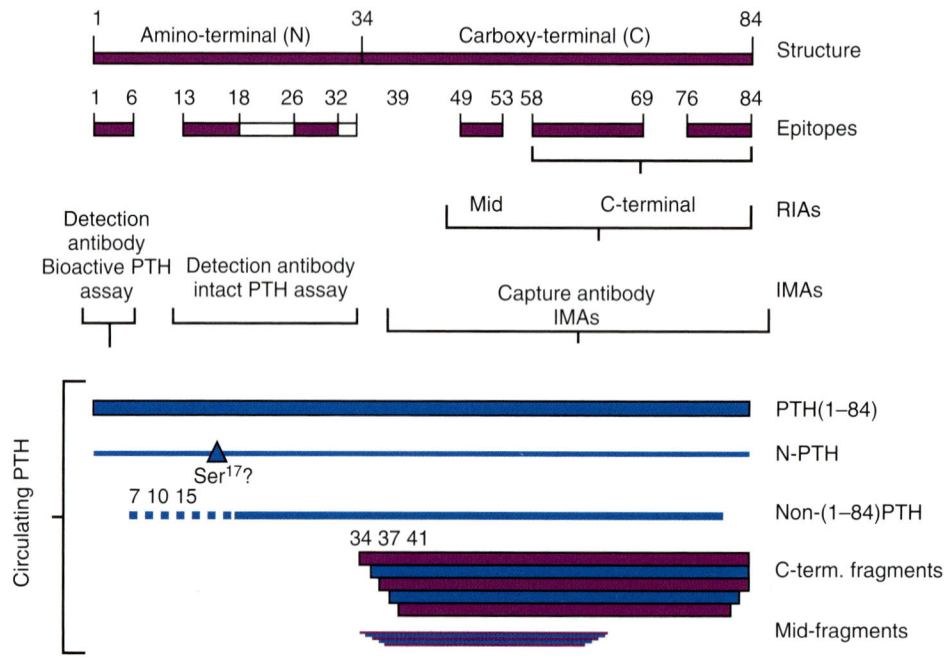

Figure 55.14 **PTH assays.** Schematic presentation of PTH(1-84) and the relationship between parathyroid hormone (PTH) assays, PTH assay epitopes, and PTH molecular forms detected in the circulation. The **upper panel** depicts the structure of human PTH and the epitopes detected by various PTH assays. First-generation PTH assays detect full-length PTH (1-84) in addition to PTH fragments. These assays include radioimmunoassays (RIAs) that use antisera specific to the amino-terminal (N-RIA), middle (MID-RIA), or carboxyl-terminal (C-RIA) regions of PTH. Second-generation "intact PTH" assays detect full-length PTH (1-84) and non(1-84)–PTH fragments. Third-generation PTH assays (biointact PTH) detect only full-length PTH (1-84). The **bottom panel** depicts PTH molecular forms present in the circulation. IMA, Immunometric assay; N-PTH, amino-terminal PTH; term., terminal. (From Henrich LM, Rogol AD, et al: Persistent hypercalcemia after parathyroidectomy in an adolescent and effect of treatment with cinacalcet HCl. *Clin Chem.* 52:2286-2293, 2006.)

active PTH(1-84) (see Figure 55.14). This difference may be important because C-terminal fragments (lacking small or large portions of the N terminus) are most abundant, representing approximately 80% of circulating PTH in healthy individuals and 95% in patients with CKD.[167] This finding may in part explain why PTH levels are "normal" in CKD yet are increased in comparison with values in patients without CKD. The second-generation intact assays are commonly used on automated platforms. Although each assay has a reasonable coefficient of variation, the standards for

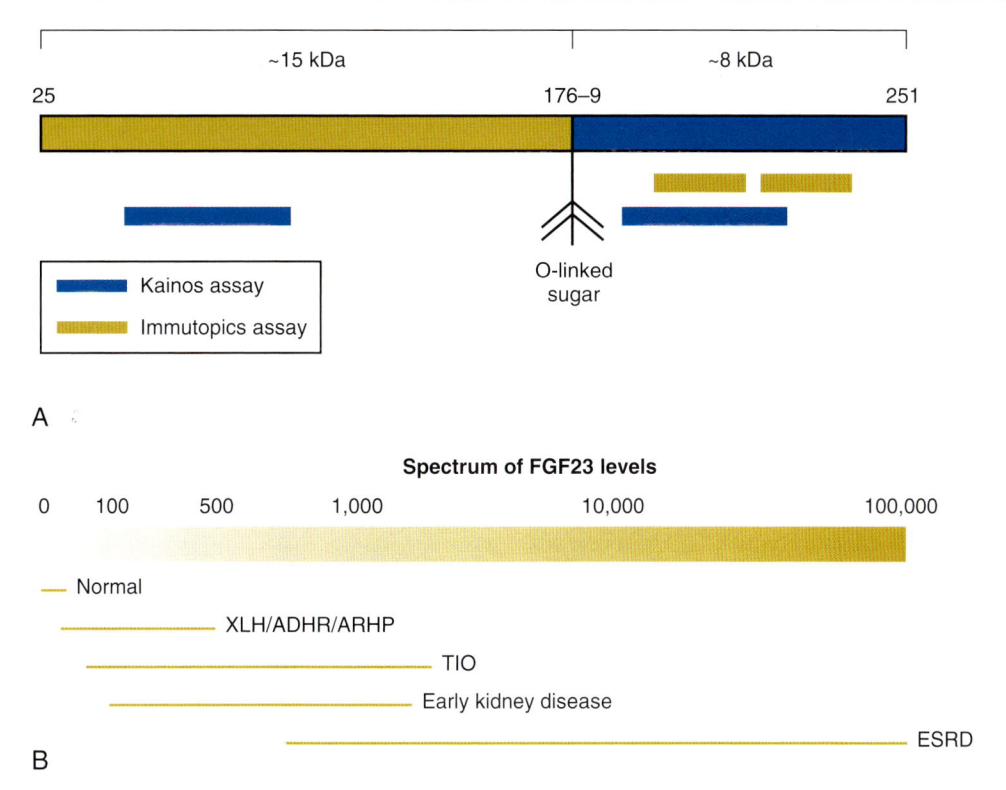

Figure 55.15 FGF-23 assays. A, Fibroblast growth factor 23 (FGF-23) O-glycosylation site and epitopes recognized by antibodies used in current assays. **B,** Spectrum of serum FGF-23 levels in early chronic kidney disease and end-stage kidney disease (ESRD) compared with the normal reference range and levels associated with different disorders affecting FGF-23. ADHR, Autosomal dominant hypophosphatemic rickets; ARHP, autosomal recessive hypophosphatemia; TIO, tumor-induced osteomalacia; XLH, X-linked hypophosphatemia. (Reprinted with permission from Block GA, Ix JH, Ketteler M, et al: Phosphate homeostasis in CKD: report of a scientific symposium sponsored by the National Kidney Foundation. *Am J Kidney Dis.* 62:457-473, 2013.)

the commercially available assays are not uniform and the detection antibodies do not all bind at the same sites. Thus, the kit-to-kit variability can be high.[168] This is the reason the Kidney Disease: Improving Global Outcomes (KDIGO) guidelines recommended using the same assay every time and evaluating trends rather than targeting precise levels.[169]

VITAMIN D

Calcidiol levels are generally measured by immunoassays, although the gold standard for calcidiol measurement is high-performance liquid chromatography (HPLC), which is not widely available clinically. Unlike in PTH assays, the sample handling in calcidiol IMAs has little impact on results. However, vitamin D circulates as both D_2 and D_3, and some laboratory kits measure only D_2, others measure only D_3, and still others measure both (expressed as 25-hydroxyvitamin D). The rationale for distinguishing D_2 from D_3 is controversial, because it is unclear how differentiating the forms of vitamin D affects management or patient level outcomes. As with PTH, there is some assay-to-assay variability, which could affect the classification of insufficiency/deficiency or sufficient levels of calcidiol.[170] Fortunately, current initiatives are under way to standardize these assays.[171] The half-life of calcidiol is long and thus represents total body stores.

In contrast, $1,25(OH)_2D$ levels are generally measured only in the setting of hypercalcemia. The half-life is comparatively short, and the assay more expensive and difficult.

FGF-23

FGF-23 is currently measured primarily with two different assays (Figure 55.15). The first uses two antibodies directed against the C-terminal end and thus measures the intact as well as C-terminal fragments (results are reported in RU/mL). The second assay uses one antibody directed against an epitope within the N-terminal region and a second antibody directed against an epitope within the C-terminal region of the molecule, and thus detects intact molecules (results are reported in picograms per milliliter). Although these two assays appear comparable in the association with clinical events at this time, they have poor agreement because of differences in FGF-23 fragment detection, antibody specificity, and calibration. Such analytical variability does not permit direct comparison of FGF-23 measurements made with different assays, a fact that probably, at least in part, accounts for some of the inconsistencies noted among observational studies.[172] From a clinical perspective, more data are required prior to the use of FGF-23 measurements for routine clinical management.

SOLUBLE KLOTHO

It is unclear whether the circulating or soluble α-klotho levels reflect tissue level expression of klotho. Some studies have found that low circulating levels were associated with progression of CKD,[173] but other studies have failed to confirm this finding.[174] Klotho can be detected in urine,[175] suggesting its levels may be altered by residual renal function. The different assay kits give variable results.[69,176]

SCLEROSTIN

Circulating sclerostin levels are elevated in CKD[177] and rise with progressive disease. However, sclerostin does not appear to be renally excreted,[178] suggesting that the rising levels reflect underlying biology. The role of sclerostin in clinical diagnosis of CKD remains exploratory, although elevated sclerostin values are associated with arterial calcification[179] and increased osteoblast number in human bone biopsy specimens.[180]

BONE-SPECIFIC ALKALINE PHOSPHATASE

Bone specific alkaline phosphatase (BALP) is not cleared renally. BALP concentration has relatively good correlation with bone formation in CKD and may be additive to the interpretation of PTH measurements.[169] However, its concentration has limited ability as an independent measurement.[166,181]

COLLAGEN-BASED BONE BIOMARKERS

Osteoblasts secrete C- and N-terminal cleavage products of type I procollagen called secreted procollagen type IN propeptide (s-PINP) and secreted procollagen type IC propeptide (s-PICP), which are markers for bone formation. In contrast, serum C-terminal cross-linking telopeptide of type 1 collagen (s-CTX) and serum N-terminal cross-linking telopeptide of type I collagen (s-NTX) are measured as fragments of cross-links that are released when bone is resorbed. With the exception of the S-PICP, all of these markers are renally excreted, making interpretation of their measurements difficult.[182] In cross sectional analyses, higher levels are associated with increased odds of fracture.[182a]

TARTRATE-RESISTANT ACID PHOSPHATASE 5b

Tartrate-resistant acid phosphatase 5b (TRAP5b) is released by osteoclasts during bone resorption and thus may be a good marker of bone resorption.[183] However, studies relating this biomarker to bone in patients with CKD-MBD are limited.[182]

BONE BIOPSY ASSESSMENT OF BONE IN CKD-MBD

Abnormalities of bone quality and quantity are common in CKD-MBD (Figure 55.16), leading to fractures and impaired growth in children. *Renal osteodystrophy* is defined as an alteration of bone morphology in patients with CKD that is quantifiable by bone histomorphometry.[1]

HISTOMORPHOMETRY IN PATIENTS WITH CKD

The clinical assessment of bone remodeling is best performed with a bone biopsy of the trabecular bone, usually at the iliac crest. The patient is given a tetracycline derivative approximately 3 to 4 weeks prior to the bone biopsy and a different tetracycline derivative 3 to 5 days prior. Tetracycline binds to hydroxyapatite and emits fluorescence, thereby serving as a label for the bone. A core of predominantly trabecular bone is collected and embedded in a plastic material, and then sectioned. The sections can be visualized with special stains under fluorescent microscopy

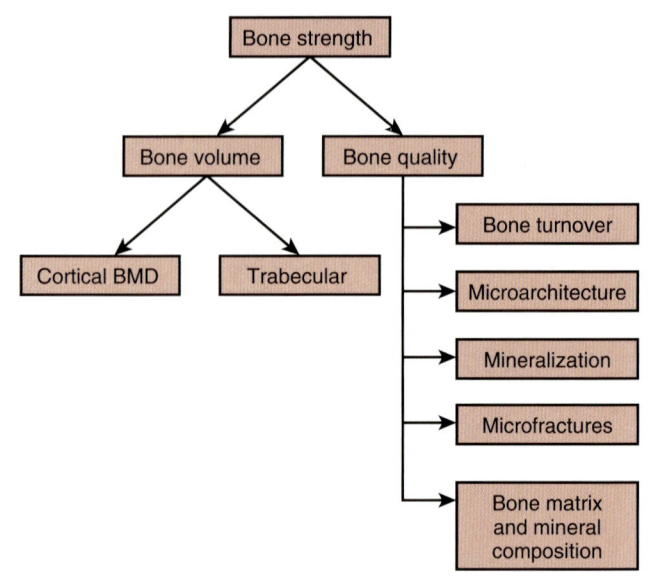

Figure 55.16 Determinants of bone strength. Bone strength comprises both bone density and bone quality. *Bone quality* refers to bone turnover, microarchitecture, microfractures, and mineralization as well as the composition of the mineral matrix. *Trabecular microarchitecture* involves trabecular thickness, the ratio of plates and rods, and their connectivity and spacing. *Cortical microarchitecture* consists of cortical thickness, porosity, and bone size. Composition of the mineral matrix includes changes in the cross-linking of type I collagen and alterations in the size and structure of bone mineral. Bones accumulate microfractures over time even with normal physical activity. The ability to repair them affects bone quality. BMD, Bone mineral density. (Reprinted with permission from Moorthi R, Moe S: Recent advances in the noninvasive diagnosis of renal osteodystrophy. *Kidney Int.* 84:866-894, 2013.)

to determine the amount of bone between administrations of the two tetracycline labels, or that formed in the interval. This dynamic parameter assessed with bone biopsy is the basis for evaluating bone turnover, which is key in discerning types of renal osteodystrophy. In addition to dynamic indices, bone biopsies can be analyzed by quantitative histomorphometry for static parameters as well. The nomenclature for these assessments has been standardized.[184]

Clinically, bone biopsies are most useful for differentiating bone turnover as well as bone volume and mineralization. However, with the advent of several new markers of bone turnover, the use of bone biopsy has been reserved primarily for the diagnosis of renal osteodystrophy and for research purposes. Sherrard and colleagues proposed a classification system for renal osteodystrophy that utilized the parameters of osteoid (unmineralized bone) area as a percentage of total bone area and fibrosis.[185] These two static parameters, together with the dynamic bone turnover assessed by bone formation rate or activation frequency, have been used to distinguish the various forms of renal osteodystrophy over the past 30 years[185]; however, this evaluation has been replaced by the KDIGO TMV system (see later).[1]

Figure 55.17 illustrates bone histology utilizing the original classification scheme. Normal bone is illustrated in Figure 55.17A. The histologic features of high-turnover disease (predominant hyperparathyroidism or osteitis fibrosa cystica) are characterized by increased rate of bone formation, increased bone resorption, extensive osteoclastic and osteoblastic activity, and progressive increase in endosteal peritrabecular fibrosis (Figure 55.17B). High osteoblast activity is manifested by an increase in unmineralized bone matrix. The number of osteoclasts is also increased as well as the total resorption surface. There may be numerous dissecting cavities through which the osteoclasts tunnel into individual trabeculae. In osteitis fibrosa cystica, the alignment of strands of collagen in the bone matrix has an irregular woven pattern, unlike the normal lamellar (parallel) alignment of strands of collagen in normal bone. Although woven bone may appear to be thicker, the disorganized collagen structure may render the bone physically more vulnerable to stress.

The histologic features of low-turnover (adynamic) bone disease (Figure 55.17C) is characterized histologically by absence of cellular (osteoblast and osteoclast) activity, osteoid formation, and endosteal fibrosis. It appears to be essentially a disorder of decreased bone formation accompanied by a secondary decrease in bone mineralization. Although low-turnover disease is common in the absence of aluminum, it was initially described as a result of aluminum toxicity. Aluminum bone disease is diagnosed with special staining that demonstrates the presence of aluminum deposits at the mineralization front (Figure 55.17D). Frequently, aluminum disease is associated with osteomalacia. Osteomalacia is characterized by an excess of unmineralized osteoid, which manifests as wide osteoid seams and a markedly decreased mineralization rate (Figure 55.17E). The presence of increased unmineralized osteoid per se does not necessarily indicate a mineralizing defect, because greater quantities of osteoid appear in conditions associated with high rates of bone formation when mineralization lags behind the increased synthesis of matrix. Other features of osteomalacia are the absence of cellular activity and the absence of endosteal fibrosis.

Mixed uremic osteodystrophy is the term that has been used to describe bone biopsies that have features of secondary hyperparathyroidism together with evidence of a mineralization defect (Figure 55.17F). There is extensive osteoclastic and osteoblastic activity and increased endosteal peritrabecular fibrosis coupled with more osteoid than expected, and tetracycline labeling uncovers a concomitant mineralization defect. Unfortunately, mixed uremic osteodystrophy, in particular, as well as high- and low-turnover bone diseases, have been inconsistent and poorly defined.

THE SPECTRUM OF BONE HISTOMORPHOMETRY IN CKD

The prevalence of different forms of renal osteodystrophy has changed over the past decade. Whereas osteitis fibrosa cystica due to severe hyperparathyroidism had previously been the predominant lesion, the prevalence of mixed uremic osteodystrophy and adynamic bone disease has increased. However, the overall percentage of patients with high bone formation compared to low bone formation has not changed dramatically over the last 20 to 30 years, although osteomalacia has been essentially "replaced" by adynamic bone disease. There are differences in prevalence of mixed uremic osteodystrophy in patients not yet undergoing dialysis, which appears to depend on the level of GFR and the country in which the study was performed.[186] Two large analyses of patients undergoing long-term dialysis revealed a relatively high incidence of low bone turnover; one study of 489 biopsy specimens in predominantly Caucasian subjects revealed low turnover in 59%,[166] whereas in another study of 630 patients, low turnover disease was noted in 62% of Caucasian but only 32% of African American subjects.[187] The prevalence of mineralization defect or osteomalacia was relatively low at only 3%.[187] Thus, these data demonstrate that histologic abnormalities of bone begin very early in the course of CKD and that differences in bone turnover may be based on racial differences.

In contrast, low-turnover bone disease has diverse pathophysiology. In the 1980s, aluminum-induced osteomalacia was common. The potential toxicity of aluminum was initially recognized by Alfrey, who identified a fatal neurologic syndrome in dialysis patients consisting of dyspraxia, seizures, and electroencephalographic abnormalities in association with high brain aluminum levels on autopsy.[188] The source of aluminum in these severe cases was believed to be elevated concentrations in dialysate water. Subsequently, aluminum-containing phosphate binders were also identified as a source. The additional symptoms of fractures, myopathy, and microcytic anemia were described several years after the initial reports of the neurologic syndrome.[188,189] Fortunately, exposure to aluminum is greatly limited, and the incidence of aluminum bone disease is relatively rare. However, the diagnosis of aluminum-induced bone disease can be difficult, because aluminum toxicity is due to tissue burden, not serum levels. Thus, if aluminum bone disease is suspected, bone biopsy remains the gold standard for making the diagnosis.[190,191]

In adynamic bone disease, there is a paucity of cells with resultant low bone turnover (Figure 55.17C). Unlike in osteomalacia, in adynamic bone there is no increase in osteoid or unmineralized bone. The lack of bone cell activity led to the initial description of the disease as "aplastic" bone disease. Early investigators believed that the disease was due to aluminum, but it was later identified in the absence of aluminum. The etiology of adynamic bone disease is likely multifactorial, and major contributory factors include diabetes, aging, and malnutrition.[192]

Proposed pathophysiologic mechanisms of low bone turnover are listed in Table 55.4. Increases in both sclerostin and Dickkopf-1 (dkk-1), which are soluble inhibitors of wnt signaling that inhibit osteoblastic bone formation, likely play a role in development of adynamic bone disease.[95,193,194] Circulating fragments of PTH (7-84 amino acid fragments) may also be antagonists to PTH,[195] resulting in an effective resistance to 1-84 amino acid at the level of bone. There is evidence that markedly elevated concentrations of FGF-23 may be associated with decreased osteoblastic activity.[196] Also, abnormal regulation of cell differentiation in the presence of renal failure may explain, in part, the relative paucity of cells in adynamic bone, although this possibility remains to be proven. In rats, the administration of bone morphogenic protein-7 (BMP-7) can restore normal cell function, supporting that a failure of normal cell differentiation, likely due to a number of causes, may be critical.[197] Although most patients with low-turnover bone disease are asymptomatic, they are at increased risk of fracture owing to impaired remodeling[196,198,199] and at risk of vascular

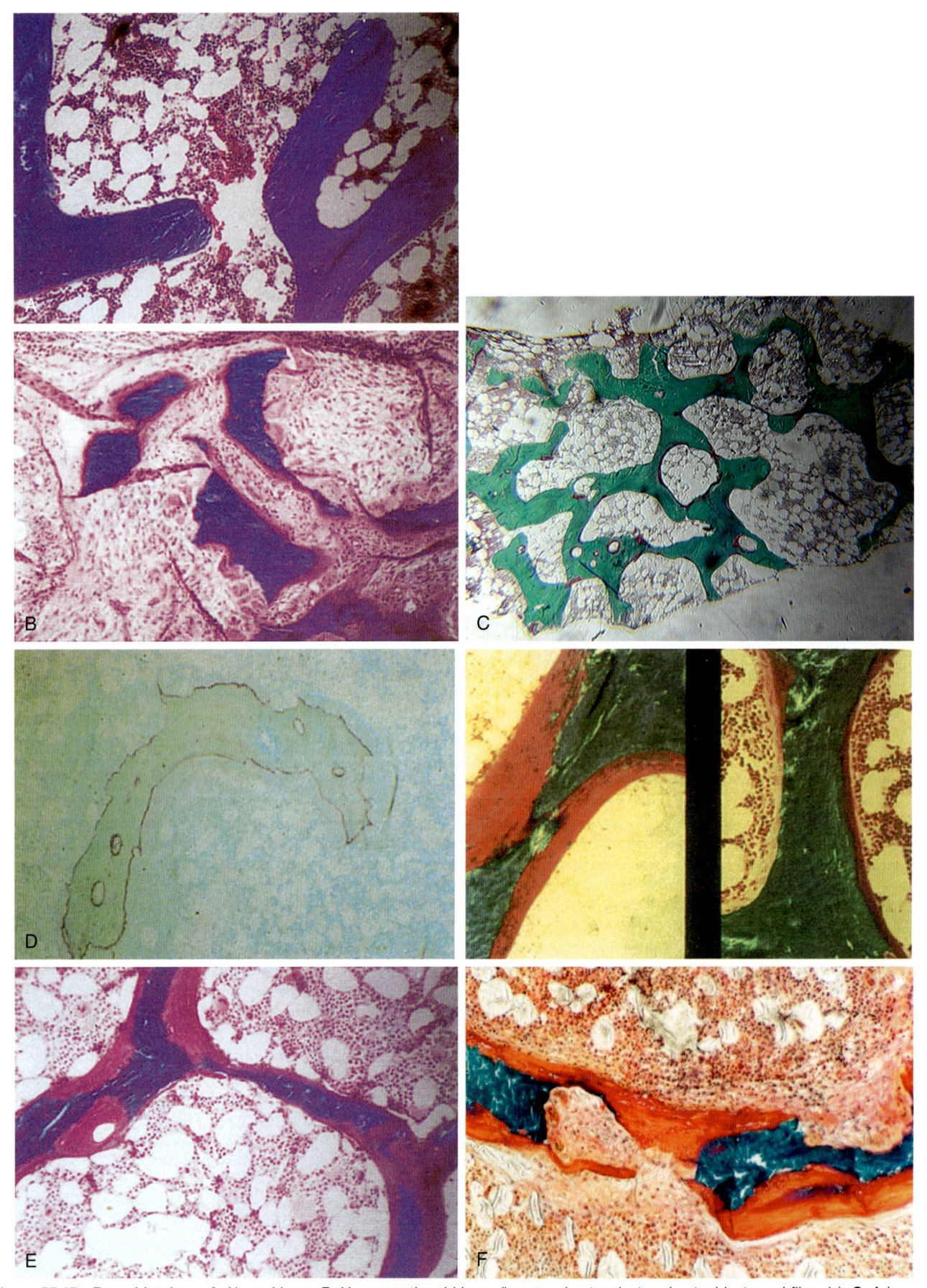

Figure 55.17 Bone histology. **A,** Normal bone. **B,** Hyperparathyroid bone (increased osteoclast and osteoblasts and fibrosis). **C,** Adynamic bone (no cellular activity and no osteoid). **D,** Aluminim bone disease (left aluminum staining at mineralization front) and right two panels show accumulation of osteoid (orange-red stain). **E,** Osteomalacia (increased unmineralized osteoid in pink/red). **F,** Mixed uremic osteodystrophy presence of increase osteoid (orange red) indicating mineralization defect, and increased osteoclast activity. (**A, B, D [right],** and **E,** Courtesy S.L. Teitelbaum, MD; **D [left],** courtesy D. J. Sherrard, MD.)

Table 55.4	Causes and Proposed Mechanisms of Decreased Bone Formation in Patients with Chronic Kidney Disease
	Mechanism of Decreased Osteoblast Activity
Low serum 1,25-vitamin D	↓Osteoblast differentiation ↓Osteoblast life span
Metabolic acidosis	↓1,25-vitamin D production ↓Collagen synthesis
High serum phosphate	↓1,25-vitamin D production
Calcium loading/hypercalcemia	↓1,25-vitamin D production and ↑1,25-vitamin D degradation (mediated by calcium-sensing receptor)
High serum interleukins 1 and 6, tumor necrosis factor	↓Osteoblast life span
Low serum insulin-like growth factor-I (IGF-I) activity	↓IGF-I and IGF binding protein 5 (IGFBP5) levels ↑Inhibitory IGFBP (2, 4, 6) levels ↓Osteoblast life span
Sclerostin	↓Wnt/β-catenin signaling ↓Osteoblastic activity
Dickkopf-1 (dkk-1)	↓Wnt/β-catenin signaling ↓Osteoblastic activity
Malnutrition, proteinuria	↓IGF-I; 25-hydroxyvitamin D levels
Diabetes	↓25-hydroxyvitamin D and 1,25-vitamin D levels ↑Advanced glycation end products (AGEs) ↓Osteoblast life span
Age-related	↑AGEs ↓Osteoblast life span
Hypogonadal	
Women (↓ estrogen and ↑ sex hormone–binding globulin (SHBG)	↓Osteoblast life span
Men (↓ testosterone and ↑SHBG)	↓Osteoblast life span
Uremic toxins (uric acid)	↓1,25-vitamin D production ↓Vitamin D receptor (VDR) activity ↓Osteoblast proliferation
Aluminum toxicity	↓Osteoblast activity

↓, Decreased; ↑, increased.

Table 55.5	TMV Classification System for Renal Osteodystrophy	
Turnover	**Mineralization**	**Volume**
Low	Normal	Low
Normal		Normal
High	Abnormal	High

From Moe S, Drüeke T, Cunningham J, et al: Definition, evaluation, and classification of renal osteodystrophy: a position statement from Kidney Disease: Improving Global Outcomes (KDIGO). Kidney Int 69:1945-1953, 2006.

calcification because of the inability of bone to buffer a sudden calcium load.[196,200,201]

TMV CLASSIFICATION

As previously mentioned, the KDIGO recommends that the definition of renal osteodystrophy be limited to describing the alterations of bone morphology in patients with CKD and is one measure of the skeletal component of the systemic disorder of CKD-MBD that can be quantifiable by histomorphometry.[1] Historically, *renal osteodystrophy* often included disorders of bone mineral metabolism in addition to histomorphometric changes in bone. As our understanding of bone biology progresses, there is greater appreciation of the diverse physiologic processes leading to similar bone biopsy findings. In addition, information on bone volume as an independent parameter is available.[202] Thus, the previous classification was updated by KDIGO to use three key histologic descriptors—bone turnover, mineralization, and volume (TMV system), with any combination of each of the descriptors possible in a given specimen (Table 55.5).[1] The TMV classification scheme provides a clinically relevant description of the underlying bone pathology as assessed by histomorphometry, which in turn helps define the pathophysiology and thereby guide therapy.

Turnover reflects the rate of skeletal remodeling, which is normally the coupled process of bone resorption and bone formation. It is assessed with histomorphometry by dynamic measurements of osteoblast function using double-tetracycline labeling, as previously described. Bone formation rate (BFR) and activation frequency (Ac.f) represent acceptable parameters for assessing bone turnover. Bone turnover is affected mainly by hormones, cytokines, mechanical stimuli, and growth factors that influence the recruitment, differentiation, and activity of osteoclasts and osteoblasts. It is important to clarify that although bone formation rate is frequently similar to bone resorption rate, which cannot be measured directly, it is not always so. Imbalance in these processes can affect bone volume. For example, if resorption exceeds formation, negative bone balance and decreased bone volume result.

Mineralization reflects how well bone collagen becomes calcified during the formation phase of skeletal remodeling. It is assessed with histomorphometry by static measurements of osteoid volume and osteoid thickness and by dynamic, tetracycline-based measurements of mineralization lag time and osteoid maturation time. Causes of impaired mineralization include inadequate vitamin D nutrition, mineral (calcium or Pi) deficiency, acidosis, and bone aluminum toxicity.

Volume indicates the amount of bone per unit volume of tissue. It is assessed with histomorphometry by static measurements of bone volume in cancellous bone. Determinants of bone volume include age, gender, race, genetic factors, nutrition, endocrine disorders, mechanical stimuli, toxicities, neurologic function, vascular supply, growth factors, and cytokines.

The KDIGO classification is consistent with the classically used classification system[185] but provides more information on parameters other than turnover. Two large-scale analyses utilizing the updated TMV system revealed that this classification system provides clinically relevant information.[166,187] Low bone volume and low bone turnover are more common than heretofore appreciated, whereas defective mineralization is relatively rare in adult patients with CKD stage 5.

Clinically, serum PTH concentration is used as a surrogate biomarker to predict bone turnover. However, as detailed earlier, studies evaluating the ability of the serum concentration of intact PTH to predict both low- and high-turnover bone diseases have been disappointing. The ability to reliably predict the presence of high-turnover bone disease is poor until intact PTH levels become greater than 500 pg/mL. Primarily on the basis of earlier studies utilizing the Allegro intact PTH assay, the K/DOQI guidelines recommend a target intact PTH level of 150 to 300 pg/mL.[189] Unfortunately, these studies that correlate intact PTH concentration with bone histology were performed with an assay no longer available. Use of the currently available assays have shown that the intact PTH value between 150 to 300 pg/mL is not predictive of underlying bone histology.[203] However, an analysis of 610 biopsy specimens found that although the intact PTH value could not predict underlying bone histology, it was able to discriminate low-turnover from non–low-turnover bone diseases and high-turnover from non–high-turnover bone diseases.[166]

NONINVASIVE ASSESSMENT OF BONE

DUAL-ENERGY X-RAY ABSORPTIOMETRY

Dual-energy x-ray absorptiometry (DXA) measures areal bone mineral density (aBMD) in g/cm^2 using minimal radiation and rapid scan times. BMD assessment by DXA has good reproducibility (<1%-2% coefficient variation) and reliable reference ranges for age, gender, and race. In the general population, aBMD measured by DXA can be used clinically to define osteoporosis and is an accepted surrogate end point after prospective studies demonstrated an age-dependent predictive value of DXA for fractures.[204] However, the discordance between changes in DXA findings and antifracture efficacies of drugs has led to appreciation of the importance of bone quality, which is not assessed by DXA. This observation has forced the use of fractures as end points for approval of new therapeutics for the treatment of osteoporosis.

The KDIGO CKD-MBD guideline recommends DXA to assess fracture risk in patients with stage 1 through early stage 3 CKD, as long as biochemical testing does not suggest CKD-MBD.[169] However, for patients with CKD stages 3b through 5, the guideline did not recommend DXA owing to the lack of definitive data demonstrating that DXA predicts fracture in CKD-MBD. A meta-analysis was performed to determine whether DXA measurements at the femoral neck, spine, and radius were associated with spine and/or non-spine fractures in patients undergoing dialysis.[205] On the basis of results of six studies with 683 subjects, lower BMD levels in the spine and distal radius, but not in the femoral neck, were associated with fractures. Although BMD levels may have been lower in patients with CKD and a history of fracture, there is considerable overlap in BMD levels such that BMD provides poor fracture discrimination in individuals. Since the publication of KDIGO guidelines, studies have demonstrated fracture prediction value of DEXA in CKD subjects at least equivalent to that in the general population.[206,207] These data therefore support that DXA can predict fracture risk in patients with CKD. DXA is an inexpensive and widely available technique that can be easily standardized among sites, so it may be a good tool in longitudinal CKD research studies for the serial assessment of BMD in response to interventions. Unfortunately, to date, treatment studies utilizing DXA as an end point in patients with CKD are limited.

QUANTITATIVE COMPUTERIZED TOMOGRAPHY TECHNIQUES

Quantitative CT (QCT) allows three-dimensional (3D) imaging of cross sections of the central and axial skeleton to provide spatial or volumetric bone mineral density (vBMD). It also allows distinction between cortical and trabecular compartments. In CKD, QCT measures of trabecular bone density at the spine have been correlated with trabecular bone volume histomorphometry.[208] Peripheral QCT (pQCT) avoids the large dose of ionizing radiation exposure for patients by focusing on the tibia and distal radius, and in one study, it was predictive of fracture.[209] Although from a single study, these results are in line with expected associations between loss of bone quality and fracture risk in patients undergoing dialysis.

High-resolution peripheral computerized tomography (HRpQCT) has greater resolution than pQCT and allows evaluation of trabecular microarchitecture (bone volume fraction, trabecular thickness, separation, and number). HRpQCT of the radius and tibia was found to be able to discriminate between patients with CKD with and without fracture.[210,211] However, the power of the various HRpQCT parameters to individually discriminate between those with and without fractures by receiver operating curve (ROC) analyses was less than 0.75. When patients with the longest duration of CKD were considered, the area under the receiver operating curve improved to more than 0.8 for multiple parameters, including radial cortical thickness, radial total vBMD, and cortical vBMD. Interestingly, aBMD by DXA of the ultra-distal radius performed similarly in its ability to discriminate prevalent fractures in this subpopulation with the longest duration of kidney disease.[212] In another study areal BMD by DXA at the ultra-distal radius was superior to HRpQCT measures for fracture discrimination.[213] Therefore, high-resolution CT techniques do provide assessment of bone architecture, but their use at this time is limited to research centers and their additive value over distal radius DXA has not yet been proven.

MICRO–COMPUTED TOMOGRAPHY AND MICRO–MAGNETIC RESONANCE IMAGING

Resolution of micro-techniques is as low as 8 mm, compared with about 100 μm for HRpQCT, thus providing spatial resolution almost that of an actual bone biopsy. Micro-CT was used to assess the effects of severe high-turnover renal osteodystrophy on trabecular and cortical architecture in growing rats. The technique demonstrated irregular trabecular thickening and loss of trabecular connectivity in the femoral neck and greater endocortical porosity in the femoral shaft, consistent with biopsy findings in high-turnover osteodystrophy.[214] Unfortunately, this technique is currently limited to in vitro studies. In an evaluation of 17 patients undergoing hemodialysis who had secondary hyperparathyroidism, micro–magnetic resonance imaging (MRI) demonstrated disruptions of the distal tibial trabecular network.[215] There have not been subsequent confirmatory studies or studies comparing this technique with other imaging methods in the ability to predict fractures in CKD.

ASSESSMENT OF VASCULAR CALCIFICATION

Arterial calcification can be detected in humans through a number of techniques. Plain radiographs can be used to assess the presence or absence, and thus prevalence, of vascular calcification. Scoring methods utilizing the number of aorta segments calcified along the lumbar spine can also allow reproducible quantification during longitudinal follow-up,[216] although the sensitivity is less than with CT-based imaging. Although some distinction can be made between medial and intimal calcification on plain radiographs,[217] the reproducibility among multiple research sites of this method for differentiation of calcification type has not been evaluated. Ultrasonography of the carotid arteries can be used to assess intimal-medial thickness, which correlates well with atherosclerosis and cardiovascular events. In a later study, intravascular ultrasonography of the coronary arteries was found to be able to detect atherosclerotic lesions and calcification. This technique, although invasive, can detect circumferential lesions, and external remodeling of atherosclerosis—lesions that invade the internal elastic artery into the medial layer rather than protrude into the vessel lumen. The latter luminal lesion is all that is detected on angiography, leading some to question the use of angiography as the "gold standard."[218] Finally, technologic advances have led to ultra-fast CT scans—electron beam CT (EBCT) and multi-slice CT (MSCT)—that use electrocardiography gating to allow imaging only in diastole, thus avoiding motion artifact of the heart. These techniques have allowed reproducible quantification of coronary artery and aorta calcification and therefore serve as excellent research end points. Unfortunately, these techniques do not allow differentiation of medial from intimal calcification, and the radiation dose with their use is large.

A study in each of 140 prevalent patients undergoing hemodialysis compared a lateral radiograph of the lumbar abdominal aorta, an echocardiogram, and measurement of pulse pressure with EBCT results.[219] Calcification of the abdominal aorta was scored as 0 through 24 divided into tertiles, echocardiograms were graded as 0 through 2 for absence or presence of calcification of the mitral and aortic valves, and pulse pressure was divided in quartiles. The researchers found that the likelihood ratio (95% confidence interval [CI]) of coronary artery calcification score on EBCT of 100 or higher was 1.79 (1.09 to 2.96) for calcification of either valve on echocardiography and 7.50 (2.89 to 19.5) for participants with a lateral abdominal radiographic score greater or equal to 7. Verbeke and colleagues confirmed this predictive value of lateral abdominal radiographs in more than 1000 dialysis recipients.[220]

On the basis of observational studies, calcification detected on all of these imaging studies is predictive of mortality in patients with CKD. Bellasi and Raggi analyzed multiple such studies and calculated the positive predictive value to be between 19% and 52% and the negative predictive value to be between 68% and 100%.[221] The addition of the clinical variables age and dialysis vintage to abdominal calcification, called the cardiovascular calcification index (CCI), was linearly associated with death, with a 12% increase in hazard ratio for each point increase in the CCI.[222]

CLINICAL CONSEQUENCES OF THE ABNORMALITIES IN CKD-MBD

BIOCHEMICAL ABNORMALITIES

PHOSPHORUS AND CALCIUM

Epidemiologic data suggest that serum Pi levels above the normal range are associated with increases in morbidity and all-cause and cardiovascular mortality in patients with CKD. These studies differ in their sample size, analyses, and chosen reference ranges, and most evaluate only patients undergoing dialysis. In patients with CKD stages 2 to 5, higher levels of serum Pi, even within the normal range, have been associated with increased risk of all-cause or cardiovascular mortality in one study[223] but not in other studies.[224,225] However, in patients undergoing dialysis, nearly all studies demonstrate an association of elevated Pi with mortality, although there are slight differences in the inflection point or range at which Pi becomes significantly associated with increased all-cause mortality. Furthermore, several studies have demonstrated that treatment of patients undergoing dialysis with Pi binders is associated with a 20% to 40% lower risk of death.[226-228] In patients with CKD stages 3 to 5, there are no data to support an increased risk of mortality or fracture with rising serum calcium concentrations. However, as with Pi, there are several studies in dialysis recipients demonstrating rising mortality with hypercalcemia and in patients with very low calcium levels.

PARATHYROID HORMONE

Although PTH has long been considered a surrogate marker for bone disease, it also has systemic effects, including effects on endothelial, cardiac, and skeletal health. As with other biochemical measures of CKD-MBD, observational studies have found an association of all-cause mortality with various levels of PTH, with inflection points ranging from more than 400 to 600 pg/mL. On the basis of these observational data and the assay limitations, the KDIGO guidelines consider levels of intact PTH less than 2 and more than 9 times the upper limit of normal for the PTH assay (<130 and >585 pg/mL for most kits with an upper normal limit of 65 pg/mL) are abnormal and that values within that range should be interpreted by evaluation of trends. Intervention should occur if the trends are consistently going up or down.[169] However, it is important to recognize that there are no randomized clinical trials demonstrating that treatment to achieve specific PTH level results in improved outcomes, with the exception of the Evaluation Of Cinacalcet Hydrochloride (HCl) Therapy to Lower CardioVascular Events (EVOLVE) trial discussed in Chapter 63.

A Cochrane meta-analysis found that Pi and calcium levels, but not PTH level, were associated with cardiovascular and all-cause mortality.[229]

COMBINATION OF ABNORMALITIES OF CALCIUM, PHOSPHORUS, AND PARATHYROID HORMONE

The relationship of calcium, Pi, and PTH with outcomes is further complicated by the clinical reality that these laboratory parameters do not move in isolation from one another, but rather change depending on the levels of other parameters and treatments. For example, Stevens and colleagues assessed various biochemical combinations and found that the relative risk for mortality was greatest when serum levels of calcium and Pi were elevated and the PTH level was low and was lowest when serum levels of calcium and Pi were normal and the PTH level was high.[230] In addition, duration of dialysis significantly impacted the results. A Dialysis Outcomes and Practice Patterns Study (DOPPS) trial also evaluated combinations of serum parameters of mineral metabolism and reached slightly different conclusions.[231] The researchers found that in the setting of an elevated serum PTH (>300 pg/mL), hypercalcemia (>10 mg/dL) was associated with increased mortality risk even with normal serum Pi levels. Block and associates, analyzing average values over 4 months from more than 26,000 patients undergoing dialysis, categorized them according to whether serum levels of calcium, Pi, and PTH were below, within, or above target ranges. In only 20% of subjects were all three variables within reference ranges. Those patients with high PTH (>300 pg/mL) and high calcium had consistently higher mortality.[232] It is important to remember that abnormalities in mineral metabolism are common. Ultimately, we need prospective randomized controlled trials that demonstrating that treatments or combinations of treatments to achieve specific biochemical end points affect mortality in patients undergoing dialysis.

FIBROBLAST GROWTH FACTOR 23

Elevations of FGF-23 (greater than 100 RU/mL) were observed in 70% and 100% of patients with estimated GFRs of 50 and less than 20 mL/min, respectively, in the Chronic Renal Insufficiency Cohort study.[71] FGF-23 levels continue to rise throughout progressive CKD, presumably to maintain normal levels of Pi and calcium. In CKD, elevations of FGF-23 are associated with death,[233] progression of CKD,[233,234] left ventricular hypertrophy,[76,235,236] and cardiovascular events,[237,238] independent of Pi and PTH levels. Once patients need dialysis, levels of FGF-23 can be 1000-fold greater, and such levels have been associated with poor survival in incident patients in some studies[239] but not in smaller studies.[240,241] In prevalent patients undergoing dialysis, FGF-23 was also associated with increases in mortality[242] and left ventricular mass index.[241] In a secondary analyses of nearly 2000 hemodialysis patients treated with cinacalcet, a reduction of FGF-23 by 30% or greater was associated with reduced cardiovascular events.[243]

NUTRITIONAL VITAMIN D DEFICIENCY

Although, traditionally the term *vitamin D* has been used to indicate the active metabolite, $1,25(OH)_2D$, the correct use of the term is for the precursor molecule, calcidiol or $25(OH)D$. In the general population, calcidiol levels are accepted as the standard measures of nutritional uptake because they correlate best with end-organ effects. The conversion of vitamin D_2 and vitamin D_3 to $25(OH)D$ by CYP27A1 is essentially unregulated, and therefore levels of $25(OH)D$ are a reliable indicator of the vitamin D status of a given individual. However, controversy exists as to what constitutes adequate stores. Although there is no absolute level of calcidiol that defines deficiency, a level less than 10 ng/mL (25 nmol/L) is typically used, because it is associated with rickets in children and osteomalacia in adults. The term *vitamin D insufficiency* has been used to describe less severe calcidiol-deficient states. Although controversial, the typical range of "insufficient" calcidiol levels is 10 to 30 ng/mL (25 to 75 nmol/L). In contrast to the severity of bone disease observed with deficiency, insufficiency is associated with elevated PTH and osteoporosis.[244] Unfortunately, despite supplementation of calciferol in various foods such as milk, calcidiol insufficiency is relatively common in the general population, particularly in some at-risk groups such as African Americans, hospitalized patients, nursing home residents, and people living in northern climates.[245] The Institute of Medicine convened a panel whose report, released in November 2010, recommended that vitamin D levels of 20 ng/mL are adequate and that the adult recommended dietary allowance is 600 IU/day, with an upper level intake of 4000 IU/day.[246] The Endocrine Society has subsequently recommended a vitamin D level higher than 30 ng/mL, further suggesting that 40 to 60 ng/mL is ideal and that up to 100 ng/mL is safe.[247] Either vitamin D_2 or vitamin D_3 can be used for vitamin D supplementation. Although there has been controversy regarding the use of D_3 or D_2 for achieving and maintaining higher serum vitamin D levels, most analyses have found them to be equally effective in raising and maintaining serum vitamin D levels in patients without CKD.[248]

The importance of vitamin D in health and disease is suggested by a number of studies, with the effects of local cellular (autocrine) conversion thought responsible for the nonendocrine effects. Vitamin D deficiency (<20 ng/mL) is likely to be an important etiologic factor in the pathogenesis of many chronic diseases, including autoimmune diseases (e.g., multiple sclerosis, type 1 diabetes), inflammatory bowel disease (e.g., Crohn's disease), infections, immune deficiency, cardiovascular diseases (e.g., hypertension, heart failure, sudden cardiac death), cancer (e.g., colon cancer, breast cancer, non-Hodgkin's lymphoma), and neurocognitive disorders (e.g., Alzheimer's disease).[247,249-254] Two relatively large cohort studies demonstrated increased mortality with low vitamin D levels. Using data from the third National Health and Nutrition Examination Survey (NHANES III), the investigators found that in comparison with subjects with vitamin D levels in the highest quartile, those with the lowest quartile (< 17.8 ng/mL) had a 26% higher rate of all-cause mortality, with a population-attributable risk percentage of 3.1%.[249] Similarly, analysis of a German cohort of about 10,000 women and men aged 50 to 74 years showed that vitamin D deficiency significantly increased general and cardiovascular mortality during a median follow-up of 9.5 years. The vitamin D levels and overall mortality demonstrated a pronounced nonlinear inverse association, with increased mortality risk beginning at vitamin D levels below 30 ng/mL. Vitamin D deficiency was also associated with significantly higher rates of death due to cancer and respiratory diseases.[254]

The results of randomized trials demonstrating efficacy of vitamin D supplementation on fractures and falls have been mixed. One of the reasons is the concomitant use of calcium in most studies, and another is the wide differences in dose of vitamin D utilized. According to the latest update of the *Cochrane Review* analysis of vitamin D and vitamin D analogs for prevention of fractures in postmenopausal women and older men, vitamin D alone is unlikely to prevent fractures in the doses and formulations tested so far. However, supplements of vitamin D and calcium may prevent hip or any type of fracture. A small but significant increase in gastrointestinal symptoms and renal disease was associated with vitamin D and calcium. The researchers found no evidence of an increased risk of death from taking calcium and vitamin D.[255]

Vitamin D deficiency (<20 ng/mL) and insufficiency (<30 ng/mL) are common in patients with CKD, only 29% and 17% of those with stage 3 and 4 disease, respectively, having sufficient levels in one study.[256] This prevalence of deficiency and insufficiency in an ambulatory CKD population is similar to that in non-CKD nursing home residents, hospitalized patients, and elderly women with hip fractures. However, the prevalences of frank deficiency (<10 mg/mL) were 14% and 26% in patients with stage 3 and 4 CKD, respectively.[256] Several other investigators have similarly found widespread vitamin D insufficiency in patients with CKD, although not all investigators have identified a relationship with CKD stage.[256-259]

Evidence from epidemiologic studies suggests that vitamin D deficiency as well as supplementation of vitamin D plays a role in survival outcomes in patients with CKD regardless of dialysis status.[260-265] A meta-analysis of prospective studies demonstrated a significant decrease, 14%, in mortality risk for every 10–ng/mL increase in vitamin D level.[266] Furthermore, the survival benefit with vitamin D supplementation appears to be independent of changes in serum calcium, Pi, and PTH levels. Although there is no direct explanation for the apparent survival benefits associated with vitamin D, indirect supportive evidence can be derived from studies showing an association of low levels of vitamin D and calcitriol with cardiovascular risk factors, including higher renin activity, hypertension, left ventricular hypertrophy, inflammation, insulin resistance, diabetes mellitus, and albuminuria.[267-269]

In animal studies, activated vitamin D inhibits renin production.[270,271] Human studies have demonstrated an inverse relationship between the level of vitamin D and degree of albuminuria.[272,273] Several trials in patients with CKD reported that the use of an active vitamin D analog, paricalcitol, resulted in a significant reduction in proteinuria.[274-276] Evaluation of patients with CKD not undergoing dialysis found a correlation between decreasing vitamin D levels and worsening brachial artery flow-mediated dilation as a marker of endothelial dysfunction.[277] Other studies have demonstrated that patients undergoing hemodialysis who have received cholecalciferol supplements have decreased inflammatory parameters, as indicated by increased serum albumin and reduction of both C-reactive protein and interleukin-6, as well as improved cardiac function, as reflected by lower brain natriuretic peptide levels and decreased left ventricular mass index.[278,279] In a prospective placebo-controlled study in patients who have not started dialysis, paricalcitol failed to demonstrate a reduction in ventricular mass index at the end of 48 weeks in patients with mild to moderate left ventricular hypertrophy. There was, however, a decrease in hospitalizations, a secondary end point.[280] The lack of effect may have been a function of the relatively high dose of paricalcitol, which may have further raised FGF-23 levels, because multiple studies have shown a link between FGF-23 and left ventricular hypetrophy.[76,235,281] Further studies evaluating whether treatment with vitamin D leads to improvement in clinical outcomes are still required.

FRACTURE

In patients with CKD not yet on dialysis, there is an increased incidence of fractures.[169,282-284] The incidence of fractures has been found to rise as CKD progresses,[285] suggesting that kidney disease is associated with progressive bone deterioration. However, another study did not confirm increased rates of hip, wrist, and vertebral fractures in patients with CKD independent of age and sex.[286]

In patients undergoing dialysis, the studies are very consistent and demonstrate a higher prevalence of hip fracture in patients undergoing dialysis than in the general population in all age groups.[198,287] Dialysis recipients in their 40s have a relative risk of hip fracture 80-fold higher than the relative risk in age- and sex-matched controls.[287] Patients undergoing hemodialysis may have a 50% higher rate of hip fractures than patients undergoing peritoneal dialysis.[288] Furthermore, hip fractures in patients on dialysis were found to be associated with a doubling of the mortality observed in hip fractures in patients not on dialysis.[198,289] Depending on the study, 10% to 52% of prevalent patients undergoing dialysis have fractures.[169] Unfortunately, most of these studies are of cross-sectional design or were cohort studies with limited follow-up.

Elevated PTH values are known to cause abnormal bone remodeling, especially of cortical bone. HRpQCT shows a rapid decline in cortical bone in patients on dialysis.[290] In prevalent patients undergoing dialysis who have secondary hyperparathyroidism, clinical fractures are predominantly cortical in location.[290a] However, the association of PTH with fracture has been inconsistent,[169] perhaps because both high and low PTH values are associated with fractures. Other risk factors associated with CKD include older age, female sex, low serum albumin, prior kidney transplantation, and peripheral vascular disease.[291-294] Falls are also increased in patients with CKD and predispose to fracture. The increased falls in patients undergoing dialysis may be due to peripheral vascular disease,[287] low muscle strength, impaired neuromuscular function,[295] and the administration of psychoactive medications.[292]

In summary, the abnormalities of bone, in terms of both quality and quantity, variable biochemical abnormalities, and multiple comorbid conditions likely all contribute to the pathogenesis of fractures in ESKD. This complexity also may limit generalizability of therapies routinely used in the general population to patients with the disease.

EXTRASKELETAL CALCIFICATION

Arterial calcification has a multitude of clinical manifestations. Intimal calcification (in association with atherosclerotic disease) can lead to myocardial infarction from stenosis and acute thrombus or to ischemia in both coronary and peripheral arteries. Medial calcification (or circumferential calcification) can lead to arterial stiffening, with reduced compliance of the artery and an inability to appropriately dilate in the setting of increased stress. In the coronary arteries, similar symptoms of ischemia can develop, and in theory could lead to arrhythmias and sudden death. In the larger arteries such as the aorta, calcification can lead to increased pulse wave velocity and elevated pulse pressure and is commonly associated with systolic hypertension in the elderly, a known risk factor for cardiovascular disease in the general population. In addition, the premature return of wave reflections during systole (instead of diastole) can lead to altered coronary perfusion with subsequent left ventricular hypertrophy. Lastly, calcification of the arterioles of the skin and other organs can lead to localized infarction and ischemia, including ischemic bowel and calciphylaxis.

VASCULAR CALCIFICATION IN PATIENTS WITH CKD

The high prevalence of vascular calcification in patients with CKD is not a new observation. In 1979, Ibels and colleagues demonstrated that both renal and internal iliac arteries of patients undergoing renal transplantation had greater atherogenic/intimal disease and increased calcification (detected by biochemical methods) than transplant donors.[296] In addition, the medial layer was thicker and more calcified in uremic patients than in the donors.[296] A study comparing histologic changes in coronary arteries from patients undergoing dialysis at autopsy were compared with non-dialysis, age-matched patients who had died from a cardiac event, found similar magnitudes of atherosclerotic plaque burden and intimal thickness, but with more calcification in the dialysis recipients.[297] In addition, morphometry of the arteries demonstrated increased medial thickening.[297] When these same investigators evaluated more distal segments of the coronary arteries, they found medial calcification.[298] Studies of the inferior epigastric artery of patients undergoing kidney transplantation demonstrated calcification in 31% of patients, with histology demonstrating isolated medial calcification without evidence of atherosclerotic or intimal changes, and both medial and intimal calcification in the same artery without disruption of the internal elastic lamina.[299] Thus, there is histologic evidence of (1) increased arterial calcification in coronary, renal, and iliac arteries of patients who undergo dialysis than in those who do not and (2) the presence of both intimal and medial calcification in patients undergoing dialysis, and this can occur independently of each other suggesting unique inciting factors. As noted previously, it is likely that calcification of plaque (atherosclerosis) and calcification of medial layer occur by similar mechanisms. However, the initiating event is clearly different.

Braun and colleagues first demonstrated that coronary artery calcification as detected by EBCT increased with advancing age in patients on dialysis and that the calcification scores were twofold to fivefold higher in patients on dialysis than in age-matched individuals with normal renal function and angiographically proven coronary artery disease.[300] Nearly 50% to 60% of patients starting hemodialysis have evidence of coronary artery calcification,[301] with higher prevalence in patients with diabetes.[302] The prevalence of detectable coronary or peripheral artery calcification is 51% to 93% in prevalent patients undergoing dialysis and 47% to 83% in patients with CKD stages 3 through 5. Valvular calcification is similarly common, occurring in 20% to 47% of patients on dialysis.[169] Studies that have evaluated the natural history of coronary calcification demonstrate that once it is present, the course is progressive. In contrast, many patients without calcification remain free of it for several years.[169,303,304] The presence of calcification in the coronary arteries, valves, and peripheral arteries is associated with increased mortality.[221] Given the high prevalence of calcification, it is currently uncertain whether routine imaging offers clinical utility or whether it can help stratify patients whose calcification will and will not respond to specific therapies.

There is an inverse relationship between bone mineralization and vascular calcification in patients on dialysis. There are several different, not mutually exclusive, mechanisms by which disturbances in the bone metabolism may cause or accelerate vascular calcification.[300,305] Interestingly, it appears to be low-turnover bone disease that leads to greatest risk of vascular calcification. London and colleagues evaluated patients on hemodialysis who underwent assessment of vascular calcification by ultrasonography with semiquantitative scoring and by bone biopsy with histomorphometry. Those patients with lowest bone formation rates and decreased osteoblast surfaces had the greatest degree of peripheral artery calcification, and this relationship held true in patients with and without previous parathyroidectomy.[306] Another study found that patients with low-turnover bone disease on biopsy were more likely to have progression of coronary artery calcification over 1 year as assessed by serial multislice CT than those with high-turnover bone disease.[203] Abnormalities in both cortical and trabecular bone on HRpQCT were associated with coronary artery calcification.[307] The likely mechanism for these findings is that adynamic bone cannot incorporate an acute calcium load, whereas actively remodeling bone can, as demonstrated by Kurz and associates using radiolabeled calcium.[200] In contrast to evidence in low-turnover bone disease, data are less robust as to the effects of high-turnover bone disease on vascular calcification, perhaps because the treatments for high-turnover bone disease confound the effects of calcification.

CKD-MBD IN KIDNEY TRANSPLANT RECIPIENTS

Bone and mineral disorders are universal complications in patients with CKD prior to transplantation. Ideally, all of these complications would be improved with successful kidney transplantation. Unfortunately, in many cases, kidney transplantation achieves milder forms of CKD (as opposed to normal kidney function), and thus transplant recipients still suffer from disorders associated with CKD-MBD. In addition, disorders of mineral metabolism occur following successful transplantation, including the effects of medications (steroids and calcineurin inhibitors), persistence of underlying disorders (hyperparathyroidism and vitamin D deficiency), development of hyperphosphaturia with hypophosphatemia, and the recurrence of varying degrees of CKD, which, unfortunately persists after transplantation.

BIOCHEMICAL CHANGES AFTER TRANSPLANTATION

Biochemical changes of mineral metabolism are common in patients after kidney transplantation.[308-311] Decreased calcidiol levels are common in kidney transplant recipients, with reported prevalence of up to 81%.[309] The causes are multifactorial, and may include nutritional deficiency, malabsorption, and decreased sun exposure. However, the improvement in kidney function results in an increase in CYP27B1 activity, resulting in greater conversion of calcidiol to calcitriol, which subsequently causes a gradual decrease in PTH concentrations during the first 3 to 6 months after transplantation. However, persistent hyperparathyroidism exists in about 33% and 20% of patients at 6 and 12 months, respectively.[312] FGF-23 concentrations decrease immediately after transplantation, although they remain inappropriately elevated for the prevailing serum Pi concentration. By about 3 months after transplantation, FGF-23 concentrations are reduced by 89%, and at 12 months FGF-23 concentrations appear to be similar to those in patients without transplantation who have comparable stages of CKD.[309] The elevated FGF-23 inhibits CYP27B1 and contributes to the low calcitriol concentrations observed in the early posttransplantation period, likely contributing to the persistent hyperparathyroidism seen after transplantation. The elevated FGF-23 and PTH concentrations combined with the low calcitriol concentrations likely contribute to hypophosphatemia observed in many transplant recipients.[312,313]

Serum calcium levels typically drop very early after transplantation, as a result of cessation of therapy with calcitriol and its analogs and/or calcium-containing phosphate binders. After that initial drop, however, calcium concentrations progressively increase, with hypercalcemia developing in a substantial number of patients during the first to third month after transplantation. Hypercalcemia can be transient, resolving by 6 to 8 months in some cases but lasting for many years in others. Hypercalcemia is typically associated with hyperparathyroidism and results from enhanced renal tubular reabsorption of calcium under the influence of PTH in the functioning allograft, the effects of calcitriol on the gastrointestinal absorption of calcium, and, potentially, a direct effect of PTH in causing calcium efflux from bone. Low bone turnover with relatively low PTH may also result in hypercalcemia because the bone is not able to act as a buffer for the circulating calcium pool.[308,309]

BONE CHANGES AFTER TRANSPLANTATION

These disorders of mineral metabolism and the associated bone disease lead to the development of fractures following transplantation, which occur after up to 44% of successful transplantations.[308] This fracture risk appears to be less than that observed with other solid organ transplants.[308] The combination of a kidney-pancreas transplantation raises fracture risk above that associated with kidney transplantation alone.[314,315] In a retrospective analysis of 68,814 patients, fracture developed in 22.5% within 5 years.[316] In a study of first-time kidney transplant recipients between 1997 and 2010, the incidence of hip fracture was 3.8 per 1000 person-years. The risk of fracture in 2010 was 0.56 (95% confidence interval, 0.47 to 0.77) in comparison with that in 1997, indicating a decrease over the 13-year period, presumably due to changes in immunosuppression therapy.[317] Factors associated with greater fracture risk during the first 5 years included female gender, age greater than 45 years, Caucasian race, recipient of a deceased donor kidney, increased human leukocyte antigen mismatches, diabetes, pretransplantation dialysis, steroid use, and an aggressive induction regimen.[316] Importantly, even with the use of steroid-sparing regimens, total (all sites) fractures have occurred in up to 50% of kidney transplant recipients at 6 years.[317,318] In contrast, a recent study from Canada evaluated 4821 kidney transplant recipients and found the 10-year cumulative incidence of hip fracture was 1.7%.[318a]

Studies evaluating bone histology in recipients of kidney transplants are limited. The main alteration is an uncoupling of bone remodeling, which results in a decrease of bone formation with persistent bone resorption and net bone loss. In a small cohort of young patients who underwent transplantation prior to the initiation of dialysis and were treated predominantly with corticosteroids, bone biopsies revealed a mineralization defect as early as 6 months after transplantation.[319] Another study evaluating the early histologic changes after transplantation revealed that osteoid volume, osteoid thickness, osteoid resorption surface, and osteoclast surface were above the normal range before transplantation and remained increased approximately 35 days afterwards. However, osteoid and osteoblast surfaces, which also were increased before transplantation, were significantly decreased approximately 35 days after transplantation.[320] Both bone formation and mineralization were also inhibited after transplantation. An important observation was that although none of the pretransplantation biopsy specimens showed evidence of apoptosis, 45% of posttransplantation specimens showed significant apoptosis after an average of only 35 days. Thus, early posttransplantation apoptosis and a decrease in osteoblast number and osteoblast surface play a role in the pathogenesis of posttransplantation bone disease that may be related directly to the use of glucocorticoids.[320] The few evaluations that examined the longer-term effect of transplantation on bone histology generally demonstrate low bone turnover and histology consistent with adynamic bone disease.[321,322] Lehmann and colleagues performed a retrospective study of 57 patients after approximately 54 months after kidney transplantation.[322] Seven histologic subgroups were identified: normal, osteitis fibrosa cystica, mild osteitis fibrosa, mixed uremic bone disease, osteomalacia, adynamic bone disease, and osteoporosis. Given the limited number of patients in the study, no significant correlations were observed. However, this study did show a variable degree of histologic abnormalities following transplantation that could not have been predicted by biochemical testing and confirmed that preexisting bone disease lesions persist in the posttransplantation period.

The effect of other immunosuppressive agents on bone histology has also been examined. Bone biopsies performed approximately 10 years after transplantation in patients whose treatment included cyclosporine monotherapy, azathioprine and prednisone, or triple therapy revealed no differences among the immunosuppressant regimens.[323,324] A subgroup analysis of 21 patients with normal PTH levels showed that cyclosporine monotherapy was associated with a more pronounced decrease in bone thickness than the other regimens.[324] In addition, the cyclosporine group showed a lower trabecular appositional than the azathioprine and prednisone group. Multiple regression analysis showed that sex and time after transplantation were the most significant factors predicting bone volume and mineralizing surface. Predictive factors for eroded bone surface and osteoclast number included age and time on dialysis before transplantation.[323,324]

Initial studies examining bone mineral content by densitometry show severe and rapid bone loss.[319] However, later studies have not found the dramatic decrease initially described, perhaps because of the current practice of using lower steroid dosages or steroid-free immunosuppression regimens.[308,325] The use of corticosteroids is the major determinant of low bone mineral content, because these agents impair calcium absorption from the gastrointestinal tract and inhibit bone cell recruitment and function.[308] Cueto-Manzano and associates also evaluated bone densitometry as a function of immunosuppressive therapy.[323,324] In comparison with age- and sex-matched controls, none of the treated groups showed a significant reduction in BMD in the lumbar spine or femoral neck. However, in comparison with young normal controls, osteopenia was detected in the femoral neck, except in premenopausal women. There was no significant difference in bone density related to immunosuppressant regimen, sex, or menopausal status.

Although reductions in bone density have been associated with an increased fracture rate in postmenopausal women and in men treated with glucocorticoids, as well as in heart or liver transplant recipients, very little data support its role in predicting fractures after kidney transplantation. In the one study that demonstrated low bone density to be predictive of fracture risk, 283 kidney transplant recipients with varying degrees of kidney function underwent 670 bone density examinations of the hip. An absolute bone density value less than 0.9 g/cm^2 was associated with an increased risk of fracture.[326] A study evaluating patients with early steroid withdrawal after kidney transplantation found a preservation of bone mineral content by DXA but continued loss at the ultra-distal radius. The latter finding was confirmed by HRpQCT to be predominantly cortical loss, which was associated with persistent hyperparathyroidism.[327] As indicated earlier in this chapter, abnormal bone turnover may alter the predictive value of bone densitometry in patients with CKD, and thus, preexisting rate of bone turnover likely affects the assessment and outcomes of bone disease in transplant recipients. In addition, for lumbar spine assessment of bone densitometry by DXA, existing aortic calcification may confound the measurement.

VASCULAR CALCIFICATION CHANGES AFTER TRANSPLANTATION

Most transplant recipients enter their posttransplant course with a preexisting burden of vascular calcification; as in patients with CKD, vascular calcification strongly predicts cardiovascular events and all-cause mortality. Unfortunately there are few studies of the impact of vascular calcification in transplant recipients. Although preexisting calcifications progress after transplantation, they appear to do so at a much slower rate than prior to transplantation.[328,329] A review of 13 clinical studies of the impact of vascular calcifications on kidney transplant recipients shows that as in the CKD population, the association of both traditional and nontraditional risk factors is variable in patients who have undergone transplantation.[330] There is a strong association between baseline coronary artery calcification score and progression. A significant improvement in secondary hyperparathyroidism after transplantation favorably affects the progression of coronary artery calcification. Independent risk factors of coronary artery calcification include low levels of calcidiol, fetuin-A, and MGP. Although diabetes is a risk factor for the presence of coronary artery calcification in transplant recipients, it has not been independently associated with progression of coronary artery calcification. The data on the effects of immunosuppressive drugs as factors in progression are few and inconclusive; however, it does appear that mycophenolate mofetil may have a beneficial effect because its antiproliferative action may inhibit smooth muscle cell proliferation, thus having a favorable effect on endothelial cell activity.[330] In the general population and in patients with ESKD, there is an inverse relationship between coronary artery calcification and bone density. This association has not been shown in kidney or kidney-pancreas transplant recipients.[331]

SUMMARY

In summary, kidney transplantation results in persistence of some abnormalities of CKD-MBD. With changing immunosuppressive protocols and persistence of CKD of varying degrees, the treatment is difficult. Later reviews have highlighted the importance of treatment before transplantation to ensure better outcomes and have called for more studies in both children and adults.[310,311,332]

Complete reference list available at ExpertConsult.com.

KEY REFERENCES

1. Moe S, Drueke T, Cunningham J, et al: Definition, evaluation, and classification of renal osteodystrophy: a position statement from Kidney Disease: Improving Global Outcomes (KDIGO). *Kidney Int* 69:1945–1953, 2006.
7. Hill KM, Martin BR, Wastney ME, et al: Oral calcium carbonate affects calcium but not phosphorus balance in stage 3-4 chronic kidney disease. *Kidney Int* 83:959–966, 2013.
22. Bindels RJ: 2009 Homer W. Smith Award: Minerals in motion: from new ion transporters to new concepts. *J Am Soc Nephrol* 21:1263–1269, 2010.
25. Brennan SC, Thiem U, Roth S, et al: Calcium sensing receptor signalling in physiology and cancer. *Biochim Biophys Acta* 1833:1732–1744, 2013.
32. Rodriguez-Ortiz ME, Canalejo A, Herencia C, et al: Magnesium modulates parathyroid hormone secretion and upregulates parathyroid receptor expression at moderately low calcium concentration. *Nephrol Dial Transplant* 29:282–289, 2014.
49. Raggi P, Chertow GM, Torres PU, et al: The ADVANCE study: a randomized study to evaluate the effects of cinacalcet plus low-dose vitamin D on vascular calcification in patients on hemodialysis. *Nephrol Dial Transplant* 26:1327–1339, 2011.
55. Sprague SM, Moe SM: The case for routine parathyroid hormone monitoring. *Clin J Am Soc Nephrol* 8:313–318, 2013.

58. Jones G: Extrarenal vitamin D activation and interactions between vitamin D(2), vitamin D(3), and vitamin D analogs. *Annu Rev Nutr* 33:23–44, 2013.
59. Chanakul A, Zhang MY, Louw A, et al: FGF-23 regulates CYP27B1 transcription in the kidney and in extra-renal tissues. *PLoS One* 8:e72816, 2013.
69. Hu MC, Shi M, Zhang J, et al: Renal production, uptake, and handling of circulating α klotho. *J Am Soc Nephrol* 2015 May 14. [Epub ahead of print.]
71. Isakova T, Wahl P, Vargas GS, et al: Fibroblast growth factor 23 is elevated before parathyroid hormone and phosphate in chronic kidney disease. *Kidney Int* 79:1370–1378, 2011.
72. Hu MC, Kuro-o M, Moe OW: Renal and extrarenal actions of Klotho. *Semin Nephrol* 33:118–129, 2013.
76. Faul C, Amaral AP, Oskouei B, et al: FGF23 induces left ventricular hypertrophy. *J Clin Invest* 121:4393–4408, 2011.
84. de Borst MH, Vervloet MG, ter Wee PM, et al: Cross talk between the renin-angiotensin-aldosterone system and vitamin D-FGF-23-klotho in chronic kidney disease. *J Am Soc Nephrol* 22:1603–1609, 2011.
92. Baron R: Kneissel M: WNT signaling in bone homeostasis and disease: from human mutations to treatments. *Nat Med* 19:179–192, 2013.
101. Rhee Y, Lee EY, Lezcano V, et al: Resorption controls bone anabolism driven by parathyroid hormone (PTH) receptor signaling in osteocytes. *J Biol Chem* 288:29809–29820, 2013.
133. Giachelli CM: The emerging role of phosphate in vascular calcification. *Kidney Int* 75:890–897, 2009.
141. Ketteler M, Bongartz P, Westenfeld R, et al: Association of low fetuin-A (AHSG) concentrations in serum with cardiovascular mortality in patients on dialysis: a cross-sectional study. *Lancet* 361:827–833, 2003.
147. Ketteler M, Rothe H, Brandenburg VM, et al: The K-factor in chronic kidney disease: biomarkers of calcification inhibition and beyond. *Nehrol Dial Transplant* 29:1267–1270, 2014.
163. Lavi-Moshayoff V, Wasserman G, Meir T, et al: PTH increases FGF23 gene expression and mediates the high-FGF23 levels of experimental kidney failure: a bone parathyroid feedback loop. *Am J Physiol Renal Physiol* 299:F882–F889, 2010.
164. Rodriguez-Ortiz ME, Lopez I, Munoz-Castaneda JR, et al: Calcium deficiency reduces circulating levels of FGF23. *J Am Soc Nephrol* 23:1190–1197, 2012.
166. Sprague SM, Bellorin-Font E, Jorgetti V, et al: Diagnostic accuracy of bone turnover markers and bone histology in patients with chronic kidney disease treated by dialysis. *Am J Kidney Dis* 2015 (in press).
169. Bellorin-Font E, Ambrosoni P, Carlini RG, et al: KDIGO Clinical Practice Guidelines for the diagnosis, evaluation, prevention, and treatment of chronic kidney disease-mineral and bone disorder (CKD-MBD). *Kidney Int* 76:S1–S130, 2009.
182. Moorthi R, Moe S: Recent advances in the non-invasive diagnosis of renal osteodystrophy. *Kidney Int* 84:886–894, 2013.
185. Sherrard DJ, Hercz G, Pei Y, et al: The spectrum of bone disease in end-stage renal failure—an evolving disorder. *Kidney Int* 43:436–442, 1993.
188. Alfrey AC: Aluminum and renal disease. *Contrib Nephrol* 102:110–124, 1993.
189. National Kidney Foundation: K/DOQI clinical practice guidelines for bone metabolism and disease in chronic kidney disease. *Am J Kidney Dis* 42:S1–S201, 2003.
196. Ott SM: Bone disease in CKD. *Curr Opin Nephrol Hypertens* 21:376–381, 2012.
203. Barreto DV, Barreto Fde C, Carvalho AB, et al: Association of changes in bone remodeling and coronary calcification in hemodialysis patients: a prospective study. *Am J Kidney Dis* 52:1139–1150, 2008.
212. Nickolas TL, Stein E, Cohen A, et al: Bone mass and microarchitecture in CKD patients with fracture. *J Am Soc Nephrol* 21:1371–1380, 2010.
217. London GM, Guerin AP, Marchais SJ, et al: Arterial media calcification in end-stage renal disease: impact on all-cause and cardiovascular mortality. *Nephrol Dial Transplant* 18:1731–1740, 2003.
222. Bellasi A, Block GA, Ferramosca E, et al: Integration of clinical and imaging data to predict death in hemodialysis patients. *Hemodial Int* 17:12–18, 2013.
229. Palmer SC, Hayen A, Macaskill P, et al: Serum levels of phosphorus, parathyroid hormone, and calcium and risks of death and cardiovascular disease in individuals with chronic kidney disease: a systematic review and meta-analysis. *JAMA* 305:1119–1127, 2011.
233. Isakova T, Xie H, Yang W, et al: Fibroblast growth factor 23 and risks of mortality and end-stage renal disease in patients with chronic kidney disease. *JAMA* 305:2432–2439, 2011.
239. Gutierrez OM, Mannstadt M, Isakova T, et al: Fibroblast growth factor 23 and mortality among patients undergoing hemodialysis. *N Engl J Med* 359:584–592, 2008.
246. Ross AC, Manson JE, Abrams SA, et al: The 2011 report on dietary reference intakes for calcium and vitamin D from the Institute of Medicine: what clinicians need to know. *J Clin Endocrinol Metab* 96:53–58, 2011.
259. Levin A, Bakris GL, Molitch M, et al: Prevalence of abnormal serum vitamin D, PTH, calcium, and phosphorus in patients with chronic kidney disease: Results of the study to evaluate early kidney disease. *Kidney Int* 71:31–38, 2007.
265. Zheng Z, Shi H, Jia J, et al: Vitamin D supplementation and mortality risk in chronic kidney disease: a meta-analysis of 20 observational studies. *BMC Nephrol* 14:199, 2013.
276. de Zeeuw D, Agarwal R, Amdahl M, et al: Selective vitamin D receptor activation with paricalcitol for reduction of albuminuria in patients with type 2 diabetes (VITAL study): a randomised controlled trial. *Lancet* 376:1543–1551, 2010.
290. Nickolas TL, Stein EM, Dworakowski E, et al: Rapid cortical bone loss in patients with chronic kidney disease. *J Bone Miner Res* 28:1811–1820, 2013.
294. Nickolas TL, Cremers S, Zhang A, et al: Discriminants of prevalent fractures in chronic kidney disease. *J Am Soc Nephrol* 22:1560–1572, 2011.
298. Gross ML, Meyer HP, Ziebart H, et al: Calcification of coronary intima and media: immunohistochemistry, backscatter imaging, and x-ray analysis in renal and nonrenal patients. *Clin J Am Soc Nephrol* 2:121 134, 2007.
309. Alshayeb HM, Josephson MA, Sprague SM: CKD-mineral and bone disorder management in kidney transplant recipients. *Am J Kidney Dis* 61:310–325, 2013.
310. Haffner D, Schuler U: Metabolic bone disease after renal transplantation. *Curr Opin Pediatr* 26:198–206, 2014.
317. Sukumaran Nair S, Lenihan CR, Montez-Rath ME, et al: Temporal trends in the incidence, treatment and outcomes of hip fracture after first kidney transplantation in the United States. *Am J Transplant* 14:943–951, 2014.
327. Iyer SP, Nikkel LE, Nishiyama KK, et al: Kidney transplantation with early corticosteroid withdrawal: paradoxical effects at the central and peripheral skeleton. *J Am Soc Nephrol* 25:1331–1341, 2014.
330. Cianciolo G, Capelli I, Angelini ML, et al: Importance of vascular calcification in kidney transplant recipients. *Am J Nephrol* 39:418–426, 2014.
332. Sgambat K, Moudgil A: Optimization of bone health in children before and after renal transplantation: current perspectives and future directions. *Front Pediatr* 2:13, 2014.

56 Cardiovascular Aspects of Kidney Disease

Richard Haynes | David C. Wheeler | Martin J. Landray | Colin Baigent

CHAPTER OUTLINE

THE SPECTRUM OF CARDIOVASCULAR PATHOLOGIC PROCESSES IN PATIENTS WITH CHRONIC KIDNEY DISEASE, 1855
Arterial Disease, 1855
Cardiac Disease, 1857
Clinical Manifestations of Cardiovascular Disease in Chronic Kidney Disease, 1859
EPIDEMIOLOGY OF CARDIOVASCULAR DISEASE IN CHRONIC KIDNEY DISEASE, 1860
Association Between Kidney Function and Cardiovascular Disease, 1860
Association Between Albuminuria and Cardiovascular Disease, 1860
DOES KIDNEY DISEASE CAUSE CARDIOVASCULAR DISEASE? 1861
Blood Pressure, 1861
Dyslipidemia, 1863
Other Direct Risk Factors, 1863
INDIRECT RISK FACTORS: CAUSES OF BOTH KIDNEY AND CARDIOVASCULAR DISEASE, 1865

Diabetes Mellitus, 1865
Obesity, 1865
CARDIOVASCULAR RISK PREDICTION, 1866
Basic Risk Prediction Scores, 1866
Role of Estimated Glomerular Filtration Rate in Risk Prediction, 1866
Use of Imaging and Other Assessments of Cardiovascular Function in Risk Prediction, 1866
CARDIOVASCULAR RISK PREVENTION, 1867
Smoking Cessation, 1867
Blood Pressure Reduction, 1867
Reduction of Low-Density Lipoprotein Cholesterol Level, 1868
Tight Glycemic Control, 1871
Correction of Anemia, 1871
Reduction of Homocysteine Level, 1872
Correction of Chronic Kidney Disease–Mineral Bone Disorder, 1872
Antiplatelet Therapy, 1873
CONCLUSIONS, 1873

The expanding availability of dialysis and kidney transplantation in developed countries has led to improvements in the prognosis of patients with end-stage kidney disease (ESKD). However, the life expectancy of patients receiving such renal replacement therapy (RRT) remains considerably lower than that of age- and sex-matched healthy controls with normal or near normal kidney function, and the risks for both cardiovascular and noncardiovascular causes of mortality are increased at all ages.[1] This chapter will focus on the pathology, epidemiology, and treatment of cardiovascular disease in patients with chronic kidney disease (CKD).

The first description of a link between diseases of the kidneys and the cardiovascular system is attributable to Richard Bright, who described cardiac hypertrophy in patients with small kidneys at postmortem examination over 170 years ago.[2] The problem became more obvious with the advent of dialysis, since patients survived long enough after ESKD to develop clinical manifestations of cardiovascular disease. In the early 1970s, clinicians were alarmed at the high incidence of cardiovascular events in young patients receiving RRT and presumed that either kidney disease or the dialysis process itself led to "accelerated atherosclerosis".[3] Twenty years later, a task force report published by the U.S. National Kidney Foundation focused the attention of the nephrology community on the problem of increased cardiovascular disease risk associated with CKD.[4] Research over the last 10 years or so has improved our understanding of the cardiovascular consequences of impaired kidney function and has helped to suggest appropriate treatment strategies. For example, the nature of the cardiac and arterial changes that complicate CKD are now better described. Although atherosclerosis contributes to arterial pathologic processes, in advanced CKD, nonatherosclerotic changes, including arterial wall thickening and calcification, are the dominant pathologic feature.[5] While an increased risk for cardiovascular events associated with atherosclerotic plaque rupture is recognized in patients with CKD,[6] the clinical consequences of structural heart disease (heart failure and sudden dysrhythmic death) appear to be a more important cause of morbidity and mortality than are the complications of atherosclerotic disease.[7] However, our understanding remains incomplete.

Although the problem of premature cardiovascular disease was first recognized in dialysis populations, patients with lesser degrees of impaired kidney function are also at increased risk for cardiovascular events.[8] Numerous studies have shown an inverse association between estimated glomerular filtration rate (eGFR) and cardiovascular risk.[9] The nature of both cardiac and arterial disease may change with declining kidney function, and this might have implications for the development of optimal management strategies. It has also become clear that albuminuria is associated with an increased risk for cardiovascular disease, whether or not GFR is reduced.[9,10]

It follows that assessment and management of cardiovascular diseases should start early in the course of CKD in an effort to reduce morbidity and mortality, bearing in mind that most patients in whom CKD is diagnosed early do not progress to ESKD. Those who do may have well-established structural cardiac and vascular damage by the time they commence RRT.[11,12] This is particularly important when considering a patient's suitability for transplantation, and most clinicians will screen such patients (or at least those they consider to be at high risk) for cardiovascular disease before transplant listing in an effort to reduce perioperative morbidity and mortality and to optimize the results of organ allocation.[13] Despite such screening strategies, patients who receive a kidney transplant remain at higher risk than age- and sex-matched controls without kidney disease.[4]

At present, there is much uncertainty about how to reduce cardiovascular risk in patients with CKD. Epidemiologic relations among recognized cardiovascular risk factors and particular clinical outcomes are often confounded by other factors associated with ill health in CKD, such as inflammation and malnutrition,[14,15] and it may not be possible to account for them accurately or completely. Consequently, it may be more appropriate to approach the problem of preventing cardiovascular disease in CKD by defining the types of pathologic conditions observed in patients with CKD and then considering what is known about the treatment or prevention of such pathologic conditions from studies among individuals without CKD (which provide more reliable information on the effectiveness of particular drugs in specific disease processes). Another possible strategy, which is applicable where treatments that modify a particular risk factor are available, is to conduct randomized trials of such treatments, which can yield unconfounded and less biased assessments of the causal relevance of that risk factor for particular types of cardiovascular disease.

Table 56.1 Characteristics of Cardiovascular Diseases in Chronic Kidney Disease
Arteries
Increased wall thickness
Arterial stiffness
Endothelial dysfunction
Arterial calcification
Heart
Altered cardiac geometry
Myocardial fibrosis
Left ventricular dysfunction
Valvular disease
Dysrhythmia and conduction defects

THE SPECTRUM OF CARDIOVASCULAR PATHOLOGIC PROCESSES IN PATIENTS WITH CHRONIC KIDNEY DISEASE

Cardiovascular changes observed in patients with CKD can be divided broadly into those that involve the blood vessels (specifically the arteries) and those that involve the heart (Table 56.1). Although a wide spectrum of cardiovascular pathologic changes is recognized in CKD, much less is known about the association between particular pathologic processes and specific cardiovascular risk factors in the CKD population. It is likely that any associations between a given risk factor and particular cardiovascular pathologic changes will vary in their strength (and possibly direction), so careful phenotyping of cardiovascular outcomes is essential in epidemiologic studies.

ARTERIAL DISEASE

The term "arteriosclerosis" (derived from the Greek meaning "hardening of the arteries") is generally used to describe a range of pathologic processes. Strictly, arteriosclerosis encompasses three different lesions: atherosclerosis, arteriolosclerosis, and Mönckeberg's medial calcific sclerosis (or Mönckeberg's sclerosis).[16] Atherosclerosis, a word derived from the Greek "atheroma" (gruel-like material), is characterized by the development of lipid-enriched plaques in the intimal layer of the artery. Calcification is an important feature of atherosclerosis, and its presence or absence is relevant in determining the stage of the lesion.[17] Distinct from atherosclerosis, the phenomenon of noncalcified, nonatheromatous stiffening of smaller muscular arteries was first described in patients with Bright's disease in 1868 and soon came to be known as "arteriolosclerosis." Thirty-five years later, in 1903, Mönckeberg reported what he considered to be a third distinct form of arterial disease involving the media of the artery and characterized by medial thickening and heavy calcification without the presence of atheroma.[18]

Patients with CKD may exhibit all these features of arteriosclerosis. The exact nature of arterial disease in any given individual patient is likely to depend on multiple factors, including the patient's age and exposure to risk factors and the duration of CKD. For example, a patient with preexisting atherosclerosis who develops CKD as a result of atherosclerotic renovascular disease may have a rather different spectrum of arterial pathologic changes than a patient with a similar level of kidney function due to kidney damage from glomerulonephritis. The various structural and functional arterial abnormalities associated with CKD are covered in more detail later.

ARTERIAL WALL THICKENING

One of the few autopsy studies examining arterial pathologic processes in ESKD reported that there was more pronounced medial thickening in sections of coronary artery than in equivalent sections from age- and gender-matched non-CKD patients known to have had coronary artery disease.[5] Thickening of the arterial wall can be measured noninvasively by assessing the combined width of the intima and media of the carotid artery on ultrasonography (carotid intima-media thickness [CIMT]) and has been found to be increased in populations at high risk for cardiovascular disease such as older adults[19] and patients with type 2 diabetes mellitus.[20] Studies in patients receiving hemodialysis dating back to the mid-1990s have indicated higher arterial intima-media thickness values for carotid and femoral sites as compared to healthy controls.[21] More recent studies suggest increased CIMT is also found in patients with less advanced CKD and indicate that eGFR independently predicts carotid diameter (which increases wall stress).[22] CIMT has also been shown to be a strong predictor of death from cardiovascular causes in patients with CKD, independent of other risk factors.[23,24]

ARTERIAL STIFFENING

Stiffening is thought to be a functional consequence of artery wall thickening (and calcification) and is readily assessed noninvasively by measuring the velocity of propagation of a pulse wave through the arterial tree (pulse wave velocity).[25] Stiffening may represent an early feature of CKD-associated arterial disease and can be detected in pediatric populations receiving dialysis as early as the first decade of life.[26] Stiffness has prognostic significance: both carotid[27] and aortic[28] stiffness independently predict death in adult patients on hemodialysis, as in other high-risk groups such as patients with diabetes mellitus[29] and older adults.[30]

Another method of measuring arterial stiffness is to assess the pulse waveform in an accessible artery (e.g., the carotid artery). A parameter derived from the pulse waveform, the augmentation index, provides a measure of the interaction between outgoing and reflected pulse waveforms at the point of measurement and in part reflects the stiffness of the arterial tree.[31] Augmentation index assessed at the common carotid artery has been found to predict mortality in one study of ESKD[32] but not another.[33] A further study comparing different methods of measuring arterial stiffness found that higher pulse wave velocity, but not augmentation index, predicted an increased risk for cardiovascular disease outcomes in patients with CKD.[34]

A third method, measurement of carotid artery stiffness parameter β, which is determined by monitoring pulsatile changes in the artery during echo-tracking sonography,[35] was used in a prospective cohort study examining the independent predictive value of arterial stiffness in 423 patients receiving hemodialysis. This measurement of stiffness independently predicted cardiovascular events even after adjustments had been made for arterial thickness, possibly implicating distinct roles for stiffening and thickening in the development of arterial complications in patients with CKD.[36]

ENDOTHELIAL DYSFUNCTION

The vascular endothelium plays a key role in maintaining arterial tone, predominantly through the continuous production of nitric oxide. Nitric oxide is a vasoactive compound that contributes to the resting tone of the artery and protects against the development of arterial disease by inhibiting vascular smooth muscle cell proliferation, platelet aggregation, and monocyte adhesion.[37] Production of nitric oxide is stimulated by hypoxia, increased sheer stress, or by locally released mediators such as acetylcholine.

Endothelial function can be measured by assessing the vasodilatory response of an artery to endothelial stimulation. This can be achieved by directly infusing compounds into an artery (usually the brachial) or by monitoring the response to reactive hyperemia following temporary arterial occlusion. Arterial vasodilation can be assessed by measuring changes in forearm size using strain-gauge plethysmography (which works on the principle that the rate of distension of a forearm is proportional to the rate of arterial inflow) or by measuring the diameter of the arterial lumen using high-resolution ultrasonography.[38]

Studies in patients with stage 4 or 5 CKD have consistently demonstrated impairment of endothelial function using invasive[39] and noninvasive approaches.[40] One possible mechanism for endothelial dysfunction in the context of CKD is the accumulation of asymmetric dimethyl arginine (ADMA), an endogenous inhibitor of the enzyme nitric oxide synthetase.[41] ADMA inhibits nitric oxide synthetase and thereby limits the bioavailability of nitric oxide, which is essential for normal endothelial function.[42] Blood concentrations of ADMA are elevated in CKD, are inversely proportional to GFR,[41,43] and also appear to be associated with an increased risk for cardiovascular disease in the general population in some, but not all, studies.[44] At present there is no intervention that can selectively reduce ADMA concentrations, so the causal relationship (and clinical relevance) of this risk factor remains unclear.

ARTERIAL CALCIFICATION

Arterial calcification is a recognized feature of two of the pathologic processes that are prevalent in patients with CKD, namely atherosclerosis[17] and Mönckeberg sclerosis (see "Arterial Disease" section).[18] The pattern observed in atherosclerosis is of patchy intimal calcification in association with lipid deposits, whereas in Mönckeberg disease there is a linear pattern of medial calcium deposition (Figure 56.1).[45] Both are closely linked to disturbances in calcium and phosphate homeostasis and to associated abnormalities in bone metabolism (see Chapter 55).

Autopsy studies have indicated a greater degree of arterial calcification in patients with ESKD than controls with known coronary artery disease.[5] In life, calcification can be detected by both ultrasonographic and x-ray–based techniques.[46] Studies using electron beam computerized tomography, a technique that allows rapid image acquisition, thereby "freezing" the heart during diastole,[47] have indicated that, compared to patients known to have cardiovascular disease, patients undergoing dialysis have much higher calcification scores.[48] Furthermore, calcification develops at a younger age in CKD than in non-CKD populations,[49] being detectable even in children and adolescents.[50]

Some investigators have attempted to distinguish the two patterns of arterial calcification on the basis of imaging studies.[51] Although they may represent a continuum of the same pathologic process,[52] patchy calcium deposition (suggestive of an atherosclerotic pattern) was more common in older patients with a clinical history of cardiovascular events

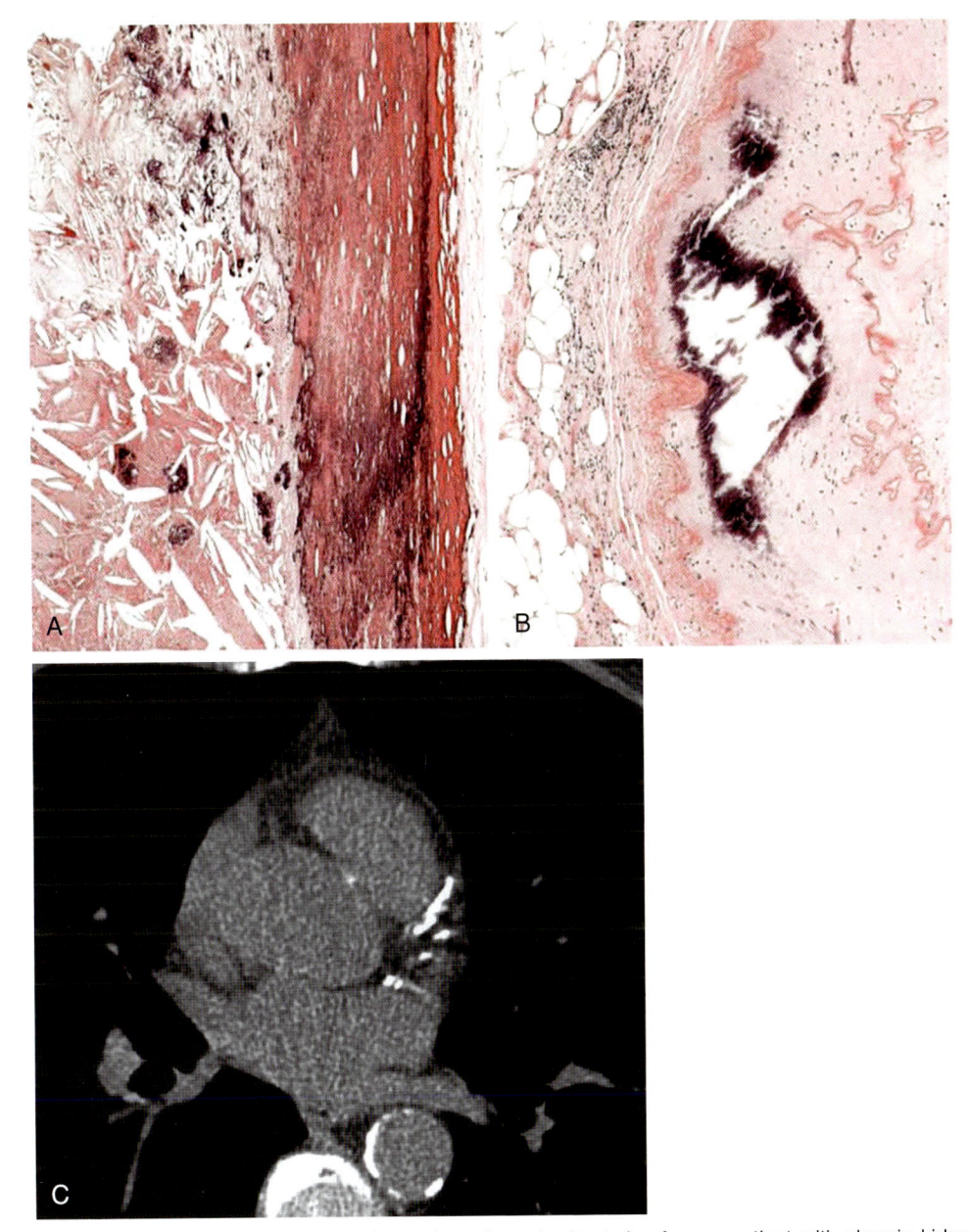

Figure 56.1 Arterial calcification in CKD. Cross sections of medium-sized arteries from a patient with chronic kidney disease showing deposition of calcium (*black*) in the intima **(A)** and media **(B)** in association with atherosclerosis (von Kossa stain). Calcium deposits may be visible on computed tomographic scanning of the heart as depicted in **C**, where calcification is visible in the left anterior descending and left circumflex coronary artery as well as the descending aorta. (Courtesy of Professor A.J. Howie.)

before starting dialysis.[51] The physiologic consequences of arterial calcification may include stiffening of the artery,[53] but it is unclear whether calcification has a positive or negative impact on plaque stability.[54]

CARDIAC DISEASE

Echocardiographic studies performed in the mid-1990s indicated a high prevalence of structural heart abnormalities in patients starting dialysis, with 74% having increased left ventricular mass in one study.[11] Left ventricular remodeling occurs well before the initiation of dialysis[55] and is detectable even in patients with stage 2 or 3 CKD.[56,57] Although adaptive in the early stages, such structural changes may eventually lead to functional impairment, including reduced compliance of the left ventricular wall during diastole (diastolic dysfunction) and impaired myocardial contractility (systolic dysfunction), or both.[58] In addition to these changes in left ventricular geometry, histologic changes such as fibrosis and calcification occur in the myocardium,[59] and valvular calcification is also frequently observed.[60]

ALTERED CARDIAC GEOMETRY

Left ventricular hypertrophy is generally classified according to the predominant pattern of abnormality on echocardiogram. In one study of 3487 patients with CKD, the prevalence of left ventricular hypertrophy was 32%, 48%,

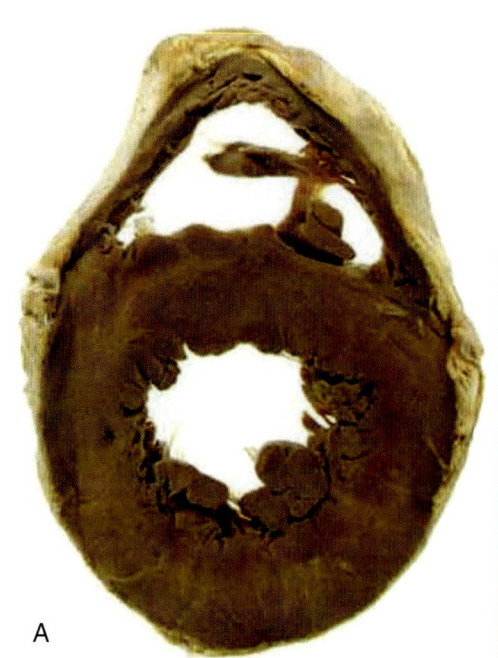

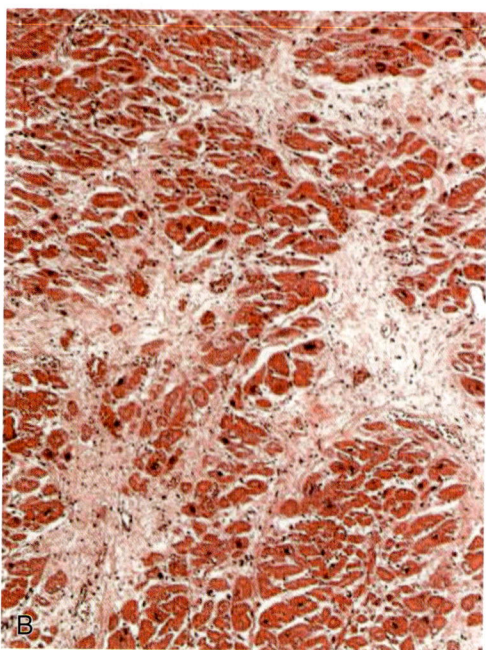

Figure 56.2 Myocardial disease in CKD. Postmortem cross section of a heart from a patient with long-standing chronic kidney disease showing concentric left ventricular hypertrophy **(A)**. Histologic analysis **(B)** often reveals myocardial fibrosis (*pale staining*) disrupting the normal architecture of cardiac myocytes. (**A**, Courtesy of Professor A.J. Howie; **B**, Courtesy of Dr. M. Rubens.)

57%, and 75% for eGFR categories 60 or higher, 45 to 59, 30 to 44, and less than 30 mL/min/1.73 m². [56] After adjustment for numerous potential confounders, the odds of having left ventricular hypertrophy were more than double among patients with eGFR of less than 30 mL/min/1.73 m² compared to those with eGFR of 60 mL/min/1.73 m² or higher (odds ratio [OR], 2.2; 95% confidence interval [CI], 1.4 to 3.4). Recognizing that categorization is complicated by volume changes related to dialysis, Foley and associates found that 44% of patients had predominantly left ventricular wall thickening (concentric hypertrophy) and 30% predominantly increased cavity volume (eccentric hypertrophy) in a study of patients starting dialysis.[11] Such changes are likely to represent adaptations to volume and pressure overload.[61] Volume overload increases left ventricular filling pressure and thereby stretches the ventricular wall. The heart adapts by lengthening existing myocytes, thus enlarging the internal dimensions of the left ventricular cavity. This process is usually accompanied by wall thickening, a further adaptive response that reduces wall stress. Thus volume overload results in a ventricle with a thickened wall and enlarged cavity, but with a normal ratio of wall thickness to internal diameter (eccentric hypertrophy). In contrast, pressure overload increases wall stress during systole, leading to myocyte proliferation and wall thickening with preservation or reduction of cavity volume (concentric hypertrophy; Figure 56.2). These adaptive responses, which may be reversible in the early stages, are essentially beneficial, at least initially. Dilation permits increased cardiac output for a similar level of energy expenditure, while wall thickening redistributes increased tension over a larger area and reduces energy consumption per myocyte.[62]

Cardiac magnetic resonance studies have allowed the geometry of the heart to be assessed in a volume-independent manner. Such studies have identified two major types of cardiomyopathy in patients with advanced CKD.[63] Gadolinium-based contrast studies have shown that over two thirds of patients have left ventricular hypertrophy with preserved systolic volume and function, which is associated with diffuse myocardial fibrosis. Left ventricular dilation and impaired systolic function were observed in another 15% of patients, but, by contrast, this was associated strongly with traditional atherosclerotic risk factors and a higher burden of coronary artery disease on angiography.[63] However, the recognition of gadolinium-induced nephrogenic systemic fibrosis has meant such studies can no longer be conducted until a safer contrast agent is identified.

MYOCARDIAL FIBROSIS

In the longer term, excess myocyte work leads to cell death and interstitial cardiac fibrosis.[59] Such maladaptive changes may be exacerbated by ischemia. Even in the absence of occlusive coronary artery lesions, there may be a reduction in capillary density to hypertrophied cardiac myocytes, which exacerbates local hypoxia.[64] Furthermore, stiffening of conduit arteries leads to a fall in diastolic pressure, which in turn may compromise coronary artery perfusion during diastole. Finally, it is possible that repetitive myocardial ischemia induced by hemodialysis exacerbates myocyte injury.[65] A mismatch in oxygen supply and demand to the myocardium might explain the well-recognized clinical observation that patients receiving dialysis are prone to develop angina, even in the absence of occlusive lesions in the major epicardial coronary arteries (i.e., "demand ischemia").[66]

An alternative explanation for the changes described earlier is that patients develop a distinct uremic cardiomyopathy, defined as a primary disease of cardiac muscle associated with CKD and causing systolic dysfunction.[67] Characteristic histologic changes include interstitial myocardial fibrosis. Such pathologic changes may occur early in the course of CKD[68] and could be the result of metabolic changes, rather than a response to changes in left ventricular geometry.[69]

CHANGES TO LEFT VENTRICULAR FUNCTION

In the early stages of left ventricular remodeling, indices of systolic function may be preserved by the Starling mechanism and increased sympathetic activity.[59] However, in the longer term, impaired myocardial contractility ensues, together with a reduction in ejection fraction (or systolic dysfunction). Echocardiographic studies suggest that systolic dysfunction is present in approximately 20% of patients on maintenance dialysis.[70] The disease is clinically silent in the early stages, but in due course patients may develop symptoms suggestive of congestive cardiac failure. Furthermore, symptoms may result from diastolic dysfunction (see later) in patients with a well-preserved ejection fraction.[71] Severe systolic dysfunction may lead to a fall in systolic blood pressure in a previously hypertensive patient, a phenomenon that may help to explain the association between lower systolic pressure and mortality in patients undergoing dialysis (see the "Blood Pressure" section under "Does Kidney Disease Cause Cardiovascular Disease?").[72] Observational studies suggest that systolic dysfunction improves following successful kidney transplantation, even in patients with severe disease.[73] Thus, the practice of excluding such individuals from transplant waiting lists should be questioned, particularly if prolonged dialysis or CKD exacerbates myocardial dysfunction.[74]

The histologic changes to the myocardium described earlier undoubtedly contribute to diastolic dysfunction, which is characterized by impaired ventricular relaxation and reduced ventricular compliance. Compared to systolic dysfunction, diastolic dysfunction is more likely to lead to clinical manifestations—typically heart failure. A patient with a stiff left ventricle may be particularly sensitive to tachyarrhythmia (e.g., atrial fibrillation) or an increase in intravascular volume and pulmonary edema, while intravascular volume depletion results in reduced ventricular filling (with a risk for syncope) and hemodynamic instability on dialysis.[75] Diastolic dysfunction is more common than systolic dysfunction in patients undergoing dialysis, being present in approximately 50% of prevalent patients,[76] and may be associated with an even worse prognosis than systolic dysfunction.[77]

VALVULAR DISEASES

Calcification of the mitral and/or aortic valve is four times more common in patients receiving dialysis than in matched controls and is associated with increased intima-media thickening and arterial calcification, perhaps suggesting a common pathogenic mechanism.[60] Consequences of valvular calcification include acceleration of aortic sclerosis (and possible progression to symptomatic aortic stenosis and consequent pressure overload of the left ventricle)[78] and incompetence of the mitral valve (exacerbated by left ventricular dilation), which further contributes to volume overload of the left ventricle.

DYSRHYTHMIA

CKD is associated with impaired intracardiac conduction, manifest as prolongation of the PQ and QRS intervals.[79] In critically ill patients[80] and infarct survivors[81] an eGFR of less than 60 mL/min/1.73 m^2 has been consistently associated with 2- to 3-fold increases in the risk for arrhythmias such as atrial fibrillation, ventricular tachycardia, and ventricular fibrillation. The contribution that these abnormalities make to the increased risk for sudden death among patients undergoing dialysis and after transplantation is not known.

Most of the studies of electrophysiology in patients with CKD have been conducted in the population receiving hemodialysis and therefore represent one extreme of the CKD phenotype. Hemodialysis is associated with particular risk factors that are known to trigger dysrhythmias, such as large changes in extravascular volume and rapid electrolyte shifts.[82] The excess of deaths around the first dialysis session of the week (i.e., after the typical longer interdialytic interval) also suggest these hemodialysis-specific factors are important,[83] but perhaps not generalizable to other patients with CKD. However, other findings in this population do suggest that features associated with CKD per se, such as the presence of autonomic neuropathy and reduced heart rate variability,[84,85] predispose to dysrhythmias.

Atrial fibrillation is also more common among patients with CKD.[86,87] The development of atrial fibrillation can reduce cardiac output in patients with left ventricular hypertrophy (who may rely on atrial contraction to fill the left ventricle). Furthermore, CKD is also a risk factor for thromboembolic complications of atrial fibrillation.[88] However, there is uncertainty about anticoagulation because the absolute excess of bleeding events is larger, so the risk/benefit balance is unproven. Furthermore, synthesis of matrix Gla protein (an important endogenous calcification inhibitor) is vitamin K dependent; thus, vitamin K antagonists may lead to excess vascular calcification.[87]

CLINICAL MANIFESTATIONS OF CARDIOVASCULAR DISEASE IN CHRONIC KIDNEY DISEASE

Whereas coronary artery disease explains over half of cardiovascular mortality in the general population,[89] studies have shown that coronary artery disease accounts for less than one fifth of cardiovascular mortality in patients undergoing dialysis.[90-92] At some point, therefore, in the natural history of CKD, nonatherosclerotic cardiovascular disease evolves to become the dominant pathologic process.

As GFR falls there is an increasing burden of arterial stiffness and structural heart disease.[56,61,93] The clinical picture in patients with structural heart disease but normal kidney function includes heart failure, arrhythmias, and sudden cardiac death (SCD).[94] Similar syndromes are also observed in patients with advanced CKD. Data from the United States suggest that the annual incidence of SCD in the CKD population is 2.8%, which is five times that in the general population.[95] In the U.S. dialysis population, SCD accounts for over half of all cardiac mortality.[95,96] Strategies that target nonatherosclerotic disease are required, and randomized trials of these should be a high priority.

Although atherosclerotic disease may account for a smaller proportion of cardiovascular events among persons with advanced CKD, the absolute risk for atherosclerotic events is high: the risk for myocardial infarction among such patients is around 2% to 3% per annum.[90,91] Strategies that target atherosclerotic disease may therefore be effective at reducing the burden of cardiovascular disease in advanced CKD.[95]

EPIDEMIOLOGY OF CARDIOVASCULAR DISEASE IN CHRONIC KIDNEY DISEASE

Although the association between CKD and cardiovascular disease first became apparent from observations in young patients undergoing dialysis, it is now recognized that the increased risk starts much earlier in the natural history of CKD.

ASSOCIATION BETWEEN KIDNEY FUNCTION AND CARDIOVASCULAR DISEASE

Numerous studies have shown that there is an inverse association between kidney function (at least as measured by GFR or an estimate thereof) and cardiovascular risk.[8,97-103] Studies that have assessed the relation between kidney function and cardiovascular risk generally fall into three categories: community-based prospective epidemiologic studies, observational data from randomized controlled trials, and analyses of health care management databases. Despite differences in the populations studied and adjustment for confounding variables, the results are surprisingly consistent. A meta-analysis of 19 creatinine-based studies (including over 160,000 events) has shown that for each 20 mL/min/1.73 m² reduction in eGFR, the risk for major vascular events (which includes both nonfatal and fatal events) increases by approximately 50% (hazard ratio [HR], 1.49; 95% CI, 1.38 to 1.61).[104]

The Chronic Kidney Disease Prognosis Consortium combined the results of 19 studies in the general population.[9] After adjustment for age, sex, ethnicity, diabetes, blood pressure, total cholesterol level, smoking, and history of cardiovascular disease, lower eGFR was associated with an increased risk for death from any cardiovascular cause as compared to the reference group (eGFR 90 to 104 mL/min/1.73 m²) (Figure 56.3).

However, very few of the available studies have sought to assess the nature of any associations between reduced eGFR and *particular types* of cardiac events, such as coronary artery disease, heart failure, and cardiac arrhythmia. A community-based prospective study from Iceland demonstrated an inverse relation between eGFR and coronary artery disease specifically, but few participants had CKD, and if present it was mild (mean eGFR in CKD group 58.7 mL/min/1.73 m²).[103] Such information will be essential if we are to develop a better understanding of the reasons why reduced kidney function is associated with an excess risk for the aggregate of deaths from any cardiovascular cause.

ASSOCIATION BETWEEN ALBUMINURIA AND CARDIOVASCULAR DISEASE

Data from the Chronic Kidney Disease Prognosis Consortium indicate that among persons without known kidney disease, a higher level of albuminuria is associated with an increased risk for cardiovascular disease, and there is no apparent threshold below which lower albuminuria is not associated with lower risk.[9] In another meta-analysis of 26 cohorts with over 7000 coronary events, there was a continuous association between the degree of albuminuria and risk for coronary artery disease.[105] Compared to "normal" levels of albuminuria (i.e., < 2.5 mg/mmol in men or < 3.5 mg/mmol in women), microalbuminuria (i.e., < 30 mg/mmol) was associated with a 50% increase in risk for coronary artery disease (HR, 1.47; 95% CI, 1.30 to 1.66) and macroalbuminuria (≥30 mg/mmol) was independently associated with a doubling of risk (HR, 2.17; 95% CI, 1.87 to 2.52). The association between albuminuria and cardiovascular risk appears to be independent of GFR.[9,10,106]

Since leakage of albumin into the extravascular space may occur due to endothelial dysfunction, it has been suggested that some albuminuria may represent a renal manifestation of progressive, diffuse arterial disease.[107,108] If true, this could imply that some or all of the observed association between albuminuria and cardiovascular disease is attributable to residual "confounding by disease," in which unmeasured vascular disease (manifest as endothelial dysfunction) is both a cause of albuminuria and of cardiovascular events. Since available treatments that reduce albumin leakage also exert other salutary effects on cardiovascular risk, it is unlikely that the multiple benefits of these therapies could be disentangled. It therefore remains unclear whether reducing albuminuria per se will reduce the risk for vascular

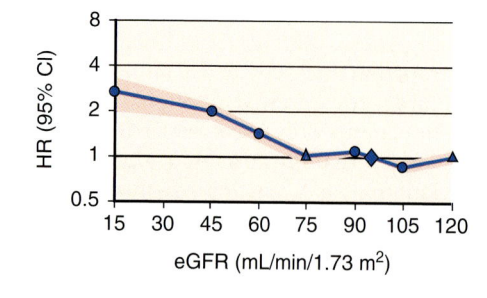

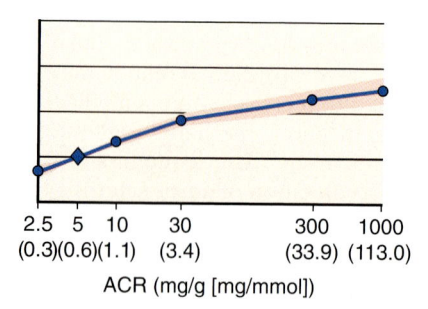

Figure 56.3 Association between estimated glomerular filtration rate (eGFR) (*left*) and albuminuria (*right*) and cardiovascular mortality. This meta-analysis included data from 1,234,182 participants in 21 cohorts from the general population. Albumin to creatinine ratio (ACR) was available from 14 studies of 105,872 participants. *Diamonds* represent reference group (eGFR 95 mL/min/1.73 m² and ACR 5 mg/g [0.6 mg/mmol], respectively); *circles* represent statistically significant; and *triangles* represent not significant. CI, Confidence interval; HR, hazard ratio. (From Matsushita K, van der Velde M, Astor BC, et al: Association of estimated glomerular filtration rate and albuminuria with all-cause and cardiovascular mortality in general population cohorts: a collaborative meta-analysis. *Lancet* 375:2073-2081, 2010.)

disease. Indeed, trials of more-intensive versus less-intensive albuminuria reduction strategies (such as adding angiotensin-converting enzyme or direct renin inhibitors to angiotensin receptor blockers) have not shown additional cardiovascular protection (although their statistical power to do so was limited).[109,110]

DOES KIDNEY DISEASE CAUSE CARDIOVASCULAR DISEASE?

As described in earlier chapters, the kidneys are responsible for a wide variety of physiologic processes including clearance of metabolic waste products, salt and water balance, blood pressure regulation, and hormone production. Even mild kidney disease has direct effects on the regulation of these processes and could therefore potentially lead to disturbed function and metabolism in other systems, including the cardiovascular system. It is of considerable interest therefore to consider to what extent the excess risk for cardiovascular disease in CKD could be explained by such disturbances.

In this section and the next, we suggest a framework for considering the evolution of cardiovascular risk in CKD, as illustrated in Figure 56.4. We consider two main types of risk factors:

1. *Direct risk factors* (e.g., hypertension) that arise as a direct consequence of kidney damage and are associated with one or more types of cardiovascular disease (this section) (Table 56.2)
2. *Indirect risk factors* (e.g., diabetes mellitus, obesity) that cause both kidney disease and one or more types of cardiovascular disease

In general, observational studies of particular risk factors among persons with kidney disease may not provide quantitatively reliable information about any associations that might exist because of the difficulty of adjusting for confounding by disease, also known as "reverse causality".[15] For example, reduced left ventricular function among patients undergoing dialysis may lead to lower blood pressure, yielding an apparent association between lower blood pressure and cardiovascular mortality which is not one of cause and effect.[15] Paradoxically, therefore, it may be more appropriate to rely chiefly on epidemiologic studies performed in nonrenal populations when assessing the potential relevance of particular risk factors to the etiology of the various types of cardiovascular disease observed in CKD.

BLOOD PRESSURE

The kidney is centrally involved in blood pressure regulation. Even relatively mild kidney damage can raise blood pressure, mediated by salt and water retention (and hence intravascular volume expansion), sympathetic overactivity, activation of the renin angiotensin aldosterone system and accumulation of endogenous vasopressors.[111] In turn, hypertension can damage the kidneys further, leading to a vicious cycle of rising blood pressure (with arterial hyalinosis and vascular stiffening) and declining GFR. Evidence from kidney donors (who are selected for being healthy and in particular having preserved kidney function) suggests that a 10 mL/min reduction in GFR leads directly (i.e., causally) to a 5 mm Hg increase in systolic blood pressure (which may be an underestimate because elevations in blood pressure are likely to be treated in this population).[106]

Hypertension is strongly associated with several different types of cardiovascular disease in the general population. Prospective epidemiologic studies have indicated that there is a log-linear association between higher blood pressure and an increased risk for coronary artery disease, ischemic and hemorrhagic stroke, and congestive heart failure. The Prospective Studies Collaboration showed in a meta-analysis of 61 prospective studies (which included a total of 1,000,000 adults without prior cardiovascular disease with roughly 56,000 cardiovascular deaths) that a prolonged 20 mm Hg increment in usual systolic blood pressure was associated with a more than twofold higher risk for stroke-related death, and a twofold higher risk for death due to coronary artery disease and of death due to heart failure.[112]

That these associations are causal has been established reliably by randomized trials showing that lowering systolic blood pressure reduces the risk for stroke, coronary artery disease, and other cardiovascular diseases, with every 5 mm Hg reduction associated with a reduction of approximately one fifth in risk.[113] The results are broadly similar for different classes of antihypertensive treatment, although there is some evidence to suggest that inhibitors of the renin angiotensin aldosterone system may have particularly beneficial effects on the risk for heart failure.[114]

Since hypertension appears very early in the natural history of CKD, a patient who has progressed to stage 3 CKD will generally have been exposed to a prolonged increase in blood pressure, which, depending on the degree of treatment received, would be expected to contribute substantially to his or her subsequent risk for both nonatherosclerotic and atherosclerotic cardiovascular disease. For example, a 5 mm Hg difference resulting from a mild reduction in GFR (e.g., from 90 to 80 mL/min) could translate into an increase of approximately one quarter for the risk for stroke death and one fifth for the risks of coronary artery disease–associated death and other cardiovascular death. These relative risks may be substantially larger in younger individuals (in whom the association between blood pressure and cardiovascular death is stronger than in older individuals).[112]

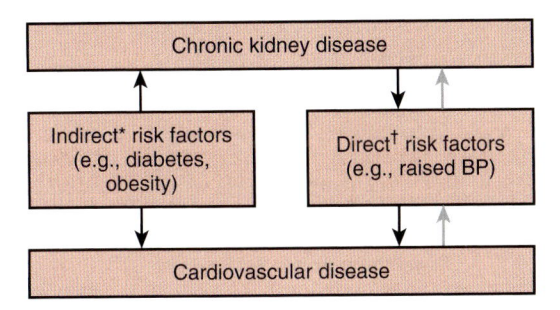

Figure 56.4 The relationship between chronic kidney disease and cardiovascular disease mediated by direct and indirect risk factors. *Indirect risk factors are those that cause both renal disease and one or more types of cardiovascular disease. †Direct risk factors are those that arise as a direct consequence of kidney damage and are associated with one or more types of cardiovascular disease. BP, Blood pressure.

Table 56.2 Direct Risk Factors Linking Chronic Kidney Disease and Cardiovascular Disease

Risk Factor	Estimated Change for Each 10 mL/min/1.73 m² lower eGFR*	Approximate Stage of CKD at Which Abnormality Manifests	Approximate Relative Risk†	Causal?	Comment
Coronary Artery Disease					
Systolic blood pressure	↑5 mm Hg	1-2	1.2	Yes	Reliable data from large-scale observational studies[112] and RCTs[113] support causal relationship.
HDL cholesterol	↓0.2-0.4 mmol/L	3	1.2	Possible	Large-scale observational studies support inverse association with coronary disease.[120] Genetic studies and randomized trials inconclusive.
Lipoprotein (a)	↑0.2-0.4 µmol/L	3	<1.5	Possible	Genetic studies support causal association with coronary disease.[128] Requires confirmation in trials.
Phosphate	↑0.3 mmol/L	3b-4	1.4	Possible	Observational studies in general population[158] suggest possible causal link. Requires confirmation in trials.
PTH	↑3 pmol/L	3	1.3	Possible	Observational studies in general population suggest possible causal link.[177,187]
Anemia	↓0.2-0.5 g/dL	3b-4	—	No	RCTs in CKD population do not show that correcting anemia improves cardiac outcomes.[188]
Homocysteine	↑0.5 µmol/L	3	<1.5	No	RCTs do not demonstrate reduced CHD risk with reduction in homocysteine.[149]
Congestive Heart Failure					
Systolic blood pressure	↑5 mm Hg	1	1.2	Yes	Reliable data from large-scale observational studies[112] and RCTs[113] support causal relationship.
Phosphate	↑0.3 mmol/L	3b-4	1.4	Possible	Observational studies in general population[158] suggest possible causal link. Requires confirmation in trials.
PTH	↑3 pmol/L	3	1.3	Possible	Observational studies in general population suggest possible causal link.[177,187]
Anemia	↓0.2-0.5 g/dL	3b-4	—	No	Although observational data support link between anemia and structural heart disease,[135] randomized trials do not show that correcting anemia improves cardiac outcomes.[188]
FGF-23	↑10-30 RU/mL	1-2	<1.5	Possible	Supportive experimental and observational data in CKD and general population.[168]
Stroke					
Systolic blood pressure	↑5 mm Hg	1-2	1.3	Yes	Reliable data from large-scale observational studies[112] and RCTs[113] support causal relationship.
HDL cholesterol	↓0.2-0.4 mmol/L	3	1.1	Possible	Weak inverse association in observational studies.[120]
Phosphate	↑0.3 mmol/L	3b-4	1.4	Possible	Observational studies in general population[158] suggest possible causal link.
Anemia	↓0.2-0.5 g/dL	3b-4	—	No	No supportive observational data in general population.[189] RCTs in CKD population suggest that correcting anemia with ESA may *cause* stroke.[190]
Homocysteine	↑0.5 µmol/L	3	<1.5	No	RCTs do not demonstrate reduced stroke risk with reduction in homocysteine.[149]

The table shows typical differences in risk factors for coronary artery disease, stroke, and congestive heart failure between patients with mild renal impairment and middle-aged healthy general population.

*See text for justification of change in risk factor assumed. Relative risk estimated from observational studies (where available) of association between long-term exposure to risk factor and outcome. Estimates for congestive heart failure based on data for coronary artery disease if specific data not available.

†Associated with change in risk factor induced by 10 mL/min reduction in GFR.

CHD, Coronary heart disease; CKD, chronic kidney disease; eGFR, estimated glomerular filtration rate; ESA, erythropoietin-stimulating agent; FGF-23, fibroblast growth factor 23; HDL, high-density lipoprotein; PTH, parathyroid hormone; RCT, randomized controlled trial; RU, rat unit.

DYSLIPIDEMIA

The characteristic lipid profile resulting from impaired kidney function beyond approximately stage 3 CKD is an accumulation of partially catabolized triglyceride-rich very low-density lipoprotein and intermediate-density lipoprotein, leading to an elevated serum triglyceride concentration, with lower high-density lipoprotein (HDL) cholesterol concentrations. Low-density lipoprotein (LDL) cholesterol concentration in CKD is similar to or lower than the population average, except that nephrotic-range proteinuria leads to an increase in LDL cholesterol level.[115] Cholesterol continues to be progressively removed from these particles and triacylglycerol is added, leading to an excess of small dense LDL particles that may be more atherogenic.[116] HDL function may also be impaired in CKD.[117] In addition, lipoprotein (a) (Lp[a]) concentrations are increased in association with CKD (and, again, this abnormality is a direct result of impaired kidney function since it can be normalized by kidney transplantation).[118,119]

Based on what is known from epidemiologic studies in persons without CKD, it remains unclear whether the typical dyslipidemia seen in CKD would be expected to result in a large increase in the risk for atherosclerotic events in patients with (nonnephrotic) CKD. Although it is clear from epidemiologic studies[89,120] and large-scale randomized trials[121] that elevated LDL cholesterol level is a contributing cause of atherosclerotic events, the observed incidence of atherosclerotic events in CKD cannot be caused chiefly by increased LDL cholesterol concentrations because such an abnormality occurs in a minority of patients, usually in association with severe proteinuria. Similarly, it is unlikely that hypertriglyceridemia contributes much to an increase in the risk for atherosclerotic events, since a meta-analysis of prospective studies has shown that, once proper adjustment is made for HDL cholesterol level and other confounders, there is no clear association between higher triglyceride levels and atherosclerotic events such as myocardial infarction and ischemic stroke.[120]

On the other hand, HDL cholesterol level is generally reduced in CKD. In one study, for example, patients on hemodialysis had a mean HDL cholesterol level of 0.89 mmol/L compared to 1.4 mmol/L in healthy controls.[122] Prospective studies have shown that a 0.4-mmol/L (15-mg/dL) higher HDL cholesterol level is associated with a one-fifth reduction in coronary events (HR, 0.78; 95% CI, 0.74 to 0.82),[120] while the association with ischemic stroke is less clear.[120,123] However, trials of drugs that can raise HDL cholesterol level have so far not shown clear benefit, and genetic studies have also been inconclusive.[124-127] Thus, it remains unclear whether reduced HDL cholesterol level is of causal relevance in either the general or the CKD population.

It is also possible that elevated Lp(a) level might contribute to an increase in risk. Modest reductions in GFR are associated with an increase of 0.2 to 0.4 µmol/L in Lp(a) concentrations,[118] and genetic data strongly suggest that there is a causal association between Lp(a) concentration and coronary artery disease in the general population.[128] However, it is difficult to predict the effect of CKD-induced changes in Lp(a) concentration because the distribution is very skewed and very dependent on the subpopulation of patients with CKD being studied.[119]

In summary, it is unclear whether the dyslipidemia typically found in association with CKD contributes materially to the excess risk for atherosclerotic cardiovascular disease that is observed in CKD. However, in the general population, reducing LDL cholesterol level reduces the risk for atherosclerotic events even among people with average or low LDL cholesterol levels,[121] and this strategy has also proven effective in reducing atherosclerotic risk in CKD (see the "Reduction of Low-density Lipoprotein Cholesterol Level" section under "Cardiovascular Risk Prevention").

OTHER DIRECT RISK FACTORS

In addition to increased blood pressure, which has an established association with cardiovascular disease in the general population, several other metabolic disturbances caused by kidney disease may contribute to some of the increased risk for cardiovascular disease.

COAGULATION DEFECTS

CKD is associated with raised fibrinogen concentrations, which in turn would increase plasma viscosity and modulate coagulation in a procoagulant direction.[129,130] CKD also increases factor VIII and von Willebrand factor concentrations.[131] Although increases in fibrinogen concentrations are not well characterized in CKD, a 1-g/L increase in fibrinogen concentration has been reported in one study.[131] Epidemiologic studies in the general population suggest that, after adjustment for potential confounders, such an increase is associated with a 1.8-fold excess risk for coronary disease, stroke, and other cardiovascular events.[132] However, the lack of an association between genetic variants that determine fibrinogen concentrations and cardiovascular risk make it less plausible that raised fibrinogen concentration itself is a cause of atherosclerotic disease, so the relevance of any such increase in CKD is uncertain.[133]

ANEMIA

Anemia in CKD is caused by a combination of factors that include erythropoietin deficiency, functional iron deficiency, and chronic inflammation (see Chapter 57). The effects of chronic anemia on the cardiovascular system are not well studied in the general population because anemia is generally associated with disease. In CKD, however, anemia is associated with left ventricular hypertrophy. In one study a 0.5-g/dL lower hemoglobin concentration was associated with a 30% higher frequency of increased left ventricular mass (defined as 20% greater than baseline),[134] while in another study of patients undergoing dialysis each 1-g/dL decrease in hemoglobin level was associated with a 50% increased risk for left ventricular dilation and a 25% increased risk for cardiac failure.[135]

Although some small nonrandomized studies have suggested that partial correction of anemia reduces left ventricular mass index in patients with CKD,[136,137] randomized trials have not shown that complete correction of anemia (compared to partial correction) leads to a reduction in left ventricular mass.[138-140] It is therefore unclear whether anemia is a cause of structural heart disease in CKD, but, since it does not appear until a significant amount of kidney function is lost (e.g., eGFR below approximately 40 mL/min/1.73 m^2),[141] it seems unlikely that it could contribute substantially to the excess risk for cardiovascular disease observed among those with higher eGFR. The results of randomized trials of treatments to increase hemoglobin concentration that involved assessment of cardiovascular end points are discussed later in the "Correction of Anemia" section.

HOMOCYSTEINE

The observation that homocystinuria (which results in a very large increase in plasma homocysteine concentrations) is associated with premature cardiovascular disease led to interest in whether more moderate increases in homocysteine might be associated with an increased risk for coronary artery disease.[142] Homocysteine concentrations have a strong inverse association with GFR, and, since they are reduced by kidney transplantation, the rise in homocysteine concentration is a direct result of impaired kidney function.[143] However, the mechanism(s) underlying hyperhomocysteinemia in CKD are complex and not fully understood. They are not attributable to reduced clearance, because renal homocysteine excretion accounts for less than 1% of its elimination, so they must instead involve metabolic disturbances in remethylation and transsulfuration pathways.[144] Moderate reductions in GFR are associated with a 5-μmol/L increase in total plasma homocysteine concentration.[145]

A meta-analysis of prospective observational studies showed that a 25% lower than usual homocysteine concentration (approximately 3 μmol/L) was associated with an 11% lower risk for coronary disease and a 19% lower risk for stroke.[146] The earliest genetic studies of mutations in the methylenetetrahydrofolate reductase gene (MTHFR) appeared consistent with this association being causal,[147] but subsequent meta-analysis of all available genetic data has indicated that such an association is unlikely to reflect causality.[148] Large-scale randomized trials of folate and B vitamins, which reduce plasma homocysteine concentration, have also failed to demonstrate a benefit of lowering homocysteine concentration (see the "Homocysteine" section under "Cardiovascular Risk Prevention").[149-151]

CHRONIC KIDNEY DISEASE–MINERAL BONE DISORDER

Impaired kidney function causes a complex disorder of calcium and phosphate metabolism, including effects on vitamin D and parathyroid hormone (PTH) (see Chapter 55 for a detailed description), which becomes especially marked after stage 3b CKD. Since such abnormalities are uncommon in persons without CKD, the information we have available to us is derived mostly from observational studies conducted in patients with CKD, which, because of the likelihood of residual confounding, severely limits their interpretation.

Phosphate

Serum phosphate concentrations rise once the kidney's ability to excrete the dietary phosphate load is exceeded.[141] Multiple homeostatic processes are in place to maintain serum phosphorus concentrations in the normal range despite diminished excretion with impaired kidney function, and hence a serum phosphate concentration within the reference range does not necessarily imply normal phosphate metabolism.[152] Higher serum phosphate concentrations are associated with increased vascular stiffness[153,154] and calcification,[155,156] perhaps because hyperphosphatemia can induce vascular smooth muscle cells to develop an osteoblastic phenotype.[157] Such vascular stiffness could plausibly increase the risk for structural heart disease and thereby for heart failure and cardiac arrhythmias.[71]

At least within the range of concentrations observed in the general population there is an association between higher serum phosphate concentration and increased risk for cardiovascular events and mortality.[158,159] In the Framingham Offspring Study, for example, a 1-mg/dL (0.32-mmol/L) increment in serum phosphate concentration was associated with an increase in the risk for cardiovascular disease (namely, coronary artery disease, stroke, peripheral arterial disease, or heart failure) of approximately one third (HR, 1.30; 95% CI, 1.05 to 1.63) after adjustment for conventional cardiovascular risk factors and eGFR.[158] However, there were too few events to allow the association with heart failure to be assessed separately from typical atherosclerosis-related events.

Randomized trials of treatments that lower serum phosphate concentration (such as phosphate binders) are required to determine whether hyperphosphatemia, or the counterregulatory processes that are activated in CKD, are causally related to cardiovascular disease. The issue is complicated by the possibility of adverse effects of calcium-containing phosphate binders, which may contribute to vascular calcification by inducing a positive calcium balance, which results in deposition of calcium in the vasculature rather than bone.[160]

Fibroblast Growth Factor 23

Fibroblast growth factor 23 (FGF-23) concentrations rise earlier in CKD than the serum concentrations of phosphate or even PTH[161] and help maintain a normal serum phosphate concentration via a phosphaturic effect. The association of FGF-23 with mortality was first demonstrated in patients undergoing maintenance hemodialysis,[162] and since then, other studies have found associations between FGF-23 concentrations and subsequent all-cause and cardiovascular mortality in patients with CKD.[163-165] More recently, FGF-23 was studied in a population without prior cardiovascular disease and over 10 years' follow-up; in this study it was again independently associated with all-cause mortality (HR per doubling, 1.25; 95% CI, 1.14 to 1.36) and incident heart failure events (697 events; HR, 1.41; 95% CI, 1.23 to 1.61) but not incident atherosclerotic events (797 events; HR, 1.12; 95%, CI 0.98 to 1.29).[166]

Unlike phosphate concentrations, serum FGF-23 concentrations do not correlate with arterial calcification.[167] Experimentally FGF-23 has been shown to induce left ventricular hypertrophy in the absence of its coreceptor Klotho; furthermore, FGF-23 and left ventricular mass are positively associated among patients with CKD and those with normal renal function.[168,169] Assuming these associations are causal, the biologic mechanisms linking FGF-23 with cardiovascular diseases may be different from those for serum phosphate.

Vitamin D

As discussed in more detail in Chapter 55, vitamin D is activated (via 1α-hydroxylation) by the kidney, and therefore fully active 1,25-dihydroxyvitamin D concentrations decline early in the progression of CKD.[141,170] In addition, rising FGF-23 concentrations also inhibit activation of vitamin D. There is also an association between "native" vitamin D (usually measured as 25-hydroxyvitamin D) concentration and GFR.[170] However, this may reflect poorer nutrition in patients with chronic disease. Vitamin D deficiency (and subsequent hypocalcemia) removes negative feedback from the parathyroid glands, and PTH concentrations therefore rise as GFR falls.[141]

Some observational studies in the general population have suggested that there is an inverse association between 25-hydroxyvitamin D concentrations and subsequent cardiovascular events, whereas others have not.[171] A meta-analysis demonstrated inverse associations between 25-hydroxyvitamin D and all-cause mortality (and its components, including vascular, cancer, and other nonvascular causes).[172] Randomized trials of vitamin D supplementation in the general population have not demonstrated a reduction in cardiovascular events.[171] However, it is possible that these trials used doses of vitamin D that were too low to induce a potent enough effect. Some studies have suggested that vitamin D deficiency predisposes patients to diabetes mellitus and raises blood pressure, but again these data are not conclusive.[171] It is unclear whether disturbed vitamin D metabolism could plausibly contribute to the observed excess risk for cardiovascular disease in CKD.

Parathyroid Hormone

PTH concentrations rise as a direct result of declining GFR early in the progression of CKD; secondary hyperparathyroidism (sHPT) can be found in one fifth of patients with CKD stage 1 or 2.[141] PTH level rises because of lack of negative feedback from declining 1,25-hydroxyvitamin D and calcium concentrations and rising concentrations of serum phosphate (even within the population reference range). PTH has been implicated in atherogenesis (and in calcification of atherosclerotic lesions) and also in modifying cardiac fibrosis in animal models.[173,174] There are case reports of improved myocardial metabolism and structure after parathyroidectomy, suggesting that high concentrations of PTH may damage the heart.[175] There does not appear to be a clear association between PTH and all-cause and cardiovascular mortality in patients with CKD.[176] However, studies in the general population (which may be less prone to confounding) have suggested that there is an independent association between elevated PTH concentrations and both fatal and nonfatal cardiovascular disease.[177] A meta-analysis of 12 such studies showed that the risk for cardiovascular disease was 50% (HR, 1.50; 95% CI, 1.18 to 1.92) higher among patients in the groups with highest PTH concentration compared to those in the lowest.[177]

OXIDATIVE STRESS AND INFLAMMATION

Oxidative stress is defined as tissue injury resulting from an excess of oxidant compounds and is important in protecting against infection and tissue repair. Oxidative stress leads to a reduction in nitric oxide bioavailability and thus to endothelial dysfunction[178] and may also contribute to left ventricular remodeling and fibrosis, and oxidation of lipoproteins.[179] CKD is associated with oxidative stress,[180] although precise quantification is difficult. In the general population, dietary intake or plasma concentrations of antioxidant vitamins (vitamins A [β-carotene], C, and E) are inversely related to cardiovascular disease incidence and mortality,[181] but randomized trials of antioxidant treatments indicate that, at least in the doses studied, use of these drugs does not reduce the risk for cardiovascular disease.[182]

Patients with CKD have increased measures of inflammation compared to age- and sex-matched controls.[129] Genetic data from the general population suggest that inflammation is causally associated with coronary disease, although the mechanism remains unclear.[183,184] Trials of antiinflammatory therapies are ongoing in the general population, which will help to clarify the potential utility of such therapies in CKD.[185,186]

INDIRECT RISK FACTORS: CAUSES OF BOTH KIDNEY AND CARDIOVASCULAR DISEASE

DIABETES MELLITUS

Diabetes mellitus is a common disease that affects approximately 150 million people worldwide. The overall prevalence is increasing—driven in part by a rise in the prevalence of obesity and an aging population—and it has been estimated that there will be over 300 million persons globally with type 2 diabetes by 2025.[191]

Diabetic nephropathy is caused by glycation of structural proteins within the kidney, beginning with the glomerular basement membrane but later causing mesangial and interstitial matrix expansion (see Chapter 39). Approximately 40% of patients new to dialysis in the United States have diabetic nephropathy, and diabetes mellitus is present as a comorbid illness in an additional 10% of patients (in other words, diabetes mellitus is present but is thought not to be the primary cause of ESKD).[95] Strict glycemic control and blood pressure control (with renin angiotensin aldosterone system inhibitors) both appear to retard the progression (and perhaps development) of diabetic nephropathy.[192-196] Patients with diabetes (either type 1 or type 2) are at increased risk for mortality, and approximately two thirds of deaths can be attributed to cardiovascular causes.[197] Prospective data from a meta-analysis of 102 studies with information on fatal and nonfatal outcomes demonstrated that the presence of diabetes mellitus doubled the risk for coronary heart disease (HR, 2.00; 95% CI, 1.83 to 2.19).[198] The risk for ischemic stroke was increased by approximately half (HR, 1.56; 95% CI, 1.56 to 2.09), hemorrhagic stroke by around four fifths (HR, 1.84; 95% CI, 1.54 to 2.13), and other vascular deaths (including heart failure) by approximately three quarters (HR, 1.73; 95% CI, 1.51 to 1.98). These estimates were not significantly affected by adjustment for traditional cardiovascular risk factors (e.g., lipids and blood pressure) but were also unaffected by adjustment for kidney function.[198] Among patients with CKD, therefore, the presence of diabetes mellitus seems likely to contribute additional risk over and above any risk arising from direct risk factors associated with impaired kidney function (see Figure 56.4).

OBESITY

In the general population, observational studies have shown that obesity is associated with an increased risk for cardiovascular disease above a body mass index (BMI) of 25 kg/m², with each 5 kg/m² associated with an increase in risk for cardiovascular mortality of approximately 40% (HR, 1.41; 95% CI, 1.37 to 1.45).[199] This association is probably causal and mediated by the known adverse effects of adiposity on blood pressure, lipoproteins, and glucose intolerance.

Obesity is also known to increase the risk for death from nonneoplastic kidney disease by approximately 60% (HR, 1.59; 95% CI, 1.27 to 1.99) per 5 kg/m² above a BMI of 25 kg/m².[199] A systematic review indicates that, as compared to a BMI between 18 and 25 kg/m², being overweight (BMI ≥ 25 < 30 kg/m²) is associated with a 40% (HR, 1.40; 95% CI, 1.30 to 1.50) increase in the risk for kidney disease, while being obese (BMI ≥ 30 kg/m²) is associated with an 80% increased risk (HR, 1.83; 1.57 to 2.13).[200] This association may be mediated by effects on blood pressure and diabetes, but kidney biopsies of overweight individuals (without diabetes or hypertension) can show typical signs of hyperfiltration, a known cause of premature decline in kidney function.[201] Furthermore, weight loss can reduce blood pressure and proteinuria.[202]

CARDIOVASCULAR RISK PREDICTION

Risk prediction models in the CKD population are desirable because they may help to target therapies to those most at risk. Most people with stage 4 or 5 CKD are at high risk for atherosclerotic disease and so would be suitable candidates for effective treatments, but at earlier stages of CKD the risk for cardiovascular events may be lower, and so models are needed to assess whom to treat. Models that involve demographic variables (e.g., age and sex), basic clinical measurements (e.g., blood pressure, anthropometric measurements), and simple blood and urine biomarkers (e.g., lipid fractions, albuminuria) have now been developed, and there are also versions that incorporate imaging or other measurements (such as pulse wave velocity).

BASIC RISK PREDICTION SCORES

Equations have been developed in the general population that can be used to predict cardiovascular events based on knowledge of a few basic parameters. For example, the Framingham risk score requires knowledge of the patient's age, sex, smoking status, total and HDL cholesterol levels, and systolic blood pressure.[203,204] However, such equations are inaccurate and generally underestimate the incidence of cardiovascular events in patients with CKD.[205]

ROLE OF ESTIMATED GLOMERULAR FILTRATION RATE IN RISK PREDICTION

Estimated GFR equations were developed to assess kidney function without the need for invasive direct measurements. Since their introduction the association between eGFR and cardiovascular risk has been the subject of much research. The most widely used filtration marker is creatinine, but its inadequacies in terms of measuring kidney function are well recognized (including dependence on muscle mass and significant tubular secretion at low GFR). However, nonrenal determinants of creatinine and other filtration markers such as cystatin C may improve cardiovascular risk prediction,[206] as they incorporate information on other cardiovascular risk factors such as diabetes mellitus.[207] Indeed, combining filtration markers may provide better risk prediction.[208]

USE OF IMAGING AND OTHER ASSESSMENTS OF CARDIOVASCULAR FUNCTION IN RISK PREDICTION

Blood markers of myocardial damage and dysfunction, such as cardiac troponin and brain ("B-type") natriuretic peptide, strongly predict cardiovascular risk among patients with CKD,[209] including those undergoing dialysis.[210,211] Furthermore, numerous studies have demonstrated that echocardiographic measures can provide useful prognostic information. This includes both static measures (e.g., left ventricular mass) and dynamic measures (dobutamine stress echocardiography). For example, left ventricular mass predicts mortality in patients undergoing dialysis,[67,212-214] and the presence of systolic dysfunction can provide further information.[215] Echocardiography is therefore recommended for routine use in patients undergoing dialysis,[216] but its additional value over more simple risk stratification tools has not been studied in detail.

CIMT has been used in the general population to predict risk for cardiovascular events, but variation in the technique used makes comparison of studies difficult. Although CIMT appears to predict risk for coronary and cerebrovascular events in the general population, it does not appear to provide additional prognostic information to a standard score such as that derived from the Framingham equation.[217] In the CKD population it is unclear whether CIMT provides independent prognostic information: one study of 203 Chinese patients with stage 3 or 4 CKD found that CIMT was independently associated with outcome,[218] whereas another study of 315 patients with stage 4 or 5 CKD did not find this relation.[34]

Vascular calcification can also be assessed using x-ray–based methods, and its presence is independently associated with subsequent cardiovascular events.[219,220] However, in the general population the value of coronary calcification scores is uncertain because they may not usefully add information to traditional scores.[221] The incremental predictive value of calcium scoring has not been studied in detail in CKD populations. Similarly, the functional equivalent of calcification (i.e., vascular stiffness) independently predicts risk for subsequent cardiovascular events in some studies,[34] but the method used may be important (see "Arterial Stiffening" section).

The purpose of risk prediction is to identify a high-risk group of patients who will benefit most from interventions. It is important to note that treatment decisions should not be based solely on the risk factor that will be modified by the treatment in question. For example, decisions on whether to lower LDL cholesterol level should not be based on measured LDL cholesterol level, but rather on a holistic risk assessment that considers all available data. Treatment decisions based on single risk factors would lead to the undertreatment of the highest-risk patients. The next section will discuss the available evidence from randomized trials of treatments for cardiovascular disease in the CKD population.

CARDIOVASCULAR RISK PREVENTION

In general, individual treatments for the prevention of cardiovascular events are at best only moderately effective, yielding relative risk reductions of at most a quarter, and so the detection of such effects can only be reliably achieved through large-scale randomized trials.[222] Observational studies are prone to at least moderate biases that may obscure or mimic treatment effects.[223] Since the pathophysiology of cardiovascular disease may be qualitatively different once patients reach stages 3 to 5 CKD, with a higher proportion of events attributable to structural heart disease, extrapolation of the results of trials conducted in the general population may not be appropriate. It is necessary therefore to consider what information is available from subgroup analysis of large trials, as well as from trials conducted exclusively among patients with CKD, before determining whether to extrapolate results obtained in studies in the general population to patients with varying stages of CKD.

SMOKING CESSATION

In the general population, cigarette smoking is associated with an increased risk for cardiovascular disease,[224] and the beneficial effects of smoking cessation provide strong evidence that the association is one of cause and effect.[204,225] Substantial numbers of patients with CKD smoke tobacco,[226,227] and data demonstrate that the hazards are similar in patients with CKD to the general population.[228] As a consequence, the *absolute* excess cardiovascular (and noncardiovascular) risks attributable to smoking are likely to be greater in smokers with CKD than in similarly aged smokers without CKD, and therefore the potential benefits of cessation are substantial.

BLOOD PRESSURE REDUCTION

Among persons without CKD, randomized trials have shown clearly that lowering blood pressure reduces the risk for subsequent cardiovascular events.[113] Although there may be subtle differences in efficacy among different antihypertensive regimens, the major determinant of benefit is the absolute magnitude of any blood pressure reduction that is achieved.[114] After standardizing for the amount of blood pressure reduction, the relative reduction in risk appears to be approximately independent of the initial blood pressure level, suggesting that antihypertensive treatments will reduce the risk for cardiovascular events in people even without obviously elevated blood pressure, but who are at increased risk for other reasons.[229]

Information about the effects of lowering blood pressure among persons with CKD stages 1 to 3 is available from trials conducted largely in people without known kidney disease. For example, the Perindopril Protection Against Recurrent Stroke Study (PROGRESS) included 1757 participants with stage 3 or higher CKD among the 6105 participants with prior cerebrovascular disease who had been enrolled.[230] Assignment to active therapy was associated with a 35% reduction in the risk for stroke in subjects with CKD (HR, 0.65; 95% CI, 0.50 to 0.83), which was similar to the risk reduction observed in the whole study population. Because subjects with CKD had a higher background risk for cardiovascular events, the absolute treatment effect was 1.7-fold greater than for patients without CKD.[231] Similarly, in a post hoc analysis of the Heart Outcomes and Prevention Evaluation (HOPE) study, 980 patients with impaired kidney function (serum creatinine level > 124 μmol/L or 1.4 mg/dL) were studied,[232] and the proportional reduction in cardiovascular death, myocardial infarction, and stroke resulting from allocation to ramipril 10 mg daily was similar in patients with impaired kidney function and those without (HR, 0.79 versus HR, 0.80, $P > 0.2$ for heterogeneity). An individual patient data meta-analysis of 26 trials, which included 152,290 participants, showed that the benefits of reducing blood pressure among patients with eGFR of less than 60 mL/min/1.73 m^2 were similar to those among patients with higher eGFR.[233] However, most participants with CKD had stage 3a, and only 1% of participants had eGFR of less than 30 mL/min/1.73 m^2.

Less information is available about the effects of lowering blood pressure on cardiovascular outcomes among patients with more advanced CKD, with most studies involving CKD stages 3b to 5 and primarily assessing kidney end points. The Irbesartan Diabetic Nephropathy Trial compared the effects of irbesartan 300 mg daily, amlodipine 10 mg daily, and placebo among 1715 subjects with type 2 diabetes mellitus and serum creatinine level 1.0 to 3.0 mg/dL in women and 1.2 to 3.0 mg/dL in men, principally to assess the effects of each regimen on CKD progression. Irbesartan was shown to be effective at preventing the composite kidney outcome of doubling of serum creatinine level, dialysis, or death.[195] However, neither irbesartan nor amlodipine was superior to placebo in preventing the composite cardiovascular outcome of cardiovascular death, myocardial infarction, congestive heart failure, stroke, or coronary revascularization, despite a 6/3 mm Hg reduction in blood pressure in the irbesartan group and a 4/3 mm Hg reduction in the amlodipine group.[195] Similarly, the Reduction in Endpoints in NIDDM with the Angiotensin II Antagonist Losartan (RENAAL) study failed to demonstrate a reduction in cardiovascular morbidity and mortality (defined as myocardial infarction, stroke, first hospitalization for unstable angina or heart failure, arterial revascularization, or cardiovascular death).[196] Both of these studies had limited power for detecting moderate effects on cardiovascular outcomes, but additional information on the effects of lowering blood pressure among people with advanced CKD is available from meta-analyses of trials conducted exclusively among patients undergoing dialysis, with one including a total of 1202 patients from five trials[234] and the other, 1679 patients from eight trials.[235] Both analyses concluded that blood pressure lowering–therapy reduced cardiovascular event rates and cardiovascular death in patients receiving dialysis when compared to controls. In the more complete meta-analysis, a reduction of 4 to 5 mm Hg in mean systolic and 2 to 3 mm Hg in diastolic blood pressure was associated with a 29% reduction in both cardiovascular events and cardiovascular mortality when compared to control regimens (HR, 0.71; 95% CI,

0.55 to 0.92),[235] which is comparable to the effect that would be expected from a blood pressure reduction of this magnitude in the general population.

Although a number of randomized controlled trials of blood pressure lowering–interventions have been conducted in kidney transplant recipients, these have almost exclusively examined transplant-related outcomes such as graft loss, change in GFR, and proteinuria and have not assessed cardiovascular end points.[236]

Thus, based on our present knowledge, it is sensible to treat hypertension in patients with CKD, although there is still much to be learned about the optimal timing of blood pressure measurements, the thresholds for treatment, and the safest method to achieve the largest possible reduction in blood pressure.[237] Older guidelines, including those published by the U.S. National Kidney Foundation, recommend a target blood pressure of less than 130/80 mm Hg in patients with CKD.[238] However, since there are few studies that have addressed the optimal blood pressure goal in CKD, this target is largely based on data from other high-risk groups, such as patients with diabetes mellitus or congestive heart failure. A systematic review of 11 trials that assessed different targets in patients with advanced CKD suggests that achieving a blood pressure of less than 140/90 mm Hg may be adequate in patients without proteinuria with no additional outcome benefits associated with tighter blood pressure control.[239] The results of the Action to Control Cardiovascular Risk in Diabetes (ACCORD) blood pressure trial,[240] in which few patients with CKD were enrolled, did not identify a significant benefit on a cardiovascular composite outcome when targeting systolic blood pressure to 120 mm Hg rather than 140 mm Hg, although there was a significant reduction in the risk for stroke (a secondary outcome) and an increased risk for adverse effects with the 120 mm Hg target. That trial lacked statistical power, however, and an ongoing trial (the Systolic Blood Pressure Intervention Trial [SPRINT]) is comparing the same systolic blood pressure targets (120 versus 140 mm Hg) in approximately 9300 patients without diabetes mellitus, polycystic kidney disease, or a history of stroke, approximately 30% of whom have stage 3 CKD.[241] In observational studies, current targets are achieved in fewer than half of CKD patients, possibly in part because more intensive blood pressure control is associated with an increased number of adverse events.[242]

An international guideline published by Kidney Disease: Improving Global Outcomes (KDIGO) in 2012 recommends aiming for a blood pressure of less than 140/90 mm Hg in patients without proteinuria with CKD who are not receiving dialysis.[243] If proteinuria (>3 mg/mmol) is present, the guideline recommends a lower blood pressure target of less than 130/80 mm Hg, although this is based on post hoc analysis and long-term follow-up of cohorts previously randomized to different blood pressure targets. Data from the general population support more intensive blood pressure lowering and suggest that the potential benefits among patients with CKD are substantial. Therefore, the uncertainty surrounding the optimal target should not distract nephrologists from making efforts to reduce blood pressure in patients (especially the very large number of patients with systolic blood pressures well above 140 mm Hg) who frequently are undertreated and therefore left at unnecessary risk.[242]

REDUCTION OF LOW-DENSITY LIPOPROTEIN CHOLESTEROL LEVEL

Other than in the presence of nephrotic-range proteinuria, blood LDL cholesterol concentration is not normally raised in patients with CKD. Nevertheless, randomized trials in the general population have clearly shown that reducing LDL cholesterol level reduces the risk for myocardial infarction or death from coronary artery disease, ischemic stroke, and coronary revascularization even among people with average or low blood cholesterol levels.[121] Therefore, even though dyslipidemia is probably not the main contributor to an increased risk for atherosclerosis in CKD as compared to persons without CKD (see the "Dyslipidemia" section under "Does Kidney Disease Cause Cardiovascular Disease?"), reducing blood LDL cholesterol level may be an effective strategy for reducing such risk, and a number of randomized trials have addressed this hypothesis.

Among persons without established kidney disease, post hoc analyses of randomized trials conducted in the general population have shown that the proportional reduction in the risk for a myocardial infarction or coronary artery disease death, stroke, or coronary revascularization is independent of kidney function.[121] As discussed in the "Epidemiology of Cardiovascular Disease in Chronic Kidney Disease" section, however, by the time patients reach stages 4 and 5 CKD the pathophysiology of cardiovascular disease may have been modified by the "uremic" milieu, and, as well as an increased risk for atherosclerotic events, there is an increased risk for cardiac arrhythmia and heart failure related to arteriosclerosis.

Two randomized trials have examined the effects of lowering LDL cholesterol level with statin therapy on cardiovascular outcomes, specifically among patients receiving dialysis. In the Die Deutsche Diabetes Dialyse Studie (4D) randomized trial of atorvastatin, 20 mg daily versus placebo among 1255 patients on maintenance hemodialysis with type 2 diabetes, lowering LDL cholesterol level by an average of approximately 39 mg/dL (1.0 mmol/L) for a median of 4 years yielded a nonsignificant 8% reduction in the prespecified primary outcome of cardiac death, nonfatal myocardial infarction, or stroke.[91] In A Study to Evaluate the Use of Rosuvastatin in Subjects on Regular Hemodialysis: An Assessment of Survival and Cardiovascular Events (AURORA) randomized trial of rosuvastatin 10 mg daily versus placebo among 2776 patients on maintenance hemodialysis (with and without type 2 diabetes mellitus), lowering LDL cholesterol level by an average of approximately 43 mg/dL (1.1 mmol/L) for a median of 4 years yielded a nonsignificant 4% reduction in the primary outcome of cardiovascular death, nonfatal myocardial infarction, or stroke.[90] A high proportion of cardiac deaths in these trials were not attributable to coronary artery disease, and there was no evidence in either trial of a reduction in the risk for such deaths (Figure 56.5).[90,91] However, although lowering LDL cholesterol level with statin therapy among patients with ESKD did not yield statistically significant reductions in the primary outcomes in these trials, there were promising proportional reductions of 18% (RR, 0.82; 95% CI, 0.68 to 0.99; $P = 0.03$)

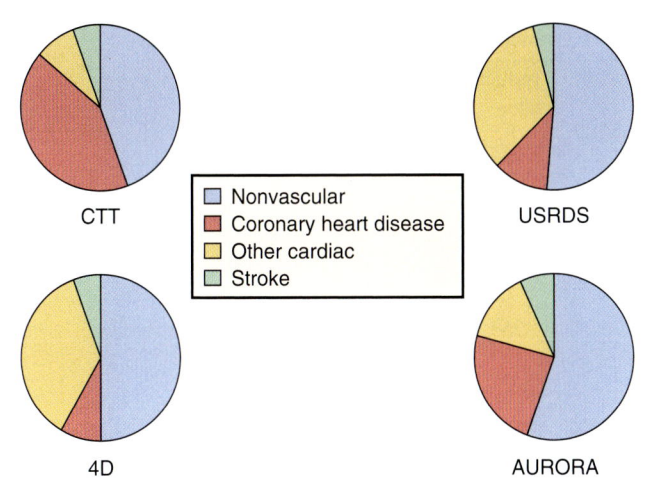

Figure 56.5 Causes of death in individuals with and without end-stage kidney disease. A group of patients without overt kidney disease recruited into trials of statin therapy (Cholesterol Treatment Trialists' Collaboration [CTT][96]) compared to patients with end-stage kidney disease as recorded by the United States Renal Data System (USRDS)[95] or recruited into the Die Deutsche Diabetes Dialyse Studie (4D)[91] or A Study to Evaluate the Use of Rosuvastatin in Subjects on Regular Hemodialysis: An Assessment of Survival and Cardiovascular Events (AURORA).[90] Note the declining contribution of coronary artery disease and increasing proportion of other cardiac disease in the end-stage kidney disease population.

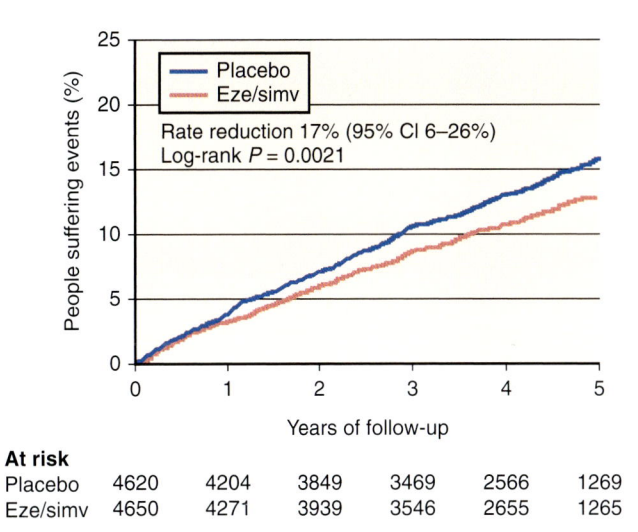

Figure 56.6 Life table plot of effects of allocation to ezetimibe/simvastatin (Eze/simv) on major atherosclerotic events in the Study of Heart and Renal Protection (SHARP).[92] CI, Confidence interval.

in major cardiac events in the 4D trial and of 16% (RR, 0.84; 95% CI, 0.64 to 1.11; $P = 0.2$) in nonfatal myocardial infarction in the AURORA trial.[90,91] These findings raised the possibility of small, but meaningful, proportional benefits on atherosclerotic outcomes among patients receiving dialysis.

Subsequently, the Study of Heart and Renal Protection (SHARP) trial assessed the safety and efficacy of reducing LDL cholesterol level among patients with stages 3 to 5 CKD, including many who were receiving dialysis. In order to achieve an average reduction in LDL cholesterol level of approximately 1 mmol/L without using high statin doses (which are associated with an increased risk for myopathy,[244] especially in patients with impaired renal function[245]), a low dose of a statin (simvastatin 20 mg daily) was combined with a cholesterol-absorption inhibitor[9] (ezetimibe 10 mg daily); the biochemical efficacy and tolerability of this regimen was first confirmed in the United Kingdom Heart and Renal Protection (UK-HARP) pilot studies.[246,247]

Overall, 9270 patients were randomized to ezetimibe/simvastatin versus placebo, and allocation to ezetimibe/simvastatin yielded an average LDL cholesterol level difference of 0.85 mmol/L (with approximately two-thirds adherence) during a median follow-up of 4.9 years, and produced a 17% proportional reduction in major atherosclerotic events (526 [11.3%] ezetimibe/simvastatin versus 619 [13.4%]; RR, 0.83; 95% CI, 0.74 to 0.94; log-rank $P = 0.0021$; Figure 56.6).[92]

There was a nonsignificant reduction in nonfatal myocardial infarction or coronary death (213 [4.6%] versus 230 [5.0%]; RR, 0.92; 95% CI, 0.76 to 1.11; $P = 0.37$), and significant reductions in nonhemorrhagic stroke (131 [2.8%] versus 174 [3.8%]; RR, 0.75; 95% CI, 0.60 to 0.94; $P = 0.01$) and revascularization procedures (284 [6.1%] versus 352 [7.6%]; RR, 0.79; 95% CI, 0.68 to 0.93; $P = 0.0036$). Allocation to ezetimibe/simvastatin was not associated with a significant excess risk for myopathy, hepatitis, or gallstones, and there were no significant excesses of any type of cancer, death from cancer, or death from other noncardiovascular causes.

SHARP did not have sufficient power to assess the effects on major atherosclerotic events separately in the 3000 patients receiving dialysis and 6000 patients not receiving dialysis at baseline, but within the SHARP trial there was no evidence to suggest that the proportional benefit on the composite outcome differed significantly in these two groups of patients. Observational studies have suggested that the association between LDL cholesterol level and coronary disease risk weakens as kidney function worsens,[248] but SHARP found no evidence of a trend toward smaller proportional benefits among patients with lower eGFR.

At first sight, the findings of SHARP might appear to be inconsistent with the findings of 4D and AURORA, as well as the nonsignificant reduction in the primary end point of the Assessment of Lescol in Renal Transplantation (ALERT) trial among kidney transplant recipients.[249] However, the proportional effects on particular cardiovascular outcomes in these three trials and SHARP were statistically compatible for nonfatal myocardial infarction, for nonfatal hemorrhagic stroke, for coronary revascularization (which was not part of the primary outcomes of the 4D and AURORA trials), and for any cardiovascular death (heterogeneity tests all showed a nonsignificant P value) (Figure 56.7).

Moreover, the effects on particular cardiovascular outcomes in these four renal trials were compatible with those observed in the trials of statin therapy in nonrenal populations that were included in the meta-analysis of the Cholesterol Treatment Trialists' Collaboration.[121] Hence, the failure to achieve statistical significance in the previous trials involving patients undergoing dialysis and kidney transplant recipients may derive from both the much smaller number and the much smaller proportion of modifiable cardiovascular events in the respective primary composite outcomes:

	Events (% pa)		
Outcome	Allocated LDL-C reduction	Allocated control	Risk ratio (RR) per mmol/L LDL-C reduction

Outcome	LDL-C reduction events (% pa)	Control events (% pa)	RR (95% CI)
Nonfatal MI			
4D	33 (1.91)	35 (2.02)	
ALERT	54 (1.03)	65 (1.24)	
AURORA	91 (1.97)	107 (2.33)	
SHARP	134 (0.71)	159 (0.85)	
Subtotal: 4 renal trials	312 (1.02)	366 (1.21)	0.83 (0.70–0.98)
23 other trials	3307 (0.97)	4386 (1.29)	0.73 (0.70–0.76)
All trials	**3619 (0.97)**	**4752 (1.29)**	**0.74 (0.70–0.77)**

Heterogeneity between renal trials: $\chi^2_3 = 0.3$ ($P = 0.96$)
Difference between renal and nonrenal trials: $\chi^2_1 = 2.2$ ($P = 0.14$)

Nonfatal nonhemorrhagic stroke			
4D	31 (1.80)	29 (1.67)	
ALERT	51 (0.97)	40 (0.76)	
AURORA	46 (0.99)	39 (0.84)	
SHARP	97 (0.51)	128 (0.68)	
Subtotal: 4 renal trials	225 (0.73)	236 (0.77)	0.95 (0.78–1.17)
23 other trials	1624 (0.48)	2052 (0.61)	0.78 (0.73–0.83)
All trials	**1849 (0.50)**	**2288 (0.62)**	**0.79 (0.74–0.84)**

Heterogeneity between renal trials: $\chi^2_3 = 6.4$ ($P = 0.09$)
Difference between renal and nonrenal trials: $\chi^2_1 = 3.4$ ($P = 0.07$)

Nonfatal hemorrhagic stroke			
4D	2 (0.12)	3 (0.17)	
ALERT	–	–	
AURORA	7 (0.15)	6 (0.13)	
SHARP	19 (0.10)	17 (0.09)	
Subtotal: 4 renal trials	28 (0.11)	26 (0.10)	1.08 (0.60–1.98)
23 other trials	154 (0.05)	136 (0.04)	1.05 (0.83–1.34)
All trials	**182 (0.05)**	**162 (0.04)**	**1.06 (0.85–1.33)**

Heterogeneity between renal trials: $\chi^2_2 = 0.3$ ($P = 0.87$)
Difference between renal and non-renal trials: $\chi^2_1 = 0.0$ ($P = 0.93$)

Coronary revascularization			
4D	55 (3.31)	72 (4.29)	
ALERT	52 (1.00)	60 (1.15)	
AURORA	55 (1.20)	70 (1.53)	
SHARP	149 (0.79)	203 (1.09)	
Subtotal: 4 renal trials	311 (1.02)	405 (1.34)	0.74 (0.63–0.87)
23 other trials	5191 (1.54)	6605 (1.99)	0.75 (0.72–0.78)
All trials	**5502 (1.50)**	**7010 (1.94)**	**0.75 (0.72–0.77)**

Heterogeneity between renal trials: $\chi^2_3 = 0.8$ ($P = 0.85$)
Difference between renal and nonrenal trials: $\chi^2_1 = 0.0$ ($P = 0.91$)

Vascular death			
4D	151 (8.52)	167 (9.36)	
ALERT	66 (1.23)	73 (1.36)	
AURORA	324 (6.87)	324 (6.86)	
SHARP	361 (1.82)	388 (1.97)	
Subtotal: 4 renal trials	902 (2.85)	952 (3.01)	0.94 (0.85–1.04)
23 other trials	3679 (1.05)	4230 (1.21)	0.85 (0.81–0.89)
All trials	**4581 (1.20)**	**5182 (1.36)**	**0.86 (0.83–0.90)**

Heterogeneity between renal trials: $\chi^2_3 = 0.9$ ($P = 0.82$)
Difference between renal and nonrenal trials: $\chi^2_1 = 3.8$ ($P = 0.05$)

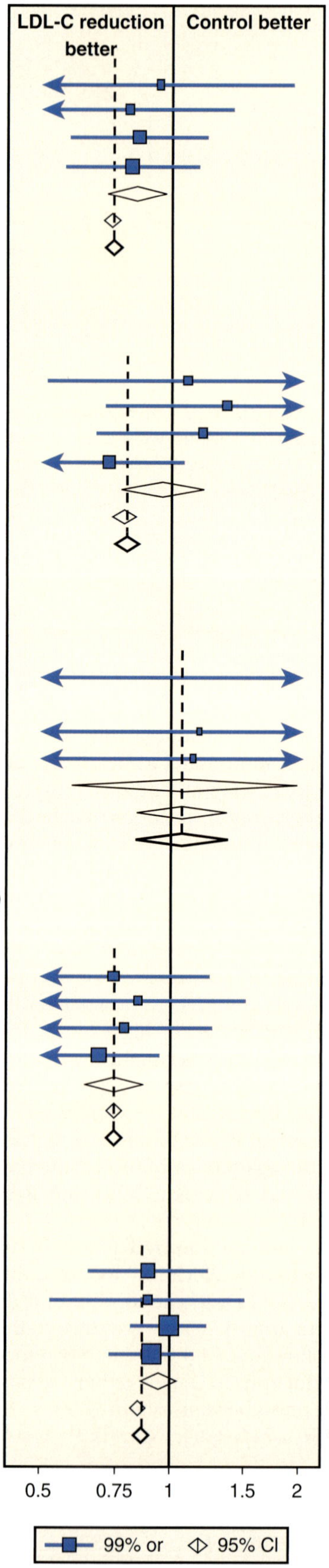

■ 99% or ◇ 95% CI

Figure 56.7 Effects of therapy to lower low-density lipoprotein cholesterol (LDL-C) on particular vascular outcomes in four trials among patients with chronic kidney disease and 23 trials among other types of patients. ALERT, Assessment of Lescol in Renal Transplantation; AURORA, A Study to Evaluate the Use of Rosuvastatin in Subjects on Regular Hemodialysis: An Assessment of Survival and Cardiovascular Events; CI, Confidence interval; 4D, Die Deutsche Diabetes Dialyse Studie; MI, myocardial infarction; SHARP, Study of Heart and Renal Protection.

whereas over half of the primary outcomes in 4D and AURORA were cardiovascular deaths (for which there were nonsignificant benefits), approximately three quarters in SHARP were nonfatal atherosclerotic events (for which there were significant benefits). Several meta-analyses of the effects of statins in patients with CKD have been published since then, and, although all agree there is good evidence of benefit among patients not receiving dialysis, their conclusions differ on the efficacy of statins among patients undergoing dialysis.[250-252] An international guideline published by KDIGO in 2013 recommends using statins or statin-based lipid-lowering regimens in patients with stages 3 to 5 CKD over 50 years of age and in those under 50 years with additional risk factors.[253] However, the guideline does not recommend initiating statin therapy in patients receiving dialysis (although such therapy should be continued if started before dialysis).[253] Even if the relative risk reduction is slightly smaller among patients receiving dialysis, the very high absolute risk among such patients means that even modest relative risk reductions would translate into substantial absolute benefits.

Guidelines have emphasized the importance of treating overall risk rather than individual risk factors.[253,254] Given the safety and current costs of generic statin-based therapy, the risk threshold at which LDL-lowering therapy should be considered has fallen (to 7.5% over 10 years in American guidelines[254]). Although most risk calculators have not been validated in CKD populations, most patients with CKD will have an atherosclerotic risk that warrants treatment, even if their LDL cholesterol level is average or even below average. The potential benefits are substantial and suggest that widespread use of LDL-lowering therapy in patients with CKD would result in a worthwhile reduction in cardiovascular disease complications.

TIGHT GLYCEMIC CONTROL

Among patients without established CKD, strict glycemic control has been shown in randomized trials to reduce the risk for microvascular disease outcomes (including development of albuminuria). In type 1 diabetes, a strategy of more intensive glycemic control reduced the development of microalbuminuria by 39% (95% CI, 21 to 52).[192] In type 2 diabetes the use of a gliclazide-based strategy to reduce hemoglobin A_{1c} (HbA_{1c}) below 6.5% was associated with a reduction in the development of nephropathy (HR, 0.79; 95% CI, 0.66 to 0.93; $P = 0.003$).[193] Individual trials in the general population have not shown a clear benefit in terms of cardiovascular risk reduction with stricter glycemic control in either type 1 or type 2 diabetes, and indeed some have even suggested a hazard.[255] However, a meta-analysis of the available randomized trials supported the hypothesis that stricter glycemic control (with HbA_{1c} lower, on average, by 0.9%) reduces the risk for cardiovascular events (OR, 0.85; 95% CI, 0.77 to 0.93), albeit modestly.[256]

It is very likely that the existing trials included a significant proportion of patients with diabetic kidney disease, but the results among such patients have not been reported as a specific subgroup analysis. Therefore the available data suggest that it would be reasonable to aim for tight glucose control among patients with CKD, but with due regard for the potential hazards of too rapid a reduction in HbA_{1c} and hypoglycemia,[255] as well as the altered pharmacokinetics of hypoglycemic agents in CKD.[257]

CORRECTION OF ANEMIA

Four large trials have assessed the impact on mortality and cardiovascular events of partial or full correction of anemia. The first three of these studies investigated the effect of two different erythropoietin regimens, normalization of hemoglobin level versus partial correction, on cardiovascular outcomes. Only the Trial to Reduce Cardiovascular Events with Aranesp Therapy (TREAT) trial (see later) was placebo controlled.

The first study randomized 1233 patients undergoing hemodialysis with clinical features suggestive of ischemic heart disease or heart failure. The trial was stopped early (after a median follow-up of 14 months) predominantly because of an excess risk for vascular access thrombosis with higher hemoglobin concentrations. At this point, 33% of patients had died or experienced a nonfatal myocardial infarction in the group randomized to a hemoglobin target of 14.0 g/dL as compared to 27% of those randomized to the 10.0 g/dL target (RR, 1.3; 95% CI, 0.9 to 1.9).[258]

Results of the Correction of Hemoglobin and Outcomes in Renal Insufficiency (CHOIR) study, which recruited 1432 patients with CKD not receiving dialysis and naive to erythropoietin-stimulating agent (ESA) therapy, supported this observation. The trial was terminated because patients randomized to achieve a hemoglobin level of 13.5 g/dL were more likely to reach a primary end point (death, myocardial infarction, hospitalization to treat heart failure) than those in the 11.3 g/L target group (HR, 1.34; 95% CI, 1.03 to 1.74).[259] The findings of the Cardiovascular Risk Reduction by Early Anemia Treatment with Epoetin Beta (CREATE) trial conducted among patients with stage 3 or 4 CKD were similar. No benefit was demonstrated for targeting a normal hemoglobin level (13.0 to 15.0 g/dL) compared to a subnormal hemoglobin level (10.5 to 11.5 g/dL), and numerically more cardiovascular events occurred in the normal hemoglobin level group, although the primary composite end points in the two trials differed, as did the distribution of events.[260] It has long been recognized that ESAs can increase blood pressure and blood viscosity (particularly when hemoglobin changes are rapid), and it was predicted over 20 years ago that hemodynamic and rheologic effects may offset cardiovascular benefits of correcting anemia.[261] Thus in TREAT, the first large randomized controlled trial to compare an ESA to placebo, the protocol was designed to avoid rapid changes to hemoglobin concentrations.[190] In this study, 4038 patients with type 2 diabetes, CKD, and anemia received either darbepoietin alfa in an effort to achieve a target hemoglobin level of 13 g/dL or placebo with "rescue" therapy if hemoglobin level fell below 9 g/dL. The primary end point of death or nonfatal cardiovascular event occurred in 31.4% of patients assigned to the active treatment and 29.7% of patients assigned to placebo (HR, 1.05; 95% CI, 0.94 to 1.17). There was a twofold increase in the risk for stroke in darbepoietin alfa–treated group, which was nominally significant (101 versus 53 strokes; HR, 1.92; 95% CI, 1.38 to 2.68).

Taken together, the results of these four key trials do not support the concept that correction of anemia using ESAs reduces cardiovascular risk in patients with CKD—whether receiving or not receiving dialysis.[188] However, the current data do not exclude the possibility that small corrections in hemoglobin level (e.g., fixed low-dose ESAs) are beneficial in the context of CKD. The use of ESAs probably improves health-related quality of life among patients with debilitating symptoms of anemia (although the trials to date are inconclusive on this[188]) and, by reducing transfusion requirements, also reduces the risk for sensitizing potential transplant recipients to nonself HLA antigens (discussed in more detail in Chapters 57 and 71).

REDUCTION OF HOMOCYSTEINE LEVEL

Randomized trials of folate and B vitamins in both the general population and patients with CKD have shown that reducing homocysteine level does not reduce the risk for cardiovascular events.[149] The Homocysteinemia in Kidney and End Stage Renal Disease (HOST) trial randomized 2056 adults with an eGFR of less than 30 mL/min/1.73 m^2 (n = 1305) or ESKD (n = 751) to a regimen of folic acid and B group vitamins or placebo.[262] Despite a 25.5% reduction in plasma homocysteine level, there was no difference in mortality (448 deaths in the treated group versus 436 in the placebo) (HR, 1.04; 95% CI, 0.91 to 1.18), nor was there a reduction in cardiovascular events, including myocardial infarction, stroke, and amputation of the lower extremity, which were all components of the secondary end point.

In addition, the Folic Acid for Vascular Outcome Reduction in Transplantation (FAVORIT) trial randomized 4110 kidney transplant recipients with elevated homocysteine levels and an eGFR of 30 mL/min/1.73 m^2 or greater to either a multivitamin tablet containing folic acid, vitamin B$_6$, and vitamin B$_{12}$ or to a low-dose vitamin B$_6$/B$_{12}$ regimen.[263] Despite the expected reduction in homocysteine levels in the treated group, there was no difference in a composite cardiovascular end point (adjusted HR, 1.0). A meta-analysis of all trials of folic acid in CKD populations found a similar null result.[151] These results are consistent with the totality of evidence in the general population.[149]

CORRECTION OF CHRONIC KIDNEY DISEASE–MINERAL BONE DISORDER

Although interventions aimed at correcting the biochemical and endocrinologic manifestations of CKD-MBD were initially driven by the need to prevent the associated debilitating bone pathologic processes, the suggestion that there might be a link between bone and vascular health in CKD has led to a greater focus on assessing the effects of interventions on cardiovascular outcomes.

REDUCING SERUM PHOSPHATE LEVEL

Numerous observational studies have demonstrated a link between raised serum phosphate level and mortality. However, there have been no placebo-controlled trials investigating the benefits of lowering phosphate level.[264] It is therefore impossible to know whether current guideline recommendations to maintain serum phosphate concentrations below certain targets are beneficial or harmful. Current therapies only reduce serum phosphate modestly, although the effects on phosphate balance (as indicated by changes in urinary phosphate excretion) may be larger than suggested by serum phosphate concentration alone.[265]

The most widely used phosphate binders are calcium based, and there are some data to suggest that their use contributes to vascular calcification. Patients with advanced CKD and ESKD taking calcium-based phosphate binders are in positive calcium balance; only such patients with ample residual kidney function on loop diuretic agents remain in neutral or possibly negative calcium balance. The availability of non–calcium-based phosphate binders (e.g., sevelamer, lanthanum, and newer iron-based compounds) has allowed this hypothesis to be tested, but trials designed to assess whether sevelamer retards the progression of vascular calcification as compared to calcium-based phosphate binders have yielded conflicting results.[160,266-268] A relatively large outcomes trial was fraught with high patient dropout and missing data; while there were some signals indicating potential benefit, results were decidedly inconclusive.[267] It is therefore unclear whether to treat elevated serum phosphorus concentrations and, if so, with what agent and to what target.

Reducing serum phosphate concentrations might be expected to reduce FGF-23 concentrations. However, a randomized trial comparing sevelamer, lanthanum, and calcium-based phosphate binders found that, overall (i.e., data pooling all binders ["active therapy"] versus placebo), reducing serum phosphate concentration by 0.3 mg/dL had no effect on FGF-23 concentration.[265] However, whereas FGF-23 concentration increased in patients assigned calcium-based binders (median increase 28 pg/mL; P = 0.03), it decreased in patients assigned sevelamer (median decrease 24 pg/mL) and was unchanged in patients assigned lanthanum.

Niacin also reduces serum phosphate concentration by approximately 0.4 mg/dL via inhibition of the intestinal sodium-phosphate transporter.[269] However, randomized trials have shown that niacin does not reduce cardiovascular risk despite multiple potentially beneficial effects (lipid modification and blood pressure reduction in addition to effects on phosphate balance) and indeed has a number of harmful effects.[126,270] These trials do not therefore support the use of niacin for reducing serum phosphate concentration or for other indications to reduce cardiovascular risk in CKD or ESKD.

VITAMIN D

1,25-Dihydroxyvitamin D (calcitriol) and its synthetic analogues (collectively termed "active" vitamin D derivatives) have been used to correct vitamin D deficiency in the context of CKD for many years. These compounds replenish calcitriol, which is produced by the kidney and suppress levels of PTH, preventing the development of sHPT.[271] More recently, attention has focused on deficiency of parent vitamin D (usually measured indirectly as 25-hydroxyvitamin D [25(OH)D], the hydroxylated compound produced in the liver). Over 80% of patients with CKD have vitamin D insufficiency or frank deficiency.[272] In patients not receiving dialysis, low levels of 25(OH)D are more strongly associated with progression to ESKD and death than calcitriol (1,25[OH]$_2$D) levels.[273] To date, no trials of vitamin D (in any form) have been designed specifically to investigate clinical outcomes such as fractures, cardiovascular events, or mortality among patients with CKD, and a meta-analysis of 76 randomized trials of vitamin D found that insufficient data were available on cardiovascular outcomes to assess any possible reduction in the risk for such events.[274] Despite observational data suggesting that vitamin D supplementation may be beneficial, there is no randomized trial evidence to support recommending such treatment for the reduction of cardiovascular events among patients with CKD.

CALCIMIMETICS

Calcimimetic treatment reduces serum PTH and calcium concentrations.[275] The Evaluation of Cinacalcet Hydrochloride Therapy to Lower Cardiovascular Events (EVOLVE) trial compared a cinacalcet-based regimen with a non–cinacalcet-based regimen (including a placebo) in 3883 patients receiving hemodialysis with moderate to severe sHPT.[276] The primary composite outcome was time to death, nonfatal myocardial infarction, hospitalization for unstable angina, heart failure, or a peripheral vascular event. In the intention-to-treat analysis, allocation to cinacalcet was associated with a nonsignificant 7% reduction in the primary outcome (HR, 0.93; 95% CI, 0.85 to 1.02; $P = 0.11$).[277] However, the randomization process was only stratified for country and diabetes status, and by chance the two groups were imbalanced for age (median age 55.0 years among those allocated cinacalcet versus 54.0 years among those allocated placebo). After adjustment for age, allocation to cinacalcet was associated with a nominally significant reduction in the primary outcome (HR, 0.88; 95% CI, 0.79 to 0.97; $P = 0.008$) and all-cause mortality alone (HR, 0.86; 95% CI, 0.78 to 0.96; $P = 0.006$).

The treatment effect was similar on all components of the primary outcome and on both vascular and nonvascular mortality. Taking all fatal and nonfatal cardiovascular events combined, randomization to cinacalcet was associated with a 16% (95% CI, 4 to 26) lower hazard of nonatherosclerotic cardiovascular events. While the hazard of atherosclerotic events was also numerically lower in patients randomized to cinacalcet (95% CI, −1 to 24), this difference was not significant. Although derived from post hoc analysis, these data support the hypothesis that mineral bone disease disturbances contribute to nonatherosclerotic cardiovascular disease.

Cinacalcet reduces PTH level in patients with CKD not undergoing dialysis.[278] However, the associated reduction in serum calcium concentration is more marked than in patients receiving dialysis (with 62% of those assigned cinacalcet having a serum calcium concentration of less than 8.4 mg/dL compared to 6% of those assigned placebo), leading to safety concerns that have limited the provision of cinacalcet to patients undergoing dialysis, or rarely to patients with other parathyroid disorders (e.g., parathyroid carcinoma, primary HPT in a patient unsuitable for surgery).[278]

ANTIPLATELET THERAPY

Antiplatelet therapy reduces the risk for occlusive cardiovascular disease among patients at high risk for such disease, and these benefits greatly outweigh any risks for bleeding,[279] but patients with CKD are at increased risk for bleeding,[280] so it is unclear whether the balance of benefit and hazard remains beneficial among such patients. The meta-analysis by the Antithrombotic Trialists' Collaboration of trials of antiplatelet therapy among patients at high risk for occlusive vascular disease included 14 trials conducted among 2632 patients on maintenance hemodialysis after placement of a dialysis graft or fistula. Overall, antiplatelet therapy yielded a 41% proportional reduction in the risk for nonfatal myocardial infarction, nonfatal stroke, or vascular death, which was consistent with the proportional benefit observed among other high-risk patients studied, but there were insufficient data on bleeding risk to assess safety.[279] Based on event rates among patients receiving dialysis in SHARP (and applying the summary risk ratios for aspirin from the meta-analysis by the Antithrombotic Trialists' Collaboration),[281] treating 1000 patients receiving dialysis *with* vascular disease with aspirin for 5 years is projected to cause an additional 19 intracranial bleeds and 53 serious extracranial bleeds. There is, therefore, substantial uncertainty about the relative benefits and harms of antiplatelet therapy in ESKD.

There have been no appropriately sized trials of aspirin with clinical end points in the population with CKD that does not require dialysis. Among patients with early-stage CKD, post hoc analysis of the Hypertension Optimal Treatment trial showed that the benefits of aspirin were similar in the 470 patients with a serum creatinine concentration above 117 µmol/L (1.5 mg/dL) to those with a lower serum creatinine concentration but did not report information on any additional bleeding risks.[282] However, there is very little information about the effects of aspirin on those with more severe CKD. One pilot study has demonstrated that aspirin increases the risk for minor bleeding in patients with CKD, but there was no detectable increase in the risk for major bleeding.[246,279] Randomized trials will be required to evaluate the relative risks and benefits of antiplatelet therapy at different stages of CKD.

CONCLUSIONS

Patients with CKD are at increased risk for both atherosclerotic and nonatherosclerotic heart disease, as well as stroke and peripheral arterial disease. The increased risk for cardiovascular disease begins early in the natural history of CKD, so an understanding of that excess risk should begin with an assessment of the magnitude of any early changes in known causal risk factors. Hypertension seems likely to be the most important such risk factor as its control is disturbed early in the development of CKD. With CKD progression, other abnormalities, including disorders of mineral metabolism (elevated levels of FGF-23 and PTH and altered calcium and phosphate metabolism) appear and may contribute to the rising risk for cardiovascular disease, but there is a lack of evidence about the mechanism by which these processes might occur.

Observational studies of particular risk factors among patients with advanced CKD cannot be expected to produce reliable information, because, as in other sick populations (such as very old patients), the observed associations are distorted by confounding and may yield findings that are misleading. For example, there are numerous observational studies suggesting that cholesterol level is inversely associated with major outcomes among patients receiving dialysis, and yet in the randomized SHARP trial an *unconfounded* assessment of the effects of reducing cholesterol levels has indicated that reducing LDL cholesterol level is beneficial. For many of the risk factors considered in this chapter, whether they are established as causal (e.g., hypertension) or are of uncertain relevance (e.g., disorders of mineral metabolism), there are no adequately powered randomized trials that assess whether currently available (and often widely used) treatments that modify these abnormalities can safely reduce the risk for cardiovascular events. Studies such as SHARP, TREAT, and EVOLVE have shown that international collaboration can yield really large and informative trials, but many more of comparable size are now needed if effective strategies for reducing the risk for cardiovascular disease are to be identified.

Complete reference list available at ExpertConsult.com.

KEY REFERENCES

4. Foley RN, Parfrey PS, Sarnak MJ: Clinical epidemiology of cardiovascular disease in chronic renal disease. *Am J Kidney Dis* 32:S112–S119, 1998.
9. Matsushita K, van der Velde M, Astor BC, et al: Association of estimated glomerular filtration rate and albuminuria with all-cause and cardiovascular mortality in general population cohorts: a collaborative meta-analysis. *Lancet* 375:2073–2081, 2010.
15. Baigent C, Burbury K, Wheeler D: Premature cardiovascular disease in chronic renal failure. *Lancet* 356:147–152, 2000.
42. Vallance P: Importance of asymmetrical dimethylarginine in cardiovascular risk. *Lancet* 358:2096–2097, 2001.
63. Mark PB, Johnston N, Groenning BA, et al: Redefinition of uremic cardiomyopathy by contrast-enhanced cardiac magnetic resonance imaging. *Kidney Int* 69:1839–1845, 2006.
89. Lewington S, Whitlock G, Clarke R, et al: Blood cholesterol and vascular mortality by age, sex, and blood pressure: a meta-analysis of individual data from 61 prospective studies with 55,000 vascular deaths. *Lancet* 370:1829–1839, 2007.
90. Fellstrom BC, Jardine AG, Schmieder RE, et al: Rosuvastatin and cardiovascular events in patients undergoing hemodialysis. *N Engl J Med* 360:1395–1407, 2009.
91. Wanner C, Krane V, Marz W, et al: Atorvastatin in patients with type 2 diabetes mellitus undergoing hemodialysis. *N Engl J Med* 353:238–248, 2005.
92. Baigent C, Landray MJ, Reith C, et al: Randomised trial of the effects of lowering LDL-cholesterol with ezetimibe/simvastatin in patients with chronic kidney disease: the Study of Heart and Renal Protection (SHARP). *Lancet* 377:2181–2192, 2011.
104. Mafham M, Emberson J, Landray MJ, et al: Estimated glomerular filtration rate and the risk of major vascular events and all-cause mortality: a meta-analysis. *PLoS ONE* 6:e25920, 2011.
112. Lewington S, Clarke R, Qizilbash N, et al: Age-specific relevance of usual blood pressure to vascular mortality: a meta-analysis of individual data for one million adults in 61 prospective studies. *Lancet* 360:1903–1913, 2002.
113. Turnbull F: Effects of different blood-pressure-lowering regimens on major cardiovascular events: results of prospectively-designed overviews of randomised trials. *Lancet* 362:1527–1535, 2003.
148. Clarke R, Bennett DA, Parish S, et al: Homocysteine and coronary heart disease: meta-analysis of MTHFR case-control studies, avoiding publication bias. *PLoS Med* 9:e1001177, 2012.
162. Gutierrez OM, Mannstadt M, Isakova T, et al: Fibroblast growth factor 23 and mortality among patients undergoing hemodialysis. *N Engl J Med* 359:584–592, 2008.
176. Palmer SC, Hayen A, Macaskill P, et al: Serum levels of phosphorus, parathyroid hormone, and calcium and risks of death and cardiovascular disease in individuals with chronic kidney disease. *JAMA* 305:1119–1127, 2011.
190. Pfeffer MA, Burdmann EA, Chen CY, et al: A trial of darbepoetin alfa in type 2 diabetes and chronic kidney disease. *N Engl J Med* 361:2019–2032, 2009.
209. Landray MJ, Emberson J, Blackwell L, et al: Prediction of end-stage renal disease and death among people with chronic kidney disease: the Chronic Renal Impairment in Birmingham (CRIB) study. *Am J Kidney Dis* 56:1082–1094, 2010.
222. Collins R, MacMahon S: Reliable assessment of the effects of treatment on mortality and major morbidity. I. Clinical trials. *Lancet* 357:373–380, 2001.
225. Pirie K, Peto R, Reeves GK, et al: The 21st century hazards of smoking and benefits of stopping: a prospective study of one million women in the UK. *Lancet* 381:133–141, 2013.
233. Blood Pressure Lowering Treatment Trialists Collaboration, Ninomiya T, Perkovic V, et al: Blood pressure lowering and major cardiovascular events in people with and without chronic kidney disease: meta-analysis of randomised controlled trials. *BMJ* 347:f5680, 2013.
274. Palmer SC, McGregor DO, Macaskill P, et al: Meta-analysis: vitamin D compounds in chronic kidney disease. *Ann Intern Med* 147:840–853, 2007.
281. Baigent C, Blackwell L, Collins R, et al: Aspirin in the primary and secondary prevention of vascular disease: collaborative meta-analysis of individual participant data from randomised trials. *Lancet* 373:1849–1860, 2009.

Hematologic Aspects of Kidney Disease

57

Carlo Brugnara | Kai-Uwe Eckardt

CHAPTER OUTLINE

ANEMIA OF KIDNEY DISEASE, 1875
Definition and Prevalence of Anemia in Chronic Kidney Disease, 1875
Pathobiology of Anemia in Chronic Kidney Disease, 1878
Anemia of Chronic Kidney Disease, 1884
Association of Anemia with Adverse Outcomes, 1888
Erythrocytosis of Patients with Kidney Disease, 1888
Treatment of Renal Anemia, 1889

DISORDERS OF HEMOSTASIS IN CHRONIC KIDNEY DISEASE, 1904
Bleeding and Chronic Kidney Disease, 1904
Hypercoagulability and Chronic Kidney Disease, 1906
Heparin-Induced Thrombocytopenia, 1909
WHITE CELL FUNCTION IN CHRONIC KIDNEY DISEASE, 1909
Leukocyte (Monocyte) Activation, 1909
Leukocyte Functional Impairment, 1909
Markers of Leukocyte Activation, 1910

ANEMIA OF KIDNEY DISEASE

Reduced erythrocyte mass, or anemia, is one of the regular consequences of chronic kidney disease (CKD) because of the central role played by erythropoietin (EPO) in the regulation of erythropoiesis. Anemia can manifest itself early in the course of CKD, and its severity and prevalence go *pari passu* with the progression of kidney disease. Given the significant effect of severe anemia on quality of life among patients with kidney failure, anemia is considered one of the most clinically significant complications of this disease. Nevertheless, the direct consequences of CKD-related anemia and the degree to which anemia should be corrected in patients with CKD remain controversial.

DEFINITION AND PREVALENCE OF ANEMIA IN CHRONIC KIDNEY DISEASE

Anemia is a state characterized by a reduced mass of red blood cells (RBCs) and hemoglobin (Hgb) concentration in blood, resulting in reduced oxygen-carrying capacity and delivery to the body's tissues and organs.[1-3] Because direct measurements of red cell mass are cumbersome and not readily available, *anemia* is defined as a reduction below the normal range for Hgb concentration and hematocrit (Hct); these values depend on sex, race, and age with an increased prevalence of anemia in the elderly population.[4-7] The definition of anemia is somewhat arbitrary. The World Health Organization (WHO) defines anemia as an Hgb concentration below 13.0 g/dL for adult men and below 12.0 g/dL for adult women.[8] This definition has been adopted in the clinical practice guideline for anemia in CKD developed by Kidney Disease: Improving Global Outcomes (KDIGO),[9] whereas previous guidelines have proposed a slightly higher threshold in men (13.5 g/dL).[10,11] Persons living at higher altitudes are characterized by a larger red blood cell mass and reduced Hgb oxygen affinity, compensatory changes required to maintain tissue oxygen delivery in the reduced ambient oxygen tension at such altitudes.[12-18]

The prevalence of anemia in patients with CKD has been widely studied. In general, anemia is more frequent at lower levels of kidney function, becoming almost universal in end-stage kidney disease (ESKD) (Figures 57.1 and 57.2).[19,20] The prevalence reported in different studies depends on the definition of anemia and the target population. The most useful analyses are those that were community based, avoiding biases inherent in studies of clinic-based populations. Hsu and coworkers studied 12,055 adult ambulatory subjects from health clinics in Boston, using the Cockcroft-Gault equation to estimate creatinine clearance and the Modification of Diet in Renal Disease (MDRD) formula to estimate the glomerular filtration rate (GFR) indexed to body surface area.[21] They found that mean Hct values were progressively lower with creatinine clearance below 60 mL/min in men and below 40 mL/min in women. Moderately severe anemia (Hct < 33%) was present in more than 20% of patients when GFR was below 30 mL/min in women and below 20 mL/min in men.[21] Similar results have been obtained in different populations: In Japan, a study of 54,848 subjects identified an estimated GFR (eGFR)

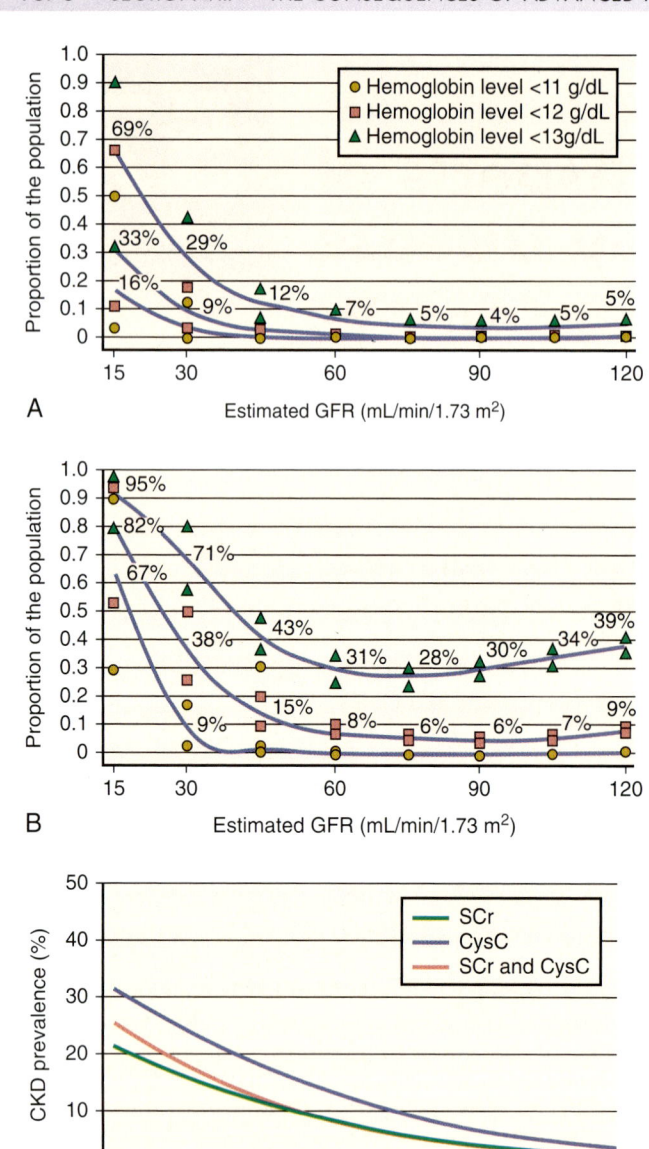

Figure 57.1 Prevalence of hemoglobin (Hgb) level less than 11 g/dL, 12 g/dL, and 13 g/dL among men (**A**) and women (**B**) 20 years and older from the Third National Health and Nutrition Examination Survey (NHANES III) (1988-1994). All values are adjusted to the age of 60 years. **C,** Predicted prevalence of chronic kidney disease (CKD) (defined as estimated glomerular filtration rate [eGFR], 1-59 mL/min/1.73 m²) using different GFR-estimating methods in U.S. adults age 20 years or older by hemoglobin. Estimated GFR are based separately on serum creatinine (SCr), serum cystatin C (CysC), and combined serum creatinine and cystatin C (SCr and CysC). Prevalence curves are truncated when the number of relevant participants is less than 30. (**A** and **B** adapted from Astor B, Muntner P, Levin A, et al: Association of kidney function with anemia. *Arch Intern Med.* 162:1401-1408, 2002; **C** from Estrella MM, Astor BC, Köttgen A, et al: Prevalence of kidney disease in anaemia differs by GFR-estimating method: the Third National Health and Nutrition Examination Survey [1988-94]. *Nephrol Dial Transplant* 25:2542-2548, 2010.)

threshold of 60 mL/min per 1.73 m² for both sexes, below which anemia prevalence increased significantly, and a threshold of 45 mL/min for the association of anemia with complications.[22]

Hsu and coworkers conducted a second study, using the third National Health and Nutrition Examination Survey (NHANES III) (1988-1994) of 15,971 adults aged over 18 years, with measurements of serum creatinine, Hgb, and iron indices. Creatinine clearance was estimated using the Cockcroft-Gault formula.[23] A statistically significant lower mean Hgb was found in men and women with creatinine clearances below 70 mL/min and 50 mL/min, respectively, than in those with creatinine clearances greater than 80 mL/min. However, a mean decrease of 1.0 g/dL was found only for those with creatinine clearances less than 30 mL/min. Astor and colleagues studied the same NHANES III data as Hsu and coworkers but restricted analysis to a different age range, selecting 15,419 participants 20 years and older.[20] Anemia according to the WHO definition was present in 7.3% of all participants (see Figure 57.1). Functional iron deficiency and absolute iron deficiency were found to be important predictors of anemia.[20] Another study on the same dataset showed that Hgb values below 11 g/dL were present in 42.2% of subjects with eGFRs below 30 mL/min/1.73 m² and in 3.5% of subjects with eGFRs between 30 and 60 mL/min/1.73 m² (MDRD formula).[24] Stauffer and Fan, using the 2007-2008 and 2009-2010 NHANES dataset, estimated that 14.0% of the U.S. adult population had CKD, with anemia having a twofold greater prevalence in CKD than in the general population (15.4% vs. 7.65%).[25]

The worldwide prevalence of anemia associated with CKD rose from 1990 to 2010, and CKD is currently the sixth leading cause of anemia in women and the ninth in men worldwide.[26]

Anemia is more common among women and non-Hispanic blacks: In the latter population, the risk for anemia was generally more than twice that in non-Hispanic whites in one study.[23] Another study reported a 3.3-fold higher prevalence of anemia in blacks than in whites, with CKD being less common in anemic blacks than in anemic whites (22% vs. 34%), suggesting a higher prevalence of non–CKD-related anemia as well.[27] The investigators extrapolated the data to the general U.S. population and estimated that approximately 1,590,000 Americans with creatinine clearances less than 50 mL/min are anemic, with Hgb concentrations lower than 12 g/dL.[23] A targeted community-based screening program for CKD has confirmed a threefold higher likelihood of anemia in African Americans than in whites, as well as a twofold higher prevalence of anemia in this higher-risk population than in NHANES population surveys (see Figure 57.2).[28] The same study reported a lower prevalence of anemia in smokers than in nonsmokers (see Figure 57.2), which has been attributed to an enhanced stimulation of erythropoiesis due to relative hypoxia. It has been advocated that the traditionally accepted eGFR threshold of 60 mL/min to define "CKD" should be modified to higher levels in African Americans, in whom metabolic abnormalities and anemia are more common and present at higher eGFR values than in whites.[29] In a large retrospective analysis, anemia was associated equally among African Americans and whites with ESKD.[30] However, in patients on

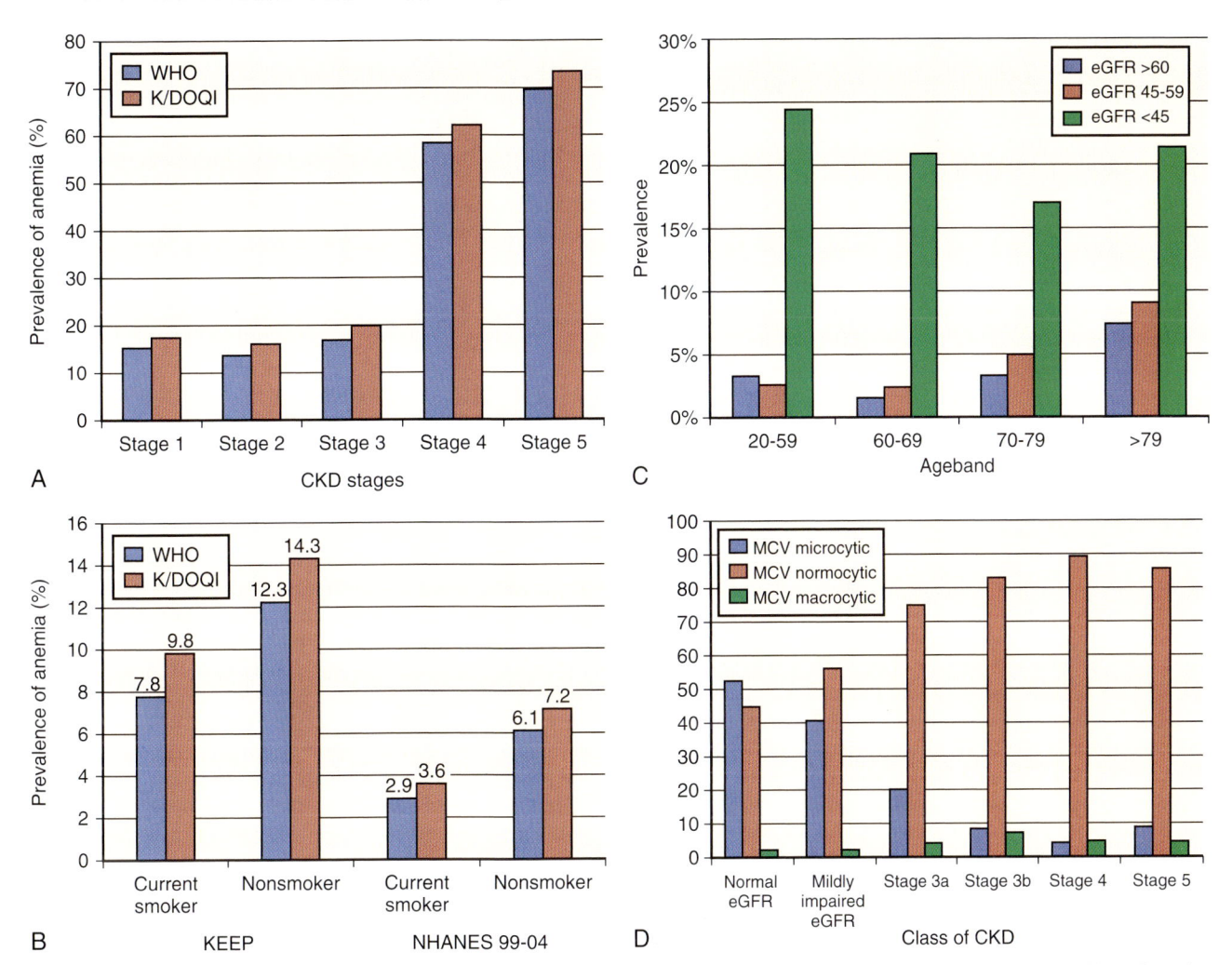

Figure 57.2 **A,** Prevalence of anemia by stage of chronic kidney disease (CKD) in the Kidney Early Evaluation Program (KEEP). **B,** Prevalence of anemia by smoking status. K/DOQI, Kidney Disease Outcomes Quality Initiative; NHANES, National Health and Nutrition Examination Survey; WHO, World Health Organization. **C,** Age-specific prevalence of anemia in CKD according to estimated glomerular filtration rate (eGFR). **D,** Rates of microcytic, normocytic, and macrocytic anemia for each stage of CKD. MCV, Mean corpuscular volume. (**A** and **B** from McFarlane SI, Chen SC, Whaley-Connell AT, et al: Prevalence and associations of anemia of CKD: Kidney Early Evaluation Program [KEEP] and National Health and Nutrition Examination Survey [NHANES] 1999-2004. *Am J Kidney Dis.* 51[Suppl]:S46-S55, 2008; **C** and **D** from Dmitrieva O, de Lusignan S, Macdougall IC, et al: Association of anaemia in primary care patients with chronic kidney disease: cross sectional study of quality improvement in chronic kidney disease [QICKD] trial data. *BMC Nephrol* 14:24, 2013.)

dialysis, the Hgb threshold below which higher mortality rates are observed is higher in African Americans than in whites (11 g/dL vs. 10 g/dL).[31] In any case, observations on race/ethnicity cannot be interpreted in isolation but must take into consideration socioeconomic status as well as cultural and behavioral differences.[32]

For people with eGFRs of 30 to 59 mL/min/1.73 m², low concentrations of 25-hydroxyvitamin D [25(OH)D] and elevations in C-reactive protein (CRP) were independently associated with Hgb concentrations below 12 g/dL.[33] Other studies have also reported an independent association of high-sensitivity CRP results with anemia in patients with eGFRs less than 60 mL/min/m².[34]

Anemia develops earlier in the course of CKD, and its magnitude tends to be more severe, in patients with diabetes mellitus than in patients without diabetes.[7,35-42] El-Achkar and colleagues studied 5380 community-dwelling patients surveyed as part of the Kidney Early Evaluation Program (KEEP), a community-based screening initiative for patients at high risk for kidney disease.[41] Anemia was more prevalent among patients with diabetes and developed earlier than in patients without diabetes mellitus. In patients with CKD stage G3 (GFR 30-59 mL/min), 22.2% of those with diabetes were anemic; in patients with CKD stage G4 (GFR 15-29 mL/min/1.73 m²), the prevalence was 52.4%. The difference among patients with and without diabetes was most prominent in patients with CKD stage G3, in which the prevalence of anemia was nearly threefold greater among those with diabetes. Men with diabetes were particularly prone to anemia, more so than women.

The prevalence of anemia in persons with diabetes and normal kidney function can be as high as 32%, with aggravating factors being advanced age and thiazolidinedione ("glitazone") therapy.[43] Symeonidis and coworkers explored the mechanism for anemia in diabetes by studying 694 anemic individuals, of whom 237 had diabetes.[42] Serum

EPO concentrations were found to be lower in subjects with diabetes, particularly in relation to the degree of anemia present, with a significant inverse correlation between serum EPO and the fraction of glycosylated Hgb. Thomas and associates studied the contribution of proteinuria to anemia among 315 Australian patients with type 1 diabetes.[40] The prevalence of anemia was found to be higher in patients with macroalbuminuria than in those with microalbuminuria or with no albuminuria (52% vs. 24% vs. 8%, respectively). A large study of 79,985 adults with diabetes mellitus showed a higher risk of anemia in black subjects and a lower one in Asian subjects in comparison with white subjects.[44]

With aging, kidney function tends to progressively decline. The interaction of aging and loss of kidney function might be expected to raise the prevalence of anemia. In actuality, the relation is more complex. Men with CKD tend to have higher prevalence of anemia with older age, but among women with CKD, anemia is more frequent at younger ages.[23] It is likely that the high prevalence of iron deficiency in menstruating women accounts for this difference. If analysis is limited to older men and women, the association between older age and anemia is clearer. Ble and colleagues studied 1005 community-living elderly in Italy (InCHIANTI study).[45] The prevalence of anemia was found to increase with age in both sexes. By multivariate analysis, much of the risk for anemia segregated to individuals with creatinine clearance less than 30 mL/min, who also had lower mean serum EPO concentrations. Another InCHIANTI analysis showed that lower than normal total and bioavailable testosterone concentrations resulted in significantly higher risk for development of anemia at 3-year follow-up for both men and women.[46] In a study of 6200 nursing home residents (mostly Caucasian women), prevalences of anemia and CKD were 60% and 43%, respectively.[47] Age was an important determinant of anemia in the absence of CKD, whereas this effect was lost in the presence of CKD, which became the strongest determinant of anemia.[47,48] One third of the anemias found in elderly adults (older than 65 years) may be unexplained, but significant associations are present between anemia and low EPO concentrations and low lymphocyte counts.[49] In this setting, RBC distribution width (RDW) becomes a very powerful predictor of mortality.[50]

Hemoglobin values in patients with advanced CKD are frequently confounded by the use of erythropoiesis-stimulating agents (ESAs; see later) and iron. Although there had been an increase in ESA use before initiation of dialysis and in patients on dialysis in the past, this trend has reversed after publication of the results of randomized controlled trials (RCTs), changes in prescribing instructions, and new guidelines (see later). In fact, there has now been a steady decline in the use of ESAs before initiation of dialysis (Figure 57.3). The Hgb concentration at initiation of dialysis has been declining since 2007, and in half of patients beginning hemodialysis in the United States Hgb is now below 10 g/dL[51]:

Taken together, the findings of the studies discussed previously led to the following conclusions regarding the prevalence of anemia in CKD:

1. Anemia is relatively uncommon in earlier stages (stages G1-3) of CKD.
2. The prevalence of anemia begins to increase significantly with eGFR below 60 mL/minute/1.73 m^2 but anemia is generally not a frequent or severe complication of CKD until GFR is below 30 mL/min × 1.73 m^2.
3. Anemia is a more significant problem for younger women, older men, and African Americans.
4. Anemia occurs earlier in the course of disease and is often more severe among patients with CKD and diabetes mellitus.
5. Screening for anemia (measurement of Hgb) should generally begin at CKD stage G3.

PATHOBIOLOGY OF ANEMIA IN CHRONIC KIDNEY DISEASE

NORMAL ERYTHROPOIESIS

The delivery of oxygen to peripheral tissues is a highly regulated process: A crucially important determinant is red blood cell mass, which is determined by the dynamic balance between the removal of older cells from the circulation and the production of newer cells by the bone marrow. Under normal conditions, approximately 1% of the circulating erythrocytes is replaced daily, corresponding to about 250 billion erythrocytes, with 2.5 to 3.0 million erythrocytes being produced each second.[52] The control of red blood cell mass is based on a classic negative feedback loop mediated by changes in the production of the hormone EPO. EPO is mainly produced in the kidney and regulates the production of erythrocytes by interaction with specific EPO receptors (EPO-R) on bone marrow erythroid progenitors. For this mechanism, to function properly, several other cofactors, like iron, vitamin B_{12} and folic acid, are also required.

Erythropoietin

EPO, the major regulatory hormone of erythrocyte production, is a 30.4-kDa glycoprotein. Its production in the kidney is modulated by the delivery of oxygen from the circulating erythrocytes. When the mass of the circulating erythrocytes decreases, from decreased production, enhanced destruction, or loss of erythrocytes, the reduction in oxygen delivery results in increased production of this hormone. The first recognition of the linkage between hypoxia and erythrocyte quantity arose from astute nineteenth-century observations on the effects of living at higher altitude.[53,54] Carnot and Deflandre first postulated that a humoral factor (a "hemopoietin") might regulate erythropoiesis.[55] They injected serum from anemic rabbits into normal animals, resulting in increased reticulocyte counts, and these investigators termed the circulating factor hematopoietin. However, in retrospect, their observation was probably an artifact, because the amount of serum transferred was too low and attempts to confirm their results were unsuccessful.[56]

Forty-four years later, Reissmann rekindled interest in the field with ingenious experiments in parabiotic rats (i.e., artificial conjoined animals).[57] In this model, rats were joined by skin and muscle, ear to tail, living for 3 months in parabiosis. When one animal breathed air with low oxygen tension and the other breathed normal air, both animals demonstrated increased bone marrow erythropoiesis. This finding provided strong evidence that a humoral factor was

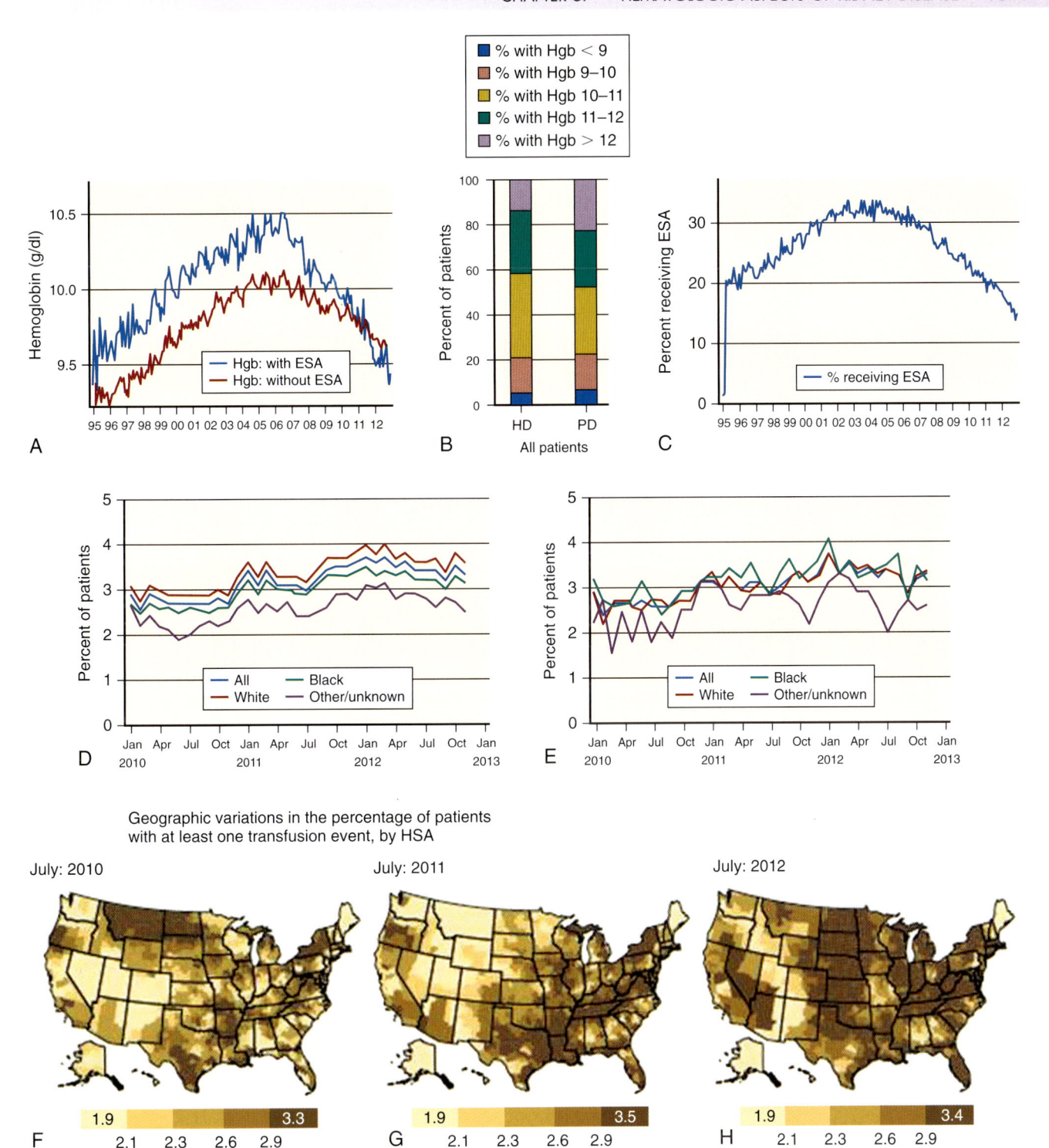

Figure 57.3 Anemia and treatment in end-stage kidney disease (ESKD). **A,** Trend in hemoglobin (Hgb) levels among incident patients with ESKD, 1995-2012. **B,** Clinical indicators: percentage distribution of achieved mean hemoglobin (Hgb) among prevalent patients on hemodialysis (HD) and peritoneal dialysis (PD). **C,** Trend in the percentage of patients who received pre-ESRD erythropoiesis-stimulating agent (ESA) treatment, among incident ESKD patients, 1995-2012. **D,** Percentage of adult patients receiving HD with one or more claims for a red blood cell (RBC) transfusion in a month (from Medicare claims data, by race: monthly time trend from 2010-2012). **E,** Percentage of patients on PD 18 years or older with one or more claims for RBC transfusion in a month (from Medicare claims data, by race: monthly time trend from 2010-2012). **F-H,** Geographic variations in the percentage of patients with at least one transfusion, by Health Service Area (HSA). The ESKD bundled Prospective Payment System (PPS) was implemented in January, 2011, and appears to have directly affected the use of erythropoietin (EPO) and other injectable therapeutics. In 2011 **(G),** for example, the transfusion rate for dialysis patients was 2.9% nationwide and averaged 3.5% in the upper quintile, which included patients residing in Texas, Louisiana, and the eastern third of the country. In 2012 (1 year after implementation of the bundle) **(H),** the likelihood of a transfusion event was far more widespread geographically, averaging 3.0% nationwide and 3.4% in the upper quintile, which included the eastern two thirds of the nation as well as parts of Arizona, Nevada, and California. ESA, Erythropoiesis-stimulating agents. (**A** through **E** from United States Renal Data System: *2014 Annual data report: an overview of the epidemiology of kidney disease in the United States,* Bethesda, MD, 2014, National Institutes of Health, National Institute of Diabetes and Digestive and Kidney Diseases; **F** through **H** from United States Renal Data System: *2013 USRDS annual data report: atlas of chronic kidney disease and end-stage renal disease in the United States,* Bethesda, MD, 2013, National Institutes of Health, National Institute of Diabetes and Digestive and Kidney Diseases.)

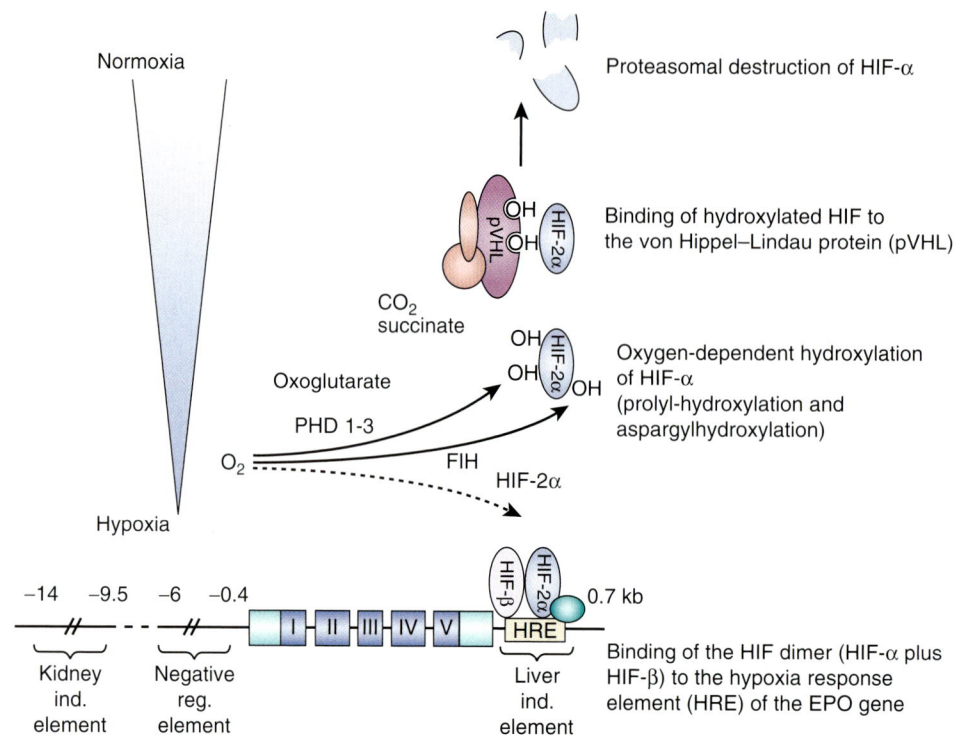

Figure 57.4 Schematic presentation of hypoxia-inducible factor (HIF) signaling and the oxygen-dependent control of erythropoietin (EPO) gene expression. HIF consists of one of two oxygen-dependent α-subunits (HIF-1α and HIF-2α) and a constitutive β-subunit. For EPO regulation, HIF-2α is the relevant isoform. In the presence of oxygen (normoxia), HIF-α is hydroxylated at two prolyl and one asparagyl residues through prolyl-hydroxylases (PHDs 1-3) and an asparagyl-hydroxylase (factor-inhibiting HIF [FIH]), enzymes that require oxoglutarate as a cosubstrate. Hydroxylation of the asparagyl-residue inhibits binding of the transcriptional coactivator p300 and hydroxylation of the prolyl-residues enables binding to the von Hippel–Lindau protein, which represents the recognition component of an E3 ubiquitin ligase. Thus, hydroxylated HIF-α is targeted for proteasomal destruction, and hydroxylated HIF that escapes destruction is not transcriptionally active. Under hypoxia, there is no substrate (oxygen) for the hydroxylation reactions and, thus, HIF-α is stabilized, can bind to hypoxia-responsive elements of its target genes, and can induce or enhance their transcription. The hypoxia response element (HRE) of the EPO gene is located at 5′ of the gene; other regulatory elements determine the tissue specificity of its expression, limiting EPO expression mainly to liver and kidneys. ind., Inducible; reg., regulatory.

the stimulus for erythropoiesis. In 1953, Erslev definitively demonstrated the erythropoietic role of the serum factor, now termed *erythropoietin*.[58] He infused 100 to 200 mL of plasma from bled anemic rabbits into normal rabbit recipients. Reticulocyte count increased rapidly, with a fourfold rise in cell count within 4 days of infusion.[58,59] In 1957, Jacobson and coworkers provided indirect evidence to suggest that the kidneys were the primary source of EPO.[60] After demonstrating that removal of a variety of different organs did not affect EPO production after phlebotomy, they showed that nephrectomized rats and rabbits failed to increase EPO production (incorporation of iron-Fe 59 into erythrocytes) after blood loss.[60] Further studies by Koury and associates and Lacombe and associates demonstrated that the cells responsible for EPO production were peritubular interstitial cells,[61,62] which were subsequently identified as peritubular fibroblasts, located within the renal cortex.[63-65] Although the nature of these cells has still not been fully clarified, they have been suggested to be derived from the neural crest[66] and share characteristics of pericytes.[67]

It has also been shown that with growing severity of anemia, the number of EPO-producing peritubular cells increases. This recruitment was found mostly in the inner cortex but appeared also throughout the renal cortex when the anemia was particularly severe.[68,69] Epo production is regulated by a specific hypoxia-sensing mechanisms that is based on transcription factors stabilized by hypoxia, called *hypoxia-inducible factors* (HIFs, Figure 57.4).[70] This regulatory mechanism is not unique to EPO and is based on the capability of two separate helix-loop-helix components, HIF-α and HIF-β, to bind as a complex to specific hypoxia-responsive DNA elements, which regulate the transcription of hypoxia-inducible genes.[71] The concentrations of the β-subunit do not respond to hypoxia.[72,73] The α-subunits (1α, 2α, and 3α) are produced constitutively but are rapidly degraded in the presence of oxygen by the ubiquitin-proteasome system.[74-78] In hypoxic conditions, degradation of the α-subunits is inhibited, leading to rapid increases in HIF-α concentrations and to the formation of the HIF transcription complex. For EPO regulation HIF-2 appears to be the important HIF isoform.[79-84] Renal HIF-2 is required for hypoxia-driven EPO production; in the absence of renal HIF-2, hepatic HIF-2 becomes the main regulator of EPO production.[70,79] HIF-2α, together with HIF-β, hepatocyte nuclear factor-4 (HNF-4), and p300, binds to a 120–base pair (bp) enhancer located at the 3′ end of the human EPO polyadenylation signal.[52,73,85-87] This interaction results in rapid EPO transcription followed by translation and secretion of the EPO glycoprotein.[88-91]

The rapid degradation of HIF-α in the presence of oxygen depends on binding of the tumor suppressor protein von Hippel–Lindau (VHL), a process that results in tagging of the molecule for proteasomal degradation via polyubiquitination by ubiquitin ligase.[92,93] This regulatory mechanism is based on the hydroxylation of two proline residues, which are critical for the recognition of HIF-α by VHL, and an additional hydroxylation of one asparagine residue is required for HIF binding with p300.[94-98] Hydroxylation at these three sites depends on the presence of oxygen as molecular substrate for specific hydroxylase enzymes, placing these enzymes in a central role for sensing oxygen and detecting hypoxia. A mutation in the VHL protein that impairs the degradation of HIF-α and increases EPO production causes so-called Chuvash congenital polycythemia, an autosomal recessive disorder endemic in the mid–Volga River region.[99] HIF-2α but not HIF-1α displays a typical iron response element (IRE) in its 5′ untranslated region (UTR), which has been shown in mice to constitute an important regulatory loop for HIF-2α messenger RNA (mRNA) translation in the presence of either hypoxia or iron loading.[100] This regulatory system in conditions of reduced iron availability would allow iron response protein 1 (IRP1) to bind with high affinity to IRE, inhibit mRNA translation, and decrease HIF-2α synthesis and EPO production. When cellular iron is abundant, IRP1 loses its RNA-binding activity and becomes a cytosolic aconitase, resulting in de-repression of mRNA translation, which increases both HIF-2α synthesis and EPO production.

Purification and identification of EPO is credited to Miyake and coworkers.[101] From 2550 L of urine from patients with aplastic anemia and using multiple isolation steps, they obtained a small quantity of pure glycoprotein.[101] Purification of human EPO led to successful cloning of the gene, reported in 1985 by Lin and associates.[102] They found that the gene encodes a protein of 193 amino acids, including a 27–amino acid leader sequence and a terminal single amino acid that are cleaved during processing, resulting in a 165–amino acid, mature EPO molecule. When these investigators introduced the gene into Chinese hamster ovary cells, EPO with full biologic activity was produced.[102] These findings were confirmed by an almost simultaneous report by Jacobs and colleagues.[103] These findings led in short order to the development of techniques to produce recombinant human EPO (rhEPO). By 1989, clinical trials of rhEPO had demonstrated its remarkable efficacy,[104-107] leading to regulatory approval and routine clinical use of EPO as replacement treatment.

EPO itself is a member of the family of class 1 cytokines.[108] The carbohydrate moiety is important for molecular stability, whereas the 165–amino acid protein component is critical for receptor binding.[109-111] There are four discrete carbohydrate chains, three N-linked, and one O-linked, each of them having two to four branches, most of which end with a negatively charged sialic acid.[109,112-116] The physiologic role of the carbohydrate chains is complex: They seem to be required for the in vivo biologic activity of EPO but are not essential for in vitro receptor binding or growth stimulation of cells in culture.[117] There is considerable heterogeneity in the glycosylation of EPO, resulting in multiple isoforms with different numbers of sialic acid residues: Isoforms with higher sialic content have a prolonged half-life in the circulation and induce greater stimulation of erythropoiesis despite having a lower affinity for the EPO receptor (EPO-R).[118] A hyperglycosylated recombinant EPO, called novel erythropoiesis-stimulating protein (NESP) or darbepoetin, carries two additional N-linked carbohydrate chains with up to 22 sialic acid residues; the endogenous EPO has a maximum of 14.[119] Despite a lower (approximately fivefold) affinity for the EPO-R, NESP exhibits a halflife in the circulation approximately three times longer than that of EPO.[120,121] Gross and Lodish have developed an in vitro model accounting for the prolonged bioactivity of NESP.[118] They found that NESP and EPO have similar rates of internalization when bound to the EPO-R, with similar degradation and re-secretion, but that EPO dissociates at a much slower rate from the EPO-R than NESP, so more EPO is internalized and degraded.

EPO is produced primarily by the liver in the fetal period; after birth, the kidneys become the major source of production.[63,64,108,122-125] Clearance of circulating EPO occurs by mechanisms that have not yet been fully elucidated. The liver, kidneys, and bone marrow have all been studied as possible sources of EPO elimination. A small fraction of either endogenous or exogenous EPO appears to be cleared by filtration into the urine.[126] EPO degradation products can be found in urine, but the location and mechanisms responsible for this degradation are not known.[113]

An important determinant of the fate of the circulating EPO is its binding to the EPO-R on erythroid cells[127]; the relative abundance of erythroid precursors (i.e., the size of the pool of erythroid progenitors) is known to modulate serum EPO concentrations.[128] The EPO-R is a 55-Da transmembrane protein that belongs to the cytokine receptor superfamily.[129-134] It is present on erythroid progenitors from the colony-forming unit–erythroid (CFU-E) stage to late basophilic erythroblasts.[129] The number of receptors has been estimated to be around 1000 per cell. The molecular signaling cascade activated upon binding of EPO to EPO-R has been studied in great detail. The first event seems to be the homodimerization of the receptor, which also undergoes a conformational change. This is followed by the generation of the intracellular signal by clathrin-mediated endocytosis and proteolysis of the whole ligand-receptor complex, which ultimately determines the clearance of EPO from the circulation.[118,135-140]

Rather than intrinsic enzymatic activity, the EPO-R signal transduction pathway depends on the activation of Janus tyrosine kinases-2 (JAK2), which are physically associated with the receptor and become phosphorylated when the conformation of the receptor is changed by the binding of EPO.[141-148] Activated JAK2 phosphorylates several of the eight tyrosine molecules of the cytoplasmic side of the EPO-R, exposing SH2 (src homology 2) binding sites for key signaling proteins.[149,150] The result is a cascade of signal transduction, with activation of multiple pathways, including Ras/MAP kinase, JNK/p38 MAP kinase, JAK/STAT, the p85 regulatory subunit of phosphoinositide 3-kinase (PI3K), and AKT.[151-156] Both JAK2 and the tyrosines on the cytoplasmic portion of the EPO-R seem to play a role in the internalization process:[157] Familial/genetic forms of polycythemia due to truncations in the EPO-R with absence of key tyrosines such as Y429 and Y431 have been shown to result in defective internalization of the EPO-R complex, prolonged signal transduction, and increased EPO sensitivity.[157] The EPO-R endocytic machinery is critically dependent on a Cbl/p85/epsin-1 pathway, which ultimately leads to receptor downregulation.[158]

The interaction of JAK2 with important intermediaries in signal transduction, STATs (signal transducers and activators of transcription), has been extensively studied. After phosphorylation, STAT5 becomes activated and undergoes homodimerization and may translocate to the nucleus, where it activates EPO-inducible genes.[159] In transgenic mice lacking both STAT5a and STAT5b, fetal anemia develops, with increased apoptosis of erythroid progenitors due to decreased survival of early erythroblasts.[160,161]

The signaling induced by the binding of EPO to the EPO-R eventually results in an increased number of erythroid progenitors and precursors, in particular the CFU-E,[162] and at the same time in the activation of parallel molecular pathways that eventually suppress the signaling of the receptor via tyrosine phosphatases, which dephosphorylate and inactivate JAK2, downregulate the EPO-R on the cell surface, and induce negative regulators such as CIS/SOCS (cytokine-inducible SH2-containing protein/suppressor of cytokine signaling).[163-171]

An important aspect of the overall mechanism of action of EPO has been elucidated by Koury and associates, who demonstrated that EPO does not directly stimulate erythroid proliferation but, rather, prevents the programmed death (apoptosis) of the erythroid progenitors (Figure 57.5).[162,172-174] Burst-forming units–erythroid (BFU-Es), named for their capacity to generate multiclustered colonies of cells, are the earliest cell type exclusively committed to the erythrocyte line.[175] It is believed that these cells

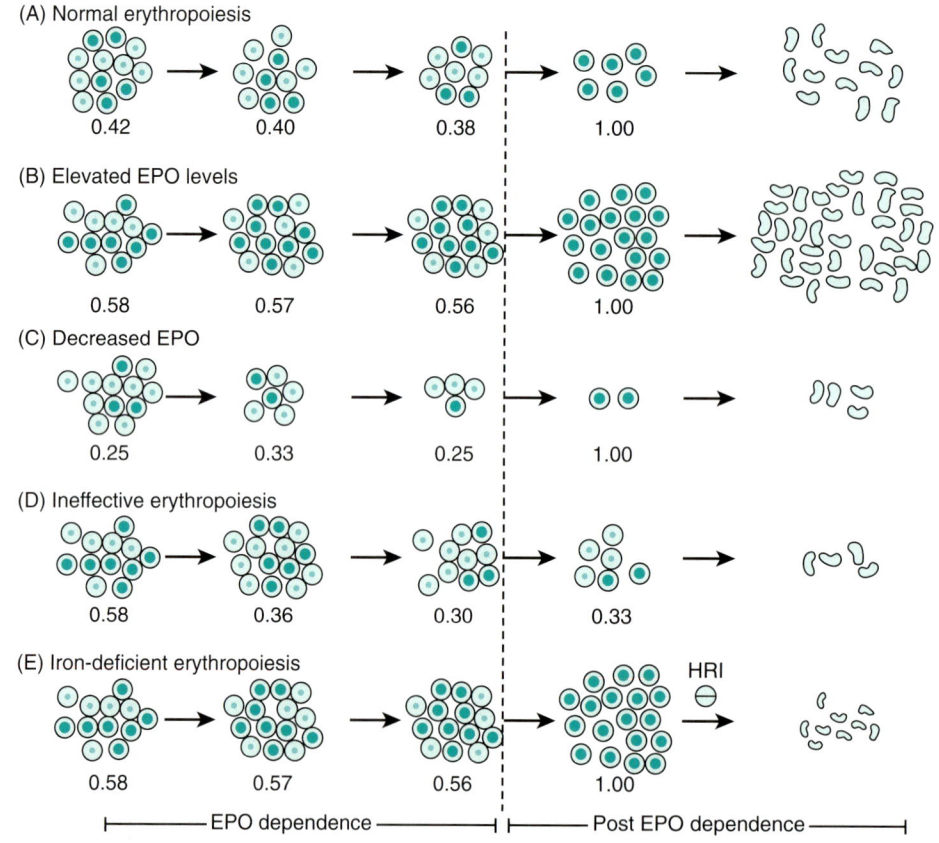

Figure 57.5 Model of erythropoiesis based on suppression of programmed cell death (apoptosis) by erythropoietin (EPO) and heterogeneity in EPO dependence among erythroid cells. **A,** Normal erythropoiesis with an average survival rate of 40% in each of the EPO-dependent generations. Normal erythropoiesis produces about 250 billion new erythrocytes daily even though a minority of all potential erythroid cells survive the EPO-dependent period. **B,** Elevated EPO levels as found after acute blood loss or hemolysis increase average survival rates to 57% in each EPO-dependent generation. Daily erythrocyte production increases to three times the normal amount. **C,** Decreased EPO levels as found in renal failure decrease average survival rate to 28% in each EPO-dependent generation. Daily erythrocyte production is one third of normal. **D,** Ineffective erythropoiesis with high EPO levels increases rates of apoptosis caused by a pathologic process such as folate or vitamin B_{12} deficiency. High EPO levels are the response to decreased erythrocyte production and expand surviving cells in the early EPO-dependent generation, but the increased rates of apoptosis in the late EPO-dependent and post–EPO-dependent stages decrease daily erythrocyte production to one-third normal. **E,** Iron-deficient erythropoiesis with elevated EPO levels, resulting in a similar increase to an average of 57% survival as seen in **B,** but in the post–EPO-dependent period, when hemoglobin is synthesized, heme-regulated inhibitor (HRI) prevents apoptosis by inhibiting protein synthesis. The inhibited protein synthesis decreases the size of the erythrocytes produced and reduces daily erythrocyte production to three fourths of the normal numbers. (From Koury M: Red cell production and kinetics. In Simon T, Snyder EL, Solheim BG, et al, editors: *Rossi's principles of transfusion medicine*, Hoboken, NJ, 2009, Blackwell Publishing.)

are produced stochastically from pluripotent stem cells. Only a minority of BFU-Es, 10% to 20%, are in cell cycle at any given time; the rest remain an inert reserve of progenitor cells. Cells then begin to take on the characteristics of CFU-Es.[176] BFU-Es contain only small quantities of GATA-1, a key transcription factor for erythroid development, whereas CFU-Es have much higher concentrations.[177,178] CFU-Es begin to express some attributes of mature erythrocytes, including blood group and Rh antigens.[179,180] It is at the CFU-E stage that EPO exerts its greatest influence; CFU-E cells express the highest surface concentration of EPO-Rs of any erythrocyte precursor.[175,181,182] Without EPO present, these cells are rapidly lost to programmed cell death.[183-185] EPO is an essential survival factor for erythroid progenitors from the CFU-E stage all the way to basophilic erythroblasts. There is substantial heterogeneity in the responsiveness of erythroid progenitors to EPO within a certain tissue and differentiation stage, possibly related to the number of EPO-Rs, their functional status, or both.[186] This diversity in EPO responsiveness corresponds to the 3 log units' range of serum EPO concentrations that can be measured in human patients.

The quantity of EPO is traditionally expressed in units, with 1 unit representing the same erythropoietic effect in animals as occurs after stimulation with 5 mmol cobalt chloride.[108] Steady-state production of small amounts of EPO maintains the serum EPO concentration at approximately 10 to 30 U/L, enough to stimulate sufficient production of erythrocytes to replace those lost to senescence.[85,108] When anemia or hypoxia is present, serum EPO concentrations increase rapidly to as much as 10,000 U/L.[88-90] Human studies indicate a sustained increase in serum EPO concentrations after phlebotomy, with values remaining elevated for several weeks.[187,188] With chronic anemia, as occurs with pure red cell aplasia (PRCA) and aplastic anemia, serum EPO remains chronically elevated, with values as much as 1000-fold higher than normal in very severe aplastic anemias.[189-193]

Koury and associates have incorporated these basic physiologic concepts into a model that explains how EPO regulates erythropoiesis in a variety of pathologic conditions (see Figure 57.5).[52,162,194] The EPO-dependent phase of erythropoiesis encompasses in this model three generations (from CFU-E through early erythroblasts), with each generation having a certain proportion of surviving cells and the remaining cells being lost by apoptosis. Owing to their reduced EPO responsiveness (or greater EPO dependence) most of the cells at the CFU-E become victims of apoptosis, so the erythropoietic production flow in a normal subject is produced by a relatively small fraction of progenitors that have escaped apoptosis. When EPO concentrations increase in response to hypoxia, blood loss, or hemolysis, additional progenitors are allowed to escape apoptosis, and resulting in the generation a few days later of an increased absolute number of reticulocytes and ultimately of RBCs. If this response is sufficient to compensate for the decreased oxygen-carrying capacity of blood, EPO concentrations decline and so does erythropoiesis. When EPO production is impaired, such as in CKD, a much greater number of cells become apoptotic, and EPO concentrations are insufficient to maintain an adequate pool of differentiating progenitors, resulting in impaired reticulocyte production and ultimately anemia.

It has become apparent that erythropoiesis does not happen in a vacuum and thus critically depends on the interaction of erythroblasts with the macrophages at the center of the erythroblastic island in the marrow. A still undetermined fraction of basal and EPO-stimulated erythropoiesis requires the contact between erythroblasts and central macrophages.[195,196] Macrophages play a role not only in the proliferation and final enucleation of erythroblasts but also possibly in supplying ferritin and iron to the erythroblast.[197] In chronic inflammatory conditions, negative regulation of erythropoiesis may be mediated locally by macrophage-produced cytokines such as tumor necrosis factor-α (TNF-α), transforming growth factor-β (TGF-β), interferon-γ (INF-γ), and interleukin-6 (IL-6). Osteoblasts are another important component of the hematopoietic microenvironment in bone. They are able to produce EPO, and this local production can modulate the response to systemic anemia.[198]

The Role of Iron, Folate, and Vitamin B_{12} in Erythropoiesis

Because of the continuous proliferative activity of the erythroid tissue and the associated production of large amounts of hemoglobin, adequate nutritional supplies of folate, vitamin B_{12}, and iron are essential for proper erythropoietic function. If any of these three components is inadequate, erythropoiesis becomes unable to meet both baseline and stimulated demands.

Inefficient erythropoiesis is a distinguishing feature of megaloblastic anemias, with the inability of erythroid progenitors to progress through the cell cycle and escape apoptosis, owing to impaired DNA synthesis and repair. Work by Koury and associates has shown that the erythroid differentiation stage most affected by either folate or B_{12} deficiency is the one coinciding with the end of the EPO-dependent effects and the initiation of Hgb synthesis.[199,200] The expansion of erythroid progenitors induced by EPO creates a large pool of progenitors (CFU-Es and pro-erythroblasts), which are extremely susceptible to apoptosis. The inefficient erythropoiesis of megaloblastic anemias is characterized by a reduced number of reticulocytes and increased serum bilirubin and lactic dehydrogenase (LDH), and accelerated iron turnover. In the case of B_{12} deficiency, thymidine and purine synthesis are impaired because of unavailability of methylenetetrahydrofolate and formyltetrahydrofolate, respectively, and the trapping of folate as methyltetrahydrofolate.[201] Folate deficiency affects several key coenzymes that are involved in the transfer of single carbon units for synthesis of pyrimidines and purines and for amino acid metabolism.

A regulated iron supply capable of matching the iron needs of the erythroid marrow is key for proper erythropoiesis. Intracellular availability of iron, heme, and globin chains have to be perfectly matched, because excess of any of these constituents is toxic for the cell. One mg of iron can be adsorbed daily from the intestine, approximately 5% to 10% of the 14 mg of iron contained in the average daily Western diet. The large majority of iron used for erythropoiesis comes from recycling of iron contained in aged RBCs via macrophages. Each milliliter of blood contains on average 0.5 mg of iron. Small, long-term blood losses result eventually in the depletion of body iron stores and development of iron-deficient erythropoiesis and anemia. Iron deficiency suppresses HIF-2alpha synthesis which in turn reduces EPO production, resulting in decreased erythropoiesis and inappropriately low reticulocyte counts for the degree of anemia.[201a,201b] Heme-regulated eIF-2α (eukaryotic initiation factor 2 eIF-2α) kinase (HRI) is a key master controller of globin synthesis based on iron/heme availability.[202] In iron-sufficient states, free heme binds to HRI and inhibits the phosphorylation of eIF-2α, allowing globin synthesis to proceed. In iron-deficient states, HRI phosphorylates eIF-2α, which in turn decreases protein synthesis and erythropoiesis, with production of microcytic erythrocytes without ineffective erythropoiesis. In macrophages, HRI acts as a positive modulator of cytokine and hepcidin production, thus affecting both inflammation and iron metabolism.[203]

ANEMIA OF CHRONIC KIDNEY DISEASE

Anemia in CKD can develop because of any of the diseases or deficiencies that may affect individuals without kidney disease such as iron deficiency, vitamin B_{12}[204,205] or folic acid deficiency,[204] and chronic blood loss.[206] But the form of anemia most common in CKD is a normocytic, normochromic or slightly hypochromic[207] anemia with insufficient production of erythrocytes (see Figure 57.2).[208-211] The etiology is multifactorial, contributors such as relative EPO deficiency, iron deficiency, blood loss, hemolysis, chronic inflammation, drugs like nonsteroidal antiinflammatory drugs (NSAIDs), and other factors, which may include circulating inhibitors of erythropoiesis.[211-214] The preponderance of evidence demonstrates that EPO deficiency is the major cause of anemia in CKD.[215-218] Ultimately, the greatest proof of the primacy of EPO deficiency in the pathogenesis of renal anemia has been the consistent success of treatment with rhEPO or its derivatives. Other contributing causes to anemia should be considered if the severity of anemia is much greater than expected, if higher than usual doses of rhEPO are needed, and in the presence of leukopenia or thrombocytopenia.

ERYTHROPOIETIN PRODUCTION AND KIDNEY DISEASE

In normal persons, serum EPO concentrations rise in response to a reduction in red cell mass, in other words, anemia. In patients with CKD, EPO concentrations are inappropriately low for the degree of anemia but may still be similar to or even higher than those in normal, nonanemic subjects.[219-223] The adequacy of EPO production in response to anemia appears to decline in rough proportion to the degree of reduction in nephron mass.[224-226] Radtke and coworkers measured serum EPO in 135 patients with CKD and 59 normal subjects.[227] At all stages of CKD, serum EPO values were found to be higher than in nonanemic normal subjects, but the relation between Hgb and serum EPO depended on the severity of CKD. Among patients with mild-to-moderate CKD, the correlation was inverse, with lower Hgb concentrations being associated with higher serum EPO concentrations. However, among patients with creatinine clearances below 40 mL/min, mean serum EPO concentrations were severely depressed and uncorrelated with the degree of anemia, but directly correlated with creatinine clearance, indicating a parallel loss of renal excretory and endocrine function.[227] Fehr and associates studied 395 patients undergoing coronary angiography, 84% of whom had reduced creatinine clearance values.[228] Like Radtke and colleagues, Fehr and associates found that serum EPO concentrations were higher in patients with lower Hgb, except when creatinine clearance was below 40 mL/min.[227,228]

Why EPO production by diseased kidneys is inadequately low remains incompletely understood. Some evidence suggests that EPO production is reduced because of the transformation of peritubular fibroblasts into myofibroblasts.[229,230] On the other hand, it has been demonstrated that pharmacologic stabilization of HIF with inhibitors of the prolylhydroxylases results in significant EPO secretion from renal and extrarenal tissues even in patients undergoing dialysis.[231] On the basis of these findings and other circumstantial evidence, it appears that a disturbed oxygen-sensing mechanism rather than destroyed production capacity for EPO is the primary cause of renal anemia. In fact, despite the severely diminished EPO response with advanced CKD, some degree of sustained feedback remains. Radtke and colleagues found that during the 6 months prior to the start of dialysis, as anemia worsened, serum EPO concentrations increased, and that in the 6 months after the start of dialysis, the opposite occurred.[227] This continued response to anemia in patients with advanced CKD was also demonstrated by Walle and coworkers, who found that serum EPO increased after hemorrhage and declined after blood transfusion in patients on dialysis.[232] Other workers also reported that hypoxia can increase EPO production significantly in anemic patients with CKD.[233,234] Consistent with such observations and a relevant capacity for endogenous EPO secretion in patients with CKD, a large analysis in the United States revealed that with increasing altitude—and thus lower blood oxygen content for any given Hgb concentration—higher achieved Hgb was observed even though lower doses of ESA were used.[235]

Taken together, studies in the literature indicate that in patients with CKD:

1. Serum EPO concentrations are generally equal to or higher than those in patients without CKD.
2. Mean serum EPO concentrations increase with worsening anemia in mild-to-moderate CKD (although to an insufficient degree).
3. Mean serum EPO concentrations become more a function of GFR than of Hgb concentration when the GFR drops below around 40 mL/min.
4. Even with advanced CKD, the ability to produce EPO is preserved and some responsiveness to lower Hgb is retained.

The pronounced breakdown of EPO production in response to anemia when creatinine clearance is below 40 mL/min fits well with the observation that clinically relevant anemia becomes common only with moderate-to-advanced CKD (see earlier discussion and Figures 57.1 and 57.2).[20,23]

SHORTENED RED BLOOD CELL SURVIVAL

Although there are several published reports on reduced RBC survival in CKD,[19,209,236] it is not clear how much it contributes to the anemia of CKD. Several abnormalities have been described in uremic erythrocytes, which may result in their increased premature destruction. An abnormal externalization of phosphatidylserine (PS), a phospholipid normally present only on the inside of the RBC membrane, has been associated with increased erythrophagocytosis and anemia in CKD.[237] Uremic RBCs have been reported to become more fragile in response to osmotic stimuli,[238] although this finding was not confirmed in pediatric patients undergoing peritoneal dialysis.[239] The rheologic properties of uremic erythrocytes are altered owing to changes in RBC shape and decreased deformability.[240] Uremic erythrocytes may not be able to mount an effective response to oxidative stress,[241-243] possibly because of glutathione deficiency,[244] and may benefit from the antioxidant effects of vitamin E bound to dialysis membranes.[243,245] Carnitine deficiency may also contribute to the reduced survival of uremic erythrocytes.[246,247] An abnormal deposition of complement onto erythrocytes in CKD could also play a role in their premature removal from the circulation.[248] Because the contribution to shortened RBC life span of each of these factors is variable from patient to patient and not easily quantifiable, and because there are no simple, reliable methods to measure RBC survival, it is extremely difficult to identify anemic patients who are particularly affected, unless they have a preexisting RBC disorder.

BLOOD LOSS

Excessive bleeding has long been recognized as a common and significant complication of CKD. The coagulopathy of CKD, discussed in the final section of this chapter, is thought to play a major role in the occult blood loss via gastrointestinal bleeding of patients with CKD.[249] In addition, blood loss due to the dialysis procedure and associated laboratory studies is also significant. A classic paper published 30 years ago estimated the blood loss due to hemodialysis to be between 1 and 3 liters per year.[250] Subsequent improvements in dialysis techniques and clinical laboratory testing methodology have reduced this loss considerably. Later estimates of the blood lost within the whole extracorporeal circuit for each dialysis session vary from a range of 0.5 to 0.6 mL[251] to a median of 0.98 mL (range 0.01 to 23.9 mL).[252] Each milliliter of blood contains approximately 0.5 mg of iron, so an important consequence of blood loss is the loss of iron and the development of iron deficiency (see later).

UREMIC "INHIBITORS" OF ERYTHROPOIESIS

Although a variety of uremic toxins have been identified in CKD,[253,254] including some with hematologic effects such as quinolinic acid[255] and N-acetyl-seryl-aspartyl-lysyl-proline (AcSDKP),[256] there is no convincing demonstration that any of them plays a significant role in the anemia of CKD. Nevertheless, the response to ESAs can be improved with dialysis, and the EPO doses used to treat patients with anemia in CKD are much greater than the amounts endogenously produced in normal individuals, indicating reduced responsiveness. Apart from factors associated with anemia, it is likely that inhibition of erythropoiesis in CKD also occurs through the concomitant chronic inflammatory state, which is characteristic for the anemia of chronic disease (ACD). Contributing factors include decreased EPO production or responsiveness plus hepcidin-induced reduction in iron availability or absorption.[257] No significant reduction in the dose of ESAs used to manage anemia was observed for patients undergoing frequent hemodialysis (six times per week) in comparison with those on the conventional three times per week schedule.[258]

IRON METABOLISM, HEPCIDIN, AND ANEMIA OF CHRONIC DISEASE

Patients with CKD are in negative iron balance due to increased blood loss (see earlier), which frequently cannot be adequately compensated. In the absence of chronic inflammation, blood loss leads to a reduction of serum ferritin and serum iron, and a progressive increase in the desaturation of transferrin, below the 16% threshold that guarantees a normal supply of iron to the erythroid marrow.[259] Some studies have reported reduced intestinal iron absorption in patients on maintenance dialysis,[260,261] mostly due to the concomitant inflammation. However, other studies have shown it to be upregulated by EPO administration and not substantially impaired in comparison with that in normal subjects.[262,263] The chronic inflammatory state frequently accompanying CKD creates additional constraints to the proper absorption and utilization of iron.[257]

The identification of hepcidin as a key regulator of iron homeostasis in normal conditions and in ACD has redefined our understanding of iron homeostasis in CKD (Figure 57.6).[264-271] Hepcidin, a 25–amino acid peptide produced and secreted by the liver,[272] modulates iron availability by promoting the internalization and degradation of ferroportin,[273] a key iron transporter (so far the only identified mammalian iron exporter) that is essential for both iron absorption in the duodenum and recycling of iron/iron efflux by macrophages.[274,275] High hepcidin concentrations turn off both duodenal iron absorption and release of iron from macrophages; low hepcidin concentrations promote iron absorption and heme iron recycling/iron mobilization from macrophages. Thus, hepcidin concentrations are expected to be high in iron overload states and diminished in iron deficiency states. In normal subjects, an oral iron load produces a measurable increase in hepcidin concentrations.[276] A hepcidin knockout mice model shows increased iron absorption, increased liver iron concentration, and decreased reticuloendothelial iron stores.[265] Hepcidin overexpression in mice leads to severe iron deficiency.[277] Some of the genetic forms of hemochromatosis, like juvenile hemochromatosis, are caused by mutations in the hepcidin gene.[278] Hepcidin production can be induced by type II acute inflammatory reactions, which are mediated by IL-6 but not IL-1 or TNF-α,[279,280] thus providing a mechanism for inflammation to affect iron availability and causing the ACD. Anemia, EPO administration, and hypoxia increase iron absorption and mobilization by decreasing hepcidin production,[281,282] although hepcidin is not a direct target gene of HIF.[283] Erythroferrone (ERFE) has been identified as the key mediator of the erythropoietic regulation of iron metabolism: ERFE production rises with increased erythropoietic activity, leading to hepcidin suppression and mobilization of the iron stores.[284,285]

Urinary and serum concentrations of hepcidin have been measured with mass spectrometry.[286-288] An immunoassay for serum human hepcidin has been developed, with a lower limit of detection of 5 ng/mL, yielding a normal range for

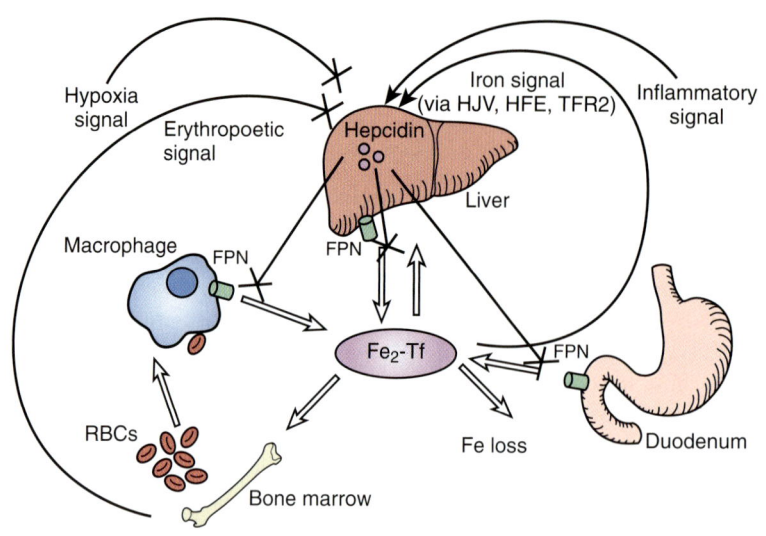

Figure 57.6 Hepcidin is a central regulator of systemic iron homeostasis. Serum iron concentrations are determined by the balance of iron entry from intestinal absorption; macrophage iron recycling; and mobilization of hepatocyte stores versus iron utilization, primarily by erythroid cells in the bone marrow. A peptide hormone secreted by the liver, hepcidin controls iron release into the plasma by downregulating cell-surface expression of the iron export protein ferroportin (FPN) on absorptive enterocytes, macrophages, and hepatocytes. Hepcidin production is inhibited by erythropoietic drive and hypoxia to ensure iron availability for erythropoiesis. Hepcidin production is stimulated by iron (through human hemochromatosis protein [HFE], hemojuvelin [HJV], and transferrin receptor 2 [TFR2]) as a negative feedback loop to maintain steady-state iron concentrations. Hepcidin production also is stimulated by inflammation, thereby sequestering iron from invading pathogens in the setting of infection but also causing the hypoferremia of anemia of chronic disease. FE_2-Tf, Transferrin-bound iron; RBC, red blood cell. (From Babitt JL, Lin HY: Molecular mechanisms of hepcidin regulation: implications for the anemia of CKD. *Am J Kidney Dis* 55:726-741, 2010.)

serum hepcidin of 29 to 254 ng/mL in men and 16 to 288 ng/mL in women.[276] The assay has enough sensitivity to detect changes in serum hepcidin due to diurnal variation and in response to oral iron. Measurements of prohepcidin, the precursor of the biologically active 25–amino acid hepcidin, seem to be poorly correlated with those of hepcidin and are unresponsive to known hepcidin regulators.[289] Several studies have measured hepcidin concentrations in CKD but have at times produced conflicting results.[290] A proper interpretation of these studies' findings must consider the following caveats: First, in the presence of anemia, hepcidin concentrations are reduced in persons with normal kidney function; thus, a normal hepcidin concentration in CKD can be still inappropriately high for the level of anemia. Second, hepcidin concentrations in healthy persons are reduced by 70% to 75% 24 hours after EPO administration.[291]

Residual kidney function, iron stores, erythropoiesis status, and inflammation all seem to be related to the hepcidin concentrations observed in CKD.[292] Hepcidin concentrations were found in one study to be elevated in patients on dialysis but were not correlated with either IL-6 concentrations or responsiveness to treatment, although they decreased after initiation of EPO therapy.[293] Progression or severity of anemia in patients with non-dialysis requiring CKD (ND-CKD) seems to be associated with higher serum hepcidin concentrations.[294,295] Elevated serum hepcidin has also been observed in anemic patients with combined renal (GFR 20-70 mL/min) and cardiac failure[296] and in association with both fatal and nonfatal cardiovascular events in patients receiving maintenance hemodialysis.[297] EPO therapy leads to a reduction in serum hepcidin that correlates with the bone marrow response.[296] Elevated serum hepcidin concentrations in pediatric and adult patients with CKD have been found to be associated with elevated ferritin and/or CRP concentrations and with stage 5 CKD.[276,298] Serum hepcidin assessment by surface-enhanced laser desorption/ionization–time-of-flight (SELDI-TOF) mass spectrometry did not seem to offer any advantage as predictor of iron needs over the established, traditional markers for adult patients on hemodialysis and maintenance ESA therapy.[299] Serum hepcidin concentrations are reduced following dialysis treatment.[300,301] Hepcidin concentrations also may vary in patients on hemodialysis owing to the presence of concomitant HFE mutations, the presence of which results in reduced hepcidin production.[302] Other studies have reported normal concentrations of hepcidin in CKD but did not address the caveats mentioned previously.[300,303] Although it has been suggested that hepcidin may improve the identification of iron deficiency in CKD prior to transplantation,[304] more work is needed to define the role of hepcidin in the assessment of iron status in CKD. In iron-deficient persons without CKD, elevated hepcidin levels have been shown to predict nonresponsiveness to oral iron therapy.[305]

Given the central role played by hepcidin in ACD, pharmacologic modulation of its production or bioavailability has potential as a new therapeutic modality.[306] In particular, the use of anti-hepcidin compounds may restore iron availability in ACD and improve the effectiveness of ESA therapy.[307] Strategies targeting hepcidin production, neutralizing hepcidin with specific peptides, or interfering with the binding of hepcidin to ferroportin or with the hepcidin-induced endocytosis of ferroportin are under consideration.[306] For conditions of iron overload, hepcidin mimetics (mini-hepcidin) have shown effectiveness in vivo in animal models,[308] and stimulators of hepcidin production are also under study.

Another regulator of iron homeostasis, growth differentiation factor 15 (GDF15), is induced by hypoxia and iron depletion,[309] and down modulates hepcidin, thus contributing to iron overload in conditions with significant expansions of the bone marrow and inefficient erythropoiesis, such as severe β-thalassemias.[310] However, in patients with ACD, there seems to be no association between GDF15 and hepcidin concentrations, suggesting that this regulatory loop may not be active in the presence of inflammation.[310]

Transmembrane serine protease 6 (TMPRSS6) may act as a cell membrane sensor of iron deficiency, which in turn suppresses hepcidin production and allows increased intestinal absorption of iron.[311] Mutations in *TMPRSS6* have been associated with iron-refractory iron deficiency anemia (IRIDA),[312] and population studies have identified a *TMPRSS6* allele associated with lower serum iron and Hgb concentrations.[313-317] It is likely that iron metabolism in patients with CKD may be similarly affected by genetic polymorphism of *TMPRSS6*.

INFLAMMATION AND ANEMIA OF CHRONIC DISEASE

Inflammation may also impact on erythropoiesis independent of its effects on iron metabolism and RBC survival. Responsiveness to EPO declines in patients with CKD in the presence of acute inflammation, bacterial infections, and cancer.[318] A chronic inflammatory state with elevated serum cytokine concentrations and decreased lymphocytes and CD4+ T cell counts has been described in patients on dialysis.[319] Serum CRP has been used to monitor or predict the hematologic consequences of inflammation.[320] Inflammatory cytokines can induce anemia either via impaired production of EPO, via impaired erythropoietic response to EPO with suppression of erythroid progenitor differentiation, and proliferation and possibly also via reduced RBC survival. TNF-α is known to directly inhibit erythropoiesis[321] as well as to reduce EPO production[322]: Antibody-mediated blockade of TNF-α produces an improvement of anemia in rheumatoid arthritis[323] and in inflammatory bowel disease.[324] Cytokines such as TNF-α, IL-1, IL-8, IL-12, and INF-γ may impair erythroid proliferation via multiple mechanisms, including cytokine-induced apoptosis,[325] downregulation of EPO-Rs, impaired production of other factors such as stem cell factor, and direct toxic effects on progenitors.[326,327] It has also been proposed that inflammation may promote the release of soluble EPO-Rs, which may inhibit EPO signaling and increase EPO resistance.[328] Sotatercept, a novel therapeutic agent that targets activin A and possibly other receptors of the TGF-β superfamily, is currently under investigation for both prevention of vascular calcification and improvement of anemia in CKD.[329]

FOLIC ACID, VITAMIN D, AND ZINC DEFICIENCIES

A net loss of folate is associated with dialysis, although the deficit is typically compensated for by a normal diet and/or routine supplementation of water-soluble vitamins. Folate status is best assessed by measuring RBC folate, because the plasma assay is affected by recent dietary intake and overestimates the true prevalence of folate deficiency.[330] Changes in RBC parameters (increases in mean corpuscular/cell volume [MCV] and mean corpuscular/cell hemoglobin [MCH] from baseline) are helpful in identifying folate deficiency states in patients on dialysis.[331,332]

Vitamin D deficiency is an independent predictor of anemia in early CKD[33,333] as well as in normal subjects,[334] but whether vitamin D directly affects erythroid proliferation[335] or is just a marker remains to be demonstrated.[336] Vitamin D supplementation (50,000 IU/month) in patients on dialysis did not result in changes in Hgb concentrations in one study, although a possible EPO-sparing effect was reported.[337]

Low plasma zinc (Zn) concentration has been reported with variable incidence in patients undergoing hemodialysis.[338-340] A zinc supplementation trial showed measurable improvements in Hgb concentrations.[341]

ALUMINUM OVERLOAD

In past years, aluminium was commonly used in patients on dialysis for its effects as a potent intestinal binder of phosphate. Although calcium-containing and non–calcium-containing phosphate binders have largely supplanted aluminium, the effects of aluminium toxicity on hematopoiesis are of historical interest. Parenteral aluminium exposure, either via dialysate contamination[342] or through other routes,[343] is still observed. The erythropoietic effects of aluminum toxicity are characterized by altered iron metabolism,[344] direct inhibition of erythropoiesis,[345,346] and disruption of RBC membrane function and rheology.[347-349] In dialyzed patients, the most notable hematologic effect of aluminum overload is microcytic anemia,[350,351] which improves with either the use of deionized water to reduce the aluminum content of the dialysate[352] or chelation therapy with desferrioxamine.[353] EPO responsiveness is reduced in patients receiving dialysis who have higher serum aluminum concentrations either at baseline or after a desferrioxamine challenge[354] and can be restored with desferrioxamine treatment.[355] Improvement of anemia has also been shown in patients with the use of chelation therapy with desferrioxamine even in the absence of overt aluminum toxicity.[356,357] Interestingly, HIF destabilization requires iron as a cofactor, and iron chelation with desferrioxamine can induce HIF, providing a possible alternative explanation for an improvement in anemia.

HORMONES, PARATHYROID HORMONE, AND MARROW FIBROSIS

The inhibitory effects of parathyroid hormone (PTH) on erythropoiesis are primarily indirect and a consequence of myelofibrosis.[358] Secondary hyperparathyroidism is associated with diminished responsiveness to EPO.[359] Moreover, PTH levels were identified as effect modifiers of the erythropoietic response to EPO in adult CKD patients on hemodialysis.[360] However, in pediatric patients no association was found between serum intact PTH and Hgb concentrations.[361] An increase in EPO levels and improvement in anemia have been reported after parathyroidectomy.[362,363]

DRUGS

Use of renin angiotensin aldosterone system (RAAS) inhibitors may induce or worsen anemia[364] for several reasons. Angiotensin II has direct facilitating effects on erythroid progenitor cells, which are inhibited by these compounds.[365] *N*-acetyl-seryl-lysyl-proline (AcSDKP), an endogenous inhibitor of erythropoiesis, accumulates in patients treated with angiotensin-converting enzyme (ACE) inhibitors.[256] Endogenous EPO production may also be reduced through the hemodynamic effects of angiotensin II inhibition. Because angiotensin II leads to preferential constriction of efferent glomerular arterioles, it increases the ratio of filtered sodium—the main determinant of renal oxygen consumption—to peritubular blood flow and thus oxygen supply, thereby presumably lowering peritubular oxygen tension. RAAS inhibitors reverse these effects and therefore have the potential to mitigate renal hypoxia and the signal for EPO production.[366] It has also been postulated that RAAS inhibitors may promote anemia and EPO resistance via a reduction in testosterone serum concentrations in men younger than 60 years.[367] Myelosuppressive effects of immunosuppressants may further contribute to anemia, especially in the posttransplantation setting.[368-370]

ASSOCIATION OF ANEMIA WITH ADVERSE OUTCOMES

The availability of rhEPO greatly increased interest in the role that anemia plays with respect to health-related quality of life (HRQOL) and prognosis of patients with CKD. A large number of observational studies have consistently shown that even modest reductions in Hgb concentrations are associated with adverse outcomes. This statement applies to mortality in patients on dialysis[10,371] and patients with CKD not on dialysis[372] as well as individuals in the general population[373] or with other complex chronic diseases, such as heart failure.[374] A large study of 159,720 patients undergoing hemodialysis and receiving epoetin therapy showed that the duration of anemia, rather than the Hgb concentration per se, was the most powerful predictor of short-term mortality, with Hgb concentrations less than 11g/dL for 3 months or longer being associated with an increased risk of death.[375,376] However, there is no agreement on how to best study Hgb variability effects on mortality, with various methods having been applied to describe Hgb variability[377] and with significant confounding attributable to variations in Hgb concentrations among dialysis centers[378] and the effects of ESA dosing and iron therapy.[379]

A systematic review supported the notion that Hgb concentrations below an *a priori* established reference range (Hgb 9-10 g/dL in some studies and 11-12 g/dL in others) are generally associated with increased all-cause mortality in dialysis recipients. Similar findings have been reported in pediatric patients on peritoneal dialysis.[380] In patients with ND-CKD, the severity of anemia is also associated with the rate of decline in kidney function,[381] consistent with the concept that anemia may aggravate intrarenal hypoxia.[382,383] Moreover, anemia was found to be a strong risk factor for the development of left ventricular hypertrophy,[384,385] an established surrogate for mortality and cardiovascular events. An increase in cardiac output as part of the compensatory mechanisms that maintain oxygen delivery in anemia has been considered as a possible reason for the link between anemia and cardiac geometry.[384]

Other specific complications, such as proliferative retinopathy in patients with diabetes, were found to be associated with anemia.[386] In a relatively large (21,899) cohort of dialyzed patients in the United States, Hgb concentrations below 8 g/dL were associated with a twofold increase in the odds of death in comparison with those for Hgb concentrations between 10 and 11 g/dL; several laboratory parameters related to iron status and nutrition as well as dose of dialysis were also associated with Hgb concentrations.[207] There was no association with mortality when Hgb was above 11 g/dL in this cohort study, but other studies suggested that the relationship among Hgb, comorbidities, and outcomes extends into the normal range of Hgb, leading to the hypothesis that normalization of Hgb might be associated with best outcomes. However, RCTs failed to confirm this suggestion (see later). Therefore, although it is undisputable that anemia is a sensitive risk marker for adverse outcomes, its role as a causal risk factor has not been established.

ERYTHROCYTOSIS OF PATIENTS WITH KIDNEY DISEASE

Although anemia is a typical complication of advanced CKD, irrespective of its etiology, there are few circumstances under which disorders of renal structure and function can also result in abnormally high rates of RBC production, that is, erythrocytosis. The pathogenesis of these disorders remains incompletely understood but they probably all result from *increased* production of renal EPO.

(POLY)CYSTIC KIDNEY DISEASE

The degree of anemia in patients with autosomal dominant polycystic kidney disease (ADPKD) is usually somewhat less severe than for other etiologies of CKD, although patients with ADPKD on dialysis usually require treatment with ESAs. Occasionally patients with ADPKD may become polycythemic.[387] Erythrocytosis may also develop in patients on hemodialysis with acquired renal cysts and single cysts.[388,389] Serum EPO concentrations in patients with ADPKD are, on average, up to twofold greater than in patients with CKD from other causes,[234,390,391] and significant arteriovenous concentration differences for EPO have been found in polycystic kidneys.[392] In the cyst walls of patients with ADPKD, interstitial cells have been shown to express EPO mRNA, and cysts derived from proximal but not distal tubules contain increased concentrations of bioactive erythropoietin.[392] In a later study, continuous activation of HIF was demonstrated in cyst walls of patients with ADPKD and in a rat model of cystic kidney disease.[393] The physiologic distinction between HIF-1α expression in tubular cells and HIF-2α expression in peritubular cells is maintained in the cyst walls. The genetic defects underlying ADPKD do not lead to HIF activation. However, cyst expansion results in pericystic hypoxia, and hypoxic stimulation of pericystic angiogenesis is believed to play an important role in cyst progression.[394,395] Therefore, the enhanced production of EPO in cystic kidneys is probably due to local hypoxia and mediated via HIF activation. It is possible that factors other than EPO, induced through this pathway, contribute to cyst growth. Regional hypoxia also appears to stimulate cyst growth, primarily via increased fluid secretion into the cyst lumen.[396]

POSTTRANSPLANTATION ERYTHROCYTOSIS

Kidney transplantation is usually followed by full correction of renal anemia.[374,397,398] Interestingly, a regular increase in EPO production is not related to the presence of the transplant but does correlate with the onset of graft function,[399] providing further evidence for the role of excretory kidney function in EPO regulation. Some 10% to 20% of patients manifest overcorrection and demonstrate erythrocytosis, usually within the first 6 months following transplantation.[400-402] Graft failure is associated with anemia, and therefore polycythemia is more likely to occur in patients with normal kidney function.[374,390]

Increased plasma EPO concentrations have been reported in patients with posttransplantation erythrocytosis.[403] Selective venous catheterization studies and the response to removal of the native kidneys suggest that the native kidneys are the main source of increased EPO production.[403,404] Although this suggestion clearly indicates that a sufficient production capacity for EPO may be preserved in diseased kidneys, it is unclear how the secretion rate is enhanced after transplantation. Improvement of the uremic state has been speculated to play a role. Moreover, given that inflammatory cytokines can inhibit erythropoietin production, the application of immunosuppressive agents could theoretically enhance EPO formation. Interestingly, the prevalence of posttransplantation erythrocytosis seems to be elevated in combined kidney and pancreas transplantation,[405] but whether the erythrocytosis is related to enhanced EPO formation or to insulin-stimulated pathways remains unclear. In some patients with posttransplantation polycythemia, the circulating EPO concentrations are normal or reduced, and it may be that in these cases there is an increased sensitivity of the erythroid progenitor cells to EPO or loss of other feedback control mechanisms.

The most effective therapy of posttransplantation erythrocytosis consists of agents blocking the RAAS.[401,406-408] There is no evidence that angiotensin acts directly on EPO-producing cells, but there are several ways through which RAAS blockade may inhibit erythropoiesis (see earlier). Alternative therapeutic strategies to reduce increased RBC concentrations after transplantation include the discontinuation of diuretics, application of theophylline,[407] and phlebotomies, which, however, can lead to iron deficiency.

RENAL ARTERY STENOSIS

Although renal artery stenosis reduces the oxygen supply to the kidneys it is only rarely associated with erythrocytosis.[409-412] The data on EPO production in this situation are contradictory. In experimental animals enhancement of EPO production after renal artery stenosis has been demonstrated by some, but not all, investigators.[413] A study performed in rats showed that graded reduction of renal blood flow to 10% of the control value caused a maximal threefold increase in serum EPO concentrations.[414] Therefore, renal EPO production appears rather insensitive to changes in renal blood flow. Because the ratio of oxygen demand and delivery determines local oxygen tension in the area of EPO-producing cells, it is possible that the two are equally reduced after a reduction in renal blood flow, thus not resulting in sufficient hypoxia to stimulate *EPO* gene expression. It has been argued that the indirect coupling of oxygen demand to supply makes the kidney an ideal site for the oxygen sensing that controls RBC production.[415]

RENAL TUMORS

Up to 5% of patients with renal carcinomas have erythrocytosis,[416] and conversely, approximately a third of tumor-associated erythrocytosis is caused by renal cancer.[417] Conflicting data have been reported concerning serum EPO concentrations in patients with renal tumors, but at least in some patients, raised EPO concentrations have been found.[418] Furthermore, overexpression of EPO mRNA has been demonstrated in renal tumors.[419] In situ hybridization revealed that accumulation of EPO mRNA occurs in epithelial tumor cells but not in interstitial cells of the tumor stroma.[419] The majority of clear cell renal carcinomas—the most frequent type of renal cancer—are associated with mutations of the *VHL* gene that interfere with its ability to target HIF for proteasomal degradation (see earlier).[420] Indeed, clear cell renal carcinomas contain high concentrations of HIF.[421-424] Although stabilized HIF in renal tumors appears to be functionally active in inducing HIF target genes, it is yet unclear why overexpression of EPO is confined to about one third of these tumors.[425] Although activation of HIF appears necessary for *EPO* gene expression in renal cell carcinoma, it is clearly not the only determinant. The fact that erythrocytosis occurs far less frequently than overexpression of EPO in renal cancer is probably due to a variety of mechanisms causing anemia in patients with cancer, which include inhibition of the effect of EPO and reduced iron availability. There is some albeit controversial evidence suggesting that EPO has autocrine or paracrine tumor growth promoting effects.[426,427]

TREATMENT OF RENAL ANEMIA

ERYTHROPOIESIS-STIMULATING AGENTS

Recombinant human erythropoietin was developed in the 1980s with support from an orphan drug program. At that time it was unclear to what extent the anemia of patients with kidney disease could be influenced by application of the hormone as well as how many patients might benefit from this kind of therapy. The initial clinical studies revealed an unexpected efficacy in patients receiving dialysis, with both high response rates and evidence that hemoglobin concentrations could not just be increased to some extent but virtually be normalized.[105,107] In the subsequent years, the use of recombinant EPO in patients on maintenance dialysis became routine in most parts of the world. The indication was subsequently extended to the much larger group of patients with ND-CKD as well as to several other patient groups with anemia, including those whose cancer was treated with chemotherapy. Over the years, efficacy of the therapy and presumed benefits led to a gradual increase in Hgb concentrations in virtually all patient groups that were treated (see Figure 57.3). Data from the U.S. Renal Data System indicate a substantial increase in the use of these agents (as well as intravenous [IV] iron and blood transfusion) in older (>67 years) adults with ESKD.[428] Not surprisingly the expanded clinical use resulted in an extraordinary commercial success. Although investigators originally intended to copy the endogenous molecule as closely as possible, patent and marketing considerations together with concepts for improving patient management resulted in the development of a number of derivatives of the EPO molecule with altered pharmacokinetic properties and, later, the development of different molecules that can directly or indirectly stimulate the EPO-R. Discussions about the appropriate terminology for all these compounds have not been settled, but erythropoiesis-stimulating agents (ESA) is increasingly used to describe the heterogeneous class of drugs that stimulate erythropoiesis through stimulation of the erythropoietin receptor.

Epoetin

The term epoetin is usually applied to rhEPO preparations, produced by means of overexpression of the human EPO gene in mammalian cell lines. Production in mammalian cells rather than bacteria is required, because EPO is a highly glycosylated molecule and bacteria lack the ability to generate glycoproteins. Epoetin alfa and epoetin beta are the two compounds first developed by two different companies. Both are produced in Chinese hamster ovary (CHO) cells and show a high degree of similarity, with identical protein backbones of 165 amino acids and one O-linked and three N-linked glycosylation sites each, but with subtle differences in their carbohydrate composition.[429] Although the amino acid sequence unequivocally determines glycosylation sites, the precise composition of the sugar side chains is also determined by the repertoire and activity of glycating enzymes, which may vary among cell lines and under different tissue culture conditions. Glycosylation of the EPO molecule is not required for binding or activation of its receptor[117]; in fact the in vitro activity of deglycosylated erythropoietin is enhanced.[430] However, in vivo deglycosylated EPO is inactive owing to rapid clearance from the circulation, and the carbohydrate chains are thus responsible for its pharmacokinetic properties.

Early clinical trials in patients on hemodialysis used IV epoetin administered thrice weekly; subsequently the intraperitoneal (IP), subcutaneous (SC), and intradermal routes of administration were also investigated.[431,432] After IV administration, plasma EPO concentrations decay monoexponentially, with an elimination half-life of approximately 4 to 11 hours.[433] The apparent volume of distribution of EPO is about one to two times the plasma volume, and the total body clearance is lower than for other protein hormones, such as insulin, glucagon, and prolactin. The IP route was investigated as a potential means of administering EPO to patients on peritoneal dialysis, but the bioavailability of intraperitoneal epoetin is disappointingly low, at 3% to 8%. This application has therefore not been pursued.[431,434,435]

With SC. administration, peak serum concentrations of about 4% to 10% of an equivalent IV dose are obtained at around 12 hours, and thereafter they decay slowly such that concentrations greater than baseline are still present at 4 days.[432,433] The bioavailability of SC epoetin is around 20% to 25%. Nevertheless, SC application is even more efficient than IV application, allowing a dose reduction of approximately 30% to maintain the same hemoglobin concentration.[436,437] Presumably, the early peak concentrations of epoetin after IV injection are inefficient, and the more prolonged elevation of hormone concentrations following SC application allows a more sustained stimulation of RBC production. Thrice-weekly administration has remained the most popular dosage frequency for both IV and SC administration, although once-weekly,[438] twice-weekly, and seven-times-weekly (once-daily) dosing have all been used.[439] With IV epoetin, once-weekly administration is associated with much lower efficacy, and twice- or thrice-weekly dosing is required. In 2012, the mean weekly dose of EPO in adult HD patients in the United States was below 10,000 units per week (Figure 57.7).

A number of additional epoetin preparations have been developed all over the world. Some have distinct differences in the production process—for example, epoetin delta was produced in a human cell line through increased transcription of the endogenous EPO gene,[440] but this product is currently not being distributed. Other epoetins are so-called bio-similars, generic drugs that are designed as copies of epoetin alfa or beta and are being licensed on the basis of a more limited clinical trial program after expiration of the patents for the originator compounds in Europe.[441] Additional epoetins are available in other parts of the world but are not necessarily produced to the same regulatory standards as the preparations marketed in the United States and Europe and may show variable product characteristics.[442]

The importance of the formulation of epoetins was highlighted in 2002 with an upsurge in cases of antibody-mediated PRCA in association with the SC use of epoetin alfa marketed outside the United States after a change to an albumin-free formulation. Patients affected by this complication develop neutralizing antibodies against both rhEPO and the endogenous hormone, resulting in severe anemia and transfusion dependence.[443] The cause of this serious complication remains obscure, although circumstantial evidence suggested that rubber stoppers of prefilled syringes used for the albumin-free epoetin alfa formulation may have released organic compounds that acted as immunologic adjuvants.[444] Factors such as breach of the cold storage chain may also have played a role. In anti-EPO antibody cases observed so far, the subcutaneous application route was usually a prerequisite. Although the unfortunate combination of adverse factors leading to a temporary increase in antibody-induced PRCA was specific for one product, a low baseline rate of PRCA also occurs with use of epoetin beta and darbepoetin alfa (see later).

Darbepoetin Alfa

Darbepoetin alfa is an EPO derivative with a further two N-linked glycosylation sites, created by site-directed mutagenesis in order to prolong its plasma survival time (as discussed earlier).[119] Each of these glycosylation sites can carry an additional four sialic acid residues. Thus, this molecule (called darbepoetin alfa or novel erythropoiesis-stimulating protein [NESP]) contains five N-linked and one O-linked glycosylation chains, and has the capacity to carry up to 22 sialic acid residues, compared with a maximum of 14 sialic acid residues for original rhEPO. The additional glycosylation on darbepoetin alfa results in a molecule weighing 37.1 kDa, compared with 30.4 kDa for epoetin. As intended, darbepoetin alfa has a longer half-life in vivo than rhEPO: 25.3 hours versus 8.5 hours after IV administration.[121] The elimination half-life after SC administration is around 48 hours, which is approximately twice that previously reported for epoetin alfa or beta. A number of studies have examined once-weekly and every-other-week dosing.[445] Darbepoetin alfa can both correct and maintain Hgb at these dosing frequencies, and its side effect profile is very similar to that of epoetin alfa or beta.[431,446] Several "conversion" studies suggested that an appropriate conversion factor for switching patients on epoein alfa or beta to darbepoetin alfa is

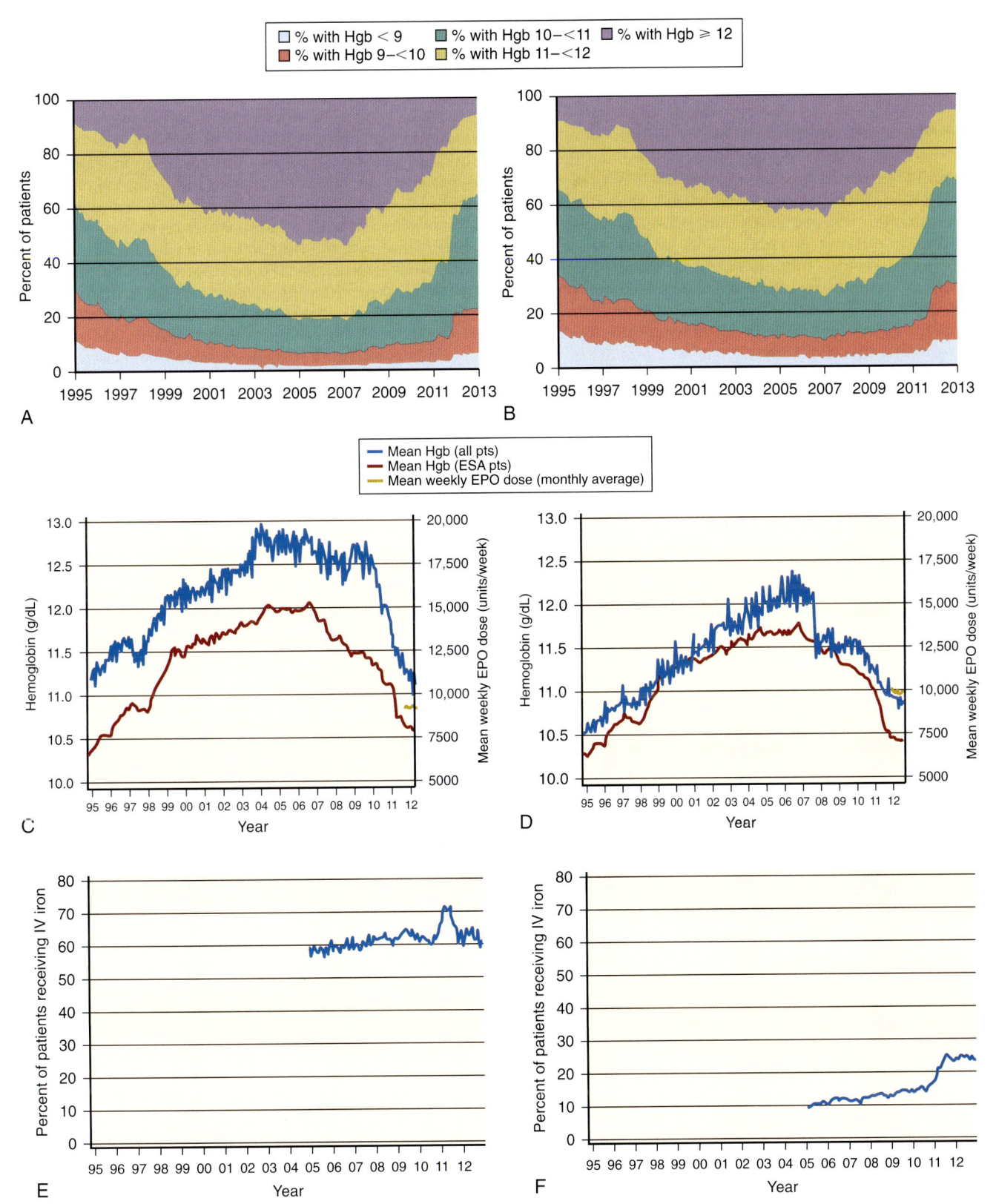

Figure 57.7 Anemia, erythropoiesis-stimulating agents (ESAs) and intravenous (IV) iron in patients undergoing hemodialysis and peritoneal dialysis. **A,** Distribution of monthly hemoglobin (Hgb) (g/dL) levels in ESA-treated adult patients on hemodialysis (HD) for 90 days or more. **B,** Distribution of monthly Hgb (g/dL) levels in ESA-treated adult (≥18 years of age) patients on peritoneal dialysis (PD) for 90 days or more. **C,** Mean monthly Hgb level and mean weekly erythropoietin (EPO) dose (monthly average, expressed in units/week) in adult patients on HD for 90 days or more. **D,** Mean monthly Hgb level and mean weekly EPO dose (monthly average, expressed in units/week) in adult patients on PD for 90 days or more. **E,** Monthly percentage of adult HD patients receiving IV iron for 90 days or more. **F,** Monthly percentage of adult PD patients receiving IV iron for 90 days or more. (From United States Renal Data System: *2014 annual data report: an overview of the epidemiology of kidney disease in the United States,* Bethesda, MD, 2014, National Institutes of Health, National Institute of Diabetes and Digestive and Kidney Diseases.)

200 units of epoetin to 1 μg of darbepoetin alfa. In contrast to epoetin alfa or beta, the dose requirements for darbepoetin alfa do not differ significantly between IV and SC administration routes.

Methoxypolyethylene Glycol Epoetin Beta

Alternative bioengineering techniques to prolong the half-life of EPO further resulted in the development of methoxypolyethylene glycol epoetin beta (also called continuous erythropoietin receptor activator [CERA]), which is a PEGylated derivative of epoetin beta with an elimination half-life of around 130 hours when administered either IV or SC.[447-449] A methoxypolyethylene glycol polymer chain is integrated through amide bonds between the N-terminal amino group or the ε-amino group of lysine (predominantly lysine-52 or lysine-45), with a single succinimidyl butanoic acid linker. The molecular weight of CERA is twice that of epoetin (approximately 60 kDa). Phase III studies showed that, because of the longer half-life time of CERA, less frequent injections were sufficient to maintain stable hemoglobin concentrations. CERA given IV once every 2 weeks was found to be as safe and effective as epoetin given thrice weekly for correcting anemia in patients on hemodialysis.[450] A larger study also showed that CERA given at 4-week dosing intervals was not inferior to epoetin given thrice weekly in terms of maintaining Hgb concentrations.[451]

Other Erythropoiesis-Stimulating Agents

Several other ESAs have been developed or are currently in clinical development.[452-454] These include EPO polymers, EPO fusion proteins, EPO-mimetic molecule, and the so-called HIF stabilizers, which induce endogenous EPO formation. The ability of molecules, which are structurally unrelated to EPO, to dimerize the EPO-R and activate the intracellular signaling cascade was first described 20 years ago.[455] Peginesatide is an EPO-mimetic peptide that was subsequently developed for treatment of anemia. Its amino acid sequence is completely unrelated to that of native or rhEPO although it shares the same properties with EPO with respect to EPO-R activation.[456,457] The potential advantages of this compound included greater ex vivo stability, allowing storage at room temperature; prolonged pharmacodynamic action, allowing once-monthly administration; and a simple manufacturing process involving synthetic peptide chemistry. In addition, because peginesatide is structurally unrelated to EPO, it does not cross-react with anti-EPO antibodies, allowing effective treatment of anti–EPO antibody–mediated PRCA.[458] Two phase 3 studies demonstrated that peginesatide was not inferior to conventional epoetin in correcting anemia in CKD.[459,460] However, for reasons that remain unclear, peginesatide increased the risk of a combined cardiovascular end point in patients with ND-CKD.[459] Accordingly, it was approved in the United States for use in patients on dialysis only. Only slightly more than 6 months after its introduction, the drug was recalled as a result of postmarketing reports of serious hypersensitivity reactions—including fatal reactions in approximately 0.02% of patients—that occurred within 30 minutes of the first IV dose and had not been reported during clinical trials.[461]

The HIF stabilizers are competitive inhibitors of HIF prolyl-hydroxylases and asparaginyl-hydroxylase, enzymes involved in the degradation of HIF and suppression of its transcriptional activity, respectively (as discussed earlier).[70] The HIF stabilizers, therefore, cause an increase in endogenous EPO production.[462] These drugs are orally active. They have been shown to effectively stimulate erythropoiesis in monkeys[463] and are currently being tested in phase 2 and 3 studies in patients with CKD.[464,465] A phase 1/2 single-dose study comparing erythropoietin formation in small groups of patients on dialysis with native kidneys and after bilateral nephrectomy provided evidence that EPO production can be stimulated in both extrarenal sites (presumably the liver) and the diseased, nonfunctioning, fibrotic kidneys.[231] These data provide proof for the concept that a disturbance of the renal oxygen-sensing mechanism rather than a loss of EPO-producing cells is the main cause of renal anemia. There is much discussion about whether HIF stabilizers upregulate not only EPO gene expression but also other HIF target genes, such as those involved in iron metabolism and neoangiogenesis. Although some of these effects may facilitate an increase in hemoglobin concentrations, the long-term consequences—good or bad—of these other effects have not been established. Interestingly, genetic causes of impaired degradation of HIF, potentially comparable to long-term pharmacologic inhibition of HIF degradation, have been identified as causes of rare polycythemias.[99,466,467]

Initiation and Maintenance of Therapy

Following commencement of regular therapy with ESAs, a significant increase in the reticulocyte count to around two to three times baseline is usually evident at 1 week, and an increase in Hgb concentration is seen by 2 to 3 weeks. The increase is dose dependent, and most physicians aim for an increment of not more than 1 g/dL/month in order to minimize the risk of adverse effects. In the majority of patients, ESA therapy is initiated at the outset of dialysis therapy, and according to the U.S. Renal Data System report, peak doses of ESA are being administered at month 2 after initiation of dialysis.

The increase in Hgb concentration following ESA therapy is associated with an increase in RBC count. No significant changes in either leukocyte or platelet counts are usually seen, although a moderate increase in the platelet count has been documented in some studies. There is usually a marked decline in the serum ferritin concentration and/or the transferrin saturation value after start of ESA therapy, unless iron stores are being replenished in parallel, because large quantities of iron are used up in the manufacture of new RBCs (see later).

Radioisotopic blood volume studies confirmed that there is an increase in RBC mass after treatment with ESAs and it is associated with a compensatory reduction in plasma volume so that the whole blood volume remains unchanged. Early ferrokinetic studies indicated that epoetin therapy induces a twofold increase in marrow erythropoietic activity, as evidenced by a doubling of marrow and RBC iron turnover.[233,468] There is little or no change in mean RBC life span after epoetin therapy; thus the increased RBC mass is largely accounted for by the production of greater numbers of RBCs rather than any significant change in their survival.

IRON MANAGEMENT

Iron is the fourth most common element—after oxygen, silicon, and aluminium—in the Earth's crust and the most abundant transitional metal in the human body. Although it plays an essential role in multiple biologic processes, such as transport of oxygen, transfer of electrons, DNA synthesis, and heme-based enzymatic reactions, iron is also highly susceptible to undergoing transition from the ferrous state (Fe^{2+}) to the ferric (Fe^{3+}) state and to generate reactive oxygen species (ROS) via the Haber-Weiss-Fenton reaction, thus requiring the presence of multiple systems to prevent or control this potentially harmful transition.[469]

The metabolism of iron is geared toward conservation and recycling, with the gastrointestinal absorption of iron in adults being tightly regulated to compensate for the daily losses and keep the total iron pool in the body constant in the range of 35 to 45 mg per kg body weight. Of the iron pool, approximately two thirds is contained in the RBC pool as Hgb, with the remaining fraction stored in macrophages and the reticuloendothelial system (RES), liver, and muscle (myoglobin).

Multiple factors induce a negative iron balance in patients with CKD, including reduced intake/absorption, chronic losses due to occult and overt blood loss, and reduced bioavailability of iron due to the chronic inflammatory state and increased hepcidin production (see earlier). Iron losses in patients with CKD can be up to 5 to 6 mg iron daily (1 mg iron daily in normal subjects) and cannot be adequately compensated with oral iron supplements, because gastrointestinal absorption is limited by the chronic inflammatory state and hepcidin. In addition, in patients with CKD treated with ESAs, insufficient amounts of iron are released from the body stores to meet the greater demand of ESA-driven erythropoiesis.[470] Similar evidence was provided for normal subjects when erythropoiesis was increased by an intensive blood donation schedule and EPO, or EPO alone, despite concomitant oral iron supplementation.[471-473]

Markers of Iron Status

When hematologic signs of iron-deficient erythropoiesis—reduced Hgb with abnormally low MCV and MCH, inadequate reticulocyte response, and low reticulocyte Hgb content—are associated with biochemical markers of low iron stores (abnormally low serum ferritin), the diagnosis of absolute iron deficiency is straightforward. However, straightforward determination of iron deficiency is the exception rather than the rule in patients with CKD, in whom iron may be present in storage form but not readily available for erythropoiesis and serum ferritin concentrations are increased owing to the concomitant inflammatory state. Thus, the diagnosis of iron deficiency in CKD must rely on a variety of markers both biochemical and hematologic and, in the most challenging cases, on the erythroid response to IV iron (see later for the significant limitations of bone marrow biopsy). These markers are determined in individual patients over time: markers with high biologic/analytical variability, such as transferrin saturation and ferritin, are less suitable to assess iron status than markers with low variability, such as Hgb, Hct, and reticulocyte Hgb content.[474,475]

Serum Ferritin. Serum ferritin values higher than 200 µg/L are recommended for patients on dialysis,[10,11] and values of 100 µg/L should be considered the lower limit of normal for patients with ND-CKD.[476] The sensitivity for ruling out iron deficiency was reported to be 90% for a ferritin cutoff of 300 µg/L and 100% for 500 µg/L.[477,478] Concerns about iron toxicity/overload have resulted in several guidelines setting an upper limit for ferritin of 500 µg/L,[9-11,476] above which IV iron is not recommended. However, this recommendation is not evidence based.[479] Additional factors that elevate serum ferritin are hyperthyroidism, liver disease (associated with hepatitis C virus [HCV] and other conditions), alcohol consumption, and oral contraceptives, whereas vitamin C deficiency and hypothyroidism decrease ferritin concentrations.[480]

Serum Iron, Transferrin, and Transferrin Saturation. The biochemical markers serum iron, transferrin, and transferrin saturation (TSAT) are routinely used in the diagnosis of iron deficiency states but have some important limitations: Serum iron concentrations and TSAT values are sensitive to diurnal variations and to dietary intake, with serum iron concentrations being higher early in the day, increased by greater iron intake with food or dietary supplements, and decreased in the presence of infection and inflammation.[481] Some of the biochemical methods used to measure iron are sensitive to hemolysis and produce falsely elevated iron values,[482] whereas other serum iron assays have been shown to perform poorly in patients on dialysis.[483] Serum transferrin can be elevated by the use of oral contraceptives and reduced with inflammation or infection. Several studies have shown that these traditional biochemical iron parameters perform poorly in CKD and are inferior to some of the newer hematologic parameters described later.[484-487] However, a lower serum iron concentration has been shown to be an independent predictor of mortality and hospitalization in dialysis recipients,[488] and a higher TSAT value has been associated with lower mortality.[489] A TSAT of 20% is generally considered a threshold value below which iron therapy is indicated.[10,11] In one study using data from the National Health and Nutritional Examination Survey (NHANES), more than 50% of the non-institutionalized adult U.S. population were found to have values below the "CKD thresholds" for ferritin (100 ng/mL) and TSAT (20%).[490] Overall, women were far more likely to have laboratory-based evidence of iron deficiency. Men with CKD had higher prevalence of iron deficiency than men without CKD, whereas the prevalences in women with and without CKD were similar (Figure 57.8). Serum transferrin and total iron-binding capacity (TIBC) are dual markers of iron status as well as of nutritional status and protein balance: Lower baseline TIBC value or its decrease over time in dialyzed patients is associated with higher mortality and with the presence of protein-energy wasting and inflammation.[491]

Serum Transferrin Receptor. Serum transferrin receptor (sTfR) concentration is a marker of iron status that has shown promise in the evaluation of iron deficiency in patients with CKD. Transferrin receptors are shed from the membrane of maturing erythroblasts and reticulocytes, either in soluble form or as vesicles.[492-494] Concentration of sTfR is abnormally elevated in iron deficiency states and has been shown to be a valuable parameter in several different clinical conditions, including ACD.[495-499] Although sTfR concentration is not affected by inflammation, it is an expression of the size of the pool of maturing erythroblasts; also,

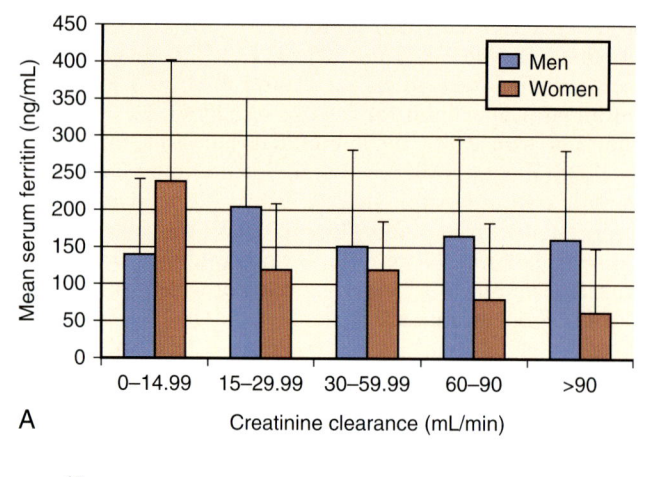

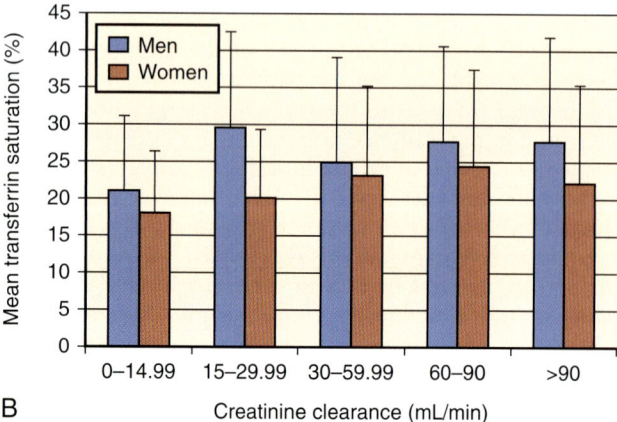

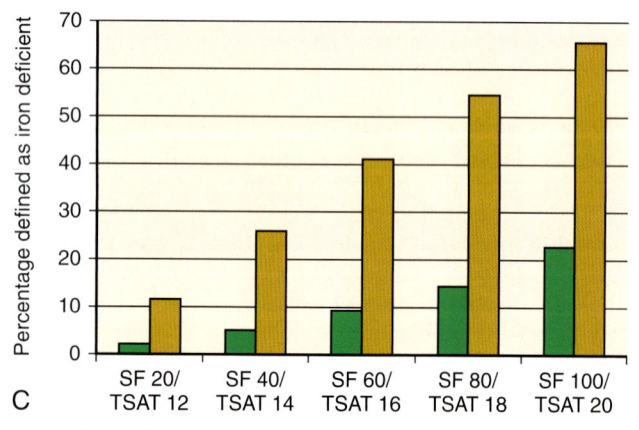

Figure 57.8 Mean **(A)** serum ferritin and **(B)** transferrin saturation (TSAT) as a function of creatinine clearance (CrCl) for the combined National Health and Nutrition Examination Survey (NHANES) cohorts (*error bars* are standard deviation [SD]). The trend for both TSAT and ferritin is not significant (NS) for men, but for women, $P < .0001$ for serum ferritin and $P < .02$ for TSAT. National Kidney Foundation (NKF) chronic kidney disease (CKD) stages relative to CrCl (mL/min) are stage 5, 0 to 14.99; stage 4, 15 to 29.99; and stage 3, 30 to 59.99. Patients with CrCl 60 to 90 mL/min and patients with CrCl > 90 mL/min may have CKD stage 1 or 2, respectively, if other renal abnormalities are present. **C,** Percentage of individuals defined as iron deficient with the use of different threshold combinations of serum ferritin (SF) and TSAT. The NKF Kidney Disease Outcomes Quality Initiatives (KDOQI) thresholds of serum ferritin 100 ng/mL and TSAT 20% are different from indices of iron deficiency in the non-CKD population, in which lower thresholds are generally used. The *green bars* indicate AND logic, both test results below the specified threshold, and the *yellow bars* indicate OR logic, with either test result being below the threshold. (From Fishbane S, Pollack S, Feldman HI, et al: Iron indices in chronic kidney disease in the National Health and Nutritional Examination Survey 1988-2004. *Clin J Am Soc Nephrol* 4:57-61, 2009.)

independently of iron status, this parameter increases in hyperproliferative anemias and with the use of ESAs.

The STfR assay is not yet widely available, and a single reference standard has been established only recently,[500] with different methods still reporting different units and normal ranges. A study in patients on dialysis with anemia showed that sTfR concentrations lower than 6 mg/L (which rule out iron deficiency; normal value 3.8-8.5) were associated with responsiveness to initiation of EPO therapy.[501] However, because increased erythropoiesis by itself raises the sTfR concentration, sTfR measurement could not reliably detect functional iron deficiency in patients on maintenance EPO therapy. Other studies have failed to show a predictive value for sTfR in CKD anemia management.[502,503] A decline in sTfR concentration may reflect increases in iron availability when IV ascorbic acid is used to mobilize iron stores.[504] Race-ethnicity, smoking, alcohol consumption, and body mass index have been shown to be associated with sTfR values.[505,506] One can correct the sTfR for the value of iron stores by also accounting for serum ferritin: The sTfR/ferritin ratio provides an accurate assessment of iron status and of the need for iron supplementation.[493,507,508] However, to date, there is limited evidence to support the clinical use of this or similar ratios in patients on dialysis.[509-511]

Erythrocyte Ferritin Concentration. Some studies in the 1990s had suggested a potential value for using erythrocyte ferritin concentration as a marker of iron status in patients on dialysis.[478,512-514] Although this assay can be run on automated analyzers using the regular serum ferritin methodology,[515] the method is cumbersome, requires complete removal of white blood cells to avoid measuring leukocyte ferritin,[516] is insensitive to dynamic changes in iron status, and is rarely available to clinicians.

Erythrocyte Zinc Protoporphyrin Concentration. The determination of erythrocyte zinc protoporphyrin (ZPP) concentrations had shown some promise to identify patients on maintenance dialysis who require iron replacement therapy.[517-520] This marker is elevated in the presence of iron-deficient erythropoiesis, with Zn replacing iron in the heme precursor protoporphyrin.[521] Erythrocyte ZPP concentration is also elevated in the presence of lead poisoning. However, the diagnostic value of erythrocyte ZPP concentration appears to be inferior to that of RBC or reticulocyte parameters.[485,522] In addition, because whole blood ZPP concentration is falsely elevated in patients undergoing dialysis and in the presence of bilirubin and various drugs, careful washing of the RBCs is required to remove these interferences, rendering this assay not suitable for routine clinical care.[523,524]

Percentage of Hypochromic Red Blood Cells. A distinguishing characteristic of iron-deficient erythropoiesis is the production of hypochromic, microcytic erythrocytes. Iron-deficient erythropoiesis results in an increase in the percentage of hypochromic erythrocytes (%HYPO), defined as the percentage of erythrocytes with mean corpuscular hemoglobin concentration (MCHC) lower than 28 g/dL, for hematology analyzers produced by Siemens Medical Solutions.[525,526] Similar parameters (low hemoglobin density [LHD%] and DF-Hypo XE, respectively) are available in Beckman-Coulter and Sysmex instruments, respectively.[527,528] A classic study by

Macdougall and colleagues showed that functional iron deficiency induced by epoetin treatment and the response to IV iron could be detected by changes in %HYPO.[470] Several studies have confirmed that an increased %HYPO is a sensitive and early indicator of iron deficiency.[485,529-533] A European study found %HYPO to be the only independent predictor of mortality among various iron status parameters, with a twofold higher mortality risk for values higher than 10% than for values lower than 5%.[534] According to the European Best Practice Guidelines for the Management of Anaemia in Patients with Chronic Renal Failure, patients with %HYPO values higher than 6% are most likely to show response to IV iron therapy.[476] A clinical study tested the previous European Best Practice Guidelines for anemia management, which recommended a %HYPO target of less than 10%, by prospectively raising the delivered dose of IV iron to 228 patients to achieve a %HYPO value lower than 2.5% and a serum ferritin concentration of 200 to 500 ng/mL.[533] In this study, the median %HYPO value decreased from 8% to 4%, median serum ferritin concentration increased from 188 to 480 ng/mL, and median rhEPO dose decreased from 136 to 72 IU/kg/wk, showing that a strategy aimed at achieving %HYPO values much lower than 10% could be cost-effective, but it also resulted in serum ferritin values in some patients much higher than those recommended by guidelines.

Contrary to the European studies, North American studies have failed to show value for %HYPO in assessing iron availability in dialysis recipients.[535,536] The reasons for this discrepancy are not clear. It is worth noting that %HYPO progressively increases with storage of the blood sample, owing to the concomitant increase in MCV and reduction in MCHC, and is therefore best measured within 4 hours. In addition, %HYPO increases with reticulocytosis, because reticulocytes have lower MCHCs than mature RBCs.[537]

Reticulocyte Hemoglobin Content. After being released from the marrow, reticulocytes spend 18 to 36 hours in the circulation before becoming mature erythrocytes. Studies of the cellular characteristics of reticulocytes thus provide a real-time assessment of the functional state of the bone marrow. Automated analyzers can determine with great precision not only the absolute number of reticulocytes but also their size and Hgb concentration and content.[538,539] The reticulocyte Hgb content (CHr or RetHe), expressed in pg/cell, has been extensively studied, especially in patients treated with rhEPO.[540,541] A reduction in CHr is the most sensitive indicator of functional iron deficiency: Healthy subjects with normal iron stores who were treated with rhEPO produced a substantial fraction of hypochromic, low–Hgb content reticulocytes when their baseline serum ferritin levels were below 100 μg/L.[472] When IV iron was used in conjunction with EPO in normal subjects, the production of hypochromic reticulocytes was abolished.[542] Several small studies have described the value of CHr in identifying iron deficiency in dialysis recipients, mostly based on the subsequent response to IV iron.[487,535,536,543] A sensitivity of 100% and specificity of about 70% to 80% were reported in one study,[536] although other studies reported lower values.[487,543]

These initial studies led to additional large clinical trials that tested the values of CHr in managing the dosing of IV iron and rhEPO in dialysis recipients. Fishbane and colleagues randomly assigned 157 patients to two different IV iron management strategies: one based on CHr, in which IV iron was started if CHr fell below 29 pg/cell, and one in which IV iron was started if the serum ferritin concentration fell below 100 ng/mL or the TSAT value below 20%.[486] A significant reduction in exposure to IV iron was obtained in the CHr-based management, with no differences in weekly EPO dosing between the two groups.[486] Tessitore and coworkers[485] compared the diagnostic precision of a variety of hematologic and biochemical markers to identify subjects who exhibit an increase in Hgb in response to IV iron. A combination of %HYPO higher than 6% and CHr less than 29 pg/cell showed the best diagnostic efficiency for iron deficiency (80%) based on the Hgb response to IV iron. Other studies have provided additional confirmation of the diagnostic value of CHr,[544,545] although one has questioned its superiority to TSAT,[546] and only one study showed that use of IV iron in patients with low CHr resulted in decreased weekly usage of rhEPO.[547]

Several studies have also validated reticulocyte Hgb measurements (RET-He and Ret-Hb) generated by analyzers produced by Sysmex.[474,528,548-550] The current availability of the reticulocyte Hgb parameter on several analytical platforms may allow a wider utilization of this parameter. However, reticulocyte Hgb cannot be used to assess iron availability in the presence of either thalassemia traits (alpha or beta) or megaloblastic erythropoiesis.

Bone Marrow Iron. Although iron staining of a bone marrow biopsy is regarded as the gold standard method of assessing iron stores, widely divergent estimates of the prevalence of iron deficiency have been generated by this invasive, potentially painful procedure.[551-554] A study in 100 patients with ND-CKD showed that evaluation of iron stores by iron staining of a bone marrow sternal aspirate was no better than either TSAT or ferritin in correctly identifying "responders" to IV iron therapy.[555] Some patients with CKD have been found to have no stainable iron evident on sternal bone marrow biopsy, despite the presence of normal to elevated serum ferritin concentrations.[554,556] Bone marrow studies also have no value in identifying patients at risk for development of functional iron deficiency with EPO therapy.

Liver Magnetic Resonance Imaging. Hepatic magnetic resonance imaging (MRI) provides a noninvasive tool to estimate liver iron deposition and is regarded as the gold standard methodology for monitoring patients with iron overload disorders. However, the number of studies applying this technology in CKD is still very limited.[557-559] In the largest of these studies, conducted in 119 patients undergoing hemodialysis and receiving IV iron in a single center according to current guidelines, 84% had evidence of hepatic iron deposition and 30% had hepatic MRI findings consistent with severe iron overload.[559] These data raise concerns that the use of IV iron and current thresholds for laboratory parameters may be too liberal, especially considering the increased use of IV iron in the United States since 2011 (see Figure 57.7). On the other hand, it has not yet been demonstrated that the observed increases in hepatic iron are of any functional significance and/or associated with clinically relevant adverse outcomes.

Iron Balance Considerations. As already mentioned, 1 mL of blood normally contains 0.5 mg of iron and proportionately less when the Hgb concentration is reduced. An estimated annual blood loss of 2 L in a dialysis recipient with moderate anemia (20% reduction in Hgb) therefore roughly corresponds to 0.8 g of iron loss. Irrespective of all parameters of iron metabolism, IV iron supplementation in excess of this amount results in positive iron balance unless blood loss (and thereby iron loss) is more pronounced than anticipated. When patients were categorized according to their level of hepatic iron deposition, the average monthly iron dose was 150 mg and 283 mg in those with signs of mild and moderate iron overload, respectively, compared with 100 mg in those without.[559]

Intravenous Iron Therapy

There is general agreement that oral iron therapy is insufficient to properly support the functional needs of EPO-stimulated erythropoiesis in patients with ESKD. A systematic review and meta-analysis have shown that the Hgb response is much more potent with IV iron than with oral iron, with this effect being more substantial in patients on dialysis and of a lower magnitude in patients with ND-CKD.[560,561] Similar data were obtained in a systematic Cochrane analysis, which identified significant associations of IV iron therapy with increased Hgb, ferritin, and transferrin saturation values as well as reduced ESA requirements, with no differences in mortality.[562] Cost-effectiveness of IV iron therapy has also been demonstrated under the assumption that a higher mortality risk is associated with Hgb levels less than 9.0 g/dL.[563]

Nevertheless, oral iron may be effective in patients with ND-CKD. The FIND CKD (Ferinject assessment in patients with iron deficiency anemia and Non-Dialysis-dependent Chronic Kidney Disease) study compared the efficacy and safety of oral iron with IV administration of ferric carboxymaltose targeting two different serum ferritin ranges, 100 to 200 μg/L and 400 to 600 μg/L.[564] Although the IV therapy targeting the higher ferritin range showed greater efficacy, there was no difference in Hgb concentration or the need to switch to other anemia therapy between the IV arm targeting the lower ferritin range and the oral iron therapy arm.[565] Ferric citrate (Zerenex, Keryx Biopharmaceuticals, New York, NY) a newly developed iron-containing phosphate binder, was shown to reduce serum phosphate and increase TSAT values and to moderately increase Hgb levels in comparison with placebo in patients with ND-CKD, providing support for the potential use of this product as an oral iron supplement in this patient group.[566] However, the U.S. Food and Drug Administration (FDA) has approved the product only as a phosphate binder and placed a safety warning for a potentially excessive elevation of iron stores.

Several IV iron preparations are available for clinical use, most of them containing iron associated with a carbohydrate shell. The strength or lability of this association is crucial for dosing, with the most stable preparations, like iron dextran, being suitable for large dose replacements, and the more labile preparations, like iron gluconate, requiring multiple dosing with a single-dose maximum of approximately 100 mg. Intravenous iron infusion may lead to some immediate binding of the infused iron to transferrin, resulting in its complete saturation and the generation of free iron, which has vasoactive effects and can produce hypotensive and/or anaphylactoid reactions. This risk involves mainly semilabile iron-sugar complexes like iron sucrose and iron gluconate, and not more stable complexes like ferric carboxymaltose, ferumoxytol, and iron dextran.

Several preparations of IV iron are meanwhile available in the United States and European market (Table 57.1):

Lower-molecular-weight iron dextran, produced by PharmaCosmos, Holbaek, Denmark, is in use both in the United States (INFeD, Actavis, Dublin) and Europe (Cosmofer, Pharmacosmos, Holbaek, Denmark; Ferrisat, H.A.C. Pharma, Caen, France); it has a significantly better tolerability and fewer side effects than the higher-molecular-weight product, which has now been removed from U.S. and European markets.[567-573]

Iron sucrose (Venofer, produced by Vifor, St. Gallen, Switzerland, and marketed in the United States by American Regent Laboratories, Inc., Shirley, NY) is used worldwide in the treatment of renal anemia and is the most used parenteral iron preparation in the United States.[574] Allergic reactions have been reported in less than 1/100,000 infusions. IV injection into rats of three different commercial preparations of iron sucrose resulted in different degrees of inflammation and oxidative stress, suggesting that the stability of the iron complex may differ from one iron sucrose preparation to another.[575]

Ferric gluconate (Ferrlecit, marketed in the United States by Sanofi Aventis US, Bridgewater, NJ) is the second most commonly prescribed IV iron preparation in the United States and is frequently used worldwide in patients on hemodialysis.[576]

Ferric carboxymaltose (Ferinject, Vifor; Injectafer, American Regent Inc., Luitpold Pharmaceuticals, Shirley, NY) is the newest iron preparation registered in both Europe and the United States.[577] A significant advantage of this preparation is the possibility of infusing up to 750 mg of iron in a short time (15 min) with minimal side effects.[578,579] Transient hypophosphatemia has been reported in patients without CKD and in those with ND-CKD treated with ferric carboxymaltose, possibly mediated by a decreased tubular reabsorption of phosphate.[580,581]

Ferumoxytol (Feraheme, AMAG Pharmaceuticals, Inc., Lexington, MA) is an iron oxide nanoparticle with polyglucose sorbitol carboxymethylether coating designed to minimize immunologic sensitivity and release of free iron, allowing a rapid injection (17 to 60 sec, currently approved infusion time >15 min) of a large dose (510 mg) of iron, which can be repeated after 3 to 8 days.[582-585] Efficacy and adverse events in patients with CKD were found to be similar to those of iron sucrose.[586] Ferumoxytol is the only IV iron preparation possessing super magnetic properties, similar to MRI contrast agents, which may alter MRI findings for up to 3 months owing to its uptake into the reticuloendothelial system.[583] On the basis of the studies used for FDA registration, 0.2% of treated subjects experienced anaphylaxis or anaphylactoid reactions, and 3.7% had hypersensitivity-type reactions (pruritus, rash, urticaria, or wheezing); 1.9% of patients had hypotension, and 3 patients experienced serious hypotensive reactions.[583] The development of nephrogenic systemic fibrosis following gadolinium use

Table 57.1 Intravenous Iron Preparations

			FDA Approved			Not FDA Approved
Generic Name	Iron Dextran	Iron Sucrose	Na Ferric Gluconate	Ferric Carboxymaltose	Ferumoxytol	Iron Isomaltoside 1000
Trade Name USA (marketed by)	INFed (Actavis)	Venofer (American Regent Inc., Luitpold Pharmaceuticals, Inc.)	Ferrlecit (Sanofi/Aventis), Nulecit (Actavis)	Injectafer (Luitpold/American Regent, Inc.)	Feraheme (AMAG Pharmaceuticals, Inc.)	Monofer (Pharmacosmos A/S)
Trade Name(s) Europe	Cosmofer, Uniferon, Ferrisat	Venofer, Idafer, FerroLogic, Ferion, Venotrix, Fermed, Netro-Fer	Ferrlecit, Ferlixit	Injectafer, Ferinject	Rienso	Monofer, Monover, Monoferro, Diafer
Carbohydrate	Dextran polysaccharide (LMW)	Sucrose	Gluconate	Carboxymaltoside	Polyglucose sorbitol carboxymethylether	Isomaltoside
Molecular weight (kDa)	165	34-60	289-444	150	750	150
Iron, mg/mL	50	20	12.5	50	30	50 or 100
Hemodialysis, mg/session	100	100	125	—	510	100-200 (UK)
Peritoneal dialysis	100	1 × 300 mg 1 × 300 mg after 14 d 1 × 400 mg after 14 d		—	510	
CKD, nondialysis	100	200 mg or 500 mg		750 mg	510	
TDI possible?	Yes	No	No	Yes	No	Yes
Maximum approved dose	100 mg	400	125 mg	750 mg for body weight > 50 kg	510 mg	Up to 20 mg/kg (UK)
Maximum safe dose	TDI over 1-4 hr	400 mg over 2 hr	250 mg over 1 hr	750 mg over 15 min	510 mg in > 15 min	20 mg/kg over 15 min
Premedication?	No	No	No	No	No	No
Test dose required?	Yes	No	No	No	No	No
"Black Box" warning (FDA)?	Yes	No	No	No	Yes	NA
Adverse reaction(s)				Hypophosphatemia	Alteration of magnetic resonance imaging findings	
Preservative	None	None	Benzyl alcohol	None	None	None

CKD, Chronic kidney disease; FDA, U.S. Food and Drug Administration; NA, not applicable; TDI, tolerable daily intake.
FDA warnings: Iron dextran and Ferumoxytol, fatal allergic reactions.

has prompted the use of ferumoxytol as an alternative MRI contrast agent in patients with CKD stage 4 or 5, and in dialysis-dependent CKD.[587,588]

Ferric isomaltoside (Monofer, Pharmacosmos A/S) is based on a nonbranched carbohydrate, which does not form the typical spheroidal iron carbohydrate nanoparticle like other IV iron preparations and seems to be associated with lower immunogenic potential. Monofer can be administered in a single dose, with dosages up to 20 mg/kg. Monofer is currently approved and marketed in 28 countries, including 21 European Union members, but not in the United States.

A study on IV iron use for the period 1994 through 2002 in the United States indicated that iron sucrose and ferric gluconate were the predominant forms of IV iron used in CKD, with 84.4% of hemodialysis and 19.3 of peritoneal dialysis patients having some form of IV iron therapy.[589]

Parenteral iron administration has increased substantially in the United States, most likely because of a shift in reimbursement practices toward a bundled/capitated model (see Figure 57.7). Data from the Dialysis Outcomes and Practice Patterns Study (DOPPS) show IV iron use increasing from 55% to 66% to 68% of patients on hemodialysis between 2010 and 2012.[590] Similar trends have been reported for European countries, Japan, Australia, and New Zealand.[591] A ferritin threshold of 800 ng/mL is now commonly used for prompt withholding of IV iron therapy in patients on maintenance dialysis.

Side Effects of IV Iron. Iron sucrose, lower-molecular-weight iron dextran, and ferric carboxymaltose have excellent track records for both safety and tolerability. Hypersensitivity reactions (erythematous rash and urticaria) are rare and their intensity is usually mild or moderate. Lack of recurrence after rechallenge indicates that most of these events are not due to immunologic reactions. Severe life-threatening allergic reactions are a major problem with the higher-molecular-weight iron dextran, prompting its removal from European and U.S. markets. The use of a test dose is still required for iron dextran in the United States, but the European Medicines Agency no longer recommends it.[592] A retrospective study by Chertow and colleagues examining more than 50 million doses of IV iron demonstrated the higher risk of reactions with higher-molecular-weight iron dextran and found that rates of serious events associated with lower-molecular-weight iron dextran were similar to those seen with the other forms of IV iron (≈1/200,000).[568,569] A study from the FDA,[593] using data obtained from the administration's Adverse Event Reporting System (AERS) and other U.S. databases, was unable to provide firm data on the relative safety of the four IV preparations marketed in the United States owing to incomplete brand information on these reports, but it did confirm that allergic reactions have been reported for all brands.[594] Chertow and colleagues estimated absolute rates of life-threatening reaction per million doses of 0.6 for iron sucrose, 0.9 for sodium ferric gluconate complex, 3.3 for lower-molecular-weight iron dextran and 11.3 for higher molecular weight iron dextran.[569] However, a later systematic review highlighted the lack of properly conducted and powered studies comparing adverse events rates between lower-molecular-weight iron dextran and iron sucrose.[595] The amount of labile iron, which differs among the various IV iron preparations, is likely an important determinant of possible oxidative and nitrosative stress.[596]

Infection Risk and Intravenous Iron Therapy. In vitro data seem to support the notion that iron can promote bacterial growth and at the same time impair leukocyte function.[522,597-600] IV injection of iron sucrose in dialyzed patients has been associated with the dose-dependent appearance of markers of oxidant damage in lymphocytes and a decrease in plasma ascorbate and alpha tocopherol in some studies[601] but not in others.[602-604] In addition, studies have not accounted for the fact that the capability of leukocytes to cope with oxidant damage is markedly affected by polymorphisms in glutathione S-transferase M1.[605] Although there is indirect and inconclusive evidence for an association between iron stores and bacteremia,[597] most studies have failed to show an association of IV iron therapy with an increased risk of infection in dialyzed patients.[522,599-600] Many studies attempting to link iron status and risk of bacterial infection have used serum ferritin, an unreliable marker of iron status in CKD, as discussed previously.[597,606-610] One study showed that in patients receiving more than 10 vials of 100 mg iron dextran over 6 months, there was an increased risk of death and hospitalization.[611] One uncontrolled retrospective study reported a higher incidence of bacteremia with iron sucrose than with ferric gluconate.[612] Other studies have failed to show a significant effect of IV iron dosing or iron status (using serum ferritin) on bacteremia, mortality, infection, or hospitalization.[522,600,613,614] On the other hand, a later observational study using a very large database found that bolus administration of higher doses of IV iron was associated with higher risks for infection-related hospitalizations and death, particularly in patients undergoing dialysis with catheters rather than arteriovenous fistulas or grafts.[615] Despite the lack of proof of significant effects on the rates of infections, cardiac events, and mortality, long-term toxicities and, in particular, the possible consequences of oxidant damage due to free radical generation are still a concern.[604,616] Unfortunately no large outcome studies have been performed so far to prospectively test the efficacy and safety of iron replacement strategies, either in the short or the long term.[617] An ongoing trial in the United Kingdom, comparing proactive high-dose IV iron therapy with reactive low-dose therapy in 2080 patients new to dialysis, will assess the impact of both regimens on mortality and cardiovascular events.[618]

Iron Therapy in Patients with CKD. Iron therapy in CKD should be guided by iron status test results and clinical considerations and needs to take into account the potential benefits of avoiding or minimizing blood transfusions, ESA use, and anemia-related symptoms against the risk of potential harm (Table 57.2).[9] Iron tests should be performed monthly in the initial phase of ESA treatment and every 3 months thereafter.[10,11] As discussed in detail previously, a target of serum ferritin concentration higher than 200 ng/mL and TSAT value greater than 20% or a CHr value higher then 29 pg/cell has been used for patients on dialysis.[10,11] The KDIGO guideline recommends using IV iron if an

Table 57.2 Current Anemia Guidelines and Position Statements Regarding Iron Administration

KDIGO Clinical Practice Guideline (International)	2.1.1: When prescribing iron therapy, balance the potential benefits of avoiding or minimizing blood transfusions, ESA therapy, and anemia-related symptoms against the risks of harm in individual patients (e.g., anaphylactoid and other acute reactions, unknown long-term risks). *(Not Graded)* 2.1.2: For adult CKD patients with anemia not on iron or ESA therapy we suggest a trial of IV iron (or in CKD ND patients alternatively a 1-3 month trial of oral iron therapy) if (2C): • An increase in Hb concentration without starting ESA treatment is desired* and • TSAT is ≤30% and ferritin is ≤500 ng/mL (≤500 µg/L) 2.1.3: For adult CKD patients on ESA therapy who are not receiving iron supplementation, we suggest a trial of IV iron (or in CKD ND patients alternatively a 1-3 month trial of oral iron therapy) if (2C): • An increase in Hb concentration† or a decrease in ESA dose is desired‡ and • TSAT is ≤30% and ferritin is ≤500 ng/mL (≤500 µg/L)
KDOQI Commentary (United States)	• We believe that the degree of caution expressed by KDIGO is not supported by the available evidence and could have negative effects, such as sustained iron deficiency anemia, higher ESA dose requirements, and increased blood transfusions. • We therefore believe that a therapeutic trial of IV iron could be considered when TSAT is low (≤30%), even if ferritin concentration is above 500 ng/mL. • There is insufficient evidence upon which to base a recommendation for an upper ferritin limit above which IV iron must be withheld. • A decision to administer iron in the setting of high ferritin would require weighing potential risks and benefits of persistent anemia, ESA dosage, comorbid conditions, and health-related QoL. In accordance with KDIGO recommendations, Hb response to iron therapy, TSAT, and ferritin should be monitored closely and further iron therapy titrated accordingly.
CSN Commentary (Canada)§	• There is good evidence (1B) to support the administration of iron in adult CKD patients when the TSAT and ferritin thresholds are above 20% and 200 ng/mL. A therapeutic trial of iron can be considered in those where an increase in Hb or reduction of ESA or avoidance of ESA and transfusion is desired, while recognizing that an increase in hemoglobin is less likely when TSATs are >30% and ferritins are >500 ng/mL. • However, as opposed to the KDIGO anemia guideline, the CSN anemia work group feels the current evidence does not permit a clear delineation for an upper limit of TSAT or ferritin levels.

*Based on patient symptoms and overall clinical goals, including avoidance of transfusion, improvement in anemia-related symptoms, and after exclusion of active infection.
†Consistent with Recommendations #3.4.2 and 3.4.3.
‡Based on patient symptoms and overall clinical goals including avoidance of transfusion and improvement in anemia-related symptoms, and after exclusion of active infection and other causes of ESA hyporesponsiveness.
§Quoted material is excerpted to focus on hemodialysis; ferritin units for CSN commentary converted to ng/mL.
CKD, Chronic kidney disease; CKD ND, non–dialysis-dependent CKD; CSN, Canadian Society of Nephrology; ESA, erythropoiesis-stimulating agent; Hb, hemoglobin; IV, intravenous; KDIGO, Kidney Disease: Improving Global Outcomes; KDOQI, Kidney Disease Outcomes Quality Initiative; QoL, quality of life; TSAT, transferrin saturation.
From Weiner DE, Winkelmayer WC: Commentary on "The DOPPS practice monitor for US dialysis care: update on trends in anemia management 2 years into the bundle": iron(y) abounds 2 years later. Am J Kidney Dis.62:1213-1220, 2013; quoted material from Kidney Disease Improving Global Outcomes (KDIGO) Anemia Work Group: KDIGO clinical practice guideline for anemia in chronic kidney disease. Kidney Int Suppl. 2:279-335, 2012; Kliger AS, Foley RN, Goldfarb DS, et al: KDOQI US Commentary on the 2012 KDIGO clinical practice guideline for anemia in CKD. Am J Kidney Dis. 62:849-859, 2013; and Moist LM, Troyanov S, White CT, et al: Canadian Society of Nephrology commentary on the 2012 KDIGO clinical practice guideline for anemia in CKD. Am J Kidney Dis 62: 860-873, 2013.

increase in Hgb concentration or a decrease in ESA requirements is aimed for, if serum ferritin ≤ 500 ng/mL and TSAT ≤ 30%.[9] For patients with ND-CKD and patients undergoing peritoneal dialysis, target values of more than 100 ng/mL for serum ferritin and higher than 20% for TSAT should be used. The objective of iron therapy in CKD is to abolish overt and/or functional iron deficiency, because it reduces erythropoietic response to and effectiveness of ESAs. The response to ESAs can be optimized by the simultaneous use of IV iron, which enables a significant reduction in ESA dosing.[619] Several studies conducted in the early and late 1990s demonstrated that IV iron therapy is associated with significant ESA dose reductions.[562,603,620-628] The DRIVE (Dialysis Patients Response on IV Iron with Elevated Ferritin) studies showed that an intensive IV iron administration protocol (125 mg ferric gluconate with each of eight hemodialysis sessions) can significantly reduce ESA dosing requirements.[629,630] A Cochrane systematic review has provided additional support to the ESA-sparing effects of IV iron.[562] Shirazian and associates have noted that ESA-sparing effects of IV iron could easily be demonstrated when there was a high prevalence of iron deficiency and low usage of IV iron.[619] However, they suggest that most of the benefits of IV iron in reducing ESA use have already been achieved, given that 60% to 80% of patients on dialysis in the United States are being treated with IV iron and that it is not clear how much additional ESA dose reduction could be obtained with more intensive IV iron regimens.

Given the potential adverse effects of ESAs (see later) the latest KDIGO anemia guideline mentions explicitly that the desire to avoid or minimize ESAs can influence the decisions about iron use[9] (see Table 57.2).[9]

As shown in Table 57.1, several forms of IV iron are available worldwide. Although they have important differences in formulation and dosing, no convincing evidence has been provided about superiority of one form over the others in the setting of CKD. The REPAIR-IDA trial demonstrated that a regimen of two doses of 750 mg of ferric carboxymaltose in 1 week was not inferior to up to five infusions of iron sucrose in 14 days for anemic subjects with ND-CKD.[581] Use of larger doses of IV iron rather than lower maintenance doses does not appreciably affect cardiovascular morbidity and mortality in hemodialyzed patients.[631]

Some studies have suggested that the addition of ascorbic acid to the therapeutic regimen of patients treated with ESA and iron has beneficial effects, although none was rigorously conducted to provide definitive evidence.[632,633] Limited evidence suggests that ascorbic acid may be pro-oxidant and may increase cytokine levels.[634] A systematic review and meta-analysis concluded that there is evidence, in a limited number of small studies, that use of ascorbic acid results in increased Hgb concentrations, improves transferrin saturation, and reduces EPO utilization.[635] However, use of ascorbic acid is not recommended in either the KDOQI or KDIGO guidelines.[10]

EFFICACY AND SAFETY OF ANEMIA MANAGEMENT WITH ESAS AND IRON

The change in the condition of patients on maintenance dialysis following the advent of rhEPO was impressive and obviously advantageous. Transfusion requirements declined, iron overload due to previous RBC transfusions gradually resolved, and patients could easily be maintained at Hgb values above those that had to be accepted when rRBC transfusions were the only viable option of anemia management. Androgen therapy, which had been associated with significant side effects, could also be abolished. Because of these obvious benefits, the use of epoetin soon became routine and the workup for anemia is considered part of the management program of patients in all stages of CKD (Figure 57.9). If the workup reveals no reasons for anemia other than EPO deficiency associated with CKD and in particular has ruled out iron deficiency, ESA therapy provides an option to correct anemia in almost all patients. However, despite the apparent advantages, formal evidence of a positive long-term benefit has never been established.

Several lines of indirect evidence suggested that correcting or ameliorating anemia could reduce or at least mitigate the rate of left ventricular hypertrophy, a frequent complication in CKD clearly associated with poor prognosis (see preceding discussion). Together with the apparent lack of adverse effects of ESA therapy and the contention that higher Hgb concentrations might lead to improved HRQOL and physical function, this evidence led to an increase in Hgb target values. In addition, treatment was expanded to those patients not yet on dialysis, in whom anemia is generally less severe than in those on dialysis, because avoidance of anemia rather than late correction was intuitively considered the most appropriate strategy to improve prognosis and quality of life. Unfortunately, however, for a long time the true nature of the relationship between long-term reductions in Hgb concentrations and adverse outcomes was not adequately tested in prospective interventional trials. Few studies have actually compared ESAs against placebo, and those trials testing two different Hgb target ranges have usually been inadequately powered.[598]

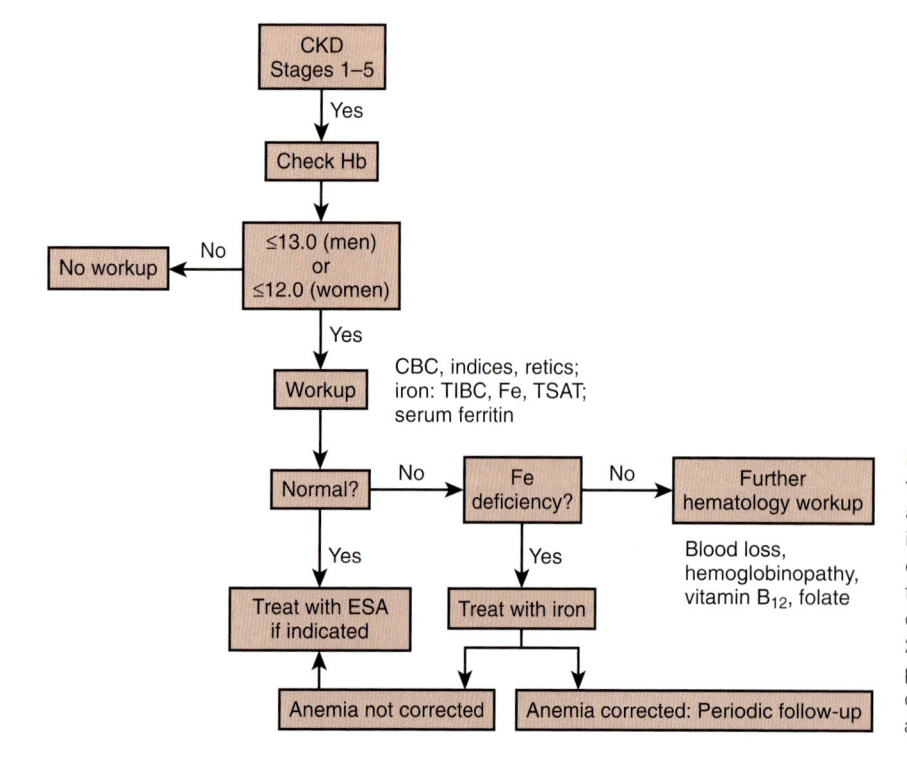

Figure 57.9 Flowchart for the evaluation of the patient with chronic kidney disease (CKD) and anemia. CBC, Complete blood count; Fe, iron; Hb, hemoglobin; TIBC, total iron-binding capacity; TSAT, transferrin saturation. (Modified from Lankhorst CE, Wish JB: Anemia in renal disease: diagnosis and management. *Blood Rev* 24:39-47, 2010. Adapted from K/DOQI clinical practice guidelines and clinical practice recommendations for anemia in chronic kidney disease in adults. *Am J Kidney Dis* 47[Suppl 3]:S1-145, 2006.)

Meanwhile, evidence from several larger RCTs became available,[635a] suggesting that normalization of Hgb concentrations with ESAs is associated with limited benefit and relevant harm.

Trial Overview

Since 1989 slightly more than 25 RCTs using ESAs in patients with CKD have been published, in which either different target Hgb concentrations were compared or ESA treatment was compared with placebo. Approximately half of these trials were conducted in patients on dialysis, the other half in patients with ND-CKD. Overall approximately 11,000 patients have been enrolled in these trials, more than 4000 of whom were involved in one study, the Trial to Reduce Cardiovascular Events with Aranesp Therapy (TREAT).[636] The number of patients in the other trials varied between fewer than 20 to approximately 1400.[10,11] Several small trials conducted until 1997 compared ESA therapy with placebo. Thereafter, only treatment strategies testing two different ESA regimens were performed until TREAT was designed as the first large trial to compare ESA therapy with placebo in patients with diabetes and CKD who were not undergoing dialysis.

Large Randomized Controlled Trials. The U.S. Normal Hematocrit Trial was the first to test whether normalization of hemoglobin concentrations improves the prognosis of patients on dialysis.[637] It was hypothesized that any presumed benefit would be most obvious in patients with cardiac disease and, therefore, the trial enrolled slightly more than 1200 hemodialysis recipients who had congestive heart failure or ischemic heart disease. The target hematocrit in the higher arm was 42%, and in the lower arm 30%. The primary end point was a composite of death and first nonfatal myocardial infarction. The study was terminated early after 29 months because more patients in the higher arm had reached the primary end point. Although the difference did not reach statistical significance, study termination was recommended because it was obvious that the original hypothesis, that the higher hematocrit target was of benefit, could not be proven. In addition, the incidence of vascular access thrombosis was significantly higher in the higher target hematocrit arm. Self-reported physical function score improved at higher hematocrits, but importantly there was no significant difference between the two treatment arms for this parameter. A later analysis, which included end point events that the data safety monitoring committee had not yet considered when recommending termination of the study, also did not reveal a significant difference, and the rates of events occurring during 1-year of follow-up after study termination were similar in the two treatment arms.[638]

A second large trial in ESKD included almost 600 patients new to hemodialysis without symptomatic heart disease and left ventricular dilation.[639] Patients were randomly assigned in a double-blind fashion to an Hgb treatment target of either 13.5 to 14.5 g/dL or 9.5 to 11.5 g/dL. The primary end point was a change in left ventricular volume index, on the assumption that raising the Hgb concentration would prevent the progression of left ventricular hypertrophy. However, changes in left ventricular volume index were similar for the two treatment groups. The only difference among a number of secondary outcomes was a better 36-Item Short Form Health Survey (SF-36) vitality score in the higher Hgb than in the lower Hgb group. Adverse event rates were also similar, except that rates of skeletal pain, surgery, and dizziness were higher in the lower arm, whereas those of headache and cerebrovascular events were slightly higher in the higher arm.

Thus, neither trial provided any evidence in favor of normalization of hemoglobin concentrations in patients on dialysis. However, because the prognosis, extent of comorbidities, and hemodynamic and metabolic milieu of patients receiving dialysis are so different from those of patients with ND-CKD, the benefit of anemia correction was further tested in ND-CKD in three other studies.

The CREATE (Cardiovascular Risk Reduction by Early Anemia Treatment with Epoetin Beta) trial was conducted in Europe, Mexico, and Taiwan.[640] It enrolled approximately 600 patients with an eGFR of 15 to 35 mL/min and an Hgb concentration of 11 to 12.5 g/dL. Patients were randomly assigned to a treatment arm in which epoetin beta therapy was started immediately to achieve Hgb concentrations of 13 to 15 g/dL or to an arm in which treatment with epoetin was not initiated before Hgb had dropped to below 10.5 g/dL; the target Hgb in this second arm was 10.5 to 11.5 g/dL. The primary end point was a composite of eight cardiovascular events, which included "the time to a first cardiovascular event, including sudden death, myocardial infarction, acute heart failure, stroke, transient ischemic attack, angina pectoris resulting in hospitalization for 24 hours or more or prolongation of hospitalization, complication of peripheral vascular disease (amputation or necrosis), or cardiac arrhythmia resulting in hospitalization for 24 hours or more."[640] The study did not show a significant difference in the time to event between the treatment arms. Some dimensions of HRQOL were improved in the arm with earlier treatment and higher target, but unexpectedly, time to dialysis was significantly shorter in this treatment arm. One of the limitations of the trial was that the observed event rate was much lower than the anticipated event rate, yielding lower than expected statistical power.

The CHOIR (Correction of Hemoglobin and Outcomes in Renal Insufficiency) study, conducted in the United States, had a similar design but enrolled patients with more comorbid disease and yielded different conclusions.[641] More than 1400 patients with eGFR values 15 to 50 mL/min and Hgb concentrations below 11 g/dL were randomly allocated to receive epoetin alfa to achieve one of two different target Hgb values, 13.5 or 11.3 g/dL. The primary end point was a composite of death, myocardial infarction, hospitalization for congestive heart failure, and stroke. The trial was terminated when significantly more patients in the higher Hgb arm experienced at least one cardiovascular event. Separate analysis of the four components of the combined end point revealed trends for more frequent hospitalizations for heart failure and more frequent deaths but no difference in the rates of myocardial infarction or stroke. In addition, there was a trend toward more rapid progression of kidney disease in the higher Hgb target group. However, a meta-analysis of available studies support an effect of ESA on the progression of CKD.[642] Unlike in the CREATE trial, twofold to threefold higher doses of epoetin were needed in the CHOIR study to achieve and maintain similar Hgb values. Interestingly, a post hoc analysis showed that the risks associated with the higher Hgb target were not apparent among subgroups with higher mortality risk.[643]

In contrast to the other four large trials, the TREAT (Trial to Reduce Cardiovascular Events with Aranesp Therapy) was designed to test the effect of ESA in comparison with placebo in a sufficiently powered study. More than 4000 patients with CKD (eGFR 20 to 60 mL/min/1.73 m^2) and type 2 diabetes, and an Hgb concentration below 11 g/dL were randomly assigned to receive either darbepoetin with a treatment target of 13 g/dL or placebo.[636] In order to avoid development of severe anemia in the placebo-treated group, a rescue protocol was established, according to which darbepoietin was administered when Hgb fell below 9 g/dL. The study was double blinded. There were two primary end points, a cardiovascular composite end point and a renal composite end point, including death or initiation of maintenance dialysis. The trial showed no difference in the composite renal or cardiovascular end points, but analysis of the components of the primary end point revealed a significant, twofold higher risk of stroke in the darbepoetin arm. As an additional safety signal, the number of deaths attributed to cancer tended to be higher in the treatment arm, albeit not significantly, and in a subgroup of approximately 350 patients with a history of malignancy, all-cause mortality tended to be higher and significantly more deaths were attributed to cancer. These findings were consistent with some findings in ESA RCTs in patients with cancer, which showed higher mortality and more rapid progression of malignancy in patients treated with ESA for chemotherapy-related anemia.[644] Patients in the darbepoetin arm of the TREAT received fewer transfusions and showed a larger mean change in the Functional Assessment of Cancer Therapy: Fatigue (FACT-F) score.

Risk/Benefit Relationship and Target Hemoglobin Recommendations. In summary, evidence from well-designed, larger RCTs indicate that raising Hgb to normal or near-normal values with ESAs does not enhance survival or reduce the rate of cardiovascular events in patients with ND-CKD or ESKD but is associated with risk for harm.[645] These results are consistent also with another large trial in patients with heart failure, many of whom had CKD.[646] Almost all studies showed increased rates of thromboembolic events, but for unknown reasons, other risks are not consistent across different studies. Although the CHOIR study, for example, suggested a mortality risk,[641] this finding was not confirmed in TREAT.[636] Also, a negative impact on the time to dialysis, as found in the CREATE trial,[640] was not found in the TREAT. The TREAT, on the other hand, found an increased incidence of stroke,[639] and although another study had previously reported a slightly higher number of strokes in a higher Hgb treatment arm,[646] neither the CREATE trial nor the CHOIR study found differences in stroke rates.[640,641] These inconsistencies may point toward important yet unrecognized factors that determine the side effect profile of ESAs. Despite intensive investigation, it has not been possible so far to identify characteristics that distinguish patients in whom stroke developed during ESA therapy in the TREAT.[647] Whether any of the observed adverse events are related to the actual achieved Hgb values, to indirect effects of an increase in erythropoiesis, or to direct, hemoglobin-independent effects of ESAs is unknown.[643]

Any benefit of higher Hgb for HRQOL appears modest on average once Hgb concentrations above about 10 g/dL are reached. Transfusion rates are lower with higher Hgb,[648,649] but it is also clear that attempts to normalize Hgb by no means eliminate transfusion requirements. Moreover, the actual benefit from avoiding RBC transfusions is difficult to determine in individual patients, although the risk of sensitization in prospective transplant recipients should be strongly considered.[650]

Whether the balance of the risks and benefits of ESA therapy depends on the patient's responsiveness remains unclear. In treatment protocols driven by a target Hgb range, hyporesponsiveness leads to the use of higher doses and is associated with a greater likelihood of adverse events, but whether ESAs play a causal role remains unclear. A secondary analysis of the CHOIR study suggested that high ESA doses rather than high Hgb concentrations are associated with poor outcomes.[379,643] In the TREAT, the response to the first two weight-based doses of darbepoetin was a significant predictor of poor prognosis, with patients in the lowest quartile of ESA responsiveness having higher rates of the composite cardiovascular end point or death.[651] However, because "hyporesponders" could be identified only among the treated patients, it is unclear whether their poor prognosis was affected by ESA therapy.

The global KDIGO guideline for anemia in CKD takes these considerations into account.[9] Careful balancing of the risks and benefits of ESA and iron therapy is an overarching recommendation. In patients not undergoing dialysis the guideline recommends that a drop of Hgb value to less than 9 g/dL be avoided by initiation of ESA when the Hgb is between 9 and 10 g/dL. In general, ESA should not be used to maintain Hgb concentrations above 11.5 g/dL, and there is a strong recommendation against intentionally raising the Hgb above 13 g/dL. However, individualization appears appropriate, as some patients may have improvements in quality of life with Hgb values above 11.5 g/dL and are prepared to accept an increased risk.

In the United States, a major change in payment for dialysis and related services has resulted in bundling of payments for laboratory services and IV medications and their oral equivalents. Together with the previously mentioned results from clinical trials and subsequent changes in drug labeling from the FDA, these payment changes have produced measurable reductions in the use of ESAs and Hgb levels and have resulted in higher rates of transfusion in patients on maintenance dialysis.[652] The U.S. experience may not be directly applicable to other countries.[653]

RED BLOOD CELL TRANSFUSION

When large RCTs questioned the safety and overall benefit of ESAs and of targeting higher Hgb concentrations, an appreciable increase was observed in the proportion of patients having Hgb values less than 10 g/dL, which, in conjunction with stable transfusion rates for this patient subgroup, translated into an increase in the absolute number of transfusions.[648] As shown in Figures 57.3 and 57.10, transfusion rates for U.S. patients on maintenance dialysis were 2.9% in 2011 and 3.0% in 2012. Interestingly, transfusion rates in patients with ND-CKD also rose significantly from 2002-2003 to 2008 (see Figure 57.10).[649]

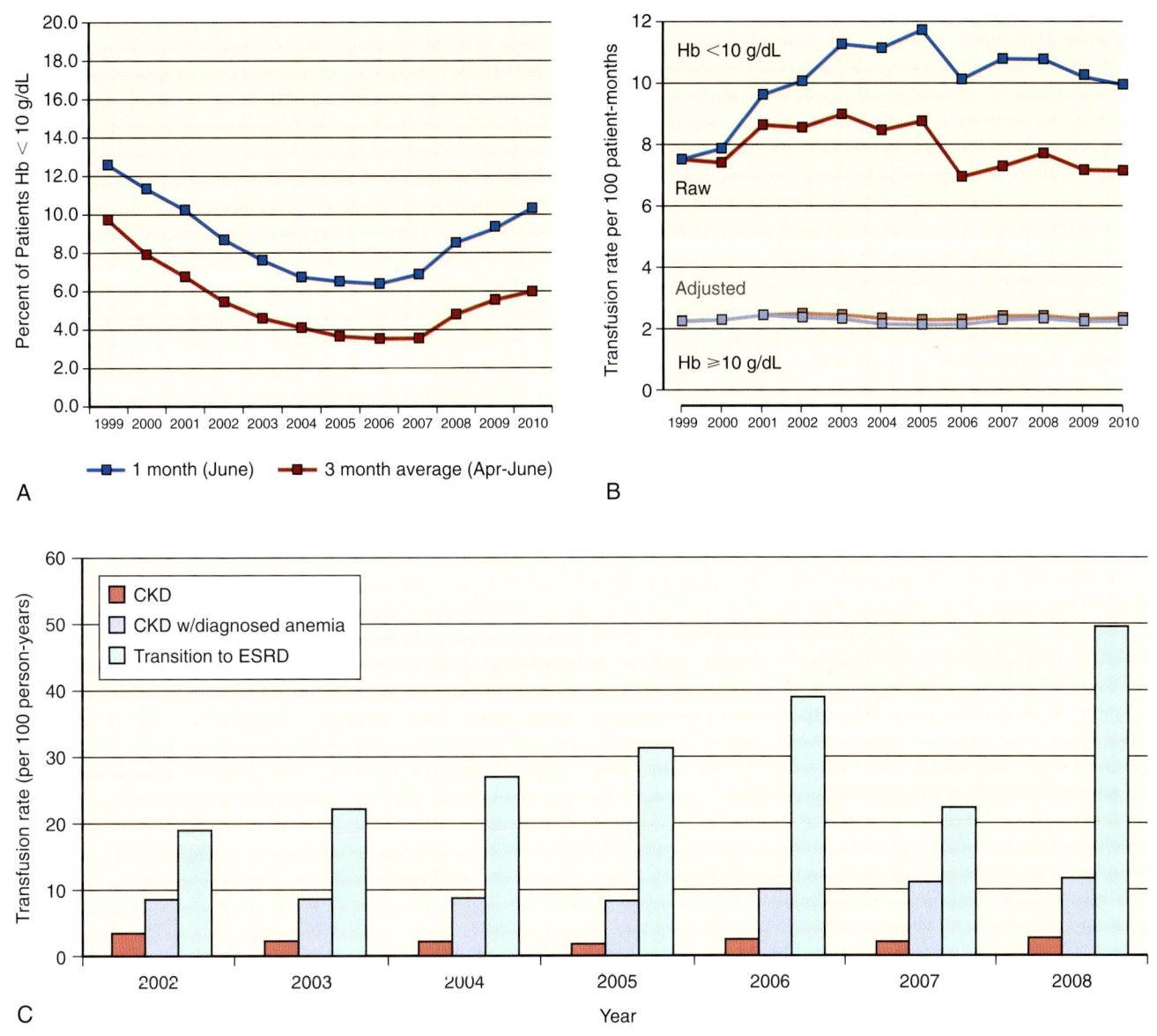

Figure 57.10 Red blood cell transfusion in chronic kidney disease (CKD). **A,** Proportion of patients with a single monthly or 3-month average hemoglobin (Hb) concentration of ≤10 g/dL, 1999-2010. **B,** Unadjusted and adjusted (for age, sex, race, primary cause of end-stage kidney disease, hospitalization days, and dose of erythropoiesis-stimulating agent) 6-month transfusion rates for patients with Hb levels less than 10 and equal to or greater than 10 g/dL (1999-2010). **C,** Annual red blood cell transfusion rates per 100 person-years (2002–2008) for patients with CKD; patients with CKD and diagnosed anemia, and patients with CKD transitioning to end-stage renal disease (ESRD) during each follow-up year. (**A** and **B** from Gilbertson DT, Monda KL, Bradbury BD, et al: RBC transfusions among hemodialysis patients (1999-2010): influence of hemoglobin concentrations below 10 g/dL. *Am J Kidney Dis.* 62:919-928, 2013; **C** from Gill KS, Muntner P, Lafayette RA, et al: Red blood cell transfusion use in patients with chronic kidney disease. *Nephrol Dial Transpl* 28:1504-1515, 2013.)

Transfusion is associated with development of alloantibodies and HLA sensitization,[654] which has important negative consequences for donor matching of patient candidates for renal transplantation. HLA sensitization also increases graft rejection and diminishes graft survival. It is unlikely that blood transfusion has any benefit on subsequent allograft function. Although the published literature seems to have mixed results, patients who received transfusions and who developed alloantibodies were less likely to undergo transplantation. It is unreasonable and potentially misleading to compare patients who received transfusions and did not develop alloantibodies with all patients who did not receive transfusions. We agree with the current consensus that blood transfusion should be avoided if possible.[650] Because transplantation waiting times exceed life expectancy throughout most of the United States and much of the developed world, patients can ill afford a procedure (i.e., transfusion) that offers modest if any benefit and that can further lower the likelihood of ever receiving a kidney transplant.

Relatively common complications of RBC transfusions are febrile or urticarial/allergic (immediate hypersensitivity) reactions. Less common complications include acute and delayed hemolytic transfusion reactions, hypotensive transfusion reactions, transfusion-associated dyspnea, transfusion-associated circulatory overload, transfusion-related acute lung injury, posttransfusion purpura, and transfusion-associated graft-versus-host disease. Additional complications of RBC transfusion include potential transmission of known and unknown infectious agents, and iron overload.

DISORDERS OF HEMOSTASIS IN CHRONIC KIDNEY DISEASE

BLEEDING AND CHRONIC KIDNEY DISEASE

Excessive bleeding has long been recognized as an important complication of the uremic state.[655-657] This was particularly true prior to the advent of dialysis and the availability of rhEPO. Events may be as minor as epistaxis, excessive bleeding with tooth brushing, and easy bruisability. More severe, clinically relevant bleeding episodes tend to occur with trauma or after invasive procedures rather than spontaneously.[658] Before the availability of routine dialysis, catastrophic gastrointestinal hemorrhage was the major cause of death with uremia.[655] Bleeding is frequently a predictor of increased mortality risk or complications.[659]

PATHOPHYSIOLOGY

Traumatic disruption of the endothelial lining of blood vessels results in a complex and coordinated response aimed to maintain vascular integrity and prevent bleeding. The first line of defense in hemostasis is represented by platelets, which specifically interact with ligands exposed as a consequence of endothelial damage. These ligands, which include collagen, fibronectin, laminin, thrombospondin, and von Willebrand factor (vWF), promote the adhesion of platelets to subendothelium and their activation. Activated platelets further release adhesive ligands stored in their α-granules, such as vWF, fibrinogen, thrombospondin, fibronectin, and vitronectin, and promote the activation of additional platelets by releasing aggregating agents such as thromboxane A_2 (TXA_2) and adenosine diphosphate (ADP). An occlusive plug is eventually formed by deposition of platelets on collagen fibers. The surfaces of platelets play an essential role in supporting the coagulation cascade in plasma, which results in the activation of thrombin, conversion of fibrinogen to fibrin, and formation of the fibrin plug, which is stabilized by factor XIIIa. Generation of thrombin further enhances the activation of platelets and upregulates glycoprotein (GP) receptors like those for GPIb-IX-V and GPIIb-IIIa. Several systems play an important role in limiting the extent of coagulation activation and thrombus formation. Nitric oxide (NO) and prostacyclin limit the activation of platelets. Tissue factor pathway inhibitor (TFPI), the protein C and S system, and antithrombin turn off activated coagulation factors at various steps of the coagulation cascade. The fibrinolytic system is also crucial in both limiting the growth of thrombi and promoting their organization and removal. Fibrin digestion is mediated by plasmin, which is circulating in plasma as plasminogen, an inactive precursor. Conversion of plasminogen to plasmin is promoted by tissue plasminogen activator (t-PA) and inhibited by plasminogen activator inhibitors (PAI-1 and PAI-2).[660,661]

Several factors contribute to increase the risk of bleeding in patients with CKD (Figure 57.11).[662] It has long been noted that bleeding in uremic patients occurs despite normal or elevated circulating values of coagulation factors.[655] This observation suggested that platelet abnormalities are the primary cause of the bleeding diathesis. The function of platelets is often impaired (thrombasthenia) whereas the number of circulating platelets is generally normal, with perhaps a tendency to decrease the longer patients have been undergoing dialysis.[663] Thrombopoietin values are elevated in patients who are on maintenance hemodialysis and being treated with rhEPO but do not correlate with platelet counts.[663,664] Evidence for platelet dysfunction includes elevated bleeding time,[655] diminished aggregation response to ADP and epinephrine,[665] reduced ristocetin-induced platelet agglutination,[666] and prolonged closure time with the Platelet Function Analyzer (PFA, Siemens Medical Solutions).[667,668]

The most consistent abnormality in platelet function in uremia is an impaired interaction of platelets with the vascular subendothelium.[655] As a result, platelet adhesion and aggregation are hindered. The cause of this dysfunction is incompletely understood and could be related to abnormalities of the vessel wall, platelets, or plasma constituents. As for the vessel wall, it appears that its function may be altered in uremia. In particular, endothelial production of NO, a powerful platelet inhibitor, has been noted to be increased,[669-671] resulting in higher concentrations of cyclic guanosine monophosphate and reduction of platelet responsiveness. In uremic rats, treatment with an NO inhibitor partially restores platelet function.[672] Interestingly, guanidinosuccinic acid, long postulated to play a role in uremic platelet dysfunction, has been found to upregulate NO production by the vascular endothelium.[673] Prostaglandin I_2 (PGI_2), which is released by endothelium, is increased in patients with CKD and increases bleeding times[674] and probably plays a role in reducing platelet aggregability.[674]

The platelet itself is intrinsically altered in uremia. For example, the content of serotonin and ADP is reduced in uremic platelet granules.[665] Secretion of mediators may also be impaired, although this effect may be a function of repeated activation during hemodialysis.[675] Platelet receptors that play a critical role in adhesion to the vessel wall and aggregation, like those for GP1b and GPIIb-IIIa, are probably not significantly reduced in quantity in uremia.[676] However, interaction of the receptors with vessel wall proteins may be abnormal.[677] In particular, activation of GPIIb-IIIa to facilitate its adhesion to vWF may be impaired.[678] The platelet cytoskeleton may be altered, with diminished actin incorporation and suboptimal intracellular trafficking of molecules.[679-681]

Although the platelet itself is not entirely normal in uremia, it appears that a more important pathogenic factor in platelet dysfunction may be the effect that uremic plasma has on platelet responsiveness. Platelets from normal individuals develop impaired adhesive function on exposure to uremic plasma.[682] In contrast, platelets from uremic subjects regain some function on exposure to normal plasma.[682] Certain molecules with molecular weights that preclude adequate clearance with hemodialysis accumulate in uremia and may contribute to platelet dysfunction.[683] A variety of toxins, including quinolinic acids and guanidine substances,

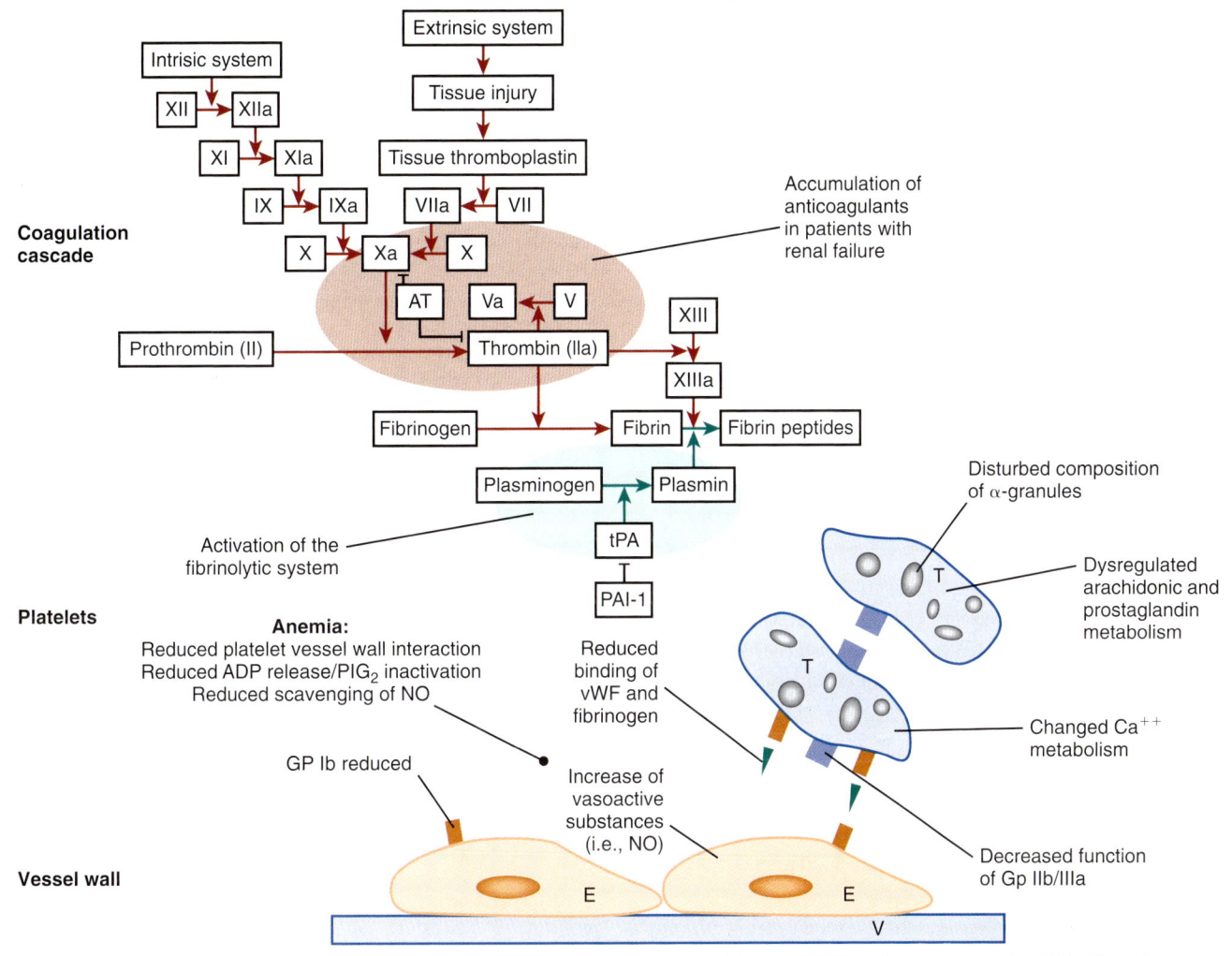

Figure 57.11 Factors involved in the increased risk of bleeding in patients with renal failure. *Roman numerals with/without lower case letters* indicate clotting factors; ADP, adenosine diphosphate; AT, Anti-thrombin; Ca^{++}, calcium ion; E, endothelium; GP, glycoprotein; NO, nitric oxide; PIG2, prostaglandin I 2; T, thrombocyte; tPA, tissue-type plasminogen activator; V, vessel; vWF, von Willebrand factor. (From Lutz J, Menke J, Sollinger D, et al: Haemostasis in chronic kidney disease. *Nephrol Dial Transpl* 29:29-40, 2014.)

have been implicated.[655] In addition, a role for hyperparathyroidism has been suggested. Benigni and colleagues found parathyroid hormone to impair platelet aggregation induced by a variety of substances.[684] Hyperparathyroidism may affect platelet function by elevating intracellular calcium concentrations via channels that are sensitive to calcium channel blockers like nifedipine.[685]

It is generally accepted that dialysis reduces uremic platelet dysfunction and the risk for bleeding. But dialysis does not completely eliminate the problem. Moreover, hemodialysis may induce a transient worsening in platelet function. Sloand and Sloand measured a variety of indicators of platelet function immediately before and after treatments and noted a transient decrease of platelet membrane expression of GPIb after hemodialysis. Ristocetin responsiveness was impaired after hemodialysis and normalized the day after treatment.[686] Other potential detrimental consequences of hemodialysis might include the enervating effect of repeated platelet activation,[687,688] removal of younger platelets with greater function,[689-691] and impairment of platelet function from a secondary effect of activated leukocytes.[692]

Anemia is an important contributor to uremic platelet dysfunction.[693] During normal circulation, erythrocytes tend to force the flow of platelets radially, away from the center of flow and toward the endothelial surfaces. When vascular injury occurs, platelets are in closer apposition to the vessel wall, facilitating platelet adherence and activation by vessel wall constituents such as collagen. With anemia, more platelets circulate in the center of the vessel, further from endothelial surfaces, hindering efficient platelet activation.[693] In addition, anemia may contribute to platelet dysfunction because release of ADP by erythrocytes normally stimulates platelet interaction with collagen.[694,695] Treatment of anemia may help reverse platelet dysfunction, as both transfusion of blood[693,696] and ESA therapy[697] have been found to be beneficial.

The plasma content of the major adhesive proteins, vWF and fibrinogen, are normal in uremia. One study showed a normal distribution of VWF multimers[666] while another one reported a reduction in high-molecular-weight VWF multimers.[698] The functional properties of vWF are altered, however, mostly at the level of the interaction with the

GPIb-IX-V platelet receptors, a key step in the signaling pathways, which ultimately lead to TxA$_2$ production.[699-702]

Platelet-derived procoagulant microparticles have been described in CKD,[703,704] but owing to inconsistent and unreliable methodologies to measure microparticles in plasma, it is not possible at this time to determine their clinical relevance.

DIAGNOSTIC STUDIES

Despite abundant evidence that the bleeding time is an unreliable test which has limited value in predicting bleeding complications,[705] use of this test is still reported in CKD.[662] More reliable tests are available, such as platelet aggregation and platelet function analyzer (PFA), although their value in predicting and managing bleeding complications is not yet proven. Thrombin generation assays may help in assessing both hypo- and hyper-coagulable states, but there are so far only limited studies in patients with CKD.[706]

TREATMENT

The treatment of patients with renal failure experiencing bleeding episodes requires (1) an assessment of the severity of blood loss, (2) hemodynamic stabilization, (3) replacement of blood products as needed, (4) identification of the bleeding source and etiology, and (5) correction of platelet dysfunction and other factors contributing to the bleeding diathesis (Figure 57.12). The first four aspects are routine components of clinical care and are not discussed further here; the fifth extends from the previous discussion on the pathobiology of uremic bleeding. It should be clear, however, that the intensity of interventions to correct uremic platelet dysfunction hinges on the degree of bleeding severity.

The first aspect of treatment to correct uremic platelet dysfunction is provision of adequate dialysis. Initiation of dialysis will lead to some improvement in thrombasthenia and bleeding risk.[665,707] The PFA closure time improves in 25% of patients after a dialysis session.[708] No studies have fully elucidated the relative effectiveness of hemodialysis versus other dialytic modalities, but platelet activation measured by CD62 expression was increased by hemodiafiltration while PLT degranulation products were increased in hemodialysis.[709] In any case anticoagulation must be minimized. The relation of dose of dialysis with improvement of platelet function has not been well studied.

Treatment of anemia with ESAs may be the most effective treatment of uremic platelet dysfunction (see above). Cases and associates found that treatment with epoetin alfa, 40 U/kg intravenously resulted in improvement in several parameters of platelet function as the Hgb rose.[710] Others have found the same salutary effect of ESA treatment.[105,697] Improved platelet function following EPO treatment is most likely related to the associated changes in blood flow, with platelets moving closer to the vessel walls. However, it is also possible that EPO treatment itself may directly affect platelet function. Tassies and colleagues found that platelet function improved in some patients after epoetin treatment was initiated, before Hgb values increased.[711] The authors attributed this effect to an increase in young circulating forms of platelets, with improved functional characteristics. Other potential direct beneficial effects of ESA include improved platelet intracellular calcium mobilization,[712] increased expression of GPIb,[655,713] and repaired platelet signal transduction.[714]

Desmopressin (1-deamino-8-d-arginine vasopressin, DDAVP) is a synthetic form of antidiuretic hormone that is often used to treat uremic bleeding. The drug has little vasopressor activity and only rarely induces hyponatremia. The mechanism of improved platelet function is not completely known, but enhanced release of larger vWF multimers by endothelial cells probably plays an important role.[715,716] Other factors may include improved platelet aggregation on contact with collagen and increased concentrations of platelet glycoprotein Ib/IX.[717] Given the unreliability of the bleeding time, it is not a surprise that IV infusion of 0.3 mcg/kg desmopressin (or 3.0 mcg/kg subcutaneously) produced inconsistent results.[715,718-720] DDAVP infusion improves platelet function in vitro and increases plasma concentrations for both VWF and Factor VIII.[667] DDAVP may also be administered by the intranasal route, at a dose approximately tenfold greater than that given intravenously.[721-723] Repeated administrations of DDAVP may result in a diminished response with development of tachyphylaxis, caused by the depletion of the endothelial stores of vWF multimers.[724,725]

Other treatments for uremic bleeding include infusion of cryoprecipitate, a plasma product rich in vWF and fibrinogen.[726,727] There is very little published evidence to support the use of cryoprecipitate, and response appears to be highly variable. In one study of five patients with active bleeding, only two had normalization of bleeding time and a favorable clinical outcome after treatment.[728] Cryoprecipitate use should be reserved for life-threatening bleeding due to the risk for infectious complications and limited availability.

Estrogens improve platelet function in both men and women.[729-731] After IV infusion, Livio and associates found the beneficial effect of conjugated estrogens to begin early and last for up to 2 weeks.[732] The mechanism of action of estrogen treatment is not fully known, but it may be related to inhibition of vascular NO production, by decreasing production of its precursor, L-arginine.[733]

Short-term (6 days) and long-term (3 months) treatments with the fibrinolytic inhibitor tranexamic acid were associated with a reduction in the bleeding time and improved platelet function.[734,735] Tranexamic acid may also be beneficial in the treatment of acute upper gastrointestinal bleeding episodes.[736]

HYPERCOAGULABILITY AND CHRONIC KIDNEY DISEASE

Although bleeding is the most clinically relevant manifestation of the effects of advanced CKD on hemostasis, several lines of evidence indicate the presence of a prothrombotic, hypercoagulable state, which may play a role in the atherosclerotic/cardiovascular complications. Deep venous thrombosis (DVT) seems to affect predominantly CKD patients in younger age, of African American or Hispanic background, in association with cardiovascular disease and prior surgical interventions.[737] The incidence of symptomatic venous thromboembolism is moderately increased in mild-to-moderate CKD (based on eGFR and albuminuria) as shown by a study pooling three European and two U.S.-based community-based cohorts,[738,739] as well as by a

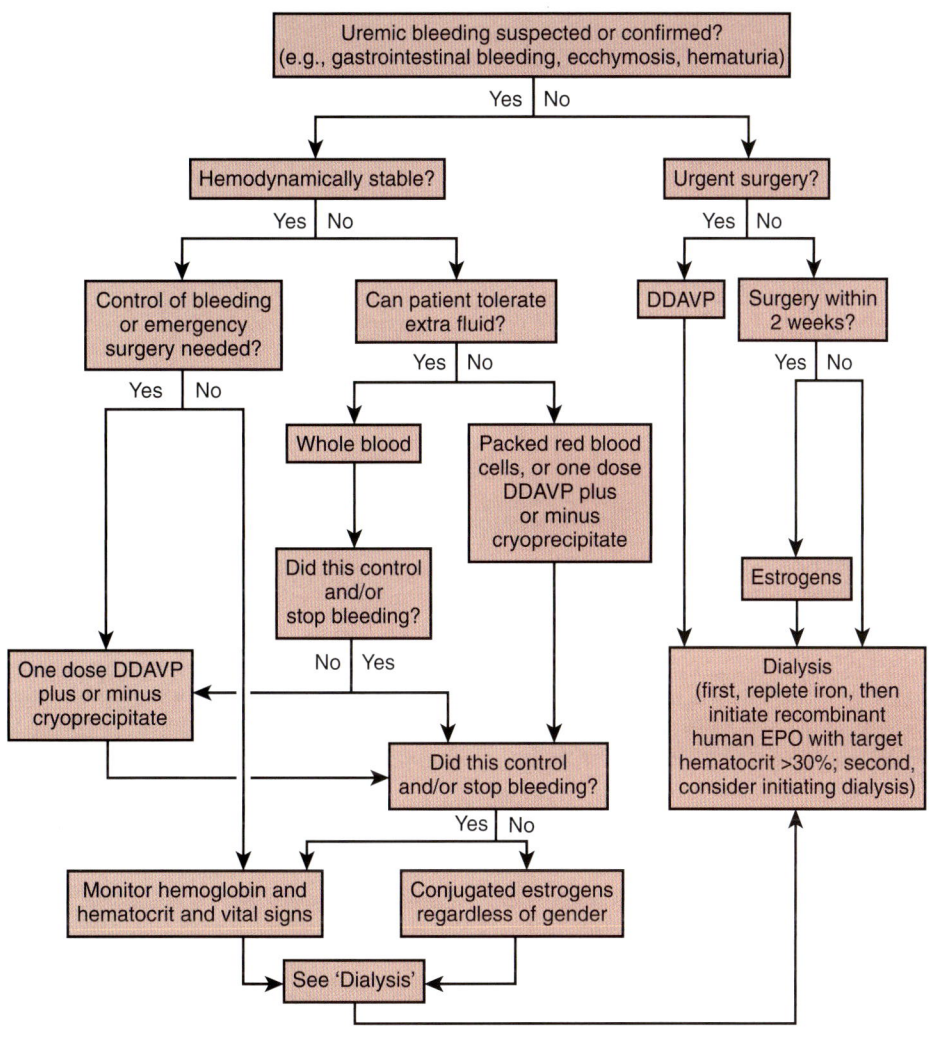

Figure 57.12 Algorithm for the management of patients with uremic platelet dysfunction. If at any stage in the algorithm the patient with uremic platelet dysfunction starts to actively bleed, the clinician should return to the top of the algorithm. This algorithm is not intended to replace sound clinical judgment or prevent additional consideration of patient factors that could influence management decisions. DDAVP, desmopressin (1-deamino-8-D-arginine vasopressin; single doses of 0.3-0.4 μg/kg body weight intravenous); EPO, erythropoietin. (From Hedges SJ, Dehoney SB, Hooper JS, et al: Evidence-based treatment recommendations for uremic bleeding. *Nat Clin Pract Nephrol* 3:138-153, 2007.)

large population-based study in Denmark.[740] The incidence of pulmonary embolism in CKD and ESKD is not precisely known (it may be particularly common after vascular access procedures—see Chapter 65), but mortality rates for pulmonary embolism are substantially higher in patients on dialysis than in the general population.[741] As described above ESA therapy may further increase thromboembolic complications.

EVIDENCE FOR HYPERCOAGULABILITY IN CKD

As outlined in Figure 57.13, several pathways are altered toward hypercoagulability and increased risk of thrombosis in CKD.[662] Activated/hypercoagulable platelets have been reported in patients with impaired or declining kidney function,[742,743] while other studies have shown increases in soluble markers of activated coagulation and fibrinolysis.[744,745] Several markers for thrombin activation (prothrombin fragment F1.2 and thrombin-antithrombin complex) and fibrinolysis (D-dimer and plasmin-antiplasmin complex) are abnormally elevated in dialyzed CKD patients, with erythrocyte membrane phosphatidylserine externalization possibly playing a role in this procoagulant state.[746-749] Phosphatidylserine externalization may be mediated by uremic toxins, since it improves after dialysis treatment.[750] Despite the functional platelet defects described above, abnormalities in the soluble coagulation cascade and in some of the natural anticoagulant systems like fibrinolysis generate a hypercoagulable state which may facilitate cardiovascular and thrombotic complications in dialyzed patients.[751,752] Complement activation may take place during dialysis, with increased expression of tissue factor on peripheral neutrophils and increased production of granulocyte colony-stimulating factor (G-CSF) resulting in a hypercoagulable state.[753]

PHARMACOLOGIC INTERVENTIONS

Treatment of hypercoagulability may expose patients to additional bleeding complications. A systematic review of bleeding rates in patients with CKD treated with antiplatelet drugs showed that these agents are effective in reducing arteriovenous fistula and central venous catheter, but not

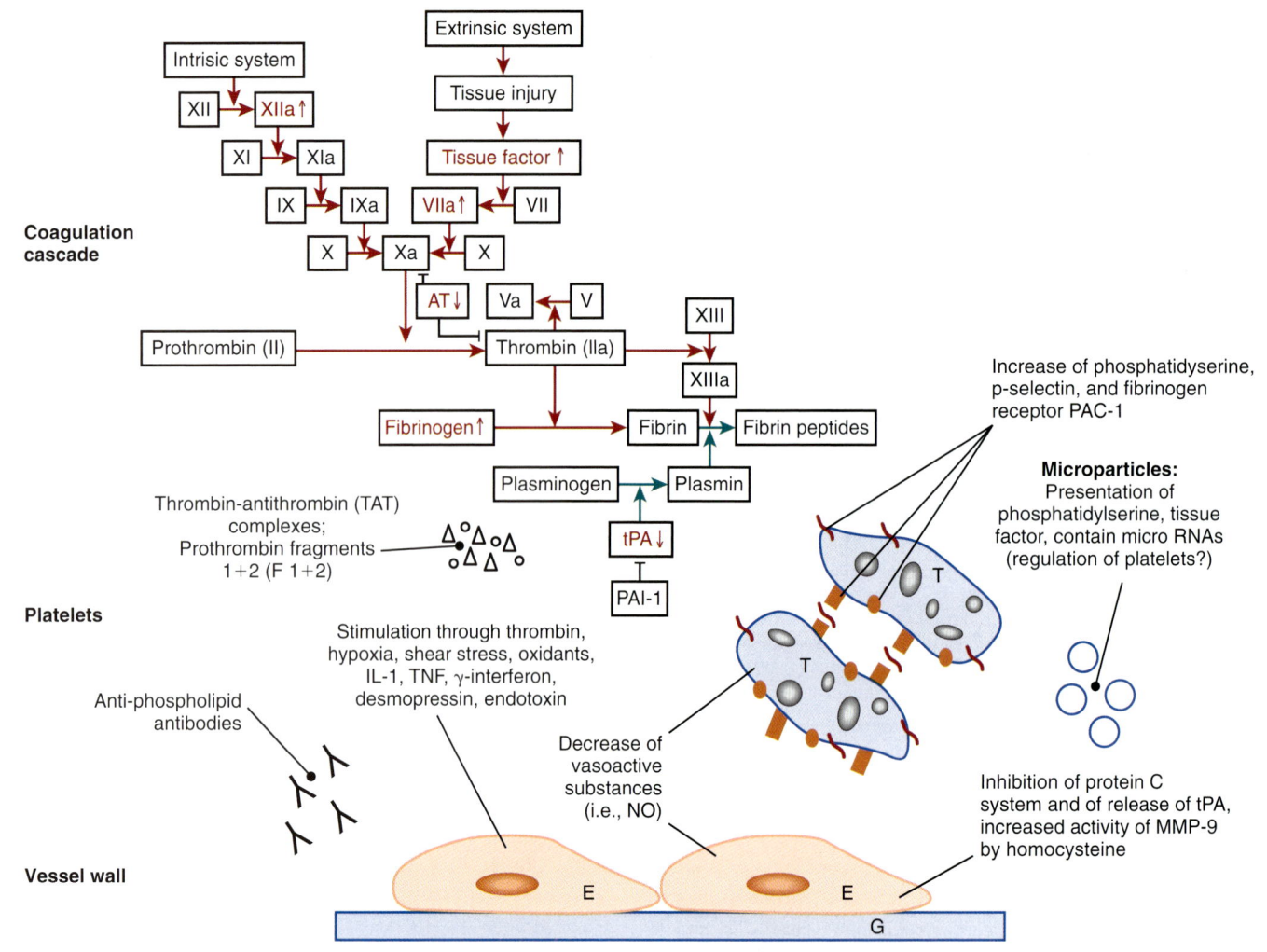

Figure 57.13 Factors involved in the increased risk of thrombosis in patients with renal failure. *Roman numerals with/without lower case letters* indicate clotting factors; AT, Anti-throbin; E, endothelium; G, sub-endothelial connective tissue; IL-1, interleukin-1; MMP-9, matrix metalloproteinase 9; NO, nitric oxide; PAC-1, monoclonal antibody specific for the activated form of GPIIb-IIIa; PAI-1, plasminogen activator inhibitor-1; T, thrombocytes; TNF, tumor necrosis factor; tPA, tissue-type plasminogen activator; vWF, von Willebrand factor; ↓, decreased; ↑, increased. (From Lutz J, Menke J, Sollinger D, et al: Haemostasis in chronic kidney disease. *Nephrol Dial Transpl* 29:29-40, 2014.)

arteriovenous graft thrombosis.[754] No firm conclusions could be reached about possible increases in bleeding rates in patients treated with a single agent, while there was an apparent increase in bleeding risk for combination therapy.[754] In patients treated for ischemic stroke, presence of CKD was associated with a two-fold increased frequency of clopidogrel resistance (by VerifyNow P2Y12 Assay).[755]

Atrial fibrillation is a relatively common occurrence in patients with CKD and ESKD. The optimal approach to prevention of stroke and other embolic complications is unknown. There are concerns that chronic treatment with vitamin K antagonists may worsen vascular calcification.[756] Warfarin dosing is complicated in CKD and ESKD by drug-drug interactions, variability in dietary intake and frequent administration of antibiotics. The risk-benefit balance of warfarin for stroke prevention in advanced CKD and ESKD is unknown. A recent study showed no reduction in the risk of stroke and higher bleeding risk in dialyzed CKD patients with atrial fibrillation treated with warfarin.[757] However, warfarin use to treat atrial fibrillation in patients with CKD post myocardial infarction (MI) was associated with lower mortality and lower incidence of MI and ischemic stroke with no substantial higher risk of bleeding complications.[758] A Danish registry study has shown that in high-risk CKD patients treatment of atrial fibrillation with warfarin resulted in measurable reductions in all-cause mortality and in hospitalization for stroke/bleeding.[759]

Novel oral anticoagulants have been approved for use in the general population with studies including a variable fraction (7 to 21%) of subjects with impaired kidney function (eGFR < 50 mL min^{-1}).[760] A systematic review and meta-analysis showed no significant differences in either thrombo-embolic or hemorrhagic complications in CKD patients treated with either warfarin or novel anticoagulants.[761] A similar study showed significant reduction (compared with warfarin) for bleeding complications in patients with impaired renal function only for agents with lower renal excretion (<50%, i.e. apixaban, rivaroxaban and edoxaban).[760] However, until properly controlled, randomized trials are conducted in patients with end stage renal disease, it seems premature to recommend replacing warfarin therapy with these newer agents.[762]

Dabigatran,[763] a direct thrombin inhibitor, apixaban[764] and rivaroxaban,[765] two factor Xa inhibitors, have been used in patients with CKD. Limited experience is available for newer agents, like the indirect factor Xa inhibitor fondaparinux.[766,767] While low molecular weight (LMW) and unfractionated heparin (UFH) can be reversed with administration of protamine sulphate, newer agents like fondaparinux have no specific antidotes, although recombinant factor VIIA and antithrombin have been used to reverse novel anticoagulant overdoses.[768-770]

The safety of omitting heparinization when dialyzing patients on chronic anticoagulation therapy with vitamin K antagonists has recently been demonstrated.[771]

HEPARIN-INDUCED THROMBOCYTOPENIA

HIT can be seen in patients receiving hemodialysis due to their repeated and frequent exposure to heparin.[772,773] The presence of antibodies to the platelet factor 4-heparin (PF4-H) complex has been associated with arterial and venous thrombosis and increased mortality,[774,775] but other studies have found no correlation between the presence of these antibodies and either reduction in platelet counts,[776] or clinical complications,[773,777] or vascular access thrombosis.[778] An acute thrombotic event in a thrombocytopenic patient on maintenance hemodialysis or unexpected occlusions of the extracorporeal circuit,[779] should prompt a search for possible HIT. However, the isolated presence of PF4-H antibodies should not by itself lead to either a diagnosis of HIT or institution of specific anti-HIT therapies. The presence of oversulfated chondroitin sulfate as a purposeful contaminant of heparins produced in China, which resulted in a large number of adverse events, has also been associated with increased prevalence of PF4-H antibodies but no thrombocytopenia.[780] If the presence of HIT is confirmed based on established criteria,[773] all heparin-based therapies should be discontinued and the use of direct thrombin inhibitors (pelirudin and argatroban) or factor Xa inhibitors (danaparoid) should be considered. Warfarin should not be considered until the resolution of thrombocytopenia and neither should be prophylactic platelet transfusions.

WHITE CELL FUNCTION IN CHRONIC KIDNEY DISEASE

CKD is accompanied by a chronic inflammatory state of complex pathogenesis, which is believed to be at least in part due to an increased generation of oxygen radicals and associated activation of monocytes. Uremic toxins have been blamed as a likely cause of this dysfunctional state, however with no specifically proven connections.[253,254,781,782] For more specific information on the biological significance of uremic toxins, see Chapter 54, or the European Uremic Solutes database (EUTox-db): http://eutoxdb.odeesoft.com/index.php. The use of particular dialyzers and dialysates has been associated with intradialytic leukocyte activation and enhanced oxidant stress, which exacerbate the underlying activated inflammatory state. Activation of platelets adhering to dialysis membranes may contribute to leukocyte activation and production of reactive oxygen species (ROS).[783-789] Different types of synthetic dialysis membranes have been shown to induce different degrees of oxidative stress (measured in serum with the surrogate marker malondialdehyde).[790]

LEUKOCYTE (MONOCYTE) ACTIVATION

Several studies have shown elevations in markers of leukocyte and monocyte activation in patients receiving dialysis,[788,791-793] as well as increased heterotypic aggregation for both leukocytes and lymphocytes.[794] Advanced oxidation protein products (AOPP) carried mostly by serum albumin have been identified in the serum of patients receiving dialysis.[795] These AOPPs are believed to be end-products of protein oxidation, whose concentrations are correlated with the severity of uremia, the extent of monocyte activation (assessed by serum neopterin)[796,797] and to the generation of myeloperoxidase by neutrophils in dialysis patients but not in predialysis conditions.[798] AOPP can trigger neutrophil activation and respiratory burst, which can be reduced *in vitro* by N-acetylcysteine.[799] Leukocyte 8-hydroxy-2′-deoxyguanosine (8-OHdG) is a marker of oxidant-induced DNA damage, which is particularly elevated in patients carrying a Glutathione S-transferase M1 (GST M1) polymorphic dysfunctional variant.[605]

Evidence for leukocyte activation and ROS generation has also been found in patients with ND-CKD.[800] Degranulation of neutrophils results in release of a variety of enzymes and proinflammatory mediators;[801,802] some of these mediators, such as heparanase,[803] an endoglycosidase involved in the degradation of extracellular matrix, have been linked to the generation of atherosclerotic lesions; others, like myeloperoxidase generate hypochlorous acid potent microbicidal and oxidant compound. Hypochlorous acid may play a role in activating monocytes, which produce a whole array of inflammatory cytokines (IL-6, TNF-α, and IL-1β).

LEUKOCYTE FUNCTIONAL IMPAIRMENT

Granulocytes of patients receiving hemodialysis exhibit impaired adhesion to fibronectin, which is more prominent in conditions of malnutrition.[804] Prominent apoptosis is observed in monocytes of patients with CKD,[805] and changes in monocyte subpopulations (CD16+) are associated with increased soluble proinflammatory markers such as chemokine (C-X3-C motif) ligand 1, or CX(3)CL1.[806] Increased production of ROS and accumulation of toxic products associated with uremia[253,254] are likely but not yet proven culprits in the generation of a dysfunctional immune response in patients with CKD. Enhanced susceptibility to bacterial or viral infections on the one hand and reduced response to hepatitis B vaccine on the other have been described.[807] Functional abnormalities in monocytes and T lymphocytes[808-810] as well as in natural killer cells[811] have been reported. It has been suggested that such abnormalities may be representative of a myeloid shift of erythropoiesis similar to that observed with aging.[812] New dialysis membranes designed to reduce immune dysfunction are being developed, with encouraging but still preliminary results.[813]

MARKERS OF LEUKOCYTE ACTIVATION

Elevations in either serum CRP or myeloperoxidase have been associated with higher mortality risk in hemodialyzed patients.[814] Expression studies with oligonucleotide microarray chips have identified distinct patterns of inflammatory/oxidative stress responses in dialyzed patients,[815] with some evidence suggestive for a possible pathogenetic role of an impairment of the mitochondrial respiratory system.[816] IV administration of vitamin C in a small cohort of patients produced changes in markers of oxidant stress.[817] Vitamin C supplementation in hemodialysis is a controversial issue because of the requirements for IV administration, prolonged therapy, and the risk of hyperoxaluria.[818]

A better identification of the pathogenesis and clarification of disease modifier genes will allow us to design better focused and more personalized treatment approaches for the inflammatory state associated with CKD.[819,820]

Complete reference list available at ExpertConsult.com.

KEY REFERENCES

9. Kidney Disease: Improving Global Outcomes (KDIGO) Anemia Work Group: KDIGO clinical practice guideline for anemia in chronic kidney disease. *Kidney Int Suppl* 2:279–335, 2012.
10. KDOQI Clinical Practice Guideline and Clinical Practice Recommendations for anemia in chronic kidney disease: 2007 update of hemoglobin target. *Am J Kidney Dis* 50:471–530, 2007.
11. K/DOQI clinical practice guidelines and clinical practice recommendations for anemia in chronic kidney disease in adults. *Am J Kidney Dis* 47(Suppl 3):S11–S145, 2006.
19. Eschbach JJ, Funk D, Adamson J, et al: Erythropoiesis in patients with renal failure undergoing chronic dialysis. *N Engl J Med* 276:653–688, 1967.
20. Astor B, Muntner P, Levin A, et al: Association of kidney function with anemia. *Arch Intern Med* 162:1401–1408, 2002.
28. McFarlane SI, Chen SC, Whaley-Connell AT, et al: Prevalence and associations of anemia of CKD: Kidney Early Evaluation Program (KEEP) and National Health and Nutrition Examination Survey (NHANES) 1999-2004. *Am J Kidney Dis* 51:S46–S55, 2008.
58. Erslev AJ: Humoral regulation of red cell production. *Blood* 8:349–357, 1953.
63. Bachmann S, Le Hir M, Eckardt KU: Co-localization of erythropoietin mRNA and ecto-5′-nucleotidase immunoreactivity in peritubular cells of rat renal cortex indicates that fibroblasts produce erythropoietin. *J Histochem Cytochem* 41:335–341, 1993.
64. Maxwell PH, Osmond MK, Pugh CW, et al: Identification of the renal erythropoietin-producing cells using transgenic mice. *Kidney Int* 44:1149–1162, 1993.
69. Eckardt KU, Koury ST, Tan CC, et al: Distribution of erythropoietin producing cells in rat kidneys during hypoxic hypoxia. *Kidney Int* 43(4):815–823, 1993.
70. Haase VH: Hypoxic regulation of erythropoiesis and iron metabolism. *Am J Physiol Renal Physiol* 299(1):F1–F13, 2010.
101. Miyake T, Kung CK, Goldwasser E: Purification of human erythropoietin. *J Biol Chem* 252:5558–5564, 1977.
104. Eschbach JW, Kelly MR, Haley NR, et al: Treatment of the anemia of progressive renal failure with recombinant human erythropoietin. *NEJM* 321:158–163, 1989.
162. Koury MJ, Bondurant MC: Erythropoietin retards DNA breakdown and prevents programmed death in erythroid progenitor cells. *Science* 248:378, 1990.
194. Koury MJ, Bondurant MC: Control of red cell production: the roles of programmed cell death (apoptosis) and erythropoietin. *Transfusion* 30:673–674, 1990.
198. Rankin EB, Wu C, Khatri R, et al: The HIF signaling pathway in osteoblasts directly modulates erythropoiesis through the production of EPO. *Cell* 149:63–74, 2012.
207. Madore F, Lowrie EG, Brugnara C, et al: Anemia in hemodialysis patients: variables affecting this outcome predictor. *J Am Soc Nephrol* 8:1921–1929, 1997.
211. Dmitrieva O, de Lusignan S, Macdougall IC, et al: Association of anaemia in primary care patients with chronic kidney disease: cross sectional study of quality improvement in chronic kidney disease (QICKD) trial data. *BMC Nephrol* 14:24, 2013.
230. Souma T, Yamazaki S, Moriguchi T, et al: Plasticity of renal erythropoietin-producing cells governs fibrosis. *J Am Soc Nephrol* 24:1599–1616, 2013.
231. Bernhardt WM, Wiesener MS, Scigalla P, et al: Inhibition of prolyl hydroxylase increases erythropoietin production in ESRD. *J Am Soc Nephrol* 21:2151–2156, 2010.
271. Zhao N, Zhang A-S, Enns CA: Iron regulation by hepcidin. *J Clin Invest* 123:2337–2343, 2013.
273. Nemeth E, Tuttle MS, Powelson J, et al: Hepcidin regulates cellular iron efflux by binding to ferroportin and inducing its internalization. *Science* 306:2090–2093, 2004.
276. Ganz T, Olbina G, Girelli D, et al: Immunoassay for human serum hepcidin. *Blood* 112:4292–4297, 2008.
284. Kautz L, Jung G, Valore EV, et al: Identification of erythroferrone as an erythroid regulator of iron metabolism. *Nat Genet* 46:678–684, 2014.
305. Bregman DB, Morris D, Koch TA, et al: Hepcidin levels predict nonresponsiveness to oral iron therapy in patients with iron deficiency anemia. *Am J Hematol* 88:97–101, 2013.
436. Kaufman JS, Reda DJ, Fye CL, et al: Subcutaneous compared with intravenous epoetin in patients receiving hemodialysis. Department of Veterans Affairs Cooperative Study Group on Erythropoietin in Hemodialysis Patients [see comments]. *NEJM* 339:578–583, 1998.
451. Levin NW, Fishbane S, Canedo FV, et al: Intravenous methoxy polyethylene glycol-epoetin beta for haemoglobin control in patients with chronic kidney disease who are on dialysis: a randomised non-inferiority trial (MAXIMA). *Lancet* 370:1415–1421, 2007.
471. Brugnara C, Chambers LA, Malynn E, et al: Red-blood-cell regeneration induced by subcutaneous recombinant erythropoietin—iron-deficient erythropoiesis in iron-replete subjects. *Blood* 81:956–964, 1993.
481. Brugnara C: Iron deficiency and erythropoiesis: new diagnostic approaches. *Clin Chem* 49:1573–1578, 2003.
486. Fishbane S, Shapiro W, Dutka P, et al: A randomized trial of iron deficiency testing strategies in hemodialysis patients. *Kidney Int* 60:2406–2411, 2001.
490. Fishbane S, Pollack S, Feldman HI, et al: Iron indices in chronic kidney disease in the National Health and Nutritional Examination Survey 1988-2004. *Clin J Am Soc Nephrol* 4:57–61, 2009.
541. Brugnara C, Mohandas N: Red cell indices in classification and treatment of anemias: from M. M. Wintrobes's original 1934 classification to the third millennium. *Curr Opin Hematol* 20:222–230, 2013.
559. Rostoker G, Griuncelli M, Loridon C, et al: Hemodialysis-associated hemosiderosis in the era of erythropoiesis-stimulating agents: a MRI study. *Am J Med* 125:991.e1–999.e1, 2012.
565. Macdougall I, Bock A, Carrera F, et al: FIND-CKD: a randomized trial of intravenous ferric carboxymaltose versus oral iron in patients with chronic kidney disease and iron deficiency anaemia. *Nephrol Dial Transplant* 29:2075–2084, 2014.
629. Coyne DW, Kapoian T, Suki W, et al: Ferric gluconate is highly efficacious in anemic hemodialysis patients with high serum ferritin and low transferrin saturation: results of the Dialysis Patients' Response to IV Iron with Elevated Ferritin (DRIVE) Study. *J Am Soc Nephrol* 18:975–984, 2007.
636. Pfeffer MA, Burdmann EA, Chen CY, et al: A trial of darbepoetin alfa in type 2 diabetes and chronic kidney disease. *N Engl J Med* 361:2019–2032, 2009.
637. Besarab A, Bolton WK, Browne JK, et al: The effects of normal as compared with low hematocrit values in patients with cardiac disease who are receiving hemodialysis and epoetin. *N Engl J Med* 339:584–590, 1998.
639. Parfrey PS, Foley RN, Wittreich BH, et al: Double-blind comparison of full and partial anemia correction in incident hemodialysis patients without symptomatic heart disease. *J Am Soc Nephrol* 16:2180–2189, 2005.

640. Drueke TB, Locatelli F, Clyne N, et al: Normalization of hemoglobin level in patients with chronic kidney disease and anemia. *N Engl J Med* 355:2071–2084, 2006.
641. Singh AK, Szczech L, Tang KL, et al: Correction of anemia with epoetin alfa in chronic kidney disease. *N Engl J Med* 355:2085–2098, 2006.
650. Macdougall IC, Obrador GT: How important is transfusion avoidance in 2013? *Nephrol Dial Transplant* 28:1092–1099, 2013.
651. Solomon SD, Uno H, Lewis EF, et al: Erythropoietic response and outcomes in kidney disease and type 2 diabetes. *NEJM* 363:1146–1155, 2010.
665. Di Minno G, Martinez J, McKean ML, et al: Platelet dysfunction in uremia: multifaceted defect partially corrected by dialysis. *Am J Med* 79:552–559, 1985.
695. Valles J, Santos MT, Aznar J, et al: Erythrocytes metabolically enhance collagen-induced platelet responsiveness via increased thromboxane production, adenosine diphosphate release, and recruitment. *Blood* 78:154–162, 1991.
732. Livio M, Mannucci PM, Vigano G, et al: Conjugated estrogens for the management of bleeding associated with renal failure. *N Engl J Med* 315:731–735, 1986.
738. Mahmoodi BK, Gansevoort RT, Næss IA, et al: Association of mild to moderate chronic kidney disease with venous thromboembolism: pooled analysis of five prospective general population cohorts. *Circulation* 126:1964–1971, 2012.
754. Hiremath S, Holden RM, Fergusson D, et al: Antiplatelet medications in hemodialysis patients: a systematic review of bleeding rates. *Clin J Am Soc Nephrol* 4:1347–1355, 2009.
757. Shah M, Tsadok MA, Jackevicius CA, et al: Warfarin use and the risk for stroke and bleeding in patients with atrial fibrillation undergoing dialysis. *Circulation* 129:1196–1203, 2014.
758. Carrero JJ, Evans M, Szummer K, et al: Warfarin, kidney dysfunction, and outcomes following acute myocardial infarction in patients with atrial fibrillation. *JAMA* 311:919–928, 2014.

58 Endocrine Aspects of Chronic Kidney Disease

Juan Jesús Carrero | Peter Stenvinkel | Bengt Lindholm

CHAPTER OUTLINE

PANCREATIC HORMONAL DISORDERS: INSULIN RESISTANCE, 1912
Causes of Uremic Insulin Resistance, 1913
Insulin Resistance is a Risk Factor for CKD, 1914
Insulin Resistance and Cardiovascular Risk, 1914
Treatment of Insulin Resistance in CKD, 1914
HYPOTHALAMO-PITUITARY AXIS, 1915
Thyroid Hormonal Alterations, 1915
GROWTH HORMONE, 1916
Resistance to Growth Hormone in CKD, 1918
Growth Failure in Children with CKD, 1918
Growth Hormone Treatment in Adult Patients with CKD, 1918

The GH/IGF-I System and Kidney Function, 1918
PROLACTIN, 1919
ADRENAL GLANDS, 1919
Adrenocorticotropic Hormone, 1919
Aldosterone and Cortisol, 1919
Adrenal Androgens, 1920
GONADAL DYSFUNCTION, 1920
In Women, 1920
In Men, 1921
VITAMIN D, PARATHYROID HORMONE, AND KIDNEY DISEASE, 1923
Vitamin D and Parathyroid Hormone: Metabolism and Actions in CKD, 1923
Vitamin D Deficiency in CKD, 1924
Vitamin D Supplementation in CKD, 1924

The kidney is a potent endocrine organ, a key modulator of endocrine function, and an important target for hormonal action. Thus, alterations in signal-feedback mechanisms and in production, transport, metabolism, elimination, and protein binding of hormones occur rather commonly in conditions affecting the kidney. As a direct consequence, chronic kidney disease (CKD), end-stage kidney disease (ESKD), and kidney transplantation are all associated with abnormalities in the synthesis or action of many hormones. The purpose of this chapter is to overview specific endocrine abnormalities that manifest as a consequence of kidney disease.

PANCREATIC HORMONAL DISORDERS: INSULIN RESISTANCE

Insulin resistance (IR) is a common feature of CKD—regardless of underlying etiology—that describes a clinical condition in which there is a reduced biologic effect for any given blood concentration of insulin.[1] The body's resistance to the actions of insulin results in a compensatory increase in production and secretion of insulin by the pancreas and leads to hyperinsulinemia in order to maintain euglycemia. If there is a concomitant inadequate secretion of insulin, this condition is manifested as abnormal glucose tolerance and if severe as diabetes mellitus. In CKD, both hyperparathyroidism and vitamin D deficiency may mediate insulin secretory abnormalities. Indeed, treatment of hyperparathyroidism[2] and pharmacologic doses of vitamin D[3] have been reported to correct glucose tolerance. The "gold standard" for determining IR is the euglycemic hyperinsulinemic clamp method.[4] However, because the clamp method is complex, expensive, and impractical to perform in large population studies, several surrogate methods (such as the homeostasis model assessment [HOMA]) have been developed. Unfortunately, all surrogate methods of determining insulin resistance suffer important limitations, including poor precision, and oral glucose tolerance test (OGTT)–derived insulin sensitivity indices may be preferred to fasting samples–derived indices.[5] Insulin resistance is seen as the common denominator for a number of metabolic disturbances, including hyperinsulinemia, impaired glucose tolerance, fatty liver, abdominal obesity, hyperuricemia, elevated triglycerides, low high-density lipoprotein (HDL) cholesterol, and hypertension.[6]

CAUSES OF UREMIC INSULIN RESISTANCE

The seminal study by DeFronzo and colleagues demonstrated that impaired tissue sensitivity to insulin is the primary cause of insulin resistance in uremia, implying a post-receptor defect in peripheral skeletal muscle.[7] Still, the molecular site of the post-receptor defect in humans has not been clearly established.[8] A reduced level of insulin receptor phosphorylation mediated by inflammation has been observed, both in animal models of diabetes and in patients with type 2 diabetes.[9] Whether the same mechanism is operative in CKD is unknown. Studies in animal models of uremia have reported failure of insulin to activate pyruvate dehydrogenase,[10] downregulation of insulin receptor substrate 1 (IRS-1)–associated phosphoinositol 3-kinase (PI3K), and upregulation of the IRS-2–associated PI3K activity.[11] In the uremic milieu, the etiology of IR is likely multifactorial, and many metabolic alterations may contribute concurrently (Table 58.1).

One hallmark of advanced CKD is low levels of 1,25-dihydroxyvitamin D (1,25[OH]$_2$ D), a pleiotropic vitamin with multiple noncalcemic functions. Evidence of an important role for vitamin D in uremic IR was provided in an international study of patients receiving dialysis in whom 1,25(OH)$_2$ D infusion corrected glucose intolerance and IR in the absence of changes in parathyroid hormone (PTH).[12] Although many studies in the general population have demonstrated that low serum 25-hydroxyvitamin D concentrations are associated with IR and diabetes risk,[13] the precise mechanism(s) by which vitamin D supplementation improves IR is unknown. Metabolic acidosis is another common complication in advanced CKD, also associated with IR, and 2 weeks of oral sodium bicarbonate supplementation in patients receiving dialysis have been found to improve insulin sensitivity.[12] As in the general population without kidney disease, fat mass seems to be an important risk factor for IR in CKD.[14] Considering the obesity epidemic, the possible role of high fructose intake in the development of metabolic syndrome, and possibly CKD, definitely needs to be highlighted. Later evidence suggests that fructose not only induces metabolic syndrome, hyperuricemia, and weight gain[15] but also exerts direct adverse effects on renal tubular cells.[16]

Persistent inflammation and protein-energy wasting (PEW) are two frequent and interrelated features of advanced CKD that also may mediate IR. Loss of skeletal muscle mass results in abnormal glucose disposal, so it seems logical that treatment of PEW with intravenous nutrition improved IR in a study of surgical patients.[17] Elevated circulating proinflammatory cytokine values may also mediate IR.[18] Indeed, metabolic syndrome seems associated with inflammatory markers[19] and leukocyte count[20] in patients with CKD. Among inflammatory mediators, tumor necrosis factor (TNF) (partially produced by fat tissue) especially influences the ability of insulin to stimulate glucose transport.[21] Blockade of interleukin-1 (IL-1) with anakinra (an IL-1 receptor antagonist) in patients with type 2 diabetes is associated not only with less inflammation but also improved glycemic control.[22] It has been shown that the suppressors of cytokine signaling (SOCS) family of proteins not only exacerbate IR but also inhibit insulin signaling and insulin-like growth factor (IGF) signaling.[23] On the basis of these findings, and from the fact that SOCS-1 knockout mice have a low blood glucose level and increased insulin signaling,[23] the SOCS proteins have been suggested to represent an important link between elevations of cytokines and IR. Indeed, in patients with type 2 diabetes, high (IL-6) levels are associated with increased SOCS-3 expression in skeletal muscle, and IL-6–induced SOCS-3 expression inhibits insulin signaling in human differentiated myotubes grown in vitro.[24] In CKD, few studies have yet examined the links between inflammation and IR. However, an inflammatory response during hemodialysis (HD) is linked to elevated SOCS-3 values and IR.[25]

In uremic mice, urea-induced generation of reactive oxygen species (ROS) has been suggested to induce IR,[26] although the mechanism thereof remains to be proven in humans. Additional factors that may contribute to uremic IR include physical inactivity and anemia. Correction of anemia by erythroid-stimulating agents (ESAs) was reported to reverse IR in patients undergoing HD independently of iron overload.[27] Furthermore, a small study in nonobese, nondiabetic, stable patients undergoing dialysis demonstrated the beneficial effect of ESA treatment on IR.[28] The observation that IR is associated with reduced responsiveness to ESA in patients receiving dialysis may, in part, be attributed to the presence of persistent inflammation in both conditions.[29]

Finally, IR in patients receiving peritoneal dialysis (PD) merits discussion because the dialysis procedure itself, in addition to the uremic state, appears to modulate the magnitude of IR.[30] IR may be exacerbated by the intraperitoneal presence of glucose-containing dialysate.[31,32] PD has significantly higher IR than HD, which may reflect the presence of glucose-based dialysate in the peritoneal cavity.[33,34]

Table 58.1 Multiple Causes and Consequences of Insulin Resistance and Abnormalities of Insulin Secretion in Chronic Kidney Disease

Causes	Insulin secretion abnormalities:
	Hyperparathyroidism
	Vitamin D deficiency
	Insulin resistance:
	Uremic toxins
	Anemia
	Metabolic acidosis
	Inflammation
	Oxidative stress
	Muscle loss
	Increased fat mass
	Physical inactivity
Consequences	Dyslipidemia
	Sodium retention
	Vascular calcification
	Muscle wasting
	Hyperuricemia
	Renin activation
	Hypertension and cardiovascular disease

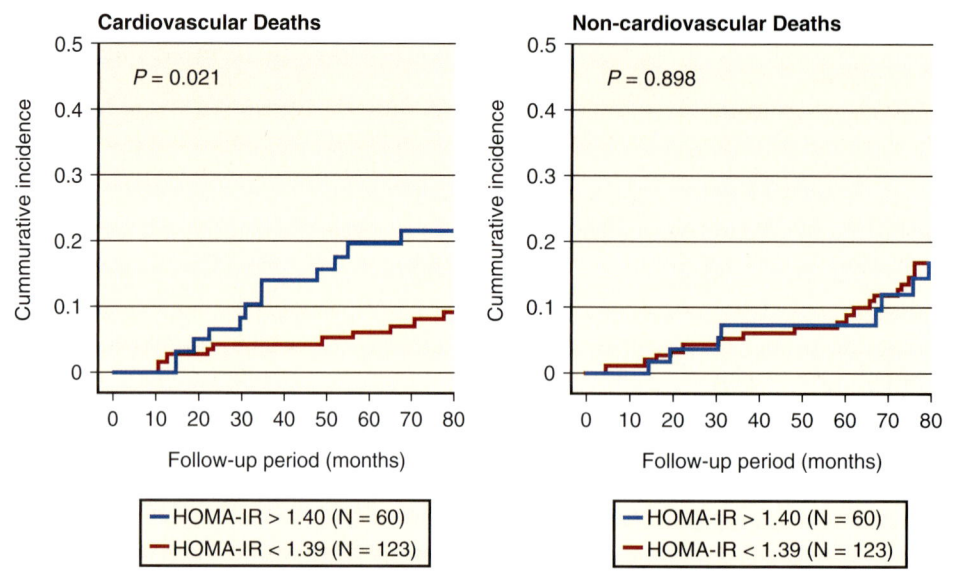

Figure 58.1 Kaplan-Meier curves showing the association between the homeostasis model assessment (HOMA)–estimated insulin resistance (HOMA-IR) and mortality in 183 nondiabetic patients with end-stage kidney disease (ESKD) treated with maintenance hemodialysis. (Redrawn from Shinohara K, Shoji T, Emoto M, et al: Insulin resistance as an independent predictor of cardiovascular mortality in patients with end-stage renal disease. *J Am Soc Nephrol* 13:1894-1900, 2002.)

INSULIN RESISTANCE IS A RISK FACTOR FOR CHRONIC KIDNEY DISEASE

Whether IR (and the metabolic syndrome) is an antecedent of CKD or merely a consequence of impaired kidney function has been debated. Large population-based studies have shown that the metabolic syndrome is associated with an increased risk for incident CKD.[35,36] A "dose-response" relationship was documented between the number of metabolic syndrome traits and the prevalence of microalbuminuria.[36] Furthermore, a smaller-scale study of nondiabetic patients with CKD showed that IR estimated by HOMA was more than 2.5 times more prevalent in patients with CKD than in controls. Finally, a Japanese study in nondiabetic patients with hypertension and stage 3 CKD showed that IR (estimated by both HOMA and IR index) is a significant risk factor for the deterioration of kidney function.[37] The cross-sectional design of these studies precludes causal inferences, and mechanistic/intervention studies are needed to resolve whether the metabolic syndrome is a cause or a consequence (or both) of CKD. However, insulin has potent growth-stimulating properties and may have proliferative effects on glomerular and mesangial cells, and it also stimulates transforming growth factor β (TGF-β) and the renin angiotensin aldosterone system (RAAS). Although insulin may also promote fibrosis,[38] it is not clear whether therapy directed to tackle the metabolic syndrome will delay, or even halt, the progression of CKD.

INSULIN RESISTANCE AND CARDIOVASCULAR RISK

In a prospective observational study of nondiabetic patients with ESKD, IR was associated with cardiovascular mortality (Figure 58.1) independent of Quételet's (body mass) index (BMI), hypertension, and dyslipidemia.[39] Thus, as in the general population, IR and ensuing hyperinsulinemia may be independent risk factors for cardiovascular complications in patients with ESKD. Hyperinsulinemia promotes tubular sodium retention,[40] decreases urinary uric acid clearance, and upregulates the RAAS,[41] all established risk factors for hypertension. Another atherogenic link between IR and CVD is uremic dyslipidemia, which is typically characterized by hypertriglyceridemia, reduced HDL cholesterol, increased very low-density lipoprotein (VLDL), and small dense low-density lipoprotein (LDL) particles. Of note, uremic lipid abnormalities improved concomitantly with the correction of IR and glucose intolerance after intravenous administration of $1,25(OH)_2 D$ therapy.[12]

Because insulin accelerates calcium deposition in human vascular smooth muscle cells,[42] it has been speculated that although the beneficial metabolic and vasomotor effects of insulin are impaired in IR, the mitogenic signals are enhanced, and the resulting imbalance can promote vascular calcification.[43] Finally, the role of insulin in protein turnover merits attention, particularly given that altered protein turnover may have a role in CKD, cardiovascular disease (CVD), and PEW. Animal models of insulin deficiency suggest that the effect of insulin on protein turnover is mediated through the activation of the ubiquitin proteasome pathway.[44] In accordance, patients with ESKD and type 2 diabetes who are undergoing dialysis have increased skeletal muscle protein breakdown in comparison with their nondiabetic counterparts.[45]

TREATMENT OF INSULIN RESISTANCE IN CKD

Management of IR in uremia should be multifaceted. In addition to attention to and treatment of the many uremic metabolic alterations that may lead to IR and/or impaired insulin secretion, other more specific treatment options should be discussed with the patient. Regular exercise should be an integral part of the management of IR, although a small interventional trial in patients receiving HD did not show IR improvements after 3 months of aerobic exercise training.[46] As angiotensin-converting enzyme (ACE) inhibitor treatment appears to improve insulin sensitivity and may reduce the risk of type 2 diabetes mellitus in patients with essential hypertension,[47] the effect of ACE inhibitors or angiotensin receptor blockers (ARBs) on IR needs to be tested in patients with advanced CKD. The Diabetes REduction Assessment with ramipril and rosiglitazone Medication (DREAM) trial,[48] involving participants without CVD but with impaired levels of fasting glucose, showed that ramipril did not reduce the incidence of diabetes or death but that it did facilitate regression of glucose elevations to normoglycemia.

In a later evaluation of new users of oral hypoglycemic medication monotherapy in patients with type 2 diabetes mellitus, higher risk of mortality was associated with glibenclamide, glipizide, and rosiglitazone than with metformin.[49] Because rosiglitazone was found to substantially reduce the incidence of type 2 diabetes mellitus and also increased the likelihood of regression to normoglycemia,[50] thiazolidinedione ("glitazone") treatment was thought to be an attractive treatment option for patients with CKD. However, subsequent studies provided conflicting results. A cross-sectional evaluation showed significantly higher (>38%) cardiovascular and all-cause mortality in rosiglitazone users,[51] consistent with a systematic review of trials in patients with type 2 diabetes mellitus that showed increased risk of myocardial infarction and a borderline increased risk of death from cardiovascular causes.[52] In any case, thiazolidinedione treatment in ESKD cannot currently be advocated until its efficacy has been demonstrated in randomized controlled trials. A later randomized clinical trial in patients with CKD showed that short-term rosiglitazone therapy reduced IR but had no effect on arterial function and stiffness.[53]

The insulin sensitizer metformin is associated with both attenuation of the metabolic syndrome and cardiovascular protection. However, metformin is cleared by the kidneys so there is a risk of metformin accumulation and associated lactic acidosis in CKD. Clinical practice guidelines suggest that the drug should be used with caution when estimated glomerular filtration rate (eGFR) is less than 60 mL/min and stopped when eGFR falls below 30 mL/min. Some writers believe, however, that there is a disproportionate fear surrounding the safety of metformin in CKD that may not be valid if patients are counseled and monitored carefully. A retrospective comparative effectiveness study of oral antidiabetic drugs showed that in comparison with metformin, treatment with sulfonylureas increased the risks of a decline in eGFR, ESKD, and death.[54] Many of the sulfonylureas should be avoided in CKD owing to the risk of hypoglycemia; others should be used with caution. Newer approaches to improving IR, such as the provision of sodium glucose cotransporter 2 (SGLT-2) inhibitors and/or incretin-based therapies, could provide novel potential strategies to prevent excess mortality in this patient group. Although dipeptidyl peptidase IV inhibitors are well tolerated in general, dosage adjustments according to kidney function are needed to avoid side effects.

HYPOTHALAMO-PITUITARY AXIS

THYROID HORMONAL ALTERATIONS

Although thyroid hormones are necessary for growth and development of the kidney and for the maintenance of water and electrolyte homeostasis, the kidney is involved in the metabolism and clearance of these hormones. Thus, a decline of kidney function is accompanied by a characteristic disturbance in thyroid physiology (Table 58.2).

CAUSES OF THYROID HORMONE DISTURBANCES IN CKD

The kidney contributes to the clearance of iodide. Plasma iodide retention in CKD favors thyroidal iodide uptake and potentially blocks thyroid hormone production by a negative feedback mechanism.[55,56] Serum free triiodothyronine (T_3) concentrations in uremia may be additionally low, serving as an appropriate compensatory response aimed at reducing energy expenditure and minimizing protein catabolism in the presence of PEW.[57] Metabolic acidosis[58,59] and systemic inflammation[60-62] are additional features of uremia that can further contribute. Medications that are able to suppress thyroid hormone metabolism include corticosteroids, amiodarone, propranolol, and lithium.[63,64]

Serum thyrotropin (thyroid-stimulating hormone [TSH]) concentrations are usually normal or elevated in CKD, but the response to TSH-releasing hormone (TRH) is generally diminished.[65] Both TSH circadian rhythm and TSH glycosylation are altered in CKD. The latter may compromise TSH bioactivity. Because serum TSH concentrations are frequently in the normal range, uremic patients are often considered euthyroid. Free and total thyroxine (T_4) concentrations may be normal or slightly reduced, mainly as a result of impaired hormone binding to serum carrier proteins. Circulating thyroid hormones are normally bound to thyroid hormone-binding globulin (TBG) and, to a lesser extent, to prealbumin (transthyretin) and albumin. Retained

Table 58.2 Thyroid Abnormalities in Chronic Kidney Disease

Hypothalamus	Normal or high TSH
	Altered TSH circadian rhythm
	Altered TRH and TSH clearance
Pituitary gland	Increased thyroid volume
	Higher prevalence of goiter and hypothyroidism
	Low or normal total T_3 and total T_4
	Low or normal free T_3 and free T_4
	Impaired T_3 conversion from T_4
	Normal total rT_3 and elevated free rT_3
	Alteration in binding proteins
	Elevated serum iodine due to reduced renal excretion
Cell	Reduced thyroid hormone cell uptake
	Impaired binding of thyroid hormone receptor to DNA

rT_3, Reverse triiodothyronine level; T_3, triiodothyronine; T_4, thyroxine; TRH, TSH-releasing hormone; TSH, thyroid-stimulating hormone.

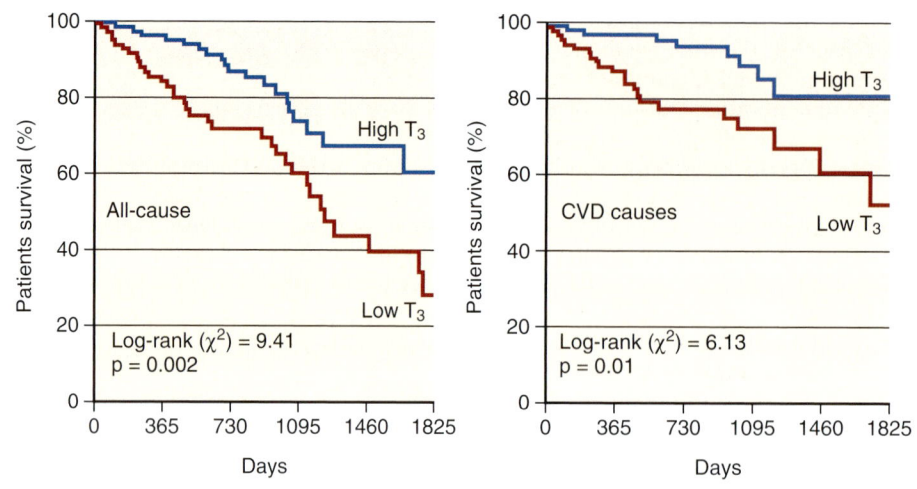

Figure 58.2 Thyroid alterations and outcome of chronic kidney disease (CKD). The "low T_3 syndrome" is linked to a survival disadvantage in the end-stage kidney disease (ESKD) population. The figures represent mortality risk, for all causes **(left)** and cardiovascular (CVD) causes **(right)**, according to the presence or absence of low triiodothyronine (T_3) values in a cohort of euthyroid patients with ESKD. (Redrawn from Carrero JJ, Qureshi AR, Axelsson J, et al: Clinical and biochemical implications of low thyroid hormone levels (total and free forms) in euthyroid patients with chronic kidney disease. J Intern Med 262:690-701, 2007.)

substances in CKD may inhibit hormone binding to these proteins. For example, urea, creatinine, indoles, and phenols all strongly inhibit protein binding of T_4. The transient elevation in plasma T_4 levels that occurs during the HD procedure may be due to the effect of heparin used to prevent clotting in the hollow-fiber dialyzer and associated tubing, because heparin inhibits binding of T_4 to its binding proteins.[66] Most patients with ESKD have decreased plasma levels of free T_3 (low T_3 syndrome), which primarily reflects diminished conversion of T_4 (thyroxine) to T_3 in the periphery.[67] This peculiar hormonal profile, however, is not associated with increased conversion of T_4 to the metabolically inactive reverse T3 (rT_3) because plasma rT_3 levels are typically normal in uremia. Such finding differentiates the uremic patient from patients with other chronic illnesses.

In addition, bioavailability and cell uptake of thyroid hormones may be partially blunted in uremia, leading to a state of thyroid resistance. This possibility is important to take into consideration because serum TSH may not be an accurate measure of the *cellular* action of thyroid hormone. In normal rat hepatocytes, treatment with serum from uremic patients reduced T_4 uptake by 30%.[68] Uremic plasma from patients undergoing HD inhibited the binding of thyroid hormone receptor to DNA and impaired T_3-dependent transcriptional activation.[69] Because dialysis per se corrected these abnormalities, the investigators suggested that a dialyzable substance was involved.[69]

As a consequence, CKD is associated with a higher prevalence of primary hypothyroidism, mainly subclinical, but not with hyperthyroidism.[70,71] The prevalence of the low T_3 syndrome (reduced T_3 in the presence of normal levels of TSH and T_4) is in comparison remarkably high, being reported in more than 70% of patients with ESKD.[72,73]

CLINICAL IMPLICATIONS AND CONSEQUENCES OF THYROID HORMONE ALTERATIONS IN CKD

Because kidney function in hypothyroid patients was reported to be maintained or improved after thyroid hormone supplementation,[74-76] it has been speculated that thyroid disorders may impair kidney function and vice versa. Two observational studies with longitudinal design in patients with subclinical hypothyroidism and preexisting CKD showed that thyroxine supplementation attenuated the decline in kidney function over time.[77,78] The previously mentioned studies may be limited by confounding by indication, but their findings justify the need to explore this interesting possibility.

Subclinical hypothyroidism or the low T_3 syndrome may instead constitute an intermediate link between the inflammatory stress, subsequent PEW, and impaired cardiovascular response in CKD. A number of studies have consistently shown that low T_3 concentrations are inversely correlated with markers of systemic inflammatory response and are an independent predictor of mortality in euthyroid patients with ESKD (Figure 58.2)[79] and in dialysis populations,[80-82] having a stronger association with cardiovascular death.[83] Low T_3 has been additionally linked to impaired cardiac function and geometry,[84,85] coronary artery calcification,[86,87] increased intima-media thickness,[87] flow-mediated vasodilatation (FMD),[88] and measures of systemic arterial stiffness.[89] Low T_3 levels before kidney transplantation are associated with decreased graft survival.[90] The observational nature of the studies reporting these results emphasizes the importance of verifying whether uremic patients without primary thyroid dysfunction would benefit from thyroid hormone therapy. So far, there is insufficient evidence to recommend routine provision of thyroid hormone replacement in CKD with low T_3 alone. Because of potential unfavorable effects of thyrotoxicosis, such as tachycardia and loss of skeletal muscle and bone, the key therapeutic approach for the successful management of nonthyroidal illness in CKD might be to simply restore thyroid hormone deficiencies and maintain thyroid hormones within the normal range.

GROWTH HORMONE

The growth hormone (GH)/insulin-like growth factor-I (IGF-I) system is of key importance for anabolism, body growth, and body composition. It regulates a range of

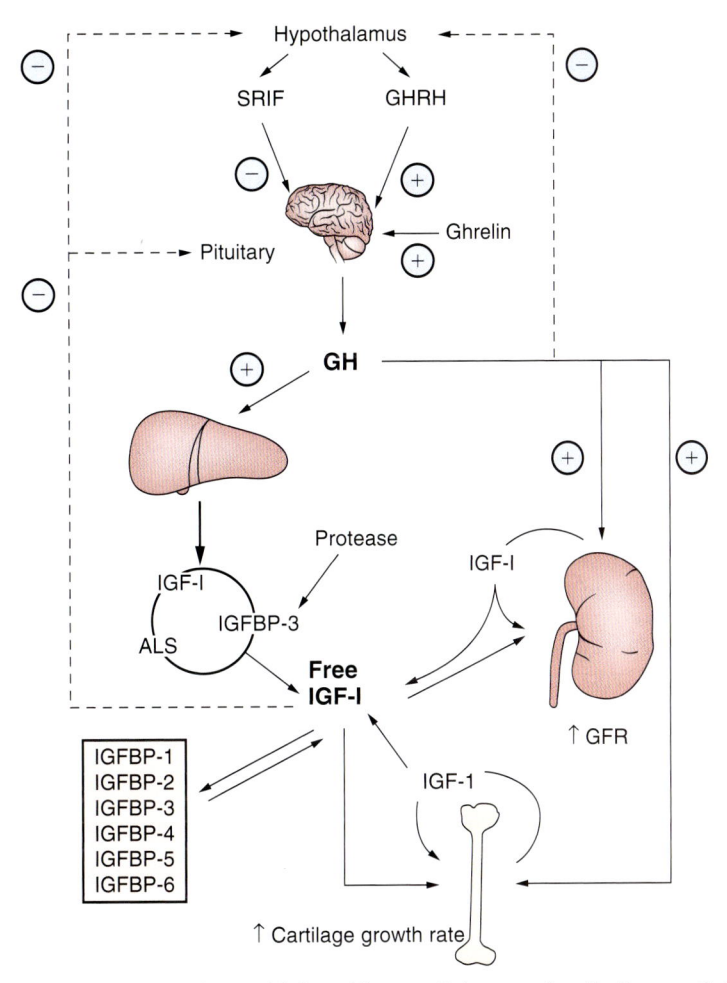

Figure 58.3 Deranged somatotropic axis in chronic renal failure. The growth hormone/insulin-like growth factor-I (GH/IGF-I) axis in chronic kidney disease (CKD) is markedly different from the normal axis. In CKD, the total concentrations of the hormones in the GH/IGF-I axis are not reduced, but there is reduced effectiveness of endogenous GH and IGF-I, which probably plays a major role in reducing linear bone growth. The reduced effectiveness of endogenous IGF-I likely is due to decreased levels of free, bioactive IGF-I as levels of circulating inhibitory IGF binding proteins (IGFBPs) are increased. ALS, Acid-labile subunit protein; GFR, glomerular filtration rate; GHRH, growth hormone–releasing hormone; SRIF, somatotropin release-inhibiting factor. (Redrawn from Roelfsema V, Clark RG: The growth hormone and insulin-like growth factor axis: its manipulation for the benefit of growth disorders in renal failure. *J Am Soc Nephrol* 12:1297-1306, 2001.)

metabolic processes that are needed for the growth of cells and tissues in the body during all phases of life but with the most profound effects during childhood. The metabolism and secretion of GH, a 22-kDa 191–amino acid protein produced in the pituitary gland, are inhibited by somatostatin and stimulated by GH-releasing hormone, but many other factors are also involved, such as fatty acids and other nutrients and factors linked to nutrient intake, such as ghrelin, leptin, and neuropeptide Y. In general, nutrient intake regulates GH secretion so that body protein stores rather than fat tissue are preserved, especially during energy restriction. Fasting as well as insulin-induced hypoglycemia increases GH secretion, whereas a glucose load decreases circulating GH by reducing somatostatin release. On the other hand, supply of protein and amino acids, especially arginine, increases GH secretion. During CKD many of these pathways may be disturbed.[91-93]

Growth hormone is an anabolic hormone stimulating protein synthesis, bone growth, calcium retention, bone mineralization, and lipolysis with decrease in body fat (Figure 58.3). Although the effects of GH may vary according to whether the patient is fasting or fed, GH reduces hepatic glucose uptake and promotes gluconeogenesis and lipolysis, thereby opposing the glucose-lowering actions of insulin. GH released from the pituitary acts in an endocrine fashion on hepatic GH receptors to trigger the synthesis and release of IGF-I from the liver. IGF-1 circulates free (biologically active) or bound to proteins (IGF-binding proteins [IGFBPs] 1-6). The binding of IGF-I to specific muscle receptors induces muscle synthesis, inhibits muscle proteolysis, promotes the delivery of amino acids and glucose to myocytes, and stimulates myoblast proliferation.[91-93] Disturbances in the GH/IGF-I system may therefore contribute to many complications in CKD, such as growth retardation, PEW/sarcopenia, and progression (i.e., loss of kidney function in CKD); GH deficiency is associated with decreases in GFR and renal plasma flow. Low circulating levels of IGF-I are associated with increased mortality in patients with CKD stage 5 at the time of dialysis initiation.[94] Whereas therapeutic use of GH to promote growth in growth-retarded children with advanced CKD is an accepted therapy, administration of GH or IGF-I might also improve nutritional status in adults with CKD. Furthermore, increased circulating levels of GH and IGF-I may acutely improve kidney function in children and adults.[95-97] However, it should be noted that experimental studies in mice suggest that GH and IGF-I may increase the risk of glomerular sclerosis and thereby could contribute to progression of CKD.[98,99]

RESISTANCE TO GROWTH HORMONE IN CKD

Because growth retardation is common even though serum GH concentrations are normal or even elevated in children with CKD, a state of GH resistance and possibly also IGF-I resistance has been proposed.[91,100,101] Insensitivity to GH is the consequence of multiple defects in the GH/IGF-I system including, at the molecular level, a defect in JAK/STAT phosphorylation that may be due in part to concurrent inflammation.[102,103] One clinical implication of this resistance to GH and IGF-I is that children with advanced CKD whose growth has been impaired often require very large doses of GH to achieve normal or near-normal body growth.

Resistance to the actions of GH and IGF-I is typically present also in adult patients with advanced CKD.[92] It may be due to decreased GH receptors and/or post–GH receptor defects as well as to decreased IGF-I synthesis. Evidence also suggests that IGF-I bioavailability may be reduced, because of (1) reduced synthesis of IGF-I receptors in the muscle[104]; (2) inactivation of IGF-I due to increased binding to IGFBPs; and (3) increased hepatic production of IGFBPs (IGFBP-1 and IGFBP-2) and reduced excretion of IGFBPs in general, leading to a larger proportion of inactive IGF-I despite normal total serum IGF-I concentrations.[105,106] Newer treatment modalities targeting GH resistance with recombinant human IGF-I (rhIGF-I), recombinant human IGFBP3 (rhIGFBP3), and IGFBP displacers may prove to be more effective in treating growth failure in CKD.[92] Finally, it was elegantly shown that resistance to pharmacologic doses of GH may be related not to uremia per se but rather to an increased inflammatory state associated with uremia.[107] Abnormalities in the interaction of these pathways with those that involve other molecules, such as ghrelin, myostatin, and the SOCS family, may also be important.[91]

GROWTH FAILURE IN CHILDREN WITH CKD

Recombinant human GH (rhGH) is an approved treatment for growth failure in children with kidney failure that has proved to be safe and efficacious. Identifying and addressing growth failure early on is an important component in the treatment of children with CKD. Treatment with rhGH is used in approximately 15% of all children undergoing dialysis in the United States.[108] Unfortunately many children with CKD and growth retardation still do not receive adequate GH treatment for their growth failure. Growth hormone therapy should be considered in children with CKD who have a height less than two standard deviations (SD) below the mean. Unusual causes for poor growth, such as hypothyroidism, should be investigated. Early institution of GH therapy is likely to improve the final achieved height. Recombinant human GH is administered as a daily subcutaneous injection. Once treatment is initiated, monitoring of growth, pubertal stage, nutritional state, funduscopic examination (to detect papilledema due to intracranial hypertension), and blood examination should occur every 3 to 4 months, to determine whether growth is adequate and whether dose adjustments are needed. In patients younger than 3 years, the head circumference should be routinely monitored as well. Later studies have shown that rhGH treatment is most effective when started at an early age and that the growth response is affected by the degree of impairment of kidney function.[109]

Even though rhGH has been shown to improve "catch-up" growth, the final adult height may still be below the genetic target. After kidney transplantation, growth retardation may persist because of multiple factors, such as corticosteroid use, decreased kidney function, and an abnormal GH/IGF-I axis.[92] Although there have been concerns that long-term therapy with rhGH may have various adverse effects, rhGH is generally very well tolerated and does not seem to be associated with increased incidence of glucose intolerance, pancreatitis, progressive deterioration of kidney function, acute allograft rejection, or fluid retention.[110,111] Newer formulations of rhGH are undergoing experimental testing, with the hope that adverse effects could be reduced, efficacy increased, and the administration schedule might be more convenient in comparison with currently available formulations.

GROWTH HORMONE TREATMENT IN ADULT PATIENTS WITH CKD

Many studies have explored a possible therapeutic role of rhGH and rhIGF-I therapy in the CKD population.[112] Among patients receiving dialysis, evidence suggests that rhGH stimulates protein synthesis, decreases urea generation, and improves nitrogen balance,[100] effects that appear to be dose dependent.[113] IGF-I enhances intracellular transport of glucose and amino acids, stimulates protein synthesis, suppresses protein degradation, and stimulates bone growth and enlargement of many organs.[93,114] Whereas the use of rhGH or rhGH plus rhIGF-I in patients receiving dialysis has been generally well tolerated[113-115] and long-term GH replacement may even improve cardiovascular mortality and morbidity in GH-deficient adults,[116,117] rhGH treatment in patients with an acute critical illness may result in increased mortality.[118] Among reported adverse reactions to GH treatment are a higher risk of benign intracranial hypertension, hyperglycemia, and fluid retention. In obese adults, rhGH therapy leads to a decrease in visceral adiposity and increase in lean body mass as well as beneficial changes in the lipid profile, without inducing weight loss, despite increases in fasting plasma glucose and insulin levels.[119]

THE GH/IGF-I SYSTEM AND KIDNEY FUNCTION

Receptors for GH and IGF-I are expressed in the kidney and influence kidney structure and function,[95] and short-term rhGH treatment in CKD is linked to a general improvement of capillary blood flow.[120] Regarding kidney function, GH may increase renal hemodynamics and filtration rate, whereas rhIGF-I can enhance GFR and renal plasma flow when administered short-term to humans with ESKD.[96] In connection with this, GFR and renal plasma flow rates are elevated in patients with acromegaly, whereas kidney function is usually low in GH-deficient states. GH increases GFR with a delay of many hours up to a day, consistent with induction of IGF-I synthesis. Endogenous IGF-I may contribute to the physiologic regulation of GFR.[121] Several studies have assessed the potential of rhGH and/or rhIGF-1 administration to improve kidney function: Whereas GH resulted in no or only a modest and transitory increase of GFR in adults with advanced CKD and in children with growth failure,[95] IGF-I produced a more sustained increase in GFR and renal plasma flow.[96] A regimen using rhIGF-I in patients with advanced CKD was well tolerated and resulted in a sustained improvement in kidney function.[97] Transgenic mice expressing GH developed increased mesangial proliferation followed by progressive mesangial sclerosis, which was not seen in transgenic mice expressing IGF-I[98,99] and there has been a concern that GH/IGF-I therapy could contribute to progression of CKD. However, prolonged treatment with GH in children with CKD has not been reported to lead to more rapid progression of CKD.[110,111]

PROLACTIN

Prolactin's normal function in women is to promote lactation, but its function in men is not fully established. Serum prolactin concentrations are usually elevated in patients with CKD, and the prevalence of hyperprolactinemia in ESKD ranges between 30% and 65%.[122-124] Hyperprolactinemia in CKD is understood as a consequence of both reduced renal clearance[124] and increased production due to suppressed dopaminergic activity.[125] Thus, antidopaminergic medications (such as neuroleptics, metoclopramide, or cimetidine), which can further stimulate prolactin production, should be minimized or avoided if possible. The consequences of hyperprolactinemia in CKD and ESKD are reflected in the commonly observed reproductive abnormalities resulting from the associated inhibition of gonadotropin secretion: Hyperprolactinemic patients eventually experience galactorrhea and infertility due to the inhibition of gonadotropin secretion; in women amenorrhea may concur, whereas in men erectile dysfunction and hypogonadism often appear concomitantly. Although bromocriptine treatment has proved to decrease prolactin levels in uremic men and women,[126] the previously mentioned symptoms do not fully disappear, suggesting that other factors may contribute in parallel. Therapy with erythropoiesis-stimulating agents (ESAs) has been suggested to decrease serum prolactin levels[127] and to improve sexual function.[128] Thus, it has been postulated that prolactin may contribute to the severity of anemia associated with CKD.

It is possible that prolactinemia may have previously underrecognized effects independent of its effects on the gonads. Studies in patients with CKD report a strong association between prolactinemia, endothelial dysfunction, arterial stiffness and cardiovascular outcomes, in men and women.[129] These associations may be explained as a consequence of (1) the inhibition of gonadotropic hormones, which may link per se to increased cardiovascular risk (discussed later); (2) decreased dopaminergic activity; (3) other risk factors affecting prolactin production such as hypercytokinemia[130]; or (4) yet unknown mechanisms.

Advancement in the understanding of prolactin physiology reveals additional functions such as a regulation of the immune system and serving as a growth and anti-apoptotic factor. As a growth factor, prolactin influences hematopoiesis, angiogenesis, and blood clotting. Prolactin modulates the inflammatory response, stimulates the adhesion of mononuclear cells to endothelium, and enhances vascular smooth muscle cell proliferation.[131-134] Prolactin also induces regional vasoconstriction through the β_2-adrenergic and nitric oxide mechanisms.[135] Some small studies have evaluated the effects of bromocriptine therapy in CKD, describing a reduction in blood pressure and the regression of left ventricular hypertrophy in patients receiving dialysis.[136-138] Another randomized-controlled trial in patients with diabetes mellitus and stage 4 CKD tested bromocriptine supplementation for 6 months versus placebo,[139] observing a decrease in blood pressure and left ventricular mass index. Whether these effects were, at least partly, mediated by prolactin reduction is unknown.

ADRENAL GLANDS

Because symptoms of hypercortisolism and hyperaldosteronemia are common in CKD, it has been proposed that the hypothalamic-pituitary-adrenal (HPA) axis may be upregulated.[140] This proposal is plausible, given that both glucocorticoid and aldosterone metabolites are excreted by the kidneys and that cortisol metabolism is partly regulated by the kidneys. Nonetheless, few studies to date have addressed adrenal gland disorders in CKD, an issue in part hampered by the prescription of medication interfering with the RAAS and cortisol system.

ADRENOCORTICOTROPIC HORMONE

Adrenocorticotropic hormone (ACTH) was used 60 years ago for the treatment of nephrotic syndrome in children but was gradually replaced by synthetic glucocorticoid analogs. In addition to its role in controlling steroidogenesis, ACTH stands as a physiologic agonist of the melanocortin system. Clinical and experimental evidence suggests that ACTH may have antiproteinuric, lipid-lowering, and renoprotective properties, which are not fully explained by its steroidogenic effects.[141,142]

ALDOSTERONE AND CORTISOL

Over and above the classical effect on sodium reabsorption, aldosterone may exert other effects on renal and cardiovascular damage. Aldosterone increases oxidative stress and promotes vascular inflammation[143,144] and impairs vascular reactivity by limiting the bioavailability of nitric oxide.[145] In the presence of salt overload, aldosterone causes hypertrophy and fibrosis in the heart, both of which are prevented by the administration of mineralocorticoid receptor (MR) antagonists.[146] The MR binds aldosterone and cortisol with similar affinities. Under normal conditions cortisol is incapable of activating the MR because cortisol is converted into the inactive metabolite cortisone by 11β-hydroxysteroid dehydrogenase type 2 (11β-HSD2).[147] Thus, it may be hypothesized that the beneficial effects of MR antagonists may result from blocking the action of both aldosterone and cortisol. In an observational analysis in patients with type 2 diabetes mellitus undergoing maintenance HD,[148] the joint presence of high serum aldosterone and high serum cortisol concentrations was associated with sudden cardiac death. Whether the use of MR antagonists decreases the risk of sudden death in such patients must be examined in future trials.

ADRENAL ANDROGENS

Dehydroepiandrosterone (DHEA) and dehydroepiandrosterone sulfate (DHEA-S) are secreted from the zona reticularis of the adrenal gland. DHEA and DHEA-S are interconverted, and DHEA serves as a precursor of sex hormones. In a population-based study of young adults, serum DHEA concentrations were inversely associated with kidney function.[149] Low circulating serum concentrations of DHEA-S were also associated with the progression of glomerular injury in men with type 2 diabetes mellitus.[150] This finding is in line with those of two studies showing that serum DHEA-S was significantly reduced in male patients on maintenance HD and was associated with all-cause and CVD-related mortality.[151,152] Like concentrations of other hormones, the reduced DHEA-S concentration may be a surrogate of disease severity, being suppressed in critical illness. However, DHEA-S may have protective functions against atherosclerosis and CVD, given that DHEA supplementation improves endothelial function and insulin sensitivity in men.[153] DHEA-S may have other functions as a peroxisome proliferator–activated receptor α (PPARα) activator that can modulate immune function, inflammation, and oxidative stress.[154] Finally, one should not forget that DHEA-S may be an intermediate in the pathways of both prolactin (upstream) and testosterone (downstream), thus mediating the risk.

GONADAL DYSFUNCTION

Disturbances in the hypothalamic-pituitary-gonadal axis are common in patients with CKD and play an important role in the development of sexual dysfunction (Table 58.3). Sexual dysfunction in these patients should be thought of as a multifactorial problem that is affected by a variety of physiologic and psychological factors as well as comorbid conditions. In addition to a number of endocrine alterations described later, diabetes and vascular disease, for instance, can interfere with the ability of the male patient to achieve an erection and the female patient to achieve sexual arousal. Various psychological factors, such as depression, can significantly and adversely affect sexual function in both sexes.

IN WOMEN
ENDOCRINE ABNORMALITIES

Elevated serum concentrations of prolactin (see earlier discussion), follicle-stimulating hormone (FSH), and luteinizing hormone (LH) are usual findings in uremic women. Disturbances in menstruation and fertility are commonly encountered, usually leading to amenorrhea by the time the

Table 58.3 Endocrine Abnormalities Leading to Sexual Dysfunction in Chronic Kidney Disease

Men	Decreased production of testosterone
	Blunted increase in serum luteinizing hormone (LH)
	Decreased amplitude of LH secretory burst
	Variable increase in follicle-stimulating hormone (FSH)
	Increased prolactin
Women	Anovulatory menstrual cycles
	Lack of midcycle surge in LH
	Increased prolactin

patient is diagnosed with ESKD. The menstrual cycle typically remains irregular after the initiation of dialysis. Ovarian dysfunction in women undergoing dialysis is characterized by the absence of cyclic gonadotropin and estradiol release, which results in the lack of progestational changes in the endometrium.[155] Midcycle LH surge cannot be mitigated with endogenous administration of estrogen, confirming a central hypothalamic derangement.[156] As a consequence, anovulation and subsequent infertility are probably the major menstrual abnormalities in uremic women, together with decreased libido and reduced ability to reach orgasm.[157] Therefore, successful conception with pregnancy is rare in ESKD. Pathologic endometrium morphology is very common in uremic women of reproductive age undergoing HD, with proliferative changes in 30% and atrophic changes in almost 25%. However, it seems that the endometrium has preserved normal reactivity to circulating estrogens.[158]

CLINICAL MANIFESTATIONS

Young uremic women usually experience premature menopause, approximately 4.5 years earlier on average than their healthy counterparts. Hypogonadism in women has been linked with sleep disorders, depression, urinary incontinence, and, in the long term, with osteoporosis, impaired cognitive function, and increased cardiovascular risk.[159] Up to 65% of women undergoing dialysis report problems with sexual function, and up to 40% no longer engage in sexual intercourse.[160] Loss of libido may also contribute to infertility.

Finally, megestrol acetate has successfully been used in patients with ESKD as an effective therapy to treat PEW.[161-164] This finding, together with the observation of an attenuation of the symptoms associated with uremic anorexia in women in comparison with men,[165] suggests the existence of a yet uncharacterized pleiotropic role for sex hormones in the regulation of nutrient homeostasis in uremia.

TREATMENT

General principles of treatment include education about sexual function in the setting of CKD, adequate dialysis delivery, and treatment of underlying depression. Changes in lifestyle, such as smoking cessation, strength training, and aerobic exercises, may decrease depression, enhance body image, and have positive effects on sexuality.[156] Limited evidence indicates that CKD alters the pharmacokinetics of estradiol. Free and total estradiol plasma concentrations are higher in women with ESKD after an oral estradiol dose, but no change occurs in estrone concentrations. Neither estradiol nor estrone is removed in the dialysate.[166] Steady-state pharmacokinetics of oral estradiol shows that women with ESKD should receive approximately 50% of the typically prescribed dosages.[167] No information is available on the pharmacokinetics of any of the progestins in CKD.

Chronic anovulation and lack of progesterone secretion in uremic women may be treated with oral progesterone. Because ongoing menses can contribute to the anemia of CKD, particularly in patients with menorrhagia, administration of progesterone at the end of the menstrual cycle is preferred. At present, it is not clear whether unopposed estrogen stimulation (due to anovulatory cycles) predisposes women with CKD to endometrial hyperplasia or endometrial cancer. Thus, routine gynecologic follow-up is recommended in such patients. Low estradiol levels in amenorrheic women undergoing dialysis can lead to vaginal atrophy and dyspareunia; topical estrogen cream and vaginal lubricants may be helpful in these patients. Uremic women who are menstruating normally should be encouraged to use birth control. Estradiol hormonal replacement therapy was able to restore regular menses and improve sexual function in premenopausal estrogen-deficient women undergoing dialysis[168] and to improve bone histomorphometry in animal models of uremia.[169] Estrogen administration may positively affect sexual desire and prevent bone mass loss in postmenopausal women with ESKD.[170,171] Hypoactive sexual desire disorder is the most commonly reported sexual problem in women with CKD, and testosterone replacement therapy has shown effectiveness in patients without renal disease.[172,173] Nonetheless, successful kidney transplantation is clearly the most effective means to restore normal sexual desire in women with CKD.

FEMALE SEX HORMONES AND PROGRESSION OF CKD

Because the progression rate of renal disease is in general faster for men than for women,[174] it has been suggested that this sex dimorphism may be explained by the interaction of circulating steroids with specific receptors in the kidney. In experimental animal models, endogenous estrogens have shown antifibrotic and anti-apoptotic effects in the kidney,[175,176] and exogenous estradiol in ovariectomized rats attenuated glomerulosclerosis and tubulointerstitial fibrosis[177] by protecting podocytes against injury through upregulation of estrogen receptor β.[178] A direct extrapolation from these animal studies would suggest that exogenous estrogen administration may slow CKD progression. However, clinical evidence in this regard is elusive, with evidence suggesting that both estrogen replacement therapy and oral contraceptives are associated with albuminuria, increased creatinine clearance, and loss of kidney function.[179-183] The implications of these studies need to be carefully considered in the context of their observational and, in the majority of the cases, retrospective nature. It should also be noted that in general, hormone replacement therapy is prescribed less frequently to postmenopausal patients with ESKD than to the general population,[184] possibly incurring a selection and underrepresentation bias.

IN MEN

ENDOCRINE ABNORMALITIES

The occurrence of testosterone deficiency is estimated to vary from 6% to 9.5% in community-dwelling men aged 40 to 75 years, rising to 15% to 30% in diabetic or obese men.[185,186] In CKD this prevalence is much higher, ranging between 50% and 75%.[187-190] This deficiency is true for both free and total serum testosterone, although the binding capacity and levels of sex hormone-binding globulin seem within normal range. Causes of hypogonadism in CKD are multiple and must be sought within hyperprolactinemia (see preceding discussion), comorbid conditions (such as PEW, obesity, diabetes mellitus, and hypertension), and medications that may influence gonadal function (such as ACE inhibitors/angiotensin receptor blockers, spironolactone, ketoconazole, and glucocorticoids, statin, and cinacalcet).

The plasma concentration of LH is typically elevated in men with uremia, mainly owing to changes in the pulsatile release of gonadotropin-releasing hormone and LH itself, diminished feedback inhibition of LH production (because of low testosterone levels), and impaired renal clearance. FSH secretion is also increased in men with CKD, although to a more variable degree such that the LH/FSH ratio is typically increased. Feedback inhibition of FSH is impaired because of a decrease in the peptide inhibin, which is produced by the Sertoli cells.[156] All of these disturbances can be detected with only moderate reductions in GFR and progressively worsen in parallel with progression of CKD. These disorders rarely normalize with initiation of dialysis. Instead, they often progress. A well-functioning kidney transplant is likely to restore normal sexual activity, although some features of reproductive function may remain impaired.

CLINICAL MANIFESTATIONS

Symptoms and signs of hypogonadism in men depend on the stage in life at which hypogonadism develops and its duration. In adults with ESKD, hypogonadism, low testosterone levels, and hyperprolactinemia are likely responsible for decreased libido, erectile dysfunction, oligospermia and infertility, osteopenia, and to some extent osteoporosis and anemia. Erectile dysfunction has been reported in 70% to 80% of men with CKD and ESKD.[191] Additional risk factors that increase the probability of erectile dysfunction are advanced age, diabetes, hypertension, dyslipidemia, smoking, and anxiety. Semen analysis typically shows a decreased volume of ejaculate, either low sperm count or complete azoospermia, and a low percentage of motility. Medications frequently used in treating patients with CKD, such as diuretics, antihypertensive and antidepressant agents, and histamine H_2 blockers, can contribute to erectile dysfunction. Other drugs, such as spironolactone, ketoconazole, glucocorticoids, and cimetidine, can interfere directly with the synthesis of sex hormones.[192] Autonomic nervous system dysfunction, a frequent finding in patients with CKD (especially those with diabetes mellitus), likely also contributes to sexual abnormalities in CKD.[193] Disturbances in the pelvic autonomic nervous system can decrease sensation and arousal of stimuli during sexual activity. Autonomic neuropathy can also interfere with the complex

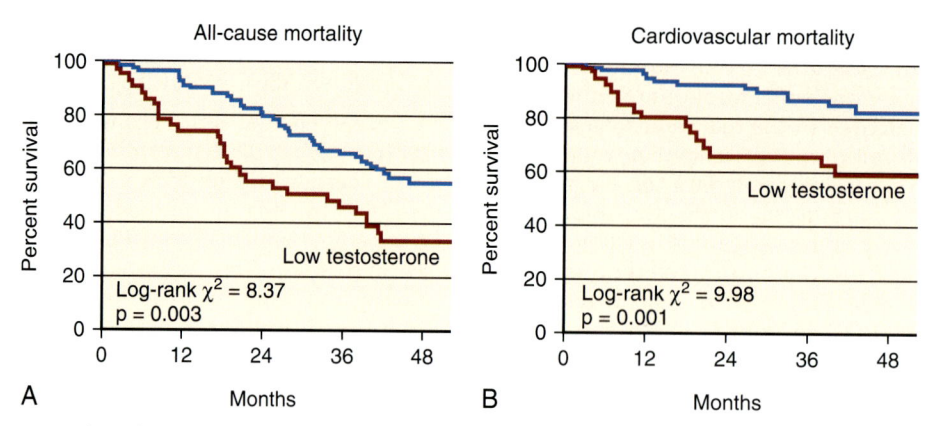

Figure 58.4 Sex-hormone alterations and outcome of chronic kidney disease (CKD). Reduced testosterone levels in male patients undergoing hemodialysis have been linked to increased mortality risk, especially that from cardiovascular causes. (Redrawn from Carrero JJ, Qureshi AR, Parini P, et al: Low serum testosterone increases mortality risk among male dialysis patients. *J Am Soc Nephrol* 20:613-620, 2009.)

neurologic axis that is necessary for achievement of an adequate erection.

Uremic hypogonadism may contribute to sarcopenia. In physiologic conditions, testosterone is an anabolic hormone that plays an important role in inducing skeletal muscle hypertrophy by promoting nitrogen retention, stimulating fractional muscle protein synthesis, inducing myoblast differentiation, and augmenting the efficiency of amino acid reuse by the skeletal muscle.[194] Consequently, positive associations between serum free and total testosterone levels with creatinine and handgrip strength have been reported in men receiving dialysis,[195] and endogenous testosterone in men with CKD stages 3 to 4 emerged as an important determinant of both muscle mass and strength.[196] Interventional studies with nandrolone decanoate (a testosterone synthetic agonist) in dialysis populations have shown significant improvements in muscle mass and strength as well as in nutritional status.[197,198]

Testosterone is known to exert a stimulatory effect on erythropoiesis[199] by inducing the growth of differentiated stem cells and enhancing the sensitivity of erythroid progenitors to circulating erythropoietin (EPO).[200,201] Because CKD is more common in the elderly, it is likely that both an age-associated decline in testosterone and the endocrine CKD abnormalities that encompass male hypogonadism contribute to some extent to a decline in erythroid mass and may contribute to anemia. For this reason, testosterone deficiency was proposed as an additional cause of anemia in ESA-naïve nondialyzed male patients with CKD and as an additional cause of resistance to ESAs in men treated with ESA undergoing HD.[202] Before the clinical introduction of recombinant human EPO (rhEPO) in 1989, androgens were the main pharmacologic intervention for correcting the anemia of ESKD. Reciprocally, anemia in patients with ESKD has been associated with a reduction of libido and endothelial dysfunction,[203] and rhEPO therapy has led to an increase in sexual desire and performance and an improvement in erectile function in some but not all patients.[204,205] Correction of anemia, improved sense of well-being, and direct endocrine effects may play a role in this result.[157] In addition, studies evaluating change in health-related quality of life in response to rhEPO therapy have noted significant improvements in physical and social functioning, overall mental health, and satisfaction with sexual activity.[206]

Finally, hypogonadism in men with non–dialysis-requiring CKD has been associated with arterial stiffness, endothelial dysfunction, and risk of cardiovascular events.[207] In patients receiving dialysis, hypogonadism has also been linked to increased mortality risk[190,195,208] (Figure 58.4), arterial stiffness,[209] worse quality of life,[187] and heightened inflammation.[189] The links between testosterone and cardiovascular complications may be explained by its association with risk factors such as dyslipidemia, obesity, diabetes mellitus, and metabolic syndrome, which may per se contribute to endothelial dysfunction and atherosclerosis. However, testosterone may also have direct atheroprotective effects in the cardiovascular system.[100] Transdermal testosterone therapy improved exercise-induced myocardial ischemia during an exercise stress test in men with stable angina,[101] and men with prostate cancer undergoing androgen deprivation therapy experienced an increase in central arterial pressure.[102] In animal models, testosterone supplementation inhibits neointimal plaque development,[103] stimulates endothelial progenitor cells,[104] increases nitric oxide release from vascular endothelial cells,[105] and enhances myocardial perfusion.[106,107]

The gonadal axis is suppressed by inflammatory cytokines,[210,211] and therefore any inflammatory disease may induce testosterone deficiency. Thus, low testosterone could be considered a biomarker of chronic inflammatory disease. In support of this contention, studies depict a strong inverse association between endogenous testosterone and surrogates of inflammation in various CKD populations.[189,195,208,209] However, it is also possible that testosterone has immunomodulatory actions per se, as suggested by the suppression of cytokine production in hypogonadal men with diabetes mellitus, coronary heart disease, and metabolic syndrome after supplementation with testosterone.[212-214]

TREATMENT

General principles of treatment of hypogonadism in men include optimal delivery of dialysis and adequate nutritional intake, as well as screening for depressive symptoms. A study compared the pharmacokinetics of a testosterone patch in patients with ESKD and in hypogonadal men with normal kidney function.[215] The researchers found that the half-life of testosterone after withdrawal of the patch was not different between the groups, nor was the minimum or maximum serum testosterone concentration during the period of patch application. Thus, it is likely that usual doses of testosterone replacement can be used in men with ESKD, with the usual monitoring of serum testosterone concentrations with dose adjustments as needed. Data on the use of testosterone in ESKD are limited; some studies suggest that erectile function in ESKD does not improve with testosterone supplementation,[216] and others indicate that normalization of endogenous testosterone by topical gels in hypogonadal men with advanced CKD improve sexual function.[217] Daily administration of 100 mg of 1% testosterone gel for 6 months in 40 hypogonadal men with CKD neither increased serum testosterone concentrations nor had an effect on ESA requirements.[218] It is possible that higher testosterone dosages may be required to achieve a clinical benefit in this patient group. Alternative modes of administration, such as intramuscular injection, may ease compliance and bioavailability. The response of testosterone in this setting may be modulated by the patient's nutritional status, activity level, and GH (and GH-binding protein) status. Because psychosocial factors may also take part in the pathophysiology of erectile dysfunction, nocturnal penile tumescence testing may be used to differentiate organic and psychological causes of impotence.

Whether testosterone deficiency may constitute a new pathophysiologic pathway in CKD-related complications such as anemia, PEW, and cardiovascular risk deserves further attention. Androgen therapy in supraphysiologic dosages has been linked to adverse effects.[25,137] Isolated cases of increase in blood pressure and clinically significant edema in healthy older men have been reported[25,128,129] as has fluid retention in men undergoing HD.[65] Treated patients must be closely monitored, but again, restoration of deficiencies and maintenance of total and free testosterone concentrations within the normal range may be the key to successful treatment.

MALE SEX HORMONES AND PROGRESSION OF CKD

In line with the finding that CKD progression is faster in men than in women, animal models of kidney injury have shown that orchidectomy attenuates glomerular and tubular damage, kidney fibrosis, and proteinuria.[219,220] Furthermore, animal studies describe proinflammatory, proapoptotic, and profibrotic effects of supraphysiologic dosages of testosterone during acute and chronic kidney injury.[176,221,222] On the other hand, it is difficult to reconcile such experimental findings with clinical observations, given that testosterone production decreases with progressive CKD and that both incidence and progression of CKD occur mainly in the elderly, who have lower testosterone concentrations on average. In line with this thinking, a population-based study of men reported that impaired kidney function and low serum testosterone concentrations were additive (and independent) mortality risk factors.[223] Thus, evidence has accumulated suggesting that testosterone may be protective to the kidney. A large case-control study involving more than 10,000 men newly diagnosed with nonmetastatic prostate cancer demonstrated that androgen deprivation therapy increased the risk of acute kidney injury.[224] Potential protective mechanisms include inducing vasodilation in renal vessels and enhancing the production of nitric oxide.[225] Thus, the use of androgen deprivation therapy might antagonize testosterone, raising the risk of damage to the glomerulus. An additional explanation for the role of hypogonadism on kidney injury was demonstrated in male rats subjected to renal ischemia followed by reperfusion.[226] In this setting, testosterone concentrations decreased dramatically after only 3 hours. Infusion of testosterone 3 hours after reperfusion attenuated the 24-hour increase in plasma creatinine and urinary kidney injury molecule-1 (KIM-1), prevented the reduction in outer medullary blood flow, and attenuated the 48-hour increase in intrarenal inflammation. Castration caused greater rises in plasma creatinine and KIM-1, and treatment with anastrozole (an aromatase inhibitor) plus testosterone almost normalized these markers.[226]

VITAMIN D, PARATHYROID HORMONE, AND KIDNEY DISEASE

The endocrine system of vitamin D and parathyroid hormone (PTH) is crucial for the homeostasis of calcium and phosphorus and for maintaining a healthy bone status. Altered levels of serum phosphate, calcium, vitamin D, PTH, and fibroblast growth factor 23 (FGF-23) contribute to the complex multiorgan syndrome of CKD–mineral and bone disorder (CKD-MBD), which leads to osteoporosis, fractures, CVD, and other complications.[227-229] Whereas abnormalities in PTH and the consequences of hyperparathyroidism are well recognized clinical problems in the management of CKD-MBD,[230] the awareness of the importance of vitamin D deficiency has also increased.[227-229] Indeed, the expression of vitamin D receptors (VDRs) by many different tissues and cells suggests a multifaceted role for this system.[231,232] Physiology and management of these hormonal alterations are discussed in more detail in Chapter 55.

VITAMIN D AND PARATHYROID HORMONE: METABOLISM AND ACTIONS IN CKD

The vitamin D family includes the biologically inert fat-soluble prohormones—vitamin D_2 (or ergocalciferol) and vitamin D_3 (or cholecalciferol). These prohormones are obtained mainly from sun exposure (by photochemical conversion of 7-dehydrocholesterol in the skin), food (especially fatty fish), and nutritional supplements. These prohormones are converted by hydroxylation in the liver to 25-hydroxyvitamin D, and by a second hydroxylation step (performed by the 1α-hydroxylase) to its active form, 1,25-dihydroxyvitamin D (calcitriol). The kidney is the most abundant source (but not exclusive) of 1α-hydroxylase in the body, and therefore CKD coincides with natural deficiencies in calcitriol.[228,229]

In normal conditions, the renal production of calcitriol is tightly regulated by PTH and by serum calcium and phosphorus levels. FGF-23, which is secreted from the bone, suppresses calcitriol synthesis, as does metabolic acidosis. Extrarenal calcitriol is converted in other tissues, including the skin, colon, prostate, and macrophages, but the regulatory processes for this conversion are not well understood. Calcitriol has a half-life of only 4 to 6 hours, and the circulating levels are low. Calcitriol, which is transported to various target organs by the vitamin D–binding protein (VDBP), mobilizes calcium into the bloodstream by promoting absorption of calcium and phosphorus from food in the intestines, and reabsorption of calcium in the kidneys. Calcitriol also promotes bone mineralization, bone growth, and bone remodeling by osteoblasts and osteoclasts, and prevents hypocalcemia. Vitamin D deficiency has been linked to multiple disorders, including growth retardation, skeletal abnormalities (osteopenia, osteoporosis, and increased risk of fractures), muscle weakness, left ventricular hypertrophy, as well as increased susceptibility to cancer, diabetes, and autoimmune and infectious diseases.[230,233-235] In the kidney, vitamin D may be important for maintaining podocyte function, preventing epithelial-to-mesenchymal transformation, and suppressing renin gene expression and inflammation.[236] Vitamin D also appears to be protective in models of diabetic nephropathy through targeting of the RAAS and the nuclear factor-kappaB (NF-κB) pathway.[237]

Parathyroid hormone has a key role in calcium and phosphate homeostasis. It stimulates excretion of phosphate by the renal tubular cells and indirectly modulates intestinal calcium absorption by stimulating the activation of calcitriol synthesis. As vitamin D deficiency progresses, the parathyroid glands are maximally stimulated, causing secondary hyperparathyroidism. Thus, levels of 25-hydroxyvitamin D are inversely associated with PTH levels, and calcitriol inhibits PTH expression. PTH increases the metabolism of 25-hydroxyvitamin D to calcitriol, further exacerbating the vitamin D deficiency. Hyperparathyroidism has been implicated in left ventricular hypertrophy as well as in the metabolic syndrome contributing to impaired glucose tolerance and dyslipidemia.[238] Parathyroid hormone and serum phosphate are well-established biomarkers of CKD-MBD, and FGF-23 is gaining increased attention.[239] However, the value of PTH[240] as well as FGF-23,[241] among others, in clinical monitoring has been questioned owing to their wide (and assay-dependent) biologic variability.

VITAMIN D DEFICIENCY IN CKD

Insufficient to deficient levels of 25-hydroxyvitamin D have been reported in the majority of individuals with CKD, including patients undergoing maintenance dialysis and others with non–dialysis-requiring CKD.[242,243] Vitamin D deficiency seems to be more pronounced in black individuals.[244] The circulating levels of 25-hydroxyvitamin D and calcitriol decrease with diminishing kidney function.[243,245] Because 25-hydroxyvitamin D has a longer half-life than calcitriol (approximately 3 weeks), it is considered the best measure of vitamin D status.[246] On these premises, vitamin D insufficiency is commonly defined as 25-hydroxyvitamin D levels lower than 30 ng/mL, whereas deficiency starts at the threshold of less than 15 ng/mL. Although there are known seasonal, geographic, ethnic, and age-related variations, the desirable level of vitamin D in patients with CKD has not yet been defined; nevertheless, it is recommended to maintain serum concentrations of 25-hydroxyvitamin D above 30 ng/mL.[230] Most commercial assays for 25-hydroxyvitamin D are thought to be acceptable for detecting vitamin D deficiency.[228] However, it should be noted that there are considerable between-laboratory and interassay variations in assays for measurement of circulating concentrations of 25-hydroxyvitamin D and PTH.[247]

1,25-Dihydroxyvitamin D assay should not be used to detect vitamin D deficiency in CKD because 25-dihydroxyvitamin D levels are usually low as a consequence of reduced 1α-hydroxylase activity in this disease, but they could also be normal, or even elevated, as a result of secondary hyperparathyroidism.

VITAMIN D SUPPLEMENTATION IN CKD

Providing children and adults with at least 800 IU of 25-hydroxyvitamin D_3 per day or its equivalent should guarantee vitamin D sufficiency. Unless a person eats oily fish frequently, it is difficult to provide that much vitamin D_3 on a daily basis from dietary sources. Thus, moderate sun exposure and/or provision of supplements are needed to fulfill the vitamin D requirement in patients with CKD.[242] Pharmacologic doses of vitamin D can be administered in the form of nutritional supplements or active vitamin D agents. The National Kidney Foundation Kidney Disease Outcomes Quality Initiative (K/DOQI) guidelines recommends starting with nutritional vitamin D supplements *before* using activated vitamin D derivatives in those patients with concurrent hyperparathyroidism associated with vitamin D insufficiency.[242,246] Although epidemiologic studies have generally indicated a survival benefit associated with the provision of activated vitamin D derivatives in all CKD stages[242,248-251] and 27% lower associated mortality risk has been found in patients receiving calcitriol or analogs,[252] the studies are subject to confounding by indication, and recommendations regarding nutritional vitamin D supplements are thus largely opinion based. There are no large interventional studies testing the effects of nutritional vitamin D supplementation on outcomes in CKD.[242]

Complete reference list available at ExpertConsult.com.

KEY REFERENCES

7. DeFronzo RA, Alvestrand A, Smith D, et al: Insulin resistance in uremia. *J Clin Invest* 67:563–568, 1981.
19. Beddhu S, Kimmel PL, Ramkumar N, et al: Associations of metabolic syndrome with inflammation in CKD: results from the Third National Health and Nutrition Examination Survey (NHANES III). *Am J Kidney Dis* 46:577–586, 2005.
25. Raj DS, Dominic EA, Pai A, et al: Skeletal muscle, cytokines, and oxidative stress in end-stage renal disease. *Kidney Int* 68:2338–2344, 2005.
36. Chen J, Muntner P, Hamm LL, et al: The metabolic syndrome and chronic kidney disease in U.S. adults. *Ann Intern Med* 140:167–174, 2004.
39. Shinohara K, Shoji T, Emoto M, et al: Insulin resistance as an independent predictor of cardiovascular mortality in patients with end-stage renal disease. *J Am Soc Nephrol* 13:1894–1900, 2002.
45. Pupim LB, Flakoll PJ, Majchrzak KM, et al: Increased muscle protein breakdown in chronic hemodialysis patients with type 2 diabetes mellitus. *Kidney Int* 68:1857–1865, 2005.
46. Mustata S, Chan C, Lai V, et al: Impact of an exercise program on arterial stiffness and insulin resistance in hemodialysis patients. *J Am Soc Nephrol* 15:2713–2718, 2004.
51. Ramirez SP, Albert JM, Blayney MJ, et al: Rosiglitazone is associated with mortality in chronic hemodialysis patients. *J Am Soc Nephrol* 20:1094–1101, 2009.
54. Hung AM, Roumie CL, Greevy RA, et al: Comparative effectiveness of incident oral antidiabetic drugs on kidney function. *Kidney Int* 81:698–706, 2012.
79. Carrero JJ, Qureshi AR, Axelsson J, et al: Clinical and biochemical implications of low thyroid hormone levels (total and free forms)

in euthyroid patients with chronic kidney disease. *J Intern Med* 262:690–701, 2007.
80. Zoccali C, Mallamaci F, Tripepi G, et al: Low triiodothyronine and survival in end-stage renal disease. *Kidney Int* 70:523–528, 2006.
86. Meuwese CL, Carrero JJ, Cabezas-Rodriguez I, et al: Nonthyroidal illness: a risk factor for coronary calcification and arterial stiffness in patients undergoing peritoneal dialysis? *J Intern Med* 274:584–593, 2013.
91. Mak RH, Cheung WW, Roberts CT, Jr: The growth hormone–insulin-like growth factor-I axis in chronic kidney disease. *Growth Horm IGF Res* 18:17–25, 2008.
92. Mahesh S, Kaskel F: Growth hormone axis in chronic kidney disease. *Pediatr Nephrol* 23:41–48, 2008.
101. Ding H, Gao XL, Hirschberg R, et al: Impaired actions of insulin-like growth factor 1 on protein synthesis and degradation in skeletal muscle of rats with chronic renal failure: evidence for a postreceptor defect. *J Clin Invest* 97:1064–1075, 1996.
103. Sun DF, Zheng Z, Tummala P, et al: Chronic uremia attenuates growth hormone-induced signal transduction in skeletal muscle. *J Am Soc Nephrol* 15:2630–2636, 2004.
104. Wang H, Casaburi R, Taylor WE, et al: Skeletal muscle mRNA for IGF-IEa, IGF-II, and IGF-I receptor is decreased in sedentary chronic hemodialysis patients. *Kidney Int* 68:352–361, 2005.
107. Garibotto G, Russo R, Sofia A, et al: Effects of uremia and inflammation on growth hormone resistance in patients with chronic kidney diseases. *Kidney Int* 74:937–945, 2008.
110. Fine RN, Ho M, Tejani A, et al: Adverse events with rhGH treatment of patients with chronic renal insufficiency and end-stage renal disease. *J Pediatr* 142:539–545, 2003.
113. Feldt-Rasmussen B, Lange M, Sulowicz W, et al: Growth hormone treatment during hemodialysis in a randomized trial improves nutrition, quality of life, and cardiovascular risk. *J Am Soc Nephrol* 18:2161–2171, 2007.
114. Guebre-Egziabher F, Juillard L, Boirie Y, et al: Short-term administration of a combination of recombinant growth hormone and insulin-like growth factor-I induces anabolism in maintenance hemodialysis. *J Clin Endocrinol Metab* 94:2299–2305, 2009.
129. Carrero JJ, Kyriazis J, Sonmez A, et al: Prolactin levels, endothelial dysfunction, and the risk of cardiovascular events and mortality in patients with CKD. *Clin J Am Soc Nephrol* 7:207–215, 2012.
139. Mejia-Rodriguez O, Herrera-Abarca JE, Ceballos-Reyes G, et al: Cardiovascular and renal effects of bromocriptine in diabetic patients with stage 4 chronic kidney disease. *Biomed Res Int* 2013:104059, 2013.
142. Gong R: The renaissance of corticotropin therapy in proteinuric nephropathies. *Nat Rev Nephrol* 8:122–128, 2012.
148. Drechsler C, Ritz E, Tomaschitz A, et al: Aldosterone and cortisol affect the risk of sudden cardiac death in haemodialysis patients. *Eur Heart J* 34:578–587, 2013.
151. Kakiya R, Shoji T, Hayashi T, et al: Decreased serum adrenal androgen dehydroepiandrosterone sulfate and mortality in hemodialysis patients. *Nephrol Dial Transplant* 27:3915–3922, 2012.
156. Anantharaman P, Schmidt RJ: Sexual function in chronic kidney disease. *Adv Chronic Kidney Dis* 14:119–125, 2007.
157. Palmer BF: Sexual dysfunction in uremia. *J Am Soc Nephrol* 10:1381–1388, 1999.
166. Anderson GD, Odegard PS: Pharmacokinetics of estrogen and progesterone in chronic kidney disease. *Adv Chronic Kidney Dis* 11:357–360, 2004.
170. Hernandez E, Valera R, Alonzo E, et al: Effects of raloxifene on bone metabolism and serum lipids in postmenopausal women on chronic hemodialysis. *Kidney Int* 63:2269–2274, 2003.
180. Agarwal M, Selvan V, Freedman BI, et al: The relationship between albuminuria and hormone therapy in postmenopausal women. *Am J Kidney Dis* 45:1019–1025, 2005.
188. Carrero JJ, Stenvinkel P: The vulnerable man: impact of testosterone deficiency on the uraemic phenotype. *Nephrol Dial Transplant* 27:4030–4041, 2012.
189. Carrero JJ, Qureshi AR, Nakashima A, et al: Prevalence and clinical implications of testosterone deficiency in men with end-stage renal disease. *Nephrol Dial Transplant* 26:184–190, 2011.
191. Palmer BF: Outcomes associated with hypogonadism in men with chronic kidney disease. *Adv Chronic Kidney Dis* 11:342–347, 2004.
195. Carrero JJ, Qureshi AR, Parini P, et al: Low serum testosterone increases mortality risk among male dialysis patients. *J Am Soc Nephrol* 20:613–620, 2009.
197. Johansen KL, Painter PL, Sakkas GK, et al: Effects of resistance exercise training and nandrolone decanoate on body composition and muscle function among patients who receive hemodialysis: a randomized, controlled trial. *J Am Soc Nephrol* 17:2307–2314, 2006.
198. Johansen KL, Mulligan K, Schambelan M: Anabolic effects of nandrolone decanoate in patients receiving dialysis: a randomized controlled trial. *JAMA* 281:1275–1281, 1999.
202. Carrero JJ, Barany P, Yilmaz MI, et al: Testosterone deficiency is a cause of anemia and reduced responsiveness to erythropoiesis stimulating agents in men with chronic kidney disease. *Nephrol Dial Transplant* 27:709–715, 2012.
230. Kidney Disease: Improving Global Outcomes (KDIGO) CKD-MBD Work Group: KDIGO clinical practice guideline for the diagnosis, evaluation, prevention, and treatment of Chronic Kidney Disease–Mineral and Bone Disorder (CKD-MBD). *Kidney Int Suppl* 113:S1–S130, 2009.
236. Agarwal R: Vitamin D, proteinuria, diabetic nephropathy, and progression of CKD. *Clin J Am Soc Nephrol* 4:1523–1528, 2009.
240. Garrett G, Sardiwal S, Lamb EJ, et al: PTH—a particularly tricky hormone: why measure it at all in kidney patients? *Clin J Am Soc Nephrol* 8:299–312, 2013.
243. Ravani P, Malberti F, Tripepi G, et al: Vitamin D levels and patient outcome in chronic kidney disease. *Kidney Int* 75:88–95, 2009.
252. Duranton F, Rodriguez-Ortiz ME, Duny Y, et al: Vitamin D treatment and mortality in chronic kidney disease: a systematic review and meta-analysis. *Am J Nephrol* 37:239–248, 2013.

59 Neurologic Aspects of Kidney Disease

Manjula Kurella Tamura

CHAPTER OUTLINE

STROKE, 1926
Epidemiology of Stroke in Chronic Kidney Disease, Dialysis, and the Transplant Population, 1927
Risk Factors for Stroke in Chronic Kidney Disease and End-Stage Kidney Disease, 1928
Stroke Prevention, 1930
Management of Acute Stroke in Chronic Kidney Disease and End-Stage Kidney Disease, 1933
DISORDERS OF COGNITIVE FUNCTION, 1934
Delirium Syndromes, 1934

Syndromes of Chronic Cognitive Impairment, 1935
NEUROPATHY, 1939
Uremic Polyneuropathy, 1939
Mononeuropathy, 1939
Autonomic Neuropathy, 1939
SLEEP DISORDERS, 1939
Prevalence of Sleep Complaints, 1939
Sleep Apnea, 1939
Restless Legs Syndrome, 1940
Periodic Limb Movements of Sleep, 1940

Neurologic aspects of chronic kidney disease (CKD) encompass a diverse spectrum of clinical disorders and syndromes. Indeed, clinical uremia was first described principally as a neurologic illness manifested by disturbances of cognitive, somatosensory, neuromuscular, and autonomic dysfunction.[1] Renal replacement therapy attenuates these features of the uremic syndrome, suggesting a central role for a retained solute (or solutes) in the pathogenesis of the neurologic manifestations of uremia. However, identification of the responsible solute(s) has proven difficult, in part due to the vast array of solutes that are retained in CKD. Earlier recognition and treatment of CKD and aging of the CKD population has changed the clinical presentation of neurologic illness in kidney disease, further complicating efforts to identify the causative factors. Dialysis therapy itself is also associated with neurologic complications, including dialysis dysequilibrium, a syndrome of delirium associated with the initiation of dialysis therapy, and dialysis dementia, a progressive disorder linked to aluminum toxicity. Fortunately, these disorders have sharply decreased in incidence.

Cerebrovascular disease, now recognized as a major cause of morbidity and mortality in patients with CKD, is an equally important part of the spectrum of neurologic illness associated with CKD. Stroke rates are increased 6- to 10-fold and stroke mortality 2- to 3-fold in patients on dialysis. While there has been substantial progress in the identification, treatment, and prevention of stroke in the general population, evidence-based treatment strategies for patients with CKD are still lacking. Interestingly, subclinical cerebrovascular disease is not only a major risk factor for stroke and a marker for future cardiovascular events; it may also play an important role in the cognitive manifestations of CKD.

This chapter reviews the epidemiology, pathophysiology, and treatment approach for stroke, disorders of cognitive function and sleep, and neuropathy in patients with kidney disease.

STROKE

Stroke is the third leading cause of death and a major cause of disability in the United States.[2] Acute stroke is characterized by a sudden onset of focal neurologic symptoms, such as dysphasia, dysarthria, hemianopia, weakness, ataxia, sensory loss, and neglect, resulting from an interruption in blood supply to a corresponding area of the brain. Symptoms are typically unilateral, and consciousness is generally preserved except in the case of some posterior circulation strokes. By convention, neurologic deficits persisting longer than 24 hours are classified as stroke, whereas deficits persisting less than 24 hours are classified as transient ischemic attack (TIA). With widespread use of brain imaging, it is now apparent that 15% to 20% of persons with symptoms lasting less than 24 hours have evidence of a brain infarct; thus, some authorities have proposed modifying the TIA definition to clinical symptoms lasting less than 1 hour and without evidence of infarction.[3] Over 30% of persons with

TIA subsequently suffer from stroke, most occur within weeks of the TIA event.[4]

Strokes can be classified as ischemic, resulting from occlusion of a blood vessel, and hemorrhagic, resulting from rupture of a blood vessel. In the U.S. and European general population, 80% of strokes are caused by ischemia, and 20% of strokes are caused by hemorrhage.[5] It is useful to classify ischemic strokes based on the mechanism of injury—large artery atherosclerosis, cardiogenic embolism, small vessel occlusive disease, and other or undetermined cause,[6] and the location of infarct—anterior circulation versus posterior circulation, since these distinctions have important therapeutic implications. In the general population, cardiogenic embolism accounts for 25% of ischemic stroke, followed by large artery atherosclerosis and small vessel occlusive disease; however, these rates vary by sex and race/ethnicity. Men and whites are reported to have a higher incidence of large artery atherosclerosis as compared to women and blacks, respectively.[7-9] Hemorrhagic stroke can also be divided into two subtypes: intracerebral hemorrhage, accounting for the majority of hemorrhagic strokes, and subarachnoid hemorrhage. Intracerebral hemorrhage is most frequently attributed to hypertension, amyloid angiopathy, septic embolism, mycotic aneurysm, and bleeding diatheses, while subarachnoid hemorrhage is most often due to rupture of an arterial aneurysm or vascular malformation.

The presence of CKD, defined as an estimated glomerular filtration rate (eGFR) of less than 60 mL/min/1.73 m^2, has several important implications for the detection, management, and prevention of stroke. Persons with CKD have a different risk factor profile and stroke epidemiology compared to persons in the general population, and they are at higher risk for stroke events and stroke-related mortality. Furthermore, several stroke detection, management, and prevention strategies may have lower efficacy and/or safety in patients with CKD.

EPIDEMIOLOGY OF STROKE IN CHRONIC KIDNEY DISEASE, DIALYSIS, AND THE TRANSPLANT POPULATION

Stroke is the third leading cause of cardiovascular disease death among persons with end-stage kidney disease (ESKD) on dialysis.[10] As compared with the general population, stroke event rates and stroke mortality rates are increased 6- to 10-fold among patients on dialysis (Figure 59.1).[11,12] As in the general population, ischemic stroke is more common than hemorrhagic stroke.[11,13] Among U.S. patients on dialysis, cardioembolic stroke is most common, followed by small vessel occlusion, and then by large artery stroke (Table 59.1).[12] Among Japanese patients, small vessel occlusion is more common, followed by cardioembolic stroke.[13] Posterior circulation strokes involving the vertebrobasilar system occur more commonly in patients on dialysis than in the general population.[13] This distribution pattern suggests screening for carotid artery disease may not be as effective as stroke prevention strategy in patients on dialysis relative to the general population. Kidney transplantation is associated with 30% lower risk for stroke or TIA compared with patients remaining on the transplant waiting list, whereas allograft failure increases the risk for stroke or TIA by 150%.[14]

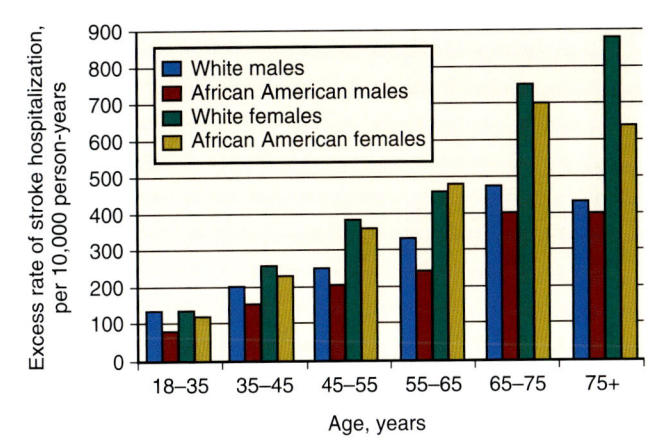

Figure 59.1 Excess rate of stroke hospitalization in patients on dialysis compared to the general population (per 10,000 person-years). (Adapted with permission from Seliger SL, Gillen DL, Longstreth WT, Jr, et al: Elevated risk of stroke among patients with end-stage renal disease. *Kidney Int* 64:603-609, 2003.)

Table 59.1 Stroke Subtypes in the General Population and in the Incident Dialysis Population

Stroke Subtype	U.S. General Population Prevalence (%)	U.S. Incident Dialysis Population (N = 176) Prevalence (%)	U.S. Incident Dialysis Population (N = 176) Case Fatality Rate (%)
Ischemic stroke	80	87	28
Large artery	7-18	10	29
Cardioembolism	15-27	24	36
Small vessel occlusion	11-21	17	17
Multiple causes	3-7	16	41
Other/undetermined	35-42	20	19
Hemorrhagic stroke	20	13	90

Data from U.S. general population adapted from references 7, 8, and 9. Data from incident dialysis population adapted from reference 12.

The extent to which less advanced stages of CKD increase stroke risk independent of traditional risk factors remains unclear, and most guidelines from professional societies do not include CKD as a stroke risk factor. For example, in a pooled analysis of U.S. community-based studies, CKD was not significantly associated with an increased risk for all-cause stroke after adjustment for traditional risk factors, such as diabetes mellitus, hypertension, hypercholesterolemia, smoking, and alcohol use.[15] However, other studies have reached different conclusions.[16-18] In a meta-analysis of 33 cohort studies, CKD was associated with a 1.4-fold higher risk for stroke.[19] One limitation of this analysis is that it did not account for proteinuria. Some, but not all, studies have reported racial variation in stroke risk, with CKD being associated with a heightened risk for stroke among blacks

Table 59.2 Modifiable Stroke Risk Factors and Prevention Strategies in Chronic Kidney Disease, End-Stage Kidney Disease, and Kidney Transplant Recipients

Risk Factor	Cohort Studies			Randomized Trials		
	CKD	ESKD	Transplant	CKD	ESKD	Transplant
Traditional Risk Factors						
Hypertension	+	+	ND	+	ND	ND
Diabetes	+	+	+	ND	ND	ND
Smoking	−	−	+	ND	ND	ND
Cardiovascular disease	+	+	+	ND	ND	ND
Dyslipidemia	+	−	ND	+	+/−	+/−
Carotid stenosis	ND	ND	ND	+	ND	ND
Atrial fibrillation	+	+	ND	ND	ND	ND
Nontraditional Risk Factors						
Proteinuria	+	NA	ND	ND	NA	ND
Malnutrition or inflammation	+	+/−	ND	ND	ND	ND
Anemia	+	+	ND	−	−	ND
Hyperhomocysteinemia	+	+	ND	−	−	ND
Hemodialysis	NA	+/−	NA	NA	ND	NA

+, Significant association or positive trial result; −, nonsignificant association or negative trial result; CKD, chronic kidney disease; ESKD, end-stage kidney disease; NA, not applicable; ND, no data.

more so than among whites.[20] Relative to the general population, CKD is associated with a 2- to 3-fold increase in the risk for death and disability following stroke.[21]

Neuroimaging studies suggest that persons with CKD and ESKD have a substantial burden of cerebrovascular disease even in the absence of clinical stroke. For example, up to 50% of patients receiving dialysis without a history of clinical stroke have evidence of an infarct with brain magnetic resonance imaging (MRI), and these patients are at increased risk for future cardiovascular events.[22,23] Brain white matter lesions, a marker of small vessel disease, are also highly prevalent among patients on dialysis,[24,25] as well as among patients with mild or moderate CKD not requiring dialysis.[26-28] Among patients who experienced an intracerebral hemorrhage, patients with CKD had a 2- to 3-fold higher likelihood of cerebral microbleeds, a marker of lipohyalinosis or amyloid angiopathy, compared to patients without CKD.[29] This association was stronger among blacks than among whites.

RISK FACTORS FOR STROKE IN CHRONIC KIDNEY DISEASE AND END-STAGE KIDNEY DISEASE

The vascular beds of the kidney and the brain are quite similar—both are low-resistance end organs that receive a high blood volume.[30] The pathologic correlates of brain white matter disease (or microbleeds) and nondiabetic CKD, namely arteriolar intima-media thickening and hyalinosis, are also quite similar. Thus the high prevalence of cerebrovascular disease in CKD may reflect a shared risk factor or factors and the similarity of their vascular supply. Epidemiologic studies have attempted to account for many shared risk factors, notably hypertension and prevalent cardiovascular disease, but may not sufficiently reflect cumulative risk factor exposure and severity of vascular injury, and this may explain the inconsistency of epidemiologic findings. Conversely, the risk factor profile for stroke may differ in patients with CKD. The relationship of traditional stroke risk factors such as hypertension and hyperlipidemia may be altered by CKD or confounded by the presence of protein energy wasting, heart failure, and other comorbid conditions. In addition, kidney disease may directly contribute to cerebrovascular disease through a number of novel mechanisms listed in Table 59.2 and discussed later.

HYPERTENSION

Hypertension is a major risk factor for both ischemic and hemorrhagic stroke. In the general population, stroke risk doubles for each 20 mm Hg increase in systolic blood pressure or 10 mm Hg increase in diastolic blood pressure above 115/75 mm Hg.[31] In the dialysis population, each 10 mm Hg increase in mean blood pressure is associated with an 11% increased risk for stroke.[32] A J-shaped association of systolic blood pressure with stroke incidence has been reported in some, but not all, studies of CKD and ESKD.[32-34] For example, in a community-based sample of persons with CKD, systolic blood pressure of less than 120 mm Hg was associated with a doubling of stroke risk as compared to individuals with systolic blood pressure of 120 to 129 mm Hg (Figure 59.2A).[33] However, this finding was not replicated in analyses of the Perindopril Protection Against Recurrent Stroke Study (PROGRESS).[34] In these post hoc analyses, blood pressure lowering with an angiotensin-converting enzyme inhibitor (ACEI) was associated with a 25% risk reduction for stroke events among the subgroup of persons with CKD (Figure 59.2B). These findings were consistent for both systolic and diastolic blood pressure lowering and for both ischemic and hemorrhagic

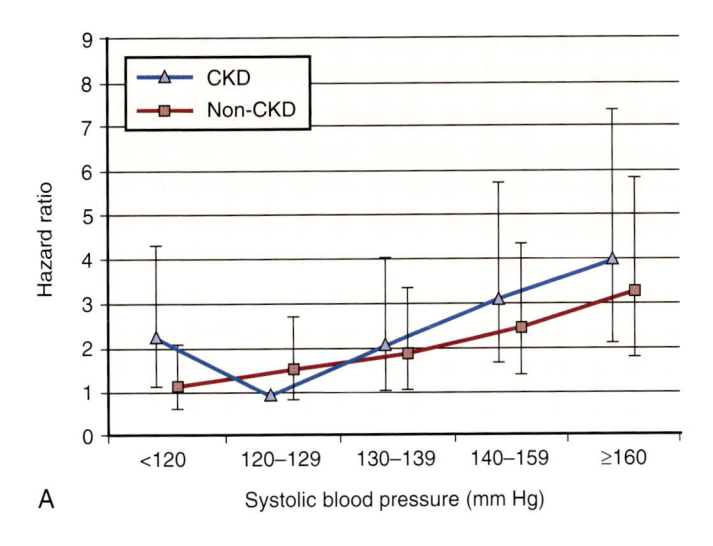

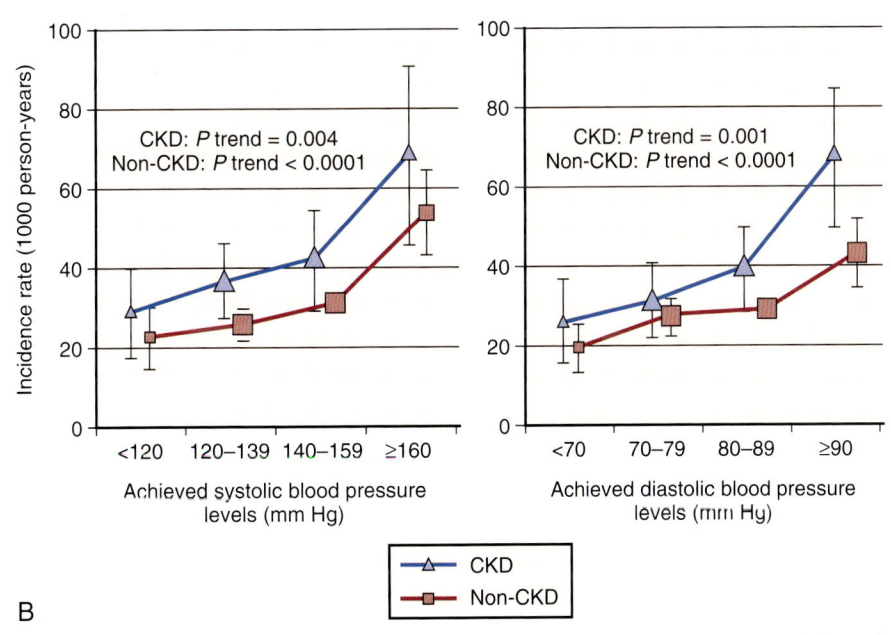

Figure 59.2 **A,** Adjusted hazard ratio of incident stroke according to systolic blood pressure and chronic kidney disease (CKD) status in a community sample of 20,358 individuals. **B,** Age- and sex-adjusted incidence rate of total stroke, according to follow-up blood pressure levels and CKD status in the Perindopril Protection Against Recurrent Stroke Study. (**A** adapted with permission from Weiner DE, Tighiouart H, Levey AS, et al: Lowest systolic blood pressure is associated with stroke in stages 3 to 4 chronic kidney disease. *J Am Soc Nephrol* 18:960-966, 2007; **B** adapted with permission from Ninomiya T, Perkovic V, Gallagher M, et al: Lower blood pressure and risk of recurrent stroke in patients with chronic kidney disease: PROGRESS trial. *Kidney Int* 73:963-970, 2008.)

stroke. Thus, available evidence currently supports blood pressure lowering in high-risk individuals with CKD to prevent cerebrovascular disease events.

DIABETES MELLITUS

Diabetes mellitus increases the risk for a first stroke by roughly 2- to 6-fold in the general population,[2] and this relationship appears to be similar in the CKD and ESKD populations. For example, in analyses of a community-based sample of U.S. adults, diabetes was associated with an 89% increased risk for stroke among persons with CKD.[35] In patients starting dialysis, diabetes was associated with a 35% increased risk for stroke.[32] No studies to date have evaluated the association of glycemic control with stroke risk in patients with CKD and ESKD.

ATRIAL FIBRILLATION

In the general population, atrial fibrillation is a potent risk factor for stroke, especially among older adults. The presence of nonvalvular atrial fibrillation increases the risk for stroke by 2.5- to 4.5-fold.[36] In patients with atrial fibrillation associated with valvular heart disease, stroke risk and prevention strategies depend on the underlying type of valvular lesion. The prevalence and incidence of atrial fibrillation are increased in the setting of CKD and ESKD, with prevalence rates ranging from 7% to 27% and incidence rates ranging from 13 per 1000 person-years among patients of all ages on dialysis, up to 148 per 1000 person-years among patients over age 65 on dialysis.[37] Among transplant recipients the incidence of atrial fibrillation is approximately 6 per 1000 person-years.[38-42] In the United States the risk for stroke associated with atrial fibrillation in patients receiving dialysis appears to have diminished over the last decade, though reasons for this remain unclear.[37]

PROTEINURIA

In a meta-analysis of stroke cohort studies involving more than 140,000 participants from several continents, proteinuria was associated with a 50% to 70% increased risk for stroke, independent of traditional stroke risk factors such as hypertension and diabetes.[43] The link between proteinuria and stroke was consistently observed across categories of sex, ethnicity, and diabetes subgroups, and for stroke subtypes. In a later study of 30,000 black and white adults in the United States, albuminuria was associated with an increased risk for incident stroke among blacks but not among whites. This relationship was independent of traditional stroke risk factors and present at levels of albuminuria below 30 mg/g.[44] In two studies, proteinuria, but not eGFR, was associated with an increased risk for stroke.[44,45] Furthermore, in one study, proteinuria largely explained the higher risk for death and disability following stroke among patients with CKD.[46] Thus, the presence and degree of proteinuria may be a more important determinant of stroke risk than solute clearance.

NUTRITIONAL FACTORS

In the general population, higher sodium and lower potassium intakes are linked to a heightened risk for stroke in epidemiologic studies. These associations appear to be mediated in part by blood pressure, as higher sodium intake tends to increase blood pressure in a dose-dependent manner, while higher potassium intake blunts the pressor effects of sodium.[47-49] Some evidence suggests that dietary sodium and potassium intake affect stroke risk through blood pressure–independent mechanisms.[50]

In addition to specific dietary factors, the syndrome of malnutrition and inflammation is strongly linked with atherosclerosis and cardiovascular events in patients on dialysis, but the association of malnutrition or inflammation syndromes with stroke is not as clear. For example, in a large sample of U.S. patients on dialysis, subjective assessment of malnutrition was associated with an increased risk for hemorrhagic and ischemic stroke,[32] while serum albumin concentration and body weight have not yielded consistent associations with stroke risk. In a large community sample of adults with CKD, lower serum albumin concentration, lower body weight, and other markers of inflammation were associated with a significantly higher risk for stroke.[35]

ANEMIA

Anemia is a common complication of CKD and linked with increased risk for cardiovascular events, including stroke, in many epidemiologic studies of CKD. One study noted a fivefold increased risk for stroke in CKD when accompanied by anemia; conversely, stroke risk was modestly and not significantly increased in CKD in the absence of anemia.[51] In another study of patients on dialysis, anemia was associated with a 22% increased risk for stroke.[32]

HOMOCYSTEINE

Numerous observational studies in the general population have identified hyperhomocysteinemia as a risk factor for stroke.[52-54] A single-nucleotide polymorphism in the gene methylenetetrahydrofolate reductase (MTHFR) reduces activity of the enzyme that metabolizes homocysteine, resulting in an increase in serum homocysteine concentration and a corresponding increase in stroke risk among persons with the homozygous genotype.[2] Homocysteine levels are increased in the setting of CKD, and up to 90% of patients on dialysis have elevated serum homocysteine concentrations.[55] The causes for elevated homocysteine levels in CKD and ESKD are thought to be altered homocysteine metabolism (either renal or nonrenal) and folate deficiency, as renal elimination of homocysteine appears to have a minor contribution to plasma concentrations.[55,56] Epidemiologic data in patients on dialysis have demonstrated strong associations of hyperhomocysteinemia with cardiovascular events, including stroke,[56-58] although genetic association studies have produced conflicting results.[59,60]

DIALYSIS-ASSOCIATED FACTORS

A number of dialysis-associated factors have been speculated to increase the risk for stroke. Even absent intradialytic hypotension, hemodialysis has been shown to cause cerebral hypoperfusion and may predispose to stroke. Overcorrection of anemia, especially in the setting of ultrafiltration, may lead to vascular stasis and thrombosis. Conversely, anticoagulation used for hemodialysis has also been speculated to contribute to hemorrhagic stroke risk during dialysis. Clinical evidence supporting these hypotheses is conflicting. Some studies note an increased risk for stroke during or immediately after hemodialysis treatments,[13] and one study found an increased rate of stroke during the months immediately before and after dialysis initiation compared to the prior year.[61] However, others have found no association between hemodialysis treatments and timing of stroke events[12] or the type of stroke events. Similarly, there is a paucity of data regarding dialysis modality and stroke risk.

STROKE PREVENTION

HYPERTENSION

Treatment of hypertension in the general population reduces stroke risk by an average of 40%; this benefit has been confirmed in a number of large randomized controlled trials.[2,62-64] Several antihypertensive drug classes, including ACEIs, angiotensin receptor blockers (ARBs), β-blockers, calcium channel blockers, and thiazide diuretics reduce stroke risk.[65] However, there are few data comparing drug classes head to head. In the Losartan Intervention for Endpoint Reduction in Hypertension Study (LIFE), which included 9193 subjects with hypertension and left ventricular hypertrophy, the relative risk for stroke was reduced by 26% (95% confidence interval [CI], 0.63 to 0.88) comparing losartan to atenolol, despite similar reductions in blood pressure.[66] Aside from the isolated findings observed in the LIFE trial, there is a lack of compelling evidence favoring one drug class over another vis-à-vis stroke reduction. Thus other indications should be taken into account when choosing initial therapy. For example, ACEIs or ARBs are preferred in the setting of proteinuria, reduced ejection fraction, or diabetes. To achieve blood pressure targets, most patients with CKD will require treatment with two or more agents.[67]

Dietary modification is an overlooked but efficacious strategy for lowering blood pressure. For example, the Dietary Approaches to Stop Hypertension (DASH) diet, rich in vegetables, fruits, and low-fat dairy products, when combined with reduced sodium intake, lowers blood pressure by an average of 11.5 mm Hg systolic in hypertensive subjects.[47] In persons without CKD, the Institute of Medicine and clinical practice guidelines recommend less than 2300 mg sodium (5.8 g sodium chloride) intake.[68] Whether intake of sodium should be lower (<1500 mg sodium [3.8 g sodium chloride]) in subpopulations with salt-sensitive hypertension, including persons with CKD, is controversial.[69]

DIABETES

In patients with diabetes, a number of studies support the benefits of blood pressure lowering to reduce stroke risk.[70,71] Multicomponent interventions targeting hypertension, dyslipidemia, proteinuria, and behavioral risk factors also reduce stroke risk in persons with diabetes by 50%.[72] While intensive glycemic control conclusively reduces microvascular complications, a similar benefit has not been demonstrated for macrovascular diseases, including stroke, a conclusion confirmed by two large randomized trials in subjects with type 2 diabetes comparing standard glycemic control (glycosylated hemoglobin [HbA_{1c}] 7% to 7.9%) to more intensive glycemic control ($HbA_{1c} < 6\%$ to 6.5%).[70,73-75] Notably, fewer than 30% of participants in these studies had CKD, and most with CKD had moderate reductions in glomerular filtration rate (GFR) (stage 3).

DYSLIPIDEMIA

In patients with preexisting cerebrovascular or coronary artery disease, 3-hydroxy-3-methylglutaryl–coenzyme A (HMG-CoA) reductase inhibitor (statin) therapy reduces the risk for stroke by 25% to 30%.[76-78] Many of the large randomized trials of lipid lowering for primary or secondary prevention of cardiovascular events largely excluded, or attempted to exclude, individuals with CKD.[79] Nevertheless, some patients with CKD were included in these trials, since exclusion was typically based on serum creatinine rather than eGFR criteria. A subsequent meta-analysis of statin trials evaluating results in patients with moderate (stage 3) CKD concluded that statins appear to have a beneficial effect for reducing cardiovascular event rates in patients with CKD, with no greater risk for adverse events such as elevated liver enzyme levels or rhabdomyolysis.[80] Stroke event rates were not analyzed separately. Nonstatin lipid-lowering agents such as niacin or gemfibrozil appear to have similar benefits as in the general population,[81] though there are fewer data regarding use of these agents for stroke prevention.

Since these studies were published, results from several randomized trials in patients with CKD or ESKD or in kidney transplant recipients have been reported. In the Die Deutsche Diabetes Dialyse Studie (4D study) of 1255 subjects with type 2 diabetes on maintenance hemodialysis, atorvastatin resulted in no difference in the primary cardiovascular composite end point as compared with placebo, despite lowering low-density lipoprotein cholesterol by an average of 42%.[82] There was a twofold increase in fatal stroke events in the atorvastatin group (relative risk [RR], 2.03; 95% CI, 1.03 to 3.93), primarily attributable to an increase in ischemic stroke events. There was no difference in the rate of nonfatal strokes. In A Study to Evaluate the Use of Rosuvastatin in Subjects on Regular Hemodialysis: An Assessment of Survival and Cardiovascular Events (AURORA), a trial of 2776 subjects on hemodialysis, rosuvastatin yielded no benefit in reducing the composite cardiovascular end point compared with placebo,[83] despite favorable changes in lipid and inflammatory surrogate markers. Unlike the 4D study, there was no increase in the incidence of stroke in AURORA; however, a marginal increase in the risk for *hemorrhagic* stroke was noted among subjects with diabetes mellitus.

In the Study of Heart and Renal Protection (SHARP), involving over 9000 persons with CKD, including approximately one third who were receiving dialysis, treatment with ezetimibe plus simvastatin resulted in a statistically significant 17% reduction in the primary composite cardiovascular end point, incidence of first major vascular event, and a 28% reduction in the incidence of ischemic stroke, one of the secondary end points.[84] There was a nonsignificant increase in the rate of hemorrhagic stroke. In a trial of 2102 kidney transplant recipients treated with fluvastatin or placebo, active treatment yielded a trend toward benefit on the primary composite cardiovascular end point (RR, 0.83; 95% CI, 0.64 to 1.06).[85] There was no statistically significant (or nominally significant) benefit for stroke reduction.

ANTIPLATELET AGENTS

In patients with noncardioembolic stroke or TIA, guidelines recommend antiplatelet agents to reduce the risk for recurrent stroke. Four antiplatelet agents have been approved by the U.S. Food and Drug Administration (FDA) for this indication—aspirin, dipyridamole plus aspirin, ticlopidine, and clopidogrel. Guidelines for the general population recommend aspirin for primary prevention of stroke when the risk for stroke is sufficiently high (10-year incidence > 6%) such that benefits outweigh risks of treatment.[2] Studies of aspirin for secondary prevention of stroke indicate relative risk reductions of 20% to 30%.[86] High and low doses of aspirin appear to have similar efficacy, though higher doses have increased rates of adverse events.

The Kidney Disease: Improving Global Outcomes (KDIGO) 2012 guidelines on management of CKD recommend offering antiplatelet agents to adults with CKD at risk for atherosclerotic events unless there is an increased risk for bleeding. These recommendations are based on post hoc analysis of the Hypertension Optimal Treatment trial. In this analysis it was estimated that for every 1000 persons with eGFR of less than 45 mL/min/1.73 m^2 treated with aspirin for 3.8 years, 54 all-cause deaths and 76 major cardiovascular events would be prevented, while 27 excess episodes of major bleeding would occur.[87]

Similarly, in one observational study of patients with ESKD, aspirin use was associated with an 18% reduction in cerebrovascular events[88] and no significant increase in the risk for hemorrhagic complications.[88,89] Short-term studies of aspirin use in the setting of acute coronary syndromes also seem to confirm the safety of aspirin in patients with CKD and ESKD.[90,91] Nevertheless, prescription rates for aspirin among patients with ESKD and a previous cerebrovascular event are relatively low (19% to 30%).[88]

In the Clopidogrel versus Aspirin in Patients at Risk for Ischaemic events (CAPRIE) trial, clopidogrel reduced the risk for recurrent vascular events with a similar or better safety profile compared to aspirin[92]; however, patients with CKD were not included in this trial. In post hoc analyses of patients receiving clopidogrel versus placebo after percutaneous coronary intervention, subjects with CKD receiving clopidogrel had no increased risk for bleeding compared to subjects with normal kidney function, but also no benefit.[93] In a study of clopidogrel plus aspirin for prevention of arteriovenous graft thrombosis in patients with ESKD, combination therapy increased the risk for bleeding by twofold.[94] In a subsequent larger study of clopidogrel alone versus placebo to facilitate maturation of arteriovenous fistulas, treatment with clopidogrel did not increase the risk for hemorrhage.[95] The combination of dipyridamole plus aspirin has been evaluated in several studies for stroke prevention. Combination therapy reduces the rate of recurrent stroke by 23% to 38% when compared to either agent alone or to placebo.[96] In a study of dipyridamole plus aspirin versus placebo for prevention of graft thrombosis in persons with ESKD, active therapy did not increase the risk for adverse events[97]; thus, this combination appears to be relatively safe for use in patients with ESKD. American Stroke Association guidelines recommend selection of antiplatelet agents for stroke prevention based on evaluation of individual risk factors and comorbid conditions. For persons with CKD or ESKD, aspirin alone because of its low cost, safety, and over-the-counter availability is a reasonable choice. Aspirin plus dipyridamole may be considered in high-risk patients, and clopidogrel may be considered for those intolerant to aspirin or with a recent acute coronary syndrome or stenting.

ANTICOAGULATION FOR ATRIAL FIBRILLATION

A number of prospective clinical trials have demonstrated that high-risk patients with nonvalvular atrial fibrillation treated with warfarin have a reduced risk for stroke and a relatively low risk for bleeding (approximately one to three events per 100 patient-years of warfarin exposure) when targeting an international normalized ratio (INR) of 2.0 to 3.0.[98-100] The $CHADS_2$ score is a clinical prediction rule for estimating stroke risk in patients with nonvalvular atrial fibrillation and can be used to determine appropriate therapy (i.e., aspirin versus warfarin),[101] and one study suggests that the $CHADS_2$ score may be useful for predicting stroke risk in patients on dialysis.[102] Many factors complicate decision making regarding warfarin use in patients with advanced CKD and atrial fibrillation. First, the efficacy of warfarin for stroke prevention in this population is unclear, and observational data in patients with CKD or ESKD are conflicting, ranging from substantial benefit to substantial harm associated with warfarin use.[40,102-104] Second, patients on dialysis experience higher risks for bleeding associated with warfarin use compared to the general population. In a systematic review of warfarin use in ESKD, the risk for bleeding was estimated at 10 to 54 events per 100 patient-years of warfarin exposure.[105] Another study of patients new to dialysis reported that stroke risk was higher with higher INR levels and among those who did not receive INR monitoring in the first 90 days of dialysis.[102] Third, warfarin use in the setting of ESKD is associated with a theoretical risk for vascular calcification, owing to inhibition of matrix Gla protein and growth arrest–specific gene 6 (GAS6).[106] The magnitude of this risk is unknown. Clinicians have begun to prescribe some of the novel oral anticoagulant agents, though safety and efficacy are not yet established in the ESKD or advanced CKD population.[107,108]

CAROTID ENDARTERECTOMY

In the general population, carotid endarterectomy (CEA) has been demonstrated to be beneficial in patients with symptomatic atherosclerotic carotid stenosis of 70% or greater.[109-111] Uncertainty exists about the benefits of CEA among patients with symptomatic stenosis of 50% to 69%, and several studies indicate no benefit of surgery in patients with stenosis of less than 50%. In a post hoc analysis of the North American Symptomatic Carotid Endarterectomy Trial, which randomized patients with symptomatic high-grade stenosis (70% to 99%), including 524 patients with CKD, to CEA versus medical management; event rates were higher in patients with CKD relative to those without CKD. Notably, the risk for ipsilateral stroke was reduced by 82% in patients with CKD who underwent CEA. Perioperative stroke and death risk were not increased. In analyses of U.S. veterans undergoing CEA, veterans with CKD had increased risks for cardiovascular and pulmonary complications following CEA surgery compared to persons without CKD, as well an increased risk for postoperative mortality among those with stage 4 CKD. A limitation is that postoperative stroke rates were not reported.[112] Thus, CEA should be considered for most patients with CKD with symptomatic severe carotid stenosis after optimization of their cardiac risk factors.

B VITAMIN SUPPLEMENTATION

Despite substantial encouraging data in observational studies, clinical trials of homocysteine lowering with B vitamin supplementation have produced disappointing results. In the Vitamin Intervention for Stroke Prevention (VISP) trial conducted in patients with a previous stroke, high-dose vitamin B failed to reduce the risk for recurrent stroke.[113] In three trials involving patients with CKD, including two trials among patients receiving dialysis and one among kidney transplant recipients, homocysteine lowering with B vitamin supplementation did not reduce mortality or cardiovascular events,[114,115] including analyses limited to stroke events. Thus, high-dose folic acid and vitamin B in patients with CKD and ESKD with hyperhomocysteinemia is not recommended to reduce stroke risk.

ERYTHROPOIETIN

While there are epidemiologic data to support a role for anemia as a risk factor for stroke in persons with CKD, in several large randomized controlled trials in patients with CKD and anemia (including those on and not on dialysis), complete or partial correction of anemia with erythropoietin increased adverse events and did not reduce mortality or cardiovascular events, including in subgroup analyses of stroke events.[116-118] Similarly, in a trial comparing darbepoetin versus placebo in patients with type 2 diabetes, CKD, and hemoglobin level of less than 11 g/dL, darbepoetin resulted in no difference in the primary composite cardiovascular outcome and a twofold increase in the risk for stroke, one of the secondary outcomes.[119] Post hoc analysis failed to identify factors associated with the increase in stroke events, including blood pressure, dose of darbepoetin, or hemoglobin levels. An observational study of U.S. veterans found that a higher risk for stroke among patients with CKD starting erythropoietin was primarily observed among patients with cancer, who required significantly higher doses of erythropoietin compared to patients with CKD without cancer.[120] Based on these data, KDIGO 2012 guidelines recommend using erythropoietin-stimulating agents with caution, if at all, in patients with CKD with a history of stroke.[121]

MANAGEMENT OF ACUTE STROKE IN CHRONIC KIDNEY DISEASE AND END-STAGE KIDNEY DISEASE

INITIAL EVALUATION

The first step in the diagnostic evaluation of stroke is to confirm that the patient's symptoms are due to stroke, and not another systemic or neurologic illness, and to distinguish ischemic from hemorrhagic stroke. Presentation with severe headache, vomiting, coma, a systolic blood pressure above 220 mm Hg, or history of warfarin use is associated with a higher likelihood of hemorrhage,[122] but symptoms alone do not have sufficient diagnostic accuracy, and brain imaging is warranted to definitively distinguish hemorrhagic stroke from ischemic stroke. The next step is to determine the appropriateness of thrombolytic therapy. Timing of symptom onset, history of recent medical events (especially any history of trauma, surgery, or cardiovascular events), and use of antiplatelet agents or anticoagulants should be ascertained. The National Institutes of Health Stroke Scale can be used to estimate prognosis and determine the risk for hemorrhage with thrombolytic therapy, although it should be recognized that the scale has not been validated in patients on dialysis and therefore may underestimate hemorrhage risk.[123]

NEUROIMAGING

Neuroimaging plays a central role in the acute management of stroke in the era of thrombolytic therapy. Neuroimaging provides information on the size, location, and vascular distribution of the infarction, as well as the presence of bleeding, and, depending on the technique used, may also provide information on the degree of reversibility and the integrity of intracranial vessels. Non–contrast media–enhanced computed tomography (CT) of the brain is the most common neuroimaging modality used for the initial diagnostic evaluation because it can usually be performed urgently, it reliably distinguishes infarction from hemorrhage, and it identifies other causes for neurologic symptoms, with the caveat that CT is relatively insensitive for detecting small cortical or subcortical infarctions, especially in the posterior fossa. Intravenous contrast media administration is usually unnecessary for acute stroke evaluation but in some cases may be indicated if there is a high suspicion for brain tumors or infection. In these cases the risk for radiocontrast media–associated nephropathy must be weighed against the potential benefits, and prophylactic measures should be considered (see Chapter 28). The American Stroke Association recommends that candidates for thrombolytic therapy have a completed CT scan within 25 minutes of arrival at the emergency department.[124]

Standard MRI techniques are not sufficiently sensitive to detect the acute changes of ischemic stroke, and therefore MRI is not usually indicated in routine evaluation. Imaging of the cerebral vasculature with angiography, CT angiography, or MR angiography is not usually a standard part of the initial evaluation but may become more common if intraarterial thrombolysis is more widely adopted. In these cases the risks for radiocontrast media–associated nephropathy associated with intravenous radiocontrast media or nephrogenic systemic fibrosis associated with gadolinium-enhanced MR angiography must be carefully weighed against the potential benefits of the imaging procedure. If these imaging procedures are utilized in patients with CKD or ESKD, appropriate procedures to reduce risk should be instituted. For intravenous radiocontrast media administration, this should include administration of intravenous saline or bicarbonate before the procedure. For gadolinium administration, this should include minimization of the contrast media volume and consideration for immediate postprocedure hemodialysis in patients with vascular access.[125]

INTRAVENOUS THROMBOLYSIS

In carefully selected patients in the general population treated within 3 hours of symptom onset, intravenous administration of recombinant tissue plasminogen activator (rt-PA) improves stroke outcomes[124]; however, the safety, efficacy, and practicality of thrombolytic therapy in the setting of CKD and ESKD remain unclear. Despite frequent contact of patients on dialysis with health care professionals, the median time from symptom onset to presentation among patients on dialysis is 8 hours, thus precluding consideration for thrombolytic therapy for most patients.[12] In trials of thrombolytic therapy conducted in the setting of acute myocardial infarction, patients with CKD were two to four times as likely to experience major bleeding, including intracranial hemorrhage, compared to those without CKD, with hemorrhage rates of 3% to 4% depending on the severity of CKD.[126,127] Similar findings have been noted in patients with stroke who received thrombolytic therapy.[128,129] The same study noted a high rate of recurrent ischemic stroke among patients with CKD receiving rt-PA, calling into question the efficacy of intravenous thrombolytics for acute ischemic stroke in this setting. Based on these findings, caution should be exercised before considering thrombolysis in a patient with advanced CKD or ESKD. If utilized, anticoagulants or antiplatelet agents should be withheld for 24 hours following rt-PA administration.

SUPPORTIVE CARE

Hypertension is common preceding and following acute stroke, but optimal management remains unclear. While there are theoretical reasons to treat hypertension following acute stroke, overly aggressive treatment of hypertension may lead to reduced perfusion and infarct expansion. In patients without CKD, hypertension typically resolves spontaneously; however, spontaneous resolution of hypertension may be less likely to occur in patients with CKD, as hypertension in patients with CKD tends to be more severe and difficult to control than in persons with normal or near normal kidney function. In patients who are not candidates for thrombolytic therapy, consensus guidelines recommend blood pressure lowering for systolic blood pressure above 220 mm Hg or diastolic blood pressure above 120 mm Hg, or if there is other evidence for end-organ damage.[124] The threshold for treatment is lowered to above 185 mm Hg systolic or above 110 mm Hg diastolic in candidates for thrombolytic therapy. When indicated, the use of parenteral agents that can be titrated easily, such as nicardipine or labetalol, is recommended. The timing of hemodialysis treatments in the setting of acute stroke should be individualized based on consideration of fluid and metabolic control. It seems prudent to avoid aggressive ultrafiltration during hemodialysis or to consider slower rates of ultrafiltration if fluid overload is present in the acute stroke period. Dialysis-related anticoagulation should be held after hemorrhagic stroke and held or minimized following ischemic stroke.

DISORDERS OF COGNITIVE FUNCTION

Changes in modern ESKD epidemiology and practice have greatly altered the presentation, significance, and risk factor profile for cognitive disorders among persons with ESKD. Neurocognitive symptoms were among the first described symptoms of the uremic syndrome and were later proposed as sensitive indicators of dialysis adequacy or, in some cases, side effects of dialysis therapy. However, with the aging of the population with ESKD and changes in dialysis practice, including earlier initiation of dialysis and elimination of aluminum contamination of dialysate water, the relation between neurocognitive disorders and uremia per se is less clear. Patients with neurocognitive disorders are at higher risk for death, hospitalization, and dialysis withdrawal. These disorders are also likely to reduce health-related quality of life and hinder adherence with the complex dietary and medication regimens prescribed to patients with CKD. This section will review the evaluation and management of delirium, dementia, and chronic cognitive impairment among persons with CKD and ESKD.

DELIRIUM SYNDROMES

Delirium is an acute confusional state characterized by a recent onset of fluctuating awareness, impairment of memory and attention, and disorganized thinking that can be attributable to a medical condition, intoxication, or medication side effect. Delirium is typically precipitated by an acute or subacute event such as a neurologic disorder, infection, electrolyte disorder, or intoxication (Table 59.3). Older patients with cognitive or sensory impairment, chronic diseases, or those taking multiple medications are thought to be most vulnerable for delirium; thus, it is not surprising that delirium would occur commonly in patients with ESKD. Several syndromes of delirium specific to patients with ESKD are described in more detail in the following section.

Table 59.3 Differential Diagnosis of Delirium in End-Stage Kidney Disease

- Cerebrovascular disorder (stroke, subdural hematoma, hypertensive encephalopathy)
- Seizure
- Infection (sepsis, meningitis)
- Electrolyte disorder (hypoglycemia, hyponatremia or hypernatremia, hypercalcemia)
- Intoxication (alcohol, drugs, aluminum, star fruit, sugihiratake mushrooms)
- Alcohol withdrawal
- Nutritional deficiency (thiamine)
- Hepatic encephalopathy
- Uremic encephalopathy or inadequate dialysis
- Dialysis disequilibrium
- Dialysis-associated hypotension

UREMIC ENCEPHALOPATHY

Clinical Features

Uremic encephalopathy is a syndrome of delirium seen in untreated or inadequately treated ESKD. It is characterized by lethargy and confusion in early stages and can progress to seizures and/or coma. It may be accompanied by other neurologic signs, such as tremor, myoclonus, or asterixis. Electroencephalographic abnormalities correspond with clinical symptoms and improve with treatment of uremia.[1,130] Conversely, the degree of azotemia alone correlates poorly with the presence or degree of encephalopathy.

Radiologic and pathologic studies in the setting of uremic encephalopathy are sparse. While the available studies report white matter lesions suggestive of small vessel cerebrovascular disease (see previous section), it is unclear whether these pathologic abnormalities play a role in the development of uremic encephalopathy since most studies did not conduct simultaneous neurophysiologic or neuropsychiatric testing. In a study of 30 patients on hemodialysis and controls without CKD, cognitive impairment was associated with more extensive enlargement of the third ventricle and temporal horns, but not with the presence of cerebrovascular disease lesions.[24] Brain perfusion studies have demonstrated reduced perfusion in the frontal cortex among patients on hemodialysis compared with controls, although these findings did not correlate with cognitive performance.[131] MRI studies utilizing diffusion-weighted imaging to detect changes in brain water have noted findings consistent with brain edema in uremic encephalopathy.[132,133]

Pathophysiology

A number of biochemical changes have been reported in acute and chronic uremic encephalopathy, including alterations in water transport and brain edema, disturbances of the blood-brain barrier, and changes in cerebral metabolism.[134-139] The significance of these changes on neurotransmitter release and neuronal function are unclear.

Studies contrasting animal models of uremic encephalopathy in acute kidney injury with hepatic encephalopathy have demonstrated an increase in brain inflammation in conjunction with an increase in vascular permeability in uremic encephalopathy.[140] Kidney injury may activate cytokines that cross the blood-brain barrier or activate other messengers that contribute to neuronal dysfunction. Alternatively, the retention of uremic solutes may trigger both the inflammatory reaction and neuronal dysfunction. A large number of solutes are retained in uremia (Chapter 54), and several may have direct neurotoxicity or contribute indirectly to the pathogenesis of uremic encephalopathy by altering the blood-brain barrier. For example, the guanidine compounds are low-molecular-weight solutes with deleterious effects on immune and neurologic function in vivo. Levels of guanidinosuccinic acid and methylguanidine are increased 100-fold in uremic brain tissue and cerebrospinal fluid,[141] and several guanidine compounds, including guanidinosuccinic acid, methylguanidine, and homoarginine, induce seizures, possibly through their effects on N-methyl-D-aspartate (NMDA) receptors and/or by modulating calcium channels.[142-144] Another guanidine compound, asymmetric dimethyl arginine (ADMA), is a potent endogenous inhibitor of nitric oxide synthesis and causes cerebral vasoconstriction by impairing endothelial relaxation.[145] Human studies have noted associations of ADMA with cerebral small vessel disease and dementia.[146-148] Phenolic compounds, such as quinolinic acid and the indole indoxyl sulfate, have also been linked with direct neuronal damage in vivo.[149,150]

In addition to uremic retention solutes, anemia and secondary hyperparathyroidism may play distinct roles in the pathogenesis of uremic encephalopathy. Epidemiologic studies link anemia with impaired cognitive function in persons with ESKD and in other chronic conditions, including heart failure and cancer.[151] Further, in uncontrolled short-term studies, administration of erythropoietin is associated with improved performance on cognitive function and electrophysiologic testing.[152-154] Parathyroid hormone is known to have central nervous system effects in persons with primary hyperparathyroidism,[155] and cognitive function has been reported to improve after parathyroidectomy in persons with primary hyperparathyroidism and normal kidney function.[156,157] Animal models of uremia have noted an increase in brain calcium content and electroencephalographic abnormalities with administration of parathyroid hormone, a finding that can be prevented by parathyroidectomy.[138] These alterations in brain calcium content may in turn disrupt cerebral function by interrupting neurotransmitter release or cerebral metabolism.

Treatment

Once other causes of delirium have been ruled out, prompt treatment of uremic encephalopathy with initiation or intensification of renal replacement therapy is indicated. Resolution of symptoms typically occurs within days. Correction of anemia may also be of benefit. Dietary protein restriction is another adjunctive measure used to delay the development of uremic symptoms, though there are few published data supporting its use for the purpose of improving cognitive function. Nevertheless, with proper instruction and follow-up, modest dietary protein restriction may be appropriate in certain settings.

DIALYSIS DYSEQUILIBRIUM

Clinical Features

This syndrome of delirium is attributable to the dialysis procedure itself and seen during or shortly after the first several dialysis treatments. It is most likely to occur in pediatric or older adult patients, patients with severe azotemia, and patients undergoing high-efficiency hemodialysis; however, it has also been reported in patients undergoing peritoneal dialysis and maintenance hemodialysis.[158,159] Dialysis dysequilibrium is characterized by symptoms of headache, visual disturbance, nausea, or agitation, and, in severe cases, delirium, lethargy, seizures, and even coma. The incidence and severity of this syndrome are felt to be declining because of earlier initiation of dialysis and institution of preventative measures in high-risk patients, including reducing the efficiency dialysis, increasing the dialysate sodium concentration, and administering mannitol.[160] Symptoms are usually self-limited.

Pathophysiology

The clinical features of dialysis dysequilibrium syndrome are primarily attributable to brain edema, although the nature and cause of the edema remain uncertain. Two hypotheses have been suggested to explain the development of brain edema. In the first, rapid removal of urea (and other water-soluble, rapidly diffusible solutes) by dialysis leads to a solute gradient between the blood and brain, in turn leading to influx of water into the brain. This theory is supported by animal studies in which the brain-to-plasma urea gradient induced by rapid hemodialysis accounted for the increase in brain water.[161] In the second theory, a decrease in intracellular pH and formation of idiogenic osmoles (osmolytes) within the brain contributes to the development of edema when an osmolar gradient is developed during dialysis.[134]

SYNDROMES OF CHRONIC COGNITIVE IMPAIRMENT

Dementia is a chronic confusional state characterized by impairment in memory and at least one other cognitive domain, such as language, orientation, reasoning, or executive functioning. The impairment in cognitive function must represent a decline from the patient's baseline level of cognitive function and must be severe enough to interfere with daily activities and independence. "Dialysis dementia" is a term reserved to describe a syndrome of progressive dementia related to aluminum intoxication and first described several decades ago in the setting of aluminum contamination of dialysate. While aluminum-based phosphate binders were often blamed for this syndrome, the aluminum moiety is so inefficiently absorbed, only parenteral exposure was likely relevant. There is growing awareness that many patients with CKD have a syndrome of chronic cognitive impairment unrelated to aluminum intoxication. This entity has various names in the literature, including "mild cognitive impairment," "subclinical dementia," "residual syndrome,"[162] and "chronic dialysis-dependent encephalopathy," reflecting an unknown but probable multifactorial origin.

DIALYSIS DEMENTIA

Dialysis dementia was first described in the 1970s, and among adults it occurred almost exclusively among patients on hemodialysis rather than peritoneal dialysis.[163,164] Epidemic, sporadic, and childhood forms of dialysis dementia have been reported. Epidemic forms occur in geographic clusters and are strongly associated with aluminum contamination of dialysate. The relation of aluminum intoxication to the sporadic and childhood forms of dialysis dementia is less clear. Some early studies revealed an increase in brain aluminum content 11-fold higher than in healthy persons and 3- to 4-fold higher than in patients requiring hemodialysis without dementia[165] and speculated that use of aluminum-containing phosphate binders might be involved. Clinical manifestations include a variety of neuropsychiatric symptoms, osteomalacia, myopathy, and anemia. Symptoms may be exacerbated by hemodialysis or by administration of deferoxamine or desferrioxamine, presumably due to mobilization and redistribution of tissue aluminum into the brain. If aluminum intoxication is confirmed, the dialysate should be checked for aluminum contamination, and any other sources of parenteral aluminum exposure should be explored. Chelation therapy is indicated despite the caveats noted earlier because there is no other effective method for removal of aluminum.[166]

CHRONIC COGNITIVE IMPAIRMENT
Epidemiology
The epidemiology of chronic cognitive impairment among patients with CKD remains only partly defined, owing to the lack of a standard definition of cognitive impairment and relatively few longitudinal studies of cognition. Fukunishi and associates were among the first investigators to describe an increased incidence of dementia in ESKD. In this study the annual incidence of dementia was 2.5% among patients with ESKD, double that of the general population.[167] Among U.S. patients the incidence of dementia is estimated at 1% to 2% for patients under age 65 years, reaching up to 6% to 8% for patients over age 85 years.[168] The prevalence of moderate-to-severe cognitive impairment based on neurocognitive testing ranges from 16% to 38% depending on the sample and the definition of impairment (Figure 59.3A).[169-172]

The incidence and prevalence of cognitive impairment are also increased among patients with CKD that does not require dialysis. The prevalence of cognitive impairment rises relatively early in the course of CKD and is higher at lower eGFR, reaching 20% for persons with an eGFR of less than 20 mL/min/1.73 m^2 (Figure 59.3B).[173] Neurocognitive deficits have also been described among children with CKD and ESKD. For example, among children with CKD that does not require dialysis, 21% to 40% fall below normative values for academic achievement, attention regulation, and executive function, though GFR is not a consistent correlate of cognitive performance.[174] In a cohort of community-dwelling older adults, CKD was associated with a 37% increased risk for dementia, attributable to an increased incidence of vascular dementia.[175] Similarly, several other studies, primarily in older adult cohorts, have described an independent association between CKD and cognitive decline.[176] However, not all studies have confirmed such an association.[177,178] Whether this is due to differences in cohort risk for dementia, misclassification of CKD, or confounding factors, such as proteinuria, remains unclear. For example, cystatin C, a purportedly more sensitive marker of CKD in patients with low muscle mass, is associated with an increased risk for cognitive decline among patients with normal creatinine-based eGFR.[179] In some studies, albuminuria, but not eGFR, has been associated with an increased risk for cognitive decline.[177]

Risk Factors and Mechanisms
Microvascular disease appears to be a major contributing factor to chronic cognitive impairment in CKD. Patients with CKD and ESKD have a high prevalence of subclinical stroke, white matter hyperintensities (thought to represent chronic ischemia), and cerebral microbleeds identified by neuroimaging. In the general population these lesions are linked with a higher risk for dementia and cognitive decline. Among patients with CKD or ESKD, stroke and symptoms of stroke have been linked to poorer cognitive function.[169,172,180] Finally, changes in kidney function appear to parallel changes in cognition,[177] suggesting shared risk factors for the decline in kidney function and cognition (Figure 59.4).

Novel factors may also contribute to chronic brain ischemia and cognitive decline in patients with CKD. For example, anemia, vitamin D deficiency, vascular calcification, inflammation, and oxidative stress are common among patients with CKD and have been linked with cognitive decline in the general population, though further study is needed to confirm their importance in patients with CKD.[181-183]

Retention of uremic solutes may contribute to chronic cognitive impairment despite the fact that dialysis appears "adequate" by conventional criteria (usually urea kinetics). Support for the "uremic solute" hypothesis comes from studies demonstrating improvement in cognitive function among children and middle-aged adults who undergo transplantation compared to matched patients on the transplant waiting list.[184,185] Recurrent brain ischemia from circulatory stress induced by the hemodialysis process has also been implicated as a contributing factor to chronic cognitive impairment. Some, though not all, studies have found that cognitive function varies according to the weekly dialysis schedule among patients requiring hemodialysis, but not among patients requiring peritoneal dialysis. One study reported reduced cerebral blood flow among patients requiring hemodialysis compared to healthy controls; however, intradialytic measurements were not reported.[131] These observations suggest a potential role for frequent hemodialysis to attenuate cognitive decline in patients with ESKD. In a randomized clinical trial of frequent in-center hemodialysis, frequent dialysis resulted in no significant improvement in most cognitive domains relative to thrice-weekly hemodialysis over the course of 12 months, including in the primary and secondary cognitive function measures. Improvements were noted in domains of memory and verbal fluency, but the significance of these findings remains to be determined. A trial of frequent home-based nocturnal hemodialysis found no improvement in several cognitive domains; however, these negative results are possibly confounded by sleep disturbance.[186]

Evaluation
History taking, ideally from the patient and caregiver, should focus on the duration and severity of cognitive and

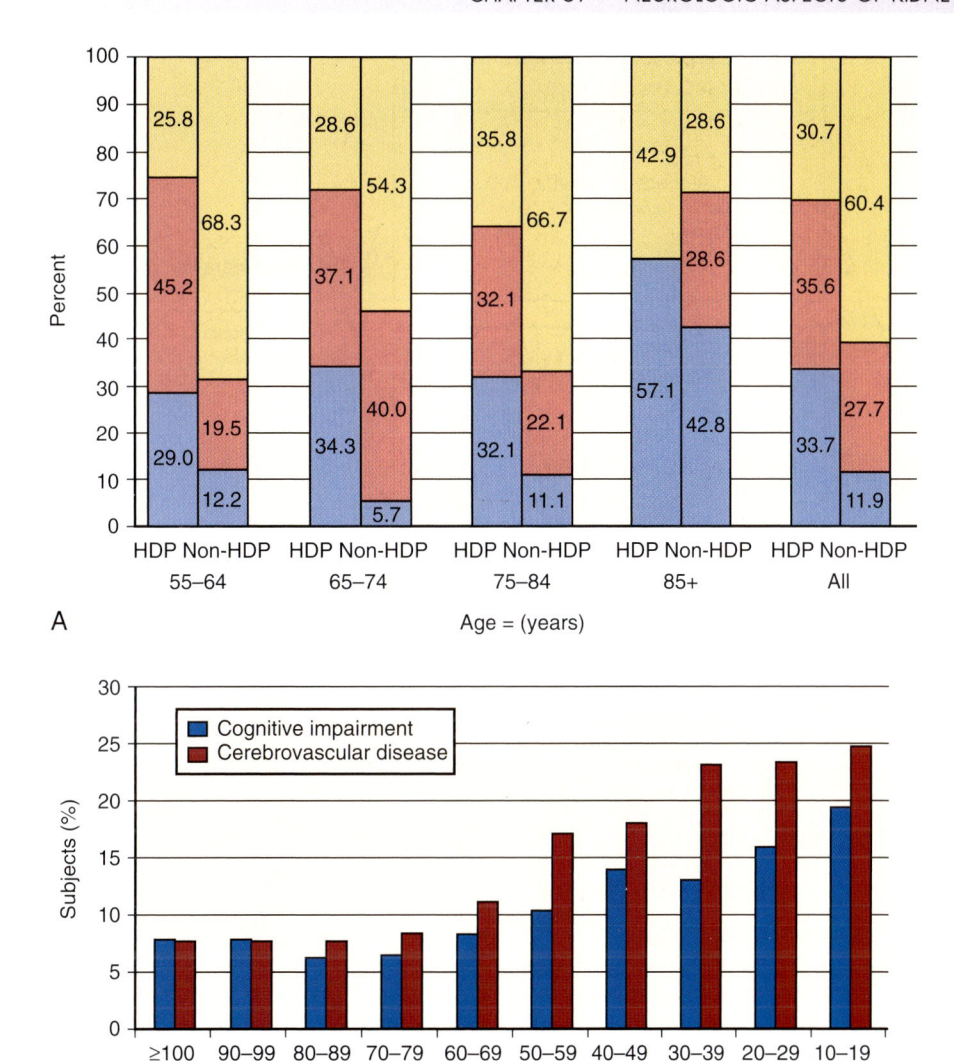

Figure 59.3 **A,** Frequency of cognitive impairment in 101 hemodialysis patients (HDP) and 101 nonhemodialysis patients (Non-HDP) according to age group. *Yellow bars* indicate normal to mild impairment, *red bars* indicate moderate impairment, and *blue bars* indicate severe cognitive impairment. **B,** Unadjusted prevalence of cognitive impairment in 23,405 black and white U.S. adults, according to estimated glomerular filtration rate (eGFR). (**A** adapted from Murray AM, Tupper DE, Knopman DS, et al: Cognitive impairment in hemodialysis patients is common. *Neurology* 67:216-223, 2006; **B** adapted with permission from Kurella Tamura M, Wadley V, Yaffe K, et al: Kidney function and cognitive impairment in US adults: the Reasons for Geographic and Racial Differences in Stroke [REGARDS] Study. *Am J Kidney Dis* 52:227-234, 2008.)

behavioral deficits, as well as use of medications that might interfere with cognitive function such as antihistamines, antipsychotics, and anticholinergics. The value of routine screening for dementia in the general population is controversial. Given the high prevalence of cognitive impairment in the CKD population and its implications for disease management, screening for cognitive impairment in older patients with CKD seems warranted. A large number of screening tests are available with a range of administration times and diagnostic accuracy; thus, there is no single best screening test. The Mini-Mental State Examination (MMSE) is perhaps the best known cognitive test for dementia screening and requires 7 to 10 minutes to administer, but it may miss impairments in executive function. Other cognitive tests that can be administered in 5 minutes or less, such as the clock-drawing task, the Mini-Cog (consisting of the clock-drawing task plus uncued recall of three words), or the Short Portable Mental Status Questionnaire, have similar performance characteristics in the general population.[187] Impairments in executive function, which can be assessed by the clock-drawing task, may be particularly important to identify, since impairments in this domain are strongly linked with adherence to therapy, functional status, and ability to live independently. Screening tests of cognitive function may also be useful for identifying patients who lack capacity to provide informed consent for medical procedures.

Delirium and depression frequently coexist with dementia; however, it is important to exclude these conditions as the sole cause of cognitive impairment before establishing a diagnosis of dementia. In practice, differentiating delirium and depression from dementia can be difficult, since unresolved uremia and subtle dialysis dysequilibrium can contribute to temporal fluctuations in cognitive

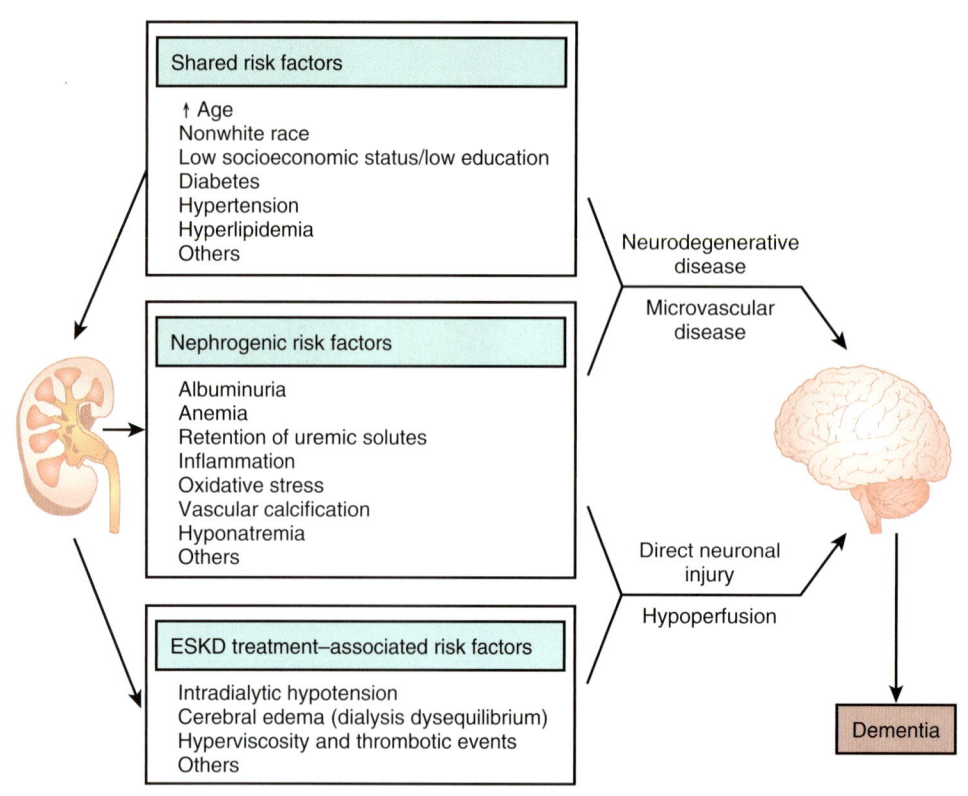

Figure 59.4 Proposed mechanisms of chronic cognitive impairment in chronic kidney disease. (Adapted from Kurella Tamura M, Yaffe K: Dementia and cognitive impairment in ESRD: diagnostic and therapeutic strategies. *Kidney Int* 79 (1):14-22, 2011.)

function.[188,189] As such, the optimal timing of cognitive function testing for patients on hemodialysis is unknown. Neuropsychologic testing on a nondialysis day can be useful if the diagnosis is uncertain or when testing is performed to establish capacity or potential reversibility (e.g., before kidney transplantation). In addition to cognitive function testing, laboratory testing for vitamin B_{12} deficiency and hypothyroidism is recommended for all patients with suspected dementia. In patients with ESKD, inadequate dialysis, severe anemia, and aluminum toxicity should be ruled out. There are conflicting recommendations from guideline panels regarding the routine use of structural neuroimaging in the work-up of chronic cognitive impairment.[190] The role of testing for genetic markers of dementia risk (e.g., apolipoprotein E variants) is controversial.

Management

The management of patients with CKD and ESKD with chronic cognitive impairment not meeting criteria for dementia is uncertain. While kidney transplantation is optimal therapy for most patients with ESKD, many patients with chronic cognitive impairment may not be eligible for transplantation due to coexisting illness. Further, the extent to which transplantation reverses cognitive impairment, especially in frail patients with coexisting illness, is uncertain. Some studies report improvements in cognitive function after transplantation among young or middle-aged patients,[191] but a few cross-sectional studies note high rates of cognitive impairment even after transplantation.[184] Intensification of the dialysis regimen is not routinely recommended due to nondefinitive findings from two clinical trials. There may be a subset of patients with cognitive impairment who benefit from these strategies, such as those without underlying microvascular disease; however, this remains speculative. Homocysteine lowering with B vitamin supplementation has failed to show benefit for reducing the risk for cognitive decline in the general population and in CKD or ESKD.[192]

For patients with dementia, two classes of medications are now available for treatment of both Alzheimer's type and vascular dementia. Cholinesterase inhibitors are approved for treatment of mild-to-moderate dementia, while memantine, an NMDA receptor antagonist, is approved for treatment of moderate-to-severe Alzheimer's dementia and may also have some efficacy in treatment of vascular dementia. The clinical benefit of both classes of agents appears to be modest, and the effect of treatment on long-term outcomes such as nursing home placement remains unclear. There are no published data on safety or efficacy of these agents in patients on dialysis; thus, therapy decisions should be individualized.

Behavioral symptoms such as agitation or hallucinations should be treated with a stepped approach, beginning with nonpharmacologic approaches such as removal of precipitating factors (e.g., pain, excessive noise), followed by psychosocial interventions (e.g., caregiver education), and pharmacologic therapy as a last step. A key aspect of dementia management is the assessment of patient safety and ability to perform self-care functions, comply with medical regimens, and participate in medical decision making. Patients on dialysis with dementia have a higher incidence of all-cause mortality and withdrawal from dialysis[193]; therefore, goals of care should be discussed early in the course of disease when possible.

NEUROPATHY

UREMIC POLYNEUROPATHY

Uremic neuropathy is a distal, symmetric, mixed sensorimotor polyneuropathy. It typically involves the lower extremities more than the upper extremities, and sensory symptoms typically precede motor symptoms. Motor involvement usually indicates advanced disease. Some authorities consider restless legs syndrome (RLS) part of the clinical spectrum of uremic polyneuropathy. Differentiating uremic polyneuropathy from other systemic diseases that contribute to ESKD and also affect nerve function, such as diabetes, amyloidosis, and systemic lupus erythematosus, can be difficult. Abnormalities in motor nerve conduction velocity parallel the decline in GFR and improve substantially after kidney transplantation.[194,195] Nerve conduction abnormalities have been reported in up to 60% of patients receiving dialysis.[196] Other manifestations of uremic polyneuropathy include symmetric muscle weakness, areflexia, and loss of vibratory sense. Similar to uremic encephalopathy, retention of a number of uremic solutes, including parathyroid hormone, myoinositol, and other "middle molecules," have been correlated with motor nerve conduction velocity. Nerve excitability studies demonstrate alterations in membrane potential and have suggested that hyperkalemic depolarization may underlie the development of uremic neuropathy rather than middle molecules.[197]

MONONEUROPATHY

Mononeuropathy syndromes typically involve compression or ischemia of the ulnar or median nerves and are most often attributable to dialysis-related (β_2-microglobulin) amyloidosis or ischemic mononeuropathy associated with an arteriovenous fistula.

AUTONOMIC NEUROPATHY

The existence of an autonomic neuropathy attributable to uremia is controversial. Manifestations include orthostatic or dialysis-associated hypotension and impotence. A study of 25 patients with ESKD who were not on dialysis and 8 healthy controls conducted extensive testing of autonomic function. Function of the efferent sympathetic pathway was similar in patients with ESKD who were not on dialysis and controls. In contrast, function of the efferent parasympathetic pathway and baroreceptor sensitivity were abnormal in patients with ESKD who were not on dialysis compared to controls.[198] Among the 8 patients who initiated hemodialysis, autonomic function was unchanged after 6 weeks of dialysis. In contrast, among the 12 patients who underwent kidney transplantation, autonomic function improved a mean of 24 weeks after transplantation.

SLEEP DISORDERS

PREVALENCE OF SLEEP COMPLAINTS

Sleep complaints are common among patients on dialysis with and without associated sleep disorders. In some series, sleep complaints are present in more than 80% of patients on dialysis.[199] Disruption of the sleep-wake cycle is a characteristic feature of uremia, with both excessive daytime sleepiness and insomnia noted in clinical studies.[200,201] Complaints of daytime sleepiness are present in 30% to 67% of patients on dialysis,[199,202,203] while complaints of insomnia are reported in 50% to 73%.[202,204] Using multiple sleep latency testing, an objective measure of daytime sleepiness, the prevalence of daytime sleepiness is lower than prevalence estimates using sleep questionnaires, but still abnormally elevated.[202-204] Sleep disorders (e.g., sleep apnea, RLS, and periodic limb movements of sleep [PLMS]) have been correlated with complaints of excessive daytime sleepiness in some but not all studies, and therefore, other factors associated with uremia, such as altered melatonin metabolism or disrupted regulation of body temperature related to use of dialysate, have been suggested as potential etiologic mechanisms.[205]

SLEEP APNEA

Sleep apnea is characterized by the repetitive cessation of respiration during sleep, resulting in oxygen desaturation and arousal. Apnea associated with continued respiratory effort is classified as obstructive, whereas apnea associated with an absence of respiratory effort is classified as central. Clinical symptoms include loud snoring, repetitive awakening from sleep with feelings of breathlessness, nocturia, excessive daytime sleepiness, and cognitive impairment.

EPIDEMIOLOGY

Utilizing polysomnography to diagnose sleep apnea, the prevalence of this disorder in the ESKD population is estimated at 50%, substantially higher than the recently estimated 10 to 20% in the U.S. population.[206] Some of this difference is explained by differences in age and other chronic diseases that predispose to sleep apnea. In one study the prevalence of sleep apnea was fourfold higher in patients on dialysis compared with age-, sex-, race-, and body mass index–matched controls, suggesting factors specific to ESKD may be implicated in the pathogenesis of this condition.[207] While obstructive sleep apnea is the predominant presentation in the general population, the presentation varies in patients with ESKD with a broad distribution of obstructive, central, and mixed types of apnea.

PATHOPHYSIOLOGY

Based on the distribution of apnea subtypes in this population, both upper airway occlusion and disturbances of central ventilatory control have been implicated in the pathophysiology of sleep apnea in ESKD. Pharyngeal narrowing has been demonstrated in patients on dialysis compared with healthy controls, which in turn may predispose to upper airway occlusion.[208] Upper airway occlusion has been attributed to pharyngeal water content and rostral overnight fluid shifts, as well as to impaired upper airway muscle tone resulting from uremic neuropathy.[209] Impairment of central ventilatory control may be a consequence of hypocapnia resulting from adaptation to chronic metabolic acidosis. In a study of 58 patients requiring hemodialysis, patients with sleep apnea demonstrated augmented

> **Table 59.4 The International Restless Legs Syndrome Study Group Criteria**
>
> 1. An urge to move the legs, usually accompanied or caused by uncomfortable and unpleasant sensations in the legs.
> 2. The urge to move or unpleasant sensations begin or worsen during periods of rest or inactivity, such as lying or sitting.
> 3. The urge to move or unpleasant sensations are partially or totally relieved by movement, such as walking or stretching, for at least as long as the activity continues.
> 4. The urge to move or unpleasant sensations are worse in the evening or night than during the day or only occur in the evening or night.
>
> All four criteria are required for the diagnosis.
> From Allen RP, Picchietti D, Hening WA, et al: Restless legs syndrome: diagnostic criteria, special considerations, and epidemiology. A report from the restless legs syndrome diagnosis and epidemiology workshop at the National Institutes of Health. Sleep Med 4:101-119, 2003.

responsiveness of central and peripheral chemoreflexes, which in turn may destabilize ventilatory control.[210] Infusion of branched-chain amino acids, which are depleted in ESKD, may improve ventilation and sleep architecture.[211]

TREATMENT

In the general population, continuous positive airway pressure (CPAP) is the primary therapy for sleep apnea, and small studies suggest this therapy has similar efficacy in patients with ESKD.[212] CPAP therapy improves symptoms of daytime sleepiness, quality of life, and hypertension and may also attenuate other cardiovascular risk factors in the general population[213,214]; however, compliance with CPAP is often less than optimal, and up to one third of patients will not tolerate CPAP. Nonpharmacologic approaches, such as weight loss, have noted limited success. Several clinical studies have suggested nocturnal hemodialysis or kidney transplantation may have salutary effects on sleep apnea. For example, in a study of 14 patients requiring hemodialysis before and after conversion from conventional thrice-weekly dialysis to nocturnal dialysis, sleep apnea severity improved substantially.[215] Subsequent studies have suggested that improvements in sleep apnea severity associated with nocturnal dialysis are associated with improvements in pharyngeal narrowing and chemoreflex responsiveness.[216,217]

RESTLESS LEGS SYNDROME

RLS is characterized by an urge to move the legs associated with feelings of discomfort or paresthesias. Symptoms occur during periods of inactivity and are alleviated by movement. The diagnosis of RLS is based on clinical criteria (Table 59.4). The reported prevalence of RLS in ESKD varies widely.[199,204,218,219] The clinical consequences are substantial. RLS impairs health-related quality of life and is associated with an increased risk for all-cause mortality and dialysis withdrawal.[219,220]

The pathogenesis of RLS is associated with disrupted dopaminergic function in the brain. Iron is a cofactor for dopamine production in certain brain regions, and iron deficiency has been implicated as an important contributing factor. Comorbid conditions, immobility, and specific medications may also contribute to the development of RLS in patients with ESKD. To date, no specific uremic risk factors have been identified.

For patients with mild or moderate symptoms, lifestyle modification, such as the practice of good sleep hygiene and elimination of exacerbating substances such as antidepressant medications, caffeine, nicotine, and alcohol, is recommended. For patients with more severe symptoms, dopaminergic therapy is recommended as first-line therapy. Levodopa and the dopamine receptor agonists pramipexole or ropinirole are effective in reducing symptoms of RLS.[221] These agents appear to be safe and effective in short-term studies of patients on dialysis,[222-225] although side effects such as daytime worsening of symptoms may occur with continuous use. Anticonvulsants, such as carbamazepine or gabapentin, and benzodiazepines may be second-line agents for RLS treatment but, with the exception of gabapentin, have not been studied as extensively. Intravenous iron infusion is associated with improvement in RLS symptoms in ESKD.[226,227] Kidney transplantation and short daily hemodialysis, but not conventional dialysis, appear to have a beneficial effect on symptoms.[228,229] Finally, in a clinical trial of 25 patients requiring hemodialysis, RLS symptoms were reduced with intradialytic exercise.[230]

PERIODIC LIMB MOVEMENTS OF SLEEP

PLMS are characterized by sudden and repetitive jerking movements of the lower extremities during sleep. This disorder is diagnosed by sleep testing. Like other sleep disorders, PLMS is common among patients on dialysis and associated with daytime sleepiness, low quality of life, and, in one study, an increased risk for mortality.[231] The pathogenesis of PLMS remains unknown; however, kidney transplantation has been reported to reduce the frequency of PLMS and improve symptoms of daytime sleepiness.[232]

Complete reference list available at ExpertConsult.com.

KEY REFERENCES

1. Teschan PE, Ginn HE, Bourne JR, et al: Quantitative indices of clinical uremia. *Kidney Int* 15(6):676–697, 1979.
11. Seliger SL, Gillen DL, Longstreth WT, Jr, et al: Elevated risk of stroke among patients with end-stage renal disease. *Kidney Int* 64(2):603–609, 2003.
12. Sozio SM, Armstrong PA, Coresh J, et al: Cerebrovascular disease incidence, characteristics, and outcomes in patients initiating dialysis: the Choices for Healthy Outcomes in Caring for ESRD (CHOICE) Study. *Am J Kidney Dis* 54(3):468–477, 2009.
21. Yahalom G, Schwartz R, Schwammenthal Y, et al: Chronic kidney disease and clinical outcome in patients with acute stroke. *Stroke* 40(4):1296–1303, 2009.
22. Naganuma T, Uchida J, Tsuchida K, et al: Silent cerebral infarction predicts vascular events in hemodialysis patients. *Kidney Int* 67(6):2434–2439, 2005.
26. Seliger SL, Longstreth WT, Jr, Katz R, et al: Cystatin C and subclinical brain infarction. *J Am Soc Nephrol* 16(12):3721–3727, 2005.
30. Seliger SL, Longstreth WT, Jr: Lessons about brain vascular disease from another pulsating organ, the kidney. *Stroke* 39(1):5–6, 2008.
34. Ninomiya T, Perkovic V, Gallagher M, et al: Lower blood pressure and risk of recurrent stroke in patients with chronic kidney disease: PROGRESS trial. *Kidney Int* 73(8):963–970, 2008.

43. Ninomiya T, Perkovic V, Verdon C, et al: Proteinuria and stroke: a meta-analysis of cohort studies. *Am J Kidney Dis* 53(3):417–425, 2009.
47. Sacks FM, Svetkey LP, Vollmer WM, et al: Effects on blood pressure of reduced dietary sodium and the Dietary Approaches to Stop Hypertension (DASH) diet. DASH-Sodium Collaborative Research Group. *N Engl J Med* 344(1):3–10, 2001.
61. Murray AM, Seliger S, Lakshminarayan K, et al: Incidence of stroke before and after dialysis initiation in older patients. *J Am Soc Nephrol* 24(7):1166–1173, 2013.
84. Baigent C, Landray MJ, Reith C, et al: The effects of lowering LDL cholesterol with simvastatin plus ezetimibe in patients with chronic kidney disease (Study of Heart and Renal Protection): a randomised placebo-controlled trial. *Lancet* 377(9784):2181–2192, 2011.
104. Olesen JB, Lip GY, Kamper AL, et al: Stroke and bleeding in atrial fibrillation with chronic kidney disease. *N Engl J Med* 367(7):625–635, 2012.
112. Sidawy AN, Aidinian G, Johnson ON, 3rd, et al: Effect of chronic renal insufficiency on outcomes of carotid endarterectomy. *J Vasc Surg* 48(6):1423–1430, 2008.
114. Jamison RL, Hartigan P, Kaufman JS, et al: Effect of homocysteine lowering on mortality and vascular disease in advanced chronic kidney disease and end-stage renal disease: a randomized controlled trial. *JAMA* 298(10):1163–1170, 2007.
119. Skali H, Parving HH, Parfrey PS, et al: Stroke in patients with type 2 diabetes mellitus, chronic kidney disease, and anemia treated with darbepoetin alfa: the Trial to Reduce Cardiovascular Events with Aranesp Therapy (TREAT) experience. *Circulation* 124(25):2903–2908, 2011.
120. Seliger SL, Zhang AD, Weir MR, et al: Erythropoiesis-stimulating agents increase the risk of acute stroke in patients with chronic kidney disease. *Kidney Int* 80(3):288–294, 2011.
130. Teschan PE, Bourne JR, Reed RB, et al: Electrophysiological and neurobehavioral responses to therapy: the National Cooperative Dialysis Study. *Kidney Int Suppl* 13:S58–S65, 1983.
134. Arieff AI, Massry SG, Barrientos A, et al: Brain water and electrolyte metabolism in uremia: effects of slow and rapid hemodialysis. *Kidney Int* 4(3):177–187, 1973.
165. Alfrey AC, LeGendre GR, Kaehny WD: The dialysis encephalopathy syndrome. Possible aluminum intoxication. *N Engl J Med* 294(4):184–188, 1976.
169. Murray AM, Tupper DE, Knopman DS, et al: Cognitive impairment in hemodialysis patients is common. *Neurology* 67(2):216–223, 2006.
174. Hooper SR, Gerson AC, Butler RW, et al: Neurocognitive functioning of children and adolescents with mild-to-moderate chronic kidney disease. *Clin J Am Soc Nephrol* 6(8):1824–1830, 2011.
175. Seliger SL, Siscovick DS, Stehman-Breen CO, et al: Moderate renal impairment and risk of dementia among older adults: the Cardiovascular Health Cognition Study. *J Am Soc Nephrol* 15(7):1904–1911, 2004.
177. Helmer C, Stengel B, Metzger M, et al: Chronic kidney disease, cognitive decline, and incident dementia: the 3C Study. *Neurology* 77(23):2043–2051, 2011.
185. Harciarek M, Biedunkiewicz B, Lichodziejewska-Niemierko M, et al: Continuous cognitive improvement 1 year following successful kidney transplant. *Kidney Int* 79(12):1353–1360, 2011.
186. Kurella Tamura M, Unruh ML, Nissenson AR, et al: Effect of more frequent hemodialysis on cognitive function in the frequent hemodialysis network trials. *Am J Kidney Dis* 61(2):228–237, 2013.
194. Bolton CF: Electrophysiologic changes in uremic neuropathy after successful renal transplantation. *Neurology* 26(2):152–161, 1976.
195. Bolton CF, Baltzan MA, Baltzan RB: Effects of renal transplantation on uremic neuropathy. A clinical and electrophysiologic study. *N Engl J Med* 284(21):1170–1175, 1971.
201. Perl J, Unruh ML, Chan CT: Sleep disorders in end-stage renal disease: "markers of inadequate dialysis"? *Kidney Int* 70(10):1687–1693, 2006.
207. Unruh ML, Sanders MH, Redline S, et al: Sleep apnea in patients on conventional thrice-weekly hemodialysis: comparison with matched controls from the Sleep Heart Health Study. *J Am Soc Nephrol* 17(12):3503–3509, 2006.
215. Hanly PJ, Pierratos A: Improvement of sleep apnea in patients with chronic renal failure who undergo nocturnal hemodialysis. *N Engl J Med* 344(2):102–107, 2001.
226. Sloand JA, Shelly MA, Feigin A, et al: A double-blind, placebo-controlled trial of intravenous iron dextran therapy in patients with ESRD and restless legs syndrome. *Am J Kidney Dis* 43(4):663–670, 2004.
227. Benz RL, Pressman MR, Hovick ET, et al: A preliminary study of the effects of correction of anemia with recombinant human erythropoietin therapy on sleep, sleep disorders, and daytime sleepiness in hemodialysis patients (the SLEEPO study). *Am J Kidney Dis* 34(6):1089–1095, 1999.
229. Jaber BL, Schiller B, Burkart JM, et al: Impact of short daily hemodialysis on restless legs symptoms and sleep disturbances. *Clin J Am Soc Nephrol* 6(5):1049–1056, 2011.

60 Dermatologic Conditions in Kidney Disease

Christine J. Ko | Shawn E. Cowper

CHAPTER OUTLINE

SKIN MANIFESTATIONS SECONDARY TO KIDNEY DYSFUNCTION, 1942
Signs and Symptoms, 1942
Manifestations Somewhat Specific to Kidney Disease, 1944
Manifestations Specific to Kidney Disease, 1947
NAIL CHANGES ASSOCIATED WITH KIDNEY DISEASE, 1949
Lindsay's (Half-and-Half) Nail, 1949

SELECTED CONDITIONS WITH SKIN AND RENAL INVOLVEMENT, 1950
Lupus Erythematosus, 1950
Leukocytoclastic Vasculitis, 1950
Henoch-Schönlein Purpura, 1951
GENODERMATOSES, 1951
DERMATOLOGIC CONDITIONS THAT MAY LATER INVOLVE THE KIDNEYS, 1953
Impetigo/Streptococcal Skin Infection, 1953

Most, if not all, patients with end-stage renal disease (ESRD) have associated skin manifestations.[1,2] In addition, skin findings may specifically direct an astute clinician to check for concomitant renal dysfunction. This chapter summarizes different dermatologic conditions that may be seen in patients with kidney disorders. Because of the large number of diseases falling into this category (see Tables 60.1 to 60.6), emphasis is placed on the more commonly encountered entities.

SKIN MANIFESTATIONS SECONDARY TO KIDNEY DYSFUNCTION (Table 60.1)

SIGNS AND SYMPTOMS

PRURITUS

Pruritus is more common in patients with ESRD disease than in those with acute kidney injury (AKI). Up to 90% of patients undergoing hemodialysis may experience pruritus, and patients receiving hemodialysis are more commonly affected than patients receiving peritoneal dialysis.[2] Sleep and mood are negatively affected.[3] Patients with severe pruritus have a poor outcome compared with patients undergoing hemodialysis without severe pruritus.[4]

Patients complaining of pruritus may or may not have skin changes. Pruritus can be defined as at least three episodes of itch in a 2-week period that cause difficulty for the patient, or as itch that occurs over a 6-month period in a regular pattern.[3] Pruritus can be localized or generalized.[5] When present, skin manifestations are secondary, with excoriations (Figure 60.1) being the main finding. Lichenified skin, prurigo nodularis, and koebnerization may also be seen. Pruritus tends to be prolonged, frequent, and intense.[3] Exacerbating factors include heat, nighttime, dry skin, and sweat.[3]

The cause of pruritus in renal failure is unclear and may be multifactorial. Risk factors include male gender and high levels of blood urea nitrogen, β_2-microglobulin, calcium, and phosphate.[4,6] Patients treated with angiotensin-converting enzyme inhibitors are more likely to have pruritus than those receiving furosemide.[3] Decreasing urine output, secondary hyperparathyroidism, abnormal levels of magnesium and aluminum, increased levels of histamine and vitamin A, increased numbers of mast cells,[7] xerosis,[8] and iron deficiency anemia are other proposed factors.[9,10]

Pruritus is transmitted through C fibers in the skin.[11] Known stimulants of C fibers include cytokines, histamine, serotonin, prostaglandins, neuropeptides,[5] and enzymes.[12] Because cytokines can stimulate nerve fibers,[12] one major theory regarding the pathogenesis of pruritus in renal failure is that it involves systemic inflammation.[13] Markers of inflammation, such as C-reactive protein and interleukin-6, show elevated levels in pruritus associated with renal disease.[13,14] An imbalance of inflammatory proteins may somehow lead to pruritus. This theory is supported by the fact that ultraviolet light treatments, which can decrease the levels of inflammation markers,[15] often ameliorate pruritus.

Another major theory focuses on the opioid system. Opioids can stimulate C fibers.[12] Central µ-opioid receptor stimulation in mice leads to scratching, and this can be prevented by central κ-opioid receptor stimulation.[16]

Table 60.1 Skin Manifestations Secondary to Renal Disease

Nonspecific

Pruritus
Xerosis
Acquired ichthyosis
Pigmentary alteration
    Pallor (secondary to anemia)
    Hyperpigmentation
    Dyspigmentation (yellow tint)
Infections (fungal, bacterial, viral)
Purpura

Somewhat Specific

Acquired perforating dermatosis
Calciphylaxis
Metastatic calcification
Blistering disorders
    Porphyria cutanea tarda
    Pseudoporphyria
Eruptive xanthomas
Pseudo–Kaposi's sarcoma

Specific

Nephrogenic systemic fibrosis
Dialysis-associated steal syndrome
Metastatic renal cell carcinoma
Dialysis-related amyloidosis
Arteriovenous shunt dermatitis
Uremic frost

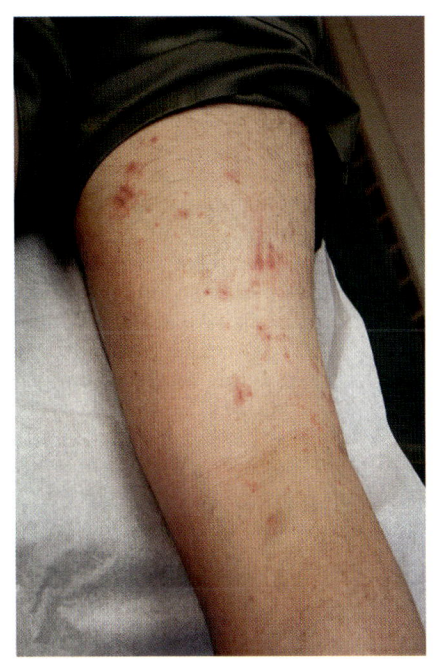

Figure 60.1 Pruritus. Patient with linear excoriations. (Courtesy Oscar Colegio, MD.)

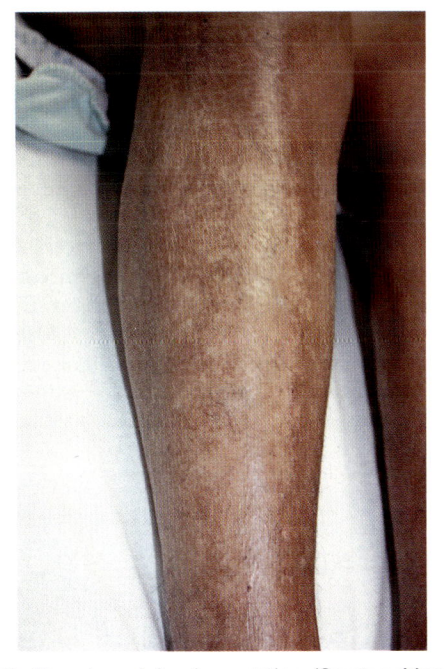

Figure 60.2 Xerosis and dyspigmentation. (Courtesy Marcus McFerren, MD.)

Successful treatment of patients with opioid antagonists also supports the involvement of the opioid system in pruritus.[17,19]

Treatment of pruritus must be tailored to the individual patient. In general, antihistamines are not effective.[20] Any condition that can exacerbate pruritus, like xerosis, should be treated.[21] Symptoms may be alleviated by optimization of hemodialysis[1] and administration of erythropoietin.[22] For more localized areas of pruritus, topical corticosteroids, pramoxine,[23] and capsaicin[5,24] may be used. In addition, twice-weekly ultraviolet light phototherapy is effective.[25] Oral treatments include naltrexone,[17,18] cholestyramine,[26] gabapentin,[27,28] thalidomide,[29] and activated charcoal.[30] Opioid κ-receptor agonists like nalfurafine may be helpful.[19] Kidney transplantation may effectively "cure" patients,[31] as may parathyroidectomy.[32]

A therapeutic ladder has been proposed, based on efficacy and safety considerations.[31] The first rung of the ladder consists of emollients and capsaicin. If pruritus is not relieved, ultraviolet light treatments can be added. If light treatments fail or are not feasible for the patient, oral gabapentin or intravenous nalfurafine may be considered.

XEROSIS

Xerosis, or "dry skin," is quite common in the general population. The skin appears dry, rough, or shiny. It may be scaly or fissured with a cracked appearance. Xerotic skin may or may not be pruritic.[21] If it is pruritic, there may be excoriations. Skin involvement may be diffuse but is often most prominent over the extensor surfaces of the lower extremities (Figure 60.2).[1]

The cause of xerosis is unknown. Decreased stratum corneum hydration[21] and abnormal eccrine gland function[33] are two proposed mechanisms. The mainstay of treatment is hydration of the skin. For pruritic cases, direct treatment of the pruritus may be helpful.

ACQUIRED ICHTHYOSIS

Ichthyosis is related to xerosis but is more than just dry skin, because the skin develops patterned scale. Histopathologic features include hyperkeratosis and occasionally epidermal hypogranulosis. The pathogenesis of acquired ichthyosis in renal failure is unknown. Treatment consists of hydration of the skin.

PIGMENTARY ALTERATION

Seventy percent or more of patients undergoing dialysis may have pigmentary changes of the skin.[2,34] The most common alteration is the development of a yellowish tint. This is more common among patients undergoing hemodialysis than those on peritoneal dialysis.[2] Hyperpigmentation may be secondary to increased melanin production as a result of elevated levels of β-melanocyte–stimulating hormone.[35] Pallor of the skin secondary to anemia has also been described.[1]

MANIFESTATIONS SOMEWHAT SPECIFIC TO KIDNEY DISEASE

ACQUIRED PERFORATING DERMATOSIS

Acquired perforating dermatosis is an umbrella term for perforating disorders in adults with kidney dysfunction and/or diabetes mellitus. This term is often used in place of older nomenclature (e.g., perforating folliculitis, Kyrle's disease, reactive perforating collagenosis). Pruritus is generally severe.[36] Lesions are distributed predominantly on the legs and arms, although the trunk and head may also be involved. Individual lesions are crateriform, umbilicated, or centrally hyperkeratotic papules and nodules (Figure 60.3). They may develop in crops and commonly resolve with scarring after 6 to 8 weeks. Histopathologic evidence of extrusion of dermal material through an epidermal channel is necessary for the diagnosis (Figure 60.4).

The pathogenesis of this disorder is unknown but may be related to increased fibronectin,[37] pruritus and scratching,[36] epidermal dysmaturation, and dermal deposition of substances not excreted in renal failure.[38,39] Patients with diabetes and renal failure are more likely to manifest acquired perforating dermatosis than are patients without diabetes.[1,36] Other associations include hepatitis and hypothyroidism.[39] Patients who are otherwise healthy may also develop acquired perforating dermatosis.[39] Treatment of this disorder is difficult, with some relief afforded by topical steroids, keratolytics, lubrication, and topical or oral retinoids.[38] Narrowband ultraviolet B light may also be helpful.[40] Patients with severe and generalized pruritus may benefit from treatments specifically directed at pruritus.

CALCIPHYLAXIS (CALCIFIC UREMIC ARTERIOLOPATHY)

Calciphylaxis is most often seen in patients with ESRD who are on hemodialysis, generally with associated hyperparathyroidism or an elevated calcium phosphate product. An incidence of approximately 4% of patients per year at one dialysis center has been reported.[41] Morbidity and mortality are high, especially once ulceration develops.[41] Involvement of the trunk and buttocks is associated with high mortality.[42] Importantly, in the absence of ESRD and hyperparathyroidism, other risk factors include female gender,[41]

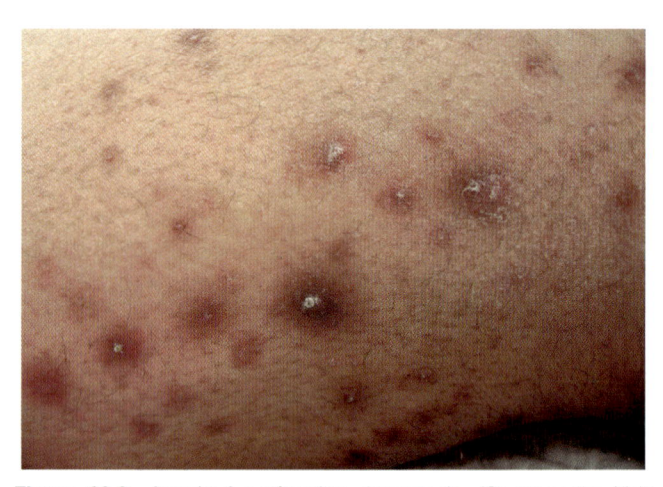

Figure 60.3 Acquired perforating dermatosis. (Courtesy the Yale Residents' Collection.)

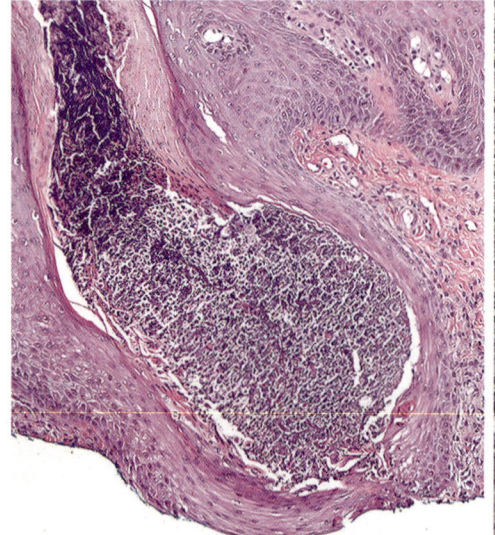

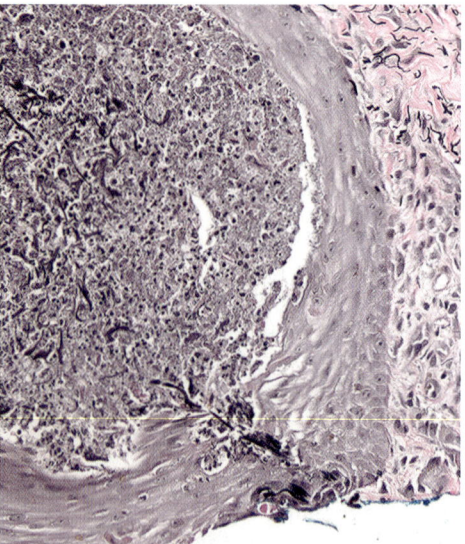

Figure 60.4 Acquired perforating dermatosis. There is an epidermal channel with extrusion of dermal elastic material and inflammatory cells. (**Left,** Hematoxylin and eosin stain, ×40; **right,** elastic van Gieson stain, ×100.)

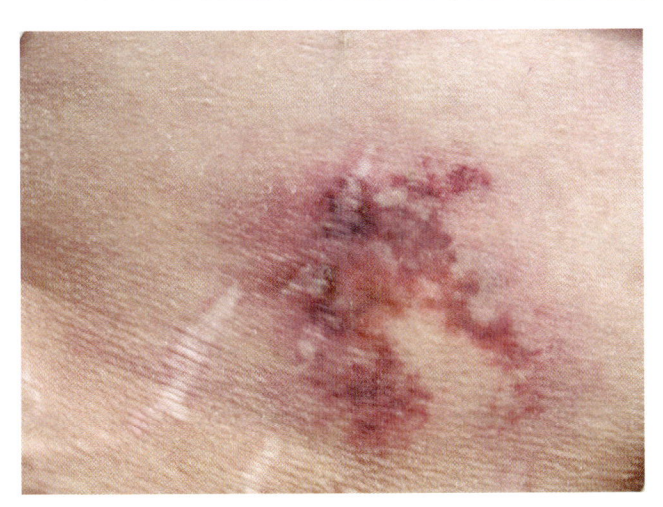

Figure 60.5 Calciphylaxis. Early lesion with retiform purpuric appearance.

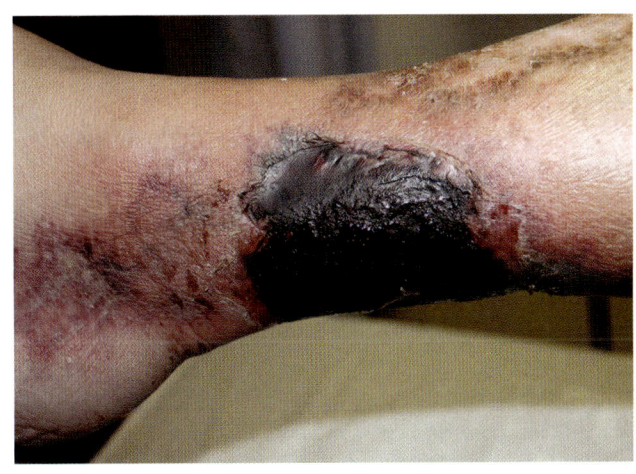

Figure 60.6 Calciphylaxis. Ulcerated lesion with black eschar. (Courtesy the Yale Residents' Collection.)

diabetes,[41] obesity, hypoalbuminemia,[43] malignancy, administration of systemic steroids, warfarin use,[43] chemotherapy, systemic inflammation, hepatic cirrhosis, rapid weight loss, protein C or S deficiency, and infection.[44]

The precise mechanism of calciphylaxis is unclear. The classical model, as described by Selye in rats, hypothesized a predisposing factor with a secondary, inciting factor.[45] This model has been criticized as not being fully reflective of calciphylaxis in humans, because Selye's rats displayed only soft tissue calcification and not skin necrosis.[46,47] Although the calcium phosphate product level is elevated in most patients, it is not by itself sufficient to cause disease.[47] Some suggest that an imbalance of inhibitors and inducers of vascular calcification leads to calciphylaxis. Evidence for this hypothesis includes the observation of elevated levels of osteopontin and bone morphogenic protein 2 (inducers of calcification) and decreased levels of matrix Gla protein, fetuin-A, and pyrophosphate (inhibitors of calcification)[48] among those affected. The final common pathway seems to involve nuclear factor-κB.[47] Abnormal metal deposition, especially of aluminum, may also be a factor in inciting inflammation.[47]

Clinically calciphylaxis most commonly affects the fatty areas of the thighs, abdomen, and buttocks symmetrically. Lesions may also affect the lower extremities.[41] Early lesions may be firm with a pink or mottled color or retiform purpura (Figure 60.5). These may progress to painful ulcers with a black eschar (Figure 60.6). Occasionally bullae, plaques, and nodules may be seen. Surrounding the ulcers, there may be skin mottling with reticulate dyspigmentation. The skin may be tender. Histopathologic findings supportive of calciphylaxis include calcification of medium-sized vessels (Figure 60.7) with intimal hyperplasia and thrombosis. Radiographic studies may also show linear calcium deposits in the skin.

Supportive and preventive measures are the mainstay of treatment, including hyperbaric oxygen therapy,[49] debridement, wound care, and antibiotic therapy. For nonulcerated lesions, systemic steroids may lead to rapid healing.[41] Parathyroidectomy is helpful in resolving lesions in some patients.[41,46] If parathyroidectomy is not possible, oral cinacalcet and phosphate binders may be helpful.[50] Use of low-calcium dialysate and non–calcium-based phosphate binders may also have a positive effect.[51] Intravenous sodium thiosulfate, a calcium chelator, is reportedly successful.[52] Bisphosphonates may also be useful.[53] Many of these treatments focus on lowering calcium and phosphate levels. Because elevated calcium and phosphate levels are not the root cause of calciphylaxis, however, optimal treatment may be to focus on other possible mechanisms, such as reduction of vascular thrombosis with anticoagulation.[47]

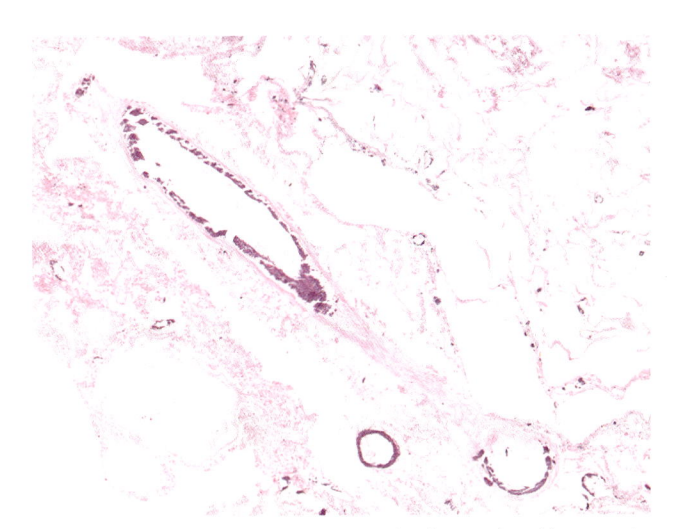

Figure 60.7 Calciphylaxis. Medium-sized vessels with extensive calcium deposition. (Hematoxylin and eosin stain, ×40.)

METASTATIC CALCIFICATION

An abnormal calcium phosphate product, with or without hyperparathyroidism, can lead to metastatic calcification of the skin. Clinically, lesions are hard, yellow to bluish papules and nodules, which most commonly affect periarticular areas and the fingertips.[51] A biopsy specimen from a nodule should reveal calcium deposits in the tissue. Importantly, not all calcification in the skin is secondary to metastatic calcification. Trauma may result in so-called dystrophic calcification. Some systemic diseases, such as dermatomyositis,

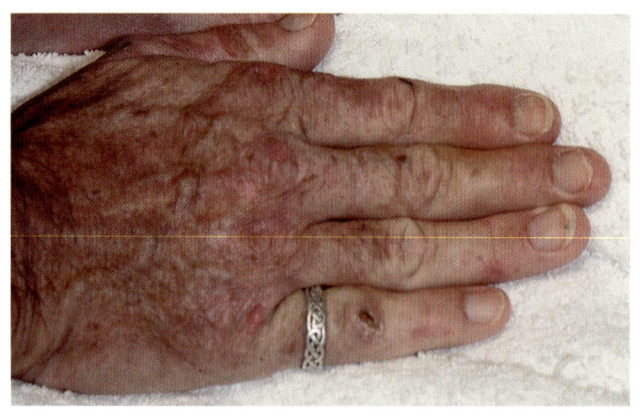

Figure 60.8 Porphyria cutanea tarda. Eroded blisters and crusts. (Courtesy the Yale Residents' Collection.)

Figure 60.9 Eruptive xanthomas. Small yellowish-orange papules over the knees. (Courtesy the Yale Residents' Collection.)

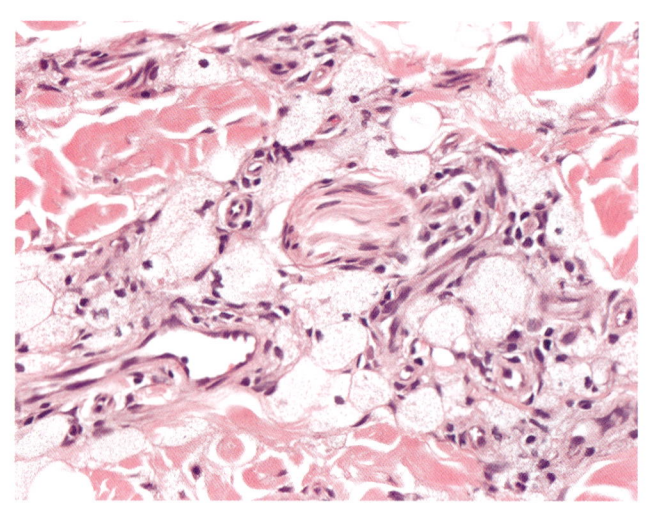

Figure 60.10 Eruptive xanthoma. Lipid-containing foamy macrophages within the dermis. (Hematoxylin and eosin stain, ×40.)

may be associated with calcification of the skin. Calcification may also be idiopathic.

Treatment of metastatic calcification focuses on normalizing calcium and phosphate levels. If hyperparathyroidism is present, parathyroidectomy may be beneficial. Use of phosphate binders and reduction of dietary phosphate are important. Foods that should be avoided include milk and milk products, certain vegetables (broccoli, brussels sprouts), oysters, salmon, beer, nuts, and wheat germ.[51] If particular lesions are symptomatic, surgical removal may be considered.

PORPHYRIA CUTANEA TARDA

Up to 18% of patients with renal failure may have porphyria cutanea tarda, with a deficiency of uroporphyrinogen decarboxylase. These patients have elevated levels of urinary uroporphyrin (if not anuric) and fecal isocoproporphyrin. The pathogenesis of porphyria cutanea tarda in renal patients is unclear. Serum aluminum level may be a contributing factor.[54] Other risk factors for the development of porphyria cutanea tarda include hepatitis B and C, estrogen administration, excess alcohol intake, and human immunodeficiency virus infection.

Cutaneous findings include noninflamed blisters, erosions, and crusts (Figure 60.8), especially those involving the dorsal hands and forearms. Blisters may heal with scarring or milia. There may be notable hypertrichosis on the face. Hyperpigmentation and sclerodermoid plaques have also been described. A biopsy specimen from a blister in porphyria cutanea tarda shows a subepidermal cleft with minimal inflammation. There may be festooning of the papillary dermis at the base of the cleft. Thickened vessel walls may be present. Direct immunofluorescent studies in porphyria cutanea tarda show granular to linear staining of immunoglobulin G (IgG) and C3 at the dermoepidermal junction and sometimes around vessels.

Treatment includes sun avoidance and sun protection. Concomitant exacerbating factors (alcohol, estrogens, iron, hepatitis) should be avoided or treated. Because iron overload can exacerbate the disease, small-volume phlebotomy may be helpful, although anemia needs to be carefully monitored. Deferoxamine, an iron chelator, is also sometimes used. If a patient is not anuric, chloroquine may be used cautiously.[51]

PSEUDOPORPHYRIA

In pseudoporphyria, patients have a presentation that is similar to that in porphyria cutanea tarda, with noninflamed blisters on the extremities, especially the hands and forearms and other sun-exposed areas. Milia, scarring, and hyperpigmentation may result.[55] Hypertrichosis is seen in a minority of patients.[55] Plasma uroporphyrin and red blood cell protoporphyrin levels may be elevated.[54] The separation of pseudoporphyria from porphyria cutanea tarda is clearer when these levels are normal.[55] Concomitant use of drugs such as tetracycline, furosemide, naproxen, amiodarone, and nalidixic acid may be involved in the development of pseudoporphyria.[55] Histologic findings are similar to those of porphyria cutanea tarda.[55] Although the pathogenesis of pseudoporphyria is unclear, elevated aluminum levels were found in a small study.[54]

ERUPTIVE XANTHOMAS

Eruptive xanthomas are yellowish-orange smooth papules and plaques (Figure 60.9) that rapidly appear on the buttocks and proximal extremities. Histopathologic examination of a lesion reveals extracellular lipid and foamy macrophages (Figure 60.10). These lesions are associated with hyperlipidemia, either familial or due to other causes

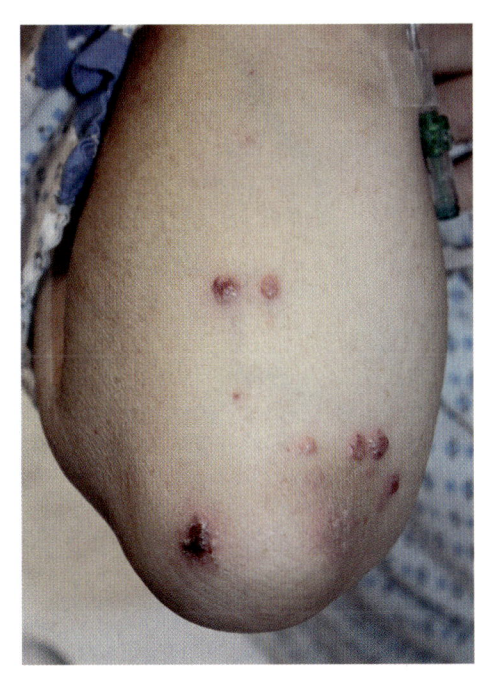

Figure 60.11 Iododerma. Translucent papules and crusted plaques on the elbow. (Courtesy Oscar Colegio, MD, and Christine Warren, MD.)

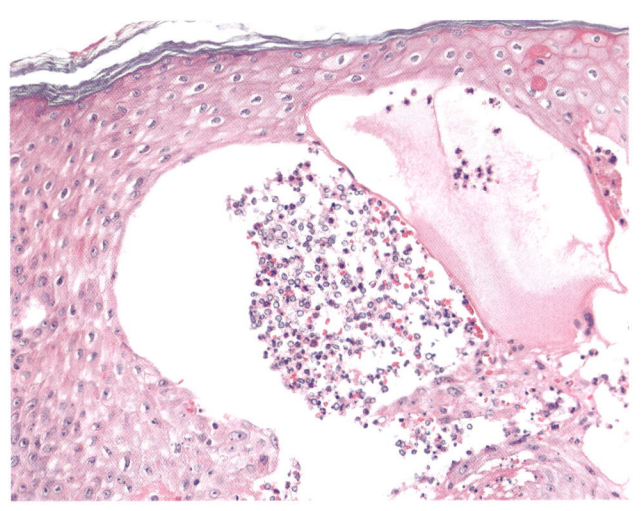

Figure 60.12 Iododerma. Epidermal hyperplasia with intraepidermal pustules. (Hematoxylin and eosin stain, ×200.)

Table 60.2 Post–Renal Transplantation Skin Conditions*
Lymphoproliferative disease
Infections
Squamous cell carcinoma and other skin cancers

*See Chapter 72.

such as hypothyroidism and nephrotic syndrome. In nephrotic syndrome the xanthomas are likely secondary to various lipid abnormalities, including elevated levels of cholesterol and triglycerides, elevated lipoprotein synthesis, diminished level of lipoprotein lipase, and elevated apolipoprotein B-100 level with diminished hepatic uptake of lipoproteins.[56] Generally, eruptive xanthomas resolve spontaneously once lipid levels are normalized.

PSEUDO–KAPOSI'S SARCOMA

Very rarely, patients may develop a vascular proliferation that mimics Kaposi's sarcoma near or over an arteriovenous shunt.[57]

IODODERMA

Often in the setting of renal insufficiency/failure, patients who receive iodide in the form of intravenous contrast may develop translucent papulonodular or vegetative lesions of iododerma (Figure 60.11).[58] Histopathologically there is marked epidermal hyperplasia with intraepidermal pustules of neutrophils and sometimes eosinophils (Figure 60.12). Clinical and histopathologic exclusion of infectious causes is required.

MANIFESTATIONS SPECIFIC TO KIDNEY DISEASE (Table 60.2)

NEPHROGENIC SYSTEMIC FIBROSIS

The first case of nephrogenic systemic fibrosis (NSF), originally described under various terms, including *scleromyxedema-like changes in renal failure* and *nephrogenic fibrosing dermopathy*,[59] was identified in 1997. Although the cause of NSF was long debated, exposure to gadolinium-based magnetic resonance imaging contrast agents in patients with abnormal renal function is now considered the precipitating factor.[60,61] Gadolinium, an element highly toxic to tissues in its unbound state, is present in a chelated form in contrast agents such as Omniscan (GE Healthcare, United Kingdom) and Magnevist (Bayer HealthCare Pharmaceuticals, Berlin, Germany). Impaired excretion of gadolinium-based contrast may allow more time for gadolinium atoms to dissociate from their proprietary ligand molecule. Unbound gadolinium is theorized to bind to other available anions (chiefly phosphates) and deposit peripherally, perhaps inducing long-standing effects on local tissue fibroblasts and/or circulating matrix stem cells termed *circulating fibrocytes*. Gadolinium has been detected in tissues of patients with NSF and in in vivo animal studies, findings that corroborate the postulated effects of prolonged gadolinium exposure.[62]

Clinically, patients with NSF have bound-down, indurated skin on the extremities (Figure 60.13), although truncal involvement is also reported. The skin may have a cobblestone appearance (Figure 60.14). Early in NSF, patients may have edema and erythema that mimics cellulitis. Joint contractures (Figure 60.15; see Fig. 60-13) and yellow scleral plaques (Figure 60.16) are common. Histopathologically, increased dermal and/or subcutaneous fibroblast-like cells are seen (Figure 60.17). The cells stain with procollagen I and CD34 by immunohistochemical methods. It is postulated that these cells are circulating fibrocytes.[63] Mucin deposition may also be observed. The clinical and histopathologic differentials are broad, and overlap with some more common entities, such as lipodermatosclerosis and morphea. Clinicopathologic correlation is essential to reach an accurate diagnosis.[64]

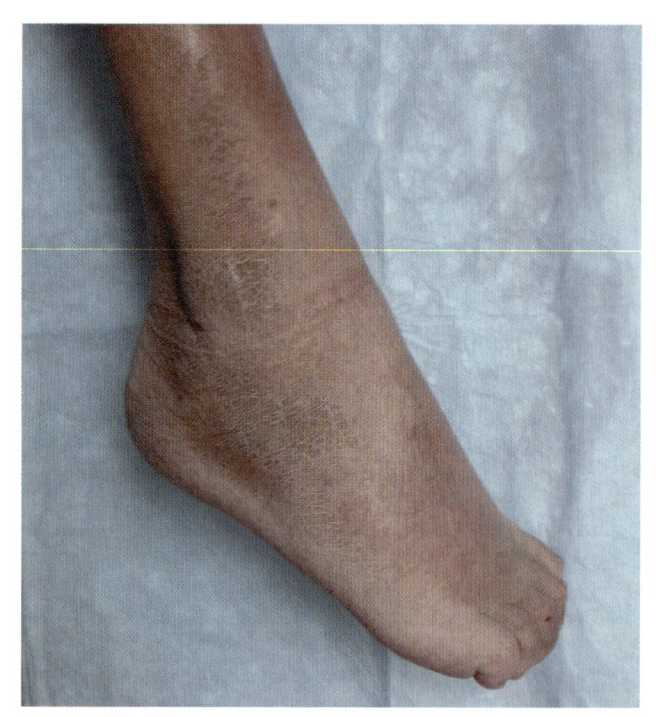

Figure 60.13 Nephrogenic systemic fibrosis. Lower leg with indurated, bound-down skin and contractures of the toes. (From Cowper SE, Rabach M, Girardi M: Clinical and histological findings in nephrogenic systemic fibrosis. *Eur J Radiol* 66[2]:191-199, 2008; courtesy Michael Girardi, MD.)

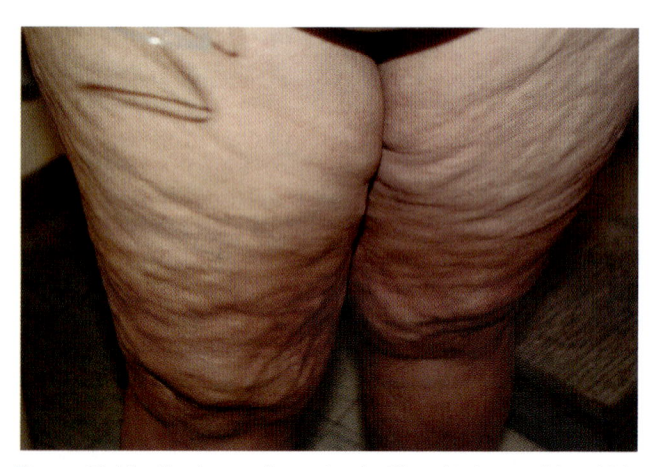

Figure 60.14 Nephrogenic systemic fibrosis. Legs with cobblestone appearance of indurated skin. (From Girardi M: Nephrogenic systemic fibrosis: a dermatologist's perspective, *J Am Coll Radiol* 5[1]:40-44, 2008; courtesy Michael Girardi, MD.)

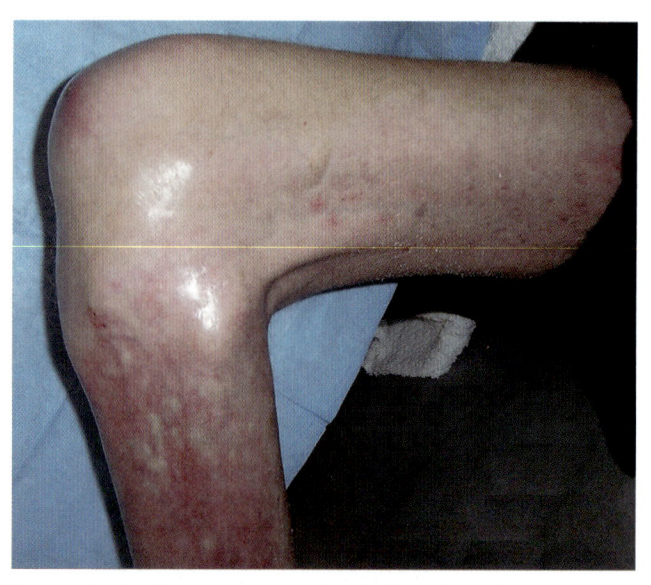

Figure 60.15 Nephrogenic systemic fibrosis. Joint contracture. (From Girardi M: Nephrogenic systemic fibrosis: a dermatologist's perspective, *J Am Coll Radiol* 5[1]:40-44, 2008; courtesy Michael Girardi, MD.)

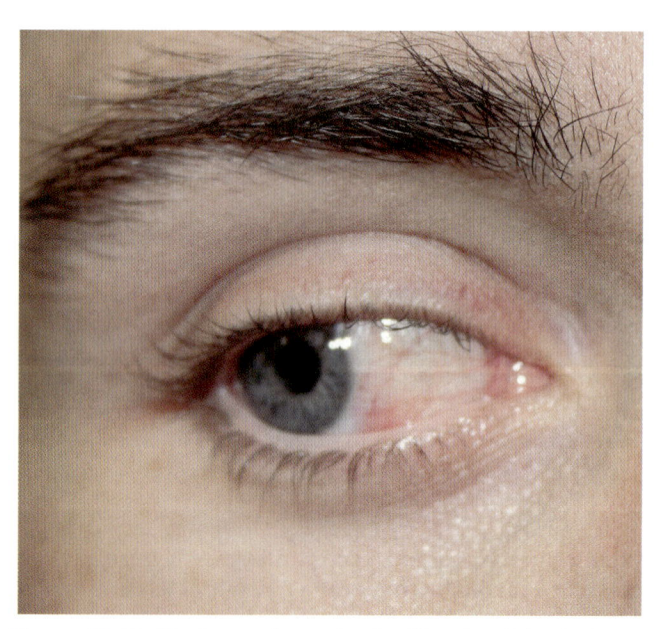

Figure 60.16 Nephrogenic systemic fibrosis. Scleral plaque. (From Cowper SE, Rabach M, Girardi M: Clinical and histological findings in nephrogenic systemic fibrosis. *Eur J Radiol* 66[2]:191-199, 2008; courtesy Michael Girardi, MD.)

Prevention of NSF by avoiding the administration of gadolinium-containing agents to patients with renal failure is key, because there is no reliable treatment for the disease. Changes in the labeling of gadolinium-containing contrast agents and careful screening of patients for underlying kidney disease have been successful preventive measures. In patients who develop the disorder, renal transplantation is sometimes helpful in halting progression and occasionally reverses the disease. Extracorporeal photopheresis may also be useful. Physical therapy may ameliorate some symptoms for patients. Reports of imatinib treatment are encouraging.[65]

DIALYSIS-ASSOCIATED STEAL SYNDROME

Dialysis-associated steal syndrome is a rare complication of fistula construction.[66] This syndrome most commonly involves the brachial area in patients with diabetes. There may be associated pallor or a reticulated pink to blue discoloration of the skin surrounding necrosis, ulceration, or gangrene (Figure 60.18). Altered hemodynamics secondary to the fistula result in decreased distal perfusion. Associated risk factors are diabetes, vascular stenosis, neuropathic disease, and calcifying sclerosis. Effective treatment involves fistula ligation and/or banding.

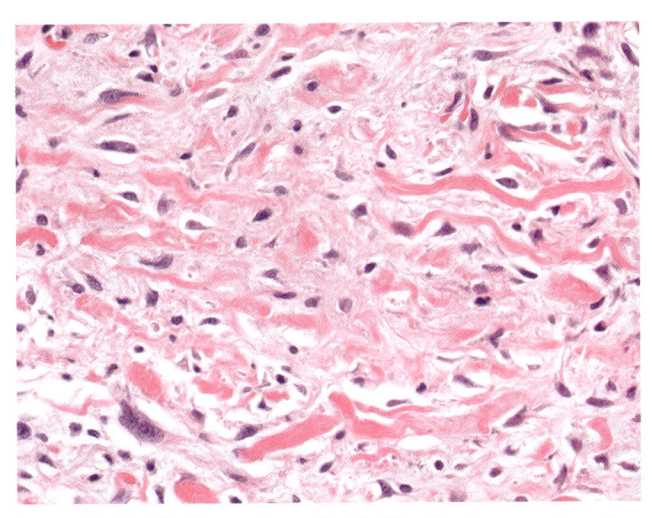

Figure 60.17 Nephrogenic systemic fibrosis. Increased numbers of fibroblast-like cells, preserved elastic tissue, and increased space between collagen bundles, suggestive of mucin deposition. (Hematoxylin and eosin stain, ×200.)

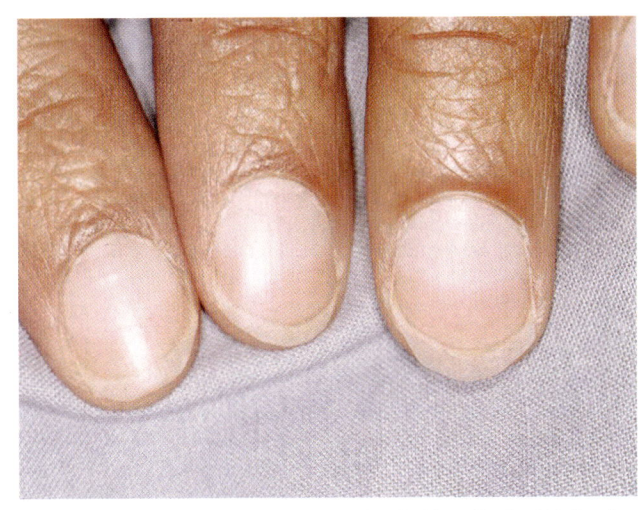

Figure 60.19 Lindsay's (half-and-half) nail. (From Butler DF: Pruritus. In Schwarzenberger K, Werchniak A, Ko C, editors: *General dermatology, Requisites in dermatology series*, Philadelphia, 2009, Saunders, pp 17-22; courtesy David F. Butler, MD.)

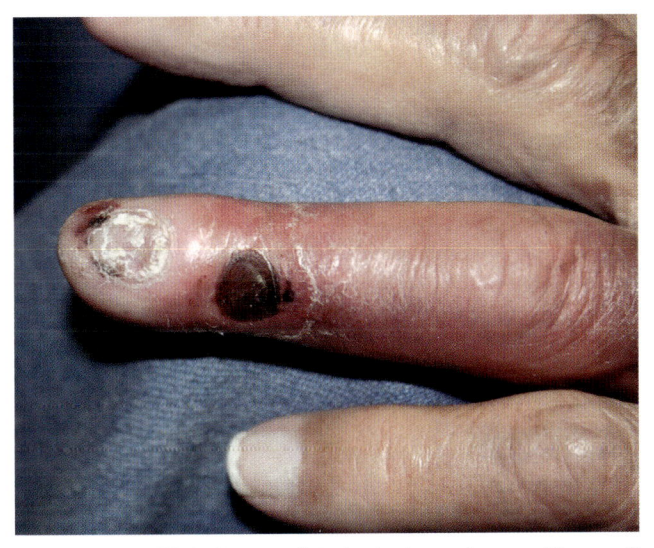

Figure 60.18 Dialysis-associated steal syndrome. Ulcer with overlying crust with surrounding erythema, distal pallor, and nail atrophy. (From Kravetz JD, Heald P: Bilateral dialysis-associated steal syndrome, *J Am Acad Dermatol* 58:888-891, 2008.)

Table 60.3 Nail Changes Associated with Kidney Disease

Lindsay's (half-and-half) nail
Triangular lunulae (nail-patella syndrome)
Splinter hemorrhages
Onychomycosis
Koilonychia
Onycholysis
Mees' lines
Muehrcke's lines
Beau's lines

METASTATIC RENAL CELL CARCINOMA

Although approximately 4.6% of cutaneous metastases originate from the kidney, only 3% to 4% of renal cell carcinomas metastasize to the skin.[67] Metastases may occasionally precede the diagnosis of the primary tumor, but often they are a late manifestation.[68] The prognosis is poor, with a 5-year survival of less than 5%. Common cutaneous sites for metastatic renal cell carcinoma are the trunk and scalp.[68] Nodules may be flesh colored, violaceous, or pink-red. Histopathologic examination often shows a tumor with clear cells and prominent hemorrhage.

DIALYSIS-RELATED AMYLOIDOSIS

Dialysis-related amyloidosis is secondary to β_2-microglobulin deposition. Unlike amyloid L, skin involvement is unusual, and the more common presentations involve carpal tunnel syndrome and destructive arthropathy. However, there are rare reports of immobile dermal nodules secondary to β_2-microglobulin deposition, most often affecting the buttocks.[69,70]

ARTERIOVENOUS SHUNT DERMATITIS

In one study, 7 of 88 patients on long-term hemodialysis developed an irritant contact dermatitis over their shunts.[71] None of the patients had an allergic component to the rash. Substituting normal saline for the cleansers (soaps, disinfectants, and alcohol) used to clean the skin before hemodialysis was helpful in alleviating the skin rash. Use of a mild topical steroid was also helpful.

NAIL CHANGES ASSOCIATED WITH KIDNEY DISEASE (Table 60.3)

LINDSAY'S (HALF-AND-HALF) NAIL

Up to 40% of patients with renal dysfunction have half-and-half nails (Figure 60.19).[2] The condition may resolve spontaneously and is likely secondary to melanin deposition in the nail bed and plate. Fingernails are affected more

Table 60.4	Selected Conditions with Concurrent Skin and Renal Involvement
More Common	
Lupus erythematosus	
Leukocytoclastic vasculitis	
Henoch-Schönlein purpura	
Mixed cryoglobulinemia	
Diabetes mellitus	
Systemic vasculitis	
Less Common	
Nail-patella syndrome	
Hemolytic-uremic syndrome	
Toxic shock syndrome	
Mixed connective tissue disease	
Dermatomyositis	
Rheumatoid arthritis	
Sjögren's syndrome	
Dermatitis herpetiformis	
Sarcoidosis	
Systemic sclerosis	
Ulcerative colitis	
Amyloidosis	
Toxic epidermolysis	
Hypothyroidism	
Graves' disease	
Fabry's disease	
Neurofibromatosis	
Hurler's syndrome	
Castleman's disease	
Infectious endocarditis	
Staphylococcal scalded skin syndrome (in adults)	

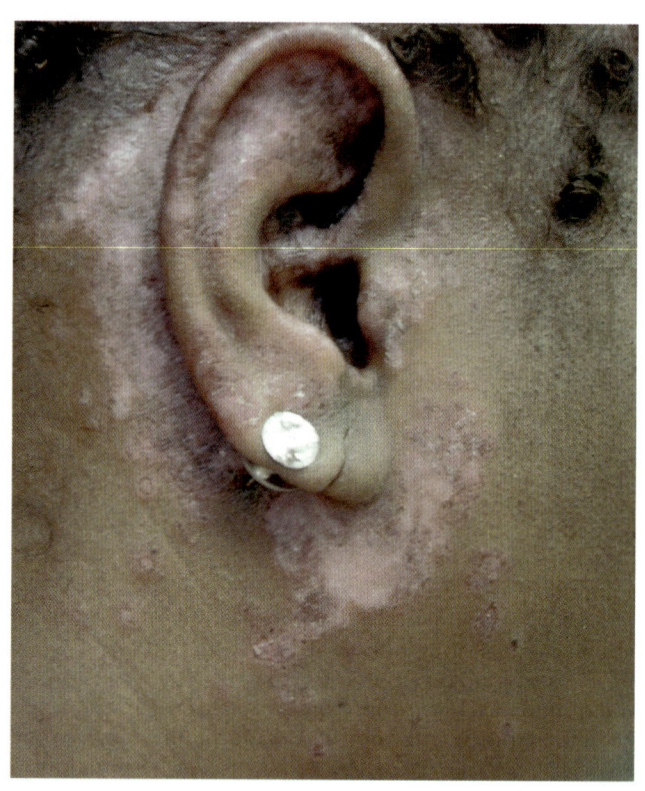

Figure 60.20 Discoid lupus erythematosus. (Courtesy the Yale Residents' Collection.)

commonly than toenails. The nails have a white to normal proximal half and a red-brown distal half.

SELECTED CONDITIONS WITH SKIN AND RENAL INVOLVEMENT (Table 60.4)

LUPUS ERYTHEMATOSUS

The skin manifestations of lupus erythematosus are varied. Acute skin changes include the classic malar rash. Annular plaques and papules with scale and erythema are typical of subcutaneous lupus erythematosus. These lesions generally resolve without scarring. In discoid lupus erythematosus, coin-shaped to oval plaques heal with dyspigmentation and scarring. There is often adherent scale within the lesions that, when lifted off, has a "carpet tack" appearance on the underside. Such discoid lesions in the conchal bowl of the ear are characteristic of lupus erythematosus (Figure 60.20). Neonates with lupus erythematosus may occasionally have annular, erythematous plaques in sun-exposed areas. In addition to these skin lesions, patients may complain of photosensitivity, oral ulcers, or alopecia.

The different skin manifestations of lupus look similar histopathologically. There are vacuolar changes at the dermoepidermal junction with a variable infiltrate of lymphocytes. There is often a superficial and deep perivascular and periadnexal lymphocytic infiltrate as well. Mucin may be increased. Direct immunofluorescent testing may show a discontinuous linear band of IgG, C3, IgA, and/or IgM at the dermoepidermal junction.

The pathogenesis of lupus erythematosus involves autoantibodies that can form immune complexes that deposit in end organs, causing damage.[72] Animal models of lupus suggest that inhibition of oxidative stress and production of nitric oxide via inactivation of the nuclear factor-κB pathway may be important in modulating disease.[73]

Currently the skin findings of lupus erythematosus are treated with steroids (oral or topical), antimalarials, and/or other immunosuppressants.

LEUKOCYTOCLASTIC VASCULITIS

Leukocytoclastic vasculitis, clinically known as *palpable purpura*, may be seen in a variety of clinical situations. Characteristically the lesions are found on the lower extremities as nonblanching to partially blanching papules and plaques (Figure 60.21). Histopathologically there is leukocytoclasia, fibrin thrombi within vessels, extravasated erythrocytes, and swollen endothelial cells. If direct immunofluorescence testing is performed on the skin, deposits of IgG, IgM, and/or C3 may be seen around the vessels.

Associated diseases include Henoch-Schönlein purpura, infections (streptococcal, mycoplasmal, viral), systemic vasculitis (granulomatosis with polyangitis [formally designated Wegener's granulomatosis], eosinophilic granulomatosis with polyangiitis [formally designated Churg-Strauss syndrome], polyarteritis nodosa), inflammatory bowel disease, and malignancy.[74] Lesions may also be drug induced. In

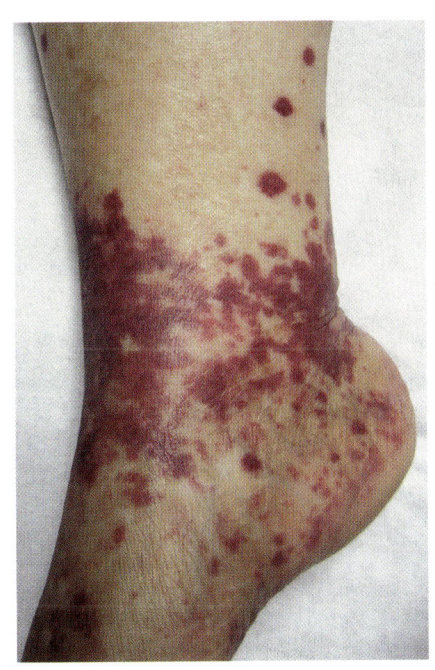

Figure 60.21 Leukocytoclastic vasculitis. (Courtesy the Yale Residents' Collection.)

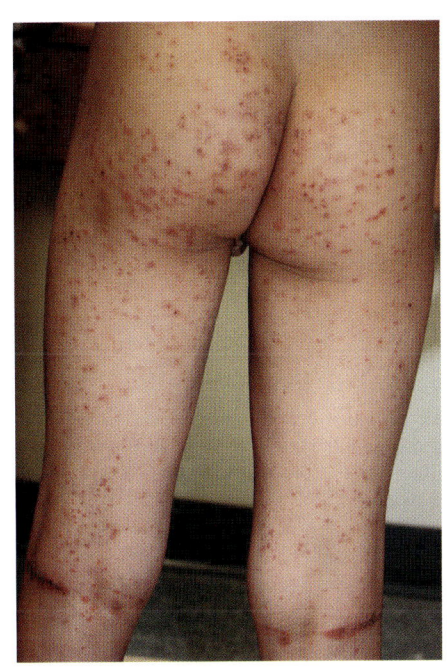

Figure 60.22 Henoch-Schönlein purpura. Nonblanchable macules and papules distributed over the buttocks and lower extremities.

Henoch-Schönlein purpura the skin lesions are often seen in association with gastrointestinal pain, joint pain, and renal involvement. Mixed cryoglobulinemia is another disorder that can present with palpable purpura in the skin and a membranoproliferative glomerulonephritis.[75] Other skin manifestations include ulcers and dyspigmentation. Many cases of mixed cryoglobulinemia are associated with hepatitis C infection; however, a variety of other infections, systemic diseases, or lymphoproliferative processes may also be associated.

HENOCH-SCHÖNLEIN PURPURA

Henoch-Schönlein purpura classically involves the skin (Figure 60.22), the joints, the gastrointestinal tract, and the kidneys.[76] Children between the ages of 3 and 10 years are most commonly affected. In one series, 82% of affected children had joint pain, 63% had abdominal pain, 33% had gastrointestinal bleeding, and 40% had nephritis.[77] In a cohort of 250 adults, 61% had arthritis, 48% had gastrointestinal involvement, and 32% had renal insufficiency (indicated by proteinuria or hematuria).[78]

Skin involvement is manifested as palpable purpura involving the lower extremities and occasionally the upper extremities, buttocks, and trunk. Biopsy specimens from skin lesions show leukocytoclastic vasculitis, and direct immunofluorescence testing may reveal deposits of IgA, and sometimes C3 and IgG, within vessel walls. The skin findings generally fade without treatment. Ankles and knees tend to be more painful than other joints. Pain, nausea, vomiting, melena, and hematochezia herald gastrointestinal involvement.

Kidney involvement may manifest only as microscopic hematuria and proteinuria, although some patients develop nephrotic syndrome. Renal involvement can be the most severe aspect of Henoch-Schönlein purpura.[77] In children, renal function generally returns to normal with treatment,[79] but in a cohort of 250 adults, 11% developed ESRD and another 27% developed chronic moderate to severe renal insufficiency.[78] A retrospective study of patients with Henoch-Schönlein purpura showed increased renal morbidity to be associated with nephrotic syndrome, decreased factor XIII levels, hypertension, and certain biopsy findings (crescents, mesangial macrophages, and tubulointerstitial disease). Kidney biopsy specimens generally show glomerulonephritis, often with IgA deposits in the mesangium and vessel walls.[80] The association of IgM deposition in the skin with renal involvement in adults is unclear.[81,82]

The pathogenesis of Henoch-Schönlein purpura is unknown. In one series, 62% of affected children had increased serum IgA levels.[77] Abnormal antigenic stimulation, possibly due to an infectious agent, may be a factor.[77] Elevated levels of vascular endothelial growth factor and endothelin have been reported,[83,84] as have decreased levels of factor XIII.[85] Abnormal cytokine levels (elevated tumor necrosis factor-α and interleukin-1β) have been described.[86] High titers of IgA anti–endothelial cell antibodies are seen in patients with more severe renal involvement.[87]

Most patients do not need treatment because the disease is self-limited. Joint pain may be ameliorated with analgesics. Severe gastrointestinal pain may benefit from systemic steroid treatment. Plasmapheresis and administration of steroids, intravenous immunoglobulin, and other immunosuppressants may decrease morbidity from renal involvement.[76,77]

GENODERMATOSES (Table 60.5)

Several genodermatoses have prominent skin and renal findings. In Birt-Hogg-Dubé syndrome,[88,89] patients have numerous flesh-colored to slightly tan, smooth papules

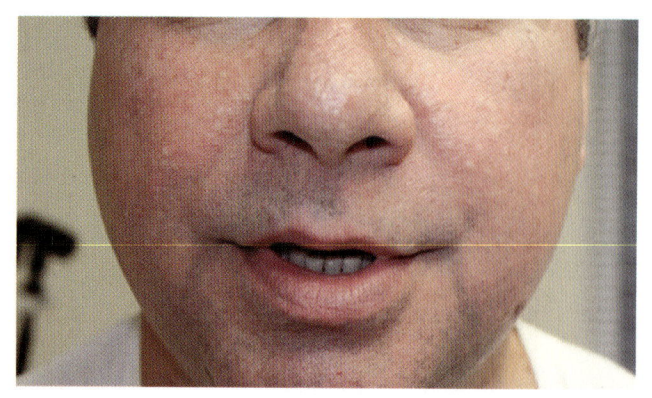

Figure 60.23 Birt-Hogg-Dubé syndrome. Multiple whitish smooth-surfaced papules (identified as fibrofolliculomas on biopsy) are present on the face. (Courtesy the Yale Residents' Collection.)

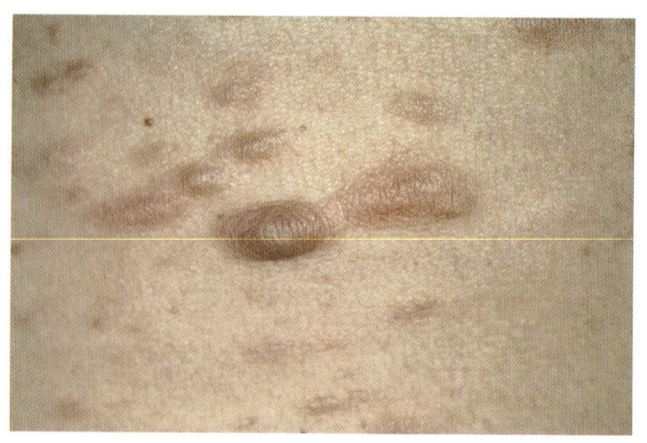

Figure 60.24 Multiple piloleiomyomas in a patient with Reed's syndrome. (Courtesy the Yale Residents' Collection.)

Table 60.5 Genodermatoses with Associated Skin and Kidney Tumors

Syndrome	Skin Findings	Renal Findings
Birt-Hogg-Dubé syndrome	Fibrofolliculoma Trichodiscoma Skin tag–like lesion	Renal cell carcinoma Cysts
Tuberous sclerosis	Adenoma sebaceum Cysts	Angiomyolipoma
Von Hippel–Lindau syndrome	Port-wine stain Cysts	Clear cell renal cell carcinoma
Muir-Torre syndrome	Sebaceous neoplasia	Genitourinary carcinoma, including renal
Hereditary leiomyomatosis and renal cell carcinoma syndrome	Leiomyoma	Carcinoma

on the face (Figure 60.23) that histopathologically are fibrofolliculomas or trichodiscomas. Skin tag–like lesions may also be seen in the axillary areas.[90] Angiofibromas and perifollicular fibromas are other potential cutaneous lesions.[91] This autosomal dominant disorder is associated with renal cell carcinoma (chromophobe, hybrid, oncocytic, and rarely clear cell types) and cysts, with a defect in folliculin, a product of the *BHD* gene on chromosome 17. Folliculin likely functions as a tumor suppressor, and haploinsufficiency may be sufficient to lead to skin tumor formation.[92] Other manifestations include spontaneous pneumothorax.

In tuberous sclerosis,[93] another autosomal dominant disorder that is sometimes sporadic, there are also numerous facial papules clustered in the nasolabial areas and over the nose—so-called adenoma sebaceum or angiofibromas. Lesions are erythematous and smooth and may resemble acne. These lesions have histopathologic features similar to those of fibrous papules of the nose, with dilated vessels, stellate fibroblasts, and onion-skin fibrosis around vessels and adnexal structures. Other skin findings include ash leaf–shaped hypopigmented macules and patches; small, hypopigmented macules in a confetti-like pattern in the axillary areas; and periungual fibromas. Renal angiomyolipomas, cysts, or carcinoma may be seen. Patients may also have seizures or mental retardation. Genetic mutations are found in tuberin and hamartin, tumor suppressor proteins.

In von Hippel–Lindau syndrome, port-wine stains of the skin (seen in a minority of patients) are associated with ocular, cerebellar, medullary, and spinal hemangioblastomas, clear cell renal cell carcinoma and cysts, pheochromocytoma, pancreatic tumors and cysts, and testicular cysts. The disease has an autosomal dominant inheritance pattern, and ocular evaluation should begin at birth. Neurologic, otologic, and endocrine evaluation with abdominal ultrasonographic screening may be initiated at age 8, or earlier if symptoms are present. The defective gene is *VHL*, a tumor suppressor gene on chromosome 3.[94] The VHL protein regulates hypoxia-inducible factors 1α and 2α, and dysregulation leads to vascular proliferation.

In hereditary leiomyomatosis and renal cell carcinoma syndrome, cutaneous (Figure 60.24) and uterine leiomyomas are associated with an aggressive renal cell carcinoma. Inheritance may be autosomal dominant, and mutations are in fumarate hydratase, a Krebs cycle enzyme that, when defective, may lead to dysregulation of the same hypoxia-inducible factors as in von Hippel–Lindau syndrome.[95]

In Fabry's disease,[96] numerous bright red, sometimes hyperkeratotic, papules are seen distributed in the bathing suit–trunk area. Such lesions may also be a manifestation of other genetic disorders such as fucosidosis and other lipid storage disorders. Histopathologically these lesions, termed *angiokeratomas,* are composed of dilated vessels that abut the undersurface of the epidermis. Other associated findings include paroxysmal pain, cornea verticillata, strokes, seizures, heart disorders, and chronic kidney failure. The defect is in α-galactosidase A, a product of the *GAL* gene on the X chromosome.

In Muir-Torre syndrome, multiple keratoacanthomas or a single sebaceous neoplasm (adenoma, carcinoma, or epithelioma) is associated with an internal malignancy. Most commonly, patients have a colorectal carcinoma, but carcinomas of the renal pelvis, ureter, and bladder are also associated. Muir-Torre syndrome is an autosomal dominant

Table 60.6	Dermatologic Conditions That May Later Involve the Kidneys

Impetigo/streptococcal skin infection
Metastatic melanoma

disorder with mutations described in *MSH2*, *MSH1*, and rarely *MSH6*.[97]

Alport's syndrome is the association of hematuric nephropathy, hearing defects, and ocular abnormalities. Although there are no skin findings, it is important to note that a simple skin biopsy can aid in the diagnosis. In Alport's syndrome there are mutations in the genes encoding type IV collagen. An absence of collagen IV may be seen in skin biopsy specimens from patients with X-linked Alport's syndrome.[98]

DERMATOLOGIC CONDITIONS THAT MAY LATER INVOLVE THE KIDNEYS (Table 60.6)

IMPETIGO/STREPTOCOCCAL SKIN INFECTION

Although poststreptococcal glomerulonephritis is more commonly associated with a preceding streptococcal pharyngitis, streptococcal skin infections can be the initiating event. The renal symptoms may present 2 to 3 weeks or more after the skin infection, by which time the skin findings have generally resolved.

Complete reference list available at ExpertConsult.com.

KEY REFERENCES

3. Zucker I, Yosipovitch G, David M, et al: Prevalence and characterization of uremic pruritus in patients undergoing hemodialysis: uremic pruritus is still a major problem for patients with end-stage renal disease. *J Am Acad Dermatol* 49:842–846, 2003.
4. Narita I, Alchi B, Omori K, et al: Etiology and prognostic significance of severe uremic pruritus in chronic hemodialysis patients. *Kidney Int* 69:1626–1632, 2006.
12. Etter L, Myers SA: Pruritus in systemic disease: mechanisms and management. *Dermatol Clin* 20:459–472, vi–vii, 2002.
13. Kimmel M, Alscher DM, Dunst R, et al: The role of microinflammation in the pathogenesis of uraemic pruritus in haemodialysis patients. *Nephrol Dial Transplant* 21:749–755, 2006.
14. Melo NC, Elias RM, Castro MC, et al: Pruritus in hemodialysis patients: the problem remains. *Hemodial Int* 13:38–42, 2009.
17. Peer G, Kivity S, Agami O, et al: Randomised crossover trial of naltrexone in uraemic pruritus. *Lancet* 348:1552–1554, 1996.
18. Pauli-Magnus C, Mikus G, Alscher DM, et al: Naltrexone does not relieve uremic pruritus: results of a randomized, double-blind, placebo-controlled crossover study. *J Am Soc Nephrol* 11:514–519, 2000.
19. Wikström B, Gellert R, Ladefoged SD, et al: Kappa-opioid system in uremic pruritus: multicenter, randomized, double-blind, placebo-controlled clinical studies. *J Am Soc Nephrol* 16:3742–3747, 2005.
20. Weisshaar E, Dunker N, Rohl FW, et al: Antipruritic effects of two different 5-HT3 receptor antagonists and an antihistamine in haemodialysis patients. *Exp Dermatol* 13:298–304, 2004.
21. Morton CA, Lafferty M, Hau C, et al: Pruritus and skin hydration during dialysis. *Nephrol Dial Transplant* 11:2031–2036, 1996.
22. De Marchi S, Cecchin E, Villalta D, et al: Relief of pruritus and decreases in plasma histamine concentrations during erythropoietin therapy in patients with uremia. *N Engl J Med* 326:969–974, 1992.
23. Young TA, Patel TS, Camacho F, et al: A pramoxine-based anti-itch lotion is more effective than a control lotion for the treatment of uremic pruritus in adult hemodialysis patients. *J Dermatol Treat* 20:76–81, 2009.
24. Tarng DC, Cho YL, Liu HN, et al: Hemodialysis-related pruritus: a double-blind, placebo-controlled, crossover study of capsaicin 0.025% cream. *Nephron* 72:617–622, 1996.
25. Gilchrest BA, Rowe JW, Brown RS, et al: Relief of uremic pruritus with ultraviolet phototherapy. *N Engl J Med* 297:136–138, 1977.
31. Patel TS, Freedman BI, Yosipovitch G: An update on pruritus associated with CKD. *Am J Kidney Dis* 50:11–20, 2007.
32. Jovanovic DB, Pejanovic S, Vukovic L, et al: Ten years' experience in subtotal parathyroidectomy of hemodialysis patients. *Ren Fail* 27:19–24, 2005.
33. Park TH, Park CH, Ha SK, et al: Dry skin (xerosis) in patients undergoing maintenance haemodialysis: the role of decreased sweating of the eccrine sweat gland. *Nephrol Dial Transplant* 10:2269–2273, 1995.
34. Lai CF, Kao TW, Tsai TF, et al: Quantitative comparison of skin colors in patients with ESRD undergoing different dialysis modalities. *Am J Kidney Dis* 48:292–300, 2006.
36. Hong SB, Park JH, Ihm CG, et al: Acquired perforating dermatosis in patients with chronic renal failure and diabetes mellitus. *J Korean Med Sci* 19:283–288, 2004.
39. Saray Y, Seckin D, Bilezikci B: Acquired perforating dermatosis: clinicopathological features in twenty-two cases. *J Eur Acad Dermatol Venereol* 20:679–688, 2006.
41. Fine A, Zacharias J: Calciphylaxis is usually non-ulcerating: risk factors, outcome and therapy. *Kidney Int* 61:2210–2217, 2002.
44. Kalajian AH, Malhotra PS, Callen JP, et al: Calciphylaxis with normal renal and parathyroid function: not as rare as previously believed. *Arch Dermatol* 145:451–458, 2009.
47. Weenig RH: Pathogenesis of calciphylaxis: Hans Selye to nuclear factor kappa-B. *J Am Acad Dermatol* 58:458–471, 2008.
54. Gafter U, Mamet R, Korzets A, et al: Bullous dermatosis of end-stage renal disease: a possible association between abnormal porphyrin metabolism and aluminium. *Nephrol Dial Transplant* 11:1787–1791, 1996.
55. Schanbacher CF, Vanness ER, Daoud MS, et al: Pseudoporphyria: a clinical and biochemical study of 20 patients. *Mayo Clin Proc* 76:488–492, 2001.
56. Tsimihodimos V, Dounousi E, Siamopoulos KC: Dyslipidemia in chronic kidney disease: an approach to pathogenesis and treatment. *Am J Nephrol* 28:958–973, 2008.
57. Goldblum OM, Kraus E, Bronner AK: Pseudo–Kaposi's sarcoma of the hand associated with an acquired, iatrogenic arteriovenous fistula. *Arch Dermatol* 121:1038–1040, 1985.
59. Cowper SE, Su LD, Bhawan J, et al: Nephrogenic fibrosing dermopathy. *Am J Dermatopathol* 23:383–393, 2001.
61. Grobner T: Gadolinium—a specific trigger for the development of nephrogenic fibrosing dermopathy and nephrogenic systemic fibrosis? *Nephrol Dial Transplant* 21(4):1104–1108, 2006.
62. Bucala R: Circulating fibrocytes: cellular basis for NSF. *J Am Coll Radiol* 5:36–39, 2008.
64. Girardi M, Kay J, Elston DM, et al: Nephrogenic systemic fibrosis: clinicopathologic definition and workup recommendations. *J Am Acad Dermatol* 65:1095–1106, 2011.
66. Kravetz JD, Heald P: Bilateral dialysis-associated steal syndrome. *J Am Acad Dermatol* 58:888–891, 2008.
69. Shimizu S, Yasui C, Yasukawa K, et al: Subcutaneous nodules on the buttocks as a manifestation of dialysis-related amyloidosis: a clinicopathological entity? *Br J Dermatol* 149:400–404, 2003.
71. Goh CL, Phay KL: Arterio-venous shunt dermatitis in chronic renal failure patients on maintenance haemodialysis. *Clin Exp Dermatol* 13:379–381, 1988.
72. Bagavant H, Fu SM: Pathogenesis of kidney disease in systemic lupus erythematosus. *Curr Opin Rheumatol* 21(5):489–494, 2009.
75. Ferri C: Mixed cryoglobulinemia. *Orphanet J Rare Dis* 3:25, 2008.
77. Saulsbury FT: Henoch-Schönlein purpura in children. Report of 100 patients and review of the literature. *Medicine (Baltimore)* 78:395–409, 1999.
78. Pillebout E, Thervet E, Hill G, et al: Henoch-Schönlein purpura in adults: outcome and prognostic factors. *J Am Soc Nephrol* 13:1271–1278, 2002.

80. Kawasaki Y, Suzuki J, Sakai N, et al: Clinical and pathological features of children with Henoch-Schoenlein purpura nephritis: risk factors associated with poor prognosis. *Clin Nephrol* 60:153–160, 2003.
88. Adley BP, Smith ND, Nayar R, et al: Birt-Hogg-Dubé syndrome: clinicopathologic findings and genetic alterations. *Arch Pathol Lab Med* 130:1865–1870, 2006.
91. Toro JR, Wei MH, Glenn GM, et al: BHD mutations, clinical and molecular genetic investigations of Birt-Hogg-Dubé syndrome: a new series of 50 families and a review of published reports. *J Med Genet* 45:321–331, 2008.
93. Rosser T, Panigrahy A, McClintock W: The diverse clinical manifestations of tuberous sclerosis complex: a review. *Semin Pediatr Neurol* 13:27–36, 2006.
94. Seizinger BR, Rouleau GA, Ozelius LJ, et al: Von Hippel–Lindau disease maps to the region of chromosome 3 associated with renal cell carcinoma. *Nature* 332:268–269, 1988.
95. Sudarshan S, Pinto PA, Neckers L, et al: Mechanisms of disease: hereditary leiomyomatosis and renal cell cancer—a distinct form of hereditary kidney cancer. *Nat Clin Pract Urol* 4:104–110, 2007.
96. Masson C, Cisse I, Simon V, et al: Fabry disease: a review. *Joint Bone Spine* 71:381–383, 2004.
97. Abbas O, Mahalingam M: Cutaneous sebaceous neoplasms as markers of Muir-Torre syndrome: a diagnostic algorithm. *J Cutan Pathol* 36(6):613–619, 2009.
98. Heidet L, Gubler MC: The renal lesions of Alport syndrome. *J Am Soc Nephrol* 20:1210–1215, 2009.

SECTION IX

CONSERVATIVE MANAGEMENT OF KIDNEY DISEASE

61 Dietary Approaches to Kidney Diseases

Denis Fouque | William E. Mitch

CHAPTER OUTLINE

JUSTIFICATION OF DIETARY SUPPORT DURING CHRONIC KIDNEY DISEASE, 1956
Dietary Influences of Protein on Kidney Function, 1958
Dietary Protein, Renal Inflammation, and Oxidant Stress, 1958
Responses of Kidney Function to Different Sources of Dietary Proteins, 1959
TURNOVER OF NITROGENOUS PRODUCTS IN CHRONIC UREMIA, 1959
Urea, 1959
Creatinine, 1961
Uric Acid, 1961
Ammonia, 1962
Other Nitrogenous Compounds in Urine, 1962
Fecal Nitrogen, 1962
Total Nonurea Nitrogen Excretion, 1962
Skin Nitrogen Losses, 1963
Other Middle Molecules and Gastrointestinal Microbiota, 1963
Summary, 1963
FACTORS INCREASING DIETARY PROTEIN REQUIREMENTS, 1963
Metabolic Acidosis, 1963
Ubiquitin-Proteasome System, 1964
Caspase-3 and Muscle Protein Losses, 1965
Signals Triggering Muscle Atrophy, 1965
External Losses of Protein, 1968
Altered Electrolyte Balance, 1968
Hyperparathyroidism, 1968
ASSESSMENT OF PROTEIN STORES IN CHRONIC KIDNEY DISEASE, 1968
Nitrogen Balance, 1968
Urea Nitrogen Appearance Rate, 1969
Serum Albumin and Malnutrition, 1969
Diet, Lipids, and Cardiovascular Risk, 1970
Serum Transferrin, Prealbumin, Complement, and Insulin-like Growth Factor-1, 1970
Anthropometrics, 1971
Early Initiation of Dialysis, 1971
Free Plasma Amino Acid and Ketoacid Levels, 1971
SPECIFIC DIETARY CONSTITUENTS AND KIDNEY DISEASE, 1973
Energy, 1973
Dietary Factors, 1974
Proteins, Phosphates, and Fiboblast Growth Factor-23, 1977
Randomized Controlled Trials, 1979
Meta-Analyses of Low-Protein Diets and Progression of Chronic Kidney Disease, 1981
Nutritional Impact and Safety of Modified Diets in Chronic Kidney Disease, 1982
Vitamins and Trace Elements in Uremia, 1983
CONCLUSION, 1984

JUSTIFICATION OF DIETARY SUPPORT DURING CHRONIC KIDNEY DISEASE

There is evidence from the United States, as well as the well-known increase in diabetes throughout the world, that the incidence of chronic kidney disease (CKD) continues to rise. What can be done about this frightening future and why are nutritional considerations so important for the management of patients with CKD? Obviously, if we do nothing, patients die or begin dialysis therapy. However, patients with CKD generally also have high blood pressure and inadequate treatment of hypertension, which can lead to diffuse vascular complications. Even if patients take the recommended first step in treating hypertension (i.e., diuretic therapy) but do not reduce their salt intake, the blood pressure–lowering effect of diuretics will be lost.[1] Patients with CKD accumulate waste products arising from the metabolism of protein, and these compounds exert toxic effects. This is relevant because it is well established that controlling protein intake will help reduce metabolic abnormalities.[2,3] Finally, it was reported that the beneficial influence of inhibiting the renin angiotensin aldosterone system (RAAS) on the progression of CKD is eliminated if intakes of phosphate and salt are unrestricted.[4,5] Again, successful treatment of CKD patients requires knowledge of dietary factors and controlling their excesses. The goal of this chapter is to provide the reader with an understanding of the metabolic aberrations associated with CKD and provide insights about how to manage these issues. We will provide the reader with concrete demonstrations that controlling protein intake is an effective step in treating problems associated with CKD.

There remains uncertainty about the influence of dietary modification on the progressive loss of kidney function that is characteristic of CKD.[6] However, arresting or slowing progression is not the sole reason to design and implement a practical and efficacious diet for patients with CKD. Other reasons include correcting acidosis, reducing the loss of protein stores, suppressing uremic bone disease, improving the treatment of hypertension, and reducing the accumulation of waste products derived from foods being eaten or arising from the breakdown of protein in muscle and other organs. In short, dietary modification may or may not slow the loss of the glomerular filtration rate (GFR) but designing a diet and providing instruction about dietary manipulation reduces the accumulation of waste products, which alone could delay the start of dialysis.

How does selective nutritional intervention affect health and disease? There are countries and regions of the world that have a long history of expertise in cuisine and a well-developed history of education about diet and its role in health and disease. In other countries, there is minimal attention to dietary education. For example, individuals in some countries manifest little interest in the control of accumulation of phosphates, which is paramount for the development of uremic bone disease, even though there has been a dramatic increase in phosphate additives to processed food over the past 10 years.[7-11] Similarly, there has been a lack of attention to the addition of sodium (salt) to foods, even though blood pressure in patients with CKD is poorly controlled and there are ongoing challenges in managing hypertension, despite the availability of a panoply of medications.[12] In addition, there is an undeniable link between the consumption of specific diets and mortality but limited attention to nutritional regimens that could protect patients. For example, the French paradox and the Mediterranean diet are among the dietary patterns demonstrated to exert positive nutritional benefits, yet these diets are understudied in terms of elucidating mechanisms that could positively affect the health of the population.[13] Other examples of a protective effect of diets include a limited but daily intake of certain wines and so-called anticancer nutrients. We do not know whether or how these factors lower the risk of mortality and whether this benefit will extend to patients with different types of diseases. Can we develop diets that take advantage of the mechanisms underlying these problems? For example, in patients with CKD, there is strong evidence that the excretion of uremic waste products is impaired and that these waste products accumulate, producing uremic symptoms. This problem can be addressed because high levels of these metabolic products are sharply reduced by simply limiting dietary protein. Even more easily understood are the beneficial effects of correcting metabolic acidosis. It arises because meat-rich diets generate acid, which is poorly excreted by the damaged kidney,

and it has been shown that simply correcting the serum bicarbonate level improves protein and calcium metabolism in patients with CKD; there is even evidence that reducing dietary acid generation slows the progression of CKD.[14-19] Therefore, attention to the diet of patients with CKD is not just an intellectual exercise but can produce rapid and sustained benefits for patients as long as attention is taken to ensure overall adequacy of the diet.[20]

As an example of the importance of dietary manipulation, consider the Mediterranean diet. This diet is rich in fruit, vegetables, fish, and olive oil and includes limited red wine consumption with meals. The diet is also low in red meat and animal fat; its benefits include reduced susceptibility to cardiovascular disease (CVD), with increased longevity. There is now accumulating evidence that this diet might be involved in producing other protective actions. For example, despite marked differences in dietary preferences in countries such as those in Latin America, China, and India, meat consumption has been associated with a higher risk of dementia, and substituting fish for meat in the diet may prevent dementia.[21] In addition to meat, the Mediterranean diet possesses antiinflammatory properties that could be of value for patients with diabetes and/or obesity.[22] For example, olive oil consumption is associated with a reduction in the carotid artery intima-media thickness that carries a high risk of developing CVD, in part because the diet reduces levels of C-reactive protein and oxidized low-density lipoprotein (LDL) cholesterol.[23,24] In fact, a systematic review of more than 500,000 adults has shown that adherence to a Mediterranean diet reduces overall mortality by 9%, cardiovascular mortality by 9%, mortality from cancer by 6%, and Parkinson's and Alzheimer's diseases by 13%.[25] Positive benefits also occur with an increased intake of fish. He and colleagues have reported that for each increase in fish intake of 20 g/day, there is a 7% reduction in the risk of cardiovascular mortality.[26] In contrast, an increase in red meat and/or processed meat consumption in the United States is associated with an increase in overall mortality, including a rise in the mortality from cancer and/or CVD by 10% to 30% (comparing the lowest with the highest quintile of meat intake).[27-29] In an analysis of the Nurse's Health Study in the United States, patients who had preexisting CVD and were switched to a Mediterranean-style diet had lower all-cause mortality.[28] Similar beneficial effects have been reported from results obtained from a Swedish cohort of older men: eating a Mediterranean-style diet was associated with a lower likelihood of developing CKD and, for patients with preexisting CKD, survival was enhanced.[29] Together, these findings demonstrate how important nutrient choices can be in terms of improvement in the health of patients with and without CKD. In this chapter, we will address how a specialized renal diet may protect patients with CKD from the consequences of metabolic abnormalities and progressive loss of kidney function. We also will address methods of monitoring compliance and safety of the diets.

The need to manipulate the diet and the approaches used to accomplish this goal will depend on the patient's level of renal insufficiency or CKD stage. This raises the question of how to measure or assess the degree of CKD. The most widely used classification was developed by the National Kidney Foundation (NKF) Kidney Disease

Table 61.1	Stages of Kidney Dysfunction	
CKD Stage	Description	GFR (mL/min/1.73 m²)
1	Kidney damage (e.g., albuminuria) with normal or increased GFR	≥90
2	Kidney damage (e.g., albuminuria) with mildly reduced GFR	60-89
3	Moderately reduced GFR	30-59
4	Severely reduced GFR	15-29
5	Kidney failure	<15

CKD, Chronic kidney disease; GFR, glomerular filtration rate.
Adapted from National Kidney Foundation: K/DOQI clinical practice guidelines for chronic kidney disease: evaluation, classification, and stratification. Am J Kidney Dis 39(Suppl 1):S1-S266, 2002.

Outcomes Quality Initiative (KDOQI) Committee (Table 61.1). Notably, even individuals who have a low risk of developing progressive CKD can develop some of its complications.[30] Baseline results from the multicenter Modification of Diet in Renal Disease (MDRD) study were reviewed to develop a method of assessing the degree of kidney damage in patients with CKD. First, kidney damage was defined as persistent abnormal albuminuria on two occasions; second, it became necessary to measure GFR or estimate it from equations based on results of the MDRD study or derived from creatinine or even cystatin C.[31,32] The variables used to estimate GFR are based on equations that account for differences in measured GFR by age, serum creatinine, gender, and race, but the accuracy of this method improves sharply when the estimated GFR (eGFR) is less than 60 mL/min/1.73 m².[32] While this staging approach is useful, it has several limitations. First, the equation was derived from individuals in the United States with established kidney disease, so it might not apply to patients in other regions of the world. For example, it was shown to be inaccurate when Chinese patients were examined.[33,34] Second, the accuracy of the MDRD equation is poor for eGFR values of 60 mL/min/1.73 m² or higher. Third, the boundaries for the stages of CKD in the categories are somewhat arbitrary. Like other continuous biologic functions, such as blood pressure, there is no absolute threshold. Fourth, certain treatments may acutely reduce the eGFR (e.g., starting a diuretic to treat hypertension), yielding an inaccurate determinant of the stage of CKD for the patient, even though there has been no long-term damage to the kidney. Nonetheless, the NKF KDOQI classification system is easy to use and should help identify individuals for whom interventions, including dietary modification, might lead to an improvement in their overall health outcomes.

DIETARY INFLUENCES OF PROTEIN ON KIDNEY FUNCTION

There is ample evidence that increasing protein intake or amino acid infusion alters renal hemodynamics, which could impair kidney function in animals with experimental kidney disease.[35-39] Hemodynamic responses to changes in dietary protein have been attributed to a number of mechanisms that increase GFR, induce and/or increase proteinuria, and lead to glomerulosclerosis and renal insufficiency. Among the potential determinants involved are hormones (e.g., glucagon, insulin, insulin-like growth factor-1, angiotensin II [Ang II]), cytokines (e.g., prostaglandins), and kinins.[40-43] Intrarenal sodium transport may also be involved via the proximal Na–amino acid cotransporter; the activity of this transporter is enhanced in response to increases in filtered amino acids, and this stimulates tubuloglomerular feedback, with an increase in GFR.[44] Alternatively, dietary protein restriction in rats reduces or corrects many of the changes in glomerular hemodynamics observed after 5/6 nephrectomy.[45] This is relevant because micropuncture studies have provided evidence that the increase in the single-nephron glomerular filtration rate and increase in glomerular capillary and transcapillary pressures found with CKD explain the acceleration of the glomerular lesion.[45] Studies in rats with smaller degrees of renal ablation have shown that a low-protein diet consistently reduces hyperfiltration and delays the onset of proteinuria and glomerular fibrosis.[38,46] The proposed mechanism for this response is that a diet with only 6% protein reduces glomerular hypertension via constriction of the afferent arteriole, resulting in decreased glomerular plasma flow and the degree of proteinuria.

DIETARY PROTEIN, RENAL INFLAMMATION, AND OXIDANT STRESS

Protein intake and protein trafficking through the kidney cause hypermetabolism and oxidant stress.[47,48] Dietary restriction to 12% protein decreases oxygen consumption and ammonia production by about 50% compared to a diet consisting of 40% protein.[48,49] This response has been attributed to a decrease in net sodium reabsorption. In the kidney, a low-protein diet has the potential to exert an antifibrotic effect. For example, Nakayama and associates have reported that the expression of fibronectin and transforming growth factor-β (TGF-β) in the kidneys of adriamycin-treated rats is dramatically reduced when the diet is 6% protein compared to results from littermate rats eating the standard 20% protein diet.[50]

TGF-β, a potent profibrotic agent, is decreased by feeding a low-protein diet. In addition, it was reported that an L-arginine supplement augmented the propensity of a low-protein diet (6%) to reduce the glomerular expression of TGF-β, fibronectin, and plasminogen activator inhibitor 1 (PAI-1) in a model of immune glomerulonephritis.[51] Notably, this response occurred independently of nitric oxide metabolism. Moreover, maximal Ang II blockade with angiotensin-converting enzyme inhibitors (ACEIs) or Ang II receptor antagonists caused only a 45% decrease in TGF-β gene expression and urinary protein, while a low-protein diet caused a further 20% reduction in TGF-β expression and production.[51] There was a similar decrease in fibronectin and PAI-1 expression and activation. Thus, a reduction in profibrotic mediators is associated with a concomitant decrease in proteinuria.

Tovar-Palacio and coworkers studied obese Zucker rats to determine the effects of different amounts and types of protein intake on kidney function.[52] For 2 months, rats with normal kidney function were fed casein or soy protein in amounts of 20%, 30%, or 45% of their food intake. Urine excretion of hydrogen peroxide, a marker of oxidative stress, increased parallel to increases in protein intake. For the same amount of dietary protein, changes in kidney function were consistently lower with vegetable sources of protein versus animal-derived dietary proteins. Proteinuria was lowest in the 20% soy protein diet, and renal expression of genes involved in inflammation (e.g., interleukin-6 [IL-6], tumor necrosis factor-α [TNF-α]), lipid metabolism (e.g., sterol regulatory element–binding protein-1 [SREBP-1], fatty acid synthase [FAS]), matrix accumulation (e.g., type IV collagen), and fibrosis (e.g., transforming growth factor-β [TGF-β]) were at the lowest level with the 20% soy diet and highest in the 45% casein diet. These results strongly support the deleterious effects of a high casein intake and a nephroprotective impact occurring in response to low dietary protein from vegetable sources.[52]

RESPONSES OF KIDNEY FUNCTION TO DIFFERENT SOURCES OF DIETARY PROTEINS

Based on the observation that vegetarians have lower GFRs than omnivores, Margetts, Wiseman, and Williams and colleagues tested different sources of protein of animal or vegetable origin (casein or soy) in rats with stable kidney function.[53-55] Both regular (24%) and moderately low (12%) protein intakes of each protein source was studied. After 3 months, glomerulosclerosis and tubular dilation were found to be significantly more pronounced in the casein- versus the soya-fed rats. The degree of proteinuria was greatest with the 24% and 12% casein diets but lower in the 24% soya group and lowest in the 12% soya-fed rats. There were no significant differences in the severity of the proteinuria or histologic lesions in the 24% versus the 12% soya groups.[55] Although these results are convincing, there are differences in the digestibility of protein, making it possible that the absorption of vegetable proteins was simply less (≈10% lower) in rats fed that diet. This would reduce the true amount of protein compared with the results with the casein-based diets. Digestibility and fiber content from vegetarian diets in humans may also change phosphorus absorption, phosphorus excretion, and serum levels of fibroblast growth factor 23 (FGF-23), factors that may cause renal impairment, as shown by Moe and associates.[56] This is also relevant to problems of patients with CKD because the fiber content of the diet may be related to systemic inflammation. Participants in the National Health and Nutrition Evaluation Survey III (NHANES III) with CKD were found to have a high intake of dietary fiber and, importantly, a reduction in all-cause mortality.[57]

TURNOVER OF NITROGENOUS PRODUCTS IN CHRONIC UREMIA

By definition, adults in neutral protein balance have equal rates of protein synthesis and protein degradation, while growing children have a positive protein balance, so their protein synthesis exceeds protein degradation. Nitrogen balance therefore provides information about protein metabolism throughout the body. It is calculated as the difference between the intake and excretion of nitrogen in subjects with normal kidney function. In patients with CKD, however, the accumulation of nitrogen-containing products in body fluids must also be measured. These products are not converted into proteins but can accumulate in the body, causing uremic symptoms, a conclusion supported by the observation that reducing waste product accumulation by restricting dietary protein or by dialysis results in symptomatic improvement.[58] Thus, CKD is a state of protein intolerance because symptom-producing waste products are generated by the catabolism of dietary protein and/or body protein stores.

UREA

Urea is the major waste product accumulating in patients with CKD.[59] Once produced, urea (or other waste products) has three fates—it is excreted, it accumulates in body fluids, or it is degraded. Since protein intake is directly and closely correlated with the production of urea, the severity of uremia can be estimated from the steady-state serum concentration of urea nitrogen (BUN [blood urea nitrogen]).[60] BUN is calculated by rearranging the clearance formula in the following fashion. The production of urea minus its degradation yields the steady-state BUN when the difference is divided by the urea clearance.[61] Alternatively, the steady-state BUN can be estimated from dietary protein. This is possible because protein is 16% nitrogen (average value). If the nonurea nitrogen (0.031 g N/kg/day) is subtracted from dietary nitrogen, the difference, divided by urea clearance, yields the steady-state BUN.[61] The calculation assumes that urea clearance is independent of the plasma concentration, which is a reasonable assumption for CKD.

The steady-state BUN is useful because it expresses the severity of impaired kidney function in terms of accumulated nitrogenous waste products. The key concept is that the steady-state concentration in blood of any nitrogen-containing waste product (derived from dietary protein or protein catabolism) will increase in parallel to the increase in BUN.[59,61-63] Since urea nitrogen excretion by normal persons varies directly with protein intake, the net production of urea or the urea appearance rate is the principal quantity to consider when prescribing a diet for patients with CKD (Figure 61.1). In this figure, nitrogen balance and urinary urea are presented as functions of nitrogen intake in patients with CKD fed varying quantities of dietary protein, from about 12 to 90 g protein/day. Patients who were fed less than 4 g of nitrogen/day were determined as being in neutral or negative nitrogen balance. In patients fed more than 4 g of nitrogen/day, the steady-state urea nitrogen excretion is equal to the increment in nitrogen intake above the amount required to achieve neutral nitrogen balance.

Urea appearance is calculated as the sum of urea excreted and accumulated.[59,61-63] It provides a method for estimating the intake of nitrogen (principally protein) in persons with or without kidney disease. For patients undergoing dialysis, urea turnover has been labelled as urea generation or protein catabolic rate (PCR).[64] It is calculated as the sum of urea excreted and removed by dialysis plus changes in the body pool of urea. These factors are similar to those of the

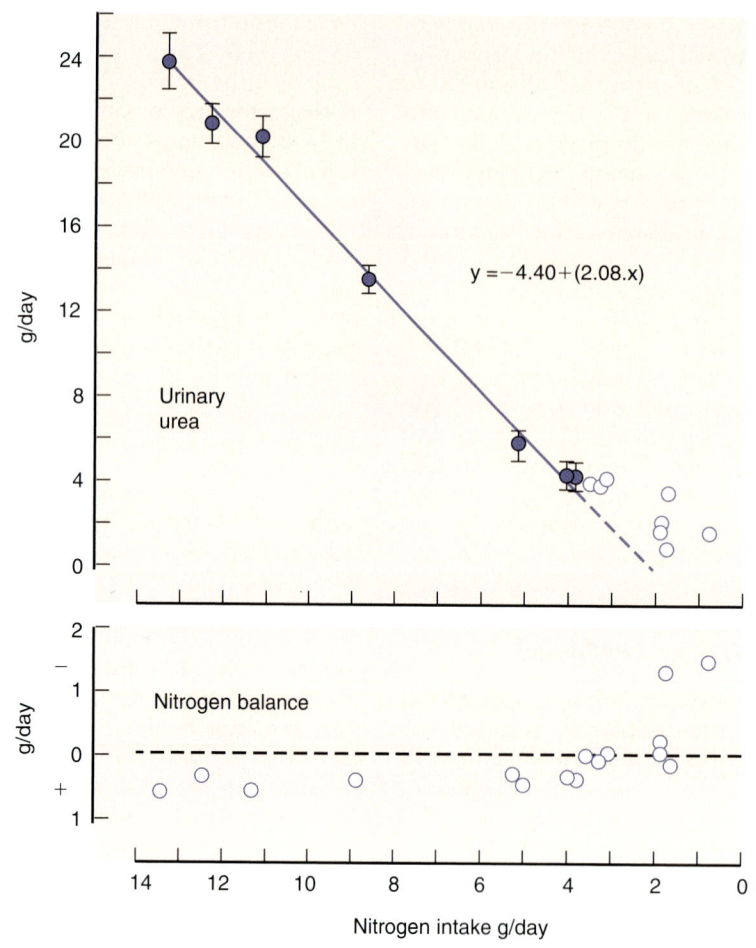

Figure 61.1 Nitrogen balance and urinary urea as a function of nitrogen intake in chronically uremic subjects fed varying quantities of dietary protein. All subjects receiving less than 4 g of nitrogen/day were in neutral or negative nitrogen balance, and urea excretion tends to plateau at a low value. In subjects receiving more than 4 g of nitrogen/day, the steady-state urea nitrogen excretion is equal to the increment in nitrogen intake above the amount required to achieve neutral nitrogen balance. (From Cottini EP, Gallina DK, Dominguez JM: Urea excretion in adult humans with varying degrees of kidney malfunction fed milk, egg, or an amino acid mixture: assessment of nitrogen balance. *J Nutr* 102:11-10, 1973.)

urea appearance rate. The protein catabolic rate is a misleading term, however, because the rate of protein catabolism is far greater than the urea appearance rate. Specifically, the daily processes of protein synthesis and degradation in cells amounts to 45 to 55 g of nitrogen/day.[65,66] This amount of protein is equivalent to the synthesis and degradation of 280 to 350 g/day of protein or more than 1 kg of muscle (muscle is assumed to be 20% protein). Thus, PCR does not measure whole-body protein catabolism, even though the principle of conservation of mass indicates that the nitrogen arising from dietary nitrogen plus the difference between whole-body protein synthesis and degradation yields the amount of waste nitrogen produced each day. In addition to protein in the diet, factors influencing urea metabolism include volume depletion with diuretics, which produces passive reabsorption of urea.[67] Second, sodium depletion causes urea appearance to rise in animals and humans.[67,68] The mechanism for stimulation of urea production with sodium depletion is unknown but apparently it does not require glucocorticoids.[68]

UREA PRODUCTION AND DEGRADATION

Accurate rates of urea production and degradation require measurement of the plasma disappearance of ^{14}C- or ^{15}N-urea. With these techniques, the rate of urea production exceeds the steady-state rate of urea excretion in normal and uremic subjects. The difference is due to degradation of urea by bacterial ureases in the gastrointestinal tract.[69] Interestingly, the rate of urea degradation in normal adults eating a diet of about 90 g protein/day averages 3.6 g/day of nitrogen, a value similar to that in patients with CKD. Another means of evaluating urea degradation is to express it as extrarenal urea clearance, which is calculated as the rate of urea degradation divided by the plasma concentration of urea. Notably, for normal adults, the extrarenal urea clearance averages about 24 L/day.[69,70] If the same value of clearance were present in patients with a high BUN, the amount of ammonia derived from urea production would be very high. High values of ammonia do not occur in CKD (see below).[71] This means that the extrarenal clearance of urea in patients with CKD must be greatly reduced. For example, in patients being treated with low-protein diets supplemented with amino acids or their α-keto or α-hydroxy analogues, the extrarenal clearance averages less than 4 L/day.[71,72] Since the amount of nitrogen available from urea degradation is not large, chronic uremia presumably changes the gut mucosa and limits access of urea to the bacterial ureases. It remains possible that a rapid elevation of plasma urea, as occurs in patients with acute kidney failure, might increase the rate of urea degradation.

CREATININE

Creatinine is formed by a nonenzymatic process that dehydrates creatine and creatine phosphate to form creatinine. The major pool of creatine and creatine phosphate is in muscle, and it is large because creatine is accumulated intracellularly by an active transport system. Since creatinine production is a nonenzymatic process, the turnover rate of the creatine pool is only 1.7%/day. Practically, this means that a change in the rate of creatinine production does not reach a new steady state for 41 days.[73,74] The slowness of the turnover of the creatine–creatine phosphate is a major reason why the 24-hour creatinine excretion rate serves as an index of lean body mass. For unknown reasons, however, the rate of creatinine excretion is highly variable. For example, it was necessary to obtain three consecutive 24-hour collections of urine for measuring creatinine excretion before a reliable estimate of lean body mass was obtained.[75-77] Another reason for the variation in calculation of lean body mass by creatinine excretion is that meat in the diet changes creatinine excretion: with creatine-free diets, creatinine excretion falls about 15%.[77] Interestingly, creatinine excretion does not decrease even more than 15% with meat-free diets because creatine production is stimulated by diets that are low in creatine content.[78]

In addition to dietary creatine-creatinine and variations in lean body mass, age is an important factor affecting creatinine excretion in normal adults.[79] In order of descending importance, the relationship between age and creatinine excretion results from reduced lean body mass and muscle as a fraction of weight (aging is associated with increased body fat) and from a decrease in meat intake with aging.[77] Notably, patients with advanced CKD have a creatinine excretion rate that is lower than predicted by changes in their lean body mass. This deficit is caused by creatinine degradation.[74,80,81] However, this ignores creatinine degradation and, when the rate of creatinine production was formally measured in patients with CKD, it was found to be virtually the same as that predicted for normal subjects of the same age, gender, and weight.[80] Thus, the difference between normal creatinine production and decreased creatinine excretion is due to degradation of creatinine.

Definitive evidence for creatinine degradation was reported by Jones and Burnett, who measured the disappearance of ^{14}C-labeled creatinine in uremic patients.[82] They detected radioactivity in products of creatinine metabolism, including sarcosine (N-methylglycine), N-methylhydantoin, creatine, and carbon dioxide. The breakdown of creatinine is most likely due to its degradation by intestinal bacteria since it has been demonstrated that flora obtained from the intestines of normal subjects or patients with CKD readily degrade creatinine.[83] We measured creatinine metabolism in uremic subjects given oral antibiotics and found no suppression of creatinine degradation.[80] Thus, the site of creatinine degradation is controversial.[80]

There is evidence that creatinine degradation is correlated with serum creatinine levels. In fact, in patients with CKD, we found that creatinine degradation, like that of urea, was directly correlated with serum creatinine and creatinine production.[80] Notably, the rate of extrarenal creatinine clearance we measured averaged only 0.039 L/kg/day, explaining why creatinine metabolism becomes clinically important only when the serum creatinine concentration is high. A low extrarenal clearance also could explain why creatinine degradation has not been detected in humans or animals with normal serum creatinine levels and creatinine clearance values.

Physiologically, the finding that creatinine is degraded, and that there is a decline in creatinine excretion in patients with CKD, means that creatinine excretion is not a reliable index of lean body mass in patients with CKD. The slow turnover rate has another physiologically important consequence. It means that conclusions about the influence of the diet on changes in progression of CKD are invalid when they are based on serum creatinine concentration unless at least 4 months (three half-lives of creatine turnover) have elapsed following changes in dietary protein.[84]

URIC ACID

The fractional clearance of uric acid rises markedly at GFR values below 15 mL/min/1.73 m^2 because there is increased secretion and reduced reabsorption of urate.[85] In addition to this adaptation, the steady-state level of uric acid excretion by patients with advanced CKD falls to about 100 to 300 mg/day (normal rate, 400 to 600 mg/day). If production is constant, this finding should be accompanied by a major increase in the serum uric acid level. However, a serum uric acid level above 10 mg/dL is unusual in patients with CKD and, as with urea and creatinine, the explanation for these findings is that there is extrarenal degradation of uric acid.[86]

For example, Sorensen[87] has reported results of uric acid turnover experiments following intravenous injection of radiolabelled uric acid. It was calculated that extrarenal urate clearance accounts for as much as 65% of uric acid produced by patients with renal insufficiency. Intestinal bacteria are probably responsible for uric acid degradation because the fraction of urate degraded was reduced from 22% to 3% in patients given oral doses of neomycin and streptomycin.[87] Since many compounds are produced during uric acid degradation (e.g., ammonia, urea, allantoin), extrarenal clearance of urate or other compounds does not eliminate nitrogen but simply results in the accumulation of other compounds.[88] Degradation of urate, however, does contribute to the fact that there is a low incidence of gouty arthritis or nephropathy (defined as urate deposits surrounded by inflammatory cells and fibrous tissue) in the kidneys of patients with CKD. These deposits are mainly found in the renal medulla of patients with long-standing CKD. There is inferential evidence that a high uric acid concentration contributes to a progressive loss of kidney function, mainly based on experimental studies in rodents.[89] However, the efficacy of long-term allopurinol therapy as a method of slowing the progression of CKD in patients with hyperuricemia is still unsettled. Early studies found no benefit while other studies observed slower progression with the administration of allopurinol.[90,91] This finding might be linked to a pathogenic role of uric acid in producing vascular disease.[92]

Johnson and coworkers[92] have report that humans have a higher serum uric acid concentration than other animals because people have a null mutation in the uricase gene (uricase initiates uric acid degradation). Experimentally, the investigators demonstrated that a higher uric acid level is associated with the development of hypertension of the salt-sensitive type and that it leads to vascular disease.[93,94] When the investigators treated rats with oxonic acid, which blocked uricase activity, the serum uric acid level increased to about 2 mg/dL, and the rats developed progressive renal insufficiency, which was linked to the development of glomerular hypertrophy and pathologic changes in arterioles of the kidney. These pathologic changes were substantially ameliorated by the administration of allopurinol or treatment with a uricosuric diuretic. From these results, it is interesting to note that Fessel eliminated patients with severe hypertension when he analyzed the effects of high levels of uric acid.[95] In the remaining subjects, the clinical course of 113 patients with asymptomatic hyperuricemia and 168 patients with gout were examined, some of whom had mild renal insufficiency. Only when the serum uric acid level exceeded 10 mg/dL in women or 13 mg/dL in men was there a loss of residual kidney function. It is still undetermined whether patients with hypertension develop vascular damage and progressive CKD because of a hyperuricemia or whether hypertension or CKD causes hyperuricemia. A recent meta-analysis of 11 randomized controlled trials, with a total of 753 patients with hyperuricemia, led the investigators to conclude that lowering serum uric acid levels by prescribing benzbromarone, losartan, allopurinol, febuxostat, rasburicase, or pegloticase is associated with a decrease in serum creatinine levels or other measures of improved renal function. Consequently, the potential for a beneficial influence of treating hyperuricemia in patients with CKD will have to be confirmed in adequately powered, randomized controlled trials (RCTs).[96]

Other problems associated with hyperuricemia are relatively uncommon in patients with CKD. For example, uric acid stones occurred in only 1.0% to 2.6% of 113 patients with normal kidney function, despite asymptomatic hyperuricemia during at least 8 years.[95] Based on these data, the widespread use of allopurinol cannot be recommended until more data have demonstrated that treatment with allopurinol slows the progression of CKD.

AMMONIA

The loss of renal mass reduces the capacity to excrete ammonia, even in response to metabolic acidosis (see Chapter 17). A major source of blood ammonia is the bacterial degradation of urea, amino acids, peptides, and protein in the intestine; there also is conversion of glutamine to ammonia in small intestinal mucosal cells. Fortunately, the intestine-derived ammonia is readily converted to urea in the liver, so blood ammonia levels in patients with CKD should be normal. Occasionally, a slightly high blood level of ammonia has been reported, but the mechanism for this finding and its clinical importance are unknown.[97] Isolated cases of hyperammonemia occurring in patients with CKD and apparently normal liver function could result from problems such as partial defects in urea cycle enzymes or other inherited disorders, high-dose chemotherapy, infections, or abscesses.[98,99] Fortunately, these metabolic disorders are unusual.

OTHER NITROGENOUS COMPOUNDS IN URINE

The difference between total urinary nitrogen and urea nitrogen in urine is termed *nonurea nitrogen*, and it includes the nitrogen in uric acid, peptides, protein, and creatinine.[61,63] In patients with proteinuria, albumin clearance expressed as a fraction of GFR varies from 0.3% to 3.0% or more and, in general, protein clearance falls as GFR decreases, but other factors can change this ratio (e.g., glomerular damage).[100-102] For example, raising dietary protein intake tends to increase proteinuria in patients with nephrotic syndrome, while dietary protein restriction reduces proteinuria.[101,103-106] Drugs also affect the degree of proteinuria; proteinuria generally falls when blood pressure is reduced, especially with ACEIs or angiotensin receptor blockers.[104-112]

FECAL NITROGEN

Patients with CKD frequently develop occult intestinal blood loss; in one study, it averaged 6 mL/day, and values this low may be difficult to detect by guaiac testing.[113] Other causes for a change in fecal nitrogen in normal adults include variations in dietary roughage, fermentable carbohydrates, and nitrogen.[61,114,115] Maroni and colleagues made extensive measurements and concluded that fecal nitrogen varies with body weight but not with protein intake.[61] Masud and associates reported on 52 adult patients with CKD who were not being dialyzed and were eating various diets.[63] In these patients, there was no relationship between dietary nitrogen and fecal nitrogen excretion.

TOTAL NONUREA NITROGEN EXCRETION

Nonurea nitrogen excretion consists of the nitrogen in feces plus all other forms of nitrogen excreted in urine except urea (e.g., urinary creatinine, uric acid, ammonium, peptides). Maroni and coworkers measured the average nonurea nitrogen excretion of 19 patients with CKD who were in neutral or nearly neutral nitrogen balance.[61] These patients were eating diets with as much as 94 g protein/day or low-protein diets supplemented with ketoacids. Despite the wide range of dietary protein intake, nonurea nitrogen was related to body weight (BW), averaging 0.031 g/kg/day of nitrogen. Using this value, Maroni and colleagues found that the estimated nitrogen balance did not differ statistically from the measured nitrogen balance. Interestingly, 0.031 g/kg/day of nitrogen (Figure 61.2) is similar to the value for nonurea urinary nitrogen plus fecal nitrogen excreted by normal subjects or patients on dialysis. Thus, the major factor for planning the protein content of dietary therapy is the urea nitrogen. Protein intake can be estimated as the sum of urea nitrogen appearance (see below) plus the estimated nonurea nitrogen excretion of 0.031 g nitrogen/kg BW/day.[61]

The relationships among dietary protein, urea nitrogen appearance, and nonurea nitrogen can be used to assess adherence to the amount of prescribed dietary protein. Kopple and associates have reported that fecal nitrogen is

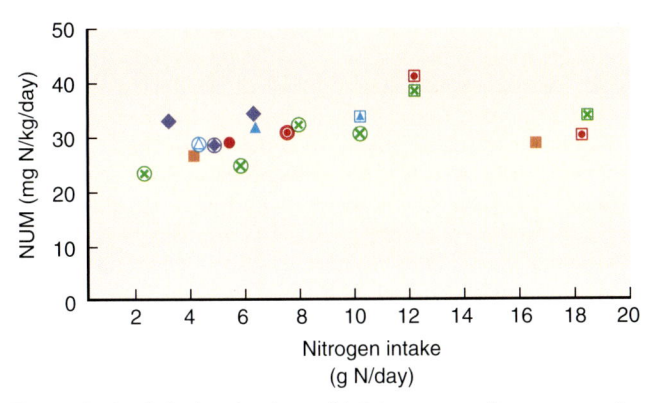

Figure 61.2 Calculated values of total nonurea nitrogen excretion (NUN) in normal subjects (▲, ●, ■) and patients with chronic renal failure being treated with nutritional therapy (◆, ⊗, ◉) or by hemodialysis or continuous ambulatory peritoneal dialysis (☒). (From Maroni BJ, Steinman TI, Mitch WE: A method for estimating nitrogen intake of patients with chronic renal failure. *Kidney Int* 27:58-65, 1985.)

directly correlated with nitrogen intake, but also noted that total nonurea nitrogen excretion does not increase with higher dietary protein intake or BW.[62] They concluded that nonurea nitrogen excretion was roughly the same for all persons and proposed an equation for dietary protein equal to 1.204 times the urea appearance value plus 1.74 g nitrogen/day. We examined 80 nitrogen balance measurements performed on 52 patients with CKD while the patients were ingesting varying levels of dietary protein.[61,63] Neither fecal nitrogen nor nonurea nitrogen was associated with nitrogen intake, and nonurea nitrogen excretion averaged 0.031 g nitrogen/kg BW/day. The formulas of Kopple's group were similar to Maroni and coworkers' method, exhibiting a somewhat lower error in documenting protein intake.[61-63] Importantly, estimates of protein intake are based on the assumption that the patient is in neutral nitrogen balance—that is, nitrogen excretion equals nitrogen intake. In patients who are highly catabolic or are receiving intravenous hyperalimentation or totally digestible diets, the estimates of nonurea nitrogen excretion are incorrect, and the method only yields estimates of protein intake.[116]

SKIN NITROGEN LOSSES

In otherwise normal adults, the average loss of nitrogen from skin and other unmeasured sources averages 0.5 g nitrogen/day. This amount should be used when calculating nitrogen balance. In addition, the concentration of urea in sweat is proportional to the plasma urea concentration, so there can be increased nitrogen losses in uremic patients who perspire heavily.

OTHER MIDDLE MOLECULES AND GASTROINTESTINAL MICROBIOTA

A product of the metabolism of the amino acid tyrosine by gut bacteria, *p*-cresol, is rapidly absorbed, leading to conjugation with sulfates to form *p*-cresyl sulfate (PCS). Unfortunately, this compound cannot be eliminated by the failing kidney, resulting in excessive accumulation of PCS. Among the metabolic consequences of PCS accumulation is insulin resistance, which has been documented in adipocyte cultures exposed to PCS and in normal rats injected with PCS to reach levels at roughly the concentration found in patients with CKD.[117] Introduction of a low-protein diet or possibly changing the intestinal flora with probiotics could reduce PCS generation, thus improving insulin resistance.

SUMMARY

Nitrogen excretion by normal or uremic subjects can be categorized as urea nitrogen appearance plus all other forms of nitrogen, known as nonurea nitrogen. The production of urea nitrogen is closely related to protein intake while the excretion of nonurea nitrogen is related to body weight. These categories of nitrogen excretion can be used to estimate dietary protein intake, with the caveats that the patient should be in neutral or in near-neutral nitrogen balance and not receiving intravenous hyperalimentation.

FACTORS INCREASING DIETARY PROTEIN REQUIREMENTS

METABOLIC ACIDOSIS

Metabolic acidosis exerts adverse metabolic responses and may even affect the progression of CKD.[19,118-120] Acidosis stimulates the catabolism of amino acids and protein in normal adults as well as in patients with CKD and aggravates bone disease. The adverse responses to metabolic acidosis are relevant because they block the ability of normal adults or patients with CKD to adapt successfully to a decrease in protein intake, resulting in a loss of protein stores. The activating mechanism involves stimulation of cellular signaling pathways, which increases the activity of branched-chain ketoacid dehydrogenase and the ubiquitin-proteasome system (UPS) in muscle. Acidosis not only increases the activity of both pathways but also stimulates transcription of the genes encoding components of the pathways. There is evidence that eliminating these responses will benefit the nutritional status of the patient with CKD in the following manner: (1) when the acidosis of CKD is corrected, there is decreased elimination of branched-chain amino acids and they are used in protein synthesis and other metabolic pathways[121,122]; (2) correction of metabolic acidosis in patients with CKD or patients being treated by dialysis also decreases the degradation of proteins, thus preserving muscle protein.[14,123,124] The most persuasive proofs of a benefit for correcting acidosis included results of a randomized, yearlong clinical trial of eliminating acidosis in patients treated with continuous ambulatory peritoneal dialysis (CAPD); patients experienced significant weight gain and an increase in muscle mass.[125] Using a similar design in a study of shorter duration, correction of acidosis was shown to increase levels of mRNA encoding ubiquitin in muscle, consistent with activity of the UPS being suppressed.[126] Since nutritional therapy with low-protein diets prevents metabolic acidosis, amelioration of acid production is one mechanism whereby dietary modification can improve amino acid and protein metabolism.[127,128] Experimentally, the association between excess dietary protein and development of acidosis is well-established. After subtotal nephrectomy, rats were fed diets containing 6% protein, 17% protein, or an excess of protein (30%). The most efficient use of dietary protein for growth was achieved with 8% protein while the most robust growth was in rats fed 17% protein; rats with CKD fed 30% protein developed acidosis and had poor growth plus low plasma values of branched-chain amino acids.[129]

Proposed mechanisms for the catabolic responses to acidosis include changes in intracellular pH and abnormal response to hormones. Bailey and coworkers used nuclear magnetic resonance (NMR) to measure the intracellular pH in muscle of rats.[130] Rats were made acidotic by intravenous infusion of acid or by subtotal nephrectomy and, in both cases, the serum bicarbonate level and blood pH fell sharply, but the pH in muscle cells scarcely changed. Moreover, there was no abnormality in the recovery of muscle cell pH in rats with CKD following nerve stimulation to produce tetany and reduce the cell pH. In rats fed a high-acid diet for 5 days, there was a small decrease in muscle cell pH, and no mechanisms were uncovered to explain the changes in metabolism induced by acidosis.

One factor causing acidosis-induced loss of protein stores (as with other catabolic conditions) is an increase in glucocorticoid production. In normal animals, pharmacologic doses of glucocorticoids will suppress protein synthesis and accelerate muscle protein breakdown.[131,132] In contrast, physiologic levels of glucocorticoids do not cause catabolism. The status of glucocorticoids is discussed because May and Bailey and colleagues noted that muscle protein breakdown in rats with metabolic acidosis and normal kidney function required an increase in glucocorticoid production; the same dose of glucocorticoids alone did not increase muscle protein breakdown.[133-135] The relevance to CKD is that with or without metabolic acidosis, rats with CKD have increased rates of glucocorticoid production.[134,135] Experimentally, a similar interaction between acidification and glucocorticoids raises the activity of branched-chain keto-acid dehydrogenase to break down branched-chain amino acids.[136,137] Thus, one of the complications of CKD, acidosis, increases glucocorticoid production, which exerts a permissive effect to degrade protein and essential amino acids (EAAs).[138-140]

The mechanism for the permissive effect of glucocorticoids has been identified. When physiologically relevant doses of glucocorticoids activate the glucocorticoid receptor, insulin, and insulin-like growth factor 1 (IGF-1), intracellular signaling is reduced because the activated glucocorticoid receptor directly interacts with phosphatidylinositol-3-kinase (PI3K). The sequestration of PI3K away from the cell membrane prevents normal insulin and IGF-1 signaling, which would lead to suppression of protein breakdown in muscle. Therefore, glucocorticoids are required for stimulating muscle protein loss.[141,142]

In addition to stimulating glucocorticoid production, acidosis can influence the activity of other hormones. For example, acidosis impairs the ability of growth hormone to stimulate the release of IGF-1, the major mediator of growth hormone action.[143] Acidosis also reduces thyroid hormone levels and stimulates parathyroid hormone release while impairing the activation of $1,25(OH)_2$ vitamin D_3.[16,144-146] How these changes in hormone activity specifically change muscle protein metabolism has not been determined. In contrast, much is known about the mechanism whereby insulin/IGF-1 signaling changes muscle protein loss. First, insulin resistance can be detected at moderate stages of CKD.[147] Second, impaired insulin and IGF-1 signaling results in decreased activity of insulin receptor substrate-1 (IRS-1)–associated PI3K, which stimulates the breakdown of muscle protein.[148] Third, the increase in endogenous glucocorticoid production present in CKD impairs IRS-1–associated PI3K activity.[141,149] These catabolic responses stimulate the expression and activity of enzymes that break down muscle protein. To avoid these problems, acidosis should be corrected in all patients with stages 3 to 5 CKD.

UBIQUITIN-PROTEASOME SYSTEM

The UPS has been identified as the pathway that degrades the bulk of protein in all cells; the importance of this function was recognized when the 2004 Nobel Prize was awarded to Hershko, Ciechanover, and Rose "for the discovery of ubiquitin-mediated protein degradation" (http://nobelprize.org/chemistry/laureates/2004). Regarding the influence of CKD on the UPS, it is well known that a sharp rise in UPS activity occurs in muscles of animal models of many catabolic conditions, including CKD.[66,150] The rise in UPS activity in muscle occurs in response to certain complications of CKD, including metabolic acidosis, decreased insulin and IGF-1 signaling, inflammation, and high levels of Ang II.[118,142,151-155] In addition, evidence for activation of the UPS has also been found in muscles of patients who have accelerated muscle atrophy from CKD, cancer, trauma, sepsis, or other catabolic events.[150]

Three enzymes sequentially link ubiquitins (Ubs) to proteins destined for degradation: a single Ub-activating enzyme (E1); one of at least 40 Ub carrier or conjugating proteins (E2); and one of a group of 500 to 1000 Ub-protein ligase enzymes (E3). The E3 enzymes are the key to specificity of the degradation of proteins because each E3 enzyme recognizes a specific protein or a specific class of proteins and catalyzes the transfer of the activated Ub to these substrate proteins. These steps not only require specific enzymes but also adenosine triphosphate (ATP).[150] Following conjugation of four or five Ubs to the substrate protein, the Ub-protein complex is recognized by the proteasome. The proteasome is a very large structure that not only recognizes the chain of Ubs conjugated to a protein but the proteasome also removes the Ubs, linearizes the substrate protein, and injects it into the proteasome, where the protein is degraded. The specificity of the degradation of proteins depends on the activity of the E3 Ub-ligases and not the proteasome. Thus, the sequence of events from the recognition of a protein that is to be degraded to conjugation of Ub to the substrate protein and, ultimately, to its degradation in the proteasome results in loss of muscle proteins.[135,156]

The activity of the UPS affects critical functions of organs because the UPS regulates the expression of proteins with short half-lives (e.g., regulatory enzymes, transcription factors), immune surveillance processes, and the regulation of long-lived proteins, including muscle proteins.[66,150] However, the UPS also affects other functions. For example, an inhibitor of the UPS was found to cause beneficial responses in patients with multiple myeloma and, potentially, other types of cancer.[150] In CKD, however, activation of the UPS causes muscle protein loss. This occurs because the loss of muscle mass from kidney failure in experimental animals or humans results in only a small decrease in protein synthesis but a sharp increase in rates of protein degradation.[135,157] This is relevant because the rate of protein turnover in humans is very high (3.5 to 4.5 g protein/kg/day) and, consequently, even a small increase in proteolysis causes muscle atrophy; most of the protein loss occurs because there is activation of the UPS.[66,126,135] For example, in rodent models of CKD, the UPS is activated, causing accelerated muscle proteolysis—a response that is associated with higher levels of mRNAs encoding certain components of the UPS. Notably, similar changes signaling activation of the UPS occur in rodent models of starvation, diabetes, cancer, or muscle denervation.[158,159] Similarly, humans afflicted with catabolic conditions also activate the UPS in muscle, as determined by increases in the mRNAs encoding Ubs and proteasome subunits.[126,160-162] The protein degradation occurs principally in muscle, indicating that there is specificity to the mechanism that causes muscle atrophy. The specificity of muscle protein losses occurs because there is activation of two critical E3 Ub-ligases, atrogin-1 (also known as MAFbx) and MuRF-1. The expression of these enzymes in muscle increases dramatically (8- to 20-fold) in catabolic states. This is relevant because an increase of atrogin-1/MAFbx in muscle results in the loss of proteins that regulate muscle protein synthesis while an increase in MuRF-1 catalyzes the breakdown of myofibrillar proteins in muscle.[163] In short, expression of these E3 enzymes in muscles impairs protein synthesis and accelerates protein degradation, causing muscle atrophy. In experimental animals, the development of muscle atrophy can be blocked with inhibitors of the proteasome.[135,151,164] Therefore, there are two potential strategies for blocking muscle wasting—suppression of the pathways that activate the UPS and direct inhibition of the proteasome. Studies have suggested that the pathway leading to activation of the UPS can be suppressed and, hence, there is a potential method for preventing muscle wasting by the UPS (see later).

CASPASE-3 AND MUSCLE PROTEIN LOSSES

Myofibrillar proteins are attacked by the UPS only slowly and, since there is loss of muscle protein, other proteases must initially disassemble the myofibril into its component proteins (actin, myosin, troponin, or tropomyosin). When these proteins are cleaved by another protease, they can be rapidly degraded by the UPS. We have shown that caspase-3 is at least one protease that performs this initial cleavage of the complex structure of proteins in muscle. Caspase-3 in muscle has been found to be activated in several catabolic conditions. The pathway activating caspase-3 can include circulating TNF-α and other inflammatory cytokines, as well as the development of insulin resistance.[165-167] Specifically, we found that caspase-3 cleaves actomyosin in vitro and when it is activated in cultured muscle cells. The initial cleavage of muscle proteins by caspase-3 produces substrates that are rapidly degraded by the UPS. Interestingly, the initial cleavage of muscle proteins in catabolic conditions can be monitored by examination of muscle biopsies. This is possible because the cleavage of muscle proteins by caspase-3 leaves a footprint of its action, a 14-kDa fragment of the C terminus of actin, which is accumulated in the insoluble fraction of muscle cells.[168] In rodent models of muscle wasting due to CKD, diabetes, or Ang II–induced hypertension, there is accumulation of the 14-kDa actin fragment. Also, in patients, the development of muscle atrophy caused by inflammation from osteodystrophy or muscle wasting related to hemodialysis or burn injury, the 14-kDa action fragment accumulates in muscle. It accumulates in proportion to the rate of protein degradation; in patients undergoing hemodialysis, the level of the 14-kDa actin fragment decreases in response to a successful exercise program (e.g., stationary cycling).[169]

In addition to the interaction between caspase-3 and muscle proteolysis via the UPS, there is another link to muscle protein breakdown. Wang and associates have found that the process of accelerated muscle protein degradation in the UPS includes an increase in the activity of the 26S proteasome.[170] We determined that this response is mediated by caspase-3–induced cleavage of specific subunits of the 19S proteasome, leading to accelerated muscle protein degradation in the UPS. This increase in proteasome activity acts as a feed-forward mechanism to degrade large amounts of protein in muscles.[153,154,169,171]

SIGNALS TRIGGERING MUSCLE ATROPHY

Complications of CKD that trigger proteolytic activity of the UPS in muscle include metabolic acidosis, impaired insulin action, increased glucocorticoids, high levels of Ang II, and inflammation.[135,151,154,155,172] As noted, the process of protein degradation involves coordinated changes in the expression of a set of genes in muscle, which suggests that there is a common cellular signaling pathway involving the UPS and caspase-3.[158,159] The regulation of signaling pathways involves decreases in protein synthesis with increases in proteolysis in muscle, and these responses are linked through decreased PI3K and Akt.[150,173] Specifically, a decrease in PI3K activity suppresses the activity of the serine-threonine kinase Akt, and this in turn leads to reduced rates of muscle protein synthesis (Figure 61.3). In addition, suppressed activity of Akt reduces forkhead transcription factors (FOXO); the dephosphorylated FOXO transcription factors enter the nucleus to stimulate the expression of the E3 Ub ligases atrogin-1/MAFbx and MuRF-1.[150] As noted above, the substrates for atrogin-1/MAFbx include regulators of protein synthesis while substrates of MuRF1 include myofibrillar proteins.[163] Decreased protein synthesis and increased protein degradation cause muscle atrophy.[174]

Another CKD-induced defect in muscle protein metabolism, impaired activity of satellite cells, has been determined. Satellite cells are present under the sarcolemmal membrane of myofibers and, in response to muscle injury, they proliferate and fuse with myofibers to repair the injury.[175] They also promote muscle growth and recovery from muscle atrophy by increasing the production of myofibrillar proteins. We found that satellite cell function is markedly impaired by CKD, and this abnormality can be improved in a model of resistance exercise.[176] The decrease in satellite function that contributes to muscle atrophy in CKD is similar to changes induced by defective IGF-1 signaling.[177] Abnormalities in the

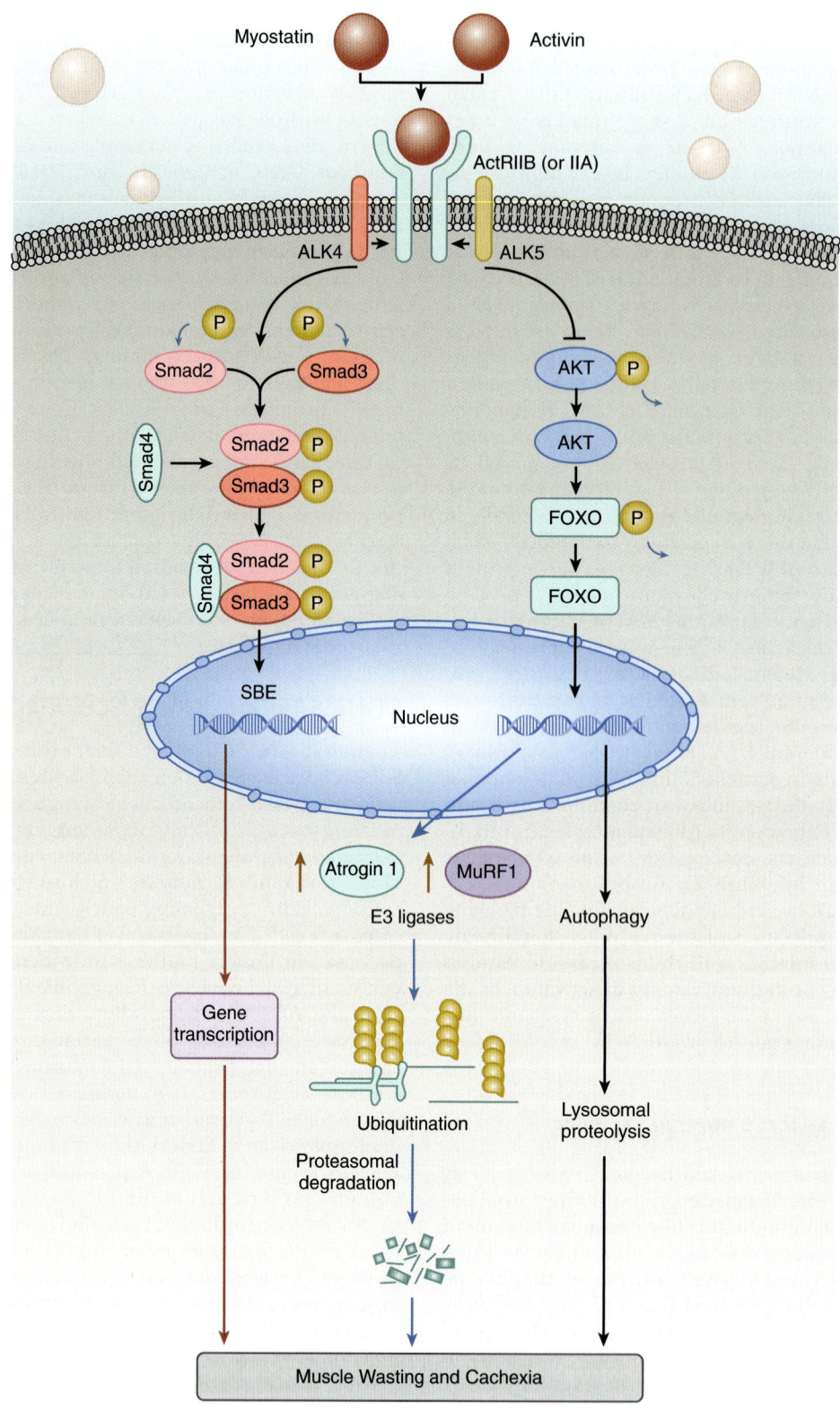

Figure 61.3 Myostatin-activin signaling and muscle protein (P) loss. Myostatin or activin binds to type IIB activin receptors (ActRIIB) on the muscle membrane, forming dimers. The dimers recruit and activate the activin receptors transmembrane kinases, ALK4 or ALK5. The kinases phosphorylate Smad2 and Smad3 and recruit Smad4 to form a Smad complex that translocates into the nucleus and stimulates transcription of genes, which results in muscle wasting. Activated ActRIIB receptors also reduce AKT activity and consequently reduce the phosphorylation of FOXO. Dephosphorylated FOXO transcription factors enter the nucleus and activate transcription of atrophy-specific E3 ligases, MuRF1, atrogin-1/MAFbx, and other atrogenes, resulting in muscle protein wasting via activation of the ubiquitin-proteasome system or autophagy. (From Han HQ, Zhou X, Mitch WE, Goldberg AL: Myostatin/activin pathway antagonism: molecular basis and therapeutic potential. *Int J Biochem Cell Biol* 45:2333-2347, 2013.)

function of isolated satellite cells are largely corrected by treatment with IGF-1.

Abnormalities in insulin–IGF-1 signaling occur frequently in CKD and are linked to abnormalities in carbohydrate and protein metabolism in muscle.[178,179] Experimentally, insulin deficiency or the induction of insulin resistance activates the UPS to degrade muscle proteins.[151,153,153] Thus, two events cause an increase in muscle proteolysis—resistance to insulin (or diabetes) causing impaired insulin–IGF-1 signaling and the presence of physiologic levels of glucocorticoids.[141] The importance of these two events was highlighted in results from a study of the inflammation induced by Ang II infusion.[155] In response to Ang II, there was an increase in the endogenous production of glucocorticoids, which stimulated the degradation of IRS-1 to impair insulin–IGF-1 signaling. Interestingly, the response to Ang II was augmented by an increase in the production of serum amyloid A (SAA), an acute phase reactant protein. The rise in SAA levels potentiated the increase in muscle protein degradation, indicating that acute phase reactant proteins can have a physiologic role beyond serving as indicators of inflammation.

A potentially important factor causing loss of protein stores in patients with CKD is their sedentary lifestyle. Although the hormonal and cellular signaling mechanisms causing muscle atrophy in the absence of exercise are not clear, Davis and colleagues have found that exercise training of rats with CKD leads to an increase in the sensitivity of muscle to insulin, thereby improving glucose uptake and suppressing muscle protein breakdown.[180] In patients with CKD, Storer and associates have found that endurance training (e.g., stationary bicycling) improves muscle function and cardiopulmonary measures in patients requiring dialysis.[181] In contrast, Johansen and coworkers have reported that resistance training improves the cross-sectional area of muscles from patients on hemodialysis, although they did not find an increase in lean body mass.[182] We recommend exercise training because it could suppress the activation of caspase-3 and the UPS and a reduction in the activities of PI3K and Akt.[169,171,183,184]

Indirect evidence has suggested that a high level of glucagon could stimulate muscle catabolism.[185] For example, administration of glucagon to fasting obese subjects increased urinary ammonia levels and, possibly, urea excretion.[186,187] Experimentally, muscle proteolysis is unaffected by glucagon, except at unphysiologically high levels.[188] Thus, the role of hyperglucagonemia in augmenting nitrogen requirements in uremia is uncertain.

The possibility that abnormalities in the metabolism of fatty acids can stimulate protein breakdown in muscle was evaluated by Li and Wassner.[189] They found no abnormalities in muscle protein turnover of rats with CKD but an increase in muscle loss with fasting.[189] The latter resulted from the breakdown of myofibrillar muscle proteins, which were inversely correlated with body fat stores. There was no change in protein synthesis, and the pathway responsible for the degradation of muscle protein was not identified.

MYOSTATIN

Myostatin, also known as growth differentiating factor 8, suppresses the genesis of new myofibrils, preventing the growth of muscle mass. Myostatin is a member of the TGF-α family of secreted proteins and is predominantly expressed in skeletal muscle, although cardiac muscle and adipose tissues contain low levels of myostatin. In skeletal muscle, the parent molecule is prepromyostatin, which is cleaved to produce promyostatin and an inactive, latent protein complex that contains myostatin. Myostatin is released from the promyostatin complex by proteolysis or in response to free radicals. Myostatin can then bind to ActRIIB, the high-affinity, type IIB activin A receptor that is present on muscle membranes (see Figure 61.3). The interaction leads to the activation of serine kinases, ALK4 or ALK5, which phosphorylate Sma- and Mad-related (SMAD) proteins 2 and 3. Following activation, SMADs translocate into the nucleus to bind to specific DNA elements and change gene transcription.[190,191]

The importance of myostatin is that it regulates skeletal muscle mass and functions. For example, in mice, deletion of the myostatin gene results in a dramatic increase in the size and number of skeletal muscle fibers.[192,193] Similarly, transgenic mice that overexpress a dominant negative receptor for myostatin or the presence of proteins that block myostatin function produce phenotypes with huge amounts of muscle tissue that is almost exclusively protein-based.[191] Specifically, a massive increase in muscle mass associated with the absence or dysfunction of myostatin has been observed in cattle, sheep, dogs, horses, and at least one child. Based on these interactions, it is not surprising that the inhibition of myostatin has been shown to increase muscle mass in animal models of catabolic disorders, including CKD and cancer.[194,195] Parenthetically, deletion of one copy of the myostatin gene improves athletic performance. In dog races, whippets bearing a single copy of the mutated myostatin gene are among the fastest dogs, but those with two mutated copies have such massive muscles that they are barely mobile.[191] Thoroughbred race horses with myostatin polymorphism also exhibit a strong association between decreased expression of myostatin and exercise tolerance—loss of one gene leads to increased physical performance while loss of both genes produces muscle hypertrophy.

Catabolic Conditions Activate Myostatin in Muscles

Myostatin and the myostatin-activin signaling pathway are upregulated in muscle wasting conditions, which include aging, responses to prolonged bed rest or to AIDS, CKD, or heart failure.[191,196,197] Moreover, in animal models of cancer cachexia, glucocorticoid administration, burn injury, and mechanical unloading of muscles, as well as responses to outer space flight, myostatin expression is increased in muscle and is associated with loss of muscle mass. Similarly, administration of myostatin or activin A experimentally leads to about a 30% decrease in muscle mass, documenting its importance as a catabolic factor in muscle.[191,192]

To examine if inhibition of myostatin might have clinical utility by improving muscle mass, three strategies have been used: (1) administration of antibodies to myostatin, including a peptibody (a genetically engineered myostatin-neutralizing peptide fused to a humanized Fc fragment); (2) administration of the myostatin propeptide to bind myostatin; or (3) administration of soluble ActRIIB receptors to soak up or block the influence of myostatin on its membrane receptor. With each strategy, muscle mass is increased in normal animals.[191]

Blocking Myostatin in Chronic Kidney Disease Improves Muscle Mass

As detailed in the preceding discussion, CKD and its complications cause progressive loss of muscle mass and increases in circulating markers of inflammation plus impaired insulin–IGF-1 signaling.[192] The development of insulin–IGF-1 resistance is due to a decrease in p-Akt.[135,148] Specifically, the low level of p-Akt suppresses phosphorylation of the forkhead transcription factors FOXO1 and FOXO3, allowing them to enter the nucleus, stimulating the expression and activity of the UPS and resulting in loss of muscle mass. Bailey and Thomas and colleagues studied a mouse model of CKD (subtotal nephrectomy followed by feeding a high-protein diet) using a pair feeding regimen.[148,149] One mouse of each pair was injected subcutaneously with the antimyostatin peptibody every other day; the paired mouse was injected with the diluent. The peptibody reduced myostatin in muscles and prevented the loss of BW and muscle mass that occurs with CKD.[195] The mechanisms for the improvement in muscle mass included an increase in protein synthesis and a decrease in protein degradation. The myostatin peptibody also increased p-Akt and led to improvements in satellite cell function. Finally, the inhibition of myostatin in mice with CKD suppressed circulating levels of inflammatory cytokines, including IL-6. These results formed the basis for initial trials in patients with CKD.

EXTERNAL LOSSES OF PROTEIN

Digestion of proteins following gastrointestinal bleeding will lead to reabsorption of amino acids and augmentation of urea production, plus depletion of body stores of hemoglobin and plasma proteins.[113] The impact of the nephrotic syndrome on body protein stores is discussed subsequently.

ALTERED ELECTROLYTE BALANCE

In patients with advanced CKD, defects in ion transport in blood cells have been demonstrated, and there is an increase in intracellular sodium in muscle. In rats with CKD, there are defects in cation transport in skeletal mass and adipocytes but the mechanism whereby acidification or other transport abnormalities directly stimulate catabolism is unknown.[198] For example, depletion of potassium in muscle occurs in patients with CKD, even in those with a normal or increased serum potassium concentration.[199] This is relevant because potassium deficiency and hyperkalemia are intertwined with abnormalities in intracellular acid-base changes as well as abnormalities in the metabolic responses to insulin or IGF-1.[200,201] It is possible that these abnormalities could increase nitrogen catabolism but, to date, the connection between hyperkalemia and catabolism has not been convincingly demonstrated.

HYPERPARATHYROIDISM

Parathyroid hormone (PTH) administration has been reported to augment urea production in normal subjects and in patients with hyperparathyroidism.[202] However, not all investigators found that adding PTH to isolated muscle increases the rate of protein degradation.[203,204] Hyperparathyroidism can also inhibit insulin release, and low levels of insulin cause muscle protein degradation in vivo. Still, evidence for a direct effect of PTH on protein metabolism has not be established.

ASSESSMENT OF PROTEIN STORES IN CHRONIC KIDNEY DISEASE

In treating patients with CKD, the goal of minimizing the accumulation of potentially toxic waste products and ions must be balanced against the need to supply enough EAAs to build protein and prevent loss of body protein. Consequently, the optimal diet is one in which protein synthesis equals protein degradation. In this case, the urea appearance rate approaches zero. and hence the accumulation of nitrogen-containing waste products will be minimal. The daily rates of protein synthesis and degradation are very high, so even a small increase in protein degradation or decrease in protein synthesis persisting for several weeks can cause a marked loss of lean body mass.[60,66,205,206] The gold standard for evaluating protein stores is determination of nitrogen balance, but this is difficult to calculate, requiring careful measurement of food eaten and of all the nitrogen that is excreted and accumulated. Notably, results of measured nitrogen balance do not identify whether protein synthesis or degradation is abnormal nor does it give insights into mechanisms that can cause loss of protein stores. Consequently, plasma proteins and indirect indices have been used to assess protein stores. Hypoalbuminemia is among the most frequently cited indicator of decreased protein stores, but the serum albumin concentration can be confounded by many factors. Thus, the serum albumin level is reduced by inflammation, acidosis, and urinary or other losses of albumin, but the presence of a low serum albumin level does not elucidate which fraction of the protein stores has been lost.[207,208] Other serum proteins such as prealbumin have similar shortcomings.

NITROGEN BALANCE

Nitrogen balance is calculated as the difference between nitrogen intake and excretion plus accumulation of nonprotein nitrogen, principally urea. The half-life of urea disappearance in a normal adult is about 7 hours, so even a large load of urea (e.g., in gastrointestinal bleeding) is virtually completely excreted over 24 hours. For this reason, changes in the urea pool of normal adults can be ignored when their nitrogen balance is being calculated. This is not the case for patients with CKD because the half-life of urea is prolonged, and a response to changes in the diet, or even gastrointestinal bleeding, may not reach equilibrium for several days. Consequently, the accumulation or loss of urea nitrogen in the body must be taken into account in the calculation of the nitrogen balance of patients with CKD. Fortunately, changes in the pool of urea nitrogen can be estimated because the concentration of urea is equal throughout body water, and it can be assumed that the urea space is equivalent to 60% of BW (body water in nonedematous persons averages 60% of BW[61,209]). When body water (in liters) is multiplied by BUN (in g/L), the result is the size of the urea nitrogen pool. Notably, the precision of measuring BUN can dominate the nitrogen balance calculation; a change in BUN from 140 to 150 mg/dL, which may be within the coefficient of variation of the BUN measurements, represents about 4 g of nitrogen in a 70-kg person. Because a change in BW or in the BUN affects calculation of the nitrogen balance, it is more accurate to estimate the urea space on a given day and then calculate the urea pool size each day (i.e., BUN times the body water plus any change in BW).[61,63] The average change in the size of the urea pool is added to the amount of urea nitrogen excreted plus the excretion of all other nitrogen-containing compounds. The calculation assumes that water accounts for all changes in BW during short periods. It is more precise to measure the urea space using ^{15}N- or ^{14}C-labeled urea. If the urea space is subtracted from BW, the calculated value is an estimate of solid tissues.[61,72,210]

Other sources of nonprotein nitrogen that may accumulate in patients with CKD, such as creatinine, can be ignored because they are a small fraction of retained nitrogen. When the serum creatinine level rises from 10 to 15 mg/dL, the retained nitrogen increases by only 0.3 g in a 70-kg adult.[80] Unfortunately, the volumes of distribution of many nitrogen-containing compounds are unknown; hence, the degree of accumulation or excess cannot be calculated.

UREA NITROGEN APPEARANCE RATE

Since the major nonprotein source of nitrogen in the body is urea, the urea nitrogen appearance rate should be calculated and included in estimates of nitrogen balance. The urea appearance equals the sum of urinary urea nitrogen excretion plus its accumulation (positive or negative). In patients with CKD, the urea appearance rate provides a quantitative measurement of the parameter that nutritional therapy seeks to minimize—that is, the accumulation of nitrogen-containing compounds. Stated explicitly, the most efficient use of protein in the diet of patients with CKD is associated with the lowest value of the urea appearance rate. Cottini and associates demonstrated this relationship when they assessed the nitrogen balance of patients with CKD.[59] They found that a diet containing 3 to 4 g nitrogen/day was associated with neutral nitrogen balance in patients with CKD and, at the same time, was associated with the lowest value of urea nitrogen excretion (see Figure 61.1).

SERUM ALBUMIN AND MALNUTRITION

A low serum albumin concentration is widely used to support a diagnosis of malnutrition.[211] This is largely incorrect because the serum albumin level arises from the balance between synthesis and degradation of albumin plus albumin losses (e.g., in nephrotic syndrome) and dilution of albumin by changes in body water.[212] Careful measurements of albumin turnover in patients on hemodialysis have revealed that serum albumin is directly correlated with BW, suggesting that variations in albumin synthesis are the critical factor controlling serum albumin levels.[207] Subsequent studies have shown that an even more important determinant of the serum albumin concentration is variability in albumin catabolism related to evidence of inflammation.[207,213] Others have reported that metabolic acidosis will decrease serum albumin levels.[214]

Although a surfeit or deficiency of dietary protein or calories may influence serum albumin levels, this is not sufficient to diagnose malnutrition. Malnutrition is defined as a complex of abnormalities due to an inadequate or unbalanced diet.[212] In addition to diet, however, there are many CKD-induced metabolic abnormalities that contribute to the uremic syndrome. This syndrome includes symptoms such as fatigue plus a loss of lean body mass and a decrease in serum albumin and other plasma protein levels. The following factors must be considered before concluding that a patient with CKD and a low serum albumin level has malnutrition. First, there are the metabolic abnormalities of uremia (e.g., metabolic acidosis, impaired insulin–IGF-1 signalling, inflammation), which stimulate losses of protein stores. Second, in the absence of these metabolic abnormalities, a poor diet (or even starvation in the short term) does not cause a meaningful change in serum albumin. Third, correcting a low serum albumin level by increasing dietary protein and calories has been difficult to establish.[212] For example, when patients with anorexia nervosa were compared with age- and height-matched subjects, the serum albumin concentrations of patients were not statistically different, even though patients with anorexia nervosa had an approximately 34% lower BW and 22% lower values of muscle mass.[215] In summary, the serum albumin level is affected by several factors other than an inadequate diet.

Notably, many of the abnormalities associated with the loss of protein stores in CKD are ameliorated, not exacerbated, by restricting dietary protein (e.g., acidosis, insulin resistance)[128,216]:

1. Low-protein diets were found to cause minimal evidence of malnutrition in participants of the MDRD study; on average, those prescribed the lowest amount of dietary protein had a small but statistically significant increase in their serum albumin level.[217]
2. Patients eating very low-protein diets supplemented with ketoacids and EAAs over periods of at least 1 year had normal serum albumin levels.[3,127,128,218]
3. The serum albumin level responds relatively slowly to changes in protein stores because it has a half-life of about 20 days; thus, its use in identifying malnourished patients is compromised during trials of protein refeeding.[219]

Inflammation in patients with CKD is frequent and can be detected by high circulating values of acute phase reactant proteins. In fact, chronic inflammation is a major cause of morbidity and mortality in dialysis patients. Kaysen and coworkers[207] have shown that albumin synthesis falls sharply in patients on hemodialysis with inflammatory illnesses (i.e., albumin functions as a negative acute phase reactant). Second, there is an association between the presence of hypoalbuminemia in patients on dialysis and higher serum concentrations of the acute phase reactant proteins SAA and C-reactive protein (CRP).[220] It is not clear that the changes in serum albumin levels and nutritional status are linked. For example, Kaysen and colleagues reported that a high level of CRP in one month did not predict a decrease in the serum albumin level in the subsequent month.[207] The group did find, however, that there is a relationship between an increase in the blood levels of longer-lived acute phase reactant proteins (e.g., ceruloplasmin, α_1-acid glycoprotein) and a decrease in serum albumin levels.[213] Specifically, their results showed that high serum concentrations of the longer-lived acute phase reactant proteins present in one month could be used to predict the development of a lower serum albumin level in the succeeding month. Changes in dietary protein estimated by urea kinetics have indicated that changes in the diet protein have minimal impact on changes in serum albumin levels. The authors concluded that responses to inflammatory cytokines but not changes in dietary protein were the major factors producing hypoalbuminemia in patients undergoing hemodialysis.[207]

The other reason to assess acute phase reactant proteins in patients with CKD and low serum albumin concentrations is that high levels of circulating inflammatory cytokines are associated with the presence of atherosclerosis.[172,220,221] The association between high levels of inflammatory cytokines and atherosclerosis in patients with CKD was designated a syndrome of malnutrition, inflammation, and atherosclerosis—the MIA syndrome.[172] From the foregoing discussion, it is clear that malnutrition (reduced levels of dietary protein) is not necessarily the dominant cause of hypoalbuminemia. Instead, inflammatory cytokines and acute phase reactant proteins can actually initiate loss of muscle protein.[155] For example, it is well known that Ang II levels are frequently high in patients with CKD. It also has been found that Ang II activates the UPS and caspase-3 to cause muscle wasting. Activation of muscle proteolysis was shown to occur because Ang II increased the production of IL-6 SAA, which blocked insulin–IGF-1 intracellular signalling. Since feeding more protein or calories does not eliminate inflammation or reduce atherosclerosis in patients with CKD, the designation of the MIA syndrome should be discarded.[212,222]

DIET, LIPIDS, AND CARDIOVASCULAR RISK

A search for the mechanisms underlying the high incidence of CVD in patients with CKD has indicated that many patients with CKD exhibit an increase in serum total triglyceride levels, subnormal concentrations of high-density lipoprotein (HDL) cholesterol, and increased very LDL (VLDL) and intermediate-density lipoprotein (IDL) cholesterol fractions, along with abnormalities in serum apoproteins. Since the prevalence of CVD in patients on dialysis is high, these abnormalities have been vigorously treated in some settings, but evidence of a treatment benefit is limited.[223]

In patients with CKD, especially those with hypercholesterolemia or low HDL cholesterol concentrations, the National Cholesterol Education Program (NCEP)–American Heart Association step 1 diet can be instituted. With this diet, 30% of total calories from fat is recommended; saturated fat should not exceed 20% of total calories, and cholesterol intake should be below 300 mg/day. If high levels of triglycerides are present, the exclusion of purified sugars should be reduced in the diet and the patient should be evaluated for type 2 diabetes and/or insulin resistance. For patients with persistently high serum LDL, VLDL, or IDL cholesterol or very high serum triglyceride levels, a more aggressive dietary restriction is needed. This should include withdrawal of alcohol and intake of complex carbohydrates instead of purified sugars. Weight reduction is obligatory for obese patients; many patients with insulin resistance who are not obese but exhibit mild-to-moderate weight excess may also benefit from caloric restriction and other dietary modifications. Medications that can reduce hypertriglyceridemia include a supplement of ω-3 fatty acids, fibric acid derivatives, and nicotinic acid. The optimal dose of ω-3 fatty acids for patients with CKD is unknown, however, and a high intake of ω-3 fatty acids (e.g., up to 6 g/day) should be avoided as it can lead to increased oxidant stress, even though the plasma lipid profile may improve. Fibrates undergo altered pharmacokinetics in patients with CKD; the dose must be reduced to avoid muscle cramps or even rhabdomyolysis.

If elevated LDL cholesterol levels are not normalized by dietary counselling (i.e., above 100 mg/dL or the upper limit of normal values), or if there is proteinuria (a condition independently associated with an increased cardiovascular risk), a 3-hydroxy-3-methylglutaryl-coenzyme A (HMG-CoA) reductase inhibitor (statin) may be added.[224] These drugs have been associated with important reductions in cardiovascular morbidity and mortality in the general population. On the other hand, statin administration to patients on dialysis may not be useful because large randomized trials have not revealed a beneficial influence on survival in hemodialysis patients, including patients with and without type 2 diabetes mellitus.[225-229] Fibrates should not be used in conjunction with most statins owing to a heightened risk of rhabdomyolysis.

Notably, prescription of a low-protein diet normally includes a reduction of protein from animals (e.g., meat and dairy products); this in turn leads to a reduced intake of saturated lipids and potentially, a healthier serum lipid profile. For example, a reduction in protein intake from 1.1 to 0.7 g/kg/day induced an increase in serum apolipoprotein AI (apo AI) and the apo AI/apo B ratio over a 3-month period.[230] Initiation of a low-protein diet improved oxidative status as marked by decreasing red cell malondialdehyde content and increasing plasma polyunsaturated fatty acid concentrations, particularly C22:4 and C22:5.[231] In an RCT over 18 months, Nanayakkara and associates evaluated responses to combining pravastatin, vitamin E, and homocysteine-lowering vitamins. A 25% decrease in serum LDL cholesterol levels were observed in the treatment group, and there was an improvement in carotid intima-media thickness, arterial vasodilation properties, and proteinuria.[232] As detailed below, institution of a low-protein diet can exert a secondary benefit on the lipid pattern because it will reduce the degree of proteinuria (see later), an independent risk factor for the development of CVD.

In the general population, a high plasma homocysteine level is associated with the development of atherosclerosis and mortality.[233,234] Similarly, an increase in plasma homocysteine levels has been linked to accelerated atherosclerosis in patients with CKD,[235] although randomized trials of homocysteine-lowering therapies have proven ineffective at lowering mortality or cardiovascular events.[236]

SERUM TRANSFERRIN, PREALBUMIN, COMPLEMENT, AND INSULIN-LIKE GROWTH FACTOR-1

Serum transferrin has been used as a marker of protein nutrition because its level decreases with dietary protein deficiency and because it has a shorter half-life (≈10 days) than albumin. However, serum transferrin levels change in response to nondietary factors; the serum transferrin level rises when iron stores are depleted and, with chronic inflammatory disorders, transferrin can decrease by as much as 50%, producing artificially low values in patients with inflammation. Interestingly, erythropoietin therapy causes no significant change in serum transferrin concentrations, at least in patients on dialysis, nor does it change nutritional status in terms of serum albumin levels, anthropometry, or muscle protein content.[237,238]

Prealbumin (also known as transthyretin) has a half-life of about 2 days, and it changes more rapidly than serum albumin when there are variations in nutritional status.[239] Unfortunately, factors that change serum albumin (e.g., inflammation) also affect serum prealbumin, so its utility in evaluating nutritional status is at best controversial.

IGF-1 is the major hormone that mediates the effects of growth hormone. Changes in IGF-1 levels have been studied in uremic patients for three reasons. First, administration of growth hormone is associated with a remarkable improvement in the growth of children, and preliminary results have indicated that growth hormone may improve the nutritional status of hemodialysis and CAPD patients.[240-242] Second, IGF-1 administration has been proposed as a means of augmenting kidney function in patients with advanced CKD.[243] Finally, administration of IGF-1 has been proposed as a means of inhibiting catabolism of muscle protein.[244] Reduced mRNA levels of IGF-1 can be found in models of uremia but normal or increased levels of IGF-1 and IGF-II were found in muscle biopsies obtained from patients on hemodialysis.[245] This is relevant because acute administration of IGF-1 can improve muscle protein synthesis in normal or uremic patients, suggesting that there is reduced responsiveness to IGF-1 in patients on hemodialysis, possibly due to a postreceptor defect in the action of IGF-1.[246-248] This is a complicated area of research because the action of IGF-1 is influenced not only by the concentration of IGF-binding proteins, but also by the circulating levels of amino acids.[249-251] Evidence that circulating IGF-1 levels are influenced by nutritional status, which includes the report that a diet containing an insufficient amount of protein reduces IGF-1 levels, as does the presence of chronic malnutrition.[251] In uremic patients, IGF-1 levels change minimally when protein intake is reduced by as much as 40%.[249] Thus, it is difficult to link IGF-1 to nutritional status. However, serum IGF-1 concentrations do decrease in response to acidosis and there is evidence that a low serum IGF-1 level is associated with poor outcomes in patients on hemodialysis.[143,252,253] Clearly, more work is needed to understand the metabolic implications of variations in serum IGF-1 levels.

ANTHROPOMETRICS

Evaluation of anthropometry in patients with CKD has limited utility because most reports are based on a single evaluation, and the results are compared to those from normal adults.[60] For example, it is difficult to interpret reports that serum protein levels are normal but that anthropometric measurements demonstrate loss of muscle mass.[254] Not surprisingly, there is a high incidence of anthropometric abnormalities in cross-sectional studies of patients but attributing them to malnutrition is questionable, particularly when tissue hydration may strongly confound anthropometric results.[212,225-257]

EARLY INITIATION OF DIALYSIS

Some have suggested that dialysis should be initiated early to avoid malnutrition in patients with CKD while improving their prognosis.[258,259] There are several reasons to reject this suggestion. Most importantly, when the influence of early dialysis on mortality was analyzed, it was concluded that early dialysis does not prolong life.[128,260,261] In fact, patients with more advanced CKD when they began dialysis tended to have a lower mortality, even after correcting for age, gender, BW, diabetes, leukocyte count, dialysis type, or dialysis access. Moreover, it was proposed that patients with CKD have a decrease in protein intake that causes malnutrition, but long-term results of patients eating low-protein diets have indicated that BW and serum protein and blood biochemistry levels are well maintained, even when kidney function is very low.[3,127,128,218] Thus, a well-planned diet does not cause malnutrition and can actually improve the biochemical markers used to estimate nutritional status.[20]

FREE PLASMA AMINO ACID AND KETOACID LEVELS

During fasting, patients with CKD have many abnormalities of plasma amino acids, including an increase in 3-methylhistidine and 1-methylhistidine, apparently caused by reduced renal clearance of these amino acids. Plasma valine is usually low, and leucine and isoleucine levels are lower, but to a more modest extent.[262-265] At least two mechanisms contribute to low levels of branched-chain amino acids (BCAAs). A low protein intake can reduce plasma concentrations of BCAAs and can lead to impaired gastrointestinal absorption.[266] Unfortunately, the contribution of the diet to changes in plasma amino acid levels is unpredictable; rats with experimental CKD fed excess protein had the most abnormal BCAAs in blood.[129] In addition, a high-protein diet causes metabolic acidosis, which can accelerate BCAA catabolism.[136,267-269] Not surprisingly, there is a correlation between plasma bicarbonate levels and free valine content in skeletal muscle of patients on hemodialysis.[14,121,122] Importantly, correction of metabolic acidosis increased the concentrations of all three BCAAs in the muscles of patients on hemodialysis.[121]

Other abnormalities in plasma amino acids include an increased citrulline concentration, attributable to impaired conversion of citrulline to arginine by the diseased kidney. Alternatively, experiments in cultured cells or rats with experimental CKD have indicated that the mechanism underlying high citrulline levels is probably more complex.[270] There also are unexplained increases in cystine, homocysteine, and aspartate levels, decreased tyrosine level, reflecting impaired hydroxylation of phenylalanine, high glycine level, and low or low-normal serine level, perhaps related to diminished production of serine from glycine by the diseased kidney.[271] The free tryptophan level is normal but total tryptophan is low because of reduced plasma protein binding.[272] Threonine and lysine concentrations are low for unknown reasons. Thus, the EAAs, with some exceptions,

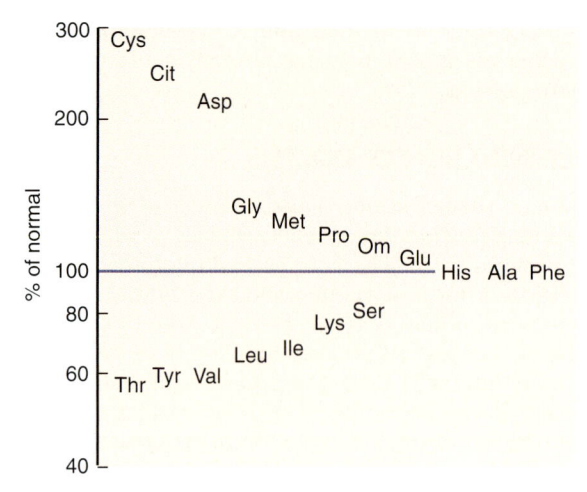

Figure 61.4 Plasma amino acids in patients with chronic renal failure treated by protein restriction alone. Results are calculated as percentages of normal values. A logarithmic scale is used, so decreases are emphasized as much as increases. The most abnormal values are shown on the left. Statistical significance cannot be evaluated in view of the variety of sources of the data. Note that not all essential amino acids are subnormal.

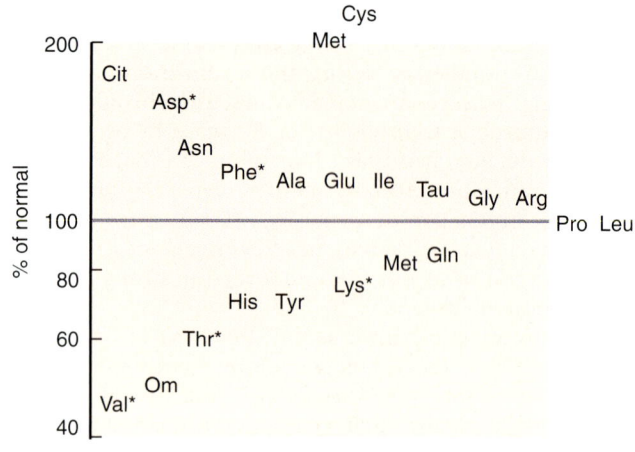

Figure 61.5 Intracellular free amino acid concentrations in muscle of chronically uremic patients treated by protein restriction alone. A logarithmic scale is used, so decreases are emphasized as much as increases. Asterisks indicate statistically significant differences. (Data from Bergström J, Fürst P, Norée L-O, et al: Intracellular free amino acids in muscle tissue of patients with chronic uraemia: Effect of peritoneal dialysis and infusion of essential amino acids. *Clin Sci Mol Med* 54:51-61, 1978.)

tend to be reduced in plasma, whereas some of the nonessential amino acids tend to be increased (Figure 61.4). Decreased EAAs are similar to the pattern seen in patients with protein malnutrition, but in patients with CKD eating an adequate diet, the same abnormalities can persist after a large meal of meat.[264,273] Thus, there is evidence that the low levels of BCAAs, decreased essential/nonessential and valine/glycine ratios, as well as the degree of increase in cystine, citrulline, and methylhistidine concentrations, are all inversely correlated with GFR, suggesting that they result from metabolic defects caused by CKD.

There is growing evidence that the concentrations of sulfur-containing amino acids (e.g., methionine, cysteine, cystine, taurine, homocysteine) are very abnormal in uremic patients, but the mechanisms accounting for these abnormalities have not been defined.[274] This is relevant because patients with CKD can have very high levels of homocysteine, which is associated with atherosclerosis (see earlier). One abnormality is that binding of homocysteine to albumin seems be abnormal, while abnormal intracellular levels of free sulfur-containing amino acids can aggravate the high plasma levels of these amino acids.[274,275]

CKD is also associated with changes in the disposal of amino acids; after an intravenous infusion of amino acids to patients on hemodialysis, the removal of valine and phenylalanine were found to be subnormal, while histidine removal was increased.[276] It is not known whether this observation contributes to the high plasma levels of histamine found in uremic patients, especially those with pruritus.[277]

In general, the degree of abnormalities in amino acids is inversely correlated with GFR, and more severe abnormalities tend to be associated with uremic symptoms.[278] Although the degree of abnormalities tends to worsen with an inadequate protein intake (e.g., there is a direct correlation between the valine/glycine ratio and protein intake), there are also abnormalities in the breakdown of amino acids and in their distribution between cells and extracellular fluid, except for values in erythrocytes or cerebrospinal fluid.[262,279-282] Bergstrom and coworkers[280] measured the intracellular concentration of amino acids in muscle of patients with non–dialysis-requiring CKD and found abnormalities that differed somewhat from those seen in plasma (Figure 61.5); levels of BCAA were subnormal and ornithine was low, as were histidine, threonine, lysine, and arginine. In an evaluation of controls and patients with non–dialysis-requiring CKD patients, Divino Filho and colleagues reported that the BCAAs valine, isoleucine, and leucine in muscle were normal.[283] The authors pointed out that metabolic acidosis was almost absent, so they did not expect that the levels would be low, as found in patients on dialysis with metabolic acidosis.[121,122]

Metabolites of amino acids, including those containing sulfur as well as a number of small peptides and amines (e.g., polyamines, guanidines, other nitrogenous compounds), accumulate in the blood.[81,284] Abnormalities in amino acid metabolites are not reviewed because the genesis of these abnormalities is largely unknown, and there is no specific therapy for them. Generally, their concentrations decrease when protein intake is reduced and urea appearance falls (see Chapter 54).

It should be emphasized that without proper dietary education, the prognosis for patients with CKD is bleak. In one report, patients who had a serum creatinine level above 5 mg/dL also were found to have serum bicarbonate concentrations below 15 mmol/L, serum phosphorus levels above 7 mg/dL, and BUN values above 120 mg/dL.[285] To emphasize one troubling aspect of this report, consider the acidosis. Because the degree of acidosis is related to creatinine clearance and intake of protein, it is not surprising to find the serum bicarbonate level so low unless it is properly addressed by restricting the amount of protein in the diet or by supplementation with oral sodium bicarbonate.[286] Correcting acidosis is not a trivial concern because many of the metabolic abnormalities caused by CKD can be ameliorated by dietary protein restriction, and correcting metabolic acidosis can reduce the progressive loss of kidney function.[19,120] There are also serious consequences of tolerating high serum phosphorus levels (see Chapter 54). The important point is that many consequences of CKD are correctable by providing education about dietary factors. Obviously, this is most easily accomplished via consultation with a dietician.

SPECIFIC DIETARY CONSTITUENTS AND KIDNEY DISEASE

ENERGY

Energy intake and energy requirements of patients with chronic CKD are important considerations.

ENERGY INTAKE

In patients entering dialysis therapy, anthropometric abnormalities, including suboptimal BW, are frequently present and could result from inadequate intake of energy-rich foods.[287-289] The dietary energy requirement can be estimated by measuring the energy expended during a patient's average activity and adding this amount to the patient's resting energy expenditure (REE). The energy required during daily activities is measured by indirect calorimetry over relatively brief periods and then extrapolating the result to 24 hours. This yields a factor that when multiplied by the REE accounts for an individual's activities. The 1981 recommendations for energy intake by the Food and Agriculture Organization of the United Nations (FAO), World Health Organization (WHO), and United Nations University (UNU) were based on approximately 11,000 REE determinations in healthy subjects.[290] The regression equations used to derive energy requirements had considerable variability, and there is a potential source of error from estimating the time spent in various physical activities and intensity of the activities. Notably, healthy subjects adapt to an inadequate nutrient intake by decreasing the value of REE.[291] In otherwise normal, semistarved adults, the REE was found to decrease by about 15% over 3 weeks, leading to a loss of lean body mass.[290] For well-nourished adults, energy balance can be obtained with only 50% of the usual caloric intake as long as physical activity is decreased, but this may result in loss of lean body mass.[289]

ENERGY REQUIREMENTS OF PATIENTS WITH CHRONIC KIDNEY DISEASE

There have been few evaluations of the caloric requirements of patients with CKD and the capacity of these individuals to adapt to a reduced-calorie intake. Monteon and associates examined the energy expenditures of normal controls and patients with CKD during rest and exercise and found no differences between the groups.[292] However, when caloric intake was reduced, energy expenditure did not decrease in either group, indicating that patients with CKD do not respond with the normal adaptive responses to calorie restriction. This leads to the development of calorie malnutrition and possibly negative nitrogen balance, with loss of protein stores. The authors concluded that on average, the energy expenditure of patients on dialysis is no different from that of normal subjects.[292] However, other investigators have reported that energy expenditure on dialysis and nondialysis days was 7% higher in patients undergoing hemodialysis compared to adults without CKD.[293] This latter report suggests that uremia per se increases energy expenditure because CKD-induced metabolic factors that impair energy utilization (e.g., insulin resistance) could reduce the ability of patients with CKD to improve protein metabolism when caloric intake is limited. For example, even modest CKD (serum creatinine ≅ 2.4 mg/dL) or the presence of obesity or metabolic acidosis contributes to insulin resistance and impairs energy utilization.[147,166,294,295] Fortunately, a low-protein diet does not complicate the task of consuming sufficient calories because low-protein diets improve insulin resistance and hence the efficiency of using calories.[2,3,296,297] Rigalleau and coworkers[297] found that insulin responses of patients with CKD eating 0.3 g protein/kg/day plus a supplement of EAAs and ketoacids led to lower plasma glucose and insulin levels plus an improvement in glucose oxidation and nonoxidative disposal (mainly glycogen synthesis). Results from the MDRD study and other reports have indicated that patients with CKD frequently have energy intakes below the recommended levels of 30 to 35 kcal/kg/day and may even reach 21 kcal/kg/day.[217,257,288] When interpreting these data, it is important to note that energy intake in the MDRD study was estimated using dietary interviews and diaries, which may underestimate caloric intake.[298,299]

There is no simple remedy for patients with CKD who have low caloric intake. One possibility is to increase the pasta content of meals as these are complex carbohydrates and will not aggravate diabetes as much as increasing simple sugars. There also needs to be careful monitoring because providing extra calories may only create more body fat rather than increase protein stores.[300] Ensuring that calories do reach the recommended levels is beneficial, and Hyne and colleagues have noted that the nitrogen balance of uremic patients fed a diet of 20 g/day of high-quality protein improved as caloric intake was raised.[301] This finding is similar to a study that found that normal adults eating a diet with only barely adequate amounts of EAAs experienced an improvement in nitrogen balance and hence protein stores when caloric intake was increased.[302] Bergstrom and associates studied patients with CKD who were eating 16 to 20 g/day of protein plus a supplement of EAAs and found no deficits in nitrogen balance when energy intake was varied between 22 and 50 kcal/kg/day.[303] The authors concluded that caloric intake is not critical unless nitrogen and EAA intakes are barely adequate. Not all reports are in agreement. Kopple and coworkers[304] fed six CKD patients a constant, minimal protein intake of 0.55 to 0.6 g/kg/day and measured the nitrogen balance while the caloric intake was varied from 15 to 45 kcal/kg/day.[304] By extrapolation of the measurements, they concluded that nitrogen equilibrium was present when each of the six patients was eating 35 kcal/kg/day (Figure 61.6). We believe that the caloric intake of patients with CKD who are below their ideal BW or are eating a protein-restricted diet should be 35 kcal/kg/day.[304,305] However, overweight patients should have their calories restricted because a caloric intake in excess of energy requirements causes obesity, which aggravates insulin resistance and impairs the utilization of protein and calories.[295,299,300]

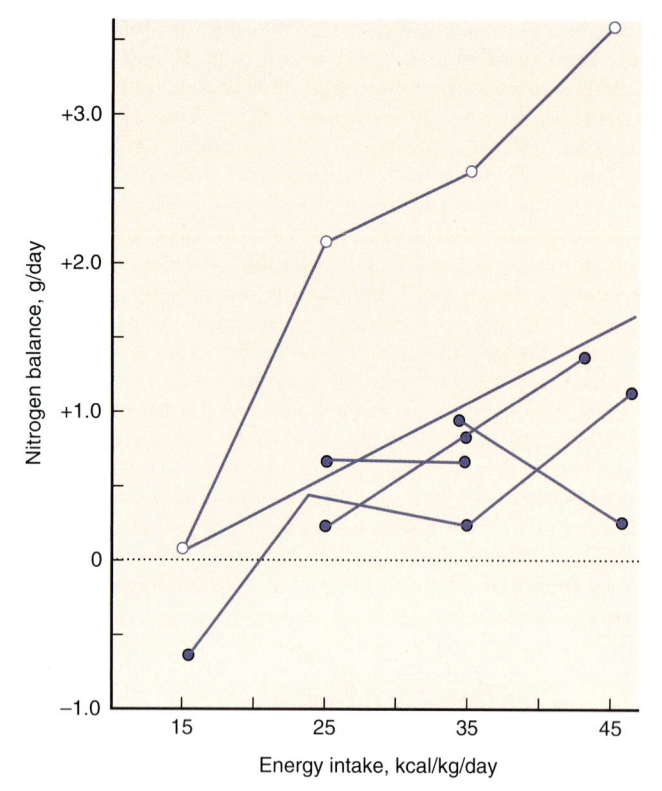

Figure 61.6 Correlation between nitrogen balance and energy intake in six clinically stable, nondialyzed, chronically uremic patients. The *open circle* represent the patient who had the lowest resting energy expenditure. The *solid line* is the regression line derived from the individual results. (From Kopple JD, Monteon FJ, Shaib JK: Effect of energy intake on nitrogen metabolism in nondialyzed patients with chronic renal failure. *Kidney Int* 29:734-742, 1986.)

DIETARY FACTORS

SALT

The ability to achieve salt balance rapidly permits normal subjects to maintain an extracellular fluid volume that changes by less than 1 L (1 kg of BW) and a change in blood pressure of less than 10%, despite wide variations in daily salt intake. If blood pressure rises when the salt intake increases, a patient is labelled salt-sensitive, and he or she will achieve neutral salt balance more slowly. In contrast, persons who are salt-resistant rapidly excrete additional salt and do not have an increase in blood pressure. This is relevant because salt sensitivity has several negative features, such as the following: (1) it precedes established hypertension; (2) constitutes a cardiovascular risk factor; (3) complicates antihypertensive therapy; and (4) contributes to progressive loss of kidney function by exacerbating proteinuria and diminishing antiproteinuric responses.[306,307] For these reasons, managing salt intake is an essential component of the treatment of patients with hypertension, CKD, and/or cardiovascular risk factors. It should also be emphasized that treatment with diuretics alone will fail if salt intake is unrestricted because the excess salt will overcome the effectiveness of the diuretic.[1] Unfortunately, managing salt intake is difficult because so much salt is added to foods: it is estimated that at least 75% or more of the daily sodium intake is included in prepared foods, indicating that patients should seek low-sodium food (and, in particular, should be encouraged to prepare foods at home) rather than be hounded about use of the salt shaker.[308,309]

A daily intake of 2 g of sodium is equivalent to about 84 mEq of sodium, while a so-called no-added-salt diet contains about 4 g, or 168 mEq of sodium. Consequently, a diet based on no added salt will often exacerbate hypertension and cause edema in patients with moderate-to-advanced CKD. The recommended sodium intake for hypertensive patients with CKD is approximately 2 g/day, a diet that can be reasonably easily achieved with appropriate dietary planning. This recommendation comes from WHO and the Joint National Commission on Prevention, Detection, Evaluation, and Treatment of High Blood Pressure (JNC) in their recommendations for the treatment of patients with pre- or established hypertension.[308] Unfortunately, processed foods and fast foods contain substantial amounts of salt, and a skilled dietitian is needed to achieve the recommended salt intake.

Patients with hypertension and CKD frequently have salt sensitivity, detected as an increase in blood pressure of more than 10% when a low-salt diet is switched to a high salt intake. The frequency of salt-sensitive hypertension is rather high, especially in African Americans, and the frequency increases with age, especially when kidney function declines.[309,310] Most patients with advanced CKD are salt sensitive, with the possible exception of those with primary tubulointerstitial disease, because these patients can excrete salt more readily and tend to have normal blood pressure.[311] With CKD, hypertension is closely related to the progression of CKD, especially in patients with proteinuria.[311] Unfortunately, relying on diuretics to reduce salt accumulation is often futile. For example, with furosemide treatment, normal adults experience a sharp increase in sodium excretion, producing an initial negative sodium balance. However, over the remaining 18 to 20 hours, dietary salt and fluid are retained, counteracting the effectiveness of the diuretic.[1] Patients who consume excess salt experience no net loss of sodium, despite furosemide-induced natriuresis. We recommend that diuretic therapy must be accompanied by restricting salt intake to 2 g sodium/day. Salt restriction is especially important for hypertensive or CKD patients because antihypertensive agents (with the possible exception of calcium channel blockers) are less effective in reducing blood pressure unless salt intake is restricted.[312] Drug-resistant hypertension is almost always due to a high level of salt intake. For example, the effectiveness of ACEIs or angiotensin receptor blockers (ARBs) declines sharply unless dietary salt is controlled; these agents are also less effective in suppressing protein excretion.[312] The ideal sodium intake for healthy normotensive individuals is 80 to 120 mmol (i.e., 2 to 3 g sodium/day). If there is hypertension, daily salt intake should be less than 100 mmol (<2.5 g sodium) and, if edema or proteinuria is present, the restriction should be 84 mmol/day of sodium (~2 g sodium). Since 95% of sodium ingested is excreted by the kidneys, a 24-hour sodium excretion is the best indicator of sodium intake. Other estimates are less accurate because sodium excretion fluctuates widely during the day. Consequently, a spot urine to measure the sodium/creatinine ratio is not useful for assessing salt intake. With fever, strenuous exercise, or diarrhea, and especially for patients with an ileostomy, there can be significant extrarenal sodium losses. It is important to note that patients accustomed to a high salt intake can experience salt craving when they begin reducing salt intake; this lasts about 2 weeks, so patients should be reassured that the craving will disappear with time.[308,313] Salt substitutes may be judiciously used in the absence of hyperkalemia or treatment with RAAS inhibitors.

In summary, a cornerstone of designing diets for CKD patients is to establish appropriate goals for blood pressure and salt intake. Optimally, home blood pressure recording or ambulatory 24-hour blood pressure recordings should be obtained to assess the effectiveness of therapy. Treatment must include plans for altering dietary salt intake, and the effectiveness of the plan should be assessed by a 24-hour urine collection for sodium excretion. The same collection can be used to determine creatinine clearance and estimate protein intake and the excretion of microalbumin and other minerals. Once the goals of dietary salt and blood pressure have been met, blood pressure values and periodic measurements of 24-hour sodium excretion are necessary to assess long-term compliance. If sodium excretion is excessive and blood pressure increases, visits to the nutritionist and repeating measurements of 24-hour urine sodium excretion will make dietary planning easier.

POTASSIUM

Guidelines from the Institute of Medicine have recommended that the general population should have a daily intake of potassium of 4.7 g/day.[314] With advanced renal insufficiency, acidosis, or other chronic conditions, the ability to excrete potassium can be impaired because of loss of functional nephron mass (indicated by a decrease in GFR), possibly abnormal responses to protective hormones (e.g., aldosterone), and impairment in function that occurs with inhibitors of RAAS (e.g., ACEIs), ARBs, and mineralocorticoid antagonists. Counteracting these problems are adaptations that increase the excretion of potassium via the kidney and gut.[209] This is fortunate because patients with progressive kidney disease find it difficult to comply with both sodium and potassium restriction.

There is substantial evidence that diets rich in potassium, particularly when the intake of fruits and vegetables is high, have a reduced likelihood of developing chronic diseases such as coronary heart disease and diabetes. Clinically important reductions in blood pressure have also been documented in subjects with normal blood pressures or mild hypertension, as long as they consume a potassium-rich diet. Results of a key randomized trial, the DASH (Dietary Approaches to Stop Hypertension) study, concentrated on modifying the diet to raise potassium intake. In this study, 459 subjects with a systolic blood pressure lower than 160 mm Hg and diastolic blood pressure of 80 to 95 mm Hg were randomly assigned to different diets.[315] Initially, all subjects were fed a control diet that was low in fruits, vegetables, and dairy products but with a typical fat content. Subsequently, subjects were randomly assigned to one of three diets for 8 weeks: (1) the control diet, rich in fruits and vegetables; (2) a combined diet, rich in fruits and vegetables, with limited dairy products; and (3) a diet with reduced content of saturated and total fats. For all three groups, sodium intake and body weight were maintained at constant levels. Compared to the control diet, the mean reductions in systolic and diastolic blood pressures associated with the combination diet were 5.5 and 3.0 mm Hg, respectively. For the 133 subjects who were hypertensive, the results were more pronounced; systolic and diastolic pressures were lowered by 11.4 and 5.5 mm Hg, respectively. The blood pressure–lowering effects of the DASH diet were more pronounced in black participants (systolic and diastolic BP reductions of 6.9 and 3.7 mm Hg) than in whites (3.3 and 2.4 mm Hg).[316] While this type of study does not directly demonstrate that high potassium intake is beneficial, it does demonstrate that a potassium-rich diet is beneficial.

Regarding the amount of dietary potassium for patients with CKD, the NKF's expert panel recommended potassium restriction to 2 g/day or less for individuals with advanced CKD (e.g., stage 4 CKD and estimated GFR values < 30 mL/min/1.73 m^2).[317] Unfortunately, for patients with more advanced CKD, potassium stores are low, even though the serum potassium level is high.[318,319] When dealing with patients who have a high serum potassium concentration, the initial search should be for nondietary causes of hyperkalemia before restricting dietary potassium. This is recommended because a diet restricted in potassium and sodium is difficult to achieve. Thus, drugs that reduce potassium excretion should be eliminated, acidosis should be corrected, and constipation should be relieved (the gut becomes an alternative organ removing potassium in patients with CKD). Clearly, more studies are needed to determine the usefulness and dangers of increasing (or limiting) dietary potassium in patients with CKD.

PROTEIN

Protein Intake

Nitrogen balance (NB) is the gold standard for assessing dietary protein requirements because a neutral or positive NB indicates that the body's protein stores are being maintained or increased. Unfortunately, measuring NB is time consuming and technically demanding, so there have been few examinations of NB as a method for examining protein requirements of patients with CKD. For healthy adults who are engaging in moderate amounts of physical activity and are consuming sufficient calories, NB measurements indicate that the average protein requirement is approximately 0.6 g protein/kg ideal BW/day. This level of dietary protein is recommended because it was derived from subjects who were fed variable amounts of protein; therefore, by extrapolation, WHO investigators determined that the average protein intake required to maintain neutral NB was 0.6 g protein/kg BW/day. This level of diet protein plus 2 SDs (standard deviations) of the measurements led to a recommended level of 0.75 g protein/kg BW/day; this value was designated as the safe level of intake and meets the dietary protein requirements of 97.5% of healthy adults.[290]

There are two caveats. First, this amount of dietary protein is not needed by all subjects as some will require less than this amount and others require more. In adults, eating more than this amount does not improve body protein stores because the catabolic pathways described earlier stimulate losses of protein stores. Instead, dietary protein in excess of the safe level of intake is converted to waste, including potential by-products of metabolism (sometimes referred to as toxins) that are excreted by patients with normal kidney function.[66] Even with a diet containing more than 1 g protein/kg BW/day, the daily rates of protein synthesis and degradation are much greater than protein intake, emphasizing the dynamic metabolic processes occurring throughout the day.[66] For example, in response to fasting, there is a reduction in the level of plasma insulin, and body protein stores (principally skeletal muscle) are degraded to amino acids, which are converted to glucose in the liver. A principal modulator of changes in protein turnover in patients with diabetes or CKD is insulin because it suppresses protein degradation in normal or diabetic subjects.[320,321] The important role of insulin in determining protein metabolism (and hence NB) is emphasized because insulin resistance occurs in patients with CKD, even when the serum creatinine level is as low as 2.4 mg/dL; insulin resistance also occurs with complications of CKD, such as metabolic acidosis.[147,166] In summary, healthy adults successfully adapt to dietary protein restriction by suppressing catabolism of EAAs and by suppressing protein degradation while stimulating protein synthesis. The principal anabolic factor, insulin, mediates metabolic responses to eating and fasting and, since CKD is associated with insulin resistance, the initiation of CKD-induced losses of protein stores could be linked to insulin resistance.

PROTEIN REQUIREMENTS

Patients with Chronic Kidney Disease

Patients with advanced but uncomplicated CKD are remarkably efficient in adapting to dietary protein restriction, even when the estimated GFR is 5 to 15 mL/min/1.73 m².[322] Specifically, the subjects reduce amino acid oxidation and protein degradation, just as that which occurs in normal adults who restrict their dietary protein from 1.0 to 0.6 g/kg/day. Similarly, these adaptive metabolic responses occur when the diet is restricted to only 0.3 g/kg/day and a supplement of EAAs or their nitrogen-free analogues (ketoacids). Both these diets can maintain neutral NB and indices of adequate nutrition for more than 1 year of observation.[218,323,324] The specific metabolic adaptations that occur with dietary protein restriction include a stimulation of the oxidation of amino acids, resulting in a lower requirement for and more efficient utilization of EAAs (Figure 61.7).

Second, when protein or amino acid intakes are barely sufficient, neutral NB is achieved by a postprandial suppression of whole-body protein degradation; there may be an accompanying increase in protein synthesis. However, if protein (or amino acid) intakes are inadequate, these compensatory response(s) cannot fully compensate for the inadequate diet, and a negative NB causes loss of lean mass. When considering low-protein diets for diabetic patients, some caution is needed because there are reports that diabetic patients cannot activate the adaptive changes to dietary protein restriction that occur in normal adults and CKD patients. These dietary protein requirements are summarized in Table 61.2.

Patients with Nephrotic Syndrome

Patients with hypercholesterolemia, edema, and more than 3 g urinary protein/day (i.e., patients with the nephrotic

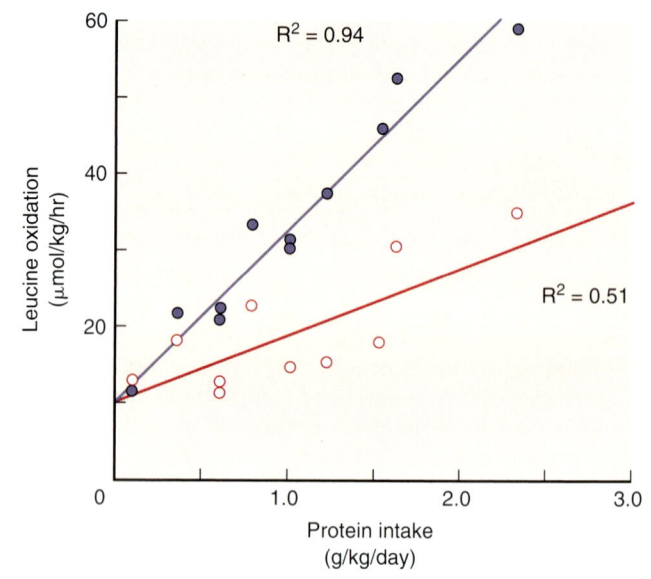

Figure 61.7 Relationships between different levels of dietary protein and rates of leucine oxidation in normal subjects and chronic kidney disease patients during fasting (*open circles*) and feeding (*closed circles*). There is a significant correlation between the amount of dietary protein and leucine oxidation during fasting and feeding, showing the adaptive response to dietary protein changes. (From Tom K, Young VR, Chapman T, et al: Long-term adaptive responses to dietary protein restriction in chronic renal failure. *Am J Physiol* 268:E668-E677, 1995.)

Table 61.2 Dietary Requirements for Patients with Chronic Kidney Disease

Patients	Protein Requirement	Comments
Normal adults or those with uncomplicated CKD	RDA, 0.8 g protein/kg/day	30-35 kcal/kg/day needed to use dietary protein efficiently
Symptomatic CKD patients, those with complications	Minimum, 0.6 g protein/kg/day or 0.3 g/kg/day + ketoacids or a mixture of essential amino acids	Adjustments for specific problems (e.g., diabetes, hyperphosphatemia)
CKD patients with loss of muscle mass	0.8 g protein/kg/day	
CKD patients with proteinuria	<0.8 g protein/kg/day + 1 g protein/g proteinuria	This is the maximum needed. Even less dietary protein may be sufficient.

CKD, Chronic kidney disease; RDA, recommended daily allowance.

syndrome) have an increased risk for developing loss of body protein stores. Notably, the defect cannot be corrected by giving nephrotic patients a protein-rich diet. In fact, such a diet increases proteinuria in patients with nephrotic syndrome and patients with many other disorders causing CKD.[103,325] A well-designed, low-protein diet (LPD) can decrease proteinuria and often can increase serum albumin levels relative to a higher protein diet, especially when examined in patients with heavy proteinuria. Because the degree of proteinuria is closely related to the risk for progressive kidney and cardiovascular diseases, the initiation of an LPD might be used to counteract the risks associated with progressive loss of kidney function. Regarding safety of protein restricted diets, patients with the nephrotic syndrome who were fed adequate calories and an LPD (0.8 g/kg/day plus 1 g/day of protein for each gram of urinary protein excreted over 5 g/day) had a neutral NB and improved components of protein turnover when compared to responses of patients with nephrotic syndrome who were fed a diet containing 1.6 g protein/kg BW/day, plus the same supplement for excess proteinuria and 35 kcal/kg/day. Moreover, patients with nephrotic syndrome fed a modest LPD suppressed amino acid oxidation and protein degradation, leading to neutral or positive NB.[206] Notably, there is evidence that an LPD (<0.6 g/kg BW/day) does not increase the risk of protein wasting in patients with the nephrotic syndrome.[109] In summary, patients with uncomplicated CKD, including those with nephrotic-range proteinuria, activate normal compensatory responses to dietary protein restrictions by suppressing EAA oxidation and reducing protein degradation. Consequently, NB is neutral and lean body mass is maintained during long-term dietary therapy.

BENEFICIAL RESPONSES TO REDUCED DIETARY PROTEIN IN CHRONIC KIDNEY DISEASE OR AFTER KIDNEY TRANSPLANTATION

To determine if the decreased loss of kidney function found in animals fed LPDs also occurs in humans, clinical trials have examined the benefits of reducing dietary protein on nutritional status and the progressive loss of kidney function in patients with CKD. Unfortunately, some of the published studies are of low methodologic quality because they were retrospective studies with only a small number of patients or serious design flaws. Based on standards of adequate quality, we examined more than 80 trials from which 10 RCTs[326-335] and five meta-analyses[336-340] were identified. With these data, we addressed the question of whether dietary protein restriction slows the progression of CKD.[339] In discussing these reports, we will use the more general term *slowed progression of kidney disease* rather than *slowed the loss of kidney function*. The GFR (the gold standard of kidney function) was determined in just a few studies. Instead, outcomes in reported trials were based on estimating differences in changes in serum creatinine levels or the degree of proteinuria.

PROTEINS, PHOSPHATES, AND FIBROBLAST GROWTH FACTOR-23

It is well known that hyperphosphatemia contributes to bone disease (and, more broadly, CKD-MBD [mineral and bone disorder]) but there are at least two reasons for reevaluating the influence of phosphate intake and CKD. First, phosphates are added to prepared or processed foods to prevent spoilage.[9,10,341] Second, there are complex relationships among protein and phosphorus intakes and excretion, plus the influences of changes in serum phosphorus levels, parathyroid hormone status, and bone metabolism. The responses to FGF-23 have added yet another level of complexity to our understanding of the complicated metabolic pathways regulating calcium and phosphate metabolism and bone disease.[57] Even the terminology is confusing. There are different types of phosphate anions, and the proportions of these anions depend critically on the blood pH and other factors, making the interpretation of the plasma phosphates complex. Because of the marked influence of pH on the different types of phosphates, clinical laboratories do not report phosphate concentrations but report the serum concentration of phosphorus, which represents the concentration of all types of phosphates. Therefore, patients and physicians concentrate on regulating the amount of phosphorus in the diet, even though all physiologically important reactions are based on phosphate metabolism.

The intake of phosphates is linked to dietary protein by a predictable relationship—approximately 1 g of protein contains 13 mg of phosphate—and, consequently, variations in the amount of protein eaten will predictably change phosphorus intake. The serum phosphorus level, therefore, is influenced by the amount of protein in the diet as well as processes that regulate phosphate metabolism, including the intestinal absorption of dietary phosphates, excretion of phosphates by renal tubules, and changes in bone metabolism.

In CKD, it is axiomatic that phosphorus retention initiates the well-established metabolic disturbances described in Chapter 55. A rise in the serum phosphate concentration is often recognized at a late stage of CKD because there are physiologic adaptations in earlier stages of CKD that prevent excessive phosphorus retention. Perhaps the most prominent adaptation is the stimulation of PTH release because this hormone increases phosphate excretion (or, more accurately, reduces phosphate absorption) by proximal tubule cells. The epidemiology of the relationships among a loss of kidney function (measured as a decrease in ^{51}Cr-EDTA clearance), the retention of phosphorus, and a compensatory increase in PTH levels has been examined in more than 1000 CKD patients.[342] At eGFR values below 49.5 mL/min/1.73 m^2, a rise in serum PTH levels above 60 pg/mL was detectable, but serum phosphate concentrations more than 4.3 mg/dL (1.38 mmol/L) were not observed until eGFR values were less than 37 mL/min/1.73 m^2. This finding suggests that phosphate retention is not a prominent reason for the development of secondary hyperparathyroidism (see Chapters 55), but there are flaws in this suggestion. The serum phosphorus level is generally measured after an overnight fast, so the absence of a protein- and phosphorus-rich meal plus the phosphaturia induced by the response to a higher PTH level yields normal or even low values of serum phosphorus. Nevertheless, it is generally agreed that the pathophysiology of hyperparathyroidism depends on phosphate retention due to lost kidney function. Moranne and colleagues have found other associations. First, the likelihood that PTH would be increased in patients with CKD was 70% higher in black patients compared to white patients.[342] Secondly, hyperphosphatemia was somewhat more likely to be present in patients with tubulointerstitial diseases compared to patients with CKD caused by other types of kidney disorders. The reasons for these associations were not identified.

Another factor affecting serum phosphorus levels is FGF-23, a phosphatonin synthesized by osteoblasts.[343] When the FGF-23 level is increased, especially in the presence of Klotho (a FGF-23 co-factor), there is a brisk phosphaturia. Activation of the proximal tubule receptor by FGF-23 and Klotho also suppresses activity of the 1-α-hydroxylase, blocking synthesis of calcitriol in the proximal tubule. Therefore, FGF-23 will reduce serum phosphorus levels despite CKD because there are two counteracting mechanisms—phosphate excretion is stimulated and calcitriol production is reduced, resulting in the suppression of intestinal phosphate absorption. The physiologic relevance of these reactions in CKD is suggested by the finding that serum levels of FGF-23 are high, even before the serum PTH level rises. There is much to learn about FGF-23 and any adverse effects it generates. Presumably, the toxic responses to FGF-23 arise in patients with CKD because of the very high levels of FGF-23. In the serum of 6 healthy adults, FGF-23 was reported to be 40 U/mL while in 20 CKD patients, FGF-23 values were as high as 2000 U/mL. In 33 hemodialysis patients, the levels were as high as 60,000 U/mL.[344] Notably, it is reported that very high levels of serum FGF-23 are associated with an increased risk of mortality, which is seemingly independent of the serum phosphorus level.[345] We recognize that these associations are difficult to interpret because such patients are also very likely to have high PTH levels and manifest problems arising from the accumulation of uremic toxins. Since phosphorus accumulation is linked to protein intake in CKD patients, and since uremic toxins are mainly derived from dietary protein, high serum phosphorus and FGF-23 levels are usually found in patients eating excessive amounts of protein.[346] This conclusion is supported by the finding that even high levels of FGF-23 do not correct hyperphosphatemia in patients with advanced CKD. The inability to stimulate phosphate excretion sufficiently to avoid phosphate accumulation occurs when the eGFR is less than 35 mL/min/1.73^2, despite the phosphaturic action of FGF-23 and PTH.[342] At this stage of CKD, phosphorus intake must be limited or adverse consequences will occur, including secondary hyperparathyroidism, renal bone disease, and soft tissue calcification.[347]

How do dietary phosphates influence the regulation of the FGF-23 and PTH? In healthy adults, FGF-23 expression can be directly regulated by varying dietary phosphate levels.[348] When otherwise normal adults were given 1 g phosphate daily for 5 days, serum FGF-23 levels increased by about 30% while serum PTH levels did not change. However, the increase in FGF-23 led to a higher value of urinary phosphates plus a decrease in serum calcitriol levels.[349] There are data highlighting the fact that FGF-23 concentrations are influenced by the restriction of dietary phosphorus.[349] Also, in healthy men, the FGF-23 concentration responds to dietary phosphorus intake. For example, reducing the dietary phosphorus intake of 13 healthy men from 1500 to 625 mg/day yielded a 32% decrease in serum FGF-23 levels, suggesting that phosphorus intake directly affects FGF-23 expression.[349] The responses of patients with CKD to dietary phosphorus restriction differ somewhat because phosphate loading causes an increase in FGF-23, even if the FGF-23 level is already high.[344] Still, these reports must be considered as preliminary because the high levels of FGF-23 found in CKD may represent partially degraded FGF-23 proteins that are recognized by the antibody (similar to the different forms of PTH in serum; see Chapter 55).

A discussion about the control of phosphorus retention is relevant to CKD because of the associated risk of cardiovascular disease in subjects with phosphorus retention, a phenomenon that has been recognized even in adults with normal or near-normal kidney function.[350] First, dietary phosphate was shown to be positively associated with left ventricular hypertrophy in the Multi-Ethnic Study of Atherosclerosis.[351] Second, an association between serum phosphate level and mortality was found in a review of data from the Framingham Study. Over a 16-year period of observation, it was found that healthy adults with serum phosphate concentrations above 3.5 mg/dL experienced a graded increase in the risk of cardiovascular morbidity and mortality.[350] Those persons who were in the highest quartile of serum phosphorus had a 55% higher risk of cardiovascular events when compared to those in the lowest quartile. Notably, an even higher mortality risk was observed in CKD. In a retrospective analysis of 7000 Veterans' Affairs patients with CKD, Kestenbaum and associates found that each 1-mg/dL increase in the serum phosphate concentration was associated with a 23% increase in mortality.[352] They also found that when the eGFR values fell below 30 mL/min/1.73 m^2, serum phosphorus levels increased, as did mortality. Menon and coworkers analyzed the associations of serum phosphate levels and mortality in patients who had enrolled in the MDRD study, a prospective RCT of the influence of different prescriptions of dietary protein and different degrees of hypertension control of progression of CKD (among other outcomes; see earlier discussion).[353] Although there was a trend toward an increase in mortality for subjects with higher serum phosphorus concentrations, the differences were not statistically significant. It was also noted that the mortality rate extrapolated over a 10-year period after the MDRD study was stopped was remarkably low; variations in serum phosphorus levels did not explain this observation. In a retrospective analysis of CKD patients by the Veterans Administration, 985 patients evaluated between 1995 and 2005 were examined to determine the frequency of a composite outcome, which included end-stage kidney disease (ESKD) and doubling of serum creatinine levels.[354] After making multiple adjustments, the authors concluded there was a 29% higher hazard ratio (HR) for the loss of kidney function when the serum phosphorus level increased by 1 mg/dL, which was above the reference level (3.3 mg/dL). This increase in risk was also present when variations in the calcium-phosphate product were examined. These results are similar to those provided by Voormolen and colleagues, who studied 448 patients with advanced CKD (stages 4 and 5) in a prospective evaluation of outcomes between 1999 and 2003.[355] The patients with more severely impaired kidney function (mean eGFR = 13 ± 5 mL/min/1.73 m^2) had a 60% increase in the HR for mortality for each increase of 1 mg/dL of serum phosphorus ($P = 0.04$). It was also found that an increase in the serum phosphorus level was associated with a faster rate of loss of kidney function ($P < 0.001$) compared to results from patients who did not experience an increase in their serum phosphorus level.

One important point is the contribution of protein structure to phosphorus metabolism. Although dietary phosphorus is strongly linked to dietary protein, phosphorus can be bound in larger molecules, such as phytates, in vegetable proteins. The human intestine does not express the phytase enzyme to digest the accompanying phosphates. Therefore, phosphorus from vegetable protein is less readily absorbed compared with phosphorus from animal protein. This issue was recently illustrated by Moe and associates, who conducted a short, randomized crossover study of patients with stage 3 CKD. Study subjects received two 800-mg/day phosphorus diets, one from vegetable sources and one from casein.[56] There was a lower degree of phosphaturia and lower serum phosphorus level in subjects during the vegetable protein phase, suggesting that intestinal phosphorus absorption was lower. Interestingly, serum FGF-23 levels varied in opposite directions from baseline—serum FGF-23 concentrations decreased during the vegetable protein phase and increased during the casein phase, underlining the importance of dietary intake in FGF-23 metabolism.

Klotho, the FGF-23 co-receptor responsible for tubular phosphate reabsorption, is an important molecule that has been linked to longevity. Circulating Klotho gradually decreases during CKD progression. The primary decrease in Klotho expression observed during CKD may be partly responsible for a reduction in FGF-23 activity and thus of the subsequent well-described FGF-23 elevation. Although there are few data on the relationship between Klotho and dietary intake as of yet, a recent experimental study has shown that reducing phosphorus intake in mice can partly restore the decline in Klotho observed in the CKD mouse model.[356]

Another important point about phosphorus and diet relates to phosphate additives. Until recently, there has been a sustained, industry-wide trend to add inorganic phosphorus during food processing.[341] There are many reasons for this addition—phosphorus extends product shelf life, enhances taste and color, and increases water content of food by 10% to 15%, the latter facilitating higher pricing. There is no incentive for manufacturers to disclose added inorganic phosphates. While the generally recommended daily phosphorus intake for patients with moderate-to-advanced CKD is roughly 800 mg/day, it is noteworthy that inorganic phosphates added to processed foods can add 1000 mg/day or more to the daily intake, thwarting other well-intentioned dietary restrictions.

This discussion emphasizes why it is important to control the dietary habits of patients with CKD. Specifically, the key to achieving a goal of maintaining serum phosphate levels within the population reference range must include a phosphorus-restricted diet. The amount of dietary phosphorus should be no more than roughly 800 mg phosphorus/day, a level that will permit enough dietary variety while preventing excessive phosphate accumulation or the triggering of a CKD-MBD biochemical spiral (e.g., rising FG-F23, PTH levels) that may contribute to bone disease, vascular and valvular heart disease and, potentially, death.

RANDOMIZED CONTROLLED TRIALS

NONDIABETIC CHRONIC KIDNEY DISEASE

Locatelli and the Northern Italian Cooperative Study Group analyzed 456 patients designated as stage 3 or 4 CKD during a period of at least 2 years.[330] Patients were randomly prescribed 0.6 g/kg/day (LPD) or 1 g/kg/day (control group); the actual amount of dietary protein was determined from urea nitrogen excretion.[61,63] The control group ingested an average of 0.90 g protein/kg/day while the low-protein group ingested an average of 0.78 g/kg/day; there also was substantial overlap in dietary protein ingested by the two patient groups. Obviously, the trial did not test the hypothesis that eating a low-protein diet will slow the loss of kidney function. Not surprisingly, the primary outcome of renal survival, as defined as the start of dialysis or the doubling of serum creatinine levels during the study, had only a borderline difference between control and LPD groups ($P = 0.059$). Slightly fewer patients assigned to the LPD group reached the end point.

The MDRD study reported the effects of different levels of protein intake and two levels of blood pressure control in a 2×2 factorial design.[331] In study A (stage 3 or 4 CKD), 585 patients were randomly assigned to a standard diet of more than 1 g protein/kg/day or a diet containing 0.6 g protein/kg/day, with targeted mean arterial blood pressures of 105 or 92 mm Hg, respectively. In study B, 255 patients with stage 4 CKD were randomly assigned to diets including 0.6 or 0.3 g protein/kg/day supplemented with a ketoacid-EAA mixture; blood pressure goals were the same as in study A. The average actual protein intakes based on urea nitrogen excretion were 1.11 or 0.73 g protein/kg/day in study A patients and 0.69 or 0.46 g protein/kg/day in study B patients, respectively (plus the ketoacids-EAAs provided to one group of study B patients).[61,63] It was concluded that there was no difference in the rate of loss of GFR between the two groups in study A. In study B patients, the average rate of GFR loss was slightly higher in the group ingesting 0.69 g protein/kg/day compared to the rate of loss function in subjects assigned to eat 0.46 g protein/kg/day plus ketoacids and EAAs ($P = 0.07$). At first glance, these results indicate a negative intervention, but there are caveats to this conclusion. First, during the first 4 months in study A, there was an initial decrease in GFR in the group assigned to the restricted protein intake. It was ascribed to a physiologic reduction in glomerular hemodynamics, which is a well-documented effect of dietary protein restriction.[357] Subsequently, there was a slower loss of GFR in patients in the LPD group compared to those with the higher intake (1.11 g protein/kg/day). Consequently, calculating the rate of loss of GFR from the initial 4 months until the last measurements of GFR would have yielded a significantly lower value in patients assigned to the protein-restricted group; there also was a significant improvement in kidney survival ($P = 0.009$). Second, the rate of loss of GFR was lower than predicted; additional follow-up time might have resulted in greater separation of kidney function curves. Consider the Diabetes Control and Complications Trial (DCCT), which examined the influence of strict blood glucose control on kidney function. Initially, there was no protective effect of intensive insulin therapy on the progression of kidney disease. After 2 years of observation, a benefit began to emerge, and after 4 years of strict glycemic control, the development of microalbuminuria or macroalbuminuria was significantly reduced.

Secondary analyses of the MDRD trial, although arguably less robust, have suggested slowing of progression with dietary protein restriction.[358] For example, when the results were analyzed according to the measured (rather than prescribed) protein intake, an LPD reduced the rate of loss of GFR in study B patients ($P = 0.011$) and reduced the frequency of renal death (death or initiation of dialysis; $P = 0.001$).[359] For every reduction in 0.2 g/kg/day of protein intake, a 1.15-mL/min/year reduction in the rate of loss of GFR was documented. There also was a 49% reduction in the frequency of renal deaths. These secondary results from the MDRD study suggest that there may be a benefit of reducing the dietary protein on progression of CKD.

Another caveat in the interpretation of the MDRD study is that no apparent benefit of restricting dietary protein or controlling blood pressure occurred in patients with polycystic kidney disease. This raises questions about the interpretation of results of the MDRD study since patients with polycystic kidney disease constituted about 25% of patients in the MDRD study. Thus, it is possible that the inclusion of results from this group may have obscured beneficial responses on the progression of CKD in patients with other types of kidney disease.[331]

In a smaller study lasting only 18 months, Williams and coworkers analyzed the effects of three dietary interventions in 95 patients with stage 4 or 5 CKD.[328] Patients were randomly prescribed one of three diets: 0.6 g protein/kg/day and 800 mg phosphate intake; 1000 mg phosphate/day plus phosphate binders; and no specified dietary protein level or a combined protein and phosphate unrestricted diet. Compliance assessments revealed protein intake as 0.7, 1.02, and 1.14 g protein/kg/day plus 815, 1000, and 1400 mg phosphorus/day, respectively. There was a minor weight loss in the low-protein and low-phosphate groups (−1.3 and −1.6 kg for the LPD and low-phosphate groups, respectively), but no differences in the decline in creatinine clearance among the three groups.

Cianciaruso and colleagues studied two different levels of protein intake, 0.55 versus 0.80 g/kg/day in patients with stage 4 or 5 CKD during 18 months.[334] In this study, 212 patients were randomly assigned to receive the lower protein intake and 211 patients were prescribed the higher level of dietary protein. Based on urea excretion, the protein-restricted group ate 0.72 g protein/kg/day; the higher protein group ate an average of 0.92 g protein/kg/day ($P < 0.05$).[61] Urinary excretion of urea, sodium, and phosphate were all reduced in subjects assigned to the low-protein diet group. Importantly, the authors found no alteration in body composition or nutritional indices (principally, serum albumin) in either group. When the results were evaluated using an intention to treat analysis, 13 patients assigned to 0.8 g protein/kg/day versus 9 patients assigned to 0.55 g protein/kg/day died or had to begin dialysis during the study.

Di Iorio and associates evaluated how a very low protein intake supplemented with ketoacids might affect the efficiency of erythropoietin therapy in 20 patients over 2 years.[333] Actual protein intakes of two randomly chosen groups were 0.49 g/kg/day plus a supplement of ketoacids versus 0.79 g/kg/day. In those assigned to the very low-protein diet plus ketoacids, only 2 patients had to begin dialysis compared to 7 subjects in the higher dietary protein group ($P < 0.05$). Erythropoietin responsiveness improved in subjects prescribed the very low protein-ketoacid regimen; this improvement was inversely related to the serum PTH level and to decreased phosphorus intake or a decrease in the serum phosphate concentration.[333]

Ihle and coworkers[329] studied 72 Australian patients with stage 4 or 5 CKD. They were randomly assigned to a diet of unlimited protein or 0.4 g protein/kg/day for 18 months. Actual protein intakes based on urea excretion were 0.6 g/kg/day for the dietary protein-restricted group and 0.8 g/kg/day for the control group. The GFR (^{51}Cr-EDTA clearance) was measured every 6 months and demonstrated a progressive decline only in the control patients. The number of patients who had to begin dialysis was higher in those assigned to the unrestricted dietary protein group ($P < 0.05$).[329]

Malvy and colleagues studied a very low protein-restricted intake diet (0.3 g protein/kg/day) supplemented with keto-analogues (Ketosteril; 0.17 g/kg/day) in comparison with a diet containing 0.65 g protein/kg/day; 50 stage 4 or 5 CKD patients were randomly assigned one of two diets.[332] The design included measuring the time until a patient's creatinine clearance decreased below 5 mL/min/1.73 m^2 or until a patient had to begin dialysis. The authors found no significant difference in renal survival between the two diets. They did report that patients in the very low protein-ketoacid group lost 2.7 kg during the 3-year study, and that weight loss included a loss of fat and lean body mass. Weight loss and changes in body composition were not found in patients prescribed the 0.65 g-protein/kg/day diet. The half-life until renal death was 9 months in the diet of 0.65 g protein/kg/day but 21 months for those eating the more restricted diet (0.3 g protein/kg/day).

Mircescu and associates observed the clinical course of 53 patients with stage 4 or 5 CKD over a period of 60 weeks[335]; 26 patients were randomly assigned to a diet of 0.6 g protein/kg/day and 27 were assigned to a diet containing only 0.3 g protein/kg/day supplemented with ketoacids. Actual protein intakes were estimated to be 0.59 ± 0.08 and 0.32 ± 0.07 g protein/kg/day, respectively. There were no deaths, and 7 of the 26 patients assigned to the 0.6 g-protein/kg/day diet reached the point of requiring dialysis compared to only 1 of 27 in the very low protein-ketoacid group ($P = 0.06$). Serum phosphate concentrations decreased from an initial value of 1.91 ± 0.68 to 1.45 ± 0.66 mM ($P < 0.05$) in patients eating the very low protein-ketoacid diet.

Rosman and coworkers evaluated the influence of dietary protein restriction in 247 stages 3 to 5 CKD patients and reported the outcomes after 2 or 4 years of observation.[326,360] The control group ate an unrestricted diet while patients with stage 3 CKD had a protein intake of 0.90 to 0.95 g/kg/day; patients with stage 4 or 5 CKD had a diet of 0.70 to 0.80 g protein/kg/day. After 2 years of follow-up, there was significant slowing of the loss of kidney function but only in male patients and, again, patients with polycystic kidney disease received no measurable benefit to the protein-restricted diet. After 4 years of follow-up, there was a survival improvement in patients treated with the protein-restricted diet calculated as kidney survival and/or the percentage of

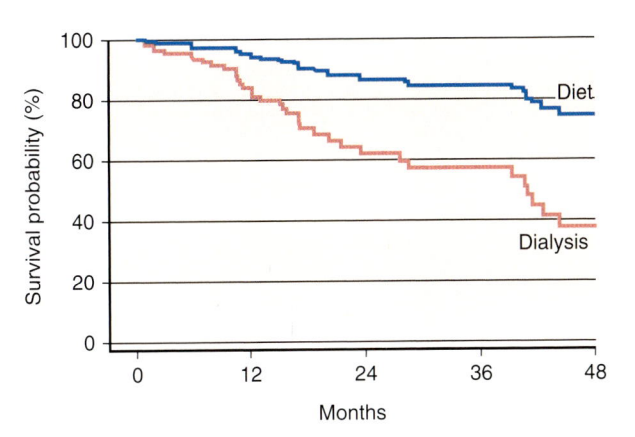

Figure 61.8 Survival of older CKD patients (stage V) who were randomly assigned at month 0 to begin dialysis treatment or to eat a very low-protein diet supplemented with ketoanalogues. As analyzed, the adjusted Cox model revealed a difference in survival ($P = 0.01$). (From Brunori G, Viola BF, Parrinello G, et al: Efficacy and safety of a very-low-protein diet when postponing dialysis in the elderly: a prospective randomized multicenter controlled study. Am J Kidney Dis 49:569-580, 2007.)

patients who did not require dialysis (60% vs. 30%; $P < 0.025$).[326] The authors concluded that compliance to the diets was fairly good and was sustained but did not cause signs of protein energy wasting.[326]

Brunori and colleagues examined 56 older Italian patients with stage 5 CKD who were randomly assigned to begin dialysis therapy or to be treated with a very low-protein diet (0.3 g protein/kg/day) supplemented with ketoacids.[361] After 1 year of observation, the survival rate was 83.7% and 87.3% in the dialysis and low-protein diet groups, respectively ($P = 0.6$). By an intention to treat analysis, the investigators found a continuous benefit of the protein-restricted diet. Patients assigned to dialysis had a 50% higher degree of hospitalization. The authors concluded there was no difference in the life span of subjects assigned to the low-protein diet plus ketoacids versus those treated by maintenance dialysis (Figure 61.8).

DIABETIC KIDNEY DISEASE

In patients with CKD and diabetes mellitus, the benefits achieved by dietary protein restriction are less clear. This was because most clinical trials of patients with CKD and diabetes mellitus assigned to different dietary regimens were too brief to identify differences in renal survival of patients prescribed the control versus experimental diets. Consequently, the analyses were largely based on surrogate criteria to determine the efficacy of protein-restricted diets in terms of progression of CKD or changes in nutritional factors. Surrogate outcomes used included a reduction in the degree of microalbuminuria or proteinuria and/or changes in creatinine clearance or serum creatinine (converted into eGFR). Unfortunately, in many of the early trials, ACEIs were not distributed equally and there were important differences in blood pressure control.

Zeller and associates compared a diet containing 1 or 0.6 g protein/kg/day in 36 type 1 diabetic CKD patients during a follow-up period averaging 35 months.[362] The outcome included measured changes in creatinine clearance and GFR (iothalamate clearance); actual protein intake, based on urea excretion, were 1.08 g versus 0.72 g protein/kg BW/day. The low-protein dietary regimen induced a significant ($P < 0.02$) reduction in the rate of decrease in GFR in patients with a GFR higher than 45 mL/min/1.73 m^2 compared to results with those on the control diet.

Hansen and coworkers reported results from the longest randomized trial of patients with type 1 diabetes and CKD.[363] Patients were prescribed their usual protein intake or assigned to a diet containing 0.6 g protein/kg/day during a 4-year trial. Actual protein intakes over the duration of the trial were 1.02 versus 0.89 g/kg/day. The degree of proteinuria was no different but the frequency of renal death (ESKD) was 36% lower in patients consuming the moderately protein-restricted diet. When renal deaths were analyzed to adjust for CVD by Cox analysis, the benefits of the low-protein diet were also statistically significant ($P = 0.01$).

META-ANALYSES OF LOW-PROTEIN DIETS AND PROGRESSION OF CHRONIC KIDNEY DISEASE

In a meta-analysis examining the impact of low-protein diets on renal function, Kasiske and colleagues pooled trials based on results from more than 1900 patients to determine if there was a renal protective effect for patients assigned to a low-protein diet. It was concluded that the protein restriction prevented a loss of 0.53 mL/min GFR/year ($P < 0.05$).[338]

Following a meta-analysis of a subgroup of patients with diabetes, Pedrini and associates showed that a combined outcome measure of microalbuminuria and renal function was improved by 44% ($P < 0.001$) in patients assigned to low-protein diets.[337] Pan and coworkers analyzed eight randomized trials that included 519 patients, 253 in the low-protein diet group and 266 in the control group.[340] Changes in GFR or creatinine clearance, hemoglobin A$_{1c}$ (HbA$_{1c}$) levels, degree of proteinuria, and serum albumin levels were recorded but no definitive outcome about differences in death or dialysis were uncovered. The dietary protein gradient between control and reduced protein intakes was 0.35 g/kg/day (1.27 to 0.91 g protein/kg/day; $P = 0.04$). Proteinuria did decrease significantly ($P = 0.003$). Glycosylated hemoglobin improved in seven of eight studies (mean reduction, 0.31%; $P = 0.005$). These results confirm that reducing protein intake in patients with diabetes and CKD improves insulin sensitivity, decreases HbA$_{1c}$, and reduces proteinuria and independent factors associated with renal protection.

We performed a meta-analysis based on 10 randomized controlled trials of low-protein diets in nondiabetic CKD patients.[339] The gender of patients and the types of their kidney diseases were equally distributed between the control and diet-restricted patient groups. Our results are shown in Figure 61.9. The outcomes of 1002 patients assigned to dietary protein restriction were compared to the outcomes of 998 patients assigned to higher protein intakes. In the low-protein groups, 113 renal deaths occurred compared to 168 in patients in the control group. These outcomes lead to a 0.68 odds ratio for renal death in the low-protein group compared to the control group; the 95% confidence interval (CI) was 0.55 to 0.84 ($P < 0.001$). The interpretation of this analysis is that a low-protein diet can result in a 32%

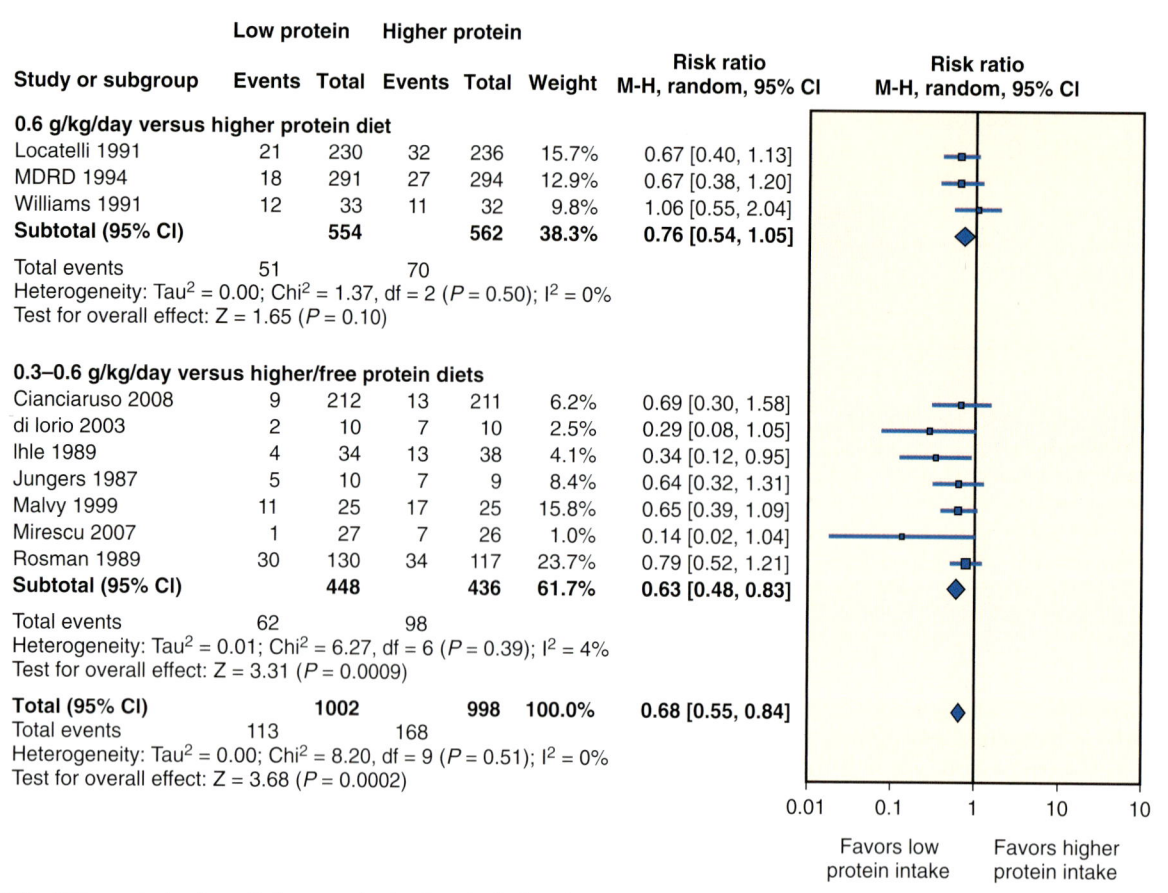

Study or subgroup	Low protein Events	Total	Higher protein Events	Total	Weight	Risk ratio M-H, random, 95% CI	Risk ratio M-H, random, 95% CI
0.6 g/kg/day versus higher protein diet							
Locatelli 1991	21	230	32	236	15.7%	0.67 [0.40, 1.13]	
MDRD 1994	18	291	27	294	12.9%	0.67 [0.38, 1.20]	
Williams 1991	12	33	11	32	9.8%	1.06 [0.55, 2.04]	
Subtotal (95% CI)		554		562	38.3%	0.76 [0.54, 1.05]	
Total events	51		70				
Heterogeneity: Tau^2 = 0.00; Chi^2 = 1.37, df = 2 (P = 0.50); I^2 = 0%							
Test for overall effect: Z = 1.65 (P = 0.10)							
0.3–0.6 g/kg/day versus higher/free protein diets							
Cianciaruso 2008	9	212	13	211	6.2%	0.69 [0.30, 1.58]	
di Iorio 2003	2	10	7	10	2.5%	0.29 [0.08, 1.05]	
Ihle 1989	4	34	13	38	4.1%	0.34 [0.12, 0.95]	
Jungers 1987	5	10	7	9	8.4%	0.64 [0.32, 1.31]	
Malvy 1999	11	25	17	25	15.8%	0.65 [0.39, 1.09]	
Mirescu 2007	1	27	7	26	1.0%	0.14 [0.02, 1.04]	
Rosman 1989	30	130	34	117	23.7%	0.79 [0.52, 1.21]	
Subtotal (95% CI)		448		436	61.7%	0.63 [0.48, 0.83]	
Total events	62		98				
Heterogeneity: Tau^2 = 0.01; Chi^2 = 6.27, df = 6 (P = 0.39); I^2 = 4%							
Test for overall effect: Z = 3.31 (P = 0.0009)							
Total (95% CI)		1002		998	100.0%	0.68 [0.55, 0.84]	
Total events	113		168				
Heterogeneity: Tau^2 = 0.00; Chi^2 = 8.20, df = 9 (P = 0.51); I^2 = 0%							
Test for overall effect: Z = 3.68 (P = 0.0002)							

0.01 0.1 1 10 10
Favors low protein intake   Favors higher protein intake

Figure 61.9 Meta-analysis of results from randomized controlled studies of the influence of low-protein diets in delaying progression of chronic kidney disease (CKD). A *square* denotes the odds ratio (treatment, control) for each trial, and the *diamond* indicates the combined results of all the trials; 95% confidence intervals are represented by *horizontal lines*. The designation 1.1.1 is from three studies. including a moderately reduced protein intake (0.6 g protein/kg/day) and a higher protein intake compared to self-selected diets. The designation 1.1.2 is the result of seven studies that included a more reduced protein intake (0.3 to 0.6 g protein/kg/day) compared to a greater amount of dietary protein or a free diet. Overall, the common odds ratio = 0.68 (95% CI, 0.55 to 0.84; P = 0.0002). (From Fouque D, Laville M: Low protein diets for chronic kidney disease in nondiabetic adults. *Cochrane Database Syst Rev* 3:CD001892, 2009, with permission.)

reduction for death or the need to start dialysis therapy when compared to unlimited protein intake.[339]

Results summarized in the preceding discussion provide insights into the potential benefits of protein-restricted diets but cannot be considered as demonstrating a cause and effect relationship. The levels of protein intake were different among the studies. but the finding that the analysis uncovers significant benefits indicates that the main therapeutic benefit is due to a gradient of protein intake, so that the lower protein intake is more likely to yield slowing of the loss of kidney function. In the foregoing analyses, only two studies actually measured GFR; those of Ihle and colleagues uncovered a protective effect while Klahr and associates concluded that a protein-restricted diet had only a slightly significant benefit (P = 0.07).[329,331]

NUTRITIONAL IMPACT AND SAFETY OF MODIFIED DIETS IN CHRONIC KIDNEY DISEASE

A critical issue in the evaluation of outcomes with long-term dietary modification is whether a low-protein diet is nutritionally sound and safe for patients with CKD. The MDRD study enrolled 840 patients with different stages of CKD, providing the largest number of patients to study to address this question.[331] Patients were examined for an average of 2.2 years, and a large number of measurements of nutritional status (e.g., body weight and anthropometrics, serum protein levels, dietary adherence) were obtained. Kopple and coworkers evaluated these results and assessed the safety of the different dietary regimens.[217] Their analysis led to the conclusion that there was some decrease in estimated protein intake in subjects with advanced kidney disease, and there appeared to be a decrease in caloric intake (the latter may be inaccurate because the analysis depended on collecting diet histories).[298,299] Importantly, only 2 of the 840 participants had to stop participating in the MDRD study because of concerns about their nutritional status.

In contrast to these rather positive outcomes from the MDRD study, Menon and colleagues reported outcomes based on an analysis of results from the U.S. Renal Data System (USRDS).[364] They compiled the numbers of patients entering dialysis or receiving a transplant and studied all-cause mortality following the 2.2 years of the MDRD study. They concluded that assignment to a very low-protein diet plus ketoacid therapy was associated with an increased risk of death. Unfortunately, they provided no information about compliance of patients during the MDRD study nor about dietary factors after the study ended. There also was no information about the effect of issues such as other illnesses, dialysis-related factors, or treatments following the end of the study. The authors speculated that patients may have persistently remained with a protein-restricted diet after beginning dialysis or there may have been an unidentified toxin from the ketoacid therapy. Regarding the former, it has been reported that patients trained in low-protein diets can have a delay of 3 months after initiation of dialysis therapy before their dietary protein increases.[365]

On the other hand, investigators with extensive experience with dietary manipulation found no delay in increasing protein intake after dialysis therapy begins.[366] Regarding the possibility that the increased risk of death resulted from accumulation of an unidentified toxin, no such substance was identified and, more importantly, the ketoacid supplements were discontinued at the end of the MDRD study, making it unlikely that toxic factors persisted for many years despite withdrawal of the ketoacid supplement. Other problems with the analysis of Menon's group have been detailed.[367] In contrast to this report, the results compiled by Chauveau and associates detailed the long-term survival of 220 stage 4 or 5 CKD patients who had been treated with 0.3 g protein/kg/day plus a mixture of ketoacids.[3] These patients had been treated for an average of 33 months (range, 4 to 230 months) before starting dialysis or undergoing transplantation. The authors analyzed patient survival and compared it to a larger cohort of patients who were not treated with a low-protein diet but were treated concurrently by the same investigators. At 1 year after beginning dialysis, they concluded that the survival of dialysis patients was 97% and, after 5 years, it was 60%. For the transplanted patients, the survival at 5 and 10 years was 97% and 95%, respectively. When compared to the survival of U.S. patients, these results are excellent.[368] Since the number of patients treated and analyzed by Chauveau and Menon and coworkers are similar, these widely disparate results are unexplained. Because details of treatment and outcomes are provided in Chauveau and colleagues' report but absent in the analysis by Menon and associates, it may be concluded that in selected patients who are carefully examined, a ketoacid-supplemented, very low-protein diet is neither harmful nor does it increase mortality in patients who progress to the degree of functional kidney loss requiring replacement therapy.

VITAMINS AND TRACE ELEMENTS IN UREMIA

The micronutrients—vitamins and trace elements—are required for energy production, organ function, and cell growth and protection (e.g., from oxygen free radicals) but only small amounts are needed; hence, the term *micronutrients*.[2,20,369] In addition to an insufficient amount of vitamins and minerals in the diet, micronutrient deficiency can occur in nephrotic patients because of losses of protein-bound elements or decreased intestinal absorption of micronutrients, impaired cellular metabolism, circulating inhibitors, or increased losses during dialysis treatments.[370] Since many factors can change the requirements for micronutrients, and since there are serious methodologic difficulties in measuring these vitamins and trace minerals, there is very little information about the minimum requirements or recommended daily allowance (RDA) for these nutrients in CKD patients. Evaluations of the effects of dialysis are present for some micronutrients; these will be considered because of the paucity of well-controlled studies in CKD patients. Meats and dairy products are rich in these nutrients but these foods are frequently restricted for CKD patients.[370]

Regarding individual micronutrients, long-term administration of supplemental vitamin B_6 and folate reportedly improve the responses to erythropoietin.[371,372] Diuretic therapy or hemodialysis can accelerate vitamin B_1 (thiamine) deficiency but it is unlikely that patients with CKD will develop beriberi from thiamine deficiency. However, there have been no long-term evaluations of providing thiamine supplements. Thiamine deficiency can mimic some of the cardiovascular and neurologic symptoms in patients with CKD, so we recommend a daily supplement containing the RDA of the water-soluble vitamins (vitamins B_1, B_6, B_{12}, and C, folate, and niacin).[373]

Riboflavin is necessary to maintain flavin mononucleotide and flavin adenine dinucleotide levels, which participate in numerous energy pathways. It is present in meats and dairy products but these are often restricted in the diet of patients with CKD. Riboflavin is a water-soluble vitamin that when deficient, produces sore throat, stomatitis and glossitis, which may be mistaken for uremic symptoms. Folic acid is required for the synthesis of nucleic acids and carbon transfer reactions, including those involved in amino acid metabolism (e.g., homocysteine).[370] Folic acid is found in fruits and vegetables but cooking can destroy it, leading to folate deficiency, which impairs erythropoietin therapy. Vitamin B_6 (pyridoxine) is necessary for amino acid metabolism via transaminase-catalyzed reactions. It is contained in meats, vegetables, and cereals, and restricted diets may lead to deficiency, with symptoms of peripheral neuropathy. Vitamin B_{12} is required for the transfer of methyl groups among different metabolic compounds and is necessary for the synthesis of nucleic acids. The major sources of vitamin B_{12} are meat and dairy products. Deficiency is unusual because vitamin B_{12} is stored in the liver, is protein bound, and its gastrointestinal absorption is carefully regulated by gastric production of intrinsic factor.[370] Vitamin C (ascorbic acid) protects tissues against antioxidant reactions and is involved in hydroxylation of proline during the formation of collagen. Symptoms of vitamin C deficiency are subtle and include poor wound healing and periodontal disease, similar to symptoms of uremia. Since high doses of vitamin C are metabolized to oxalate, which precipitates in soft tissues (including the kidney), vitamin C supplements should be limited to supplying the RDA.

The remaining water-soluble vitamins—biotin, niacin, and pantothenic acid—have been less well studied. Biotin functions as a coenzyme in bicarbonate-dependent carboxylation reactions and is produced by intestinal microorganisms. Consequently, a deficiency state is unusual. Niacin (nicotinic acid) is an essential component of the nicotinamide adenine dinucleotide phosphate coenzyme. It is synthesized from the EAA tryptophan; a deficiency state produces diarrhea, dermatitis, or increased triglycerides. Niacin supplements have been used to treat hyperlipidemic conditions that include a high LDL level, but this may be difficult to accomplish because niacin supplements can be associated with flushing symptoms. Pantothenic acid is involved in the function of coenzyme A and, hence, in the metabolism of fatty acids, steroid hormones, and cholesterol. Because so little is known about the efficacy and consequences of prescribing these vitamins, the use of supplements should be reserved for identified deficiency states and should not contain more than the RDA amount.

The requirements for fat-soluble vitamins have not been established, and these vitamins might generate complications of CKD. Thus, fat-soluble vitamins should be given only when there is a well-defined indication, and multivitamin preparations should not be prescribed unless there is evidence for a deficiency condition. For example, plasma vitamin A (retinol) levels are usually increased in patients with CKD because the level of retinol-binding protein is high. This makes it likely that vitamin A tissue levels are normal or increased, even if the unbound or free retinol in plasma is within a normal range.[370] The danger of excess vitamin A is based on its contribution to anemia, dry skin, pruritus, and especially hepatic dysfunction in uremic patients.[374]

The requirements for vitamin E also are not established. Based on a potential for suppressing oxidative injury, vitamin E was given to experimental models of CKD; it reduced renal injury in rats with experimental immunoglobulin A (IgA) nephropathy or subtotal nephrectomy or diabetes.[375-378] However, there is no evidence for a similar benefit in patients with progressive CKD.[370] Vitamin E may combat the lipid peroxidation and oxidant stress but more information is needed before prescribing vitamin E to patients with CKD.[379] For the complex relationships between vitamin D and CKD, see Chapters 19 and 55.

Recommendations for prescribing supplements of trace elements for uremic patients are even more controversial. There are several reasons for caution—it is very difficult to determine if body stores are sufficient or excessive or to prove that symptoms are reversed solely by providing more trace elements.[370] For example, plasma and leukocyte zinc levels are reported to be decreased and associated with endocrine abnormalities, such as high plasma prolactin levels.[380] Supplements of zinc have been suggested to increase B lymphocyte counts, granulocyte motility, and taste and sexual dysfunction.[370] However, these improvements have not been tested in a controlled trial. The influences of the trace element aluminum have been studied more extensively because aluminum-containing antacids have been used to control serum phosphorus and bone uremic disease (see Chapters 19 and 55). In patients with stable CKD, the administration of aluminum-based antacids were shown to accumulate and even affect serum iron levels, contributing to resistance to erythropoietin therapy.[381-383] The metabolism and metabolic effects of other trace elements have been studied very little in CKD patients, and we do not recommend giving supplements of trace elements unless there is documentation (or at least a high degree of suspicion) that trace element deficiency is responsible for a complication. The exception would be patients requiring long-term parenteral or enteral nutrition because they can develop deficiencies of vitamins and minerals.

CONCLUSION

The primary conclusion we reached in this chapter is that CKD causes a large variety of metabolic and nutritional disorders that participate in the syndrome of uremia. We highlighted the importance of integrating nutritional principals in the care of patients with CKD and presented detailed methods for monitoring compliance with prescribed diets. Since the failing kidney cannot eliminate metabolic waste products efficiently, prevention of complications of CKD should be attacked by limiting an excessive intake of nutrients to reduce the generation of toxic metabolites (e.g., uric acid, nitrogen-containing compounds, phosphates, sodium, potassium). We have discussed how the role of these potential toxins is altered with kidney disease because of impaired metabolic processes, such as creatinine production, urea metabolism, amino acid and protein metabolism, responses to accumulation of waste products, and generation of inflammation.

An important conclusion is that these metabolic disorders and the symptoms they produce will not be overcome or corrected simply by increasing the size of meals. Instead, there has been evidence for at least 145 years that manipulating the intake of dietary factors such as protein, salt, and phosphates can reduce or eliminate the consequences of CKD.[58] However, this requires repeated monitoring of nutrition, just as managing hypertension requires attention to different drugs. For example, a patient may view dietary change as an unwanted form of restriction, especially when terms such as *protein-restricted diet* are used. A more appropriate approach is to emphasize how a dietary change can benefit metabolism and relieve the complications of CKD, which is likely to be more successful. Specifically, the approach should be to work with a patient and the dietician or nutritionist to provide an optimal renal diet (Figure 61.10). We recognize that this approach is difficult, in part because of the difficulty in achieving dietary compliance. The strategy is difficult because diets of U.S. CKD patients generally include 1 g or more of protein/kg/day, even when they reach stage 5 CKD.[384] Nevertheless, a well-planned diet can avoid some of the complications of CKD. Moreover, adherence to the diet can delay the time until dialysis or transplantation becomes necessary. Patients with CKD should be offered this option to delay the time to dialysis.

A second factor that can make it easier for patients to make necessary adaptations to their diet is the need to change dietary requirements when it is necessary to begin dialysis or during the stages of kidney transplantation. The concentration cannot be only on adjusting dietary protein but should include training in, for example, the risks of salt intake with hypertension and dyslipidemia following transplantation. Moreover, the dietician or nutritionist and nephrologist will have to adjust the diet to focus on nutrients that are spontaneously reduced with anorexia, including energy sources and calcium, plus some vitamins and trace elements. An important role is played by the dietitian who specializes in kidney disease but this individual, like the nephrologist, will have to include continuous education so the patient can understand and develop the expertise needed to combat the consequences of lost kidney function.

Finally, additional basic and clinical investigations are needed to understand more fully the role of dietary factors in producing or ameliorating the complications of kidney disease. Recently published clinical trials and meta-analyses with a high level of methodologic evidence have indicated

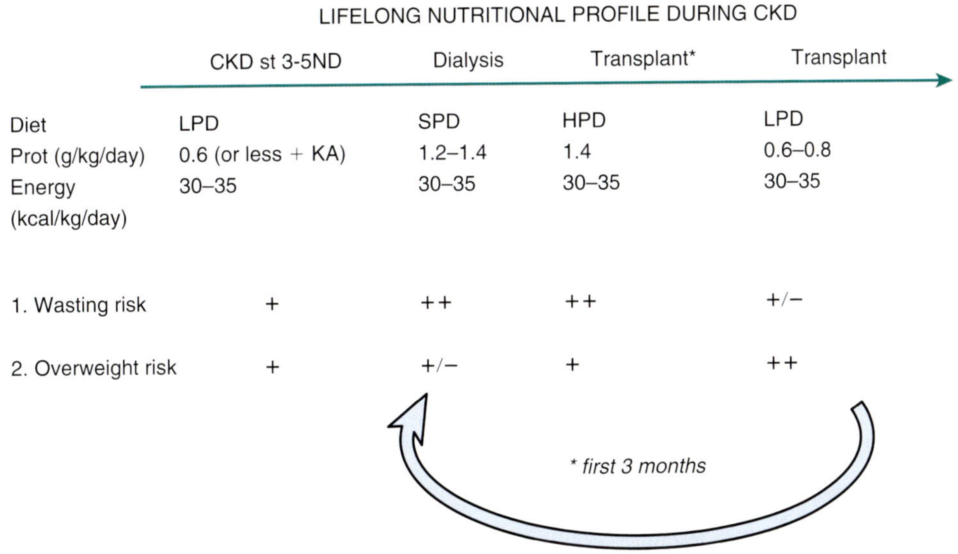

LIFELONG NUTRITIONAL PROFILE DURING CKD

	CKD st 3-5ND	Dialysis	Transplant*	Transplant
Diet	LPD	SPD	HPD	LPD
Prot (g/kg/day)	0.6 (or less + KA)	1.2–1.4	1.4	0.6–0.8
Energy (kcal/kg/day)	30–35	30–35	30–35	30–35
1. Wasting risk	+	++	++	+/−
2. Overweight risk	+	+/−	+	++

* first 3 months

Figure 61.10 Lifelong need for nutritional counseling during stages of chronic kidney disease (CKD). Each stage exhibits nutritional profiles requiring specific changes in diet and hence specific dietary training. Risks of lost protein stores or risks of obesity differ at each stage; efforts are required to reduce the risks of protein wasting or obesity. The *arrow* indicates changes that occur when patients must return to dialysis after loss of function of the transplanted kidney. HPD, High-protein diet; KA, ketoacids; LPD, low-protein diet; SPD, standard protein diet.

that reducing protein intake is associated with improvements in metabolism, control of blood pressure and proteinuria and, importantly, a delay in the need to start dialysis. At the same time, understanding the complex interactions among the intake of various nutrients with declining kidney function and the metabolic consequences of CKD could lead to more effective therapy. At this point, however, it has been demonstrated that a properly designed diet is nutritionally sound and safe in terms of prolonging life after beginning dialysis and preventing protein-energy wasting or reducing survival. Determining whether there is an impact on a patient's quality of life has not been sufficiently evaluated, and not addressing the topic will lead to increasing hypertension, hyperphosphatemia, and a very high serum urea nitrogen concentration while aggravating anemia.[2,3,283]

Complete reference list available at ExpertConsult.com.

KEY REFERENCES

3. Chauveau P, Couzi L, Vendrely B, et al: Long-term outcome on renal replacement therapy in patients who previously received a keto acid-supplemented very-low-protein diet. *Am J Clin Nutr* 90:969–974, 2009.
4. Vegter S, Perna A, Postma MJ, et al: Sodium intake, ACE inhibition, and progression to ESRD. *J Am Soc Nephrol* 23:165–173, 2012.
5. Zoccali C, Ruggenenti P, Perna A, et al: Phosphate may promote CKD progression and attenuate renoprotective effect of ACE inhibition. *J Am Soc Nephrol* 22:1923–1930, 2011.
6. Mitch WE, Buffington GA, Lemann J, et al: A simple method of estimating progression of chronic renal failure. *Lancet* 2:1326–1328, 1976.
19. de Brito-Ashurst I, Varagunam M, Raftery MJ, et al: Bicarbonate supplementation slows progression of CKD and improves nutritional status. *J Am Soc Nephrol* 20:2075–2084, 2009.
20. Mitch WE, Remuzzi G: Diets for patients with chronic kidney disease, still worth prescribing. *J Am Soc Nephrol* 15:234–237, 2004.
37. Brenner BM, Meyer TW, Hostetter TH: Dietary protein intake and the progressive nature of kidney disease: the role of hemodynamically mediated glomerular injury in the pathogenesis of progressive glomerular sclerosis in aging, renal ablation, and intrinsic renal disease. *N Engl J Med* 307:652–659, 1982.
56. Moe SM, Zidehsarai MP, Chambers MA, et al: Vegetarian compared with meat dietary protein source and phosphorus homeostasis in chronic kidney disease. *Clin J Am Soc Nephrol* 6:257–264, 2011.
61. Maroni BJ, Steinman T, Mitch WE: A method for estimating nitrogen intake of patients with chronic renal failure. *Kidney Int* 27:58–65, 1985.
62. Kopple JD, Gao X, Qing DP: Dietary protein, urea nitrogen appearance and total nitrogen appearance in chronic renal failure and CAPD patients. *Kidney Int* 52:486–494, 1997.
66. Mitch WE, Goldberg AL: Mechanisms of muscle wasting: the role of the ubiquitin-proteasome system. *N Engl J Med* 335:1897–1905, 1996.
80. Mitch WE, Collier VU, Walser M: Creatinine metabolism in chronic renal failure. *Clin Sci* 58:327–335, 1980.
91. Siu YP, Leung KT, Tong MK, et al: Use of allopurinol in slowing the progression of renal disease through its ability to lower serum uric acid level. *Am J Kidney Dis* 47:51–59, 2006.
106. Aparicio M, Bouchet JL, Gin H, et al: Effect of a low-protein diet on urinary albumin excretion in uremic patients. *Nephron* 50:288–291, 1988.
108. Gansevoort RT, De Zeeuw D, De Jong PE: Additive antiproteinuric effect of ACE inhibition and a low-protein diet in human renal disease. *Nephrol Dial Transplant* 10:497–504, 1995.
117. Koppe L, Pillon NJ, Vella RE, et al: p-Cresyl sulfate promotes insulin resistance associated with CKD. *J Am Soc Nephrol* 24:88–99, 2013.
122. Bergstrom J, Alvestrand A, Furst P: Plasma and muscle free amino acids in maintenance hemodialysis patients without protein malnutrition. *Kidney Int* 38:108–114, 1990.
125. Stein A, Moorhouse J, Iles-Smith H, et al: Role of an improvement in acid-base status and nutrition in CAPD patients. *Kidney Int* 52:1089–1095, 1997.
128. Aparicio M, Chauveau P, De Precigout V, et al: Nutrition and outcome on renal replacement therapy of patients with chronic renal failure treated by a supplemented very low protein diet. *J Am Soc Nephrol* 11:719–727, 2000.
135. Bailey JL, Wang X, England BK, et al: The acidosis of chronic renal failure activates muscle proteolysis in rats by augmenting transcription of genes encoding proteins of the ATP-dependent, ubiquitin-proteasome pathway. *J Clin Invest* 97:1447–1453, 1996.
149. Thomas SS, Dong Y, Zhang L, et al: Signal regulatory protein-alpha interacts with the insulin receptor contributing to muscle wasting in chronic kidney disease. *Kidney Int* 84:308–316, 2013.

151. Price SR, Bailey JL, Wang X, et al: Muscle wasting in insulinopenic rats results from activation of the ATP-dependent, ubiquitin-proteasome pathway by a mechanism including gene transcription. *J Clin Invest* 98:1703–1708, 1996.
155. Zhang L, Du J, Hu Z, et al: IL-6 and serum amyloid A synergy mediates angiotensin II-induced muscle wasting. *J Am Soc Nephrol* 20:604–612, 2009.
169. Workeneh B, Rondon-Berrios H, Zhang L, et al: Development of a diagnostic method for detecting increased muscle protein degradation in patients with catabolic conditions. *J Am Soc Nephrol* 17:3233–3239, 2006.
190. Han HQ, Zhou X, Mitch WE, et al: Myostatin/activin pathway antagonism: molecular basis and therapeutic potential. *Int J Biochem Cell Biol* 45:2333–2347, 2013.
195. Zhang L, Rajan V, Lin E, et al: Pharmacological inhibition of myostatin suppresses systemic inflammation and muscle atrophy in mice with chronic kidney disease. *FASEB J* 25:1653–1663, 2011.
197. Zhang L, Pan J, Dong Y, et al: Stat3 activation links a C/EBPdelta to myostatin pathway to stimulate loss of muscle mass. *Cell Metab* 18:368–379, 2013.
206. Maroni BJ, Staffeld C, Young VR, et al: Mechanisms permitting nephrotic patients to achieve nitrogen equilibrium with a protein-restricted diet. *J Clin Invest* 99:2479–2487, 1997.
212. Mitch WE: Malnutrition: a frequent misdiagnosis for hemodialysis patients. *J Clin Invest* 110:437–439, 2002.
218. Tom K, Young VR, Chapman T, et al: Long-term adaptive responses to dietary protein restriction in chronic renal failure. *Am J Physiol* 268:E668–E677, 1995.
260. Beddhu S, Samore MH, Roberts MS, et al: Impact of timing of initiation of dialysis on mortality. *J Am Soc Nephrol* 14:2305–2312, 2003.
297. Rigalleau V, Combe C, Blanchetier V, et al: Low protein diet in uremia: effects on glucose metabolism and energy production rate. *Kidney Int* 51:1222–1227, 1997.
304. Kopple JD, Monteon FJ, Shaib JK: Effect of energy intake on nitrogen metabolism in nondialyzed patients with chronic renal failure. *Kidney Int* 29:734–742, 1986.
322. Goodship THJ, Mitch WE, Hoerr RA, et al: Adaptation to low-protein diets in renal failure: leucine turnover and nitrogen balance. *J Am Soc Nephrol* 1:66–75, 1990.
326. Rosman JB, Langer K, Brandl M, et al: Protein-restricted diets in chronic renal failure: a four year follow-up shows limited indications. *Kidney Int* 36:S96–S102, 1989.
327. Jungers P, Chauveau P, Ployard F, et al: Comparison of ketoacids and low protein diet on advanced chronic renal failure progression. *Kidney Int* 22:67–71, 1987.
329. Ihle BU, Becker GJ, Whitworth JA, et al: The effect of protein restriction on the progression of renal insufficiency. *N Engl J Med* 321:1773–1777, 1989.
330. Locatelli F, Alberti D, Graziani G, et al: Prospective, randomised, multicentre trial of effect of protein restriction on progression of chronic renal insufficiency. *Lancet* 337:1299–1304, 1991.
331. Klahr S, Levey AS, Beck GJ, et al: The effects of dietary protein restriction and blood-pressure control on the progression of chronic renal failure. *N Engl J Med* 330:878–884, 1994.
333. Di Iorio BR, Minutolo R, De Nicola L, et al: Supplemented very low protein diet ameliorates responsiveness to erythropoietin in chronic renal failure. *Kidney Int* 64:1822–1828, 2003.
334. Cianciaruso B, Pota A, Pisani A, et al: Metabolic effects of two low protein diets in chronic kidney disease stage 4-5—a randomized controlled trial. *Nephrol Dial Transplant* 23:636–644, 2008.
339. Fouque D, Laville M: Low protein diets for chronic renal failure in non-diabetic adults. *Cochrane Database Syst Rev* (3):CD001892, 2009.
340. Pan Y, Guo LL, Jin HM: Low-protein diet for diabetic nephropathy: a meta-analysis of randomized controlled trials. *Am J Clin Nutr* 88:660–666, 2008.
341. Fouque D, Horne R, Cozzolino M, et al: Balancing nutrition and serum phosphorus in maintenance dialysis. *Am J Kidney Dis* 64:143–150, 2014.
352. Kestenbaum B, Sampson JN, Rudser KD, et al: Serum phosphate levels and mortality risk among people with chronic kidney disease. *J Am Soc Nephrol* 16:520–528, 2005.
359. Levey AS, Adler S, Caggiula AW, et al: MDRD Study Group: Effects of dietary protein restriction on the progression of advanced renal disease in the Modification of Diet in Renal Disease Study. *Am J Kidney Dis* 27:652–663, 1996.
361. Brunori G, Viola BF, Parrinello G, et al: Efficacy and safety of a very-low-protein diet when postponing dialysis in the elderly: a prospective randomized multicenter controlled study. *Am J Kidney Dis* 49:569–580, 2007.
362. Zeller KR, Whittaker E, Sullivan L, et al: Effect of restricting dietary protein on the progression of renal failure in patients with insulin-dependent diabetes mellitus. *N Engl J Med* 324:78–83, 1991.
363. Hansen HP, Tauber-Lassen E, Jensen BR, et al: Effect of dietary protein restriction on prognosis in patients with diabetic nephropathy. *Kidney Int* 62:220–228, 2002.
384. Moore LW, Byham-Gray LD, Scott PJ, et al: The mean dietary protein intake at different stages of chronic kidney disease is higher than current guidelines. *Kidney Int* 83:724–732, 2013.

A Stepped Care Approach to the Management of Chronic Kidney Disease

Damian G. Fogarty | Maarten W. Taal

CHAPTER OUTLINE

ESTIMATED GLOMERULAR FILTRATION RATE AND STAGING OF CHRONIC KIDNEY DISEASE: CAVEATS AND IMPLICATIONS FOR STEPPED CARE, 1989
Stratifying Risk in Patients with Chronic Kidney Disease: The Importance of Risk Factors, 1990
INTERVENTIONS FOR SLOWING PROGRESSION OF CHRONIC KIDNEY DISEASE, 1990
Mechanisms of Disease Progression and the Rationale for Interventions to Achieve Renoprotection, 1990
Lifestyle Interventions, 1990
Antihypertensive Therapy, 1995
Pharmacologic Inhibition of the Renin Angiotensin Aldosterone System, 1998
Hyperuricemia, 2004
Treatment of Metabolic Acidosis, 2004
Proteinuria as a Therapeutic Target, 2004
Time Course for Proteinuria Response, 2005
Monitoring and Safety Considerations, 2005
Strategy for Maximal Renoprotection: Aiming for Remission of Chronic Kidney Disease, 2006

INTERVENTIONS TO REDUCE CARDIOVASCULAR RISK ASSOCIATED WITH CHRONIC KIDNEY DISEASE, 2008
Association between Chronic Kidney Disease and Cardiovascular Disease, 2008
Antihypertensive Agents and Cardiovascular Protection, 2009
Treatment of Dyslipidemia, 2011
Antiplatelet Therapy, 2012
INTERVENTIONS TO MANAGE COMPLICATIONS OF CHRONIC KIDNEY DISEASE, 2013
Anemia, 2013
Mineral and Bone Disorder, 2013
A STEPPED CARE APPROACH TO CHRONIC KIDNEY DISEASE, 2014
Stages 1 and 2, 2014
Stage 3, 2015
Stage 4, 2015
Stage 5, 2016

Chronic kidney disease (CKD) is a collective term covering a number of primary disease processes that result in structural or functional kidney abnormalities, or both, persisting for at least 3 months. Abnormal urinalysis results with proteinuria or hematuria and abnormal kidney structure or histologic features, with or without a decreased glomerular filtration rate glomerular filtration rate (GFR) < 60 mL/min/1.73 m^2, are the defining manifestations.[1] CKD is subdivided into five stages according to the GFR (Table 62.1), which reflects the observation that in the majority of cases, CKD progresses slowly through the stages before reaching end-stage kidney disease (ESKD) that necessitates renal replacement therapy (RRT). The CKD staging system has two important implications: First, it suggests that if CKD is detected at an early stage, intervention may be possible to prevent or slow progression to more advanced stages.[2] Second, it reflects the observation that as GFR declines, the risk profile of patients and associated complications changes. Thus, the staging system provides a useful framework for structuring therapy and prioritizing interventions to produce a comprehensive strategy for the management of CKD. The CKD classification system was revised in 2012 to include categories for albuminuria to reflect a growing body of evidence that albuminuria is important for risk stratification (Figure 62.1; see "Stratifying Risk in Patients with Chronic Kidney Disease" section).[3,4]

This chapter describes in detail the interventions that should be used at early stages of CKD to reduce the risk of CKD progression, as well as the risk of cardiovascular disease, and the interventions that become more salient when CKD reaches more advanced stages. This description is followed by discussion of a stepped care approach with priorities determined by the stage.

Table 62.1 Overview of Chronic Kidney Disease Management by Stage

Features	Stages 1 and 2	Stage 3a	Stage 3b	Stage 4	Stage 5
Estimated GFR	≥60 mL/min/1.73 m² + albuminuria or hematuria or structural kidney damage	45-59 mL/min/1.73 m²	30-44 mL/min/1.73 m²	15-29 mL/min/1.73 m²	<15 mL/min/1.73 m²
Laboratory testing	Annual electrolytes and estimated GFR Annual urine ACR (or other estimate of proteinuria) Baseline anemia and mineral and bone profiles Glucose, lipids, and HbA$_{1c}$ See Table 62.3 for causes of AKI after initiation of ACE inhibitor or ARB therapy.				Check electrolytes and estimated GFR 1 week after new use or higher doses of ACE inhibitors or ARBs; otherwise, assess electrolytes/estimated GFR, mineral and bone, and anemia profiles every 3 to 6 months, depending on GFR decline.
Blood pressure targets	BP target <130/80 mm Hg with proteinuria BP target <140/90 mm Hg without proteinuria if no clinical or radiologic evidence of ARVD or previous episodes of AKI				Risk of AKI is increased in elderly patients (>75 years), those with CHF, and those with ARVD; 140/90 may be more appropriate for these groups.
Blood pressure agents	ACE inhibitor or ARB if urine ACR ≥30 mg/g Most patients need two to four agents in total to achieve these targets, in a combination of ACE inhibitors or ARBs and one or more of the following: a diuretic (all classes), a calcium channel blocker, and a β-blocker. The use of dual RAAS-inhibiting agents or spironolactone can help reduce proteinuria, but careful monitoring of GFR and potassium is required.				Loop diuretics are now usually required for BP and edema control.
Cardiovascular prevention	Statin if CVD risk ≥20% over 10 years HbA$_{1c}$ < 7.0% unless at risk for severe hypoglycemia			Consider statin for all patients.	Both the benefits and bleeding risks of aspirin increase as the GFR falls.
Bone and anemia complications	If PTH level rises progressively, commence phosphate restriction and then consider therapy with vitamin D or analog. If anemia is out of keeping with GFR, confirm or rule out gastrointestinal blood loss				Give intravenous iron before ESA if hemoglobin count <10 g/dL. Maintain target hemoglobin count of 10 to 11.5 g/dL.
Lifestyle and nutritional management	Smoking cessation Moderate exercise up to 30 to 60 min/day 4 to 7 days/wk Target weight with BMI < 25 kg/m² Reduced salt intake as per DASH diet <5 g/day				Limit dietary potassium excess. Weigh at each clinic and assess fluid overload, anorexia, physical function.
Specific RRT planning steps	Education regarding progression and role of conservative management with regard to blood pressure targets and specific primary renal disease treatment if indicated Hepatitis B vaccination if risk of progression is high			Education on RRT types and palliative care if CKD is progressing or patient is at high risk of progression Hepatitis B vaccination	AVF creation PD catheter insertion Enter on list for transplant.
Referral guidance from primary care physician to nephrologist	Progressive or abrupt fall in estimated GFR Proteinuria (urine protein levels >0.5 g/day; ACR > 300 mg/g or >30 mg/mmol)			Refer unless patient is terminally ill.	Refer unless patient is terminally ill.

ACE, Angiotensin-converting enzyme; ACR, albumin to creatinine ratio; AKI, acute kidney injury; ARB, angiotensin receptor blocker; ARVD, atherosclerotic renovascular disease; AVF, arteriovenous fistula; BMI, body mass index; BP, blood pressure; CHF, congestive heart failure; CKD, chronic kidney disease; CVD, cardiovascular disease; DASH, Dietary Approaches to Stop Hypertension; ESA, erythropoietin-stimulating agent; GFR, glomerular filtration rate; HbA$_{1c}$, hemoglobin A$_{1c}$; PD, peritoneal dialysis; PTH, parathyroid hormone; RAAS, renin angiotensin aldosterone system; RRT, renal replacement therapy.

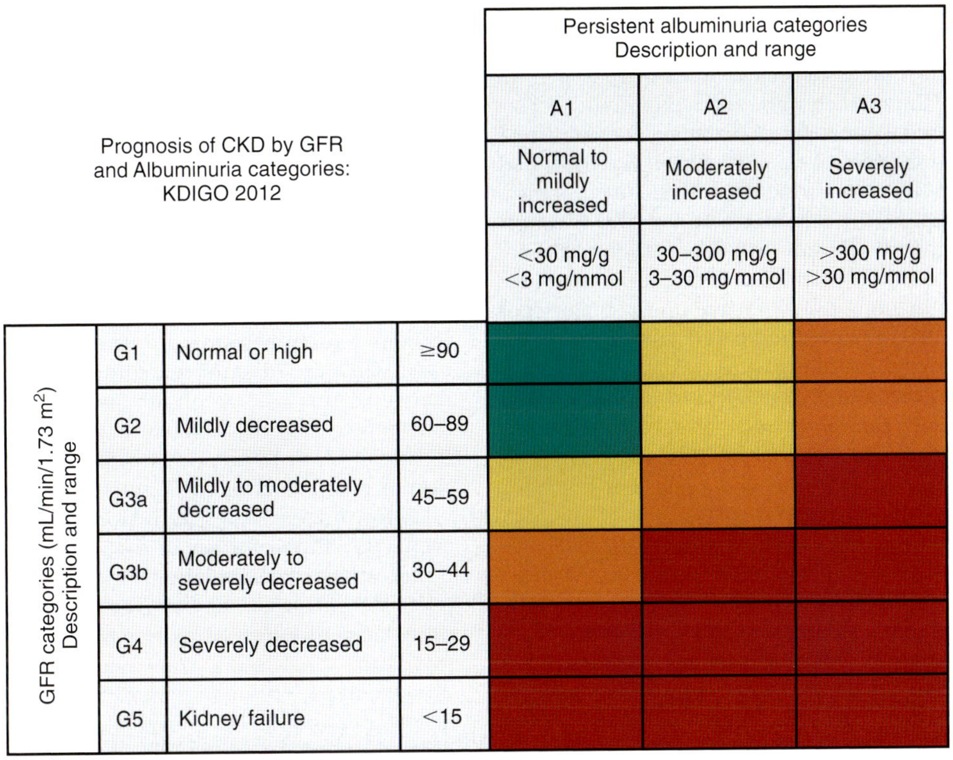

Prognosis of CKD by GFR and Albuminuria categories: KDIGO 2012			Persistent albuminuria categories Description and range		
			A1 Normal to mildly increased <30 mg/g <3 mg/mmol	A2 Moderately increased 30–300 mg/g 3–30 mg/mmol	A3 Severely increased >300 mg/g >30 mg/mmol
GFR categories (mL/min/1.73 m²) Description and range	G1	Normal or high ≥90	Green	Yellow	Orange
	G2	Mildly decreased 60–89	Green	Yellow	Orange
	G3a	Mildly to moderately decreased 45–59	Yellow	Orange	Red
	G3b	Moderately to severely decreased 30–44	Orange	Red	Red
	G4	Severely decreased 15–29	Red	Red	Red
	G5	Kidney failure <15	Red	Red	Red

Green: low risk (if no other markers of kidney disease, no CKD)
Yellow: moderately increased risk
Orange: high risk
Red: very high risk

Figure 62.1 Current classification system and nomenclature proposed by Kidney Disease: Improving Global Outcomes (KDIGO) in 2012. Chronic kidney disease (CKD) is defined as abnormalities of kidney structure or function, present for 3 months, with implications for least 3 months with implications for health. CKD is classified based on cause, glomerular filtration rate (GFR) category, and albuminuria category. (Reproduced with permission from Kidney Disease: Improving Global Outcomes CKD Work Group: KDIGO 2012 clinical practice guideline for the evaluation and management of chronic kidney disease. *Kidney Int* 3(Suppl):1-150, 2013.)

Within this context, there are four broad aims:

1. Attenuate GFR decline and thus prevent or delay the need for dialysis. It is perhaps self-evident, but the earlier that CKD progression can be halted, the greater is the possibility of maintaining kidney function as close to normal as possible.
2. Prevent premature cardiovascular death at all stages of CKD.
3. Recognize and manage complications of CKD as they arise, particularly in stages 4 and 5 CKD.
4. Plan for RRT or conservative palliative care.

Before the management of patients with CKD is considered, it is important to place in context the role of estimated glomerular filtration rate (eGFR) testing, as well as the natural history of CKD and the associated risks.

ESTIMATED GLOMERULAR FILTRATION RATE AND STAGING OF CHRONIC KIDNEY DISEASE: CAVEATS AND IMPLICATIONS FOR STEPPED CARE

Before the use of eGFR, a high proportion of patients treated with dialysis had been referred late to nephrologists for want of a more easily interpreted test of kidney function than that of an elevated serum creatinine level.[5-7] In multiple studies, patients referred later had persistently higher rates of morbidity and even mortality than did patients whose condition was diagnosed at least 6 to 12 months before dialysis initiation.[8]

Although there was widespread acceptance of the consensus statements from Kidney Disease: Improving Global Outcomes (KDIGO) regarding CKD, there remained some criticism of the use of eGFR; specifically, it was recognized that in many patients, stage 3 CKD did not progress further. Some commentators questioned the utility of CKD staging, suggesting that the high prevalence of CKD reflects a normal aging process.[9,10] Despite this, the CKD staging system originally proposed by Kidney Disease Outcomes Quality Initiative (KDOQI), was accepted by nephrology societies across the world, in recognition that the need to identify patients with early CKD overrides these caveats. Furthermore, there is emerging evidence that since the introduction of this staging system, late presentation of CKD—just before or even when dialysis is needed—has been reduced.[11]

An additional issue with the KDOQI classification was that CKD stage was not related to primary underlying renal disease, to age, or to severity of proteinuria.[12] Regardless of age, sex, and degree of proteinuria or albuminuria, all patients with CKD were considered to have moderate disease when GFR was 59 to 30 mL/min/1.73 m². An important limitation of this broad definition, lacking specific clinical characteristics, is that in the major trials of relevance to patients with CKD, the subjects were defined by clinical criteria such as primary renal disease (e.g., diabetes) or creatinine/albuminuria–based degrees of renal function; few trials had clear definitions of GFR that translate easily into the classification system. In addition, the evidence base for CKD management includes a majority of trials with age inclusion criteria. Thus, this evidence must be applied with caution to older patients (>75 years in general), who make up the majority of those affected by CKD in population-based studies.

Despite these caveats, we, along with many other nephrologists, believe that the utility of eGFR and a CKD staging system far outweigh the perceived risks of labeling of patients, over-referral, and overtreatment of some.

STRATIFYING RISK IN PATIENTS WITH CHRONIC KIDNEY DISEASE: THE IMPORTANCE OF RISK FACTORS

It is clear from the results of large cohort studies that CKD is a heterogeneous condition and that outcomes with regard to progression to ESKD or death vary widely, depending on baseline characteristics. For example, in a cohort of 10,184 Canadian subjects aged 66 years or older, the decline in kidney function was assessed and adjusted for age, sex, presence of diabetes mellitus, and comorbidity. Subjects with diabetes mellitus had the largest average annual decline in eGFR, of 2.1 and 2.7 mL/min/1.73 m² in women and men, respectively. The average rates of eGFR decline for women and men without diabetes mellitus were 0.8 and 1.4 mL/min/1.73 m² per year. Women and men with stage 4 CKD experienced the largest annual decline in eGFR: 3.0 and 4.3 mL/min/1.73 m², respectively. The annual declines were larger for both women and men with diabetes mellitus and stage 4 CKD: 6.5 and 5.0 mL/min/1.73 m², respectively.[13]

It is therefore critical that the approach to managing a patient with CKD include an assessment of the individual's risk of CKD progression, as well as cardiovascular risk. One weakness of the CKD classification system originally proposed by KDOQI was that it did not necessarily reflect an individual's risk status. Based on a large body of evidence that identified albuminuria and GFR as independent risk factors for adverse outcomes in people with CKD,[14] KDIGO therefore modified the system to add categories for albuminuria. As shown in Figure 62.1, the categories in the KDIGO CKD classification system reflect an individual's risk status, and the system therefore provides a first step in risk stratification to guide initial priorities in management.[3,4] In addition, considerable progress has been made in identifying a relatively small number of additional risk factors for CKD progression that can be combined into a risk prediction tool.[15] In the largest of these studies, progression from stages 3 to 5 CKD to ESKD was predicted with a remarkable 90% accuracy in patients attending Canadian nephrology outpatient clinics. The risk prediction equation included age, male sex, eGFR, albuminuria, serum calcium, serum phosphate, serum bicarbonate, and serum albumin (area under receiver operating characteristic [ROC] curve, 0.917). External validation was performed with data from a separate cohort of 4942 patients with stages 3, 4, and 5 CKD (British Columbia CKD Registry).[16] The authors have produced an electronic risk calculator and smartphone app (available free at www.qxmd.com/calculate-online/nephrology/kidney-failure-risk-equation) that reports an estimated risk of ESKD at 2 and 5 years. Further external validation of this risk equation was conducted by independent investigators from the Multifactorial Approach and Superior Treatment Efficacy in Renal Patients with the Aid of Nurse Practitioners (MASTERPLAN) study. In a cohort of 595 people from the Netherlands with stages 3, 4, and 5 CKD, the model again performed well with the eight-variable equation giving an area under the ROC curve of 0.89.[17] Further research is required to evaluate the performance of this risk prediction tool in diverse populations, but there is already sufficient evidence to support its use in secondary care populations with CKD. For further discussion of risk factors in CKD, see Chapter 22.

Unfortunately, risk prediction tools for cardiovascular events developed for use in the general population tend to underestimate risk in patients with CKD, and new tools that take CKD into account are urgently required. Because relatively large numbers of people are affected by CKD, efforts to reduce renal and cardiovascular risk factors should be directed at patients at high risk. On the other hand, patients at low risk should be spared the anxiety and unnecessary cost of intensive intervention or specialist referral.

INTERVENTIONS FOR SLOWING PROGRESSION OF CHRONIC KIDNEY DISEASE

MECHANISMS OF DISEASE PROGRESSION AND THE RATIONALE FOR INTERVENTIONS TO ACHIEVE RENOPROTECTION

It has long been appreciated that regardless of the primary renal disease, kidney damage tends to progress toward ESKD, especially if more than half of glomeruli have been lost. This suggests that a common pathway of mechanisms may promote kidney damage and establish a vicious circle of nephron loss. In research efforts since the 1960s, investigators have identified glomerular hemodynamic factors (glomerular hypertension and hyperfiltration), multiple effects of angiotensin II, proteinuria, and proinflammatory and profibrotic molecules as key elements of this pathway (discussed in detail in Chapter 52). A common pathway underlies progressive kidney damage from kidney diseases of diverse causes, and recognition of this pathway has been vital in informing strategies to achieve renoprotection. Thus, the interventions to slow CKD progression discussed in the following sections are each aimed at attenuating mechanisms of progression. In view of the redundancy that is characteristic of most biologic systems, it has become clear that in order to achieve optimal renoprotection, attempts should be made to inhibit the vicious circle of common pathway mechanisms at multiple points (Figure 62.2).

LIFESTYLE INTERVENTIONS

All national guidelines support healthy lifestyle advice for patients with CKD, citing the substantial literature that

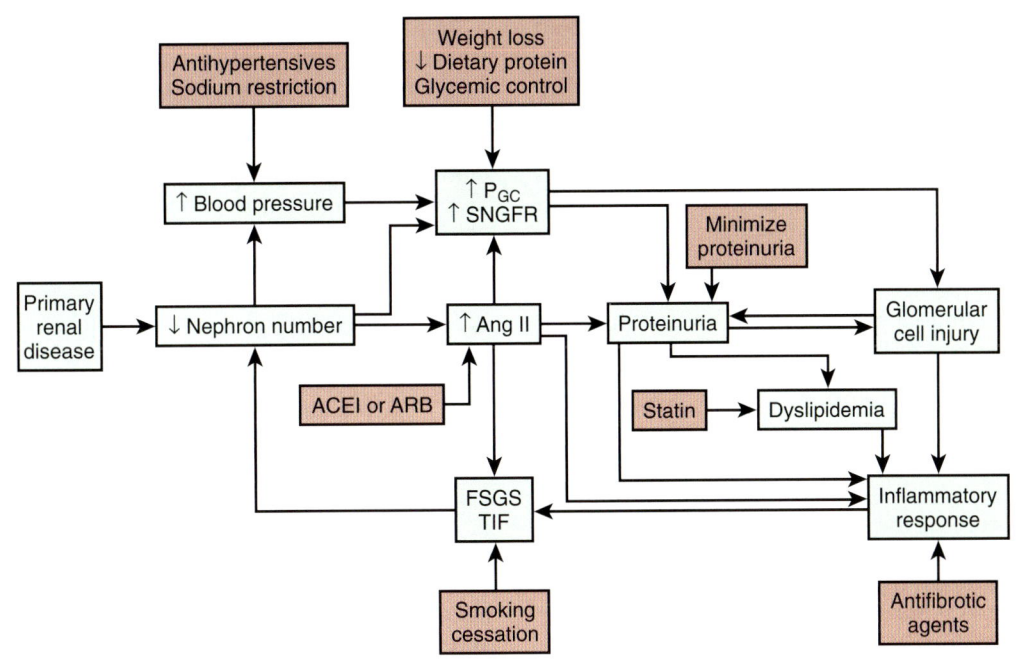

Figure 62.2 A common pathway of mechanisms that result in a vicious circle of nephron loss in chronic kidney disease (CKD). Interventions (in red) for achieving renoprotection are directed at inhibiting the common pathway at multiple points to slow CKD progression. ACEI, Angiotensin-converting enzyme inhibitor; Ang II, angiotensin II; ARB, angiotensin receptor blocker; FSGS, focal segmental glomerulosclerosis; P_{GC}, glomerular capillary hydraulic pressure; SNGFR, single nephron glomerular filtration rate; TIF, tubulointerstitial fibrosis.

exists largely for the general population. The benefit/risk ratio for pharmaceutical agents is a major factor in this recommendation, and it underlies the idea that if patients can change diet, smoking, and exercise habits, they may, over many years, substantially lessen their risks of CKD progression and of cardiovascular events. A major issue for nephrologists and physicians managing CKD is that the available randomized controlled trials (RCTs) of the effect of lifestyle interventions rarely enrolled patients with CKD. Moreover, lifestyle changes require considerable effort from patients and may take years to be effective. In the prospective observational Chronic Renal Insufficiency Cohort (CRIC) Study, regular physical activity, nonsmoking, and a body mass index (BMI) 25 kg/m² or higher were associated with lower risk of adverse outcomes, including a 50% decrease in eGFR or ESKD, atherosclerotic events, and all-cause mortality,[18] but there are potential biases in such observational studies because cardiovascular diseases and CKD may themselves result in low physical activity (reverse causality). Evidence does exist for the value of lifestyle intervention with regard to treating hypertension and preventing cardiovascular events. Although specific studies of lifestyle interventions in patients with CKD are still lacking, it is reasonable to assume that a similar relative (and greater absolute) benefit might be gained.

SMOKING CESSATION

Tobacco use is the most common cause of avoidable cardiovascular mortality worldwide; therefore, not surprisingly, smoking cessation is one of the most popular methods in management of cardiovascular risk in the general population and in patients with CKD. Smoking is estimated to contribute as much as 36% and 19% of the population-attributable fraction or risk for myocardial infarction and stroke, respectively.[19,20] Whereas many national guidelines mention the role of smoking cessation, the continued high rate of smoking in many dialysis populations suggests that there are still gains to be made from a focus on this area, particularly in patients with CKD who do not require dialysis and in patients with diabetes, who carry the highest risks.[21] For example, in the UK Renal Registry data, the smoking rate among patients receiving RRT was 21.3% in 2001 and fell slowly to 14.5% in 2008.[22] In persons with no known coronary heart disease (CHD), there is consistent reduction in cardiovascular event rates associated with smoking cessation, in the range of 7% to 47%. In addition, patients who have a cardiovascular event benefit from smoking cessation, with reduced rates of mortality after myocardial infarction.[23] In a meta-analysis of 12 studies in the general population, the combined odds ratio for death after myocardial infarction in those who quit smoking was 0.54; all studies demonstrated benefits, ranging from 15% to 61% in risk reduction. The number needed to quit smoking to save one life is 13, if the mortality rate among continuing smokers is assumed to be 20%.[24]

Evidence that smoking cessation helps prevent CKD progression is emerging.[25] In the Multiple Risk Factor Intervention Trial (MRFIT), smoking was significantly associated with an increased risk for ESKD[26]; in the Prevention of Renal and Vascular End-stage Disease (PREVEND) study, the rate of urine albumin excretion was correlated with the number of cigarettes smoked.[27] Smoking has been identified as a risk factor for the development of microalbuminuria and overt proteinuria and for the progression of CKD in patients with type 1 and type 2 diabetes.[21,28,29] In a large Swedish study, the risk for disease-specific types of CKD among smokers was compared with that among people who had never smoked. Overall, the association was modest, but an important finding was that the risk increased with high daily consumption (>20 cigarettes/day), long duration (>40 years), and a high cumulative "dose" (>30 pack-years) in comparison to subjects who had never smoked. Smoking increased risk most strongly for patients with CKD classified as nephrosclerosis and also glomerulonephritis.[30]

Smoking has been described as a risk factor for progression in various forms of nondiabetic CKD. Of patients with adult polycystic kidney disease, immunoglobulin A (IgA) nephropathy, and lupus nephritis, those who were smokers had a substantially increased risk of progression to ESKD in comparison with nonsmokers.[29,31] RCTs on the effect of smoking cessation on CKD progression have yet to be published, and few prospective data are available, but in one study of patients with diabetes, smoking cessation was associated with less progression to macroalbuminuria (proteinuria) and a slower rate of GFR decline in comparison to patients who continued smoking.[32] Further prospective studies are required, but the evidence just described strongly suggests that the kidney is another organ that may be adversely affected by smoking.

Smoking is the largest risk factor for the development of peripheral artery disease of the lower extremity in the general population.[33] Because peripheral artery disease is five times more prevalent among the population with CKD than among the general population, the well-established benefits of smoking cessation for prevention of cardiovascular and malignant disease must be a major focus for managing patients with CKD.

Pharmacotherapy to assist in smoking cessation is now well established. A meta-analysis of RCTs in the general population (69 trials involving a total of 32,908 patients) showed that varenicline, bupropion, and five nicotine replacement therapies were all more efficacious than placebo at promoting smoking abstinence at 6 and 12 months. In comparison with patients taking placebo, persons treated with these agents were 1.5 to 2.5 times more likely to quit smoking, depending on the specific agent.[23] Indeed, combining varenicline and a nicotine replacement patch achieved an impressive higher continuous abstinence rate at 12 weeks (55.4% versus 40.9%) and 6-month point prevalence abstinence rate of 65.1% versus 46.7% compared with varenicline treatment alone.[34] An important finding is that people who smoke are more likely to stop smoking if offered a combination of interventions, such as behavioral support and pharmacotherapy. Multicomponent interventions are now part of many public health guidelines. We see no reason to exclude people with CKD from this advice.

WEIGHT LOSS

Obesity is the dominant risk factor for type 2 diabetes and is also a major risk factor for hypertension and progression of CKD. Evidence linking the metabolic syndrome and CKD has emerged; each element of the metabolic syndrome is associated with increased prevalence of CKD and microalbuminuria. In animal models (obese Zucker rats with type 2 diabetes), early progressive podocyte damage and macrophage infiltration is associated with hyperlipidemia and antedates both the development of glomerulosclerosis and tubulointerstitial damage.[35,36] In humans, there was a graded relationship between the number of components of the metabolic syndrome present and the corresponding prevalence of CKD or microalbuminuria.[37]

Epidemiologic studies have identified obesity as a risk factor for CKD,[38,39] and in one study, obesity was an independent risk factor for progression of IgA nephropathy.[40] Furthermore, the largest such study to assess risk of CKD in association with obesity demonstrated a very strong biologic gradient: increasing BMI was associated with increasing risk of ESKD. In comparison to patients with an "ideal" BMI (18.5 to 24.9 kg/m^2), the relative risk of ESKD was 3.6-fold for those with a BMI of 30 to 34.9 kg/m^2, sixfold for those with BMI of 35 to 39.9 kg/m^2, and seven-fold for those with BMI of 40 kg/m^2 or higher. Controlling for baseline blood pressure and presence of diabetes attenuated the associations, but the gradient between increasing body size and ESKD risk remained strong.[41]

Because these components are major factors in the initiation and progression of CKD, respectively, patients with CKD would probably benefit from weight loss and reversal of the features of the metabolic syndrome, as observed in the general population.[42] Results of early studies support this assertion, inasmuch as weight loss in humans with obesity demonstrated reversal of glomerular hyperfiltration and albuminuria.[43]

Moreover, there is evidence that weight loss of as little as 10 lbs (4.5 kg) reduces blood pressure, prevents hypertension, or does both in a large proportion of overweight persons, although the ideal is to maintain normal body weight.[44] In the Framingham Heart Study, weight loss of 5 lbs (2.25 kg) or more was associated with reductions in cardiovascular risk of about 40%[45] for both men and women and thus should be a clear goal for patients with CKD who are overweight. It also appears that the degree of weight loss, regardless of method (lifestyle changes or bariatric surgery), dictates the benefits of lowering of blood pressure and reduction in glycemic markers.[46] However, according to longer term studies of lifestyle modification and of patients after bariatric surgery, the blood pressure–lowering benefits regress somewhat over time, although the vascular outcomes continue to be better than those in control groups.[42,47,48]

Renoprotective effects associated with weight loss interventions (dietary caloric restriction, exercise, anti-obesity medications, and bariatric surgery) were reported in a meta-analysis of data from 522 subjects in five controlled and eight uncontrolled trials.[49] In patients undergoing intervention to lose weight, persons with proteinuria had a mean reduction of urine protein levels of 1.7 g/day; even among persons with microalbuminuria, mean reduction of urinary albumin excretion was 14 mg/day. Although these reductions were modest in comparison to those in patients with overt proteinuria, results of other studies of blood pressure and glycemic control interventions in microalbuminuria suggest that they will have long-term benefit in such patients. Each 1-kg weight loss was associated with a corresponding 110-mg decrease in proteinuria and a 1.1-mg decrease in microalbuminuria, which were independent of blood pressure changes.[49] In other small studies, researchers have reported improvement or stabilization of kidney function[50] or reduction in proteinuria[51] after bariatric surgery in persons with CKD. A further systematic review of 31 studies analyzed the effects of weight loss achieved by bariatric surgery, medication, or diet and found that in the majority of studies, weight loss was associated with reductions in proteinuria. In people with glomerular hyperfiltration, GFR tended to decrease with weight loss, and in those with reduced GFR, it tended to increase.[52]

Further large interventional studies of weight loss in patients with CKD are required because gastric bypass surgery is associated with renal risks,[53] and treatment with orlistat is associated with acute kidney injury (AKI) as well as CKD.[54] On the basis of the available data, we recommend weight loss in obese patients with CKD through a combination of increased exercise and reduced caloric intake.

SODIUM RESTRICTION

There is substantial evidence from epidemiologic, migration, intervention, genetic, and animal studies that salt intake plays an important role in regulating blood pressure. Essential hypertension is observed primarily in societies in which the average sodium intake exceeds 100 mEq/day (2.3 g sodium or ≈6 g sodium chloride) and is rare in societies in which the average sodium intake is less than 50 mEq/day (1.2 g sodium or 3 g sodium chloride).[55] This relationship between sodium intake and population levels of hypertension is strong and consistent. Of importance is that sodium restriction produces a significant reduction in blood pressure.[56,57] Salt (sodium chloride) intake in many countries is 9 to 12 g/day. The World Health Organization's current recommendation for adults is to reduce salt intake to 5 g/day or less.

A meta-analysis of RCTs with a duration of at least 4 weeks concluded that reducing salt intake by 3 g/day is predictive of a linear fall in blood pressure of, on average, 3.6 to 5.6 mm Hg (systolic blood pressure [SBP]) and 1.9 to 3.2 mm Hg (diastolic blood pressure [DBP]) in hypertensive patients and of 1.8 to 3.5 mm Hg (SBP) and 0.8 to 1.8 mm Hg (DBP) in normotensive subjects.[58] The effect may be doubled with a 6 g/day reduction, and estimates suggest that reducing salt intake by 9 g/day (e.g., from 12 to 3 g/day) would reduce strokes by approximately 33% and ischemic heart disease by 25%. Weight loss and reduced sodium intake are particularly beneficial in older people. In the Trial of Nonpharmacologic Interventions in the Elderly (TONE), reducing sodium intake to 80 mEq (2 g) per day reduced blood pressure over 30 months, and about 40% of subjects on the low-salt diet were able to discontinue their antihypertensive medications.[59]

In many patients with CKD, especially those with glomerular disease and severe proteinuria, the disease behaves in a salt-sensitive manner. Several small studies have been conducted to investigate the effect of dietary sodium intake on CKD progression. One systematic review of 16 studies concluded that marked heterogeneity between the studies precluded meta-analysis.[60] Nevertheless, the general trend observed was that increasing sodium intake is associated with worsening albuminuria. Only two studies reported no benefit from reducing dietary sodium, but both were of low methodologic quality.

High dietary sodium intake has also been shown to negate the antiproteinuric effects of treatment with angiotensin-converting enzyme (ACE) inhibitors.[61] In a prospective, randomized, placebo-controlled crossover study, dietary sodium restriction increased the antihypertensive and antiproteinuric effects of therapy with angiotensin receptor blockers (ARBs), as monotherapy or in combination with a thiazide diuretic, in patients with nondiabetic CKD (Figure 62.3).

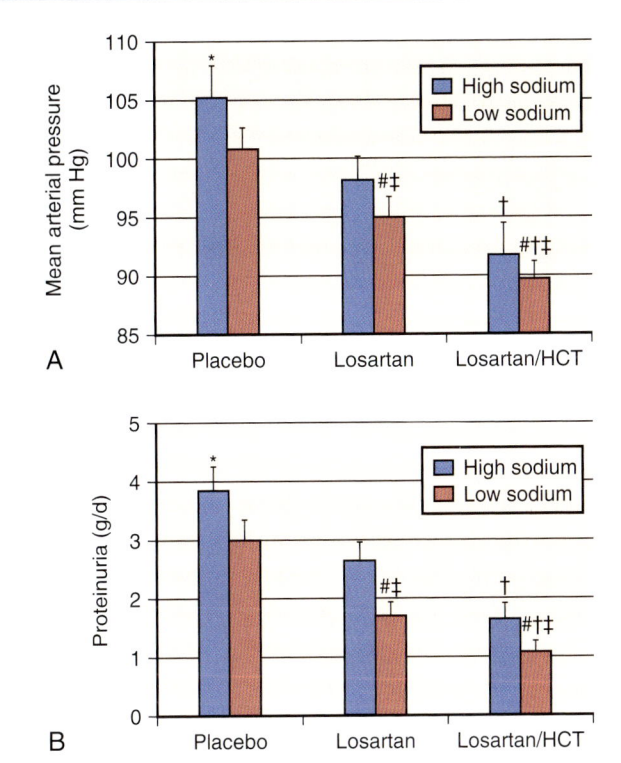

Figure 62.3 Results of a prospective randomized crossover trial showing the effect of dietary sodium restriction on the antihypertensive **(A)** and antiproteinuric **(B)** effects of treatment with an angiotensin receptor blocker as monotherapy or in combination with a thiazide diuretic. *$P < 0.05$ versus all periods; #$P < 0.05$ versus same treatment on high-salt diet (effect of low-salt diet); †$P < 0.05$ versus losartan treatment on same diet (effect of hydrochlorothiazide [HCT]); ‡$P < 0.05$ versus placebo on same diet. (From Vogt L, Waanders F, Boomsma F, et al: Effects of dietary sodium and hydrochlorothiazide on the antiproteinuric efficacy of losartan. *J Am Soc Nephrol* 19[5]:999-1007, 2008.)

Whereas the protocol aimed to restrict dietary salt intake to less than 50 mEq/day (1.2 g of sodium or 3 g of sodium chloride), these impressive results were observed with achieved sodium restriction of only 92 mEq/day.[62] Furthermore, a post hoc analysis of data from the first and second Ramipril Efficacy in Nephropathy (REIN) trials found that medium and high sodium intake were associated with significant increases in the incidence of ESKD versus low sodium intake. Each 100-mEq/g increase in 24-hour urinary sodium/creatinine excretion was associated with a 1.61-fold (95% confidence interval [CI], 1.15 to 2.24) higher risk of ESKD, independent of blood pressure.[63] In a small randomized placebo-controlled crossover study (achieved using low sodium diet of 60 to 80 mmol/day plus sodium chloride tablets [120 mmol/day] or placebo) in 20 people with stage 3 or stage 4 CKD, low sodium intake was associated with an average 10/4 mm Hg reduction in blood pressure as well as reductions in albuminuria and proteinuria.[64] Further long-term randomized trials are needed to define the role of sodium restriction in renoprotective strategies, but even the incomplete evidence available supports a recommendation for moderate dietary sodium restriction to less than 5 g/day of salt in patients with CKD.

Food processing drastically changes the cationic content of natural foods, increasing sodium content and decreasing potassium content. On average, approximately 10% of dietary sodium chloride originates naturally in foods, whereas approximately 80% is the result of food processing, the remainder being discretionary (added during cooking or at the table). We advocate assessment of salt intake in individuals with CKD and advise reducing salt intake with the assistance of a dietitian to less than 5 g/day (<90 mmol/day of sodium) as recommended by KDIGO.[3]

DIETARY PROTEIN RESTRICTION

Dietary protein restriction is based on the notion that reducing the excretory burden on the kidneys would slow the rate of progressive injury. Accordingly, dietary protein restriction was among the first interventions proposed to slow CKD progression. Experimental studies showed that a low-protein diet normalized glomerular hemodynamics in the remnant kidney model[65] and resulted in effective long-term renoprotection.[66] Unfortunately, clinical studies to date have failed to provide unambiguous evidence to support the use of protein restriction in human CKD. The proposal of nomenclature and diagnostic criteria for protein-energy wasting in AKI and CKD was an important step in planning future studies.[67] The suggested criteria for diagnosing protein-energy wasting include the presence of reduced body mass (specifically muscle mass) and serum evidence of low albumin, prealbumin, or cholesterol levels.

The Modification of Diet in Renal Disease (MDRD) study was designed to provide a definite answer to the question of whether dietary protein restriction slows the progression of CKD. The study had two components: In study A, 585 patients with mostly nondiabetic CKD (GFR, 25 to 55 mL/min/1.73 m^2) were randomly assigned to follow either a diet with "usual" protein levels (1.3 g/kg/day) or a diet "low" in protein (0.58 g/kg/day); in study B, 255 patients with GFRs of 13 to 24 mL/min/1.73 m^2 were randomly assigned to follow either a diet "low" in protein (0.58 g/kg/day) or a diet "very low" in protein (0.28 g/kg/day). After a mean follow-up period of 2.2 years, there was no difference in the rate of GFR decline in study A and only a trend toward slower decline in the "very low" protein group in study B.[68] Further analysis indicated, however, that the desired protein intake was not achieved in the randomized groups, and secondary analysis based on achieved dietary protein intake demonstrated that a reduction in protein intake of 0.2 g/kg/day was correlated with a 1.15-mL/min/yr reduction in the rate of GFR decline, equivalent to a 29% reduction in mean rate of GFR decline.[69] In addition, a post hoc two-slope analysis, in which presumptive acute effects of dietary protein restriction were taken into account, suggested a modest long-term benefit. Long-term follow-up of the cohort in MDRD study A has also yielded disappointingly inconclusive results.[70]

This issue was also examined in two meta-analyses of smaller randomized studies. Pedrini and associates[71] summarized findings on 1413 patients with nondiabetic CKD from five studies (including those from study A of the MDRD trial). Low-protein diet was associated with a relative risk (RR) of 0.67 (95% CI, 0.50 to 0.89) for ESKD or death. Similarly, among 108 patients with type 1 diabetes from five studies, low-protein diet significantly slowed the increase in albuminuria or the decline in GFR or creatinine clearance (RR, 0.56; 95% CI, 0.40 to 0.77). Kasiske and colleagues[72] pooled the results of 13 RCTs (1919 patients) and found that dietary protein restriction reduced the rate of decline in eGFR by 0.53 mL/min/yr.

Larger effects were observed in subjects with diabetes, and so the findings of a more recent meta-analysis of low-protein diet in patients with diabetes are important. In this study, Pan and colleagues[73] assessed eight RCTs. In contrast to a previous meta-analysis, they found that in comparison with a normal-protein diet, treatment with a low-protein diet was not associated with a significant improvement in kidney function (assessed by GFR). However, in only two of these trials, there was a significant but marginal decrease in proteinuria or albuminuria in the subjects following the low-protein diet. Of importance was that patients following the low-protein diet had lower serum albumin levels and poorer glycemic control, both of which are relevant to outcomes and their assessment.

Finally, Fouque and Laville[74] performed a Cochrane Database systematic review of all randomized studies, comparing two different levels of protein intake in adult patients suffering from moderate to severe CKD. A total of 2000 nondiabetic patients were identified in 10 studies (of a total of 40 studies) in which follow-up lasted at least 1 year. There were 281 renal deaths (progression to ESKD) recorded, 113 among subjects following the low-protein diet and 168 among those following the higher protein diet (RR, 0.68; 95% CI, 0.55 to 0.84; $P = 0.0002$). The authors concluded that reducing protein intake in patients with CKD reduces the occurrence of renal death by 32% in comparison with higher or unrestricted protein intake.

The caveats for these low-protein trials are that most trials were of short duration, the largest trial (MDRD) mostly excluded patients with diabetes, and compliance with low-protein diets was a factor in interpretation in some of the results. In addition to possible renoprotective effects, dietary protein restriction results in reduced intake of sodium, phosphate, and acid; reductions of all of these may be beneficial in CKD.[75] Although these results do not rule out the possibility that a low-protein diet is beneficial for patients with diabetes, the benefit with regard to kidney function does not seem to be strong, and the potential for harm from malnutrition should not be ignored. The risk of malnutrition associated with dietary protein restriction is particularly important because protein-energy wasting is evident in more than 50% of patients with stages 3, 4, and 5 CKD.[76] The early signs of muscle wasting (sarcopenia) are associated with other comorbid conditions (and so may not be causally related to CKD per se); however, in view of the strength of the associations among parameters of nutritional status and outcomes in dialysis,[77] we believe that the risk/benefit ratio of low-protein diets must be considered carefully on an individual basis and with the assistance of a trained renal dietitian.

The benefits are more apparent in patients with proteinuria, and the risks are greater in those at risk of malnutrition, such as elderly patients (age >75 years); those with below-average BMI (<20 kg/m^2), muscle wasting, or myopathic symptoms; and those with evidence of protein-energy wasting. The 2012 KDIGO guidelines recommend reducing dietary protein intake to less than 0.8 g/kg/day in adults with stages 4 and 5 CKD, and avoiding a high-protein diet (>1.3 g/kg/day) in adults with CKD who are considered to be at risk of progression.[3] For further discussion of dietary aspects in kidney disease, see Chapter 61.

GLYCEMIC CONTROL IN PATIENTS WITH DIABETES

The role of glycemic control in protecting the kidneys in patients with diabetes is discussed fully in Chapter 39. In summary, the benefit of tight glycemic control in ameliorating diabetic nephropathy seems to decrease as CKD progresses; the greatest benefits are observed in stages 1 and 2 CKD. In addition to the renoprotective effects, however, there is clear evidence that improving glycemic control can reduce the risk of developing other microvascular and macrovascular complications such as blindness and cardiovascular disease.[78] Of importance is that these benefits were maintained for up to 10 years after the trial, even though intensive control regressed to standard control levels.[79] Achieving optimal glycemic control should therefore be an important goal for all patients with diabetes and CKD but should be balanced against the risk of developing hypoglycemia, which may be increased in the elderly and those with CKD. The KDIGO guidelines recommend a target hemoglobin A_{1c} of 7.0% (53 mmol/mol) to prevent or delay progression of microvascular complications, including diabetic kidney disease, unless patients have multiple comorbidities, have reduced life expectancy, or are at risk of hypoglycemia.[3]

ANTIHYPERTENSIVE THERAPY

Interventions to slow the progression of kidney disease and thus prevent the need for dialysis have been the major focus in CKD initiatives around the world.[80] The treatment of systemic hypertension was the first intervention shown to significantly slow the rate of CKD progression and remains fundamental in renoprotective strategies. Mogensen[81] and Parving and colleagues[82] pioneered the role of blood pressure control in studies of patients with type 1 diabetes, in whom the initiation of antihypertensive therapy significantly slowed the rate of GFR decline.

Similar observations were subsequently reported among patients with nondiabetic forms of CKD.[83-85] In one of the earliest meta-analyses in nephrology, Kasiske and colleagues[86] studied 100 controlled and uncontrolled studies that provided data on kidney function, proteinuria, or both before and after treatment with an antihypertensive agent in people with diabetes. Multiple linear regression analysis indicated that ACE inhibitors decreased proteinuria independently of changes in blood pressure, treatment duration, type of diabetes or stage of nephropathy, and study design ($P < 0.0001$). Reductions in proteinuria from other antihypertensive agents could be attributed entirely to changes in blood pressure. Furthermore, blood pressure reduction was associated with a relative increase in GFR (3.70 ± 0.92 mL/min for each 10-mm Hg reduction in mean arterial pressure [MAP]; $P = 0.0002$), but in comparison with other agents, ACE inhibitors had an additional favorable effect on GFR that was independent of blood pressure changes (3.41 ± 1.71 mL/min; $P = 0.05$).

ANTIHYPERTENSIVE DRUGS

Data from the Antihypertensive and Lipid-Lowering Treatment to Prevent Heart Attack Trial (ALLHAT) have been misinterpreted by some as implying that the choice of antihypertensive drug does not affect renal outcomes in patients with CKD. It is important to note that ALLHAT was designed to investigate the effect of antihypertensive drugs on cardiovascular rather than renal outcomes in patients who had hypertension and at least one cardiovascular risk factor. There was no significant difference in the incidence of the primary outcome of fatal or nonfatal myocardial infarction among patients randomly assigned to receive treatment with a thiazide diuretic, a calcium channel blocker, or an ACE inhibitor.[87] Whereas a post hoc analysis also showed no difference in the secondary outcome of ESKD or more than a 50% decrease in GFR, patients with serum creatinine levels exceeding 2 mg/dL (>170 µmol/L) were specifically excluded from the study, and therefore only a minority (5662 of 33,357) had CKD, mostly in stages 1 to 3. Furthermore, the presence of proteinuria was not assessed.[88] In contrast, a large body of evidence supports the use of ACE inhibitors or ARB agents as first-line antihypertensive therapy in patients with CKD (see the "Pharmacologic Inhibition of the Renin Angiotensin Aldosterone System" section under "Interventions for Slowing Progression of Chronic Kidney Disease").

Despite the importance of ACE inhibition and ARB therapy in achieving renoprotection, thiazide and other diuretics are valuable and sometimes essential as additional antihypertensive agents to achieve optimal blood pressure control. Studies have shown that high dietary sodium intake may abrogate the antiproteinuric effect of ACE inhibitor treatment, but addition of a thiazide diuretic restores the antiproteinuric effect despite ongoing high sodium intake.[61] Similarly, addition of a thiazide diuretic to ARB treatment reduced blood pressure and proteinuria in patients with IgA nephropathy.[89] We therefore recommend a thiazide diuretic as second-line antihypertensive therapy in patients who have not achieved adequate blood pressure control with an ACE inhibitor or an ARB alone. In patients with advanced CKD, thiazide diuretics are considered less likely to be effective, although a recent review of published literature suggests that they may still be beneficial in stage 4 CKD.[90] In those who do not respond to a thiazide diuretic, a loop diuretic should be considered instead.

There is some evidence that, despite their efficacy as antihypertensive drugs, dihydropyridine calcium channel blockers (DCCBs) may have adverse effects with regard to CKD progression. In experimental studies, DCCB treatment was observed to allow greater transmission of systemic blood pressure to glomerular capillaries and was associated with more rapid progression of renal injury than was ACE inhibitor treatment in the 5/6 nephrectomy model.[91] Whereas one relatively small study revealed no difference between the renoprotective effects of the DCCB nifedipine and the ACE inhibitor captopril,[92] two larger studies demonstrated adverse outcomes associated with the use of DCCB agents. A secondary analysis of data from the Ramipril Efficacy In Nephropathy (REIN) study revealed that among participants not randomly assigned to receive ACE inhibitor treatment who failed to achieve a MAP of less than 100 mm Hg, the DCCB agents nifedipine and amlodipine were associated with a higher magnitude of proteinuria and more rapid GFR decline than were other antihypertensives.[93] Observations from the African American Study of Kidney Disease and Hypertension (AASK) provoked even greater concern.[94] In this study, patients with CKD and hypertension were randomly assigned to receive either treatment with an ACE inhibitor or amlodipine (DCCB) or treatment with a β-blocker and diuretic in combination. The amlodipine arm of the study was stopped prematurely because recipients exhibited a more rapid decline in GFR than did subjects receiving the β-blocker or ACE inhibitor, particularly among those with urine protein levels higher than 1 g/day. The Ramipril Efficacy In Nephropathy 2 (REIN-2) study revealed no additional renoprotection when a DCCB was added to ACE inhibitor treatment in patients with nondiabetic CKD, but there was also no adverse effect.[95] In contrast, treatment with nondihydropyridine calcium channel blockers (NDCCBs) ameliorated glomerular hypertension, reduced proteinuria, and afforded renoprotection in some experimental studies.[96] In one clinical study, the combination of ACE inhibition and NDCCB treatment resulted in greater reduction of proteinuria than did either of these treatments alone in patients with type 2 diabetes and overt nephropathy.[97] Furthermore, a meta-analysis of data from 28 RCTs revealed a 2% increase in proteinuria with DCCB treatment, in contrast to a 30% reduction with NDCCB treatment, despite similar effects on blood pressure in hypertensive patients with proteinuria.[98]

On the basis of the evidence just described, we recommend that DCCBs be avoided in patients with CKD unless they are used in combination with ACE inhibition or ARB treatment to achieve adequate blood pressure control. If possible, NDCCBs should be used in preference over DCCBs. Most of the trials in patients with CKD have established that between two and four agents is the median number of antihypertensive agents required for the respective target blood pressures. Therefore, third-line agents are needed by a substantial proportion of patients with CKD. We recommend that the choice of third- and fourth-line agents be based on factors other than renoprotection. Therefore, after blockade of the renin angiotensin aldosterone system (RAAS), diuretic therapy, and NDCCBs, we suggest use of β-blockers, α-blockers, and central nervous system agents, depending on other comorbid conditions, side effect profile, convenience, and cost.

INTENSIVE VERSUS USUAL BLOOD PRESSURE–LOWERING TRIALS

Despite the importance of blood pressure control in achieving renoprotection, the optimal blood pressure remains uncertain, particularly in elderly patients and those with mild proteinuria. In several RCTs, researchers have investigated whether blood pressure targets lower than previously recommended afford greater renoprotection than "usual" blood pressure control, but these studies have not provided a conclusive answer. In the MDRD study, primary analysis showed no significant difference in the rate of GFR decline between (1) patients randomly assigned to achieve a target MAP of less than 92 mm Hg (equivalent to less than 125/75 mm Hg), or less than 98 mm Hg for subjects aged 61 years or older, and (2) those assigned a MAP target of less than 107 mm Hg (equivalent to 140/90 mm Hg), or MAP less than 113 mm Hg for subjects aged 61 years or older. Subjects assigned to achieve the lower blood pressures, however, evidenced an early rapid decrease in GFR, probably as a result of associated renal hemodynamic effects, that obscured a later slower rate of GFR decline. Furthermore, secondary analysis did show benefit associated with the lower blood pressure target among patients with more severe baseline proteinuria (urine protein level >1 g/day). Further secondary analysis revealed that lower achieved blood pressure was also associated with a slower GFR decline, an effect that was more marked among patients with more severe baseline proteinuria.[68] The authors concluded by recommending a blood pressure goal of less than 125/75 mm Hg (MAP, 92 mm Hg) for patients with CKD whose urine protein levels exceed 1 g/day, and a goal of less than 130/80 mm Hg (MAP, 98 mm Hg) for those with urine protein levels of 0.25 to 1.0 g/day.[99]

Findings of prolonged follow-up of the patients in the MDRD study suggest that the benefits of lower blood pressure may become evident only over a longer period. Analysis after almost 10 years revealed a significant reduction in either the risk of ESKD (adjusted hazard ratio [HR], 0.68) or a combined end point of ESKD or death (adjusted HR, 0.77) among patients randomly assigned to achieve the lower blood pressure targets. The only caveat is that treatment and blood pressure data were not available beyond the 2.2 years of the original trial.[100] In AASK, no significant difference in the rate of GFR decline was observed among subjects randomly assigned to achieve a MAP goal of 92 mm Hg or lower versus a goal of 102 to 107 mm Hg. One possible explanation for this outcome is that subjects in AASK generally had milder baseline proteinuria (mean urine protein excretion, 0.38 to 0.63 g/day).[101] The results are therefore consistent with those of the MDRD study, which showed benefit only in patients with significant proteinuria. Likewise, in the REIN-2 trial, additional blood pressure reduction (total blood pressure of <130/80 mm Hg versus DBP of <90 mm Hg, regardless of SBP) failed to produce additional renoprotection in patients with nondiabetic CKD who were already receiving ACE inhibitor treatment.[95] Possible explanations are that the degree of additional blood pressure reduction was modest (4.1/2.8 mm Hg) and that in the group undergoing intensive blood pressure reduction, the number of subjects with moderate to heavy proteinuria was small.

Because not all the patients in the MDRD or AASK study received ACE inhibitor treatment, it remained unclear how important the level of blood pressure attained was in patients with CKD who were receiving an ACE inhibitor or an ARB. Several studies have sought to address this issue. Among patients with type 1 diabetes and established nephropathy who were receiving ACE inhibitor treatment, attainment of a "low" (MAP, 92 mm Hg) versus "usual" (MAP, 100 to 107 mm Hg) target blood pressure was associated with significantly milder degrees of proteinuria after 2 years, but there was no significant difference in GFR.[102] The Effect of Strict Blood Pressure Control and ACE Inhibition on the Progression of Chronic Renal Failure in Pediatric Patients (ESCAPE) trial was conducted to investigate the role of blood pressure control in children with CKD who were receiving treatment with an ACE inhibitor. Attainment of a lower blood pressure target was associated with a significantly reduced risk of reaching ESKD or doubling of serum creatinine concentration.[103] This is an important trial inasmuch as the primary end point (time to 50% decline in GFR or progression to ESKD) was not as affected by the competing mortality effects that complicate studies in older patients. A total of 30% of the patients who received intensified treatment for blood pressure control reached the primary end point, in comparison with 42% of those who received conventional treatment for blood pressure control (HR, 0.65; 95% CI, 0.44 to 0.94; $P = 0.02$). Urine protein excretion gradually rebounded during ongoing ACE inhibition after an initial 50% decrease, despite persistently good blood pressure control. Achievement of blood pressure targets and a decrease in proteinuria were significant independent predictors of delayed progression of CKD.

Results of secondary analyses of other studies also indicate that lower blood pressure is associated with more effective renoprotection in patients receiving ACE inhibitors or ARB treatment. In the Irbesartan in Diabetic Nephropathy Trial (IDNT), greater renoprotection was observed in patients who achieved lower blood pressure: An achieved SBP greater than 149 mm Hg was associated with a 2.2-fold increased risk of developing ESKD or of serum creatinine doubling, in comparison with an achieved SBP less than 134 mm Hg, independent of ARB treatment.[104] Progressive lowering of SBP to 120 mm Hg was associated with improved renal outcome and improved rates of patient survival, an effect independent of baseline GFR. However, the lower blood pressure observed was not a primary aim of these studies, and it cannot be assumed that this observed association (between lower blood pressure and improved renal and patient outcomes) is causative. Nonetheless, in a meta-analysis of 11 randomized trials (1860 patients), the lowest risk of progression of nondiabetic CKD with persistent proteinuria (levels exceeding 1 g/day) was associated with an achieved SBP of 110 to 129 mm Hg, independently of ACE inhibitor treatment (Figure 62.4).[105] This interpretation remains the best available until other investigators examine different blood pressure targets in a randomized manner, particularly in elderly patients, as well as those with milder proteinuria, for whom the risks of lower blood pressure targets may outweigh benefits in some subgroups.

Several sources indicate that excessive lowering of blood pressure may be associated with adverse effects in patients with CKD. In the meta-analysis just mentioned,[105] an achieved SBP lower than 110 mm Hg was associated with an increased risk of CKD progression (RR, 2.48; 95% CI, 1.07 to 5.77) (see Figure 62.4), and in IDNT, an achieved SBP lower than 120 mm Hg was associated with increased rates of all-cause mortality and no further improvement in renal outcomes.[104] In addition, secondary analysis of data from the Ongoing Telmisartan Alone and in Combination with Ramipril Global Endpoint Trial (ONTARGET) revealed that hypertensive patients with risk factors for cardiovascular disease who achieved an SBP of less than 120 mm Hg had a significantly higher rate of cardiovascular mortality than did those who achieved an SBP of 120 to 129 mm Hg.[106] Similarly, the Action to Control Cardiovascular Risk in Diabetes (ACCORD) blood pressure study reported no difference in primary cardiovascular outcomes (nonfatal myocardial infarction, nonfatal cerebrovascular accident, or cardiovascular death) among patients with diabetes randomly assigned to achieve an SBP target of less than 120 mm Hg, in comparison with a conventional control target of less than 140/80 mm Hg. During follow-up, the mean SBP was 119.3 mm Hg in the patients undergoing intensive therapy and 133.5 mm Hg in those undergoing standard therapy. Patients undergoing intensive therapy demonstrated a slightly lower stroke rate (annual rates of 0.32% vs. 0.53%) but a higher rate of treatment-related adverse events (3.3% vs. 1.3%). Specifically, there were significantly more instances of an eGFR of less than 30 mL/min/1.73 m² among patients receiving intensive therapy than among those receiving standard therapy (99 vs. 52 events; $P < 0.001$) and no difference in the primary cardiovascular composite outcome.[107]

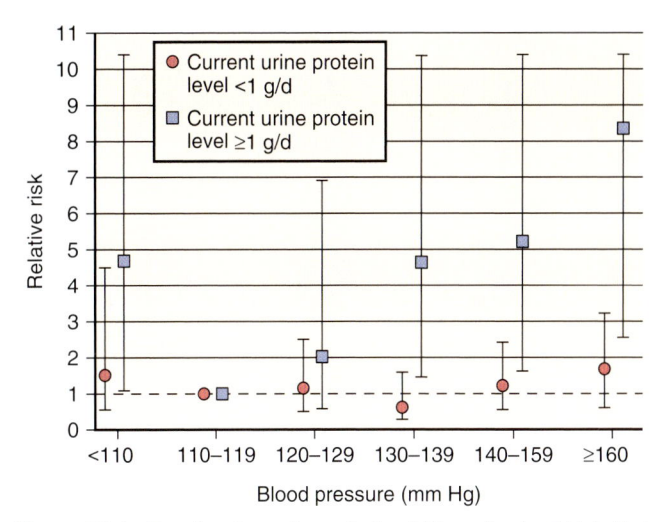

Figure 62.4 Results of a meta-analysis of 11 randomized trials that included 1860 patients with nondiabetic chronic kidney disease (CKD), showing the relationship between relative risk for kidney disease progression (doubling of serum creatinine level or end-stage kidney disease [ESKD]) and achieved systolic blood pressure in two groups according to the magnitude of proteinuria. (From Jafar TH, Stark PC, Schmid CH, et al: Progression of chronic kidney disease: the role of blood pressure control, proteinuria, and angiotensin-converting enzyme inhibition: a patient-level meta-analysis. *Ann Intern Med* 139[4]:244-252, 2003.)

The randomized trials in which "low" and "usual" blood pressure targets were compared among patients with CKD have not yielded unequivocal results, but overall, lower blood pressure targets were associated with more effective renoprotection, particularly among patients with significant proteinuria. Due to the lack of unequivocal evidence, guidelines differ somewhat in their recommendations for blood pressure targets. The KDIGO guidelines recommend an SBP of 140 mm Hg or less and DBP of 90 mm Hg or less for diabetic and nondiabetic adults with CKD and urine albumin excretion of less than 30 mg/day (or equivalent). For adults with diabetic or nondiabetic CKD and albumin excretion of at least 30 mg/day, the target values are 130 mm Hg or lower and 80 mm Hg or lower for SBP and DBP, respectively.[3] The Joint National Committee (JNC8) concluded that adults with CKD should be treated to reach the goal of SBP lower than 140 mm Hg and DBP lower than 90 mm Hg. They were unable to make a recommendation for a BP goal for people aged 70 years or older with GFR less than 60 mL/min/1.73m² due to the lack of evidence and the fact that estimating equations for GFR were not developed in populations with significant numbers of people older than 70 years.[108]

Care should be taken to avoid potentially dangerous hypotension, and SBP should not be lowered below 120 mm

Table 62.2 Summary of Studies Showing the Renoprotective Effects of Angiotensin-Converting Enzyme Inhibitors and Angiotensin Receptor Blockers in Diabetic and Nondiabetic Patients with Chronic Kidney Disease

CKD Type	Trial Outcome	Reference
Angiotensin-Converting Enzyme Inhibitors		
Type 1 DM + CKD	↓ Risk of dialysis or death	Lewis et al[113]
		Lindholm and Davies[321]
		Mathiesen et al[324]
Type 1 DM + microalbuminuria	↓ Risk of overt nephropathy	Lewis et al[113]
		Mathiesen et al[324]
		Laffel et al[325]
		Viberti et al[326]
Type 1 DM + normoalbuminuria	No significant benefit	Ravid et al[126]
		EUCLID Study Group[327]
Type 2 DM + CKD	Benefit in 1 study only	Bakris et al[115]
Type 2 DM + microalbuminuria	↓ Risk of overt nephropathy	Ravid et al[122,123,125]
		Ahmad et al[124]
Type 2 DM + normoalbuminuria	↓ Risk of developing microalbuminuria	Ravid et al[125,126]
Nondiabetic CKD	↓ Doubling of creatinine level/ESKD	Ruggenenti et al[328]
Angiotensin Receptor Blockers		
Type 1 DM + normoalbuminuria	Small ↑ in albuminuria or no benefit	Bilous et al[146]
Type 2 DM + normoalbuminuria	↓ Risk of developing microalbuminuria (small ↑ rate of cardiovascular mortality)	Sano et al[119]
		Trevisan and Tiengo[120]
		Agardh et al[121]
Type 2 DM + microalbuminuria	↓ Risk of overt nephropathy	Parving et al[145]
Type 2 DM + CKD	↓ Risk of doubling of creatinine level	Yusuf et al[141]
	↓ Risk of ESKD	Brenner et al[143]

CKD, Chronic kidney disease; DM, diabetes mellitus; ESKD, end-stage kidney disease.

Hg, particularly in elderly patients with labile blood pressure or atherosclerosis, which result in decreased vascular compliance. In particular, the association of excess cardiovascular mortality with a low DBP (e.g., 60 to 70 mm Hg), indicative of a wide pulse pressure, should be kept in mind when patients with coronary atherosclerosis are treated. In most studies whose data are used for hypertension guidelines, recruited patients were predominantly younger than 75 years, and, in addition, exclusion criteria were strict.[109] Although the benefits of blood pressure reduction on cardiovascular events are pronounced in elderly patients, as demonstrated in the Systolic Hypertension in the Elderly Program (SHEP) and Hypertension in the Very Elderly Trial (HYVET),[110,111] concerns remain because these and other trials excluded patients with moderate CKD. It is hoped that further data to inform blood pressure targets in CKD will be provided by the Systolic Blood Pressure Intervention Trial (SPRINT; NCT01206062 at www.clinicaltrials.gov), an RCT modeled after the ACCORD study, in which SBP targets of 120 and 140 mm Hg are being compared. It is projected that 4300 of the planned 9250 subjects will be persons with stage 3 or early stage 4 CKD. Patients with diabetes, polycystic kidney disease, and a history of stroke are excluded.[112]

PHARMACOLOGIC INHIBITION OF THE RENIN ANGIOTENSIN ALDOSTERONE SYSTEM

A large number of published clinical trials and meta-analyses provide clear evidence to support the use of pharmacologic inhibitors of the RAAS as an essential component of any strategy aiming to achieve maximal renoprotection in patients with CKD (Table 62.2).

ANGIOTENSIN-CONVERTING ENZYME INHIBITORS
Diabetic Nephropathy

In 1993 the Captopril Collaborative Study Group published results of the first large prospective RCT to clearly show specific renoprotection attributable to ACE inhibitor treatment, a landmark event in the development strategies for achieving renoprotection in patients with diabetes and CKD.[113] Patients (N = 409) with type 1 diabetes and established nephropathy (urine protein excretion > 0.5 g/day; serum creatinine levels < 2.5 mg/dL) were randomly assigned to receive captopril or placebo, and a blood pressure goal of less than 140/90 mm Hg was set for both groups. After a median follow-up period of 3 years, captopril treatment was associated with a 50% reduction in the risk of the combined end point of death, dialysis, and renal transplantation and a 48% reduction in the risk of serum creatinine doubling (Figure 62.5). Because blood pressure control was not statistically different between the groups, the additional renoprotection was not attributable simply to the antihypertensive effects of ACE inhibitors.

These results prompted several further studies to investigate whether ACE inhibitors may also benefit patients with early-stage nephropathy characterized by microalbuminuria. A meta-analysis of 12 such studies, including 689

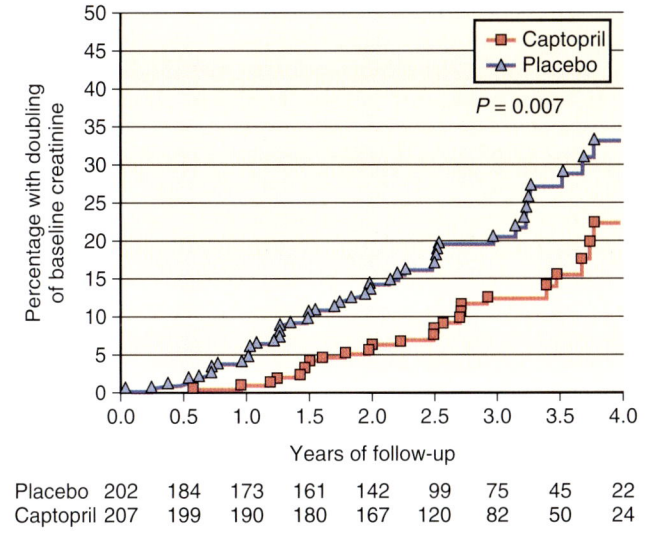

Figure 62.5 Results of the first randomized controlled trial to show the renoprotective effects of angiotensin-converting enzyme inhibitor treatment, independent of blood pressure lowering. Patients with type 1 diabetes and nephropathy were randomly assigned to receive treatment with captopril or placebo, and blood pressure was matched between the groups. The graph shows that the cumulative incidence of the primary end point, doubling of serum creatinine level, was significantly lower in the patients who received captopril treatment. (From Lewis EJ, Hunsicker LG, Bain RP, et al: The effect of angiotensin-converting-enzyme inhibition on diabetic nephropathy. *N Engl J Med* 329:1456-1462, 1993.)

patients with type 1 diabetes who were monitored for at least 1 year, revealed that ACE inhibitor treatment was associated with a significant reduction in the risk of progression to overt nephropathy (odds ratio [OR], 0.38) and three times the incidence of normalization of the microalbuminuria.[114]

Data regarding the renoprotective effects of ACE inhibitors in patients with type 2 diabetes are, to some extent, equivocal. Comparisons of ACE inhibitors and other antihypertensives among patients with overt nephropathy have included relatively small numbers of patients, and only one[115] demonstrated greater reduction in GFR decline in association with ACE inhibitor treatment.[116-118] Evidence of renoprotective benefit at earlier stages of nephropathy is more consistently supportive. Several studies, including the diabetic subgroup analysis of the Heart Outcomes Prevention Evaluation (HOPE) study, demonstrated beneficial effects of ACE inhibitor treatment among patients with type 2 diabetes in decreasing microalbuminuria[119-121] or in reducing the number of patients progressing from microalbuminuria to overt proteinuria (risk reduction, 24% to 67%).[122-125] In addition, the HOPE study reported a 25% reduction in the combined primary end point of myocardial infarction, stroke, or cardiovascular death in ramipril-treated patients with type 2 diabetes and risk factors for cardiovascular disease.

Two studies revealed a beneficial role for ACE inhibitor treatment in primary prevention of nephropathy in patients with type 2 diabetes. Among 156 normotensive, normoalbuminuric patients, ACE inhibitor treatment was associated with a 12.5% absolute risk reduction for microalbuminuria,[125,126] and in 1204 hypertensive normoalbuminuric patients, the addition of ACE inhibitor treatment to verapamil was associated with a lower incidence of microalbuminuria than was placebo plus verapamil.[127] On the other hand, one relatively large study demonstrated no renoprotective benefit of ACE inhibitors over β-blocker treatment among hypertensive patients with type 2 diabetes with normoalbuminuria or microalbuminuria,[128] and another revealed no reduction in the incidence of microalbuminuria in patients with type 1 diabetes randomly assigned to receive treatment with an ACE inhibitor versus placebo.[129]

Three meta-analyses were conducted to investigate the effect of ACE inhibitor treatment in patients with diabetic nephropathy. One analysis included only studies of type 2 diabetes with albuminuria or proteinuria as an outcome; it revealed statistically significant reductions in albuminuria in association with ACE inhibitor treatment versus placebo.[130] A second, larger analysis combined data from studies of type 1 and type 2 diabetes and revealed weak evidence of a reduced risk of serum creatinine doubling (RR, 0.60; 95% CI, 0.34 to 1.05) or reduced incidence of ESKD (RR, 0.64; 95% CI, 0.40 to 1.03) and stronger evidence of reduced risk of progression of microalbuminuria to macroalbuminuria (RR, 0.45; 95% CI, 0.28 to 0.71) with ACE inhibitor treatment versus placebo. All-cause mortality was significantly reduced in patients receiving ACE inhibitors (RR, 0.79; 95% CI, 0.63 to 0.99).[131] The third meta-analysis involved data from 16 studies of the effect of ACE inhibitor treatment on reducing the risk of microalbuminuria in type 1 and type 2 diabetes. This meta-analysis revealed a significantly reduced risk of developing microalbuminuria with ACE inhibitors in comparison with placebo (RR, 0.60; 95% CI, 0.43 to 0.84) or calcium channel blocker treatment (RR, 0.58; 95% CI, 0.40 to 0.84).[132]

On the basis of the data just described, we recommend ACE inhibitor treatment as first-line therapy for all patients with type 1 diabetes and microalbuminuria or overt nephropathy. At present, data are insufficient to support the use of ACE inhibitors to prevent nephropathy in normoalbuminuric patients with type 1 diabetes, but it seems reasonable to recommend them as the treatment of choice in those with hypertension. There is, however, sufficient evidence to recommend the use of ACE inhibitors to reduce progression to overt nephropathy in patients with type 2 diabetes and microalbuminuria or to prevent microalbuminuria in those with hypertension. There is no clear evidence of specific benefit associated with ACE inhibitors in slowing the progression of overt nephropathy in patients with type 2 diabetes; this lack of evidence may be ascribable to the lack of adequately powered studies. Finally, because cardiovascular disease is the most common cause of morbidity and mortality among patients with type 2 diabetes, ACE inhibitor treatment should be considered for the reduction of cardiovascular risk. The KDIGO guidelines recommend treatment with an ACE inhibitor or ARB in all adults with diabetes and urine albumin excretion 30 mg/day or more (or equivalent).[3] For further discussion of the management of diabetic nephropathy, see Chapter 39.

Nondiabetic Chronic Kidney Disease

After reports of renoprotection with ACE inhibitor treatment in diabetic nephropathy, researchers in further studies sought to investigate the renoprotective potential of ACE

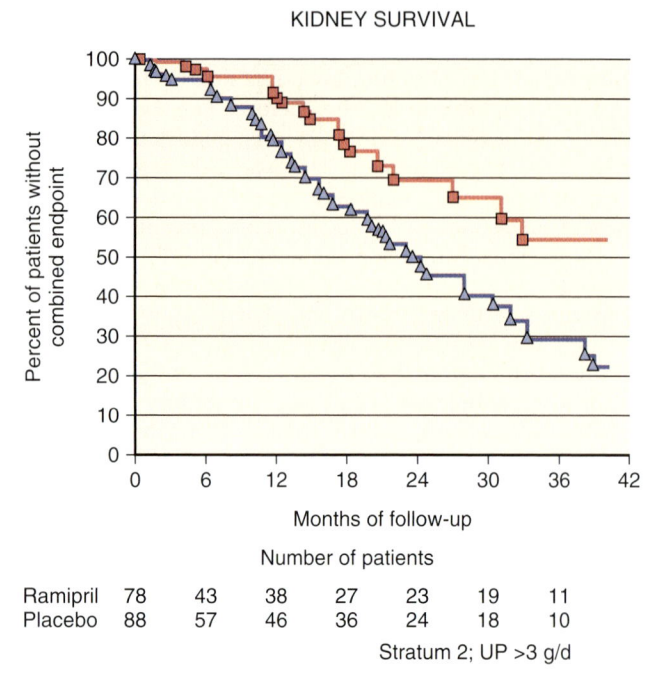

Figure 62.6 Kaplan-Meier plot showing the cumulative incidence of the primary end point of doubling of serum creatinine level or end-stage kidney disease in patients with nondiabetic chronic kidney disease and urine protein (UP) levels exceeding 3 g/day. Patients were randomly assigned to receive treatment with ramipril *(squares)* or placebo *(triangles)*; the graph shows improved renal survival in the ramipril recipients. (From Gruppo Italiano di Studi Epidemiologici in Nefrologia [GISEN]: Randomised placebo-controlled trial of effect of ramipril on decline in glomerular filtration rate and risk of terminal renal failure in proteinuric, non-diabetic nephropathy. *Lancet* 349:1857-1863, 1997.)

inhibitors in nondiabetic forms of CKD. One early study demonstrated a 53% reduction in risk of the composite end point (serum creatinine doubling or ESKD) in association with ACE inhibitor treatment, but a significantly lower blood pressure in patients receiving ACE inhibitors versus placebo made it impossible to separate the beneficial effects of lowering blood pressure from any unique effects of ACE inhibitor treatment.[133] In contrast, in the REIN study of 352 patients with nondiabetic CKD and urine protein levels exceeding 1 g/day, similar control of blood pressure was achieved in the patients randomly assigned to receive an ACE inhibitor or placebo. Among patients with at least 3 g/day of urine protein at baseline, the study was stopped early because the rate of decline in GFR in patients receiving the ACE inhibitor was significantly lower (0.53 vs. 0.88 mL/min/month)[134]; further analysis showed a significantly lower risk of the combined end point (serum creatinine doubling or ESKD) in the subjects taking ACE inhibitors (RR, 1.91 for the placebo recipients; Figure 62.6).

One hundred eighty-six patients from the REIN study who had less than 3 g/day of urine protein were monitored for a median of 31 months after randomization. In findings similar to those of patients with more severe proteinuria, ACE inhibitor treatment significantly reduced the incidence of ESKD (for placebo recipients, RR, 2.72; 95% CI, 1.22 to 6.08), particularly among those with a GFR of less than 45 mL/min at baseline.[135] After the randomized phase of the study, patients who had received placebo were switched to ACE inhibitors, and those taking ACE inhibitors continued treatment. In a finding consistent with those of the first phase of the study, there was a significant reduction in the rate of decline in GFR of patients switched to ACE inhibitors. In addition, patients continuing with ACE inhibitor treatment showed a further reduction in the rate of GFR decline. Patients who had received ACE inhibitors from the start of the REIN study had a significantly lower risk of reaching ESKD than did those who switched to ACE inhibitors after the initial phase (for placebo recipients, RR, 1.86; 95% CI, 1.07 to 3.26). In fact, from 36 to 54 months of follow-up, no additional patients in the former group experienced ESKD.[136] Of interest is that a small number of patients who continued taking ACE inhibitors exhibited an increase in GFR after prolonged treatment.[137]

One RCT confirmed that the renoprotective benefits of ACE inhibitor treatment may be observed even in advanced stages of CKD. Among 244 patients with a serum creatinine level of 3.1 to 5.0 mg/dL at baseline, random assignment to ACE inhibitor treatment was associated with a 52% reduction in urine protein levels and a 43% reduction in the risk of the primary end point (serum creatinine doubling, ESKD, or death).[138] A meta-analysis of 11 studies that included 1860 patients with nondiabetic CKD[139] revealed that ACE inhibitor treatment was associated with significantly lower risks of ESKD (RR, 0.69; 95% CI, 0.51 to 0.94) and with the composite end point of serum creatinine doubling or ESKD (RR, 0.70; 95% CI, 0.55 to 0.88). Moreover, the benefits of ACE inhibitor treatment were greater in patients with more severe baseline proteinuria but were inconclusive in patients with urine protein levels of less than 0.5 g/day. A further analysis restricted to patients with autosomal dominant polycystic kidney disease showed greater reduction in proteinuria with ACE inhibitor treatment, but overall evidence of slowing CKD progression was inconclusive and was limited to patients with more severe proteinuria.[140]

In addition to the renoprotective benefits of ACE inhibitor treatment, the HOPE study reported substantial reductions in overall mortality (RR, 0.84) and cardiovascular mortality (RR, 0.74) among 9297 participants who were at increased risk of cardiovascular disease receiving an ACE inhibitor versus placebo.[141] Although the HOPE study did not include large numbers of patients with nondiabetic CKD, cardiovascular disease remains the most widespread cause of morbidity and mortality among these patients, and the data therefore provide further support for the use of ACE inhibitor therapy in patients with CKD.

In view of the unequivocal data regarding renoprotection and the probable reduction in cardiovascular risk, we recommend ACE inhibitor treatment for all patients with CKD and urine protein levels greater than 0.5 g/day (albumin to creatinine ratio [ACR] > 30 mg/mmol; protein to creatinine ratio [PCR] > 50 mg/mmol) unless there are specific contraindications. The KDIGO guidelines recommend treatment with an ACE inhibitor or ARB in adults with CKD and urine albumin excretion exceeding 300 mg/day (or equivalent).[3]

ANGIOTENSIN RECEPTOR BLOCKERS

ARBs inhibit the RAAS by blocking angiotensin II subtype 1 (AT_1) receptors. Although ACE inhibitors and ARBs differ

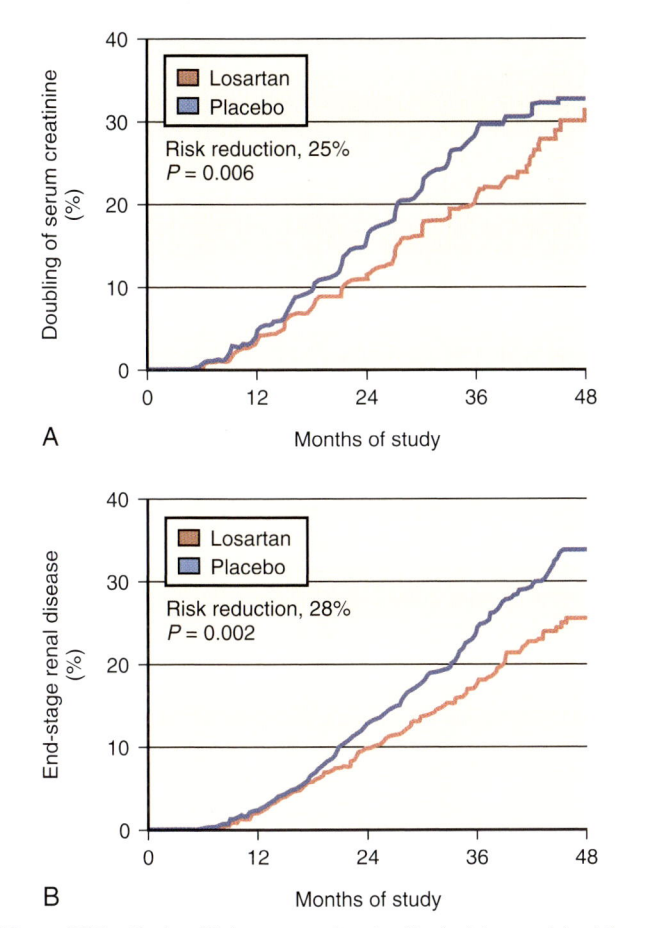

Figure 62.7 Kaplan-Meier curves showing the incidence of doubling of serum creatinine level **(A)** and the incidence of end-stage kidney disease **(B)** in patients with type 2 diabetes and nephropathy who were randomly assigned to receive treatment with losartan or placebo. (From Brenner BM, Cooper ME, de Zeeuw D, et al: Effects of losartan on renal and cardiovascular outcomes in patients with type 2 diabetes and nephropathy. *N Engl J Med* 345[12]:861-869, 2001.)

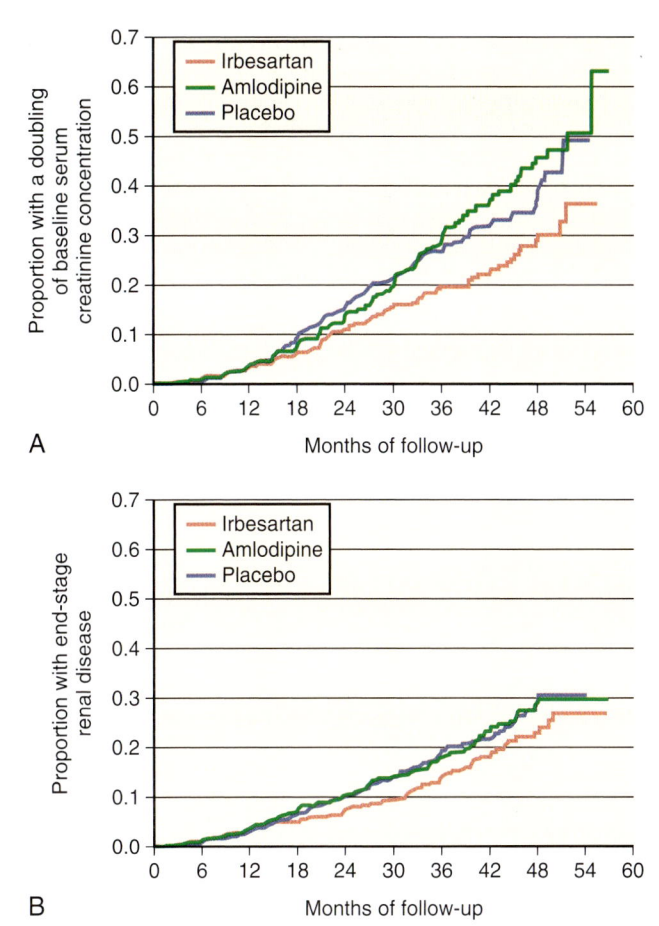

Figure 62.8 Kaplan-Meier curves showing the incidence of doubling of serum creatinine levels **(A)** and end-stage kidney disease **(B)** in patients with type 2 diabetes and nephropathy who were randomly assigned to receive treatment with irbesartan, amlodipine, or placebo. (From Lewis EJ, Hunsicker LG, Clarke WR, et al: Renoprotective effect of the angiotensin-receptor antagonist irbesartan in patients with nephropathy due to type 2 diabetes. *N Engl J Med* 345:851-860, 2001.)

significantly in their effects on the RAAS in ways that may be therapeutically relevant, experimental studies indicate that both treatments produce similar changes in glomerular hemodynamics (for a given blood pressure change) and afford equivalent renoprotection in a variety of CKD models.[142] Three large RCTs published simultaneously established a clear role for ARB therapy in achieving renoprotection for patients with type 2 diabetes. In the Reduction of Endpoints in NIDDM with the Angiotensin II Antagonist Losartan (RENAAL) trial, 1513 patients with overt diabetic nephropathy were randomly assigned to receive ARB treatment or placebo and were monitored for a mean of 3.4 years.[143] ARB treatment was associated with significant reductions in the incidence of serum creatinine doubling (relative risk reduction, 25%) and in ESKD (relative risk reduction, 28%) (Figure 62.7).

In IDNT, 1715 patients with overt diabetic nephropathy were randomly assigned to receive treatment with the ARB irbesartan, amlodipine, or placebo.[144] After a mean of 2.6 years, the risk of serum creatinine doubling was 33% lower with irbesartan than with placebo and 37% lower with irbesartan than with amlodipine. ARB treatment was associated with a 23% reduction in the risk of ESKD in comparison with placebo and amlodipine, but this reduction was not statistically significant (Figure 62.8). Of importance is that close matching of achieved blood pressure between groups in both these trials implies that, as with the ACE inhibitor studies, the additional renoprotective effects of ARB treatment could not be attributed merely to their antihypertensive effects.

In a third study, investigators examined the renoprotective effects of an ARB (irbesartan) in 590 patients with type 2 diabetes, hypertension, and microalbuminuria.[145] Patients were randomly assigned to receive irbesartan at one of two different dosages (300 or 150 mg/day) or placebo. After 2 years, there were significant differences in the incidence of overt proteinuria (5.2%, 9.7%, 14.9%), and the higher dose of irbesartan was associated with substantial reduction in the risk of overt nephropathy (HR, 0.30; 95% CI, 0.14 to 0.61) in comparison with placebo. This dose-dependent effect indicates that when ARBs are used to treat diabetic microalbuminuria, the dose should be titrated up to the maximum antihypertensive dose.

A meta-analysis confirmed the results of individual trials by showing significant reductions in the risk of ESKD (RR, 0.78; 95% CI, 0.67 to 0.91) and in doubling of serum creatinine level (RR, 0.79; 95% CI, 0.67 to 0.93), as well as a reduction in risk of progression from microalbuminuria to macroalbuminuria (RR, 0.49; 95% CI, 0.32 to 0.75) among diabetic patients treated with ARB versus placebo.[131] Of interest is that there was no reduction in all-cause mortality.

Several RCTs have been conducted to investigate the potential role of ARB treatment to prevent the development of microalbuminuria in patients with diabetes. In the Renin Angiotensin System Study (RASS), normotensive patients with type 1 diabetes randomly assigned to receive treatment with losartan evidenced a significantly higher incidence of microalbuminuria than did the subjects receiving placebo (17% vs. 6%; $P = 0.01$),[129] and in the Diabetic Retinopathy Candesartan Trials (DIRECT), mainly normotensive patients with type 1 or type 2 diabetes randomly assigned to receive treatment with candesartan evidenced no reduction in the incidence of microalbuminuria in comparison with subjects receiving placebo.[146] On the other hand, when hypertensive patients with type 2 diabetes were studied in the Randomized Olmesartan and Diabetes Microalbuminuria Prevention (ROADMAP) trial, those who received treatment with olmesartan evidenced a 23% delay in the time to onset of microalbuminuria in comparison with subjects who received placebo. A small but significantly higher incidence of death from cardiovascular causes was observed, however, particularly in patients with a previous history of cardiovascular disease and in those with the greatest reduction in blood pressure.[147]

In summary, there is sufficient evidence to support the use of ARB treatment to achieve renoprotection in patients with type 2 diabetes and overt nephropathy. ARB treatment is also effective in preventing progression from microalbuminuria to overt diabetic nephropathy in patients with type 2 diabetes. Data from the ROADMAP trial show that ARB treatment delays the onset of microalbuminuria in hypertensive patients with type 2 diabetes, but the associated increase in death from cardiovascular disease remains a concern. It seems reasonable to recommend ARB treatment for hypertensive patients with type 2 diabetes in the absence of cardiovascular disease. On the other hand, no renoprotective benefit is associated with ARB treatment in normotensive patients with type 1 or 2 diabetes. The KDIGO guidelines recommend treatment with an ACE inhibitor or ARB in all adults with diabetes and urine albumin excretion 30 mg/day or higher (or equivalent).[3]

ANGIOTENSIN-CONVERTING ENZYME INHIBITORS VERSUS ANGIOTENSIN RECEPTOR BLOCKER TREATMENT

Despite differences in their mode of action, the renoprotective effects of ACE inhibitors and ARB treatment have been directly compared in few studies. In a mixed group of patients with type 2 diabetes and microalbuminuria or macroalbuminuria, there was no significant difference between ACE inhibitors and ARB treatment in the primary outcome of change in GFR or a secondary outcome of urine ACR.[148] According to a meta-analysis of small trials in which ACE inhibitors were compared with ARB treatment in patients with diabetic CKD, benefits were similar with regard to incidence of ESKD, serum creatinine doubling, and progression of microalbuminuria to macroalbuminuria.[149] Similarly, in ONTARGET, there was no difference in cardiovascular or renal end points between patients randomly assigned to receive treatment with an ACE inhibitor and those assigned to receive an ARB.[150] On the other hand, in the RASS trial, ARB treatment was associated with a higher incidence of microalbuminuria than was placebo in patients with type 1 diabetes, whereas ACE inhibitors were not significantly different from placebo in this regard.[129]

Most national and international guidelines therefore recommend ACE inhibitor or ARB treatment for all forms of diabetic and nondiabetic CKD and leave the choice to individual physicians. One advantage of ARBs over ACE inhibitors is their more favorable side effect profile.[151] In clinical trials, ARBs have been reported to have side effect profiles similar to those of placebo[152,153] and, in particular, are not associated with the cough that may occur in up to 20% of patients receiving an ACE inhibitor. Among patients who switched from ACE inhibitors to ARB therapy, cough recurred significantly less often than in patients rechallenged with an ACE inhibitor.[154,155]

In choosing between ACE inhibitor and ARB therapy for patients with type 2 diabetes and diabetic nephropathy, physicians have to consider evidence of proven renoprotection with ARB treatment versus a mortality benefit associated with ACE inhibitor treatment (in patients without established diabetic nephropathy). One meta-analysis suggested a modestly increased risk of new cancer occurrence in patients on ARB treatment; this finding has created some controversy.[156] However, two long-term antihypertensive cohort studies linked to cancer registries, which can explore competing risk, showed no increased cancer risk from long-term hypertension therapy and RAAS blockade.[157,158] A large network meta-analysis of 70 RCTs of antihypertensive therapy in 324,168 patients recorded no difference in risk of cancer between the subjects receiving treatment (including ARBs) and control subjects.[159]

Another meta-analysis called into question the value of RAAS inhibition for renoprotection. Data from trials of ACE inhibitor and ARB treatment were pooled, and when studies of diabetic and nondiabetic CKD were considered together, the analysis revealed a benefit in reducing the risk of ESKD (RR, 0.87; 95% CI, 0.75 to 0.99) and albuminuria (mean urine albumin level, −15.7 mg/day; 95% CI, −24.7 to −6.7 mg/day) but no significant benefit in reducing the risk of serum creatinine doubling (RR, 0.71; 95% CI, 0.49 to 1.04). When data from studies of diabetic and nondiabetic CKD were considered separately, no significant benefits were evident with regard to incidence of ESKD or serum creatinine doubling, but the benefit for albuminuria reduction persisted. The authors concluded that the renoprotective effects of ACE inhibitor or ARB therapy probably result only from their antihypertensive effects.[160] This meta-analysis is, however, flawed in our opinion, and its conclusions have been rejected by many other investigators.[161] The principal weaknesses were inclusion of data from the large ALLHAT study, in which only a minority of patients (5662 of 33,357) actually had CKD[88]; heterogeneity across trials that should not have been pooled; and lack of patient-level data.[162]

COMBINATION TREATMENT WITH ANGIOTENSIN-CONVERTING ENZYME INHIBITORS AND ANGIOTENSIN RECEPTOR BLOCKERS

The differing mechanisms of ACE inhibitors and ARBs on the RAAS imply that in combination, they may have additive or synergistic effects. The added antihypertensive effects of combination therapy have, however, made it difficult to separate the benefits of additional blood pressure lowering from added renoprotection directly attributable to dual blockade of the RAAS. In several small studies, researchers reported additional lowering of urine protein excretion with combination therapy of ACE inhibitors and ARBs, in comparison with monotherapy; when pooled in three meta-analyses, all data indicate that there is greater antiproteinuric effect with combination RAAS inhibition therapy.[163-165] Only one RCT yielded results indicating benefit associated with ACE inhibitor and ARB combination therapy in CKD with respect to serum creatinine doubling or ESKD incidence. Publication of that study was, however, withdrawn because of concerns about the conduct of the study and integrity of the data.[166]

Furthermore, the results of the ONTARGET trial cast doubt on the benefit of dual therapy.[150] In ONTARGET, 25,620 patients with hypertension and additional cardiovascular risk factors were randomly assigned to receive therapy with an ACE inhibitor alone, an ARB alone, or a combination of both. The primary aims were to determine whether ARB treatment was inferior to ACE inhibitor treatment and whether combination therapy was superior in preventing vascular events.[167] The primary analysis revealed no difference in cardiovascular events between the randomized groups, but the number of events for the composite renal outcome—need for dialysis, doubling of serum creatinine level, and death[150]—was increased with combination therapy (n = 1233, or 14.5%; HR, 1.09; 95% CI, 1.01 to 1.18; P = 0.037) versus monotherapy (ARB: n = 1147, or 13.4%; ACE inhibitor: n = 1150, or 13.5%). This excess was attributable predominantly to more acute dialysis and to the combination of all types of dialysis and serum creatinine doubling. In addition, hyperkalemia (K > 5.5 mmol/L) was more frequent with combination therapy (ACE inhibitor, 3.2%; ARB, 3.3%; combination, 5.6%; $P < 0.001$ for combination versus ACE inhibitor). However, subjects were recruited on the basis of cardiovascular risk profile, and the majority did not have reduced GFR (mean baseline eGFR, 74 mL/min/1.73 m^2) or proteinuria (13% had microalbuminuria and 4% had macroalbuminuria; geometric mean of urine ACR ranged from 0.81 to 0.83 mg/mmol). In addition, participants were elderly (mean age 66.5 years) and predominantly male (73%). They had substantial vascular disease: coronary artery disease (75%), previous myocardial infarction (50%), angina (35%), unstable angina (15%), and peripheral vascular disease (13%). Angiographic studies[168] suggest that approximately 10% to 15% of this cohort would be expected to have atheromatous renal vascular disease in large vessels, and many more would have small vessel disease.

The ONTARGET results support a recommendation that combination ACE inhibitor and ARB therapy should not be used by older patients with risk factors for cardiovascular disease or previous cardiovascular disease. This recommendation is further supported by data from a population-based observational study that revealed a significantly higher incidence of the combined end point of serum creatinine doubling, ESKD, or death in elderly patients (older than 65 years) receiving combination therapy with ACE inhibitors and ARBs than among those receiving monotherapy (5.2 vs. 2.4 events per 1000 patients per month; adjusted HR = 2.36; 95% CI, 1.51 to 3.71). The incidence of hyperkalemia was also higher with combination therapy (2.5 vs. 0.9 events per 1000 patients per month; adjusted HR, 2.42; 95% CI, 1.36 to 4.32).[169] A further study in 1448 people with type 2 diabetes and urine ACR of at least 300 mg/g also found no benefit with respect to the primary outcome of CKD progression, ESKD, or death in participants randomized to combination ACE inhibitor and ARB therapy versus monotherapy, but those receiving combination therapy evidenced a significantly higher incidence of AKI and hyperkalemia.[170] In a meta-analysis of 59 RCTs comparing the efficacy and safety of combination versus single RAAS inhibitor therapy in CKD, combination therapy was associated with significant improvement in urine albumin and protein excretion as well as blood pressure control. These beneficial effects, however, were associated with a net 1.8 mL/min/1.73 m^2 decline in GFR, a significant increase in serum potassium level (3.4% higher rate of hyperkalemia), and a 4.6% higher rate of hypotension. There was no effect on doubling of the serum creatinine level, hospitalization, or mortality.[171] The KDIGO guidelines do not recommend the use of combination ACE inhibitor and ARB therapy for renoprotection,[3] but further RCTs with hard renal end points are necessary to investigate the role of combination ACE inhibitor and ARB therapy in achieving optimal renoprotection in proteinuric, nondiabetic CKD.

ALDOSTERONE ANTAGONISM

Aldosterone has been identified as an important mediator of progressive renal injury through hemodynamic and profibrotic actions. Treatment with spironolactone and other aldosterone antagonists has produced renoprotective effects in experimental[172] and small clinical studies.[173] One meta-analysis of their use in comparison with other RAAS-inhibiting agents included data from 10 trials and 845 patients. In comparison with ACE inhibitor or ARB plus placebo, nonselective aldosterone antagonists added to ACE inhibitor or ARB treatment significantly reduced proteinuria (weighted mean difference, −0.80 g/day; 95% CI, −1.23 to −0.38) and blood pressure, but these developments did not translate into an improvement in GFR (weighted mean difference, −0.70 mL/min/1.73 m^2; 95% CI, −4.73 to 3.34). There was a significant increase in the risk of hyperkalemia with the addition of an aldosterone antagonist (RR, 3.06; 95% CI, 1.26 to 7.41).[173b] A further meta-analysis of 27 studies also found that treatment with an aldosterone antagonist alone or in combination with an ACE inhibitor or ARB was associated with reduction in proteinuria and blood pressure but no clear evidence of reduction in cardiovascular events or ESKD.[174] Further studies are therefore required to evaluate the long-term effects of these agents on renal outcomes, mortality, and safety.

DIRECT RENIN INHIBITORS

Direct renin inhibitors inhibit the RAAS at its rate-limiting step (the conversion of angiotensinogen to angiotensin I) and may therefore achieve more complete blockade of the RAAS than do ACE inhibitors or ARBs. Direct renin inhibitors are effective antihypertensive drugs and reduced proteinuria in experimental models of CKD[175,176] and RCTs.[177,178] However, a large randomized trial that included 8561 people with type 2 diabetes and albuminuria or cardiovascular disease was stopped prematurely after the second interim efficacy analysis. Despite greater lowering of blood pressure and albuminuria with combination direct renin inhibitor and ARB therapy, no benefit was observed with respect to the composite primary end point of cardiovascular event, CKD progression, ESKD, or death versus ARB monotherapy, but combination therapy was associated with a higher incidence of hyperkalemia and hypotension.[179,180] There is currently therefore no evidence that direct renin inhibitor therapy, alone or in combination with ACE inhibitor therapy, affords more effective renoprotection than ACE inhibitor or ARB therapy alone.

HYPERURICEMIA

A number of studies have highlighted the fact that an elevated level of uric acid is a risk factor for the development and progression of CKD.[181,182] It has also been associated with excess cardiovascular risk and hypertension in a cohort of community-based patients.[183] Whether it is an independent risk factor for these outcomes in CKD or a marker of more severe renal and cardiovascular outcomes is an issue of ongoing debate.[184] In animal studies, an elevated level of uric acid decreases nitric oxide production, which provokes endothelial dysfunction, increases blood pressure, promotes fibrosis, and causes the release of proinflammatory cytokines and thereby results in T cell activation. A meta-analysis of eight small trials investigating the potential benefits of lowering uric acid in CKD with allopurinol included data from 476 participants. In three studies that reported serum creatinine levels, allopurinol treatment was associated with a lower creatinine level than was placebo, but in five studies that reported eGFR, there was no significant difference between groups treated with allopurinol or placebo. In five trials that measured proteinuria, no benefit was observed. Progression to ESKD was reported in only two studies and was not different between treatment groups, although the incidence was too low to allow robust conclusions to be made.[185] One randomized trial of allopurinol in 113 patients with CKD (included in the above meta-analysis) reported a 47% reduction in risk of CKD progression (defined as decrease in eGFR of >0.2 mL/min/month) in participants treated with allopurinol after multivariable Cox proportional hazards analysis, as well as a 71% reduction in risk of new cardiovascular events and 62% reduction in risk of hospitalization.[186] Long-term follow-up of these participants reported further benefit with a 68% reduction in risk of a renal event (initiation of RRT or 50% reduction in GFR or doubling of serum creatinine) and a 57% reduction in risk of cardiovascular event.[187] Nevertheless, in the absence of larger trials, uric acid–lowering therapy should not routinely be used in people with CKD unless there is clinical evidence of gout.

TREATMENT OF METABOLIC ACIDOSIS

As the number of functioning nephrons declines, CKD leads to net retention of hydrogen ions, which begins when GFR falls below 40 to 50 mL/min/1.73 m^2.[188] Among patients in whom GFR decreases from 90 to less than 20 mL/min/1.73 m^2, the prevalence of metabolic acidosis rises from 2% to 39% and is higher among younger patients and those with diabetes.[189] As the patient approaches ESKD, the plasma bicarbonate concentration tends to stabilize between 15 and 20 mEq/L. Chronic metabolic acidosis has multiple adverse consequences, including increased protein catabolism, increased bone turnover, induction of inflammatory mediators, insulin resistance, and increased production of corticosteroids and parathyroid hormone. Several observational studies, including the CRIC study, have identified low serum bicarbonate as a risk factor for CKD progression.[190]

The first study to show convincing renoprotection with bicarbonate supplementation was from a single center and involved 134 patients with advanced CKD (creatinine clearance rates between 15 and 30 mL/min/1.73 m^2) and baseline serum bicarbonate concentrations of 16 to 20 mEq/L. The patients were randomly assigned to receive treatment with oral bicarbonate or no treatment.[191] After 2 years of follow-up, there was a lower mean rate of decline in creatinine clearance (1.88 vs. 5.93 mL/min/1.73 m^2) and a lower risk of ESKD among the patients who received the bicarbonate treatment than among the controls (6.5% vs. 33%). A subsequent study reported similar renoprotective benefits in early CKD. In a randomized, placebo controlled trial in subjects with a mean eGFR of 75 mL/min/1.73 m^2, treatment with sodium bicarbonate for 5 years was associated with a slower rate of decline in eGFR (derived from plasma cystatin C measurements) compared with placebo or treatment with sodium chloride.[192] Western diets are typically acid producing, but the addition of significant portions of fruits and vegetables can move this to a base-producing state. Further studies have reported that correction of acidosis with a diet rich in fruits and vegetables was as effective as sodium bicarbonate in ameliorating kidney damage in early (stage 1 or 2 CKD)[193] and more advanced (stage 4 CKD) disease.[194] Furthermore, a recent trial has reported benefit even in people with mild acidosis. People with stage 3 CKD and serum bicarbonate 22 to 24 mmol/L were randomized to oral bicarbonate supplementation, a diet rich in fruits and vegetables, or "usual care." All participants received treatment with an RAAS inhibitor, and SBP was controlled to lower than 130 mm Hg. Both interventions achieved an increase in serum bicarbonate and were associated with a decrease in urinary angiotensinogen. After 3 years, both interventions were associated with less albuminuria and GFR decline than the "usual care" group.[195] The KDIGO guidelines recommend bicarbonate supplementation for patients with levels below 22 mEq/L,[3] but further studies are required to further investigate whether this may also be beneficial in the setting of less severe acidosis.

PROTEINURIA AS A THERAPEUTIC TARGET

Proteinuria is a marker of glomerular filtration barrier integrity, and the magnitude of proteinuria has therefore been used as an indicator of the severity of glomerulopathy. This view has been confirmed by several observations that the severity of proteinuria at baseline is the most important independent predictor of renal outcomes in randomized trials of patients with diabetic nephropathy[196,197] and nondiabetic nephropathy.[14,198,199] In addition, it has been proposed that proteinuria per se contributes to progressive renal injury[200] and that amelioration of proteinuria should therefore be viewed as a therapeutic goal.

Support for this hypothesis is derived from a number of sources. In the MDRD study, reduction in urine protein levels, independent of blood pressure, was associated with slower progression of CKD, and the degree of benefit achieved through blood pressure lowering was dependent on the extent of baseline proteinuria.[99] Furthermore, several other investigators have observed that the percentage reduction in urine protein level after initiation of ACE inhibitor or ARB treatment and the magnitude of proteinuria during treatment (residual proteinuria) are strong independent predictors of the subsequent rate of decline in GFR among patients with diabetic and nondiabetic CKD.[196,197] A meta-analysis that included data from 1860 patients with nondiabetic CKD confirmed these findings and showed that during antihypertensive treatment, the achieved level of urine protein was a powerful predictor of the combined end point of serum creatinine doubling or onset of ESKD (RR, 5.6 for each 1.0-g/day increase in achieved level of proteinuria).[139] A further meta-analysis of 21 randomized trials of drug treatment in CKD that included 78,342 participants found that for each 30% initial reduction in albuminuria on treatment, the risk of ESKD decreased by 23.7% (95% CI, 11.4% to 34.2%) independent of the class of drug used for treatment.[201]

One RCT provided direct evidence that the extent to which proteinuria is lowered determines subsequent prognosis. In the Renoprotection of Optimal Antiproteinuric Doses (ROAD) study, 360 nondiabetic patients with proteinuria and CKD were randomly assigned to receive a conventional dosage of benazepril (10 mg/day), a conventional dosage of losartan (50 mg/day), an upward titration of benazepril (range of 10 to 40 mg/day), or an upward titration of losartan (range of 50 to 200 mg/day).[202] In upward titration, the dosage of the RAAS-inhibiting agent was increased to maximize the antiproteinuric effect. After a median of 3.7 years, titration of benazepril and losartan to the maximum antiproteinuric dose, in comparison with the fixed conventional dosages, reduced the risk of serum creatinine doubling by 49% and 50%, respectively, and the risk of ESKD by 47% in both groups (Figure 62.9). Both agents provided similar overall relative risk reductions at optimal antiproteinuric dosages. Reduction of urine protein levels at 3 months (approximately 50% decrease with the upward-titration strategy) was closely correlated with the subsequent rate of GFR decline. Subjects in all conditions of the study had similar reductions in blood pressure. Regardless of whether proteinuria contributes directly to renal injury, the strong association between achieved reduction in urine protein and renoprotection in clinical studies implies that amelioration of proteinuria should be regarded as an important therapeutic goal in renoprotective strategies. We recommend a goal of reducing proteinuria to less than 0.5 g/day (equivalent urine ACR of ≈300 mg/g or 30 mg/mmol).

TIME COURSE FOR PROTEINURIA RESPONSE

In most patients, the reduction of proteinuria takes several weeks to achieve its maximal effect, which should be considered when dosages are titrated.[203] In patients in earlier stages of CKD (with diabetes and microalbuminuria, for instance) the effects are observed more promptly and tend to parallel the time course and fall in blood pressure.[204]

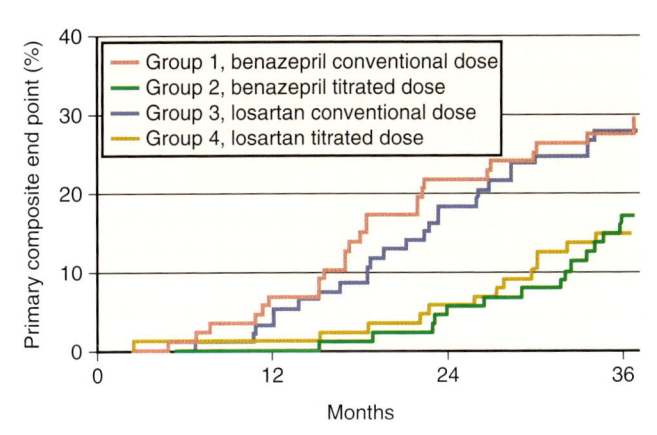

Figure 62.9 Kaplan-Meier curves showing the incidence of the combined end point of doubling of serum creatinine level or end-stage kidney disease in patients with nondiabetic chronic kidney disease and urine protein levels exceeding 1 g/day. Patients in group 1 were randomly assigned to receive standard doses of angiotensin-converting enzyme (ACE) inhibitors; those in group 3 received standard doses of angiotensin receptor blockers (ARBs); those in group 2 received ACE inhibitors titrated upward to the maximum antiproteinuric levels; and those in group 4 received ARBs titrated upward similarly. (From Hou FF, Xie D, Zhang X, et al: Renoprotection of Optimal Antiproteinuric Doses [ROAD] study: a randomized controlled study of benazepril and losartan in chronic renal insufficiency. *J Am Soc Nephrol* 18:1889-1898, 2007.)

MONITORING AND SAFETY CONSIDERATIONS

Regular monitoring is essential for optimizing therapeutic interventions to slow CKD progression and ensure safety. Kidney function is best assessed with the use of eGFR, derived from a serum creatinine measurement with the MDRD equation or Chronic Kidney Disease Epidemiology Collaboration (CKD-EPI) equation, recommended by KDIGO.[3] This strategy allows direct monitoring of the rate of GFR decline and assessment of the therapeutic goal to reduce this decline to less than 1 mL/min/yr, a rate associated with normal aging. The majority of laboratories now facilitate this monitoring by reporting eGFR with every serum creatinine measurement. In addition, monitoring allows for the detection of side effects of drug treatment and, in particular, of electrolyte disorders (hyperkalemia and hyponatremia), as well as acute changes in kidney function related to volume depletion.

Renal Dysfunction and Hyperkalemia Induced by Inhibitors of the Renin Angiotensin Aldosterone System

The appropriate frequency for monitoring of subjects with CKD should depend on the CKD stage, previous rate of GFR decline, risk of future GFR decline, and use of medication that may cause acute deteriorations in GFR or electrolyte disorders (especially RAAS inhibitors and diuretics). Despite clear trial evidence of the renoprotective and cardioprotective effects of ACE inhibitors and ARBs, some physicians remain cautious about prescribing these drugs to patients

> **Table 62.3** Causes of Acute Kidney Injury after Initiation of Therapy with Angiotensin-Converting Enzyme Inhibitor or Angiotensin Receptor Blocker
>
> Blood pressure insufficient for adequate renal perfusion
>   Poor cardiac output
>   Low systemic vascular resistance (e.g., as in sepsis)
>   Volume depletion (gastrointestinal loss, poor oral intake, excess diuretic use)
> Presence of renal vascular disease*
>   Bilateral renal artery stenosis
>   Stenosis of dominant or single kidney
>   Afferent arteriolar narrowing (caused by hypertension, cyclosporine)
>   Diffuse atherosclerosis in smaller renal vessels
> Vasoconstrictor agents (NSAIDs, cyclosporine)
>
> *Clinical features of renal vascular disease include vascular bruits (areas of the epigastric, femoral, and carotid arteries), prior rise in serum creatinine level of more than 30%, fall in estimated glomerular filtration rate (eGFR) of more than 20% after beginning of treatment with an angiotensin-converting enzyme (ACE) inhibitor or angiotensin receptor blocker (ARB), and a history of flash pulmonary edema.
> NSAID, Nonsteroidal antiinflammatory drug.

with stages 3 and 4 CKD. This caution results from concerns about renal dysfunction induced by these drugs, with a potential rise in serum creatinine or potassium level (reviewed by Schoolwerth et al[205] and Palmer[206]). General guidance on risk factors for AKI and frequency of monitoring are given in Table 62.1 and Table 62.3.

The initiation of therapy with RAAS inhibition may provoke an acute decline in GFR or hyperkalemia in patients with CKD, particularly in those with volume depletion, those with poor cardiac status, elderly patients, those with stage 4 or 5 disease, and any patient with or at risk for atherosclerotic renovascular disease. GFR and electrolytes should therefore be checked before and 1 week after treatment is started or a dosage is increased. A rapid rise in serum creatinine level or a more gradual increase of greater than 30% should prompt discontinuation of therapy and consideration of further investigation to exclude renovascular disease (see Chapter 48).

However, it should be remembered that AKI can occur even if RAAS inhibition therapy has been successful for months or years, usually when provoked by factors such as volume depletion or nephrotoxic medications. In the Studies of Left Ventricular Dysfunction (SOLVD), impaired kidney function (defined as a rise in serum creatinine level of 0.5 mg/dL [44 μmol/L] from baseline) was noted in 16% of patients randomly assigned to receive enalapril, in comparison with 12% of patients receiving placebo. This absolute 4% excess of GFR decline was associated with older age, diuretic therapy, and diabetes. Of note was that β-blocker therapy and a higher ejection fraction were renoprotective. A progressive rise in serum creatinine level is much less common in younger patients (younger than 70 years) and in those without renovascular disease.

As evidence for this, patients in the second Evaluation of Losartan in the Elderly (ELITE II) study of heart failure (average age of 73.5) showed relatively high rates of creatinine elevation during the 50-week follow-up period.[207] The incidence of persistent renal dysfunction did not differ between the losartan and captopril recipients (both 10.5%), and less than 2% of patients discontinued the RAAS agent for this reason. However, slightly more than 25% of the losartan and captopril recipients experienced at least one rise in creatinine level of 26.5 μmol (0.3 mg); this finding indicates that vigilance is needed for older patients with other comorbid conditions.

It is important to appreciate that an initial increase in serum creatinine probably results from the renal hemodynamic effects of ACE inhibitors or ARBs and in fact is predictive of greater renoprotective efficacy, particularly in patients with proteinuria and the most benefit to gain.[208] Thus, if the increase is less than 30% and is not progressive, an initial rise in serum creatinine should not be regarded as an indication for discontinuing ACE inhibitor therapy.

The dosage of ACE inhibitor or ARB should be started at a low level and titrated upward, with monitoring of creatinine and potassium levels 5 to 7 days after each dosage increase. To avoid compromise from intravascular volume depletion, patients should be counseled to omit ACE inhibitor or ARB treatment during vomiting or diarrheal illnesses and to seek medical advice if these illnesses do not resolve within 48 hours. Likewise, it is important to ensure adequate hydration, to omit or reduce diuretics for 48 to 72 hours if clinically appropriate, and to avoid nonsteroidal antiinflammatory drugs (NSAIDs) before starting a RAAS inhibitor. In general, we strongly advise discontinuation of NSAIDs because these are potent causes of AKI in patients with CKD.

Discontinuation of therapy because of uncontrolled hyperkalemia has been reported in only up to 4% of patients with CKD in trials, and the overall incidence was no different from that among patients taking ACE inhibitors versus non–ACE inhibitor treatment when data from six studies were combined.[209] However, the subjects were highly selected patients in trials with lower AKI risk than is observed in the general population. This important issue was highlighted by the observation of higher rates of hyperkalemia after publication of results of the Randomized Aldactone Evaluation Study (RALES), in which spironolactone was used in addition to ACE inhibitors for heart failure.[210,211] The discontinuation of potassium supplements, avoidance of potassium-sparing diuretics, and dietary advice to avoid high-potassium foods may all help reduce the incidence of hyperkalemia.

STRATEGY FOR MAXIMAL RENOPROTECTION: AIMING FOR REMISSION OF CHRONIC KIDNEY DISEASE

The earlier that interventions to slow CKD progression start, the more kidney function there is to protect and preserve. The best chance of achieving maximal renoprotection is therefore when therapy is established as early as possible, preferably in stage 1 or 2 disease. The concepts of "remission" and "regression" have been applied to renoprotection. *Remission* indicates that therapy has been optimized to the point that there is no evidence of active disease and GFR declines by no more than expected with aging. *Regression* implies that there is recovery of renal function with improving GFR.

The fact that remission of kidney disease can be achieved was demonstrated in one of the first follow-up studies from the Captopril Collaborative Study Group in 1994.[212] Of the 409 patients recruited into that study, 108 had nephrotic-range proteinuria (urine protein levels > 3.5 g/day) at study entry. Remission of nephrotic-range proteinuria occurred in 7 of 42 patients randomly assigned to receive captopril (16.7%) and in 1 of 66 patients randomly assigned to receive placebo (1.5%). Of importance is that over the follow-up period, those achieving remission had the largest fall in mean urine protein levels (from 5.0 g/day to 0.9 g/day, in contrast to 6.2 to 5.1 g/day in subjects who did not reach remission), lower SBP (135 to 119 mm Hg in the patients in remission; 145 to 143 mm Hg in those not in remission), and stable serum creatinine levels (baseline vs. final serum creatinine measurement: 1.5 mg/dL to 1.6 mg/dL for patients in remission; 1.5 to 3.2 mg/dL for those not in remission). Similarly, Hovind and colleagues[213] reported remission in 31% and regression (in this case, defined as GFR decline similar to that in normal aging) in 22% of 301 consecutive patients with type 1 diabetes and nephropathy who were monitored with annual measurements of isotopic GFR for 7 years. Hovind and colleagues also reported increasing prevalence of remission and regression with lower achieved blood pressure (Figure 62.10).

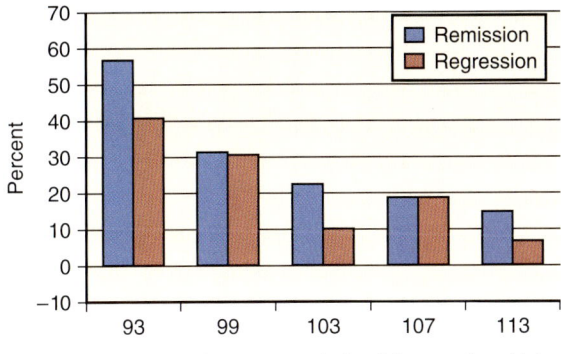

Nevertheless, it is clear that even in the setting of a randomized trial, treatment with the most active agents (RAAS inhibition therapy) is no guarantee that remission will occur; each renoprotective intervention discussed slows the rate of CKD progression by 50% at best. In order to achieve maximal long-term renoprotection, it is therefore necessary to use a comprehensive strategy with multiple interventions directed at different aspects of the pathogenesis of progressive renal injury (see Figure 62.2).[214-216] Moreover, once treatments have been introduced, frequent monitoring of blood pressure, proteinuria, and GFR is essential so that therapy can be escalated until therapeutic goals have been achieved (see Tables 62.1 and 62.4). In this regard, our approach is analogous to that applied in modern oncology chemotherapeutic strategies, in which multiple agents are used and treatment is directed toward correcting all signs of disease activity until the patient is said to be in "remission."

Data from a small number of patients suggest that if remission can be maintained over the long term, some recovery of kidney function or regression of kidney disease may be achieved.[137] Limited data indicate that significant improvements in renoprotection can be achieved with this strategy. Among 160 patients with type 2 diabetes and microalbuminuria, intensive therapy resulted in a marked reduction in the risk of overt nephropathy (OR, 0.27).[216-218] Similarly, 26 of 56 patients with resistant nephrotic-range proteinuria and CKD who were referred to a "remission clinic" achieved reduction of urine protein levels to less than 1 g/day and stabilization of renal function after application of a similar intensive therapy protocol. Furthermore, the rate of GFR decline was significantly slower than that observed in 56 matched historical controls, and only 3.6% reached ESKD, in contrast to 30.4% of the controls.[219] This strategy is based on currently available interventions, and the measurements required for monitoring are already widely used. Thus, a comprehensive approach to renoprotection is an achievable goal for all patients with CKD. Although it has been argued that there is a need for new renoprotective agents, it is also true that these available therapies are not yet applied to all patients with CKD.[220,221] If widely implemented, a comprehensive renoprotective strategy may not only delay the need for dialysis in many patients but may also substantially reduce the number of patients progressing to ESKD.

The different incidence rates of ESKD across the similarly developed nations Norway and the United States,[222] despite similar CKD prevalence rates, suggest that lower rates of progression to ESKD is a realistic goal of CKD treatment. The risk for progression in general was higher for U.S. white patients than for Norwegians. Of a population of 100,000 with stage 3 or 4 CKD, 610 progress to ESKD in the United States and 240 in Norway, a 2.5-fold excess that, after adjustment, was twofold higher among nondiabetic U.S. patients and 2.8-fold higher among diabetic U.S. patients with stages 3 and 4 CKD. In addition, white U.S. patients were referred later to a nephrologist. These results also underscore the need for public health systems to target or screen populations at high risk. In the United Kingdom, a pay-for-performance system for primary care family physicians has had dramatic impacts on the screening and management of

Figure 62.10 Results from a prospective observational cohort study in which 301 consecutive patients with type 1 diabetes and diabetic nephropathy were monitored with isotopic glomerular filtration rate (GFR) measurements annually and who underwent aggressive lowering of blood pressure. Thirty patients (10%) remained normotensive (blood pressure <140/90) during this period and did not receive prolonged antihypertensive agents. Seventeen percent of the patients received monotherapy; 47% received two agents, 30% three agents, and 6% four or more agents. *Remission* was defined in this study as urine albumin levels lower than 200 μg/min sustained for at least 1 year and a decrease of at least 30% from levels before remission (surrogate end point). *Regression* was defined as a rate of decline in GFR equal to that in the natural aging process: less than 1 mL/min/yr during the entire observation period (principal end point). Remission and regression may have occurred in the same patients. (Modified from Hovind P, Rossing P, Tarnow L, et al: Remission and regression in the nephropathy of type 1 diabetes when blood pressure is controlled aggressively. *Kidney Int* 60:277-283, 2001.)

Table 62.4 Comprehensive Strategy and Therapeutic Goals for Achieving Maximal Renoprotection in Patients with Chronic Kidney Disease

Intervention	Goals
ACE inhibitor or ARB treatment	Urine protein level < 0.5 g/day GFR decline < 1 mL/min/yr
Additional antihypertensive therapy	BP < 130/80 if urine albumin excretion > 30 mg/day BP < 140/90 if urine albumin excretion < 30 mg/day
Weight loss if patient is obese	Aim for 5% weight loss
Dietary salt restriction	<5 g/day (equivalent to 90 mEq sodium/day)
Dietary protein restriction	Avoid high protein intake >1.3 g/kg/day In stages 4 and 5 CKD, consider reducing intake to 0.8 g/kg/day
Tight glycemic control	HbA_{1c} < 7.0% unless considered high risk for hypoglycemia
Smoking cessation	Complete cessation
Lipid-lowering therapy	Total cholesterol <200 mg/dL (5.2 mmol/L) LDL cholesterol <100 mg/dL (2.6 mmol/L)

BP, Blood pressure; ACE, angiotensin-converting enzyme; ARB, angiotensin receptor blocker; CKD, chronic kidney disease; GFR, glomerular filtration rate; HbA_{1c}, hemoglobin A_{1c}; LDL, low-density lipoprotein.

diabetes; both levels of care for diabetes and testing rates for nephropathy have increased.[223,224] In addition, pay for performance was associated with improved control of blood pressure in patients with CKD.[225] Patient self-management is a further strategy that should be pursued, as highlighted by an RCT showing improved blood pressure control in participants with hypertension and cardiovascular disease, diabetes, or CKD randomized to self-management versus usual care.[226] Reports of a decline in the incidence of new patients starting dialysis therapy in the United States indicate that strategies to improve renoprotection may be starting to have an effect[227,228] (Table 62.4).

INTERVENTIONS TO REDUCE CARDIOVASCULAR RISK ASSOCIATED WITH CHRONIC KIDNEY DISEASE

ASSOCIATION BETWEEN CHRONIC KIDNEY DISEASE AND CARDIOVASCULAR DISEASE

It has long been recognized that there are excess cardiovascular deaths among patients on maintenance dialysis. In a seminal study in the early 1970s, Lindner and colleagues[229] described accelerated atherosclerosis in patients receiving maintenance hemodialysis, which caused CHD. This observation was prescient, inasmuch as the relationship between kidney disease and excess cardiovascular disease has remained an important focus of research. Increased cardiovascular mortality is expressed early in the course of CKD—for example, in the setting of microalbuminuria in patients with diabetes[230] and when the GFR starts to decline[231] in stage 3 CKD. Furthermore, the rate of mortality associated with CKD is substantial, so that reduced eGFR has gained a reputation of being an effective marker of premature cardiovascular disease, not dissimilar to that associated with a diagnosis of diabetes.

In a longitudinal U.S. study, the outcome of 27,998 patients with eGFR of less than 90 mL/min/1.73 m² was assessed over a 5-year period. RRT was initiated in 1.1%, 1.43%, and 19.9% of subjects with baseline stages 2, 3, and 4 CKD, respectively.[232] In contrast, the mortality rates were 19.5%, 24.3%, and 45.7% for these stages, indicating that for many people with CKD, the risk of premature mortality substantially outweighs the risk of ESKD. In the largest meta-analyses to date, baseline eGFR and albuminuria were related to mortality in 1,128,310 participants with almost 5 million person-years of follow-up.[233] The median age of participants was approximately 61 years. Risk of mortality was lowest among those with an eGFR in the range of 75 to 105 mL/min/1.73 m² and was increased at lower eGFRs. In comparison with a reference eGFR of more than 95 mL/min/1.73 m², the hazard ratios for all-cause mortality were 1.18 for eGFR less than 60 mL/min/1.73 m², 1.57 for eGFR less than 45 mL/min/1.73 m², and 3.14 (2.39 to 4.13) for eGFR less than 15 mL/min/1.73 m².

Similar findings were observed for cardiovascular and noncardiovascular mortality. The risk for all-cause mortality became significant at an eGFR of less than 45 mL/min/1.73 m², and the risk for cardiovascular mortality became significant at an eGFR of less than 60 mL/min/1.73 m² (Figure 62.11). A rapid decline in kidney function may confer an increased risk for CHD that is independent of baseline kidney function and age. According to data from the Atherosclerosis Risk in Communities (ARIC) study, individuals with the greatest decline in eGFR (annual decline > 5.65%) were at greater risk for CHD and all-cause mortality than were those with a more modest decline of 0.33 to 0.47%.[234] Likewise, in an analysis of the Cardiovascular Health Study, a rapid decline in kidney function during the first 7 years of the study was associated with increased risk for heart failure, myocardial infarction, and peripheral arterial disease during a subsequent 8-year follow-up period. Both these studies revealed this effect even after adjustment for baseline kidney function, age, and other traditional cardiovascular risk factors.[235]

These observations suggest that risk factors shared between early kidney disease and cardiovascular disease account for much of the future cardiovascular risk observed in patients with CKD. The classic risk factors for CHD are highly prevalent in patients with CKD. The so-called big three risk factors for CHD in the general population (high total cholesterol, high blood pressure, and cigarette smoking) accounted for at least 80% of major CHD events in middle-aged men when analyses were adjusted for regression dilution bias.[236] Hypertension was the most important risk factor with regard to stroke, contributing 35% of population-attributable risk, and the third most important with regard to acute myocardial infarction (18% population-attributable risk) in the INTERSTROKE[20] and INTERHEART[19] studies, respectively. In addition to a high

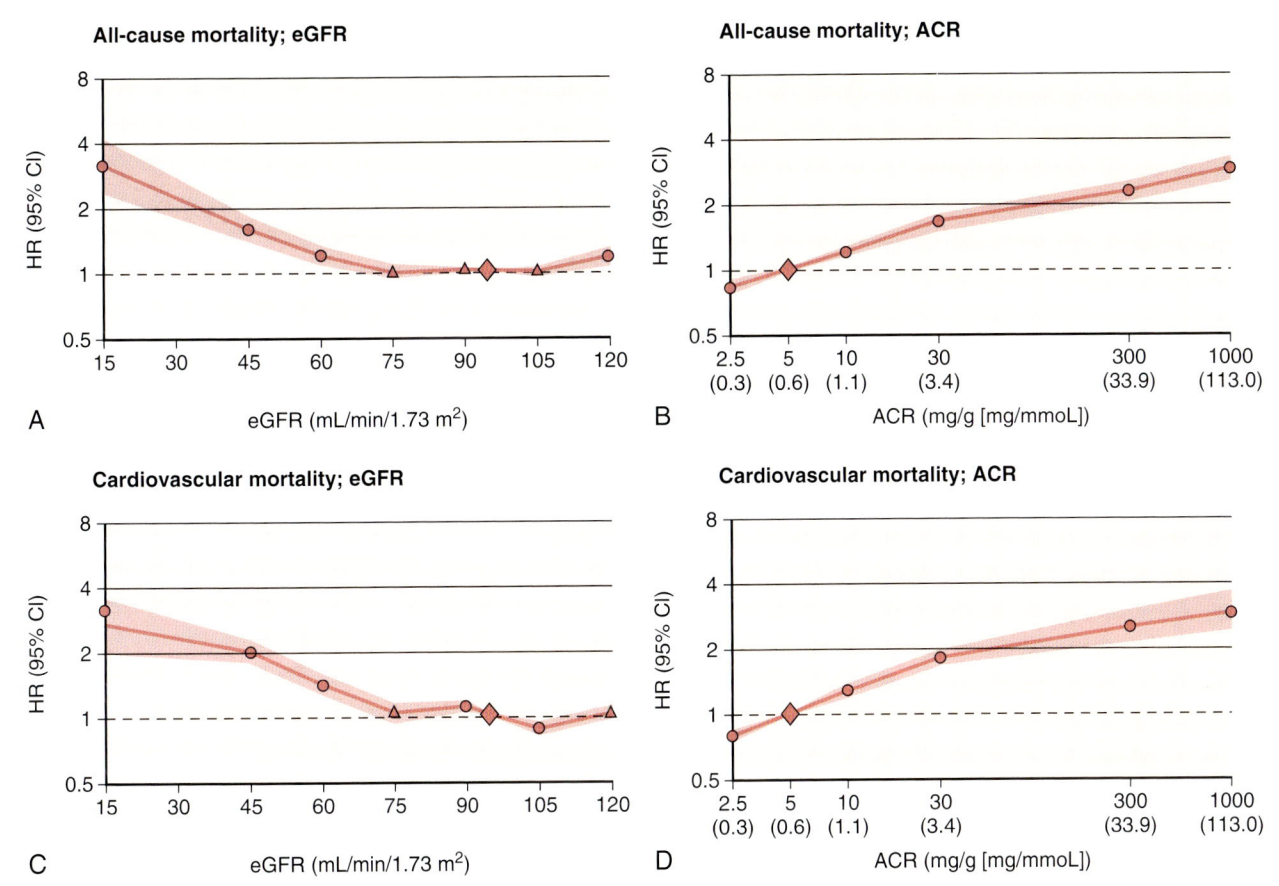

Figure 62.11 All-cause and cardiovascular mortality associated with estimated glomerular filtration rate (eGFR) and albuminuria. Hazard ratios (HRs) and 95% confidence intervals (CIs) for all-cause and cardiovascular mortality according to spline eGFR and urine albumin to creatinine ratio (ACR). Hazard ratios and 95% CIs *(shaded areas)* are shown according to eGFR **(A, C)** and ACR **(B, D)**, adjusted for each other, age, sex, ethnic origin, history of cardiovascular disease, systolic blood pressure, diabetes, smoking, and total cholesterol. The references *(diamond)* were eGFR of 95 mL/min/1.73 m² **(A, C)** and ACR of 5 mg/g (0.6 mg/mmol) **(B, D)**. *Circles* represent statistical significance, and *triangles* represent nonsignificance. ACR plotted in milligrams per gram (to convert to milligrams per millimoles, multiply by 0.113). Approximate conversions to milligrams per millimoles are shown in parentheses. (From Chronic Kidney Disease Prognosis Consortium: Association of estimated glomerular filtration rate and albuminuria with all-cause and cardiovascular mortality in general population cohorts: a collaborative meta-analysis. *Lancet* 375[9731]:2073-2081, 2010.)

prevalence of these traditional risk factors for cardiovascular disease, it is increasingly recognized that CKD is associated with a number of nontraditional risk factors for cardiovascular disease, including arterial stiffness and calcification, elevated levels of asymmetric dimethyl arginine, and accumulation of advanced glycation end products.[237] Whether these risk factors are modifiable and whether their modification is effective in reducing cardiovascular risk must be further investigated with RCTs.[237] Nontraditional risk factors become more important as CKD progresses to more advanced stages, and traditional risk factors remain the most important factors in stages 1 to 3 CKD.

CKD as evidenced by reduced GFR is now considered to be a CHD risk equivalent by both the National Kidney Foundation and the American College of Cardiology/American Heart Association. Proteinuria appears to confer additional risk.[238,239] Not surprisingly, then, several intervention studies with blood pressure–lowering agents that ameliorate CKD progression also show proportional benefit in preventing cardiovascular events. In the RENAAL trial, ARB treatment provided protection against heart failure along with renoprotection, but there was no effect on overall cardiovascular morbidity and mortality rates.[240] In an interesting parallel, the reduction in proteinuria by the intervention was predictive of the cardiovascular benefit as well as the renoprotective effect (Figure 62.12).

ANTIHYPERTENSIVE AGENTS AND CARDIOVASCULAR PROTECTION

Blood pressure targets for reducing cardiovascular risk are generally the same as those for achieving optimal renoprotection (see previous discussion). According to a growing body of evidence, however, the target blood pressure recommended for preventing cardiovascular events and CKD progression may need to be revised for older patients, for whom the evidence base is much less secure. For example, a post hoc analysis of the International Verapamil-Trandolapril Study (INVEST) trial, in which different blood pressure agents were administered to 22,576 patients with known CHD, revealed that in the elderly patients (2180 older than 80 years), there was an increased risk of death in association with lower blood pressures; the SBP associated with the lowest mortality rate was 140 mm Hg (Figure 62.13).[241]

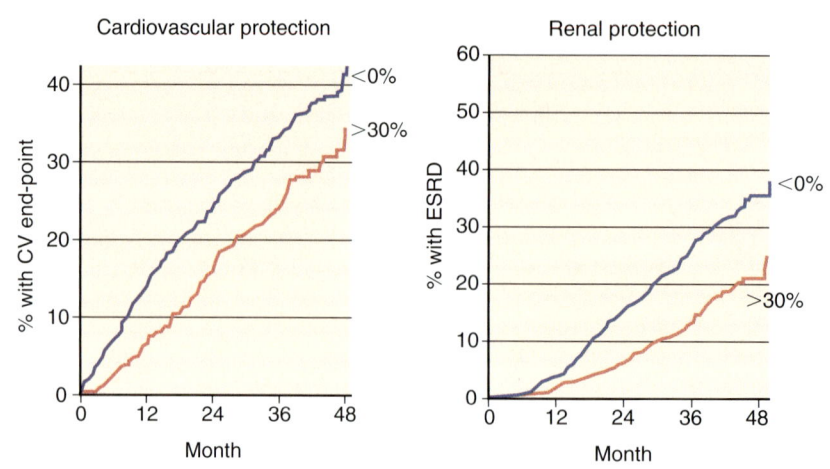

Figure 62.12 Benefits of reduced proteinuria on outcomes. Composite illustration shows the correspondence of cardiovascular (CV) and renal risk reduction in relation to antiproteinuric effect in the Reduction of Endpoints in NIDDM with the Angiotensin II Antagonist Losartan (RENAAL) study. Kaplan-Meier curves of risk for cardiovascular end points **(left)** and end-stage kidney disease (ESKD) **(right),** according to change in urine protein levels at 6 months after baseline measurements. (Adapted with permission from de Zeeuw D, Remuzzi G, Parving HH, et al: Proteinuria, a target for renoprotection in patients with type 2 diabetic nephropathy: lessons from RENAAL. *Kidney Int* 65:2309-2320, 2004.)

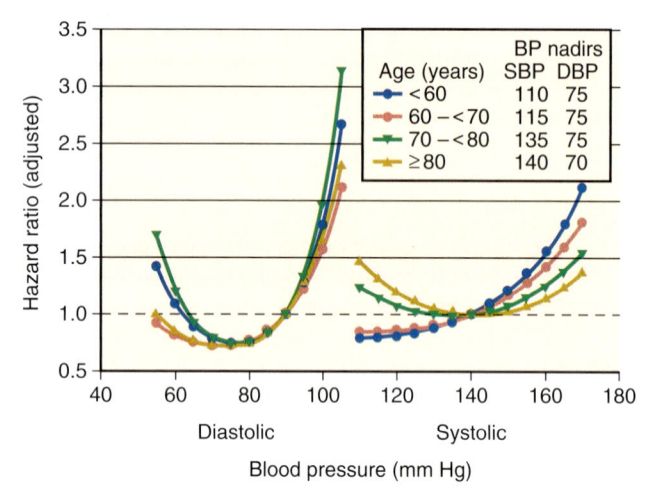

Figure 62.13 Blood pressure and mortality in very old patients with hypertension and coronary artery disease: determination of achieved blood pressures associated with lowest mortality. Adjusted hazard ratio for mortality as a function of age (in 10-year increments), systolic blood pressure (SBP), and diastolic blood pressure (DBP). The reference SBPs and DBPs for hazard ratio are 140 and 90 mm Hg, respectively. Blood pressures (BPs) shown are the on-treatment average of all post-baseline recordings. The quadratic terms for both SBPs and DBPs were statistically significant in all age groups ($P < 0.001$, except for DBP in subjects aged 60 to 70, for whom $P < 0.006$). The adjustment was based on sex, race, history of myocardial infarction, heart failure, peripheral vascular disease, diabetes, stroke/transient ischemic attack, renal insufficiency, and smoking. (From Denardo SJ, Gong Y, Nichols WW, et al: Blood pressure and outcomes in very old hypertensive coronary artery disease patients: an INVEST substudy. *Am J Med* 123:719-726, 2010.)

cardiovascular disease was compared in 147 randomized trials.[242] The five main classes of blood pressure–lowering drugs (thiazides, β-blockers, ACE inhibitors, ARBs, and calcium channel blockers) were similarly effective in preventing CHD events and strokes, except that calcium channel blockers had a greater preventive effect on stroke (RR, 0.92; 95% CI, 0.85 to 0.98). The percentages of reductions in CHD events and stroke were similar in people with and without cardiovascular disease and regardless of blood pressure before treatment (down to 110 mm Hg SBP and 70 mm Hg DBP).[242]

With regard to dose, the same investigators assessed the value of low-dose combination treatment with blood pressure–lowering drugs in an analysis of 354 randomized trials.[243] All five categories mentioned previously produced similar reductions in blood pressure (9.1 mm Hg in SBP and 5.5 mm Hg in DPB) at standard dosage and 20% less reduction at half the standard dosage (7.1 mm Hg in SBP and 4.4 mm Hg in DBP). The drugs reduced blood pressure from all pretreatment levels, more so from higher levels, so that for each initial blood pressure 10 mm Hg higher, the reduction was 1.0 mm Hg (SBP) and 1.1 mm Hg (DBP) greater. The blood pressure–lowering effects of different categories of drugs were additive. In terms of tolerance, symptoms attributable to thiazides, β-blockers, and calcium channel blockers were strongly dose related, whereas symptoms caused by ACE inhibitors (mainly cough) were not dose related. ARBs caused no excess of symptoms.[243]

There are few data regarding the relative efficacy of different combinations of antihypertensive drugs. In the Avoiding Cardiovascular Events through Combination Therapy in Patients Living with Systolic Hypertension (ACCOMPLISH) trial, patients with hypertension and risk factors for cardiovascular disease were randomly assigned to receive combination therapy with an ACE inhibitor and calcium channel blocker. These patients evidenced a significantly lower incidence of major cardiovascular events than did those randomly assigned to receive combination therapy with ACE inhibitor plus thiazide diuretic.[244] Subsequent analysis also

In choosing which antihypertensive agent or agents to use for preventing cardiovascular disease, clinicians should take account of the efficacy, side effects, and convenience of these medications because they usually need to be taken for many years. In one large meta-analysis, the use of different blood pressure–lowering drugs in the prevention of

revealed a lower incidence of serum creatinine doubling or ESKD in the subjects who received ACE inhibitors plus calcium channel blockers.[245] However, commentators have pointed out that this outcome was largely driven by the serum creatinine doubling component of the end point, which in turn was attributable to an initial increase in GFR in the subjects who took ACE inhibitors plus calcium channel blockers, in contrast to an initial decline in GFR in the subjects who took ACE inhibitors plus thiazide. The subsequent rates of decline in GFR were similar between the groups.[246]

These data accord well with observational studies in which the proportion of patients continuing ARB treatment was larger than those taking other agents.[247-250] In these studies, the next highest rate of persistence was observed with ACE inhibitors. In a large U.K.-based study of 109,454 patients, the overall rate of antihypertensive drug discontinuation was 20.3% at 6 months and 28.5% at 1 year. The median time to discontinuation of antihypertensive class was longest for ARBs (2.90 years), followed by ACE inhibitors (2.24 years), calcium channel blockers (1.86 years), β-blockers (1.50 years), thiazides (1.50 years), α-antagonists (1.35 years), potassium-sparing diuretics (0.40 year), and miscellaneous (0.39 year). One-year discontinuation rates ranged from 29.4% (95% CI, 28.0 to 30.7) for ARBs to 64.1% (95% CI, 62.1 to 66.3) for potassium-sparing diuretics.[250] Of importance is that patients with CKD have a significant medication "burden"; most investigators have noted a median of more than three antihypertensive agents. This, coupled with the higher blood pressure that patients with CKD experience, is a major factor contributing to the lack of control of blood pressure that has been documented in population-based studies.[251]

TREATMENT OF DYSLIPIDEMIA

CKD is commonly associated with abnormalities of plasma lipids characterized by elevated levels of the triglyceride-rich low-density lipoprotein (LDL) and very low-density lipoprotein and by reduced levels of high-density lipoprotein.[252] In addition to increasing the risk of cardiovascular disease in patients with CKD, these lipid abnormalities may also accelerate the progression of CKD. In the MDRD study, low serum level of high-density lipoprotein cholesterol was an independent predictor of more rapid decline in GFR[199]; in another study, elevated levels of triglyceride-rich apolipoprotein B were correlated significantly with the rate of deterioration of kidney function.[253] Hypercholesterolemia has been associated with more rapid progression among patients with diabetic CKD[126,254,255] and nondiabetic CKD.[256]

Early clinical intervention studies demonstrated conflicting results regarding whether statin treatment resulted in a reduction in proteinuria.[257,258] According to a meta-analysis of 15 placebo-controlled trials in which the effect of statins on proteinuria were specifically examined, there was an overall beneficial effect among 440 patients with urine albumin levels of 30 mg/day or higher.[259] In relation to placebo, there was a 48% reduction in urine albumin levels with statins, an effect noted with or without concurrent RAAS inhibition. The Prospective Pravastatin Pooling project combined data from three trials in which pravastatin was compared with placebo: Cholesterol and Recurrent Events (CARE), West of Scotland Coronary Prevention Study (WOSCOPS), and Long-Term Intervention with Pravastatin in Ischaemic Disease (LIPID).[260] ACE inhibitor use and blood pressure at baseline and follow-up were similar in the subjects taking pravastatin and those taking placebo. The overall rate of decline of GFR was reduced by 34% (absolute difference of 0.2 mL/min/yr) in the pravastatin recipients. These benefits were most evident in those with lower GFR and more severe proteinuria at baseline.

Strippoli and colleagues[261] performed a meta-analysis and a meta-regression analysis, using data from 50 trials and slightly more than 30,000 patients. Eleven of these trials were performed with patients on dialysis, 26 with patients who had nondialysis-requiring CKD, and 17 on kidney transplant recipients. The reported GFR in the CKD studies were wide ranging, but the majority of patients had eGFRs higher than 60 mL/min/1.73 m². Only one study recruited patients with lower GFRs (mean, <30 mL/min/1.73 m²). In comparison with placebo, statins significantly reduced total cholesterol (weighted mean difference, −42.28 mg/dL [−1.10 mmol/L]) and LDL cholesterol (weighted mean difference, −43.12 mg/dL [−1.12 mmol/L]). Statin treatment was associated with reductions in cardiovascular events, both fatal (RR, 0.81) and nonfatal (RR, 0.78). Meta-regression analysis showed that treatment effects did not vary significantly with stage of CKD. The side effect profile of statins was similar to that of placebo. Most of the available studies were small and of suboptimal quality; mortality data were provided only by a few large trials.

These results suggest that the effects of statins may be specific to patients with less advanced CKD or more severe proteinuria. In support of this is the lack of effect of statin treatment in two randomized trials performed with patients on dialysis. Die Deutsche Diabetes Dialyse Studie (the 4D study), which enrolled only patients with type 2 diabetes, showed no significant reduction in cardiovascular events (RR, 0.92; 95% CI, 0.77 to 1.10).[262] Similarly, the A Study to Evaluate the Use of Rosuvastatin in Subjects on Regular Hemodialysis: An Assessment of Survival and Cardiovascular Events (AURORA) trial demonstrated effective reduction in serum cholesterol (as did the 4D study), but there was no reduction in the composite primary end point of death from cardiovascular causes, nonfatal myocardial infarction, or nonfatal stroke.[263]

The Study of Heart and Renal Protection (SHARP), the largest CKD-specific trial to date, involved 9438 participants aged 40 or older with CKD (3191 of whom were dialysis dependent) recruited from 380 hospitals in 18 countries. Participants were randomly assigned to receive either cholesterol-lowering therapy with ezetimibe, 10 mg daily, and simvastatin, 20 mg daily or placebo, for an average of 5 years. In the treatment group, LDL cholesterol was lowered by a mean of 32% from baseline, and this lowering was associated with a 17% reduction in the relative risk of major atherosclerotic events.[264] Lipid-lowering therapy was not, however, associated with any reduction in the incidence of ESKD.[265] Pending the results of further trials in patients with CKD, these data support a policy of active dietary and drug intervention to correct dyslipidemia in patients with earlier stages of CKD to the levels recommended for other patients at high cardiovascular risk (LDL cholesterol level < 100 mg/dL [<2.6 mmol/L]).

ANTIPLATELET THERAPY

Aspirin used in dosages of 75 to 150 mg/day produces statistically significant and clinically important reductions (22% relative risk reduction) in the risk of subsequent myocardial infarction, stroke, and vascular death in many patients who have survived an occlusive cardiovascular disease event (secondary prevention).[266] Many commentators have correctly asserted that the risk of cardiovascular events in patients with stages 3 to 5 CKD is so high that such patients should be considered to be in the highest risk category (i.e., a CHD equivalent).[267] Nevertheless, because results of studies have cast doubt on the role of aspirin in primary prevention of cardiovascular events in patients with diabetes—in whom the assumption was that the benefits must outweigh risks—it has become important to establish the role of aspirin in primary prevention in patients with CKD.[268] There are, however, only limited data regarding the benefits and risks of aspirin in patients with CKD.

Inconsistent findings have been noted in post hoc analyses and in retrospective studies. In a secondary analysis of the Hypertension Optimal Treatment (HOT) trial, in which patients with diastolic hypertension were randomly assigned to receive aspirin or placebo, the benefit afforded by aspirin was significantly greater for subjects with low eGFR.[269] Risk reductions for major cardiovascular events were 9% (HR, 0.91; 95% CI, 0.76 to 1.09) for patients whose eGFR was higher than 60 mL/min/1.73 m^2; 15% (HR, 0.85; 95% CI, 0.61 to 1.17) for those whose eGFR was 45 to 60 mL/min/1.73 m^2; and 66% (HR, 0.34; 95% CI, 0.17 to 0.67) for those whose eGFR was lower than 45 mL/min/1.73 m^2 (for the interaction, $P = 0.03$). Risk reductions for mortality also increased with decreasing eGFR: 0% (95% CI, −20% to 17%) for patients whose eGFR was higher than 60 mL/min/1.73 m^2; 11% (95% CI, −31% to 40%) for patients whose eGFR was 45 to 60 mL/min/1.73 m^2; and 49% (95% CI, 6% to 73%) for patients whose eGFR was lower than 45 mL/min/1.73 m^2 (for the trend, $P = 0.04$). The incidence of adverse events was also related to GFR and there was a nonsignificant trend toward a greater risk of major bleeding with lower eGFR: HR, 1.52 (95% CI, 1.11 to 2.08) for patients whose eGFR was higher than 60 mL/min/1.73 m^2; HR, 1.70 (95% CI, 0.74 to 3.88) for patients whose eGFR was 45 to 60 mL/min/1.73 m^2; and HR, 2.81 (95% CI, 0.92 to 8.84) for patients whose eGFR was lower than 45 mL/min/1.73 m^2 (for the trend, $P = 0.30$). Among patients whose eGFR was less than 45 mL/min/1.73 m^2, the risks versus benefits were such that for every 1000 people treated for 3.8 years, 76 major cardiovascular events and 54 all-cause deaths would be prevented, but 27 excess major bleeding episodes would occur.

In the first U.K. Heart and Renal Protection (UK-HARP-1) study, patients with CKD were randomly assigned to receive 1 year of treatment with aspirin, 100 mg/day, or placebo, primarily to assess safety. There was no difference in risk of major bleeding between the groups (2% vs. 3%, respectively) but aspirin treatment was associated with a threefold excess of minor bleeding episodes (15% vs. 5%; $P = 0.001$).[270] A retrospective observational analysis from the Dialysis Outcomes and Practice Patterns Study (DOPPS) reported that aspirin treatment was associated with a decreased risk of stroke (RR, 0.82; $P < 0.01$) but increased risks of myocardial infarction (RR, 1.21; $P = 0.01$) and cardiac events (RR, 1.08; $P < 0.01$) in the whole cohort of 28,320 patients on dialysis, as well as in a subgroup with previous coronary artery disease. There was no increase in gastrointestinal bleeding.

Chan and colleagues[271] reviewed the association of mortality with use of warfarin, clopidogrel, or aspirin, or a combination of these, in 41,425 patients with incident disease who were on hemodialysis. All agents were associated with increased mortality rates, but this observation should be interpreted with caution because this study was observational and there was probably substantial confounding by indication for therapy despite various maneuvers to adjust for this.

These studies further reflect the need for randomized trials to determine definitively the risk and benefit of these medications. The uncertainty translates into a wide variation in the use of aspirin in dialysis patients: from 8% of Japanese patients to 41% of Australian/New Zealand patients. Bleeding rates in patients on dialysis are hard to associate with aspirin directly, but in one detailed review of 255 patients on hemodialysis, an overall incidence of major bleeding episodes was reported to be 2.5% per person per year. The incidence was increased among patients administered warfarin (3.1% per person-year), aspirin (4.4%), and the combination of aspirin plus warfarin (6.3%).[272] Further RCTs are needed to assess the safety and efficacy of aspirin treatment in patients with CKD.

Clopidogrel is an alternative treatment with an effect similar to that of aspirin in patients with ischemic cerebrovascular disease. The side effect profile of clopidogrel is more favorable than that of aspirin, with a lower frequency of gastric upset or gastrointestinal bleeding. This makes it a potentially attractive alternative for patients with CKD, who may be regarded as being higher risk for bleeding episodes than is the general population. However, a post hoc analysis of results of the Clopidogrel for the Reduction of Events During Observation (CREDO) trial suggests that this benefit was lost in patients with mild CKD (eGFR = 60 to 89 mL/min) and moderate CKD (eGFR < 60 mL/min) in comparison with those with normal GFR.[273] Bleeding risk was similar across the three groups.

More recently, a post hoc analysis of results of the Clopidogrel for High Atherothrombotic Risk and Ischemic Stabilization, Management, and Avoidance (CHARISMA) trial showed that clopidogrel might actually be more harmful than placebo (increased cardiovascular and overall mortality) in patients with diabetic nephropathy; this finding reinforces the need for additional studies to investigate this possible interaction.[274] Because of the higher rates of mortality in the cross-sectional dialysis study mentioned previously,[271] it is apparent that the use of clopidogrel, like that of aspirin, should be evaluated in RCTs in patients with CKD. Such evaluation may be considered more pressing in view of the results of the Dialysis Access Consortium (DAC) Fistula study,[275] which suggested that clopidogrel might increase the likelihood of short-term patency of arteriovenous fistulas, a high priority for patients and providers.

In summary, there is a shortage of RCTs concerning the efficacy and safety of interventions to reduce risk of cardiovascular disease in patients with CKD. Available evidence supports recommendations that patients with CKD should stop smoking, achieve excellent blood pressure control (but avoid an SBP less than 120 mm Hg), and receive statin therapy for dyslipidemia. The results of the SHARP study suggest that all patients with CKD may benefit from lipid-lowering therapy. Further RCTs are required to determine the relative safety and efficacy of aspirin and other platelet inhibitors.

The benefit of a combined approach to minimizing cardiovascular risk through multiple interventions was also shown in the Steno study, in which patients with type 2 diabetes and microalbuminuria were randomly assigned to receive an intensive program of cardiovascular risk reduction (blood pressure control to <130/80 mm Hg, RAAS inhibitors for all, total cholesterol controlled to <5 mmol/L, aspirin for those with a history of cardiovascular disease, smoking cessation, dietary advice to reduce fat intake, regular exercise, vitamin supplements) or to receive standard therapy. After a mean of almost 8 years' follow-up, patients who received intensive management evidenced a 53% reduction in the incidence of major cardiovascular events (HR, 0.47; 95% CI, 0.24 to 0.73), as well as significant reductions in the incidence of nephropathy (HR, 0.39; 95% CI, 0.17 to 0.87), retinopathy (HR, 0.42; 95% CI, 0.21 to 0.86), and autonomic neuropathy (HR, 0.37; 95% CI, 0.18 to 0.79).[218] This benefit persisted after the trial had been completed, and it translated into a 46% reduction in all-cause mortality (HR, 0.54; 95% CI, 0.32 to 0.89; $P = 0.02$), a 57% reduction in risk of death from cardiovascular causes (HR, 0.43; 95% CI, 0.19 to 0.94; $P = 0.04$), and a 59% reduction in risk of all major cardiovascular events (HR, 0.41; 95% CI, 0.25 to 0.67; $P < 0.001$) in the patients who had originally received intensive intervention more than 13 years later.[216] The mechanisms that contribute to the pathogenesis of cardiovascular disease in patients with CKD as well as management are discussed in greater detail in Chapter 56.

INTERVENTIONS TO MANAGE COMPLICATIONS OF CHRONIC KIDNEY DISEASE

ANEMIA

The anemia of CKD results principally from reduced renal erythropoietin production (a presumed reflection of the reduction in functioning renal mass) and, to a lesser degree, from shortened red blood cell survival and functional iron deficiency. Anemia—defined as a hemoglobin count lower than 13 g/dL in men and lower than 12 g/dL in women[3]—can develop well before the onset of uremic symptoms. Among over 15,000 participants in the Third National Health and Nutrition Examination Survey (NHANES III), the prevalence of anemia increased from 1% at an eGFR of 60 mL/min/1.73 m^2 to 9% at an eGFR of 30 mL/min/1.73 m^2 and to 33% to 67% at an eGFR of 15 mL/min/1.73 m^2.[276]

If left untreated, the anemia of CKD is associated with several adverse effects. These include deterioration in cardiac function, decreased cognition and mental acuity, and fatigue. In cross-sectional studies, associations between anemia and an increased risk of morbidity and mortality, caused principally by cardiac disease and stroke, have been described in patients on dialysis.[277] In addition, anemia may influence the progression of CKD. The effects of anemia on glomerular hemodynamics have been studied in various rat models of CKD.[278] In each of these models, anemia was associated with a reduction in hydraulic pressure in the glomerular capillaries (P_{GC}) and amelioration of glomerulosclerosis. In contrast, prevention of anemia in the remnant kidney model by administration of erythropoietin resulted in increased systemic and glomerular blood pressures and markedly increased glomerulosclerosis (see Chapter 52 for more detailed discussion).

Despite the apparently favorable hemodynamic effects of anemia in experimental models of CKD, some human studies suggest that anemia may in fact accelerate CKD progression. In patients with inherited hemoglobinopathies, chronic anemia is associated with glomerular hyperfiltration that eventuates in proteinuria, hypertension, and ESKD.[279] In several longitudinal studies, lower hemoglobin value was identified as a risk factor for CKD progression[280,281] and ESKD.[282] Whether this reflects more severe occult kidney disease in patients with lower hemoglobin values or more rapid progression secondary to low hemoglobin value and oxygen carriage per se is unclear.

Two small randomized studies revealed renoprotective benefit when anemia was corrected with erythropoietin.[283,284] On the other hand, enthusiasm for the normalization of hemoglobin has been tempered by the results of several large RCTs that revealed no benefit or adverse effects. In two studies in which effect on left ventricular mass was the primary end point, as well as the Trial to Reduce Cardiovascular Events with Aranesp Therapy (TREAT),[285] there was no effect of higher versus lower hemoglobin target on rate of decline in GFR.[286,287] Moreover, in the Cardiovascular Risk Reduction by Early Anemia Treatment with Epoetin Beta (CREATE) study, achievement of a higher hemoglobin target (13 to 15 mg/dL) was associated with a shorter time to initiation of dialysis than was achievement of the lower target (10.5 to 11.5 mg/dL).[288] Further concern was provoked by serious adverse effects associated with higher hemoglobin targets, including increased rate of mortality[289] and increased risk of stroke.[285] Current KDIGO recommendations are therefore to treat symptomatic anemia in CKD with erythropoietin or iron supplementation, or both, to partially correct the hemoglobin and achieve a range of 10 to 11.5 mg/dL.[290] Hemoglobin value should not exceed 13 g/dL.[290] The pathogenesis and treatment of anemia in CKD are discussed further in Chapter 57.

MINERAL AND BONE DISORDER

Numerous cohort studies have shown strong associations between disorders of mineral metabolism and fractures, cardiovascular disease, and mortality (reviewed by the KDIGO CKD-MBD work group[291]) (see also Chapter 55). A number of caveats are relevant here. Most of the studies describing observational data and relationships between individual parameters and clinical outcomes have been performed in dialysis populations. The limited data regarding the prevalence of biochemical and hormonal abnormalities in stages 3 to 5 CKD often do not include analyses by primary disease, which can influence the natural history of mineral and bone disorder. Furthermore, the studies are often based on data from referred populations, which probably differ from data from those not referred yet in terms of age; the major effects are on fracture and cardiovascular risk.

Changes in mineral metabolism and bone structure are detectable much earlier in CKD than had previously been considered. There is a slow decline in levels of 1,25-dihydroxyvitamin D and 25-hydroxyvitamin D, starting once the GFR is in the range of 60 to 70 mL/min. 1,25-Dihydroxyvitamin D values were correlated positively with GFR and negatively with the log of plasma parathyroid hormone and serum phosphorus concentrations. The plasma parathyroid hormone concentration rises later in the progression of CKD but more exponentially when GFR falls below 45 mL/min/1.73 m^2.[292] Calcium and phosphorus values do not generally become abnormal until GFR falls below 40 mL/min/1.73 m^2, and this occurs more commonly below 20 mL/min/1.73 m^2.[293]

In the community-based Kidney Early Evaluation Program (KEEP) and NHANES cohorts, there is evidence that parathyroid hormone levels increased early in patients with stage 3 CKD, typically while calcium and phosphorus levels remained normal.[293,294] These findings highlight the importance of monitoring parathyroid hormone along with calcium and phosphorus in individuals with eGFR less than 60 mL/min/1.73 m^2. Investigators have also described an earlier biomarker of altered mineral and bone disorder in patients with CKD. Fibroblast growth factor 23 (FGF-23) regulates phosphorus metabolism and is associated with mortality in patients on dialysis.[295] High levels of this growth factor, defined as being above 100 reference units (RU)/mL, were more common than secondary hyperparathyroidism and hyperphosphatemia at all levels of eGFR in a cohort of almost 4000 patients with stages 2 to 4 CKD.[296] Further analysis in the same cohort identified elevated FGF-23 levels as an independent risk factor for progression to ESKD and mortality.[297] However, testing for this early marker is not routinely available, and so we recommend monitoring according to the KDIGO guidelines.[298]

Thus, monitoring of serum levels of calcium, phosphorus, and parathyroid hormone and of alkaline phosphatase activity should begin in stage 3 CKD. Few patients with mineral and bone disorder in CKD develop symptomatic disease until they have stage 5 CKD; therefore, the main reason for monitoring is to implement early preventive treatment to suppress secondary hyperparathyroidism. In the majority of patients with CKD who do not require dialysis, treatment of mineral and bone disorder is based initially on dietary phosphate restriction, followed by oral phosphate binders in order to maintain phosphorus in the normal range, although there is no evidence from RCTs that this affects clinical outcomes.

In patients with stages 3 to 5 CKD who are not on dialysis, the optimal level of parathyroid hormone is unknown. However, it is suggested that patients with levels of intact parathyroid hormone above the upper normal limit of the assay be first evaluated for hyperphosphatemia, hypocalcemia, and vitamin D deficiency.[1] If parathyroid hormone level is progressively rising and remains persistently above the upper limit of normal for the assay despite correction of modifiable factors, we suggest treatment with calcitriol or vitamin D analogs (once phosphate is under control). Treatment with the vitamin D analog paricalcitol has been reported to reduce albuminuria in patients with diabetic nephropathy already receiving treatment with an ACE inhibitor or an ARB,[299] but further studies are needed to investigate the renoprotective potential of vitamin D therapies. Detailed discussion of the pathogenesis and treatment of mineral and bone disorder in CKD, which is beyond the scope of this chapter, is presented in Chapters 55 and 63.

A STEPPED CARE APPROACH TO CHRONIC KIDNEY DISEASE

For a summary of the stepped care approach, see Table 62.1.

STAGES 1 AND 2

At these stages of CKD, the diagnosis is based on the presence of albuminuria, hematuria or structural kidney disease, and an eGFR above 60 mL/min/1.73 m^2. Stage 1 disease is defined by a GFR greater than 90 mL/min/1.73 m^2 (5.7% of the total U.S. population) and stage 2 by a GFR between 60 and 89 mL/min/1.73 m^2 (5.4% of the U.S. population).[300] These statistics indicate that CKD of all stages affected an estimated 16.8% of adults aged 20 years during the period 1999 to 2004, an increase from the recalculated NHANES III (1988 to 1994) estimate of 14.5%.[301]

Patients with stages 1 and 2 disease do not have specific symptoms or complications of renal failure such as renal anemia or metabolic renal or bone disease. Patients with symptoms may have a multisystem disease with secondary glomerular or interstitial disease (see Chapters 33 and 36). The majority of patients with stages 1 and 2 CKD are detected by routine or health care insurance–mandated screening and are visiting primary care or other physicians; in many countries only a small proportion are ever evaluated by a nephrologist. With increased access to radiologic imaging, more patients are now identified with structural abnormalities such as polycystic kidney disease or single kidney.

The emphasis at these early stages should be on identification of specific renal diseases when present, appropriate referral to a nephrologist, and reduction of cardiovascular risk. A detailed family history is important because patients with a positive family history need more detailed investigation to allow early detection of inherited renal disease and, in particular, adult polycystic kidney disease. The following initial investigations are appropriate for assisting with risk assessment and for informing decisions about referral to a nephrologist or urologist (see also Chapters 25 and 26):

1. Estimation of urinary albumin or protein excretion is of paramount importance. We recommend a random measurement of ACR or PCR because it is quick to perform and the findings are predictive of outcomes as well as, if not better than, timed collections.[18] Patients with a urine protein measurement equivalent to 0.5 g/day (ACR, 300 mg/g or 30 mg/mmol) should be referred for investigation by a nephrologist.[3]
2. Further urinalysis is needed to detect hematuria. For painless but visible hematuria, serious urologic causes—such as bladder, renal cell, and, less often,

Table 62.5 Recommended Frequency of Monitoring* by Stage of Chronic Kidney Disease

Variable	Stage 1 and 2	Stage 3	Stage 4	Stage 5
GFR and electrolytes	Every 12 months	Every 3-12 months	Every 3-6 months	Every 1-3 months
Proteinuria with ACR or PCR testing	Every 12 months	Every 3-12 months	Every 3-6 months	Every 3-6 months
Blood pressure	Each visit	Each visit	Each visit	Each visit
Calcium and phosphate levels	Every 12 months	Every 12 months	Every 3-6 months	Every 3 months
Parathyroid hormone level	—	Every 12 months	Every 3-6 months	Every 3-6 months[†]
Hemoglobin	Every 12 months	Every 12 months	Every 3-6 months	Every 1-3 months[†]

*Monitoring should be individualized according to previous rate of GFR decline, risk assessment of future GFR decline (particularly high if heavy proteinuria, >1 g/day or equivalent), and current drug therapy.
[†]Monitoring of parathyroid hormone and anemia should depend on the previous results and specific treatment, if any, for these conditions. Stable values with no specific treatment require less monitoring as indicated.
ACR, Albumin to creatinine ratio; GFR, glomerular filtration rate; PCR, protein to creatinine ratio.

prostatic cancers—must be confirmed or ruled out. Patients older than age 50, smokers, and those with a family history of renal tract malignancy need particular attention. They should generally be assessed by a urologist or nephrologist who has experience in screening for these conditions. Painless microscopic hematuria (nonvisible hematuria) is much more likely to be caused by glomerular disease, but referral to a urologist may be necessary to confirm or rule out renal tract malignancy in patients at increased risk.[302] There are several national guidelines for the investigation of hematuria.[302,303] Initial blood tests include measurements of creatinine, eGFR, urea, electrolytes (Na^+, K^+, HCO_3^-, Cl^-), bone and liver profiles, blood glucose, glycosylated hemoglobin, blood cell count, erythrocyte sedimentation rate, and (in men) prostate-specific antigen. Serologic screening for underlying myeloma, antineutrophil cytoplasmic antibody (ANCA)–associated vasculitis, anti–glomerular basement membrane disease, and systemic lupus erythematosus may be indicated, depending on symptoms and the results of other investigations.

3. Abdominal ultrasonography to exclude structural abnormalities and determine the bipolar diameter of the kidneys is indicated if urinalysis results are abnormal, if there is a strong family history of CKD, or if there is significant hypertension. Asymmetry with regard to renal size may be suggestive of atherosclerotic renovascular disease, and angiography (computed tomography or magnetic resonance angiography) may therefore be helpful if this is suspected.

In general, patients with stages 1 and 2 CKD, who do not have a specific renal disease or significant proteinuria, require only annual monitoring of blood pressure, eGFR, and proteinuria. Those who develop an abrupt or sustained decline in GFR should be referred to a nephrologist for further investigation and optimization of therapy.[3]

STAGE 3

In stage 3 CKD, GFR is between 30 and 59 mL/min/1.73 m². This is a significant stage because it represents the majority of patients in whom CKD is identified (stages 1 and 2 often remain undetected until GFR declines) and because many of the complications start to manifest once the GFR drops below 45 mL/min/1.73 m². In addition, the rate of cardiovascular mortality increases substantially among patients with a GFR lower than 45 mL/min/1.73 m².[231,304] Some national guidelines and the KDIGO guidelines have therefore split this stage into two: 3A, defined by reduced GFR of 45 to 59 mL/min/1.73 m², and 3B, defined by reduced GFR of 30 to 44 mL/min/1.73 m².[3,305,306] Stage 3 CKD may be appropriately managed by a collaboration of primary care with a nephrology service. The aims of management at this stage are to identify specific renal disease, correct reversible causes of renal dysfunction, prevent or slow the progression of CKD, reduce cardiovascular risk, and treat the complications of CKD (usually in stage 3B CKD). Referral criteria are the same as for earlier stages of CKD, with the addition of anemia and mineral and bone disorder, which may necessitate specialist treatment. Monitoring of blood pressure, eGFR, and serum biochemistry profile, as well as complete blood cell count and evaluation for proteinuria, should be performed every 3 to 12 months, depending on risk profile and clinical circumstances (Table 62.5).

STAGE 4

Patients with stage 4 CKD have a high cumulative risk of cardiovascular death and progression to ESKD. Almost 66% of such patients experience either a renal or a cardiovascular event over the 5 years after diagnosis. In a population-based study,[232] the proportions of patients who needed RRT over the 5-year observation period were 1.1%, 1.3%, and 19.9%, respectively, for stages 2, 3, and 4, and the respective mortality rates were 19.5%, 24.3%, and 45.7%. Not surprisingly, patients with stage 4 disease often make up a large proportion of those attending outpatient nephrology clinics. Achieving renoprotection remains an important goal to delay the onset of RRT for as long as possible, as does minimizing cardiovascular risk. Blood pressure, eGFR, and serum biochemistry profile, including level of parathyroid hormone as well as complete blood cell count, should be monitored every 3 to 6 months.

As the GFR declines to below 20 mL/min/1.73 m², the focus should change to treating the complications of CKD and planning for RRT.[307] Effective preparation for RRT requires input from multiple staff disciplines (medical, nursing, pharmacy, dietetics, psychology, and social work) and is best delivered in a multidisciplinary clinic. There is emerging evidence that patients prefer this approach to preparation and that such clinics are associated with better outcomes, at least in observational studies.[308,309]

It is clear that late referral (less than 3 months before initiation of dialysis) for dialysis preparation is associated with significantly higher rates of mortality[7] and lower quality of life.[310] Results of a Canadian study also indicated that even when referral was appropriately timed, there was a 53% higher rate of reaching the composite end point of death, need for transfusion, or subsequent hospitalization in those without an optimal start to RRT.[311]

The need for timely preparation for dialysis is clear and is emphasized in the majority of national guidelines. However, not all patients with stage 4 CKD progress to stage 5, and unnecessary preparation may do harm. Patients with stage 4 CKD should therefore undergo a formal assessment of their risk of progression to ESKD (see the "Stratifying Risk in Patients with Chronic Kidney Disease" section under "Kidney Disease: Caveats and Implications for Stepped Care"). Preparation for initiation of dialysis requires multiple interventions to deal with both medical and psychosocial aspects. Patients require adequate counseling to assist them in the choice of dialysis modality and in coping with the psychosocial effects of starting dialysis. Elderly patients are often more accepting of dialysis than are younger patients, who may still be working or have family commitments. One large U.S. study confirmed that social support is important for patients on hemodialysis and peritoneal dialysis in terms of greater satisfaction, higher quality of life, and fewer hospitalizations.[312] Timely formation of vascular access, ideally a forearm arteriovenous fistula, is important to allow adequate maturation, modification if necessary, and repeat surgery in case of primary site failure. Peritoneal catheter insertion requires less maturation time but should be performed early enough to allow time for adequate training for peritoneal dialysis. See Chapters 65, 66, and 70 for further discussion of preparation for dialysis and vascular access.

HEPATITIS B VACCINATION

Patients on hemodialysis have a small but significantly increased risk of exposure to hepatitis B and other blood-borne viruses. Severe outbreaks of hepatitis B in hemodialysis units have resulted in considerable morbidity and even mortality among susceptible patients and staff. Therefore, patients with CKD in whom dialysis is anticipated should be screened for hepatitis B and C, as well as human immunodeficiency virus (HIV) infection. Patients who are seronegative for hepatitis B surface antigen and hepatitis B surface antibody should be immunized and their antibody levels measured after vaccination. Because seroconversion rates decrease with GFR,[313] immunization should ideally occur in stage 3 in patients with a high risk of progression; however, in view of the large number of patients and lack of precision in predicting outcomes, it is usually delayed until stage 4. Seroconversion rates are low once dialysis has commenced, particularly in elderly patients.[314] Results of a meta-analysis of 12 studies indicated that increased seroconversion rates can be achieved by administering multiple doses of vaccine and preferably by the intradermal route.[315] The mechanism is unclear, but this finding is consistent with the observed increased immunogenicity of other vaccinations after intradermal administration in patients with CKD and the rare cases of pure red blood cell aplasia after subcutaneous administration of recombinant erythropoietin.[316,317]

PREEMPTIVE RENAL TRANSPLANTATION

Assessment and preparation for possible renal transplantation should be undertaken before initiation of dialysis. The increase in death rates among waitlisted patients in comparison with transplant recipients is consistent although still debated in view of methodologic issues, such as lead-time bias and unmeasured differences confounding these analyses.[318] There are clear benefits to the recipients beyond the medical gains and significant economic drivers to planning more preemptive transplantation. Many countries and centers now permit donation and surgery when the recipient's GFR is less than 15 to 20 mL/min/1.73 m^2 and if renal function has decreased progressively over the previous 6 to 12 months.[319] The optimal timing of preemptive kidney transplantation remains unclear. Neither higher nor lower pretransplantation GFR appears to be associated with superior allograft survival.[320]

STAGE 5

Once GFR declines to below 15 mL/min/1.73 m^2, priorities include maintaining optimal health and function as well as achieving a planned and uncomplicated initiation of RRT. If patients have been referred in a timely manner, preparation for RRT should already be complete, but ongoing psychosocial support is often necessary as patients come to terms with the imminent need to start therapy. The optimal time to initiate RRT remains a topic of debate.[321] A retrospective analysis of data from 896,546 patients commencing dialysis revealed a higher mortality rate among those commencing dialysis "early" (GFR > 15 mL/min/1.73 m^2) and a lower mortality rate among those commencing "late" (GFR < 5 mL/min/1.73 m^2), although the authors conceded that the results may have been affected by unaccounted confounding and selection, as well as lead-time bias.[322] In a landmark RCT, patients with stage 5 CKD were randomly assigned to "early" (GFR = 10 to 14 mL/min/1.73 m^2) or "late" (GFR = 5 to 7 mL/min/1.73 m^2) initiation of dialysis. After a median of 3.59 years of follow-up, there was no difference in rate of survival or adverse events (cardiovascular events, infections, or complications of dialysis) between the groups.[323]

We therefore recommend that the initiation of RRT should be individualized but in general should occur when the GFR falls below 10 mL/min/1.73 m^2 but before significant uremic symptoms or malnutrition occurs. In order to facilitate this timing, the frequency of monitoring of GFR, serum biochemistry, and hemoglobin, together with clinical assessment, should increase to every 1 to 3 months. Patients who decline RRT should continue to be treated for complications of CKD to optimize their quality of life and, if necessary, be referred to a palliative care service to allow adequate planning of their care once they develop symptomatic uremia.

Complete reference list available at ExpertConsult.com.

KEY REFERENCES

3. Kidney Disease: Improving Global Outcomes CKD Working Group: KDIGO 2012 clinical practice guideline for the evaluation and management of chronic kidney disease. *Kidney Int* (Suppl 3):1–150, 2013.
4. Stevens PE, Levin A: Evaluation and management of chronic kidney disease: synopsis of the Kidney Disease: Improving Global Outcomes 2012 clinical practice guideline. *Ann Intern Med* 158(11):825–830, 2013.
14. Gansevoort RT, Matsushita K, van der Velde M, et al: Lower estimated GFR and higher albuminuria are associated with adverse kidney outcomes in both general and high-risk populations. A collaborative meta-analysis of general and high-risk population cohorts. *Kidney Int* 80:93–104, 2011.
16. Tangri N, Stevens LA, Griffith J, et al: A predictive model for progression of chronic kidney disease to kidney failure. *JAMA* 305(15):1553–1559, 2011.
17. Peeters MJ, van Zuilen AD, van den Brand JA, et al: Validation of the kidney failure risk equation in European CKD patients. *Nephrol Dial Transplant* 28(7):1773–1779, 2013.
18. Ricardo AC, Anderson CA, Yang W, et al: Healthy lifestyle and risk of kidney disease progression, atherosclerotic events, and death in CKD: findings from the Chronic Renal Insufficiency Cohort (CRIC) Study. *Am J Kidney Dis* 65(3):412–424, 2015.
20. O'Donnell MJ, Xavier D, Liu L, et al: Risk factors for ischaemic and intracerebral haemorrhagic stroke in 22 countries (the INTERSTROKE study): a case-control study. *Lancet* 376(9735):112–123, 2010.
25. Jain G, Jaimes EA: Nicotine signaling and progression of chronic kidney disease in smokers. *Biochem Pharmacol* 86(8):1215–1223, 2013.
34. Koegelenberg CF, Noor F, Bateman ED, et al: Efficacy of varenicline combined with nicotine replacement therapy vs varenicline alone for smoking cessation: a randomized clinical trial. *JAMA* 312(2):155–161, 2014.
41. Hsu C, McCulloch CE, Iribarren C, et al: Body mass index and risk for end-stage renal disease. *Ann Intern Med* 144(1):21–28, 2006.
52. Bolignano D, Zoccali C: Effects of weight loss on renal function in obese CKD patients: a systematic review. *Nephrol Dial Transplant* 28(Suppl 4):iv82–iv98, 2013.
57. Sacks FM, Svetkey LP, Vollmer WM, et al: Effects on blood pressure of reduced dietary sodium and the Dietary Approaches to Stop Hypertension (DASH) diet. DASH-Sodium Collaborative Research Group. *N Engl J Med* 344(1):3–10, 2001.
63. Vegter S, Perna A, Postma MJ, et al: Sodium intake, ACE inhibition, and progression to ESRD. *J Am Soc Nephrol* 23(1):165–173, 2012.
64. McMahon EJ, Bauer JD, Hawley CM, et al: A randomized trial of dietary sodium restriction in CKD. *J Am Soc Nephrol* 24(12):2096–2103, 2013.
90. Agarwal R, Sinha AD: Thiazide diuretics in advanced chronic kidney disease. *J Am Soc Hypertens* 6(5):299–308, 2012.
108. James PA, Oparil S, Carter BL, et al: 2014 evidence-based guideline for the management of high blood pressure in adults: report from the panel members appointed to the Eighth Joint National Committee (JNC 8). *JAMA* 311(5):507–520, 2014.
110. Beckett NS, Peters R, Fletcher AE, et al: Treatment of hypertension in patients 80 years of age or older. *N Engl J Med* 358(18):1887–1898, 2008.
112. Ambrosius WT, Sink KM, Foy CG, et al: The design and rationale of a multicenter clinical trial comparing two strategies for control of systolic blood pressure: the Systolic Blood Pressure Intervention Trial (SPRINT). *Clin Trials* 11(5):532–546, 2014.
131. Strippoli GF, Craig M, Deeks JJ, et al: Effects of angiotensin converting enzyme inhibitors and angiotensin II receptor antagonists on mortality and renal outcomes in diabetic nephropathy: systematic review. *BMJ* 329(7470):828, 2004.
150. Mann JF, Schmieder RE, McQueen M, et al: Renal outcomes with telmisartan, ramipril, or both, in people at high vascular risk (the ONTARGET study): a multicentre, randomised, double-blind, controlled trial. *Lancet* 372(9638):547–553, 2008.
170. Fried LF, Emanuele N, Zhang JH, et al: Combined angiotensin inhibition for the treatment of diabetic nephropathy. *N Engl J Med* 369(20):1892–1903, 2013.
171. Susantitaphong P, Sewaralthahab K, Balk EM, et al: Efficacy and safety of combined vs. single renin-angiotensin-aldosterone system blockade in chronic kidney disease: a meta-analysis. *Am J Hypertens* 26(3):424–441, 2013.
174. Bolignano D, Palmer SC, Navaneethan SD, et al: Aldosterone antagonists for preventing the progression of chronic kidney disease. *Cochrane Database Syst Rev* (4):CD007004, 2014.
177. Parving HH, Persson F, Lewis JB, et al: Aliskiren combined with losartan in type 2 diabetes and nephropathy. *N Engl J Med* 358(23):2433–2446, 2008.
179. Parving HH, Brenner BM, McMurray JJ, et al: Cardiorenal end points in a trial of aliskiren for type 2 diabetes. *N Engl J Med* 367(23):2204–2213, 2012.
184. Jalal DI, Chonchol M, Chen W, et al: Uric acid as a target of therapy in CKD. *Am J Kidney Dis* 61(1):134–146, 2013.
185. Bose B, Badve SV, Hiremath SS, et al: Effects of uric acid-lowering therapy on renal outcomes: a systematic review and meta-analysis. *Nephrol Dial Transplant* 29(2):406–413, 2014.
187. Goicoechea M, Garcia de Vinuesa S, Verdalles U, et al: Allopurinol and progression of CKD and cardiovascular events: long-term follow-up of a randomized clinical trial. *Am J Kidney Dis* 65(4):543–549, 2015.
190. Dobre M, Rahman M, Hostetter TH: Current status of bicarbonate in CKD. *J Am Soc Nephrol* 26(3):515–523, 2015.
191. de Brito-Ashurst I, Varagunam M, Raftery MJ, et al: Bicarbonate supplementation slows progression of CKD and improves nutritional status. *J Am Soc Nephrol* 20(9):2075–2084, 2009.
192. Mahajan A, Simoni J, Sheather SJ, et al: Daily oral sodium bicarbonate preserves glomerular filtration rate by slowing its decline in early hypertensive nephropathy. *Kidney Int* 78(3):303–309, 2010.
193. Goraya N, Simoni J, Jo C, et al: Dietary acid reduction with fruits and vegetables or bicarbonate attenuates kidney injury in patients with a moderately reduced glomerular filtration rate due to hypertensive nephropathy. *Kidney Int* 81(1):86–93, 2012.
194. Goraya N, Simoni J, Jo CH, et al: A comparison of treating metabolic acidosis in CKD stage 4 hypertensive kidney disease with fruits and vegetables or sodium bicarbonate. *Clin J Am Soc Nephrol* 8(3):371–381, 2013.
195. Goraya N, Simoni J, Jo CH, et al: Treatment of metabolic acidosis in patients with stage 3 chronic kidney disease with fruits and vegetables or oral bicarbonate reduces urine angiotensinogen and preserves glomerular filtration rate. *Kidney Int* 86(5):1031–1038, 2014.
201. Lambers Heerspink HJ, Kropelin TF, Hoekman J, et al: Drug-induced reduction in albuminuria is associated with subsequent renoprotection: a meta-analysis. *J Am Soc Nephrol* 26:2055–2064, 2015.
202. Hou FF, Xie D, Zhang X, et al: Renoprotection of Optimal Antiproteinuric Doses (ROAD) study: a randomized controlled study of benazepril and losartan in chronic renal insufficiency. *J Am Soc Nephrol* 18(6):1889–1898, 2007.
216. Gaede P, Lund-Andersen H, Parving HH, et al: Effect of a multifactorial intervention on mortality in type 2 diabetes. *N Engl J Med* 358(6):580–591, 2008.
219. Ruggenenti P, Perticucci E, Cravedi P, et al: Role of remission clinics in the longitudinal treatment of CKD. *J Am Soc Nephrol* 19(6):1213–1224, 2008.
225. Karunaratne K, Stevens P, Irving J, et al: The impact of pay for performance on the control of blood pressure in people with chronic kidney disease stage 3-5. *Nephrol Dial Transplant* 28(8):2107–2116, 2013.
226. McManus RJ, Mant J, Haque MS, et al: Effect of self-monitoring and medication self-titration on systolic blood pressure in hypertensive patients at high risk of cardiovascular disease: the TASMIN-SR randomized clinical trial. *JAMA* 312(8):799–808, 2014.
233. Chronic Kidney Disease Prognosis Consortium: Association of estimated glomerular filtration rate and albuminuria with all-cause and cardiovascular mortality in general population cohorts: a collaborative meta-analysis. *Lancet* 375(9731):2073–2081, 2010.
244. Jamerson K, Weber MA, Bakris GL, et al: Benazepril plus amlodipine or hydrochlorothiazide for hypertension in high-risk patients. *N Engl J Med* 359(23):2417–2428, 2008.
264. Baigent C, Landray MJ, Reith C, et al: The effects of lowering LDL cholesterol with simvastatin plus ezetimibe in patients with

chronic kidney disease (Study of Heart and Renal Protection): a randomised placebo-controlled trial. *Lancet* 377(9784):2181–2192, 2011.
265. Haynes R, Lewis D, Emberson J, et al: Effects of lowering LDL cholesterol on progression of kidney disease. *J Am Soc Nephrol* 25(8):1825–1833, 2014.
285. Pfeffer MA, Burdmann EA, Chen C, et al: A trial of darbepoetin alfa in type 2 diabetes and chronic kidney disease. *N Engl J Med* 361(21):2019–2032, 2009.
290. Kidney Disease: Improving Global Outcomes Anemia Working Group: KDIGO clinical practice guideline for anemia in chronic kidney disease. *Kidney Int* (Suppl 2):279–335, 2012.
295. Gutierrez OM, Mannstadt M, Isakova T, et al: Fibroblast growth factor 23 and mortality among patients undergoing hemodialysis. *N Engl J Med* 359(6):584–592, 2008.
296. Isakova T, Wahl P, Vargas GS, et al: Fibroblast growth factor 23 is elevated before parathyroid hormone and phosphate in chronic kidney disease. *Kidney Int* 79(12):1370–1378, 2011.
297. Isakova T, Xie H, Yang W, et al: Fibroblast growth factor 23 and risks of mortality and end-stage renal disease in patients with chronic kidney disease. *JAMA* 305(23):2432–2439, 2011.
323. Cooper BA, Branley P, Bulfone L, et al: A randomized, controlled trial of early versus late initiation of dialysis. *N Engl J Med* 363(7):609–619, 2010.

63

Therapeutic Approach to Chronic Kidney Disease–Mineral Bone Disorder

L. Darryl Quarles

CHAPTER OUTLINE

MULTISYSTEM ABNORMALITIES UNDERLYING THE PATHOGENESIS OF DISORDERED MINERAL METABOLISM, 2019
Guiding Therapeutic Principles, 2020
Gastrointestinal Phosphate-Binding Agents, 2021
CALCIUM, VITAMIN D RECEPTOR AGONISTS, AND CALCIUM-SENSING RECEPTOR ALLOSTERIC MODULATORS (CALCIMIMETIC AGENTS), 2023
Calcium Supplements, 2023
Treatment with Vitamin D Analogs, 2023
Calcium-Sensing Receptor Allosteric Modulators (Calcimimetic Agents), 2026

OVERVIEW OF CLINICAL MANAGEMENT OF CHRONIC KIDNEY DISEASE–MINERAL BONE DISORDER, 2028
Therapeutic Goals, 2028
TREATMENT OF CHRONIC KIDNEY DISEASE–MINERAL BONE DISORDER IN END-STAGE KIDNEY DISEASE, 2029
TREATMENT OF PATIENTS WITH STAGES 2, 3, AND 4 CHRONIC KIDNEY DISEASE, 2029
General Considerations, 2029
Phosphate-Binding Agents, 2031
Vitamin D Sterols, 2031
Calcimimetic Agents, 2032

MULTISYSTEM ABNORMALITIES UNDERLYING THE PATHOGENESIS OF DISORDERED MINERAL METABOLISM

Overviews of the physiology and pathophysiology of disordered mineral metabolism in chronic kidney disease (CKD) have been presented elsewhere (see Chapters 19 and 55). Abnormalities in mineral homeostasis occur early in CKD (Figure 63.1). CKD results in reduced clearance of phosphate and abnormalities in hormonal and cytokine pathways that lead to disturbances in mineral metabolism, including hypocalcemia, hyperphosphatemia, hyperparathyroidism, elevated circulating fibroblast growth factor 23 (FGF-23) concentrations, and reductions in 25-hydroxyvitamin D (25[OH]D) and 1,25 dihydroxyvitamin D (1,25[OH]$_2$D$_3$) concentrations. Increases in circulating levels of parathyroid hormone (PTH), a key calcemic and phosphaturic hormone, and FGF-23, another phosphaturic hormone that suppresses 1,25(OH)$_2$D production, are early adaptive responses in the course of CKD. Simplistically, loss of kidney function results in a positive phosphate balance and adaptive increments in FGF-23, leading to enhanced renal phosphate excretion and suppression of 1,25(OH)$_2$D$_3$, which limits gastrointestinal calcium and phosphate absorption.[1] The negative calcium balance in turn leads to secondary increments in PTH, which attempts to increase serum calcium level and further enhance phosphate excretion[2] (see Figure 63.1). Thus both PTH and FGF-23 have phosphaturic actions. PTH and FGF-23 have opposite effects on the activity of cytochrome P450 enzymes 27B1 and 24A1 (CYP27B1 and CYP24A1). Parathyroid hormone stimulates the production of 1,25(OH)$_2$D$_3$ and inhibits its degradation, whereas FGF-23 inhibits 1,25(OH)$_2$D$_3$ production[3-5] and increases its degradation.[4]

Both FGF-23 and PTH increase progressively in an effort to maintain normal calcium and phosphorus levels and balance, unless treatment is initiated, and contribute to the abnormalities in bone and vitamin D metabolism observed in CKD.[1,6,7] The clinical hallmarks of disordered mineral metabolism in CKD are the following: (1) parathyroid gland disease, which manifests initially by increased secretion of PTH (i.e., secondary hyperparathyroidism), but chronically by the insidious hyperplasia that can lead to autonomous gland function and tertiary hyperparathyroidism; (2) metabolic bone disease, ranging from high- to low-turnover states and impaired mineralization; (3) additional hormonal abnormalities, including elevated FGF-23 and decreased 25(OH)D and 1,25(OH)$_2$D$_3$ concentrations; (4) extraskeletal calcification; (5) derangements of immune and cardiovascular functions; and (6) activation of the oxidative stress response pathways that are associated with these myriad

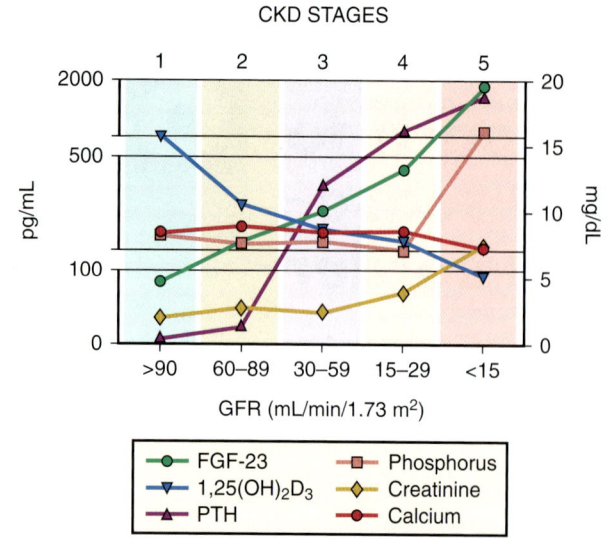

Figure 63.1 Alterations in serum fibroblast growth factor 23 (FGF-23), parathyroid hormone (PTH), 1,25-dihydroxyvitamin D (1,25[OH]$_2$D$_3$), calcium, and phosphorus as a function of chronic kidney disease (CKD) stage. Results represent a theoretical time course derived from cross-sectional studies in humans and serial analysis in animal models of CKD. (Adapted from Martinez I, Saracho R, Montenegro J, et al: The importance of dietary calcium and phosphorus in the secondary hyperparathyroidism of patients with early renal failure. *Am J Kidney Dis* 29:496-502, 1997.)

metabolic, inflammatory, and mineral homeostatic disorders.[8,9] *CKD-mineral bone disorder* (CKD-MBD) has been proposed as a term to describe this complex pathologic spectrum.[10]

The initial adaptive increments in FGF-23 and PTH levels become maladaptive as the CKD progresses. Increments in FGF-23 level are associated with greater severity of hyperparathyroidism,[11] progression of CKD,[12] and increased mortality in end-stage kidney disease (ESKD).[13] Increments in PTH are also associated with increased mortality (levels > 600 pg/mL), metabolic bone disease (high-turnover renal osteodystrophy), and fractures and reflect progressive disease of the parathyroid glands because of hypertrophy and hyperplasia, ultimately leading to adenomatous transformation and in some individuals, so-called tertiary hyperparathyroidism requiring parathyroidectomy. Hyperphosphatemia and hypocalcemia develop late in stage 5 CKD (see Figure 63.1), when these adaptive mechanisms are inadequate to compensate for the loss of kidney function, with ensuing positive phosphate balance and extraskeletal calcifications. Several reports have linked disturbances in phosphorus metabolism to adverse clinical outcomes, including cardiovascular disease and death among patients undergoing maintenance dialysis.[14,15]

Complex and poorly understood pathogenic pathways link disordered vitamin D and mineral metabolism, cardiovascular disease, inflammation, and oxidative stress in CKD. The primary focus of this chapter is to review the therapeutic options for managing these disorders among patients with CKD, which currently focus predominantly on correcting the abnormal phosphate and vitamin D homeostasis, and to discuss the specific objectives of treatment, including their benefits and risks.

GUIDING THERAPEUTIC PRINCIPLES

When viewed from the physiologic perspective of restoring phosphate, calcium, and vitamin D homeostasis in CKD, there are three major classes of drugs used to manage CKD-MBD. These include phosphate-binding agents, vitamin D analogs, and calcimimetic agents. Treatments are directed toward specific molecular targets (Table 63.1).[16,17] Vitamin D sterols and calcimimetic agents thus interact with the vitamin D receptor (VDR) and the calcium-sensing receptor (CaSR), respectively, to elicit predictable biologic responses.[16,17] Other therapeutic measures, such as phosphate-binding agents and oral calcium supplements, are less specific, and they affect mineral metabolism more broadly with divergent biologic effects, some of which are adverse (see Table 63.1). To a considerable extent, the safety and efficacy of strategies to manage bone disease and mineral metabolism among patients with CKD are determined not only by their therapeutic specificity but also by the frequency and severity of untoward side effects. Table 63.1 summarizes the differences among the various therapeutic agents. Disordered mineral metabolism in CKD cannot be cured, short of successful kidney transplantation, but it can be managed, through successful pharmacologic treatments that target multiple components of the disorder pathways. Drug combinations are typically needed to manage the multiple abnormalities of CKD-MBD, including concomitant administration of phosphate binders, vitamin D analogs, calcium, and calcimimetics.

Ideally, therapeutic decisions should be based on evidence derived from prospective, randomized controlled trials. At present, critical trials comparing the different treatment paradigms involving various combinations of phosphate binders, vitamin D analogs, calcimimetic agents, and frequency and duration of dialysis are limited. There are prospective trials comparing different phosphate binders and other randomized studies comparing use of high-dose vitamin D analogs to regimens using cinacalcet and low-dose vitamin D analogs. These studies are insufficient to reach a consensus on the optimal treatment strategies. Several clinical observations, however, have established important guiding concepts that can be used to make predictions about therapy with vitamin D analogs, phosphate binders, and calcimimetics.

There is also a general agreement that bone disease, vascular calcifications, and mortality are interconnected. There is a U-shaped relationship between bone remodeling and serum calcium and phosphate levels related to the ability of remodeling bone to buffer calcium and phosphate loads, on the one hand, and release calcium and phosphate, on the other. Consequently, low bone remodeling states that occur in adynamic bone disease result in the inability to tolerate calcium loads. In this regard, patients with adynamic bone disease have a higher prevalence of vascular calcifications. Conversely, high bone remodeling states, as occur in osteitis fibrosa cystica caused by high PTH levels, can lead to a bone-mediated increase in serum calcium and phosphate levels. In this setting, parathyroidectomy or use of calcimimetic agents can lower the serum calcium and phosphate concentrations. Although the ability to accurately diagnose adynamic bone disease is lacking, patients with low bone mineral density, evidence of vascular

Table 63.1 Therapeutic Interventions for Treating Chronic Kidney Disease–Mineral Bone Disorder

Agent	Target	Effects on Serum Biochemistries				Cost	Risk
		PTH	FGF-23	Calcium	Phosphorus		
Calcium-based binders							
Calcium carbonate						Lowest	Hypercalcemia
Calcium acetate						Low	Vascular calcifications
Calcium-free binders							
Sevelamer HCl	Intestinal Phosphate Absorption					High	Acidosis
							GI intolerance
Sevelamer carbonate						High	GI intolerance
Lanthanum carbonate						High	Lanthanum retention*
Aluminum hydroxide						Low	Aluminum retention
Aluminum carbonate							
Vitamin D sterols†	VDR					High	Hypercalcemia
Cinacalcet HCl	CaSR					Highest	Hypocalcemia
							Nausea/vomiting

*No toxicities have been demonstrated.
†Vitamin D sterols, calcitriol, paricalcitol, and so on.
CaSR, Calcium-sensing receptor; FGF-23, fibroblastic growth factor 23; GI, gastrointestinal; PTH, parathyroid hormone; VDR, vitamin D receptor.

calcifications, underlying diabetes mellitus, or serum calcium concentrations that are increased without treatment, and low PTH concentrations may be at risk from calcium-based binders.

There is a general consensus that hyperphosphatemia must be treated because elevations of serum phosphorus level are associated with decreased survival.[18,19] The mechanisms responsible for the excess in cardiovascular disease associated with hyperphosphatemia are not understood fully, but they may involve the process of vascular calcification, which is quite common among patients with CKD, and/or linkage between elevated phosphate levels and FGF-23 and inflammation.[9,20] The concept that high dietary phosphorus intake and hyperphosphatemia in CKD increases mortality has been further validated and extended to persons without CKD, where phosphate intake exceeding 1400 mg/day is associated with increased mortality.[21] New ideas supporting a role of calciproteins, consisting of calcium-phosphate crystals bound to fetuin A,[22] and the propensity of serum to promote formation of calciproteins provide new mechanisms whereby hyperphosphatemia stimulates vascular calcifications and inflammatory responses in CKD.[23]

GASTROINTESTINAL PHOSPHATE-BINDING AGENTS

Phosphate is absorbed in the small intestines by passive diffusion and by active transport mediated by the sodium-dependent phosphate transporter NaPi-IIb. Intestinal phosphate absorption is potently stimulated by $1,25(OH)_2D_3$,[24] and concurrent treatment with vitamin D analogs confounds the management of hyperphosphatemia in ESKD.[25] The ability to restrict dietary phosphate is limited to approximately 900 mg/day to provide adequate protein and nutrition; such restriction is difficult to achieve because of low adherence. Presently there are no approved agents to inhibit either the passive or active transepithelial phosphate transport in the intestine, although antibodies and drugs to block the intestinal phosphate transporter are being explored. Niacin (nicotinic acid) and its metabolite nicotinamide, which have been shown to inhibit intestinal phosphate transport via inhibition of the NaPi-IIb transporter in animal models, have been shown to reduce serum phosphate levels, increase high-density lipoprotein levels, and induce thrombocytopenia in patients undergoing hemodialysis.[26] The magnitude of the effect of niacin or nicotinamide on serum phosphate concentrations is small. In addition, tenapanor, which inhibits intestinal Na^+-H^+-exchanger isoform 3 (NHE3), reduces serum phosphate concentrations through mechanisms that remain to be established.[27] Therefore phosphate-binding agents, which diminish intestinal phosphate absorption by forming poorly soluble complexes with phosphorus in the intestinal lumen, are the mainstay of therapy.

Prevention of a positive phosphate balance by the use of drugs that bind to and prevent the absorption of dietary phosphorus remains a major goal of therapy in CKD, although the optimal type of phosphate binder remains controversial. Phosphate binders are most effective when ingested with meals to permit admixture with foods and to optimize phosphorus binding. Phosphate binders are used in combination with dietary phosphate restriction, the latter of which is difficult, given the variable bioavailability of phosphate in foods.[28] Studies have confirmed the efficacy of phosphate binders to reduce serum phosphorus concentrations in CKD, but when data from multiple phosphate binders were pooled in one pilot trial, active therapy with phosphate binders (compared to placebo) increased vascular calcification and did not decrease serum FGF-23 level.[29] All phosphate binders may have the capacity to increase calcium absorption by increasing the bioavailability of diffusible calcium in the gastrointestinal tract, which is greater with the use of calcium-containing binders and concomitant treatment with active vitamin D analogs. Meta-analyses also found no difference in coronary artery calcium progression[30] or a significant decrease in all-cause mortality, hospitalizations, or end-of-treatment serum calcium-phosphate product levels with sevelamer compared to calcium binders.[31] The risk for hypercalcemia was reduced with sevelamer and increased with calcium-binder treatment, but calcium binders were more effective than sevelamer in suppressing serum PTH. There were more pronounced gastrointestinal side effects associated with sevelamer use compared to calcium binders. Lanthanum carbonate resulted in similar end-of-treatment phosphorus levels compared to other binders but is reported to require a lower pill burden compared to sevelamer.[32] Several trials deserve special mention. Dialysis Clinical Outcomes Revisited (DCOR), which was a multicenter, randomized, open-label, parallel design trial in 2103 patients receiving hemodialysis that compared the effects of sevelamer and calcium-based binders, found no significant difference in all-cause and cause-specific mortality (cardiovascular, infection, and other) between the sevelamer and calcium-binder groups.[33] The Calcium Acetate Renagel Evaluation-2 (CARE-2) study randomized 203 prevalent patients on hemodialysis with hyperphosphatemia to receive calcium acetate plus atorvastatin or sevelamer without atorvastatin for 12 months. This study found no difference in the progression of calcification between the calcium binder and sevelamer groups provided that serum lipid levels were kept within the same range.[34]

There are three major classes of phosphate binders currently in use, including calcium-containing binders, resin binders, and noncalcium-nonresin binders, such as lanthanum carbonate, aluminum-containing binders, magnesium salts, and iron compounds. Currently available oral phosphate binders vary in cost, phosphate-binding efficacy, and side effect profiles, but available data from limited randomized controlled trials do not show the superiority of any one binder over the other with regard to control of serum phosphate level or effects on mortality or other outcomes.[32]

CALCIUM-CONTAINING BINDERS

Calcium-containing salts are effective in lowering serum phosphorus concentrations among patients with advanced CKD, but large, potentially unsafe, doses are typically required.[17] Calcium-based binders (acetate and carbonate) are effective (in terms of lowering serum phosphate concentration) and relatively inexpensive, but their administration results in positive calcium balance and hypercalcemia, especially when coadministered with vitamin D analogs, and exacerbates the progression of vascular calcification.[35] Calcium acetate is more effective in binding intestinal phosphate, per millimole of administered elemental calcium, than calcium carbonate, but the clinical significance of this difference is not certain. Calcium carbonate costs considerably less than calcium acetate, and no study has demonstrated a clinical advantage of one over the other. Calcium citrate has also been used as a phosphate-binding agent, but citrate can enhance intestinal calcium, as well as aluminum absorption,[36,37] and therefore is used infrequently as a phosphate binder (and more often as a calcium supplement in patients without CKD).

A major concern regarding use of calcium binders is the potential for cumulative positive calcium balance and soft tissue calcifications. The use of very large oral doses of calcium as a phosphate-binding agent has been associated with evidence of soft tissue and vascular calcification among patients undergoing long-term dialysis.[38-40] Calcium binder use may also be a risk factor for the syndrome of calciphylaxis and for progressive vascular calcification among patients receiving maintenance dialysis.[41,42] Treatment with calcium-containing compounds in patients with adynamic renal osteodystrophy (which is characterized by abnormally low bone remodeling rates) may be problematic because of the more limited buffering capacity. However, the continuous administration of large amounts of calcium to patients with stage 5 CKD can lower plasma PTH concentrations and diminish bone remodeling. Although the fractional absorption of calcium is limited in patients with ESKD with low endogenous $1,25(OH)_2D_3$ concentrations, and patients with high bone remodeling have a high capacity to buffer calcium, current guidelines recommend avoiding exposure to large doses of calcium-containing binders.

Based on these observations, alternative phosphate-binding strategies that limit total calcium intake to 1500 to 2000 mg/day from both dietary and medicinal sources have been proposed.[42]

ALUMINUM AND LANTHANUM SALTS

Aluminum-containing binders, such as aluminum hydroxide and aluminum carbonate, are the most potent phosphate-binding compounds, but their long-term use led to aluminum retention and aluminum toxicity (including encephalopathy and osteomalacia) because of ongoing intestinal aluminum absorption and (more importantly) concomitant exposure to aluminum-contaminated dialysate.[43] Although no studies have assessed the risk for aluminum toxicity in the era of more carefully monitored and uniformly mixed dialysate, aluminum-based agents are used sparingly to manage phosphorus retention in patients with CKD because of the fear of aluminum toxicity. When used, the duration of treatment is typically limited to periods of 2 to 3 months, the doses kept as low as possible, and concurrent administration of citrate-containing compounds avoided.[36,44] Plasma aluminum concentrations should be monitored regularly in patients who are given aluminum-containing phosphate binders.

Lanthanum carbonate is a potent phosphate-binding agent available for clinical use among patients undergoing dialysis.[45] The capacity of this compound to bind phosphorus in vitro is similar to that of aluminum hydroxide and appears to be more potent than calcium acetate, calcium carbonate, and sevelamer.[46] Clinical trials with lanthanum carbonate using doses as high as 3000 mg/day demonstrate its efficacy in lowering serum phosphate concentrations among patients undergoing dialysis.[47-50] A very small fraction of ingested lanthanum is absorbed from the gastrointestinal tract, and trace amounts are detectable in various tissues, including liver and bone. Histologic studies of bone in biopsy specimens obtained after 1 year of treatment with lanthanum carbonate show no adverse effects on skeletal mineralization or on bone remodeling.[51] Safety and efficacy have been documented among patients treated for as long as 3 years.[50]

PHOSPHATE-BINDING RESINS

Resins are becoming the preferred phosphate binders in CKD and currently consist of sevelamer (linked with either hydrochloride or carbonate), a hydrogel of cross-linked poly-allylamine, and colestilan, a 2-methylimidazole containing synthetic polymers that bind phosphorus within the lumen of the gastrointestinal tract and reduce its absorption.[52-55] Compared with other binders, sevelamer hydrochloride has a relatively low affinity for phosphate anions, thereby requiring a high pill burden. In longer-term studies, total daily doses averaging 5 to 6 g were sufficient to maintain serum phosphorus levels at approximately 5.8 to 6.0 mg/dL, or 1.8 to 2.0 mmol/L, among patients undergoing maintenance hemodialysis.[56] Larger doses may be required to achieve the more stringent therapeutic targets for serum phosphorus levels outlined in the National Kidney Foundation Kidney Disease Outcomes Quality Initiative (NKF KDOQI) guidelines. Plasma bicarbonate concentrations decrease modestly during treatment with sevelamer hydrochloride, a biochemical change that is probably caused by the release of protons from the resin during phosphate binding[57]; the carbonate compound ameliorates this problem.[58] Sevelamer also binds several drugs, including furosemide, cyclosporine, and tacrolimus, rendering them less effective.[59] Interestingly, the serum concentrations of total cholesterol and low-density lipoprotein cholesterol decrease by 20% to 30% during treatment with sevelamer or colestilan, whereas high-density lipoprotein levels tend to increase.[52,56,60] These biochemical changes represent potentially favorable side effects of therapy in patients at high cardiovascular risk. Colestilan also has glucose-lowering effects.[61]

OTHER PHOSPHATE-BINDING AGENTS (MAGNESIUM AND IRON)

Magnesium-containing medications have also been used as phosphate binders in patients undergoing hemodialysis, but these agents are limited by diarrhea and hypermagnesemia.[62] Polymeric complexes of iron and starch have also been shown to bind phosphate and reduce serum phosphate concentrations in patients on hemodialysis.[63]

The most recent advance is the emergence of other iron-based phosphate binders, including sucroferric oxyhydroxide and ferric citrate, agents approved for treatment of hyperphosphatemia in adult patients receiving dialysis. A trial comparing sucroferric oxyhydroxide with sevelamer carbonate found equal efficacy in reducing serum phosphate concentrations, but differences in side effect profiles, with sucroferric oxyhydroxide associated with diarrhea and discolored stools, and sevelamer carbonate associated with nausea and constipation.[64] Treatment with sucroferric oxyhydroxide does not yield substantial iron absorption, whereas ferritin and transferrin saturation increases significantly after treatment with ferric citrate; the choice of one of these iron-based phosphate binders should take laboratory parameters and co-interventions (especially the use of intravenous iron and erythropoietin-stimulating agents) into account.[65,66]

Currently there are insufficient data to establish the comparative superiority of non–calcium-based binding agents over calcium-containing phosphate binders. Nevertheless, concern remains regarding the potential of calcium overload and consequent exacerbation of vascular calcification with the use of calcium-based binders. Although no survival advantage has been demonstrated with the use of the resin binder sevelamer compared to calcium-based binders in randomized clinical trials, and all phosphate binders may increase intestinal calcium absorption to some degree,[67] most treatment regimens minimize the use of calcium-based binders.

The limitation of phosphate binders has led to new ways to prevent gastrointestinal phosphate absorption. Phosphate restriction or using agents to reduce gastrointestinal phosphate absorption, however, are by themselves not sufficient to normalize circulating FGF-23 or PTH concentrations in either animal models or clinical studies of CKD. Thus differing views are emerging regarding the inciting factors in CKD-MBD and what combinations of drug therapies are best used to treat this disorder (Figure 63.2).

CALCIUM, VITAMIN D RECEPTOR AGONISTS, AND CALCIUM-SENSING RECEPTOR ALLOSTERIC MODULATORS (CALCIMIMETIC AGENTS)

Three approaches are used to lower PTH concentration in ESKD: the administration of calcium to increase serum calcium level, vitamin D analogs to both raise serum calcium level and activate VDR-dependent gene regulation, and calcimimetic agents to directly target the CaSR without raising serum calcium level. Calcium is the natural ligand, and calcimimetic agents are allosteric modulators of CaSR in parathyroid chief cells, which suppresses PTH secretion, production, and hyperplasia. Vitamin D analogs directly target the VDR in the parathyroid gland to predominately suppress PTH production, and through their effects on the gastrointestinal tract to increase serum calcium level, which secondarily activates CaSR. There are several generalizations that can be made regarding these agents.

CALCIUM SUPPLEMENTS

Calcium is effective in suppressing PTH but results in a positive calcium balance, which has potential for adverse effects. Thus the current practice is to limit the amount of calcium supplementation, although little is known about whether calcium supplementation alone, in the absence of concomitant therapy with vitamin D analogs, can be safely administered to correct abnormalities in bone and mineral metabolism.[68]

TREATMENT WITH VITAMIN D ANALOGS

Like the preference for noncalcium phosphate binders to treat hyperphosphatemia, and in spite of the introduction of calcimimetics (see later), vitamin D analogs remain the drug most often used to treat secondary hyperparathyroidism.

$1,25(OH)_2D_3$ functions systemically as a calcium-regulating hormone, acting primarily through genomic mechanisms. The classical genomic actions of vitamin D are initiated by the binding of $1,25(OH)_2D$ to its receptor in the cytoplasm of cells expressing the VDR.[69,70] The ligand-bound VDR subsequently localizes to the cell nucleus, where it forms a heterodimer with the retinoid X receptor that binds to vitamin D response elements (VDREs) in target gene

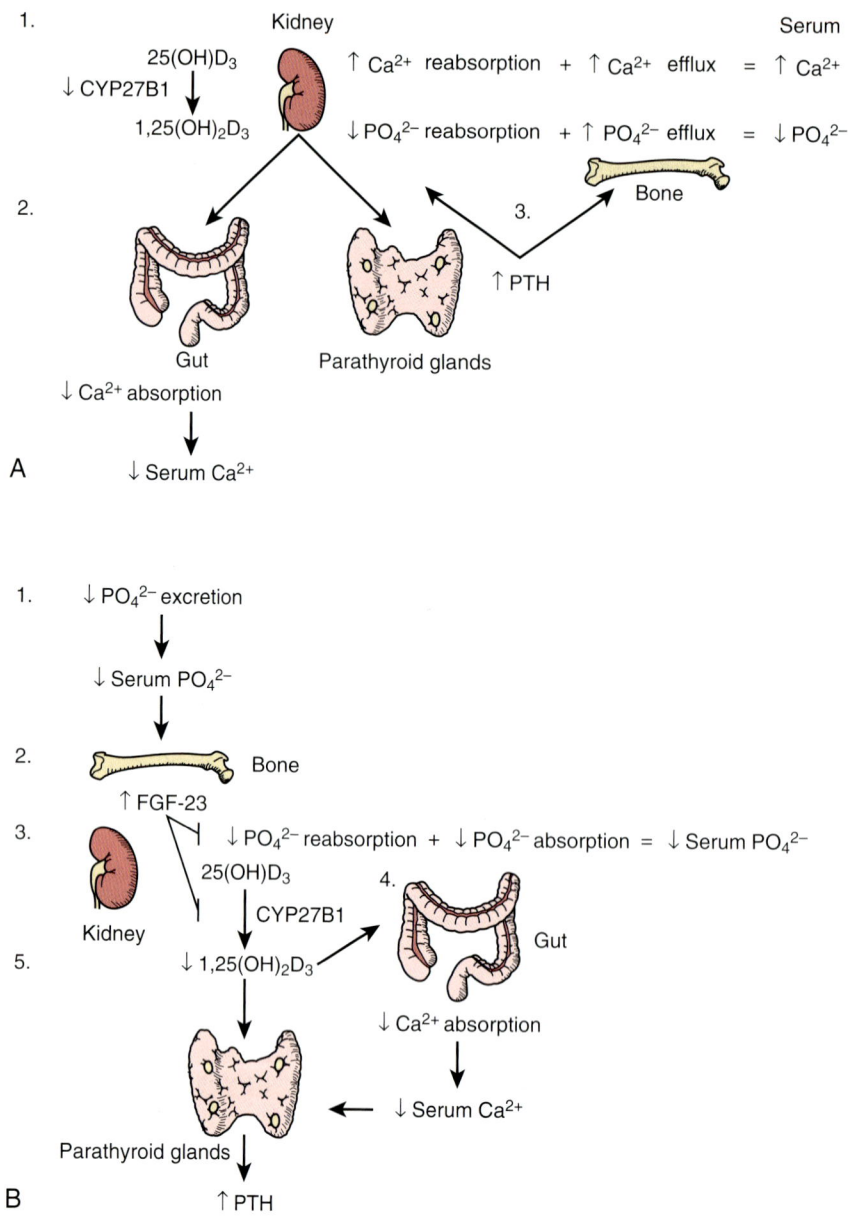

Figure 63.2 Alternative paradigms to explain secondary hyperparathyroidism (SHPT) in chronic kidney disease (CKD). **A,** Traditional paradigm: (1) primary decrease in 1,25-dihydroxycholecalciferol (1,25[OH]$_2$D$_3$) occurs because of loss of functional kidney mass and concomitant cytochrome P450 enzyme 27B1 (CYP27B1) activity; (2) reductions in 1,25-dihydroxyvitamin D (1,25[OH]$_2$D$_3$) cause development of SHPT both indirectly, by decreased gastrointestinal calcium absorption, and directly, by loss of suppressive effect on the parathyroid glands; (3) increased parathyroid hormone (PTH) levels target the kidney to increase CYP27B1 activity, increase renal calcium reabsorption, decrease renal phosphate reabsorption, and also target the bone to increase calcium and phosphate efflux; the net effect is to preserve serum calcium levels while reducing serum phosphate levels. **B,** Alternative paradigm: (1) primary decrease in renal phosphate excretion caused by loss of functioning kidney mass; (2) increased fibroblast growth factor 23 (FGF-23) secretion from bone; (3) increased FGF-23 levels target the kidney to inhibit renal phosphate reabsorption and reduce 1,25(OH)$_2$D$_3$ production; (4) phosphate homeostasis restored by the effects of both decreased 1,25(OH)$_2$D$_3$ levels, which diminish gastrointestinal absorption, and increased FGF-23 levels, which increase renal phosphate excretion; (5) reductions in 1,25(OH)$_2$D$_3$ lead to increased PTH as in the traditional paradigm, but as a late event; FGF-23 suppresses PTH during the earlier phases of CKD. (Modified from Wetmore JB, Quarles LD: Calcimimetics or vitamin D analogs for suppressing parathyroid hormone in end-stage renal disease: time for a paradigm shift? *Nat Clin Pract Nephrol* 5:24-33, 2009.)

promoters (see Figure 63.2).[71-73] Key target tissues that participate in the regulation of calcium metabolism and that are affected directly by 1,25(OH)$_2$D$_3$ include kidney, intestine, bone, and parathyroid. In response to hypocalcemia, increased PTH stimulates 1,25(OH)$_2$D$_3$ production, which in turn acts as a hormone that principally targets the small intestines to increase active calcium and phosphate absorption but also has direct effects on bone and parathyroid glands to regulate mineral homeostasis.

There are several noteworthy caveats regarding therapy with vitamin D. First, there appear to be no clinically important differences in either efficacy or side effects of the available active vitamin D analogs in CKD.[74] Indeed, in a randomized trial paracalcitol and $1,25(OH)_2D_3$ were found to be equivalent with respect to both suppressing PTH levels and increasing serum calcium and phosphate concentrations.[75] Reviews of available randomized controlled trials of different vitamin D analogs, including $1,25(OH)_2D_3$, alfacalcidol, doxercalciferol, and paricalcitol, found no data to support the use of one agent over the other.[10,76,77]

Second, the pharmacokinetics of administered vitamin D, however, may influence hormonal responses. While oral and intravenous administrations appear to be equally effective, there may be a trend for induction of less hypercalcemia and hyperphosphatemia by some of the newer analogs at low doses. These differences, however, disappear at doses required to suppress PTH long-term, and most, if not all, vitamin D analogs have the potential to cause hypercalcemia and hyperphosphatemia and to increase FGF-23 concentrations in patients with ESKD. A possible exception is a slow-release form of calcifediol that can suppress circulating PTH without increasing FGF-23 concentrations.[78]

Third, although abnormalities in vitamin D metabolism are a key feature of CKD-MBD, it is not clear if the observed changes in $25(OH)D$ and $1,25(OH)_2D_3$ circulating concentrations, which are both decreased in advanced CKD, solely represent primary deficiencies, due to poor nutrition in the case of low circulating $25(OH)D$ and renal parenchyma loss of function that leads to decreased $1,25(OH)_2D_3$ synthesis.[2] Increased catabolism due to excess FGF-23 stimulation of CYP24A1 activity may contribute to this decrease in $25(OH)D$ and $1,25(OH)_2D_3$ circulating concentrations, especially in early CKD. Nevertheless, replacement with cholecalciferol can lower PTH levels in early-stage CKD where residual activity of vitamin D metabolizing enzymes remains, while cholecalciferol does not lower PTH levels significantly in ESKD.[79]

Fourth, low circulating levels of $1,25(OH)_2D_3$ are associated with increased mortality, likely caused by effects on innate immunity and cardiovascular function and possibly other effects unrelated to its function to regulate mineral metabolism.[80,81] VDR is expressed in nearly all cell types, and at least 500 genes have been identified with VDREs, suggesting that multiple genes in many tissues are regulated by vitamin D. Calcitriol thus serves as an important modifier of gene transcription even in tissues that are not involved directly in maintaining calcium homeostasis. These nonclassical actions are important in regulating cell proliferation and differentiation, as well as other functions, such as innate immunity, insulin sensitivity, and bone and cardiovascular health. There is a resurgence of diagnosis and treatment of vitamin D deficiency in the general population with normal kidney function, as well as evidence that treatment with active vitamin D analogs improves survival of patients with ESKD undergoing hemodialysis.[82,83] In one report, mortality rates after 3 years of follow-up were lower among patients with CKD undergoing hemodialysis who were given paricalcitol compared to $1,25[OH]_2D_3$.[82] In another report, survival after 2 years was higher among patients who received paricalcitol during the first 12 months of treatment with hemodialysis as compared with those who received no vitamin D during this interval.[83] In multivariable analyses, the association of paricalcitol treatment with survival persisted irrespective of the serum concentrations of calcium or phosphorus. Such findings are notable and potentially important, but they are limited by residual confounding (indication bias).

The potential benefit of vitamin D supplementation remains unproven. While there is an association with treatment with vitamin D analogs and survival in patients with ESKD, benefits have not been confirmed in prospective studies. Moreover, a meta-analysis of 76 clinical trials provides an opposing viewpoint on the use of vitamin D therapy in patients with CKD,[84] finding that vitamin D compounds do not reduce the risk for death or vascular calcification, and that $1,25[OH]_2D_3$, when compared with placebo, increased the risks for hypercalcemia and hyperphosphatemia while inconsistently reducing PTH levels. Most disappointing, in a randomized trial, patients with CKD that did not require dialysis who were treated with paricalcitol for up to 48 weeks did not show improvement of cardiac structure, function, or left ventricular mass, compared to patients treated with placebo.[85] Thus justification for use of vitamin D analogs to prevent cardiovascular complications in CKD patients not yet on hemodialysis is lacking. In addition, active vitamin D analogs have been shown to increase FGF-23 concentrations in patients with ESKD,[86] and studies have found that elevated FGF-23 concentration is an independent predictor of mortality in patients with ESKD.[13]

Although the benefits from replacing vitamin D have not been established in patients with CKD taking $1,25[OH]_2D_3$ or other vitamin D analogs, Kidney Disease: Improving Global Outcomes (KDIGO) recommends measuring $25(OH)D$ levels to identify and treat superimposed nutritional vitamin D deficiency in ESKD. This recommendation is primarily based on the safety and low cost of nutritional vitamin D supplementation and the possibility that providing the substrate for 1α-hydroxylase will lead to the local production of $1,25(OH)_2D_3$ in peripheral tissues, where it may have a salutary effect on organ function. Studies indicate that cholecalciferol doses of 20,000 IU per week for 9 months achieved recommended levels of $25(OH)D$ greater than 75 nmol/L in only 57% of patients with ESKD, suggesting higher doses may be required than in the general population.[87] There are several studies indicating that cholecalciferol or ergocalciferol supplementation has biologic effects in ESKD, either through residual production and systemic effect of $1,25(OH)_2D_3$ produced by the kidney or through effects derived from local production of $1,25(OH)_2D_3$ in peripheral tissues.[88] Aggressive treatment with active vitamin D analogs may lead to hypercalcemia and hyperphosphatemia. Thus high-dose nutritional vitamin D supplements or use of activated vitamin D analogs for the treatment of secondary hyperparathyroidism in patients with CKD may have risks that offset potential benefits. Additional prospective clinical trials are needed to determine the optimal use of vitamin D in CKD.[89]

Finally, economic considerations influence the management of patients with ESKD. For example, intravenous synthetic vitamin D analogs administered three times a week are commonly used in the United States, whereas oral vitamin D analogs are more commonly used in other countries.[90] The End-Stage Renal Disease Prospective Payment System by the Centers for Medicare and Medicaid Services, which includes both oral and intravenous medications in a bundled payment system, has fostered the greater use of oral medications, as well as shift to home-based dialysis. The implications are several. First, increased frequency of dialysis results in a greater cumulative phosphate removal, possibly reducing the need for phosphate binders to maintain neutral phosphate balance. For example, a standard dialysis treatment removes approximately 900 mg of phosphate.[91] Studies found that the total weekly phosphorus removal with nocturnal hemodialysis six times per week is more than twice that removed by in-center hemodialysis done three times per week.[92] Indeed, nocturnal dialysis performed six times per week results in lowering of the serum phosphate level and discontinuation of phosphate binder therapy compared to patients on standard hemodialysis administered three times a week.[93] Second, these new rules will place greater emphasis on the cost-effectiveness and clinical trials comparing the relative effectiveness of different treatments.

The removal of financial incentives for the use of high-dose intravenous vitamin D analogs has resulted in a shift to less expensive oral forms of active vitamin D administration in ESKD.[94,95]

SPECIFIC VITAMIN D STEROLS

1,25(OH)D and the prodrug alfacalcidol, as well as synthetic vitamin D analogs, including paricalcitol, doxercalciferol, and maxacalcitol, have all been shown to lower plasma PTH concentrations in patients with secondary hyperparathyroidism (SHPT) receiving dialysis. Among patients undergoing maintenance hemodialysis, intravenous doses given three times a week during each dialysis session are used most often. Treatment with daily oral doses of alfacalcidol or $1,25(OH)_2D_3$ is utilized more frequently outside the United States. The estimated equivalent doses of $1,25(OH)_2D_3$, paricalcitol, and doxercalciferol are 0.5 mg, 2 mg, and 1 mg, respectively.[96] Studies to assess the differences in the efficacy of daily oral, intermittent oral, or intravenous doses of any of these agents have not demonstrated major differences between the routes of administration on measurable outcomes other than compliance. Thus the evidence supporting the common practice of large intermittent intravenous doses of vitamin D sterols over oral therapies of $1,25(OH)_2D_3$ derivatives for managing SHPT among patients with ESKD is limited.[97-100] Although short-term controlled studies suggested that paricalcitol and doxercalciferol may have a greater therapeutic window for lowering PTH level without raising serum calcium and phosphate concentrations, later studies suggest that all vitamin D analogs have the potential to cause hypercalcemia and hyperphosphatemia.

Parenteral vitamin D therapy is generally started using small initial doses, assuming that serum calcium and phosphate concentrations are not elevated. Doses are raised subsequently in increments to lower plasma PTH level. The use of larger initial doses of paricalcitol has been suggested to be a safe alternative among patients with severe disease and markedly elevated plasma PTH level.[101] Among patients who respond favorably to treatment, plasma PTH concentrations decline progressively over several months. The primary therapeutic objective is to maintain plasma PTH concentrations within a range of 150 to 300 pg/mL. Lowering plasma PTH level further increases the likelihood of episodes of hypercalcemia, and it can lead to the development of adynamic renal osteodystrophy.[102] Use of vitamin D analogs can also increase the requirement for phosphate binders. Thus doses of vitamin D sterols that can be given safely to control plasma PTH levels are determined by monitoring serum calcium and phosphorus concentrations during therapy. Values often increase during treatment, and these biochemical changes often necessitate a reduction in the dose of vitamin D analogs.

The NKF KDOQI guidelines advise against initiating treatment with vitamin D sterols or continuing vitamin D therapy when serum calcium levels exceed 9.5 to 10.0 mg/dL or when serum phosphate concentrations exceed 5.5 mg/dL. Although definitive evidence to support these recommendations is not available, data from epidemiologic studies of patients undergoing maintenance hemodialysis indicate that mortality risk increases progressively as serum calcium and phosphate concentrations rise above these values[14,103]; however, KDIGO recommendations raise the upper limit of calcium concentration to that of the general population but more stringently control serum phosphate concentration (2.5 to 4.5 mg/dL).

Downward adjustments to the concentration of calcium in dialysate have been used to permit treatment with larger oral doses of calcium-containing compounds to control serum phosphate concentrations or to allow the continued use of vitamin D sterols to manage SHPT among patients with persistently elevated serum calcium concentrations.[104,105] There is little evidence to support these measures. Dialysate calcium concentrations below the normal physiologic concentration of ionized calcium in blood will provoke PTH secretion during each hemodialysis session and thus provide ongoing and recurrent stimuli for PTH secretion and parathyroid gland hyperplasia. As such, the use of dialysis solutions containing calcium concentrations lower than 2.5 mEq/L, or 1.25 mmol/L, may aggravate SHPT among patients receiving hemodialysis.[106]

CALCIUM-SENSING RECEPTOR ALLOSTERIC MODULATORS (CALCIMIMETIC AGENTS)

Calcimimetic agents are small organic molecules that function as allosteric activators of the CaSR, the molecular mechanism that mediates calcium-regulated PTH secretion by parathyroid cells.[107,108] Cinacalcet hydrochloride is the only approved member of this new class of agents to be available to treat SHPT among patients undergoing dialysis. Calcimimetic agents bind reversibly to the membrane-spanning portion of the CaSR and lower the threshold for receptor activation by extracellular calcium ions.[109] In parathyroid tissue, activation of CaSR inhibits PTH secretion directly and lowers plasma PTH levels by a mechanism distinct from that of the vitamin D sterols.[110,111] Cinacalcet hydrochloride is a hydrophobic compound that is absorbed rapidly from the gastrointestinal tract after oral administration.[112] Peak plasma levels are attained 60 to 90 minutes after oral doses, and these correspond temporally to the maximum biologic effect, as judged by reductions in plasma PTH.[112-114]

There is evidence that the calcimimetic target CaSR is more important than VDR in regulating parathyroid gland function. CaSR regulates PTH secretion, PTH gene transcription,[108,115] and parathyroid cell proliferation.[116] In humans with severe congenital neonatal hyperparathyroidism[117] and in the analogous homozygous *Casr* knockout mice,[118] there are increases in serum PTH and calcium concentrations, and hyperplasia of the parathyroid gland, in spite of marked elevations in circulating $1,25(OH)_2D_3$ concentrations. Ablation of the VDR in mice also results in SHPT and parathyroid gland hyperplasia, but normalization of serum calcium level is sufficient to fully correct abnormal parathyroid gland function in this model, unlike in the *Casr* knockout mice or in cases of severe neonatal hyperparathyroidism.[119] The fact that $1,25(OH)_2D_3$ is ineffective in suppressing PTH production in the absence of CaSR, but calcium is sufficient to normalize parathyroid gland function in the absence of VDR, indicates that CaSR is the dominant regulator of parathyroid gland function.[110,120-122] The principal direct function of the VDR in the parathyroid gland, then, is to suppress PTH gene transcription; in addition, the VDR has an indirect action on the parathyroid gland through stimulation of gastrointestinal calcium absorption and elevation of serum calcium levels, which serves to affect parathyroid gland function via the CaSR.

Cinacalcet is a very effective agent for reducing serum PTH concentrations in patients with ESKD without raising serum calcium concentrations.[123] Plasma PTH concentrations fall abruptly after single oral doses of cinacalcet in patients with SHPT receiving hemodialysis, reaching a nadir after 2 to 4 hours. The magnitude of the initial decrease in plasma PTH concentration is largely dose dependent.[124] Although plasma PTH concentrations decrease invariably following the administration of calcimimetic agents,[125] the degree of suppression correlates with the severity of SHPT.[113,114,126,127] Cinacalcet treatment causes PTH values to decrease by 80% when baseline PTH values are between 300 and 500 pg/mL, by 60% when baseline PTH values are 500 to 880 pg/mL, and 22% when baseline PTH values are greater than 800 pg/mL.[112] Plasma PTH concentrations increase subsequently, however, toward predose concentrations during the remainder of the day as the concentration of cinacalcet in plasma decreases and as the level of CaSR activation diminishes.[112,124] Because plasma PTH concentrations decrease substantially but increase subsequently after oral doses of cinacalcet, variations in the interval between drug administration and the collection of blood samples for measurements of plasma PTH levels will affect the values obtained.[110] In this regard, all clinical trials reported thus far among patients with CKD have used plasma PTH concentrations obtained 24 hours after the preceding dose of cinacalcet to assess the biochemical efficacy of treatment and to guide decisions about dosage adjustments.[15,110,125,128] When using cinacalcet for the clinical management of patients with SHPT, it is generally recommended that plasma PTH levels be measured at least 12 hours after the preceding dose. Such an approach thus provides biochemical information similar to that used in published clinical trials to guide decisions about dosage adjustments and to judge therapeutic efficacy.[15,110] Adequate calcium-dependent signaling through the CaSR may be particularly important in preventing the development of SHPT and in retarding the progression of parathyroid gland hyperplasia.[129-131] Indeed, treatment with cinacalcet was associated with reductions in the rate of parathyroidectomy in patients with ESKD.[132] Cinacalcet may not cause regression of parathyroid gland hyperplasia, since discontinuation of cinacalcet results in rapid rebound of serum PTH concentrations to pretreatment levels.

Apart from reducing plasma PTH concentrations, treatment with calcimimetic agents lowers serum calcium concentrations.[126] Therefore cinacalcet should not be started unless the serum calcium concentration is greater than 8.4 mg/dL. Pooled analysis for phase III clinical studies found that serum calcium levels less than 8.4 mg/dL developed in 66% of patients treated with cinacalcet.[133] Serum total and blood ionized calcium levels decrease during the first 12 to 24 hours after treatment is begun, changes that temporally follow an abrupt initial decline in plasma PTH level as described previously.[124] Such findings thus underscore the crucial role of short-term variations in PTH secretion by the parathyroid glands in maintaining the level of ionized calcium in blood. Reductions in serum calcium concentration are thus a predictable, physiologic response to treatment with calcimimetic agents.

To minimize the effects of hypocalcemia, the initial dose of cinacalcet is 30 mg/day, and subsequent doses are increased every 2 to 3 weeks in 30-mg increments until a maximum dose of 180 mg/day is achieved.[15,110] The safety of this approach has been documented in large clinical trials in which symptomatic hypocalcemia did not occur.[15] All of these studies have found that calcimimetic agents suppress PTH and optimize serum calcium and phosphate concentrations in patients resistant to standard therapy alone.[15,123,134] The effects of cinacalcet are independent of concomitant vitamin D analog therapy, and later studies have demonstrated that cinacalcet can be used in treatment paradigms that reduce the dosage of vitamin D analogs.[135,136] Concomitant treatment with active vitamin D analogs, however, typifies most clinical trials and may attenuate hypocalcemia. Thus combination treatment is the standard of care for most patients with moderate to severe SHPT. The seminal Evaluation of Cinacalcet Hydrochloride Therapy to Lower Cardiovascular Events (EVOLVE) study confirmed that treatment regimens that include the calcimimetic agent result in better control of secondary hyperparathyroidism and lead to a reduction in the incidence of parathyroidectomy. The primary analysis of the trial—an unadjusted intention-to-treat approach—showed no significant effect of cinacalcet on mortality or a composite end point of death or major cardiovascular events. Analyses adjusting for baseline factors (there was an imbalance in age across randomized groups) showed nominally significant reductions in the primary composite end point as well as mortality.[137] Treatment with vitamin D sterols or calcium supplements rather than cinacalcet is recommended for patients with hypocalcemia owing to the calcium-lowering effect of calcimimetic agents.[110] Patients should be monitored for signs of hypocalcemia (i.e., tetany), and cinacalcet should be used with caution in subjects with a preexisting seizure disorder. The most frequent side effects of cinacalcet are nausea and vomiting.

In summary, vitamin D analogs and cinacalcet, which have different molecular targets (namely the VDR and CaSR, respectively), have different potency for suppression of PTH (cinacalcet more than vitamin D analogs) and different effects on calcium (cinacalcet decreases and vitamin D analogs increase) and phosphate (cinacalcet a neutral

Table 63.2 Recommended Ranges for Selected Biochemical Parameters According to Stage of Chronic Kidney Disease (CKD) as Summarized in the NKF KDOQI and KDIGO Clinical Practice Guidelines for Bone Metabolism and Disease in CKD—Recommended Serum Values

CKD Stage	GFR Range (mL/min/1.73 m^2)	Phosphorus (mg/dL)	Calcium (Corrected)(mg/dL)	Ca × P	Intact PTH (pg/mL)
3	30-59	2.7-4.6	8.4-10.2		35-70
KDOQI KDIGO			Same range as general population		
4	15-29	2.7-4.6	8.4-10.2		70-110
KDOQI KDIGO			Same range as general population		
5	<15, dialysis	3.5-5.5	8.4-9.5	<55	150-300
KDOQI KDIGO	Normal range	Normal range Avoid hyperphosphatemia	Normal range Avoid hypercalcemia	Use not endorsed	Avoid PTH < 2 or >9 times the upper normal limit

Ca, Calcium; GFR, glomerular filtration rate; KDIGO, Kidney Disease: Improving Global Outcomes; KDOQI, Kidney Disease Outcomes Quality Initiative; NKF, National Kidney Foundation; P, phosphorus; PTH, parathyroid hormone.
Modified from National Kidney Foundation: DOQI kidney disease outcomes quality initiative. *Am J Kidney Dis* 43:S1-S201, 2004; and National Kidney Foundation and Kidney Disease: Improving Global Outcomes (KDIGO).

effect and vitamin D analogs increase serum phosphate). Vitamin D analogs, cinacalcet, or combinations of vitamin D analogs and cinacalcet can be used to suppress PTH in ESKD. Serum calcium and phosphate concentrations, as well as the severity of PTH elevation, may influence the drug selection (e.g., cinacalcet would be used preferentially over vitamin D analogs in patients with elevated calcium and phosphate concentrations).

OVERVIEW OF CLINICAL MANAGEMENT OF CHRONIC KIDNEY DISEASE–MINERAL BONE DISORDER

Clinical management of CKD-MBD is based on repeated measurement of circulating laboratory values, specifically PTH, calcium, and phosphorus concentrations, and therapeutic interventions using combinations of phosphate binders, cholecalciferol and 1,25(OH)$_2$D$_3$ and vitamin D analogs, and calcimimetic agents that are dose adjusted to keep these biochemical parameters within specific target ranges, while minimizing potential side effects of the various therapies. Treatment considerations also depend on the stage of CKD, the mechanism of action and targets of the various therapeutic agents, potential toxicities associated with various treatments, and cost and reimbursement of the various therapies. Finally, successful treatment involves patient education and a multidisciplinary approach involving nephrologists, dietitians, and nurses.

THERAPEUTIC GOALS

The overall goals of therapy are to (1) regulate serum PTH concentrations within an acceptable range and prevent the progression of parathyroid hyperplasia to autonomous parathyroid gland function (i.e., prevent tertiary hyperparathyroidism); (2) prevent hyperphosphatemia and hypercalcemia and minimize vascular calcifications by maintaining neutral phosphate and calcium balance; (3) maintain normal bone remodeling and bone health (i.e., prevent both high and low bone turnover rates and reduce fracture risks); (4) provide adequate vitamin D supplementation to optimize innate immune functions and other biologic actions of vitamin D not related to mineral metabolism functions; and (5) reduce the morbidity and mortality risks associated with disordered mineral metabolism.

The 2009 and 2012 KDIGO guidelines and the 2010 KDOQI have made recommendations regarding the optimal timing of assessment and desirable range for biochemical markers of CKD-MBD (Table 63.2).[138] Monitoring of serum calcium, phosphorus, PTH, 25(OH)D, and alkaline phosphatase activity is recommended when the estimated glomerular filtration rate (GFR) is less than 45 mL/min/1.73 m^2 (GFR category G3b) In CKD before initiating dialysis (i.e., G3b to G4), it is recommended to maintain serum phosphate concentrations in the normal range and to treat PTH concentrations above the normal range by correcting hyperphosphatemia, hypocalcemia, and/or vitamin D deficiency. There are currently no recommendations to prescribe phosphate binders or vitamin D supplements or analogs in the absence of hyperphosphatemia or documented vitamin D deficiency.

In patients with ESKD, it is recommend that calcium and phosphorus be measured at 1 to 3 months, PTH at 3 to 6 months, and 25(OH)D at the initiation of dialysis. Moreover, achieving a serum PTH range, from the previously recommended (KDOQI) range of 150 to 300 pg/mL to the more "relaxed" KDIGO recommended range of approximately two to nine times the upper limit of the assay (or roughly 130 to 600 pg/mL), is desirable as is following trends in serum PTH concentrations and intervening to prevent progressive increases in PTH values within this range. A serum phosphate level from the previously recommended range of 3.5 to 5.5 mg/dL to "toward the reference range" has been recommended to permit greater flexibility, and a calcium level from between 8.4 and 9.5 mg/dL to maintaining calcium within the normal reference range. The more "relaxed" KDIGO guidelines, along with the ESKD prospective payment system in the United States, which bundled the payment for intravenous drugs used in dialysis that had oral equivalents, has resulted in an increase in mean PTH concentrations by approximately 30%. The U.S. Dialysis Outcomes and Practice Patterns Study (DOPPS) Practice Monitor found that the percentage of facilities reporting an upper PTH target level of 600 pg/mL or higher and serum calcium level greater than 10.5 mg/dL increased from less than 7% before 2011 to 40% in 2012 and from less than 26% before 2011 to 37% in 2012. The phosphorus target exceeded 5.5 mg/dL with no clear trend over time.[95]

TREATMENT OF CHRONIC KIDNEY DISEASE–MINERAL BONE DISORDER IN END-STAGE KIDNEY DISEASE

The goals of therapy are to prevent the progression of parathyroid disease, optimize bone health, normalize phosphate balance, minimize the risk for vascular calcifications, and reduce the mortality risks attributed to disordered mineral metabolism. This requires the use of these agents in various combinations that differ as a function of severity of CKD.

For patients with ESKD on dialysis, either hemodialysis or peritoneal dialysis, therapy consists of a combination of dietary phosphate restriction, calcium-containing and non–calcium-containing phosphate binders, nutritional and active vitamin D analog supplementation, and calcimimetic agents. There are many factors that influence the approaches used to treat disordered mineral metabolism in ESKD. A variety of treatment combinations are possible, which include use of a phosphate binder to treat hyperphosphatemia and either titration of vitamin D analogs or cinacalcet to suppress PTH (Figure 63.3). Efforts to control serum phosphate concentrations with dietary phosphate restriction (with adequate protein intake) and phosphate binders to maintain serum phosphate between 3.5 and 5.5 mg/dL are common to all approaches. Because there are no prospective outcome studies to separate the different binders, one can choose from among calcium-, resin-, lanthanum-, or iron-based binders.

Correcting hyperphosphatemia with phosphate-binding agents may lower plasma PTH concentrations modestly among patients with SHPT, but this does not represent a definitive and reliable pharmacologic intervention for controlling the disorder. Vitamin D sterols that target the VDR and calcimimetic agents that target the CaSR are the two pharmacologic interventions currently available that act specifically to modify parathyroid gland function and lower plasma PTH concentrations definitively. Either or both can be used to treat SHPT when plasma PTH concentrations remain elevated after measures have been implemented to control serum phosphate concentrations and optimize calcium balance.

Use of escalating doses of vitamin D analogs to suppress PTH typically requires the provision of noncalcium phosphate binders to minimize hyperphosphatemia, whereas use of cinacalcet in combination with vitamin D analogs may allow more liberal use of calcium-based binders to prevent hypocalcemia. At present, titration of vitamin D analogs and noncalcium phosphate binders is the most commonly used treatment strategy in ESKD, with cinacalcet added in approximately 30% of the patients due to progression of SHPT.[139] Algorithms comparing high-dose vitamin D analogs with low-dose active vitamin D analogs in combination with cinacalcet as first-line combined therapy found better control of serum phosphate in the combination group.[140]

Combined use of vitamin D analogs and cinacalcet is necessary to optimally treat CKD-MBD. The Open-Label, Randomized Study Using Cinacalcet to Improve Achievement of KDOQI Targets in Patients with End-Stage Renal Disease (OPTIMA)[141] found more pronounced reductions in mean intact PTH levels and a higher percentage of patients achieving target serum phosphate concentrations (<5.5 mg/dL) in the cinacalcet-treated group compared to the unrestricted conventional care group. The ACHIEVE study in patients with PTH concentrations of more than 300 pg/mL and serum calcium concentrations of 8.4 mg/dL or higher, however, found no difference between paricalcitol and cinacalcet-based therapies in attaining the primary end point of suppressing PTH to a target range of 150 to 300 pg/mL.[142] In the Improved Management of iPTH with Paricalcitol-Centered Therapy versus Cinacalcet Therapy with Low-Dose Vitamin D in Hemodialysis Patients with Secondary Hyperparathyroidism (IMPACT SHPT) study, patients receiving hemodialysis with SHPT were randomized to receive either intravenous or oral paricalcitol versus cinacalcet first-line therapy. Paricalcitol treatment yielded more suppression of PTH and favorable changes in bone turnover markers, but increased FGF-23 levels compared to cinacalcet-centered therapy.[143] Thus at present there are insufficient data to support one treatment approach over another. Regardless of which paradigm is initiated, most patients will ultimately require combinations of calcium and noncalcium phosphate binders, vitamin D analogs, and cinacalcet to optimally manage the biochemical abnormalities present in ESKD. Either starting cinacalcet or increasing vitamin D analog dose can improve control of PTH levels; starting cinacalcet and decreasing the dose of active vitamin D analogs can achieve better control of serum phosphorus concentrations.[144]

Recognizing that there are no high-quality trials showing either net beneficial or harmful effects of any of these therapies, it seems reasonable to use these agents at doses that minimize their recognized toxicities, namely, hypercalcemia and hyperphosphatemia with vitamin D analogs, and hypocalcemia and a tendency to oversuppress PTH with calcimimetic agents, while taking advantage of their different molecular targets and biologic actions (e.g., cinacalcet targets CaSR and is a more potent suppressor of PTH, whereas vitamin D analogs target the widely expressed VDR, which has potential effects on both mineral homeostasis and other biologic processes, such as innate immunity and cardiovascular function).

TREATMENT OF PATIENTS WITH STAGES 2, 3, AND 4 CHRONIC KIDNEY DISEASE

GENERAL CONSIDERATIONS

Stages 2, 3, and 4 CKD represent a progressive magnitude of reductions in GFR (60 to 89, 30 to 59, and 15 to 29 mL/min/1.73 m^2, respectively). Because the patients have residual kidney function and because the severity of SHPT, vascular calcifications, and bone disease is typically less severe,

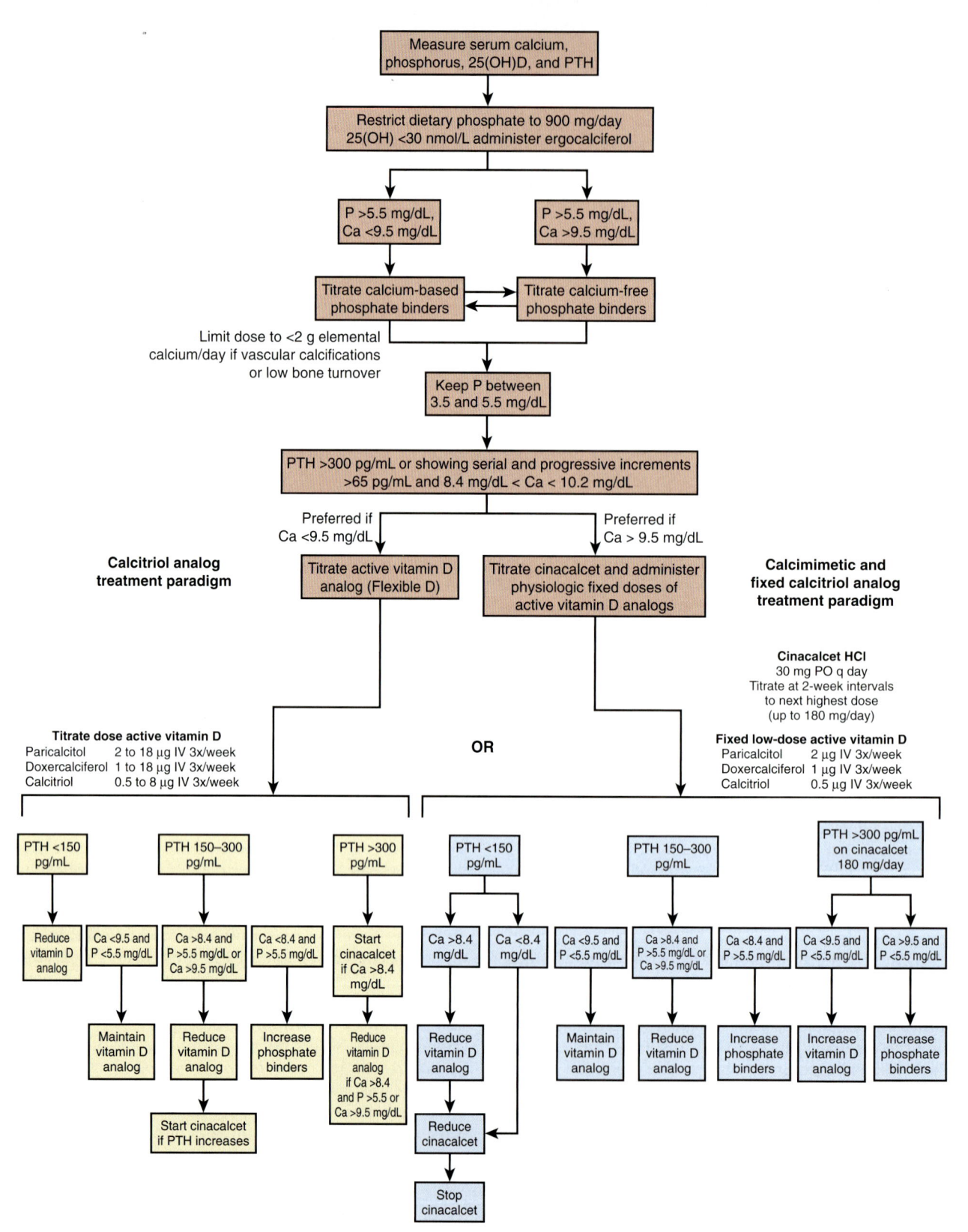

Figure 63.3 Algorithm for management of chronic kidney disease–mineral bone disorder (CKD-MBD) in stage 5 chronic kidney disease (CKD). Restricting dietary phosphate intake and normalizing serum 25-hydroxyvitamin D (25[OH]D) by administration of ergocalciferol is the initial step in management. The next step is the administration of oral phosphate binders to limit the absorption of dietary phosphate. The major modalities that are currently available are calcium salts, which are preferred in patients with low serum calcium level and the non–calcium-containing phosphate binders for patients with higher serum calcium levels. At present, there are no data evaluating clinically important outcomes that clearly favor non–calcium-containing phosphate binders over calcium-containing binders or that favor sevelamer over lanthanum. The next step is to choose between titration of active vitamin D analogs or cinacalcet to reduce parathyroid hormone (PTH) levels. Use of escalating doses of active vitamin D analogs (traditional approach) is limited by hyperphosphatemia and hypercalcemia. Upward adjustments of noncalcium phosphate binders and reductions of vitamin D analog doses are based on the changes in serum biochemical values in accord with the National Kidney Foundation Kidney Disease Outcomes Quality Initiative (NKF KDOQI) guidelines. There are no clinical data showing clinically important differences between calcitriol, paricalcitol, and doxercalciferol. Use of escalating doses of cinacalcet and fixed physiologic dose of active vitamin D analogs is more effective than the traditional approach in attaining control of serum biochemical values but is more expensive. Cinacalcet doses are titrated up to a daily dose of 180 mg. Side effects are hypocalcemia and nausea and vomiting, which may limit therapy. Concomitant vitamin D analog and phosphate-binder doses are adjusted to attain target ranges for calcium, phosphorus, and PTH (see Table 63.2). Ca, Calcium; IV, intravenously; P, phosphorus; PO, orally; PTH, parathyroid hormone.

interventions in this group differ from those in patients with ESKD.[145-147]

Treatment approaches differ among patients with ESKD, who are receiving renal replacement therapy, and patients with stages 3 to 5 CKD, who have sufficient residual kidney function. For patients with stages 3 to 5 CKD, use of phosphate binders and correction of nutritional vitamin D deficiency are the major interventions, with the possible addition of active vitamin D analogs or calcimimetic agents in patients demonstrating a progressive increase in serum PTH concentration.

It is not clear whether patients with stage 2 CKD (i.e., GFR between 60 and 89 mL/min/1.73 m^2) require treatment, but consideration should be given to dietary phosphate restriction and/or phosphate binders, because adaptive changes in FGF-23 and PTH concentrations are already occurring with mild decrements in GFR. Serum calcium, phosphate, PTH, 25(OH)D, and possibly urinary calcium and FGF-23 levels should be monitored yearly in stage 3 CKD and more frequently (every 3 to 6 months) as kidney function declines. The goal of therapy in stages 3 to 4 CKD is to maintain serum biochemical values in the same range as the general population and to prevent positive phosphate balance. There are several differences in the conceptual framework for treating earlier stages of CKD compared to patients with ESKD

PHOSPHATE-BINDING AGENTS

Dietary phosphorus restriction and the use of phosphate-binding agents are the first therapeutic interventions recommended by the KDOQI guidelines for achieving reductions in plasma PTH concentrations among patients with stages 2 to 4 CKD, even when serum phosphorus concentrations remain within the normal range.[148] Frank hypocalcemia and hyperphosphatemia occur late in the course of CKD. Phosphorus-restricted diets mandate that the intake of dairy products be limited substantially. The calcium content of such diets is often in the range of 500 to 600 mg. Calcium excretion in the urine is reduced in most patients with stage 3 or 4 CKD, a finding that reflects an overall decrease in the efficiency of intestinal calcium absorption.[149,150] Calcium balance tends to be positive in most patients with stage 3 or 4 CKD.[151] The regular provision of loop diuretics augments calciuria and can result in negative calcium balance leading to, or increasing the severity of, SHPT.[152]

Phosphate restriction is of greater importance, because phosphate restriction per se, especially in stages 2 and 3 CKD, can increase endogenous production of 1,25(OH)$_2$D$_3$ and delay the development of SHPT.[153] Several reports indicate that serum phosphate concentrations are directly associated with mortality risk among persons with CKD who do not require dialysis.[154,155]

Dietary phosphate restriction should be started early, certainly in stage 3 CKD but possibly in late stage 2 CKD. The Modification of Diet in Renal Disease equation is frequently used to estimate GFR, but it tends to underestimate GFR in the early stages of CKD; the Chronic Kidney Disease Epidemiology Collaboration equation may yield more accurate estimates of GFR in these ranges.[156,157] Greater attention to measurement of early serum markers, including elevations of FGF-23 (possibly the earliest) and PTH concentrations and fractional excretion of phosphate and calcium, may be needed to guide the timing and intensity of therapy.

Although theoretically there may be a justification for and more flexibility in choice of phosphate binder in patients with residual kidney function, use of phosphate binders in patients with CKD who are not receiving maintenance dialysis is controversial. On the one hand, urinary calcium concentration is lower in patients with CKD, and the patients exhibit inappropriate postprandial calciuria,[158] suggesting that they may have greater tolerance for calcium-based phosphate binders. Calcium-based phosphate binders are effective in lowering serum phosphorus levels and can be used as the initial binder therapy in stages 2, 3, and 4 CKD. In addition, oral doses of calcium in such patients may thus serve to maintain serum calcium concentrations, correct overt hypocalcemia, and avert compensatory secretory responses by the parathyroid glands to maintain calcium homeostasis as kidney function declines. The efficacy of such an approach has not been examined critically, however, in prospective clinical trials among patients with mild to moderate CKD. Calcium excretion in the urine should be measured periodically among patients treated with oral calcium supplements, and doses should be adjusted to avoid hypercalciuria. Although hyperphosphatemia is uncommon among patients with mild to moderate CKD, plasma PTH level is often elevated.[80,145] The PTH-lowering effect of calcium-containing compounds in this clinical context is caused, in part, by increases in intestinal calcium absorption and increases in overall calcium balance. Additional effects mediated indirectly through enhancements in renal 1,25[OH]$_2$D$_3$ synthesis as intestinal phosphorus absorption diminishes and through phosphorus-dependent changes in PTH messenger RNA stability probably also contribute.[153,159,160]

On the other hand, sevelamer hydrochloride resulted in a lower rate of progression of coronary artery calcifications in patients with CKD compared to treatment with phosphate restriction and calcium-based binders.[161,162] In contrast, phosphate binder administration to CKD patients, although lowering serum and urinary phosphorus excretion, increased coronary artery calcification.[29] Currently, phosphate-binding agents are not approved for CKD stages 2, 3, or 4 (or stage 5 not requiring dialysis), although off-label use is fairly common.[163]

VITAMIN D STEROLS

The use of vitamin D analogs in stages 3 and 4 CKD needs to undergo more careful scrutiny, in light of potential conflicting beneficial effects of nutritional vitamin D replacement for low circulating 25(OH)D levels and adverse effects of active vitamin D analogs to enhance phosphate balance and stimulate FGF-23. The dietary intake of vitamin D alone is not sufficient to sustain serum 25(OH)D levels in many groups, including chronically ill patients with CKD.[164,165] The new KDIGO guidelines recommend correction of vitamin D deficiency and insufficiency using treatment strategies recommended for the general population. If 25(OH)D levels are low, treatment with ergocalciferol or cholecalciferol should be considered to restore adequate vitamin D nutrition. Progress has been made in understanding the role of FGF-23 in suppressing 1,25(OH)$_2$D$_3$ production and increasing 25(OH)D and 1,25(OH)$_2$D$_3$ degradation in early

CKD; however, reduction in 25(OH)D and 1,25(OH)$_2$D$_3$ in CKD may be mediated by FGF-23 and designed to attenuate the effects of vitamin D to increase phosphate accumulation.[79] Indeed, cholecalciferol treatment of patients with CKD with low 25(OH)D and elevated FGF-23 concentrations resulted in increases in serum 25(OH)D concentrations that were less than in subjects with normal renal function and were associated with elevated degradative 24,25(OH)D$_2$ levels.[79] Also, the fact that 1,25(OH)$_2$D$_3$ stimulates FGF-23 and the emerging data that elevated FGF-23 concentration may have untoward effects, including progression of CKD,[12] severity of hyperparathyroidism,[11] cardiac function,[166] and increased mortality,[13] suggest that use of high-dose vitamin D analogs in this setting should be limited to patients who have failed phosphate-binder therapy. Also, proteinuria, which results in ongoing losses of vitamin D–binding protein together with vitamin D in the urine, increases the likelihood of vitamin D deficiency among patients with CKD. Serum 25(OH)D levels are thus often reduced markedly in patients with nephrotic-range proteinuria, particularly among patients with diabetes, who may have substantial urinary losses of protein.[167,168]

Ergocalciferol (vitamin D$_2$) and Cholecalciferol (vitamin D$_3$) are derived from plants and animals, respectively. Although there is some data that ergocalciferol is less bioactive, these differences are not clinical relevant. A possible treatment regimen in CKD consists of ergocalciferol at 50,000 IU/wk for 12 weeks and then once monthly for a total of 6 months.[169] With this approach 25(OH)D concentrations are reported to significantly increase (mean concentrations from 16 to 27 ng/mL), while plasma PTH levels decrease (mean concentrations from 231 to 192 ng/dL) in patients with stage 3 CKD. After initiating treatment, serum calcium and phosphorus levels should be monitored quarterly to test for possible overtreatment. In addition, treatment should continue for 6 months, and continued need for supplementation with ergocalciferol should be reevaluated annually.

In patients with persistent SHPT despite phosphate binders and nutritional vitamin D supplementation, consideration can be given to low-dose therapy with active vitamin D analogs. The comparative effects of the different active oral vitamin D analogs in patients with CKD that does not require dialysis have not been studied; consequently there are no data to support use of one of the available active oral agents over another (1,25[OH]$_2$D$_3$, alfacalcidol, doxercalciferol, or paricalcitol).

Daily doses of 0.25 to 0.5 μg of 1,25(OH)$_2$D$_3$ have generally proven to be safe.[170] Marked clinical and biochemical improvements were observed during treatment with 1,25(OH)$_2$D$_3$ among patients with mild to moderate CKD. Bone pain often diminished, muscle strength improved, and plasma PTH concentrations decreased.[171-173] Histologic features of hyperparathyroidism in bone improved,[174,175] and the rate of bone loss from the appendicular skeleton diminished as measured by dual-energy x-ray absorptiometry (DXA).[175] Similar favorable biochemical and histologic responses were reported during treatment with daily oral doses of 1α-hydroxyvitamin D$_3$, or alfacalcidol, which undergoes 25-hydroxylation in the liver to form 1,25(OH)$_2$D$_3$.[176,177]

Treatment with oral doses of doxercalciferol or paricalcitol is an alternative to 1,25(OH)$_2$D$_3$ therapy among patients with SHPT associated with stages 3 and 4 CKD.[149,150] Results from clinical studies in humans and from work in experimental animal models suggest that these compounds are less potent than 1,25(OH)$_2$D$_3$ in promoting intestinal calcium and phosphorus absorption and in raising serum calcium and phosphorus concentrations.[178-181] Both doxercalciferol and paricalcitol effectively lower plasma PTH levels when used to treat SHPT among patients with stages 3 and 4 CKD.[149,150] The effect of treatment with either agent on bone histology has yet to be reported, and the effect of treatment with either doxercalciferol or paricalcitol on bone mass among patients with mild to moderate CKD has not yet been determined. In contrast, the use of daily oral doses of alfacalcidol as compared with placebo controlled plasma PTH levels and was associated with higher bone mass, as measured by DXA, after 18 months of follow-up among patients with stages 3 to 5 CKD.[182] Additional work is needed to characterize adequately the skeletal response to treatment with vitamin D analogs among patients with mild to moderate CKD.

CALCIMIMETIC AGENTS

Unlike in ESKD, where cinacalcet has been shown to be effective in suppressing PTH, calcimimetic agents are not approved for treating SHPT in patients with stages 3 and 4 CKD, where experience with this therapeutic approach is quite limited. Treatment with cinacalcet in patients with stages 3 and 4 CKD has been shown to effectively lower plasma PTH levels, but serum phosphorus concentrations increase and serum calcium concentrations are lowered, thus the resulting hypocalcemia may limit the doses that can be used safely to control SHPT.[133,183,184] As such, concurrent treatment with phosphate-binding compounds may be required to control serum phosphorus levels adequately. The opposing effects of cinacalcet and vitamin D sterols on serum calcium concentrations may permit the use of cinacalcet in patients receiving therapy with active vitamin D analogs. At present, however, cinacalcet should be considered for patients with CKD that does not require dialysis only when severe secondary hyperparathyroidism is present that is refractory to therapy with vitamin D analogs, calcium supplements, and phosphate binders. Cinacalcet may also be used in kidney transplant recipients with hypercalcemia caused by persistent, posttransplantation hyperparathyroidism. In this population, treatment with cinacalcet corrected hypercalcemia and increased serum phosphate concentration.[185]

Complete reference list available at ExpertConsult.com.

KEY REFERENCES

1. Quarles LD: Endocrine functions of bone in mineral metabolism regulation. *J Clin Invest* 118(12):3820–3828, 2008.
2. Wetmore JB, Quarles LD: Calcimimetics or vitamin D analogs for suppressing parathyroid hormone in end-stage renal disease: time for a paradigm shift? *Nat Clin Pract Nephrol* 5(1):24–33, 2009.
3. Krajisnik T, Bjorklund P, Marsell R, et al: Fibroblast growth factor-23 regulates parathyroid hormone and 1alpha-hydroxylase expression in cultured bovine parathyroid cells. *J Endocrinol* 195(1):125–131, 2007.
4. Shimada T, Hasegawa H, Yamazaki Y, et al: FGF-23 is a potent regulator of vitamin D metabolism and phosphate homeostasis. *J Bone Miner Res* 19(3):429–435, 2004.

5. Perwad F, Zhang MY, Tenenhouse HS, et al: Fibroblast growth factor 23 impairs phosphorus and vitamin D metabolism in vivo and suppresses 25-hydroxyvitamin D-1alpha-hydroxylase expression in vitro. *Am J Physiol Renal Physiol* 293(5):F1577–F1583, 2007.
6. Larsson T, Nisbeth U, Ljunggren O, et al: Circulating concentration of FGF-23 increases as renal function declines in patients with chronic kidney disease, but does not change in response to variation in phosphate intake in healthy volunteers. *Kidney Int* 64(6):2272–2279, 2003.
7. Imanishi Y, Inaba M, Nakatsuka K, et al: FGF-23 in patients with end-stage renal disease on hemodialysis. *Kidney Int* 65(5):1943–1946, 2004.
8. Goodman WG: The consequences of uncontrolled secondary hyperparathyroidism and its treatment in chronic kidney disease. *Semin Dial* 17(3):209–216, 2004.
9. Goodman WG, London G, Amann K, et al: Vascular calcification in chronic kidney disease. *Am J Kidney Dis* 43(3):572–579, 2004.
10. Kidney Disease: Improving Global Outcomes (KDIGO) CKD-MBD Work Group: KDIGO clinical practice guideline for the diagnosis, evaluation, prevention, and treatment of chronic kidney disease-mineral and bone disorder (CKD-MBD). *Kidney Int Suppl* 113:S1–S130, 2009.
11. Nakanishi S, Kazama JJ, Nii-Kono T, et al: Serum fibroblast growth factor-23 levels predict the future refractory hyperparathyroidism in dialysis patients. *Kidney Int* 67(3):1171–1178, 2005.
12. Fliser D, Kollerits B, Neyer U, et al: Fibroblast growth factor 23 (FGF23) predicts progression of chronic kidney disease: the Mild to Moderate Kidney Disease (MMKD) study. *J Am Soc Nephrol* 18(9):2600–2608, 2007.
13. Gutierrez OM, Mannstadt M, Isakova T, et al: Fibroblast growth factor 23 and mortality among patients undergoing hemodialysis. *N Engl J Med* 359(6):584–592, 2008.
14. Block GA, Hulbert-Shearon TE, Levin NW, et al: Association of serum phosphorus and calcium x phosphate product with mortality risk in chronic hemodialysis patients: a national study. *Am J Kidney Dis* 31(4):607–617, 1998.
15. Block GA, Martin KJ, de Francisco AL, et al: Cinacalcet for secondary hyperparathyroidism in patients receiving hemodialysis. *N Engl J Med* 350(15):1516–1525, 2004.
16. Martin KJ, Gonzalez EA: Strategies to minimize bone disease in renal failure. *Am J Kidney Dis* 38(6):1430–1436, 2001.
17. Goodman WG: Recent developments in the management of secondary hyperparathyroidism. *Kidney Int* 59(3):1187–1201, 2001.
18. Block C: Association of serum phosphorus and calcium x phosphorus product with mortality risk in chronic hemodialysis patients: a national study. *Am J Kidney Dis* 31:607–617, 1998.
19. Yamada S, Tokumoto M, Tatsumoto N, et al: Phosphate overload directly induces systemic inflammation and malnutrition as well as vascular calcification in uremia. *Am J Physiol* 306:F1418–F1428, 2014.
20. Kovesdy CP, Quarles LD: The role of fibroblast growth factor-23 in cardiorenal syndrome. *Nephron* 123:194–201, 2013.
21. Chang AR, Lazo M, Appel LJ, et al: High dietary phosphorus intake is associated with all-cause mortality: results from NHANES III. *Am J Clin Nutr* 99:320–327, 2014.
22. Kuro-o M: Calciprotein particle (CPP): a true culprit of phosphorus woes? *Nefrologia* 34:1–4, 2014.
23. Smith ER, Ford ML, Tomlinson LA, et al: Serum calcification propensity predicts all-cause mortality in predialysis CKD. *J Am Soc Nephrol* 25:339–348, 2014.
24. Williams KB, DeLuca HF: Characterization of intestinal phosphate absorption using a novel in vivo method. *Am J Physiol Endocrinol Metab* 292(6):E1917–E1921, 2007.
25. Tentori F, Hunt WC, Stidley CA, et al: Mortality risk among hemodialysis patients receiving different vitamin D analogs. *Kidney Int* 70(10):1858–1865, 2006.
26. Shahbazian H, Zafar Mohtashami A, Ghorbani A, et al: Oral nicotinamide reduces serum phosphorus, increases HDL, and induces thrombocytopenia in hemodialysis patients: a double-blind randomized clinical trial. *Nefrologia* 31(1):58–65, 2011.
27. Labonte ED, Carreras CW, Leadbetter MR, et al: Gastrointestinal inhibition of sodium-hydrogen exchanger 3 reduces phosphorus absorption and protects against vascular calcification in CKD. *J Am Soc Nephrol* 26:1138–1149, 2015.
28. Gutierrez OM, Wolf M: Dietary phosphorus restriction in advanced chronic kidney disease: merits, challenges, and emerging strategies. *Semin Dial* 23(4):401–406, 2010.
29. Block GA, Wheeler DC, Persky MS, et al: Effects of phosphate binders in moderate CKD. *J Am Soc Nephrol* 23:1407–1415, 2012.
30. Zhang Q, Li M, Lu Y, et al: Meta-analysis comparing sevelamer and calcium-based phosphate binders on cardiovascular calcification in hemodialysis patients. *Nephron* 115:c259–c267, 2010.
31. Navaneethan SD, Palmer SC, Craig JC, et al: Benefits and harms of phosphate binders in CKD: a systematic review of randomized controlled trials. *Am J Kidney Dis* 54(4):619–637, 2009.
32. Hutchison AJ: Oral phosphate binders. *Kidney Int* 75(9):906–914, 2009.
33. Suki WN, Zabaneh R, Cangiano JL, et al: Effects of sevelamer and calcium-based phosphate binders on mortality in hemodialysis patients. *Kidney Int* 72(9):1130–1137, 2007.
34. Qunibi W, Moustafa M, Muenz LR, et al: A 1-year randomized trial of calcium acetate versus sevelamer on progression of coronary artery calcification in hemodialysis patients with comparable lipid control: the Calcium Acetate Renagel Evaluation-2 (CARE-2) study. *Am J Kidney Dis* 51(6):952–965, 2008.
35. Delmez JA, Slatopolsky E: Hyperphosphatemia: its consequences and treatment in patients with chronic renal disease. *Am J Kidney Dis* 19(4):303–317, 1992.
36. Molitoris BA, Froment DH, Mackenzie TA, et al: Citrate: a major factor in the toxicity of orally administered aluminum compounds. *Kidney Int* 36(6):949–953, 1989.
37. Bakir AA, Hryhorczuk DO, Berman E, et al: Acute fatal hyperaluminemic encephalopathy in undialyzed and recently dialyzed uremic patients. *ASAIO Trans* 32(1):171–176, 1986.
38. Goodman WG, Goldin J, Kuizon BD, et al: Coronary-artery calcification in young adults with end-stage renal disease who are undergoing dialysis. *N Engl J Med* 342(20):1478–1483, 2000.
39. Guerin AP, London GM, Marchais SJ, et al: Arterial stiffening and vascular calcifications in end-stage renal disease. *Nephrol Dial Transplant* 15(7):1014–1021, 2000.
40. Sperschneider H, Gunther K, Marzoll I, et al: Calcium carbonate (CaCO3): an efficient and safe phosphate binder in haemodialysis patients? A 3-year study. *Nephrol Dial Transplant* 8(6):530–534, 1993.
41. Zacharias JM, Fontaine B, Fine A: Calcium use increases risk of calciphylaxis: a case-control study. *Perit Dial Int* 19(3):248–252, 1999.
42. Block GA, Port FK: Re-evaluation of risks associated with hyperphosphatemia and hyperparathyroidism in dialysis patients: recommendations for a change in management. *Am J Kidney Dis* 35(6):1226–1237, 2000.
43. Coburn JW, Norris KC, Nebeker HG: Osteomalacia and bone disease arising from aluminum. *Semin Nephrol* 6(1):68–89, 1986.
44. Froment DP, Molitoris BA, Buddington B, et al: Site and mechanism of enhanced gastrointestinal absorption of aluminum by citrate. *Kidney Int* 36(6):978–984, 1989.
45. Joy MS, Finn WF: Randomized, double-blind, placebo-controlled, dose-titration, phase III study assessing the efficacy and tolerability of lanthanum carbonate: a new phosphate binder for the treatment of hyperphosphatemia. *Am J Kidney Dis* 42(1):96–107, 2003.
46. Hutchison AJ: Calcitriol, lanthanum carbonate, and other new phosphate binders in the management of renal osteodystrophy. *Perit Dial Int* 19(Suppl 2):S408–S412, 1999.
47. Al-Baaj F, Speake M, Hutchison AJ: Control of serum phosphate by oral lanthanum carbonate in patients undergoing haemodialysis and continuous ambulatory peritoneal dialysis in a short-term, placebo-controlled study. *Nephrol Dial Transplant* 20(4):775–782, 2005.
48. Hutchison AJ, Maes B, Vanwalleghem J, et al: Efficacy, tolerability, and safety of lanthanum carbonate in hyperphosphatemia: a 6-month, randomized, comparative trial versus calcium carbonate. *Nephron Clin Pract* 100(1):C8–C19, 2005.
49. Finn WF, Joy MS: A long-term, open-label extension study on the safety of treatment with lanthanum carbonate, a new phosphate binder, in patients receiving hemodialysis. *Curr Med Res Opin* 21(5):657–664, 2005.
50. Hutchison AJ, Maes B, Vanwalleghem J, et al: Long-term efficacy and tolerability of lanthanum carbonate: results from a 3-year study. *Nephron Clin Pract* 102(2):C61–C71, 2006.

64 Drug Dosing Considerations in Patients with Acute Kidney Injury and Chronic Kidney Disease

Gary R. Matzke | Frieder Keller

CHAPTER OUTLINE

EFFECTS OF AKI AND CKD ON DRUG DISPOSITION, 2035
Absorption, 2035
Distribution, 2036
Metabolism, 2037
PHARMACOGENOMICS, 2039
PHARMACODYNAMICS, 2040
ASSESSMENT OF KIDNEY FUNCTION, 2041
Pediatrics, 2043
Acute Kidney Injury, 2043
Patients Receiving Dialysis, 2044
DRUG DOSING CONSIDERATIONS, 2044
Patients with Chronic Kidney Disease, 2044
Patients with Acute Kidney Injury, 2046
Patients Undergoing Hemodialysis, 2046
Patients Receiving Continuous Renal Replacement Therapy, 2048
Patients Undergoing Peritoneal Dialysis, 2049
CLINICAL BOTTOM LINE, 2049

Acute kidney injury (AKI) and chronic kidney disease (CKD) can affect multiple organ systems, and these physiologic changes have been associated with profound alterations in the pharmacokinetics (PK) and pharmacodynamics (PD) of many drugs.[1,2] Clinicians must assess kidney function and consider how kidney function alters the disposition of drugs and their active or toxic metabolites. The number of patients with AKI and CKD and end-stage kidney disease (ESKD) has increased in the last 10 years.[3,4] Independent of injury or disease, kidney function tends to decrease with age, and older patients constitute an ever-increasing group for whom the optimization of drug therapy is crucial.[5] The widespread use of alternative renal replacement therapies for treating AKI (e.g., continuous venovenous hemodiafiltration) and ESKD (frequent and/or nocturnal hemodialysis or hemodiafiltration) during the last decade mandate an understanding of their influences on drug disposition.[6] When comparing outcomes of different dialytic modalities, rarely has the effect on drug disposition been considered.[3,6-8] Although innovation in peritoneal dialysis has been more modest, few studies have examined the effects of newer adequacy targets, or the use of nondextrose-containing peritoneal dialysates on drug disposition.

Data on the use of many drugs in patients with CKD, as well as the impact of dialysis, are often limited or absent at the time of regulatory approval. Patients with moderate to advanced CKD are typically excluded from participation in major safety and efficacy studies required for drug registration. Although regulatory authorities now require a pediatric investigation plan as a routine part of drug development, they have not yet responded to the challenge of ensuring robust data for patients with impaired kidney function.[1] Indeed, significant differences exist with respect to the means of assessment and classification of the degree of impaired kidney function.[9] Thus, some recommendations are not concordant as to whether drug dose adjustment is necessary at all.[10] The availability of robust and readily applicable information to guide prescribing for patients with kidney disease remains imprecise and relies on interpolation, extrapolation, and estimation.[11,12] Optimization of CKD and AKI patient care is dependent on the clinician's knowledge of basic biochemical and physiologic understanding of drug disposition as well as individual experience with the effects of renal replacement therapies (RRTs) on drug and metabolite removal.

In the 1970s, with the advent of specific and sensitive analytic techniques, the pharmaceutical industry began to investigate the relationship of kidney function to the pharmacokinetics and pharmacodynamics of the drugs they had in development. Until the 1990s, there remained no

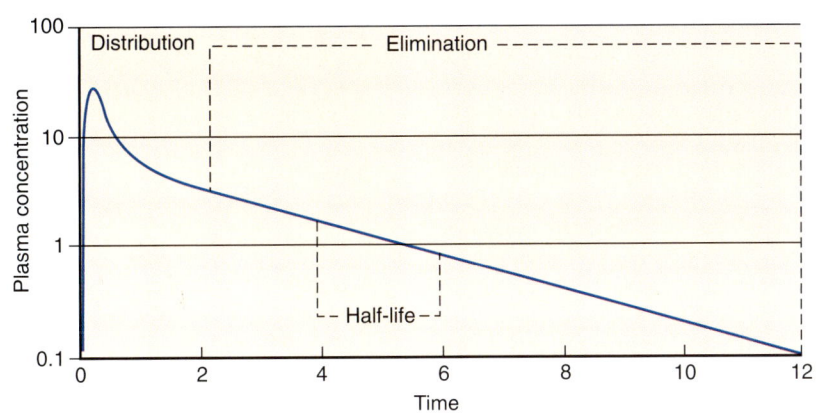

Figure 64.1 Distribution and elimination of a drug after intravenous administration.

regulatory guidance or clinical consensus for when investigations should be conducted and with what degree of rigor. Thus, much of the data on the PK of drugs in patients with kidney disease was the result of clinician-initiated, postmarketing studies. These resulted in the publication of inconsistent and, in some cases, conflicting recommendations regarding adjustments in drug dose or frequency of administration.[1] Critical issues include characterization of the degree of impact of AKI or CKD on a drug's disposition, pharmacodynamics, and/or dependence on pharmacogenetics, identification of the most reliable index of kidney function for drug dosing, determination of the desired therapeutic endpoints, significance of risks associated with the accumulation of drug and/or metabolite concentrations, predictive performance of various methodologies to calculate the desired dosage regimen, and quantification of the influence of RRTs on drug disposition.

In this chapter, the influence of AKI and CKD on drug pharmacokinetic properties is characterized, and a guide for individualizing drug therapy in patients with AKI and CKD is presented, along with dosage recommendations for many commonly used drugs. The role of pharmacodynamic measures alone or in combination with pharmacokinetics, as well as pharmacogenetic testing in drug dosage regimen design, is discussed. The impact of maintenance dialysis for ESKD and continuous RRT (CRRT) for patients with AKI on drug disposition are discussed, and dosage recommendations for most critical drugs are presented.

EFFECTS OF AKI AND CKD ON DRUG DISPOSITION

Pharmacokinetics describes the time course of drug absorption, distribution, metabolism, and elimination. Pharmacodynamics provides a characterization of the complex interaction of drug concentrations, receptor-drug interactions, mechanism of action, and clinical factors, such as concurrent diseases and degree of organ dysfunction on patients' response to drug therapy. The combination of PK and PD drug characteristics allows clinicians with foundational information to make rational prescribing decisions.

When given intravenously (IV), a rapid decrease in the plasma concentration follows an initial high drug concentration. This decrease occurs as the drug distributes from the plasma into the extravascular space and beyond. During the terminal elimination phase, drug concentrations in plasma are in equilibrium with concentrations in body tissues (Figure 64.1). The rate and extent of drug absorption and distribution and rate of drug elimination may be ascertained by mathematical analysis of the serum or plasma concentration data collected over an appropriate time interval. The terminal elimination half-life of a drug is the time required for the plasma concentration to decline by 50%; this it can be determined from the slope of the elimination phase of the plot of serum or plasma drug concentration versus time after the drug is ingested or injected. By comparing PK data from patients with normal kidney function with data from patients with impaired kidney function, rational drug dosing regimens may be proposed.[11-13]

ABSORPTION

Drugs given IV enter the central circulation directly and generally have a rapid onset of action. Drugs given by other routes must first pass through important organs of elimination before entering the systemic circulation; thus, a smaller proportion of the drug reaches the systemic circulation. In many cases, only a fraction of the administered dose may reach the circulation and become available at the site of drug action. Even drugs given IV and by inhalation must pass though the lungs before reaching arterial blood. Similar to other organs, the lungs remove substantial amounts of some agents. For drugs administered orally, the rate and extent of gastrointestinal (GI) absorption are important considerations. Absorption has been characterized by determining the maximum attained serum or plasma concentration (C_{max}), as well as the time after ingestion when the C_{max} was observed (T_{max}). Differences in these two parameters among patient groups were historically considered evidence of altered GI absorption when actually the bioavailability may have been unchanged.[14] The bioavailability of a drug depends on the extent of metabolism during its first pass through the GI tract and liver before reaching the systemic circulation. The absolute bioavailability is determined by comparing the area under the serum/plasma concentration-time curve (AUC) after oral administration to that observed after IV administration.

When this measure of bioavailability was assessed, there were very few drugs shown to be affected by the presence of CKD or AKI.[15]

First-pass biotransformation may also occur in the gut; bioflavonoids in grapefruit juice can inhibit cytochrome P 450 (CYP) 3A4 and noncompetitively inhibit the metabolism of drugs metabolized by this enzyme. This grapefruit juice–CYP3A4 interaction was first noted with the calcium channel blocker felodipine.[16] This interaction also increases the bioavailability of cyclosporine by as much as 20%.[17] A wide variety of other drugs are similarly affected, including several medications used for depression and anxiety (e.g., selective serotonin reuptake inhibitors [SSRIs], serotonin-norepinephrine reuptake inhibitors [SNRIs]) and statins.[18] Herbal medicine (e.g., hypericin) can activate the adenosine triphosphate (ATP)–binding cassette (ABC) transporter or P-glycoprotein (multidrug resistance) transporter in gut mucosa, leading to reduced drug absorption.[19]

Although GI symptoms are common in patients with ESKD, little specific information about alimentary function is available. The salivary concentration of urea increases when urea accumulates in plasma. Ammonia forms from urea in the presence of gastric urease and buffers gastric acid, increasing gastric pH. The ammonia is absorbed and converted to urea again by the liver. The gastric alkalinizing effect of this internal urea-ammonia cycle decreases the absorption of drugs that are best absorbed in an acidic environment. Drug malabsorption may be further aggravated by the increased use of various therapies to reduce gastric acidity and/or reduce phosphate absorption, especially in patients who are dialysis-dependent.[14,20,21] The resultant chelation and formation of nonabsorbable complexes reduce the bioavailability of some drugs, including several antibiotics and digoxin.

The processes of GI drug absorption are complex, may be saturable and dose-dependent, and are more variable in patients with ESKD than in those with normal kidney function.[22] Gastroparesis, commonly observed in patients with diabetes mellitus, many of whom also have CKD, prolongs gastric emptying and delays drug absorption; that is, T_{max} is observed to be delayed. Conversely, diarrhea decreases gut transit time (T_{max} is shortened and diminishes drug absorption by the small bowel). Gut mucosal integrity becomes impaired across the spectrum of CKD, as evidenced by increasing levels of circulating translocated endotoxins.[23]

DISTRIBUTION

The volume of distribution of a drug does not necessarily correspond to a specific anatomic space. Rather, the volume of distribution is a mathematical construct based on the plasma concentration achieved following the IV administration of a given dose of a drug. Agents that are highly protein-bound and those that are water-soluble tend to be restricted to the vascular compartment and extracellular fluid (ECF) space, respectively, and thus have volumes of distribution less than 0.20 L/kg. Highly lipid-soluble drugs and those extensively bound to tissues often exhibit volumes of distribution in excess of 1 L/kg. The drug distribution volume of highly water-soluble or protein-bound drugs may be increased in patients with AKI or CKD if edema and/or ascites is present (Table 64.1).[2,5,13,15,24] Drug distribution is one of the most important and complicated factors to quantify in patients with AKI. There is a fine balance between detrimental fluid overload and adequate hydration to preserve and optimize perfusion and function. Critically ill patients should be managed in a slightly negative fluid balance after initial adequate fluid resuscitation has been achieved.[25-29] If patients are volume-expanded, the administration of the usual doses of many drugs will result in inadequately low plasma concentrations.

The distribution volume of drugs may be altered by fluid removal during dialysis.[30] Changes in body cell mass (nonfat, nonwater, nonbone mineral mass) commonly occur over time in patients on dialysis,[31] resulting in sarcopenia. Failure to detect a reduction in body cell mass may lead to inappropriate maintenance of the same dry weight and drug dosage regimen, despite a real increase in total body water[32] (and thus the distribution volume of several drugs).

Finally, the method used to calculate the volume of distribution may be influenced by impaired kidney function. The three most commonly used volume of distribution terms are volume of the central compartment (V_c), volume of the terminal phase (V_β and V_{area}), and volume of distribution at steady state (V_{ss}). The V_c for many drugs approximates extracellular fluid volume and thus may be increased or decreased by acute changes. Oliguric acute renal failure is often accompanied by fluid overload and a resultant increased V_c for many drugs. The V_{area} or V_β represents the proportionality constant between plasma concentrations in the terminal elimination phase and the amount of drug remaining in the body. V_β is affected by distribution characteristics and by the terminal elimination rate constant. V_β

Table 64.1 Volume of Distribution of Selected Drugs in Patients with Normal Kidney Function and Those on Dialysis

Drug	Normal (L/kg)	Stage 5 CKD (L/kg)	Change from Normal (%)
Increased			
Amikacin	0.20	0.29	45
Cefazolin	0.13	0.17	31
Cefoxitin	0.16	0.26	63
Ceftriaxone	0.28	0.48	71
Cefuroxime	0.20	0.26	30
Doripenem	0.25	0.47	88
Dicloxacillin	0.08	0.18	125
Erythromycin	0.57	1.09	91
Furosemide	0.11	0.18	64
Gentamicin	0.20	0.32	60
Isoniazid	0.6	0.8	33
Minoxidil	2.6	4.9	88
Phenytoin	0.64	1.4	119
Trimethoprim	1.36	1.83	35
Vancomycin	0.64	0.85	33
Decreased			
Chloramphenicol	0.87	0.60	−31
Digoxin	7.3	4.0	−45
Ethambutol	3.7	1.6	−57

Data from references 2, 5, 13, and 15.

PROTEIN BINDING DEFECT IN UREMIA

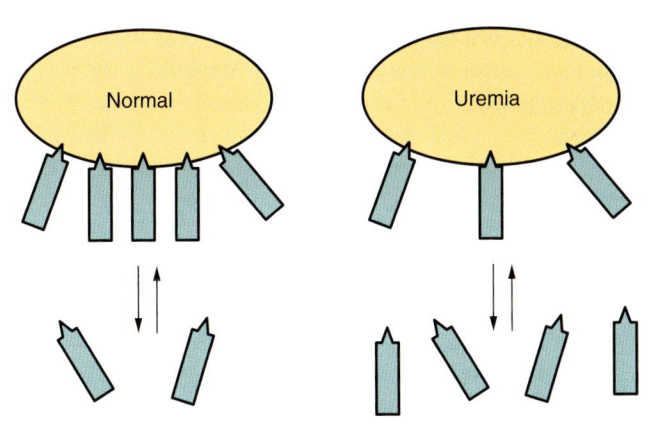

Figure 64.2 Protein-binding defect in uremia. Displacement of the drug from its binding site by an accumulation of undefined uremic toxins or a uremia-induced conformational change in the binding site geometry results in more free drug in the plasma.

Table 64.2 Unbound Fraction of Selected Drugs in Patients with Normal Kidney Function and End-Stage Kidney Disease (ESKD)

Drug	Normal Patient	ESKD Patient	Change from Normal (%)
Acidic Drugs			
Abecarnil	4	15	275
Azlocillin	62.5	75	20
Cefazolin	16	29	81
Cefoxitin	27	59	119
Ceftriaxone	10	20	100
Clofibrate	3	9	200
Dicloxacillin	3	9	200
Diflunisal	12	44	267
Doxycycline	12	28	133
Furosemide	4	6	50
Methotrexate	57.2	63.8	12
Metolazone	5	10	100
Moxalactam	48	64	33
Pentobarbital	34	41	21
Phenytoin	10	21.5	115
Salicylate	8	20	150
Sulfamethoxazole	34	58	71
Valproic acid	8	23	188
Warfarin	1	2	100
Basic Drugs			
Decreased			
Bepridil	0.3	0.1	−67
Clonidine	55.6	47.6	−14
Disopyramide	32	28	−13
Propafenone	3.4	2.4	−29
Increased			
Amphotericin B	3.5	4.1	17
Chloramphenicol	45	64	42
Clonazepam	13.9	16	15
Diazepam	2	8	300
Fluoxetine	5.5	6.5	18
Ketoconazole	1	1.5	50
Prazosin	6	10.1	68
Rosiglitazone	0.16	0.22	38
Triamterene	19	43	126

and V_{ss} will often be similar in magnitude, with V_β being slightly larger. Because V_{ss} has the advantage of being independent of drug elimination, it is the most appropriate volume term to use when it is desirable to compare drug distribution volumes between patients with renal insufficiency and those with normal renal function.[33]

Alterations of plasma protein binding in patients with CKD can also affect drug action. The volume of distribution of a drug, quantity of unbound drug available for action, and degree to which the agent is eliminated by hepatic or renal excretion are all influenced by protein binding. Drugs that are protein-bound attach reversibly to albumin or α1-glycoprotein in plasma (Figure 64.2). Whereas organic acids bind to a single binding site, organic bases probably have multiple sites of attachment.[34,35]

Protein-bound organic acids such as hippuric acid, indoxyl sulfate, and 3-carboxy-4-methyl-5-propyl-2-furanpropionic acid (CMPF) accumulate in advanced CKD and decrease the protein binding of many acidic drugs.[36-38] A combination of decreased serum albumin concentration and reduction in albumin affinity for the drug reduces protein binding in dialysis-dependent patients. Even when the plasma albumin concentration is normal, the protein-binding defect of some drugs correlates directly with the level of azotemia and may be corrected with dialysis.[5,8,34] Binding affinity is influenced by changes in the structural orientation of the albumin molecule or by the accumulation of endogenous inhibitors of protein binding that compete with drugs for their binding sites.[34]

The unbound fraction of several acidic drugs are increased in CKD because of impaired plasma protein binding. Toxicity can occur if the total plasma concentration of these drugs is pushed into the therapeutic range by increasing the dose, wherein the free (active) concentration may be in the supratherapeutic range. For such drugs, unbound plasma concentrations should be measured to guide therapy. The need to measure unbound drug concentrations applies especially to drugs with very narrow therapeutic ranges, such as phenytoin.[39] Predicting the clinical consequences of altered protein binding is difficult. Although decreased binding results in more unbound drug being available at the site of drug action or toxicity, the distribution volume is increased, resulting in lower plasma concentrations after a given dose. More unbound drug is available for metabolism and excretion, which increases the clearance and decreases the half-life of the drug in the body. Drugs with decreased protein binding in patients on dialysis are listed in Table 64.2.

METABOLISM

The disposition of drugs metabolized by the liver may be altered by changes in plasma protein binding. The systemic clearance of a highly protein-bound drug with a low hepatic extraction ratio depends on the simultaneous effects of AKI or CKD on protein binding and intrinsic metabolic drug clearance. Because the effects of severe CKD on these two factors offset each other in terms of total systemic clearance, the lowest total systemic clearance is not seen in patients with ESKD but rather occurs in patients with moderate to severe CKD. The systemic clearance of drugs with a high hepatic extraction ratio is not thought to be as susceptible to the effect of CKD as that of drugs with a low extraction ratio.[40]

Many active or toxic metabolites depend on the kidneys for their removal from the body. The accumulation of these metabolites in patients with impaired kidney function (AKI and CKD) can explain in part the high incidence of adverse drug reactions in this patient population. For example, although the liver usually rapidly metabolizes morphine, it is excreted mainly in the urine because its active metabolites, morphine-3-glucuronide (M3G) and morphine-6-glucuronide (M6G) readily cross the blood-brain barrier and bind to opiate receptors, exerting strong analgesic effects. In patients with CKD, morphine itself is metabolized more slowly, and these active metabolites increase, making prolonged narcosis and respiratory depression more likely.[41,42] Similarly, the biotransformation of meperidine results in the production of normeperidine, a more polar metabolite that is normally rapidly excreted in the urine. Normeperidine has little to no analgesic activity but lowers the seizure threshold. In patients with impaired kidney function, repeated doses of meperidine may result in the accumulation of this potentially toxic metabolite, with resultant seizures.[43] Table 64.3 lists some drugs that form active or toxic metabolites in CKD patients and have been associated with adverse outcomes.

ALTERATIONS OF CYTOCHROME P450 ENZYME ACTIVITY

A decrease in the renal clearance of drugs in patients with CKD is well appreciated. However, there is now preclinical and emerging clinical evidence suggesting that advanced CKD (stages 4 and 5) may lead to reductions in the nonrenal clearance of many medications as the result of alterations in the activities of uptake and efflux transporters, as well as CYP enzymes, in the liver and other organs (Table 64.4).[35,44-49] The effect(s) of AKI and CKD on nonrenal drug clearance appear to depend on whether the reduction in renal function is acute or chronic in nature—and likely stronger in CKD.

Preservation of nonrenal metabolic clearance has been observed early in the course of AKI,[50-53] and thus drug dosing schemes extrapolated from those with stable CKD may therefore result in ineffectively low drug concentrations. Furthermore, failure to appreciate that changes in serum creatinine levels are not an accurate marker of the glomerular filtration rate (GFR) early in AKI may lead to further dosing errors. The first reports of nonrenal clearance of drugs being affected by AKI came from the observation that the residual nonrenal clearances for vancomycin, meropenem, and imipenem were higher in patients with AKI compared to patients with CKD, who had comparable creatinine clearance (CrCl).[51-53]

Most of the direct evidence on metabolism in the presence of AKI has been derived from investigations in animal models. A number of drugs have been studied in a variety

Table 64.3 Drugs with Pharmacologically Active Metabolites that May Affect Efficacy or Toxicity in Patients with Severe Chronic Kidney Disease

Parent Drug	Metabolite	Pharmacologic Activity of Metabolites
Acetaminophen	N-Acetyl-p-benzo-quinoneimine	Responsible for hepatotoxicity
Allopurinol	Oxipurinol	Metabolite primarily responsible for suppression of xanthine oxidase
Azathioprine	Mercaptopurine	All immunosuppressive activity resides in the metabolite.
Cefotaxime	Desacetyl cefotaxime	Similar antimicrobial spectrum, but 10% to 25% as potent
Chlorpropamide	2-Hydroxychlorpropamide	Similar in vitro insulin-releasing activity
Clofibrate	Chlorophenoxyisobutyric acid	Primarily responsible for hypolipidemic effect and direct muscle toxicity
Codeine	Morphine-6-glucuronide	Possibly more active than parent compound; may contribute to prolonged narcotic effect in renal failure patients
Imipramine	Desmethylimipramine	Similar antidepressant activity
Ketoprofen	Ketoprofen glucuronide	Accumulation of acyl glucuronide may worsen toxic effects (GI disturbances, impairment of kidney function)
Meperidine	Normeperidine	Less analgesic activity than parent, but more central nervous system stimulatory effects, epileptogenic
Morphine	Morphine-6-glucuronide	Possibly more active than parent compound; may contribute to prolonged narcotic effect in ESKD
Mycophenolic acid	Mycophenolic acid glucuronide	Lacks pharmacologic activity but may be associated with dose-limiting (GI) side effects
Procainamide	N-Acetyl procainamide	Distinct antiarrhythmic activity; mechanism different from that of parent compound
Sulfonamides	Acetylated metabolites	Devoid of antibacterial activity; elevated concentrations associated with increased toxicity
Theophylline	1,3-Dimethyl uric acid	Cardiotoxicity has been demonstrated.
Zidovudine	Zidovudine triphosphate	Primarily responsible for antiretroviral activity

Table 64.4 Major Pathways of Nonrenal Drug Clearance (Cl$_{NR}$)

Cl$_{NR}$ Pathway	Selected Substrates
Oxidative Enzymes	
CYP1A2	Polycyclic aromatic hydrocarbons, caffeine, imipramine, theophylline
CYP2A6	Coumarin
CYP2B6	Nicotine, bupropion
CYP2C8	Retinoids, paclitaxel, repaglinide
CYP2C9	Celecoxib, diclofenac, flurbiprofen, indomethacin, ibuprofen, losartan, phenytoin, tolbutamide, S-warfarin
CYP2C19	Diazepam, S-mephenytoin, omeprazole
CYP2D6	Codeine, debrisoquine, desipramine, dextromethorphan, fluoxetine, paroxetine, duloxetine, nortriptyline, haloperidol, metoprolol, propranolol
CYP2E1	Ethanol, acetaminophen, chlorzoxazone, nitrosamines
CYP3A4/5	Alprazolam, midazolam, cyclosporine, tacrolimus, nifedipine, felodipine, diltiazem, verapamil, fluconazole, ketoconazole, itraconazole, erythromycin, lovastatin, simvastatin, cisapride, terfenadine
Conjugative Enzymes	
UGT	Acetaminophen, morphine, lorazepam, oxazepam, naproxen, ketoprofen, irinotecan, bilirubin
NAT	Dapsone, hydralazine, isoniazid, procainamide

Data from references 35, 44-49.

of AKI models. AKI is a heterogenous insult that is often part of multisystem failure of cellular respiration and can have in various consequences.[54-57] CYP enzymes are affected by AKI, and the extent of these effects may depend on the mechanism of experimental AKI. Definitive conclusions on the pharmacokinetics of metabolized medications in AKI remain hampered by the clinical complexity and potential confounders; hypoxia, decreased protein synthesis, competitive inhibition from concomitant medications, and decreased hepatic perfusion could also contribute to the reduced clearance.

In humans with CKD, the activities of CYPs appear to be relatively unaffected.[46,49,58] It has been reported that CYP3A4 activity is reduced,[45-47,49] but recent studies have indicated that organic anion transporting polypeptide (OATP) uptake activity is decreased. Thus, the perceived changes in CYP3A4 activity were likely due to altered transporter activity, not to an alteration in CYP activity. The reduction of nonrenal clearance of several drugs that exhibit overlapping CYP and transporter substrate specificity in patients with stage 4 or 5 CKD supports this premise. These studies must be interpreted with caution, however, because concurrent drug intake, age, smoking status, and alcohol intake were often not taken into consideration. Furthermore, pharmacogenetic variations in drug-metabolizing enzymes that may have been present in the individual before the onset of AKI or CKD must also be considered.

RENAL EXCRETION

Renal clearance (Cl$_R$) of a drug is the composite of the GFR, tubular secretion, metabolism, and reabsorption [(Cl$_R$ = (GFR × f$_u$) + (Cl$_{secretion}$ + Cl$_{metabolism}$ − Cl$_{reabsorption}$)], where f$_u$ is the fraction of the drug unbound to plasma proteins. Drug elimination by filtration occurs by a pressure gradient, whereas tubular secretion and reabsorption are bidirectional processes that involve carrier-mediated renal transport systems.[49,59-61] Renal transport systems have been broadly classified on the basis of substrate selectivity into anionic and cationic renal transport systems, which are responsible for the transport of a number of organic acidic and basic drugs, respectively.[35,49] Several drugs are actively secreted by one or more of these transporter families, including organic cationic (e.g., famotidine, trimethoprim, dopamine), organic anionic (e.g., ampicillin, cefazolin, furosemide), nucleoside (e.g., zidovudine), and P-glycoprotein transporters (e.g., digoxin, vinca alkaloids, steroids).[52,60] Alterations in filtration, secretion, or reabsorption secondary to CKD may have a dramatic effect on drug disposition. For drugs that are primarily filtered, a reduction in GFR will result in a proportional decrease in renal drug clearance.

PHARMACOGENOMICS

Over the last 2 decades, genome-wide analyses have identified genetic variants that are associated with the risk of several diseases,[62,63] although most confer a very low relative risk and have low discriminatory and predictive values.[64,65] The variability in how patients respond to drug treatments is a consequence of alterations in pharmacokinetics and pharmacodynamics, as outlined in this chapter, as well as differences in their genotypes and/or phenotypes.[63,66-72] The validity of phenotyping cocktails and their correlation with genotyping data are still in need of clarification.[73] Genotyping information is becoming more widely available than phenotyping data by clinicians and patients and this is bringing in demands for a more individualized approach to pharmacotherapy. Genotypic characterization now serves as the basis for dosing recommendations for some drugs,[74-77] and more than 120 U.S. Food and Drug Administration (FDA)–approved drugs have pharmacogenomic information in their labeling, including fluoropyrimidines, codeine, SSRIs, tricyclic antidepressants, β-blockers, opiates, neuroleptics, antiarrhythmic agents, and statins.[78] However, the promise of pharmacogenomics has not always translated into improvements in patient care because of the inaccuracy of results and the complexities involved.[79,80] In late 2013, FDA approved four diagnostic, high-throughput, gene-sequencing devices, which represents a significant step forward in the ability to generate genomic information that will ultimately improve patient care.[81] As Collins and Hamburg from the National Institutes of health (NIH) and FDA have stated, "There are many challenges ahead before personalized medicine can be considered truly embedded in health care. We need to continue to uncover variants within the genome that can be used to predict disease onset, affect progression, and modulate drug response."[80] New genomic findings need to be validated before they can be integrated into medical decision making. Physicians and other health care professionals will need support in interpreting genomic data, integrating it into clinical decision making, and applying the results to individual patients. With the right information and support, patients will be able to participate with their physicians in making more informed decisions.

As an example of the complexity of individualizing drug therapy on the basis of genomic information, the commonly prescribed anticoagulant, warfarin, may be considered. Two recently published trials raise significant questions regarding the value of genomic data to guide the initial dosing of this agent.[82,83] A genotype-guided approach to warfarin dosing failed to improve anticoagulation control during the first 4 weeks of treatment, according to the first of the articles.[82] Among 1015 patients assigned to usual care or usual care plus genotype, international normalized ratio (INR) results showed that the mean percentage of time in the therapeutic range at 4 weeks was 45.2% in the genotype-guided group and 45.4% in the usual care group. Moreover, rates of the combined outcome of any INR of 4 or more, major bleeding, or thromboembolism did not differ significantly according to dosing strategy.

The second study reported conflicting results in that pharmacogenetic-based dosing was associated with a slightly but significantly higher percentage of time in the therapeutic INR range, with significantly fewer incidences of excessive anticoagulation (INR ≥ 4.0) in the genotype-guided group. Thus, at present, there are insufficient data indicating a therapeutic benefit related to genomic information in persons with normal kidney function, much less those with CKD or AKI.[84]

PHARMACODYNAMICS

The fundamental concept of pharmacodynamics is described by the Hill equation. This model has been extensively used to optimize the effects of most antimicrobial agents.[85] The principles are applicable to guide the dosing of medications in patients with CKD, as well as those with normal kidney function. In the patient with CKD, the concentration time profile of many drugs is altered, so the dosage regimen predicted will likely be different than the normal regimen. This is because of the prolonged elimination half-life, which results in an increased area under the concentration-time curve. Only rarely has there been evidence of an alteration in the concentration effect relation in patients with AKI or CKD; pharmacokinetic changes predominantly contribute to the need for a modified dosing regimen.

The concentration (C) is the primary driving force that obligates altered dosage regimens to achieve the desired pharmacodynamic targets. The actual effect is a function of the maximum effect and the concentration producing the half-maximum effect. The Hill coefficient (H) is a measure of the sigmoidicity of the effect-concentration correlation:

$$E = \frac{E_{max}}{1 - \left(\frac{CE_{50}}{C}\right)^H}$$

From this equation, the threshold concentration, which produces 5% of the maximum effect, and the ceiling concentration, which is associated with 95% of the maximum effect, can be derived. The higher the Hill coefficient, the higher the threshold concentration and the narrower is the range of lower and upper target concentrations; this is because the ceiling concentration comes down close to the concentration producing the half-maximum effect (Figure 64.3):

$$CE_{05} = 19^{\frac{-1}{H}} \bullet CE_{50}$$

$$CE_{95} = 19^{\frac{1}{H}} \bullet CE_{50}$$

The difference between the ceiling and threshold concentrations can be measured by multiples of the respective elimination half-life. The ceiling concentration is the upper limit of the targeted peak concentration ($C_{peak} < CE_{95}$), whereas the threshold concentration marks the lower limit

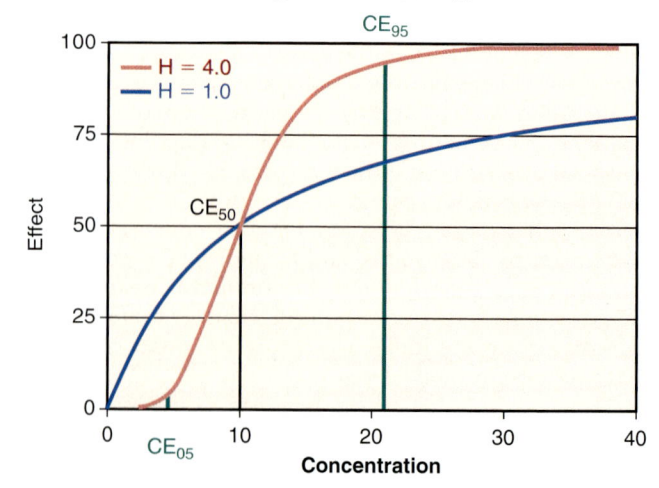

Figure 64.3 Threshold concentration, CE_{05}, producing 5% of the maximum effect and ceiling concentration, CE_{95}, producing 95% of the maximum effect. With a Hill coefficient of H = 1.0, CE_{05} = 0.5 and CE_{95} = 190, whereas for H = 4.0, the threshold is higher, with CE_{05} = 6.0, but the ceiling is much less, with CE_{95} = 21 mg/L.

of effective trough concentration ($Ct_{rough} > CE_{05}$). For a drug with a short half-life ($t_{1/2}$) and a high Hill coefficient, the therapeutic range of target concentrations can be very small (see Figure 64.3):

$$CE_{05} = CE_{95} \bullet \exp\left(-\frac{\ln(2)}{t_{1/2}} \bullet t\right)$$

$$t_{ceiling-threshold} = t_{1/2} \bullet \frac{2}{H} \bullet \frac{\ln(19)}{\ln(2)}$$

$$t_{ceiling-threshold} = t_{1/2} \bullet \frac{8.5}{H}$$

For the β-lactam ceftazidime, with a short half-life of 2.1 hours in patients with normal kidney function but with a high Hill coefficient of 3.7,[86] the peak to trough or ceiling to threshold time of 5 hours indicates that ceftazidime should be given at least every 6 hours to maximize efficacy. In contrast, and in agreement with the postulated postantibiotic effect, the maximum peak to trough time is estimated as 13 hours for gentamicin, with a half-life of 2 hours but a Hill coefficient of 1.3.[86]

The most important progress in anti-infective dosing has been achieved with the differentiation of drugs with time-dependent actions from drugs with concentration-dependent actions.[87,88] Specific examples are the β-lactam-antibiotics and antiviral drugs with a known time-dependent effect, whereas aminoglycosides and quinolones have a concentration-dependent activity. The threshold and ceiling concentrations are specific functions of the concentration producing the half-maximum effect and the Hill coefficient. Both explain the observation that anti-infective drugs with a time-dependent effect have a significantly higher Hill coefficient than those with a concentration-dependent action.[86] A high Hill coefficient is associated with a high threshold concentration but, simultaneously, with a relatively low ceiling concentration. Thus, it makes no sense to increase the dose of time-dependent anti-infective drugs above the ceiling concentration. In contrast, a low Hill coefficient is associated with a high ceiling concentration and low threshold concentration. Thus, it might increase the effect of concentration-dependent anti-infective drugs to give a high single dose but it is not so critical to extend the administration interval, as proposed for aminoglycosides.[89] Practically, it is necessary to administer anti-infective drugs with a time-dependent action more frequently, whereas anti-infective drugs with a concentration-dependent action should be given with a higher maintenance dose to increase efficacy (Figure 64.4).

Usual measures of the antimicrobial effect, such as the time over minimal inhibitory concentrations (MICs), AUC over MIC, time over MIC, or peak over MIC, can be unified to the following concept. The target concentration should not be less than the threshold concentration for time-dependent effects, but the target concentration could be as high as the ceiling concentration for concentration-dependent effects. A close correlation of the MIC and concentration producing the half-maximum effect has been shown.[86] It was obvious, however, that for concentration-dependent antimicrobial action, the MIC could fall considerably below the concentration producing

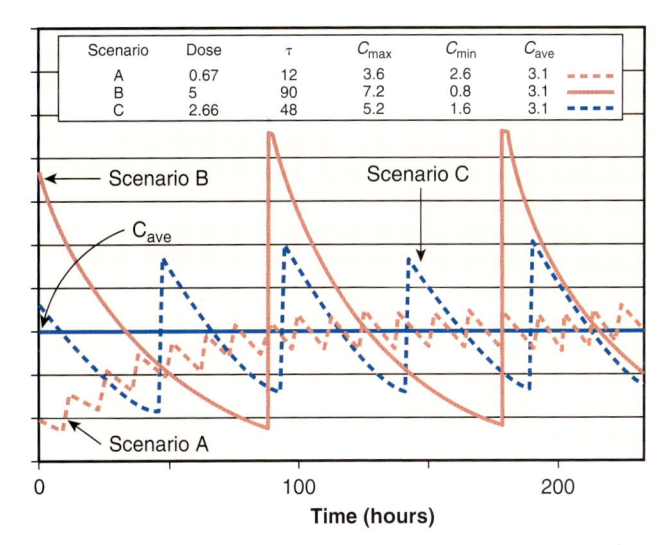

Scenario	Dose	τ	C_{max}	C_{min}	C_{ave}
A	0.67	12	3.6	2.6	3.1
B	5	90	7.2	0.8	3.1
C	2.66	48	5.2	1.6	3.1

Figure 64.4 Although the average steady-state concentrations (C_{ave}) are identical regardless of which dosage adjustment strategy one decides to use, the concentration-time profile will be markedly different if one changes the dose and maintains the dosing interval (τ) constant (Scenario A), versus changing the dosing interval and maintaining the dose constant (Scenario B) or changing both (Scenario C).

the half-maximum effect (MIC ≪ CE_{50}). Consequently, it might be more reasonable to compare the bacteriologic MIC with the pharmacodynamic parameter of a threshold concentration:

$$CE_{threshold} = CE_{05} = MIC$$

From the Hill coefficient, one can postulate that the time-dependent action and concentration-dependent action are only the extreme positions of a continuum. Every drug can be considered as concentration-dependent and time-dependent. To overcome resistance, a higher dose might be necessary, because relative resistance can be seen in cases in which a high concentration is required to produce the half-maximum effect. The potency is the inverse concentration producing the half-maximum effect:

$$Potency = \frac{1}{CE_{50}}$$

This concept distinguishes a relative resistance from an absolute drug resistance. A pathogen with a relative resistance can be made sensitive by increasing the dose.[90-92] Thus, for example, it has been recommended to treat severe infections with resistant strains by increasing the standard meropenem dose to 2000 mg/day, three times daily,[93] or the daptomycin dose to more than 8 mg/kg/day,[94] with careful monitoring of side effects.

ASSESSMENT OF KIDNEY FUNCTION

The standard measure of kidney function for decades has been the GFR.[61] The GFR can be measured using many

Table 64.5 Equations for Estimation of Creatinine Clearance or Glomerular Filtration Rate in Adults with Stable Renal Function

Reference	Equation
Cockcroft and Gault (1976)	Men: CrCl = (140 − age)IBW/(sCr × 72) Women: CrCl × 0.85
Jelliffe (1973)	Men: CrCl = 98 − [0.8 (age − 20)]/sCr Women: CrCl × 0.9
MDRD6 (1999)	eGFRcr = 170 × (sCr)$^{-0.999}$ × (age)$^{-0.176}$ × (0.762 if patient is female) × (1.180 if patient is black) × (BUN)$^{-0.170}$ × (Alb)$^{0.318}$
MDRD4 (2000)	eGFRcr = 186 × (sCr)$^{-1.154}$ × (age)$^{-0.203}$ × (0.742 if patient is female) × (1.210 if patient is black)
MDRD4-IDMS (2007)	eGFRcr = 175 × (sCr)$^{-1.154}$ × (age)$^{-0.203}$ × (0.742 if patient is female) × (1.210 if patient is black)
CKD-EPI (2009)	eGFRcr = 141 × min(sCr/κ, 1)^α × max(sCr/κ, 1)$^{-1.209}$ × 0.993^{age} × (1.018 if patient is female) × (1.159 if patient is black) • κ is 0.7 for females and 0.9 for males. • α is −0.329 for females and −0.411 for males.. • min is the minimum of sCr/κ or 1. • max is the maximum of sCr/κ or 1.
Larsson et al (2004)	eGFRcys = 77.24 × (CysC [in mg/L])$^{-1.2623}$
Macdonald et al (2006)	Log$_{10}$ eGFRcys = 2.222 + (−0.802 × $\sqrt{CysC\ in\ \frac{mg}{L}}$) + (0.009876 × LM)
CKD-EPI cystatin C equation (2012)	eGFRcys = 133 × min(sCys/0.8, 1) − 0.499 × max(sCys/0.8, 1) − 1.328 × 0.996^{age} (× 0.932 if female) • sCys is serum cystatin C. • min is the minimum of sCys/0.8 or 1. • max indicates the maximum of sCys/0.8 or 1.
CKD-EPI creatinine-cystatin C equation (2012)	eGFRcr-Cys = 135 × min(sCr/κ, 1)α × max(sCr/κ, 1) − 0.601 × min(sCys/0.8, 1) − 0.375 × max(sCys/0.8, 1) − 0.711 × 0.995^{age} (× 0.969 if female) (× 1.08 if black) • κ is 0.7 for females and 0.9 for males. • α is −0.248 for females and −0.207 for males. • min indicates the minimum of sCr/κ or 1. • max indicates the maximum of sCr/κ or 1.

Alb, Albumin; CrCl, creatinine clearance in mL/min; IBW, ideal body weight (kg); LM, lean mass; sCr, serum or plasma creatinine (mg/dL). For SI conversion purposes, serum or plasma creatinine is converted from μmol/L to mg/dL by multiplying by 0.0113; conversion from creatinine clearance conventional units of mL/min to SI units of mL/s requires multiplication by 0.0167

Equations compiled from references 95-107.

---

exogenous substances; however, the administration of exogenous substances is not practical for routine individual drug dose calculations in clinical practice because the procedures are not timely and not uniformly available.

Although GFR has been estimated based on the measured urinary clearance of creatinine (mCrCl) derived from a 24-hour urine collection, estimated creatinine clearance (eCrCl) or estimated GFR (eGFR; Table 64.5) are the means predominantly determined in clinical practice from the serum creatinine (sCr) and/or cystatin C (CysC) concentrations and patient factors.[95-101] The advantage of these methods are that timely results are available for routine clinical practice and that for most people, they provide an acceptable assessment of measured GFR (mGFR) or mCrCl, respectively. The variation in sCr assays led to differences in reported serum creatinine values among as well as within laboratories.[102] To address this issue, in 2005, the National Institute of Standards and Technologies released materials that are traceable to the certified reference materials for creatinine whose value was assigned using isotope dilution mass spectroscopy (IDMS).[96,103] It is now estimated that most laboratories currently report creatinine values traceable to this reference method. The use of IDMS creatinine assays will likely lead to less variation in kidney function estimates and theoretically more consistent drug dosing recommendations across institutions and clinical settings. Estimated GFRs based on current creatinine assays are likely to yield different drug dosage recommendations from those intended by the original study, even if the same estimating equation is used due to this change in analytic methodology. It is not possible or practical to repeat all the PK studies with standardized creatinine-determined eCrCl or eGFR, and therefore it is still reasonable to use drug dosing adjustments that appear in FDA- and European Medicines Agency (EMA)–approved product labeling.

Traditionally, drug dosing was based on estimation of creatinine clearance (eCrCl) using the Cockcroft and Gault (CG) formula.[9,100] For implementation in the chemical laboratory report, the CG equation is not suitable because body weight is usually not available in the electronic health record. The Modification of Diet in Renal Disease (MDRD) equations, which do not require body weight, were developed from an extensive sample of patients with CKD, all of whom had a measured GFR (i.e., iothalamate clearance) of less than 90 mL/min/1.73 m^2).[98,104] They were initially used by clinical laboratories, although they were only validated for patients with a GFR less than 60 mL/min. Therefore, the new CKD-EPI equation was developed to allow estimation of GFR throughout the full range of the chronic kidney disease.[99] The CKD-EPI (Chronic Kidney Disease Epidemiology Collaboration) eGFR equation has recently replaced the MDRD equation as the primary index for the staging of CKD, and values are now reported throughout the GFR range by Quest and LabCorp, the two largest laboratory service providers in the United States. For classifying kidney function into one of the five stages of chronic kidney disease, the standardized CKD-EPI formula is currently preferred.[105] Both the MDRD and CKD-EPI equations estimate the GFR for a standard 1.73 m^2 body surface area (BSA); thus, for an individual patient, the BSA must be determined separately so that the eGFR can be expressed in milliliters per minute (mL/min).

Serum cystatin C has been proposed as an alternative marker to estimate GFR, rather than serum creatinine. Multiple equations have been proposed to estimate GFR from age, weight, gender, race, and muscle mass based on serum cystatin C measurements.[106] The combined use of both serum markers, cystatin C and creatinine, allows an even more accurate estimate of kidney function than either of them alone.[107] Adjusting drug doses based on the measurement of cystatin C appears to be an effective and valid tool in the limited number of applications (mainly relating to chemotherapy and antibiotic dosing) for which it has been studied.[108-111]

Few studies have examined the role of alternative GFR estimating equations on drug dosing. In general, when considered against chromium-EDTA measurement of GFR, the MDRD formula tends to underestimate GFR relative to the CG formula.[112-115] Gill and colleagues[114] demonstrated that in a multiethnic and older CKD population, these equations were not interchangeable for the calculation of drug dosing. Discordance between the CG and MDRD equations occurred in 60% of older patients. When MDRD was used instead of CG, 20% fewer patients qualified for a reduction in the dose of amantadine, potentially resulting in an inappropriately high cumulative dose.[114]

PEDIATRICS

The original equation to estimate GFR, as described by Schwartz and colleagues,[116] is dependent on the child's age and length:

$$GFR = (length [cm] \times k)/sCr \text{ (in mg/dL)}$$

where k is defined by age group: infant (1 to 52 weeks) = 0.45; child (1 to 13 years) = 0.55; adolescent male = 0.7; and adolescent female = 0.55. The serum creatinine level in µmol/L can be converted to mg/dL by multiplication using 0.0113 as the conversion factor. A newer version of the Schwartz equation[117] was developed from a population of 349 children (age 1-19 years) with mild to moderate CKD enrolled in the Chronic Kidney Disease in Children (CKiD) study:

$$GFR = 0.41 \times (length \text{ in cm})/sCr \text{ in mg/dL}$$

Lee and associates[118] have recently reported that this new Schwartz equation performed better than the original Schwartz equation for patients with moderate CKD, but was less accurate in patients with mild CKD. In pediatric patients, methods incorporating cystatin C have several advantages for evaluating kidney function.[119] The most recent eGFR equation evaluated in pediatrics includes use of cystatin C, blood urea nitrogen (BUN), serum creatinine level (in mg/dL) and demographic data derived from over 600 pediatric patients enrolled in the CKiD study[120]:

$$eGFR \text{ (mL/min/1.73 m}^2)$$
$$= 39.8 \times (ht [m]/sCr)^{0.456} \times (1.8/cystatin\ C)^{0.418}$$
$$\times (30/BUN)^{0.079} \times 1.076^{male} \times (ht [m]/1.4)^{0.179}$$

This equation had the highest R^2 value (0.863) and highest frequency of values within 30% of iohexol-measured GFR (91.3%) when compared to seven other GFR estimating equations.

ACUTE KIDNEY INJURY

At present, the staging of acute kidney injury is based on sequential measurement of the serum creatinine level and urine output.[121-125] Because the GFR is inferred from the serum creatinine or cystatin C, all estimates of kidney function lag the real-time GFR. Although several methods have been proposed to estimate GFR in this patient population, none have been rigorously evaluated, and their use in clinical practice is extremely limited.[119,126-129] The latest proposed method to estimate GFR in patients with AKI is the kinetic GFR (kinetGFR), which is based on age (years), weight (kg), and serum creatinine (µmol/L) and holds true for increasing and decreasing kidney function.[130]

$$kinetGFR = \frac{[150 - age(years)] \bullet weight(kg)}{Cr_2(\mu mol/L)}$$
$$\bullet \left[1 - \frac{Cr_2 - Cr_1}{t_2 - t_1} \bullet \frac{24(hours)}{200(\mu mol/L)}\right]$$

This approach is based on an estimate of the creatinine production similar to the CG equation.[95] The kinetic eGFR incorporates changing creatinine values over specified time intervals as well as the actually measured serum creatinine values, similar to the earlier approaches of Jelliffe,[127] Brater,[126] and Chiou and Hsu.[128] It relates the increase in serum creatinine within a specified time interval to the maximum increase in creatinine level in 1 day. Because creatinine excretion in the urine corresponds to creatinine production, the maximum increase in sCr is about 200 µmol/L if the patient's actual GFR is 0. Thus, the kinetic eGFR predicts what subsequently will be measurable but in fact is already the case with kidney function. The kinetic eGFR solves the problem that there is always a delay between rapidly changing kidney function and measurable variables, namely sCr or urine output. The calculation of a patient's kinetic eGFR may allow one to use the eCrCl- or eGFR-based dose adjustment recommendations derived from patients with CKD and applicable in part for those with AKI.[130] Rigorous independent studies will be needed to confirm its validity and utility in clinical practice.

PATIENTS RECEIVING DIALYSIS

Some patients on dialysis or on continuous renal replacement therapy (CRRT) have residual kidney function that substantially contributes to the elimination of drugs and their metabolites. Unfortunately, estimating residual kidney function in patients undergoing dialysis is challenging because the serum creatinine concentration reflects not only residual kidney function, but also the efficiency of dialysis and role of muscle mass on creatinine generation. Creatinine clearance measurements are less reliable as a measure of GFR in patients on hemodialysis (HD) or CRRT than in those with earlier stages of CKD because of the following: (1) the volume of urine output is heavily influenced by changing hydration status during the cyclic changes that are inherent as a result of intermittent ultrafiltration; (2) the serum creatinine concentration changes over the duration of the clearance measurement; and (3) tubular secretion of creatinine contributes to its clearance. Estimation of residual kidney function in patients on HD or CRRT is often done by calculating the mean of a measured urea and creatinine clearance. Measuring the elimination of iohexol after an IV dose has been reported to be an accurate and safe measure of residual kidney function in patients on dialysis and can inform drug dosing.[131]

Which one of the many eCrCl or eGFR equations should be used to determine the degree of adjustment of drug dosage regimens for patients with AKI or CKD? The pros and cons of the various GFR estimating equations have been extensively reviewed.[112-115] Moreover, there is a body of evidence on drug dosing methodology that has been derived based on measured creatinine clearance or eCrCl using the CG equation.[132] The MDRD and CKD-EPI equations significantly overestimated CrCl (mCrCl and CG) in older individuals.[114] This has led to dose calculation errors for many drugs, particularly in individuals with severe CKD. Thus, we have concluded that eGFR equations should not be substituted in place of the CG equation in older adults for the purpose of renal dosage adjustments.

It is the advantage of the CG equation that body weight is considered as a determinant of drug distribution volume. The choice of the optimal GFR estimating equation is of utmost importance for drugs with a narrow therapeutic index for which dosing individualization is often continuous rather than categoric. Finally, because most pharmacokinetic studies in patients with CKD conducted over the last 40 years have used estimated or measured CrCl as the estimate of GFR, the CG method in adults and the latest Schwartz method in children remain the criteria to be used. However, for patients with AKI, there is no obvious best choice for GFR estimation to guide drug dosing.

DRUG DOSING CONSIDERATIONS

PATIENTS WITH CHRONIC KIDNEY DISEASE

Despite the availability of numerous guidelines regarding drug dosing for patients with impaired kidney function, there is insufficient evidence as to which, if any, is preferred.[5,13,35,133-135] Occasionally, recommendations derived from postmarketing studies conflict with the information in these reports, as well as the official FDA or EMA product labeling. Prior to 1998, there were no official guidelines regarding when and how to characterize the relationship between the pharmacokinetics and pharmacodynamics of a drug and kidney function. The FDA guidelines issued in May 1998[136] and the 2010 proposed revision,[137] and the EMA guidelines of 2004,[138] have provided frameworks for which drugs should be evaluated and guidance regarding study design, data analysis, interpretation of study results, and recommendations for the incorporation of data into product labeling.

GOALS OF THERAPY

The desired goal is typically the maintenance of a similar peak, trough, or average steady-state drug concentration or, for antibiotics, an optimized pharmacodynamic measure, such as the time above the MIC or the ratio of the drug area under the AUC to the MIC, as would be optimal for persons with normal kidney function[8,86,139] (see earlier, "Pharmacodynamics," for more detail). When there is a significant relationship between drug concentration and clinical response[86] (e.g., aminoglycosides) or toxicity[39] (e.g., phenytoin), attainment of the specific target values becomes critical. If, however, no specific PK or PD target values have been reported, a regimen goal of attaining and maintaining the same average steady-state concentration may be appropriate.

INDIVIDUALIZATION OF THE DRUG DOSAGE REGIMEN

Most dosage adjustment guidelines have proposed the use of a fixed dose or interval for patients with broad ranges of kidney function.[35,134,135,140-143] The mild, moderate, and severe CKD categories vary among reference sources, so the recommended regimen may not be optimal for all patients whose kidney function lies within the range, especially for agents with a narrow therapeutic index.[9] The approach to developing drug dosage adjustment recommendations for the patient with CKD is predicated on attainment of the desired exposure goal at steady state. To achieve the desired goal in a timely fashion, a stepwise approach that includes multiple considerations (Table 64.6) for each individual drug should be considered.[135] The following considerations may help guide individualization of therapy.

The initial or loading dose (LD), which in many patients with AKI will be larger than the typical maintenance dose, should be calculated to achieve the desired C_{max} therapeutic drug concentration. An LD should be used for most patients with stage 4 or 5 CKD to achieve the desired steady-state concentration rapidly and in which the volume of distribution (V_D) of a drug is significantly increased in patients with AKI and CKD relative to those with normal kidney function.

Table 64.6 Stepwise Approach to Adjust Drug Dosage Regimens for Patients with Impaired Kidney Function

Step	Process	Assessment
1	Obtain history and relevant demographic and clinical information.	Record demographic information, obtain past medical history. including history of renal disease, and record current laboratory information (e.g., serum creatinine).
2	Estimate creatinine clearance.	Use Cockcroft-Gault equation to estimate creatinine clearance, or calculate creatinine clearance from timed urine collection.
3	Review current medications.	Identify drugs for which individualization of the treatment regimen will be necessary
4	Calculate individualized treatment regimen.	Determine treatment goals (see text); calculate dosage regimen based on pharmacokinetic characteristics of the drug and patient's renal function.
5	Monitor.	Monitor parameters of drug response and toxicity; monitor drug levels if available or applicable.
6	Revise regimen.	Adjust regimen based on drug response or change in patient status (including renal function), as warranted.

Adapted from Mohammad RA, Matzke GR. Drug dosing in renal failure. In DiPiro J, Talbert R, Yee G, et al, editors: Pharmacotherapy: a pathophysiologic approach, *ed 9, New York, 2014, McGraw-Hill.*

If the relationship between V_D and CrCl has been characterized, then the V_D should be estimated from that relationship. If no LD is prescribed, four half-lives of the drug must pass before the desired steady-state plasma concentration is achieved; however, doing so may contribute to therapeutic failure. The proportion of the LD given affects the magnitude of the steady-state plasma concentration and how rapidly plasma concentrations are achieved. An LD equivalent to the dose given to a patient with normal kidney function should be given to patients with impaired kidney function if the drug's half-life is especially long and if the physical examination suggests normal ECF volume. If the patient has marked volume expansion or evidence indicates that the V_D of the drug is larger in patients with CKD, then a higher dose can be calculated from the following expression:

$$LD = V_D \times C_{max} \times IBW$$

where V_D is the drug's volume of distribution (in liters per kilogram of IBW in those with CKD), IBW is the patient's ideal body weight (in kilograms), and C_{max} is the desired steady-state maximum plasma drug concentration.

The primary reference for information regarding the maintenance dose for patients with CKD should be the FDA and/or EMA official product labeling. If no official drug dosing guidance is available, one may need to search the literature to find a recommendation strategy derived from nonregulatory or postmarketing clinical investigations. If no such resource is found, one can consult online or published tertiary references that have developed dosing recommendations based on the Dettli or Tozer method, initially published in 1974.[11,12] They used similar foundational PK characteristics and approaches to calculate the maintenance dose for a patient with a given eCrCl. In essence, either the dose (D) should be reduced or the interval (τ) extended. When the dose is reduced, the C_{max} will be lower and the trough concentrations will be higher than those observed in persons with normal kidney function. When the administration interval is extended, the peak and trough concentrations are kept constant but the dosing frequency decreases (see Figure 64.4).

To maintain the normal dose interval in patients with impaired kidney function, the amount of each dose after the loading dose can be estimated from the following equation:

$$D_f = D_n \times Q$$

where D_f is the dose for the patient with impaired kidney function to be given at the normal dosing interval, D_n is the normal dose, and Q is the dosage adjustment factor. The dosage adjustment factor (Q) can be calculated as:

$$Q = 1 - (f_e[1 - KF])$$

where f_e is the fraction of the drug eliminated unchanged renally in a patient with normal renal function, KF is the ratio of the patient's CrCl or GFR to the assumed normal value of 120 mL/min (equivalent to 2.00 mL/sec). Thus, for a drug that is 85% eliminated unchanged by the kidneys, the Q factor in a patient who has a CrCl of 10 mL/min (0.17 mL/sec) would be as follows:

$$\begin{aligned} Q &= 1 - (0.85[1 - 10/120]) \\ &= 1 - (0.85[0.92]) \\ &= 1 - 0.78 \\ &= 0.22 \end{aligned}$$

If one desires to give the same maintenance dose, a factor that may be required because of the limited availability of alternative formulations, the dosing interval at which the normal dose should be administered can be calculated as follows:

$$\tau_f = \tau_n / Q$$

The decision to extend the dosing interval beyond a 24-hour period should be based on the need to maintain therapeutic peak or trough levels. The dosing interval may be prolonged if the peak level is most important. Prolonging the dose interval in patients on dialysis is frequently a convenient method to modify the drug dosage regimen. This method is particularly useful for drugs with a long plasma half-life. In general, drugs removed by dialysis given once daily should be given after the dialysis treatment, with aminoglycosides a notable exception.[144-146]

A third alternative that is especially helpful when the calculated dose or dosing interval is impractical is to select the administration interval according to the target trough concentration while the peak is kept constant:

$$\tau_{target} = (t_{1/2}/0.693) \times \ln(C_{peak}/C_{trough-target})$$

$$D = LD \times (1 - C_{trough-target}/C_{peak})$$

Alternatively, one can calculate the adjusted dose (D_p) to be given at the predetermined practical dosage interval (τ_p or $\tau_{ptarget}$) as follows:

$$D_p = (D_n \times \tau_p \times Q)/\tau_n$$

where τ_f is the estimated dosing interval, as calculated from the above equation for $\tau_{ptarget}$, or the clinically practical value for the renally impaired patient (e.g., 12, 18, 24, 36, 48 hours). These approaches, which use a combination of the dose reduction and interval prolongation methods, are often the most clinically practical. When in doubt, clinicians should consult an experienced pharmacist, preferably one with extensive experience in evaluating patients with CKD and altered body composition (e.g., fluid overload).

MEASUREMENT OF THERAPEUTIC DRUG LEVELS

Measuring drug concentrations is one way to optimize therapeutic regimens and account for changes among and within individuals. Therapeutic drug monitoring requires availability of rapid, specific, and reliable assays and known correlations of drug concentration to therapeutic and toxic outcomes. Hypoalbuminemia may influence interpretation of drug concentrations because the total drug concentration may be reduced, even when the active unbound drug concentration generally is not. Unbound drug concentrations are often not clinically available, so clinicians must empirically consider the influence of hypoalbuminemia in their interpretation of measured total drug concentrations, as in the case of phenytoin and several antibiotics (e.g., daptomycin).[39,147,148]

PATIENTS WITH ACUTE KIDNEY INJURY

Critically ill patients frequently develop AKI; depending on the definition, from 5% to 15% of all non–same-day hospitalization care is complicated by AKI.[25,149] In most cases, drug dosing is based on drug disposition information derived from studies in stable patients with CKD. Unfortunately, there are large gaps in knowledge of drug metabolism and disposition in patients with AKI; thus, patients may be at significant risk for underdosing as well as overdosing. More than 30 definitions of AKI have been published in the literature.[121-125] The lack of a consensus definition and classification of AKI reflects the wide range of causes and severity with which it presents. The presentation can vary from part of multiorgan dysfunction in critically ill patients to isolated AKI.[150] As a result, AKI-related, in-hospital mortality rates vary from 70% in intensive care unit (ICU) patients[151] to 35% in other hospitalized patients.[152]

The potential effects of AKI on drug dosing are of major consequence because AKI patients are often critically ill and require multiple drug therapies, some of which may be nephrotoxic or require dose modification in the setting of AKI. The pharmacokinetic changes in absorption, distribution, metabolism, and excretion presented earlier in this chapter and in other sources are foundational to optimal patient care.[26,153] The clinician needs to appreciate these factors and realize that they may worsen and improve over the period of evolution or recovery of the AKI episode. Critically ill patients with AKI typically have minimal oral intake of food and liquids and commonly require parenteral administration of drugs otherwise given orally (e.g., antihypertensives, immunosuppressives).

There is a paucity of dosing algorithms to guide pharmacotherapy, derived from investigations of the PK and PD of medications in patients with AKI. Most of the critical care literature and almost all FDA or EMA product labeling contain drug dosage recommendations derived from observations of patients with CKD and ESKD. The limited data available in the setting of AKI have predominantly been developed by clinicians; rarely is this information incorporated into official product labeling. The principles of drug dosage regimen modification described earlier for use in CKD thus remain the foundation for therapy optimization in patients with AKI.

LOADING DOSE

Many patients with AKI are overhydrated, and the distribution volume is much larger than under normal conditions. Thus, the LD may need to be higher than the normal starting dose for persons with normal kidney function. Because the V_D of many drugs, especially hydrophilic antibiotics, including β-lactams, cephalosporins, and carbapenems, are significantly increased in the presence of AKI, the administration of proactive loading doses (25% > normal) are highly recommended.

MAINTENANCE DOSE

Forecasting the degree and rate of change in kidney function and fluid volume status is extremely challenging. Thus, maintenance dosing regimens for many drugs, especially antimicrobial agents, should be initiated at normal or near-normal dosage regimens and adjustments made based on the relationship between drug pharmacokinetic characteristics and kidney function, as described earlier. Prospective measurement of serum drug concentrations and analysis using state of the art PK and PD approaches should be used whenever possible.

PATIENTS UNDERGOING HEMODIALYSIS

The optimization of pharmacotherapy for patients receiving maintenance hemodialysis and emergent hemodialysis are both critically dependent on the availability of reliable information from well-designed pharmacokinetic studies.[154-157] The impact of hemodialysis on drug therapy is dependent on the drug characteristics and dialysis prescription. Drug-related factors include molecular weight (MW) or size, degree of protein binding, and distribution volume.[135] The vast majority of hemodialysis filters in use up until the mid-1990s were generally impermeable to drugs with a molecular weight greater than 1 kDa.[155-157] Dialysis membranes in the twenty-first century are predominantly composed of semisynthetic or synthetic materials, which have larger pore sizes, and this allows the ready passage of drugs that have a MW up to 20 kDa.

Drug clearance during dialysis can occur by three different processes.[6,156,157] Drug removal by conventional HD occurs primarily by diffusion down a concentration gradient from the plasma to the dialysate. Removal of low-MW drugs is enhanced by increasing blood and dialysate flow rates and by using large surface area dialyzers. Larger molecules require more porous membranes for increased removal. The clearance of a drug by conventional HD can be estimated from the unbound fraction (f_u) and the following relationship:

$$Cl_{HD} = f_u \times Cl_{urea} \times (60/MW_{drug})$$

where Cl_{HD} is the drug's clearance by HD, Cl_{urea} is the dialyzer clearance of urea, and MW_{drug} is the MW of the drug. The urea clearance for most conventional dialyzers varies between 150 and 200 mL/min and is markedly less than values reported with high-flux hemodialyzers.[157] With high-flux hemodialysis, the volume of distribution and degree of protein binding of the drug become more important determinants of dialyzer clearance. The hemodialyzer clearance of drugs that are not highly protein-bound and have relatively small volumes of distribution runs in parallel to urea clearance, despite their large molecular mass.[158-160] The convective transport and removal of drugs during high-flux HD depends primarily on filtration pressure gradient, treatment time, blood, and dialysate flow rates. Despite the widespread adoption of high-flux hemodialysis in certain parts of the world, there are sparse quantitative data on drug clearance.

Small solute removal is more efficient if the frequency of hemodialysis is increased. Daily and nocturnal dialysis therapies yield different clearance values compared with thrice-weekly, high-flux, in-center hemodialysis, and also differ from each other. There has been very little investigation of the effects of frequent or more intensive hemodialysis regimens on drug disposition or comparison among modalities. As a result, drug dosing in patients should be guided by drug level monitoring when possible. One of the few studies to investigate drug clearance by one of these variants focused on the aminoglycoside antibiotic gentamicin. Slow nocturnal dialysis required a significant increase in gentamicin dosage to achieve therapeutic levels compared with conventional thrice-weekly dialysis.[161] The variability in drug clearance was high and did not correlate with small solute clearance. Drugs with a molecular size of 500 to 5000 Da appear to be particularly likely to have an increased clearance with this modality. Studies of modeled clearance have suggested that frequent hemodialysis regimens would be associated with enhanced clearance (and the potential of underdosing) of daptomycin.[147,148,162,163] This enhanced clearance was confirmed in the setting of AKI when the PK associated with extended daily dialysis were investigated. These findings should be transferable to maintenance HD, with a degree of caution about the effects on distribution volumes that might arise in the setting of acute septic shock.[164,147] One of the other effects of prolonged HD appears to be a reduction in rebound of drug concentrations after the termination of dialysis.[165,166] This is probably because the rate of transfer from the peripheral to central compartment relative to the rate of diffusive removal is lower.

There were more than 100 different dialysis or hemofilters available in the United States in 2013, and at least four distinct variants of hemodialysis are currently being used.[6] The effect of hemodialysis or hemofiltration on the disposition of a drug may vary markedly and, because dialyzer or hemofilter clearance is rarely evaluated more than once, clinicians have to extrapolate data from one procedure to another.[167,168] The enhanced efficiency of twenty-first century dialyzers means that most of the literature for medications developed prior to 2000 probably reflects an underestimation of the impact of hemodialysis.[1,155] Consequently, the dosage may need to be empirically increased by 25% to 50%. Therapeutic drug monitoring should be used for drugs with narrow therapeutic indices to optimize safety and efficacy.

ASSESSMENT OF THE IMPACT OF HEMODIALYSIS

The most commonly used means for assessing the effect of hemodialysis is to calculate the dialyzer clearance of a drug (Cl^p_D) from plasma, as follows:

$$Cl^p_D = Q_p([A_p - V_p]/A_p)$$

where Q_p is plasma flow through the dialyzer, A_p is the concentration of drug in plasma going into the dialyzer, and V_p is the plasma concentration of drug leaving the dialyzer.[135,166] This equation tends to underestimate hemodialysis clearance for drugs that readily partition into and out of erythrocytes. In addition, venous plasma concentrations may be artificially high if extensive ultrafiltration is performed, so thus Cl^p_D will be lower than it really is. Because of these limitations, the recovery clearance approach remains the benchmark for the determination of dialyzer clearance and can be calculated as follows[135]:

$$Cl^r_D = R/AUC_{0-t}$$

where R is the total amount of drug recovered unchanged in the dialysate and AUC_{0-t} is the area under the predialyzer plasma concentration-time curve during the period of time that the dialysate was collected. The hemodialysis clearance values reported in the literature may vary significantly, depending on which of these methods were used.[135,156]

It is common practice in most hemodialysis units to administer drugs after dialysis to minimize the loss of drug that would result from the additional clearance during hemodialysis. However, performing hemodialysis immediately after dosing might be a good option for removal of toxic antibiotics[139,144-146,164,169] and high-dose, anticancer therapy. For anticancer drugs, the predialysis administration of a normal dose makes sense when the patient undergoes hemodialysis 2 to 12 hours later. This strategy delivers the desired maximum plasma concentration effect while minimizing the toxic drug or metabolic effects[170-183] (Table

64.7). Emerging PK and PD considerations suggest that administration after hemodialysis may not be the optimal approach for several other agents, such as aminoglycosides and vancomycin.[139,144-146,164,169] High-bolus dosing immediately before or during the last hour of dialysis has been proposed for some antibiotics, but there have been few clinical studies.

If the drug is given after dialysis, the postdialysis dose (D_{HD}) should first replace the amount eliminated during the interval between dialysis sessions (D_{fail}) that is the result of clearance by the patient's residual renal function and nonrenal clearance. Also, the fraction of drug removed by hemodialysis (FR) should be estimated and a supplementary dose calculated (D_{suppl}). The dose the patient should receive after HD would thus be the sum of these two doses (Figure 64.5):

$$D_{HD} = D_{fail} + D_{suppl} = D_{fail} + (FR \times (D_{start} - F_{fail}))$$

PATIENTS RECEIVING CONTINUOUS RENAL REPLACEMENT THERAPY

CRRT and hybrid RRTs are commonly used to manage patients with AKI in ICUs.[184] CRRT seems to provide less of a challenge for drug dosing than intermittent HD because its continuous nature is analogous with drug removal by native kidneys and potentially amenable to the use of standard, first-order drug clearance equations to calculate dosing. However, in practice, CRRT rarely proves as continuous as planned. The CRRT modality and details of the therapy prescription can also have significant effects on drug clearance. MW, membrane characteristics (highly variable between systems), blood flow rate, and dialysate flow rate determine the rate and extent of drug removal.[185-189] Because most drugs are less than 1.5 kDa, drug removal by CRRT does not depend greatly on MW. The use of higher hemofiltration volumes, especially if infused prefilter, can also affect clearance. The removal of urea, creatinine, and vancomycin were increased by 15% to 25% by the predilution modality.[190-192]

CRRT clearances have been noted to decline because the time the hemofilter has been in use increases due to the accumulation of protein on the dialysis membrane. Clotting within the hemofilter's hollow fibers also reduces the overall surface area for clearance. Although these factors have received little direct investigation, it appears that they do affect drug clearance.[192]

Drug protein binding also affects how much is removed during CRRT because only unbound drug is available for elimination by CRRT. Protein binding of more than 80% provides a substantial barrier to drug removal by convection or diffusion. During continuous venovenous hemofiltration,

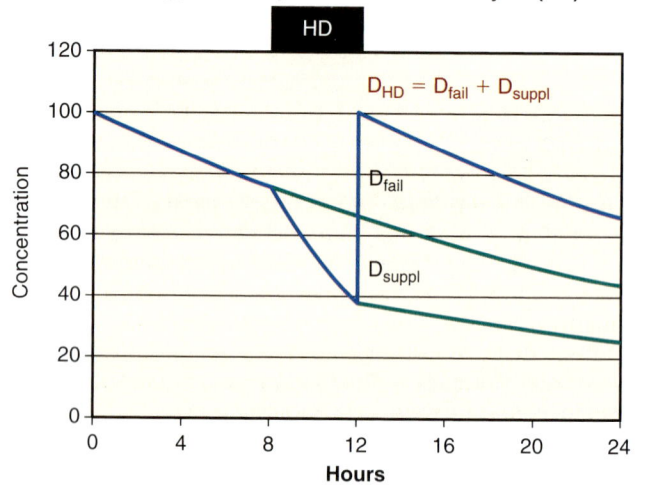

Figure 64.5 To maintain therapeutic target concentrations, a supplementary dose must be given after hemodialysis to replace the removed fraction of the dose. The dose after dialysis (D_{HD}) combines both, the adjusted maintenance dose (D_{fail}) and supplementary dose (D_{suppl}).

Table 64.7 Drugs Best Administered Prior to Hemodialysis

Drug Class	Examples	Drug Fraction Removed by One Dialysis Session (FR)	Reference
Anticancer	Carboplatin	20%	Chatelut et al[170]; Kamata et al[171]; Yoshida et al[172]; Oguri et al[173]
	Cisplatin	85%	Watanabe et al[174]
	Oxaliplatin	65%	Katsumata et al[175]
	Cyclophosphamide	22% (M % unknown)	Haubitz et al[176]
	Ifosfamide	70% to 87% (M, 72% to 77%)	Carlson et al[177]
	Capecitabine (FBAL)	50%	Walko and Lindley[178]
	Gemcitabine (dFdU)	50%	Koolen et al[179]
	Methotrexate	36%	Garlich and Goldfarb[180]
	Cytosine arabinoside	39% (M, 52% to 63%)	Radeski et al[181]
	Topotecan	50%	Herrington et al[182]
Aminoglycoside	Gentamicin	75%	Veinstein et al[164]
	Tobramicin	80%	Kamel et al[146]
Contrast agent	Gadolinium	65% to 74%	Rodby[183]

M, Metabolite.

drug clearance generally approximates the ultrafiltration rate. The addition of diffusion by continuous venovenous hemodiafiltration increases drug clearance and is dependent on the ultrafiltration and dialysate flow rates. As is the case during high-flux dialysis, drug removal often parallels the removal of urea and creatinine. Thus, the simplest method for estimating drug removal during CRRT is to estimate urea or creatinine clearance.[8,154,190-192]

Hybrid RRTs, including sustained or slow low-efficiency dialysis (SLED), extended daily dialysis (EDD), continuous SLED (c-SLED), slow low-efficiency daily dialysis (SLEDD), and slow low-efficiency daily hemodiafiltration (SLEDD-f), which use higher dialysate flow rates and shorter treatment periods (6 to 12 hours in duration), are frequently used as well.[193-198] To date, hybrid RRT pharmacokinetic data have been published for fewer than 20 drugs.[1] The improvement of RRT machines and filters has rendered old dosing guidelines for drugs, especially antibiotics, obsolete and potentially hazardous. Although there are only a few FDA or EMA official drug dosing recommendations for patients receiving CRRT, several published dosing guidelines are widely used.[8,168,190-192] Unfortunately, these recommendations have generally not been prospectively evaluated, and their influence on patient outcomes is largely unknown.

In the absence of FDA or EMA recommendations, tertiary reference sources, or any published studies relating to the handling of a drug by CRRT (common with agents that are new to the market), may be necessary for the clinician to formulate a dosing regimen using the PK principles presented in this chapter. If the volume of distribution is large (>1 L/kg), there is a low likelihood that CRRT will substantially remove it. The use of a high-flux dialyzer or hemofilter allows for drugs with a MW below 20 kDa to be readily removed. If the clearance of the drug by CRRT or hybrid RRT is less than 25% of the patient's estimated total body clearance, a dosing adjustment is probably unnecessary. On the other hand, if CRRT or hybrid RRT results in an augmentation of drug clearance by 25% to 50%, an LD based on the patient's estimated volume status should be given, and maintenance doses similar to that given to a patient with a CrCl of 30 to 50 mL/min can be used. Such estimates obviously have to take into account changing volume status and be supplemented by regular drug concentration measurements, if technically feasible.

PATIENTS UNDERGOING PERITONEAL DIALYSIS

Peritoneal dialysis, as practiced in 2014, is very unlikely to enhance total body clearance of any drug by more than 10 mL/min because most typical peritoneal dialysis prescriptions can achieve a urea clearance of about 10 mL/min or lower. Because most drugs are larger than urea, their clearance is even less; thus, it is very likely to be from 5 to 7.5 mL/min or less. Many studies performed in the 1970s and 1980s showed that drug clearances by peritoneal dialysis were in this very low range, so one can conclude that peritoneal dialysis does not enhance drug removal to a degree that would require a special dosage regimen modification.[199-202] Thus, oral or IV drug therapy recommendations for patients with an eCrCl or eGFR less than 15 mL/min are likely clinically useful.

Intraperitoneal drug administration is well accepted for the treatment of peritoneal dialysis–associated peritonitis and other infections.[203-205] Administration intervals depend on the half-life of the drug, which is mainly determined by residual renal and extrarenal metabolic clearance. Long-standing experience with intermittent antibiotic administration exists for the glycopeptides vancomycin and teicoplanin, which can be administered at 5- to 7-day intervals, as well as for aminoglycosides and cephalosporins, which are suitable for once-daily dosing.[204,206]

Patients treated by automated peritoneal dialysis (APD), with frequent short-dialysis cycles, may achieve higher plasma concentrations as compared to antibiotic loading in a single extended dwell period in patients on continuous ambulatory peritoneal dialysis (CAPD). Conversely, the higher dialysate flow and small-molecule clearance achieved with APD regimens may lead to a greater peritoneal clearance of antibiotic in the intervals between dosing.[204]

Because most pharmacokinetic studies establishing peritoneal antibiotic doses have used 4- to 8-hour loading periods, it is recommended to perform antibiotic loading by an extended cycle both in CAPD and APD patients. For intermittent maintenance dosing, a long nighttime dwell time should be used in CAPD patients and a long daytime dwell time in APD patients. In clinical practice, intraperitoneal antibiotic dosing has not been unequivocally successful in eradicating bacterial growth, partially questioning the concept of antibiotic back diffusion into the peritoneal cavity.

CLINICAL BOTTOM LINE

Recommendations for dosing selected drugs in patients with CKD and AKI are given in Table 64.8. These are meant only as a guide and do not imply the safety or efficacy of a recommended dose in an individual patient. A loading dose equivalent to the usual dose in patients with normal kidney function should be considered for drugs with half-lives longer than 12 hours. No controlled clinical trials have established the efficacy of these dosage recommendations. The effect on drug removal of HD, ambulatory peritoneal dialysis, and CRRT is variable and the values in the table are more qualitative than quantitative. Most of these recommendations were established before high-efficiency HD treatments were practical, continuous cycling nocturnal peritoneal dialysis was common, and diffusion was added to hemofiltration in CRRT.

Complete reference list available at ExpertConsult.com.

Table 64.8 Recommendations for Dosing Selected Drugs in Patients with Chronic Kidney Disease or Acute Kidney Injury

Drug	Degree of Drug Dose Reduction or Interval Prolongation			Dosage Recommendations for Patients Receiving Renal Replacement Therapy		
	GFR > 50 mL/min	GFR = 10-50 mL/min	GFR < 10 mL/min	HD	CAPD	CRRT
Acebutolol	100%	50%	25%	Dose as GFR < 10	Dose as GFR < 10	Dose as GFR 10-50
Acetaminophen	q4h	q6h	q8h	Dose as GFR < 10	Dose as GFR < 10	Dose as GFR 10-50
Acetazolamide	q6h	q12h	q24h	Dose as GFR < 10	Dose as GFR < 10	Dose as GFR 10-50
Acetohexamide	Avoid	Avoid	Avoid	Avoid	Avoid	Avoid
Acetohydroxamic acid	100%	100%	Avoid	Unknown	Unknown	Unknown
Acetylsalicylic acid	q4h	q4-6h	Avoid	As normal GFR	As normal GFR	Dose as GFR 10-50
Acrivastine	8 mg q6h	8 mg q8-12h	8 mg q12-24h	Dose as GFR < 10	Dose as GFR < 10	Dose as GFR 10-50
Acyclovir	5 mg/kg q8h	5 mg/kg q12-24h	2.5-5 mg/kg q24h	Dose as GFR < 10	Dose as GFR < 10	Dose as GFR 10-50
Allopurinol	100%	50%	33%	Dose as GFR < 10	Dose as GFR < 10	Dose for GFR 10-50
Amantadine	q24h	q48-72h	q7days	Dose as GFR < 10	Dose as GFR < 10	Dose as GFR 10-50
Amikacin*	5-6 mg/kg q12h	3-4 mg/kg q24h	2 mg/kg q24-48h	5 mg/kg after HD	15-20 mg/L/day	7.5 mg/kg q24h
Amiloride	100%	50%	Avoid	NA	NA	NA
Amoxapine	100%	100%	100%	Unknown	Unknown	Unknown
Amphotericin	q24h	q24h	q24h	Dose as GFR < 10	Dose as GFR < 10	Dose as GFR 10-50
Amphotericin B	q24h	q24h	q24h	Dose as GFR < 10	Dose for GFR < 10	Dose for GFR 10-50
Amphotericin B lipid	q24h	q24h	q24h	Dose as GFR < 10	Dose as GFR < 10	Dose as GFR 10-50
Ampicillin	250 mg-2 g q4-6h	250 mg-2 g q6h	250 mg-1 g q6h	250-500 mg q8h	Dose as GFR < 10	Dose as GFR 10-50
Atenolol	100% q24h	50% q24h	25% q24h	Dose as GFR < 10	Dose as GFR < 10	Dose as GFR 10-50
Auranofin	6 mg q24h	3 mg q24h	Avoid	Avoid	Avoid	Avoid
Azathioprine	100%	75%-100%	50%-100%	Dose as GFR < 10	Dose as GFR < 10	Dose as GFR 10-50
Aztreonam	100%	50%	25%	Dose as GFR < 10	Dose for GFR < 10	Dose as GFR 10-50
Benazepril	100%	50%-75%	25%-50%	Dose as GFR < 10	Dose as GFR < 10	Dose as GFR 10-50
Bezafibrate	50%-100%	25%-50%	Avoid	200 mg q72h	200 mg q72h	200 mg q24-48h
Bisoprolol	100%	100%	50%	Dose as GFR < 10	Dose as GFR < 10	Dose as GFR 10-50
Bleomycin	100%	75%	50%	Dose as GFR < 10	Dose as GFR < 10	Dose as GFR 10-50
Bretylium	100%	25%-50%	25%	Dose as GFR < 10	Dose as GFR < 10	Dose as GFR 10-50
Bupropion	100% q24h	100% q24h	100% q24h	Dose as GFR < 10	Dose as GFR < 10	Dose as GFR 10-50
Butorphanol	100%	75%	50%	Unknown	Unknown	As normal GFR
Capreomycin	q24h	q24h	q48h	Dose as GFR < 10	Dose as GFR < 10	Dose as GFR 10-50
Captopril	100% q8-12h	75% q12-18h	50% q24h	Dose as GFR < 10	Dose as GFR < 10	Dose as GFR 10-50
Carboplatin	100%	50%	25%	Dose as GFR < 10	Dose as GFR < 10	Dose as GFR 10-50
Carteolol	100%	50%	25%	Dose as GFR < 10	Dose as GFR < 10	Dose as GFR 10-50
Cefaclor	100%	100%	50%-100%	250-500 mg q8h	250 mg q8-12h	Dose as GFR 10-50
Cefadroxil	q12h	q12h	q24h	0.5-1.0 g after HD	0.5 g/day	Dose as GFR 10-50
Cefamandole	q6h	q6-8h	q8-12h	0.5-1.0 g q12h	0.5-1.0g q12h	Dose as GFR 10-50
Cefazolin	q8h	q12h	q24-48h	15-20 mg/kg after HD	Dose as GFR 10-50	As normal GFR
Cefepime	q12h	50%-100% q24h	25%-50% q24h	Dose as GFR < 10	Dose for GFR < 10	Dose as GFR < 10
Cefixime	100%	75%-100%	50%	Dose as GFR < 10	Dose for GFR < 10	1-2 g q12h
Cefotaxime	q6h	q6-12h	1g q8-12h	Dose as GFR < 10	Dose as GFR < 10	Dose as GFR 10-50
Cefotetan	q12h	q24h	q48h	1 g after HD	1 g q24h	1-2 g q12h
Cefoxitin	q6-8h	q8-12h	q24-48h	1 g after HD	1 g q24h	Dose as GFR 10-50
Cefpodoxime	100%	100%	100-200 mg q24-48h	Dose as GFR < 10	Dose as GFR < 10	As normal GFR
Cefprozil	100%	50% q12h	50% q12h	250 mg after HD	Dose as GFR < 10	Dose as GFR < 10
Ceftazidime	100%	1-2 g q24h	0.5-1 g q48h	1 g after HD	0.5-1g q24h	1-2 g q12h
Ceftibuten	100%	50%	25%	400 mg after HD	Dose as GFR < 10	Dose as GFR 10-50

Drug				
Ceftizoxime	q8h	q12h	q24h	Dose as GFR 10-50
Cefuroxime (IV)	100% q8h	q8-12h	750 mg q12h	Dose as GFR 10-50
Celiprolol	100%	100%	75%	As normal GFR
Cephalexin	250-500 mg q6h	250-500 mg q8-12h	250-500 mg q12-24h	Dose as GFR 10-50
Cephradine	100%	50%	25%	As normal GFR
Cetirizine	100%	100%	50%	As normal GFR
Chloroquine	100%	100%	50%	Avoid
Chlorpropamide	50%	Avoid	Avoid	Unknown
Chlorthalidone	q24h	Avoid	Avoid	Avoid
Cibenzoline	100% q12h	100% q12h	66% q24h	Dose as GFR 10-50
Cidofovir	50%-100%	Avoid	No data	No data
Cilazapril	75% q24h	50% q24-48h	10%-25% q72h	Dose as GFR 10-50
Cimetidine	100%	50%	50%	Dose as GFR 10-50
Ciprofloxacin	100%	50%-100%	50%	200 mg IV q12h
Cisplatin	100%	75%	50%	Dose as GFR 10-50
Clarithromycin	100%	75%	50%-75%	Dose as GFR 10-50
Clodronate	100%	50%	Avoid	Dose as GFR 10-50
Clofazimine	100%	100%	100%	Dose as GFR 10-50
Clofibrate	q6-12h	q12-18h	Avoid	Dose as GFR 10-50
Clomipramine	100%	Start at lower dose, monitor effect	Start at lower dose, monitor effect	Dose as GFR 10-50
Clonidine	q12h	q12-24h	q24h	As normal GFR
Clopidogrel	100%	100%	100%	Dose as GFR < 10
Codeine	100%	75%	50%	As normal GFR
Colchicine	100%	100%	50%	Dose as GFR < 10
Cyclophosphamide	100%	75%-100%	50-75%	Dose as GFR < 10
Cycloserine	q12h	q12-24h	q24h	Dose as GFR < 10
Dapsone	100%	100%	50%	Dose as GFR < 10
Daunorubicin	100%	75%	50%	Dose as GFR < 10
Didanosine	50%-100%	33%-50%	25%	Dose as GFR < 10
Diflunisal	100%	50%	50%	Dose as GFR < 10
Digitoxin	100%	100%	50%-75%	Dose as GFR < 10
Digoxin*	100% q24h	25%-50% q24h	10-25% q24-48h	Dose as GFR < 10
Disopyramide	q8h	q12h	q48h	As normal GFR
Dobutamine	100%	100%	100%	Unknown
Doxacurium	100%	50%	50%	Unknown
Dyphylline	75%	50%	25%	Dose as GFR < 10
Emtricitabine	q24h	q48-72h	q96h	Dose as GFR < 10
Enalapril	100%	50%-100%	25%	Dose as GFR < 10
Ertapenem	100%	100%	50%	Dose as GFR < 10
Erythromycin	100%	100%	50%-75%	As normal GFR
Ethambutol	q24h	q24-36h	q48h	NA
Ethchlorvynol	100%	Avoid	Avoid	Dose as GFR < 10
Ethionamide	100%	100%	50%	Dose as GFR < 10
Ethosuximide	100%	100%	75%-100%	As normal GFR
Etoposide	100%	75%	50%	Dose as GFR < 10
Famciclovir	100%	q12-24h	50% q24-48h	Dose as GFR < 10
Famotidine	100%	50%	20 mg q24h	Dose as GFR < 10
Fentanyl	100%	75%	50%	Dose as GFR < 10
Fexofenadine	q12h	q12-24h	q24h	Dose as GFR < 10

Continued on following page

Table 84.8 Recommendations for Dosing Selected Drugs in Patients with Chronic Kidney Disease or Acute Kidney Injury (Continued)

Drug	Degree of Drug Dose Reduction or Interval Prolongation			Dosage Recommendations for Patients Receiving Renal Replacement Therapy		
	GFR > 50 mL/min	GFR = 10-50 mL/min	GFR < 10 mL/min	HD	CAPD	CRRT
Flecainide	100%	50%	50%	Dose as GFR < 10	Dose as GFR < 10	Dose as GFR 10-50
Fluconazole	100%	100%	50%	Dose as GFR < 10	Dose as GFR < 10	Dose as GFR 10-50
Flucytosine	50 mg/kg q12h	50 mg/kg q24h	50 mg/kg q24-48h	Dose as GFR < 10	Dose as GFR < 10	Dose as GFR 10-50
Fludarabine	75%-100%	75%	50%	Dose as GFR < 10	Dose as GFR < 10	Dose as GFR 10-50
Foscarnet	28 mg/kg/q8h	15 mg/kg/q8h	6 mg/kg/q8h	Dose as GFR < 10	Dose as GFR < 10	Dose as GFR 10-50
Fosinopril	100%	100%	75%-100%	Dose as GFR < 10	Dose as GFR < 10	Dose as GFR 10-50
Gabapentin	400 mg q8h	300 mg q12-24h	300 mg q48h	As normal GFR	As normal GFR	As normal GFR
Gallamine	75%	Avoid	Avoid	NA	NA	Avoid
Ganciclovir	2.5-5 mg/kg q12h	1.25-2.5 mg/kg q24h	1.25 mg/kg q24h	Dose as GFR < 10	Dose as GFR < 10	2.5 mg/kg q24h
Gemfibrozil	100%	75%	50%	Dose as GFR < 10	Dose as GFR < 10	Dose as GFR 10-50
Gentamicin*	5-7 mg/kg/day	2-3 mg/kg/day by levels	2 mg/kg q48-72h by levels	3-4 mg/kg after HD	3-4 mg/L/day by levels	Dose as GFR 10-50
Gliclazide	50%-100%	20-40 mg/day	20-40 mg/day	Dose as GFR < 10	Dose as GFR < 10	Dose as GFR 10-50
Glipizide	100%	50%	50%	Dose as GFR < 10	Dose as GFR < 10	Dose as GFR < 10
Guanadrel	q12h	q12-24h	q24-48h	Dose as GFR < 10	Dose as GFR < 10	Dose as GFR 10-50
Guanethidine	q24h	q24h	q24-36h	Unknown	Unknown	Dose as GFR 10-50
Hydralazine	q8h	q8h	q8-12h	Dose as GFR < 10	Dose as GFR < 10	Dose as GFR 10-50
Hydroxyurea	100%	50%	20%	Dose as GFR < 10	Dose as GFR < 10	Dose as GFR 10-50
Hydroxyzine	100%	50%	50%	Dose as GFR < 10	Dose as GFR < 10	Dose as GFR 10-50
Idarubicin	100%	75%	50%	Dose as GFR < 10	Dose as GFR < 10	Dose as GFR 10-50
Ifosfamide	100%	75%	50%	Dose as GFR < 10	Dose as GFR < 10	Dose as GFR 10-50
Iloprost	100%	100%	100%	Dose as GFR < 10	Dose as GFR < 10	Dose as GFR 10-50
Imipenem	100%	50%	25%	Dose as GFR < 10	Dose as GFR < 10	Dose as GFR 10-50
Indapamide	100%	100%	50%	Dose as GFR < 10	Dose as GFR < 10	Dose as GFR 10-50
Indobufen	100%	50%	25%	NA	NA	NA
Isoniazid	100%	100%	75%-100%	Unknown	Unknown	Unknown
Kanamycin*	7.5 mg/kg q12h	7.5 mg/kg q24-72h	7.5 mg/kg q48-72h	Dose as GFR < 10	Dose as GFR < 10	As normal GFR
Ketorolac	100%	50%	50%	50% the normal dose	15-20 mg/L/day	Dose as GFR 10-50
Lamivudine	100%	50-150 mg q24h	25-50 mg q24h	Dose as GFR < 10	Dose as GFR < 10	Dose as GFR 10-50
Lepirudin	100%	25%-50%	Avoid	Dose as GFR < 10	Dose as GFR < 10	50 mg q24h
Levofloxacin	100%	50%	25%-50%	Avoid	Avoid	Avoid
Lincomycin	q6h	q6-12h	q12-24h	Dose as GFR < 10	Dose as GFR < 10	Dose as GFR 10-50
Lisinopril	100%	50%-75%	25%-50%	Dose as GFR < 10	Dose as GFR < 10	Dose as GFR 10-50
Lithium carbonate*	100%	50%-75%	25%-50%	Dose as GFR < 10	Dose as GFR < 10	Dose as GFR 10-50
Lomefloxacin	100%	50%-100%	50%	Dose as GFR < 10	Dose as GFR < 10	Dose as GFR 10-50
Loracarbef	q12h	q24h	q3-5days	Dose as GFR < 10	Dose as GFR < 10	Dose as GFR 10-50
Melphalan	100%	75%	50%	Dose as GFR < 10	Dose as GFR < 10	Dose as GFR 10-50
Meperidine	100%	75%	50%	Avoid	Avoid	Avoid
Meprobamate	q6h	q9-12h	q12-18h	Dose as GFR < 10	Dose as GFR < 10	Dose as GFR 10-50
Meropenem	500 mg-2 g q8h	500 mg-1 g q12h	500 mg-1 g q24h	Dose as GFR < 10	Dose as GFR < 10	Dose as GFR 10-50
Metformin	100%	50%-avoid	Avoid	Avoid	Avoid	Avoid
Methadone	100%	100%	50%-75%	Dose as GFR < 10	Dose as GFR < 10	Dose as GFR 10-50
Methotrexate	100%	50%	Contraindicated	Contraindicated	Contraindicated	Dose as GFR 10-50
Methyldopa	q8h	q8-12h	q12-24h	Dose as GFR < 10	Dose as GFR < 10	Dose as GFR 10-50
Metoclopramide	100%	75%	50%	Dose as GFR < 10	Dose as GFR < 10	Dose as GFR 10-50

Drug				
Metocurine	75%	50%	Unknown	Dose as GFR 10-50
Mexiletine	100%	100%	Dose as GFR < 10	As normal GFR
Midazolam	100%	50%	Dose as GFR < 10	As normal GFR
Midodrine	5-10 mg q8h	2.5-10 mg q8h	Dose as GFR < 10	Dose as GFR 10-50
Milrinone	100%	50%-75%	Dose as GFR < 10	Dose as GFR 10-50
Mitomycin C	100%	75%	No data	As normal GFR
Mivacurium	100%	50%	Dose as GFR < 10	Dose as GFR 10-50
Morphine	100%	50%	Dose as GFR < 10	Dose as < 10
Mycophenolate mofetil	100%	50%-100%	Dose as GFR < 10	As normal GFR
N-Acetylcysteine	100%	75%	Dose as GFR < 10	Dose as GFR 10-50
Nadolol	q24h	q24-48h	Dose as GFR < 10	Dose as GFR 10-50
Nalidixic acid	100%	Avoid	Avoid	Avoid
Neostigmine	100%	50%	Dose as GFR < 10	Dose as GFR 10-50
Netilmicin*	4-7.5 mg/kg/day	3-7.5 mg/kg/day	2 mg/kg after each	IV: 2 mg/kg q48h
Nicotinic acid	100%	50%	Dose as GFR < 10	Dose as GFR 10-50
Nitroprusside	100%	100%	Avoid	Dose as GFR 10-50
Nitrosoureas	100%	75%	25%-50%	Unknown
Nizatidine	75%-100%	50%	25%	Dose as GFR 10-50
Norfloxacin	q12h	q12-24h	q24h	Dose as GFR 10-50
Ofloxacin	100%	50%	25%	Dose as GFR 10-50
Oxcarbazepine	100%	75%-100%	50%	Dose as GFR 10-50
Pancuronium	100%	50%	25%	Dose as GFR 10-50
Paroxetine	100%	50%-75%	50%	Dose as GFR 10-50
Paraamino salicylic acid (PAS)	100%	50%-75%	50%	Dose as GFR 10-50
Penicillamine	100%	Avoid	Avoid	Avoid
Penicillin G	100%	75%	20%-50%	Dose as GFR 10-50
Pentamidine	q24h	q24h	q24-36h	Dose as GFR 10-50
Pentazocine	100%	75%	50%	Unknown
Pentopril	100%	50%-75%	50%	Dose as GFR 10-50
Pentoxifylline	q8-12h	q12-24h	q24h	Dose as GFR 10-50
Perindopril	2 mg q24h	2 mg q24-48h	2 mg q48h	Does as GFR < 10
Phenobarbital	q8-12h	q8-12h	q12-16h	Dose as GFR 10-50
Phenylbutazone	100%	50%	Avoid	Avoid
Pipecuronium	q6h	50%	25%	Dose as GFR 10-50
Piperacillin	100%	q6-12h	q12h	Dose as GFR 10-50
Plicamycin	100%	75%	50%	Unknown
Pregabalin	100% q8-12h	50% q8-12h	25% q24h	Dose as GFR 10-50
Primidone	q12	q12-24h	q24h	Dose as GFR 10-50
Probenecid	100%	Avoid	Avoid	Avoid
Procainamide	q4h	q6-12h	q8-24h	Follow levels
Propoxyphene	100%	100%	Avoid	Avoid
Propylthiouracil	100%	75%	50%	Dose as GFR 10-50
Pyrazinamide	100%	100%	50%-100%	Dose as GFR 10-50
Pyridostigmine	100%	35%	20%	Dose as GFR 10-50
Quinapril	100%	2.5-5 mg q24h	2.5 mg q24h	Dose as GFR 10-50
Quinine	q8h	q8-12h	q24h	Dose as GFR 10-50
Ramipril	100%	50%	25%	Dose as GFR 10-50
Ranitidine	100%	100%	50%	Dose as GFR 10-50
Ribavirin	100%	Avoid	Avoid	Avoid

Continued on following page

Table 84.8 Recommendations for Dosing Selected Drugs in Patients with Chronic Kidney Disease or Acute Kidney Injury (Continued)

Drug	Degree of Drug Dose Reduction or Interval Prolongation			Dosage Recommendations for Patients Receiving Renal Replacement Therapy		
	GFR > 50 mL/min	GFR = 10-50 mL/min	GFR < 10 mL/min	HD	CAPD	CRRT
Rifampin	100%	50%-100%	50%-100%	Dose as GFR < 10	Dose as GFR < 10	As normal GFR
Rivaroxaban	100%	Avoid	Avoid	Avoid	Avoid	Avoid
Simvastatin	100%	100%	10 mg q24h	Dose as GFR < 10	Dose as GFR < 10	As normal GFR
Sitagliptin	100%	50%	25%	Dose as GFR < 10	Dose as GFR < 10	Dose as GFR 10-50
Sotalol	100%	25%-50%	25%	Dose as GFR < 10	Dose as GFR < 10	Dose as GFR 10-50
Spironolactone	100%	50%	Avoid	Avoid	Avoid	Avoid
Stavudine	100%	50% q12-24h	50% q24h	Dose as GFR < 10	Dose as GFR < 10	Dose as GFR 10-50
Streptomycin*	q24h	q24-72h	q72-96h	Dose as GFR < 10	20-40 mg/L/day	Dose as GFR 10-50
Streptozocin	100%	75%	50%	Unknown	Unknown	Unknown
Sulfamethoxazole	q12h	q18h	q24h	1 g after dialysis	1 g/day	Dose as GFR 10-50
Sulfinpyrazone	100%	100%	Avoid	Avoid	Avoid	Dose as GFR 10-50
Sulfisoxazole	q6h	q8-12h	q12-24h	2 g after dialysis	3 g/day	NA
Sulindac	100%	50%-100%	50%-100%	Dose as GFR < 10	Dose as GFR < 10	Dose as GFR < 10
Sulotroban	50%	30%	10%	Unknown	Unknown	Unknown
Tazobactam	100%	75%	50%	Dose as GFR < 10	Dose as GFR < 10	Dose as GFR 10-50
Teicoplanin	q24h	q24-48h	q48-72h	Dose as GFR < 10	Dose as GFR < 10	Dose as GFR 10-50
Temocillin	q12-24h	q24h	q48h	Dose as GFR < 10	Dose as GFR < 10	Dose as GFR 10-50
Terbutaline	100%	50%	Avoid	Avoid	Avoid	Avoid
Tetracycline	100%	100%	50%	Dose as GFR < 10	Dose as GFR < 10	Dose as GFR 10-50
Thiazides	100%	100%	Avoid	Dose as GFR < 10	Dose as GFR < 10	NA
Thiopental	100%	100%	75%	NA	NA	NA
Ticarcillin	50-75 mg/kg q6h	50-75 mg/kg q8h	50-75 mg/kg q12h	Dose as GFR < 10	Dose as GFR < 10	Dose as GFR 10-50
Tobramycin*	5-7 mg/kg/day	2-3 mg/kg/day	2 mg/kg q48-72h	3 mg/kg after HD	3-4 mg/L/day	Dose as GFR 10-50
Tolvaptan	100%	100%	Avoid	Avoid	Avoid	Avoid
Topiramate	100%	50%	25%	Dose as GFR < 10	Dose as GFR < 10	Dose as GFR 10-50
Topotecan	75%	50%	25%	Dose as GFR < 10	No data	No data
Tramadol	100%	50-100 mg q8h	50 mg q8h	Dose as GFR < 10	Dose as GFR < 10	Dose as GFR 10-50
Tranexamic acid	50%	25%	10%	Dose as GFR < 10	Dose as GFR < 10	Dose as GFR 10-50
Trazodone	100%	100%	Avoid/50%	Dose as GFR < 10	Dose as GFR < 10	Dose as GFR 10-50
Triamterene	100%	Avoid	Avoid	Avoid	Avoid	Avoid
Trimethoprim	q12h	q12h	q24h	Dose as GFR < 10	Dose as GFR < 10	Dose as GFR 10-50
Trimetrexate	100%	50%-100%	Avoid	No data	No data	Dose as GFR 10-50
Tubocurarine	75%	50%	Avoid	Unknown	Unknown	Dose as GFR 10-50
Valganciclovir	50%-100%	450 mg q24-48h	450 mg Q72-96	Avoid	Avoid	450 mg q48h
Vancomycin*	1 g q12-24h	1 g q24-96h	1 g q4-7d	Dose as GFR < 10	Dose as GFR < 10	Dose as GFR 10-50
Venlafaxine	100%	50%	50%	Dose as GFR < 10	Dose as GFR < 10	Dose as GFR 10-50
Vigabatrin	100%	50%	25%	Dose as GFR < 10	Dose as GFR < 10	Dose as GFR 10-50
Zalcitabine	100%	q12h	q24h	Dose as GFR < 10	No data	Dose as GFR 10-50
Zidovudine (AZT)	100% q8h	100% q8h	50% q8h	Dose as GFR < 10	Dose as GFR < 10	Dose as GFR 10-50
Zileuton	100%	100%	100%	Dose as GFR < 10	Unknown	Dose as GFR 10-50

*Adjust dose to achieve desired serum concentrations using measured serum concentrations and pharmacokinetic modeling principles.
CAPD, Continuous ambulatory peritoneal dialysis; CRRT, continuous renal replacement therapy; HD, hemodialysis; NA, not applicable.

KEY REFERENCES

1. Matzke GR, Aronoff GR, Atkinson AJ, Jr, et al: Drug dosing consideration in patients with acute and chronic kidney disease—a clinical update from Kidney Disease: Improving Global Outcomes (KDIGO). *Kidney Int* 80:1122–1137, 2011.
7. Hoste EA, Dhondt A: Clinical review: Use of renal replacement therapies in special groups of ICU patients. *Crit Care* 16:201–211, 2012.
8. Heintz BH, Matzke GR, Dager WE: Antimicrobial dosing concepts and recommendations for critically ill adult patients receiving continuous renal replacement therapy or intermittent hemodialysis. *Pharmacotherapy* 29:562–577, 2009.
9. Dowling TC, Matzke GR, Murphy JE, et al: Evaluation of renal drug dosing: prescribing information and clinical pharmacist approaches. *Pharmacotherapy* 30:776–786, 2010.
19. Borst P, Schinkel AH: P-glycoprotein ABCB1: a major player in drug handling by mammals. *J Clin Invest* 123:4131–4133, 2013.
21. Maton PN, Burton ME: Antacids revisited: a review of their clinical pharmacology and recommended therapeutic use. *Drugs* 57:855–870, 1999.
29. Bagshaw SM, Brophy PD, Cruz D, et al: Fluid balance as a biomarker: impact of fluid overload on outcome in critically ill patients with acute renal injury. *Crit Care* 12:169, 2008.
32. Chan C, McIntyre C, Smith D, et al: Combining near-subject absolute and relative measures of longitudinal hydration in hemodialysis. *Clin J Am Soc Nephrol* 4:1791–1798, 2009.
33. Koup J: Disease states and drug pharmacokinetics. *J Clin Pharmacol* 29:674–679, 1989.
34. Meijers BKI, Bremmers B, Verbeke B, et al: A review of albumin binding in CKD. *Am J Kidney Dis* 51:839–850, 2008.
35. Verbeeck RK, Musuamba FT: Pharmacokinetics and dosage adjustment in patients with renal dysfunction. *Eur J Clin Pharmacol* 65:757–773, 2009.
46. Momper JD, Venkataramanan R, Nolin TD: Nonrenal drug clearance in CKD: searching for the path less traveled. *Adv Chronic Kidney Dis* 17:384–391, 2010.
49. Naud J, Nolin TD, Leblond FA, et al: Current understanding of drug disposition in kidney disease. *J Clin Pharmacol* 52:10S–22S, 2012.
53. Vilay AM, Churchwell MD, Mueller BA: Clinical review: drug metabolism and clearance in acute kidney injury. *Crit Care* 12:235, 2008.
58. Joy MS, Frye RF, Nolin TD, et al: In vivo alterations in drug metabolism and transport pathways in patients with chronic kidney diseases. *Pharmacotherapy* 34:114–122, 2014.
60. Masereeuw R, Russel FGM: Therapeutic implications of renal anionic drug transporters. *Pharmacol Ther* 126:200–216, 2010.
63. Godman B, Finlayson AE, Cheema PK, et al: Personalizing health care: feasibility and future implications. *BMC Med* 11:179–202, 2013.
67. Drozda K, Müller DJ, Bishop JR: Pharmacogenomic testing for neuropsychiatric drugs: current status of drug labelling, guidelines for using genetic information, and test options. *Pharmacotherapy* 34:166–184, 2014.
68. Patel JN: Application of genotype-guided cancer therapy in solid tumors. *Pharmacogenomics* 15:79–93, 2014.
71. Kawaguchi-Suzuki M, Frye RF: The role of pharmacogenetics in the treatment of chronic hepatitis C infection. *Pharmacotherapy* 34:185–201, 2014.
77. U.S. Food and Drug Administration: *Table of pharmacogenomic biomarkers in drug labeling.* Available at: www.fda.gov/drugs/scienceresearchareas/pharmacogenetics/ucm083378.htm. Accessed February 25, 2014.
82. Kimmel SE, French B, Kasner SE: A pharmacogenetic versus a clinical algorithm for warfarin dosing. *N Engl J Med* 369(24):2283–2293, 2013.
83. Pirmohamed M, Burnside G, Eriksson N: A randomized trial of genotype-guided dosing of warfarin. *N Engl J Med* 369(24):2294–2303, 2013.
85. Czock D, Markert C, Hartman B, et al: Pharmacokinetics and pharmacodynamics of antimicrobial drugs. *Expert Opin Drug Metab Toxicol* 5:475–487, 2009.
88. Eyler RF, Mueller BA: Antibiotic dosing in critically ill patients with acute kidney injury. *Nat Rev Nephrol* 7:226–235, 2011.
92. Gould IM, Miró JM, Rybak MJ: Daptomycin: The role of high-dose and combination therapy for Gram-positive infections. *Int J Antimicrob Agents* 42:202–210, 2013.
96. Earley A, Miskulin D, Lamb EJ, et al: Estimating equations for glomerular filtration rate in the era of creatinine standardization. *Ann Intern Med* 156:785–795, 2012.
105. Matsushita K, Mahmoodi BK, Woodward M, et al, Chronic Kidney Disease Prognosis Consortium: Comparison of risk prediction using the CKD-EPI equation and the MDRD study equation for estimated glomerular filtration rate. *JAMA* 307:1941–1951, 2012.
107. Inker LA, Schmid CH, Tighiouart H, et al, CKD-EPI Investigators: Estimating glomerular filtration rate from serum creatinine and cystatin C. *N Engl J Med* 367:20–29, 2012.
113. Golik MV, Lawrence KR: Comparison of dosing recommendations for antimicrobial drugs based on two methods for assessing kidney function: Cockcroft-Gault and modification of diet in renal disease. *Pharmacotherapy* 28:1125–1132, 2008.
115. Hermsen ED, Maiefski M, Florescu MC, et al: Comparison of the Modification of Diet in Renal Disease and Cockcroft-Gault equations for dosing antimicrobials. *Pharmacotherapy* 29:649–655, 2009.
120. Schwartz GJ, Schneider MF, Maier PS, et al: Improved equations estimating GFR in children with chronic kidney disease using an immunonephelometric determination of cystatin C. *Kidney Int* 82:445–453, 2012.
122. Mehta RL, Kellum JA, Shah SV, et al, Acute Kidney Injury Network: Acute Kidney Injury Network: report of an initiative to improve outcomes in acute kidney injury. *Crit Care* 11:R31, 2007.
129. Bouchard J, Macedo E, Soroko S, et al: Comparison of methods for estimating glomerular filtration rate in critically ill patients with acute kidney injury. *Nephrol Dial Transplant* 25:102–107, 2010.
130. Chen S: Retooling the creatinine clearance equation to estimate kinetic GFR when the plasma creatinine is changing acutely. *J Am Soc Nephrol* 24:877–888, 2013.
132. Dowling TD, Wang E, Ferrucci L, et al: Glomerular filtration rate equations overestimate creatinine clearance in older individuals enrolled in the Baltimore longitudinal study on aging: impact on renal drug dosing. *Pharmacotherapy* 33:912–921, 2013.
139. Fish DN, Kiser TH: Correlation of pharmacokinetic/pharmacodynamic-derived predictions of antibiotic efficacy with clinical outcomes in severely ill patients with *Pseudomonas aeruginosa* pneumonia. *Pharmacotherapy* 33:1022–1034, 2013.
146. Kamel OHM, Wahba IM, Watnick S, et al: Administration of tobramycin in the beginning of the hemodialysis session: a novel intradialytic dosing regimen. *Clin J Am Soc Nephrol* 2:694–699, 2007.
147. Kielstein JT, Eugbers C, Bode-Boeger SM, et al: Dosing of daptomycin in intensive care unit patients with acute kidney injury undergoing extended dialysis—a pharmacokinetic study. *Nephrol Dial Transplant* 25:1537–1541, 2010.
155. Matzke GR: Status of hemodialysis of drugs in 2002. *J Pharm Pract* 15:405–418, 2002.
161. Manley HJ, Bailie GR, McClaran ML, et al: Gentamicin pharmacokinetics during slow daily home hemodialysis. *Kidney Int* 63:1072–1078, 2003.
164. Veinstein A, Venisse N, Badin J, et al: Gentamicin in hemodialyzed critical care patients: early dialysis after administration of a high dose should be considered. *Antimicrob Agents Chemother* 57:977–982, 2013.
168. Decker BS, Mueller BA, Sowinski KM: Drug dosing considerations in alternative hemodialysis. *Adv Chronic Kidney Dis* 14:e17–e26, 2007.
185. Joy MS, Matzke GR, Frye RF, et al: Determinants of vancomycin clearance by continuous venovenous hemofiltration and continuous venovenous hemodialysis. *Am J Kidney Dis* 31:1019–1027, 1998.
186. Mueller BA, Pasko DA, Sowinski KM: Higher renal replacement therapy dose delivery influences on drug therapy. *Artif Organs* 27:808–814, 2003.
188. Uchino S, Cole L, Morimatsu H, et al: Clearance of vancomycin during high-volume haemofiltration: impact of pre-dilution. *Intensive Care Med* 28:1664–1667, 2002.
191. Schetz M: Drug dosing in continuous renal replacement therapy: general rules. *Curr Opin Crit Care* 13:645–651, 2007.
196. Bogard KN, Peterson NT, Plumb TJ, et al: Antibiotic dosing during sustained low-efficiency dialysis: special considerations in adult critically ill patients. *Crit Care Med* 39:560–570, 2011.
202. Taylor CA, 3rd, Abdel-Rahman E, Zimmerman SW, et al: Clinical pharmacokinetics during continuous ambulatory peritoneal dialysis. *Clin Pharmacokinet* 31:293–308, 1996.
203. Li PKT, Szeto CC, Piraino B, et al: Peritoneal dialysis-related infections recommendations: 2010 update. *Perit Dial Int* 30:393–423, 2010.
204. Manley HJ, Bailie GR: Treatment of peritonitis in APD: pharmacokinetic principles. *Semin Dial* 15:418–421, 2002.

DIALYSIS AND EXTRACORPOREAL THERAPIES

SECTION X

65 Hemodialysis

Jane Y. Yeun | Daniel B. Ornt | Thomas A. Depner

CHAPTER OUTLINE

THE HEMODIALYSIS POPULATION, 2059
Incidence and Prevalence, 2059
Causes of End-Stage Kidney Disease, 2060
Mortality, 2060
Transition from Chronic Kidney Disease Stage 5, 2063
VASCULAR ACCESS, 2064
Background, 2064
Types of Vascular Access, 2064
Maintenance of Vascular Access Function, 2066
Hemodialysis Catheters, 2067
GENERAL PRINCIPLES OF HEMODIALYSIS: PHYSIOLOGY AND BIOMECHANICS, 2068
Native Kidney versus Artificial Kidney, 2069
Clearance, 2069
Clearance versus Removal Rate, 2070
Serum Urea Concentration versus Urea Clearance, 2070
Factors That Affect Clearance in a Flowing System, 2070
Dialysance, 2071
Determinants of Clearance, 2072
Dialyzer Clearance versus Whole Body Clearance, 2072
COMPONENTS OF THE EXTRACORPOREAL CIRCUIT, 2074
Blood Circuit, 2075
Hemodialyzers, 2075
Dialysate Circuit, 2078
Online Monitoring, 2079
Dialysate, 2080
Water Treatment, 2080
HEMODIALYSIS ADEQUACY, 2082
Historical Perspectives, 2082
Uremia: The Syndrome Reversed by Dialysis Therapy, 2083
Measuring Hemodialysis Adequacy, 2083

Alternative Measures of Dialysis, 2085
Comparison of Hemodialysis and Peritoneal Dialysis Doses, 2087
Standard Clearance and Standard Kt/V, 2088
Nocturnal Hemodialysis, 2088
Short Daily Hemodialysis, 2088
Accounting for Native Kidney Function, 2089
THE DIALYSIS PRESCRIPTION, 2089
Goals of Hemodialysis, 2089
Dialysis Duration and Frequency, 2090
Dialyzer Choice, 2090
Blood and Dialysate Flow Rates, 2091
Anticoagulation, 2091
Dialysate Composition, 2092
Dialysate Temperature, 2095
Ultrafiltration Rate and Dry Weight, 2095
Reuse, 2096
MANAGEMENT OF PATIENTS ON MAINTENANCE HEMODIALYSIS, 2097
End-Stage Kidney Disease, 2097
Anemia, 2097
Nutrition, 2098
Cardiovascular Disease, 2100
Mineral Metabolism–Related Issues, 2102
Hypertension, 2103
Immune Disorders and Infection, 2104
Primary Care Management, 2105
COMPLICATIONS FOR PATIENTS ON MAINTENANCE HEMODIALYSIS, 2105
Hypotension, 2105
Dialysis Disequilibrium Syndrome, 2106
Muscle Cramps, 2107
Cardiac Events, 2107
Reactions to Dialyzers, 2108
Other Complications, 2108
THE FUTURE OF RENAL REPLACEMENT THERAPY, 2018

Hemodialysis (HD) sustains life for more than 2.6 million people worldwide. Without it, most would die within a few weeks.[1,2] The life sustaining nature of the treatment requires caregivers to possess detailed technical knowledge of the dialysis procedure itself in addition to an understanding of the pathophysiology of the uremic state (see Chapter 54). This chapter reviews the history of dialysis; the epidemiology of the HD patient population; the physical, chemical, and clinical principles of HD as they relate to the treatment of patients with uremia; and the complications associated with this treatment.

HD has been applied routinely to preserve life in patients with end-stage kidney disease (ESKD) for only the past 40 years. Several early pioneers laid the foundation. Graham (1805-1869), a Scottish professor of chemistry, invented the fundamental process of separating solutes in vitro using semipermeable membranes and coined the term *dialysis*.[3] In 1916, Abel dialyzed rabbits and dogs with a "vividiffusion" device using celloidin membranes and a leech extract, hirudin, as an anticoagulant.[4] He was the first to dialyze a living organism and to use the term artificial kidney. In 1924, in Germany, Haas was the first to dialyze a human,[5] but he was only marginally successful because of toxicity from his crude anticoagulant.

In 1944, Willem Kolff and colleagues succeeded in using extracorporeal dialysis to support patients with acute kidney failure.[6] Their success was partly attributable to the invention of cellophane, the discovery of antibiotics, and the availability of heparin. Kolff was often called the "father of hemodialysis," and his method became the standard for temporary replacement of kidney function in patients with short-lived acute renal failure.[7,8] However, HD could not support patients with prolonged or permanent loss of kidney function because of the difficulty with vascular access, which was subsequently solved by the creation of the arteriovenous (AV) fistula (see "Vascular Access" section).

Although it had become technically feasible, HD remained expensive and inefficient and was offered only to those who were free of comorbid conditions, gainfully employed, and better educated. Because dialysis was so successful in preventing death from kidney failure, the U.S. Congress, after much debate, passed a law in 1973 approving public funding for dialysis and kidney transplantation regardless of a patient's means, education, employment, and comorbidities.[9] This law paved the way to life-sustaining kidney replacement for virtually all U.S. patients.

THE HEMODIALYSIS POPULATION

INCIDENCE AND PREVALENCE

According to the U.S. Renal Data System (USRDS), 615,899 patients in the United States had ESKD at the end of 2011, the latest year of data reporting.[10] Of these patients, 30% had functioning transplants, and the remainder were managed with maintenance dialysis, 93% with HD. Although the prevalent number of patients with ESKD has continued to grow from 535,166 in 2008, the 1-year growth rate of 3.4% at the end of 2011 represents the smallest in 30 years. In 2011, ESKD developed in 115,643 U.S. patients, 91% were started on HD, and 2.5% underwent preemptive transplantation. Figure 65.1A shows that the incidence of ESKD in the United States steadily increased from 1987 to 2002, most likely as a result of aging of the population and growing acceptance of dialysis for older patients as part of their Medicare entitlement. However, later USRDS data revealed a leveling off of the incidence of ESKD from 2002 through 2006 and a decline since 2006, with the largest decrease, 3.8%, in 2011 (see Figure 65.1B). Both the prevalence and the incidence of ESKD vary widely with age (Figure 65.2), sex (Figure 65.3), and ethnicity (Figure 65.4), with a predilection for older age, men, African Americans, Latinos, and Native Americans. However, over the past few years, the incidence of ESKD has declined in persons older than 45 (Figure 65.2B), and in African Americans, Latinos, and

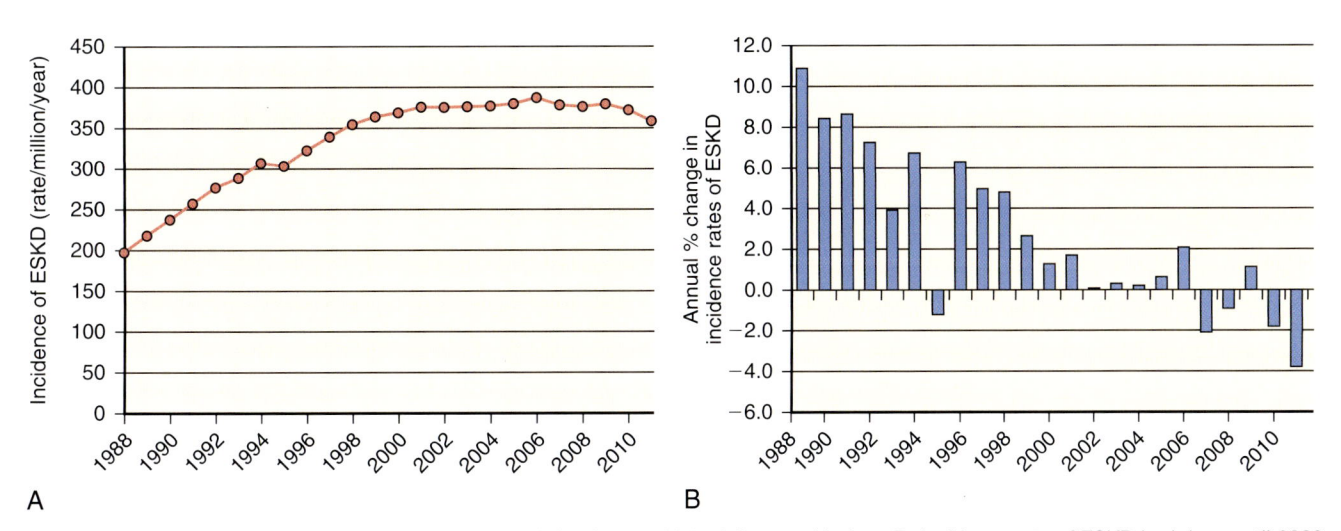

Figure 65.1 **A,** Incidence of end-stage kidney disease (ESKD) in the United States with time. **B,** Incidence rate of ESKD had risen until 2002, leveled off from 2002 to 2006, and declined from 2006 through 2011. (Adapted from U.S. Renal Data System: *USRDS 2010 annual data report: atlas of chronic kidney disease and end-stage renal disease in the United States*, Bethesda, MD, 2010, National Institutes of Health, National Institute of Diabetes and Digestive and Kidney Diseases.)

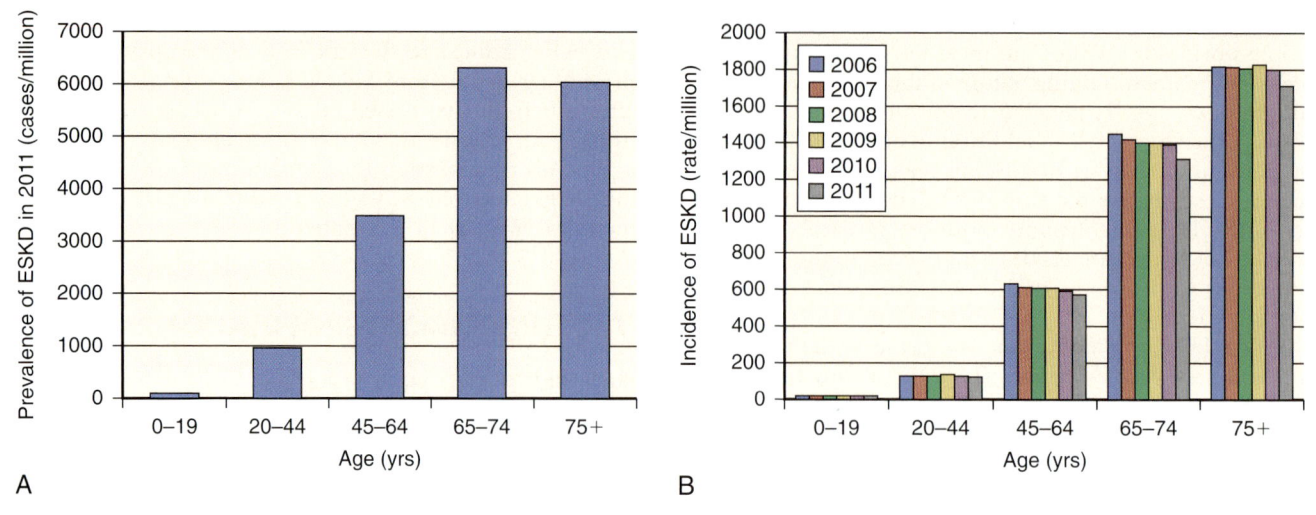

Figure 65.2 Prevalence **(A)** and incidence **(B)** of end-stage kidney disease (ESKD) with age. (Adapted from U.S. Renal Data System: *USRDS 2010 annual data report: atlas of chronic kidney disease and end-stage renal disease in the United States*, Bethesda, MD, 2010, National Institutes of Health, National Institute of Diabetes and Digestive and Kidney Diseases.)

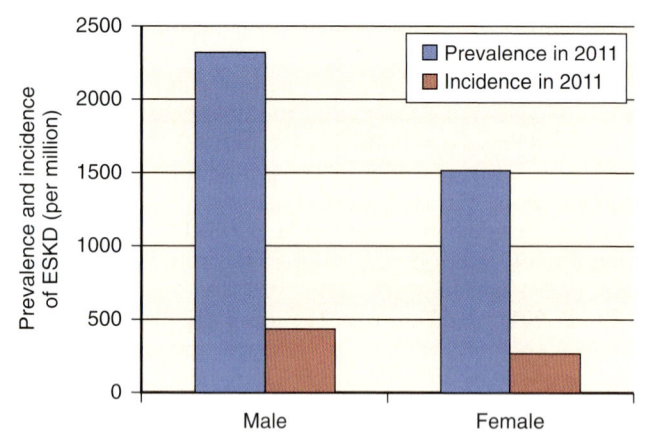

Figure 65.3 Prevalence and incidence of end-stage kidney disease (ESKD) according to gender. (Adapted from U.S. Renal Data System: *USRDS 2010 annual data report: atlas of chronic kidney disease and end-stage renal disease in the United States*, Bethesda, MD, 2010, National Institutes of Health, National Institute of Diabetes and Digestive and Kidney Diseases.)

Native Americans (Figure 65.4*B*). The high ratio of incidence to prevalence reflects a high mortality rate, especially in older age groups.

Worldwide in 2011, Mexico had the highest incidence rate for ESKD, at 527 per million population, followed closely by the United States, Taiwan, and Japan at 362, 361 (2010 data), and 295 per million population, respectively.[10] The highest prevalence rate for ESKD is found in Taiwan, at 2584 per million population (2010 data), followed by Japan and the United States (prevalence rates of 2309 and 1924 per million population, respectively). These high numbers reflect the policies of these nations to provide open access to maintenance dialysis therapy and nearly universal health care for patients with ESKD. However, the worldwide prevalence of ESKD varies greatly, with the lowest rate reported in the Philippines, at 159 per million population. The broad ranges of reported ESKD prevalence likely result from variable access to treatment. Countries that offer preventive and maintenance health care to a larger segment of their populations also may have a higher prevalence rate partly because more patients survive to have ESKD. Longitudinal follow-up data from patients with chronic kidney disease (CKD) in the United States show that most do not survive to have ESKD.[10]

CAUSES OF END-STAGE KIDNEY DISEASE

The causes of ESKD in the United States are listed in Table 65.1. Beginning in 1980, the percentage of patients with diabetic kidney disease increased, from near 0% to 44% of patients starting dialysis in 2011 (Figure 65.5), primarily because of greater acceptance of patients with diabetes into dialysis programs. Although the incidence rate of ESKD from diabetes in 2011 was 9.3% lower than that in 2006 (172.9/million population in 2006 compared with 156.8/million in 2011) (see Figure 65.5), diabetes remains the most common cause of ESKD in the United States and in many other countries,[10] exceeding 40% of cases in Israel, the Republic of Korea, Hong Kong, Taiwan, the Philippines, Japan, the United States, and New Zealand and reaching as high as 60% in Singapore, Mexico, and Malaysia. In comparison with patients without diabetes, mortality rates for dialysis recipients with diabetic kidney disease tend to be higher and worsen with time on dialysis (Figure 65.6).

MORTALITY

The survival of dialysis recipients in the United States has slowly improved in the past 20 years despite increasing comorbidity (Figure 65.7). If 1-year mortality rates of incident patients (those beginning dialysis) in 2000 and 2010, all-cause mortality has declined by 22%, cardiovascular mortality by 38%, and death due to infections by 50%.[10] Similarly, the overall mortality rate for prevalent patients receiving HD has decreased by 26% since 1985 and by 21% since 2000.[10] However, mortality remains very high. Patients starting hemodialysis in 2006 had 76% 1-year, 63% 2-year, and 36% 5-year survival rates (see Figure 65.7).[10] Compared with age-matched persons without kidney disease, patients with ESKD or undergoing dialysis have a sixfold to eightfold

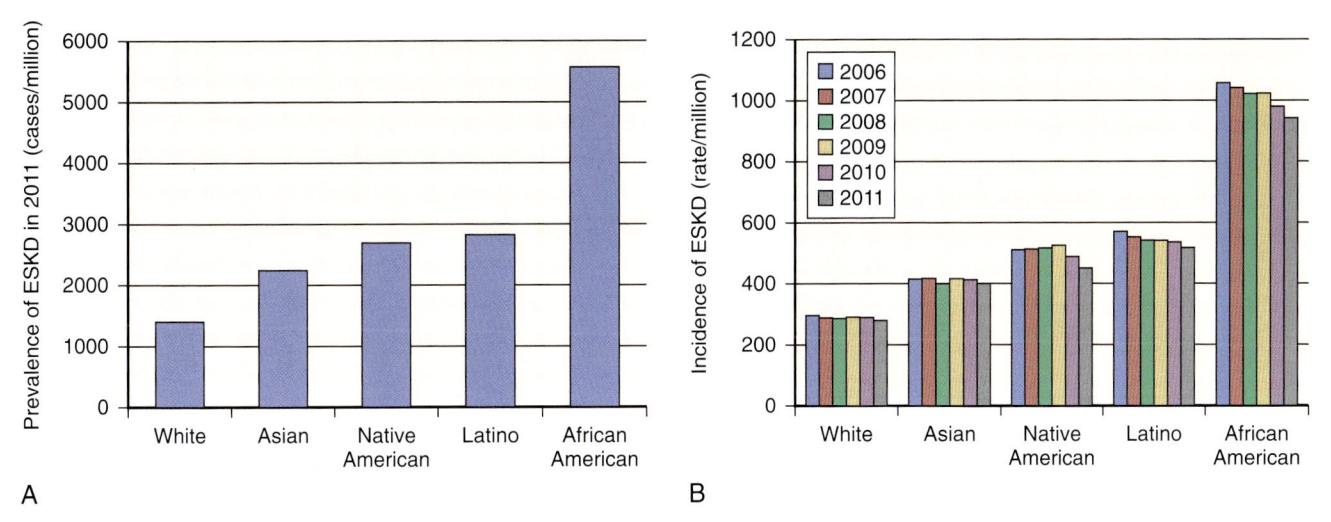

Figure 65.4 Prevalence **(A)** and incidence **(B)** of end-stage kidney disease (ESKD) according to ethnicity. (Adapted from U.S. Renal Data System: *USRDS 2010 annual data report: atlas of chronic kidney disease and end-stage renal disease in the United States*, Bethesda, MD, 2010, National Institutes of Health, National Institute of Diabetes and Digestive and Kidney Diseases.)

Table 65.1 Causes of End-Stage Kidney Disease in Incident and Prevalent Patients in the United States in 2011

Primary Kidney Disease	Incident Patients		Prevalent Patients	
	N	% Total	N	% Total
Diabetes mellitus	49,603	42.9	228,114	37
Hypertension	31,831	27.5	151,317	24.6
Glomerulonephritis	7215	6.2	86,307	14
Cystic kidney disease	2502	2.2	28,932	4.7
Other	24,492	21.2	121,229	19.7
Total	115,643	100	615,899	100

Data from USRDS; excerpts from U.S. Renal Data System: USRDS 2013 annual data report: atlas of chronic kidney disease and end-stage renal disease in the United States, Bethesda, MD, 2013, National Institutes of Health, National Institute of Diabetes and Digestive and Kidney Diseases.

Figure 65.5 Causes of end-stage kidney disease (ESKD) in the United States. (Adapted from U.S. Renal Data System: *USRDS 2010 annual data report: atlas of chronic kidney disease and end-stage renal disease in the United States*, Bethesda, MD, 2010, National Institutes of Health, National Institute of Diabetes and Digestive and Kidney Diseases.)

higher mortality (Figure 65.8A) and markedly reduced life expectancy (Figure 65.8B). At age 60 years, a healthy person can expect to live for about 20 years, but the average life expectancy of a 60-year-old patient starting HD is closer to 4 or 5 years (see Figure 65.8B).[10] Remarkably, mortality of patients with ESKD is higher than that of patients with heart failure and most types of cancer (Figure 65.8C).

Causes of death are listed in Table 65.2. Not surprisingly, mortality rates increase with age, but the relative contributions of different causes to mortality appear to be similar across the age groups except for withdrawal from dialysis. About 40% of deaths are attributed to cardiovascular disease, compared with 50% a few years ago, but the relative contributions from the uremic milieu, coexisting medical illnesses, and/or dialysis itself to cardiovascular disease remain unclear (see Chapter 56). Infections account for another 10% to 20% of deaths.[11] Overall, voluntary withdrawal from dialysis because of failure to thrive, intervening medical complications, or poor quality of life accounts for another 10% of deaths, with disproportionate representation from older patients. Sixteen percent of deaths in patients older than 75 years of age were due to withdrawal from dialysis, compared with 6% and 11% in patients 45 to 64 and 65 to 74 years of age, respectively (see Table 65.2),[10] likely reflecting the burden of comorbidities and decreased reserve, resulting in more medical complications and poorer quality of life, in older patients. In addition, insufficient exploration of goals of care in the elderly prior to embarking on maintenance hemodialysis may be a major contributor to the higher withdrawal rate.[12,13]

The cause of the higher ESKD-related mortality documented in the United States than in other countries remains incompletely understood. Although more liberal acceptance of patients for dialysis, including those with diabetes

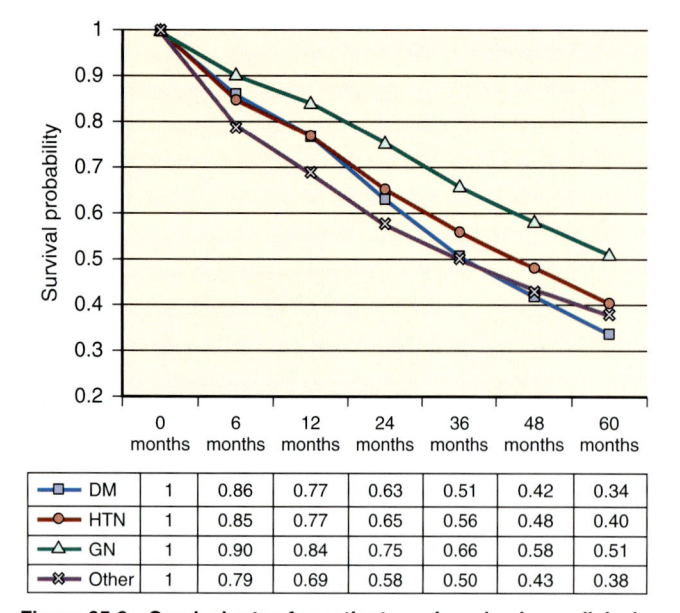

Figure 65.6 Survival rates for patients undergoing hemodialysis. Compared to patients without diabetes, survival rates tend to be lower for patients with diabetes (DM). GN, Glomerulonephritis; HTN, hypertension. (Adapted from U.S. Renal Data System: *USRDS 2010 annual data report: atlas of chronic kidney disease and end-stage renal disease in the United States*, Bethesda, MD, 2010, National Institutes of Health, National Institute of Diabetes and Digestive and Kidney Diseases.)

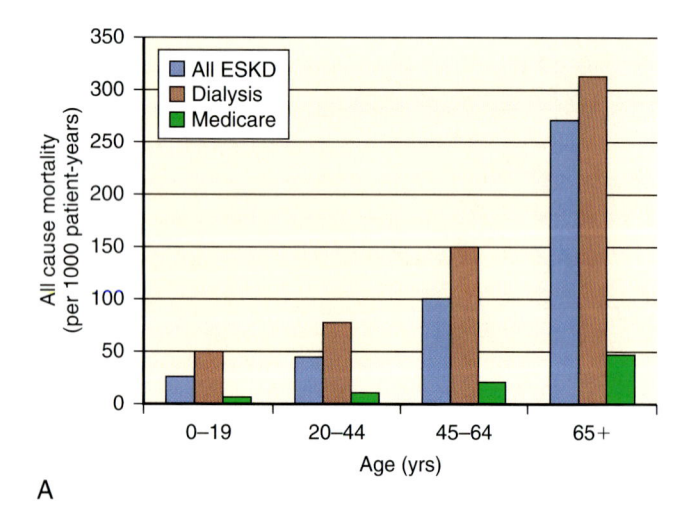

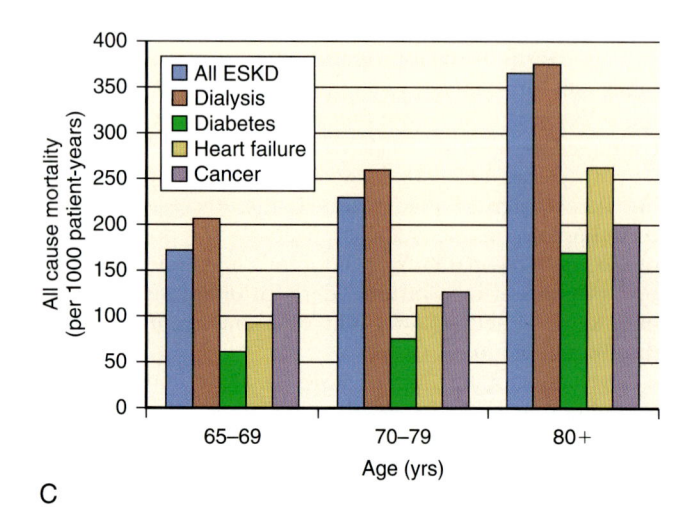

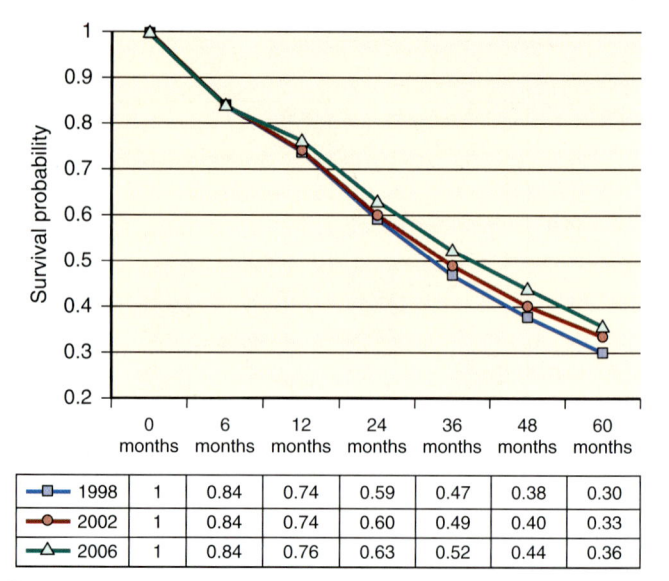

	0 months	6 months	12 months	24 months	36 months	48 months	60 months
DM	1	0.86	0.77	0.63	0.51	0.42	0.34
HTN	1	0.85	0.77	0.65	0.56	0.48	0.40
GN	1	0.90	0.84	0.75	0.66	0.58	0.51
Other	1	0.79	0.69	0.58	0.50	0.43	0.38

Figure 65.7 Probability of survival for patients undergoing hemodialysis. The likelihood of survival of patients on hemodialysis has improved slightly from 1998 to 2006. (Adapted from U.S. Renal Data System: *USRDS 2010 annual data report: atlas of chronic kidney disease and end-stage renal disease in the United States*, Bethesda, MD, 2010, National Institutes of Health, National Institute of Diabetes and Digestive and Kidney Diseases.)

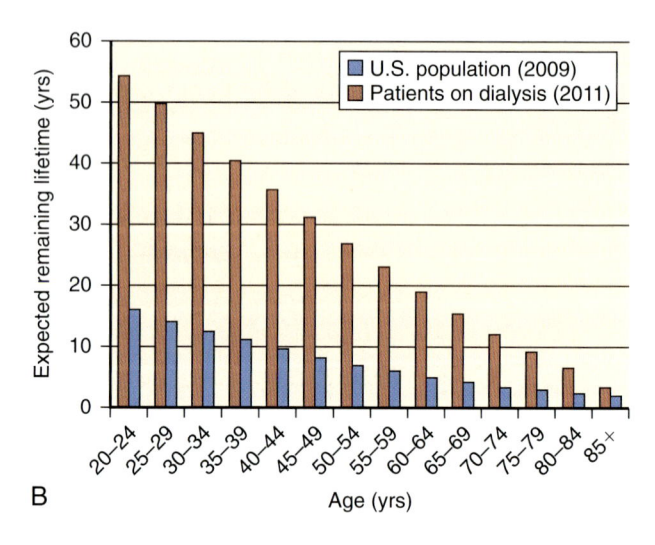

	0 months	6 months	12 months	24 months	36 months	48 months	60 months
1998	1	0.84	0.74	0.59	0.47	0.38	0.30
2002	1	0.84	0.74	0.60	0.49	0.40	0.33
2006	1	0.84	0.76	0.63	0.52	0.44	0.36

Figure 65.8 All-cause mortality rates for patients with end-stage kidney disease (ESKD) in 2010. Patients with ESKD or on dialysis have a higher mortality rate **(A)** and a markedly reduced life expectancy **(B)** in comparison with the general population. These patients' mortality rate is even higher than that of patients with cancer and heart failure **(C)**. (Adapted from U.S. Renal Data System: *USRDS 2010 annual data report: atlas of chronic kidney disease and end-stage renal disease in the United States*, Bethesda, MD, 2010, National Institutes of Health, National Institute of Diabetes and Digestive and Kidney Diseases.)

Table 65.2 Causes of Death for Prevalent Patients on Hemodialysis 2009-2011

Cause of Death	Mortality Rates per 1000 Patient-Years at Risk and Percentage of Total Mortality by Patient Age Range					
	45-64 Years		65-74 Years		75+ Years	
Cardiac arrest	38.7	26.5%	59.7	24.4%	84.4	21.7%
Acute myocardial infection	7.4	5%	11.9	4.9%	15.9	4.1%
Cardiac arrhythmia	4.9	3.3%	7.3	3%	11.1	2.9%
Other cardiac	4.6	3.1%	9.4	3.8%	16.7	4.3%
Cerebrovascular	5.2	3.6%	7.1	2.9%	9.3	2.4%
Infection	16.3	11.1%	25	10.2%	37.1	9.6%
Malignancy	5.9	4%	11.3	4.6%	13.7	3.5%
Cachexia	1.7	1.2%	4.3	1.8%	11.2	2.9%
Withdrawal from dialysis	9.5	6.5%	26	10.6%	62.9	16.2%
Other causes	52.2	35.7%	82.3	33.8%	125.8	32.4%
All cause	146.4	100%	244.3	100%	388.1	100%

Data from USRDS; excerpts from U.S. Renal Data System: USRDS 2013 annual data report: atlas of chronic kidney disease and end-stage renal disease in the United States, *Bethesda, MD, 2013, National Institutes of Health, National Institute of Diabetes and Digestive and Kidney Diseases.*

and advanced age, remains a potential contributor, other contributors appear to be the lower use of AV fistulas as vascular access, later referral to nephrologists, shorter duration of HD sessions with resultant higher ultrafiltration rates, less frequent and shorter nephrologist-patient contact time, decreased patient adherence to treatment recommendations, and international and regional differences in background health and cardiovascular mortality of the general population.[14-22]

TRANSITION FROM CHRONIC KIDNEY DISEASE STAGE 5

The high mortality of patients receiving HD results in part from the many comorbid conditions, including cardiovascular disease and diabetes. These comorbid conditions extract a toll on patients with CKD before ESKD develops and they require dialysis. The relative risk of death is two to three times higher in patients with CKD, diabetes, and cardiovascular disease than in patients without these conditions, those with CKD stage 4 to 5 having the highest mortality risk.[10] A patient with stage 4 to 5 CKD who has an acute myocardial infarction (MI) has a 2-year mortality rate of 70%, compared with 43% in those without CKD.[10] Reducing the burden of comorbid disease is critical in caring for patients with CKD (see Chapters 56 and 62).

In addition, close attention to replacing hormone deficiencies such as erythropoietin (see Chapter 57) and calcitriol (see Chapters 55 and 63) and preventing complications of uremia such as malnutrition (see Chapter 61) and renal osteodystrophy (see Chapters 55 and 63) are essential. Another critical element in preparing the patient with CKD for ESKD care is preemptive planning for potential transplantation as well as for a permanent vascular access to support HD (see later), beginning when the estimated glomerular filtration rate (GFR) has declined to 20 to 25 mL/min.

Psychologic support is another important but often overlooked and poorly understood part of caring for a patient on HD. About 25% to 44% of patients experience depression,[23-25] and another 60% to 90% experience fatigue, which is frequently disabling.[26,27] Severe restless leg syndrome, leg cramps, insomnia, anxiety, and prolonged recovery time from dialysis also occur commonly.[28-33] These symptoms are associated with poorer quality of life, with persistent depression, and with increased comorbidities, including malnutrition, anemia, poor sleep quality, low level of physical function, presence of inflammation, and impaired immune function[23,24,30,32] as well as hospitalization[34-40] and death.[24,33-37,39-43] Although depression is associated with significant morbidity and mortality, fewer than one third of depressed patients undergoing dialysis receive treatment.[25,39] Later studies suggest that certain serotonin-selective reuptake inhibitors,[44,45] daily HD,[44,46,47] cognitive behavior therapy,[44,48-50] and exercise[44,51] may be effective in reducing depressive symptoms, sleep disturbances, and postdialysis recovery time and improving quality of life.

Because of the multifaceted care required before the start of HD, timely referral to a nephrologist is important. Studies have documented higher rates of hospitalization,[52] symptoms of depression,[53] morbidity,[52,54,55] and mortality[52,56-59] when referral of patients with CKD to nephrologists is delayed, although these results may be confounded by the reasons underlying late referral, such as patient nonadherence, multiple comorbidities, and advanced age.[60,61] Later studies demonstrate that even with earlier referral, initiation of dialysis may still be suboptimal, which is defined as a need for hospitalization or use of a central venous catheter, both of which are associated with a higher 6-month mortality rate.[62,63] Not meeting the Kidney Disease Outcomes Quality Initiative (KDOQI) guideline goals—use of AV fistula or graft, hemoglobin (Hgb) 11 g/dL or higher, and/or serum albumin goal (4 g/dL or higher with bromcresol green assay, 3.7 g/dL or higher with bromcresol purple assay)—at dialysis initiation has also been found to result in a higher 1-year mortality.[64] Clinical practice guidelines and practical recommendations are now available internationally with the ultimate goal of improving the quality of life and reducing mortality for patients with CKD.[65-69]

Current clinical practice guidelines suggest that dialysis be initiated when patients become symptomatic from uremia, a change that often occurs at an estimated GFR between 5 and 10 mL/min/1.73 m^2.[69] In some patients, volume overload and hyperkalemia not responsive to conservative medical management with diuretics and dietary potassium restriction and unexplained progressive decline in nutritional status despite aggressive dietary intervention may dictate earlier initiation of dialysis. The goal for patients with kidney failure is a smooth transition from CKD to ESKD, avoiding the complications of overt uremia. The results of several later studies support these clinical practice guidelines.[70-73] The IDEAL (Initiating Dialysis Early and Late) study,[70] the only randomized controlled trial, reported comparable survival and clinical outcomes in patients randomly assigned to "early start" (estimated GFR higher than 10 mL/min/1.73 m^2 by the Cockcroft-Gault equation) and "late start" of dialysis (GFR 5 to 7 mL/min/1.73 m^2). Of note, 75% of the late-start patients initiated dialysis when the estimated GFR was above 7 mL/min/1.73 m^2 because of intervening symptoms suggestive of uremia, volume overload, or nutritional decline. A potential weakness of the study is the use of the Cockcroft-Gault equation to estimate GFR, although secondary analysis of the data using the MDRD (Modification of Diet in Renal Disease) and the CKD-EPI (Chronic Kidney Disease–Epidemiology) formulas to estimate GFR also demonstrated no effect of timing of dialysis initiation on survival.[74] Earlier initiation of dialysis is not cost effective[75] and may potentially be harmful.[76-78] Potential explanations for the higher mortality in patients who start dialysis early are an accelerated loss of residual kidney function, more frequent use of dialysis catheters, myocardial stunning, depression, and provider inexperience at a time when life-saving benefits from dialysis are low.[78,79] Until the risks leading to increased mortality are better understood and can be modified, trends toward earlier start of dialysis in the absence of uremic complications should be discouraged.

VASCULAR ACCESS

BACKGROUND

Innovative techniques in vascular surgery truly paved the way for the availability of maintenance HD as a viable approach to the management of ESKD. Although the external AV device, the Quinton-Scribner shunt (named for the designers), led in 1960 to a more viable tool for access to the circulation for HD, thrombosis and infection limited the longevity of the device, and the placement procedure required permanent sacrifice of major arteries and veins.[80] Brescia and colleagues developed the procedure to create an endogenous AV fistula in 1966, ushering in the viability of HD as a long-term therapy for ESKD.[81] Described in detail later, this procedure was relatively simple, totally subcutaneous, and preserved arterial flow to the hand. The advent of procedures using vein grafts allowed the patient with ESKD who was not a candidate for the Brescia-Cimino fistula to receive a subcutaneous access.[82,83] The 1970s brought the development of artificial material made of expanded polytetrafluoroethylene (ePTFE), which took the place of natural vein grafts and greatly expanded the use of AV access for patients on maintenance HD. Unfortunately, the use of synthetic graft material does not provide the same success as the Brescia-Cimino procedure or other procedures to create an autogenous AV fistula with respect to duration of function and incidence of complications (see later). The arm is clearly the preferred site for fistulas or grafts; however, in some patients, the leg becomes a necessary alternative.[84] The radiocephalic AV (Brescia-Cimino) fistula to this day remains by far the access of choice for patients with ESKD anticipating or receiving HD.

Table 65.3 Characteristics of an Ideal Vascular Access

High blood flow rates
Instant usability
No needles
Long survival
Low thrombosis rates
Low infection rates
Patient comfort
Minimal cosmetic effect

Procedures that allowed safe placement of wide-bore catheters in large-diameter veins such as the femoral were developed in the 1970s. First single-lumen and then double-lumen catheters led to the use of these devices to support patients on maintenance HD who lacked AV access. The creation of more flexible plastics and the advent of cuffed catheters inserted through subcutaneous tunnels led to the use of so-called permanent catheters, which offer longevity of use that makes them practical for maintenance HD. In the United States, the availability of these catheters has allowed patients to receive maintenance HD despite inadequate vasculature to support endogenous AV access. However, there is growing concern that these catheters are used inappropriately.

A list of qualifications for the "ideal vascular access" has been proposed (Table 65.3), and the failure to meet these qualifications in the creation of an access continues to make vascular access the Achilles' heel for maintenance HD.[85] Complications of access alone continue to account for a major portion of the morbidity and mortality within the HD population. There are well-recognized associations between type of vascular access and the mortality and cost in patients with ESKD.[86] Data from the USRDS 2008 *Annual Report* demonstrate the relationship of total health care costs per patient per year to the type of vascular access (Figure 65.9). As the role of more frequent hemodialysis treatments is fully established, there is some evidence that this practice will pose even greater challenges for maintaining vascular access.[87]

TYPES OF VASCULAR ACCESS

ARTERIOVENOUS FISTULAS

The AV fistula, the preferred type of vascular access, is created by connecting a vein to an artery, which requires that the two vessels be in proximity to each other. Both artery and vein must have adequate lumens for the procedure to be successful. The original procedure described by Brescia and colleagues was a side-to-side AV fistula using the radial artery and the cephalic vein at the wrist; and has become the preferred access when these vessels are adequate (Figure 65.10).[81] The advantage of the side-to-side anastomosis and the alternative end-to-side connection, in which the vein is transected, is the maintenance of distal flow in the artery. An additional advantage of the end-to-side procedure is the avoidance of venous hypertension, which can occur distally with the side-to-side approach. Data supporting the benefit of a fistula have raised the question of whether some radiocephalic fistulas are being unwisely attempted in patients with known higher failure rates, including smaller women and people with diabetes and obesity.[88] Systematic use of preoperative ultrasonographic imaging ("vein mapping") to examine both arterial and venous anatomy may increase the success rate of AV fistulas.[89,90]

The upper arm veins provide alternatives when a distal fistula has failed or when distal vessels are inadequate. Both the cephalic and the basilic veins lend themselves to fistula creation; however, the basilic vein requires an additional procedure of transposition because it courses the upper arm in deep fascia. The brachiobasilic fistula can be performed in stages, a feature that is particularly advantageous in children, with anastomosis first followed by the transposition surgery after the vein has matured.[91] Even in adults, this procedure appears to have advantages over an AV graft.[92] The basilic vein has also been transposed to the forearm with successful outcomes.[93]

Focus on the superiority of fistulas over other forms of access appears to be increasing the prevalence of fistulas in the United States. In Europe, the prevalence of fistulas for maintenance HD has long been higher than that in the United States. Data from the Dialysis Outcomes and Practice Patterns Study (DOPPS) have demonstrated a marked difference in the training of surgeons in Europe and the United States.[94] The much higher number of procedures completed by European surgeons in training may lead to greater expertise or facility in performing fistula procedures. However, a meta-analysis of more than 12,000 patients found that the failure rate for fistulas may be increasing, causing concern about overly aggressive "fistula first" approaches.[95] New approaches to improve primary patency of AV fistulas include balloon-assisted maturation and localized far infrared exposure of new fistulas.[96,97]

ARTERIOVENOUS GRAFTS

Vascular access using ePTFE has become the most prominent type of AV vascular access in the United States. The high prevalence of ePTFE accesses or AV grafts is at least

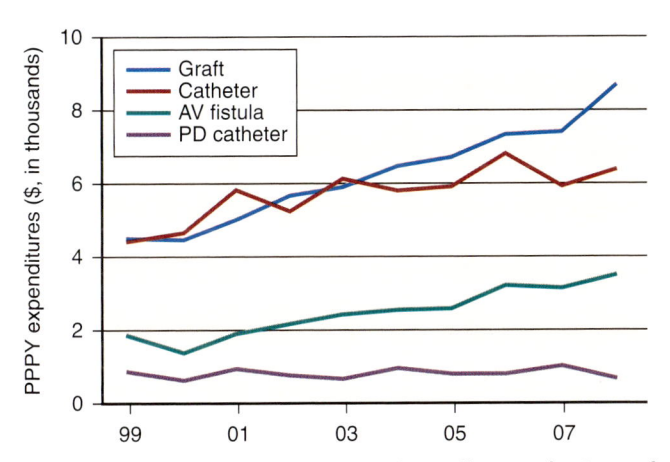

Figure 65.9 Health care costs vary depending on the type of dialysis access. Total health care costs per person per year (pppy) vary with the type of dialysis access, peritoneal dialysis (PD) catheters being the most economical and arteriovenous (AV) grafts and dialysis catheters being the most expensive to maintain. (Adapted from U.S. Renal Data System: *USRDS 2010 annual data report: atlas of chronic kidney disease and end-stage renal disease in the United States*, Bethesda, MD, 2010, National Institutes of Health, National Institute of Diabetes and Digestive and Kidney Diseases.)

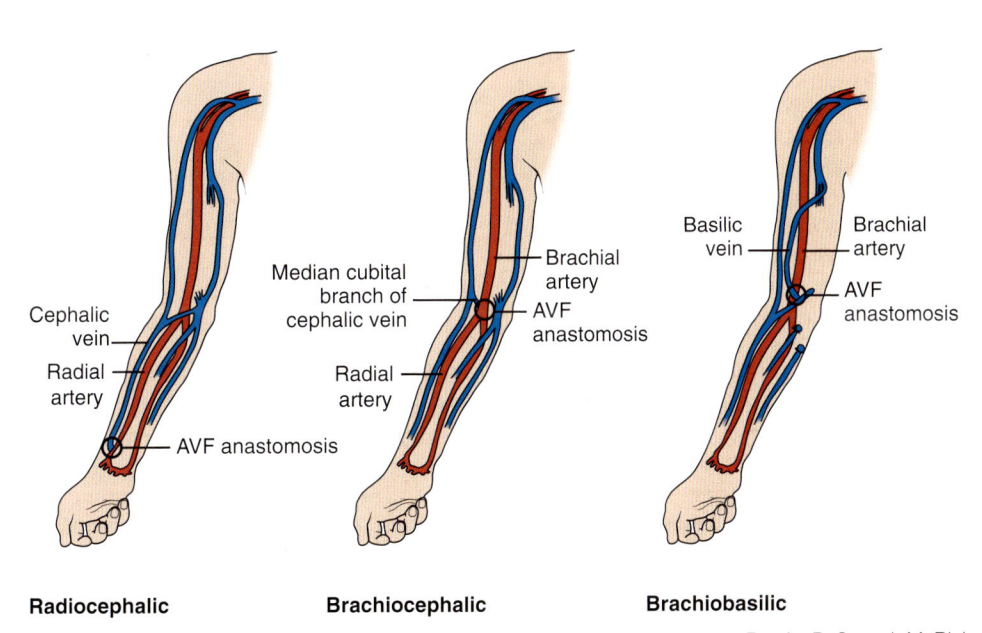

Figure 65.10 Types of autogenous fistulas. AVF, Arteriovenous. (Reproduced with permission from Pereira B, Sayegh M, Blake P, editors: *Chronic kidney disease, dialysis, and transplantation*, 2nd ed, Philadelphia, 2005, Saunders, p 344.)

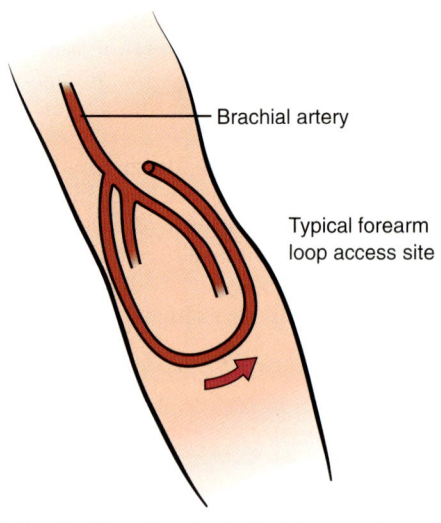

Figure 65.11 Configuration for typical forearm loop graft. *Arrow* indicates direction of blood flow (arterial to venous). (Modified from Kapoian T, Kaufman JL, Nosher J, Sherman RA: Dialysis access and recirculation. In Henrich WL, editor: *Dialysis as treatment of end-stage renal disease*, vol 5, Philadelphia, 1999, Current Medicine & Blackwell Science.)

partly attributable to the ease of placement and the short time required between the placement of an AV graft and initiation of cannulation. Placement of an AV graft is perceived as advantageous by many nephrologists and surgeons because it does not require an adequate vein in the forearm yet provides a forearm site for access placement (Figure 65.11). Although the recognized low thrombosis rate for grafts is an early advantage, this low rate does not persist, and the primary patency rate at 12 months is only around 50%.[98] The graft material has a high risk for development of infection, although an infected graft can occasionally be salvaged by resection of the infected section and replacement with new graft material. Other approaches to placement are available when vascular anatomy or previous access prohibits placement in the forearm. The thigh often becomes the only remaining site for graft placement but is thought to pose too great a risk of infection; however, one report suggests that a thigh graft may be a better alternative than a tunneled catheter.[99] A new device for patients with very limited vascular access options uses typical graft material at the arterial end and throughout the length of potential needle cannulation sites but then attaches to catheter material that is tunneled to achieve central venous drainage: the Hemodialysis Reliable Outflow (HeRO) system.[100]

A complex biologic response develops within the lumen and in the distal native vein after an AV graft is surgically placed. A host of immune responses occur in addition to cellular growth, which develops within the lumen itself and distally. The resulting hyperplasia leads to a high incidence of stenosis, which is the leading cause of graft failure.[101] The vast majority of stenoses that develop are at the venous anastomosis or beyond. As discussed later, the high incidence of stenosis certainly is a rationale for monitoring graft flow in hopes of preventing eventual thrombosis. The documented inflammatory response and hyperplasia within grafts have focused attention on devices and drugs that may prevent or reduce the eventual stenosis. In addition to angioplasty, stents are frequently used as tools to prevent restenosis and maintain patency. Whether drug-eluting stents will have a role in AV graft survival has yet to be determined. Use of drug elution from graft material itself is also under investigation in animals and may offer promise in the future.[102] Later work has redefined the concept of grafts by constructing a totally biologic graft, using artificial materials as the initial skeleton for a conduit over which autologous fibroblasts are grown, after which the lumen is seeded with autologous endothelial cells.[103] This technology may eventually offer biologic grafts that are less vulnerable to thrombosis and infection.

MAINTENANCE OF VASCULAR ACCESS FUNCTION

After some form of vascular access is achieved, the goal of maintaining adequate function becomes paramount. Numerous strategies have been explored to accomplish this goal. Cannulation methods have received some attention, with speculation that methods such as the buttonhole technique might provide advantages over other methods. One nonrandomized study compared the rope-ladder technique (70 patients), in which cannulation occurs along the entire length of the fistula, with the buttonhole procedure (75 patients), in which repeated cannulation occurs in the exact spot, over 9 months.[104] Unsuccessful cannulation occurred more frequently in the buttonhole group, but this group had fewer complications, including hematoma and aneurysm formation, than the rope-ladder group. Data from a later study suggest that the buttonhole technique is associated with a higher rate of infection of the fistula without evidence of improved fistula survival.[105] Guidelines for needle insertion were created through the National Kidney Foundation's effort to develop management standards, but these guidelines do not include definitive recommendations regarding this question of cannulation methodology.[69]

Other strategies are generally divided into the following basic approaches: (1) methods of monitoring the access for early signs of potential failure, (2) treatments to prevent access loss, and (3) interventions to fix problems such as occlusion after they have occurred. There is an accepted nomenclature for access failure that categorizes access as having primary or secondary patency. The definition of *primary access patency* is an access capable of supporting adequate HD without any intervention since the time of original placement. After an intervention has occurred for any reason (reduced flow or total thrombosis), *secondary patency* is then invoked to characterize the status of the vascular access.

MONITORING AND SURVEILLANCE

The natural history of vascular access loss suggests that observable and physiologic changes in access venous pressure or total blood flow occur before and predict impending loss of function. If detectable change in either pressure or flow were observed reliably, intervention to prevent emergency loss of access function would be theoretically possible. The question is whether salvaging the access before total loss of function offers any advantage. Currently, vascular access pressure can be monitored by measuring either static or dynamic venous pressure with several methods, and equipment now exists that allows routine measurement of actual blood flow within an access.

Despite this theoretic gain with monitoring, the impact of aggressive surveillance programs on maintenance of vascular access is controversial.[106] A nonrandomized report of a comparison of three monitoring schemes in a single dialysis program demonstrated significant improvement in short-term graft and fistula survival with use of blood flow monitoring over either dynamic pressure monitoring or no monitoring.[107] In addition to access survival, fewer HD sessions were missed and overall patient costs were reduced when the blood flow monitoring protocol was used. The overall goal of surveillance protocols, however, is to prolong duration of function of the AV access. The unfortunate natural history of access failure, especially with AV grafts, is the occurrence of restenosis after intervention procedures such as angioplasty. There may be no difference in eventual access survival whether the approach is preemptive intervention or responding to a thrombosis event when it occurs. A detailed review of surveillance trials does not support routine monitoring of HD access.[108]

Whether the additional intervention of stent placement improves access survival has received a great deal of attention. A randomized trial of 190 patients undergoing HD provides evidence that use of a stent is superior to balloon dilation alone with stenosis at the venous end of an AV graft.[109] New materials for manufacturing stents are under investigation, and the place for drug-eluting stents, although well studied in other vascular systems, needs to be addressed in AV access.[106] Likely in relation to the frequency of access failures and the need for timely treatment, a new field has emerged in renal medicine, interventional nephrology. With support of the specialty from the creation of the American Society of Diagnostic and Interventional Nephrology, reports have documented the quality and safety of the care delivered by interventional nephrologists.[110,111] These physicians are reporting experience with AV access as well as additional experience with other related arterial diseases, such as subclavian and renal artery stenosis, and peripheral vascular disease.[112] See Chapter 70 for a further discussion of interventional nephrology.

PROPHYLACTIC THERAPY FOR ACCESS MAINTENANCE

Access loss occurs from the combined pathologic events of thrombosis and hyperplasia leading to stenosis. Strategies to prevent both of these pathologic processes have been used with the goal of prolonging access survival, so far with no clear prevention regimen established. Thrombosis may be the final pathway to access failure, but so far, agents well known to prevent thrombosis in other vascular diseases have not affected access survival consistently. In fact, a large, multicenter trial in the Veterans Administration Heath System with the newer agent clopidogrel plus aspirin had to be discontinued because of bleeding problems in the treatment group.[113] The Dialysis Access Consortium (DAC) Study Group reported that although clopidogrel reduced the early thrombosis rate of new AV fistulas, it did not increase the number of usable fistulas.[114] Some small randomized trials have suggested that the use of agents such as fish oils may be effective in reducing thrombosis in grafts, but this approach has yet to receive further study and widespread application.[115,116] The DAC Study Group graft study provided support for the use of dipyridamole and low-dose aspirin started immediately after placement of an AV graft,[117] although the incremental extension of time with a functional graft was modest and relatively few patients are treated with these agents currently.

The myointimal proliferation and resulting stenosis that occur particularly with AV grafts has also been a focus of prevention, especially because the process may be the ultimate source of access failure.[118] Strategies to prevent this cellular proliferation have resulted from focus on this process in other vascular diseases, such as cardiac disease. For example, a retrospective study using angiotensin-converting enzyme (ACE) inhibitors in patients with AV grafts suggested a lower risk for graft loss in such patients than in patients not receiving this class of medication.[119] Interventions that have been shown to reduce proliferation in other vascular diseases are being studied. Brachytherapy has been used for some time and has been shown to be safe and to have promise in reducing stenosis in AV grafts.[120] Far-infrared therapy, which improves endothelial function, was shown in a randomized trial to improve patency rates of new AV fistulas when administered repeatedly[96] and may become a tool to improve AV graft survival in the future.[121] Experimental grafts created by biologic, autologous materials, as already described, may eventually provide one solution for access maintenance.

Finally, personalized medicine may eventually become part of vascular access protocols as genetic studies uncover possible predictors of higher risk for access loss. One such study has suggested that polymorphism in the methylenetetrahydrofolate reductase gene *(C677T)* may be a predictor of access thrombosis, presumably through the impact on homocysteine.[122] Another study suggests that the complex relationship between transforming growth factor β_1 and polymorphisms in the plasminogen activator inhibitor type 1 gene may identify patients at risk for access thrombosis.[123] Advance knowledge of genetic determinants may allow tailored prophylactic therapy to be administered in the future to patients at risk.

HEMODIALYSIS CATHETERS

Technology has greatly advanced the use of external connections for HD, providing HD with venous access alone and removing the need to sacrifice an artery as required with the use of shunts. Initially, large, single-lumen catheters supported HD through single veins. Later, improved plastic materials allowed the construction of large double-lumen catheters that greatly improved HD efficiency over that with single-lumen catheters. Further advances resulted in catheters made of softer material, and the development of the cuff provided catheters that could be used for markedly longer durations. Clearly, this technology has been a blessing and a curse, because the ease of insertion and the duration of use have resulted in the cuffed catheter's being a viable access for patients on maintenance HD. Some patients would face death from kidney failure without the availability of this catheter technology. However, the data suggest an inappropriately high utilization of catheters as a means of vascular access. In fact, DOPPS data have suggested that the high prevalence of catheter use in the United States may explain a major portion of the higher mortality rate in the US HD population than in similar patients in Europe.[124] A report of a large cohort of incident patients in 2007 demonstrated continued high prevalence of catheters in the United States.[125] Hence, the elevated mortality risk and frequent complications associated with catheters create major challenges for nephrologists.[126]

Thrombosis with loss of catheter function is a frequent complication leading to the need for intervention. No uniform solution to prevent these events has been established. Catheters are routinely "locked" with installation of high-dose heparin solutions injected into both lumens, but this procedure does not completely prevent the problem. The use of heparin for locking may occasionally result in bleeding through an error in dose or failure to remove the heparin solution before use. Even the addition of systemic therapy with low-dose warfarin did not prevent thrombosis in a clinical trial setting and led to an increase in complications.[127] Some small studies have explored alternatives to heparin, such as locking catheters with citrate-containing or other solutions.[128] One such study demonstrated that locking the catheter with recombinant tissue plasminogen activating factor once a week and heparin the other 2 days, in comparison with heparin 3 days a week, reduced thrombosis and also the incidence of bacteremia.[129,130] Infection isolated to the catheter itself or systemic infection with the catheter as a source is a substantial complication of catheter use, resulting in morbidity and costly hospitalizations as well as mortality. The frequency of bacteremia associated with HD catheters has been estimated to be 2 to 4 episodes per 1000 patient-catheter days,[131] a frequency 10- to 20-fold higher than estimated rates of infection in patients with AV fistulas. These catheter-related infections can result in more complex infections, such as osteomyelitis, endocarditis, and septic arthritis, despite antibiotic therapy.

Careful management of catheter-related infection is critical, including an adequate duration of antibiotic treatment (3-week minimum) and an aggressive approach to catheter removal and replacement, with replacement delayed until the patient is symptom free (so-called line holiday).[132-134] When there is evidence for an isolated exit site infection or when the tunnel is thought not to be involved, studies suggest that catheter exchange can be successfully undertaken. Attempting to treat infected catheters with antibiotics alone usually results in failure, although infection with some organisms (e.g., *Staphylococcus epidermidis*) may clear with that approach. The combined use of antibiotic installation into catheters and systemic antibiotics may increase success in preserving the existing catheter.

Several approaches to prevention of infection with catheters have demonstrated potential promise. The use of mupirocin ointment at the exit site may reduce the incidence of infection.[135,136] Locking catheters with antibiotic-containing solutions may be helpful also in reducing the incidence of catheter-related infections.[134,136,137] Use of catheters impregnated with antibacterial agents so far has not been as promising in preventing infection.[138]

Even if the thrombosis and infection problems could be solved, catheters generally yield less efficient solute clearance in comparison with fistulas and grafts and may not provide "adequate" dialysis in a sizable fraction of patients. In the end, the catheter must remain an interim solution or the access of last resort for the patient undergoing maintenance HD.

GENERAL PRINCIPLES OF HEMODIALYSIS: PHYSIOLOGY AND BIOMECHANICS

Therapeutic HD removes solutes principally by diffusion and to a lesser extent by convection across a semipermeable membrane. The driving force for solute diffusion is the transmembrane concentration gradient (Figure 65.12A), and the driving force for convection, commonly called *ultrafiltration*, is the transmembrane hydrostatic pressure (see Figure 65.12B). Selective removal of solutes is achieved by restricting the pore size in the membrane to admit small molecules and reject large molecules and by including

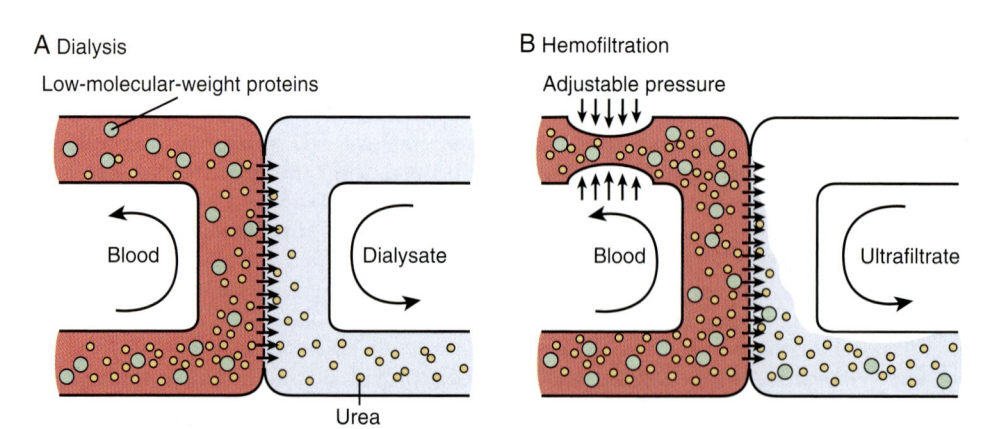

Figure 65.12 Diffusion versus convection. **A,** Diffusion across a semipermeable membrane. The driving force for solute diffusion is the transmembrane concentration gradient. Small solutes with higher concentrations in the blood compartment, such as potassium, urea, and small uremic toxins, diffuse through the membrane into the dialysate compartment. Dialysis dissipates this concentration gradient (i.e., the molecular concentration gradient decreases with dialysis). Larger solutes and low-molecular-weight proteins such as albumin diffuse poorly across the semipermeable membrane. **B,** Convection (hemofiltration) across a semipermeable membrane. The driving force for convection, commonly called ultrafiltration, is the transmembrane hydrostatic pressure. When applied to the blood compartment, solvent flows across the membrane into the dialysate compartment, bringing along solutes. For solutes with a sieving coefficient close to 1, there is no change in concentrations in the blood compartment with time. (Reproduced with permission from Meyer TW, Hostetter TH: Uremia. *N Engl J Med* 357:1316-1325, 2007.)

desirable solutes in the dialysate, effectively preventing their removal.

NATIVE KIDNEY VERSUS ARTIFICIAL KIDNEY

Separation of solutes based on molecular size appears to be a major function of native kidneys, and the dialyzer attempts to mimic that function. Most of the soluble large molecules found in the blood are the products of complex intracellular synthetic energy-requiring processes. Most continue to be active, serving to signal and regulate processes in distant organs. Their loss by filtration through the kidneys would be a liability best avoided. Loss is first prevented by the bilipid cell membrane barrier, which keeps many of the most precious molecules in a sequestered intracellular location. Those that are secreted or leak out of the cell are often bound to serum macromolecules, most notably serum albumin, a well-known transport protein. Although the glomerular membrane is highly permeable in comparison with cell membranes in general, albumin and its bound ligands as well as other macromolecules are poorly filtered and thus are protected from loss. Small proteins and peptides that leak through the filter are efficiently reabsorbed by the proximal tubule, where they are broken down and their subunits reutilized.

Smaller molecules are often end products of metabolism or ingested intruders that the kidney effectively eliminates by filtration without reabsorption. Precious small molecules are reclaimed after filtration by selective reabsorptive mechanisms in the renal tubules. Dialyzers lack the latter vital functions, so losses are prevented by including some of these measurable small solutes in the dialysate, effectively eliminating the gradient for diffusive loss. Fortunately, most of these small solutes are abundant and can be relatively inexpensively added to the dialysate.

Although both the native or natural kidney and the artificial kidney are excretory "organs" and both use semipermeable membranes to separate small from large particles, they operate on different principles. The natural kidney is a selective filtration or convection device driven by blood pressure generated by the heart with highly selective reabsorption and secretion downstream. In contrast, the dialyzer separates molecular species primarily by simple diffusion without the need for pressure generation or reabsorption. Urea, for example, is highly reabsorbed after filtration by the glomerulus, but selective reabsorption plays no role within hemodialyzers. The rapid equilibration of urea across red blood cell (RBC) membranes facilitates urea removal during dialysis but plays no role during glomerular filtration. In contrast, creatinine and most other water-soluble compounds are poorly reabsorbed by the native kidney and exhibit slow or no transport across RBC membranes within the short time frame that blood transits through the dialyzer. As a consequence, native kidney clearance rates of creatinine are higher and dialyzer clearance rates are lower than their clearances of urea.

The artificial hollow-fiber kidney contains 8000 to 10,000 fibers, each approximately 200 µm in diameter and 250 mm in length, providing a surface area for exchange of about 1.5 m^2. Each of the 1 to 2 million functioning nephrons in the two native kidneys has a proximal tubule diameter of about 40 µm and a length of about 14 mm, providing a minimum surface area for proximal reabsorption of approximately 3 m^2 (if one ignores microvilli). The native kidneys also perform several known and probably other unknown synthetic functions such as the regulated synthesis of erythropoietin and activation of vitamin D.

For endogenous solutes, the first pathway on the route to elimination is diffusion through intracellular and extracellular pathways, including passive or facilitated diffusion across membranes. Thus, diffusion is a vital transport mechanism for the function of both native and artificial kidneys. Because removal of small solutes appears to be the major function of both excretory methods, dialyzer clearance of small solutes can be compared with similar clearances by the native kidney as a reasonable first step toward assessing hemodialyzer adequacy.

CLEARANCE

The goals of dialysis are straightforward: removal of accumulated fluid and by-products of metabolism, sometimes referred to as "toxins." With respect to toxins, the ultimate goal is to maintain concentrations below the threshold at which uremic symptoms and signs begin to appear. However, the levels of retained toxic solutes are not used as performance measures for dialysis because their identities are unknown and because their generation rates probably vary from patient to patient and from time to time (see later). Instead, performance of dialysis is judged from the *clearance* of representative solutes.

As already noted, the most representative solutes are small. Small solute clearance can be used to measure the most important dialyzer function, which is to lower the concentration of small toxic solutes in the patient. This is an inescapable conclusion based on the observation that dialysis works extremely well to rapidly reverse life-threatening uremia. The mechanism for this life-giving property of dialysis is not mysterious; it is simply the result of solute removal by diffusion across the semipermeable dialysis membrane. Although effective in reversing uremia, earlier cellulose-based dialyzer membranes removed solutes with molecular weights above 3000 Da very poorly, so small solutes are the obvious main culprits accounting for the uremic syndrome and the primary targets for dialyzer clearance. It is therefore reasonable to use the clearance of a representative small solute as a measure of this fundamental dialysis function.

Clearance is recognized as the best measure of first-order processes such as diffusion and filtration. A zero-order process such as urea generation by the liver is uninfluenced by the solute concentration, but first-order removal processes use the concentration as the driving force for diffusion, rendering the removal rate directly proportional to the concentration. Clearance (K) is the proportionality constant:

$$K = \text{Removal rate/Concentration} \quad (1)$$

K has value as an expression of first-order processes that is independent of either the solute removal rate or its concentration. For intermittent dialysis, the main advantage of the clearance expression is that it tends to remain constant despite rapid changes in both the solute concentration and the removal rate during the procedure.

In a simple flowing system, the removal rate is the difference between the inflow concentration (C_{in}) and the outflow concentration (C_{out}) multiplied by flow (Q). From equation 1, clearance can also be expressed as the *extraction ratio* (E) multiplied by flow:

$$E = (C_{in} - C_{out})/C_{in} \quad (2)$$

$$K = Q \cdot E \quad (3)$$

For a constant-flow system, the extraction ratio is also constant over time despite marked changes in concentration. E is the fraction of total inflow (Q), and K is the absolute flow that is completely cleared of the solute; both tend to remain constant during dialysis. Clearance is affected by the flow of both blood and dialysate as well as other variables such as the convective filtration rate (see later) but is independent of concentration.

Although clearance is independent of solute concentration, the converse is not true (i.e., concentrations depend on clearance, and solute concentrations are used to measure clearance). During a period of steady-state kinetics, in which generation equals removal, if the generation rate of a solute is fixed, its concentration is inversely proportional to its clearance. Because dialysis is simpler than native kidney function and removes solutes primarily by diffusion, the calculation of clearance is nearly the same for all easily dialyzed substances if one assumes that these solutes are distributed in a single mixed pool within the patient. Application of this principle allows selection of an easily measured solute (e.g., urea) to assess dialyzer performance, with the expectation that the measured clearance will correlate inversely with patient levels of similar easily dialyzed solutes. The measured solute need not be toxic, but it must behave like the toxic solutes. Generation rates of various solutes differ, but if each is relatively constant from week to week (e.g., creatinine generation), then the measured clearance of a representative solute can be used to reflect the effectiveness of the dialysis for clearing all easily dialyzed solutes. This principle, which forms the basis of established standards for measuring and prescribing HD, has logical merit, but its applicability has been challenged and may require modification for solutes that are strongly sequestered in remote body compartments (see later).[68,69,139,140] In addition, after adjustment for body size and possibly gender (see later), all patients appear to require the same weekly clearance. Furthermore, the dose requirement or need for dialysis does not seem to vary from time to time in the same (anuric) patient, provided that a minimum threshold clearance is delivered during each treatment.

Native kidneys appear to clear small solutes at a rate far above the minimum required to sustain life. For example, removal of a kidney for transplantation can be done without adverse consequences in the donor. Although the reason for this surplus function is unknown, it helps to explain how modern intermittent HD, which achieves a continuous equivalent small solute clearance that is only about 10% to 15% of the normal GFR, is able to sustain life (see "Continuous Equivalent Clearance" section).

CLEARANCE VERSUS REMOVAL RATE

The clearance of a solute must be distinguished from its absolute removal rate. Clearance is best envisioned as a measure of removal expressed as a fraction of the remaining solute and is therefore independent of the concentration. Two substances may have the same clearance, but if one is present at half the concentration of the other, the one's removal rate will also be half the other's. In practical terms, it is impossible to compare dialyzers by measuring removal rates alone because removal depends on the solute concentration. Measurement of clearance eliminates this requirement, allowing use of a single term to make valid comparisons among purgative instruments.

Similarly, finding a lower concentration of a solute within a patient does not indicate that the clearance is higher; it may simply reflect a lower generation rate. If a steady state exists in which input equals output, the removal rate of a substance is simply a measure of its generation rate, revealing little about the effectiveness of the dialyzer. If the clearance decreases and the generation rate does not change, the patient's solute concentration increases until a new steady state is reached, at which point the removal rate again matches the generation rate.

SERUM UREA CONCENTRATION VERSUS UREA CLEARANCE

The serum urea concentration has proved to be a poor surrogate for uremic toxicity. The determinants of urea concentration are generation and clearance. Whereas urea clearance by the dialyzer should correlate with the clearance of other small (dialyzable) solutes that are presumably responsible for uremic toxicity, the generation of urea as an end product of protein catabolism correlates poorly with uremic toxicity. In fact, patients with higher urea generation rates have better outcomes, probably as a reflection of better appetite and higher protein intake.[141] It is difficult to dissect the clearance factor from the generation factor in a single blood urea nitrogen (BUN) measurement, but as explained later, this dissection can be accomplished by modeling the change in BUN during a dialysis treatment. For purposes of measuring the dose of dialysis and dialysis adequacy, only the relative change in urea concentration during dialysis is used to model clearance; the absolute concentrations are ignored. Thus, despite urea's lack of intrinsic toxicity and the poor correlation with overall uremic toxicity, urea measurements during dialysis can be used to assess dialysis effectiveness and adequacy. The change in urea concentration during dialysis, which reflects its clearance, is used as a surrogate for the clearance of other small easily dialyzed solutes, some of which must be toxic or dialysis would not reverse the life-threatening component of uremia. This logic justifies use of urea clearance as an index of dialysis adequacy while acknowledging that isolated urea concentrations cannot be used for this purpose.

FACTORS THAT AFFECT CLEARANCE IN A FLOWING SYSTEM

Diffusive clearance in a flowing system depends on the rates of blood and dialysate flow as well as the targeted solute's membrane permeability. The biomaterials used to make the hollow-fiber dialyzer, together with the pore size and thickness of the membrane, determine its clearance, or the *membrane permeability constant* (K_0), for a given solute. Multiplying K_0 by the surface area for diffusion (A) yields the

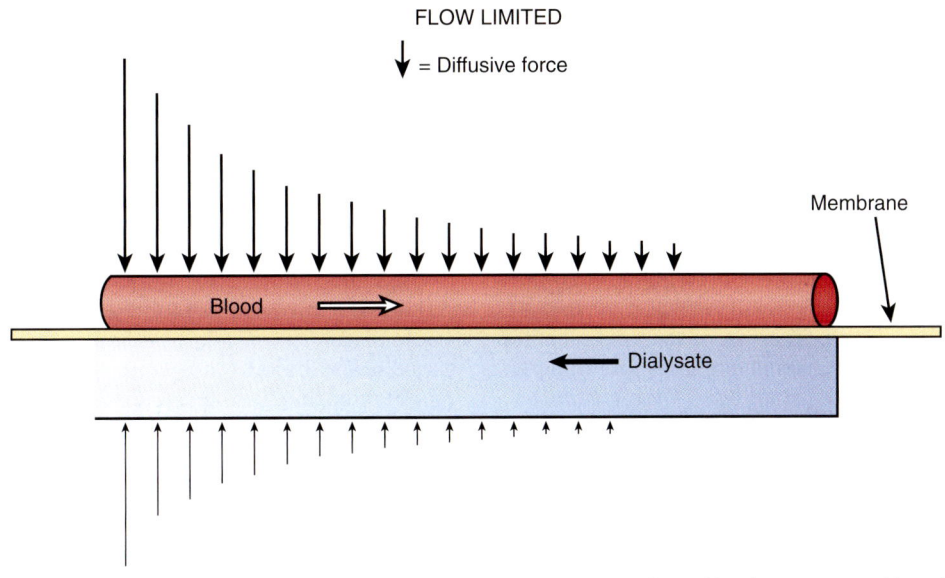

Figure 65.13 Flow-limited clearance. A logarithmic decline in solute concentrations, indicated by the *arrows* on either side of the membrane, is depicted from dialyzer inlet on the *left* to blood outlet on the *right*. This predictable decline is attributable to relatively rapid diffusion of solute across the membrane and forms the basis for Equation 5. Flux is equal to the product of membrane-solute mass transfer area coefficient (K_0A) and the log mean gradient. Solute flux and removal are maximized by countercurrent flow of blood and dialysate.

permeability or *mass transfer area coefficient* (K_0A) of an entire dialyzer. K_0A is expressed in milliliters per minute and, like clearance, is independent of solute concentration. The predictable exponential decline in concentration gradient along the dialyzer membrane from blood inflow to outflow (Figure 65.13) is the basis for calculation of K_0A from the blood and dialysate flow rates and is widely used in mathematical models of solute kinetics. For countercurrent dialysate and blood flow,[142] where K_d is dialyzer clearance:

$$K_0A = \frac{Q_bQ_d}{Q_b-Q_d} \times \ln\left(\frac{Q_d(Q_b-K_d)}{Q_b(Q_d-K_d)}\right) \quad (4)$$

Analogous to clearance, which expresses the dialyzer removal rate normalized to the inflow solute concentration, K_0A is an expression of dialyzer performance normalized to blood and dialysate flow rates (Q_b and Q_d, respectively). K_0A, which is sometimes called the "intrinsic clearance" of a dialyzer, can be viewed as the maximum clearance possible for a particular solute and dialyzer at infinite Q_b and Q_d. Note that K_0A is both dialyzer specific and solute specific. It is the best parameter for comparing dialyzers, with higher values indicating more efficient solute removal.

A useful rearrangement of Equation 4 provides a measure of clearance at any blood and dialysate flow rate, as follows:

$$K_d = Q_b\left[\frac{e^{K_0A\left(\frac{Q_d-Q_b}{Q_dQ_b}\right)}-1}{e^{K_0A\left(\frac{Q_d-Q_b}{Q_dQ_b}\right)}-\frac{Q_b}{Q_d}}\right] \quad (5)$$

The preceding expression of clearance does not include the contribution of convective solute removal by ultrafiltration (Q_f) during therapeutic HD. Convective clearance results from bulk movement of solute across the membrane driven by hydrostatic pressure. Simultaneous filtration across the same membrane used for dialysis removes additional solute, but the amount removed is inversely related to the efficiency of the dialysis. For example, if the dialyzer removes solute very efficiently by diffusion, with an extraction ratio approaching 100%, addition of ultrafiltration adds very little or nothing to the removal rate, which cannot exceed 100% of the inflow. The effect of ultrafiltration on clearance is expressed as follows[143]:

$$K_d = Q_b(C_{in} - C_{out})/C_{in} + Q_f(C_{out}/C_{in}) \quad (6)$$

where Q_b is the blood inflow rate, C_{in} is the inflow concentration, C_{out} is the outflow concentration, and Q_f is the ultrafiltration rate in millimeters per minute. As C_{out} approaches zero, the dialysis component of clearance maximizes, and the Q_f component extinguishes.

DIALYSANCE

For peritoneal dialysis (PD), after the infusion of fresh dialysate, solute begins to accumulate in the peritoneal fluid. As the level increases, the concentration gradient from blood to dialysate decreases, causing the removal rate and the clearance to decrease, both eventually falling to zero as equilibrium is reached. However, the flux of solute per unit of concentration gradient, also known as *dialysance* (D), remains constant:

$$D = (\text{Removal rate})/(\text{Concentration gradient}) \quad (7)$$

Dialysance can be formulated as the initial clearance when the dialysate concentration is zero or, in a flowing HD system, as the solute removal rate per mean solute gradient along the membrane (blood minus dialysate concentration) and is equivalent to the dialyzer's K_0A for the measured solute.

DETERMINANTS OF CLEARANCE

A number of variables affect clearance during dialysis (Table 65.4). Solute-related variables include the physical and chemical properties of the substance to be removed and its distribution in the body. Treatment-related variables include the permeability of the membrane to solutes of various sizes, dialysis treatment time, membrane surface area, and flow rates of blood and dialysate (see preceding equations).

Molecular size and membrane permeability together limit the rate of movement for individual molecular species. In flowing systems, the concentrations of larger molecules tend to remain constant along the length of the dialyzer, uninfluenced by blood and dialysate flow. Their clearances, which are low because of their large size, are limited by the size and permeability of the membrane alone and are independent of flow rates (Figure 65.14). Smaller molecules tend to be cleared at the proximal end of the dialyzer, leaving the more distal end for further enhancement of clearance as flow is increased (see Figure 65.13). In this situation, clearance is said to be flow limited. Note that flow-limited clearance for small solutes and membrane-limited clearance for larger solutes may occur at the same time within a dialyzer. The relationship between flow and clearance is shown graphically in Figure 65.15 for both limiting scenarios.

The molecular activity of a solute determines its capacity for movement across the dialysis membrane. Because water-soluble solutes are active only in the water phase of the blood, only the water component (≈90% of normal blood volume) participates in the dialysis process. Blood flow through the dialyzer for water-soluble solutes (nearly all) should be expressed as blood water flow or about 90% of whole blood flow. Similarly, blood concentrations should be expressed as blood water concentrations, which are about 7% higher than whole serum concentrations. Note that BUN is a misnomer; *serum* urea nitrogen is actually measured. For charged molecules, the Donnan effect acts in the opposite direction, reducing the effective blood activity.[144] Correcting for this reduced activity, the effective sodium concentration on the blood side of the membrane is about 3 mEq/L lower than its actual concentration. The Donnan effect for blood equilibrated with dialysate is attributable to nondialyzable plasma proteins, mostly albumin, which has a net negative charge (≈17 mEq/mmol albumin). The asymmetric charge distribution across the membrane effectively "captures" a small fraction of the positively charged sodium ions on the plasma side, reducing their potential for diffusion.

The size of the molecule is the most important intrinsic physical feature governing its removal (Figure 65.16). In general, the rate of movement or flux (J) of smaller molecules is higher than the flux of larger molecules. Other factors, such as binding to plasma proteins, shape, charge, and sequestration in the intracellular compartment, must be considered in the prediction of clearance (see Figure 65.16).

DIALYZER CLEARANCE VERSUS WHOLE BODY CLEARANCE

A distinction must be made between clearance across the dialyzer and clearance across the patient. For each of these, the removal rate (Equation 1) is the same, but the

Table 65.4 Factors Influencing Effective Clearance

Solute-related	Molecular size
	Molecular charge
	Macromolecular binding
	Body distribution and sequestration
Treatment-related (in order of importance):	
Small molecules	Blood and dialysate flow
	Membrane surface area
	Treatment time
	Membrane permeability
Large molecules	Membrane permeability
	Treatment time
	Membrane surface area
	Blood and dialysate flow

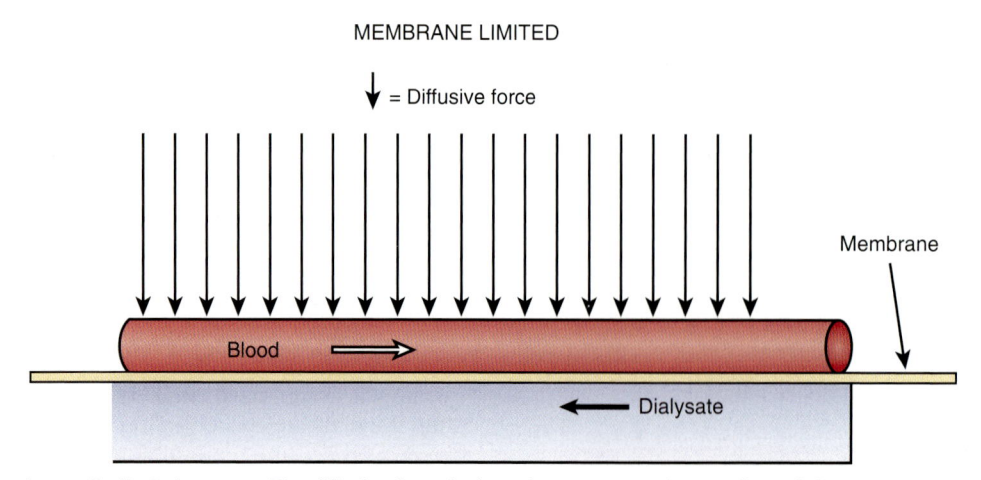

Figure 65.14 Membrane-limited clearance. The diffusive force is the solute concentration gradient. Solute concentrations along the membrane from dialyzer inflow to outflow for both blood and dialysate are relatively constant because transport across the membrane is limiting and relatively low.

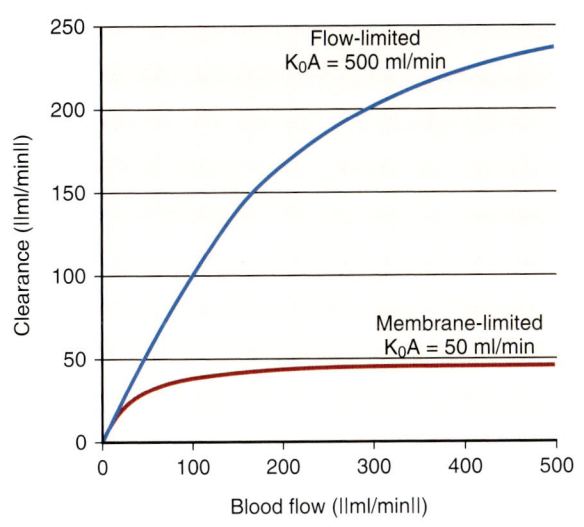

Figure 65.15 Flow-limited versus membrane-limited clearances. Flow limits clearance when the membrane is not fully exposed to inflow solute concentrations (see Figure 65.13). This typically occurs for small, easily dialyzed solutes. In contrast, larger solutes tend to saturate the membrane along its entire length at lower blood (or dialysate) flow rates (see Figure 65.14). For these less easily dialyzed solutes, further increases in flow have no influence on clearance. K_0A, Mass transfer area coefficient.

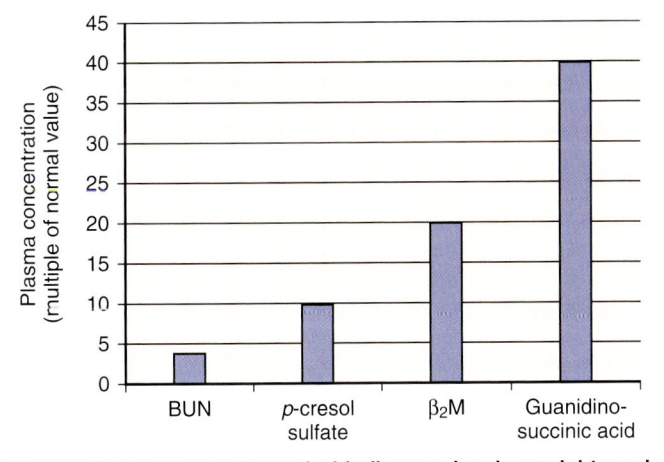

Figure 65.16 Effect of protein binding, molecular weight, and sequestration on solute concentrations in hemodialysis (HD) recipients. Conventional thrice-weekly dialysis is very effective at removing blood urea nitrogen (BUN), resulting in an average urea level of about four times the normal value in a patient undergoing HD. Binding of p-cresol to albumin and the large molecular size of β₂-microglobulin limit their removal with conventional dialysis, so their levels are about 10 and 20 times normal, respectively. Plasma guanidinosuccinic acid levels are even higher (about 40 times normal) because of increased production in kidney failure and intracellular sequestration, making it difficult to remove during dialysis. Although the plasma levels of these other solutes are several orders of magnitude higher than normal, their absolute levels are much lower than that of urea, and it is unclear whether they exert any toxicity. (Adapted from Meyer TW, Hostetter TH: Uremia. *N Engl J Med* 357:1316-1326, 2007.)

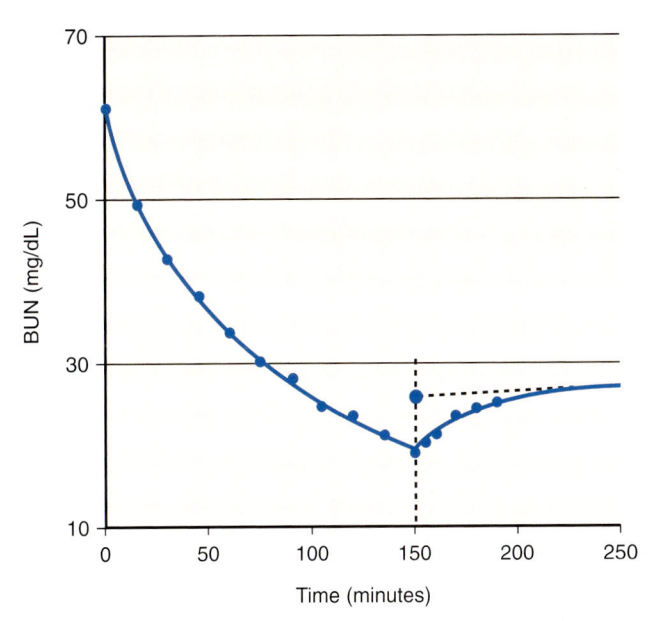

Figure 65.17 Equilibrated postdialysis blood urea nitrogen (BUN), the basis for estimated dialysis efficiency (eKt/V). Precise measurements of BUN every 15 minutes during a typical patient's 2.5-hour hemodialysis shows a logarithmic decrease in concentration during the treatment and a rapid rebound that is complete approximately 1 hour later. The double-pool model shown in Figure 65.22 and the *solid line* in the graph predict the concentrations accurately. The equilibrated postdialysis BUN is an extrapolated value shown as the *large solid circle*.

denominator differs. Dialyzer clearance is an expression of solute removal as a fraction of the blood concentration (adjusted for blood water content) at the dialyzer inflow port. In contrast, whole-body clearance is an expression of removal as a fraction of average concentrations throughout the body. The average "whole-body concentration" is substituted for dialyzer inflow concentration in the denominator of the standard clearance formula (Equation 1). Whole-body concentrations are higher than serum concentrations during dialysis because of *solute disequilibrium,* so whole-body clearances are always lower than dialyzer clearances. Higher concentrations throughout the body result from *solute sequestration* or a delay in diffusive movement of solute from remote body compartments to the patient's blood, which is the immediately dialyzed compartment.

Typical solutes that exhibit disequilibrium distribute preferentially in the intracellular compartment and diffuse slowly across the cell membrane to the extracellular compartment. Such solutes are sometimes labeled as "difficult to dialyze." For example, therapeutic dialysis is not recommended for removal of digoxin in patients with digoxin intoxication[145] even though the substance is water soluble and easily removed in vitro with a high clearance across the dialyzer membrane. Removal in vivo, however, is limited by sequestration in remote tissue compartments. Solutes such as digoxin have an apparent large distribution, often larger than total body water volume.

Even urea, one of the most diffusible solutes, exhibits disequilibrium during HD. Whole-body urea clearance can be calculated by substituting the equilibrated postdialysis BUN (Figure 65.17) for the immediate postdialysis BUN in the modeling equations. Experience has shown that urea sequestration can be predicted from the rapidity or rate of solute removal. This observation led to development of simplified equations to estimate the equilibrated Kt/V (eKt/V) from single-pool Kt/V (spKt/V),[146,147] where Kt/V is dialyzer clearance × time over volume:

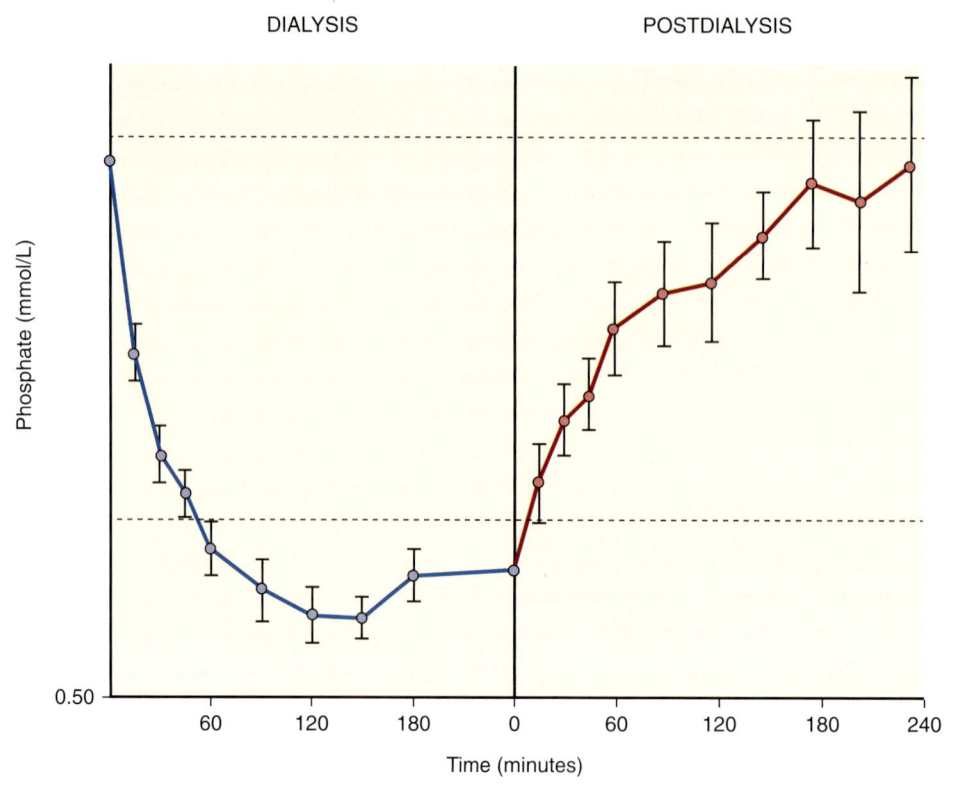

Figure 65.18 Effect of sequestration on serum phosphate levels and removal during dialysis. Measurements of serum inorganic phosphorus concentrations were taken at 15-minute intervals during both high-flux and standard hemodialysis. The rapid flux of phosphorus due to its relatively high mass transfer area coefficient caused levels to fall into the hypophosphatemic range (below the lower *dotted line*) during most of the 4-hour dialysis. A marked rebound continued for 4 hours after dialysis ended. The two *dotted lines* indicate the normal serum phosphate range. (Adapted from DeSoi CA, Umans JG: Phosphate kinetics during high-flux hemodialysis. *J Am Soc Nephrol* 4:1214-1218, 1993.)

$$eKt/V = spKt/V - 0.6spK/V + 0.03 \quad (8)$$

$$eKt/V = spKt/V[t/(t+35)] \quad (9)$$

When eKt/V is the chosen standard of care, these equations allow its calculation without requiring the patient to wait 30 to 60 minutes after dialysis has stopped for the equilibrated BUN to be measured.

EFFECT OF RED BLOOD CELLS PASSING THROUGH THE DIALYZER

Within the blood compartment, solutes may diffuse slowly or not at all out of RBCs during transit through the dialyzer.[148,149] For example, creatinine and uric acid are small molecules with clearances similar to that of urea when measured in a saline solution in vitro. Measured in vivo, however, their clearances are lower than urea clearance because their movement out of the RBC as it passes through the dialyzer is much slower than urea's movement, being limited by lack of specific urea-like transporters in the RBC membrane.[150-152]

Sequestration in Remote Compartments

Other solutes such as potassium and phosphorus are cleared easily in vitro, but their removal is limited by cellular and bone sequestration within patients, explaining the need for dietary restriction and for use of phosphate binders to control the toxic effects of these solutes. Phosphorus is rapidly removed from the intravascular compartment, causing hypophosphatemia during HD in most conventionally treated patients. However, for 2 to 4 hours after dialysis, the serum phosphorus concentration increases relatively rapidly, returning to near predialysis levels (Figure 65.18). Thus, sequestration and its consequent postdialysis rebound account for the failure of conventional HD alone to normalize interdialysis levels of this easily dialyzed molecule. Low blood phosphate levels generated during dialysis may also account for at least part of the postdialysis disequilibrium syndrome, discussed elsewhere in this chapter. Extrapolating further, one can speculate that the magnitude of sequestration of the toxic solutes responsible for the reversible life-threatening aspect of uremia cannot be as great as for phosphorus; otherwise, HD would not be successful.

COMPONENTS OF THE EXTRACORPOREAL CIRCUIT

The HD system for a single patient in the 1940s was about the size of a twin bed. Modern HD machines are about the size of a three- to four-drawer filing cabinet. Central to the dialysis delivery system is the artificial kidney or dialyzer, which acts as the point of exchange between blood and dialysate. The system is designed to deliver blood and properly constituted dialysate to the dialyzer, where diffusion and convection occur. Technologic advances have allowed the development of online monitors that accurately monitor and regulate the blood flow and dialysate flow rates, circuit pressures, and dialysate composition and temperature.

Additional advances include automated safety mechanisms designed to detect blood leaks and air in the circuit and online devices that monitor vascular access, hematocrit, and dialysis adequacy during each treatment.

BLOOD CIRCUIT

During dialysis, the steady flow of blood required may be obtained from a central venous catheter or from an AV fistula or graft. If a catheter is used, blood enters the extracorporeal circuit from the ports along the sides of the double-lumen catheter ("arterial" lumen) and returns through the port at the distal tip ("venous" lumen). Alternatively, the graft or fistula is cannulated with two needles, with blood flowing from the "arterial" needle into the blood tubing and dialyzer and returning to the patient through the "venous" needle. The driving force for the blood circuit is a peristaltic roller pump, which sequentially compresses the pump segment of the tubing against a curved rigid track, forcing blood from the tubing. Elastic recoil refills the pump tubing after the roller has passed, readying it for the next roller. Because of the elastic recoil and because most pumps have only two or three rollers, blood flow through the dialyzer is pulsatile. Increasing the number of rollers makes the flow less pulsatile but increases the risk of hemolysis and damage to the pump segment.

An alternative configuration of the dialysate delivery system allows the use of a single needle in the vascular access or a single-lumen catheter for dialysis.[153,154] This arrangement uses either one blood pump and two pressure-controlled blood-line clamps or two pressure-controlled blood pumps. The advantage is less trauma to the vascular access, especially during initial cannulation of a new fistula, and potentially reduced dialysis catheter use after surgical revision of a vascular access.[154] However, recirculation and hemolysis may be increased and the efficiency of solute clearance may be compromised.[153,155,156] Raising the effective blood flow rate to 250 mL/min, increasing the length of the dialysis session, or using a larger dialyzer may improve the efficiency of solute clearance, but careful monitoring of "adequacy" and for complications remains essential.[155]

Pressure monitors are located proximal to the blood pump and immediately distal to the dialyzer. The proximal or *arterial pressure monitor* guards against excessive suction on the vascular access site by the blood pump. Accepted ranges for arterial inflow pressures are −20 to −80 mm Hg, but may be as low as −200 mm Hg when blood flow rate (Q_b) is high. The distal or *venous pressure monitor* gauges the resistance to blood return in the vascular access, and acceptable values range from +50 to +200 mm Hg. When the upper or lower limits of arterial or venous pressures are exceeded, an alarm sounds, and the blood pump turns off. Excessively low arterial pressures may be caused by kinks in the tubing, improper arterial needle position, hypotension, or arterial inflow stenosis. Blood clotting in the dialyzer, kinking or clotting in the venous blood lines, improperly positioned venous needles, infiltration of a venous needle, or venous outflow stenosis can cause high venous pressures. Accurate measurements of both the arterial and venous pressures are essential to determining the transmembrane pressure (TMP), which partly determines the ultrafiltration rate. Excessively high pressures anywhere in the blood compartment may rupture the dialyzer membrane or disconnect the blood circuit, leading to an abrupt decrease in pressure in the blood circuit. The automatic shutoff of the blood pump in this circumstance is potentially lifesaving.

Two additional safety devices, the *venous air trap* and the *air detector*, are located in the blood line distal to the dialyzer. Air may enter the blood circuit through loose connections, improper arterial needle position, or the saline infusion line. The venous air trap prevents any air that may have entered the blood circuit from returning to the patient. If air is still detected in the venous line after the air trap, the machine alarms, and a relay switch turns off the blood pump. Excessive foaming of blood also triggers the air detector. These safety features prevent air embolism, which carries a high mortality rate, especially if not immediately recognized.[157] If air embolism is suspected, additional interventions must include clamping the venous line leading back to the patient and placing the patient immediately in the Trendelenburg position with the left side down, sequestering the air in the right ventricle and allowing it to be reabsorbed. However, microbubbles formed during dialysis may escape detection and lodge in organs such as the brain and lungs, possibly contributing to the higher incidence of pulmonary hypertension and cognitive decline observed in dialysis recipients.[158,159] Ensuring a high blood level in the venous air trap may reduce such microemboli.[160]

HEMODIALYZERS

A *hemodialyzer*, or *dialyzer*, is often called an "artificial kidney." Its configuration allows blood and dialysate to flow, preferably in opposite directions, through individual compartments separated by a semipermeable membrane. By convention, blood entering the hemodialyzer is designated *arterial*, and blood leaving the hemodialyzer is *venous*. The many available hemodialyzers differ mainly in the composition, configuration, and surface area of the membrane. Hemodialyzers influence the efficiency and the quality of dialysis through their membranes, which determine their K_0A value, and through the blood and dialysate flow rates, which determine the clearance values (see also Factors that Affect Clearance in a Flowing System) (Table 65.5).

Virtually all of the commercial dialyzers available in the United States are *hollow-fiber dialyzers*. Such hemodialyzers are constructed with a cylindrical plastic casing (usually polycarbonate) that encloses several thousand hollow-fiber semipermeable membranes stretched from one end to the other and anchored at each end by a plastic *potting compound*, usually polyurethane. The blood compartment or fiber bundle volume of the hollow fiber dialyzer ranges from 60 to 150 mL, and in contrast to that in older dialyzer designs, does not expand during dialysis. Each fiber has an inside diameter of approximately 200 μm. Along with the semipermeable membrane, the potting compound separates the blood compartment from the dialysate compartment, where dialysate flows between and around each fiber. Blood flows to or from the open end of each fiber through a removable *header* attached to the blood tubing. Apart from lowering blood priming volume, the hollow-fiber design also improves the efficiency of solute exchange by increasing the contact area between blood and dialysate. Additional maneuvers to maximize surface area include insertion

Table 65.5 Key Factors That Affect the Solute Clearance of a Hemodialyzer

	Key Factors	Effect on Clearance
Properties of the membrane	Membrane porosity	↑
	Membrane thickness	↓
	Membrane surface area	↑
	Membrane charge	Varies
	Membrane hydrophilicity	↑
Properties of the solute	Molecular weight and size	↓
	Charge	Varies
	Lipid solubility	↓
	Protein binding	↓
Blood side	Unstirred blood layer	↓
	Blood flow	↑
Dialysate side	Dialysate channeling and unstirred layer	↓
	Dialysate flow	↑
	Countercurrent direction of flow	↑

↑, Increases; ↓, decreases.

of spacer yarns between fibers and wavy moiré configuration of the fibers to prevent loss of surface area through fiber-to-fiber contact.[161] Arterial port design also influences the distribution of blood flow through the hollow fibers and can reduce dialysis efficiency.[162] Thrombosis and the need for potting compound are major disadvantages of the hollow-fiber design. The potting compound absorbs chemicals used to disinfect newly manufactured dialyzers (e.g., ethylene oxide) or reprocessed dialyzers (e.g., formaldehyde, peracetic acid, glutaraldehyde) and acts as a reservoir for these chemicals, allowing them to leach out slowly during dialysis into the patient's blood.[163]

MEMBRANE COMPOSITION

The biomaterials used to make the hollow-fiber dialyzer dictate its clearance and ultrafiltration characteristics as well as its biocompatibility. Two major classes of membrane material are available commercially: (1) cotton fiber, or *cellulose-based membranes*, and (2) *synthetic membranes*. KDOQI guidelines discourage the use of unmodified cellulose-based membranes because they contain many free hydroxyl groups, which are thought to be responsible for their bioincompatibility and propensity to activate WBCs, platelets, and serum complement via the alternate pathway (see later).[68] Treating the cellulose polymer with acetate and tertiary amino compounds improves membrane biocompatibility, presumably through covalent binding of the hydroxyl groups to form acetylated cellulose and aminated cellulose (such as hemophane).[164,165]

The major polymers in synthetic membranes are polyacrylonitrile, polysulfone, polycarbonate, polyamide, polyethersulfone, and polymethylmethacrylate. Although these membranes are thicker, they can be rendered more permeable than the cellulose membranes, yielding greater fluid and solute removal. Because the pore sizes in the synthetic membranes are larger, higher-molecular-weight substances, such as β_2-microglobulin (β_2M), can be removed more efficiently.[166-168] Some membranes, such as those of polyacrylonitrile, polyamide, and polymethylmethacrylate, have low hydrophilicity, providing significant protein adsorption and enhancing protein removal.[169] Synthetic membranes also are more biocompatible.[168,169] Since the cost of synthetic hemodialyzers has declined, they are increasingly preferred for the preceding reasons.

MEMBRANE BIOCOMPATIBILITY

Dialyzer membranes may interact with blood components during dialysis to activate WBCs, platelets, and the complement cascade via the alternative pathway with generation of the anaphylatoxins C3a and C5a.[168-171] The degree to which the membrane activates blood components determines its *biocompatibility*. Through activation of WBCs, platelets, and the complement cascade, bioincompatible membranes may cause allergic reactions, hypoxemia, transient neutropenia, altered immunity, tissue damage, anorexia, protein catabolism, or an inflammatory state. Because dialysis is repetitive, the effects of low-grade subclinical membrane interactions during each treatment may be cumulative, eventually resulting in adverse clinical outcomes such as infection, accelerated atherosclerosis, frequent hospitalization, and death.

In addition to the capacity of the membrane to activate blood elements, its absorptive capacity can influence its biocompatibility. Some synthetic membranes, such as polyacrylonitrile, are more hydrophobic, bind proteins to a greater extent, and may ameliorate bioincompatible inflammatory reactions through their ability to bind anaphylatoxins such as C3a and C5a and cytokines.[168,169] Therefore, measurements of these elements in blood may not accurately reflect the true capacity of a membrane for inciting the complement cascade, producing cytokines, and inducing an inflamed state.[168] In general, however, synthetic membranes and modified or substituted cellulose membranes are more biocompatible than unmodified cellulose membranes.

Because bacterial contaminants in product water also can activate complement and leukocytes if they come in contact with blood (see "Water Treatment" section), it is difficult to determine the relative contributions of bioincompatible membrane and contaminated water to the inflamed state seen in dialysis recipients. With increasing use of modified cellulose and synthetic membranes and closer attention to water quality, the distinction has become even more difficult. Studies evaluating the relative biocompatibility of substituted cellulose versus synthetic membranes reported no difference.[165,172,173] Ongoing efforts to improve biocompatibility include coating the membrane with heparin or vitamin E.[174,175]

MEMBRANE PERMEABILITY AND SURFACE AREA

Dialyzers perform two important functions: elimination of unwanted solutes and removal of excess fluid. The thickness, porosity, composition, and surface area of a membrane determine its ability to clear solutes and remove water. In general, the thinner and more porous the membrane, the more efficient is the transport of solutes and fluid across it. The urea K_0A (or clearance) of the dialyzer describes its ability to eliminate low-molecular-weight substances; the vitamin B_{12} and β_2-microglobulin (β_2M) K_0A (or clearance), its capacity to remove higher-molecular-weight substances;

Table 65.6 Characteristic Values for Standard, High-Efficiency, and High-Flux Dialyzers*

	Standard	High Efficiency	High Flux
Blood flow rate (mL/min)	250	≥350	≥350
Dialysate flow rate (mL/min)	500	≥500	≥500
K_0A urea	300-500	≥600	Variable
Urea clearance (mL/min)	<200	>210	Variable
Urea clearance/body weight (mL/min/kg)	<3	>3	Variable
Vitamin B_{12} clearance (mL/min)	30-60	Variable	>100
$β_2$-microglobulin clearance (mL/min)	<10	Variable	>20
Ultrafiltration coefficient (mL/hr/mm Hg)	3.5-5.0	Variable	>20
Membrane	Cellulose	Variable	Variable

*See text.

and the ultrafiltration coefficient (Kf), its ability to remove water (Table 65.6).

Most hemodialyzers have a membrane surface area of 0.8 to 2.1 m². The desirable increase in solute transport associated with larger membranes can be achieved by increasing the length, increasing the number, or decreasing the diameter of the hollow fiber,[176] but each maneuver has undesirable effects when carried too far. Lengthening the fiber increases the shear rate and resistance to blood flow, magnifying the pressure decrease between blood entering and exiting the dialyzer. Increasing the shear rate can damage RBCs, and the higher pressure can raise the ultrafiltration rate. However, the higher filtration rate at the arterial inflow end of the dialyzer is partially offset by the dissipation of pressure at the venous end, reducing the contribution of ultrafiltration to solute clearance and offsetting this potential advantage of greater surface area.[161] Increasing the number of hollow fibers enlarges surface area but expands the extracorporeal blood volume, a change that can compromise the patient's hemodynamic stability. Smaller-diameter fibers can offset this disadvantage, but as the fiber diameter decreases, resistance to blood flow increases, enhancing not only filtration but also backfiltration and clotting.[177] As fibers become thrombosed, the effective surface area for diffusion decreases and solute clearances decrease. Because of these adverse effects, the minimal acceptable internal fiber diameter is 180 μm.[177] The design and geometry of the hollow-fiber dialyzer represent a delicate balance among these factors.

HIGH-EFFICIENCY AND HIGH-FLUX DIALYZERS

Historically, low dialyzer membrane permeability limited the efficiency of HD, requiring more than 6 hours for each treatment. As dialyzer design improved, treatment times were shortened progressively. In the late 1980s, with the advent of more permeable dialyzer membranes, improved techniques to reduce bacteriologic contamination of bicarbonate dialysate (see later), more precise ultrafiltration control, and more reliable vascular access to achieve adequate blood flow, treatment times decreased to 2 to 3 hours three times weekly in the United States. These substituted cellulose and synthetic membranes ushered in the era of the high-efficiency and high-flux dialysis.

The distinction between *high-efficiency* and *high-flux* dialyzers is imprecise, and sometimes these terms are used interchangeably. In essence, both types of dialyzers have improved solute and fluid clearance over that with standard hemodialyzers and take advantage of higher blood and dialysate flow rates to reduce dialysis time while maintaining an adequate dose. High-efficiency dialyzers have a higher K_0A and a higher clearance of small molecules, such as urea, than standard dialyzers (see Table 65.6). High-flux dialyzers have a highly permeable membrane for larger molecules, such as vitamin B_{12} and $β_2M$, and have a higher Kf than high-efficiency dialyzers, but not necessarily high urea clearances (see Table 65.6). As evident from the foregoing discussion, the two dialyzer designs frequently overlap, hence the imprecision (see Table 65.6).

High-efficiency and high-flux dialyzers contain either substituted cellulose or a synthetic membrane. Both membranes improve dialyzer permeability because substituted cellulose membranes can be made thinner to increase porosity and surface area, and synthetic membranes can be manufactured with more and larger pores. Both high-efficiency and high-flux types of dialysis require the use of bicarbonate dialysate and volume-controlled filtration. When acetate was used as a base, its rate of diffusion into blood exceeded the metabolic capacity of the body, leading to acidosis, vasodilation, and intradialytic hypotension (see "Dialysate Composition" section). The high Kf of these dialyzers creates the potential for hemodynamic collapse with pressure-controlled filtration because it is less precise in controlling volume removal (see "Dialysate Circuit" section).

Because of their greater porosity, high-flux dialyzers can remove larger molecules such as $β_2M$ that are not removed at all by standard cellulosic dialyzers.[166-168] Removal of $β_2M$ reduces the risk of carpal tunnel syndrome in patients undergoing long-term dialysis.[166,178,179] Initial results suggested that removal of other large molecules might offer additional benefits such as a greater response to erythropoietin[180]; a higher leptin removal, possibly leading to a better appetite[181]; and perhaps lower mortality and hospitalization rates.[179,182] However, potential adverse consequences include more thorough removal of amino acids,[183] albumin,[184] and drugs such as vancomycin.[185] Theoretically, the backfiltration that occurs during high-flux dialysis can increase the exposure of patients to endotoxin from the dialysate, but this theoretical concern has not been verified clinically.[186,187]

Despite early promise, randomized controlled or crossover trials comparing high-flux with standard hemodialysis found no difference in the incidence of hypotension and intra-dialysis symptoms,[166,188] control of blood pressure,[189] neuropsychological function,[190] Hgb concentration and use of erythropoiesis-stimulating agents (ESAs),[191-193] or markers of inflammation, oxidative stress and nutritional status.[192] Three large randomized controlled trials, the Hemodialysis (HEMO) Study,[194,195] the Membrane Permeability Outcome

(MPO) Study,[196] and the EGE Study (Multiple Interventions Related to Dialysis Procedures in Order to Reduce Cardiovascular Morbidity and Mortality in HD Patients),[197] detected no significant difference in mortality or morbidity between patients treated with standard and high-flux membranes. *Post hoc* subgroup analyses demonstrated that high-flux dialysis reduced cardiovascular events in patients with longer dialysis vintage in the HEMO Study,[194,195] enhanced survival in patients with low serum albumin concentrations (<4.0 g/dL) and diabetes in the MPO Study,[196] and decreased cardiovascular mortality in patients with an arteriovenous fistula or diabetes in the EGE study.[197] A meta-analysis of available data concluded that high-flux hemodialysis may reduce cardiovascular mortality by 15% but does not alter infection-related or all-cause mortality.[198]

Convection versus Diffusion

Further increases in dialyzer flux may not improve middle molecule clearance or outcomes because some solutes that accumulate in kidney failure are protein bound or sequestered inside the cell.[199] Because of slow diffusion caused by low free concentrations of protein-bound solutes and delayed diffusion across cell membranes, the removal of such solutes remains time dependent. Initial experience suggested that hemofiltration (HF) and hemodiafiltration (HDF) may augment removal of larger molecules and protein-bound solutes through increased convective clearance.[199-201] However, randomized controlled studies comparing HF and HDF with HD found no difference in Hgb level or ESA resistance,[202,203] phosphate level,[204] health-related quality of life,[205] cardiovascular parameters such as left ventricular mass and pulse-wave velocity,[206] or intradialytic hypotension,[207,208] although some studies reported less intradialytic hypotension with HDF.[209,210] Two of the three largest randomized controlled studies, the Convective Transport Study (CONTRAST)[211] and the Turkish Online Haemodiafiltration (OL-HDF) Study,[208] reported no difference in cardiovascular and all-cause mortality, but subgroup analyses suggested a benefit in patients treated with larger convective and replacement volumes (>22 L and 17.4 L, respectively, so-called high-efficiency HDF). The ESHOL (Estudio de Supervivencia de Hemodiafiltracion On-Line) Study,[210] which achieved about 23 L of convective volume per session, reported lower rates of cardiovascular mortality, all-cause mortality, and hospitalization in patients randomly assigned to receive HDF. The latest meta analyses conclude that convective therapies may reduce intradialytic hypotension[201,212,213] and cardiovascular mortality,[201,213] but additional high-quality randomized and controlled studies addressing the effect of convective volume on outcomes are needed.

DIALYSATE CIRCUIT

Another major function of the HD system is the preparation and delivery of dialysate to the dialyzer. Most dialysis clinics use a *single-pass* delivery system, which discards the dialysate after a single passage through the dialyzer, and a *single-patient* delivery system, which prepares dialysate individually and continuously at each patient station by mixing liquid concentrates with a proportionate volume of purified water. To ensure that the dialysate concentrates are diluted safely and accurately, the delivery system has many built-in safety monitors. Some clinics use a central multipatient delivery system. In this design, either the dialysate is mixed in an area separate from patient care and then piped to each patient station or the concentrate is piped to each station before mixing. These centralized systems lower patient care costs and reduce staff back injuries from carrying the individual concentrate jugs. However, a major disadvantage is the inability to modify the dialysate concentration of electrolytes such as calcium and potassium for individual patients.

The dialysis machine warms purified water to physiologic temperatures and then deaerates it under vacuum. Because the patient is exposed to 100 to 200 L of dialysate during each treatment, the dialysate must be warmed to avoid hypothermia. In practice, the dialysate temperature is maintained at 35° to 37° C. If the dialysate is too hot, protein denaturation (>42° C) and hemolysis (>45° C) occur. To ensure safety, the *temperature monitor* within the dialysate circuit alarms and a bypass valve diverts the dialysate directly to the drain, automatically bypassing the dialyzer if the dialysate temperature is outside of the limits of 35° to 42° C. Without *deaeration*, dissolved air would come out of solution as negative pressure is applied during dialysis, creating air bubbles in the dialysate, which would lead to malfunction of the blood leak detector and the conductivity detector, increased channeling, masking of parts of the membrane, and reduced effective membrane surface area.

The heated and deaerated product water is then mixed proportionately with the concentrate to produce dialysate. Improperly proportioned dialysate may cause severe electrolyte disturbances in the patient and lead to death. Because the primary solutes in the dialysate are electrolytes, the electrical conductivity of the dialysate varies directly with the concentration of solutes. On the basis of this principle, the *conductivity monitor* downstream from the proportioning pump continuously measures the electrical conductivity of the product solution to ensure proper proportioning. This monitor has a narrow range of tolerance, is usually redundant, and must be calibrated periodically with use of standardized solutions or by laboratory measurements of electrolytes in the dialysate. Changes in temperature, the presence of air bubbles, or malfunction of the sensor (usually an electrode) can alter the dialysate conductivity.

The *dialysate pump*, located downstream from the dialyzer, controls dialysate flow and dialysate pressure. Although many dialyzers require a negative dialysate pressure for filtration, the circuit also must be able to generate positive dialysate pressures within the dialyzer because positive pressure is required to limit filtration with use of dialyzers with high Kf or under conditions that increase pressure in the blood compartment. The dialysate circuit regulates the pressure by controlled constriction of the dialysate outflow tubing while maintaining a constant flow rate. In addition, the dialysate delivery system controls the filtration rate, either indirectly by altering the TMP (*pressure-controlled* ultrafiltration) or directly by modifying the actual filtration rate (*volume-controlled* ultrafiltration). Earlier systems used manual pressure-controlled filtration, requiring dialysis personnel to calculate and enter the TMP, closely monitor the filtration rate, and recalculate and adjust the TMP as needed. For dialyzers with Kf greater than 6 mL/hr/mm Hg, dialysate delivery systems with built-in balance chambers and servomechanisms that accurately control the volume of the fluid removed during dialysis (volume-controlled filtration)[214] are mandatory to prevent excessive fluid gain or removal.

When blood is detected in the dialysate, the *blood leak monitor* located in the dialysate outflow tubing sounds an alarm and shuts off the blood pump. Presence of blood in the dialysate usually indicates membrane rupture and may be caused by a TMP exceeding 500 mm Hg or by damage to a dialyzer membrane from the bleach or heat disinfection used to reprocess dialyzers for repeated use. Although a rare complication, membrane rupture can be life threatening because it allows blood to come into contact with nonsterile dialysate.

ONLINE MONITORING

In addition to delivering dialysate to the dialyzer and the many built-in safety features described previously, modern-day dialysis machines also are able to record and store such varied, real-time data as patient vital signs, blood and dialysate flows, arterial and venous pressures, delivered dialysis dose, plasma volume, thermal energy loss, and access recirculation. Linking computerized medical information systems with dialysis delivery systems can facilitate and improve patient care by allowing integration of patient data while maintaining treatment records.

MONITORING CLEARANCE

Online monitoring of clearance may provide the best assessment of dialysis adequacy.[215-219] Online monitors record urea clearances by measuring urea concentration in the dialysate either continuously or periodically[215,220,221]; dialyzer sodium clearance by pulsing the dialysate with sodium and measuring dialysate conductivity at the dialyzer inlet and outlet (ionic dialysance) (Gambro, Stockholm, Sweden; Fresenius, Bad Homburg, Germany),[215,217,222,223]; or clearance of uremic solutes by measuring ultraviolet light absorbance of spent dialysate (Hospal, Medolla, Italy).[215,224] Most online methods for monitoring urea or sodium kinetics provide Kt/V on the basis of whole-body clearance in addition to dialyzer clearance.[217,222] Online urea monitoring has not gained popularity possibly because of the need for repeated calibration and the added expense for additional disposable supplies. Online clearance monitoring removes the expense and risks of blood sampling, reduces dialysis personnel time, allows more frequent determination of delivered dose, and provides real-time measurements for instant feedback.[217-219] However, reported clearance values may differ depending on the online equipment used and adjustments applied by the instrument's software to more closely match urea Kt/V.[223,224] Drawbacks of online clearance monitoring include the need for multiple measurements of K_d to obtain an average for the entire dialysis, accurate monitoring of treatment time, the need still for blood urea sampling to allow determination of protein catabolic rate (a marker of nutrition), and the need to measure or estimate V to allow calculation of Kt/V from the online K_d measurements.[225]

MONITORING HEMATOCRIT AND RELATIVE BLOOD VOLUME

The hematocrit can be measured online during dialysis with the use of an ultrasound determination of plasma protein concentration[226] or an optical measure of Hgb or hematocrit concentration.[215,218,219,227] Of these, the optical technique is more widely available. In theory, patients treated with dialysis who are prone to hypotension and cramping may benefit from online monitoring of hematocrit because their symptoms are often caused by a decrease in circulating blood volume when the ultrafiltration rate exceeds intravascular refilling from the interstitium and the intracellular space.[215,218,219,227,228] The degree of hemoconcentration reflects the magnitude of intravascular volume depletion and allows determination of changes in blood volume, or *relative blood volume*. Theoretically, monitoring the hematocrit online and altering the filtration rate during dialysis to minimize excessive hemoconcentration may reduce the occurrence of symptoms during dialysis and optimize the dry weight.[215,219,229] In practice, using just the relative blood volume to guide filtration rate has not been very successful in ameliorating symptoms,[215,219,227,228,230,231] likely because of inaccuracies in the measurements, the varied compensatory cardiovascular response to volume depletion within and among individual patients, and a dialysis-induced reduction in arteriolar tone and left ventricular function (*myocardial stunning*).[227,228,232-235] Online determination of relative blood volume varies significantly among devices and underestimates the true decline in blood volume because of "intravascular translocation" of blood from the microcirculation (capillaries and venules), which has a lower hematocrit, to the larger vessels.[227,228] Because of these limitations, identifying the pattern of the relative blood volume decline and using a computer-controlled biofeedback system to modify the filtration rate continuously during dialysis (see later), in combination with clinical assessments such as symptoms and bioelectrical impedance analysis (BIA), have shown more promise.[215,218,219,236-238] The absolute or total blood volume may be more predictive of intradialytic symptoms, but automated online monitoring of this parameter is not available currently, although mathematical models may allow derivation of total blood volume from relative blood volume.[228,239,240]

COMPUTER CONTROLS

Solute removal during HD reduces plasma osmolarity, favoring fluid shift into the cells and thwarting efforts to achieve net fluid removal.[241] Raising the dialysate sodium concentration (sodium ramping) helps preserve plasma osmolarity and may allow continued fluid removal but leads to increased thirst, excessive interdialytic weight gain (IDWG), and hypertension,[218,242-247] although the last is not a consistent finding.[248-250] Computer-controlled sodium modeling changes the dialysate sodium concentration automatically during dialysis, usually starting at 150 to 155 mEq/L and stepping down to 135 to 140 mEq/L near or at the end of dialysis, and offers the theoretic benefit of fewer intradialytic symptoms (hypotension and cramps) while minimizing thirst, IDWG, and hypertension. In practice, however, thirst, increased IDWG, and hypertension persist because of predialysis hyponatremia (on average, 134 to 136 mEq/L) and an overall positive sodium balance during dialysis despite the stepdown.[218,242-244,251,252] Instead, individualizing dialysate sodium to maintain a sodium gradient of 0 to −2 mEq/L with respect to predialysis plasma sodium concentration results in less thirst, lower IDWG, improved blood pressure control, and perhaps fewer intradialytic symptoms because of lower ultrafiltration requirements.[242-244,249] Such individualization may be accomplished through the use of online conductivity monitoring[242-244] or by estimating each patient's inherent plasma sodium concentration (sodium set point)[252] using an average predialysis sodium concentration, either measured with direct potentiometry or mathematically corrected for the Gibbs-Donnan effect (unavailability of sodium for diffusion because of trapping by negatively charged proteins).[242-244] To complicate matters further, data from DOPPS suggest a differential effect of dialysate sodium on outcome: HD recipients with the lowest predialysis plasma levels have lower mortality when they undergo dialysis against a high dialysate sodium, despite an increase in IDWG.[246] Given our incomplete understanding of the effects of altering dialysate sodium on morbidity and mortality, indiscriminate use of dialysate sodium ramping and sodium modeling in its current form should be abandoned, and individualization of dialysate sodium employed cautiously.[235,253,254]

Ultrafiltration modeling, like sodium modeling, provides a variable rate of fluid removal during dialysis according to a preprogrammed profile (linear decline, stepwise changes, or exponential decline of ultrafiltration rate with time). Theoretically, altering the ultrafiltration rate during dialysis allows time for the blood compartment to refill from the interstitial compartment, leading to less hypotension and cramping. Also like sodium modeling, stand-alone ultrafiltration modeling is crude, and altering the ultrafiltration rate in response to blood volume monitoring may be of more benefit (see "Monitoring Hematocrit and Relative Blood Volume" section). The effects of sodium modeling and ultrafiltration modeling may be difficult to separate because they are often used together, although the latter does not result in positive sodium balance.[215,218,219,251]

Technological advances include the development of dialysis machines with *biofeedback systems*, allowing for computer-controlled adjustments of treatment parameters based on real-time input from the online monitors. The most common system in use monitors the blood volume (see earlier) and adjusts the ultrafiltration rate and dialysate conductivity to prevent it from decreasing below a preset value during dialysis.[215,218,219,236] Small studies have demonstrated that this device ameliorates symptoms in both patients who are prone to hypotension and those who are not.[215,218,219,236,244,255] Although the ability to monitor plasma conductivity throughout dialysis may ensure sodium balance despite constant modifications of the dialysate conductivity and may reduce the problem of thirst, IDWG, and hypertension,[215] most authorities advise against sodium modeling even with a feedback control system (see preceding discussion).[68,218,219,244,256] Instead, automated control of dialysate temperature to maintain isothermic dialysis (constant body temperature) shows promise and is superior to thermoneutral dialysis (using lower but constant dialysate temperature) in reducing intradialytic hypotension without incurring a sodium load.[215,219,257-259] Although these online monitors and automated biofeedback systems are expensive, they have the potential to reduce hypotension, detect vascular access dysfunction,[260,261] and increase dialysis efficiency while minimizing blood sampling. By improving patient care, they may prove to be cost effective in the long run.

Table 65.7	Solutes Present in the Dialysate
Solute	**Concentration (mEq/L)**
Sodium	135-145
Potassium	0-4.0
Chloride	102-106
Bicarbonate	30-39
Acetate	2-4
Calcium	0-3.5
Magnesium	0.5-1.0
Dextrose	11
pH	7.1-7.3

DIALYSATE

During HD, blood flows in the blood compartment in one direction, and isosmotic dialysate flows in the opposite direction in the dialysate compartment (see Figure 65.12*A*). This countercurrent flow optimizes the concentration gradient for solute removal. Preparation of the dialysate and its composition is critical to the success of dialysis. The solution must be prepared from properly treated water (see later) that includes reducing the concentration of endotoxin to prevent pyrogenic reactions in the patient. Sterility is not required because the semipermeable membrane excludes large particles such as bacteria and viruses. The concentrations of vital solutes added to the dialysate reflect those normally maintained in the body by the native kidneys (Table 65.7). The dialysate is essentially a physiologic salt solution that creates a gradient for removal of unwanted solutes and maintains a constant physiologic concentration of extracellular electrolytes (see later).

WATER TREATMENT

Because patients receiving HD are exposed to as much as 600 L of dialysate water a week, treating the water used to generate dialysate is essential to avoid exposure to harmful substances such as aluminum, chloramines, fluoride, endotoxin, and bacteria.[262-266] Technical advances such as high-flux dialyzers, reuse or reprocessing of dialyzers, and bicarbonate-based dialysate have made high water quality even more imperative. To avoid these complications, tap water is softened, exposed to charcoal to remove contaminants such as chloramine, filtered to remove particulate matter, and then filtered under high pressure (reverse osmosis) to remove other dissolved contaminants (Figure 65.19). A complete review of this topic is beyond the scope of this chapter, and readers are referred to reviews on the topic.[262-266] Highlights are discussed here.

HAZARDS ASSOCIATED WITH DIALYSIS WATER

Improperly treated water contains potentially harmful substances and can cause injury or death.[262-268] Accumulation of aluminum in the body may cause osteomalacia, microcytic anemia, and dialysis-associated encephalopathy (dialysis dementia and movement disorders).[269-271] Treating water to keep aluminum levels below 10 mg/L has markedly reduced aluminum-associated diseases.[272] Chlorine is added to

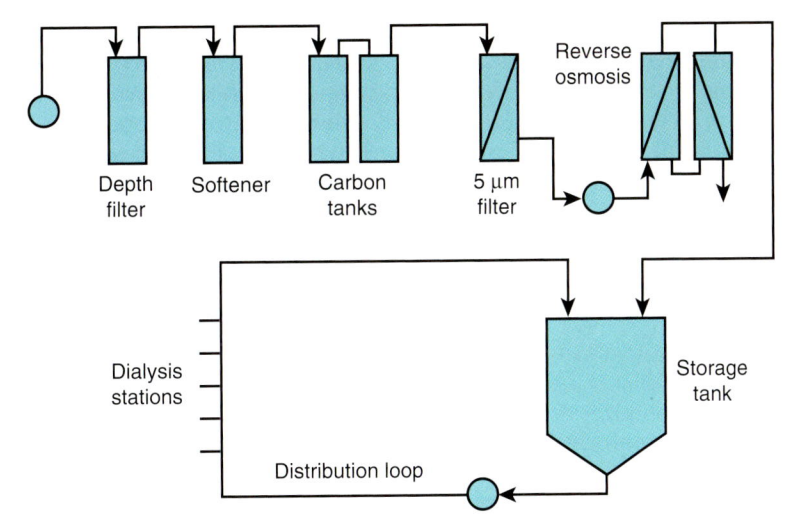

Figure 65.19 Schematic of the typical configuration of a reverse osmosis water treatment system. Tap water undergoes filtration to remove gross particulate matter and then is softened before exposure to charcoal (in carbon tanks) to remove contaminants such as chloramine. A second filtration process removes particulate matter as well as microbiologic organisms. Finally, water is filtered under high pressure to remove dissolved contaminants such as aluminum (reverse osmosis). Product water is then either stored in a water tank or piped directly to each dialysis station.

municipal water as a bactericidal agent and interacts with organic material in the water to form chloramines. Alternatively, chloramine may occur naturally or may be added directly to municipal water as a bactericidal agent. Unfortunately, unlike the beneficial effects of chlorine, direct exposure of the blood to chloramine causes acute hemolysis and methemoglobinemia.[265,266,273-275] Fluoride can cause cardiac arrhythmias and death in the short term[276,277] and osteomalacia over the long term.[278] Excess calcium and magnesium have been linked to the "hard water syndrome," consisting of a constellation of symptoms including nausea, vomiting, weakness, flushing, and labile blood pressures.[279] Close communication between the dialysis center and water suppliers is critical to anticipate changes in feed water quality from added chemicals, environmental conditions such as flooding, or contamination, because alterations in the water purification process may be required.[265,267] With the advent of large-pore high-flux membranes, efforts at improving water purity have focused on further reducing bacterial endotoxin, which can cause febrile reactions, hypotension, and chronic inflammation (see later).[263,265-267]

ESSENTIAL COMPONENTS OF WATER PURIFICATION

Temperature-blending valves proportion incoming supplies of hot and cold tap water to yield a water temperature of about 77° F, the optimal temperature for the carbon tank and most reverse osmosis membranes. Water temperatures below 77° F reduce the flow rate and thus the efficiency of the reverse osmosis system, and temperatures above 100° F may damage the membrane. *Multimedia depth filters* then remove particulate matter from the water (see Figure 65.19). Using cation-exchange resins that contain sodium, the *water softener* then removes calcium, magnesium, and other polyvalent cations from the feed water, preventing these cations from depositing on and damaging the reverse osmosis membrane. Next, *granular activated carbon* in the carbon filtration tank absorbs chlorine, chloramines, and other organic substances from the water. Activated carbon is very porous and has a high affinity for organic material, but if not serviced properly or exchanged frequently, it can be contaminated with bacteria. Downstream, the water is then filtered through a 5-μm cartridge filter to prevent carbon particles from fouling up the reverse osmosis pump and membrane. Finally, the water is delivered to the *reverse osmosis unit*, which applies high hydrostatic pressure to force water through a highly selective semipermeable membrane that rejects 90% to 99% of monovalent ions, 95% to 99% of divalent ions, and microbiologic contaminants larger than 200 Da. The water exiting the reverse osmosis unit is termed the *permeate* or *product water* and, in most clinics, can be used safely for dialysis.

When there is heavy ionic contamination of feed water, however, the product water from the reverse osmosis unit is further "polished" with a *mixed-bed ion-exchange system* (deionization system) and then passed through an ultrafilter to remove any bacterial contamination from the ion exchanger. The cationic resin exchanges hydrogen ions for other cations in descending order of affinity: calcium, magnesium, potassium, sodium, and then hydrogen. The anionic resin exchanges hydroxyl ions for other anions in descending order of affinity: nitrites, sulfates, nitrates, chloride, bicarbonate, hydroxyl, and fluoride. When the resin is exhausted, previously adsorbed ions, especially those of lower affinity, can elute into the effluent, resulting in levels that are more than 20 times their usual concentration in tap water and cause severe toxicity and even death.[276,280] Because of this danger, the deionization system is rarely used alone in treating water for dialysis and requires stringent monitoring of product water.

MICROBIOLOGY OF HEMODIALYSIS SYSTEMS

Despite municipal treatment of tap water and the extensive water treatment system described previously, water used for dialysis still can become contaminated with bacteria and endotoxins,[262,263,265-268,281-283] principally with water-borne gram-negative bacteria and nontuberculous mycobacteria. Such contamination arises because the system removes the normally protective chlorine and chloramine as already described and then low-flow and stagnation points in the water treatment circuit predispose to biofilm deposition. Although nontuberculous mycobacteria do not produce endotoxins, they are more resistant to germicides than gram-negative bacteria and can survive and multiply in product water that contains little organic matter.[284-287] In 1984, the U.S. Centers for Disease Control and Prevention (CDC) found nontuberculous mycobacteria in the water of 83% of surveyed dialysis centers.[285]

In addition to treating water to remove potentially harmful chemicals, routine disinfection and surveillance of the water treatment equipment, product water, and dialysate are critically important to optimize dialysis water quality.[262,265-268,282] Because of dialyzer reprocessing and the use of high-flux dialyzers, the patient may be exposed to bacterial and endotoxin contaminants in improperly handled product water either through direct contact of product water with the blood compartment during reprocessing or through backleak of endotoxin into the blood compartment during dialysis. Therefore, stricter standards for water quality as well as high-level disinfection to kill all microorganisms (except bacterial spores) are necessary. The Association for the Advancement of Medical Instrumentation (AAMI) adopted the International Organization for Standardization (ISO) guidelines for dialysis water quality in 2009, recommending a lower maximal level of 100 colony-forming units per milliliter (CFU/mL) for bacteria and a maximal concentration of less than 0.25 endotoxin units per milliliter (EU/mL) for endotoxin (compared with 200 CFU/mL and 2 EU/mL previously), with action levels (levels at which corrective measures must be taken to prevent adverse outcomes) of 25 CFU/mL and 0.125 EU/mL, respectively.[288,289] In addition to routine scheduled disinfection, the water treatment equipment and system and affected dialysis machines must be disinfected when action levels are detected on scheduled monitoring. For *ultrapure dialysate*, even more stringent criteria are in place, including a bacterial count less than 0.1 CFU/mL and an endotoxin level less than 0.03 EU/mL.[290] A meta-analysis reported that use of ultrapure dialysate is associated with less inflammation and oxidative stress, higher serum albumin and Hgb levels, and lower ESA requirement.[291] The only randomized controlled trial to evaluate the effect of ultrapure dialysate on fatal and nonfatal cardiovascular events found no benefit, although the power of the study to detect a difference may have been reduced by a lower than expected endotoxin level (0.15 ± 0.22 EU/mL) in the conventional dialysate group.[197]

Water contaminated with bacteria and endotoxin can lead to pyrogenic reactions, characterized by shaking chills, fever, and hypotension in a previously afebrile and asymptomatic patient.[262,264,266,282,292] Headache, myalgia, nausea, and vomiting also may be present. Typically, the symptoms begin 30 to 60 minutes into the dialysis treatment. The source of the reaction is unlikely to be the microorganisms per se, because they are too large to cross an intact dialyzer membrane. Instead, bacterial pyrogens such as lipopolysaccharide, peptidoglycans, exotoxin, and their fragments are thought to be the culprits.[262,264,266,282,293] Pyrogenic reactions are typically seen in association with reprocessing of dialyzers because contaminated water gains direct access to the blood compartment during reprocessing.[163,292,294,295] In the absence of reuse, pyrogenic reactions are rare and occur only with high-level bacterial contamination of the dialysate or bicarbonate. Although the larger pore size in hi-flux dialyzers may increase backfiltration and allow endotoxins to enter the blood compartment from the dialysate, synthetic membranes also adsorb endotoxin, thereby attenuating the effect of moderately contaminated dialysate.[163,262,282] However, even in the absence of pyrogenic reactions, low levels of dialysate contamination with microbes may result in chronic inflammation, manifested as higher C-reactive protein levels, increased oxidative stress, lower albumin and Hgb levels, and ESA resistance,[291] which can be reversed by use of ultrapure dialysate (see earlier).

MONITORING WATER QUALITY

Because of the potential complications that can occur when improperly treated water is used for dialysis, monitoring of water quality is crucial. The source water and the product water must be assayed routinely to ensure that product water meets standards for heavy metal and other ionic contaminants. In the United States, the AAMI has adopted ISO water standards for dialysis, as already discussed. The frequency of scheduled testing depends on the quality of the water source, the type of water treatment system used, and the seasonal variation in chemicals added to municipal water to ensure its potability.

At least monthly, samples of source water, water obtained from critical points in the water treatment system, product water, dialysate, and bicarbonate solution must be cultured to ensure that bacterial contamination is below the limits set forth by AAMI standards. In addition, water is tested with the Limulus amoebocyte lysate (LAL) assay to determine the degree of endotoxin contamination. Although the most common test used, the LAL assay may not detect endotoxin fragments that are small enough to cross even low-flux membranes to cause pyrogenic reactions. The cytokine induction assay using mononuclear cells may allow improved detection of these low-molecular-weight substances.[263,282,296]

HEMODIALYSIS ADEQUACY

HISTORICAL PERSPECTIVES

In 1973, when Medicare in the United States began to fund dialysis for any citizen regardless of age, little attention was paid to the adequacy of dialysis. If the patient was awake and functioning at any level, the dialysis was deemed successful. As dialysis evolved and its prophylactic aspect was better appreciated, concern raised about adequacy led to a meeting in Monterey, California in 1974 that served to launch the National Cooperative Dialysis Study (NCDS) to provide guidelines for clinicians.[297] Sponsored by the National Institutes of Health (NIH), this first clinical trial of HD adequacy aimed to control the average BUN at 50 mg/dL versus 100 mg/dL, but the ultimate finding was a strong correlation between Kt/V and outcome.[298] Subsequent observational studies have repeatedly confirmed the higher risk of mortality when the fractional clearance during each dialysis, expressed as Kt/V, falls below 1.2.[299-301] Another controlled trial of dialysis dose and adequacy sponsored by the NIH in the late 1990s showed no further benefit from increasing the dialyzer single-pool Kt/V above 1.3 per treatment three times weekly[195] and showed that previously reported benefits from doses above 1.3 observed in uncontrolled studies were subject to bias from regression to the mean and from a newly recognized "dose targeting bias."[302-304] Failure to achieve the targeted dose is apparently a risk factor in itself, independent of the actual dose. Together, these findings led the medical community and the Medicare sponsor to issue guidelines for HD adequacy that have become standards of care in the United States and later in other countries.[66,67,305,306] The persistently high mortality rates in the dialysis population, although often unrelated to the dialysis itself, have spurred interest in dialysis adequacy and its methods of measurement over the years. This section reviews the rationale and methods for measuring dialysis adequacy, focusing on mathematical models of solute kinetics that have been effectively put into clinical practice in nearly all HD clinics.

In light of discussions about the scope of dialysis adequacy, it is important to distinguish the adequacy of the treatment itself (i.e., removal of accumulated solutes and water) from global kidney replacement therapy. The clinician must treat the whole patient, including giving such treatments as psychotherapy for depression, management of anemia, nutrition, blood cholesterol, and application of new methods for prophylaxis and treatment of cardiovascular risk factors. However, it is important to put proper emphasis on the primary reason for the patient's attendance at the dialysis clinic, the dialysis itself. Although it remains possible that some aspects of the dialysis (e.g., high-molecular-weight solute flux) may impact factors that otherwise seem independent of the dialysis itself (e.g., anemia or cardiovascular disease) and may therefore be considered part of dialysis adequacy, erythropoietin replacement or parathyroidectomy cannot cure uremia. Similarly, replacement of activated vitamin D, although certainly a vital part of kidney replacement therapy, is not dialysis. The focus of the following discussion is on solute and water removal; standards established for other aspects of kidney replacement are discussed in the section "Management of Patients on Maintenance Hemodialysis."

UREMIA: THE SYNDROME REVERSED BY DIALYSIS THERAPY

The clinical syndrome resulting from kidney failure is a toxic state caused by accumulation of solutes normally excreted by the kidney (see also Chapter 54). The relationship between the syndrome and kidney disease was not obvious in antiquity, and even after the relationship was known, loss of non-excretory functions of the kidney could be equally implicated as the cause, especially because urine volume and content, which reflect oral intake, differ little from normal as the disease progresses. When urea was discovered more than 200 years ago, investigators began to find elevated concentrations of urea and other organic solutes in the patients' serum that are normally found in urine. This development confirmed suspicions of an accumulation disease, but it was not until dialysis reversed the syndrome that this hypothesis could be considered proven. Similar to fulfilling Koch's postulates, clinicians can be confident that the immediate life-threatening aspect of uremia is a toxic state caused by small-molecule accumulation because it is rapidly reversed by HD, a process that does little else than to remove small solutes by diffusion across a semipermeable membrane.

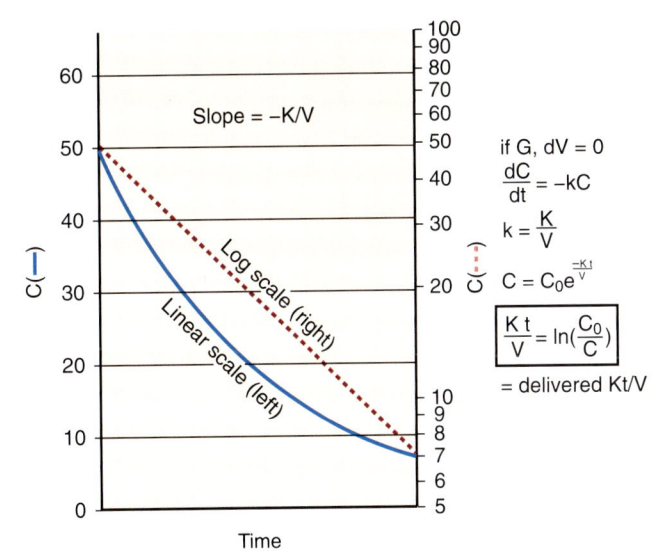

Figure 65.20 Intradialysis urea kinetics: origin of Kt/V. **Left,** The nonlinear decrease in blood urea nitrogen during dialysis (*solid line*) becomes a straight line when plotted on a log scale (*dashed line*). The fractional rate of decrease is a constant, $k = K/V$, where k is the elimination constant, K is the clearance, and V is the urea distribution volume. **Right,** The solution to the equation describing first-order kinetics shows that delivered Kt/V primarily depends on the predialysis and postdialysis blood urea nitrogen values (see text and legend for Figure 65.21 for definition of variables shown). This oversimplified equation is expanded in Figure 65.21 to include the other important variables.

$$\text{if } G, dV = 0$$
$$\frac{dC}{dt} = -kC$$
$$k = \frac{K}{V}$$
$$C = C_0 e^{\frac{-Kt}{V}}$$
$$\boxed{\frac{Kt}{V} = \ln\left(\frac{C_0}{C}\right)}$$
$$= \text{delivered } Kt/V$$

MEASURING HEMODIALYSIS ADEQUACY

As noted in the discussion of the general principles of hemodialysis, measuring dialyzable solute levels in the blood as a method for assessing the effectiveness or adequacy of dialysis treatments has been replaced by measuring the clearance of the marker solute urea. Clearance can be measured instantaneously across the dialyzer or as an integrated parameter over time. For native kidney function, the latter is achieved by collecting timed urine specimens. For intermittent HD, collection of dialysate is impractical, so advantage is taken of the perturbations in serum urea levels that allow estimation of the urea clearance simply through the sampling of blood before and after dialysis. The magnitude of the reduction in urea concentrations during each HD session can be translated to a urea clearance much like the decrease in drug levels after a loading dose can be used to measure the drug's clearance. Application of well-established pharmacokinetic principles to urea kinetics provides an estimate of the elimination constant for urea (K/V), which is essentially the slope of the decrease in concentration expressed on a logarithmic scale, as shown in Figure 65.20. K is the urea clearance and V is the volume of urea distribution, which is the patient's total body water volume. If one incorporates the treatment time element and ignores fluid removal and generation of urea during dialysis, the log ratio

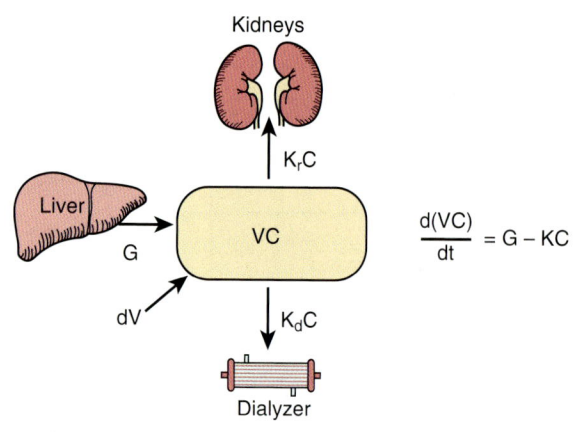

Figure 65.21 Single-pool model of urea mass balance in a hemodialysis (HD) recipient. When the patient is not receiving dialysis (most of the time for conventional HD), K_d is zero, and removal is determined solely by K_r. V is the urea distribution volume, equated to body water space, C is urea concentration, and dV is the rate of fluid gain (negative during dialysis, positive between dialyses). During HD, total clearance (K) is the sum of K_d and K_r. An explicit solution is available to the differential equation that describes the rate of urea accumulation or loss (dVC/dt) as the difference between generation (G) and removal (KC).

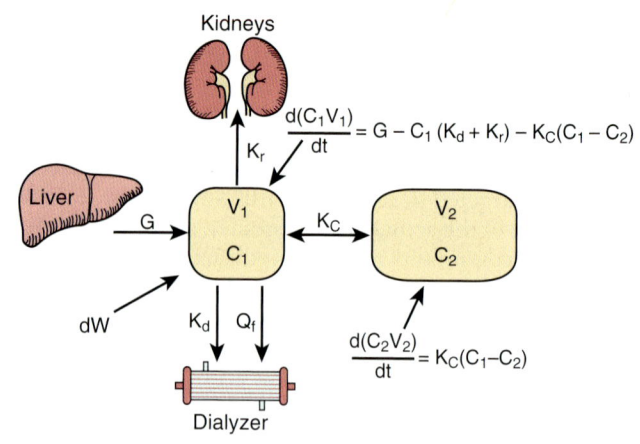

Figure 65.22 Double-pool model of urea mass balance in a hemodialysis recipient. Addition of a second compartment to the diffusion model of urea mass balance shown in Figure 65.21 accounts for the postdialysis rebound in urea concentration shown in Figure 65.17 and in general is considered a more accurate model. K_C is the coefficient of mass transfer between compartments, analogous to dialyzer K_0A. Solution of the differential equation requires numerical analysis and is not commonly applied in dialysis clinics.

of the predialysis to postdialysis BUN values can be simply translated to Kt/V, as shown in Figure 65.20.

Because substantial volumes of fluid are removed as part of therapeutic HD and a significant amount of urea is generated especially during longer treatments, a more formal model of urea mass balance, shown in Figure 65.21, is required to accurately measure Kt/V. In addition to the change in urea volume and urea generation, this model can be extended to include the interdialysis interval and the effects of residual kidney function (K_r). The latter, in contrast to the dialyzer clearance, is a continuous clearance that has little effect during dialysis but provides a marked benefit between treatments when the dialyzer clearance is zero. Solute sequestration or delayed transport of dialyzed solutes within the patient during dialysis, as discussed before, causes postdialysis rebound (see Figure 65.17) and can be incorporated in the model if a second compartment is included as shown in Figure 65.22. The single-compartment model shown in Figure 65.21, however, remains the standard for measuring dialysis in most dialysis clinics, primarily because of the complexities of the two-compartment model that requires numerical analysis to solve, but also because the errors in the single-compartment model caused by ignoring two-compartment effects tend to cancel one another.[143] The two models give similar results for Kt/V in the usual clinical range of Kt/V when dialysis is provided three times weekly.[143,307] A two-compartment model with formal numerical analysis has been made available on the Internet and may become useful for measuring nonstandard dialysis schedules such as daily or nocturnal dialysis or for more prolonged treatments given three times weekly.[308,309]

IMPORTANCE OF THE POSTDIALYSIS CONCENTRATION

Accurate measures of predialysis and postdialysis BUN are required to reliably measure the delivered dose of dialysis (see Figure 65.20). Predialysis sampling of blood is straightforward, but the postdialysis BUN is a moving target, and measurement errors are more significant when the BUN is low.[310,311] Although it decreases more slowly toward the end of dialysis, the BUN rebounds rapidly as soon as the blood pump is stopped. The early rapid phase of upward rebound is determined by both access recirculation and cardiopulmonary recirculation. Efforts should be made to sample after access-related rebound is complete but before cardiopulmonary rebound begins. KDOQI guidelines recommend slowing the blood pump to 100 mL/min for 10 seconds (to permit access rebound) and then stopping the pump before sampling.[68] Access recirculation dilutes the postdialysis BUN, causing a falsely high Kt/V, which can endanger the patient because of inadequate dialysis. Sampling after cardiopulmonary rebound has begun gives a falsely low Kt/V.

SOLUTE GENERATION

In addition to measuring the dose of dialysis, urea modeling allows measurement of two patient parameters that independently influence the patient's risk of mortality: urea generation (G) and the patient's volume of urea distribution (V). Accumulation of urea in the patient results from both amino acid catabolism, a measure of protein nutrition, and failure of renal excretion. Although these dual effects on urea concentrations complicate interpretation of any single measured level, mathematical modeling of urea mass balance allows both separation of the two and an estimate of urea distribution volume. Both higher urea generation rates and higher urea volumes have been associated with lower patient mortality.[312,313] For patients who undergo dialysis three times weekly, diurnal variations in urea generation have little effect, but for nocturnal dialysis, the reduction in urea generation at night can cause a significant error, an overestimation of Kt/V, and underestimation of V if G is modeled as a constant.[314]

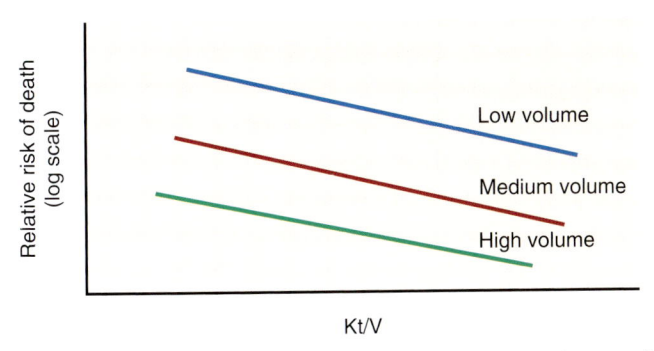

Figure 65.23 Risk of death as a function of dialysis dose and body size. The risk of death in patients undergoing hemodialysis decreases with increased dialysis dose (Kt/V) and may be further stratified by urea volume as a measure of body size. Larger patients in general have a lower death risk.

Toxic solute concentration levels are the net effect of solute generation and elimination. If one attributes uremic toxicity to the concentrations of accumulated solutes (concentration-dependent toxicity), then it might seem logical that the clearance (Kt/V) should sufficiently balance the generation rate to maintain a safe low concentration. However, during the NCDS, attempts to demonstrate this relationship by reducing the dose of dialysis in patients who ate poorly caused an unfortunate vicious circle of uremia-induced anorexia and malnutrition that eventually led to early discontinuation of the study.[315,316] Similarly, observational studies have consistently shown an improved survival in patients who eat more, even when Kt/V is held constant, and patients who generate more creatinine have a similar improved survival.[141,317] It appears that the relationship between diet and uremic toxin generation/elimination is complex and poorly understood. Control of solute concentrations by dialysis clearly improves outcomes, but control by limiting of dietary intake is often ill advised. Consuming a vegetarian or high-fiber diet may alter intestinal flora and reduce the generation of gut-derived toxins.[318-323]

UREA VOLUME

Urea modeling essentially provides a measure of the urea elimination constant, which can be considered the fractional rate of urea disappearance during HD (K/V). To calculate K, one must know V or vice versa. Because the prescribed K should be the same as the delivered K, and prescribed K can be determined from Equation 5, modeled V is easily determined. By convention, V is expressed after dialysis because it is less variable. Comparison of modeled V from dialysis to dialysis can be used as a quality assurance measure, and values should not differ by more than 15%.[143,324] Causes of a discrepancy include access recirculation, dialyzer malfunction (e.g., from clotting), blood pump variances, and blood sampling and measurement errors.[325,326]

Several studies have shown that various measures of body size, including V, correlate independently with patient mortality (Figure 65.23).[312,313,327,328] Survival rates in larger patients are higher than in smaller patients for reasons that are not entirely clear but may be related to nutrition and the caloric buffer afforded by muscle and fat. Because body size expressed as V is the size-normalizing factor for urea clearance in the Kt/V expression, larger patients require higher clearances and are therefore at higher risk for underdialysis. However, correction for the favorable influence of large size on mortality tends to mitigate this risk, as shown in Figure 65.24.[313] Figure 65.24 also shows that Kt/V is a more powerful predictor of mortality than body size and that correction of Kt/V for the independent (and opposing) risk associated with body size renders it an even more powerful predictor of mortality.

The HEMO Study uncovered a potential size-independent effect of gender on the response to higher doses of Kt/V. Although mortality was not affected by administering a higher dialysis dose for the 1846 randomized patients as a whole, when women were analyzed separately, a borderline significant improvement in mortality and secondary outcomes was seen at the higher dose.[329] The counterbalancing effect was a nonsignificant higher mortality in men, especially African American men. However, gender was difficult to separate from size because the two are so closely linked, especially with regard to V. If body surface area is considered the more appropriate denominator for dosing of dialysis,[330] women would clearly require more dialysis than men when the dose is measured as Kt/V,[331,332] as shown in Figure 65.25.[333] Similarly, malnourished patients who lose weight have an automatic increase in Kt/V unrelated to the effort of dialysis but simply because the denominator in the Kt/V expression decreases. This dose increase in patients at higher risk of death may explain the reverse J-shaped relationship between Kt/V and survival in observational studies.[334]

TREATMENT TIME

Attempts by patients to shorten their HD treatments reflect the discomfort they experience toward the end of the procedure. Muscle cramps, fatigue, and general malaise increase in intensity as more fluid and solute are removed. Paradoxically, shortening the treatment accentuates these symptoms because the rate of removal must increase if the patient is to remain in solute and water balance. Extending treatment time (Td) or increasing the dialysis frequency tends to alleviate these symptoms. Many hours have been spent by nephrologists and dialysis nurses in attempts, often unsuccessful, to persuade patients that extending Td would be beneficial. Sometimes a temporary trial of either an extended Td or increased frequency is sufficient to persuade the patient.

Although the NCDS showed only a borderline significant effect of Td, most population studies have shown that longer Td is associated with longer survival time.[335-338] Like the NCDS, the HEMO Study failed to show a significant benefit for longer Td but it, too, did not specifically target Td, and the range of treatment times within the study was limited.[195] No clinical trials specifically targeting long versus short conventional treatments has been done, but prospective observational studies and clinical experience favor more prolonged and slower treatments, including slower ultrafiltration rates.[304,337,339-341]

ALTERNATIVE MEASURES OF DIALYSIS

UREA REDUCTION RATIO

The U.S. Centers for Medicare and Medicaid Services requires that participating dialysis clinics report urea

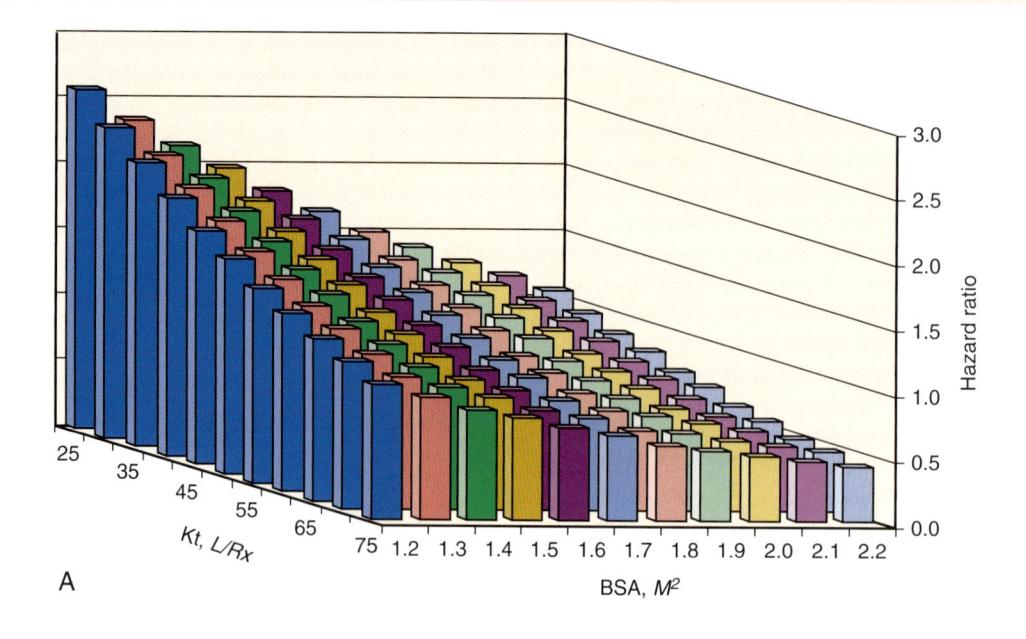

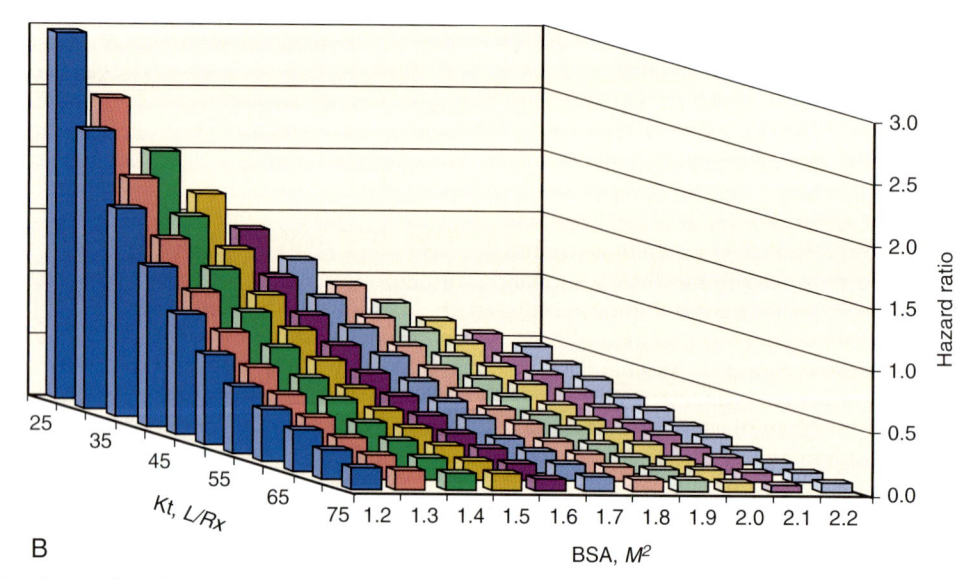

Figure 65.24 Risk of mortality related to body size as well as dialysis dose. These data were obtained from a large observational study of 43,334 patients. **A,** Hazard ratio analysis was adjusted for case mix. **B,** Hazard ratio analysis included an interaction term between Kt and body mass index and was adjusted for case mix. BSA, Body surface area; L/Rx, liters per treatment. (From Lowrie EG, Li Z, Ofsthun N, et al: Body size, dialysis dose and death risk relationships among hemodialysis patients. *Kidney Int* 62:1891-1897, 2002.)

reduction ratios (URRs), as defined here, monthly for each patient:

$$URR = (C_0 - C)/C_0 \qquad (10)$$

where C_0 is the predialysis BUN and C is the postdialysis BUN.

URR has the advantage of simplicity, but it is the least accurate measure of HD. For example, as the frequency of dialysis increases and presumably its efficiency improves, URR diminishes. It is not possible to add URR values to show a cumulative weekly effect, and as the frequency extends to continuous dialysis, URR extinguishes to zero. URR is also reduced by interdialysis fluid accumulation, urea generation, and residual renal function, and the additional clearance afforded by fluid removal during dialysis is not incorporated in URR. On the positive side, however, in addition to its simplicity, URR has a curvilinear relationship with Kt/V, as shown in Figure 65.26, paralleling the relationship between outcome and Kt/V. For example, if Kt/V doubles from 1.5 to 3.0 per dialysis three times a week, URR increases only from 0.75 to 0.85.

Although efforts have been made to convert Kt/V to a URR equivalent[342] or to use the solute removal index, a more reliable index of dialysis dose,[343] these approaches have not been popular. Other efforts to report the reciprocal of Kt/V as a concentration equivalent,[344] targeting low concentrations instead of high clearances, has not been applied, partly because Kt/V has become ingrained in the practice of dialysis quantification. Although mathematically inexact, because URR is the ratio of postdialysis to

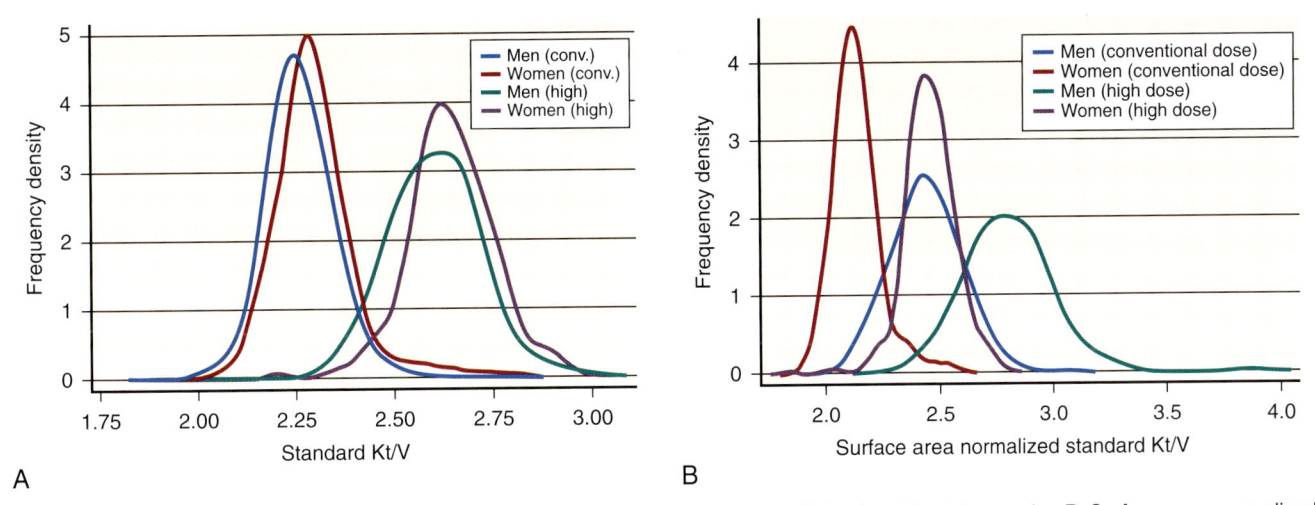

Figure 65.25 **A,** Standard Kt/V in the conventional and high-dose Hemodialysis (HEMO) Study subjects by gender. **B,** Surface area–normalized standard Kt/V in the conventional and high-dose HEMO Study subjects by gender. Conversion to surface area was based on an anthropometric estimate of V in each patient (see references 333 and 347). (From Daugirdas JT, Greene T, Chertow GM, Depner TA: Can rescaling dose of dialysis to body surface area in the HEMO study explain the different responses to dose in women versus men? *Clin J Am Soc Nephrol* 5:1628-1636, 2010.)

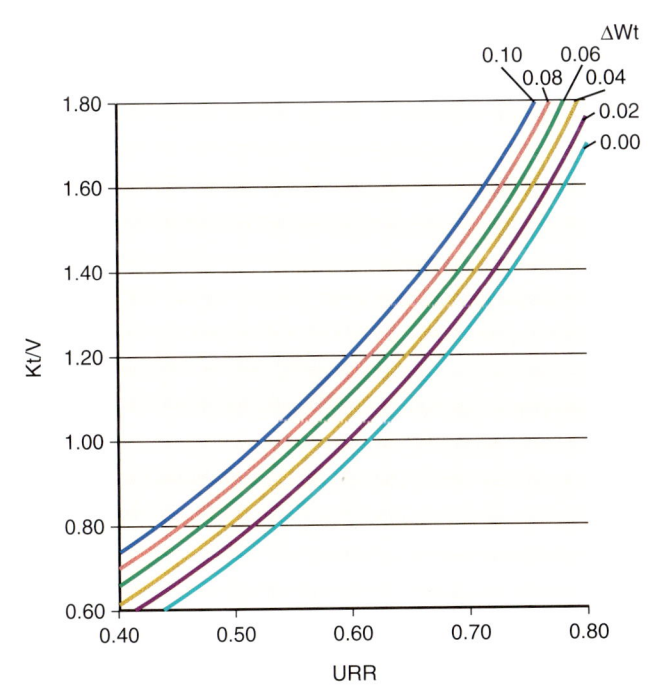

Figure 65.26 Curvilinear relationship between urea reduction ratio (URR) and Kt/V, stratified by degree of ultrafiltration during dialysis. Whereas the urea reduction ratio (see text) falls with increasing fluid removal during dialysis (ΔWt) from 0% to 10% of body weight, Kt/V increases. The latter more appropriately accounts for the increase in clearance caused by ultrafiltration. Curves are derived from formal urea modeling.

predialysis BUN values (URR = 1 – Cpost/Cpre), instead of predialysis to postdialysis values, it correlates better than Kt/V with small (toxic) solute concentrations, and its relationship with outcome is more linear.

Conductivity Clearance

The average clearance of small (dialyzable) solutes is easily derived from measurement of the predialysis and postdialysis BUN, as explained previously. The instantaneous clearance of small solutes is also easily measured from the dialyzer inlet and outlet BUN values, but it can also be derived from measurement of the change in electrical conductivity of dialysate before and after an abrupt change in the dialysate concentration (conductivity clearance).[345,346] Because the major electrically conducting ion in the dialysate is sodium, conductivity clearance is primarily a measure of sodium clearance, which is equivalent to urea clearance. This method requires multiple measurements during the dialysis to obtain the treatment average, as well as an adjustment for cardiopulmonary recirculation, but it has the advantage that no blood specimens are required and the result is available immediately. The clearance is expressed in milliliters per minute and must be adjusted to body size through the use of either an estimate of V for comparison with Kt/V or an estimate of surface area.[330,331,347,348] Surface area as a denominator is more consistent with measures of native kidney clearance and may reduce or eliminate the potential gender error already discussed.[328,332,333]

COMPARISON OF HEMODIALYSIS AND PERITONEAL DIALYSIS DOSES

The minimum recommended weekly dose of PD expressed as Kt/V is 1.7 (see Chapter 66 for discussion of PD adequacy). This dose compares with a cumulative 3.6 per week for HD (1.2/dialysis three times per week). Although the minimum HD dose is more than twice the minimum PD dose, outcomes are similar or better even when adjusted for the lower average comorbidity in PD recipients.[349-351] Furthermore, solute kinetic analyses have shown that the dialysis efficiency improves with increased frequency of treatments (Figure 65.27). These observations, together with acknowledgment of little or no benefit from more intense or more prolonged intermittent dialysis,[195] have led to the conclusion that intermittent treatments are less efficient than continuous treatments and have stimulated efforts to define a continuous equivalent clearance expression for HD.

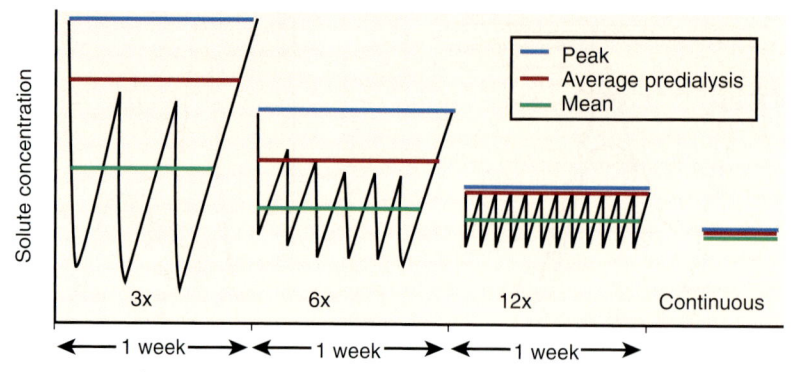

Figure 65.27 Effect of frequency on peak and average solute concentrations. Two-compartment formal kinetic modeling of a solute with low K_c predicts that both peak and mean concentrations decrease significantly as the frequency of treatments increases even though there is no change in the weekly dialyzer clearance × treatment time (Kt).

STANDARD CLEARANCE AND STANDARD K_T/V

These efforts have produced a continuous equivalent expression for urea clearance as G/TAC,[143,352] where TAC is the time-averaged urea concentration, and a more profound adjustment defined as "standard K" and "standard Kt/V."[343,353] The latter redefines *clearance* as the removal rate factored for the predialysis concentration, placing more emphasis on the predialysis BUN as a risk factor for uremia. Because the predialysis BUN is always higher than the mean BUN, standard Kt/V is always lower than the continuous urea clearance and is comparable to fractional clearances achieved with continuous PD. Despite its somewhat arbitrary definition, the matching of doses with PD has generated interest in standard Kt/V (stdKt/V) as an expression of dialysis dose that is independent of frequency. Increasing interest in clinical applications of HD given more frequently than three times per week has generated a need for quantification that accounts for the improved efficiency of more frequent treatments. For patients in a steady state of urea, mass balance in which generation equals removal and dialyzed according to any schedule of treatments, standard Kt/V is defined as follows:

$$\text{stdKt/V} = \frac{\text{Urea removal rate}}{\text{Peak concentration}} = \frac{G}{\text{Average predialysis BUN}} \quad (11)$$

G is the patient's urea generation rate, derived from formal urea modeling. KDOQI guidelines call for a minimum stdKt/V of 2.0 per week, significantly higher than the minimum PD dose but considered safe in the absence of controlled trials of dialysis frequency.[68] An explicit mathematical formula for calculating standard Kt/V based on spKt/V has greatly simplified the calculation,[354] and subsequent refinements allow inclusion of the effects of ultrafiltration during dialysis and the patient's residual native kidney clearance, as follows[355]:

$$\text{stdKt/V} = \frac{10{,}080 \dfrac{1 - e^{-eKt/V}}{t}}{\dfrac{1 - e^{-eKt/V}}{eKt/V} + \dfrac{10{,}080}{Nt} - 1} \quad (12)$$

where N is the number of dialysis treatments per week.

Because urea is relatively nontoxic, peak levels probably do not mediate uremic toxicity, so an alternative explanation for the inefficiency of infrequent HD was developed on the basis of sequestration of compartmentalized solutes other than urea. A two-compartment model that accounts for sequestration gives a pattern of average clearances that closely match standard Kt/V values,[356] as shown in Figure 65.28, providing further theoretical support for the clinical application of standard Kt/V in recipients of frequent dialysis.

NOCTURNAL HEMODIALYSIS

In an approach intended to provide HD treatments more frequently than three times per week while controlling the cost and patient burden, patients have been trained to dialyze themselves at home each night while sleeping (nocturnal HD).[357-361] This approach allows the patient freedom during the day to conduct normal life activities unfettered by dialysis and symptoms of disequilibrium. Several studies have shown improvements in blood pressure, nutrition, stamina, and quality of life, which are presumably responsible for patient acceptance of a procedure that places considerably more burden on the patient than standard in-center HD.[358,362,363] Later controlled studies have confirmed improvements in left ventricular mass, blood pressure, need for phosphate binders, and some aspects of quality of life with nocturnal HD.[362,364-366] However, recruitment of patients for home training was difficult, more vascular access interventions were required, and the nocturnal group of patients in the study experienced a more rapid decline in residual kidney function.[359,365-367]

SHORT DAILY HEMODIALYSIS

The incentive to shorten the treatment time (Td) is often patient-generated, as noted previously, but when shortened Td is combined with an increase in frequency, outcomes might be improved, as suggested in Figure 65.28. Controlled studies of short daily dialysis have shown improvements in cardiac hypertrophy, quality of life, and cardiac function.[362,364,365] All studies of short daily dialysis have shown decreases in interdialysis weight gain and predialysis blood pressure, but such changes are to be expected when the interdialysis treatment time is shortened to nearly half that of thrice-weekly dialysis. The NIH daily in-center HD study,

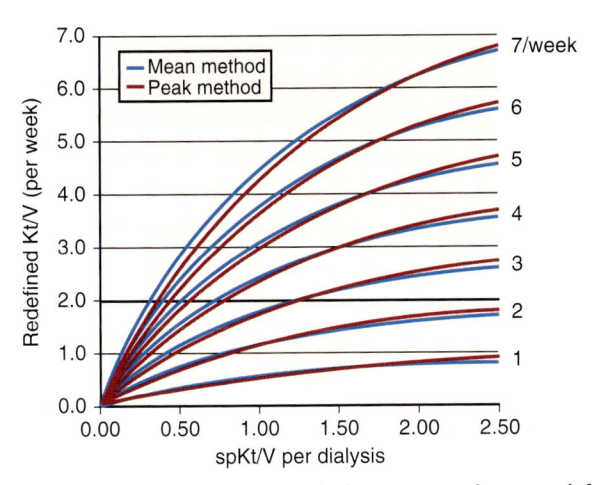

Figure 65.28 Effect of increased dose versus increased frequency on effective clearance. The effective clearance, expressed as "standard Kt/V" on the *vertical axis*, tends to plateau despite increases in dialyzer clearance, expressed as "single pool (sp) Kt/V" on the *horizontal axis*. Two different models of solute kinetics show similar diminishing returns as the delivered dose increases. A marked increase in effective clearance can be achieved only by increasing the frequency of treatments.

the largest randomized and controlled trial to date, showed improvements in left ventricular mass, self-reported physical health, predialysis phosphorus concentration, and predialysis systolic blood pressure in comparison with conventional thrice-weekly dialysis.[365] However, the study was unable to demonstrate improvements in mortality, hospitalization rates, predialysis albumin, or erythropoietin dose.

ACCOUNTING FOR NATIVE KIDNEY FUNCTION

Clearance of small solutes, the principal metric of dialyzer function, is augmented by clearance of the same solutes by the patient's remnant native kidney. Addition of the two urea clearances (K_d and K_r) seems reasonable except in intermittent dialysis recipients, in whom the two clearances do not occur simultaneously. Because, as noted previously, continuous clearances are more efficient than intermittent clearances, an adjustment is required before the two clearances can be added. This adjustment consists either of inflation of K_r or deflation of K_d. As noted previously, conversion to stdKt/V effectively deflates K_d to the equivalent of a continuous clearance, allowing simple addition. For example, if the patient's stdKt/V determined by Equation 12 is 2.2/week, the native kidney urea clearance is 4 mL/min, and the patient's urea volume is 35 L, the two can be added, as follows:

$$2.2/\text{week} \times 35{,}000\text{ mL}/(10{,}080\text{ min/week}) + 4\text{ mL/min} \\ = 11.6\text{ mL/min continuous urea clearance} \quad (13)$$

or

$$4\text{ mL/min} \times (10{,}080\text{ min/week})/35{,}000\text{ mL} \\ + 2.2/\text{week} = 3.4/\text{week stdKt/V} \quad (14)$$

If the dialyzer stdKt/V is determined by formal urea modeling, care must be taken to avoid inappropriate deflation of K_r when stdKt/V is calculated from the predialysis and postdialysis BUN values.[355]

Alternatively, K_r can be inflated to add to K_d as originally described by Gotch[368] and later outlined in the KDOQI guidelines.[68]

Residual kidney function confers a survival advantage far in excess of that associated with the dialyzer's urea clearance.[369] Despite near complete destruction by the patient's disease, the native kidney continues to eliminate by secretion solutes that are eliminated poorly if at all by dialysis, helps maintain salt and water balance, and may supply reduced synthetic functions.[370-372] Preservation of K_r is therefore an important goal of kidney replacement therapy.

THE DIALYSIS PRESCRIPTION

GOALS OF HEMODIALYSIS

The goal of HD is to replace the kidneys' excretory function. To accomplish this goal, blood and dialysate are circulated in opposite directions (countercurrent) on opposite sides of a semipermeable membrane in the dialyzer (see Figure 65.12A), allowing unwanted solutes such as potassium, urea, and phosphorus to diffuse from the blood into the dialysate and permitting addition of solutes such as bicarbonate and calcium from the dialysate into blood. The concentrations of the solutes added to the dialysate mirror those normally maintained in the body by the native kidneys (see Table 65.7). An additional goal is the elimination of excess extracellular water volume via ultrafiltration, accomplished by controlling the hydrostatic pressure gradient across the semipermeable membrane (see "Dialysate Circuit" section).

A secondary goal of HD is the replacement of hormones normally produced by the kidney. The failing kidneys produce lower levels of 1,25-dihydroxyvitamin D (calcitriol), an activated form of vitamin D produced by the renal proximal tubular cells, resulting in osteomalacia, secondary hyperparathyroidism, and renal osteodystrophy (see Chapters 55, 58 and 63 and later discussion). Erythropoietin, a hormone uniquely synthesized by the kidneys and responsible for activation of bone marrow erythroid precursors, is also deficient in kidney failure, leading to the anemia of kidney failure (see Chapter 57 and later). Replacing vitamin D with calcitriol, its analogs, or calcimimetic agents has allowed nephrologists to prevent or ameliorate CKD bone and mineral disorder and to suppress parathyroid hormone (PTH) levels without causing hypercalcemia. Administering erythropoietin synthesized with recombinant DNA technology and its analogs (or ESAs) has markedly diminished transfusion dependency for nearly all patients and improved health-related quality of life for most patients, at least in part by raising the average blood Hgb concentration, although later studies raise concern about increased morbidity and mortality with high doses (see later).

Nutritional counseling is also important, primarily to prevent malnutrition, a major yet potentially reversible risk for morbidity and mortality. Counseling on limiting fluid intake helps limit fluid gains between dialysis sessions, potentially reducing risks for hypertension and heart failure.

Table 65.8	Components of the Dialysis Prescription

Duration
Frequency
Vascular access
Dialyzer (membrane, configuration, surface area, sterilization method)
Blood flow rate
Dialysate flow rate
Ultrafiltration rate
Dialysate composition (see Table 65.7)
Anticoagulation
Dialysate temperature
Intradialytic medications

Dietary phosphate restriction is critical in controlling hyperphosphatemia and the attendant risks for renal osteodystrophy and vascular calcification because phosphate is sequestered intracellularly and is removed poorly by conventional HD. Limiting potassium ingestion reduces the life-threatening risk of hyperkalemia.

The rate of accumulation of solutes and fluid in each patient varies and depends on his or her nutritional and metabolic status and adherence with dietary restrictions. The response to calcitriol, its analogs, a calcimimetic agent, and ESAs also varies among patients. Thus, the HD prescription must be individualized to achieve these goals for each patient. The separate components of the HD prescription that may be manipulated on the basis of the clinical assessment are listed in Table 65.8.

DIALYSIS DURATION AND FREQUENCY

The clearance of any solute, such as urea, can be increased by extending the dialysis session length or increasing session frequency. After optimization of blood and dialysate flows and selection of a dialyzer with a large mass transfer coefficient, the dialysis session can be lengthened to augment solute clearance. However, because diffusive solute clearance depends on solute concentration on the blood side, the efficiency of solute removal declines over the course of the dialysis procedure, leading to "diminishing returns" for total solute removal as measured by urea concentrations, with dialysis treatments longer than 4 to 5 hours (see "Dialysis Adequacy" section). Conversely, shortening treatment times to less than 3 hours accentuates the effects of intermittence, exacerbates solute disequilibrium (see "Dialyzer Clearance versus Whole Body Clearance" section and Figure 65.18), reduces clearance of larger molecules such as $\beta_2 M$ for which removal is more time dependent, increases the ultrafiltration rate, and raises the potential for hypotension and myocardial stunning.[166,167,188,373-377] Providing dialysis more frequently lessens the impact of declining solute concentrations and improves clearance but involves greater expense and use of resources, higher chance of vascular access dysfunction, and, potentially, patient "burnout."[87,373,374]

Additional benefits of longer or more frequent hemodialysis sessions include optimal volume homeostasis and improved removal of high-molecular-weight, sequestered, or protein-bound solutes (see "Dialysis Adequacy" section).[373,374,377-383] Longer or more frequent dialysis allows the accumulated fluid to be removed over a longer time and may reduce intradialytic symptoms such as nausea, vomiting, cramping, and hypotension (see "Complications of Dialysis" section); decreases postdialysis fatigue; improves blood pressure control; and ameliorates myocardial stunning.[364-366,384] Sequestered solutes such as phosphate have more time to equilibrate among the various volume compartments, leading to improved total removal and lower serum concentrations. More frequent dialysis also may mitigate the higher cardiovascular morbidity and mortality rate observed at the end of the long interdialytic interval in patients receiving conventional thrice-weekly dialysis.[378,385-387]

The Frequent Hemodialysis Network (FHN) study, the largest randomized controlled study to compare thrice-weekly in-center HD with 6-day-a-week in-center HD, confirmed that more frequent dialysis improved blood pressure and phosphate control, decreased left ventricular mass and left ventricular end-diastolic volume, and reduced the composite end points of death with either increase in left ventricular mass or decline in self-reported physical health.[365,384] However, more frequent dialysis did not improve cognitive function, measures of depression, or serum albumin concentrations or reduce the need for, or dose of, ESAs. The FHN and Canadian studies comparing frequent nocturnal HD with thrice-weekly HD, hampered by the relatively small number of study subjects, demonstrated only a beneficial effect on blood pressure and phosphate control and possibly left ventricular mass.[364,366]

Because of the increased cost and greater use of resources with longer or more frequent HD sessions, the inability of randomized controlled trials to demonstrate improved survival and quality of life, and the adverse effect of more frequent HD on vascular accesses and residual kidney function,[87,367] the common practice in the United States is to prescribe dialysis three times a week for 3 to 4 hours each session.[373] Longer session length or more frequent dialysis is employed currently for large patients, patients with severe hypertension not responding to maximal antihypertensive treatment, and patients with volume overload and intradialytic hypotension preventing fluid removal. Extending session length to more than 3 hours and switching to alternate-day HD to eliminate the long interdialytic period may be the most cost-effective and least disruptive way to improve dialysis therapy for our patients, reaping benefit from a slight improvement in frequency and duration without incurring the potential costs of declining residual kidney function and vascular access dysfunction.[373,374]

DIALYZER CHOICE

In the choice of a dialyzer, the most important determinants are (1) its capacity for solute clearance, (2) its capacity for fluid removal, and (3) the potential of the dialyzer membrane to interact with components of the blood, or the degree of biocompatibility.[164] The ideal hemodialyzer membrane would have high clearance of low-molecular-weight and middle-molecular-weight uremic toxins, adequate ultrafiltration, high biocompatibility, and a low blood volume compartment to maximize the efficiency of and reduce the adverse metabolic and hemodynamic effects of the HD procedure.

In the evaluation of dialyzer solute clearance characteristics, urea is the solute most often used because of its relevance to kinetic models of dialysis adequacy (see earlier). In clinical practice, physicians rely on industry-derived determinations of in vitro dialyzer clearance of low-molecular-weight and middle-molecular-weight solutes. Gibbs-Donnan effects, membrane adsorption of solute, protein binding of solute, and solute aggregation are not taken into account in determining in vitro dialyzer clearances and will reduce in vivo clearances. The variable relationship between the diffusive and the convective clearances of a solute further complicates the determination of solute clearance of different dialyzers. Solutes larger than 300 daltons have lower diffusive clearance than smaller solutes such as urea and potassium and may rely primarily on convective clearance. For patients with large interdialytic weight gains requiring more ultrafiltration during each dialysis session, simple comparisons of the in vitro diffusive solute clearances may be misleading.

Another factor in the selection of a hemodialyzer is its ultrafiltration coefficient, which describes the capacity of a dialyzer to remove fluid and is expressed in units of mL/min/mm Hg. As with solute clearances, the manufacturer performs in vitro tests to determine the ultrafiltration coefficient of each dialyzer model. In vivo values may vary by as much as 10% to 20%.

As already discussed, dialyzer membranes vary in their capacity to activate the coagulation cascade and formed blood elements, with synthetic membranes, in general, being the most "inert" and hence the most biocompatible,[165,168-171] but even synthetic membranes vary in degree of biocompatibility.[388,389] In addition to the issues of biocompatibility and cytokine release, activated thrombin adsorbs on the dialyzer membrane, creating a nidus for platelet adhesion and further thrombin deposition.[390] The propensity of a dialyzer for thrombogenesis may be another important factor in selection of a dialyzer, especially when anticoagulation during dialysis is not feasible. It is unclear whether dialyzers bonded with heparin will reduce the incidence of thrombosis during heparin-free dialysis. A randomized crossover study suggested that such dialyzers are superior to both saline flushes and infusion in preventing intradialytic thrombosis,[391] but other studies found comparable thrombotic rates with use of saline flushes and a polysulfone membrane.[392,393]

An additional consideration in hemodialyzer selection is whether it will be reused for subsequent dialysis sessions, because the chemicals used in reprocessing dialyzers may damage some of the membranes.[163] Bleach, which is commonly used to strip protein off the membrane and to improve the appearance of the dialyzer, may increase the pore size of some synthetic membranes after repeated use, resulting in loss of plasma proteins during each dialysis session that rivals the loss seen in nephrotic patients. Heat disinfection may result in cracks in the headers of the dialyzers.

BLOOD AND DIALYSATE FLOW RATES

Configuring the dialysate flow *countercurrent* to blood flow maximizes the concentration gradient between the two throughout the length of the dialyzer (see Figure 65.12A and Table 65.5). When flows are in the same direction *(cocurrent)*, small solute clearance decreases by about 10%. Increasing the dialysate flow (Q_d) reduces the accumulation of waste products in the dialysate and provides a higher solute gradient between blood and dialysate for optimal diffusion. Higher Q_d also decreases *boundary layers* and *streaming effects* in the dialysate. Dialysate flowing along the membrane tends to adhere to it to create an unstirred layer, or *boundary layer*, reducing the rate of diffusion across the membrane.[169,394] Dialysate also tends to move along the path of least resistance or channel *(streaming effect)*, resulting in non-uniform flow and bypassing some of the membrane area. As dialysate flow increases or turbulence is produced at the membrane surface, the unstirred layer becomes thinner, channeling is minimized,[395] and K_0A increases,[396] although the in vivo effect is less than the in vitro effect.[397,398] These findings prompted an increase in Q_d from 500 to 800 mL/min when dialyzer blood flow rate (Q_b) was prescribed at 350 to 500 mL/min. Advances in hemodialyzer technology led to modification of hollow fiber shape and insertion of inert spacer yarns, reducing channeling and unstirred layers and further improving dialyzer performance.[161,399] With these newer dialyzers, raising Q_d above 600 mL/min has yielded minimal increases in urea, phosphate, and $\beta_2 M$ clearance[400,401] but may still have a significant impact on clearance of protein-bound solutes.[402,403]

Dialyzer blood flow (Q_b) is driven by a roller pump and usually ranges from 200 to 500 mL/min, depending on the type of vascular access. Blood flow influences the efficiency of solute removal (see Table 65.5). As Q_b rises, more solute is presented per minute to the membrane and solute removal increases. Urea removal increases steeply as Q_b rises to 300 mL/min, but the rate of increase is less steep as Q_b approaches 400 to 500 mL/min because of greater resistance to and turbulence of flow within the hollow fibers, resulting in nonlinear flow and reduced clearance. Unlike dialysate, the boundary layer and streaming effects are less prominent on the blood side of hollow fibers because of the geometric advantages of flow within hollow fibers, the scrubbing effects of RBCs, and less variance in Q_b. For larger molecules, sequestered solutes, and protein-bound solutes, removal is slower and more time dependent than flow dependent because of limited diffusion across the membrane and protein binding, as discussed previously.[372-374,381-383]

ANTICOAGULATION

Blood clotting during dialysis results in patient blood loss and reduces solute clearance through decreasing dialyzer surface area.[404] To prevent clotting, an anticoagulant is usually delivered into the blood circuit before the dialyzer via a peristaltic pump or syringe pump.

Heparin, the most commonly used anticoagulant, may be given as a bolus at the start of dialysis (1000-5000 U or 50 U/kg bolus) followed by a continuous infusion (1000-1500 units/hr) until 15 to 60 minutes before the end of dialysis or as intermittent boluses as needed during dialysis.[404-407] Disadvantages of the bolus method include longer nursing time and episodic over-anticoagulation and under-anticoagulation. In patients at risk of bleeding (Table 65.9), low-dose heparin (500-1000 U bolus followed by 500-750 U/hr),

Table 65.9	Guidelines for Anticoagulation in Hemodialysis Recipients at High Risk for Serious Bleeding
Anticoagulation for Hemodialysis	**Clinical Condition**
No anticoagulation or regional anticoagulation	Actively bleeding Significant risk for bleeding Major thrombostatic defect Major surgery within 7 days Intracranial surgery within 14 days Biopsy of visceral organ within 72 hours Pericarditis
Low-dose heparin	Major surgery beyond 7 days Biopsy of visceral organ beyond 72 hours Minor surgery 8 hours prior Minor surgery within 72 hours
Low-dose heparin or no anticoagulation	Major surgery 8 hours prior

regional anticoagulation, dialyzers coated with heparin, or no anticoagulation may be appropriate.[404,406,407]

In regional anticoagulation, the anticoagulant is infused into the blood circuit (arterial line) before the hemodialyzer, followed by infusion of a neutralizing agent into the venous line (after the dialyzer). Regional citrate anticoagulation, a common strategy in the acute dialysis setting, uses citrate as the anticoagulant and calcium as the neutralizing agent, with the dialysate being calcium free.[406-409] Citrate binds calcium in the blood, an important cofactor in the coagulation cascade, thereby inhibiting clotting in the dialyzer. Infusion of calcium after the dialyzer restores the ability of blood to clot. Regional anticoagulation also may be accomplished with heparin as the anticoagulant and protamine as the reversing agent.[410,411] Both methods are labor intensive and prone to error in inexperienced hands, requiring frequent monitoring of ionized calcium level with the citrate-calcium combination or of partial thromboplastin time, with the heparin-protamine combination. Citrate anticoagulation also may result in hypocalcemia and death if calcium replacement is inadequate and in metabolic alkalosis as citrate is metabolized.[407-409] However, in intermittent short-duration HD, metabolic alkalosis may not be an issue.[408] Rebound in anticoagulation may be seen after the completion of dialysis with regional heparinization because heparin has a longer half-life than protamine. Because of the close monitoring required and the risk of serious complications, regional anticoagulation is not commonly used in the outpatient dialysis setting, being employed more in the intensive care unit for continuous renal replacement therapy. However, if a simplified treatment protocol can be perfected,[412] regional citrate anticoagulation may become more feasible and desirable in the outpatient setting,[409,413] because citrate may reduce inflammation,[409,414] lower bleeding risk, and improve clearance because of less dialyzer clotting in comparison with heparin.[415,416] Currently, low-dose heparin and anticoagulation-free dialysis remain the more commonly used strategies in outpatients.

During anticoagulation-free dialysis, several strategies may help to prevent clotting: (1) rinsing the circuit before dialysis with heparinized saline, (2) using a less thrombogenic dialyzer, (3) flushing the circuit with 100 to 200 mL of 0.9% sodium chloride every 30 minutes during dialysis, (4) avoiding blood and platelet transfusions through the circuit, (5) maintaining a high blood flow rate to decrease sludging of blood in the hollow fibers, and (6) limiting ultrafiltration as feasible because hemoconcentration within the hollow fibers increases thrombotic risk. In a patient with a hypercoagulable state or the situation in which higher blood flow rates and limited ultrafiltration are not possible, these measures are unlikely to prevent clotting. Remaining options, then, are regional citrate anticoagulation and the use of heparin-coated dialyzers,[407,417] although the latter may be inferior to the former in reducing dialyzer clotting.[393,417]

Alternatives to anticoagulation with heparin and citrate include low-molecular-weight heparin (LMWH),[407,418-420] hirudin, prostacyclin, dermatan sulfate, and argatroban.[406,407,421-423] Of these, LMWH is becoming widely used in Europe,[407,420] but the complexity of use, expense, lack of sufficient experience, and equivalency to heparin have deterred the widespread use of the other anticoagulants. For the rare patient with confirmed heparin-induced thrombocytopenia, LMWH, lepirudin, bivalirudin, argatroban, and citrate anticoagulation are viable alternatives.[407,423,424] Finally, substituting citric acid for acetic acid in the dialysate may augment the effect of heparin use, improve clearance, and increase dialyzer reuse, presumably because of decreased clotting.[425-427]

DIALYSATE COMPOSITION

The composition of dialysate is crucial to attaining the desired blood purification and to achieving body fluid and electrolyte homeostasis.[243,428,429] To accomplish these end points, dialysate contains the solutes listed in Table 65.6 in concentrations comparable to those in plasma. Addition of electrolytes and glucose to the dialysate reduces or eliminates their concentration gradients and prevents excessive removal during dialysis. Potassium, calcium, and bicarbonate concentrations may be individualized, but most other solute concentrations in the dialysate are fairly standard (see Table 65.7). Because dialysate glucose concentration is comparable to plasma glucose concentration, osmotic forces do not drive fluid removal, unlike in PD. Reducing the dialysate concentration of potassium provides a gradient for its removal from blood, and providing bicarbonate or a bicarbonate precursor at higher concentrations enhances its accumulation in the patient and corrects the acidosis of kidney failure.

SODIUM

Because sodium is the major determinant of tonicity of extracellular fluids, dialysate sodium concentration influences cardiovascular stability during HD. Historically, the dialysate sodium concentration was kept lower than blood sodium concentration (130 to 135 mEq/L) to facilitate diffusive sodium loss during dialysis and to prevent interdialytic hypertension, exaggerated thirst, and excessive interdialytic weight gain.[241,243] However, with the advent of high-flux dialyzers and more efficient solute removal, headaches, nausea, vomiting, seizures, hypotension, and cramps became more common and were attributed to the hyponatric dialysate,[241,243,428,430] although they were more likely due to use of acetate as a source of base (see later). This development prompted the progressive increase in sodium concentration in dialysate first to that in plasma and subsequently to higher than that in plasma, with an improvement in symptoms.[241,243,428,431] The pendulum now has swung back, and high-sodium dialysate has resulted in thirst with polydipsia, increased weight gains, and hypertension, leading to a resurgent interest in reducing dialysate sodium concentrations and abandoning the use of sodium modeling or "ramping" (see earlier) in most patients.[243-247,428,432] A computer-controlled biofeedback system using conductivity to lower plasma sodium to 135 mEq/L or routine monitoring of predialysis serum sodium concentration to individualize dialysate sodium and reduce the dialysate-to-plasma sodium gradient may offer the added benefits of decreased extracellular water, improved blood pressure control, and lower interdialytic weight gains without sacrificing hemodynamic stability.[242,249,432] However, these methods add complexity and/or increase demand on staff time; a reasonable alternative may be to apply a constant dialysate sodium of 137 to 138 mEq/L to achieve the same ends, because many dialysis recipients tend to be hyponatremic.[252]

POTASSIUM

Unlike sodium, only 2% of the 3000 to 3500 mEq of potassium is distributed in the extracellular space. In patients with ESKD, potassium accumulates in the plasma in between dialysis treatments and can become life threatening. Use of a dialysate potassium concentration lower than that of plasma removes excess potassium during dialysis, mainly through diffusion down its concentration gradient.[218,243,428,433-435] However, potassium flux from the intracellular to the extracellular compartment is usually slower than the efflux of potassium into the dialysate, potentially creating significant intradialytic hypokalemia followed by a 30% rebound in the potassium concentration 3 to 4 hours after completion of dialysis.[433,436] Life-threatening levels of intradialytic hypokalemia typically occur during the first 2 hours of dialysis, when a high predialysis potassium level favors efficient removal and a precipitous decline in its concentration, leading to arrhythmias through QT prolongation and increase in ventricular late potentials.[243,428,433-435]

Minimizing the risk for intradialytic hypokalemia and postdialysis rebound is made even more complex by the highly variable efficiency of potassium removal among patients (≤70% variability) and between treatments for each patient (≤20%) despite an identical dialysis prescription.[437] The intracellular distribution of potassium leads to a variable volume of distribution such that the greater the total body potassium content, the lower the volume of distribution and the higher the fractional decline in potassium concentration during dialysis. During dialysis, amelioration of acidosis, stimulation of insulin release by dialysate glucose, release of catecholamines in response to hemodynamic events, and decline of plasma tonicity all favor the shift of potassium into cells, thus reducing the gradient for its removal.[243,428,433-435] The extent to which each of these factors is present varies considerably among patients.

Two large epidemiologic studies found an increased risk for sudden death when HD patients undergo dialysis against a low dialysate potassium concentration, variably defined as less than 2 mEq/L by Pun and colleagues using the DaVita database[438] and less than 3 mEq/L by Jadoul and associates with DOPPS data,[387] especially in patients with predialysis serum potassium levels less than 6 mEq/L and 5 mEq/L in the respective studies. To add to the complexity, Kovesdy and associates reported that predialysis hyperkalemia (≥5.6 mEq/L), alone and in concert with a higher dialysate potassium, is associated with higher mortality even after adjustments for comorbidities.[439] The optimal predialysis potassium level was 4.6 to 5.3 mEq/L in this study, and the effect of dialysate potassium on mortality for patients with predialysis potassium concentration lower than 5.6 mEq/L was not explored. Individualizing dialysate potassium concentration for the unique situation of each patient may be crucial in navigating between increased mortality from predialysis hyperkalemia and sudden death from hypokalemia in the 12 hours during and after each dialysis session.[433-435]

Prescribed dialysate potassium concentration, then, is guided by the serum concentration before dialysis and the preceding considerations.[433-435] Because of the higher incidence of sudden death during and after dialysis, presumably due to rapid decline in serum potassium levels, dialysate concentrations of 0 mEq/L should be abandoned. Most patients should undergo dialysis against a dialysate potassium of 2 to 3 mEq/L. Patients with increased total body potassium from diet, medications, hemolysis, tissue breakdown, catabolism, or gastrointestinal bleeding may require a lower dialysate potassium concentration. Because of the higher risk of arrhythmias and death, however, concentrations of 1 mEq/L are used only when a compelling reason exists and only after all efforts targeting dietary potassium restriction have been exhausted and medications that interfere with aldosterone production and gastrointestinal elimination of potassium (e.g., ACE inhibitor, angiotensin receptor blocker, aldosterone antagonist) have been discontinued. Use of oral sodium polystyrene sulfonate to control hyperkalemia remains controversial, although an analysis of DOPPS data suggests that it may be safe and effective, associated only with increased IDWG and higher serum bicarbonate and phosphorus levels.[440] In particular, patients taking digoxin must undergo dialysis against a dialysate potassium of at least 2 mEq/L because of the greater propensity for digoxin toxicity and death in the setting of predialysis potassium levels lower than 4.3 mEq/L[441] and intradialytic hypokalemia. Potassium modeling with gradual stepdown in dialysate potassium concentration, thus keeping the blood-to-dialysate potassium gradient constant, during each dialysis session may optimize potassium removal and minimize the risk of arrhythmias.[243,428,433-435,442] However, experience with and data in favor of this approach are scant and consist of small studies using the electrocardiogram (ECG) to monitor for conduction abnormalities or to determine the presence of dispersion of action potential (e.g., prolonged QT interval or QT dispersion) as a surrogate marker for sudden death. Also, the validity of these tools as surrogate markers for life-threatening arrhythmias have been called into question in the cardiology literature.[435,443,444] Large randomized studies are needed.

CALCIUM

Historically, patients with ESKD underwent dialysis against a higher calcium concentration (3 to 3.5 mEq/L) to help control hyperparathyroidism and to prevent calcium and subsequent bone mineral loss.[428,429,445] However, the increased use of calcium-containing phosphate binders and vitamin D analogs, the resulting hypercalcemia, and the subsequent recognition that these medications are associated with accelerated vascular calcification in dialysis recipients have prompted the KDOQI to recommend a dialysate calcium concentration of 2.5 to 2.6 mEq/L (1.25 to 1.3 mmol/L).[428,429] In contrast, international guidelines recommend a concentration of 2.5 to 3 mEq/L (1.25 to 1.5 mmol/L).[445,446] The differing opinions reflect the poor understanding of calcium mass balance in dialysis recipients.[445-448] Scant data suggest that 2.5 mEq/L is the "fulcrum" for dialysate calcium concentration, below which calcium is removed from the patient and above which calcium diffuses into the patient during dialysis, although there is wide variability among patients. In the few studies available, interdialytic calcium balance is not accounted for, and a calcium kinetic model suggests that interdialytic calcium mass balance is positive in most patients undergoing dialysis, especially when they are treated with calcium-containing phosphate binders and vitamin D analogs.[448] Thus, raising the dialysate calcium concentration as suggested by KDIGO guidelines may result in positive calcium balance and further acceleration of vascular calcification as well as adynamic bone disease.[447,448]

The dialysate calcium concentration may also affect hemodynamic stability during dialysis through lowering ionized calcium levels and thus impairing left ventricular contractility and peripheral vasoconstriction.[243,428,445,447,449] A large observational study reported that a dialysate calcium concentration less than 2.5 mEq/L or a larger serum-to-dialysate calcium gradient is associated with an increased risk of intradialytic hypotension as well as sudden death.[449] In patients who are prone to hypotension or at risk for sudden death, then, raising the dialysate calcium concentration to 3 to 3.5 mEq/L may ameliorate the hypotension, although this approach is largely opinion driven. Further validation of the calcium kinetic model may render it a useful tool for individualizing dialysate calcium and taking into account the myriad factors already described—the use of differing phosphate binders and vitamin D analogs, the type of renal osteodystrophy, the serum calcium concentration, the degree of vascular calcification, and the propensity for arrhythmias and intradialytic hypotension.[447,448] In the absence of such a tool, the goal should be to maintain neutral calcium mass balance,[447] and the most commonly employed dialysate calcium concentrations in the United States currently are 2.25 to 2.5 mEq/L (1.12 to 1.25 mmol/L).

MAGNESIUM

As with potassium, only 1% to 2% of magnesium is in the extracellular compartment.[428] Because two thirds is in bone, magnesium flux during HD is difficult to predict. Conventional dialysis with magnesium-free dialysate removes about 10 mmol of magnesium each session, an amount lower than the daily dietary intake of 10 to 15 mmol of magnesium on the average North American diet.[428] However, most dialysis clinics use a dialysate magnesium concentration of 0.5 to 1 mEq/L because magnesium-free dialysate is associated with severe muscle cramps and intradialytic hypotension.[428,429,450]

BICARBONATE

Correction of metabolic acidosis during dialysis is achieved through an increase in the dialysate concentration of a base equivalent to promote its diffusion into the blood. Historically, bicarbonate was introduced into the dialysate by bubbling carbon dioxide through it to lower pH and to prevent the precipitation of calcium and magnesium salts.[6,428] In the 1960s, acetate was introduced as a source of base and became the standard for two decades.[243,428] Acetate offered the advantages of a low incidence of bacterial contamination, a lack of precipitation with calcium and magnesium, and ease of storage. However, it became a hemodynamic stressor when high-efficiency and high-flux dialysis was introduced in the 1980s because the higher rate of acetate diffusion into blood exceeded the metabolic capacity of the liver and skeletal muscle.[243,428] Acetate accumulation led to acidosis, vasodilation, and hypotension. These complications prompted the resurgence of bicarbonate-based dialysate.

The major complications of bicarbonate dialysate are bacterial contamination and precipitation of calcium and magnesium salts. Gram-negative halophilic rods thrive in bicarbonate dialysate because they require sodium chloride or sodium bicarbonate to grow.[451,452] With regular disinfection of bicarbonate containers, these bacteria have a latency period of 3 to 5 days, an exponential growth phase at 5 to 8 days, and maximal growth rate at 10 days,[451] which compare favorably with a latency of 1 day, exponential growth at 2 to 3 days, and maximal growth by 4 days in a contaminated container. Therefore, disinfecting the containers and mixing the bicarbonate daily help prevent bacterial contamination. Use of commercially available dry powder cartridges offers an alternative solution to this problem.[451,452] Recognizing the risks of microbiologic contamination and taking steps to prevent bacterial contamination have greatly reduced the incidence of pyrogenic reactions reported with early high-flux dialysis. Although the risk for pyrogenic reactions is increased theoretically by backfiltration during high-flux dialysis, during which contaminants from the dialysate can diffuse into blood, few reports of this complication have appeared.[186,453]

To minimize formation of insoluble calcium and magnesium salts with bicarbonate, bicarbonate and the acid concentrate, which contains all solutes other than bicarbonate, are separated until use.[428] The acid concentrate derives its name from the small amount of acetic acid (typically 4 mEq/L in the final dilution) used to ensure the solubility of divalent cations. The dialysate delivery system draws up the two components separately and mixes them proportionately with purified water to form the final dialysate. This technologic advance allowed the widespread reintroduction of bicarbonate as a dialysate buffer in the 1970s. Because some precipitation of calcium and magnesium salts still occurs, the dialysate delivery system must be rinsed periodically with an acid solution to eliminate any buildup.

In many dialysis centers, the bicarbonate concentration is fixed at 35 or 39 mEq/L to accommodate the use of a central bicarbonate delivery system in which the bicarbonate concentrate is piped from a centrally located tank to the individual patient stations. The advantage of a centralized delivery system is fewer back injuries among the dialysis personnel, but a major disadvantage is the inability to individualize dialysate bicarbonate concentration. As already mentioned, dry powder cartridges placed in line at each patient station or individual bicarbonate containers at each station allow individualized dialysate bicarbonate prescriptions.[428]

Although correction of metabolic acidosis is desirable to reduce protein catabolism, bone demineralization, inflammation, and insulin resistance, overcorrection to generate metabolic alkalosis during dialysis could theoretically predispose patients to hemodynamic instability, reduced cerebral blood flow, paresthesias, muscle twitching, and cramping, possibly through alkalosis-induced lowering of serum potassium and ionized calcium concentrations as well as increased calcium phosphate deposition in tissues.[428,454,455] Several large observational studies reported that very low (<17 mEq/L) and very high (>27 mEq/L) predialysis serum bicarbonate concentrations were associated with increased rates of mortality and hospitalization, but after adjustment for case-mix and markers of inflammation and malnutrition, only the association between very low bicarbonate concentrations and adverse outcomes remained.[454,456-458] Patients with moderate acidosis (serum bicarbonate 20 to 23 mEq/L) appear to have the best survival, presumably because mild acidosis reflects better nutritional status.[455-459] Although lowering dialysate bicarbonate concentrations for patients with predialysis hyperbicarbonatemia is prudent, intervention should target malnutrition and inflammation.[455,459] Whether patients with very low serum bicarbonate concentrations benefit from raising dialysate bicarbonate concentrations is unclear, because analysis of the DOPPS database demonstrated that high dialysate bicarbonate concentration is associated with higher mortality and hospitalization rates, even in patients with very low predialysis serum bicarbonate concentrations.[454,460] The validity of this finding has been questioned, however, because the increased deaths were from infectious and not cardiovascular causes as would be expected if potassium and ionized calcium changes were responsible; and because inaccurate reporting of comorbidities, and variability of serum bicarbonate measurements, may have influenced the data analysis.[460] It may be that the increased mortality risk is related to a high dialysate-to-blood bicarbonate gradient and that abrupt changes in serum bicarbonate levels are detrimental, as speculated for potassium and sodium (discussed previously). Until a definitive answer is available, oral bicarbonate supplementation may be preferable to raising the dialysate bicarbonate to correct very low predialysis serum bicarbonate concentrations (<17 mEq/L).

GLUCOSE

Historically, dialysate glucose concentrations were high (>320 mg/dL) to provide osmotic pressure for fluid removal and to prevent hypoglycemia. However, high dialysate glucose concentrations can lead to hyperglycemia and can reduce potassium removal through stimulation of insulin production and consequent potassium shift to the intracellular space.[428] With technologic advances to allow alteration of hydrostatic pressure to enhance ultrafiltration, use of a glucose-free dialysate or a lower glucose dialysate concentration, 100 to 200 mg/dL, has become the current standard.[428,429] Most nondiabetic and non–insulin-dependent diabetic patients tolerate glucose-free dialysis well despite losing 25 to 30 g of glucose during each dialysis. However, this glucose loss may result in subclinical hypoglycemia and stimulate protein catabolism during dialysis, thereby increasing the intradialytic loss of free amino acids. Physiologic dialysate glucose concentrations (100 to 200 mg/dL) have few adverse effects but may aggravate hyperglycemia and induce insulin production, the latter in nondiabetic patients.[428,461]

DIALYSATE TEMPERATURE

Dialysate temperature is generally maintained between 35° and 37° C at the inlet of the dialyzer (see "Dialysate Circuit" section). If dialysate temperature is kept constant at 37° C or at the patient's core body temperature at the start of dialysis ("thermoneutral" dialysis, in which no heat energy is transferred through the dialysis circuit), the patient's core temperature rises during dialysis. The reason behind this rise is incompletely understood, but may in part be reduced heat loss from the skin through vasoconstriction in response to fluid removal and blood volume contraction.[256,257,259,462] With progressive heat accumulation, a reflex dilation of the peripheral blood vessels occurs, leading to a reduced peripheral vascular resistance and intradialytic hypotension. Arbitrary lowering of dialysate temperature to 35° to 36° C may keep patients "isothermic" (no intradialytic change in core temperature) and lead to improved hemodynamic stability in hypotension-prone patients,[256,257,259] although true isothermic dialysis requires use of a blood temperature monitor with computer-controlled modulation of dialysate temperature.[463] Computer-controlled isothermic dialysis has an effect similar to that of sodium modeling and high dialysate sodium concentration in maintaining hemodynamic stability without the undesirable side effects of positive sodium balance and may reduce the shivering and complaints of coldness seen with empiric lowering of the dialysate temperature.[215,219,259,462] It also allows for further cooling of core temperature by 0.5° C during dialysis, which may contribute to better maintenance of central blood volume and hemodynamic stability.[463]

ULTRAFILTRATION RATE AND DRY WEIGHT

Another main goal of HD is to maintain fluid balance, accomplished through establishing a dry weight and applying ultrafiltration during each dialysis to remove the interdialytic weight gain. Ultrafiltration is a process of convection, in which fluid moves across the dialyzer membrane because of positive pressure in the blood compartment of the dialyzer combined with "negative" subatmospheric pressure created within the dialysate compartment. These two separate pressures combine to create the TMP, which can approach 400 mm Hg. Adjusting the amount of negative pressure within the dialysate compartment controls the total level of TMP, and the higher the TMP, the higher the ultrafiltration rate.

Traditionally, *dry weight* is defined as the lowest body weight a patient can tolerate without becoming hypotensive, with clinical examination and evaluation used as a crude estimate.[464,465] A more rigorous definition is the body weight at which extracellular volume is physiologic,[464] because both volume depletion and volume overload are associated with significant morbidity and mortality.[464,466] However, a physiologically appropriate extracellular volume and body weight are difficult to assess clinically, especially because patients requiring HD vary widely in the response to fluid removal.

Most patients can tolerate up to 0.35 mL/min/kg of filtration (1.5 L/hr in a 70-kg person) without experiencing nausea, cramping, or hypotension.[376] Although healthy individuals can tolerate a loss of 20% of their circulating blood volume before becoming hypotensive, the tolerance of patients undergoing dialysis is highly variable, with some able to tolerate up to a 29% decline of their blood volume but others becoming symptomatic with as little as a 2% decline.[256] This wide patient variability results from the differing response to blood volume depletion and the disparate rate of vascular refilling from the interstitial and intracellular spaces.[256] Autonomic dysfunction, diastolic dysfunction, increased core temperature, intradialytic hypocalcemia, hypokalemia, alkalosis (see earlier), and myocardial stunning may all lead to impairment of both cardiac response and constriction of resistance and capacitance vessels during volume depletion.[256] Dialytic removal of solutes, malnutrition, and inflammation may retard vascular refilling through decreased osmotic pressure, reduced oncotic pressure, and increased vascular permeability.[256] Hence, a patient undergoing HD may become symptomatic before his or her physiologic weight is reached, and clinically determined "dry weight" is an unreliable measure of physiologic weight. The presence or absence of pedal edema and hypertension are unreliable tools to assess "dry weight" because they correlate poorly with volume status measured by multifrequency BIA.[467]

Newer technologies to help determine optimal dry weight and to improve tolerance of dialysis include continuous online blood volume determination during dialysis coupled with computer-controlled ultrafiltration rates (see "Online Monitoring" section), ultrafiltration modeling (see "Online Monitoring" section), and BIA.[464-468] Although continuous blood volume determination may reduce hypotensive episodes during dialysis, it is unable to accurately assess the extracellular volume compartment or to identify patients with impaired vascular refilling and therefore is less useful for determining an optimal dry weight.[465] BIA shows promise in establishing dry weight and in reducing intradialytic symptoms but is not widely used because of the underlying complex principles and the lack of a gold standard method of determining dry weight to allow its full validation.[466] In this evaluation, an electrical current is applied to the body and the resistance (opposition to flow of the current) and reactance (opposition to passage of the current) are measured. The resistance is used to estimate the volume of extracellular fluid, and the reactance is used to estimate the volume of intracellular compartments. Data from a euvolemic population (typically derived from a nonuremic population) is required to interpret the results.[466,469] Segmental multifrequency BIA of the calf may be the best method because it does not require normative values for interpretation, it continuously monitors changes in the calf extracellular volume during dialysis, and the calf more closely resembles a cylinder (an assumption made in the measurement) than the body. Dry weight is achieved when there is no further reduction in extracellular volume despite ultrafiltration.[464,466,468,469]

Current strategies to determine dry weight rely on clinical evaluation, with periodic empiric challenge of the patient's end-dialysis weight by 0.2 to 1 kg when evidence for weight loss is present. In hypotension-prone patients, the following actions may be beneficial: use of ultrafiltration modeling; avoiding intradialytic hypocalcemia, hypomagnesemia, and alkalosis; lowering dialysate temperature; increasing the duration or frequency of dialysis; and, possibly, separating ultrafiltration from diffusive clearance during dialysis.[256,467] Sequential ultrafiltration and diffusive clearance provide initial isolated ultrafiltration with isoosmotic removal of fluid followed by diffusive clearance with or without additional fluid removal. Maintaining constant plasma osmolarity during ultrafiltration prevents further depletion of the blood volume from fluid shifts into the interstitial and intracellular spaces, although sequential ultrafiltration was found to be inferior to sodium modeling and dialysate cooling in preventing intradialytic hypotension.[470]

Two randomized controlled studies involving 156 and 131 patients have demonstrated that multifrequency BIA is superior to clinical evaluation in determining physiologic dry weight, as evidenced by improvements in blood pressure control, left ventricular mass index and arterial stiffness, and lower mortality with use of the method.[471,472] Instances of intradialytic hypotension and access thrombosis were comparable in the BIA and clinical evaluation groups, but the percentage of patients with residual kidney function declined from 20% to 10% in the BIA group.[471] Although this method is promising, the potentially deleterious effects from loss of residual kidney function require further study.[473]

REUSE

Initially, hemodialyzers were reprocessed for repeated use (*reuse*) because of the potential benefits of improving biocompatibility. Subsequently, the higher cost of better-quality dialyzers continued to provide an impetus for this practice.[163,474] Automated devices that reprocess the dialyzers are safer and result in lower incidences of febrile reactions than manual reprocessing.[163] During the cleaning process, bleach or hydrogen peroxide is used to improve its aesthetics, but bleach also strips proteins off the dialyzer membrane and negates the improved biocompatibility afforded by the protein-coated membrane. After cleaning, dialyzer integrity is assessed by measurement of the volume of the fiber bundle in the blood compartment (fiber bundle volume) and pressurizing of the dialyzer to ensure the fibers are structurally intact (pressure test). For a dialyzer to be accepted for reuse, the fiber bundle volume must be greater than 80% of the initial value, and the dialyzer should hold greater than 80% of the maximal operating pressure.

After being deemed suitable for reuse, the dialyzer is packed with chemical disinfectants such as peracetic acid, formaldehyde, or glutaraldehyde. Over the past four decades, peracetic acid has gained popularity over formaldehyde in centers that practice reuse, increasing from being used in 5% of such centers in 1983 to 72% in

2002. Formaldehyde fell from use from 95% to 20% of such centers by 2002.[306] A small percentage of clinics use heat disinfection with or without citrate.

Close scrutiny of the safety of dialyzer reuse practices has yielded conflicting results in comparisons of reuse and non-reuse and evaluations of the various disinfectants, largely because the studies were nonrandomized and uncontrolled.[163,474,475] Overall, however, the data suggest that the various disinfectants are comparable when their use complies with AAMI standards and that facilities that reuse dialyzers have a risk-adjusted mortality rate similar to that of facilities not reusing dialyzers.[163,474,475] Concerns remain that long-term exposure to chemical disinfectants and the potential for infectious or pyrogenic reactions may be detrimental to the health of both patients and health care staff,[163,474] prompting a decline in the relatively stable prevalence of reuse, from 76% to 80% during 1997 to 2001 to 60% in 2002, with an even lower estimate of 40% by 2005.[474] This sharp decline in the prevalence of reuse is largely attributable to a change in practice patterns in some large dialysis chain providers favoring single use. A further impetus for the decline in reuse comes from the wide availability and lower cost of dialyzers constructed with synthetic membranes, rendering the medical and financial justification for dialyzer reuse to improve biocompatibility while controlling cost less compelling.[163,474] However, the amount of dialyzer-related polymer waste has been estimated at more than 10,000 tons per year if none of the U.S. dialysis facilities were to employ reuse compared with 500 tons per year if all facilities reused each dialyzer 20 times.[474] Research on best management of the medical waste associated with dialysis is needed, especially with the decline in reuse and the potential rise in more frequent dialysis.

MANAGEMENT OF PATIENTS ON MAINTENANCE HEMODIALYSIS

END-STAGE KIDNEY DISEASE

End-stage kidney disease (ESKD) is considered the level of kidney function at which a patient should initiate renal replacement therapy. If HD is the therapy of choice, the patient begins a therapy that, as described in detail in this chapter, removes numerous solutes and water. In some aspects, the process of HD can be viewed as the glomerular component of kidney function, during which water and smaller solutes cross a membrane, limited in part by its molecular size. Unfortunately, the analogy ends because the filtering surface in HD is only an artificial membrane with no biologic function (e.g., charge discrimination). Furthermore, dialysis lacks a tubular component to reclaim or further excrete specific solutes as well as the "metabolic" capacity of the kidneys to synthesize critical proteins. Therefore, HD is a complex therapy in which beneficial solutes such as amino acids cross the dialysis membrane and are "excreted" but larger substances that may be toxic are not removed at all. Some of the renally synthesized proteins can be replaced (e.g., erythropoietin), but others cannot or may not as yet be recognized. The long hunt for the "uremic toxin" continues, but the evidence is clear that there is not just a single agent.[372,476,477] Focus on p-cresol sulfate and indoxyl sulfate demonstrates the complexity of the problem because these solutes are of a size that could be cleared by HD but protein binding markedly reduces their clearance.[372,477] HD remains a lifesaving therapy but is far from full renal replacement. Thus, kidney transplantation should be considered as a superior therapeutic option in most patients with ESKD.

ANEMIA

The kidney is the major source of endogenous erythropoietin. (See Chapters 57 and 62 for a full discussion of anemia in advancing CKD and its management. In this chapter, we focus on the management of anemia in patients undergoing maintenance HD.) Before the advent of recombinant erythropoietin, severe anemia with Hgb below 7 g/dL was common in HD recipients, leading to frequent transfusions and iron overload in many. Now, with erythropoietin and optimal management of CKD, patients should begin HD therapy with Hgb concentrations in the targeted range.

PRINCIPLES OF ERYTHROPOIETIN USE

Before the advent of erythropoietin in 1989, initiation of HD only partially corrected anemia, presumably by improving erythrocyte survival and reducing erythropoietin resistance. Recombinant human erythropoietin was extremely effective in raising Hgb concentrations in the vast majority of patients,[478] but controversy remains regarding the optimal Hgb concentration (see later and Chapter 57). The positive clinical effects of higher Hgb concentrations are numerous: enhanced exercise capability, presumably in part from improved cardiac function with reduction in ventricular hypertrophy[479-484]; a better quality of life with improved physical performance, work capacity, and cognitive capacity[485-487]; improved sexual function[488]; and reduced rates of hepatitis and iron overload because of fewer transfusions.

The original preparation of human erythropoietin (epoetin) was produced by recombinant methods in Chinese hamster ovary cells. It differed from the endogenous protein in glycosylation, which may explain the development of neutralizing antierythropoietin antibodies and pure red cell aplasia (PRCA) in a small number of patients. Reports of PRCA first surfaced in 1998, peaked in 2002, and continue to appear periodically.[489,490] Its cause remains elusive despite extensive investigations. The most promising theory suggests that substituting polysorbate 80 for albumin during manufacturing destabilized the epoetin and, in conjunction with prolonged and improper storage and exposure to contaminants such as tungsten, lead to increased epoetin aggregation, resulting in antibody production with subcutaneous administration.[489,490] Unfortunately, these neutralizing antibodies react to epoetin (native erythropoietin) as well as to darbepoetin-α.[489,490] Affected patients are treated with withdrawal of erythropoietin and immunosuppression,[489,490] and they may tolerate rechallenge with novel ESAs such as epoetin-ζ and peginesatide, a synthetic, peptide-based erythropoietin receptor agonist.[489,491-493] Studies report that these new preparations of ESAs do not appear to induce or to cross react with neutralizing antibodies to erythropoietin,[491,492] although drug-specific antibodies to peginesatide did develop in 12 patients (≈1%) with some evidence for ESA resistance in 10 patients.[491]

The optimal route of administration of ESAs remains controversial. Original studies in patients on HD used the intravenous (IV) route solely. As their use broadened to include patients receiving PD as well as patients with advanced, non–dialysis-requiring CKD, subcutaneous administration gained interest, but this route may increase the risk for development of neutralizing erythropoietin antibodies.[489,490] Studies have demonstrated that ESA bioavailability with subcutaneous dosing may be reduced, but the overall pharmacodynamics are more favorable.[494]

HEMOGLOBIN TARGET

The therapeutic goal for Hgb concentrations in patients with ESKD has received substantial attention since the advent of ESAs. The initial Hgb goal was 10 to 11 g/dL, which increased to 11 to 12 g/dL by the mid-1990s. Observational studies suggested that higher Hgb targets were associated with improvements in a variety of physiologic and cognitive functions, prompting the nephrology community to consider normalizing Hgb levels to 14 g/dL. Although smaller studies demonstrated that normalization of Hgb resulted in an improved health-related quality of life with neutral effects on cardiovascular morbidity,[495,496] a large randomized trial of more than 1200 HD recipients with underlying cardiovascular disease was terminated because of safety concerns about a higher mortality rate in the higher hematocrit group (42% vs. 30%), as well as significantly higher rates of vascular access thrombosis.[497] Three large randomized controlled studies in the predialysis CKD population reported that in comparison with Hgb less than 11.5 g/dL, normalization of Hgb may improve health-related quality of life, but increases headaches, hypertension, and risk for cardiovascular events.[498-500] Careful reviews concluded that in patients on HD, no data supported an Hgb goal above 12 g/dL and that normalization of Hgb is associated with an increased risk of stroke, hypertension, and vascular access thrombosis, and probably with increased risk of death and serious cardiovascular events as well.[501-503] These conclusions led KDIGO to recommend 11.5 g/dL as the preferred Hgb goal.[503] Results of a large metaregression analysis of more than 12,000 patients suggest that higher doses of ESAs may increase mortality risk independent of the Hgb level.[504]

IRON THERAPY

The role of iron in the management of anemia for patients on maintenance HD has been a fascinating saga. Before ESAs, frequent transfusion requirements in severely anemic patients resulted in iron overload and hemosiderosis, requiring iron chelation with desferoxamine to prevent hemochromatosis and other complications. The complex protocols required to ensure intradialytic removal of the chelated iron and the greater risk of infection further complicated the delivery of dialysis.[505] However, the widespread use of ESAs has completely transformed the problem from a risk of iron overload to one of insufficient iron stores to respond to ESAs.

Patients undergoing HD who are receiving ESAs have substantial requirements for iron.[503] The challenge is to identify the markers that would indicate most accurately the need for iron replacement.[506] Serum iron and total iron-binding capacity, the accepted markers in otherwise healthy persons with iron deficiency, lack sensitivity and specificity in patients on dialysis. A multicenter trial demonstrated that in patients with anemia despite ESAs, serum ferritin levels higher than 700 ng/mL and transferrin saturation values of 25% or less, intravenous (IV) iron replacement raises Hgb levels.[507]

Post hoc analysis of the Normal Hematocrit Cardiac Trial and observational data suggested that administration of substantial doses of iron may lead to increased rates of hospitalization.[497,508] Theoretically, IV iron may raise the risk of cardiovascular disease and infection by exacerbating oxidative stress, enhancing bacterial growth, and impairing phagocytic cell function.[509-511] However, whether these effects translate into clinically relevant events is unknown.[512] Observational data suggest that IV doses of up to 400 mg per month are actually associated with better survival than no iron.[513] Even in anemia secondary to cancer and chemotherapy with no evidence for iron deficiency, iron administration improved response to ESAs without higher rates of adverse events.[514] However, none of these studies was randomized or controlled.

Resistance to ESAs may be due to inadequate iron stores, presence of inflammation, secondary hyperparathyroidism, inadequate dialysis, nutrient deficiencies, or underlying bone marrow diseases.[515,516] Inflammation states may interfere with erythropoiesis and response to ESAs beyond their impact on iron availability.[517] Serum albumin is strongly associated with the responsiveness to ESAs, likely because it serves as a marker of inflammation. Maneuvers that reduce inflammation, such as use of ultrapure water (see earlier), may improve response to ESAs.[516] Although more frequent dialysis was thought to improve ESA response in early trials, a later randomized trial did not confirm this finding.[518]

NUTRITION

The complex relationship between protein metabolism and body composition in kidney disease is discussed elsewhere. Nutritional status in patients undergoing dialysis are influenced by factors related to kidney failure and the HD treatment itself (Table 65.10). There is strong evidence that nutritional status affects overall morbidity and mortality in the dialysis population, highlighting the need to evaluate patients for malnutrition and devise strategies to improve their nutritional status. Growing evidence suggests the problem is not simply protein malnutrition but protein energy wasting (PEW), similar to the cachexia seen with

Table 65.10 Factors Causing Malnutrition*

Inadequate protein or calorie intake
Increased energy expenditure
Metabolic acidosis
Hormonal alterations
Comorbidities or hospitalizations
Dialytic nutrient losses
Dialysis-induced catabolism
Infection

*For a comprehensive discussion on the factors causing malnutrition, see Chapter 61.

inflammation.[519-521] Hence, simply adding protein supplements will not reverse the wasting.

MARKERS OF NUTRITIONAL STATUS

No single assessment of nutritional status seems to be optimal. Serum albumin concentration is a strong predictor of mortality in observational studies, but it is influenced by both protein intake and acute illness and inflammation, in opposite directions.[522-524] Because of its shorter half-life, serum prealbumin, an important transport protein, has been suggested as another potential marker of overall nutritional status. However, the kidneys are the primary source of clearance for prealbumin, rendering interpretation of its level difficult in the setting of CKD.[520] Prealbumin may be an even stronger predictor of overall mortality than albumin.[520]

Another potential marker for PEW in patients on maintenance HD is insulin-like growth factor-1 (IGF-1). IGF-1 is produced primarily in the liver and found in the circulation. Its levels are lower in settings of protein malnutrition and, in patients on maintenance HD, decline along with other markers of malnutrition.[525,526] In 207 incident HD patients in one study, low serum IGF-1 concentrations at initiation and 1 year were a marker of body composition and were associated with mortality.[527] Ghrelin, a hunger-stimulating peptide produced in the gut, is also associated with PEW[528] and increased appetite when administered daily to 12 malnourished dialysis recipients.[529] BUN and serum creatinine are also affected by the level of dietary protein intake and overall nutrition but, as individual measures, are insufficient reflections of nutritional status. On the other hand, using urea concentrations to calculate the protein catabolic rate (PCR) (also known as protein nitrogen appearance, or PNA) yields a useful marker of dietary protein intake.[530,531]

Anthropometric techniques may be useful in assessing nutritional status. These measurements appear deceptively easy to perform but must be taken carefully and may be inaccurate in patients on HD owing to varying tissue hydration and because standardization was undertaken in healthy volunteers.[532,533] Therefore, changes over time may be more reliable than isolated values. Additional methodologies to measure or estimate body composition, such as dual-energy x-ray absorptiometry (DEXA) and BIA are available.[534-536] However, DEXA does not differentiate intracellular from extracellular water, and extracellular fluid is "counted" as part of the lean (nonfat) body mass, potentially overestimating lean body mass in edematous patients. In addition, DEXA is relatively expensive and usually requires traveling to larger centers with access to the technology.

Although BIA has been available for years, it remains mainly a research tool. As the technology has progressed from single-frequency to dual-frequency and now multifrequency, its accuracy in estimating total body water and lean body mass has improved, but equipment cost and complexity have increased as well, making multifrequency BIA less practical.[535] Results obtained with BIA correlate with DEXA results[536] but, as with other body composition technologies, are most reliable when completed after dialysis.[537] The increased use of BIA in clinical trials may eventually inform its optimal use in the clinical setting.[472,538] Protocols using multifrequency BIA to estimate changes in extracellular fluid in the calf during HD may become a tool for establishing an optimal dry weight (see also "Ultrafiltration and Dry Weight" section).[468,469]

MANAGEMENT OF PROTEIN ENERGY WASTING

The management of HD recipients in whom PEW develops is unclear because the many markers previously described are also influenced by inflammation. In addition, cytokine release during inflammation can lead to muscle wasting, anorexia, and cachexia, which are difficult if not impossible to distinguish from poor nutritional status with our current tools. Nevertheless, if PEW is present, it should respond to increased nutritional support. Use of the enteral route to provide nutrition in patients with adequate gastrointestinal function can improve serum albumin or prealbumin levels and measures of overall function such as the subjective global assessment,[521,539,540] even in those with inflammation[541] and when oral supplements are provided only during dialysis.[542,543] When oral enteral supplementation is unsuccessful, tube feeding has been attempted in some cases, especially in younger patients for whom nutrition is so critical for growth and development.[543,544] Parenteral nutrition has been considered in patients on HD when enteral feeding is not possible, mainly during each dialysis session to ameliorate the obvious challenge of large fluid volume requirements. Providing intradialytic parenteral nutrition to patients with hypoalbuminemia increased serum albumin in some study subjects.[543,545] Whether any of these approaches has a salutary effect in the long term has yet to be answered with a large randomized study, especially when PEW is intertwined with inflammation.[521,539,543,546]

Pharmacologic intervention to reverse the anorexia so often seen in patients on maintenance HD has received increased attention.[543] Agents such as megestrol acetate, used in other settings of chronic disease, led to weight gain and an improved ability to exercise in a small pilot study.[547] Providing specific replacement of deficient branched-chain amino acids or ghrelin may also improve appetite and nutritional status.[529,548,549] Unfortunately, no large clinical trials to guide optimal treatment of PEW in patients on HD have been conducted.[543,549]

VITAMINS AND TRACE ELEMENTS

Vitamin supplementation for patients on maintenance HD is a complex issue. Vitamin D is covered in detail in Chapters 55 and 63, along with the complex interactions among the kidney, bone, and calcium and phosphorus metabolism. Retrospective studies suggest that vitamin D deficiency may be associated with cardiovascular mortality and is a growing problem in the general population as well as in patients on HD,[550,551] but it is not clear whether vitamin D supplementation or repletion will reduce cardiovascular mortality.

Because most trace elements are excreted by the kidneys, their levels rise as kidney function declines and may contribute to uremic toxicity. Exceptions are selenium and zinc, which have the most consistently low levels.[450,552,553] Selenium is an important cofactor in certain antioxidant enzymes, and its deficiency is associated with cardiovascular disease in patients without kidney disease. Zinc deficiency is associated with immune deficiency, anorexia, dysgeusia, and impotence. No clear data exist that zinc supplements are beneficial in dialysis recipients,[554,555] but they may improve appetite and nutritional status.[556] Selenium supplementation is controversial because it has a narrow therapeutic index and may result in selenosis with nausea, vomiting, peripheral neuropathy, and loss of hair or nails.[450,552] Water-soluble vitamins are recommended for patients undergoing HD because dietary intake of these vitamins is low as a result of dietary potassium restriction and because the dialysis process itself removes these vitamins, especially folic acid.[557] The antioxidant effects of vitamins C and E have generated interest regarding their ability to reduce oxidative injury (see later).

CARDIOVASCULAR DISEASE

TRADITIONAL CARDIOVASCULAR RISK FACTORS

Cardiovascular disease is the number one cause of mortality in patients undergoing dialysis, accounting for roughly half of the deaths. The complex relations among CKD and vascular and cardiac complications are described in detail in Chapter 56. The high prevalence of traditional cardiac risk factors (e.g., diabetes, hypertension, lipid abnormalities) in patients with CKD and their interactions with nontraditional cardiac risk factors, such as inflammation, oxidative stress, retained metabolites to include advanced glycation end products, and PEW, combine to lead ultimately to severe cardiomyopathy, ischemic heart disease, and death.[558,559] In the general population, intervention to ameliorate cardiac risk factors such as hyperlipidemia, inflammation, diabetes, hypertension, smoking, sedentary lifestyle, and obesity reduces cardiovascular morbidity and mortality. However, in the HD population, the classic risk factors do not have the same predictive value and seem to lead to paradoxical findings: Obesity is "protective" and high levels of low-density lipoproteins (LDLs) do not predict mortality.[558,560-562]

Of the multiple lipid abnormalities in patients on maintenance HD, low levels of high-density lipoprotein (HDL) and elevated levels of lipoprotein (a) [Lp(a)] are key predictors of cardiovascular disease.[560,563] A complex relation exists between the level of Lp(a) and the size of the constituent glycoprotein, apolipoprotein (a) [Apo(a)], which is determined by genetic polymorphisms. The larger the Apo(a), the lower the level of Lp(a), and both low Apo(a) and high Lp(a) levels predict mortality in HD recipients, with Apo(a) isoform exerting a stronger estimated effect.[560,563-565] An in vivo turnover study suggests that ions of Lp(a) in the HD population are caused by decreased clearance rather than overproduction.[566]

Left ventricular hypertrophy (LVH) is a risk factor for cardiovascular events in the general population.[567] It is prevalent in the majority of patients on HD and may represent a major risk factor for cardiac events not specifically related to traditional atherosclerosis.[568,569] Multiple factors have been invoked for the high prevalence of LVH in the HD population, including anemia, hypoalbuminemia, volume expansion, and systolic hypertension.[570] AV access with prolonged and severe high output may also contribute to the frequency of left ventricular disease,[571,572] although this issue is debated.[573] Cardiac magnetic resonance imaging (CMRI) may be better for measuring left ventricular mass than traditional echocardiography in patients undergoing HD, because it abrogates confounding of findings by volume overload[574,575]; and LVH demonstrated by CMRI was associated with systolic blood pressure, predialysis pulse pressure, and calcium × phosphorus product.[575]

NONTRADITIONAL CARDIOVASCULAR RISK FACTORS

Inflammation has gained growing appreciation as an important factor in cardiovascular disease in both the CKD and general populations.[558,576,577] Plasma levels of C-reactive protein (a marker of inflammation) and interleukin-6 (a proinflammatory cytokine) are strong predictors of cardiovascular and all-cause mortality in the ESKD population.[578-580] Numerous factors predispose patients on HD to the burden of endogenous inflammation compared with the general population: Kidney failure, the dialysis process, genetic predisposition, chronic periodontitis, type of vascular access, and other as yet unidentified factors all act in concert to contribute to oxidative stress, endothelial dysfunction, carbonyl stress, and accumulation of advanced glycation end products.[86,558,578,581] The critical role that inflammation plays in cardiovascular disease led to the hope that statins, which lower lipid levels and reduce vascular inflammation,[582] would ameliorate cardiovascular risk in dialysis recipients, but several large randomized controlled studies have yielded disappointing results (see "Diagnosis and Treatment" section).[583,584]

Homocysteine concentrations are elevated in patients undergoing HD and correlate with cardiovascular risk,[585-587] presumably through induction of endothelial dysfunction and a prothrombotic state. Because homocysteine is largely protein bound, poor nutritional status may confound the relationship, leading to the findings that HD recipients with cardiovascular disease paradoxically had lower homocysteine concentrations than those without.[587] An alternative explanation for this paradox may be that malnutrition and inflammation are more important cardiovascular risk factors than hyperhomocysteinemia. Although small studies in the HD population have suggested a potential benefit from folic acid and methylcobalamin administration to lower homocysteine levels and cardiovascular risk,[586,588] the bulk of data in both the general population[589,590] and patients on HD[591,592] suggests that lowering homocysteine levels with folic acid and B vitamins does not reduce the risk of cardiovascular events. However, the power of individual studies to detect a benefit may have been reduced by the widespread pre-study folic acid fortification in dialysis recipients, because a meta-analysis of seven trials involving around 3800 patients suggested a benefit to folic acid supplementation and lowering of homocysteine levels.[593] Regardless, prescribing folic acid to HD recipients to prevent nutritional deficiency and to facilitate hematopoiesis is still advocated.

Oxidative stress from kidney failure or the dialysis process itself may contribute to the high risk of cardiovascular disease.[594,595] Biomarkers of oxidative stress (thiobarbituric acid–reactive substances, protein carbonyl content, and the ratio of nitrite to nitrate levels) in patients on HD are difficult to quantify accurately but seem to correlate with carotid intimal media thickness (CIMT), a surrogate marker for cardiovascular disease.[596] Increased oxidation of LDL results and promotes the production of foam cells, an early event in the atherosclerotic process. Strategies to reduce oxidative stress include oral administration of antioxidants such as D-tocopherol and N-acetylcysteine, which reduced the rate of cardiac events but not all-cause mortality in small controlled trials.[594,597-599] Impregnating the dialysis membrane with vitamin E to reduce intradialytic oxidative stress lowered biomarkers of oxidative stress and improved CIMT in a small number of patients,[175,600,601] but did not improve response to ESAs in a large randomized study.[602] Use of ultrapure dialysate or a process of "electrolyte reduction" to treat the water reduced markers of inflammation and oxidative stress.[291,603,604] Advances in treating oxidative stress are hampered by the difficulty in quantifying oxidative stress and the lack of large randomized controlled trials.

Novel biomarkers such as the proteins paraoxonase (PON1) and fibroblast growth factor 23 (FGF-23) also are associated with cardiovascular disease. HDL-associated PON1 protects LDLs against oxidation. Reduced PON1 activity, determined by genetic factors in concert with several environmental factors to include smoking, correlates inversely with markers of inflammation and cardiovascular mortality in patients undergoing HD.[605,606] Elevations of FGF-23 in CKD may directly influence LVH and cardiovascular risk, independent of the factor's relationship to phosphorus.[607]

Sleep apnea appears to be four times more common in patients undergoing HD than in the general population, affecting up to 70% of HD recipients.[608,609] Small studies in the CKD population suggest that sleep apnea alters muscular composition, reduces physical functional capacity,[610] impairs cognitive function,[611] and may increase oxidative stress and the risk for cardiovascular disease.[612,613] Because patients on HD tend to have more sleep disturbances despite fewer stereotypical symptoms (snoring, witnessed apnea during sleep, unrefreshing sleep, and morning headaches) and a lower body mass index,[31,614] a high index of suspicion for this condition is crucial.

DIAGNOSIS AND TREATMENT

Unique factors in the HD population complicate the diagnosis and treatment of cardiovascular disease. A classic example is the reduced rate of symptoms, especially in patients with diabetes, despite substantial angiographic evidence of coronary disease.[615,616] Conflicting data exist regarding the utility of the various screening tests for coronary artery disease in HD recipients.[616-618] In general, tests that require the patient to exercise or that rely on electrocardiographic (ECG) findings for diagnosis are less reliable because of reduced exercise tolerance and abnormal resting ECG findings in HD recipients. Various pharmacologic stress imaging tests, such as dobutamine stress echocardiography and dipyridamole exercise thallium imaging, have better sensitivity and specificity.

Elevated plasma values of several different measures of troponin can be found even in asymptomatic patients on HD and are associated variably with cardiovascular risk,[619] LVH and subsequent mortality,[620] and increased risk for an acute coronary event in the subsequent 3 years.[621] Studies suggest that cardiac troponin T (TnT) may be the most accurate prognostic indicator of future cardiovascular events in patients on HD,[622] but TnT and to a lesser extent troponin I levels poorly predict obstructive coronary artery disease and acute coronary syndrome.[623,624] The seeming discrepancy in the predictive value of TnT for future cardiovascular events but not coronary artery disease may be explained by the observation that arrhythmias, not atherosclerotic disease per se, account for the largest proportion of cardiovascular deaths in dialysis recipients.[625-627] A myriad of factors contribute to the risk for sudden death, including ischemic cardiomyopathy, peridialytic electrolyte shifts, LVH and diabetes with subendocardial ischemia, divalent cation abnormalities, hyperkalemia, volume overload, increased sympathetic activity, inflammation, and dialysis-induced myocardial stunning.[235,377,628,629] Elevated TnT value, then, may serve as an indicator of non–atherosclerosis-mediated myocardial injury. In fact, elevated TnT values during and after dialysis correlate with echocardiographic evidence of regional wall motion abnormalities that develop during dialysis[235,629] and seem to be markers of dialysis-induced myocardial ischemia and stunning. The value of measuring any of the cardiac troponins routinely in patients on hemodialysis remains unclear.

Unlike clinical trials in the prevention of cardiovascular disease in the general population, trials in patients on dialysis are limited in size and number. Of the trials that do explore therapeutic interventions in the HD population, many have surrogate end points that may not truly reflect an effect on mortality. Randomized controlled trials that have been undertaken have often had disappointing conclusions. For example, despite the promise of statins to potently reduce LDL cholesterol concentrations and perhaps inflammation in the HD population, two large randomized placebo-controlled trials of statin use in patients on maintenance HD reported no improvement in rates of cardiovascular deaths and nonfatal cardiovascular events despite a 42% to 43% reduction in LDL cholesterol concentrations.[583,630,631] Subsequent reviews of these trials highlighted the presence of underlying cardiomyopathy in patients on HD, the increased incidence of sudden death, and the altered lipid profile with higher levels of Lp(a) and modified LDL particles—all of which may, in part, explain the lack of benefit from statins in this population.[632,633]

As mentioned previously, sudden cardiac death appears to be the leading cause of death among patients receiving hemodialysis.[625-627] A myriad of factors may increase the risk for arrhythmias and sudden death in patients on dialysis (see earlier),[235,377,628,629,634] with the presence of LVH being one of the most prominent[635] and coronary artery disease playing a minor role. Reducing the rate of LVH remains a major therapeutic focus (see later), but without clear evidence that doing so would improve survival. The dialysis prescription itself poses additional risks for sudden death (see also "Dialysis Duration and Frequency" and "Dialysate Composition" sections), including short treatment time, large ultrafiltration volume, and low dialysate potassium, which are potentially modifiable practices that may improve outcomes.[387] The timing of sudden death appears to cluster around the long interdialytic interval in patients undergoing dialysis three times per week or less (either Monday or Tuesday),[385,387] a pattern not seen with more frequent therapy or peritoneal dialysis.[636] The high incidence of sudden death has focused attention on the role of implantable defibrillators to improve survival in the dialysis population, but indications for implantation may differ from those in the general public, risks may be higher, and benefit is uncertain.[627,637,638]

In the general population, LVH is a cardiovascular risk factor that may be modified by treatment to reduce ventricular mass, such as with an ACE inhibitor.[639,640] For the HD population, an extensive review found very limited evidence to support the use of pharmacologic treatment for cardioprotection.[641] The only reported controlled trial for ACE inhibitors in patients on HD demonstrated improved blood pressure control but no reduction of risk.[642] Patients on HD with a recent MI may benefit more specifically from classic cardioprotective medications such as ACE inhibitors and β-blockers.[641] More frequent HD reduces LVH significantly,[364,384] but whether this effect translates into lower mortality is not clear.

The growing emphasis on health has focused attention on behavioral interventions that may reduce cardiovascular risk by modifying traditional risk factors. For example, smoking is a risk predictor even in the HD population.[247,643] However, little is known regarding the impact of smoking cessation on cardiovascular risk in patients on HD, as the only data available in this patient population explored only the pharmacokinetics of various smoking cessation aids in the setting of kidney impairment.[644] Exercise has received growing attention, especially intradialytic exercise, which may improve adherence and appears to improve self-reported physical function measures[645] and cardiac functional measures such as aerobic capacity, heart rate variability, late potentials, and T-wave alternans.[646] Although physical activity is associated with survival in observational studies,[647,648] evidence that increasing exercise lowers mortality is still lacking. However, in patients on HD who have undergone cardiac intervention such as coronary artery bypass grafting (CABG), exercise through a cardiac rehabilitation program is beneficial and cost effective.[649] Finally, substantial epidemiologic data link poor oral health and the presence of periodontal disease to systemic inflammation and cardiovascular risk in the general population,[650] and some data for the link exist in patients on HD,[581,651,652] but causality has not been established. Whether diminishing periodontal disease burden would reduce mortality remains to be seen.[651]

Data suggest that patients undergoing HD in whom acute coronary syndromes develop are managed less aggressively than members of the general population. They are less likely to receive thrombolytic therapy[653,654] and to undergo diagnostic coronary angiogram and revascularization[655] despite epidemiologic data suggesting that revascularization improves survival.[654,656] Optimal management of HD recipients with coronary artery disease remains controversial[657,658] because of the propensity of patients on dialysis to present with atypical symptoms and nondiagnostic ECG findings,[657,659] their higher early mortality after CABG than in the general population (9%-12% vs. 2%-3%),[660-662] the lack of randomized studies comparing percutaneous intervention with CABG in this population,[663] and their markedly elevated 5-year mortality rate after coronary revascularization in comparison with patients without CKD (>50% vs. 10%).[658,664] Several epidemiologic studies and meta-analyses have suggested better outcomes (lower risks of late cardiac deaths, sudden death, myocardial infarction, and repeat coronary revascularization) with surgery than with a percutaneous approach,[661,662,664-667] although drug-eluting stents placed percutaneously may be superior to metal stents and comparable to CABG in the HD population.[667,668]

Cardiovascular disease remains the number one cause of death in patients undergoing HD despite substantial progress in understanding the natural history of this disease through all the stages of CKD. Part of the reason for the lack of success in preventing cardiovascular deaths in this population may be that the vast burden of disease already exists at initiation of HD. Another contribution is the complex interplay among inflammation, oxidative stress, malnutrition, retention of uremic solutes, the dialysis process itself, and cardiovascular disease that remains poorly understood but renders traditional cardiac risk factors and treatment less effective in predicting and ameliorating cardiovascular mortality and morbidity in the HD population.[583,632,658,659] Finally, the transition from atherosclerosis-induced cardiovascular events in patients with CKD for which traditional therapies such as statins do improve outcomes to the predominance of sudden cardiac deaths in dialysis recipients likely accounts in part for the persistently high cardiovascular mortality once patients are on dialysis. For now, applying established therapeutic approaches to amelioration of traditional risk factors earlier in the course of CKD while awaiting more evidence to support alterations in management of HD and treatment of nontraditional risk factors in the HD population would seem prudent. Increasing frequency of dialysis, prolonging treatment times, limiting rapid ultrafiltration, and modifying dialysate potassium, bicarbonate, and calcium concentrations may reduce the rate of intradialytic myocardial stunning and the risk for sudden death (also see earlier).[364,376,384,669,670]

MINERAL METABOLISM–RELATED ISSUES

The complex influence of kidney disease on bone and mineral metabolism is covered in detail in Chapters 55 and 63. Although maintaining a normal or near-normal serum phosphorus concentration may be one of the most challenging goals for patients on maintenance HD (see Chapter 63), growing evidence suggests its importance, because serum phosphorus concentrations correlate highly with mortality.[671] Several complications thought to be related to calcium and phosphorus perturbations in kidney failure present particular challenges in managing patients on HD and are highlighted here briefly.

VASCULAR CALCIFICATION

Although atherosclerosis is a major cause of cardiovascular mortality in the general population, growing evidence suggests that diffuse vascular calcification may be an equally or more important contributor to cardiovascular mortality and morbidity in the HD population. Vascular calcification in advanced CKD appears to differ from "garden variety" atherosclerosis and disproportionately involves the medial portion of the vessel in association with disorganized vascular smooth muscle cells (VSMCs) and expression of bone matrix protein.[672-674] This process is evident even in young children on dialysis.[675] The molecular mechanisms underpinning vascular calcification involve a complex balance among inhibitors and potentiators of calcification.[673,676-680] Inhibitors of calcification, such as fetuin-A and matrix Gla protein, are reduced or inactivated in vessel walls.[676,681] A careful study of blood vessels in patients with CKD and ESKD suggests that although significant calcium loading of vessels is present in patients with CKD, dialysis appears to trigger an increased rate of apoptosis of VSMCs, which then leads to vascular calcification.[682]

The exact signals responsible for inducing VSMC apoptosis have yet to be identified. Serum phosphorus, calcium, and PTH concentrations correlate with the degree of vascular calcification, making control of phosphorus and PTH levels and avoidance of calcium logical targets for reducing cardiovascular risk.[674,678] Use of calcium-free phosphorus binders ameliorated vascular calcification in some studies[683,684] but not others,[685,686] and did not appear to be associated with lower rates of all-cause or cause-specific (infectious or cardiovascular) mortality in HD patients than calcium-containing binders.[687,688] In addition, a prospective cohort study of more than 10,000 patients found that those who received phosphorus binders during the first 90 days of HD therapy had a lower 1-year all-cause mortality than those not taking binders[689] regardless of the type of binder and the serum phosphate concentration. Similarly, improved control of hyperparathyroidism with cinacalcet in patients on dialysis[690] and with paracalcitol in patients with CKD[691] did not significantly reduce mortality or morbidity, although off-protocol use of the study drug in control subjects may have reduced the power of these studies to detect significant differences.[692] Clearly, additional controlled trials addressing the effect of phosphate and/or PTH control with different classes of phosphate binders and PTH-lowering agents on hard clinical end points are needed.

CALCIFIC UREMIC ARTERIOLOPATHY

Calcific uremic arteriolopathy (CUA), previously referred to as "calciphylaxis," is a devastating condition characterized by painful ischemia of the skin and subcutaneous tissues, manifesting as symmetric, violaceous patches early on and progressing more commonly to subcutaneous plaques as a result of infarction[693] and less so to necrotizing, nonhealing skin ulcers.[694-697] The name suggests a connection to substantial kidney impairment, but rarely, cases are seen in nonuremic patients.[698] Lesions tend to occur in areas of high adipose content and more commonly involve the abdominal wall, breasts, buttocks, and thighs, but they can develop on the calves and forearms as well as the hands, feet, and face. When the lesions are isolated to more distal sites, the prognosis may be better than with predominant involvement of proximal areas.[699,700] Pathologically, subcutaneous calcification with ischemic epidermolysis is the common lesion but it must be distinguished from conditions that cause necrosis with secondary calcification. The presence of diffuse calcification of the media and internal elastic lamina of small to medium-sized arteries and arterioles with atrophy of smooth muscle cells is an important diagnostic finding; only rarely are the vessels totally occluded.[694,695,697,701] Because of the poor healing associated with CUA, disagreement exists over the indications for skin biopsy.[693]

The pathogenesis of CUA is controversial.[694-697] Recognized risk factors include type 2 diabetes mellitus, obesity, female sex, white race, hyperphosphatemia, use of calcium-containing phosphate binders and vitamin D, hyperparathyroidism, and the use of vitamin K antagonists (e.g., warfarin). The extent to which disorders of mineral metabolism contribute to CUA is unclear, because severe cases appear to resolve after parathyroidectomy in some reports but not others, and PTH and phosphate values seem to be elevated to the same degree in patients with and without CUA, suggesting that other factors are at play. Analysis of pathologic specimens from a small number of patients with CUA demonstrated deposits of iron and aluminum in the lesions but none in adjacent normal tissue or in tissue from CKD controls, suggesting a potential role for metal deposition in the pathogenesis.[702,703] Histologic studies have also revealed the presence of an active osteogenic process in CUA lesions, to include increased expression of bone morphogenic protein 2 and osteopontin.[672,704]

Therapy for CUA is focused on reducing serum calcium and phosphate concentrations and controlling high PTH levels,[694-697] although the role of parathyroidectomy remains controversial.[693,695,699,701] Discontinuing or avoiding calcium-containing phosphate binders and vitamin D seems prudent. When ulcerations occur, aggressive local wound care and antibiotics to prevent wound infections are important. Case reports and small case series have introduced novel therapies that may aid in healing: hyperbaric oxygen,[701,705,706] cinacalcet,[700,707,708] bisphosphonates,[695,708] and sodium thiosulfate,[700,706,707,709-711] with many writers advocating a "multimodal" treatment approach to include more frequent dialysis.[705] Sodium thiosulfate therapy appears to be the most promising and may offer benefit through both chelation of calcium and amelioration of inflammation.[700,706,711]

HYPERTENSION

The complex relationship between blood pressure and the kidneys and the management of hypertension are discussed in detail in Section VII. It is important to provide a brief discussion here of the unique challenges of blood pressure evaluation and management in patients on maintenance HD. Paradoxically, low blood pressure in the HD population, as opposed to high blood pressure, is associated strongly with risk of death.[562] Explanation for this paradox is that low blood pressure acts as a potential indicator of underlying cardiac disease and poor nutritional status. To add further complexity, patients on dialysis whose systolic blood pressures rose from less than 120 mm Hg before dialysis by more than 10 mm Hg during dialysis had a higher mortality rate.[712] Pulse pressure (the difference between systolic and diastolic pressure), in contrast to absolute blood pressure levels, may be a better predictor of mortality in the HD population.[713]

The management of blood pressure in the HD population is complicated by the vast variation in predialysis, intradialytic, postdialysis, and interdialytic blood pressures in any given patient and their clinical significance.[714,715] Peridialysis blood pressures are influenced significantly by volume status and correlate less well with mortality risks than interdialytic blood pressures. Ambulatory blood pressure monitoring may yield a more realistic picture of blood pressure control and offer more prognostic information,[716,717] but because of its cost and inconvenience to patients, combining intradialytic blood pressure values with both predialysis and postdialysis blood pressure measures may be a good predictor of overall blood pressure status.[718]

The pharmacologic approach to management of blood pressure has been presented and applies to the HD population, although a small randomized study comparing antihypertensives administered thrice weekly in HD patients with

LVH suggested that atenolol was superior to lisinopril in reducing cardiovascular morbidity and all-cause hospitalization.[719] The role of volume regulation in controlling blood pressure complicates hypertension management in the HD population, and the challenge for nephrologists is to determine the optimal dry weight for each patient at which the blood pressure is controlled with the fewest medications and the patient can tolerate the ultrafiltration required to achieve that goal weight.[720] Achieving optimal dry weight through more frequent HD treatments per week[365] or through gradual, protocol-driven reduction in weight for patients receiving conventional thrice-weekly HD[721] markedly improves blood pressure control and supports volume regulation as a critical element in blood pressure management (see also "Dialysis Duration and Frequency" section). Blood pressure control continues to be important, although the best method for establishing dry weight, the optimal use of antihypertensives, the target for blood pressure control, and the observed blood pressure "paradox" in dialysis require further research.[714,715,720]

IMMUNE DISORDERS AND INFECTION

Infection is the second leading cause of death and hospitalization for patients on maintenance HD, after cardiovascular disease, accounting for nearly one quarter of deaths and one third of hospitalizations.[722,723] The mortality rate from sepsis may be as high as 300 times that of the general population.[724,725] One fifth of the infections are access related, with pulmonary, soft tissue, and genitourinary infections accounting for the rest.[722,723] Likely reasons for the increased infection risk can be divided into two categories, those related to the HD treatment itself and those endogenous to the patient and the uremic milieu.

ROLE OF THE VASCULAR ACCESS AND HEMODIALYSIS PROCEDURE

Leading the factors related to the HD treatment is the universal presence of some form of vascular access. As discussed earlier, the use of catheters is a significant cause of sepsis in the HD population (see "Vascular Access" section).[135,722] Biofilm, which seems to develop on all indwelling artificial surfaces, appears to play an important role in the pathogenesis of these infections.[726] Although indwelling catheters are clearly the major source of vascular access infection, the repeated percutaneous needle insertions required with AV access also contribute, with AV grafts implicated more frequently than AV fistulas.[86] Infections in AV grafts often require removal of the ePTFE graft.

The HD treatment itself presents a risk of bacterial or viral infection from the dialysis machine, the dialyzer, or the dialysate because of exposure to nonsterile water in the dialysate and through reuse (see "Water Treatment" section). In addition, microbe-generated impurities such as endotoxins in water may cross the dialyzer membrane and stimulate an endogenous inflammatory response. As discussed previously, strict standards have been established for purifying water, disinfecting HD machines, and handling dialyzers, particularly if reuse is practiced. Growing evidence suggests that impurities in the water may be a significant cause of the inflammatory responses in patients on HD,[268] and efforts are under way to find more sensitive assays and improved methods of treating water to allow detection and removal of these impurities.[282,291,296]

UREMIA-INDUCED IMMUNE DISORDER

The uremic milieu gives rise to both immune activation and immune deficiency, which contribute to the high risk and severity of infections, the reduced response to vaccines, a state of chronic inflammation, and, indirectly, cardiovascular disease.[727-729] Both innate and adaptive immune systems are altered. Monocytes, neutrophils, and dendritic cells exhibit decreased endocytosis and impaired maturation but enhanced production of interleukin-12p70 (a T cell–stimulating factor) and allogeneic T-cell proliferation.[730] The expression of Toll-like receptor 4, which detects lipopolysaccharides (LPSs) from gram-negative bacteria and leads to activation of the innate immune system, is reduced constitutively in infection-prone patients with CKD not yet on HD.[731] Monocytes from these patients, when challenged with LPSs, demonstrate reduced synthesis of tumor necrosis factor-α and several interleukins. This relative acquired immune deficiency state from chronic immune activation leads to inflammation and also may explain the high failure rates of vaccinations in the HD population as well as the viral infections endemic in this population.[728,729,732]

INFECTIONS AND RESPONSE TO VACCINATION

Hepatitis viruses have presented management challenges in the HD population since maintenance therapy became available. The risk of hepatitis B transmission has been greatly reduced by less need for blood transfusions, common isolation procedures, and vaccination, although the hepatitis vaccine is less effective than in the general population, especially if administration is delayed until after initiation of dialysis.[728,729,733] With the wane of hepatitis B, hepatitis C has been a major concern in HD clinics since the discovery that this virus explained much of the non-A, non-B hepatitis in patients on HD. The prevalence of hepatitis C is extremely variable depending on the location of the dialysis clinic and ranges from 4% to 70% worldwide.[734] The natural history of the disease is also variable and depends on the severity of underlying liver disease and the presence or absence of known complications, such as hepatocellular carcinoma. In a large meta-analysis, the presence of anti–hepatitis C antibodies was associated independently with a 34% increase in all-cause mortality.[735] Treatment of hepatitis C in patients on HD is complicated by reduced renal excretion of the drugs used and their side effects. Although treatment with pegylated interferon and ribavirin has been controversial in HD recipients, later studies have demonstrated the critical importance of these two agents as well as some success.[736-738] Current recommendations to control hepatitis C transmission in the dialysis clinic include strict adherence to universal precautions, careful attention to hygiene and sterilization of dialysis machines, and routine serologic testing and surveillance for hepatitis C infection, but they do not require isolation of the affected patient or dialysis machine.[739]

The prevalence of human immunodeficiency virus (HIV) in the HD population remains unknown because routine screening is not practiced. Estimates published in 2000 by the CDC of rates of HIV infection and acquired immunodeficiency syndrome (AIDS) in patients on HD were about 1.5% and 0.4%, respectively.[740] There is substantial experience with the treatment of HIV and AIDS in the HD population,[741] and the survival of patients on HD who are infected with HIV improved significantly during the latter half of the 1990s.[742]

Pneumonia is a particularly common infection in the HD population, with an incidence of 21% within 12 months of starting dialysis in an analysis of more than 289,000 incident patients.[743] More than 80% of patients diagnosed with pneumonia have no specified microbial etiology, and nearly half die over the subsequent 12 months.[743,744] Although the contribution of pneumococcal pneumonia to the incidence and mortality of pneumonia in HD patients is unclear, administering the pneumococcal vaccine to such patients may be prudent in light of the very high mortality rate. However, because of the reduced acquired immunity, patients on HD may have an impaired antibody response to vaccines, and measurable antibody levels may wane quickly,[745] raising the question about the best approach for revaccination.

Current recommendations are for all patients on dialysis to receive the full vaccine series for hepatitis B, the pneumococcal vaccine, the appropriate seasonal influenza vaccine, and the H1N1 flu vaccine when recommended by the CDC. Although impaired immunity may contribute to the low rate of seroconversion and the need for revaccination, studies also reveal a low rate of adherence to vaccination recommendations. For example, in a survey of 683 dialysis clinics, only 44% of the patients had received the pneumococcal vaccine.[746] The low adherence rate may be due to the paucity of data supporting the efficacy of vaccinations in the HD population.[747] The observed poor response rate to hepatitis B vaccine in the HD population mandates vaccination as early in the course of CKD as possible, careful follow-up, and revaccination when indicated. Appropriate surveillance for hepatitis B should continue, with booster vaccination for low titers of anti–hepatitis B surface antigen. Vaccination for herpes zoster infection is now available to minimize the impact of zoster infections, particularly in elderly adults,[748] although its use has been limited worldwide even in the general population.[749] New approaches to vaccination and to prevention of infections in the HD population are needed, because mortality and morbidity in the HD population from infections remain high with current practice.

PRIMARY CARE MANAGEMENT

In providing care for patients on HD, nephrologists must address numerous management issues related to the disease or the treatment itself. However, patients on HD need routine preventive health care just like the general population, including routine surveillance services such as colonoscopy. Of 158 patients surveyed in a suburban HD clinic, only 56 had a primary care physician, and patients just starting HD were more likely to have a primary care physician than those who had been receiving HD for more than a year.[750] A Canadian survey demonstrated the importance of communication among family physicians, nephrologists, and patients, because duplication or omission of important health care services was common.[751]

Serious clinical depression is an underrecognized illness in HD patients and correlates strongly with mortality and morbidity (see also "Transition from CKD Stage 5" section).[37,40,43] Hence, depression is another important health care issue that should be addressed by the primary care physician, the nephrologist, or, optimally, both. It is paramount that nephrologists know whether each patient has a primary care physician and communicate regularly with this physician.

COMPLICATIONS FOR PATIENTS ON MAINTENANCE HEMODIALYSIS

In light of the physiologic events occurring during a routine 3- to 4-hour HD treatment and the more than 300,000 patients undergoing 50 million treatments per year in the United States alone, the severe adverse events that actually develop during treatments are remarkably infrequent. The safety of the treatment is largely attributable to improved water treatment, more physiologic dialysate, and improvements in the equipment and procedures used to perform HD. Despite the obvious absence of readily available technical help, home HD is safe with infrequent adverse events, but when adverse events occur, careful re-evaluation of policies and procedures is important.[752]

HYPOTENSION

To maintain sodium and water balance, excess fluid must be removed during HD. The amount of fluid to be removed depends largely on residual urine output and interdialytic sodium and fluid intake and contributes to the frequency of hypotensive events, in conjunction with female gender, older age, and compromised heart function. Depending on the definition used, the population studied, and the era of the report,[467,753] hypotensive events may occur in 15% to 30% up to 50% of treatments. Additional discussion of this topic from a more technical perspective is available in the "The Dialysis Prescription" and "Computer Controls" sections.

ULTRAFILTRATION

For successful ultrafiltration, *vascular refilling* of the intravascular compartment from the extravascular space must occur. To avoid hypotension, both heart rate and total systemic vascular resistance increase during fluid removal. Both of these processes may be affected adversely by the diffusion that also occurs during HD, acting to reduce intravascular osmolarity (see later) and transfer heat from dialysate to the patient. A physiologic response to heat transfer is vasodilation, which counteracts the corrective response to intravascular volume reduction.

DIALYSATE FACTORS

As discussed in the "Dialysate Composition" section, technologic advances that allow replacement of acetate with bicarbonate as a source of base in the dialysate reduced hypotension during HD. However, debate continues as to the appropriate sodium and calcium concentrations in dialysate.

During HD, solute removal decreases the plasma osmolality and favors a shift in volume from the intravascular to the extravascular space. This volume loss is additive to the loss from ultrafiltration and may be reduced by using a dialysate sodium of 140 mEq/L. With this approach, however, most patients complete dialysis with a higher sodium level, especially because the predialysis serum sodium levels tend to be lower than 140 mEq/L consistently, leading to thirst, greater fluid gains, and more intradialytic symptoms. Sodium modeling protocols, with the dialysate sodium programmed to start high and decrease throughout the treatment, were designed to prevent a positive sodium balance but still resulted in higher interdialytic weight gains and hypertension.[244,248,249,251,252,754] A more individualized dialysis prescription with dialysate sodium approximating the endogenous sodium level may be preferred.[244]

Dialysate calcium concentration is no less controversial. A dialysate calcium concentration of 3.5 mEq/L may improve cardiac function and reduce hypotension during HD but may also accelerate vascular calcification. In the United States, dialysate calcium concentration is typically set at 2.25 to 2.5 mEq/L, but some authorities have recommended an individualized approach to dialysate calcium prescription to include modeling protocols.[447,448]

MANAGEMENT

The first approach to managing hypotension during HD is to establish the pattern of the hypotensive episodes. Isolated episodes of hypotension may not require any alteration in the dialysis prescription other than treating the acute event. Modest declines in blood pressure are addressed by temporary reduction in the ultrafiltration rate alone or in combination with placing the patient in a supine or Trendelenburg position. For significant hypotension, the preceding maneuvers should be combined with fluid replacement, usually 100 to 250 mL of normal saline and sometimes albumin or mannitol. In most patients the response is quick, but if blood pressure does not improve after several minuets or continues to decrease, a second saline bolus should be given. When an episode does not reverse quickly, the dialysis staff must consider more complex causes for the event such as myocardial injury or pericardial disease, administer oxygen, and reduce the blood flow. Persistent hypotension requires discontinuation of the treatment.

Preventing further episodes of hypotension becomes the goal after the acute episode has resolved. The timing of the episode within the treatment may provide some insight into a prevention strategy. Hypotension that occurs late in the treatment may reflect a fluid removal goal that is either incorrect or excessive, and the patient should be carefully evaluated to reassess the ideal postdialysis weight. No simple method exists to determine the ideal dry weight, and the utility of the physical examination for this purpose is questioned.[467] More technical tools that estimate total body water are not readily available and do not yield an exact dry weight, although BIA shows promise and may become easier to use and more accurate in the future.

Not infrequently, the target weight may be correct but the interdialytic fluid gain is too large to remove during a single treatment in the time allotted. In this circumstance, the hypotensive episode may occur earlier in the treatment because vascular refilling cannot match the required ultrafiltration rate. The focus in such a case must be reduction of sodium and water intake, although lowering the dialysate sodium concentration to prevent a positive sodium balance,[244] reducing dialysate temperature,[257,259,755] prolonging treatment duration, and providing more frequent dialysis[756,757] also may ameliorate intradialytic hypotension, especially in the hypotension-prone patient. In addition to offering greater hemodynamic stability during dialysis, lowering the dialysate temperature may reduce dialysis-induced left ventricular dysfunction and myocardial stunning.[258,758] Patients with persistent hypotension despite these maneuvers or with autonomic insufficiency may have a response to midodrine, an oral α_1-adrenergic agonist, at a dose of 5 to 10 mg given 30 to 60 minutes before HD. However, the risk for supine hypertension has led the U.S. Food and Drug Administration (FDA) to place an interim "black-box" warning on midodrine's packaging; its eventual fate will depend on the results of ongoing trials to determine its efficacy.[755,759]

Antihypertensive and pain medications render patients more susceptible to hypotension during HD,[467] especially the shorter-acting antihypertensive medications, which should be avoided before HD if possible. Longer-acting antihypertensive medications are preferred and should be taken daily at the same time, to coincide with time after dialysis on treatment days. The challenge is to control the blood pressure while allowing a safe HD treatment.

Other tools to improve ultrafiltration tolerance include sequential ultrafiltration[470,760] and computer-controlled ultrafiltration modeling. Separating filtration from diffusion may improve hemodynamic tolerability[760] but is difficult to achieve in the outpatient setting because of time constraints. Advances in technology now allow continuous monitoring of intravascular volume and/or sodium concentration with automated control of ultrafiltration rate but as yet have not solved this complication in HD, because most methods monitor relative and not absolute blood volume.[227,228,230,237,761]

DIALYSIS DISEQUILIBRIUM SYNDROME

The occurrence of severe dialysis disequilibrium syndrome, characterized by mental status changes, generalized seizures, and coma, has declined, in part because of earlier initiation of maintenance HD.[762,763] A milder form of the syndrome, with much less dramatic symptoms including nausea and vomiting, headaches, fatigue, and restlessness, is still evident.

The etiology for the disequilibrium syndrome is likely multifactorial, but the major suspect is the rapid reduction in solute levels over a relatively short time.[763,764] Animal studies suggest that a transient urea concentration gradient may be created between plasma and the cerebrospinal fluid (CSF) during dialysis,[762,763] which is exacerbated in uremia because of a reduced expression of urea transporters combined with an increased expression of aquaporins in the brain.[765] The resulting delay in urea egress and enhancement of water uptake increase water influx into brain cells during dialysis and promote brain swelling. In addition, provision of bicarbonate in the dialysate may lead to paradoxic acidosis in the CSF through diffusion of carbon dioxide across the blood-brain barrier, further compromising the ability of the brain to regulate solute and water transport.[762,763]

Awareness of the potential for disequilibrium is critical when patients are started on maintenance HD. As noted, timely initiation of dialysis is the key to preventing this syndrome. Several maneuvers can be used to reduce clearance and hence the risk for disequilibrium during the first two or three HD treatments: (1) using a dialyzer with a small surface area; (2) maintaining a low blood flow rate throughout the treatment; and (3) reducing or using cocurrent (vs. countercurrent) dialysate flow. Increasing dialysate sodium concentration or administering mannitol may also help prevent disequilibrium.[762,763] If an acute, serious event with significant mental status changes or seizures occurs, immediate termination of treatment and use of mannitol are recommended.

MUSCLE CRAMPS

Unfortunately, muscle cramps occur frequently during HD as well as in the interdialytic period, are quite painful, and reduce health-related quality of life. The cause is not well understood. Cramps occurring during HD may be related to excessive or too rapid fluid removal with or without simultaneous hypotension but may also be triggered by electrolyte shifts. Accumulation of as yet unidentified uremic solutes may predispose to interdialytic muscle cramps.

No clear method or agent universally prevents or reduces the frequency of painful cramping during HD, but strategies targeting ultrafiltration rate may be effective in reducing cramps, depending on the pattern of onset. When muscle cramps precede or occur during hypotensive episodes, giving careful attention to ultrafiltration rates, reassessing dry weight, increasing the frequency or duration of dialysis, or educating the patient to reduce interdialytic fluid gains can prevent cramps in some cases. A variety of agents may reverse intradialytic muscle cramps, including normal saline as a bolus, hypertonic (23%) saline infusion in small volumes, and 50% dextrose solution, with normal saline being the most commonly used. L-Carnitine deficiency has been proposed as a cause of intradialytic muscle cramping, and a meta-analysis suggested that administration of L-carnitine may be beneficial.[766] Quinine was often prescribed in maintenance HD recipients to treat intradialytic as well as nocturnal cramps in past years, but the occurrence of adverse events and controversy over its effectiveness led the FDA to remove quinine from the over-the-counter market, restrict its availability, and place a "black box" warning against its use for muscle cramps on its packaging. Vitamin E has been suggested as a viable alternative despite its variable efficacy.[767]

CARDIAC EVENTS

ARRHYTHMIA, MYOCARDIAL STUNNING, AND DEATH

Underlying cardiac disease with LVH, coronary vascular disease, and disordered calcium and phosphate metabolism with possible calcific deposits in the conduction system predispose patients to arrhythmias and even cardiac arrest during HD.[768,769] The high propensity for arrhythmias is partly attributable to the HD-induced shifts in solute from cellular and extracellular fluid, especially when the removal rate exceeds the ability of the solutes to diffuse out of the intracellular compartment. Alterations in serum potassium during dialysis may be the major factor, although changes in serum calcium, magnesium, and pH may also contribute (see "Dialysate Composition" section). The challenge resides in the need to remove sufficient potassium while avoiding critical reductions in extracellular potassium and is complicated further with the use of digoxin to manage patients with arrhythmias or congestive heart failure. In patients at risk, programmed potassium removal during dialysis (potassium "modeling") may be advantageous.[442]

Cardiac arrest may be the most concerning occurrence in an outpatient HD clinic. One center reported 102 cardiac arrests over a 14-year period with the vast majority occurring during treatment; 72 of the episodes were related to ventricular tachycardia.[770] Although the availability of easy-to-use external defibrillators may have a positive impact on the outcomes of such arrests, the 1-year survival rate is poor, at 15%.[770] Internal defibrillators still leave HD recipients with a 2.7-fold higher risk of death than patients in the general population with the devices.[771,772]

In addition to ventricular arrhythmias, atrial arrhythmias and frank cardiac ischemia may occur during HD. Atrial fibrillation is common in patients on HD with a prevalence rate of 13% to 27%. Compared with the general population, patients receiving dialysis could theoretically benefit more from anticoagulation because of the higher risk of stroke from atrial fibrillation, but they also experience more bleeding complications, complicating management decisions and requiring individualized risk/benefit analysis.[773] Ischemia occurs during dialysis even in the absence of chest pain, as demonstrated by the release of troponin during HD, the onset of regional left ventricular dysfunction on echocardiogram, and reduced myocardial blood flow on positron emission tomography.[235,628,629,768,774] Ultimately, such alterations in myocardial blood flow lead to myocardial stunning, and the HD procedure itself may contribute significantly to overall cardiac mortality.

PERICARDIAL DISEASE

Pericardial disease is a well-recognized complication in patients with ESKD. Before the availability of renal replacement therapy, Bright found postmortem evidence for pericardial disease in 8% of patients with uremia and concluded that pericarditis is a complication of terminal uremia.[775] Occasionally, pericarditis develops in patients with stage 5 CKD before they start dialysis, likely because of an inappropriate delay in therapy. Pericarditis that occurs within 8 weeks of initiation of dialysis is considered "uremic" disease and requires intensification of dialysis.[776] Pericarditis in patients on maintenance HD is likely multifactorial and may not be directly attributable to uremia because most patients are receiving sufficient solute clearance to avoid uremic complications. However, some patient characteristics (e.g., catheter as vascular access, recirculation within a graft or fistula, larger body size, poor adherence or early "sign-off") are associated with pericarditis in spite of the provision of hemodialysis; in these patients, an intensification of hemodialysis (i.e., longer session length or more frequent sessions) is reasonable. In other patients receiving dialysis, pericarditis does not respond to more frequent dialysis and is likely related to another condition (e.g., viral infection or autoimmune disease).[777] Complications of pericarditis in patients receiving dialysis include cardiac tamponade and constrictive disease. Approaches to treating pericarditis that does not improve with intensification of dialysis range from antiinflammatory medication (both systemic and intrapericardial) to surgery when pericardial disease leads to hemodynamic compromise.[777]

REACTIONS TO DIALYZERS

Historically, reactions to hemodialyzer membranes or residual sterilants frequently occurred during the HD treatment. The classic "first-use" syndrome occurs early in the treatment when a dialyzer is used for the first time, resembles an anaphylactic episode, and can result in profound hypotension and death. These reactions are likely caused by immunoglobulin E (IgE) antibodies to ethylene oxide, a sterilizing agent that leaches out slowly from the potting compound, which acts as a reservoir (see also "Hemodialyzers" section).[778]

The advent of more biocompatible membrane material, careful rinsing of the dialyzer before each dialysis session, and availability of nonchemical methods to sterilize dialyzers has greatly reduced the frequency of these events. Newer synthetic membrane materials such as polyacrylonitrile and polysulfone cause less complement activation and are better tolerated. However, one specific membrane, polyacrylonitrile (AN69), confers a unique risk when used in patients receiving ACE inhibitors. Bradykinin that is stimulated by AN69-induced activation of Hageman factor accumulates in the presence of ACE inhibitors (ACE degrades bradykinin) and predisposes to episodes of hypotension.[779,780] The differential diagnosis for reactions to dialyzers includes sensitization to sterilants with IgE antibodies directed against ethylene oxide or formaldehyde and exposure to contaminated water used to reprocess the dialyzer or to prepare the dialysate (see "Water Treatment and Reuse" section). Treatment of patients with any severe suspected dialyzer reaction includes saline for hypotension, epinephrine for severe reductions in blood pressure, urgent cessation of HD without blood return, and possibly corticosteroid use.

OTHER COMPLICATIONS

Hypoglycemia is a rare event during HD because of the common use of dialysate with a glucose concentration of 100 to 200 mg/dL. When it is observed, reduction of predialysis insulin dose may be warranted. Studies now suggest that dialysate glucose concentrations greater than 100 mg/dL predispose to hyperglycemia and increased vagal tone in patients with diabetes, possibly contributing to intradialytic hypotension.[461,781]

Hemorrhage during dialysis is an obvious risk, given the need for anticoagulation in most patients. When hemorrhage occurs, the high blood flow rates necessary for HD further raise the risk of a serious event. Mechanical events such as blood tubing disconnection and needle displacement are usually detected by safety technology within the HD machine (see "Components of the Extracorporeal Circuit" section) but rarely may be recognized too late, resulting in fatal blood loss. Exposure of the access during HD should be the practice in every clinic, increasing the likelihood that dialysis staff will promptly identify and address bleeding from the vascular access or blood circuit.

When the dialyzer membrane separating blood from dialysate is disrupted, the patient's blood is contaminated with nonsterile dialysate, and pyrogenic reactions may ensue. The HD machine is designed to detect such blood leaks, signal an alarm, and turn off the blood pump to stop dialysis. The dialysis staff must test the dialysate directly to confirm the blood leak, because administration of cyanocobalamin may trigger the blood leak alarm in some dialysis machines.[782]

Intradialytic hemolysis likely occurs to some degree during every HD treatment because of mechanical trauma to RBCs.[783] More profound acute hemolysis during dialysis may result from mechanical problems such as defective dialysis tubing and roller pumps,[784] which lead to excessive RBC fragmentation; improper proportioning of the dialysate concentrate, which leads to osmotically induced hemolysis; overheating of the dialysate; and contamination of dialysate from chemicals such as formaldehyde, chloramines, bleach, and copper. This degree of hemolysis will likely trigger the blood alarm, and patients may experience chest tightness, back pain, and shortness of breath with acute pigmentation of the skin.[785] In such an event, treatment should be discontinued immediately without returning the blood to the patient, and serum potassium concentration should be determined. The diagnosis can be confirmed by assaying for free Hgb and examining the peripheral smear. The dialysate should be screened for contaminants, and the blood tubing inspected to determine the proximate cause.

THE FUTURE OF RENAL REPLACEMENT THERAPY

HD has been called the most successful medical treatment to be introduced during the past century. In contrast to antibiotics, considered by some to be equal to or greater in scope and success, HD always works. It gives indefinite and useful life to anephric persons otherwise facing certain death, usually within a few days. Were it not for the onus of unending dependency on a machine, dialysis therapy would have been considered an unequivocal winner in this best therapy contest. The real and psychologic burden of treatment has been greatly relieved over the past four decades but not eliminated, and in later years, the real burden has actually increased for those seeking the benefits of more frequent treatments. For many of these patients, improvement in health-related quality of life and overall well-being seem to outweigh the increased burden, leading investigators to pursue more objective evidence to sway providers of dialysis therapy. In addition to reducing the burden, the challenges of the future include controlling the accessible risks—including reducing cardiovascular disease, preventing vascular access infections, and managing the legacy of comorbid conditions that affect every patient as he or she initiates long-term dialysis therapy. These conditions differ for each patient, and most require additional and varied treatments that cannot be delivered in the dialysis clinic itself. The physician must partner with multiple specialists, including primary care physicians, who must not be afraid to manage the special needs of dialysis recipients.

One of the challenges is the sheer number of patients in need of kidney replacement. The ever-growing population with CKD in the United States and worldwide who are likely to require HD in the future presents a challenge to health care providers, who must develop systems to deliver treatments to larger populations in the most cost-effective manner while optimizing treatment outcomes. Achieving the desired improvement in mortality rates would increase the prevalence, thus compounding the problem with numbers of patients despite no change or even a decrease in the incidence of ESKD. These statistical considerations underscore the importance of preventive measures to reduce the prevalence of CKD, thereby allowing limited public resources to better manage patients who need kidney replacement. No one envisioned the massive industry that would spring up from the successes of dialysis therapy and that is sometimes accused of stifling innovation and falling prey to corporate functional fixedness. The challenges to the dialysis industry and provider organizations are to be brave and creative, to ignore the fears of investors and economic advisors, and to put the needs of the patients at the forefront.

The pioneering efforts of Belding Scribner and Willem Kolff were rewarded in 2002 by their joint reception of the Albert Lasker Award for clinical medical research "for the development of renal hemodialysis, which changed kidney failure from a fatal to a treatable disease, prolonging the useful lives of millions of patients." Innovative efforts have also been made in the direction of more compact and more easily managed systems that can be handled by the patient at home.[786,787] Other workers have sought a much more compact system that can be carried or worn by the patient during dialysis. Advances in sorbent technology, partially from the aerospace industry, have spurred this effort, which could lead to smaller, more compact systems for delivery of both HD and PD.[788-791]

Successes in the transplantation arena are equally if not more welcome and could change the role of dialysis therapy from that of replacement to that of a bridge to transplantation for many incident recipients. Paired donation and application of extended donor criteria may help extend the availability of transplants to patients previously considered ineligible.

With regard to the measurement and purported adequacy of HD, the Kt/V for urea and its variant measures of small solute clearance remain the most convenient validated measure of the main function of dialysis, which is removal of small solutes. However, dialyzer clearance is not the only determinant of outcome. Multiple factors, including preexisting cardiovascular disease, diabetic microvascular disease, blood pressure control, severe anemia, patient compliance, genetic risk factors, and the patient's vascular access, affect survival and health-related quality of life. While we seek to improve dialysis itself, the other modifiable comorbidities must be addressed if outcomes are to improve. Lacking at present is an understanding of how relatively infrequent (thrice-weekly) short applications of artificial clearances compare with continuous native kidney clearances of the same solutes, especially when the solutes are sequestered or protein bound. Likely, the fluctuating and relatively high concentrations of solute and fluid volumes in the patient and the inefficient removal of sequestered or protein-bound solutes contribute to the sluggish immune and inflammatory responses, impaired growth, and susceptibility to malignancies that contribute to morbidity and mortality in today's HD recipients. Sorting out the relative roles of solute toxicity, fluid balance, and unrelated comorbidities remains a major challenge for the next generation.

Complete reference list available at ExpertConsult.com.

KEY REFERENCES

11. de Jager DJ, Vervloet MG, Dekker FW: Noncardiovascular mortality in CKD: an epidemiological perspective. *Nat Rev Nephrol* 10:208–214, 2014.
13. Germain MJ, Davison SN, Moss AH: When enough is enough: the nephrologist's responsibility in ordering dialysis treatments. *Am J Kidney Dis* 58:135–143, 2011.
44. Hedayati SS, Yalamanchili V, Finkelstein FO: A practical approach to the treatment of depression in patients with chronic kidney disease and end-stage renal disease. *Kidney Int* 81:247–255, 2012.
47. Jaber BL, Schiller B, Burkart JM, et al: Impact of short daily hemodialysis on restless legs symptoms and sleep disturbances. *Clin J Am Soc Nephrol* 6:1049–1056, 2011.
52. Smart NA, Titus TT: Outcomes of early versus late nephrology referral in chronic kidney disease: a systematic review. *Am J Med* 124:1073–1080, 2011.
68. National Kidney Foundation: K/DOQI clinical practice guidelines and clinical practice recommendations for 2006 Updates: Hemodialysis adequacy. *Am J Kidney Dis* 48(Suppl 1):S2–S90, 2006.
72. Rosansky S, Glassock RJ, Clark WF: Early start of dialysis: a critical review. *Clin J Am Soc Nephrol* 6:1222–1228, 2011.
86. Ravani P, Palmer SC, Oliver MJ, et al: Associations between hemodialysis access type and clinical outcomes: a systematic review. *J Am Soc Nephrol* 24:465–473, 2013.
87. Suri RS, Larive B, Sherer S, et al: Risk of vascular access complications with frequent hemodialysis. *J Am Soc Nephrol* 24:498–505, 2013.
95. Al-Jaishi AA, Oliver MJ, Thomas SM, et al: Patency rates of the arteriovenous fistula for hemodialysis: a systematic review and meta-analysis. *Am J Kidney Dis* 63:464–478, 2014.
108. Paulson WD, Moist L, Lok CE: Vascular access surveillance: an ongoing controversy. *Kidney Int* 81:132–142, 2012.
109. Haskal ZJ, Trerotola S, Dolmatch B, et al: Stent graft versus balloon angioplasty for failing dialysis-access grafts. *N Engl J Med* 362:494–503, 2010.
117. Dixon BS, Beck GJ, Vazquez MA, et al: Effect of dipyridamole plus aspirin on hemodialysis graft patency. *N Engl J Med* 360:2191–2201, 2009.
132. Allon M: Treatment guidelines for dialysis catheter-related bacteremia: an update. *Am J Kidney Dis* 54:13–17, 2009.
136. James MT, Conley J, Tonelli M, et al: Meta-analysis: antibiotics for prophylaxis against hemodialysis catheter-related infections. *Ann Intern Med* 148:596–605, 2008.
168. Vanholder R, Glorieux G, Van Biesen W: Advantages of new hemodialysis membranes and equipment. *Nephron Clin Pract* 114:c165–c172, 2010.
197. Asci G, Tz H, Ozkahya M, et al: The impact of membrane permeability and dialysate purity on cardiovascular outcomes. *J Am Soc Nephrol* 24:1014–1023, 2013.
212. Wang AY, Ninomiya T, Al-Kahwa A, et al: Effect of hemodiafiltration or hemofiltration compared with hemodialysis on mortality and cardiovascular disease in chronic kidney failure: a systematic review and meta-analysis of randomized trials. *Am J Kidney Dis* 63:968–978, 2014.
228. Thijssen S, Kappel F, Kotanko P: Absolute blood volume in hemodialysis patients: why is it relevant, and how to measure it? *Blood Purif* 35:63–71, 2013.
235. McIntyre CW: Haemodialysis-induced myocardial stunning in chronic kidney disease—a new aspect of cardiovascular disease. *Blood Purif* 29:105–110, 2010.
244. Santos SF, Peixoto AJ: Revisiting the dialysate sodium prescription as a tool for better blood pressure and interdialytic weight gain management in hemodialysis patients. *Clin J Am Soc Nephrol* 3:522–530, 2008.
245. Hecking M, Karaboyas A, Saran R, et al: Predialysis serum sodium level, dialysate sodium, and mortality in maintenance

hemodialysis patients: the Dialysis Outcomes and Practice Patterns Study (DOPPS). *Am J Kidney Dis* 59:238–248, 2012.
266. Coulliette AD, Arduino MJ: Hemodialysis and water quality. *Semin Dial* 26:427–438, 2013.
291. Susantitaphong P, Riella C, Jaber BL: Effect of ultrapure dialysate on markers of inflammation, oxidative stress, nutrition and anemia parameters: a meta-analysis. *Nephrol Dial Transplant* 28:438–446, 2013.
365. Chertow GM, Levin NW, Beck GJ, et al: In-center hemodialysis six times per week versus three times per week. *N Engl J Med* 363:2287–2300, 2010.
366. Rocco MV, Lockridge RS, Jr, Beck GJ, et al: The effects of frequent nocturnal home hemodialysis: the Frequent Hemodialysis Network Nocturnal Trial. *Kidney Int* 80:1080–1091, 2011.
373. Hakim RM, Saha S: Dialysis frequency versus dialysis time, that is the question. *Kidney Int* 85:1024–1029, 2014.
385. Zhang H, Schaubel DE, Kalbfleisch JD, et al: Dialysis outcomes and analysis of practice patterns suggests the dialysis schedule affects day-of-week mortality. *Kidney Int* 81:1108–1115, 2012.
387. Jadoul M, Thumma J, Fuller DS, et al: Modifiable practices associated with sudden death among hemodialysis patients in the Dialysis Outcomes and Practice Patterns Study. *Clin J Am Soc Nephrol* 7:765–774, 2012.
406. Davenport A: What are the anticoagulation options for intermittent hemodialysis? *Nat Rev Nephrol* 7:499–508, 2011.
433. Labriola L, Jadoul M: Sailing between Scylla and Charybdis: the high serum K-Low dialysate K quandary. *Semin Dial* 27:463–471, 2014.
455. Lisawat P, Gennari FJ: Approach to the hemodialysis patient with an abnormal serum bicarbonate concentration. *Am J Kidney Dis* 64:151–155, 2014.
467. Reilly RF: Attending rounds: a patient with intradialytic hypotension. *Clin J Am Soc Nephrol* 9:798–803, 2014.
474. Upadhyay A, Sosa MA, Jaber BL: Single-use versus reusable dialyzers: the known unknowns. *Clin J Am Soc Nephrol* 2:1079–1086, 2007.
477. Dobre M, Meyer TW, Hostetter TH: Searching for uremic toxins. *Clin J Am Soc Nephrol* 8:322–327, 2013.
489. Macdougall IC, Roger SD, de Francisco A, et al: Antibody-mediated pure red cell aplasia in chronic kidney disease patients receiving erythropoiesis-stimulating agents: new insights. *Kidney Int* 81:727–732, 2012.
509. Vaziri ND: Understanding iron: promoting its safe use in patients with chronic kidney failure treated by hemodialysis. *Am J Kidney Dis* 61:992–1000, 2013.
520. Kovesdy CP, Kalantar-Zadeh K: Accuracy and limitations of the diagnosis of malnutrition in dialysis patients. *Semin Dial* 25:423–427, 2012.
543. Kalantar-Zadeh K, Cano NJ, Budde K, et al: Diets and enteral supplements for improving outcomes in chronic kidney disease. *Nat Rev Nephrol* 7:369–384, 2011.
593. Qin X, Huo Y, Langman CB, et al: Folic acid therapy and cardiovascular disease in ESRD or advanced chronic kidney disease: a meta-analysis. *Clin J Am Soc Nephrol* 6:482–488, 2011.
599. Coombes JS, Fassett RG: Antioxidant therapy in hemodialysis patients: a systematic review. *Kidney Int* 81:233–246, 2012.
627. Green D, Roberts PR, New DI, et al: Sudden cardiac death in hemodialysis patients: an in-depth review. *Am J Kidney Dis* 57:921–929, 2011.
664. Marui A, Kimura T, Nishiwaki N, et al: Percutaneous coronary intervention versus coronary artery bypass grafting in patients with end-stage renal disease requiring dialysis (5-year outcomes of the CREDO-Kyoto PCI/CABG Registry Cohort-2). *Am J Cardiol* 114:555–561, 2014.
688. Jamal SA, Vandermeer B, Raggi P, et al: Effect of calcium-based versus non-calcium-based phosphate binders on mortality in patients with chronic kidney disease: an updated systematic review and meta-analysis. *Lancet* 382:1268–1277, 2013.
692. Moe SM, Thadhani R: What have we learned about chronic kidney disease-mineral bone disorder from the EVOLVE and PRIMO trials? *Curr Opin Nephrol Hypertens* 22:651–655, 2013.
710. Nigwekar SU, Brunelli SM, Meade D, et al: Sodium thiosulfate therapy for calcific uremic arteriolopathy. *Clin J Am Soc Nephrol* 8:1162–1170, 2013.
714. Agarwal R, Flynn J, Pogue V, et al: Assessment and management of hypertension in patients on dialysis. *J Am Soc Nephrol* 25:1630–1646, 2014.
736. Fabrizi F, Aghemo A, Messa P: Hepatitis C treatment in patients with kidney disease. *Kidney Int* 84:874–879, 2013.
762. Patel N, Dalal P, Panesar M: Dialysis disequilibrium syndrome: a narrative review. *Semin Dial* 21:493–498, 2008.
773. Reinecke H, Brand E, Mesters R, et al: Dilemmas in the management of atrial fibrillation in chronic kidney disease. *J Am Soc Nephrol* 20:705–711, 2009.

Peritoneal Dialysis

Ricardo Correa-Rotter | Rajnish Mehrotra | Anjali Saxena

CHAPTER OUTLINE

PERITONEAL MEMBRANE ANATOMY AND STRUCTURE, 2111
PERITONEAL TRANSPORT PHYSIOLOGY, 2112
EVALUATION OF PERITONEAL TRANSFER RATE, 2113
THE PERITONEAL CATHETER AND ACCESS, 2114
CATHETER-RELATED COMPLICATIONS, 2116
PERITONEAL DIALYSIS SOLUTIONS, 2117
Icodextrin Peritoneal Dialysis Solution, 2118
Glucose-Based Solutions Low in Glucose Degradation Products, 2118
Bicarbonate-Based Peritoneal Dialysis Solution, 2119
Glucose-Sparing Regimens, 2119
PERITONEAL DIALYSIS MODALITIES, 2119
DIALYSIS ADEQUACY, 2120
Indicators to Evaluate Dialysis Adequacy, 2120
Determinants of Solute Clearance and Fluid Removal In Peritoneal Dialysis, 2121
CLEARANCE TARGETS AND CLINICAL OUTCOMES, 2122
NUTRITION AND PERITONEAL DIALYSIS, 2124
Nutritional Counseling and Nutrient Supplements, 2124
Dialysis Solutions with Amino Acids, 2125
Reversible Causes of Anorexia, 2125
L-Carnitine, 2125
INFLAMMATION AND PERITONEAL DIALYSIS, 2125
RESIDUAL KIDNEY FUNCTION AND PERITONEAL DIALYSIS, 2126
Measures to Preserve Residual Kidney Function, 2126
CARDIOVASCULAR DISEASE IN PERITONEAL DIALYSIS, 2127
Management of Cardiovascular Disease in Peritoneal Dialysis, 2127
PERITONITIS, 2128
Definition, Diagnosis, and Clinical Course, 2128
Treatment, 2129
Catheter Removal, 2131
Prevention, 2131
Noninfectious Complications of Peritoneal Dialysis, 2131
PATIENT OUTCOMES WITH PERITONEAL DIALYSIS, 2133
ECONOMICS AND COST-EFFECTIVENESS OF PERITONEAL DIALYSIS, 2134

PERITONEAL MEMBRANE ANATOMY AND STRUCTURE

The peritoneum, a serous, semipermeable membrane composed of a thin layer of connective tissue covered by a mesothelial cell monolayer covers most of the abdominal wall and intraabdominal organs. This mesothelium derives from mesenchymal cells that form a basement membrane and develop tight junctions and desmosomes.[1] At the peritoneal cavity side, the mesothelial cells have abundant cytoplasmic extensions (*microvilli*), which have anionic fixed charges, and play a role in the transmembrane transfer of small charged molecules as well as plasma proteins.[1-5] The surface area of the human adult peritoneum is variable and ranges from 1.6 to 2.0 m^2, yet mesothelial microvilli seem to increase effective peritoneal surface up to 40 m^2.[6] Loss of microvilli is a common morphologic change of the peritoneal membrane in patients receiving peritoneal dialysis (PD). When the peritoneal membrane is injured and mesothelial cells are undergoing apoptosis, surface anionic charges are reduced.[7]

The peritoneal microvessels and mesothelium are thought to function by either a two- or three-pore size model of capillary permeability.[8-10] The three-pore model pore sizes are: more than 150 Å for large pores, up to 40 to 45 Å for small pores, and 2 to 5 Å for ultra-small pores. The main pathway for exchanges across the microvascular wall is the junctions between capillary endothelial cells.

Mesothelial cells of the peritoneum have glucose transporters that play an active role in solute transport.[11] In addition, mesothelial cells express aquaporin channels, which correspond physiologically to the ultra-small pores. These channels may be modulated by diverse types of stimuli, both osmotic and non-osmotic.[10] Desmosomes have also been observed near the cellular luminal front and gap junctions.[12,13]

Mesothelial cells with stomata of 4 to 12 μm that communicate between the abdominal cavity and the submesothelial diaphragmatic lymphatics have been demonstrated.[14-16] Transport through this pathway of very large particles, as large as red blood cells (RBCs), malignant cells, bacteria, and others, have been demonstrated.[17,18] Actin-like filaments of stomatal mesothelial cells, their channels, and lymphatic endothelial cells induce cell contraction and allow the passage of macromolecules and cells.

Under the mesothelial cell layer of the peritoneum there is a monolayered structure called the basement membrane, which has anionic charges along both the lamina rara externa and lamina rara interna.[1,3,19] After long-term treatment with PD this submesothelial basement membrane may be duplicated; this phenomenon may also be induced by cell death and by a local environment exposed to a high glucose concentration.[20,21]

The peritoneal interstitium (variable in thickness from 1 to 30 μm) is composed mainly of fibroblasts, collagen fibers, and an amorphous proteinaceous substance (glycosaminoglycans, mainly hyaluronic acid) that displays anionic charges. Additionally, macrophages and mast cells are often, and monocytes rarely, present in this structure.[3,22] Solute transport across the interstitial tissue is modified by diverse factors including thickness of the interstitium in that specific site as well as molecular weight, shape, and electric charge of the molecule.[23,24] To modulate the flow of water from plasma to lymph and to prevent interstitial edema, the local interstitial pressure is usually low and, at times, negative (0 to −4 mm Hg).[25,26] Transfer of small solutes along the interstitium is in general diffusive, and convective transport contributes in the parietal peritoneum.[27] Intraabdominal pressure plays an important role in the movement of fluid from the cavity to the interstitium. During PD, a positive intraabdominal pressure between 4 and 10 cm H_2O drives fluid and solutes from the cavity to the interstitium, and fluid loss is directly proportional to intraabdominal pressure.[28]

A thin basement membrane of the endothelial capillaries separates them from the connective tissue of the interstitium. Capillaries with fenestra are present in the peritoneum, and these structures as well as intercellular junctions play an important role in their permeability.[29,30] Tight junctions (zonula occludens) link the endothelial cells in a monolayer structure.[31] In addition, the arteriolar endothelium typically exhibits gap junctions. There is significant controversy about which is the main pathway for water as well as for small and large solutes across the peritoneal membrane. Although some writers consider the intercellular cleft the main pathway, others believe that tight junctions offer a paracellular barrier that regulates movement of water, solutes, and even immune cells between the interstitial space and the microvascular compartment.[32-34]

When the presence of aquaporin-1 channels was demonstrated, it was clear that water transport occurs through several pathways. In addition to its transport via the paracellular pathway through intercellular junctions at the endothelial level, transcellular water transport was confirmed, and a significant proportion of water transport is now known to flow through these ultra-small transcellular pores.[35,36]

PERITONEAL TRANSPORT PHYSIOLOGY

In PD, solute transport occurs through both diffusion and convection. Diffusion takes place from the presence of a concentration gradient across a semipermeable membrane. The first law of Fick (the transfer rate of a solute is determined by the diffusive permeability of the membrane to that solute, the surface area available for transport, and the concentration) governs diffusion across the peritoneal membrane. A second mechanism that plays a role in solute transport is convection, which takes place during ultrafiltration. This type of transport is determined by the mean concentration of the solute, water flux, and the specific solute reflection coefficient of the membrane.[37] An important factor that influences transport across the peritoneal membrane is the effective surface area available for this process to happen, which is strongly determined by the number of capillaries and the proportion of the peritoneal membrane in contact with the dialysate. In addition, the peritoneal membrane has a defined intrinsic permeability, which determines the ability of solutes to be transported.[38,39]

The peritoneum poses several barriers to solute transport.[40,41] Peritoneal capillaries are the main barrier. A two-pore theory proposed the presence of abundant small pores, 40 to 50 Å, and few larger pores, up to 150 Å.[42] The presence of transcellular (endothelial cells) ultra-small pores (aquaporin-1 channels, 3 to 5 Å), through which around 50% of the transcapillary ultrafiltration occurs, has been confirmed.[36,43] This development led to the proposal of a three-pore model, in which around 50% of the transcapillary ultrafiltration occurs through aquaporin-1 channels and the remaining mostly through small pores.[44-46] The interstitium constitutes a significant barrier to water and solute transport across the peritoneal membrane.[47-49] In order to describe the kinetics of water and solute movement during PD, several distributed models have been proposed.[48,50-53]

Solute transport over time is highly dependent on the ultrastructural characteristics of peritoneal capillaries. Transport of low-molecular-weight (LMW) and medium-molecular-weight (MMW) solutes depends mostly on their size and the surface area available for transport and to a lesser degree on changes in the permeability of the peritoneum.[54,55] Transport of larger molecules is size-selective; therefore it depends on several variables, including effective membrane surface area, permeability of the membrane itself, and importantly, the molecular size of the solute.[44,56] Although in animal models the anionic negative charge at the peritoneal barrier may restrict macromolecular clearance, this finding has not been demonstrated in humans.[4,56-58] In order to calculate the mass transfer area coefficient (MTAC), which is the theoretical instantaneous maximal clearance at time 0 without ultrafiltration, models of variable complexity have been proposed.[53,59] For PD clinical practice, simple procedures that correlate appropriately with MTAC have been developed. For example, a 24-hour clearance or a 4-hour dialysate/plasma (D/P) ratio of LMW solutes is clinically used to evaluate dialysis efficiency.[60] As described previously, diffusive transport accounts for removal of the large majority LMW solutes (e.g., potassium, urea, and creatinine), and convection represents a small proportion of solute transport.[61,62]

Peritoneal water transport is driven mostly through an osmotic gradient artificially generated by additives of the PD solution, such as glucose and icodextrin. The normal peritoneal membrane also presents a small and continuous amount of transcapillary ultrafiltration to the peritoneal cavity through differences in hydrostatic and colloid osmotic pressures and via small and ultra-small pores. Coupled to this transcapillary ultrafiltration is reabsorption of water from the peritoneal cavity through transcapillary back-filtration and peritoneal lymphatics.[63] Given these physiologic pathways of water transport, the net ultrafiltration achieved in a PD exchange is the balance between the transcapillary ultrafiltration into the cavity and back absorption through capillaries and lymphatics.

As already described, the osmotic reflection coefficient of a given dialysate solution determines its effectiveness to induce ultrafiltration. Large molecules such as proteins are not permeable and have a reflection coefficient of 1, whereas very small solutes have a reflection coefficient of 0 or close to 0. The reflection coefficient may differ according to the size of the pores; therefore that for glucose through "small pores" is very low and close to 0, while that through aquaporin-1's ultra-small pores is very high (value of 1 and impermeable).[64-66]

Water transport during a standard glucose-based dialysate can be described as follows[61,63]: When the dialysate is infused (time 0), glucose concentration in the dialysate is the highest and therefore, crystalloid osmotic pressure and ultrafiltration rate are also highest. Glucose is absorbed from the dialysate over time (almost two thirds of glucose content of a solution over a 4-hour period), and the crystalloid pressure and ultrafiltration diminish.[67] Ultrafiltration volume accumulates within the peritoneal cavity and peaks at the time of osmotic equilibrium between serum and dialysate. This diminution takes place along with a progressive reduction in transcapillary ultrafiltration rate, to the point at which it is equal to the lymphatic rate and back absorption rate of the capillaries. From then on and if the lymphatic and back absorption rates exceed the transcapillary ultrafiltration rate, intraperitoneal volume diminishes. Patients display individualized transport characteristics that can be explored with a clinical peritoneal transport test (see following section).[61]

EVALUATION OF PERITONEAL TRANSFER RATE

In patients with end-stage kidney disease (ESKD), maintenance dialysis allows for the removal of solutes and water that would otherwise be excreted by the kidneys. The efficiency of solute and water removal depends, in part, on the characteristics of the dialysis membrane. In patients treated with PD, the naturally occurring peritoneal barrier serves as the dialysis membrane. It has long been recognized that there is a large interindividual variability in the efficiency of transfer of solutes and water across the peritoneal barrier and that in a significant proportion of individuals the efficiency changes over time with exposure to PD solutions.[61,68] Hence, it is imperative to characterize the peritoneal solute and water transfer rate to individualize the dialysis prescriptions. This is often done at the time of start of PD and is repeated if clinically indicated.

Several approaches have been developed to characterize the rate of solute and water transfer in patients undergoing PD. These include the peritoneal equilibration test (PET), the standard permeability analysis (SPA), the peritoneal dialysis capacity (PDC) measurement, and the dialysis adequacy and transport test (DATT).[61,67,69,70] Each of these tests allow for a standardized assessment of solute transfer and ultrafiltration capacity of the peritoneum, information that is critical to fashioning effective PD prescription (Table 66.1). Often, this capacity as assessed by each of these tests is not the same as a precise measure of diffusion and convection across the peritoneum. Common to each of these approaches is that each step of the procedure is performed in a standardized way. This standardization is critical in ensuring the reproducibility of the results essential for its clinical application.

The PET is the most widely used assessment of peritoneal solute and water transfer rates because of overall ease of use and interpretation in day-to-day clinical practice. The key elements of the process that were standardized when the test was first described included having a long preceding overnight exchange (8-12 hours), method to completely drain the overnight exchange prior to start of test (sitting position, over 20 minutes), volume and concentration of dialysate instilled (2 L of 2.5% dextrose), rate of infusion (400 mL per 2 minutes; total infusion time, 10 minutes), total dwell time (240 minutes), timing of collection of dialysate (0, 30, 60, 120, 180, and 240 minutes), time for venipuncture (120 minutes), and the way the results of the test are expressed (4-hour dialysate creatinine concentration to 2-hour plasma creatinine concentration [D/P creatinine], and similar for other solutes; 4-hour to 0-hour dialysate glucose concentrations [D_4/D_0 glucose]; and ultrafiltration

Table 66.1 Parameters Obtained from Standardized Tests to Evaluate Peritoneal Membrane Function

Test	Solute	Fluid Removal
Peritoneal equilibration test	D/P creatinine, D_t/D_0 glucose	Drain volume
Standard permeability analysis	Mass transfer area coefficient, creatine	Drain volume, D/P sodium
Peritoneal dialysis capacity	Area parameter	Ultrafiltration coefficient
Dialysis adequacy and transport test	24-hour D/P creatinine	24-hour drain volume

D_t/D_0, ratio between dialysate concentrations of a solute at a particular dwell time (t) and zero dwell time; D/P, ratio of dialysate concentration to plasma concentration for a solute.

volume).[61] Since the first description of the test, the standardized test has been modified for collection of dialysate at 0, 120, and 240 minutes (modified PET). A large number of other variations of this initial description of the modified PET have been described—variation in length of preceding exchange, dwell time (60 minutes), or tonicity of dialysate (4.25% dextrose), or the use of biocompatible PD solutions.[71-77] Yet, the overwhelming majority of patients starting treatment still undergo the modified PET with 2 L 2.5% dextrose.

As mentioned earlier, there is large interindividual variability in the rate of transfer of solute and water across the peritoneum, which is the primary reason for the need to assess peritoneal function in each patient. Even though the PET can describe the rate of transport of virtually any solute, the 4-hour D/P creatinine is most widely used for both clinical and research purposes. Large population-based studies suggest that, on average, the concentration of creatinine in the dialysate at 4 hours is about two thirds that in the blood (or 4-hour D/P creatinine is 0.67).[61] It is conventional to assign patients a "transport" type based on the results of the PET as being low, low-average, high-average, or high (or slow, slow-average, fast-average, and fast) transporters.[61] Individuals assigned as having an average transport are the ones that are within one standard deviation of the mean, and the ones with slow or fast transport are more than one standard deviation below or above the mean, respectively.

The variability in the peritoneal solute transfer rate likely reflects, for the most part, the density of peritoneal capillaries per unit surface area. Simplistically speaking, the 4-hour D/P creatinine value could be considered a measure of the effective peritoneal surface area. The reason for the large interindividual variability in peritoneal solute transfer rate is not clear. Demographic and clinical variables (age, gender, race, diabetes, cardiovascular disease [CVD]) explain only a very small fraction of this variability.[78] Preliminary studies indicate that some of the variability is, in part, genetically determined.[79-85] There also is compelling evidence that intraperitoneal inflammation, as measured by dialysate interleukin-6 (IL-6) levels, is an important determinant of peritoneal solute transfer rate; this may, in part, also be genetically determined.[79,86,87] Large population-based genome-wide association studies are currently underway that could help clarify the genetic underpinnings in the variability of peritoneal solute transfer rate; this clarification, in turn, could help us better understand peritoneal biology and pathobiology.

The information obtained from a PET could be used as a guide to optimize PD prescription; several validated software programs based on urea kinetic modeling have been developed that use the data from the PET to optimize prescriptions.[88,89] The slower the peritoneal solute transfer rate, the greater the challenge with solute removal, particularly in large, muscular anuric individuals; inadequate ultrafiltration is rarely, if ever, a concern. Individuals with slower rates need longer dwell times to achieve adequate solute removal, which can be done with either continuous ambulatory PD (CAPD) or automated PD (APS). In contrast, the faster the solute transport is, the greater the challenge with fluid removal, particularly with loss of residual renal function; achieving an adequate dose of dialysis is rarely, if ever, a concern. Individuals with faster rates generally need shorter dwell times with a cycler at night and extreme care in limiting long dwells with dextrose-based solutions. The long dwells can be optimized with either complete or partially "dry" days in individuals with significant residual kidney function (RKF), or with addition of day exchange or icodextrin in individuals without RKF.

In addition, a large number of studies have examined the association of peritoneal solute transfer rate with meaningful patient outcomes. The preponderance of evidence seems to suggest that patients with a higher peritoneal solute transfer rate have a higher risk of death.[90-95] The evidence for other meaningful outcomes, such as risk of transfer to hemodialysis or protein-energy wasting, is inconsistent. Several hypotheses have been put forth to explain the higher risk of death in high/fast transporters; they include a higher prevalence of protein-energy wasting from greater protein losses and/or suppression of appetite from greater absorption of glucose, systemic inflammation, or comorbid condition. However, there is an emerging consensus that the higher risk for death in high/fast transporters is from inadequate ultrafiltration with conventional PD prescriptions, particularly with CAPD.[96] Even though the risk is mitigated with use of automated PD with shorter nighttime dwells, it is not completely abrogated.[97] Thus, care must be observed in the design of prescriptions that optimize fluid removal in high/fast transporters.

THE PERITONEAL CATHETER AND ACCESS

Successful PD therapy depends on permanent and safe access to the peritoneal cavity. A good catheter provides obstruction-free access to the peritoneum; additionally, it should not be a source of peritoneal infection. Mechanical catheter problems cause transfer to hemodialysis in nearly 20% of prevalent PD recipients; peritoneal infections, which are often catheter-related, are responsible for another 30% to 50% of PD technique failures.[98,99] Therefore, proper catheter selection and placement are imperative to the success of PD.

Globally, the most widely used catheter is the standard Tenckhoff catheter, followed by the swan neck catheter.[100] Catheters are made of either polyurethane or silicone rubber. Polyurethane is a stronger material than silicone rubber that allows creation of a thinner catheter wall, resulting in a larger catheter lumen, which in turn allows faster flow rates (3.1 mm internal diameter for polyurethane vs. 2.6 mm for traditional silicone). Some manufacturers have begun offering larger-diameter silicone catheters in some countries (e.g., Flex-neck catheter, Cardiomed). Polyurethane catheters, which are most often found outside the United States, can degrade with the routine use of ointments and povidone-iodine at the exit site, whereas silicone catheters have been reported to degrade with exposure to povidone-iodine but not ointments such as mupirocin.[101]

PD catheters have essentially three segments: intraperitoneal, tunneled, and extraperitoneal. The intraperitoneal segment is the portion of the catheter that resides inside the peritoneal cavity; side holes along its length deliver and drain dialysate. The extraperitoneal segment passes through a subcutaneous tunnel within the abdominal wall (intramural), exits through the skin, and has an external (outside

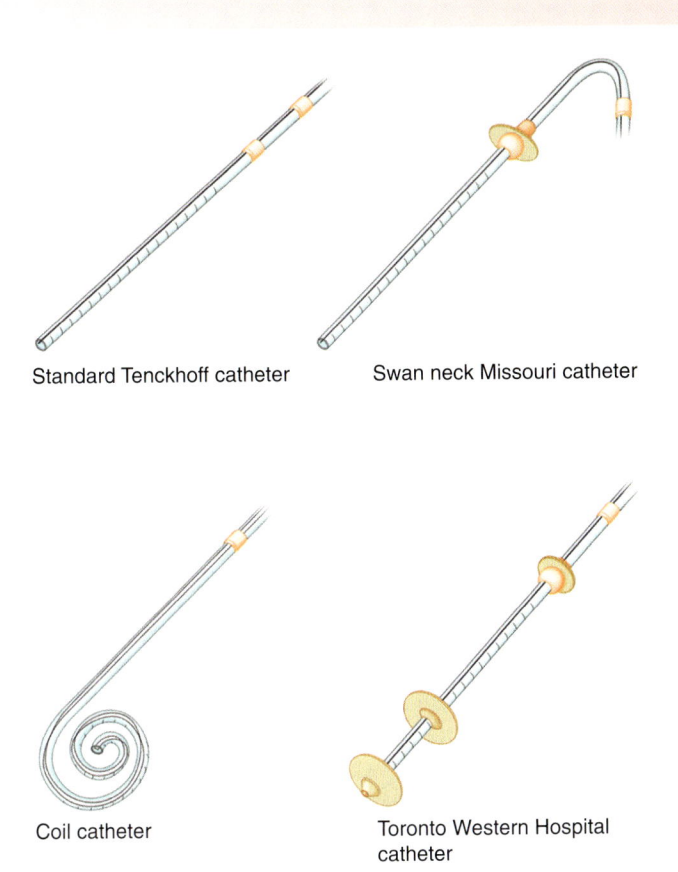

Figure 66.1 Intraperitoneal and extraperitoneal designs of currently available peritoneal catheters.

the body) segment. The catheter may contain one or two polyester cuffs, typically 1 cm long, referred to as the internal (preperitoneal) and external (subcutaneous) cuffs. Figure 66.1 shows different intraperitoneal and extraperitoneal designs of currently available peritoneal catheters.

The straight double-cuff Tenckhoff catheter is available in variable lengths but is most often used in either the 42-cm or 47-cm length, with an intraperitoneal segment length of 15 cm in the former and 20 cm in the latter; each has an intramural segment about 5 to 7 cm long, and an external segment about 20 cm long.[102,103] The intraperitoneal segment has multiple 0.5-mm side openings along its course, which measures 10 to 15 cm depending on the total catheter length. The coiled Tenckhoff catheter is also available in variable lengths between 57 cm and 72 cm with a coiled, perforated intraperitoneal end that is 19.5 cm long in all coiled catheters. It is important to select the proper catheter length for each patient individually to avoid malposition of the catheter in the peritoneum; too-short catheters pose the risk for incomplete drainage and entrapment from hanging omentum, whereas too-long catheters can cause inflow pain most often in the rectal or perineal region. Most Tenckhoff catheters have a barium-impregnated radiopaque stripe throughout the catheter length to assist in radiologic visualization.

There are also several other different configurations of peritoneal catheters. The swan neck catheter, a modified Tenckhoff catheter, features a preformed 180-degree bend between the two cuffs.[100,104] This catheter can be placed in an arcuate tunnel such that both external and internal segments of the tunnel can easily be directed downwards. The preformed angle between cuffs keeps rubber "shape memory" from causing the catheter to straighten over time, thus potentially reducing the risk for catheter tip migration and external cuff extrusion. Swan neck catheters are available with three different intraperitoneal configurations: straight, coiled, and straight with two intraperitoneal silicone disks (also called the Toronto Western Hospital or Oreopoulos-Zellerman catheter). The coiled and silicone-disk configurations were each developed to help reduce omental wrapping and to maintain catheter position in the pelvis. The Toronto Western Hospital and Missouri catheters also differ from the Tenckhoff catheter in that they replace the internal cuff with a felt disk–silicone bead combination; the disk, which is sutured to the rectus muscle just outside the peritoneum, serves as an anchor for the catheter and the bead, which is placed just inside the peritoneum, serves as a physical barrier to prevent peritoneal fluid leakage. All of the aforementioned catheters are available with the traditional subcutaneous cuff that is optimally placed 2 cm proximal to the catheter exit site.

Presternal catheters, another modification of catheter design, enter the peritoneum in the traditional location and are then tunneled subcutaneously up to the chest wall, where they finally exit the skin. The unique design of the presternal catheter offers several benefits over standard abdominal catheters in certain settings. Presternal exit sites are easily visible even in the obese patient with a large pannus or other obstruction to visualizing the lower abdominal skin. Patients with limited flexibility who cannot easily bend to see a traditional exit site also benefit from the easy visibility of a presternal exit site. The presternal catheter allows patients with abdominal ostomies and pediatric patients in diapers to utilize PD without risk of exit site cross-contamination. Presternal catheters potentially reduce the risk of catheter trauma (a risk factor for exit site infection) because the chest is a rather rigid structure with minimal wall motion. A long catheter tunnel, combined with three cuffs, may reduce pericatheter bacterial contamination of the peritoneal cavity and hence lower the chance of peritonitis.[105]

The presternal catheter is composed of two silicone rubber tubes, cut to an appropriate length and connected end to end at the time of implantation. The intraperitoneal tube is available in the dual cuff or the Missouri catheter configuration, whereas the upper tube is a variation on the swan neck catheter. A titanium connector connects the two components at the time of implantation. The catheter should be tunneled ipsilaterally to the peritoneal insertion point so that implantation directly over the sternum is avoided, thereby preventing catheter damage during any cardiac surgery that necessitates sternotomy. Outcomes with the presternal catheter have been favorable in experienced hands.[105]

The Moncrief-Popovich (embedded) catheter is a modified swan neck coiled catheter with a longer subcutaneous cuff (2.5 cm instead of 1 cm) that is implanted normally except that the external portion of the catheter is buried subcutaneously at the time of placement. This catheter is inserted months before it is needed, typically before the patient requires dialysis. The embedded catheter heals in a sterile environment so there is low risk for early bacterial catheter colonization, in turn reducing the risk of exit site or peritoneal infection.[106,107] When dialysis is needed, the external portion of the catheter is exteriorized and connected to an external catheter extender in a short outpatient procedure. Full inflow volumes can be used immediately without increased risk of catheter leak because the catheter has healed fully over the preceding months while embedded. A futility rate of approximately 10% has been reported with embedded catheters (futility due to transplantation, death, or treatment with hemodialysis instead of PD). Nevertheless, embedded catheters that are needed tend to work well. Early catheter drain problems have been reported to occur in 5% to 29% of exteriorized embedded catheters, are most often due to fibrin, and can be readily corrected without catheter removal.[108-111]

Other catheters in use include the T-fluted catheter; the self-locating catheter; the Cruz catheter; the Ash (Life) catheter; the column disc catheter; and the Gore-Tex peritoneal catheter.[100]

Rigid catheters for acute dialysis, rarely used in developed nations, are still used in some countries. Complications of rigid catheter insertion include minor bleeding, leakage of dialysis solution, extravasation of fluid into the abdominal wall particularly in patients who have had a previous abdominal operation or multiple catheter insertions, and inadequate drainage as a result of omental wrapping, loculation, or misplacement of the catheter in the upper abdomen. Loss of a part or all of rigid catheter after manipulation of a poorly functioning rigid catheter has been reported. The incidence of peritonitis varies widely with rigid catheters; the rate may depend on the duration of dialysis and the history of catheter manipulation, among other factors.[112,113]

For long-term use, standard nonrigid PD catheters can be inserted by nonsurgical or surgical methods. PD catheter placement can occur promptly at the patient's bedside with the Seldinger technique (blind insertion); however, this method incurs a nontrivial risk of bowel trauma. Peritoneoscopic assisted catheter placement, often used by nephrologists, allows visualization of the peritoneum before catheter insertion, thus limiting the risk of bowel trauma but does not allow simultaneous visualization while the catheter is physically inserted. A modified percutaneous approach using fluoroscopic and ultrasound guidance at the time of catheter placement allows both avoidance of bowel and confirmation of catheter placement. An experienced nephrologist, interventional radiologist, or surgeon should be the operator in such approaches.

Surgical catheter placement has historically been performed using open surgical techniques (minilaparotomy), but technologic advances have led to increased utilization of laparoscopic catheter placement techniques, which offer the advantage of direct peritoneal visualization. Basic laparoscopically guided PD catheter placement allows proper catheter placement in the lower pelvis. Surgical placement via open mini-laparotomy has also been increasingly replaced by surgical laparoscopic catheter placement because the latter allows visualization and correction of hernias, adhesions, and low-hanging omentum at the time of catheter insertion; additionally, laparoscopy ensures correct catheter tip placement in the pelvis.[114] Advanced laparoscopic techniques such as rectus sheath tunneling, selective prophylactic omentopexy, and selective prophylactic adhesiolysis provide additional benefits at the time of catheter placement and in experienced hands have resulted in a 2-year catheter survival rate of 99.5%.[114] The details of these insertion techniques are beyond the scope of this chapter.[115,116]

CATHETER-RELATED COMPLICATIONS

The most common complications of PD catheters are exit site and tunnel infection, impaired flow, external cuff extrusion, dialysate leaks, and infusion pain. Catheter-related infections can result from improper catheter placement, poor wound healing at the exit site, external catheter trauma, interference of the normal healing process during and after catheter placement, and inadequate routine exit site care. Exit site infections have been shown to be a result of sinus tract bacterial colonization, so it is imperative that a new exit site be allowed to heal in a sterile environment as long as possible. One way to achieve this goal is by keeping the original postoperative dressing in place for 5 to 7 days after catheter placement, removing it only in the case of frank bleeding or drainage; trained PD personnel should be the first to uncover the original catheter dressing, and they should always wear masks while inspecting the exit site in this perioperative period. After the exit site is well healed, trauma to the external segment of the catheter predisposes to infection by allowing bacterial colonization of the sinus tract and exit site and impairing normal tissue regeneration.[117-120] Certain cleansing agents (e.g., iodine, bleach, alcohol) can also impair normal skin cell turnover and should be avoided.

Impaired dialysate flow can be seen during drainage, inflow, or both. Impaired catheter drainage is often associated with constipation, when stool-filled bowel loops either obstruct catheter side holes or cause loculated fluid collections that are not readily accessible for drainage. A successful laxative regimen, imposed over the course of 1 day, is often successful in restoring proper catheter drainage; abdominal radiographs can confirm constipation when the clinical picture is unclear. Abdominal radiographs are also useful to detect PD catheter tip migration, which is another cause of impaired dialysate drainage. Catheter repositioning can be attempted noninvasively with the use of guidewire manipulation under fluoroscopic guidance; if it is unsuccessful, laparoscopic catheter repositioning typically succeeds in improving catheter function when performed by an experienced surgeon. As described earlier, the swan neck catheter configuration may reduce the risk of catheter migration over time.[121]

Entrapment, or "capture," of the catheter by the active omentum may cause outflow obstruction in the post-implantation period. Omental "capture" as a late event is rare. From time to time in some patients, drainage slows as a result of catheter translocation, obstruction by omentum, or fibrin clot formation. Laxatives or addition of heparin, 500 U per liter of dialysis solution, or both may be successful in restoring good dialysate flow. In other patients, catheters have migrated out of the true pelvis. If the catheter continues to function appropriately, repositioning is not necessary. If the catheter fails to function after simple maneuvers are implemented, however, more aggressive measures (e.g., laxatives, forced flushing) may be tried. When these measures fail, laparoscopic repositioning of the catheter tip back to the true pelvis and anchoring may be necessary. The Toronto Western Hospital catheter has two silicone discs in the intraperitoneal segment that hinder the free movement of catheter tip out of the pelvis after placement.[117]

The catheter tip, as it rests against the pelvic wall or intraabdominal organs, may cause localized pain from irritation.[119] The jet effect of rapidly flowing dialysis solution may also cause abdominal pain. In some rare instances, compartmentalization from adhesion formation around the catheter may cause severe abdominal pain.[116] Coiled catheters are designed to reduce infusion-related abdominal pain by avoiding a direct jet effect of solution against the bowel.

Extrusion of the external synthetic cuff can be prevented by creating the tunnel in a shape similar to that of the catheter and placing this cuff approximately 2 to 3 cm under the skin. In the absence of catheter infection, shaving off the extruded external cuff may help prolong the life of the catheter.[115]

Insertion of the deep cuff into the center of the rectus muscle, as opposed to midline placement, has significantly reduced the incidence of early leakage of pericatheter dialysis solution.[117,119] Pericatheter leaks are rare with catheters that have a bead and polyester flange at the deep cuff (Toronto Western Hospital catheter, swan neck Missouri catheter, swan neck presternal peritoneal catheter). In contrast to early leaks, which are usually external, late leaks infiltrate the abdominal wall through prior healed incisions. PD catheters may make minor tears in small vessels or, on occasion, may erode into the mesenteric vessels, leading to hemoperitoneum. In rare cases, a peritoneal catheter damages the internal organs, causing intraabdominal bleeding. Transvaginal leakage of peritoneal fluid is rare, but the possibility should be considered in an appropriate clinical setting.[117,119]

PERITONEAL DIALYSIS SOLUTIONS

The dialysate used to perform PD can be considered to have three components: (1) an osmotic agent to induce ultrafiltration; (2) a buffer to correct uremic metabolic acidosis; and (3) a combination of electrolytes to optimize diffusive removal of solutes. The various options for each of these components among the solutions that are commercially available are listed in Table 66.2. The most widely used formulation comprises dextrose as an osmotic agent (1.5%, 2.5%, or 4.25%), lactate as the buffer (usually 40 mEq/L), and a physiologic concentration of calcium (2.5 mEq/L), at a pH of 5.4. Even though several decades of use support the general efficacy and safety of conventional PD solutions for the long-term treatment of ESKD, concerns about the formulation's limitations or about each of its components has driven the quest for better solutions.

Conventional PD solutions contain dextrose (or glucose monohydrate) as the *osmotic agent*; three different strengths of solution are commercially available, at 1.5%, 2.5%, or 4.25% dextrose (or 1.36%, 2.25%, and 3.86% glucose, respectively). The suprapysiologic concentration of glucose in PD solutions exerts a high osmotic force across the peritoneal barrier to generate brisk ultrafiltration.[63] Yet there are two major limitations. First, glucose is absorbed across the peritoneum, thereby reducing the osmotic force driving ultrafiltration over the course of an intraperitoneal dwell. Hence, ultrafiltration volume is often inadequate with glucose-based PD solutions with longer dwell times, such as the overnight dwell in patients undergoing CAPD or the day dwell in patients treated with APD.[122] Second, a wide range of glucose degradation products form during heat sterilization of glucose-based PD solutions.[123,124] Many of these degradation products (GDPs) either are directly cytotoxic or accelerate the formation of advanced glycosylation end products and are thought to underlie the structural and functional changes seen in the peritoneum with long-term PD.[125] These limitations have led to development of solutions that contain either an osmotic agent better suited for longer dwell times (such as icodextrin) or glucose-based solutions with undetectable concentrations of GDPs (biocompatible PD solutions).

Lactate is the most commonly used *buffer* in PD solutions. During PD, bicarbonate in the blood moves into the dialysate, and lactate is absorbed systemically, each along its concentration gradient. Lactate is metabolized in the liver into bicarbonate, resulting in correction of uremic metabolic acidosis. There are few, if any, adverse consequences of the use of lactate as a buffer. However, with the recognition that lactate is not a physiologic buffer, bicarbonate-based solutions have been developed. Such solutions have two compartments that separate calcium and magnesium from bicarbonate; this arrangement precludes precipitation of bicarbonate salts during heat sterilization of PD solutions. The two compartments are separated by a thin membrane that is disrupted prior to infusion of dialysate into the peritoneal cavity. The resultant solution has a physiologic pH, unlike the dextrose- or icodextrin-based solutions in single-chamber bags.

Conventional PD solutions also have a combination of other *electrolytes*, such as sodium, calcium, magnesium, and chloride. The concentration of sodium in PD solutions (132 mEq/L) is lower than in the dialysate used for hemodialysis (138-142 mEq/L), allowing for a somewhat greater diffusive removal of sodium. In order to further enhance sodium removal, PD solutions with significantly lower concentrations of sodium have been tested. Such low-sodium PD solutions require higher concentration of glucose to ensure an adequate osmotic force across the peritoneal barrier and achieve greater sodium removal with resultant better control of blood pressure than conventional

Table 66.2 Components of Different Peritoneal Dialysis Solutions Available Commercially

	Osmotic Agent	Buffer	pH
Conventional	Dextrose	Lactate	5.2
Low-glucose degradation product	Dextrose	Lactate or bicarbonate	7.0-7.4
	Dextrose	Lactate and bicarbonate	7.4
Icodextrin	Icodextrin	Lactate	5.2
Amino acids	Amino acids	Lactate	6.4

PD solutions.[126] The older formulation of PD solutions contained a higher concentration of calcium (3.5 mEq/L). This put patients, particularly those treated with calcium-containing phosphate binders or activated vitamin D, at risk for hypercalcemia and oversuppression of parathyroid hormones. In order to mitigate this risk, most of the PD solutions used in contemporary clinical practice contain physiologic concentrations of calcium (2.5 mEq/L).[127,128]

The following sections provide an overview of three different PD solutions (icodextrin, low-GDP solution, and bicarbonate-based solution) and the role for glucose-sparing regimens; the clinical experience with amino acid solutions is discussed along with other considerations for management of protein-energy wasting.

ICODEXTRIN PERITONEAL DIALYSIS SOLUTION

Icodextrin is a polymer in which molecules of glucose are linked by α-(1-4) bonds.[129] It is derived from hydrolysis of corn starch, each chain has variable number of molecules of glucose, and the average molecular weight is about 16,000 Da.[129] It is available commercially as a 7.5% solution with lactate as a buffer, calcium concentration of 3.5 mEq/L, and pH of 5.4. The solution is isosmotic to normal plasma, and icodextrin exerts oncotic pressure across the peritoneum to induce ultrafiltration. Given the high molecular weight, icodextrin is not absorbed across the peritoneal barrier but is removed slowly from the peritoneal cavity via the lymphatics. Only about one third of the icodextrin is absorbed, on an average, over 12 hours. This proportion, in turn, maintains the oncotic pressure for ultrafiltration for longer dwell periods and is optimally suited for use during either the overnight dwell of patients treated with CAPD or day dwell for patients undergoing nighttime APD.[130] The icodextrin that is absorbed is metabolized by circulating amylase into oligosaccharides of varying length, with maltose being the dominant circulating compound in patients treated with icodextrin-based dialysate.[131] Maltose readily enters the cells and is metabolized by maltase, found in lysozymes of many cells, into glucose.

A large number of clinical trials have tested the efficacy of icodextrin.[132-139] In patients with high-average or high transport, icodextrin generates greater ultrafiltration volume than either 2.5% or 4.25% dextrose during the long dwells of either CAPD or APD.[132,133,137] This volume is associated with higher ultrafiltration efficiency and a larger volume per gram of absorbed carbohydrate.[132,137] The greater ultrafiltration volume results in a reduction in total body water and a higher likelihood of euvolemia than dextrose-based solutions.[138] Perhaps as a result of achieving euvolemia, patients undergoing CAPD with icodextrin have been shown to have regression of left ventricular hypertrophy in comparison with 1.5% dextrose.[134] Despite a reduction in total body water, treatment with icodextrin has no significant effect on RKF.[140] In addition to improvement in hypervolemia, there is evidence for potential benefits with the use of icodextrin in metabolic milieu, such as improved glycemic control as well as lipid levels.[141] An observational study has also demonstrated potentially beneficial effects on maintenance of peritoneal membrane function in comparison with the increase in peritoneal solute transport rate over time with conventional PD solutions.[142] Moreover, a small clinical trial has demonstrated that diabetic patients treated with icodextrin have a lower probability for transfer to in-center hemodialysis.[136] Finally, an observational study has shown a lower risk of death in patients treated with icodextrin.[143]

On the basis of the accumulated body of evidence, it is recommended that icodextrin be used in a single exchange during the long dwell in patients in whom ultrafiltration is inadequate with dextrose-based solutions—most likely in individuals with high-average and high transport. At least two studies have examined the use of two daily exchanges with icodextrin and demonstrated a higher ultrafiltration volume and improvement in other clinically relevant parameters.[144,145] However, such use remains investigational. Hybrid solutions containing both icodextrin and glucose have also been tested and shown to have substantially higher ultrafiltration volumes; however, no hybrid solutions are commercially available.[146]

Rash is the most commonly reported adverse effect of the use of icodextrin.[133,140] The rash is typically an exfoliating one that involves the palms and soles, is reported to occur 2 to 3 weeks after the start of exposure to the solution, and resolves completely after cessation of exposure. In addition, glucometers that use glucose dehydrogenase pyrroloquinoline quinone overestimate the blood glucose levels secondary to the accumulation of maltose.[147] Care needs to be exercised to ensure that a diagnosis of hypoglycemia is not missed. Episodes of aseptic peritonitis have also been reported in patients treated with icodextrin. This complication has been traced to the presence of peptidoglycan in the solution from hydrolysis of corn starch, and the problem has been substantially minimized with changes in manufacturing processes such that the commercially available solution does not have any detectable peptidoglycan.[148]

GLUCOSE-BASED SOLUTIONS LOW IN GLUCOSE DEGRADATION PRODUCTS

A dual-chamber PD solution commercially available in some parts of the world comprises glucose as the osmotic agent and lactate as the buffer but has a physiologic pH and undetectable levels of GDPs. A large number of clinical trials have examined the potential clinical benefits with such biocompatible solutions, but the evidence base consists of studies with heterogeneous results.[149-160]

The primary impetus for the development of these solutions was laboratory studies demonstrating that glucose degradation products contributed to damage to the integrity and long-term health of the peritoneum and precluded long-term treatment with PD. Post hoc analyses of data from the balANZ trial suggest that the peritoneal solute transfer rate does not change over time in patients treated with these solutions, in contrast to the progressive increase in the transfer rate and the associated decrease in ultrafiltration capacity seen in patients treated with conventional PD solutions.[161] However, there is no evidence that this steady solute transfer rate translates into a clinically meaningful benefit, such as lower risk of transfer to in-center hemodialysis in patients treated with these solutions.[159]

An early crossover study demonstrated that patients had a higher urine volume when treated with this biocompatible PD solution, which decreased upon restart of treatment with conventional PD solutions.[162] Even though some writers have proposed a hemodynamic effect of such solutions with lower ultrafiltration volume and consequent volume expansion leading to natriuresis, the mechanism for higher urine volume with biocompatible PD solutions is currently not known.[163] The results of the studies examining the effects of this solution on RKF are heterogenous, but the summary evidence seems to suggest a higher urine volume particularly with long-term treatment.[159]

At least one large clinical trial has shown a significantly lower risk for peritonitis in patients treated with a PD solution with a low concentration of GDPs[155]; however, this finding has not been validated in any other clinical trial.[157,160,164-166] Even though observational studies have shown a lower risk of death in patients treated with biocompatible PD solution, no such benefit in terms of risk for death is evident in a systematic review of clinical trials.[159,167] This finding may, in part, be related to small sample sizes and short follow-up periods in the clinical trials performed to date. Nevertheless, there is no evidence for harm with the use of this solution, and the decision to use it is dictated by both the availability and the cost of the solution.

BICARBONATE-BASED PERITONEAL DIALYSIS SOLUTION

The bicarbonate-based PD solution, a dual-chamber PD solution commercially available in some parts of the world, contains glucose as the osmotic agent and bicarbonate as the buffer and has a physiologic pH and low concentrations of GDPs. The development of this solution was also driven by the laboratory evidence demonstrating risk to the health and integrity of the peritoneum with the use of bioincompatible PD solutions. There is no evidence for better preservation of structural or functional integrity of the peritoneum in humans treated with a bicarbonate-based solution. However, this solution results in a more complete correction of metabolic acidosis and reduces infusion pain.[168,169] There is no evidence that this solution reduces the risk for transfer of PD patients to hemodialysis. An observational study has demonstrated a lower risk for death in patients treated with this solution,[143] but no clinical trial has validated this finding. The use of this solution, thus, is dictated by its availability and cost, as there is no clear-cut evidence for any clinically meaningful benefit.

GLUCOSE-SPARING REGIMENS

A large number of studies have raised concern about the local and systemic effects of glucose in patients treated with PD.[170] There have, thus, been studies that have examined the efficacy and safety of PD regimens that systematically reduce the exposure to glucose with PD solutions through the course of the day. Central to such glucose-sparing regimens is substitution of one glucose-based exchange with icodextrin for the long dwell. The glucose exposure can be further reduced by substituting a second glucose-based exchange with amino acid solution. Such glucose-sparing regimens have been shown to result in improvement in glycemic control in individuals with diabetes treated with PD, along with improvement in lipid parameters.[139,141,171-173] However, there is a higher risk for adverse events in patients treated with these regimens,[141] which is thought to result from a greater risk of volume overload with reduction in glucose exposure. Moreover, it remains unclear whether glucose-sparing regimens will reduce the cardiovascular risk of patients treated with PD.[174] Given the higher cost of glucose-sparing regimens, the decision to use them should be made on a case-by-case basis.

PERITONEAL DIALYSIS MODALITIES

PD allows flexibility in regimen such that the prescription can be individualized to meet the lifestyle considerations of each patient while reducing the burden of treatment. Broadly speaking, PD prescriptions (1) can be continuous or intermittent and (2) can either involve manual exchanges or be automated using a cycler. Continuous regimens are the ones in which there is intraperitoneal dialysate 24 hours a day, 7 days a week. Continuous regimens may involve either only manual exchanges (CAPD and continuous cyclic peritoneal dialysis [CCPD]). The most widely used intermittent regimens involve the use of a cycler to deliver PD for a part of the day—either at night (nocturnal intermittent PD [NIPD]) or day (diurnal intermittent PD). Such intermittent regimens are appropriate only for individuals with significant RKF.[175] Rarely, intermittent PD is delivered by performing frequent exchanges over 10 to 36 hours every few days. It is used either as a bridge for individuals in the immediate postoperative period (such as "urgent start" PD) or as palliative therapy as part of end-of-life care.[176,177]

Arguably, patients with slower peritoneal solute transfer rates (slow or low transporters) would require longer dwell times, as are typical with CAPD regimens for adequate solute removal. Similarly, patients with faster peritoneal solute transfer rates (fast or high transporters) could benefit with shorter nighttime dwells to optimize daily ultrafiltration. However, most patients can be successfully treated with either CAPD or APD, particularly if they have RKF.

A large number of observational studies have examined the potential effects of treatment with CAPD or APD on clinically meaningful outcomes, and the evidence has been summarized in a narrative review.[178] In the early days of PD, use of the cycler involved fewer connections and disconnections during the course of the day than with CAPD. Studies from this period showed a lower risk of peritonitis in patients treated with APD. However, there has been a widespread adoption of flush-before-fill, twin-bag systems as well as of disconnect systems for APD, and in contemporary practice, there is no difference in risk for peritonitis between patients treated with CAPD and those treated with APD.[178]

Concern has been raised that the total daily sodium and water removal may not be adequate in patients treated with APD.[179-182] This has been attributed to sieving of sodium during short nighttime dwells and reabsorption of fluid during the long daytime dwell that are typical for APD prescriptions. However, such comparative studies have typically not taken into account the overfill for the flush-before-fill step that is common in bags used for CAPD.[183] As a result, the studies may have overestimated sodium and water removal with CAPD. This possibility is consistent with the observation that there is no difference in the prevalence of volume overload or blood pressure control between patients treated with CAPD and those treated with APD.[184]

Despite the reduction in burden of treatment, there is no evidence that patients treated with APD have a better health-related quality of life or lower risk for transfer to in-center hemodialysis.[185-189] Similarly, there is no consistent evidence for a difference in the risk for death between patients treated with these two PD modalities.[186-188] Hence, there is no evidence of a meaningful difference in any clinically relevant outcome between patients treated with CAPD and those treated with APD.[178] The differential use of the two PD modalities is likely to continue to be driven by lifestyle and cost considerations, with a likely greater use of APD in many countries such as United States and those in Western Europe.

The use of PD for acute kidney injury (AKI) is outside the scope of the present chapter, yet it is important to point out that such use is becoming increasingly important, particularly in some environments where patients have limited access to hemodialytic therapies.[190]

DIALYSIS ADEQUACY

The concept of an optimal or adequate dialysis dose for PD has evolved in the last decade. What we currently consider an "adequate" PD dialysis dose has been strongly influenced by results of randomized controlled trials and a better understanding of the multiplicity of factors affecting PD patients with little or no RKF.[191-193] Before the Adequacy of Peritoneal Dialysis in Mexico (ADEMEX) study and the Hemodialysis (HEMO) study, there was a generally accepted notion that an increase in small solute clearances would lead to increased survival and better clinical results.[191,192,194] The current concept of adequate dialysis now encompasses attention to a multiplicity of clinical variables, including RKF, cardiovascular effects of blood pressure control, ultrafiltration and volume overload, mineral metabolism, nutrition, and individual psychologic as well as quality-of-life indicators (Table 66.3).[191,194]

Adequate dialysis is defined as the administration of an effective dosage of dialysis solution capable of keeping a patient clinically asymptomatic and active and maintaining a good enough correction of the altered metabolic and homeostatic components secondary to the loss of kidney function.[195] *Optimal dialysis* is defined as either (1) the dose capable of reducing morbidity and mortality associated with ESKD and with the dialytic procedure itself or (2) the dose above which an increase does not justify the greater burden of treatment.[196,197]

INDICATORS TO EVALUATE DIALYSIS ADEQUACY

The amount of dialytic treatment prescribed is widely based on the presence or absence of symptoms related to uremia (e.g., nausea, vomiting, dysgeusia, sleeping disorders).[198] Nevertheless, this procedure is highly subjective and prone to dosage underestimation. Although clinical indicators should not be ignored, therapeutic decisions should not be based solely on them.[199] Clearance of urea is now typically used as marker of dialysate dosage. In PD, the preservation of RKF in addition to the peritoneal clearance obtained by the dialytic procedure itself is of utmost importance, because RKF usually tends to be maintained in PD for a longer period than in hemodialysis and may account for a significant proportion of the total clearance.[197,200,201]

Urea is the traditional solute to quantitate dialysis because its concentration is increased in chronic kidney disease and it has a low molecular weight (60 kDa), which allows rapid diffusion between body compartments and therefore application of a single-pool model for approximation. In addition, its volume of distribution is the total body water, it easily diffuses across the dialysis membrane, and it is easy to measure.[201] After results of the National Cooperative Dialysis Study (NCDS) were published in the early 1980s, the urea kinetic model took on a prominent role in dosage prescription in PD, notwithstanding the fact that it was created for hemodialysis and that its application to PD was accomplished only through inferences and analogies.[202]

The fractional clearance of urea is expressed as Kt/V_{urea}, which is the clearance of urea (K) per time unit (t) in relation to its volume of distribution or total body water (V). Peritoneal Kt is calculated by collecting a 24-hour amount of effluent dialysate and determining its urea concentration (D_{urea}); this in turn is divided by the plasma urea concentration (D/P_{urea}). To compare clearance values among patients, these values are normalized to a function of patient size: For urea, the metric is typically the volume of urea distribution (V). In PD practice, Kt/V_{urea} can be expressed as a total (sum of peritoneal Kt/Vurea [pKt/V_{urea}] and renal urea clearances) or as each of its fractions independently. Renal Kt is calculated similarly, with a 24-hour urine collection.

Creatinine clearance (both peritoneal and residual renal) has also been used for dosage prescription in PD; this value is also obtained from a 24-hour collection of dialysate, to which is added the average of the renal creatinine and urea nitrogen clearances. Kt/V_{urea} and creatinine clearance may be expressed as daily values but are usually multiplied by 7 and expressed as weekly values. This change was made to allow comparisons between PD and hemodialysis delivered dosages; yet these comparisons are not useful, given the intermittent nature of hemodialysis and the continuous nature of PD (Table 66.4).[203,204] The urea kinetic model, which has been repeatedly validated for hemodialysis prescription, has been applied to PD, but its validity is questionable. If the same dosing principles employed for hemodialysis were used for CAPD, patients on PD would be considered grossly underdialyzed because their Kt/V_{urea} values would be much lower in absolute numbers, but this is clearly not the case: Most patients undergoing PD do not have more uremic

---

Table 66.3 Considerations for Adequate Dialysis

Clinical manifestations: fluid balance, systemic blood pressure control, and cardiovascular risk
Residual kidney function
Acid-base homeostasis
Nutritional status
Calcium-phosphorous metabolism homeostasis
Inflammation
Small solute clearance
Middle molecule clearance
Psychologic and quality-of-life indicators

Table 66.4 Calculations for Dosage of Dialysis Solution

Fractional urea clearance (Kt/V_{urea})	Daily total Kt/V_{urea} = peritoneal Kt/V_{urea} + renal Kt/V_{urea} Weekly Kt/V_{urea} = 7 × {[(24-hr urea D/P × 24-hr EV)/V] + [(U_{urea}/P_{urea}) × 24-hr UV)]}
Total body water (Watson's formula)*	Male: V = 2.447 − (0.3362 × weight) − (0.1074 × height) − (0.09516 × age) Female: V = −2.097 + (0.2466 × weight) + (0.1069 × height)

*In Watson's formulas, age is in years, height is in centimeters, and weight is in kilograms.

D/P, Ratio of dialysate concentration to plasma concentration for a solute; EV, dialysate effluent volume; Kt, clearance of urea (K) per time unit (t); P_{urea}, plasma urea; U_{urea}, urine urea; V, total body water volume of distribution; V_{urea}, volume of distribution for urea.

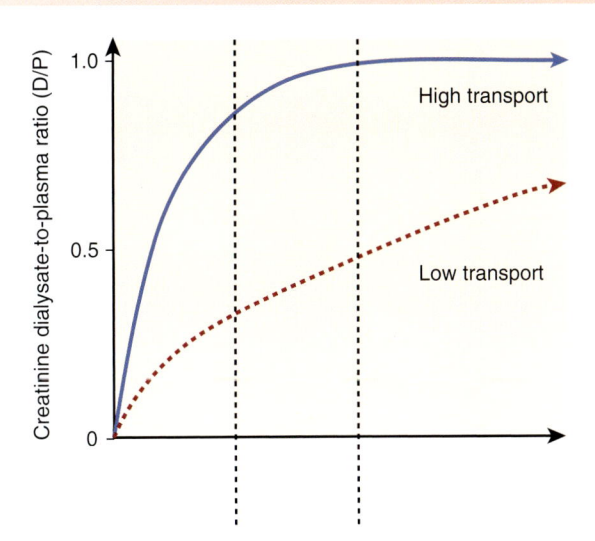

Figure 66.2 The ratio of dialysate-to-plasma ratio for creatinine (D/P_{Cr}) plotted against dwell time of a dialytic exchange in conditions of high and low peritoneal transport.

Table 66.5 Determinants of Solute Clearance and Fluid Removal in Peritoneal Dialysis

Patient-related factors	Renal residual function Body mass index Peritoneal transport type
Prescription-related factors	Dialytic modality Frequency of exchanges per day Volume of each exchange Dwell time Dialysis fluid tonicity

manifestations, higher rates of morbidity, or higher rates of mortality than patients on hemodialysis.

DETERMINANTS OF SOLUTE CLEARANCE AND FLUID REMOVAL IN PERITONEAL DIALYSIS

The initial PD prescription is defined empirically; a series of factors that influence clearance of solutes and fluid removal are taken into account. Some of these factors are modifiable and others are nonmodifiable (Table 66.5).[204-206]

PATIENT-RELATED FACTORS

RKF contributes significantly to fluid removal and variably to solute clearance in PD patients. In these patients, RKF is best estimated by measuring the weekly renal component of the Kt/V_{urea}. Each milliliter per minute of urea clearance accounts for the addition of 0.25 L to the total weekly Kt/V_{urea}.[198] Estimation of RKF enables physicians to plan the PD prescription, but during follow-up, RKF should be evaluated periodically because it tends to diminish over time; the dialysis prescription should be modified to compensate.

VOLUME OF DISTRIBUTION AND BODY SURFACE AREA

The volume of distribution of urea is equivalent to the total body water, which can be estimated by the Watson or Hume formula, but these formulas may underestimate total body water in patients on dialysis and potentially overestimate dialysate dosage.[207,208] An equation has specifically been developed for patients undergoing maintenance dialysis and has been validated to provide superior prediction of total body water in patients on hemodialysis and, potentially, also in patients on PD.[209]

Peritoneal Transport Type

Figure 66.2 displays the ratio between dialysate and plasma creatinine concentrations (D/P_{Cr}) plotted against dwell time of a dialytic exchange in conditions of high and low peritoneal transport. The D/P_{Cr} equilibrium (ratio of 1.0) is achieved earlier in high peritoneal transport; therefore, a shorter dwell time is preferred for patients with higher peritoneal transport rates, and a longer dwell time is required to augment solute clearance in patients with lower transport rates (Figure 66.3). In comparison, patients with lower peritoneal transport achieve higher ultrafiltration volumes, whereas patients with higher peritoneal transport rates reabsorb larger quantities of glucose, an occurrence that reduces the gradient to ultrafiltration and generates net fluid reabsorption with longer dwell times (see Figure 66.3).[61,112] Patients with higher peritoneal transport rates obtain better ultrafiltration and adequate clearance of small molecules with techniques that involve short dwell times, such as APD, prescribed with multiple short exchanges. In contrast, patients with lower transport rates benefit from longer exchange dwell times to augment removal of small molecules while preserving the ultrafiltration capability. Of importance is that most patients have intermediate transport rates, so individualized evaluation is required to prescribe the best regimen.[61,112]

In addition to the discussed relationship between transport type with ultrafiltration and solute clearance, it is important to consider that the smaller the solute, the faster the diffusive equilibrium reached. Urea, with a molecular weight of 60 Da, reaches equilibrium much faster than creatinine, with a molecular weight of 112 Da. These conditions influencing small-molecule solute clearance may not

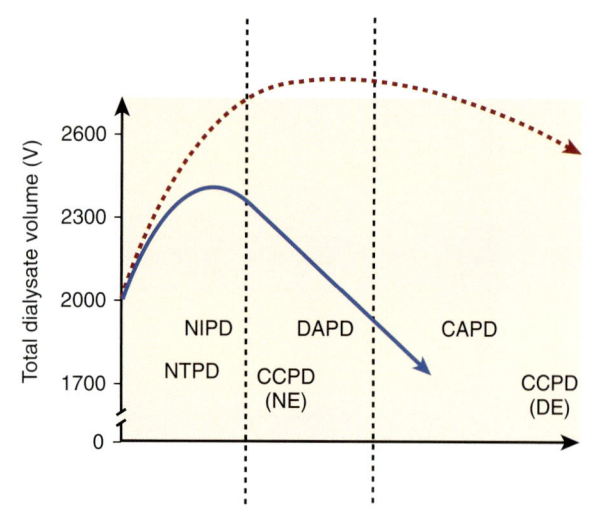

Figure 66.3 Differences in ultrafiltration and net fluid reabsorption between patients with lower peritoneal transport (*red line*) and patients with higher peritoneal transport (*blue line*). CAPD, Continuous ambulatory peritoneal dialysis; CCPD, continuous cycling peritoneal dialysis; DAPD, daytime ambulatory peritoneal dialysis; DE, daytime exchanges; NE, nocturnal exchanges; NIPD, nocturnal intermittent peritoneal dialysis; NTPD, nightly tidal peritoneal dialysis.

be relevant to clearance of large-molecule, charged, or protein-bound solutes. A more detailed discussion of uremic solutes and the limitations of using urea as a solute marker is provided in Chapter 54.

PRESCRIPTION-RELATED FACTORS

The main factors in PD prescription that can be modified to attain recommended goals are frequency of exchanges, volume of PD fluid exchanges, and tonicity of solutions.

Frequency of Exchanges

Traditional CAPD prescription is based on a four exchanges of 1.5 to 3.0 L every day. Yet some patients with small body surface area or significant RKF may start their treatment with three or fewer exchanges per day; this modality has been defined as incremental, because with time patients are expected to require an increase in dosage. Creatinine is a larger molecule than urea, so an increase in exchange frequency is less effective than an increase in fluid volume per exchange for removal of creatinine, particularly in patients with low transport rates.[198] In APD, an increase in frequency of exchanges also induces an increase in solute clearance because the concentration gradient between dialysate and blood is maximized, but this increase in exchange frequency in a given period may require that a large proportion of the total treatment time be dedicated to infusion and drainage. Therefore, there is a point at which the number of exchanges may be counterproductive in relation to both clearance attained and costs. This "break even" point is variable from patient to patient and is related in part to the peritoneal transport rate.[204]

The best way to increase clearance in NIPD is to add a daytime exchange, which increases Kt/V_{urea} by 25%. The main drawback is that a long daytime exchange often leads to net fluid reabsorption, particularly in patients with high and high-average peritoneal transport rates. A way to avoid this problem is to individually tailor the daily exchange time for each patient according to the clinical behavior.[192] In some patients, additional clearance may be obtained by adding a second or third daytime exchange or by switching to CAPD.

Increase in Volume Exchange

An increase in fill volume is a more effective means of increasing small-molecule solute clearance than an increase in exchange frequency. Therefore, it is one of the main prescription actions to achieve goals for CAPD as well as for APD. Volume exchange is limited to peritoneal cavity size, body surface area, patient tolerance of and risk for complications with PD fluid leaks and hernias.[204-206]

Increase in Solution Osmolality

A dialysate with a higher tonicity, which induces an increase in ultrafiltration volume, is employed mainly to avoid or control the hypervolemia often observed in patients without RKF independent of their transport type, in patients with high and high-average transport rates, and in nonadherent patients who ingest large amounts of salt or water. These dialysates may also induce a convection-driven, quantifiable increase in solute clearance. It is important to point out that use of hypertonic glucose solutions has potential adverse metabolic consequences: hyperglycemia, dyslipidemia, obesity, and long-term peritoneal membrane injury. The use of polyglucose solutions (icodextrin) allows greater ultrafiltration with a lower risk of inducing metabolic complications.[204]

CLEARANCE TARGETS AND CLINICAL OUTCOMES

When outcomes of patients on PD were assessed in the prospective Canada-USA cohort study of adequacy in PD (CANUSA), there was an inverse correlation between Kt/V_{urea} and mortality.[200] This finding led to the implementation of "evidence-based" recommendations by the Kidney Disease Outcomes Quality Initiative (KDOQI) that the weekly dose of CAPD achieve a Kt/V_{urea} of at least 2.0 for all patients and that the total creatinine clearance rate be at least 60 L/week/1.73 m² for those with high and high-average transport rates and 50 L/week/1.73 m² for those with low and low-average transport rates.[198] In a reanalysis of their data, the CANUSA investigators noted that one conclusion was erroneous[210]: In the first analysis of CANUSA, the equivalence of renal and peritoneal clearances was assumed, and therefore they were merely added. For every 5-L/week/1.73 m² increase in residual creatinine clearance, there was a 12% decrease in the relative risk of death; no such association with peritoneal creatinine clearance was evident. The observed survival advantage with higher small-solute clearances could be accounted for by RKF.[210] This fact was further supported by the findings of other investigators who have stressed the utmost importance of RKF.

Other studies were unsuccessful in evaluating the effect of peritoneal clearance on patient.[211-213] As previously mentioned, the ADEMEX study was a prospective, randomized clinical trial to evaluate the effect of an increase in peritoneal clearance on patient survival.[191] The study involved 960 patients with incident and prevalent renal disease (>50%

Table 66.6 Adequacy Targets in Peritoneal Dialysis (PD)

Index Measure	Adequacy Index		
	European Renal Association (2005)	Kidney Disease Dialysis Outcomes Quality Initiative (2006)	International Society of Peritoneal Dialysis (2006)
Total urea clearance (Kt/V$_{urea}$)			
Continuous ambulatory PD	1.7	1.7	1.7
Automated PD	1.7	1.7	1.7

anuric) who were receiving CAPD with four 2-L exchanges and had peritoneal creatinine clearance rates less than 60 L/week/1.73 m^2 at 24 centers in Mexico. Subjects were monitored for more than 2 years. A control group received a standard prescription (four 2-L exchanges), and for the experimental group, the prescription was changed to achieve a peritoneal creatinine clearance of 60 L/week by increasing dwell volumes and, when necessary, adding a fifth automated night exchange. The control group achieved a peritoneal creatinine clearance rate of 46 L/week/1.73 m^2 and a peritoneal Kt/V$_{urea}$ of 1.62 per week, whereas the experimental group achieved a peritoneal creatinine clearance rate of 56 L/week/1.73 m^2 and a Kt/V$_{urea}$ of 2.13 per week. No differences were observed between the two groups in primary (risk of death) and secondary (technique failure, hospitalization, nutritional status) outcomes.[191] These results support the hypothesis that increases in creatinine and urea clearance with higher PD dosage, within the studied ranges, do not enhance patient survival.

Data from several subgroups—including younger and older subjects, those with or without RKF, those with or without diabetes, and those with larger and smaller body surface areas—were analyzed and, again, showed no differences in mortality or other outcomes by randomized group among these subgroups. Control subjects were more likely to drop out of the study because of uremia. The results of the ADEMEX study may not be generalizable, however, as the participants were smaller in size, younger, and apparently more undernourished that other PD populations.[214] However, these arguments do not preclude the external validity of the study, inasmuch as comorbid conditions, general survival rates, and causes of mortality were similar to those observed in all other studies, including the CANUSA study.[200]

Results of the ADEMEX study were supported by those of Lo and colleagues in a randomized clinical trial of 320 patients with incident renal disease who were receiving CAPD and whose baseline renal Kt/V$_{urea}$ values were less than 1.0.[193] Patients were randomly assigned to three target groups: In group A, Kt/V$_{urea}$ ranged from 1.5 to 1.7; in group B, Kt/V$_{urea}$ ranged from 1.7 to 2.0; and in group C, Kt/V$_{urea}$ exceeded 2.0. Total Kt/V$_{urea}$ values of the three groups were significantly different, and this difference was mostly attributable to peritoneal Kt/V$_{urea}$. There were no differences in patient survival, serum albumin level, or hospitalization rates among the three groups; however, more patients from group A required erythropoietin and were withdrawn from the study by their physicians. Thus, patients with total Kt/V$_{urea}$ values below 1.7 had more anemia and clinical complications, and yet there was no difference in survival or other outcomes for groups B and C, with Kt/V$_{urea}$ either between 1.7 and 2.0 or above 2.0. Results of this and the ADEMEX study support the notion that a total Kt/V$_{urea}$ of 1.7 or higher is an appropriate target. Lo and colleagues did not recommend reduction in dialysate dosage for patients who achieved higher clearance rates, but they did demonstrate that within the studied ranges, there were no significant differences among groups in mortality and in most other secondary end points.[193] In addition, these investigators performed a 10-year retrospective survival analysis of 150 anuric patients on PD, according to the baseline peritoneal Kt/V$_{urea}$ at time of documentation of anuria and of the latest PD prescription (based on Kt/V$_{urea}$).[215] Baseline Kt/V$_{urea}$ was not an independent risk factor overall; nevertheless, patients with peritoneal Kt/V$_{urea}$ values lower than 1.67 had poorer survival rates. Survival rates did not differ among patients with Kt/V$_{urea}$ either higher or lower than 1.80. The survival rate was best among female patients with Kt/V$_{urea}$ values of 1.67 to 1.86, followed by those with Kt/V$_{urea}$ higher than 1.86, and was lowest in those with Kt/V$_{urea}$ lower than 1.67. Peritoneal Kt/V$_{urea}$ below 1.67 was consistently associated with lower survival rates. Reliable information linking dialysis dose in APD with survival is scarce, and controlled trials are required.

In the last few years, clinical practice guidelines for PD prescription have been adjusted on the basis of the available evidence. According to most of these documents, Kt/V$_{urea}$ is still the best available index of "adequacy" and a value of total Kt/V$_{urea}$ of 1.7 or more can be considered adequate (Table 66.6).[202,205,206,216] Overemphasis on urea kinetic modeling has resulted in the neglect of several relevant issues. Long-term overhydration has major negative consequences, and CVD is the most frequent cause of morbidity and mortality in patients with ESKD in general and in those on PD specifically.[217] The adverse effects of overhydration may trump the marginal benefits of enhanced solute clearance if the latter is attended to in lieu of the former. Salt and water overload have to be closely monitored and corrected, through dietary restrictions, dialysis ultrafiltration, pharmacologic interventions, or a combination of these measures.

Renal clearance is not equivalent to peritoneal clearance, inasmuch as the kidney provides benefits that are not achieved with PD, including better middle-molecule clearance, volume control, and metabolic and endocrine benefits. Hyperphosphatemia and other abnormalities of mineral metabolism are strong predictors of cardiovascular morbidity and mortality.[217] Protein-energy wasting should also receive close attention because it is present in many patients with chronic kidney disease (see Chapter 61). Protein-energy wasting, a negative prognostic indicator to be considered even before the need of dialysis, is also discussed in the "Nutritional Counseling and Nutrient Supplements" section of this chapter. Attention to nontraditional risk factors, particularly inflammation, almost always present in patients with renal disease, is important; inflammation is also discussed in more detail in the "Inflammation and Peritoneal Dialysis" section. Social and psychologic factors are also important for the care of the patient on PD.

At present, it is clear that volume status constitutes a major determinant of PD patient survival and of an adequate prescription. Volume overload has a major impact on cardiovascular morbidity as well as mortality in PD recipients. Therefore, it is of upmost importance to consider normovolemia as a major target of dialysis adequacy.[205,206,218] Determination of optimal volume status is a complex issue, and studies with bioimpedance spectroscopy have proven useful for this purpose.[219,220]

NUTRITION AND PERITONEAL DIALYSIS

Protein-energy wasting is often present in patients on PD and correlates directly with time on PD.[221-224] A deficient nutritional status in the PD recipient is strongly associated with morbidity and mortality.[225-228] Multiple variables are employed to assess the nutritional status of the patient on PD, including serum albumin level, prealbumin level, lean body mass, total body nitrogen level, creatinine excretion, anthropometric indices, subjective global assessment, and composite nutritional scores. In order to better evaluate and monitor the nutritional status of a PD recipient, the use of multiple tools is required, as no single measure provides a complete evaluation.[229]

The cause of protein-energy wasting in patients on PD is multifactorial and complex (Table 66.7). Nutrient losses during dialysis, low nutrient intake, comorbid conditions, chronic inflammation, metabolic acidosis, loss of RKF, uncorrected uremia, and a variety of endocrine disorders contribute to the deficient nutritional status.[230-233] Some studies have shown that patients with high peritoneal membrane permeability could be at higher risk for protein-energy wasting; however, association studies between peritoneal transport rate and nutritional status have shown contradictory results.[234,235] It has been long said that patients on dialysis may have at least two different types of protein-energy wasting.[236] The first type is related to low nutrient intake, and a second type is associated with inflammation and CVD. These types of protein-energy wasting often coexist in the clinical setting.

A diversity of therapeutic strategies has been suggested to treat or prevent improper nutritional status in the PD recipient. They include nutritional counseling for adequate nutrient intake, treatment of reversible causes of anorexia, and correction of catabolic factors (inflammation, correctable comorbidities, uremia, and acidosis; see Table 66.7).

NUTRITIONAL COUNSELING AND NUTRIENT SUPPLEMENTS

Nutritional counseling is the first-line intervention to achieve adequate nutrient intake.[237] The usually recommended daily energy intake for patients on maintenance PD

Table 66.7 Etiology of Protein-Energy Wasting in Patients on Peritoneal Dialysis

Causes of Malnutrition	Possible Management Strategies
Nutrient losses:	
Amino acids	Nutritional counseling
Peptides	30-35 kcal/kg/day
Proteins	1.2 g of protein/kg/day
Water-soluble vitamins	Nutrient and vitamin supplements
Other bioactive compounds	Dialysis solutions with amino acids
Low nutrient intake:	
Anorexia	Treatment of reversible causes of anorexia
Impaired gastric emptying	Increasing the dosage of dialysis solution
Altered taste sensation	Prokinetic agents
Unpalatable diet	Nutritional counseling
Inadequate clearance of anorexigens	30-35 kcal/kg/day
Intercurrent illness	1.2 g of protein/kg/day
Emotional distress	Nutrient and vitamin supplements
Impaired ability to procure, prepare, or ingest food	Dialysis solutions with amino acids
Comorbidity	Treatment of comorbid illnesses
Chronic inflammation	Extracellular fluid volume control
	Antiinflammatory drugs (in the future)
Metabolic acidosis	Correction of acidosis
Loss of residual kidney function	Renin angiotensin aldosterone system inhibitors
	High-dose furosemide (urine volume)
	Avoidance of nephrotoxins
Conditions with possible role(s):	
Endocrine disorders of uremia	Recombinant growth hormone
Fast peritoneal membrane transport	Correction of anemia and comorbid conditions
Occult gastrointestinal bleeding	

is 35 kcal per kilogram of body weight per day for those younger than 60 years and 30 to 35 kcal/kg/day for those 60 years or older.[229] Nevertheless, the presence of obesity may modify our prescription accordingly, because in some PD recipients a reduced intake is preferred in order to limit overweight increase or even to induce weight loss. Energy intake in patients on PD, in addition to dietary intake, should take in account glucose absorbed from the dialysate, which depends on factors such as peritoneal transport, volume, dwell time, and glucose concentration. Energy from dialysate on average is around 20% of the total energy intake, corresponding to 3 to 13 kcal/kg/day.[238] In relation to protein intake, no less than 1.2 g/kg (≥50% of proteins with high biologic value) is the daily recommendation for adults on PD, and in some specific instances of severe protein-energy wasting it should be higher.[229] It is important to point out that actual protein and energy intake of PD recipients is often considerably lower than recommended and that anorexia and dysgeusia could be contributing to this situation.[229]

Intensive nutritional support may be of value during hypercatabolic conditions, including episodes of peritonitis. However, the effect of counseling on the nutritional status of affected patients remains largely untested. One report suggested that nutritional counseling, as an isolated measure, may maintain nutritional status despite a decrease in RKF and higher rates of systemic inflammation.[239] Administration of oral nutritional supplements may contribute to improvement of nutritional status; however, published data are scarce, and very few controlled clinical trials have involved commercially available supplements or dry egg albumin–based supplements as a nutritional intervention.[240-243] Major drawbacks of commercial oral nutrient supplements are the cost and difficulty to ensure sustained adherence, which may preclude their long-term and broad use.

DIALYSIS SOLUTIONS WITH AMINO ACIDS

Management of protein-energy wasting with the available PD solutions has been poorly explored and seems to require a personalized prescription.[244] The use of amino acids has been explored, and in few randomized trials conducted to date, anthropometric and biochemical measures have been better preserved in some but not all treated patients.[245] The potential benefits of amino acid–based dialysate may be greater when it is combined with provision of sources of energy, either orally or with glucose in dialysate. However, hard end points such as technique survival, hospitalization, and quality of life have yet to be studied in well-designed trials.

REVERSIBLE CAUSES OF ANOREXIA

Increasing the dosage of dialysis solution to correct anorexia is an approach often attempted but found to be ineffective in large randomized trials.[191,213,221] Gastroparesis is a frequent complication in patients on PD, particularly, but not exclusively among those with diabetes[246]; correction of gastroparesis may increase dietary intake and reduce nausea and vomiting. The use of prokinetic agents (e.g., metoclopramide, erythromycin) has been reported to increase serum albumin concentration in hypoalbuminemic patients on dialysis with delayed gastric emptying.[247]

METABOLIC ACIDOSIS

Given that acidosis induces protein catabolism, correction of acidosis with oral alkali has been a measure to improve nutritional status (see Chapter 61). In a randomized trial conducted among patients on PD, oral sodium bicarbonate supplementation resulted in a significant increase in the plasma bicarbonate concentration along with improvements in some anthropometric measurements and nutritional status (evaluated by subjective global assessment); this response in turn was associated with shorter hospitalization period and reduced morbidity.[248]

ANABOLIC HORMONES

An anabolic strategy is to administer recombinant growth hormone. Its administration has been reported to be effective in improving nutritional parameters in short-term studies and seems to be particularly appealing for children; however, its use is limited by cost and the development of hyperglycemia and other side effects.[249] Similar results have been observed with the use of insulin-like growth factor-1.[250] In addition, in small randomized trials, androgenic (anabolic) steroids have been shown to improve some parameters of nutritional status, yet significant risks and side effects preclude their use in clinical practice.[251] Ghrelin is a protein hormone synthesized by gastric endocrine cells and involved in regulation of food ingestion and energy metabolism. Patients on PD have lower ghrelin concentrations than patients on hemodialysis or controls.[252] Although ghrelin, administered subcutaneously, enhances short-term food intake in patients with mild to moderate protein-energy wasting, further studies are necessary to determine the therapeutic role of this hormone.[253] Other hormones and cytokines, such as leptin, tumor necrosis factor-α (TNF-α), and IL-6, all of which have been found to be elevated in patients undergoing maintenance dialysis, could participate in the loss of appetite present in patients on PD.[254]

L-CARNITINE

Advanced chronic kidney disease is associated with abnormal L-carnitine metabolism. Although results of some studies have suggested that L-carnitine has an erythropoietin-sparing effect in the management of anemia in patients on hemodialysis, data demonstrating a salutary effect of L-carnitine on nutritional status are insufficient.[255-257] In the case of PD, it is currently unclear whether the abnormalities in L-carnitine metabolism have a role in the genesis or treatment of protein-energy wasting. DeVecchi and associates review the role of L-carnitine in PD as a nutritional supplement and offer extensive discussion of its role as a potential osmotic agent.[258]

INFLAMMATION AND PERITONEAL DIALYSIS

An inflammatory phenomenon evidenced by increased proinflammatory cytokines and acute phase reactants is observed in 12% to 65% of patients with chronic kidney disease before they start dialysis, and it is aggravated with both PD and hemodialysis.[259,260] Systemic inflammation is strongly related to atherosclerosis and protein-energy wasting.[259] Local intraperitoneal inflammation induces important structural alterations, including thickening and cubic transformation of mesothelial cells, fibrin deposition, fibrous capsule formation, perivascular bleeding, and interstitial fibrosis, and is associated with peritoneal solute transfer rate.[87] These structural alterations induce clinical and functional changes, including ultrafiltration failure, which can occur in a large proportion of patients on long-standing PD.[261]

In the stable patient on PD without active peritonitis or other infection, several conditions may be implicated in the origin of systemic inflammation, including the use of biocompatible dialysis solutions.[262] Additional factors, such as rapid peritoneal membrane transport, reduced RKF, and overhydration, have also been associated with inflammation.[86,263,264] The interaction among uremia, protein-energy wasting, CVD, and loss of RKF and peritoneal membrane function, however, continues to be incompletely understood.[265] It is clear, and there is a universal consensus, that systemic inflammation, independently or in combination with all the variables mentioned previously, is an important factor in predicting morbidity and mortality.[232,262,266,267]

There is a strong association among fluid overload, cardiac natriuretic hormones, and proinflammatory cytokines.[268] Adequate control of the hypervolemia may reduce a heightened inflammatory state, particularly in patients with high transport rates. When hypervolemia was ameliorated by NIPD in PD recipients with high and high-average transport rates, a reduction of serum C-reactive protein and IL-6 was observed.[269]

Results of small studies indicate that agents such as thiazolidinediones and statins may have relevant antiinflammatory effects, but the effect is modest.[270,271] Angiotensin-converting enzyme (ACE) inhibitors may suppress C-reactive protein and oxidized low-density lipoprotein (LDL) cholesterol in patients with diabetes, but they do not appear to reduce inflammation in patients on hemodialysis.[272,273] In contrast, some evidence has been generated to support the idea that inhibition of the renin angiotensin aldosterone system (RAAS) may have an antiinflammatory effect on the peritoneal membrane.[274]

At present, there are no studies testing the impact of treatment for chronic non–dialysis-related infections (*Chlamydia pneumoniae, Helicobacter pylori,* dental-gingival infections, and viral hepatitis) on the inflammatory status of PD recipients. The development of drugs targeting specific mediators of the inflammatory response, such as IL-6 and TNF, may hold promise for the future.

RESIDUAL KIDNEY FUNCTION AND PERITONEAL DIALYSIS

PD is associated with preservation of RKF and has been consistently shown to preserve RKF longer than hemodialysis.[275] PD may be better at preserving RKF in part because, in comparison with hemodialysis, PD is associated with less hemodynamic instability and less frequent volume depletion, and its use avoids the extracorporeal system of hemodialysis that serves as sources of systemic inflammation, oxidative stress, and subsequent kidney injury. The use of ultrapure dialysate and biocompatible membranes in hemodialysis may reduce sources of inflammation during hemodialysis and are two strategies that could be employed to help attenuate the decline in RKF observed in hemodialysis.[276] Some factors that have been associated with a loss of RKF in PD are female sex, presence of diabetes mellitus, and nonwhite race; the associated comorbid conditions include congestive heart failure, poorly controlled hypertension, coronary artery disease, and, probably, long-term aminoglycoside use.[277-280]

Multiple cohort studies have confirmed a positive association between the presence and degree of RKF and survival in patients on PD.[210,281,282] Subsequent studies have consistently shown an association between loss of RKF and increased risk for volume overload, left ventricular hypertrophy, and congestive heart failure, all of which are considered surrogate end points for survival.[283,284] The improved survival observed in PD recipients with better-preserved RKF has been postulated to result from several factors, including renal clearance of circulating proinflammatory cytokines and middle molecular weight uremic toxins (e.g., *p*-cresol) that are otherwise poorly removed with dialysis alone; improved anemia management due to persistent endogenous erythropoietin production; and preserved renal salt and water excretion, which allows better maintenance of euvolemia and normotension.[283,284] Additionally, preserved RKF allows for better maintenance of normal bone mineral metabolism; RKF loss in PD recipients is associated with higher serum phosphate concentrations and higher serum fibroblast growth factor 23 (FGF-23) levels (independent of serum phosphorus), both of which have been implicated in increased arterial stiffening and valvular calcification and, hence, increased cardiovascular mortality.[285] Loss of RKF per se is associated with greater valvular calcification and cardiac hypertrophy.[286]

Nutritional status, which is strongly related to the presence of inflammation, is better maintained in the presence of RKF.[232,287] Appetite and intake of both macronutrients and micronutrients are linked to better-preserved RKF.[232,267] Moreover, anuric patients seem to have higher resting energy expenditure than patients with RKF, which may partially explain the superior nutritional status seen in the latter group.[288] Better nutrition has been linked to a stronger immune system, and indeed, incident PD recipients with RKF have been shown to have lower rates of peritonitis and peritonitis-related mortality than anuric patients.[287,289] The strategy of preferentially using PD as the initial dialysis modality in patients with RKF is intriguing and deserves additional investigation; small studies seem to show a survival advantage for some patients who initiate PD therapy and subsequently transfer to hemodialysis therapy in comparison with matched hemodialysis-only patients.[290-292]

MEASURES TO PRESERVE RESIDUAL KIDNEY FUNCTION

The effect of PD modality (i.e., CAPD versus APD) on RKF preservation has been investigated in numerous studies.[178] Although some reports suggest that APD is associated with a more rapid decline of RKF than CAPD, in spite of similar peritoneal ultrafiltration volumes, the preponderance of evidence suggests that PD modality has no effect on RKF.[178]

High-dose furosemide has been shown to preserve urinary volume, increase sodium removal, and decrease weight gain better than placebo, without an independent effect on RKF per se.[293] On the other hand, hypovolemia and hypotension have been shown to be independent risk factors for the RKF loss; thus special care is needed to achieve a safe balance between extracellular fluid volume overload and the hypovolemia caused by overzealous diuresis and ultrafiltration.

Biocompatible PD fluids have been hypothesized to be less glomerulotoxic than conventional glucose-based solutions because they contain fewer GDPs and lead to less formation of advanced glycosylation end products (AGEs) than traditional PD solutions. Circulating GDPs and their byproducts, AGEs, are mediators of inflammation, fibrosis, and glomerular injury in diabetic nephropathy and a similar process is thought to induce kidney injury in PD recipients who are exposed to GDP-containing glucose-based PD solutions. When intraperitoneal GDPs and AGEs lead to increased levels of circulating AGEs, kidney injury and RKF decline follow.[294] Several studies comparing low-GDP/neutral pH PD solutions with standard PD solutions found higher renal clearance rates and higher urine volumes in patients exposed to the former. Importantly, three of these studies reported less peritoneal ultrafiltration with the low-GDP than with the standard PD solution, suggesting that increased urine volumes in the former resulted from hypervolemia, which in turn resulted from decreased peritoneal ultrafiltration volumes.[162,164,295] The results of the studies examining the effects of this solution on RKF are heterogenous, but the summary evidence seems to suggest a higher urine volume, particularly with long-term treatment.[159] The impact of icodextrin on RKF is less controversial, in that summary evidence suggested no effect of treatment with this solution on RKF.[140]

In patients with chronic kidney disease, RAAS blockade has an established role in slowing progression of renal disease. In prevalent patients on PD, two small randomized controlled trials have shown that use of ACE inhibitors and angiotensin receptor blockers (ARBs) promote preservation of RKF in comparison with control conditions.[296,297] Avoidance of nephrotoxins such as nonsteroidal antiinflammatory drugs and aminoglycosides seems logical for maintenance of RKF. One small prospective observational study showed a greater decline in RKF after at least 3 days of aminoglycoside use for peritonitis treatment, in comparison with no aminoglycoside.[298] A subsequent observational study in a larger group of patients was unable to find any significant difference in RKF decline between those patients who did and did not receive an aminoglycoside for peritonitis treatment[299]; similarly, no adverse effect of aminoglycosides on RKF was found in a randomized control trial of netilmicin versus ceftazidime for the treatment of peritonitis.[280] Studies on the effect of intravenous contrast dye on RKF in PD patients have also shown limited evidence for harm to RKF.[300]

CARDIOVASCULAR DISEASE IN PERITONEAL DIALYSIS

Cardiovascular disease—including new-onset cardiac failure, peripheral vascular disease, ischemic heart disease, sudden cardiac death, and stroke—is common among patients with ESKD.[301] Moreover, patients on PD have a remarkably high risk of dying from myocardial infarction, arrhythmias, and valvular disease and for sudden cardiac death.[302] Vascular and valvular calcification, volume overload with resultant left ventricular hypertrophy, inflammation, and accelerated atherosclerosis all contribute to cardiovascular mortality in patients with ESKD.[303]

The interplay of many pathways may underlie the development of CVD in patients on PD. These pathways include traditional risk factors (diabetes mellitus, hypertension, dyslipidemia, sedentary lifestyle, left ventricular hypertrophy, smoking, male sex, insulin resistance), uremia-specific factors (anemia, phosphate retention, vascular calcification, uremic toxins, volume overload, hyperparathyroid), novel risk factors (inflammation, oxidative stress, endothelial dysfunction, activation of the sympathetic nervous system, wasting, carbamylation of proteins, epigenetic changes), and genetic factors.[304] Additionally, there are factors specific to PD that increase cardiovascular risk. For example, hypokalemia (more common with PD than hemodialysis) has been demonstrated to confer an increased risk of death in PD recipients; similarly, overhydration and loss of RKF have each been associated with increased risk for CVD in patients on PD.[94,191,210,281,306,307]

MANAGEMENT OF CARDIOVASCULAR DISEASE IN PERITONEAL DIALYSIS

Hypertension is a well-recognized risk factor for CVD in the general population. The relationship between hypertension per se and CVD in dialysis recipients is complex owing to the myriad comorbidities seen in the ESKD population. Although short-term studies have found a weak or even inverse relationship between hypertension and CVD in ESKD, longer-term studies have found benefit in control of hypertension in PD recipients.[308,309] Volume overload is a major cause of hypertension in such patients, particularly when ultrafiltration capacity is insufficient to maintain normotension after RKF declines. It is thus of utmost importance to routinely monitor urine volumes over time and to adjust PD prescriptions promptly when needed to compensate for loss of RKF. Patients with high peritoneal membrane transport rates should be evaluated for cycler therapy and/or icodextrin use during the long dwell time, to reduce the risk of volume overload.

Glucose-containing PD solutions contribute to CVD both by increasing a patients' exposure to GDPs (and hence, circulating AGEs) and by possibly inducing insulin resistance, which is associated with greater cardiovascular morbidity.[310,311] Thiazolidinediones can be used to modulate insulin resistance, but the published evidence in favor of their use is still scarce.[312] Exercise including strength training may improve glucose tolerance in ESKD with impaired glucose tolerance.[313,314] Non-glucose PD solutions are another potential solution to this problem: lower serum insulin levels and increased insulin sensitivity have been reported with Icodextrin.[315,316] The role of glucose-sparing regimens is discussed earlier in the chapter.

Hyperlipidemia due to systemic glucose absorption and peritoneal protein losses potentially contribute to the observation of higher levels of total and LDL cholesterol, apolipoprotein B, lipoprotein (a), and triglycerides and lower levels of high-density lipoprotein (HDL) cholesterol in patients on PD than in patients on hemodialysis.[317] As in the general population, statins safely decrease cholesterol levels in dialysis but their efficacy in reducing the cardiovascular mortality rate has not yet been proven.[318] However, the Study of Heart and Renal Protection (SHARP) included patients who were undergoing treatment with PD at the time of enrollment or initiated therapy with the modality during the course of the trial.[319] The study demonstrated a lower risk for cardiovascular events in patients treated with simvastatin-ezetimibe but no effect on cardiovascular mortality.[319] Further studies should provide more insight about the efficacy of statins in reducing mortality among dialysis recipients, particularly in those on PD, for whom virtually no information is available.

Vascular calcification, affecting the arterial media, atherosclerotic plaques, myocardium, and heart valves, is a common feature in patients with ESKD and is associated with CVD and mortality in patients on dialysis, including those treated with PD.[320] Moreover, cardiac valve calcifications are more frequent in patients on PD who have inflammation and are associated with a sixfold higher risk of cardiovascular death.[321] In patients on hemodialysis, therapy with sevelamer, a non-calcium phosphate binder, results in smaller increases in vascular calcification scores in comparison with calcium-based binders, although the long-term effect on patient survival is uncertain.[322]

Genetic factors may also affect the risk of vascular complications and outcome in the PD population. Examples are (1) the finding that a single nucleotide polymorphism in the IL-6 gene is associated with higher plasma levels of IL-6, higher diastolic blood pressure, and higher left ventricular mass and (2) the finding that non–BB allele variants of the BsmI polymorphism of the vitamin D receptor gene are associated with increased risk of hypercalcemia.[323,324] The clinical relevance of these associations, however, remains uncertain at this time.

PERITONITIS

DEFINITION, DIAGNOSIS, AND CLINICAL COURSE

The presence of a cloudy peritoneal effluent is often the earliest sign of peritonitis, although abdominal pain precedes it in some patients. A diagnosis of peritonitis in the patient on PD can be established when at least two of the following manifestations are present: abdominal pain, positive result of a peritoneal fluid culture, and more than 100 white blood cells (leukocytes) per mm^3 of the dialysis effluent.[325,326] Although turbid effluent is not always associated with peritonitis, its presence should always be considered a sign of possible infection until proven otherwise. When the peritoneal fluid culture result is negative and the effluent leukocyte count is normal, other causes for the cloudy effluent should be considered, including fibrin, chylous ascites, malignancy, chemical or eosinophilic peritonitis, and a specimen taken from a dry peritoneum.[326-331] The presence of more than 10% eosinophils in a cloudy effluent is diagnostic of eosinophilic peritonitis. The condition may manifest early after catheter placement or may be associated with mycotic infections, allergic reactions, and exposure to drugs such as vancomycin.[332,333]

The most common pathway for invasion of the peritoneal cavity by infectious agents is through the catheter's lumen; the next most common is the periluminal route.[334] Transmural bacterial migration has been implicated as another cause of PD-related peritonitis in patients with constipation, diarrhea, recent colonoscopy, diverticulitis, or other bowel pathology. Carriage of *Staphylococcus aureus* in the nasal mucosa and skin is linked to exit site and catheter-related infections.[335] When purulent exudate is present at the exit site, a swab culture should be performed. Other less common routes of infection are hematogenous spread, due to either active bacteremia or transient bacteremia after periodontal procedures, and ascending bacterial spread from the female genital tract. The incubation period of a peritonitis episode varies depending on the route of infection and the specific organism; for example, touch contamination has been reported to cause symptoms between 6 and 48 hours later.[336] The severity of clinical manifestations is also variable and may be related to the specific causal agent. *Staphylococcus epidermidis* infections in general cause milder symptoms than infections with gram-negative organisms, *S. aureus*, and mycotic organisms.[325,337] Unlike surgical or spontaneous peritonitis, PD-related peritonitis is rarely associated with bacteremia.

Bacterial peritonitis typically manifests as a peritoneal effluent leukocyte count exceeding 100 cells/mm^3 with a leukocyte predominance (effluent neutrophils account for more than 50% of the total leukocyte count). Adequate cultures of peritoneal effluent samples should yield positive results in more than 80% of cases. If a high rate of culture-negative peritonitis is present in a dialysis center, peritoneal culture methods should be reviewed and optimized. The simplest way to obtain peritoneal fluid cultures is by inoculating 5 to 10 mL of effluent directly into a blood culture bottle; the sample should be sent to the laboratory within 6 hours or less for best results. Another culture method involves inoculating 50 mL of centrifuged dialysate into a solid culture media; conflicting reports are unable to confirm which method leads to lower rates of culture-negative peritonitis.[338-340]

Gram stain preparations of PD effluent are notoriously insensitive methods of detecting bacteria, being useful mainly for early identification of yeast (see later discussion of fungal peritonitis).[336] Inadequate effluent collection can cause low leukocyte counts despite clinical symptoms of peritonitis; this occurrence is more common in APD owing to short dwell times. If indicative symptoms are present without effluent leukocytosis, cultures and cell counts should be repeated after a dwell period of at least 2 hours. The differential diagnosis of culture-negative peritonitis with dialysate leukocytosis includes inadequate sample collection or laboratory processing, previous antibiotic treatment, and the presence of fungi or mycobacteria.[325]

In spite of double-bag systems substituting for spike connections, the most prevalent organism in most reported series is still gram-positive bacteria, particularly *S. epidermidis* acquired through touch contamination. Pathogenic flora may vary significantly according to geographic and other environmental circumstances.[334,341,342] The second most frequent bacterial cause of PD peritonitis is *S. aureus*, often associated with tunnel or exit site infection; compared with peritonitis due to *S. epidermidis*, that due to *S. aureus* may cause more severe disease and more often lead to catheter loss and the need to transfer temporarily or permanently to hemodialysis.[343,344] Enterococci are the third most commonly encountered agents of gram-positive peritonitis; they typically respond to antimicrobial treatment, but care must be taken to review bacterial sensitivity patterns because vancomycin-resistant strains are not uncommon.[345] Constipation and other bowel pathology may predispose to enterococcal infections, which frequently cause recurrent and relapsing peritonitis.[346]

Although gram-positive organisms are the most common cause of PD peritonitis, the proportion of infections due to gram-negative organisms has increased over the past 20 years.[347,348] A variety of organisms derived from bowel, skin, urinary tract, water sources, and animal contact have been reported to cause gram-negative peritonitis. *Escherichia coli* strains and other Enterobacteriaceae such as *Klebsiella* and *Proteus* species pose a serious problem, particularly in developing nations, but in most cases they respond to antibiotic regimens. *Pseudomonas* peritonitis accounts for approximately 8% to 10% of gram-negative peritonitis cases and frequently necessitates catheter removal. Early catheter removal, temporary transfer to hemodialysis with peritoneal cavity rest, and dual-antipseudomonal antibiotic coverage are all associated with better outcomes. *Pseudomonas* species are also commonly associated with exit site and tunnel infections.[336,349-351]

Multiorganism gram-negative peritonitis should prompt consideration of a primary abdominal pathologic process, such as diverticulitis or an intraabdominal abscess; however, most patients with polymicrobial peritonitis do not have an underlying abdominal catastrophe.[352] In cases of bowel perforation, fecal effluent may be evident and anaerobes are often present. The mortality rate in cases secondary to an abdominal catastrophe may be as high as 50% and is correlated with the primary event as well as with delays in diagnosis and surgery.[353]

Fungal peritonitis occurs rarely but is always feared because of high mortality rates; early removal of the peritoneal catheter is required.[354] The species most frequently involved is *Candida albicans*; the concurrent presence of bowel obstruction and abdominal pain portend worse outcomes. It has been postulated that current or recent antibacterial treatment may increase the risk for fungal peritonitis; systemic antibiotics (for peritonitis or even non-PD infections) are thought to suppress normal bowel flora, allowing intestinal overgrowth of fungi; fungal peritonitis then results in some patients after fungal mural transmigration into the peritoneum.[355]

Peritonitis due to mycobacteria is very rare; in most instances, it is initially diagnosed as culture-negative peritonitis. Diagnosis requires adequate culture techniques and a high index of suspicion. In mycobacterial infections, leukocyte counts may exhibit a predominance of monocytes or lymphocytes in the peritoneal effluent.[325,356] Acid-fast smear preparations are notoriously insensitive, and mycobacterial cultures require days to weeks of incubation time. Polymerase chain reaction techniques have been useful in detecting tuberculous gene products in peritoneal fluid, and there are reports of retrospective diagnosis either after peritoneal biopsy (at the time of catheter removal) or after empirical antimycobacterial therapy led to a clinical resolution of the infection. In areas that are endemic for tuberculosis, tuberculosis peritonitis may account for up to 4% of all infections and carries a high morbidity, particularly in patients with protein-energy wasting.[357,358]

TREATMENT

Empirical antibiotic treatment should be started as soon as infectious peritonitis is diagnosed. Peritoneal fluid leukocytosis is sufficient cause to initiate antimicrobial therapy, and treatment should start without delay even if culture results are pending.[325] Antibiotic regimens should be tailored to culture and sensitivity reports once available; center-specific bacterial sensitivity patterns should be taken into consideration in the choice of antimicrobial therapy. Cloudy effluent and abdominal pain usually improve early in the course of treatment and may disappear within 48 to 72 hours. Persistent clinical manifestations of peritonitis may indicate a nonresponding bacterial organism, necessitating prompt change in antibiotic treatment or consideration of catheter removal.[325] Follow-up effluent cell counts are useful tools to evaluate treatment response because prolonged peritoneal fluid leukocytosis is associated with a higher rate of treatment failure and need for catheter removal.[359-361]

INITIAL EMPIRICAL THERAPY

Ideal empirical peritonitis treatment should provide broad antimicrobial coverage for the most common causes, should be convenient to administer, and should not favor the development of resistant organisms.[362] Such a perfect regimen does not exist. Selection of empirical therapy should be center-specific, depending on the local history of sensitivities of organisms. Empirical antibiotics must cover both gram-positive and gram-negative organisms. The latest international guidelines, based on evidence when available, include a regimen containing a cephalosporin or vancomycin for gram-positive bacteria together with either a third-generation cephalosporin, such as ceftazidime or cefepime, or an aminoglycoside; the latter may be preferable in patients with no RKF because the nephrotoxic effects of aminoglycosides may be a concern, although some reports suggest that short-term may not harm RKF (see preceding section on RKF).[325] Vancomycin is highly effective against most gram-positive bacteria, but its use has raised discussions about whether it favors the appearance of vancomycin-resistant staphylococci and enterococci.[363] Drug-resistant *S. aureus* and *Enterococcus* strains may necessitate administration of newer agents, such as linezolid, quinupristin/dalfopristin, imipenem/cilastatin, and daptomycin.[364]

Changing microbiologic features, toxic effects of drugs, or difficulties administering therapy may lead individual groups to tailor the initial antimicrobial regimen to their own patients' needs. There is evidence from several prospective studies that monotherapy with different agents (aztreonam, oral quinolones, cefepime) may be efficacious, but results are controversial.[364]

Antibiotic dosages should be determined from the patient's weight and RKF; when dosages are not adjusted for these factors, there is a considerable risk for underdosing with resulting treatment failure.

ROUTE AND SCHEDULE OF ADMINISTRATION

Antibiotics can be administered by different routes (e.g., oral, intraperitoneal, intravenous). Intraperitoneal (IP) administration is preferred to intravenous (IV) infusion; IP administration produces a greater concentration of antibiotics locally at the infection site, is easy to administer, and has been demonstrated to be superior in a meta-analysis of randomized controlled trials (Table 66.8).[364] According to this analysis, intermittent administration (once a day in a long dwell of at least 6 hours) and continuous administration (dosage with each exchange) of antibiotics are equally efficacious in CAPD, and there is no benefit for routine peritoneal lavage or use of urokinase.[365] Antibiotic dosing and interval

Table 66.8 Intraperitoneal Antibiotic Dosing Recommendations for Patients on Continuous Ambulatory Peritoneal Dialysis*

Drug	Intermittent (per Exchange, Once Daily)	Continuous (mg/L†; All Exchanges)
Aminoglycosides		
Amikacin	2 mg/kg	LD 25, MD 12
Gentamicin, netilmicin, or tobramycin	0.6 mg/kg	LD 8, MD 4
Cephalosporins		
Cefazolin, cephalothin, or cephradine	15 mg/kg	LD 500, MD 125
Cefepime	1000 mg	LD 500, MD 125
Ceftazidime	1000-1500 mg	LD 500, MD 125
Ceftizoxime	1000 mg	LD 250, MD 125
Penicillins		
Amoxicillin	ND	LD 250-500, MD 50
Ampicillin, oxacillin, or nafcillin	ND	MD 125
Azlocillin	ND	LD 500, MD 250
Penicillin G	ND	LD 50,000 U, MD 25,000 U
Quinolones		
Ciprofloxacin	ND	LD 50, MD 25
Other Antibacterials		
Aztreonam	ND	LD 1000, MD 250
Daptomycin[117]	ND	LD 200, MD 20
Linezolid[41]	Oral 200-300 mg qd	
Teicoplanin	15 mg/kg	LD 400, MD 20
Vancomycin	15-30 mg/kg every 5-7 days	LD 1000, MD 25
Antifungals		
Amphotericin	NA	1.5
Fluconazole	200 mg intraperitoneally every 24-48 hours	
Combinations		
Ampicillin/sulbactam	2 g every 12 hours	LD 1000, MD 100
Imipenem/cilastatin	1 g bid	LD 250, MD 50
Quinupristin/dalfopristin	25 mg/L in alternate bags‡	
Trimethoprim/sulfamethoxazole	Oral 960 mg bid	

*For dosing of drugs with renal clearance in patients with residual renal function (defined as >100 mL/day urine output), dosage should be empirically increased by 25%.
†Except as noted.
‡Given in conjunction with 500 mg intravenously twice daily.
LD, Loading dose; MD, maintenance dose; NA, not applicable; ND, no data.
From Li PK-T, Szeto CC, Piraino B, et al: Peritoneal dialysis-related infections recommendations: 2010 update, Perit Dial Int. 30:393-423, 2010.

Table 66.9 Intermittent Administration of Antibiotics in Automated Peritoneal Dialysis

Drug	Intraperitoneal Dosage
Cefazolin	20 mg/kg every day, in long daytime dwell[69]
Cefepime	1 g in one exchange per day
Fluconazole	200 mg in one exchange per day every 24-48 hours
Tobramycin	Loading dose, 1.5 mg/kg in long dwell; then 0.5 mg/kg each day in long dwell[69]
Vancomycin	Loading dose, 30 mg/kg in long dwell; repeat 15 mg/kg in long dwell every 3-5 days (aim to keep serum trough levels above 15 µg/mL)

of administration in APD have not been sufficiently studied for all available regimens. The latest guidelines acknowledge the lack of evidence for adequate antibiotic prescription in APD, and guidelines are available for intermittent dosing of antibiotics for APD recipients (Table 66.9); nevertheless, they propose continuous dosing particularly of cephalosporins for this modality.[325] Cephalosporins and aminoglycosides could be administered intermittently in the long-dwell daytime exchange.[366,367] Vancomycin is administered intermittently every 3 to 6 days according to the patient's own drug metabolism, and blood levels may be monitored to guide therapy. Because vancomycin efficacy is time dependent, care should be taken to keep therapeutic blood levels above the bacteria's minimum inhibitory concentration (MIC) for as long as possible during the entire dosing interval. Researchers recommend keeping the peak blood drug value at five to eight times the MIC and the trough blood drug value one to two times the MIC.[368]

SPECIFIC ANTIBIOTIC TREATMENT

Once the results of the peritoneal effluent culture are known, if the initial empirical treatment is inadequate, it should be adjusted and the response monitored.

Gram-Positive Bacteria

Coagulase-negative staphylococci usually respond rapidly to treatment and are adequately eradicated with the initially prescribed cefazolin or vancomycin administered for 2 weeks.[325] Treatment of *S. aureus* peritonitis can continue with a first-generation cephalosporin if the organism is methicillin sensitive, or with vancomycin if it is methicillin resistant. In the rare occurrence of vancomycin-resistant *S. aureus*, linezolid, daptomycin, or quinupristin/dalfopristin should be prescribed. *S. aureus* infections should be treated for 3 weeks, even if a clinical response is seen early in the infection's course. In the presence of an exit site infection by the same microorganism, the catheter often must be removed.[325,343-345] If enterococcal peritonitis is diagnosed, intraperitoneal ampicillin and an aminoglycoside are indicated, or vancomycin in the case of ampicillin-resistant enterococci.[325]

Gram-Negative Bacteria

Nonpseudomonal gram-negative enterobacteria usually respond to third-generation cephalosporins or aminoglycosides; dual-antibiotic coverage may reduce the relapse and recurrence rate of certain gram-negative peritoneal infections.[349,351] *Pseudomonas aeruginosa* peritonitis should be treated with two antibiotics for 3 weeks; if clinical improvement is not seen promptly, catheter removal is indicated. In individuals with coexisting exit site infection with the same organism, catheter removal is recommended because of a high incidence of relapse even if there is clinical improvement with antibiotics alone.[325] Intraperitoneal aminoglycosides and third-generation cephalosporins, oral quinolones, and intravenous piperacillin have been employed with success in pseudomonal peritonitis.[353]

Polymicrobial Peritonitis

In the presence of multiple enteric organisms, catastrophic intraabdominal pathologic processes such diverticulitis and appendicitis should be considered, and if any is diagnosed, surgery should be performed.[353] Antibiotic treatment should include an aminoglycoside, a third-generation cephalosporin or carbapenem, and anaerobic coverage with metronidazole or clindamycin. Treatment should continue for at least 3 weeks.

Fungal Peritonitis

Fungal peritonitis is a highly lethal infection that responds poorly to antifungal agents if the catheter is not removed because the organism easily forms biofilm on the catheter, thus resulting in a permanent reservoir for the fungus.[354,355] Occasionally, patients with fungal peritonitis may be too ill for surgery or may refuse catheter removal. Small case reports describe successful treatment of fungal peritonitis without catheter removal through the use of a combination of systemic and IP antifungal therapy plus continuous high-dose intracatheter amphotericin B.[369] With regard to selection of antifungal agents, a combination of flucytosine and amphotericin B has traditionally been recommended; development of resistance is high with flucytosine so this agent should never be used alone. Newer and less toxic antifungal agents (e.g., voriconazole, fluconazole, and caspofungin) may be successful when chosen according to fungal culture results and antifungal sensitivity reports; infectious disease consultation can be helpful in choosing proper antifungal therapy in complicated situations.[325,355] Treatment typically continues for 2 weeks if the catheter is removed, or longer if the catheter is not removed.[325] Intraperitoneal abscess and adhesion formation are the most common reasons patients cannot return to PD after microbiologic cure.[370] Some authorities have advocated keeping the catheter in place for a short period to reduce the chance of adhesion formation.

Mycobacterial Peritonitis

Treatment of mycobacterial peritonitis requires a complex antibiotic regimen consisting of isoniazid, pyrazinamide, ofloxacin, and intraperitoneal rifampicin. Catheter removal may be required, and treatment with the four agents should commence as soon as possible, but definitely within 4 to 6 weeks of initial presentation, to produce the best outcomes. Treatment should continue for 6 to 9 months, incorporating an initial intense treatment with four drugs followed by a maintenance period with two antimycobacterial agents.[356,357]

CATHETER REMOVAL

In addition to fungal peritonitis, intraabdominal disease, and refractory tunnel and/or exit site infections, two other conditions warrant catheter removal: (1) relapsing peritonitis, defined as an episode with the same organism that caused the preceding episode of peritonitis, or one sterile peritonitis within 4 weeks after the end of the initial course of antibiotics, and (2) refractory peritonitis, defined as the failure to respond within 5 days of appropriate antibiotics. Catheter removal with simultaneous placement of a new catheter is most successful for exit site or tunnel infections and for relapsing infections but should not be done in refractory peritonitis or severe peritoneal infections.[371] Success is most common in infections that do not involve *S. aureus*, *Pseudomonas*, mycobacteria, or fungi; in these cases the patient should undergo hemodialysis until peritonitis is resolved (usually 3 to 4 weeks), and a new catheter placed at that time.[325]

PREVENTION

Adequate catheter placement is relevant for peritonitis prevention. Exit site placement and prophylactic antibiotic therapy at the time of placement, usually with a first-generation cephalosporin, is used to prevent postoperative infections. Postoperative care of the exit site is also important. Only when the exit site is healed should the patient take over its care. Mupirocin cream applied to the exit site has proved useful in preventing local *S. aureus* infection. Mupirocin applied to the nares 5 days a month is also effective in reducing *S. aureus* exit site infection. The use of local gentamicin has been shown to reduce rates of *Pseudomonas* and other gram-negative infections at the exit site as well as of peritonitis.[372] Adequate patient training is very important in preventing peritonitis episodes. The training of patients should include teaching them how to identify contamination and notify the dialysis facility that it has occurred; episodes of contamination can be managed with a change of peritoneal dialysis transfer set with or without administration of prophylactic antibiotics.[373] The use of double-bag systems in ambulatory patients and a flush-before-fill step after connection of the tubing to the solution bags in automated procedures are highly efficacious in preventing peritonitis episodes.[373-377]

NONINFECTIOUS COMPLICATIONS OF PERITONEAL DIALYSIS

MECHANICAL COMPLICATIONS

Intraperitoneal instillation of dialysate causes an increase in intraabdominal pressure, and the amount of intraabdominal pressure varies according to several factors, including age, body mass index, volume of dialysate, and patient position (intraabdominal pressure is greatest in the sitting position, less when standing, and least in the supine position).[378,379] Additionally, certain maneuvers, such as coughing, straining during defecation, and lifting, may further raise intraabdominal pressure. The major risks associated with increased intraperitoneal pressure are the development of hernias, pericatheter leaks, diaphragmatic leaks, restriction of pulmonary expansion with resultant dyspnea, gastroesophageal reflux, abdominal discomfort, and pain.[380]

Hernias occur in more than 10% of peritoneal dialysis patients and are related to increased intraperitoneal pressure of PD. Many hernias, particularly in the inguinal or periumbilical region, are present prior to start of PD and become more apparent with the intraperitoneal instillation of dialysate. There are several different types of hernias: umbilical, abdominal (ventral), incisional, and indirect inguinal. A preexisting but previously undetected patent processus vaginalis can suddenly become apparent as an inguinal hernia after initiation of PD owing to new dialysate flow into the hernia, causing genital swelling.[381] New hernias can form *de novo* at the catheter incision site, umbilicus, ventral abdominal wall, or inguinal area. Most hernias require surgical repair; however, a conservative treatment may be indicated for some, particularly in elderly patients. Surgical repair may be performed without temporary transfer to hemodialysis if the patient can be treated with low-volume supine exchanges; however, the need for surgery must be judged and decided on an individual basis.[381-383]

Pericatheter leaks may occur after dialysis initiation and are more common in obese patients. They may manifest as an external dialysate leak or as abdominal or genital edema. Conservative treatment, often successful, consists of reduction of inflow volume per exchange, NIPD, temporary PD postponement, and, if needed, temporary transfer to hemodialysis.[380,381,383-387] If leakage recurs, the catheter may require reinsertion.[383,351] A 3- to 4-week *break-in period,* defined as the time between catheter insertion and initial use, significantly reduces the risk of pericatheter leaks.[380,383]

Diaphragmatic leaks, due to preexisting diaphragmatic stoma, are uncommon and typically become clinically apparent soon after initiation of PD. The diagnosis of pleuroperitoneal fistula may be made with imaging techniques whereby contrast dye or radioactive isotope is instilled into the dialysate solution and is later found in the pleural space. Upright daytime-only dialysis (with an empty peritoneum at night) can be performed for very temporary relief, but ultimately, surgical correction or pleurodesis is needed to continue PD.

METABOLIC COMPLICATIONS

The most relevant metabolic complications associated with PD are related to the consequences of systemic glucose absorption. Absorption of glucose from PD solutions may provide 500 to 800 kcal/day.[387-391] Glucose absorption may induce hyperglycemia in previously nondiabetic PD patients with impaired glucose tolerance.[391] Treatment of hyperglycemia may be a complex clinical problem. Biguanides are contraindicated, as in all patients with ESKD, but other hypoglycemic agents, including some sulfonylureas and thiazolidinediones, may be used.[389] The latter have been associated with reduction of fibrosis through inhibition of inflammation and regulation of the transforming growth factor/SMAD signaling pathway.[392] Intraperitoneal insulin has been used in diabetic patients with CAPD because it appears convenient and physiologically beneficial, but it poses an important risk of contamination in the process of bag injection. Use of non–dextrose-containing PD fluids has been associated with improved glycemic control, as previously discussed in the section "Glucose-Sparing Regimens."

A second metabolic condition highly prevalent in patients on PD is the presence of hyperlipidemia, accompanied by high levels of LDL cholesterol and apolipoprotein B; this lipid profile may be atherogenic and may potentially contribute to the high cardiovascular mortality among patients on PD, although direct evidence of a link is lacking.[393] Patients may be treated with fibrates if hypertriglyceridemia is severe; statins are also used to lower levels of LDL cholesterol.[394] Combined use of these two agents is usually not recommended because of risk for rhabdomyolysis and hepatotoxicity, frequent side effects in patients with ESKD.

Mineral metabolism abnormalities are present in patients on PD, as in all patients with ESKD, but there are some differences in calcium and phosphate handling between patients on PD and those on hemodialysis. Hypercalcemia may occur in PD because of vitamin D use, high calcium levels in some peritoneal fluids (i.e., 3.5 mEq/L), and ingestion of calcium-based phosphate binders; this in turn may induce suppression of parathyroid hormone secretion, resulting in adynamic bone disease, a condition that has been reported to occur more frequently in PD than in hemodialysis.[370,395,396] The increased use of lower calcium dialysate (i.e., 2.5 mEq/L) and the use of non-calcium phosphate binders appears to have reduced the incidence of hypercalcemia in later PD cohorts. Phosphate control tends to be better in PD than in hemodialysis, probably because of better adherence to diet and/or binders in patients who have additionally assumed the responsibility for their own dialysis, the continuous nature of the dialytic procedure, and prolonged maintenance of RKF.[395-397] Nevertheless, similar associations between hyperphosphatemia and mortality are observed among patients on PD and hemodialysis.[398]

Among all dialysis recipients, patients on PD uniquely experience the complication of hypokalemia. Hypokalemia is not uncommon owing to the continuous nature of PD and the use of potassium-deficient dialysate; additionally, some clinicians advocate that low potassium intake and/or high doses of loop diuretics in PD recipients with RKF also contribute to hypokalemia. Hypokalemia has been identified as an adverse prognostic factor in patient survival and therefore should be corrected.[305,399] Fortunately, nearly all patients on PD can achieve normal serum potassium levels by increasing dietary intake of potassium-containing foods and/or oral potassium supplements. Hyperkalemia is less commonly encountered in PD than hypokalemia and is usually related to RAAS blockade, missed dialysis, or dietary excess. It is usually self-limited and not severe, as long as the patient is compliant with the dialysis prescription.

Hyponatremia is a common finding in patients on PD, partly because of fluid overload and the low dialysate sodium concentration, usually 132 mmol/L. Severe hyponatremia is infrequent and may be associated with hyperglycemia, protein-energy wasting, or water overload.[400,401] Hypernatremia is very rarely observed but may be present in older patients who have lost the sense of thirst or have limited access to water; a long series of frequent exchanges with very short dwell times using hypertonic dialysate can also lead to hypernatremia through the mechanism of sodium sieving, discussed earlier. This complication is easily avoided by allowing some longer dwell times throughout the 24-hour cycle, thus allowing sodium to reequilibrate between blood and dialysate.

ENCAPSULATING PERITONEAL SCLEROSIS

Encapsulating peritoneal sclerosis (EPS), one of the most feared complications of PD, is an uncommon but serious entity that is most often associated with longer time on PD; the cumulative incidence varies between 0.5% and 4.4%.[402,403] In this condition, massive sclerosis of the peritoneal membrane ensues, resulting in encapsulation of the intestines. Encapsulating peritoneal sclerosis is responsible for severe disturbances of intestinal function, manifesting as motility disorders that cause impaired nutrient absorption, obstructive ileus, hemorrhagic ascites, anorexia, weight loss, and progressive clinical deterioration. Systemic inflammation is usually present, manifested by low-grade fever, hypoalbuminemia, elevations of serum C-reactive protein, and other inflammatory markers. The diagnosis requires both clinical features of intestinal obstruction or disturbed gastrointestinal function and either radiologic or pathologic evidence of bowel encapsulation. Computed tomography (CT) has emerged as a reliable tool that in experienced hands can be used to confirm a diagnosis of EPS in an appropriate clinical setting.[404-408] Pathologic confirmation is available when patients are subjected to surgery for treatment or catheter removal.[409-411] However, care should be exercised because accidental injury to bowel may result in the formation of enterocutaneous fistula.

The cause of EPS is unknown, but a number of factors that may contribute or predispose to its development have been identified. Contributing factors can be divided into those directly related to PD (time on PD, peritonitis, plasticizers, bio-incompatible dialysate, discontinuation of PD) and those that are not (idiopathic, β-blockers, autoimmune diseases, cancer, talc or other particulate substances, genetic predisposition).[409,410] Unknown factors render patients more susceptible, inasmuch as the disease never develops in some patients even after continuous exposure to multiple predisposing conditions. The reported incidence is higher in some countries, particularly Japan and Australia, and an apparent increase in incidence has been reported in the European Union.[409,410,412] This increase may be related to ethnic or genetic factors, greater longevity of PD technique in certain areas, longer waiting times for kidney transplantation, or improved diagnosis and awareness of the disease. Among patients with a confirmed diagnosis, the mortality rate is very high, varying from 20% to more than 90%.[410,412] However, the survival in later cohorts appears considerably higher than in earlier reports.[403] This difference may be related to a greater recognition of the disease entity and diagnosis at an earlier stage than in previous years.

Treatment for EPS is often not successful and could even be described as ineffective, particularly if it is not implemented early in the course of the disease. There is no defined treatment of choice. Surgical treatment, which involves releasing or lysing adhesions of the small bowel, requires precision and expertise to avoid morbid outcomes such as enterocutaneous fistula.[413] Medical treatments are either supportive or therapeutic, the latter aimed at ameliorating the inflammatory and profibrotic processes in EPS. Total parenteral nutrition and discontinuation of PD with subsequent transfer to hemodialysis are often required; in some (but not all) instances, such treatment may induce regression of the pathogenic process.[409,410,412,414,415] One promising therapeutic option in EPS is the antifibrotic agent tamoxifen.[416] More than 14 published reports provide most of the available information regarding tamoxifen use in EPS but the majority of these are small case series[417]; randomized controlled trials are clearly needed although difficult to perform owing to the infrequency with which EPS occurs.[417] Prevention of EPS is not yet possible because clinicians do not understand the process that leads to this condition; nevertheless, early identification may be of great importance because early intervention is more effective than treatment later in the disease process.[409,412,414,415]

PATIENT OUTCOMES WITH PERITONEAL DIALYSIS

Optimal comparison of two therapies, such as hemodialysis and PD, requires adequately powered randomized controlled clinical trials. One such trial was attempted in the Netherlands but had to be abandoned because more than 90% of eligible patients refused to undergo randomization to different modalities.[418] Currently there is an ongoing clinical trial comparing the outcomes with these two dialysis modalities in China (clinicaltrials.gov identifier: NCT01413074). Until the results of this trial are available, the information available is based mainly on retrospective registries and a few prospective cohorts from around the world.[419-429]

Results of these studies are not conclusive, and discrepancies can be attributed to multiple factors, including methodologic issues such as use of intent-to-treat versus as-treated analysis, level of case-mix adjustments, use of proportional versus nonproportional hazards models, and assessment of prevalent versus incident patients.[430-432] In general, when these differences are accounted for, similar results for the two modalities are found among registry studies and, to a lesser degree, among prospective cohort studies.[426,428,429]

Nondiabetic and younger patients treated with PD have an equal or lower risk for death than those treated with hemodialysis; among older diabetic patients, results vary by country.[430] For example, the Canadian registry shows no difference in risk for death between PD and hemodialysis among older diabetic patients, whereas in the United States, older diabetic patients treated with hemodialysis have a lower risk for death than those treated with PD.[426] In Danish populations, one study demonstrates a lower risk for patients undergoing PD, which could be related to a cohort effect and to the mode of dialysis initiation.[433] In a large population-based study performed in Korea, patients with ESKD and CVD or diabetes who were treated with PD had a lower survival rate than those undergoing hemodialysis.[434] A recently published analysis of the French Renal Epidemiology and Information Network (REIN) Registry demonstrated that patients with congestive heart failure treated with hemodialysis had a lower risk for death than the ones treated with PD.[435] Similarly, the study of Wang and coworkers demonstrated that PD was associated with poorer survival among patients with ESKD and either CVD or diabetes mellitus in comparison with hemodialysis.[434] Despite the disparate findings, it remains unclear whether the differences in risk for death are a result of differences in patients treated with the two modalities or of a direct benefit (or harm) of the therapy itself.[431,432] Hence, these survival studies should inform but should not be central to the selection of dialysis modality for a particular patient.[436]

Multiple studies have demonstrated a time-dependent trend in the relative risk of death, whereby PD is generally associated with equivalent or better survival rates during the first 1 or 2 years of dialysis. An interesting European study has reported that PD recipients have a survival advantage during the first year and hemodialysis recipients have this advantage in the next 2 years of dialysis, yet the overall survival rates in the two groups were similar and influenced by age, presence or absence of diabetes mellitus, and dialysis center size.[437] Results of later studies seem to suggest that some of these differences occur from bias. Many patients who start treatment with hemodialysis have had inadequate preparation for dialysis, which in turn, is an independent risk factor for death.[438] When this source of bias is accounted for in data analysis, there does not seem to be significant differences in early survival between patients treated with PD and those treated with hemodialysis.[426,439,440]

In relation to long-term survival, results vary according to the nature of the study and to different subgroups within studies. Although subgroup analyses in the cohort studies have the advantages of being prospective and providers of more clinical and laboratory details, they are usually limited by smaller numbers of patients in comparison with larger registry-based studies.[423,441,442] On the other hand, large registry-based studies, although offering adequate statistical power for subgroup analyses, may be "overpowered" for detecting differences between the whole population of subjects on PD and those on hemodialysis. For instance, the overall relative risk of death in PD versus hemodialysis was 1.04 (95% confidence interval [CI], 1.03 to 1.06; $P < 0.001$) for U.S. Medicare recipients who initiated dialysis between 1995 and 2000[420]; this difference was statistically significant, in being powered by nearly 400,000 patients studied. However, this relative risk of 1.04 translates into an adjusted 3-year survival difference between hemodialysis and PD of only 1 month.[430] A general improvement in survival among patients with renal replacement therapy has been observed; these improvements seem to be greater for patients undergoing PD than for those treated with hemodialysis.[425,443] According to the United States Renal Data System (USRDS) *Annual Data Report 2013*, there is a continued trend to an improvement in survival in patients who began either hemodialysis or PD in comparison with those beginning therapy between 1993 and 1997 as well as for those beginning therapy between 1998 and 2002.[444] Data from other countries, in particular Japan those in Europe, have demonstrated better survival than data from the USRDS, results that were initially attributed to higher quality of treatment; however, multiple factors, including patients' comorbidities, age, and other factors, undoubtedly play an important role in these differences, making comparisons quite difficult.

In relation to technique failure, it is clear that this situation is more common in PD than in hemodialysis. According to data not accounting for transplantation and death, 7% to 15% of prevalent patients on PD experienced technique failure annually, most often because of peritonitis, catheter malfunction, "burn-out," and, in some long-term patients, ultrafiltration failure; such patients are transferred to hemodialysis.[445,446] This fact should not be regarded as a limitation of PD, because in an appropriate renal replacement therapy program, patients must be able to be readily transferred from one modality (PD, hemodialysis, or transplantation) to another according to medical and other needs.

In summary, to date there is no conclusive evidence that one modality is superior to the other in terms of survival rate for all patients with ESKD, yet some subpopulations seem to perform better with PD and others in general with hemodialysis. It is important to point out that an individualized and educated decision is of importance in choosing a renal replacement modality and may play a role in survival.[447] Appropriate clinical judgment, consideration of cultural factors, and informed patient's choice are factors that should be always taken into account in the choice of dialytic modality.

ECONOMICS AND COST-EFFECTIVENESS OF PERITONEAL DIALYSIS

ESKD is a growing global health concern, the treatment of which constitutes a financial challenge even for the developed world. According to the 2011 USRDS report, the overall Medicare expenditure for CKD treatment reached $34.3 billion.[430] The economics of dialysis is very complex, and dialysis cost may become or already is a threat to the health care systems of many countries.[448] In the industrialized world, PD has been shown to be less expensive than hemodialysis.[449-451] Most of the studies are either limited cost analyses or consider costs in relation to survival. Some studies have also shown that the cost-utility ratio is most favorable for PD.[452] In general, the cost continuum, from most to least expensive, is as follows: in-center hemodialysis, out-of-center hemodialysis (satellite, or self-care hemodialysis) similar to APD, home hemodialysis, and CAPD.

Several reasons may explain the lower cost of PD, including the fact that the patient or a helper administers dialysis, whereas hemodialysis must be performed by trained staff, which is relatively expensive. In addition, PD requires fewer physical resources than hemodialysis. Therefore, in countries with predominantly public dialysis providers, such as government-run hospitals (Great Britain, Canada, New Zealand, Hong Kong, and Mexico), the use of PD is much higher than in countries with mainly private providers, such as physicians' offices and franchise dialysis centers (United States, France, Germany, and Japan), in order to constrain ESKD expenditure.

Following are additional questions which may have a decisive economicaly based clinical impact. If PD is less costly, why do private providers prescribe it in a small percentage of cases? A number of factors may explain this phenomenon, but the underlying argument is that the economic drivers of modality selection in countries with mainly private providers are determined by the local economic features of the system and not by actual costs (hemodialysis is better reimbursed and more profitable).[453] In this situation, it is important to consider the following: (1) Once a hemodialysis unit is set up, there is economic pressure to maximize its efficiency by operating it at full capacity; (2) PD may cost less, but the payer (frequently the government) may reimburse expenses at a correspondingly lower level; and (3) in many countries with mainly private providers, hemodialysis offers more opportunity to bill for additional procedures (e.g., provision and administration of intravenous erythropoietin, vitamin D analogs, and iron).[453] An analysis of reimbursement policies and regulations in seven developed nations gives further insight into the complexity and diversity of factors that may influence dialysis modality selection and further stresses the need for better research in this area.[454] Changes in ESKD reimbursement policies in the United States, in which a system is in place that provides a bundled payment per person, per treatment, are expected to encourage an increase in the use of PD.[455]

An additional factor that significantly reduces the use of PD in some regions is a lack of adequate PD education and training in some nephrology programs, as a result of lack of expertise, interest, or economic incentive to promote PD growth. This situation has been reported as a significant factor that is limiting the development of PD in the United States.[456]

The economics of dialysis in developing nations differs from that of industrialized nations.[448] The lack of well-conducted economic evaluations in these countries makes it difficult to accurately understand the real basis of dialysis modality distribution. In developing nations, where labor is relatively inexpensive and the cost of imported equipment and solutions is high, PD may be more expensive than hemodialysis. A further negative aspect for PD therapy in developing nations is that treatment may still entail outdated intermittent systems, and sometimes transfer sets are even reused, with the consequent high rates of peritonitis, higher costs, and high dropout rates. Nevertheless, several published analyses disavow this perception, showing that PD treatment may be less expensive than hemodialysis in developing nations[457]; in fact, the local production of PD fluids and competition between different providers may influence the lowering of PD costs. Thus, the perception that PD is not a viable option for developing countries may be inappropriate. In countries where the cost of PD is lower than that of hemodialysis, an increased use of clinically appropriate PD provides an opportunity to substantially lower the overall cost of ESKD treatment, as is being demonstrated in some nations.[458,459]

Complete reference list available at ExpertConsult.com.

KEY REFERENCES

37. Krediet R: The physiology of peritoneal solute, water, and lymphatic transport. In Khanna R, Krediet R, editors: *Nolph and Gokal's textbook of peritoneal dialysis*, New York, 2009, Springer, pp 137–172.
41. Flessner M, Henegar J, Bigler S, et al: Is the peritoneum a significant transport barrier in peritoneal dialysis? *Perit Dial Int* 23:542–549, 2003.
57. Krediet RT, Struijk DG, Koomen GC, et al: Peritoneal transport of macromolecules in patients on CAPD. *Contrib Nephrol* 89:161–174, 1991.
61. Twardowski ZJ, Nolph KD, Khanna R, et al: Peritoneal equilibration test. *Perit Dial Bull* 7:138–148, 1987.
67. Pannekeet MM, Imholz AL, Struijk DG, et al: The standard peritoneal permeability analysis: a tool for the assessment of peritoneal permeability characteristics in CAPD patients. *Kidney Int* 48:866–875, 1995.
72. Mujais S, Nolph K, Gokal R, et al: Evaluation and management of ultrafiltration problems in peritoneal dialysis. International Society for Peritoneal Dialysis Ad Hoc Committee on Ultrafiltration Management in Peritoneal Dialysis. *Perit Dial Int* 20(Suppl 4):S5–S21, 2000.
87. Lambie M, Chess J, Donovan KL, et al: Independent effects of systemic and peritoneal inflammation on peritoneal dialysis survival. *J Am Soc Nephrol* 24:2071–2080, 2013.
94. Brown EA, Davies SJ, Rutherford P, et al: Survival of functionally anuric patients on automated peritoneal dialysis: the European APD Outcome Study. *J Am Soc Nephrol* 14:2948–2957, 2003.
118. Werner S, Grose R: Regulation of wound healing by growth factors and cytokines. *Physiol Rev* 83:835–870, 2003.
125. Perl J, Nessim SJ, Bargman JM: The biocompatibility of neutral pH, low-GDP peritoneal dialysis solutions: benefit at bench, bedside, or both? *Kidney Int* 79:814–824, 2011.
127. Weinreich T, Passlick-Deetjen J, Ritz E: Low dialysate calcium in continuous ambulatory peritoneal dialysis: a randomized controlled multicenter trial. The Peritoneal Dialysis Multicenter Study Group. *Am J Kidney Dis* 25:452–460, 1995.
140. Qi H, Xu C, Yan H, et al: Comparison of icodextrin and glucose solutions for long dwell exchange in peritoneal dialysis: a meta-analysis of randomized controlled trials. *Perit Dial Int* 31:179–188, 2011.
142. Davies SJ, Brown EA, Frandsen NE, et al: Longitudinal membrane function in functionally anuric patients treated with APD: data from EAPOS on the effects of glucose and icodextrin prescription. *Kidney Int* 67:1609–1615, 2005.
155. Johnson DW, Brown FG, Clarke M, et al: Effects of biocompatible versus standard fluid on peritoneal dialysis outcomes. *J Am Soc Nephrol* 23:1097–1107, 2012.
161. Johnson DW, Brown FG, Clarke M, et al: The effect of low glucose degradation product, neutral pH versus standard peritoneal dialysis solutions on peritoneal membrane function: the balANZ trial. *Nephrol Dial Transplant* 27:4445–4453, 2012.
170. Mehrotra R, de Boer IH, Himmelfarb J: Adverse effects of systemic glucose absorption with peritoneal dialysis: how good is the evidence? *Curr Opinion Nephrol Hypertens* 22:663–668, 2013.
178. Bieber SD, Burkart J, Golper TA, et al: Comparative outcomes between continuous ambulatory and automated peritoneal dialysis: a narrative review. *Am J Kidney Dis* 2014.
188. Mehrotra R, Chiu YW, Kalantar-Zadeh K, et al: The outcomes of continuous ambulatory and automated peritoneal dialysis are similar. *Kidney Int* 76:97–107, 2009.
190. Cullis B, Abdelraheem M, Abrahams G, et al: Peritoneal dialysis for acute kidney injury. *Perit Dial Int* 34:494–517, 2014.
191. Paniagua R, Amato D, Vonesh E, et al: Effects of increased peritoneal clearances on mortality rates in peritoneal dialysis: ADEMEX, a prospective, randomized, controlled trial. *J Am Soc Nephrol* 13:1307–1320, 2002.
192. Eknoyan G, Beck GJ, Cheung AK, et al: Effect of dialysis dose and membrane flux in maintenance hemodialysis. *N Engl J Med* 347:2010–2019, 2002.
199. Vanholder RC, Ringoir SM: Adequacy of dialysis: a critical analysis. *Kidney Int* 42:540–558, 1992.
205. Peritoneal Dialysis Adequacy Work Group: Clinical practice guidelines for peritoneal dialysis adequacy. *Am J Kidney Dis* 48(Suppl 1):S98–S129, 2006.
209. Chertow GM, Lazarus JM, Lew NL, et al: Development of a population-specific regression equation to estimate total body water in hemodialysis patients. *Kidney Int* 51:1578–1582, 1997.
214. Churchill DN: The ADEMEX Study: make haste slowly. *J Am Soc Nephrol* 13:1415–1418, 2002.
216. Lo WK, Bargman JM, Burkart J, et al: Guideline on targets for solute and fluid removal in adult patients on chronic peritoneal dialysis. *Perit Dial Int* 26:520–522, 2006.
217. Moran J, Correa-Rotter R: Revisiting the peritoneal dialysis dose. *Semin Dial* 19:102–104, 2006.
223. Tan SH, Lee EJ, Tay ME, et al: Protein nutrition status of adult patients starting chronic ambulatory peritoneal dialysis. *Adv Perit Dial* 16:291–293, 2000.
232. Kalantar-Zadeh K, Kopple JD: Relative contributions of nutrition and inflammation to clinical outcome in dialysis patients. *Am J Kidney Dis* 38:1343–1350, 2001.
235. Kang DH, Yoon KI, Choi KB, et al: Relationship of peritoneal membrane transport characteristics to the nutritional status in CAPD patients. *Nephrol Dial Transplant* 14:1715–1722, 1999.
236. Stenvinkel P, Heimburger O, Lindholm B, et al: Are there two types of malnutrition in chronic renal failure? Evidence for

247. Silang R, Regalado M, Cheng TH, et al: Prokinetic agents increase plasma albumin in hypoalbuminemic chronic dialysis patients with delayed gastric emptying. *Am J Kidney Dis* 37:287–293, 2001.
260. Arici M, Walls J: End-stage renal disease, atherosclerosis, and cardiovascular mortality: is C-reactive protein the missing link? *Kidney Int* 59:407–414, 2001.
280. Lui SL, Cheng SW, Ng F, et al: Cefazolin plus netilmicin versus cefazolin plus ceftazidime for treating CAPD peritonitis: effect on residual renal function. *Kidney Int* 68:2375–2380, 2005.
291. Van Biesen W, Vanholder RC, Veys N, et al: An evaluation of an integrative care approach for end-stage renal disease patients. *J Am Soc Nephrol* 11:116–125, 2000.
302. Prichard S: Cardiovascular risk in peritoneal dialysis. *Contrib Nephrol* 82–90, 2003.
308. Heerspink HJ, Ninomiya T, Zoungas S, et al: Effect of lowering blood pressure on cardiovascular events and mortality in patients on dialysis: a systematic review and meta-analysis of randomised controlled trials. *Lancet* 373:1009–1015, 2009.
324. Akcay A, Ozdemir FN, Sezer S, et al: Association of vitamin D receptor gene polymorphisms with hypercalcemia in peritoneal dialysis patients. *Perit Dial Int* 25(Suppl 3):S52–S55, 2005.
345. Huen SC, Hall I, Topal J, et al: Successful use of intraperitoneal daptomycin in the treatment of vancomycin-resistant enterococcus peritonitis. *Am J Kidney Dis* 54:538–541, 2009.
364. Furgeson SB, Teitelbaum I: New treatment options and protocols for peritoneal dialysis-related peritonitis. *Contrib Nephrol* 163:169–176, 2009.
383. Crabtree JH: Rescue and salvage procedures for mechanical and infectious complications of peritoneal dialysis. *Int J Artif Org* 29:67–84, 2006.
384. Stuart S, Booth TC, Cash CJ, et al: Complications of continuous ambulatory peritoneal dialysis. *Radiographics* 29:441–460, 2009.
386. Del Peso G, Bajo MA, Costero O, et al: Risk factors for abdominal wall complications in peritoneal dialysis patients. *Perit Dial Int* 23:249–254, 2003.
402. Brown MC, Simpson K, Kerssens JJ, et al: Encapsulating peritoneal sclerosis in the new millennium: a national cohort study. *Clin J Am Soc Nephrol* 4:1222–1229, 2009.
417. Guest S: Tamoxifen therapy for encapsulating peritoneal sclerosis: mechanism of action and update on clinical experiences. *Perit Dial Int* 29:252–255, 2009.
421. Huang CC, Cheng KF, Wu HD: Survival analysis: comparing peritoneal dialysis and hemodialysis in Taiwan. *Perit Dial Int* 28(Suppl 3):S15–S20, 2008.
425. Chang YK, Hsu CC, Hwang SJ, et al: A comparative assessment of survival between propensity score-matched patients with peritoneal dialysis and hemodialysis in Taiwan. *Medicine* 91:144–151, 2012.
426. Mehrotra R, Chiu YW, Kalantar-Zadeh K, et al: Similar outcomes with hemodialysis and peritoneal dialysis in patients with end-stage renal disease. *Arch Intern Med* 171:110–118, 2011.
427. McDonald SP, Marshall MR, Johnson DW, et al: Relationship between dialysis modality and mortality. *J Am Soc Nephrol* 20:155–163, 2009.
440. Perl J, Wald R, McFarlane P, et al: Hemodialysis vascular access modifies the association between dialysis modality and survival. *J Am Soc Nephrol* 22:1113–1121, 2011.
442. Murphy SW, Foley RN, Barrett BJ, et al: Comparative mortality of hemodialysis and peritoneal dialysis in Canada. *Kidney Int* 57:1720–1726, 2000.

Critical Care Nephrology   67

Ron Wald | Kathleen Liu

CHAPTER OUTLINE

ACUTE KIDNEY INURY IN THE CONTEXT OF CRITICAL ILLNESS, 2137
Sepsis, 2137
Fluid Management and its Impact on AKI, 2138
AKI in the Context of Pulmonary Dysfunction, 2138
AKI in the Context of Liver Dysfunction, 2139
AKI in the Setting of Cardiac Dysfunction, 2139
RENAL REPLACEMENT THERAPY IN THE INTENSIVE CARE UNIT, 2139
Goals of Care, 2139
INDICATIONS FOR COMMENCING RENAL REPLACEMENT THERAPY, 2140
RENAL REPLACEMENT MODALITY, 2140

Intermittent Hemodialysis, 2140
Continuous Renal Replacement Therapy, 2141
Sustained Low Efficiency Dialysis, 2142
The Impact of Modality on Clinical Outcomes, 2142
MODE OF CLEARANCE, 2142
INTENSITY OF RENAL REPLACEMENT THERAPY, 2142
ANTICOAGULATION, 2144
FLUID BALANCE, ULTRAFILTRATION, AND MAINTENANCE OF HEMODYNAMIC STABILITY, 2144
VASCULAR ACCESS CONSIDERATIONS, 2145
DRUG DOSING CONSIDERATIONS, 2145

Studies now suggest that 25% to 40% of patients in intensive care units (ICUs) have acute kidney injury (AKI).[1-3] A substantial fraction have severe AKI that requires renal replacement therapy (RRT). Short-term mortality among critically ill patients with acute AKI who require RRT is in excess of 50%,[4] and among survivors, quality of life is poor.[5] AKI, as well as electrolyte and acid-base abnormalities, may occur in the setting of a number of different types of critical illness. In some cases, the management of the underlying disease itself has important renal implications. In this chapter, we first discuss AKI in the context of a number of different types of critical illness: sepsis, the acute respiratory distress syndrome, acute liver failure, and acute decompensated heart failure. We then review RRT for AKI in critically ill patients and some of the special considerations that distinguish RRT in this setting from the setting of chronic kidney disease. Of note, we do not discuss acute brain injury, which is typically associated with dysnatremias (including the syndrome of inappropriate secretion of antidiuretic hormone, cerebral salt wasting, and central diabetes insipidus) but not AKI. The reader is referred to Chapters 15 and 16 for further discussion of these disorders.

ACUTE KIDNEY INJURY IN THE CONTEXT OF CRITICAL ILLNESS

SEPSIS

AKI, a common complication of sepsis, occurs through multiple mechanisms, including hypotension leading to hypoperfusion, inflammation, and oxidative stress.[6,7] There are no specific treatments for AKI or for sepsis itself (apart from source control and treatment with appropriate antimicrobial agents) at present. With regard to inflammatory mediators in sepsis, there has been significant interest in the use of high-volume hemofiltration to remove proinflammatory cytokines, but studies to date have not shown any benefit.[8] Later studies have focused on the use of adsorptive (polymyxin B) columns to enhance cytokine removal,[9] and multicenter randomized clinical trials are ongoing.[10]

The role of fluid management in the management of patients with sepsis has been a topic of controversy. After the publication of the pivotal study by Rivers and colleagues,[11] there has been a major shift in clinical practice towards early goal-directed therapy in which inotropes and packed red blood cell transfusions are used in addition to early volume resuscitation and vasopressors in patients with septic shock. However, results of a clinical trial suggested no benefit of early goal-directed therapy, which included early recognition of sepsis and timely antibiotic administration, over standard therapy.[12] The ProCESS (Protocol-Based Care for Early Septic Shock) trial randomly allocated 1341 patients to protocol-based early goal-directed therapy, protocol-based standard therapy, or usual care. There was no difference in 60-day, 90-day, or 1-year mortality between the treatment arms (60-day mortality 21% in the protocol-based early goal-directed therapy arm, 18.2% in the protocol-based standard therapy arm, and 18.9% in the usual care arm). Patients in the protocol-based standard therapy and usual care arm received fewer packed red blood cell transfusions and less dobutamine than patients in the other two arms, suggesting that these interventions are of limited benefit in a general population with sepsis.

FLUID MANAGEMENT AND ITS IMPACT ON AKI

Indeed, studies of fluid management in critically ill patients have suggested that fluid overload may be in and of itself deleterious, particularly in the context of AKI. Fluid overload is associated with a number of adverse consequences, including decreased gastrointestinal absorption and impaired wound healing.[13] In patients with AKI, fluid overload has been independently associated with an increased risk of new sepsis as well as with an increased short- and long-term risk of death.[14-17] However, many of these studies are observational in nature and therefore subject to confounding (e.g., patients who are sicker are more likely to be hypotensive and receive fluid boluses and consequently more likely to become fluid overloaded). Furthermore, total body fluid overload may dilute serum creatinine concentration and consequently mask AKI.[18,19]

An adverse consequence of fluid overload that has gained significant interest is intraabdominal hypertension and the abdominal compartment syndrome.[20] *Intraabdominal hypertension* is defined as an intraabdominal pressure greater than 12 mm Hg. This pressure is typically measured by instilling a fixed volume of water (30 mL) into the urinary bladder via Foley catheter and using pressure tubing to transduce a bladder pressure from the Foley catheter tubing. The *abdominal compartment syndrome* is defined as an intra-abdominal pressure greater than 20 mm Hg and the presence of end-organ dysfunction. AKI results from intraabdominal hypertension via two mechanisms. The main mechanism of renal dysfunction is thought to be compression of the inferior vena cava, which results in impaired venous return and venous stasis throughout the abdominal cavity, including the renal veins.[21,22] In addition, impaired venous return leads to decreased cardiac output and increased sympathetic and renin angiotensin aldosterone system signaling, resulting in renal artery vasoconstriction. The result is a functional prerenal state, characterized by low urinary sodium concentration and oliguria. Decompression of the abdominal compartment (typically via a surgical approach) may be required, and newer guidelines suggest that consideration should be given to decompression in patients with intraabdominal hypertension before the abdominal compartment syndrome develops.[20] However, this is an area of ongoing research, and further studies are needed.

In addition to the amount of fluid, there is significant interest in the type of fluid administered and its impact on renal function. It has been suggested that chloride-rich solutions may be associated with greater renal vasoconstriction and exacerbation of medullary hypoxia.[23] In a small crossover study of human volunteers, administration of chloride-rich solutions was associated with greater fluid retention and reduced renal perfusion than administration of balanced salt solutions.[24] A number of observational studies have suggested that the use of chloride-rich solutions is associated with higher risk of AKI than balanced salt solutions.[25,26] The largest of these studies was a single-center, prospective, open-label sequential study.[26] During the control period, patients received normal saline or chloride-rich colloids for resuscitation. During the intervention period that followed, patients received Plasmalyte or chloride-restricted colloids for resuscitation. During the intervention period, the incidence of Risk, Injury, Failure, Loss and End-stage kidney disease (RIFLE) stage I and stage F[27] AKI decreased (from 14% to 8.4%; $P < 0.001$). Challenges to the interpretation of these findings include the larger than expected effect size, concurrent changes made to other aspects of fluid management, and other practice changes that may have reduced the risk of AKI. For example, the use of RRT in this study dropped from 10% to 6.3% ($P = 0.005$) in the intervention period; one explanation for this difference is that the concomitant hyperchloremic metabolic acidosis from chloride-rich fluid administration may lead to an earlier requirement for RRT to control metabolic acidosis. On the other hand, the use of RRT continued to decline over the next several years in the study experience described, suggesting the presence of a secular trend that may not have been related to the change in the content of intravenous solutions.

AKI IN THE CONTEXT OF PULMONARY DYSFUNCTION

In the context of acute lung injury and the acute respiratory distress syndrome (ARDS), a fluid, conservative management strategy has been associated with improved outcomes and no adverse renal consequences.[28] The mainstay of supportive care for patients with ARDS is low tidal volume, lung-protective ventilation, which has led to a significant reduction in mortality and is associated with decreased levels of proinflammatory cytokines.[29] As part of the lung-protective ventilation strategy, permissive hypercapnia is encouraged to minimize ventilator-associated lung injury. In the setting of normal renal function, compensatory metabolic alkalosis will ensue. However, in the setting of renal dysfunction (either acute or chronic), the metabolic acidosis that arises and the inability to compensate for the respiratory acidosis associated with permissive hypercapnia may trigger the initiation of RRT for correction of the acid-base imbalance or the use of boluses of sodium bicarbonate. In patients with severe ARDS in whom ventilation is markedly impaired because of alveolar injury (as reflected by a high dead space fraction and impaired respiratory carbon dioxide excretion), bolus doses of bicarbonate may paradoxically worsen arterial pH through an abrupt increase in $PaCO_2$ and conversion to carbonic acid.[30] Therefore, continuous RRT (CRRT) may be the preferred modality to slowly correct pH and compensate for respiratory acidosis.

Studies in animal models suggest there is significant crosstalk between the kidney and the lung—that is, injury to one organ results in injury to the other.[31-34] For example, kidney injury is associated with elevations of proinflammatory cytokines and worse lung injury in mice[35]; in one study, concentrations of interleukin-6 and interleukin-8 were higher in children with AKI after cardiopulmonary bypass surgery than in controls (children without AKI) and were associated with a longer duration of mechanical ventilation.[36]

AKI IN THE CONTEXT OF LIVER DYSFUNCTION

In the setting of acute liver failure, a major cause of death is cerebral edema resulting in elevated intracranial pressure and brainstem herniation.[37] Elevated intracranial pressure occurs in up to 35% of patients with grade III encephalopathy (stupor, incoherent speech, sleeping but wakes with stimulation) and 75% of patients with grade IV encephalopathy (coma, unresponsiveness).[38] Thus, a significant component of the management of acute liver failure is prevention and management of cerebral edema. Patients with acute liver failure are at risk for AKI from either hepatorenal syndrome or acute tubular necrosis. Acute tubular necrosis may be caused by hypotension, sepsis (a common complication of acute liver failure), or ingestion of a substance that is both hepatotoxic and nephrotoxic (for example, acetaminophen, *Amanita* mushrooms). CRRT is often used for meticulous control of volume status in these patients, given the high risk of cerebral edema and frequent high obligate intake in the form of infusions (*N*-acetylcysteine, vasopressors, and blood products, including fresh-frozen plasma). Hyponatremia is a common complication of liver failure and may further exacerbate cerebral edema.

AKI IN THE SETTING OF CARDIAC DYSFUNCTION

Finally, it is clear that cardiac function affects renal function and vice versa. The following five clinical subtypes of the cardiorenal syndrome (CRS) have been proposed[39,40]:

Acute CRS (type 1), in which acute worsening of heart function leads to AKI
Chronic CRS (type 2), in which chronic abnormalities in heart function result in kidney dysfunction
Acute renocardiac syndrome (type 3), in which AKI precedes cardiac dysfunction
Chronic renocardiac syndrome (type 4), in which CKD leads to cardiac dysfunction
Secondary CRS (type 5), in which systemic conditions such as sepsis result in simultaneous cardiac and renal dysfunction

With type 1 CRS in particular, volume overload and consequent venous congestion may result in renal dysfunction via several mechanisms, including renal venous hypertension, development of ascites with intraabdominal hypertension, and perhaps inflammation.[41,42] Consequently, the use of diuretics to improve volume overload in acute decompensated heart failure may actually improve renal function as renal venous hypertension in particular improves. However, over-diuresis and volume depletion may lead to AKI and can result in significant electrolyte and acid-base abnormalities.

There has been significant interest in the optimal management of volume overload in the context of acute decompensated heart failure. Several studies have compared the use of continuous versus intermittent bolus dosing of loop diuretics,[43,44] on the basis of the hypothesis that continuous infusion results in more effective diuresis by avoiding periods of "rebound" sodium retention between bolus doses. However, no clear benefit to continuous infusions over bolus dosing has been demonstrated to date.

Extracorporeal ultrafiltration has been proposed as an alternative to diuretic management for volume overload in acute decompensated heart failure and has been tested in a number of randomized clinical trials. The Cardiorenal Rescue Study in Acute Decompensated Heart Failure (CARESS-HF) trial compared the safety and efficacy of ultrafiltration (with a target fluid removal of 200 mL/hour) to stepped pharmacologic therapy (target urine output of 3-5 L/day) in patients with acute CRS type 1 (Figure 67.1).[45] The primary end point was the bivariate change from baseline in serum creatinine level and body weight. The trial was terminated early owing to a lack of benefit in the ultrafiltration group (serum creatinine increased slightly in comparison with a slight decrease in the pharmacologic group, and change in weight was the same in the two groups), combined with an increased risk of adverse events, including bleeding and catheter-related complications. On the basis of this experience, ultrafiltration is no longer favored as a first-line therapy for patients with acute *decompensated* heart failure and cardiorenal syndrome. Nonetheless, ultrafiltration may be required in patients with acute decompensated heart failure that fails to respond to intravenous diuretics and other pharmacotherapy, particularly in the presence of CKD and/or AKI.

RENAL REPLACEMENT THERAPY IN THE INTENSIVE CARE UNIT

GOALS OF CARE

Regardless of etiology, when severe AKI develops, the consideration of RRT arises. Broadly speaking, optimal renal support in critically ill patients revolves around management of the fluid and metabolic abnormalities of AKI in a manner that facilitates and promotes recovery from the underlying illness. RRT should ideally be performed with minimal complications of and disruption to the broader care that the patient is receiving. Philosophically, one may debate whether RRT is merely supportive or confers an additional therapeutic benefit that may enhance survival. Specifically, with the exception of dialysis dose, it remains unclear whether modulating various aspects of the RRT prescription can improve survival. A further goal of RRT is maximizing the likelihood of kidney recovery among surviving patients. This goal is associated with the growing recognition that AKI survivors are at high risk for CKD.[46,47] RRT protocols should be designed to minimize iatrogenic injury to the kidney (e.g., injury due to hypotension and/or hypovolemia) in the hope that dialysis independence can be

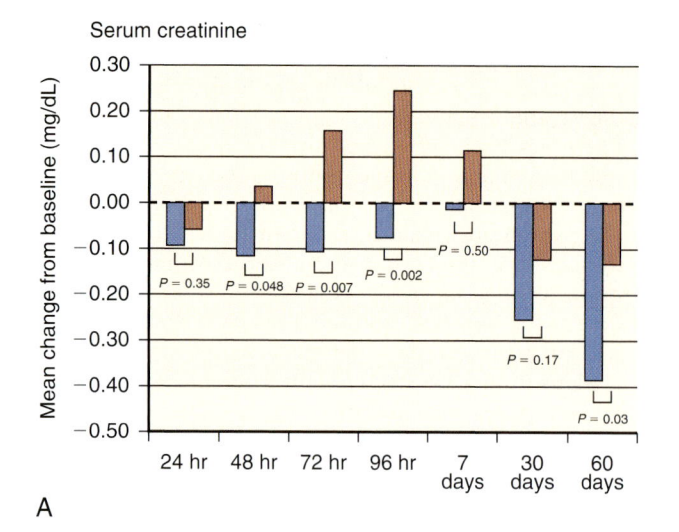

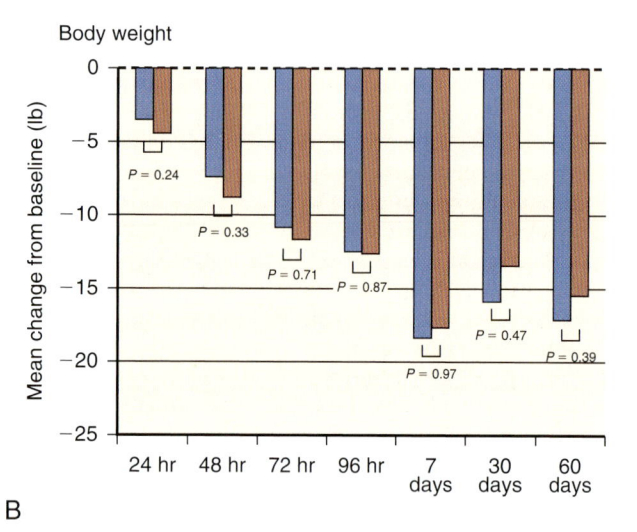

Figure 67.1 Role of ultrafiltration in decompensated heart failure. Changes from baseline in **(A)** serum creatinine and **(B)** body weight at various time points, according to treatment group. The *P* values were calculated with the use of a Wilcoxon test. (Reproduced with permission from Bart BA, Goldsmith SR, Lee KL, et al: Heart Failure Clinical Research Network: Ultrafiltration in decompensated heart failure with cardiorenal syndrome. *N Engl J Med.* 367:2296-2304, 2012.)

achieved, as well, ideally, as an eventual return to the level of kidney function that preceded the acute illness. At present, no specific maneuvers have been shown to enhance kidney recovery after an episode of AKI.

INDICATIONS FOR COMMENCING RENAL REPLACEMENT THERAPY

The decision to initiate RRT is unambiguous when AKI is complicated by hyperkalemia or pulmonary congestion refractory to medical maneuvers or in the setting of a concomitant intoxication with a dialyzable toxin.[48] However, in the absence of a life-threatening complication, the timing of RRT initiation is more controversial. Proponents of early or preemptive initiation of RRT have suggested progressive volume overload and the toxicity of uncontrolled uremia as arguments to commence RRT.[49,50] A meta-analysis and systematic review of early versus later initiation of renal support in critically ill patients suggested a 55% reduction in 28-day mortality (odds ratio [OR], 0.45; 95% confidence interval [CI], 0.28 to 0.72) with early initiation but no significant association with kidney recovery.[51] One multicenter cohort study in the United States showed that patients who started RRT with a serum blood urea nitrogen concentration higher than 76 mg/dL, which was considered to reflect later RRT initiation, had a twofold higher risk of death.[52] On the other hand, results of a study comparing patients with AKI who started RRT matched with nondialyzed patients with AKI suggested that RRT conferred a survival benefit only when serum creatinine exceeded 3.8 mg/dL at dialysis initiation.[53]

Virtually all of the completed studies in this area are subject to confounding by indication, and the definitions around timing of RRT are variable and arbitrary. For example, whether higher urea or creatinine concentrations are appropriate surrogates of AKI duration, and hence can be used as barometers of timing, is debatable, particularly because these measures are also influenced by CKD, muscle mass, and nutritional status. The only significant clinical trial in this area randomly assigned 106 critically ill patients with oliguric AKI to either initiation of RRT within 12 hours or deferral of RRT until a clinical complication was apparent.[54] Although patients in the late initiation arm started RRT about 36 hours after those in the early RRT arm, there was no significant survival difference; however, the trial was underpowered and hence the results inconclusive.[54]

An aggressive approach to RRT initiation has conceivable shortcomings. Spontaneous renal recovery is frequently observed, and the widespread adoption of earlier RRT could result in the unnecessary exposure of patients to the risks associated with vascular access placement and the RRT procedure itself (e.g., hypotension, arrhythmia, electrolyte abnormalities, and compromised antibiotic concentration). At present, a more aggressive approach to RRT initiation is limited by the inability to predict which patients will have progressive AKI. Optimally, a clinical prediction rule applied during the early phases of AKI, possibly enhanced by novel biomarkers, would permit the targeted initiation of renal support in those who are most likely to have progressive disease and therefore more likely to experience benefit.

RENAL REPLACEMENT MODALITY

A variety of RRT modalities are available for the treatment of critically ill patients, each with a unique set of advantages and shortcomings (Table 67.1). However, no single modality has been shown to confer improved survival. As a result, logistic factors such as costs, local availability, and staff expertise can be justified as factors that determine the availability of RRT modalities. Furthermore, there may be center-to-center variation in the application of each modality, although practice guidelines now established may stimulate more standardized care.[55]

INTERMITTENT HEMODIALYSIS

Intermittent hemodialysis (IHD) is classically defined as the application of technology designed for patients with

Table 67.1 Advantages and Shortcomings of Renal Replacement Therapy Modalities

	Intermittent Hemodialysis	Sustained Low-Efficiency Dialysis	Continuous Renal Replacement Therapy
Advantages	Familiarity to nursing staff Widespread availability Low cost of disposables Delivery with no anticoagulation feasible	Low cost of disposables Delivery with no anticoagulation feasible Reasonable hemodynamic tolerability	Greater hemodynamic tolerability Ability to rapidly adjust prescription to evolving patient needs Possibility of improved kidney survival among survivors
Shortcomings	Challenges with hemodynamic instability Limitations of fluid removal	Limited data on appropriate dosing of antimicrobials Lack of random controlled trials comparing efficacy with that of other modalities	High cost of disposables Greater logistic complexity Challenging to administer without anticoagulation

end-stage kidney disease to patients with AKI. However, some modifications are needed for the ICU. Water purification is generated by portable reverse osmosis machines. Due to the lower blood flow rates typically achieved with temporary dialysis catheters and the high catabolic rates of critically ill patients, session durations up to 5 hours may be required.[56] Heparin is often omitted owing to the bleeding risks that are frequently seen in critically ill patients (see later discussion of anticoagulation). Blood flow ranges from 200 to 400 mL/min, with lower blood flows used in initial sessions for patients who are believed to be at risk for dialysis disequilibrium. In hemodynamically unstable patients, a hypertonic dialysate sodium (e.g., 145 mmol/L) may promote stability by enhancing fluid movement from the extracellular to intracellular space. Although hyperkalemia is often a trigger for RRT initiation, excessive potassium removal may result in hypokalemia and may precipitate arrhythmias. The goal of acute RRT should be reducing serum potassium to the safe range (<5.5 mmol/L) rather than complete normokalemia, and hence, a dialysate potassium concentration less than 2 mmol/L should be prescribed with caution. Critically ill patients may become hypophosphatemic, especially after receiving prolonged RRT, which may be associated with additional complications in this population, including weakness. Critically ill patients may have an array of risks for hypoglycemia, thereby mandating the uniform inclusion of dextrose in the dialysate.

In order to achieve euvolemia in a population that is generally fluid overloaded,[15,17] the prescribed ultrafiltration volume must address the patient's expected intake from infusions and nutrition while achieving net fluid removal. The key challenge of IHD is the need to ultrafilter relatively large volumes in a short time in the patient with hemodynamic compromise, who has a tendency to poor refilling from the interstitium. In addition to modification of the dialysate sodium concentration, intradialytic hypotension can be prevented by lowering the dialysate temperature or initiating or escalating the doses vasopressors. However, if a patient requires escalating doses of vasopressors to tolerate fluid removal via IHD, modalities that permit a slower pace of fluid removal should be considered, as described in the next two sections. The application of more frequent IHD sessions (e.g., daily versus alternate day) or exclusive ultrafiltration alternating with IHD may permit a lower ultrafiltration volume per session, thereby enabling the achievement of euvolemia with less hemodynamic instability.

CONTINUOUS RENAL REPLACEMENT THERAPY

CRRT enables the slow removal of fluid and solutes using dialysis and hemofiltration, in isolation or in combination (see later section on clearance mode). In comparison with IHD on a unit-time basis, CRRT is an inefficient form of RRT and thus would not be considered optimal when the goal is the rapid removal of a dangerous solute (e.g., potassium, ingested toxin). The efficacy of CRRT, and its putative benefits, is thus realized only when it is applied throughout the 24-hour period with minimal interruption. Technical factors (e.g., frequent clotting) and time away from the ICU for procedures may hamper CRRT delivery. Clinical practice guidelines from Kidney Disease/Improving Global Outcomes (KDIGO) suggest using CRRT and intermittent forms of RRT in a complementary fashion.[55] Although this recommendation opens the door to flexibility in clinical practice, the general approach is to employ CRRT for patients who are hemodynamically unstable and IHD for patients who are more stable, with the understanding that variability in hemodynamics will affect the modality used.

The administration of CRRT must be highly protocolized. Ordering clinicians must determine the optimal intensity of RRT to be administered (see later section on dose/intensity). Fluid balance is frequently managed on an hourly basis; because volume overload is virtually ubiquitous in the critically ill patient with AKI, achievement of a net fluid removal mandates that hourly ultrafiltration exceed the patient's overall fluid balance during the preceding hour. As an example, one may consider a net ultrafiltration goal of 50 mL/hour being prescribed to an anuric patient. If the patient received 30 mL from parenteral nutrition and 40 mL from a variety infusions and lost 30 mL from a variety of postoperative drains (net balance + 40 mL), the actual ultrafiltration volume needs to be 90 mL. CRRT offers the unique flexibility of altering ultrafiltration volumes on an hourly basis according to the variability of intake/losses and the patient's ability to tolerate ultrafiltration, which may be of significant benefit because volume overload is virtually ubiquitous in critically ill patients with AKI.

SUSTAINED LOW-EFFICIENCY DIALYSIS

Sustained low-efficiency dialysis (SLED), also known as extended daily dialysis (EDD) and prolonged intermittent renal replacement therapy (PIRRT), is a hybrid modality that utilizes conventional hemodialysis devices with an extension of therapy to 8 to 12 hours in the hopes of achieving the putative hemodynamic benefits of continuous dialysis. SLED has gained currency owing to the absence of mortality benefit with CRRT (see later), the high costs associated with the application of CRRT,[57,58] and the concomitant desire to provide safe RRT to hemodynamically unstable patients. Initial reports showed that SLED was generally associated with reasonable solute control and an achievement of planned ultrafiltration goals.[59-61] SLED was also associated with hemodynamic stability comparable to that of CRRT.[61-63] Further practical advantages of SLED include the delivery of therapy without anticoagulation and administration during nighttime hours in order to minimize interruptions by clinical procedures.

THE IMPACT OF MODALITY ON CLINICAL OUTCOMES

CONTINUOUS RRT VERSUS INTERMITTENT HEMODIALYSIS

Despite the theoretical benefits attributed to CRRT, randomized trials have not demonstrated enhanced survival in comparison with IHD. The largest of such trials, randomly allocated 360 patients (the vast majority of whom were catecholamine-dependent and mechanically ventilated) to IHD or CRRT and demonstrated a 60-day survival of approximately 32% in both groups.[64] A Cochrane review involving seven clinical trials showed no benefit for CRRT over IHD with respect to short-term hospital mortality (risk ratio [RR], 1.01; 95% CI, 0.92 to 1.12) or RRT independence (RR, 0.99; 95% CI, 0.92 to 1.07).[65]

If the putative benefits of CRRT are in hemodynamics and the prevention of iatrogenic renal ischemia, one would expect that benefits to kidney function would be observed in survivors of the acute phase of illness. A meta-analysis of predominantly observational studies demonstrated a lower risk of dialysis dependence among CRRT recipients.[66] A study from Ontario, Canada, showed that among patients who survived to 90 days after initiation of acute RRT, the risk of long-term dialysis dependence over 2 years of follow-up was 25% lower among CRRT recipients than in matched controls whose initial modality was IHD.[67] The possible nephroprotective benefits seen with CRRT, if borne out by clinical trials, are potentially relevant because the cost utility of applying RRT in AKI is closely tied to patients who achieve dialysis independence and survive for longer than 1 year.[68] Although the in-hospital costs of CRRT are higher than for IHD, this initial cost increment may be neutralized if CRRT reduces the risk of long-term dialysis among surviving patients.[57]

CONTINUOUS RRT VERSUS SUSTAINED LOW-EFFICIENCY DIALYSIS

The emergence of SLED has been accompanied by limited evidence. A single-center trial randomly assigned 232 patients with AKI admitted to a surgical ICU to either SLED (target 12 hours/session) or CRRT.[69] The primary outcome of 90-day mortality did not differ between the groups (49.6% vs. 55.6% in SLED and CRRT recipients, respectively; $P = 0.43$). However, inferences from these results are limited by the small sample size and limited statistical power of this trial. Furthermore, the mean duration of SLED treatments was longer than expected (15 hours), and the mean duration of CRRT sessions was shorter than expected (16 hours). Two studies evaluated SLED recipients in comparison with historical controls (patients treated with CRRT); in one study, the introduction of SLED was associated with improved outcomes,[70] and in the other, outcomes were comparable.[71] Thus, the available data suggest that SLED is well tolerated by critically ill patients with hemodynamic compromise and appears safe, but whether or not there is any benefit (beyond potential cost savings) is unknown.

MODE OF CLEARANCE

As in long-term RRT, solute removal in patients with AKI may be mediated by diffusive and/or convective mechanisms. The relative contributions of diffusive clearance and convective clearance to the administered therapy may vary and ultimately define the clearance mode (hemodialysis, hemofiltration, or hemodiafiltration). In hemodialysis, a concentration gradient is generated by the countercurrent flow of dialysate and blood across a semipermeable membrane. The diffusive clearance that ensues is the essence of hemodialysis. However, solutes may also be removed as a consequence of convective clearance, whereby the ultrafiltration of large volumes of plasma water down a pressure gradient forces concomitant "drag" of solutes across the membrane pores. In hemofiltration, a balanced electrolyte solution devoid of the unwanted solutes then replaces the ultrafiltrate in an isovolemic fashion. Hemodialysis and hemofiltration are equally effective in the removal of low-molecular-weight substances (e.g., creatinine, urea, electrolytes). However, because diffusion is size-related, slower-moving, larger molecules are less efficiently cleared by dialysis. With hemofiltration, in contrast, clearance of any substance of interest is related to the size of the molecule in relation to the size of the membrane's pores. Depending on the porosity of the membrane, larger molecules, which include potentially toxic cytokines, might be better removed by hemofiltration than by hemodialysis.

Hemofiltration may be provided in tandem with hemodialysis (hemodiafiltration) or as the exclusive mode of clearance. It can be applied in the context of continuous (as in continuous venovenous hemofiltration [CVVH] or continuous venovenous hemodiafiltration [CVVHDF]) or intermittent forms of RRT.[72] Despite its theoretical benefits, there is no evidence that hemofiltration ameliorates clinical outcomes.[73] The largest trial to date on this topic, a comparison of CVVH and CVVHD, enrolled only 75 patients and did not find a difference in 60-day mortality rates.[74]

INTENSITY OF RENAL REPLACEMENT THERAPY

Small clinical trials suggested that the escalation of RRT intensity or dose, defined as increased effluent volume in

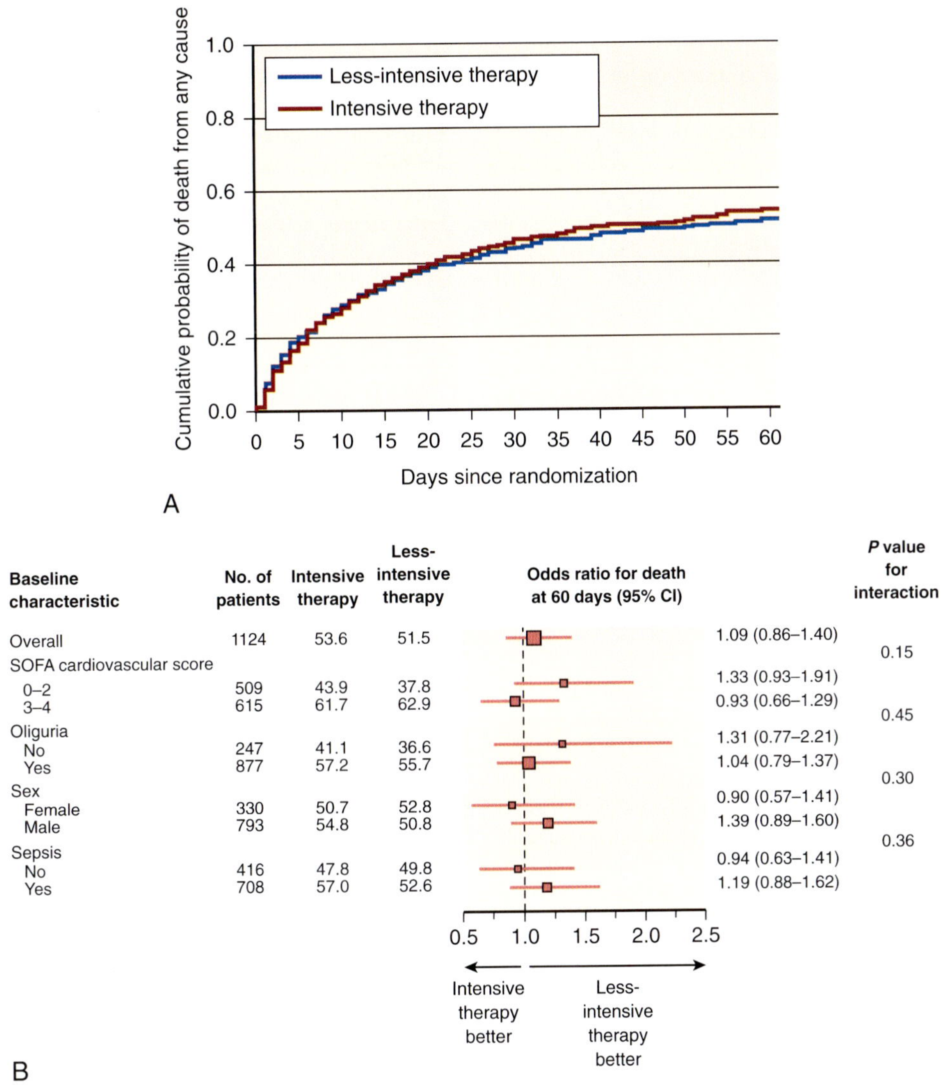

Figure 67.2 Effect of intensity of renal support in critically ill patients with acute kidney injury. Kaplan–Meier plot of cumulative probabilities of death (**A**) and odds ratios for death at 60 days, according to baseline characteristics (**B**) from the VA/NIH Acute Renal Failure Trial Network. **A** shows the cumulative probability of death from any cause in the entire study cohort. **B** shows odds ratios (and 95% confidence intervals [CIs]) for death from any cause by 60 days in the group receiving the intensive treatment strategy in comparison with the group receiving the less intensive treatment strategy, as well as P values for the interaction between the treatment group and baseline characteristics. P values were calculated with the use of the Wald statistic. Higher Sequential Organ Failure Assessment (SOFA) scores indicate more severe organ dysfunction. There was no significant interaction between treatment and subgroup variables, as defined according to the prespecified threshold level of significance for interaction ($P = 0.10$). (Reproduced with permission from Palevsky PM, Zhang JH, O'Connor TZ, et al: Intensity of renal support in critically ill patients with acute kidney injury. *N Engl J Med.* 359:7-20, 2008.)

CRRT[75] or increased session frequency in IHD,[76] could lead to enhanced survival. These findings stimulated two large-scale trials to definitively address whether dialysis intensification could improve survival in AKI. The American Acute renal failure Trials Network (ATN) trial randomly assigned 1124 critically ill patients with AKI to two strategies of RRT intensity; in this study, modality of therapy varied within each group depending on a patient's evolving hemodynamics (Figure 67.2).[56] Intensive therapy consisted of CVVHDF at 35 mL/kg/hr or SLED 6 days/week when the patient was hemodynamically unstable and IHD 6 days/week when the patient was hemodynamically stable; the less intensive strategy was CVVHDF at 20 mL/kg/hr or SLED 3 days/week during hemodynamic instability and IHD 3 days/week during hemodynamic stability. For patients receiving IHD, Kt/V (treatment adequacy) was measured per protocol and the IHD prescription was altered as needed to target a Kt/V of 1.2. The intensive RRT strategy was not associated with lower mortality at 60 days (53.6% versus 51.5% in the less intensive arm) or a higher likelihood of kidney recovery. The Randomized Evaluation of Normal Versus Augmented Level of Replacement Therapy (RENAL) was conducted in Australia and New Zealand during roughly the same period and compared CVVHDF given at 40 and 25 mL/kg/hr.[77] Higher CRRT intensity did not lead to improved survival at 90 days. No specific advantage of intensive therapy was observed in either study with respect to pre-specified patient subgroups such as those with sepsis. Studies of ultra-high CRRT doses (i.e., up to 70-85 mL/kg/hr) have also shown no benefit.[8,78] Ultimately, it remains unclear whether the improved control of harmful solutes afforded by high-intensity RRT is counterbalanced by the removal of beneficial solutes such as essential nutrients, endogenous antiinflammatory cytokines, and antibiotics.

The results of the aforementioned trials have prompted clinical practice guidelines to recommend a target RRT dose of 20 to 25 mL/kg/hr in CRRT and a Kt/V of 3.9/week in patients receiving SLED or IHD.[55] The recommendations for SLED and IHD are extrapolated from the long-term dialysis setting and the ATN trial.[56] With regard to CRRT, a provocative observational study did not demonstrate inferior outcomes among patients receiving a mean CRRT dose of 14 mL/kg/hr in comparison with those receiving a mean dose of 20 mL/kg/hr,[79] highlighting that the lowest safe dose remains unknown. However, pending further data on "low-dose CRRT," a target RRT dose of 20 to 25 mL/kg/hr is recommended for routine clinical practice.

ANTICOAGULATION

Anticoagulation of the extracorporeal circuit is widely prescribed in order to counter the propensity of blood to clot when it comes in contact with an artificial membrane. Other factors that must be considered in the selection of an anticoagulant for RRT include the presence of parallel indications for anticoagulation, the patient's propensity for bleeding and thrombosis, and the chosen RRT modality.

For patients who require anticoagulation for alternative indications (e.g., mechanical heart valves, deep vein thrombosis), systemically infused unfractionated heparin provides adequate anticoagulation of the RRT circuit. In patients with heparin-induced thrombocytopenia, systemically infused argatroban is an appropriate alternative.[80]

However, in the common scenario in which systemic anticoagulation is contraindicated or undesirable, regional citrate anticoagulation (RCA) has emerged as an effective and safe anticoagulation strategy.[81,82] When infused into the extracorporeal circuit, citrate chelates calcium, a required cofactor in the clotting cascade, and extracorporeal hypocalcemia (0.25-0.45 mmol/L) prevents circuit clotting. Systemic calcium level is maintained in the normal range through a concurrent calcium infusion. In comparison with use of unfractionated heparin, RCA confers a lower risk of bleeding.[83] Because citrate is converted to bicarbonate in the liver, RCA strategies often lead to metabolic alkalosis, which can be corrected by modifying the bicarbonate content of the replacement solution or dialysate. In the setting of impaired hepatic function, citrate accumulation may occur, theoretically manifesting as a wide anion gap metabolic acidosis and hypocalcemia. With judicious monitoring, however, RCA can be safely used in patients with hepatic failure.[84] Although RCA is recommended by the KDIGO guidelines, it remains unclear whether, in the absence of a higher bleeding propensity, RCA is the preferred anticoagulation strategy for CRRT recipients.[55] Some trials have reported a longer filter survival time with RCA,[85,86] but this finding was not borne out in a meta-analysis of six trials that compared RCA and use of unfractionated heparin.[83]

Though heparin is traditionally the default anticoagulant in SLED and IHD, RRT with both modalities can be readily administered without anticoagulation. The risk of clotting may be mitigated by administering a continuous saline infusion that is added to blood entering the dialyzer, thereby lowering intradialyzer blood viscosity. Accelerating the blood flow also reduces the risk of clotting. RCA protocols have been successfully deployed in patients treated with SLED or IHD who experience frequent clotting without anticoagulation and in whom systemic heparinization is contraindicated.[87,88]

FLUID BALANCE, ULTRAFILTRATION, AND MAINTENANCE OF HEMODYNAMIC STABILITY

The achievement of euvolemia is one of the central goals of any RRT strategy, especially in light of emerging data suggesting the harms of fluid overload.[13] Extracellular volume expansion is often substantial at RRT initiation and has been associated with adverse outcomes.[14-17] In addition, persistent fluid overload while patients are receiving RRT is associated with higher mortality. Although the relationship between fluid overload and death is likely confounded by a host of factors, an effective ultrafiltration strategy may have many benefits, including reduction in pulmonary edema (which may facilitate ventilator weaning) and mitigation of peripheral edema (which might help the mobilization process).

The achievement of effective ultrafiltration presents two challenges. The first is performing a valid assessment of the patient's volume status. Standard physical examination maneuvers (assessment of the jugular venous pressure, chest auscultation, peripheral edema) may be difficult to apply in the critical care setting and may be complemented by a search for pulmonary congestion on chest radiograph or information gleaned from a transduced central venous pressure. However, given the limitations of all these tools,[89,90] emerging technologies such as bedside point-of-care ultrasonography (for assessment of lung fluid[91] and inferior vena cava diameter[92,93]) and bioelectric impedance analysis[94] may prove to be useful adjuncts to standard volume assessment techniques.

In the setting of volume overload, the clinician is presented with the challenge of achieving net fluid removal while avoiding iatrogenic RRT-associated hypotension. Such hypotension occurs, even in patients with bona fide extracellular volume expansion, through inadequate refilling of the intravascular space from the interstitium to compensate for fluid that was removed. The proclivity for hypotension is further enhanced by impairment of vascular tone, which may result from the underlying illness, medications, or dialysis-induced rise in core body temperature.[95] Continuous therapies have been advocated in patients with hemodynamic instability who might benefit from the low yet consistent ultrafiltration rate afforded by this modality. For patients receiving intermittent modalities, modifications to the dialysate prescription as described previously might mitigate iatrogenic hypotension.[96] In addition, novel biofeedback technology, including blood volume monitoring, appears promising but has not been definitively proven to reduce intradialytic hypotension.[97]

VASCULAR ACCESS CONSIDERATIONS

The initiation of acute RRT mandates placement of a dedicated dual-lumen central venous catheter with the goal of sustaining an adequate blood flow with minimal recirculation in order to ensure adequate solute clearance. To maximize RRT efficiency, the distal catheter tip should reside in a large vein, necessitating the use of a catheter with an adequate length. An internal jugular catheter tip should be at the atriocaval junction, thereby requiring a catheter length of 15 to 20 cm; a catheter placed in the femoral veins must reach the inferior vena cava and so have an optimal length of at least 20 to 25 cm.[98] To minimize mechanical and infectious complications of central venous catheters, ultrasound-guided insertion[99] and adherence to strict aseptic technique[100] are recommended.

Though subclavian catheters may be associated with a lower rate of infection,[101] they are generally avoided, owing to the associated higher rate of central vein stenosis, which might preclude the future creation of a permanent vascular access in the ipsilateral arm among individuals who will require permanent dialysis.[102,103] Stenosis is believed to result from contact of the catheter with the vessel wall, and the tortuosity of the vessel makes it more prone to stenosis; this is most problematic when catheters are placed in the subclavian or the left internal jugular vein.

A randomized clinical trial showed similar rates of catheter colonization among those receiving internal jugular and femoral catheters overall, and no difference in catheter associated-bacteremia.[104] A secondary analysis of these data suggested a trend for less catheter dysfunction among catheters placed in the right internal jugular vein than in the femoral vein; however, the rate of dysfunction was highest for catheters in the left internal jugular vein.[105] Accordingly, the KDIGO Clinical Practice Guidelines for AKI suggest the right internal jugular vein (which flows in a direct line with the superior vena cava) as the preferred access site for patients with AKI, followed by the femoral veins, the left internal jugular vein, and, as a last resort, the subclavian vein on the dominant side.[55] Because of their ease of insertion at the bedside, temporary noncuffed catheters are preferred in critically ill patients with AKI. However, it would seem reasonable that even well-functioning nontunneled catheters should be replaced with cuffed tunneled catheters, which are associated with a lower risk of infection, if the need for RRT appears to be prolonged.

DRUG DOSING CONSIDERATIONS

In critically ill patients with AKI, medications must be reviewed frequently and meticulously. There are three principal issues of concern: (1) the perpetuation of kidney injury through the administration of nephrotoxins; (2) the administration of agents that accumulate and cause extrarenal toxicity in the setting of impaired kidney function; and (3) drug dosing considerations when patients are receiving RRT. Consultation with the ICU pharmacist and updated medication compendia are recommended.

In patients with established AKI, irrespective of cause, avoidance of nephrotoxic medications is a fundamental component of any AKI management strategy. Nephrotoxic agents that are frequently used in the ICU include antimicrobials such as aminoglycosides and amphotericin B, phosphate-based enemas, and radiocontrast agents.[106] Later trials have highlighted the potential nephrotoxicity of hydroxyethyl starches used as volume expanders.[107,108] Alternative agents and imaging modalities should be considered.

As glomerular filtration rate (GFR) changes during AKI, otherwise safe drugs may accumulate, with adverse consequences.[109] When the serum creatinine concentration rises rapidly, the absence of a steady state limits the applicability of GFR estimating equations.[109] If the serum creatinine concentration is increasing, the GFR calculated from an estimating equation would overestimate GFR. In contrast, if AKI is improving, the calculated GFR would underestimate GFR.

Specific medications that may accumulate with acute or chronic kidney function impairment include morphine, which has a metabolite that accumulates in the setting of a decreased GFR. Hydromorphone is preferable in this setting owing to decreased renal metabolism.[110] Novel oral anticoagulants such as dabigatran may rapidly accumulate in the setting of AKI, with dangerous implications for bleeding.[111,112] The accumulation of sulfonylurea may precipitate hypoglycemia, and metformin might contribute to lactic acidosis.[113] Finally, the accumulation of gabapentin and pregabalin can cause sedation and myoclonus.[114,115]

Dosing adjustments in the setting of AKI are fraught with challenges because much of the available data about such adjustments are from patients with stable CKD. Even in the setting of a comparable GFR, critical illness and AKI have unique implications for pharmacokinetics. Volume overload may markedly inflate the volume of distribution, necessitating higher loading doses. Once a drug is in the bloodstream, its concentration may be altered by fluctuations in hepatic and renal metabolism. Finally, drug excretion, predominantly of water-soluble drugs, is impaired in the setting of AKI. Thus, although published recommendations can be used as a starting point for drug dosing, careful monitoring, by following drug levels when available or by clinical assessment for evidence of toxicity, is warranted.

When RRT is initiated, dosing strategies must further account for the extracorporeal clearance of medications. Drug characteristics (e.g., volume of distribution, molecular weight, extent of protein binding), RRT prescription (e.g., blood flow, session duration, proportion of convective and diffusive clearances) and dialyzer features (e.g., porosity or flux, surface area) are important determinants of medication clearance. In some instances, RRT may have a more subtle impact on drug clearance by enhancing extrarenal drug metabolism, perhaps through the removal of uremic toxins.[109] For recipients of intermittent dialysis, medications should be administered after dialysis whenever feasible with consideration of a supplemental dose. With the current predominant use of high-flux filters, which enhance drug clearance, dosing recommendations that were derived for use with low-flux filters typically need to be increased by 25% to 50%.[109]

The advent of SLED poses a further challenge because extracorporeal clearance is augmented by this modality for an extended time, resulting in a longer period of increased drug clearance during which blood concentrations of some vital drugs might become inadequate. To date, drug dosing guidance with SLED is available for only a few agents.[116] As a general rule, drug doses should probably be higher than those administered to patients receiving standard IHD, and where feasible, their use should be accompanied by careful drug level monitoring.[117] In patients receiving CRRT, total effluent flow and the relative breakdown of convective and diffusive therapy will affect drug removal and subsequent dosing changes. The initiation of CRRT at usual doses, assuming that there are no interruptions to the therapy, will begin to approximate endogenous kidney function, and more frequent drug dosing is generally required than with IHD or SLED. For a more detailed discussion of this topic, the reader is referred to Chapter 64.

Complete reference list available at ExpertConsult.com.

KEY REFERENCES

2. Odutayo A, Adhikari NK, Barton J, et al: Epidemiology of acute kidney injury in Canadian critical care units: a prospective cohort study. *Can J Anaesth* 59:934–942, 2012.
3. Vaara ST, Pettila V, Kaukonen KM, et al: The attributable mortality of acute kidney injury: a sequentially matched analysis. *Crit Care Med* 42:878–885, 2014.
4. Uchino S, Kellum JA, Bellomo R, et al: Beginning, ending supportive therapy for the kidney. I: acute renal failure in critically ill patients: a multinational, multicenter study. *JAMA* 294:813–818, 2005.
7. Zarjou A, Agarwal A: Sepsis and acute kidney injury. *J Am Soc Nephrol* 22:999–1006, 2011.
11. Rivers E, Nguyen B, Havstad S, et al: Early goal-directed therapy in the treatment of severe sepsis and septic shock. *N Engl J Med* 345:1368–1377, 2001.
12. Angus DC, Yealy DM, Kellum JA, et al: Protocol-based care for early septic shock. *N Engl J Med* 371:386, 2014.
13. Prowle JR, Echeverri JE, Ligabo EV, et al: Fluid balance and acute kidney injury. *Nat Rev Nephrol* 6:107–115, 2010.
14. Sutherland SM, Zappitelli M, Alexander SR, et al: Fluid overload and mortality in children receiving continuous renal replacement therapy: the prospective pediatric continuous renal replacement therapy registry. *Am J Kidney Dis* 55:316–325, 2010.
15. Bouchard J, Soroko SB, Chertow GM, et al: Fluid accumulation, survival and recovery of kidney function in critically ill patients with acute kidney injury. *Kidney Int* 76:422–427, 2009.
16. Mehta RL, Bouchard J, Soroko SB, et al: Sepsis as a cause and consequence of acute kidney injury: Program to Improve Care in Acute Renal Disease. *Intensive Care Med* 37:241–248, 2011.
17. Heung M, Wolfgram DF, Kommareddi M, et al: Fluid overload at initiation of renal replacement therapy is associated with lack of renal recovery in patients with acute kidney injury. *Nephrol Dial Transplant* 27:956–961, 2012.
19. Liu KD, Thompson BT, Ancukiewicz M, et al: Acute kidney injury in patients with acute lung injury: Impact of fluid accumulation on classification of acute kidney injury and associated outcomes. *Crit Care Med* 2011.
20. Kirkpatrick AW, Roberts DJ, De Waele J, et al: Intra-abdominal hypertension and the abdominal compartment syndrome: updated consensus definitions and clinical practice guidelines from the World Society of the Abdominal Compartment Syndrome. *Intensive Care Med* 39:1190–1206, 2013.
24. Chowdhury AH, Cox EF, Francis ST, et al: A randomized, controlled, double-blind crossover study on the effects of 2-L infusions of 0.9% saline and Plasma-Lyte(R) 148 on renal blood flow velocity and renal cortical tissue perfusion in healthy volunteers. *Ann Surg* 256:18–24, 2012.
26. Yunos NM, Bellomo R, Hegarty C, et al: Association between a chloride-liberal vs chloride-restrictive intravenous fluid administration strategy and kidney injury in critically ill adults. *JAMA* 308:1566–1572, 2012.
27. Bellomo R, Ronco C, Kellum J, et al for the Acute Dialysis Quality Initiative Workgroup: Acute renal failure: definition, outcome measures, animal models, fluid therapy and information technology needs. The Second International Consensus Conference of the Acute Dialysis Quality Initiative Group. *Crit Care* 8:R204–R212, 2004.
28. Wiedemann HP, Wheeler AP, Bernard GR, et al: Comparison of two fluid-management strategies in acute lung injury. *N Engl J Med* 354:2564–2575, 2006.
29. Ventilation with lower tidal volumes as compared with traditional tidal volumes for acute lung injury and the acute respiratory distress syndrome. The Acute Respiratory Distress Syndrome Network. *N Engl J Med* 342:1301–1308, 2000.
32. Faubel S: Pulmonary complications after acute kidney injury. *Adv Chronic Kidney Dis* 15:284–296, 2008.
33. Grams ME, Rabb H: The distant organ effects of acute kidney injury. *Kidney Int* 81:942–948, 2012.
38. Lee WM, Stravitz RT, Larson AM: Introduction to the revised American Association for the Study of Liver Diseases Position Paper on acute liver failure 2011. *Hepatology* 55:965–967, 2012.
39. Ronco C, Haapio M, House AA, et al: Cardiorenal syndrome. *J Am Coll Cardiol* 52:1527–1539, 2008.
40. McCullough PA, Kellum JA, Haase M, et al: Pathophysiology of the cardiorenal syndromes: executive summary from the eleventh consensus conference of the Acute Dialysis Quality Initiative (ADQI). *Contrib Nephrol* 182:82–98, 2013.
45. Bart BA, Goldsmith SR, Lee KL, et al: Heart Failure Clinical Research N. Ultrafiltration in decompensated heart failure with cardiorenal syndrome. *N Engl J Med* 367:2296–2304, 2012.
47. Chawla LS, Eggers PW, Star RA, et al: Acute kidney injury and chronic kidney disease as interconnected syndromes. *N Engl J Med* 371:58–66, 2014.
48. Tolwani A: Continuous renal-replacement therapy for acute kidney injury. *N Engl J Med* 367:2505–2514, 2012.
51. Karvellas CJ, Farhat MR, Sajjad I, et al: A comparison of early versus late initiation of renal replacement therapy in critically ill patients with acute kidney injury: a systematic review and meta-analysis. *Crit Care* 15:R72, 2011.
52. Liu KD, Himmelfarb J, Paganini E, et al: Timing of initiation of dialysis in critically ill patients with acute kidney injury. *Clin J Am Soc Nephrol* 1:915–919, 2006.
53. Wilson FP, Yang W, Machado CA, et al: Dialysis versus nondialysis in patients with AKI: a propensity-matched cohort study. *Clin J Am Soc Nephrol* 9:673–681, 2014.
55. Kidney Disease/Improving Global Outcomes: KDIGO clinical practice guideline for acute kidney injury. *Kidney Int Suppl* 2:1–138, 2012.
56. Palevsky PM, Zhang JH, O'Connor TZ, et al: Intensity of renal support in critically ill patients with acute kidney injury. *N Engl J Med* 359:7–20, 2008.
59. Marshall MR, Golper TA, Shaver MJ, et al: Sustained low-efficiency dialysis for critically ill patients requiring renal replacement therapy. *Kidney Int* 60:777–785, 2001.
64. Vinsonneau C, Camus C, Combes A, et al: Continuous venovenous haemodiafiltration versus intermittent haemodialysis for acute renal failure in patients with multiple-organ dysfunction syndrome: a multicentre randomised trial. *Lancet* 368:379–385, 2006.
65. Rabindranath K, Adams J, Macleod AM, et al: Intermittent versus continuous renal replacement therapy for acute renal failure in adults. *Cochrane Database Syst Rev* (2):CD003773, 2007.
67. Wald R, Shariff SZ, Adhikari NK, et al: The association between renal replacement therapy modality and long-term outcomes among critically ill adults with acute kidney injury: a retrospective cohort study*. *Crit Care Med* 42:868–877, 2014.
74. Wald R, Friedrich JO, Bagshaw SM, et al: Optimal mode of clearance in critically ill patients with Acute Kidney Injury (OMAKI): a pilot randomized controlled trial of hemofiltration versus hemodialysis: a Canadian Critical Care Trials Group project. *Crit Care* 16:R205, 2012.
77. Bellomo R, Cass A, Cole L, et al for the Randomized Evaluation of Normal Versus Augmented Level of Replacement Therapy (RENAL) Study Investigators: Intensity of continuous renal-replacement therapy in critically ill patients. *N Engl J Med* 361:1627–1638, 2009.

81. Morabito S, Pistolesi V, Tritapepe L, et al: Regional citrate anticoagulation for RRTs in critically ill patients with AKI. *Clin J Am Soc Nephrol* 9:2173–2188, 2014.
82. Tolwani A, Wille KM: Advances in continuous renal replacement therapy: citrate anticoagulation update. *Blood Purif* 34:88–93, 2012.
83. Wu MY, Hsu YH, Bai CH, et al: Regional citrate versus heparin anticoagulation for continuous renal replacement therapy: a meta-analysis of randomized controlled trials. *Am J Kidney Dis* 59:810–818, 2012.
89. Shippy CR, Appel PL, Shoemaker WC: Reliability of clinical monitoring to assess blood volume in critically ill patients. *Crit Care Med* 12:107–112, 1984.
90. Marik PE, Baram M, Vahid B: Does central venous pressure predict fluid responsiveness? A systematic review of the literature and the tale of seven mares. *Chest* 134:172–178, 2008.
98. Wilson P, Lertdumrongluk P, Leray-Moragues H, et al: Prevention and management of dialysis catheter complications in the intensive care unit. *Blood Purif* 34:194–199, 2012.
99. Prabhu MV, Juneja D, Gopal PB, et al: Ultrasound-guided femoral dialysis access placement: a single-center randomized trial. *Clin J Am Soc Nephrol* 5:235–239, 2010.
100. Pronovost P, Needham D, Berenholtz S, et al: An intervention to decrease catheter-related bloodstream infections in the ICU. *N Engl J Med* 355:2725–2732, 2006.
104. Parienti JJ, Thirion M, Megarbane B, et al for the Cathedia Study Group: Femoral vs jugular venous catheterization and risk of nosocomial events in adults requiring acute renal replacement therapy: a randomized controlled trial. *JAMA* 299:2413–2422, 2008.
105. Parienti JJ, Megarbane B, Fischer MO, et al for the Cathedia Study Group: Catheter dysfunction and dialysis performance according to vascular access among 736 critically ill adults requiring renal replacement therapy: a randomized controlled study. *Crit Care Med* 38:1118–1125, 2010.
106. Perazella MA: Drug use and nephrotoxicity in the intensive care unit. *Kidney Int* 81:1172–1178, 2012.
108. Perner A, Haase N, Guttormsen AB, et al for the 6S Trial Group and Scandinavian Critical Care Trials Group: Hydroxyethyl starch 130/0.42 versus Ringer's acetate in severe sepsis. *N Engl J Med* 367:124–134, 2012.
109. Matzke GR, Aronoff GR, Atkinson AJ, Jr, et al: Drug dosing consideration in patients with acute and chronic kidney disease: a clinical update from Kidney Disease: Improving Global Outcomes (KDIGO). *Kidney Int* 80:1122–1137, 2011.
116. Bogard KN, Peterson NT, Plumb TJ, et al: Antibiotic dosing during sustained low-efficiency dialysis: special considerations in adult critically ill patients. *Crit Care Med* 39:560–570, 2011.
117. Heintz BH, Matzke GR, Dager WE: Antimicrobial dosing concepts and recommendations for critically ill adult patients receiving continuous renal replacement therapy or intermittent hemodialysis. *Pharmacotherapy* 29:562–577, 2009.

68 Plasmapheresis

Ernesto Sabath | Bradley M. Denker

CHAPTER OUTLINE

HISTORICAL PERSPECTIVE, 2148
GENERAL PRINCIPLES, 2148
PLASMAPHERESIS APPLICATIONS IN KIDNEY DISEASE, 2149
　Anti–Glomerular Basement Membrane Disease, 2149
　Rapidly Progressive Glomerulonephritis, 2150
　Lupus Nephritis, 2151
　Mixed Cryoglobulinemia, 2152
　Kidney Failure Associated with Multiple Myeloma and Other Hematologic Disorders, 2152
　Hemolytic Uremic Syndrome and Thrombotic Thrombocytopenic Purpura, 2154
KIDNEY TRANSPLANTATION, 2155
　Recurrent Focal Segmental Glomerulosclerosis, 2155
PLASMAPHERESIS AND NONRENAL DISEASE, 2157
　Guillain-Barré Syndrome, 2158
　Chronic Inflammatory Demyelinating Polyneuropathy, 2158
　Myasthenia Gravis, 2158
　Catastrophic Antiphospholipid Antibody Syndrome, 2158
　Familial Hypercholesterolemia, 2159
　Removal of Toxins, 2159
PREGNANCY AND PLASMAPHERESIS, 2159
TECHNICAL ASPECTS, 2159
　Plasma Separation Techniques, 2160
　Venous Access, 2161
　Anticoagulation, 2162
　Replacement Fluid, 2162
COMPLICATIONS, 2162
CONCLUSION, 2164

The therapeutic plasma exchange (TPE) or plasmapheresis (PE) procedure involves the therapeutic removal of macromolecules from the plasma of patients with various medical conditions. This chapter will review the history of plasmapheresis and the major conditions (renal and nonrenal) for which it has therapeutic benefit and concludes with technical aspects and details of the plasmapheresis process.

HISTORICAL PERSPECTIVE

The term *plasmapheresis* is derived from the Greek word *apheresis*, which means "taking away," or removal. It is unclear when the notion of therapeutic removal of blood components first originated, but it was flourishing even before Hippocrates in the fifth century BC. Bloodletting to remove evil humors was commonplace in medical practice, in part due to lack of understanding of disease processes and the paucity of effective therapies. By the Middle Ages, surgeons and barbers were specializing in this bloody and often painful practice and, even as late as the nineteenth century, bloodletting was used for nearly every infectious and malignant malady afflicting patients in the United States and Europe.[1] The first true plasmapheresis procedure involving the removal of so-called bad blood and replacement with a clean solution was performed in 1914 by Abel, Rowntree, and Turner at the Johns Hopkins Hospital. The procedure was termed *vivi-diffusion* and demonstrated the principle that the blood of a living animal could be dialyzed outside the body and then returned to the circulation.[2,3] In 1960, Schwab and Fahey performed the first therapeutic manual plasmapheresis to reduce elevated globulin levels in a patient with macroglobulinemia.[4]

In the early days, the utility of plasmapheresis was based on anecdotal or uncontrolled studies. In recent years, the number of clinical indications for plasmapheresis has been growing. However, the number of clinical conditions that have been rigorously studied with prospective randomized controlled trials remains small, and decisions about the implementation of plasmapheresis (an invasive and potentially dangerous procedure) often still rests on anecdotal experience and uncontrolled studies.

GENERAL PRINCIPLES

The mechanism for the clinical improvement of kidney diseases by plasmapheresis depends on the pathophysiologic

Table 68.1 Pathologic Factors Removed by Plasmapheresis
ADAMTS 13 (metalloproteinase)
Autoantibodies
Complement products
Cryoglobulins
Immune complexes
Lipoproteins
Myeloma proteins
Protein-bound toxins

Table 68.2 Summary of Renal Diseases Treated with Plasmapheresis	
Disease	Category*
Anti–glomerular basement membrane disease	I
Rapidly progressive glomerulonephritis	II
Hemolytic uremic syndrome	III
Thrombotic thrombocytopenia purpura	I
Renal transplant rejection	IV
Desensitization for renal transplantation	II
Recurrent focal and segmental glomerulosclerosis	III
Cryoglobulinemia	II
Systemic lupus erythematosus	III

*Category I, standard primary therapy; category II, supportive therapy; category III, when evidence of benefit is unclear; category IV, when there is no current evidence of benefit or for research protocols.

features of the underlying disease. Plasmapheresis should be considered when the pathogenic factor is a substance with a large molecular weight or when the patient has a deficiency of a plasma component. However, hemodialysis and hemofiltration are more efficient procedures for the removal of small molecules and toxins with large volumes of distribution. In treating any disease characterized by the accumulation of toxic proteins or antibodies, the success of plasmapheresis depends on the interaction of two general variables: (1) the rate of production of the abnormal protein or antibody; and (2) the efficiency of removal by plasmapheresis. This balance determines whether an abnormal component can be removed rapidly enough to provide clinical benefit, typically assessed by the prevention of, or improvement in, end-organ damage. The ultimate benefit of the procedure is strongly dependent on a rapid and efficient reduction in plasma levels of the toxic substance. As a result, plasmapheresis is rarely used in isolation but is most often used with other immunosuppressive strategies to decrease abnormal protein or antibody production and reduce inflammation.

Table 68.1 lists the pathologic factors that may be removed with plasmapheresis. The molecular weight complexes suitable for plasmapheresis are usually abnormal proteins (typically autoantibodies present in numerous diseases), monoclonal immunoglobulins present in plasma cell dyscrasias, and potentially high-grade immune complexes present in some forms of acute glomerulonephritis. In addition to removal of toxic proteins or replacement of deficient ones with plasma exchange, there may be additional benefits, including reversal of impaired splenic function to remove immune complexes,[5] removal of fibrinogen, and replacement of humoral factors.

PLASMAPHERESIS APPLICATIONS IN KIDNEY DISEASE

The clinical indications for plasmapheresis in the treatment of kidney diseases are summarized in Table 68.2.

ANTI–GLOMERULAR BASEMENT MEMBRANE DISEASE

Anti–glomerular basement membrane (anti-GBM) disease is a disorder in which circulating antibodies are directed against the noncollagenous domain (NC1) of the α3 chain of type IV collagen, resulting in rapidly progressive glomerulonephritis (RPGN). Goodpasture's syndrome is classically defined by the triad of pulmonary hemorrhage, RPGN, and circulating anti-GBM antibodies. More than 90% of patients have circulating anti-GBM antibodies, and the titer of circulating antibodies correlates with disease activity.[6,7] Approximately 60% to 70% of patients will have pulmonary disease in addition to RPGN and, rarely, a patient may present with pulmonary hemorrhage and no renal involvement. Before the use of current therapies, the mortality rate exceeded 90%, with a mean survival time of less than 4 months. Currently, with the combination of plasmapheresis, corticosteroids, and cyclophosphamide, the mortality rate has been reduced to less than 20%. The role of plasmapheresis in anti-GBM diseases is rapid removal of the pathogenic antibodies, whereas the cyclophosphamide and corticosteroids are essential to prevent additional antibody synthesis and reduce inflammation. A rapid reduction in anti-GBM antibody levels is necessary in view of the speed of glomerular damage, which cannot be achieved by drug therapy alone.

Plasmapheresis was first used for the treatment of anti-GBM disease in 1975,[8] and numerous uncontrolled studies and case series published in the last 30 years have suggested the beneficial effects of plasmapheresis on overall survival and preservation of kidney function. Some of the major studies are summarized in Table 68.3 and, although none were prospective randomized trials, the use of plasmapheresis is now considered standard therapy. In an early uncontrolled study of 20 patients with anti-GBM disease,[9] 8 patients were treated with plasmapheresis and immunosuppression, 4 patients with immunosuppression alone, and 8 patients with nonspecific therapy. The patients treated with plasmapheresis had less severe renal failure, shorter duration of alveolar hemorrhage, and a lower rate of mortality. In the only randomized trial published, Johnson and colleagues[10] compared the effect of therapy with immunosuppression alone with that of immunosuppression plus plasmapheresis on the clinical course in 17 patients with anti-GBM disease. Only 2 of 8 patients who received plasmapheresis became dependent on dialysis, in comparison with 6 of 9 who received immunosuppression alone; thus, the addition of plasmapheresis showed a trend toward a better outcome. However, the initial serum creatinine level and number of

Table 68.3 Renal Recovery in Patients with Anti–Glomerular Basement Membrane Antibody Disease*

Study (Year)	No. of Patients in Study	Patients with Independent Renal Function at 1 Year		Treatment
		Initial Cr Concentration <5.7 mg/dL	Initial Cr Concentration ≥5.7 mg/dL[†]	
Bouget et al (1990)[171]	13	50%	0%	Most patients received PE.
Herody et al (1993)[172]	29	93%	0%	Most patients received PE.
Merkel et al (1994)[173]	32	64%	3%	25 patients received PE.
Andrews et al (1995)[174]	15	NA	7%	All patients had Cr concentration ≥600 mmol/L; only 8 patients received treatment.
Daly et al (1996)[175]	40	20%	0%	23 patients received PE.
Levy et al (2001)[11]	71	94%	15%	All patients received PE, C, and CFM.
Saurina et al (2003)[176]	32	71%	18%	24 patients received treatment with C, CFM, and PE.

*According to initial creatinine concentration.
[†]Or dialysis-dependent.
C, Corticosteroids; CFM, cyclophosphamide; Cr, creatinine; PE, plasmapheresis.

fibrocellular crescents were also major factors associated with outcome.

The largest study to date was uncontrolled and reported long-term outcomes in 71 patients with anti-GBM disease.[11] All patients received a standard immunosuppressive regimen of plasmapheresis, oral prednisolone, and oral cyclophosphamide. Plasma exchange (50 mL/kg up to a maximum of 4 L) was performed with a centrifugal cell separator daily for at least 14 days or until anti-GBM antibody levels were undetectable. Human albumin (5%) with added calcium and potassium was used as replacement fluid, and fresh-frozen plasma (FFP; 150 to 300 mL at the end of the exchange) was used in patients who had recently undergone surgery or kidney biopsy and in those with pulmonary hemorrhage. Patients who had a creatinine concentration less than 5.7 mg/dL (n = 19) had 100% patient survival and 95% renal survival at 1 year. In patients who had a creatinine concentration higher than 5.7 mg/dL (n = 13) but did not require immediate dialysis, patient and renal survival were 83% and 82% at 1 year, respectively. In patients who presented with dialysis-dependent renal failure (n = 39), patient and renal survival were 65% and 8% at 1 year, respectively. All patients who required immediate dialysis and who had 100% crescents on renal biopsy remained dialysis-dependent.

The conclusion was that all patients with anti-GBM antibody disease and severe renal failure who do not require immediate dialysis should be treated with an aggressive immunosuppressive regimen and intensive plasmapheresis. Because pulmonary hemorrhage is associated with a high risk of mortality, plasmapheresis should be initiated in such patients, regardless of the severity of the kidney failure.

Outcomes with kidney transplantation after anti-GBM disease have been excellent. Most patients with anti-GBM disease have no recurrence of the disease in the allograft, although up to 50% may show linear immunoglobulin G (IgG) staining of the glomerular basement membrane.[12] The delay of kidney transplantation for 12 or more months after the disappearance of anti-GBM antibodies and the degree of the immunosuppression necessary to maintain a functioning allograft are thought to be the main reasons why recurrences are very rare.[13]

RAPIDLY PROGRESSIVE GLOMERULONEPHRITIS

RPGN is characterized by rapid deterioration in kidney function occurring over a period ranging from a few days to a few weeks. Untreated RPGN usually leads to end-stage kidney disease (ESKD). RPGN is characterized by severe inflammation and necrosis of most glomeruli and, frequently, by fibrocellular crescents (crescentic glomerulonephritis). There are three major subgroups of RPGN: (1) anti-GBM disease and Goodpasture's syndrome (discussed above); (2) immune complex–mediated processes in which immune deposition occurs, usually as a result of autoimmune diseases (e.g., systemic lupus erythematosus, postinfectious processes, mixed cryoglobulinemia, IgA nephropathy); and (3) pauci-immune diseases that are usually (in about 80% of patients) associated with antineutrophil cytoplasmic antibody (ANCA), including granulomatosis with polyangiitis (GPA; formerly known as Wegener's granulomatosis) or microscopic polyangiitis (MPA). A therapeutic role for plasmapheresis in anti-GBM disease is discussed above, although its role in immune complex–mediated processes is still uncertain (see below).

ANTINEUTROPHIL CYTOPLASMIC ANTIBODY–ASSOCIATED VASCULITIS

Crescentic glomerulonephritis induced by ANCA is associated with progressive impairment of kidney function and often involves other organs. Aggressive treatment is required to avoid end-organ damage and potentially fatal complications.[14] The rationale for using plasmapheresis in pauci-immune ANCA-associated diseases (GPA and MPA) was initially based on similarities in renal histopathology between these disorders and anti-GBM disease. The first use of plasmapheresis for the treatment of GPA-associated RPGN was reported in 1977, when the combination of plasmapheresis, oral prednisolone, and cyclophosphamide was associated with rapid recovery of kidney function in five of nine patients.[15]

In an early controlled trial of 48 patients with focal necrotizing glomerulonephritis, 25 patients received plasmapheresis and drug therapy (prednisolone, cyclophosphamide, azathioprine), and 23 patients received drug therapy alone. The number of plasmapheresis exchanges was determined by the clinical response, and a mean of nine exchanges were performed (range, 5 to 25). Replacement fluid was with 5% albumin. In patients not requiring dialysis, the response to immunosuppressive therapy alone was excellent; the addition of PE provided no additional benefit, nor did it prevent some patients from progressing to the need for dialysis. However, this study was the first to suggest that some patients who were dialysis dependent might be able to discontinue dialysis after treatment of the vasculitis, and the proportion of patients coming off dialysis was higher in the PE group (10 of 17 vs. 3 of 8 in the drug therapy–alone group).[16]

More recent studies have suggested that plasmapheresis improves prognosis in patients with ANCA-associated glomerulonephritis. Frasca and colleagues[17] retrospectively analyzed 26 patients with acute renal failure due to ANCA vasculitis. They reported that patients who received immunosuppressive treatment plus plasmapheresis experienced a more favorable outcome than patients who received immunosuppressive treatment alone. Results from the multicenter European Vasculitis Study Group have supported this conclusion.[18,19] In this study, 137 patients with ANCA-associated systemic vasculitis (kidney biopsy–confirmed) and serum creatinine level higher than 5.7 mg/dL were randomized to receive seven plasmapheresis exchanges (n = 70) or 3 g of methylprednisolone in divided doses (n = 67). Both groups received oral cyclophosphamide and oral prednisolone as maintenance therapy. Dialysis independence at 3 months was the primary end point; 33 of 67 of methylprednisolone-treated patients (49%) were alive and independent of dialysis compared with 48 of 70 patients (69%) who received plasmapheresis ($P = 0.02$). When compared with methylprednisolone, plasmapheresis was associated with a reduction in risk for progression to ESKD of 24% at 1 year. A meta-analysis summarizing nine trials with 387 patients has shown that PE confers a significant benefit to patients with RPGN by reducing the number of patients requiring dialysis at 12 months from diagnosis. It has been estimated that the number of patients requiring dialysis may be reduced by 50% with this intervention.[20,21] Therefore, plasmapheresis is the best complement to immunosuppressive therapy for patients with ANCA vasculitis and advanced kidney disease.[22] Some patients present with antibodies to both ANCA and GBM. Plasmapheresis is recommended in such cases in addition to any patient with either of these disorders who also has diffuse pulmonary hemorrhage.[23-25]

IDIOPATHIC RAPIDLY PROGRESSIVE GLOMERULONEPHRITIS AND OTHER VASCULITIDES

The Canadian Apheresis Study Group randomized 32 patients with idiopathic RPGN to receive intravenous methylprednisolone, followed by oral prednisolone and azathioprine, with or without plasmapheresis (10 exchanges in the first 16 days). Again, there was no demonstrable benefit of plasmapheresis in the non–dialysis-dependent patients; however, a nonsignificant trend in benefit was seen in the dialysis-dependent patients, with 3 of 4 patients receiving plasmapheresis coming off dialysis compared with only 2 of 7 in the control group.[26] In 62 patients with Churg-Strauss syndrome or polyarteritis nodosa, there was no additional benefit seen in patients who received plasmapheresis in addition to cyclophosphamide and steroids.[27] Zauner and associates[28] performed a prospective, randomized multicenter study that compared 39 patients with RPGN treated with immunosuppression alone or immunosuppression and plasmapheresis. They found that the addition of plasmapheresis had no significant effect on renal or patient survival independent of age, gender, or serum creatinine concentration at the time of diagnosis.

There is little evidence for the use of plasmapheresis for those with other causes of RPGN, although there has been one report of benefit in children with RPGN from Henoch-Schönlein purpura (HSP).[29,30] One study has suggested that plasmapheresis may be beneficial in kidney transplant recipients with recurrent HSP nephritis, but there are no prospective studies or protocols indicating the optimal therapeutic regimen for these patients.[31]

LUPUS NEPHRITIS

Acute and chronic kidney disease are common and potentially serious complications of systemic lupus erythematosus (SLE). Traditionally, active lupus nephritis was treated with corticosteroids, azathioprine, and intravenous cyclophosphamide, but safer and more effective therapies have been sought. More recent studies have shown that mycophenolate mofetil[32] is an alternative to intravenous cyclophosphamide in patients with active proliferative disease. Although promising in uncontrolled studies, the role of rituximab in treating lupus nephritis remains to be determined.[33]

The use of plasmapheresis for patients with proliferative lupus nephritis was first reported in the 1970s, but it was not until 1992 that the Lupus Nephritis Collaborative Study Group undertook a randomized study to examine systematically the safety and efficacy of plasmapheresis. The Lupus Nephritis Collaborative Study Group[34] was a large, randomized, controlled multicenter trial comparing a standard-therapy regimen of prednisone and cyclophosphamide with a regimen of standard therapy plus plasmapheresis in patients with severe lupus nephritis. In this study, 46 patients were randomly assigned to receive standard therapy, and 40 were randomly assigned to receive plasmapheresis. Histologic categories included lupus nephritis types III, IV, and V. Plasmapheresis was carried out three times per week for 4 weeks, and drug therapy was standardized. The mean follow-up period was 136 weeks. Although patients treated with plasmapheresis experienced more rapid reduction of antibodies to double-stranded DNA and cryoglobulins, the addition of plasmapheresis did not improve clinical outcomes. Of the 46 patients who received standard therapy, 8 (17%) developed kidney failure and 6 (13%) died; in comparison, of the 40 patients who received plasmapheresis, 10 (25%) developed kidney failure and 8 (20%) died. Results were similar in magnitude and direction after an extended follow-up of 277 weeks. Another small trial confirmed these findings. Wallace and coworkers[35] randomly assigned 9 patients to receive 6 months of intravenous cyclophosphamide and prednisone and 9 patients to receive plasmapheresis before each infusion of cyclophosphamide. In each group, 2 patients developed ESKD, and 3 patients achieved renal remission at 24 months. Together, the results of these studies indicate that addition of plasmapheresis to conventional treatment for lupus nephritis does not appear to improve the prognosis of lupus nephritis, despite more rapid reduction in circulating autoantibodies.

Despite these results, other small studies have suggested that plasmapheresis is beneficial in a select group of patients with aggressive lupus nephritis. Euler and Guillevin[36] administered plasmapheresis and pulse intravenous cyclophosphamide, followed by oral cyclophosphamide and prednisone, in an uncontrolled study of 14 patients with severe SLE and lupus nephritis. All 14 patients responded, and 8 were able to discontinue therapy for 5 to 6 years. One patient had a major relapse, and 2 others had a minor relapse at 2 and 3 years. The main adverse effects were herpes zoster, and 4 women developed irreversible amenorrhea. Danieli and colleagues[37] compared two groups of patients with proliferative lupus nephritis at 4 years of follow-up. The first group (12 patients) received synchronized therapy with plasmapheresis and cyclophosphamide, whereas the second group (16 patients) received intermittent cycles of cyclophosphamide. At the end of the follow-up period, patients who received synchronized plasmapheresis and cyclophosphamide therapy achieved remission faster than patients who received intermittent cycles of cyclophosphamide alone, although renal outcomes were not superior at longer-term follow-up. Yamaji and associates[38] reported a retrospective analysis of 38 patients; they found that synchronized therapy with plasmapheresis and cyclophosphamide might be superior to plasmapheresis or cyclophosphamide alone in achieving complete remission of lupus nephritis and in minimizing the risk of relapse. However, the proportion of patients with class IV disease differed among the three groups—synchronized therapy, 39%; cyclophosphamide alone, 69%; and plasmapheresis alone, 0%.

Thus, the available published evidence does not support the addition of plasmapheresis to immunosuppressive therapy for lupus nephritis. As a result, the American Society for Apheresis has considered plasmapheresis as a category IV treatment (no evidence) for use of plasmapheresis for lupus.[39] However, most studies have included patients with classes III, IV, and V lupus nephritis, so it remains unknown whether there may be a narrow role for plasmapheresis in refractory class IV patients. Immunoadsorption with protein A, protein C1q, or dextran sulfate cellulose columns may hold future promise; a small case series has shown benefit in treating refractory lupus nephritis.[40]

MIXED CRYOGLOBULINEMIA

Cryoglobulinemia is the presence of serum proteins that precipitate at temperatures below 37° C and redissolve on rewarming. More than 80% of patients with mixed cryoglobulinemia are infected by hepatitis C virus, and cryoglobulinemia can often be found in patients with membranoproliferative glomerulonephritis related to this virus. The glomerular injury is the consequence of the glomerular deposition of immune complexes, and the renal manifestations range from isolated proteinuria to overt nephritic or nephrotic syndrome, with variable progression toward ESKD.[41] The use of plasmapheresis for cryoglobulinemia has not been studied in randomized controlled trials. However, the hypothesis that plasmapheresis may remove pathogenic cryoglobulins is rational, and numerous anecdotal case reports and uncontrolled studies have demonstrated that plasmapheresis may benefit patients with severe active disease manifested by progressive kidney failure, severe or malignant hypertension, purpura, and advanced neuropathy.[42,43] In the treatment of severe acute flares of cryoglobulinemia with glomerulonephritis or vasculitis, one approach is combination antiviral therapy with peginterferon (pegylated interferon alfa-2a) and ribavirin for 48 weeks, plus corticosteroids and cyclophosphamide as needed to control severe symptoms. In the most severe cases, the addition of plasmapheresis (exchanges of 3 L of plasma three to four times per week for 2 to 3 weeks) can be helpful. In uncontrolled studies with more than five patients, plasmapheresis induced rapid reduction in the cryocrit, improved kidney function in 55% to 87% of patients, and improved survival ($\approx$25% mortality rate) in comparison to historical data ($\approx$55% mortality rate).[44] It is unclear whether there will be a role for plasmapheresis in the management of hepatitis C–related cryoglobulinemia with newer treatment regimens for hepatitis C, including sofosbuvir, and combination regimens of sofosbuvir-ledipasvir or dasabuvir-ombitasvir-ritonavir.

Due to the unique characteristics of cryoglobulins, the plasmapheresis technique has been modified to enhance their removal. Cryofiltration cools the plasma in an extracorporeal circuit, allowing for more efficient removal of the pathogenic proteins. However, this technique is most efficiently performed by a continuous process that requires a specialized machine designed for this purpose. An alternative protocol is a two-step procedure in which the patient's own plasma can be reinfused after incubation in the cold to cause the abnormal proteins to precipitate out.[45]

KIDNEY FAILURE ASSOCIATED WITH MULTIPLE MYELOMA AND OTHER HEMATOLOGIC DISORDERS

Kidney disease is a common finding in multiple myeloma; in 20% to 50% of affected patients, the plasma creatinine concentration exceeds 1.5 mg/dL (133 µmol/L). Kidney injury is a serious complication associated with a poor prognosis. The mechanisms of injury are thought to be mediated by the toxic and inflammatory effects of monoclonal free light chains (FLCs) on kidney proximal tubule cells and by the formation of intratubular casts through interaction with Tamm-Horsfall proteins. Other factors frequently implicated in myeloma-associated kidney failure include hypercalcemia, hyperuricemia, amyloidosis, hyperviscosity, infections, and chemotherapeutic agents (Figure 68.1).[46,47]

Although trials of plasma exchange to remove the nephrotoxic light chains have shown a disappointing lack of benefit, high cutoff dialysis removes larger quantities of light chains; therefore, some studies have been investigating whether this approach can improve the renal prognosis independently of chemotherapy.[48,49] An early study of 29 patients with multiple myeloma and acute kidney injury included 24 patients on dialysis and an additional 5 with serum creatinine concentrations higher than 5 mg/dL. The patients were randomly assigned to one of two groups; 15 patients received plasmapheresis plus standard therapy, and 14 patients received standard therapy alone. Of the 15 patients who received plasmapheresis, 13 patients recovered kidney function (serum creatinine concentration < 2.5 mg/dL), in contrast to only two of the 14 who received standard therapy.[50] However, in a study of 21 patients who were randomly assigned to receive plasmapheresis plus chemotherapy or chemotherapy alone, Johnson and coworkers[51] reported no difference in patient survival or in recovery of kidney function. The mortality rate at 6 months was 20% in each group, which increased to 60% to 80% at 12 months.

In the largest study to date, 104 patients (of whom 97 completed follow-up) with multiple myeloma and acute kidney injury (kidney biopsies were not used to confirm cast nephropathy) were randomly assigned to receive conventional therapy alone or conventional therapy plus five to seven plasma exchanges (5% human serum albumin) of 50 mL/kg of body weight for 10 days. The primary end point (death, dialysis, or glomerular filtration rate < 30 mL/min) occurred in 33 of 58 patients (56.9%) who received plasmapheresis and in 27 of 39 control subjects (69.2%).[52] This lack of efficacy may not be surprising; light chains are small proteins (25 to 50 kDa) that equilibrate between intravascular and extravascular compartments so that the intravascular compartment may contain only 20% of the total body burden. Therefore, a standard series of 3.5-L plasma exchanges might only remove 65% of intravascular free light chains and therefore have little impact on the total body burden. Together, the results of these studies leave the role of plasmapheresis in the management of cast nephropathy unresolved. Questions remain about subgroups of patients who may benefit; in general, these results suggest that caution should be used when plasmapheresis is considered for patients with acute kidney injury in association with multiple myeloma (Table 68.4).[53]

High-cutoff dialyzers have been tested in patients with myeloma kidney. These dialyzers have membranes with very large pores through which light chains can pass. An early analysis of this method has suggested that up to 90% of light chains could be removed during 3 weeks of extended daily dialysis. However, this success rate is dependent on the plasma cell clone responding to chemotherapy. Hutchison and colleagues studied the efficacy of immunoglobulin free light chain removal by high-cutoff hemodialysis as an adjuvant treatment to chemotherapy in 67 patients with kidney injury and multiple myeloma; 32 of 38 (85%) patients who had undergone kidney biopsy had cast nephropathy.[54] The median number of high-cutoff dialyzer sessions was 11 (range, 3 to 45), and two thirds of those in the study had a sustained reduction in serum free light chain concentrations by day 12. In total, 63% of patients became independent of dialysis; the most important factors that predicted independence from dialysis were the degree of free light chain reduction and the time to initiation of high-cutoff hemodialysis.

Waldenström's macroglobulinemia is a B cell disorder resulting from the accumulation of clonally related IgM-secreting lymphoplasmacytic cells. The morbidity associated with Waldenström's macroglobulinemia is typically mediated by tissue infiltration by neoplastic cells and by the physicochemical and immunologic properties of the monoclonal IgM. Due to the large molecular weight of IgM (>950 kDa), hyperviscosity can be a major issue. In affected patients with symptomatic hyperviscosity, cryoglobulinemia, or moderate-to-severe cytopenia as a result of bone marrow infiltration by lymphoplasmacytic cells, the burden of plasma paraproteins should be reduced rapidly and, in these cases, plasmapheresis should be performed. Typically, two to three sessions of plasmapheresis are necessary to reduce serum IgM levels by 30% to 60%. Treatment should

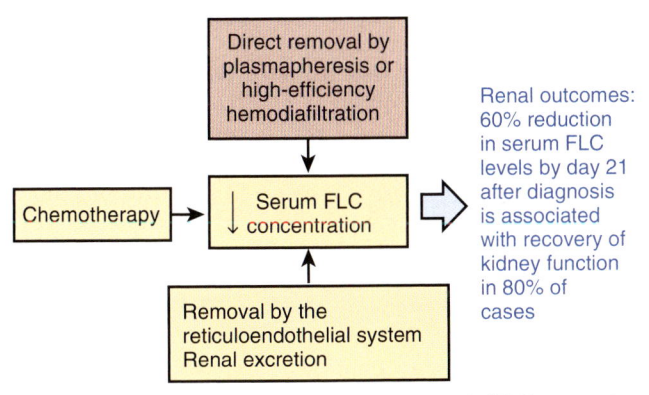

Figure 68.1 Factors that influence free light chain (FLC) concentration and outcome in myeloma kidney. (From Cockwell P, Cook M: The rationale and evidence base for the direct removal of serum-free light chains in the management of myeloma kidney. *Adv Chronic Kidney Dis* 2012;19:324-332.)

Study (Year)	Renal Biopsy	No. of Patients	Dialysis (%)	PE Sessions	Chemotherapy	Outcome	Results
Zucchelli et al (1988)[177]	17	29	82.8	5-7	Melphalan and PDN or VAD	Recovery—renal function	13/15 PE group 2/14 control group
Johnson et al (1990)[51]	21	21	57.1	3-12	Melphalan and PDN	Recovery—if dialysis-independent	3/7 PE group 0/5 control group
Clark et al (2005)[52]	Not Stated	104	29.9	5-7	Melphalan and PDN or VAD	Death or dialysis at 6 mo	33/57 PE group 27/39 control group

Table 68.4 Randomized Controlled Trials of Plasmapheresis (PE) in Treatment of Multiple Myeloma

CFM, Cyclophosphamide; PDN, prednisone; VAD, vincristine, adriamycin, dexamethasone.

be initiated as soon as possible with a regimen that includes bortezomib, dexamethasone, and rituximab to achieve more rapid disease control.[55]

Plasmapheresis has been widely used in hematologic and oncologic diseases; however, only the following disorders are considered category I (standard primary therapy) by the American Society for Apheresis: (1) leukocytosis and thrombocytosis (cytapheresis); (2) thrombotic thrombocytopenic purpura (TTP; see next section); (3) posttransfusion purpura (plasmapheresis); (4) sickle cell disease (red blood cell exchange); (5) ABO-incompatible bone marrow transplantation (red blood cell removal from the marrow; plasmapheresis in the recipient to eliminate ABO antibodies is considered category II [supportive therapy]); (6) hyperviscosity in monoclonal gammopathies; and (7) cutaneous T cell lymphoma (photopheresis; see Table 68.2).[56]

HEMOLYTIC UREMIC SYNDROME AND THROMBOTIC THROMBOCYTOPENIC PURPURA

TTP and hemolytic uremic syndrome (HUS) share a spectrum of abnormalities in numerous organ systems and are characterized by the presence of thrombocytopenia and microangiopathic hemolytic anemia. In HUS, the prominent features are hemolytic anemia, thrombocytopenia, and advanced acute or chronic kidney disease. The finding of neurologic symptoms with fever and perhaps less severe kidney failure is classically considered TTP. However, these designations are artificial, and both syndromes are characterized by pathologic changes of endothelial injury and platelet microthrombi. With two exceptions, the causes for these disorders remain unknown and can be viewed as complications of drug therapy (mitomycin, cyclosporine, ticlopidine), autoimmune disorders (SLE, antiphospholipid antibody syndrome), and pregnancy.[57] Shiga toxin–producing–O157:H7 enterohemorrhagic Escherichia coli (STEC/EHEC) is one of the most common causes of HUS; however, the 2011 outbreak in Northern Europe was the first to be caused by the serotype O104:H4. In this disease, the enterotoxin induces colonic vascular injury, which leads to systemic absorption and activation of numerous signaling pathways and results in endothelial cell damage over several days. Platelet microthrombi are particularly prominent in the glomerular capillaries and often cause severe renal failure. Infection with E. coli O157:H7 can be asymptomatic or may manifest as nonbloody diarrhea, hemorrhagic colitis, HUS, thrombocytopenia, and death.[58]

Treatment of infection with enterohemorrhagic E. coli strains, including E. coli O157:H7, is mainly based on supportive therapy, particularly rehydration. The use of antimotility agents, which inhibit peristalsis and delay clearance of the organism, may worsen HUS. The disease is often self-limited in children, and a role for plasmapheresis is not clear. However, in adults and in patients with severe or persistent disease, plasmapheresis is often used. One of the first uncontrolled trials for plasmapheresis in E. coli–associated HUS was in 22 patients in Scotland with confirmed E. coli O157:H7 infection. Plasmapheresis was performed in 16 patients, of whom 5 (31%) died, compared to 5 of 6 patients (83%) who did not receive plasmapheresis.[59] In 2011, there was an outbreak of Shiga toxin–producing E. coli STEC O104:H4, with 855 confirmed hemolytic–uremic syndrome (HUS) cases in Germany. Most patients with HUS (87%) underwent plasmapheresis, and the mean number of sessions was 6.3/patient. Analysis of the outcomes of this outbreak found that mortality was higher in patients who received supportive care without plasmapheresis (10.6%) when compared to patients treated with plasmapheresis (3.7%) or plasmapheresis plus eculizumab (2.6%).[60] Although this was not a controlled study, this large outbreak has given additional support to the recommendation for the use of plasmapheresis in Shiga toxin–producing, E. coli–related HUS. The role of plasmapheresis for Shiga toxin–producing, E. coli–related HUS in children is not clear. In the 2011 German outbreak, only 12% of patients were in children. Loos and associates reported the outcomes of 90 children with HUS; only 1 patient (1.1%) died in the acute phase.[61] Most patients (67 of 90 [74%]) received supportive care only. Renal replacement therapy was required in 64 of 90 (71%) children. Neurologic complications, mainly seizures and altered mental status, were present in 23 of 90 patients (26%). Ten patients received plasmapheresis, 6 eculizumab, and 7 a combination of both. Plasmapheresis was performed in 17 of 90 patients (19%), mainly for neurologic complications ($n = 16$), but also for severe renal involvement ($n = 1$). Exchange was done with albumin ($n = 12$) or FFP ($n = 5$), with a median of four exchanges (range, two to seven). Treatment with plasmapheresis included 7 patients with neurologic complications for whom additional subsequent treatment with the anti-C5 antibody eculizumab was used.

Atypical hemolytic uremic syndrome (aHUS) is a rare form of thrombotic microangiopathy associated with genetic or acquired disorders that leads to dysregulation of the alternative pathway of complement. Atypical HUS is strongly associated with mutations or polymorphism in proteins implicated for activation or regulation of the alternative pathway of complement, with factor H heterozygous mutations representing the major cause of aHUS. Plasmapheresis has been recommended by the Apheresis Guidelines for the treatment of aHUS and in guidelines produced in 2009 by the European Pediatric Study Group for HUS. They recommended "urgent and empirical" plasma exchange once Shiga toxin enterocolitis and invasive pneumococcus have been excluded.[62] Dragon-Durey and coworkers reported the outcome of 45 patients with aHUS; 15 received plasmapheresis alone and 3 were treated with immunosuppressive treatments (steroids plus cyclophosphamide or mycophenolate mofetil).[63] None of the 3 patients treated by plasmapheresis and immunosuppression relapsed, and all of them fully recovered without relapse at up to 12 months of follow-up. Late-relapsing patients were treated conservatively (2 of 6; 33%), FFP infusion (5 of 6; 83.3%), or plasmapheresis alone (6 of 15; 40%). Sinha and colleagues studied a multicenter cohort of 138 Indian children with anticomplement factor H antibody–associated HUS (aHUS) and found that prompt use of immunosuppressive agents and plasmapheresis are useful for improving outcomes and renal survival.[64,65]

The mechanism of TTP is now partially understood and reveals why plasmapheresis with plasma exchange is beneficial. Genetic studies of congenital TTP have led to the identification of defects in the metalloproteinase, von Willebrand factor (vWF)–cleaving protease (ADAMTS13—a *d*isintegrin-like *a*nd *m*etalloprotease with *t*hrombospondin type 1 repeats).[66] TTP can result from the accumulation of ultra-large vWF. Multimers of vWF normally accumulate on the endothelial cell membrane and are rapidly cleaved into normal-sized multimers by the ADAMTS13 protease. In some patients, ADAMTS13 deficiency leads to the accumulation of ultra-large vWF multimers, resulting in platelet microthrombus formation and subsequent microangiopathic hemolytic anemia. An inhibitory autoantibody to the ADAMTS13 metalloproteinase has been found at varying titers in a high percentage of patients with the idiopathic form of this disease.[67,68] By removing autoantibodies to ADAMTS13 and replacing with normal plasma (containing ADAMTS13 activity), plasmapheresis can reverse the TTP syndrome caused by ADAMTS13 deficiency. However, ADAMTS13 deficiency may be necessary but is not sufficient to account for many cases of TTP. Furthermore, enzyme activity is significantly reduced in numerous other conditions, including infection, cancer, cirrhosis, uremia, SLE, and disseminated intravascular coagulation.

Before the introduction of plasma infusion and plasmapheresis, the disease rapidly progressed and was almost uniformly fatal (90% mortality).[69] In 1977, it was discovered that infusion of FFP or plasmapheresis with FFP replacement could reverse the course of disease.[70,71] The efficacy of plasma exchange in the treatment of TTP-HUS in adults was demonstrated in two trials that included 210 patients.[72,73] Plasma exchange with FFP was more effective than plasma infusion alone. At 6 months, the remission rate was 78% versus 31% and the survival rates with these two procedures were 78% and 50%, respectively. Patients treated with plasma exchange received approximately three times as much plasma as those treated with plasma infusion alone (the amount of plasma administration was limited by the risk of volume overload). Therefore, it is possible that the benefit observed with plasma exchange may have resulted from infusion of more plasma rather than from the removal of a toxic substance. There is also evidence from a single report of 60 patients that plasmapheresis improves outcomes with ticlodipine-associated HUS-TTP (24% mortality vs. 50% in patients not treated with plasmapheresis).[74] However, there is no evidence for a beneficial role of plasmapheresis in patients with HUS-TTP secondary to cancer chemotherapy or bone marrow transplantation.[75]

The optimal duration of plasmapheresis in HUS-TTP is not known but, in our opinion, it should be performed daily until the platelet count has risen to near normal and evidence for hemolysis (schistocytes, lactate dehydrogenase [LDH] elevation) has resolved. A wide range of exchanges (3 to 145) have been reported; on average, 7 to 16 daily exchanges are generally necessary to induce remission.[69,72,73,75] The American Association of Blood Banks has recommended daily plasmapheresis until the platelet count is above 150,000/L for 2 to 3 days, and the American Society for Apheresis has recommended daily plasmapheresis until the platelet count is above 100,000/L and the serum LDH level is nearly normal.[76] When present, neurologic symptoms rapidly improve, and the serum LDH level tends to improve over the first 1 to 3 days. The platelet count may not rise for several days, and improvements in kidney function often take longer. Patients requiring dialysis at presentation may be able to recover enough function to discontinue dialysis, but many patients have residual chronic kidney disease. When a normal platelet count has been achieved, plasma exchange may be gradually tapered by increasing the interval between treatments. Many patients (one third to one half) abruptly develop recurrent thrombocytopenia and increased evidence of hemolysis when daily plasma exchanges are tapered or stopped. Some of these patients may benefit from the addition of prednisone or some other immunosuppressive therapy (e.g., cyclosporine, rituximab) although data in support of these strategies are sparse.[57]

KIDNEY TRANSPLANTATION

Plasmapheresis has been used in several different clinical scenarios involving kidney transplantation. These include recurrent focal glomerulosclerosis (FSGS) in the transplant, ABO blood group–incompatible transplants, positive T cell cross-match, and acute humoral rejection.

RECURRENT FOCAL SEGMENTAL GLOMERULOSCLEROSIS

FSGS is a relatively common cause of ESKD, and recurrent primary FSGS occurs at a rate of 20% to 30% in kidney transplant recipients. The risk of relapse is particularly high (80% to 90%) in patients with a prior history of allograft loss resulting from recurrent FSGS. Additional factors associated with an increased risk of recurrence are rapid progression to ESKD, mesangial hypercellularity, and younger age. The time on dialysis and the immunosuppressive regimen are not proven risk factors. The mechanisms of recurrent FSGS after kidney transplantation are unclear, but the early reappearance of proteinuria suggests that a circulating factor that alters glomerular permeability may be present.[77,78] Removal of a circulating factor by immunoadsorption or plasma exchange may account for the remission of the disease in some patients.[79] The potential circulating factor may be a nonimmunoglobulin protein with a molecular weight less than 100 kDa, although there are discrepancies in the characteristics of this permeability factor.[77-79] An alternative hypothesis is that nephrotic patients lack one or more factors necessary for the maintenance of normal glomerular permeability, and a factor in normal serum (e.g., clusterin) may be lost or diminished.[80-82] However, at this time, the mechanisms of recurrent proteinuria and FSGS remain unknown. New advances in understanding FSGS include identification of the soluble podocyte urokinase receptor (sPAR) as a circulating factor leading to the development and recurrence of FSGS after transplantation.[83] However, it remains to be determined whether plasmapheresis will be proved clinically effective in patients with sPAR as a circulating factor.[84]

The currently available treatments for recurrent FSGS are immunosuppressive drugs (e.g., cyclophosphamide, methylprednisolone), plasmapheresis and, according to some reports, rituximab.[85] However, the management of patients with recurrent FSGS is difficult and controversial, and none of the multiple approaches currently available has been shown to be consistently beneficial. Zimmerman[86] first reported a 38-year-old patient with recurrent FSGS who was successfully treated with plasmapheresis. Cochat and associates[87] studied 3 patients with recurrent FSGS in a prospective uncontrolled trial in which early plasmapheresis was used in combination with methylprednisolone pulses and cyclophosphamide over a 2-month period. All 3 patients achieved remission within 12 to 24 days, which suggests that plasma exchange instituted early in the course of recurrent nephrotic syndrome may be beneficial in some patients with FSGS. Dantal and coworkers[88] treated 9 patients within 1 week of the onset of proteinuria; 7 had a mean reduction in protein excretion from 11.5 to 0.8 g/day, and these remissions were sustained for up to 27 months. Deegens and colleagues analyzed data from 23 patients with recurrent FSGS, of whom 13 were treated with plasmapheresis and 10 were historical controls.[89] After a median follow-up of 3.5 years, 2 patients (15%) who had been treated with plasmapheresis had lost their allografts in comparison with all 10 controls. In patients with recurrent proteinuria, FSGS recurred within 4 weeks after transplantation (77%), and plasmapheresis was initiated within 14 days of recurrence (85%). In most studies, researchers reported a remission rate between 70% and 80%, but 33% of patients relapsed after the end of the treatment.[90] Nevertheless, retrospective evaluations of patients managed without plasmapheresis have indicated that early rates of graft failure were as high as 80%; therefore, plasmapheresis is indicated as initial therapy for recurrent FSGS.

Beneficial results have also been reported in children with recurrent FSGS after kidney transplantation who were treated with plasmapheresis and cyclophosphamide. In a study of 11 children with recurrent FSGS posttransplantation, 9 were treated with plasmapheresis (6 to 10 times over 15 to 24 days) and 7 had a persistent remission after a follow-up of 32 months.[91] Similarly, Cheong and associates reported the treatment of 6 children with recurrent FSGS with plasmapheresis plus cyclophosphamide, treatment which resulted in complete or partial remissions in all 6 patients.[92] Some reports have suggested that for high-risk individuals, preemptive treatment with plasmapheresis in the pretransplantation or perioperative period may alter or even prevent disease recurrence. Ohta and associates[93] reported on 15 patients who received preoperative plasmapheresis; FSGS recurred in 5, whereas in the 6 who did not receive preoperative plasmapheresis, 4 developed recurrence. Gohh and coworkers[94] reported on 10 patients at high risk for FSGS recurrence because of rapid progression to renal failure ($n = 4$) or prior posttransplantation recurrence of FSGS ($n = 6$). Patients underwent a course of eight plasmapheresis treatments in the perioperative period. Seven patients, including all 4 with first grafts and 3 of 6 with prior recurrence, were free of recurrence at follow-up (238 to 1258 days), and the final serum creatinine concentration in the 8 patients with functioning kidneys averaged 1.53 mg/dL. Therefore, the use of preoperative and prophylactic postoperative plasmapheresis may be warranted in patients at high risk, but the optimal approach is unknown. Given such poor results in untreated patients, randomized trials with and without plasmapheresis are unlikely to be performed at this juncture.

Rituximab is an anti-CD20 monoclonal antibody approved for the treatment of B cell lymphoma that has also been used to treat autoimmune disorders. Increasingly, rituximab is being used in transplant recipients to decrease anti-HLA and anti-ABO antibodies. Pediatric patients with posttransplantation lymphoproliferative disorder and recurrent FSGS have been reported to achieve remission of nephrotic syndrome after treatment with rituximab. However, the role of rituximab in recurrent FSGS to induce remission of nephrotic syndrome in pediatric patients is still controversial. Yabu and colleagues[95] administered rituximab to four consecutive patients with early recurrent FSGS refractory to or dependent on plasmapheresis; none of the patients treated with rituximab achieved remission in proteinuria, and one patient experienced early graft loss. Meyer and associates[96] reported one case in which addition of rituximab to plasmapheresis induced remission of proteinuria, and Hickson and coworkers[97] reported four pediatric patients in whom rituximab was effective in inducing remission. To date, the literature supporting the use of rituximab in recurrent FSGS is limited, and reports of success have tended to involve younger patients.

In summary, the duration and intensity of treatment with plasmapheresis in patients with recurrent FSGS has not been studied rigorously. In most reports, plasmapheresis has shown promise for reducing proteinuria, although there is concern for publication bias that excludes negative studies. The role of other adjuvant therapies for this condition remains to be established.[98]

ABO-INCOMPATIBLE KIDNEY TRANSPLANTATION

The ABO blood group antigen system was discovered on red blood cells by Landsteiner in 1901. These antigens are expressed throughout the body and, in the kidney, they are found in the distal tubules, collecting tubules, and vascular endothelium of peritubular and glomerular capillaries. ABO antibodies (isoagglutinins) are produced in the first years of life by sensitization to environmental substances such as food, bacteria, and viruses and are usually of the IgM type.[99] These antibodies against ABO antigens generally preclude kidney transplantation across ABO barriers and are the key mediators of antibody-mediated rejection. In the early days of kidney transplantation, results with ABO-incompatible (ABOi) organs were disappointing. In 1981, Slapak and colleagues[100] described a patient with blood group O who inadvertently received a mismatched kidney from a donor of blood group A; 2 days after transplantation, the patient experienced acute rejection, which was treated successfully with plasmapheresis. Twenty months after transplantation, the patient had normal kidney function. From 1982 to 1989, Squifflet and associates[101] performed 39 ABO-incompatible kidney transplantations and were the first group to attempt renal transplantation with ABO incompatibilities. The protocol to prepare the living donor recipient included two to five plasmapheresis sessions, pretransplantation immunosuppressive treatment, and splenectomy to remove antibodies. Graft survival rates appeared to be better among the group of patients younger than 15 years (89% at 5 years) than in those older than 15 years (77% at 5 years).

In Japan, ABO-incompatible kidney transplantation flourished in the 1990s, and the outcomes to date have been excellent. Takahashi and coworkers[102] reported the outcomes of 441 ABO-incompatible kidney transplantations performed at 55 centers across Japan from 1989 to 2001. The rates of graft survival were 84% in the first year and

59% at 9 years of follow-up; these survival rates were not statistically different in comparison with historical controls (recipients of ABO-compatible living donor organs). The therapy used to prepare the recipient consisted of four components: (1) extracorporeal immunomodulation with plasmapheresis or immunoadsorption to remove AB antibodies before transplantation; (2) use of immunosuppressive drugs; (3) splenectomy; and (4) anticoagulation therapy. The goal was to decrease pretransplantation serum AB titers by 8- to 16-fold. Antibody removal was usually not performed after transplantation. The same group treated 876 patients from 2001 to 2007 and achieved a relatively high graft survival rate of 86% at 5 years after transplantation.[64]

The Japanese literature had emphasized the need for splenectomy at the time of transplantation, but the Johns Hopkins group established a preconditioning protocol of plasmapheresis, cytomegalovirus (CMV) hyperimmune globulin (CMVIg), and anti-CD20 (rituximab) to enable the success of ABO-incompatible renal transplantation without splenectomy. The treatment protocol requires four to five preoperative sessions of plasmapheresis to remove anti-A or anti-B antibodies, and each session is followed by the administration of CMVIg. After achieving a pretransplantation A or B antibody titer less than 1:16, a single dose of rituximab is given 1 or 2 days prior to transplantation. Thereafter, immunosuppression with tacrolimus and mycophenolate mofetil is initiated, followed by steroids and daclizumab after transplantation. Postoperative treatment included another three sessions of plasmapheresis and CMVIg on days 1, 3, and 5. The 5-year graft survival rate for a cohort of 60 consecutive patients was 88.7%.[103,104] Recently, Lawrence and colleagues[105] reported the experience of an ABO-incompatible kidney transplantation program to define the likelihood of achieving transplantation dependent on ABO antibody titers. Transplantation proceeded when the ABO titer reached 1:4 or lower, and 51 of 56 patients (91%) underwent transplantation after 8.3 ± 5 plasmapheresis sessions. However, 5 patients with high ABO titers were not transplanted, despite extensive plasmapheresis procedures.

OTHER APPLICATIONS OF PLASMAPHERESIS IN TRANSPLANTATION

Plasmapheresis has been used with methylprednisolone for the treatment of acute antibody-mediated rejection in patients with ABO-incompatible renal transplants. Gloor and associates treated five patients with acute antibody-mediated rejection after ABO-incompatible kidney transplantation with plasmapheresis and steroids, and three demonstrated improvement in renal function.[106,107]

In another study, investigators compared high-dose intravenous immune globulin (IVIG) desensitization with two plasmapheresis protocols and found that among patients who received plasmapheresis, cross-matches were more likely to be negative.[108] However, the number of patients was small (13 to 32 in each group), the study was not randomized, and other differences in treatment limited comparisons among the groups.

POSITIVE T CELL CROSS-MATCH

High sensitization to HLA indicates positive T cell cross-matches, with multiple potential donors. The degree of sensitization is quantified as the percentage of the donor pool with which the serum of the patient had positive T cell cross-matches. This is commonly referred to as the panel reactive antibody status, or PRA. Those patients with PRA persistently higher than 50% are generally considered highly sensitized; primary sensitization results from exposure to foreign HLA antigens through transplantation, transfusion, or pregnancy, although infection and other conditions can also alter sensitization status. Patients with preformed antibodies against HLA antigens have a lower probability of receiving a matched kidney from a deceased or living donor. Furthermore, presensitized recipients experience less favorable outcomes after deceased-donor kidney transplantation and are at increased risk for hyperacute or acute antibody-mediated rejection and graft loss. Successful transplantation in these patients often requires a protocol of desensitization (either to a specific donor or more generally) to reduce the risk of hyperacute rejection and immediate graft loss.[109] The general approach is to reduce HLA antibodies with the use of high-dose IgG and plasmapheresis. Plasmapheresis is performed to remove anti-HLA antibodies and is followed by infusion of low doses of IgG during hemodialysis. The rationale is that low-dose IgG has beneficial immunomodulating effects. Concurrently with plasmapheresis initiation, patients are treated with tacrolimus, mycophenolate mofetil, steroids, and antimicrobial prophylaxis. Plasmapheresis is continued three times weekly until the T cell cross-match is negative, and transplantation usually takes place within 24 hours. Plasmapheresis and low-dose IgG are usually repeated several times during the first 2 weeks after transplantation to remove any rebounding antibody. Plasmapheresis-based protocols are usually not suitable for highly sensitized patients awaiting deceased-donor transplantation because the availability of suitable organs is unpredictable, and plasmapheresis is difficult and very expensive to continue indefinitely; if plasmapheresis is stopped, anti-HLA antibody titers rebound.[110,111]

ACUTE HUMORAL REJECTION

Acute humoral rejection is characterized by severe allograft dysfunction in association with the presence of circulating donor-specific antibodies. Very poor outcomes are observed with acute humoral rejection, and treatment with pulse steroids and antilymphocyte therapy is often ineffective.[112] Removal of the donor-specific antibodies with plasmapheresis has been successful when this treatment is combined with tacrolimus and mofetil mycophenolate.[113] It has been proposed that the combination of plasmapheresis and IVIG may lead to short-term recovery from acute antibody-mediated rejection in more than 80% of cases.[114,115] Rituximab and the proteasome inhibitor bortezomib have been used in some studies as a rescue treatment when patients failed to respond to plasmapheresis and IVIG.[116]

PLASMAPHERESIS AND NONRENAL DISEASE

According to several national registries, TTP, myasthenia gravis, chronic inflammatory demyelinating polyneuropathy, Waldenström's macroglobulinemia, and Guillain-Barré syndrome are the most frequent indications for plasmapheresis; results of randomized controlled trials have shown benefit for patients with these disorders.[117] There are now almost 100 rational indications for plasmapheresis and, in 2013, the American Society for Apheresis published an exhaustive review of the experimental data supporting the different indications for plasmapheresis.[56] In many clinical settings, the nephrologist is asked to initiate plasmapheresis. Therefore, it is essential that nephrologists be generally familiar with the literature supporting the use of plasmapheresis for these conditions.

Plasma exchange is a well-established therapeutic procedure commonly used for many neurologic disorders of autoimmune origin. It is thought that the beneficial effects of plasmapheresis occur through the removal of inflammatory mediators, including autoantibodies, complement components, and cytokines. Guillain-Barré syndrome, myasthenia gravis, chronic inflammatory demyelinating polyneuropathy, and demyelinating polyneuropathy with IgG-IgA are considered category I indications by the American Society for Apheresis.[56]

GUILLAIN-BARRÉ SYNDROME

Guillain-Barré syndrome has become the most frequently occurring clinical paralytic disorder, with an annual incidence of 2 cases/100,000 persons. Guillain-Barré syndrome is dangerous; 10% to 23% of affected patients require mechanical ventilation, and up to 1 in 20 patients may die from complications of the disease. In about 60% of cases, Guillain-Barré syndrome develops shortly after an infection, usually caused by *Campylobacter jejuni*. A large number of diverse antibodies against different glycolipids, including GM1, GD1a, and GQ1b, have been described.[118] The disorder is characterized by symmetric weakness, paralysis, and distal paresthesias that usually start with the lower limbs, followed by rapid progression to the proximal limbs and trunk over several days. A typical diagnostic feature is the finding of an increased concentration of cerebrospinal fluid protein in the absence of pleocytosis.[119] Plasmapheresis is a well-established treatment for Guillain-Barré syndrome. The advantages over supportive care have been demonstrated in two large randomized, controlled, nonblinded, multicenter trials. Substantial benefit has been documented for the time to recover the ability to ambulate with assistance, reduction of the proportion of patients who needed assisted mechanical ventilation, more rapid recovery of motor function, and time to recover the ability to walk with and without assistance. The French Cooperative Group on Plasma Exchange in Guillain-Barré Syndrome[120] has established the optimal number of plasmapheresis sessions for the treatment of this disease—two sessions for patients with mild disability and four for patients with moderate or severe disability. Plasmapheresis is considered as efficacious as IVIG therapy, but combined treatment of plasmapheresis and IVIG does not seem to yield additional benefit.[121]

CHRONIC INFLAMMATORY DEMYELINATING POLYNEUROPATHY

Chronic inflammatory demyelinating polyneuropathy (CIDP) has an estimated prevalence of about 1 to 2/100,000 adults. Symmetric weakness in proximal and distal muscles that progressively increases for more than 2 months is the pivotal symptom in the diagnosis of this disease. CIDP is associated with impaired sensation, absence or diminishment of tendon reflexes, an elevated protein level in cerebrospinal fluid, demyelinating nerve findings in conduction studies, and signs of demyelination in nerve biopsy specimens. The presence of autoantibodies against various proteins and glycolipids of the peripheral nerve in samples of serum and cerebrospinal fluid from patients with CIDP may provide a rationale for the therapeutic use of plasmapheresis. The treatments most widely used for CIDP consist of IVIG, plasmapheresis, and corticosteroids. According to published data, there appears to be no difference in efficacy among these three main therapies. Therapy should be initiated early in the course of the disease to prevent continued demyelination and secondary axonal loss, which lead to permanent disability.[122,123] Nephrologists should be particularly aware of CIDP, as it may be easily confused for uremic neuropathy and vice versa.

MYASTHENIA GRAVIS

Myasthenia gravis is an autoimmune-mediated disorder of the neuromuscular junction, clinically characterized by fluctuating muscle weakness and fatigability. The most common variant of the disease is mediated by circulating autoantibodies against the nicotinic acetylcholine receptor (AChR). Mechanisms responsible for loss of functional nicotinic AChR that compromise neuromuscular transmission include the degradation of the receptor, complement-mediated lysis of the receptor, and interference with neurotransmitter binding. In subgroups of patients negative for nicotinic AChR antibody, antibodies against the receptor tyrosine kinase can be detected.[124] The treatment of myasthenia gravis includes thymectomy, acetylcholine esterase inhibitors, corticosteroids, immunosuppressive agents, plasmapheresis, and IVIG. It is presumed that by eliminating circulating nicotinic AChR antibodies and other humoral factors, plasmapheresis leads to the observed beneficial effects.

Indications for plasmapheresis include situations that necessitate rapid clinical improvement, such as myasthenic crisis, impending crisis, and preoperative stabilization; patients for whom long-term control of symptoms is suboptimal with other forms of therapy also benefit from plasmapheresis. On occasion, patients require long-term outpatient exchange to achieve adequate control of myasthenia gravis symptoms. Treatment consists of four to six exchanges, each removing 3 to 5 L of plasma, performed daily or every other day. Plasmapheresis provides major improvement in symptoms for up to 2 to 3 weeks in 65% of cases, and any degree of improvement lasts less than 3 months in 68% of cases. Sometimes patients enjoy a more prolonged response.[125-127]

CATASTROPHIC ANTIPHOSPHOLIPID ANTIBODY SYNDROME

Catastrophic antiphospholipid antibody syndrome (CAPS) is a rapidly progressive and life-threatening disease that results in thrombosis in multiple organs in the presence of antiphospholipid antibodies. Rapid-onset thromboses in multiple organs and extensive involvement of small and medium-sized vessels in atypical locations are the general characteristics of CAPS. Treatment with anticoagulation, corticosteroids, and plasmapheresis or IVIG can be initiated. Plasmapheresis can remove pathologic antiphospholipid antibodies, as well as cytokines, tumor necrosis factor-α, and complement products. Although plasmapheresis improves outcomes in patients with CAPS, most reports have used FFP as the replacement fluid. FFP contains natural anticoagulants (e.g., antithrombin III, protein C), as well as clotting factors, so it is unknown whether plasmapheresis per se or the FFP replacement provides the benefits to patients with CAPS. No randomized controlled studies of plasmapheresis use in this condition are available, and none are currently under way.[128,129]

FAMILIAL HYPERCHOLESTEROLEMIA

Familial hypercholesterolemia has been successfully treated with plasmapheresis. The first report in 1975 was followed by additional studies showing that long-term repetitive plasmapheresis had a beneficial effect on aortic and coronary atherosclerosis and significantly prolonged survival in comparison with untreated siblings. However, although plasmapheresis is still used in some centers to treat severe hypercholesterolemia, low-density lipoprotein (LDL) apheresis is now accepted as the treatment of choice for patients with homozygous familial hypercholesterolemia and for heterozygotes with cardiovascular disease refractory to lipid-lowering drug therapy. Current methods of LDL apheresis use immunoadsorption with columns containing polyclonal sheep antibodies to human apolipoprotein B100 (apoB100) coupled with agarose (Sepharose 4B gel) or adsorption to dextran sulfate-cellulose, which covalently and selectively binds very LDL and LDL but not high-density lipoprotein (HDL).[130]

LDL apheresis is indicated for patients with homozygous familial hypercholesterolemia from the age of 7 years unless their serum cholesterol level can be reduced by more than 50% or decreased to less than 9 mmol/L (350 mg/dL) by drug therapy. It is also indicated for individual patients with heterozygous familial hypercholesterolemia or family history of premature cardiac death and progressive coronary disease. In addition, patients in whom LDL cholesterol remains higher than 5.0 mmol/L or is decreased by less than 40% with maximal drug therapy should be treated with LDL apheresis. Apheresis is also occasionally indicated for patients with severe, progressive coronary disease and whose lipoprotein (a) and LDL cholesterol levels are higher than 60 mg/dL (150 nmol/L) and 3.2 mmol/L (124 mg/dL), respectively, despite maximal drug therapy.[131,132]

REMOVAL OF TOXINS

Plasmapheresis has also been used to remove toxins, depending on the effective clearance, plasma protein binding, and volume of distribution of the toxic substance. Plasmapheresis is used to treat mushroom intoxication by *Amanita phalloides*, but some reports have suggested that forced diuresis is the treatment of choice.[133,134] There is controversy about the beneficial effect of plasmapheresis in the treatment of life-threatening intoxications with tricyclic antidepressants, benzodiazepines, quinine, and phenytoin. Other drugs, such as L-thyroxine, verapamil, diltiazem, carbamazepine, and theophylline, as well as heavy metals, are effectively removed by plasmapheresis, but the overall change in total body toxin level is usually not clinically significant. Because of the lack of controlled studies, it is difficult to make recommendations with respect to plasmapheresis for the treatment of poisonings and overdoses.[135,136]

PREGNANCY AND PLASMAPHERESIS

Plasmapheresis can be performed safely during pregnancy, and introduction of plasmapheresis during pregnancy for appropriate disorders has improved maternal and fetal survival rates. Plasmapheresis has been safely carried out in patients with myasthenic crisis, Guillain-Barré syndrome, anti-GBM disease, acute fatty liver of pregnancy, and TTP. Plasmapheresis has been tried with varied degrees of success in acute hypertriglyceridemia-induced pancreatitis in pregnancy and also as a prophylactic measure for the prevention of pancreatitis in pregnant women with known hypertriglyceridemia. Until the effectiveness of plasmapheresis was recognized, the rate of mortality from TTP was 95%; in cases of pregnancy-related TTP, maternal survival was rare, and the fetal mortality rate approached 80%. Since 1990, numerous reports have revealed the efficacy of plasma exchange, and TTP has become a curable disease, with a response rate of about 80% and minimal or no sequelae.

Hemolytic disease of the fetus and newborn (HDFN) occurs when maternal plasma contains an alloantibody against a red blood cell antigen carried by the fetus. Maternal IgG crosses the placenta and causes hemolysis of the fetal red blood cells, leading to fetal anemia and, if severe, possible fetal death (hydrops fetalis). Usually, HDFN is secondary to Rh incompatibility (anti-D) disease (Rh-positive fetus and Rh-negative mother), but it can also be caused by a variety of red blood cell alloantibodies (e.g., anti-K, anti-C, anti-PP1Pk, anti-E). Plasmapheresis removes the maternal red blood cell alloantibody that causes HDFN. By decreasing the maternal antibody titer, the amount transferred to the fetus is reduced, and the magnitude of HDFN is reduced. In severe cases of HDFN treated with plasmapheresis, IVIG, or both before intrauterine transfusion, the rate of survival is about 70%.

Plasmapheresis can result in premature delivery due to the removal of essential hormones needed to maintain pregnancy. Other complications can result from hypovolemia, allergy, transitory cardiac arrhythmias, nausea, and impaired vision. During the exchanges, hypotension must be carefully monitored and corrected and, in the second or third trimester, it is preferable to place the patient on her left side to avoid compression of the inferior vena cava by the gravid uterus.[137-139]

TECHNICAL ASPECTS

The plasmapheresis technique involves the withdrawal of venous blood through a peripheral or central venous catheter to allow separation of blood cells from plasma by centrifugation or membrane filtration. The separated cells plus autologous plasma or another replacement solution are reinfused. For most conditions, the goal of the procedure is the removal of pathologic autoantibodies or toxins; the initial treatment target is to exchange 1 to 1.5 times the plasma volume per plasmapheresis procedure. This will lower plasma macromolecule levels by 60% to 75%, respectively. The following formula can be used to estimate plasma volume in an adult[140]:

$$\text{Estimated plasma volume (L)} = 0.07 \times \text{weight (kg)} \times (1 - \text{hematocrit [Hct]})$$

The ultimate clinical success of the procedure depends on the abundance of the abnormal protein in plasma and its rate of production. Unless the removal of the protein by plasmapheresis is combined with additional therapies (usually immunosuppressive or cytotoxic) to eliminate or reduce the source of the abnormal protein(s), the procedure is unlikely to provide clinical benefit. The time required to suppress abnormal protein production can take several weeks, thus necessitating daily (or almost daily) apheresis for prolonged periods.

PLASMA SEPARATION TECHNIQUES

The two major modalities to separate the plasma from the blood during a plasmapheresis procedure are centrifugation and membrane filtration (Figure 68.2).

CENTRIFUGATION

The centrifugation method uses centrifugal force to separate whole blood into plasma and cellular fractions according to their density. The centrifugation process can be intermittent or continuous.

Intermittent Centrifugation

In intermittent centrifugation, sequential volumes of whole blood are removed and centrifuged; the cellular fraction is returned to the patient, and the process is repeated until the desired volume of plasma is removed. The blood is pumped from the patient at a flow rate of up to 100 mL/min into the processing unit, which consists of a bell-shaped bowl that rotates at high speed. The denser cellular blood components are centrifuged against the lateral walls while the plasma is removed through a central outlet on the top of the bowl. Each cycle removes about 500 to 700 mL of plasma, and usually it is necessary to perform the process five or six times to achieve the goal of 2.5 to 4.0 L (1 to 1.5 plasma volumes) during a session. At the conclusion of each segment, the packed cells are emptied from the bowl and returned to the patient. The advantages of intermittent centrifugation include the relative simplicity of operation, portability of machines, and convenience of a single-needle peripheral venipuncture. The disadvantages include the time involved (the procedure typically takes more than 4 hours) and relatively large extracorporeal volume removed each time.

Continuous Flow Centrifugation

In the continuous flow centrifugation system, the blood is pumped continuously into a rapidly rotating bowl, where plasma and cells are separated. Plasma is removed at a specified rate, and the cells plus replacement fluid are returned to the patient in a continuous manner. This method is faster and more suitable for hemodynamically unstable patients; however, it is more costly and requires two venipunctures or insertion of a dual-lumen central venous catheter.

MEMBRANE FILTRATION

The membrane filtration technique uses a synthetic membrane filter composed of different pore sizes. Similar to a hemodialysis filter, the plasmapheresis filter is composed of many hollow fiber tubes made of a membrane material with a relatively large pore size (0.2 to 0.6 μm in diameter) and arranged in parallel. Blood is pumped through the hollow fiber tubes; the large pores are sufficient to allow passage of plasma (proteins and plasma water) while retaining cells within the hollow fiber lumen. The plasma is drained off while the cells are returned to the patient through a typical hemodialysis circuit. This technique can be done using conventional or continuous hemodialysis equipment, with a blood flow rate of 100 ± 20 mL/min and an optimal transmembrane pressure of less than 70 mm Hg. Plasma is removed at a rate of 30 to 50 mL/min; the infusion rate of replacement fluid is adjusted to maintain intravascular volume. Potential disadvantages of membrane filtration include activation of complement and leukocytes by the artificial membrane, and the need for a central catheter to obtain adequate blood flow rates. If severe acute renal failure is also present, and dialysis is required, the membrane filtration method can be done in combination with conventional hemodialysis.

Both centrifugation and membrane filtration are safe and efficient plasmapheresis techniques; the main differences lie in the cost and expertise needed to operate.[141-143] The double-filtration plasmapheresis technique (DFPP; also called cascade filtration) is another variation of membrane plasmapheresis; the plasma that has been separated by the membrane flows again through membranes with different pore diameters and filtration and adsorption characteristics. High-molecular-weight proteins are discarded and small-molecular-weight substances, including valuable albumin, are returned to the patient. Small amounts of substitution fluid such as albumin may be added.[144]

OTHER SEPARATION MODALITIES

In recent years, these basic techniques have been modified and/or coupled to other separation modalities. Cytapheresis is the removal of leukocytes or platelets in hematologic conditions with hyperleukocytosis or thrombocytosis. Cytapheresis can also be performed for sickle cell crisis; in this setting, the goal is the removal of more than 50% of hemoglobin S and replacement with normal allogenic red cells. When the plasma filtration is done above normal physiologic temperature, the process is termed *thermofiltration*. This technique is performed on patients with severe dyslipidemia, whereas cryofiltration is used when the procedure is done with the temperature below normal; it is used to remove immunoglobulin and immune complexes (cryoglobulins; see above). Alternatively, absorption columns for plasma or immunoglobulins can be used for separation. For example, protein A, binds and removes IgG antibodies and immune complexes. Chemical affinity columns such as dextran sulfate have negative charges and are used to remove antibodies or other positively charged plasma

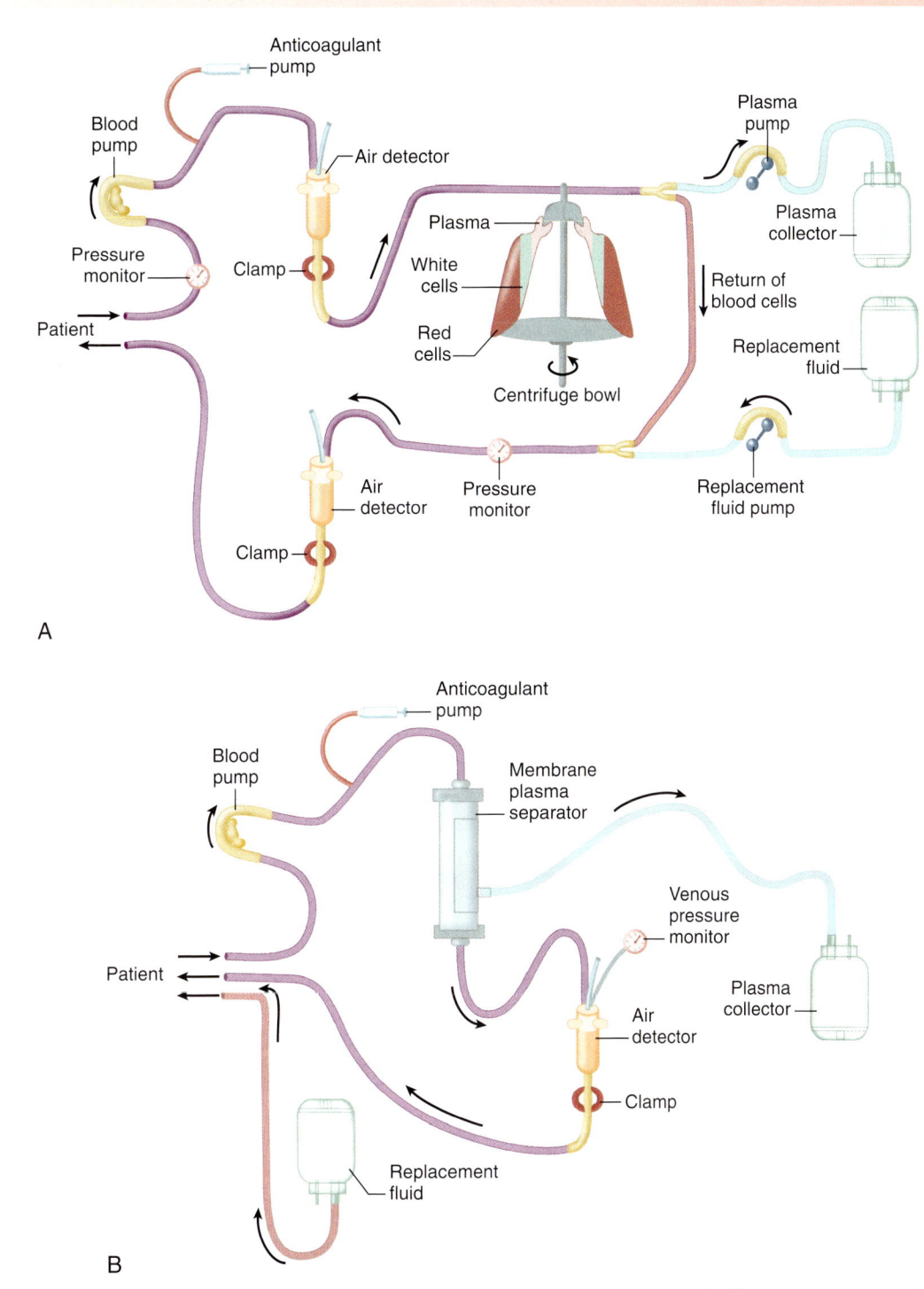

Figure 68.2 Centrifugal separator (**A**) and membrane filtration systems (**B**) for plasma exchange. **A,** Blood is pumped into the separator container. As the centrifuge revolves, different blood components are separated into discrete layers, which can be harvested separately. Plasma is pumped out of the centrifuge into a collection chamber. Red blood cells, leukocytes, and platelets are returned to the donor, along with replacement fluid. **B,** Blood is pumped into a biocompatible membrane that allows the filtration of plasma while retaining cellular elements. (From Madore F, Lazarus JM, Brady HR: Therapeutic plasma exchange in renal diseases, *J Am Soc Nephrol* 7:367-386, 1996.)

substances, such as LDL and very low-density lipoproteins (VLDLs).[145]

VENOUS ACCESS

Successful implementation of the plasmapheresis procedure requires reliable venous access. The clinical scenario, especially the possibility for long-term venous access and type of plasmapheresis being used, are important factors to consider in deciding whether to use peripheral or central venous access. A peripheral vein allows a maximum flow of about 50 to 90 mL/min, so a single venous access is adequate for intermittent centrifugation. Continuous centrifugation techniques require two venous access sites; for short-term procedures, this may be adequate, but recurrent use of intravenous catheters and phlebotomy in chronically ill patients can lead to loss of venous access. If long-term plasmapheresis (>1 to 2 weeks) is planned, a central venous catheter should be used. When the membrane filtration technique is used, a central venous catheter is necessary to sustain blood flows higher than 70 mL/min. Central venous access can be achieved through the femoral, internal jugular, or subclavian vein; the femoral vein should be avoided if the patient will be ambulatory during treatment.[146] In patients who require lifelong therapy such as LDL apheresis, an arteriovenous fistula or arteriovenous graft should be considered. Central venous catheters are associated with numerous long-term complications, including catheter thrombosis, catheter infection, pneumothorax, central vein thrombosis, and vein stenosis.

ANTICOAGULATION

To prevent activation of the coagulation system within the extracorporeal circuit, the plasmapheresis procedure requires anticoagulation. For centrifugation procedures, a solution of citric acid, sodium citrate, and dextrose in water (one ninth the volume of solute per volume of solution), given as a continuous intravenous infusion, is the anticoagulant most frequently used. The infusion rate is adjusted according to the blood flow rate (target ratios range from 1:10 to 1:25). When the venous flux and infusion rate of citrate are slow, the risk for catheter clotting is increased. In this circumstance, heparin (if not contraindicated) can be used alone or in combination with citrate. For membrane filtration plasmapheresis, the use of standard unfractionated heparin is preferred, and the required dose of heparin is about twice that needed for hemodialysis because a significant amount of infused heparin is removed along with the plasma. However, heparin may enhance systemic anticoagulation more than is expected because of the additional effect of dilution of clotting factors by the nonplasma replacement solutions. The initial loading dose of heparin (40 U/kg) is usually administered intravenously, followed by a continuous infusion (20 U/kg/hr), adjusted to maintain adequate anticoagulation in the circuit.[141,142] For patients who are receiving standard oral anticoagulants, additional low-dose anticoagulation should be achieved by regional anticoagulation—within the plasmapheresis circuit only, not systemically—with citrate or heparin. The heparin dose can usually be reduced by at least 50% in this situation.[147] In critically ill patients with coagulation abnormalities, the use of regional citrate is preferred.[148] Hirudin and lepirudin (thrombin inhibitors) are effective and safe alternatives for patients at increased risk for thrombosis but who have contraindications to heparin administration.[149,150]

REPLACEMENT FLUID

The choice of replacement fluid includes 5% albumin, FFP (or other plasma derivatives [e.g., cryosupernatant]), crystalloids (e.g., 0.9% saline, Ringer's lactate), and synthetic plasma expanders (e.g., hydroxyethyl starch).[151] Albumin is the replacement most commonly used in plasmapheresis and is generally combined with 0.9% saline in a 1:1 ratio. Albumin solutions do not contain calcium or potassium and also lack coagulation factors and immunoglobulins. They have never been associated with transmission of hepatitis viruses or HIV.[152] FFP contains complement and coagulation factors and is the replacement fluid of choice for patients with TTP because the infusion of normal plasma may contribute to the replacement of the deficient plasma factor ADAMTS13 (see above). Plasma may also be preferable when there is a heightened risk of bleeding (e.g., in patients with liver disease, disseminated intravascular coagulation, or after kidney biopsy), or when intensive therapy is required (e.g., daily exchanges for several weeks) because frequent replacements with albumin solution eventually result in postplasmapheresis coagulopathy and a large net loss of immunoglobulins. The disadvantages of using FFP include the risk of infectious disease transmission and potential for citrate overload.

Replacement fluid using colloidal starch is well tolerated, interaction with other drugs is minimal, the potential for disease transmission is absent, and it is cost-effective in comparison with human albumin.[153] Hydroxyethyl starch is a polysaccharide colloid widely used as an agent for plasma volume expansion and for enhancement of granulocyte yields during leukapheresis. Its pharmacologic and safety profiles have been well established. When used in moderate amounts in humans and animals, hydroxyethyl starch produces relatively minor changes in coagulation, and overt bleeding is rare. Although the mechanisms leading to changes in coagulation are unknown, it has been ascribed, at least in part, to hemodilution. In plasmapheresis, the effects of hydroxyethyl starch on coagulation factor levels and activity are comparable with those of other replacement fluids. Hydroxyethyl starch can be used safely for short-term plasmapheresis in patients with an albumin level higher than 30 g/dL[154]; longer exposure to hydroxyethyl starch (130 L within 20 months) can lead to adverse side effects (e.g., sensory polyneuropathy, weight loss) and diffuse tissue infiltration with hydroxyethyl starch–laden foamy macrophages. Excessive exposure to hydroxyethyl starch in patients with impaired kidney function can result in acquired lysosomal storage disease; thus, hydroxyethyl starch should be avoided in chronic plasmapheresis procedures. Contraindications for using starches in plasmapheresis are congestive heart failure, renal or liver failure, coagulopathy, hyperviscosity, allergic reactions to starches, pregnancy, and breast feeding and in pediatric patients.[155,156]

COMPLICATIONS

Plasmapheresis is a generally well-tolerated and relatively safe procedure. Although adverse events are common, most are modest and death is rare, occurring in less than 0.1% of all procedures.[157] There are fewer adverse reactions when albumin is administered as volume replacement than with procedures using FFP (1.4% vs. 20%). Risk factors for developing an adverse event during plasmapheresis include hypotension, active bleeding, severe bronchoconstriction, severe anemia, pregnancy, and conditions requiring continuous nursing support.[158] Table 68.5 summarizes the most common complications related to the plasmapheresis procedure. The Swedish registry of therapeutic apheresis has reported more than 14,000 procedures from 1996 to 1999. Adverse events

Table 68.5	Complications of Plasmapheresis
Modality	Complications
Vascular access	Hematomas
	Pneumothorax
	Catheter infections
Replacement fluids	Anaphylactoid reactions to fresh-frozen plasma
	Coagulopathies
	Transmission of viral infections
	Hypocalcemia
	Hypokalemia
Other modalities	Hypotension
	Dyspnea
	Thrombocytopenia
	Removal of erythropoietin and drugs bound to plasma proteins

occurred in 4.2% of procedures, and no fatalities were reported; 1% of all the apheresis procedures had to be interrupted due to an adverse event. The most common adverse effects reported were paresthesias (0.52%), hypotension (0.5%), urticaria (0.34%), shivering, and nausea. Events were most frequent in patients with Goodpasture's syndrome (12.5%), TTP-HUS (10.5%), and Guillain-Barré syndrome (11.0%).[159] Kiprov and coworkers[160] reported on 17,940 procedures performed on 3,583 patients; adverse events occurred in 3.9% of all procedures. The following adverse reactions were documented: reactions related to citrate toxicity (3%); vasovagal reactions and hypotension (0.5%); vascular access–related complications (0.15%); reactions related to FFP (0.12%); hepatitis B from FFP (0.06%); arrhythmias (0.01%); hemolysis due to inappropriate dilution of 25% albumin (0.01%); and one death (from underlying disease) during plasmapheresis (0.006%). No significant bleeding complications were observed, and patients receiving FFP had significantly higher rates of adverse reactions than patients receiving other exchange fluids.

One of the most frequent complications of plasmapheresis is hypocalcemia related to citrate infusion as anticoagulant for the extracorporeal system or in the FFP administered as a replacement fluid. Citrate binds to free calcium to form soluble calcium citrate, thereby lowering the free but not total serum calcium concentration. Hypocalcemia is manifested by perioral and distal extremity paresthesias. Symptoms can be prevented by administration of intravenous or oral calcium if the plasmapheresis therapy will last longer than 1 hour. The administration of oral calcium carbonate or addition of calcium gluconate to the infused fluids is a useful maneuver to prevent hypocalcemia. The incidence of hypocalcemic symptoms is reduced with the prophylactic administration of calcium; without calcium prophylaxis, the incidence of symptoms was 9.1% (6 in 66 treatments), whereas with calcium prophylaxis, the incidence was reduced to 1% (6 in 633 treatments).[161,162] Marques and colleagues[163] reported a 3% incidence of hypocalcemia when calcium gluconate was infused in 5% albumin. Another complication of citrate administration is the development of metabolic alkalosis, but critical levels of serum bicarbonate higher than 35 mmol/L are rarely seen. Risk factors are use of FFP and patients with concurrent acute or chronic renal failure. The excess citrate generates bicarbonate in the setting of normal liver function, and excretion of the bicarbonate is limited when kidney function is absent or severely impaired. Replacement regimens using saline and albumin solutions can result in a 25% reduction in the plasma potassium concentration in the postapheresis period; hypokalemia can be minimized by adding 4 mEq/L potassium to the infused fluids. Hypokalemia is also a consequence of metabolic alkalosis.[163]

Plasmapheresis can lead to a reduction in blood pressure that is usually due to a decrease in intravascular volume. As the volume of extracorporeal whole blood is higher with intermittent centrifugation techniques, episodes of hypotension are more common than with continuous modalities. Hypotension can also occur in response to complement-mediated reactions to the membrane filter or sensitivity to the ethylene oxide that is used to sterilize the membrane. FFP is also associated with anaphylactoid reactions, but rarely resulting in death. FFP reactions are usually characterized by fever, rigors, urticaria, wheezing, and hypotension. The development of dyspnea suggests the presence of pulmonary edema due to fluid overload; noncardiogenic edema can rarely occur as a component of anaphylactic reactions. Another cause of acute-onset dyspnea is the presence of massive pulmonary emboli; this has been reported when the reinfused blood components are not adequately anticoagulated.

Plasma exchange with albumin replacement produces a predictable decrease in clotting factors that may predispose to bleeding (Table 68.6). A single plasma volume exchange increases the prothrombin time by 30% and the partial thromboplastin time by 100%; these changes return toward normal within several hours but, with repeated plasmapheresis sessions, these abnormalities can persist. The most significant change reported is on fibrinogen levels[164]; Keller and associates[165] have reported that fibrinogen levels were lowered to 25% of preapheresis levels and recovered to baseline after 2 to 3 days. Therefore, 1 L or more of FFP (3 to 4 U/L) should be substituted as the replacement fluid each week or sooner in patients at risk for bleeding. Thrombocytopenia is also a consequence of large-volume plasma removal. The mean platelet reduction following a plasmapheresis procedure ranges from 9.4% to 52.6%. Clinical bleeding associated with plasmapheresis is rarely reported and, when plasmapheresis-related hemorrhage is present, it is more likely a consequence of thrombocytopenia or inadequate heparin neutralization.[166,167]

Removal of immunoglobulins and complement could result in an immunodeficient state. However, in a randomized controlled trial of plasmapheresis in patients with lupus nephritis, TTP, or multiple myeloma, patients receiving plasmapheresis were not more prone to infection than the other patients.[168] Nevertheless, repeated apheresis treatments with albumin replacement will deplete the patient's reserve of immunoglobulins for several weeks. If an infection occurs, a single infusion of 100 to 400 mg/kg of intravenous immune globulin will restore the plasma immunoglobulin concentration toward normal. Although estimates for the risk of viral transmission by the use of FFP are low, the large volumes from multiple donors increase the risk in patients receiving long-term plasmapheresis therapy. Use of large-volume plasma units collected from a single donor and use

Table 68.6 Decrease of Clotting Factors Following Plasmapheresis

Factor	Decrease from Baseline (%)	Factor Level 24 Hr After Plasmapheresis	Factor Level 48-96 Hr After Plasmapheresis
V	50-71	RTB	RTB
VII	69-82	62	RTB
VIII	50-82	62, RTB	RTB
IX	26-55	RTB	RTB
X	67-84	RTB	RTB
XI	50-66		RTB
XII	66		RTB
Antithrombin III	58-84	70, RTB	82%, RTB
Fibrinogen	50-78	60	63%, RTB

RTB, Return to baseline.

of hepatitis B vaccine may reduce the risk of virally transmitted infections.

Flushing, hypotension, abdominal cramping, and other gastrointestinal symptoms have been reported during plasmapheresis in patients receiving angiotensin-converting enzyme inhibitors (ACEIs). In one report of 299 consecutive patients undergoing plasmapheresis, these atypical symptoms occurred in all 14 patients receiving an ACEI versus only 7% of those not treated with these agents.[169] The administration of an ACEI may prolong the half-life of bradykinin, which permits a clinically significant concentration in the plasma to be reached. It is recommended to withhold ACEIs 24 hours prior to plasmapheresis.[170] Finally, substantial drug removal by plasmapheresis occurs for drugs that are highly protein bound and therefore primarily limited to the vascular space. Among drugs used to treat renal diseases, prednisone is not substantially removed while cyclophosphamide and azathioprine are removed to some extent. By administering these drugs after the plasma exchange treatment, this important disadvantage can be avoided.

CONCLUSION

The use of plasmapheresis to treat a variety of kidney diseases has expanded significantly since the 1990s. In some cases, the rationale and benefit are supported by data from clinical studies but, for many conditions, data are sparse. Nevertheless, the rationale of removing plasma-containing pathogenic antibodies is now well established. When used with caution, the risk/benefit ratio of plasmapheresis in several life-threatening and kidney-threatening diseases is quite favorable.

Complete reference list available at ExpertConsult.com.

KEY REFERENCES

11. Levy JB, Turner AN, Rees AJ, et al: Long-term outcome of antiglomerular basement membrane antibody disease treated with plasma exchange and immunosuppression. *Ann Intern Med* 134:1033–1042, 2001.
13. Khandelwal M, McCormick BB, Lajoie G, et al: Recurrence of anti-GBM disease 8 years after renal transplantation. *Nephrol Dial Transplant* 19:491–494, 2004.
14. Buhaescu I, Covic A, Levy J: Systemic vasculitis: still a challenging disease. *Am J Kidney Dis* 46:173–185, 2005.
18. de Lind van Wijngaarden RA, Hauer HA, Wolterbeek R, et al: Clinical and histologic determinants of renal outcome in ANCA-associated vasculitis: a prospective analysis of 100 patients with severe renal involvement. *J Am Soc Nephrol* 17:2264–2274, 2006.
19. Jayne DR, Gaskin G, Rasmussen N, et al: Randomized trial of plasma exchange or high-dosage methylprednisolone as adjunctive therapy for severe renal vasculitis. *J Am Soc Nephrol* 18:2180–2188, 2007.
20. Walters G, Willis NS, Craig JC: Interventions for renal vasculitis in adults. *Cochrane Database System Rev* 3:CD003232, 2008.
21. Walsh M, Catapano F, Szpirt W, et al: Plasma exchange for renal vasculitis and idiopathic rapidly progressive glomerulonephritis: a meta-analysis. *Am J Kidney Dis* 57:566–574, 2011.
23. Gallagher H, Kwan JT, Jayne DR: Pulmonary renal syndrome: a 4-year, single-center experience. *Am J Kidney Dis* 39:42–47, 2002.
31. Lee J, Clayton F, Shihab F, et al: Successful treatment of recurrent Henoch-Schonlein purpura in a renal allograft with plasmapheresis. *Am J Transplant* 8:228–231, 2008.
34. Lewis EJ, Hunsicker LG, Lan SP, et al: A controlled trial of plasmapheresis therapy in severe lupus nephritis. The Lupus Nephritis Collaborative Study Group. *N Engl J Med* 326:1373–1379, 1992.
38. Yamaji K, Kim YJ, Tsuda H, et al: Long-term clinical outcomes of synchronized therapy with plasmapheresis and intravenous cyclophosphamide pulse therapy in the treatment of steroid-resistant lupus nephritis. *Ther Apher Dial* 12:298–305, 2008.
39. Shaz BH, Linenberger ML, Bandarenko N, et al: Category IV indications for therapeutic apheresis: ASFA fourth special issue. *J Clin Apher* 22:176–180, 2007.
41. Ferri C, Sebastiani M, Giuggioli D, et al: Mixed cryoglobulinemia: demographic, clinical, and serologic features and survival in 231 patients. *Semin Arthritis Rheum* 33:355–374, 2004.
47. Batuman V: The pathogenesis of acute kidney impairment in patients with multiple myeloma. *Adv Chronic Kidney Dis* 19:282–286, 2012.
48. Hutchison C, Sanders PW: Evolving strategies in the diagnosis, treatment, and monitoring of myeloma kidney. *Adv Chronic Kidney Dis* 19:279–281, 2012.
50. Zucchelli P, Pasquali S, Cagnoli L, et al: Controlled plasma exchange trial in acute renal failure due to multiple myeloma. *Kidney Int* 33:1175–1180, 1988.
51. Johnson WJ, Kyle RA, Pineda AA, et al: Treatment of renal failure associated with multiple myeloma. Plasmapheresis, hemodialysis, and chemotherapy. *Arch Intern Med* 150:863–869, 1990.
52. Clark WF, Stewart AK, Rock GA, et al: Plasma exchange when myeloma presents as acute renal failure: a randomized, controlled trial. *Ann Intern Med* 143:777–784, 2005.
56. Schwartz J, Winters JL, Padmanabhan A, et al: Guidelines on the use of therapeutic apheresis in clinical practice-evidence-based approach from the Writing Committee of the American Society for Apheresis: the sixth special issue. *J Clin Apher* 28:145–284, 2013.

57. Salvadori M, Bertoni E: Update on hemolytic uremic syndrome: diagnostic and therapeutic recommendations. *World J Nephrol* 2:56–76, 2013.
58. Rahal EA, Kazzi N, Nassar FJ, et al: Escherichia coli O157:H7-Clinical aspects and novel treatment approaches. *Front Cell Infect Microbiol* 2:138, 2012.
59. Dundas S, Murphy J, Soutar RL, et al: Effectiveness of therapeutic plasma exchange in the 1996 Lanarkshire Escherichia coli O157:H7 outbreak. *Lancet* 354:1327–1330, 1999.
60. Kielstein JT, Beutel G, Fleig S, et al: Best supportive care and therapeutic plasma exchange with or without eculizumab in Shiga-toxin-producing E. coli O104:H4 induced haemolytic-uraemic syndrome: an analysis of the German STEC-HUS registry. *Nephrol Dial Transplant* 27:3807–3815, 2012.
61. Loos S, Ahlenstiel T, Kranz B, et al: An outbreak of Shiga toxin-producing Escherichia coli O104:H4 hemolytic uremic syndrome in Germany: presentation and short-term outcome in children. *Clin Infect Dis* 55:753–759, 2012.
62. Ariceta G, Besbas N, Johnson S, et al: Guideline for the investigation and initial therapy of diarrhea-negative hemolytic uremic syndrome. *Pediatr Nephrol* 24:687–696, 2009.
64. Egawa H, Tanabe K, Fukushima N, et al: Current status of organ transplantation in Japan. *Am J Transplant* 12:523–530, 2012.
66. Levy GG, Nichols WC, Lian EC, et al: Mutations in a member of the ADAMTS gene family cause thrombotic thrombocytopenic purpura. *Nature* 413:488–494, 2001.
72. Bell WR, Braine HG, Ness PM, et al: Improved survival in thrombotic thrombocytopenic purpura-hemolytic uremic syndrome. Clinical experience in 108 patients. *N Engl J Med* 325:398–403, 1991.
73. Rock GA, Shumak KH, Buskard NA, et al: Comparison of plasma exchange with plasma infusion in the treatment of thrombotic thrombocytopenic purpura. Canadian Apheresis Study Group. *N Engl J Med* 325:393–397, 1991.
83. Wei C, El Hindi S, Li J, et al: Circulating urokinase receptor as a cause of focal segmental glomerulosclerosis. *Nat Med* 17:952–960, 2011.
90. Pardon A, Audard V, Caillard S, et al: Risk factors and outcome of focal and segmental glomerulosclerosis recurrence in adult renal transplant recipients. *Nephrol Dial Transplant* 21:1053–1059, 2006.
98. Keith DS: Therapeutic apheresis rescue mission: recurrent focal segmental glomerulosclerosis in renal allografts. *Semin Dial* 25:190–192, 2012.
102. Takahashi K, Saito K, Takahara S, et al: Excellent long-term outcome of ABO-incompatible living donor kidney transplantation in Japan. *Am J Transplant* 4:1089–1096, 2004.
103. Gloor J, Stegall M: ABO-incompatible kidney transplantation with and without splenectomy. *Transplantation* 82:720, 2006.
104. Montgomery RA, Locke JE, King KE, et al: ABO incompatible renal transplantation: a paradigm ready for broad implementation. *Transplantation* 87:1246–1255, 2009.
105. Lawrence C, Galliford JW, Willicombe MK, et al: Antibody removal before ABO-incompatible renal transplantation: how much plasma exchange is therapeutic? *Transplantation* 92:1129–1133, 2011.
108. Stegall MD, Gloor J, Winters JL, et al: A comparison of plasmapheresis versus high-dose IVIG desensitization in renal allograft recipients with high levels of donor-specific alloantibody. *Am J Transplant* 6:346–351, 2006.
109. Thielke JJ, West-Thielke PM, Herren HL, et al: Living donor kidney transplantation across positive crossmatch: the University of Illinois at Chicago experience. *Transplantation* 87:268–273, 2009.
110. Magee CC: Transplantation across previously incompatible immunological barriers. *Transplant Int* 19:87–97, 2006.
116. Roberts DM, Jiang SH, Chadban SJ: The treatment of acute antibody-mediated rejection in kidney transplant recipients—a systematic review. *Transplantation* 94:775–783, 2012.
119. van Doorn PA, Ruts L, Jacobs BC: Clinical features, pathogenesis, and treatment of Guillain-Barre syndrome. *Lancet Neurol* 7:939–950, 2008.
120. The French Cooperative Group on Plasma Exchange in Guillain-Barre Syndrome: Appropriate number of plasma exchanges in Guillain-Barre syndrome. *Ann Neurol* 41:298–306, 1997.
123. Brannagan TH, 3rd: Current treatments of chronic immune-mediated demyelinating polyneuropathies. *Muscle Nerve* 39:563–578, 2009.
127. Mandawat A, Mandawat A, Kaminski HJ, et al: Outcome of plasmapheresis in myasthenia gravis: delayed therapy is not favorable. *Muscle Nerve* 43:578–584, 2011.
128. Bucciarelli S, Erkan D, Espinosa G, et al: Catastrophic antiphospholipid syndrome: treatment, prognosis, and the risk of relapse. *Clin Rev Allergy Immun* 36:80–84, 2009.
131. McGowan MP: Emerging low-density lipoprotein (LDL) therapies: management of severely elevated LDL cholesterol—the role of LDL-apheresis. *J Clin Lipidol* 7:S21–S26, 2013.
151. Le Conte P, Nicolas F, Adjou C, et al: Replacement fluids in plasmapheresis: cross-over comparative study. *Intensive Care Med* 23:342–344, 1997.
154. Hanafusa N, Noiri E, Nangaku M: Differences in reduction of coagulation factor XIII (F13) between immunoadsorption plasmapheresis and double filtration plasmapheresis. *Ther Apher Dial* 17:241–242, 2013.
158. Lu Q, Nedelcu E, Ziman A, et al: Standardized protocol to identify high-risk patients undergoing therapeutic apheresis procedures. *J Clin Apher* 23:111–115, 2008.
161. Kaplan A: Complications of apheresis. *Semin Dial* 25:152–158, 2012.

69

Elimination Enhancement of Poisons

Marc Ghannoum | Karine Mardini | Paul Ayoub

CHAPTER OUTLINE

OVERVIEW OF CORPOREAL TREATMENTS FOR ENHANCED ELIMINATION OF POISONS, 2167
Forced Diuresis, 2167
Manipulation of Urinary pH, 2168
Fecal Elimination Enhancement, 2168
PRINCIPLES AND FACTORS INFLUENCING POISON REMOVAL DURING EXTRACORPOREAL TREATMENTS, 2169
Poison-Related Factors, 2169
Extracorporeal Treatment–Related Factors, 2169
AVAILABLE EXTRACORPOREAL TREATMENTS TO ENHANCE ELIMINATION OF POISONS, 2170
Hemodialysis, 2170
Hemoperfusion, 2170
Hemofiltration, 2170
Combination Therapy, 2171
Continuous Renal Replacement Therapy, 2171
Peritoneal Dialysis, 2171
Therapeutic Plasma Exchange and Plasmapheresis, 2171
Exchange Transfusion, 2171

Extracorporeal Liver Assist Devices (Albumin Dialysis), 2171
GENERAL INDICATIONS FOR EXTRACORPOREAL REMOVAL OF POISONS, 2172
Technical Considerations, 2173
POISONS AMENABLE TO EXTRACORPOREAL ELIMINATION, 2173
The Toxic Alcohols: Ethylene Glycol, Methanol, Isopropanol, 2173
Salicylic Acid, 2178
Lithium, 2180
Valproic Acid, 2181
Carbamazepine, 2182
Barbiturates, 2183
Phenytoin, 2183
Metformin, 2184
Paraquat, 2185
Theophylline, 2186
Acetaminophen, 2187
Methotrexate, 2188
Others, 2189
CONCLUSION, 2189

Poisonings are a major contributor to morbidity and mortality, in addition to being responsible for significant health care expenditure worldwide. According to the National Poison Data System data compiled by the American Association of Poison Control Centers, nearly 2.2 million human exposures to poisoning were reported in the United States in 2013.[1] Approximately 75% of reported cases were unintentional (e.g., food poisoning, therapeutic error), 15% were intentional (e.g., suicide, abuse), and 3% were adverse reactions. Despite the majority of reported exposures having occurred in the pediatric population, the majority of fatalities involve adults. The classes of drugs accounting for the majority of fatal cases were sedatives, cardiovascular agents, opioids, antidepressants, and stimulants. Table 69.1 presents the 2013 U.S. statistics of the incidence and outcomes related to various poisons that may require the care of a nephrologist.

All toxic exposures should initially be considered life-threatening. The general approach to the poisoned patient necessitates prompt resuscitation and stabilization, clinical and laboratory evaluation, antidote administration, and gastrointestinal decontamination if appropriate; these are reviewed extensively elsewhere.[2,3] In certain clinical circumstances, poison elimination can be enhanced through various techniques. Elimination enhancement modalities can be divided between corporeal treatments, occurring inside the body, and extracorporeal treatments (ECTRs), occurring in a circuit outside the body.[4] Because the prognosis for most toxic exposures remains excellent with supportive measures, only a small minority of poisonings benefit from active elimination enhancement. The frequency of use of elimination enhancement techniques in poisonings is outlined in Figure 69.1.

Because of the inherent difficulties of studying poisoned patients (heterogeneous baseline characteristics, urgent condition, consent issues) and because of the ethical problems limiting study of ECTRs to control, evidence-based treatment recommendations from randomized trials are lacking. Current evidence is mostly derived from animal studies, cohort observations plagued by confounders, and human case reports. Fortunately, consensus-based recommendations derived from available data and endorsed by international toxicology and nephrology societies are now becoming available for both corporeal[5,6] and extracorporeal treatments.[7-16] The treating physician must have a working knowledge of the characteristics of a poison, its clinical effects, its pharmacokinetics, and its potential removal by various techniques. The purpose of this chapter is to review fundamental concepts of poison elimination, to review available elimination enhancement modalities, and to present poisonings that the nephrologist is most likely to encounter in practice.

Table 69.1 Exposures to Common Dialyzable Toxins (2013)

Poison	Total Exposures*	Deaths
Ethylene glycol	6,600	16
Methanol	1,988	8
Isopropanol	16,944	3
Lithium	6,744	6
Valproic acid	7,776	2
Carbamazepine	3,946	1
Phenytoin	2,850	1
Gabapentin	13,163	3
Barbiturates	2,127	3
Theophylline	210	0
Paraquat	96	5
Salicylates	40,461	31
Acetaminophen	188,267	188
Metformin	8,229	12

*Includes co-ingestions and mixed formulations.
Data from Mowry JB, Spyker DA, Cantilena LR Jr, et al: 2013 Annual report of the American Association of Poison Control Centers' National Poison Data System (NPDS): 31st annual report. Clin Toxicol 52(10):1032-1283, 2014.

OVERVIEW OF CORPOREAL TREATMENTS FOR ENHANCED ELIMINATION OF POISONS

FORCED DIURESIS

The physiologic mechanisms involved in the elimination of xenobiotics by the kidney include (1) glomerular filtration, (2) active secretion in the proximal tubule, and (3) passive reabsorption in the distal tubule. Historically, forced diuresis through volume expansion with isotonic fluids (0.9% NaCl or lactated Ringer's solution), with or without concomitant diuretics, has been used to enhance renal elimination of poisons. Unfortunately, results of early studies failed to show any significant benefit of forced diuresis but rather showed that it is associated with complications such as volume overload, pulmonary edema, cerebral edema, and electrolyte disturbances (e.g., hyponatremia, hypokalemia). At present, forced diuresis is not recommended in the management of acute poisonings. However, aggressive volume repletion remains warranted for some poisons, to correct hypotension and/or to overcome proximal tubular reabsorption of some offending agents (e.g., lithium) during volume contraction (explained later).

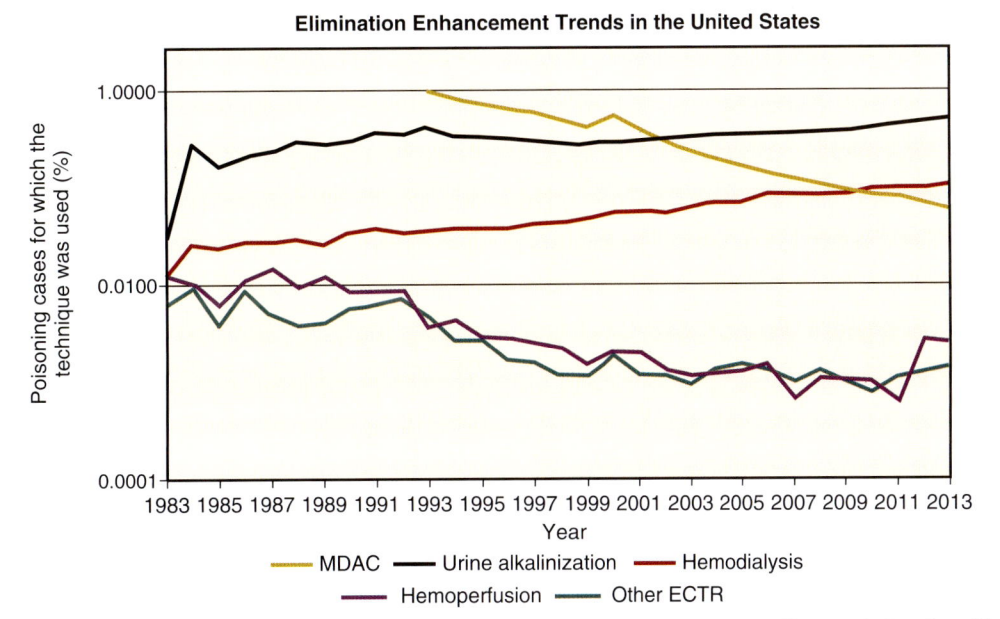

Figure 69.1 Use of elimination enhancement techniques in the United States from 1983 to 2013. The y-axis is a logarithmic scale. ECTR, Extracorporeal treatment; MDAC, multiple-dose activated charcoal.

MANIPULATION OF URINARY pH

Manipulation of urinary pH can enhance renal elimination of selected poisons. The underlying mechanism is based on the concept of *ion trapping*; because cell membranes are generally more easily permeated by non-ionized molecules, the goal of manipulating urinary pH is to favor the formation of an ionized form in the tubular lumen that cannot be passively reabsorbed. The ionized poison becomes "trapped" in the tubular lumen and is then eliminated in the urine. The dissociation of a weak acid or base into its ionized state is determined by its dissociation constant (K_d) (i.e., the pH at which it is 50% ionized and 50% non-ionized). For example, the K_d of salicylic acid is 3, that is, when the urinary pH is 3, salicylate exists in a 1:1 ratio of the ionized to non-ionized forms. Alkalinization of the urine to a pH of 7.4 increases the ratio to 20,000:1 in favor of the ionized form, which is more readily eliminated in urine.

The clinical efficacy of urine alkalinization is dependent on the relative contribution of kidney clearance to the total body clearance of active poison; if only 1% of the ingested poison is excreted unchanged in the urine, even a 10-fold increase in renal elimination will have no clinically significant effect.[6] Criteria that determine whether a poison is amenable to urinary alkalinization are as follows: (1) it is eliminated unchanged by the kidneys, (2) it is distributed primarily in the extracellular fluid compartment, and (3) it is weakly acidic (i.e., with a K_d of 3.0 to 7.0). Urine alkalinization enhances kidney excretion of xenobiotics such as salicylates, phenobarbital, chlorpropamide, 2,4-dichlorophenoxyacetic acid, methylchlorophenoxypropionic acid, diflunisal, fluoride, and methotrexate (Table 69.2).[6]

Urine alkalinization can be achieved with intravenous administration of sodium bicarbonate, beginning with a 1-ampule bolus (50 mEq), followed by 5% dextrose in water with 2 to 3 ampules of sodium bicarbonate added to each liter at 250 mL/hr, although the rate of infusion should be adapted to the volume status of the patient. During urine alkalinization, serum electrolyte levels and urinary pH must be closely monitored every 2 to 3 hours; the target pH range for urine is between 7.5 and 8.5. Complications can include hypokalemia, hypernatremia, fluid overload, pulmonary edema, cerebral edema, and alkalemia. The degree of hypokalemia may be profound because of both intracellular potassium shifts and urinary potassium losses. Moreover, normokalemia is a prerequisite for urine alkalinization to be effective; in the setting of hypokalemia, potassium is reabsorbed at the distal tubule in exchange for a hydrogen ion. Therefore, if hypokalemia remains uncorrected during urine alkalinization, not only is the nephron unable to produce alkaline urine, but the patient is also at higher risk for the development of alkalemia. Carbonic anhydrase inhibitors (e.g., acetazolamide) can alkalinize urine but at the serious expense of exacerbating systemic metabolic acidosis and thus are never recommended.

In the past, urinary acidification (goal of urinary pH < 6.0) was used to enhance renal elimination of weak bases such as amphetamines, phencyclidine, and quinine but no longer has a role in poisoning because of lack of efficacy and potential complications.

FECAL ELIMINATION ENHANCEMENT

Activated charcoal, when given in multiple doses, can enhance elimination of certain poisons. Multiple-dose activated charcoal (MDAC) promotes clearance of poisons by interrupting their enterohepatic circulation and by promoting passive diffusion down a concentration gradient from the intestinal capillaries to the intraluminal gut space, a process often referred to as "gut dialysis." Multiple regimens exist for MDAC: it can be given every 4 hours at a dose of 1 g/kg or every 2 hours at 0.5 g/kg until improvement in clinical status. Ideal properties of poisons amenable to MDAC include a small volume of distribution (V_d), a prolonged half-life, and a low intrinsic clearance. Contraindications to MDAC include an altered level of consciousness with an unprotected airway, protracted vomiting unresponsive to antiemetic therapy, and intestinal occlusion. Complications such as aspiration pneumonitis, appendicitis, or charcoal bezoar with MDAC are infrequently reported, and their incidence increases with the amount of activated carbon doses given. Present guidelines recommend MDAC for poisoning due to theophylline, dapsone, carbamazepine, phenobarbital, and quinine,[5] although there may also be some benefit of use in poisoning from oleander seed[17] and phenytoin (see Table 69.2).[18]

Ion-exchange resins may also attract poisons from the gut capillaries to the lumen. Sodium polystyrene sulfonate (Kayexalate) has long been used for the treatment of hyperkalemia, and there is current evidence that it can also reduce the half-life of lithium.[19] Prussian blue can be used

Table 69.2 Poisons Whose Elimination May Be Enhanced by Corporeal Techniques			
Urine Alkalinization	Multiple-Dose Activated Charcoal	Sodium Polystyrene Sulfonate	Prussian Blue
Salicylates	Theophylline	Potassium	Thallium
Fluoride	Dapsone	Lithium	Radiocesium
Phenobarbital	Quinine		
Chlorpropamide	Phenobarbital		
2,4-Dichlorophenoxyacetic acid	Carbamazepine		
Mecoprop	Salicylates		
Diflunisal	Phenytoin		
Methotrexate	Oleander seed		

to enhance fecal elimination of radiocesium and thallium (see Table 69.2).[20]

PRINCIPLES AND FACTORS INFLUENCING POISON REMOVAL DURING EXTRACORPOREAL TREATMENTS

The elimination of a poison depends on its physicochemical and pharmacologic properties as well as the extracorporeal technique chosen. Extracorporeal elimination of a poison is only possible if all of the following are present: (1) it can be extracted from the plasma compartment, (2) a significant proportion of its body stores can be eliminated, and (3) extracorporeal clearance contributes to a significant extent to total clearance. The first condition is dependent on the molecular size and protein binding of the poison, and it is correlated to the extraction ratio (ER) and extracorporeal clearance (CL_{ECTR}). ER can be calculated as (A-V)/A, where A represents the inflow (or prefilter) plasma concentration and V represents the outflow (or postfilter) plasma concentration. An extraction ratio of 1.0 implies complete elimination of a substance from the plasma after a single pass through the extracorporeal circuit (i.e., V = 0). Extracorporeal plasma clearance may be calculated as: $CL_{ECTR} = Q_B \times (1 - Hct) \times ER$, where Q_B is the blood flow and Hct the hematocrit. CL_{ECTR} can also be calculated by quantifying poison in spent ultrafiltrate and/or dialysate and dividing by averaged plasma concentration of the poison over time. The second condition relates to its V_d, and the third depends on its endogenous clearance (explained later).

Therapy-specific factors to consider include the process of poison removal (e.g., diffusion, adsorption, convection), as well as the parameters chosen for a specific technique such as the dialysis membrane (dialyzer surface area, membrane pore structure), characteristics of the filter or cartridge, rate of blood flow, and rate of effluent flow.[21]

POISON-RELATED FACTORS

MOLECULAR SIZE

Poisons with a molecular size below 1000 Da will be removed by any of the three processes but best by diffusion. Solutes in excess of 1000 Da will be better removed by convection or adsorption,[22] although present-day hemodialysis (HD) is usually capable of clearing poisons with an upper limit of approximately 10,000 Da. Hemofiltration can remove poisons up to 50,000 Da. Poisons with very high molecular sizes (>100,000 Da) can be removed only by adsorption or by centrifugation/separation.

PROTEIN BINDING

The extent of a poison's binding to plasma proteins will also determine its removal. Hemofiltration and HD can only remove unbound poison, because the poison-protein complex size exceeds the capacity of the hemofilter or dialyzer. Hemoperfusion, however, may be more effective in these cases, inasmuch as the adsorbent (activated carbon or resin) competes with plasma proteins and is dependent purely on the affinity of the adsorbent for the poison.

The degree of protein binding can be influenced by alterations in plasma poison or protein concentration and the presence of different pathologic states.[23] For example, as a result of hypoalbuminemia, less protein is available for binding, and accumulation of organic acids in uremia leads to a reduction in binding sites for some xenobiotics (e.g., salicylates, warfarin, and phenytoin). Furthermore, in toxic concentrations, there may be saturation of the protein binding sites (e.g., valproic acid), increasing the fraction of unbound in relation to its total concentration, which then provides a larger pool of poison that is removable by ECTR.

VOLUME OF DISTRIBUTION

The V_d of a drug is the apparent volume into which it is distributed at equilibrium and before metabolic clearance begins. V_d may be calculated by dividing the total drug in the body by its concentration. This mathematical relationship assumes that the body is a single compartment of homogeneous water into which the drug is distributed.

Drugs that distribute extensively in tissue (e.g., tricyclic antidepressants) have a high V_d; conversely, drugs that distribute in total body water (e.g., methanol) have a V_d of 0.6 L/kg. Poisons exclusively confined to the blood compartment (e.g., rituximab) have a V_d of approximately 0.06 L/kg. Because ECTRs only remove poisons from the intravascular space, the elimination of poisons with a high V_d will not be significantly enhanced. For example, due to its low protein binding (25%) and relatively low molecular size (780 Da), digoxin easily crosses the dialyzer; however, because of its high V_d (7 L/kg), less than 5% of total body burden of digoxin will be removed in a 6-hour dialysis session. Many publications still erroneously conclude that a poison with a high V_d is amenable to extracorporeal clearance solely based on a high clearance or a rapid reduction of serum concentrations.[24,25]

ECTR may be considered for very toxic xenobiotics despite a high V_d (e.g., thallium) if a patient presents early after exposure; in these cases, it is anticipated that the poison has not yet distributed into various tissues and may be successfully removed by dialysis.[9]

ENDOGENOUS CLEARANCE

Extracorporeal removal will not be useful if endogenous clearance of a poison (via metabolism and native elimination routes) far outweighs that which can be obtained via ECTR (usually < 200 mL/min).[26] This explains why HD is not indicated for poisons like cocaine or toluene. Similarly, the decisional threshold to initiate dialysis will certainly be lower if there is presence of kidney impairment in a patient poisoned by a toxin exclusively eliminated by kidneys (e.g., lithium).

EXTRACORPOREAL TREATMENT–RELATED FACTORS

Factors specific to the ECTR that affect poison elimination include the process of poison removal, characteristics of the dialysis membrane (i.e., material, surface area, porosity), concentration gradient across the membrane, and blood/dialysate/ultrafiltration flow rates. Some hemoperfusion (HP) cartridges become saturated after a few hours and need to be replaced.[27] These characteristics are discussed later in this chapter, where the different extracorporeal modalities will be further described.

AVAILABLE EXTRACORPOREAL TREATMENTS TO ENHANCE ELIMINATION OF POISONS

Numerous techniques exist to facilitate removal of poison. These can usually be classified by their process: diffusion (HD, peritoneal dialysis), convection (hemofiltration), adsorption (HP), centrifugation/separation (plasma exchange).[28,29]

HEMODIALYSIS

During HD, poison diffuses from the blood compartment to a dialysate flowing in a countercurrent direction, separated by a semipermeable dialysis membrane. The same principles that dictate solute removal in HD also apply to poison elimination (see Chapter 65 for a detailed discussion). Characteristics of a xenobiotic that favor efficient poison removal by HD are low molecular size (10,000 Da), low V_d (2 L/kg), low protein binding (<80%), low endogenous clearance (<4 mL/min/kg), and high water solubility/low lipid solubility.

Specific components of the dialysis system will affect poison clearance; these include membrane type, its surface area, and blood and dialysate flow rates (Table 69.3). Poison elimination is limited by the pore size of the dialysis membrane. However, even if the poison size is below that of the membrane's cutoff, larger molecules do not diffuse as freely as smaller ones. The advent of newer synthetic high-flux membranes and catheters now permit removal of larger poisons that were considered nondialyzable 20 years ago.[22] Increasing both the rates of dialysate and especially blood flow result in greater diffusion and elimination of the poison and should therefore always be maximized in poisoning situations.[29]

HD has several distinct advantages over other extracorporeal modalities in the management of acute poisonings[30]: Both poison and volume removal occur rapidly, and dialysis also corrects complications associated with severe poisonings—acute kidney injury (AKI), volume overload, acid-base abnormalities, electrolyte disturbances, and even hypothermia.

The most common acute complication of HD is systemic hypotension, and this is most prevalent in patients with AKI or end-stage kidney disease (ESKD) who require fluid removal. Because poisoned patients rarely require net ultrafiltration, the true incidence of dialytic hypotension in the toxicology setting is unknown but is more likely related to the effect of the poison rather than the treatment itself.

HEMOPERFUSION

During HP, blood circulates through an extracorporeal circuit equipped with a charcoal or a resin cartridge onto which poison can be adsorbed.[31] Unlike diffusion, adsorption is not as limited in regard to molecular size, lipid solubility, or protein binding of the poison. Alcohols and most metals, however, are poorly adsorbed to HP columns. Although certain exchange resins (XAD-4) are effective in the removal of organic solutes and nonpolar, lipid-soluble drugs, they are no longer available in the United States.

Current HP devices have improved their biocompatibility over the years; coating of the sorbent material minimizes direct contact between the adsorbent and the blood constituents, thereby greatly reducing the risk for embolization, without impairing their adsorptive capacity. The circuit requires more generous systemic anticoagulation than dialysis. Blood flows are limited to less than 350 mL/min to minimize the risk for hemolysis.[32]

Complications of HP are mostly related to the nonselective adsorption of certain cells and important molecules, in particular a fall in the concentration of platelets (≈30% to 50%), white blood cells (≈10%), serum fibrinogen, fibronectin, calcium, or glucose.[33,34] Although these complications are reversible and were more common with earlier devices, HP still carries a higher risk for complications than does HD.[35] Furthermore, a cartridge costs several-fold higher than a performant dialyzer and needs to be replaced every 2 to 4 hours, as it becomes saturated.

Although clearances for many poisons were superior with HP compared to dialysis 20 years ago, with the technologic advancements of dialysis, this is no longer necessarily true. For example, the clearances for both theophylline and phenobarbital, poisons for which HP was historically considered superior to dialysis, are now considered comparable.[31,35,36] In addition, HP does not allow for rapid correction of electrolyte or acid-base disturbances, cannot remove fluid, and is less readily available. For these reasons, HD is generally preferred in almost all settings where HP is indicated.[31] These considerations are reflected by the trends in ECTR choice for poisonings (see Figure 69.1).[37-39]

HEMOFILTRATION

During hemofiltration, solute and solvent are removed by solvent drag, a process known as convection, and replaced by a physiologic solution. Ultrafiltration is dependent on the sieving coefficient of the membrane. The sieving coefficient is the ratio of the solute filtrate concentration to the respective solute plasma concentration. A sieving coefficient of 1 indicates unrestricted transport, whereas there is no transport at all at when the coefficient is 0. Drug elimination by hemofiltration is dependent on factors comparable to HD (diffusion) with a few differences; convective transport allows removal of toxins with larger molecular size (<50,000 Da) but performs slightly worse for smaller molecules.[29] Because most poisons possess a low molecular size (<1000

Table 69.3 Factors That May Enhance Poison Clearance during Hemodialysis

Larger surface area of dialysis membrane
High-flux dialyzer
High blood and dialysate flow
Increased ultrafiltration rate (with replacement solution)
Increased time on dialysis
A vascular site that has less recirculation
Two dialyzers in series
Two distinct extracorporeal circuits

Da), hemofiltration does not offer any advantage over HD for the majority of poisonings.

COMBINATION THERAPY

Clinicians sometimes combine more than one mechanism for poison removal. For example, adsorption and diffusion (HD and HP) are sometimes used concurrently, in series, to maximize poison clearance. Although there is evidence that this combination approach may yield the best results, the kinetic benefits of two procedures are usually not additive and may also increase the incidence of complications. Diffusion and convection (hemodiafiltration) are also commonly combined.

CONTINUOUS RENAL REPLACEMENT THERAPY

Most ECTRs can be offered intermittently or continuously. Continuous renal replacement therapies (CRRTs) are particularly popular in the critical care setting in the management of AKI, and they are available in various forms (see Chapters 31 and 65): continuous arteriovenous hemodialysis, continuous venovenous hemodialysis, continuous arteriovenous hemofiltration, continuous venovenous hemofiltration, continuous arteriovenous hemodiafiltration, and continuous venovenous hemodiafiltration. Their role in the management of acute poisonings remains uncertain.[40] The solute clearance with continuous modalities is usually much lower than those with intermittent ones because of lower blood, dialysate, and ultrafiltrate flow rates. Continuous modalities present an advantage in AKI, in which rapid fluid and solute fluxes may be undesirable in hemodynamically unstable patients. However, in poisoned patients, because net fluid removal is rarely required, and because removal of the offending agent is urgent, intermittent therapies are usually favored. Although it has been suggested that CRRT may be preferred to avoid the sudden increase in poison concentration seen after discontinuation of intermittent therapies ("rebound"), the benefit of this remains uncertain (see later).

Sustained low-efficiency dialysis (SLED) is a hybrid technique that is described as an alternative to intermittent HD and CRRT.[41,42] Although used in anecdotal reports,[43] the same reservations described for CRRT apply (i.e., lower poison clearance).

PERITONEAL DIALYSIS

There is little role for peritoneal dialysis in acute poisoning. It is an inefficient method of toxin elimination, achieving a maximum clearance of 10 to 15 mL/min (less than one-tenth of that achievable by HD).[28] Peritoneal dialysis has no advantages over the other ECTRs in poisoning situations.

THERAPEUTIC PLASMA EXCHANGE AND PLASMAPHERESIS

Plasmapheresis is a process in which plasma is separated either by filtration or centrifugation from withdrawn blood, and formed elements are retransfused back to the patient. In therapeutic plasma exchange (TPE), the removed plasma is discarded and replaced by 5% albumin, fresh-frozen plasma, cryoprecipitate-poor plasma, or stored plasma. Clearance during TPE is limited by the plasma removal rate, which cannot readily exceed 50 mL/min.[28,44] The role of TPE in the treatment of acute poisoning is not well defined, but this method should only be considered for poisons that are very highly protein bound (>95%) or in very large poisons that are over the cutoffs accepted for hemofiltration or HP (>50,000 Da), such as rituximab.[45-47] Adverse outcomes from TPE involve complications associated with placement of the vascular access, bleeding, hypocalcemia, and hypersensitivity reactions to the replacement plasma proteins.[48,49]

EXCHANGE TRANSFUSION

Exchange transfusion is a treatment in which apheresis is used to remove the patient's red blood cells and replace them with transfused blood products. Its role in poisoning is unclear but may be considered in poisons that cause massive hemolysis (e.g., sodium chlorate) or in infants, because it is technically less cumbersome to use than HD in this population.

EXTRACORPOREAL LIVER ASSIST DEVICES (ALBUMIN DIALYSIS)

Albumin dialysis is a relatively new ECTR and is sometimes used for liver replacement in the context of severe acute hepatitis and cirrhosis. Theoretically, these devices can remove albumin-bound xenobiotics and endogenous substances (bile acids, bilirubin) better than classical diffusive and convective techniques. However, preliminary clearance data do not show any superiority of these techniques in poisonings from theophylline, valproic acid, or phenytoin[50-52]; the application of extracorporeal liver assist devices in poisoning appears most pertinent for toxin-induced hepatotoxicity, especially to *Amanita* mushrooms and acetaminophen.[53-56] The advantages of albumin dialysis are more apparent for its liver replacement support, especially as a bridge to liver transplantation or remission, rather than for its capacity to eliminate poison.

Many devices exist, but the following are among the better known:

- Single-pass albumin dialysis (SPAD) is a technique similar to HD but with the added difference that albumin is supplemented in the dialysate, which is thereafter discarded after its contact with the filter.
- The Molecular Adsorbent Recirculating System (MARS) is identical to SPAD, but the albumin-enhanced dialysate (with the adsorbed xenobiotics) is recycled after going through a dialysis filter, a resin, and a charcoal cartridge.
- The Prometheus system combines albumin adsorption with high-flux HD after selective filtration of the albumin fraction through a polysulfone filter.

Whether these expensive (>$8000 per treatment in the United States), complicated, and nonspecific procedures would offer any advantage over HD, HP, or TPE is not currently known.

Table 69.4 summarizes the various ECTRs available for poison removal.

Table 69.4 Summary of Extracorporeal Treatments

	Process	Molecular Size Cutoff (Da)	Protein-Binding Cutoff	Relative Cost	Complications	Comments
Hemodialysis	Diffusion	<10,000	<80%	+	+	Correction of uremia and acid-base/E+ disorders
Hemoperfusion	Adsorption	<50,000	<95%	++	+++	Saturation of cartridge
Hemofiltration	Convection	<50,000	<80%	++	+	Correction of uremia and acid-base/E+ disorders
Plasma exchange	Centrifugation/separation, filtration	<1,000,000	None	+++	+++	
Albumin dialysis	Diffusion, adsorption	<300,000	<95%	++++	++	Liver replacement support
Exchange transfusion	Centrifugation/separation, filtration	None	None	++	++	Easier in neonates; Correction of hemolysis
Peritoneal dialysis	Diffusion	<5,000	<80%	++	++	

All extracorporeal treatments in the table are less likely to be useful for poisons that have a high V_d or a high endogenous clearance.
E+, Electrolyte; V_d, volume of distribution.

GENERAL INDICATIONS FOR EXTRACORPOREAL REMOVAL OF POISONS

The EXTRIP (EXtracorporeal TReatments In Poisoning, http://www.extrip-workgroup.org/) workgroup[7,8] is currently drafting guidelines for the use of blood purification for 16 key toxins.[9-14,16] These recommendations should help to standardize management for patients exposed to these toxins and propose future research direction.[8] The decision to initiate any form of blood purification must take into account the patient's clinical status, the benefit expected from ECTRs, and poison-related factors.

Absolute indications for ECTR include the following (all must be present)[30]:

1. **The poisoning exposure must be severe.** The exposure to a specific poison must be significant enough to warrant the complications and cost associated with ECTR. Obviously, a patient with life-threatening clinical signs (repeated seizures, respiratory depression, dysrhythmias) will be classified as severe. A proper risk assessment of the exposure, which includes close collaboration with a poison control center, may help estimate the risk for any specific patient. In rare cases a poison may produce delayed effects (methanol, paraquat); monitoring of levels might therefore predict future clinical compromise and would prompt *prophylactic* ECTR (i.e., before the appearance of toxic symptoms).
2. **There must be an absence of life-saving alternatives.** Rarely, an antidote may either amend or prevent the apparition of toxic symptoms related to a poison. ECTR then becomes less crucial or indicated. This is the case for acetaminophen poisoning, when *N*-acetylcysteine (NAC) is available. Because ECTR is somewhat invasive and may require transfer to a specialized center, its benefit and cost should be weighed against those of the antidote.
3. **The ECTR must be capable of removing the poison from the blood compartment.** The poison should permeate readily through the dialysis membrane or the column. This relates to a high extraction ratio and a high extracorporeal clearance (see earlier).
4. **ECTR must be expected to significantly contribute to total body clearance.** As shown previously, if a poison is mostly confined outside of the intravascular space (high V_d), or if it is extensively and rapidly metabolized by endogenous routes, ECTR will likely not be removing poison from the body to a proportion that justifies its initiation.

To decide whether blood purification is indicated for a specific poisoning, the clinician must anticipate which benefits are expected from the procedure; some exposures can cause death (e.g., salicylates at high ingestions, paraquat), whereas others may cause irreversible tissue damage (e.g., blindness for methanol). The advantages of ECTR in those circumstances would largely outweigh the complications and costs of the procedure. In other situations, the poisoning itself may not cause irreversible injury, but the patient may be subjected to prolonged coma and immobilization, requiring mechanical ventilation and tight surveillance in the intensive care unit. This is the case for poisons that can produce central nervous system (CNS) depression (e.g., barbiturates, anticonvulsants). Finally, there may be situations in which ECTR will likely not affect outcome but may reduce hospitalization and associated costs (e.g., dialysis versus fomepizole in a methanol-poisoned patient without metabolic acidosis).[57,58] The clinician should therefore assess the risk of the specific exposure and consider the cost/benefit ratio of ECTR in this context. Complications associated with ECTR are minimal and are usually limited to the traumatic insertion of a vascular access (which can be minimized with ultrasonographic guidance)[59]; more rarely, ECTR can potentiate elimination of certain antidotes[60] and precipitate withdrawal symptoms if drug levels fall below the therapeutic range.[61] Costs of a single dialysis, including equipment and nursing and physician fees, are minor compared to the cost of a day in the intensive care unit. In the absence of any clinical outcome data, studies should demonstrate, at a minimum, significant drug removal.

TECHNICAL CONSIDERATIONS

Patients presenting with poisonings are different from patients with AKI or ESKD; it is therefore normal that the prescription of any ECTR for the purpose of poison removal reflects these differences.

- **Vascular access:** A double-lumen central catheter is required for administering most forms of ECTR. Because time is usually a concern, a temporary catheter is preferred, using ultrasonographic guidance to limit complications and ensure patency.[62] The femoral line is simpler for insertion and does not require radiographic placement confirmation but has more recirculation than subclavian or jugular insertion sites.[63] There has been some experience in the use of dual catheter sites and circuits to maximize poison clearance.[64,65]
- **Choice of hemodialyzer/filter/adsorber:** For dialysis, high-flux, high-efficiency dialyzers with the largest surface area should be used. The dialyzer or hemofilter should have a molecular size cutoff above that of the poison that needs to be removed. With respect to HP, the only column available in the United States is the Gambro Adsorba 300C, a coated activated charcoal cartridge.[31]
- **Heparinization:** Heparinization of the dialysis circuit is usually done with unfractionated heparin or low-molecular-weight heparin to prevent clotting and maintain patency of the circuit. In patients at high risk for bleeding, saline flushes can be substituted for heparin. For HP, heparin is also used to reduce the risk for hemolysis[32] and is usually required in greater quantities than for HD.
- **Blood, dialysate, and effluent flow:** They should all be maximized according to the capabilities of the machine to maximize clearance.[29]
- **Dialysate composition:** As mentioned earlier, poisoned patients may not share the same metabolic characteristics as those with renal failure. Bicarbonate, sodium, calcium, and magnesium levels need to be adjusted in the dialysate bath (or replacement fluid) to the requirement of the poisoned patient to avoid dangerous imbalances. Phosphate may also be added to the bath to avoid hypophosphatemia. It is also recommended that periodic measurement of serum biochemistry be performed and the content of the dialysate be adapted if needed.
- **Duration of ECTR:** A single 6-hour ECTR will usually suffice to substantially lower blood levels of most xenobiotics. When significant toxicity is present or suspected to be prolonged, there is little risk in extending this for several more hours (HP cartridges may need to be replaced because of saturation). Obviously, more time will be required if a less efficient therapy (CRRT, peritoneal dialysis, SLED) is used.
- **Patient disposition:** Many poisoned patients die before initiation of dialysis.[66] If the risk analysis on a suspected toxic exposure suggests that a patient may require dialysis, prompt communication with a dialysis unit and even prophylactic transfer to one may be required, even if the patient does not yet meet criteria for blood purification. Because significant delay may occur between the time a decision is made to perform ECTR and the time when it is initiated, a dialysis nurse should be rapidly contacted and a temporary dialysis catheter installed as early as possible. Logistics and clinical status may require transfer of the patient to the intensive care unit.[30]
- **Rebound:** Rebound is defined as a sudden increase in poison concentration after discontinuation of the ECTR, and it occurs more typically after intermittent therapies. Rebound may be either due to redistribution of poison from deep compartments (e.g., tissues and intracellular space) to the plasma (such as seen with lithium[67] and methotrexate[68]), especially in poisons with a large V_d, or due to ongoing absorption of the poison. It is important for the clinician to identify which of these is causing the rise. In the former case, the elevation of the serum concentration comes at the expense of a concomitant decrease in poison concentration from the toxic compartments, a phenomenon that would therefore not be worrisome but rather even desirable,[69] and that would present an added opportunity to remove more poison with a subsequent treatment. In the situation of ongoing absorption of the poison, the increase in serum concentration can cause recurrence of toxic symptoms. To address rebound, clinicians may choose to repeat a session, switch to a continuous therapy, or extend the intermittent therapy longer than the typical 4- to 6-hour treatment duration without added risk.[70] Following ECTR, serial poison concentration and clinical status should be monitored for a period long enough to account for redistribution or ongoing absorption ($\approx$12 to 24 hours). The catheter should remain in place until the physician is convinced that additional sessions are unnecessary.

POISONS AMENABLE TO EXTRACORPOREAL ELIMINATION

In the large majority of poisoning cases, ECTRs are not required. In fact, the drugs or poisons that are most commonly responsible for poisoning-related fatalities (e.g., tricyclic antidepressants, short-acting barbiturates, stimulants, and "street drugs") are not effectively amenable to extracorporeal removal. The remainder of this chapter focuses on the clinical characteristics of intoxicants that may be responsive to extracorporeal removal.

THE TOXIC ALCOHOLS: ETHYLENE GLYCOL, METHANOL, ISOPROPANOL

Toxic alcohols share many similar molecular characteristics and toxicity and will therefore be grouped within this section. In its pure form, ethylene glycol is colorless, odorless, syrupy, and sweet-tasting, which makes it attractive to young children. It is commonly found in antifreeze, radiator fluid, solvents, hydraulic brake fluid, deicing solutions, detergents, lacquers, and polishes. Methanol, also known as wood alcohol, is the simplest of alcohols. It is a light, volatile, flammable liquid with a distinctive odor similar to ethanol.

Table 69.5 Physiochemical Characteristics and Toxicokinetics of Various Poisons

	Molecular Size (Da)	Protein Binding	Volume of Distribution (L/kg)	Endogenous Clearance in Healthy Adults (mL/min/kg)
Methanol	32	0%	0.6	0.7
Ethylene glycol	62	0%	0.6	1.8
Isopropanol	60	0%	0.6	1.2
Theophylline	180	60%	0.5	0.7
Lithium	7	0%	0.8	0.4
Salicylic acid	138	80%*	0.2	1.5
Valproic acid	144	90%*	0.2	0.1
Metformin	166	5%	5	10
Phenytoin	252	90%	0.6	0.4
Carbamazepine	236	75%	1.2	1.3
Acetaminophen	151	20%	1	5
Phenobarbital	232	40%	0.7	0.2
Paraquat	186	5%	1.0	8
Methotrexate	454	50%	0.8	1.5

*Protein binding saturation occurs at high concentration.

It is used as a solvent, as an intermediate of chemical synthesis during various manufacturing processes, or as an octane booster in gasoline. The solvents that contain methanol include windshield- or glass-cleaning solutions, enamels, printing solutions, stains, dyes, varnishes, thinners, fuels, and antifreeze additives for gasoline. Isopropanol (i.e., isopropyl alcohol or 2-propanolol) is a clear, colorless and volatile liquid with a faint odor of acetone and bitter taste. It is commonly found in "rubbing alcohol," skin lotion, hair tonics, aftershave lotion, denatured alcohol, solvents, cements, cleaning products, and the manufacturing process of acetone and glycerin. Although the parent alcohols themselves cause minor toxicity (usually no more than moderate inebriation), their metabolites can induce life-threatening toxicity.

TOXICOCOLOGY AND TOXICOKINETICS

Molecular characteristics of major xenobiotics, including toxic alcohols, are shown in Table 69.5. Ethylene glycol, methanol, and isopropanol are all small molecules, unbound to protein, and distribute in total body water (V_d = 0.6 L/kg). Intoxication of these alcohols occurs rapidly after exposure and usually results from oral ingestion, although inhalation of vapors[71,72] and cutaneous absorption have been reported, especially in children.[73,74]

Approximately 20% of ethylene glycol is excreted unmetabolized by the kidney. The remaining 80% is oxidized to glycoaldehyde by alcohol dehydrogenase in the liver and then rapidly converted to glycolic acid by aldehyde dehydrogenase, which is followed by the slow conversion of glycolic acid to glyoxylic acid, the rate-limiting step (Figure 69.2A). The final end products include oxalic acid, glycine, and oxalomalic acid. Metabolic acidosis is caused by the formation and accumulation of glycolic acid, glycoaldehyde, and glyoxylic acid.[75,76] Lactic acidosis may also be present, as the decrease in the ratio of oxidized nicotinamide adenine dinucleotide (NAD^+) to reduced nicotinamide adenine dinucleotide (NADH) promotes the reduction of pyruvate to lactate. The remainder of the toxicity of ethylene glycol is precipitated by systemic calcium oxalate deposition in various tissues such as the kidneys.

Methanol is metabolized principally by alcohol dehydrogenase (85%) to formaldehyde in the presence of NAD^+ and then quickly oxidized by formaldehyde dehydrogenase to formic acid. Small amounts are excreted unchanged by the lungs (10%) and the kidneys (5%). In a folate-dependent step, formic acid is then transformed to water and carbon dioxide (see Figure 69.2B). Methanol follows zero-order kinetics elimination at low serum concentration and first-order kinetics at higher concentration, which may relate to pulmonary clearance.[77]

Formic acid is the metabolite most responsible for the toxic symptoms of methanol, because it inhibits cytochrome c oxidase in the cell mitochondria, interferin with cellular oxidative metabolism.[78] Energy production is shifted toward anaerobic glycolysis with production of lactate. There is also a shift of the NAD^+/NADH ratio when methanol is converted to formaldehyde, which promotes further the conversion of pyruvate to lactate. As the cellular pH falls, inhibition of cytochrome c oxidase by formic acid is increased, exacerbating the acidosis, eventually leading to cell hypoxia and cell death.[79]

The metabolism of isopropanol is illustrated in Figure 69.2. Approximately 80% is metabolized to acetone via alcohol dehydrogenase, and the remainder is eliminated unchanged in urine, with very small amounts excreted by the lungs.[80] Isopropanol displays first-order elimination kinetics with an elimination half-life of 3 to 8 hours,[81,82] whereas that of acetone is 10 hours.[83,84] Alcohol dehydrogenase inhibitors markedly increase the half-life of isopropanol but have little effect on that of acetone.[85] Most of the CNS depressant effects are attributed to isopropanol, whereas acetone likely has a minor effect.[81]

Any pure ethylene glycol ingestion over 0.1 mL/kg requires medical treatment. The lethal dose of ethylene glycol is approximately 1.4 mL/kg, but deaths have been reported with ingestions as low as 30 mL. The minimum lethal dose of methanol is estimated at 10 mL, although this

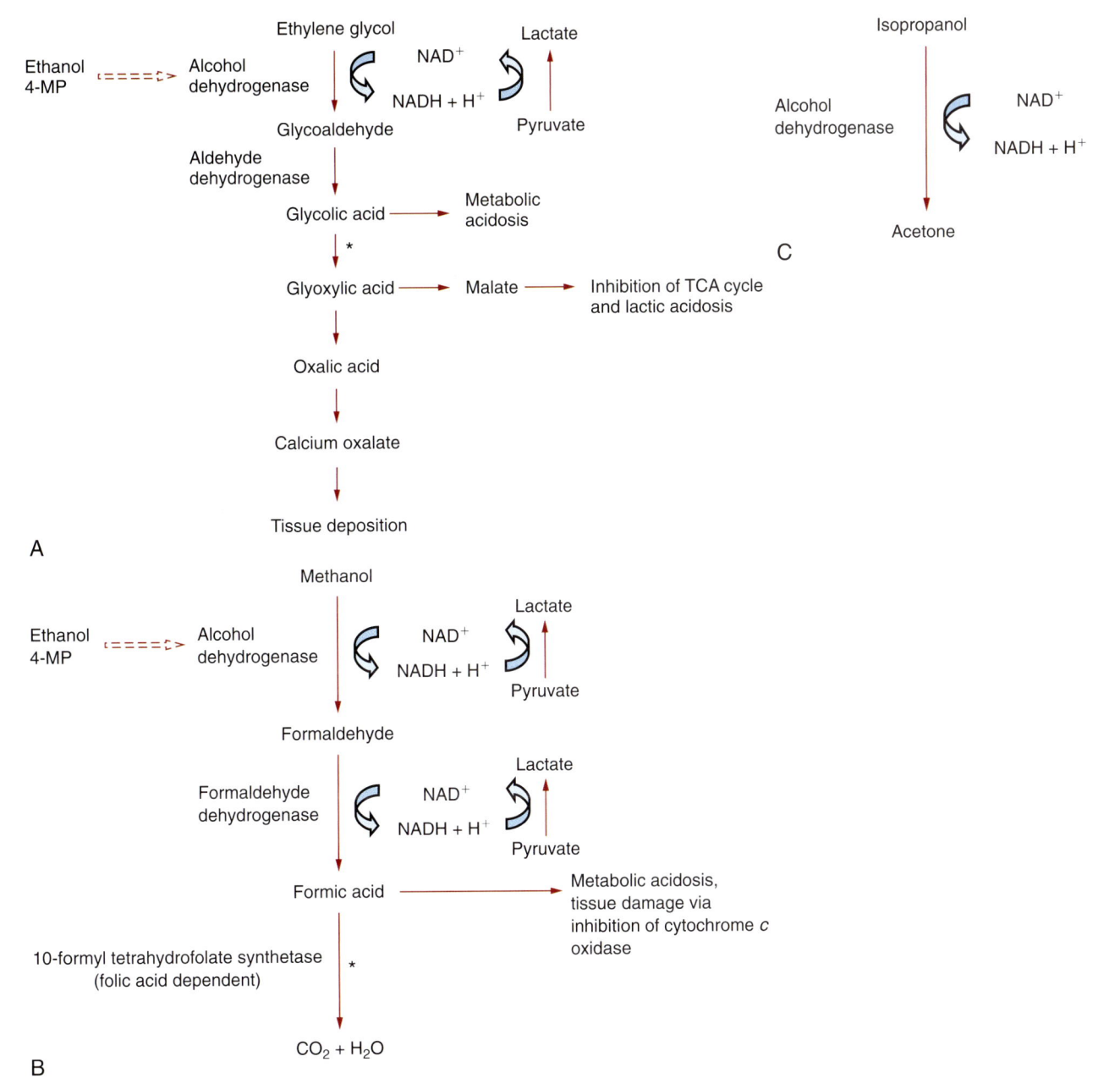

Figure 69.2 **A,** Metabolism of ethylene glycol. The *broken arrow* points to site of action of ADH inhibitors; the *asterisk* denotes the rate-limiting step. In the presence of the electron acceptor, NAD⁺, ethylene glycol is oxidized to glycoaldehyde by alcohol dehydrogenase. Aldehyde dehydrogenase then rapidly converts glycoaldehyde to glycolic acid, which is followed by the slow conversion of glycolic acid to glyoxylic acid (the rate-limiting step). The final end products include oxalic acid, glycine, and oxalomalic acid, which are all effectively removed by hemodialysis. **B,** Metabolism of methanol. The *broken arrow* points to site of action of ADH inhibitors; the *asterisk* denotes the rate-limiting step. **C,** Metabolism of isopropanol. 4-MP, Fomepizole; NAD⁺, oxidized nicotinamide adenine dinucleotide; NADH, reduced nicotinamide adenine dinucleotide; TCA, tricarboxylic acid.

is highly variable.[86] The lethal dose of pure isopropanol is 100 to 250 mL.[87]

CLINICAL PRESENTATION

Following ingestion, the symptoms of ethylene glycol poisoning follow a three-stage progression, the severity of which depends on certain factors, such as the ingested dose, concurrent ingestion of ethanol, and timing of treatment.[88] Stage 1 is the neurologic stage, which occurs 30 minutes to 12 hours after ingestion and is due to the parent alcohol causing inebriation, similar to ethanol but without the typical breath. Altered consciousness may progress to coma and seizures. Cerebral edema, nystagmus, ataxia, myoclonic jerks, and hyporeflexia have been described. New onset of cranial nerve defects (in particular the seventh) should make a clinician suspect ethylene glycol ingestion. Gastrointestinal irritation may lead to vomiting, hematemesis, and aspiration pneumonia.

Stage 2 is the cardiopulmonary stage, occurring 12 to 24 hours after ingestion, and results from the accumulation of newly formed organic acids. During this stage, calcium oxalate crystals deposit in the vasculature, myocardium, and lungs.[89] Hypertension or hypotension, dysrhythmias, myocarditis, pneumonitis, and noncardiogenic pulmonary edema have all been reported as potential cardiopulmonary complications. This phase is also associated with severe high anion gap metabolic acidosis. Most deaths occur during this stage.

Stage 3 is the renal stage, occurring 24 to 72 hours after ingestion, and develops as calcium oxalate crystals precipitate in the kidney, resulting in flank pain, hematuria, crystalluria, and AKI. The pathogenesis of AKI is unclear but may relate to interstitial nephritis, cortical necrosis, direct renal cytotoxicity, or obstruction. However, because the degree of renal injury does not correlate with the extent of calcium oxalate deposition in the kidney, it has been suggested that glycolic acid or other metabolites may be primarily responsible for the development of AKI.[90] In addition, low calcium concentrations in the blood may occur and cause overactive muscle reflexes and QT-interval prolongation.

Methanol intoxication should always be suspected in a patient presenting with neurologic, visual, and gastrointestinal symptoms in the presence of high anion gap metabolic acidosis with increased osmolal gap. CNS presentation may include inebriation, headaches, dizziness, nausea, and seizures and may progress to cerebral edema. Methanol can produce Parkinson-like syndrome by damage to putamen and subcortical white matter of the basal ganglia.[91,92] Gastrointestinal symptoms include anorexia, nausea, vomiting, gastritis, and abdominal pain from acute pancreatitis. Metabolic acidosis, caused by accumulation of formate and lactate, can be severe. Visual changes are the hallmark of methanol poisoning and usually occur 6 to 30 hours after exposure, depending on whether ethanol is co-ingested; symptoms may include blurred vision (flashes or snowstorm), central scotoma, impaired papillary response to light, decreased visual acuity, photophobia, visual field defect, and progression to complete blindness.[93,94] The mechanisms of visual defects are not very well understood but are thought to be caused by the inhibition of mitochondrial function in the optic nerve. Because the optic nerve cells possess few mitochondria and low cytochrome oxidase levels, they are extremely susceptible to the toxic effects of formic acid. Visual abnormalities are permanent in one-fourth of cases. Death is usually caused by cardiovascular shock and respiratory arrest.

The diagnosis of isopropanol overdose should be suspected in any patient with altered sensorium, a "fruity" acetone breath, an increased osmolal gap without an increase in anion gap, and the presence of acetonemia or acetonuria in the absence of hyperglycemia, glycosuria, or acidosis. Isopropanol poisoning mainly affects the CNS, with symptoms ranging from mild inebriation to lethargy, stupor, respiratory depression, and even coma. Isopropanol is also a gastrointestinal tract irritant and can cause nausea, vomiting, gastritis, and abdominal pain. Finally, isopropanol is directly toxic to myocytes and can induce severe hypotension, which is the strongest predictor of mortality in isopropanol overdose.[86] AKI may develop because of severe hypotension or myoglobinuria. Other systemic findings include hypoglycemia from impaired gluconeogenesis, hypothermia, and hemolytic anemia.

Table 69.6 Conversion of Toxic Alcohol Concentration from mmol/L to mg/dL

Toxic Alcohol	Conversion from mmol/L to mg/dL
Ethanol	×4.61
Ethylene glycol	×6.21
Isopropanol	×6.01
Methanol	×3.20
Diethylene glycol	×10.61
Propylene glycol	×7.61
Acetone	×5.81

DIAGNOSTIC TESTING

Because specific measurement of toxic alcohols (by colorimetric and enzymatic assays or chromatographic methods) is not widely available, treatment should begin immediately if exposure to toxic alcohols is suspected.[95] Ethylene glycol and methanol poisoning should be considered in any patient presenting with a high anion gap metabolic acidosis and a high osmolar gap, even in the absence of symptoms.[96] Because toxic alcohols are osmotically active compounds, the osmolal gap, calculated as the difference between measured osmolality (by freezing point depression) and calculated osmolality, can be used as an approximation of the toxic alcohol concentration (in mmol/L), which can then be converted to mg/dL (Table 69.6). This estimation can be monitored serially during admission and especially during dialysis, when precise serum levels are unavailable.[97,98] The calculated osmolality is based on the concentrations of sodium, glucose, blood urea nitrogen (BUN), and ethanol (if co-ingested), as follows:

$$\begin{aligned}
&\text{Toxic alcohol concentration (mmol/L)} \\
&\cong \text{Osmolal gap} - \text{ethanol} \\
&= \text{Osmolality}_{meas} - \text{Osmolality}_{calc} - \text{ethanol (mmol/L)} \\
&= \text{Osmolality}_{meas} - (2\,[\text{Na (mEq/L)}] \\
&\quad + \text{glucose (mg/dL)}/18 + \text{BUN (mg/dL)}/2.8 \\
&\quad - \text{ethanol (mg/dL)}/4.6
\end{aligned}$$

The normal osmolal gap is less than 10 to 12 mOsm/kg H$_2$O. An osmolal gap over 25 mOsm/kg suggests the presence of ethylene glycol, methanol, ethanol, isopropanol, propylene glycol, or acetone.[99] In isopropanol poisoning, both isopropanol and acetone contribute to the osmolal gap.[100] However, it is important to recognize that a normal osmolal gap does not exclude the diagnosis of toxic alcohol poisoning, if the patient presents late after ingestion, once the parent alcohol already has undergone oxidation (glycolic acid and formic acid do not contribute to the osmolal gap).[101,102]

Similarly, the anion gap can be used to estimate the glycolic acid and formic acid concentrations. The anion gap is the difference between measured cations (Na$^+$ and K$^+$) and measured anions (Cl$^-$ and HCO$_3^-$), representing the difference between unmeasured anions and unmeasured cations, all values being in mmol/L. Lactate can also contribute to the anion gap (AG) and needs to be factored in the following equation:

Glycolic acid/Formic acid concentration
$= \Delta AG - \Delta Lactate$
$= ((Na + K) - (Cl + HCO_3) - 16\ [AG\ upper\ reference\ limit])$
$\quad - (Lactate\ (mmol/L) - 2\ [lactate\ upper\ reference\ limit])$
$= Na + K - Cl - HCO_3 - Lactate - 14$

Studies have showed a good correlation between the level of metabolites and the anion gap.[99] The absence of an anion gap suggests either early presentation after ethylene glycol or methanol exposure (before metabolism), co-ingestion of ethanol, or the presence of another alcohol (isopropanol, propylene glycol).

Urinalysis can provide supporting evidence of ethylene glycol exposure; calcium oxalate crystals (monohydrate and dihydrate forms) may be present in the urine sediment and are birefringent when viewed under polarized light. These crystals appear 4 to 8 hours after ingestion and are found in approximately 50% of patients.[103,104] The presence of the monohydrate form is not specific for ethylene glycol poisoning because it is also seen in individuals who ingest large amounts of vitamin C or food containing high levels of oxalate. The dihydrate form, which is octahedral, or tent shaped, is present only under conditions of high urinary calcium and oxalate levels, therefore more specific for ethylene glycol poisoning. Urine that fluoresces under Wood lamp illumination is another unique feature of ethylene glycol poisoning. Many types of antifreeze contain sodium fluorescein, a fluorescent dye used as a marker to detect radiator leaks. For up to 6 hours after ingestion, sodium fluorescein can be detected in the urine.[105,106] Other laboratory abnormalities commonly found are hypocalcemia, leukocytosis, and elevated protein level in cerebral spinal fluid.

Characteristic test findings of isopropanol exposure include increased osmolality, the absence of metabolic acidosis (except if lactic acidosis is present), ketonemia, ketonuria, and normoglycemia. Acetonemia or acetonuria can be suspected by a positive sodium nitroprusside reaction in plasma or urine. Low concentration of serum ketones 2 hours after isopropanol ingestion (in the absence of alcohol dehydrogenase inhibition) generally excludes substantial ingestion.[81] Ketoacidosis from starvation, alcoholism, or diabetes mellitus can be differentiated from isopropanol poisoning by the presence of metabolic acidosis.

TREATMENT

In case of toxic alcohol poisoning, rapid decision making is critical because most clinicians have to proceed without a drug level confirmation. Management can be divided into supportive care, correction of the metabolic acidosis, antidotal therapy, and enhanced elimination with ECTRs.

Initial management, as for all poisonings, is directed toward stabilization and providing appropriate supportive care, which may include airway management, volume resuscitation, seizure management, and vasopressors. High minute ventilation should be maintained if significant acidemia is present. Because toxic alcohols are rapidly absorbed from the gastrointestinal tract, and because mucosal irritation is often present, gastrointestinal decontamination is seldom performed in this context.

Acidemia should be corrected with the administration of intravenous sodium bicarbonate,[107] which enhances deprotonation of acid metabolites, making them less likely to penetrate end-organ tissues (retina and kidney) and more likely to be excreted by the kidneys. An initial intravenous bolus (1 to 2 mEq/kg), followed by a perfusion if necessary, should be given to maintain an arterial pH no less than 7.35. Asymptomatic hypocalcemia is not routinely treated in the setting of ethylene glycol poisoning because it can potentially exacerbate calcium oxalate crystal formation and deposition.

Pyridoxine, thiamine, and magnesium are co-factors in the metabolism of ethylene glycol, and their supplementation is recommended in patients who may be malnourished (e.g., alcoholics) or in those with known deficits.[96] Because the rate-limiting step of methanol metabolism is mediated by 10-formyltetrahydrofolate synthetase, which is folic acid dependent, folic acid supplementation is recommended in methanol poisoning. The suggested dose is 50 mg intravenously every 4 hours for five doses and then once daily.

The cornerstone of the treatment of ethylene glycol or methanol poisoning is to delay their metabolism into toxic metabolites by use of antidotal agents (ethanol or fomepizole), which inhibit the actions of alcohol dehydrogenase.

Indications for use of these antidotes are as follows[96,108]:

1. Serum concentration of ethylene glycol above 20 mg/dL or methanol above 20 mg/dL
2. Documented recent (hours) ingestion of toxic amount of ethylene glycol or methanol and osmolal gap higher than 10 mOsm/L
3. A history or strong clinical suspicion of ethylene glycol or methanol poisoning, and at least two of the following: arterial pH less than 7.3, serum bicarbonate less than 20 mEq/L, osmolal gap greater than 10 mOsm/L, or presence of oxalate crystal in the urine

Antidote treatment is not recommended in isopropanol poisoning because the metabolite acetone does not cause metabolic acidosis and is eliminated by endogenous routes; if fomepizole were used, the CNS depressant effect of isopropanol could be prolonged.[109] Because alcohol dehydrogenase has greater affinity for ethanol than for either methanol or ethylene glycol, it has been the traditional antidote to prevent the formation of toxic metabolites. Ethanol can be given orally, intravenously, or via the dialysate. The intravenous formulation has the advantages of immediate bioavailability and avoiding gastrointestinal distress. Target serum ethanol concentrations for alcohol dehydrogenase competition are between 100 and 150 mg/dL[110]; below this concentration, alcohol dehydrogenase inhibition would not maximally inhibit metabolite formation, whereas above this range, CNS and respiratory depression might appear.[108] More predictable serum ethanol concentrations can be obtained during HD by adding 475 mL of 65% ethanol in the 4.5 L–acid bath of the dialysate.[110]

Fomepizole (4-methylpyrazole, Antizol) is a newer U.S. Food and Drug Administration (FDA)–approved antidote for both ethylene glycol and methanol poisoning. Compared to ethanol, fomepizole has multiple advantages: (1) more potent alcohol dehydrogenase inhibition, (2) simple dosing, (3) predictable pharmacokinetics, (4) no blood monitoring, (5) few side effects and no CNS depression, and (6) longer duration of action. Its main drawback is the cost ($5000 in the United States). Whichever antidote is chosen,

Table 69.7 Antidote Dosage during Toxic Alcohol Poisoning			
	Absolute Ethanol	**10% Intravenous Ethanol***	**Fomepizole**
Loading dose[†]	600 mg/kg	7.6 mL/kg	15 mg/kg IV
Maintenance dose	66 mg/kg/hr (nondrinker)	0.83 mL/kg/hr (nondrinker)	10 mg/kg q12hr × 4 doses, then
	154 mg/kg/hr (chronic drinker)	1.96 mL/kg/hr (chronic drinker)	15 mg/kg q12hr
Maintenance dose during HD	169 mg/kg/hr (nondrinker)	2.13 mL/kg/hr (nondrinker)	Same dose but q4hr or a constant
	257 mg/kg/hr (chronic drinker)	3.26 mL/kg/hr (chronic drinker)	infusion of 1.0-1.5 mg/kg/hr

*Equivalent to 7.9 g ethanol per deciliter.
[†]Assumes initial ethanol concentration is zero; dose is independent of chronic drinking status.
HD, Hemodialysis; IV, intravenous.

it is usually continued until ethylene glycol or methanol levels are below 20 mg/dL and the patient is asymptomatic with a normal arterial pH. Table 69.7 presents dosage of ethanol and fomepizole during toxic alcohol poisonings.

ECTRs, especially HD, are extremely efficient at removing alcohols and their toxic metabolites, as well as rapidly correcting acidosis. When dialysis parameters are optimized (see earlier), clearance of alcohols and metabolites can reach 250 mL/min.

The increasing availability of fomepizole has modified the indications and pertinence of ECTR because of its great efficacy at preventing new formation of metabolites. For example, patients who are poisoned with ethylene glycol, but who neither are acidotic nor have renal impairment, may be treated with fomepizole alone, whatever the concentration of ethylene glycol.[58,111] The same applies for methanol; however, endogenous clearance of methanol is extremely low when fomepizole is used. Assuming a methanol half-life of 54 hours under fomepizole,[112] a patient with an initial methanol concentration of 320 mg/dL would need to be hospitalized 9 days for methanol concentration to be considered safe (under 20 mg/dL). Dialysis might therefore be instituted to reduce hospitalization costs and antidote requirement for patients poisoned with either ethylene glycol or methanol.[57,113] The situation is altogether different if either a metabolic acidosis or an increased anion gap, both suggestive of accumulation of toxic metabolites, is present. In these cases, alcohol dehydrogenase inhibition should not be used alone but in association with some form of extracorporeal purification.

Indications for HD for ethylene glycol and methanol poisoning are the following[14,52,56]:

1. Serum ethylene glycol or methanol concentration above 50 mg/dL if fomepizole is not used
2. Metabolic acidosis (pH less than 7.2) or an anion gap greater than 24 mEq/L
3. Coma or seizures
4. Visual changes secondary to methanol
5. AKI or chronic kidney disease

The expected duration of dialysis can be estimated using this formula: $T(hours) = [-V \ln (5/A)/0.06 k]$, where V is the total water in liters, A is the initial alcohol concentration in mmol/L, and k is 80% of the dialyzer urea clearance in mL/min at the observed blood flow rate.[114,115] However, serial monitoring of alcohol concentration or osmolal gap is recommended to confirm the estimation. HD should be continued until the parent alcohol levels are less than 20 mg/dL and metabolic acidosis is corrected. Other modalities, such as CRRT, would not offer comparable clearance but may be considered if intermittent dialysis is unavailable.[116]

HD can also effectively remove both isopropanol and acetone, although it is only indicated when the isopropanol level is above 400 mg/dL or there is prolonged coma, hypotension, myocardial depression, tachydysrhythmias, or AKI.[117-119] Other modalities would not offer comparable clearances.[120]

Phosphate addition in the dialysate is often required during HD. The use of heparin should be minimized or altogether avoided in methanol-poisoned patients, because they are at higher risk for intracerebral hemorrhage.

SALICYLIC ACID

Salicylates are widely used as analgesics and antiinflammatory medications. Salicylic acid produces its antiinflammatory effects by suppressing the expression of cyclo-oxygenase (COX), which induces the production of proinflammatory mediators such as prostaglandins. Salicylic acid also uncouples oxidative phosphorylation, which leads to increased ratios of adenosine diphosphate to adenosine triphosphate and adenosine monophosphate to adenosine triphosphate in cells. Aspirin (acetylsalicylic acid) is commonly prescribed as an antiplatelet therapy. Salicylic acid is used as a topical keratolytic agent and wart remover; bismuth subsalicylate (Pepto-Bismol; 236 mg of salicylate per 15 mL) is used for reflux disease, and methyl salicylate (oil of wintergreen; 98% salicylate; 1 teaspoon contains 7 g of salicylates) is used for pain relief and as a flavoring agent.[121,122] Because many over-the-counter formulations exist and because serious toxicity can occur with relatively minor exposures, salicylates are among the substances most commonly involved in human poisoning.[1] Because of modification in packaging and availability of nonsteroidal antiinflammatory alternatives, fewer exposures to salicylates are reported yearly in the United States.

TOXICOLOGY AND TOXICOKINETICS

Salicylates in general are rapidly absorbed by the gastrointestinal tract. Peak serum concentrations are reached within an hour, unless enteric-coated products are used. In acute overdose, bezoar formation and pylorospasm may delay appearance of symptoms.[123,124]

Within the therapeutic range, salicylic acid (molecular size, 138.1 Da; V_d, 0.2 L/kg) is 90% protein bound and undergoes first-order hepatic metabolism. Salicylate and aspirin are rapidly hydrolyzed by the liver to salicylic acid and subsequently oxidized or conjugated to glucuronic acid or glycine. Normally, less than 10% of salicylate is excreted unchanged by the kidneys, and its elimination half-life is between 2 and 4 hours.[125,126] In acute overdose, the protein binding falls to 50%, the V_d increases, and major pathways of metabolism become saturated; elimination kinetics change from first order to zero order, and more salicylic acid is eliminated by the kidneys. Salicylic acid is filtered at the glomerulus, actively secreted in the proximal tubule, and reabsorbed passively in the distal tubules. These modifications result in a major increase in the elimination half-life (>30 hours).[127-129]

Salicylic acid is a weak acid with a K_d of 3.0. It exists in an ionized and a non-ionized state in the plasma:

$$H^+ + Sal^- \rightleftharpoons HSal$$

Uncharged particles, such as non-ionized salicylic acid, cross the blood-brain barrier and other tissues more easily. Acidemia drives this reaction to the right, therefore causing more CNS toxicity.[130] Elimination is similarly influenced by urinary pH; an increase in tubular lumen pH drives the reaction toward the ionized form and limits its uptake by renal tubular cells and favors its elimination in urine. This provides the rationale for urinary alkalinization to enhance elimination of salicylates.

CLINICAL PRESENTATION AND DIAGNOSTIC TESTING

Salicylate poisoning can be acute or chronic. Acute ingestions over 150 mg/kg usually present with mild-to-moderate toxicity; over 300 mg/kg, patients usually have severe clinical features, and exposures over 500 mg/kg are potentially lethal. The therapeutic range is 10 to 30 mg/dL. In concentrations greater than 40 mg/dL, toxic symptoms may appear. Concentrations over 75 mg/dL are associated with significant severity.

Acute salicylate ingestion often causes nausea and vomiting as a result of gastritis and direct stimulation of the chemoreceptor trigger zone in the medulla. Hemorrhagic ulcers, decreased gastric motility, and pylorospasm are also seen. A variety of acid-base abnormalities may occur with salicylate poisoning, but the classical finding is mixed respiratory alkalosis and high anion gap metabolic acidosis. Salicylate stimulates the respiratory center in the brainstem independently of the aortic and carotid chemoreceptors, leading to an early fall in carbon dioxide pressure and respiratory alkalosis.[131-133] Metabolic acidosis is induced by a variety of factors but is primarily caused by the accumulation of organic acids (the salicylate anion itself has a minor effect on the anion gap). Increased minute ventilation promotes lactic acid production.[131,134] In addition, salicylates uncouple mitochondrial oxidative phosphorylation and interrupt glucose and fatty acid metabolism in the Krebs cycle, leading to an increase in the production of tissue carbon dioxide, lactic acid, and ketoacids.[134]

Salicylates cause a variety of central nervous system effects, either directly or through the selective reduction of brain glucose concentration. Cerebral edema, perhaps secondary to capillary leak, may also play a role in alterations in mental status.[134] Neurologic manifestations include tinnitus, central hyperthermia, vertigo, altered mental status (hyperactivity, agitation, delirium, hallucination), or coma.[135,136] As stupor progresses, there may be blunting of the respiratory response, which may decrease pH and increase salicylate entry in the CNS.[130,137] Tinnitus occurs at salicylate concentration of 30 mg/dL and may lead to decreased auditory acuity and even deafness.[138] Early salicylate poisoning may present with hyperglycemia resulting from glycogenolysis, gluconeogenesis, and decreased peripheral use. Hypoglycemia occurs later with heightened cellular energy demand and uncoupling of oxidative phosphorylation.[139]

Chronic poisoning may be seen in patients who are treated on prolonged salicylate therapy (for chronic disease), often in the setting of reduced kidney clearance. Symptoms in this setting are often more prominent than after an acute ingestion for a same salicylate concentration; such patients are often misdiagnosed as having delirium, encephalopathy, or fever of unknown origin, and they have a high mortality.[140,141] Noncardiogenic pulmonary edema, a classical albeit rare finding, may occur as a result of local release of vasoactive peptides and increased capillary permeability, which further limits the application of urine alkalinization.[142,143]

The diagnosis of salicylate intoxication is usually suspected from the history, classical clinical findings, and metabolic abnormalities described earlier. An elevated anion gap with concomitant respiratory alkalosis should prompt confirmation of salicylate exposure. Bedside urine ferric chloride testing can confirm the presence of salicylate exposure but is not specific for poisoning. Quantitative serum salicylate levels can generally be obtained rapidly in many centers. Because absorption may be erratic or prolonged, serial measurements (every 2 to 4 hours) are required. The magnitude of the level is less important in patients with significant symptoms because treatment will be initiated regardless. In these cases the salicylate level is most useful for monitoring the effectiveness and determining the duration of therapy. The Done nomogram, which was an attempt to correlate salicylate levels with toxicity, is no longer in clinical use because of its poor predictive value.[144]

TREATMENT

General principles of poisoning management apply to salicylates. Special consideration should be geared toward respiratory support. Patients are dependent on maintaining a high minute ventilation and a higher serum pH to prevent salicylate entry into the CNS. Endotracheal intubation should therefore be performed only if absolutely necessary and by an experienced clinician to avoid prolonged periods of apnea, during which many deaths are reported.[145] Ventilator settings should try to replicate the patient's respiratory pattern before intubation, although this is usually difficult because of auto–positive end-expiratory pressure (auto-PEEP).

Once the patient is stabilized, further therapy is aimed toward decreasing absorption and increasing elimination of salicylates. Activated charcoal remains the preferred decontamination technique.[146,147] MDAC can enhance elimination of salicylates, but it is considered less efficacious and more cumbersome to perform than urine alkalinization.[5,6,148,149] Nevertheless, MDAC should be considered, especially in patients who may still have a significant burden of unabsorbed salicylate in the gastrointestinal tract.

Serum and urine alkalinization is a crucial component of treatment. As mentioned previously, alkalinization will drive salicylate to be dissociated, which will prevent both its diffusion through the blood-brain barrier and its tubular reabsorption (ion trapping). Because K_d is a logarithmic function, small changes in urine will have a large effect on salicylate elimination.[150] Urinary clearance of salicylate is enhanced several-fold with alkalinization when compared to forced diuresis alone; in one small series the percentage of the salicylate dose excreted in urine increased from 2% under acidic conditions to 30% under alkaline conditions.[151] The bicarbonate infusion is titrated to reach a urinary pH of 7.5 or until salicylate concentration is below 30 mg/dL. Because an alkaline urine cannot be produced in the presence of severe hypokalemia (kidney reabsorption of potassium occurs via the H^+-K^+-exchange pump in the distal tubule), potassium levels should be monitored and aggressively corrected. Alkalinization may be contraindicated in patients with AKI or pulmonary edema; in these cases HD may be preferred over the risk for precipitating respiratory failure and requirement of mechanical ventilation. Acetazolamide is absolutely contraindicated because it lowers arterial pH and promotes salicylate movement into the CNS and other tissues.

The first article ever published on diffusion-based techniques showcased removal of salicylates from animal subjects in 1913 by Abel and colleagues.[152] Salicylate displays properties of a highly dialyzable compound because of its low V_d, small molecular size, and low protein binding at high concentration.[153-155] HD is the best ECTR because it can remove salicylate while correcting the acid-base and volume status of patients with salicylate poisoning. Although peritoneal dialysis,[156,157] exchange transfusion,[144] HP,[158-160] and CRRT[161-163] all provide interesting clearances, none of them match the efficacy of intermittent HD. HD remains underutilized in salicylate poisoning; the availability of alternative treatments (MDAC, urinary alkalinization) may lure the clinician into a false sense of security, and so most deaths still occur before ECTR is initiated.[66]

Indications for ECTR include neurologic symptoms (confusion, coma), pulmonary edema, pH below 7.20, AKI, clinical deterioration despite appropriate treatment, and serum salicylate levels above 100 mg/dL in acute poisoning. Patients chronically poisoned are more toxic at lower salicylate concentration; they usually present with symptoms that will prompt HD and are therefore not as reliant on an absolute serum concentration for ECTR initiation. Extracorporeal purification should be maintained until salicylate levels are below 20 mg/dL. Although some authors suggest continuing urinary alkalinization during ECTR, dialysis would likely alkalinize a patient much more quickly and more reliably than an intravenous perfusion of bicarbonate.[164]

LITHIUM

Lithium, the lightest metal on the periodic table, was used therapeutically for gout in the nineteenth century and later in soft-drinks preparation. Its use became widespread in the 1950s, when it became a first-line therapy for the treatment of bipolar disorder.[165]

Although generally considered a safe drug, lithium has a narrow therapeutic range (0.7 to 1.2 mmol/L) and can induce major side effects when serum levels become supratherapeutic. Lithium may also cause long-term metabolic and renal effects, such as dysthyroidism, hyperparathyroidism, nephrogenic diabetes insipidus, and progressive decline of glomerular filtration rate (GFR), which are beyond the scope of this chapter.[166]

The mechanism of action and toxic effects of lithium are incompletely understood; lithium is thought to stabilize cell membranes, reduce neural excitation, and reduce synaptic transmission. Potential mechanisms include depletion of CNS inositol,[167] inhibition of intracellular signaling pathways involved in neuroprotection,[168,169] and modulation of nitric oxide, glutamate, and other neurotransmitters.[170]

TOXICOLOGY AND TOXICOKINETICS

The pharmacokinetic parameters of lithium are well known. Lithium is a 7-Da monovalent cation, orally administered as a carbonate (capsule) or citrate (liquid). Oral absorption is rapid and complete, and its bioavailability is not affected by food. Peak blood levels are reached within 1 to 2 hours for immediate-release formulation and within 4 to 6 hours for the sustained-release form, but these can be extended several-fold in poisoning. Lithium is unbound to proteins and has a V_d of 0.7 to 0.8 L/kg. Its distribution into tissues is variable—lithium diffuses into the liver and kidneys rapidly, but its transfer into bone, muscle, and brain is much slower, which explains the delay in peak CNS levels after an acute overdose.[171] Lithium also predominantly distributes into the intracellular compartments by active transport. Lithium is eliminated almost exclusively by the kidney, where it is freely filtered; 80% of filtered lithium is reabsorbed (three-fourths in the proximal tubule, one-fourth in the distal tubule). Total body clearance is therefore approximately 20% of GFR. Lithium reabsorption follows that of sodium, and therefore sodium-avid states (e.g., volume depletion, nonsteroidal antiinflammatory drug use, congestive heart failure, cirrhosis) markedly increase lithium retention. The half-life of lithium is approximately 18 to 24 hours for normal subjects but can be prolonged in older patients, chronic lithium users, and patients with impaired GFR.[172,173]

CLINICAL PRESENTATION AND DIAGNOSTIC TESTING

Lithium overdose may be defined as "acute" when it occurs after a single massive exposure and as "chronic" when it occurs after adjustments in dosing or in situations in which lithium clearance becomes impaired.[174] Severity of symptoms does not correlate closely with serum lithium concentration; acutely poisoned patients may be completely asymptomatic at lithium concentrations of 4.0 mmol/L, whereas there may be evident clinical signs in chronic poisonings with levels near the therapeutic range.[173,175] Acute poisoning is predominantly manifested by gastrointestinal symptoms (nausea, vomiting, or diarrhea) and with nonspecific cardiac conduction delay, although life-threatening dysrhythmias are uncommon. Neurologic findings are especially prominent in chronic poisoning and may range from mild symptoms (e.g., coarse tremor or dysarthria) to more severe presentation such as lethargy, seizures, hyperthermia, coma, and death.[176,177] A protracted neurologic course is sometimes seen after severe poisoning,[172] and some patients develop a syndrome of irreversible lithium-effectuated neurotoxicity, which may last years.[178]

TREATMENT

Therapy should be guided not only by lithium levels but also by symptoms, underlying kidney function, and a proper patient-specific risk assessment.[175]

Initial supportive care should target the specific manifestations of lithium toxicity, including treatment of hyperthermia, dysrhythmias, and seizures. Volume contraction favors proximal lithium reabsorption and should therefore be promptly corrected. Although isotonic saline (0.9%) is preferred, it may need to be replaced by hypotonic solutions or free water with 5% dextrose if lithium-induced nephrogenic diabetes insipidus and hypernatremia become a concern.

Gastrointestinal decontamination may be required in massive oral ingestions, although oral activated charcoal does not bind lithium and therefore has no role in isolated lithium poisoning.[179] Whole-bowel irrigation with polyethylene glycol can be considered for sustained-release formulations.[180] Oral sodium polystyrene sulfonate, a cation-exchanger commonly used for the treatment of hyperkalemia, has been shown to bind unabsorbed lithium from the gastrointestinal tract and enhance elimination of absorbed lithium in both animals and humans.[19,181,182] It should be considered in patients who have mild-to-moderate symptoms for whom dialysis is delayed or is not considered as a treatment option.[19]

Lithium has ideal properties for extracorporeal removal (small size, negligible protein binding, small V_d, low endogenous clearance). However, it is unknown if enhancement of lithium removal by ECTR translates into clinical benefit; in one retrospective underpowered comparative study, clinical outcome was similar in one group that received HD to another that did not, although cohorts were not comparable at baseline.[183]

Intermittent HD is the modality of choice when extracorporeal elimination is required. Clearances in excess of 180 mL/min can be obtained with modern filters.[184-187] Serum lithium levels often rebound after HD termination,[172,188] but, as mentioned earlier, this may not be concerning, because lithium CNS levels actually decrease during redistribution,[69] unless there is ongoing absorption of lithium from the gut. CRRT provides inferior clearance and removal rates compared to intermittent HD.[185,189-191] Lithium clearance with peritoneal dialysis is even inferior to that of functioning kidneys.[192,193]

Despite the controversies, accepted indications for HD include the following[16]:

1. The presence of severe neurologic features (central hyperthermia, seizures, and/or depressed consciousness)
2. A serum lithium concentration higher than 5 mmol/L regardless of the clinical status
3. The presence of kidney impairment
4. The presence of life-threatening dysrhythmias

The threshold for dialysis initiation should be lower in patients who cannot tolerate volume repletion.[172,194]

VALPROIC ACID

Valproic acid is used for the treatment of absence seizures, complex partial seizures, migraine, and mood disorders. Although acute valproic acid intoxication generally results in mild, self-limited CNS depression, serious toxic effects and death are reported.[195]

TOXICOLOGY AND TOXICOKINETICS

Valproic acid (molecular size = 144.21 Da, V_d = 0.2 L/kg) is available in immediate- and sustained-release formulations, both of which have high bioavailability. Serum concentrations typically peak 1 to 13 hours after ingestion, depending on the preparation.[196] Therapeutic serum concentrations range from 50 to 100 µg/mL.

Protein binding of valproic acid depends on its concentration; typically 90% is protein bound to albumin at therapeutic concentration, but progressively decreases to 35% when concentrations reach 300 µg/mL.[197] Liver disease, renal impairment, human immunodeficiency virus infection, and hyperlipidemia can also decrease protein binding.[198,199]

Valproic acid is rapidly metabolized by the liver. It undergoes glucuronic acid conjugation (70%) and β- and ω-oxidation to various metabolites, whereas less than 3% is normally excreted unchanged in the urine.[197] In overdose, more of its metabolism undergoes cytochrome P450 (CYP)–mediated ω-oxidation, the metabolites of which are thought to be responsible for some of the toxic effect of valproic acid, such as 5-OH-VPA and 4-en-VPA.

CLINICAL PRESENTATION AND DIAGNOSTIC TESTING

Most toxic valproic acid exposures are well tolerated. Toxicity only becomes evident in ingestions over 200 mg/kg.[200,201] Acute poisoning is typically manifested by gastrointestinal distress (nausea, vomiting, diarrhea), CNS abnormalities (confusion, obtundation, coma with respiratory failure), hypotension, and elevated transaminase levels. Free and total valproic acid serum concentrations are poorly correlated with severity of intoxication, but most patients with levels greater than 180 µg/mL develop some degree of CNS depression.[202]

Hyperammonemia is commonly seen at therapeutic and toxic valproate concentrations,[203] and although it is usually asymptomatic, when severe, it can cause encephalopathy, cerebral edema, and death. The mechanism by which valproic acid leads to hyperammonemia is incompletely understood; inhibition of carbamoyl phosphate synthetase and carnitine-dependent β-oxidation, both leading to inhibition of the urea cycle, are postulated theories.[203]

At very high serum levels (>1000 µg/mL), complications include high anion gap metabolic acidosis, elevated osmolality (valproic acid levels greater than 1500 µg/mL may raise the osmolar gap by 10 mOsm/L or more), hypernatremia, hypocalcemia, pancreatitis, noncardiogenic pulmonary edema, bone marrow suppression, and AKI.[204,205] Diagnosis of valproic acid intoxication is based on history of exposure, typical toxic symptoms, and confirmation with determination of the serum valproate level.

TREATMENT

Treatment consists of initial stabilization of respiratory and cardiovascular function. Gastrointestinal decontamination should be administered if the patient presents within 1 hour of exposure. Because the excretion of valproic acid by the kidney is limited, urine elimination enhancement is ineffective. Patients with hyperammonemic-induced encephalopathy may respond to L-carnitine; in one retrospective study of severe valproate-induced hepatotoxic effects, patients who received intravenous carnitine therapy had a marked survival advantage.[206] If used, intravenous L-carnitine should be administered with a loading dose of 100 mg/kg followed by 15 mg/kg every 4 hours, up to a maximum of 6 g/day.

The small molecular size and low V_d of valproic acid are conducive for extracorporeal elimination. Although HD has little effect on the elimination of valproic acid at usual serum concentrations because of its extensive protein binding, significant clearance can be obtained at supratherapeutic drug levels when plasma proteins become saturated.[196,207] HD has the added advantage of clearing ammonia and reversing metabolic acidosis.[196] In a multicenter study, patients with peak valproic acid concentrations exceeding 850 μg/mL were more likely to develop coma, respiratory depression, or metabolic acidosis; therefore current recommendations support the early initiation of HD in these cases.[208] Rebound of valproic acid levels is often observed 5 to 13 hours following high-flux dialysis cessation, requiring additional sessions.[197] Charcoal HP has been successfully used in cases but is limited by early column saturation.[195] Tandem, or "in-series" HD-HP, may be the most effective technique but probably offers marginal advantage over HD to offset the added cost of the technique.[209] Intermittent hemodiafiltration has been used successfully in two reports,[210,211] but there is insufficient evidence to determine whether this technique offers additional benefit over HD alone. Continuous renal replacement techniques, however, appear considerably less effective than intermittent alternatives and should only be used if HD is unavailable.[212] Albumin dialysis, slow low-efficiency dialysis with filtration, TPE, and peritoneal dialysis are inferior therapeutic options in valproate poisoning and are not recommended.[213,214]

CARBAMAZEPINE

Carbamazepine is a widely used anticonvulsant agent that is also used increasingly for pain management and bipolar disorders.

TOXICOLOGY AND TOXICOKINETICS

The structure of carbamazepine (molecular size = 236 Da) is similar to tricyclic antidepressants. The therapeutic effect of carbamazepine results from binding to sodium channels, inhibiting neuronal depolarization and decreasing glutamate release. It also has anticholinergic effects at high concentration. Carbamazepine is available in various immediate- and modified-release formulations. Its rate of dissolution is slow, resulting in erratic and incomplete absorption, which is worsened in overdose because of the formation of pharmacobezoars and potentiated by the presence of ileus secondary to the anticholinergic properties of carbamazepine.[215] The therapeutic concentration range of carbamazepine is 4 to 12 μg/mL. Carbamazepine is lipophilic and has a V_d of 1.2 L/kg, with a protein binding of approximately 75%, which does not decrease much in overdose.[216] It undergoes hepatic metabolism, mainly through CYP3A4 into many metabolites, the most important being carbamazepine-10,11-epoxide, which is active. Carbamazepine induces its own metabolism with chronic use.

CLINICAL PRESENTATION AND DIAGNOSTIC TESTING

Carbamazepine toxicity frequently presents with neurologic, cardiovascular, and anticholinergic symptoms, which may be delayed in onset because of its erratic absorption. Mild toxicity (≈30 μg/mL) presents as drowsiness, nystagmus, tachycardia, hyperreflexia, or dysmetria. In more severe exposures (>40 μg/mL), lethargy, seizure, coma, QRS prolongation, hypotension, and pronounced anticholinergic symptoms (especially ileus) may develop. Agranulocytosis and syndrome of inappropriate antidiuretic hormone secretion are associated with chronic use and are not typically seen in acute poisonings. Death remains unusual.

The diagnosis of carbamazepine toxicity relies on the presence of typical clinical findings, as well as drug testing. Serum carbamazepine concentrations should be followed serially because time to peak concentration may be significantly delayed. Levels should be obtained every 4 to 6 hours until a definite downward trend is seen.

TREATMENT

Most patients poisoned with carbamazepine can be managed with supportive care alone, including ventilatory support, benzodiazepines for seizure control, vasopressors for hypotension, and sodium bicarbonate for sodium channel blockade. Gastrointestinal decontamination may be required if the patient presents early after ingestion or if a large bulk of carbamazepine is thought to remain in the gastrointestinal tract, but it is contraindicated if ileus is present. No antidote exists to reverse the toxicity of carbamazepine. MDAC can enhance carbamazepine clearance and may even reduce the duration of coma and need for mechanical ventilation.[217] MDAC is recommended by the latest guidelines for carbamazepine toxicity,[5] but again its efficacy is reduced by decreased gastrointestinal motility.[5,217-220]

Severe carbamazepine poisonings can be managed by ECTRs, which can provide better and more predictable clearance than MDAC.[221-223] Historically, charcoal or resin HP was the ECTR of choice because of extensive protein binding by carbamazepine. However, with high-flux filters, high blood flows, and larger catheters, carbamazepine clearance with HP and HD are comparable and can both exceed 100 mL/min.[222-230] Because of the greater availability, lower cost, and lower complication rate, HD is therefore preferred. There are limited data on the ECTR clearance of the toxic metabolite carbamazepine-10,11-epoxide, but it also appears to be dialyzable because its protein binding is inferior to that of carbamazepine (50% versus 75% to 90%).[216,227,231,232] CRRT, TPE, and albumin dialysis have been used in carbamazepine poisoning but do not provide comparable removal rates.[233,234] Indications for ECTR include prolonged coma, seizures, cardiovascular instability, symptoms unresponsive to supportive care, rising concentrations despite MDAC, and the carbamazepine concentration is higher than 45 μg/mL.[13]

BARBITURATES

Barbiturates are CNS depressants and are used as sedatives, hypnotics, anxiolytics, and anticonvulsants. They are all derived from barbituric acid. Barbiturates were extremely popular agents until the arrival of benzodiazepines in the 1960s. Although their use has steadily decreased over the years, barbiturates, especially those that are long acting, are still a concern.[1] Phenobarbital is by far the most commonly available barbiturate worldwide and is most often implicated in poisoning, although others are seen in developing countries.[235]

TOXICOLOGY AND TOXICOKINETICS

Barbiturates are weak acids. Their two principal mechanisms of action are potentiating the effect of the γ-aminobutyric acid (GABA) receptor and blocking the α-amino-3-hydroxy-5-methyl-4-isoxazolepropionic acid (AMPA) receptor (a subtype of glutamate receptor); both contribute to the CNS effects.[236] They are usually categorized by their duration of action: short-acting (>3 to 4 hours; pentobarbital, secobarbital), intermediate-acting (>4 to 6 hours; amobarbital, butabarbital), or long-acting (≥ 6 to 12 hours; barbital, primidone, phenobarbital).[235] Absorption is variable and is influenced by the dose ingested, ileus, and concomitant ingestion of other drugs. The ability of a particular barbiturate to penetrate the blood-brain barrier will determine its clinical effects. Barbiturates are small molecules with a protein binding usually below 50%, although long-acting barbiturates are less protein bound than short-acting ones. The metabolism of barbiturates is mostly hepatic, but there may be renal excretion for those that are less lipophilic. There may be enzymatic induction and higher barbiturate clearance for patients who are chronically taking these medications. The following discussion will focus only on phenobarbital, although it shares many properties similar to other long-acting and short-acting barbiturates. Recommendations also apply to primidone because it is metabolized to phenobarbital.[237] An oral dose of 1 g of most barbiturates will cause serious toxicity in most adults, whereas death can result with ingestions of over 2 g,[238] or with a concentration above 80 μg/mL.[239]

CLINICAL PRESENTATION AND DIAGNOSTIC TESTING

Phenobarbital has a slow onset of action, but its clinical effects can be prolonged.[240,241] In mild exposures, toxicity usually manifests as altered level of consciousness. Moderate poisonings will produce apnea and circulatory collapse. More severe cases present as areflexia, cutaneous bullae, hypotension, hypothermia, and coma.[235,238] Concomitant AKI, cardiac disease, or pulmonary disease may increase the clinical sensitivity to barbiturates.[242] Early deaths after barbiturate ingestion are caused by respiratory and cardiovascular arrest, whereas delayed deaths are caused by acute lung injury, ventilator-acquired pneumonia, cerebral edema, or multiorgan system failure. Although positive results of serum screening for barbiturates may confirm recent exposure, a specific level is difficult to interpret as to whether a patient is naive or not to barbiturates and whether the level follows an acute ingestion or not. Specific serum sampling of most barbiturates other than phenobarbital are not systematically available.

TREATMENT

Supportive measures, including passive rewarming, hydration, and vasopressors, are usually sufficient to manage most barbiturate poisoning. Patients may be profoundly comatose and require prolonged mechanical ventilation. There is no direct antidote for barbiturate overdose.

If an airway is secured, MDAC can facilitate clearance of phenobarbital.[243] Because barbiturates are weak acids, urinary alkalinization can also increase phenobarbital renal clearance at least 2- to 3-fold.[244,245] However, because renal clearance of phenobarbital is already low (<3 mL/min), alkalinization would have little effect on total body clearance.[244] MDAC has a greater impact on clearance than alkalinization.[245,246] Surprisingly, the duration of coma was shown to be reduced by urine alkalinization in one study[247] but not by MDAC in a small randomized trial.[248] Nevertheless, MDAC is preferred to urine alkalinization in the latest recommendations.[5,6]

An animal study has shown a very significant and clear decrease in mortality in dogs and rats that underwent HP after a lethal phenobarbital infusion[153] compared to those who did not. No studies have evaluated the effect of ECTR in humans, although the mortality rate appeared lower in an uncontrolled group that underwent HP.[249] HP and HD are particularly appealing for toxicity to long-action barbiturates, because endogenous clearance for these drugs is low, especially in those patients who are naive to barbiturates and have no autoinduction.[235] Endogenous half-life for short-acting barbiturates is short and therefore would not benefit as much from extracorporeal removal. Patients presenting with severe hepatic and/or renal dysfunction or chronic respiratory disease are particularly susceptible to toxicity. Modern high-flux dialyzers provide clearances at least equal to HP. Indications for ECTR include coma, respiratory depression, hypotension, and an inefficiency of MDAC at reducing the concentration of the barbiturate.[10,235] Clinical deterioration following initial improvement from ECTR may occur when ECTR is terminated, because of drug redistribution into the central circulation.[250-253] This may be minimized by repeating treatment sessions or by using continuous techniques.[250,254-257]

A particular concern in the use of ECTR is the risk for precipitating barbiturate withdrawal in chronic users when concentrations fall below the therapeutic range, which can manifest as seizures and/or delirium after approximately 48 to 72 hours.[61,258-260] Consequently, ongoing monitoring of patients undergoing ECTR to promptly detect rebound toxicity or withdrawal is essential, especially for short-acting barbiturates and chronic users.

PHENYTOIN

Phenytoin is an anticonvulsant drug used as a first-line treatment of epilepsy, both for status epilepticus and for seizure prevention. Phenytoin toxicity is relatively frequent considering its narrow therapeutic range, although phenytoin-related deaths are rare.

TOXICOLOGY AND TOXICOKINETICS

Phenytoin stabilizes neuronal membranes and decreases seizure activity possibly by producing a voltage-dependent blockade of membrane sodium channels implicated in the action potential leading to seizures.[261] Phenytoin has a molecular size of 252 Da and a high protein binding (90% to 95%), which decreases to 70% in the presence of renal failure or hypoalbuminemia, although surprisingly remains almost unchanged in overdose. Only the unbound fraction of phenytoin has biologic effect.

Phenytoin is available in various forms and has erratic bioavailability,[262] especially in overdose.[263] Most of the metabolism of phenytoin consists of hepatic hydroxylation through CYP2C9. Phenytoin is then eliminated in the bile as an inactive metabolite, reabsorbed from the intestinal tract, and excreted in the urine. Elimination is of the first order at low serum concentration and becomes zero order at higher concentrations. The elimination half-life of oral preparations ranges between 14 and 22 hours. Therapeutic serum levels range between 10 and 20 mg/L. The lethal dose in adults is estimated at 2 to 5 g.

CLINICAL PRESENTATION AND DIAGNOSTIC TESTING

Most of the toxic manifestations of phenytoin are neurologic, the severity of which are loosely correlated with its serum concentration; between 20 and 40 mg/L, symptoms include nystagmus, ataxia, dysarthria, and mild CNS depression.[264] Over 40 mg/L, lethargy, confusion, hypotension, coma, and seizures may be observed. Death is usually caused by respiratory or circulatory depression but is rare. Cardiovascular toxicity is unusual with oral formulations, but atrioventricular delays and bradycardia may be occasionally seen with rapid intravenous infusion,[264] possibly due to the diluent propylene glycol.

Total serum phenytoin concentration should be obtained in all suspected overdose cases. There are conditions that may alter protein-binding capacity, such as hypoalbuminemia, uremia, extremes of age, or concomitant use of agents that displace phenytoin from its albumin binding site (e.g., salicylates, sulfonamides, tolbutamide, and valproic acid). Free phenytoin fraction should therefore be obtained in such cases, if available (toxicity is apparent at levels above 2.1 mg/L).[265] Because hepatic function may alter phenytoin's toxicokinetics, and because elevation of liver enzymes is an independent variable for morbidity in phenytoin toxicity,[266] this parameter should also be monitored.

TREATMENT

Treatment of phenytoin poisoning is mostly supportive because most patients have an excellent outcome. Furthermore, there is a concern that an abrupt lowering of serum phenytoin level may precipitate withdrawal symptoms and rebound seizures in epileptic patients.

Benzodiazepines can be given for seizures. Gastrointestinal decontamination can limit the systemic burden of phenytoin. There exists no specific antidote to phenytoin toxicity. MDAC has been shown to significantly reduce the elimination half-life of phenytoin in healthy and poisoned patients,[18,267,268] although improvement in morbidity and mortality has yet to be demonstrated. MDAC can be considered in cases where serum phenytoin levels escalate or remain elevated, if the airway is protected.[5]

Experience with ECTRs remains anecdotal. In theory, given the high protein binding of phenytoin, HP or TPE have been historically favored, and they both have been used successfully in this context.[269-276] Surprisingly, despite phenytoin's high protein binding, there is some evidence that HD may also enhance its elimination, perhaps because of its low dissociation constant to albumin, which ensures a constant pool of freely diffusible unbound phenytoin.[277,278] This finding is attributable to newer high-flux, high-efficiency dialyzers—older obsolete dialysis apparatus did not have any effect on phenytoin clearance.[279]

The combination of HP and HD could potentially maximize clearance and has been used in a few reports,[275,280,281] although it remains unclear if the combination is superior to either technique used alone. Neither peritoneal dialysis nor CRRT have any role in phenytoin poisoning,[282-285] whereas the data are still uncertain for albumin dialysis.[51] In summary, the outcome of most phenytoin poisonings is inconsequential and favorable. Supportive care alone is usually sufficient. In the rare case of prolonged neurologic toxicity, HD or HP can be considered.

METFORMIN

Metformin, a biguanide, is a first-line drug for the treatment of type 2 diabetes, particularly in overweight patients. Metformin improves insulin sensitivity and decreases insulin resistance in patients and is now the most popular antidiabetic drug in the world. The related biguanide, phenformin, was withdrawn in 1978 because of the high incidence of lactic acidosis.

TOXICOLOGY AND TOXICOKINETICS

Metformin is a small molecule (165 kDa) and unbound to proteins but has a large V_d (3 L/kg) because of its ability to diffuse into the intracellular compartment and bind to microsomes. Its bioavailability is incomplete. It does not undergo hepatic metabolism and is eliminated unchanged by renal tubular secretion (renal clearance ≅ 500 mL/min), hence the concern in patients with kidney impairment. The toxic dose is not well established but can be seen over 100 mg/kg.

CLINICAL PRESENTATION AND DIAGNOSTIC TESTING

Toxicity to metformin can manifest itself in various ways: gastrointestinal symptoms (e.g., abdominal pain, diarrhea, nausea and vomiting), lactic acidosis, hypotension, and respiratory failure are the hallmarks of metformin intoxications. Hypoglycemia, hypothermia, altered mental status, and acute pancreatitis have also been reported.[286,287] Metformin-associated lactic acidosis (MALA) usually occurs in the presence of underlying conditions, particularly acute or chronic kidney disease. MALA is defined as an arterial pH of 7.35 or less and lactate concentration above 5 mmol/L[288,289] and can happen with acute or chronic toxicity. There is controversy about the association between metformin and lactic acidosis; some sources claim that the association is coincidental and due to other factors such as sepsis and heart failure,[290,291] whereas others suggest that metformin itself directly causes lactic acidosis. The finding of asymptomatic patients who develop toxicity shortly after an acute toxic ingestion of metformin appears to give credence to the latter hypothesis,[292-294] which is occasionally named metformin-induced lactic acidosis. The true prevalence of MALA and metformin-induced lactic acidosis is unknown, but severe life-threatening acidosis is estimated at 0.05 cases per 1000 patient-years.[295]

The physiopathology of MALA is not entirely understood but seems to be related to the suppressing of hepatic gluconeogenesis impairment of lactate utilization. Mitochondrial binding of metformin membranes in overdose can shift energy use toward anaerobic metabolism, which in turn yields large quantities of lactate.[296] The increase in lactic acid production is often compounded by a defect in lactate clearance by kidneys or liver.

Because serum metformin measurements are not usually available in a clinically useful time frame, the diagnosis of metformin poisoning must be suspected in every patient presenting with severe metabolic lactic acidosis. There is evidence that the clinical outcome is correlated with the metformin concentration, the lactate concentration, serum pH, or a combination of these.[290]

TREATMENT

Given the absence of a specific antidote to metformin, the established mainstay of management for metformin toxicity is supportive care—more specifically, normalizing the acid-base imbalance, eliminating the offending medication, and treating concomitant and exacerbating conditions. Decontamination with activated charcoal should be considered after a large ingestion of metformin. Patients who develop lactic acidosis, hypoglycemia, or other signs of metformin toxicity should be admitted to an intensive care unit.

Severely acidotic patients (pH ≤ 7.1) should receive intravenous sodium bicarbonate in bolus and/or perfusion. However, treatment is often limited by hypernatremia, volume overload, and AKI. Dichloroacetate acts by stimulating pyruvate dehydrogenase and has been used to treat type A lactic acidosis.[297-299] It has been shown to improve pH and lactate levels without increasing patient survival,[300] although there are no data concerning its use in MALA.

Renal replacement therapies often become necessary to control volume overload and uremia. Furthermore, ECTRs can correct acidosis much more quickly than intravenous bicarbonate and can also help clear lactate. In fact, the dramatic improvement described in some acutely poisoned patients within moments of dialysis initiation suggests that the benefit might be attributed more to pH correction than metformin removal.[301] One study compared patients who underwent dialysis to those who did not, and the mortality rate did not differ between the two groups (although the HD group was sicker at baseline).[288] There is some evidence that ECTRs can remove metformin, especially when kidney function is impaired[302-304]: in AKI, metformin distributes in a smaller apparent volume[305] and is thus more available for extracorporeal removal. Indications for ECTR include a lactate concentration over 135 mg/dL (15 mmol/L), an arterial pH less than 7.1, failure of supportive therapy, or the presence of cardiac instability, impaired kidney function, or coma.

Hourly metformin clearance during CRRT is much lower than during intermittent HD[64]; lactate removal is also greater during a 6-hour session of HD than during 24 hours of continuous venovenous hemodiafiltration,[306] although it is likely that ECTR lactate removal remains negligible compared to endogenous production.[307] Optimal surrogate markers for ECTR cessation should be complete normalization of pH and lactate. Shortened sessions can result in life-threatening rebound in MALA.[308] Occasionally an initial high-efficiency intermittent dialysis session followed by subsequent CRRT can be performed.[309] HP should never be used without HD in MALA, because it will not correct the patient's acid-base imbalance.[309]

PARAQUAT

Paraquat (1,1' dimethyl-4-4'-bipyridinium dichloride) is among the most commonly used herbicides in the world. It is available in various formulations, is nonselective, and fast acting and becomes biologically inactive on contact with soil, making it an extremely convenient weed killer.

Because it is generally not absorbed across intact skin, and because the droplets generated from the aerosol spray are large, toxicity from direct contact or inhalation is rarely problematic. However, accidental or intentional oral ingestion of paraquat is extremely toxic with high rate of morbidity and mortality (50% to 90%). The use of paraquat is restricted in the United States and European countries but remains a major health issue in many Third World and the Asia-Pacific countries.[310]

TOXICOLOGY AND TOXICOKINETICS

Paraquat (molecular size, 186 Da; protein binding, 5%) has an oral bioavailability that is less than 30%. Peak concentrations are generally reached 2 hours after ingestion, but maximal tissue distribution occurs during the next 6 hours.[311,312] Paraquat distributes to most organs, especially the lungs, kidney, and liver, with a V_d of approximately 1.0 L/kg. Most of its elimination is via the kidneys; elimination half-life is 12 hours if renal function is intact, but it can increase to more than 48 hours as GFR fails.[312,313]

Paraquat catalyzes the formation of reactive oxygen species, more specifically the superoxide free radical, by oxidation-reduction cycling. It is reduced by an electron donor such as reduced nicotinamide adenine dinucleotide phosphate and later oxidized by an electron receptor such as dioxygen. Because this process can be sustained by the extensive supply of electrons and oxygen in the lungs, the resultant oxidative stress causes cell injury and a profound inflammatory reaction.[311,314,315]

CLINICAL PRESENTATION AND DIAGNOSTIC TESTING

The presentation and the clinical course of a patient with paraquat poisoning depend largely on the dose ingested and timing of presentation to a health care facility after exposure. Ingestions of less than 20 mg/kg may not cause symptoms other than oral ulceration, vomiting, and diarrhea. Ingestions between 20 and 40 mg/kg will usually cause multiple organ failure with death occurring between 1 week and several weeks after exposure. Patients who ingest over 40 mg/kg usually die within 3 days from accelerated multiorgan failure and/or from the corrosive effects of paraquat.[316-319]

Most paraquat-related deaths are caused by respiratory failure. Type I and II alveolar epithelial cells take up paraquat via an energy-dependent polyamine transporter.[311,320] Patients develop a presentation similar to that of acute respiratory distress syndrome, which ultimately progresses to irreversible pulmonary fibrosis. In the kidneys, paraquat causes acute tubular necrosis. Other clinical manifestations include severe upper gastrointestinal tract ulcerations, hepatic injury, and shock. Paraquat does not readily cross the blood-brain barrier and therefore does not typically cause CNS effects.

Serum paraquat concentration predicts the mortality risk, and nomograms have been validated to correlate with clinical outcome.[321,322] Unfortunately, few laboratories have the ability to perform quantitative paraquat assay.[323-326] A rapid and inexpensive qualitative test for urine paraquat can be obtained by adding sodium dithionite to urine. If the color of urine changes from yellow to blue, it confirms the presence of recent paraquat exposure (the more intense the blue, the higher the paraquat exposure). A negative test result rules out significant paraquat ingestion.

TREATMENT

The dismal prognosis related to paraquat poisoning has prompted the use of several experimental treatments. Alas, none of them has proven to alter the outcome significantly. Any suspected paraquat exposure warrants prompt assessment and aggressive management. After initial stabilization, volume resuscitation should be aggressively provided. Oxygen should be used only if required for hypoxemic patients, because it may promote further cellular damage induced by the oxidation-reduction cycling. Paraquat is absorbed quickly, which limits the efficacy of usual decontamination techniques, especially because there may be paraquat-induced caustic injury present. Many paraquat formulations already contain a pro-emetic and an alginate to reduce its absorption.[327] Forced diuresis does not increase the renal clearance of paraquat,[313] and no antidote is available.

Because paraquat is a small molecule, is unbound to protein, and has a reasonably small V_d, its content in plasma is removable by standard ECTRs (clearance in excess of 120 mL/min). However, paraquat distributes quickly to tissues, especially lungs, a compartment from which paraquat does not easily diffuse back to the blood. Furthermore, once the toxicodynamic process involving free-radical generation is initiated, it is unlikely that any elimination enhancement could blunt its progression. This concept has been confirmed in animal studies: half of the dogs exposed to a lethal dose of paraquat survived with HP when it was initiated 2 hours after exposure, whereas 100% mortality occurred when it was initiated at 12 hours.[328]

HD or HP is mostly reserved for patients presenting early after ingestion, especially within 4 hours, after confirmation from a urine dithionite test.[329] In that scenario, all resources should be pooled to initiate ECTR as quickly as possible.[330] Other ECTRs, including peritoneal dialysis, are of no utility.[313] Rebound is usually observed following ECTR treatment.[313,331-336]

Several other treatments have been tried with variable degrees of success, including antioxidants (vitamin C or E, superoxide dismutase, deferoxamine, selenium, niacin, NAC, sulfite, thiosulfate), salicylate, colchicine, D-propranolol, corticosteroids, cyclophosphamide, and radiotherapy.

Of note, the combination of cyclophosphamide and corticosteroids is no longer recommended, because a large randomized controlled trial failed to report a statistical benefit.[337] The palliative care team should also be precociously integrated in the treatment plan given the disastrous outcome of most patients.

THEOPHYLLINE

Theophylline (1,3-dimethylxanthine) is a methylxanthine bronchodilator traditionally used in the treatment of asthma, chronic obstructive pulmonary disease, and infant apnea. Its use has dramatically declined over the years in favor of inhaled corticosteroids, anticholinergics, and β_2-adrenergic agonists.[1]

TOXICOLOGY AND TOXICOKINETICS

Theophylline (molecular size = 180.2 Da, protein binding = 40%) acts as a nonselective inhibitor of phosphodiesterase and a nonselective antagonist of the adenosine receptor. This results in smooth muscle relaxation, catecholamine release, bronchodilation, and peripheral vasodilatation, as well as inotropic and chronotropic activation.[338]

Theophylline is available in immediate- and slow-release formulations and is completely absorbed by the gastrointestinal tract. It distributes in a volume smaller than that of water (0.5 L/kg). Theophylline is metabolized by the liver, primarily by the isozyme CYP1A2 of CYP, whereas only 10% is excreted by the kidneys.

The pharmacokinetics and metabolism of theophylline are influenced by age, sex, body weight, concurrent illness (e.g., congestive heart failure, liver disease, infection), cigarette smoking, and medication affected by the CYP1A2 isozyme.[339] Endogenous metabolism is slow. At therapeutic range (10 to 20 µg/mL), theophylline exhibits first-order kinetics; however, at toxic levels, the kinetics change to zero order, and a small increase in dosage can lead to a dramatic increase in serum concentration.[340]

CLINICAL PRESENTATION AND DIAGNOSTIC TESTING

Theophylline intoxication may result from acute ingestion (from attempted suicide or medication error) or chronic use (when theophylline clearance decreases from impairment in its metabolism). For the same serum theophylline level, symptoms of chronic toxicity are more severe than those following acute intoxication.[341] Caffeine, which is an active metabolite of theophylline, shares many of its toxic effects. The therapeutic index is very narrow; even at therapeutic concentrations, nearly one-third of patients may exhibit signs of mild intoxication. At serum concentrations between 20 and 30 µg/mL, more than 50% of affected patients are likely to demonstrate symptoms, and at serum concentrations over 30 µg/mL, more than 90% are clinically toxic.

Early symptoms of toxicity consist of transient caffeine-like effects such as nausea, vomiting, diarrhea, irritability, tremor, headache, insomnia, and tachycardia. Patients with moderate intoxication may be lethargic and disoriented, and they may develop supraventricular tachycardia and frequent premature ventricular contractions. Severe intoxication includes life-threatening symptoms such as seizure activity, hyperthermia, hypotension, ventricular tachycardia, rhabdomyolysis, and AKI. Irreversible brain injury may follow seizures if not addressed promptly. Death is most often the result of cardiorespiratory collapse or hypoxic encephalopathy following cardiac dysrhythmias or generalized seizures.[341-343] Hypokalemia, caused by $β_2$-adrenergic receptor–induced transcellular potassium shifts, can be severe and is most often seen following acute overdose.[342,344]

TREATMENT

Aggressive supportive measures are required in severe theophylline poisoning. Hypotension usually responds to volume repletion and vasopressors. Tachycardia can be corrected by β-adrenergic antagonists, such as propranolol or esmolol, but should be used with caution in patients susceptible to bronchospasm.[345,346] Theophylline-associated seizures can be particularly difficult to control; benzodiazepines are first-line therapy, but propofol, barbiturates, and neuromuscular paralysis may be required in refractory cases. Multiple-dose oral activated charcoal increases clearance of theophylline but is sometimes limited by profound and intractable emesis in severely intoxicated patients.[347-349]

Because of its small molecular size, low protein binding, low endogenous clearance, and low V_d, theophylline is an ideal candidate for extracorporeal elimination. There are numerous reports of successful treatment with HP and HD; in one observational retrospective cohort study, a group treated with HP or HD had a significantly shorter duration of clinical toxicity compared to a group only managed with supportive care, despite being sicker at presentation.[350] Extracorporeal clearances can surpass 150 mL/min.[351-353] HD has been shown to provide clearances comparable to HP with fewer complications in one retrospective study[35]; because of this and because of its usual advantages over HP (including correction of hypokalemia), HD is preferred.

Continuous techniques have also been reported in the management of theophylline intoxication with acceptable results despite the inferior clearances they provide.[354,355] Peritoneal dialysis and TPE are not useful alternatives. Exchange transfusion is an option for neonates.[356]

Indications for ECTR can be summarized as follows:

1. Serum theophylline level greater than 100 μg/mL
2. Chronic poisoning with serum theophylline concentration greater than 60 μg/mL
3. The presence of refractory seizures, shock, life-threatening dysrhythmias, incapacity to administer charcoal because of intractable vomiting, or extremes of age (<6 months or >60 years)[341,342,350,357]

The ECTR should be continued until clinical improvement is achieved and the serum level is less than 15 μg/mL. Rebound is usually minor (levels may re-increase up to 10 μg/mL) and must be monitored after blood purification.

ACETAMINOPHEN

Acetaminophen (*N*-acetyl-*p*-aminophenol) is an analgesic and antipyretic, which has been available in the United States since 1955. Because it is available without prescription in various forms and combinations, acetaminophen is a major contributor to acute voluntary poisoning.

TOXICOLOGY AND TOXICOKINETICS

The actions of acetaminophen remain incompletely understood but appear to predominantly inhibit COX activity, primarily COX-2. Analgesic and antipyretic activity occur at serum acetaminophen levels between 10 and 20 μg/mL.[358] Acetaminophen is available in immediate- and extended-release preparations and has high oral bioavailability. Serum concentrations, even in overdose, usually peak within 4 hours of ingestion.

Protein binding (≈20%) and V_d (0.8 L/kg) of acetaminophen do not change in overdose. Once absorbed, acetaminophen is extensively metabolized (90%) by the liver through conjugation to form inactive metabolites, with an irrelevant fraction excreted unchanged in urine and the remaining fraction oxidized mostly by CYP2E1 into *N*-acetyl-*p*-benzoquinoneimine (NAPQI). Glutathione combines with NAPQI to form a nontoxic complex that is eliminated in the urine. In overdose, however, glutathione becomes depleted and NAPQI accumulates; NAPQI is very reactive and will covalently bind vital proteins and nucleic acids in hepatocytes, leading to cellular injury and subsequent liver cell necrosis.[359] The lowest toxic dose is considered to be 7.5 g for adults and 150 mg/kg for children.[360]

CLINICAL PRESENTATION AND DIAGNOSTIC TESTING

Acetaminophen poisoning cases are difficult to recognize at early stages. Patients can remain clinically asymptomatic up to a day after ingestion, and initially only nonspecific symptoms, including nausea, vomiting, anorexia, malaise, or abdominal pain, are evident. Hepatic injury typically occurs approximately 24 hours after ingestion, by which time initiation of antidotal treatment will have diminished efficacy. The severity of the injury can vary and is most commonly detected by elevation of serum transaminase level, which generally peaks 2 to 3 days after ingestion. Hepatotoxicity is defined as peak serum transaminase level above 1000 IU/L.[361] More severe cases can evolve to fulminant liver failure with encephalopathy, coagulopathy, hypoglycemia, and death for those who cannot receive a liver transplant. AKI may also occur because of tubular susceptibility to NAPQI by various possible mechanisms, which include the CYP pathway, prostaglandin synthetase, and *N*-deacetylase enzymes.[362]

The assessment of the risk associated with acute acetaminophen poisoning can be largely estimated by timing the exposure to a serum acetaminophen concentration and plotting this on the Rumack-Matthew nomogram.[363] A point below the "treatment line" can reliably prognosticate that a patient will not develop hepatotoxicity. This nomogram has been validated as such for over 30 years, despite some limitations, which are outside the scope of this chapter. For example, a serum acetaminophen concentration of 160 μg/mL at 4 hours after ingestion indicates the need for NAC treatment.

TREATMENT

A comprehensive management of acetaminophen toxicity is reviewed elsewhere.[364] The majority of cases are evaluated and treated in the emergency department in collaboration with the regional poison control center and intensivists, without the involvement of a nephrologist. Most of the specific management of acetaminophen toxicity is centered on the timely administration of the antidote, NAC.[365] NAC serves as a glutathione precursor and substitute, increasing its availability, therefore increasing the capacity to detoxify NAPQI and limiting its formation.[366] It is most efficacious when initiated within 8 hours of an acute overdose. NAC is usually prescribed if there is evidence of hepatic injury or if acetaminophen concentration is above the treatment line on the Rumack-Matthew nomogram.

Although acetaminophen is amenable to extracorporeal removal (low V_d, small molecule, low protein binding), ECTR is rarely necessary, given the safety, low cost, efficacy, and availability of NAC. HD or CRRT can be considered for patients developing AKI or occasionally in those presenting following massive ingestions with a pattern of mitochondrial toxicity (i.e., coma, lactic metabolic acidosis, and cardiovascular instability).[12,367,368] These patients can be distinguished by early-onset presentation (as opposed to the delayed hepatic features described earlier). In these cases the potential removal of NAC by ECTR can be overcome by at least doubling its perfusion.[60] Liver replacement therapies like MARS and SPAD have been used for liver support as bridges to liver transplantation or pending native liver recovery.[369-373] However, limited availability of these techniques, as well as major bleeding complications associated with them and their high cost, warrant further investigation.

METHOTREXATE

Methotrexate is a folate analogue used to treat a variety of cancers and rheumatologic and dermatologic diseases. Methotrexate inhibits dihydrofolate reductase, an enzyme necessary for the synthesis and replication of RNA and DNA.

TOXICOLOGY AND TOXICOKINETICS

The oral absorption of methotrexate is limited by a saturable intestinal absorption mechanism for doses over 30 mg/m²; high serum concentrations are therefore best achieved by parenteral administration. Methotrexate does not sufficiently penetrate the blood-brain barrier with oral or parenteral administration and must therefore be given intrathecally to achieve CNS penetration. Methotrexate (molecular size = 454 Da) has a small V_d (0.4 to 0.8 L/kg) and is 50% bound to plasma proteins, regardless of serum concentration. Methotrexate is primarily excreted unchanged (80% to 90%) in the urine by passive glomerular filtration and active tubular secretion; renal clearance varies greatly and decreases at higher doses. It undergoes hepatic and intracellular metabolism to active metabolites.

In the presence of renal failure, methotrexate can rapidly accumulate in the serum and tissue cells. A toxic concentration of methotrexate is defined as greater than 5 to 10 µmol/L at 24 hours, 1 µmol/L at 48 hours, and 0.1 µmol/L at 72 hours.[374,375] These concentrations are predictive of renal, gastrointestinal, mucosal, and bone marrow toxicity in patients receiving chemotherapy. Methotrexate levels in patients being treated for indications other than cancer should not surpass 0.01 µmol/L.[376]

CLINICAL PRESENTATION AND DIAGNOSTIC TESTING

At high concentrations, methotrexate and its metabolites can precipitate in renal tubules, causing crystal nephropathy and AKI. Methotrexate can also cause bone marrow suppression, mucositis and stomatitis, liver damage, and neurotoxicity. The onset of the toxicity is generally rapid; nausea and vomiting typically begin 2 to 4 hours after high-dose therapy (>1000 mg/m²). Mucositis and pancytopenia will manifest approximately 1 to 2 weeks after exposure. CNS toxicity usually follows approximately 12 hours after high-dose intravenous methotrexate therapy or intrathecal administration.

TREATMENT

Gastrointestinal decontamination should be performed if a patient presents within 1 hour after an oral overdose. Cholestyramine can interrupt the enterohepatic circulation of methotrexate,[377] but MDAC has no role for enhancing its elimination.[5,378]

Aggressive hydration is indicated for patients presenting with methotrexate toxicity. Because methotrexate is a weak acid ($K_d = 5$), and because it is eliminated largely unchanged in the urine, urinary alkalinization with intravenous sodium bicarbonate (target urine pH ≅ 8) will enhance methotrexate elimination and may help to prevent AKI.[6,379]

Leucovorin (folinic acid; an active form of folate) can limit the bone marrow and gastrointestinal toxicity of methotrexate by bypassing its effect on dihydrofolate reductase. Leucovorin "rescue" is most beneficial when administered promptly after methotrexate exposure and should always be given to patients after high doses. Other supportive measures include transfusion of blood components, antiemetics, and nutritional support for stomatitis. Dose recommendations and precise application are covered elsewhere.[380]

Carboxypeptidase G_2 (glucarpidase), a recombinant bacterial enzyme, is also a rescue agent that catabolizes methotrexate to inactive metabolites; it is used in combination with leucovorin because it cannot access intracellular stores of methotrexate. It decreases serum methotrexate concentration within 1 hour following administration. This FDA-approved antidote is available for use only in patients with a serum methotrexate concentration of more than 1 µmol/L with delayed methotrexate clearance (AKI) or under investigational protocol for intrathecal overdoses (100 mg intrathecal methotrexate). Because it is expensive (>$50,000) and either unavailable or restricted in most countries, its precise application remains uncertain.

Intrathecal overdoses of methotrexate may require special measures, including cerebrospinal fluid drainage and exchange, and administration of corticosteroids in addition to leucovorin/glucarpidase. Methotrexate can be removed by ECTRs; high clearances can be achieved by various modalities, especially charcoal HP and high-flux HD.[374] CRRT, as usual, provides lesser removal rates,[381] and peritoneal dialysis and TPE are ineffective.[382-384] ECTR clearance is usually below endogenous clearance in patients with intact kidney function and is therefore most beneficial for patients with AKI. The indication for ECTR, especially with the arrival of carboxypeptidase G_2, remains to be defined but may be related to cost and availability factors. ECTR seems to be indicated if serum methotrexate levels are above the following: 1600 to 2200 µmol/L at the end of infusion, 30 to 300 µmol/L at 24 hours, 3 to 30 µmol/L at 48 hours, and over 0.3 µmol/L at 72 hours. ECTR protocols are usually continued until methotrexate concentrations are below 0.1 µmol/L.[385] Rebound in serum methotrexate concentration, attributable to redistribution, often follows ECTR.

OTHERS

There are other conditions and poisoning situations in which extracorporeal elimination enhancement may reduce the duration of toxicity. Although space restriction does not permit presenting them in detail, there are reports of successful extracorporeal removal of the following poisons: propylene glycol,[386] diethylene glycol,[387] gabapentin,[388] pregabalin,[389] isoniazid,[390] metronidazole,[391] dapsone,[392] gentamycin,[393] vancomycin,[394] cefepime,[395] aluminum,[396] thallium,[397] cibenzoline,[398] baclofen,[399] bromate,[400] *Amanita phalloides*,[401] barium,[402] fluoride,[403] carambola,[404] iodine,[405] and dabigatran.[406,407]

CONCLUSION

General supportive care is sufficient to manage most poisoned patients. In a small selection of cases, extracorporeal blood purification, usually consisting of intermittent HD, can reduce the toxic effects of a poison. An understanding of poison toxicokinetics can help a clinician discern the timely conditions and circumstances when ECTRs are most likely to be beneficial.

ACKNOWLEDGMENT

The authors would like to acknowledge the contribution of previous authors to this section: James P. Smith and Ingrid J. Chang. We would also thank Andrea Palumbo and Monique Cormier for proofreading this chapter.

Complete reference list available at ExpertConsult.com.

KEY REFERENCES

1. Mowry JB, Spyker DA, Cantilena LR, Jr, et al: 2013 Annual Report of the American Association of Poison Control Centers' National Poison Data System (NPDS): 31st Annual Report. *Clin Toxicol (Phila)* 52:1032–1283, 2014.
5. Vale J, Krenzelok EP, Barceloux VD: Position statement and practice guidelines on the use of multi-dose activated charcoal in the treatment of acute poisoning. American Academy of Clinical Toxicology; European Association of Poisons Centres and Clinical Toxicologists. *J Toxicol Clin Toxicol* 37:731–751, 1999.
6. Proudfoot AT, Krenzelok EP, Vale JA: Position paper on urine alkalinization. *J Toxicol Clin Toxicol* 42:1–26, 2004.
7. Ghannoum M, Nolin TD, Lavergne V, et al: Blood purification in toxicology: nephrology's ugly duckling. *Adv Chronic Kidney Dis* 18:160–166, 2011.
8. Lavergne V, Nolin TD, Hoffman RS, et al: The EXTRIP (Extracorporeal Treatments In Poisoning) workgroup: guideline methodology. *Clin Toxicol (Phila)* 50:403–413, 2012.
9. Ghannoum M, Lavergne V, Nolin TD, et al: The utility of extracorporeal treatment for acute thallium poisoning: the first recommendation from the Extracorporeal Treatment in Poisoning Workgroup. *Clin Toxicol* 50:574–720, 2012.
10. Mactier R, Laliberte M, Mardini J, et al: Extracorporeal treatment for barbiturate poisoning: recommendations from the EXTRIP Workgroup. *Am J Kidney Dis* 64:347–358, 2014.
11. Yates C, Galvao T, Sowinski KM, et al: Extracorporeal treatment for tricyclic antidepressant poisoning: recommendations from the EXTRIP Workgroup. *Semin Dial* 27:381–389, 2014.
12. Gosselin S, Juurlink DN, Kielstein JT, et al: Extracorporeal treatment for acetaminophen poisoning: recommendations from the EXTRIP workgroup. *Clin Toxicol (Phila)* 52:856–867, 2014.
13. Ghannoum M, Yates C, Galvao TF, et al: Extracorporeal treatment for carbamazepine poisoning: systematic review and recommendations from the EXTRIP workgroup. *Clin Toxicol (Phila)* 52:993–1004, 2014.
14. Roberts DM, Yates C, Megarbane B, et al: Recommendations for the role of extracorporeal treatments in the management of acute methanol poisoning: a systematic review and consensus statement. *Crit Care Med* 43:461–472, 2014.
15. Lavergne V, Ouellet G, Bouchard J, et al: Guidelines for reporting case studies on extracorporeal treatments in poisonings: methodology. *Semin Dial* 27:407–414, 2014.
16. Decker BS, Goldfarb DS, Dargan PI, et al: Extracorporeal treatment for lithium poisoning: systematic review and recommendations from the EXTRIP workgroup. *Clin J Am Soc Nephrol* 10(5):875–887, 2015.
26. Schreiner GE: The role of hemodialysis (artificial kidney) in acute poisoning. *Arch Intern Med* 102:896–913, 1958.
28. Ouellet G, Bouchard J, Ghannoum M, et al: Available extracorporeal treatments for poisoning: overview and limitations. *Semin Dial* 27:342–349, 2014.
29. Bouchard J, Roberts DM, Roy L, et al: Principles and operational parameters to optimize poison removal with extracorporeal treatments. *Semin Dial* 27:371–380, 2014.
30. Ghannoum M, Roberts DM, Hoffman RS, et al: A stepwise approach for the management of poisoning with extracorporeal treatments. *Semin Dial* 27:362–370, 2014.
31. Ghannoum M, Bouchard J, Nolin TD, et al: Hemoperfusion for the treatment of poisoning: technology, determinants of poison clearance, and application in clinical practice. *Semin Dial* 27:350–361, 2014.
35. Shannon MW: Comparative efficacy of hemodialysis and hemoperfusion in severe theophylline intoxication. *Acad Emerg Med* 4:674–678, 1997.
37. Holubek WJ, Hoffman RS, Goldfarb DS, et al: Use of hemodialysis and hemoperfusion in poisoned patients. *Kidney Int* 74:1327–1334, 2008.
38. Shalkham AS, Kirrane BM, Hoffman RS, et al: The availability and use of charcoal hemoperfusion in the treatment of poisoned patients. *Am J Kidney Dis* 48:239–241, 2006.
39. Mardini J, Lavergne V, Roberts D, et al: Case reports of extracorporeal treatments in poisoning: historical trends. *Semin Dial* 27:402–406, 2014.
40. Kim Z, Goldfarb DS: Continuous renal replacement therapy does not have a clear role in the treatment of poisoning. *Nephron Clin Pract* 115:c1–c6, 2010.
49. Perino GC, Grivet V: Hemoperfusion and plasmapheresis complications. *Minerva Urol Nefrol* 39:161–163, 1987.
53. Kantola T, Koivusalo AM, Hockerstedt K, et al: Early molecular adsorbents recirculating system treatment of *Amanita* mushroom poisoning. *Ther Apher Dial* 13:399–403, 2009.
54. Sein Anand J, Chodorowsk Z, Hydzik P: Molecular adsorbent recirculating system—MARS as a bridge to liver transplantation in *Amanita phalloides* intoxication. *Przegl Lek* 62:480–481, 2005.
55. Lionte C, Sorodoc L, Simionescu V: Successful treatment of an adult with *Amanita phalloides*-induced fulminant liver failure with molecular adsorbent recirculating system (MARS). *Rom J Gastroenterol* 14:267–271, 2005.
58. Ghannoum M, Hoffman RS, Mowry JB, et al: Trends in toxic alcohol exposures in the United States from 2000 to 2013: a focus on the use of antidotes and extracorporeal treatments. *Semin Dial* 27:395–401, 2014.

66. Fertel BS, Nelson LS, Goldfarb DS: The underutilization of hemodialysis in patients with salicylate poisoning. *Kidney Int* 75:1349–1353, 2009.
69. Amdisen A, Skjoldborg H: Haemodialysis for lithium poisoning. *Lancet* 2:213, 1969.
96. Barceloux DG, Krenzelok EP, Olson K, et al: American Academy of Clinical Toxicology practice guidelines on the treatment of ethylene glycol poisoning. Ad hoc committee. *J Toxicol Clin Toxicol* 37:537–560, 1999.
108. Barceloux DG, Bond GR, Krenzelok EP, et al: American Academy of Clinical Toxicology practice guidelines on the treatment of methanol poisoning. *J Toxicol Clin Toxicol* 40:415–446, 2002.
130. Hill JB: Experimental salicylate poisoning: observations on the effects of altering blood pH on tissue and plasma salicylate concentrations. *Pediatrics* 47:658–665, 1971.
150. Proudfoot AT, Krenzelok EP, Brent J, et al: Does urine alkalinization increase salicylate elimination? If so, why? *Toxicol Rev* 22:129–136, 2003.
152. Abel JJ, Rowntree LG, Turner BB: On the removal of diffusible substances from the circulating blood by dialysis. *Trans Assoc Am Physicians* 58:51–54, 1913.
164. Dargan PI, Wallace CI, Jones AL: An evidence based flowchart to guide the management of acute salicylate (aspirin) overdose. *Emerg Med J* 19:206–209, 2002.
183. Bailey B, McGuigan M: Comparison of patients hemodialyzed for lithium poisoning and those for whom dialysis was recommended by PCC but not done: what lesson can we learn? *Clin Nephrol* 54:388–392, 2000.
185. Leblanc M, Raymond M, Bonnardeaux A, et al: Lithium poisoning treated by high-performance continuous arteriovenous and venovenous hemodiafiltration. *Am J Kidney Dis* 27:365–372, 1996.
207. Singh SM, McCormick BB, Mustata S, et al: Extracorporeal management of valproic acid overdose: a large regional experience. *J Nephrol* 17:43–49, 2004.
235. Roberts DM, Buckley NA: Enhanced elimination in acute barbiturate poisoning—a systematic review. *Clin Toxicol (Phila)* 49:2–12, 2011.
277. Ghannoum M, Troyanov S, Ayoub P, et al: Successful hemodialysis in a phenytoin overdose: case report and review of the literature. *Clin Nephrol* 74:59–64, 2010.
288. Peters N, Jay N, Barraud D, et al: Metformin-associated lactic acidosis in an intensive care unit. *Crit Care* 12:R149, 2008.
289. Luft D, Deichsel G, Schmulling RM, et al: Definition of clinically relevant lactic acidosis in patients with internal diseases. *Am J Clin Pathol* 80:484–489, 1983.
321. Proudfoot AT, Stewart MS, Levitt T, et al: Paraquat poisoning: significance of plasma-paraquat concentrations. *Lancet* 2:330–332, 1979.
341. Shannon M: Predictors of major toxicity after theophylline overdose. *Ann Intern Med* 119:1161–1167, 1993.
350. Woo OF, Pond SM, Benowitz NL, et al: Benefit of hemoperfusion in acute theophylline intoxication. *J Toxicol Clin Toxicol* 22:411–424, 1984.
363. Rumack BH, Peterson RC, Koch GG, et al: Acetaminophen overdose. 662 cases with evaluation of oral acetylcysteine treatment. *Arch Intern Med* 141(3 Spec No.):380–385, 1981.
368. Wu ML, Tsai WJ, Deng JF, et al: Hemodialysis as adjunctive therapy for severe acetaminophen poisoning: a case report. *Zhonghua Yi Xue Za Zhi (Taipei)* 62:907–913, 1999.
381. Vilay AM, Mueller BA, Haines H, et al: Treatment of methotrexate intoxication with various modalities of continuous extracorporeal therapy and glucarpidase. *Pharmacotherapy* 30:111, 2010.
385. Wall SM, Johansen MJ, Molony DA, et al: Effective clearance of methotrexate using high-flux hemodialysis membranes. *Am J Kidney Dis* 28:846–854, 1996.

Interventional Nephrology

70

Timmy Lee | Ivan D. Maya | Michael Allon

CHAPTER OUTLINE

OVERVIEW OF VASCULAR ACCESS AND EPIDEMIOLOGY FOR DIALYSIS, 2191
RATIONALE FOR INTERVENTIONAL NEPHROLOGY, 2192
RADIATION AND PERSONAL SAFETY, 2194
BIOLOGY AND PATHOGENESIS OF VASCULAR ACCESS STENOSIS IN ARTERIOVENOUS FISTULAS AND ARTERIOVENOUS GRAFTS, 2194
PROCEDURES INVOLVING ARTERIOVENOUS GRAFTS, 2194
Surveillance for Graft Stenosis, 2194
Angioplasty of Arteriovenous Graft Stenosis, 2198
Deployment of Stents for Arteriovenous Graft Stenosis and Thrombosis, 2202
PROCEDURES INVOLVING ARTERIOVENOUS FISTULAS, 2203
Preoperative Vascular Mapping, 2203
Salvage of Immature Arteriovenous Fistulas, 2206
Percutaneous Transluminal Angioplasty of Arteriovenous Fistulas, 2209
Percutaneous Mechanical Thrombectomy and Thrombolysis of Arteriovenous Fistulas, 2210

NOVEL TECHNIQUES FOR TREATMENT OF SEVERE STENOTIC LESIONS, 2212
Cutting Balloon, 2212
Cryoplasty Balloon, 2212
Local Perivascular Modalities, 2212
CENTRAL VEIN STENOSIS, 2212
ACCESS-INDUCED HAND ISCHEMIA, 2214
INDWELLING HEMODIALYSIS CATHETERS, 2214
Nontunneled Temporary Hemodialysis Catheters, 2214
Tunneled Hemodialysis Catheters, 2216
Less Common Locations for Tunneled Hemodialysis Catheters, 2218
Exchange of Tunneled Hemodialysis Catheters, 2219
PERITONEAL DIALYSIS CATHETER PROCEDURES, 2220
PERCUTANEOUS KIDNEY BIOPSY, 2222
Technical Procedure: Percutaneous Kidney Biopsy Under Real-Time Ultrasound Guidance, 2223

OVERVIEW OF VASCULAR ACCESS AND EPIDEMIOLOGY FOR DIALYSIS

Most patients with end-stage kidney disease (ESKD) use hemodialysis as their renal replacement modality of choice three times weekly to optimize their survival, minimize medical complications, and enhance quality of life.[1] Thus, the hemodialysis vascular access is the lifeline for the patient receiving hemodialysis care. A reliable and durable vascular access is a critical requirement for providing adequate hemodialysis. The ideal vascular access would be easy to place, ready to use as soon as it is placed, deliver high blood flows indefinitely, and be free of complications. None of the existing types of vascular access achieves this ideal. Among the three types of vascular access currently available, native arteriovenous (AV) fistulas are superior to AV grafts, which in turn are superior to dialysis catheters. Recognizing the relative merits of the vascular access types, the 2006 Kidney Disease Outcomes Quality Initiative (KDOQI) guidelines for vascular access recommended placement of AV fistulas in at least 65% and catheter use in only 10% of prevalent patients.[2] The Dialysis Outcomes and Practice Patterns Study (DOPPS), an international observational study, reported that fistulas from 2005 to 2007 were used by only 47% of U.S. patients receiving hemodialysis.[3] In comparison, prevalent fistula rates were 91% in Japan, 83% in Italy, 80% in Germany, 74% in France, 70% in Spain, 67% in England, 57% in Belgium, 59% in Sweden, and 77% in Australia and New Zealand.[3] However, the proportion of patients receiving hemodialysis in the United States using a fistula has increased progressively from 2003 to 2012; this has been in response to the KDOQI guidelines and the Fistula First initiative of the Centers for Medicare & Medicaid Services (CMS)

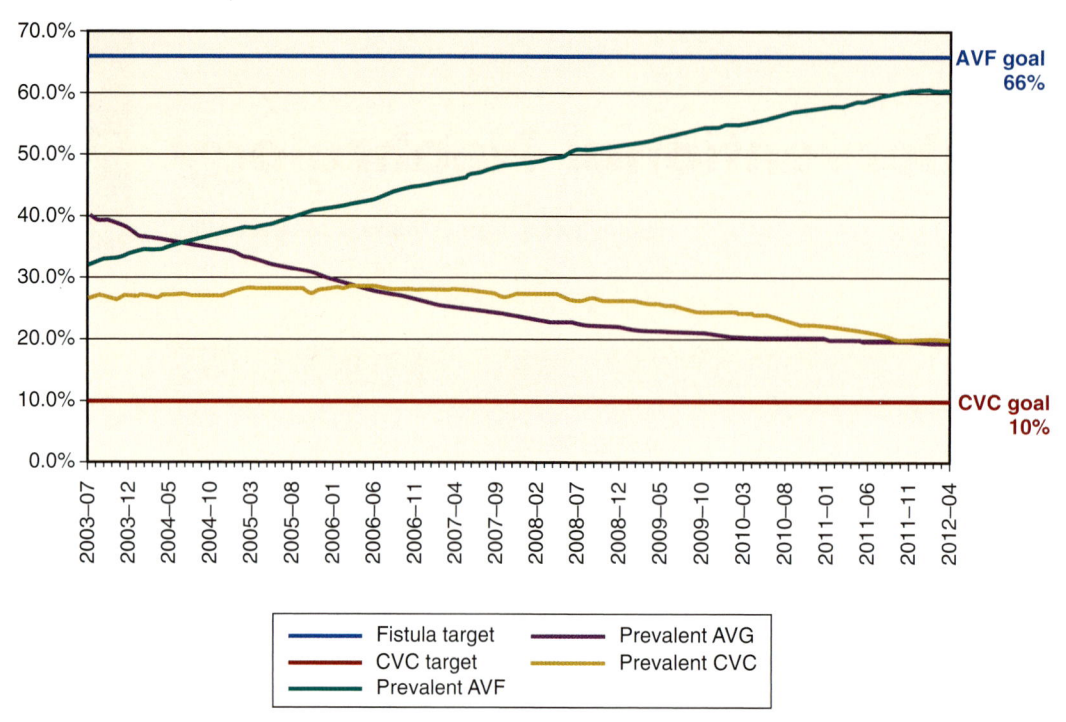

Figure 70.1 Impact of Fistula First Breakthrough Initiative (FFBI). Since the initiation of FFBI, there has been an increase in AV fistula use (AVF) and reduction in AV graft (AVG) use. However, there has been only a modest reduction in central venous catheter (CVC) use. (Adapted from *Fistula First Breakthrough Initiative Dashboard*. Available at: www.fistulafirst.org. Accessed December 1, 2013.)

(Figure 70.1).[4] Unfortunately, there has been only a modest improvement in catheter reduction, from 27% in 2003 to 20% in 2012, well above the KDOQI target of 10% of patients.[4] More recently, Fistula First has increased the bar to a target of 66% fistulas. The distribution of vascular accesses from April 2012 among prevalent hemodialysis patients in the United States was approximately 61% fistulas, 19% grafts, and 20% dialysis catheters (see Figure 70.1).[4] However, despite substantial improvements in prevalent fistula rates, rates in patients new to dialysis have not improved in a similar fashion. The current distribution of vascular accesses from April 2012 among patients new to dialysis is 18% fistulas, 10% grafts, and 72% catheters.[4]

Vascular access procedures and their subsequent complications represent a major cause of morbidity, hospitalization, and cost for patients on maintenance hemodialysis.[5-9] More than 20% of hospitalizations in these U.S. patients are vascular access–related, and the annual cost of vascular access morbidity is close to $1 billion.[8] AV grafts are prone to recurrent stenosis and thrombosis and often require multiple interventions to ensure their long-term patency. AV fistulas have a much lower incidence of stenosis and thrombosis than grafts and require fewer interventions to maintain long-term patency for dialysis.[8-10] Incorporating data from the Dialysis Access Consortium (DAC) Fistula Trial, Dember and colleagues reported that U.S. fistula nonmaturation rates were approximately 60%,[11] even among centers of excellence participating in a high-profile, National Institutes of Health (NIH)–sponsored clinical trial. Tunneled dialysis catheters have the highest frequency of infection and thrombosis but are a necessary evil, either as a bridge device in patients waiting for a fistula to mature or a graft to heal, and as access for emergent dialysis, or as an access of last resort in patients who have exhausted all or almost all fistula or graft options.[12,13] As compared to patients who continue to dialyze with catheters, those who switch from a catheter to a fistula or graft have a substantially lower mortality risk,[14] as well as improvements in serum albumin level and erythropoietin responsiveness.[15]

Even with ongoing efforts to meet KDOQI guideline targets, it is likely that all three types of vascular access will remain in use for the foreseeable future. Thus, substantially more clinical research will be necessary to learn how to minimize complications of, and optimize outcomes associated with, each type of vascular access. Basic research studies will also be needed to elucidate the pathophysiology of vascular access dysfunction failure with each respective vascular access and develop novel and targeted therapies.

RATIONALE FOR INTERVENTIONAL NEPHROLOGY

Patients with advanced chronic kidney disease (CKD) are regularly seen by their nephrologist and referred to different subspecialists, including vascular surgeons and interventional radiologists, for vascular access placement for hemodialysis or peritoneal dialysis. For patients who choose hemodialysis, a vascular access plan becomes a very important aspect of care, ideally completed well before hemodialysis initiation. The goal is to have a functioning fistula in the large majority of patients at the time of hemodialysis initiation. However, many patients undergo frequent placement of temporary or tunneled hemodialysis catheters, revision of a permanent access, surgical or percutaneous thrombectomy, and other related endovascular procedures during the course of their vascular access history. For many years, nephrologists took a passive role in this critically important area of dialysis care. However, during the past decade, nephrologists have strived to improve the quality and timely provision of these services. As a consequence, there has been a growing interest in having such procedures performed by appropriately trained nephrologists who know the patients extremely well and are focused on these procedures without being obligated to attend to other major vascular (e.g., aortic repair) or interventional radiology–directed procedures.[16] In response to this clinical need, organizations such as the American Society of Diagnostic and Interventional Nephrology (ASDIN) were founded and provide guidelines for training, quality assurance, and certification in what is known as interventional nephrology.[17]

Vascular access treatment and research were largely neglected in the past. Interventional techniques were underused, and care of the dysfunctional access was primarily surgical. However, this topic has received growing prominence during the last decade since publication of the initial KDOQI guidelines in 1997 and its subsequent updates. Several nephrologists became directly involved in providing vascular access procedures for their patients. Interventional nephrology was pioneered by Gerald Beathard[18] and subsequently adopted by nephrologists at other medical centers.[19-24] The approval of a number of devices (e.g., mechanical thrombectomy devices, angioplasty balloons, hemodialysis catheters) over the past 25 years has expanded the repertoire of percutaneous interventions for vascular access.[25] Charles O'Neill pioneered an academic program to train nephrologists in the use of ultrasonography for the diagnosis of kidney diseases and facilitate safe and successful kidney biopsies.[26] Finally, Prabir Roy-Chaudhury has been a pioneer in investigating the biology and pathobiology of vascular access dysfunction.[27]

In 2000, a group of interventional nephrologists and radiologists, under the leadership of Dr. Beathard, formed the ASDIN. This organization provides certification to interventional nephrologists and accreditation to the institutions involved in the practice and teaching of interventional procedures in the nephrology specialty.[22] Certification and accreditation are given for diagnostic ultrasonography, peritoneal dialysis insertion, and endovascular procedures on AV fistulas and grafts and central venous catheters for hemodialysis. Comprehensive training is required to achieve dexterity and knowledge. The ASDIN has been actively involved in teaching and promoting the performance of vascular, peritoneal, and ultrasound procedures by well-trained nephrologists, with the goal of providing optimal vascular and peritoneal care to patients receiving dialysis.[28] Several academic and nonacademic centers in the United States already train practicing nephrologists and nephrology fellows in the techniques and procedures pertinent to interventional nephrology. These training centers are located in a freestanding interventional facility or in a hospital-based radiology suite.

A comprehensive list of procedures typically performed by interventional nephrologists is provided in Table 70.1. A given interventional nephrology program may provide only a subset of these procedures, depending on the local needs and arrangements with other medical and surgical subspecialties. A solo nephrologist may decide to perform selected procedures necessary to provide an immediate dialysis access (such as insertion of dialysis catheters), thus eliminating delays resulting from scheduling difficulties. On the other hand, a nephrology group practice may designate one or two nephrologists to be fully trained to perform a spectrum of interventional procedures.

At present, it is not uncommon to find well-trained nephrologists in community and academic settings actively involved in performing various imaging and interventional dialysis procedures. Depending on the degree and depth of their training, interventional nephrologists may provide a range of procedures, including placement of dialysis catheters, ultrasonography, and biopsy of kidneys, preoperative vascular mapping, and postoperative interventions for the maintenance of long-term patency of the vascular access. A decrease in hospitalizations for vascular access–related complications and missed outpatient hemodialysis sessions has been documented at one dialysis center when nephrologists performed interventional access procedures.[24] Furthermore, interventional nephrologists in the United States have also begun creating native AV fistulas in outpatient centers where vascular access procedures are performed.[29,30]

At the University of Alabama at Birmingham (UAB), a unique multidisciplinary model has been adopted to streamline vascular access management. This model consists of a joint interventional radiology and nephrology program, with interventional nephrologists and interventional radiologists sharing the same radiology suites and working side by side to perform all dialysis access procedures. This program has been successful by using all existing technical, clinical, imaging, and surgical talents at the same institution. Recent publications from other academic medical centers have also highlighted the opportunity of interventional nephrology to serve as a model for training, research, and patient care.[31-33]

A key element of any successful interventional program, whether it involves radiologists or nephrologists, is to have actively involved nephrology and dialysis program directors tracking the outcomes of the procedures and implementing timely quality improvement initiatives to improve outcomes. This can be best accomplished by having dedicated vascular

Table 70.1 Procedures Performed by Interventional Nephrologists

Diagnostic renal ultrasonography
Percutaneous renal biopsy
Placement of nontunneled and tunneled dialysis catheters
Exchange of tunneled dialysis catheters
Implantation of subcutaneous dialysis devices
Preoperative vascular mapping
Surveillance for stenosis
Diagnostic fistulograms of grafts and fistulas
Angioplasty of peripheral and central stenosis
Deployment of endoluminal stents for peripheral and central stenosis
Thrombectomy of grafts and fistulas
Sonographic and angiographic assessment of immature fistulas
Salvage procedures for immature fistulas
Placement of peritoneal dialysis catheters

access coordinators who maintain prospective computerized records of all procedures performed.[34]

RADIATION AND PERSONAL SAFETY

Understanding basic radiation safety is very important to protect the patient, physician, and staff involved in the care of the patient. Unnecessary radiation exposure is harmful and can be easily prevented. The U.S. Food and Drug Administration (FDA) oversees the rules and regulations for the use of x-ray equipment. The Occupational Safety and Health Administration (OSHA) regulates the radiation exposure of workers. Each state has its own regulatory office to ensure that workers do not exceed a predetermined radiation dose.

Exposure is the amount of ionizing radiation reaching a subject, and is measured in roentgen units (R). The amount of energy absorbed by a material when exposed to ionizing radiation is measured as rad units. The absorbed dose is always lower than the exposure because the tissue does not absorb all the energy from the radiation. An absorbed dose equivalent is used to relate the amount of biologic damage; it is measured in rem units. The OSHA occupational dose limit for the whole body is 1.25 rem/calendar quarter; for the extremities it is 18.75 rem/calendar quarter. A dosimeter must be worn at all times on the outside of the lead apron, and the absorbed dose is measured monthly. To protect against radiation, the interventionist should minimize the time of exposure to radiation, minimize the use of magnification imaging, use collimators and field filters properly, maximize the distance between the source of radiation and personnel involved with the procedure, minimize the use of cineangiography and continuous fluoroscopy, and use proper shielding, including lead aprons, thyroid collars, leaded glasses, and lead shields.

Knowledge of these facts and the application of appropriate safeguards is particularly important in hemodialysis access procedures, especially those involving vascular access interventions in the upper extremity. The operator's proximity to the x-ray tube and difficulty in shielding increases his or her radiation exposure

BIOLOGY AND PATHOGENESIS OF VASCULAR ACCESS STENOSIS IN ARTERIOVENOUS FISTULAS AND ARTERIOVENOUS GRAFTS

The most common cause of vascular access dysfunction in AV grafts is development of venous neointimal hyperplasia at the vein-graft anastomosis.[35,36] In AV grafts, the stenosis usually results from progressive development of venous neointimal hyperplasia and is characterized by myofibroblasts and extracellular matrix components within the neointima.[35] Furthermore, angiogenesis within the adventitia and a macrophage layer lining the perigraft region that is also present develops in AV grafts.[35]

In AV fistulas, neointimal hyperplasia has been shown to be the most common histology in early and late fistula failures; the predominant cellular phenotypes present within the neointima are myofibroblasts[36-40] (Figure 70.2). However, in AV fistula nonmaturation, inadequate vasodilation (inward remodeling), in addition to neointimal hyperplasia, plays an important role in AV fistula maturation.[36,41,42]

The pathogenesis of neointimal hyperplasia after AV fistula creation or graft creation placement involves a cascade of events that are best divided into upstream and downstream events. Upstream events are characterized as the initial injuries to the vascular endothelium and smooth muscle cells and include the following[36,39,41]: (1) surgical trauma at the time of AV access creation; (2) hemodynamic sheer stress at the vein-artery or vein-graft anastomosis; (3) inflammatory response to the polytetrafluoroethylene (PTFE) grafts; (4) injury from vessel cannulation; (5) effects of uremia on the veins and arteries, leading to endothelial dysfunction; and (6) angioplasty-related injury. Downstream events represent the vascular biologic response to these upstream vascular injuries. An inappropriate downstream response will lead to activation, proliferation, and migration of fibroblasts, smooth muscle cells, and myofibroblasts, ultimately leading to the development of neointimal hyperplasia.[36,39,41,42] In AV fistulas, vasodilation is a necessary downstream response for maturation in addition to the inhibition of neointimal hyperplasia.[41,42]

Recent investigations from experimental models have provided valuable insight into the downstream biology of AV fistula nonmaturation. These studies have shown that the proper balance of expression of protective factors, such as heme oxygenase 1 (HO-1) and nitric oxide synthase (endothelial nitric oxide synthase [eNOS] and inducible nitric oxide synthase [iNOS]), and inhibition of chemokines and mediators, such as monocyte chemoattractant protein-1 and matrix metalloproteinases 1 and 2 (MMP-2 and MMP-9), are crucial to increasing fistula blood flow and vasodilation and inhibiting venous neointimal hyperplasia and stenosis after AV fistula creation.[43-45] From clinical studies, gene polymorphisms in HO-1[46] and factor V Leiden[47] have been found to be associated with AV fistula failure.

In recent years, the health of the vein and artery at the time of access creation and its impact on AV graft and fistula outcomes has been an area of emerging interest. Several studies have shown that preexisting venous neointimal and arterial neointimal hyperplasia are present in the large majority of vessels collected at the time of new vascular access surgery.[48-51] Preexisting arterial intimal hyperplasia and arterial microcalcification have been associated with early AV fistula failure.[51,52] However, no studies to date have reported an association of preexisting venous neointimal hyperplasia and AV fistula outcomes. In fact, a recent study by Allon and coworkers has demonstrated that preexisting venous neointimal hyperplasia was not associated with early postoperative AV fistula stenosis.[53] This suggests the possibility that outward remodeling after AV fistula creation plays a more important role in the maturation process.

PROCEDURES INVOLVING ARTERIOVENOUS GRAFTS

SURVEILLANCE FOR GRAFT STENOSIS

About 80% of AV graft failures are due to thrombosis, whereas 20% are due to infection.[54,55] Thus, improving AV

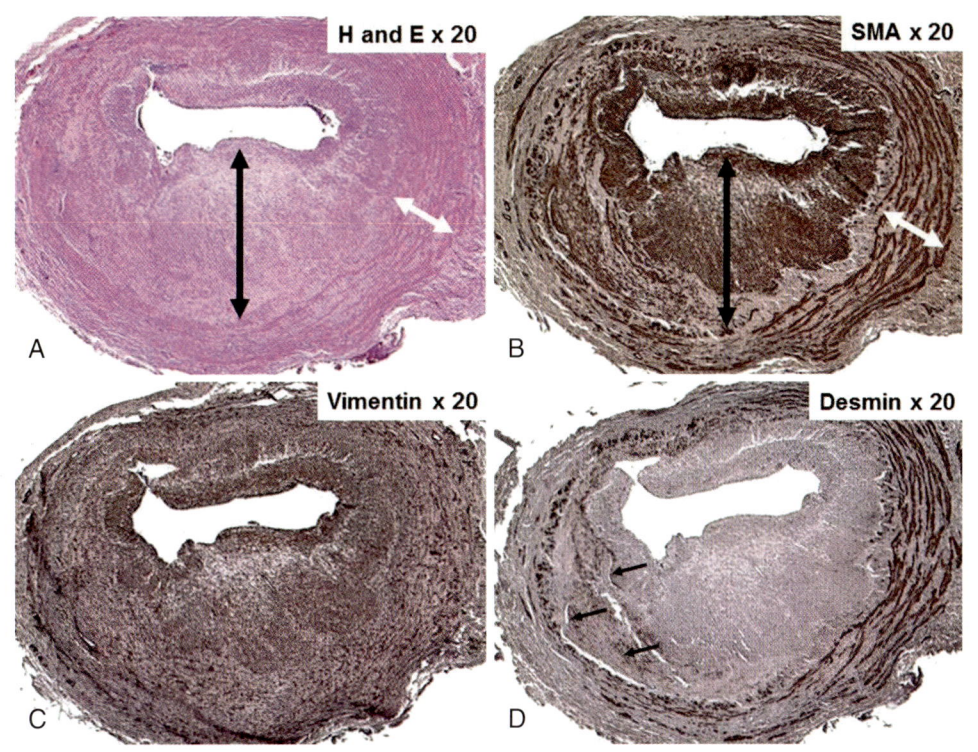

Figure 70.2 Venous neointimal hyperplasia. Shown are hematoxylin and eosin (**A**), smooth muscle actin (SMA; **B**), vimentin (**C**), and desmin (**D**) stains on sequential sections of the venous segment of an AV fistula with maturation failure (**A-D** magnification, ×20). Note the very significant degree of neointimal hyperplasia (*black double-headed arrows*), with relatively less medial hypertrophy (*white double-headed arrow*). Note also that although most of the cells within the region of neointimal hyperplasia appear to be SMA-positive, vimentin-positive, and desmin-negative myofibroblasts, there are also some SMA-positive, desmin-positive contractile smooth muscle cells present within the neointima (*small black arrows* in **D**). (Adapted from Roy-Chaudhury P, Arend L, Zhang J, et al: Neointimal hyperplasia in early arteriovenous fistula failure. *Am J Kidney Dis* 50:782-790, 2007.)

graft longevity requires implementing measures to reduce the frequency of AV graft thrombosis. Reports from the U.S. Renal Data System (USRDS) have shown that the number of angioplasties and thrombectomies ("declots") for AV grafts has substantially increased, from 0.49 to 1.10 and 0.15 to 0.48 (rate/patient-year), respectively, from 1998 to 2007.[1] When thrombosed AV grafts are referred for thrombectomy, a significant underlying stenosis is frequently observed, usually at the venous anastomosis, recipient or draining vein, or central veins.[56-58] This observation suggests that prophylactic angioplasty of hemodynamically significant AV graft stenosis may reduce the frequency of AV graft thrombosis, thereby increasing cumulative AV graft survival.

A seminal study by Schwab and associates was the first to provide evidence supporting this approach.[59] They performed measurements of dynamic venous pressures during consecutive hemodialysis sessions under carefully standardized conditions. They discovered that a persistent elevation in venous pressure measured at a low blood flow was associated with hemodynamically significant stenosis. They then instituted a program of clinical monitoring for AV graft stenosis, with referral for prophylactic angioplasty if there was a suspicion of AV graft stenosis. As compared to the historical control period, a regimen of stenosis monitoring and prophylactic angioplasty reduced the frequency of AV graft thrombosis by about two thirds, from approximately 0.6 to 0.2 events/year. This landmark study stimulated a large volume of subsequent clinical research directed at two fundamental issues: (1) identifying a variety of noninvasive methods to screen for AV graft stenosis; and (2) evaluating whether stenosis surveillance and prophylactic angioplasty improved AV graft outcomes.

A variety of methods have been validated for detection of hemodynamically significant AV graft stenosis (Table 70.2). Clinical monitoring consists of using information that is readily available from physical examination of the AV graft, abnormalities experienced during the dialysis sessions (difficult cannulation or prolonged bleeding from the needle puncture sites), or unexplained decreases in the dose of dialysis, urea reduction ratio (URR), or volume-indexed clearance-time product (Kt/V).[56,57,60] AV graft surveillance uses noninvasive tests requiring specialized equipment or technician training that are not determined as part of the routine dialysis treatment. These include measurement of static dialysis venous pressure (normalized for the systemic pressure),[61,62] measurement of the access blood flow,[63-66] and Duplex ultrasonography to evaluate for evidence of stenosis directly.[67-70] Each of these monitoring or surveillance tools has been reported to have a positive predictive value for AV graft stenosis from 70% to 100% (Table 70.3). The negative predictive value has not been studied systematically because it would require obtaining routine angiograms (fistulograms, or "graft-o-grams") in patients whose screening test was negative. However, the negative predictive value can be inferred from the proportion of AV graft thromboses not preceded by abnormalities of AV graft surveillance (~25%).[66]

Table 70.2 Methods of Stenosis Monitoring

Clinical Monitoring

Physical examination (abnormal bruit, absent thrill, distal edema)
Dialysis abnormalities (prolonged bleeding from needle sites, difficult cannulation)
Unexplained decrease in Kt/V

Surveillance

Static dialysis venous pressure (adjusted for systemic pressure)
Access blood flow
  Qa < 600 mL/min
  Qa decreased by >25% from baseline
Doppler ultrasonography

Kt/V, Volume-indexed clearance-time product; Qa, arterial blood flow.

Table 70.3 Positive Predictive Value of Monitoring Methods for Graft Stenosis

Surveillance Method and Reference	No. of Measurements	Positive Predictive Value (%)
Clinical Monitoring		
Cayco et al, 1998[73]	68	93
Robbin et al, 1998[69]	38	89
Safa et al, 1996[60]	106	92
Maya et al, 2004[57]	358	69
Robbin et al, 2006[70]	151	70
Static Venous Pressure		
Besarab et al, 1995[61]	87	92
Flow Monitoring		
Schwab et al, 2001[84]	35	100
Moist et al, 2003[78]	53	87
Ultrasonography		
Robbin et al, 2006[70]	122	80

In contrast, the predictive value of surveillance methods for AV graft thrombosis is much less impressive. Thus, when AV grafts with abnormal monitoring criteria suggestive of stenosis are observed without preemptive angioplasty, only about 40% of the AV grafts clot over the next 3 months.[71,72] In practice, this means that in any program of AV graft monitoring, about 50% of preemptive angioplasties performed may be unnecessary. Unfortunately, there are no reliable tests to distinguish between the subset of AV grafts with stenosis that will progress to thrombosis from those that will remain patent without any intervention.

Several observational studies have documented that the introduction of a monitoring or surveillance program for AV graft stenosis with preemptive angioplasty lowers the frequency of AV graft thrombosis by 40% to 80%, as compared to the historical control period during which there was no monitoring program (Table 70.4).[34,59-61,73,74] The promising findings from multiple observational studies have led the KDOQI work group to recommend implementing a programs of graft surveillance and preemptive angioplasty in all dialysis centers, with the goal of reducing the frequency of AV graft thrombosis.[75]

Only in the last few years has the value of AV graft stenosis surveillance been subjected to rigorous testing in randomized clinical trials. To date, there have been six such trials evaluating surveillance with access flow monitoring, static dialysis venous pressure, or ultrasonography (Table 70.5). Only one of the six randomized trials has demonstrated a benefit of ultrasound AV graft surveillance[67]; the other five studies showed no benefit of surveillance, despite a substantial increase in the frequency of preemptive angioplasty in the surveillance group.[68,70,76-78] For example, one study randomized patients with grafts to standard clinical monitoring alone or to a combination of clinical monitoring and ultrasound surveillance for stenosis. The patients in the ultrasound group underwent a 66% higher frequency of preemptive angioplasty, yet there was no difference between the two randomized groups in terms of frequency of AV graft thrombosis, time to first thrombosis, or likelihood of AV graft failure (Figure 70.3).[70] Because the randomized trials were relatively small in size, it is possible that they were inadequately powered to detect a modest benefit of AV graft surveillance. However, a meta-analysis of the randomized studies has suggested that the benefit of surveillance with preemptive angioplasty, if present, is likely to be quite small, with a reduction of AV graft thrombosis not exceeding 23% and a reduction in AV graft failure no greater than 17%.[79]

Table 70.4 Effect of Surveillance on Graft Thrombosis: Observational Studies

		Thrombosis Rate (per graft-yr)		
Reference	Surveillance Method	Historical Control	Surveillance Period	Reduction (%)
Schwab et al, 1989[59]	Dynamic dialysis venous pressure	0.61	0.20	67
Besarab et al, 1995[61]	Static dialysis venous pressure	0.50	0.28	64
Safa et al, 1996[60]	Clinical monitoring	0.48	0.17	64
Allon et al, 1998[34]	Clinical monitoring	0.70	0.28	60
Cayco et al, 1998[73]	Clinical monitoring	0.49	0.29	41
McCarley et al, 2001[74]	Flow monitoring	0.71	0.16	77

Table 70.5 Randomized Clinical Trials of Graft Surveillance

Reference	Surveillance Method	No. of Subjects		PTA/yr		Thrombosis-free Survival (at 1 yr)		Cumulative Survival (at 1 yr)	
		con	surv	con	surv	con	surv	con	surv
Lumsden et al, 1997[245]	Doppler US	32	32	0	1.5	0.51	0.47	N/A	N/A
Ram et al, 2003[68]	Access flow	34	32	0.22	0.34	0.45	0.52	0.72	0.80
	Doppler US		35		0.65		0.70		0.80
Moist et al, 2003[78]	Access flow	53	59	0.61	0.93	0.74	0.67	0.83	0.83
Dember et al, 2004[76]	Static DVP	32	32	0.04	2.1	N/A	N/A	0.74	0.56
Malik et al, 2005[67]	Doppler US	92	97	N/A	N/A	N/A	N/A	0.73	0.93
Robbin et al, 2006[70]	Doppler US	61	65	0.64	1.06	0.57	0.63	0.83	0.85

con, Control: DVP, dialysis venous pressure; PTA, percutaneous transluminal angioplasty; surv, surveillance; US, ultrasonography.

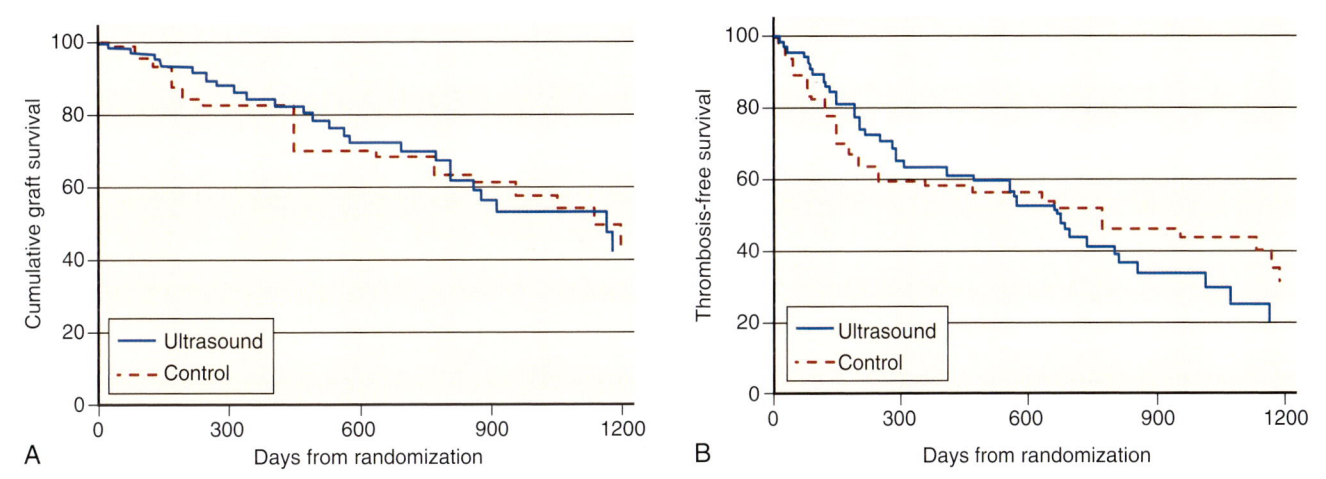

Figure 70.3 **A,** Comparison of cumulative graft survival between randomized patients with clinical monitoring versus clinical monitoring plus regular ultrasound surveillance of grafts ($P = 0.93$ by the log rank test). **B,** Comparison of thrombosis-free graft survival between randomized patients with clinical monitoring versus clinical monitoring plus regular ultrasound surveillance of grafts ($P = 0.33$ by the log rank test). (Reproduced with permission from Robbin ML, Oser RF, Lee JY, et al: Randomized comparison of ultrasound surveillance and clinical monitoring on arteriovenous graft outcomes. *Kidney Int* 69:730-735, 2006.)

A large-scale, multicenter study trial, which takes into account multiple factors involved in access thrombosis, would be required to provide a definitive answer to this controversial question. In the meantime, the value of surveillance of AV graft stenosis and preemptive angioplasty in improving graft outcomes remains controversial.[80-83]

If underlying AV graft stenosis is an important predictor of AV graft thrombosis, why is preemptive angioplasty not more successful in reducing AV graft thrombosis? The fundamental problem appears to be the short-lived efficacy of angioplasty to relieve AV graft stenosis. When serial access blood flows have been used as a surrogate marker of successful angioplasty, 20% of AV grafts were found to have recurrent stenosis within 1 week of angioplasty and 40% within 1 month of angioplasty.[78,84] In another study, the mean vascular access blood flow following angioplasty increased from 596 to 922 mL/min. However, 3 months later, the mean flow had decreased to 672 mL/min.[85] In addition, there is published evidence suggesting that the injury from balloon angioplasty can actually accelerate neointimal hyperplasia, thereby resulting in recurrent stenosis.[86] Not surprisingly, patients undergoing angioplasty for AV graft stenosis require frequent re-interventions because of recurrent stenosis. The median intervention-free patency following AV graft stenosis is only about 6 months.[56,57]

Finally, AV graft surveillance is likely to be most useful in new AV grafts (within 3 months of their creation).[87] Unfortunately, a large proportion of AV grafts fail before there has been adequate opportunity for surveillance to be performed and for hemodynamically significant stenosis to be detected and treated.[88] A recent study has evaluated drug-coated balloon angioplasty with paclitaxel to evaluate the effects of minimizing endothelial injury.[89] Initial results from this study have shown that cumulative target patency at 6 months, defined as angiographic evidence of a patent lesion or circuit with less than 50% angiographic restenosis and without requiring any repeat procedures during the follow-up period, was significantly higher in the drug-coated balloon group (70% in the drug-coated balloon group vs. 25% in the standard balloon angioplasty group).[89]

The pathophysiology of AV graft stenosis involves proliferation of vascular smooth muscle cells (neointimal hyperplasia), with progressive encroachment of the lesion into the AV graft lumen.[90] To improve the patency of AV grafts following angioplasty, some investigators have attempted stent deployment. The rationale is that the rigid scaffold of the stent helps keep the vascular lumen open.[91] There has also been ongoing interest in pharmacologic approaches to the prevention of neointimal hyperplasia. Two small, single-center, randomized clinical trials have documented a beneficial effect of dipyridamole and fish oil in preventing AV graft thrombosis.[92,93] A multicenter, randomized, double-blinded study compared clopidogrel plus aspirin to placebo for the prevention of AV graft thrombosis. The study was terminated early due to an excess of bleeding complications in the intervention group; there was no difference in the rate of AV graft thrombosis between the two randomized groups.[94] Similarly, a randomized clinical trial found that low-intensity warfarin posed a substantial risk of major hemorrhagic complications without reducing the frequency of AV graft thrombosis.[95]

The Dialysis Access Consortium was a larger multicenter, randomized, double-blinded clinical trial comparing long-acting dipyridamole plus low-dose aspirin (Aggrenox) to placebo for the prevention of AV graft failure.[88] There was a modest but statistically significant improvement in primary unassisted AV graft survival in patients receiving dipyridamole-aspirin as compared with those treated with placebo (28% vs. 23%, at 1 year; $P = 0.03$). Cumulative AV graft survival did not differ between the two treatment arms. Most recently, a double-blinded, randomized controlled study evaluating fish oil on polytetrafluoroethylene (PTFE) AV graft patency and cardiovascular outcomes has reported that fish oil does not decrease loss of native patency (time from creation to first intervention) of AV grafts at 12 months, but overall AV graft patency and cardiovascular outcomes show improvement.[96] A more detailed discussion of pharmacologic approaches to prophylaxis of AV graft stenosis and thrombosis is beyond the scope of this chapter, but has been reviewed rather recently.[97]

ANGIOPLASTY OF ARTERIOVENOUS GRAFT STENOSIS

As just described, patients with patent AV grafts are frequently referred for elective angioplasty when hemodynamically significant stenosis is detected by clinical monitoring or by one of several methods of AV graft surveillance. The goal of elective angioplasty is to correct the stenotic lesion that impairs optimal delivery of dialysis and hopefully delay AV graft thrombosis. The most common location of the stenosis by angiography is the venous anastomosis, followed by the peripheral draining vein, central vein, and intragraft (Table 70.6). Inflow (arterial anastomosis) stenosis has been rare (<5%) in most series. However, one study, using retrograde angiography with manual occlusion of the venous limb, documented an inflow stenosis (>50%) in 29% of grafts referred for diagnostic angiography, although all these patients also had venous anastomosis stenosis.[98]

A number of published series have documented the short-lived primary patency (time to next radiologic or surgical intervention) of AV grafts following elective angioplasty (Table 70.7), with only 50% to 60% patent at 6 months and 30% to 40% patent at 1 year. This means that on average, each AV graft requires two angioplasties per year. The primary patency is shorter after angioplasty of central vein stenosis as compared with other stenotic locations. In one study, the primary patency at 6 months was only 29% for central vein stenosis as compared with 67% for stenosis at the venous anastomosis.[58] Most studies have documented progressively shorter patency after each consecutive angioplasty, although one investigator found a comparable primary patency for the first and subsequent AV graft angioplasties.[58]

The primary patency of AV grafts following elective angioplasty is not affected by patient age, race or ethnicity, diabetes, or peripheral vascular disease.[57] However, the patency tends to be shorter in women than in men.[57] The primary patency after angioplasty is also not influenced by the location of the AV graft or number of concurrent stenotic lesions found.[56]

The technical success of an angioplasty procedure may be assessed in several ways. The first is visual inspection of the fistulogram before and after the procedure to determine whether the magnitude of the stenosis (percent stenosis relative to the normal vessel diameter) has been reduced. The degree of stenosis of each lesion can be quantified with calipers or electronic quantitative vascular angiography (QVA) or graded semiquantitatively using the following scale: grade 1, no stenosis (<10%); grade 2, mild stenosis (10% to 49%); grade 3, moderate stenosis (50% to 69%);

Table 70.6 Location of Stenosis in Patients with Grafts Undergoing Angioplasty

Reference	No. of All Stenotic Lesions (%)				
	VA	VO	CV	IG	AA
Beathard, 1992[58]	42	34	4	20	0
Lilly et al, 2001[56] (elective PTA)	55	22	15	6	2.5
Lilly et al, 2001[56] (thrombectomy)	60	14	9	10	7
Maya et al, 2004[57]	62	16	8	12	1.5

AA, Arterial anastomosis; CV, central vein; IG, intragraft; PTA, percutaneous transluminal angioplasty; VA, venous anastomosis; VO, venous outflow.

Table 70.7 Primary Graft Patency after Elective Angioplasty

Reference	No. of Procedures	Primary Patency at		
		3 mo	6 mo	12 mo
Beathard et al, 1992[58]	536	79	61	38
Kanterman et al, 1995[246]	90		63	41
Safa et al, 1996[60]	90	70	47	16
Turmel-Rodrigues et al, 2000[150]	98	85	53	29
Lilly et al, 2001[56]	330	71	51	28
Maya et al, 2004[57]	155	79	52	31

and grade 4, severe stenosis (70% to 99%).[56,57] A second approach is to measure the intragraft pressure before and after the procedure, and normalize it for the systemic blood pressure. A third approach is to measure the change in access blood flow before and after the procedure. Each of these measures has been shown to be predictive of the primary patency of AV grafts following elective angioplasty. In one large series, following elective angioplasty, the median intervention-free survival of AV graft with no residual stenosis was 6.9 months as compared with 4.6 months of any degree of residual stenosis.[56] Similarly, the median primary patency of AV grafts following angioplasty was inversely related to the intragraft-to-systemic pressure ratio—7.6, 6.9, and 5.6 months—when this ratio was less than 0.4, 0.4 to 0.6, and more than 0.6, respectively.[56] Finally, a failure to increase the access blood flow significantly after angioplasty is observed in 20% of AV grafts at 1 week and in 40% by 1 month,[78,84] confirming the short-lived benefit of this intervention.

Measurements of the degree of stenosis are not always feasible, nor are they entirely objective. Caliper measurement or eyeballing are, to various degrees, subjective. Even QVA is not reliable in detecting the various densities and edges of the normal vessels and requires operator adjustment of detected vascular edges (a subjective intervention). AV graft loops originating from the brachial artery and anastomosis at a 90-degree angle with the basilic vein are hardest to image in profile, which is necessary to obtain an accurate measurement of stenosis. We routinely perform intragraft pressure measurement during angiography and percutaneous transluminal angioplasty (PTA) to add a hemodynamic parameter to the visual assessment of fistulograms.

TECHNICAL PROCEDURE: PERCUTANEOUS GRAFT ANGIOPLASTY

The AV graft is accessed with a micropuncture single needle at the arterial limb of the AV graft toward the venous outflow. The needle is exchanged for a 4-Fr introducer. A digitally subtracted antegrade angiogram is taken through the catheter to visualize the venous limb of the AV graft, draining vein, and central vessels. After applying pressure to the venous outflow, retrograde angiography is performed to visualize the arterial anastomosis. The presence or absence of stenotic lesions and their number and location, arterial anastomosis, intragraft, venous anastomosis, draining vein, and central vein are reported. The degree of stenosis of each lesion is quantified with calipers or graded semiquantitatively.[56,57] Lesions with at least 50% stenosis are considered to be hemodynamically significant and undergo angioplasty. If a stenotic lesion is encountered, then the 4-Fr catheter is exchanged for a 6-Fr sheath. An angioplasty balloon is introduced through the sheath. Balloon sizes vary from 7 to 12 mm in diameter to 20 to 80 mm in length, depending on the vessel to be treated. The chosen balloon is usually selected to be 1 mm larger than the size of the AV graft or vessel to be treated. The balloon is placed within the stenotic lesion and inflated to its nominal pressure for 30 to 90 seconds (Figures 70-4 and 70-5). Most anastomotic lesions require higher pressure than that required for peripheral arterial angioplasty. Therefore, high-pressure balloons, with minimal burst pressure more than 15 atm are routinely used.[99] The patient's intragraft and systemic pressures are measured before and immediately after the intervention. In addition to angiographic findings, we rely on a reduction of intragraft-to-systemic pressure ratio to confirm technical success and hemodynamic improvement. If a residual stenosis (>30%) is found, prolonged angioplasty (5-minute inflation), higher pressure balloons (up to 30 atm), and occasionally stent or covered stent deployment may be required to treat these lesions.

The major complication of this procedure is vessel extravasations and rupture of the vessel after the angioplasty treatment. Deploying a covered stent (endograft) can treat these complications. Surgical repair is indicated if the rupture is not corrected by stent placement.

THROMBECTOMY OF GRAFTS

Most graft failures are due to thrombosis, which usually occurs in the context of underlying stenosis at the venous anastomosis.[55,56] For this reason, successful graft thrombectomy requires resolution of the clot and correction of the underlying stenotic lesion. The primary patency of AV grafts after thrombolysis or thrombectomy and angioplasty (Table 70.8) ranges from 30% to 63% at 3 months and 11% to 39% at 6 months. These outcomes are considerably worse than the primary patency observed after elective angioplasty (see Table 70.7), which is 71% to 85% at 3 months and 47% to 63% at 6 months.

The primary AV graft patency is similar for mechanical thrombectomy and pharmacomechanical thrombectomy.[100] A large series comparing the outcomes of both types of radiologic procedures at one institution found that the primary patency was only 30% at 3 months for clotted AV grafts, as compared with 71% for patent AV grafts undergoing elective angioplasty (Figure 70.6A).[56] The discrepancy was still apparent when the analysis was restricted to the subset of procedures in which there was no residual stenosis, with a median primary patency of 2.5 months after thrombectomy, as compared with 6.9 months after elective angioplasty (see Figure 70.6B).[56]

Table 70.8 Primary Graft Patency After Thrombectomy

Reference	No. of Procedures	Primary Patency at	
		3 mo	6 mo
Valji et al, 1991[247]	121	53	34
Trerotola et al, 1994[248]	34	45	19
Beathard, 1994[100]	55 mech	37	
	48 pharm	46	
Cohen et al, 1994[249]	135	33	25
Sands et al, 1994[250]	71		11
Beathard, 1995[251]	425	50	33
Beathard et al, 1996[252]	1176	52	39
Trerotola et al, 1998[253]	112	40	25
Turmel-Rodrigues et al, 2000[150]	58	63	32
Lilly et al, 2001[56]	326	30	19

mech, Mechanical; pharm, pharmacomechanical.

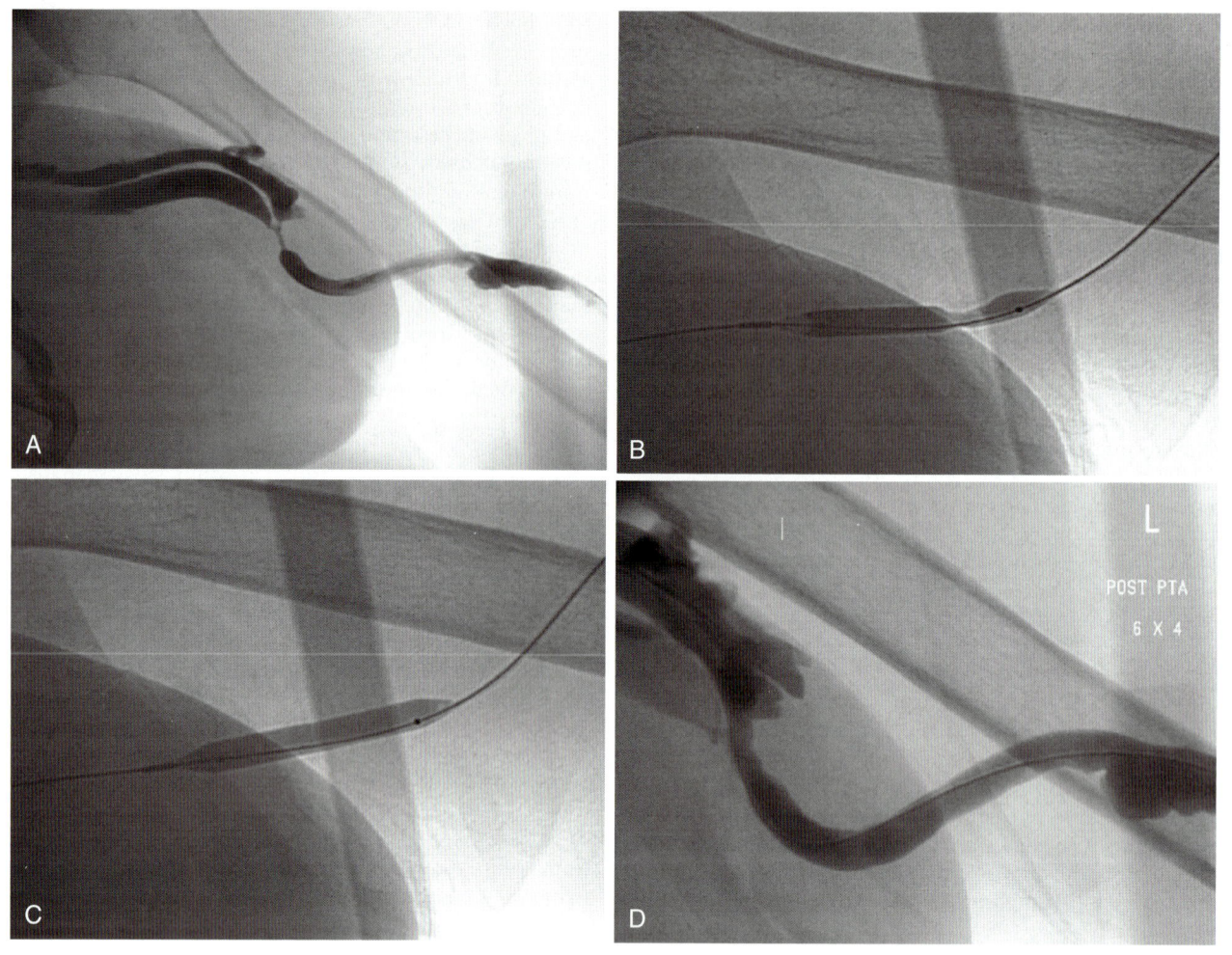

Figure 70.4 **A,** Left upper arm AV graft angiogram showing a severe (95%) stenotic lesion at the level of the venous anastomosis. **B,** Left upper arm AV graft stenotic lesion at the venous anastomosis with the angioplasty balloon partially inflated. **C,** Left upper arm AV graft stenotic lesion at the venous anastomosis with the angioplasty balloon fully inflated. **D,** Final postangioplasty left upper arm AV graft angiogram showing a treated lesion with minimal residual stenosis.

The duration of AV graft patency following thrombectomy does not appear to differ among patients with and without diabetes mellitus. AV graft patency is also generally unrelated to the graft location or number of concurrent AV graft stenoses found.[56] However, similar to the observations obtained after elective angioplasty, the primary patency of AV grafts after thrombectomy is inversely proportional to the magnitude of residual stenosis at the end of the procedure.[56]

TECHNICAL PROCEDURE: PERCUTANEOUS ARTERIOVENOUS GRAFT THROMBECTOMY

The AV graft is initially accessed with a single-wall needle at the level of the arterial limb of the graft. A guidewire is passed up to the venous outlet, and the needle is exchanged for a 6-Fr sheath. A catheter is placed beyond the clotted AV graft, and venography of the venous outflow and central circulation is performed. Extreme caution is exercised not to pressure-inject contrast into the AV graft because it can dislodge a clot and cause arterial emboli. Because more than 60% of stenotic lesions are located at the venous anastomosis, an angioplasty balloon, usually 8 × 40 mm, is placed at that site and inflated to its nominal pressure (15 atm).

The balloon is removed and a mechanical thrombectomy can be achieved by one of several methods: manual aspiration of the clots; infusion of a thrombolytic agent (tissue plasminogen activator [t-PA]; Urokinase); use of a clot buster device (e.g., Angiojet, Arrow-Trerotola, Cragg thrombolytic brush, Hydrolyser, Prolumen, Amplatz thrombectomy device); or a combination of any of these (Figure 70.7). Pure mechanical thrombectomy is sufficient, and thrombolysis is rarely necessary. The AV graft is accessed for a second time with a single-wall needle at the venous limb of the AV graft, toward the arterial anastomosis. The needle is exchanged over a wire for a 6-Fr catheter sheath. A guidewire is passed into the arterial circulation. A Fogarty balloon is passed beyond the arterial anastomosis and pulled back to dislodge the arterial plug, if present. Aspiration of the clots through both sheaths is performed; the clot buster device is used again to clear all residual debris from the AV graft. Once blood flow in the AV graft is restored, as assessed by physical examination, small amounts of contrast are injected to check for residual clots and flows. Finally, antegrade and retrograde angiograms of the AV graft are obtained to assess for patency and look for other stenotic lesions. Angioplasty of any residual hemodynamically

Figure 70.5 **A,** Digital subtraction angiography (DSA) of a left upper arm AV graft showing a moderate stenotic lesion at the level of the arterial limb of the graft. **B,** Spot film showing the stenotic lesion being angioplastied. **C,** Final postangioplasty DSA image showing excellent results.

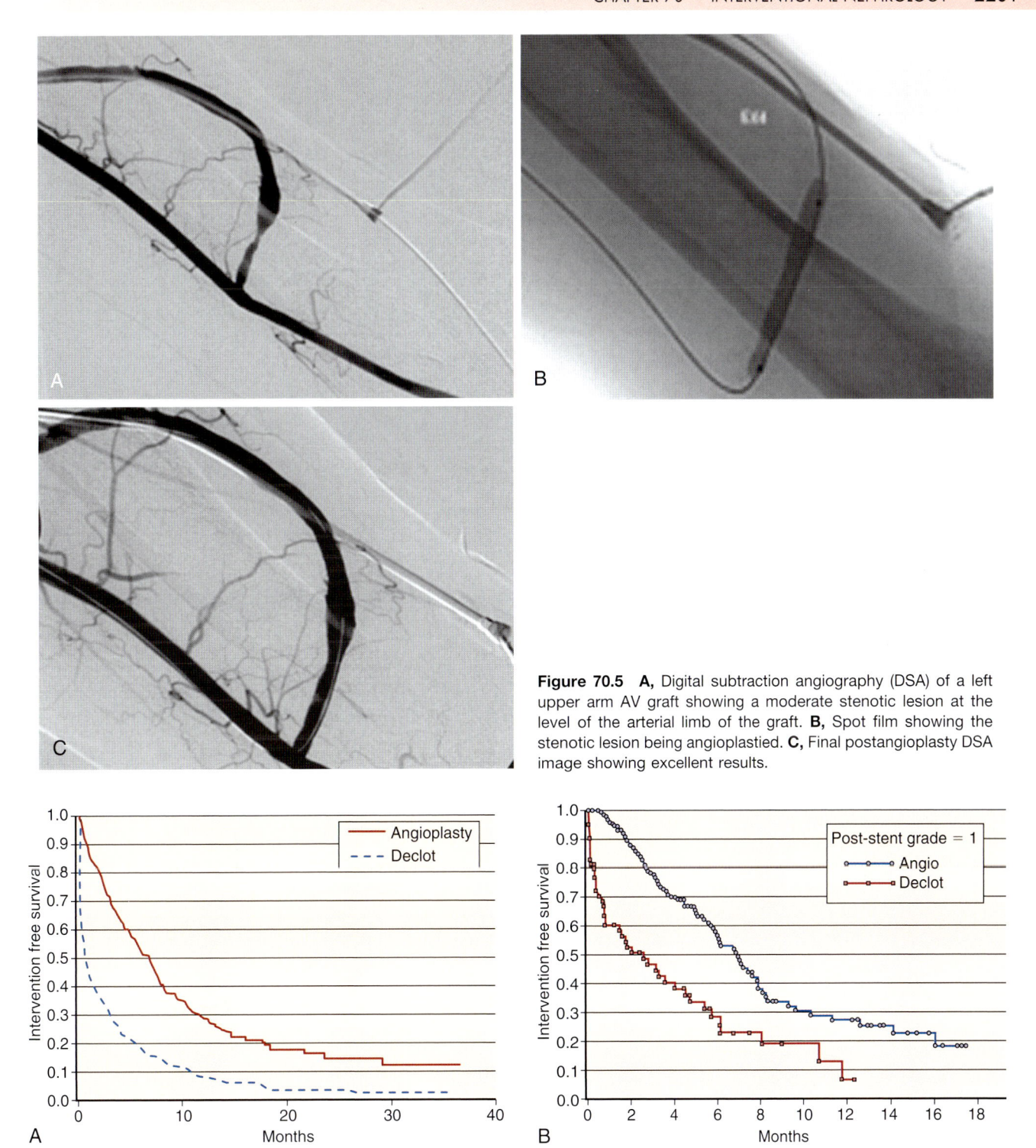

Figure 70.6 **A,** Intervention-free graft survival following elective angioplasty *(solid line)* or thrombectomy plus angioplasty *(dotted line)*. Graft survival was calculated from the date of the initial intervention to the date of the next intervention (angioplasty, declot, or surgical revision). **B,** Intervention-free graft survival following elective angioplasty *(circles)* or thrombectomy plus angioplasty *(squares)* in the subset of procedures with no residual stenosis. Graft survival was calculated from the date of the initial intervention to the date of the next intervention (angioplasty, declot, or surgical revision). $P < 0.001$ for the comparison between the two groups. (From Lilly RZ, Carlton D, Barker J, et al: Clinical predictors of arteriovenous graft patency following radiologic intervention in hemodialysis patients. *Am J Kidney Dis* 37:945-953, 2001.)

significant stenotic lesion in the vascular access circuit is performed. Intra-access pressure and systemic pressure (measured inside the AV graft by occluding the venous outflow) are measured. The ratio is calculated to confirm acceptable angioplasty results. High intragraft pressures indicate residual venous anastomotic obstruction, whereas extreme low pressures indicate obstruction at the arterial inflow.

Major complications of the thrombectomy procedure are vessel extravasations (Figure 70.8) and rupture of the vein,

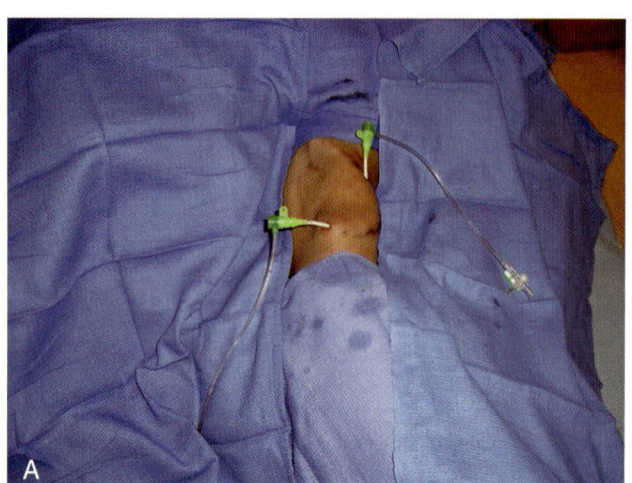

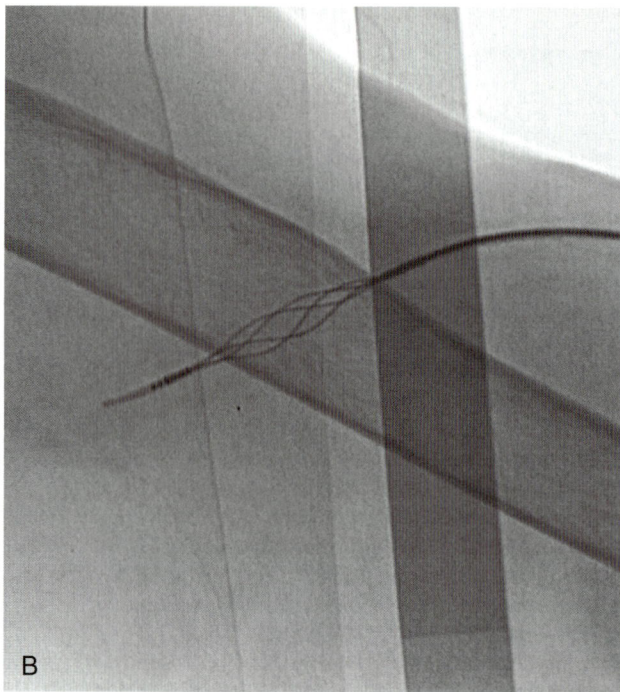

Figure 70.7 **A,** Percutaneous mechanical thrombectomy. A left upper arm AV graft site is prepped and two 6-Fr sheaths are in place. **B,** Percutaneous mechanical thrombectomy. This spot film shows the use of a percutaneous thrombectomy device (PTD; Arrow-Trerotola).

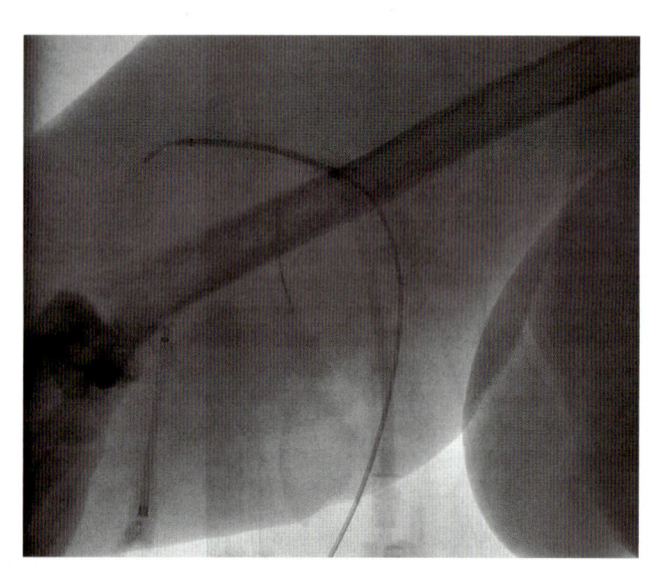

Figure 70.8 Mechanical thrombectomy complication—extravasation of contrast at the middle portion of the arteriovenous graft.

either because of wire manipulation or as a result of the angioplasty. Small extravasations are self-limited and may be observed; otherwise, stent deployment is the treatment of choice. Arterial emboli distal to the arterial anastomosis may occur and, if encountered, intervention or surgical embolectomy is required. One interventional method to treat this complication is back bleeding; this refers to an occlusion of the artery before its anastomosis to the AV graft, causing retrograde blood flow that brings the clot into the AV graft. A Fogarty balloon to remove the clot and thrombolytic agents can also be used to treat this complication.[101] There have been very few published studies evaluating the frequency of pulmonary embolism following thrombectomy. One study has reported that pulmonary embolism is common (~35%) in patients undergoing AV graft thrombectomy.[102]

DEPLOYMENT OF STENTS FOR ARTERIOVENOUS GRAFT STENOSIS AND THROMBOSIS

As noted, the primary patency of AV grafts following angioplasty is short-lived, and there is evidence that the vascular injury from angioplasty may actually accelerate neointimal hyperplasia.[86] In view of these considerations, there has been considerable interest in technical modifications to improve the patency of AV grafts following angioplasty. Endoluminal stents work by forming a rigid scaffold, which prevents elastic recoil and helps keep the vascular lumen open. Therefore, although neointimal hyperplasia recurs, layering a thickness of 1 mm on the wall of a stent is less likely to cause significant stenosis of the vascular lumen of an 8-mm stent. Stent placement has been attempted for the treatment of rapidly recurrent stenosis. A stenosis that is highly resistant to balloon angioplasty and cannot be expanded with a balloon is a contraindication for stent placement because the stent will be as narrow as the original stenosis. On rare occasions, when trying to overcome such resistant stenoses with very high pressure, angioplasty may result in venous rupture and extravasation. Surgery is not necessary in these situations because the complication can be converted to success by using stents or stent grafts (endograft).

The KDOQI Clinical Practice Guidelines for Vascular Access have recommended stent deployment only when there is acute elastic recoil of the vein (>50% stenosis) after angioplasty, when stenosis recurs within a 3-month period, or to treat vascular rupture complicating the angioplasty.[103]

Several small series have reported outcomes following stent deployment for refractory vascular access stenosis.[104-110] Most of these studies have been limited by retrospective data collection, absence of a suitable control group, lumping together of patent and thrombosed accesses, and combining grafts with fistulas.[111] A small randomized study comparing stents with conventional angioplasty found no difference in primary graft patency following the intervention.[105] However, this study enrolled a mixture of clotted and patent grafts, and the stenotic lesions were at a variety of locations, thus limiting the interpretation of the findings.

Because primary AV graft patency is particularly short-lived in clotted AV grafts undergoing thrombectomy, those AV grafts may experience better patency after stent deployment. One series reported the outcomes of 34 clotted AV grafts undergoing thrombectomy with stent placement at the venous anastomosis.[108] The primary patency following intervention in this homogeneous group of AV grafts was 63% at 6 months. Although there was no matched control group treated with angioplasty alone, the primary graft patency was much higher than that reported previously (11% to 39% at 6 months; see Table 70.8). A nonrandomized study comparing outcomes of clotted AV grafts treated with thrombectomy and stent placement at the venous anastomosis with matched control patients treated with only thrombectomy and angioplasty found a significantly longer primary patency in AV grafts treated with a stent as compared with those treated with angioplasty alone.[112] Similarly, a retrospective study of 48 patients found longer AV graft patency after elective treatment of stenosis with stent deployment as compared with angioplasty alone.[113] A definitive randomized clinical trial is warranted to evaluate whether the patency of AV grafts following thrombectomy is enhanced by stent deployment.

There are a number of stent types available, including covered and noncovered stents and balloon- or self-expandable stents. Balloon-expandable stents are susceptible to be crushed under pressure if used peripherally and may only be used centrally. A variety of self-expanding, nitinol-based stents are available for use outside the coronary circulation. Although they appear similar, there are subtle differences that may favor one stent over another in a particular circulation. However, there have been no published clinical trials comparing the outcomes among stent types used for dialysis access. The use of a drug-eluting stent (DES) in the coronary circulation has significantly reduced recurrent stenosis from 20% to 23% to less than 10%. DESs were implicated in cases of acute and late thrombosis, which led to the routine and obligatory administration of antiplatelet agents (aspirin and Clopidogrel) for at least 1 year from stent implantation. It is also possible that the administration of antiplatelet agents after stent placement, use of a DES (e.g., sirolimus), or both may further improve the primary patency of AV grafts following angioplasty and/or thrombectomy but, again, there are no definitive data available at this time. However, a pilot study in 32 patients with graft dysfunction randomly assigned to a paclitaxel DES or standard balloon angioplasty reporting a trend toward improvement in mean primary patency (163 vs. 104 days; $P = 0.16$).[114] Future studies should help resolve the question of whether a DES is truly superior to balloon angioplasty in managing vascular graft failure.

Finally, stent grafts, which consist of a metallic stent covered with graft material, have been used successfully to treat and exclude large pseudoaneurysms in the AV graft and complications such as rupture and extravasation. However, a multicenter, randomized clinical trial allocated 190 patients with more than 50% AV graft stenosis at the venous anastomosis to treatment with stent grafts or balloon angioplasty, with follow-up protocol angiography performed at 2 and 6 months.[115] AV graft patency at 6 months was significantly higher in patients randomized to stent grafts, but AV graft thrombosis was no different in the two treatment arms. Despite the cost of these endografts or covered stents, they may become quite valuable if long-term patency proves superior to angioplasty and bare metal stents.

TECHNICAL PROCEDURE: PERCUTANEOUS DEPLOYMENT OF STENT

Percutaneous mechanical thrombectomy is carried out as described in the previous section. If a severe elastic recoil is seen on the final angiogram, or a large residual stenosis (>30%) is seen at the level of the original stenotic lesion, a stent could be deployed.[101] Self-expanding stent sizes vary from 6 to 14 mm in diameter, and 10 to 80 mm in length. The most commonly used stents are nitinol or nitinol covered with expanded PTFE (e-PTFE). The appropriate size and length are determined by grading the stenotic lesion at the time of placement. Usually, the stent is selected to be 1 mm larger than the size of the AV graft or the vessel to be treated, and the length is 5 mm longer than the stenotic lesion on each side. The stent comes already mounted in a device that is inserted through the sheath located at the arterial limb of the AV graft. A "road map" contrast injection of the stenotic lesion is performed. The stent is placed at the site of the stenotic lesion and deployed under fluoroscopic guidance (Figure 70.9). A postdeployment angioplasty with an appropriate-sized balloon is usually necessary to re-expand recoiled lesions. A final angiogram is obtained to assess for patency and proper placement of the stent.

Complications of stent deployment include those related to angioplasty. In addition, underestimation of the required stent size may result in stent migration to the systemic circulation. If the stent is placed at a site where another vessel joins the main venous outlet, that vessel may be completely or partially occluded. The stent can fracture (Figure 70.10) and occasionally thrombose (Figure 70.11). Finally, a potential long-term complication is intrastent restenosis or thrombosis, which may require multiple and frequent re-interventions.

PROCEDURES INVOLVING ARTERIOVENOUS FISTULAS

PREOPERATIVE VASCULAR MAPPING

The need to increase placement of native AV fistulas has been highlighted by the KDOQI guidelines[75] and by the Fistula First initiative (www.fistulafirst.org). There is widespread consensus among nephrologists and surgeons about

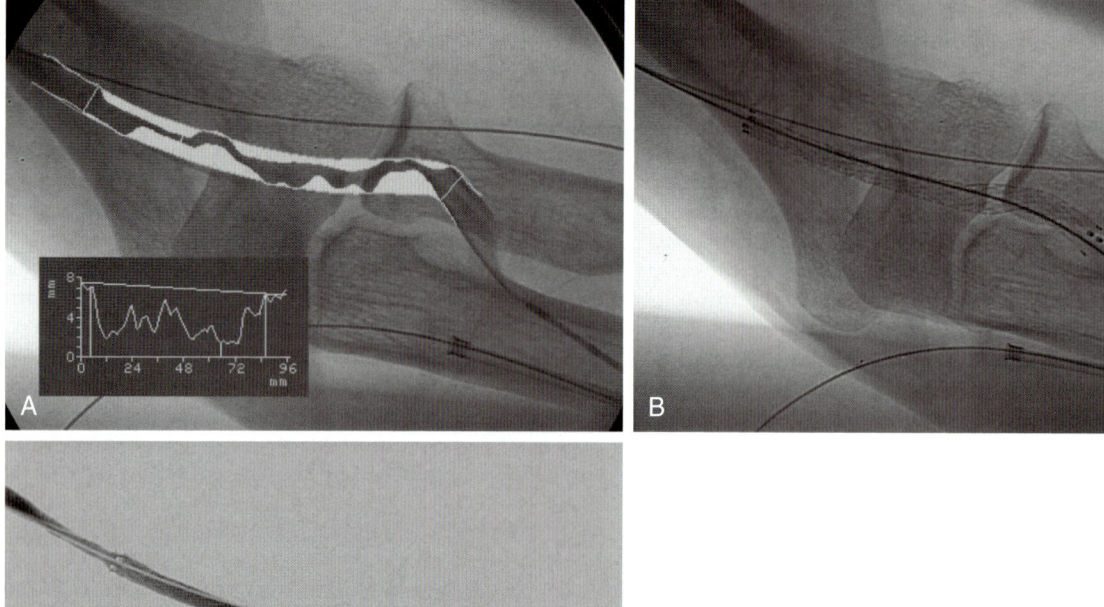

Figure 70.9 **A,** Angiogram demonstrating a severe stenotic lesion at the level of the venous anastomosis and the draining vein of a left forearm AV graft. The stenotic lesion was graded before stent deployment. **B,** The stent is fully deployed. **C,** Digital subtraction angiography (DSA) image of the left forearm AV graft shows excellent results after stent deployment

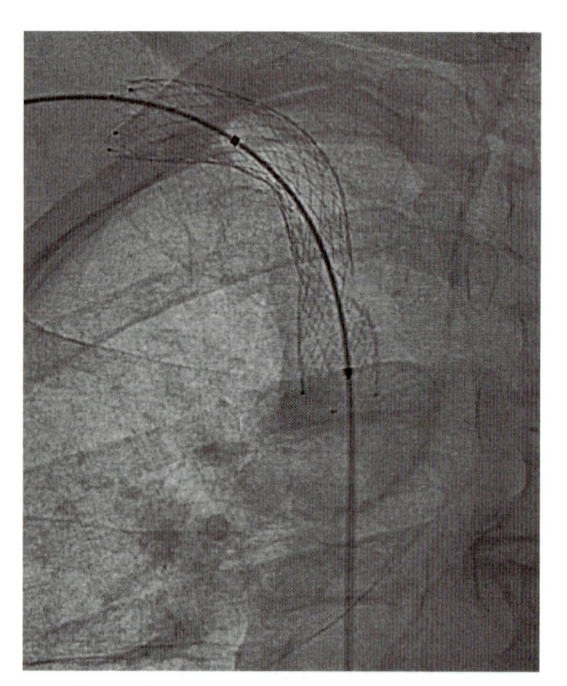

Figure 70.10 Fracture stent at the level of the right subclavian vein and right innominate vein.

the importance of maximizing functional AV fistula prevalence in patients undergoing hemodialysis. Achieving this goal, however, requires overcoming a number of obstacles, including timely referral of the patient with CKD to the nephrologist and access surgeon, timely placement of an AV fistula, adequate maturation of new AV fistulas, and successful cannulation of the AV fistula for dialysis.[9] In the past, the surgeon's decision about the type and location of vascular access was determined by physical examination of the extremity, with and without a tourniquet. This approach had the potential for substantial errors. The surgeon may not be able to visualize the veins in obese patients adequately. As a result, the surgeon might place an AV graft when an AV fistula could have been feasible. In other patients, the surgeon may decide to place a radiocephalic AV fistula after visualizing a large-diameter cephalic vein at the wrist. However, an unsuspected stenosis or thrombosis in a proximal portion of that vein could doom the outcome of such an AV fistula.

The use of preoperative sonographic vascular mapping has been shown to increase substantially the proportion of patients receiving an AV fistula rather than an AV graft. A prospective pilot study at UAB compared the surgeon's decision about access placement in 70 consecutive patients with CKD before and after the results of preoperative vascular mapping were provided to the surgeon.[116] In almost one third of the patients, the surgeon changed her or his mind about the intended access procedure after receiving the mapping results. In most of these cases, the surgeons decided to place an AV fistula rather than an AV graft or changed their mind about the location of the AV fistula.[116] On the basis of these promising results, a program of routine preoperative vascular mapping was implemented. The results were dramatic; as compared to the historical control period, the proportion of patients having an AV fistula

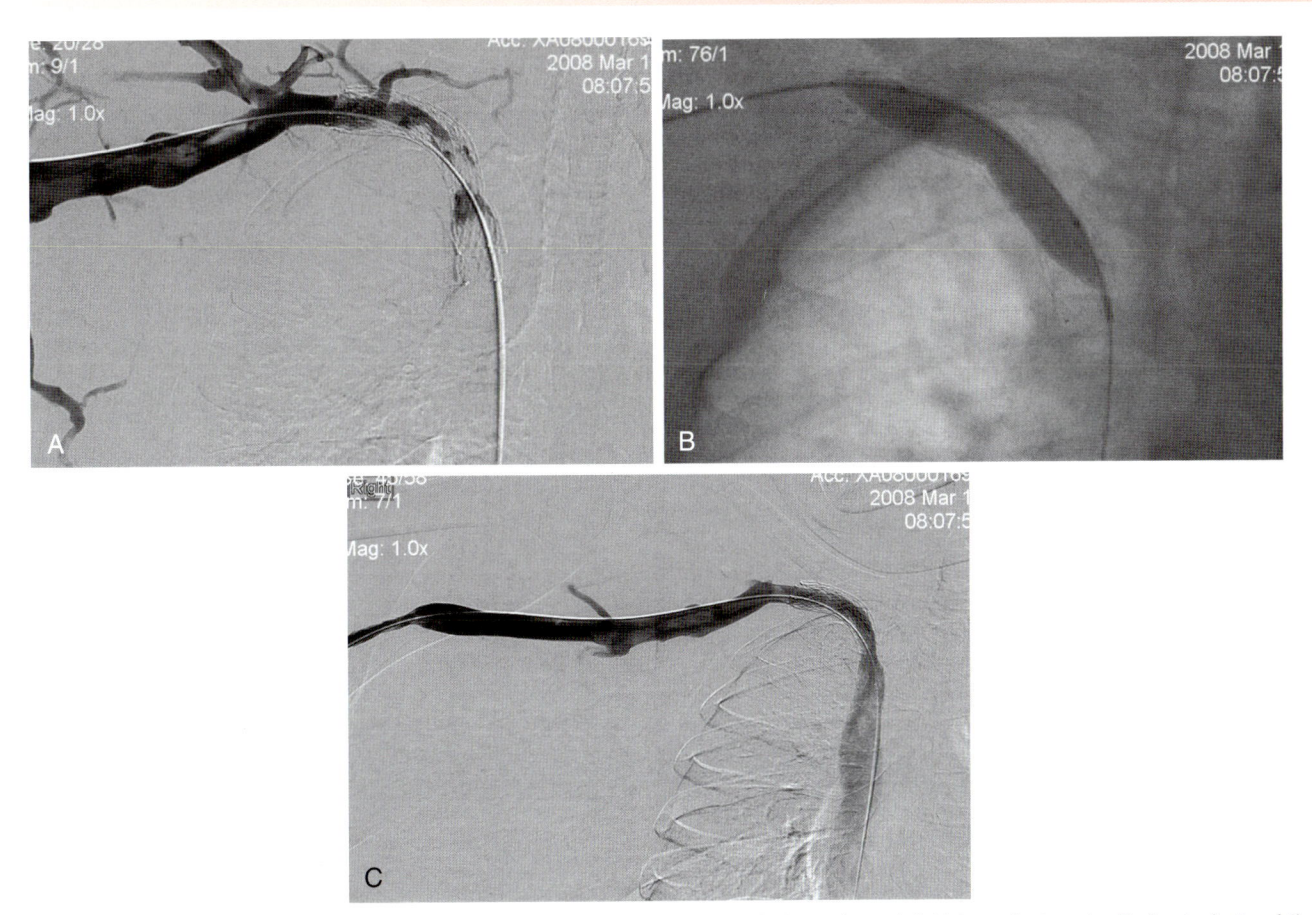

Figure 70.11 **A,** Thrombosed and fractured stent at the level of the right subclavian vein and right innominate vein. **B,** Angioplasty of the stenotic intrastent lesion, which caused the thrombosis of the access circuit. **C,** Restoration of blood flow of the thrombosed stent.

placed increased from 34% to 64%. Moreover, the proportion of patients dialyzing with an AV fistula doubled, from 16% to 34%.[117] Similar increases in AV fistula placement following the introduction of preoperative vascular mapping have been documented by other investigators (Table 70.9), although a reduction in primary AV fistula failure has not been a consistent finding in all studies.[117-121] Two randomized clinical trials have compared outcomes of new AV fistulas placed after preoperative ultrasound vascular mapping to those placed after clinical evaluation alone. In a Turkish study of 70 patients, the two treatment groups had similar primary and secondary AV fistula survival.[122] In a British study of 218 patients, the patients undergoing a preoperative sonogram had a lower incidence of immediate AV fistula failure (4% vs. 11%; $P = 0.03$). Primary (intervention-free) AV fistula survival was no different between the two groups (65% vs. 56%; $P = 0.081$), but the assisted primary (thrombosis-free) AV fistula survival was superior in the group undergoing preoperative ultrasound mapping (80% vs. 65%; $P = 0.01$).[123]

Although most centers have used sonographic vascular mapping, some have used conventional venography.[124] In patients with stage 4 CKD who have not yet started dialysis, there is a theoretical concern of radiocontrast-associated nephropathy precipitating the need for initiation of dialysis. However, in a series of 25 patients with a mean glomerular filtration rate of 13 mL/min, none developed acute renal failure after undergoing angiography with 10 to 20 mL of low-osmolality contrast material.[125] Another potential risk of venography is that direct venography may injure the very veins required for future AV fistula creation. One advantage of venography is the ability to image the central vessels to exclude central vein stenosis. Venipuncture should be performed in the hand veins, if at all possible, and the cephalic vein should be avoided. Prospective studies are needed to define further which preoperative vascular mapping techniques are most useful in optimizing fistula maturation and to delineate specific situations.

TECHNICAL PROCEDURE: SONOGRAPHIC PREOPERATIVE VASCULAR MAPPING

Vascular measurements are performed with the patient in a seated position, with the arm resting comfortably on a Mayo stand. All measurements are performed in the anteroposterior dimension in the transverse plane (Figure 70.12). The minimum vein diameter for a native arteriovenous fistula is 2.5 mm.[126] The minimum vein diameter for graft placement is 4.0 mm.[126] The minimum arterial diameter for fistula or graft placement is 2.0 mm.[126] Veins are assessed for stenosis, thrombus, and sclerosis (thickened walls).

First, the radial artery diameter at the wrist is measured. A tourniquet is then placed at the mid to upper forearm. The veins above the wrist are percussed for 2 minutes, with special emphasis on the cephalic vein area. Sequential measurements are made of the cephalic vein at the wrist and mid and cranial forearm. Any other dorsal or volar veins at

Table 70.9 Effect of Preoperative Vascular Mapping on Vascular Access Outcomes

Reference	No. of Fistulas Placed (%)		No. of Primary Fistula Failures (%)		Prevalence of Fistula Use (%)	
	Pre-VM	Post-VM	Pre-VM	Post-VM	Pre-VM	Post-VM
Silva et al, 1998[120]	14	63	36	8	8	64
Ascher et al, 2000[118]	0	100	N/A	18	5	68
Gibson et al, 2001[119]	11	95	18	25	N/A	N/A
Allon et al, 2001[117]	34	64	54	46	16	34
Sedlacek et al, 2001[254]	N/A	62	N/A	25	N/A	N/A
Mihmanli et al, 2001[255]			25	6		
Miller et al, 1997[256]	N/A	76				
Kakkos et al, 2011[121]	12	53	32	18		

N/A, Not available; VM, preoperative vascular mapping.
From Allon M, Robbin ML. Increasing arteriovenous fistulas in hemodialysis patients: problems and solutions. Kidney Int 62:1109-1124, 2002.

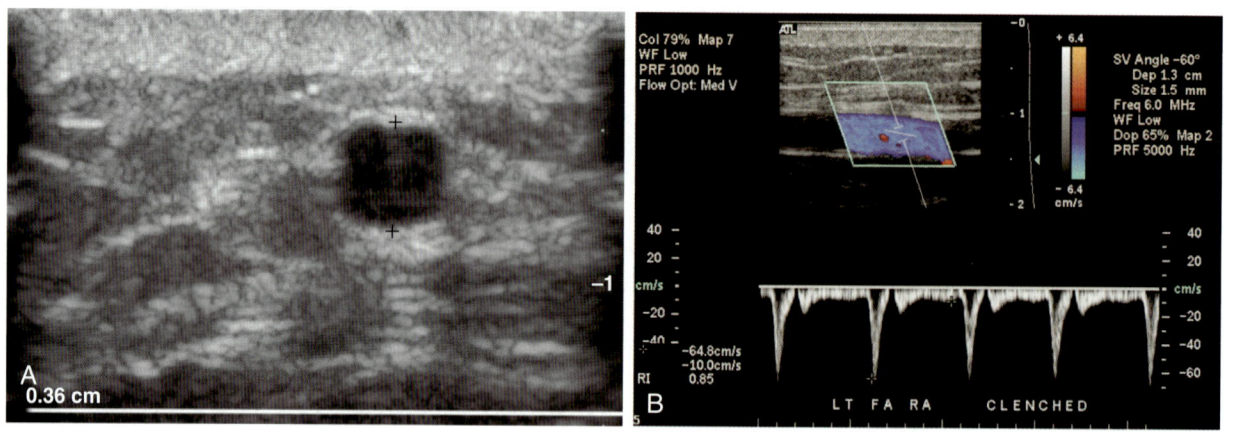

Figure 70.12 **A,** Venous mapping. This venous sonogram shows a transverse section of a cephalic vein being measured (0.36 cm). **B,** Venous mapping. Doppler flow measurements and color Doppler sonogram show a longitudinal section of a left forearm radial artery that is 1.3 cm deep and 1.5 mm in diameter.

the wrist are also measured and followed up the arm, according to established diameter criteria. The tourniquet is sequentially moved up the arm and cephalic, basilic, and brachial vein diameters are measured.

After the tourniquet is removed, the subclavian and jugular veins are assessed for stenosis and thrombus. Evidence of a more central stenosis is determined by analysis of the spectral Doppler waveform for respiratory phasicity and transmitted cardiac pulsatility. If there is a clinical or sonographic suspicion of central vein stenosis, venography or magnetic resonance venography (MRV) is performed.

Measurements are recorded on a worksheet. The sonographic measurements are used by the surgeon to select the most appropriate vascular access on the basis of the following (agreed on by nephrologists, radiologists, and vascular surgeons), from most desirable to least desirable[126]:

1. Nondominant forearm, cephalic vein AV fistula
2. Dominant forearm, cephalic vein AV fistula
3. Nondominant or dominant upper arm, cephalic vein AV fistula
4. Nondominant or dominant upper arm, basilic vein transposition AV fistula
5. Forearm loop, AV graft
6. Upper arm, straight AV graft
7. Upper arm loop, AV graft (axillary artery to axillary vein)
8. Thigh, AV graft

SALVAGE OF IMMATURE ARTERIOVENOUS FISTULAS

As compared with AV grafts, AV fistulas require a much lower frequency of intervention (angioplasty or thrombectomy) to maintain their long-term patency for dialysis.[126] However, AV fistulas have a substantially higher primary failure rate (AV fistulas that are never usable for dialysis). Similar to AV grafts, the rate of angioplasty use (from USRDS data) has increased from 0.16 to 0.47 (rate/patient-year) from 1998 to 2007,[1] likely due to the increasing frequency of treating primary AV fistula failures. The proportion of AV fistulas with primary failure has ranged from 20% to 50% in multiple recent series, even when routine preoperative vascular mapping was used.[9] A landmark multicenter randomized controlled trial reported a primary AV fistula failure rate of 60% in the United States.[11] Primary AV fistula failures fall into two major categories, early thrombosis and failure to mature.[127-129] Early thrombosis refers to AV fistulas that thrombose within 3 months of their creation, before they have been used for dialysis. Failure to mature refers to AV fistulas that never develop adequately to be cannulated reproducibly for dialysis. Nonmaturation is less common with upper arm than forearm AV fistulas.[9] Among upper arm AV fistulas, nonmaturation is less likely with transposed brachiobasilic AV fistulas than with brachiocephalic AV fistulas.[130]

Native AV fistulas are created by performing a direct anastomosis between a high-pressure artery and a low-pressure vein. Exposure of the vein to the high arterial pressure causes it to dilate and increase its blood flow. To be used reproducibly for dialysis, a fistula must have a large enough diameter to be safely cannulated with large-bore dialysis needles and a sufficiently high-access blood flow to permit a blood flow rate of 350 mL/min or more. It also must be superficial enough for the landmarks to be easily appreciated by the dialysis staff performing the cannulation. Increases in blood flow and draining vein diameter occur fairly rapidly following AV fistula creation. Whereas blood flow in a normal radial artery is only 20 to 40 mL/min, it increases more than 10-fold within a few weeks of fistula creation. In one study, the mean access blood flow in successful AV fistulas was 634 mL/min 2 weeks postoperatively[131]; in a second study, it was 650 mL/min 12 weeks following AV fistula creation.[132] Moreover, the mean access blood flows and AV fistula diameters are not significantly different in the second, third, and fourth months following AV fistula creation.[133] This implies that determination of whether a new AV fistula is likely to be used successfully for dialysis should be possible within 4 to 6 weeks of the initial surgery.

In some patients, maturation of the AV fistula can be easily assessed by clinical evaluation by the nephrologist, surgeon, or an experienced dialysis nurse. In less straightforward cases, duplex ultrasonography may be useful in predicting whether a new AV fistula can be used successfully for hemodialysis. One pilot study used a combination of two simple sonographic criteria to assess AV fistula maturation, AV fistula diameter and access blood flow.[133] When the sonogram documented a draining vein diameter of 4 mm or more and an access blood flow of 500 mL/min or more, 95% of the AV fistulas were subsequently usable for dialysis. In contrast, when neither criterion was met, only 33% of the AV fistulas achieved adequacy for dialysis. The likelihood of AV fistula adequacy for dialysis was intermediate (~70%) when only one of the two criteria was met.

Failure of an AV fistula to mature can be related to one of several anatomic defects, which can be identified by sonography or angiography.[134] Stenosis at the anastomosis or in the draining vein is one such problem. Another possibility is that the draining vein has one or more large side branches. With these tributary veins, the arterial blood flow is distributed among two or more competing veins, thereby limiting the increase in blood flow in each vein. A third scenario may be observed in obese patients, in whom the fistula has adequate caliber and blood flow but is simply too deep to be cannulated safely by the dialysis staff. In most patients, these anatomic problems can be corrected by radiologic or surgical intervention. Stenotic lesions can be treated by angioplasty or surgical revision. Superficial side branches can be ligated by a suture through the skin; deeper branches can be embolized. Finally, the surgeon can superficialize fistulas that are too deep to be cannulated safely.

In immature AV fistulas with one or more of these anatomic lesions, specific interventions to correct the underlying lesion may promote subsequent AV fistula maturation. Several published series have evaluated the ability to salvage immature AV fistulas to those that are subsequently usable for dialysis. A number of studies using only radiographic procedures (e.g., angioplasty of stenotic lesions, obliteration of side branches) in immature AV fistulas have had a high success rate (Table 70.10).[124,135-139] An initial salvage (ability to use the AV fistula for dialysis) was accomplished in 80% to 90% of patients, with a subsequent 1-year primary patency of 39% to 75%. In another study using a combination of radiologic and surgical salvage procedures in an unselected dialysis population, the salvage rate was more modest, at 44%.[129] Of interest, the frequency of a salvage procedure for immature AV fistulas in that study was twice as high in women than in men. A retrospective study has found that immature AV fistulas with an anatomic abnormality that was corrected percutaneously or surgically are much more likely to achieve suitability for dialysis, as compared with similar fistulas that did not undergo a salvage procedure.[140] A novel approach to enhance AV fistula maturation, balloon-assisted maturation (BAM), has been

Table 70.10 Effect of Salvage Procedures on Immature Fistulas

Reference	No. of Patients	Type of Intervention	No. Usable for Dialysis (%)	Primary Patency at 1 yr
Beathard et al, 1999[135]	63	PTA, vein ligation	82	75
Turmel-Rodrigues et al, 2001[137]	69	PTA, vein ligation	97	39
Miller et al, 2003[129]	41	PTA, vein ligation, surgical revision	44	N/A
Beathard et al, 2003[136]	100	PTA, vein ligation	92	68
Asif et al, 2005[124]	24	PTA, vein ligation	92	N/A
Nassar et al, 2006[138]	119	PTA, vein ligation	83	65
Singh et al, 2008[140]	32	PTA, vein ligation, surgical revision	78	NA
Han et al, 2013[139]	141	PTA	87	72

N/A, Not available; PTA, percutaneous transluminal angioplasty.

described.[141] In this procedure, repeated long-segment angioplasty procedures are used to dilate the perianastomotic venous segment sequentially, converting it at times into a collagen tube.[141] Other recent articles have described the use of intraoperative primary balloon angioplasty at the time of surgery, with or without BAM, which could allow for AV fistulas to be created in patients with small arteries and veins (artery <2 mm; vein <2.5 mm).[142,143] None of these studies evaluated their techniques with a control group, and all suggested that a large number of postmaturation angioplasties are needed to maintain patency.

In summary, aggressive percutaneous or surgical interventions are worthwhile because they can often convert immature AV fistulas to those that are suitable for dialysis. However, there are no randomized studies comparing different types of interventions or different timing of interventions in terms of their effect on AV fistula maturation. Finally, a recent study has observed that immature AV fistulas requiring two or more interventions to achieve maturity have significantly shorter cumulative patency and require more interventions to maintain patency as compared with AV fistulas achieving maturation with no or one intervention(s) (Figure 70.13).[144]

TECHNICAL PROCEDURE: SALVAGE OF IMMATURE ARTERIOVENOUS FISTULAS

Angioplasty of Stenotic Lesions

The stenosis at the juxta-arterial anastomosis can be treated with sequential balloon dilations. This requires two to five treatments until the size of the anastomosis is appropriate. Long segments of stenotic lesions at the level of the most proximal part of the venous outlet near the anastomosis are amenable to balloon angioplasty and sometimes may require several follow-up interventions.

Immature AV fistulas are by definition small and could be difficult to access; therefore, it is best if evaluation can be done with high-resolution sonographic guidance to avoid several stick, extravasation, and vein damage. The AV fistula is initially accessed at its most proximal portion with a 21-gauge micropuncture needle. A Cope mandril wire is passed into the venous circulation, and a 4-Fr catheter sheath is exchanged for the needle. Subtracted digital angiograms of the venous outlet and central circulation and a reflux retrograde arteriogram are obtained. Once the lesion is identified, the proper technique is selected. This initial fistulogram could be skipped altogether if reliable information is obtained from a surveillance sonogram indicating the presence of a stenosis near or at the arterial anastomosis.

If the lesion is at the juxta-arterial anastomosis, a second access is achieved by inserting a micropuncture needle from the most distal portion of the AV fistula toward the AV anastomosis. The needle is exchanged for a 5-Fr catheter sheath; a wire (0.014 to 0.018 inch) is passed into the AV fistula and through the arterial anastomosis into the arterial circulation. An arteriogram of the arteriovenous anastomosis is obtained, and the stenotic lesion is evaluated and graded. Depending on the severity of the stenosis, a balloon is selected that is 2 to 6 mm in diameter and 10 to 40 mm in length. The balloon is introduced into the stenotic lesion and inflated carefully up to its nominal pressure. Subsequent angiograms are performed for a postangioplasty grading of the lesion (Figure 70.14). Intrafistular and systemic pressures are taken before and after the angioplasty, and the corresponding ratios are calculated. At UAB, patients are brought back to the intervention suite 2 to 4 weeks later for a second-look angiogram of the AV fistula.

If the lesion is located in the proximal part of the AV fistula or at the central vessels, the initial venous access is appropriate. The initial 4-Fr catheter is exchanged for a 4- to 6-Fr sheath, and a guidewire is passed into the central venous circulation. The balloon is selected depending on the severity of the lesion and its location. Sizes can be from 4 to 8 mm in the peripheral venous circulation and up to 14 mm in the central circulation. Once the angioplasty is completed, digitally subtracted angiograms are obtained for postangioplasty grading of the lesion. Intrafistular and systemic pressures are measured. Patients are followed at their local dialysis center and, if the AV fistula does not mature or the nursing personnel are still having problems cannulating the AV fistula, a second-look angiogram of the AV fistula is indicated.

Ligation of Accessory Veins

Accessory veins can be treated by surgical ligation or endovascular coil deployment. Treatment of these lesions requires a well-trained interventionist because of the difficult technical approach to these lesions. Accessory veins are treated depending on their size, location, and number (Figure 70.15). Some interventionists advocate percutaneous ligation of superficial accessory veins at the time of the initial angiography of the AV fistula.[145] If the accessory vein is deep and has a good lumen size, surgical ligation is indicated. If

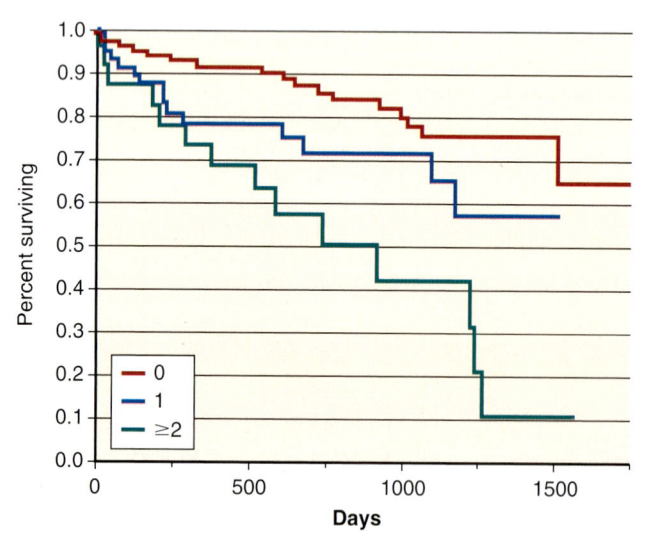

Figure 70.13 Interventions to promote AV fistula maturation. Cumulative survival, defined from the time of access cannulation to permanent failure, is shorter in patients receiving two or more interventions before AVF maturation compared with those with zero interventions (hazard ratio [HR], 2.07; 95% confidence interval [CI], 1.21 to 2.94; $P = 0.0001$). (From Lee T, Ullah A, Allon M, et al: Decreased cumulative access survival in arteriovenous fistulas requiring interventions to promote maturation. *Clin J Am Soc Nephrol* 6:575-581, 2011, with permission from the American Society of Nephrology.)

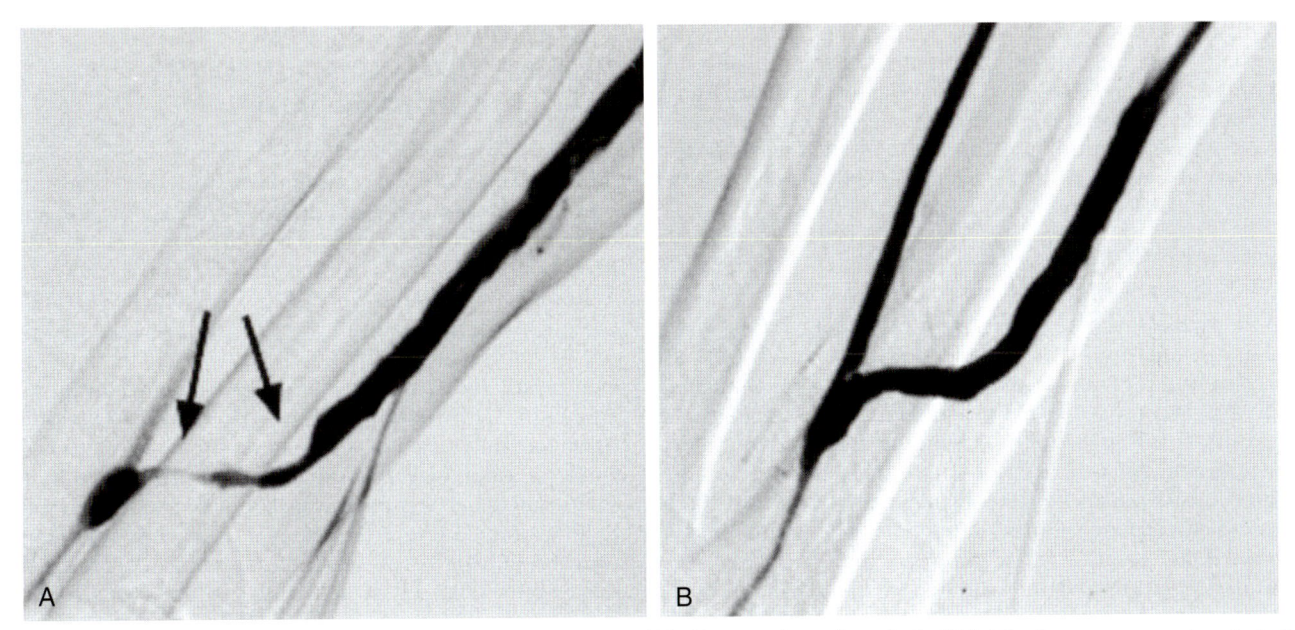

Figure 70.14 **A,** Fistula salvage. This digital subtraction angiography (DSA) image of a radiocephalic AV fistula shows a severe stenotic lesion at the level of the juxta-arterial anastomosis *(arrows)*. **B,** Fistula salvage. This postangioplasty DSA image of a radiocephalic fistula shows radiologic improvement of the stenotic lesion at the level of the juxta-arterial anastomosis.

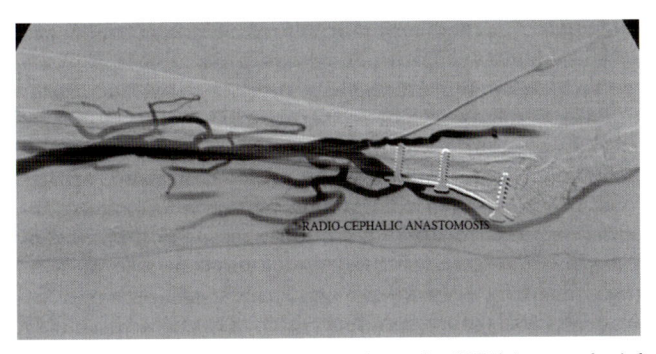

Figure 70.15 Digital subtraction angiography (DSA) image of a left radiocephalic AV fistula showing multiple collaterals. There is a metallic plate from a prior open reduction and internal fixation of a radius bone fracture.

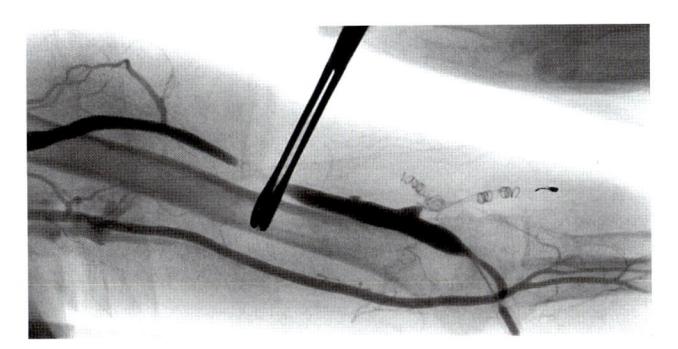

Figure 70.16 Coil deployed in a collateral vein of an upper arm arteriovenous fistula.

Table 70.11 Primary Patency after Elective Angioplasty: Fistulas versus Grafts

Reference	Primary Access Patency at 6 mo (%)	
	Grafts	Fistulas
Safa et al, 1996[60]	43	47
Turmel-Rodrigues et al, 2000[150]	53	67
McCarley et al, 2001[74]	37	34
Van der Linden et al, 2002[146]	25	50
Maya et al, 2004[57]	52	55

the accessory vein is deep but has a small lumen size, a coil deployment should be considered (Figure 70.16).

The AV fistula is accessed and, depending on its size, an appropriate sheath is introduced. A selective catheter is introduced in each accessory vein, and an appropriate-sized coil is deployed. A final angiogram of the AV fistula is taken to ascertain proper coil deployment and occlusion of all collateral veins.

PERCUTANEOUS TRANSLUMINAL ANGIOPLASTY OF ARTERIOVENOUS FISTULAS

Although the frequency of interventions is several-fold lower in AV fistulas than grafts,[9] fistulas are also susceptible to developing stenosis and thrombosis. Most studies have documented a comparable primary patency of fistulas and grafts following elective PTA (Table 70.11), although one study observed a higher primary patency in fistulas.[146] As is the case with angioplasty of grafts, the primary patency of AV fistulas following PTA is inversely related to the magnitude of postangioplasty stenosis, as well as the magnitude of the postangioplasty intra-access-to-systemic pressure ratio.[57] It should be noted that highly matured and developed AV fistulas dilate and elongate significantly over the years, forming aneurysmal dilation. With fixed points at the wrist and elbow or elbow and shoulder, they become tortuous, and significant kinks develop at certain points between dilated segments at certain intervals, which appear as significant stenoses. Many of these are not flow-limiting; however, some are truly flow-limiting but are unlikely to respond to PTA and may require surgical intervention. Age, race, presence of diabetes mellitus or peripheral vascular disease, access location, and number of stenotic sites have not been associated with the likelihood of vascular access patency after PTA.[57]

TECHNICAL PROCEDURE: ANGIOPLASTY OF ARTERIOVENOUS FISTULAS

The AV fistula is accessed at its most proximal portion with a 21-gauge micropuncture needle. A Cope mandril wire is passed into the venous circulation. The needle is exchanged for a 4-Fr catheter. An initial digitally subtracted angiogram of the AV fistula is obtained, including the venous outlet and central circulation. Lesions with more than 50% stenosis are considered to be hemodynamically significant and undergo angioplasty. Once the stenotic lesion has been identified and graded, a guidewire is introduced to the central circulation and the catheter exchanged for a 6-Fr catheter sheath. An angioplasty balloon is introduced through the catheter sheath. Balloon sizes vary, depending on the vessel to be treated. The balloon is placed at the level of the stenotic lesion and inflated to its nominal pressure for 30 to 90 seconds. High pressures (>20 atm) are frequently needed in AV fistulas.[99] A final digitally subtracted angiogram is obtained to assess for residual stenosis and further treatment of the stenotic lesion (Figure 70.17). The patient's intrafistular pressure and systemic pressure are measured before and immediately after the intervention, and a reduction in the intrafistular-to-systemic pressure ratio is used to confirm hemodynamic improvement.

The major complications of this procedure are vessel extravasations and rupture of the vessel after the angioplasty (Figure 70.18). Deploying a covered stent can treat these complications. Surgical repair is indicated if the rupture is not corrected by stent placement.

PERCUTANEOUS MECHANICAL THROMBECTOMY AND THROMBOLYSIS OF ARTERIOVENOUS FISTULAS

Dealing with thrombosed AV fistulas is one of the most challenging aspects in interventional nephrology.[147] Thrombectomy of aneurysmally dilated AV fistulas is the most technically difficult. The most common cause of fistula thrombosis is an underlying stenotic lesion in the venous outflow circulation (peripherally or centrally). Less common causes include needle infiltration,[148] excessive manual pressure for hemostasis at the needle insertion site, and severe and prolonged hypotension. Successful restoration of patency in a thrombosed AV fistula requires expeditious thrombectomy. Several series have reported on the outcomes of radiologic thrombectomy of AV fistulas.[147,149-156] The immediate technical success has been fairly high, ranging from 73% to 93%. The primary patency of these AV fistulas following thrombectomy has ranged from 27% to 81% at 6 months and 18% to 70% at 1 year (Table 70.12). In one study, the primary patency following thrombectomy was lower in upper arm AV fistulas as compared to those in the forearm.[150] However, with additional interventions, the secondary patency of these AV fistulas has been 44% to 93% at 1 year. A recent study over a 2-year period evaluated 140 consecutive patients with thrombosed immature AV fistulas who underwent attempts at salvage via thrombectomy procedures.[157] All AV fistulas had thrombosed following access creation and had never been used for hemodialysis. Thrombectomy was successful in 119 immature clotted AV fistulas (85%), and hemodialysis adequacy was achieved in 111 AV fistulas (79%). The average maturation time from thrombectomy to cannulation for dialysis was 46.4 days, with an average of 2.64 interventions per patient. There were five cases of angioplasty-induced rupture (3.5%), all of which were treated with stent placement. Clinically significant pseudoaneurysm formation occurred in four patients

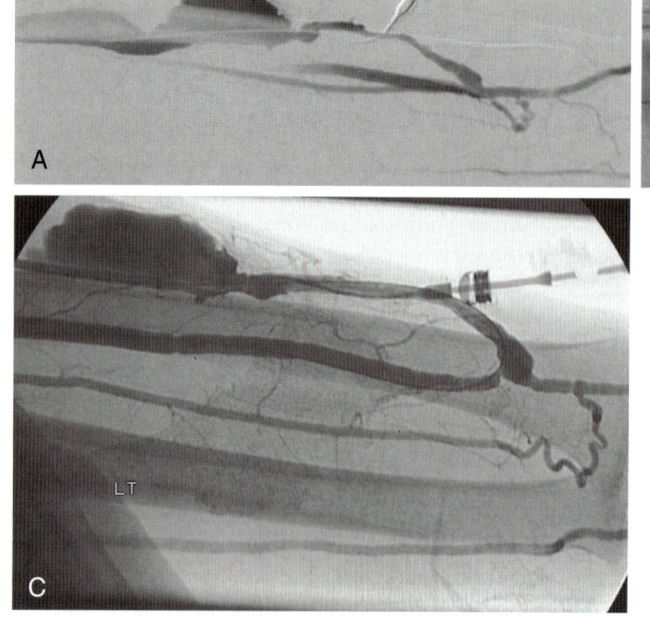

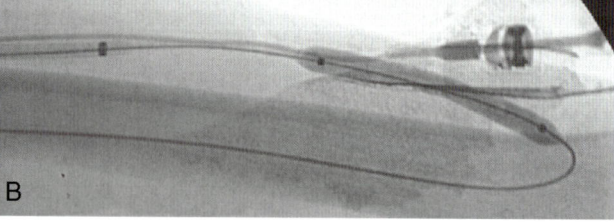

Figure 70.17 **A,** Digital subtraction angiography (DSA) image of a left radiocephalic AV fistula showing a long severe segment of stenosis distal to the arterial anastomosis, followed by a pseudoaneurysm of the fistula. **B,** Spot film of a left radiocephalic AV fistula showing the segment of stenosis being angioplastied. **C,** Postangioplasty DSA image showing a successful treatment. The pseudoaneurysm is unchanged.

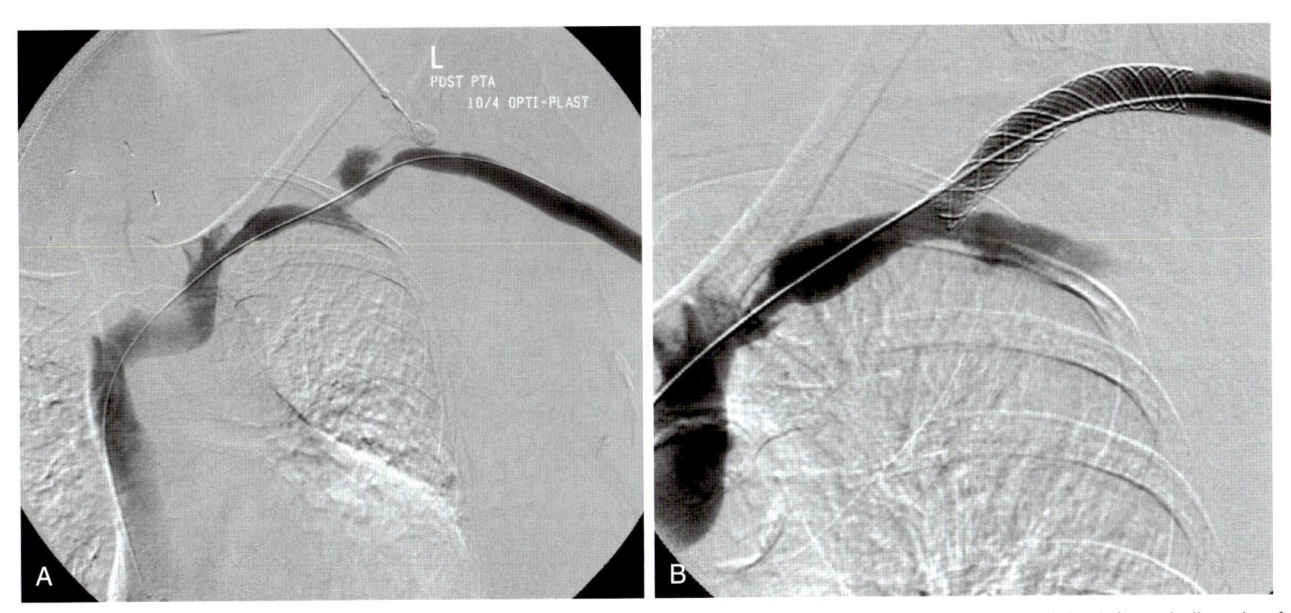

Figure 70.18 **A,** Angioplasty complication. This digital subtraction angiography (DSA) image shows a rupture of the left cephalic vein after aggressive percutaneous transluminal angioplasty. There is a coexisting stenosis of the left subclavian. **B,** Angioplasty complication. This DSA image shows salvage and correction of the complication by deploying a covered stent (wall graft).

Table 70.12 Primary Fistula Patency after Thrombectomy*

Reference	No. of Procedures	Primary Patency at 6 mo	Primary Patency at 12 mo
Haage et al, 2000[149]	54		27
Turmel-Rodrigues et al, 2000[150]	54 forearm	74	47
	9 upper arm	27	27
Rajan et al, 2002[154]	30	28	24
Liang et al, 2002[153]	42	81	70
Shatsky et al, 2005[155]	44	38	18
Jain et al, 2008[156]	41	20	—
Miller et al, 2011[157]	140	—	59

*Series with fewer than 25 procedures not included.

(2.8%). At 12 months, secondary access patency of salvaged accesses was 90%. Considering that the alternative would be to abandon the thrombosed fistula and proceed with placement of a new AV fistula, concerted efforts to salvage thrombosed AV fistulas are extremely worthwhile.

TECHNICAL PROCEDURE: PERCUTANEOUS THROMBECTOMY OF ARTERIOVENOUS FISTULAS

Although more challenging than graft thrombectomy, AV fistulas can also be declotted successfully. There are few contraindications, including concurrent infection, fistula immaturity, and very large aneurysms. The technical challenges include difficulty in the initial cannulation of a thrombosed fistula, complete removal of large thrombi, and successful treatment of recalcitrant stenotic lesions.

The AV fistula is accessed at its most distal portion toward the arterial anastomosis with an 18-gauge needle, either blind or by guided ultrasonography. A guidewire is introduced, and a catheter is placed over the guidewire. A thrombolytic agent, 2 to 4 mg of tissue plasminogen activator (t-PA, Alteplase), is infused and left to dwell in the AV fistula for 1 hour. The patient is taken back to the intervention suite, the guidewire is reinserted into the arterial circulation, and the catheter is replaced with a conventional 6-Fr sheath. A percutaneous thrombectomy over-the-wire device can be used (e.g., Angiojet). After a successful thrombolysis of the AV fistula, a Fogarty balloon is passed beyond the arterial anastomosis and pulled back to dislodge the plugging clot. Once the thrombus is cleared and blood flow re-established, a digitally subtracted angiogram of the AV fistula is taken to evaluate for stenotic lesions along the venous outlet track or central circulation. If a lesion is encountered in the upstream or central circulation, a second access is placed, and the lesion is angioplastied.

Manual aspiration without the use of thrombolytic agents is another approach. A sheath is placed to gain access to the venous outflow. A guide catheter with a large lumen is introduced through the sheath. The aspiration is performed with a 50-mL syringe connected to the guide catheter while the catheter is removed with back-and-forth movements. The contents of the syringe are flushed, and the aspiration maneuver is repeated several times to remove all the thrombus. A second sheath is introduced toward the arterial anastomosis, and the same aspiration technique is performed to aspirate the rest of the thrombus located between the introducer and anastomosis. A Fogarty balloon is passed beyond the arterial anastomosis and pulled back to dislodge the arterial plug clot. Digitally subtracted anterograde angiograms of the AV fistula are obtained to assess for patency and look for stenotic lesions. Angioplasty of any hemodynamically stenotic lesion in the vascular access circuit is performed. A final digitally subtracted angiogram of the AV fistula is obtained and the patient's intra-access and systemic pressures are measured before and immediately after the intervention. The pressure ratio is calculated to confirm improvement in blood flow, as noted earlier.

The major complications of this procedure are vessel extravasations and rupture of the vessel after the angioplasty. Pulmonary embolism is generally of greater concern with AV fistula thrombectomy as compared with AV graft thrombectomy due to the larger volume of thrombus. Finally, arterial emboli distal to the AV anastomosis may occur with higher frequency than for AV grafts.

NOVEL TECHNIQUES FOR TREATMENT OF SEVERE STENOTIC LESIONS

CUTTING BALLOON

Despite the use of angioplasty with high-pressure balloons and prolonged inflations, some lesions remain severely stenotic. The use of cutting balloons has been advocated as a tool to treat these lesions by creating a controlled rupture of the vessel wall. The cutting balloon catheter is a balloon with four blades arranged along the balloon. When the balloon is inflated, it exposes the blades to the offending lesion; this will create a controlled rupture of the intima or hyperplastic fibrous tissue. A regular angioplasty balloon can be used afterward to shape the vessel and expand it to the desired diameter. It has been used in lesions at all levels, from intragraft to central lesions. Preliminary reports have suggested that cutting balloons may result in superior outcomes as compared with conventional angioplasty.[158,159] In one series of nine patients, grafts with a high-grade venous anastomosis stenosis were treated with a cutting balloon plus stent deployment.[158] The patients maintained a functional graft during short-term follow-up (up to 20 months in one patient). However, a multicenter randomized clinical trial comparing use of the cutting balloon with conventional angioplasty for treatment of AV graft stenosis observed no advantage to use of the cutting balloon. The primary patency at 6 months was 48% in grafts treated with a cutting balloon as compared with 40% for AV grafts treated with angioplasty. Device-related complications occurred in 5% of the patients in the cutting balloon group (primarily vein rupture or dissection) as compared with none of the patients whose AV grafts were treated with angioplasty alone.[160] The considerable additional cost of cutting balloons is substantial and precludes their routine use.

CRYOPLASTY BALLOON

Cryotherapy with the cryoballoon is a novel therapy for patients with intractable stenoses at the venous anastomosis of AV grafts. This technique uses cold temperatures at the balloon site to cause apoptosis of the intima layer. Rifkin and coworkers reported the outcomes of five patients with recurrent stenotic lesions at the venous anastomosis who were treated with the cryoballoon. The primary patency increased from 3 weeks after angioplasty alone to more than 16 weeks after cryoplasty.[161] There have been no published randomized trials comparing the outcomes of AV graft stenosis treated with cryoplasty compared with angioplasty alone.

LOCAL PERIVASCULAR MODALITIES

Some investigations have evaluated prophylaxis of access stenosis in animal models by using local perivascular drug delivery to the site of neointimal hyperplasia. Antiproliferative drugs are injected locally during access creation or introduced by DESs or wraps. These novel pharmacologic therapies remain investigational, but offer promise for the future. Detailed discussion of these potential therapies is beyond the scope of this chapter, but this topic has been reviewed.[27,97]

CENTRAL VEIN STENOSIS

Central vein stenosis is a frequent occurrence in patients on hemodialysis.[13,162] Acute or chronic trauma of the central vessels by temporary or permanent dialysis catheters is the major cause.[163] Stenosis leads to impairment of venous return on the ipsilateral extremity and, in turn, might result in malfunction or thrombosis of the vascular access. Although it may be asymptomatic, patients with central vein stenosis usually present with ipsilateral upper extremity edema. In some patients, a previously unappreciated central vein stenosis becomes evident clinically following the creation of an ipsilateral AV fistula or graft. The diagnosis can be confirmed by angiography, ultrasonography, or MRV.

The most commonly encountered location of central vein stenosis is at the junction of the cephalic vein with the subclavian vein (not catheter injury–related). Other central veins that may be affected (often related to injury from a previous catheter injury) include the subclavian vein, brachiocephalic vein, and superior vena cava (Figure 70.19). In patients with tunneled femoral catheters, central vein

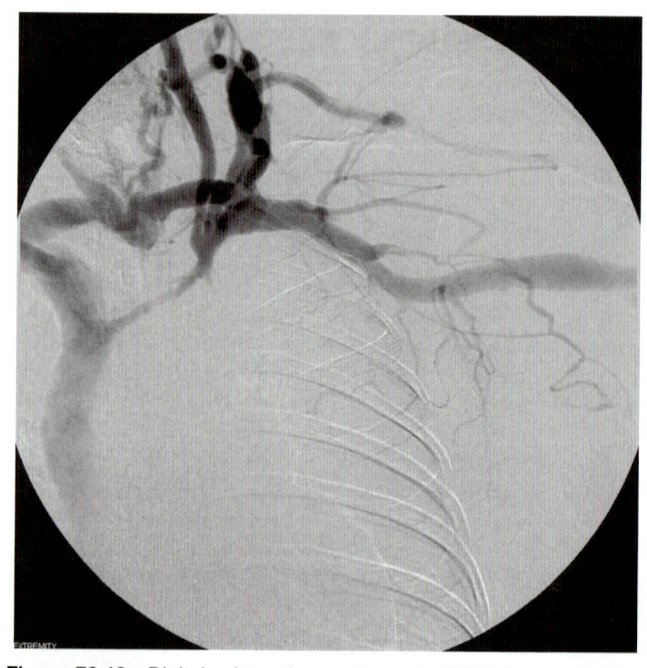

Figure 70.19 Digital subtraction angiography (DSA) image showing a severe stenosis of the left innominate vein. There are multiple ipsilateral and across the neck collaterals draining into a normal right innominate vein.

stenosis may occur in the external iliac vein, common iliac vein, or inferior vena cava (Figure 70.20), resulting in ipsilateral lower extremity edema. The stenotic lesion is an aggressive neointimal proliferation or there is clot and fibrin sheath formation around indwelling dialysis catheters that is organized and incorporated into the vessel wall.

These may progress over time to complete occlusion of the venous circulation (Figure 70.21). If left untreated, central vein stenosis will cause increased retrograde pressure and formation of venous collaterals (Figure 70.22). In some patients, the collaterals are sufficiently well developed to permit adequate venous drainage, which prevents the formation of edema (Figure 70.23).

The treatment of choice of symptomatic central vein stenosis is PTA of the stenotic lesion.[77,164-170] Unfortunately, the long-term success of PTA of central venous stenosis is poor because of a combination of elastic recoil and aggressive neointimal hyperplasia. In one study, the primary patency was substantially shorter after angioplasty of a central vein stenosis as compared to stenoses at more peripheral

Figure 70.20 Digital subtraction angiography (DSA) image showing a severe stenosis of the intrahepatic portion of the inferior vena cava with some intrahepatic collaterals.

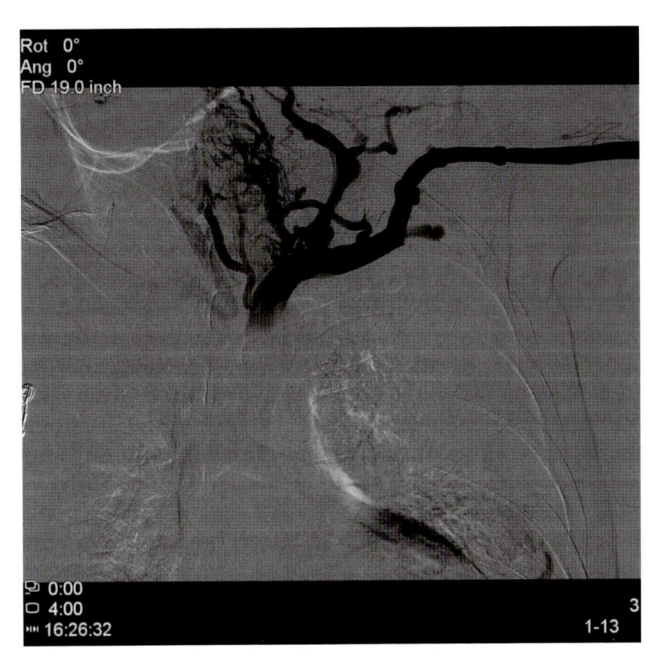

Figure 70.21 Digital subtraction angiography (DSA) image showing a complete occlusion of the left innominate vein.

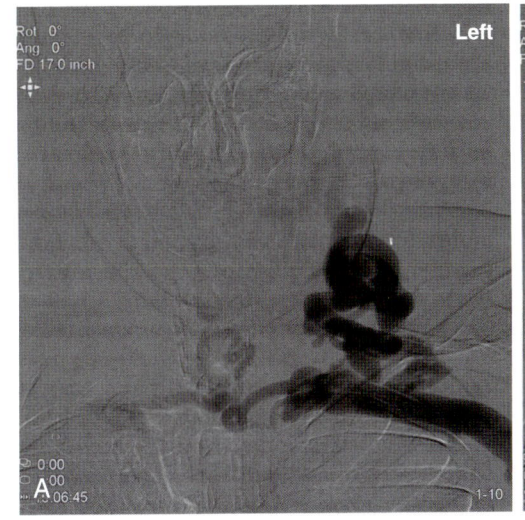

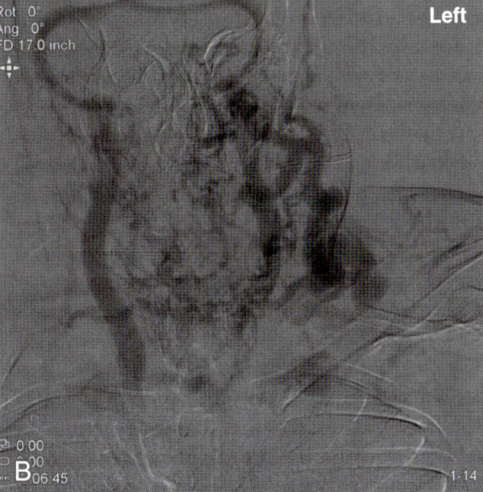

Figure 70.22 **A,** Digital subtraction angiography (DSA) image showing complete occlusion of the left innominate vein, with severe enlargement of the left internal jugular, and multiple ipsilateral and across the neck collaterals draining into a normal right innominate vein. **B,** DSA image of the same patient showing the drainage of the left internal jugular to the right internal jugular across the cavernous veins.

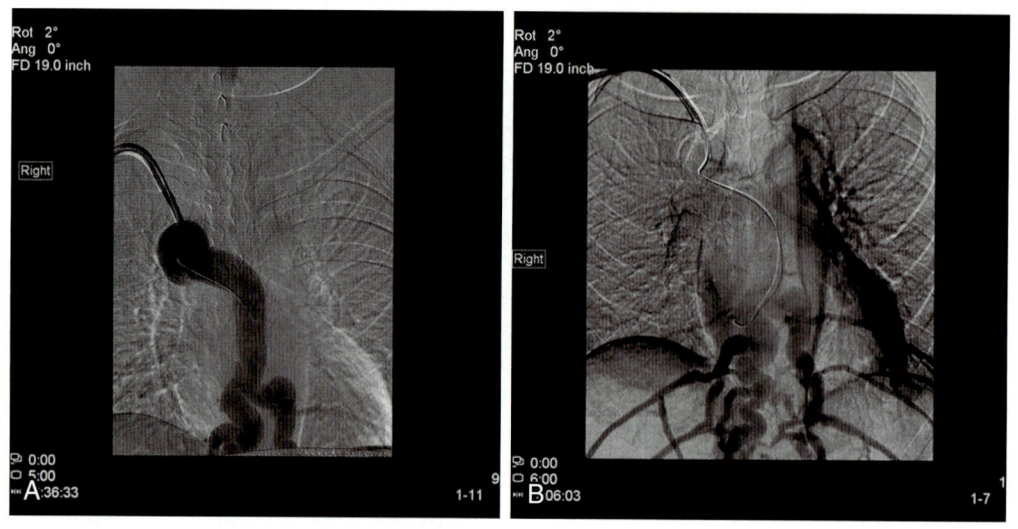

Figure 70.23 **A,** Digital subtraction angiography (DSA) image showing complete occlusion of the superior vena cava, with severe augmentation of the azygos vein. **B,** DSA image of the same patient showing the drainage of the azygos vein into the lumbar and intercostal vein.

locations.[58] As a result, patients with central vein stenosis may require multiple angioplasties to treat recurrent lesions.

Stent placement has been attempted in the management of refractory central vein stenosis caused by elastic recoil (Figure 70.24). Several small series have reported the outcomes of stent placement for refractory central venous stenotic lesions. These studies have been limited by their retrospective study design, small numbers of patients, and absence of a control group. In two uncontrolled series, the primary patency following stent deployment for central vein stenosis was 42% to 50% at 6 months and only 14% to 17% at 1 year.[77,164] Although there have been no published randomized studies comparing stent deployment with angioplasty of central vein stenosis, the primary patency using stents appears no better than that achieved with angioplasty alone.[171] In patients with ipsilateral vascular access and persistent upper extremity edema despite attempted angioplasty, the only recourse may be ligation of the vascular access, creation or placement of a contralateral arteriovenous access, transition to peritoneal dialysis, or urgent kidney transplantation.

ACCESS-INDUCED HAND ISCHEMIA

The clinical manifestations of access-induced hand ischemia can vary widely, ranging from mild (hand pain) to severe (tissue necrosis, with loss of digits). Vascular accesses have a normal retrograde blood flow, which does not cause hand ischemia. There are three recognized mechanisms for access-induced hand ischemia: (1) true arterial steal (with complete retrograde blood flow toward the graft or fistula); (2) arterial stenosis distal to the arterial anastomosis; and (3) generalized arterial calcification (usually seen in patients with diabetes mellitus), with distal digital occlusions (Figure 70.25). Because all three mechanisms may coexist in a single patient, *distal hypoperfusion ischemic syndrome* is the preferred term.[172] Other causes of hand pain, such as carpal tunnel syndrome, arthropathies, diabetic neuropathy, ischemic monomelic neuropathy, and reflex sympathetic dystrophy syndrome, should be excluded before making a definitive diagnosis of vascular access–induced hand ischemia.

Physical examination is the most important tool to diagnose access-induced hand ischemia. Pale cold digits during and between hemodialysis sessions are seen in almost 90% of cases. There are several additional diagnostic tools, including digital brachial index measurement, digital plethysmography, duplex ultrasonography, and transcutaneous oxygen saturation. If these noninvasive tests are suggestive of access-induced hand ischemia, a complete angiogram of the vascular access, including the feeding artery, should be obtained.

Management of access-induced hand ischemia is directed at alleviating the underlying cause. Treatment options range from angioplasty of the stenosis distal to the anastomosis to ligation of the vascular access. Other interventions that have been successful in relieving the ischemia while maintaining patency of the AV fistula include banding or plication of the AV fistula, graft interposition, and distal revascularization with interval ligation (DRIL).[173]

INDWELLING HEMODIALYSIS CATHETERS

NONTUNNELED TEMPORARY HEMODIALYSIS CATHETERS

Temporary hemodialysis catheters are indicated for acute dialysis treatments. They are made of polyurethane, polyethylene, or PTFE, have a double lumen, and are semirigid and relatively easy to place in the internal jugular (preferably on the right side), femoral and, rarely, subclavian veins. Each site has its advantages and disadvantages, but if they are placed in the femoral vein, the catheter should not be left for longer than 72 hours, and the internal jugular vein catheters not longer than 1 week, because of the high risk of bacteremia with longer dwell times.[174] The subclavian vein is generally used only if there is no other access available because it is more difficult and a higher risk stick (pneumothorax); also, there is increased risk for central

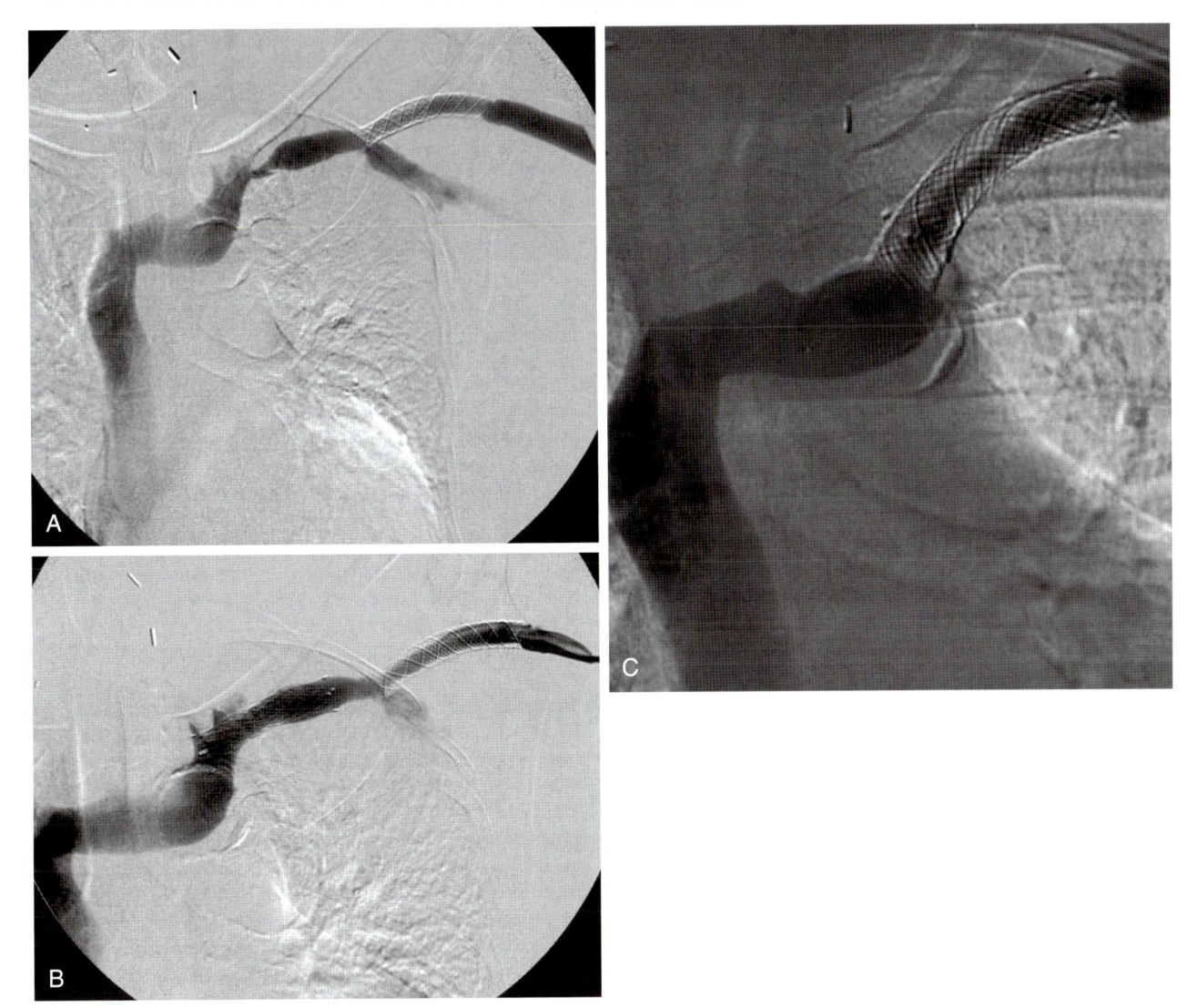

Figure 70.24 **A,** Digital subtraction angiography (DSA) image showing a severe stenotic lesion of the left subclavian vein. There is also a stent in the left cephalic vein. **B,** DSA image showing a stent deployed at the severe stenotic lesion of the left subclavian vein, with excellent initial results. **C,** DSA image taken 12 months after the initial placement of a stent in the left subclavian vein showing intrastent stenosis due to significant myointimal hyperplasia.

venous stenosis and occlusion of the central vessels, which can compromise creation or placement of future AV fistulas or grafts.[163] If the upper vessels are used, the catheter should be long enough to have its tip at the junction of the right atrium and superior vena cava; if the femoral vein is used, the catheter's tip should be located in the inferior vena cava. If the patient is expected to remain catheter-dependent for a longer period, a tunneled catheter should be placed. Temporary hemodialysis catheters can be placed blindly or by sonographic or fluoroscopic guidance. A chest radiograph should always be obtained immediately following placement of a central vein dialysis catheter in the chest before hemodialysis is initiated; it is not needed after placement of a femoral dialysis catheter.

TECHNICAL PROCEDURE: INSERTION OF TEMPORARY DIALYSIS CATHETERS

The procedure is usually performed at the patient's bedside, but occasionally done in the interventional suite. Strict sterile technique and use of local anesthesia are indicated. Access to the femoral or internal jugular vein may be done blindly or by real-time ultrasound guidance. Real-time ultrasonography is highly recommended because it decreases the number of attempts at vein cannulation and minimizes the risk of inadvertent arterial cannulation. An 18-gauge needle is generally used for initial access to the vein. Once the vein has been cannulated, a J-wire is introduced through the needle and advanced into the venous circulation. The needle is exchanged for a series of dilators and a temporary dialysis catheter (13 to 20 cm in length) is introduced and sutured in place. The lumens are flushed and generally filled with heparin or another lock solution.

Potential complications at the time of placement at the upper vessels include pneumothorax, vein or arterial perforation, mediastinal or pericardial perforation (with the possibility of hemothorax and cardiac tamponade), air embolism, and local hematoma, with possible extension into the soft subcutaneous tissue of the neck and external

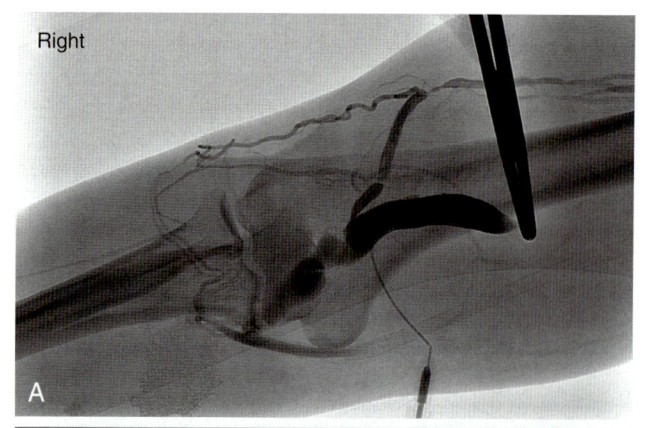

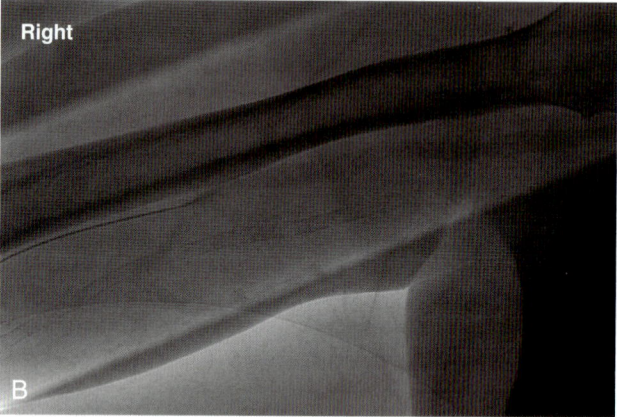

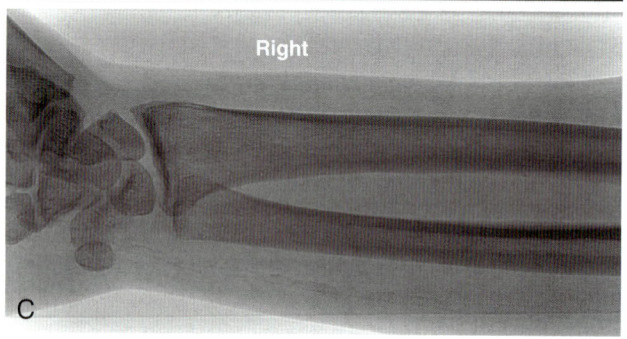

Figure 70.25 **A,** Angiogram of a right upper arm fistula demonstrating an arterial steal syndrome in a patient with generalized arterial disease. **B,** Spot film of the same patient showing a calcified brachial artery. **C,** Spot film of the same patient showing a calcified ulnar artery.

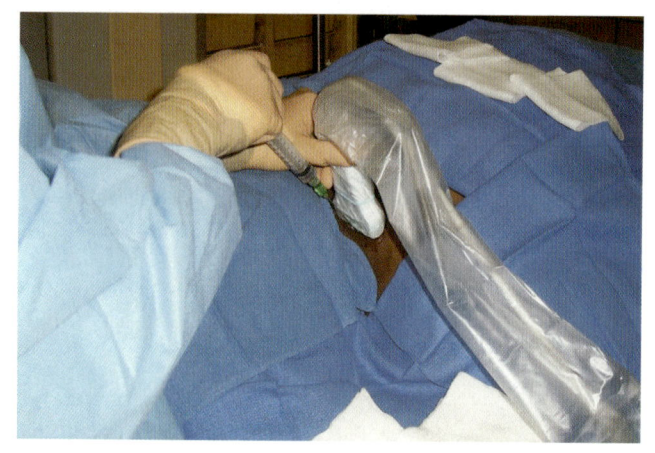

Figure 70.26 Access to the right internal jugular vein guided by real-time ultrasonography.

obstruction of the airways. Long-term complications include development of stenotic lesions along the trajectory of the catheter, which may preclude the use of the ipsilateral limb for future creation of a vascular access. If the patient already has a documented stenotic lesion of the central vessels, placement of an indwelling catheter may cause life-threatening acute central vessel occlusion. Exit site infections and catheter-related bacteremia are frequent complications of temporary dialysis catheters. Development of catheter-related bacteremia requires the institution of systemic antibiotics and removal of the nontunneled dialysis catheter.

The complications at the femoral site are less dramatic, but vein or arterial perforation and formation of an AV fistula are possible. Deep vein thrombosis (related to the catheter itself or to immobilization related to prescribed bed rest), local hematomas, exit site infections, and bacteremia are other important complications.

TUNNELED HEMODIALYSIS CATHETERS

Tunneled hemodialysis catheters are also commonly used for temporary vascular access in patients waiting for maturation of a permanent vascular (AV fistula or graft). They are also required for long-term access in patients who have exhausted the options for placement of a permanent access in all four extremities. Tunneled dialysis catheters are usually placed in a central vein in the chest, usually through the internal jugular vein and rarely in the subclavian vein. They have the same characteristics as temporary catheters, but are longer and have a Dacron cuff located in the tunneled portion of the catheter in the subcutaneous tissue. An inflammatory response around the cuff results in scar tissue, creating a mechanical barrier that prevents the introduction of infection from the exit site into the bloodstream. As a result, the frequency of catheter-related bacteremia is lower with tunneled dialysis catheters as compared with acute nontunneled catheters.[175,176]

TECHNICAL PROCEDURE: INSERTION OF TUNNELED HEMODIALYSIS CATHETERS

Strict sterile technique, topical local anesthesia (1% lidocaine [Xylocaine]), and conscious sedation are used. Access to the internal jugular vein is guided by real-time ultrasonography (Figure 70.26). A 21-gauge micropuncture needle is used for access. Once the vein has been cannulated, a 0.018-inch guidewire is introduced through the needle and advanced under fluoroscopic guidance. The needle is removed and exchanged for a 4-Fr catheter. The guidewire and inner dilator are removed, and a stiff 0.035-inch wire is passed through the catheter, down into the inferior vena cava (IVC), under fluoroscopic guidance. A skin pocket of about 1 cm is created at this location. The permanent indwelling hemodialysis catheter is attached to a tunneler device and a tunnel is created laterally, down and approximately 5 to 7 cm from the initial needle insertion. The catheter is pulled through and buried under the skin (Figure 70.27). At this point, the tunneler device is

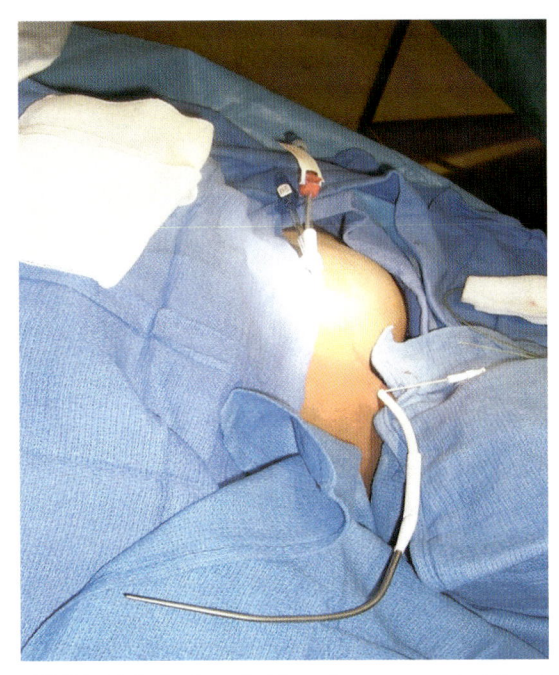

Figure 70.27 Catheter tunneled from the upper part of the chest to the internal jugular site entrance.

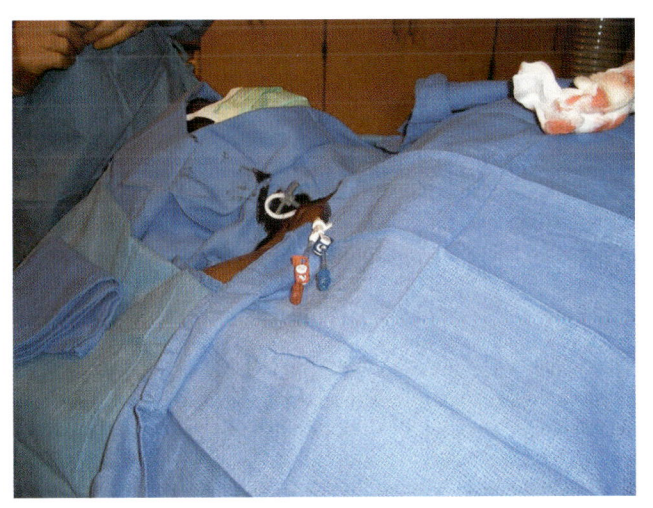

Figure 70.28 Catheter is introduced into the opening of the peel-away sheath and fed up to the junction of the superior vena cava (SVC) and right atrium.

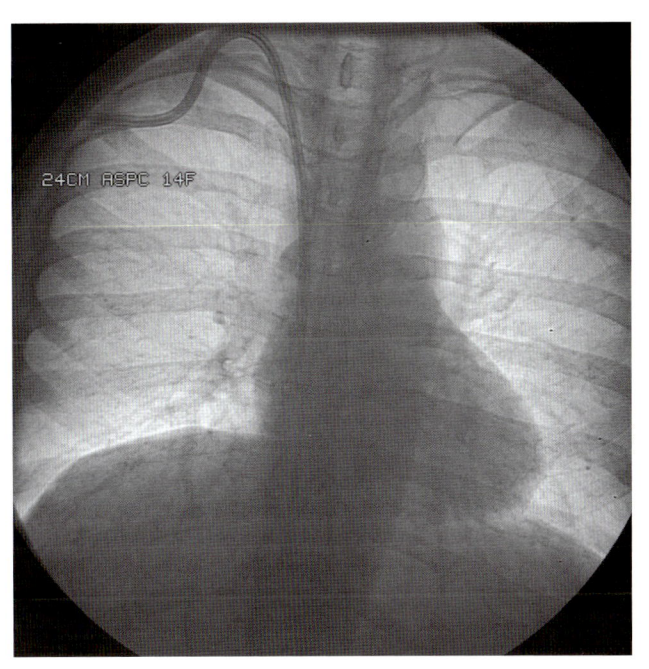

Figure 70.29 Spot film of appropriate placement of a right internal jugular vein–tunneled chronic dialysis catheter.

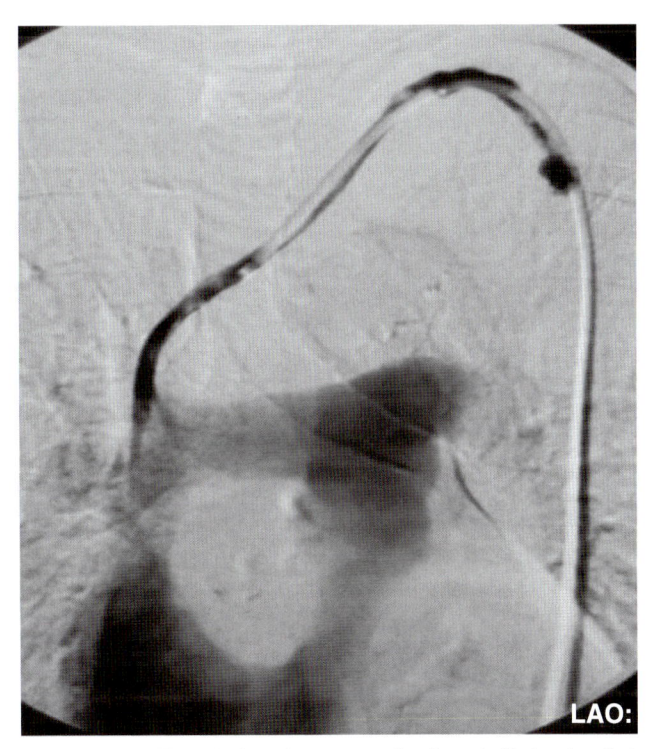

Figure 70.30 Tunneled catheter complication. A fibrin sheath is around the left internal jugular vein catheter.

discarded and a series of dilators are passed over the wire under fluoroscopic guidance, leaving a peel-away catheter sheath and inner dilator in place. The inner dilator and wire are removed, leaving the peel-away sheath behind. The tip of the catheter is introduced into the opening of the sheath and fed up to the junction of the superior vena cava (SVC) and right atrium (Figure 70.28). The peel-away sheet is then removed. A final radiograph is taken to assess for kinks of the catheter and for placement (Figure 70.29). Sutures are placed at the initial skin incision and at the entry site of the catheter. The catheter lumens are filled with heparin. The catheters are 14.5- or 15-Fr, with lengths of 24 cm for the right internal jugular, 28 cm for the left internal jugular, and 36 to 42 cm for femoral veins.

Complications at the time of placement are similar to those associated with temporary catheters (Figures 70.30 to 70.33). Internal jugular thrombosis develops in about 25% of tunneled catheters, but is usually asymptomatic.[177] Other long-term complications include dysfunction due to intraluminal thrombosis or fibrin sheaths, exit site infections, tunnel infections, and catheter-related bacteremia.[13]

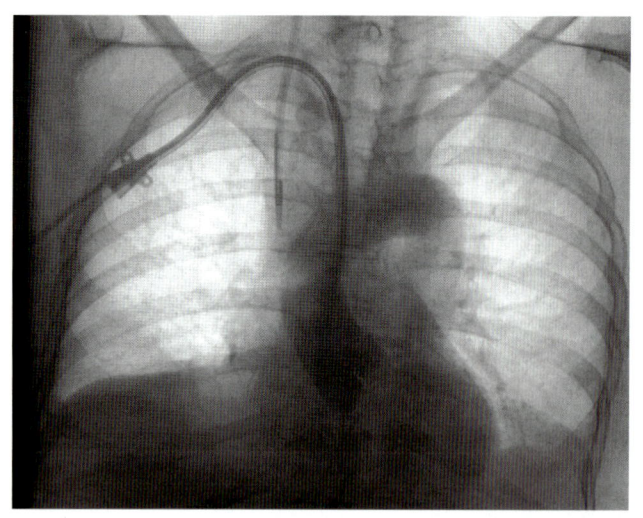

Figure 70.31 Tunneled catheter complication. The catheter was placed in the right carotid artery, with the tip near the aortic valves. Contrast demonstrates the aortic arch.

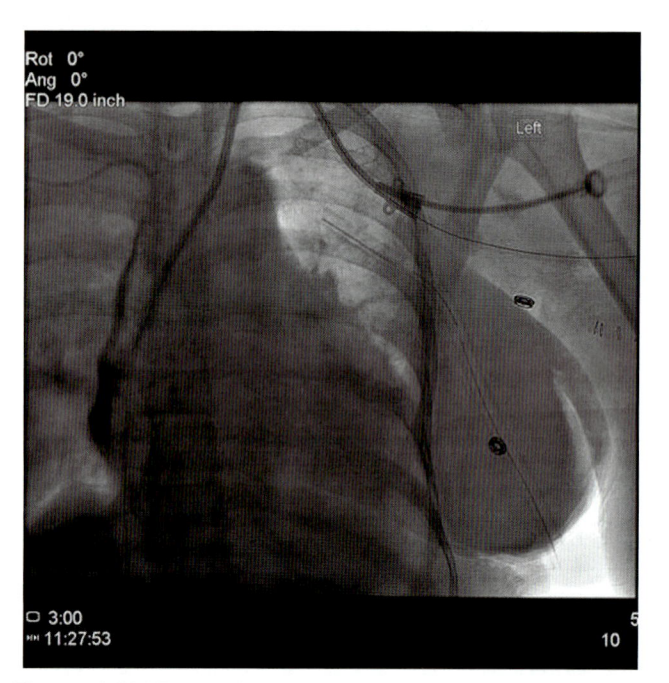

Figure 70.32 Tunneled catheter complication—left internal jugular vein catheter with its tip located in the pericardial sac. Contrast demonstrates the outer lining filling defect that corresponds to the lower part of the adventitia of the superior vena cava and upper part of the pericardium.

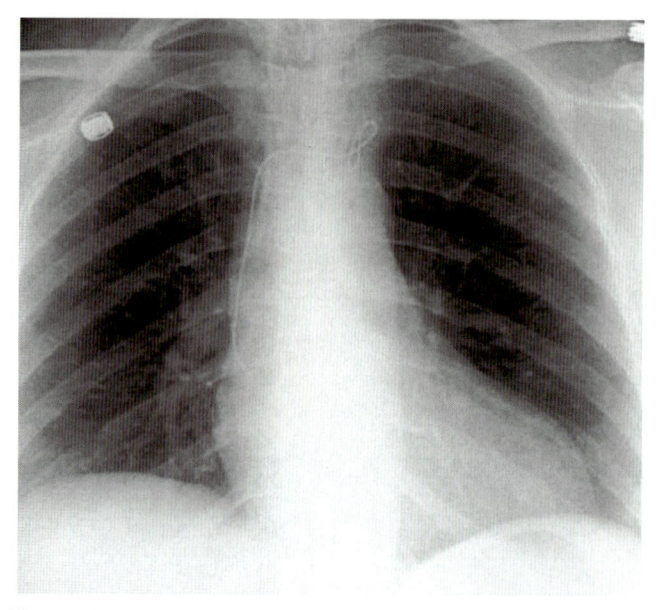

Figure 70.33 Tunneled catheter complication. Shown is a foreign body (metallic wire) that was left behind after an attempt for internal jugular vein catheter placement.

LESS COMMON LOCATIONS FOR TUNNELED HEMODIALYSIS CATHETERS

If prolonged use of an upper extremity dialysis catheter leads to bilateral central vein occlusion, it becomes necessary to place a tunneled catheter in the femoral vein.[178,179] The procedure for placement of a tunneled femoral catheter is similar to that for a tunneled internal jugular vein catheter, except that a longer catheter (36 to 42 cm) is required, and the catheter tip is placed in the proximal inferior vena cava or right atrium (Figure 70.34).[178] The subcutaneous tunnel is created in the anterior upper thigh.

The primary patency of tunneled femoral catheters is significantly worse than that of tunneled internal jugular catheters.[178] Presumably, some failures are due to kinking of the catheter in the groin when the thigh is flexed. However, the frequency of catheter-related bacteremia is similar for patients with femoral and internal jugular dialysis catheters. The likelihood of catheter-related bacteremia is proportionate to the duration of catheter use.[180] There is a high frequency (~25%) of symptomatic ipsilateral deep vein thrombosis after placement of a tunneled femoral catheter.[178] Fortunately, this complication can be treated with long-term anticoagulation, thereby permitting continued use of the catheter. In patients on hemodialysis in whom the central veins in the chest and groin have been exhausted, the placement of tunneled dialysis catheters at unconventional sites (e.g., translumbar, transhepatic) has been described. Catheters at these locations should be considered as last resort options because they are associated with a substantial risk for complications.

For translumbar catheters, there are essentially two tunnels. One tunnel extends from the access site in the back toward the IVC and the second from the abdomen to the access site in the back. The patient is placed on the angiography table in a lateral position, with his or her left side down. The initial access site is in the right lower back posterolaterally, just above the iliac wing. The needle is directed toward the inferior vena cava under fluoroscopic guidance; once venous access is achieved, a guidewire is placed. A tunnel is created from a lower abdominal site approximately 10 cm from the initial needle access around the waist toward the initial needle access. The permanent hemodialysis catheter is advanced through the tunnel and the cuff is buried into the adjacent subcutaneous tissue (Figure 70.35).[181,182] Dilation followed by peel-away sheath insertion is done from the back access to the IVC. The dialysis catheter is then inserted through the sheath to the IVC, preferably over the guidewire, which is passed in a retrograde fashion all the

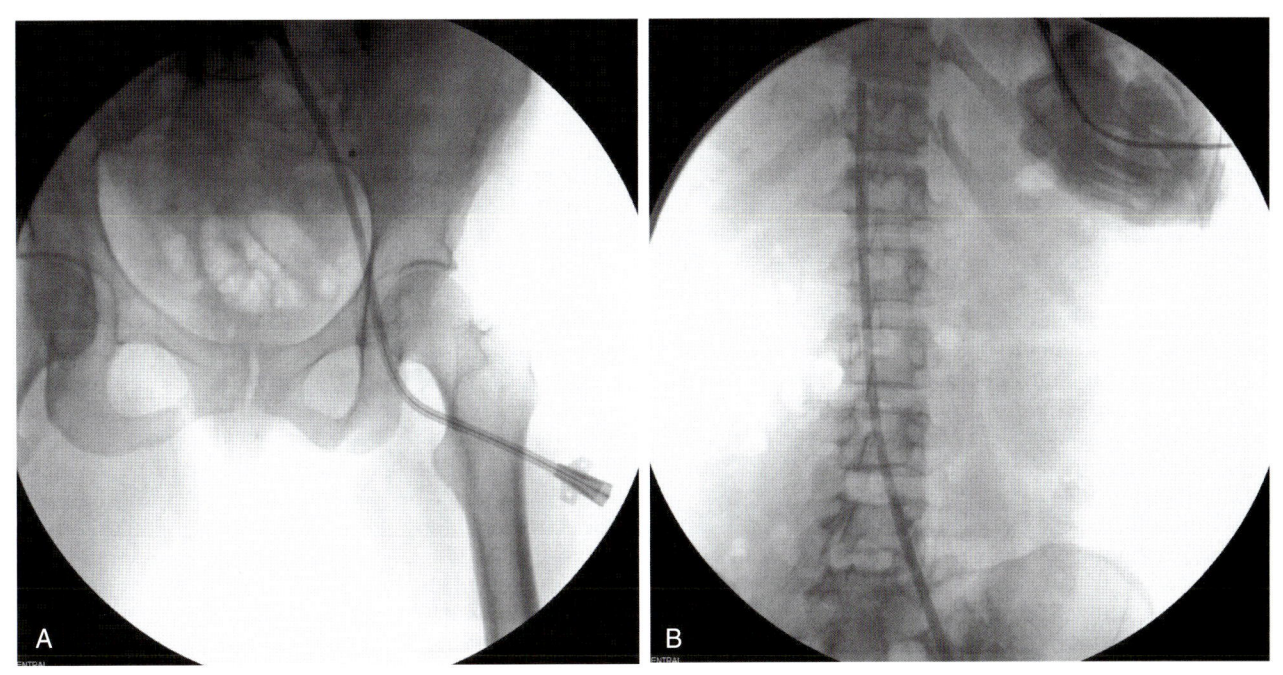

Figure 70.34 **A, B,** Spot films of appropriate placement of a left femoral vein–tunneled chronic dialysis catheter.

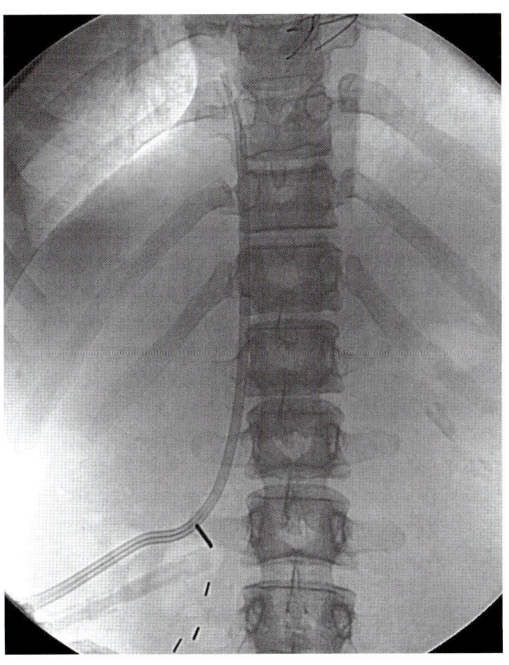

Figure 70.35 Spot film of appropriate placement of a translumbar-tunneled chronic dialysis catheter.

way through the catheter. The access site is sutured, and the catheter is secured in place.

Placement of tunneled translumbar hemodialysis catheters requires higher expertise in interventional techniques than jugular or femoral access, especially because ultrasound guidance is not possible. The risk of bleeding and retroperitoneal hematoma is considerably higher than that associated with tunneled femoral vein catheters. The most common complication of translumbar catheters in one series of 10 patients was partial dislodgment of the catheters.[182]

Interventional radiologists at some centers have placed transhepatic catheters. The right upper quadrant is prepped and draped in the usual manner; a 21-gauge needle is placed halfway through the liver in a direction parallel to the right of the middle hepatic veins under fluoroscopic guidance, contrast material is injected through the needle, and the needle withdrawn until a hepatic vein is visualized. Once a suitable vein is accessed, a guidewire is placed and advanced to the right atrium. A subcutaneous tunnel is created inferiorly to the insertion site, and a dual-lumen cuffed hemodialysis catheter is placed.[183-185] The major complications are bleeding and perihepatic hematoma. Hepatic vein thrombosis is likely, and dislodgment of the catheter because of liver excursion movement with breathing is frequent. Stavropoulos and colleagues have reported a series of 36 transhepatic dialysis catheters placed in 12 patients.[184] The mean survival of these catheters was only 24 days. The thrombosis rate was 2.40 per 100 catheter-days, with the poor catheter patency rates being associated with a high rate of late thrombosis.

EXCHANGE OF TUNNELED HEMODIALYSIS CATHETERS

There are two major indications for catheter exchange, dysfunction and infection. Catheter dysfunction is diagnosed when blood cannot be aspirated from the catheter lumen at the time of dialysis initiation or, more commonly, if it is not possible to achieve consistently a blood flow required to yield sufficient urea and other solute clearance (>250 mL/min). In catheters that were previously delivering an adequate blood flow, intraluminal thrombus was the most common cause for dysfunction, although a fibrin sheath may be the culprit in some patients. This problem is usually treated empirically in the dialysis unit by instilling t-PA into the catheter lumens[186]; t-PA instillation is successful in about 70% to 80% of catheters, but problems with poor flow frequently recur within 2 or 3 weeks. If the thrombolytic agent does not improve the catheter flow, the patient is referred for catheter exchange.

An exit site infection usually resolves with topical antimicrobial agents or oral antibiotics and is not usually an indication for catheter removal. However, if the patient has a tunnel track infection, catheter removal is mandatory.

Finally, catheter-related bacteremia (CRB) is a common indication for catheter replacement.[12] In one series, the cumulative risk of CRB among catheter-dependent patients was 35% at 3 months and 48% at 6 months.[180] CRB is suspected when a catheter-dependent patient experiences fever or chills and is confirmed by blood cultures from the catheter and a peripheral vein growing the same organism.[12] When a single set of blood cultures is positive, CRB is still the most likely diagnosis in the absence of clinical evidence of an alternative source of infection.

The clinical management of CRB has evolved in the past few years.[12] In the subset of patient whose fever persists after 48 to 72 hours of appropriate systemic antibiotics (~10% to 15% of patients with CRB), removal of the infected catheter is mandatory. For the remaining patients, there are several management options. The first is to continue systemic antibiotics without removal of the infected catheter. Unfortunately, infection is infrequently eradicated with this approach—once the course of systemic antibiotics has been completed, bacteremia recurs in 63% to 78% of patients.[187-191] Moreover, delays in removing an infected catheter may result in metastatic infection, such as endocarditis, septic arthritis, or epidural abscess.[192] Prompt removal of the catheter removes the source of infection. However, to continue delivering dialysis to the patient, it is necessary to place a temporary (nontunneled) dialysis catheter. Once the bacteremia has resolved, a new tunneled catheter is placed. In an effort to reduce the number of required access procedures, a number of investigators have evaluated the strategy of exchanging the infected catheter for a new one over a guidewire. Several reports have documented the safety and efficacy of this approach.[190,193-196]

In the past few years, there has been a growing recognition of the central role of bacterial biofilms in causing CRB. Biofilms develop on the inner surface of the lumens of central vein catheters in as little as 24 hours and are relatively refractory to conventional plasma concentrations of antibiotics.[197-199] Instillation of a concentrated antibiotic solution into the catheter lumen after each dialysis session (termed *antibiotic lock*) can frequently kill the bacteria in the biofilm. This approach can potentially remove the source of the infection (the biofilm) while permitting catheter salvage. The use of antibiotic locks, in conjunction with systemic antibiotics, has been shown to eradicate infection and salvage the catheter in about two thirds of patients.[12,200-203] This strategy is not associated with an increased risk of metastatic infections as compared to prompt catheter removal or exchange of the infected catheter over a guidewire. At our institution, implementation of an antibiotic lock protocol has dramatically reduced the frequency of catheter exchanges caused by infection. The overall success rate of an antibiotic lock in curing an episode of CRB is about 70%.[204] However, it varies considerably depending on the bacterial organism, being highest for gram-negative infections, intermediate for *Staphylococcus epidermidis* and *Enterococcus* infections, and lowest for *Staphylococcus aureus* infections.[202,203,205-207] Catheter-related candidemia always requires catheter exchange in conjunction with antifungal therapy.[208] The catheter should be removed or exchanged over a guidewire in patients with persistent fever or bacteremia despite a trial of an antibiotic lock.[12]

The thrombus inside the catheter may act as a nidus for the catheter biofilm. Heparin coating of the catheters may prevent bacterial adherence.[209] Two randomized clinical trials with short-term, nontunneled central vein catheters found a lower rate of CRB in patients with heparin-coated catheters than in those with noncoated catheters.[209,210] A recent retrospective study observed fewer infections in patients with heparin-coated catheters as compared with those using a coated catheter.[211] However, a randomized clinical trial is needed to confirm this benefit. A recent study by Hemmelgarn and colleagues has reported that instillation of recombinant t-PA (rt-PA) instead of heparin into the dialysis catheter lumen once weekly, as compared with the standard use of heparin locks three times a week, significantly reduces the incidence of catheter malfunction and bacteremia,[212] suggesting that rt-PA may prevent thrombosis and biofilm development.

TECHNICAL PROCEDURE: EXCHANGE OF TUNNELED HEMODIALYSIS CATHETERS

Patients are brought to the interventional suite for the exchange of permanent indwelling hemodialysis catheters. Strict sterile technique, topical local anesthesia (1% lidocaine), and conscious sedation are provided. Under fluoroscopic guidance, an extra-stiff 0.03-inch wire is passed through one of the lumens of the catheter and advanced to the inferior vena cava. The catheter cuff located near the exit site in the subcutaneous tissue is dissected, and the catheter is pulled out, leaving behind the wire. The exit site and wire are cleaned and wiped with antibacterial soap. The operators' gloves are exchanged. A new, permanent hemodialysis catheter is then prepped and advanced over the wire into place. The tip of the catheter is advanced to the inferior vena cava for the femoral catheter or to the junction of the SVC and right atrium for the internal jugular vein. Finally, the wire is removed, and the catheter is sutured in place. The lumens of the catheter are filled with heparin.

PERITONEAL DIALYSIS CATHETER PROCEDURES

Peritoneal dialysis (PD) is an alternative to hemodialysis in patients with ESKD. Although it is widely used in many countries, fewer than 10% of the U.S. dialysis population is treated by this modality.[213] Peritoneal catheters can be placed into the abdominal cavity by surgeons,[214-216] interventional radiologists,[217] or interventional nephrologists.[218] There are several techniques, such as the blind (Seldinger),[219] peritoneoscopic,[220] laparoscopic,[221] and Moncrief-Popovich techniques,[222] surgical placement,[214] and fluoroscopic insertion.[218] Incorporation of PD catheter placement in an established interventional nephrology program increases the utilization of this dialysis modality.[223] A modified fluoroscopic technique, which adds real-time ultrasound visualization, avoids the risk of inadvertent epigastric artery injury.[224]

Peritoneal catheters are made of silicone rubber or polyurethane. The Tenckhoff catheter is still the most common type of PD catheter placed. The intraperitoneal portion of the catheter can be straight, coiled, or T-fluted or with a silicone disc.[225] The extraperitoneal portion of the catheter may be straight or have a swan neck design, with single or double inner cuffs or a combination of a single cuff and silicone disc. The most widely used PD catheter is the double-cuff, swan neck, coiled Tenckhoff design. This design has been shown to decrease mechanical complications (e.g., inflow and outflow problems). The coiled catheter design also decreases pain during infusion and is less likely to migrate. The swan neck design was introduced to avoid cuff extrusions.[226] The intraperitoneal portion of the catheter should be placed between the visceral and parietal peritoneum, near the pouch of Douglas. The inner cuff should be inserted in the abdominal wall musculature (rectus muscle) to prevent leaks. The outer cuff should be located in the subcutaneous tissue to create a dead space in between the two cuffs, which is thought to prevent the migration of infections coming from the exit site. The subcutaneous tract and exit site should face downward and laterally to avoid exit site infection. The exit site should be determined and marked prior to the insertion while the patient is in the upright position. The belt line, prior surgical sites, and abdominal midline should be avoided. Postoperative catheter care is very important. The catheter should be covered with a nonocclusive dressing and should not be used for 10 to 14 days. The catheter should be flushed at least two or three times per week with saline or dialysate solution until the patient is ready to start PD.[227] Usually, PD is started between 2 to 4 weeks after placement of the catheter to allow for wound healing and securing of the catheter cuff. Providing sufficient time for healing helps avoid leaks, which can increase the risk of infection and are discouraging to patients. Low-volume PD may be attempted within 24 hours of catheter placement if no other dialysis access is available.[228]

Two studies comparing swan neck and straight Tenckhoff catheters have shown a similar risk for peritonitis and exit infection, but less cuff extrusion with the swan neck design. The lower incidence of cuff extrusion enhances the survival of swan neck catheters.[229-231] A modified technique, which places the swan neck catheter in a presternal exit site location, has been reported by Twardowski and associates[232,233] and has shown an increase in access survival up to 95% at 2 years. The presternal exit site modification has been shown to decrease the incidence of peritonitis and exit site infection. They advocated the use of the presternal catheters in obese patients, patients with ostomies, and children wearing diapers and/or with fecal incontinence. Gadallah and coworkers demonstrated that placement of PD catheters by a peritoneoscopic approach had a longer survival rate (survival defined as inflow-outflow obstruction, persistent dialysate leak, and persistent peritonitis, or exit site or tunnel infection requiring catheter removal) than those placed surgically, and that the rates of exit infection and leak were lower.[234] Moncrief and colleagues described a technique in which the extraperitoneal portion of the catheter is buried in the abdominal subcutaneous tissue until the patient is ready for PD. It appears that the Montcrief modification may lower the risk of initial infection of the tract.[222]

A major complication during placement of the PD catheter is bowel perforation. It is infrequent with all techniques except for blind placement but, once identified, requires bowel rest, intravenous (IV) antibiotic therapy and, rarely, surgical exploration.[214,223] Tip migration is a very common late complication (up to 35%), which could cause problems with draining of the PD fluid. It can be fixed with radiologic or surgical manipulation.[235,236] PD leaks around the catheter have been reported to be as high as 10%, but the use of double-cuff, swan neck catheters has decreased the likelihood of migration.[237] Perioperative infection and bleeding are very rare; prophylactic antibiotics are usually given.[236]

TECHNICAL PROCEDURE: INSERTION OF PERITONEAL CATHETERS BY FLUOROSCOPIC AND ULTRASOUND TECHNIQUES

The abdomen is prepped and draped in a sterile fashion. Conscious sedation is administered with midazolam hydrochloride and fentanyl citrate. A nurse obtains vital signs and administers conscious sedation during the procedure. The insertion site is selected to be 2 cm to the left or right and below the umbilicus. An ultrasound machine with a 5- to 12-MHz transducer and a sterile cover is used to guide a 21-gauge needle into the peritoneum. Under ultrasound guidance, the needle penetrates through the skin, subcutaneous tissue, outer fascia of rectus muscle, muscle fibers, inner fascia, and parietal layer of peritoneum. Radiocontrast, 3 to 5 mL, is injected into the peritoneal cavity under fluoroscopic guidance to ensure the correct location; a radiologic pattern of outer bowel delineation is indicative of good placement. A Cope mandril wire, 0.018 inch, is introduced through the needle. The needle is exchanged for a 6-Fr catheter sheath. A 2-cm incision is made on the skin, and the subcutaneous tissue is digitally dissected up to the rectus muscle. A series of dilators (8-, 12-, and 14-Fr) are passed over a stiff guidewire, and an 18-Fr peel-away sheath is placed. A double-cuff, swan neck, Tenckhoff peritoneal dialysis catheter is introduced over the stiff guidewire into the peritoneal cavity. The coiled intraperitoneal portion is placed in the lower intraabdominal area. The inner cuff is pushed into the muscle before removing the peel-away sheath. Alternatively, the tunnel can be created before catheter insertion into the peritoneum. A tunnel is created with an exit site located distally, laterally, and below the initial incision, with the outer cuff buried in the subcutaneous tissue. A final fluoroscopic image is obtained to verify placement of the Tenckhoff catheter (Figure 70.36). Inflow and outflow of the PD catheter are tested with 500 mL of normal saline. The PD catheter is flushed with 10 to 15 mL of heparin. The subcutaneous tissue and skin are sutured, and the site is dressed.

TECHNICAL PROCEDURE: INSERTION OF PERITONEAL CATHETERS BY PERITONEOSCOPIC TECHNIQUE

Peritoneal catheters placed peritoneoscopically are implanted through the rectus muscle using a percutaneous laparoscopic (Y-TEC) technique. It has the same initial preparation as for the fluoroscopic or ultrasound technique. Under local anesthesia, a 2-cm skin incision is made. The subcutaneous tissue is dissected up to the rectus muscle. A

Figure 70.36 **A,** Spot film demonstrating free flow of contrast injection into the peritoneal cavity. **B,** Spot film showing a peel-away sheath in place during insertion of a Tenckhoff catheter. **C,** Spot film showing appropriate placement of a Tenckhoff catheter.

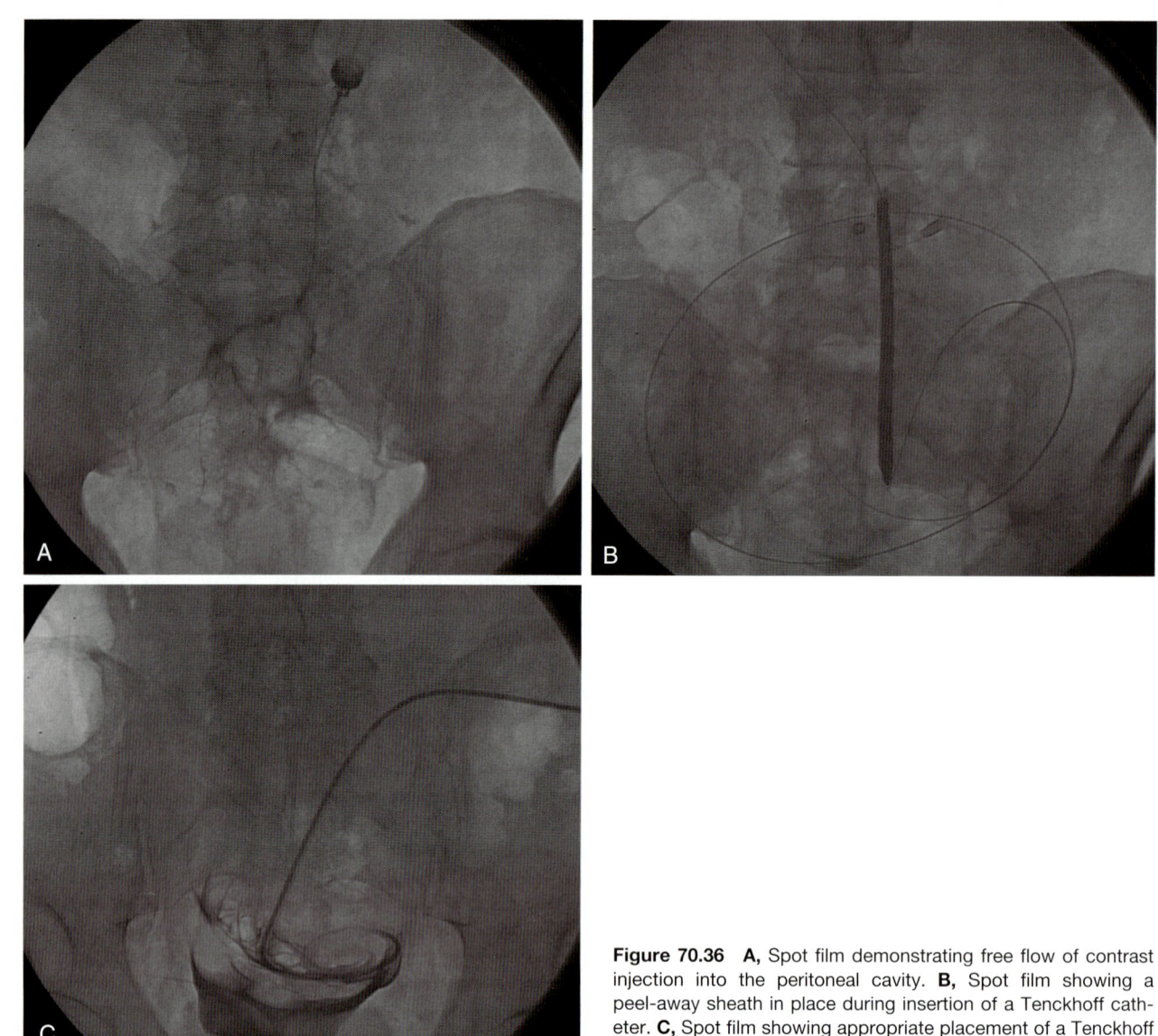

catheter guide is inserted into the abdomen, and the Y-TEC peritoneoscope is inserted into the catheter to assess initial entry to the peritoneal cavity. The scope is removed, and 500 mL of air is infused into the cavity. The scope is again replaced and advanced to the pelvic area. This area is inspected for adhesions and bowel loops. The scope is again removed, and the peritoneal catheter is introduced through the catheter with the help of a stainless steel stylette. The catheter is advanced to the pelvic area. The stylette is removed, and the inner cuff is buried into the musculature. The exit location is determined, and the catheter is tunneled to that location.

TECHNICAL PROCEDURE: INSERTION OF PERITONEAL CATHETERS BY PRESTERNAL CATHETER PLACEMENT

The peritoneal catheter implantation technique is the same as peritoneoscopic insertion, except that the PD catheter has a straight design instead of a swan neck. After the PD catheter is placed, a second catheter is tunneled from the midabdomen up to the chest wall. The two catheters are connected by a titanium joint piece. The second catheter has a swan neck design and two cuffs. The exit site is located lateral to the midsternal line.

PERCUTANEOUS KIDNEY BIOPSY
(see also Chapter 29)

A percutaneous kidney biopsy is an important procedure in the diagnosis of acute and chronic kidney disease. The results of a kidney biopsy are helpful in guiding medical therapy and providing a prognosis. The goal of a kidney biopsy should be to maximize the yield of adequate tissue while minimizing the risk of complications. Percutaneous kidney biopsies have evolved from a blind procedure to a real-time, ultrasound-guided needle biopsy. At some institutions, radiologists perform kidney biopsies under computed tomography (CT) guidance. Although some nephrologists still use the Franklin-Silverman and Tru-Cut needles for blind biopsy, several authors have documented that the use of real-time ultrasonography, along with the use of an automatic biopsy gun, minimizes complications and provides a

Table 70.13 Adequacy of Kidney Tissue Retrieval and Complications*

Reference	No. of Biopsies	Adequate Tissue (%)	Major Complications (%)†
Dowd et al, 1991[257]	23	95.5	<0.5
Doyle et al, 1994[258]	86	99	0.8
Hergesell et al, 1998[259]	1090	98.8	<0.5
Donovan et al, 1991[260]	192	97.8	<1
Burstein et al, 1993[240]	200	97.5	5.6
Cozens et al, 1992[238]		93	N/A
Marwah et al, 1996[239]	394		6.6
Maya et al, 2007[261]	65	100	0

*By real-time, ultrasound-guided percutaneous renal biopsy.
†Definitions of major complications differed among studies.

high yield of adequate tissue for pathologic diagnosis (Table 70.13). Cozens and coworkers[238] retrospectively compared a 15-gauge, Tru-Cut renal biopsy with ultrasound localization and marking to the use of an 18-gauge, spring-loaded gun renal biopsy under real-time ultrasound guidance. They reported a 79% yield of adequate renal tissue with the blind technique (15 gauge) as compared with 93% with real-time ultrasound guidance (18 gauge). Similarly, two other studies reported a higher mean number of glomeruli from biopsies obtained under real-time ultrasonography as compared to those performed blindly.[239,240]

Major complications of kidney biopsies, including gross hematuria or retroperitoneal hematoma requiring blood transfusion, invasive procedure, or surgical intervention, have been reported in fewer than 1% of biopsies in some series and 5% to 6% by others (see Table 70.13). The likelihood of major complications was not associated with patient age, blood pressure, or serum creatinine level in one large series.[239] In patients with major complications, the time interval from biopsy to diagnosis of the complication was 4 hours or less in 52%, 8 hours or less in 79%, and 12 hours or less in 100% of patients.[239] Thus, the minimal period of observation following a renal biopsy should be 12 hours. A recent prospective study of 100 consecutive patients has shown that outpatient, real-time, ultrasound-guided percutaneous renal biopsy is safe and minimizes the need for postbiopsy hospitalization.[241] Minor complications, including transient gross hematuria and perinephric hematoma not requiring transfusion or intervention, occurred after 6.6% of biopsies in one series.[239] Ultrasonigraphy or CT can be used to diagnose perinephric hematomas.[242] Most hematomas resolve spontaneously within a few weeks, with no significant sequelae. Major bleeding complications that do not resolve with conservative measures require further intervention. In the past, this entailed urgent surgical nephrectomy. However, selective renal arteriography with embolization of the bleeding arteriole can often stop the bleeding in most cases. A review article reported major complications in only 0.3% of cases, with death in fewer than 0.1% among 9595 percutaneous kidney biopsies performed over the last 50 years.

For patients at high risk of bleeding complications or liver disease with coagulopathy for whom a kidney biopsy is indicated, a transjugular kidney biopsy may be performed by an interventional radiologist or nephrologist. Thompson and colleagues have reported 91% adequate tissue retrieval, with an average of nine glomeruli for light microscopy, in 23 patients undergoing transjugular renal biopsy. A capsular perforation was encountered in 17 patients (74%), of whom six (26%) required coil embolization of the bleeding vessel. Two major complications were reported—one arteriocalyceal system fistula and one renal vein thrombosis 6 days after the biopsy.[243] Abbott and associates have reported a series of nine patients who had a transjugular renal biopsy. Adequate tissue was obtained from all patients. Capsular perforation occurred in 90% of patients, and two patients developed gross hematuria requiring transfusion.[244] The very high rate of capsular perforation casts real doubts on any advantage of transjugular over percutaneous kidney biopsy.

A bleeding disorder is an absolute contraindication to performing a percutaneous kidney biopsy. However, if it can be corrected medically, and if the potential benefit of doing a biopsy outweighs the potential risk, the biopsy can still be performed. Relative contraindications to kidney biopsy include a solitary kidney, pyelonephritis, perinephric abscess, uncontrolled hypertension, hydronephrosis, polycystic kidney disease, severe anemia, pregnancy, renal masses, and renal artery aneurysms.

TECHNICAL PROCEDURE: PERCUTANEOUS KIDNEY BIOPSY UNDER REAL-TIME ULTRASOUND GUIDANCE

A complete blood count, prothrombin time, and partial thromboplastin time are checked before the procedure. The patient is taken to the ultrasound suite and placed in the prone position. An initial ultrasound examination is performed to confirm the presence of two kidneys. Sterile technique is observed, and a sterile cover is placed over the ultrasound probe. The lower pole of the left kidney is preferred for right-handed operators. The skin and subcutaneous tissue are anesthetized with 1% lidocaine. A small incision is made with a scalpel at the site of needle insertion. Under real-time ultrasound guidance, a biopsy needle gun is advanced up to the capsule of the kidney (Figure 70.37AB). The patient is asked to hold her or his breath, and the spring-loaded gun is activated. The gun is retrieved, and the specimen is placed in a container with media. There are different types of needle biopsy guns—full-core, half-core, and ¾ of a core. Sizes vary from 14- to 18-Fr, with lengths from 10 to 20 cm. Also, the throw of the device (amount of tissue that the gun can obtain) can be adjusted from 13 to 33 mm. Usually, two or three biopsy pieces are taken in one setting to provide enough tissue for light microscopy, immunofluorescence, and electron microscopy studies. After the biopsy is completed, a second-look ultrasound examination

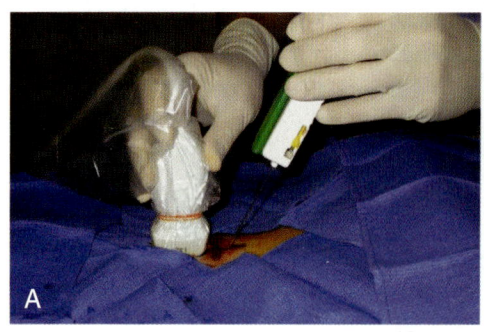

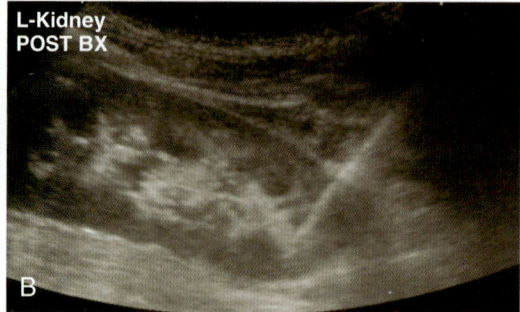

Figure 70.37 **A,** Operator showing the technique of a real-time ultrasound kidney biopsy. **B,** Kidney ultrasound image showing a biopsy needle located at the lower pole of the kidney.

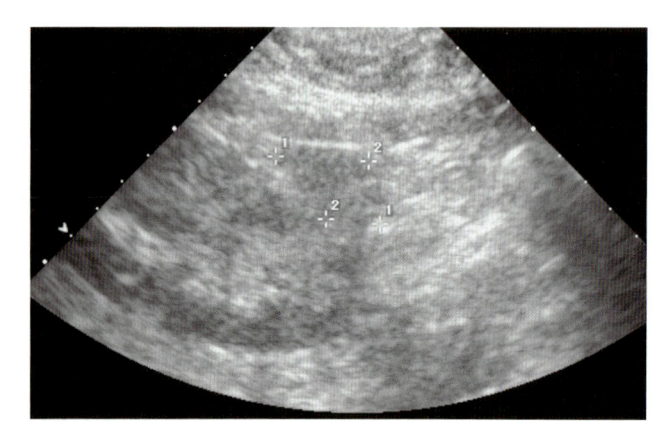

Figure 70.38 Postbiopsy kidney ultrasound image of a perinephric hematoma.

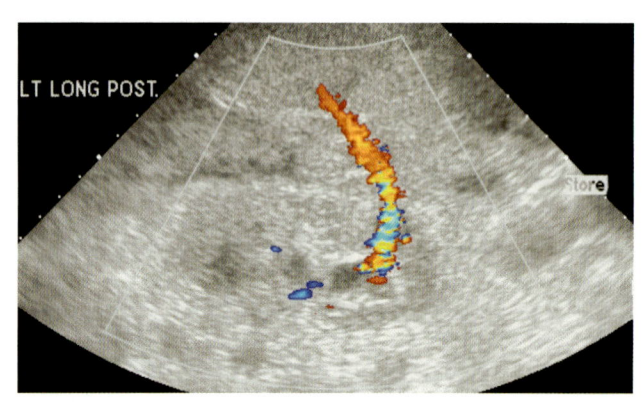

Figure 70.39 Postbiopsy kidney color Doppler ultrasound image showing active bleeding.

is performed to assess for perinephric hematomas (Figure 70.38). A color Doppler ultrasound postbiopsy surveillance imaging examination would also be helpful to localize any active bleeding (Figure 70.39). Vital signs are obtained frequently in the first hour and then every 2 to 4 hours. Hematocrit levels are checked every 6 hours for the next 24 hours.

Complete reference list available at ExpertConsult.com.

KEY REFERENCES

3. Ethier J, Mendelssohn DC, Elder SJ, et al: Vascular access use and outcomes: an international perspective from the Dialysis Outcomes and Practice Patterns Study. *Nephrol Dial Transplant* 23:3219–3226, 2008.
8. Feldman HI, Kobrin S, Wasserstein A: Hemodialysis vascular access morbidity. *J Am Soc Nephrol* 7:523–535, 1996.
9. Allon M, Robbin ML: Increasing arteriovenous fistulas in hemodialysis patients: problems and solutions. *Kidney Int* 62:1109–1124, 2002.
10. Schwab SJ: Vascular access for hemodialysis. *Kidney Int* 55:2078–2090, 1999.
11. Dember LM, Beck GJ, Allon M, et al: Effect of clopidogrel on early failure of arteriovenous fistulas for hemodialysis: a randomized controlled trial. *JAMA* 299:2164–2171, 2008.
12. Allon M: Dialysis catheter-related bacteremia: treatment and prophylaxis. *Am J Kidney Dis* 44:779–791, 2004.
14. Allon M, Daugirdas JT, Depner TA, et al: Effect of change in vascular access on patient mortality in hemodialysis patients. *Am J Kidney Dis* 47:469–477, 2006.
17. Asif A, Besarab A, Roy-Chaudhury P, et al: Interventional nephrology: from episodic to coordinated vascular access care. *J Nephrol* 20:399–405, 2007.
19. Asif A, Byers P, Vieira CF, et al: Developing a comprehensive diagnostic and interventional nephrology program at an academic center. *Am J Kidney Dis* 42:229–233, 2003.
23. O'Neill WC: Renal ultrasonography: a procedure for nephrologists. *Am J Kidney Dis* 30:579–585, 1997.
24. Mishler R, Sands JJ, Osfsthun NJ, et al: Dedicated outpatient vascular access center decreases hospitalization and missed outpatient dialysis treatments. *Kidney Int* 69:393–398, 2006.
27. Roy-Chaudhury P, Sukhatme VP, Cheung AK: Hemodialysis vascular access dysfunction: a cellular and molecular viewpoint. *J Am Soc Nephrol* 17:1112–1127, 2006.
34. Allon M, Bailey R, Ballard R, et al: A multidisciplinary approach to hemodialysis access: prospective evaluation. *Kidney Int* 53:473–479, 1998.
35. Roy-Chaudhury P, Kelly BS, Miller MA, et al: Venous neointimal hyperplasia in polytetrafluoroethylene dialysis grafts. *Kidney Int* 59:2325–2334, 2001.
39. Lee T, Roy-Chaudhury P: Advances and new frontiers in the pathophysiology of venous neointimal hyperplasia and dialysis access stenosis. *Adv Chronic Kidney Dis* 16:329–338, 2009.
41. Lee T: Novel paradigms for dialysis vascular access: downstream vascular biology—is there a final common pathway? *Clin J Am Soc Nephrol* 8:2194–2201, 2013.
48. Lee T, Chauhan V, Krishnamoorthy M, et al: Severe venous neointimal hyperplasia prior to dialysis access surgery. *Nephrol Dial Transplant* 26:2264–2270, 2011.
53. Allon M, Robbin ML, Young CJ, et al: Preoperative venous intimal hyperplasia, postoperative arteriovenous fistula stenosis, and clinical fistula outcomes. *Clin J Am Soc Nephrol* 8:1750–1755, 2013.
58. Beathard GA: Percutaneous transvenous angioplasty in the treatment of vascular access stenosis. *Kidney Int* 42:1390–1397, 1992.
66. Smits JHM, Van der Linden J, Hagen EC, et al: Graft surveillance: venous pressure, access flow, or the combination? *Kidney Int* 59:1551–1558, 2001.
67. Malik J, Slavikova M, Svobodova J, et al: Regular ultrasound screening significantly prolongs patency of PTFE grafts. *Kidney Int* 67:1554–1558, 2005.
68. Ram SJ, Work J, Caldito GC, et al: A randomized controlled trial of blood flow and stenosis surveillance of hemodialysis grafts. *Kidney Int* 64:272–280, 2003.

69. Robbin ML, Oser RF, Allon M, et al: Hemodialysis access graft stenosis: US detection. *Radiology* 208:655–661, 1998.
70. Robbin ML, Oser RF, Lee JY, et al: Randomized comparison of ultrasound surveillance and clinical monitoring on arteriovenous graft outcomes. *Kidney Int* 69:730–735, 2006.
71. Dember LM, Holmberg EF, Kaufman JS: Value of static venous pressure for predicting arteriovenous graft thrombosis. *Kidney Int* 61:1899–1904, 2002.
76. Dember LM, Holmberg EF, Kaufman JS: Randomized controlled trial of prophylactic repair of hemodialysis arteriovenous graft stenosis. *Kidney Int* 66:390–398, 2004.
86. Chang CJ, Ko PJ, Hsu LA, et al: Highly increased cell proliferation activity in restenotic hemodialysis vascular access after percutaneous transluminal angioplasty: implication in prevention of stenosis. *Am J Kidney Dis* 43:74–84, 2004.
88. Dixon BS, Beck GJ, Vazquez MA, et al: Effect of dipyridamole plus aspirin on hemodialysis graft patency. *N Engl J Med* 360:2191–2201, 2009.
91. Haskal ZJ, Trerotola S, Dolmatch B, et al: Stent graft versus balloon angioplasty for failing dialysis-access grafts. *N Engl J Med* 362:494–503, 2010.
94. Kaufman JS, O'Connor TZ, Zhang JH, et al: Randomized controlled trial of clopidogrel plus aspirin to prevent hemodialysis access graft thrombosis. *J Am Soc Nephrol* 14:2313–2321, 2003.
96. Lok CE, Moist L, Hemmelgarn BR, et al: Effect of fish oil supplementation on graft patency and cardiovascular events among patients with new synthetic arteriovenous hemodialysis grafts: a randomized controlled trial. *JAMA* 307:1809–1816, 2012.
98. Asif A, Gadalean FN, Merrill D, et al: Inflow stenosis in arteriovenous fistulas and grafts: a multicenter, prospective study. *Kidney Int* 67:1986–1992, 2005.
108. Sreenarasimhaiah VP, Margassery SK, Martin KJ, et al: Salvage of thrombosed dialysis access grafts with venous anastomotosis stents. *Kidney Int* 67:678–684, 2005.
116. Robbin ML, Gallichio ML, Deierhoi MH, et al: US vascular mapping before hemodialysis access placement. *Radiology* 217:83–88, 2000.
124. Asif A, Cherla G, Merrill D, et al: Conversion of tunneled hemodialysis catheter-consigned patients to arteriovenous fistula. *Kidney Int* 67:2399–2406, 2005.
125. Asif A, Cherla G, Merrill D, et al: Venous mapping using venography and the risk of radio-contrast-induced nephropathy. *Semin Dial* 18:239–242, 2005.
132. Wong V, Ward R, Taylor J, et al: Factors associated with early failure of arteriovenous fistulae for hemodialysis access. *Eur J Vasc Endovasc Surg* 12:207–213, 1996.
144. Lee T, Ullah A, Allon M, et al: Decreased cumulative access survival in arteriovenous fistulas requiring interventions to promote maturation. *Clin J Am Soc Nephrol* 6:575–581, 2011.
150. Turmel-Rodrigues L, Pengloan J, et al: Treatment of stenosis and thrombosis in haemodialysis fistulas and grafts by interventional radiology. *Nephrol Dial Transplant* 15:2029–2036, 2000.
162. Agarwal AK, Patel BM, Haddad NJ: Central vein stenosis: a nephrologist's perspective. *Semin Dial* 20:53–62, 2007.
166. Kovalik EC, Newman GE, Suhocki PV, et al: Correction of central vein stenoses: use of angioplasty and vascular Wallstents. *Kidney Int* 45:1177–1181, 1994.
190. Saad TF: Bacteremia associated with tunnneled, cuffed hemodialysis catheters. *Am J Kidney Dis* 34:1114–1124, 1999.
201. Krishnasami Z, Carlton D, Bimbo L, et al: Management of hemodialysis catheter-related bacteremia with an adjunctive antibiotic lock solution. *Kidney Int* 61:1136–1142, 2002.
212. Hemmelgarn BR, Moist LM, Lok CE, et al: Prevention of dialysis catheter malfunction with recombinant tissue plasminogen activator. *N Engl J Med* 364:303–312, 2011.
217. Degesys GE, Miller GA, Ford KK, et al: Tenckhoff peritoneal dialysis catheters: the use of fluoroscopy in management. *Radiology* 154:819–820, 1985.
219. Zappacosta AR, Perras ST, Closkey GM: Seldinger technique for Tenckhoff catheter placement. *ASAIO J* 37:13–15, 1991.
224. Maya ID: Ultrasound/fluoroscopy-assisted placement of peritoneal dialysis catheters. *Sem Dial* 20:611–615, 2007.
229. Eklund BH, Honkanen EO, Kala AR, et al: Catheter configuration and outcome in patients on continuous ambulatory peritoneal dialysis: a prospective comparison of two catheters. *Perit Dial Int* 14:70–74, 1994.
259. Hergessel O, Felten H, Andrassy K, et al: Safety of ultrasound-guided percutaneous renal biopsy—retrospective analysis of 1090 consecutive cases. *Nephrol Dial Transplant* 13:975–977, 1998.
261. Maya ID, Maddela P, Barker J, et al: Percutaneous renal biopsy: comparison of blind and real-time ultrasound-guided technique. *Semin Dial* 20:355–358, 2007.

KIDNEY TRANSPLANTATION

SECTION XI

71 Transplantation Immunobiology

Mohamed H. Sayegh | Leonardo V. Riella | Anil Chandraker

CHAPTER OUTLINE

CHARACTERISTICS OF THE ALLOGENEIC IMMUNE RESPONSE, 2228
Tolerance and Immunity: Self-Nonself Discrimination, 2229
Antigen Recognition, 2229
Immune Tolerance, 2229
TRANSPLANTATION ANTIGENS, 2230
The Major Histocompatibility Complex, 2231
HLA Molecules: Class I, 2231
HLA Molecules: Class II, 2233
Inheritance of HLA, 2233
HLA Typing, 2234
Relative Strengths of HLA Loci, 2235
Non-HLA Antigens, 2236
ABO Blood Group Antigens, 2236
Effects of Blood Transfusions, 2237
THE IMMUNE RESPONSE TO ALLOGRAFTS, 2237
T CELL–ANTIGEN-PRESENTING CELL INTERACTIONS, 2237
T Cell Receptor Complex, 2237
CD4 and CD8 T Cells, 2239
Adhesion Molecules, 2239
Costimulatory Molecules, 2240
Cytokines and Chemokines, 2241
HELPER T CELLS AND THEIR ROLE IN THE ALLOIMMUNE RESPONSE, 2241
B Cells and Antibody Production, 2242
EFFECTOR MECHANISMS OF ALLOGRAFT REJECTION, 2242
ACUTE CELLULAR AND HUMORAL REJECTION, 2244
CHRONIC REJECTION, 2244
MECHANISMS OF IMMUNOSUPPRESSION, 2245
Corticosteroids, 2245
Azathioprine, 2245
Mycophenolic Acid, 2245
Cyclosporine, 2246
Tacrolimus, 2247
Mammalian Target of Rapamycin Inhibitors, 2247
Polyclonal Immune Globulins, 2247
Monoclonal Antibodies, 2248
Genomics and Proteomics, 2249
TOLEROGENIC PROTOCOLS IN TRANSPLANTATION, 2249

CHARACTERISTICS OF THE ALLOGENEIC IMMUNE RESPONSE

The term *allogeneic* refers to the genetic relationship between two individuals of the same species, in contrast to *xenogeneic* for different species, and *syngeneic* for human monozygous twins or completely inbred animals of the same genetic background or strain. The immune system evolved to protect us from invading microorganisms. It appears also to play a protective role in surveillance for altered normal cells, such as ones that have undergone malignant transformation or those that become reactive to self-tissue such as in autoimmune diseases. The components of the immune system that are recruited when there is a threat to body integrity are multiple, and they vary according to the nature of the threat (e.g., viral versus bacterial) and the anatomic location of the insult (e.g., skin or gastrointestinal tract). Many important components of immunity that are ancient in evolutionary time are described as components of natural or innate immunity. These include phagocytic cells, natural killer (NK) cells, complement, and some cytokines and chemokines. Tissue injury from any cause can activate the innate immune system. In contrast, immune reactants that specifically recognize foreign molecules or antigens from the microbial world are generated as a result of an adaptive immune response. The main components of such antigen-specific adaptive immunity are immunoglobulins, which are made by B cells, and (thymus-dependent) T cells. In transplantation immunity, recognition of donor antigens is crucial in developing antigen-specific clones of T and B cells, which then direct an even larger array of cellular and humoral responses, many of which do not use specific antigen receptors in the effector phase. Fundamentally, the "firestorm" of allograft rejection does not occur in the absence of cell-mediated immune responses initiated by specific T lymphocytes, but the full force of the rejection uses components of both innate and adaptive immunity. The innate immune response, initially triggered by ischemia-reperfusion injury associated with transplantation, is capable of driving immune cells to the target injury site and augmenting the antigen-specific immune response, thus contributing ultimately to graft destruction.

The first successful kidney transplantation was performed in 1954 at the Peter Bent Brigham Hospital in Boston, Massachusetts, between identical twins. In the 1960s, recognition of the immunosuppressive properties of azathioprine in combination with corticosteroids made it possible to successfully perform transplant surgeries between nonidentical donors and recipients. Improvements in surgical techniques and the development of newer immunosuppressive agents, including cyclosporine, tacrolimus, mycophenolic acid (MPA), and mammalian target of rapamycin (mTOR) inhibitors, as well as polyclonal and specific monoclonal antibodies, have reduced the incidence and intensity of acute rejection, but the problem of chronic allograft dysfunction has remained as a persistent obstacle. Because transplantation was a very rare event until modern times, the immune system clearly did not evolve to mediate allograft rejection. It was the investigation of the alloimmune response to transplanted tissues that led to the identification of the major histocompatibility complex (MHC) molecules, also called HLA antigens. This investigation, in turn, provided crucial insights into the process of immune recognition, leading to the discovery that MHC molecules play a central role in presenting foreign antigenic peptides molecules to T cells in a way that they can be recognized by the antigen-specific T cell receptors (TCRs). MHC molecules exhibit a large degree of polymorphism between different individuals and therefore become an important target for immune recognition by the recipient upon transplantation. Although there are many similarities between immune recognition of conventional antigen and the recognition of allogeneic transplantation antigens, the major difference is the markedly increased frequency of responding T cells against donor MHC molecules in the allogeneic response. T cells do not contact allo-MHC or foreign MHC molecules during development in the thymus and thus escape the deletion (negative selection) imposed by interaction with self-MHC. The molecular basis for the high frequency of T cells responding to an allogeneic stimulus remains incompletely understood; however, the high frequency of alloantigen-specific T cells contributes to the vigorous nature of the immune response that causes early acute allograft rejection, and it is the major initial obstacle to successful organ transplantation.

TOLERANCE AND IMMUNITY: SELF-NONSELF DISCRIMINATION

The principal tenet of immune recognition is that the immune system must discriminate self from nonself. This process has been viewed as being dependent on two components. First, the immune system must not respond to any self-antigens, which it does principally through the mechanisms of self-tolerance. Second, nonself (foreign) antigens derived from numerous sources, including pathogens and tumor cells, must be effectively recognized to prevent infection and malignancy. In this paradigm, the immune system simply recognizes transplanted tissues as nonself, causing allograft rejection. In reality, it now seems that auto recognition of self-antigens is not uncommon, but only rarely results in autoimmune disease. The key resides in an effective immunoregulatory system that is more complex than was previously imagined. The ultimate goal of clinical transplantation is to develop protocols to induce specific tolerance to the graft, so that the immune system is regulated to accept the allograft as self without maintenance immunosuppression.

ANTIGEN RECOGNITION

T and B cells are capable of recognizing a foreign antigen through antigen-specific receptors—and B cell antigen receptor (BCR), respectively. While the TCR recognizes peptide fragments of processed antigen only when they are bound to MHC molecules expressed on the surface of antigen-presenting cells (APCs), immunoglobulins or the B cell receptor can bind directly to peptide fragments or to the same peptide sequences in the intact native molecule. In the early days of study of MHC antigens, investigators wondered why hematopoietic cells, especially B cells, dendritic cells, and monocyte-macrophages, have high expression of MHC molecules. It is now quite clear that the true role of the MHC is to present potentially immunogenic peptides of foreign antigens to T lymphocytes. Whereas the T cell response to a conventional antigen can be experimentally detected only after previous immunization, an allogeneic response, as assayed in a mixed lymphocyte culture in vitro, can be readily detected in previously unimmunized (naive) lymphocytes. At least part of the basis for the greater magnitude of the allogeneic response is the increased frequency of responding cells. For example, the frequency of specific T cells to conventional antigens is approximately 1 in 10^4 to 10^5, whereas the frequency responding during allogeneic stimulation can be as high as 1%. The allograft, which includes donor bone marrow–derived APCs, usually expresses several class I and class II MHC molecules that differ from the recipient's MHC molecules and can directly stimulate recipient T cells (direct allorecognition). Alternatively, donor antigens can be processed and peptide fragments presented by the host MHC molecules on self-APCs, indirectly stimulating the recipient T cells (indirect allorecognition) by way of the same pathway used for responses to microbial antigens (see "T-Cell–Antigen-Presenting Cell Interactions" section). Relevant to clinical transplantation, the greater intensity of an allogeneic response can produce vigorous episodes of acute allograft rejection that can be difficult to control and may require large doses of immunosuppressive agents (see Chapter 72).

IMMUNE TOLERANCE

Immune tolerance is a state of unresponsiveness to specific antigens derived from either self-proteins or nonself-proteins.

From numerous studies it is clear that maintenance of immune tolerance to self-antigens involves multiple mechanisms. First, tolerance can occur at the level of either T or B lymphocytes.[1] Second, tolerance can be induced in either immature lymphocytes during the early steps of differentiation or in mature lymphocytes after they have migrated to the peripheral lymphoid tissues, including lymph nodes and spleen.[2] Third, tolerance, or immune unresponsiveness, can be mediated by several mechanisms, including clonal deletion of antigen-specific lymphocytes, anergy (inactivation of lymphocytes that nevertheless remain viable), and suppression involving regulatory processes among different subsets of lymphocytes. Evidence from human studies and animal models indicates that maintenance of self-tolerance involves many, if not all, of these mechanisms.

The major mechanism of self-tolerance is the elimination of potentially autoreactive T cells at an immature stage of development during maturation in the thymus by a process called "negative selection."[3] It is estimated that more than 95% of thymocytes die because of a high-affinity encounter with self-MHC before they migrate to the peripheral lymphoid organs.[4] Thymocyte clones that are positively selected for differentiation into mature peripheral T lymphocytes have receptors that are less avid for self-MHC and also possess the necessary repertoire to recognize a large number of peptide configurations when bound to self-MHC, and by cross reaction (molecular mimicry), to the intact surfaces of allo-MHC. Although negative selection is a major mechanism for maintaining self-tolerance, the process of negative selection is not complete, and potentially self-reactive T cells are able to escape and emigrate to the periphery. The immune system has therefore evolved mechanisms to maintain tolerance in the periphery.[5]

TRANSPLANTATION ANTIGENS

Normal persons maintain a state of self-tolerance to self-tissues. Allografts, however, express nonself antigens to which the recipient is not tolerant, and they cause an anti-allograft immune response that initiates rejection. Several types of transplantation antigens have been characterized, including the MHC molecules, minor histocompatibility antigens, ABO blood group antigens, and monocyte and endothelial cell antigens. The antigenic stimulus for initiation and progression of the rejection response to allografted tissue is provoked by cell surface molecules that are polymorphic (i.e., vary in structure from individual to individual and are treated as foreign intruders that the body must recognize and destroy). The most important transplantation antigens are those of the MHC (Figures 71.1 and 71.2), which can trigger a strong immune response without priming. In animals and humans, this series of linked genes provides the strongest incompatibilities for any sort of tissue and organ transplantation. The MHC antigens were originally discovered during tumor transplants between different inbred strains of mice, but their evolutionary conservation is based on defense against the microbial world. The minor histocompatibility antigens are processed antigens in the form of small peptides that are presented by MHC molecules but are not derived from the MHC molecules. T cells recognize a combination of the antigen and MHC complexes through a trimolecular interaction involving the TCR, MHC molecule, and processed antigen in the form of a short peptide. The minor histocompatibility antigens require priming and can be detected only in a secondary immune response.

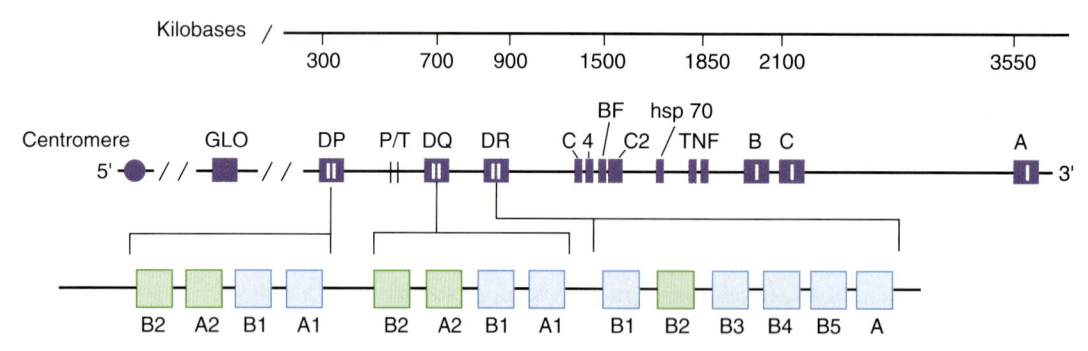

Figure 71.1 Schematic map of the HLA region on the short arm of chromosome 6. Distances are shown in kilobases derived from sequencing of DNA nucleotides. The centromere is to the left (5′). The boxes along the central line represent coding regions for the HLA polypeptides expressed on cell surfaces. GLO is a polymorphic red blood cell enzyme more than 4000 kilobases from HLA. On the right are the HLA-A, HLA-B, and HLA-C loci for the three sets of class I heavy chains, and on the left are the loci for the three sets of class II molecules, HLA-DP, HLA-DQ, and HLA-DR. The latter are composed of two chains, α and β, each the product of linked genes of the DP, DQ, or DR subregions. The *DRA* gene, for example, encodes the α-chain, and several *DRB* genes encode the β-chains, of the heterodimeric HLA-DR molecules. In the case of DR, DRA is not polymorphic, so all the antigenicity lies with DRB. As shown in the expansion at the bottom, each subregion contains tandem sets of exons for one or more α- and β-chains. The gene for DR private specificities is *HLA-DRB1*; the more public HLA-DR51, HLA-DR52, and HLA-DR53 are encoded by the other B genes (see text). Pseudogenes, which are not expressed on the cell surface, are shown as *white boxes*. The HLA-DP and HLA-DQ molecules are also heterodimers, and both the α- and β-chains are polymorphic. Genes involved in proteolysis of proteins and the intracellular transport of peptides to meet up with class I molecules are in the class II region near DQ (shown as P/T). Between the class I and II loci are genes for the complement components C2, BF (factor B), and C4. The genes for tumor necrosis factor-α (TNF-α) and tumor necrosis factor-β (TNF-β), and heat shock protein 70 (hsp70), have been mapped between the complement region and HLA-B. (From Carpenter CB: Histocompatibility systems in man. In Ginns LC, Cosimi AB, Morris PJ, editors: *Transplantation*, Boston, 1999, Blackwell Science, p 61.)

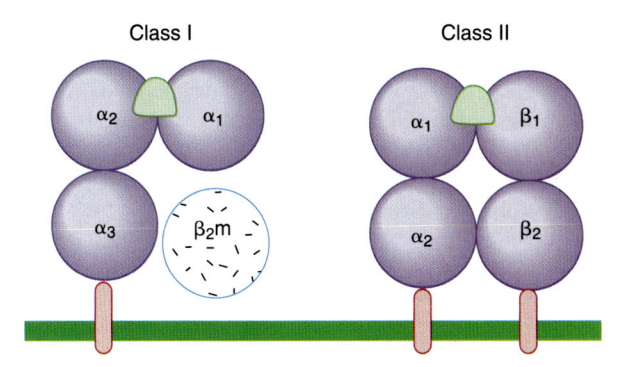

Figure 71.2 Class I and class II HLA molecules on a cell membrane as seen from the side of the molecules. In the class I HLA molecule, the 44-kDa α-chain is inserted through the lipid bilayer of the membrane and has three domains (α_1, α_2, α_3) formed in part by disulfide bonding. β_2-Microglobulin, encoded by a gene on chromosome 15, is noncovalently bound and is not membrane inserted. The α_2 and α_1 domains from the β-strands and α-helices form the base and sides, respectively, of the groove that binds a potentially immunogenic peptide. The variable amino acids that confer the antigenic differences between individual HLA types are arrayed along this groove. Class II molecules consist of one α-chain (34 kDa) and one β-chain (28 kDa), each having two domains, and each is membrane inserted. A similar peptide-binding groove is formed by the α_1 and β_1 domains. (From Carpenter CB: Histocompatibility systems in man. In Ginns LC, Cosimi AB, Morris PJ, editors: *Transplantation*, Boston, 1999, Blackwell Science, p 62.)

THE MAJOR HISTOCOMPATIBILITY COMPLEX

The MHC was first defined in the mouse as the agent of rapid rejection of tumor transplants between inbred strains of mice.[6,7] This antigen system was called H-2 and was found to function in rejection of normal tissues as well. Rejection elicits serum antibodies that are used for typing of H-2 antigens. It was subsequently shown that cytotoxic T cells also arise in response to H-2 differences and that the H-2 genes are all clustered in a single region on chromosome 17.[8] Except for some details of the ordering of genes, the human (HLA) and rat (RT1) MHC regions are quite homologous to H-2 of the mouse.[9] The species' chromosome numbers are different only because they have not been numbered in a manner that reflects the locations of actual genes. Transplants compatible for the MHC antigens can still be rejected because of minor antigen (e.g., H-1, H-3, H-4) incompatibilities, but not with the same intensity as with MHC-incompatible allografts. Modification of rejection by drugs or other means is more readily accomplished when the donor and recipient MHC antigens are matched. Extensive work in the mouse skin allograft model with a large number of different major (H-2) and minor incompatibilities has shown that, in general, the sum total of multiple non–H-2 (minor) incompatibilities, once the recipient has become immunized to such antigens, can be equal to the strength of the H-2 barrier alone in the unimmunized, or first-set, rejection response.[10] For both MHC and non-MHC barriers, placement of a second allograft from the same donor is rejected at an accelerated rate (second-set rejection). The distinction of first- and second-set rejection phenomena in humans was first made by Holman in 1924 with skin allografts in patients with burns.[11] During World War II, the problem of extensive burn injuries prompted fundamental studies of skin allografting by Medawar[12] and laid the groundwork for the development of clinical transplantation in the second half of the twentieth century.

The ability to produce an efficient immune response to many antigens is inherited in a mendelian autosomal dominant fashion, and the controlling genes, called "Ir" (for immune response), are of the MHC. In fact, the failure to mount a response to a peptide antigen may be attributed to a genetically determined inability to bind properly the antigenic fragment to MHC molecules.[13] The complex of antigen and MHC provides an efficient mode of presentation to clones of T lymphocytes that bear the appropriate antigen receptors. Indeed, it is clear that the TCR recognizes the total configuration of self-MHC plus the antigen fragment (peptide), and not antigen alone. Many experimental systems have demonstrated this MHC restriction phenomenon; that is, T cells, in order to respond, must share MHC antigens with the APCs. The combined recognition of self-MHC plus antigen (self plus X hypothesis) has been visualized at the molecular level (see later).

The HLA region on the short arm of chromosome 6 (see Figure 71.1) contains more than three million nucleotide base pairs. It encodes two structurally distinct classes of cell surface molecules, termed *class I* and *II* (see Figure 71.2). The term *MHC antigen* has been traditionally applied to the product of a given locus that displays polymorphism in a population of individuals. Now that the sequence and structure of molecules bearing MHC antigens have been extensively elucidated, it is known that the polymorphic, or antigenic, portions of MHC molecules are, indeed, quite small, often involving only one to four amino acid substitutions in regions of sequence hypervariability. In an MHC molecule, the specific substituted area that causes a change in antigenicity is called an *epitope*. Normal pregnancy induces antibodies against the HLA antigens of the fetus derived from the father's genes. The first appreciation of the HLA system came from the studies of Dausset on blood transfusion reactions caused by antileukocyte antibodies.[9] Subsequent studies showed that such antibodies marked a codominantly expressed antileukocyte system that segregated in a mendelian distribution in families. International workshops on the HLA system began in 1962, and today they continue to accelerate progress in the definition and technical aspects of typing for the polymorphic antigens of this chromosome region.

Class I and II molecules show some structural homology to immunoglobulins, the T cell antigen receptor, and to molecules bearing the T cell differentiation antigens CD4 and CD8 (see later). The latter are part of the system whereby T cells interact preferentially with class II or class I molecules, respectively, on APCs or on cells that are targets for immune destruction. This family of cell surface and extracellular recognition and interaction structures may have evolved from the same progenitor gene, diversifying by duplication and mutation, and in the process the new genes have moved to multiple chromosome sites. All mammalian species studied thus far have structural and functional representations of this "immunoglobulin supergene" family.

HLA MOLECULES: CLASS I

Class I HLA molecules consist of two polypeptide chains in noncovalent association on cell surfaces. The heavy chain

(44 kDa) is inserted into the plasma membrane and contains the antigenic portions. The light chain (12 kDa) is β_2-microglobulin, encoded by a gene on chromosome 15. There are three domains of the class I heavy chain, formed in part by disulfide bonding to make loops (see Figure 71.2). The amino acid sequence variable regions are on the first (α_1) and second (α_2) domains. Class I molecules are expressed on almost all nucleated body cells, including the endothelium of blood vessels. Tissue typing is performed on peripheral blood, lymph node, or spleen lymphocytes, all of which strongly express HLA class I. Platelets are not commonly used for typing, but they are useful for absorbing anti–class I antibodies from serum, as they do not express class II antigens. Some organ-specific anatomic variations occur in endothelial expression, and in states of active inflammation the density of class I can be locally increased. There are three class I heavy chain loci, *HLA-A, HLA-B,* and *HLA-C* (see Figure 71.1). Each locus product in a given individual bears a unique—so-called private—antigenic epitope plus additional *public* epitopes that are shared more widely among the population. Traditionally HLA epitopes were recognized by serologically typing, identifying HLA antigens through their reactivity to defined anti-HLA antibodies. More recently HLA alleles have been defined by DNA typing, which will likely become the standard for tissue typing in the near future.

Currently over 8000 class I alleles have been defined by DNA techniques, although the majority of these may not be clinically relevant in solid organ transplantation, as they are not expressed or are expressed at low levels on the cell surface or are of low antigenicity.

The first MHC molecule to be crystallized was HLA-A2, and the structure of this class I allele was determined by x-ray diffraction studies to a resolution of 3.5 Å (Figure 71.3). This accomplishment afforded visualization of how the amino acid sequence relates to the folding of the chains into a three-dimensional structure. The two distal membrane domains, α_1 and α_2, form a groove along the top surface of the molecule facing away from the cell membrane. The margins of the groove are formed by α-helices, and the base is floored by a series of eight parallel β-strands, with the α_1 and α_2 domains contributing more or less equally

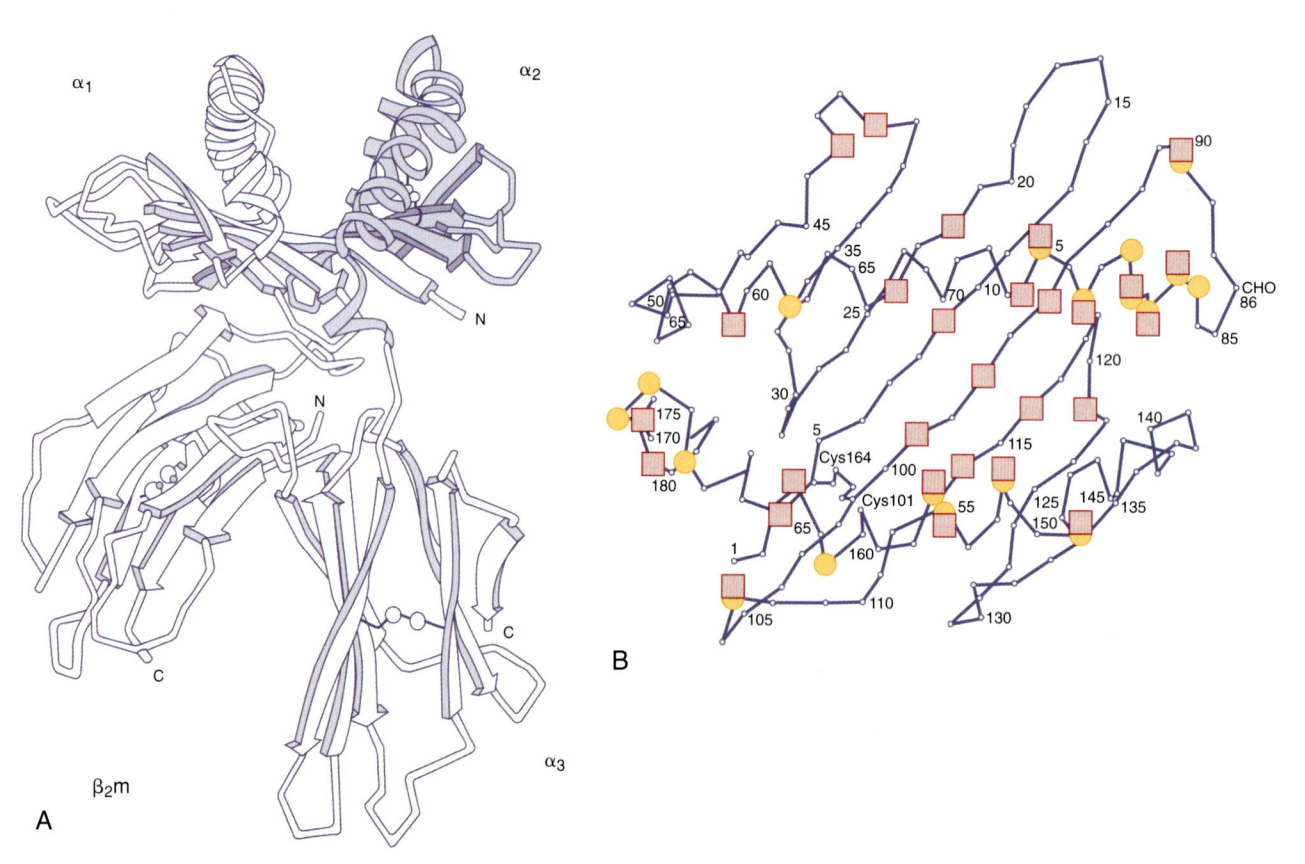

Figure 71.3 The structure of the HLA-A2 molecule derived from x-ray crystallographic study. **A,** The flat ribbons represent the β-sheets or β-strands, and the spiral areas at the top (membrane distal) are the α-helices, which form the sides of a groove approximately 10 Å wide and 25 Å long. The floor of the groove is formed by eight parallel β-sheets. The COOH-terminal end of the α_3 domain is inserted in the membrane. **B,** This view looks down on the top of the molecule, so that the groove goes from left to right. Diagrammed is the core structure of the amino acid sequence, consecutively numbered from 1 (*bottom left*) to 180 (*center left*). The symbols show the variable amino acid substitutions that have been identified in different human or mouse haplotypes as relating to sites of reactivity to alloreactive T cells (*squares*) or to monoclonal antibodies (*circles*). Sites that relate to both are shown as dual symbols. Whereas the antibody sites are on the external surface of the helices, many of the T cell sites are at the base of the groove. The variable sites determine which peptide sequences can be bound by a given major histocompatibility complex allele (see text). (**A** from Bjorkman P, Saper M, Samroui B, et al: Structure of the human class I histocompatibility antigen, HLA-A2, *Nature* 329:506-512, 1987; **B** modified from Bjorkman P, Saper M, Samroui B, et al: The foreign antigen binding site and T cell recognition regions of class I histocompatibility antigens, *Nature* 329:512-518, 1987.)

to each side of the structure. In the crystallographic study, the groove, approximately 25 Å long and 10 Å wide, contained an unidentified molecule that in subsequent studies was shown to represent the bound peptide fragment, eight to nine amino acids long. These peptides have an extended linear core structure, and binding is to a large measure determined by side-chain interactions. When the locations of amino acid variations, already known from study of sequences and interactions with antibodies or cytotoxic T cells, are related to the crystal structure, it is remarkable that the HLA variable sites lie along the α-helical and β-strand surfaces that form the margins of the groove (see Figure 71.3). In other words, the polymorphisms serve to define the shape of the binding groove on MHC molecules and thus determine which peptides will be bound and recognized by T cells. The sites that determine whether or not a given peptide binds may also confer a conformational change on the fragment. The result is that the TCR binds to the unique topography of the MHC surface formed by a given MHC and peptide combination.[14] The TCR has two chains, α and β, which form a heterodimer. The membrane distal surface of the assembled TCR has six variable loops, called $CDR\alpha_1$, $CDR\alpha_2$, and $CDR\alpha_3$, and $CDR\beta_1$, $CDR\beta_2$, and $CDR\beta_3$, which provide the specificity of binding to the MHC α-helices and bound-peptide antigen.[15] Additional human and mouse class I molecules have been crystallized, and the hypothesis that allelic polymorphisms determine binding of different peptide sequences has been confirmed. Peptides found in eluates from class I crystals or purified molecules are usually eight or nine residues in length. Their origin is in the intracellular pool of polypeptides derived from metabolic turnover of housekeeping proteins or intracellular infections such as viruses. There is selective proteolysis and transmembrane transport from lysosomal compartments into the Golgi, where octamer or nonamer peptides are placed in class I binding sites before transport to the cell surface. Some of the genes that control this process are in the class II region of the MHC (see Figure 71.1).[16]

HLA MOLECULES: CLASS II

Class II HLA molecules consist of two membrane-inserted and noncovalently associated glycosylated polypeptides, called α (34 kDa) and β (28 kDa) (see Figure 71.2). Each of these chains has two domains, and, again, the polymorphic regions are mostly on the outer, NH2-terminal domains. The region of *HLA* encompassing class II genes is generally referred to as *HLA-D*. More than 2000 alleles can be identified using DNA-typing techniques. Although three class II molecules, HLA-DP, HLA-DQ, and HLA-DR, are generally recognized on cell surfaces, the situation is not entirely analogous to class I because the α- and β-chains of each class II molecule are encoded by separate, closely linked genes (see Figure 71.1). Although α- and β-chains of different parental haplotypes can associate, such hybrid associations are restricted to products of the same *DP, DQ,* or *DR* subregion. The naming of *HLA-D*–region genes is based on knowledge of the biochemistry of expressed antigens and on the growing database of DNA nucleotide sequencing. The gene that encodes the HLA-DR α-chain, for example, is called *DRA*. It has no sequence variation (i.e., it is monomorphic). All the variability of different alleles lies in the HLA-DRB chains: *HLA-DRB1* encodes the private DR antigens 1 to 21, and *HLA-DRB3*, *HLA-DRB4,* and *HLA-DRB5* encode α-chains for HLA-DR52, HLA-DR53, and HLA-DR51. The *HLA-DQ* subregion contains the genes *HLA-DQA1, HLA-DQB1, HLA-DQA2,* and *HLA-DQB2*. The latter two are nonexpressed pseudogenes; the products of the first two, DQα and DQβ, are both polymorphic. *HLA-DP* is similarly organized and has polymorphisms on both chains. Study by the Southern blot technique to determine restriction fragment length polymorphisms (RFLPs) of DNA digested with various nucleases and hybridized to complementary DNA probes specific for the *HLA* genes has proved to be an alternative detection technique that has been particularly informative for class II genes.[17] More rapid and precise detection of actual DNA sequences can now be accomplished by selective polymerase chain reaction amplification of polymorphic gene regions, followed by hybridization with short oligonucleotide probes specific for a given HLA sequence or by RFLP analysis of the amplified product.[8] Comparative studies in ongoing workshops have demonstrated a strong correlation between serologically defined polymorphisms and those identified by T cell clones reactive to class II molecules.

Analysis of crystals of class II HLA-DR1 shows a remarkable similarity to class I molecules in the peptide-binding region (see Figure 71.3). The α-helical and β-stranded core structures of class I and II are virtually superimposable. The main difference is at the ends of the groove, which in class II are more open, allowing for binding of longer peptides. Typically, the length of eluted peptides from class II molecules is 13 to 26 residues, and there is protrusion of the linearly arrayed peptide at both ends of the groove.[18,19] Class II antigens are limited in expression to B lymphocytes, monocytes and macrophages, dendritic cells, and activated T lymphocytes. Human endothelium generally does not express class II, but inflammation in the vicinity can result in endothelial expression of class II antigens. In addition, epithelial cells of skin, intestine, and renal proximal tubule can synthesize and express class II molecules in response to injury and inflammation.

Peptides bound to class II molecules are derived from proteolysis in acidic endosomal compartments and represent endocytosed proteins or microorganisms coming from outside the APC. Thus the extracellular compartment, in contrast to the intracellular compartment for class I, is the responsibility of the typical class II–positive APC. When foreign polypeptide antigens are added to cultured APCs, peptide fragments appear on class II (but not on class I) molecules in a matter of minutes. Peptide fragments of self-MHC classes I and II are found in the eluates from class II molecules,[19] indicating that there is representation of intracellularly synthesized products on class II at the cell surface or that secreted molecules reenter the cell by the endocytic pathway.

INHERITANCE OF HLA

Because chromosomes are paired, each person has two sets of HLA antigens, one set from each parent. The genetically linked antigens of the entire HLA region inherited from one parent collectively are called a *haplotype*, and, according to the rules of simple mendelian dominant inheritance, any

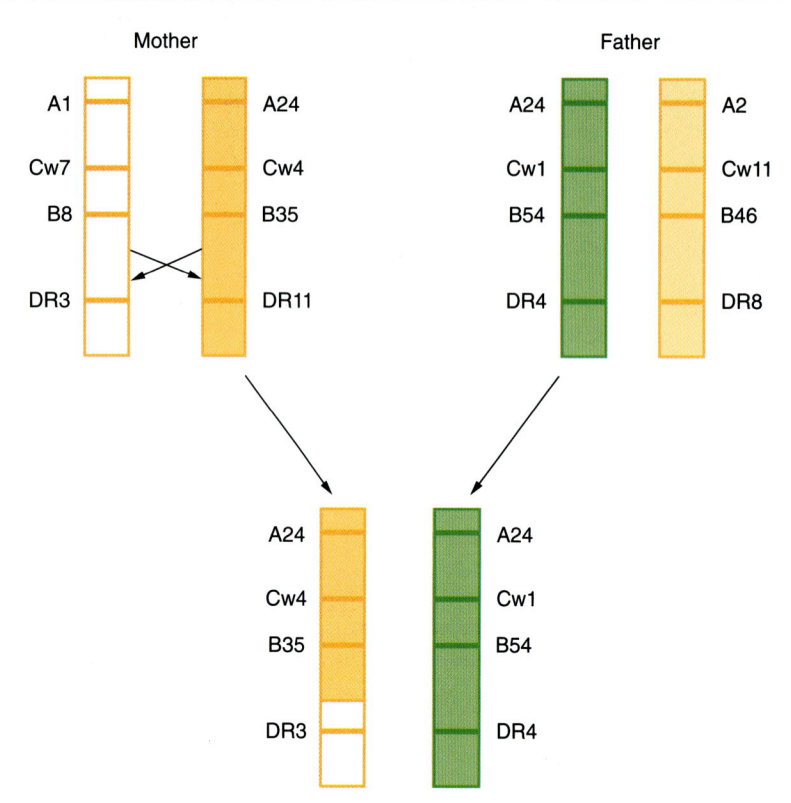

Figure 71.4 Inheritance of HLA haplotypes. The *HLA-A*, *HLA-Cw*, *HLA-B*, and *HLA-DR* genes are shown to represent the entire region. Children inherit one of each of the parental HLA haplotypes, and they are inherited as a block unless a recombination has occurred during meiosis of an ovum or sperm, shown here as an *arrow* between B and DR in the mother. Such events occur less than 1% of the time for HLA. The chances of an HLA-identical sibling or an entirely nonmatching pair in a family is 1:4. Haploidentical siblings occur with odds of 1:2, and all children are haploidentical with each parent.

sibling pair has a 25% chance of inheriting the same two parental haplotypes, a 50% chance of sharing one haplotype, and a 25% chance of having two completely different haplotypes (Figure 71.4). The main evidence that HLA is the major transplantation barrier in humans originally came from the observation that, in kidney transplantation, HLA-identical sibling donor kidneys provided the best long-term transplant survival and required the least aggressive immunosuppression. In the absence of a recombination (crossover), the entire *HLA-A* to *HLA-DP* region is expressed with each inherited haplotype. Recombination rates within the region are in the vicinity of less than 1%; thus, generally, it is not necessary to "type" for the expressed products of all the loci to identify haplotypes within a family. Rarely, when recombination has occurred or when several common antigens are present on both sides of a family, complete molecular typing of HLA may be necessary.

The distribution of HLA antigens in the general population is not random. Some are more common than others, and racial and ethnic patterns are well known. Furthermore, within a given racial or ethnic group, certain HLA haplotypes or portions thereof are likely to be found with higher frequency than one would predict by random distribution. For example, HLA-A1, HLA-B8, and HLA-DR3 very often occur on the same haplotype in northern Europeans. These alleles are not in equilibrium and thus are said to be in "linkage disequilibrium." When entire, so-called extended haplotypes are found in apparently unrelated persons, it is likely that they were inherited from a common and relatively recent ancestor. When alleles of adjacent loci of the HLA region (e.g., *B* and *DR*) are in linkage disequilibrium, the possibility exists that selective pressures were exerted over many generations to sustain the coexpression of a combination that favors defense against infectious diseases. Review of the associations of HLA alleles with a number of diseases is beyond the purpose of this chapter,[20] but the existence of linkage disequilibrium is relevant to considerations of HLA antigen distribution throughout the general population, a matter of direct concern when matching donors for transplantation.

HLA TYPING

Traditionally the main sources of antibodies for typing come from large-scale screenings of thousands of serum samples from multiparous women. Immunizations among humans yield the most highly specific antibodies to private HLA determinants. Anti–class I (HLA-A, HLA-B, HLA-C) antibodies react with both B and T lymphocytes, whereas anti–class II antibodies react with B, but not T, cells. Generally, a positive reaction is marked by cell lysis in the presence of rabbit complement. In addition, more broadly reactive antisera, originally thought to contain several antibodies in mixture, may have reactivity to the public determinants. For example, HLA-B molecules contain at least three immunogenic regions, one for private and two for public polymorphisms. Monoclonal antibodies derived from the immunization of mice or rats with human lymphocytes only occasionally bind to the same antigenic sites defined by human antibodies. Although there are several examples of monoclonal antibodies that may substitute for human antisera, a large number of monoclonal antibodies react in a "public" fashion, but not necessarily in the same patterns that human antisera do.

The mixed lymphocyte reaction (MLR) occurs when lymphocytes of one individual are cultured with those of another. Proliferation occurs over 5 to 7 days and is measured by the incorporation rate of 3H-thymidine into newly replicated DNA.[21] Usually one population of cells is irradiated to prevent proliferation; then the readout represents the response of nonirradiated helper T (T_H) cells to the class II antigens present on stimulator B cells or macrophages or dendritic cells. Genetic identity for HLA yields a negative, nonproliferating MLR; similarity is revealed by weak proliferation. Before the HLA-DP, HLA-DQ, and HLA-DR subregions were clearly defined, incompatibility for the MLR was attributed entirely to "HLA-D." The MLR is rarely used now as a clinical test, because the complexity of HLA-D can be fully assessed by typing. HLA-DR determinants provide the strongest MLR stimulus, whereas DQ plays a lesser role, although it is increasingly recognized as the target for anti-HLA antibodies involved in antibody-mediated rejection in kidney transplantation. HLA-DP is recognized only by primed (i.e., previously immunized) cells. The MLR itself is a complex series of cellular responses. Helper cell clones are first activated to proliferate but then induce the proliferative burst of $CD8^+$ cytotoxic T cells. The latter are generally directed to class I incompatibilities and injure appropriate target cells after direct cell-to-cell contact is initiated by T cell–antigen receptors. When cytotoxic T cells are tested against a large number of individuals typed by classical serologic techniques, a good, but not perfect, correlation is observed overall. Some antigenic sites, or epitopes, recognized by T cells are actually different from those on the same class I molecule that are recognized by antibodies. This is explained by the fact that immunoglobulins can recognize small epitopes on intact whole molecules with tertiary structures, whereas T cells "see" only the complex surface made up of a peptide fragment bound in the MHC-binding groove. Further, there is more than one diversity site per HLA molecule that provides targets for rejection. The private specificities are, by definition, most immunogenic in the human antihuman alloresponse, but a given specificity usually involves a composite of small amino acid differences at more than one site in an HLA molecule.

The marked superiority of HLA haplotype–identical sibling donors for organ and bone marrow transplantation has been demonstrable since the early 1970s.[22] The technology of HLA typing need not be absolutely accurate for selection of HLA-identical sibling donors, but, conversely, true definition of a zero-mismatched cadaver donor for HLA-A, HLA-B, and HLA-DR may require molecular DNA typing. It is fair to say that widespread competency in both class I and class II serologic typing has been achieved only in the past decade, but it is still imperfect, and there is direct evidence that technical difficulties with HLA serologic methods can account for poor correlations with grafting results. Pooled information from a large number of collaborating centers, and that include tens of thousands of cases, provides strong evidence of the role of HLA phenotypic matching in the success of deceased donor kidney transplantation.

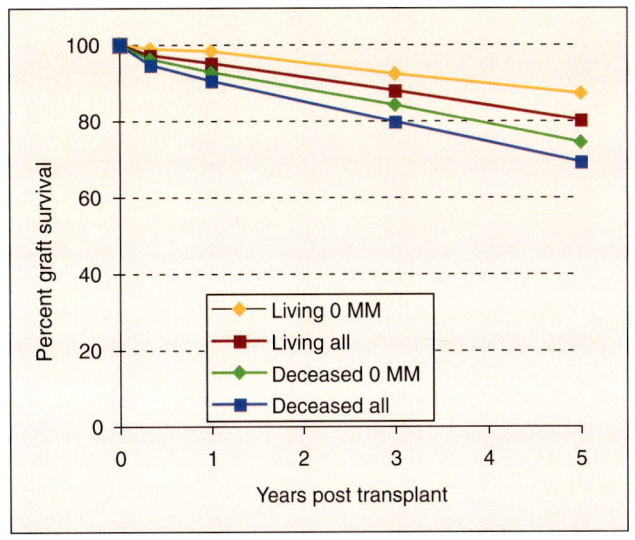

Figure 71.5 Long-term graft survival as a function of donor source and HLA matching. Data are from the Scientific Registry of Transplant Recipients. Recipients of living kidney transplants have improved short- and long-term outcomes compared with recipients of deceased donor grafts, indicating the influence of the ischemic insult that deceased donor kidneys are exposed to during harvesting and transportation. The survival for randomly matched living-donor kidneys (*Living all*) is still superior to zero HLA-mismatched deceased donor kidneys (*Deceased 0 MM*). (Survival curves drawn from Scientific Registry of Transplant Recipients data, www.srtr.org.)

There is rather strong evidence that long-term allograft survival is improved by avoiding HLA mismatches. Log-linear plots of allograft survival always show a straight-line decline after the first year, which makes it possible to calculate a half-life and to project survival rates over time. The rate of allograft survival at 5 years is higher for zero HLA antigen mismatch compared to six-antigen mismatch kidneys for living (88% vs. 79%), deceased standard criteria donor (75% vs. 66%), and deceased extended criteria donor (60% vs. 55%), respectively[23] (Figure 71.5). Avoiding ischemic and storage injury of organs from living donors certainly enhances outcomes as compared with those from deceased donors.

There is considerable opportunity both for matching more cases and for avoiding completely mismatched allografts. It is worth noting that current projections give the same, or better, 10-year allograft survival rates to deceased donor organs that are not mismatched with recipients for HLA-A, HLA-B, and HLA-DR as with HLA haplotype–identical family donors. It is for this reason that the United Network for Organ Sharing (UNOS) has a mandatory share policy for zero-mismatched deceased donor kidneys. Because of the size of the national pool available, approximately 15% to 20% of deceased donor kidneys are now shared on this basis.

RELATIVE STRENGTHS OF HLA LOCI

Clinical data do not support the simple assumption that each mismatch for antigens of various loci has equal weight in causing allograft loss. The major impact comes from the effects of B and DR antigens; little additional effect comes from the A locus. Transplant data from the United Kingdom show that DR matching has a much greater effect than matching of A or B. As compared with the results when no mismatches are present for A, B, or DR, the addition of a single mismatch for A, B, or DR increases the chances of allograft loss twofold for A, threefold for B, and fivefold for DR. The UNOS system uses as the mandatory sharing criterion of a zero mismatch for HLA-A, HLA-B, and HLA-DR. There also appears to be a temporal effect of HLA-A, HLA-B, and HLA-DR mismatching: HLA-DR matching is the most important in the first 6 months after transplantation, the HLA-B effect emerges during the first 2 years, and HLA-A matching does not show an effect before 3 years. These findings are similar to those of Opelz,[23a] who found that during the first posttransplantation year, the class II HLA-DR locus had a larger impact than the class I HLA-A and HLA-B loci. In subsequent years, however, the influence on allograft survival of the three loci was found to be roughly equivalent and additive. This would indicate that, in the absence of prior sensitization, HLA-A mismatches have a deleterious effect only on long-term allograft survival.

The more effective immunosuppressive therapy in common use today produces 1-year deceased donor allograft survival rates as high as those associated with one-haplotype matched living, related donors. The short-term results are approximately 95% allograft survival for first allografts at 1 year (see Figure 71.5). These results are in keeping with the steady increase in early allograft survival and late allograft survival with newer and more powerful immunosuppressive agents. Although 1-year allograft survival rate has steadily improved to more than 95% over the past few decades with better immunosuppressant strategies, this has not been successfully translated to improved long-term kidney allograft survival. Five-year overall adjusted allograft survival of extended criteria donor, non–extended criteria donor, and living donor kidney recipients is only 57%, 72%, and 81%, respectively.[23] The association of HLA matching with long-term allograft survival is less apparent. Patients experiencing an acute rejection episode have shorter long-term allograft survival. Acute rejections were of less importance when donor and recipient were HLA matched. It should be noted that the degree of mismatch was not in itself directly predictive of early rejection, but it did predict the prognosis once a rejection episode had occurred. Acute vascular rejection has poorer long-term outcome than less severe tubulointerstitial rejection. Multiple acute rejection episodes are associated with a higher risk for chronic allograft injury. A poor long-term outcome is significantly more common in patients who had more than one acute rejection episode compared to those with only one episode (34.8% vs. 8.9%, respectively). Likewise, a single, late acute rejection episode (occurring >3 months after transplantation) carries a much higher risk for allograft failure than early (<3 months) acute rejections. Studies have shown that patients with acute rejection episodes who recovered their baseline kidney function to more than 95% at 1 year post transplantation had significantly higher 6-year allograft survival compared with their counterparts who had less than 75% baseline recovery. Intrinsic responsiveness of individual patients may to a large extent determine the rejection rate, but in those patients who do reject, the HLA barrier becomes important to short-term survival rates. Alternatively, the rejection tempo may be intrinsically more powerful with more mismatched antigens.

The question of defining intrinsic responsiveness remains open. Failure to reject may reflect the patient's susceptibility to immunosuppressive agents, or it may be related to different donor-recipient histocompatibility combinations. One example would be a patient who does well with a second transplantation after vigorously rejecting a first allograft, with different HLA antigens.

The use of cross-reactive groups (CREGs) (for serologically cross-reacting groups) has been suggested as an alternative to exact HLA matching to increase the potential pool of donors for any given recipient. CREGs classify HLA antigens more broadly into families of structurally related HLA antigens that share public antigenic sites. In addition, novel findings in HLA epitope matching have suggested that this technique may permit identifying mismatches with greater potential to trigger an immune response, including antibody production, which therefore could be avoided during organ allocation.

NON-HLA ANTIGENS

Occasionally allografts undergo hyperacute rejection, despite appropriate ABO matching and negative cross-matches for HLA antibodies. Some of these rejection episodes have been attributed to additional non-HLA antigens, and the importance of these antigens in triggering rejection and alloantibody production has been increasingly recognized. These antigenic targets are expressed on cells of the allograft, including endothelium and epithelium, and are classified as alloantigens, such as the MHC class I chain–related gene A (*MICA*) or B (*MICB*), or tissue-specific autoantigens such as vimentin, cardiac myosin, collagen V, and angiotensin II receptor type 1 (AT_1R). The presence of antibodies against AT_1R has been associated with a higher rate of antibody-mediated kidney graft rejection and worse graft survival. In addition, patients with both anti-AT_1R and donor-specific antibodies had lower graft survival than those with donor-specific antibodies alone. Therefore it seems that a break in self-tolerance may be elicited after transplantation, leading to the generation of these autoantibodies. On the other hand, *MICA* and *MICB* are highly polymorphic genes that are located near the HLA-B locus and are strongly implicated in innate immunity. They are expressed on the cell surface of a restricted number of cell types, including endothelial cells, epithelial cells, fibroblasts, dendritic cells, and activated T and B lymphocytes. An association of anti-MICA antibodies with graft loss has been reported, though few studies have questioned this finding. Lastly, some specific assays looking at anti–endothelial cell antibodies using donor-derived endothelial cells are under development with the promise of expanding the cross-match to non-HLA endothelium antigens and helping better risk stratify patients.

ABO BLOOD GROUP ANTIGENS

The ABO blood group antigens were initially identified as the cause of transfusion reactions during red blood cell transfusions. The A and B groups are glycosylated differentially, whereas group O lacks the enzymes necessary for glycosylation. The antigens are readily recognized by natural antibodies, termed *hemagglutinins* because they cause red cell agglutination. They are relevant to transplantation because they are also expressed on other cell types, including the endothelium. Thus they may cause hyperacute rejection of vascular allografts because of preformed natural antibodies. Specifically, individuals with group A or B types produce natural antibodies to the opposite type, and those with group O produce antibodies to both A and B. However, because group O does not express the glycosylated moiety, both A and B fail to produce antibodies to group O. Allograft rejection because of red blood cell type mismatching can be readily prevented by routine blood typing before transplantation. The rhesus (Rh) factor and other red cell antigens are of little concern, because they are not expressed on endothelial cells. In recent years, a variety of desensitization protocols have been developed to enable ABO-incompatible pairs to proceed with transplantation. The currently recommended protocol involves plasmapheresis, pooled intravenous immunoglobulin, and monoclonal anti-CD20 antibody; long-term graft outcomes of patients desensitized with this regimen have been excellent.[24]

EFFECTS OF BLOOD TRANSFUSIONS

Blood transfusions are associated with a 20% risk for sensitization to incompatible HLA antigens, even with the use of leukocyte-reduced irradiated blood. With the introduction of erythropoietin-stimulating agents, the need for blood transfusions before transplantation has dramatically diminished, and this has helped in the reduction of sensitization in potential transplant recipients.

THE IMMUNE RESPONSE TO ALLOGRAFTS

Acute allograft rejection in an unsensitized host is characterized by a lymphocytic infiltration into the allograft. The vast majority of these cells are not alloantigen specific. Immune cells, as part of the immune surveillance process, pass from the circulatory system through the endothelium and into tissues before returning via the lymphatic system into the circulation. The inevitable tissue damage that occurs during transplantation results in a non–antigen-specific inflammatory response, which greatly increases leukocyte recruitment (including T cells). This in turn is mediated through interactions between surface molecules (known as adhesion molecules) and their receptors on endothelial cells and leukocytes, and also through the secretion and binding of small soluble proteins known as chemokines. The site of alloantigen recognition had been believed to be to the allograft itself, but data seem to indicate that antigen recognition may occur in lymphoid tissues.[25] Unique to the transplant setting, T cells may also recognize foreign MHC and antigen through a process of "molecular mimicry," where the foreign MHC and antigen complex resemble the intended receptor of the TCR and activate the T cell. After T cell interaction with APC through the TCR, a number of other cellular interactions between the cells stabilize the interaction and lead to full T cell activation. The context of antigen presentation, most strongly defined by the type of cell that presents antigen, is also increasingly recognized as important in whether the T cell mounts an aggressive or passive response to the antigen.

T CELL–ANTIGEN-PRESENTING CELL INTERACTIONS

There are two fundamental questions in allorecognition that must be clarified. First, why is the frequency of alloreactive T cells so high? Second, how can positively selected (in the thymus) self-MHC restricted T cells recognize foreign antigens as well as allo-MHC? For one thing, it is apparent that there are at least two distinct, but not necessarily mutually exclusive, pathways of allorecognition.[26] In the so-called direct pathway, T cells recognize intact allo-MHC molecules on the surface of donor or stimulator cells. In the indirect pathway, T cells recognize processed alloantigen as peptides in the context of self-APCs, which is the normal route of T cell recognition of foreign antigens. Both pathways have been shown in experimental animals to contribute independently to allograft rejection.

The relative contributions of the direct and indirect pathways of allorecognition to allograft rejection in humans are under investigation, although data in cardiac, renal, and lung transplant recipients suggest that indirect allorecognition of donor HLA peptides may play a key role in chronic rejection (Figure 71.6).

Direct recognition of intact MHC molecules, though focused on the polymorphic MHC epitopes, is strongly influenced by the presence of peptide in the MHC groove. MHC molecules "empty" of peptide generally are not recognized unless the missing self-peptides are reconstituted. It has also been shown that changing the bound peptide can alter the allorecognition of a given MHC molecule. These observations have provided the rationale for studying the immunomodulatory functions of synthetic peptides, particularly MHC peptides in vitro and in vivo.

The basic premise for indirect allorecognition as a mechanism for initiation or amplification of allograft rejection is that donor alloantigens are shed from the allograft, taken up by recipient APCs, and presented to CD4$^+$ T cells.[27] Indeed, it has been demonstrated that intact HLA molecules are present in the circulation of renal transplant recipients. Therefore, during transplantation, shed fragments of allo-MHC could be processed by host APCs and presented as allopeptides to T cells on self-MHC. This indirect pathway of allorecognition may lead to activation of T_H, which secrete lymphokines and provide the necessary signals for the growth and maturation of effector cytotoxic T lymphocytes, B cells, and monocytes and macrophages, leading to allograft rejection (see Figure 71.6). Other important yet poorly understood mechanisms that may contribute to allograft destruction include nonspecific tissue injury and repair and allograft cell apoptosis. Ischemia-reperfusion injury of the allografted organ leads to upregulation of MHC class II and costimulatory molecules, which in turn increase the "immunogenicity of the allograft" and amplify the immune response to it. The clinical syndromes of rejection are described in detail in Chapter 72.

T CELL RECEPTOR COMPLEX

T cell recognition of alloantigens on APCs is the primary and central event that initiates allograft rejection. The interactions among T lymphocytes and APCs involve multiple T cell surface molecules and their counter-receptors expressed

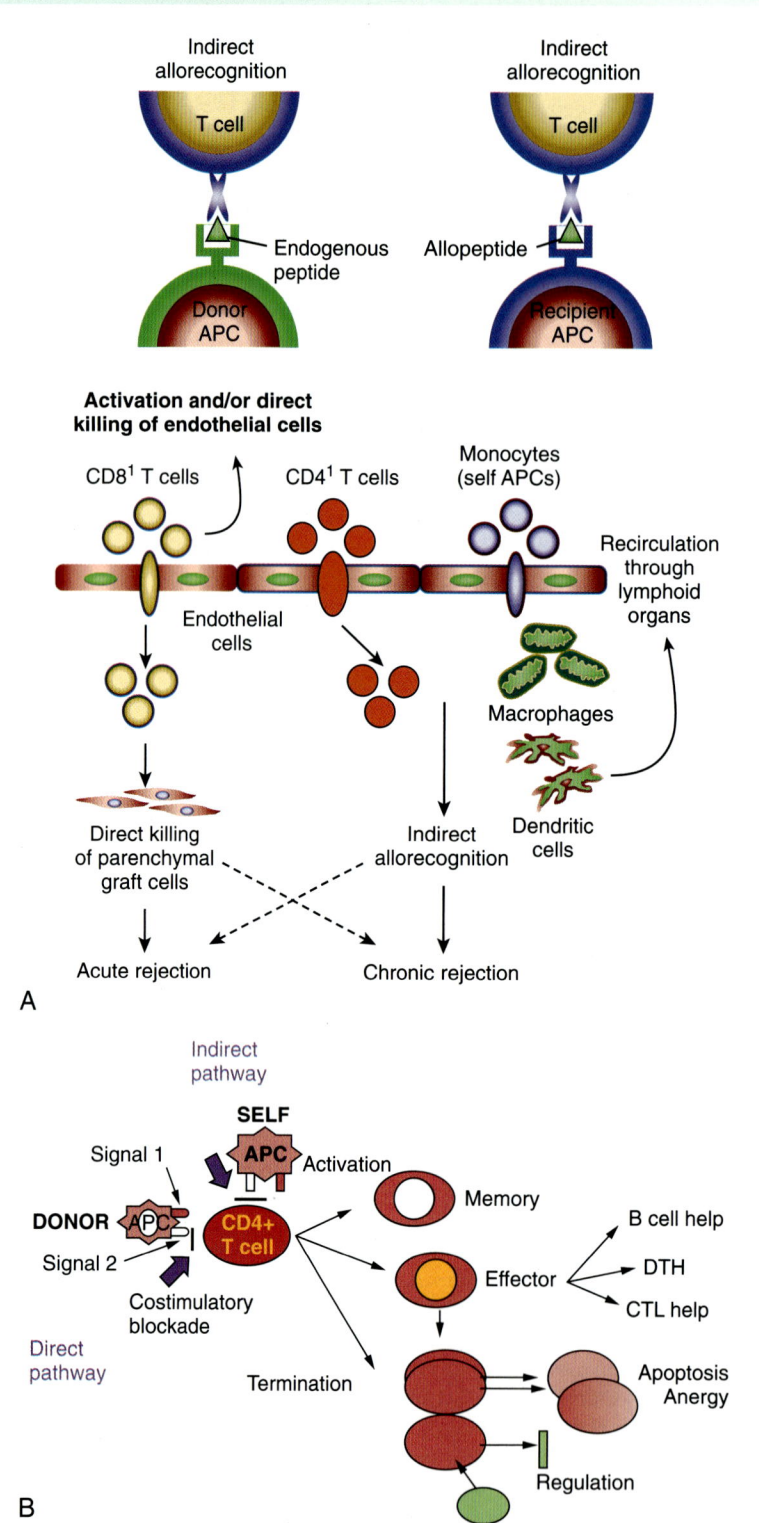

Figure 71.6 **A,** Mechanisms of allorecognition and T cell response. T cells recognize antigen through direct and indirect pathways. In the direct pathway, T cells recognize intact major histocompatibility molecules on donor antigen-presenting cells (APCs). In the indirect pathway, T cells recognize processed alloantigen in the form of peptides presented by recipient APCs. Recipient monocytes are recruited by endothelial cells to the graft tissue. They are also transformed to become highly efficient antigen-presenting dendritic cells that recirculate to peripheral lymphoid organs for maturation. The dendritic cells and intragraft macrophages present donor peptides by way of the indirect pathway to recruited CD4+ T cells. CD8+ T cells, conversely, are activated by donor endothelial cells and can either directly kill endothelial cells or traverse the endothelium and kill parenchymal graft cells. **B,** The alloreactive T cells can undergo a number of different fates. They may provide help for macrophages, B cells, and monocytes by secreting cytokines and by cell-cell contact-dependent mechanisms or kill graft cells in an antigen-specific manner through the release of toxic agents and by Fas-mediated apoptosis. As a process of activation, some T cells undergo cell death or become unresponsive (anergic) to antigenic stimulation through either regulation soluble factors or direct cell contact. Yet others may become memory T cells and await antigenic restimulation to provide a recall response. CTL, Cytotoxic T lymphocyte; DTH, delayed-type hypersensitivity. (**A** from Briscoe DM, Sayegh MH: Rendezvous before rejection: where do T cells meet transplant antigens? *Nat Med* 8:220-222, 2002; **B** from Salama AD, Remuzzi G, Harmon WE, Sayegh MH: Challenges to achieving clinical transplantation tolerance, *J Clin Invest* 108:943-948, 2001.)

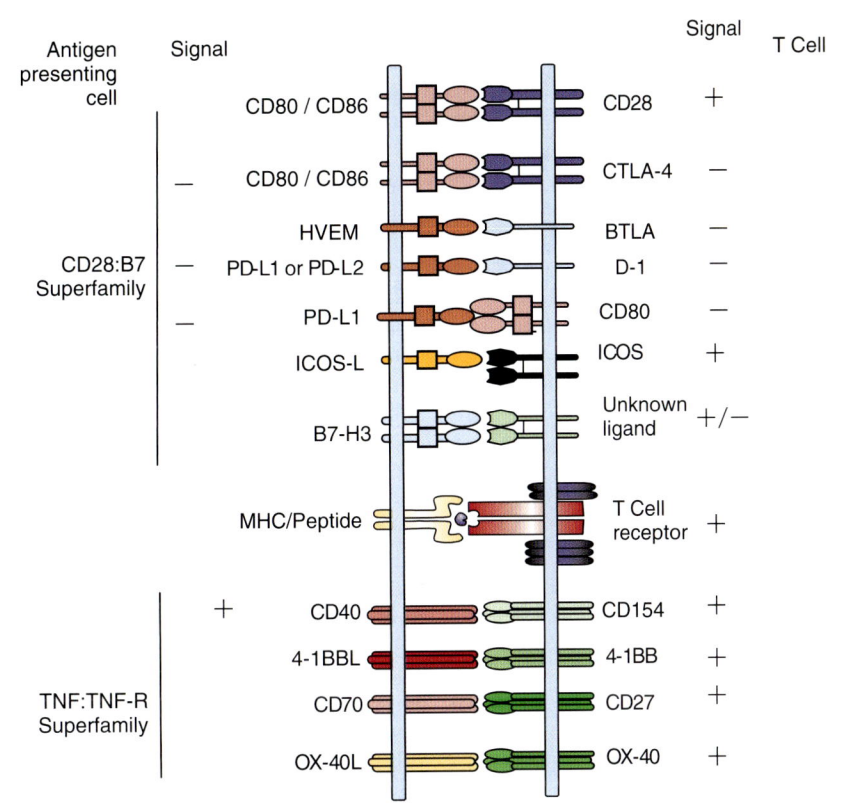

Figure 71.7 CD28:B7 and TNF:TNF-R T cell costimulatory superfamilies. Following ligation of the receptor-ligand pair there is a net stimulatory (+) or inhibitory (−) signal transduced. In some cases, there is bidirectional signaling, and for certain pairs both the ligand and receptor are expressed on the same cell constitutively or more commonly following activation. The expression of ligands is also not limited to professional antigen-presenting cells and may also be observed on endothelial and parenchymal cells. (From Clarkson MR, Sayegh MH: T cell costimulatory pathways in allograft rejection and tolerance. *Transplantation* 80:555-563, 2005.)

by APCs (Figure 71.7). Antigen specificity is determined by the TCR, which recognizes processed antigen in the form of short peptides bound to an MHC molecule. The specificity of antigen recognition is exquisitely precise; the alteration of a single amino acid in the peptide antigen or MHC molecule can alter recognition by the TCR. Thus T cell recognition of antigen involves a trimolecular interaction involving the TCR on the surface of the T cell, the MHC molecule on the surface of the APC, and the antigenic peptide bound to the MHC molecule. While the T cell receptor is responsible for antigen recognition, the invariant proteins CD3 and ζ-chain (which are noncovalently bound to the TCR) are responsible for signal transduction through the activation of protein tyrosine kinases associated with the cytoplasmic tails of CD3 and other TCR-associated receptors. This interaction provides "signal 1" of T cell activation (see later). Binding of the TCR to a peptide-MHC complex is of itself usually insufficient to cause T cell activation. Provision of signal 1 alone leads instead to a state of T cell unresponsiveness or "anergy."

CD4 AND CD8 T CELLS

The two major subsets of T cells, *cytotoxic* CD8⁺ T cells and *helper* CD4⁺ T cells, recognize processed antigen on MHC class I and II molecules, respectively. Although not directly involved in antigen recognition, the CD4 and CD8 coreceptors bind to nonpolymorphic regions of the MHC molecules. Thus the specificity of class I versus class II recognition is determined by whether a T cell expresses CD4 or CD8 in conjunction with the specificity of the TCR. In addition, CD4 and CD8 promote and stabilize the immunologic synapse between the T cell and the APC. The cytoplasmic tails of CD4 and CD8 molecules are associated with the tyrosine kinase p56lck, which plays an important role in T cell activation. Binding of the CD4 or CD8 coreceptor approximates the cytoplasmic tail to immunoreceptor tyrosine-based activation motifs on the CD3 complex. This in turn leads to the phosphorylation of a series of intracellular proteins, resulting in the activation of a variety of enzymes, including calcineurin (the target of the immunosuppressive drugs cyclosporine and tacrolimus), and the activation of transcription factors, such as nuclear factor of activated T cells (NFAT) and nuclear factor κ light-chain enhancer of activated B cells (NF-κB). These transcription factors are responsible for the increased and, in some cases, decreased expression of a variety of gene products associated with T cell activation. This signaling process is also dependent on the binding of T cell costimulatory or coinhibitory receptors with their specific ligands present on APCs.

ADHESION MOLECULES

Cells of the immune system infiltrate the allograft from nearby lymphoid organs and the bloodstream through a three-step process. First, they roll along the vessel wall through interactions between selectins on the endothelium and receptors on immune cells. Second, they adhere to vessel endothelium. Third, chemoattractant cytokines (chemokines) are released. Adhesion molecules and chemokines are important regulators of rejection and appear to be targets for immunotherapy. Adhesion molecules on T cells include lymphocyte function–associated antigen-1 (LFA-1), which interacts with intercellular adhesion molecule-1 (ICAM-1) and intercellular adhesion molecule-2 (ICAM-2); CD2, which interacts with CD58 (lymphocyte function–associated antigen-3 [LFA-3]); and very late activation antigen-4 (VLA-4) ($\alpha_4\beta_1$-integrin, CDw49d, CD29), which interacts with vascular cell adhesion molecules (VCAM-1, CD106). These receptors are of two large structural families. The integrins, including LFA-1 and VLA-4, are made up of α, β heterodimers, whereas members of the immunoglobulin superfamily, including CD2, LFA-3, VCAM-1, and the ICAMs, are made up of disulfide-linked "receptor" domains. Some of these receptors have also been shown to transduce signals and thus are more appropriately called *accessory molecules*. The inhibition of adhesion or accessory cell function has been shown to attenuate the alloimmune response. Previous studies in a primate model showed increased allograft survival with anti–ICAM-1 monoclonal antibodies, although clinical trials have failed to demonstrate benefit in human renal transplant recipients. Similarly, alefacept (LFA-3 immunoglobulin [Ig]) promoted allograft survival in a kidney primate transplant model; however, it did not improve patient or graft survival in humans and was associated with increased cancer risk in a randomized controlled study.

COSTIMULATORY MOLECULES

Classical understanding of T cell function is based on Bretscher and Cohn's two-signal hypothesis of T cell activation. One signal is transduced by the antigen-specific TCR when it recognizes processed antigen bound to an MHC molecule on the surface of an APC (see earlier). The second signal is mediated by a costimulatory molecule that is independent of antigen. The TCR and costimulatory signal transduction pathways are distinct and use different second messengers. At the level of the regulation of transcription, as shown for the interleukin-2 gene (*IL2*), the two pathways interact by poorly understood mechanisms to control gene expression. By controlling the level of expression of *IL2* and other genes, the TCR and costimulatory pathways can regulate T cell activation and function. The best-characterized costimulatory molecule is CD28, which is constitutively expressed on the surface of essentially all $CD4^+$ and approximately 50% of $CD8^+$ peripheral T lymphocytes.[28] CD28 binds a family of counter-receptor cell types termed *B7* (B7-1 and B7-2 or CD80 and CD86, respectively), which are expressed by APCs. T cell cosignaling pathways may also downregulate T cell responses. Following activation, cytotoxic T lymphocyte activation antigen 4 (CTLA4), which also binds B7 but with greater affinity than CD28, is expressed by the T cell. CTLA4 interaction with B7 transduces a "negative" signal to the T cell, resulting in physiologic termination of the immune response (see Figure 71.7). CTLA4-deficient mice exhibit severe lymphoproliferative disease, with infiltration of activated T cells to various organs and death within a few weeks of birth.[29] Ise and associates elegantly showed that this phenomenon is not an autonomous T cell proliferation but rather an autoantigen-dependent and tissue-specific T cell response. As an example, pancreatic T cell infiltration was driven by a pancreatic acinar autoantigen called protein disulfide isomerase-associated 2 (PDIA2). Interestingly, the infiltration of self-reacting T cells is enhanced by CTLA4 deficiency on either PDIA2-specific effector T cells or regulatory T (T_{reg}) cells, suggesting a critical role of CTLA4 in the immune regulation of both effector and T_{reg} cells. Furthermore, use of anti-CTLA4 antibody prevents maintenance of tolerance in an experimental model of tolerance.[30] Reinforcing those findings, autoimmunity is attenuated in mice expressing transgenic TCR or in mice lacking positive costimulatory signals through CD28:B7. In addition, T_{reg} cell–specific depletion of CTLA4 is not sufficient to fully rescue the autoimmune phenotype, suggesting a role of CTLA4 in effector function. In summary, CTLA4 plays a major role in immune homeostasis in mice. Interestingly, in humans CTLA4 polymorphisms are associated with type 1 diabetes and other autoimmune diseases.

Signaling via the TCR plus the CD28 costimulatory molecule is sufficient to activate T cells. In contrast, signaling via the TCR alone without costimulation induces long-term T cell unresponsiveness (i.e., anergy) or ignorance. Experimental analysis of the minimal signal transduction event necessary to induce anergy showed that an increase in intracellular calcium concentration was sufficient. Because increased intracellular calcium is produced by signaling via the TCR, these results are consistent with the observation that anergy can be induced by monoclonal antibodies to the TCR or by APCs expressing the appropriate MHC molecule but lacking the costimulatory counter-receptor. In vivo, anergy is defined as failure of T cell clonal expansion after immunization with antigen. Anergic T cells remain viable but are unresponsive for at least several weeks in experimental murine models in vitro and in vivo. In vitro, some anergic states can be reversed by cytokines such as interleukin-2 (IL-2). The fate and function of anergic T cells in vivo remain undetermined; however, evidence from experimental models suggests that anergic T cells can be reactivated by some processes (e.g., viral infections). These observations suggest that anergy is a reversible state, and that therapeutic use of anergy during clinical transplantation, although potentially very useful, will require thorough evaluation and careful monitoring. Certain anergic states may not be reversible and may be associated with T cell death by apoptosis. Strategies targeted at inducing such states in vivo are clinically desirable. Inhibition of costimulation with soluble receptors to (e.g., CTLA4- Ig) or monoclonal antibodies against the B7 molecules has been shown to dramatically prolong allograft survival and induce tolerance in some animal models. However, the fact that blockade of the CD28-B7 pathway alone does not appear to be effective at inducing tolerance in the more stringent models of transplantation, including primate models, has lead to speculation that other pathways are capable of providing T cell costimulation.

Additional members of the CD28 family with costimulatory or coinhibitory function have been recognized. Inducible T cell costimulator (ICOS) is a homologue of CD28 and binds to B7h. It does not interact with B7-1 and B7-2, and in contrast to CD28 it is not constitutively expressed but is upregulated on activated T cells. Blocking this pathway leads to increased allograft survival in experimental models. Programmed death 1 (PD-1), which binds to its ligands PD-L1 and PD-L2, is one of the more recently recognized members of the CD28 family.[31] PD-1–deficient C57BL/6 mice develop lupus-like autoimmune disease or autoimmune dilated cardiomyopathy. However, compared to CTLA4-deficient mice, PD-1–deficient mice exhibit a much milder phenotype of disease, particularly in autoimmune-prone mouse backgrounds.[31]

PD-1 is known to regulate both central and peripheral tolerance. In the thymus, PD-1/PD-L1 is important for the maturation of T cells from double negative to double positive population. In the periphery, PD-1 signaling controls peripheral tolerance both through inhibition of effector T cell function and induction of peripheral T_{reg} (iT_{reg}) cells. PD-1 on peripheral APC restrains initial activation or reactivation of self-reactive effector T cells. PD-1 signaling enhances peripheral iT_{reg} cells in several ways. First, PD-L1–expressing DCs induce the conversion of naive T cells to Foxp3$^+$ iT_{reg} cells, and conversely, signaling from iT_{reg} cells into PD-L1–expressing DCs may promote APC tolerogenicity.[32] Consistently, in the presence of anti-CD3 and transforming growth factor-β (TGF-β), PD-L1-Ig can induce a profound increase in the de novo generation of CD4$^+$Foxp3$^+T_{reg}$ cells from naive CD4 T cells in the periphery via attenuation of the Akt-mTOR pathway. In addition, PD-L1 on endothelial cells restricts extravasation of T cells into target organs. The importance of the PD-1 pathway in peripheral tolerance is shown in several animal models of autoimmune disease such as in the NOD mouse model of autoimmune T cell mediated diabetes and an experimental autoimmune encephalomyelitis model of human multiple sclerosis. In sum, it appears that the PD-1–PD-L1/PD-L2 pathway regulates the generation and functions of peripheral T_{reg} cells.

A separate family of costimulatory molecules that belong to the TNF:TNF-R family of molecules also play a role in T and B cell activation. CD40 and its ligand CD40L (CD154) were the first members of this family to have demonstrable costimulatory function. CD40 is expressed on B cells and other APCs, including dendritic cells and endothelial cells, and belongs to the TNF superfamily of molecules. Its ligand, CD40L (CD154), is expressed early on activated T cells. CD40 is critical in providing cognate T cell help for B cell immunoglobulin production and class switching. A defect in CD154 expression is responsible for the hyper-IgM syndrome, where there is failure to switch from IgM to IgG, seen in humans. Blockade with anti-CD154 antibodies has been shown to be effective at prolonging allograft survival in rodent and primate models of transplantation. There is evidence that CD154 acts "directly" to transduce a costimulatory signal to the T cell or "indirectly," by ligation of CD40 on APCs and induction of B7 expression, thus enhancing CD28-B7 costimulation. Other members of the group include the CD134-CD134L, CD30-CD30L, CD27-CD70, and the 4-1BB–4-1BBL pathways (see Figure 71.7). In summary, costimulatory signals are critical to fully activating T cells, and modulating this pathway has become an attractive target for the prevention of rejection and promotion of tolerance.

CYTOKINES AND CHEMOKINES

In addition to cell-to-cell interactions, cell function can be directed through proteins produced by a variety of cell types. These factors can function as growth, activation, and differentiation factors (cytokines) or as chemoattractants (chemokines) of inflammatory cells to a site of immune responses. They can act locally or systemically through signaling cell surface receptors that result in changes in gene expression of the cell. Cytokines are produced by cells that participate in the immune response, including T cells, B cells, and APCs. In addition, nonimmune cells, such as endothelial cells, also produce lymphokines that can modulate an immune response. Thus, complex regulatory networks of lymphokines that are incompletely understood modulate the antiallograft immune response.

Chemokines (chemoattractant cytokines) are structurally related by amino acid homologies, in particular the placement of cysteines. The nomenclature of chemokines is becoming increasingly complex; four chemokine families are now recognized, of which most members belong to the C-C chemokine family, represented by RANTES (regulated on activation, normal T expressed, and secreted), or the C-X-C chemokine family, typified by IL-8. In general C-C chemokines attract monocytes and T lymphocytes, and C-X-C chemokines attract granulocytes. Receptors on the surface of immune cells are named after the family of chemokines with which they interact and can bind with a variety of chemokines in that family. For example CCR1 and CCR5 can respectively bind with the chemokines monocyte chemoattractant protein-3 (MCP-3) and macrophage inflammatory protein-1α (MIP-1α), and both can bind RANTES and MIP-1α. They act to create a chemoattractant gradient across tissues to move cells into sites of inflammation. Detection of altered chemokine messenger RNA (mRNA) in experimental models of rejection suggests that they play an important role in this process; however, because of redundancy and differences in the function of chemokines among rodents and humans, the exact role individual chemokines play in an alloimmune response remains unclear, although data suggest that expression of CCR5 is associated with acute allograft rejection.

HELPER T CELLS AND THEIR ROLE IN THE ALLOIMMUNE RESPONSE

Upon alloantigen encounter, naive effector CD4$^+$ T_H cells are activated and differentiate into distinct subsets, such as T_H1, T_H2, T_H17, follicular helper T cells (T_{FH}), and T_{reg} cells. The differentiation decision is influenced by a number of factors, including the prevailing cytokine milieu and the nature of the costimulatory molecules providing the second signal to the TCR complex.[17]

In experimental models of transplantation, altering the T cell response from T_H1 to T_H2 has been shown to prevent acute allograft rejection. Except for blockade of the interleukin-2 receptor (IL-2R), therapeutic strategies that modulate lymphokines have not proved highly effective in human transplantation. This may be caused by the pleiotropic effects of each lymphokine and by the complex interactions exhibited by regulatory networks of multiple lymphokines. It has also been suggested that a T_H1 profile is associated with rejection, whereas a T_H2 phenotype promotes tolerance. However, this paradigm has been challenged by several investigators, although it may hold true in cases of lower mismatched allografts. For example, IL-2 has been shown by several criteria to promote allograft rejection, and blockade of the IL-2R has been shown to promote allograft survival. However, knockout mice, which do not express any IL-2 owing to inactivation of the *Il2* gene by homologous recombination, reject allografts as easily as do normal mice. Rejection in animals that lack IL-2 is likely mediated by other lymphokines that compensate for the IL-2 deficit by having overlapping functions. Furthermore, studies with specific T_H1 or T_H2 cytokine gene knockout animals indicate the complexity of the T_H1-T_H2 paradigm in allograft rejection and tolerance. Interesting data from animal and human studies have shown that T_H2 clones propagated from patients with stable kidney transplant function, or animals tolerant to kidney transplants, can regulate a proliferative response from T_H1 clones isolated from patients or animals undergoing active rejection. Therefore, although manipulation of lymphokine functions may hold promise as a therapeutic modality, we will have to better understand the role of lymphokines under physiologic conditions if we are to develop novel, more effective treatments to prevent rejection and/or induce tolerance.

In summary, cell-to-cell interactions between T cells and APCs can be mediated by five classes of receptors: the antigen-specific TCR, the CD4 or CD8 coreceptor, costimulatory molecules, accessory or adhesion molecules, and lymphokine receptors. Therapeutic or experimental manipulation of members of each class of receptors has been shown to prolong allograft survival. The most effective in clinical studies to date have been thymoglobulin and antibodies targeting the IL-2R complex. Interaction of alloreactive T cells and alloantigen does not uniformly lead to an aggressive T cell response. While T_H1 and T_H17 have been linked with allograft rejection, T_H2 cells and T_{reg} cells are believed to favor long-term graft survival. Furthermore, T_{FH} cells have been identified as key supporters of B cells in the generation of an alloantibody response. T_{FH} cells enter the germinal center via an ICOS-dependent signal and support the affinity maturation, isotype class–switching, and memory responses of antigen-specific B cells. The challenge in the transplant setting is to drive the immune response toward regulatory phenotypes (e.g., T_{reg} cells) and away from effector T cells such as T_H1, T_H17, T_{FH}, and cytotoxic $CD8^+$ T cells.

B CELLS AND ANTIBODY PRODUCTION

B lymphocytes develop from hematopoietic precursor cells in the bone marrow. After undergoing immunoglobulin rearrangement and deletion of autoreactive B cells, immature B cells then migrate to the spleen and differentiate into follicular or marginal zone B cells. Mature, naive B cells ($CD20^+$, $CD19^+$, $CD27^-$, IgD^+, and IgM^+) are able to recognize cognate antigen via B cell receptor and become activated in either a T cell independent or dependent process. The latter is capable of supporting the generation of early memory B cells and the formation of germinal centers that lead to immunoglobulin class switch and B cell differentiation into long-lived plasma cells. B cells may participate in the immune response through different roles, including antibody production, as well as enhancing T cell response via antigen presentation, costimulatory signal delivery, and/or cytokine production.

Long-lived plasma cells are nondividing terminally differentiated cells with no expression of surface immunoglobulin and major function of antibody secretion. This cell subtype is the one responsible for the production of high-affinity anti-HLA antibodies.[33] They are located early in the immune response in secondary lymphoid organs and later migrate to the bone marrow, where their survival is tightly regulated by the microenvironment composed of macrophages, eosinophils, and prosurvival signals such as IL-6, APRIL (a proliferation-inducing ligand), and BAFF (B-cell activating factor of the TNF family; or also known as BLyS, B lymphocyte-stimulating factor). The presence of long-lived plasma cells is in particular demonstrated by the maintenance of stable anti-HLA levels for years in previously sensitized patients.

EFFECTOR MECHANISMS OF ALLOGRAFT REJECTION

Cellular (delayed-type hypersensitivity [DTH] responses, cell-mediated cytotoxicity) and humoral components contribute to transplant rejection. Once fully activated, $CD4^+$ T_H cells produce cytokines that orchestrate various effector arms of the alloimmune response (see Figure 71.6). T_H1 cytokines activate macrophages, and both $CD4^+$ T_H1 cells and activated macrophages effect DTH responses. Although initiated by a specific immune response, DTH results in nonspecific tissue injury and repair. Although the exact mechanisms by which DTH leads to allograft destruction remain unclear, it is hypothesized that some of the cytokines produced by T cells and macrophages (TNF-α) mediate apoptosis of allograft cells. It has been suggested that DTH responses, presumably initiated by indirect allorecognition, are particularly important in the pathogenesis of chronic rejection.

Several effector mechanisms that participate in allograft destruction have been identified (see Figure 71.6). Adaptive immune responses mediated by B and T cells play a significant role in allograft destruction as evidenced by the fact that inhibiting these cell types can often prevent allograft destruction. T cells mediate destruction of allografts by direct lysis of donor tissues via $CD8^+$ cytotoxic T lymphocytes and by the production of proinflammatory cytokines via $CD4^+$ T cells, as occurs in DTH. Alloantigen-specific antibodies produced by B cells are able to mediate endothelial cell activation leading to allograft loss, as well as mediate lysis of allogenic cells within the allograft by activating the complement cascade. Innate immune responses also play a role, although they are insufficient to mediate allograft rejection in the absence of an adaptive response. $CD8^+$ precytolytic T lymphocytes recognize specific HLA class I antigens on the surface of donor cells, and in the presence of helper T cytokines (IL-2, IL-4, and IL-5), differentiate and divide. Mature cytotoxic T lymphocytes damage target cells displaying foreign HLA class I by at least two mechanisms (Figure 71.8). A secretory pathway involves

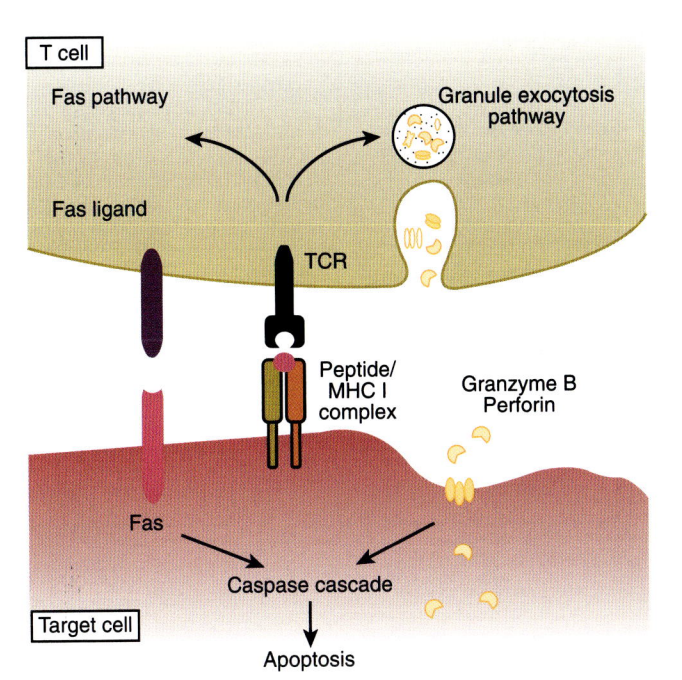

Figure 71.8 Mechanisms of CD8⁺ T cell–mediated killing. Cytotoxic T cells (*top*) activated through the class I major histocompatibility peptide complex can cause target cell killing by two pathways. One involves granule exocytosis, releasing perforin and granzyme B, which in turn cause membrane damage and cell lysis by osmotic dysregulation and activation of caspase cascade, giving rise to programmed cell death (apoptosis). The second involves expression of Fas ligand on activated T cells. When Fas on target cells interacts with its ligand on activated T cells, the target cell undergoes apoptosis by activation of caspase cascade. MHC, Major histocompatibility complex; TCR, T cell receptor.

granule-mediated exocytosis of soluble factors, including granzymes (serine esterases) and a complement-like molecule, perforin. These proteins induce cell death by means of both DNA degradation and osmotic lysis secondary to pore formation in the target cell membrane. Detection of both the perforin and granzyme mRNA from cells isolated from the allograft, peripheral blood lymphocytes of urinary lymphocytes, have been shown to predict whether acute rejection is ongoing within the allograft. A second cytolytic pathway involves interaction between Fas (CD95), a TNF-like protein, and Fas ligand. Fas ligand is induced on cytotoxic T lymphocytes through triggering of the TCR. Fas-expressing target cells undergo apoptosis when Fas ligand is engaged. It is possible to demonstrate ex vivo specific cytotoxicity against donor cells in rejecting animals and humans. In addition, passive transfer of specific "killer" T cell clones to naive animals induces allograft rejection, particularly skin allografts. In humans, both CD8 and CD4 cells play an important role in rejection, with CD8 cells being most important early after transplant, while CD4 T cells are critical for indirect allorecognition and for providing help to antibody production by B cells later in the transplant course.

Alloantibody response against the allograft represents another effector mechanism that contributes to allograft injury. Naive B cells circulate through the follicles of peripheral lymphoid tissues; at some point they encounter antigen either presented by dendritic cells or in soluble form. B lymphocytes express clonally restricted antigen-specific cell surface receptors, immunoglobulins that together with Igα and Igβ make up the BCR complex. Igα and Igβ are the B cell equivalent to the CD3 and ζ molecules that make up the TCR complex. When cell surface immunoglobulin binds specific antigen in the context of soluble helper factors such as IL-4, IL-6, and IL-8, B cells are activated. In addition to initiating B cell proliferation and differentiation, these events also prepare the B cells for subsequent interactions with T cells by upregulating cell surface expression of MHC and costimulatory molecules and cytokine receptors. To ensure direct interaction between T and B cells, activated T cells upregulate CXCR5, a chemokine receptor that allows it to home toward the B cell–rich primary follicles of the lymph node. Simultaneously, B cells upregulate CCR7 to respond to T cell zone chemokines CCL19 and CCL21. In addition to antigen stimulation, naive B cells also need to bind to B cell survival regulators such as BAFF and APRIL. Once activated, B cells differentiate, divide, and become plasma cells, which secrete soluble forms of antigen-specific antibodies that are displayed on their cell surfaces. These antibodies in turn can bind allogeneic target antigens and induce allograft damage by fixing complement, triggering Fc-dependent cellular cytotoxicity, and/or direct cell injury. IgM and IgG alloantibodies can be detected in the serum and in the allografts (of animals and humans) that are being rejected. Preformed anti-HLA class I antibodies, and occasionally antiendothelial antibodies, play an important role in hyperacute rejection and accelerated vascular rejection observed in previously sensitized transplant recipients. In xenotransplantation, naturally occurring xenoreactive antibodies play a critical role in hyperacute rejection of allografts. Finally, alloantibodies, particularly IgG, play important pathogenic roles in the development of chronic rejection and allograft arteriosclerosis. CD4 T cells are also able to mediate allograft rejection through a mechanism that is most similar to DTH. CD4 T cells activated following recognition of alloantigen produce a variety of cytokines that are able to recruit other cell types to the allograft site, including CD8⁺ lymphocytes, B cells, and macrophages. Resulting inflammation leads to allograft destruction by production of cytokines such as TNF-α.

Other effector mechanisms include cell death through NK cells. NK cells express cell surface receptors called *killer inhibitory receptors* that recognize HLA class I molecules. Although the role of NK cell–mediated cytotoxicity in allograft rejection remains controversial, NK cells seem to play an important role in antibody-mediated injury.

It has become apparent that a relatively recently defined IL-17–producing T cell lineage, T_H17 cells, may play a role in rejection responses. It has been shown that when T_H1 responses are avoided, such as in Tbet-deficient mice, alloimmune responses by T_H17 cells can mediate chronic rejection. Tbet knockout animals, which lack T_H1 cells, have a strong T_H17 cell response and reject transplanted organs faster than wild-type mice. Rejection seems to be at least partially dependent on IL-17 production. These observations open up the possibility that altering the response of T cell lineages, in this case T_H1 cells, may allow for other T cell lineages to participate in mounting a rejection response. Interestingly, blocking the interaction of T cell immunoglobulin mucin-1 (TIM-1) with its ligand inhibited the secretion of IL-17 by T_H17 cells. Although costimulation blockade is ineffective in preventing rejection in Tbet knockouts by T_H17 cells, combining costimulation and TIM-1 blockade can prevent rejection. Thus the discovery of new T cell subsets able to participate in rejection responses has made it apparent that old strategies capable of preventing rejection may need to be expanded.

ACUTE CELLULAR AND HUMORAL REJECTION

Acute rejection is the clinical syndrome that occurs as the result of an alloimmune response against a transplanted organ and can be caused by either a cellular or humoral response. An acute cellular rejection normally occurs in the first 3 months after transplant surgery in an unsensitized recipient but can occur in an accelerated fashion if this is the result of a secondary immune response and previously primed T cells are present. In addition, the tempo of rejection has changed after the introduction of induction therapy leading to significant T cell depletion, delaying acute rejection episodes to later time points. Clinically, acute cellular rejection is characterized by a mononuclear cellular interstitial infiltrate, edema, and tubulitis. A humoral response, by definition, requires $CD4^+$ T cells and preformed anti-HLA antibodies that have long been recognized as a cause of accelerated rejection. The ability to detect evidence of antibody-mediated injury through peritubular C4d staining within the allograft and the characteristic histologic changes of neutrophilic infiltration of the peritubular capillaries and the detection of circulating anti-HLA antibodies have led to increasing awareness of acute antibody-mediated rejection. The clinical aspects of acute rejection are covered in more detail in Chapter 72.

CHRONIC REJECTION

Chronic rejection is the slow progressive deterioration in kidney function characterized clinically by an increase in serum creatinine level, increasing proteinuria, and progressive hypertension and histologically by tubular atrophy, interstitial fibrosis, and fibrous neointimal thickening of arterial walls; it is an almost universal finding in renal transplant recipients (Figure 71.9). Previously the terminology most commonly used to describe these changes was *chronic allograft nephropathy*. The term *chronic rejection* is more commonly used to denote an immunologic cause of injury. The Banff classification system for renal allograft injury has adopted the term *interstitial fibrosis and tubular atrophy* (IFTA) to describe these changes. In addition to these pathologic findings, allografts may demonstrate peritubular C4d staining, suggesting a role for antibody-mediated injury, whereas a subset of transplanted kidneys may have changes of transplant glomerulopathy characterized by swollen glomeruli, infiltration of the glomeruli with mononuclear cells, mesangial matrix expansion, mesangiolysis, and splitting of the glomerular basement membrane with a subendothelial deposition of electron lucent material. Transplant glomerulopathy with IFTA is an almost universal finding in transplanted kidneys over time. Serial protocol biopsy studies

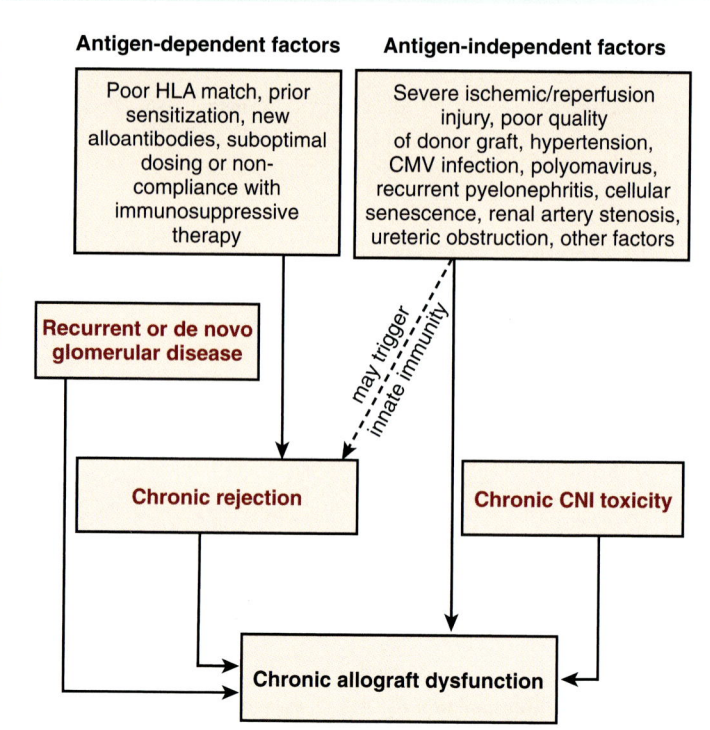

Figure 71.9 Mechanisms of chronic allograft dysfunction. Many different forms of injury can contribute to the development of chronic allograft dysfunction. Immunologically mediated injury, in the form of cellular and/or humoral rejection, may lead to chronic graft injury and shorten graft survival. This injury is most likely mediated by indirect alloreactivity, in which recipient T cells recognize allopeptides present on recipient antigen-presenting cells and trigger antibody- and cellular-mediated injury. Antigen-independent factors, such as ischemic injury at the time of transplantation, are thought to be important by triggering innate immunity and enhancing the alloimmune response through upregulation of cell surface molecules involved in antigen presentation and secretion of chemokines that mediate immune cell trafficking to the allograft. CMV, Cytomegalovirus; CNI, calcineurin inhibitor.

have shown that rejection and glomerular disease accounted for more than 50% of graft loss with the remaining due to infections such as BK virus, recurrent pyelonephritis, ureteral obstruction, and medical or surgical complications. A minority of cases was due to isolated calcineurin inhibitor (CNI) toxicity.[34]

A number of different antigen-independent or so-called nonimmunologic factors have been associated with progression of allograft dysfunction. These include factors present before transplantation, such as ischemia-reperfusion injury suffered by the kidney at the time of transplantation, brain death in the donor, and nonspecific factors associated with donor age, hypertension, and diabetes. Posttransplantation factors have also been shown to accelerate the course of chronic allograft injury, including reduced functional nephron mass, CNI toxicity, hypertension in the recipient, BK virus infection, and cytomegalovirus infection. In many cases, the innate immunity is activated, leading to increased MHC expression on donor tissue augmenting the adaptive immunity. In nearly every transplant, there is a degree of tissue incompatibility, whether this is a mismatch of the minor histocompatibility antigens alone or in combination with the MHC. Figure 71.5 shows that the half-life of death-censored allograft survival differs greatly when comparing HLA-identical to HLA-nonidentical living transplant recipients. The same effector mechanisms that are responsible for acute rejection are thought to be active chronically, although the relative importance of each may be different. Indirect, as opposed to direct, allorecognition is thought to play an important role in the process. The evidence for this comes from a number of studies that have shown that donor MHC–derived peptides are capable of eliciting an immune response long after donor-derived APCs (the main target of the direct alloimmune response) have disappeared from the allograft. Alloantibodies have always been thought to be important in the development of chronic rejection, and studies have supported this hypothesis.

The overall pathways involved in development of fibrosis and tissue remodeling in transplanted kidneys have not been elucidated as yet. However, a number of studies have shed some light on individual components that influence this process. TGF-β has been shown to play an important role in the development of fibrosis in native kidney disease; however, it is well known that TGF-β has both immunosuppressive and profibrotic properties, and while the tolerance and immunosuppressive aspects of TGF-β production are desirable in transplantation, the remodeling and fibrosing are damaging. Data have shown that anti–TGF-β antibody in high doses can abrogate long-term allograft survival induced by cyclosporine administration in a cardiac rat transplant model, indicating the importance of TGF-β in mediating the immunosuppressive properties of cyclosporine. In the same model both high and low doses of anti–TGF-β antibodies prevent cyclosporine-related fibrotic renal injury. TGF-β has also been shown to be crucial in the regulation of transplantation and other forms of tolerance. In rodent models of transplantation tolerance, induction does not prevent the development of chronic rejection, and a transplanted animal can exhibit tolerance to a second donor-specific allograft and have evidence of chronic allograft dysfunction within the original allograft simultaneously. Regulation of TGF-β–associated fibrosis has been achieved by a variety of inhibitors that inhibit TGF-β expression or signaling, including decorin, pirfenidone, relaxin, and bone morphogenetic protein 7 (Bmp7), or by agents that interfere with TGF-β–associated profibrotic pathways, including angiotensin II, endothelin-1, and connective tissue growth factor. Of particular interest is epithelial-mesenchymal transition (EMT). This describes the process of phenotypic change that cells of a variety of origins, including mesenchymal cells, resident fibroblasts, and epithelial cells, undergo, leading to fibrosis. Both Bmp7 and hepatocyte growth factor have been used to reduce TGF-β–associated EMT in experimental models of renal fibrosis.

Clinically, prevention of chronic allograft injury is focused on preventing alloantibody formation, minimization of CNI nephrotoxicity, and optimal control of blood pressure and blood glucose levels. Numerous approaches have been studied in clinical trials, including substitution of CNIs with the mTOR inhibitors everolimus and sirolimus, as well as the use of belatacept, a modified CTLA4-Ig fusion protein that blocks T cell CD28 costimulation. However, because multiple factors have been shown to contribute to the development of chronic graft injury, it is unlikely that the modification of one factor, such as CNI-associated toxicity, will result in a complete solution to this problem. There has been growing evidence that the humoral response plays an important role in chronic rejection. Studies have shown that development of anti-HLA antibodies after transplantation is associated with a substantial decrease in transplant survival.[35] Whether intervening to decrease donor-specific antibodies may improve long-term graft survival remains to be determined.

MECHANISMS OF IMMUNOSUPPRESSION

CORTICOSTEROIDS

Most immunosuppressive drug regimens use an adrenocorticosteroid, such as prednisone, in combination with other immunosuppressive agents. Corticosteroids modulate the immune response by regulating gene expression. The steroid molecule enters the cytosol, where it binds the steroid receptor, inducing a conformational change in the receptor. The complex then migrates to the nucleus and binds regulatory regions of DNA called *glucocorticoid response elements*, which regulate the transcription of many genes, including the genes for IL-1, IL-2, IFN-γ, TNF-α, and IL-6 (Figure 71.10). Thus the many effects of corticosteroids on multiple cell types account for both their efficacy and the diverse array of complications (see Chapter 72).

AZATHIOPRINE

Azathioprine is a purine analog that in vivo is enzymatically converted to 6-mercaptopurine and other derivatives, which are molecules that function as antimetabolites. After metabolic conversion, it has multiple activities, including incorporation into DNA, inhibition of purine nucleotide synthesis, and alteration of RNA synthesis (see Figure 71.10). The major immunosuppressive effect is thought to be caused by blocking of DNA replication, which prevents lymphocyte proliferation after antigenic stimulation. Although it is useful for inhibiting primary immune responses, azathioprine has little effect on secondary responses or the reversal of acute allograft rejections, which are not dependent on lymphocyte proliferation. Azathioprine also decreases the number of migratory mononuclear and granulocytic cells while inhibiting proliferation of promyelocytes in bone marrow. As a result, the number of circulating monocytes capable of differentiating into macrophages is decreased. Among the possible deleterious effects of azathioprine administration are severe leukopenia and occasionally thrombocytopenia, gastrointestinal disturbances, hepatotoxicity, and increased risk for neoplasia.

MYCOPHENOLIC ACID

In most centers, mycophenolate mofetil or mycophenolate sodium has replaced azathioprine in standard immunosuppression protocols for new kidney and pancreas-kidney transplantation. Both mycophenolate mofetil and mycophenolate sodium are metabolized into MPA, which is the active agent. The rationale for this switch is that MPA is a selective inhibitor of the pathway of de novo purine synthesis. In the normal mammalian cell, guanine and adenine nucleotides

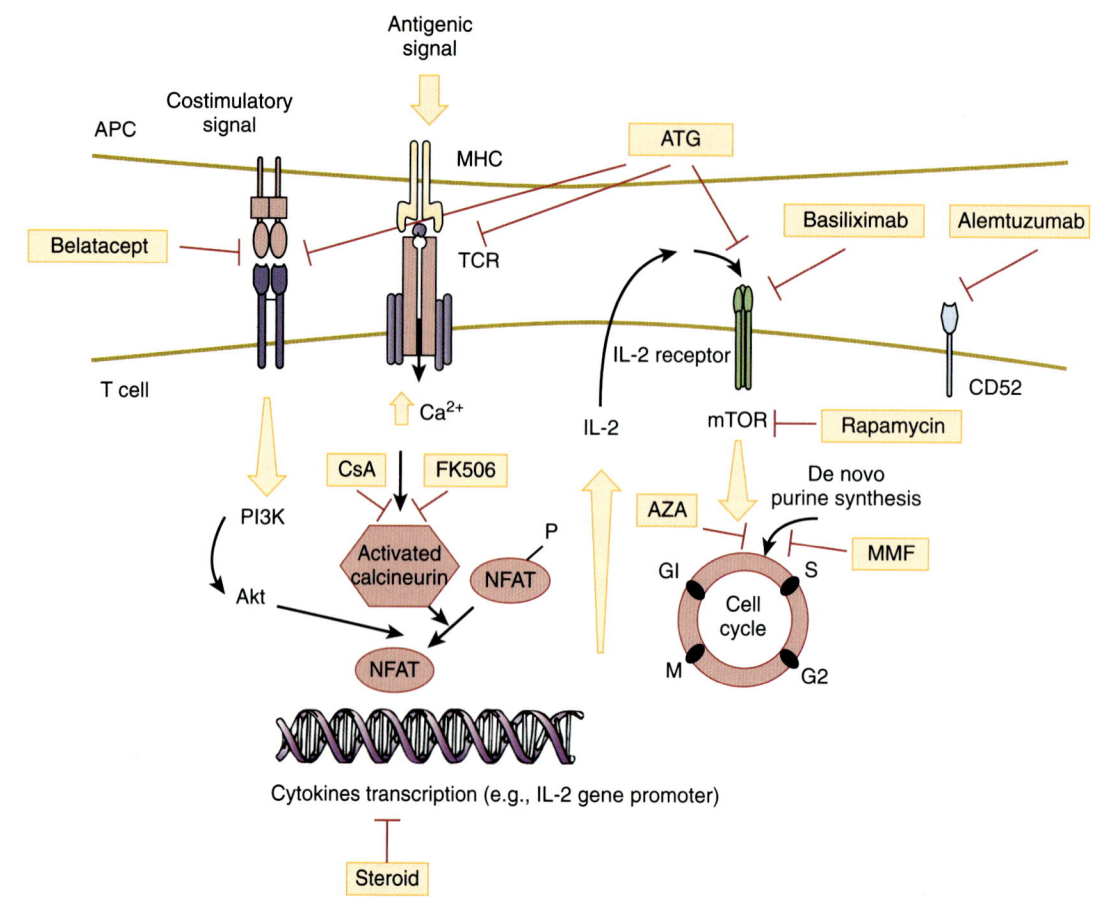

Figure 71.10 Mechanisms of action of immunosuppressive agents viewed as a function of inhibiting T cell activation. Signal 1: The calcium-dependent signal induced by T cell receptor (TCR) stimulation results in calcineurin activation, a process inhibited by cyclosporine (CsA) and tacrolimus. Calcineurin dephosphorylates nuclear factor of activated T cells (NFAT), enabling it to enter the nucleus and bind to the interleukin-2 (IL-2) promoter. Corticosteroids bind to cytoplasmic receptors, enter the nucleus, and inhibit cytokine gene transcription in both T cells and the antigen-presenting cells (APCs). Corticosteroids also inhibit nuclear factor κ light-chain enhancer of activated B cells (NF-κB) activation (not shown). Signal 2: Costimulatory signals are necessary to optimize T cell IL-2 gene transcription, prevent T cell anergy, and inhibit T cell apoptosis (belatacept target). Signal 3: IL-2 receptor stimulation induces the cell to enter the cell cycle and proliferate. Signal 3 may be blocked by IL-2 receptor antibodies (basiliximab) or by mammalian target of rapamycin (mTOR) inhibitors (such as rapamycin), which inhibits S6 kinase activation. Following progression into the cell cycle, azathioprine (AZA) and mycophenolate mofetil (MMF) interrupt DNA replication by inhibiting purine synthesis. Antithymocyte globulin (ATG) has multiple targets, including IL-2R, CD3, and CD28, leading to T cell depletion. Alemtuzumab selectively targets CD52 receptor on T cells. MHC, Major histocompatibility complex; PI3K, phosphatidylinositol-3-kinase.

are manufactured to form smaller precursors through two mechanisms, a de novo pathway or a salvage pathway (where purine bases are recycled). Mycophenolate is a reversible inhibitor of inosine monophosphate dehydrogenase, which is the rate-limiting enzyme in the de novo synthesis of guanosine nucleotide and nucleosides. Inhibition of this enzyme results in the selective inhibition of T and B lymphocyte proliferation (see Figure 71.10). MPA has minimal effects on other cell populations because proliferation of T and B cells is dependent on the de novo pathway for purine synthesis, whereas other cells are capable of using a salvage pathway. The main active metabolite of mycophenolate is mycophenolic acid glucuronide (MPAG), which is excreted into bile and undergoes enterohepatic recirculation. Cyclosporine, but not FK506 (tacrolimus), inhibits MPAG excretion into bile and thereby decreases circulating levels of MPA, which would suggest that lower doses of mycophenolate are required when used in combination with FK506.

CYCLOSPORINE

Cyclosporine, a small cyclic peptide of fungal origin, has played a major role in preventing allograft rejection and has improved allograft survival rates. Although highly effective in blocking the initiation of an immune response, cyclosporine, like azathioprine, is of limited value in treating acute allograft rejection. Its primary action is to block the expression of cytokine genes produced by T cells, including the genes for IL-2, IL-3, IL-4, IFN-γ, and TNF-α, but it does not interfere with IL-1, TNF-α, or TGF-β produced by APCs, including macrophages. There is likewise no evidence that NK cells are affected by cyclosporine. In the presence of cyclosporine, T cell proliferation is indirectly inhibited owing to the absence of cytokines; however, the addition of exogenous IL-2 has been shown to restore T cell proliferation.

It is now understood that cyclosporine blocks the calcium-dependent component of the TCR signal transduction pathway (see Figure 71.10). Cyclosporine binds to a family of cytoplasmic molecules termed *cyclophilins*, and the complex then inhibits calcineurin, which is a cytoplasmic serine threonine phosphatase. After T cell activation in the absence of cyclosporine, calcineurin dephosphorylates the cytosolic component of NFAT. After dephosphorylation, NFAT is translocated from the cytosol to the nucleus, where it forms a complex with other DNA-binding proteins, including FOS and JUN. The complex of DNA-binding proteins regulates gene transcription, including the gene for IL-2. During treatment with cyclosporine, the inhibition of the formation of the NFAT complex has been shown to prevent transcription of the gene for IL-2,[36] and a similar complex has been shown to regulate TNF-α gene transcription. The net result is a reduction of IL-2 and resultant T cell activation. Clinically, a reduction in IL-2 concentrations minimizes the immune response associated with allograft rejection. Patients maintained on therapeutic levels of cyclosporine experience approximately a 50% reduction in calcineurin activity, allowing the patient to retain a degree of immune responsiveness sufficient enough to maintain host defenses. It is likely that identical or similar DNA-binding complexes regulate the transcription of multiple lymphokine genes. The mechanism of action of cyclosporine in cells other than lymphocytes remains poorly understood; however, it has been shown that nontoxic analogs of cyclosporine also lack immunosuppressive effects. These findings suggest that the toxic and immunosuppressive effects are mediated by similar signal transduction mechanisms. The differential susceptibility to cyclosporine of lymphocytes, as compared with other cell types, may be caused by differential levels of expression of calcineurin and the cyclophilins.

TACROLIMUS

Tacrolimus (FK506), another CNI, is a potent immunosuppressive agent that inhibits T cell activation in vitro. In contrast to cyclosporine, tacrolimus is a macrolide antibiotic produced by fungi, yet the immunosuppressive effects on T cells are similar. Because of structural differences, tacrolimus binds a family of cytosolic proteins termed *FK506-binding proteins* (FKBPs), which are different from the cyclosporine-binding cyclophilins. Interestingly, both FKBP and cyclophilin have peptidylprolyl isomerase activity and collectively are called *immunophilins*; however, the similar immunosuppressive properties of the two drugs are attributable to the fact that both agents inhibit the phosphatase activity of calcineurin (see Figure 71.10).[37] Thus, although tacrolimus and cyclosporine have different structures and binding partners, their immunosuppressive effects are mediated through a common final pathway. Thus it is not surprising that both drugs block the induction of lymphokine mRNA, including IL-2, inhibit lymphokine production, and indirectly inhibit T cell proliferation. The side-effect profiles of tacrolimus and cyclosporine are similar, with certain exceptions such as hirsutism and gingival hyperplasia caused by cyclosporine and alopecia and neurotoxicity caused by tacrolimus. In experimental studies, the combination of tacrolimus and cyclosporine show additive increases in toxicity and in efficacy. Therefore, in clinical transplantation, immunosuppressive protocols involving multiple drugs use either cyclosporine or tacrolimus, though the latter is currently the preferred agent based on its stronger immunosuppressive effect.

MAMMALIAN TARGET OF RAPAMYCIN INHIBITORS

Rapamycin (sirolimus) was first used as an immunosuppressive drug through a search for drugs with a similar structure to FK506. Like FK506, it is a macrolide antibiotic and binds to the same family of FKBP isomerase proteins.

However, whereas cyclosporine and tacrolimus inhibit calcineurin in the calcium-dependent component of the TCR signal transduction pathway, rapamycin binds to mTOR and prevents phosphorylation of p70 S6 kinase in the CD28 costimulatory and IL-2R signal transduction pathways (see Figure 71.10). In functional studies, activation of T cells by monoclonal antibodies to the TCR was inhibited by either cyclosporine or tacrolimus but not rapamycin. Conversely, the activation of T cells by exogenous IL-2 plus protein kinase C stimulation with a phorbol ester was inhibited by rapamycin but not by cyclosporine or tacrolimus. Similarly, T cell activation by monoclonal antibodies to the CD28 costimulatory molecule plus protein kinase costimulation with a phorbol ester was also inhibited by rapamycin but not by cyclosporine or tacrolimus. Cell-cycle analysis shows that rapamycin blocks T cell proliferation during late G1 phase of the cell cycle and before S phase. Thus rapamycin inhibits late signals in T cell activation that are transduced by either the IL-2R or CD28 costimulatory signal transduction pathways.[38] In contrast, cyclosporine and tacrolimus inhibit an early signal in T cell activation that is transduced by the TCR signal transduction pathway. Despite interacting with the same binding proteins as tacrolimus, there is no competitive inhibition of these drugs, as the binding proteins are present in great excess compared to the tacrolimus and rapamycin. In experimental models the combination of rapamycin with a CNI results in a synergistic effect. Everolimus (RAD) is a rapamycin derivative and has a similar mode of action to sirolimus. The mTOR inhibitors have been shown to be potent inhibitors of vascular endothelial growth factor, which may explain their role in preventing progression of many forms of cancer. Because the mTOR inhibitors have powerful immunosuppressive properties, they are also being used as CNI-sparing agents in transplant recipients (see Chapter 72).

POLYCLONAL IMMUNE GLOBULINS

Polyclonal antithymocyte globulin (ATG) preparations have been available for approximately 2 decades and have proven more effective than steroids alone for reversing acute renal allograft rejection. Polyclonal immune globulins are produced by injecting animals such as horses or rabbits with human thymocytes to obtain the purified γ-globulin fractions of the resulting immune sera. Polyclonal immune globulin may exert its immunosuppressive effect by several mechanisms, including classical complement-mediated lysis of lymphocytes, clearance of lymphocytes through reticuloendothelial uptake, masking of T cell antigens, and the possible expansion of regulatory cells. Administration of immune globulins produces prompt and profound lymphopenia. It soon abates, however, and the number of circulating T cells gradually increases, even while treatment continues, but the proliferative response continues to be impaired. It has been suggested that regulatory cells may be responsible for the prolonged immunosuppressive effect that persists after the resolution of lymphopenia. Thus the resolution of cell-mediated allograft rejection results from elimination of circulating T cells, and the subsequent inhibition of proliferative responses sustains the immunosuppressive effect.

Each polyclonal immune globulin preparation has different constituent antibodies. Because of the unpredictable nature of the antibody mixtures, treatment is associated with variable efficacy and risks for adverse reactions, though batch standardization has improved lately. Unwanted antibodies could cause thrombocytopenia, granulocytopenia, serum sickness, or glomerulonephritis. Although polyclonal immune globulins are potent immunosuppressive agents, the major concern is the potential for excessive immunosuppression, which not infrequently results in opportunistic infections and higher risk for long-term malignancies. Therefore caution is the rule when combining immune globulins with other immunosuppressive agents. There has been an increased interest in the use of ATG as induction therapy in renal transplantation, partially because of the suggested benefit in protecting against delayed graft function by postponing the introduction of CNI and allowing steroid elimination from maintenance immunosuppressive regimens.

MONOCLONAL ANTIBODIES

The development of monoclonal antibodies to T cell surface molecules offers the advantage of homogeneous preparations and more predictable therapeutic agents. A number of monoclonal antibodies have been shown in clinical trials to be effective immunosuppressive agents. One of the most effective monoclonal antibodies was muromonab-CD3 (OKT3), which binds the CD3 of the TCR complex; however, this drug has fallen out of favor because of its significant adverse drug reactions. The TCR is a complex of six or seven polypeptides, including the polymorphic α- and β-chains, which provide the antigen-recognition component, and the γ-, δ-, and ε-chains, plus a ζζ-homodimer or ζη-heterodimer, which provide the signal transduction function of the receptor. Muromonab-CD3 binds to the TCR ε-chain, which is a pan–T cell nonpolymorphic component of the antigen receptor. Immunosuppression with muromonab-CD3 blocks both $CD4^+$ and $CD8^+$ T cell function.

Chimeric and humanized antibodies targeted against the IL-2R have also been developed. They are created by splicing together the DNA encoding the antigen-recognition portion of the murine antibody and human immunoglobulin DNA. Humanized antibodies contain 90% human and 10% murine antibody sequences. Chimeric antibodies are composed of mouse light and heavy chains and the human Fc portion. Anti–IL-2R antibodies bind to the α subunit of the high-affinity IL-2R, which is only expressed on activated lymphocytes.[6] This agent competitively inhibits the IL-2 activation of lymphocytes. Therapy with IL-2R antibodies results in a highly specific inhibition of the lymphocytic immune response of activated T cells, therefore suppressing T cell activity against the allograft. However, in patients 10% to 15% of T cells are IL-2R positive; therefore use of IL-2R antibodies may also have more of a generalized antiinflammatory effect. These antibodies are indicated for prophylaxis rather than treatment of acute allograft rejection.

Alemtuzumab (Campath) is a lymphocyte-depleting antibody (anti-CD52) that has been approved for use in leukemia. It has been used for induction therapy in kidney transplantation with low-dose cyclosporine, sirolimus, or alone with variable results. One of the major advantages of alemtuzumab is the requirement of only a single dose, significantly reducing the cost of the induction therapy and possibly shortening the number of admission days. Interestingly, a high rate of acute rejection rates, including humoral rejection, was reported when the antibody was used alone or with sirolimus monotherapy.[39] In addition, a study found that 30% of patients treated with alemtuzumab for multiple sclerosis developed autoimmune disease. Thymoglobulin and alemtuzumab administration led to similar patient and graft outcomes in a randomized trial, though late rejections were more common in the alemtuzumab group.

T cell costimulatory blockade, in the form of CTLA4-Ig (belatacept)[40] was approved for use in transplantation by the U.S. Food and Drug Administration (FDA) in 2011 as a CNI-sparing agent (see Chapter 72). Belatacept, which prevents the interaction of CD28 on T cells with CD80/86 (B7) on APCs, is the first agent available for use in transplantation that specifically blocks a signal II pathway. Two other costimulatory pathways that are also being looked at as potential targets are the CD40-CD154 pathway and the LFA-3–CD2 pathway. A study using an anti-CD154 agent in kidney transplant recipients was prematurely terminated because of the development of thromboembolic events in the patients. This was thought to be related to the upregulation of CD154 on human platelets, an unforeseen side effect that was not predicted from the animal models. Agents targeting the CD40 end of this pathway are being tested in preclinical trials. In humans, unlike in many of the animal models of transplantation, the memory immune response plays an important role in allograft rejection. The fusion protein alefacept blocks interaction of LFA-3 with its ligand CD2.[41] Memory T cells have a high expression of CD2, and alefacept has been shown to be particularly effective at inhibiting, as well as depleting, the memory T cell response. However, alefacept in a randomized controlled trial did not improve graft survival or decrease the rate of rejection.

Other agents that have been FDA approved for other indications are been increasingly used in the kidney transplant setting, especially for the treatment or prevention of antibody-mediated rejection. Bortezomib, a proteasome inhibitor that selectively targets dividing metabolically active cells, such as plasma cells, has been used as an effective therapy for multiple myeloma. In the transplant setting it has been shown to reduce the number of plasma cells and alloantibody production. Eculizumab, a C5a inhibitor approved for use in treatment for paroxysmal nocturnal hemoglobinuria, has been used as a last-resort therapy in severe antibody-mediated rejection.[42] Unlike other therapies aimed at interrupting antibody-mediated rejection, eculizumab inhibits the complement activation cascade triggered by anti-HLA antibodies and as such would either need to be given continuously or combined with other agents that would reduce antibody levels.

GENOMICS AND PROTEOMICS

Completion of a draft of the sequence of the human genome,[43] in addition to concurrent technologic advances, have made the simultaneous analysis of tens of thousands of genes feasible. The application of DNA microarrays to the analysis of transplantation is evolving. A study of rejection in human recipients of kidney allografts analyzed gene expression in biopsy specimens of renal allografts from patients on triple immunosuppression with a confirmed diagnosis of acute rejection.[3] Expression of gene transcripts from seven renal biopsy specimens with histopathologic evidence of acute cellular rejection were compared to tissue from three normal renal biopsy specimens. Using a minimum threshold of fourfold induction, four genes were identified in each acute rejection sample: human monokine induced by interferon-γ (a CXC chemokine crucial for murine acute allograft rejection), TCR active β-chain protein, IL-2–stimulated phosphoprotein (expressed predominantly in T cells), and RING4 (important in intracellular antigen processing). Murine cardiac allografts analyzed for the expression of approximately 6500 genes and ESTs (expressions sequenced tagged) following transplantation identified 181 genes with significantly modulated expression in at least one of the experimental groups of ischemia, stress, innate, or adaptive immunity. In an additional study, differentially expressed genes were identified using self-organizing maps; 29 genes were upregulated as early as 6 hours after transplantation. These genes included those encoding the interleukin-1 receptor (IL-1R), IL-6, and haptoglobin, all of which have been associated with the acute phase response. In addition, studies from Halloran and colleagues have demonstrated the potential benefit of using microarrays from biopsy specimens to more accurately diagnose antibody-mediated rejection.[37] In current clinical practice, acute rejection is typically diagnosed solely by histologic analysis of allograft biopsy specimens. The application of these newer technologies could produce a molecular profile of each biopsy specimen that could provide more precise diagnostic criteria.

Although the study of genomics has given us insight into the upregulation of genes that occur in certain circumstances such as allograft rejection, genomic data alone do not provide the whole picture because distinct genes may be upregulated in different cells, and proteins are subject to a variety of modifications during translation. The corollary study of the entire complement of proteins has been dubbed the *proteome*. Many investigators are actively working on correlating the various forms of rejection with the study of proteomics using mass spectrometry.

TOLEROGENIC PROTOCOLS IN TRANSPLANTATION

Since the original work in tolerance by Medawar in the 1940s, multiple attempts have been made to achieve tolerance in human organ transplantation. Tolerance is infrequently achieved outside of liver transplantation in humans and is encountered rarely in patients who have become noncompliant with their medications or in cases for which physicians have withdrawn immunosuppression for severe adverse effects or malignancy. In clinical practice, operational tolerance is defined as "*a well-functioning graft lacking histological signs of rejection, in the absence of any immunosuppressive drugs (for at least 1 year), in an immunocompetent host.*"[44]

There are multiple proposed strategies to promote tolerance in transplantation, including the induction of central tolerance through a combined bone marrow–kidney transplant or the development of peripheral tolerance through cellular therapy with regulatory cells. Chimerism is the concept that cells of different donor origins can coexist in the same organism and is generally described as mixed or full chimerism. Mixed chimerism is defined as the presence of both donor and recipient cell lineages coexisting in the recipient bone marrow. Full chimerism implies complete elimination of recipient hematopoietic lineages and population of the recipient bone marrow by 100% donor cells. Full chimerism is associated with significant higher morbidity and mortality from the effects of myeloablative therapy and risk for graft-versus-host disease (GVHD). In addition, full chimerism often leads to defects in the immune response since these patients lack a supply of peripheral recipient APCs to present antigens optimally to donor T cells that are positively selected on recipient thymic epithelial MHC molecules. In the absence of MHC sharing between donor and recipient, T cells do not efficiently recognize peptides presented by donor APCs, which are the only ones available in full chimeras. Therefore mixed-chimerism strategies have been the main focus of tolerance protocols in transplantation.

Bone marrow transplantation is able to promote mixed chimerism through a combination of nonmyeloablative conditioning and infusion of a certain amount of donor-derived bone marrow cells. Multiple successful attempts have been made to achieve mixed chimerism,[45-47] though inability to obtain a sustained chimerism and toxicity related to conditioning protocol have been significant limitations. In one study, 12 living-donor HLA-matched kidney transplant recipients received a donor-cell infusion of 5 to 16 × 10^6 CD34$^+$ cells per kilogram mixed with 1 to 10 × 10^6 CD3$^+$ T cells per kilogram after conditioning with total lymphoid irradiation and five doses of rabbit ATG.[47] Eight of these patients are now more than 2 years after transplant off immunosuppression, while four recipients developed rejection and were maintained on some immunosuppression. None of the patients developed GVHD. In another study, patients underwent combined kidney and bone marrow transplantation after conditioning with cyclophosphamide, thymic irradiation, anti-CD2 monoclonal antibody, rituximab, and a short course of CNI and steroids after transplantation.[45] All recipients developed transient chimerism and reversible capillary leak syndrome, but only four patients could be maintained off immunosuppression long-term. The other six patients developed rejection or recurrence of original disease, with two patients losing their graft. A phase II clinical trial investigated the use of hematopoietic stem cell transplantation in combination with facilitating cell infusion to promote the development of chimerism and subsequent tolerance in eight HLA-mismatched living-donor kidney transplant recipients.[46] Similar to prior studies, all patients initially developed chimerism, though only half showed stable persistent chimerism over time and could be withdrawn from immunosuppression. One patient with persistent chimerism developed a severe viral infection that led to graft loss. In sum, combined bone marrow and kidney transplantation is an interesting strategy to promote central tolerance, though the toxicity of the conditioning protocol and the partial maintenance of chimerism long-term are major limitations to the broad application of this approach.

The development of peripheral tolerance has been proposed through the use of cellular therapy with T_{reg} cells, mesenchymal stem cells, or tolerogenic APCs, as well as with agents that promote regulatory cells such as low-dose IL-2. The idea is based on the clear importance of the peripheral regulatory immune system in maintaining self-tolerance, and therefore expanding this arm of the immune system may permit downregulation of the effector alloimmune response. There has been a successful trial using low-dose IL-2 to promote T_{reg} cells in bone marrow transplantation resolving refractory cases of chronic GVHD, and preclinical trials have suggested a potential benefit of adoptive transfer of regulatory cells in solid organ transplantation.[44] Several larger clinical studies are being conducted in Europe and the United States to address the potential benefit of tolerance induction strategies in solid organ transplantation. There are a number of difficult questions still to be answered, including the optimal type of regulatory cell (T_{reg} cells, mesenchymal stem cells, or myeloid-derived suppressor cells), timing and location of administration, and the longevity and fate of these cells after infusion.

Though our knowledge has significantly expanded since the initial work from Medawar more than 70 years ago, achieving tolerance remains a major challenge based on the heterogeneous outcome of trials and the lack of stability of this immunologic state. Rather than achieving tolerance, a more realistic approach is to develop protocols that allow minimization of immunosuppression and therefore limiting the frequency and severity of side effects from drugs and potential long-term consequences of over-immunosuppression such as increased malignancy risk.

Complete reference list available at ExpertConsult.com.

KEY REFERENCES

2. Shevach EM: CD4+ CD25+ suppressor T cells: more questions than answers. *Nat Rev Immunol* 2(6):389–400, 2002.
4. Murphy KM, Weaver CT, Elish M, et al: Peripheral tolerance to allogeneic class II histocompatibility antigens expressed in transgenic mice: evidence against a clonal-deletion mechanism. *Proc Natl Acad Sci U S A* 86(24):10034–10038, 1989.
6. Nossal GJ: Negative selection of lymphocytes. *Cell* 76(2):229–239, 1994.
7. Fry AM, Jones LA, Kruisbeek AM, et al: Thymic requirement for clonal deletion during T cell development. *Science* 246(4933):1044–1046, 1989.
12. Medawar PB: The behaviour and fate of skin autografts and skin homografts in rabbits: a report to the War Wounds Committee of the Medical Research Council. *J Anat* 78(Pt 5):176–199, 1944.
14. Gorer PA: The genetic and antigenic basis of tumor transplantation. *J Pathol Bacteriol* 44:691, 1937.
15. Snell GD: Methods for the study of histocompatibility genes. *J Genetics* 49:87, 1948.
18. Dausset J: [Platelet antibodies]. *Acta Haematol* 20(1–4):185–194, 1958.
19. Graff RJ, Silvers WK, Billingham RE, et al: The cumulative effect of histocompatibility antigens. *Transplantation* 4(5):605–617, 1966.
20. Holman E: Protein sensitization in iso-skin grafting. Is the latter of practical value? *Surg Gynecol Obstet* 38:100, 1924.
21. Medawar PB: The behaviour and fate of skin autografts and skin homografts in rabbits: a report to the War Wounds Committee of the Medical Research Council. *J Anat* 78(Pt 5):176–199, 1944.
22. Germain RN: MHC-dependent antigen processing and peptide presentation: providing ligands for T lymphocyte activation. *Cell* 76(2):287–299, 1994.
27. Davis MM, Bjorkman PJ: T-cell antigen receptor genes and T-cell recognition. *Nature* 334(6181):395–402, 1988.
28. Garboczi DN, Ghosh P, Utz U, et al: Structure of the complex between human T-cell receptor, viral peptide and HLA-A2. *Nature* 384(6605):134–141, 1996.
30. Patel SD, Monaco JJ, McDevitt HO: Delineation of the subunit composition of human proteasomes using antisera against the major histocompatibility complex-encoded LMP2 and LMP7 subunits. *Proc Natl Acad Sci U S A* 91(1):296–300, 1994.
33. Higuchi R, von Beroldingen CH, Sensabaugh GF, et al: DNA typing from single hairs. *Nature* 332(6164):543–546, 1988.
35. Brown JH, Jardetsky TS, Gorga JC, et al: Three dimensional structure of the human class II histocompatibility antigen HLA-DR1. *Nature* 364:33, 1993.
36. Chicz RM, Urban RG, Gorga JC, et al: Specificity and promiscuity among naturally processed peptides bound to HLA-DR alleles. *J Exp Med* 178(1):27–47, 1993.
39. Thorsby E: HLA-associated disease susceptibility. Which genes are involved? *Immunologist* 3:41, 1995.
41. Bach FH, van Rood JJ: The major histocompatibility complex—genetics and biology (third of three parts). *N Engl J Med* 295(17):927–936, 1976.
42. Human Renal Transplant Registry: Report No. 12. *JAMA* 233:787, 1995.
45. U.S. Renal Data System: USRDS: *2011 annual data report: atlas of chronic kidney disease and end-stage renal disease in the United States*, Bethesda, MD, 2013, National Institutes of Health, National Institute of Diabetes and Digestive and Kidney Diseases. Available at: http://www.usrds.org, (Accessed February 2, 2014).

Clinical Management of the Adult Kidney Transplant Recipient

72

Colin R. Lenihan | Stéphan Busque | Jane C. Tan

CHAPTER OUTLINE

TRANSPLANTATION SURGERY PROCEDURE, 2251
Live Donor Nephrectomy, 2252
Handling and Preservation of Donor Kidney, 2252
Complications of Transplantation Procedures, 2253
IMMUNOSUPPRESSIVE AGENTS USED IN KIDNEY TRANSPLANTATION, 2253
Overview, 2253
Immunosuppressive Drugs, 2255
Immunosuppression Protocols, 2259
EVALUATION OF RECIPIENT, 2259
Immediately Before Transplantation, 2259
Medical Status, 2259
Immunologic Status, 2260
Desensitization, 2261
Immediately After Transplantation, 2261
MANAGEMENT OF ALLOGRAFT DYSFUNCTION, 2261
Immediate Posttransplantation Period (First Week), 2261
Early Posttransplantation Period (First 6 Months), 2265
Late Posttransplantation Period, 2271
Drug and Radiocontrast Nephrotoxicity, 2273
Late Allograft Dysfunction and Late Allograft Loss, 2273
ASSESSING OUTCOMES IN KIDNEY TRANSPLANTATION, 2276
Actual and Actuarial Allograft and Patient Survival, 2276
Survival Benefits of Kidney Transplantation, 2276
Factors Affecting Kidney Allograft Survival, 2276
Improving Kidney Allograft Outcomes: Matching Kidney and Recipient Risk, 2280
MEDICAL MANAGEMENT OF TRANSPLANT RECIPIENTS, 2281
Electrolyte Disorders, 2281
Bone Disorders After Kidney Transplantation, 2281
Posttransplantation Diabetes Mellitus, 2283
Cardiovascular Disease, 2283
Cancer After Kidney Transplantation, 2284
Infectious Complications of Kidney Transplantation, 2286
TRANSPLANTATION ISSUES IN SPECIFIC PATIENT GROUPS, 2288
Patients with Diabetes, 2288
Kidney-Pancreas Transplantation, 2289
Patients with Human Immunodeficiency Virus Infection, 2289
Pregnant Kidney Transplant Recipients, 2289
Surgery in the Kidney Transplant Recipient, 2290
Patients with a Failing Kidney, 2290
TRANSPLANTATION AND IMMUNOSUPPRESSION: THE FUTURE, 2290
CONCLUSION, 2290

TRANSPLANTATION SURGERY PROCEDURE

The kidney allograft is placed in the extraperitoneal iliac fossa (Figure 72.1). A curvilinear incision is made in the right or left lower quadrant, the retroperitoneal space is widened, and the iliac vessels exposed. The external iliac artery and vein are mobilized, and surrounding lymphatic vessels are ligated and divided. End-to-side anastomoses are performed between the renal vein and external iliac vein, followed by the renal artery and external iliac artery.

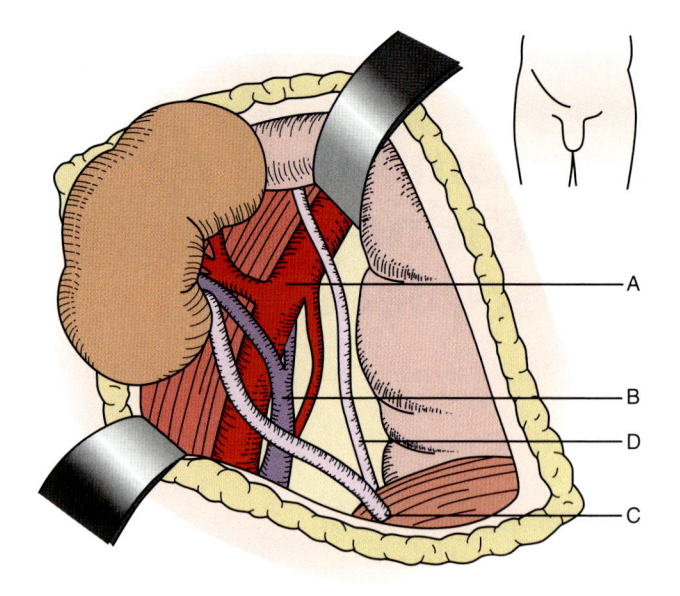

Figure 72.1 Anatomy of a typical first kidney transplant. *A*, External iliac artery; *B*, external iliac vein; *C*, implanted donor ureter; *D*, native ureter.

Alternate techniques for the renal artery are end-to-side anastomosis to the common iliac artery or end-to-end anastomosis to the mobilized internal iliac artery. The site of anastomosis is chosen after examining the length, size, and quality of the donor and recipient vessels. The Lich-Gregoir implantation of the ureter to the bladder, a technique designed to minimize urinary reflux into the ureter, has become the preferred technique for neoureterocystostomy. A double-J ureteric stent can be inserted either routinely or selectively for higher risk candidates. It is usually retrieved 2 to 4 weeks after transplantation in the outpatient setting. A recent Cochrane review has suggested that the incidence of urine leak and ureteric stenosis are significantly reduced with prophylactic uretic stenting.[1] A low-pressure suction drain can also be used and retrieved within the first week after surgery. While the surgical techniques for deceased and living donor kidney transplant are similar, attention is given to preserving longer stretches of the donor vessels with deceased donor allografts. The renal artery or arteries are procured along with an aortic patch; this technique facilitates the vascular anastomosis and reduces the risk of post-transplant renal artery stenosis.

LIVE DONOR NEPHRECTOMY

Traditionally, the procurement of kidneys from live donors has been performed through a right or left flank incision. In 1995, a laparoscopic approach for kidney donation was introduced as an alternative that would reduce postoperative pain, wound morbidity, and recovery time associated with the traditional donor nephrectomy.[2] The laparoscopic approach is now the procedure of choice, and is performed in over 90% of live kidney donations in the United States.[3] Initial concern regarding ureteral complications and graft dysfunction has mostly subsided with the improvement of surgical technique and experience.[4,5] Pure laparoscopic, hand-assisted, robotic-assisted, and single-port access are variants of the laparoscopic donor nephrectomy. All these techniques avoid flank incision by intraabdominal mobilization of the kidney after establishing the pneumoperitoneum. A periumbilical or infraumbilical small incision, which spares transection of muscle tissue, is used to retrieve the kidney. The hand-assisted variant is the most popular approach. A small periumbilical or infraumbilical incision of 8 cm allows the surgeon to insert one hand inside the abdomen with the help of a device that seals the pneumoperitoneum. The hand is used to help with retraction of the kidney and also allows faster retrieval of the kidney, reducing the warm ischemia by 50% compared to a pure laparoscopic approach. The left kidney is preferred even more than with the open nephrectomy because the laparoscopic instrument used to secure the renal vein effectively reduces its length by 0.5 to 1 cm. When the open nephrectomy surgical technique is used, an incision is made from the rectus muscle in direction of the tip of the 12th rib on the right or left side. This operation is retroperitoneal, as opposed to the laparoscopic approach, which is transperitoneal. Smaller incisions and muscle sparing are now used to improve the postoperative recovery of this operation.

HANDLING AND PRESERVATION OF DONOR KIDNEY

The basic principle of organ preservation is to prevent damage from ischemia by replacing the circulating blood with a preservation solution and by retrieving and cooling the organs expediently. The composition of preservation solutions vary, but all have ingredients designed to: (1) minimize cell edema; (2) preserve the energy and integrity of cells and tissue; and (3) buffer free radicals.

The two cold storage preservation solutions most widely used in the United States are the University of Wisconsin solution (Viaspan, UW) and histidine-tryptophan-ketoglutarate (HTK) solution (Custodiol). The UW solution has an electrolyte composition similar to that of the intracellular fluid, with a high concentration of potassium (120 mmol/L). Among other additives, lactobionate and raffinose prevent cellular edema, and hydroxyethyl starch buffers free radicals. Its viscosity is three times that of water, making it relatively difficult to flush. The HTK solution is a low-viscosity solution. The concentration of potassium is low (15 mmol/L), and this decreases the risk of hyperkalemia after transplantation. Histidine serves as a strong buffer, and tryptophan and mannitol are free radical scavengers.

The UW solution had been the preservation solution of choice since its introduction in 1988 for multiorgan deceased donor recovery. However, HTK is used by a growing number of organ procurement organizations (OPOs). One of the major advantages of HTK is its relatively low cost. Two small randomized studies comparing UW to HTK preservation solutions found no difference in delayed graft function or graft survival between groups.[6,7] However, a large retrospective (nonrandomized) study comparing HTK versus UW preservation found that HTK use was associated with an increased risk of late death-censored graft loss.[8] For living donor kidneys with short ischemia times, the use of simple and inexpensive solutions such as heparinized lactated

Ringer's with procaine has been proposed[9]; however, we prefer to use a preservation solution such as HTK.

Machine perfusion is an alternative to static cold preservation of the deceased donor kidney. Following standard retrieval and flushing of the kidney allograft, the renal artery is connected to a perfusion pump that circulates a preservation solution, maintained at 1° to 10° C. Perfusion parameters can also be used to determine the quality of the graft. Machine perfusion compared to static cold storage has been associated with a reduction of delayed graft function and an improvement of graft survival at 1 year.[10]

COMPLICATIONS OF TRANSPLANTATION PROCEDURES

SURGICAL COMPLICATIONS

Advances in donor and recipient surgical technique, anesthesia, organ preservation, and perioperative care have all likely contributed to improvements in 1-year patient and graft survival rates. However, early recognition and management of surgical complications remain important. Specific vascular and urologic complications are described more fully later (see "Management of Allograft Dysfunction" section). A brief description of these complications is presented here.

VASCULAR COMPLICATIONS

Hemorrhagic Complications

Acute and life-threatening hemorrhagic complications in the immediate postoperative course usually involve the anastomotic site. Bleeding can be brisk and requires immediate surgical exploration. Perirenal hematomas can result from both venous and small arterial bleeding or be related to the incision or retroperitoneal dissection. Unless small and stable, perirenal hematomas require surgical exploration to ensure adequate hemostasis. Large hematomas should be evacuated to reduce the risk of subsequent infection.[11]

Arterial Thrombosis

Renal artery thrombosis of the allograft is rare (0.5% to 1%). Acute thrombosis is usually related to an anastomotic problem or kink in the renal artery. Recipient arteriosclerosis, multiple arteries, vasospasm, and hypotension are also significant risk factors. Sudden anuria should raise suspicion for arterial thrombosis. Arterial thrombosis results in immediate warm ischemia. Delays associated with confirming the diagnosis and preparing the patient for surgical exploration usually exceed the time required to reestablish arterial flow to the kidney, resulting in prolonged warm ischemia, hypoxia and often permanent loss of function.

Venous Thrombosis

Renal vein thrombosis usually presents with local swelling, pain, and hematuria. The ultrasound Doppler findings reveal the persistence of an arterial flow to the kidney, however, no diastolic flow or even reversal flow during the diastole is seen. Venous flow is usually not detectable. The causes of venous thrombosis include problems with the surgical anastomosis, extrinsic compression by a lymphocele or a hematoma, and a deep venous thrombosis that extends from the iliac vein at the level of the venous anastomosis. Surgical exploration with thrombectomy followed by anticoagulation can be attempted; however, it is rarely successful. Contributing factors, such as thrombophilia, should be evaluated and corrected, if possible.[12]

Pseudoaneurysm of the arterial anastomosis is a rare infectious complication that leads almost invariably to graft loss and is associated with significant mortality and morbidity. Depending on its severity, noninvasive treatment with covered stenting can be attempted; however, usually transplantation nephrectomy, vascular reconstruction, or excision with extraanatomic bypass is required. Limb loss due to distal thrombosis or dissection of the femoral artery at the time of transplant is a rare but reported vascular complication, and usually associated with preexisting vascular disease in the recipient.[13]

Lymphocele

A lymphocele is a lymphatic fluid collection originating from the severed iliac lymphatics or lymphatic drainage of the renal allograft itself. Most lymphoceles are asymptomatic. However, some may compress the ureter, causing hydronephrosis, or obstruct lower limb venous return, resulting in unilateral edema. Large lymphoceles may present as an abdominal mass. Analysis of aspirated fluid will typically show a high lymphocyte count and creatinine concentration similar to that of serum. This contrasts with urinoma fluid, which has a creatinine concentration much higher than serum. Percutaneous drainage alone is often associated with persistent drainage or recurrence but has been successful in some cases, particularly those associated with injection of a sclerosing agent. The preferred and more definitive treatment is internal drainage of the lymphocele into the peritoneal cavity. In many centers, a laparoscopic transabdominal approach has replaced the traditional open approach that uses the kidney transplant incision site.[14]

IMMUNOSUPPRESSIVE AGENTS USED IN KIDNEY TRANSPLANTATION

OVERVIEW

The immunosuppressive drugs commonly used in clinical transplantation are summarized in Table 72.1, and their mechanisms of action are illustrated in Figure 72.2. T lymphocytes play a central role in the recognition of the allograft as foreign and in the initiation of the rejection process. The T cell immune response is described as requiring three distinct signaling events (the three-signal model). Briefly, antigen-presenting cells (APCs—dendritic cells, macrophages, activated endothelium), most likely of donor origin, migrate to the secondary lymphoid organs of the recipient where a foreign antigen or major histocompatibility (MHC) complex is presented to the (recipient) T cell receptor (signal 1). A costimulatory T cell–APC interaction (signal 2) is then required for downstream signal transduction to occur. The ensuing activation of the T cell calcineurin-nuclear factor of activated T cells (NFAT), mitogen-activated protein (MAP) kinase, and nuclear factor-kappa B (NF-κB) signaling pathways results in the production of cytokines (e.g., interleukin-2 [IL-2], IL-15) and surface molecules (e.g., the IL-2 receptor). IL-2 and other

Table 72.1 Drugs Used for Maintenance Immunosuppression

Drug	Mechanism of Action	Adverse Effects
Corticosteroids	Block synthesis of several cytokines including IL-2; multiple antiinflammatory effects	Glucose intolerance, hypertension, hyperlipidemia, osteoporosis, osteonecrosis, myopathy, cosmetic defects; growth suppression in children
Cyclosporine	Inhibits calcineurin-induced synthesis of IL-2 and other molecules critical for T cell activation	Nephrotoxicity (acute and chronic), hyperlipidemia, hypertension, glucose intolerance, cosmetic defects
Tacrolimus	Similar to cyclosporine, although binds to different cytoplasmic protein (FKBP)	Broadly similar to cyclosporine; diabetes mellitus more common; hypertension, hyperlipidemia, and cosmetic defects less common
Azathioprine	Inhibits purine biosynthesis, inhibiting lymphocyte replication	Bone marrow suppression; rarely, pancreatitis, hepatitis
MMF	Inhibits de novo pathway of purine biosynthesis, inhibiting lymphocyte replication	Bone marrow suppression, gastrointestinal upset; invasive CMV disease more common than with azathioprine
Sirolimus	Sirolimus-FKBP complex inhibits mTOR blocking the lymphocyte proliferative response	Bone marrow suppression, hyperlipidemia, interstitial pneumonitis; enhances nephrotoxicity of cyclosporine-tacrolimus
Belatacept	Blocks T cell costimulation	PTLD in EBV-seronegative patients, PML (rare), reactivation of TB

CMV, Cytomegalovirus; EBV, Epstein-Barr virus; FKBP, FK-binding protein; IL-2, interleukin-2; MMF, mycophenolate mofetil; PML, progressive multifocal leukoencephalopathy; PTLD, posttransplantation lymphoproliferative disorder; TB, tuberculosis; TOR, target of rapamycin.

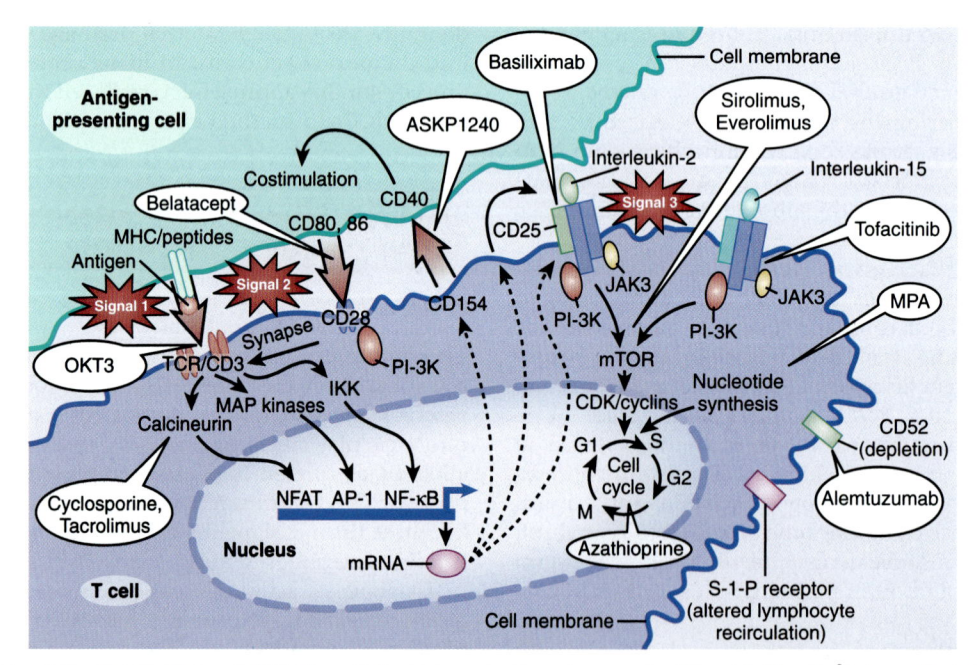

Figure 72.2 Stages of T cell activation—multiple targets for immunosuppressive agents. *Signal 1,* The Ca^{2+}-dependent signal induced by T cell receptor (TCR) stimulation results in calcineurin activation, a process inhibited by the calcineurin inhibitors (CNIs). Calcineurin dephosphorylates nuclear factor of activated T cells (NFAT), enabling it to enter the nucleus and bind to the interleukin-2 (IL-2) promoter. Corticosteroids bind to cytoplasmic receptors, enter the nucleus, and inhibit cytokine gene transcription in the T cell and antigen-presenting cell (APC). Corticosteroids also inhibit the activation of the transcription factor, nuclear factor-κB. *Signal 2,* Costimulatory signals, such as those between CD28 on the T cell and CD80 or CD86 on the APC, are necessary to optimize T cell transcription of the IL-2 gene, prevent T cell anergy, and inhibit T cell apoptosis. *Signal 3,* IL-2 receptor stimulation induces the cell to enter the cell cycle and proliferate. IL-2 and related cytokines have autocrine and paracrine effects. Signal 3 may be blocked by IL-2 receptor antibodies or by sirolimus. Further downstream, azathioprine and mycophenolate mofetil (MMF) inhibit progression into the cell cycle by inhibiting purine and therefore DNA synthesis. (From Halloran PF: Immunosuppressive drugs for kidney transplantation. *N Engl J Med* 351:2715-2729, 2004.)

cytokines then stimulate T cell proliferation (signal 3) via the phosphatidylinositol-3-kinase (PI3K)/Akt/mammalian target of rapamycin (mTOR), Janus kinase 3 (JAK3)/signal transducer and activator of transcription 5 (STAT5), and MAP kinase signaling pathways.[15] Most immunosuppressive agents either deplete lymphocytes (depleting agents) or act at the level of, or downstream from, one or more of the three T cell immune activation signals.

Immunosuppressive strategies can also be divided into induction and maintenance therapy. Induction of immunosuppression is defined as the rapid achievement of profound immunosuppression, usually at the time of transplantation, with the use of depleting agents. Maintenance immunosuppression is achieved by the combination of oral agents that take advantage of additive or synergistic immunosuppressive effects of different drug categories to minimize their nonimmunosuppressive side effects. Dosage is usually greater during the first 3 months after transplantation and decreases afterward. A combination of a calcineurin inhibitor (CNI), antiproliferative agent, and corticosteroid is the most common regimen.

IMMUNOSUPPRESSIVE DRUGS

DEPLETING AGENTS

Rabbit antithymocyte globulin (Thymoglobulin), horse antithymocyte globulin (Atgam), and muromonab-CD3 (Orthoclone OKT3) are agents approved in the United States for the treatment of acute rejection. Alemtuzumab (Campath) is approved for the treatment of B cell chronic lymphocytic leukemia but has to be used off label for the induction of immunosuppression.

POLYCLONAL ANTIBODY PREPARATIONS

Polyclonal antibodies against human T cells, antithymocyte globulins (ATGs), are prepared by immunization of animals with human lymphoid cells. Available products include Thymoglobulin (globulin derived from rabbits inoculated with human thymocytes), ATG-Fresenius (globulin derived from rabbits inoculated with Jurkat T cells; not available in the United States), and Atgam (gamma globulin derived from horses inoculated with human thymocytes). For Thymoglobulin, the resulting purified globulin includes antibodies that target more than 20 different T cell epitopes. Antibodies at higher concentrations include TCR, CD2, CD3, CD5, CD6, CD8, CD11A, CD49, and β_2-microglobulin.[16,17] The mechanism of T cell depletion is thought to involve complement-dependent lysis, mostly in the blood compartment, and apoptosis and phagocytosis in the peripheral lymphoid tissue. Antibodies against adhesion molecules that are present in the ATG preparation may also play a role by modulating leukocyte function.[18]

A number of randomized controlled trials (RCTs) have compared ATG induction with other strategies. A study from the late 1970s compared a 1-month induction using horse ATG with no induction treatment in patients treated with azathioprine and a steroid-based immunosuppression regimen and found a significantly improved 2-year graft survival in the ATG-treated group.[19] Rabbit ATG (ATG-Fresenius) induction resulted in an equivalent 1-year graft survival but a lower rate of acute rejection and infection- and noninfection-related complications compared to OKT3 in patients treated with cyclosporine, azathioprine, and steroid maintenance immunosuppression.[20] A long-running randomized trial comparing horse ATG to rabbit ATG induction therapy demonstrated the superiority of rabbit ATG in terms of reduction of the composite of death, graft loss, or rejection.[21] In sensitized patients, defined as a current or peak panel reactive antibody (PRA) more than 30% or 50%, respectively, rabbit ATG induction was associated with significantly lower rate of biopsy proven acute rejection and steroid resistant rejection in the first year posttransplantation but no difference in 1-year survival compared to daclizumab induction.[22] In another study of kidney transplant recipients with risk factors for delayed graft function or acute rejection, rabbit ATG resulted in a lower acute rejection rate than basiliximab induction but no difference in delayed graft function or 1 year graft survival. A 5-year follow-up of this study showed sustained superiority of rabbit ATG in terms of acute rejection.[23,24] Notably, infectious complications were more common in the rabbit ATG groups of both trials which compared the agent with IL-2 receptor antagonizing antibodies. In immunologically high-risk kidney transplant recipients randomly assigned to rabbit ATG or alemtuzumab induction, no differences were seen in acute rejection rates between the groups followed up to 3 years posttransplantation,[25] although infectious complications were more common in rabbit ATG–treated subjects.

ATG also has an important role in the treatment of severe or steroid-resistant acute cellular rejection. A randomized study has shown superiority of rabbit ATG compared to horse ATG in the treatment of acute rejection in terms of rejection reversal and 90-day recurrence rates.[26] In another study, rabbit ATG and OKT3 were shown to be similarly efficacious in the treatment of steroid-resistant acute rejection; however, rabbit ATG had the advantage of a more favourable side-effect profile.[27] Given a more favorable side-effect profile, rabbit ATG has now replaced OKT3 as the second-line therapy for acute rejection. OKT3 still may still have had a role as a potential rescue therapy in "ATG-resistant" rejection; however, the agent is no longer available in the United States.[28]

Rabbit ATG is given at a dosage of 1.5 mg/kg/day. The initial regimen of 7 to 14 days of treatment is rarely used today because a shorter course of treatment (5 days) has been demonstrated to be efficacious.[23] Infusion-related side effects, such as fever, chills, hypotension and, less frequently, cardiovascular events, are usually mild, particularly if coadministered with adequate steroid and antihistamine premedication are infused slowly. These reactions are more likely to occur during the first few infusions and become rare with subsequent infusions. Serum sickness, characterized by fever, rash, and arthralgia, occurring 10 to 15 days after treatment, have been reported as well,[29] possibly more frequently in patients not receiving steroid prophylaxis.

MONOCLONAL ANTIBODIES

Muromonab-CD3 is a mouse antihuman monoclonal antibody against the T cell receptor–associated CD3 antigen that was first approved for clinical use in 1986. OKT3 results in apoptosis and rapid depletion of T cells from the circulation. The cytotoxic effect is preceded by a transient, antibody-induced T cell activation and cytokine surge, an effect responsible for many of the undesired side-effects associated with OKT3. T cell number and function usually return to normal limits 1 week after completion of treatment. Cytokine release syndrome is present, usually after the first infusion. It is most frequently reported to be mild, self-limited, flulike illness; however, severe life-threatening reactions, such as serious cardiovascular and central nervous system manifestations, have been reported.[30] Noncardiac pulmonary edema has also been seen, particularly if the patient is fluid-overloaded pretransplantation. Patients may develop anti–mouse-neutralizing antibodies rapidly, which may limit efficacy of the treatment and prevent retreatment.[31] The efficacy of OKT3 as an induction agent and in the treatment of acute rejection has been well established.[30,32] As a result of its side effects, the use of OKT3 decreased considerably following the emergence of alternative immunosuppressive agents, such as ATG and IL-2 blockers.[33]

Alemtuzumab (Campath) is a humanized monoclonal antibody against CD52 that was originally developed to treat refractory B cell chronic lymphocytic leukemia. Alemtuzumab treatment results in profound and long-lasting depletion of T and B lymphocytes. Evidence for the efficacy of alemtuzumab as an induction agent was provided by an RCT that compared a single 30-mg dose of alemtuzumab to induction with basiliximab in immunologically low-risk patients and to rabbit ATG in immunologically high-risk patients. Alemtuzumab treatment proved superior to basiliximab and equivalent to rabbit ATG in terms of biopsy-confirmed acute rejection followed up to 3-years posttransplantation, although the overall rate of late biopsy-proven rejection (from 1 to 3 years posttransplantation) was significantly higher in the alemtuzumab group.[25] Infectious complications were higher with alemtuzumab than basiliximab, but lower with alemtuzumab than rabbit ATG. Alemtuzumab may cause an infusion first-dose reaction, which can be avoided if the subcutaneous route is used.[34] Neutropenia and anemia are also seen. Concern about the development of autoimmune disease (especially thyroid-related) following alemtuzumab treatment was initially raised after publication of data from a study comparing the agent with interferon-β for the treatment of multiple sclerosis.[35] The development of autoimmune diseases has also been reported in solid organ transplant recipients treated with alemtuzumab induction.[36,37] Potential advantages of alemtuzumab include the simplicity of a single-dose treatment and lower cost compared to other induction agents.

INTERLEUKIN-2 RECEPTOR ANTAGONIST

Daclizumab is a humanized monoclonal antibody, and basiliximab is a chimeric monoclonal antibody. Both are IgG1 (immunoglobulin G1) antibodies directed against the α-chain of the IL-2 receptor (CD25 antigen), which is expressed on activated T lymphocytes. Blockade of the IL-2 receptor inhibits a key T lymphocyte proliferation signaling pathway, thereby blunting the cellular immune response. These agents reduce the rate of rejection by about 30% to 40% compared to placebo when used in combination with conventional immunosuppression.[38-40] Rabbit ATG and alemtuzumab are both more effective in reducing the rate of rejection but incur a higher infectious risk than the IL-2 receptor blockers.[22,25,23] Advantages of IL-2 receptor blockers include minimization of injection-related side effects and lack of risk of infection or cancer compared to placebo.[39,40] Daclizumab was "retired" from the market by the manufacturer at the end of 2009, and thus basiliximab is the only IL-2 blocker currently available in the United States. The treatment regimen consists of two infusions of 20 mg, the first at the time of transplantation and the second 3 to 4 days posttransplantation. The pharmacokinetics of that dose regimen provides prophylaxis for 30 days posttransplantation. Few data exist regarding the use of IL-2 receptor antagonists (IL-2 RAs) for the treatment of acute rejection.

ANTI-CD20 MONOCLONAL ANTIBODY

Rituximab (Rituxan) is a chimeric, anti-CD20, cytolytic monoclonal antibody that has been approved for the treatment of non-Hodgkin's lymphoma, chronic lymphocytic leukemia, and rheumatoid arthritis. Rituximab was initially used in the transplant population for the treatment of posttransplantation lymphoproliferative disease.[41] It interferes with the humoral alloresponse by specifically targeting normal B lymphocytes. Rituximab has become an important element in many successful desensitization protocols (see later, "Desensitization" section).[42,43] Rituximab has also been used successfully in combination with plasmapheresis and/or intravenous Ig (IVIg) for the treatment of acute humoral rejection.[44,45] It is typically administered intravenously at 375 mg/m² or 1 g twice over 2 weeks. Steroid and antihistamine premedication and administration over 6 hours result in a lower incidence of infusion-related side effects. Notably, an RCT comparing induction with rituximab versus daclizumab was stopped early because of an excess of acute rejection in the rituximab group.[46]

MAINTENANCE IMMUNOSUPPRESSIVE AGENTS

Calcineurin Inhibitors

Calcineurin is a calcium-dependent, serine-threonine phosphatase involved in a diverse range of cellular functions, including T cell signal transduction.[47] In brief, the binding of foreign antigen to the T cell receptor, when accompanied by a costimulatory signal, triggers the cytosolic influx of calcium and downstream activation of calcineurin. Activated calcineurin dephosphorylates the transcription factor, NFAT, which then translocates to the nucleus and activates a host of target genes, including the cytokine IL-2.[48] IL-2 then binds to its receptor and initiates T cell expansion.[15] CNIs have contributed to a significant improvement in kidney transplantation survival and to the expansion of transplantation of extrarenal organs. Despite considerable toxicity, CNIs remain the cornerstone of immunosuppression in clinical transplantation. CNI-associated nephrotoxicity certainly contributes to the reduction of long-term graft survival and to nephrotoxicity among recipients of extrarenal solid organs.[49,50] The magnitude of graft failure attributable to CNI-toxicity is still hotly debated.

Cyclosporine

Cyclosporine is a lipophilic amino acid cyclic peptide that binds to cytoplasmic cyclophilin and forms a complex that inhibits calcineurin. The introduction of cyclosporine in the early 1980s heralded a new era in kidney transplantation. European and American clinical trials demonstrated the superiority of cyclosporine, alone or with steroid, over the standard immunosuppression regimen of azathioprine and steroid.[51,52] The original oil-based formulation of cyclosporine (Sandimmune) was associated with erratic gastrointestinal absorption and highly variable bioavailability. The subsequent development of a microemulsion formulation of cyclosporine (Neoral) significantly improved the drug's absorption and pharmacokinetic profile.[53] Cyclosporine is now also available in a generic microemulsion formulation. Gengraf is an alternative water-based microemulsion that many patients find more palatable.[54] Care should be taken to avoid nonmicroemulsion generic cyclosporine formulations without the prescriber's knowledge, as they are associated with unpredictable absorption and may expose the patient to an increased risk of rejection or toxicity.

Therapeutic drug monitoring of cyclosporine is most commonly performed using 12-hour trough levels, although monitoring blood levels 2 hours after ingestion of cyclosporine (C2 level) actually has a better correlation with drug exposure.[55] The side effects of cyclosporine include hypertension, hyperlipidemia, gingival hyperplasia, hypertrichosis, tremors, and nephrotoxicity. Cyclosporine is also associated with the development of posttransplantation diabetes mellitus (PTDM) and, rarely, hemolytic uremic syndrome.

Tacrolimus

Tacrolimus (Prograf) is a macrolide antibiotic that binds FK506 binding protein (FKBP12). The resulting drug-protein complex inhibits calcineurin activity. Many trials have demonstrated reduced rates of rejection compared to cyclosporine,[56] particularly the original formulation of cyclosporine. The toxicity profile is slightly different than that of cyclosporine; tacrolimus is not associated with gingival hyperplasia, hypertrichosis, or hyperlipidemia. However, it is associated with greater neurotoxicity, higher incidence of PTDM, and gastrointestinal toxicity. Hypertension and nephrotoxicity appear to be milder than with cyclosporine. The exposure to mycophenolate acid is increased by approximately 40% with tacrolimus as compared to cyclosporine (see below).[57] Tacrolimus is now also available in generic formulation. An extended-release formulation of tacrolimus (Astagraf) has also been approved in the United States. This once-daily tacrolimus formulation may be advantageous in terms of compliance.[58] Notably, an increase in the total daily tacrolimus dose is frequently required to achieve equivalent drug exposure following the switch from the twice-daily to once-daily tacrolimus formulation.[59] Therefore, close monitoring of drug levels, especially in early posttransplantation patients, is recommended following formulation changeover.

Voclosporin

Voclosporin (ISA247) was developed by modification of the functional group on the amino acid residue at position 1 of the cyclosporin A (CsA) molecule. This small modification results in a conformational change associated with tighter binding to calcineurin and a consequent increase in the inhibition of phosphatase activity. In addition, the number of inactive metabolites available to compete for binding to calcineurin is significantly smaller. As a result, voclosporin can achieve a higher inhibition of calcineurin at doses 4 to 10 times lower than cyclosporine. A 6-month, phase 2 randomized trial comparing low, medium, and high doses of voclosporin to tacrolimus in immunologically low-risk kidney transplant recipients showed voclosporin to be non-inferior in terms of episodes of rejection and kidney function. Notably, rates of PTDM were significantly lower in the low-dose voclosporin group.[60] Recently, the development of voclosporin for kidney transplantation maintenance immunosuppression was halted due to lack of funding. The drug remains under investigation for the treatment of lupus nephritis.

ANTIPROLIFERATIVE AGENTS

Azathioprine

Azathioprine (Imuran) is a prodrug whose metabolites exert a number of actions, including the following: (1) the incorporation of thioguanine purine analogs into DNA and RNA, resulting in cell death; (2) inhibition of de novo purine synthesis by methylthioinosine monophosphate; and (3) T cell apoptosis via inhibition of the Rho family GTPase, Rac1.[61] Azathioprine, in combination with prednisone, was the mainstay of transplant immunosuppression from the early 1960s until the introduction of cyclosporine in the early 1980s, at which point it maintained its role as an adjuvant medication to cyclosporine. Azathioprine has now been largely replaced by mycophenolate mofetil (MMF; see later) in most new immunosuppressive protocols,[62] although many older vintage kidney transplant recipients remain on the drug. Also, azathioprine is commonly substituted for MMF in female transplant recipients who are planning to conceive. The most important side effect of azathioprine is myelosuppression. Individuals with reduced thiopurine methyltransferase (TPMT) enzyme activity tend to accumulate active drug metabolites and are predisposed to myelosuppression. By some estimates, 10% of the population has reduced TPMT activity and 0.3% has absent TPMT activity.[63] Notably, coadministration of allopurinol with azathioprine also shifts azathioprine metabolism toward the production of metabolically active substrates and may lead to potentially serious toxicity.

Mycophenolate Acid

MMF is a prodrug that releases mycophenolate acid, an inhibitor of inosine monophosphate dehydrogenase (IMPDH) required for the de novo pathway synthesis of guanosine from inosine. The effects of MMF are relatively lymphocyte-specific because, lacking a purine salvage pathway, T and B cells rely exclusively on de novo purine synthesis. By limiting the pool of available guanine triphosphate, MMF prevents T and B lymphocyte replication and suppresses the cellular and humoral immune responses. Clinical trials have demonstrated that MMF reduces acute rejection rates by 50% compared to azathioprine or placebo.[64] A meta-analysis of 19 trials has shown that MMF is associated with a reduction of acute rejection and improved graft survival compared to azathioprine.[62] Cyclosporine inhibits the enterohepatic recirculation cycle of the metabolism of MMF, reducing the exposure by approximately 40%. Tacrolimus and sirolimus do not interfere with the metabolism of MMF.[57] The side effects of MMF predominate as gastrointestinal symptoms (diarrhea, epigastric pain, nausea). MMF can also cause neutropenia and, less frequently, anemia. However, it is not associated with nephrotoxicity, hyperlipidemia, or hypertension. MMF is associated with an increased risk of major fetal malformations, and patients planning pregnancy should be switched to azathioprine at least 6 weeks before conception.[65] Despite the high inter- and intra-individual variability of its pharmacokinetics, routine therapeutic drug monitoring of MMF has not been established. MMF is approved at a dose of 1 g twice daily when used in conjunction with a CNI and steroids. The excellent results obtained with a standard dosing regimen and the poor correlation of a single time point to the AUC (area under the concentration-time curve, particularly when used in combination with cyclosporine A [CsA]) supports a fixed-dose regimen.[15,66] However, the emergence of calcineurin and/or steroid-minimizing strategies have contributed to a growing interest in MMF therapeutic drug monitoring and optimization of early exposure. Mycophenolate mofetil is now also available in a generic formulation in the United States.

Mycophenolate sodium (Myfortic) is an enteric-coated, slow-release formulation of mycophenolic acid that was developed to decrease the gastrointestinal side effects of MMF. Multiple randomized trials have demonstrated a similar efficacy and side effect profile to that of MMF.[67]

TARGET OF RAPAMYCIN INHIBITORS

Sirolimus (Rapamune) is a macrocyclic antibiotic that has immunosuppressive properties. Even though it shares its cytoplasmic binding protein with tacrolimus (FKBP12), the resulting complex does not interfere with calcineurin. Rather, it binds with the mammalian target of rapamycin (mTOR). The resulting inhibition of mTOR prevents the propagation of IL-2–mediated cell proliferation signaling through the PI3K/AKT/mTOR pathway.[68] Sirolimus inhibits cellular proliferation of T and B lymphocytes and reduces antibody production.[15] Its immunosuppressive effects have been demonstrated in preclinical studies to be synergistic with those of CsA and tacrolimus.[69,70] Side effects of sirolimus include hyperlipidemia, thrombocytopenia, anemia, delayed wound healing, diarrhea, pneumonitis, mouth ulcers, proteinuria, and peripheral edema. High drug withdrawal rates due to side effects have been a common theme in many of the sirolimus trials.

Sirolimus has been studied in a number of different immunosuppression protocols, including as de novo maintenance immunosuppression in combination with a CNI and steroid or an antimetabolite and steroid, in early CNI withdrawal protocols, or as replacement for a CNI in patients with chronic allograft dysfunction or cancer. Sirolimus/MMF versus cyclosporine/MMF combined with rabbit ATG induction and 6 month of steroids resulted in similar 12-month survival and rejection rates, although adverse drug events and discontinuation rates were significantly higher in sirolimus-treated subjects.[71] Another study that compared sirolimus/tacrolimus withdrawn at 3 months, sirolimus/MMF and tacrolimus/MMF in patients treated with daclizumab induction and steroid maintenance reported significantly higher acute rejection rates with sirolimus/MMF treatment, prompting early withdrawal of the group from the trial. Impaired wound healing and dyslipidemia were both more common in the sirolimus-treated groups, as was drug withdrawal.[72] In another study, switching from tacrolimus to sirolimus at 3 months posttransplantation (vs. staying on tacrolimus) was associated with similar graft function but a higher rate of acute rejection.[73]

An RCT with median follow-up of 8 years reported increased acute rejection rates and lower glomerular filtration rates (GFRs) in cyclosporine/sirolimus and tacrolimus/sirolimus– versus tacrolimus/MMF–treated subjects. Tacrolimus/sirolimus treatment was also associated with an excess in death with a functioning graft compared to the other groups. A trend toward a worse GFR in CNI/sirolimus treatment combinations (especially cyclosporine) is consistent with animal studies showing that sirolimus cotreatment potentiates CNI nephrotoxicity.[74,75]

Late conversion from CNI to sirolimus has shown some promise in improving or stabilizing kidney function in patients with chronic allograft dysfunction, with the caveat that the development of nephrotic- or subnephrotic-range proteinuria following conversion to sirolimus is relatively common and requires cessation of the treatment. The presence of proteinuria before conversion is predictive of a poor response and should be screened for prior to considering a switch to sirolimus.[76] Finally, conversion from a CNI to sirolimus is associated with regression of Kaposi's sarcoma and reduction in the development of squamous cell skin cancers.[77,78] Sirolimus use peaked at just under 20% of kidney transplants in the early 2000s, but its use has since declined to the low single digits.

Everolimus (Zortress) is derived from sirolimus and has a shorter half-life. It has been approved in the United States for prophylaxis against rejection in kidney and heart transplant recipients. It has also been approved for the treatment of advanced renal cell carcinoma (Afinitor).

JAK3 Inhibitor

Tofacitinib (formerly CP-600550) is an oral agent that inhibits JAK3-induced phosphorylation and activation of its downstream signal transducing molecule, STAT5. Inhibition of JAK3 blocks the signaling of the γ-chain subfamily of cytokines (IL-2, -4, -7, -9, -15, and -21), resulting in immunosuppression. In contrast to mTOR, JAK3 expression is restricted to T, B, and natural killer (NK) cells, and this level of specificity may improve the toxicity profile. A phase 2 RCT that compared two doses of tofacitinib with cyclosporine, both combined with MMF and steroid, showed equivalent rejection rates, higher GFR, and better kidney histology in the tofacitinib groups. However, the rates of posttransplant lymphoproliferative disease (PTLD) and serious infection, particularly BK virus and cytomegalovirus (CMV) infection, were higher in the tofacitinib groups.[79] Tofacitinib (Xeljanz) has been approved for the treatment of rheumatoid arthritis. The development of the drug for kidney transplantation has been halted.

COSTIMULATORY SIGNAL BLOCKERS

Belatacept is a selective costimulation blocker. This human fusion protein binds the ligands CD80 and CD86 on APCs and prevents their interaction with the costimulation receptor on the T cells (CD28). Blockade of the costimulation signal prevents T cell activation. Belatacept is given as an IV infusion. Two studies randomized recipients of living or standard deceased donor (Benefit) and expanded criteria for deceased donor kidneys (Benefit-Ext) to higher dose belatacept, lower dose belatacept, or cyclosporine, with all subjects receiving IL-2 antagonist induction, MMF, and steroid concurrently. Results at 1 year showed similar graft and patient survival across the groups but significantly higher GFR in belatacept-treated subjects. Acute rejection was significantly higher in those treated with belatacept in the Benefit study but not in Benefit-Ext.[80,81] The calculated GFR remained approximately 22 and 11 mL/min/1.73 m² higher with belatacept versus cyclosporine treatment at 5-year follow-up of the Benefit and Benefit-Ext trials respectively.[82,83] The incidence of PTLD (mostly central nervous system) was higher in patients treated with belatacept in both trials and was associated with pretransplantation Epstein-Barr virus (EBV) seronegativity. The current package insert recommends use of belatacept only in kidney transplant patients who are documented as anti-EBV antibody seropositive because of the risk of PTLD.

An anti-CD40 antibody, ASKP1240, that blocks CD40/CD154 costimulatory signaling, is currently under investigation in a phase 2a randomized trial with three arms—basiliximab-tacrolimus-MMF-steroid versus basiliximab-ASKP1240-MMF-steroid versus basiliximab-tacrolimus-ASKP1240-steroid. The drug has shown some promise in preclinical studies.[84]

CORTICOSTEROIDS

Since the early days of clinical transplantation, corticosteroids have played an important role in the immunosuppressive management of transplant recipients and remain first-line treatment for acute rejection. Corticosteroids have antiinflammatory and immunosuppressive properties. The antiinflammatory effects of steroids are mediated by the reduction of proinflammatory molecules, including platelet-activated factor (PAF), prostaglandins, and leukotrienes and reduction of the release of tumor necrosis factor-α (TNF-α). Immunosuppressive properties of steroids include prevention of T cell proliferation, inhibition of cytokine production, including IL-2, and interference with antigen presentation. Some of these effects are mediated through the inhibition of the transcription factor NF-κB. The chronic use of steroids potentiates lymphocyte apoptosis, results in lymphopenia, and interferes with leukocyte trafficking.[11] These various mechanisms of action acting in concert make steroids potent and versatile immunosuppressive drugs. However, side effects related to their chronic use are also extensive (e.g. diabetes, hypertension, hyperlipidemia, osteoporosis, avascular necrosis, truncal obesity, hypertrichosis, acne, cataracts). The emergence of new, more potent immunosuppressive drugs has allowed the successful implementation of steroid-sparing protocols—avoidance, minimization, or withdrawal.[85,86] This is reflected by a significant trend toward decreased steroid use, with just over 60% compared to 90% of U.S. kidney transplant recipients maintained on steroids in 2011 and 1995, respectively.

The reported benefits of steroid-sparing strategies are manifold and include improvements in blood pressure, glycemic and lipid control, reduced posttransplantation weight gain, and better bone mineral density, growth, and physical appearance.[87-90] A Cochrane review of 30 randomized trials of steroid avoidance (<2 weeks of exposure) and steroid withdrawal (>2 weeks of exposure) has demonstrated that such steroid-sparing strategies are not associated with an increase in mortality or all-cause graft loss but are associated with an increase in death-censored graft loss and acute rejection. However, the increased risk of acute rejection was seen in those treated with cyclosporine but not tacrolimus-based immunosuppressive regimens.[91] Steroid-sparing strategies are a reasonable option for low immunologic risk patients treated with modern era immunosuppressive regimens (e.g., tacrolimus/MMF). Most steroid withdrawal protocols wean steroids within 3 to 6 months of transplantation. Late withdrawal from steroid use (>1 year posttransplantation) has been associated with increased acute rejection rates and deterioration in graft function in studies from the cyclosporine-azathioprine era.[92,93] While late withdrawal may be safer in the tacrolimus-MMF era, ongoing caution is recommended with this approach.[94]

IMMUNOSUPPRESSION PROTOCOLS

CNI-associated nephrotoxicity represents a major drawback of current immunosuppression protocols[95] and, as such, the last several years has seen a greater focus on strategies to minimize CNI exposure. Data from two RCTs from the late 2000s have supported the efficacy and safety of lower dose cyclosporine and tacrolimus-based regimens in immunologically low-risk patients.[96,97] However, the importance of CNI in kidney transplantation was emphasized by a recent study that withdrew tacrolimus at 6 months in stable, immunologically low-risk patients maintained on steroid and MMF. The study was discontinued due to an unacceptably high rate of acute rejection (6 of 14 patients) and donor-specific antibody development in the withdrawal group.[98] To date, belatacept probably represents the best available option for calcineurin avoidance.[80]

The vast majority of kidney transplant recipients in the United States are maintained on tacrolimus and MMF, with about two thirds of patients also treated with maintenance steroids. The greatest source of intraprogram variability in an immunosuppressive regimen is the choice of induction therapy and patient selection for, and method of, steroid withdrawal. When deciding on a regimen for a given recipient, the following factors are taken into consideration: (1) the patient's immunologic risk; (2) the baseline quality of the allograft; and (3) the anticipated vulnerability profile to specific side effects of immunosuppression. Familiarization with local challenges (e.g., regional distribution of patient risk factors, organ attribution scheme) is essential for successful optimization of immunosuppression protocols for any given patient.

EVALUATION OF RECIPIENT

IMMEDIATELY BEFORE TRANSPLANTATION

The general pretransplantation workup is reviewed in Chapter 64.

MEDICAL STATUS

The potential recipient should be evaluated to ensure that there are no new contraindications to general anesthesia and transplantation surgery. This is more relevant for recipients of deceased donor allografts for whom the date of surgery cannot be planned. Special emphasis should be placed on cardiovascular and infectious risks. With longer waiting periods for transplantation, it is common for a potential recipient's cardiovascular risk profile to have changed since the time of his or her last evaluation. The need for hemodialysis prior to surgery should be assessed. In general, preoperative hemodialysis is advisable if the plasma potassium level is greater than 5.5 mmol/L or severe volume overload is present. The threshold for preoperative dialysis should be lower when delayed or slow graft function is anticipated or patients are of higher cardiovascular risk. A short session of 1.5 to 2 hours without anticoagulation usually suffices. Patients on peritoneal dialysis need to have instilled peritoneal dialysis fluid drained out before surgery; if the patient is hyperkalemic, several rapid exchanges can be performed. If there is a history of coronary artery disease, β-blockers should be administered before and after surgery.[99]

IMMUNOLOGIC STATUS

DONOR IMMUNE STATUS AND CROSS-MATCH

The presence of preformed recipient antibody against the donor ABO blood group or donor HLA will frequently result in hyperacute rejection. The past 50 years have seen huge advances in the laboratory detection of recipient anti-HLA antibody. The complement-dependent lymphocyte cytotoxicity (CDC) assay, in which donor lymphocytes are incubated with recipient serum, was first developed in the 1960s.[100] Preformed recipient antibody to donor lymphocytes (subsequently identified as anti-HLA antibody) resulted in lymphocyte death in vitro and predicted rapid (hyperacute) graft failure in vivo. The assay has been refined in many respects and is now performed as separate assays with donor T lymphocytes, which exclusively express HLA class I antigen, and to donor B lymphocytes, which express both HLA class I and II antigens. The addition of antihuman globulin to the CDC assay increases its sensitivity. A positive CDC T cell cross-match is an absolute contraindication to transplantation. A negative B cell cross-match is reassuring. However, the assay has a high false-positive rate due to the binding of non-HLA antibody or autoantibody, therefore a positive result should always be interpreted in combination with other HLA antibody detection techniques.

The flow cytometric cross-match (FXM) test is a more sensitive assay for detecting donor anti-HLA antibody. Donor T lymphocytes (T cell flow) or B lymphocytes (B cell flow) are mixed with recipient serum and a fluorescent anti-IgG antibody. Any recipient antibody that binds to donor HLA on the lymphocyte cell surface will be tagged by the fluorescent IgG and subsequently detected using flow cytometry. The FXM assay detects low-titer and non–complement-binding, anti-HLA antibody and may be positive when a CDC cross-match is negative. A negative CDC cross-match but positive T cell FXM is associated with poor short-term transplantation outcomes and is a relative contraindication to transplantation.[101]

Solid-phase technologies such as the Luminex single antigen bead (SAB) anti-HLA antibody assay permit detection and quantification of a wide array of anti-HLA antibodies. Multiple color-coded beads coated with a broad range of HLA antigens are incubated with recipient serum. The binding of antibody to a bead coated with a specific HLA antigen results in a distinct fluorometric signal that is then detected by flow cytometry. Molecular (e.g., polymerase chain reaction [PCR]) HLA typing techniques have now superseded serologic identification of HLA type for donors and recipients. Accurate molecular donor HLA typing and SAB-based recipient anti-HLA antibody screening can be combined to perform a virtual cross-match. Many centers will now proceed with a deceased donor transplant in low immunologic risk patients based on a negative virtual cross-match. For high immunologic risk donors, virtual cross-matching has assisted in the identification of potentially compatible donors and has improved transplantation rates for sensitized donors.[102] Computerized virtual cross-match algorithms have also been central to the success of kidney paired donor exchange and transplant chains.[103,104] In the United States, wait-listed kidney transplantation candidates usually have SAB-based HLA-antibody screening performed every 2 months. Transplantation centers regularly update each candidate's antibody status on UNet, a centralized computer database that virtually matches candidates with potential donors. HLA antigens against which a candidate has antibody are listed as unacceptable HLA antigens or "avoids" on the system.

The calculated panel reactive antibody (cPRA) replaced the measured PRA in the United States in 2009 as the main measure of immune sensitization. The cPRA is calculated using an algorithm that correlates donor anti-HLA antibody (as measured by SAB assay) with the population frequency of HLA antigens to generate a percentage score. A candidate with no anti-HLA antibody will have a cPRA of 0, whereas a sensitized candidate with a cPRA of 85% will be immunologically incompatible with 85% of the donor population. The choice of predonation cross-match depends mostly on a donor's immunologic risk (Table 72.2). Intended recipients should be specifically asked if they have recently received a blood transfusion because this could cause a surge in alloantibodies.[105]

Donor-specific anti-HLA antibody (DSA) may be present pretransplantation or develop de novo posttransplantation. De novo DSA development frequently follows acute cellular rejection episodes and is also associated with patient noncompliance.[106] Preformed and de novo DSAs are both associated with an increased risk of antibody-mediated rejection and poor graft outcomes.[107,108] DSAs may also be measured using a variation on the SAB technique, the Luminex C1q assay, which detects anti-HLA antibodies that bind and activate complement. The development of posttransplantation C1q-binding DSA is strongly associated with poor graft outcomes.[109]

DSA may be accompanied by the following: (1) normal renal function and histology; (2) normal renal function and

Table 72.2 Recipient Risk Factors for Acute Rejection

Previous blood transfusions, particularly if recent
Previous pregnancies, particularly if multiple
Previous allograft, particularly if rejected early
African ancestry (e.g. African-American)
History of high panel reactive antibody (>20%)
Donor-specific antibody (current or historic)

antibody-mediated rejection (AMR) histology (subclinical AMR); (3) overt AMR; or (4) chronic AMR (transplantation glomerulopathy). Posttransplantation DSA monitoring practices vary from center to center, but DSA screening is certainly warranted in immunologically high-risk recipients and at the time of "for clinical indication" biopsy. Treatment of DSA depends on accompanying clinical and histologic findings. Isolated de novo DSA warrants intensification of immunosuppression and, in some centers, will be trigger specific therapies, such as IVIg. Treatment of DSA accompanied by AMR is discussed separately. There is currently no effective therapy for chronic AMR transplantation glomerulopathy.

DESENSITIZATION

The number of highly sensitized patients (PRA > 80%) wait-listed for kidney transplantation is growing.[3] Difficulty in finding a compatible match for highly sensitized patients results in low transplantation rates; for patients who are close to 100% sensitized, the likelihood of finding a successful transplant match, in the absence of intervention, is very low.[3,110] The last decade has seen significant growth in desensitization protocols that aim to lower anti-HLA antibody titers in sensitized kidney transplant candidates sufficiently to create an immunologic window for successful transplantation. Desensitization protocols among centers but fall broadly into two categories: (1) high-dose IVIg/anti-CD20-based[43] and (2) low-dose IVIg/plasmapheresis-based[110] regimens. High-dose IVIg has been used as a monotherapy and effectively lowers donor-specific antibody titers and permits successful transplantation.[111] However, a number of studies have suggested that IVIg alone (vs. IVIg plus plasmapheresis and rituximab or IVIg plus rituximab) is associated with a posttransplantation rebound in DSA titers and increased incidence of AMR.[112] Recent reports have also described good results with the incorporation of newer agents such as the 26S proteasome inhibitor, bortezomib, and the complement inhibitor, eculizumab,[113,114] into desensitization protocols. Other novel agents that are currently being investigated for desensitization are tocilizumab, a monoclonal antibody against the IL-6 receptor, and IdeS (for *I*gG-*d*egrading *e*nzyme of *S*treptoccus *pyogenes*), an enzyme that cleaves and inactivates IgG.

Desensitization may be performed in patients who have an identified living donor or may be timed to coincide with the candidate being positioned at the top of the deceased donor waiting list. In addition, desensitization may be facilitated by identifying more immunologically favorable donor candidates through living donor paired exchange.[115,116] Desensitization greatly increases the prospect of sensitized patients receiving a transplant and is associated with good medium-term graft survival rates and a survival advantage compared to remaining on dialysis.[42,110,117] However, AMR rates are high,[42,118] and few data are available about long-term graft survival in desensitized patients.

IMMEDIATELY AFTER TRANSPLANTATION

The nephrologist should carefully review the donor history and operating room notes, with particular emphasis on cold and warm ischemia times, technical difficulties encountered, intraoperative fluids administered, blood pressure, and urine output. An immediate excellent urine output, which should always be the case with living donor transplants, greatly simplifies management. The management of the oligoanuric recipient can be complicated and is discussed later.

MANAGEMENT OF ALLOGRAFT DYSFUNCTION

In the current era of surgical technique and immunosuppression, major postoperative complications are rare. The focus of clinical management has shifted from improving short-term outcomes to long-term outcomes. Early detection and treatment of early graft dysfunction is an important factor in preserving long-term allograft function. Because early signs of graft dysfunction rarely manifest as detectable symptoms, routine surveillance laboratory testing is a cornerstone of posttransplantation management. Surveillance laboratory testing should be performed, regardless of the difficulty of the immediate postoperative course. In general, surveillance is performed frequently in the early posttransplantation period and progressively less frequently with time. While there may be variations to this schedule among different centers, a typical schedule for routine surveillance laboratory testing is shown in Table 72.3.

Management is discussed here for three time periods—immediate, early, and late posttransplantation.

IMMEDIATE POSTTRANSPLANTATION PERIOD (FIRST WEEK)

Patients can be divided into three groups based on allograft function in the first posttransplantation week—those with

Table 72.3 Routine Surveillance Laboratory Testing After Transplantation

Test	<6 Months After Transplantation		>6 Months After Transplantation	
	q 2 wk	q mo	q 2 mo	q 12 mo
CBC	x	x	x	
Electrolytes, glucose, BUN	x	x	x	
Creatinine	x	x	x	
Drug level*	x	x	x	
Albumin, calcium, phosphate, uric acid†	x	x	x	
Liver enzymes	x	x	x	
Urinalysis	x	x	x	
Lipid profile				
BK virus‡				x§

*Depending on the immunosuppressive regimen, to include tacrolimus, cyclosporine, and mycophenolic acid.
†Posttransplantation parathyroid hormone (PTH) monitoring frequency determined by individual PTH and calcium levels.
‡Frequency per individual transplant center.
§Once at 2-3 months post-transplant then annually.
BUN, Blood urea nitrogen; CBC, complete blood count.

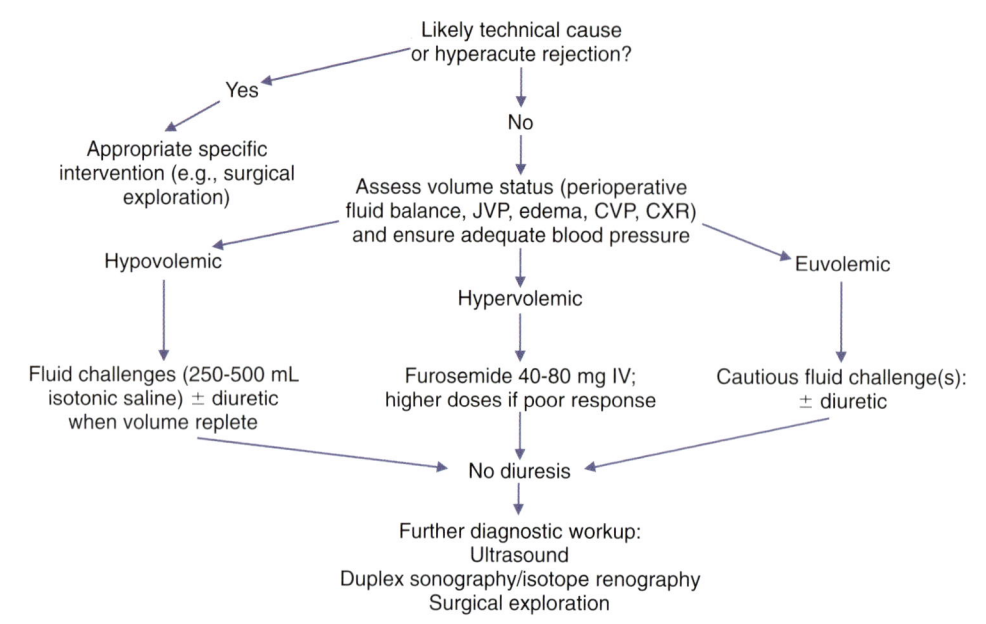

Figure 72.3 Management of kidney allograft nonfunction and oliguria immediately after transplantation. CVP, Central venous pressure; CXR, chest x-ray; JVP, jugular venous pressure.

excellent graft function, delayed graft function (DGF), and slow graft function (SGF). Excellent allograft function is manifest by an ample urine output and rapidly falling plasma creatinine concentration. Management of patients with excellent allograft function (almost all living donor recipients and a highly variable percentage of deceased donor allograft recipients) is relatively straightforward. Routine imaging studies are not required.

DGF is usually defined by the need for one or more dialysis treatments within the first posttransplantation week. SGF defines a group of recipients with moderate early graft dysfunction. One commonly used definition of SGF is a plasma creatinine level higher than 3 mg/dL at 1 week posttransplantation; the causes, management, and outcomes of SGF are similar to those of DGF (see below).[119] Interventions that simply convert DGF to SGF appear to have little effect on allograft outcomes. A scheme for managing allograft dysfunction in the immediate posttransplantation period is depicted in Figure 72.3.

DELAYED GRAFT FUNCTION

The definition of DGF as the requirement for dialysis within 1 week of transplantation is somewhat arbitrary. The designation excludes some patients with residual native kidney function, such as those undergoing preemptive transplantation who have DGF per se but do not require dialysis. There is also likely significant intracenter variation in the use of dialysis posttransplantation. The incidence of DGF, by the conventional definition, varies widely, depending on the donor source. Recent Scientific Registry of Transplant Recipients data reported a 3%, 23%, and 31% incidence of DGF in living donor, standard deceased donor, and expanded criteria donor (ECD) allografts, respectively.[3] Although the causes of DGF include prerenal, intrarenal, and postrenal insults, ischemic acute tubular necrosis (ATN) is the most common cause of DGF.

Risk factors for DGF include recipient factors such as male gender, black race, longer dialysis vintage, higher PRA status, and greater degree of HLA mismatching. Donor factors include use of deceased donor kidneys (especially with ECD or donation after cardiac death [DCD]), older donor age, and longer cold ischemia time. Most of these factors mediate their effects through ischemia-reperfusion injury as well as immunologic mechanisms. Older studies have suggested that CNIs prolong or worsen DGF. However, a French RCT comparing delayed versus immediate introduction of cyclosporine posttransplantation showed no difference in DGF rates or graft function at 3 months but did show a numeric trend toward increased acute rejection in the delayed cyclosporine group.[120]

The diagnosis of the underlying cause of DGF is based on clinical, radiologic, and histologic findings. Careful review of the donor history and of the retrieval and transplantation procedures provides clues about the cause of DGF. Notably, interpretation of the posttransplantation urine output requires knowledge of the residual (native) urine output. Prerenal and postrenal causes (e.g., volume depletion, urinary catheter malposition or obstruction) should be excluded. If such simple steps fail to improve urine output, further investigation is warranted. Standard ultrasonography is commonly used to assess potential surgical complications in the immediate postoperative period. Ultrasonography can be performed quickly, is inexpensive and noninvasive, and is usually effective in identifying postrenal causes of kidney failure. Duplex sonography is also useful in assessing the graft's arterial and venous blood flow. The resistive index (RI) is often reported in transplant kidney ultrasounds and is elevated in the setting of intrarenal graft dysfunction. However, a raised RI does not discriminate between ATN and rejection and is therefore of limited diagnostic utility.[121]

The evaluation and management of DGF is patient context–dependent. Persistent oliguria in a living donor

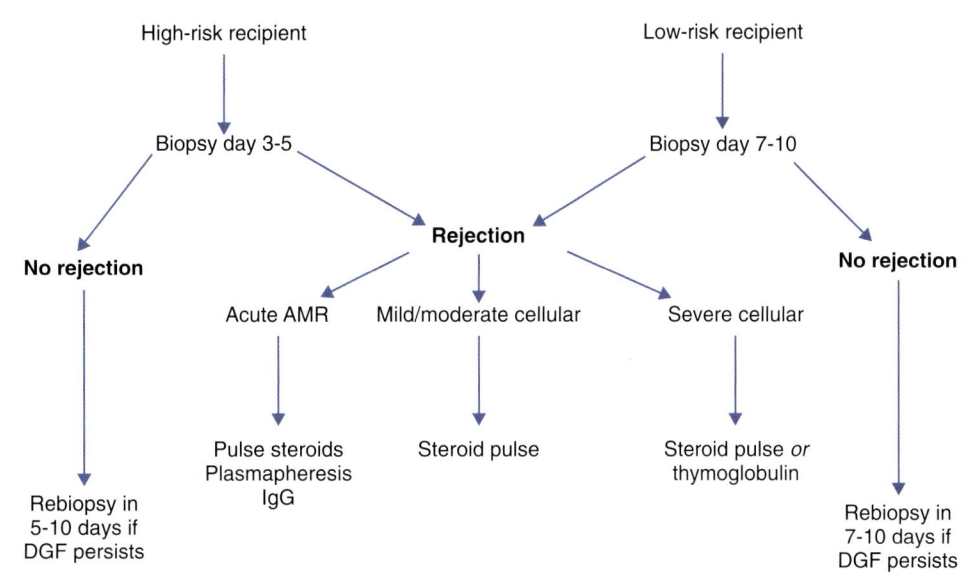

Figure 72.4 Algorithm for management of persistent delayed graft function. The presence of antidonor human leukocyte antigen (HLA) antibodies should prompt immediate biopsy in this setting. AMR, Antibody-mediated rejection; DGF, delayed graft function.

Table 72.4 Risk Factors for Delayed Graft Function
Prerenal
Severe hypovolemia, hypotension
Renal vessel thrombosis
Intrarenal
Ischemic ATN
Hyperacute rejection
Accelerated or acute rejection superimposed on ATN
Acute CNI nephrotoxicity (±ATN)
Postrenal
Urinary tract obstruction/leakage
ATN, Acute tubular necrosis; CNI, calcineurin inhibitor.

Table 72.5 Causes of Ischemic Damage to the Deceased Donor Kidney Allograft
Preharvest Donor State
Shock syndromes
Endogenous and exogenous catecholamines
? Brain injury
Nephrotoxic drugs
Organ Procurement Surgery
Hypotension
Trauma to renal vessels
Organ Transport and Storage
Prolonged storage (cold ischemia time)
Pulsatile perfusion injury
Transplantation of Recipient
Prolonged second warm ischemia time
Trauma to renal vessels
Hypovolemia/hypotension
Postoperative Period
Cyclosporine, tacrolimus
Acute heart failure (myocardial infarction)
? Hemodialysis

kidney is much more likely to be a major surgical complication than ATN. However, in many cases, prerenal and postrenal causes of DGF are excluded in deceased donor kidney transplant recipients (KTRs) who are at high risk of ischemic ATN. In the absence of a high suspicion for an alternative diagnosis (such as rejection), expectant management for 7 to 10 days posttransplantation is a reasonable approach. A typical algorithm for managing persistent DGF is shown in Figure 72.4.

Causes of Delayed Graft Function

Ischemic Acute Tubular Necrosis. Ischemic ATN is the most common cause of DGF in deceased donor kidney recipients. At multiple steps during the surgical transplantation procedure, the allograft is at risk of ischemia-reperfusion injury (Table 72.4).[122]

There are no clinical or radiologic features unique to early posttransplantation ATN. As is the case with acute kidney injury (AKI) in native kidneys, posttransplant ATN should be a diagnosis of exclusion. Several of the risk factors identified in Table 72.5 may be present. Intact allograft perfusion and the absence of obstruction should be confirmed with renal imaging. Histology, if available, shows tubular cell damage and necrosis. Patchy interstitial mononuclear cell infiltrates, but not tubulitis, may be present. The natural history of uncomplicated ATN is spontaneous resolution. Usually, improvements in urine output begin from 5 to 10 days after transplantation, but ATN may persist for weeks.

Management of the patient during this period is supportive. When early hemodialysis is required, minimal anticoagulation should be used to reduce the risk of postsurgical bleeding. Intradialytic hypotension should also be avoided to prevent further exacerbation of ischemic kidney injury. Peritoneal dialysis may be successfully continued posttransplantation, although it should be avoided if the peritoneum was violated at the time of surgery. Early postoperative treatments should be performed with low-volume exchanges.

A major concern in the management of the patient with posttransplantation ATN is that evidence of new surgical or medical complications involving the allograft may be masked. Rejection, for example, may be easily missed. In fact, acute rejection occurs more frequently in allografts with delayed as opposed to immediate function. The postulated mechanism is that ischemia-reperfusion injury increases the immunogenicity of the allograft, thereby predisposing to acute rejection. Experimental animal models have demonstrated that ischemic ATN is associated with increased expression or production of class I and II MHC molecules, costimulatory molecules, proinflammatory cytokines, and adhesion molecules within the kidney parenchyma.[122] Such an altered local milieu could amplify the alloimmune response. Therefore, a high degree of suspicion for additional complications related to the allograft must be maintained. The possibility of accelerated acute rejection must be considered, particularly in the high-risk recipient. We recommend a low threshold for performing a kidney biopsy in patients with DGF. Radiologic evaluation of the graft should also be repeated if there is suspicion of new urinary or vascular complications.

Hyperacute Rejection. Hyperacute rejection has become a rare cause of immediate graft nonfunction because of modern tissue-typing technology. However, the increased prevalence of desensitization protocols has once again made this diagnosis clinically relevant. Hyperacute rejection is caused by preformed recipient antibodies reacting with antigens on the endothelium of the allograft, resulting in activation of the complement and coagulation cascades. These antibodies are usually directed against antigens of the ABO blood group system or against HLA class I antigens. Anti-HLA class I antibodies are formed in response to previous transplantation, blood transfusion, or pregnancy. Less commonly, hyperacute rejection is caused by antibodies directed against donor HLA class II antigens or endothelial or monocyte antigens (the last two are not detected in the standard cross-match). In classic hyperacute rejection, cyanosis and mottling of the kidney and anuria occur minutes after the vascular anastomosis is established. Disseminated intravascular coagulopathy may occur. Histology shows widespread, small-vessel endothelial damage and thrombosis, usually with neutrophils incorporated into the thrombus. There is no effective treatment, and transplant nephrectomy is indicated. Screening for recipient-donor ABO or class I HLA incompatibility (the presence of the latter is often termed a *positive T cell cross-match*) has ensured that hyperacute rejection is now uncommon. Rare cases occur because of clerical errors or the presence of other preformed antibodies (described earlier) that are not detected by routine screening methods.

Accelerated Rejection Superimposed on Acute Tubular Necrosis. Accelerated acute rejection refers to rejection occurring roughly 2 to 5 days after transplantation. Accelerated rejection occurs in recipients with pretransplantation sensitization to donor alloantigens and is frequently associated with the presence of historic or low-titer pretransplantation anti-donor antibodies. Rapid posttransplantation antibody production by memory B cells underlie this phenomenon.[123]

Accelerated acute rejection may be superimposed on ischemic ATN, in which case there may be no signs of rejection. Diagnosis is made by kidney biopsy in conjunction with cross-match findings and DSA titers. Histology usually shows evidence of antibody rather than cell-mediated immune damage. The diagnosis and management of these two forms of rejection are discussed in detail below.

Acute Cyclosporine or Tacrolimus Nephrotoxicity Superimposed on Acute Tubular Necrosis. Cyclosporine and tacrolimus, especially in high doses or by the intravenous route of administration, may result in an acute decrease in the GFR through renal vasoconstriction, particularly of the afferent glomerular arteriole. Such vasomotor effects may potentially exacerbate ischemic ATN. Acute CNI toxicity is now rare with the targeting of lower CNI levels. However, caution should be taken in the context of drug interactions that raise CNI levels (discussed later).

Vascular and Urologic Complications of Surgery. Renal vessel thrombosis, urinary leaks, and obstruction are rare but important causes of DGF. These complications may also cause allograft dysfunction in the early postoperative period and are discussed later in this chapter.

Outcome and Significance of Delayed Graft Function

In most cases, recovery of kidney function is sufficient to become independent of dialysis. Renal recovery fails to occur in less than 5% of cases, resulting in primary nonfunction (PNF). Most studies have suggested that DGF has a negative impact on long-term kidney allograft survival.[122] Patients with DGF require longer hospitalization and more investigations and are at higher risk of occult rejection. Postoperative fluid and electrolyte management are more difficult.

Therefore, measures that limit the incidence and duration of DGF are important. Graft injury may occur in the following settings: (1) prior to donation; (2) at retrieval; (3) during transport; (4) during transplantation surgery; or (5) postoperatively.

Prior to donation, heart-beating donors are potentially exposed to various renal insults that may affect future graft function. Good intensive care unit (ICU) management of the potential deceased donor is of great importance in mitigating many of these factors. Treating the brain dead donor with dopamine prior to organ harvesting has been shown to reduce the rate of DGF.[124] However, other specific donor interventions, including desmopressin and steroids, have not been shown to improve subsequent graft function.[125,126]

Meticulous surgical technique, rapid transport of retrieved allografts, and use of optimum preservation solutions are also of extreme importance. Data regarding machine

| Table 72.6 | Advantages and Disadvantages of Induction Regimens in the Setting of Delayed Graft Function |

	Polyclonals	OKT3	Interleukin-2 Receptor
Effectiveness in preventing early acute cellular rejection	+++	+++	++
Increased risk of opportunistic infection	++	++	0
Increased risk of neoplasia	++	++	0
Cytokine release syndrome	+	++	0
Sensitization, affecting future use of product	?	++	0
Cost	+++	+++	+++

| Table 72.7 | Causes of Allograft Dysfunction in the Early Postoperative Period |

Prerenal

Hypovolemia, hypotension
Renal vessel thrombosis
Drugs: ACE inhibitors, NSAIDs
Transplantation renal artery stenosis

Intrarenal

Acute rejection
Acute CNI nephrotoxicity
CNI-induced thrombotic microangiopathy
Recurrence of primary disease
Acute pyelonephritis
Acute interstitial nephritis

Postrenal

Urinary tract obstruction, leakage

ACE, Angiotensin-converting enzyme; CNI, calcineurin inhibitor; NSAIDs, nonsteroidal antiinflammatory drugs.

perfusion have been somewhat conflicting. A study that randomly assigned one kidney from 336 consecutive deceased donors to machine perfusion and the other to cold storage showed a reduction in DGF and an improvement in 1-year graft survival in the machine perfusion group.[10] However, machine perfusion was associated with no benefit compared to cold storage in kidneys donated after cardiac death in the United Kingdom.[127] The major disadvantages of machine perfusion are its relative expense and complexity compared to standard cold perfusion techniques.

Cold ischemia time (CIT) is an important risk factor for DGF.[128] Measures designed to decrease CIT include faster identification of potential recipients, establishment of a list of patients in each transplant region who would quickly accept ECD kidneys, and a consensus on allocation and management of DCD organs.[129,130] Nationwide organ sharing of zero–HLA-mismatched organs also results in the prolongation of CIT in some cases. However, the small increase in CIT, associated with national organ sharing, is offset by the substantial immunologic benefits of zero– HLA-mismatched transplantation.[131]

Intraoperative mean arterial pressure should be maintained greater than 70 mm Hg in the recipient. In cases in which DGF is expected, antilymphocyte antibody preparations are often used and may have benefits beyond acute rejection prophylaxis. In experimental models, ATGs directly ameliorate ischemia reperfusion injury through modulation of adhesion molecule expression and of the inflammatory response.[132] Intraoperative (vs. postoperative) thymoglobulin administration was associated with reduced DGF in one randomized study.[133] Another study demonstrated reduced DGF with thymoglobulin over daclizumab.[22] The advantages and disadvantages of antibody therapy in the setting of DGF are summarized in Table 72.6.

Despite theoretical benefits, peritransplantation erythropoietin treatment showed no effect on DGF in two RCTs.[134,135]

Calcium channel blockers have been shown in experimental models to prevent ischemic injury and attenuate CNI-mediated renal vasoconstriction. These properties suggest that their administration to recipients or the donor before organ retrieval might reduce the incidence and duration of ischemic ATN. A Cochrane review that included 13 trials suggested a reduced risk of ATN and delayed graft function associated with perioperative calcium channel blocker use, but no difference in graft loss or mortality.[136] Early reports of a randomized study comparing p53 small interfering RNA (siRNA) infusion with placebo at the time of ECD transplantation suggested a benefit in terms of reduced DGF in the treatment group and may represent an important therapy in the future.[137]

EARLY POSTTRANSPLANTATION PERIOD (FIRST 6 MONTHS)

Table 72.7 shows the causes of allograft dysfunction during the early posttransplantation period. Despite its known limitations, the primary measure of early and late transplant function remains the plasma creatinine concentration. Prerenal and postrenal causes of graft dysfunction should be systematically excluded. An algorithm for the management of allograft dysfunction in the early posttransplantation period is shown in Figure 72.5.

PRERENAL KIDNEY DYSFUNCTION

Hypovolemia and Drugs

Hypovolemia may develop secondary to excessive diuresis from the transplanted kidney or from diarrhea. Diarrhea is a common adverse effect of MMF, especially when used with tacrolimus. Angiotensin-converting enzyme inhibitors (ACEIs), angiotensin receptor blockers (ARBs), and nonsteroidal antiinflammatory drugs (NSAIDs) should be avoided in the early posttransplantation period because of the risk

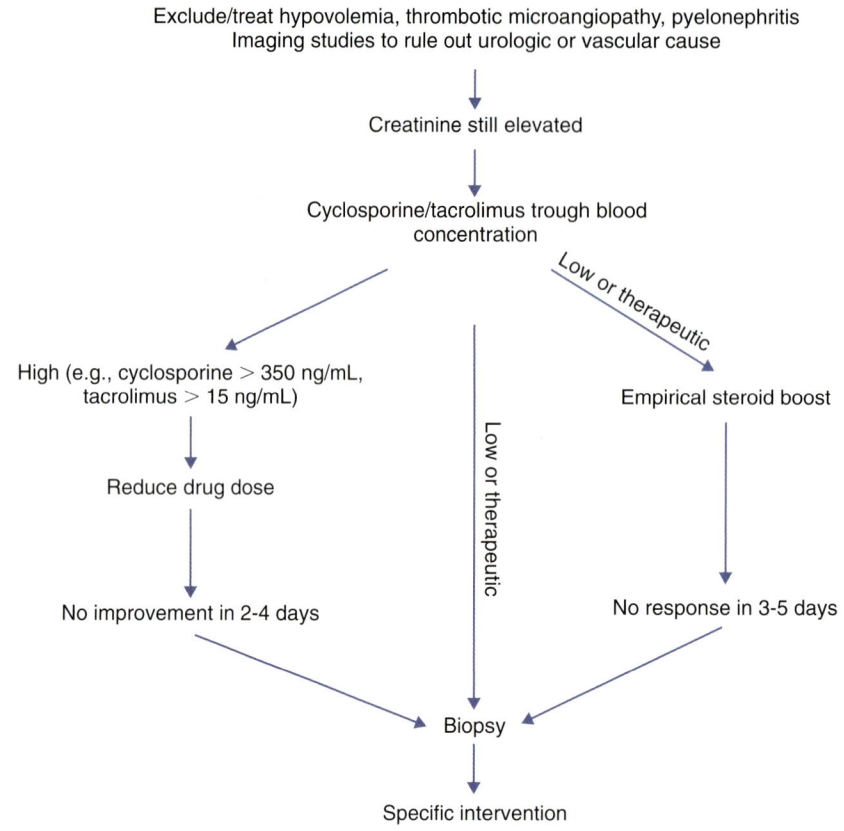

Figure 72.5 Algorithm for management of allograft dysfunction in early posttransplantation period.

of prerenal failure, a risk that may be potentiated by the renal vasoconstrictive effects of CNIs.

Renal Vessel Thrombosis

Transplant renal artery or renal vein thrombosis usually occurs in the first 72 hours but may be delayed for up to 10 weeks. Acute vascular thrombosis is the most common cause of allograft loss in the first week. Although poor surgical technique is a factor in some cases, there is now a greater appreciation of the role of hypercoagulable states.[12]

Renal artery thrombosis presents with abrupt onset of anuria (unless there is a native urine output) and rapidly rising plasma creatinine level, but often with negligible graft pain. Duplex studies show absent arterial and venous blood flow. Renography or magnetic resonance (MR) angiography shows absent perfusion of the transplanted kidney. Removal of the infarcted kidney is indicated.

Renal vein thrombosis also manifests with anuria and a rapidly increasing plasma creatinine level. Pain, tenderness, swelling in the graft, and hematuria are more pronounced than in renal artery thrombosis. Severe complications such as pulmonary embolus, graft rupture, or hemorrhage may occur. Duplex studies show absent renal venous blood flow and characteristic renal arterial waveforms. MR venography demonstrates thrombus in the vein. Transplant nephrectomy is usually indicated. If the venous thrombosis extends beyond the renal vein, anticoagulation is necessary to reduce the risk of embolization. There are reports of salvaging kidney function after early diagnosis of renal vessel thrombosis and its treatment with thrombolysis or thrombectomy. In almost all cases, however, infarction occurs too quickly to make this treatment worthwhile. Furthermore, thrombolysis is relatively contraindicated in the early posttransplantation period because of the high risk of graft-related bleeding.

INTRARENAL DYSFUNCTION

Acute Rejection

Acute rejection is characterized by a decline in kidney function mediated by a recipient immune reaction against the allograft. Although acute rejection can occur at any time, it is most common in the first 6 months posttransplantation. Fortunately, the incidence of acute rejection has decreased dramatically in the past 20 years; it is now around 10% in the first 12 months posttransplantation in the United States.[138]

In the era of modern immunosuppression, symptoms and signs of acute rejection are rarely pronounced, but low-grade fever, oliguria, and graft pain or tenderness may occur. Most cases of acute rejection are identified through surveillance monitoring of graft function. However, the creatinine level is a rather late and insensitive marker of renal injury. There is, therefore, a growing interest in the development of early biomarkers of immune system activation.

Acute rejection may involve both cellular and/or humoral immune components. Clinical transplantation has traditionally been focused on cell-mediated responses. However, AMR has been receiving more attention because of improvements in diagnostic techniques and the increased transplantation of immunologically high-risk candidates. Differences between acute cellular rejection (ACR) and AMR are summarized in Table 72.8.

Table 72.8 Differences Between Pure Forms of Acute Cellular Rejection (ACR) and Acute Antibody-Mediated Rejection (AMR)

Parameter	ACR	Acute AMR
Clinical onset	>5 days	>3 days
Donor-specific antibody in serum	Usually absent	Present
Tubulitis	Present	Absent
Neutrophil polymorphs in glomerular and peritubular capillaries	Absent	Present
C4d staining of peritubular capillaries	Absent	Present
Primary therapy	Pulse steroids	Plasmapheresis, IVIg, pulse steroids, rituximab

IgG, Immunoglobulin G.

Acute Cellular Rejection. The modified Banff classification (Table 72.9) is a widely used schema for classifying rejection. Histologic findings characteristic of ACR include the following: (1) mononuclear cell infiltration of the interstitium, mainly with T cells but also with some macrophages and plasma cells; (2) tubulitis (infiltration of tubule epithelium by lymphocytes); and (3) arteritis, which manifests as infiltration of mononuclear cells beneath the endothelium. Vascular involvement reflects more severe rejection.

Focal infiltrates of mononuclear cells without tubulitis or arteritis may occur in the presence of stable allograft function, and treatment is not required. Conversely, histologic evidence of rejection can also be seen in the presence of stable allograft function (subclinical rejection). Some studies have reported improvement of graft function with treatment of subclinical rejection,[139] but no benefit was found in a larger multicenter trial.[140] The presence of eosinophils in the infiltrate suggests severe rejection, but allergic interstitial nephritis should also be considered. Note that

Table 72.9 Banff 2009 Diagnostic Categories for Renal Allograft Biopsies

1. **Normal**
2. **Antibody-mediated changes (may coincide with categories 3, 4, 5, and 6)**
Due to documentation of circulating antidonor antibody, C4d, and allograft pathology
   (a) **C4d deposition without morphologic evidence of active rejection**
   C4d+, presence of circulating antidonor antibodies, no signs of acute or chronic T cell–mediated rejection (TCMR) or ABMR (i.e., g0 (no glomerulitis), cg0 (no chronic transplantation glomerulopathy), ptc0 (no peritubular capillaritis), no ptc lamination (<five layers by electron microscopy), no ATN-like minimal inflammation). Cases with simultaneous borderline changes are considered as indeterminate.
   (b) **Acute antibody-mediated rejection**
   C4d+, presence of circulating antidonor antibodies, morphologic evidence of acute tissue injury, such as type or grade
   I. ATN-like minimal inflammation
   II. Capillary and or glomerular inflammation (ptc/g > 0) and/or thromboses
   III. Arterial (v3)
   (c) **Chronic active antibody-mediated rejection**
   C4d+, presence of circulating antidonor antibodies, morphologic evidence of chronic tissue injury, such as glomerular double contours and/or peritubular capillary basement membrane multilayering and/or interstitial fibrosis/tubular atrophy and/or fibrous intimal thickening in arteries
3. **Borderline changes**—suspicious for acute TCMR (may coincide with categories 2, 5, and 6) This category is used when no intimal arteritis is present, but there are foci of tubulitis (t1, t2, or t3) with minor interstitial infiltration (i0 or i1) or interstitial infiltration (i2, i3) with mild (t1) tubulitis
4. **TCMR (may coincide with categories 2, 5, and 6)**
   (a) Acute TCMR (type, grade)
   IA. Cases with significant interstitial infiltration (>25% of parenchyma affected, i2 or i3) and foci of moderate tubulitis (t2)
   IB. Cases with significant interstitial infiltration (>25% of parenchyma affected, i2 or i3) and foci of severe tubulitis (t3)
   IIA. Cases with mild to moderate intimal arteritis (v1)
   IIB. Cases with severe intimal arteritis comprising >25% of the luminal area (v2)
   III. Cases with transmural arteritis and/or arterial fibrinoid change and necrosis of medial smooth muscle cells with accompanying lymphocytic inflammation (v3)
   (b) Chronic active TCMR
   Chronic allograft arteriopathy (arterial intimal fibrosis with mononuclear cell infiltration in fibrosis, formation of neointima)
5. **Interstitial fibrosis and tubular atrophy, no evidence of any specific cause** (may include nonspecific vascular and glomerular sclerosis, but severity graded by tubulointerstitial features)
   Grade
   I. Mild interstitial fibrosis and tubular atrophy (<25% of cortical area)
   II. Moderate interstitial fibrosis and tubular atrophy (26%-50% of cortical area)
   III. Severe interstitial fibrosis and tubular atrophy/loss (>50% of cortical area)
6. **Other**—changes not considered to be due to rejection, acute and/or chronic*

*Includes calcineurin nephrotoxicity, chronic hypertension, viral infection, pyelonephritis, recurrent or de novo glomerulonephritis.
Adapted from Sis B, Mengel M, Haas M, et al: Banff '09 meeting report: antibody-mediated graft deterioration and implementation of Banff working groups. Am J Transplant 10:464-471, 2010.

polyoma virus infection may also cause tubulointerstitial nephritis.

Uncomplicated ACR is generally treated with a short course of high-dose steroids. There is a 60% to 70% response rate to this regimen, but the dose and duration of treatment have not been standardized. Typically, methylprednisolone, 250 to 500 mg, is given intravenously for 3 to 5 days. After completion of pulse therapy, the dose of oral steroids can be tapered back or resumed immediately after the maintenance dose. If the patient has been on a steroid-free regimen, adding a maintenance dose should be considered as an episode of acute rejection suggests that prior immunosuppression may have been inadequate. The patient's compliance with prescribed medications should be reviewed. If there are no contraindications, baseline immunosuppression should be increased or changed, at least in the short term. Lymphocyte-depleting antibodies are highly effective in treating first rejection episodes but, because of toxicity and cost, these agents are usually reserved for steroid-resistant cases or when there is severe rejection on the initial biopsy.[141]

Steroid-resistant ACR, defined somewhat arbitrarily as failure of improvement in urine output or plasma creatinine level within 5 days of starting pulse treatment, is usually treated with depleting antibodies. If steroid treatment was based on an empirical rather than a histologic diagnosis, allograft biopsy should be performed to confirm this diagnosis before starting treatment with depleting antibody agents. A higher grade of ACR with endothelial involvement (Banff II or III) is more likely to be steroid-resistant, and many centers use depleting antibody therapy as an initial treatment. The advantage of this approach is prompt and effective treatment of the ACR in higher risk patients. The disadvantage is cost, inconvenience, and exposure of the patients to potentially serious complications of therapy, such as infection and cancer. However, in steroid-resistant rejection, the benefits of lymphocyte-depleting agents outweigh their risks. ATG is better tolerated than OKT3 and is the most commonly used depleting agent.[27]

Refractory Acute Cellular Rejection. Refractory ACR is generally defined as ACR resistant to treatment with antilymphocyte antibody. By definition, the patient has already received aggressive immunosuppression; the risks and benefits of further amplifying immunosuppression should be very carefully considered. Renal histology is helpful in this regard. Therapeutic options include the following: (1) continuing maintenance immunosuppression in the hope that kidney function will slowly improve; (2) repeating a course of antilymphocyte antibody therapy; or (3) switching from cyclosporine to tacrolimus, if not already done.[142] If there is a component of acute AMR, this can be treated as discussed below.

Acute Antibody-Mediated Rejection. AMR is increasingly recognized as a cause of allograft dysfunction and has been reported in 3.5% to 9% of for-cause biopsies.[143,144] Increased recognition of AMR is partly a result of improved diagnostics (in particular, C4d staining and DSA detection[145]) and the expansion of immunologically high-risk and incompatible transplantation.[146] The diagnosis of acute AMR requires allograft dysfunction and at least two of the following: (1) histologic features, including peritubular capillaritis, glomerulitis, thrombi in glomerular capillaries, arterioles or small arteries, and arterial fibrinoid necrosis; (2) diffusely positive staining of peritubular capillaries for C4d; and (3) serologic evidence of antibody against donor HLA or ABO antigens.[147] Acute AMR typically occurs early after transplantation but can also occur late, especially in the setting of reduced immunosuppression or noncompliance. Acute AMR may occur alone or with ACR. In addition, subclinical AMR is commonly present on surveillance biopsies of immunologically high-risk KTRs and is associated with poor graft outcome.[148]

The prognosis of acute AMR is poorer than that of ACR. The optimal treatment of AMR is currently unknown.[149] Strategies that have been used to treat AMR include combinations of plasma exchange to remove DSA and/or intravenous immunoglobulins and anti-CD20 monoclonal antibody to suppress DSA.[150]

Significance of Acute Rejection

Although acute rejection is frequently reversed, retrospective studies have shown that it is strongly associated with the development of chronic rejection and poorer allograft survival. Poorer allograft outcome also correlates with the severity of rejection and with rejection occurring after 6 months posttransplantation.[151] Whatever the outcome is in terms of allograft function, treatment involves exposing the patient to supplemental immunosuppression and its attendant risks. Reducing the incidence of acute rejection has been a major goal in kidney transplantation.

Acute Calcineurin Inhibitor Nephrotoxicity. The CNIs, especially in high doses, cause an acute decrease in GFR by renal vasoconstriction, particularly of the afferent glomerular arteriole. This is manifested clinically as a dose- and blood concentration–dependent acute reversible increase in the plasma creatinine level. Because acute CNI nephrotoxicity is mainly hemodynamic in origin, histology is frequently normal. However, with prolonged CNI toxicity, tubular cell vacuolization and hyaline arteriolar thickening may be seen.[152] The treatment of acute CNI nephrotoxicity is dose reduction.

Distinguishing Acute Calcineurin Inhibitor Nephrotoxicity and Acute Rejection. Distinguishing acute CNI nephrotoxicity and acute rejection clinically can be difficult. Low and high blood concentrations in the presence of rising creatinine levels suggest but do not imply rejection and drug nephrotoxicity, respectively. Both syndromes can coexist. Indicators of a diagnosis of acute CNI nephrotoxicity are severe tremor (neurotoxicity), a moderate increase in plasma creatinine (>25% over baseline), and high trough blood CNI concentrations (e.g., cyclosporine levels >350 ng/mL or tacrolimus levels >20 ng/mL). Indicators of a diagnosis of acute rejection are low-grade fever, allograft pain and tenderness (although, with current drug regimens, these symptoms or signs are uncommon), rapid, nonplateauing increases in plasma creatinine levels, and low drug concentrations. Fever and symptoms localized to the allograft do not occur with CNI toxicity but do not necessarily imply rejection; acute pyelonephritis must also be considered.

If acute CNI nephrotoxicity is suspected, our practice is to reduce the CNI dose and repeat serum creatinine and drug level monitoring within 48 to 96 hours. If graft function has not improved or plateaued at this point, we usually go on to kidney biopsy. The threshold for biopsy is lower in high-risk patients—those who are highly sensitized, have previously rejected an allograft, or are at high risk of early recurrent primary kidney disease (see later). In certain cases, where kidney biopsy is deemed high risk, we will empirically treat with a steroid pulse for a presumptive diagnosis of acute rejection. However, failure of graft function to improve rapidly with this strategy will usually prompt a biopsy.

Most transplant centers provide rapid biopsy and processing of tissue, with basic histology available within 5 to 6 hours. Since a delay of 6 hours in initiating specific therapy should not be detrimental to the graft, a biopsy-proven diagnosis is the preferred approach. In addition to determining the degree and type of rejection in the allograft, histology also occasionally reveals unexpected pathology, such as thrombotic microangiopathy (TMA) or polyoma virus infection. Biopsy results alone should not dictate management; rather, the combination of clinical and histologic findings should be used to determine a treatment plan.

Immune Monitoring. Signs and symptoms of graft dysfunction often occur late, after significant graft injury. Thus, monitoring of serum electrolyte and immunosuppressive drug levels is an essential part of posttransplantation management. Serum creatinine levels, basic chemistry panel, liver function tests, and complete blood count (CBC) are routinely checked to screen for graft dysfunction and manifestations of drug toxicity. Drug levels for CNI, MMF, and mTOR are also monitored for adjustment of immunosuppressive drug dosing. The frequency of monitoring is greater immediately posttransplantation and is gradually decreased. At our institution, we monitor routine blood levels twice weekly during the first month, once a week during the second month, and once every 2 weeks during the third to sixth months posttransplantation. Thereafter, we require monitoring on a monthly basis. The frequency of monitoring is increased if there is graft dysfunction and subsequent treatment.

Most patients are on CNIs. CsA levels can be measured using trough (C_0) levels, 2-hour postdose (C_2) levels, or through abbreviated AUCs. C_0 is the measured level after the dosing interval (e.g., 12 hours after dosing if given every 12 hours), C_2 is the measured level 2 hours after dosing, and AUC is the area under the curve during the first 4 hour after dosing. C_2 levels correlate more closely with the AUC, but no significant differences have been found in the incidence of acute rejection, graft loss, or adverse events between patients monitored using C_0 or C_2 levels.[153] The standard target level for CsA is a C_0 level of 150 to 300 ng/mL early and 100 to 200 ng/mL late posttransplantation,[154] or a C_2 level of 1400 to 1800 ng/mL early and 800 to 1200 ng/mL later after transplantation.[155] Tacrolimus C_0 levels correlate better with AUC,[156,157] and measuring the C_0 tacrolimus level is usual practice. The standard target level for tacrolimus C_0 is 10 (5 to 15) ng/dL. A low-dose level with a C_0 of 5 ng/mL (range, 3 to 7 ng/mL) has also been used successfully.[97,158] Note that these levels serve as guidelines based on case series and multicenter randomized controlled studies, but the optimal level for any given patient depends on multiple factors, such as level of risk for rejection and degree of side of effects from drugs.

Biopsies have remained the gold standard for diagnosing intrarenal allograft dysfunction. Ongoing efforts are being made to identify noninvasive serum or urine biomarkers, which could aid in early detection of graft dysfunction or obviate the need for biopsy. Biomarkers that have been investigated include cytokines, IL-2 receptors, adhesion molecules, and other inflammatory markers, such as complement and acute phase proteins. Urinary mRNA levels of perforin and granzyme B have been shown to be associated with acute rejection.[159] While levels of FOXP3 mRNA in urinary cells have been demonstrated to predict the reversibility of acute rejection and identify patients at high risk for graft loss after an episode of acute rejection.[160] A urinary mRNA signature has been reported to show good discrimination for acute rejection, with the test preempting acute rejection episodes by up to 10 days.[161] There is also increasing interest in the use of donor-derived, cell-free DNA as a biomarker of acute allograft injury.[162,163]

The use of molecular diagnostic tools, such as the molecular microscope, which use a microarray-based approach to measure differential gene expression in renal biopsy tissue has shown great promise. They may prove particularly useful in the diagnosis and prognosis of AMR.[164]

Acute Thrombotic Microangiopathy

Acute TMA after kidney transplantation is a rare but serious complication.[165] It usually occurs in the early posttransplantation period and is accompanied by increasing plasma creatinine and lactate dehydrogenase levels, thrombocytopenia, falling hemoglobin level, schistocytosis, and low haptoglobin concentrations. This diagnosis can be overlooked because thrombocytopenia and anemia commonly occur after transplantation in the setting for induction therapy. The diagnosis is confirmed by allograft biopsy, which shows endothelial damage and, in severe cases, thrombosis of glomerular capillaries and arterioles.

Causes include CNIs,[166] OKT3, AMR,[167] viral infections such as CMV, and recurrence of primary disease. The presence of hepatitis C and anticardiolipin antibodies increases the risk.[168] Early diagnosis of TMA is essential to salvage kidney function. There are no controlled trials of therapy for TMA after transplantation. Suggested measures are cessation of CNIs and other implicated drugs and control of any hypertension present. Although plasma exchange has been used, the benefit is unclear.[169] Eculuzimab, which blocks the complement activation cascade at the level of C5, has also been successfully used.[170]

Acute Pyelonephritis

Urinary tract infections (UTIs) may occur at any period but are most frequent shortly after transplantation because of catheterization, stenting, and aggressive immunosuppression.[171] Other risk factors for UTIs are anatomic abnormalities and a neurogenic bladder. Fortunately, acute pyelonephritis is less common since the widespread use of prophylactic sulfamethoxazole-trimethoprim (SMX-TMP). Fever, allograft pain and tenderness, and leukocytosis are usually more pronounced in acute pyelonephritis than in acute rejection. Diagnosis requires urine culture, but empirical antibiotic treatment should be started immediately.

Delay in treatment can lead to rapid clinical decline in the immunosuppressed patient. The most commonly implicated microorganisms are gram-negative bacilli, coagulase-negative staphylococci, and enterococci. Kidney function usually returns to baseline quickly with antimicrobial therapy and volume expansion. Recurrent pyelonephritis requires investigation to exclude underlying urologic abnormalities. A voiding cystourethrogram (VCUG) should be considered to evaluate for reflux into the transplant allograft.

Acute Allergic Interstitial Nephritis

In the setting of kidney transplantation, acute allergic interstitial nephritis is a diagnosis of exclusion. Distinguishing acute allergic interstitial nephritis and ACR is very difficult. In fact, the pathogenesis is somewhat similar in both cases, and mainly involves cell-mediated immunity. While fever and rash after ingestion of a new drug favor the former, these clinical features are rarely seen. Mononuclear cell and eosinophil infiltration of the transplanted kidney may occur with either condition, but endothelialitis implicates rejection. Polyomavirus infection must also be considered in the differential diagnosis. Acute allergic interstitial nephritis and ACR usually respond to steroids; of course, the suspected drugs must be stopped. SMX-TMP is the drug most commonly implicated in causing allergic interstitial nephritis in KTRs; other antibiotics, including penicillins, cephalosporins and quinolones, can also be implicated.

Early Recurrence of Primary Disease

Several kidney diseases may recur early and cause acute allograft dysfunction. These may be classified into three groups: (1) glomerulonephritides; (2) metabolic diseases such as primary oxalosis; and (3) systemic diseases such as hemolytic uremic syndrome/thrombotic thrombocytopenia purpura (HUS/TTP). Primary focal segmental glomerulosclerosis (FSGS) is considered in more detail in the following section because of its relatively high frequency of recurrence and its propensity to cause severe graft injury.

Primary Focal Segmental Glomerulosclerosis. The recurrence of primary FSGS is variable. The sporadic variety is reported to be about 30%,[172] but recurrence of familial FSGS is rare. Risk factors for recurrence include non-African ancestry recipient, younger recipient, rapidly progressive FSGS in the recipient's native kidneys, and recurrence of disease in a previous allograft. Most cases become manifest (as proteinuria) hours to weeks after transplantation. This rapidity of recurrence suggests the presence of a pathogenic circulating plasma factor.[173] Because of the poor prognosis associated with delayed treatment, patients with primary FSGS should be monitored after transplantation for new-onset proteinuria. Early biopsy is exhibit in those who develop proteinuria; this may not show FSGS lesions per se but may exhibit diffuse foot process effacement on electron microscopy. Treatment options include plasmapheresis or immunoadsorption, high-dose CNIs, ACEIs, high-dose corticosteroids, cyclophosphamide, and rituximab, but controlled studies are lacking.[174] A recent case series reported successful treatment of recurrent FSGS with the costimulation blocker abatecept in patients who had positive immunostaining for the costimulatory molecule B7-1 (CD80) on their podocytes.[175] Because of the high risk of recurrence in those who have had previous recurrences, subsequent living donor transplantation in such individuals is often discouraged.

Antiglomerular Basement Membrane Disease. Before transplantation, patients with end-stage kidney disease (ESKD) due to antiglomerular basement membrane (GBM) disease should generally be on dialysis for at least 6 months and have negative anti-GBM serology.[176] If these criteria are fulfilled, posttransplantation recurrence is rare. De novo anti-GBM disease can occur in recipients with Alport's syndrome. Here, the recipient with abnormal type IV collagen produces antibodies against the previously unseen normal α_5-chain NC1 domain in the basement membrane of the transplanted kidney. Patients with allograft dysfunction should be treated with plasmapheresis and cyclophosphamide.[176]

Hemolytic Uremic Syndrome/Thrombotic Thrombocytopenia Purpura. The causes of TMA after kidney transplantation have been discussed earlier. Recurrence of classic (diarrhea-associated) HUS/TTP is uncommon. However, transplantation should still be deferred until the disease is quiescent for at least 6 months. In contrast, recurrence of atypical (non–diarrhea-associated) HUS/TTP, particularly if inherited, has been reported to be as high as 80%.[177] Certain genetic disorders of complement regulation (such as of factor H) are associated with high risks of severe recurrence, so it is very useful to define these risks, if possible, before proceeding with transplantation.[178] The prognosis of disease recurrence had previously been considered very poor; however, the complement inhibitor eculizumab has recently been shown to halt recurrent atypical HUS successfully.[170]

POSTRENAL DYSFUNCTION

Most urologic complications are secondary to technical factors at the time of transplantation and manifest themselves in the early postoperative period, but immunologic factors may play a role in some cases.

Urine Leaks

Leaks may occur at the level of the renal calyx, ureter, or bladder. Causes include infarction of the ureter due to perioperative disruption of its blood supply and breakdown of the ureterovesical anastomosis. Severe obstruction may also result in rupture of the urinary tract with leakage. Clinical features include abdominal pain and swelling; the plasma urea and creatinine levels increase due to resorption of solutes across the peritoneal membrane. If a perirenal drain is being used, however, a urine leak may present with high-volume drainage of fluid. Ultrasound may demonstrate a fluid collection (urinoma); aspiration of fluid from the collection (or from the drain bag) by sterile technique allows comparison of the fluid and plasma creatinine level. When the excretory function of the kidney is good, the creatinine concentration in the urinoma greatly exceeds that in the plasma.

In cases in which ultrasound diagnosis is difficult, renal scintigraphy may be useful in demonstrating extravasation of tracer from the urinary system, provided there is adequate kidney function. Rough localization of the site of the leak is sometimes possible by this technique. Antegrade pyelography allows precise diagnosis and localization of proximal urinary leaks. Cystography is the best test to demonstrate a bladder leak.

The clinical features may mimic those of acute rejection. Whenever urine leakage is suspected, a bladder catheter should be immediately inserted to decompress the urinary tract. Selected patients may do well with a bladder catheter or endourologic treatment. Many cases, however, require urgent surgical exploration and repair. The type of repair depends on the level of the leak and viability of involved tissues.

Urinary Tract Obstruction

Although urinary tract obstruction can occur at any time after transplantation, it is most common in the early postoperative period. Intrinsic causes include poor implantation of the ureter into the bladder, intraluminal blood clots or slough material, and fibrosis of the ureter due to ischemia or rejection. Extrinsic causes include an enlarged prostate in older men (causing bladder outlet obstruction) and compression by a lymphocele or other fluid collection. Rarely, calculi cause transplantation urinary tract obstruction.

Urinary tract obstruction is often asymptomatic and should always be considered in the differential diagnosis of allograft dysfunction in the early transplantation period. Ultrasound often demonstrates hydronephrosis. However, some dilation of the transplant urinary collecting system is often seen in the early postoperative period, and serial scans showing worsening hydronephrosis may be needed to confirm the diagnosis. Renal scintiscanning with diuretic washout is useful in equivocal cases. Percutaneous antegrade pyelography is the best radiologic technique for determining the site of obstruction and can be combined with interventional endourologic techniques. In expert hands, endourologic techniques (e.g., balloon dilation, stenting) may be effective in treating ureteric stenosis and stricture. More complicated cases require open surgical repair. Extrinsic compression requires specific intervention, such as draining or fenestration of the lymphocele.

Obstruction in the early postoperative period due to an enlarged prostate should be managed with bladder catheter drainage and drugs such as tamsulosin.

LATE POSTTRANSPLANTATION PERIOD

LATE ACUTE ALLOGRAFT DYSFUNCTION

The causes and evaluation of late acute allograft dysfunction (defined as occurring >6 months posttransplantation) include those of early acute dysfunction. Acute prerenal failure may occur at any time; the causes are similar to those seen with native kidneys, such as shock syndromes, and may be further exacerbated by the hemodynamic effects of concurrent ACEI or NSAID use. Urinary tract obstruction must also be considered in the differential diagnosis. In contrast to the early posttransplantation period, the causes of obstruction are similar to those associated with native kidney disease (e.g., stones, bladder outlet obstruction, neoplasia). Ureteric obstruction due to BK virus infection has also been described. Several causes of late acute allograft dysfunction are reviewed in more detail below.

LATE ACUTE REJECTION

Acute rejection is less common after the first 6 months. Late acute rejection should alert the physician to prescription of inadequate immunosuppression or patient noncompliance.[179] Withdrawal of steroids or CNIs by the physician may be initiated due to side effects of these medications, but when carried out later in the posttransplantation period, may be associated with a high risk of acute rejection.[180,181] Therefore, the plasma creatinine level must be carefully monitored in this setting. AMR has been increasingly recognized as an important cause of late acute allograft dysfunction, especially many years posttransplantation; in a recent study, over 50% of 173 subjects biopsied for acute graft dysfunction, a mean of 7 years posttransplantation, had evidence of AMR.[182]

Acute rejection can also occur when CNI levels are subtherapeutic in the setting of newly prescribed medications that are known to decrease CNI levels (Table 72.10).

Table 72.10 Agents That May Induce Acute Kidney Injury in Kidney Transplant Recipients

Class of Drug	Increase Level	Decrease Level
Drugs That Interact with CNIs and Sirolimus		
Calcium channel blocker	Diltiazem, verapamil	
Antibiotics	Erythromycin, azithromycin, clarithromycin	Nafcillin
Antifungals	Fluconazole, ketoconazole, itraconazole, voriconazole	
Antituberculin		Rifampin, rifabutin
Antiviral	Ritonavir, nelfinavir, saquinavir	Efavirenz, nevirapine
Antiseizure		Phenytoin, phenobarbital, carbamazepine, primidone
Antidepressant	Fluoxitine, nefazodone, fluvoxamine	
Foods and Herbal Preparations That Interact with CNIs		
Food	Grapefruit juice	
Herb		St. John's wort

CNIs, Calcineurin inhibitors; INH, isoniazid.

Common agents that decrease CNI levels include antituberculin medications and antiseizure medications. CNI levels should be measured more frequently, and dose adjustments should be made when prescribing or withdrawing these medications.

Treatment is the same as for early acute rejection (whether ACR, acute AMR, or both) but responses are poorer, with a greater negative impact on allograft survival than early acute rejection or DGF. Risk factors for noncompliance include adolescence, more immunosuppressant adverse effects, poor social support and psychologic stress or illness.[183] Closer monitoring, simplification of the drug regimen, and social worker assistance may aid in the management of patients with a high risk of nonadherence.

LATE ACUTE CALCINEURIN INHIBITOR NEPHROTOXICITY

Although lower doses of CNIs are generally prescribed after the first 6 to 12 months, acute CNI toxicity may occur at any time after transplantation. This may occur in the setting of taking new medications that impair the metabolism of the CNIs (see Table 72.10). Patients should be made aware of common medications that interact with CNI. CNI levels should be monitored closely, and dose adjustments should be made when such medications are prescribed.

TRANSPLANT RENAL ARTERY STENOSIS

Renal Artery Stenosis

Transplant renal artery stenosis (TRAS) is the most common transplant vascular complication and is associated with reduced long-term allograft survival.[184,185] TRAS can arise at any time after transplantation, although the mean time to diagnosis is 0.83 ± 0.81 years posttransplantation.[186] The reported incidence varies widely.[185] TRAS may be a consequence of an inadequate arterial anastomosis, inherent vascular disease of the recipient, or preexisting renovascular disease of the donor. Immune-mediated or infection-related damage to the transplant renal artery also plays an important role in some patients; new posttransplantation DSAs and CMV infection are both associated with the development of TRAS.[187,188]

Luminal narrowing of more than 70% is probably required to render a stenosis functionally significant. The stenosis may occur in the donor or recipient artery or at the anastomotic site. Stenosis of the recipient iliac artery may also compromise renal arterial flow. Worsening or difficult to control hypertension, an unexplained deterioration in kidney function, or azotemia associated with the introduction of an ACE or ARB should raise suspicion of TRAS.[185,189,190] Clinical examination may also reveal a new vascular bruit over the graft. Ultrasound with Doppler, magnetic resonance, and computed tomography (CT) angiography can support a diagnosis but direct angiography is usually required for confirmation. CO_2 or minimal contrast angiography can be used to reduce the risk of radiocontrast injury.[191] Good outcomes have been reported with primary angioplasty and stent placement in terms of blood pressure control and renal function.[192,193] If the diagnosis is made in the early postoperative period, a surgical approach with revision of the anastomosis may be preferred.[185]

INFECTIONS CAUSING LATE ACUTE ALLOGRAFT DYSFUNCTION

Human Polyomavirus Infection

The polyomaviruses are DNA viruses, the best known of which are the BK virus, JC virus, and SV40 virus. BK virus causes a mild self-limiting upper respiratory tract infection in healthy individuals (mostly in childhood). Around 80% of the adult population have serologic evidence of prior BK infection. Following primary infection, the virus remains dormant in the urothelium. In immunosuppressed states, the virus may reactivate and replicate. Viral reactivation may result in viral shedding into the urine, viremia, cystitis, ureteritis, or interstitial nephritis (BK nephropathy).

Over the past 20 years, BK virus has been increasingly recognized as an important cause of kidney allograft dysfunction and loss. This probably reflects improved recognition and reporting of the disease and the use of more potent maintenance MMF and tacrolimus-based immunosuppression regimens. BK nephropathy is most common in the first 2 years posttransplantation. Around 30% to 40% of renal transplant recipients develop viruria, around 25% of those patients (10% to 20%) will become viremic, and about 50% of those viremic patients (0% to 10%) will manifest BK nephropathy on biopsy.[194] Because viruria and viremia almost always precede BK nephropathy, urine or plasma viral screening offers the opportunity to screen for early infection and instigate measures to clear the virus before nephropathy occurs.[195] Many centers advocate biopsy when plasma viral titers reach a predefined threshold (usually >10^4 copies/mL), while others, such as our own, treat empirically and reserve biopsy for patients with evidence of new graft dysfunction.

Approaches to screening vary and are influenced by local prevalence and economic factors. Many transplantation centers now screen all new transplant recipients at intervals over the first 2 years posttransplantation. Protocols for screening include testing the urine by light microscopy for decoy (infected) cells or by PCR quantification of urinary or plasma viral load. KDIGO guidelines recommend quantitative plasma PCR testing as follows: (1) monthly for the first 3 to 6 months after transplantation; (2) then every 3 months until the end of the first posttransplantation year; (3) whenever there is an unexplained rise in serum creatinine level; and (4) after treatment of acute rejection.[149]

Allograft biopsy is required for the diagnosis of BK interstitial nephritis. Adequate sampling is needed, as the interstitial nephritis can be patchy. The presence of intranuclear tubule cell inclusions by light microscopy should raise suspicion; diagnosis is confirmed by immunohistochemistry using antibodies against BK viral proteins (SV40). The excellent performance of immunohistochemical stains and concurrent measurement of BK viral titers at the time of for-cause biopsy mean that BK nephropathy is no longer frequently mistaken for and treated as acute cellular rejection.

The mainstay of treatment is reduction in immunosuppression.[195] Our usual practice has been to first discontinue the antimetabolite (usually MMF) in response to significant viremia or biopsy evidence of nephropathy. If this measure fails to result in a favorable viral response, we reduce the dose of CNI by 30% to 50% and continue to monitor viral titers. There are a number of adjunct therapies that may be considered in subjects who fail to respond to immunosuppression reduction or for whom very aggressive immunosuppression reduction is unattractive because of their immune risk status. Leflunomide is a tyrosine kinase inhibitor, approved for the treatment of rheumatoid arthritis, that has antiviral effects in vitro. A number of small series have suggested that treatment with leflunomide (usually as a substitute for an antimetabolite) results in enhanced BK viral clearing, although in the absence of clinical trials its efficacy remains contentious.[196,197] The antiviral cidofovir has also, by some reports, been associated with a reduction in BK viral load, but note that prudent dosing is important in view of the drug's potential nephrotoxicity.[198] Finally, hopes for fluoroquinolones as a treatment for BK virus were considerably dashed by a recent small RCT showing that a 30-day course of levofloxacin cleared BK virus no better than placebo.[199]

Hepatitis C

Treatment options for hepatitis C virus (HCV) infection in the general population have greatly improved with the recent emergence of the NS3-4A protease and NS5B polymerase inhibitors, permitting successful interferon-α (IFN-α)–free treatment of the virus.[200] There are currently no data on the use of these new agents in KTRs, although we expect this to change soon. Currently, IFN-α–based treatment of HCV is relatively contraindicated posttransplantation because of the associated increased risk of graft rejection.[201,202] Treatment is therefore limited to reduction in immunosuppression, reserving rescue interferon treatment for patients with rapidly worsening liver failure. Dialysis patients on the transplant waiting list may currently be treated with interferon monotherapy. The addition of ribavirin, which is renally excreted, improves viral clearance but has traditionally been avoided because of the risk of developing hemolytic anemia. However, recent trial data have suggested that ribavirin may be safely used at reduced doses in dialysis patients.[203]

Both membranoproliferative glomerulonephritis (MPGN) and membranous nephropathy are more commonly seen in HCV-positive compared with HCV-negative KTRs. MPGN is often associated with cryoglobulinemia, although severe systemic vasculitis is rare. An association of TMA with anticardiolipin antibodies in HCV-positive patients has also been reported.[168] KTRs with HCV also have a higher risk of posttransplantation diabetes mellitus.[204]

DRUG AND RADIOCONTRAST NEPHROTOXICITY

Drugs that cause nephrotoxicity in the native kidney will also adversely affect the kidney allografts. Drug-related nephrotoxic effects that are more common in the setting of transplantation are listed in Table 72.10. Special attention should be paid to drugs that interact with CNIs. CNIs are metabolized by the cytochrome P450 isoenzyme CYP3A5, and drugs that interact with CYP3A5 will affect its plasma level. When prescribing diltiazem, verapamil, ketoconazole, and the macrolide antibiotics, particularly erythromycin, the dosage of CNI should be reduced and levels should be followed. Conversely, rifampin, phenobarbital, and phenytoin lower the CNI level, so the CNI should be increased.

Drugs with known nephrotoxic effects, such as aminoglycosides, amphotericin, and NSAIDs, probably have enhanced toxicity when used concomitantly with a CNI. Nevertheless, they are sometimes required in transplant recipients. Use of the liposomal preparation of amphotericin is preferable because it is less nephrotoxic than the standard preparation (amphotericin B).

Plasma creatinine levels can be increased with high-dose SMX-TMP by inhibiting tubular secretion of creatinine (GFR per se is not compromised, and the plasma creatinine level decreases within 5 days of stopping SMX-TMP). Rarely, SMX-TMP can provoke allergic interstitial nephritis.

Not surprisingly, ACEIs or ARBs have been implicated in precipitating acute renal failure (ARF) in the presence of TRAS. Overall, if carefully prescribed, these agents are well tolerated. The use of ACEIs or ARBs in the immediate posttransplantation period, when volume status and CNI dosages are fluctuating, is not recommended.

The risk of developing AKI after administration of radiocontrast to KTRs has not been well defined. Single-center studies point toward a higher prevalence in KTRs.[205] Presumably, risk factors for contrast nephrotoxicity are similar to those in patients who have not undergone transplantation surgery. Thus, the same preventive measures should be used.

LATE ALLOGRAFT DYSFUNCTION AND LATE ALLOGRAFT LOSS

Preventing late allograft loss remains a major challenge. Death with a functioning graft accounts for approximately half of graft losses. Important causes of death-censored late graft loss include acute rejection, recurrent or de novo glomerular disease, AKI related to sepsis or hypotension, and pyelonephritis.[206] Most of the remaining late graft failures, with features of interstitial fibrosis and tubular atrophy (IF/TA) on histology, were conventionally attributed to an amalgam of immune and non–immune-mediated fibrosis and vascular injury, termed *sclerosing/chronic allograft nephropathy*. More recently, improved pathologic and immunologic diagnostic tools (e.g., C4d stain, DSA) mean that underlying chronic AMR is increasingly recognized in biopsies with IF/TA. The Banff 2005 update added the term *chronic active antibody-mediated rejection*, currently defined as positive C4d staining, presence of circulating antidonor antibodies, morphologic evidence of chronic tissue injury, such as glomerular double contours and/or peritubular capillary basement membrane multilayering and/or IF/TA and/or fibrous intimal thickening in arteries. The term IF/TA without evidence of any specific cause is reserved for cases without evidence of chronic immune injury. In addition, any biopsy with IF/TA may be further supplemented to include features suggestive of nonimmune causes of IF/TA, such as CNI toxicity, chronic hypertension, obstruction, pyelonephritis, viral infection, and recurrent or de novo glomerular disease (see Table 72.9). Increasing attention is also being paid to the presence of subclinical inflammation accompanying fibrosis (often below the Banff threshold for ACR), as it appears to portend a poor prognosis.[207,208] Figure 72.6 illustrates factors thought to contribute to the development of late allograft failure.

The causes of late dysfunction are summarized in Table 72.11 and further discussed in the following sections.

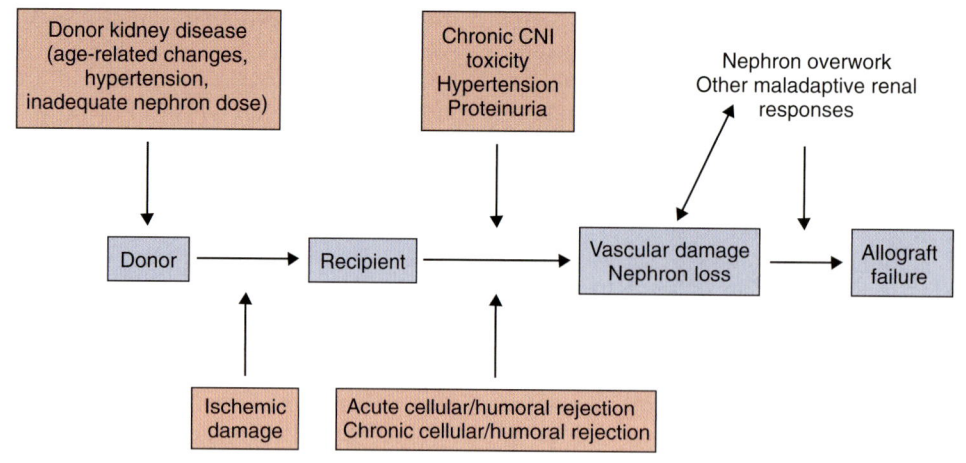

Figure 72.6 Immune and non-immune factors that contribute to the pathogenesis of chronic allograft injury. CNI, Calcineurin inhibitor.

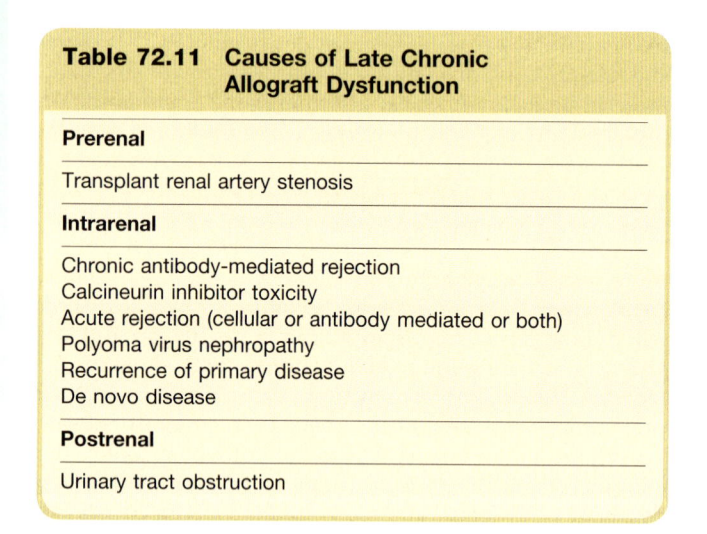

Table 72.11	Causes of Late Chronic Allograft Dysfunction
Prerenal	
Transplant renal artery stenosis	
Intrarenal	
Chronic antibody-mediated rejection	
Calcineurin inhibitor toxicity	
Acute rejection (cellular or antibody mediated or both)	
Polyoma virus nephropathy	
Recurrence of primary disease	
De novo disease	
Postrenal	
Urinary tract obstruction	

The diagnosis is supported by positive peritubular capillary immunostaining for the complement split product, C4d, and the presence of DSA.

Chronic AMR, commonly accompanied by transplantation glomerulopathy on histology, is clinically characterized by a slow decline in kidney function, hypertension, and often heavy proteinuria. Treatment options are limited. A single-center study of 23 consecutive KTRs with AMR diagnosed at least 6 months posttransplantation, nearly half of whom had some evidence of transplantation glomerulopathy on biopsy, observed minimal benefit in response to therapies that included plasmapheresis, IVIg, rituximab, and bortezomib.[210] Our approach is largely supportive, with the use of ACE inhibitors or ARBs, control of hypertension, and modification of cardiovascular risk factors. Most of our patients already take tacrolimus and MMF; we do not aggressively escalate immunosuppression.[211]

CALCINEURIN INHIBITOR TOXICITY

Over 30 years after CNI-associated nephropathy was first described in heart transplant recipients, there remains debate about the importance of CNI in late graft failure.[212] Nankivell and colleagues reported longitudinal histologic data on 120 diabetic KTRs (119 were simultaneous pancreas-kidney [SPK] recipients) who underwent sequential kidney transplantation biopsies from the time of transplantation up to 10 years posttransplantation.[49] The study identified histologic evidence of CNI toxicity, defined as the presence of striped cortical fibrosis or new-onset arteriolar hyalinosis (not from renal ischemia or preexisting hyalinosis in the allograft) supported by tubular microcalcification (without preceding acute tubular necrosis) in over 50% of biopsies at 5 years and 100% of biopsies at 10 years posttransplantation. Based on the pathologic findings, the authors attributed most of the late graft dysfunction to CNI toxicity. In contrast, newer studies have suggested a much lower prevalence of interstitial fibrosis at 5 years postbiopsy and question the specificity of arteriolar hyalinosis for the diagnosis of CNI toxicity.[206,213] This, combined with increased evidence for immune-mediated injury in many cases of late allograft failure, has led many to deemphasize the importance of chronic CNI toxicity.

Certain causes such as TRAS and urinary tract obstruction have been discussed earlier.

CHRONIC ANTIBODY-MEDIATED REJECTION

Several studies have recently shown that an antibody-mediated process frequently accompanies late graft injury. In one study, 99 of 173 patients (57%) who underwent for-cause biopsy, a mean of 7 years posttransplantation, had evidence of an AMR, indicated by C4d positivity, DSA, or both.[182] Another study that evaluated all death-censored graft losses in 1317 KTRs, irrespective of time since transplantation, found evidence for chronic AMR in 18% (with histologic evidence of transplantation glomerulopathy or IF/TA). The probability of AMR on for-cause biopsies rises from around 10% at 6 months to 35% at 5 years posttransplantation, is associated with medication nonadherence, and augurs poor graft survival.[209]

The histopathologic changes of chronic AMR are seen in the tubulointerstitium, vessels, and glomeruli and include glomerular double contours with variable mesangial matrix expansion, peritubular capillary basement membrane multilayering, IF/TA, and fibrous intimal thickening in arteries.

We remain believers in CNI toxicity as a cause of graft dysfunction. If the clinical and histologic picture suggests a significant component of chronic CNI nephrotoxicity without evidence of rejection, we dose-reduce the CNI. Substituting CNI with sirolimus has also been used successfully, although the development of proteinuria (and other issues noted above) is a problem.[76] The use of sirolimus should probably be avoided in those with baseline proteinuria or a GFR of less than 40 mL/min.[214] The significant difference in GFR between belatacept- and cyclosporine-treated patients 5 years posttransplantation in the Benefit trial lends credence to the nephrotoxic effects of CNIs and the emphasizes the potential merits of developing CNI-free immunosuppression regimens.[82]

RECURRENCE OF PRIMARY DISEASE

Diseases that recur early in the posttransplantation period have been addressed earlier. The incidence of late recurrence is difficult to estimate for several reasons: the original cause of ESKD is often unknown; transplant kidney biopsies are not always performed; and most relevant studies are small and retrospective, with variable follow-up periods. In one large study of patients who underwent transplantation after developing ESKD from glomerulonephritis, recurrence was the third most frequent cause of graft loss at 10 years (after chronic rejection and death).[215] Recurrence can present as decreasing GFR, proteinuria, or hematuria.

IgA Glomerulonephritis

Studies with longer follow-up times have shown that histologic recurrence of this condition is common. The reported incidence varies from 13% to 53%[216] and likely reflects the varying threshold for biopsies among different centers. The estimated 10-year incidence of graft loss due to recurrence was 9.7%.[215] The risk of recurrence is higher if a previous graft was lost to recurrent disease.[217] As with the treatment of native disease, ACEIs and ARBs can be used.[218]

Lupus Nephritis

Allograft and patient survival overall had been thought to be similar in patients with ESKD due to lupus nephritis compared with those with ESKD from other causes,[219] but analysis of the U.S. Renal Data System (USRDS) database has shown worse outcomes of deceased donor transplant recipients with ESKD due to lupus nephritis.[220] Recurrence of severe systemic lupus erythematosus (SLE), systemically or within the graft, is uncommon. Low rates of recurrence in SLE probably reflect patient selection, disease activity burning out on maintenance dialysis, and the effects of powerful posttransplantation immunosuppression. A recent analysis of nearly 7000 KTRs with ESKD from SLE suggested that acute rejection (affecting 26%) had a more important impact on graft failure than recurrent disease (affecting 3%).[221] As with other glomerular diseases that may recur, transplantation should be deferred until SLE is clinically quiescent. Many centers prefer a 6- to 12-month period of clinical quiescence before proceeding with transplantation to reduce the risk of recurrence. If the patient is receiving anticoagulation for antiphospholipid syndrome (APS) before transplantation, anticoagulation should be resumed as soon as safely possible (initially with intravenous heparin) after transplantation surgery. This procedure is used to reduce the risk of thrombosis of the allograft or other sites.

Granulomatosis with Polyangitis and Microscopic Polyangiitis

Renal and extrarenal recurrences of these diseases have been described. In a pooled series of 127 patients, antineutrophil cytoplasmic antibody (ANCA)–associated small vessel vasculitis recurred in 17% of cases, renal involvement recurred in 10% of cases, and the recurrence rate was not lower with cyclosporine therapy.[222] A lower incidence (7%) of recurrence has been reported in a more recent study.[223] These studies have found that positive ANCA serology at the time of transplantation does not predict relapse. Patients with ESKD secondary to ANCA-associated vasculitis should not undergo transplant surgery until the disease is clinically quiescent. Recurrences usually respond to cyclophosphamide.

Membranoproliferative Glomerulonephritis

MPGN has recently been reclassified based on the deposition of C3 alone (the C3 nephritides) versus C3 and immunoglobulin on immunofluorescence.[224] The C3 nephritides (dense deposit disease and C3 nephritis) are driven by an underlying defect in regulation of the alternative complement pathway. The recent classification change means that there are limited data on the recurrence rate of the C3 nephritides; however, 5-year graft survival in 75 patients with ESKD from MPGN type II (now termed *dense deposit disease*) was reported to be significantly worse than other pediatric KTRs, and recurrence was documented in 12 of the 18 patients biopsied.[225] Limited success has been reported in treating posttransplantation recurrence of the C3 nephritides with the complement inhibitor ecluzimab.[226,227] MPGN associated with glomerular deposition of C3 and immunoglobulin should trigger the evaluation and treatment of underlying causes such as infection (especially hepatitis C), autoimmune diseases, and plasma cell dyscrasias.

Membranous Nephropathy

Membranous nephropathy may recur after transplantation or arise de novo.[228] The associated clinical features vary from minimal to nephrotic syndrome. De novo membranous nephropathy is often associated with IF/TA. As with native kidney disease, hepatitis B virus (HBV) and HCV infection and other conditions associated with membranous nephropathy should be excluded. The recurrence of primary IgG4 anti-PLA2R1 antibody–associated disease is more likely in patients with persistently detectable posttransplantation titers and may be related to the intensity of posttransplantation immunosuppression.[229] Management includes treatment of the underlying cause and supportive measures. The recurrence of primary membranous nephropathy has been successfully treated with rituximab.[230]

Diabetic Nephropathy

Recurrence of diabetic nephropathy in the allograft has not been well studied. This reflects the relatively poor long-term survival of diabetic KTRs; the duration of exposure to the diabetic milieu is often insufficient to allow development of severe diabetic nephropathy. PTDM can also result in diabetic nephropathy,[231] and histologic evidence of this may occur rapidly after transplantation.[232]

ASSESSING OUTCOMES IN KIDNEY TRANSPLANTATION

The most convenient and widely used method for assessing outcomes after kidney transplantation is measurement of allograft survival. Other important measures include allograft function (typically measured by plasma creatinine level), patient survival, number of rejection episodes, days of hospitalization, and quality of life indices. Registry data from the USRDS, Collaborative Transplant Study (CTS), and Australia and New Zealand Dialysis and Transplant Registry (ANZDATA) have all proved extremely useful in assessing these outcomes.

ACTUAL AND ACTUARIAL ALLOGRAFT AND PATIENT SURVIVAL

Allograft survival is calculated from the day of transplantation to the day of reaching a defined end point (e.g., return to dialysis, retransplantation, or death). The most widely accepted measure of outcome is the Kaplan-Meier probability estimate of patient and graft survival. One-year, 5-year, and 10-year actuarial survival rates are frequently presented, but actual survival may ultimately not be as impressive as projected survival.[233] Another actuarial measure commonly used is allograft half-life (median allograft survival).

Traditionally, allograft survival is assessed under two distinct time phases, early and late. Early allograft loss refers to loss within the first 12 months, and late loss refers to any time thereafter. This distinction is empirical but makes clinical sense. In the first 12 months, the most common causes of allograft loss are technical complications and rejection. After 12 months, the incidence is lower and generally stable over time. Frequently, analysis of long-term survival is restricted to allografts that have survived to 12 months after transplantation. Patient death is, in essence, equivalent to allograft loss, but allograft survival is also sometimes calculated after censoring for patient death (death-censored allograft survival).

SURVIVAL BENEFITS OF KIDNEY TRANSPLANTATION

Comparison of survival between the general dialysis population and transplanted patients is greatly affected by selection bias, as only relatively healthy patients are referred (and listed) for transplantation. Thus, comparisons among patients on the waiting list who do or do not receive a transplant are usually performed instead. Such analyses assume that the two groups (those who have undergone transplantation surgery and those still on the list) can otherwise be matched; this is not necessarily true.

One USRDS study found that during the first 106 days after transplantation, the risk of death after transplantation was higher than the corresponding risk while remaining on the waiting list (on dialysis). This mainly reflected the risks associated with the transplantation procedure itself. Thereafter, transplantation conferred a survival benefit. On the basis of 3 to 4 years of follow-up, transplantation was found to reduce the risk of death overall by 68%.[234]

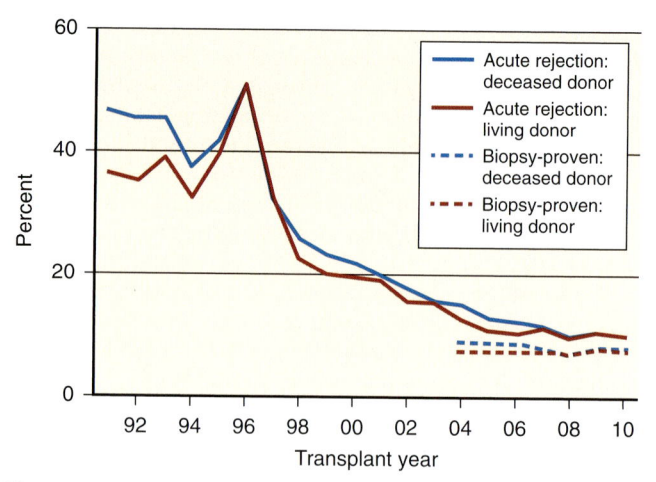

Figure 72.7 Secular trends in acute rejection in the first year posttransplantation.

SHORT-TERM OUTCOMES

The acute rejection rate has fallen substantially over the past 20 years. The rate of acute rejection in the first year posttransplantation is currently around 10%. Figure 72.7 illustrates the decline in rates of acute rejection in the first posttransplantation year from 1992 to 2010.[138] The same period has seen a significant improvement in short-term graft survival. One-year graft survival in 2010 was 91% for deceased donor transplants and 97% for living donor transplants. Figures 72.8 and 72.9 illustrate 1-year graft survival by donor type between 1992 and 2010. The principal causes of allograft loss in the first posttransplantation year are acute rejection, thrombosis, primary nonfunction, and patient death.

LONG-TERM OUTCOMES

There has also been an improvement in long-term allograft survival (see Figures 72.8 and 72.9). Recently, this increase has occurred mainly in higher-risk patients, such as those receiving retransplants. When first deceased donor transplants alone are assessed, recent improvements are less impressive. These findings indicate that improving long-term allograft survival is not just a matter of preventing early acute rejection.[235]

Beyond the first posttransplantation year, the principal causes of kidney allograft loss are patient death and chronic allograft injury (CAI); less common causes are late acute rejection and recurrent disease.[206] The primary cause of death remains cardiovascular disease, followed by infection and malignancy (Figure 72.10). In children, however, death is a much less common cause of allograft loss; conversely, in older adults, death is more common.

FACTORS AFFECTING KIDNEY ALLOGRAFT SURVIVAL

Prospective studies and analyses of registry data have shown that many variables influence kidney allograft survival. These can be considered as donor, recipient, and

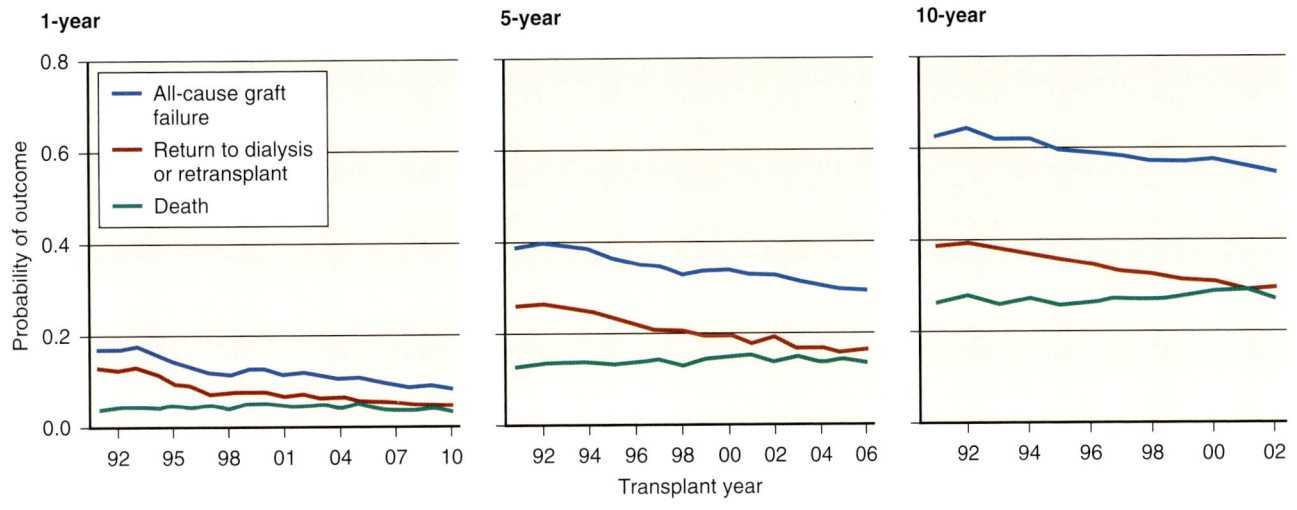

Figure 72.8 Secular trends in 1-, 5-, and 10-year mortality and graft failure for first-time adult deceased donor transplant recipients.

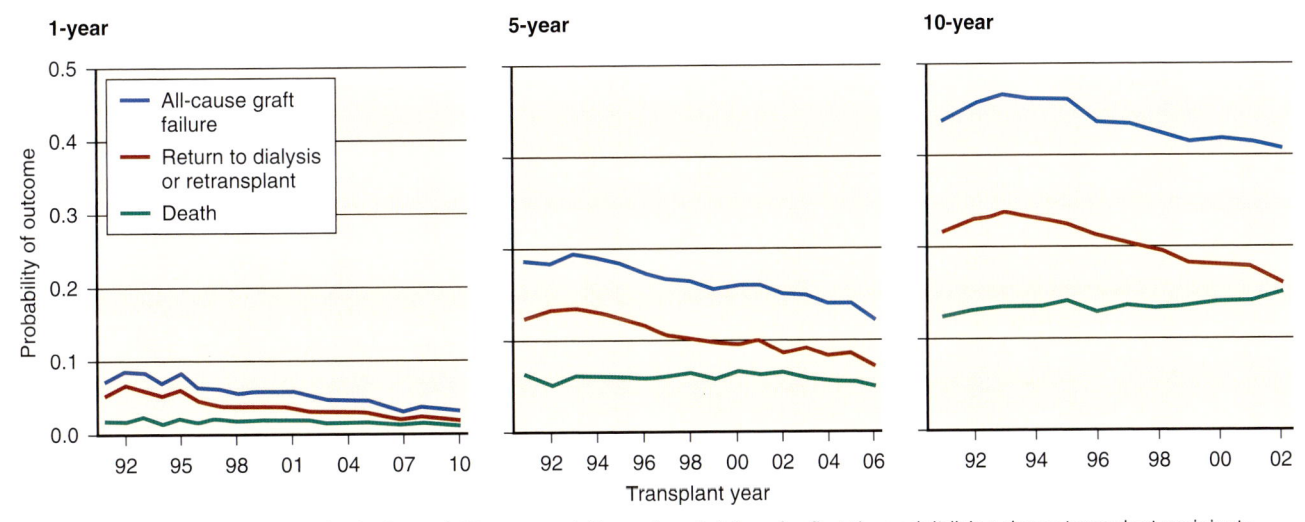

Figure 72.9 Secular trends in 1-, 5-, and 10-year mortality and graft failure for first-time adult living donor transplant recipients.

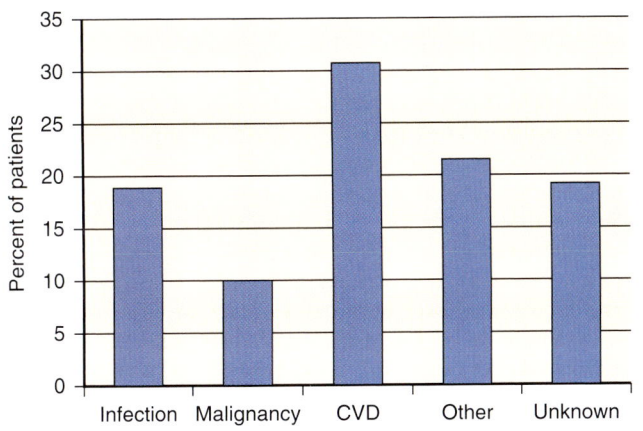

Figure 72.10 Causes of death with a functioning graft in adult first-time kidney transplant recipients, 2007 to 2011. CVD, Cardiovascular disease.

donor-recipient factors. Many of them contribute to the development of chronic allograft injury and have been discussed above.

DONOR-RECIPIENT FACTORS

Delayed Graft Function

DGF is associated with poorer allograft and patient survival and poorer allograft function.[236] Registry data have shown that DGF reduces allograft half-life by 30%, a larger effect than early acute rejection.[237] Even though CITs have steadily decreased from 24 to 18 hours over the past 20 years, the incidence of DGF in deceased donor transplants has remained at approximately 25%.[3]

Human Leukocyte Antigen Matching

Registry data have demonstrated that even with current immunosuppression regimens, better HLA-matched allografts have better survival.[238,239] This benefit applies to living and deceased donor kidneys. The difference in

10-year graft survival between the best and worst HLA matches was 10%, with half-lives from 11.6 to 8.6 years. Evidence suggests that the benefits of HLA matching are diminishing in deceased donor recipients and are much less pronounced in living donor recipients, although a large survival advantage is still seen in those with two haplotype matches.[240] In the 11% of living donor transplants that were HLA-matched 10-year graft survival was 74% compared to 58% for HLA-mismatched transplants. The half-lives for HLA-matched and HLA-mismatched living donor transplants were 27 and 15 years, respectively.

Cytomegalovirus Status of Donor and Recipient

Registry data have shown a small but definite association of donor and recipient CMV serologic status with kidney allograft and recipient survival (hazard ratio, 1.1).[241] Donor-negative–recipient-negative pairings have the best outcomes, whereas donor-positive–recipient-negative pairings have the worst. Cytomegalovirus probably affects graft outcomes through overt infection, but subclinical effects on immune function may also be important.

Timing of Transplantation

In the case of living donor transplantation, there is evidence that preemptive (before initiation of dialysis) transplantation is associated with a lower risk of acute rejection and allograft failure.[242] Other retrospective studies have shown that longer time on dialysis is independently associated with poorer graft and patient survival.[243,244] In 2012, 15% of all living donor transplantations were preemptive. Minimizing time on dialysis has many potential benefits; this strategy should thus be pursued whenever possible.[3,245]

Center Effect

Not surprisingly, reported outcomes have varied among transplantation centers.[246] This reflects normal statistical variance as well as center expertise. Outcomes are confounded by many donor and recipient factors that differ across centers.[247] USRDS data have suggested minimal difference in outcomes among small and large U.S. transplantation centers.[248]

DONOR FACTORS

The quality of the kidney immediately before transplantation has a major impact on long-term graft function and the risk of developing chronic allograft injury.

Donor Source: Deceased Versus Living Donor

The donor source is one of the most important predictors of short- and long-term allograft outcomes. In general, living donor allografts are superior to deceased donor allografts (see Figures 72.8 and 72.9). This benefit applies across all degrees of HLA mismatching. The better outcomes reflect several factors, such as the good health of living donors, absence of brain death, benefits of elective as opposed to semiemergency surgery, minimization of ischemia-reperfusion injury, higher nephron mass, and the effects of a shorter time on or complete avoidance of dialysis. Excellent results also occur with living unrelated kidney transplantation.[239] Potential donors must be fully informed of the donation process in all its aspects..[249] Overall, the relationship of outcome to transplant kidney donor source further emphasizes the importance of the healthy transplant kidney effect. Allograft outcomes are superior from deceased donors with trauma as opposed to nontrauma being the cause of death.[250]

Donor Age

Older kidney donor age is associated with reduced kidney transplant survival. A donor age effect is apparent among deceased and living donor transplants.[3,251] These results are thought to reflect a higher incidence of DGF and nephron underdosing. Allografts from older donors have fewer functioning nephrons because of the aging process[252] as well as donor-related conditions such as hypertension and atherosclerosis. However, because of the organ donor shortage, older deceased donor kidneys are being increasingly used. Donor age younger than 5 years is also associated with poorer outcomes, reflecting higher rates of technical complications and probably nephron underdosing (see later). En bloc transplantation (two kidneys) from donors aged 0 to 5 years significantly improves survival, however.

Donor Gender

There is evidence that allografts from female donors have slightly poorer survival.[253] Again, this probably reflects a nephron underdosing effect (see later), because women have a smaller kidney mass than men. However, female recipients of male kidneys may have poorer graft survival related to the immune response to antigens encoded by the Y chromosome,[254-256]

Donor Population Ancestry and Ethnicity

Deceased donor allografts from African Americans are at greater risk of loss.[257] There is increasing evidence that much of the increased risk of graft loss associated with African American donated kidneys is attributable to the presence of the apolipoprotein L1 (APOL1) high-risk variant (16% of African American donors in one study). African American–donated kidneys from donors lacking the APOL1 high-risk variant have outcomes comparable to those of non-African American–donated kidneys.[258,259]

Donor Nephron Mass

An imbalance between the metabolic and excretory demands of the recipient and the functional transplant mass has been postulated to play a role in the development and progression of chronic allograft injury (see Figure 72.6). Nephron underdosing, exacerbated by perioperative ischemic damage and postoperative nephrotoxic drugs, might lead to nephron overwork and eventual failure, similar to the mechanisms occurring in native, progressive, kidney disease. Thus, kidneys from small donors transplanted into recipients with a large body surface area or large body mass index would be at highest risk of this problem. There is support for this hypothesis from animal[260] and retrospective human studies.[261-263]

Cold Ischemia Time

Prolonged CIT is associated with higher risk of DGF and poorer allograft survival.[128,264] Registry data have suggested that a CIT longer than 24 hours is particularly deleterious to the graft.

Expanded Criteria Donors and Kidney Donor Profile Index

As the discrepancy between the numbers of patients awaiting kidney transplantation and available organs increases, many centers worldwide are now using ECD allografts. ECD kidneys are defined by donor characteristics associated with a 70% greater risk of allograft failure when compared to a reference group of nonhypertensive donors aged 10 to 39 years whose cause of death was not a cerebrovascular accident (CVA) and whose terminal creatinine level is less than 1.5 mg/dL.[265] ECD kidneys are defined as kidneys from all donors who are 60 years of age or older, or donors aged 50 to 59 years who also meet two of the following criteria: (1) CVA as cause of death; (2) history of hypertension; or (3) terminal creatinine level more than 1.5 mg/dL. ECD kidneys are associated with a 70% greater risk of allograft failure when compared to nonhypertensive donors aged 10 to 39 years whose cause of death is not a cerebrovascular accident (CVA) and whose terminal creatinine level is less than 1.5 mg/dL.[265] Survival of ECD kidneys is, on average, shorter for two general reasons: (1) the baseline GFR of these kidneys is likely lower; and (2) ECD kidneys tend to be transplanted into older recipients, who have higher rates of posttransplantation death. However, older patients have a higher risk of mortality while awaiting transplantation and have been shown to benefit from ECD kidney transplantation.[266]

In the United States, a new allocation system has recently replaced the previous standard and expanded criteria deceased donor categories, with a single pool of kidneys graded using the kidney donor profile index (KDPI). The KDPI score is calculated using 10 donor characteristics and is a modified version of the predictive tool first described by Rao and associates.[257] The KDPI is expressed as a percentile score, with 0 and 100% signifying excellent quality and marginal organs, respectively. To maximize the utility of the deceased donor organ supply, deceased donor kidneys with a KDPI less than 20% will be allocated to candidates with the highest posttransplantation life expectancy, as judged by the four-variable, estimated posttransplantation survival (EPTS) score. Older candidates, for whom long waiting times represent a barrier to transplantation, who would previously have agreed to receipt of an ECD kidney, may now choose to accept deceased donor kidneys with a high KDPI value (>85%).

Donation after Cardiac Death (DCD)

There has been a significant increase in the use of DCD kidneys.[267] DCD donors can be subclassified as uncontrolled or controlled. Uncontrolled donors are those who are unsuccessfully resuscitated or present dead on arrival to hospital, while controlled donors suffer a cardiac arrest following the withdrawal of life support in the controlled environment of the ICU or operating room immediately prior to donation. The duration of warm ischemia time is likely to be significantly greater in the setting of uncontrolled donation.[268] Protocols for managing DCD kidneys vary from center to center. In uncontrolled donation, isolated perfusion of the kidneys with cold preservation solution can be achieved using double-balloon aortic catheterization, with balloons inflated in the aorta above and below the renal arteries, to minimize warm ischemia time. Short-term outcomes (e.g., rates of DGF, primary nonfunction) are inferior to those of brain-dead donors. However, long-term outcomes of DCD organs (from donors < 50 years old) are similar to those from standard deceased donors.[269]

RECIPIENT FACTORS

Recipient Age

In general, allograft survival rates are poorer in those at the extremes of age—that is, younger than 18 or older than 65 years of age.[3,270] In the very young, technical causes of graft loss such as vessel thrombosis are relatively more common. Acute rejection is also a more common cause of allograft loss; conversely, death with a functioning graft is relatively rare. Death with a functioning allograft is a much more common cause of graft loss in older adults (responsible for >50% of graft failures). Conversely, acute rejection may be less common. Thus, although RCTs are not available to inform practice definitively, it seems reasonable, in general, to use less aggressive immunosuppression in older patients.[271]

Recipient Race and Ethnicity

African American recipients have poorer allograft survival compared with that of whites.[272] This probably reflects multiple factors, including higher incidence of DGF, higher incidence of acute and late acute rejection, stronger immune responsiveness, predominantly white donor pool (with resultant poorer matching of HLA and non-HLA antigens), altered pharmacokinetics of immunosuppressive drugs, and higher prevalence of hypertension. Socioeconomic factors, including the ability to pay for transplantation medications and access to high-quality medical care, unfortunately may also play a role.[273] There is some evidence that African Europeans have equivalent outcomes to whites in Europe.[274] Asian and Hispanic recipients have superior outcomes to whites; the reasons for this are unknown.[272] Strategies that may improve outcomes in African American recipients include diligent use of higher doses of immunosuppression and attention to social factors that may limit access to health care or medications.[275] Increasing living donations from African American donors is also desirable. Predonation screening for the ApoL1 high-risk genotype in donors of African descent may improve African American living donor safety and recipient outcomes.[258]

Recipient Gender

Registry studies of the association of recipient gender with transplantation outcomes have yielded differing results. In the CTS database, female recipients had slightly better allograft survival than male recipients of deceased donor kidneys or HLA-identical living donor kidneys.[253] Data from U.S. transplant centers have shown better allograft survival in male as opposed to female recipients of living donor kidneys.[276] An important difference between female and male transplantation candidates is the higher degree of sensitization of the former to HLA antigens, as well as to non-HLA antigens. Women tend to be more sensitized because of pregnancy and possibly as a result of more blood transfusions because of anemia related to menstruation. An immune response to H-Y antigens by female recipients may play a role, although the generally larger nephron dose in male donors may be a confounding factor in registry analyses.

Recipient Sensitization

Patients who are highly sensitized generally have poorer early and late graft survival compared with nonsensitized recipients. This is mainly related to an increased incidence of complications in the early posttransplantation period, such as DGF and acute rejection. The principle reasons for sensitization are previous transplants, pregnancy, and blood transfusion. Thus, allograft survival is poorer in recipients of subsequent transplants compared with recipients of a first transplant.[277] Highly sensitized patients have longer wait times until transplantation and are usually given more intensive immunosuppression. Improvements in desensitization protocols have offered such patients better access to transplantation.[278,279]

Acute Rejection

Acute rejection remains a significant risk factor for allograft loss. Even when acute rejection is successfully treated, some irreversible graft injury has likely occurred. Such damage accentuates the effects of poor-quality donor tissue, perioperative ischemic injury, and nephron underdosing. Acute rejection refractory to steroids, acute rejection with a humoral component, and late acute rejection have particularly negative impacts on allograft and patient outcomes.[233] Although current immunosuppressive regimens have steadily decreased rates of acute rejection, major improvements in long-term allograft survival have not been observed.[233]

Recipient Immunosuppression

Undoubtedly, improvements in the acute rejection rate and allograft survival reflect the effectiveness of modern antirejection drugs, such as the CNIs and MMF. The contribution of long-term calcineurin nephrotoxicity, particularly with currently used maintenance doses, to chronic kidney allograft dysfunction and loss remains controversial (see earlier, "Late Allograft Dysfunction and Late Allograft Loss"). For now, CNIs remain the cornerstone of immunosuppression.[280] Registry data have shown that the most common immunosuppression regimen used in the United States is tacrolimus and MMF with or without steroid.

Recipient Compliance

Poor compliance with the immunosuppressive regimen markedly increases the risk of acute rejection (particularly late acute rejection) and allograft loss.[281] Allograft loss has been reported to be sevenfold higher in nonadherent patients.[282] Efforts are being made to improve strategies to prevent nonadherence.[283] Noncompliance is a particularly difficult problem in pediatric transplantation.[281,284]

Recipient Body Size

Morbid obesity (grade 2 or higher), corresponding to a Quételet body mass index (BMI) of 35 kg/m^2 or greater, is associated with more transplantation surgery–related complications, more DGF, and poorer allograft survival.[285,286] Even grade 1 obesity (BMI = 30 to 34.9 kg/m^2) is a risk factor for allograft failure. Poorer long-term graft survival probably reflects the effects of DGF, nephron overwork, and more difficult dosing of immunosuppressive drugs. Nevertheless, a study of patients with a BMI greater than 30 kg/m^2 has suggested that transplantation provides a survival benefit over remaining on the waiting list (on dialysis), at least up to a BMI of 41 kg/m^2.[287] Bariatric surgery prior to transplantation is an option for morbidly obese patients.[288] The issue of nephron underdosing has been discussed in regard to donor factors (see earlier) but also relates to its interaction with the recipient's size. Body surface area (BSA) has been used as a surrogate measure for donor nephron mass and recipient metabolic demand. Gross mismatch (i.e., low donor BSA and high recipient BSA) has been associated with poorer long-term allograft survival.[262,263]

Recipient Cause of End-Stage Kidney Disease

Diabetes mellitus as the primary cause of ESKD is a risk factor for allograft failure due to death with a functioning graft.

Recipient History of Hepatitis C

Hepatitis C antibody positivity is a risk factor for allograft failure due to premature graft failure and death with a functioning graft.[289]

Recipient Hypertension

Good blood pressure control (systolic blood pressure <140 mm Hg) is important for graft survival. It is associated with improved allograft and patient survival.[290]

RECURRENCE OF PRIMARY DISEASE

As discussed earlier, determining the incidence and prevalence of recurrent or de novo kidney disease is difficult. An Australian study of patients with biopsy-proven glomerulonephritis found a 10-year incidence of graft loss from recurrence of 8.4%.[215] However, patients whose primary kidney disease was biopsy-proven glomerulonephritis had allograft survival comparable to patients with nonglomerulitis causes. As kidney allograft survival improves, recurrent or de novo disease is being increasingly diagnosed and is recognized as an important cause of late graft loss.[206]

PROTEINURIA

Proteinuria, even when modest, is associated with poorer allograft survival.[291]

IMPROVING KIDNEY ALLOGRAFT OUTCOMES: MATCHING KIDNEY AND RECIPIENT RISK

The number of kidney transplant candidates far outweighs the number of available organs. First, maximizing the number of deceased and living organs available for transplantation is a key goal for national transplantation programs. Organ donor cards, education of medical staff and family members, and expanded criteria donor and DCD programs have all positively influenced deceased donor rates. Unfortunately, in the United States, living donation rates have fallen despite increased access to donor exchange programs[292] and desensitization protocols.[279]

A second parallel goal is to maximize the life span of donated organs. In this respect, the criteria used for allocation of deceased donor allografts can have an important effect on overall allograft survival. A purely utilitarian approach to maximize allograft survival would direct organs only to the youngest and healthiest, maximizing the life years from transplantation (LYFT) gained.[293] In practice, a balance must be struck between utility and equity, ensuring that anyone medically fit for a transplant has a reasonable chance of obtaining one. In many countries, this balance is achieved by means of a point system, with points being awarded for characteristics such as fewer HLA mismatches and time on the waiting list. There is evidence that preferential allocation of organs of younger donors to younger recipients (as opposed to the current system, where some organs of younger donors are transplanted into older patients) would significantly improve overall allograft survival.[294] In the United States, a new allocation system was instituted in late 2014. This system will match the 20% highest quality deceased donor kidneys with the top 20% of candidates to maximize the usefulness of the best organs (see earlier, "Expanded Criteria Donors and Kidney Donor Profile Index").

MEDICAL MANAGEMENT OF TRANSPLANT RECIPIENTS

More emphasis is being placed on the general medical management of patients who have received a transplant. Comprehensive practice guidelines on the care of KTRs were published by the American Society of Transplantation and European Best Practice Guidelines Expert Group in 2000 and 2002, respectively.[295,296] More recently, KDIGO (Kidney Disease: Improving Global Outcomes) has published its evidenced-based *2009 KDIGO Clinical Practice Guideline for the Care of Kidney Transplant Recipients.*[149] Reflecting the paucity of quality evidence, only 25% of the KDIGO graded guidelines were level 1 ("we recommend") and 75% were level 2 ("we suggest"). The evidence supporting the guidelines was of low or very low quality in almost 85%. There is much opportunity for improving our understanding and management of transplant recipient care.

Transplantation is generally preferable to dialysis, but there is an increased appreciation that the posttransplantation state is often one of chronic kidney disease (CKD). The management of common electrolyte, endocrine, and cardiovascular complications posttransplantation is discussed in the following sections.

ELECTROLYTE DISORDERS

HYPERCALCEMIA AND HYPOPHOSPHATEMIA

Hypercalcemia is common and is due mainly to persistent hyperparathyroidism or the overzealous administration of calcium and vitamin D. The management of posttransplantation hyperparathyroidism is discussed later. Hypophosphatemia is also common in the early posttransplantation period, particularly when allograft function is excellent. This is due to a combination of reduced phosphate absorption (vitamin D depletion is common) and urinary phosphate wasting, which is a consequence of high fibroblast growth factor 23 (FGF-23) and parathyroid hormone (PTH) levels and the tubular effects of CNIs, sirolimus, and high-dose steroids.[297] Rarely, phosphate depletion is severe enough to cause profound muscle weakness, including respiratory muscle weakness. Phosphate normalizes in most patients by 1 year posttransplantation, mirroring posttransplantation declines in the fractional excretion of phosphate, PTH, and FGF-23.[298] In the longer term, persistent negative phosphate balance likely contributes to posttransplantation bone disease. Treatment involves a diet high in phosphorus (e.g., inclusion of low-fat dairy products) and vitamin D replacement. Overaggressive replacement of phosphate posttransplantation can lower calcium and vitamin D levels and potentially exacerbate hyperparathyroidism.[299] In addition, acute phosphate nephropathy has been reported in posttransplantation recipients on phosphate replacement.[300] We tend to reserve oral phosphate supplements for patients with a phosphate level lower than 1 to 1.5 mg/dL or symptomatic hypophosphatemia.

HYPERKALEMIA

Mild hyperkalemia is common, even with good allograft function. The principle cause is CNI-induced impairment of tubular potassium secretion. A recent study has suggested that tacrolimus activates the thiazide-sensitive, renal sodium-chloride cotransporter (NCC), resulting in hypertension and reduced renal potassium excretion.[301] Hyperkalemia may be exacerbated by poor allograft function, ingestion of excess potassium, hyperglycemia, and medicines such as ACEIs and β-blockers. Because the hyperkalemia is usually not severe and typically improves with reduction in CNI dosage, additional treatment is often not required; exacerbating factors should be minimized. In an occasional case, treatment with the mineralocorticoid fludrocortisone will be necessary. Hyperkalemia can also be caused by an amiloride-like effect of trimethoprim, a component of TMP-SMX, that is frequently used for prophylaxis against *Pneumocystis jiroveci*.

METABOLIC ACIDOSIS

Mild metabolic acidosis is also common and often associated with hyperkalemia. In most cases, it has the features of a distal (hyperchloremic) renal tubular acidosis. This reflects tubular dysfunction caused by CNIs, rejection, or residual hyperparathyroidism (and the effect of TMP, as above). Alkali repletion with oral bicarbonate may be necessary.

OTHER ELECTROLYTE ABNORMALITIES

Hypomagnesemia is common and due to a magnesuric effect of the CNIs, as well as to residual hyperparathyroidism, and is usually asymptomatic. Magnesium supplements are sometimes prescribed when the plasma magnesium level is less than 1.5 mg/dL. However, their effectiveness is limited, they can cause diarrhea, and they add more complexity to the multidrug regimen of the transplant recipient.

BONE DISORDERS AFTER KIDNEY TRANSPLANTATION

Bone disease in the ESKD patient is multifactorial and involves varying degrees of hyperparathyroidism (osteitis fibrosa cystica), vitamin D deficiency, low bone turnover, aluminum intoxication (osteomalacia), and amyloidosis (see Chapter 55). Unfortunately, bone disease can remain a problem after transplantation owing to persistence of the conditions discussed above and the superimposed effects of immunosuppressants on bone.

HYPERPARATHYROIDISM

Residual hyperparathyroidism is very common in the first posttransplant year, but can persist for years. One study found elevated serum PTH levels in 23 of 42 (54%) normocalcemic patients with plasma creatinine levels less than 2 mg/dL more than 2 years after transplantation.[302] Not surprisingly, the main risk factors for posttransplant hyperparathyroidism are the degree of pretransplant hyperparathyroidism and duration of dialysis.[303] Inadequate vitamin D stores and poor allograft function (de novo secondary hyperparathyroidism) probably contribute to persistence of the condition in some patients.

Typically, posttransplant hyperparathyroidism is manifest by a low plasma phosphate level and a mild to moderate elevation in the plasma calcium level. The serum PTH level is inappropriately high for the level of plasma calcium. Posttransplant hyperparathyroidism is often asymptomatic and tends to improve with time. Therapy with paricalcitol has been shown to increase the likelihood of resolution of hyperparathyroidism at 1 year posttransplantation.[304] However, active vitamin D analogs must be used with caution and stopped if the plasma calcium level rises above the normal range or complications of hypercalcemia occur. The calcimimetic cinacalcet has been shown to lower serum PTH and calcium levels safely and effectively and raise serum phosphate concentrations in a placebo-controlled study of KTRs with persistent hyperparathyroidism.[305]

There are two main indications for posttransplantation parathyroidectomy: (1) severe symptomatic hypercalcemia (in the early posttransplantation period, now rare, and usually managed medically with cinacalcet and/or bisphosphonate); and (2) persistent, moderately severe hypercalcemia (serum calcium level ≥ 12.0 to 12.5 mg/dL) for more than 1 year after transplantation or calcific uremic arteriolopathy (calciphylaxis), a rare complication following transplantation. Subtotal parathyroidectomy is the procedure of choice.

GOUT

The most important cause of hyperuricemia and gout after transplantation are the CNIs, particularly cyclosporine. The CNIs impair renal uric acid clearance. Approximately 80% of CNI-treated KTRs develop hyperuricemia, and about 13% develop new-onset gout.[306] Diuretic use may exacerbate hyperuricemia and precipitate a gout attack.

Acute gout should be treated with colchicine or high-dose steroids; NSAIDs should generally be avoided. Colchicine-induced neuromyopathy is more common in patients with impaired kidney function and in cyclosporine-treated (and presumably tacrolimus-treated) patients due to an increase in colchicine levels. Therefore, the lowest effective dose of colchicine should be used, and patients should be monitored for muscle weakness. For prevention of further gouty attacks, allopurinol is generally used. Note that the metabolism of azathioprine is inhibited by allopurinol. Ideally, these drugs should not be coprescribed. If azathioprine must be used in conjunction with allopurinol, then the azathioprine dose should be reduced by at least 75% of the original dose and the CBC closely monitored. A safer alternative is to change azathioprine to MMF; no adjustment of MMF is required. The newer xanthine oxidase inhibitor febuxostat has also been successfully used in hyperuricemic kidney transplantation patients.[307] The packaging insert for febuxostat warns against concurrent azathioprine use. In cases of severe recurrent gout, it may be worthwhile to stop CNIs altogether. The uricouric agent probenecid may be cautiously used in KTRs with excellent renal function. The uricase pegloticase remains untested in the transplantation population.

CALCINEURIN INHIBITOR–ASSOCIATED BONE PAIN

A syndrome of severe bone pain in the lower limbs has been associated with CNI use. This is uncommon and thought to represent a vasomotor effect of the CNIs. Osteonecrosis and other common bone lesions should be excluded before the diagnosis is made. Symptoms usually respond to reduction in CNI dosage and administration of calcium channel blockers. Magnetic resonance imaging (MRI) of the involved bones may show bone marrow edema.[308]

OSTEONECROSIS

Osteonecrosis (avascular necrosis) is a serious bone complication of kidney transplantation. The pathogenesis is not well understood, but high doses of steroids are one risk factor. Up to 8% of KTRs develop osteonecrosis of the hips[309]; this figure is falling with lower dose steroid protocols.[310] The most commonly affected site is the femoral head; other sites are the humeral head, femoral condyles, proximal tibia, vertebrae, and small bones of the hand and foot. Many patients have bilateral involvement at the time of diagnosis. The principal symptom is pain; signs are nonspecific. Diagnosis is made by imaging studies—MRI is the most sensitive, plain radiography is the least sensitive, and scintigraphy is intermediate. However, MRI abnormalities do not always imply clinically significant osteonecrosis. Treatment remains controversial. Options include resting the joint, decompression, and joint replacement.

OSTEOPOROSIS

Osteoporosis is a common bone disorder characterized by a parallel reduction in bone mineral and bone matrix so that bone mass is decreased but is of normal composition. The most commonly used definition is that based on the World Health Organization scoring system. Osteoporosis is defined as bone density greater than 2.5 SDs (standard deviation) below the mean bone density of gender-matched, young adults (T-score); osteopenia is defined as 1.0 to 2.5 SDs below the T-score. In the general population, reduced bone mineral density is strongly associated with fracture risk.

Reduction in bone mineral density is now recognized as a very common complication of kidney transplantation. Most bone loss occurs in the first 6 months posttransplant.[311] Risk factors for posttransplant osteoporosis include steroid use, ongoing hyperparathyroidism, vitamin D deficiency or resistance, and phosphate depletion. Diabetes mellitus is also associated with an increased risk of posttransplant fracture. The risk of hip fracture in KTRs is as high at 3.3 to 3.8 events/1000 person-years; KTRs have a 34% increased risk of fracture early posttransplantation when compared to dialysis patients on the transplant waiting list. The risk of hip fracture in wait-listed dialysis patients and transplant recipients subsequently equalizes by 2 years posttransplant.[312]

Bone mineral density (BMD), as measured by dual energy X-ray absorptiometry (DEXA), has been shown to predict fractures in the general population.[313] Surprisingly, the effects of steroid avoidance and minimization protocols on BMD and fracture rates in the kidney transplant population have been somewhat contradictory, with some studies finding an association with reduced fracture rates and improved BMD, while others have identified no beneficial association.[310,314-316] Treatment with bisphosphonates early posttransplantation has been shown to prevent bone loss when compared to controls but may exacerbate preexisting adynamic bone disease.[317] Perhaps as a consequence, bisphosphonates have not been shown to reduce fracture rates in KTRs.[318] Notably, bisphosphonates are not recommended in patients with a GFR lower than 30 mL/min/1.73 m^2. A number of studies have shown a favorable effect for vitamin D derivatives, with or without calcium supplementation, on BMD in KTRs.[319,320] In patients with persistent posttransplantation hyperparathyroidism and hypercalcemia, cinacalcet treatment may improve BMD in addition to serum calcium and PTH levels.[321]

Current KDIGO guidelines recommend monitoring of calcium, phosphate, and PTH levels posttransplantation. DEXA scanning is recommended in the first 3 months posttransplantation for patients on steroids or with risk factors for osteoporosis and a GFR higher than 30 mL/min/1.73 m^2. For KTRs within 1 year of transplantation, with a GFR higher than 30 mL/min/1.73 m^2 and low BMD, treatment with vitamin D, vitamin D, calcitriol or alfacalcidol, or bisphosphonate should be considered.[149]

POSTTRANSPLANTATION DIABETES MELLITUS

PTDM, formerly referred to as new-onset diabetes after transplantation (NODAT), is common after kidney transplantation. First-time KTRs in the United States from 2004 to 2008 had a 3-year cumulative incidence of posttransplantation diabetes of over 40%. Risk factors include older age, obesity, positive HCV antibody, CMV infection status, nonwhite ethnicity, family history, steroids, CNIs (especially tacrolimus), and episodes of acute rejection. Strategies to prevent and treat PTDM include steroid minimization, avoidance of tacrolimus, and lifestyle modification. The adoption of steroid-free immunosuppression regimens at discharge after kidney transplantation has been shown to reduce the odds of developing PTDM.[322,323] A small Austrian study reported a reduction in PTDM at 1 year in patients whose blood glucose level was strictly maintained with insulin immediately posttransplantation versus those who received standard management of their blood glucose level.[324]

Unfortunately, PTDM is associated with reduced graft and patient survival.[325] PTDM may require treatment with oral agents or insulin. Metformin is probably the drug of choice in KTRs with an adequate GFR because it is the most effective in reducing complications of type 2 diabetes mellitus, but its propensity for inducing lactic acidosis in the setting of impaired kidney function, albeit rare, must be considered.[231] Targeting a hemoglobin A$_{1c}$ (HbA$_{1c}$) level of 7.0% to 7.5% and avoiding HbA$_{1c}$ of 6.0% or less is recommended based on recent trials in the general diabetic population, which showed no cardiovascular benefit and more frequent complications related to intensive glucose-lowering therapy.[149]

CARDIOVASCULAR DISEASE

Cardiovascular disease is a leading cause of death in KTRs.[326] Despite pretransplantation screening, the cumulative incidences of myocardial infarction (MI), stroke, and de novo peripheral arterial disease are 11%, 7%, and 24%, respectively.[327-329] De novo congestive heart failure is also common.[330] The KTR population is enriched with traditional cardiovascular risk factors such as smoking, diabetes mellitus, and hypertension and are also burdened with nontraditional CKD-related and transplantation-associated risk factors.[331,332] Aspirin is an effective therapy for the primary and secondary prevention of cardiovascular disease in the general population[333,334] However, one study has shown marked variability in the use of cardioprotective medications, including aspirin, in KTRs.[335]

SMOKING

Tobacco smoking should be strongly discouraged; there is evidence that it affects allograft function as well as recipient survival.[336]

HYPERTENSION

The prevalence of hypertension in the CNI era is at least 60% to 80%.[149] Causes include use of steroids, CNIs, weight gain, allograft dysfunction, native kidney disease, and TRAS. The complications of posttransplantation hypertension are presumed to be a heightened risk of cardiovascular disease and allograft failure.

The new Joint National Committee Guidelines (JNC 8) revised its recommended blood pressure target for patients with CKD to 140/90 mm Hg or lower.[337] A recent post hoc analysis of the FAVORIT (Folic Acid for Vascular Outcome Reduction in Transplantation) trial found that each increase of 20 mm Hg in baseline systolic blood pressure was associated with 32% and 13% increases in the adjusted relative risks of cardiovascular events and death, respectively. In contrast, each 10-mm Hg drop in diastolic blood pressure below 70 mm Hg was associated with a 31% increase in the relative risks of cardiovascular events and death, possibly due to the association of pulse pressure with vascular stiffness and the association of vascular stiffness with left ventricular hypertrophy, arrhythmia, and sudden death. The highest risk was seen in patients with a systolic blood pressure higher than 140 mm Hg and diastolic blood pressure lower than 70 mm Hg.[338]

Nonpharmacologic measures such as weight loss, reduced sodium intake, reduced alcohol intake, treatment of obstructive sleep apnea, and increased exercise should be encouraged. The dosage of steroids and CNIs should be minimized. However, antihypertensive drug therapy is still frequently required. There is little evidence for one antihypertensive drug class over another. Results from retrospective studies in the kidney transplantation population have been conflicting regarding the benefits of angiotensin receptor blockade.[339,340] We routinely use ACEIs and ARBs, especially in patients with proteinuria, diabetes, or other cardiovascular indications (Table 72.12). KDIGO guidelines have suggested the use of any class of antihypertensive medication,

Table 72.12 Recommended Antihypertensive Agents in the Transplant Recipient

Indication	β-Blockers	ACEI	ARB	Diuretic	Calcium Channel Blocker
Hypertension only		X	X	X	X
CHF	X	X	X		
Post-MI	X	X	X		
CAD	X	X	X		
Diabetes		X	X		

ACEI, Angiotensin-converting enzyme inhibitor; ARB, angiotensin receptor blocker; CAD, coronary artery disease; CHF, congestive heart failure; MI, myocardial infarction.

Adapted from James PA, Oparil S, Carter BL, et al: 2014 evidence-based guideline for the management of high blood pressure in adults: report from the panel members appointed to the Eighth Joint National Committee (JNC 8). JAMA 311:507-520, 2014.

provided that adverse side effects and potential drug-drug interactions are monitored closely.[149]

HYPERLIPIDEMIA

The prevalence of hyperlipidemia after transplantation is very high.[341] Steroids, CNIs (cyclosporine more than tacrolimus), and sirolimus are the principal causes. Some studies have suggested that hyperlipidemia is associated with poorer allograft outcomes, although no causal relationship has been established. The American Heart Association guidelines (for the general population) have deemphasized the importance of cholesterol level on the decision to treat with statin and highlighted the importance of assessing cardiovascular risk. High-intensity statin is recommended for the following: (1) patients between 21 and 75 years of age with atherosclerotic cardiovascular disease; (2) patients with a low-density lipoprotein (LDL) level higher than 190 mg/dL (moderate intensity is recommended those older than 75 years or those who are not candidates for high-intensity statin); and (3) those aged 40 to 75 years with diabetes mellitus and an estimated 10-year cardiovascular risk higher than 7.5%. Moderate intensity statin is recommended for the following: (1) persons aged 40 to 75 years with diabetes mellitus and an estimated 10-year cardiovascular risk lower than 7.5%; (2) nondiabetics 40 to 75 years of age with an estimated 10-year cardiovascular risk higher than 5%; and (3) those patients older than 75 years with atherosclerotic cardiovascular disease..[342] The application of a risk-guided statin treatment algorithm in the kidney transplantation population seems like a reasonable approach. The only caveat is that the starting dose of a statin should be reduced in KTRs because the CNIs (especially cyclosporine) increase statin blood levels and may predispose to statin-related toxicities.[343]

The main RCT of statin therapy in KTRs showed no benefit in the primary outcome—composite of cardiac death, nonfatal MI, or coronary intervention procedure.[344] However, follow-up after an additional 2 years of statin therapy showed a significantly reduced risk of major cardiac events.[345] As in the general population, statin use is associated with an increased risk hyperglycemia in KTRs.[346]

Hypertriglyceridemia can be a problem posttransplantation. Strategies for lowering triglyceride levels include lifestyle modification, substitution of sirolimus for an alternative agent (e.g., MMF), and treatment with ezetimibe.

The high prevalence of metabolic syndrome, a consequence of dysregulation of glucose and vascular metabolism, is being increasingly recognized in KTRs.[347] Better recognition and management of metabolic syndrome, including control of obesity, glucose, hyperlipidemia, and blood pressure, are expected to decrease the morbidity and mortality of KTRs.

HYPERHOMOCYSTEINEMIA

As in the general population, hyperhomocysteinemia has been proposed as a risk factor for cardiovascular disease in KTRs. Plasma homocysteine concentrations typically fall after transplantation but do not normalize. Based on the results of well-performed RCTs in the general and CKD populations, current interventions to lower homocysteine levels cannot be recommended.[348]

CANCER AFTER KIDNEY TRANSPLANTATION

A number of studies have linked transplant and cancer registry data, giving good insight into posttransplant cancer incidence. Data from the United States and the United Kingdom have shown that KTRs are at considerably greater risk for certain cancers when compared to the general population (Table 72.13).[349-351]

There are several reasons why reported cancer incidence has increased. First, immunosuppression inhibits normal tumor surveillance mechanisms, allowing unchecked proliferation of spontaneously occurring neoplastic cells. There is also experimental evidence that cyclosporine has tumor-promoting effects mediated by its effects on transforming growth factor-β (TGF-β) production[352] and expression of the angiogenic, cytokine, vascular endothelial growth factor (VEGF).[353] Second, immunosuppression allows uncontrolled proliferation of oncogenic viruses (Table 72.14). Third, factors related to the primary kidney disease (analgesic abuse, certain herbal preparations, HBV or HCV infection) or the ESKD milieu (acquired renal cystic disease) might promote neoplasia.

It is believed that the cumulative amount of immunosuppression rather than a specific drug is the most important factor increasing the cancer risk. However, there is evidence that the routine use of CNIs has increased the risk of skin cancers[354]; fortunately, these are usually not fatal. The long-term impact of currently used powerful

Table 72.13 Cancers Categorized by Standard Incidence Rate (SIR) for Kidney Transplant Patients and Cancer Incidence

Standard Incidence Rate	Common Cancers	Common Cancers in Transplant Population	Rare Cancers
High SIR (>5)	Kaposi's sarcoma (with HIV)	Kaposi's sarcoma, vagina, non-Hodgkin's lymphoma, kidney, skin cancer, nonmelanoma, lip, thyroid, penis, small intestine	Eye
Moderate SIR (>1 to 5; $P < 0.05$)	Lung, colon, cervix, stomach, Hodgkin's disease (liver)	Oronasopharynx, esophagus, bladder, leukemia, lymphoma	Melanoma, larynx, multiple myeloma, anus
No increased risk shown	Breast, prostate	Rectum	Ovary, uterus, pancreas, brain, testis

Adapted from Kasiske BL, Zeier MG, Chapman JR, et al: Kidney disease: Improving global outcomes: KDIGO clinical practice guideline for the care of kidney transplant recipients: a summary. Kidney Int 77:299-311, 2010.

Table 72.14 Viral Infections Associated with Development of Cancers in Kidney Transplant Patients

Virus	Neoplasm
HBV	Hepatocellular cancer
HCV	Hepatocellular cancer
EBV	PTLD
HPV	Squamous cell cancers of anogenital area and mouth
HHV-8	Kaposi's sarcoma

EBV, Epstein-Barr virus; HBV, hepatitis B virus; HCV, hepatitis C virus; HHV-8, human herpes virus-8; HPV, human papillomavirus; PTLD, posttransplantation lymphoproliferative disorder.

immunosuppression regimens on cancer incidence is unknown but is certainly of concern. The single most important measure to prevent cancers is to minimize excess immunosuppression. A general rule is that when cancer occurs, immunosuppression should be greatly decreased. In some cases, rejection of the allograft may result, but the risks and benefits of immunosuppression must be judged on a case-by-case basis.

SKIN AND LIP CANCERS

Squamous cell carcinoma, basal cell carcinoma, and malignant melanoma are all more common in KTRs. The incidence of nonmelanomatous skin cancer in KTRs is 13 times greater than in the general population.[350] Risk factors include time after transplantation, cumulative immunosuppressive dose, exposure to ultraviolet light, fair skin, and human papillomavirus infection. Primary and secondary prevention is important; patients should be specifically counselled on minimizing exposure to ultraviolet light and to self-screen for skin lesions.[149] Retinoids are sometimes used in high-risk patients.[355] Suspicious skin lesions should be surgically excised. In patients with posttransplant squamous cell carcinoma, switching from a CNI to sirolimus reduces the risk of further tumors developing by 44%.

ANOGENITAL CANCERS

Cancers of the vulva, uterine cervix, penis, scrotum, anus, and perianal region are significantly more common in KTRs. Furthermore, these cancers tend to be multifocal and more aggressive than in the general population. Infection with certain human papillomavirus strains is an important risk factor. Secondary prevention measures include yearly physical examination of the anogenital area and, in women, yearly pelvic examinations and cervical histology. Suspicious lesions should be excised, and patients should be closely followed for recurrence.

KAPOSI'S SARCOMA

The incidence of Kaposi's sarcoma in transplant and non-transplant patients depends greatly on ethnic background. Those of Jewish, Arab, and Mediterranean ancestry are at much higher risk. Other risk factors are the cumulative immunosuppressive dose and human herpes virus-8 infection. Visceral (lymph nodes, lungs, gastrointestinal tract) and nonvisceral (skin, conjunctivae, oropharynx) involvement may occur. The prognosis for the former is poor, but for the latter it is good. Treatment involves various combinations of surgical excision, radiotherapy, chemotherapy, and immunotherapy. Immunosuppression, of course, should be reduced or modified. Substitution of sirolimus for CNIs has been reported to stop progression of the disease without sacrificing allograft function.[77]

POSTTRANSPLANTATION LYMPHOPROLIFERATIVE DISORDER

PTLD is one of the most feared complications of transplantation because it can occur early after transplantation and carries a high morbidity and mortality. The cumulative 3-year incidence of PTLD is 0.5% in adult and 1.5% in pediatric KTRs. More than 90% are non-Hodgkin's lymphomas, and most are of recipient B cell origin.[356] Risk factors include the following: (1) EBV-positive donor and EBV-negative recipient; (2) CMV-positive donor and CMV-negative recipient; (3) pediatric recipients (in part because children are more likely to be EBV-naive); and (4) intensity of immunosuppression.[357] Clinical trials of belatacept found high rates of PTLD in EBV-negative subjects; the drug is now contraindicated in patients who are seronegative for EBV.[80]

Table 72.15 Clinical and Pathologic Spectrum of Posttransplantation Lymphoproliferative Disorder (PTLD) and Management

	Early Disease (50%)	Polymorphic PTLD (30%)	Monoclonal PTLD (20%)
Clinical features	Infectious mononucleosis-type illness	Infectious mononucleosis type illness ± weight loss, localizing symptoms	Fever, weight loss, localizing symptoms
Pathology	Preserved architecture; atypical cells infrequent	Intermediate transformed cells	High-grade lymphoma with confluent and marked atypia
Clonality	Polyclonal	Usually polyclonal	Monoclonal
Treatment	Reduce immunosuppression; acyclovir	Reduce immunosuppression; acyclovir; if poor response, then treat as here	Reduce immunosuppression to low-dose steroids only; combination surgery, chemotherapy, radiotherapy, immunotherapy, rituximab
Prognosis	Good	Intermediate	Poor

Important in the pathogenesis of PTLD is the infection and transformation of B cells by EBV; transformed B cells undergo proliferation that is initially polyclonal, but a malignant clone may evolve. Thus, the clinical and histologic spectrum of PTLD at presentation and its treatment can vary greatly (Table 72.15). Extranodal, gastrointestinal tract, and central nervous system involvement is more common than in nontransplant-associated lymphomas. The kidney allograft may be involved. Treatment options for PTLD include immunosuppression reduction, rituximab and CHOP (cyclophosphamide, doxorubicin [Adriamycin], vincristine, and prednisone). Screening high-risk patients (EBV-positive donor/EBV-negative recipient) for EBV viremia in the first year posttransplantation with the institution of rituximab treatment for persistently viremic patients has been shown to reduce PTLD incidence in one small study.[358]

CANCER SCREENING

Since life expectancy in KTRs is significantly improved compared to patients undergoing dialysis, we recommend that patients follow cancer screening guidelines (cervical smear, mammography, colonoscopy) for the general population. We also recommend annual dermatologic screening. Screening for kidney cancer is not advised in the most recent KDIGO guidelines.[149]

INFECTIOUS COMPLICATIONS OF KIDNEY TRANSPLANTATION

The transplant procedure itself and subsequent immunosuppression increase the risk of serious infection. The principal factors determining the type and severity of infection are exposure (in the hospital and community) to potential pathogens and the state of immunosuppression.[359] Factors affecting the net state of immunosuppression include the cumulative amount of immunosuppression, recipient comorbidities (e.g., diabetes, UTI), infection of viruses that affect the immune system (e.g., EBV, CMV, human immunodeficiency virus [HIV], HCV), and the integrity of mucocutaneous barriers.

The patterns of infection after kidney transplant can be roughly divided into three time periods: 0 to 1 month, 1 to 6 months, and more than 6 months after transplantation.[359] These divisions of time serve as guidelines only. Maintenance immunosuppressive regimens are becoming more powerful, and much older patients are undergoing transplant surgery; on the other hand, antimicrobial prophylaxis is becoming more effective. An outline of the pattern of infection according to time after transplantation is shown in Table 72.16.

A general point is that whenever life-threatening infection occurs, immunosuppression should be reduced to an absolute minimum or stopped altogether (so-called stress dose steroids often are required). Prompt diagnosis (e.g., bronchoscopy in patients with pneumonitis) and therapy are essential.[359]

PATTERNS OF INFECTION

Infections in the First Month

Most infections in the first month are standard infections, as would be seen in nontransplantation patients after surgery. Thus, infections of surgical wounds, lungs, and urinary tract and infections related to vascular catheters predominate. Bacterial infections are much more common than fungal ones. Preventive measures include ensuring that donor and recipient are free of overt infection before transplantation, good surgical technique, and SMX-TMP prophylaxis to prevent UTIs.

Infections 1 to 6 Months After Transplantation

Weeks of intensive immunosuppression increase the risk of opportunistic infections. Infections with CMV, EBV, *Listeria monocytogenes*, *P. jiroveci*, and *Nocardia* spp. are relatively common. Preventive measures include antiviral prophylaxis (for 3 to 6 months) and SMX-TMP prophylaxis (for 6 to 12 months).

Infections More Than 6 Months After Transplantation

With gradual reduction in immunosuppression, the risk of long-term infection usually diminishes. However, patients can be roughly divided into two groups based on risk. Those with good ongoing allograft function and no need for late supplemental immunosuppression are at low risk for developing opportunistic infections unless exposure is intense (e.g., to *Nocardia* spp. from soil). In contrast, those with poor allograft function are at higher risk for opportunistic infection. This probably reflects poor allograft function and the fact that many of these patients have received large cumulative doses of immunosuppression.

Table 72.16 Infections After Transplantation According to Time After Transplantation

Time After Transplantation (mo)	Type of Infection
<1	Infection with antimicrobial-resistant species—MRSA, VRE, *Candida* spp. (non–*Candida albicans*); aspiration; catheter infection; wound infection; anastomotic leaks and ischemia; *Clostridium difficile* colitis; donor-derived infection (uncommon)—HSV, LCMV, rhabdovirus (rabies), West Nile virus, HIV, *Trypanosoma cruzi*; recipient-derived infection (colonization)—*Aspergillus*, *Pseudomonas*
1-6	With PCP and antiviral (CMV, HBV) prophylaxis—polyomavirus, BK infection, nephropathy; *C. difficile* colitis; HCV infection; adenovirus infection, influenza; *Cryptococcus neoformans* infection; *Mycobacterium tuberculosis* infection; without prophylaxis—*Pneumocystis jiroveci*; infection with herpesviruses (HSV, VZV, CMV, EBV); HBV infection; infection with *Listeria*, *Nocardia*, *Toxoplasma*, *Strongyloides*, *Leishmania*, *T. cruzi*
>6	Community-acquired pneumonia, UTI; infection with *Aspergillus*, typical molds, *Mucor* spp.; infection with *Nocardia*, *Rhodococcus* spp.; late viral infections—CMV infection; hepatitis (HBV, HCV); HSV encephalitis; community-acquired (SARS, West Nile virus infection); JC polyomavirus infection (PML); skin cancer, lymphoma (PTLD)

BKV, Human polyomavirus BK; CMV, cytomegalovirus; EBV, Epstein-Barr virus; HBV, hepatitis B virus; HCV, hepatitis C virus; HIV, human immunodeficiency virus; HSV, herpes simplex virus; LCMV, lymphocytic choriomeningitis virus; MRSA, methicillin-resistant Staphylococcus aureus; PCP, Pneumocystis jiroveci pneumonia; PML, progressive multifocal leukoencephalopathy; PTLD, posttransplantation lymphoproliferative disease; SARS, severe acute respiratory syndrome; UTI, urinary tract infection; VRE, vancomycin-resistant enterococcus; VZV, varicella-zoster virus.
Adapted from Fishman JA: Infection in solid-organ transplant recipients. N Engl J Med 357:2601-2614, 2007.

Late amplification of immunosuppression may increase the risk of opportunistic infection in any patient. Therefore, any patient receiving a late steroid pulse or antithymoglobulin therapy should be restarted on SMX-TMP with or without anti-CMV prophylaxis (if donor or recipient were CMV-positive). The role of EBV infection in causing PTLD has been discussed earlier; CMV and *P. jiroveci* pneumonia infection are discussed later.

CYTOMEGALOVIRUS

Exposure to CMV (as evidenced by the presence in serum of anti-CMV IgG) increases with age; more than two thirds of adult donors and recipients are latently infected before kidney transplant. Infection may arise from the following: (1) reactivation of latent recipient virus; (2) primary infection with donor-derived virus (transmitted in the allograft or less commonly via blood products); or (3) reactivation of latent donor-derived virus. CMV disease means that there is infection with symptoms, evidence of tissue invasion, or both. The risk of CMV infection or disease is highest in CMV-positive donor/CMV-negative recipient pairings, followed by CMV-positive donor/CMV-positive recipient pairings and then CMV-negative donor/CMV-positive recipient pairings. The risk is lowest with CMV-negative donor/CMV-negative recipient pairings. OKT3/polyclonal antibody therapy, particularly when prescribed for treatment of rejection, significantly increases the risk of subsequent CMV disease.

CMV disease usually arises 1 to 6 months after transplantation, although gastrointestinal and retinal involvement often occurs later. Typical clinical features are fever, malaise, and leukopenia; there may be symptomatic or laboratory evidence of specific organ involvement (Table 72.17). Urgent investigation and immediate empirical treatment are needed in severe cases. Confirmation of presumed CMV disease is by demonstration of the virus in body fluids or solid organs. CMV infection after transplant is usually associated with viremia; CMV viremia may be detected by culture, antigenemia assay, or quantitative PCR. The PCR assay is fast and sensitive and allows the monitoring of viral load in response to therapy. However, viremia may be absent in certain CMV infections, most notably the retina or gastrointestinal tract. In such cases, the CMV infection may be diagnosed by ophthalmologic examination, with or without vitreous humor CMV PCR and immunohistochemistry or culture of gastrointestinal tissue, respectively. Other procedures, such as lumbar puncture and bronchoscopy, should be aggressively pursued according to symptoms and signs. A tissue diagnosis is also required to exclude co-infection with other microbes, such as *P. jiroveci*. In addition to its direct effects, CMV may have indirect effects after transplantation, including an increased risk of infection, rejection, and PTLD.[360]

The treatment of posttransplantation CMV infection depends on disease severity and organ systems involved. Low-grade CMV viremia usually responds to a reduction in immunosuppression (usually the antimetabolite). Patients with symptomatic or significant viremia but relatively mild symptoms may be treated as outpatients, with immunosuppression reduction and oral valganciclovir. The VICTOR trial demonstrated that oral valganciclovir was noninferior to intravenous ganciclovir in the treatment of non–life-threatening CMV infection in solid organ transplantations.[361] However, patients with severe systemic CMV infection or organ-specific disease (e.g., pneumonitis, gastrointestinal, or central nervous system [CNS]) should be treated initially with intravenous ganciclovir, with a transition to oral valganciclovir as symptoms improve. For viremic patients with mild to moderate disease, some advocate continuing treatment for 2 weeks after resolution of viremia, while others treat for at least 2 weeks and discontinue

Table 72.17 Manifestations of Cytomegalovirus Disease in Kidney Transplant Recipients

Tissue Affected	Clinical Features	Comment
Systemic	Fever, malaise, myalgia	Nonspecific but very important clue to cytomegalovirus disease
Bone marrow	Leukopenia	Usually not severe; reduce azathioprine or mycophenolate mofetil; valganciclovir can also cause leukopenia
Lungs	Pneumonitis	May be life-threatening; exclude co-infection with other organisms
Gastrointestinal tract	Inflammation and ulceration of esophagus or colon	May be life-threatening; often occurs late
Liver	Hepatitis	Rarely severe
Eyes (retina)	Blurred vision, flashes, floaters	Rare in kidney transplants; if occurs, usually late

therapy. Treatment of severe or invasive disease may benefit from longer courses of treatment followed by prophylactic dose therapy.[362] Dose adjustment is required in kidney dysfunction for valganciclovir and ganciclovir. Although supportive data are unavailable, it is reasonable to add CMV hyperimmune globulin in severe cases.[363]

The prevention of CMV disease is of great clinical importance. One strategy is to give prophylaxis to all patients at risk (D+/R−, D−/R+, D+/R+ [D, donor; R, recipient]). Another strategy is to monitor for CMV viremia and begin prophylaxis only when there is evidence of active viral replication.[360] Prophylactic and preemptive strategies using valganciclovir have been shown to be comparable in terms of cost and prevention of symptomatic CMV.[364]

PNEUMOCYSTOSIS

Antimicrobial prophylaxis is very effective in preventing pneumonia due to *P. jiroveci*. The preventive agent of choice is SMX-TMP. It is generally well tolerated and quite inexpensive; furthermore, it prevents UTIs and opportunistic infections such as nocardiosis, toxoplasmosis, and listeriosis. Alternative preventive agents include dapsone and pyrimethamine, atovaquone, and aerosolized pentamadine.[365] Typical symptoms of pneumonia due to *P. jiroveci* are fever, shortness of breath, and cough. Chest radiography characteristically shows bilateral interstitial alveolar infiltrates. Diagnosis requires detection of the organism in a clinical specimen by colorimetric or immunofluorescent staining. Because the organism burden is usually lower than in HIV-infected patients, the sensitivity of induced sputum or bronchoalveolar lavage specimens is lower in KTRs; tissue should be quickly obtained if these tests are negative and clinical suspicion remains high.

The treatment of choice remains SMX-TMP.[365] High-dose SMX-TMP may increase the plasma creatinine level without affecting the GFR. There is no firm evidence to support the use of higher dose steroids during the early treatment phase of pneumocystosis in KTRs.

IMMUNIZATION IN KIDNEY TRANSPLANT RECIPIENTS

Important general rules concerning immunization in KTRs are the following: (1) immunizations should be completed at least 4 weeks before transplantation; (2) immunization should be avoided in the first 6 months posttransplantation because of ongoing high doses of immunosuppression and a risk of provoking allograft dysfunction; and (3) live vaccines are generally contraindicated after transplantation. A

Table 72.18 Recommended and Contraindicated Vaccines in Kidney Transplant Recipients

Recommended Vaccines	Contraindicated Vaccines
Diphtheria-pertussis-tetanus	Varicella zoster
Haemophilus influenzae B	BCG (Bacillus Calmette-Guérin)
Hepatitis A (for travel, occupational, or other specific risk)	Smallpox
Hepatitis B	Intranasal influenza
Pneumovax (consider booster every 3 to 5 years)	Live Japanese B encephalitis
Inactivated polio	Oral polio
Influenza types A and B, H1N1 (administer annually)	Rubella
Meningococcus (if recipient is high risk)	Measles (except during outbreak)
Typhoid V	Live oral typhoid Ty21a, yellow fever

comprehensive review of this issue has recently been published.[366] Vaccines that are recommended and contraindicated are summarized in Table 72.18. Household contacts of KTRs should receive yearly immunizations against influenza.

SUMMARY

Infections are a predictable complication of kidney transplantation. Minimizing infections requires meticulous surgical technique, antiviral prophylaxis for the first 3 to 6 months, SMX-TMP prophylaxis for the first 6 to 12 months, and avoidance of excess immunosuppression. A substantial increase in immunosuppression, no matter how long after transplantation, should trigger resumption of SMX-TMP and probably antiviral prophylaxis.

TRANSPLANTATION ISSUES IN SPECIFIC PATIENT GROUPS

PATIENTS WITH DIABETES

Although the survival rate of diabetic patients after kidney transplantation is lower than that of nondiabetic patients, the benefits of transplant are greater in younger recipients.[219] Cardiovascular disease is highly prevalent in the diabetic ESKD population and should be aggressively treated. A subset of diabetic ESKD patients are also suitable for kidney-pancreas transplantation (see the following discussion).

KIDNEY-PANCREAS TRANSPLANTATION

The benefits of pancreas transplantation are the following: (1) freedom from insulin therapy and the metabolic derangements of type 1 diabetes mellitus; and (2) potentially slowing or reversing the progression of end-organ damage from this condition. The disadvantage of pancreas transplantation is that it has a higher risk of surgical complications and the need for higher levels of immunosuppression. Thus, patients must be carefully selected for this procedure. Although select patients with type 2 diabetes can undergo pancreas transplantation, the vast majority of pancreas transplants are performed in patients with type 1 diabetes. For diabetic ESKD patients deemed suitable candidates for kidney plus pancreas transplantation, options include SPK transplantation or pancreas after kidney (PAK) transplantation (the latter allows living donor kidney transplantation). Pancreas transplant alone (PTA) is also performed in a minority of patients without ESKD. In contrast to SPK transplantation, there is some concern as to whether pancreas transplant alone or later improves patient survival. However, PAK transplantation offers the advantages of preemptive living donor kidney transplantation and better kidney allograft outcomes. Rates of pancreas transplantation have decreased somewhat over the past decade, from a peak of around 1500 procedures in 2004 to just over 1000 in 2012.

Complications of pancreatic transplantation include thrombosis, infection, rejection, and problems related to drainage of the exocrine secretions.[367] Safe drainage of the exocrine secretions is vital. Drainage of exocrine secretions into the bladder affords the advantages of sterility and of serial measurement of urinary amylase concentrations, which can aid in the early detection of pancreatic allograft dysfunction. Important disadvantages include severe cystitis, hypovolemia, and acidosis (the last two due to large losses of bicarbonate-rich fluid). Because rates of technical complications from enteric drainage have decreased, this technique is becoming more popular.[367]

The graft half-life for pancreas transplantations is over 12 years in the United States. Pancreas graft survival rates are better for recipients of SPK allografts than for PTA or PAK recipients.[368] The major causes of graft failure are technical (40%) and acute rejection (15%) in the early posttransplantation period and chronic rejection (25%) in the late posttransplantation period.[369]

PATIENTS WITH HUMAN IMMUNODEFICIENCY VIRUS INFECTION

Until recently, HIV infection was considered an absolute contraindication to kidney transplantation. This reflected fears that immunosuppression would promote severe infections and that the short survival of HIV-positive patients undergoing transplantation surgery would waste valuable allografts. With the introduction of antiretroviral agent therapy in 1996 and subsequent improvements in the survival of HIV-positive patients, many centers accept patients with HIV for transplantation. Relatively good allograft and recipient survival has been reported.[370] These patients should be referred to centers specializing in the management of transplanted HIV-positive patients because of the complexity of management (e.g., the potential for interactions between the multiple antiviral medicines, some of which inhibit and some of which induce the CYP450 system). A recent prospective, nonrandomized trial in HIV-infected patients showed very good 1- and 3-year patient survivals of 95% and 88%, respectively, and corresponding graft survivals of 90% and 75% with no increases in complications associated with HIV infection.[371] Patients selected in this study had CD4+ T cell counts of at least $200/m^3$ and undetectable viral RNA levels. A surprising finding was that rejection rates were higher than expected. Studies directed at optimizing immunotherapy in this population are needed. Successful transplantation of kidneys from HIV-positive donors to HIV-positive recipients has been reported.[372]

PREGNANT KIDNEY TRANSPLANT RECIPIENTS

Fertility is often improved after kidney transplantation.[373] Although the risks of pregnancy and childbirth are greater in KTRs compared to the general population, it is generally considered safe for the mother, fetus, and kidney allograft if the following criteria are met before conception: good general health for more than 18 months before conception, stable allograft function with a plasma creatinine level less than 2.0 mg/dL (preferably <1.5 mg/dL), minimal hypertension, minimal proteinuria, immunosuppression at maintenance doses, and no dilation of the pelvicaliceal system on recent imaging studies.[374]

A recent systematic review and meta-analysis of 50 studies, which included data on 4706 pregnancies in 3570 KTRs from 2000 to 2010, gives insight into the relative risks of pregnancy post–kidney transplantation.[375] The rate of live births was actually higher than that of the general population. However, KTR pregnancies were more likely to end with cesarean section, preterm birth (35.6 vs. 38.7 weeks), and lower birth weight (2.4 vs. 3.3 kg). Preeclampsia and gestational diabetes were both more common in KTRs than in the general population. More than 50% of KTRs were hypertensive during pregnancy. Overall, pregnancy did not appear to be associated with an increased risk of acute rejection or subsequent graft loss.

All pregnant kidney allograft recipients should be managed as high-risk obstetric cases, with nephrology involvement. Throughout the pregnancy, regular monitoring of blood pressure, proteinuria, kidney function, and urine cultures is advised. Significant kidney dysfunction occurs in a minority of cases; the principal causes are severe preeclampsia, acute rejection, acute pyelonephritis, and recurrent glomerulonephritis. Distinguishing these causes clinically may be difficult. Initial investigations should include plasma creatinine level, creatinine clearance, 24-hour urinary protein excretion, urine microscopy, urine culture, and kidney ultrasound. Acute rejection should be confirmed by allograft biopsy before instituting antirejection therapy. Pulse steroids are used to treat rejection.

There are no transplantation-specific reasons to perform a cesarean section; if it is performed (for obstetric reasons), care should be taken to avoid damaging the transplanted ureter. Kidney function should be monitored closely for 3 months postpartum because of the increased risk of HUS and possibly acute rejection.

Short-term and long-term data indicate that children born to transplant recipients using cyclosporine, steroids, or azathioprine do not have a significant increase in morbidity. Short-term data on tacrolimus are similarly reassuring. Dosages of cyclosporine and tacrolimus may need to be increased to maintain prepregnancy trough concentrations. MMF is considered to be teratogenic and should not be used in women contemplating pregnancy.[376] Sirolimus should also be avoided. Limited data regarding the paternal use of cyclosporine, steroids, azathioprine, tacrolimus, and MMF are reassuring.

SURGERY IN THE KIDNEY TRANSPLANT RECIPIENT

ALLOGRAFT NEPHRECTOMY

Allograft nephrectomy is not commonly required. Indications include the following: (1) allograft failure with ongoing symptomatic rejection causing fever, malaise, hematuria, and graft pain; (2) infarction due to thrombosis; (3) severe infection of the allograft such as emphysematous pyelonephritis; and (4) allograft rupture. The morbidity associated with allograft nephrectomy is relatively high. Ongoing rejection in a failed allograft can sometimes be controlled with steroids, but prolonged immunosuppression of a patient who is on dialysis is obviously not ideal. Rejection in this context is less likely to be controlled by small doses of steroids when it is acute and when the transplant is recent. Whether nephrectomy of the allograft after a patient returns to dialysis offers a survival advantage remains controversial. In a retrospective analysis of registry data, the authors noted a survival advantage in transplant recipients who underwent allograft nephrectomy after returning to dialysis.[377] The observed survival advantage was attributed to cessation of immunosuppressive agents and removal of a source for chronic inflammation. However, a limitation to this type of study is the effects of confounding factors and treatment biases intrinsic to such retrospective studies. The risk of surgery needs to be weighed against the risk of chronic inflammation and continued immunosuppressive therapy.

NONTRANSPLANTATION-RELATED SURGERY OR HOSPITALIZATION

Many KTRs are hospitalized or undergo surgery for nontransplant related reasons. Precautions for procedures and surgery in transplant recipients are listed in Table 72.19. Common sense measures such as maintenance of adequate volume status, avoidance of nephrotoxic medicines (including NSAIDs), and proper dosing of immunosuppressive drugs are advised. Whenever possible, immunosuppressive drugs should be given by the enteral route; if this is not possible, a regimen of intravenous steroids and intravenous CNIs usually suffices. A simple way to dose intravenous steroids is to prescribe the same milligram for milligram dose of intravenous methylprednisolone as the maintenance prednisone dose; supplemental stress dose hydrocortisone is then prescribed separately. Intravenous cyclosporine should be prescribed in slow infusion form at one third of the total daily oral dose, and intravenous tacrolimus should be at one fifth of the total daily dose.

Table 72.19 Precautions for Procedures and Surgery in Kidney Transplant Recipients

Use caution with radiocontrast exposure.
Maintain volume status and hydration.
Avoid nephrotoxic antibiotics and analgesics.
Administering stress dose steroids is not always necessary.
If enteral route of medication is contraindicated, give CNI via IV route (at one third and one fifth of total oral dose of cyclosporine and tacrolimus respectively).
Monitor allograft function, plasma potassium level, and acid-base balance daily.
Consider wound-healing impairment.

PATIENTS WITH A FAILING KIDNEY

As for native CKD, management of anemia, hyperparathyroidism, hypertension, preparation for dialysis, and creation of appropriate dialysis access are important. If there are no contraindications, patients can be listed again for another transplant. The waiting time may be prolonged, however, because of sensitization to HLA antigens. Once the patient returns to dialysis, immunosuppression should be weaned gradually. Active communication between the primary nephrologist and transplantation physician is critical to ensuring a smooth transition for the patient. In cases in which management of the patient has been primarily through a transplantation center, early referral to a primary nephrologist is important for preparation and initiation of dialysis. Conversely, patients who are managed primarily by a general nephrologist should alert the transplantation center to coordinate the modification and weaning of immunosuppressive medications. Abrupt cessation of immunosuppressive agents can precipitate acute rejection, resulting in the need for transplantation nephrectomy. Finally, patients with a failing allograft should be evaluated for repeat transplantation.

TRANSPLANTATION AND IMMUNOSUPPRESSION: THE FUTURE

Major areas of ongoing investigation include expansion of the donor pool,[292,378] optimization of immunosuppression regimens (with particular focus on individualizing immunosuppression), induction of tolerance,[379-381] and xenotransplantation. There is also growing interest in therapies that modulate B cell and plasma cell function, thus preventing or treating AMR. Some of these topics are discussed in greater detail in Chapter 71.

CONCLUSION

Improvements in short-term and to some extent long-term kidney allograft survival have been encouraging. This reflects multiple influences, including more effective immunosuppression, more frequent use of living donors, and better medical and surgical care. The focus is likely to shift somewhat toward improving other posttransplantation outcomes, such as complications of immunosuppression, chronic allograft dysfunction, and morbidity from cardiovascular disease. The availability of adequate numbers of organs for transplantation remains an ongoing problem.

Complete reference list available at ExpertConsult.com.

KEY REFERENCES

10. Moers C, Smits JM, Maathuis MH, et al: Machine perfusion or cold storage in deceased-donor kidney transplantation. *N Engl J Med* 360:7–19, 2009.
15. Halloran PF: Immunosuppressive drugs for kidney transplantation. *N Engl J Med* 351:2715–2729, 2004.
21. Hardinger KL, Rhee S, Buchanan P, et al: A prospective, randomized, double-blinded comparison of thymoglobulin versus Atgam for induction immunosuppressive therapy: 10-year results. *Transplantation* 86:947–952, 2008.
24. Brennan DC, Schnitzler MA: Long-term results of rabbit antithymocyte globulin and basiliximab induction. *N Engl J Med* 359:1736–1738, 2008.
25. Hanaway MJ, Woodle ES, Mulgaonkar S, et al: Alemtuzumab induction in renal transplantation. *N Engl J Med* 364:1909–1919, 2011.
23. Brennan DC, Daller JA, Lake KD, et al: Group TIS. Rabbit antithymocyte globulin versus basiliximab in renal transplantation. *N Engl J Med* 355:1967–1977, 2006.
39. Nashan B, Moore R, Amlot P, et al: Randomised trial of basiliximab versus placebo for control of acute cellular rejection in renal allograft recipients. CHIB 201 International Study Group. *Lancet* 350:1193–1198, 1997.
42. Riella LV, Safa K, Yagan J, et al: Long-term outcomes of kidney transplantation across a positive complement-dependent cytotoxicity crossmatch. *Transplantation* 97:1247–1252, 2014.
49. Nankivell BJ, Borrows RJ, Fung CL, et al: The natural history of chronic allograft nephropathy. *N Engl J Med* 349:2326–2333, 2003.
56. Webster AC, Woodroffe RC, Taylor RS, et al: Tacrolimus versus ciclosporin as primary immunosuppression for kidney transplant recipients: meta-analysis and meta-regression of randomised trial data. *BMJ* 331:810, 2005.
62. Knight SR, Russell NK, Barcena L, et al: Mycophenolate mofetil decreases acute rejection and may improve graft survival in renal transplant recipients when compared with azathioprine: a systematic review. *Transplantation* 87:785–794, 2009.
77. Stallone G, Schena A, Infante B, et al: Sirolimus for Kaposi's sarcoma in renal-transplant recipients. *N Engl J Med* 352:1317–1323, 2005.
78. Euvrard S, Morelon E, Rostaing L, et al: Sirolimus and secondary skin-cancer prevention in kidney transplantation. *N Engl J Med* 367:329–339, 2012.
82. Rostaing L, Vincenti F, Grinyó J, et al: Long-term belatacept exposure maintains efficacy and safety at 5 years: results from the long-term extension of the BENEFIT study. *Am J Transplant* 13:2875–2883, 2013.
91. Pascual J, Zamora J, Galeano C, et al: Steroid avoidance or withdrawal for kidney transplant recipients. *Cochrane Database Syst Rev* CD005632, 2009.
96. Ekberg H, Grinyó J, Nashan B, et al: Cyclosporine sparing with mycophenolate mofetil, daclizumab and corticosteroids in renal allograft recipients: the CAESAR Study. *Am J Transplant* 7:560–570, 2007.
97. Ekberg H, Bernasconi C, Tedesco-Silva H, et al: Calcineurin inhibitor minimization in the Symphony study: observational results 3 years after transplantation. *Am J Transplant* 9:1876–1885, 2009.
100. Patel R, Terasaki PI: Significance of the positive crossmatch test in kidney transplantation. *N Engl J Med* 280:735–739, 1969.
107. Lefaucheur C, Loupy A, Hill GS, et al: Preexisting donor-specific HLA antibodies predict outcome in kidney transplantation. *J Am Soc Nephrol* 21:1398–1406, 2010.
109. Loupy A, Lefaucheur C, Vernerey D, et al: Complement-binding anti-HLA antibodies and kidney-allograft survival. *N Engl J Med* 369:1215–1226, 2013.
122. Perico N, Cattaneo D, Sayegh MH, et al: Delayed graft function in kidney transplantation. *Lancet* 364:1814–1827, 2004.
140. Rush D, Arlen D, Boucher A, et al: Lack of benefit of early protocol biopsies in renal transplant patients receiving TAC and MMF: a randomized study. *Am J Transplant* 7:2538–2545, 2007.
149. Kasiske BL, Zeier MG, Chapman JR, et al: Kidney Disease: Improving Global Outcomes: KDIGO clinical practice guideline for the care of kidney transplant recipients: a summary. *Kidney Int* 77:299–311, 2010.
160. Muthukumar T, Dadhania D, Ding R, et al: Messenger RNA for FOXP3 in the urine of renal-allograft recipients. *N Engl J Med* 353:2342–2351, 2005.
161. Suthanthiran M, Schwartz JE, Ding R, et al: Urinary-cell mRNA profile and acute cellular rejection in kidney allografts. *N Engl J Med* 369:20–31, 2013.
164. Halloran PF, Pereira AB, Chang J, et al: Microarray diagnosis of antibody-mediated rejection in kidney transplant biopsies: an international prospective study (INTERCOM). *Am J Transplant* 13:2865–2874, 2013.
170. Zuber J, Le Quintrec M, Krid S, et al: Eculizumab for atypical hemolytic uremic syndrome recurrence in renal transplantation. *Am J Transplant* 12:3337–3354, 2012.
175. Yu CC, Fornoni A, Weins A, et al: Abatacept in B7-1-positive proteinuric kidney disease. *N Engl J Med* 369:2416–2423, 2013.
182. Gaston RS, Cecka JM, Kasiske BL, et al: Evidence for antibody-mediated injury as a major determinant of late kidney allograft failure. *Transplantation* 90:68–74, 2010.
195. Hardinger KL, Koch MJ, Bohl DJ, et al: BK-virus and the impact of pre-emptive immunosuppression reduction: 5-year results. *Am J Transplant* 10:407–415, 2010.
199. Lee BT, Gabardi S, Grafals M, et al: Efficacy of levofloxacin in the treatment of BK viremia: a multicenter, double-blinded, randomized, placebo-controlled trial. *Clin J Am Soc Nephrol* 9:583–589, 2014.
206. El-Zoghby ZM, Stegall MD, Lager DJ, et al: Identifying specific causes of kidney allograft loss. *Am J Transplant* 9:527–535, 2009.
210. Gupta G, Abu Jawdeh BG, Racusen LC, et al: Late antibody-mediated rejection in renal allografts: outcome after conventional and novel therapies. *Transplantation* 97:1240–1246, 2014.
234. Wolfe RA, Ashby VB, Milford EL, et al: Comparison of mortality in all patients on dialysis, patients on dialysis awaiting transplantation, and recipients of a first cadaveric transplant. *N Engl J Med* 341:1725–1730, 1999.
257. Rao PS, Schaubel DE, Guidinger MK, et al: A comprehensive risk quantification score for deceased donor kidneys: the kidney donor risk index. *Transplantation* 88:231–236, 2009.
258. Reeves-Daniel AM, DePalma JA, Bleyer AJ, et al: The APOL1 gene and allograft survival after kidney transplantation. *Am J Transplant* 11:1025–1030, 2011.
301. Hoorn EJ, Walsh SB, McCormick JA, et al: The calcineurin inhibitor tacrolimus activates the renal sodium chloride cotransporter to cause hypertension. *Nat Med* 17:1304–1309, 2011.
305. Evenepoel P, Cooper K, Holdaas H, et al: A randomized study evaluating cinacalcet to treat hypercalcemia in renal transplant recipients with persistent hyperparathyroidism. *Am J Transplant* 14:2545–2555, 2014.
324. Hecking M, Haidinger M, Döller D, et al: Early basal insulin therapy decreases new-onset diabetes after renal transplantation. *J Am Soc Nephrol* 23:739–749, 2012.
337. James PA, Oparil S, Carter BL, et al: 2014 evidence-based guideline for the management of high blood pressure in adults: report from the panel members appointed to the Eighth Joint National Committee (JNC 8). *JAMA* 311:507–520, 2014.
350. Collett D, Mumford L, Banner NR, et al: Comparison of the incidence of malignancy in recipients of different types of organ: a UK Registry audit. *Am J Transplant* 10:1889–1896, 2010.
351. Engels EA, Pfeiffer RM, Fraumeni JF, et al: Spectrum of cancer risk among US solid organ transplant recipients. *JAMA* 306:1891–1901, 2011.
361. Asberg A, Humar A, Jardine AG, et al: Long-term outcomes of CMV disease treatment with valganciclovir versus IV ganciclovir in solid organ transplant recipients. *Am J Transplant* 9:1205–1213, 2009.

366. Danziger-Isakov L, Kumar D, Practice AIDCo: Vaccination in solid organ transplantation. *Am J Transplant* 13(Suppl 4):311–317, 2013.
371. Stock PG, Barin B, Murphy B, et al: Outcomes of kidney transplantation in HIV-infected recipients. *N Engl J Med* 363:2004–2014, 2010.
375. Deshpande NA, James NT, Kucirka LM, et al: Pregnancy outcomes in kidney transplant recipients: a systematic review and meta-analysis. *Am J Transplant* 11:2388–2404, 2011.
377. Ayus JC, Achinger SG, Lee S, et al: Transplant nephrectomy improves survival following a failed renal allograft. *J Am Soc Nephrol* 21:374–380, 2009.
380. Scandling JD, Busque S, Dejbakhsh-Jones S, et al: Tolerance and chimerism after renal and hematopoietic-cell transplantation. *N Engl J Med* 358:362–368, 2008.

PEDIATRIC NEPHROLOGY

SECTION XII

73 Malformation of the Kidney: Structural and Functional Consequences

Norman D. Rosenblum

CHAPTER OUTLINE

CLINCAL CLASSIFICATION OF KIDNEY MALFORMATION, 2294
EPIDEMIOLOGY OF CAKUT, 2296
PATHOGENESIS OF CAKUT, 2296
Mechanisms of Inheritance, 2296
Molecular Pathogenesis, 2297
The Environment In Utero and CAKUT, 2300
Functional Consequences of CAKUT, 2301
CLINICAL PRESENTATION OF CAKUT, 2302
Clinical Presentation in the Fetus, 2302
Clinical Presentation of Specific Forms of CAKUT, 2302
CLINICAL MANAGEMENT OF CAKUT, 2304
Overall Approach to Management of CAKUT In Utero and in the Immediate Postnatal Period, 2304
Management of Specific Types of CAKUT, 2305
Long-Term Outcomes of Renal Malformation, 2305

Developmental disorders of the kidney and urinary tract comprise a spectrum of malformations ranging from complete absence of kidney tissue to minor structural abnormalities.

Kidney–urinary tract structural abnormalities are an important cause of human disease; they are the most common cause of all birth defects, making up 23% of all such defects,[1] and cause 30% to 50% of all cases of end-stage kidney disease (ESKD) in children.[2] Within the adult population, congenital anomalies of the kidney and urinary tract (CAKUT) are the cause of 2.2% of all ESKD. Adult patients with CAKUT differ from adults with other causes of chronic kidney disease in their requirement for renal replacement therapy at a mean age of 30 years compared to 61 years.[3] This chapter focuses on the classification, epidemiology, pathogenesis, and clinical management of kidney malformations.

CLINCAL CLASSIFICATION OF KIDNEY MALFORMATION

As a group, renal–urinary tract malformations have been grouped together under the rubric "congenital anomalies of the kidney and urinary tract" (CAKUT). This classification is supported by the following: (1) multiple structures within one or both kidney–urinary tract units may be affected within any given affected individual, (2) mutation in a particular gene is associated with different urinary tract anomalies in different affected individuals, and (3) mutations in different genes give rise to similar renal and lower urinary tract phenotypes. A classification of kidney and urinary tract malformations within the CAKUT rubric is as follows:

- Aplasia (agenesis), defined as congenital absence of kidney tissue
- Simple hypoplasia, defined as renal length less than two standard deviations below the mean for age, a reduced number of nephrons, and normal renal architecture
- Dysplasia with or without cysts, defined as malformation of tissue elements
- Isolated dilation of the renal pelvis or ureters or both (collecting system)
- Anomalies of position, including the ectopic and fused (horseshoe) kidney

Simple renal hypoplasia is defined by the presence of a small kidney with a decrease in the number of nephrons and normal renal architecture. Viewed through the lens of embryology, normal tissue architecture indicates that patterning of renal tissue elements is normal.

Renal dysplasia is defined as an abnormality of tissue patterning (Figure 73.1). Renal dysplasia is a polymorphic disorder. At the level of gross anatomy, the dysplastic kidney varies in size from one extreme to the other compared to

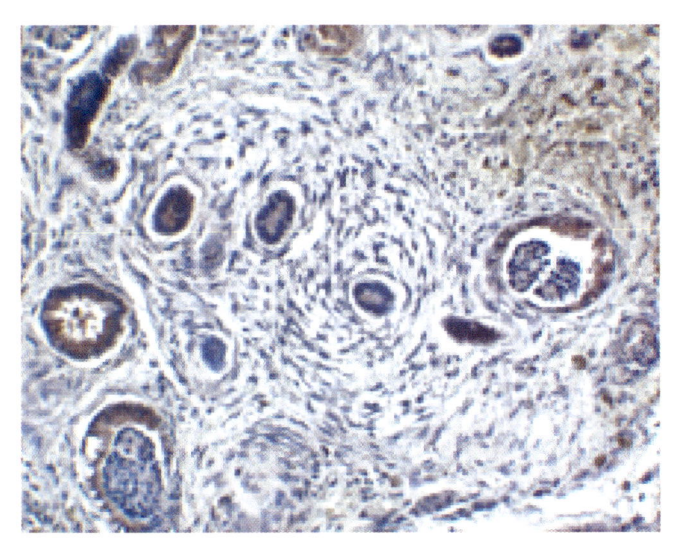

Figure 73.1 Histologic section of renal dysplastic tissue. Dysplastic renal tissue demonstrates a paucity of glomerular and tubular elements, disorganization of tissue elements, an abundance of stroma, and thickened and dilated renal tubules.

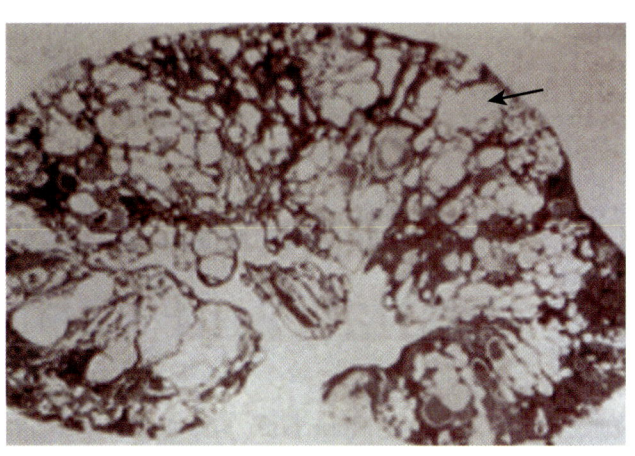

Figure 73.2 Histologic section of a multicystic dysplastic kidney. The kidney consists in large part of multiple polymorphic cysts (*arrow*). Normal renal tissue elements cannot be identified.

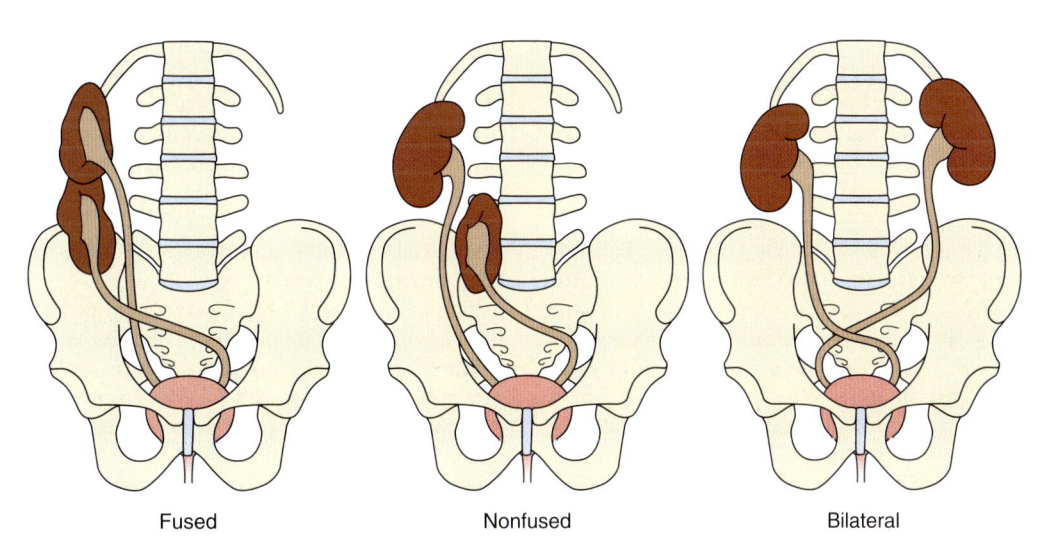

Fused　　　Nonfused　　　Bilateral

Figure 73.3 Crossed fused ectopia. Renal ectopia is classified as simple (nonfused), fused, and bilateral. A fused kidney migrates across the midline and fuses to the lower pole of the normally positioned contralateral kidney. A simple crossed (nonfused) kidney migrates across the midline, does not fuse with the normally positioned contralateral kidney, and is usually positioned at the rim of the pelvis. In bilateral ectopia, both kidneys are ectopic and cross the midline with their native ureters, which are inserted normally into the bladder.

the mean size for age. However, most dysplastic kidneys are small for age. Dysplastic kidneys also vary in the presence of epithelial cysts, the number of cysts, and cyst size. The multicystic dysplastic kidney (MCDK) is an extreme form of renal dysplasia in which large polymorphic cysts dominate kidney structure (Figure 73.2). At the level of histopathology, the dysplastic kidney (see Figure 73.1) is characterized by several primary features: (1) abnormal differentiation of mesenchymal and epithelial elements, (2) decreased nephron number, (3) loss of corticomedullary differentiation, and (4) metaplastic transformation of mesenchyme to cartilage and bone. Renal tubular dysgenesis represents a particular form of renal dysplasia and is characterized by the absence or poor development of proximal tubules and is accompanied by thickening of the renal arterial vasculature from the arcuate to the afferent arteries.[4]

An ectopic kidney is classified by its position and its relationship with an independent kidney unit (Figure 73.3). Simple non-crossed (nonfused) ectopy refers to a kidney that lies on the correct side of the body but lies in an abnormal position. Kidneys that cross the midline are referred to as crossed renal ectopy. Crossed renal ectopy can occur with and without fusion to the contralateral kidney. Ectopic kidneys that do not ascend above the pelvic brim are commonly called pelvic kidneys. Renal fusion occurs when a portion of one kidney is fused to the other. The most common fusion anomaly is the horseshoe kidney, which involves abnormal migration of both kidneys (ectopy), resulting in fusion (Figure 73.4). This differs from crossed fused renal ectopy, which usually involves abnormal movement of only one kidney across the midline with fusion of the contralateral noncrossing kidney.

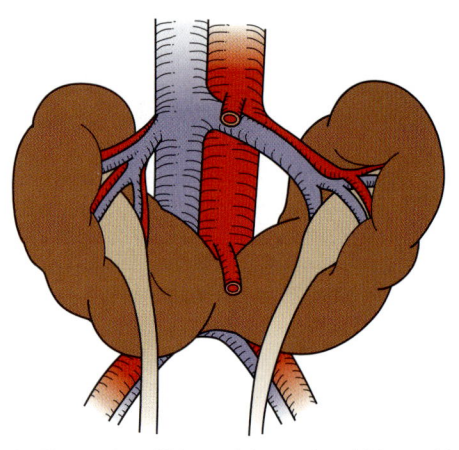

Figure 73.4 Horseshoe kidney. A horseshoe kidney with fusion of the lower poles. Note that the renal pelvis is positioned anteriorly and the ureter traverses the anterior aspect and the fused lower pole of each kidney.

EPIDEMIOLOGY OF CAKUT

CAKUT is the most frequent malformation detected in utero. The incidence of renal and urinary tract malformations identified in fetal ultrasonography is 0.3 to 1.6 per 1000 liveborn and stillborn infants.[5] Lower urinary tract abnormalities can be identified in approximately 50% of affected patients, consistent with the common origin of the kidney and ureter from the mesonephric duct. These anomalies include vesicoureteral reflux (25%), ureteropelvic junction obstruction (11%), and ureterovesical junction obstruction (11%).[6] Renal malformations, other than mild antenatal pelviectasis, occur in association with nonrenal malformations in approximately 30% of cases.[5]

The reported incidence of particular types of renal–urinary tract malformation is no doubt dependent on the ascertainment method. Most incidence rates are not based on population-based studies during pregnancy. Rather, they are based on autopsy series or studies in selected liveborn infants. Incidence rates based on methods other than population-based ascertainment may underestimate the true incidence because fetal loss may not be accounted for and because CAKUT can be clinically silent in the surviving fetus.

Complete or partial duplication of the renal collecting system is the most common congenital anomaly of the urinary tract.[7] Autopsy studies report an estimated incidence of 0.8% to 5%.[8] A similar rate was reported in a study of 13,705 fetuses with antenatal ultrasonography performed in a tertiary center in Turkey.[9] However, a study that screened 132,686 Taiwanese schoolchildren (6 to 15 years of age) found a lower incidence of 1 per 5000 children.[10] Bilateral renal agenesis occurs in 1 per 3000 to 10,000 births. Males are affected more often than females. Unilateral renal agenesis has been reported with a prevalence of 1 per 1000 autopsies. The incidence of unilateral dysplasia is 1 per 3000 to 5000 births (1 per 3640 for the MCDK) compared to 1 per 10,000 for bilateral dysplasia.[11] The male/female ratio for bilateral and unilateral renal dysplasia is 1.32:1 and 1.92:1, respectively.[12] The incidence of renal ectopia is 1 per 1000 autopsies, but the clinical recognition is estimated to be only 1 per 10,000 patients.[13] Males and females are equally affected. Renal ectopia is bilateral in 10% of cases; when unilateral, there is a slight predilection for the left side. The incidence of fusion anomalies is estimated to be approximately 1 per 600 infants.[14] The most common fusion anomaly is the horseshoe kidney, which occurs with fusion of one pole of each kidney. The reported incidence of horseshoe kidney based upon data from birth defect registries varies from 0.4 to 1.6 per 10,000 live births.[14,15]

PATHOGENESIS OF CAKUT

MECHANISMS OF INHERITANCE

The genetics of CAKUT are complex. In the majority of affected patients, congenital renal malformations occur as sporadic events. In approximately 30% of affected individuals, these malformations occur as part of a multiorgan genetic syndrome. Renal–urinary tract malformations and extrarenal malformations can go unrecognized unless a careful phenotypic examination is performed. Over 200 distinct genetic syndromes feature some type of kidney and urinary tract malformation. More than 30 genes have been identified as mutant in multiorgan syndromes with CAKUT (Table 73.1). Incomplete penetrance with variable expressivity is frequent in affected families. That is, within any particular family in which affected members carry the same mutation, the renal phenotype can vary from agenesis to dysplasia to isolated abnormalities of the collecting system (e.g., hydronephrosis).

The majority of CAKUT occurs without a clear mendelian pattern of inheritance. In probands with bilateral renal agenesis or bilateral renal dysgenesis and without evidence of a genetic syndrome or a family history, 9% of first-degree relatives were shown by ultrasonography to have some type of malformation in the kidney and/or lower urinary tract.[16] A study of CAKUT in asymptomatic first-degree relatives of patients with CAKUT in Turkey revealed a positive family history of CAKUT in 23% and ultrasonographic evidence of CAKUT also in 23% of individuals.[17] A study of 100 patients with renal hypodysplasia and renal insufficiency demonstrated a gene mutation in 16% of affected individuals. The majority of mutations were identified in *TCF2* (hepatocyte nuclear factor-1β [HNF-1β]), especially in patients with kidney cysts; mutations in *PAX2* and *EYA1* were identified in single cases.[18] Some of the mutations were de novo mutations, explaining the sporadic appearance of CAKUT. Careful clinical analysis of patients with *TCF2* and *PAX2* mutations revealed the presence of extrarenal symptoms in only 50%, which supports previous reports that *TCF2* and *PAX2* mutations can be responsible for isolated renal tract anomalies or at least CAKUT malformations with minimal extrarenal features.[19,20]

Studies suggest that polymorphic variants in genes that control renal development contribute to the pathogenesis of CAKUT. Analysis of a cohort of 168 white newborns from Montreal suggests that single nucleotide polymorphisms in *PAX2* are associated with newborn kidney size at the low end of the population spectrum.[21] Analysis of the *RET* gene in the aforementioned Montreal cohort demonstrated that a

Table 73.1 Human Gene Mutations Associated with Syndromic CAKUT

Primary Disease	Gene	Kidney Phenotype	References
Alagille's syndrome	JAG1	Cystic dysplasia	161
Apert's syndrome	FGFR2	Hydronephrosis	162
Beckwith-Wiedemann syndrome	$p57^{KIP2}$	Medullary dysplasia	77
Branchio-oto-renal (BOR) syndrome	EYA1, SIX1, SIX5	Unilateral or bilateral agenesis/dysplasia, hypoplasia, collecting system anomalies	56
Campomelic dysplasia	SOX9	Dysplasia, hydronephrosis	163, 164
Duane–radial ray (Okihiro) syndrome	SALL4	UNL agenesis, VUR, malrotation, cross-fused ectopia, pelviectasis	165
Fraser's syndrome	FRAS1	Agenesis, dysplasia	166
Isolated renal hypoplasia	BMP4, RET	Hypoplasia, VUR	22, 35
Hypoparathyroidism, sensorineural deafness, and renal anomalies (HDR) syndrome	GATA3	Dysplasia	167
Kallmann's syndrome	KAL1, FGFR1, PROK2, PROKR2	Agenesis	168
Mammary-ulnar syndrome	TBX3	Dysplasia	169
Pallister-Hall syndrome	GLI3	Agenesis, dysplasia, hydronephrosis	70, 72
Renal-coloboma syndrome	PAX2	Hypoplasia, VUR	40
Renal tubular dysgenesis	RAAS components	Tubular dysplasia	95
Renal cysts and diabetes syndrome	HNF1B	Dysplasia, hypoplasia	170
Rubinstein-Taybi syndrome	CREBBP	Agenesis, hypoplasia	171
Simpson-Golabi-Behmel syndrome	GPC3	Medullary dysplasia	172
Smith-Lemli-Opitz syndrome	DHCR7	Agenesis, dysplasia	173
Townes-Brock syndrome	SALL1	Hypoplasia, dysplasia, VUR	47
Ulnar-mammary syndrome	TBX3	Hypoplasia	169
Zellweger's syndrome	PEX1	VUR, cystic dysplasia	174

RAAS, Renin angiotensin aldosterone system; UNL, unilateral; VUR, vesicoureteral reflux.

reduction in newborn kidney volume by 9.7% was significantly associated with the single nucleotide polymorphism rs1800860, which encodes a G→A nucleotide transition at codon 1476.[22] Analyses in vitro indicate that the amount of messenger RNA (mRNA) generated from this allele is reduced consistent with decreased RET expression in affected individuals.

MOLECULAR PATHOGENESIS

The morphologic and genetic events that control kidney development are detailed in Chapter 1. Briefly summarized, formation of the human kidney is initiated at 5 weeks of gestation in the human when the ureteric duct is induced to undergo lateral outgrowth from the wolffian duct and to invade the adjacent metanephric mesenchyme. The ureteric bud then undergoes repetitive branching events, so termed because each event consists of expansion of the advancing ureteric bud branch at its leading tip, division of the ampulla resulting in formation of new branches, and elongation of the newly formed branches. Beginning with the tenth- to eleventh-branch generation, the pattern of branching becomes terminally bifid. During branching morphogenesis 65,000 collecting ducts are formed, both as cortical and medullary collecting ducts, a process that is essential to the function of the mature kidney. During the latter stages of kidney development, tubular segments formed from the first five generations of ureteric bud branching undergo remodeling to form the kidney pelvis and calyces.[23]

Genetic analyses in humans have identified mutant alleles associated with CAKUT. Studies in mice have identified genes that are required during renal development. Together, such studies have provided complementary information and critical insights into the likely functions of CAKUT-related genes during human renal morphogenesis. In this section the functions of genes mutated in human CAKUT and for which a function has been elucidated are reviewed as a framework for understanding the molecular pathogenesis of CAKUT.

URETERIC BUDDING, ROBO2, AND BMP4

The proto-oncogene RET, a tyrosine kinase receptor, and its ligand, glial cell line–derived neurotrophic factor (GDNF), regulate ureteric budding and renal branching morphogenesis. RET is expressed on the surface of ureteric cells.[24] GDNF is expressed by metanephric mesenchyme cells.[25] Homozygous deletion of either Ret or Gdnf in mice causes failure of ureteric outgrowth and renal agenesis. Patients with CAKUT have mutations in the RET-GDNF signaling pathway.[26-29] A study of 122 patients with CAKUT identified heterozygous deleterious sequence variants in GDNF or RET in 6 of 122 patients, 5%, whereas another group screened 749 families from all over the world and identified 3 families with heterozygous mutations in RET.[26] Similar findings have been reported in studies of fetuses with bilateral or unilateral renal agenesis.[27,29]

The site of ureteric bud outgrowth from the wolffian duct is normally invariant, and the number of outgrowths is limited to one. Outgrowth of more than one ureteric bud can result in renal malformations, including a double collecting system and duplication of the ureter. The position at which the ureteric bud arises from the wolffian duct relative to the metanephric mesenchyme is critical to the nature of the interactions between the ureteric bud and the metanephric mesenchyme. Ectopic positioning of the ureteric bud is associated with renal tissue malformation (dysplasia) due to abnormal ureteric bud–metanephric mesenchyme interactions and is also thought to contribute to the integrity of the ureterovesical junction. Mackie and Stephens postulated that an abnormal position of the ureteral orifice in the bladder is associated with vesicoureteral reflux in humans.[30] Consistent with this hypothesis, mutations in *ROBO2* are associated with vesicoureteral reflux in humans.[31] ROBO2, a cell surface receptor, is expressed in the nephrogenic mesenchyme.[32] Mice deficient in *Robo2* exhibit ectopic ureteric bud formation, multiple ureters, and hydroureter. Interestingly, the domain of *Gdnf* expression is expanded anteriorly in these mice, which suggests that loss of inhibition of *Gdnf* expression by *Robo2* dependent signaling expands the domain of *Gdnf* expression and results in ectopic ureteric budding.[33] Members of the bone morphogenetic protein (BMP) family of secreted proteins also negatively regulate GDNF signaling. *Bmp4* is expressed in stromal cells immediately adjacent to the wolffian duct and the ureteric bud. Mice heterozygous for *Bmp4* exhibit ectopic or duplicated ureteric buds, which suggests that BMP-4 suppresses ureteric induction by antagonizing the local effect of GDNF-RET signaling at the normal site of induction on the wolffian duct. Indeed, exogenous BMP-4 has been shown to block GDNF-induced ureteric bud outgrowth from the wolffian duct in vitro.[34] Consistent with these observations, mutations in *BMP4* have been identified in humans with CAKUT phenotypes, including renal dysgenesis and vesicoureteral reflux.[35]

URETERIC BRANCHING, *PAX2*, AND *RET*

Branching of the ureteric bud is initiated immediately following invasion of the metanephric mesenchyme by the ureteric bud. The number of ureteric bud branches elaborated is considered to be a major determinant of final nephron number because each ureteric bud branch tip induces a discrete subset of metanephric mesenchyme cells to undergo nephrogenesis (see Chapter 1). Regulation of ureteric branch number has been informed by complementary studies in humans and mice. These investigations have demonstrated an essential role for PAX2, a transcription factor of the paired box family of homeotic genes that is expressed in the mesonephros and in the metanephros during renal development.

Mutations in *PAX2* cause renal-coloboma syndrome (also named papillorenal syndrome), an autosomal dominant disorder characterized by the association of renal hypoplasia, vesicoureteric reflux, and optic nerve coloboma.[36] Although the prevalence of the syndrome is unknown, approximately 100 affected families have been reported.[37] A wide range of renal malformations is observed in renal-coloboma syndrome; these include most frequently oligomeganephronic hypoplasia, renal dysplasia, and vesicoureteral reflux.[38] Ureteropelvic junction obstruction has also been described.[18,19,38] The ocular phenotype is extremely variable. The most common finding is an optic disc pit associated with vascular abnormalities and cilioretinal arteries, with mild visual impairment limited to blind spot enlargement.[39] In other cases the only ocular anomaly is optic nerve dysplasia with an abnormal vessel pattern and no functional consequence.

The *PAX2* gene is located on chromosome 10q24-25. It encodes a transcription factor that belongs to the paired box family of homeotic genes. The vast majority of the mutations are located in exons 2 and 3 encoding the DNA-binding domain. In 1995, Sanyanusin and colleagues reported heterozygous mutations in two families with renal-coloboma syndrome.[40] Since then, more than 30 mutations have been reported, most of them lying in the second and third exons, which encode the paired domain that binds to DNA, or in exons 7 to 9, which encode the transactivation domain.[37,41]

During renal development, *Pax2* is expressed in the wolffian duct, the ureteric bud, and the metanephric mesenchyme. Studies in the 1Neu mouse strain, which is characterized by a *Pax2* mutation, demonstrated decreased ureteric branching in association with decreased nephron number. Decreased ureteric branch number and nephron number are rescued by inhibition of apoptosis in the ureteric lineage.[42,43] Studies in normal full-term newborns suggest that loss of *PAX2* function may also contribute to generating a lower number of nephrons within the range of nephron number (approximately 250,000 to 1,600,000) observed in humans.[44] Quinlan and associates hypothesized that gene polymorphisms that generate loss of PAX2 function could contribute to mild reductions in nephron number and discovered that a *PAX2* haplotype (*PAX2^{AAA}*) is associated with an approximately 10% decrease in kidney volume in a cohort of newborn infants.[21]

Ureteric branching is also mediated in large part by the GDNF-RET signaling axis. During ureteric branching, RET is expressed on the surface of ureteric tip cells and controls the number and pattern of branches elaborated.[45] The observation that *Ret$^{+/-}$* mice exhibit a 22% reduction in nephron number[46] suggested that allelic variants in *RET* associated with decreased *RET* function contribute to decreased nephron number in humans. Indeed, a *RET* allelic variant that generates a reduced amount of RET mRNA in vitro, in comparison with the predominant allele in the *RET* gene, has been associated with an approximately 10% decrease in total kidney volume, used in this case as a quantitative trait and surrogate measure of nephron number, in a cohort of newborn infants.[22]

CONTROL OF GDNF EXPRESSION IN THE METANEPHRIC MESENCHYME: *SALL1*, *EYA1*, AND *SIX1*

As discussed earlier, *Gdnf* expression by metanephric mesenchyme cells is critical to ureteric branching. In the metanephric mesenchyme, *Sall1*, *Eya1*, and *Six1* positively control *Gdnf* expression. *Sall1*, a member of the Spalt family of transcriptional factors,[47] is expressed in the metanephric mesenchyme before and during ureteric bud invasion. Mutational inactivation of *Sall1* in mice causes renal agenesis or severe dysgenesis and a marked decrease in *Gdnf* expression.[48] Mutations in *SALL1* are associated with Townes-Brock syndrome, an autosomal dominant malformation syndrome characterized by imperforate anus, preaxial polydactyly, and/or triphalangeal thumbs, external ear defects, sensorineural hearing loss, and, less frequently, kidney, urogenital, and heart malformations.[49,50] *SALL1* mutations have also been identified in patients who lack extrarenal features of Townes-Brock syndrome.[18]

EYA1, a DNA-binding transcription factor, is expressed in metanephric mesenchyme cells in the same spatial and temporal pattern as GDNF. EYA1 functions in a molecular complex with SIX1[51] to control expression of GDNF.[52] Both EYA1 and SIX1 are also expressed in developing otic and branchial tissues.[53,54] Mice with *Eya1* deficiency demonstrate renal agenesis and failure of *Gdnf* expression.[55] Mutations in *EYA1* and *SIX1* occur in humans with branchio-oto-renal (BOR) syndrome.[51,56] Classic BOR syndrome, an autosomal dominant disorder, is defined by its major features: conductive and/or sensorineural hearing loss (95% of patients), branchial defects (49% to 69% of patients), ear pits (83% of patients), and renal anomalies (38% to 67% of patients).[57,58] Renal malformations include unilateral or bilateral renal agenesis, hypodysplasia, and malformation of the lower urinary tract, including vesicoureteral reflux, pyeloureteral obstruction, and ureteral duplication. Different renal malformations can be observed in the same family. Many patients have only one or two of these major BOR syndrome features; these findings in the absence of renal findings is termed branchio-oto syndrome. Mutations in *EYA1* have been identified as well in children with CAKUT who lack any of the extrarenal features of BOR or branchio-oto syndrome.[18]

BOR syndrome is transmitted as an autosomal dominant trait with incomplete penetrance and variable expressivity. A mutation in *EYA1* has been identified in approximately 40% of patients with BOR syndrome.[58] Mutations are most commonly identified in a highly conserved region called the eyes absent homologous region encoded within exons 9 to 16. It is estimated that 5% may have a mutation in *SIX1*.[59] Molecular testing can confirm the diagnosis and provide genetic recurrence risk information to families. However, variability of the phenotype even with the same mutation does not permit accurate prediction of the disease severity. Within the same family a given mutation may be associated with renal malformation in some individuals, but not in others.

HEDGEHOG SIGNALING, GLI3 REPRESSOR, AND CAKUT

Studies in mice and humans have demonstrated a critical role for hedgehog-dependent signaling during kidney development. Hedgehog ligands function within concentration gradients. Binding of hedgehog ligand, including Sonic hedgehog (SHH), to its cognate cell surface receptor stimulates nuclear translocation of full-length GLI transcriptional activators and inhibits proteolytic processing of full-length GLI3 to a shorter transcriptional repressor.[60] Loss-of-function mutations in *SHH* have been identified in patients with holoprosencephaly and renal hypoplasia or urogenital malformations.[61] Renal malformations have also been reported in patients exhibiting deletions of chromosome 7q, encompassing the *SHH* gene locus.[62-64] Posttranslational modification of hedgehog ligand is essential for regulated diffusion of hedgehog proteins and signaling.[65] A hedgehog loss-of-function phenotype, including renal agenesis and hypodysplasia, is observed in Smith-Lemli-Opitz syndrome.

The syndrome is caused by heterozygous mutations in the *DHCR7* gene, encoding delta-7-steroid reductase, which is required in mammalian sterol biosynthesis to convert 7-dehydrocholesterol into cholesterol.[66] Reduced Hedgehog modification with cholesterol may be pathogenic in Smith-Lemli-Opitz syndrome.

Pallister-Hall syndrome is an autosomal dominant multiorgan disorder characterized by multiple renal abnormalities, including agenesis or dysplasia, hypoplasia, and hydronephrosis.[67-69] Affected individuals carry frameshift/nonsense and splicing mutations exclusively in the second-third of the *GLI3* gene. These mutations are predicted to generate a truncated protein similar in size to GLI3 repressor.[70,71] The pathogenic role of GLI3 repressor was demonstrated in mice with homozygous *Shh* deficiency in which the levels of GLI3 in kidney tissue are elevated. Remarkably, renal dysgenesis in the absence of *Shh* is completely rescued by homozygous inactivation of *Gli3*.[72] Murine deficiency of *Smo*, which encodes a cell surface protein required for Hedgehog signaling, targeted to the metanephric mesenchyme lineage, causes hydronephrosis, dyskinesia of the ureter, and absent expression of cell surface markers that characterized pacemaker cells in the renal pelvis and upper ureter. Homozygous deficiency of *Gli3* in these mutant mice rescues these abnormalities.[73]

THE MEDULLA AND GLYPICAN-3

Between the twenty-second and thirty-fourth week of human fetal gestation, the peripheral (cortical) and central (medullary) domains of the developing kidney are established. Glypican-3 (GPC3), a glycosylphosphatidylinositol–linked cell surface heparan sulfate proteoglycan, whose gene is mutated in Simpson-Golabi-Behmel syndrome, is required for normal patterning of the medulla.[74,75] Medullary dysplasia in mice deficient in *Gpc3* is associated with increased ureteric branching and cell proliferation,[74] and subsequent destruction of medullary collecting ducts due to apoptosis.[75] The defect is thought to be caused by insensitivity to inhibitors of branching morphogenesis, including BMPs, and enhanced sensitivity to the stimulatory effect of other factors, including FGF7. The finding of medullary dysplasia in humans and mice mutant for $p57^{KIP2}$, an inhibitor of cell proliferation, further suggests that regulation of cell proliferation and apoptosis is important in the renal medulla[76] and suggests a further link to human renal medullary dysplasia as observed in some patients with Beckwith-Wiedemann syndrome and $P57_{KIP2}$ mutations.[77]

TCF2, MATURITY-ONSET DIABETES TYPE 5, AND SPORADIC FORMS OF CAKUT

TCF2 encodes HNF-1β, a homeotic DNA-binding transcription factor, which is required during the development of the pancreas, kidneys, liver, and intestine. During kidney development in mice, *Tcf2* is expressed in the wolffian duct, ureteric bud, comma- and S-shaped bodies, and proximal and distal tubules.[78] Epithelial-specific inactivation of *Tcf2* in the kidney causes renal cystic disease and downregulation of several genes, inactivation of which cause renal cystic disease.[79] In humans, heterozygous mutations in *TCF2* cause maturity-onset diabetes type 5 (MODY5).[80,81] More than 50 different *TCF2* mutations have been reported, most of which are located in the first four exons that encode the

DNA-binding domain. In more than one-third of the cases, the gene is entirely deleted.[20,82] Diabetes mellitus is present in approximately 60% of all the cases reported, usually occurs before 25 years of age, and is often associated with pancreatic atrophy.[82-84] In the presence of renal cysts, the term renal cysts and diabetes syndrome, is used.

Although *TCF2* mutations were first identified in MODY5, such mutations are likely to be observed more frequently in fetuses with bilateral hyperechoic kidneys. An analysis of 62 newborns or fetuses with antenatally diagnosed bilateral hyperechogenic kidneys revealed that large genomic *TCF2* deletions were the most frequent cause (29%).[85] A complementary retrospective analysis of 377 patients with a *TCF2* mutation demonstrated that isolated hyperechogenic kidney with normal or slightly enlarged size is the most frequent phenotype observed before birth in these patients.[86] After birth, *TCF2* mutations most commonly manifest as bilateral small cortical cysts.[20] However, other manifestations of CAKUT are observed in these patients, including renal hypoplasia and dysplasia, multicystic dysplastic kidney, renal agenesis, horseshoe kidney, ureteropelvic junction obstruction, and clubbing and tiny diverticula of the calyces.[83,86-89] Patients with hyperechoic kidneys as a fetus and bilateral cortical cysts after birth and found to harbor *TCF2* mutations rarely manifest extrarenal anomalies during infancy and childhood.

TUBULAR DYSGENESIS AND MUTATIONS OF RENIN ANGIOTENSIN ALDOSTERONE SYSTEM ELEMENTS

Renal tubular dysgenesis is a severe perinatal disorder characterized by absence or paucity of differentiated proximal tubules, early severe oligohydramnios, and perinatal death. The latter is usually due to pulmonary hypoplasia and skull ossification defects.[4,90,91] This condition has also been described in clinical conditions associated with renal ischemia, including the twin-twin transfusion syndrome, major cardiac malformations, severe liver diseases, and fetal or infantile renal artery stenosis,[92] and in fetuses that are exposed in utero to angiotensin-converting enzyme (ACE) inhibitors or angiotensin II receptor blockers.[93] All of these pathophysiologic states are postulated to lead to chronic hypoperfusion of the fetal kidneys with upregulation of the renin angiotensin aldosterone system.[94] Mutations in the genes that encode components of the renin angiotensin aldosterone system have been identified in some families.[95] Mutations in the ACE and renin genes have been identified in 65.5% and 20% of cases, respectively. Mutations in angiotensinogen and in the angiotensinogen type 1 receptor genes occur much less frequently.[96]

CHD1L, CHD7, AND CHARGE SYNDROME

Chromodomain helicase DNA binding protein 1-like (CHD1L) protein is a member of the SNF2 family of helicase-related adenosine triphosphate (ATP)-hydrolyzing proteins. Like its related family member, CHD7, CHD1L contains a helicase-like region. CHD1L is expressed in early ureteric bud and comma- and S-shaped structures during human kidney development.[97] Heterozygous missense mutations in CHD1L were identified in 3 patients among 85 with CAKUT.[97] Mutations in CHD7 have also been identified in CHARGE syndrome (*c*oloboma, *h*eart defects, choanal *a*tresia, *r*etarded growth and development, *g*enital hypoplasia, *e*ar anomalies, and deafness), with 20% of these patients affected with CAKUT phenotypes, including horseshoe kidneys, renal agenesis, renal dysplasia, vesicoureteral reflux, ureterovesical junction obstruction, posterior urethral valves, and renal cysts.[98,99]

DSTYK AND CAKUT

DSTYK is a dual serine-threonine and tyrosine protein kinase that is coexpressed with fibroblast growth factor receptors in the developing mouse and human kidney in both metanephric mesenchyme and ureteric bud cells. Heterozygous mutations in DSTYK have been identified in a small number of individuals (7 of 311) with CAKUT.[100]

COPY NUMBER VARIANTS, CAKUT, AND NEUROPSYCHIATRIC DISORDERS

Copy number variants (CNVs) are stretches of DNA that are larger than 1 kb in length. Rare CNVs have been implicated in neuropsychiatric and craniofacial syndromes and in syndromes with CAKUT.[101,102] Sanna-Cherchi and colleagues examined the frequency of rare CNVs in individuals with CAKUT and identified such variants in 10% of affected individuals compared with 0.2% of population controls.[102] Deletions at the *HNF1* locus (chromosome 17q12) and the locus for DiGeorge's syndrome (chromosome 22q11) were most frequently identified, which suggests that these are "hot spots" for copy number variation. Interestingly, 90% of the CNVs associated with congenital renal malformations were previously reported to predispose to developmental delay or neuropsychiatric disease, which suggests that there are shared pathways implicated in renal and central nervous system development. Similarly, Handrigan and associates demonstrated that CNVs at chromosome 16q24.2 are associated with autism spectrum disorder, intellectual disability, and congenital renal malformations.[101]

THE ENVIRONMENT IN UTERO AND CAKUT

An increasing body of evidence, derived from human epidemiologic studies and animal models, demonstrates an important role for the intrauterine environment and fetal programming in the pathogenesis of renal hypoplasia and predisposition to later kidney disease (reviewed by Denton[103]) (Table 73.2). Low birth weight or intrauterine growth restriction is generally considered to be due to a suboptimal in utero environment. Here, the fetal kidney is particularly susceptible, which leads to reduced nephron number. In humans intrauterine growth restriction is most often due to uteroplacental insufficiency and maternal undernutrition. Modeling of these disorders in animals causes a significant reduction in nephron endowment.[104,105] Maternal dietary protein restriction results in decreased nephron number, reduced renal function, and hypertension in a variety of species, including rodents and sheep.[106-109] Although the underlying mechanisms are not well defined, some evidence suggests that the maternal diet programs the expression of critical genes required for embryonic kidney development, cell survival, and renal function.[107,110,111]

Studies in mutant mice have identified a requirement for vitamin A and its retinoic acid receptor–signaling effectors in RET expression and ureteric branching.[112] Vitamin A deficiency during pregnancy causes renal hypoplasia and

Table 73.2 Factors Influencing In Utero Environment That Are Associated with Renal Hypoplasia

Fetal Exposure To	Renal Phenotype	Reference
Uteroplacental insufficiency	Hypoplasia	104
Vitamin A deficiency	Hypoplasia, hydronephrosis/hydroureter	113
Low-protein diet	Hypoplasia	106, 108
Hyperglycemia	Agenesis, ectopic/horseshoe kidney, cystic dysplasia, hypoplasia, hydronephrosis/ureter	115
Cocaine	Agenesis, hypoplasia, hydronephrosis/hydroureter	117
Alcohol	Agenesis, ectopia/horseshoe kidney, cystic dysplasia, hypoplasia, hydronephrosis/hydroureter	118, 119
Angiotensin-converting enzyme inhibitors and angiotensin II receptor blockers	Renal dysgenesis	116

decreased glomerular number and *Ret* expression in the rodent fetus.[113] Interestingly, a single dose of retinoic acid administered at midgestation is able to normalize kidney size and nephron number in rat offspring exposed to maternal protein restriction, which raises the possibility of preventive approaches in humans.[114]

Maternal diabetes and in utero exposure to drugs and alcohol are associated with renal hypoplasia in the absence of reduced birth weight. In animal models, offspring of hyperglycemic or diabetic mothers demonstrate a significant nephron deficit.[115] Exposure of human fetuses to ACE inhibitors during the first trimester is associated with an increased risk for renal dysplasia, as well as cardiovascular and central nervous system malformations.[116] Human infants exposed to cocaine in utero have an increased risk for renal tract anomalies.[117] Similarly, infants with fetal alcohol syndrome have a higher incidence of CAKUT.[118] The pathogenic mechanisms underlying fetal alcohol exposure are beginning to be elucidated. Ethyl alcohol administration to pregnant rats at E13.5 and E14.5, stages that correspond to human E5 to E7, caused a modest decrease in nephron number but no deleterious effect on fetal kidney weight or maternal weight gain. The expression of *Gdnf* and *Wnt11*, both of which are required during ureteric branching was reduced, consistent with a decrease in nephrogenesis. Analysis of blood pressure at 6 months of age in pups exposed to ethyl alcohol in utero demonstrated a 10% increase in both males and females compared with age-matched sham-treated controls, although glomerular filtration rate (GFR) and renal vascular resistance differed between sexes.[119]

FUNCTIONAL CONSEQUENCES OF CAKUT

A growing body of evidence indicates that the number of functional nephrons formed by 32 to 34 weeks of gestation has important implications for short- and long-term renal function. Infants with simple renal hypoplasia or a moderate to severe degree of hypodysplasia exhibit renal insufficiency. A more subtle deficiency in nephron number has been associated with adult-onset hypertension.[120] The association of decreased nephron number with hypertension is consistent with the Barker hypothesis, which is based on epidemiologic evidence showing a correlation between birth weight and the incidence of cardiovascular diseases and proposes that adult-onset diseases such as hypertension have a fetal origin.[121,122] The human kidney does not exhibit a capacity to accelerate the rate of nephron formation in children born prematurely or to extend the period of nephrogenesis beyond the equivalent of 34 weeks of gestation.[123] Thus the integrity of nephron formation in utero is absolutely critical to postnatal life.

Growth of renal tubules and expansion of glomerular cross-sectional area in utero and after birth is critical to renal functional capacity. The general observation that tubule number, cross-sectional area, and cellular maturation are abnormal in renal dysgenesis is consistent with clinical observations that infants with moderate to severe renal hypoplasia or dysplasia demonstrate a limitation of GFR and tubular function. The developmental maturation of renal structures is discussed in this chapter in the context of their functions. Illustrative examples are provided for how abnormal differentiation, growth, and maturation in the malformed kidney can limit these functions. Existing knowledge has been generated, for the most part, from the study of maturing preterm and term animals. In contrast, very few data have been derived from the study of animals, such as mutant mice, with renal malformation. Thus interpretation of physiologic abnormalities in humans and experimental animals with renal malformation is largely an extrapolation from developmental studies in experimental animals with normal kidney development.

A major increase in glomerular basement surface area after birth contributes to the maturational increase in GFR during infancy, childhood, and adolescence.[124] Low GFR at birth limits excretion of free water, which increases the susceptibility of newborns to hyponatremia in association with a hypotonic fluid challenge.[125] Maximum urine concentrations achieved by preterm and term infants following fluid restriction are 600 mOsm/kg and 800 mOsm/kg, respectively.[126] An adult level of urine concentrating capacity is attained by 6 to 12 months of age.[127] Establishment of cortical and medullary domains during the twenty-second to twenty-fourth weeks of gestation is critical to urine concentration.[123] During embryogenesis the renal cortex grows along a circumferential axis with a 10-fold increase in its volume. The renal medulla expands 4.5-fold in thickness along a longitudinal axis, an increase that is mainly due to elongation of the outer medullary collecting ducts.[128] Longitudinal growth of the medulla contributes to lengthening of the loops of Henle such that they reach the inner renal medulla in the mature kidney. Elongation of the loops of Henle is important to the urine concentration mechanism because the magnitude of sodium and urea transport is greatest in longer loops, which generate steeper medullary tonicity gradients. The responsiveness of collecting duct cells to vasopressin is limited in newborns. This is thought to be due to high intrarenal levels of prostaglandins, which antagonize vasopressin.[129]

Maturation of sodium transport in the fetus and infant is dependent on growth and differentiation within the proximal tubule, loop of Henle, and distal tubule. Normal newborn infants are limited in their capacity to respond to sodium restriction by reducing urinary sodium excretion. Interruption of tubule generation, differentiation, and growth, which are hallmark features of renal dysplasia, contributes to an exaggerated limitation in the capacity to absorb sodium in affected infants and children. The proximal tubule exhibits dramatic growth and maturation during renal development. The epithelium matures from a columnar to a cuboidal epithelium, microvilli are elaborated on the apical and basal domains, and expression of sodium-potassium adenosine triphosphatase (Na^+-K^+-ATPase) and the sodium-hydrogen isoform 3 exchanger (NHE3) increase.[130-132] At birth proximal tubule length is heterogeneous between the inner and outer cortex[124]; by 1 month of life, proximal tubule length becomes uniform and tubule length and diameter have increased.[130] Maturation of tubule length is associated with the capacity to absorb sodium.[133] The loop of Henle is also characterized by increased spatial expression of transporters (Na^+-K^+-$2Cl^-$ cotransporter type 2[NKCC2], NHE3, renal outer medullary potassium [ROMK], Na^+-K^+-ATPase) key to sodium transport.[134] Similarly, expression of Na-Cl cotransporter (NCC) and epithelial sodium channel [ENaC] is low in the neonatal kidney and increases thereafter.[135]

Urinary potassium secretion is achieved predominantly by secretion of potassium in the cortical collecting duct via apical ROMK K^+ channels. In neonates, K^+ secretion is lower than in children due to the low secretory capacity of the cortical collecting duct. The postnatal increase in K^+ secretion is thought to be due to a developmental increase in the number of ROMK channels.[136] Malformation of tubules in disorders such as renal dysplasia is commonly associated with limited K^+ secretion, particularly during infancy.

CLINICAL PRESENTATION OF CAKUT

CLINICAL PRESENTATION IN THE FETUS

The majority of renal malformations are diagnosed antenatally, largely because of the widespread use and sensitivity of fetal ultrasonography. The human fetal kidney can be visualized at 12 to 15 of weeks of gestation. A screening antenatal ultrasound examination is recommended between 16 and 20 weeks of gestation, by which time renal anatomy can be imaged with considerable definition and anomalies can be detected with a sensitivity of approximately 80%.[137] Corticomedullary differentiation is distinct by 25 weeks of gestation and sometimes earlier. The fetal ureters are not normally detected by ultrasonography. Visualization of ureters may be indicative of ureteric or bladder obstruction or vesicoureteral reflux. A urine-filled bladder is normally identified at 13 to 15 weeks of gestation.[138] The bladder wall is normally thin. If the bladder wall is thick, urethral obstruction such as posterior urethral valves in a male fetus may be present.

Development of the kidney in utero is commonly assessed using fetal renal length standardized for gestational age as a surrogate marker.[139] The volume of amniotic fluid is a surrogate measure of renal function. Fetal urine production begins at 9 weeks of gestation. By 20 weeks of gestation and thereafter, fetal urine is the primary source of amniotic fluid volume.[140] A decrease in amniotic fluid volume, termed oligohydramnios, at or beyond the twentieth week of gestation is an excellent indicator of a critical defect in both kidneys, for example, bilateral renal dysplasia (or a critical defect in one kidney if a solitary kidney exists), bilateral ureteral obstruction, or obstruction of the bladder outlet. Severe oligohydramnios in the second trimester can result in lung hypoplasia because an adequate amniotic fluid volume is critical for lung development.[141] In its most severe form, oligohydramnios results in Potter's syndrome, which consists of a typical facies characterized by pseudoepicanthus, a recessed chin, posteriorly rotated and flattened ears, and flattened nose, as well as decreased fetal movement, clubfoot, hip dislocation and joint contractures, and pulmonary hypoplasia.

The composition of fetal urine is also used as a marker of kidney function. Urine levels of sodium and $β_2$-microglobulin decrease with increasing gestational age, and urine osmolality increases.[142,143] Impaired resorption occurs in fetuses with bilateral renal dysplasia or severe bilateral obstructive uropathy and results in abnormally high urine levels of sodium and $β_2$-microglobulin and low urine osmolality.[144] In general, sodium and chloride concentration greater than 90 mEq/L (90 mmol/L) and urinary osmolality less than 210 mOsmol/kg H_2O (210 mmol/kg H_2O) are indicative of fetal renal tubular impairment and poor renal prognosis.[145] In addition, urinary $β_2$-microglobulin levels greater than 6 mg/L are predictive of severe renal damage with a sensitivity and specificity of 80% and 71%, respectively.[146]

CLINICAL PRESENTATION OF SPECIFIC FORMS OF CAKUT

RENAL AGENESIS

A diagnosis of unilateral renal agenesis depends on the certainty that a second kidney does not exist in the pelvis or some other ectopic location. Because absence of one kidney induces compensatory hypertrophy in the existing kidney, the presence of a large kidney on one side supports a diagnosis of unilateral renal agenesis. Unilateral renal agenesis is generally asymptomatic. A solitary kidney is most often detected either during routine antenatal ultrasonography or during the assessment of an accompanying urinary tract abnormality, the occurrence of which has been reported in 33% to 65% of cases.[147] Vesicoureteral reflux is the most commonly identified urologic abnormality, occurring in approximately 37% of patients with unilateral renal agenesis and prompting investigation particularly in newborn infants. Other associated urologic anomalies include obstruction of the ureteropelvic junction in 6% to 7% and ureterovesical junction in 11% to 18% of patients.

RENAL DYSPLASIA

The dysplastic kidney is generally smaller than normal and is characterized with ultrasonography by increased echogenicity, loss of corticomedullary differentiation, and cysts of varied size and location. Large cystic elements can contribute to large kidney size. The multicystic dysplastic kidney is an extreme example of a large dysplastic kidney (see Figure 73.2). Renal dysplasia may be unilateral or bilateral and may be discovered during routine antenatal screening or postnatally when renal ultrasonography is performed in a dysmorphic infant. Bilateral dysplasia is likely to be diagnosed earlier than unilateral dysplasia, especially if oligohydramnios is present. Infants with bilateral dysplasia may demonstrate impaired renal function shortly after birth. Associated urinary tract abnormalities include hydronephrosis, a duplicated collecting system, megaureter, ureteral stenosis, and vesicoureteral reflux.[145] Clinical presentation may be related to complications such as urinary tract infection associated with these disorders.

The multicystic dysplastic kidney is identified by ultrasonography as a large cystic nonreniform mass in the renal fossa and by palpation as a flank mass. The multicystic dysplastic kidney is nonfunctional and usually unilateral. If the condition is bilateral, it is fatal. In unilateral multicystic dysplastic kidney, associated contralateral abnormalities occur in 25% of cases and can include rotational or positional anomalies, renal hypoplasia, vesicoureteric efflux, and ureteropelvic junction obstruction.[11] Although hypertension rarely occurs (0.01% to 0.1% of cases), blood pressure should be monitored intermittently during the first few years of life. Wilms' tumor and renal cell carcinoma have also been described, but the incidence of malignant complications is not significantly different from that in the general population.[148] The natural history of a multicystic dysplastic kidney is gradual reduction in size such that the kidney eventually cannot be detected using noninvasive imaging. At 2 years of age, an involution in size can be detected by ultrasonography in up to 60% of the affected kidneys.

DOUBLE COLLECTING SYSTEM

Complete or partial duplication of the renal collecting system is the most common congenital anomaly of the urinary tract[7] (Figure 73.5). A double collecting system is thought to result from duplication of the ureteric bud, whereby the superior bud is associated with the upper renal pole and the inferior bud with the lower renal pole. In complete duplication the kidney has two separate pelvicalyceal systems and two ureters. The ureter from the lower collecting system usually enters the bladder in the trigone, whereas the ureter from the upper collecting system can have a normal insertion in the trigone or be inserted ectopically in the bladder or elsewhere. In boys, insertion can occur in the posterior urethra, ejaculatory ducts, or epididymis; in girls, insertion can occur in the vagina or uterus. Ectopic insertion of the ureter can result in obstruction or vesicoureteral reflux. Depending upon the location of the ectopic insertion, incontinence also may be present. Partial duplication is more common than complete duplication. In these cases the kidney has two separate pelvicalyceal systems with either a single ureter or two ureters that unite before insertion into the bladder.

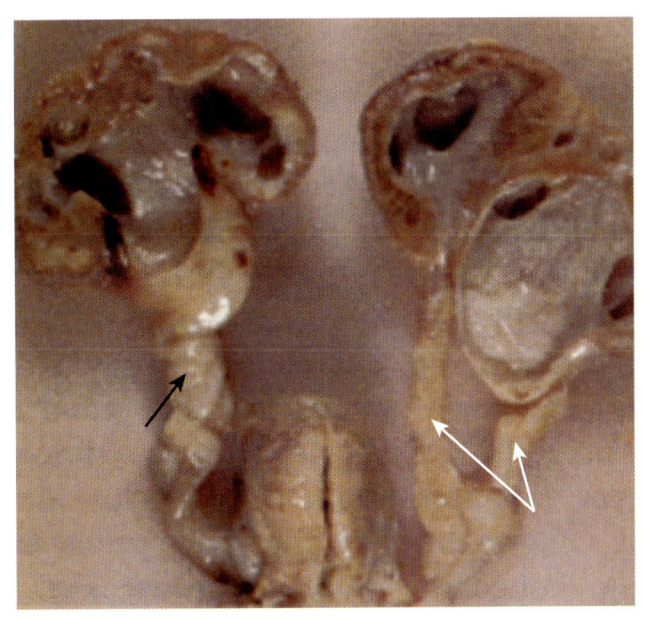

Figure 73.5 Duplicated collecting system. Duplicated ureters (*white arrows*) are shown on the right. A single dilated ureter (*black arrow*) is shown on the left. Each ureter is dilated due to obstruction at the level of the bladder.

RENAL ECTOPY

Renal ectopy (see Figures 73.3 and 73.4) results from disruption of the normal embryologic migration of the kidneys. Rapid caudal growth during embryogenesis results in migration of the developing kidney from the pelvis to the retroperitoneal renal fossa. With ascension comes a 90-degree rotation from a horizontal to a vertical position with the renal hilum finally directed medially. Migration and rotation are complete by 8 weeks of gestation. Simple congenital ectopy refers to a low-lying kidney that failed to ascend normally. It most commonly lies over the pelvic brim or in the pelvis and is termed a pelvic kidney. Less commonly, the kidney may lie on the contralateral side of the body, a state that is termed crossed ectopy without fusion. Although affected individuals are generally asymptomatic and are identified during an imaging study performed for some other indication, some patients develop symptoms due to complications, such as infection, renal calculi, and urinary obstruction.[139] The ectopic kidney is often characterized by decreased function. In a case study of 82 cases of unilateral renal ectopy, decreased renal function was detected by technetium 99m (^{99m}Tc)–labeled dimercaptosuccinic acid (DMSA) renal scan in 74 patients.[139] A high incidence of other urologic abnormalities has been associated with renal ectopy. The most frequent of these is vesicoureteral reflux, which occurs in 20% of crossed renal ectopy, 30% of simple renal ectopy, and 70% in bilateral simple renal ectopy.[139] Other associated urologic abnormalities include contralateral renal dysplasia (4%), cryptorchidism (5%), and hypospadias (5%).[13]

RENAL FUSION

Renal fusion occurs when a portion of one kidney is fused to the other (see Figure 73.4). The most common fusion anomaly is the horseshoe kidney, which involves abnormal migration of both kidneys (ectopy). The horseshoe kidney differs from crossed fused renal ectopy, which usually involves abnormal movement of only one kidney across the midline with fusion of the contralateral noncrossing kidney. In more than 90% of cases of horseshoe kidney, fusion occurs at the lower poles; as a result two separate excretory renal units and ureters are maintained. The isthmus (fused portion) may lie over the midline (symmetric horseshoe kidney) or lateral to the midline (asymmetric horseshoe kidney). Depending on the degree of fusion, the isthmus can be composed of renal parenchyma or a fibrous band. Fusion is thought to occur before the kidneys ascend between the fourth and ninth week of gestation from the pelvis to their normal dorsolumbar position. If large portions of the renal parenchyma fuse, the fusion anomaly loses its horseshoe appearance and appears as a flattened disk or lump kidney. Early fusion also causes abnormal rotation of the developing kidneys. As a result, the axis of each kidney is shifted so that the renal pelvis lies anteriorly and the ureters either traverse over the isthmus of the horseshoe kidney or the anterior surface of the fused kidney. Fusion anomalies seldom ascend to the dorsolumbar position of normal kidneys and are typically found in the pelvis or at the lower lumbar vertebral level (L4 or L5). The blood supply of the fused kidney is variable and may come from the iliac arteries, aorta, and at times the hypogastric and middle sacral arteries.[149]

The majority of patients with renal fusion are asymptomatic. Some, however develop urinary tract obstruction, which presents with loin pain, hematuria, and may be associated with urinary tract infections due to urinary stasis or vesicoureteric reflux. Renal calculi may occur in up to 20% of cases.[150] Other associated urologic anomalies include ureteral duplication, ectopic ureter, and retrocaval ureter. Investigations should include static imaging (renal ultrasonography) and functional imaging such as a ^{99m}Tc–labeled DMSA scan and voiding cystourethrography (VCUG). Renal calculi are reported to occur in 20% of cases. Obstruction resulting in urinary stasis and complicating urinary tract infection have been thought to be the major contributing factors to stone formation. Patients with a horseshoe kidney appear to have an increased risk for Wilms' tumor. This was illustrated in a retrospective review of 8617 patients from the National Wilms Tumor Study, between 1969 and 1998, that identified 41 patients with Wilms' tumor in a horseshoe kidney.[151]

In crossed fused ectopy, the ectopic kidney and ureter cross the midline to fuse with the contralateral kidney, but the ureter of the ectopic kidney maintains its normal insertion into the bladder. In most cases the ectopic kidney is positioned inferiorly to the contralateral kidney. The contralateral kidney can either retain its normal dorsolumbar position or is positioned lower in the pelvis or lower lumbar vertebral level (L4 or L5). Most patients with crossed fused ectopy are asymptomatic and are detected coincidentally, often by antenatal ultrasonography. As is true in patients with horseshoe kidney, most patients have an excellent prognosis without need for intervention. In some cases, complications can occur, including obstructive uropathy due to extrinsic ureteric compression by aberrant blood vessels or ureteropelvic junction obstruction, renal calculi, urinary tract infection, and vesicoureteral reflux.[152]

CLINICAL MANAGEMENT OF CAKUT

Because CAKUT plays a causative role in 30% to 50% of cases of ESKD in children,[153] it is important to diagnose and initiate therapy to minimize renal damage, prevent or delay the onset of ESKD, and provide supportive care to avoid complications of ESKD.

OVERALL APPROACH TO MANAGEMENT OF CAKUT IN UTERO AND IN THE IMMEDIATE POSTNATAL PERIOD

Counseling of families during pregnancy is a key element in the management of CAKUT. Coordinated consultation among professionals in the disciplines of obstetrics, pediatric nephrology, pediatric urology, and neonatology is critical. Consistent and clear clinical information regarding diagnosis and prognosis should be provided during pregnancy and after birth. The level of certainty regarding the severity of the diagnosis and prognosis has a major impact on decision making during pregnancy and in the immediate postnatal period. Intervention in utero has been designed to (1) reduce renal damage arising from urinary tract obstruction and (2) rescue pulmonary development in the face of urinary tract obstruction and oligohydramnios. To date, little evidence exists that relief of urinary tract obstruction in utero prevents the development of associated renal dysplasia or renal scarring. In contrast, insertion of a bladder–amniotic cavity shunt in the fetus with obstruction below the bladder neck can rescue oligohydramnios and pulmonary hypoplasia.[152,154] Diagnostic and therapeutic management after birth should be anticipated via the coordinated actions of obstetricians, neonatologists, pediatric nephrologists, and pediatric urologists and should include an immediate assessment in the postnatal period of the need for specialized imaging, assessment of renal function, and management of nutrition and electrolytes.

After delivery a detailed history and careful physical examination should be performed in all infants with an antenatally detected renal malformation. The examination should include the respiratory system to assess the presence of pulmonary insufficiency; the abdomen to detect the presence of a mass that could represent an enlarged kidney due to obstructive uropathy or multicystic dysplastic kidney or a palpable enlarged bladder, which could suggest posterior urethral valves; the ears, because outer ear abnormalities are associated with an increased risk for CAKUT; and the umbilicus, because a single umbilical artery is associated with an increased risk for CAKUT.

In newborns with bilateral renal malformation, a solitary malformed kidney, or a history of oligohydramnios, abdominal ultrasonography is recommended within the first 24 hours of life because an intervention such as decompression of the bladder with a transurethral catheter may be required. Newborn infants with unilateral involvement do not need immediate attention. In these infants renal ultrasonography is generally performed after 48 hours of age and within the first week of life. Ultrasonographic examination before 48 hours of age may not detect collecting system dilation because a newborn is in a relatively volume-contracted state during this period of time.[155] The serum creatinine concentration can be used to estimate the extent of renal impairment and should be measured when there is bilateral renal disease or an affected solitary kidney. The serum creatinine concentration at birth is similar to that in the mother (usually ≤1.0 mg/dL [88 μmol/L]). Thus serum creatinine concentration should be measured after the first 24 hours of life. It declines to normal values (0.3 to 0.5 mg/dL [27 to 44 μmol/L]) within approximately 1 week in term infants and 2 to 3 weeks in preterm infants.

MANAGEMENT OF SPECIFIC TYPES OF CAKUT

RENAL DYSPLASIA

Because of the frequent association of renal dysplasia with a collecting system anomaly, particularly vesicoureteral reflux, VCUG should be considered in all patients with renal dysplasia. The presence of vesicoureteral reflux or some other collecting system abnormality in the normal contralateral kidney places children with unilateral renal dysplasia at increased risk for long-term sequelae of renal scarring from recurrent urinary tract infection. A DMSA radionuclide scan can provide further information on the differential function of each kidney, which may be useful in management decisions regarding surgical interventions.

The prognosis for a patient with renal dysplasia depends on whether there is unilateral or bilateral disease. In general, the long-term outcome of unilateral renal dysplasia is excellent, particularly if there is a normal contralateral kidney. Serial ultrasonography can assess compensatory renal growth of a normal contralateral kidney and any further change in the size of the abnormal kidney.

Over time, as mentioned previously, a multicystic dysplastic kidney is gradually reduced in size to the point that the kidney eventually cannot be detected through noninvasive imaging. Renal ultrasonography is generally recommended at intervals of 3 months for the first year of life and then every 6 months up to involution of the mass, or at least up to 5 years.[156] Compensatory hypertrophy of the contralateral kidney is expected and should be monitored by renal ultrasonography. Hypertension is unusual; blood pressure should be monitored intermittently during the first few years of life. Medical therapy is usually effective in treating hypertension in the small number of affected patients, but nephrectomy may be curative in resistant cases. As mentioned earlier, Wilms' tumor and renal cell carcinoma have also been described, but the incidence of malignant complications is not significantly different from that in the general population.[148]

RENAL ECTOPY AND FUSION

Detection of an ectopic kidney provides a basis to determine renal function and any associated urinary tract anomalies. Reduced renal function in the ectopic kidney can be determined by radionuclide scan. Abdominal and pelvic ultrasonography is indicated to determine the presence of a collecting system. VCUG should be undertaken, particularly if there is hydronephrosis, given the risk for vesicoureteral reflux and urinary tract obstruction. VCUG should be performed in all patients with a horseshoe kidney because of the increased association with vesicoureteral reflux. If vesicoureteral reflux is detected, then prophylactic antibiotics should be considered, especially in patients who have a history of urinary tract infections.

Further evaluation is based upon the results of renal ultrasonography and VCUG and on the serum creatinine concentration. No further evaluation is required in the patient with a normal-appearing contralateral kidney and no evidence of hydronephrosis in the ectopic kidney. If the serum creatinine concentration is elevated or if the contralateral kidney appears abnormal, a DMSA renal scan should be performed to assess differential renal function. Diuretic renography should be performed with ^{99m}Tc–labeled mercaptoacetyltriglycine (MAG3) or ^{99m}Tc–labeled diethylenetriaminepentaacetic acid (DTPA) to detect obstruction if there is severe hydronephrosis and the VCUG findings are normal. If the hydronephrosis is mild or moderate and the VCUG findings are normal, then follow-up ultrasonography should be performed 3 to 6 months later. If there is progressive hydronephrosis, then MAG-3 or DTPA diuretic renography should be performed to detect obstruction.

LONG-TERM OUTCOMES OF RENAL MALFORMATION

Clinical outcomes in CAKUT vary widely from no symptoms whatsoever to chronic kidney disease resulting in a need for renal replacement during a period ranging from the newborn period to the fourth and fifth decades of life. Risk factors for mortality during infancy and early childhood include coexistence of renal and nonrenal disease, prematurity, low birth weight, oligohydramnios, and severe forms of renal–urinary tract malformation (agenesis, hypodysplasia).[157] In a case series of 822 children with prenatally detected CAKUT who were followed for a median time of 43 months, Quirino and coworkers reported a mortality of 1.5% and morbid conditions including urinary tract infection, hypertension, and chronic kidney disease in 29%, 2.7%, and 6% of surviving children, respectively.[158] A faster rate of decline of renal function in patients with CAKUT and chronic kidney disease has been associated with a urine albumin to creatinine ratio greater than 200 mg/mmol compared with less than 50 mg/mmol (estimated GFR [eGFR]: −6.5 mL/min/1.73 m^2/yr vs. −1.5 mL/min/1.73 m^2/yr), and with more than two (vs. less than two) febrile urinary tract infections (eGFR: −3.5 mL/min/1.73 m^2/yr vs. −2 mL/min/1.73 m^2/yr). A greater decline in eGFR occurs during puberty (eGFR: −4 mL/min/1.73 m^2/yr vs. −1.9 mL/min/1.73 m^2/yr).[159] A study examining the risk for dialysis in patients with CAKUT demonstrated a significantly higher risk for patients with a solitary kidney compared to controls without disease.[160] These results raise the possibility that the prognosis for a solitary apparently, normal kidney may not be as "normal" as previously thought. Finally, a study of CAKUT patients receiving some form of replacement therapy and registered within the European Renal Association–European Dialysis and Transplant Association registry showed that some of these patients only require renal replacement in the third, fourth, or fifth decade of life. The finding that the mean age at which patients with CAKUT require dialysis and/or transplantation is 31 years indicates that children with CAKUT are at risk for developing a requirement for dialysis and/or transplantation as adults.[3]

Complete reference list available at ExpertConsult.com.

KEY REFERENCES

1. Loane M, Dolk H, Kelly A, et al: Paper 4: EUROCAT statistical monitoring: identification and investigation of ten year trends of congenital anomalies in Europe. *Birth Defects Res A Clin Mol Teratol* 91(Suppl 1):S31–S43, 2011.
3. Wuhl E, van Stralen KJ, Verrina E, et al: Timing and outcome of renal replacement therapy in patients with congenital malformations of the kidney and urinary tract. *Clin J Am Soc Nephrol* 8:67–74, 2013.
4. Allanson JE, Hunter AG, Mettler GS, et al: Renal tubular dysgenesis: a not uncommon autosomal recessive syndrome: a review. *Am J Med Genet* 43:811–814, 1992.
5. Wiesel A, Queisser-Luft A, Clementi M, et al: Prenatal detection of congenital renal malformations by fetal ultrasonographic examination: an analysis of 709,030 births in 12 European countries. *Eur J Med Genet* 48:131–144, 2005.
12. Harris J, Robert E, Kallen B: Epidemiologic characteristics of kidney malformations. *Eur J Epidemiol* 16:985–992, 2000.
13. Guarino N, Tadini B, Camardi P, et al: The incidence of associated urological abnormalities in children with renal ectopia. *J Urol* 172:1757–1759, 2004.
16. Roodhooft AM, Jason MD, Birnholz JC, et al: Familial nature of congenital absence and severe dysgenesis of both kidneys. *N Engl J Med* 310:1341–1344, 1984.
17. Bulum B, Ozcakar ZB, Ustuner E, et al: High frequency of kidney and urinary tract anomalies in asymptomatic first-degree relatives of patients with CAKUT. *Pediatr Nephrol* 28:2143–2147, 2013.
18. Weber S, Moriniere V, Knuppel T, et al: Prevalence of mutations in renal developmental genes in children with renal hypodysplasia: results of the ESCAPE study. *J Am Soc Nephrol* 17:2864–2870, 2006.
20. Ulinski T, Lescure S, Beaufils S, et al: Renal phenotypes related to hepatocyte nuclear factor-1beta (TCF2) mutations in a pediatric cohort. *J Am Soc Nephrol* 17:497–503, 2006.
21. Quinlan J, Lemire M, Hudson T, et al: A common variant of the PAX2 gene is associated with reduced newborn kidney size. *J Am Soc Nephrol* 18:1915–1921, 2007.
23. Rosenblum ND: Developmental biology of the human kidney. *Semin Fetal Neonatal Med* 13:125–132, 2008.
26. Chatterjee R, Ramos E, Hoffman M, et al: Traditional and targeted exome sequencing reveals common, rare and novel functional deleterious variants in RET-signaling complex in a cohort of living US patients with urinary tract malformations. *Hum Genet* 131:1725–1738, 2012.
30. Mackie GG, Stephens FD: Duplex kidneys: a correlation of renal dysplasia with position of the ureteral orifice. *J Urol* 114:274–280, 1975.
31. Bertoli-Avella AM, Conte ML, Punzo F, et al: ROBO2 gene variants are associated with familial vesicoureteral reflux. *J Am Soc Nephrol* 19:825–831, 2008.
33. Grieshammer U, Le M, Plump AS, et al: SLIT2-mediated ROBO2 signaling restricts kidney induction to a single site. *Dev Cell* 6:709–717, 2004.
35. Weber S, Taylor JC, Winyard P, et al: SIX2 and BMP4 mutations associate with anomalous kidney development. *J Am Soc Nephrol* 19:891–903, 2008.
40. Sanyanusin P, Schimmenti LA, McNoe LA, et al: Mutation of the PAX2 gene in a family with optic nerve colobomas, renal anomalies and vesicoureteral reflux. *Nat Genet* 9:358–363, 1995.
45. Shakya R, Watanabe T, Costantini F: The role of GDNF/Ret signaling in ureteric bud cell fate and branching morphogenesis. *Dev Cell* 8:65–74, 2005.
47. Kohlhase J, Wischermann A, Reichenbach H, et al: Mutations in the SALL1 putative transcription factor gene cause Townes-Brocks syndrome. *Nat Genet* 18:81–83, 1998.
51. Ruf RG, Xu PX, Silvius D, et al: SIX1 mutations cause branchio-oto-renal syndrome by disruption of EYA1-SIX1-DNA complexes. *Proc Natl Acad Sci U S A* 101:8090–8095, 2004.
52. Sajithlal G, Zou D, Silvius D, et al: Eya1 acts as a critical regulator for specifying the metanephric mesenchyme. *Dev Biol* 284:323–336, 2005.
53. Xu PX, Adams J, Peters H, et al: Eya1-deficient mice lack ears and kidneys and show abnormal apoptosis of organ primordia. *Nat Genet* 23:113–117, 1999.
56. Abdelhak S, Kalatzis V, Heilig R, et al: A human homologue of the *Drosophila* eyes absent gene underlies branchio-oto-renal (BOR) syndrome and identifies a novel gene family. *Nat Genet* 15:157–164, 1997.
70. Kang S, Graham JM, Jr, Olney AH, et al: GLI3 frameshift mutations cause autosomal dominant Pallister-Hall syndrome. *Nat Genet* 15:266–268, 1997.
72. Hu MC, Mo R, Bhella S, et al: GLI3-dependent transcriptional repression of Gli1, Gli2 and kidney patterning genes disrupts renal morphogenesis. *Development* 133:569–578, 2006.
73. Cain JE, Islam E, Haxho F, et al: GLI3 Repressor controls functional development of the mouse ureter. *J Clin Invest* 121:1199–1206, 2011.
74. Cano-Gauci DF, Song HH, Yang H, et al: Glypican-3-deficient mice exhibit the overgrowth and renal abnormalities typical of the Simpson-Golabi-Behmel syndrome. *J Cell Biol* 146:255–264, 1999.
76. Zhang P, Liégeois NJ, Wong C, et al: Altered cell differentiation and proliferation in mice lacking $p57^{KIP2}$ indicates a role in Beckwith-Wiedemann syndrome. *Nature* 387:151–158, 1997.
77. Hatada I, Ohashi H, Fukushima Y, et al: An imprinted gene $p57^{KIP2}$ is mutated in Beckwith-Wiedemann syndrome. *Nat Genet* 14:171–173, 1996.
82. Bellanne-Chantelot C, Clauin S, Chauveau D, et al: Large genomic rearrangements in the hepatocyte nuclear factor-1beta (TCF2) gene are the most frequent cause of maturity-onset diabetes of the young type 5. *Diabetes* 54:3126–3132, 2005.
83. Bellanne-Chantelot C, Chauveau D, Gautier JF, et al: Clinical spectrum associated with hepatocyte nuclear factor-1beta mutations. *Ann Intern Med* 140:510–517, 2004.
85. Decramer S, Parant O, Beaufils S, et al: Anomalies of the TCF2 gene are the main cause of fetal bilateral hyperechogenic kidneys. *J Am Soc Nephrol* 18:923–933, 2007.
86. Heidet L, Decramer S, Pawtowski A, et al: Spectrum of HNF1B mutations in a large cohort of patients who harbor renal diseases. *Clin J Am Soc Nephrol* 5:1079–1090, 2010.
87. Lindner TH, Njolstad PR, Horikawa Y, et al: A novel syndrome of diabetes mellitus, renal dysfunction and genital malformation associated with a partial deletion of the pseudo-POU domain of hepatocyte nuclear factor-1beta. *Hum Mol Genet* 8:2001–2008, 1999.
90. McFadden DE, Pantzar JT, Van Allen MI, et al: Renal tubular dysgenesis with calvarial hypoplasia: report of two additional cases and review. *J Med Genet* 34:846–848, 1997.
95. Gribouval O, Gonzales M, Neuhaus T, et al: Mutations in genes in the renin-angiotensin system are associated with autosomal recessive renal tubular dysgenesis. *Nat Genet* 37:964–968, 2005.
99. Hwang DY, Dworschak GC, Kohl S, et al: Mutations in 12 known dominant disease-causing genes clarify many congenital anomalies of the kidney and urinary tract. *Kidney Int* 85:1429–1433, 2014.
100. Sanna-Cherchi S, Sampogna RV, Papeta N, et al: Mutations in DSTYK and dominant urinary tract malformations. *N Engl J Med* 369:621–629, 2013.
102. Sanna-Cherchi S, Kiryluk K, Burgess KE, et al: Copy-number disorders are a common cause of congenital kidney malformations. *Am J Hum Genet* 91:987–997, 2012.
112. Batourina E, Gim S, Bello N, et al: Vitamin A controls epithelial/mesenchymal interactions through Ret expression. *Nat Genet* 27:74–78, 2001.
116. Cooper WO, Hernandez-Diaz S, Arbogast PG, et al: Major congenital malformations after first-trimester exposure to ACE inhibitors. *N Engl J Med* 354:2443–2451, 2006.
120. Keller G, Zimmer G, Mall G, et al: Nephron number in patients with primary hypertension. *N Engl J Med* 348:101–108, 2003.
121. Barker DJ, Osmond C, Golding J, et al: Growth in utero, blood pressure in childhood and adult life, and mortality from cardiovascular disease. *BMJ* 298:564–567, 1989.
146. Morris RK, Quinlan-Jones E, Kilby MD, et al: Systematic review of accuracy of fetal urine analysis to predict poor postnatal renal function in cases of congenital urinary tract obstruction. *Prenat Diagn* 27:900–911, 2007.
156. Heymans C, Breysem L, Proesmans W: Multicystic kidney dysplasia: a prospective study on the natural history of the affected and the contralateral kidney. *Eur J Pediatr* 157:673–675, 1998.

158. Quirino IG, Diniz JS, Bouzada MC, et al: Clinical course of 822 children with prenatally detected nephrouropathies. *Clin J Am Soc Nephrol* 7:444–451, 2012.
160. Sanna-Cherchi S, Ravani P, Corbani V, et al: Renal outcome in patients with congenital anomalies of the kidney and urinary tract. *Kidney Int* 76:528–533, 2009.
165. Sakaki-Yumoto M, Kobayashi C, Sato A, et al: The murine homolog of SALL4, a causative gene in Okihiro syndrome, is essential for embryonic stem cell proliferation, and cooperates with Sall1 in anorectal, heart, brain and kidney development. *Development* 133:3005–3013, 2006.
167. Van Esch H, Groenen P, Nesbit MA, et al: GATA3 haploinsufficiency causes human HDR syndrome. *Nature* 406:419–422, 2000.

74 Diseases of the Kidney and Urinary Tract in Children

Sevcan A. Bakkaloglu | Franz Schaefer

CHAPTER OUTLINE

SPECTRUM OF KIDNEY AND URINARY TRACT DISORDERS IN CHILDREN, 2308
EVALUATION OF KIDNEY FUNCTION IN CHILDREN, 2309
Assessment of Glomerular Filtration Rate, 2309
Assessment of Proteinuria, 2310
CONGENITAL ANOMALIES OF THE KIDNEY AND URINARY TRACT, 2311
Definitions, 2311
Epidemiology, 2311
Phenotypes, 2311
Syndromic Forms of Congenital Anomalies of the Kidney and Urinary Tract, 2316
Ciliopathies, 2319
GLOMERULAR DISORDERS, 2322
Nephrotic Syndrome, 2323
Nephritic Syndrome, 2331
TUBULAR DISORDERS, 2333
Bartter-Like Syndromes, 2333
Renal Tubular Acidosis, 2335
Nephrogenic Diabetes Insipidus, 2338
Cystinosis, 2339
UROLITHIASIS AND NEPHROCALCINOSIS IN CHILDREN, 2340
Risk Factors for Stone Formation, 2340
Presentation and Treatment of Kidney Stone Disease, 2342
Genetic Kidney Stone Disease, 2344
SYSTEMIC DISORDERS AFFECTING THE KIDNEY, 2348
Childhood Vasculitides with Kidney Involvement, 2348
Hemolytic Uremic Syndrome, 2352
PEDIATRIC ASPECTS OF CHRONIC KIDNEY DISEASE, 2357
Growth, Nutrition, and Development, 2357
Cardiovascular Comorbidity in Pediatric Chronic Kidney Disease, 2359
Progression of Chronic Renal Failure in Children, 2361

SPECTRUM OF KIDNEY AND URINARY TRACT DISORDERS IN CHILDREN

The spectrum of chronic pediatric kidney disorders differs greatly from the distribution of nephropathies in adults (Figure 74.1). Approximately 70% of pediatric patients have congenital abnormalities of the kidneys and/or urinary tract. In these patients, renal failure develops if there is significant renal hypoplasia or dysplasia. Obstructive uropathies (e.g., posterior urethral valves, pelvicoureteric or distal ureteric stenosis) are often detected in the prenatal or neonatal period and then relieved surgically if functionally relevant. Chronic kidney disease (CKD) may still develop if the obstruction has caused significant renal dysplasia in utero. Inherited monogenic kidney disorders constitute another major cause of pediatric CKD, accounting cumulatively for another 15% to 20% of cases. Nephronophthisis, polycystic kidney disease, oxalosis, cystinosis, Alport's syndrome, and a large proportion of childhood cases of focal segmental glomerulosclerosis and atypical hemolytic uremic syndrome are caused by identifiable genetic abnormalities. Other causes include kidney injury following ischemic insults (most importantly, perinatal asphyxia and septicemia). In contrast, even large pediatric patient registries have not reported significant numbers of children with diabetic or hypertension attributed nephropathy, the two most common causes of CKD in adult populations. Acquired glomerulopathies leading to CKD are limited to rare cases of immunoglobulin A (IgA) nephropathy or Henoch-Schönlein nephritis and systemic vasculitides such as lupus erythematosus and Wegener's granulomatosis.

The prevalence of end-stage kidney disease (ESKD) among children younger than 15 years in Europe is currently 34 per million age-related population (pmarp) or 5.4 per million population (pmp).[1] The annual incidence is 6.5 pmarp or 1.0 pmp. When the pediatric population is defined as those up to age 19 years, the prevalence of ESKD in children and adolescents is 80 to 90 pmp and the annual incidence is 15 pmp. This is only 10% of the incidence in young

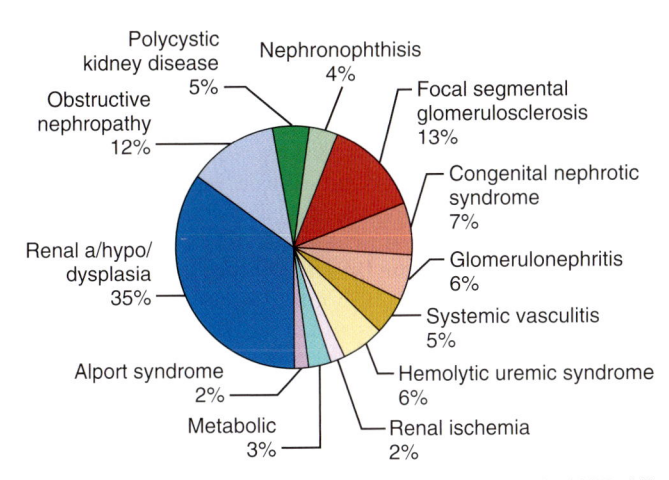

Figure 74.1 Spectrum of underlying renal diagnoses in 1367 children with end-stage kidney disease. (From the International Pediatric Peritoneal Dialysis Network Registry.)

adults and fewer than 2% of that observed in the older population. Because of the preponderance of males among those with certain urinary tract abnormalities (e.g., urethral valves), renal replacement therapy occurs almost 50% more often in males than in females. ESKD incidence is highest in adolescence (8 pmarp), lowest in middle childhood (4.6 pmarp), and intermediate in children younger than 5 years of age (6.7 pmarp).

The demographics of mild to moderate CKD in children are unknown but is likely to be similar to that in the adult population. In countries with a high prevalence of consanguineous marriages, the prevalence of pediatric CKD is estimated to be several-fold higher than in the Western countries.

Because of the predominantly genetic origin of pediatric nephropathies, CKD in children is frequently associated with a variety of extrarenal abnormalities. The prevalence of severe associated comorbid conditions appears to have been increasing because a growing number of children with severe syndromal disease are accepted into CKD and ESKD management programs. In the Registry of the International Pediatric Peritoneal Dialysis Network, 13% of children with CKD starting dialysis had a defined syndrome with one or several extrarenal manifestations. Impaired neurocognitive development was observed in 16%, cardiac anomalies in 15%, ocular abnormalities in 13%, and hearing abnormalities in 5% of patients.

Impaired neurodevelopment and sensory dysfunctions are among the most severe general disabilities interfering with psychosocial adjustment and integration in children with CKD. Some 20% to 25% of infants undergoing appropriate neurodevelopmental testing show moderate to severe developmental delays, which usually remain unchanged after successful kidney transplantation. IQ testing of children with CKD at school age usually reveals a distribution of scores that is shifted downward with respect to total verbal and performance IQs compared with healthy children. Although testing may be biased in a substantial proportion of patients due to associated sensory disorders, such as hearing loss or visual impairment, these disturbing findings clearly show a need for regular assessment of neurodevelopmental and/or neurocognitive function in all children with significant impairment in their glomerular filtration rate (GFR) and for the development of interventional programs, including individualized education programs (IEPs) to optimize developmental and educational outcomes for these children.

EVALUATION OF KIDNEY FUNCTION IN CHILDREN

ASSESSMENT OF GLOMERULAR FILTRATION RATE

Several issues need to be considered when assessing and interpreting kidney function in children. Childhood is the final extrauterine period of growth and maturation. During this phase, the metabolic needs of the organism, on the one hand, and the functional capacity of the kidneys, on the other, undergo profound, synchronized changes. From birth to adulthood, body weight increases 20-fold, body length three to fourfold, and body surface area (BSA), the closest correlate of basal metabolic rate, eightfold. By convention, the GFR is normalized to the BSA of an average-sized adult—that is, 1.73 m^2.

Although nephron formation is complete by the 30th gestational week, nephrons continue to grow in size and functional capacity after birth. In early postnatal life, nephron size and capacity increase not only in absolute terms but also relative to BSA, which results in a significant physiologic gain in normalized global renal function. The average GFR in the neonate is 20 to 30 mL/min/1.73 m^2 and increases rapidly in the first few months of life. From 18 months of age, the absolute increase in GFR precisely matches the growth in body surface area, which results in a constant normal range of BSA-indexed GFR throughout childhood and adolescence. After 2 years of age, the conventional CKD staging system, which assigns stages of CKD based on estimated GFR (eGFR) in multiples of 15 and 30 mL/min/1.73 m^2, can be used.

Regular assessments of GFR are crucial for the staging and monitoring of renal function in children with CKD. The direct measurement of GFR is a challenging task in children. Although inulin clearance is still considered the gold standard, inulin is unavailable in many countries, and formal steady-state inulin clearance studies are difficult to perform in the pediatric setting due to technical problems and ethical considerations. Radioisotope single-injection dilution studies (e.g., using chromium 51–labeled ethylenediaminetetraacetic acid [^{51}Cr-EDTA] or technetium 99–labeled diethylenetriaminepentaacetic acid [^{99}Tc-DTPA]) have been largely abandoned due to the significant radiation exposure. A simplified single-injection clearance protocol using the radiocontrast agent iohexol has been validated in children with CKD and may become a standard technique, at least for research purposes. However, even iohexol carries a small but definite risk of toxicity, and injection and timed blood collection protocols are not trivial to establish and perform regularly in busy clinical programs. Therefore, use of such protocols will depend on the availability of valid noninvasive alternatives.

The most commonly used direct GFR measurement in children is endogenous creatinine clearance, measured and normalized to a BSA of 1.73 m². Measurement of creatinine clearance requires that the child be able to control his or her voiding. A shortened protocol with a carefully timed urine collection over 3 to 6 hours in an ambulatory setting is a valid alternative to 24-hour sampling. Creatinine clearance accurately reflects GFR in patients with normal or mildly impaired renal function. As GFR declines, tubular creatinine secretion increases, which results in an overestimation of true GFR. In advanced CKD (GFR < 20 mL/min/1.73 m²), the mean of creatinine and urea clearances is a well-established estimator of actual GFR.

The need for simple and rapid GFR assessment in clinical practice has led to the development of prediction equations that allow estimation of GFR from levels of serum markers. The most widely used eGFR markers are creatinine, a product of muscle metabolism, and cystatin C, a low-molecular-weight (13-kDa) serum protein.

Creatinine generation, and consequently steady-state serum creatinine levels, strongly depend on the relative muscle mass, which in turn strongly depends on age and gender. Mean serum creatinine levels gradually increase during childhood from 0.3 to 0.4 mg/dL (26 to 35 µmol/L) in early infancy to 1.0 mg/dL in female and 1.3 mg/dL in male adolescents (88 and 115 µmol/L, respectively). Hence, Schwartz devised a formula to estimate GFR from the serum creatinine level that accounted for the developmental changes in creatinine generation. The eGFR equals the ratio of height to serum creatinine concentration multiplied by a constant, K.[2] In the original Schwartz equation, K was age- and gender-specific. Although the Schwartz formula, due to its simplicity and ready availability, has found wide acceptance in the field of pediatrics, validation studies have demonstrated poor precision and accuracy of the original equation. True GFR tends to be overestimated by 10% to 15%, and the average 95% confidence intervals typically range from −40% to +50%. Since the relationship of serum creatinine concentration to GFR is exponential, with very little change in serum creatinine level down to a GFR of 50 to 60 mL/min/1.73 m², serum creatinine–based prediction equations are particularly insensitive in detecting GFR changes for CKD stage 2. Another problem arises from changes in laboratory methodology. The original K values were validated using the Jaffé method to measure creatinine. Most laboratories currently use enzymatic assays and, more recently, an isotope dilution mass spectrometric assay was introduced to which creatinine assays are now being calibrated. Enzymatic assays and isotope dilution, mass spectrometry–calibrated assays systematically yield lower serum creatinine values, which results in GFR overestimations by 5% to 10% when the original K values are used. In a more recent study, Schwartz and colleagues validated a new equation adapted for use with enzymatic creatinine measurements.[3] The newer Schwartz formula uses a uniform K value for both genders and is valid in children from 1 to 16 years of age:

$$\text{Estimated GFR} = \text{height (cm)} \times 0.413/\text{serum creatinine (mg/dL)}$$

Cystatin C has been advocated as a serum marker of GFR. Cystatin C is produced by all nucleated cells at a relatively stable rate. The principal mode of excretion of cystatin C is via the renal route. Cystatin C is freely filtered by the glomerulus and is then metabolized after being reabsorbed in the proximal tubule. Because of this, serum cystatin C levels increase in a predictable fashion as GFR falls. The use of a cystatin C–based eGFR may be particularly advantageous in children because its production rate, after correction for BSA, is much less influenced by age than serum creatinine concentration, and its serum levels are independent of gender and muscle mass. After decreasing by approximately 50% in the first year of life, cystatin C plasma levels remain stable until about age 50 years. Cystatin C appears to be a more sensitive and reliable marker of GFR than the serum creatinine level, with an earlier increase in serum levels in patients with early stages of CKD. Filler and Lepage[4] have derived an equation to predict GFR from serum cystatin C levels in a pediatric validation study using ^{99}Tc-DTPA, single-injection clearance as the standard. The sensitivity for detecting CKD stage 2 in children was 74% for the serum cystatin C level compared with 46% for the serum creatinine level. Confidence intervals were consistently narrower for the cystatin C–based than for the creatinine-based eGFR. In children with CKD stages 3 to 5, the intrapatient coefficient of variation of cystatin C values is significantly lower than that of serum creatinine values, which suggests that cystatin C may be a better tool for longitudinal monitoring of patients with advanced CKD.[5]

Schwartz and colleagues derived a best-fitting GFR prediction equation based on height, serum creatinine level (S_{Cr}), cystatin C level, blood urea nitrogen (BUN) level, and gender.[3] Validated against iohexol clearance in North American children older than 12 months, this refined formula promises improved precision and accuracy of GFR estimation:

$$\begin{aligned}\text{Estimated GFR} = &\ 39.1\,[\text{height}/S_{Cr}]^{0.516} \\ &\times [1.8/\text{cystatin C}]^{0.294} \times [39/\text{BUN}]^{0.169} \\ &\times [1.099]^{\text{male}} \times [\text{height}/1.4]^{0.188}\end{aligned}$$

The formula is thought to be useful in the GFR range of 15 to 75 mL/min/1.73 m².

ASSESSMENT OF PROTEINURIA

Proteinuria is a common laboratory finding in children. A rapid semiquantitative assessment of proteinuria can be made using dipstick testing. The most precise quantitation is obtained by measuring protein excretion in 12- or 24-hour samples with the Coomassie blue method. However, precise urine collections are usually difficult to obtain in infants and young children. If timed urine collections are not possible, assessment of the protein/creatinine ratio in random urine samples is a valid alternative. Most healthy children excrete small amounts of protein in their urine. Physiologic proteinuria varies with the age and size of the child. When corrected for BSA, the upper normal limit of protein excretion is 300 mg/m²/day at age 1 month in full-term infants, 250 mg at 1 year, 200 mg at 10 years, and 150 mg in late adolescence. Urinary protein excretion exceeding 1.0 g/m²/day is strongly indicative of inherent kidney pathophysiology.

The upper limit of normal for the urine protein/creatinine ratio (as grams of protein/gram of creatinine) is 0.5 at age 6 months to 2 years and 0.2 in older children and adolescents.[6] A urine protein/creatinine ratio above 3.0 is consistent with nephrotic-range proteinuria, thought to reflect glomerular disease, and is often associated with systemic manifestations, such as salt and fluid retention and edema.[7]

Isolated asymptomatic proteinuria in children can occur as a transient phenomenon (e.g., caused by fever, strenuous exercise, extreme cold or heat exposure, epinephrine administration, emotional stress, congestive heart failure, abdominal surgery, seizures) or as a persistent abnormality. It can represent a benign condition (e.g., orthostatic proteinuria) or may be the manifestation of serious CKD.

Estimates of the prevalence of isolated asymptomatic proteinuria in children range between 0.6% and 6%. Orthostatic proteinuria accounts for up to 60% of all cases of asymptomatic proteinuria reported in children, with an even higher incidence in adolescents. Children with orthostatic proteinuria usually excrete less than 1 g of protein/day (urine protein/creatinine ratio < 1.0). Although patients with orthostatic proteinuria have an excellent prognosis, the long-term prognosis for children with isolated fixed proteinuria remains unknown.[7]

CONGENITAL ANOMALIES OF THE KIDNEY AND URINARY TRACT

DEFINITIONS

Kidney malformations are classified according to macroscopic and microscopic anatomic features, which are usually determined by ultrasonographic assessment in clinical practice. Renal fusion and ectopic kidney localization are general anomalies of kidney development. The congenital absence of the kidney and ureter is termed *renal agenesis*. The term *renal hypoplasia* defines a small kidney with a reduced number of nephrons but normal renal architecture. Renal dysplasia is characterized by abnormal mesenchymal and epithelial tissue differentiation, a reduced nephron number, absent corticomedullary differentiation, and the presence of dysplastic elements, including cartilage and bone. Dysplastic kidneys vary in size and may or may not contain cysts. Small dysplastic kidneys without macroscopic cysts are usually termed *hypodysplastic kidneys*. The multicystic dysplastic kidney is an extreme form of renal dysplasia. Polycystic kidneys of the recessive or dominant type and nephronophthisis are additional specific entities of dysplastic kidneys.

Common abnormalities of the lower urinary tract include vesicoureteral reflux (VUR) and obstruction of the ureteropelvic junction, ureterovesical junction, or urethra due to posterior urethral valves. Renal hypoplasia and dysplasia and malformations of the urinary tract are variably associated, constituting a spectrum of phenotypes summarized by the term *congenital anomalies of the kidney and urinary tract* (CAKUT).

EPIDEMIOLOGY

The incidence of CAKUT is 0.3 to 1.6/1000 births.[8] Abnormalities of the lower urinary tract are present in approximately 50% of children with renal malformations. Refluxive and obstructive uropathies are observed with equal frequency.[9]

Renal fusion anomalies occur in about 1 in 600 infants.[10] The incidence of renal ectopy is 1 in 1000 autopsies.[11] Bilateral agenesis occurs in 1 in 3,000 to 10,000 births, and unilateral renal agenesis has been found at a prevalence of 1 in 1,000 autopsies. The incidence of renal dysplasia is 1 in 3,000 to 5,000 births for unilateral disease and 1 in 10,000 for bilateral disease.[12] Boys are 1.3 to 1.9 times more likely to be affected than girls.[13]

PHENOTYPES

RENAL ECTOPY

During embryogenesis, the developing kidneys migrate from the pelvis to the retroperitoneal renal fossa and rotate from a horizontal to vertical position. Failure to ascend results in the pelvic kidney phenotype. Less commonly, the kidney is located on the contralateral side (crossed ectopy without fusion). Ectopic kidneys are commonly associated with urinary tract abnormalities. VUR is present in 30% of simple and in 20% of crossed ectopic kidneys. Other associated urogenital abnormalities include dysplasia of the contralateral kidney, cryptorchidism, and hypospadias in boys and malformation of the uterus and vagina in girls.[13-16] Adrenal, cardiac, and skeletal anomalies can also occur in association with renal ectopia. Ectopic kidneys are usually clinically asymptomatic and diagnosed during routine prenatal or postnatal sonography, but sometimes manifest with symptoms of urinary tract infection (UTI), hematuria, incontinence, renal insufficiency, and/or hypertension.

RENAL FUSION ANOMALIES

Fusion anomalies are believed to arise between the fourth and ninth weeks of gestation, before the kidneys ascend from the pelvis to the dorsolumbar space. The most common configuration is the horseshoe kidney, in which fusion usually occurs at the lower poles of each kidney. The fused kidney may lie symmetrically around the midline or in an asymmetric lateral position. The maximal variant of ectopic fusion is the crossed ectopic kidney, which has crossed the midline completely to fuse with the contralateral kidney. Early fusion is associated with altered ascension and rotation of the developing kidneys and is frequently accompanied by ectopy of the renal vessels, which often connect to the iliac vessels rather than to the aorta and vena cava. The ureters are frequently compressed by traversing the horseshoe isthmus, the anterior surface of the fused kidney, and/or aberrant arteries. Whereas most patients with fused kidneys are clinically asymptomatic, ureteric obstruction may sometimes cause loin pain, hematuria, and renal stasis related to UTI or renal calculi.[15] Associated urogenital abnormalities such as duplication and ectopic ending of ureters, hypospadias, cryptorchidism, and malformations of the uterus have been described, as well as extrarenal anomalies involving the gastrointestinal tract (e.g., anal atresia, Meckel's diverticulum), neural tube, and skeleton.

RENAL AGENESIS AND HYPOPLASIA

Although major disorders of kidney formation are usually diagnosed by antenatal ultrasonographic screening, subtle forms of hypoplasia may be detected incidentally at the time of abdominal ultrasonography for another indication. Bilateral renal agenesis leads to anhydramnios and the

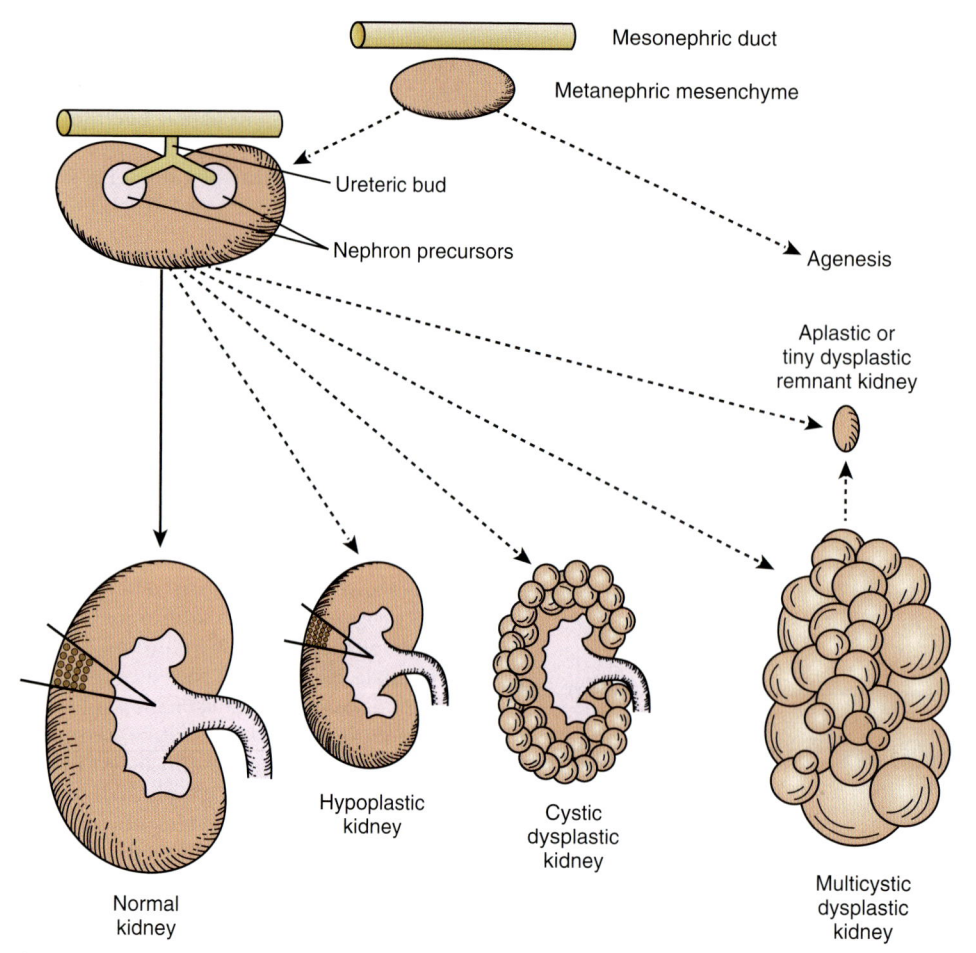

Figure 74.2 Anomalies at various stages of kidney development may lead to renal agenesis, aplasia, hypoplasia, or dysplasia. (From Kerecuk L, Schreuder MF, Woolf AS: Renal tract malformations: perspectives for nephrologists. *Nat Clin Pract Nephrol* 4:312-325, 2008.)

typical Potter's appearance with facial dysmorphic features, decreased fetal movement, joint contractures and dislocation, and pulmonary hypoplasia, usually leading to death within hours after birth. Unilateral agenesis induces compensatory hypertrophy of the contralateral kidney, the lack of which suggests a developmental abnormality of the existing kidney. In approximately one third of cases of unilateral agenesis, urinary tract abnormalities are present on the contralateral side, which necessitates careful diagnostic evaluation. Whereas unilateral agenesis or hypoplasia is usually asymptomatic, bilateral renal hypoplasia is the most common single cause of chronic kidney disease in childhood.

Oligomeganephronia, characterized by progressive proteinuric renal failure in childhood, represents a severe variant of bilateral hypoplasia in which the kidneys are 15% to 50% of normal weight.[17] Nephron numbers are reduced by 80% and the nephrons are markedly hypertrophied. Glomerular diameter is increased up to 12-fold and tubular length up to fourfold.[18]

RENAL DYSPLASIA

Dysplastic kidneys are usually diagnosed by ultrasonographic features such as increased echogenicity, loss of corticomedullary differentiation, and cortical cysts. Renal dysplasia is strongly associated with obstructive or refluxive abnormalities of the urinary tract.[19] Accordingly, imaging of the lower urinary tract should be performed to determine whether these abnormalities are present. The dysplastic kidney is typically of small size but may also be enlarged if cystic elements are present. Renal dysplasia is usually discovered incidentally by ultrasonography. Severe bilateral disease may cause oligohydramnios, pulmonary hypoplasia, and progressive renal failure soon after birth.

MULTICYSTIC DYSPLASTIC KIDNEY

The multicystic dysplastic kidney (MCDK) is an extreme phenotype of renal dysplasia that presents as a unilateral flank mass by palpation and as a large cystic nonreniform mass by ultrasonography (Figure 74.2). The ureter is atretic, which results in a nonfunctioning kidney. Abnormalities of the contralateral urinary tract are observed in 25% of cases. These include ureteropelvic junction obstruction (5% to 10% of cases), VUR, renal hypoplasia, and rotational or positional anomalies.[12]

Although a temporary increase in size may occur postnatally, the MCDK gradually shrinks in size. Complete involution of MCDK has been reported in 3% to 4% of patients at birth and in 20% to 25% at age 2 years. Therefore, many patients diagnosed with unilateral renal agenesis in later childhood or adult life may originally have had MCDK. The contralateral kidney undergoes compensatory hypertrophy. Hypertension and malignant tumors very rarely arise in the setting of MCDK and are not more common than in the normal population.[20] Hence, the management of patients with MCDK has shifted from routine nephrectomy to observation and medical therapy. Because of the risk of associated anomalies in the contralateral kidney, the possibility of VUR should be evaluated, and blood pressure should be measured. If the contralateral kidney is normal, long-term renal functional outcome is excellent. Regular ultrasonographic monitoring is recommended to document involution of the mass and compensatory hypertrophy of the contralateral kidney.

UPPER URINARY TRACT DUPLICATION

Duplex collecting systems are the most common anomaly of the upper urinary tract, with a reported incidence of 0.8%.[21] A duplex kidney is one that has two separate pelvicaliceal systems. If two separate ureteric buds originate from the mesonephric duct, two separate interactions will develop between the ureter and metanephric blastema, resulting in the formation of a duplex system. This duplex system includes two separate renal units and collecting systems, ureters, and ureteral orifices. Bifid pelvis, bifid ureters, or double ureters can be formed, depending on the level at which the ureters join. Duplication anomalies are usually asymptomatic; therefore they often remain undetected. However, a proportion of duplex kidneys may be associated with VUR or obstruction. Fetal urinary tract dilations are related to complicated renal duplication in 4.7% of cases.[22]

The final position of the ureteral orifices in the bladder follows the somewhat counterintuitive so-called Weigert-Meyer rule—the lower orifice belongs to the upper pole orifice and the higher orifice to the lower pole. To achieve these positions, the two ureters and orifices rotate 180 degrees clockwise in their longitudinal axes.[23] The orifice draining the lower moiety is commonly refluxive, whereas the ureter draining the upper moiety may end in an obstructive ureterocele that inserts into the bladder in a more distal position than normal. Ectopic insertion—for example, into the urethra—is also seen occasionally and may be a cause of primary enuresis.[24] The upper renal moiety is frequently dysplastic and may contribute only a small part of the kidney's overall function.

The routine postnatal radiologic imaging workup of abnormal duplex kidneys is based on ultrasonography and voiding cystourethrography. Voiding cystourethrography is performed to detect VUR and evaluate the ureterocele. Isotope studies are required to determine the function of the dilated renal moiety.

The presence of ureteral ectopy compromises the ability of the VUR to subside spontaneously.[24] Compared with single-system reflux, duplex-system VUR tends to be of a higher grade, with an elevated incidence of lower pole dysplasia.[22] Although deflux injection can be tried,[25] many patients with duplex systems require surgical management of the VUR if recurrent ascending infections occur.[24] Although surgery is clearly indicated for ectopic ureters, the need for surgical correction of ureteroceles depends on the degree of functional obstruction.

VESICOURETERAL REFLUX

VUR is defined as the retrograde flow of urine from the bladder into the ureter and renal pelvis.[26] Reflux into renal parenchyma is termed *intrarenal reflux*. It can be primary or secondary to obstruction or bladder dysfunction. VUR is caused by lateral-proximal dystopia of the ureteric orifice, which results from ectopic ureteric budding from the Wolffian duct during embryogenesis. The dystopic location causes a shortened submucosal tunnel, with insufficient function of the intramural muscular valve mechanism.

Epidemiology

Primary VUR is the most common entity in the CAKUT complex, with an estimated prevalence of 1% to 6%. It is characterized by a high familial occurrence, with a prevalence of around 30% in siblings and 50% to 60% in offspring of affected patients. These findings are compatible with dominant inheritance with variable penetrance, although pedigrees suggestive of recessive transmission have also been described.[27] Recently, a heterozygous deleterious mutation in TNXB (encoding tenascin XB) has been described in a family with hereditary VUR.[28] TNXB is expressed in the uroepithelial lining of the ureterovesical junction and may be important for generating tensile forces that close the ureterovesical junction during voiding.

Diagnosis

Ultrasonography is a useful initial investigation to evaluate for kidney size, presence of hydroureteronephrosis, bladder wall thickness, and extent of bladder emptying. A sonographic examination of the kidneys and urinary tract is recommended for all children with febrile UTI.[29] Micturition cystourethrography (MCUG) is still indicated as the primary diagnostic imaging procedure for VUR in boys, in whom exclusion of subvesical obstruction by a posterior urethral valve is also required.[30] In girls, MCUG should only be performed after a second febrile UTI or if abnormalities such as hydronephrosis or scarring are noted on ultrasound.[29] Contrast-enhanced micturition urosonography has been an increasingly popular alternative for diagnosing and monitoring VUR.[31] Staging systems that allow quantification of the severity of reflux (grades I through V) have been defined for both imaging approaches (Figure 74.3).

Prognosis

VUR grading is of high prognostic relevance. Spontaneous resolution of VUR is observed during the first decade of life in 100% of cases with unilateral and in 50% of those with bilateral grade III reflux and in 40% of those with bilateral grade IV reflux. The likelihood of spontaneous resolution is negatively affected by older age at diagnosis, male gender, low bladder volume and bladder dysfunction, and the presence of other CAKUT features, such as urinary tract duplication and renal hypodysplasia.[32]

VUR is usually diagnosed in children who come for treatment of a UTI. VUR is present in 30% of children with febrile UTI. The incidence of kidney injury after acute pyelonephritis in children with VUR has been estimated to be up to 6%, particularly in girls, and appears to be related to the severity of reflux.[26] However, the risk of development of postpyelonephritic parenchymal scars (reflux nephropathy) may have been overestimated in the past. Scars, which are diagnosed based on perfusion defects in dimercaptosuccinic acid (DMSA) isotope scans,

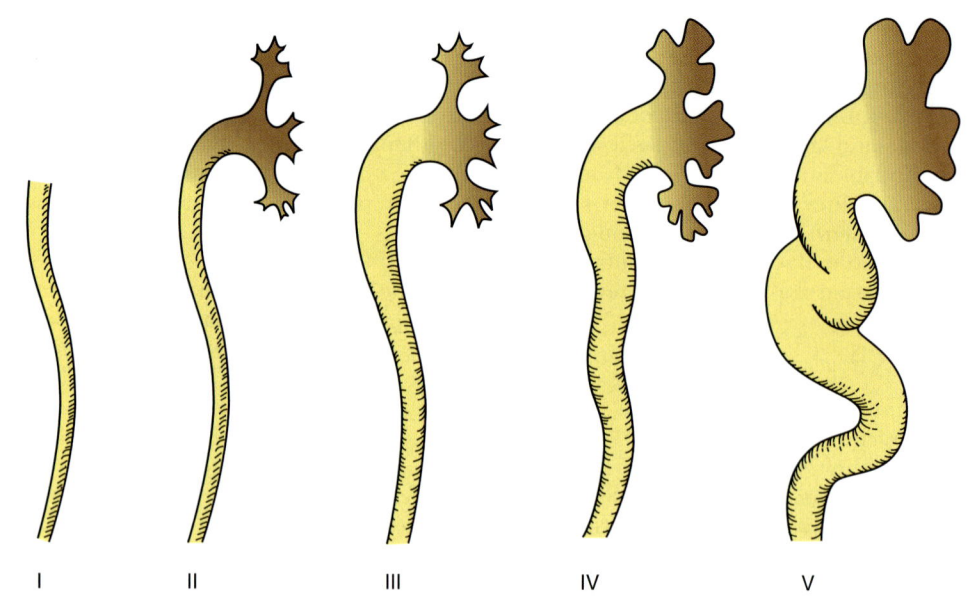

Figure 74.3 Grading scheme for vesicoureteric reflux (I to V). (From Schaefer F: Pädiatrische Nephrologie. In Mayatepek E, editor: Pädiatrie, Munich, 2007, Elsevier/Urban & Fischer, pp 683-733.)

can sometimes be visualized even in neonates with VUR, which suggests that they may reflect developmental dysplastic regions in the renal parenchyma.[18]

Management

The major goal of therapy in children with VUR should be the prevention of long-term morbidity due to recurrent UTIs and reflux nephropathy.[26] Available management options include close monitoring and early treatment of UTIs, continuous antibiotic prophylaxis, and surgical correction, which can be performed by open reimplantation of ureters or by endoscopic correction of VUR.

Continuous antibiotic prophylaxis (trimethoprim, 1 to 2 mg/kg, nitrofurantoin 1 to 2 mg/kg, or cefaclor, 10 mg/kg administered as a single evening dose) was traditionally recommended for virtually all patients with VUR but has been revisited and scrutinized in light of the results of several randomized controlled trials (RCTs) and meta-analyses demonstrating a low overall risk of developing a second febrile UTI (20%), a modest protective effect of antibiotic prophylaxis (50% risk reduction) and, most importantly, lack of beneficial effect of prophylaxis on new scar formation following UTI.[33-39] Moreover, there has been increasing concern about the emergence of resistant organisms caused by long-term antibiotic prophylaxis.[38-41] Currently, the American Urological Association guideline panel continues to recommend prophylaxis for children younger than 1 year with a history of UTI and/or VUR grade III to V. For children older than 1 year, prophylaxis is recommended only for those with documented bladder-bowel dysfunction or history of febrile UTI.[42] The optimal duration of prophylaxis has not been established; in most prospective trials, treatment has been limited to 1 to 2 years.

Although open surgical correction has a 95% technical success rate and reduces the incidence of recurrent febrile UTI, it is not superior to antibiotic prophylaxis with respect to scar formation, renal growth, and preservation of kidney function.[32,43,44] Therefore, surgical intervention is an alternative for patients with frequent symptomatic UTIs, particularly those who have difficulty adhering to a continuous antibiotic prophylactic regimen. Endoscopic techniques have recently gained wide acceptance as an early alternative to continuous prophylactic antibiotic administration in the management of reflux.[26,32] A systematic review has shown an overall success rate of dextranomer–hyaluronic acid injection of 77% per ureter after 3 months.[45] The likelihood of successful endoscopic VUR correction is inversely related to the grade of VUR.[45] A recent head-on comparison study has demonstrated similar efficacy of endoscopic intervention and antibiotic prophylaxis in reducing UTI rates.[36]

VUR management guidelines have increasingly focused on the role of bladder and bowel dysfunction (BBD) as a risk factor for VUR and recurrent UTIs.[42,46] Nearly 50% of infants with dilating VUR exhibit dysfunctional voiding characterized by overactive bladder and urge incontinence, voiding postponement, and/or underactive bladder function, with or without abnormalities of bowel function such as constipation and encopresis.[47] BBD reduces the likelihood of spontaneous resolution of VUR and the success rate of endoscopic injection therapy for VUR. Even following surgical correction, BBD is associated with a high rate of febrile UTI, irrespective of surgical success.[42,48-50] Hence, therapy of BBD should precede surgical therapy. Available treatments include biofeedback, medical therapy, and behavioral modification.

URETEROPELVIC JUNCTION OBSTRUCTION

Fetal hydronephrosis is the most common anomaly detected on antenatal ultrasonographic examination, affecting 1% to 5% of pregnancies.[51] Ureteropelvic junction obstruction is believed to account for 35% to 50% of these uropathies. It is twice as common in boys as in girls and affects the left ureter twice as often as the right ureter.[52] The narrowing of the ureteropelvic portion of the ureter is intrinsic (i.e., caused by segmental intrafascicular and perifascicular fibrosis, smooth muscle hypertrophy, and abnormal innervation) or extrinsic (i.e., related to aberrant crossing of renal pole vessels or fibrosis of adjacent tissue).[53] Obstruction of urine flow during intrauterine life leads to dilation of the renal pelvis. The spectrum of phenotypes ranges from slight pelvic dilation with normal urine flow to an almost complete obstruction with renal parenchymal damage and atrophy.[53] It is important to note that in the overwhelming majority of cases, congenital ureteropelvic junction obstruction is a transient condition. Whereas the population prevalence of pelvic dilation as determined by prenatal and neonatal ultrasonography is approximately 2.5%, it is 0.07% to 0.1% by age 2 years.[54-56]

Cause

The cause of ureteropelvic junction obstruction is poorly understood. Although most cases are isolated, ureteropelvic junction obstruction may be associated with other CAKUT features or comprise one manifestation of a complex syndrome. Polygenic inheritance as well as nongenetic pathogenic mechanisms have been invoked.[57]

Clinical Phenotype

The condition is usually asymptomatic and is mostly detected by prenatal ultrasonography. Older children occasionally complain of colicky pain episodes, typically after rapid ingestion of large fluid volumes. Concrements in the renal pelvis can also occur as a consequence of urinary stasis. In up to 10% of cases, ureteropelvic junction obstruction is associated with ipsilateral VUR. Infections are uncommon, but require urgent intervention and drainage.

Diagnosis

Ultrasonography and diuresis isotope scanning are the most important diagnostic tools. Ultrasonographically determined intrarenal and extrarenal pelvis diameter relative to established reference values can be used for longitudinal montoring.[56,58,59] The thickness of the renal parenchyma gives some indication of pressure-induced damage to kidney tissue. The definitive functional relevance of an obstructed ureteropelvic junction may be obtained by a mercaptoacetyltriglycine (MAG3) isotope scan before and after stimulation of diuresis by a defined furosemide bolus. This test can be performed once excretory function has matured, around the sixth week of life. Both the urodynamic effect of the stenosis and partial function of the affected kidney can be visualized. A more time-consuming but radiation-free alternative is dynamic magnetic resonance urography, which allows simultaneous assessment of renal morphology and partial function, as well as the dynamics of urinary drainage[58] (Figure 74.4).

Management

Patients with ureteropelvic junction obstruction are generally considered at risk of pressure-induced renal damage. However, congenital obstruction resolves spontaneously in most cases, although individual cases of late deterioration of kidney function have been reported.[59] Since valid prospective outcome studies in large populations are lacking, individual risk prediction is difficult. Currently, mild pelvic dilation on ultrasonography (<15 mm), more than 40% partial function and, most importantly, more than 50% nuclide drainage on diuresis renography are considered indicators of a low risk of renal damage. Most children are monitored using ultrasonographic studies and nuclide scans in case of ultrasonographic deterioration at 3- to 6-month intervals. Pyeloplasty is usually successful in restoring urine drainage, although urinary leaks and recurrent stenosis may occur. Laparoscopic pyeloplasty is a recently favored, minimally invasive, safe, and effective therapeutic modality associated with shorter hospital stays, reduced postoperative complications, and excellent short-term outcomes.[60]

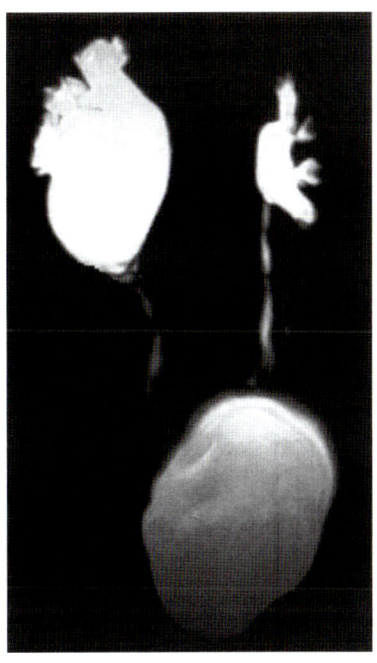

Figure 74.4 Magnetic resonance urography of bilateral pelvicoureteric junction obstruction. Mild, functionally insignificant pelvic dilation on the left side contrasts with subtotal obstruction of the right collecting system, with ballooning of the pelvis and calices. (From Schaefer F: Pädiatrische Nephrologie. In Mayatepek E, editor: *Pädiatrie*, Munich, 2007, Elsevier/Urban & Fischer, pp 683-733.)

PRIMARY MEGAURETER

Primary megaureter is defined as a ureteric width of more than 7 mm caused by a functional or anatomic abnormality involving the ureterovesical junction.[61] It is classified into four subtypes based on the presence of reflux, obstruction, or both. The term *secondary megaureter* is reserved for dilation resulting from other processes, such as neurogenic bladder, ureteroceles, or infravesical obstruction (e.g., posterior urethral valves, urethral atresia, cloacal dysgenesis).[62] Primary megaureter is the second most common cause of hydronephrosis in newborns, accounting for approximately 20% of cases, with an estimated incidence of 0.36/1000 live births.[63] Boys are affected more frequently, and the left ureter is affected more commonly than the right one.

Pathogenesis

The pathogenesis of primary megaureter is uncertain. It appears to be most commonly due to impaired or delayed smooth muscle development in the distal ureter at around 20 weeks' gestation.[64] This results in the formation of an aperistaltic segment, which leads to functional obstruction. The refluxive megaureter also has an abnormal transvesical tunnel, which allows urine to reflux up the ureter. In patients with refluxive-obstructive megaureter, the refluxed urine does not return through the ureterovesical junction.

Diagnosis

The diagnosis of primary megaureter is made by prenatal or neonatal ultrasonography. Postnatal presentation can occur at any age, with symptoms of UTI, hematuria, abdominal pain and/or mass, and sometimes uremia. Diuresis scintigraphy establishes the presence of obstruction, and voiding cystourethrography identifies VUR. Magnetic resonance urography provides excellent anatomic detail, often allowing identification of the site of obstruction.[65]

Prognosis

The prognosis of primary megaureter is generally good. Most cases resolve spontaneously within the first 3 years of life. In children with high-grade hydronephrosis or a retrovesical ureteral diameter of more than 1 cm, the condition may persist and may require surgical reinsertion of the ureter.[66] Poor renal outcome appears to be related to concomitant congenital renal hypodysplasia rather than to the megaureter per se, except in the setting of high-grade and worsening obstruction.[67]

Management

In symptomatic patients with any type of megaureter, surgical intervention to relieve the obstruction is recommended. In asymptomatic patients with nonrefluxing, nonobstructed megaureters, regular ultrasonographic monitoring and prophylactic antibiotics during the first year of life are suggested.

POSTERIOR URETHRAL VALVES

Posterior urethral valves—tissue leaflets fanning distally from the prostatic urethra to the external urinary sphincter—are the most common cause of neonatal lower urinary tract obstruction in males, occurring in 1 in 5000 to 8000 pregnancies.[68] Although the cause is not completely understood,[69] it appears that the normal embryologic development of the male urethra is disrupted between weeks 9 and 14 of gestation, which results in persistence of the urogenital membrane. Posterior urethral valves act as rigid bands or membranes and balloon into the urethral lumen with urine flow, causing obstruction and proximal dilation (dilated posterior urethra, keyhole sign).

Phenotype

Most cases are identified by prenatal ultrasonography. The enhanced urethral resistance causes detrusor hypertrophy, bladder enlargement and trabeculation, sacculation of the bladder wall, and formation of pseudodiverticuli, secondary unilateral or bilateral VUR, hydronephrosis, and (typically microcystic) renal dysplasia. The degree of renal dysplasia determines the postnatal course. Oligohydramnios and associated pulmonary hypoplasia are common.[70] Neonates and infants may present with respiratory distress, abdominal distension, urosepsis, and failure to thrive, whereas older boys typically show primary enuresis and other signs of bladder dysfunction, such as frequency, straining to void, poor urinary stream, a large urinary volume per void,[71] occasional UTIs, and eventually progressive CKD.

Diagnosis

In the developed world, the overwhelming majority of posterior urethral valve cases are identified by prenatal ultrasonography. Postnatally, the presumptive diagnosis of posterior urethral valves is made by voiding cystourethrography, which demonstrates the hallmark findings of a dilated and elongated posterior urethra, with a thin linear defect during the voiding phase (Figure 74.5). The diagnosis is confirmed by cystoscopy.

Management

Prenatal surgery (e.g., vesicoamniotic shunt placement, valve ablation, bladder marsupialization) to relieve obstructive uropathy has been explored. However, fetal interventions are associated with a high morbidity rate, and evidence that such procedures improve outcomes and reduce the risk of CKD is lacking.[72,73] Postnatally, initial management of suspected or confirmed posterior urethral valves includes drainage of the urinary tract. In neonates, this is traditionally accomplished by suprapubic catheterization followed by cystoscopic valve ablation at age 3 months. Alternatively, primary valve ablation at a neonatal age is also possible, even in premature babies.[74,75] In one third of children with secondary VUR, reflux resolves after valve ablation. If valve ablation cannot be performed within the first few months of life, vesicostomy is the next preferred procedure. Abnormal bladder function often persists, requiring intermittent catheterization and anticholinergic medication.[71]

Prognosis

Some 15% to 40% of boys with posterior urethral valves experience persistent continence problems. Due to renal dysplasia and possibly additional acquired renal damage by infections and bladder dysfunction, one third of patients develop significant CKD and 15% to 20% eventually progress to ESKD.[74,76] Most patients require surgical augmentation of bladder capacity prior to kidney transplantation.

SYNDROMIC FORMS OF CONGENITAL ANOMALIES OF THE KIDNEY AND URINARY TRACT

The following sections describe selected syndromic forms of CAKUT that are of high clinical relevance because of their prevalence, prognostic relevance, and/or mild extrarenal phenotype. For comprehensive listings of syndromic CAKUT, see Chapter 73.[27,77]

RENAL CYST AND DIABETES SYNDROME

Hepatocyte nuclear factor-1β (HNF-1β), encoded by the gene *TCF2*, is a transcription factor involved in the development of the pancreas, kidneys, liver, and intestine. Abnormalities in *TCF2* can cause a wide spectrum of renal developmental anomalies, the most consistent of which are bilateral small cortical cysts of glomerular origin.[78,79] Abnormalities in *TCF2*/HNF-1β are the most common known cause of cystic renal dysplasia, accounting for 22% to 31% of cases of ultrasonographically identified cysts or hyperechogenicity at birth.[79,80] *TCF2* gene variations have also been found in patients with noncystic renal hypoplasia and dysplasia, multicystic dysplastic kidneys, renal agenesis,

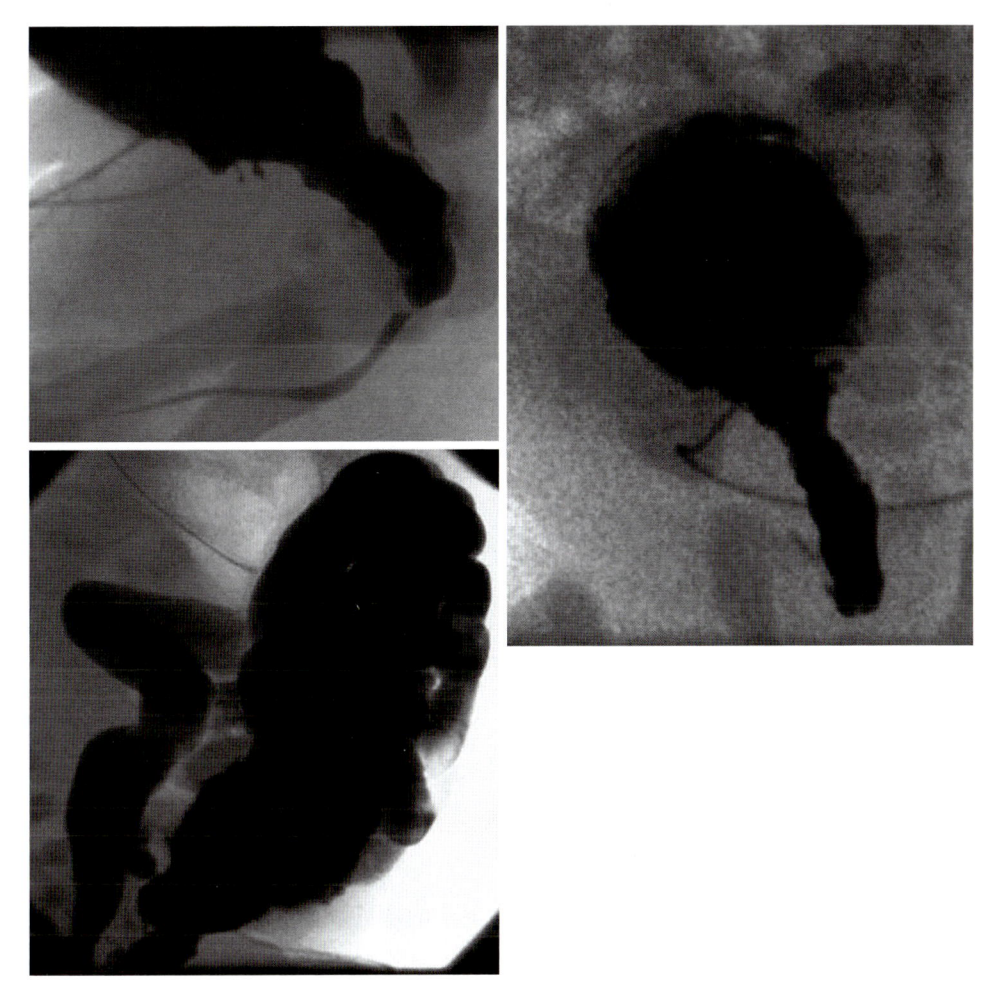

Figure 74.5 Voiding cystourethrogram of posterior urethral valve. Filiform narrowing of the posterior urethra is seen with prestenotic dilation of the prostatic urethra, trabeculated and sacculated bladder and secondary bilateral vesicoureteric reflux. (From Schaefer F: Pädiatrische Nephrologie. In Mayatepek E, editor: *Pädiatrie,* Munich, 2007, Elsevier/Urban & Fischer, pp 683-733.)

horseshoe kidneys, and pelviureteric junction obstruction, although they appear to be much less common in these entities.[81-83]

Mutations in the *TCF2* gene were initially found in patients with maturity-onset diabetes of the young (MODY) type 5.[84,85] Diabetes mellitus develops in approximately 60% of mutation carriers, usually in the third decade of life.[86-88] Subclinical deficiencies of the exocrine pancreas function have also been described. Early metabolic alterations in renal cyst and diabetes syndrome (RCAD) include impaired glucose tolerance, hyperuricemia due to reduced fractional excretion of uric acid, hyperlipidemia, and mild elevation of liver enzyme levels.

In addition to renal developmental anomalies, various genital tract malformations are found in 10% to 15% of patients with *TCF2* gene abnormalities. These include aplasia or duplication anomalies of the vagina and uterus in females and hypospadias, epididymal cysts, and agenesis of the vas deferens in males.[86]

More than 50 mutations have been reported in *TCF2,* most of which are located in the DNA-binding domain. In more than one third of cases, the gene is entirely deleted.[78,87] Because deletions are usually missed in conventional mutation screening, specific deletion screening methods are required in the molecular genetic workup of *TCF2*. Notably, more than 50% of the genetic abnormalities occur de novo. There is no genotype-phenotype correlation, and large phenotypic variability exists, even within families with the same mutation. Isolated renal cysts, diabetes, or urogenital anomalies may occur in individual family members.

The high prevalence of *TCF2* abnormalities and the associated risk of developing metabolic abnormalities, including diabetes mellitus, in early adult life make it reasonable to screen for *TCF2* abnormalities in all children with renal cysts, irrespective of family history. In children with other CAKUT phenotypes, *TCF2* screening appears to be indicated in cases of associated metabolic abnormalities, genital malformations, or family history of early-onset diabetes.

RENAL COLOBOMA SYNDROME

Renal coloboma syndrome (RCS) is an autosomal dominant congenital anomaly usually caused by mutations in *PAX2*, a gene encoding a transcription factor with key functions in kidney development. *PAX2* is expressed in the mesonephros and metanephros at the earliest stages of nephrogenesis (see Chapter 73 for details). *PAX2* mutations account for 50% of RCS cases. More than 30 mutations have been reported, most of which are located in exons 2 and 3 encoding the DNA-binding domain.

RCS is classically characterized by the association of renal hypoplasia, VUR, and optic nerve coloboma.[89] However, the range of renal malformations described in RCS includes also noncystic or multicystic renal dysplasia[82] and ureteropelvic junction obstruction.[90-92] The ocular phenotype is similarly variable, ranging from subtle optic nerve dysplasia and abnormal vascular configuration, to mild visual impairment limited to blind spot enlargement,[93] to large colobomas of the optic nerve or of the chorioretina, with severe visual impairment.[94] Apart from the metanephros and optic fissure, PAX2 is also expressed in the developing hindbrain. Consequently, disease manifestations can include sensorineural hearing loss, seizures, and the Arnold-Chiari malformation.[95-96]

The RCS phenotype is highly variable, even in patients harboring the same PAX2 mutation, which strongly suggests a role of modifier genes. PAX2 mutations were found in 7 of 100 individuals with renal hypodysplasia and mild to moderate renal insufficiency (The ocular phenotype was so subtle that it had escaped clinical detection in five of the seven children.) Given the high prevalence of PAX2 mutations in renal hypodysplasia and the frequent minimally associated ocular and otic phenotypes, thorough ophthalmologic and audiometric investigation are recommended for any child with newly diagnosed renal hypodysplasia, followed by PAX2 screening in case of abnormalities. Conversely, any patient with coloboma should undergo kidney ultrasonography.

BRANCHIO-OTO-RENAL SYNDROME

The association of branchial, otic, and renal anomalies defines BOR syndrome, an autosomal dominant disorder with incomplete penetrance and expressivity and an incidence of about 1 in 40,000 births.[97] Sensorineural or conductive hearing loss is present in 93% to 98%, branchial defects in 49% to 69%, ear pits in 82% to 84%, and renal anomalies in 38% to 67% of cases.[98,99] Renal malformations include unilateral or bilateral renal agenesis, hypodysplasia, and malformation of the lower urinary tract, including VUR, ureteropelvic obstruction, and ureteral duplication. Different renal phenotypes may occur within families, including individuals with normal kidneys (branchio-oto syndrome).

Hearing impairment usually results from cochlear hypoplasia and malformation of the internal auditory canals.[98] Less frequent abnormalities include aplasia of the lacrimal ducts, congenital cataract, and anomalies of the anterior ocular segment.[100,101] BOR syndrome is caused by abnormalities in the EYA1[102] or, less commonly, the SIX1 gene. EYA1 is a non-DNA binding transcription cofactor, and SIX1 is a transcription factor interacting with EYA1.[103] EYA1 and SIX1 control the expression of PAX2 and GDNF (glial cell line–derived neurotrophic factor) in the metanephric mesenchyme.[104] More than 50 different mutations in EYA1 have been identified. In addition, large deletions, duplications, and chromosomal rearrangements account for 20% to 25% of abnormalities in EYA1,[105] which mandates screening for DNA copy number variations if results of direct sequencing are negative. SIX1 heterozygous mutations are much less frequent than EYA1 abnormalities.[103]

The diagnostic approach to BOR syndrome is complicated by its wide phenotypic spectrum.[99] First-degree relatives should be examined for renal disease, hearing impairment, preauricular pits, and branchial cysts or fistulas. Molecular testing should be performed in patients with complete BOR syndrome and in those with an incomplete phenotype but a suggestive family history.

TOWNES-BROCKS SYNDROME AND VATER/VACTERL ASSOCIATIONS

Townes-Brocks syndrome is an autosomal dominant malformation syndrome characterized by an imperforate anus, preaxial polydactyly and/or triphalangeal thumbs, external ear defects, sensorineural hearing loss and, less frequently, kidney, urogenital, and heart malformations.[106,107] The presentation of Townes-Brocks syndrome is highly variable within and between affected families. The gene mutated in human Townes-Brocks syndrome is SALL1, a member of the Spalt family that is required for the normal development of the limbs, nervous system, kidney, and heart.[108]

Features of Townes-Brocks syndrome partially overlap with those seen in the VATER association (vertebral defects, anal atresia, tracheoesophageal fistula with esophageal atresia, and radial and renal malformations) but do not include tracheoesophageal fistula or vertebral anomalies. Ear anomalies and deafness are not typical of VATER. The VATER association is usually sporadic, and there is no recognized teratogen or chromosomal abnormality.

The VACTERL association with hydrocephalus, reported as an X-linked or autosomal recessive condition, may include radial, cardiac, and renal anomalies and imperforate anus, along with other VATER features. Some of these patients also have Fanconi's anemia.

KALLMANN'S SYNDROME

Kallmann's syndrome is defined by the presence of hypogonadotropic hypogonadism and deficiency of the sense of smell (anosmia or hyposmia).[109,110] Anosmia and hyposmia are related to the absence or hypoplasia of the olfactory bulbs and tracts. Hypogonadism is due to a deficiency in gonadotropin-releasing hormone (GnRH). The GnRH-synthesizing neurons migrate during development from the olfactory epithelium to the forebrain along the olfactory nerve pathway.[111]

About one third of individuals affected by Kallmann's syndrome exhibit unilateral renal agenesis. Other renal and urinary tract malformations such as duplex systems, hydronephrosis, and VUR have also been reported. Other facultative features of Kallmann's syndrome include a cleft lip and/or palate, selective tooth agenesis, bimanual synkinesis, and hearing impairment.[112] Kallmann's syndrome is genetically heterogeneous. Four genes with mutations in affected patients have been identified: KAL1, an X chromosome–encoded gene that gives rise to anosmin-1; FGFR1 (fibroblast growth factor receptor 1), mutated in autosomal dominant forms of Kallmann's syndrome[113]; PROK2 (prokinectin-2); and PROK2R (prokinectin-2 receptor).[114] Renal anomalies seem to be limited to patients with KAL1 mutations.[115]

PRUNE-BELLY SYNDROME

Prune-belly (Eagle-Barrett) syndrome is a congenital disorder defined by a characteristic clinical triad that includes abdominal muscle deficiency, nonobstructive dilative urinary tract malformation, renal dysplasia, and bilateral cryptorchidism. The estimated incidence is 1 in 30,000 live births.[116] Boys are primarily affected, although rare cases in females have been reported.

Cause

Prune-belly syndrome is thought to be due to a local anomaly of mesenchymal development occurring in the fourth to twelfth weeks of gestation. A primary defect in the intermediate and lateral plate mesoderm would affect embryogenesis of the musculature of the abdominal wall, the mesonephric and paramesonephric ducts, and the urinary organs.[117]

Phenotype

The characteristic multiple abdominal skin wrinkles at birth tend to smooth out as the child grows older. About 50% of children develop ESKD due to severe renal dysplasia.[118] In severe cases, oligohydramnios leads to pulmonary hypoplasia and high neonatal mortality.[119] The ureters are grossly elongated, dilated, and tortuous. The bladder is usually enlarged, and urodynamic abnormalities are present. The posterior urethra is dilated due to hypoplasia of the prostate. Hence, the urinary tract malformation resembles the pattern of posterior urethral valves but no infravesical obstruction is present. Other clinical findings may include malrotation of the midgut or anorectal malformations, skeletal abnormalities (e.g., clubfoot), and, rarely, cardiac anomalies.

Management

The management of prune-belly syndrome depends on the severity of the clinical findings. In rare cases, antenatal intervention has been performed to reduce the risk and severity of pulmonary hypoplasia. Postnatal surgical intervention may be needed to provide adequate urinary drainage and avoid UTIs in some patients.[120] Renal replacement therapy for those patients with ESKD includes dialysis and renal transplantation.[121,122] Other interventions include additional genitourinary procedures to improve bladder control and capacity, orchidopexy, abdominal wall reconstruction and, in rare cases, orthopedic surgery for skeletal deformities.

CILIOPATHIES

The identification of the primary cilia-centrosome complex of the tubular epithelial cell as the organelle centrally involved in the pathogenesis of cystic nephropathies has been an important milestone in the molecular understanding of this peculiar type of kidney malformation. The following sections describe the cilia-related dysplasias, with special reference to the diagnostic, therapeutic, and prognostic aspects of disease relevant to the pediatric nephrologist.

POLYCYSTIC KIDNEY DISEASE

The term *polycystic kidney disease* (PKD) is reserved by convention for two genetically distinct conditions, autosomal recessive PKD (ARPKD) and autosomal dominant PKD (ADPKD).

ARPKD is caused by mutations in the polycystic kidney and hepatic disease 1 gene, *PKHD1*, located on chromosome 6p21, coding for fibrocystin (also called polyductin), a protein localized to the primary cilia of epithelial cells lining the collecting ducts, thick ascending limb, and hepatic bile ducts.[123-125] The reported incidence of ARPKD is 1 in 20,000 live births. ADPKD is caused by mutations in the *PKD1* gene (85% of patients) or *PKD2* gene, which encode for polycystin 1 and polycystin 2, respectively.[126-128] These proteins are localized to the primary cilia of renal epithelial cells, and mutations cause multiple cysts in all parts of the nephron. The phenotype of ARPKD can be mimicked by mutations in *TCF2*/HNF-1β and other genes. About 2% of patients with a mutation in *PKD1* or *PKD2* (often de novo, with an unremarkable family history) exhibit an early and severe phenotype indistinguishable from that of ARPKD. Furthermore, mutations in the *ADPKD* genes can also be inherited as a recessive trait.[129] The pathogenic effects of mutations in cystoproteins have been the subject of intense research and are described in detail in Chapter 46.

Although ADPKD, occurring in 1 in 400 live births, is approximately 50 times more common than ARPKD, the two disorders are seen at comparable frequency by pediatric nephrologists because ARPKD is usually diagnosed in utero or at birth and is symptomatic at pediatric age, whereas only 2% of patients affected by ADPKD show symptoms during childhood.

Clinical Features

ARPKD is characterized by enlarged hyperechogenic kidneys with multiple microcysts, without corticomedullary differentiation. Neonates present with massively enlarged, palpable kidneys, oligohydramnios, and pulmonary hypoplasia. About 25% to 30% of affected neonates die due to respiratory insufficiency.[130] Some children with rapid kidney growth require unilateral or bilateral nephrectomy to relieve symptoms of abdominal compression and/or malignant hypertension (Figure 74.6). Those who survive the neonatal period often experience an extended period of stabilized kidney size and function. However, polyuria and electrolyte losses due to tubular dysfunction require attention, and hypertension and proteinuria herald the development of renal insufficiency.[128] Approximately 50% of individuals affected by ARPKD progress to ESKD within the first 10 to 15 years of life.[130] However, some affected patients are only diagnosed as adults, with renal function ranging from normal to ESKD.[131] In addition to the renal symptoms, hepatic involvement is commonly present; it is usually characterized by bile duct dysplasia and ectasia and progressive liver fibrosis, gradually leading to portal hypertension. In many cases, the hepatic complications are more prominent than the renal disease manifestations.

ADPKD usually remains clinically silent during the childhood years, although a small subset of patients have early disease onset, with episodes of hematuria and cyst infection and symptoms similar to those observed in ARPKD.[132] Progressive macrocystic enlargement usually starts during adolescence and is commonly associated with arterial hypertension.[133] Subclinical cardiovascular alterations such as nocturnal hypertension, increased arterial stiffness, and left ventricular hypertrophy may develop long before progressive cyst growth and CKD manifest clinically.[134,135]

Diagnosis

The diagnosis of PKD is usually based on family history, clinical and imaging findings and, if required, molecular genetic

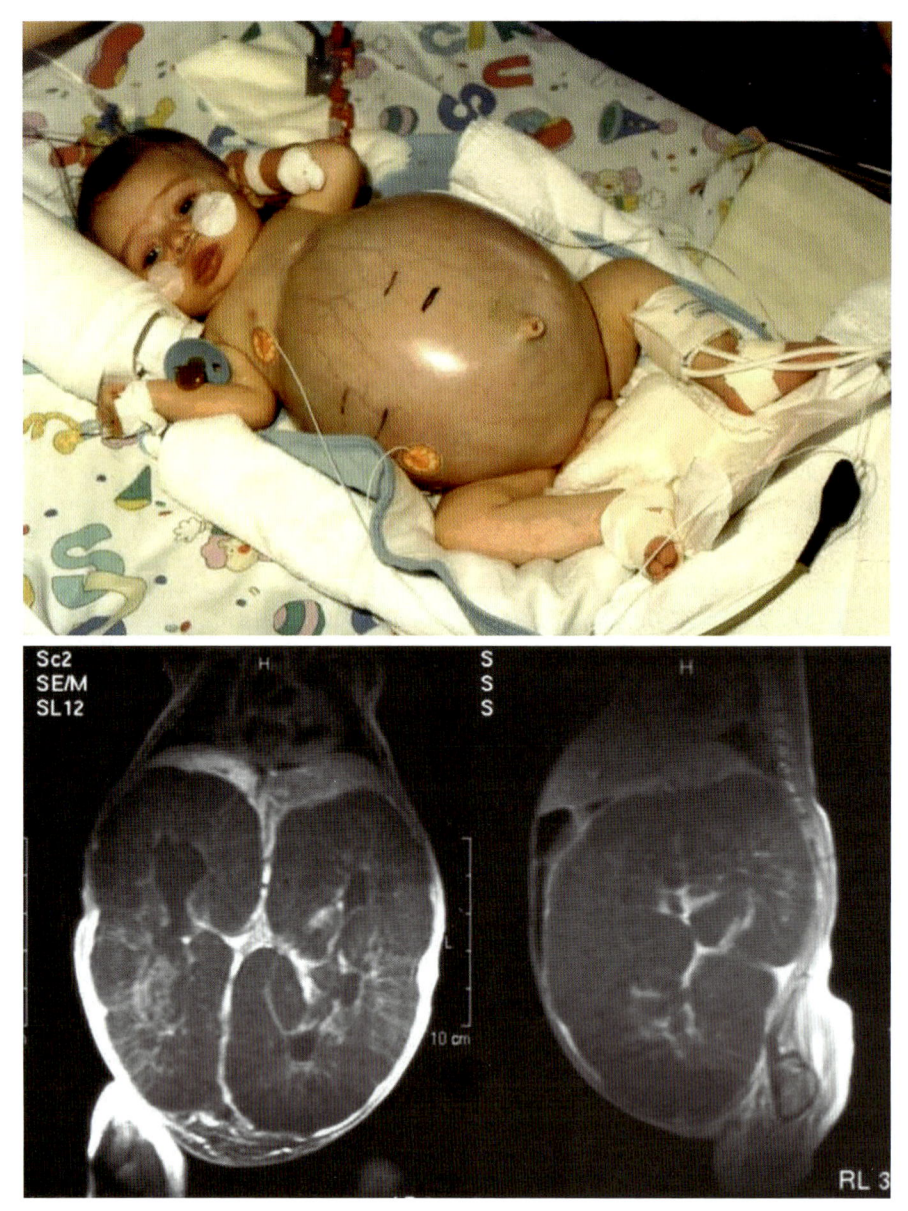

Figure 74.6 Severe nephromegaly in a 3-month-old infant with autosomal recessive polycystic kidney disease, with x-rays. (From Schaefer F: Pädiatrische Nephrologie. In Mayatepek E, editor: *Pädiatrie,* Munich, 2007, Elsevier/Urban & Fischer, pp 683-733.)

analysis. Recessive and dominant forms can usually be differentiated reliably by ultrasonographic appearance. Recent progress in genetic diagnostic testing has been accomplished by next-generation sequencing; this has made it possible to investigate all genes associated with cystic and polycystic kidney disease and other ciliopathies simultaneously, greatly facilitating diagnostic ascertainment and genetic counseling in ambiguous cases.[136] In ARPKD, knowledge of the causative mutation allows rapid screening in early pregnancy.[137]

A moderate genotype-phenotype correlation is observed in ARPKD. Severe phenotypes, such as neonatal demise, are more frequent in carriers of a truncating *PKHD1* mutation, and the presence of two truncating mutations invariably results in perinatal lethality. In contrast, amino acid substitutions are typically associated with a nonlethal presentation, and the presence of at least one amino acid substitution is required for affected individuals to survive the perinatal period. However, the phenotypic appearance varies, even within families affected by the same mutation, inviting speculation about the role of disease-modifying genes, epigenetic factors, hormonal effects, and environmental influences.[131,138]

Treatment

The treatment of ARPKD is limited to supportive therapy, including the management of respiratory distress in affected neonates, fluid and electrolyte substitution, strict blood pressure control, prevention of sequelae of CKD, and renal replacement therapy in patients who progress to ESKD. Unilateral or bilateral nephrectomy may be required, particularly in patients undergoing peritoneal dialysis and renal transplantation.

Until recently, the management of ADPKD was limited to controlling blood pressure and lowering lipid levels. Angiotensin-converting enzyme (ACE) inhibition may help stabilize GFR in young ADPKD patients.[139] An ongoing study in adults with ADPKD has been evaluating the potential benefits of rigorous blood pressure control and intensified renin angiotensin aldosterone system (RAAS) inhibition on kidney disease progression.[140] In a double-blind, placebo-controlled clinical trial in pediatric ADPKD patients, pravastatin administered in combination with ACE inhibitor therapy significantly attenuated the increase of total kidney volume within a 3-year treatment period.[141]

In recent years, the unraveling of the molecular basis of cystogenesis has yielded exciting innovative pharmacologic approaches to attenuate cyst progression and kidney volume expansion. Several new therapies with demonstrated efficacy in preclinical studies have been or are being explored in clinical trials in ADPKD patients. Clinical trials with mTOR (mammalian target of rapamycin) inhibition have yielded largely negative results.[142] Two placebo-controlled randomized trials investigating the effect of the somatostatin analog octreotide have found borderline effects on total kidney volume.[143,144] A placebo-controlled randomized trial evaluating the vasopressin type 2 receptor antagonist tolvaptan demonstrated significant reduction of cyst growth and superior preservation of GFR within a 2-year treatment period.[145] However, adverse events related to aquaresis and regarding hepatic function led to treatment discontinuation in a significant number of subjects.

Further trials evaluating epidermal growth factor receptor–specific tyrosine kinase inhibitors, and triptolide, a natural proapoptotic molecule, are currently underway.[146] Once the safety and anticystogenic efficacy of some of these drugs are demonstrated, further exploration of their nephroprotective potential will require long-term trials starting at an early stage of cyst formation—that is, during adolescence and young adulthood. Another particular pediatric interest is to test the efficacy of novel anticyst drugs in ciliopathies other than ADPKD.

Prognosis

The outcome of ARPKD depends on the degree of renal and hepatic involvement, which is usually reflected by age at presentation.[147] The mortality risk is greatest for patients with neonatal renal failure. Late liver failure occurs in a considerable proportion of children with ARPKD, which necessitates a comprehensive strategy for sequential or combined kidney and liver transplantation. Combined liver-kidney transplantation is a viable option for patients with advanced kidney disease or ESKD and recurrent cholangitis or complications of portal hypertension.[148] Simultaneous liver-kidney transplantation from the same donor provides an immunologic advantage, with a reduced risk of kidney allograft rejection and lower immunosuppression requirements.[148-150]

Children diagnosed with ADPKD are likely to have preserved renal function for decades. However, those who are symptomatic during childhood are at risk for early progression to ESKD. In such children and adolescents, transplantation of kidneys from living related donors requires exclusion of the disease in the donor relative by molecular testing.[151]

NEPHRONOPHTHISIS-RELATED CILIOPATHIES

The discovery of the crucial role of primary cilia led to the general term *ciliopathy*, which includes the polycystic kidney diseases, medullary cystic kidney disease, and the nephronophthisis-related ciliopathies (NPHP-RCs).[152] The latter term describes a group of rare autosomal recessive cystic kidney diseases typically characterized by chronic kidney disease progressing to ESKD during childhood. NPHP-RCs include isolated nephronophthisis (NPHP) and certain syndromes with additional extrarenal manifestations, including Senior-Loken syndrome (SLS), Joubert's syndrome (JBTS), Jeune's syndrome (JS), and Meckel-Gruber syndrome (MKS). More than 80 genes encoding proteins involved in ciliary structure and function have been associated with the different forms of NPHP-RCs.[153] Whereas mutations in some genes lead to distinct phenotypes, others exhibit a variable phenotypic appearance, with overlapping clinical features. To date, molecular subtypes of NPHPs are constituted by abnormalities in 16 genes— JBTS in 22, MKS in 11, JS in 11, and Bardet-Biedl syndrome in 17 genes. Nine of these genes are associated with more than one NPHP-RC (Table 74.1).[153]

NEPHRONOPHTHISIS

Nephronophthisis, an autosomal recessive disorder, is the most frequent single genetic cause of ESKD in children. In the early stage of the disease, impaired urine-concentrating ability causes polyuria and polydipsia. Subsequently progressive CKD develops, leading to severe anemia and growth failure. ESKD occurs within the first 2 decades of life.[154,155] Nephronophthisis is characterized histopathologically by microcysts at the corticomedullary border, thickening of the tubular basement membrane, and marked tubulointerstitial fibrosis. Infantile, juvenile, and adolescent disease variants are distinguished, with ESKD reached at a median age of 1, 13, and 19 years, respectively, in the three groups.[154] Nephronophthisis may also occur in association with characteristic extrarenal manifestations.

These phenotypic variants reflect mutations in distinct genes encoding for the nephrocystins, a family of proteins involved in primary ciliary function. Nephrocystins interact with one another and with other proteins (e.g., tensin, filamins, tubulins) involved in cell-cell and cell-matrix signaling. Mutations in the NPHP genes alter ciliary function via defects in intracellular signaling pathways, resulting in the inability of the ciliary mechanosensors to sense luminal flow rates, dysregulation of tissue growth, and cyst formation correctly.[154,156] The 16 genes associated with NPHP (see Table 74.1)[153] explain less than half of all cases.

NPHP1 (gene product, nephrocystin-1) is the gene most commonly involved. Deletions or mutations in *NPHP1* cause the common juvenile disease variant at an incidence of 1 in 5000, accounting for 25% of all nephronophthisis cases.[154,156] The juvenile form may also be caused by mutations in *NPHP3* to *NPHP13* and *AHI1*. Mutations in *NPHP2* (encoding inversin or nephrocystin-2) cause the infantile variant and, in mutations in *NPHP3*, the adolescent variant.

Retinitis pigmentosa is the most common extrarenal finding and occurs in approximately 20% of patients. The combination of nephronophthisis and retinitis pigmentosa is termed *Senior-Loken syndrome*.[157] The common pathophysiologic basis of the two disorders is explained by the structural equivalence of the primary cilium of renal epithelial cells and the connecting cilium of the photoreceptor cells in the retina.[157] Senior-Loken syndrome is usually caused by mutations in *NPHP5* and *NPHP6,* although mutations in most NPHP genes have been found with this syndrome.

Table 74.1 Inheritance Patterns and Defective Proteins in Ciliopathies

Disorder	Transmission	Affected Proteins*
Autosomal dominant polycystic kidney disease (types 1 and 2)	Both autosomal dominant	PKD1, PKD2
Autosomal recessive polycystic kidney disease	Autosomal recessive	PKHD1
Medullary cystic kidney disease and familial juvenile hyperuricemic nephropathy	Autosomal dominant	UMOD; REN; MUC1
Nephronophthisis types 1 to 16	Autosomal recessive	NPHP1, INVS, NPHP3, NPHP4, IQCB1, CEP290, GLIS2, RPGRIP1L, NEK8, SDCCAG8, TMEM67, TTC21B, WDR19, ZNF423, CEP164, ANKS6
Joubert's syndrome (subtypes with renal phenotype 1-7, 9-11, 14-16, 18-22)	All autosomal recessive except type 9 (X-linked inheritance)	INPP5E, TMEM216, AHI1, NPHP1, CEP290, TMEM67, RPGRIP1L, CC2D2A, OFD1, TTC21B, TMEM237, CEP41, TMEM138, TCTN3, ZNF423, TMEM231, CSPP1, PDE6
Meckel-Gruber syndrome (type 1-11)	Autosomal recessive	KS1, TMEM216, TMEM67, CEP290, RPGRIP1L, CC2D2A, NPHP3, TCTN2, B9D1, B9D2, TMEM231
Short rib–polydactyly syndrome (Jeune's syndrome; types 1-11)	Autosomal recessive	Unknown, IFT80, DYNC2H1, TTC21B, WDR19, NEK1, WDR35, WDR60, IFT140, IFT172, WDR34
Bardet-Biedl syndrome (types 1-15,17)	Autosomal recessive	BBS1, BBS2, ARL6, BBS4, BBS5, MKKS, BBS7, TTC8, PTHB1, BBS10, TRIM32, BBS12, MKS1, CEP290, Human fritz (WDPCP; C2orf86), LZTFL1
Alström's syndrome	Autosomal recessive	ALMS1
Cranioectodermal dysplasia (types 1-4)	Autosomal recessive	IFT122, WDR35, IFT43, WDR19
Oral-facial-digital syndrome (type 1)	X-linked inheritance	OFD1
Renal-hepatic-pancreatic dysplasia	Autosomal recessive	NPHP3 (nephrocystin-3); NEK8 (nephrocystin-9)

*HUGO gene Nomenclature Committee symbol.
Adapted from Devuyst O, Knoers NV, Remuzzi G, Schaefer F; Board of the Working Group for Inherited Kidney Diseases of the European Renal Association and European Dialysis and Transplant Association: Rare inherited kidney diseases: challenges, opportunities, and perspectives. Lancet 383:1844-1859, 2014.

NPHP1 deletions or mutations have also been described in association with Cogan's syndrome (nephronophthisis associated with oculomotor apraxia), MKS (see below), and in a subset of individuals with JS.[153,158,159] This overlapping phenotypic spectrum, with abnormalities in a single gene, points to the role of genetic modifiers in the nephronophthisis complex.

JOUBERT'S SYNDROME

In JS, nephronophthisis is combined with mid-hindbrain malformation and cerebellar vermis hypoplasia or aplasia, descriptively designated as a molar tooth sign on a cranial magnetic resonance imaging (MRI) scan. This anomaly results in various neurologic features, including developmental delay, intellectual disability, muscle hypotonia, ataxia, oculomotor apraxia, nystagmus, and respiratory distress. Mutations in *AHI1*, encoding jouberin, are the most common among the more than 20 genes associated with JS.[153] Jouberin is a centrosome protein interacting with nephrocystin-1.

MECKEL-GRUBER SYNDROME

MKS is an autosomal recessive, usually perinatally lethal disorder, characterized by central nervous system malformation (e.g., occipital encephalocele), bilateral renal cystic dysplasia, cleft palate, postaxial polydactyly, and ductal proliferation in the portal area of the liver.[160,161] The condition is caused by abnormalities in various genes (currently 11) encoding ciliary proteins.[153]

BARDET-BIEDL SYNDROME

Bardet-Biedl syndrome (BBS) is an autosomal recessive ciliopathy characterized by extremely variable polydactyly, obesity, mild developmental delay, hypogonadism, and an atypical retinitis pigmentosa. Variable renal abnormalities are present in up to 90% of patients, and renal failure occurs in up to 60%, usually in adulthood. Polydactyly may be the only obvious feature prenatally. The disorder is highly heterogeneous, with 17 *BBS*-associated genes identified to date. Complex genetic interactions between causal and modifying alleles of ciliary genes seem to contribute to phenotypic variability.[153,162]

GLOMERULAR DISORDERS

Glomerular disease in children may be caused by a plethora of primary kidney diseases and may also be secondary to systemic disorders such as autoimmune disease, vasculitis, or infectious disease. Many of these conditions vary in presentation from absent or mild symptoms to serious renal disease with life-threatening complications. Childhood glomerular diseases can be categorized principally according to their clinical presentation into nephritic and nephrotic phenotypes.

On histologic analysis of biopsy specimens, a nephritic pattern is seen to be associated with inflammation and presents with an active urine sediment with dysmorphic red cells, white cells, red cell and granular casts, and a variable degree of proteinuria. Acute nephritic syndrome is characterized by the sudden onset of macroscopic hematuria accompanied by hypertension, oliguria, edema, and renal insufficiency. Most cases of acute nephritic syndrome occur after an infection, most commonly a group A beta-hemolytic streptococcal infection.

By contrast, the nephrotic pattern presents with marked proteinuria and inactive urine sediment with few cells or casts, characterized histopathologically by the absence of inflammation. Children with nephrotic syndrome usually show generalized edema, including anasarca, ascites, and pleural effusion, but have a preserved GFR.

Some patients with severe kidney disease have nephritic and nephrotic features on presentation. Conversely, there are also patients with suspected glomerular disease who do not fit either category because they are likely to have a mild course of a glomerulonephritis. For example, children with mild IgA nephropathy may have recurrent gross hematuria after an upper respiratory tract infection without an active sediment or proteinuria.

The following sections focus on the most common glomerulopathies observed in childhood.

NEPHROTIC SYNDROME

The pediatric definition of nephrotic syndrome (NS) is proteinuria greater than 40 mg/m^2/hr (50 mg/kg/day) or a urine protein/creatinine ratio of more than 2.0 mg/mg, hypoalbuminemia of less than 2.5 g/dL, and the presence of edema and hyperlipidemia.[163,164]

The pathogenesis of NS has long been investigated, with an emphasis on the mechanisms of glomerular injury and proteinuria. It has been suggested that idiopathic steroid-sensitive NS, as well as a subset of steroid-resistant nephrotic syndrome (SRNS), is caused by an immunologic alteration that possibly implies the production of a circulating proteinuric factor secondary to T cell dysfunction.[165] Sera of patients with focal segmental glomerulosclerosis (FSGS) have been demonstrated to increase glomerular permeability to albumin when incubated with rat glomeruli in vitro.[166] This mechanism appears to affect adults and children, except for mutations in epithelial membrane protein-2 (EMP2), which cause childhood-onset SSNS.[167] There have been 24 mutations in podocyte-specific genes regulating foot process structure and function identified in inherited forms of SRNS, with congenital, infantile, and adolescent onset.[167-169]

In addition to primary alterations of the foot process and slit diaphragm, the glomerular basement membrane (GBM) is also likely to play a role in the pathogenesis of proteinuria. The GBM contributes to the unique charge and size selectivity of the filtration barrier restricting the filtration of macromolecules such as albumin across the glomerular capillary wall.[170] Children with minimal change glomerulopathy (MCG) show decreased anionic charges in the GBM,[170,171] without any structural damage or change to the glomerular filtration unit observed by light microscopy. In glomerular diseases other than MCG, structural injury, with podocyte loss and denudation of the GBM, allows movement of normally restricted proteins of varying sizes across the filtration barrier.

NS in children is traditionally classified into three categories: primary (also termed *idiopathic nephrotic syndrome*), secondary, and congenital NS. Idiopathic nephrotic syndrome is subcategorized according to histopathologic appearance, mainly including MCG, FSGS, membranoproliferative glomerulonephritis (MPGN), membranous nephropathy, and diffuse mesangial proliferation. The term *secondary nephrotic syndrome* refers to NS associated with an identifiable systemic disease or infection, which is often accompanied by a nephritic component. Congenital nephrotic syndrome has been defined as NS occurring within the first 3 months of life. Although this classification is useful for clinical purposes, in this chapter NS has been stratified primarily by the presence or absence of a genetic cause.

HEREDITARY NEPHROTIC SYNDROME

Inherited structural defects of the glomerular filtration barrier account for a large proportion of pediatric SRNS cases, highlighting the crucial role of the development and structural architecture of podocytes in the pathogenesis of glomerulopathies.[169,172,173] Abnormalities in genes encoding podocyte-specific proteins may lead to loss of foot processes and slit membrane integrity, disruption of cell-cell signaling at the slit diaphragm,[174] defects in foot process–GBM interaction,[175] altered podocyte motility, and mitochondrial dysfunction, resulting in glomerular protein leakage and NS.[176-179]

To date, mutations in more than a dozen genes *(NPHS1, NPHS2, NPHS3 [PLCE1], ACTN4, CD2AP, TRPC6, INF2, PTPRO, ITGA3, MYO1E, ARHGDIA, COQ2, COQ6, ADCK4)* have been implicated in nonsyndromic SRNS (Table 74.2).[169,172-175,178-183] Nephrin, podocin, and CD2-associated protein, encoded by *NPHS1, NPHS2,* and *CD2AP,* respectively, are major structural elements of the slit diaphragm.[169,172,173,180] Nephrin is a transmembrane protein and contributes to the porous structure of the slit diaphragm, forming pores of approximately 40 nm. These pores are partly responsible for the size selectivity of the slit diaphragm and filtration barrier. Nephrin also appears to participate in intracellular signaling pathways maintaining the functional integrity of the podocyte. A number of proteins within this signaling platform have been identified to interact with nephrin, among them podocin, CD2-associated protein, phospholipase Cϵ_1, and transient receptor potential cation channel, subfamily C, member 6 (TRPC6). PTPRO (protein tyrosine phosphatase receptor type O) is a membrane-bound tyrosine phosphatase involved in cell-cell signaling at the podocyte slit membrane.[174] ITGA3 (integrin alpha 3) is a key protein in foot process–GBM interaction.[175] In addition, a number of cytoskeleton-regulating proteins are expressed selectively in podocytes (e.g., *ACTN4*, encoding α-actinin-4; INF2, a member of the formin family of actin-regulating proteins; and the non-muscle class I myosin 1E [MYO1E]).[169,173,178] ARHGDIA, a regulator of Rho GTPases, indirectly regulates actin cytoskeleton-dependent cellular functions.[179] COQ2, COQ6, and ADCK4 are important components of CoQ10 biosynthesis in the mitochondria[181-183] (Figure 74.7).

In addition, syndromic forms of SRNS may be due to mutations in genes encoding the following: transcription factors *(WT1, LMX1B);* GBM components *(LAMB2, ITGB4);* lysosomal protein *(SCARB2);* a DNA-nucleosome restructuring mediator *(SMARCAL1);*[169,172,173,184] and mitochondrial proteins *(COQ6)*[181] (see Table 74.2).

All hereditary proteinuria syndromes share a common electron microscopic phenotype, which uniformly demonstrates flattening of the foot processes and loss of the slit

Table 74.2 Causative Genes and Histologic Patterns of Nephrotic Syndrome by Time of Disease Onset

	Cause	Inheritance/Locus	Gene/Protein	Histologic Features
Congenital Onset (0-3 mo)				
Isolated	Congenital nephrotic syndrome of the Finnish type (CNF)	AR	NPHS1/nephrin	Radial dilation of proximal tubule
	Recessive SRNS, type 2	AR	NPHS2/podocin	FSGS/MGC
	Recessive SRNS, type 3	AR	NPHS3/PLCE1	DMS
	Isolated DMS	AR	WT1	DMS
	Recessive SRNS	AR	COQ2	FSGS, collapsing
	Recessive SRNS + deafness	AR	COQ6	FSGS
	Dominant SRNS + deafness	AD/11q24	Unknown	FSGS
	DMS + neurologic findings	AR	ARHGDIA/Rho GDP dissociation inhibitor (GDI) alpha	DMS
	NS + lung and skin disease	AR	ITGA3/integrin alpha 3	DMS
Syndromic	Steroid-sensitive nephrotic syndrome	AR/2p12-13.2	Unknown	MGC/FSGS
	Denys-Drash syndrome	AD	WT1	DMS
	Pierson's syndrome	AR	LAMB2/laminin-β2	FSGS
	Nail-patella syndrome	AD	LMX1B/LIM homeobox transcription factor-1β	
	Frasier's syndrome	AD	WT1	FSGS
	Schimke's immunoosseous dysplasia	AR	SMARCAL1	FSGS
	Epidermolysis bullosa + FSGS	AR	ITGB4/integrin-β4	FSGS
	Galloway-Mowat syndrome	AR	Unknown	MGC to FSGS
Infancy-Childhood Onset				
Genetic	Recessive SSNS	AR	EMP2/epithelial membrane protein 2	
	Recessive SRNS	AR	NPHS2/podocin	FSGS/MGC
	Recessive SRNS	AR	NPHS1/nephrin	FSGS/MGC
	Recessive SRNS	AR	NPHS3/PLCE1	DMS
	Isolated DMS	AD	WT1	DMS
	Recessive SRNS + deafness or intellectual disability	AR	ARHGDIA	DMS
	SRNS	AR	MYOE1/nonmuscle class I myosin E	FSGS
	SRNS	AR	PTPRO/GLEPP1 protein tyrosine phosphatase receptor type O/glomerular epithelial protein-1	FSGS
Juvenile-Adult Onset				
Genetic	SRNS	AR or sporadic	NPHS2 (p.R229Q)	FSGS
	Familial SRNS	AD	INF2/formin family of actin-regulating proteins	FSGS
	FSGS, type 1	AD/19q13	ACTN4/α-actinin-4	FSGS
	FSGS, type 2	AD/11q21-22	TRPC6/transient receptor potential cation channel, subfamily C, member 6	FSGS
	FSGS, type 3	AR-AD/6p12	CD2AP/CD2-associated protein	FSGS
	SRNS	AR	PTPRO/GLEPP1 protein tyrosine phosphatase receptor type O/glomerular epithelial protein-1	FSGS
	SRNS	AR	ADCK4/aarF domain containing kinase 4	FSGS
	SRNS (no extrarenal symptoms)	AD or sporadic	LMX1B encodes homeodomain-containing transcription factor	FSGS

AD, Autosomal dominant; AR, autosomal recessive; DMS, diffuse mesangial sclerosis; FSGS, focal segmental glomerulosclerosis; MGC, minimal glomerular changes; NS, nephrotic syndrome; SRNS, steroid-resistant nephrotic syndrome.
Adapted from references 169, 172-175, 178-183.

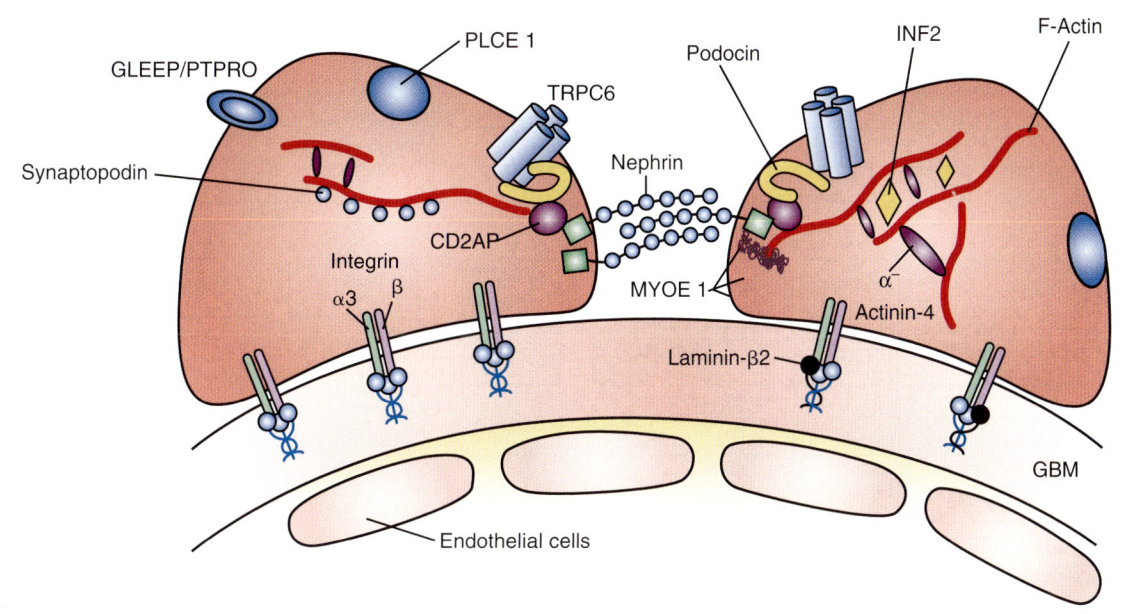

Figure 74.7 Proteins involved in the maintenance of the structure and function of podocyte foot processes and the slit diaphragm. (Modified and reproduced with permission from Weber S: Hereditary nephrotic syndrome. In Geary DF, Schaefer F, editors: *Comprehensive pediatric nephrology,* Philadelphia, 2008, Mosby, pp 219-228.)

diaphragm. However, the clinical phenotype can be diverse. The early-onset nephrotic presentation with a severe course is seen in individuals with mutations in nephrin and podocin, whereas in families with *INF2* or *ACTN4* mutations, the disorder presents in early adolescence or adulthood, typically with moderate proteinuria that is slowly progressive, often leading to ESKD in adulthood.[164,169,172,173,180,185] These distinct hereditary forms of NS are discussed in the following sections.

Early Onset

The most common subtype of congenital NS is the Finnish type (CNF), an autosomal recessive disorder that is very common in Finland (incidence of 1 in 8200 live births). Patients typically show massive proteinuria at birth, a large placenta, marked edema, enlarged kidneys, and characteristic radial dilation of the proximal tubules. The glomeruli show a slight increase of mesangial matrix and mesangial hypercellularity. Degenerative changes such as shrinking of the glomerular tuft, fibrotic thickening of Bowman's capsule, and glomerular sclerosis become evident with time.[185] Electron microscopy shows effacement of foot processes, irregularity in the GBM, and some swelling of the endothelial cells and rarefaction of tubulointerstitial capillaries.[186,187] CNF is steroid-resistant; treatment options include albumin infusions, pharmacologic interventions with ACE inhibitors and indomethacin and, ultimately, unilateral or bilateral nephrectomy. CNF generally progresses to ESKD within the first decade of life, although patients with milder forms of the disease have been described.[173,185,188]

The gene affected in CNF, *NPHS1,* was mapped in 1994 to chromosome band 19q13.1. To date, more than 140 different *NPHS1* mutations have been identified.[185] Two mutations, Fin-major (p.L41fsX91) and Fin-minor (p.R1109X), account for 78% and 16% of the mutated alleles, respectively, among Finnish patients. In non-Finnish patients with a CNF phenotype, the *NPHS1* mutation detection rate approaches 66%.[185]

Congenital NS is not synonymous with CNF, because mutations in other genes encoding slit diaphragm proteins, such as podocin (see later), can also cause early-onset NS. In one study, mutations in *NPHS2* were shown to be responsible for up to 40% of all cases of NS occurring in the first 3 months of life.[168] These patients showed histologic features similar to those of CNF. On the other hand, *NPHS1* mutations have been described in individual patients with disease onset in later childhood, and there have been even anecdotal reports of adult-onset SRNS.[189,190]

Other genes causing early-onset NS are Wilms' tumor-1 (*WT1*), phospholipase Cε_1 (*PLCE1*), laminin-β2 gene (*LAMB2*), *ARHGDIA*, and *ITGA3*.[168,171,172,175,179] These disorders have a more widespread age of onset and spectrum of clinical manifestations. Mutations in PLCE1, a cytoplasmic enzyme required for podocyte maturation, have been associated with as many as 28% of cases of congenital NS due to isolated diffuse mesangial sclerosis. Mutations in the developmental regulatory gene *WT1* are associated with forms of congenital NS caused by diffuse mesangial sclerosis with male to female sex reversal and Wilms' tumor (Denys-Drash syndrome) or gonadoblastoma (Frasier's syndrome).[191] Nail-patella syndrome, a disorder characterized by skeletal and nail dysplasia as well as NS, is caused by mutations in the *LMX1B* gene, which regulates expression of type IV collagen and the podocyte proteins nephrin, podocin, and CD2-associated protein.[152] *LMX1B* mutations can also cause isolated SRNS.[192]

Pierson's syndrome, characterized by microcoria, abnormal lens shape, cataracts, blindness, severe neurologic deficits, congenital NS, and progressive kidney failure, is caused by mutations in *LAMB2*, which codes for laminin-β2, a constituent of the GBM, retina, lens, and neuromuscular synapses.[173]

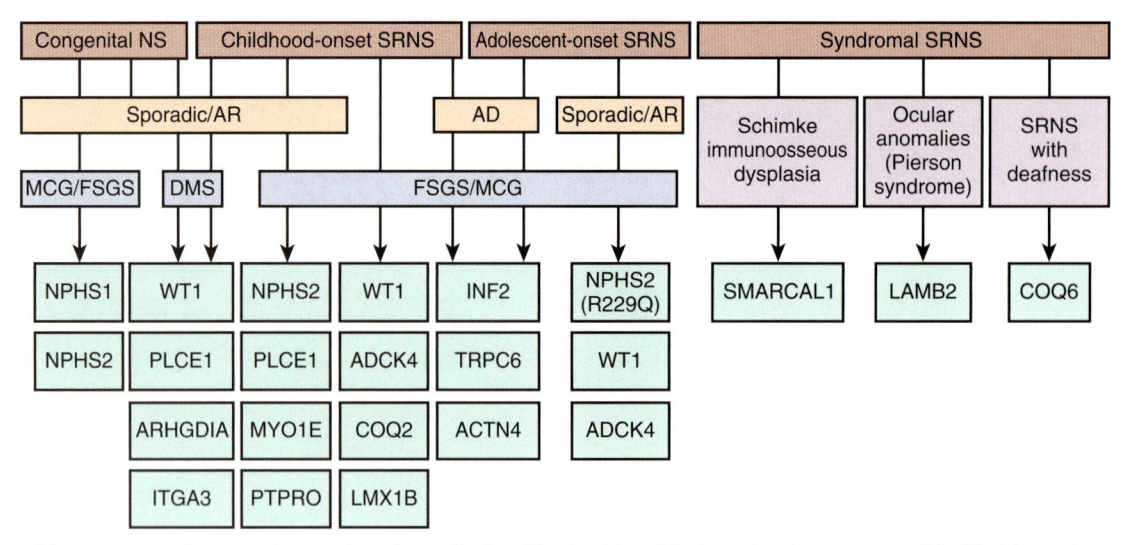

Figure 74.8 Molecular genetic screening strategy for patients with steroid-resistant nephrotic syndrome. (Modified from Podonet Registry. Available at: http://www.podonet.org/opencms/opencms/podonet/podonet_en/Algorithms/screen/diagnostics.html. Reproduced with permission.)

As many as 85% of cases that occur during the first 3 months of life can be explained by mutations in one of four candidate genes—*NPHS1*, *NPHS2*, *WT1*, and *LAMB2*.[168] Genetic screening in nonsyndromic patients with congenital NS should start with *NPHS1*, followed by *NPHS2* if results are negative. Patients with congenital NS presenting somewhat later in infancy should probably be screened initially for *NPHS2* mutations, followed by *NPHS1*. If diffuse mesangial sclerosis is revealed by kidney biopsy, genetic testing should start with *WT1*, and *PLCE1*, with *ARHGDIA* and *ITGA3* to follow[172,175,179] (Figure 74.8).

Finally, NS manifesting in the first 3 months of life may also result from congenital infections such as syphilis and cytomegalovirus infection (see Table 74.2).

Infantile and Childhood Onset

The term *infantile nephrotic syndrome* has been proposed for NS developing between the ages of 4 and 12 months, while childhood-onset usually refers to those in the 1- to 10-year-old age range. The most common genetic abnormalities found in these age groups are recessive mutations in the *NPHS2* gene, which encodes the podocyte membrane protein podocin.[169,173,184] In whites, mutations in this gene account for about 40% of familial and approximately 6% to 17% of sporadic SRNS cases.[168,193,194] Patients typically progress to ESKD before the end of the first decade of life.[168,193-195] Renal histologic findings show MCG (if biopsy is performed early) or FSGS. Podocin is part of a membrane protein complex that links the slit diaphragm to the podocyte cytoskeleton. To date, 126 pathogenic *NPHS2* mutations and 43 variants of unknown significance have been reported.[169,196] Frameshift, nonsense, and the homozygous p.R138Q missense mutations are associated with early disease manifestation.[148,166] *R138Q*, the most common mutation, causes defective protein folding and retention of the mutant protein in the endoplasmic reticulum.[196]

WT1 mutations may account for about 9% of cases of nonfamilial isolated SRNS,[197] and they have been identified in patients with isolated diffuse mesangial sclerosis, with clinical onset varying from a few days of life to 2 years of age, as well as in patients with isolated FSGS occurring at 1 to 14 years of age.[191] Similarly, mutations in *PLCE1*, the gene encoding phospholipase Cε1, have been found in some infantile- and childhood-onset SRNS cases with histologic features of diffuse mesangial sclerosis, with first disease manifestation occurring up to 4 years of age.[198-200] All patients identified to date had truncating mutations.

In addition to these relatively common genetic causes of SRNS, a rapidly increasing number of genes expressed specifically or preferentially in the podocyte are being identified; mutations in these genes cause rare recessive forms of SRNS. Truncating and splice-site mutations in *PTPRO* (protein tyrosine phosphatase receptor-type O), a receptor-like membrane protein tyrosine phosphatase expressed at the apical membrane of podocyte foot processes, caused childhood-onset SRNS in two Turkish families.[174] Mutations in *MYO1E*, encoding a nonmuscle, membrane-associated, class I myosin, have been associated with childhood- and adolescent-onset SRNS with FSGS histopathology.[178]

Finally, mutations in several mitochondrial enzymes involved in CoQ10 biosynthesis have been identified in children with SRNS. These include *COQ2*, *PDSS2*, *ADCK4*, and *COQ6*. *PDSS2* and *COQ2* mutations are typically characterized by early onset and variable extrarenal manifestations, which may include encephalopathy, lactic acidosis, myoclonic epilepsy and hypertrophic cardiomyopathy. *COQ6* (CoQ10 biosynthesis monooxygenase 6) has been identified as a cause of early-onset SRNS with sensorineural deafness. Patients with *ADCK4* mutations have a less severe phenotype, with isolated SRNS and disease onset typically at adolescence.[181-183] The early identification of genetic mitochondriopathies may be of immense clinical relevance since preliminary findings suggest that the disorders might be amenable to oral treatment with CoQ10.[181]

Newly identified *ARHGDIA* and integrin alpha 3 (*ITGA3*) mutations cause congenital NS with the histology of diffuse mesangial sclerosis (DMS) and extrarenal findings.[175,179]

Genetic screening in infantile- and childhood-onset SRNS with histologic features of MCG or FSGS should start with *NPHS2*, followed by *NPHS1* and *WT1*. Patients with histologic findings of diffuse mesangial sclerosis should be tested for mutations in *WT1* followed by *PLCE1* (see Figure 74.8).

Mutations in the *ARHGDIA*, *ACTN4*, and *TRPC6* genes (see later) have been only anecdotally reported in infants and children. These reports do not justify systematic mutational screening of these genes for patients in this age group unless there is an autosomal dominant familial history of FSGS.[172,179]

Late Onset

NS first manifesting in adolescence is commonly steroid resistant. Although most cases remain unexplained, a few genetic causes have been identified.

Compound heterozygous mutations in podocin involving one allele carrying the p.R229Q variant probably constitute the most frequent known cause of sporadic late-onset SRNS.[201,202] R229Q is a non-neutral polymorphism leading to impaired podocin-nephrin interaction. It is present in approximately 6% of the European population. In combination with another mutated allele, it causes a podocytopathy of relatively late onset and slowly progressive course.

INF2, *ACTN4*, and *TRPC6* have been identified as causing autosomal dominant familial forms of SRNS first manifesting in adolescence or adulthood, usually with moderate proteinuria and a slow progression to ESKD over decades.[172,180,203] *INF2* mutations have been shown to account for 17%, *TRPC6* mutations for 6%, and *ACTN4* mutations for 4% of autosomal dominant SRNS cases.[174-176] De novo mutations in *INF2*, *TRPC6*, and *ACTN4* are rare.[203-206] Among 227 patients with nonsyndromic familial and sporadic SRNS with adolescent disease onset, *NPHS2* mutations explained 7% and *WT1* 4% of cases, whereas *INF2* was exclusively found in familial cases. Thus, screening of *NPHS2* and exons 8 and 9 of *WT1* should be the most rational and cost-effective screening approach in sporadic, juvenile, steroid-resistant NS, whereas screening of *INF2*, *ACTN4*, and *TRPC6* can be restricted to dominant familial forms of the disease.[207]

IDIOPATHIC NEPHROTIC SYNDROME

Epidemiology and Definitions

Idiopathic nephrotic syndrome (INS) is the most common form of childhood NS. The annual incidence of INS in children in the United States and Europe is 1 to 3/100,000 children, with a cumulative prevalence of 16/100,000 children.[208] More than 90% of these cases manifest between 1 and 10 years of age.[209]

Diffuse foot process effacement on electron microscopy corresponds to MCG, FSGS, or mesangial proliferation on light microscopy. The vast majority of preadolescent children with INS (77%) show MCG on kidney biopsy.[209,210]

Of children with MCG, 90% respond to glucocorticoid treatment and have a favorable long-term prognosis,[164,210] but the 10% who do not respond to corticosteroids are at particular risk for the development of ESKD, which occurs in 30% to 40% of children with SRNS after a follow-up of 10 years.[211,212] Based on these observations, patients with INS are further classified according to their response to empirical glucocorticoid therapy.

Although the definition of steroid resistance varies in the literature, patients who fail to enter remission after 8 weeks of glucocorticoid treatment are generally categorized as having SRNS.[163,164,213] Some patients initially show a response to glucocorticoid treatment but experience a relapse, either two consecutive relapses during corticosteroid therapy or within 14 days of ceasing therapy. These patients are considered to have steroid-dependent NS (SDNS). Patients who show a response to steroids but develop relapses after discontinuation of treatment are referred to as relapsers. One relapse within 6 months of initial response or one to three relapses in any 12-month period is termed *infrequent relapse*; two or more relapses within 6 months of initial response or four or more relapses in any 12-month period is termed *frequent relapse* (FR).[214]

INS with MCG can be differentiated clinically from other causes of NS.[209] The relevant findings include age younger than 6 years, absence of hypertension, absence of hematuria, normal complement levels, and normal renal function.[209]

Pathogenesis

INS is believed to have an immune pathogenesis that remains to be fully elucidated and may not be uniform in all phenotypes. Abnormal regulation of T cell subsets has been suggested, as well as expression of a circulating glomerular permeability factor.[165,166,215] Evidence of the immune-mediated nature of INS is demonstrated by the fact that immunosuppressive agents can induce complete disease remission. Also, NS has been known to undergo remission during infection with the measles virus, which suppresses cell-mediated immunity. Improvement of posttransplantation proteinuria by plasmapheresis lends further support to the presence of one or several circulating factors.[164,215]

The association of allergic responses with NS also illustrates the role of the immune system in INS. NS has been reported to occur after various allergic reactions. Food allergy might play a role in relapses of INS. Various cytokines and growth factors have been implicated, of which interleukin-13 seems to be most consistently associated with acute disease episodes.[164,216,217]

The precise mechanism of proteinuria in MCNS remains unknown.[218,219] MCG has been recently suggested to result from a two-hit podocyte immune response. In the first step, the costimulatory membrane molecule CD80, a part of the innate immune system, is induced in podocytes by circulating cytokines, microbial products, or allergens. In the case of regulatory T cell dysfunction and/or impaired autoregulatory podocyte functions, elevated CD80 expression becomes persistent and induces proteinuria.[220,221]

Recently, soluble urokinase receptor (suPAR), the soluble form of urokinase plasminogen-type activator receptor, has been reported to be elevated in two thirds of patients with primary FSGS but not in other forms of primary glomerular diseases. Experimentally, suPAR binding and activation of β_3-integrin on podocytes led to alterations in the morphology (foot process effacement) and function of podocytes, which resulted in proteinuria and initiation of FSGS.[222] In two clinical trial cohorts, elevated suPAR levels were found in 55% of pediatric and 84% of adult patients with FSGS.[223] However, subsequent studies in adults and children with FSGS did not confirm a specific elevation of suPAR levels in FSGS patients; suPAR concentrations seemed to accumulate nonspecifically with failing renal function.[224]

Clinical Features

Edema is the presenting symptom in about 95% of children with INS. It usually appears first in areas of low tissue resistance (e.g., periorbital, scrotal, and labial regions) and progresses during the disease course. Ultimately, it becomes generalized and can be massive (anasarca). An upper respiratory tract infection, allergic reaction, or another factor (e.g., drugs, vaccination) may immediately precede the development or relapse of the disease. A history of allergy is present in approximately 30% of children.[225]

Microscopic hematuria may be seen in up to 23% of patients with MCG and in a higher percentage of patients with other histologic variants.[209] Macrohematuria develops in 3% to 4% of MCG cases. Given the increased risk of venous thrombosis in NS, renal vein thrombosis must be considered in patients with significant hematuria and in cases of acute kidney injury due to intravascular volume depletion. Other thrombotic events can have various manifestations, including tachypnea and respiratory distress (pulmonary thrombosis or embolism) and, in rare cases, seizures (e.g., sinus vein thrombosis). Symptoms of infection such as fever, lethargy, irritability, or abdominal pain due to sepsis or peritonitis should not be overlooked. Hypotension and signs of shock can be present in children with sepsis. Anorexia, irritability, fatigue, abdominal discomfort, and diarrhea are common. Gastrointestinal distress can be caused by ascites, bowel wall edema, or both. Respiratory distress can occur due to massive ascites, frank pulmonary edema, or pleural effusions.[225] Hypertension has been reported in up to 21% of children 6 years of age and younger with biopsy-confirmed MCG and may be present in up to 50% of children with other histologic types.[209]

Classification, Kidney Biopsy Indications, and Histology Patterns

The high correlation of the response to empirical glucocorticoid therapy with short- and long-term prognoses makes steroid responsiveness the first classifying criterion in childhood INS. A kidney biopsy is not indicated for the first manifestation of typical childhood INS occurring between 1 and 8 years of age unless history, physical findings, and/or laboratory results indicate the possibility of secondary NS or INS other than MCG. Thus, patients in the typical age range—and even older children with normal kidney function, no macroscopic hematuria, no symptoms of systemic disease (fever, rash, joint pain, weight loss), normal complement levels, negative results on viral screens (e.g., human immunodeficiency virus, hepatitis B and C viruses), and no family history of kidney disease—will usually be treated primarily with glucocorticoids; kidney biopsy is reserved for complicated and steroid-resistant cases.[225,226]

INS in childhood can be classified by histologic subtype. MCG is the most common form and is associated with steroid sensitivity in 90% of cases. FSGS is the most common histopathologic correlate of steroid-resistant disease with a risk of progressing to ESKD. Mesangial proliferative glomerulonephritis has an intermediate prognosis. MPGN, membranous nephropathy, IgM nephropathy, and C1q nephropathy are rather infrequent forms of INS.[226] A detailed discussion of the various types of INS and histologic findings is beyond the scope of this chapter. Briefly, the most common features are as follows.

The designation "MCG" indicates glomerular morphology that on light microscopic examination is little different from normal. Minimal mesangial hypercellularity may be present. Immune deposits are absent. Occasionally, mesangial IgM deposition may be seen. Some authors consider the presence of IgM to represent a separate entity (IgM nephropathy), whereas others consider this to be a variant of MCG. The presence of IgM may indicate a more difficult course of NS. Electron microscopy shows uniform abnormality of the podocytes, with marked effacement of the foot processes over at least 50% of the glomerular capillary surface. The cytoplasm of the cells may be enlarged, with clear vacuoles and prominence of organelles. This is accompanied by microvillous transformation along the urinary surface of the podocytes.[226]

Mesangioproliferative glomerulonephritis is characterized by generalized, diffuse mesangial cell hyperplasia involving more than 80% of the glomeruli. Increased numbers of mesangial cell nuclei are present within the mesangial matrix, which is normal or only mildly increased. Many cases of mesangioproliferative glomerulonephritis show positive granular mesangial IgM with or without C3 and, very occasionally, small amounts of C1q or IgG, although some cases have negative immunofluorescence. On electron microscopy, there is mesangial cell hyperplasia with effacement of epithelial cell foot processes and microvillous transformation of epithelial cells. Patients with diffuse mesangial proliferation have an increased incidence of steroid resistance.[226]

FSGS is the most common finding in SRNS. FSGS describes a lesion in which, as seen on light microscopy, discrete segments of the glomerular tuft reveal sclerosis (segmental); some glomeruli are involved, whereas others are spared (focal). Adhesion of the glomerular tuft to Bowman's capsule (synechiae) is observed. Glomerular hypertrophy is common. Interstitial fibrosis and tubular atrophy are often present and correlate with the severity of disease. IgM and C3 are trapped in the sclerotic areas. As in MCG, electron microscopy reveals effacement of the podocyte foot processes and obliteration of capillary lumens by fine granular and lipid deposits. Five variants of FSGS have been defined in adult patients—collapsing, cellular, tip lesion, perihilar, and "not otherwise specified." The collapsing type is associated with the highest rate of progression to ESKD, followed by the tip lesion histologic type.[226] A single pediatric study looked for clinical and histologic markers predicting the outcome of FSGS; 66 patients were followed for at least 10 years. Mesangial expansion and tip lesions were independent predictors of a favorable response to cytotoxic therapy, whereas the presence of renal impairment and extensive focal segmental sclerosis predicted an unfavorable response.[227]

MPGN is characterized by mesangial proliferation and thickening of the peripheral GBM. Typically, the thickening is due to mesangial cell interposition, with double contours of the GBM. Immunofluorescence reveals a characteristic capillary deposition of C3. Three types of MPGN can be distinguished by electron microscopy according to the location of immune deposits. Type I, the classical form of MPGN, is characterized by subendothelial deposits. The additional presence of numerous electron-dense deposits on the subepithelial side of the GBM defines type III MPGN.[228] The presence of ribbon-like, dense intramembranous deposits differentiates dense deposit disease, formerly known as MPGN type II. Recently, the group of disorders with glomerular C3 without immunoglobulin deposition has been termed the *C3 glomerulopathies,* which comprise dense deposit disease and C3 glomerulonephritis.[229] Both disorders are caused by fluid phase dysregulation of the complement cascade. They are defined by their shared pattern of immunofluorescence and distinguished on electron microscopy by the character and location of complement deposits in the glomeruli.[230,231] Genetic abnormalities in genes regulating the alternative complement pathway are found in 20% to 25% of these subjects.

Membranous nephropathy is a very rare cause of INS during childhood, identified in only approximately 1% of biopsy specimens, in contrast to the 25% to 40% prevalence observed in adult INS. See Chapters 32 and 33 for more details.

Treatment of Idiopathic Nephrotic Syndrome

First-Line Therapy. Oral glucocorticoids are the first line of treatment for a child with INS. About 90% of children who are experiencing their first episode of NS achieve remission with glucocorticoid therapy. Of those who show a response, about 95% do so after 4 weeks of daily glucocorticoid therapy and 98% after 8 weeks of glucocorticoid therapy.[209]

The recommended standard therapy for the first episode of NS is oral prednisolone, 60 mg/m^2/day (maximum, 60 mg) in three divided doses for 4 to 6 weeks, followed by 40 mg/m^2/day (maximum, 40 mg) given as a single dose for 4 to 6 weeks, with or without tapering over 2 to 5 months.[214,232,233] A Cochrane systematic review has concluded that continuation of alternate-day steroid therapy for 6 months reduces the subsequent relapse rate by 33% compared with shorter, alternate-day treatment regimens.[234] However, a recent placebo-controlled randomized clinical trial has demonstrated that extension of steroid exposure from 3 to 6 months at the same cumulative dose does not reduce relapse risk, questioning the usefulness of steroid tapering.[235]

Therapy for relapse is shorter than initial treatment. For infrequent relapses (one relapse within 6 months of initial response or one to three relapses in any 12-month period), prednisone should be administered at 60 mg/m^2/day until the child has been in complete remission for at least 3 days, followed by 40 mg/m^2 alternate-day therapy for 4 weeks. Steroids may then be stopped or gradually tapered.[214,233] In frequently relapsing disease, daily prednisone until there is remission for 3 days, followed by alternate-day prednisone at the lowest dose to maintain remission for at least 3 months, is suggested. During episodes of infection, prophylactic daily prednisone administration is suggested for children prone to relapses.[214]

Intravenous loop diuretics (e.g., furosemide 3 to 6 mg/kg/day), if necessary combined with thiazides to maximize natriuresis, are usually highly efficient in mobilizing edema and effusions. In patients with anasarca and signs of intravascular volume depletion, 20% albumin at 1 to 2 g/kg/day can be infused. However, this is controversial because albumin has a short plasma half-life but a strong transient oncotic action, which puts the child at risk of pulmonary edema if administered rapidly.[164]

Antihypertensive therapy should be administered to children with persistent hypertension. In some patients, the hypertension will respond to diuretics. ACE inhibitors or angiotensin II receptor blockers may also help reduce proteinuria but should be used cautiously in the presence of compromised kidney function or volume depletion. Calcium channel blockers and β-blockers may also be used as first-line agents.[226]

Second-Line Therapies in Steroid-Sensitive Nephrotic Syndrome. About 80% to 90% of children with steroid-sensitive NS (SSNS) develop relapses. About 50% become frequent relapsers and are at risk of adverse effects of glucocorticoid therapy. Alternative immunosuppressive agents are successfully used to prolong periods of remission in these children. However, these agents have significant potential adverse effects.

Currently, there is no consensus as to the most appropriate second-line agent for children.[236] Eight-week courses of cyclophosphamide or chlorambucil as well as maintenance cyclosporine and levamisole therapy reduce the risk of relapse in children with relapsing SSNS compared with corticosteroids alone. More recently, mycophenolate mofetil and rituximab have been applied successfully.[236]

Alkylating agents offer the benefit of sustained remission, albeit at a substantial risk of side effects. Cyclophosphamide and chlorambucil are equally efficacious.[236] Recommended dosing for cyclophosphamide is 2 mg/kg/day orally for 8 to 12 weeks (maximum cumulative dose, 168 mg/kg), and for chlorambucil it is 0.1 to 0.2 mg/kg/day for 8 weeks (limited to 11.2 mg/kg total dose).[214] Cyclophosphamide induced remission for at least 2 years in 70% of children with frequently relapsing NS (FRNS); however, it induced remission in fewer than 30% of children with SDNS. Hence, alkylating agents are recommended only for FRNS.[214] Patients should be monitored for leukopenia. After achieving remission, patients must also maintain adequate hydration and take cyclophosphamide in the morning to limit the risk of hemorrhagic cystitis.[214] The main long-term limitations of alkylating agents, however, are gonadal toxicity and carcinogenicity.[237] Irreversible azoospermia has been reported to occur with high incidence when the cumulative cyclophosphamide dose exceeds 200 to 250 mg/kg. In addition, long-term follow-up studies have suggested a potential increased risk of malignancy in patients exposed to alkylating agents during childhood.[237] Hence, second courses of alkylating agents are not suggested; alternatives to these agents are increasingly being used as second-line treatment of relapsing steroid-sensitive NS.

The calcineurin inhibitor agents cyclosporin A (CsA) and tacrolimus are now commonly considered as first-choice steroid-sparing agents in children. Complete remission is achieved by calcineurin inhibitor therapy in the vast majority of patients with steroid-sensitive disease.[214,226,236] However, maintenance therapy is required since NS tends to recur when treatment is discontinued. Relapses may also occur during extended treatment. Steroids can be discontinued in many but not all patients.[214] Kidney biopsy should be performed in children with decreasing GFR on calcineurin inhibitor therapy to rule out nephrotoxicity.[214]

Cyclosporine is usually started at 4 to 5 mg/kg/day, with recommended trough levels of 50 to 100 ng/mL or, preferably, C2 levels of 300 to 400 ng/mL.[238] Adjusted dosing of cyclosporine according to blood levels is more effective in maintaining remission than fixed-dose administration.[239] Tacrolimus is typically administered at 0.1 to 0.2 mg/kg/day, with trough levels adjusted to 3 to 8 ng/mL.[240]

Adverse effects are significant, with 4% to 13% of cyclosporine-treated children developing hypertension, 6% to 10% experiencing reduced renal function, 28% to 33% showing gum hypertrophy, and 35% to 70% developing hypertrichosis.[214,226,233,236] Since at least the cosmetic side effects occur much less frequently with tacrolimus and therapeutic efficacy is at least equivalent,[241] this drug is increasingly favored over cyclosporine in the treatment of SDNS and FRNS.[214]

Mycophenolate mofetil (MMF), an inhibitor of the de novo purine pathway with inhibitory effects on T and B lymphocyte proliferation, is increasingly being used as a steroid-sparing agent in children with FRNS or SDNS. Three prospective studies involving 76 children treated for 6 to 12 months reported a reduction in relapse rate by 50% to 75% during treatment. Prednisone dosage could be reduced in many patients and the drug discontinued in about 50% of cases.[242-244] Treatment at a dose of of 1200 mg/m^2/day for at least 12 months is recommended, as most children will relapse when MMF is stopped.[214] Trough levels of mycophenolic acid below 2.5 µg/mL were associated with a greater risk of relapse.[244] A recent randomized crossover trial comparing 1-year treatment periods with MMF or CsA in 60 children with frequently relapsing SSNS showed that MMF is less effective than cyclosporine in maintaining remission.[245] The study confirmed that relapse risk is inversely correlated to mycophenolate blood levels, indicating that therapeutic drug monitoring might improve the efficacy of MMF therapy in SSNS. Furthermore, the GFR was maintained with MMF while it decreased during CNI therapy. Another comparative trial showed MMF to be less efficacious than cyclosporine in maintaining remission following rituximab therapy in children with SDNS.[246]

The main adverse effects of MMF, gastrointestinal and hematologic alterations, have so far not limited its use in children with steroid-sensitive NS.

Levamisole is a repurposed anthelmintic agent with mild immunosuppressive activity. Administered at 2.5 mg/kg on alternate days for at least 12 months, it is an inexpensive, steroid-sparing, therapeutic alternative virtually devoid of side effects.[214] In an early randomized clinical trial, levamisole reduced relapse risk by 57%.[247] Levamisole and MMF were recently compared head to head in children with frequently relapsing or SDNS. While both drugs efficiently reduced relapse rates, levamisole was less efficacious than MMF, with 16% versus 38% of children in persistent remission after 12 months of treatment.[248]

Rituximab, a chimeric anti-CD20 antibody, is highly effective in inducing and maintaining remission in steroid-sensitive NS.[249-254] The drug causes complete depletion of circulating B lymphocytes and may thereby modulate regulatory T lymphocyte activity.[255] It has been speculated that the drug might act also directly on podocytes by stabilizing the cytoskeleton and preventing apoptosis.[256]

Rituximab is infused at a dose of 375 mg/m^2. Remission rates tend to be higher with two to four once-weekly doses (40% to 60% at 11 to 29 months) as compared to single dosing (25% to 40% at 12 to 17 months).[252,257-259]

A recent RCT of 48 patients with FRNS or SDNS showed significantly longer remission following rituximab than placebo at 1-year follow-up (267 vs. 101 days). Side effects were generally mild, and the frequency of serious adverse events did not differ between groups.[260] An excellent long-term safety profile of rituximab has been observed in thousands of adult patients treated for rheumatologic diseases over the past decade.[261] Although rituximab has little to no effect on overall infection rates, potentially increased susceptibility to *Pneumocystis* infections mandates cotrimoxazole prophylaxis.[262] Also, hepatitis B reactivation may occur, and a few cases of progressive multifocal leukoencephalopathy, a John Cunningham virus (JCV)–induced lethal condition, have been observed mainly in patients who received rituximab as part of chemotherapy, stem cell transplantation, or combined immunosuppressive protocols.[263] It is currently recommended to consider rituximab for children with relapses despite conventional steroid-sparing therapy and for patients with calcineurin inhibitor nephrotoxicity.[214] Further study is needed to explore the benefit-risk ratio of rituximab relative to other steroid-sparing therapies in SSNS.[260]

Treatment of Steroid-Resistant Nephrotic Syndrome. In children who fail to respond to standard oral glucocorticoids and intravenous methylprednisolone pulses, calcineurin inhibitors, MMF, and ACE inhibitors, administered alone or in combination, are principal therapeutic options. Cyclophosphamide is not effective in SRNS and therefore should not be used when steroid resistance has been diagnosed.[213,264-266]

Calcineurin Inhibitors. In a case series of 65 children with primary nonresponse to steroids published by the French Pediatric Nephrology Society in 1994, complete remission of proteinuria was achieved by cyclosporin A therapy in 46% of children with MCG and 30% with FSGS.[267] Subsequent RCTs confirmed that cyclosporine was significantly superior to placebo, no treatment, or intravenous cyclophosphamide in inducing remission.[212,265,266,268,269] Most previous studies had not taken into account the information that patients with SRNS who have a genetic origin to their disease are unlikely to respond to any immunosuppressive therapy.[270] A retrospective analysis of children with nongenetic FSGS observed complete remission in 84% of children receiving intravenous methylprednisolone, cyclosporine, and oral prednisone and in 64% of children treated with cyclosporine and oral prednisone alone.[270] In contrast, none of 20 children with genetic forms of SRNS experienced remission by immunosuppressive drug protocols.

Tacrolimus appears to be at least as effective as cyclosporine in inducing remission in SRNS, with 86% complete or partial remission rates for tacrolimus versus 80% for cyclosporine reported in a RCT.[271] Among patients who experienced relapses while receiving treatment, relapses were steroid-sensitive in a significantly higher fraction of the tacrolimus-treated patients.

Current guidelines recommend using a calcineurin inhibitor (CNI) as first-line therapy for children with SRNS.[213] A minimum of 6 months of treatment combined with low-dose glucocorticoid therapy is suggested to determine efficacy. If complete or partial remission is achieved by 6 months, continuation of therapy for at least 6 months more is recommended.[213]

Mycophenolate Mofetil. There has been limited treatment experience with MMF in children with SRNS. Observational studies involving a total of 42 children with SRNS who were treated for a minimum of 6 months with MMF suggested complete remission in 23% to 62%, partial remission rate in 25% to 37%, and no remission in 8% to 40%.[272,273] An RCT in 138 young patients with primary SRNS and FSGS found complete or partial remission in 46% of patients receiving cyclosporine and in 33% of patients treated with a combination of high-dose dexamethasone and MMF.[274] Hence, the role of MMF as a monotherapy or add-on therapy in SRNS is currently unclear.

Renin Angiotensin Aldosterone System Antagonists. ACE inhibitors and angiotensin II receptor blockers attenuate protein excretion by about 50% in children with proteinuric kidney disorders.[275-277] In children with moderate, mainly obesity-related proteinuria, Chandar and colleagues have demonstrated that long-term treatment with angiotensin II receptor blockers efficiently reduces proteinuria, even when administered as the sole treatment.[278] Angiotensin inhibition might yield a long-term nephroprotective effect in SRNS,[279] although evidence for such an effect from controlled trials is lacking. Small pediatric studies have supported an additional benefit of dual blockage of the RAAS in the reduction of proteinuria, with few side effects.[278,280,281] However, larger studies are necessary before dual blockage can be recommended for children, particularly in view of the negative effect of combination therapy on renal outcome, as highlighted in the Renal Outcomes with Telmisartan, Ramipril, or Both, in People at High Vascular Risk (ONTARGET) study in adults.[282]

Rituximab. There are limited data with mixed results regarding the efficacy of rituximab therapy in children with difficult to treat SRNS.[251] A recent RCT evaluating the efficacy and safety of add-on rituximab in 31 children with steroid- and CNI-resistant NS did not show a clear benefit.[283] On the contrary, the four largest case series evaluating the efficacy of rituximab, including a total of 87 patients with steroid- and CNI-resistant NS, revealed an overall remission rate of 46%, confirming previous reports of rituximab efficacy, at least in a fraction of patients with multidrug-resistant disease who are at high risk of rapid progression to ESKD.[263,284] Remission usually occurred within 4 to 6 weeks from completion of therapy and was sustained for 6 to 24 months. In the patients who achieved remission, immunosuppressive treatment could be tapered or discontinued.[250,253,285,286]

Plasma exchange is an effective and established therapy for most cases of posttransplantation disease recurrence.[287-289] Given its obvious efficacy in treating posttransplantation proteinuria recurrence,[289] it is remarkable that plasma exchange is rarely tried in patients with multidrug-resistant FSGS who are progressing toward ESKD. The few case reports and small series available to date suggest some efficacy of plasma exchange or immunoadsorption in the treatment of primary FSGS and SRNS,[290] which supports its use as maintenance therapy in selected cases of drug-resistant disease.

NEPHRITIC SYNDROME

Nephritic syndrome is a clinical condition defined by the association of hematuria, proteinuria, and often hypertension and renal failure. There is inflammation on histologic examination of biopsy specimens and an active urine sediment with red cells, often composed of red cell and other cellular casts, and a variable degree of proteinuria. Clinical presentations in childhood mainly include acute nephritic syndrome, sometimes with a rapidly progressive course, recurrent macroscopic hematuria, and chronic glomerulonephritis, although there are considerable numbers of subclinical cases.[291] Clinical presentation, family history, presence of extrarenal symptoms, results of immunologic tests, and renal histologic analysis usually identify the underlying disease. Glomerulonephritis may be isolated to the kidney (primary nephritic syndrome) or may be a component of a systemic disorder (secondary nephritic syndrome). The most common cause of nephritic syndrome in children is acute postinfectious glomerulonephritis.

ACUTE POSTINFECTIOUS GLOMERULONEPHRITIS

Glomerulonephritis caused by an immunologic response of the kidney that occurs after a nonrenal infection, often with group A streptococci and rarely with other strains of streptococci (groups C and G), staphylococci, gram-negative bacilli, mycobacteria, parasites, fungi, and viruses,[291] led to the introduction of the term *postinfectious glomerulonephritis*. This term is generally used interchangeably with *poststreptococcal glomerulonephritis*. Since acute poststreptococcal glomerulonephritis (APSGN), the prototype of postinfectious glomerulonephritis, remains the most common cause of nephritic syndrome in children in some developing countries, where it accounts for 50% to 90% of cases, this chapter focuses particularly on APSGN.[292]

Epidemiology

Although the incidence of APSGN has decreased considerably in Europe, America, and Asia, it continues to be the most common cause of acute nephritis globally.[293,294] The estimated worldwide yearly burden of APSGN is 472,000 cases; approximately 404,000 of those cases occur in children. Most of the burden of APSGN is borne by developing countries. In children from less developed countries, and in minority populations, the median incidence of disease was estimated at 24.3 cases/100,000 person-years.[295] However, the true incidence of APSGN is difficult to determine because subclinical disease is thought to be 1.5 to 19 times more common than symptomatic disease.[291,296] A few studies have examined mortality due to poststreptococcal glomerulonephritis, and these reported low mortality rates (mean, 0.028/100,000 in developing countries).[293]

In the tropics, APSGN is usually a complication of pyoderma, whereas in countries with moderate and cold climates, it typically occurs as a complication of tonsillopharyngitis during winter. Over time, the prevalence of pyoderma-associated APSGN has decreased markedly.[296]

Certain serotypes are associated with postinfectious glomerulonephritis following pyoderma, whereas others are associated with postinfectious glomerulonephritis following pharyngitis. The male/female ratio is up to 2:1.[291,297] The disease is most common in children aged 3 to 12 years, although it has been reported in infants as well.[298]

Pathogenesis

Several mechanisms have been proposed for the immunologic glomerular injury induced by group A streptococcal infection,[299] such as the following: deposition of circulating immune complexes with streptococcal antigenic components; in situ immune complex formation within the GBM; in situ formation of glomerular immune complexes that cross-react with glomerular components (molecular mimicry); and alteration of a normal renal antigen that elicits autoimmune reactivity. The available evidence suggests that the major pathogenetic mechanism is in situ immune complex formation due to deposition of streptococcal nephritogenic antigens within the glomerulus.[299]

Streptococcal glyceraldehyde phosphate dehydrogenase (nephritis-associated plasmin receptor)[298,300] and streptococcal cationic proteinase exotoxin B (nephritis strain–associated protein) have been proposed as putative antigens.[298-300] Antibodies to streptococcal glyceraldehyde phosphate dehydrogenase and streptococcal proteinase exotoxin B are found specifically in patients with APSGN and persist for at least 10 years and 1 year, respectively, after the acute attack, which indicates long-lasting immunity.[301] Streptococcal proteinase exotoxin B has also been found in the glomeruli of these patients, co-localized with complement deposition and within the subepithelial electron-dense deposits.[302,303]

Both antigens activate the alternative complement pathway, leading to low plasma C3 levels.[298,300] When deposited in glomeruli, they can interact with plasmin or plasminogen, which leads to activation of latent metalloproteinases or collagenases, with subsequent enzymatic degradation of the GBM and loss of its negative charge.[298] Immune complexes can then pass through the damaged GBM and accumulate as humps in the subepithelial space.[298,300] Damage to the GBM also causes podocyte foot process effacement and proteinuria.

Although local plasmin and complement activation by these nephritogenic antigens has been demonstrated, doubts about their pathogenic role persist. Both antigens can also be found in strains of group A streptococci that rarely cause glomerulonephritis.[304] Therefore, individual susceptibility, possibly determined by the genetic disposition of the host, might exert a major influence on the pathogenicity of the precipitating organism.[303]

Clinical Features

The clinical presentation varies from asymptomatic microscopic hematuria to full-blown acute nephritic syndrome.[291,297] There is usually a history of a group A streptococcal skin or throat infection[297,305] and edema after a latent period of a group A streptococcal infection, followed by smoky and scant urine and increasing blood pressure. Anuria and nephrotic-range proteinuria are sometimes observed. Generalized edema, caused by sodium and water retention, is present in about two thirds of patients. Severe fluid overload may lead to pulmonary edema. Gross hematuria is present in about 30% to 50% of cases. Hypertension is present in 50% to 90% and is primarily caused by fluid retention.[306,307]

APSGN is associated with a variable decline in GFR detected by a rise in the serum creatinine concentration. The severity of renal insufficiency is proportional to the degree of proliferation and crescent formation.[308,309] Although uncommon, rapid progression to oligoanuric acute renal failure may occur and requires prompt management.

Diagnosis

APSGN is usually diagnosed based on clinical findings of acute nephritis and demonstration of a recent group A streptococcal infection. Documentation of a recent streptococcal infection includes a positive finding on culture of throat or skin specimens (seen only in 25% of patients) or positive results on serologic tests (e.g., antistreptolysin A titer or the streptozyme test, which measures five different streptococcal antibodies). Positive streptococcal serologic test results are more sensitive (94.6%) than a history of recent infection (75.7%) or positive culture results (24.3%) in supporting the diagnosis.[305]

The combination of a low C3 level and normal or only slightly decreased C4 level is found in 90% of patients and indicates activation of the alternative complement pathway. In contrast, lupus nephritis is associated with activation of the classical pathway, with reductions in levels of C3 and C4. C3 levels return to normal within 4 to 8 weeks after presentation.[307]

Pathology. Renal biopsy is not routinely performed to confirm the diagnosis of APSGN since the clinical history is usually highly suggestive and resolution typically begins within 1 week of presentation. Indications for biopsy are hypocomplementemia persisting beyond 6 weeks, recurrent episodes of hematuria, and a progressive increase in the serum creatinine concentration.

Light microscopic examination of biopsy specimens shows diffuse proliferative glomerulonephritis, with prominent endocapillary proliferation and numerous neutrophils. Trichrome stain may show small subepithelial hump-shaped deposits. Crescent formation is uncommon and is associated with a poor prognosis.[308,309]

Immunofluorescence analysis commonly reveals granular deposition of complement C3, often with IgG and occasionally with IgM; IgA deposition is rare. So-called full house immunostaining (positive staining for IgG, IgA, IgM, C3, C4, and C1q) resembling the picture of lupus nephritis is frequently reported. Several histologic patterns of immunofluorescence, including mesangial, capillary wall (garland), and diffuse (starry sky) patterns, have been described. The garland pattern is more commonly associated with proteinuria and a poor prognosis.[310] The starry sky pattern is seen in crescentic forms.[311,312]

The dome-shaped, subepithelial, electron-dense deposits or humps are characteristic electron microscopic lesions. They correspond to the deposits of IgG and C3 found on immunofluorescence studies.[313,314]

Differential Diagnosis

In general, although the diagnosis of acute glomerulonephritis is straightforward, identification of the cause often is a challenge. If there is progressive disease beyond 2 weeks, hematuria or hypertension that persists beyond 4 or 6 weeks, and absence of a documented preceding group A streptococcal infection, MPGN, IgA nephropathy, glomerulonephritides, and secondary vasculitic disorders such as systemic lupus erythematosus and Henoch-Schönlein purpura need to be considered. Increased serum antistreptolysin A titers may result from previous infections unrelated to the current disorder. The differential diagnosis of a low serum C3 level includes systemic lupus erythematosus and MPGN.

Treatment

There is no specific therapy for APSGN. Management is supportive and focuses on treating the clinical manifestations of the disease, particularly complications due to volume overload. These include hypertension and, less commonly, pulmonary edema. General measures include sodium and water restriction and administration of loop diuretics. Intravenous furosemide is given at an initial dosage of 1 to 4 mg/kg/day. Control of hypertension is essential to reduce morbidity and may require the use of calcium channel blockers in addition to loop diuretics.[307,313] Although a recent systematic review has shown that better control of blood pressure is achieved with ACE inhibitors than with other antihypertensive drugs or diuretics, RAAS antagonists should be used with caution in APSGN due to the risks of acute kidney injury (AKI) and hyperkalemia.[315] Potassium exchange resin and sodium polystyrene sulfonate can be used to treat hyperkalemia. Spontaneous diuresis typically begins within 1 week, and the serum creatinine level normalizes within 3 to 4 weeks. Occasionally, acute renal failure, severe fluid retention unresponsive to diuretics, and intractable hyperkalemia necessitate hemodialysis or continuous venovenous hemofiltration. Infrequently, at presentation, patients have hypertensive encephalopathy due to severe hypertension, which requires emergency treatment.[307,313] Reversible posterior leukoencephalopathy syndrome, characterized by hyperintense signals in the parietooccipital regions on T2-weighted MRI scans, has also been observed in patients with APSGN; these patients may have decreased visual acuity, focal neurologic signs, and confusion.[316]

The urinary abnormalities disappear at differing rates. Hematuria usually resolves within 3 to 6 months. Proteinuria also falls during recovery, but at a much slower rate. A mild increase in protein excretion is still present in 15% of patients at 3 years and in 2% at 7 to 10 years.[317]

Patients with evidence of persistent group A streptococcal infection should receive a course of antibiotic therapy. Although there is no evidence from randomized studies that aggressive immunosuppressive therapy has any beneficial short- or long-term effect in patients with rapidly progressive crescentic disease,[315,318] patients with more than 30% crescents on renal biopsy specimens are commonly treated with methylprednisolone pulses and/or plasmapheresis.[309,310]

Prognosis

APSGN usually has a benign clinical course, with full recovery of renal function and a good long-term prognosis,[301,312,313,317] even in patients who have acute renal failure at presentation and crescentic glomerulonephritis on the initial renal biopsy specimen.[296,318] A review of three case series of 229 children with APSGN found that approximately 20% had abnormal urinalysis results (proteinuria and/or hematuria), but almost all (92% to 99%) had normal or only modestly reduced renal function 5 to 18 years after presentation.[294] NS or an elevated creatinine concentration at presentation, crescentic glomerulonephritis, glomerulosclerosis, and a garland immunofluorescence pattern are associated with a less favorable prognosis.[308,309,319]

A recent study in Aboriginal Australians has shown that poststreptococcal glomerulonephritis due to streptococcal A skin infections (often related to scabies) during childhood is a risk factor for albuminuria and CKD in later life in this population, which is at high general risk for CKD.[320]

TUBULAR DISORDERS

See also Chapter 45.

BARTTER-LIKE SYNDROMES

For many years, the term *Bartter's syndrome* was applied inconsistently for various salt-losing tubulopathies. More recently, the elucidation of the molecular causes and mechanisms of individual tubulopathies has allowed unambiguous classification of Bartter-like syndromes according to the underlying genetic defect and replacement of the historical typology by a pharmacologic classification consisting of three major subgroups of inherited salt-losing tubulopathies (Table 74.3)[321]:

1. Thiazide-like distal convoluted tubule (DCT) disorders, DC1, DC2, and DC3 (traditionally referred to as Gitelman's syndrome [GS]) and classical (or type III) Bartter's syndrome caused by mutations in the sodium chloride cotransporter (NCCT), basolateral chloride channel (ClC-Kb, encoded by the *CLCNKB* gene), or Kir 4.1
2. More severe polyuric and furosemide-like loop disorders, types L1 and L2 (traditionally referred to as antenatal Bartter's syndrome/HPS [hyperprostaglandin E syndrome] or Bartter's syndrome types I and II) caused by mutations in the type 2 sodium-potassium chloride cotransporter (NKCC2, encoded by the *SLC12A1* gene), or the renal outer medullary potassium channel (ROMK, encoded by the *KCNJ1* gene)
3. Combination of both tubular disorders, types L-DC1 and L-DC2 (traditionally referred to as antenatal Bartter's syndrome/HPS with sensorineural deafness [BSND], or Bartter's syndrome type IV), the most severe conditions, caused by mutations in the ClC-Ka and ClC-Kb chloride channels or their β-subunit barttin (encoded by the *BSND* gene)[321]

Bartter's and Gitelman's syndromes are autosomal recessive disorders characterized by hypokalemia, hypochloremic metabolic alkalosis, hyperreninemia, hyperplasia of the juxtaglomerular apparatus, hyperaldosteronism and, in some patients, hypomagnesemia.[322,323] The estimated prevalence is approximately 1 in 40,000 for Gitelman's syndrome and 1 pmp for Bartter's syndrome.[324]

Bartter's syndrome generally presents early in life and is often but not always associated with growth and mild mental retardation. Polyuria, polydipsia, and decreased

Table 74.3 New Terminology and Pharmacologic Classification of Salt-Losing Tubulopathies (Bartter-Like Syndromes)

Type of Disorder (Gene Product Affected)	Affected Tubular Segment	Pharmacotype	Polyhydramnios	Key Features of Clinical Presentation
Loop Disorders				
L1 type (NKCC2)	TAL	Furosemide type	+++	Polyuria, hypercalciuria, NC
L2 type (ROMK)	TAL/CCDb	Furosemide-amiloride type	+++	Polyuria, hypercalciuria, NC, transient hyperkalemia
DCT Disorders				
DC1 type (NCCT)	DCT	Thiazide type	−	Hypomagnesemia, hypocalciuria, growth retardation
DC2 type (ClC-Kb)	DCT/TALb	Thiazide-furosemide type	+	Hypochloremia, mild hypomagnesemia, FTT in infancy
DC3 type (Kir 4.1)	DCT	Thiazide type	−	Hypomagnesemia, hypocalciuria, EAST sydrome
Combined Disorders				
L-DC1 type (ClC-Ka + b)	TAL + DCT	Furosemide-thiazide type	+++	Polyuria, hypochloremia, mild hypomagnesemia, SND, CRF
L-DC2 type (barttin)	TAL + DCT	Furosemide-thiazide type	+++	Polyuria, hypochloremia, mild hypomagnesemia, SND, CRF

CRF, Chronic renal failure; DCT, distal convoluted tubule; NC, nephrocalcinosis; SND, sensorineural deafness; TAL, thick ascending limb of the loop of Henle.
From Seyberth HW, Schlingmann KP: Bartter- and Gitelman-like syndromes: salt-losing tubulopathies with loop or DCT defects. Pediatr Nephrol 26:1789-1802, 2011.

concentrating ability are also common.[323,325] Blood pressure is lower than that in the general population due to salt wasting and increased renal release of prostaglandin E_2 and prostacyclin.[326] Urinary calcium excretion is usually increased, and the plasma magnesium level is normal or mildly reduced.[325]

The genetic defects underlying the Bartter's syndrome phenotype involve several ion transport channels in the thick ascending limb of the loop of Henle and distal convoluted tubule. The process of active sodium chloride transport is mediated by the loop diuretic–sensitive NKCC cotransporter that results in sodium chloride entry into the tubular cells and by potassium channels (ROMK) that permit reabsorbed potassium to leak back into the lumen for continued sodium-potassium chloride cotransport. The chloride channels permit the chloride that has entered the cell to exit and be returned to the systemic circulation.[327]

SUBTYPES OF BARTTER'S SYNDROME

The application of genetic testing combined with clinical phenotyping currently allows us to characterize six subtypes of Bartter's syndrome. The presence of early transitory hyperkalemia suggests mutations in *KCNJ1*, whereas the presence of deafness is in most cases associated with *BSND* mutations. However, these signs might be absent at diagnosis, and the genetic classification does not perfectly match the clinical classification. Patients with mutations in the *SLC12A1* gene may become manifest beyond the neonatal period. Most mutations in the *CLCNKB* gene (type III) are responsible for classical Bartter's syndrome but can also lead to a neonatal or antenatal phenotype, as well as to a Gitelman phenotype. Clinical and biochemical criteria will guide genetic diagnostics—deafness indicates *BSND*, a neonatal history of hyperkalemia indicates *KCNJ1*, and severe hypokalemic alkalosis indicates *CLCNKB*. In ambiguous cases, genetic workup will follow the mutation frequency: *KCNJ1* > *SLC12A1* > *CLCNKB* > *BSND*.[328]

Antenatal Neonatal Bartter's and Hyperprostaglandin E Syndromes (Types I and II)

These are the most severe forms of Bartter's syndrome and are associated with maternal polyhydramnios, premature birth, intrauterine and postnatal polyuria complicated by severe dehydration episodes, recurrent vomiting, failure to thrive, and growth retardation. Hypercalciuria and nephrocalcinosis are frequent, and renal function is usually normal, although ESKD may occur. This phenotype is caused by defects in the Na-K-2Cl cotransporter or the luminal potassium channel. Familial hypomagnesemia with nephrocalcinosis can be confused with this form of antenatal BS.[327,329]

Classical Bartter's Syndrome (Type III)

The classical Bartter's syndrome phenotype first manifests in infancy or early childhood, with a variety of clinical features. These range from mild muscle weakness and cramps, chronic fatigue, constipation, and recurrent vomiting to severe polyuria and volume depletion. Nephrocalcinosis is not a constant feature. This form is caused by mutations in the basolateral chloride channel.[327,329] In the Internet-based tubulopathy registry (www.renaltube.com), classical Bartter's syndrome (19%) is the second most common tubulopathy after renal tubular acidosis (23%).[330]

Antenatal Bartter's Syndrome with Deafness (Types IV and VI)

This form is rare and disabling. The product of the affected gene, barttin, regulates the chloride channels ClC-Ka and ClC-Kb; both are also present in the inner ear, explaining the association with deafness.[331] Bartter's syndrome type VI is clinically similar to type IV but is caused by a digenic mutation affecting the genes for ClC-Ka and ClC-Kb.[329]

Hypocalcemia with Bartter's Syndrome (Type V)

This is a very rare form specifically associated with hypoparathyroidism. It is due to gain-of-function mutations in the calcium-sensing receptor (CaSR) located at the parathyroid gland and at the renal tubular basolateral membrane.[332] Clinical features include hypocalcemia, hypercalciuria, hypokalemic metabolic alkalosis, and hypomagnesemia.[333]

GITELMAN'S SYNDROME

Gitelman's syndrome (familial hypokalemia-hypomagnesemia)[334] is a more benign condition than Bartter's syndrome that is often not diagnosed until late childhood or even adulthood.[325] Mutations in the solute carrier family 12, member 3 gene *(SLC12A3)*, which encodes the thiazide-sensitive NaCl cotransporter (NCC), are found in most GS patients. A defect in this transporter can account for the magnesium wasting and often marked decrease in calcium excretion, which is the opposite of the hypercalciuria seen in classical Bartter's syndrome.[325]

Transient periods of muscle weakness and tetany, fatigue of variable degree, and occasional abdominal pain, vomiting, and fever are typical symptoms of Gitelman's syndrome. Paresthesias, especially in the face, also occur frequently. Remarkably, some patients are completely asymptomatic except for the appearance of chondrocalcinosis at adult age that causes swelling, local heat, and tenderness of the affected joints. Polyuria is usually mild or absent. Blood pressure is significantly lower than in the general population. Statural growth is generally normal but can be delayed in Gitelman's syndrome patients with severe hypokalemia and hypomagnesemia.[335] Sudden cardiac arrest has been reported occasionally due to potassium and magnesium depletion leading to ventricular arrhythmias.

The diagnosis is based on clinical symptoms and biochemical abnormalities (hypokalemia, metabolic alkalosis, hypomagnesemia, hypocalciuria) but can be confirmed by genetic testing.

TREATMENT OF BARTTER-LIKE SYNDROMES

The tubular defects in Bartter's or Gitelman's syndrome cannot be corrected. Treatment, which must be lifelong, is limited to substituting electrolytes and minimizing the effects of the secondary increases in prostaglandin and aldosterone production.

Most patients require oral potassium (1 to 3 mmol/kg/day) and magnesium supplementation. However, the restoration of normal magnesium and potassium balance is often difficult to achieve due to gastrointestinal side effects of oral electrolyte supplements (nausea, vomiting, diarrhea, constipation).

The combination of a nonsteroidal antiinflammatory drug (NSAID; indomethacin, 2 to 4 mg/kg/day) in case of elevated prostaglandin excretion with a potassium-sparing diuretic (e.g., spironolactone or amiloride, often required in higher than usual daily doses of 10 to 15 mg/kg and 0.1 to 0.3 mg/kg, respectively, to maximize blockade of distal potassium secretion) can raise the plasma potassium concentration toward normal, largely reverse metabolic alkalosis, and partially correct hypomagnesemia. ACE inhibitors may also be used to block the secondary activation of the RAAS.[329] Rehydration and/or indomethacin lead to improved statural growth (Figure 74.9).[328] Long-term studies in children treated with indomethacin and potassium supplementation have demonstrated an adequate metabolic and electrolyte balance and recovered growth velocity. In the long term, mild impairment of kidney function develops in approximately 25% of patients. Finally, a large subset of patients develops gallbladder stones.[336]

In general, the long-term prognosis of Gitelman's syndrome is excellent. Most asymptomatic patients with Gitelman's syndrome remain untreated. Lifelong supplementation of magnesium (magnesium oxide and magnesium sulfate) and a high-sodium and high-potassium diet are recommended. Since prostaglandin excretion is normal,[337] prostaglandin synthesis inhibitors are of little benefit in Gitelman's syndrome.[325]

RENAL TUBULAR ACIDOSIS

Renal tubular acidosis (RTA) is a disease state characterized by metabolic acidosis with a normal anion gap. There are inherited and acquired forms (Table 74.4). The three main forms of RTA are proximal (type 2) RTA, distal (type 1) RTA, and hyperkalemic (type 4) RTA. Mixed lesions (those with elements of types 1 and 2 RTA) are designated as type 3 RTA by some authors.[338]

Distal RTA is due to impaired distal acid secretion by α-intercalated cells that results in an inability to excrete the daily acid load. Patients with distal RTA cannot acidify their urine and thus have a urine pH of more than 5.5, despite metabolic acidosis. Acidosis can be provoked by giving oral ammonium chloride (100 mg/kg) or furosemide (40 mg) plus fludrocortisone (1 mg) and monitoring the urine pH over 8 hours or 4 hours, respectively. In distal RTA, the urine pH should not fall to less than 5.3.[339]

Patients with distal RTA may develop hypokalemia, hypercalciuria, hypocitraturia, nephrolithiasis, and nephrocalcinosis. Failure to thrive caused by chronic metabolic acidosis is the most common presenting complaint. Bone demineralization and rickets are also common. Mutations in genes that encode the chloride-bicarbonate exchanger AE1 (*SLC4A1* gene) or subunits of the H+–adenosine triphosphatase pump (*ATP6V1B1* and *ATP6V0A4* genes) cause dominant and recessive forms of distal RTA.[340] The clinical manifestations vary depending on the underlying cause. The autosomal dominant form is relatively mild, and many patients do not show manifestations of the disease until adulthood. Patients typically have mild or no acidosis, mild to moderate hypokalemia, and, rarely, bone disease or poor growth.[341] Autosomal recessive distal RTA is more severe, presents in infancy, and is often associated with deafness.[342] Acquired distal RTA may occur at any age due to renal tubular injury (see Table 74.4).

Proximal RTA is caused by a reduction in proximal bicarbonate reabsorptive capacity, which results in a fall in

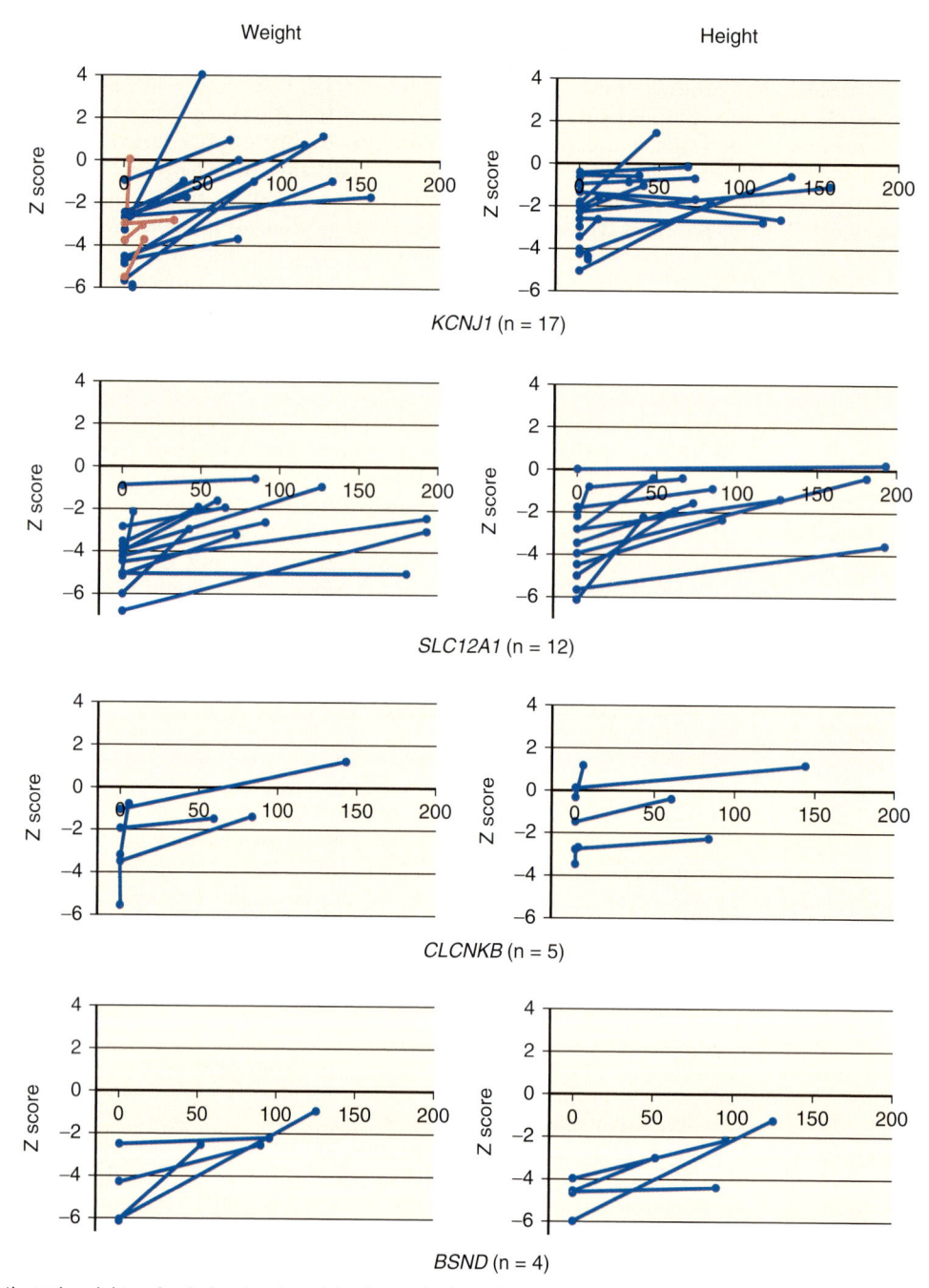

Figure 74.9 Length and weight gain during treatment (water and electrolyte substitution, indomethacin) according to the gene involved in antenatal-neonatal Bartter's syndrome. The x-axis represents observation time in months under indomethacin treatment; the y-axis represents weight or height expressed as a z score normalized to age (normal range, −2 to 2). (From Brochard K, Boyer O, Blanchard A, et al: Phenotype-genotype correlation in antenatal and neonatal variants of Bartter syndrome. *Nephrol Dial Transplant* 24:1455-1464, 2009.)

the plasma bicarbonate level. It is rarely present in isolation. In most patients, proximal RTA is part of Fanconi's syndrome, a generalized dysfunction of the proximal tubule. This leads to glycosuria, aminoaciduria, and excessive urinary losses of phosphate and uric acid. Low serum uric acid levels, glycosuria, and aminoaciduria are helpful diagnostic hints. Clinical findings include growth failure, hypovolemia, osseous abnormalities, and constipation and muscle weakness due to hypokalemia. Systemic acidosis is less severe than in distal RTA. Renal stones and nephrocalcinosis are less common, in part because of increased urinary citrate excretion, except in proximal RTA due to Fanconi's syndrome, in which rickets and osteomalacia occur because of phosphaturia and vitamin D deficiency.[343] The ability to acidify the urine is intact; therefore, untreated patients have a urine pH of less than 5.5. However, bicarbonate therapy increases bicarbonate losses in the urine and the urine pH increases. In patients with proximal RTA, bicarbonate loading to normalize serum bicarbonate concentration results in renal bicarbonate leak measured by fractional bicarbonate excretion, which will be higher than 15%.[344]

Table 74.4 Causes and Laboratory Features of Renal Tubular Acidosis (RTA)

Parameter		Type 1 RTA (Distal)	Type 2 RTA (Proximal)	Type 4 RTA (Hyperkalemic)
Primary defect		Impaired distal acidification	Reduced proximal bicarbonate reabsorption	Decreased aldosterone secretion or effect
Plasma bicarbonate		Variable, may be <10 mEq/L	Usually 12 to 20 mEq/L	>17 mEq/L
Urine pH		>5.3	Variable; >5.3 if above bicarbonate reabsorptive threshold	Usually <5.3
Plasma potassium		Usually reduced but hyperkalemic forms exist; hypokalemia corrects with alkali therapy	Reduced; hypokalemia aggravated by bicarbonaturia induced by alkali therapy	Increased
Response to acid load		No	Yes	
Cause	Primary Genetic	Idiopathic, sporadic AR dRTA with deafness, *ATP6V1B1* AR dRTA without early deafness, *ATP6V0A4* AD dRTA, *SLC4A1* (*AE1*)	Idiopathic, sporadic AR pRTA Cystinosis Tyrosinemia Fructose intolerance Galactosemia Wilson's disease Lowe's syndrome Dent's disease	Primary adrenal insufficiency Congenital adrenal hyperplasia (21-hydroxylase deficiency) Isolated aldosterone synthase deficiency Hyporeninemic hypoaldosteronism Pseudohypoaldosteronism types 1 and 2
	Secondary	Hypercalciuria, nephrocalcinosis (e.g., medullary sponge kidney) Rheumatologic (rheumatoid arthritis, Sjögren's syndrome, systemic lupus erythematosus) Drugs (ifosfamide, amphotericin B, lithium) Renal transplantation Obstructive uropathy Cirrhosis Sickle cell anemia	Drugs (ifosfamide, tenofovir, carbonic anhydrase inhibitors) Heavy metals Vitamin D deficiency Renal transplantation Amyloidosis	Drugs (heparin, angiotensin-converting enzyme inhibitors, nonsteroidal antiinflammatory drugs, cyclosporin A, trimethoprim, pentamidine, amiloride, spironolactone, triamterene) Renal (diabetic nephropathy, obstructive uropathy, tubulointerstitial disease, acute glomerulonephritis via volume expansion) Human immunodeficiency virus infection Aldosterone resistance

Mixed RTA (type 3) is a rare autosomal recessive disorder that has features of types 1 and 2 RTA. It is due to an inherited carbonic anhydrase II deficiency resulting in a syndrome with multiple clinical findings, including mixed RTA, osteopetrosis, cerebral calcification, and mental retardation. Other clinical features include bone fractures (due to increased bone fragility) and growth failure. Excessive facial bone growth leads to facial dysmorphism as well as conductive hearing loss and blindness due to nerve compression.[340,345,346]

In type 4 (hyperkalemic) RTA, the renal excretion of acid and potassium is impaired. This form is due to aldosterone deficiency or an inability of the kidney to respond to aldosterone. It is generally characterized by hyperkalemia and mild acidosis (serum bicarbonate level >17 mEq/L). The manifestations depend on the severity of aldosterone deficiency or insensitivity. In addition to inherited defects (e.g., type 1 pseudohypoaldosteronism), the most common cause of type 4 RTA is the administration of drugs that impair aldosterone release or function (e.g., heparin, NSAIDs, ACE inhibitors or angiotensin II receptor blockers, CNIs, and potassium-sparing diuretics).[344]

The treatment of RTA is empirical and mainly involves oral alkali supplementation, which is best given as potassium citrate or bicarbonate, especially when hypokalemia is present. In distal RTA, 1 to 2 mmol/kg/day of oral alkali is usually sufficient to maintain the plasma bicarbonate concentration above 20 mmol/L. Much larger amounts of oral bicarbonate (up to 10 mmol/kg/day) are necessary in proximal RTA. Correction of hypokalemia is important to prevent muscle weakness. High fluid intake is necessary for patients with distal RTA prone to stone formation. Thiazide diuretics can be used in proximal RTA to increase paracellular bicarbonate reabsorption indirectly.[344] Treatment of type 4 RTA depends on the underlying cause. Drug-induced acidosis is usually readily reversible on discontinuation of the causative agent. If withdrawal is not an option, oral mineralocorticoid administration can be useful.[344]

NEPHROGENIC DIABETES INSIPIDUS

Nephrogenic diabetes insipidus (NDI) refers to a decrease in urinary concentrating ability that results from resistance to the action of antidiuretic hormone (arginine vasopressin [AVP]). In the collecting ducts, AVP binds to its receptor V_2, which leads to the insertion of water channels (aquaporin-2 [AQP2]) in the apical membrane of the principal cells of the collecting tubule, which makes them water-permeable.[347] AQP2 channels are stored in the cytosol. Under the influence of antidiuretic hormone, they are phosphorylated and redistributed to the apical (luminal) membrane; this allows water to be reabsorbed along the tonicity gradient between the tubular fluid and hypertonic medullary interstitium, which results in urine concentration.[348,349] In NDI, mutations in AQP2 and its receptor result in an impaired response to AVP.

NDI can occur in congenital and acquired forms. Congenital forms present in the first weeks to months of life. They can be X-linked recessive due to mutations in V_2 (90%) or autosomal recessive due to mutations in AQP2 (10%).[350] In one kindred, the autosomal dominant form of NDI was mediated by deficient phosphorylation of the AQP2 water channel.[351] Acquired forms mainly result from renal causes (e.g., obstructive uropathy, acute kidney injury, tubulointerstitial nephritis, renal dysplasia, nephronophthisis, cystic kidney disease), use of certain drugs (e.g., lithium, cidofovir, foscarnet, amphotericin B, ifosfamide), and electrolyte disturbances (e.g., hypokalemia, hypercalcemia). Symptoms present much later in this form and are characterized by polyuria and frequency.[352,353]

Congenital NDI typically presents with polyuria, hypernatremic dehydration, fever, irritability, constipation, and failure to thrive. Polyhydramnios is not seen due to solute clearance via the placenta. Breast-fed infants do better than formula-fed ones, possibly because of the osmolar load of breast milk. Symptoms typically improve with increasing age. Free access to water helps self-regulation of plasma osmolality. Polyuria, bed wetting, and mental retardation can be seen in untreated patients.[347,352,353] At 5 years, 20% to 30% of children with X-linked NDI show severe growth retardation.[354]

DIAGNOSIS

A desmopressin (DDAVP) test can be used to discriminate central from nephrogenic diabetes insipidus. DDAVP can be administered via the intranasal (10-20 µg), oral (200 µg/kg), intramuscular (0.4 µg if <10 kg; 2 µg if >10 kg), or intravenous route (0.3 µg/kg). Oral or intravenous administration of DDAVP requires 2 to 4 hours of observation; administration by other routes requires 4 to 6 hours. Urine osmolality should increase to more than 800 mOsm/kg (>500 mOsm/kg in young infants). Persistently low osmolality of less than 200 mOsm/kg is diagnostic of NDI, whereas intermediate values may indicate acquired partial NDI. If intravenous DDAVP is used, systemic vasodilation causing mild hypotension and tachycardia may occur. This response is helpful in discriminating X-linked V_2 receptor defects from autosomal recessive aquaporin defects[353] because V_2 receptors mediate the antidiuretic response as well as peripheral vasodilation.[355] Molecular genetic testing is also available.[350]

TREATMENT

There is no specific therapy for NDI. Early and proper symptomatic treatment is important to prevent hypernatremic complications. High fluid intake (150 mL/kg/day) is necessary for excretion of solute load. Thiazide diuretics (hydrochlorothiazide, 2 mg/kg/day, or bendroflumethiazide 50 to 100 µg/kg/day) inhibit reabsorption of sodium and chloride in the distal convoluted tubule and increase proximal tubular reabsorption of sodium. As a result, less fluid is delivered to the collecting duct and the urine volume decreases. Amiloride (0.1 to 0.3 mg/kg/day) can also be used. Prostaglandin synthesis inhibitors (indomethacin 1 to 3 mg/kg/day) can help decrease urine output. A combination of thiazide and indomethacin, with or without amiloride, is useful during the first years of life.[353]

Several molecular therapies for NDI may become available in the foreseeable future. Mutant V_2 receptor proteins are frequently misfolded, which leads to their trapping in the endoplasmic reticulum and nability to reach the plasma membrane. Vasopressin receptor antagonists (vaptans; e.g., tolvaptan) can act as chaperones, inducing correct folding and transport of the protein to the plasma membrane. Pilot studies have shown a significant decrease in urine output with the use of these antagonists.[356] Other nonpeptide agonists have been identified that can activate mutant V_2 receptors at their intracellular sites.[357] Another experimental concept is to bypass defective vasopressin receptor signaling and promote AQP2 trafficking to the membrane via other intracellular pathways, such as activation of the cyclic adenosine monophosphate (cAMP) or cyclic guanosine monophosphate (cGMP) pathways by phosphodiesterase inhibitors (e.g., sildenafil, rolipram), prostanoid receptor agonists (e.g., butaprost) or calcitonin. Another therapeutic approach under consideration involves the use of statins, which increase expression of AQP2 at the apical membrane.[358]

CYSTINOSIS

Cystinosis is a metabolic disease characterized by an accumulation of cystine in different organs and tissues, leading to potentially severe organ dysfunction. In the kidney, the disease causes a profound global tubulopathy (Fanconi's syndrome), which progresses to a fibrosing tubulointerstitial nephropathy and eventually ESKD. Cystinosis is classified into three forms based on age at presentation and severity of symptoms—infantile (nephropathic), intermediate (juvenile, late onset), and adult (benign, ocular).[359,360]

CAUSE

Nephropathic cystinosis is an autosomal recessive disorder caused by mutations in the *CTNS* gene (17p13.3), which encodes for cystinosin, a lysosomal cystine carrier. The disease is characterized by elevated levels of intracellular cystine. The estimated incidence of the disease is 1 in 100,000 to 200,000 live births.[359] Although cystine accumulation due to altered transmembrane cystine transport is the primary pathogenetic lesion, numerous additional lysosomal functions appear to be impaired in cystinosis. Findings include accumulation of autophagosomes in cystinotic cells and increased plasma chitotriosidase activity, indicating lysosome stress in cystinotic children. The exploration of cellular pathways beyond cystine accumulation is a major challenge for cystinosis research.[361]

CLINICAL FEATURES

Infantile cystinosis is the most common and severe phenotype. Patients are usually asymptomatic at birth and develop normally during the first few months of life. Around 6 months of age, they typically show failure to thrive, vomiting, constipation, polyuria, excessive thirst, dehydration, and sometimes rickets.[360] These symptoms result from Fanconi's syndrome, which is characterized by inappropriate urinary losses of water, amino acids, phosphate, bicarbonate, glucose, sodium, potassium, low-molecular-weight proteins, and other solutes as a consequence of defective renal proximal tubular reabsorption.[359-361] Untreated patients develop CKD during early childhood, progressing to ESKD in the first decade of life. Moreover, the spontaneous course of cystinosis is characterized by numerous extrarenal complications, such as very severe growth failure, hypothyroidism, hypogonadism with delayed puberty, impaired glucose tolerance, diabetes mellitus, dysphagia, distal myopathy, progressive corneal crystal deposition and clouding, anemia related to bone marrow fibrosis, and vascular calcifications.[362,363] The severe growth failure peculiar to infantile cystinosis is multifactorial in origin. It is not only caused by decreased renal function but probably also by direct deposition of cystine crystals in the growth plates. It is further aggravated by malnutrition and electrolyte imbalances that lead to rickets and metabolic acidosis, hypothyroidism, and steroid treatment after transplantation.[363,364]

The intermediate form of cystinosis generally presents around 8 years of age, with manifestations due to renal tubular dysfunction. These patients also have a progressive decline in GFR, resulting in ESKD by 15 years of age. Adult cystinosis is the most benign form. Patients are generally asymptomatic except for photophobia or ocular discomfort due to crystal deposition in the cornea.[359,360]

Diagnostic confirmation is achieved by measuring the cystine concentration in leukocytes, which is more than 2 nmol of cystine/mg of protein in untreated cystinosis (normal level < 0.2 nmol). The presence of corneal crystals is also pathognomonic for cystinosis. Molecular genetic testing is also available.[365]

TREATMENT

Treatment consists of general measures and specific cystine-depleting therapy with cysteamine. High fluid intake, potassium and phosphate supplementation, correction of acidosis by sodium bicarbonate or sodium-potassium citrate solutions, vitamin D therapy, and growth hormone (GH) therapy are recommended.[365,366] When gross polyuria is present, a trial of indomethacin may be undertaken at a dosage of 1 to 2 mg/kg/day. It may be sufficient to provide indomethacin as a single evening dose of 1 to 2 mg/kg/day to reduce polyuria and excessive drinking.

The introduction of oral cysteamine therapy marked the advent of specific pharmacologic therapy for cystinosis. Cysteamine reacts with intralysosomal cystine to form cysteine and mixed disulfide cysteamine-cystine, both of which freely leave the cystinotic lysosome. Oral cysteamine therapy can lower intracellular cystine content by 95%. For children younger than 12 years or weighing less than 50 kg, the recommended maintenance dosage is 1.3 g/m^2/day administered in four equal divided doses. For older patients, the maximal recommended dosage is 2 g/day.[365] Cysteamine therapy should be started as early as possible after diagnosis of the disease. In infants, it is usually administered via nasogastric tube. The leukocyte cystine level should be measured regularly to monitor treatment efficacy, with a goal of less than 1 nmol of cystine/mg of protein.[365]

Recently, an enteric-coated, delayed-release cysteamine formulation for twice-daily administration (cysteamine bitartrate) has become available (Procysbi). It is as effective in lowering the leukocyte cystine level as immediate-release cysteamine.[367,368]

Kidney transplantation successfully restores kidney function. Although the disorder does not affect the kidney allograft, apart from occasional interstitial cystine crystal deposition, the complications of the metabolic defect progress in all other affected tissues.[360]

PROGNOSIS

Untreated children are at risk of life-threatening dehydration and electrolyte imbalance. They progress to ESKD around 10 years of age,[362] exhibit severe growth failure, and develop a plethora of extrarenal disease manifestations during the second and third decades of life, which used to limit life expectancy to less than 30 years. This dismal prognosis has profoundly changed with the advent of cysteamine therapy, which has proven efficacious in delaying renal glomerular deterioration, enhancing growth, preventing hypothyroidism, and lowering muscle cystine content.[363,369,370] Early initiation of cysteamine therapy is the most important predictor of preserved renal function and normal or near-normal growth in children with cystinosis[363,370] (Figure 74.10). The impressive clinical efficacy of oral cysteamine treatment makes early diagnosis and treatment of nephropathic cystinosis imperative. Every effort should be made to identify patients with this disorder in their first year of life. Careful prevention and correction of metabolic and nutritional deficits and treatment of hypothyroidism are further prerequisites for appropriate growth.[364] If cysteamine treatment, adequate nutrition, and electrolyte supplementation do not prevent growth retardation, GH treatment should be started early in the course of the disease because this has been demonstrated to be efficacious and safe in children with nephropathic cystinosis.[366]

UROLITHIASIS AND NEPHROCALCINOSIS IN CHILDREN

If the physiologic mechanisms preventing crystal formation, aggregation, and retention in the urine are overwhelmed by dietary or environmental influences or are affected by an underlying metabolic defect, the consequence is a tendency to form renal stones.[371]

Although kidney stone disease (urolithiasis or nephrolithiasis) affects approximately 3% to 5% of the general population,[372] only 2% to 3% of stone formers are children.[373] Urinary tract calculi account for 1 in 1000 to 7600 hospital admissions of children in the United States. Admission rates have been increasing, possibly due to improved radiographic techniques, increased survival of premature neonates taking medications that lead to nephrocalcinosis, changing dietary habits (e.g., increased protein and sodium intake), and increasing prevalence of obesity.[374-376]

Nephrocalcinosis, which can affect the medulla, cortex, or both, is characterized by deposits of calcium salts in the tubules, tubular epithelium, or interstitial tissue. The most common causes of nephrocalcinosis are furosemide administration, distal RTA, hyperparathyroidism, medullary sponge kidney, hypophosphatemic rickets, sarcoidosis, cortical necrosis, hyperoxaluria, prolonged immobilization, Cushing's syndrome, and hyperuricosuria.

In children, stones from the upper urinary tract are comprised of calcium oxalate in 40% to 60% of cases, calcium phosphate in 15% to 25%, mixed calcium oxalate and phosphate in 10% to 25%, magnesium ammonium phosphate in 17% to 30%, cystine in 6% to 10%, and uric acid in 2% to 10%.[377]

RISK FACTORS FOR STONE FORMATION

In children with nephrolithiasis, an underlying risk factor, such as a urinary metabolic abnormality (e.g., hypercalciuria, hyperphosphaturia, hyperoxaluria, hypocitraturia, hyperuricosuria, cystinuria, low urinary volume, defect in urinary acidification), UTI, and/or a structural renal or urinary tract abnormality, is identified in 75% to 85% of affected children.[377-379]

The cause of metabolic abnormalities and of renal stones is multifactorial and depends on the interplay of environmental, anatomic, and genetic factors. The main risk factors for renal stone formation are summarized in Table 74.5.[380] An increasing role for environmental risk factors such as dietary changes and obesity, as compared with the constant genetic predisposition, has been suggested.[380]

URINARY METABOLIC ABNORMALITIES

Hypercalciuria

Hypercalciuria, which can be diagnosed by measuring 24-hour urine calcium excretion or the calcium/creatinine ratio in a spot urine sample, is the most common metabolic abnormality associated with stone disease in children.[381] Urinary calcium excretion indices are increased in recurrent stone formers, especially when referenced to citrate.[382] The risk of urolithiasis in children with idiopathic hypercalciuria varies between 0% to 16%.[383] Of note, spot urine electrolyte/solute ratios vary inversely with age in children, whereas 24-hour excretion rates normalized to body size are constant across the pediatric age range (Table 74.6).[384-386] Hypercalciuria may be absorptive, renal, or resorptive. The primary abnormality in absorptive hypercalciuria is intestinal hyperabsorption of calcium. The term *renal hypercalciuria* refers to impaired renal tubular reabsorption of calcium. Resorptive hypercalciuria is found in patients with primary hyperparathyroidism.[383] A diagnostic algorithm for children with hypercalciuria is presented in Figure 74.11.[387]

Hyperoxaluria

Hyperoxaluria is detected in 10% to 20% of children with nephrolithiasis.[378] The cutoff values defining hyperoxaluria are given in Table 74.6.[384,385] Idiopathic hyperoxaluria is the most common cause of oxalate stones in children. Increased urinary oxalate excretion is due to increased oxalate production or enhanced gastrointestinal oxalate absorption.

The primary forms of hyperoxaluria are discussed in detail later (see "Primary Hyperoxaluria"). Secondary hyperoxaluria is more common and can be caused by increased intake of oxalate and oxalate precursors such as vitamin C, pyridoxine deficiency, and ingestion of methylene glycol or methoxyflurane, which are metabolized to oxalate.[384] Enteric hyperoxaluria is observed in conditions such as inflammatory bowel disease, extensive bowel resection, pancreatic insufficiency, and biliary disease, in which there is gastrointestinal malabsorption of fatty acids. Excess fatty acids bind calcium in the intestinal lumen, which leads to an increased fraction of free oxalate available for enteric absorption. Intensified treatment of the underlying disorder, if possible, reduction of dietary oxalate and fat, use of dietary calcium supplements, and increased fluid intake are suggested for those with these conditions.[384]

Hypocitraturia

Citrate inhibits precipitation by forming complexes with calcium, increasing the solubility of calcium in the urine,

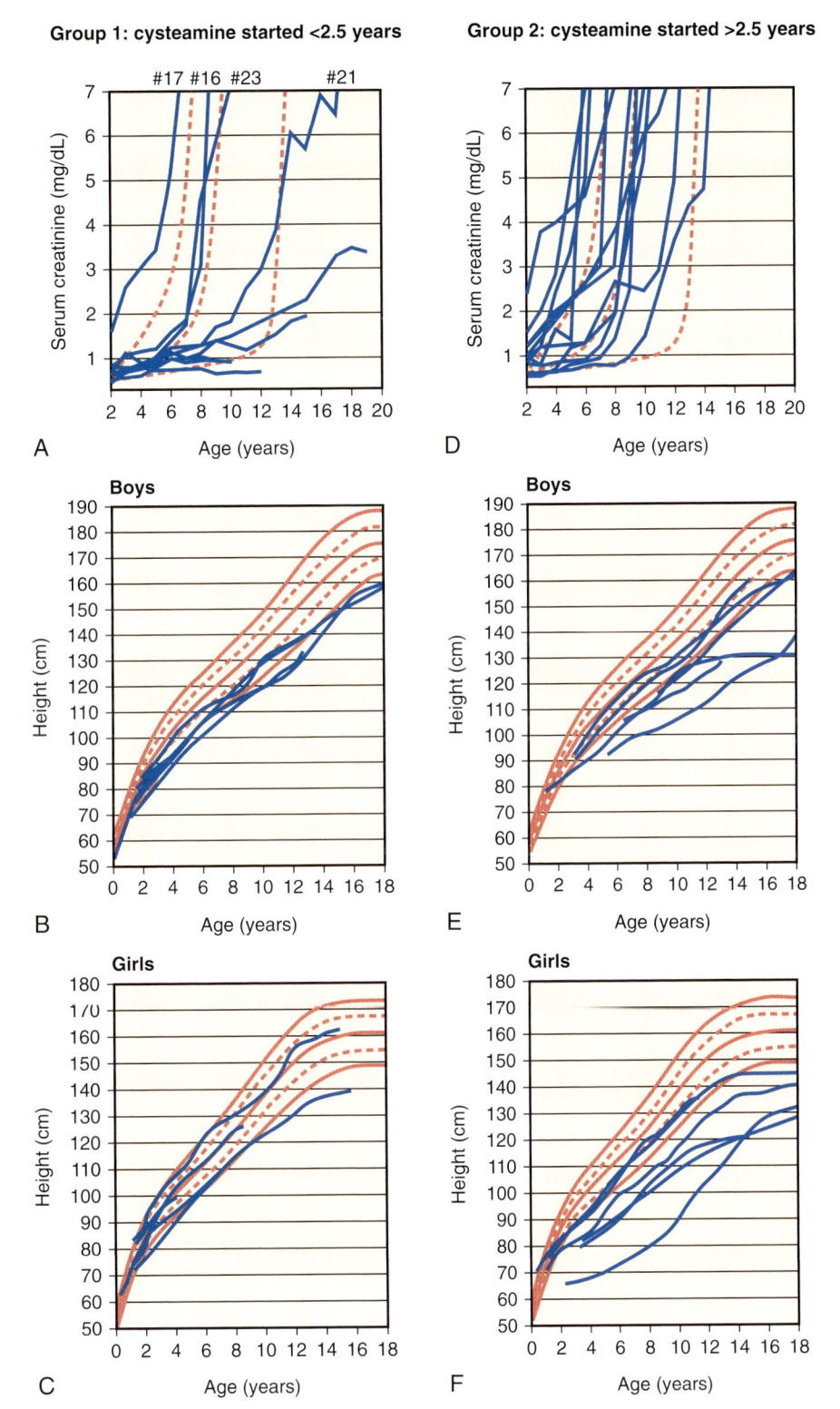

Figure 74.10 **A** and **D,** Evolution of serum creatinine concentration in children with cystinosis treated with cysteamine before or after 2.5 years of age. *Hashed lines* indicate the 3rd, 50th, and 97th percentiles of the reference population. **B, C, E,** and **F,** Growth charts for the same patients. (From Greco M, Brugnara M, Zaffanello M, et al: Long-term outcome of nephropathic cystinosis: a 20-year single-center experience. *Pediatr Nephrol* 25:2459-2467, 2010.)

Table 74.5 Major Risk Factors for Renal Stone Formation in Children

Parameter	Type of Stone	
1. Urinary Constituents, Absorption	**Calcium Stones**	
Solute excess (calcium, oxalate, uric acid, cystine)	Hypercalciuria	Horseshoe kidney
Dysregulation of urinary pH	Hyperparathyroidism	Hyperoxaluria (calcium oxalate)
Dehydration	Distal renal tubular acidosis, type 1 (calcium phosphate)	Primary hyperoxaluria types 1 and 2
Low urine volume	Sarcoidosis	Secondary hyperoxaluria (increased intake or enhanced absorption of oxalate)
Decrease in stone inhibitors (e.g., citrate, magnesium, pyrophosphate, Tamm-Horsfall protein, nephrocalcin, osteopontin/uropontin, bikunin, urinary trefoil factor 1, prothrombin fragment 1)	Furosemide administration	Enteric hyperoxaluria
Dysregulation of urinary pH	Vitamin D excess	Fat malabsorption
	Immobilization	Chronic bowel disease
	Corticosteroid administration	Cystic fibrosis
	Cushing's disease	Bowel resection
	Medullary sponge kidney	Hyperuricosuria
	Autosomal dominant polycystic kidney disease	Hypocitraturia
2. Diet, Solute Production	**Uric Acid Stones**	
High animal protein diet	Hyperuricosuria	
High-fructose diet	Lesch-Nyhan syndrome	
Excess production of uric acid	Myeloproliferative disorders	
	After chemotherapy	
	Hemolysis	
	Glycogen storage disease	
3. Anatomic Considerations	**Struvite Stones (magnesium ammonium phosphate)**	
Anomalies of the urinary tract leading to urinary tract infection	Urinary tract infection (urea-spitting microorganisms)	
	Urinary stasis (e.g., neurogenic bladder, ileal loops, megaureter, augmentation of the bladder)	
4. Enzymatic Defects	Cystine stones—cystinuria	
	Oxalate stones—primary hyperoxaluria	

Adapted from Sayer JA: Renal stone disease. Nephron Physiol 118:35-44, 2011.

and inhibiting the aggregation of calcium phosphate and oxalate crystals. Hypocitraturia has been reported in 10% of children with renal calculi[388] and may be more important than hypercalciuria in stone formation in certain regions of the world (e.g., Turkey).[389] Proposed causes include the ingestion of a high-protein diet and polygenetic factors.

Hyperuricosuria

Hyperuricosuria is detected in 2% to 8% of children with nephrolithiasis. Uric acid excretion is highest in infants and remains high in children until adolescence. In infants, the normal urinary uric acid excretion is so high that crystals may precipitate in the diaper and be misidentified as blood. Age-specific reference values are given in Table 74.6. Increased urinary excretion of uric acid can result from enhanced renal excretion or increased production of uric acid.

In childhood, pure uric acid stones are usually caused by overproduction of uric acid due to tumor lysis syndrome, lymphoproliferative disorders, or rare genetic disorders (e.g., Lesch-Nyhan syndrome, glycogen storage diseases). High dietary intake of purines and hemolysis have also been associated with uric acid nephrolithiasis in children.[384,390]

INFECTIOUS AND ANATOMIC RISK FACTORS

UTIs are associated with nephrolithiasis in 20% to 25% of children. Infection with urea-splitting organisms (most often *Proteus* spp.) leads to urinary alkalinization and excessive production of ammonia, which can result in the precipitation of magnesium ammonium phosphate (struvite) and calcium phosphate. The calculi often have a staghorn configuration, filling the calyces. These stones are often seen in children with neuropathic bladder dysfunction, particularly those who have undergone an ileal conduit procedure.[384,390] Also, obstructive uropathies leading to local urine stasis (e.g., severe pelvicoureteric junction obstruction) can predispose to stone formation.

PRESENTATION AND TREATMENT OF KIDNEY STONE DISEASE

CLINICAL FEATURES

Younger children typically have hematuria or UTI at presentation. Adolescents are more likely to develop ureteric stones and usually have renal colic[391] if the calculus is in the renal pelvis, calyx, or ureter, causing acute obstruction. If

Table 74.6 Pediatric Normal Values for Solute Urinary Excretion Rates

Solute	Solute/Cr Ratio	Solute/Cr Ratio	24-hour Urinary Excretion
Calcium	mol/mol	g/g	0.1 mmol/kg (4 mg/kg)
<1 yr	<2.2	<0.8	
1-3 yr	<2.5	<0.5	
3-5 yr	<1.1	<0.4	
5-7 yr	<0.8	<0.3	
>7 yr	<0.6	<0.2	
Oxalate	µmol/mmol	µg/mg	<0.5 mmol/1.73 m^2 (<45 mg/1.73 m^2)
<1 yr	15-260	12-207	
1-5 yr	11-120	9-96	
5-12 yr	60-150	47-119	
>12 yr	2-80	1.6-64	
Glycolate	µmol/mmol	µg/mg	<0.5 mmol/1.73 m^2 (<45 mg/1.73 m^2)
<1 yr	8-70	5-47	
1-5 yr	6-91	4-61	
5-12 yr	6-46	4-31	
>12 yr	4-40	3-27	
Glycerate	µmol/mmol	µg/mg	
0-5 yr	13-190	12-177	
>5 yr	22-123	19-115	
Cystine	mmol/mol	mg/g	<10 yr: <55 µmol/1.73 m^2
<1 mo	<85	<180	>10 yr: <200 µmol/1.73 m^2
1-6 mo	<53	<112	Adults: <250 µmol/1.73 m^2
>6 mo	<18	<38	
Uric acid	mol/mol	g/g	From age 1 yr: <815 mg/1.73 m^2/24 hr
<1 yr	<1.5	<2.2	
1-3 yr	<1.3	<1.9	
3-5 yr	<1.0	<1.5	
5-10 yr	<0.6	<0.9	
>10 yr	<0.4	<0.6	
Citrate	mol/mol	g/g	>0.8 mmol/1.73 m^2 (>0.14 g/1.73 m^2)
0-5 yr	>0.12-0.25	0.20-0.42	
>5 yr	>0.08-0.15	0.14-0.25	

Adapted from references 384-386.

the calculus is in the distal ureter, the child may have irritative symptoms of dysuria, urgency, and frequency. Bladder stones may be asymptomatic. If the stone is in the urethra, dysuria and difficulty in voiding may result.

DIAGNOSIS

The presence of colorless hexagonal cystine crystals in the urine is diagnostic of cystinuria. Massive, envelope-shaped, calcium oxalate crystals may be suggestive of hyperoxaluria. Serum levels of calcium, phosphorus, alkaline phosphatase, creatinine, uric acid, and electrolytes, as well as the anion gap should be measured, and evaluation should be performed for hypercalciuria, hyperoxaluria, hyperuricosuria, and cystinuria.

Ultrasonography, plain radiography, and noncontrast helical computed tomography (CT) can be used to visualize stones. In small children, ultrasonography should be the first option due to concerns about radiation exposure.[392] However, stones smaller than 5 mm, papillary or calyceal concrements, and ureteral stones may escape ultrasonographic detection.[393] Noncontrast helical CT is the most sensitive modality to detect small renal or ureteral radiolucent stones in children[375,394] and provides additional information about obstruction or a structural abnormality.[395]

TREATMENT

Episodes of colicky pain should be treated with analgesic agents. In a child with a renal or ureteral calculus, the decision whether to remove the stone depends on its location, size, and composition (if known) and on the presence of obstruction, infection, or both. Most stones smaller than 5 mm will pass spontaneously, even in small children. Hydration increases urinary flow and facilitates stone passage.

Administration of α-adrenergic blockers decreases ureteral pressure and decreases the frequency of the peristaltic contractions of the obstructed ureter. Also, experience in adult patients suggests that calcium channel blocking agents, with or without steroids, facilitate stone passage.[396] Although use of these agents in children with ureteral calculi has been reported anecdotally, their safety and efficacy have not been demonstrated.[397]

Interventional stone removal is suggested for children with severe debilitating pain refractory to parenteral analgesic therapy, significant urinary obstruction (immediate

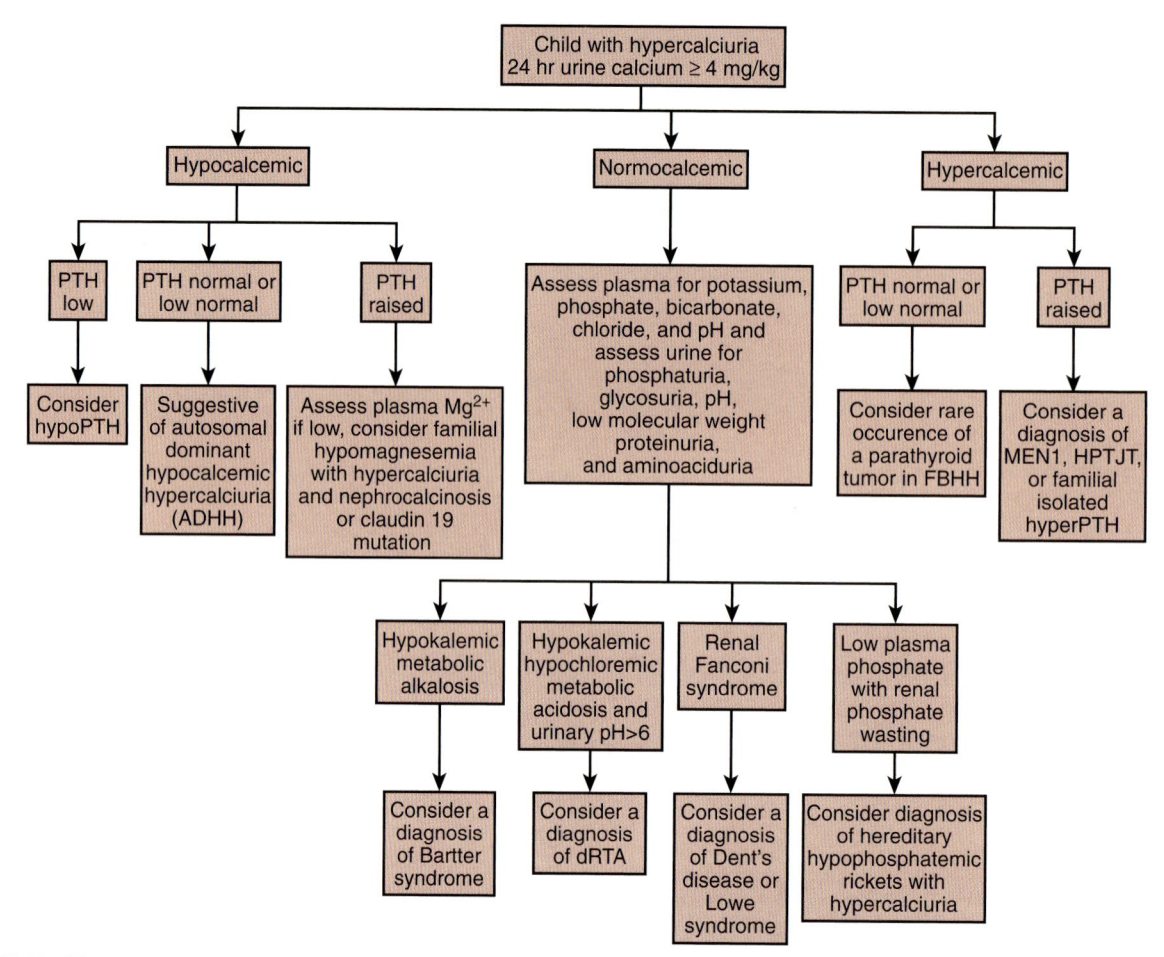

Figure 74.11 Diagnostic algorithm for hypercalciuric monogenic stone disorders. (From Stechman MJ, Loh NY, Thakker RV: Genetic causes of hypercalciuric nephrolithiasis, *Pediatr Nephrol* 24:2321-2332, 2009.)

removal is required), struvite stones, and associated UTIs and in children who fail to pass a stone within 2 weeks. Interventional treatment options include extracorporeal shock wave lithotripsy, percutaneous nephrolithotomy, and ureteroscopy. Extracorporeal shock wave lithotripsy has been successfully used in children with renal and ureteral stones smaller than 2 cm, with a success rate of more than 75%.[398] In patients with stones larger than 2 cm in diameter, ureteroscopy with lithotripsy is suggested.[399] In some cases, placement of a ureteral stent provides pain relief and dilates the ureter sufficiently to allow the calculus to pass.

Urinary alkalinization and maintenance of a high urine output are effective methods to prevent further stone formation.

In children with hypercalciuria, some reduction in calcium and sodium intake is necessary. Thiazide diuretics also reduce renal calcium excretion. Addition of potassium citrate, an inhibitor of calcium stones, at a dose of 1 to 2 mEq/kg/24 hr is beneficial. In patients with uric acid stones, allopurinol is effective.[400]

GENETIC KIDNEY STONE DISEASE

Hypercalciuria is found in approximately 40% of pediatric patients with kidney stones.[381] Up to 65% of patients with hypercalciuric nephrolithiasis have a positive family history of nephrolithiasis,[401] with inheritance as a monogenic or, more commonly, a polygenic quantitative trait. Studies of these monogenic forms of hypercalciuric nephrolithiasis in humans have helped identify a number of transporters, channels, and receptors involved in the regulation of renal tubular calcium reabsorption. In addition to these rare monogenetic hypercalciuric disorders, cystinuria and primary hyperoxaluria, the most important normocalciuric disorders leading to stone formation, will be discussed.[387]

HYPERCALCIURIC NEPHROLITHIASIS

Bartter's Syndrome

Bartter's syndrome is a heterogeneous group of disorders of electrolyte homeostasis characterized by hypokalemic metabolic alkalosis, renal salt wasting, hyperreninemic hyperaldosteronism, increased urinary prostaglandin excretion, and hypercalciuria with nephrocalcinosis.[402] Mutations of several ion transporters and channels have been associated with Bartter's syndrome, and six types are now recognized[402] (see earlier, "Bartter-Like Syndromes" and Chapter 45 for a more detailed discussion).

Dent's Disease

Dent's disease is an X-linked, recessive, renal tubular disorder characterized by hypercalciuria, nephrocalcinosis, nephrolithiasis, low-molecular-weight proteinuria, and eventual renal failure.[403] Dent's disease is also associated with renal Fanconi's syndrome. With the exception of rickets, which occurs in a minority of patients, there appear to be no extrarenal manifestations in Dent's disease.[403] The gene causing Dent's disease, *CLCN5*, encodes the chloride-proton antiporter ClC-5,[404] which is expressed predominantly in the kidney and, in particular, in the proximal tubule, thick ascending limb of Henle, and α-intercalated cells of the collecting duct. Defects in ClC-5 cause defective endocytosis within the renal tubule, which results in hypercalciuria and hyperphosphaturia, leading to calcium stone formation.[384,405]

Oculocerebrorenal Syndrome (Lowe's Syndrome)

Oculocerebrorenal syndrome (Lowe's syndrome) is an X-linked recessive disorder characterized by congenital cataracts, mental retardation, muscle hypotonia, rickets, and defective proximal tubular reabsorption of bicarbonate, phosphate, and amino acids. Hypercalciuria, nephrocalcinosis, and stones are well described.[406] Manifest disease is nearly always confined to boys, who develop renal dysfunction in the first year of life and have delayed bone age and reduced height. Later in life, progressive renal failure is typical.[407] Female carriers, who have normal neurologic and kidney function, can be identified in 80% of cases by micropunctate cortical lens opacities.

Deficiency of OCRL1 (oculocerebrorenal syndrome protein 1), the product of the Lowe's syndrome gene, leads to disruptions in lysosomal trafficking and endosomal sorting. Phosphatidylinositol-4,5-bisphosphate, the preferred substrate of OCRL1, accumulates in the renal proximal tubular cells of patients with Lowe's syndrome.[408]

Autosomal Dominant Hypocalcemia with Hypercalciuria. Autosomal dominant hypocalcemia with hypercalciuria (ADHH) is a stone disease associated with activating mutations of the calcium-sensing receptor. Patients with ADHH usually have mild hypocalcemia that is generally asymptomatic, but in some patients it may be associated with carpopedal spasm and seizures. The serum phosphate level is elevated or in the upper normal range, serum magnesium level is low or low normal, and parathyroid hormone level is low normal. Treatment with active vitamin D metabolites to correct hypocalcemia has been reported to result in marked hypercalciuria, nephrocalcinosis, nephrolithiasis, and renal impairment, which were partially reversible after cessation of the vitamin D treatment. Thus, it is important to identify ADHH patients and their families, whose hypocalcemia is due to a gain-of-function mutation in the CaSR mutation and not hypoparathyroidism, and to restrict their use of vitamin D treatment.[387,384,409]

Hereditary Hypophosphatemic Rickets with Hypercalciuria. Hereditary hypophosphatemic rickets with hypercalciuria is due to mutations in the type 2C sodium-phosphate cotransporter and presents with rickets, short stature, increased renal phosphate clearance, hypercalciuria but normal serum calcium levels, increased gastrointestinal absorption of calcium and phosphate due to elevated serum levels of 1,25-dihydroxyvitamin D, suppressed parathyroid function, and normal urinary excretion of cAMP.[384,410]

Familial Hypomagnesemia with Hypercalciuria and Nephrocalcinosis

The syndrome of familial hypercalciuria and hypomagnesemia with renal magnesium wasting (FHHNC) leads to progressive nephrocalcinosis with renal failure.[411] It is caused by a mutation of the *CLDN16* gene that encodes the tight junction protein paracellin-1 (claudin-16). The diagnosis is often missed unless the magnesium level is measured in serum and urine. No effective therapy is currently available. The risk of progressing to end stage kidney disease is high.[412] Treatment consists mostly of hydrochlorothiazide and oral magnesium supplementation; however, this does not appear to prevent early ESKD.[413] FHHNC is genetically heterogenous because mutations in another tight junction gene encoding claudin-19 cause a similar renal and skeletal phenotype.[414] In addition to FHHNC, *CLDN19* defects cause severe myopia, nystagmus, or macular coloboma, which have led to the designation of the *CLDN19*-related disease entity as FHHNC with severe ocular involvement.

NONHYPERCALCIURIC NEPHROLITHIASIS

Cystinuria

Cystinuria is a rare autosomal recessive cause of kidney stones characterized by defective reabsorption of cystine and other dibasic amino acids (e.g., ornithine, arginine, lysine) along the luminal brush border of the proximal renal tubule cells. Most cases of classical cystinuria (type A) are due to mutations in the *SLC3A1* gene. Heterozygotes have normal dibasic amino acid excretion. Mutations in *SLC7A9* are responsible for types II and III disease (type B).[384,415] Digenic inheritance (one mutated allele each in *SCL3A1* and *SLC7A9*) is not sufficient to induce stone formation.[416] Genetic differentiation offers little clinical advantage because subtypes do not appear to correlate with disease severity or treatment response.[416,417]

The median age at onset of nephrolithiasis is 12 years, but stones may occur even in infancy.[418] The diagnosis of cystinuria is typically based on family history, stone analysis, and identification of the pathognomonic hexagonal cystine crystals on urinalysis. In first-time stone formers, urine should be screened for cystine using the cyanide-nitroprusside test (Figure 74.12). A positive result indicates a cystine concentration of more than 75 mg/L,[419] and a quantitative test for cystine (colorimetric or high-performance liquid chromatography [HPLC]) should then be performed.[420] Recently, a method to estimate the potential for stone formation (cystine capacity) has been proposed as a monitoring tool.[416]

The upper limit of daily cystine excretion increases from 13 mg/1.73 m^2 in young children to 60 mg/1.73 m^2 in adults (see Table 74.6). In comparison, patients with cystinuria generally excrete more than 400 mg/day.[384,421] Heterozygotes and patients with Fanconi's syndrome excrete less than 250 mg/day and usually do not form stones because the urinary cystine concentrations remain within the range of solubility.

General measures, including high fluid intake, urinary alkalinization with potassium citrate or Shohl's solution,[422] and limitation of dietary sodium intake can be helpful in preventing the recurrence of cystine calculi.

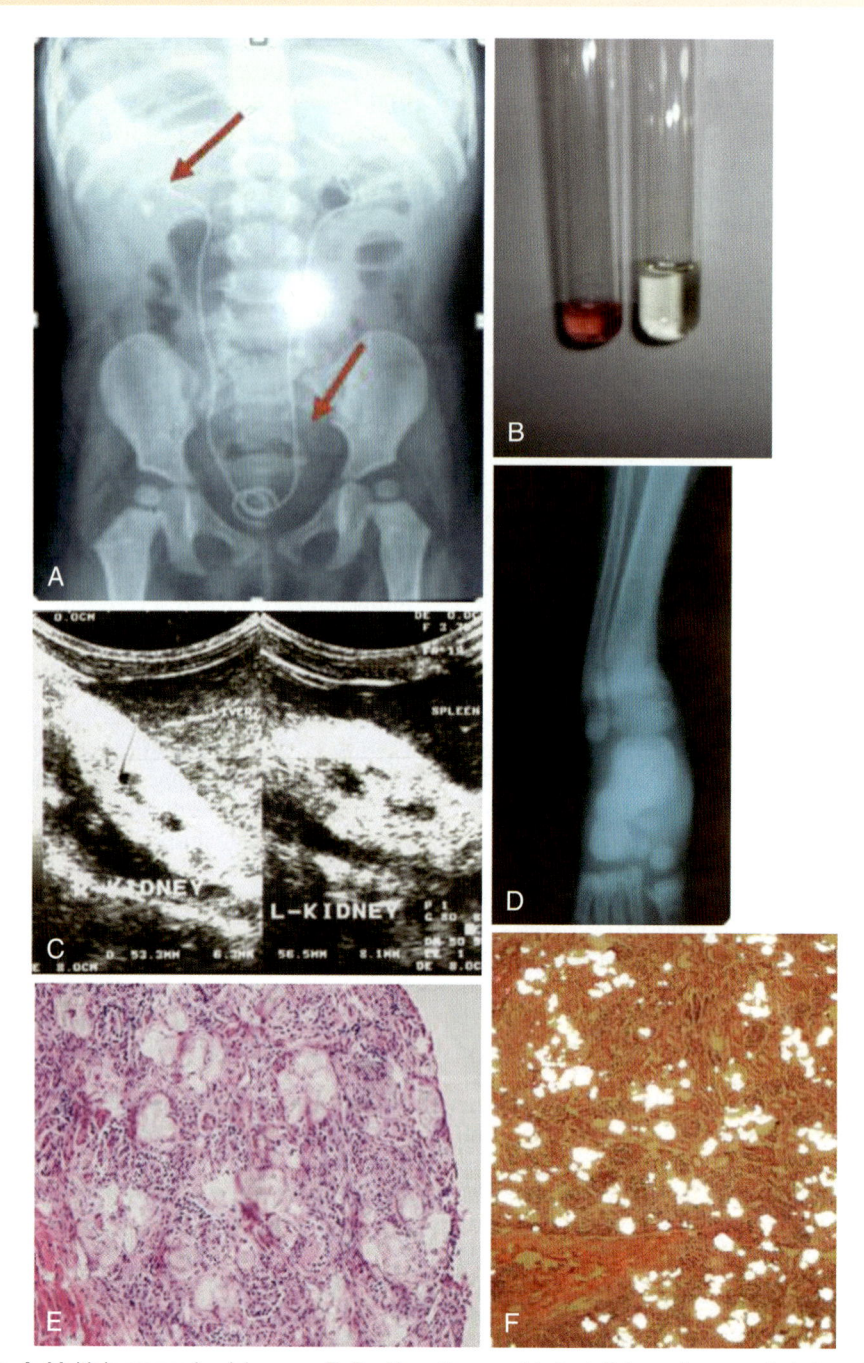

Figure 74.12 Cystinuria. **A,** Multiple stones in plain x-ray. **B,** Positive nitroprusside test. Primary hyperoxaluria type 1. **C,** Severely echogenic kidneys due to oxalosis. **D,** Angulation of tibia and fibula leading to bowing and mineralization defect in metatarsal bones. **E,** Disseminated luminal oxalate crystals in the tubules of a kidney allograft. **F,** Oxalate crystals under polarized light.

In refractory cases, α-mercaptopropionylglycine, which forms a soluble dimer with cystine, administered orally at 10 to 15 mg/kg/day, can reduce the formation of new stones and even dissolve existing calculi.[423] Another important medication is D-penicillamine, a chelating agent that binds to cysteine or homocysteine, increasing the solubility of the product. Since both compounds can cause some toxic damage to podocytes, proteinuria should be monitored. N-acetylcysteine appears to have low toxicity and may be effective, but long-term experience is lacking. Captopril also forms soluble dimers with cystine.[384] Bucillamine, a dithiol compound, is another promising alternative.[424] Because these medications have an antipyridoxine effect, supplemental vitamin B_6 should be provided.

Primary Hyperoxaluria

The primary hyperoxalurias (PHs) are rare metabolic disorders with autosomal recessive inheritance characterized by increased generation and urinary excretion of oxalate. There are three forms—PH types 1, 2, and 3. Type 1 is the most devastating form and type 3 the least severe. However, sometimes type 1 and 2 PH cannot be distinguished according to age at onset and, in some cases, PH type 2 is initially assumed to be type 1. The two forms can be distinguished biochemically by assessing the urinary excretion of glycolate and L-glyceric acid, respectively.[385,425]

Primary hyperoxaluria type 1 is caused by mutations in the gene *AGXT*, which encodes for the hepatic peroxisomal enzyme alanine-glyoxylate aminotransferase (AGT).[426,427] AGT metabolizes the oxalate precursor glyoxylate to glycine, which is further metabolized to serine. Deficient AGT activity results in failure to detoxify glyoxylate, which is oxidized to oxalate or reduced to glycolate. The presence of AGT activity in liver biopsy specimens does not rule out the diagnosis of primary hyperoxaluria type 1 because mutant enzymes may be mistargeted to mitochondria instead of peroxisome.

Primary Hyperoxaluria Type 1. Patients with primary hyperoxaluria type 1 typically develop severe nephrolithiasis and nephrocalcinosis, with progressive kidney failure. However, there is enormous phenotypic variability, which can range from neonatal nephrocalcinosis to isolated kidney stones first occurring in adulthood.[428] The first symptoms of primary hyperoxaluria type 1 occur before 1 year of age in 15% of patients and before 5 years of age in 50%.[429] Primary hyperoxaluria type 1 is responsible for approximately 1% of ESKD cases in children.[429] The rate of progression is variable. Certain *AGXT* mutations allow residual enzyme activity[430] and, in some, this residual enzyme activity can be stimulated with the co-factor pyridoxine, which promotes the conversion of glyoxylate to glycine rather than to oxalate. Primary hyperoxaluria type 1 caused by these mutations typically has a less severe clinical course. The most malignant infantile form is characterized by massive parenchymal oxalosis and nephrocalcinosis and rapid progression to ESKD within a few months, typically without stone formation.[431] Older children exhibit bilateral, radiopaque, calcium oxalate stones. In some patients, the disease is not identified until adulthood, when the patient comes for treatment of ESKD.[384,432,433]

Systemic oxalosis occurs when serum oxalate levels increase as kidney function deteriorates and oxalate clearance becomes impaired. At the stage of systemic oxalosis, calcium oxalate crystal deposition occurs in many tissues, including skeleton, heart, blood vessels, joints, retina, and skin,[384] with devastating functional consequences.

Markedly increased urinary excretion of oxalate is essential for a diagnosis of primary hyperoxaluria type 1 (>0.7 mmol [90 mg]/1.73 m^2/day). By comparison, normal urinary oxalate excretion is less than 0.5 mmol (45 mg)/1.73 m^2/day.[384,385,434] Glycolate excretion is elevated in two thirds of patients with PH type 1 but may also be increased in patients with PH type 3. Measurement of plasma levels of oxalate should be reserved for patients with stage 3b chronic kidney disease, since plasma levels remain relatively normal until kidney function is substantially impaired.[385]

Delayed diagnosis is common (40% of patients) with an average lag time of 3.4 years after the onset of symptoms.[432] The diagnosis of primary hyperoxaluria should be suspected in a patient with recurrent calcium stones, nephrocalcinosis, normal urinary calcium and uric acid excretion, calcium oxalate crystals in the urine sediment, pure calcium oxalate monohydrate stones, and marked hyperoxaluria.[384,434]

The determination of AGT enzyme activity in liver biopsy tissue used to be the gold standard for diagnosing primary hyperoxaluria type 1[435,436] but has been largely replaced by *AGXT* mutation screening. More than 180 mutations have been described to date.[385]

Medical treatment includes the following: high fluid intake (3 to 4 L/day, with the aim of keeping oxalate concentration <0.5 mmol [45 mg]/L); avoidance of high-oxalate foods such as tea, chocolate, spinach, and rhubarb; and administration of potassium citrate (0.3 to 0.5 mmol/kg per day, as long as GFR is preserved) to inhibit calcium oxalate precipitation. Oral high-dose pyridoxine (5 to 20 mg/kg/day) is helpful in a fraction of patients and should be tried empirically for 3 months. Genetic information is helpful in anticipating pyridoxine responsiveness; the Gly170Arg, Phe152Ile, and Ile244Thr genotypes are associated with a sustained reduction of urinary oxalate levels on pyridoxine administration, leading to an improved overall prognosis.[385]

These therapeutic measures are more effective if started at an early age, before significant impairment of kidney function has occurred. In a multicenter retrospective study, 20 of 22 children with primary hyperoxaluria (median age at diagnosis, 2.4 years) who were treated with medical management did not require renal replacement at a median follow-up of 8.7 years.[437]

The dialytic oxalate clearance achieved with standard hemodialysis or peritoneal dialysis is not sufficient to compensate for the enhanced oxalate synthesis in patients with PH type 1 because progressive tissue oxalosis occurs during maintenance dialysis. High-intensity dialysis protocols with more than 40 hours of hemodialysis/week and/or combined hemodialysis and peritoneal dialysis have been used in individual patients but can at best slow down the progression of systemic oxalosis. Isolated kidney transplantation is usually contraindicated in patients with systemic oxalosis, since mobilization of the large tissue oxalate pool leads to rapid deposition of oxalate crystals in the transplant (see Figure 74.12) and loss of graft function. It may be an option for select patients with residual enzyme activity responding to pyridoxine and with minimal tissue oxalate deposition[438] and possibly for adults with a late-onset form of the disease. Liver transplantation cures primary hyperoxaluria because the defective enzymes are exclusively expressed in the liver. Isolated liver transplantation is recommended if the diagnosis is made before significant impairment of kidney function has occurred (i.e., GFR > 40 to 50 mL/min/1.73 m^2). In children with CKD stage 3 or 4, a sequential transplantation strategy can be considered, with observation of the course of kidney function after liver transplantation.[439] In patients with CKD stage 5, combined liver-kidney transplantation is the treatment of choice.[439,440]

Probiotic therapy with *Oxalobacter formigenes*, an oxalate-degrading intestinal bacterium, was recently tested in a placebo-controlled randomized clinical trial for its potential to promote intestinal oxalate excretion, but with disappointing results.[441]

Primary Hyperoxaluria Type 2. PH type 2 is caused by mutations in the *GRHPR* gene, which encodes the glyoxylate reductase/hydroxypyruvate reductase (GRHPR).[442] The disease generally has a more benign clinical course than PH1. It typically first manifests with recurrent oxalate stones during adolescence. Progressive CKD occurs in approximately 10% of patients. Biochemically, hyperoxaluria is accompanied by increased excretion of L-glycerate. The diagnosis is confirmed by genetic screening of GRHPR or by the demonstration of deficient enzyme activity in liver biopsy specimens.[442] Patients with type 2 PH do not benefit from pyridoxine treatment. Because liver transplantation has not been demonstrated to correct the metabolic defect in patients with type 2 disease, and because such patients may do well with kidney transplantation alone, distinguishing between PH types 1 and 2 is especially important when managing primary hyperoxaluria patients who have renal failure.

Primary Hyperoxaluria Type 3. PH type 3 is caused by mutations in the gene encoding 4-hydroxy-2-oxoglutarate aldolase (*HOGA1* gene).[443-445] The mitochondrial enzyme is expressed in liver and kidney and catalyzes hydroxyproline metabolism from 4-hydroxy-2-oxoglutarate to glyoxylate and pyruvate. The clinical phenotype of PH3 is mild and limited to recurrent stone formation, which may even improve spontaneously over time, despite persisting hyperoxaluria. Nephrocalcinosis or the development of chronic kidney disease is uncommon.

SYSTEMIC DISORDERS AFFECTING THE KIDNEY

CHILDHOOD VASCULITIDES WITH KIDNEY INVOLVEMENT

Childhood vasculitides may occur as a primary process or secondary to an underlying disease. Clinical symptoms vary widely, depending on the type and location of the vessels involved and the extent of inflammation. The most recent classification criteria proposed by the European League Against Rheumatism, Paediatric Rheumatology International Trials Organisation, and Paediatric Rheumatology European Society is based primarily on the size of the predominantly involved arteries.[446] This section focuses on Henoch-Schönlein nephritis, childhood polyarteritis nodosa, microscopic polyangiitis, Wegener's granulomatosis, and Takayasu's arteritis.

HENOCH-SCHÖNLEIN PURPURA (IMMUNOGLOBULIN A–ASSOCIATED VASCULITIS)

Henoch-Schönlein purpura (HSP) is the most common systemic small vessel vasculitis in childhood, with an estimated annual incidence of 10 to 20/100,000 in children younger than 17 years of age.[447-449] The disorder manifests predominantly in the fall, winter, and spring. Approximately 10% of HSP cases occur in adults (incidence, 0.8 to 1.8/100 000).[450] A seasonal pattern is not seen in adults.

HSP, recently renamed as immunoglobulin A vasculitis (IgAV),[451] is an IgA-mediated small vessel leukocytoclastic vasculitis predominantly affecting the skin, joints, gastrointestinal tract, and kidneys and occasionally other organs. A diagnosis of IgAV requires the presence of purpura or petechiae (mandatory) with lower limb predominance (Figure 74.13), plus at least one of the following four signs or symptoms: (1) abdominal pain; (2) histopathologic findings showing leukocytoclastic vasculitis or proliferative glomerulonephritis with predominantly IgA-containing immune complex deposition see (see Figure 74.13); (3) arthritis or arthralgia; and (4) kidney involvement (e.g., hematuria, red blood cell casts, proteinuria).[446,452] In a review of 254 patients, the frequency of skin, joint, gastrointestinal, and renal manifestations was 100%, 66%, 56%, and 30%, respectively.[453] Testicular, ocular, pulmonary, and central and peripheral nervous system manifestations occur less frequently. The diagnosis of IgAV is usually based on clinical manifestations of the disease. No laboratory test is diagnostic for IgAV. Skin biopsy specimens show inflammation of the small blood vessels (leukocytoclastic vasculitis). Definitive confirmation is provided by the demonstration of IgA deposition in the skin or kidney.[446]

It has long been speculated that HSP nephritis and IgA nephropathy share common pathogenetic mechanisms and may represent two ends of a spectrum,[454] since both manifestations can occur consecutively in the same patient and are found in identical twins.[455] The clinical, genetic, and immunologic features of these conditions are so closely linked that one could consider HSP nephritis as the systemic form of IgA nephropathy.[456] Both conditions are characterized by the presence of galactose-deficient IgA1 in the circulation and its deposition in the glomerular mesangium.[456,457] A recent study has shown that not only pediatric patients with HSP nephritis and IgA nephropathy but also a significant fraction of their first-degree relatives exhibit increased serum levels of hypoglycosylated IgA1, which supports a common genetic basis and pathogenetic link between these disorders.[457] However, the factors leading to systemic activation of IgA-containing immune complexes in IgAV and selective activation of IgA-containing immune complexes in IgA nephropathy have not been identified.[455]

Renal Manifestations of Immunoglobulin A Vasculitis

Renal disease can develop at any time over a period of several days to several weeks, generally within a month of presentation, and is not predictably related to the severity of extrarenal involvement.[458] Some degree of renal involvement is observed in 20% to 50% of children at initial presentation,[453] ranging from asymptomatic hematuria and sometimes proteinuria to NS, hypertension, and acute renal failure.[453,459] In a systematic review assessing the course of HSP nephritis in 1133 children, renal involvement was found to occur in 34% of children; 80% of them showed isolated hematuria and/or proteinuria, and 20% had acute nephritis or NS.[458] There is a general correlation between the severity of the renal manifestations, kidney biopsy findings, and disease prognosis.[459-461]

Histopathologic Features. Light microscopic findings range from isolated mesangial proliferation to focal and segmental proliferation to severe crescentic glomerulonephritis. The diagnostic finding is dominant or codominant IgA deposition in the mesangium on immunofluorescence testing (see Figure 74.13). In addition, immunofluorescence may reveal IgG, IgM, fibrinogen, C3, and properdin in the glomeruli. By electron microscopy, dense deposits are typically found in the mesangial areas. The histologic classification of HSP nephritis distinguishes minimal or moderate glomerular lesions and absence of crescents (class I or II), extracapillary cellular proliferation of variable extent (<50% of glomeruli, class III; 50% to 75%, class IV; >75%, class V), and pseudomembranoproliferative glomerulonephritis (class VI).[462]

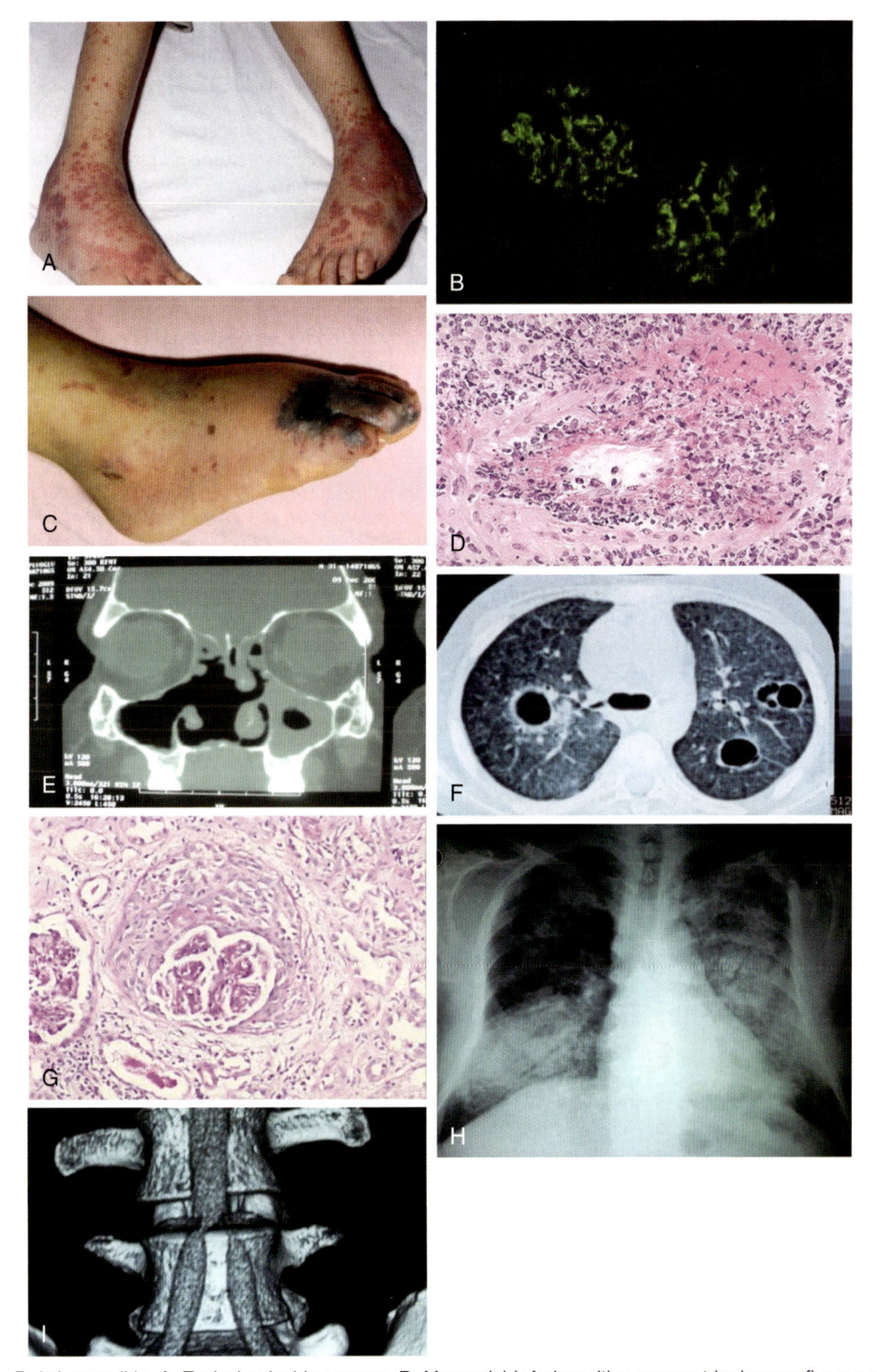

Figure 74.13 A, B, IgA vasculitis. **A,** Typical palpable purpura. **B,** Mesangial IgA deposition apparent by immunofluorescence microscopy. **C, D,** Polyarteritis nodosa. **C,** Necrotic skin lesions. **D,** Polyarteritis with disintegrated tunica muscularis of an arcuate artery wall, perivascular inflammation, and fibrinoid necrosis. **E-H,** ANCA-associated vasculitis. **E-G,** Granulomatosis with polyangiitis. **E,** Bone destruction in paranasal sinuses. **F,** Multiple pulmonary cavitary lesions. **G,** Glomerulus showing large cellular crescent, with irregular focus of fibrinoid necrosis. **H,** MPO-ANCA–positive vasculitis—diffuse infiltration due to pulmonary capillaritis. **I,** Takayasu's arteritis—narrowing abdominal aorta at the level of iliac artery bifurcation (MRI scan).

Treatment. The large majority of IgAV cases require symptomatic treatment only. There is suggestive evidence that corticosteroid therapy enhances the rate of resolution of abdominal pain. However, the evidence for a reduction in the incidence of nephritis with oral steroid administration early in HSP is conflicting.[463-467] A meta-analysis has suggested that early corticosteroid treatment reduces the risk of developing persistent renal disease.[462,464] However, two RCTs and a Cochrane review have concluded that steroids do not prevent kidney involvement in HSP.[465,466,468]

A meta-analysis of treatment of severe established kidney disease[468] and a systematic review of various reports of treatment with prednisolone, methylprednisolone, cyclophosphamide, azathioprine, cyclosporine, dipyridamole, warfarin, and plasma exchange have shown that there is insufficient evidence to guide best practice in the management of HSP nephritis.[469] A single-center, retrospective therapy review of severe (>class III) HSP and IgA nephropathy has suggested that different combinations of steroids, cyclophosphamide, and RAAS antagonists are associated with good outcomes in 54% of children with severe histologic changes on initial kidney biopsy specimens.[470] In children with crescentic disease, there is low-grade evidence from uncontrolled trials for the benefit of intense immunosuppressive therapy (pulse methylprednisolone, 250 to 1000 mg/day for 3 days) followed by oral prednisone (1 mg/kg/day) and, in these patients, steroid and immunosuppressive combination therapy is often initiated.[471,472] However, spontaneous recovery can also be observed, even in patients with crescent formation. Thus, aggressive therapies, particularly combination therapies, are suggested for clinically and histologically severe HSP nephritis (higher than class III with NS), but not for moderate to severe disease (histologic classes I to III and serum albumin level > 2.5 g/dL).[473] Plasma exchange and intravenous immunoglobulin have shown at least short-term efficacy in individual cases.[460,474] ACE inhibitors are effective in lowering proteinuria; however, their long-term benefit is unknown.[458,473]

Prognosis. The overwhelming majority of children with IgAV experience full recovery. Persistent renal involvement ensues in 1.8% of all children with IgAV, in 1.6% of those with isolated hematuria and/or proteinuria, and in 19.5% of those with nephritic syndrome and/or NS during the initial disease phase.[458] Long-term outcomes are poorest in children who initially have a mixed nephritic-nephrotic presentation,[459] with up to 33% of these children developing CKD. HSP nephritis is the underlying diagnosis in 1% to 3% of children with end-stage renal failure.[459,467] Among patients with HSP nephritis progressing to ESKD and undergoing transplantation, mild disease recurrence is seen in approximately 35% of these patients 5 years after transplantation. Approximately 10% of them experience graft loss due to recurrent disease. Disease recurrence is more likely in patients with aggressive initial disease who progressed to ESKD within fewer than 3 years.[475]

CHILDHOOD POLYARTERITIS NODOSA

Childhood polyarteritis nodosa (also termed *macroscopic polyarteritis* or *classic polyarteritis nodosa*) is a systemic necrotizing vasculitis affecting small and/or medium-sized arteries predominantly in skin, abdominal viscera, kidneys, central nervous system, and muscles.[458,476,477] The peak age of disease onset in childhood is 7 to 11 years, and no gender difference is noted.[478]

Diagnosis

The diagnosis of childhood polyarteritis nodosa requires the presence of a systemic inflammatory disease with evidence of necrotizing vasculitis or angiographic abnormalities of medium-sized and small arteries (mandatory criterion) plus one of the following: (1) skin involvement (livedo reticularis, tender subcutaneous nodules, superficial or deep skin infarctions; see Figure 74.13); (2) myalgia or muscle tenderness; (3) hypertension; (4) peripheral neuropathy; (5) renal involvement (e.g., proteinuria, hematuria, or red blood cell casts, or GFR < 50% the normal value for the patient's age).[446,452]

Pathogenesis

Infections are implicated as a triggering mechanism in a predisposed host. A number of reports have pointed to the role of streptococcal infection in childhood polyarteritis nodosa.[478] An increased frequency of polyarteritis nodosa has been suggested in patients with familial Mediterranean fever; this association may be related to the inflammatory milieu in these patients.[479,480] However, the precise mechanisms linking specific infectious agents and/or general inflammatory conditions with polyarteritis nodosa have not been elucidated to date.

Clinical Features

Childhood polyarteritis nodosa typically presents with systemic symptoms (e.g., fever, malaise, weight loss) and signs of multisystem involvement, including skin rash, myalgia, abdominal pain, and arthropathy, renal manifestations such as hematuria, proteinuria, hypertension, and acute renal failure, and neurologic features such as focal defects, hemiplegia, visual loss, and mononeuritis multiplex.[478,481-483]

Laboratory Findings

Anemia, leukocytosis, thrombocytosis, increased erythrocyte sedimentation rate, and increased C-reactive protein level are usually present in childhood polyarteritis nodosa.[481] If renal involvement is present, renal angiography or, rarely, kidney biopsy is indicated. The classical angiographic finding in polyarteritis nodosa is aneurysms affecting renal, celiac, and coronary arteries.[476] However, nonaneurysmal changes are detected more commonly on renal angiography than are aneurysms. The most reliable signs of nonaneurysmal arteriopathy are perfusion defects, presence of collateral arteries, lack of crossing of peripheral renal arteries, and delayed emptying of small renal arteries.[480,484] Kidney biopsy specimens show necrotizing arteritis characterized by fibrinoid necrosis and perivascular inflammation (see Figure 74.13). Antineutrophil cytoplasmic antibodies may be present in rare cases.

Treatment

There are no pediatric RCTs to guide treatment of polyarteritis nodosa in children. Induction of remission is usually achieved with high doses of corticosteroids and cyclophosphamide, in combination with antiplatelet doses of aspirin. Maintenance therapy with daily or alternate-day low-dose prednisolone and oral azathioprine is frequently continued for up to 18 months. Other immunosuppressive agents used in the maintenance phase include methotrexate, MMF, and cyclosporine.[458,476,485] Adjunctive plasma exchange can be used in life-threatening situations.[474] Successful treatment with biologic agents such as infliximab or rituximab in refractory cases has been reported.[474,481,486]

ANTINEUTROPHIL CYTOPLASMIC ANTIBODY-ASSOCIATED VASCULITIDES

Antineutrophil cytoplasmic antibody (ANCA)–associated vasculitides do occur in children but are less common than polyarteritis nodosa.[487] The ANCA-associated vasculitides include microscopic polyangiitis, granulomatosis with polyangiitis (GPA), formerly known as Wegener's granulomatosis, and eosinophilic granulomatosis with polyangiitis (EGPA), formerly known as Churg-Strauss vasculitis. All these disorders target the small arteries. The most accepted pathogenetic model proposes that ANCA activates cytokine-primed neutrophils, which leads to bystander damage of endothelial cells and an escalation of inflammation, with recruitment of mononuclear cells. Of the two main ANCA classes, the cytoplasmic ANCA (C-ANCA) and perinuclear or antimyeloperoxidase ANCA (P-ANCA, MPO-ANCA) types, a pathogenic role in renal vasculitis is more evident for the myeloperoxidase type. A third type of ANCA, directed against human lysosome membrane protein-2, has been described as a potentially sensitive and specific marker for renal ANCA-associated vasculitis.[488] However, other concomitant exogenous factors and genetic susceptibility also appear to be necessary for disease expression.[485]

Types of Antineutrophil Cytoplasmic Antibody-Associated Vasculitides

Microscopic Polyangiitis. Microscopic polyarteritis or polyangiitis is a nongranulomatous, necrotizing, multisystem, pauci-immune small vessel vasculitis without upper airway involvement that is often associated with a high titer of MPO-ANCA or positive P-ANCA staining.[446,452] Microscopic polyangiitis differs from classical polyarteritis nodosa in that extensive glomerular involvement is present and the pulmonary capillaries also are often involved (see Figure 74.13).[451] The typical clinical manifestations are rapidly progressive glomerulonephritis and alveolar hemorrhage, which can be difficult to distinguish from GPA.[489]

Granulomatosis with Polyangiitis. GPA is a systemic vasculitis with granulomatous inflammation of small and medium-sized arteries, typically affecting the upper and lower respiratory tracts and kidneys (see Figure 74.13). The cause of GPA is unknown, but staphylococcal infections have been postulated as a potential trigger. Nasal carriage of *Staphylococcus aureus* is a strong risk factor for relapse and may have a causative role in the pathogenesis of the disorder. Prophylactic treatment with cotrimoxazole was found to result in a 60% reduction in relapses. The role of *S. aureus* carriage can be explained in different ways. Carriage may induce low-grade infection in the upper airways, resulting in priming of neutrophils, and primed neutrophils can be further activated by proteinase 3 (PR3)-ANCA, which results in vasculitis. Alternatively, superantigens from *S. aureus* may nonspecifically activate an autoimmune response and immune complex formation in kidneys. *S. aureus* carriage might also induce antibodies to PR3 that in turn, by idiotypic–anti-idiotypic interactions, result in the development of PR3-ANCA.[490]

GPA is a rare disease in childhood. The only incidence study in children, examining a 15-year period in southern Alberta, Canda, showed an overall average annual incidence of childhood GPA of 2.75 cases/pmp (95% confidence interval [CI], 1.93 to 3.70), with a significant increase from 0.9 cases pmp in 1994 to 2003 to 6.4 cases pmp from 2004 to 2008.[491]

A diagnosis of GPA requires the presence of at least three of the following six indicators[446,452]: (1) histopathologic evidence of granulomatous inflammation; (2) upper airway involvement (chronic or recurrent purulent or bloody nasal discharge or crusting or recurrent epistaxis); (3) laryngotracheobronchial stenosis; (4) pulmonary involvement (chest radiograph or CT scan showing nodules, cavities, or fixed infiltrates); (5) ANCA positivity; (6) renal involvement (hematuria, proteinuria, or red blood cell casts or necrotizing pauci-immune glomerulonephritis).

Symptoms and signs of upper respiratory tract involvement include epistaxis, otalgia, and hearing loss. Nasal septal involvement with cartilaginous collapse results in the characteristic saddle nose deformity. Chronic sinusitis may be observed. Lower respiratory tract manifestations also include granulomatous pulmonary nodules or pulmonary hemorrhages. The typical renal lesion is a focal segmental necrotizing glomerulonephritis, with pauci-immune crescentic glomerular changes (see Figure 74.13). Involvement of other systems with atypical leading symptoms is not uncommon.[485] These may include blurred vision, eye pain, conjunctivitis, episcleritis, persistent otitis media, cranial nerve palsies, seizures, and neuropathies. Skin lesions include purpuric maculae, nodules, ulcerations, and gangrene.

Eosinophilic Granulomatosis with Polyangiitis. EGPA is defined as an eosinophil-rich granulomatous inflammation involving the respiratory tract and necrotizing vasculitis affecting small to medium-sized vessels. There is an association with asthma and eosinophilia.[451] In a review of 33 cases of childhood EGPA, all patients had significant eosinophilia and asthma.[487] ANCA positivity was found in only 25% of children with EGPA. Compared with EGPA in adults, mortality is substantial in pediatric cases, pulmonary and cardiac involvement is predominant, and peripheral nerve involvement is rare.[487]

Treatment

Treatment of pediatric ANCA-associated vasculitis (AAV) includes an induction phase with intravenous corticosteroid pulse therapy, cyclophosphamide, plasma exchange (particularly in dialysis-dependent patients and in the presence of diffuse alveolar hemorrhage[289]), and aspirin at an antiplatelet dosage. Intravenous cyclophosphamide pulses are preferred to oral cyclophosphamide since they cause fewer side effects at dosages with equal efficacy. In milder cases of AAV, methotrexate can be tried as a less toxic alternative to cyclophosphamide to induce remission. Also, MMF may be as efficient as cyclophosphamide in inducing remission. During the subsequent maintenance phase, low-dose oral corticosteroids and azathioprine are therapeutic options.[476,477,481,482,485]

In adults with severe AAV, a single course of B cell–depleting antibody rituximab is as effective as continuous conventional immunosuppressive therapy (cyclophosphamide followed by azathioprine) for the induction and maintenance of remission over the course of 18 months.[492] Rituximab has also been used successfully to achieve remission in children with AAV,[481,485,486] but randomized comparative trials are still lacking. Rituximab should be considered for the treatment of children with AAV who fail to respond to conventional induction therapy with glucocorticoids and cyclophosphamide, and also for patients with relapsing disease in whom there is particular concern regarding cumulative glucocorticoid and/or cyclophosphamide toxicity.[493]

Cotrimoxazole is routinely added for the treatment of GPA, serving both as prophylaxis against opportunistic infections and as a disease-modifying agent.

Prognosis

ANCA-associated vasculitis carries considerable morbidity and mortality, mainly due to progressive CKD or aggressive respiratory involvement. Flares of GPA occur in up to 75% of patients during weaning from treatment, and significant long-term renal impairment occurs in 17% to 40%.[494,495] Furthermore, significant treatment-related infections have been observed in 20% to 40% of patients.[494] Mortality from GPA was 12% in one pediatric series.[496] In children, severe renal involvement is more common with microscopic polyangiitis or microscopic polyarteritis than with GPA. Markedly decreased GFR, oliguria, nephrotic range proteinuria and chronic glomerular lesions at first presentation are predictors of poor outcome.[497] In children with EGPA, one report found 18% mortality, with all deaths attributed to disease rather than to therapy.[487]

TAKAYASU'S ARTERITIS

Takayasu's arteritis is a chronic inflammatory, large vessel vasculitis of unknown cause that primarily affects the aorta and its major branches (see Figure 74.13). The disease is most common in Asia. At disease onset, only 7% of patients are younger than 10 years, but 19% are 10 to 20 years old.[498]

A diagnosis of Takayasu's arteritis in childhood requires the demonstration of the typical angiographic abnormalities of the aorta or its main branches and pulmonary arteries (e.g., aneurysm or dilation, narrowing, occlusion, arterial wall thickening not due to fibromuscular dysplasia) in addition to the presence of one of the following: (1) pulse deficit (lost, decreased, or unequal peripheral artery pulses) or claudication; (2) blood pressure discrepancy in any limb; (3) bruits or thrills over the aorta and/or its major branches; (4) hypertension; (5) elevated level of acute phase reactant.[446,452]

In a series of 19 children with Takayasu's arteritis, the most common complaints at presentation were headache (84%), abdominal pain (37%), claudication of extremities (32%), fever (26%), and weight loss (10%).[499] Hypertension was present in 89%, absent pulses in 58%, and arterial bruits in 42% of patients.[499]

Treatment

Therapy for Takayasu's arteritis in children is largely empirical, with corticosteroids remaining the mainstay of treatment. In addition, methotrexate, azathioprine, MMF, and cyclophosphamide have been used. Cyclophosphamide has been used in refractory cases.[500] Steroid and cyclophosphamide induction followed by methotrexate has been suggested as effective and safe for childhood Takayasu's arteritis.[501] Anti–tumor necrosis factor therapy is a promising treatment option.[502]

In addition to pharmacologic therapy, surgical intervention is frequently required to alleviate end-organ ischemia and hypertension resulting from vascular stenoses.[503]

HEMOLYTIC UREMIC SYNDROME

Hemolytic uremic syndrome (HUS) is defined by the simultaneous occurrence of microangiopathic hemolytic anemia, thrombocytopenia, and acute renal failure.[504] The classical form, formerly known diarrhea-positive (D+) HUS, is caused by infectious agents. It accounts for 90% of all cases and is a common cause of acute kidney injury in young children. Atypical HUS (aHUS) is a rare condition that occurs without preceding diarrhea and is characterized by a recurrent course and frequent progression to ESKD.[504,505] In most patients with aHUS, genetic or acquired defects in the alternative complement pathway are found.[506-508]

SHIGA TOXIN–ASSOCIATED HEMOLYTIC UREMIC SYNDROME

Shiga toxin (Stx)–positive HUS usually occurs within 5 to 7 days of a prodromal episode of diarrhea that is frequently bloody. It is caused by infection with Stx-producing *Escherichia coli* (STEC) or *Shigella*,[509] with considerable regional variation in strain prevalence. In Argentina, where HUS is endemic, 1 in 25 children presenting with diarrhea is infected with STEC.[510] The organism is responsible for at least 70% of cases of D+ HUS in the United States, and 80% of these are caused by the O157:H7 serotype.[511] In Europe and other areas of the world, non-O157:H7 strains are emerging as important pathogens. The O111 serotype caused a large outbreak of hemorrhagic colitis and HUS in Australia and is also a common cause of disease in European children. *Shigella dysenteriae* type 1–associated HUS occurs in South Africa.[512]

Epidemiology

HUS principally affects children younger than 5 years. Only 5% to 10% of individuals infected with Stx-producing *E. coli* progress to HUS.[510,513] The incidence of D+ HUS in Germany and Austria is between 0.7 and 1/100,000 in children younger than 15 years and 1.5 to 1.9/100,000 in children younger than 5 years. Similarly, a Canadian surveillance study found an annual incidence of 1.1 cases/100,000 children younger than 16 years.[513] In Argentina, an annual incidence of 10.4 to 12.2/100,000 children younger than 5 years has been reported.[514]

Consumption of unpasteurized milk and undercooked beef is the primary cause of infection.[515] Secondary human to human contamination is also possible.[516] Although epidemics are notable, most cases of HUS due to STEC infection are sporadic. The largest STEC outbreak to date occurred in Germany in 2011, caused by contamination of sprouts with an *E. coli* strain (O104:H4) that showed features of STEC and enteroaggregative *E. coli*. 22% of the 3816 infected individuals developed HUS; of these, only 12% were children, probably due to the peculiar distribution chain of the contaminated food to restaurants.[517,518]

Pathogenesis

E. coli O157 can produce two different Shiga toxins. Stx1 is very similar to the type 1 toxin of *S. dysenteriae*. The expression of Stx2 strongly correlates with the occurrence of bloody diarrhea and HUS. Orally ingested Stx-producing bacteria attach to the intestinal mucosa and cause enterocyte effacement.[519] Stx is then transferred through the intestinal barrier and probably travels bound to leukocytes in the circulation.

Kidney biopsy specimens show a fibrin-rich glomerular microangiopathy, with apoptosis of glomerular and tubular cells.[519] The specific pathogenetic event in HUS is endothelial cell injury. Stx binds to glycosphingolipid globotriaosylceramide, a cell surface receptor present on glomerular endothelial cells, podocytes, and tubular epithelial cells. Toxins are internalized and inhibit protein synthesis by acting on the 28S eukaryotic ribosomal RNA, which results in cytokine release and apoptotic cell death.[519] Endothelial injury generates thrombin, and fibrin is deposited in the microvasculature. Concentrations of plasminogen activator inhibitor-1 rise. Plasminogen activator inhibitor-1 blocks fibrinolysis, which further accelerates the accumulation of fibrin in vessels and exacerbates the thrombotic injury.[509]

Furthermore, Stx increases endothelial cell expression of the chemokine receptor CXCR4 and its ligand stromal cell-derived factor 1 (SDF-1). Specific blockade of this ligand-receptor system ameliorates STEC-HUS in mice.[520] Plasma levels of SDF-1 are nearly fourfold higher in children with STEC enteritis who progress to HUS than in those who do not develop HUS,[520] raising hopes that SDF-1 could become a useful biomarker to predict patients prone to develop HUS.

Finally, complement activation plays a role in the pathogenesis of STEC-HUS.[521-523] Serum markers of alternative complement pathway activation are found to be increased during STEC-HUS episodes.[521] Experimentally, Stx induces activation and binding of C3 to endothelial cells, promoting thrombus formation on endothelial cells.[522] Factor B deficiency and treatment with a C3a antagonist were found to be partially protective in a murine HUS model.[522] Finally, Stx-induced activation of the alternative pathway of complement and generation of C3a promotes integrin-linked kinase signaling, leading to podocyte dysfunction and loss in Stx-HUS.[523] A mutation in the complement-regulating gene *MCP* was reported in a fatal case of STEC-HUS.[524]

Hemolytic anemia is believed to result from mechanical damage to red blood cells as they pass through the altered vasculature. Thrombocytopenia is caused by intrarenal and diffuse microvascular platelet adhesion or damage.[515]

Diagnosis

The diagnosis of Stx-associated HUS in children is based on the presence of microangiopathic hemolytic anemia, thrombocytopenia, and acute renal injury following a diarrheal prodrome (Table 74.7). About 3 days after ingestion of the organism, the patient develops diarrhea, abdominal pain, fever, and vomiting. In 80% to 90% of cases, the diarrhea turns bloody within 1 to 3 days.[509] Three criteria must be met to diagnose STEC infection: isolation of STEC strains, detection of free fecal Stx, and detection of circulating Stx antibodies.[514] Progression to HUS occurs in 5% to 15% of STEC enteritis cases. Bloody diarrhea and a high neutrophilic leukocytosis may indicate patients at increased risk of developing HUS.[510]

In the typical presentation, examination of a blood smear reveals helmet and burr cells and fragmented red blood cells (fragmentocytes). Plasma hemoglobin levels are elevated, whereas plasma haptoglobin becomes undetectable. Strikingly high levels of lactate dehydrogenase quantitatively reflect ongoing intravascular hemolysis. The Coombs test yields negative results. Significant leukocytosis is common, and thrombocytopenia is found in more than 90% of patients. The degree of anemia and thrombocytopenia do not predict disease severity.[525,526] By definition, all patients with STEC-HUS manifest some degree of renal insufficiency. Renal involvement may range from hematuria and proteinuria to oligoanuric acute renal failure. Marked hypertension is also common, and 30% to 40% of cases will require dialysis therapy; the prognosis for recovery of renal function is generally favorable. However, dialysis for more than 7 days is associated with worse long-term renal outcomes, and renal function rarely recovers substantially if the duration of dialysis is longer than 4 weeks.[527,528]

Microangiopathic lesions may also occur in organs other than the kidneys. Central nervous system symptoms (seizures, altered vision, hemiparesis) are observed in up to 25% of patients and are usually transient, although severe and even lethal courses have been reported.[529]

Treatment

No specific therapy has proven to affect the course of the disease in children. Supportive therapy during diarrhea and colitis (e.g., compensation for the electrolyte and water deficits) is most important to prevent an additional prerenal component during acute kidney injury. Use of antibiotics and antimotility drugs in children with confirmed or suspected *E. coli* O157:H7 infection during the bloody diarrheal phase is questionable due to the potentially increased risk of subsequent development of HUS. However, a meta-analysis has not shown a higher risk of HUS associated with antibiotic administration.[530] Approximately 50% of patients require dialysis during the course of the disease.[531] Peritoneal dialysis, hemodialysis, and slow dialysis–continuous renal replacement therapy appear to be equally effective.[532]

There are no published data to prove that plasma exchange positively affects the outcome of Stx-mediated HUS. A meta-analysis of seven RCTs involving 476 children with HUS concluded that supportive therapy, including dialysis, is still the most effective treatment for patients with postdiarrheal HUS.[533,534] The studied interventions included heparin and heparin with urokinase or dipyridamole, fresh-frozen plasma, glucocorticoids, and experimental therapy with a Stx-binding globotriaosylceramide receptor analog (Synsorb Pk). None of the assessed interventions was superior to supportive therapy alone as judged by all-cause mortality and the occurrence of neurologic and/or other extrarenal events, changes in renal biopsy specimens, proteinuria, or hypertension at the last follow-up visit.

Anticomplement 5 therapy with eculizumab was associated with rapid clinical improvement in three infants with fulminant STEC-HUS with extrarenal manifestations.[535]

Table 74.7 Features of Typical and Atypical Hemolytic Uremic Syndrome (HUS)

Parameter	Typical Diarrhea-Positive HUS	Atypical Diarrhea-Negative HUS
Cause	Shiga toxin–producing *Escherichia coli* or *Shigella*	Genetic (dysregulation of complement pathway due to mutations or autoantibodies) Infectious (*Streptococcus pneumoniae*) Metabolic (Cobalamin C synthase deficiency) Coagulation (von Willebrand factor–cleaving protease deficiency, DGKE) Drugs (quinine, possibly calcineurin inhibitors, ganciclovir, oral contraceptives, etc.) Rare reported associations include systemic lupus erythematosus, systemic sclerosis, bone marrow transplantation, leukemia
Age	Primarily <5 yr, but possible at any age	Preferentially infants and young children, but possible at any age
Seasonal preference	Summer	None
Onset	Sudden, mostly diarrheal prodrome	More insidious, no diarrhea, sometimes prodromal features like fever, vomiting
Outbreak	Yes, mostly sporadic	No
Clinical findings	Paleness, hematuria (microscopic) and proteinuria to severe renal failure and oligoanuria, edema, arterial hypertension, coma, and seizures	More severe clinical course (particularly renal insufficiency and hypertension)
Laboratory findings	Hemolytic anemia, hemoglobin <10 g/dL Fragmented erythrocytes Thrombocytopenia <150,000/mm^3 Increased serum creatinine Reduced serum haptoglobin Elevated lactate dehydrogenase	Laboratory findings of typical HUS plus: Low C3, elevated C3d Reduced CH50, factors H, D, I, B Mutations in genes for complement factors H, I, B, C3, membrane cofactor protein, thrombomodulin Factor H autoantibodies associated with CFHI/III gene deletions Low von Willebrand factor-cleaving protease activity/*ADAMTS13* mutations Elevated plasma homocysteine
Treatment	Mostly symptomatic (energetic fluid-electrolyte therapy, dialysis when required; rarely, plasma exchange in cases of severe clinical course with suspected complement system disorder)	Plasma exchange Eculizumab
Recurrence	Rare	Common
Prognosis	Generally favorable	Historically poor; some forms now improved with anti-C5 therapy

Eculizumab was subsequently used nonselectively without complement status testing in more than 200 adult patients during the 2011 German outbreak, but a clear short-term benefit could not be demonstrated in face of very good overall outcomes.[536,537]

Promising therapies under development include toxin binders (e.g., neutralizing monoclonal antibodies, receptor analogues, receptor synthase inhibitors), inhibitors of CXCR4/SDF-1 interaction (plerixafor [Mozobil]), and secondary therapies targeting downstream molecular events (e.g., inhibitors of caspase, mitogen-activated protein kinase, thrombin-platelet signaling).[532,538,539]

Prognosis

Spontaneous resolution usually begins 1 to 3 weeks after the onset of disease. With proper management, most patients show a favorable recovery. The hematologic manifestations of Stx HUS usually resolve within 1 to 2 weeks, and GFR returns to normal.

Overall mortality from D$^+$ HUS is around 4% to 9%, with most deaths occurring during the acute phase of the disease, mainly from extrarenal causes.[528,540] In a review encompassing 17 children who died from HUS, central nervous system involvement was the leading cause of death. Other causes included hyperkalemia, heart failure, and pulmonary hemorrhage. Patients who had lethargy, oligoanuria, dehydration, leukocyte count of more than 20,000/mm^3, and hematocrit less than 23% at presentation were at increased risk of death.[540]

The long-term renal prognosis of D$^+$ HUS was analyzed in a meta-analysis of 49 studies involving 3476 patients, with a mean follow-up of 4.4 years. The average mortality was 9%, incidence of ESKD was 3%, and incidence of residual renal damage was 25%. The latter figure included 15% of patients with proteinuria, 10% of patients with hypertension, and 8%, 6%, and 1.8% of those with a GFR of 50 to 80, 30 to 59, and 5 to 29 mL/min/1.73 m^2, respectively.[528]

The severity of the acute illness, particularly the presence of central nervous system symptoms and the need for initial dialysis, is strongly associated with a worse long-term prognosis.[528] Renal recovery will remain incomplete when dialysis is needed for longer than 4 weeks. In addition, prolonged oligoanuria (>5 days of anuria and >10 days of oliguria) and a white blood cell count of more than 20,000/mm^3 at presentation are risk factors for permanent renal dysfunction.[541]

Conversely, patients with an eGFR of more than 80 mL/min/1.73 m², are free of proteinuria, and are normotensive 1 year after having D⁺ HUS have an excellent long-term prognosis.[528] Therefore, further follow-up can probably be limited to children with proteinuria, hypertension, abnormal morphologic findings by ultrasonography, and/or impaired GFR at 1 year.[542]

ATYPICAL HEMOLYTIC UREMIC SYNDROME

Atypical HUS is an ultrarare disorder, with an estimated prevalence of 7 million children in Europe.[543] However, the condition may have been underdiagnosed in the past, and diagnosis rates appear to be increasing recently due to greater awareness and better understanding of its pathogenesis and genetic background. A wide variety of triggers have been identified, including nonenteric bacterial infections, viruses, drugs, and genetic, immunologic, and metabolic abnormalities (see Table 74.7). Atypical HUS occurs in familial and sporadic forms. Inherited and acquired alternative complement pathway regulator deficiencies are increasingly understood to have a pivotal role in the pathogenesis of the disorder.[507,526,544]

Streptococcus pneumoniae–Associated Hemolytic Uremic Syndrome

About 14% to 30% of aHUS cases occur following an infection with *Streptococcus pneumoniae*.[545,546] The clinical picture is unique and usually severe, with respiratory distress, anuria, neurologic involvement, and coma. Children with *S. pneumoniae*–associated HUS are generally younger, more likely to require dialysis, and have a higher mortality rate.[525,547] Cellular injury in *S. pneumoniae*–associated HUS is related to circulating bacterial neuraminidase, which exposes normally hidden Thomsen-Friedenreich T antigen on platelets and endothelial cell surfaces to preformed circulating IgM antibodies, with subsequent platelet aggregation and endothelial injury.[548] The outcome is strongly dependent on the effectiveness of antibiotic treatment. Plasma therapy is contraindicated because it delivers fresh antibodies against Thomsen-Friedenreich antigen, which may accelerate polyagglutination and hemolysis.[548]

Hemolytic Uremic Syndrome Due to Complement Disorders

Abnormalities affecting components of the complement regulatory system are the most common causative factor[526] in aHUS unrelated to *S. pneumoniae* infection (Figure 74.14).[515] These abnormalities are usually caused by mutations in complement system genes (components of C3 convertase [C3 and factor B] or its regulators [factor H, factor I, membrane cofactor protein, and thrombomodulin]), but autoimmune mechanisms may also be involved (anti–factor H antibodies).[549] The number of identified complement mutations has increased from 109 in 2008 to 604 in 2013.[550] Altogether, these abnormalities explain up to 70% of aHUS cases. Although the penetrance of complement mutation in aHUS is incomplete, and healthy mutation carriers are frequently found within families, genetic investigations are clinically useful because they allow the risk of posttransplantation disease recurrence, eligibility for liver transplantation and, possibly, the safety of withdrawing eculizumab treatment to be assessed.[551]

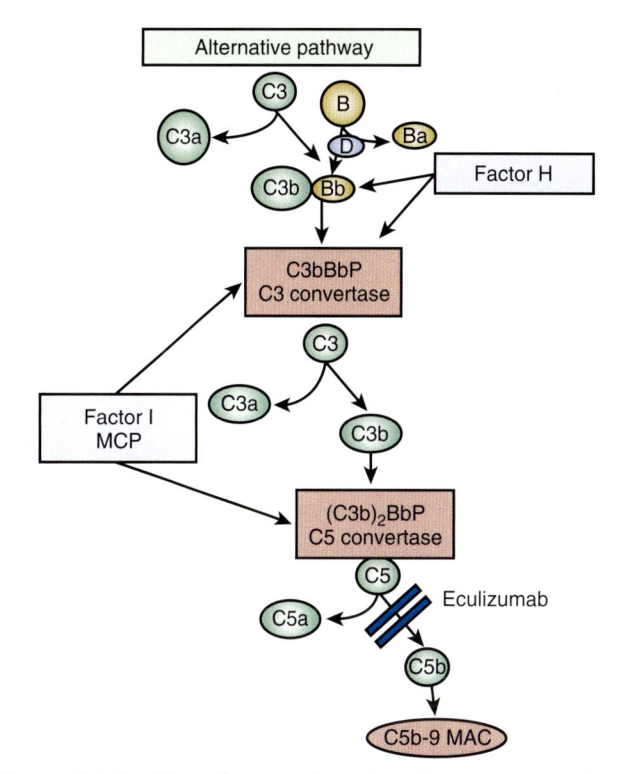

Figure 74.14 Alternative complement pathway and regulatory systems. Shown are inhibitors of the activated complement system and its action sites in the complement cascade. The inhibition site of the C5 antibody eculizumab, the first clinically available complement inhibitor, is indicated. (From Scheiring J, Rosales A, Zimmerhackl LB: Clinical practice: today's understanding of the haemolytic uraemic syndrome. *Eur J Pediatr* 169:7-13, 2010.)

The defective complement inactivation causes persistent endothelial damage after resolution of the activating event, which usually is a bacterial or viral infection, and explains the recurrent nature of aHUS. Persistently low C3 and more sensitively elevated C3d serum levels indicating alternative pathway activation are an important clue to the diagnosis of complement-mediated aHUS.[549]

The type of complement abnormality determines the clinical presentation, response to plasma therapy, and risk of recurrence before and after kidney transplantation.[526] Complement factor H is usually affected, generally by heterozygous mutations leading to altered synthesis or, more often, deficient C3-inactivating function of this circulating protein. Factor H–related aHUS usually presents during infancy or early childhood, although some cases with first manifestation in adult life have been observed.[552-554] Substitution of normal factor H by plasma exchange is effective in interrupting the disease process, but because of the short half-life of factor H (2 to 3 days), intense treatment is required, and relapses are common. More than 80% of patients with factor H–related aHUS progress to ESKD, and the risk of recurrence after transplantation is very high (30% to 100%).[526,544,554] Living donor transplantations should be avoided due to the high risk of recurrence of the disease in the patient and the potential risk of triggering the disease in the donor, who may be carrying an unrecognized genetic susceptibility factor.[506]

Neutralizing autoantibodies against factor H are an important alternative mechanism of factor H inactivation.

Factor H autoantibodies appear to arise in patients with deletions in the genes coding for complement factor H–related protein I or III.[526,555] In a multicenter cohort of 138 Indian children with anti–factor H antibody–associated HUS (56% of patients with HUS), combined plasma exchanges and induction immunosuppression comprised of prednisolone, with or without intravenous cyclophosphamide or rituximab, resulted in significantly improved renal survival and decreased antibody titers. Significant independent risk factors for adverse outcomes were an antibody titer greater than 8000 arbitray units (AU)/mL, low C3 level, and delay in plasma exchange.[554] Heterozygous and homozygous deletion of CFHR1 and CFHR3 through nonallelic homologous recombination events downstream of CFH is associated with an increased risk of aHUS.[556]

Mutations in complement factor I, the circulating co-factor for membrane co-factor protein and factor H, usually causes protein deficiency detectable by low circulating factor I levels. The clinical effect and response to plasma therapy are similar to those in factor H–mediated disease.[557]

Membrane co-factor protein is expressed on the surface of endothelial cells. The protein is part of the C3-inactivating complex. Mutations in the membrane co-factor protein gene lead to a loss of protein expression on all endothelial cell surfaces. Although plasma therapy is ineffective, the disease is often self-limited. In cases progressing to ESKD, the disease does not recur in transplanted kidneys, which have normal membrane co-factor protein expression.[557]

Atypical HUS can also be caused by mutations in complement factor C3. Since these mutations usually affect the factor H binding domain,[558] the disease course is similar to that in factor H mutations, with a recurrent progressive course and a very high risk of posttransplantation recurrence.[549]

Hemolytic Uremic Syndrome Due to von Willebrand Factor–Cleaving Protease Deficiency

Atypical HUS can also be caused by deficient activity of von Willebrand factor (vWF)–cleaving protease (ADAMTS13, a disintegrin-like metalloprotease with thrombospondin type 1 repeat motifs 13).[544,559] This protease normally degrades large vWF multimers. Accumulation of vWF multimers leads to systemic platelet activation and thrombosis.[525] Autosomal recessive vWF-cleaving protease deficiency is a very rare cause of childhood atypical HUS.[560] In adolescents and adults, autoantibodies against vWF-cleaving protease can be a cause of thrombotic microangiopathy.[561]

Hemolytic Uremic Syndrome Due to Cobalamin C Synthase Deficiency

Another important, most likely underdiagnosed, and treatable cause of atypical HUS in children is cobalamin C synthase deficiency.[562,563] This metabolic disorder is caused by mutations in the MMACHC (*m*ethyl*m*alonic *ac*iduria and *h*omocystinuria type *C* protein) gene and leads to excessively high endotheliotoxic plasma homocysteine levels. Supplementation of vitamin B_{12} and folic acid rapidly lowers plasma homocysteine to near-normal levels and reverses aHUS symptoms. Whereas initial case reports described disease onset at neonatal-onset aHUS, milder variants of the disease apparently can manifest in later childhood.[564] In view of the important therapeutic implications of diagnosing the disorder, plasma homocysteine screening should be part of the diagnostic workup of childhood atypical HUS.

Hemolytic Uremic Syndrome Due to Diacyl Glycerol Kinase ε Mutations

Recessive mutations in DGKE (encoding diacylglycerol kinase epsilon) that cosegregated with aHUS in nine unrelated kindreds were recently identified.[565] DGKE gene variants were also reported as the cause of a membranoproliferative-like glomerular microangiopathy.[566] DGKE is found in endothelium, platelets, and podocytes and attenuates intracellular protein kinase C (PKC) signaling by inactivating arachidonic acid–containing diacylglycerols. Loss of DGKE function results in a prothrombotic state. Affected individuals present with aHUS before 1 year of age. Episodes are usually self-limited, but patients develop persistent hypertension, hematuria, proteinuria (sometimes in the nephrotic range), and progressive CKD. ESKD usually occurs in the second decade of life.[565]

Treatment and Prognosis

Historically, plasma therapy has been the empirical first-line treatment in patients with aHUS.[567] Plasma exchange and sometimes even repetitive plasma infusions appear to have some beneficial effect in patients with mutations in factor H, factor I, C3, or factor B mutations.[526,557,567] However, in view of the short half-life of complement factors, plasma therapy needs to be performed at least two or three times a week to achieve and maintain sufficiently high serum concentrations.[567] In contrast, plasma therapy does not correct the underlying pathogenic defect in patients with mutations in the endothelial membrane co-factor protein (MCP) and has not been found to affect clinical outcomes in these patients.[567]

During the last 5 years, a dramatic improvement in the management of aHUS patients has been achieved by the introduction of an effective complement-inhibiting drug, the monoclonal antibody eculizumab, into clinical practice.[551] Eculizumab blocks complement activity by cleavage of the complement protein C5 and prevents the generation of the inflammatory peptide C5a and cytotoxic membrane attack complex (see Figure 74.14).[515]

In the pre-eculizumab era, patients with mutations in complement-regulating genes who showed no response to plasma therapy and/or had a recurrent course of disease were likely to progress to ESKD.[557] Historically, one third of patients died or progressed to ESKD following the initial disease manifestation, and two thirds did so within 12 months from disease onset. Eculizumab use has dramatically improved the prognosis of aHUS episodes and the disease overall.[508,551,568-571] Remarkable late improvement in renal function has been observed, even in CKD patients who had undergone chronic plasma therapy.[572] Consequently, eculizumab is now the recommended first-line therapy for children with aHUS while awaiting the results of diagnostic testing. In addition to being more effective than plasma therapy, eculizumab infusions avoid the risks and complications of plasma exchange and central venous catheters.[551]

If autoantibodies against factor H or ADAMTS13 are detected, eculizumab should be replaced by plasmapheresis using albumin substitution,[289] and immunosuppressive therapy should be initiated to prevent antibody restitution.[526]

The appropriate duration of costly eculizumab therapy in aHUS related to hereditary complement disorders is currently a matter of debate. In patients with mutations associated with poor outcomes *(CFH, C3, CFB)*, lifelong eculizumab treatment may be appropriate. By contrast, eculizumab therapy may reasonably be withdrawn in the subgroup of children with an isolated *MCP* mutation who have fully recovered from aHUS.[551]

Aytpical HUS patients undergoing kidney transplantation have a high risk of recurrence and graft loss.[549] In a series of 57 aHUS patients (two thirds confirmed complement mutation carriers) who received 71 renal allografts, death-censored 5-year graft survival was 51%.[573] For some genetic abnormalities, the recurrence risk is probably close to 100%. Consequently, patients with ESKD due to aHUS were historically often not considered candidates for transplantation. The advent of eculizumab has profoundly changed the outlook for this patient population.[508,569,570] Eculizumab is not only effective in reversing recurrent HUS after transplantation[572] but is also likely to prevent posttransplantation disease recurrence if administered prophylactically to high-risk patients.[508,569,570] Alternatively, since the bulk of circulating complement factors is synthesized by the liver, hepatic transplantation (or combined liver-kidney transplantation if ESKD is already established) may be considered for patients with confirmed genetic complement abnormalities as a curative treatment option.[549]

In patients with cobalamin C deficiency, lifelong vitamin B_{12} substitution may be required. No effective therapy exists for children with DGKE nephropathy. Since the disorder is not associated with abnormal complement activation, disease episodes are resistant to eculizumab, and the disease does not recur after transplantation.[574]

Other previously applied therapeutic modalities, such as antiplatelet agents, heparin or fibrinolytic agents, steroids, and intravenous immunoglobulins, are not effective in aHUS.[526]

PEDIATRIC ASPECTS OF CHRONIC KIDNEY DISEASE

GROWTH, NUTRITION, AND DEVELOPMENT

Impaired statural growth and sexual development are among the most obvious and important complications of CKD in childhood. Growth retardation and delayed maturation can interfere markedly with psychosocial adjustment and are mentioned most consistently by young adult survivors of childhood-onset CKD as major factors compromising their social integration and subjective quality of life.

PATTERNS OF GROWTH FAILURE IN CHRONIC KIDNEY DISEASE

The impact of uremia and its sequelae on statural growth depends on the age at first manifestation of CKD. One third of total postnatal growth occurs during the first 2 years of life. Therefore, any circumstances affecting growth rates during infancy will cause rapid and severe growth retardation. During the first year of life, as much as 1 standard deviation (SD) of relative height can be lost within 2 months of untreated uremia.[575] Between the second year of life and onset of puberty, growth inhibition is more subtle. Growth patterns typically remain stable along the normal percentiles as long as GFR remains higher than 25 mL/min/1.73 m^2 but gradually deviate from the normal range in CKD stages 4 and 5[576] (Figure 74.15). However, even in children with reduced absolute height who appear to be growing normally along a given height percentile, successful kidney transplantation may result in catch-up growth into the normal range as optimal growth conditions are restored, which suggests persistent suppression of growth potential in the uremic state.

The onset of clinical signs of puberty, as well as the start of the pubertal growth spurt, occur with a delay of up to 2 years, depending on the degree of renal dysfunction.[577] Pubertal height gain is diminished by up to 50% (from 30 to 15 cm) in adolescents with ESKD. Final adult heights below the normal range are attained by 30% to 50% of children with CKD, although a trend of improving final heights has been noted during the past decade. The duration of CKD, presence of a congenital nephropathy, and male gender are among the most important predictors of a reduced final height.[575]

CAUSES OF GROWTH FAILURE AND DEVELOPMENTAL DELAY IN CHRONIC KIDNEY DISEASE

During infancy, growth depends largely on nutritional and metabolic factors. Growth failure in infants with CKD usually is caused by inadequate spontaneous intake of nutrients due to anorexia and frequent vomiting. Reduced spontaneous energy intake resulting from uremic anorexia starts to impair growth rates when it falls below 70% to 80% of the recommended dietary allowance. The almost inevitable anorexia and wasting in infants with CKD may or may not be related to a subclinical state of microinflammation, as found in adult patients.[578] Additional factors contributing to vomiting and anorexia include the accumulation of circulating satiety factors and the frequent general retardation of psychomotor development in uremia. Gastric emptying is abnormally slow. Fluid and electrolyte losses due to tubular dysfunction in dysplastic kidney disorders and catabolic episodes related to intercurrent infections may also play a role in worsening infantile growth failure.

Metabolic acidosis, which usually occurs when GFR is below 50% of normal, contributes to CKD-associated growth failure by various mechanisms, including increased protein breakdown, suppressed secretion of GH and insulin-like growth factor-1 (IGF-1), as well as impaired GH and IGF-1 receptor expression in target tissues. Hence, metabolic acidosis in CKD induces a state of GH insufficiency and insensitivity.[575]

Independent of metabolic acidosis, the endocrine systems show a complex dysregulation in the uremic state. Circulating GH levels are normal or increased due to impaired metabolic clearance, but the actual rate of GH secretion from the pituitary is diminished.[579] GH-induced IGF-1 synthesis is impaired in uremia due to impaired activation of the GH-dependent JAK2/STAT5 (Janus kinase 2/signal transducer and activator of transcription-5) signaling

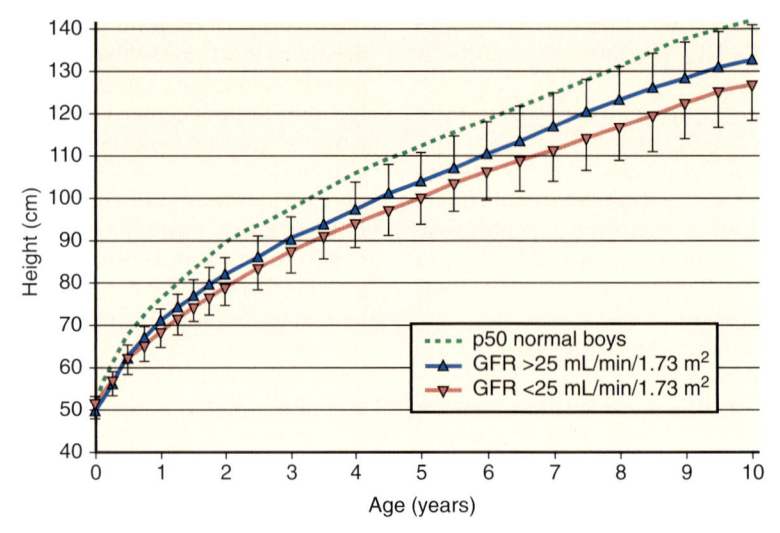

Figure 74.15 Glomerular filtration rate (GFR)–dependent growth pattern in children with chronic renal failure due to hypodysplastic renal disorders. Approximately 100 children per age interval were evaluated. Mean ± 1 standard deviation (SD) of height is shown for children with an average GFR more or less than 25 mL/min/1.73 m². (Adapted from Schaefer F, Wingen AM, Hennicke M, et al: Growth charts for prepubertal children with chronic renal failure due to congenital renal disorders. European Study Group for Nutritional Treatment of Chronic Renal Failure in Childhood. *Pediatr Nephrol* 10:288-293, 1996.)

pathway[580] (Figure 74.16). This postreceptor signaling defect may be caused by upregulation of inhibitory suppressors of STAT signaling (SOCS [suppressor of cytokine signaling] proteins), which are induced by inflammatory cytokines in the uremic state. In addition, accumulation of IGF-1–binding proteins results in a molar excess of IGF-binding proteins relative to circulating IGFs, which results in reduced IGF bioactivity. Finally, the normal or reduced GH secretion in the presence of markedly reduced IGF-1 bioactivity is compatible with an insufficient feedback activation of the somatotropic hormone axis at the hypothalamic and pituitary levels. In summary, these findings indicate multilevel homeostatic failure of the GH–IGF-1 system, which may in part be related to chronic inflammation.

The gonadotropic hormone axis is subject to a similarly impaired activation in CKD.[579] Peripubertal patients with advanced renal disease or ESKD exhibit normal or low sex steroid levels in the presence of elevated levels of circulating gonadotropins. The elevation of circulating gonadotropins is explained by impaired metabolic hormone clearance, whereas pituitary secretion rates are low, possibly due to impaired hypothalamic GnRH secretion related to increased inhibitory neurotransmitter tone. In addition to deficient central nervous activation, there is accumulation of circulating factors that inhibit GnRH release from the hypothalamus and testosterone release from Leydig cells. Finally, the crosstalk between gonadotropic and somatotropic hormones during puberty appears to be impaired, as evidenced by a blunted surge of GH secretion in response to rising sex steroid levels. Hence, uremia appears to cause a state of multiple endocrine resistance, effectively inhibiting longitudinal growth and sexual development.

PREVENTION AND TREATMENT OF GROWTH FAILURE IN CHRONIC KIDNEY DISEASE

In infants with CKD, the most important measures for avoiding uremic growth failure are the provision of adequate

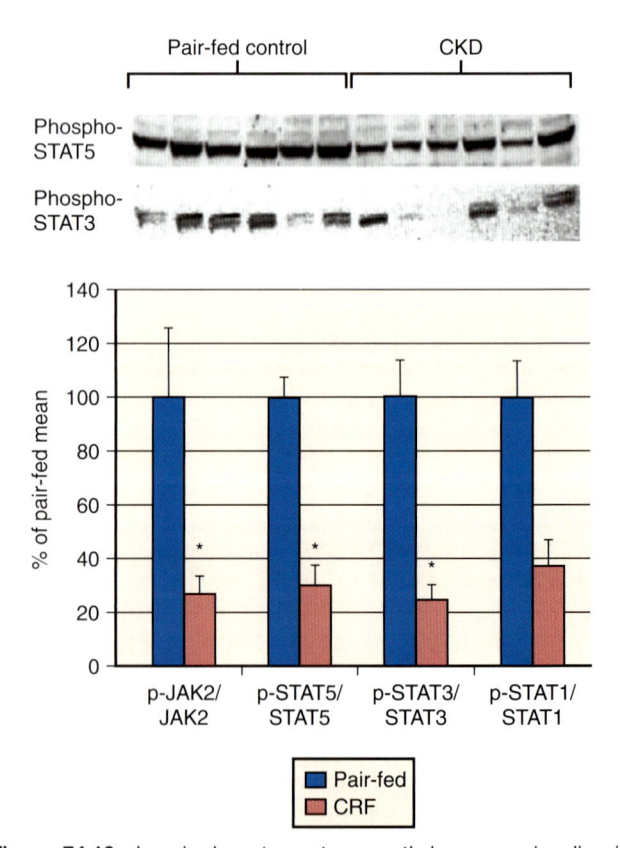

Figure 74.16 Impaired postreceptor growth hormone signaling in rats with experimental uremia. **Top,** Deficient nuclear accumulation of tyrosine-phosphorylated STAT5 (signal transducer and activator of transcription-5) and STAT3 protein on growth hormone stimulation in livers of rats with chronic kidney disease (CKD) compared with pair-fed controls. **Bottom,** Reduced hepatic phosphorylation of JAK2 (Janus kinase 2), STAT5, STAT3, and STAT1 in uremic rats. (From Schaefer F, Chen Y, Tsao T, et al: Impaired JAK-STAT signal transduction contributes to growth hormone resistance in chronic uremia. *J Clin Invest* 108:467-475, 2001.)

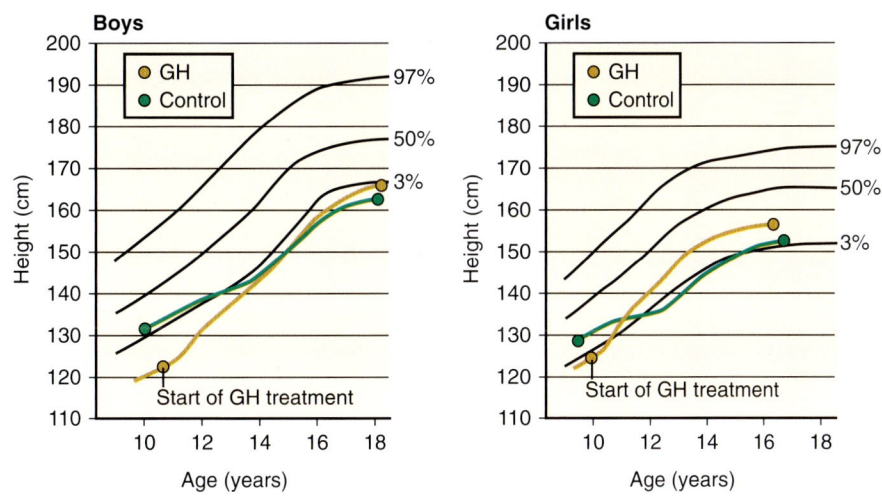

Figure 74.17 Favorable effects of long-term recombinant human growth hormone (GH) therapy on final adult height in children with chronic kidney disease (CKD). Synchronized mean growth curves are shown for 38 children (32 boys and 6 girls) with CKD who were treated with GH and for 50 control children with CKD who did not receive GH. Normal values are indicated by the 3rd, 50th, and 97th percentiles. The *circles* indicate the time of the first observation (the start of GH treatment in the treated children) and the end of the pubertal growth spurt. (Haffner D, Schaefer F, Nissel R, et al: Effect of growth hormone treatment on the adult height of children with chronic renal failure. German Study Group for Growth Hormone Treatment in Chronic Renal Failure. *N Engl J Med* 343:923-930, 2000.)

energy intake, correction of metabolic acidosis, and maintenance of fluid and electrolyte balance.[581] Supplementary feedings via nasogastric tube or gastrostomy are frequently required to achieve these targets.

Caloric intake should be targeted to provide 80% to 100% of the regular daily allowance for healthy children. Increasing caloric intake above 100% of the recommended daily allowance does not induce further catch-up growth but rather results in obesity, with a potential adverse impact on long-term cardiovascular health. Protein intake should be at least 100% of the dietary reference intake but should not exceed 140% of the dietary reference intake in patients with CKD stage 2 or 3 and 120% of the reference intake in children with CKD stage 4 or 5. Excessive protein intake should be avoided in advancing CKD to limit phosphorus and acid load in patients with failing kidney function. Moderate protein restriction is safe with respect to the preservation of growth and nutritional status.[582]

Metabolic acidosis should be rigorously treated by oral alkaline supplementation. In addition, the supplementation of water and electrolytes is essential for children with polyuria and/or salt-losing nephropathies. Water and electrolyte losses are very common and are frequently underestimated in children with hypoplastic and dysplastic renal malformations.

Early and consistent provision of supplementary nutrients, fluids, and electrolytes, with delivery ensured by enteral feeding via a nasogastric tube or percutaneous gastrostomy whenever necessary, has markedly improved the growth and development of young children with CKD.[575,583] In the postinfantile phase of childhood, nutrition, fluid, and electrolyte balance continue to be permissive factors for adequate longitudinal growth, but catch-up growth can rarely be provided by dietary and supplementary measures alone. If growth failure is imminent and/or has already occurred, despite adequate provision of nutrients, salts, and fluid, then treatment with recombinant growth hormone (rGH) is a viable option. The efficacy and safety of rGH therapy in children with CKD have been demonstrated in numerous short- and long-term trials. The administration of rGH at pharmacologic dosages (0.05 mg/kg/day subcutaneously) overcomes endogenous GH resistance and markedly increases systemic and local IGF-1 production, with only a slight effect on IGF-binding proteins. This restores normal IGF-1 bioactivity and stimulates longitudinal growth. In children with predialytic CKD, height velocity typically doubles in the first treatment year, and a steady albeit less marked catch-up growth is observed during subsequent years of therapy. Long-term studies have demonstrated mean standardized height increases of −2.6 to −0.7 SD in North American children, −3.4 to −1.9 SD in German children, and −3.0 to −0.5 SD in Dutch children after 5 to 6 treatment years.[575]

The therapeutic response to rGH in CKD patients is superior to that observed in children who are undergoing dialysis or who have undergone kidney transplantation, probably due to a more marked uremic GH resistance in ESKD and the growth-suppressive effect of glucocorticoids in renal allograft recipients. In patients receiving rGH studied at around 9 to 10 years of age and followed through puberty until attainment of final height, catch-up growth was largely limited to the prepubertal period[584] (Figure 74.17). Final height was markedly improved in comparison with an untreated control group, with an overall benefit attributable to rGH treatment of 10 to 15 cm. Total height gain was positively correlated with the duration of rGH therapy and was negatively affected by the time spent on dialysis. These experiences permit one to conclude that rGH therapy should be initiated as early as possible in the predialytic CKD period, preferentially before severe growth retardation has occurred.

CARDIOVASCULAR COMORBIDITY IN PEDIATRIC CHRONIC KIDNEY DISEASE

A common assumption in cardiovascular medicine is that high blood pressure and other risk factors identified in

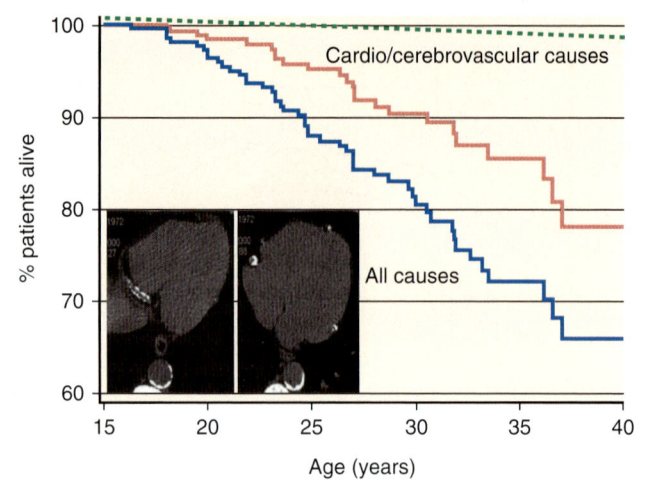

Figure 74.18 Long-term survival of 283 patients with childhood-onset ESKD. *Green dotted line,* Survival rate considering all causes of death. *Red line,* Survival rate considering cardiovascular and cerebrovascular causes of death only. *Blue line,* Survival rate in the general population. *Inset,* CT sections from 27-year-old male hemodialysis patient with extensive calcification in all three coronary arteries and aorta. (From Oh J, Wunsch R, Turzer M, et al: Advanced coronary and carotid arteriopathy in young adults with childhood-onset chronic renal failure. *Circulation* 106:100-105, 2002.)

adult populations affect only older adults. However, CKD-associated cardiovascular disease is present already in childhood and manifests relatively early in the course of CKD,[585] leading to significant morbidity and mortality from cardiovascular causes when ESKD has developed, even during childhood (Figure 74.18).[586] Among individuals younger than 19 years of age with ESKD, cardiac disease is responsible for 22 deaths/1000 patient-years, accounting for 16% of all deaths in whites and 26% in African Americans. This represents up to a 1000-fold increase in risk compared with that in the general population.

HYPERTENSION

CKD is the most common reason for arterial hypertension in childhood. The prevalence of hypertension is around 40% to 50% in children with CKD stages 2 to 4 and approaches 90% by the time ESKD has developed. High blood pressure is associated with target organ damage during childhood and is closely related to the rate of progression of renal failure.

CKD-associated hypertension develops by a variety of pathophysiologic mechanisms.[587] Fluid overload and activation of the RAAS are certainly crucial in this process, and sympathetic hyperactivation, endothelial dysfunction, and chronic hyperparathyroidism are likely to contribute to pediatric nephropathies as they do in adult kidney disorders.

The definition of arterial hypertension in the pediatric population is a challenging issue. Blood pressure increases physiologically by approximately 30 mm Hg over the course of childhood. Furthermore, at any given age, blood pressure also depends on relative body size. Due to the low mortality and long time lag to cardiovascular complications, hard clinical outcome criteria are not available to define critical cutoff blood pressure values in children. Therefore, childhood hypertension is defined based on the distribution of blood pressure in the general population matched for age, gender, and height. Hypertension is defined as a systolic and/or diastolic blood pressure that on at least three occasions is greater than or equal to the 95th percentile for age, gender, and height. Blood pressure values of more than 5 mm Hg above the 99th percentile define stage 2 hypertension. Values from the 90th to 95th percentile at any blood pressure level at or above 120/80 mm Hg are termed *prehypertension*.[588] It is important to note that children may be hypertensive at absolute blood pressure values that may not seem high by adult standards. For example, a blood pressure of 120/75 mm Hg represents severe stage 2 hypertension in a 2-year-old, stage 1 hypertension in a 7-year-old, and prehypertension in an 11-year-old of average height. Altered circadian blood pressure patterns, as described in adult patients with CKD, can be detected by ambulatory blood pressure monitoring in children.[589] Approximately 10% of children with CKD have so-called masked hypertension—that is, elevated blood pressure with 24-hour monitoring despite normal office readings, a condition associated with an increased prevalence of left ventricular hypertrophy.[590] Various online calculators are available to compare the blood pressure of a child of a given gender, age, and height with that in the normal population (e.g., www.pediatriconcall.com/fordoctor/pedcalc/bp.aspx).

Current management guidelines recommend regular blood pressure screening for all children with CKD.[591] In addition to clinic measurements, ambulatory blood pressure monitoring should be performed at least once a year and within 1 to 2 months of modification of therapy in patients receiving antihypertensive medication. Children with CKD should be considered at increased risk for cardiovascular complications, and therapeutic interventions should be initiated when blood pressure exceeds the 90th percentile for age and height. Interventions should aim at achieving a 24-hour blood pressure well below the 75th percentile.[591] Lifestyle changes such as increased physical activity, avoidance of salty foods, and reduction of weight in obese patients are also recommended for children with CKD but are rarely effective as sole measures.[587] ACE inhibitors and angiotensin receptor blockers should be the first choice of antihypertensive medications (see later, "Progression of Chronic Renal Failure in Children") and, if given at appropriate dosages (e.g., ramipril 6 mg/m^2/day[592] or candesartan 0.2 to 0.4 mg/kg/day[593]), will normalize blood pressure in most patients. If the blood pressure–lowering effect is insufficient, a loop diuretic should be added (e.g., furosemide, 2 to 4 mg/kg/day), followed by a calcium channel antagonist (e.g., amlodipine, 0.2 mg/kg/day). The timing of drug dosing should be adapted to achieve optimal blood pressure control throughout 24 hours as verified by ambulatory blood pressure monitoring.

INTERMEDIATE CARDIOVASCULAR END POINTS IN CHILDREN WITH CHRONIC KIDNEY DISEASE

Left ventricular hypertrophy (LVH) and increased carotid intima-media thickness have been demonstrated not only in hypertensive children with advanced CKD, in whom alterations of mineral metabolism and volume overload are important superimposed risk factors, but also in children with early essential hypertension and even in children with masked hypertension. LVH is the most common identifiable

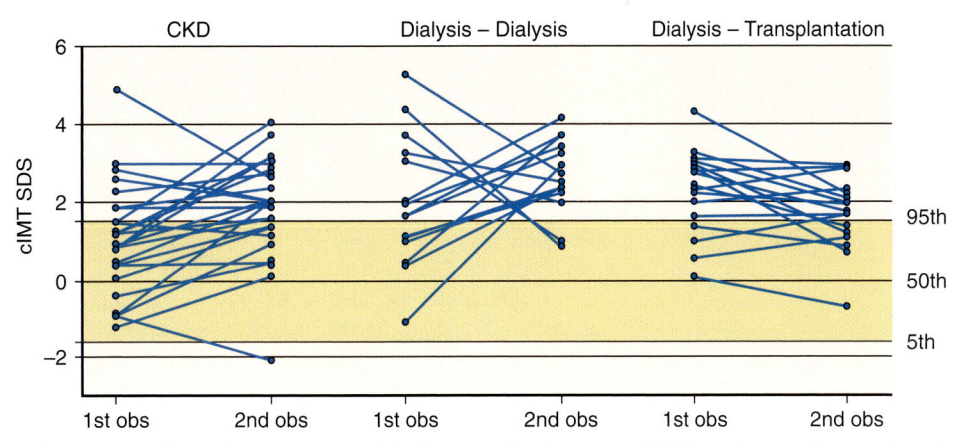

Figure 74.19 Change in sonographically determined carotid intima-media thickness (cIMT) in children with chronic kidney disease, children undergoing dialysis, and children who underwent kidney transplantation. Mean time interval between the first and second observations (obs) was 12 months. IMT is expressed as a standard deviation (SD) score normalized for age and gender. *Shaded area* denotes normal range, with SDs of −1.64, 0, and +1.64 corresponding to the 5th, 50th, and 95th percentiles. cIMT SDS, Change in Intima media thickness standard deviation score. (From Litwin M, Wühl E, Jourdan C, et al: Evolution of large-vessel arteriopathy in pediatric patients with chronic kidney disease. *Nephrol Dial Transplant* 23:2552-2557, 2008.)

cardiac alteration in CKD and the most important indicator of cardiovascular risk in adult and pediatric patients with ESKD.[594-597] LVH is believed to contribute to the high risk of sudden cardiac death in children with CKD due to lethal arrhythmias brought about by myocardial fibrosis and cellular hypertrophy. LVH is present in approximately 15% to 30% of children with stage 2 to 4 CKD,[598,599] in 50% to 75% of children undergoing dialysis,[600,601] and in 50% to 67% of renal allograft recipients.[602,603] Concentric and eccentric changes of left ventricular geometry are observed, which suggests that volume- and pressure-related pathogenic mechanisms are operative.[604] An increase in circulating volume early in CKD might be brought about by hyperactivation of the RAAS and sympathetic nervous system. Moreover, some evidence has indicated that nonhemodynamic mechanisms affect left ventricular growth and function in CKD, including hyperparathyroidism, inflammatory cytokines, and other autocrine and paracrine pathways. In addition to these morphologic changes, a subclinical impairment of left ventricular systolic function is found in about 25% of children with mild to moderate CKD.[605] Systolic dysfunction is most common in patients with concentric LVH and is associated with a low GFR and anemia.

Moreover, increasing evidence in children, as in adults, has suggested that the CKD-associated bone mineral disorder and its treatment not only affects bone and mineral metabolism but also contributes to the development of calcifying uremic vasculopathy. This is a consequence of a redistribution of mineral salts from the skeleton to the large arteries and soft tissue compartments. Coronary artery calcifications are found in individual adolescent patients undergoing dialysis[606] and in more than 90% of young adults with childhood-onset CKD[586] (see Figure 74.18). Early signs of vasculopathy, such as an increased intima-media thickness and stiffness of the carotid artery, can be detected as early as the second decade of life.[607] Both morphologic and functional alterations are progressive over time and are most marked in adolescents undergoing dialysis, but they also may be seen in children with moderate CKD and appear to improve partially after successful renal transplantation (Figure 74.19). Intima-media thickness and stiffness of the carotid artery correlate with the degree of hyperparathyroidism, serum calcium-phosphorus ion product, and cumulative dose of calcium-containing phosphate binders.

PROGRESSION OF CHRONIC RENAL FAILURE IN CHILDREN

COURSE OF RENAL FUNCTION IN CHILDREN WITH CHRONIC KIDNEY DISEASE

The course of renal function in pediatric CKD is mainly determined by the age and degree of renal failure at the time of first disease manifestation. Two thirds of children with CAKUT progress to ESKD during the first 2 decades of life.[608] The physiologic early increase in GFR is typically extended to the first 3 to 4 years of life, which potentially reflects an adaptive hypertrophy of the reduced number of functioning nephrons.[609] In approximately 50% of children, this early incremental phase is followed by a period of stable or very slowly deteriorating renal function, which usually lasts for 5 to 8 years. Around the onset of puberty, the GFR loss tends to accelerate, typically leading to ESKD in late adolescence or early adulthood (Figure 74.20). The reasons for this nonlinear progression of renal failure are incompletely understood and may include an insufficient capacity of the nephrons to adapt to the rapidly growing metabolic needs during the pubertal growth spurt, adverse renal effects of puberty-related increases in sex steroid production, and/or an accelerated sclerotic degeneration of a diminishing number of remnant hyperfiltering nephrons. In children with very severe renal hypoplasia, the early increase in GFR may be blunted, and early progression to ESKD may occur instead. About 20% of patients with renal hypoplasia maintain a stable GFR, even beyond puberty. Follow-up studies have shown that in patients with mild bilateral renal hypoplasia, progressive deterioration of GFR frequently ensues in the third decade of life.

RISK FACTORS FOR PROGRESSIVE RENAL FAILURE AND PHARMACOLOGIC NEPHROPROTECTION

Among the numerous factors predicting progressive renal failure in adult populations and in animal models,

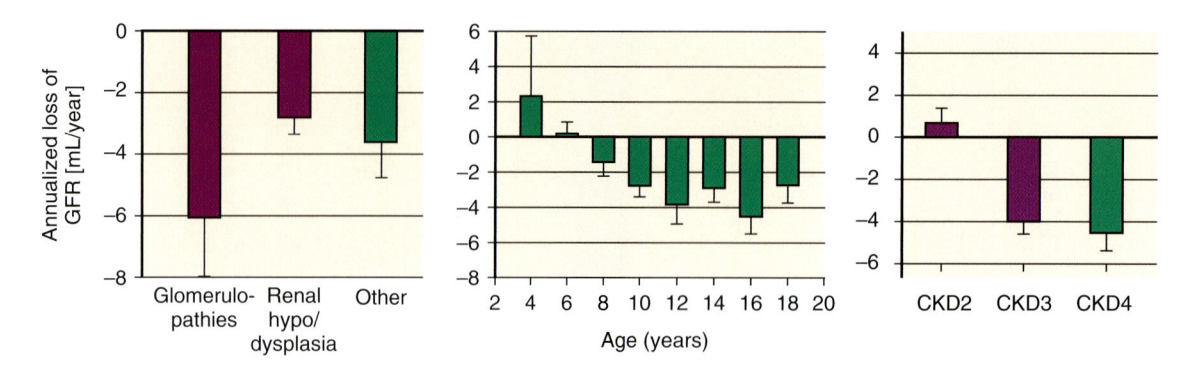

Figure 74.20 Mean spontaneous change in estimated glomerular filtration rate (GFR) in 385 children with chronic kidney disease (CKD) randomly assigned to treatment conditions in the ESCAPE trial (measured during the run-in period). The rate of renal failure progression in children depends on underlying renal disease, age, and CKD stage.

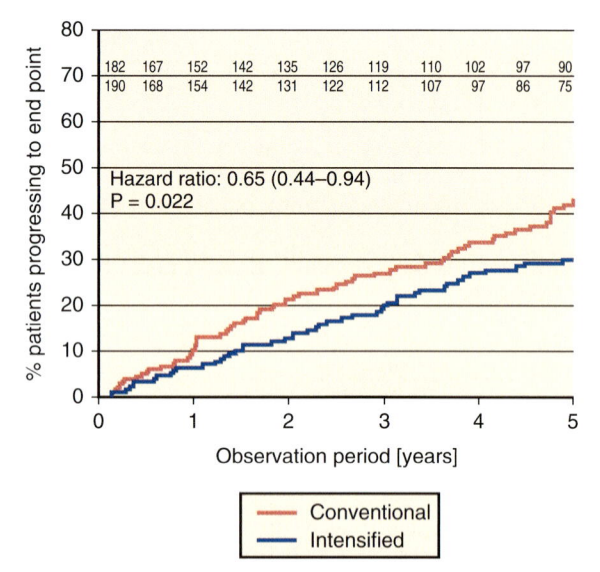

Figure 74.21 Effect of intensified blood pressure control on renal survival in children with chronic kidney disease (CKD). Within 5 years, 30% of patients randomly assigned to intensive control with a low-normal, 24-hour blood pressure target reached the end point of 50% glomerular filtration rate (GFR) loss or end-stage kidney disease (ESKD), compared with 42% of patients assigned to standard control with a conventional blood pressure target. (Data from Wühl E, Trivelli A, Matteucci MC, et al: Strict blood pressure control and progression of renal failure in children. N Engl J Med 361:1639-1650, 2009.)

hypertension and proteinuria have also been identified as consistent, modifiable, risk factors in children. In the European Study for Nutritional Treatment of Chronic Renal Failure in Childhood, a systolic blood pressure greater than 120 mm Hg was associated with a significantly faster decline of GFR.[582] The randomized, prospective ESCAPE trial (Effect of Strict Blood Pressure Control and ACE Inhibition on the Progression of CRF in Pediatric Patients) demonstrated that in children with CKD due to various disorders, intensified antihypertensive treatment forcing blood pressure into the low-normal range (<50th percentile for age) was associated with improved long-term renal survival[610] (Figure 74.21). Proteinuria is predictive of CKD progression in children, as it is in adult populations. Proteinuria predicts renal disease progression in children with renal hypodysplasia and, even in children with normal kidney function, persistent nephrotic-range proteinuria is a risk factor for progressive renal injury. In the ESCAPE trial, for children receiving fixed-dose ACE inhibitors, residual proteinuria proved to be predictive of CKD progression, despite treatment. These findings provide a strong rationale for the early and consistent application of RAAS antagonist treatment protocols.[610]

Both ACE inhibitors and angiotensin receptor blockers have been shown to be safe and effective in children with CKD. Ramipril, administered at a dosage of 6 mg/m^2/day, normalized blood pressure and lowered proteinuria by approximately 50% in the ESCAPE trial patients.[592] Similar results have been obtained with the angiotensin receptor blockers losartan,[277,611] valsartan,[612] and candesartan.[593] It should be noted, however, that the renoprotective superiority of RAAS antagonists over other antihypertensive agents has not been formally demonstrated in pediatric CKD. Data from the ItalKid registry did not show significant modification of CKD progression by ACE inhibitor treatment in children with hypodysplastic kidney disease compared with matched untreated subjects.[613] However, no information regarding the type and dosages of ACE inhibitors used and prevailing degree of proteinuria was available, and the baseline progression rate was very slow.

Another important observation in the ESCAPE trial was a gradual return of proteinuria, despite ongoing ACE inhibitor treatment. This effect was dissociated from persistently excellent blood pressure control and might limit the long-term renoprotective efficacy of ACE inhibitor monotherapy in pediatric CKD.[610]

Complete reference list available at ExpertConsult.com.

KEY REFERENCES

3. Schwartz GJ, Muñoz A, Schneider MF, et al: New equations to estimate GFR in children with CKD. *J Am Soc Nephrol* 20:629–637, 2009.
8. Wiesel A, Queisser-Luft A, Clementi M, et al: EUROSCAN Study Group: prenatal detection of congenital renal malformations by fetal ultrasonographic examination: an analysis of 709,030 births in 12 European countries. *Eur J Med Genet* 48:131–144, 2005.
18. Kerecuk L, Schreuder MF, Woolf AS: Renal tract malformations: perspectives for nephrologists. *Nat Clin Pract Nephrol* 4:312–325, 2008.
26. Wadie GM, Moriarty KP: The impact of vesicoureteral reflux treatment on the incidence of urinary tract infection. *Pediatr Nephrol* 27:529–538, 2012.

38. Williams G, Craig JC: Long-term antibiotics for preventing recurrent urinary tract infection in children. *Cochrane Database Syst Rev* (3):CD001534, 2011.
39. RIVUR Trial Investigators; Hoberman A, Greenfield SP, et al: Antimicrobial prophylaxis for children with vesicoureteral reflux. *N Engl J Med* 370:2367–2376, 2014.
46. Tekgül S, Riedmiller H, Hoebeke P, et al: European Association of Urology: EAU guidelines on vesicoureteral reflux in children. *Eur Urol* 62:534–542, 2012.
47. Elder JS, Diaz M: Vesicoureteral reflux—the role of bladder and bowel dysfunction. *Nat Rev Urol* 10:640–648, 2013.
60. Mei H, Pu J, Yang C, et al: Laparoscopic versus open pyeloplasty for ureteropelvic junction obstruction in children: a systematic review and meta-analysis. *J Endourol* 25:727–736, 2011.
133. Cadnapaphornchai MA, Masoumi A, Strain JD, et al: Magnetic resonance imaging of kidney and cyst volume in children with ADPKD. *Clin J Am Soc Nephrol* 6:369–376, 2011.
141. Cadnapaphornchai MA, George DM, McFann K, et al: Effect of pravastatin on total kidney volume, left ventricular mass index, and microalbuminuria in pediatric autosomal dominant polycystic kidney disease. *Clin J Am Soc Nephrol* 9:889–896, 2014.
153. Devuyst O, Knoers NV, Remuzzi G, et al: Board of the Working Group for Inherited Kidney Diseases of the European Renal Association and European Dialysis and Transplant Association: Rare inherited kidney diseases: challenges, opportunities, and perspectives. *Lancet* 383:1844–1859, 2014.
167. Gee HY, Ashraf S, Wan X, et al: Mutations in EMP2 cause childhood-onset nephrotic syndrome. *Am J Hum Genet* 94:884–890, 2014.
172. Benoit G, Machuca E, Antignac C: Hereditary nephrotic syndrome: a systematic approach for genetic testing and a review of associated podocyte gene mutations. *Pediatr Nephrol* 25:1621–1632, 2010.
173. Caridi G, Trivelli A, Sanna-Cherchi S, et al: Familial forms of nephrotic syndrome. *Pediatr Nephrol* 25:241–252, 2010.
175. Has C, Spartà G, Kiritsi D, et al: Integrin alpha3 mutations with kidney, lung, and skin disease. *N Engl J Med* 366:1508–1514, 2012.
177. Lal MA, Tryggvason K: Knocking out podocyte rho GTPases: and the winner is. *J Am Soc Nephrol* 23:1128–1129, 2012.
178. Mele C, Iatropoulos P, Donadelli R, et al: PodoNet Consortium: MYO1E mutations and childhood familial focal segmental glomerulosclerosis. *N Engl J Med* 365:295–306, 2011.
179. Gee HY, Saisawat P, Ashraf S, et al: ARHGDIA mutations cause nephrotic syndrome via defective RHO GTPase signaling. *J Clin Invest* 123:3243–3253, 2013.
181. Heeringa SF, Chernin G, Chaki M, et al: COQ6 mutations in human patients produce nephrotic syndrome with sensorineural deafness. *J Clin Invest* 121:2013–2024, 2011.
183. Ashraf S, Gee HY, Woerner S, et al: ADCK4 mutations promote steroid-resistant nephrotic syndrome through CoQ10 biosynthesis disruption. *J Clin Invest* 123:5179–5189, 2013.
196. Bouchireb K, Boyer O, Gribouval O, et al: NPHS2 mutations in steroid-resistant nephrotic syndrome: a mutation update and the associated phenotypic spectrum. *Hum Mutat* 35:178–186, 2014.
207. Lipska BS, Iatropoulos P, Maranta R, et al: PodoNet Consortium: Genetic screening in adolescents with steroid-resistant nephrotic syndrome. *Kidney Int* 84:206–213, 2013.
213. Lombel RM, Hodson E, Gipson DS: Kidney disease: improving global outcomes: treatment of steroid-resistant nephrotic syndrome in children: new guidelines from KDIGO. *Pediatr Nephrol* 28:409–414, 2013.
214. Lombel RM, Gipson DS, Hodson E: Kidney disease: improving global outcomes: treatment of steroid-sensitive nephrotic syndrome: new guidelines from KDIGO. *Pediatr Nephrol* 28:415–426, 2013.
231. Pickering MC, D'Agati VD, Nester CM, et al: C3 glomerulopathy: consensus report. *Kidney Int* 84:1079–1089, 2013.
236. Pravitsitthikul N, Willis NS, Hodson EM, et al: Non-corticosteroid immunosuppressive medications for steroid sensitive nephrotic syndrome in children. *Cochrane Database Syst Rev* (10):CD002290, 2013.
251. Sinha A, Bagga A: Rituximab therapy in nephrotic syndrome: implications for patients' management. *Nat Rev Nephrol* 9:154–169, 2013.
260. Iijima K, Sako M, Nozu K, et al: Rituximab for Childhood-onset Refractory Nephrotic Syndrome (RCRNS) Study Group: Rituximab for childhood-onset, complicated, frequently relapsing nephrotic syndrome or steroid-dependent nephrotic syndrome: a multicentre, double-blind, randomised, placebo-controlled trial. *Lancet* 384:1273–1281, 2014.
289. Schwartz J, Winters JL, Padmanabhan A, et al: Guidelines on the use of therapeutic apheresis in clinical practice-evidence-based approach from the Writing Committee of the American Society for Apheresis: the sixth special issue. *J Clin Apher* 28:145–284, 2013.
330. Mejia N, Santos F, Claverie-Martin F, et al: Renal Tube group: Renal Tube: a network tool for clinical and genetic diagnosis of primary tubulopathies. *Eur J Pediatr* 172:775–780, 2013.
358. Moeller HB, Rittig S, Fenton RA: Nephrogenic diabetes insipidus: essential insights into the molecular background and potential therapies for treatment. *Endocr Rev* 34:278–301, 2013.
367. Langman CB, Greenbaum LA, Sarwal M, et al: A randomized controlled crossover trial with delayed-release cysteamine bitartrate in nephropathic cystinosis: effectiveness on white blood cell cystine levels and comparison of safety. *Clin J Am Soc Nephrol* 7:1112–1120, 2012.
387. Stechman MJ, Loh NY, Thakker RV: Genetic causes of hypercalciuric nephrolithiasis. *Pediatr Nephrol* 24:2321–2332, 2009.
441. Hoppe B, Groothoff JW, Hulton SA, et al: Efficacy and safety of Oxalobacter formigenes to reduce urinary oxalate in primary hyperoxaluria. *Nephrol Dial Transplant* 26:3609–3615, 2011.
446. Ozen S, Pistorio A, Iusan SM, et al: Paediatric Rheumatology International Trials Organisation (PRINTO): EULAR/PRINTO/PRES criteria for Henoch-Schönlein purpura, childhood polyarteritis nodosa, childhood Wegener granulomatosis and childhood Takayasu arteritis: Ankara 2008. Part II: Final classification criteria. *Ann Rheum Dis* 69:798–806, 2010.
451. Jennette JC, Falk RJ, Bacon PA, et al: 2012 revised International Chapel Hill Consensus Conference Nomenclature of Vasculitides. *Arthritis Rheum* 65:1–11, 2013.
492. Specks U, Merkel PA, Seo P, et al: RAVE-ITN Research Group: efficacy of remission-induction regimens for ANCA-associated vasculitis. *N Engl J Med* 369:417–427, 2013.
493. Guerry MJ, Brogan P, Bruce IN, et al: Recommendations for the use of rituximab in anti-neutrophil cytoplasm antibody-associated vasculitis. *Rheumatology (Oxford)* 51:634–643, 2012.
510. López EL, Contrini MM, Glatstein E, et al: An epidemiologic surveillance of Shiga-like toxin-producing Escherichia coli infection in Argentinean children: risk factors and serum Shiga-like toxin 2 values. *Pediatr Infect Dis J* 31:20–24, 2012.
517. Frank C, Werber D, Cramer JP, et al: HUS Investigation Team: Epidemic profile of Shiga-toxin-producing Escherichia coli O104:H4 outbreak in Germany. *N Engl J Med* 365:1771–1780, 2011.
523. Locatelli M, Buelli S, Pezzotta A, et al: Shiga toxin promotes podocyte injury in experimental hemolytic uremic syndrome via activation of the alternative pathway of complement. *J Am Soc Nephrol* 25:1786–1798, 2014.
526. Noris M, Remuzzi G: Atypical hemolytic-uremic syndrome. *N Engl J Med* 361:1676–1687, 2009.
536. Menne J, Nitschke M, Stingele R, et al: EHEC-HUS consortium: Validation of treatment strategies for enterohaemorrhagic Escherichia coli O104:H4 induced haemolytic uraemic syndrome: case-control study. *BMJ* 345:e4565, 2012.
539. Petruzziello-Pellegrini TN, Marsden PA: Shiga toxin-associated hemolytic uremic syndrome: advances in pathogenesis and therapeutics. *Curr Opin Nephrol Hypertens* 21:433–440, 2012.
551. Zuber J, Fakhouri F, Roumenina LT, et al: French Study Group for aHUS/C3G: Use of eculizumab for atypical haemolytic uraemic syndrome and C3 glomerulopathies. *Nat Rev Nephrol* 8:643–657, 2012.
554. Sinha A, Gulati A, Saini S, et al: Indian HUS Registry: Prompt plasma exchanges and immunosuppressive treatment improves the outcomes of anti-factor H autoantibody-associated hemolytic uremic syndrome in children. *Kidney Int* 85:1151–1160, 2014.

572. Legendre CM, Licht C, Muus P, et al: Terminal complement inhibitor eculizumab in atypical hemolytic-uremic syndrome. *N Engl J Med* 368:2169–2181, 2013.
573. Le Quintrec M, Zuber J, Moulin B, et al: Complement genes strongly predict recurrence and graft outcome in adult renal transplant recipients with atypical hemolytic and uremic syndrome. *Am J Transplant* 13:663–675, 2013.

601. Bakkaloglu SA, Borzych D, Soo Ha I, et al: International Pediatric Peritoneal Dialysis Network: Cardiac geometry in children receiving chronic PD: Findings from the International Pediatric Peritoneal Dialysis Network. *Clin J Am Soc Nephrol* 6:1934–1943, 2011.

Fluid, Electrolyte, and Acid-Base Disorders in Children

75

James C. M. Chan | Fernando Santos

CHAPTER OUTLINE

SODIUM AND WATER DISORDERS, 2365
Normal Metabolism of Water and Sodium of Specific Interest to the Pediatric Age, 2365
Hyperosmolality and Hypernatremia: Pathogenesis and Classification, 2367
Hypo-osmolality and Hyponatremia: Pathogenesis and Classification, 2370
Hyponatremia in Hospitalized Children, 2372
Syndrome of Inappropriate Antidiuretic Hormone Secretion, 2372
Nephrogenic Syndrome of Inappropriate Antidiuresis, 2372
Basis of Fluid Therapy for Dehydration in Children, 2373
POTASSIUM DISORDERS, 2374
Aspects of Normal Metabolism of Potassium of Specific Interest to the Pediatric Age, 2374
Hypokalemia, 2375
Hyperkalemia, 2380

HYDROGEN ION DISORDERS, 2382
Acid-Base Equilibrium in Children, 2382
Renal Tubular Acidosis, 2383
MAGNESIUM DISORDERS, 2386
Metabolism of Magnesium, 2386
Hypomagnesemia, 2387
CALCIUM AND PHOSPHATE DISORDERS, 2389
Calcium and Phosphate Distribution and Regulation, 2389
Calcium and Phosphate Balances, 2389
Vitamin D, Parathyroid Hormone, Calcitonin, and Fibroblast Growth Factor 23, 2390
Hypocalcemia, 2391
Hypercalcemia, 2393
Hypophosphatemia, 2396
Hyperphosphatemia, 2398
CHAPTER SUMMARY AND CONCLUSION, 2400

New findings in gene mutations of channels, receptors, and transporters in renal tubular cells continue to improve our understanding of acid-base, water, and electrolyte disorders. In this esteemed textbook of nephrology, it is fitting to have a chapter on fluid-electrolyte and acid-base disorders, unique to the neonate and child.

Pediatricians have always worked with the developing child's ever-changing body size and prescribed treatment based on the body weight and other parameters related to growth from infancy to young adulthood. Many pediatric nephrologists maintain dialysis in children under an internal medicine certificate of need and have research mentors/collaborators in internal medicine. These connections are valuable in the transition of the pediatric patient to adult nephrology care.

SODIUM AND WATER DISORDERS

NORMAL METABOLISM OF WATER AND SODIUM OF SPECIFIC INTEREST TO THE PEDIATRIC AGE

The most abundant constituent of the human body is water. The relative amount of water changes with age.[1,2] In newborns and infants, total body water (TBW) constitutes a greater proportion of body weight than in adults, approximately 75% to 80% in preterm newborns, 70% in term infants, and 65% to 66% from 1 to 12 months of age. From this age on, the percentage of TBW progressively diminishes to approximately 60% to 65% of body weight in adults. Variability in TBW among individuals of similar age is related to differences in fat content because adipocytes practically do not contain water, but approximately 80% of the weight of other cells is water. Fat and water content are inversely related to each other in any given individual. Therefore obese individuals have a lower percentage of TBW. For the same reason, TBW is 5% to 10% lower in women than men. This gender-related difference in TBW is not observed before puberty.

The TBW comprises the intracellular fluid (ICF) and the extracellular fluid (ECF), which may in turn be subdivided into intravascular and interstitial fluids. The age-dependent changes in TBW that occur during infancy and childhood are mostly attributable to variations in ECF because the ICF proportion remains essentially constant after the first year of life at roughly 40% of the body weight.[1] The ECF decreases rapidly during the embryonic development stage, during the first year of life, and more slowly from 1 year of age onward.

The solute composition of the ICF and ECF differs considerably. The electroneutrality within each compartment is maintained by the balance between the sum of positive charges from cations and the sum of negative charges from anions. The major cationic electrolyte in the ECF is sodium, with smaller contributions from calcium, magnesium, and potassium. With regard to ECF anions, chloride is the most abundant, followed by bicarbonate and, in the plasma, by proteins, which are physiologically restricted by the capillary membrane from passage to the interstitial fluid. In the ICF, potassium is the predominant cation. There are significant amounts of magnesium but only a small concentration of sodium. With respect to ICF anions, proteins and organic phosphates are by far the most abundant. The potassium and sodium gradients between the ICF and the ECF compartments are maintained by membrane-bound Na^+/K^+ pumps.

Most biologic membranes are permeable to water but not to aqueous solutes. Thus water molecules free of solutes cross the cell and capillary membranes, driven by osmotic pressure gradients. The hydrostatic pressure and the intrinsic permeability of the capillary membrane also intervene in the net movement of water across the capillary barrier.

Osmolality is defined as the number of milliosmoles (mOsm) of solute per kilogram of solvent. The mOsm is a measure of the number of particles dissolved in a solution and results from the number of electrolytic particles produced by dissociation of a millimole (mmol) of a given substance. Osmolality is the property of a solution independent of any membrane and independent of the size or weight of the particles. The major extracellular osmoles are sodium and its accompanying anion, chloride. Other physiologic osmoles within the extracellular water are glucose and urea. Plasma osmolality (mOsm/kg H_2O) can be estimated for practical purposes as $2 \times Na + Urea + Glucose$ (all in mmol/L). Plasma urea and glucose concentrations often provided by clinical laboratories in mg/dL are converted to mmol/L by dividing by 2.8 and 18, respectively. In terms of the movement of water caused by the osmotic pressure gradient, urea permeates the cell membrane freely and therefore is not considered as an "effective" osmole. That is, unlike sodium, urea does not contribute to tonicity, which is the property of a solution with reference to a membrane and represents the effective osmolality of a solution (i.e., the sum of the concentrations of solutes that are able to exert an osmotic force across a semipermeable membrane). Glucose, at normal physiologic plasma concentrations, is taken up by cells via active transport mechanisms and therefore is osmotically ineffective in many, but not all, tissues. However, glucose produces an osmotic gradient in hyperglycemic conditions (e.g., diabetes mellitus) when the cellular uptake of glucose is impaired.[3]

In addition to the internal distribution of water hitherto described, water and electrolyte metabolism depends on the external balance between intake and output.[3] Children must keep a positive balance to allow body growth. A young infant gains approximately 30 g of weight per day, which means a physiologic retention of 20 mL/day of water and 2 mEq/day of sodium. On the other hand, the ratio of surface area to weight is higher in infants than adults, and the skin is more permeable in infants. This means that water loss is proportionally much greater in infants than adults, especially in children with fever.

Thirst is the body's signal to increase water consumption. Thirst is stimulated by intracellular water loss (dehydration), so small increments of plasma osmolality from 1% to 4% are able to produce a strong stimulus to drink by activating osmoreceptors located in the central nervous system (CNS). Different neural projections connect the primary osmoreceptors to brain areas responsible for arginine vasopressin (AVP) secretion (see later) and thirst. It must be kept in mind that osmoreceptor cells in the brain primarily respond to plasma tonicity rather than to total plasma osmolality. The physiologic relevance of this finding is that osmoreceptors function primarily to preserve cell volume. Elevations of solutes such as urea do not cause cellular dehydration and consequently do not activate the mechanisms that protect body fluid homeostasis.[4] Thirst can also be caused by intravascular hypovolemia. This mechanism is less sensitive because sustained reductions of at least 4% to 8% in ECF volume or blood pressure are needed to stimulate cardiovascular baroreceptors. Under physiologic conditions, plasma osmolality in humans usually does not change above the threshold required to stimulate thirst, and water balance is maintained by modifications in the effective solute-free component of urinary volume.

Urinary flow is determined by changes in the renal load of solutes and in the excretion of solute-free water. A high intake of sodium will expand the ECF volume, leading to a compensatory reduction of renal tubular reabsorption and solute-driven water excretion and therefore increased urine volume (see later). Free water excretion, which is water elimination in excess of what is needed for solute excretion, is regulated by the action of AVP (also termed *antidiuretic hormone* in reference to one of its principal functions). AVP is synthesized as a prohormone in the hypothalamus and stored in the neurohypophysis until its release. Circulating AVP activates type 2 vasopressin (V_2) receptors located in the basolateral membrane of the collecting tubule principal cells to increase water reabsorption through the insertion of water channels, aquaporin 2, into the luminal membranes of these cells (see also Chapters 10 and 11). The lower urinary concentrating capacity of young infants in comparison with older children and adults can be at least partially attributed to immaturity of expression of these water channels.[5] Pituitary AVP secretion occurs in response to small increases of only 1% or less in plasma osmolality. Accordingly, maximal urine concentration and therefore maximal antidiuresis is achieved after increases in plasma osmolality of only 5 to 10 mOsm/kg H_2O. Hypovolemia also stimulates AVP secretion, but, similar to thirst, AVP secretion is much less sensitive to changes in blood volume and blood pressure than to changes in osmolality. There are also nonosmotic stimuli to AVP secretion that probably play no role in the control of water metabolism in physiologic conditions. Thus the sensation of nausea is by far the most potent stimulus to AVP secretion known in humans and is able to elevate circulating AVP levels.

Sodium balance is mainly dependent on the modulation of renal excretion, because a specific appetite for salt has only been unequivocally observed in the presence of adrenal insufficiency. Likewise, sodium intake is not spontaneously inhibited in the setting of excess sodium and ECF volume. The renal elimination of sodium is regulated by several complex factors: glomerular filtration rate (GFR), intrarenal hemodynamic changes, aldosterone levels, and several other factors, as outlined in detail elsewhere in this book. Preterm infants have a low capacity to retain sodium, and their sodium excretion is often inappropriately high. Both full-term and preterm infants have, compared with adults, a low capacity to excrete excessive salt loads.[5] Vascular volume expansion increases renal perfusion pressure and subsequently increases fractional sodium excretion. Aldosterone production by the adrenal cortex is stimulated by angiotensin II, which is formed as the end result of renin secretion from the juxtaglomerular apparatus in response to renal hypoperfusion. Whereas hyperkalemia also increases aldosterone secretion, atrial natriuretic peptide and hyperosmolality are potent inhibitors. Aldosterone stimulates distal reabsorption of sodium with accompanying potassium excretion, by a mechanism that partly involves the epithelial sodium channels (ENaCs) at the luminal membrane of collecting tubule cells. Normal values of plasma renin activity and aldosterone increase with upright position and with sodium restriction, vary within a wide range, are higher in children than adults, and are particularly high in infants.[6] Reasons for the elevated plasma concentrations of renin and aldosterone in infancy may be low sodium intake at this age, immature proximal tubular reabsorption that allows an increased delivery of filtered sodium to the macula densa, low expression of Na^+-K^+-ATPase (which is the energy generator for salt transport), deficient dynamic regulation of Na^+-K^+-ATPase activity, low numbers of angiotensin II receptors in the vessel wall, low blood pressure, and increased renal vascular resistance. Positive, although weak, correlations have been found between resistive index measured by Doppler ultrasonography in the renal interlobar artery arteries and active plasma renin concentrations ($r = 0.158$) and plasma aldosterone concentrations ($r = 0.222$) in 169 healthy children.[7] Reference values for renin and aldosterone are scarce in the literature. Third and 97th percentiles for serum aldosterone (2.5 and 20.6 ng/dL; 1 pmol/L = 0.036 ng/dL), plasma renin activity (0.6 and 7.5 ng/mL/hr), and aldosterone renin ratio (0.8 and 13.1) have been reported in 211 normotensive children aged 4 to 16 years in the sitting position with at least a 15-minute rest.[8]

HYPEROSMOLALITY AND HYPERNATREMIA: PATHOGENESIS AND CLASSIFICATION

Hyperosmolality results from a deficiency of water relative to solutes in the ECF. The vast majority of situations leading to hyperosmolality are attributable to losses of body water in excess of body solutes caused by either insufficient water intake or excessive water excretion or both, although a minority of cases can occur as a result of excessive total-body sodium loading.[3] A detailed examination of the causal mechanisms of hyperosmolar disorders summarized in Table 75.1 allows us to appreciate just how vulnerable young infants are to developing hypernatremia. The conjunction of several factors such as lack of voluntary access to water, high physiologic insensible water loss because of a large body surface in relation to body weight, occurrence of acute diarrhea frequently associated with fever, vomiting, and intolerance of oral fluid intake all contribute to this potentially dangerous vulnerability.

Table 75.1 Pathogenesis of Hyperosmolar Disorders

Insufficient water intake
- Inability to obtain water: preambulatory infants, unconscious or disabled children, lack of water
- Abnormalities of thirst: hypodipsia secondary to CNS disorders

Net loss of water in excess of solutes
- Renal losses: central and nephrogenic diabetes insipidus
- GI losses: vomiting, diarrhea
- Cutaneous losses: sweating, burns
- Pulmonary losses: hyperventilation

High sodium intake + low intake of water free of solutes
- Excessive administration of NaCl or $NaHCO_3^-$: parenteral nutrition, cardiopulmonary resuscitation, seawater intake

CNS, Central nervous system; GI, gastrointestinal.

DEHYDRATION

It should be noted that in pediatrics the term *dehydration* is often used as the most general term, encompassing the different forms of net fluid loss, including forms in which (1) water loss exceeds solute loss, leaving the child hypertonic; (2) water and solute loss are proportionate, leaving the child normotonic; and (3) solute loss exceeds water loss, leaving the child hypotonic. Although not as strictly rigorous as the term *net fluid volume depletion*, the term *dehydration* will be retained in this chapter in order to be consistent with terminology used in everyday pediatrics.

HYPERNATREMIC DEHYDRATION

Dehydration may occur as a result of inappropriately low intake (anorexia, coma, fluid restriction) or excessive loss of fluids by gastrointestinal (GI; vomiting, diarrhea, fistula, or drains), renal (polyuric states), and/or cutaneous (heat, cystic fibrosis, burns, inflammatory skin disease) routes. Hypernatremic dehydration (plasma sodium concentration > 150 mEq/L) results from insufficient water intake or net loss of water in excess of solutes (see Table 75.1; i.e., the net fluid loss is hypotonic). In hypernatremic dehydration, water shifts from the ICF to the ECF, driven by an osmotic gradient. Thus a certain degree of extracellular and intracellular volume loss coexists. In view of the fact that many of the most commonly assessed clinical manifestations are proportional to the reduction of ECF volume, the manifestations of dehydration will be less intense for the same degree of water loss in the hypernatremic dehydration state than in other forms of dehydration (see later); therefore progressive dehydration associated with hypernatremia may be overlooked even in babies with marked weight loss.[9]

Any form of dehydration is characterized by weight loss in the child. The magnitude of acute weight loss reflects the amount of water loss and is the best clinical indicator of the degree of dehydration. Weight losses in infants of 5%, 10%, and 15% (50, 100, 150 mL/kg, respectively) classically correspond with mild, moderate, and severe degrees of dehydration.[1] Older children and adults manifest symptoms at a somewhat lower degree of fluid loss than infants because the former have relatively smaller TBW and ECF volume whereby weight losses of 3%, 6%, and 9% are better used as indicative of mild, moderate, and severe dehydration, respectively.[1]

In addition to weight loss, the reduction of ECF will cause a range of symptoms and physical signs depending on the intensity and rate of the dehydration, such as decreased skin turgor; dry mucous membranes; sunken anterior fontanelle; cool and mottled skin with poor capillary refilling; oliguria; acceleration of heart rate and pulse; decrease in blood pressure; and in the most severe cases (most commonly combined volume depletion with concomitant net sodium loss as well), hypovolemic shock. A review of the literature to find out the precision and accuracy of symptoms, signs, and basic laboratory tests for evaluating dehydration in infants and children came to the conclusion that delayed capillary refill time, reduced skin turgor, and deep respirations with or without an increase in rate were the most useful clinical signs that predicted 5% hypovolemia, and these parameters should be the basis of the initial assessment of dehydration in young children.[10] In patients with hypernatremic dehydration, the reduction of the ICF volume will also cause fever and CNS manifestations such as irritability, a high-pitched cry, seizures, and other neurobehavioral disturbances, reminiscent of febrile and neurologic illness. Hyperosmolality causes thirst and avidity for water. Elevations of hematocrit and plasma concentrations of total proteins, uric acid, and urea are biochemical indicators of dehydration, although they are not reliable parameters to assess its severity.[10] Metabolic acidosis is usually present because of frequent associated loss of bicarbonate and alkalinizing organic anions from the GI tract (non–anion gap [AG] acidosis) or anaerobic metabolism caused by poor peripheral perfusion (AG acidosis caused by lactate accumulation). A value of plasma bicarbonate below 17 mEq/L is indicative of moderate or severe hypovolemia.[10] Renal hypoperfusion leading to decreased GFR and oliguria is a compensatory mechanism to ECF volume depletion. In hypernatremic dehydration, serum osmolality is greater than 310 mOsm/kg H_2O, stimulating AVP secretion and intensifying the oliguria. Thus a variable degree of prerenal failure, with preserved structural integrity of the kidneys, occurs reactively in a patient with dehydration of nonrenal origin. Table 75.2 provides indices used in pediatrics to differentiate this situation of prerenal failure from that of established renal failure with tubular or cortical necrosis secondary to prolonged ischemia.[11]

NEPHROGENIC DIABETES INSIPIDUS

Nephrogenic diabetes insipidus (NDI) is a disease defined by renal resistance to AVP action, which results in an inability to concentrate urine adequately. It is clinically characterized by an increased risk for dehydration from polyuria and polydipsia, low urinary osmolality, persistent predisposition to hypernatremia, and serum hyperosmolality. Unlike central diabetes insipidus, NDI occurs with high or normal circulating levels of AVP and lack of response to exogenous administration of desmopressin, an AVP analog.

This chapter focuses on the primary forms of NDI. NDI may also be present in the context of other congenital and acquired tubular or interstitial disorders that interfere with the normal process of urine concentration. Thus polyuria and defective urinary concentration capacity form part of the wide spectrum of clinical manifestations of hypokalemic tubulopathies, including Bartter's syndrome, Fanconi's syndrome, distal renal tubular acidosis (RTA), interstitial cystic diseases, Bardet-Biedl syndrome, nephronophthisis complex, nephrocalcinosis, obstructive uropathy, acute interstitial nephritis, chronic kidney disease, diabetes mellitus, and hypercalcemia, as well as secondary forms caused by the ingestion of medications such as lithium, cisplatin and other antineoplastics, demeclocycline, amphotericin B, and diphenylhydantoin, among others.[12] These secondary forms of NDI are generally less severe than primary NDI. The risk for dehydration is lower because patients are able to increase urinary osmolality above plasma osmolality, although normal maximum urine osmolality between 800 and 1200 mOsm/kg H_2O is not achieved. With the exception of prolonged lithium treatment, NDI secondary to most therapeutic pharmacologic agents is usually reversible after discontinuation of the medications.[13] In polyuric states, induced by osmotic diuresis (i.e., diabetes mellitus), the urine osmolality is usually above 300 mOsm/kg H_2O, in contrast to the dilute urine typically found with the aquaretic diuresis of diabetes insipidus. Primary congenital NDI is a rare inherited disease linked to the X chromosome

Table 75.2 Urinary Indices for the Clinical Diagnosis of Prerenal and Intrinsic Renal Failure in Oliguric Children

	Prerenal Failure		Intrinsic Renal Failure	
	Children	Neonates	Children	Neonates
Urinary Na (mEq/L)	<10-20	<20-30	>30-40	>30-40
Urinary osmolality (mOsm/kg H_2O)	>400-500	>350	<350	<300
FE of Na (%)*	<1	<2.5	>2	>3
U/P osmolality	>2	>1.5	<1	<1
U/P creatinine	>40	>30	<20	<10
Renal failure index[†]	<1	<2.5	>2	>2.5

*FE of Na = Fractional excretion of Na = (Urine Na/Plasma Na) × (Plasma creatinine × 100/Urine creatinine).
[†]Renal failure index = Urine sodium/(U/P creatinine).
U/P = Urine-to-plasma ratio.
From Chim S: Acute renal failure: medical (non-dialytic) management. In Chiu MC, Yap HK, editors: Practical paediatric nephrology: an update of current practices, Hong Kong, 2005, Medcom Limited, pp 227-233.

(OMIM 304800) in approximately 90% of cases (http://www.ndif.org), with an estimated prevalence rate of four to eight cases per million, except in the Canadian provinces of Nova Scotia and New Brunswick, where the incidence is more than six times higher.[14] Carrier females may be asymptomatic or have partial defects of urine concentration ability; more rarely, they have severe polyuria, likely because the normal X chromosome is preferentially inactivated.[15] X-linked NDI is caused by loss-of-function mutations in the gene encoding the AVP type 2 receptor *(AVPR2)* located on Xq28.[16] Type 2 receptors of AVP are normally located on the basolateral membrane of the principal cells of the collecting tubule. In primary congenital NDI, five classes of molecular defects leading to defective function of the receptor have been described. The most prevalent type of mutations results in misfolding of the receptor and retention in the endoplasmic reticulum.[17]

In approximately 10% of patients, primary congenital NDI results from loss-of-function mutations in the gene encoding the aquaporin-2 water channel *(AQP2)* located on 12q13. These forms follow autosomal recessive[18] or, more rarely, autosomal dominant[19] modes of inheritance (OMIM 125800). Mutations in *AVPR2* or *AQP2* genes have not been found in some families with hereditary NDI, suggesting that mutations in other genes encoding the several proteins that take part in the development of interstitial hypertonicity in the renal medulla and in the water permeability of the collecting duct might be responsible for some cases of NDI.[20]

Clinical manifestations of congenital NDI present in male patients in the first few weeks of life. Polydipsia and polyuria with dilute urine, hypernatremia, and a high risk for dehydration are the hallmarks of the disease. Repeated episodes of brain dehydration and brain edema (brought about by attempts to rehydrate too quickly) can lead to mental retardation. Values of permanent urine output greater than 3 mL/kg/hr, greater than 80 mL/m^2/hr, or greater than 2 mL/m^2/day are considered to be polyuria. The concepts of polydipsia and polyuria are not easy to define in infants who normally ingest large amounts of liquids per kilogram of weight and eliminate high volumes of urine. A young infant receiving enough quantities of mother's milk or fed with low–solute concentration formulas may remain asymptomatic or nearly so. Later in life, as more solid food is introduced to the diet, the increased solute load causes more water excretion. Irritability, avidity for water, vomiting, constipation with emission of pebble-like hardened stools, failure to thrive related at least to a great extent to inadequate caloric intake, and intermittent bursts of fever and dehydration are common and represent major manifestations of congenital NDI. A delay in the diagnosis may lead to repeated episodes of hypernatremic dehydration, seizures, and irreversible neurologic damage. In 30 male patients with a diagnosis of NDI confirmed by mutation analysis, the median age of diagnosis was 9 months. The majority of the children (63%) were diagnosed during the first year of life, and vomiting or anorexia, growth failure, fever, constipation, and polydipsia were the most frequent presenting symptoms and signs.[21] There are infants with partial forms of congenital NDI caused by mutations in the *AVPR2* gene in whom the symptoms are milder, and the diagnosis is often missed in early infancy.[22,23] In some patients with autosomal dominant NDI, there is partial resistance to AVP, but in the recessive forms, either X-linked or autosomal, the symptoms are usually of great and similar severity. The dilatation of the urinary tract secondary to the polyuria is frequent in patients with NDI, and this manifestation often leads to the correct diagnosis.[24] Urinary symptoms associated with polyuria and hydronephrosis such as incontinence, enuresis, urine retention, or traumatic rupture of the urinary tract may be found as well as some degree of renal insufficiency, which has been attributed to bladder dysfunction.[25,26] The typical biochemical profile of infants with congenital NDI consists of hypernatremia or plasma sodium concentration at the upper normal limits, plasma hyperosmolality, normal or high values of circulating AVP, and dilute urine with osmolality below that of plasma often approaching minimal urinary osmolality values of 50 to 70 mOsm/kg H$_2$O. High plasma concentrations of urea, creatinine, uric acid, and total proteins are also found when the patient is dehydrated.

The family history as well as the clinical picture and the biochemical profile just described lead to a diagnostic workup for NDI, which should be confirmed by mutational analysis of the *AVPR2* or *AQP2* genes.[27] Low or normal plasma sodium concentration in a polyuric child is indicative of primary polydipsia. Acquired forms of NDI are usually of later onset and cause less severe urine concentration defects than congenital NDI so that urine osmolality may increase above plasma osmolality, and the risk for dehydration is low unless additional factors such as vomiting, diarrhea, or prolonged fasting are present. Polyuria in the context of other primary tubulopathies can start in the first weeks of life, such as congenital NDI, but associated clinical and biochemical findings, such as nephrocalcinosis, metabolic acidosis or alkalosis, hypokalemia, manifestations of proximal tubular dysfunction, and so on are usually present. Central diabetes insipidus results from defective synthesis or release of AVP secondary to acquired lesions of the CNS in the majority of cases. These patients have polyuria with hypernatremia, but they can be differentiated from patients with NDI by the response of urinary osmolality to exogenous AVP. Administration of intranasal (10 μg in infants; 20 μg in children) or intravenous (IV) (1 μg; maximum dose, 0.4 μg/kg infused over 20 minutes) desmopressin will increase urine osmolality over the subsequent 2 hours in patients with central diabetes insipidus so that the ratio of urine osmolality to plasma osmolality will become greater than 1.5; urine osmolality does not increase by more than 100 mOsm/kg H$_2$O over baseline in children with congenital NDI. A classical water restriction test is used in the differential diagnosis of polyuria and polydipsia. However, in infants and children with complete forms of NDI, this test is not advisable to confirm the diagnosis because of the high risk for inducing dangerous dehydration. If it is to be done, the patient should be admitted to the hospital with close medical supervision during regular daytime hours and coordinated with the clinical laboratory to obtain immediate test results as soon as possible after the sample is collected. The test must be terminated when one of the following end points is reached: urine specific gravity of 1.020 or above, urine osmolality of 600 mOsm/kg H$_2$O or above, plasma osmolality greater than 295 or 300 mOsm/kg H$_2$O, plasma sodium concentration at or greater than 147 mEq/L, or loss of 5% of body weight or signs of volume depletion. In any

Table 75.3 Summary of Typical Responses to Water Deprivation Test and Administration of Antidiuretic Hormone in Clinical Situations Characterized by Polyuria and Polydipsia

	Primary Polydipsia	Nephrogenic Diabetes Insipidus		Central Diabetes Insipidus	
		Complete	Partial	Complete	Partial
Baseline plasma sodium and osmolality	Low/normal	High/normal	Normal	High/normal	Normal
Baseline plasma AVP	Low	High/normal	High/normal	Very low	Low
Baseline urine osmolality	Low; below plasma	Very low; <100 mOsm/kg H_2O	Low; below plasma	Very low; <100 mOsm/kg H_2O	Low; below plasma
Maximum urine osmolality after water restriction	≥500-600 mOsm/kg H_2O	No elevation with respect to baseline values	Small increment with respect to baseline values; ≤45%	No elevation with respect to baseline values	Variable increment with respect to baseline values; above plasma osmolality
Maximum urine osmolality after exogenous AVP administration	No further increase	No further increase	No further increase or increment <100 mOsm/kg H_2O	Marked increment; much greater than 100%; noticeable decrease in urine volume	15%-50% increase; noticeable decrease in urine volume

AVP, Antidiuretic hormone.

case the duration of water restriction should not exceed 6 hours in infants younger than 6 months of age, 8 hours in children from 6 months to 2 years of age, or 12 hours in children older than 2 years of age. Typical responses to hydropenia and AVP administration in NDI and other polyuric disorders are summarized in Table 75.3. It is noteworthy that maximum urine concentrating ability is frequently impaired in children with primary polydipsia, likely because of the chronic washing out of the renal medulla, downregulation of AVP, and aquaporin synthesis. However, a progressive reduction of water intake over several weeks results in normalization of the urine output volume and restoration of the normal urine concentration ability.

Treatment of patients with congenital NDI is aimed at providing enough water to prevent hypernatremia and dehydration, minimizing polyuria by diminishing the solute renal load and by using pharmacologic treatments, and decreasing polydipsia to allow enough ingestion of calories and nutrients to facilitate growth and development. Patients must be allowed free access to water. Young children should be offered water every 2 hours during the day and night; in severe cases, continuous gastric feeding may be required. Infants with congenital NDI must receive human milk or the commercial milk-based formula with the lowest osmotic load; after infancy, a low-salt diet should be recommended. Prolonged treatment with thiazide diuretics (oral hydrochlorothiazide at 1 to 3 mg/kg/day twice or three times a day.) paradoxically decreases the urine output in patients with NDI on a low-salt diet, presumably through a hypovolemia-induced increase in proximal sodium and water reabsorption, thereby diminishing water delivery to the AVP-sensitive sites in the collecting tubules.[28] The addition of amiloride, 0.1 to 0.3 mg/kg/day, to block the epithelial sodium channel localized at the luminal membranes of the cortical collecting tubule enhances the antipolyuric effect of thiazides and minimizes the risk for hypokalemia and alkalosis.[29,30] Indomethacin, at dosages of 0.75 to 2 mg/kg/day given every 8 to 12 hours, has been used effectively with thiazides to reduce urine output in pediatric patients with NDI.[31] Indomethacin decreases the synthesis of prostaglandins, which has been shown to antagonize the action of AVP, and increases the availability of *AQP2* channels in the apical membrane of collecting ducts. The use of indomethacin should be reserved for patients who fail to respond to a low-salt diet and thiazides plus amiloride. Administration of desmopressin has been shown to reduce polyuria in adults and children with partial forms of NDI.[32] More interestingly, intranasal desmopressin may be useful to treat nocturnal enuresis in pediatric patients with congenital NDI even though it does not decrease the daily urine output, suggesting that the activation by this drug of CNS AVP receptors is important for the nervous regulation of bladder control.[33,34] In addition to the treatment of clinical symptoms of NDI, later studies have used new molecular strategies to restore the functionality of the mutant receptors. These innovative approaches have not been tested in children but provide a promising means of therapy in the near future.[35]

HYPO-OSMOLALITY AND HYPONATREMIA: PATHOGENESIS AND CLASSIFICATION

Hypo-osmolality indicates excess water relative to solute in the ECF. Because water moves freely between the ECF and the ICF, this also indicates an excess of TBW relative to total body solute. Hyponatremia (plasma sodium concentration < 135 mEq/L) and hypo-osmolality (plasma osmolality < 180 mOsm/kg H_2O) are used synonymously. However, high/normal osmolality with low sodium concentration may be found when effective solutes other than sodium are present in the plasma, enlarging the osmolal gap. The latter is the difference between the measured osmolality and the calculated osmolality (see earlier), which stands normally in children between 0 and 10 mOsm/kg H_2O.[36] In this respect a high osmolal gap has been found in two of six edematous children with nephrotic syndrome and marked hypoproteinemia, pointing to the existence of unidentified nonsodium and nonpotassium osmoles in the plasma of these patients.[37] An increase of 100 mg/dL in the plasma glucose concentration decreases plasma sodium concentration by approximately 1.7 mEq/L, resulting in an increase in osmolality of approximately 2.0 mOsm/kg H_2O.[38] On the other hand, pseudohyponatremia, with normal osmolality, can be produced by marked elevation of plasma lipids or proteins. Although the concentration of sodium per liter of plasma water is unchanged, the concentration of sodium per liter of plasma is decreased because of the increased nonaqueous portion of the plasma occupied by lipids or protein. Methods that measure sodium in the whole plasma (i.e., flame photometry) underestimate sodium concentration by about 2 mEq/L for an increment of 1 g/dL in triglyceride levels.[39] This does not occur with use of more modern analyzers based on techniques such as direct potentiometry, in which the water content of the sample does not affect the measurement of sodium concentration.

The normal range for plasma sodium concentration varies between different laboratories but is often quoted as 135 to 145 mEq/L. Significant hyponatremia is defined as plasma sodium concentration of less than 130 mEq/L. However, clinical symptoms are usually not noticeable until plasma sodium concentrations fall below 125 mEq/L. A major consequence of hyponatremia is the influx of water into the intracellular space, resulting in cellular swelling, which gives rise to cerebral edema and encephalopathy. Neurologic manifestations related to hyponatremia are lethargy, apathy, depressed sensorium, confusion, agitation, seizures, and even death. More than 50% of children with plasma sodium concentration below 125 mEq/L develop hyponatremic encephalopathy,[40] although the severity of the clinical manifestations depends on the degree of hyponatremia and the rate of sodium decline. Adverse outcomes are more strongly correlated with an acute decrease in serum sodium concentration (within 48 hours) than with the same absolute decrease that spans a longer period of time, allowing the brain to adapt.[41] Children are at increased risk for developing hyponatremic encephalopathy because of their relatively larger ratio of brain to intracranial volume compared with adults. The brain reaches adult size by 6 years of age, but the skull does not reach adult size until 16 years of age.[42] The average plasma sodium concentration in children with hyponatremic encephalopathy has been found to be 120 mEq/L; in adults, it is 111 mEq/L. Hypoxia is also a major risk factor for the development of hyponatremic encephalopathy because it impairs the ability of the brain to adapt to hyponatremia and hyponatremia in turn leads to a decrease in both cerebral blood flow and arterial oxygen content.[43]

Briefly, hyponatremia may result from loss of sodium in excess of water or from gain of water in excess of sodium. Both mechanisms may coexist in the same patient. Solute depletion is accompanied by some degree of secondary retention of water by the kidneys in response to the resulting intravascular hypovolemia or secondary stimulation of AVP secretion. On the other hand, water retention can lead to hypervolemia that in turn causes solute losses.[4] Patients with hyponatremia are usually classified according to the status of the ECF volume (Table 75.4). This classification is useful from the clinical point of view, although such a pathophysiologic approach may be too simplistic because the regulation of plasma sodium concentration is complex and the definite assignment of a given patient to one of the three groups is not always possible despite the use of the clinical and biochemical indexes described earlier. The measurement of urine sodium concentration is more useful in arriving at a correct classification and diagnosis of hyponatremia in a pediatric patient than in adults because the confounding effect of frequently concomitant primary sodium-retaining states may be less problematic. In the presence of ECF volume contraction, a urine sodium value less than 10 mEq/L indicates that the renal response is well preserved and suggests that the loss of solutes is of cutaneous or GI origin. Urine sodium concentration of 20 to 30 mmol/L or greater is found in most patients with euvolemic hyponatremia, unless they have become secondarily sodium depleted or are receiving a diuretic. In edematous patients with ECF expansion, low urinary sodium concentration points to avid tubular sodium reabsorption induced by secondary hyperaldosteronism.

Table 75.4 Clinical Classification of Hyponatremic Disorders in Children According to the Status of Extracellular Fluid Volume

Contracted	Normal	Expanded
Renal solute loss	Administration of hypotonic solutions	Congestive heart failure
• Diuretics (thiazides)	SIADH	Cirrhotic liver disease
• Osmotic diuresis: hyperglycemia	Nephrogenic syndrome of inappropriate antidiuresis	Nephrotic syndrome
• Salt-wasting nephropathies	Severe hypothyroidism	Advanced oliguric renal failure
• Mineralocorticoid deficiency	Glucocorticoid deficiency	Excessive water intake
• Cerebral salt wasting		
Nonrenal solute loss		
• Gastrointestinal: vomiting, diarrhea, aspiration, fistula, stoma, third space		
• Cutaneous: sweating, burns, cystic fibrosis		

SIADH, Syndrome of inappropriate antidiuretic hormone secretion.

HYPONATREMIA IN HOSPITALIZED CHILDREN

The prescription of hypotonic solutions as maintenance IV fluids in hospitalized children, according to the classical recommendations of Holliday and Segar,[44] has been challenged by a growing number of studies over the past 2 decades, which have drawn attention to the risk for severe neurologic complications and even death in hospitalized children who developed hyponatremia. The incidence of acute hospital-acquired hyponatremia has been reported to be as high as 10% in a case-control study performed in a pediatric tertiary hospital.[45] Likewise, 11% of infants with severe bronchiolitis had serum sodium levels of less than 130 mEq/L at the time of admission to the intensive care unit.[46] The retrospective incidence of postoperative hyponatremia among 24,412 pediatric patients with generally minor illnesses subjected to routine surgical procedures has been reported to be 0.34% with a mortality rate of those so affected at 8.4%.[47]

Hospital-acquired hyponatremia is usually attributed to the administration of hypotonic fluids in the presence of simultaneous impaired free water excretion resulting from elevated AVP secretion by hemodynamic (i.e., effective circulating volume depletion) and nonhemodynamic (i.e., malignancies, CNS disorders, pulmonary diseases, medications, nausea, pain, stress) stimuli.[48] Excessive fluid administration is also considered a common contributing factor.[49] Despite the general assumption that hypotonic fluids are a crucial factor in the development of hyponatremia of hospitalized children, a systematic review of studies to determine whether hypotonic solutions increase the risk for acute hyponatremia comparing hypotonic versus isotonic IV maintenance fluids in hospitalized children came to the conclusion that these studies were observational and inconclusive and that hypotonic fluid administration does not always explain the development of hyponatremia.[50] By contrast, Choong and colleagues using a similar system of literature analysis, concluded that hypotonic solutions significantly increased the risk for developing acute hyponatremia and resulted in greater patient morbidity.[51] To prevent the risk for hyponatremia, the British National Patient Safety Agency has recommended increasing the tonicity of IV fluids administered as maintenance therapy in children (see later) from 0.18% NaCl, as formerly used, to 0.45% NaCl and prescribe isotonic solutions to hospitalized children with disorders entailing high risk for elevated AVP secretion and ensuing hyponatremia.[52] This approach has been criticized on the grounds that this might cause more children to develop hypernatremia than it would help prevent children from developing hyponatremia.[53] Additional measures to decrease the risk for hyponatremia include the reduction of fluids to two thirds of the normal recommended volume except in dehydrated children.[54] Treatment of patients with symptomatic hyponatremia is described later.

SYNDROME OF INAPPROPRIATE ANTIDIURETIC HORMONE SECRETION

Syndrome of inappropriate antidiuretic hormone secretion (SIADH) is characterized by hyponatremia less than 135 mEq/L, low plasma osmolality (<275 mOsm/kg H_2O in classical descriptions), and urine osmolality that is not at minimum value of less than 100 mOsm/kg H_2O in a patient who is euvolemic. The diagnosis requires absence of clinical or biochemical signs of hypovolemia, of diuretic use, and of other causes of impaired free water excretion by the kidneys, such as hypothyroidism; adrenal insufficiency; renal, cardiac, or hepatic failure. Characteristically the patient is not edematous, and the urinary sodium concentration is greater than 20 mEq/L.

SIADH is the result of the release of endogenous AVP produced ectopically by a tumor or eutrophically by the neurohypophysis, in response to some unknown stimuli induced by a variety of illnesses and drugs. In children, CNS diseases, pulmonary infections, and postsurgery states are the leading causes of SIADH.[55] SIADH causes an absolute increase in body water that results from a degree of fluid intake in a patient who cannot dilute his or her urine sufficiently to mount a compensatory water diuresis.[56] In this syndrome, hyponatremia is initially caused by simple dilution and subsequently by natriuresis triggered by a homeostatic response to volume expansion and probably mediated, at least in part, by suppression of plasma renin activity and aldosterone secretion and an increase of plasma atrial natriuretic peptide.[56]

It is important to emphasize that the vast majority of SIADH in children is acute and transient, resolving with the passage of time or after the underlying condition improves or heals. Thus pediatricians usually do not cope with chronic states of hyponatremia. If the SIADH resolves while the patient has hyponatremia, AVP secretion will be suppressed by the hypo-osmolality, and a water diuresis will ensue. The excretion of maximally dilute urine can rapidly increase the serum sodium concentration. Therefore the treatment of choice for patients with acute SIADH is water restriction, which usually achieves the normalization of plasma sodium concentration within 2 or 3 days. In occasional patients whose plasma sodium concentration is low enough to cause neurologic symptoms, it is necessary to infuse hypertonic 3% sodium chloride to increase plasma sodium concentration to a safe range because patients with euvolemic hypo-osmolality such as SIADH do not respond to isotonic saline.[57] It is usually recommended to program and monitor the rate of infusion to achieve an increase in plasma sodium concentration by approximately 1 mEq/L/hr.[57] The sodium content of 3% sodium chloride is 0.513 mEq/mL; if we assume that the TBW of an infant is approximately 70% of body weight, an infusion of 0.7 mEq/kg/hr of sodium (1.4 mL/kg/hr of 3% sodium chloride) will increase the serum sodium concentration by 1 mEq/L, although this will depend on the simultaneous sodium losses. As mentioned previously, chronic SIADH is rarely seen in children. It requires slow correction of hyponatremia to avoid the risk for the dreaded complication demyelinating encephalopathy and may include the use of AVP receptor antagonists (vaptans) or of demeclocycline. The efficacy of urea in treating hyponatremia secondary to SIADH by inducing an osmotic water drive has been reported in a study of European children.[58]

NEPHROGENIC SYNDROME OF INAPPROPRIATE ANTIDIURESIS

In 2005 Feldman and colleagues described two male infants whose clinical and laboratory evaluations were consistent

Table 75.5 Features of Intravenous Fluids Commonly Used in Pediatrics

Solution	Osmolality (mOsm/L)	Sodium (mEq/L)	Osmolality (Compared with Plasma)	Tonicity (with Reference to Cell Membrane)
NaCl 0.9%	308	154	Isosmolar	Isotonic
NaCl 0.45%	154	77	Hyposmolar	Hypotonic
Glucose 5%	278	0	Isosmolar	Hypotonic
Glucose 10%	555	0	Hyperosmolar	Hypotonic
NaCl 0.9% with glucose 5%	586	150	Hyperosmolar	Isotonic
½ NaCl 0.9% + ½ glucose 5%*	293	77	Isosmolar	Hypotonic
⅓ NaCl 0.9% + ⅔ glucose 5%*	288	77	Isosmolar	Hypotonic
⅕ NaCl 0.9% + ⅘ glucose 5%*	285	31	Isosmolar	Hypotonic
Lactated Ringer's solution†	273	130	Hyposmolar	Isotonic
Hartmann's solution	278	131	Isosmolar	Isotonic
Human albumin 5%	260	140	Hyposmolar	Isotonic

*Fractions indicate the proportions of NaCl 0.9% and glucose 5% that form part of the whole solution.
†Lactated Ringer's solution also contains 4 mEq/L of potassium as well as 1.4 mmol/L of calcium and 28 mmol/L of lactate.

with the presence of SIADH but whose circulating AVP levels were undetectable.[59] This novel disease, termed *nephrogenic syndrome of inappropriate antidiuresis*, is caused by activating mutations of the *AVPR2* gene. Its prevalence is unknown, but some cases of patients currently diagnosed with SIADH with undetectable AVP concentrations may indeed correspond to this syndrome. The syndrome has been reported in additional pediatric cases[60–62] as well as in hyponatremic men.[63,64] Heterozygous women may have some degree of inappropriate antidiuresis when challenged with a water load, indicating penetrance of the disease in female individuals.[63] The spectrum of symptoms has been reported to vary within the same family ranging from infrequent voiding to incidentally noted hyponatremia to recurrent admissions with hyponatremic seizures.[64] Male patients meeting all criteria for a diagnosis of SIADH without any apparent cause for the disorder or if there is a family history of hyponatremia, particularly if plasma AVP levels are undetectable, require sequencing of the *AVPR2* gene.[57] Administration of oral urea as osmotic agent at a dose titrated up from 0.1 to a maximum of 2 g/kg/day given in up to four divided doses has been shown to be effective in these children.[60] Some patients harboring mutations that do not lock the receptor in an irreversible active state might respond favorably to vaptans.[65]

BASIS OF FLUID THERAPY FOR DEHYDRATION IN CHILDREN

The three steps in treating dehydration are (1) repletion of deficit, which means previous losses of fluids and can be estimated by the patient's weight loss; (2) maintenance therapy, which means physiologic requirements of fluid and electrolytes; and (3) sustained provision of continuing extraordinary losses. Replacement of the deficit was traditionally carried out slowly, over 24 to 48 hours, particularly in the presence of hyponatremia or hypernatremia. In acute processes, usually from a GI origin and when most of the fluid lost by the child comes from the ECF, current recommendations are more in favor of a policy of rapid repletion of the isotonic depletion to quickly restore the ECF volume

Table 75.6 Calculation of Intravenous Maintenance Fluid Therapy in Children

Child's Weight	Daily Metabolic Rate
3-10 kg	100 kcal/kg
10-20 kg	1000 + 50 kcal for each kilogram above 10
>20 kg	1500 + 20 kcal for each kilogram above 20

From Holliday MA, Segar WE: The maintenance need for water in parenteral fluid therapy. Pediatrics 19:823-832, 1957; Friedman A: Pediatric hydration therapy: historical review and new approach. Kidney Int 67:380-388, 2005.

on the basis of the following benefits: improved GI perfusion that allows earlier oral feeding, improved renal perfusion, and a lower morbidity and mortality rate.[54] If the child has signs of severe hypovolemia (see earlier), repletion therapy should begin with rapid IV infusion of 20 mL/kg of isotonic 0.9% saline (Table 75.5), which should be repeated as needed until adequate perfusion is restored under careful monitoring of the patient. Even in patients with less severe forms of dehydration and subtle signs of hypovolemia, administration of 20 to 40 mL/kg of 0.9% saline over 2 to 4 hours is safe.[66] Lactated Ringer's solution is a valid alternative to normal saline[54] (see Table 75.5), although its use is less common.

After extracellular volume depletion has been restored with IV fluid, fluid repletion can continue with either continued IV fluid or, if possible, oral rehydration therapy. The type of IV repletion fluid that is given in this second step of fluid therapy varies with the serum sodium concentration. Maintenance fluids can be calculated following the Holliday-Segar method,[44] which estimates physiologic losses of water scaled to the metabolic rate, as shown in Table 75.6, keeping in mind that this calculation does not apply to newborn infants; that the total volume of fluid should not exceed

Table 75.7 Approximate Electrolyte Composition of Gastrointestinal Fluids in Infants

	Sodium (mEq/L)	Potassium (mEq/L)	Chloride (mEq/L)	Bicarbonate (mEq/L)
Salivary glands	50	20	30	40
Stomach	35	10	180	—
Gallbladder	150	10	90	40
Pancreas	150	10	50	110
Small intestine	140	5	70	75
Colon (stool)	40	90	15	30

From Awazu M, Kon V, Barakat AY: Volume disorders. In Ichikawa I, editor: *Pediatric textbook of fluids and electrolytes,* Baltimore, 1990, Williams & Wilkins, pp 121-129.

2400 mL/day[67]; and that calories should be provided, usually as glucose, to supply at least 20% of the daily metabolic rate. The maintenance fluid calculation does not take into account abnormal fluid losses such as those frequently presented by dehydrated children. Fluids used to replace ongoing losses should reflect the electrolyte composition of the fluid being lost (Table 75.7), if possible by direct measurement, although in most circumstances, an isotonic solution (see Table 75.5) administered over a minimum of 24 hours is an appropriate initial option.

A bolus of 20 mL/kg represents 2% of body weight. Normal saline or lactated Ringer's solution is usually used because the sodium concentration of these solutions is comparable to that of plasma (see Table 75.5) and achieves the expansion of intravascular volume without causing major fluid shifts. After the expansion of ECF volume is accomplished, the remaining fluid deficit, if any, can be corrected in a few hours with isotonic saline if the patient is isonatremic or has mild hyponatremia.[67] However, when hypovolemia is associated with significant hyponatremia or hypernatremia or when hypovolemia and associated alterations in serum sodium concentration have evolved slowly, attention must be paid to the rate of correction of the serum sodium concentration to avoid excessive shifts of water out of the brain (too rapid treatment of hyponatremia) or into the brain (too rapid treatment of hypernatremia) that can lead to serious neurologic complications. Treatment of symptomatic hyponatremia has been described earlier. The sodium deficit is calculated by the following formula:

$$\text{Na deficit in mEq} = (\text{normal TBW} \times 140\,\text{mEq/L}) - (\text{current TBW} \times \text{plasma sodium in mEq/L})$$

In hypernatremic dehydration, no neurologic sequelae appear to occur if the plasma sodium concentration is lowered at a rate of 0.5 mEq/L/hr or less; thus the calculated deficit fluid and electrolyte requirements are typically administered in 48 hours.[68]

Rehydration therapy with oral solutions, such as World Health Organization solution (osmolality, 330 mOsm/kg H_2O; glucose, 110 mmol/L; sodium, 90 mEq/L; chloride, 80 mEq/L; bicarbonate, 30 mEq/L; potassium, 20 mEq/L), should be attempted as an alternative to IV therapy in children with mild (≤50 mL/kg over 12 to 24 hours) and moderate (25 to 50 mL/kg over 6 to 12 hours) dehydration, and good oral tolerance.[54] Even in patients with initial vomiting, oral administration of small and frequent volumes of the solution often succeeds in correcting the dehydration.

POTASSIUM DISORDERS

ASPECTS OF NORMAL METABOLISM OF POTASSIUM OF SPECIFIC INTEREST TO THE PEDIATRIC AGE

Homeostasis of potassium and its principal regulating mechanisms are extensively reviewed elsewhere in this book. The vast majority of total body potassium is intracellular, the largest fraction being located in the muscle. Although the intracellular potassium concentration (100 to 150 mEq/L) is much higher than that of the ECF (3.5 to 5.0 mEq/L), the latter is what is usually available for measurement. The circulating concentration of potassium is tightly regulated by mechanisms that control the distribution between intracellular and extracellular compartments and the external potassium balance. The distribution of potassium results from two processes: the active cellular uptake by Na^+-K^+-ATPase and the passive leak of potassium from cells. It depends on the concentration of potassium in the ECF, acid-base status, and hormones, such as insulin, insulin-like growth factor-1, catecholamines, and aldosterone. The external potassium balance depends on dietary intake versus renal and GI eliminations. In the small intestine and in the proximal tubule of the kidney and thick ascending limb of Henle's loop (TAL), reabsorption of potassium takes place in connection with water and sodium and does not appear to be the site of tight regulation. However, in the colon and in the distal nephron, both potassium reabsorption and secretion occur and are regulated by similar factors. The capacity of colonic potassium secretion is limited, and in physiologic conditions, the kidneys excrete the bulk of potassium. In the connecting tubule and cortical collecting tubule, principal cells mediate potassium secretion, and intercalated cells are responsible for potassium reabsorption. Most of the factors known to modulate potassium excretion do so by changing its secretion, which in turn is modulated by distal delivery of sodium and increased tubule fluid flow as elicited by extracellular volume expansion and administration of diuretics. Factors that stimulate potassium secretion in urine are potassium dietary intake, increased luminal electronegativity in the distal nephron as happens when urine becomes alkaline in acute metabolic and respiratory alkalosis, and increased levels of aldosterone.[69,70] The effect of aldosterone is dual because aldosterone maximizes sodium reabsorption during hypovolemia, whereas it stimulates distal potassium secretion in the presence of hyperkalemia and noncontracted ECF volume.[71]

Unlike adults, infants and children need to maintain a continual positive balance of potassium to grow normally because cellular mass depends on potassium as the major intracellular cation. Total body potassium increases from approximately 8 mEq/cm body height at birth to greater than 14 mEq/cm body height by 18 years of age, the rate of accumulation of body potassium per kilogram of weight being more rapid in infants than children and adolescents.[69] In vitro and experimental studies indicate that the capacity of neonatal kidney to secrete potassium is less than in the adult.[69] The immature kidneys are relatively insensitive to aldosterone, which in the clinical setting correlates with the higher plasma concentrations of aldosterone and potassium and the lower ratio of urinary sodium to potassium characteristic of newborns and infants.

HYPOKALEMIA

Hypokalemia is usually defined as a serum potassium concentration of less than 3.5 mEq/L. Acute changes in serum potassium concentration usually reflect modifications in the distribution of potassium between the extracellular and intracellular compartments. By contrast, alterations in the external potassium balance give rise to more chronic changes of plasma potassium concentration and lead to situations of true potassium deficit. Clinical conditions leading to sustained hypokalemia are listed in Table 75.8.

Potassium is critical for many important cell functions, so hypokalemia and potassium depletion may result in clinical manifestations in several organs and tissues (Table 75.9). In general, the same degree of hypokalemia is better tolerated when it results from a chronic potassium loss than from an acute decline, but both conditions may coexist in the same patient. Arrhythmias and marked weakness or paralysis of respiratory muscles are life-threatening symptoms that require urgent therapy. Growth retardation is a characteristic of potassium-depleted young animals and of a large, although not well-defined, percentage of children with hypokalemic tubular disorders.[72,73] Association with growth hormone (GH) deficit, reported in a few of these patients,[74] resistance to GH action, and a disturbed process of growth plate chondrocyte hypertrophy have been invoked as pathogenic factors of longitudinal growth failure in potassium depletion.[75,76] Long-standing hypokalemia leads to so-called hypokalemic nephropathy, which includes development of renal cysts; chronic interstitial nephritis; and, in the very long term, progressive loss of renal function. Polyuria resistant to the administration of AVP and polydipsia linked to both the excessive diuresis and the stimulus of the thirst center by potassium depletion via increased production of angiotensin II may be important manifestations in hypokalemic children. In rats, potassium depletion results in kidney hypertrophy.[77] Studies on kidney size in children with chronic hypokalemic disorders have not been performed.

The cause of hypokalemia is usually apparent from anamnesis and the global assessment of the patient. Excessive renal wasting of potassium can be identified by measuring potassium loss in urine collected for 24 hours or by calculating urinary indices in spot samples. Thus a child with a rate of daily urinary excretion of potassium exceeding normal potassium intake, fractional excretion of potassium [fractional excretion of potassium = [(Urine K/Plasma K) × (Plasma creatinine × 100/Urine creatinine)] above 30%, or urinary sodium to potassium ratio consistently less than 1 in the absence of renal failure is suspected of having renal potassium wasting. A urinary ratio of potassium to creatinine below 1.5 mmol/mmol has been proposed as an index of adequate renal conservation of potassium in adult patients with hypokalemia based on the assumption that patients

Table 75.8 Most Relevant Causes of Hypokalemia in Pediatric Patients

Acute redistribution of potassium to the intracellular compartment
- Metabolic alkalosis
- Insulin administration
- Hypokalemic periodic paralysis

Prolonged lack of intake

Increased renal loss
- Drugs: diuretics, antibiotics, aminoglycosides, penicillin, amphotericin B, capreomycin
- Metabolic acidosis and diabetic ketoacidosis
- Increased mineralocorticoid activity
  - Cushing's syndrome
  - Congenital adrenal hyperplasia
  - Primary or secondary hyperaldosteronism
- Primary tubulopathies
  - Bartter's syndrome
  - Gitelman's syndrome
  - Liddle's syndrome
  - Types 1 and 2 renal tubular acidosis
  - Epilepsy, ataxia, sensorineural deafness, and tubulopathy (EAST) syndrome
  - Fanconi's syndrome

Increased gastrointestinal loss
- Vomiting (hypertrophic pyloric stenosis)
- Diarrhea

Table 75.9 Main Manifestations of Hypokalemia and Potassium Deficit in Pediatric Patients

Organ System	Manifestation
Neuromuscular	- Skeletal muscle weakness - Muscular paralysis - Paralytic ileum - Muscle ischemia and rhabdomyolysis

Heart	- ECG alterations
	  - Depression of S-T segment
	  - Low amplitude of T wave
	  - Appearance of U wave
	- Arrhythmias

Nutrition and growth	- Mild glucose intolerance - Growth retardation
Kidney	- Hypokalemic nephropathy - Polyuria-polydipsia

ECG, Electrocardiographic.

with a very low potassium excretion rate eliminate 10 to 15 mmol/day and that creatinine excretion rate in adults is of 10 to 15 mmol/day.[78] This assessment needs to be validated in children. In the clinical setting the coexistence of hypokalemia of renal origin and arterial hypertension points to hyperaldosteronism, either associated (in the cases of renal vascular hypertension or coarctation of the aorta) or not with elevated plasma renin activity or expanded extracellular volume (e.g., congenital adrenal hyperplasia, Cushing's syndrome, Liddle's syndrome). If blood pressure is normal, the presence of acidosis suggests RTA, diabetic ketoacidosis, penicillin or other nonresorbable anion toxicity, and the presence of alkalosis raises the suspicion of diuretic use, administration of aminoglycosides or capreomycin, Bartter's syndrome, and Gitelman's syndrome[79,80] (Figure 75.1).

Hypokalemia secondary to internal potassium redistribution is transient and normalizes after the underlying disorder is corrected. Potassium deficit is treated with a potassium-rich diet and, if needed, oral potassium supplements, usually potassium chloride; potassium citrate is preferred in cases with concomitant acidosis. Patients with arrhythmias, respiratory paralysis, or rhabdomyolysis or those unable to take oral medications must be treated with IV potassium chloride at a maximum rate of 0.5 mEq/Kg/hour and maximum concentration of 40 mEq/L in saline solutions. Higher concentration and rate of administration can be used in life-threatening situations under intensive care control and continuous electrocardiographic monitoring.[81]

BARTTER'S SYNDROME

In 1962 Bartter and colleagues described two patients with a new syndrome characterized by hypokalemia, metabolic alkalosis, hyperaldosteronism with normal blood pressure, decreased pressor response to angiotensin II infusion, and hyperplasia of the juxtaglomerular apparatus of the kidneys.[82] It is currently appreciated that Bartter's syndrome includes several entities having different genetic mutations and diverse molecular pathophysiology but sharing the common denominator of decreased tubular transport of sodium chloride in the TAL (Table 75.10 and Figure 75.2).[83,84]

Types 1 and 2 of Bartter's syndrome have antenatal or neonatal variants, also termed *hyperprostaglandin E syndrome*,[85] caused by loss of function in the Na^+-K^+-$2Cl^-$ cotransporter type 2 (NKCC2) encoded by the *SLC12A1* gene[86,87] and in the potassium channel ROMK (renal outer medullary potassium) encoded by the *KCNJ1* gene,[88,89] respectively. Type 4 Bartter's syndrome is also a neonatal form associated with neurosensory hearing loss caused by loss of function of barttin, a protein coded by the *BSND* gene required for the insertion of chloride channels ClC-Ka and ClC-Kb in the plasma membrane.[90] These channels are expressed

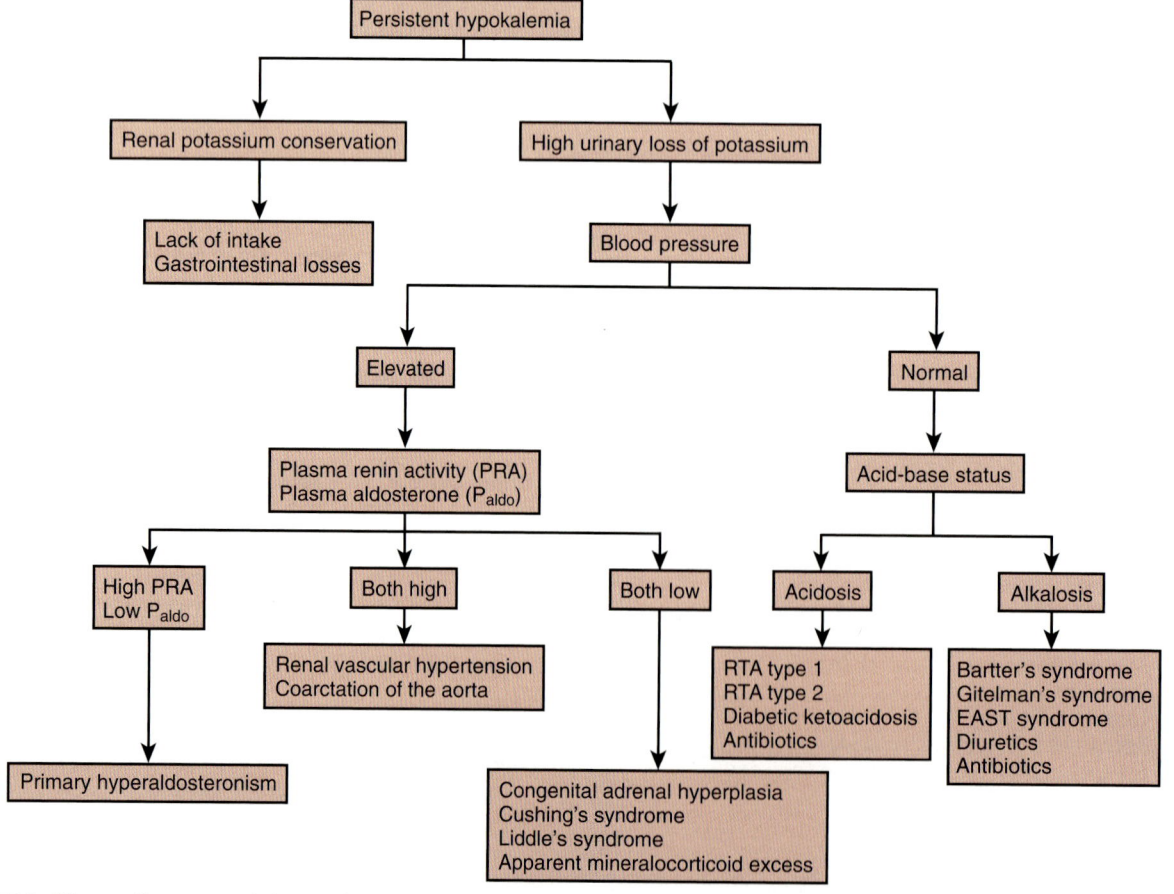

Figure 75.1 Diagnostic approach to persistent hypokalemia in children. Transient hypokalemias are usually secondary to transcellular shifts of potassium ion. EAST, Epilepsy, ataxia, sensorineural deafness, and tubulopathy; RTA, renal tubular acidosis.

Table 75.10 Distinctive Characteristics of the Four Types of Bartter's Syndrome*

	Type 1	Type 2	Type 3	Type 4
Defective gene	SLC12A1	KCNJ1	ClCNK	BSND
Abnormal protein	NKCC2 cotransporter	ROMK channel	ClC-Kb channel	Barttin
Clinical onset	Perinatal	Perinatal	0-5 yr	Perinatal
Clinical manifestations	Polyhydramnios	Polyhydramnios	Classical Bartter's syndrome	Polyhydramnios
	Premature birth	Premature birth		Premature birth
	Severe polyuria	Severe polyuria		Chronic renal failure
Associated findings	Nephrocalcinosis	Nephrocalcinosis	Calciuria	Sensorineural deafness
			Normal or mildly high hypomagnesemia	
Pharmacotype	Furosemide	Furosemide + amiloride	Thiazide + furosemide	Furosemide + thiazide

*Common features are salt-losing hypokalemic metabolic alkalosis, hyperaldosteronism with normal blood pressure, elevation of prostaglandin E_2, and autosomal recessive inheritance.
NKCC2, Na^+-K^+-$2Cl^-$ cotransporter type 2; ROMK, renal outer medullary potassium.

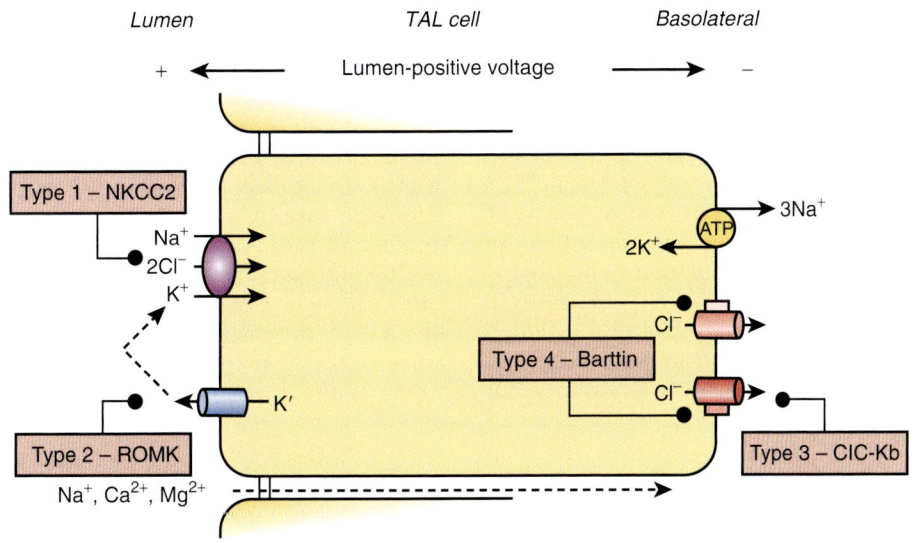

Figure 75.2 Schematic representation of a cell of the thick ascending limb of the loop of Henle (TAL) showing the transport systems disturbed in the four types of Bartter's syndrome. The bumetanide-sensitive Na^+-K^+-$2Cl^-$ cotransporter (NKCC2) and the renal outer medullary K^+ channel (ROMK) are depicted on the luminal membrane of the cell. The Na^+-K^+-ATPase and the chloride channels ClC-Ka and ClC-Kb with their barttin subunit are represented on the basolateral side. See text for description of type 5 and type 6 Bartter's syndrome. ATP, Adenosine triphosphate; ATPase, adenosine triphosphatase.

invariably, associated with their β-subunit barttin, in the nephron, where they are crucial for the reabsorption of NaCl and for the mechanisms of urine concentration.[91,92] Likewise, both the ClC-K channels and barttin participate in transcellular chloride reabsorption in the stria vascularis of the inner ear.[91] A few cases of children having renal salt wasting and deafness and no mutation in the BSND gene have been described. These patients were found to have loss-of-function mutations in the two closely adjacent genes encoding ClC-Ka (CLCNKA) and ClC-Kb (CLCNKB) on chromosome 1p36[93,94] (Bartter's syndrome type 6).

The clinical manifestations of these forms of Bartter's syndrome start during intrauterine life or immediately after birth and include polyhydramnios, premature birth, massive polyuria and loss of salt, hypercalciuria, and nephrocalcinosis. Salt wasting increases the formation of renal and systemic prostaglandin E_2 by stimulating the enzymatic activity of cyclo-oxygenase-1 and -2.[95] IV infusion of saline solutions, enteral nutrition, or both may be needed during prolonged periods of time to avoid dehydration and even death. If needed, cyclo-oxygenase inhibitors, such as indomethacin, can be used to ameliorate the polyuria and the electrolyte wasting,[95] but the physician must be aware of the risk/benefit ratio because of the high risk for toxicity, including necrotizing enterocolitis.[96] After 4 to 6 weeks of life, the vast majority of patients benefit from the combined administration of indomethacin (1 to 2 mg/kg/day) and potassium chloride. In most cases, sodium and potassium supplementation can be reduced or even discontinued by the age of 2 years.[97] Patients with type 2 Bartter's syndrome respond very well to low doses of indomethacin, less than 1 mg/kg/day, and may not need potassium supplements.[96] By contrast, patients with type 4 Bartter's syndrome are resistant to indomethacin.[98] Animal studies have shown that administration of drugs that rescue endoplasmic reticulum–retained mutant barttin ameliorates hypokalemia, metabolic alkalosis, and hearing loss, pointing to a new modality of treatment for patients with Bartter's syndrome type 4.[99] Hypercalciuria can be expected because 25% of filtered calcium is reabsorbed in the ascending loop of Henle by a mechanism of paracellular absorption facilitated by a lumen-positive voltage gradient and dependent on the adequate function of the NKCC2 cotransporter. No current treatment has succeeded in significantly decreasing the hypercalciuria and nephrocalcinosis.[96] Patients with *BSND* mutations do not have hypercalciuria or nephrocalcinosis but can be at high risk for developing early and progressive chronic kidney disease (CKD),[98] although renal function is preserved in some patients.[100,101] It is also of note that most patients with type 2 Bartter's syndrome have transient hyperkalemia during the first week of life, which is likely caused by reduced distal secretion of potassium secondary to involvement of the distal ROMK channel[102]; these neonates exhibit hyperkalemia and hyponatremia, mimicking pseudohypoaldosteronism (PHA) type 1 (PHA1). Failure to thrive is the rule in infants with neonatal forms of Bartter's syndrome, but long-term growth may be normal provided that appropriate treatment, frequent monitoring, and metabolic control are maintained.[96,97] A similarity in facial features, including a prominent forehead, a large head, triangular facies with a drooping mouth, and large eyes and pinnae has been noted in infants with Bartter's syndrome.[103-105]

Type 3 or classical Bartter's syndrome is caused by loss of function mutations in the ClC-Kb channel encoded by the *ClCNK* gene,[106,107] the p.Ala204Thr mutation being highly prevalent in Spanish families.[108] There is a large phenotypic variation in patients with type 3 Bartter's syndrome. In some cases the clinical presentation is similar to those described earlier for neonatal variants of Bartter's syndrome, but others resemble Gitelman's syndrome (see later).[109-111] Moreover, features of Bartter's syndrome have also been reported in patients with autosomal dominant hypocalcemia,[112] a disease caused by activating mutations in the calcium-sensing receptor (CaSR).[113] This form of Bartter's syndrome (type 5) likely results from inhibition of the activity of NKCC2, ROMK, and Na+-K+-ATPase by the activated CaSR, a mechanism similar to that of the hypokalemia caused by aminoglycosides or capreomycin toxicity.[80,83] The natural history of patients with type 3 Bartter's syndrome is favorable using combined treatment with indomethacin and supplements of potassium chloride; some patients require the administration of spironolactone (10 to 15 mg/kg/day) or magnesium salts to control the hypokalemia and hypomagnesemia, respectively.[96]

GITELMAN'S SYNDROME

Gitelman's syndrome is a primary tubular disorder first described by Gitelman, Graham, and Welt in 1966.[114] It is caused by a wide variety of loss-of-function mutations in the *SLC12A3* gene, located in chromosomic region 16q13, encoding the thiazide-sensitive NaCl cotransporter of the distal convoluted tubule,[115,116] which is believed to be the principal mediator of sodium and chloride reabsorption in this segment of the nephron (Figure 75.3). The disease is transmitted with an autosomal recessive inheritance pattern. Although rare, it is one of the most frequently inherited tubular disorders with an estimated prevalence of 1 in 40,000 and, accordingly, a prevalence of heterozygotes of approximately 1%.[117] The prevalence is much higher in the Roma population, who present a specific mutation intron 9+1 G>T in the *SLC12A3* gene suggestive of a founder effect in this large ethnic group.[118,119] In some patients with

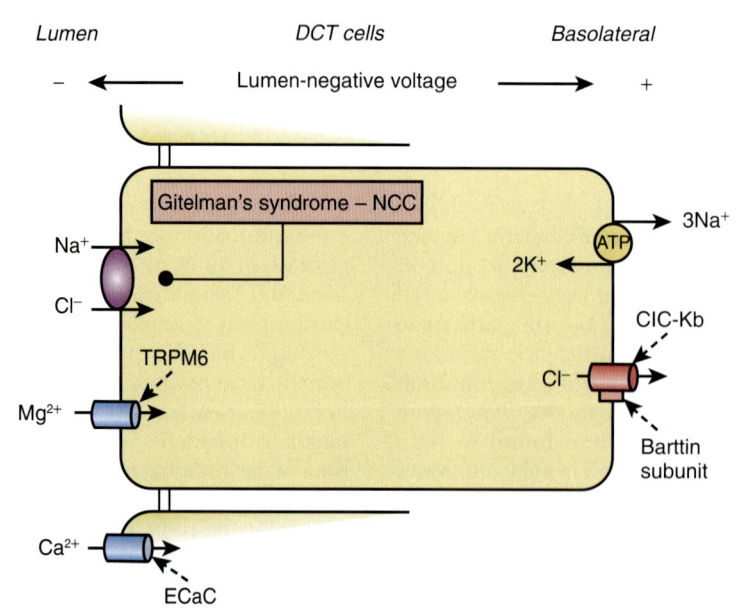

Figure 75.3 **Schematic representation of a cell of the distal convoluted tubule (DCT) showing the transport systems involved in the reabsorption of NaCl.** The thiazide-sensitive Na+-Cl− cotransporter (NCC), the magnesium transporting channel TRPM6, and the epithelial calcium channel (ECaC) are depicted on the luminal membrane of the cell. The Na+-K+-ATPase and the chloride channel ClC-Kb with their barttin subunit are represented on the basolateral side. NCC, ClC-Kb, and TRPM6 are expressed in the early downstream segment of the DCT, and ECaC is expressed in the late downstream portion of DCT. TRPM6, Transient receptor potential channel melastatin 6.

Gitelman's syndrome, only one mutation in the *SLC12A3* coding exons and flanking intronic nucleotides has been identified, suggesting that a second mutation was present in a gene region not sequenced (i.e., the promoter or the introns). The theoretical possibility of a dominant effect of some mutations is unlikely because of the lack of symptoms in the parents of affected children and in families having one of the parents and some of the offspring with Gitelman's syndrome.[120,121] High-throughput sequencing technologies now available will readily sort this out and enable a population assessment of the postulated impact of the Gitelman's syndrome carrier state with one loss-of-function copy of the *SLC12A3* mutations on protection from hypertension.[122]

Gitelman's syndrome is biochemically characterized by hypokalemic metabolic alkalosis in association with hypomagnesemia and hypocalciuria. Patients present older than 6 years of age or even as adults and may remain asymptomatic and be diagnosed as a result of a family study. The most frequent manifestations are crises of tetany, paresthesias, muscle cramps, salt craving, generalized weakness, and fatigue. Significant polyuria is generally absent.[96] Data indicate that passive calcium reabsorption in the proximal tubule and reduced abundance of the epithelial magnesium channel TRPM6 (transient receptor potential channel melastatin 6) located in the distal convoluted tubule account for the hypocalciuria and hypomagnesemia.[123] Hypomagnesemia and hypocalciuria may be absent in less than 10% of patients.[124] A tendency to mild hypophosphatemia and associated renal phosphate wasting related to the leak of potassium and chloride has also been noted.[125] Although there may be considerable phenotypic overlap among some patients with type 3 classical Bartter's and Gitelman's syndromes,[109,110] the severity of the symptoms is usually much milder in those with Gitelman's syndrome than in those with Bartter's syndrome in agreement with the fact that only 5% of filtered sodium is reabsorbed in the distal convoluted tubule in contrast with 25% to 30% in the TAL of the loop of Henle. In addition, functional clinical studies suggest that the renal sodium loss in patients with Gitelman's syndrome can be partly compensated for by the enhancement of sodium reabsorption in the cortical TAL.[126] It has also been proposed that a low fractional excretion of chloride in response to administration of hydrochlorothiazide might help differentiate Gitelman's syndrome from other hypokalemic tubular disorders.[127] There is no genotype-phenotype correlation in Gitelman's syndrome, so patients with the same mutation may exhibit a large variability of symptoms, even within the same family.[118,128,129] However, it has been reported that males and patients harboring some specific mutations exhibit more severe phenotypes, severe neuromuscular manifestations, growth retardation, and ventricula.[130] It is also of note that when responding to a questionnaire, 45% of adults with Gitelman's syndrome consider their symptoms a moderate to serious problem with significant adverse impact on their quality of life.[128] Growth retardation has been found in 20% to 30% of children with Gitelman's syndrome at diagnosis, particularly in males; height deficit improves with supplemental treatment, although not in all patients.[110,118,130] Some adult patients with Gitelman's syndrome have chondrocalcinosis, which is assumed to result from chronic hypomagnesemia. The symptoms are swelling, local heat, and tenderness over the affected joints.[117] Chronic renal failure and type 2 diabetes mellitus have been found in 6.0% and 4.3%, respectively, of adults with Gitelman's syndrome, these complications being related to the development of hypokalemic nephropathy and the inhibitory effects of potassium and magnesium deficits on the secretion of insulin and its intracellular signal transduction pathway.[124]

Patients with Gitelman's syndrome must be encouraged to maintain a diet high in sodium, potassium, and magnesium and to avoid alcoholic drinks. Oral lifelong magnesium supplementation, preferably as magnesium chloride, is recommended to prevent symptoms, particularly in the case of intercurrent processes such as vomiting and diarrhea, and to avoid the development of chondrocalcinosis.[96,117] In case of acute tetany, 20% magnesium chloride should be administered IV (0.1 mmol Mg/kg per dose) and can be repeated every 6 hours.[117] To correct the hypokalemia, some patients may need the concomitant administration of potassium chloride and potassium-sparing diuretics. Some mutations have been associated with higher requirements of potassium and magnesium and with the risk for developing arterial hypertension in adult life, likely as a result of chronic secondary hyperaldosteronism.[131]

EAST SYNDROME

The EAST syndrome (epilepsy, ataxia, sensorineural deafness, and tubulopathy), also known as SeSAME syndrome (seizures, sensorineural deafness, ataxia, mental retardation, and electrolyte imbalance),[132] is rare and was described in 2009 in five children from two consanguineous families with epilepsy, ataxia, sensorineural deafness, and normotensive hypokalemic metabolic alkalosis secondary to renal salt tubulopathy.[133] Mutations in the *KCNJ10* gene encoding a potassium channel expressed in the brain, inner ear, and basolateral membrane of the distal convoluted tubule in the kidney have been found in these children. Loss of function of this channel impairs salt reabsorption and secondarily causes hypokalemia, hypomagnesemia, and hypocalciuria.[134] The detection of these biochemical alterations, which mimic Gitelman's syndrome, in patients with any cardinal signs or symptoms of epilepsy, ataxia, or sensorineural deafness should raise the suspicion of EAST syndrome.

LIDDLE'S SYNDROME

Liddle's syndrome is a very rare autosomal dominant disorder characterized by severe hypertension and hypokalemia resulting from hyperactivity of ENaC of the principal cell of the cortical collecting tubule. The syndrome is caused by gain-of-function mutations in the *SCNN1B* or *SCNN1G* genes encoding the β- and γ-subunits of ENaC, respectively.[135,136] The exaggerated reabsorption of sodium chloride leads to extracellular volume expansion, arterial hypertension, and marked inhibition of the renin aldosterone axis. Hypokalemia and metabolic alkalosis develop in response to reabsorption of cationic sodium in the absence of an anion. This creates a lumen-negative electrical gradient, which promotes secretion of potassium and hydrogen ions into the collecting tubule.[137] Treatment must be based on a low-sodium diet and the administration of a diuretic, such as triamterene or amiloride, which is able to block ENaC.[96]

HYPERKALEMIA

Hyperkalemia is usually defined as a plasma potassium concentration exceeding 6.0 mEq/L in newborns and 5.5 mEq/L in older children. Pseudohyperkalemia refers to those conditions, mainly hemolysis caused by mechanical trauma during sample extraction, in which the elevation in the measured serum potassium concentration is caused by potassium movement out of the cells during or after the blood specimen has been drawn. It is of note that because of potassium release from clotting, serum values of potassium may be up to 0.5 mEq/L greater than the corresponding plasma values. Causes of hyperkalemia are listed in Table 75.11. Appropriate urinary potassium excretion may be identified by measuring 24-hour urinary potassium elimination, spot urine test for potassium concentration, fractional excretion of potassium (>30%), and urine K/Na ratio (>1). In the absence of advanced renal failure (GFR < 15 mL/min/1.73 m^2), reduced potassium elimination in urine points to aldosterone deficiency or aldosterone resistance in the distal nephron. These measures may not be optimal indices of the distal potassium secretion reflecting actual aldosterone action because the effect of water reabsorption, which also takes place in the distal nephron, is not taken into account.

In an attempt to overcome this limitation, the transtubular potassium concentration gradient (TTKG) is formulated. The TTKG is calculated as (Urine potassium/Plasma potassium) × (Plasma osmolality/Urine osmolality).[138] Normal values of TTKG in normokalemic children and in infants are 4.1 to 10.5 (median, 6.0) and 4.9 to 15.5 (median, 7.8), respectively.[139] In the presence of sufficient delivery of sodium to the collecting duct, a decreased TTKG suggests aldosterone deficit or insensitivity to aldosterone. The TTKG may be most helpful in the evaluation of hyperkalemia to discriminate between low aldosterone levels and aldosterone resistance. It has been suggested that in adults after a physiologic dose (0.05 mg) of 9α-fludrocortisone, the TTKG should increase to greater than 6 within 4 hours in mineralocorticoid-deficient but not in aldosterone-resistant states. There may be a delayed response (>24 hours) after a pharmacologic dose (0.2 mg) of 9α-fludrocortisone in mineralocorticoid-resistant states.[140,141]

Hyperkalemia is often asymptomatic until the plasma potassium concentration exceeds 7.0 mEq/L. The clinical consequences of hyperkalemia are related to impaired myocardial or neuromuscular transmission, and immediate therapy is warranted if characteristic progressive ECG changes (i.e., tall, peaked T waves; long PR interval; wide QRS complex; disappearance of P waves, "sine wave" pattern, ventricular fibrillation, and cardiac arrest or peripheral neuromuscular abnormalities) are encountered, regardless of the degree of hyperkalemia. Management of hyperkalemia must be based on the measures listed in Table 75.12.[142,143] In addition, treatment should be given to treat the underlying disease and to suppress the potassium ingress. In this regard the addition of sodium polystyrene sulfonate to infant formula for 1 hour has been shown to reduce markedly the content in potassium of the formula.[144]

PSEUDOHYPOALDOSTERONISM

PHA is a clinical syndrome caused by end-organ resistance to the effects of aldosterone, resulting in hyperkalemia, metabolic acidosis, and normal to high serum aldosterone levels.[145,146] PHA may be primary (hereditary) or secondary (acquired). Primary forms are subclassified into two distinct congenital syndromes: PHA1 and PHA type 2 (PHA2; Gordon's syndrome). Secondary forms (also termed PHA3) may be caused by medications or tubulointerstitial diseases (i.e., underlying urologic malformations and severe urinary tract infection).[147] This secondary PHA is transient and resolves after the infection resolves. Abnormal renal sodium handling typically is present in patients with PHA and may be characterized by either sodium wasting (PHA1) or sodium retention (PHA2).

PHA1 may be renal or systemic. The renal form is more frequent and is caused by inactivating mutations in the NR3C2 gene encoding the human mineralocorticoid receptor.[148] It follows autosomal dominant transmission, although apparent sporadic cases are also reported and intrafamilial phenotypic heterogeneity is common. The clinical manifestations start in the first weeks of life with failure to thrive and frequent episodes of vomiting and dehydration. Patients are hyponatremic, hyperkalemia is generally mild, and metabolic acidosis is not always detectable.[149] There is a state of renal salt wasting similar to that found in congenital adrenal hyperplasia but with normal genitalia, normal urinary excretion of 17-ketosteroids and pregnanetriol, normal plasma 17-OH-progesterone, and very high levels of aldosterone and renin.[96] Medical treatment consists of sodium supplementation in amounts sufficient to lower the elevated potassium levels. Sodium supplementation becomes generally

---

Table 75.11 Most Relevant Causes of Hyperkalemia in Pediatric Patients

Pseudohyperkalemia
- Improper collection of blood
- Hematologic disorders: leukocytosis, thrombocytosis, spherocytosis

Transcellular shift of potassium
- Acidosis
- Insulin deficiency
- Hyperosmolality
- Exercise with nonselective β-blockers
- Familial hyperkalemic periodic paralysis

Increased potassium load
- From exogenous origin: pharmacologic supplements
- From endogenous origin (cellular lysis): burns, trauma, intravascular hemolysis, rhabdomyolysis, tumor mass destruction

Decreased urinary excretion
- Renal failure
- Mineralocorticoid deficiency
  - Addison's disease
  - Hypoaldosteronism
- Mineralocorticoid resistance
  - Type 1 and type 2 pseudohypoaldosteronism
- Renal tubular acidosis: type 4 and hyperkalemic form of type 1
- "Hyperkalemic" drugs: potassium-sparing diuretics, trimethoprim, calcineurin inhibitors, blockers of the renin angiotensin aldsosterone system

Table 75.12 Management of Severe Hyperkalemia in Children*

	Via	Dose	Onset of Action	Comments
Stabilization of Cardiac Membranes				
Calcium gluconate, 10% solution	IV	0.5-1 mL/kg over 10 min	Immediate	Repeat one dose after 5 min if ECG changes persist; cardiac monitor.
Movement of Potassium into Cells				
Glucose + Regular insulin	IV	10% dextrose at 5 mL/kg/hr + Insulin 0.1-0.2 U/kg/hr	15-30 min	Monitor blood glucose at least hourly.
Salbutamol	Nebulized	0.1-0.3 mg/kg	20-30 min	Doses may be repeated as often as needed The effect lasts for up to 2 hr. Tachycardia is the main side effect.
	IV	4 µg/kg over 10-20 min	5-10 min	
Sodium bicarbonate	IV	2-3 mEq/kg over 30 min	15-30 min	Do not give in the same IV line as calcium; minimum effect unless the patient has acidosis.
Remove Potassium from the Body				
Cation exchange resins	PO	1 mo to 18 yr: 125-250 mg/kg (max 15 g)	1-2 hr	3-4 times daily.
	Rectal	Neonate to 18 yr: 125-25 mg/kg	1-2 hr	Repeat doses every 6 hr if needed; colonic irrigation to remove resin after 6-12 hr. Dilute 1 g resin with 5-10 mL methylcellulose or water. Do not give within 1 wk of surgery. Do not use enema with sorbitol, and keep in mind that sodium polystyrene sulfonate use, both with and without sorbitol, may be associated with fatal gastrointestinal injury.
Furosemide	IV	1-2 mg/kg	5 min	Repeat dose every 2 hr if needed; monitor fluid balance.
Hemodialysis or peritoneal dialysis				Hemodialysis is more effective.

*The measures listed here can be taken simultaneously. The choice of therapy to be used depends on the severity of the symptoms and on the particular clinical situation.
ECG, Electrocardiographic; IV, intravenously; PO, orally.

unnecessary by 1 to 3 years of age, although the high concentrations of aldosterone persist.

Systemic PHA1 follows an autosomal recessive transmission and is caused by mutations in the *SCNN1A*, *SCNN1B*, or *SCNN1G* genes encoding the α-, β-, and γ- subunits of the ENaC, respectively.[150] Mutations have been found in all three subunits, more frequently in the α-subunit, which is expressed in epithelial cells of the renal collecting ducts, respiratory airways, colon, and salivary and sweat glands.[151] Autosomal recessive PHA1 manifests in the first week of life with severe renal salt wasting, life-threatening hypovolemia, extreme hyperkalemia, metabolic acidosis, and markedly elevated plasma renin activity and aldosterone levels. Disruption of ENaC function in extrarenal epithelia causes excessive salt loss through sweat and the colon, as well as accumulation of excess fluid in respiratory airways, leading to frequent pulmonary infections, although, interestingly, no neonatal respiratory distress syndromes are reported.[149]

In patients with systemic PHA1, neonatal mortality is high, and spontaneous remissions do not occur. Patients require lifelong high salt supplementation and ion-exchange resins to control hyperkalemia.[146] Heterozygous carriers do not develop symptoms but have elevated sodium and chloride levels in sweat.[152]

PHA2 (or Gordon's syndrome or familial hyperkalemic hypertension) is an autosomal dominant disease characterized by hyperkalemia and hyperchloremic metabolic acidosis with normal to high circulating levels of mineralocorticoids. It is distinguished clinically from PHA1 by its distinct lack of sodium wasting and volume depletion. Rather, salt retention and hypertension are the hallmarks of this syndrome.[146] Consistent features of PHA2 are normal GFR, hyperkalemia between 6 and 8 mEq/L, mild metabolic acidosis, and renin consistently low in untreated individuals; aldosterone levels are more variable.[146] Less consistent features are age of clinical onset (2 weeks to 59 years) and the presence of hypertension at the time of diagnosis. The phenotypic variability is high. Hypertension is present in approximately two thirds of patients at the time of diagnosis, is often absent early in life, and is believed to develop eventually in all patients with time.[153] Hypertension and biochemical abnormalities, including hypercalciuria, which is also frequent and precedes hypertension,[154] improve with the administration of thiazides. It is of note that the PHA2 phenotype resembles a mirror image of that seen in Gitelman's syndrome.

However, no mutations of the *SLC12A3* gene leading to activation of the Na$^+$-Cl$^-$ cotransporter (NCC) have been described. Mutations in with-no-lysine (WNK) kinases *WNK1* and *WNK4*,[155] and later in *KLHL3* (encoding kelch-like 3) and *CUL3* (encoding cullin 3),[156,157] components of an E3 ubiquitin ligase complex that ubiquitinates and degrades WNK4,[158] have been found to regulate the activity of the NCC cotransporter and cause PHA2.

HYDROGEN ION DISORDERS

ACID-BASE EQUILIBRIUM IN CHILDREN

The normal mean pH of arterial blood is 7.40 and is physiologically maintained within narrow limits, between 7.36 and 7.44, by the following regulatory mechanisms: extracellular and intracellular buffering, control of the partial pressure of CO_2 (P_{CO_2}) by the respiratory system, renal tubular bicarbonate (HCO_3^-) reabsorption, and renal acid excretion. The most important extracellular buffer is bicarbonate (HCO_3^-), which reacts with H$^+$ as follows: $H^+ + HCO_3^- \rightleftharpoons H_2O + CO_2$. The equilibrium of this reaction in blood can be expressed by the Henderson-Hasselbalch equation: $pH = 6.1 + \log[HCO_3^-/(0.03 \times P_{CO_2})]$. Volatile CO_2 is produced by the complete oxidation of carbohydrates and fats, and its accumulation in the body is prevented by the respiratory exhalation. Nonvolatile acids (acids other than carbonic acid) mostly derive from the metabolism of proteins and are buffered by bicarbonate. The kidneys reabsorb the filtered bicarbonate, mostly in the proximal tubule, where 85% of filtered bicarbonate is recovered and, in the collecting duct, regenerate the plasma bicarbonate used in buffering the nonvolatile acids at the time that eliminates the H$^+$ as phosphate and ammonium.[159] Net acid excretion (NAE) is defined as the sum of titratable acid and ammonium (NH_4^+) minus urine HCO_3^-. Urine HCO_3^- is negligible at a urine pH below 6.3. Titratable acid is a function of the urine pH and the amount of H_3PO_4/NaH_2PO_4 buffer system in urine. NAE mostly depends on urinary NH_4^+. NAE per kilogram of body weight is higher in infants than adults and less in infants fed human milk than in infants fed formulas.[160]

According to the Henderson-Hasselbalch equation, alkalemia, or high blood pH, results from a process leading to increase of plasma HCO_3^-, metabolic alkalosis, or decreases of P_{CO_2} (i.e., respiratory alkalosis). Conversely, acidemia, or low blood pH, results from a process leading to decrease of plasma HCO_3^-, metabolic acidosis, or increases of P_{CO_2} (i.e., respiratory acidosis). In an attempt to avoid the deviation of pH, changes in HCO_3^- elicit compensatory modifications in P_{CO_2} and vice versa. Each mEq/L reduction in plasma HCO_3^- results in an approximately 1.0 to 1.2 mm Hg decrease in the P_{CO_2}, and each mEq/L increment in plasma HCO_3^- results in an approximately 0.7 mm Hg increase in the P_{CO_2}, limited of course by the need to oxygenate. In compensated acidosis or alkalosis, variations in HCO_3^- and P_{CO_2} temper excessive deviations in acid-base balance.

Except for the few hours after birth, the blood pH during infancy and childhood remains relatively constant, and values are equivalent to normal adult values at 3 to 5 years of age. In pediatrics, samples for acid-base measurement are often collected from arterialized capillary blood or from venous blood. The pH and P_{CO_2} of venous samples are approximately 0.05 lower and 6 mm Hg higher, respectively, than those of arterial blood in a child with well-perfused extremities, although both parameters decrease quickly after removal of the tourniquet used for blood extraction.

Metabolic acidosis results from the net loss of HCO_3^- or from the net gain of acid. It is diagnosed by low plasma HCO_3^- concentration (<22 to 24 mEq/L in children and <20 to 22 mEq/L in infants) and low blood P_{CO_2} (<40 mm Hg in children and <35 mm Hg in infants). To avoid erroneous diagnoses, it is important to note that the venous HCO_3^- concentration must be determined using a blood gas analyzer. Clinically, it is useful to classify the metabolic acidosis according to the value of the plasma or serum AG estimated by the following formula: $(Na^+ + K^+) - (Cl^- + HCO_3^-)$ (Table 75.13). The normal range varies among laboratories and with the methods used for measurement of electrolytes. Therefore it is essential that each clinician establishes the normal range of plasma AG in his or her clinical setting.[161] The most commonly cited normal range in adults is 8 to 16 mEq/L (i.e., 12 ± 4 mEq/L). The normal value in children younger than 2 years of age may be somewhat higher at 16 ± 4 mEq/L.[162] The use of autoanalyzers yields lower reference values. Modifications in the circulating concentrations of albumin and phosphate, which account for the majority of unmeasured anions, affect the AG value. The AG falls approximately 0.5 mEq/L for every 1 mg/dL reduction in serum phosphate concentration and 2.3 mEq/L for every 1 g/dL reduction in serum albumin concentration.[163] Metabolic acidosis caused by the overproduction or decreased excretion of organic acids is associated with an elevated plasma AG and can also be called *normochloremic metabolic acidosis*. If the acid that accumulates in blood is hydrochloric acid, then no change in the serum AG is expected because an equivalent number of chloride ions are retained in the blood to maintain charge neutrality when bicarbonate ions

---

Table 75.13 Metabolic Acidosis in Children According to the Serum Anion Gap

Normal serum anion gap
- Loss of bicarbonate in the stool
  - Diarrhea
  - Digestive fistulas or surgical drainage
  - Drugs: $CaCl_2$, $MgCl_2$, cationic exchange resins
- Loss of bicarbonate in urine
  - Mild to moderate renal failure (greater tubulointerstitial than glomerular damage)
  - Renal tubular acidosis
  - Extracellular volume expansion

High serum anion gap
- Advanced renal failure (uremic acidosis)
- Ketoacidosis
  - Diabetes mellitus
  - Inborn errors of metabolism
  - Prolonged fasting
- Lactic acidosis
  - Tissue hypoxia
  - Inborn errors of metabolism
  - Toxics: salicylate, methanol, ethylene glycol

are titrated by the retained protons. This type of metabolic acidosis therefore is termed *normal anion gap* or *hyperchloremic metabolic acidosis*. Likewise, the loss of bicarbonate in the urine or the stool (directly or indirectly after its metabolic conversion to another organic anion) also can produce normal AG metabolic acidosis likely because the loss of bicarbonate, along with sodium, produces volume contraction, thereby stimulating the renal tubule to retain sodium with chloride.[161]

RENAL TUBULAR ACIDOSIS

The term *renal tubular acidosis* refers to a group of clinical entities in which normal AG hyperchloremic metabolic acidosis occurs as a result of defective transport of the proximal tubular reabsorption of HCO_3^- or of the distal secretion of H^+. The GFR is normal or comparatively less impaired than is the defect in tubule function. From a pathophysiologic point of view, RTA can be classified as proximal or type 2 RTA, distal or type 1 RTA, or hyperkalemic type 4 RTA (Table 75.14). Autosomal recessive type 3 RTA occurs in association with osteopetrosis, cerebral calcification, and mental retardation in patients with loss-of-function mutations in the gene encoding carbonic anhydrase II (see later). This section focuses on the primary congenital inherited forms of RTA because they are characteristic of the pediatric age; acquired forms are more prevalent in adults.

PRIMARY PROXIMAL TYPE 2 RENAL TUBULAR ACIDOSIS

Primary proximal type 2 RTA results from a decreased reabsorption of HCO_3^- in the proximal tubule secondary to a genetic defect in some of the transporters or enzymes involved in this reabsorption (Figure 75.4). Primary forms of proximal RTA are extremely rare, the majority of cases in children being found in the context of Fanconi's syndrome.[164]

Autosomal dominant proximal RTA has been reported in only two families, and the underlying genetic and molecular defects have not yet been identified.[165,166] Autosomal recessive pure proximal RTA associated with severe short stature and ocular abnormalities (cataracts, glaucoma, and band keratopathy) is caused by mutations in the *SLC4A4* gene leading to loss of function of the Na^+-HCO_3^- cotransporter (NBC1),[167,168] which also plays a major role in overall HCO_3^- transport by the ocular lens epithelium and is indispensable not only for the maintenance of corneal and lenticular transparency but also for the regulation of aqueous humor outflow.[169] Additional features reported in patients having this form of proximal RTA are enamel defects of the permanent teeth, psychomotor retardation, impaired intellectual capacity, calcification of the basal ganglia, hypothyroidism, and hyperamylasemia.[170] Functional analysis of NBC1 mutants have suggested that approximately 50% reduction of NBC1 activity is necessary to cause severe proximal RTA with ocular abnormalities.[171]

A nonfamilial transient type of isolated proximal RTA has been reported in infants with recurrent vomiting and growth retardation,[172,173] perhaps resulting from immature Na^+-H^+ exchanger isoform 3 (NHE3), NBC1, or low carbonic anhydrase activity. A mixed form of proximal and distal RTA (type 3 RTA) secondary to carbonic anhydrase II deficiency

Table 75.14 Etiologic Classification of Renal Tubular Acidosis in Children

Proximal type 2 RTA
- Primary
  - Sporadic (transient)
  - Inherited
    - Autosomal dominant: isolated
    - Autosomal recessive: with ocular abnormalities
- Secondary
  - Component of Fanconi's syndrome: idiopathic, cystinosis, Lowe's syndrome, Wilson's disease, galactosemia
  - Other diseases: nephrotic syndrome, vitamin deficiency, renal transplantation, cyanotic congenital heart disease, paroxysmal nocturnal hemoglobinuria
  - Drugs and toxics: ifosfamide, carbonic anhydrase inhibitors, heavy metals

Distal type 1 RTA
- Primary
  - Sporadic (persistent)
  - Inherited
    - Autosomal dominant
    - Autosomal recessive: with or without sensorineural deafness
- Secondary
  - Systemic genetic diseases: osteopetrosis, elliptocytosis, Ehlers-Danlos syndrome, primary hyperoxaluria type 2
  - Acquired
    - Autoimmune diseases: Sjögren's syndrome, rheumatoid arthritis, hyperglobulinemia
    - Renal transplantation
    - Medullary sponge kidney
    - Hyperthyroidism
    - Malnutrition
    - Drugs and toxics: amphotericin B, lithium salts, amiloride, toluene

Type 3 RTA: hybrid of type 1 and type 2 RTA
- Deficiency of carbonic anhydrase II (associated with osteopetrosis and mental retardation)

Hyperkalemic type 4 RTA
- Hypoaldosteronism
- Pseudohypoaldosteronism
- Drugs and toxics: potassium salts, heparin, spironolactone, triamterene, trimethoprim, indomethacin, captopril, cyclosporin A

RTA, Renal tubular acidosis.

has been identified in children with osteopetrosis[174]; the majority of patients are of Arabic origin and come from North Africa and the Middle East.[175]

Patients with proximal RTA have a low renal HCO_3^- threshold that is normally 22 mEq/L in infants and 26 mEq/L in older children and adults. With normal concentrations of HCO_3^-, these individuals lose large amounts of HCO_3^-, greater than 15% of filtered HCO_3^-. After the circulating HCO_3^- concentration falls below the abnormally low threshold, the bicarbonaturia ceases, and because the distal mechanisms of urine acidification are intact, the urine pH decreases to less than 5.5, and the excretion of NH_4^+ increases substantially. Sustained correction of metabolic

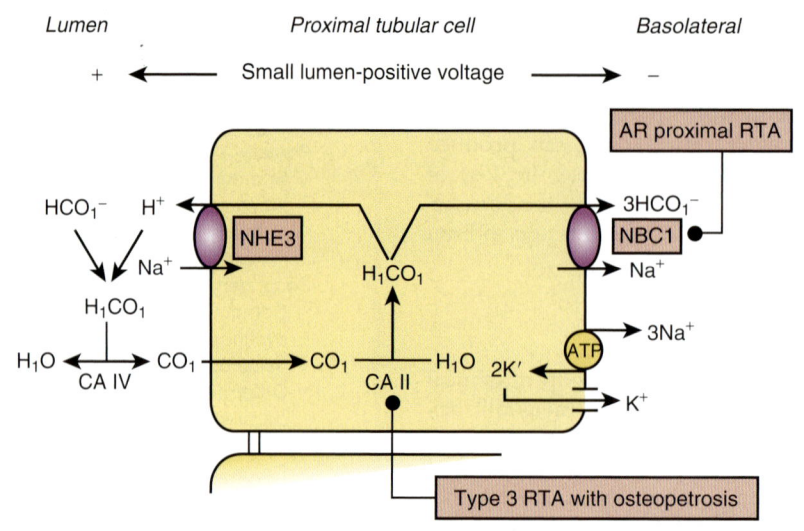

Figure 75.4 Schematic representation of the reabsorption of bicarbonate in a cell of the proximal tubule showing the transport systems involved in the genesis of primary proximal renal tubular acidosis (RTA). The Na$^+$-H$^+$-exchanger isoform 3 (NHE3) is depicted on the luminal membrane of the cell. The Na$^+$-K$^+$-ATPase and the Na$^+$-HCO$_3^-$ cotransporter (NBC1) are represented on the basolateral side. AR, Autosomal recessive; ATP, adenosine triphosphate; ATPase, adenosine triphosphatase; CA II, intracellular carbonic anhydrase; CA IV, luminal carbonic anhydrase.

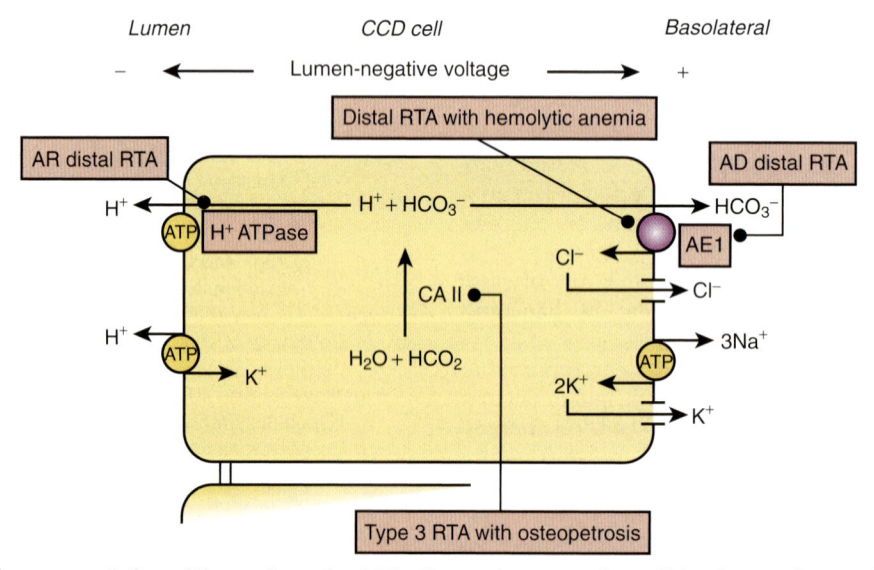

Figure 75.5 Schematic representation of the system of acidification and regeneration of bicarbonate in an α-intercalated cell of the cortical collecting duct (CCD) showing the transport systems involved in the genesis of primary distal renal tubular acidosis (RTA). The H$^+$-ATPase pump and the H$^+$-K$^+$-ATPase are depicted on the luminal membrane of the cell. The Na$^+$-K$^+$-ATPase and the Cl$^-$-HCO$_3^-$-exchanger (AE1) are represented on the basolateral side. AD, Autosomal dominant; AR, autosomal recessive; ATP, adenosine triphosphate; ATPase, adenosine triphosphatase; CA II, intracellular carbonic anhydrase.

acidosis in these patients is difficult because the needed dose of alkali is high (10 to 15 mEq/kg/day), necessitating unwieldy frequent doses every 2 to 4 hours. The leak of large amounts of bicarbonate enhances the urinary losses of potassium by increasing sodium and water delivery to the distal nephron.[176] Therefore a fraction of alkali supplementation should be given as potassium salt, usually in the form of potassium citrate. The concomitant administration of hydrochlorothiazide may facilitate the correction of acidosis with lower doses of alkali supplementation.[96]

PRIMARY DISTAL TYPE 1 RENAL TUBULAR ACIDOSIS

Primary distal type 1 RTA is the most common distal RTA found in children. It results from defective urinary acidification in the cortical collecting tubule secondary to a genetic defect in transporters involved in the elimination of H$^+$ and associated regeneration of HCO$_3^-$ (Figure 75.5). Autosomal dominant distal RTA is caused by mutations in the *SLC4A1* gene leading to loss of function by abnormal processing or trafficking of the Cl$^-$-HCO$_3^-$-exchanger (AE1) located at the basolateral surface of α-intercalated cells and in the erythrocytes.[177-181] Mutations in *SLC4A1* also cause the dominant red cell morphologic diseases hereditary spherocytosis and ovalocytosis, although the association of these entities with distal RTA is rare.[182-185] Families from several countries in Southeast Asia with distal RTA caused by mutations in AE1, either associated or not with hemolytic anemia, who follow an autosomal recessive transmission pattern have been reported.[186-189] This form of distal RTA presents in children and adults.[182,185,190,191]

The apical proton pump H+-ATPase that transfers H+ into the urine (see Figure 75.5) is composed of at least 13 different subunits.[192] Mutations in the gene *ATP6V1B1* encoding the B1-subunit of H+-ATPase are responsible for a form of autosomal recessive distal RTA associated with sensorineural deafness.[193,194] H+-ATPase containing the B1 subunit is probably required for maintaining a pH of 7.4 and low Na+ and high K+ concentrations in the endolymph. These patients have congenital and severe deafness, although in some individuals hearing impairment is delayed in onset,[195] and some hearing-impaired children harboring *ATP6V1B1* mutations are not acidotic.[196] Mutations and deletions in the gene *ATP6V0A4* encoding the a4 subunit of H+-ATPase are responsible for another form of autosomal recessive distal RTA with preserved hearing.[197,198] Long-term follow-up of patients with distal RTA caused by *ATP6V0A4* mutations demonstrate that some of them develop mild, moderate hearing loss in consonance with the expression of *ATP6V0A4* within the human cochlea.[199] Apart from the hearing impairment, the clinical expressivity of these two forms of distal RTA, secondary to *ATP6V1B1* or *ATP6V0A4*, is similar.[199]

Biochemically, distal RTA manifests normal AG hyperchloremic metabolic acidosis with simultaneous inability to acidify the urine below a pH of 5.5. Unlike proximal RTA, the amount of bicarbonate lost in urine in the presence of normal bicarbonatemia is low (i.e., <5% of filtered bicarbonate). The reduced NAE causes persistent accumulation of nonvolatile acids and buffering by bone salts leading to hypercalciuria. Urinary net charge (formerly termed urinary AG) defined as $[Na^+] + [K^+] - [Cl^-]$ can be used in the clinical setting as a crude estimate of urinary NH_4^+ concentration because direct measurement of NH_4^+ is not routinely done in many laboratories. To maintain electroneutrality, when more NH_4^+ is present in the urine, the sum of $[Na^+] + [K^+]$ decreases, but $[Cl^-]$ does not. Therefore as NH_4^+ increases, the urinary net charge decreases and, in the normal response to acidosis, becomes negative. By contrast, when elimination of NH_4^+ is abnormally low, as happens in patients with distal RTA, the urine net charge remains positive.[200]

Urinary excretion of citrate is decreased because the increased availability of hydrogen ions in the tubular lumen converts the filtered trivalent citrate anion into the divalent anion, which is more easily reabsorbed via a sodium-citrate cotransporter in the luminal membrane. Intracellular acidosis may also contribute by increasing cell citrate utilization. Coexistence of hypercalciuria and hypocitraturia leads to nephrocalcinosis and urolithiasis characteristic of these patients. Nephrocalcinosis can be identified by ultrasonography very early within the first weeks of life and is irreversible, but renal calculi are not usually detected until an older age and are preventable by adequate alkaline therapy. Progression of nephrocalcinosis may result in a reduction in GFR, which is normal at the early stages of the disease. Hypokalemia of variable degree is frequently found in patients with distal RTA; its pathogenic mechanism is not well understood, but it has been related to a low activity of the Na+-K+-ATPase pump in the collecting duct.[201] Infants with permanent distal RTA may manifest transient proximal leaks of HCO_3^-, which normalize as the child becomes older. This form of RTA was formerly termed *type 3 RTA*.[202] Two siblings with distal RTA and mutations in the *ATP6V1B1* gene and with reversible generalized proximal tubular dysfunction with hyperoxaluria have been reported.[203] In addition, it is noteworthy that the existence of incomplete forms of distal RTA has been proposed in patients with nephrocalcinosis or urolithiasis without overt metabolic acidosis but with hypocitraturia and the inability to decrease urine pH appropriately.[204] However, it should be kept in mind that urine concentration disorders, such as those seen in interstitial nephropathies, result in defective urinary acidification because of the inability to achieve high H+ concentrations and do not represent true forms of distal RTA. In the presence of elevated bicarbonaturia, low urine P_{CO_2} during alkaline loading has been proposed as a sensitive marker indicative of a low rate of H+ secretion.[205]

Primary forms of distal RTA manifest in early infancy with vomiting, polyuria and polydipsia, dehydration crisis, failure to thrive, and growth retardation. The nephrocalcinosis is usually present at diagnosis. Primary distal RTA may present in children with neuromuscular symptoms linked to potassium deficit, including hypokalemic paralysis,[203,206] although this is more common in adults with distal RTA and Sjögren's syndrome.[207] Long-term treatment with oral alkali supplementation, potassium citrate, or sodium bicarbonate at doses of 2 to 3 mEq/kg/day every 4 to 6 hours to maintain normal values of serum HCO_3^- concentration induces catch-up growth, arrests progressive nephrocalcinosis and the related development of renal failure, and may avoid the appearance of urolithiasis and bone deformities.[208,209] Normalization of urine calcium excretion follows the correction of acidosis,[202] although not always,[195] but nephrocalcinosis is irreversible. Hearing must be systematically and repeatedly tested even in patients who have *ATP6V0A4* mutations because of the risk for late and mild hearing impairment.

The progress in the knowledge of both the physiology of urinary acidification in the collecting duct and the genetic and molecular basis of primary distal RTA has facilitated understanding of the mechanisms responsible for the acidification defect in patients in whom the use of functional tests, such as the analysis of urinary pH and the kaliuretic response to furosemide or the assessment of urine P_{CO_2} in alkaline urine or after phosphate loading, to explore the underlying cause of distal RTA is not indicated or yields ambiguous results. In forms of secondary distal RTA, these tests may be needed to clarify the pathogenesis of the defective acidification that can result from the inability to create a steep lumen-to-cell H+ gradient because of increased backleak of secreted H+ (gradient defect), absence of a distal lumen-negative transepithelial difference (voltage-dependent defect), or reduced urinary NH_4^+ available to buffer the free H+. Patients with obstructive uropathy and an inability to maximally acidify the urine because of voltage-dependent defects have impaired K+ secretion and develop hyperkalemia (hyperkalemic distal RTA).[210] On the other hand, progress in genetic analysis and testing may render mutation identification more cost-effective and, importantly, more straightforward for the child and family and then be used to direct either functional testing or therapeutic intervention.[27]

TYPE 4 RENAL TUBULAR ACIDOSIS

Type 4 RTA is found together with aldosterone deficiency or aldosterone resistance. Both conditions cause hyperkalemia, low synthesis of ammonium, and ensuing low levels of urinary NH_4^+ and NAE. Patients are able to decrease urine pH well below 5.5 (because urine ammonium is deficient as a buffer of free hydrogen ions), and the proximal reabsorption of HCO_3^- in the face of normal serum HCO_3^- concentration is decreased but not as much as in type 2 RTA.[96] Type 4 RTA has been found in patients with obstructive uropathy and interstitial renal diseases usually associated with some degree of renal insufficiency.[210] In children it can be observed in patients with PHA either primary or secondary to obstructive uropathies and urinary tract infections (see earlier).

Table 75.15 summarizes the main features of primary RTA types in children.

MAGNESIUM DISORDERS

METABOLISM OF MAGNESIUM

Magnesium is the fourth most abundant mineral in the body and is the most abundant intracellular divalent cation. It is essential for a diverse range of physiologic functions.[211] Sixty

Table 75.15 Schematic Description of Major Features of the Three Types of Primary Renal Tubular Acidosis in Children*

	Type 1 RTA		Type 2 RTA		Type 4 RTA	
Genetic and Molecular Features						
Mutated gene	*ATP6V1B1*	*ATP6V0A4*	*SLC4A1*	*SLC4A4*	?	*NR3C2*	*SSCNN1A* *SCNN1B* *SCNN1G*
Defective protein	H$^+$-ATPase B1-subunit	H$^+$-ATPase a4-subunit	AE1	NBC1	?	MC receptor	α, β, γ subunits of ENaC
Inheritance	AR	AR	AD and AR	AR	AD	AD	AR
Associated extrarenal findings	Early and severe deafness	Risk for late deafness	Cases with hemolytic anemia	Ocular abnormalities	—		Systemic PHA
Comments			Most cases from Southeast Asian countries	Most type 2 RTAs are part of Fanconi's syndrome with gene, molecular defects, and inheritance being those of the primary systemic disease		Renal PHA	
	Type 3 RTA is a combined type 1 and type 2 RTA, caused by mutations in intracellular CA associated with osteopetrosis. It was also used to denominate infants with permanent type 1 RTA and transient proximal leak of bicarbonate						
Clinical and Biochemical Features Common to the Three Types of RTA							
	Vomiting, dehydration episodes, and failure to thrive when onset in infancy; polyuria; growth failure Normal serum anion gap hyperchloremic metabolic acidosis Normal or mild reduction of glomerular filtration rate						
Distinctive Clinical and Biochemical Features							
	Normokalemia or hypokalemia, hypercalciuria, hypocitraturia, nephrocalcinosis, urolithiasis		Hypokalemia		Hyperkalemia, salt wasting, hyponatremia, elevated renin and aldosterone		
Minimum urinary pH in acidosis	>5.5		<5.5		<5.5		
Urinary NH_4^+ in acidosis	Low		Normal		Low		
Urinary anion gap in acidosis as estimate of urinary NH_4^+	Positive		Negative		Positive		
FE of HCO_3^- with normal serum HCO_3^-	<5%		>15%		5%-10%		
Urine minus blood P_{CO_2} with normal serum HCO_3^- and alkaline urine	<20 mm Hg		>20-30 mm Hg		>20-30 mm Hg		

*See text for details.
AD, Autosomal dominant; AE1, Cl$^-$-HCO$_3^-$-exchanger; AR, autosomal recessive; ATPase, adenosine triphosphatase; CA, carbonic anhydrase; ENaC, epithelial Na$^+$ channel; FE, fractional excretion; MC, mineralocorticoid; NBC1, Na$^+$-HCO$_3^-$ cotransporter; PHA, pseudohypoaldosteronism; RTA, renal tubular acidosis.

percent of body magnesium is in bone, 29% is in muscle, 10% is in soft tissue, and only 1% is in the ECF. Normal values of serum total magnesium concentrations are 1.8 to 2.3 mg/dL (to convert to mmol/L, multiply by 0.4114).

Magnesium circulates free or ionized, complexed to anions and bound to proteins. The ratio of ionized magnesium to total serum magnesium in healthy children is 64.8 ± 3.1%.[212] There appears to be no demonstrable advantage to measuring ionized magnesium as opposed to total magnesium for evaluating magnesium status.[211] Serum magnesium is dependent on dietary intake, intestinal absorption, and urinary elimination.

The main site of magnesium absorption is the small bowel, where approximately one third of dietary magnesium is absorbed. Absorption in jejunum and ileum occurs via paracellular simple diffusion at high intraluminal concentrations and, at low concentrations, by active transcellular uptake via TRPM6.[213]

Regulation of serum magnesium concentration depends primarily on the kidney. Approximately 95% to 97% of filtered magnesium is reabsorbed along the nephron; 5% to 15% in the proximal tubule, although it is of note that a much larger fraction of filtered magnesium is reabsorbed in the proximal tubule in newborns; and 50% to 72% in the TAL of Henle's loop, where it diffuses passively through the paracellular pathway. Finally, 5% to 10% of Mg is reabsorbed in the early distal convoluted tubule. This segment determines the final urinary magnesium concentration by active absorption, via the TRPM6 channel. Epidermal growth factor (EGF)[214,215] and 17β-estradiol[216] stimulate the magnesium reabsorption by promoting the transcription, surface expression, or activity of TRPM6 channels. Other hormones, such as parathyroid hormone (PTH), 1,25-dihydroxyvitamin D, calcitonin, AVP, mineralocorticoids, and insulin, stimulate renal magnesium reabsorption through an unknown mechanism of action.[217] Thiazides,[193] calcineurin antagonists,[218] and cisplatin[219] downregulate TRPM6. Renal TRPM6 expression is decreased in chronic metabolic acidosis and increased in chronic metabolic alkalosis.[220]

After magnesium is absorbed by the early distal convoluted tubule cell, the mechanisms of transcellular transport and its passage through the basolateral membrane are not well defined. Findings indicate that CaSR activity reduces cell surface expression of the basolateral potassium channel Kir4.1. This channel provides potassium ions to the Na^+-K^+-ATPase, which maintains a local negative membrane potential essential for transcellular Mg reabsorption.[221]

HYPOMAGNESEMIA

In the clinical setting, low serum magnesium concentrations indicate magnesium deficiency, although values in the normal range do not rule out the possibility of a total body deficit, compensated for by the release of magnesium from the bone.[211] In the face of hypomagnesemia, normal kidneys retain magnesium by decreasing its excretion to as little as 0.5% of the filtered load. Prevalent causes of hypomagnesemia in children are listed in Table 75.16. Hypokalemic primary tubular disorders and CaSR-related diseases with associated hypomagnesemia are discussed elsewhere in this chapter.

Table 75.16 Main Causes of Hypomagnesemia in Children

Primary inherited disorders
- Familial hypomagnesemia with hypercalciuria and nephrocalcinosis
- Hypomagnesemia with secondary hypocalcemia
- Autosomal dominant hypomagnesemia
- Isolated autosomal recessive hypomagnesemia with normocalciuria
- Activating mutations of calcium-sensing receptor
- Gitelman's syndrome
- Bartter's syndrome

Secondary disorders
- Decreased gastrointestinal absorption
  - Malabsorptive syndromes
  - Vomiting and diarrhea
- Increased urinary excretion
  - Extracellular volume expansion
  - Polyuric states: obstructive uropathy, kidney transplant
  - Drugs
    - Diuretics
    - Calcineurin antagonists
    - Others: cisplatinum, aminoglycosides, amphotericin B
  - Metabolic acidosis
- Miscellaneous: "hungry bone," low-birth-weight newborn, infant of diabetic mother

Hypomagnesemia is usually asymptomatic, and clinical manifestations of magnesium deficiency are generally not manifested until serum magnesium concentration decreases below 1.0 mg/dL, although the appearance of symptoms may depend more on the rate of development of magnesium deficiency or on the total body deficit.

Magnesium depletion inhibits PTH secretion and causes resistance to PTH action, leading to hypocalcemia, neuromuscular hyperexcitability and risk for tetany and convulsions. Cardiac manifestations of hypomagnesemia include prolongation of the QT interval and a wide range of arrhythmias.

Severe manifestations related to hypomagnesemia must be treated with IV magnesium sulfate under strict monitoring. A diet rich in magnesium and oral supplements must be used in asymptomatic patients with chronic magnesium loss.

FAMILIAL HYPOMAGNESEMIA WITH HYPERCALCIURIA AND NEPHROCALCINOSIS

Familial hypomagnesemia with hypercalciuria and nephrocalcinosis (FHHNC) is an autosomal recessive primary tubulopathy caused by loss-of-function mutations in the *CLDN16*[222,223] or, less frequently, *CLDN19* genes.[224] These genes encode two proteins, claudin-16 (formerly paracellin-1) and claudin-19, members of the claudin family that constitute a 22-gene family that encodes essential structural proteins of the tight junction, which are the principal regulators of paracellular permeability.[225] These mutations prevent the claudins from reaching the surface membrane, decrease membrane residence time, or render them functionless.[226,227] Claudin-16 and claudin-19 co-localize in the TAL of Henle's loop, where the magnesium ion is absorbed paracellularly, driven by a favorable electrical gradient (see Figure 75.2). Although the precise mechanism is unknown, the interaction of both proteins is required at the tight junction to keep the lumen-positive transepithelial diffusion potential that favors the reabsorption of Mg^{2+} and Ca^{2+} via the paracellular pathway.[225]

Most common presenting manifestations of FHHNC are recurrent urinary tract infections and polyuria and polydipsia.[228,229] Hematuria, abdominal pain, sterile leukocyturia, growth failure, and seizures are also frequent. Hypomagnesemia, hypercalciuria, and nephrocalcinosis are always found, and the majority of patients have increased PTH levels, urine acidification defect, hypocitraturia, and hyperuricemia. Hypocalcemia has been reported in some patients.[230] Ocular alterations, mostly myopia, are identified in 25% of individuals with demonstrated claudin-16 mutations.[228] However, severe ocular involvement, including myopia, nystagmus, ocular colobomata, and marked visual impairment, is characteristic of patients with mutations in *CLDN19*.[224,231]

Renal failure is often present at diagnosis and is more frequently observed in patients with *CLDN19* mutations,[232] although patients with two mutations causing complete loss of claudin-16 function have been found to present early and undergo rapid progression to renal failure.[233] Family members heterozygous for *CLDN16* mutations frequently have hypercalciuria, urolithiasis, or urinary tract infections.[234]

The clinical course of FHHNC is not modified by treatment with magnesium supplements and thiazides. Hypercalciuria, hypomagnesemia, and the progression of renal failure persist despite the therapy.[228,229] Inhibitors of endocytosis might be useful for patients with mutated claudin-16 protein not retained in the plasma membrane and rapidly retrieved by internalization.[235]

FAMILIAL HYPOMAGNESEMIA WITH SECONDARY HYPOCALCEMIA

Familial hypomagnesemia with secondary hypocalcemia (HSH) is a rare autosomal recessive disorder caused by loss-of-function mutations in the *TRPM6* gene encoding the TRPM6 protein.[236-239] As already mentioned, the TRPM6 channel is essential for the intestinal and renal reabsorption of magnesium (Figure 75.6).

Accordingly, patients with HSH and complete loss of function of TRPM6 manifest a homogeneous clinical picture with onset in early infancy with generalized convulsions associated with extremely low levels of serum magnesium, hypocalcemia, and inadequately low PTH levels. Patients need acute and urgent IV magnesium supplementation to control the seizures, to avoid permanent neurologic sequelae, and to normalize calcium levels followed by lifelong oral magnesium supplementation. The renal wasting of magnesium becomes appreciable after magnesium supplementation is unable to restore serum magnesium concentrations to a normal range.[238]

AUTOSOMAL DOMINANT HYPOMAGNESEMIA

Autosomal dominant hypomagnesemia with renal magnesium wasting has been detected in a few families with a heterogeneous genetic basis and intrafamilial variability in age of onset and/or severity of symptoms (see Figure 75.6).[240-245] In families with hypomagnesemia and hypocalciuria the disease has been linked to a putative dominant-negative mutation in the gene *FXYD2* encoding the Na^+-K^+-ATPase γ-subunit, leading to defective routing of the protein.[241] The precise molecular mechanism of the renal wasting of magnesium and hypocalciuria remains to be elucidated. It has been speculated that abrogation of γ-mediated modulation of the Na^+-K^+-ATPase kinetics

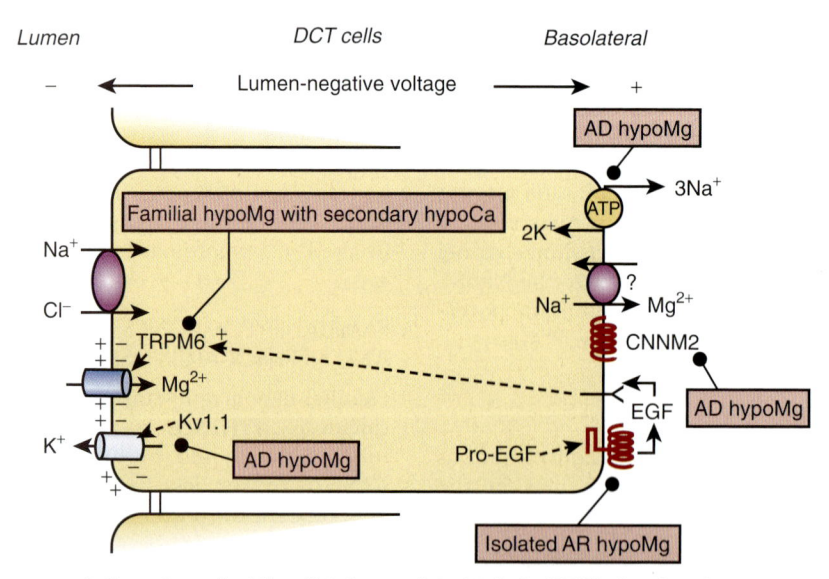

Figure 75.6 Schematic representation of a cell of the distal convoluted tubule (DCT) showing the transport systems involved in the reabsorption of magnesium and its inherited disorders. The thiazide-sensitive Na^+-Cl^- cotransporter, the magnesium transporting channel TRPM6, and the voltage-gated Kv1.1 potassium channel are depicted on the luminal membrane of the cell. The Na^+-K^+-ATPase, a putative Na^+-Mg^{++}-exchanger, the cyclin M2 protein (CNNM2), the receptor of epidermal growth factor (EGF), and the precursor of this peptide, the membrane protein pro-EGF are represented on the basolateral side (see text for details). *AD*, Autosomal dominant; *AR*, autosomal recessive; *ATP*, adenosine triphosphate; *ATPase*, adenosine triphosphatase; *hypoCa*, hypocalcemia; *hypoMg*, hypomagnesemia; *TRPM6*, transient receptor potential channel melastatin 6.

changes the electrochemical gradients of Na+ and K+ with a secondary reduction in magnesium reabsorption through the apical TRPM6 channel.[241]

Families with autosomal dominant renal magnesium loss with low or normal calciuria and no mutations in the *FXYD2* gene have also been described.[242,243] Mutations in the *KCNA1* gene encoding the voltage-gated Kv1.1 potassium channel subunit that co-expresses with the TRPM6 channel in the luminal membrane of the distal convoluted tubule have been described in a Brazilian family with dominant hypomagnesemia, normokalemia, and no alterations in serum or urinary levels of calcium.[244] The study of this family indicates that Mg^{2+} influx in the distal convoluted tubule through TRPM6 is driven by a favorable membrane voltage established by the Kv1.1 potassium channel. The ability to set this membrane potential would be impaired by *KCNA1* mutations. Mutations in the cyclin M2 (*CNNM2*) gene encoding CNNM2, a protein with high expression at the basolateral membrane of TAL and distal convoluted tubule, have been described in two families with dominant hypomagnesemia caused by renal magnesium loss.[245] The role of this protein in the regulation of magnesium tubular reabsorption is still to be defined.[246]

Hypomagnesemia has retrospectively been detected in children with dominant renal cysts and diabetes syndrome bearing heterozygous mutations in the *HNF1B* (hepatocyte nuclear factor 1B) gene, which is a transcription factor associated with abnormal renal development and that regulates the transcription of *FXYD2*, the gene linked to autosomal dominant hypomagnesemia with hypocalciuria.[247] Homozygous mutations in the *PCBD1* gene that functions as a dimerization cofactor for the transcription factor HNF1B have been shown to cause hypomagnesemia and renal magnesium loss associated or not with maturity-onset diabetes of the young.[248]

ISOLATED AUTOSOMAL RECESSIVE HYPOMAGNESEMIA WITH NORMOCALCIURIA

This is a very rare disease found in two sisters from consanguineous parents who showed psychomotor retardation and seizures with low serum magnesium concentrations and normal urinary calcium concentrations.[249] The disease was shown to be caused by a homozygous mutation in the *EGF* gene encoding the pro-EGF protein expressed in the luminal and basolateral membranes of the distal convoluted tubule cells, where it is thought to play a role in the activation of TRPM6 channels[214] (see Figure 75.6).

CALCIUM AND PHOSPHATE DISORDERS

CALCIUM AND PHOSPHATE DISTRIBUTION AND REGULATION

The 2013 Nobel Prize in Physiology or Medicine honored Thomas C. Südhof (together with James E. Rothman and Randy W. Schekman) for discovering the calcium-sensitive molecular machinery regulating the traffic of vesicle cell membrane junction. The malfunctions of such molecules give rise to tetany and other neurologic malfunctions. Calcium is central to the precision and timing of vesicle release of its cellular cargo.[250] Research into rare genetic diseases of calcium homeostasis may yield unexpected insight into basic mechanisms and possible treatments of overlapping illnesses.[251]

Serum total calcium concentrations normally range from 8.8 to 10.4 mg/dL (2.2 to 2.6 mmol/L).[252] Extracellular calcium is in three fractions: a non-ultrafiltrable protein-bound fraction and two ultrafiltrable fractions of calcium complexes and ionized calcium.

Serum inorganic phosphate concentrations normally range from 3 to 5 mg/dL (0.9 to 1.5 mmol/L) in a child or adolescent. However, in the neonatal period and infancy, the inorganic phosphate concentrations are higher, ranging from 4 to 6 mg/dL (1.3 to 1.9 mmol/L).[252]

This neonatal hyperphosphatemia may be linked to higher tubular reabsorption of phosphate, coupled with blunted tubular response to the already low circulating PTH, normally encountered in neonatal life. Finally, milk is the main nutritional intake at this age. The easily absorbable phosphate in milk is high to start with and especially so with formula milk.[253]

This high serum phosphate concentration continues to fall after infancy and reaches adult normal value by adolescence. Small seasonal variations are encountered, as well as variations with fasting and with circadian cycle.

Extracellular inorganic phosphate is bound to protein (10%), and one third is bound to sodium, calcium, and magnesium.[252]

CALCIUM AND PHOSPHATE BALANCES

To satisfy the requirements of bone mineralization and growth in the rapidly growing child, there needs to be balance between absorption and excretion of calcium and phosphate, respectively (Figures 75.7 and 75.8). The daily calcium intake (see Figure 75.7) on a North American or

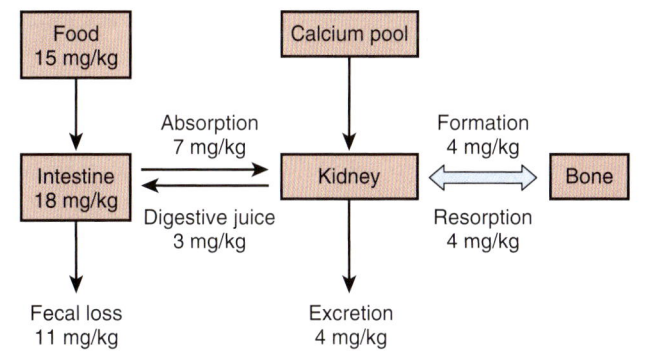

Figure 75.7 The calcium pool is sustained essentially by balance between dietary intake, intestinal absorption, and renal excretion of calcium. Every day, the skeletal system uses calcium at 4 mg/kg body weight per day to form new bone. This rate of calcium accretion in new bone formation is balanced by the same rate of calcium resorption from bone. Calcium in food is the most important source. Food provides calcium nutrition of 15 mg/kg body weight per day on a North American diet. Approximately 7 mg/kg is absorbed to augment the calcium pool. Digestive juice contributes 3 mg/kg to bring the total intestinal calcium content to 18 mg/kg body weight per day, out of which fecal loss is 11 mg/kg body weight per day. Finally, the renal excretion is 4 mg/kg body weight per day to maintain calcium balance.

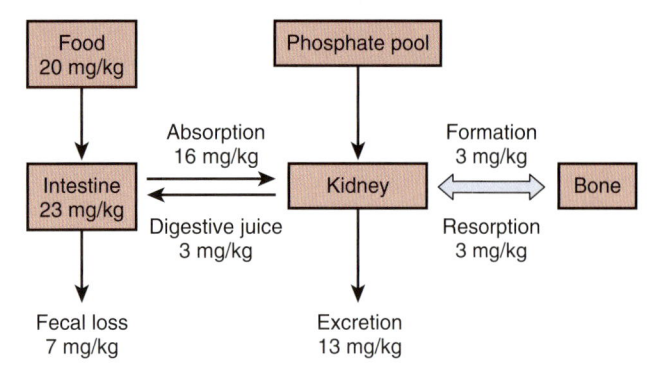

Figure 75.8 The phosphate pool is sustained essentially by dietary intake, intestinal absorption, and renal excretion of phosphate. Every day, the skeletal system uses phosphate at 3 mg/kg body weight per day to form new bone. This rate of phosphate used in new bone formation is balanced by the same amount of phosphate resorption from bone. Phosphate in food is the most important source. Food provides phosphate nutrition of 20 mg/kg body weight per day on a North American diet. Approximately 16 mg/kg body weight per day is absorbed to augment the phosphate pool. Digestive juice contributes 3 mg/kg body weight per day to bring the total intestinal phosphate content to 23 mg/kg body weight per day, out of which fecal loss is 7 mg/kg body weight per day. Finally, the renal excretion of phosphate is 13 mg/kg body weight per day to maintain phosphate balance.

European diet is 15 mg/kg body weight per day from food consumption.[254] The digestive juice internally contributes 3 mg/kg body weight per day. Total absorbed intestinal calcium is 7 mg/kg body weight per day, balanced by a urinary excretion of 4 mg/kg body weight per day and fecal excretion of 11 mg/kg body weight per day (see Figure 75.7). Finally, bone accretion of 4 mg/kg body weight per day is balanced by calcium resorption of the same amount.

It is important to recognize that depending on the calcium intake,[254] the net intestinal absorption of calcium varies widely, from 25% to 50%. For example, a North American diet, commonly referred to as a Western diet, is high in calcium from diary and meat products. In contrast, in non-Western countries, where vegan or vegetarian diets are more common, the calcium intake is low, and the intestine absorbs a higher percentage of the dietary calcium, to maintain calcium balance.

Phosphate intake in food amounts to 20 mg/kg body weight per day and digestive juices contribute 3 mg/kg body weight per day (see Figure 75.8). Thus a total of 23 mg/kg body weight per day is available in the intestine. With fecal excretion of 7 mg/kg body weight per day, the intestinal absorption of phosphate is 16 mg/kg body weight per day. The exchanges between bone formation and resorption are 3 mg/kg body weight per day. The urinary phosphate excretion is 13 mg/kg body weight per day to achieve net zero balance in the steady state.[254]

VITAMIN D, PARATHYROID HORMONE, CALCITONIN, AND FIBROBLAST GROWTH FACTOR 23

The control of calcium and phosphate homeostasis is complicated. For the purposes of this chapter, we shall focus here on four of the key regulators engaged in maintaining calcium and phosphate balance: vitamin D, parathyroid hormone, calcitonin, and fibroblast growth factor 23 (FGF-23).

Vitamin D exists in two principal forms: vitamin D_2 (ergocalciferol) from plants and vitamin D_3 (cholecalciferol) from animal tissues and by ultraviolet light activation of skin dehydrocholesterol.[255]

Cholecalciferol is carried in vitamin D–binding protein (DBP) to hepatocytes, which activate it to 25-hydroxyvitamin D [25(OH)D], by enzyme activity[256] of CYP2R1 and CYP27A1. DBP is also known as GC-globulin with three polymorphic forms: GC1F, GC1S, and GC2. Bound to DBP, 25(OH)D circulates to the proximal tubular brush border, where DBP is replaced by the receptor-associated protein, megalin (LRP2). Megalin, a transmembrane protein, facilitates internalization of megalin–25(OH)D.[257,258]

On reaching the mitochondria, megalin–25(OH)D is separated, with megalin degraded within the mitochondria. On reaching the kidney, 25(OH)D undergoes a second hydroxylation[256] by 1α-hydroxylase (CYP27B1) to produce the potent 1,25-dihydrovitamin D [$1,25(OH)_2D$].[259] At the antiluminal surface, $1,25(OH)_2D$ is again bound to DBP before entering circulation. Finally, the DBP–$1,25(OH)_2D$ complex accounts for the bulk of circulating calcitriol.

The key enzyme for $1,25(OH)_2D$ catabolism is CYP24A1. In a five-step progression, starting with 24-hydroxylation, CYP24A1 catabolizes $1,25(OH)_2D$ into a water-soluble calcitroic acid.[256]

The mitochondrial 1α-hydroxylase activity is tightly regulated, stimulated by low concentrations of circulating $1,25(OH)_2D$, calcium, and phosphate as well as high concentration of circulating PTH. The key enzyme for 1α-hydroxylase is CYP27B1.

High $1,25(OH)_2D$ concentration downregulates CYP27B1 and inhibits 1α-hydroxylase. In addition, high concentration of $1,25(OH)_2D$ stimulates the production of FGF-23 and Klotho, both of which inhibit 1α-hydroxylase.[256] Such feedback loops precisely control $1,25(OH)_2D$ production.

Klotho and FGF-23 are strong stimuli to the renal excretion of phosphate. Thus, by their downregulation of CYP27B1, phosphate homeostasis is linked to vitamin D metabolism. To maintain normal mineral balances, for example, hypocalcemia stimulates 1α-hydroxylation of 25(OH)D to $1,25(OH)_2D$, promoting active intestinal absorption and skeletal mobilization of calcium to normalize serum calcium concentration.

Similar to hypocalcemia, hypophosphatemia also stimulates the 1α-hydroxylase system and brings about the same responses. In contrast, hypercalcemia or hyperphosphatemia promotes the reverse.

Intestinal absorption of calcium[258,259] is accomplished via two major pathways: the concentration gradient–dependent, passive paracellular channel and two actively regulated calcium channels (epithelial calcium channel 1 [ECaC1] and epithelial calcium channel 2 [ECaC2]). The latter two channels are dependent on calcitriol enhancing gene transcription by nuclear vitamin D receptor (VDR) binding, promoting messenger RNA of the ECaC1 and ECaC2 proteins, thus augmenting the number of channels.[259,260]

After calcium enters the intestinal cell, it is carried by calbindin (calcium-binding protein) to the basolateral membrane and enters the circulation by a plasma membrane Ca^{2+}-ATPase (PMCA)–dependent process. Finally, PMCA gene expression is upregulated by calcitriol.

Parathyroid hormone, from the chief cells of the parathyroid glands, stimulates renal excretion of phosphate and renal retention of calcium and magnesium, while simultaneously promoting release of calcium phosphate and magnesium from bone.

Low extracellular ionized calcium concentration activates CaSR in the parathyroid chief cell, triggering uncoupling of a $G_{\alpha q}$ subunit from the G protein complex.[252] The $G_{\alpha q}$ subunit stimulates membrane-bound phospholipase C activity and phosphatidylinositol triphosphate generation. The ensuing calcium release from the endoplasmic reticulum reduces PTH secretion.

Calcitonin (CT), produced by the parafollicular cells (C cells) of the thyroid gland, inhibits calcium resorption from osteoclasts. CT operates via the same CaSR as PTH, but the action of CT is opposite to that of PTH.

FGF-23 from osteocytes is a potent phosphaturic agent. In concert with calcium, phosphate, $1,25(OH)_2D$, and parathyroid hormone, FGF-23 plays an important role in regulating phosphate homeostasis.[261]

FGF-23 decreases serum phosphate concentration by downregulating expression of sodium-phosphate transporters, both NaPi-IIa and NaPi-IIc, in the proximal tubular membrane. FGF-23 and Klotho inhibit renal 1α-hydroxylase expression. FGF-23 promotes 24-hydroxylase expression.[261] Consequently, $1,25(OH)_2D$ production is reduced, resulting in lowered phosphate absorption from the intestine and bone.

In contrast, with low serum phosphate concentration and/or low serum PTH concentration, the kidneys increase production of $1,25(OH)_2D$ (Figure 75.9). Consequently, the intestinal absorption of phosphate is increased.

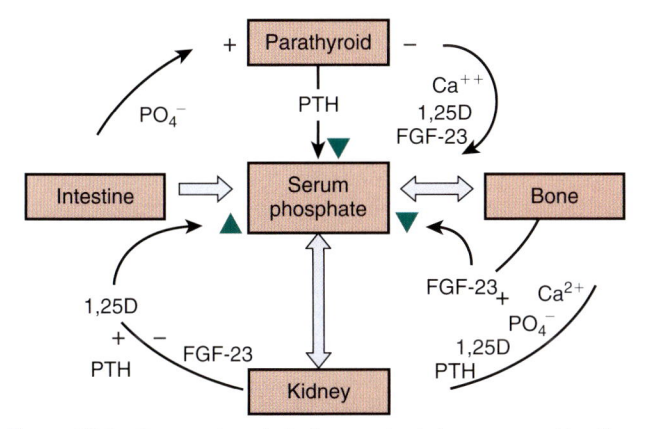

Figure 75.9 Serum phosphate homeostasis is conserved by three potent hormones: the parathyroid hormone (PTH), fibroblast growth factor 23 (FGF-23), and 1,25-dihydroxyvitamin D (1,25D). As indicated by the *green arrowheads* in the diagram, PTH and FGF-23 lower serum phosphate concentrations and 1,25D increases serum phosphate concentrations. Secretion of these hormones is regulated by reciprocal relationships and by the interaction of calcium (Ca^{2+}) and phosphate (PO_4^-). Specifically, the kidney's production of 1,25D is stimulated by low serum PO_4^- and PTH and inhibited by FGF-23. At the parathyroid gland, high PO_4^- stimulates production of PTH, which increases phosphaturia.

At the parathyroid glands, high serum phosphate concentrations stimulate PTH production, promoting phosphaturia to restore serum phosphate to normal concentrations.

In essence, PTH and FGF-23 are hypophosphatemic, whereas $1,25(OH)_2D$ is hyperphosphatemic (see Figure 75.9). These three hormones are regulated by reciprocal interaction and by the stimuli of calcium and phosphate.[262,263]

HYPOCALCEMIA

In preterm infants, hypocalcemia is defined as total serum calcium concentration of less than 7 mg/dL; in newborns, less than 8 mg/dL; and in older children less than 8.8 mg/dL. The causes of hypocalcemia are listed in Table 75.17.

Clinical presentation of mild hypocalcemia is often masked by the underlying disorders.[252] However, severe hypocalcemia strikes with symptoms of paresthesia, tetany, positive Chvostek's and Trousseau's signs, prolongation of the QT interval, QRS and ST complex changes, and eventually grand mal seizures and ventricular arrhythmias.

EARLY NEONATAL HYPOCALCEMIA

Early neonatal hypocalcemia, presenting in the first 3 days of life, is frequently seen in premature infants of diabetic mothers and in asphyxiated neonates.[252,264,265] The hypocalcemia is due to inadequate parathyroid response, compounded by hyperphosphatemia secondary to delayed phosphaturic action of PTH and by the hypomagnesemia common in diabetic pregnant mothers.

LATE NEONATAL HYPOCALCEMIA

Late neonatal hypocalcemia presents at 5 to 10 days of life and is commonly due to anticonvulsants administered to the pregnant mother.[264,265] Phenytoin and phenobarbital anticonvulsants amplify hepatic clearance of vitamin D, resulting in hypovitaminosis D, in both the mother and neonate, in that the impaired absorption of calcium gives rise to the delayed hypocalcemia. Another cause of the hypocalcemia is the reciprocal chemical relationship between calcium and phosphate concentrations. Thus hypocalcemia arises from the neonatal hyperphosphatemia, which is the result of three compounding factors: (1) the diminished phosphate excretion of the immature neonatal kidneys and the high circulating GH, (2) the low circulating PTH at this stage of life, and (3) the high phosphate load in milk.

Maternal hyperparathyroidism also causes late neonatal hypocalcemia in the first few weeks to as late as 1 year of life, due to the fact that maternal hypercalcemia leads to fetal hypercalcemia, which inhibits fetal PTH production.[266,267] The inability of maternal PTH to cross the placenta further aggravates the low circulating fetal PTH, which leads to the late neonatal hypocalcemia.

Familial hypocalciuric hypercalcemia (FHH) in the mother suppresses fetal parathyroid secretion.[266-268] Such neonates develop a transient hypocalcemia, owing to oversuppression of the parathyroid function.

INFUSIONS OF LIPID OR CITRATE BLOOD PRODUCTS

Infusions of lipid or citrate blood products cause hypocalcemia.[252,269] Fatty acids or citrates combine with ionized calcium, decreasing serum ionized calcium concentrations.

Table 75.17 Causes of Hypocalcemia

Neonatal Hypocalcemia

Early neonatal hypocalcemia (first few days of life)
- Maternal hyperparathyroidism
- Maternal diabetes mellitus
- Toxemia of pregnancy
- Sepsis
- SGA, IUGR, prematurity
- Asphyxia
- Transfusion (citrated blood products)
- Congenital rubella
- Hypomagnesemia
- Respiratory or metabolic alkalosis

Late neonatal hypocalcemia (fourth to tenth day of life)
- Vitamin D deficiency: nutritional deficiency; VDR loss-of-function mutation; deficient 1α-hydroxylase activity
- Phosphate overload: excessive intake of evaporated/whole milk
- Nutritional calcium deficiency
- Hypomagnesemia
- Hypoalbuminemia (nephrotic syndrome)
- Transfusion (citrated blood products)
- Acute/chronic kidney insufficiency
- Diuretics (furosemide)
- Organic acidemia
- Primary hypoparathyroidism: DiGeorge's syndrome; familial hypoparathyroidism; pseudohypoparathyroidism; Kenny-Caffey syndrome; partial deletion of GCMB; retardation dysmorphism syndrome; Pearson's mitochondriopathy; Kerns-Sayre mitochondropathy; PTH gene defects; CaSR-activating gene mutation

Hypocalcemia in Childhood

Parathyroid-related hypocalcemia
- Primary hypoparathyroidism: DiGeorge's syndrome; familial hypoparathyroidism; pseudohypoparathyroidism; Kenny-Caffey syndrome; Sanjad-Sakati syndrome; partial deletion of GCMB; retardation dysmorphism syndrome; Pearson's mitochondriopathy; Kerns-Sayre mitochondropathy; PTH gene defects; CaSR-activating gene mutation; Bartter's syndrome type 5
- Secondary hypoparathyroidism: radiation; surgery; infiltration (hemochromatosis, thalassemia, Wilson's disease)
- Autoimmune polyglandular syndrome type 1

Vitamin D–related hypocalcemia
- Nutritional vitamin D deficiency
- Defective 1α-hydroxylase activity
- VDR loss-of-function mutation

Nutritional calcium deficiency

Hypomagnesemia

Hyperphosphatemia: kidney failure; rhabdomyolysis; tumor lysis

Hypoalbuminemia (nephrotic syndrome)

Medications: diuretics; chemotherapy; transfusion (citrated blood)

Organic acidemia (IVA, MMA, PPA)

CaSR, Calcium-sensing receptor; GCMB, glial cell missing homolog B (a parathyroid-specific transcription factor); IUGR, intrauterine growth retardation; IVA, isovaleric acidemia; MMA, methylmalonic acidemia; PPA, propionic acidemia; PTH, parathyroid hormone; SGA, small for gestational age; VDR, vitamin D receptor.

RESPIRATORY ALKALOSIS

Finally, respiratory alkalosis causes hypocalcemia, due to a shift of ionized calcium to the protein-bound compartment.[252]

The majority of mild hypocalcemia resolves after 2 to 4 weeks of neonatal life. If hypocalcemia and hyperphosphatemia persist beyond this period of time, further workup for hypocalcemia is essential to rule out vitamin D metabolic defects, isolated hypoparathyroidism, or pseudohypoparathyroidism.[252] Finally, neonates with chronic kidney failure are expected to show hypocalcemia, hyperphosphatemia, and elevated concentrations of serum PTH, as well as urea nitrogen and creatinine.

DIAGNOSTIC WORKUP FOR HYPOCALCEMIA

Diagnostic workup for hypocalcemia in the neonate, infant, or child follows the algorithm presented in Figure 75.10 and starts with a careful history to rule out false hypocalcemia. The next steps are a determination of the serum albumin level, spot urine sample for calcium-to-creatinine ratio to delineate hypocalciuria or hypercalciuria, and then determination of values for serum PTH, magnesium, phosphate, serum creatinine, and 25(OH)D and other specific tests as dictated by the underlying disease causing the hypocalcemia (see Table 75.17). In the presence of persistent hypocalcemia and suspected maternal hypoparathyroidism or vitamin D deficiency, the mother should be tested for levels of maternal serum total and ionized calcium, magnesium and phosphate, PTH, 25(OH)D_3 and 1,25(OH)$_2$D, and spot urine examination for calcium-to-creatinine ratio.[252]

TREATMENT OF HYPOCALCEMIA

Treatment of acute, symptomatic hypocalcemia (Table 75.18) consists of 10% calcium gluconate at a dose of 1 to 2 mL/kg body weight (9 mg of elemental calcium/mL) intravenously at a slow drip of less than 1 mL/min over 10 minutes with ECG monitoring of the QT interval until symptoms vanish.[252,269] If tetany or seizures persist, calcium infusion is repeated as necessary at intervals of 6 to 8 hours until resolution of severe symptoms. Alternatively, a continuous infusion of elemental calcium, 1 to 3 mg/kg body weight per hour can be given. The addition of amiloride, 0.1 to 0.3 mg/kg/day, if serum calcium concentration fails to rise with such therapy, primary hypomagnesemia must be sought, and if proven, it requires magnesium sulfate intravenously at a dose of 0.1 to 0.2 mL/kg body weight (50% solution) under cardiacmonitoring or given intramuscularly.

Elemental calcium continuous infusion at 1 to 3 mg/kg body weight per hour to resolve symptomatic hypocalcemia may be needed to maintain serum calcium concentration above 7.5 to 8.0 mg/dL.[252,269]

Hypocalcemic infants with hyperphosphatemia may benefit from low-phosphate formula or breast milk with overall calcium to phosphate ratio of 4:1. Infants with vitamin D deficiency rickets due to maternal hypovitaminosis D respond well to oral vitamin D (1000 to 2000 U daily for 4 weeks) and elemental calcium (40 mg/kg body weight per day).

For early neonatal hypocalcemia this treatment brings about normalization in 2 to 3 days, after which the calcium

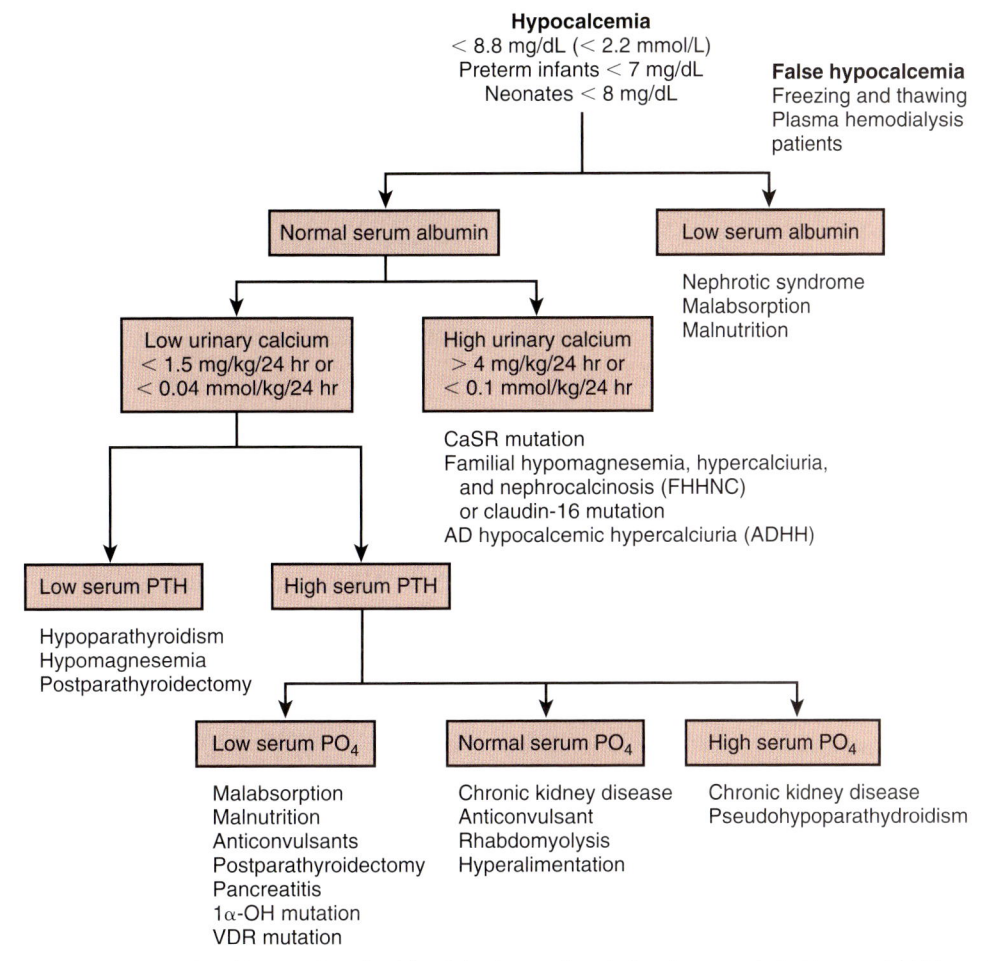

Figure 75.10 Algorithm for diagnosis of hypocalcemia. After false hypocalcemia has been excluded by careful history, the first laboratory diagnostic step is to examine serum albumin concentrations. Low serum albumin concentration points to specific disorders associated with hypocalcemia, such as nephrotic syndrome, malabsorption, and malnutrition. Normal serum albumin concentration points to an examination of urinary calcium excretion. Low urinary calcium excretion relative to low serum PTH points to hypoparathyroidism, hypomagnesemia, and postparathyroidectomy. Low urinary calcium excretion associated with high serum PTH relative to low, normal, and high serum PO_4 concentration, respectively, points to several diagnostic conditions as listed. AD, Autosomal dominant; CaSR, calcium-sensing receptor; 1α-OH, 1α-hydroxylase; PO_4, phosphate; PTH, parathyroid hormone; VDR, vitamin D receptor.

supplementation is reduced by half for 2 days and then discontinued. If prolonged calcium supplementation is required, hypoparathyroidism, pseudohypoparathyroidism, or defective vitamin D metabolism must be considered.

MONITORING OF HYPOCALCEMIA

Monitoring of hypocalcemia during treatment includes determination of fasting total and ionized serum calcium concentration, fasting serum phosphate concentration, and spot urine examination for calcium-to-creatinine ratio. Twenty-four hour urinary collection at home before the clinic visit is recommended to measure calcium and creatinine excretion.

The goal is to keep 24-hour urinary calcium excretion below 4 mg/kg body weight per day to prevent hypercalciuria and nephrocalcinosis related to the calcium supplementations and vitamin D administration. Serum PTH level is included in the monitoring if hypocalcemia is not due to PTH deficiency or resistance. Serum magnesium concentrations should be checked at least annually.

HYPERCALCEMIA

Although the range of normal for serum calcium concentrations vary between laboratories, serum calcium concentration of 12 mg/dL is usually considered mild hypercalcemia,[269] which usually is asymptomatic and resolves spontaneously. Serum calcium concentration between 12 and 13.5 mg/dL is considered moderate hypercalcemia, and the patient is invariably symptomatic.[252]

Presenting features of hypercalcemia include hypertension and GI symptoms due to its effect on increasing contractility of cardiac and smooth muscle.[269] Complaints of weakness, hypotonia, anorexia, nausea, colic, and constipation are common. The polyuria and dehydration are caused by hypercalcemia inhibiting the action of AVP on the collecting tubules. The vasoconstriction of hypercalcemia reduces renal blood flow and GFR, with the fall in GFR aggravated by the dehydration. Nephrocalcinosis ensues from prolonged hypercalcemia and dehydration. Acute pancreatitis associated with hypercalcemia is related to

Table 75.18 Treatment of Hypocalcemia

Medication	Dose	Administration
Symptomatic Hypocalcemia in the Neonate		
Calcium gluconate	IV 10% solution 1 mg/kg (9 mg elemental Ca^{2+}/mL) 1 mL/min over 10 min	Repeat dose in 8 hr
Magnesium sulfate, 50% solution	0.1 mL/kg IV or IM	
Symptomatic Hypocalcemia in the Infant		
Calcium gluconate	IV 10% solution 1 mg/kg (9 mg elemental Ca^{2+}/mL) 1 mL/min over 10 min	Repeat dose in 8 hr
Elemental Ca^{2+} continuous infusion	1 mg elemental Ca^{2+}/kg/hr	
Asymptomatic Hypocalcemia in the Infant		
Calcium carbonate PO	50 mg elemental calcium/kg/day	Divided into 4 doses per day

IM, Intramuscularly; IV, intravenously; PO, orally.

Table 75.19 Causes of Hypercalcemia

Neonatal Hypercalcemia
- Maternal hypervitaminosis D
- Idiopathic infantile hypercalcemia
- Excess calcium and vitamin D intakes
- Infantile hypothyroidism
- Neonatal Bartter's syndrome
- Williams-Beuren syndrome
- Renal tubular acidosis

PTH-Dependent Hypercalcemia
- Primary hyperparathyroidism: adenoma, hyperplasia, carcinoma
- Tertiary hyperparathyroidism
- Drug-induced: lithium
- Familial hypocalciuric hypercalcemia
- PTH receptor gain-of-function mutation (Jansen's syndrome)
- Autoimmune hypocalciuric hypercalcemia

PTH-Independent Hypercalcemia
- Immobilization
- Vitamin D excess: ingestion or topical analogues; granulomatous disease; Williams-Beuren syndrome
- Drug induced: thiazides; milk-alkali syndrome; estrogen; vitamin A intoxication; aminophylline
- Kidney insufficiency: acute kidney injury; chronic kidney disease with aplastic bone disease
- Neoplasm: multiple endocrine neoplasia types 1 and 2 ; lytic bone metastases; hyperparathyroidism-jaw tumor syndrome
- PTH receptor excess (non-neoplastic)
- Thyrotoxicosis
- Adrenal insufficiency

PTH, Parathyroid hormone.

---

microcalcinosis. How hypercalcemia induces somnolence, lethargy, stupor, and coma is poorly understood. Vasoconstriction reducing cerebral blood flow is considered a possible mechanism.

Table 75.19 lists the causes of hypercalcemia. This list is extensive, and many of the individual conditions are covered elsewhere in this book. Here we will focus on the following four conditions: idiopathic infantile hypercalcemia, Williams-Beuren syndrome, familial hypocalciuric hypercalcemia, and neonatal severe hyperparathyroidism.

IDIOPATHIC INFANTILE HYPERCALCEMIA

In Britain in the 1950s, vitamin D supplementation of infant formula and fortified milk at high doses (up to 4000 IU per day) brought about an epidemic of infantile hypercalcemia, presenting with failure to thrive, intermittent fever, vomiting, dehydration, and nephrocalcinosis. A number of fatal cases occurred. Vitamin D hypersensitivity and/or defective catabolism of vitamin D was suspected, but never resolved.

In response to such fatalities, a dramatic reduction in vitamin D supplementation to 400 IU per day was enforced, resulting in a significant drop in idiopathic infantile hypercalcemia in Britain.[256]

Later evidence[256] shows loss of function of CYP24A1, causing poor degradation of $1,25(OH)_2D$. This plays a central role in autosomal recessive idiopathic infantile hypercalcemia.

Prophylactic vitamin D is valuable in preventing rickets. But mutations in CYP24A1 in idiopathic infantile hypercalcemia stress the need for close attention to family history to identify those at genetic risk for idiopathic infantile hypercalcemia resulting from vitamin D prophylaxis.

WILLIAMS-BEUREN SYNDROME

Microdeletion at chromosome 7q11.23 gives rise to the multisystem disorder Williams-Beuren syndrome (OMIM 194050; also known as Williams syndrome), which is characterized by hypercalcemia, supravalvular aortic and pulmonary stenosis, growth retardation, and variable gradations of mental retardation.[251]

Williams-Beuren syndrome (prevalence: 1 in 10,000) is now regarded as an excellent model of contiguous gene syndrome, which may reveal genetic factors underlying calcium and cardiovascular lesions, hypertension, glucose intolerance, and anxiety disorders.

Presenting features include round, elfin face and full lips, broad forehead, strabismus, flat nasal bridge, upturned nostrils, dental malocclusion, hypodontia; early graying hair, and slight premature aging. Short stature and obesity are persistent features. Hypotonia, poor balance, and reduced coordination; scoliosis, lordosis, joint laxity, and hyperreflexia; and inguinal hernia and rectal prolapse are findings described in patients with Williams-Beuren syndrome.

A history of problematic feeding, colic, constipation, and delayed toilet training may lead to findings of gastroesophageal reflux, diverticular disease, or celiac disease. Urinary urgency and frequency, enuresis, and recurrent urinary tract infections often lead to investigations revealing structural anomalies and nephrocalcinosis.[251]

Subclinical hypothyroidism (in 15% to 30% of patients), early-onset puberty, glucose intolerance or diabetes mellitus, osteopenia, and osteoporosis present management challenges.

Hypercalcemia, once regarded as a constant feature of Williams-Beuren syndrome, is actually found in a minority of patients, varying from 5% to 50% of cases.[251] This large degree of variability in hypercalcemia is probably due to divergent study methods and diagnostic standards before the availability of the *fluorescence in situ hybridization test (FISH)* test (see later). Transient hypercalciuria usually accompanies the duration of the hypercalcemic episode. Whether the hypercalcemic episode is the result of vitamin D hypersensitivity as originally proposed or of elevated $1,25(OH)_2D$ or defective calcitonin production has not been resolved The suboptimal bone density found in 45% of patients presents a challenging concern. The long-term outcome of vitamin D prophylactics in children with Williams-Beuren syndrome remains unsettled.

Hypertension is present in 50% of patients.[251] The mechanism is unclear. Hypertension from renovascular lesions is uncommon in patients with Williams-Beuren syndrome. No general guidelines have been available on treating the hypertension of such patients. Management of hypertension has to be individualized.

The choice of surgical procedures to treat supravalvular aortic stenosis varies with the structural form and severity of the stenosis. Stent insertion and balloon angioplasty have been used.[251] However, as the child grows bigger, the stent stays the same or narrows from in-stent restenosis. There is a distinct hazard of rupture, aneurysm, and restenosis from vascular smooth muscle overgrowth. For these reasons, infants and children do not always have stents implanted. In addition, balloon angioplasty in younger children does not work well. Severe cases of supravalvular aortic stenosis are initially corrected by surgical reconstruction. When the child is older, if restenosis occurs, it will be more responsive to stent implantation or balloon angioplasty.

Unless it is severe, supravalvular pulmonary stenosis in patients with William-Beuren syndrome can be monitored without surgical intervention.

Intracranial stenosis (extremely rare) can cause strokes. There are reports of sudden death from coronary artery stenosis and outflow tract obstruction from biventricular hypertrophy. There are also increased risks when anesthesia is used in these patients. Overall, cardiovascular complications are the leading cause of death in patients with Williams-Beuren syndrome.[251]

These patients are often friendly, engaging, and endearing. Such a "cocktail personality" and attention deficit/hyperactivity mask underlying severe anxiety, phobia, obsessive-compulsive traits, and dysthymia. Cognitive impairment varies over a wide range, with IQ scores from 40 to 100 (mean IQ 55). Some patients suffer from hypersensitivity to sound, visuospatial weaknesses, and enormous learning difficulties but selective language skills. A special education curriculum is beneficial and needs to be individualized, given these multiple behavioral phenotypes and disabilities.

Overall, this syndrome encompassing growth failure, hypertension, autosomal dominant familial supravalvular aortic stenosis (OMIM 185500) results from a microdeletion of the elastin gene (*ELN*). It is not a point mutation disorder. A segment of an allele of the *ELN* gene is completely lacking. The FISH test includes *ELN*-specific probes and has become the most widely used laboratory test to establish the diagnosis of Williams-Beuren syndrome.[251]

Intense research into contiguous gene deletion involving the *ELN* gene on chromosome 7 may yield insight into a wide range of disorders from Chiari malformation and sleep disorders to the central features of hypercalcemia, vascular stenosis, hypertension, short stature, and mental retardation that characterize Williams-Beuren syndrome.

FAMILIAL HYPOCALCIURIC HYPERCALCEMIA

FHH is a rare asymptomatic autosomal dominant condition (prevalence 1 in 78,000) with mild to moderate elevation of total and ionized calcium concentration.[270]

The hypocalciuria is characterized by fractional excretion of calcium as low as 1%. Serum vitamin D concentrations are normal. Serum PTH concentrations are normal in the majority of patients, but in 15% to 20% of patients the PTH is mildly elevated. Serum magnesium concentrations are normal or slightly elevated. Serum phosphate concentrations are low or normal. Bone mineral density is normal.

FHH has been regarded as a benign condition, although a lifelong ailment, with a small risk for pancreatitis and chondrocalcinosis. Hence FHH is also known as familial *benign* hypocalciuric hypercalcemia.

Three variants of FHH have been identified, based on research into signaling pathways of CaSR,[270] as follows:

1. Type 1 FHH is due to loss-of-function mutations of CaSR, a guanyl-nucleotide-binding protein (G protein) coupled receptor. CaSR signals by means of G protein subunit $\alpha 11$ ($G_{\alpha 11}$).
2. Type 2 FHH is due to loss-of-function mutations of $G_{\alpha 11}$, encoded by the *GNA11* gene, which co-localized with the FHH type 2 loci on chromosome 19p13.3.[270]
3. Type 3 FHH is due to mutations of adaptor-related protein complex 2, σ_1-subunit (AP2S1), which modifies CaSR endocytosis.[270]

Associated with activation of CaSR, hypercalcemia stimulates G protein–dependent activation of phospholipase C, through G_q and G_{11} signal transduction. This spurs a buildup of inositol 1,4,5-triphosphate and boosts intracellular calcium concentration, which in turn reduces PTH production and stimulates renal calcium excretion. In FHH the loss-of-function mutations of CaSR weaken these CaSR-mediated signal pathways and block this renal response. Therefore, despite hypercalcemia, the hypocalciuria persists in FHH.[270]

The hypercalcemia of FHH is asymptomatic and does not need medical intervention. Occasionally a calcimimetic agent, for example cinacalcet, has been used successfully.

NEONATAL SEVERE HYPERPARATHYROIDISM

Neonatal severe hyperparathyroidism is an extremely rare autosomal recessive disorder, characterized by relentlessly symptomatic hypercalcemia, elevated PTH level, severe parathyroid hyperplasia, and hyperparathyroid bone disease. The patient inherits two copies of an allele of the CASR gene from consanguineous PHH parents, and bears inactivating mutations. The hypercalcemia of neonatal severe hyperparathyroidism is fatal without total parathyroidectomy. Postoperatively, the neonate needs lifelong vitamin D and calcium supplementation.

DIAGNOSTIC WORKUP FOR HYPERCALCEMIA

Diagnostic workup for hypercalcemia follows the algorithm presented in Figure 75.11 and starts by ruling out false hypercalcemia by careful history, to exclude laboratory error and tourniquet not released during blood sampling. Then serum PTH concentrations are examined in relation to the presence of hypercalciuria or hypocalciuria with a spot urine test to determine calcium-to-creatinine ratio. Next, in the face of a low serum PTH concentration, examination of PTH-related protein (PTHrP), followed by serum $25(OH)D_3$ and $1,25(OH)_2D_3$, is indicated. It is essential to examine the family history for FHH[270] as shown in the algorithm, and for occult neoplasms, including multiple endocrine neoplasia syndromes, and to review the history of medications (see Table 75.19) with side effects of hypercalcemia.

TREATMENT OF HYPERCALCEMIA

Treatment of patients with hypercalcemia (Table 75.20) consists of rehydration with IV normal saline at twice maintenance to restore normal circulating volume and improve GFR and calcium excretion.[252] To further augment calcium excretion, furosemide is given intravenously. To keep up with the furosemide-induced diuresis, additional fluid intake must be provided. As soon as calcium concentration falls below 12 mg/dL, furosemide is no longer needed.

Severe hypercalcemia with serum values exceeding 13.5 mg/dL requires reversal with bisphosphonate, which cuts bone reabsorption.[252] To prevent recurrent dehydration during treatment, monitoring of fluid intake and output is critical. In addition, dialysis to remove calcium has been effective. Finally, parathyroidectomy is indicated in severe hypercalcemia from primary hyperparathyroidism that fails to respond to medical therapy.

HYPOPHOSPHATEMIA

Serum phosphate concentration of 1.5 to 3.5 mg/dL (0.48 to 1.12 mmol/L) is usually accepted as mild hypophosphatemia, which usually is asymptomatic and may

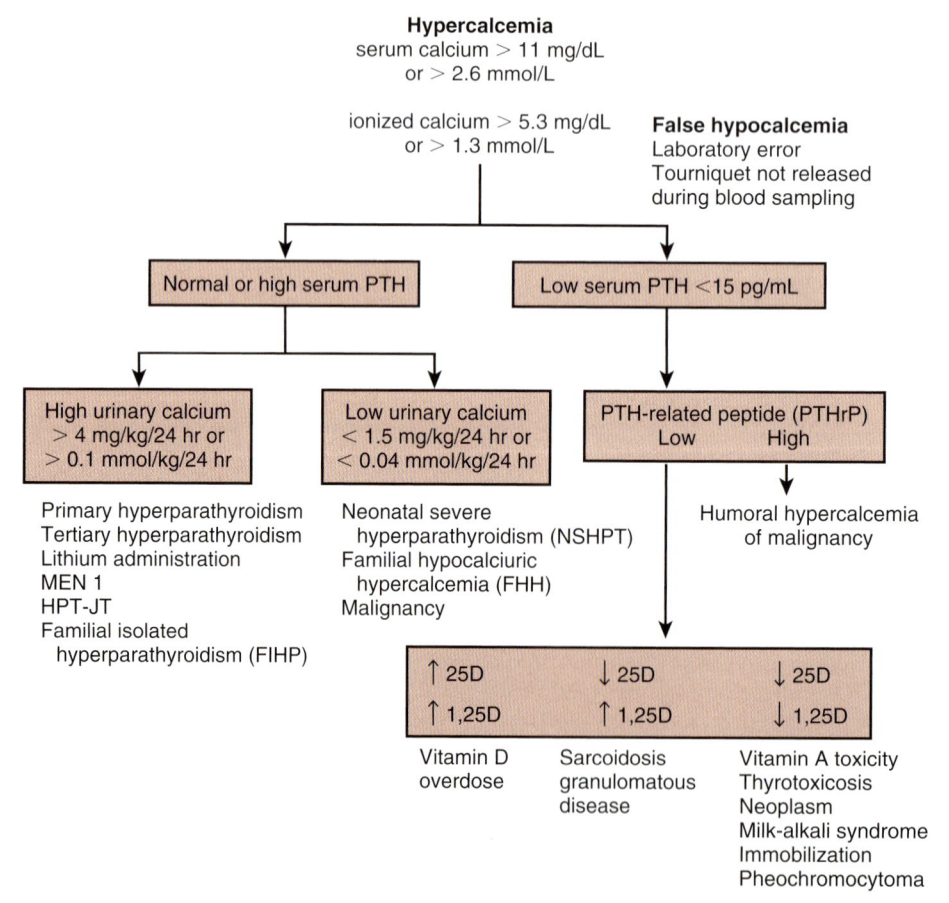

Figure 75.11 Algorithm for diagnosis of hypercalcemia. After false hypercalcemia has been excluded by careful history, the first laboratory diagnostic step is to examine serum parathyroid hormone (PTH) concentrations. Low serum PTH in relation to PTH-related peptide (PTHrP) suggests specific disorders associated with hypercalcemia and may need an examination of vitamin D metabolites: 25 hydroxyvitamin D (25D) and 1,25-dihydroxyvitamin D (1,25D) for differential diagnosis. Normal or high serum PTH concentration calls for an examination of urinary calcium excretion. High urinary calcium excretion relative to normal or high serum PTH concentration points to several diagnostic considerations. Low urinary calcium excretion with normal or high serum PTH concentration yields another set of diagnostic conditions as listed in the algorithm. HPT-JT, Hyperparathyroidism–jaw tumor syndrome; MEN, multiple endocrine neoplasia.

Table 75.20 Treatment of Hypercalcemia

Therapy	Dosage	Administration
Saline infusion	3000 mL/m²/day IV	This is twice the daily maintenance; reduce to maintenance dose as soon as serum calcium is below 12 mg/dL
Furosemide	1 mg/kg IV	q12-24 hr
Hydrocortisone	150 mg/m²/day IV	Repeat no more than 5 days
Prednisone	30 mg/m²/day PO	Repeat no more than 5 days
Bisphosphonate	1-2 mg/kg IV over 4 hr	Once
Calcitonin	4-8 IU/kg SC	q12-24 hr
Dialysis		

IV, Intravenously; PO, orally; SC, subcutaneously.

Table 75.21 Causes of Hypophosphatemia

Decreased Phosphate Intake

- Starvation, inadequate phosphate intake, chronic diarrhea, chronic alcoholism
- Total parenteral nutrition with insufficient phosphate content

Increased Loss of Phosphate

- Increased renal phosphate excretion
  - Primary hyperparathyroidism
  - Secondary hyperparathyroidism: vitamin D deficiency or resistance (including 1α-hydroxylase deficiency, VDR mutations, VDDR); imatinib
  - Excess FGF-23 or phosphatonins: X-linked hypophosphatemia, AD hypophosphatemic rickets, tumor-induced osteomalacia, epidermal nevus, McCune-Albright syndrome
  - Fanconi's syndrome, cystinosis, Wilson's disease, Dent's disease, Lowe's syndrome, multiple myeloma, amyloidosis, heavy-metal toxicity, rewarming of hyperthermia, Na/Pi-IIa and Na/Pi-IIc mutation (HHRH)
  - PTHrP-dependent hypercalcemia of malignancy
  - Hypomagnesemia
- Decreased intestinal absorption
  - Vitamin D deficiency or resistance (VDDR I and II)
  - Malabsorption
- Increased intestinal loss
  - Phosphate binding antacids used in treating peptic ulcers
- Increased loss from other routes
  - Skin: severe burns
  - Vomiting

Phosphate Shifting from Extracellular Compartment to Cells and Bones

- Diabetic ketoacidosis
- Alcohol intoxication
- Acute respiratory alkalosis, salicylate intoxication, gram-negative sepsis, toxic shock syndrome, acute gout
- Refeeding syndromes from starvation, anorexia nervosa, hepatic failure: acute intravenous glucose, fructose, glycerol
- Rapid cellular proliferation: intensive erythropoietin therapy, GM-CSF therapy, leukemic blast crisis
- Recovery from hypothermia
- Heat stroke
- Post parathyroidectomy; "hungry bone" disease: osteoblastic metastases, antiresorptive treatment of severe Paget's disease
- Catecholamine (albuterol, dopamine, terbutaline, epinephrine)
- Thyrotoxic periodic paralysis
- Hypocalcemic periodic paralysis

Miscellaneous

- Hyperaldosteronism
- Oncogenic hypophosphatemia
- Post kidney transplantation
- Post partial hepatectomy
- High-dose corticosteroids, estrogens
- Medications: ifosfamide; toluene; calcitonin; bisphosphonate; tenofovir; paraquat, cisplatin; acetazolamide and other diuretics
- Post obstructive diuresis

AD, Autosomal dominant; FGF-23, fibroblast growth factor 23; GM-CSF, granulocyte-macrophage colony-stimulating factor; HHRH, hereditary hypophosphatemic rickets with hypercalciuria; Na/Pi-II, type II sodium-dependent phosphate cotransporter; PTHrP, parathyroid hormone–related peptide; VDR, vitamin D receptor; VDDR, vitamin D–dependent rickets.

resolve spontaneously.[271] One exception is long-standing hypophosphatemia (e.g., in X-linked hypophosphatemia), in which the patients may be asymptomatic, despite low phosphate concentrations. Another exception is in early infancy, when normal serum phosphate concentrations range from 4 to 7 mg/dL. Thus, in the first 6 months of infancy, hypophosphatemia is suggested by serum concentration of 4 mg/dL or less.

CAUSES OF HYPOPHOSPHATEMIA

Serum phosphate concentration of less than 1.5 mg/dL (0.48 mmol/liter) in a child is severe and usually symptomatic, demanding prompt treatment.[252] The causes of hypophosphatemia are listed in Table 75.21.

Clinical features of severe hypophosphatemia result from reduction in intracellular adenosine triphosphate level, increasing the risks for hemolysis, rhabdomyolysis, and myopathies including respiratory and cardiac failures.[252] Paradoxically, intracellular phosphate released from cell breakdown may result in normophosphatemia or hyperphosphatemia, which may mask the true hypophosphatemia.

DIAGNOSTIC WORKUP FOR HYPOPHOSPHATEMIA

Diagnostic workup for hypophosphatemia follows the algorithm presented in Figure 75.12 and starts with serum PTH concentration and urine for calculation of the FEP, potassium concentration, and other specific tests such as PTHrP and FGF-23 as indicated.[252]

Depending on the dietary phosphate intake, FEP varies from 5% to 15% when serum phosphate concentration is normal. However, in response to hypophosphatemia, the tubular reabsorption of phosphate rises sharply as reflected in the corresponding drop in FEP. Thus, in the presence of severe hypophosphatemia, FEP persisting at 15% or higher confirms renal phosphate wasting.[271-273]

The serum calcium concentration is particularly helpful in the workup for hypophosphatemia. Because PTH is a powerful phosphaturic hormone, a high FEP accompanied by hypercalcemia points to primary hyperparathyroidism as

Hypophosphatemia
< 3 mg/dL (< 0.9 mmol/L)
Neonate < 4 mg/dL (< 1.3 mmol/L)

↑Serum PTH and ↑FEP

- Hypercalcemia: PTHrP-dependent malignancy
- Normocalcemia: Hypomagnesemia, XLH ↑FGF-23, Primary hyperparathyroidism
- Hypocalcemia: Malabsorption, Vitamin D deficiency, Secondary hyperparathyroidism

Hypokalemia
- Diabetic ketoacidosis
- Fanconi's syndrome
- Respiratory alkalosis

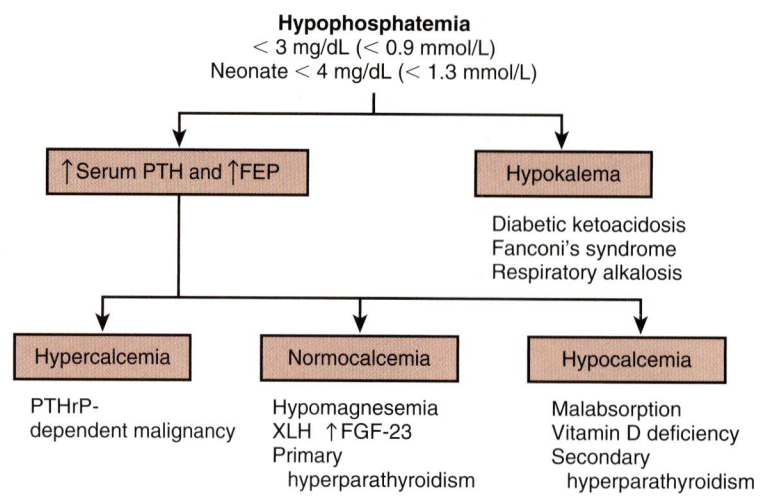

Figure 75.12 Algorithm for diagnosis of hypophosphatemia. Diagnostic workup requires examination of serum parathyroid hormone (PTH) and fractional excretion of phosphate (FEP), as well as serum potassium concentrations. Hypophosphatemia in the face of increased serum PTH and FEP requires an examination of the serum calcium concentrations. FGF-23, Serum fibroblast growth factor 23; PTHrP, PTH-related peptide; XLH, X-linked hypophosphatemia.

the cause of the hypophosphatemia. In contrast, if high FEP is accompanied by hypocalcemia, vitamin D deficiency and malabsorption must be considered. The symptoms of malnutrition may already be obvious on physical examination, but hypoalbuminemia not only supports such a diagnosis but also accounts for the hypocalcemia due to reduction of the albumin-bound fraction of serum calcium. A fall of 1 g/dL of serum albumin level accounts for a drop of 0.8 mg/dL of serum calcium concentration.

IMAGING STUDIES IN CHRONIC HYPOPHOSPHATEMIA

Imaging studies in chronic hypophosphatemia include skeletal x-ray examination to delineate osteopenia, osteomalacia, and rickets. Ultrasonography of the neck is helpful to rule out parathyroid adenoma. Finally, a scan using technetium 99m as an imaging agent may be indicated to delineate the presence of an ectopic parathyroid gland.

TREATMENT OF HYPOPHOSPHATEMIA

Treatment of hypophosphatemia from long-standing conditions, such as starvation or diabetic ketoacidosis, is complicated by the risk for rapid progression to severe, life-threatening hypophosphatemia during refeeding, as precipitated by rehydration and IV glucose infusion. Thus the concurrent use of oral phosphate supplementation (Table 75.22) is indicated. The fat and lactose content in skim milk is less than in whole milk and may be better tolerated by severely anorexic children. Intolerance to oral supplementation compels the use of IV phosphate (see Table 75.22).

Total body phosphate is depleted in diabetic ketoacidosis of many weeks' duration, in which there is a greater risk for rapid progression to severe hypophosphatemia on initiation of insulin and fluid therapy.[252] IV phosphate administered concurrently with the oral treatment is indicated for the first few days, especially if mental acuity is initially impaired. The side effects of diarrhea, diuresis, and volume depletion require close monitoring of fluid electrolyte balance, body weight, and blood pressure. IV phosphate is contraindicated in kidney failure, hypocalcemia, hypercalcemia, or hyperkalemia. Once the serum phosphate concentration returns to above 2 mg/dL, parenteral phosphate can be discontinued and the oral therapy curtailed.

Table 75.22 Treatment of Hypophosphatemia

Therapy	Dosage	Administration
Mild and Moderate Hypophosphatemia		
Low-fat milk		Phosphate 0.9 mg/mL
Buffered Na phosphate (Fleet enema)		1-3 g/day in 4 divided doses
Neutra-Phos (250 mg elemental phosphorus per capsule)		1-3 g/day in 4 divided doses
Calcitriol		30-70 ng/kg body weight per day
Asymptomatic Severe Hypophosphatemia		
Elemental phosphate	2.5 mg/kg body weight	IV over 6 hr
Symptomatic Severe Hypophosphatemia		
Elemental phosphate	5 mg/kg body weight	IV over 6 hr

IV, Intravenously.

HYPERPHOSPHATEMIA

As discussed earlier in this chapter, the hyperphosphatemia (up to 7 mg/dL or 2 mmol/L) in the neonatal period is physiologic. But beyond 2 years of age, a serum phosphate concentration higher than 5 mg/dL (1.6 mmol/L) is

```
                    Hyperphosphatemia
                    > 5 mg/dL (> 1.6 mmol/L)
                    Neonates > 7 mg/dL (> 2 mmol/L)
```

Hypercalcemia	Normocalcemia	± Hypocalcemia
Thyrotoxicosis Vitamin D toxicity		

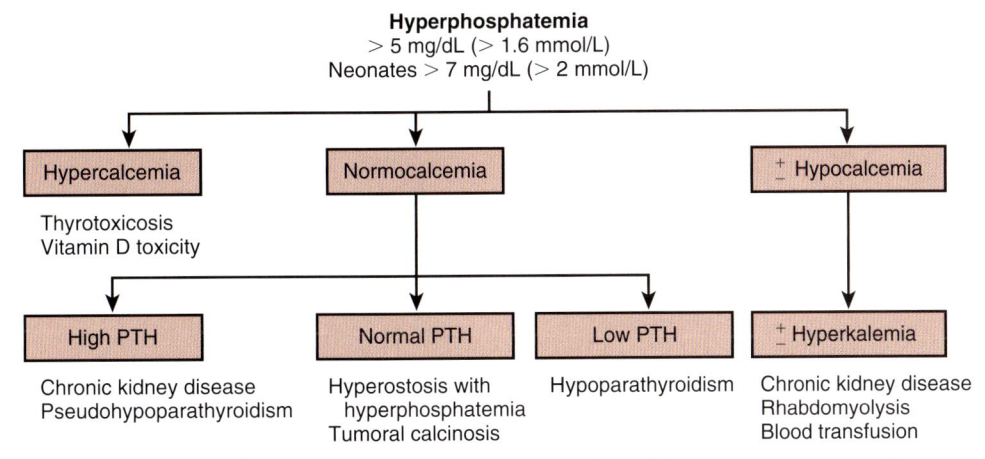

High PTH	Normal PTH	Low PTH	± Hyperkalemia
Chronic kidney disease Pseudohypoparathyroidism	Hyperostosis with hyperphosphatemia Tumoral calcinosis	Hypoparathyroidism	Chronic kidney disease Rhabdomyolysis Blood transfusion

Figure 75.13 Algorithm for diagnosis of hyperphosphatemia. The first step is to differentiate between conditions associated with hypercalcemia, normocalcemia, and hypocalcemia, respectively. Subsequently, serum parathyroid hormone (PTH) and serum potassium concentrations point to related diagnoses.

considered nonphysiologic and clinically significant hyperphosphatemia.

CAUSES OF HYPERPHOSPHATEMIA

Table 75.23 lists the causes of hyperphosphatemia. The clinical features of hyperphosphatemia are related to hypocalcemia. In view of the reverse interrelationship between these divalent ions, a high serum phosphate concentration is chemically linked to a low serum calcium concentration and vice versa.[251] Thus hyperphosphatemia becomes symptomatic from the hypocalcemia (e.g., tetany and other symptoms, discussed earlier under the section on hypocalcemia).

DIAGNOSTIC WORKUP FOR HYPERPHOSPHATEMIA

The diagnostic workup for hyperphosphatemia follows the algorithm presented in Figure 75.13 and starts with serum calcium concentration to delineate the presence of hypocalcemia, normocalcemia, or hypercalcemia. Next, concentrations of serum PTH, potassium, creatinine, and 25(OH)D are indicated. The underlying disease (see Table 75.23) causing hyperphosphatemia dictates other specific tests. Finally, spurious hyperphosphatemia results from interference with phosphate measurement by hyperlipidemia, hyperbilirubinemia, and hyperglobulinemia, requiring specific tests for each condition.[251]

IMAGING STUDIES IN HYPERPHOSPHATEMIA

Imaging studies in hyperphosphatemia depend on the underlying disease, for example, wrist x-ray examination to delineate renal osteodystrophy and magnetic resonance imaging to rule out pituitary adenoma in acromegaly.

TREATMENT OF HYPERPHOSPHATEMIA

Treatment of hyperphosphatemia includes adequate fluid intake to promote diuresis and restriction of phosphate intake[252] with the addition of phosphate binders (Table 75.24). Finally, specific treatment for the underlying disease is discussed in other chapters.

Table 75.23 Causes of Hyperphosphatemia

Impaired Renal Excretion of Phosphate
- Renal insufficiency
- Hypoparathyroidism, pseudohypoparathyroidism
- Transient parathyroid resistance of infancy
- Acromegaly
- Tumoral calcinosis
- Hyperthyroidism
- Juvenile hypogonadism
- High ambient temperature
- Heparin
- Bisphosphonate etidronate

Increased Phosphate Intake

Exogenous loads
- Phosphate salts: laxatives and enemas
- Vitamin D intoxication
- Blood transfusion
- White phosphorus burns
- Liposomal amphotericin B
- Fosphenytoin
- Parenteral phosphate

Endogenous loads
- Crush injury
- Rhabdomyolysis
- Cytotoxic therapy of neoplasms: tumor lysis
- Hemolysis
- Malignant hyperthermia
- Catabolic states
- Lactic acidosis
- Fulminant hepatitis

Transcellular Shift of Phosphate
- Cellular shift in diabetes ketoacidosis
- Metabolic acidosis
- Respiratory acidosis

Miscellaneous
- Hyperostosis

Table 75.24 Treatment of Hyperphosphatemia

Therapy	Dosage	Administration
Reduce phosphate intake	<800 mg/day	Low-phosphate milk in infants
Adequate fluid intake		Promote diuresis
Calcium carbonate	5 g/day	Given with meals to bind phosphate
Calcium acetate	5 g/day	Given with meals to bind phosphate
Parathyroidectomy		Severe hyperphosphatemia and hyperparathyroidism uncontrollable by medical means

CHAPTER SUMMARY AND CONCLUSION

We have highlighted the etiology, clinical characteristics, and management of acid-base, water, and electrolyte disorders in pediatric patients, in particular the pathogenesis and treatment of hyperosmolar and hyponatremic disorders. We have delineated how the gain or loss of function of renal tubular pathways contribute to disorders of potassium and hydrogen ion homeostasis, in particular in the different types of Bartter's syndrome and RTA.

Research into magnesium, calcium, and phosphate disorders in infancy and childhood has advanced our understanding of the sophisticated, interlinked homeostatic controls of these divalent ions, as exemplified by FHH. Finally, Williams-Beuren syndrome represents a contiguous gene syndrome, which may reveal genetic regulators key to calcium and cardiovascular lesions, hypertension, glucose intolerance, and anxiety disorders.

As the child with CKD grows older and transitions to adult medical care, nephrologists need to be cognizant that diseases once regarded as specific vulnerabilities of middle and old age may reveal risk predictors in childhood. For example, chronic hyperphosphatemia and elevated serum FGF-23 concentrations in the child with CKD forecast coronary calcification.[274] These and other considerations require intervention and coordination between pediatric and internal medicine nephrology teams.

Complete reference list available at ExpertConsult.com.

KEY REFERENCES

1. Winters RW: Regulation of normal water and electrolyte metabolism. In Winters RW, editor: *The body fluids in pediatrics*, Boston, 1973, Little, Brown & Company, pp 95–112.
3. Verbalis JG: Disorders of body water homeostasis. *Best Pract Res Clin Endocrinol Metab* 17:471–503, 2003.
8. Martinez-Aguayo A, Aglony M, Campino C, et al: Aldosterone, plasma renin activity, and aldosterone/renin ratio in a normotensive healthy pediatric population. *Hypertension* 56:391–396, 2010.
17. Moeller HB, Rittig S, Fenton RA: Nephrogenic diabetes insipidus: essential insights into the molecular background and potential therapies for treatment. *Endocr Rev* 34:278–301, 2013.
21. van Lieburg AF, Knoers NV, Monnens LA: Clinical presentation and follow-up of 30 patients with congenital nephrogenic diabetes insipidus. *J Am Soc Nephrol* 10:1958–1964, 1999.
27. Mejía N, Santos F, Claverie-Martín F, et al: RenalTube: a network tool for clinical and genetic diagnosis of primary tubulopathies. *Eur J Pediatr* 172:775–780, 2013.
44. Holliday MA, Segar WE: The maintenance need for water in parenteral fluid therapy. *Pediatrics* 19:823–832, 1957.
50. Beck CE: Hypotonic versus isotonic maintenance intravenous fluid therapy in hospitalized children: a systematic review. *Clin Pediatr (Phila)* 46:764–770, 2007.
54. Friedman A: Pediatric hydration therapy: historical review and new approach. *Kidney Int* 67:380–388, 2005.
57. Verbalis JG, Goldsmith SR, Greenberg A, et al: Diagnosis, evaluation, and treatment of hyponatremia: expert panel recommendations. *Am J Med* 126(Suppl 1):S1–S42, 2013.
59. Feldman BJ, Rosenthal SM, Vargas GA, et al: Nephrogenic syndrome of inappropriate antidiuresis. *N Engl J Med* 352:1884–1890, 2005.
60. Gitelman SE, Feldman BJ, Rosenthal SM: Nephrogenic syndrome of inappropriate antidiuresis: a novel disorder in water balance in pediatric patients. *Am J Med* 119(Suppl):S54–S58, 2006.
66. Holliday MA, Ray PE, Friedman AL: Fluid therapy for children: facts, fashions and questions. *Arch Dis Child* 92:546–550, 2007.
67. Endom EE, Somers MJ: Clinical assessment and diagnosis of hypovolemia (dehydration) in children. Available at: <www.uptodate.com:UpToDate>.
70. Giebisch G, Krapf R, Wagner C: Renal and extrarenal regulation of potassium. *Kidney Int* 72:397–410, 2007.
72. Gil-Peña H, Mejía N, Alvarez-García O, et al: Longitudinal growth in chronic hypokalemic disorders. *Pediatr Nephrol* 25:733–737, 2010.
82. Bartter FC, Pronove P, Gill JR, Jr, et al: Hyperplasia of the juxtaglomerular complex with hyperaldosteronism and hypokalemic alkalosis. A new syndrome. *Am J Med* 33:811–828, 1962.
86. Simon DB, Karet FE, Hamdan JM, et al: Bartter's syndrome, hypokalaemic alkalosis with hypercalciuria, is caused by mutations in the Na-K-2Cl cotransporter NKCC2. *Nat Genet* 13:183–188, 1996.
88. Simon DB, Karet FE, Rodriguez-Soriano J, et al: Genetic heterogeneity of Bartter's syndrome revealed by mutations in the K⁺ channel, ROMK. *Nat Genet* 14:152–156, 1996.
90. Birkenhäger R, Otto E, Schürmann MJ, et al: Mutation of BSND causes Bartter syndrome with sensorineural deafness and kidney failure. *Nat Genet* 29:310–314, 2001.
92. Krämer BK, Bergler T, Stoelcker B, et al: Mechanisms of disease: the kidney-specific chloride channels ClCKA and ClCKB, the Barttin subunit, and their clinical relevance. *Nat Clin Pract Nephrol* 4:38–46, 2008.
114. Gitelman HJ, Graham JB, Welt LG: A new familial disorder characterized by hypokalemia and hypomagnesemia. *Trans Assoc Am Physicians* 79:221–235, 1966.
115. Simon DB, Nelson-Williams C, Bia MJ, et al: Gitelman's variant of Bartter's syndrome, inherited hypokalaemic alkalosis, is caused by mutations in the thiazide-sensitive Na-Cl cotransporter. *Nat Genet* 12:24–30, 1996.
117. Knoers NV, Levtchenko EN: Gitelman syndrome. *Orphanet J Rare Dis* 3:22, 2008.
124. Tseng MH, Yang SS, Hsu YJ, et al: Genotype, phenotype, and follow-up in Taiwanese patients with salt-losing tubulopathy associated with SLC12A3 mutation. *J Clin Endocrinol Metab* 97:E1478–E1482, 2012.
132. Scholl UI, Choi M, Liu T, et al: Seizures, sensorineural deafness, ataxia, mental retardation, and electrolyte imbalance (SeSAME syndrome) caused by mutations in KCNJ10. *Proc Natl Acad Sci U S A* 106:5842–5847, 2009.
133. Bockenhauer D, Feather S, Stanescu HC, et al: Epilepsy, ataxia, sensorineural deafness, tubulopathy, and KCNJ10 mutations. *N Engl J Med* 360:1960–1970, 2009.
135. Shimkets RA, Warnock DG, Bositis CM, et al: Liddle's syndrome: heritable human hypertension caused by mutations in the beta subunit of the epithelial sodium channel. *Cell* 79:407–414, 1994.
137. Garovic VD, Hilliard AA, Turner ST: Monogenic forms of low-renin hypertension. *Nat Clin Pract Nephrol* 2:624–630, 2006.

142. Masilamani K, van der Voort J: The management of acute hyperkalaemia in neonates and children. *Arch Dis Child* 97:376–380, 2012.
145. Bonny O, Rossier BC: Disturbances of Na/K balance: pseudohypoaldosteronism revisited. *J Am Soc Nephrol* 13:2399–2414, 2002.
155. Wilson FH, Kahle KT, Sabath E, et al: Molecular pathogenesis of inherited hypertension with hyperkalemia: the Na-Cl cotransporter is inhibited by wild-type but not mutant WNK4. *Proc Natl Acad Sci U S A* 100:680–684, 2003.
156. Louis-Dit-Picard H, Barc J, Trujillano D, et al: KLHL3 mutations cause familial hyperkalemic hypertension by impairing ion transport in the distal nephron. *Nat Genet* 44:456–460, 2012.
161. Kraut JA, Madias NE: Serum anion gap: its uses and limitations in clinical medicine. *J Am Soc Nephrol* 2:162–174, 2007.
170. Igarashi T, Sekine T, Inatomi J, et al: Unraveling the molecular pathogenesis of isolated proximal renal tubular acidosis. *J Am Soc Nephrol* 13:2171–2177, 2002.
192. Karet FE: Inherited distal renal tubular acidosis. *J Am Soc Nephrol* 13:2178–2184, 2002.
224. Konrad M, Schaller A, Seelow D, et al: Mutations in the tight-junction gene claudin 19 (CLDN19) are associated with renal magnesium wasting, renal failure, and severe ocular involvement. *Am J Hum Genet* 79:949–957, 2006.
236. Schlingmann KP, Weber S, Peters M, et al: Hypomagnesemia with secondary hypocalcemia is caused by mutations in TRPM6, a new member of the TRPM gene family. *Nat Genet* 31:166–170, 2002.
244. Glaudemans B, van der Wijst J, Scola RH, et al: A missense mutation in the Kv1.1 voltage-gated potassium channel-encoding gene KCNA1 is linked to human autosomal dominant hypomagnesemia. *J Clin Invest* 119:936–942, 2009.
251. Pober BR: Williams-Beuren syndrome. *N Engl J Med* 362:239–252, 2010.
253. Lyon AJ, McIntosh N: Calcium and phosphorus balance in extremely low birth weight infants in the first six weeks of life. *Arch Dis Child* 59:1145–1150, 1984.
254. Nordin BE: *Calcium, phosphate and magnesium metabolism: clinical physiology and diagnostic procedures*, Edinburgh, 1976, Churchill Livingstone.
258. Kumar R: Vitamin D metabolism and mechanisms of calcium transport. *J Am Soc Nephrol* 1:30–42, 1990.
259. Bouillon R, van Cromphaut S, Carmeliet G: Intestinal calcium absorption: molecular vitamin D mediated mechanisms. *J Cell Biochem* 88:332–339, 2003.
262. Santos F, Fluente R, Mejia N, et al: Hypophosphatemia and growth. *Pediatr Nephrol* 28:595–603, 2013.
263. Rachez C, Freedman LP: Mechanisms of gene regulation by vitamin D_3 receptor: a network of coactivator interactions. *Gene* 246:9–21, 2000.
265. Kovacs CS: Commentary: calcium and bone metabolism in pregnancy and lactation. *J Clin Endocrinol Metab* 86:2344–2348, 2001.
270. Nesbit MA, Hannan FM, Howles SA, et al: Mutations affecting G-protein subunit $α_{11}$ in hypercalcemia and hypocalcemia. *N Engl J Med* 368:2476–2486, 2013.
273. Mount DB, Pollak MR: *Molecular and genetic basis of renal disease: a companion to Brenner & Rector's the kidney*, Philadelphia, 2008, Saunders Elsevier.

76 Renal Replacement Therapy (Dialysis and Transplantation) in Pediatric End-Stage Kidney Disease

Yaacov Frishberg | Choni Rinat | Rachel Becker-Cohen

CHAPTER OUTLINE

EPIDEMIOLOGY OF END-STAGE KIDNEY DISEASE, 2403
ETIOLOGY, 2404
CLINICAL CONSEQUENCES OF PEDIATRIC END-STAGE KIDNEY DISEASE, 2404
Nutrition and Weight, 2404
Linear Growth, 2405
Electrolyte Imbalance, 2405
Metabolic Acidosis, 2405
Anemia, 2405
Chronic Kidney Disease–Mineral Bone Disorder, 2406
Cardiovascular System, 2406
Neurodevelopment, 2408
Quality of Life, 2409
MORTALITY, 2409
Cardiovascular Mortality, 2409
MEDICATIONS, 2409
RENAL REPLACEMENT THERAPY, 2410
ADVANTAGES OF KIDNEY TRANSPLANTATION OVER LONG-TERM DIALYSIS IN CHILDREN, 2410
Survival, 2410
Quality of Life, 2410
Neurodevelopment, 2410
Exhaustion of Access Sites, 2410
Cost, 2411
COMPARING HEMODIALYSIS WITH PERITONEAL DIALYSIS, 2411
HEMODIALYSIS, 2411
Vascular Access, 2412
Dialysis Apparatus, 2413
Dose of Dialysis, 2414
Fluid Removal, 2414
Complications, 2414
PERITONEAL DIALYSIS, 2415
Access, 2415
Peritoneal Dialysis Prescription, 2415
Adequacy of Dialysis, 2416
Complications, 2416
Adherence to Treatment, 2417
Global Disparities, 2417
Change of Dialysis Modality, 2417
RENAL REPLACEMENT THERAPY FOR CHILDREN WITH INBORN ERRORS OF METABOLISM, 2417
CONTINUOUS RENAL REPLACEMENT THERAPY, 2417
Indications, 2418
Comparison to Hemodialysis and Peritoneal Dialysis, 2418
Technical Considerations, 2418
Dosing of Continuous Renal Replacement Therapy, 2418
Continuous Renal Replacement Therapy Outcomes, 2418
KIDNEY TRANSPLANTATION, 2418
Incidence, Prevalence, and Allocation, 2419
PREPARATION OF THE RECIPIENT FOR TRANSPLANTATION, 2420
Timing, 2420
Contraindications, 2420
Recipient Evaluation, 2420
TRANSPLANTATION IMMUNOLOGY, 2422
HLA Matching and Sensitization, 2422
ABO Compatibility, 2423
IMMUNOSUPPRESSION, 2423
Induction Immunosuppression, 2423

Maintenance Immunosuppression, 2424
Immunosuppression Combinations, 2426
PERIOPERATIVE MANAGEMENT, 2427
IMMEDIATE POSTOPERATIVE PERIOD, 2427
EARLY COMPLICATIONS OF KIDNEY TRANSPLANTATION, 2427
Delayed Graft Function, 2427
Acute Rejection, 2428
Infections, 2428
Recurrence of Primary Kidney Disease, 2431
CHRONIC ALLOGRAFT NEPHROPATHY, 2431
PATIENT SURVIVAL, 2431
GRAFT SURVIVAL, 2432
LONG-TERM FOLLOW-UP OF CHILDREN WITH KIDNEY TRANSPLANT, 2432
Hypertension, 2432
Cardiovascular Disease, 2432
Metabolic Syndrome and Diabetes Mellitus, 2433
Cancer, 2433
Anemia, 2434
Bone Health and Growth, 2434
Urologic Issues, 2435
Puberty and Reproduction, 2435
Nonadherence, 2436
Transition, 2436
Rehabilitation and Quality of Life, 2436

Until the middle of the twentieth century, end-stage kidney disease (ESKD) was a lethal condition, with a life expectancy of weeks to months at most. The developments over the subsequent 2 decades in both dialysis and transplantation completely transformed the lives of patients with chronic kidney disease (CKD), dramatically reducing mortality and morbidity. As technologies and surgical techniques developed, these treatments became available for children and later infants as well.

Treating pediatric patients with ESKD poses unique challenges to families, the medical team, and the health care system, which must address not only the disease itself, but the many manifestations that affect patients' lives and families. Reynolds reported 20 years ago that compared to the general population, adult survivors of pediatric ESKD were less socially mature and had lower educational qualifications, fewer had intimate relationships outside the family, and more were unemployed.[1] Two decades later, changing this unfavorable state should be one of the main goals for providers treating children with ESKD.

EPIDEMIOLOGY OF END-STAGE KIDNEY DISEASE

There are many barriers to accurate assessment of the global epidemiology of ESKD in pediatric patients. Approximately 80% of pediatric renal replacement therapy (RRT) is provided to patients who live in high-income countries, which account for only 12% of the global population. Registries, such as the North American Pediatric Renal Trials and Collaborative Studies (NAPRTCS), the European Society of Paediatric Nephrology, the European Renal Association and European Dialysis and Transplant Association (ESPN/ERA-EDTA), which can provide robust information, exist only in those developed countries. The information from developing countries is derived from surveys conducted among health care providers or from reports of patients admitted to tertiary centers. Both these methods result in underestimation, because most of the population has limited access to health services. Also, in countries in which registries exist, there are differences in the age span reported. Thus information from high-income countries shows an incidence of 9.5 per million age-related population (pmarp) in most Western European countries and Australia and 15 pmarp in the United States.[2-5] This is less than 10% of the incidence of ESKD in adults in the same countries. On the far end of the spectrum, Nepal, Nigeria, and some Eastern European countries report an incidence of less than 1 pmarp.[4-5] This very low reported incidence probably reflects underdiagnosis rather than true rarity of ESKD.

The incidence in all registries is higher in adolescents, due to both a different range of diseases in this age-group and the natural accelerated progression of CKD during adolescence because of rapid physical growth and possibly also due to hormonal factors. Higher incidence in males, due to the higher prevalence of congenital anomalies of the kidney and urinary tract (CAKUT) in boys compared to girls, is also a finding common to all registries or reports.[6-10]

The population ancestry composition of each one of the registries may also affect the incidence of ESKD reported, suggesting yet-undefined genetic susceptibility factors. In the United States, African American children have a twofold increased incidence of ESKD compared to white children.[2] In the United Kingdom the incidence was higher in patients who originated from Southeast Asia.[11] In Australia and New Zealand the incidence was higher in Aboriginal Australians, Maori, and inhabitants of the Pacific Islands.[12] In Kuwait there is a high incidence of pediatric ESKD, at 17 pmarp, probably the result of the increased incidence of autosomal recessive inherited diseases among populations with a high rate of consanguineous marriages.[13]

Over the years there has been an increase in both incidence and prevalence rates for pediatric ESKD in Western countries.[2,14] This probably does not mean that there is a real biologic change in the disease course. Instead it may result from the inclusion of patients who in previous years would not have been eligible for RRT, such as infants, thus increasing the reported incidence, together with improved survival of patients on RRT, which increases the prevalence.

ETIOLOGY

A major obstacle to accurately evaluating and comparing the various causes of ESKD worldwide is the actual definition of a given entity, which varies by reporting center (Table 76.1). This may be due to the introduction of a more accurate diagnosis based on genetic or other studies, which may be expensive and not widely available, or on the other hand, adherence to traditional dogmas that are now regarded as inaccurate. These include, for instance, focal segmental glomerulosclerosis (FSGS), which encompasses many different disease processes, and reflux nephropathy, which is better described as hypodysplastic kidneys with vesicoureteral reflux (VUR). In addition, a specific patient's diagnosis may occasionally fit more than one etiologic category; for example, autosomal dominant FSGS may be recorded under FSGS or as a hereditary disorder. A strictly defined and universally accepted CKD etiologic classification is lacking. Having said that, it is still possible to state that CAKUT is the leading primary diagnosis in pediatric patients with ESKD worldwide, responsible for 24% to 39.5% of patients with ESKD (see Table 76.1:).[2,4,6,14-19] Of note, this is proportionately lower than the incidence of CAKUT at earlier CKD stages, reflecting the relatively slow progression rate of this subgroup of diseases, at least during childhood and early adolescence. Hypoplastic-dysplastic kidneys, with or without VUR, and obstructive uropathies are the main categories of CAKUT, and the differences in listed diagnoses between various reports or registries are often semantic rather than biologic in nature. In most countries the second most frequent category is glomerulonephritis (8.3% to 30.4%), of which the most common entity is FSGS, especially in Japan and the United States (where it is the most common cause of ESKD among adolescent African Americans). Inherited diseases constitute the next category, although there are variations in which diseases are classified under this heading in different reports. The frequency varies from 6% (Australia and New Zealand) to 47.5% (Iran).[3,18] In countries where there is a high rate of consanguineous marriages, autosomal recessive inherited diseases cause a much higher proportion of ESKD. Specific diagnoses include cystinosis, familial steroid-resistant nephrotic syndrome (mostly due to mutations in *NPHS1*, *NPHS2*, and *PLCE1*), autosomal recessive polycystic kidney disease, primary hyperoxaluria type 1, nephronophthisis, and others.

CLINICAL CONSEQUENCES OF PEDIATRIC END-STAGE KIDNEY DISEASE

In children with ESKD the treatment goal is not only to prolong survival and to enable a life as normal as possible, but also to promote normal long-term growth and development.

Because life expectancy is much longer in a young child with ESKD, compared to a patient in the sixth to seventh decade of life, the child may go through the cycle of CKD-dialysis-transplantation more than once. This also has implications for the choice of treatment modalities (e.g., type of dialysis, vascular access) and the priority given in allocation of organs for transplantation.

Before describing the various modalities of RRT in children, the main medical issues of pediatric ESKD and their management will be discussed.

NUTRITION AND WEIGHT

Nutrition has a critical role in childhood. It significantly affects both linear growth and neurocognitive development.

Table 76.1 Major Causes of End-Stage Kidney Disease in Various Registries and Reports Worldwide

	USRDS	ANZDATA	Italkid	ERA-EDTA	Iran	Japan	United Kingdom
Years of data collection	2006-2010	2006-2011	1990-2000	2008-2010	1993-2006	1998	2011
Number of patients	6711	308	263	1598	120	582	675
Age	<18	<18	<20	<15	<14	<20	<16
Registry type	Prevalence	Incidence	Prevalence	Incidence	Incidence	Prevalence	Prevalence
CAKUT (%)	1580 (24%)	107 (35%)	104 (39.5%)	536 (33.5%)	32 (26.7%)	208 (35.7%)	218 (32.3%)
Hypoplasia/dysplasia ± VUR	998 (15%)	86 (28%)	27%*		21 (17.5%)	198 (34.0%)	121 (17.9%)
Obstructive uropathy	582 (9%)	21 (7%)	12%*		9 (7.5%)	10 (2%)	
Glomerulonephritis (%)	1501 (22%)	91 (30%)	28 (10.6%)	222 (13.9%)	8.3% 5.0%	177 (30.4%)	93 (13.8%)
FSGS	790 (11.8%)		16 (6.1%)			112 (19.2%)	
Hereditary (%)	631 (9%)	19 (6%)	66 (25.1%)	298 (18.6%)	57 (47.5%)	101 (17.4%)	114 (16.9%)
Autosomal recessive	455 (7%)	≈3%	57 (21.7%)		57 (47.5%)	73 (12.5%)	

*Estimated.
ANZDATA, Australia and New Zealand Dialysis and Transplant Registry; CAKUT, congenital anomalies of the kidney and urinary tract; ERA-EDTA, European Renal Association and European Dialysis and Transplant Association; FSGS, focal segmental glomerulosclerosis; USRDS, United States Renal Data System; VUR, vesicoureteral reflux.
Data adapted from references 2, 4, 6, and 14-19.

Malnutrition, which is the result of poor appetite, vomiting, and decreased intestinal absorption, is common in children with ESKD. Close monitoring is crucial when the patient is younger than 1 year (every 2 to 4 weeks), decreasing in frequency as the patient grows. Dietary intake should be assessed periodically. In patients on a formula-based diet this includes formula type, caloric value, protein content, volume, and length of each meal. Height and weight are plotted on appropriate growth curves and z scores calculated. Head circumference is measured regularly in children younger than 3 years. Normalized protein catabolic rate can be calculated for patients undergoing dialysis. The individual nutritional plan is based on Kidney Disease Outcomes Quality Initiative (KDOQI) guidelines with adjustments to achieve weight gain and linear growth targets while addressing clinical and laboratory issues. The majority of younger children fail to meet the energy and protein requirements by oral feeding alone and need supplementation by nasogastric tube or gastrostomy.

Initial recommended caloric intake is the age-related dietary reference intake (DRI), but it is adjusted according to weight gain. Protein intake recommendation is 100% to 120% of the age-related DRI, with somewhat higher intake in patients undergoing peritoneal dialysis (PD) to compensate for peritoneal losses.[20] In contrast to adults, a Cochrane review found that protein restriction has no impact on delaying progression of renal failure in children.[21,22] Another study raises concern about the detrimental influence of protein restriction on linear growth.[23]

Dietary restrictions may include fluid, sodium, phosphorus, and potassium; special infant formulas are adapted to the needs of patients with CKD. Human milk also has the adequate electrolyte composition for the infant with CKD, because it is relatively low in potassium and phosphorus. However, because the infant's diet is fluid based, it may ultimately cause volume overload. This requires in some cases concentrating the formula to achieve a higher caloric intake in a smaller volume (80 to 120 kcal/100 mL versus the usual 67 kcal/100 mL). It may also influence the dialytic modality selected or the frequency of the dialysis sessions. On the other hand, in several renal diseases (e.g., dysplastic kidneys, nephronophthisis, and cystinosis) patients may be polyuric due to a renal concentrating defect even when they reach ESKD. This makes water handling and nutrition easier.

LINEAR GROWTH

Growth is severely impaired in children with ESKD. Almost half of children with ESKD reach a final adult height below the third percentile if growth hormone (GH) is not prescribed.[24] A longer period with ESKD and short stature at disease onset are associated with decreased final height. Short stature affects body image and may have an impact on self-esteem. Patients, including young adults, are often treated as younger than their chronologic age. In the context of chronic illness this leads to overprotection, low expectations, and delayed independence and may subsequently affect socioeconomic status and forming intimate relationships.

When assessing the present stature of a patient, the clinician should remember that there are differences between races and in growth curves, with normal values available only for some (developed) countries. In countries with population heterogeneity, attempts to construct uniform growth charts for the whole population create inaccuracies, which may lead to inappropriate clinical decisions.[25]

Many factors contribute to impaired linear growth:

- Low calorie and protein intake: this is especially significant in early childhood.
- Disturbed GH/insulin-like growth factor-1 (IGF-1) axis.
- Additional factors include water and electrolyte imbalance, anemia, mineral bone disorder (MBD),[26] and metabolic acidosis. Correcting these abnormalities may improve the likelihood of achieving normal growth.

Beyond correction of the metabolic disorders and providing the best nutritional support, treatment includes recombinant GH therapy. This treatment was proved to be efficient by a study based on NAPRTCS data. Of 5122 patients receiving dialysis who are registered, 33% received GH treatment. Catch-up growth was achieved in 11% of the treated patients (compared to 27% of patients in earlier stages of CKD). The mean increase was 0.5 standard deviation score (SDS) (compared to 0.8 SDS in earlier stages).[27] In addition, a Cochrane database meta-analysis found increased height velocity (+3.9 cm/yr after 1 year), without advance in bone age.[28] In the NAPRTCS 2011 report, children younger than 6 years had improvement in z score of +0.63 compared to −0.1 in the untreated patients. Older children had less pronounced improvement of +0.26 z scores.[29]

ELECTROLYTE IMBALANCE

Hyperkalemia is commonly found in children with ESKD. Treatment includes dietary restriction and the use of sodium polystyrene sulfonate. Formula adapted for infants with CKD, low in potassium, phosphorus, and calcium, is commercially available. Further reduction in the potassium content of a formula-based diet can be achieved by pretreatment of the food with sodium polystyrene sulfonate.[30] This method is associated with increased sodium intake, which may lead to hypervolemia and hypertension.

METABOLIC ACIDOSIS

Chronic metabolic acidosis is treated in children because of its impact on bone linear growth and structure. The effect of acidosis on bone health and growth is multifactorial, including increased osteoclastic and decreased osteoblastic activity, blunted action of the GH/IGF-1 axis on bones, decreased 1,25-dihydroxyvitamin D production and hence less intestinal calcium absorption, and alteration of homeostatic relationships between vitamin D, parathyroid hormone (PTH), and ionized calcium. Metabolic acidosis is treated with bicarbonate salts, and the target serum bicarbonate levels are 20 to 22 mEq/L.

ANEMIA

Hemoglobin starts to decline in children when estimated glomerular filtration rate (eGFR) is lower than approximately 50 mL/min/1.73 m^2.[31] Diagnosis of iron deficiency may be challenging, because many patients with ESKD have low transferrin levels due to malnutrition and/or a chronic inflammatory state, causing the transferrin saturation not to reflect the low levels expected in iron deficiency. Ferritin concentrations, on the other hand, may be high because ferritin is an acute phase reactant. Additional data, including mean corpuscular volume, red blood cell width distribution index, reticulocyte count, and a blood smear, may assist in diagnosis. Other assays such as hepcidin and soluble transferring receptor are not in routine clinical use. The physiologic hemoglobin concentrations vary with age and gender as do the recommended target levels: above the fifth percentile of the specific age. Treatment includes iron supplementation and erythropoietin-stimulating agents (ESAs). Target iron levels are higher than in the healthy population: transferrin saturation greater than 20% and ferritin greater than 100 ng/mL (to optimize the effect of ESA). The relative ESA dose (units per kilogram per week) is higher in children and may even reach 1250 units/kg/wk of epoetin in infants.[32] In very young children undergoing chronic hemodialysis, there is an obligatory blood loss in the dialysis tubing, which is comparable (in absolute volume units) to the situation in adults, but when calculated per kilogram of body weight, it is much higher and may reach a total volume almost equivalent to 3 units of blood (27 mL/kg) per month.[32] Other causes for failure of ESA include osteitis fibrosa cystica, chronic inflammation, malnutrition, hemolysis, and rarely carnitine deficiency or aluminum toxicity. Studies in adults receiving dialysis found that excessive correction of anemia (even within the physiologic hemoglobin level) is associated with increased mortality, so it is recommended not to exceed hemoglobin levels of 13 g/dL. The pathophysiology of this phenomenon is unclear and has not been validated in children.

CHRONIC KIDNEY DISEASE–MINERAL BONE DISORDER

Although the pathophysiology of CKD-MBD and the pathologic types in children are similar to those in adults, both the management and the consequences are different as children grow. Monitoring of various CKD-MBD–associated parameters, including measurement of serum calcium, phosphorus, and PTH levels, is performed every 1 to 3 months, and vitamin D levels and bone radiography annually. Because normal blood concentrations and DRI are age dependent, the target levels and nutritional recommendations also vary with age. Age-adjusted hypophosphatemia should be avoided because it can result in hypophosphatemic rickets, often seen in preterm infants with insufficient phosphorus intake or in children with phosphaturia due to proximal tubulopathy. In CKD stage 5 the KDOQI 2008 guidelines recommend phosphorus restriction to 80% to 100% of the DRI, depending on blood levels.[20] This is expected to result in lower PTH and increased 1,25-dihydroxycholecalciferol (calcitriol) levels, as well as better bone morphologic characteristics and reduced risk for CKD-associated vasculopathy,[33,34] without linear growth restriction.[23,35] The choice of phosphate binders is limited in children. The first line remains calcium-based phosphate binders. Sevelamer hydrochloride was associated with increased metabolic acidosis,[36] which may impair linear growth. The newer sevelamer carbonate addresses the issue of acidosis, but it is not yet approved by the U.S. Food and Drug Administration (FDA) for use in children.[37] The use of lanthanum carbonate is not recommended in children because lanthanum deposits in bones, including growth plates, and the consequences on the developing bone are as yet unknown.

Vitamin D supplementation is important especially in CKD stages 2 to 4, whereas in CKD stage 5 active vitamin D metabolite is often added.[38,39] Pediatric studies of paricalcitol, a new vitamin D analog, have shown either equivalent efficacy to intravenous calcitriol in all parameters (PTH, calcium, phosphorus levels and calcium-phosphorus product [Ca × P]) or superiority to calcitriol only in invoking fewer episodes of increased Ca × P above 70 mg^2/dL^2.[40,41] Finally, calcimimetics, which increase the sensitivity of the parathyroid calcium receptors, are not yet approved for use in children.

The recommended KDOQI PTH levels in CKD stage 5 are 200 to 300 pg/mL. This is concordant with the international pediatric PD network,[42] but there is no consensus, and other opinions have suggested a much lower target.[43]

Deformities of the growing bone and impaired linear growth are complications that are typical in the pediatric age-group, in addition to vascular calcification (VC), which is also well described in the adult patient population. Because abnormal linear growth is attributable to a number of factors whose relative contribution remains to be determined, the consensus is to treat whatever is treatable. Of note, it has been shown that correcting active vitamin D metabolite deficiency alone can increase growth rate.[26] This was possibly achieved due to maintaining PTH levels at near normal values.[44] Skeletal deformities in CKD, similar to the phenotype of vitamin D–dependent rickets, may be very debilitating but are amenable to medical therapy with marked improvement and even complete resolution (Figure 76.1).

CARDIOVASCULAR SYSTEM

Cardiovascular system (CVS) disease is common in children with ESKD. Because clinical entities such as ischemic heart disease and valvular heart disease are rare in children, there is an opportunity to better define the development and progression of CKD-related CVS disease. There are some distinct, although interrelated, clinical features.

HYPERTENSION

Hypertension, defined as blood pressure (systolic or diastolic) above the ninety-fifth percentile for age, gender, and height percentile or treated hypertension, is found in 51% to 79% of patients with ESKD.[45-48] In one of these studies 21% of the children with hypertension were not treated at all, and 74% of the treated patients had uncontrolled hypertension. It was more frequent in patients receiving hemodialysis (HD) compared to PD or children who had received transplants (63.8%, 54.6%, and 26.6%, respectively).[47] Other risk factors for hypertension are age under 3 years, short time on RRT, acquired (as compared to congenital) kidney disease, and very low body mass index (BMI). The younger patients with hypertension are more likely to be untreated. This may be due to underestimation of the

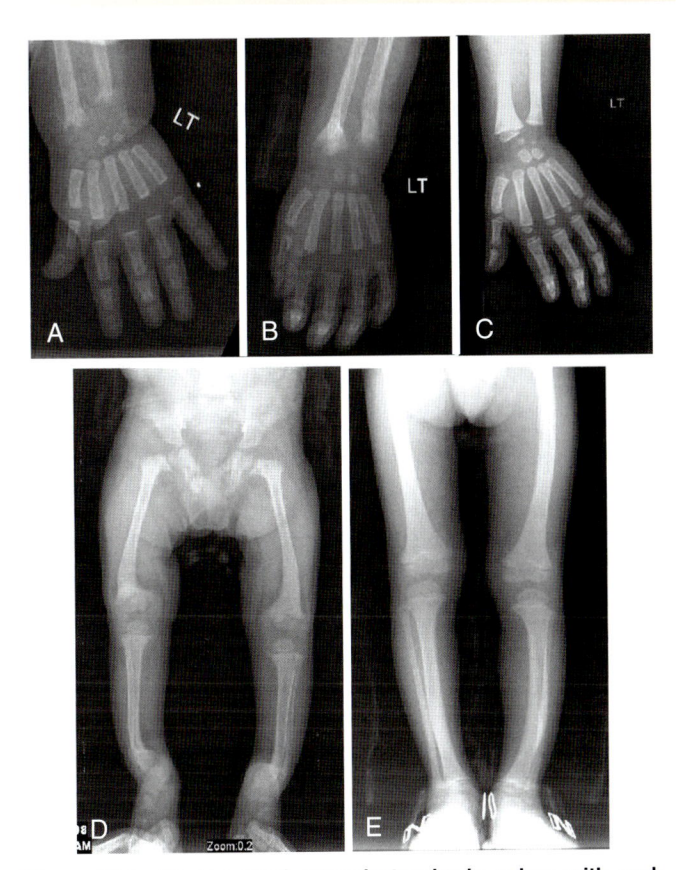

Figure 76.1 Severe renal osteodystrophy in a boy with end-stage kidney disease with resolution obtained with medical treatment. **A,** Age 1 year: severe rickets, absorption of the metaphyseal edges of the radius and ulna. Delayed bone age (6 months). **B,** Age 2 years: deformation in the radius and ulna bones, widening of the metaphyseal edges, healing rickets. **C,** Age 4 years: normal bone structure. Bone age is 3½ years. **D,** Age 2 years: deformation with angulations of the femur, tibia, and fibula bones, healing phase. **E,** Age 4: marked improvement although some angulation can still be seen.

measured blood pressure as hypertension. For example, in a 2-year-old girl of average height, the ninety-fifty percentile of blood pressure is as low as 104/59 mm Hg. Other explanations are that this group of patients tends to be hypervolemic due to a predominantly liquid diet and that correct assessment of dry weight is difficult and continually changing with the patient's growth. A short time on RRT is a risk factor for hypertension. This may be because the patient is not yet accustomed to fluid intake limitation or the follow-up is too short for adequate blood pressure control. Patients with congenital kidney diseases (mostly dysplastic kidneys) tend to be polyuric and thus normotensive. The definition of hypertension is blood pressure measurement at or above the ninetieth percentile, and the treatment goal in high-risk patients, including children with CKD, is blood pressure measurements below the ninetieth percentile.[49] Using this cutoff, more children with CKD are defined as hypertensive and may therefore be undertreated. In conclusion, hypertension, with its extreme detrimental effects (as detailed later), is frequently overlooked, undertreated, or even untreated in pediatric patients with ESKD.

VASCULAR CALCIFICATION

Milliner and colleagues first noted the high prevalence of VC as part of systemic calcinosis in autopsies of pediatric patients with ESKD undergoing dialysis or after renal transplantation: 43 of 120 patients (36%) had systemic calcinosis, 30 (70%) had VC.[50] A positive correlation was found with the use of vitamin D and peak Ca × P (but also age and male gender), now well-known risk factors.

In vivo, VC can be measured anatomically by duplex ultrasonography measuring carotid intima-media thickness or by electron beam computed tomography enabling quantification of VC. Functional studies also exist and measure arterial stiffness by various modes.[51]

In contrast to adults, in whom two different vascular-calcifying processes coexist (intimal-atherosclerotic plaque and medial), in children with CKD medial calcification is the predominant pathologic condition. VC is associated with hyperphosphatemia, high Ca × P, incremental dose of vitamin D and calcium (as phosphate binder), as well as reduced calcification inhibitors such as fetuin A, all leading to calcification and concomitant osteoblastic differentiation of vascular smooth muscle cells. There is increased vascular stiffness rather than narrowing of the arterial lumen despite the mineral deposition. These may in turn cause hypertension, increased pulse pressure, and later left ventricular hypertrophy (LVH) and relative cardiac ischemia. Carotid intima-media thickness has also been found to be elevated in children with ESKD, though not in all studies.

The primary process, endothelial dysfunction, is found in early stages of CKD in children and worsens as disease progresses. Subsequently, medial VC appears and worsens, both quantitatively and functionally, with the increase in CKD stage.[33,34,52,53] In young adults with ESKD since childhood, increased arterial stiffness is found.[54]

Possible preventive strategies include lowering Ca × P, reduction of calcium-containing phosphate binder dose, reduction of calcitriol intake, reducing PTH levels, optimal blood pressure control, and shortening of time on dialysis. This may be achieved by reducing dietary phosphate intake, using non–calcium-containing phosphate binders,[55] rarely parathyroidectomy, intense antihypertensive therapy, intensified dialysis, and early transplantation. Two studies, exploring the effects of various parameters are of special interest. Shroff and associates, in an observational rather than an interventional study, showed that patients with time-integrated PTH levels of less than twice the upper normal limit had normal vessels, measured by carotid intima-media thickness and stiffness, compared to those with higher PTH levels.[53] Hoppe and colleagues demonstrated that intensified dialysis improved all variables associated with VC, in addition to improved blood pressure control, and, surprisingly, better quality of life and school attendance.[56] Anatomic and functional VC measures were not tested.

Classic atherosclerosis has an accelerated course in adults with ESKD, and this disease process starts even among the healthy population in childhood. The only prevalent modifiable risk factor for atherosclerosis is hypertension. The dyslipidemia observed in children with ESKD is not the typical atherosclerosis risk profile (high triglyceride levels, low high-density lipoprotein [HDL] levels but usually normal total and low-density lipoprotein [LDL] cholesterol levels in CKD, as opposed to low HDL levels and high total and LDL cholesterol levels[57]), nor does it correlate with current CVS disease[58]; therefore it is not clear whether lipid-lowering therapy is appropriate.[59] Diabetes, smoking, and obesity are all rare before transplantation in children.

CARDIAC PATHOLOGIC CONDITIONS

Left Ventricular Hypertrophy

LVH is found in 30.4% to 63% of pediatric patients with ESKD.[48,57,60] It is correlated (in different studies) to systolic blood pressure, anemia, gender, and PTH levels. The pathophysiologic factors are complicated and include hypertension, volume overload, anemia, and the uremic milieu per se. Important components of the uremic milieu are the endogenous cardiotonic steroids, digitalis-like substances whose secretion is augmented in patients with CKD as an adaptation to the uremic electrolyte–water imbalance.[61] Another pathogenic factor that has been shown to induce LVH is elevated serum fibroblast growth factor 23 (FGF-23) levels. LVH by itself may lead to relative ischemia and diastolic dysfunction. In adults, LVH is considered as a mortality risk factor, although this has not been directly proven in children.

Diastolic Dysfunction

Diastolic dysfunction prevalence may be as high as 22.5% to 43.4% in patients with ESKD.[48,52] It is associated with left ventricular mass index (left ventricular mass corrected for height to power of 2.7), Ca × P, anemia, hypertension, and PTH levels.[57,60,62] The pathophysiologic features may be poor compliance of the hypertrophied left ventricle, myocardial fibrosis, and relative ischemia.

Arrhythmia

The common findings of arrhythmia are ventricular and supraventricular extrasystoles, first-degree arteriovenous (AV) block, or sinus tachycardia and transiently prolonged corrected QT interval.[63-65] The incidence of these arrhythmias is not higher than in the general pediatric population.[63] Life-threatening arrhythmia is rare and is usually associated with severe electrolyte abnormalities.

Valvular Disease

Valvular disease with incidence of 6% to 15% (depends on age and race) was reported.[63] The specific pathologic condition may be not structural but secondary to overload (mitral regurgitation) or to pulmonary hypertension (tricuspid regurgitation)—frequent findings in patients receiving hemodialysis.[66] Aortic valve calcification, without hemodynamic significance, was found in 12% to 25% of patients in a single report.[57]

NEURODEVELOPMENT

There are a number of reasons for neurodevelopmental compromise in children with ESKD. Some pediatric renal diseases are part of a syndrome or systemic disease that may have an effect on the central nervous system and on psychomotor development (e.g., Bardet-Biedl syndrome, cystinosis). Others can be associated with prematurity (congenital nephrotic syndrome of the Finnish type) or associated with oligohydramnios and hypoplastic lungs and hence possible perinatal hypoxia (autosomal recessive polycystic kidney disease). Uremic toxins, hypertension (or blood pressure fluctuations during hemodialysis), and chronic anemia can cause further damage to the developing brain. Motor skills development can also be delayed because the sick infant is not free to move and play while connected to the dialysis or feeding machine. Various catheters, feeding tube, or gastrostomy may interfere with rolling over and crawling, and there is less sensory stimulation during hospitalization or dialysis. Muscle tone is diminished, and renal osteodystrophy may be painful and prevent the needed physical activity for normal development. Some medications frequently given to patients with CKD, including aminoglycoside antibiotics and furosemide, are potentially ototoxic. Several studies over the past 30 years have shown that patients with CKD have compromised cognitive functions. This can be seen even in the early stages of CKD.[67] Specifically, studies found lower IQ levels (approximately 10 points), verbal or written language difficulties, impaired memory, decreased executive functions, and inefficiency in key neurocognitive domains.[68-72] Particularly affected are children who reached ESKD at a younger age (Figure 76.2),[69,73] children with longer dialysis vintage,[70,74,75] more severe hypertension or hypertensive crisis events,[68,74] and children with comorbid conditions.[76] Sensorineural hearing loss was found in 14% to 18% of the patients, and ischemic lesions of variable severity on magnetic resonance imaging (MRI) were seen in 18% to 33%.[74,76] Despite this, 61% to 79% of the children with ESKD attend regular school[70,74] and have academic achievement comparable with their siblings.[71] Long-term follow-up in adults treated since childhood for ESKD[75] found impaired schooling and lower IQ (9.2 to 10.4 points less than controls). Current ESKD treatment modality (dialysis or transplantation) was not associated with IQ score. However, dialysis for more than 4 years was associated with

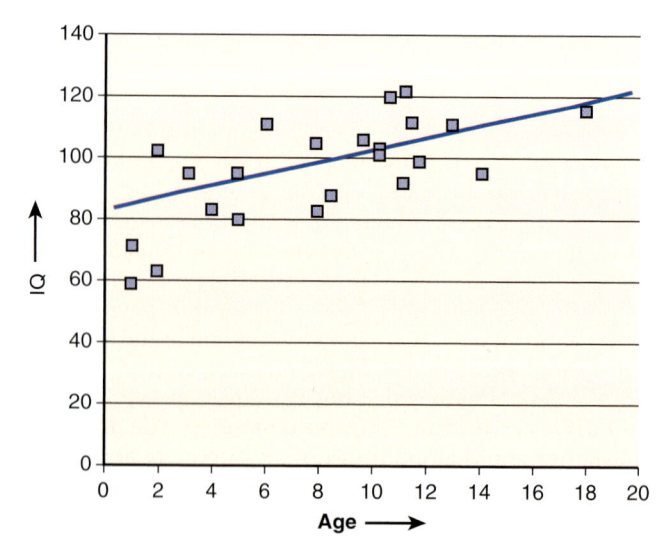

Figure 76.2 Distribution of IQ scores by age at onset of renal failure (creatinine level >2.5 mg/dL). The earlier the onset of chronic kidney disease, the lower the IQ score ($r = 0.49$; $P = 0.029$). (Adapted from Lawry KW, Brouhard BH, Cunningham RJ: Cognitive functioning and school performance in children with renal failure. *Pediatr Nephrol* 8:326-329, 1994, p 328, Figure 2.)

3.4 times higher risk for decreased IQ. The authors conclude that it is not clear whether the lower IQ and achievements are the result of lower potential or lack of school attendance.

QUALITY OF LIFE

Quality of life of children on RRT was assessed in only a few studies.[77] Quality-of-life scores are lower than the general population norms in all domains. Generally, patients perceive their quality of life as better than their parents do.[78] This may be due to the patients' not knowing any different—this has always been their reality; it may be a defense mechanism; or it may reflect parental overprotection. The disadvantage is that parents' lower rating may decrease motivation of the patients and family members or caregivers and thus may adversely affect patient outcomes.

MORTALITY

The mortality rate in pediatric patients with ESKD is 30 times higher than in the healthy age-adjusted population, with overall survival of 79% at 10 years and 66% at 20 years.[79] Factors associated with higher death rates are earlier era, younger age at initiation of RRT, and mode of treatment (mortality rate is higher for dialysis than for transplantation). These factors were repeatedly confirmed in other studies. Mortality hazard ratio (HR) was highest in younger age-groups compared to adolescents: hazard ratio 5.13 (95% confidence interval [CI], 2.62 to 10.03) in patients less than 2 years of age and 2.69 (95% CI, 1.20 to 6.02) in patients 2 to 3.99 years old.[19] In the youngest age-group most deaths occurred within the first year of life, and the mortality rate among survivors of the first year is comparable to other age groups. (In the first year the annual death rate is 14%, and then there is a marked decrease: In the second year the annual death rate is 3%; years 3 to 5, 1% per year; and in the next 5 years, 0.6% per year). Similar results are presented in the United States Renal Data System (USRDS) database: Overall 5-year survival is 79% for patients beginning RRT during the years 2001 to 2005, with the worst results for patients aged 0 to 4 years. Analysis by type of RRT found 5-year survival of 95% for patients who had undergone transplantation, 75% for patients who were receiving HD, and 81% for patients who were receiving PD. A later study[80] also found improvement in survival in the United States over time: For patients under 5 years of age the adjusted hazard ratio per 5-year increment in calendar year at ESKD initiation from 1990 to 2010 is 0.80 (95% CI, 0.75 to 0.85), and for patients more than 5 years of age, the hazard ratio is 0.88 (95% CI, 0.85 to 0.92).

The main causes of death are cardiovascular disease and infection, responsible for 45% and 21%, respectively, according to the Australia and New Zealand Dialysis and Transplant Registry (ANZDATA).[79] Similar findings in the United States showed death from cardiovascular disease of 27.1% to 39.3% and from infection 9.7% to 22.5%.[80] A decrease over time of death rates from both these causes was demonstrated. CVS mortality decreased in patients younger than 5 years from 36.3 per 1000 person-years in 1990 to 1994 to 22.6 in 2006 to 2010 (adjusted HR 0.54, 95% CI, 0.47 to 0.63) and in older patients declined from 16.2 to 9.3 per 1000 person-years (HR 0.66, 95% CI, 0.61 to 0.70). A similar trend was found for infection-related mortality. A different point of view was presented by Kramer and colleagues studying young adults who started RRT as children.[81] The 5-year survival from the eighteenth birthday was 95.1% (95% CI, 93.9 to 96.0), with average life expectancy of 63 years for young adults with a functioning graft and 38 years for those continuing to undergo dialysis.

CARDIOVASCULAR MORTALITY

CVS disease is the most frequent reported cause of death: 14% to 41% of all pediatric deaths, depending on age and race.[63,78,79,81-83] Although CVS disease has a major impact, it is conceivable that the percentages are an overestimation, and death may not be caused directly or exclusively by a disease of either the heart or blood vessels. All of the studies are inevitably retrospective and depend on reliability of physician reporting. The most frequent cause of death is "cardiac arrest" (25% to 52%), a very nonspecific diagnosis, which may well be the final common pathway of various primary causes of death.[78,81] In a single study in which the authors directly reviewed all patient files, the report includes under the heading of CVS death, CVA (58% of cardiac deaths), congestive heart failure (15%), and other diagnoses that may be the consequence of hypertension, heparinization, and volume overload.[83] In addition, most of the data available are for children who reached ESKD 2 or 3 decades ago. There has been a marked reduction not only in the absolute death rate but also in the percentage of deaths attributed to cardiac causes over the years: from 44.4% in 1972 to 1981 to 33.3% in 1992 to 1999.[83] This was also shown in the period of 1990 to 2010: In patients younger than 5 years at initiation of dialysis, CVS mortality decreased from 35.3% in 1990 to 1994 to 22.6% in 2005 to 2010.[79] More specific causes of death must be defined. This is not merely semantic, because accurate determination of causes of death can help focus efforts aimed at decreasing the death rate.

Nevertheless, to underscore the high risk for morbidity and mortality, the American Heart Association classified pediatric patients with CKD in the same high-risk group as children with homozygous familial hypercholesterolemia, type 1 diabetes mellitus, and post–orthotopic heart transplantation.[49]

MEDICATIONS

Any medication theoretically needs to be specifically approved for use in children, after testing its pharmacokinetics, pharmacodynamics, bioavailability, efficacy, dosing, and effects on growth and development at various ages. Many routinely used drugs have not been through this process, have never received such formal approval for use in children, and yet are widely used based on clinical experience accumulated and lack of alternatives. Newer medications approved for adults are often not yet adequately tested in children, for example, some long-acting ESAs, whereas others have raised concerns over safety, such as calcimimetics. Some drugs used for treatment of patients with CKD are contraindicated in children due to possible side effects specific to children (e.g., lanthanum carbonate, which has been shown to accumulate in bone growth plates).

RENAL REPLACEMENT THERAPY

All available RRT modalities can be used in children. Transplantation is the preferred long-term modality, but it is not always possible initially.

ADVANTAGES OF KIDNEY TRANSPLANTATION OVER LONG-TERM DIALYSIS IN CHILDREN

SURVIVAL

Survival is longer following kidney transplantation in all age-groups and in both genders (from 6 months after transplantation and on): The adjusted relative risk of a child who underwent transplantation compared to a child who continued to receive dialysis at 30 months is 0.26 ($P < 0.001$; 95% CI, 0.11 to 0.46)[84] (Figure 76.3).

Similar results are presented in the USRDS 2011 report: The all-cause mortality rate per 1000 patient-years is 58.2, 48.0, and 11.9 for children undergoing HD, PD, and after renal transplantation, respectively. Five-year survival in the same report is 95% for patients who have undergone transplantation, compared to 81% for patients undergoing PD and 75% for patients undergoing HD. In a report from the ANZDATA registry, hazard ratio was calculated using HD as the reference value; PD was equivalent to HD, but transplantation had a reduced hazard ratio of 0.15 to 0.30 (dependent on era tested).[79]

Several risk-associated variables are improved in children who have undergone transplantation compared to children treated with dialysis. Blood pressure values above the ninety-fifth percentile were significantly more prevalent in patients on HD compared to transplant recipients (as well as those undergoing PD) with odds ratios of 2.48 and 1.59, respectively.[47] In addition, there is slower coronary artery calcification after transplantation as compared to patients undergoing HD.[85] Carotid intima-media thickness does not progress and sometimes regresses after kidney transplantation.[86]

QUALITY OF LIFE

Parents of patients who underwent kidney transplantation (but less so the children themselves) noted a positive impact of transplantation on almost all the domains of health-related quality-of-life questionnaire.[87] Another study found that patients after kidney transplantation and their parents reported better health-related quality of life compared to patients on chronic HD.[88]

NEURODEVELOPMENT

Neurodevelopment is improved following kidney transplantation. This was shown in 1984[89] and later in a longitudinal study[90] showing improved mental processing speed and better sustained attention and in comparative studies in which patients after kidney transplantation had better language performances and school grades compared to patients undergoing dialysis.[69] Furthermore, more dialysis years was reported to correlate with worse neurocognitive outcome.[70,74]

EXHAUSTION OF ACCESS SITES

Because life expectancy is longer than the graft survival in children, pediatric age-group patients may pass more than once through the cycle of dialysis and transplantation. Being exclusively on dialysis as RRT will exhaust access sites (vascular and peritoneal) sooner.

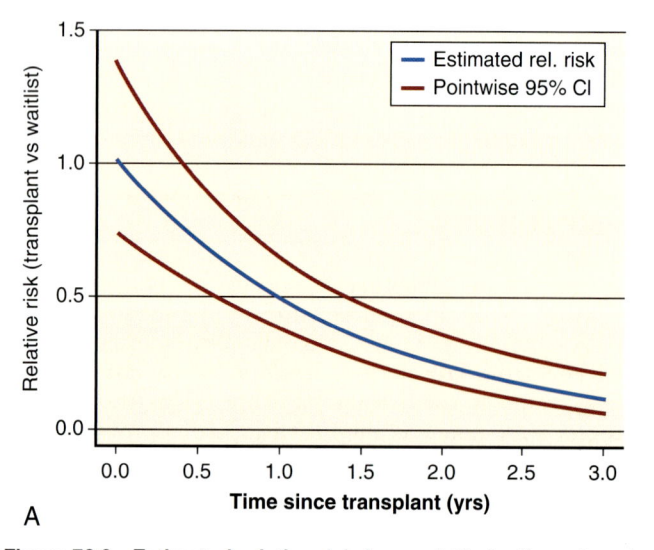

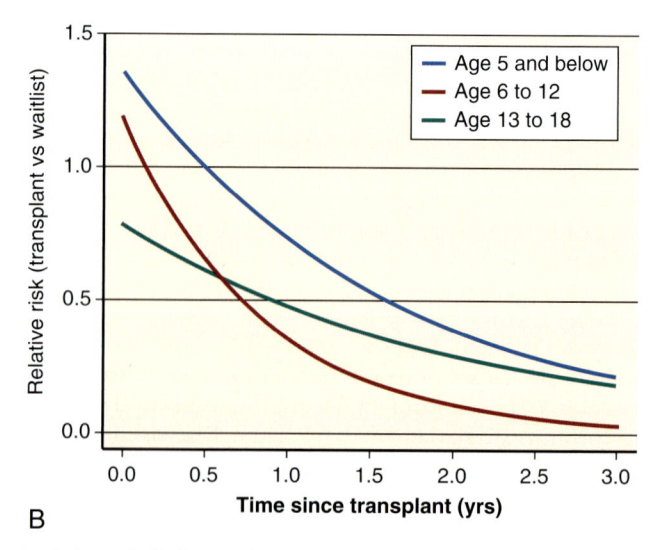

Figure 76.3 Estimated relative risk for mortality by time since transplantation. **A,** Estimates from a model including all ages. **B,** Model-based estimates stratified by age. CI, Confidence interval. (Adapted from Gillen DL, Stehman-Breen CO, Smith JM, et al: Survival advantage of pediatric recipients of a first kidney transplant among children awaiting kidney transplantation. *Am J Transplant* 8:2600-2606, 2008, p 2603, Figure 1.)

COST

Kidney transplantation is more cost effective than any other RRT modality. In a meta-analysis of articles published between 1968 and 1998,[91] after adjusting for changing price levels, in-center HD was found to be the most expensive modality (steady over the years between $55,000 and $80,000 per life-year saved) compared to kidney transplantation ($10,000 per life-year saved), becoming more cost effective over time). Another study[92] calculated cost effectiveness of RRT in Austria: The first year of treatment costs €43,600 for HD, €25,900 for PD, and €51,000 for kidney transplantation. In the third year of treatment, medical costs decline to €40,600 for HD, €20,500 for PD, and €12,900 for the patient after kidney transplantation. In some developing countries where most people do not have health insurance, dialysis is not a valid option due to its high price as well as the limited professional services. Kidney transplantation remains the only potential option, although at times with catastrophic financial ramifications for the families.[93]

Usually a minimal weight of 8.5 to 10 kg is required to achieve good surgical results, necessitating postponement of transplantation in smaller infants. Although the pediatric patient often has potential willing and suitable donors, primarily the parents, this is not always the case. Donor issues such as ABO incompatibility, positive cross-match, medical conditions or unwillingness to donate a kidney, and sometime patient size or medical reasons preclude or delay transplantation. For all these reasons in the great majority of children, dialysis is regarded as a necessary but temporary interim solution until transplantation is possible.

COMPARING HEMODIALYSIS WITH PERITONEAL DIALYSIS

If preemptive transplantation is not an option, the mode of dialysis (HD or PD) has to be selected. There are no comparative studies proving superiority of one mode over the other in the long-term outcome. The treatment burden on the patients' families is extreme, whatever dialysis mode is chosen. Parents of patients on RRT, in addition to their usual parental roles, must become high-level health care providers, able to solve problems and seek information, and have financial resources and practical skills. Caregivers are in continuous need of emotional, psychologic, and financial support.[78] All these in turn may cause fatigue, stress, and disruption of work and social life.[94] Thus, once a patient approaches ESKD, the family's abilities and socioeconomic and psychologic background have to be carefully evaluated by a multidisciplinary team, including a nephrologist, a dialysis nurse, a social worker, a psychologist, and other allied health professionals. PD enables more liberal fluid intake, which is especially important in infants with fluid-based nutrition. In-center HD mandates traveling at least three times weekly to the dialysis center, which is time consuming, costly, and in some places not available. PD enables better school attendance than HD: according to the 2011 NAPRTCS report: 74% to 85% of patients undergoing PD receive full schooling in the first 3 years (the rate is steady from initiation of dialysis to 36 months later), but only 47% to 59% of patients undergoing HD attend school regularly (and the rate steadily declines the longer the patient is receiving HD). However, with PD the treatment burden is on nonprofessional caregivers, so they have to be compliant and capable of performing dialysis at home, with the additional risk for parental stress and burnout. Taken together, the final decision is based upon center experience, patient or family choice, socioeconomic issues, compliance, and treatment availability.

The first treatment modality used for children with ESKD in developed countries according to the registries is presented in Table 76.2. Preemptive transplantation is performed in 16.6% to 26% of patients. The Norwegian RRT program, on the other hand, reports 51% preemptive transplantations (from living donors) and median duration of dialysis treatment before first transplantation of 3 months.[95] The cause of the disparities between the reports reflects differences in attitudes toward kidney donation, traditions, and religious beliefs, as well as the health care system and financial issues.

The choice of selection of HD versus PD is greatly influenced by patient age. According to the NAPRTCS 2011 report, of 927 patients initiating dialysis at the age of 0 to 1 years, 857 (92%) were receiving PD, 552 of 727 (77%) of the 2 to 5 age-group, 1373 of 2125 patients (65%) of the 6 to 12 age-group, and 1648 of 3250 (51%) in the 13 to 18 age-group. In Australia and New Zealand similar proportions are seen: 89.8% of infants were initially treated with PD, with declining percentage to 34.5% of adolescents.[96] Similar trends were noted in the United Kingdom: For age 0 to 2 years, 80% were receiving PD, and for age 16 to 18 years, only 10.4%.

The proportion of patients under the age of 1 year at initiation of dialysis has steadily increased[29] and doubled from 10% to around 20% of all pediatric patients undergoing dialysis from 1990 to 2010. This is explained by the fact that nephrologists are encouraged to treat younger patients as their survival improved. The same trend was found in the UK registry. From the 1996 to 2000 period to the 2006 to 2010 period the percentage of patients at age 0 to 2 years increased from 13.7% to 17.6% (the absolute figures are from 70 to 104 per year), whereas the age-group of 12 to 16 years decreased by 2.3%.

In the United States there is steady trend of increased use of HD instead of PD, from 34% of patients receiving HD in 1991 to 54% in 2010. This trend was not found in the United Kingdom, where a relatively constant percentage, around 30%, of pediatric patients undergoing dialysis has been receiving HD since 1996. Similarly, in Australia and New Zealand, 30% to 40% of all patients undergoing dialysis were receiving HD during the period 2006 to 2010.

HEMODIALYSIS

Given the complexity of the treatment with HD in children, a hospital providing this service needs to have a multidisciplinary team with expertise in the various facets of this modality. The specialties include pediatric nephrologists, dialysis nurses, dietitians, invasive radiologists, vascular surgeons, pediatric surgeons, a vascular laboratory, and all the subspecialties in pediatrics, as well as social workers, educators, psychologists, and other therapists.

Table 76.2 First Treatment Modality for Pediatric Patients with End-Stage Kidney Disease in the Major Registries Worldwide

	ESPN/ERA-EDTA	ANZDATA		UK Renal Registry	NAPRTCS
Year(s) of data collection	2008-2010 (incidence)	1963-2006 (incidence)	2006-2011 (incidence)	1997-2011 (prevalence)	1992-2010 (prevalence)
N	1641	1445	308	1208	9198*
Age limit	<15	<18	<18	<16	<18
Preemptive transplant	272 (16.6%)	281 (19.4%)	57 (18.5%)	24%[†‡]	26%*
HD	549 (33.5%)	473 (32.7%)	115 (37.3%)	48%[†]	46%*
PD	820 (50.0%)	691 (47.8%)	136 (44.2%)	28%[†]	26%*

*Approximate percentages and total number (N): N calculated from absolute preemptive transplants number plus number of first course of dialysis.
[†]Data for treatment at 3 months from initiation of RRT.
[‡]Preemptive transplantation includes both living (15%) and deceased donors (9%).
ANZDATA, Australia and New Zealand Dialysis and Transplant Registry; ESPN/ERA-EDTA, European Society of Paediatric Nephrology, the European Renal Association and European Dialysis and Transplant Association; HD, hemodialysis; NAPRTCS, North American Pediatric Renal Trials and Collaborative Studies; PD, peritoneal dialysis; RRT, renal replacement therapy.
Adapted from references 3, 4, 14-16, 19, and 29.

There are several modifications of the HD procedure distinct for children and several specific medical issues that have to be addressed in addition to tailoring the dialysis prescription for every child according to weight.

VASCULAR ACCESS

The main forms of vascular access are central venous catheter (CVC), AV fistula, or rarely AV graft. AV fistula is the recommended choice because of the lower rate of complications, including infection and malfunction, and longer longevity. The median survival time is 3.14 year for AV fistula (95% CI, 1.22 to 5.06) compared to 0.6 year for a CVC (95% CI, 0.2 to 1.00).[97] Additional advantages attributed to AV fistulas, including better clearance and higher albumin and hemoglobin levels, are less convincing.[98] CVCs cause more damage to blood vessels, and the resulting central venous stenosis may preclude future ipsilateral AV fistula creation. This is important in children, who are expected to require RRT for longer, and therefore blood vessel preservation is crucial. The National Kidney Foundation KDOQI guidelines therefore recommend AV fistula,[99] with the exception of children weighing less than 20 kg, for whom CVC is the better and sometimes the only option, because of the technical difficulties of vascular surgery. Although some exceptions exist, AV fistula is rarely created in patients weighing less than 15 kg.[100] When HD is planned for a short time, bridging for PD or awaiting a potential living donor to complete their evaluation, CVC should be used. However, reviewing the pediatric registries shows a different picture.

A survey in Europe found that the use of CVCs was more frequent than recommended in prevalent pediatric patients undergoing HD: 40% had AV fistula or graft versus 57% who had CVCs.[101] There were more patients with AV fistula as an access only in children over 15 years of age. In the ANZDATA 2009 registry all children under 9 years of age had CVC as their prevalent access. Although in adolescents the overall use of AV fistulas was more prevalent, there is a decreased trend over time in Australia from 78% in 2005 to only 46% in 2008.[102] According to the NAPRTCS 2011 report, the majority of patients receiving HD use CVCs. Of all pediatric patients starting HD, 78.7% have a CVC, and there is a clear increase in this trend, from 73% in 1992 to more than 90% in 2010.[29] However, this is probably due to the choice of HD using CVC access preferentially by patients who are expected to require dialysis for a short time. Time receiving dialysis is shorter in children with CVCs: At 3 months 20.7% ± 1.0% of patients with CVCs have discontinued dialysis compared to 7.2% ± 1.6% for AV fistula and 7.0% ± 2.0% for AV grafts. At 24 months the comparable figures are 71.9% ± 1.2%, 50.0% ± 3.2%, and 57.5% ± 4.3%. In addition, dialysis is terminated sooner in patients undergoing HD compared to those undergoing PD. Within 6 months 30.0% ± 1.0% of patients undergoing HD have discontinued treatment compared to only 18.9% ± 0.6% of patients undergoing PD.[29] Other reasons for increased use of CVC in pediatric HD include lack of needling experience in small HD units, the ease of achieving a functioning CVC with the advancement of invasive radiology, and the preference for painless connection to the dialysis machine. Not all centers have vascular surgeons experienced in construction and maintenance of AV fistulas in children, a factor that is crucial to fistula patency and function, and therefore CVCs may be used more often in such units.[103] An AV fistula needs time to mature before it can be used, usually longer in children than adults.[104] In the majority of cases appropriate planning can overcome this issue.

CVCs should be adjusted to patient size. Catheter diameter of 8 Fr is the smallest tunneled catheter size available and can be used even in patients as small as 3 kg in weight. This is also the smallest size that can provide long-term adequate flow to ensure sufficient solute and fluid removal, because the flow is proportional to the fourth power of the CVC diameter. The distance between the arterial and venous ends should ideally be as far as possible to reduce recirculation but close enough to ensure that both are within the right atrium, preventing sealing of the catheter ends by the venous wall. However, an 8-Fr CVC is almost the same size as the venous lumen of the small child, increasing the risk for vascular damage and stenosis. Patients weighing more than 18 to 20 kg can accommodate 10-Fr catheters. Ultrasonographic and fluoroscopic guidance are used to prevent catheter malposition, reducing the primary failure rate to almost zero. Although there are no published data in children, it is recommended to follow the experience in adults, using the internal jugular veins as the preferred access. Anecdotally, in newborns who need short-term HD as in the case of inborn errors of metabolism, the umbilical vein can be used as an access.

The main CVC complications are infections and malfunction. Infections are more common in younger patients[105,106] possibly due to close proximity of the exit site to the infection source: diapers and gastrostomy tubes. Infection rate is usually 1.5 to 4.8 per 1000 CVC days,[107-110] although an exceptionally favorable report documented a rate of 0.5 per 1000 CVC days.[111] Malfunction is the result of thrombosis, fibrin sheath formation, vascular stenosis, or mechanical damage to the CVC. If local fibrinolysis fails, the CVC must be replaced. A major complication with long-term sequelae is central venous stenosis. It occurs more often in younger patients, with small-diameter veins, with prolonged use of CVCs, with many reinsertions, and possibly also depending on CVC locations: The worst outcome is for subclavian veins, followed by left internal jugular vein, and the use of the right internal jugular vein carries the smallest chance of becoming obstructed. Clinically, stenosis is often asymptomatic until an ipsilateral AV fistula is constructed, but sometimes superior vena cava syndrome may develop.

AV fistulas, and rarely AV grafts, have a much lower complication rate, resulting in fewer hospitalizations and fewer revisions, and they have higher access longevity.[112] In a small survey, although with significant difference in ages between groups, the hospitalization rate for access-related issues was 0.44% versus 3.1% per year in the AV fistula versus the CVC groups.[113] Because fistula thrombosis or malfunction is the main complication, and this is usually the result of vessel stenosis, routine surveillance of the fistula by Doppler ultrasonography should be performed by an experienced professional. Vascular surgeons and invasive radiologists should be available to detect and treat stenosis or thrombosis.

The average AV fistula blood flow is 800 to 1200 mL/min. In adults this is significant compared to the normal cardiac output (CO): normal adult CO is 5.2 to 8.6 L/min, and the flow through an AV fistula will increase CO by 9% to 23%. A similar flow in a child, required for adequate dialysis, may increase the CO of a child with a 0.7-m² body surface area, whose normal CO is 2.1 to 3.5 L/min, by 23% to 57%. Theoretically this may lead to high-output heart failure, although this rarely becomes of clinical significance.

Pulmonary hypertension is another complication of adults receiving HD, and the presence of an AV fistula contributes, at least in part, to this process.[66] High pulmonary blood flow, a direct result of the AV fistula, may cause pulmonary hypertension.[114,115] Other contributing factors include hormonal imbalances such as high thelin-1 and low nitric oxide levels. This issue has not been tested in the pediatric HD population. Pulmonary hypertension is partially reversible after kidney transplantation, but this may have significant sequelae, including increased mortality.

DIALYSIS APPARATUS

TUBING

Tubing has to be adapted to the patient's size. The extracorporeal volume, consisting of the arterial and venous segments and the dialyzer, should not exceed 10% of the patient's blood volume. For patients weighing less than 6 kg this goal cannot be achieved with the smallest available tubing, and priming of the extracorporeal system is needed, either with whole blood, or with packed red blood cells diluted with normal saline to an estimated hematocrit of 33% to 36%. Although blood units can be divided so a single unit can be used for four HD sessions, there still is a high exposure to blood products. Iron overload does not occur because at the end of each session the blood in the extracorporeal system is not routinely washed back to the patient unless the patient requires a transfusion.

Exposing a patient to many units of blood increases the risk for infection and for HLA sensitization. However, for infants treated with chronic HD necessitating multiple transfusions, the risk for becoming highly sensitized has not been systematically studied.

The procedure of washing back blood at the end of dialysis in any patient deserves special consideration because the blood volume filling the tubing is equivalent to 0.5 to 1 weight-adjusted blood units. Even with the slowest possible pump speed the whole volume will be washed back within 2 to 3 minutes, which is exceptionally fast. This may cause an abrupt increase in the right atrial pressure, and if the patient has a patent foramen ovale, it would increase the risk for possible microthrombi paradoxical embolism. Despite this concern, as well as the known relative cognitive deficiency in patients undergoing dialysis and the frequent (18% to 33%) finding of ischemic lesions on brain MRI studies[74,76] in pediatric patients with ESKD, this point has not been explored. In adult patients receiving HD there was no proof for a faster cognitive deterioration with patent foramen ovale compared with those without patent foramen ovale, although atrial pressures during blood return at the end of dialysis may not be as high in adults.[116]

DIALYZER

The dialyzer should also be adjusted to patient size to ensure adequate clearance with minimal extracorporeal blood volume, and therefore hollow-fiber dialyzers are used. The dialyzer size is determined by patient's body surface area.

MACHINE

The HD machine to provide dialysis for children must be compatible with the use of small tubing, be adjustable to low pump speed, and have a volumetric function. The latter is crucial because the ultrafiltrate has to be measured directly, and small volumes that are negligible in adults can be removed accurately.

BLOOD FLOW

Blood flow speed is a major determinant of solute clearance, but excessively high flow can cause cardiovascular instability, which might manifest as pallor, irritability, vomiting, or altered mental status. Blood flow is determined according to body size and is usually not higher than 10% of blood volume in milliliters per minute.

DOSE OF DIALYSIS

According to the National Kidney Foundation KDOQI 2006 guidelines, dialysis should be initiated once the eGFR falls below 15 mL/min/1.73 m^2, or earlier if other metabolic derangements, volume overload, or medical signs and symptoms are refractory to conventional treatment. The recommendation states that solute clearance should be greater than that recommended for adults ((Kt/V [dialyzer urea clearance times treatment time divided by body urea volume]) > 1.2, urea reduction ratio > 65%), given that it should support higher protein intake, needed for adequate growth and development. However, there is little observational information and no randomized studies regarding the correct dose of dialysis for children. Hence HD is arbitrarily delivered three times weekly, for 3 to 4 hours each session. However, the true adequacy test is based on clinical grounds, which in children is, in the short term, optimal balance of electrolytes, blood pressure, and volume, and in the long term, adequate weight gain, linear growth, neurodevelopment, and quality of life. Several small studies suggest that delivering more dialysis can improve blood pressure control and hyperphosphatemia, obviate dietary restriction, and improve appetite and general well-being, linear growth, and even school attendance.[117-122] Intensive dialysis may also attenuate vascular disease, which is a major concern.[55] This goal can be achieved either by nocturnal home HD, performing five to seven sessions per week, hemodiafiltration, or a combination of both. The theoretical basis for these observations was established in a study by Daugirdas.[123] In the standard calculation, the dose of dialysis is scaled to urea distribution volume, which is similar to total body water. If, however, dialysis is scaled to body surface area, similar to calculation of the GFR, because body surface area is relatively higher in children, this would require increased dialysis time for smaller children. When these calculations were applied to two of the studies of intensive dialysis,[120,122] the patients were indeed found to have a much higher weekly dialysis dose. Despite this, intensive dialysis is still not widely used, and it is premature to recommend a general increase in the dose or frequency of dialysis in all pediatric patients. Randomized studies with clinical end points are necessary. Widespread changes in clinical practice would have substantial financial ramifications. Daily or nocturnal home HD is not available in most countries for children.

FLUID REMOVAL

Total body water percentage changes by age from 80% in neonates to 65% in 12-year-old children to 55% to 60% in adults (women and men, respectively). Moreover the extracellular volume falls from 52% in infancy to only 18% to 20% in the adult.[124] For this reason the allowance of interdialytic fluid gain is larger and also the tolerance of dialytic fluid removal is better in infants (up to 8% to 10% of body weight) compared to adolescents (up to 5%). Another point is that childhood growth is accompanied by expected weight gain, such that dry weight reassessment is required on a frequent basis, especially in the very young age-groups. There is no single reliable marker of the correct dry weight, and thus it is estimated as the lowest weight not causing symptomatic hypovolemia.

Infants, receiving fluid-based nutrition, often require HD 4 to 5 days weekly, to enable adequate caloric intake without volume overload.

COMPLICATIONS

Complications associated with vascular access for HD were detailed earlier and include catheter-related infections, malfunction, and in the long term, central venous stenosis. AV fistula complications include fistula malfunction and thrombosis or rarely high-output heart failure or pulmonary hypertension. In smaller children there is obligatory exposure to multiple blood products, which may increase the risk for infection or HLA sensitization.

HYPOTENSION

Hypotension is a common complication during dialysis. It is associated with excessive or rapid fluid removal, which often exceeds 5% of body weight, both in younger children on liquid diets and in adolescent patients who are not adherent to their fluid restriction requirements. Hypotension may appear without warning, particularly in infants, and manifest as pallor, irritability, vomiting, or altered mental status. Accurate measurement of ultrafiltration (UF) volume is crucial in small children, because small volumes constitute a relatively large percentage of their blood volume. Sodium profiling, osmotic agents such as mannitol, or lowering dialysate temperature can be helpful in some cases. More frequent dialysis sessions may be necessary for large interdialytic weight gain, to reach dry weight and avoid hypotension during dialysis.[125]

DISEQUILIBRIUM SYNDROME

Disequilibrium syndrome is now a rare, yet potentially dangerous complication of HD. It is usually precipitated by overly rapid urea removal causing a discrepancy between the osmolality of the plasma and that of the brain cells, causing fluid shift into the brain.[126] Seizures are more common in children with disequilibrium syndrome than in adults. Prevention is aimed at a gradual reduction of blood urea nitrogen level, especially in new patients undergoing HD and when urea level is very high. This is achieved by selection of an appropriately small dialyzer and limiting blood flow and session length for the first few treatments. Mannitol infusion, or in cases of hypertension and hypervolemia, high dialysate glucose or slightly increased dialysate sodium concentration may also be helpful, by preventing the decrease in plasma osmolality. Blood flow rate should be slowed if mild symptoms such as nausea, vomiting, or headache appear, and dialysis stopped if more significant neurologic manifestations appear.[127]

HYPOTHERMIA

Hypothermia may occur if the dialysate is not warmed, particularly in small children, because the dialysate flow is generally constant regardless of patient size.

HYPOPHOSPHATEMIA

Hypophosphatemia may be caused by HD, particularly in younger children, when renal function is normal (when HD is done as emergency treatment for inborn errors of metabolism) and when intensive dialysis is performed (for fluid removal purposes or daily dialysis for ESKD due to primary hyperoxaluria). Hypophosphatemia is attributed to excessive phosphate clearance due to high flow of dialysate relative to patient weight.[128] This can be treated either by adding phosphate, for example sodium phosphate in enema preparations to the dialysate concentrate, or by slowing the dialysate flow.

HYPOGLYCEMIA

Hypoglycemia may occur during HD as described in adults.[129] It is associated with the use of glucose-free dialysate and high dialysate flow, leading to excessive glucose clearance. Infants, especially if catabolic, may be at a higher risk for hypoglycemia, and plasma glucose should be monitored during dialysis if it is suspected.

PERITONEAL DIALYSIS

PD is the most common modality of dialysis treatment in children worldwide, especially at young ages.[2,4,29] The PD prescription can be individualized according to the patient's age, body size, residual renal function (RRF), nutritional intake, and growth-related metabolic needs. Because there are no studies comparing outcomes of children treated with HD or PD, this choice is based on the assumption that PD is better adapted to the infant's or child's lifestyle and diet. Sometimes PD is the default choice due to the lack of experienced HD personnel or equipment. However, family preference and center philosophy may direct even newborns to HD. As opposed to HD, PD efficacy is dependent on biologic properties of the patient's peritoneal membrane rather than on a synthetic dialyzer. This means the initial prescription has to be modified according to membrane characteristics (determined only after initiation of PD). The peritoneum is periodically assessed and the prescription modified according to findings, and it may also fail, precluding further PD. Assessing the membrane function is done by the peritoneal equilibration test, which is modified according to the patient's body surface area because exchange volume may affect test results.

Some contraindications are specific to the pediatric patient.[130] These include various abdominal congenital anomalies such as gastroschisis, omphalocele, diaphragmatic hernia, or bladder exstrophy, and usually polycystic kidney disease, which may literally fill the whole abdominal cavity. In addition, because PD depends on the availability of a compliant caregiver, the lack of appropriate parental support precludes using this technique. Finally, medical issues, including abdominal surgery, ventriculoperitoneal shunt, abdominal adhesions, and membrane failure may all preclude the use of PD.

ACCESS

A reliable access is critical for successful PD. A double-cuffed Tenckhoff catheter with a downward-pointing exit site is associated with a lower infection rate. Specifically in infants or children receiving PD, the catheter has to be placed as far as possible from sources of infection such as diapers or gastrostomy tubes.[130]

PERITONEAL DIALYSIS PRESCRIPTION

TYPES OF PERITONEAL DIALYSIS

All available PD modalities can be used in children. Continuous ambulatory peritoneal dialysis (CAPD) is usually reserved for special circumstances. However, in many parts of the world, if dialysis is at all available, this is the only modality used.[18] Because automated PD (APD) is easier and flexible, this is almost the exclusive modality used in developed countries. Nocturnal intermittent PD, which is APD at night, no dialysis in the daytime, can be used when there is significant RRF, because fluid removal and solute clearance are limited. The advantages are daytime convenience, lower intraperitoneal pressure, lower risk for hernia formation, less glucose absorption, and less membrane exposure to glucose. In continuous cycling PD a daytime exchange is added, thus the nocturnal intermittent PD advantages are partially abolished, although better fluid and clearance are achieved, making it more suitable for patients with low RRF or with continuous need for efficient fluid removal (e.g., infants with a fluid-based diet). Tidal PD is an option when complete drainage either causes pain or is inefficient. Only part of the fluid is removed each cycle. This makes the dialysis less efficient, but this is partially compensated for by shorter drainage time and thus more possible cycles.

PERITONEAL DIALYSIS SOLUTIONS

Solutions contain buffer to control acidosis, electrolytes, and an osmotic agent (usually dextrose at varying concentrations) to enable net fluid removal and water as a carrier. Dialysis is satisfactorily performed with standard solutions; however, long-term membrane exposure to lactate-acidic solution and high dextrose concentration are detrimental, leading to peritoneal fibrosis and reduced function.[131] This is more common in frequent and short cycles as used in APD. For this reason newer solutions have been developed and also tested in children. In addition, there are special considerations in children at varying ages. Recommendations by the European Pediatric Dialysis Working Group have been published and include the use of the lowest glucose concentration possible and fluids with reduced glucose degradation products content whenever possible.[132] In the face of the paucity of studies prospectively comparing low glucose degradation products solutions or various buffers, firm recommendations cannot yet be given, but it seems that correction of metabolic acidosis with pH-neutral bicarbonate-based fluids is superior to single-chamber, acidic, lactate-based solutions. Icodextrin (high-molecular-weight glucose polymers, with high osmotic power) may be applied once daily in a long dwell, in particular in children with insufficient UF. In addition, sodium balance needs to be closely monitored because infants receiving PD are at risk for UF-associated sodium depletion, whereas anuric adolescents may have water and salt overload. Dialysate calcium level should be adapted according to individual needs as the child grows, to maintain positive calcium balance.[130] The use of amino acid–based PD fluids (designed to compensate for excessive protein loss during PD) in children is well tolerated but has little anabolic effect.

EXCHANGE VOLUME

The volume of dialysate infused is adjusted to patient size, 1000 to 1200 mL/m^2 for patients 2 years of age or older,[130] approximately two-thirds of that volume for younger patients. As in adults, volumes that are too small can lead to rapid solute equilibration and thus inadequate UF, and too high a volume may result in increased intraperitoneal pressure, with increased lymphatic absorption (causing reduced UF), physical discomfort, dyspnea, hernia formation, and gastroesophageal reflux.

DWELL TIME

The length of each exchange depends on PD modality; it is short in APD compared to CAPD. Membrane properties, as detected by the peritoneal equilibration test, guide the subsequent adjustment of the initial prescription, shortening the dwell time in patients with higher solute transport to prevent loss of osmotic gradient due to solute equilibration and reduced UF.

ADEQUACY OF DIALYSIS

No large-scale prospective studies have been performed in children that assess the correlation between solute removal and clinical outcomes. This is due to the rarity of ESKD in children and the relatively shorter time on dialysis in children compared to the adult patient. Also, longer life expectancy in pediatric RRT precludes the assessment of the effect of dialysis prescription changes on survival. In areas where there is no pediatric data, adult clinical practice guidelines serve as a minimal standard. Clinical and laboratory assessment should be performed at least once a month (more often if clinically necessary). Kt/V should be measured 1 month after initiating PD and subsequently at least every 6 months; RRF is assessed by 24-hour urine collection every 3 months. Adequacy is evaluated clinically, seeking signs and symptoms of uremia: hypertension, pulmonary congestion, pericarditis, hyperkalemia, hyperphosphatemia, and worsening school performance and general well-being. In addition, laboratory data may indicate inadequacy of dialysis (serum solute concentrations, hemoglobin and albumin levels), and Kt/V is calculated. Target Kt/V is 1.8 per week or higher, whereas V, or total body water, should be calculated using age- and gender-specific nomograms.[130] The prescription should be modified if needed, also taking into account preservation of RRF, patient convenience (intraperitoneal pressure, time consumption), and lowest possible dialysate dextrose concentration to achieve sufficient fluid removal.[132]

COMPLICATIONS

INFECTION

Peritonitis is a major complication in patients undergoing PD, which may result in long-term membrane failure. The reported rate by NAPRTCS in 2011 is one episode per 18.8 PD months, higher in infants (1 per 15.3 months) compared to adolescents (1 per 21.2 months), probably due to close proximity to contamination sources such as diapers or gastrostomy tubes in the young ages. Similar results were found in Australia (1 per 16.9 months), however, with no correlation to age.[133] A report of the Italian Registry of Paediatric Chronic Dialysis found somewhat better results: 1 per 20.7 months in infants and 1 per 28.3 months in older children.[134] In a survey including 47 centers in 14 countries, 44% of the peritonitis events were due to gram-positive bacteria, 25% due to gram-negative bacteria, and 31% were culture negative.[135] Less than half of the patients had fever above 38°C, less than half had abdominal pain, and 70% had marked effluent cloudiness. Of 482 children, 420 (87%) made a full recovery, and 39 (8.1%) had to discontinue PD permanently because of UF problems, adhesions, uncontrolled infection, and secondary fungal infection. As such, infections are the most common reason for modality change for patients receiving PD. In another study, including 501 peritonitis events from 44 pediatric dialysis centers in 14 countries,[136] significant regional variability was found both for bacteria type and sensitivity. This makes recommendation for global treatment guidelines more complex. Permanent discontinuation of PD varied considerably, from 0 of 18 episodes (Argentina) to 9 of 46 episodes (20%) in Eastern Europe.

Other infections include exit site and tunnel infections. Preventive measures include aseptic handling of the catheter, daily cleansing, immobilization, and applying topical antibiotics.

TECHNIQUE FAILURE

Catheter Malfunction

Catheter malfunction may preclude efficient dialysis and includes catheter migration or occlusion. Technical solutions, such as the use of specific types of catheters and omentectomy at the time of catheter insertion, may reduce the incidence.

Ultrafiltration Failure

UF failure is a main cause of a technique failure and leads to volume overload. High solute transport, as detected by the peritoneal equilibration test, causes rapid dissipation of the osmotic gradient needed for UF. Peritonitis events and long-term exposure to glucose degradation products in the standard PD solutions are the main causes. Filling volume that is too high can in addition lead to UF failure due to lymphatic absorption, whereas low exchange volumes may falsely seem to be peritoneal failure, because with low volumes there is rapid solute equilibration.

Fluid Leaks

Fluid leaks secondary to high intraperitoneal pressure are more common in infants, often manifesting as hernias. Recurrent hydrothorax is due to pleura-peritoneal connections and the negative pressure produced on inhalation. Pericatheter exit site leak is usually an early event after insertion and is usually managed by postponing the start of PD or using smaller volumes initially. Leak into the abdominal wall causes subcutaneous edema.

ENCAPSULATING PERITONEAL SCLEROSIS

Encapsulating peritoneal sclerosis is a rare complication with a high fatality rate, characterized by extensive intraperitoneal fibrosis, which causes UF failure occasionally with symptoms of bowel obstruction. It was found in 14 of 712 (1.9%) pediatric patients undergoing PD registered in the Italian registry of chronic dialysis.[137] Eleven of the patients were treated with PD for longer than 5 years. Because the disease is insidious and progresses slowly, five (36%) were diagnosed when no longer receiving dialysis. In 71% of the patients, high-dextrose solutions were used over the 6 months before diagnosis. The peritonitis rate was not higher than in patients without this complication. A second study found the same rate of encapsulating peritoneal sclerosis but a higher infection rate relative to those without this complication, and no correlation to dialysate type.[138]

ADHERENCE TO TREATMENT

Patient compliance was evaluated in 51 patients in a single-center study,[139] using automatic PD device memory cards. Variables tested were number of sessions per month, duration of each session, number of cycles per session, and volume of PD solution instilled. Only 55% were adherent in all four variables; males and African Americans were less likely to be adherent. Nonadherent patients tended to skip whole sessions or instill reduced volumes more than shortening sessions or reducing the number of cycles. Apart from being aware of the gap between prescribed and provided PD treatment, this can shed light on the challenge of being compliant with complex treatment, the aspiration for some "treatment holidays," and the discomfort of large-volume instillation.

GLOBAL DISPARITIES
(see also Chapters 77 to 84)

Gross national income has a major impact not only on the availability but also on the practices of PD. In a study of the International Pediatric Peritoneal Dialysis Network Registry, close associations were found between gross national income and percentage of infants undergoing dialysis, lack of diagnosis of the primary disease, prevalence of APD and more advanced techniques such as biocompatible solutions, enteral feeding, calcium-free phosphate binders, ESAs, and vitamin D analogues.[140] Lower gross national income led to a higher death rate from infectious complication (although peritonitis incidence was not higher), lower hemoglobin and calcium levels, higher PTH levels, lower height percentile, and overall higher mortality.

CHANGE OF DIALYSIS MODALITY

The main reasons for termination of PD are transplantation, transition to HD, death, and rarely withdrawal of treatment or recovery of renal function.

The NAPRTCS 2011 report provides information about termination of 4687 PD courses in the registry (excluding deaths): 19.4% still had working access, 53.7% underwent transplantation, and 16.0% changed modality. The main reason for modality change was excessive infections (43%), 8.8% were due to family choice, 8.2% due to access failure, and 26.7% due to other medical issues.[29] The report does not address the relative role of ultrafiltration failure. It is interesting to note that in patients receiving HD, reasons for modality change were mainly family choice (43.0%) and only rarely excessive infections (7.0%). Because PD is much more demanding for caregivers, one might expect higher rates of family choice to switch modality in peritoneal dialysis, compared to hemodialysis, reflecting caregiver burnout.[29]

The answer to this may be the following. Half of patients undergoing HD that change modality do so within 3 months and two-thirds within 6 months, over a total 36-month observation period, whereas patients undergoing PD change modality at a steady pace over the time period. This means that most modality changes from HD to PD are actually planned in advance, and only insufficient time for PD catheter insertion and PD learning time mandated starting HD temporarily. In addition, some patients live very far from pediatric HD centers and therefore have no option of modality change to HD.

Several other reports from around the world demonstrate the transition of pediatric patients from PD to HD. In a report from Taiwan 8 of 29 (27.5%) changed modality: 2 due to refractory peritonitis, 3 due to inadequate dialysis, and 3 due to UF failure.[141] In Turkey, of 476 children treated with CAPD, 142 converted later to APD; 95% continued receiving PD at 1 year and 69% at 5 years,[142] whereas 13.7% changed to HD. In a report from Iran, outcomes improve by era but are still poor.[18] Between 1998 and 2001 the death rate was 60%, 13% switched to HD, 11% underwent transplantation, and only 4% continued to receive PD. In the next era (2002 to 2006) the death rate decreased to 23%, 15% switched to HD, 10% were transplanted, and 50% were still receiving PD.

RENAL REPLACEMENT THERAPY FOR CHILDREN WITH INBORN ERRORS OF METABOLISM

Some inborn errors of metabolism manifest in early infancy and may lead to death or permanent, severe neurologic damage due to accumulation of neurotoxic abnormal metabolites. Long-term outcome depends upon quick diagnosis and removal of the toxins by diet (reducing their synthesis) or medications (redirecting the toxins to alternative metabolic pathways). These modalities are frequently insufficient in the short term and necessitate more aggressive treatment to reduce metabolites to a nonhazardous range, especially in neonates.[1] All RRT modalities have been used for metabolite clearance in various diseases, such as urea cycle defects, maple syrup urine disease, and methylmalonic acidemia. In the past, acute PD was the only technologic solution for clearance of toxic metabolites, but HD, continuous venovenous HD, and continuous venovenous hemofiltration are now possible even in neonates and have been found to be superior in clearance rate.[143-146] Comparison of later outcomes to historical cohorts shows clearly better outcomes. However, due to the rarity of these diseases and their detrimental outcome, there are no comparative studies of long-term outcomes of the various treatment modalities.

CONTINUOUS RENAL REPLACEMENT THERAPY

Over the past 2 decades, continuous renal replacement therapy (CRRT) has become the preferred modality for the management of children with acute kidney injury (AKI) and volume overload, who may be hemodynamically unstable.[147,148] CRRT allows provision of diffusive and convective clearance separately or in combination. Diffusion refers to the movement of molecules down a concentration gradient across a semipermeable membrane, and convection describes the movement of dissolved solutes with water in response to transmembrane pressure. Both mechanisms provide similar clearance of small molecules, although larger ones would be better cleared by convection. The nomenclature of CRRT stems from the access type and the mode of clearance. Although CRRT was originally developed based on combined arterial and venous access, namely continuous arteriovenous hemofiltration, current practice uses pump-driven venovenous access, which, on its own, provides convective clearance through high UF rates. To prevent volume depletion, most of the ultrafiltrate is replaced by electrolyte-containing fluid. Continuous venovenous hemodiafiltration combines both diffusive and convective clearance by countercurrent infusion of dialysate and net UF to maintain euvolemia. The choice of a given modality is often center dependent.

The shift in the epidemiology of AKI in developed countries affects the use of CRRT as it is delivered to critically ill patients with AKI. During the 1980s the leading causes of AKI were primary renal diseases, including hemolytic uremic syndrome (HUS), sepsis, and burns.[149] Studies reporting on more recent periods show that most children have at least one comorbid condition such as congenital heart disease and corrective surgery, acute tubular necrosis (ATN), sepsis, and the administration of nephrotoxic agents.[150,151]

INDICATIONS

Of the Prospective Pediatric Continuous Renal Replacement Therapy (ppCRRT) registry, 46% received CRRT to treat fluid overload and electrolyte abnormalities, 29% for isolated volume overload, and 3% to obviate the need for fluid restriction and allow better intake of nutrition or the administration of blood products. An additional 6% were treated for inborn errors of metabolism, primarily hyperammonemia, or intoxications/overdose.[152]

COMPARISON TO HEMODIALYSIS AND PERITONEAL DIALYSIS

Although CRRT shares similar principles with HD, both the blood and dialysate flows are significantly slower, resulting in a lower hourly clearance rate. This is compensated for by extending the clearance time. Over 24 hours, CRRT provides solute clearance comparable to a 4-hour HD session. The main advantage of CRRT in the critically ill child is the ability to maintain hemodynamic stability. CRRT and PD are continuous in nature, but the former provides much greater daily clearance rates.

TECHNICAL CONSIDERATIONS

Double-lumen catheters are usually used, and the diameter-size is selected based on the patient's body surface area. Although femoral catheters are used four times more often than internal jugular ones, the latter result in a far better circuit survival.[153] Also, femoral catheters, unless located in the inferior vena cava (IVC), are significantly affected by patient movement and may require the patient to be sedated or even paralyzed for proper use. The recommended blood flow is 3 to 10 mL/kg/hr with a relatively higher flow in the very young child if an adult-sized device is used. Whereas in previous years, lactate-based fluids were used, resulting in lactic acidosis, cardiac dysfunction, and hypotension, bicarbonate-based dialysate and replacement fluids are currently considered standard of care.[154] Large volumes of replacement fluid, containing varying amounts of electrolytes, are administered. This requires close monitoring of the patient laboratory profile to ensure stable acid-base and electrolyte balance. Activation of the clotting cascade, affecting circuit longevity, results from the contact of blood with the artificial filter, as well as slow blood flow and the small catheters used. This mandates the administration of anticoagulants. Although a single pediatric study demonstrated that heparin and citrate are equally efficacious, with more bleeding episodes occurring with the former,[155] most adult studies favor regional citrate, together with systemic calcium infusion, for better longevity of the circuit and fewer bleeding episodes. In a multicenter pediatric survey, it was shown that citrate was used in 56% of children, compared to heparin in 37%.[152] Citrate is metabolized to bicarbonate in the liver and should be cautiously used in patients with liver failure.

DOSING OF CONTINUOUS RENAL REPLACEMENT THERAPY

There are no robust studies in children exploring the optimal CRRT dosing, but the consensus in adults is that there is no benefit to delivering high-volume CRRT reaching greater than 20 to 25 mL/kg/hr clearance.[156] Attention should be paid though to the potential discrepancy between the prescribed and the delivered doses of CRRT, particularly those that are due to technical difficulties, which are prevalent among very young patients. Higher intensity of CRRT may lead to hypophosphatemia, increased amino acid loss, and augmented drug clearance rate.

CONTINUOUS RENAL REPLACEMENT THERAPY OUTCOMES

Patient outcomes are largely dependent on the underlying disease state and comorbid conditions. According to the ppCRRT registry, overall mortality was 42%, with higher rates in children with liver failure or liver transplant, children with pulmonary disease or lung transplant, and stem cell transplant recipients, ranging from 55% to 69%.[157] Children with multiple organ dysfunction syndrome, defined as receiving one vasoactive medication and invasive mechanical ventilation, have been found in the same registry to have a higher mortality rate with an odds ratio of 4.7. Also, fluid overload at the initiation of CRRT is an independent risk factor for mortality: Patients with greater than 20% fluid overload were 8.5-fold more likely to die than those with less than 20%.[158]

KIDNEY TRANSPLANTATION

Although long-term dialysis provides clearance of uremic toxins and, together with medications and strict dietary limitations, enables long-term survival of patients with ESKD, renal transplantation offers significant advantages, particularly in children, as discussed earlier.[2] A well-functioning kidney graft can provide all the functions of a normal kidney, in addition to efficient clearance of metabolic waste products and fine tuning of water and electrolyte balance, as well as secretion of hormones involved in systemic and renal hemodynamics, ESAs, and calcitriol. Despite the need for long-term immunosuppressive medications and close monitoring, children after kidney transplantation can lead, in many cases, normal lifestyles, with improved growth, development, and rehabilitation in comparison to children treated with dialysis.

INCIDENCE, PREVALENCE, AND ALLOCATION

NAPRTCS is a voluntary database active since 1987, collecting information on pediatric patients undergoing kidney transplantation from centers in the United States (later expanded to include children with CKD). The latest report in 2010 provides data on 11,603 renal transplants performed in 10,632 pediatric patients.[159] The Organ Procurement and Transplantation Network (OPTN) contains the database of all organ transplantations in the United States since 1986, including pediatric kidney transplantation.[160] Both these registries provide current information about the status of pediatric renal transplantation in the United States, and extensive analysis has been performed on the data collected. Other registries providing information on pediatric renal transplantation include ESPN/ERA-EDTA, the Cooperative European Paediatric Renal TransplAnt INitiative (CERTAIN), the UK renal registry, ANZDATA, and others.[3,161]

As of June 2013, 919 children under the age of 18 years were on the U.S. waiting list for a kidney, out of a total of 103,574 patients listed (0.89%).[159] Table 76.3 summarizes the demographics of pediatric patients undergoing renal transplantation in the United States. Of the 16,485 kidney transplants performed in 2012, 758 were in children (4.6%), a significantly higher proportion than those wait-listed. Of these, 38% of pediatric kidney transplants were from a living donor, whereas 51.7% of the kidney transplants in the entire population were from living donors. The most frequent living donor was a parent (61% of living donors in 2012); the rest were siblings, other family members, and living unrelated donors. This is in contrast to adult living-donor transplant recipients, for whom the most common donor was a sibling, followed by a biologic child and a spouse.[160] Whereas there was an increase in living-donor kidney donation to pediatric patients between 1987 and 2001, with a peak of 64% living-donor transplantation, there has been a gradual decrease in this trend in the years between 2001 and 2012 in the United States. This may be due to a change in allocation of deceased-donor kidneys—the "Share 35" policy, giving priority to patients younger than 18 years to be offered a kidney from a deceased donor under the age of 35. Since the implementation of this policy, waiting time has shortened, and the proportion of children receiving deceased-donor kidneys increased.[159,160,163] Overall, 24% of pediatric renal transplantations were preemptive, that is, no dialysis had been performed before transplantation.[159] The majority of preemptive transplantations were from living donors.

In Europe a survey including 32 countries reported 900 kidney transplants in children in 2008, constituting 4.4% of total renal transplants. Approximately 43% were from living donors, and 27% were preemptive. Most countries implement an allocation scheme that prioritizes pediatric patients on the waiting list, in particular in regard to younger donors. The rates of pediatric kidney transplantation, waiting time, and donor source vary considerably between the different European countries. A positive correlation between the national gross domestic product per capita and the rate of pediatric kidney transplantation was noted.[164]

Table 76.3 Age, Race, Gender and Cause of End-Stage Kidney Disease at Time of Transplantation in the United States, 1987-2010

	Age 0-1 Years (%)	Age 2-5 Years (%)	Age 6-12 Years (%)	Age 13-17 Years (%)	Age ≥18 Years (%)
Transplants	5.3	14.7	32.8	39.2	8
Gender					
Male	69.2	65.5	58.7	56.4	55.9
Female	30.8	34.5	41.3	43.6	44.1
Race					
White	73.6	63	60.3	56.1	51.7
Black	8.2	14.4	14.7	19.8	25
Hispanic	11.9	16.2	18.2	17.6	15.7
Other	6.3	6.4	6.9	6.5	7.6
Primary diagnosis					
Hypoplasia/dysplasia	29	23.5	16.6	11.3	9.6
Obstructive uropathy	18.6	20.6	16	13.2	10.1
FSGS	0.7	8.4	12.3	13.2	16.6
Other	51.7	47.4	55.1	62.2	63.7

FSGS, Focal segmental glomerulosclerosis.
Adapted from North American Pediatric Renal Trials and Collaborative Studies: NAPRTCS 2010 annual transplant report. Available at: https://web.emmes.com/study/ped/annlrept/2010Report.pdf. Accessed July 10, 2013.

Kidney transplantation in infants under the age of 1 year is uncommon, with 96 transplantations in this age-group between 1987 and 2010 in the United States; however, only 10 were performed between 2004 and 2010.[159] Living-donor kidneys are associated with improved long-term graft survival in pediatric recipients, even when compared to younger deceased-donor kidneys.[165] The estimated half-life (median survival) of a graft from a living donor performed in 2010 is 15 years, in comparison to approximately 11 years for a deceased-donor kidney.[160] The added beneficial effect of a biologically related donor compared to an unrelated donor is minor.

As noted earlier, deceased-donor kidneys from younger donors are preferentially allocated to children in the United States. However, use of deceased-donor kidneys from infants under the age of 2 years in the 1980s yielded poor outcomes both in Europe and in the United States, resulting in fewer infant kidneys being used in the subsequent years.[166-168] Later data have shown good results in children receiving kidneys from small pediatric donors, either a single kidney or both donor kidneys en bloc.[169-172] One study from Europe reported a significant increase in allograft size after transplantation and superior graft function in the recipients of pediatric kidneys.[173]

PREPARATION OF THE RECIPIENT FOR TRANSPLANTATION

TIMING

In general, renal transplantation is the preferred modality of treatment for children with ESKD. There is a significant survival advantage for children with a functioning graft over children remaining on the waiting list, from 6 months after transplantation (see Figure 76.3).[84,174] If preemptive transplantation is not possible, a short period on dialysis (up to 1 to 2 years) does not significantly affect patient survival, according to a large study in European registries.[175] There is some controversy whether preemptive transplantation offers an advantage in graft survival over patients who spent time undergoing dialysis first. After adjusting for donor source, a possible small increase in graft survival may be demonstrated in preemptive transplantation compared with HD first.[176,177] However, this does not take into account other considerations, particularly morbidity on dialysis, effect on neurocognitive development, and decreased linear growth. Certain situations preclude preemptive transplantation, such as active nephrotic disease, which is also a hypercoagulable state, presenting a high risk for thrombosis during transplantation. To be a candidate for transplantation without dialysis, a patient must have sufficient urine output and balanced electrolyte levels. When the patient approaches KDOQI stage 4 CKD, preparation of the patient for transplantation and evaluation of potential living donors should be pursued. Transplantation should not be performed before the child reaches ESKD, because graft survival is not indefinite, and no benefit has been demonstrated for this practice.[178]

Two age-groups require special consideration. Very young children, in particular those weighing less than 10 kg, may have inferior results mainly because of technical difficulties and graft thrombosis. Some specialized centers, with greater experience in this age-group, have demonstrated excellent results.[179] The alternative, continuing to receive dialysis for a prolonged period of time, also carries a high morbidity and mortality, particularly in this young age-group.[32,180,181] Most units refer young patients for transplantation when they reach a weight close to 10 kg, but the risks and benefits must be carefully considered in each case. The other potentially complex age-group is adolescents. There is a higher rate of acute rejection episodes, shorter graft survival, and lower creatinine clearance in this group.[159] This is mostly due to nonadherence, which is more frequent in teenagers and may manifest as missed doses of immunosuppressive medications, more extensive "drug holidays," missed clinic visits, and other high-risk behaviors.[182,183]

CONTRAINDICATIONS

Some clinical situations may present a temporary or permanent contraindication to transplantation. Malignancy should postpone plans for transplantation until complete remission is achieved, chemotherapeutic medications are discontinued, and no relapse is evident. High-dose immunosuppressive therapy after transplantation may increase the risk for cancer recurrence, presumably due to progression from occult residual tumor and/or micrometastases. The time period between completion of therapy for cancer and listing for transplant will depend also on the type of malignancy and its characteristics.[184] Immunosuppressive medications also impair the ability to fight infection; therefore active infection is a temporary contraindication to transplantation, and latent infections should be sought out and addressed before proceeding to transplantation. Severe comorbid conditions or profound neurodevelopmental disability may render a child unsuitable for transplantation. Each child should be evaluated individually to assess the impact of transplantation on life expectancy, quality of life, and rehabilitation, taking into account the wishes of the family. Recalcitrant nonadherence to medication or dialysis schedule, diet, and clinic appointments may also be a temporary contraindication to transplantation.

RECIPIENT EVALUATION

Before transplantation an extensive evaluation of the recipient must be performed. The goals of this workup are to provide an optimal plan for each individual patient, reduce complications, and increase long-term patient and graft survival. The main elements of the pretransplant evaluation are summarized in Table 76.4. Some of the important issues are discussed in the following sections.

INFECTION

A history, physical signs, or laboratory findings suggesting active infection need to be addressed before subjecting the patient to major surgery and high-dose immunosuppression. The respiratory tract, teeth, skin, dialysis access exit site, and other sites of possible chronic infection should be carefully examined. Even a minor infection may be exacerbated by immunosuppressive therapy. Serologic testing for cytomegalovirus (CMV) and Epstein-Barr virus (EBV) to assess the risk for posttransplantation viral disease

Table 76.4 Evaluation of Pediatric Candidates for Kidney Transplantation

Medical history	ESKD cause, family history of renal or other disease, biopsy results, previous transplantation history, dialysis access and prescription, medication list, compliance with medical regimen, urologic interventions, urine output, other comorbid conditions, allergies, previous procedures, transfusions, growth charts
Physical examination	Weight, height, BMI and percentiles, blood pressure and pulse, general well-being, complete physical examination
Specialist assessments	Pediatric nephrologist, transplant surgeon, urologist, anesthesiologist, transplant coordinator, nurse, social worker, dietitian, pediatric dentist. As indicated: psychologist, cardiologist, hematologist, pulmonologist
Laboratory tests	Blood type, CBC, electrolytes, BUN, creatinine, calcium, phosphorus, liver enzymes, protein, albumin, lipids, iron, PTH, thyroid, fasting glucose and Hb A_{1c}, PT/PTT, urinalysis, 24-hour urine collection for creatinine clearance and proteinuria
Serologic tests	EBV (IgG, EBNA, and IgM), CMV (IgG and IgM), HBV (surface Ag and Ab), HCV, HIV, varicella, PPD test
Histocompatibility testing	HLA typing—class I (A, B), class II (DR, DQ), PRA, DSA, cross-match with donor (T and B cell cross-match, by CDC-AHG or flow cytometry)
Imaging	Chest x-ray examination; abdominal ultrasonography, including kidneys, bladder, and postvoiding volume; echocardiography; and ECG. Doppler study of abdominal and pelvic arteries and veins, VCUG, urodynamic testing or other if indicated
Vaccinations	DTaP, Hib, IPV, HAV, HBV, varicella, MMR, pneumococcus, influenza. Selected patients: meningococcus, HPV
Social	Evaluation of the family, support systems, financial issues, school

Ag, Antigen; Ab, antibody; BMI, body mass index; BUN, blood urea nitrogen; CBC, complete blood count; CDC-AHG, complement-dependent cytotoxicity with anti–human globulin; CMV, cytomegalovirus; DSA, donor-specific antibodies; DTaP, diphtheria and tetanus toxoids and acellular pertussis vaccine; EBNA, Epstein-Barr virus–associated nuclear antigen; EBV, Epstein-Barr virus; ECG, electrocardiography; ESKD, end-stage kidney disease; HAV, hepatitis A virus; Hb A_{1c}, hemoglobin A_{1c}; HBV, hepatitis B virus; HCV, hepatitis C virus; Hib, *Haemophilus influenzae* type B; HIV, human immunodeficiency virus; HPV, human papillomavirus; Ig, immunoglobulin; IPV, poliovirus vaccine inactivated; MMR, measles-mumps-rubella; PPD, purified protein derivative (tuberculin); PRA, panel-reactive antibodies; PTH, parathyroid hormone; PT, prothrombin time; PTT, partial thromboplastin time; VCUG, voiding cystourethrogram.

is important in planning, monitoring, and antiviral prophylaxis after transplantation. Many pediatric patients are seronegative for these viruses and should be monitored frequently while on the waiting list, to avoid inadvertently referring for transplantation during a subclinical primary infection. Vaccinations should be reviewed and completed before transplantation, because response to vaccines may be attenuated by immunosuppressive medications, and live vaccines are not recommended following transplantation.[185] The regular pediatric schedule should be given, including pneumococcus, influenza, and varicella, as well as other vaccines depending on age, gender, and exposure.[186]

MALIGNANCY

Although less common in children, a basic workup to rule out malignancy includes history, physical examination, chest x-ray examination, and abdominal ultrasonography, as well as routine laboratory tests. Children with a history of cancer should be evaluated by a pediatric oncologist to assess remission and risk for recurrence and to help determine the timing of transplantation.[184]

UROLOGIC ISSUES

The most frequent cause of ESKD in younger children is CAKUT.[159] Structural and functional evaluation of the urinary tract is important before transplantation, because the kidney allograft may be compromised by an abnormal urinary tract, with obstructed drainage, massive reflux, or a small defunctionalized bladder. Investigation should begin with ultrasonography of the kidneys and urinary tract, including imaging of the full and postvoiding bladder. In patients with an abnormal urinary tract, further tests such as a voiding cystourethrogram and urodynamic evaluation provide further information. When the child has prolonged anuria, it is sometimes difficult to assess bladder capacity and function. Surgical intervention to alleviate obstruction or correct massive reflux if needed or occasionally bladder augmentation can be performed before or during transplantation. However, a small defunctionalized bladder may increase in capacity after renal transplantation and enable normal voiding without compromising graft function, thus avoiding the need for bladder augmentation.[187] Nephrectomy of native kidneys is indicated in cases of persistent nephrotic syndrome of presumed immunologic cause to enable prompt and accurate diagnosis of recurring nephrotic syndrome, chronically infected kidneys, very large kidneys in a relatively small recipient, for example, in polycystic kidney disease (to enable more physical space for the graft and to alleviate discomfort), and sometimes for uncontrolled hypertension.[188] In cases of congenital nephrotic syndrome, particularly the Finnish type, because of the high mortality associated with this condition, bilateral nephrectomy is usually performed when the child has reached a size compatible with transplantation, even if renal function is good or even normal.[189]

CARDIOVASCULAR ISSUES

Congenital heart disease may coexist with CKD in some patients, which requires consultation with a pediatric cardiologist and consideration of surgical correction before transplantation. Hypertension is very common in ESKD, in many cases causing LVH, with diastolic and occasionally systolic dysfunction. Treatment with antihypertensive medications and avoiding chronic volume overload in patients undergoing dialysis are important, though optimal control of hypertension is often difficult to achieve. However, FGF-23, which is elevated in CKD, induces LVH independent of blood pressure. Therefore LVH may not be completely correctible as long as CKD persists.[190] Cardiomyopathy may improve significantly in children undergoing renal transplantation.[191]

Evaluation of abdominal vasculature before transplantation is beneficial in planning anastomoses and anticipating significant surgical challenges. Children who have had previous abdominal or pelvic surgery, CVCs in the lower body, including neonatal umbilical arterial or venous catheterization, and patients with hypercoagulable state should have Doppler studies of the large arteries and veins before transplantation. Abnormal study results can be followed by formal venography.[192]

RISK FOR RECURRENCE

Recurrence of the underlying disease after renal transplantation, affecting graft function, can be due to persistence of the causative immunologic or humoral factor (FSGS, membranoproliferative glomerulonephritis [MPGN] type II), enzymatic defect (primary hyperoxaluria, atypical HUS), or due to a parallel mechanism unique to a specific disease entity (proteinuria in congenital nephrotic syndrome of the Finnish type, Alport's syndrome).

Recurrence is particularly frequent in idiopathic FSGS, with a rate in children of 30% to 80% depending on the report. Nephrotic syndrome and graft dysfunction may appear immediately after transplantation, and prompt intervention is needed. In these cases pretransplantation nephrectomy of native kidneys, if the patient still has proteinuria, will assist in timely diagnosis of recurrence and enable early treatment. However, FSGS is a histologic diagnosis, which may be due to one of several underlying pathophysiologic processes. For example, genetic forms of steroid-resistant nephrotic syndrome with mutations in the gene encoding podocin, *NPHS2*, have a very low rate of recurrence in the graft.[193,194]

MPGN also carries a high risk for recurrence, which affects graft survival. The risk for graft loss at 5 years is significantly higher in children with FSGS or MPGN compared to children with renal dysplasia.[195,196] Other glomerular diseases, such as lupus nephritis and immunoglobulin A (IgA) nephropathy, may recur but are not usually associated with graft loss.

Primary hyperoxaluria type 1 is a disorder of glyoxylate metabolism in which an enzymatic defect in the liver causes overproduction of oxalate and deposition of calcium oxalate in the kidneys and in other organ systems once advanced renal failure develops. Presentation in infancy is associated with nephrocalcinosis and early CKD. Kidney transplantation alone usually results in massive oxalate deposition in the new kidney and early graft failure. In these cases, combined liver and kidney transplantation (or liver transplantation alone if renal function is not severely affected) is curative, correcting the underlying enzymatic defect.[197]

Genetic forms of atypical HUS are usually due to deficiencies of regulatory elements of the complement system, can cause ESKD, and have a high rate of recurrence in the graft. Treatment strategies have included frequent plasma infusions, plasmapheresis, or combined liver and kidney transplantation, all aimed at providing the deficient factor and preventing relapse. Treatment with the monoclonal antibody to complement factor 5, eculizumab, was found to be effective in the treatment of atypical HUS and to prevent recurrence after transplantation by inhibiting complement activation.[198] Eculizumab was FDA approved for the treatment of atypical HUS in 2011.

SENSITIZATION

Blood type, HLA typing, and panel-reactive antibodies should be tested in each transplant candidate. Donor-specific antibodies (DSA) should be identified and quantified if panel-reactive antibody test results are positive. A negative direct cross-match by complement-dependent cytotoxicity with anti–human globulin is crucial to avoid hyperacute rejection. Cross-match by the flow cytometry method is more sensitive, but the clinical implications of a positive test result are less clear cut. Ideally, blood type compatibility and close HLA matching without DSA are preferred. However, in some cases for which such a match is not available, ABO incompatibility or the presence of low titers of DSA can be overcome with special desensitization protocols, with good results, as detailed later.[199]

TRANSPLANTATION IMMUNOLOGY

HLA MATCHING AND SENSITIZATION

Chapter 71 covers the subject of transplantation immunobiology in detail. The importance of human leukocyte antigen (HLA) matching between donor and recipient was recognized in the 1960s to 1970s and became the cornerstone of deceased-donor allocation policy. A clear association between number of HLA mismatches and graft survival was shown in several large studies.[200] With the introduction of more potent immunosuppression, the significance of HLA matching may have diminished,[201] while other factors such as peak panel-reactive antibodies, cold ischemic time, and donor age retained their relative importance. However, other publications have shown that HLA mismatches continue to adversely affect renal allograft outcomes in the present era, as shown by a study from ANZDATA that included children.[202] Studies that examined the effect of HLA matching specifically in children have also shown that an increase in the number of HLA mismatches is associated with decreased graft survival.[203] Mismatch at the DR locus may be correlated with increased acute rejection.[204] The algorithm that prioritizes children in allocation of deceased-donor kidneys from younger donors shortens waiting times but deemphasizes HLA matching. Both donor age and HLA matching are important in determining deceased-donor graft survival and may be offset by each other.[205]

Most pediatric patients with CKD will need to undergo more than one transplantation over their lifetime, and HLA matching of the first kidney graft may have an impact on subsequent transplants. More HLA mismatches at the first transplantation are associated with HLA sensitization,[206] longer waiting time for a second transplant, and decreased graft survival.[207]

In addition to HLA matching, panel-reactive antibodies are measured in renal transplant candidates, and if positive, should be characterized by solid-phase assays.[208] The presence of DSA is associated with increased risk for acute antibody-mediated rejection (AMR) as well as chronic AMR and decreased graft survival. When DSA are further characterized, patients with complement-binding DSA after transplantation are at the highest risk for graft loss and AMR.[209] The deleterious impact of DSA has been demonstrated in children, even when the direct cross-match between donor and recipient is negative by flow cytometry,[210] though not in all series.[211] Although good HLA matching without DSA is desirable, not all patients will find an appropriate donor. In fact, when comparing data from 2009 to 2011 to a decade earlier, the OPTN report shows that children undergoing renal transplantation were now more likely to have panel-reactive antibody results above 80% (5.1% vs. 2.7%).[160] Desensitization protocols, including treatment with combinations of intravenous γ-globulin, plasmapheresis, and rituximab, enable transplantation for adult patients with acceptable outcomes.[212,213] Less data are available on these treatment protocols in children.[214]

De novo DSA appear in 25% of children in the first years after transplantation; the most common antibody is to HLA-DQ loci. These antibodies are associated with increased risk for AMR and graft dysfunction.[215] Serial monitoring of DSA in children after transplantation may help to identify patients at risk for adverse outcomes and guide tailoring of immunosuppression.[216]

Although it has been suggested that kidneys transplanted from mothers to their children might have a survival advantage compared to other one-haplotype–matched living related donors because of fetal-maternal microchimerism, this was not found to be the case in a study of data from the Scientific Registry of Transplant Recipients.[217]

ABO COMPATIBILITY

In the past, ABO incompatibility was considered a contraindication to transplantation, because of the high risk for hyperacute AMR. However, in the past few years there have been increasing reports of successful ABO-incompatible renal transplantation in children. According to the NAPRTCS report, 0.6% of pediatric kidney transplantations in the United States are ABO incompatible, though most of the cases are since the year 2000.[159] ABO-incompatible transplantation is more common in Japan, where deceased-donor transplants are not frequently performed. Treatment protocols include pretransplantation plasmapheresis, in order to remove anti-A and anti-B antibodies, together with splenectomy or rituximab to prevent ongoing antibody production after transplantation. With this regimen there was an increase in acute rejection episodes in comparison with ABO-compatible transplantation using conventional immunosuppression, but no significant difference in long-term graft survival.[198] The risk for AMR is associated with higher titers of anti-A or anti-B isoagglutinins, and the intensity of desensitization may be modifiable according to pre-treatment titers, thus potentially opening this option in deceased-donor transplantation as well.[218] Rituximab with antibody-specific immunoadsorption has been used, with the goal of less long-term impact on the immune system. In this study none of the patients had acute rejection, and there was no difference in graft function compared to ABO-compatible transplantation.[219] Immunoadsorption therapy for ABO-incompatible renal transplantation has been associated with surgical bleeding in some cases.[220] Late AMR in the setting of ABO incompatibility is less frequent than AMR in HLA sensitization.[208,221,222] Despite more intense immunosuppressive regimens, a study in adults did not demonstrate a higher risk for cancer in patients undergoing ABO-incompatible transplantation.[223]

IMMUNOSUPPRESSION

A wide range of immunosuppressive medications are used in pediatric renal transplantation, and they are a key factor in preventing rejection and enabling long-term graft function. In general more information is available from trials in adult patients undergoing transplantation, and specific data in children do not always exist. Special considerations in children include altered drug metabolism, as well as adverse effects particular to children, including effects on growth and development. The optimal immunosuppression regimen should minimize the risk for rejection, without causing overimmunosuppression or other side effects of medications.

INDUCTION IMMUNOSUPPRESSION

The risk for acute rejection is highest in the immediate posttransplantation period, which is why in addition to higher doses of maintenance immunosuppressive drugs, many transplantation protocols include a biologic induction agent. These antibody preparations are aimed at depleting T cells or preventing their activation and are administered in the perioperative period.

Antilymphocyte preparations are T cell–depleting agents that can be polyclonal or monoclonal. In addition to their use for induction immunosuppression, they have a role in treatment of acute cellular rejection. The polyclonal antibody antithymocyte globulin (ATG) contains antibodies to a wide variety of lymphocyte antigens in serum of animals immunized with human lymphocytes.

Monoclonal preparations include antibodies to the CD3 antigen of T cells, muromonab-CD3 (Orthoclone OKT3), and antibodies to CD52, alemtuzumab, which binds to T and B cells as well as monocytes and natural killer cells, causing cell lysis.

T cell activation induces interleukin-2 (IL-2) production causing T cell proliferation; therefore monoclonal IL-2 receptor antibodies block this pathway, preventing T cell activation without depletion. Two products were initially available in this category, daclizumab and basiliximab; however, daclizumab has been withdrawn by the manufacturer and is no longer available.

Antibody induction has been shown to improve outcomes in kidney transplantation in adults compared to conventional immunosuppression alone. However, in children there are less supportive data. Observational data from the NAPRTCS database in the late 1990s suggested a beneficial effect of T cell–depleting antibody induction, though most patients were receiving maintenance therapy consisting of azathioprine, steroids, and cyclosporine at that time.[224] Rabbit ATG (Thymoglobulin) is usually the agent of choice, with a lower rate of acute rejection than horse-derived ATG (ATGAM).[225] Another study, based on NAPRTCS, showed no advantage in graft or patient survival in children treated with muromonab-CD3 or rabbit ATG compared to children without antibody induction, and a higher risk for infection in the antibody-treated group.[226] However, this was a retrospective study that did not consider whether patients were at a higher risk and therefore more likely to receive induction therapy. Pediatric studies using the IL-2 receptor blocker basiliximab as induction therapy combined with triple-drug maintenance immunosuppression showed a good safety profile but minimal or no additional benefit.[227,228] Alemtuzumab induction has been described in several small series of children, enabling steroid avoidance or tacrolimus monotherapy, with good results. Additional data will be necessary to assess long-term graft outcomes and the risk for infection and posttransplantation lymphoproliferative disease (PTLD) associated with the use of this agent.[229,230]

According to NAPRTCS data, 50% to 60% of children receive antibody induction, a figure that did not change significantly between 1996 and 2009. Initially this was divided between rabbit ATG and muromonab-CD3; however, the use of muromonab-CD3 for induction in children declined sharply, because of its adverse effects, particularly the "first-dose reaction," which occurs in more than two-thirds of patients, and consists of fever, chills, headache, vomiting, diarrhea, hypotension, and occasionally pulmonary edema. In addition, some children may develop antibodies to muromonab-CD3. IL-2 receptor blockers were introduced in the late 1990s, and their use increased and largely replaced T cell–depleting agents in low-risk patients in the following years (Figure 76.4). However, the withdrawal of daclizumab together with data suggesting minor efficacy of basiliximab have decreased their use in the last few years.[159] On the other hand, steroid-avoidance protocols have used prolonged daclizumab dosing or rabbit ATG induction with excellent results, thus increasing the percentage of children receiving rabbit ATG.

In general, most centers use rabbit ATG induction for high-risk renal transplantation, especially in sensitized patients or in children on a steroid-free protocol. Antibody induction may be avoided in low-risk patients, though basiliximab is used in some centers.

MAINTENANCE IMMUNOSUPPRESSION

CALCINEURIN INHIBITORS

Cyclosporine

Cyclosporine was introduced as an immunosuppressant for kidney transplantation in 1982, revolutionizing the treatment of transplant recipients. Whereas in 1996, 82% of children were treated with cyclosporine 1 month after renal transplantation, this decreased to 1% in 2009, because it was largely replaced by tacrolimus.[159] Cyclosporine doses in children need to be higher per body weight, because it is more rapidly metabolized than in adults. It has been suggested that cyclosporine should therefore be divided every 8 hours in young children and infants; however, this may actually result in lower dose–normalized area under the curve (AUC) throughout the day, in addition to being a drug regimen that is more difficult to follow.[231] Drug level monitoring is important for maintaining therapeutic concentrations, while avoiding toxicity. Trough levels are usually kept at 150 to 300 µg/L initially, and 75 to 125 µg/L after the first 6 months. Monitoring AUC or 2-hour–postdrug level, as an indicator of AUC, may be more effective in avoiding toxic effects. Cyclosporine is available as capsules and oral

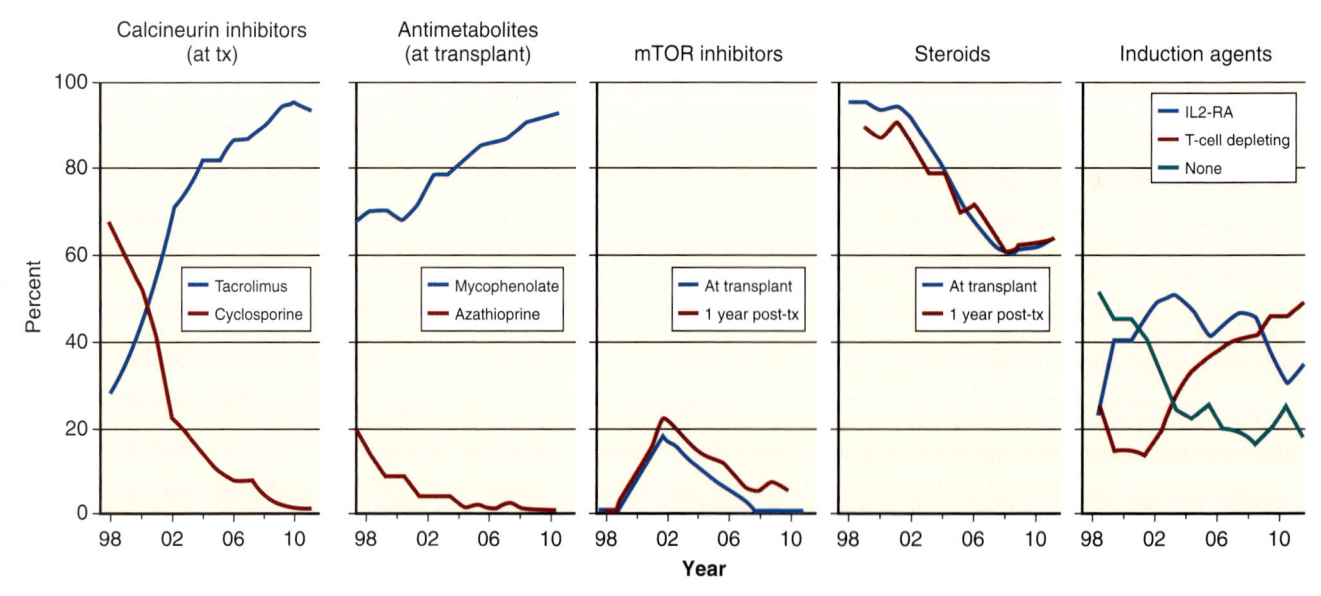

Figure 76.4 Trends in immunosuppression treatment in pediatric kidney transplant (tx) recipients in the United States in 1998-2011. IL2-RA, Interleukin-2 receptor antibodies; mTOR, mammalian target of rapamycin. (Adapted from Scientific Registry of Transplant Recipients: *OPTN/SRTR 2011 annual data report: kidney*. Pediatric transplant, pp 37-44. Available at: http://srtr.transplant.hrsa.gov/annual_reports/2011/pdf/01_kidney_12.pdf. Accessed June 29, 2013, p 42, Figure KI 8.23.)

solution. Absorption of different formulations may vary, and dosing should be guided by drug levels.

Of note, cyclosporine is nephrotoxic in a dose-dependent manner. It is associated with hypertension, hyperlipidemia, and hyperuricemia, all of which may contribute to cardiovascular disease. Cosmetic side effects are a major issue in young patients and include hirsutism, gum hyperplasia, and less frequently coarse facial features, which may contribute to nonadherence, particularly in teenagers.[232] Several drugs interact with cyclosporine, in many cases decreasing its metabolism and potentially causing toxic concentrations. Common examples in children include macrolide antibiotics or azole antifungal medications, which should be given with care, while monitoring calcineurin inhibitor levels. Ingestion of grapefruit juice may also decrease calcineurin inhibitor metabolism and should be avoided.

Tacrolimus

In the past decade, tacrolimus has been part of the immunosuppression regimen in 60% to 70% of children after kidney transplantation in the United States.[159] Metabolism varies greatly between individuals, younger children may require higher doses by weight,[233] and all patients should have regular drug level monitoring. Initial target tacrolimus levels are high (10 to 15 ng/mL), gradually decreasing to 3 to 6 ng/mL after the first 6 months. Several studies have been published comparing tacrolimus and cyclosporine in children. A NAPRTCS study comparing tacrolimus and cyclosporine, both in combination with mycophenolate mofetil and prednisone, showed no difference in rejection or graft survival at 1 and 2 years after transplantation. However, the children in the tacrolimus group were less likely to require antihypertensive treatments and had a higher GFR.[234] A similar multicenter study from Europe showed decreased frequency of acute rejection and a higher GFR in the tacrolimus group, with a similar safety profile for both drugs.[235] Long-term data showed better graft survival and GFR in the tacrolimus group, as well as lower cholesterol levels. There was no difference between the groups in regard to PTLD or diabetes mellitus.[236] A comparison of protocol biopsy results in children demonstrated more subclinical acute rejection in those treated with cyclosporine.[237]

Tacrolimus adverse effects are similar to those for cyclosporine, with a higher rate of posttransplantation diabetes mellitus and neurotoxicity for tacrolimus, manifested as tremor or seizures.[238] A frequent reason for changing treatment from cyclosporine to tacrolimus in children and adolescents is the lack of cosmetic side effects of tacrolimus. A once-daily modified-release formulation of tacrolimus has been shown to improve patient compliance.[239]

ANTIMETABOLITES

Azathioprine

Azathioprine was found to be effective in prevention of renal graft rejection in the early 1960s, especially when combined with corticosteroids. When it is given as part of triple therapy with cyclosporine, pediatric doses are generally 1 to 2 mg/kg. In the 1990s several studies comparing azathioprine with mycophenolate mofetil showed a significantly lower rate of acute rejection in patients treated with mycophenolate.[240] Whereas 20 years ago most children were treated with azathioprine as part of their immunosuppression regimen, in 2010, according to NAPRTCS, only 2.5% of children were receiving azathioprine, although it has not been proven inferior to mycophenolate in combination with tacrolimus.[159] Adverse effects of azathioprine include myelosuppression and hepatotoxicity, which might require dose reduction. The therapeutic efficacy, bone marrow toxicity, and liver toxicity of azathioprine and its active metabolite 6-mercaptopurine (6-MP) may be related to their metabolites: 6-thioguanine and 6-methylmercaptopurine. Thiopurine methyltransferase (TPMT) enzyme activity is a major factor determining azathioprine and 6-MP metabolism. Testing for TPMT genotype and enzyme activity is available and can help guide therapy. The myelosuppressive action of azathioprine is potentiated by xanthine oxidase inhibitors such as allopurinol, and if these medications are absolutely necessary, the dose of azathioprine must be reduced by 50% to 75%. Although azathioprine is still classified by the FDA as category D for use in pregnancy, suggesting positive evidence of risk to the fetus, data accumulated over the years, especially from the National Transplantation Pregnancy Registry, have shown that the incidence of birth defects is similar to that in the general population.[241] In addition, azathioprine is significantly less expensive than mycophenolate.

Mycophenolate

Mycophenolate mofetil, a reversible inhibitor of inosine monophosphate dehydrogenase, which downregulates specifically T and B cell proliferation, was developed as an alternative antimetabolite to azathioprine, with less bone marrow toxicity. It is rapidly metabolized to mycophenolic acid in vivo. It was shown to reduce the frequency of acute rejection and improve 5-year graft survival in children compared to azathioprine, in combination with cyclosporine and prednisone.[242] Some data suggest that in children with chronic allograft nephropathy (CAN), adding mycophenolate to the immunosuppressive regimen improves graft function.[243] The main adverse effects of mycophenolate mofetil are gastrointestinal, including abdominal discomfort, nausea, and diarrhea. An alternative formulation, enteric-coated mycophenolic acid, has been shown to have fewer side effects, as shown in small studies in children.[244] Mycophenolate mofetil is available as capsules, tablets, and oral suspension, as well as intravenous preparation. Enteric-coated mycophenolic acid cannot be made into a suspension, which limits its use in younger children, who may also be more susceptible to adverse gastrointestinal effects and leukopenia. However, a study did not demonstrate a higher rate of mycophenolate discontinuation due to side effects in children compared to adults.[245] Anemia and leukopenia may also necessitate dose reduction. There is debate whether mycophenolic acid monitoring is beneficial in prevention of acute rejection. At this time approximately two-thirds of children with a kidney graft in the United States are treated with mycophenolate.[159] Although initially dosing was 600 mg/m^2 body surface area twice daily, some protocols give a lower dose (300 mg/m^2) to low-risk patients, with less adverse effects.[246]

Pregnancies in patients exposed to mycophenolic acid are associated with a high rate of birth defects; therefore adolescent girls must be cautioned to use reliable contraception if sexually active while treated with mycophenolate.[247]

CORTICOSTEROIDS

Corticosteroids have been a cornerstone drug in prevention of rejection of transplanted organs for decades. However, chronic corticosteroid therapy is associated with many adverse effects, including hypertension, hyperlipidemia, cardiovascular disease, glucose intolerance, osteoporosis and aseptic bone necrosis, cataracts and glaucoma, as well as weight gain, cushingoid appearance, acne, and psychologic effects. The cosmetic effects are often a cause of nonadherence in many patients, particularly adolescents. Corticosteroids also inhibit linear growth by several mechanisms of action, including interference with the action of GH and inhibition of bone formation.[248] Efforts to reduce the adverse effects of corticosteroids in children undergoing renal transplantation have included using lower doses of prednisone, alternate-day regimens, steroid withdrawal protocols, and steroid avoidance.

Studies of steroid withdrawal protocols have shown improved linear growth and cardiovascular risk factors without increased acute rejection in low-risk children on combined cyclosporine or tacrolimus and mycophenolate.[249,250] Steroid avoidance in unsensitized pediatric renal transplantation was reported initially in a single-center nonrandomized controlled study and demonstrated improved graft function and linear growth in the steroid-free group. In this protocol, induction therapy of prolonged daclizumab followed by tacrolimus and mycophenolate was given, and 13% required conversion to steroid-based immunosuppression due to rejection.[251] A subsequent multicenter randomized controlled trial of the same protocol also showed no difference in the rate of biopsy-proven acute rejection between the steroid-free and steroid-based groups. Improved systolic blood pressure and serum cholesterol levels were seen in the steroid-free group, but improvement in linear growth was seen only in a subgroup of children under the age of 5 years.[246] As daclizumab became unavailable, this protocol was tested in a small group of higher-risk children using ATG with similar results.[252] Most centers that use rapid discontinuation of corticosteroids or steroid-free protocols now do so with ATG induction therapy.[253] Steroid avoidance protocols have not been well studied in high-risk pediatric transplant recipients, including nonwhites, patients who have undergone retransplantation, and sensitized patients. According to NAPRTCS, corticosteroid use was almost universal in children undergoing renal transplantation until the year 2000. Subsequently their use has decreased to approximately 60%, which has remained constant over the past few years (see Figure 76.4).[160] Centers that continue to use triple immunosuppression in low-risk patients generally taper corticosteroid dose within a few weeks to doses of 0.1 mg/kg or less, and many give alternate-day low-dose steroids.

MAMMALIAN TARGET OF RAPAMYCIN INHIBITORS

Mammalian target of rapamycin (mTOR) inhibitors block the proliferative response of lymphocytes to IL-2 stimulation.

Sirolimus

The first drug in this group, sirolimus, was approved for use in adult solid organ transplantation in 2000. It is available as tablets and in liquid form. In adults it is usually prescribed once daily, but it has a shorter half-life in children, usually requiring twice-daily dosing. Trough levels should be monitored and maintained at lower concentrations if used together with calcineurin inhibitors, because the combination enhances calcineurin inhibitor toxicity.

A study that used calcineurin inhibitors together with sirolimus and basiliximab induction, with the goal of steroid withdrawal in children, found a higher incidence of PTLD.[254] Sirolimus has mostly been used in place of calcineurin inhibitors, in an attempt to reduce nephrotoxicity. A protocol treating children with IL-2 receptor blocker induction, mycophenolate, sirolimus, and steroids showed a higher incidence of acute rejection, as well as more adverse effects in the sirolimus group.[255] Conversion from calcineurin inhibitor to sirolimus to treat calcineurin inhibitor–induced nephrotoxicity has also been attempted with improved GFR in some children, but with an increase in adverse events.[256,257] Adverse effects of sirolimus include impaired wound healing, which can present a problem when used immediately after transplantation, hyperlipidemia, proteinuria, decreased levels of testosterone in some adolescent males, aphthous ulcers, interstitial pneumonia (including *Pneumocystis jiroveci* infections), anemia, and thrombocytopenia.[258,259] The use of sirolimus in pediatric renal transplantation peaked in 2002 at 25% but subsequently decreased to less than 3% in the United States[159,160]; a similar trend was also seen in the Australia and New Zealand registry report.[3]

Everolimus

Everolimus has been studied in several small uncontrolled studies in children in combination with low-dose calcineurin inhibitors with good short-term graft function.[260] It may have less adverse effects than sirolimus, but there are no pediatric studies comparing the two medications.

OTHER IMMUNOSUPPRESSIVE MEDICATIONS

In most cases, new immunosuppressive agents are studied in adults before trials in children are performed. Belatacept, a costimulation inhibitor, has shown promise in adult patients undergoing renal transplantation, demonstrating improved GFR compared with cyclosporine, though with a higher incidence of acute rejection.[261] Studies in children have not been performed, and a specific concern might be the higher frequency of PTLD in the belatacept-treated patients, particularly of the central nervous system. Because more children are seronegative for EBV going into transplantation, the potential risk for PTLD could be even higher in this population.

IMMUNOSUPPRESSION COMBINATIONS

In North America the most common combination of immunosuppression for pediatric kidney transplantation in the past decade has been tacrolimus, mycophenolate, and prednisone, followed by tacrolimus and mycophenolate without corticosteroids.[159] Approximately half the children receive antibody induction therapy, most commonly ATG, followed by IL-2 receptor blocker basiliximab. Most steroid-free protocols use antibody induction therapy.[159]

PERIOPERATIVE MANAGEMENT

Pediatric renal transplantation should always be managed by an experienced team that includes pediatric transplant surgeons, nephrologists, anesthesiologists, intensive care experts, and other specialists, to ensure an optimal outcome.

Technical causes are responsible for a higher proportion of early graft loss in young children, primarily from graft thrombosis. Vascular anastomoses of the graft in very small children are usually to the aorta and the IVC, rather than the iliac vessels used in older children and adults, to provide sufficient renal perfusion, particularly when the graft is an adult-sized kidney. The donor renal artery may be the same size as the recipient aorta, and the renal vein may be significantly larger than the recipient's IVC. A straight and direct course for each renal vessel to the aorta and vena cava will avoid kinking and risk for thrombosis. A midline transperitoneal approach is often used in the youngest patients, in contrast to the usual lower abdominal extraperitoneal incision. Stenosis or thrombosis of the IVC is a rare finding but may be seen in children who have had CVCs in infancy, abdominal surgery, or a hypercoagulable state, posing a problem for graft anastomosis. This should be evaluated before transplantation by Doppler ultrasonography or venography, and in case of a significant IVC pathologic condition an alternative vein should be selected. There may be an advantage for transplanting a pediatric (deceased) donor kidney in such cases.[262]

The adult-sized kidney graft requires a major increase in CO to maintain good perfusion and avoid AKI attributed to ATN or vascular thrombosis. Even with optimal maintenance of recipient intravascular volume, blood flow to the adult-sized donor kidney is significantly reduced at transplantation. Further reduction in blood flow could result in graft ischemia; therefore blood pressure values, which may be relatively high for the young child, and high-normal central venous pressure need to be maintained during transplant surgery and postoperatively. After anastomosis is completed, release of vascular clamps will cause immediate flow of a large portion of the child's blood volume into the graft, a critical time point when intravascular volume must be controlled. Maintaining relative hypervolemia immediately after transplantation may delay weaning from mechanical ventilation for 1 to 2 days. Aggressive volume administration to optimize intravascular volume and graft blood flow is important in the following weeks and months and may require fluid supplements by the nasogastric route.[262] Avoiding AKI in the postoperative period also enables early full dosing of calcineurin inhibitors, thus preventing early acute rejection.

IMMEDIATE POSTOPERATIVE PERIOD

In the first few days after transplantation the child is usually treated in the intensive care unit. Close attention is paid to vital signs and fluid management with the goal of optimizing graft perfusion. Good urine output, particularly in a patient previously oliguric or anuric, is a useful marker of graft function. Oligoanuria or a significant decrease in urine output, on the other hand, needs to be evaluated and treated immediately. Bladder drainage must be assessed by flushing or exchanging the bladder catheter. Ultrasonography can assess the kidney, its perfusion, the presence of a fluid collection suggesting leak or bleeding, the ureter, and the bladder. Absent blood flow may be due to thrombosis and necessitates prompt surgical intervention, as does significant bleeding or a urinary leak. Intravenous fluids are given to replace insensible losses and urine output, as well as additional fluids to account for third-space losses and to keep central venous pressure on the high side of normal. This approach should maintain good graft perfusion, which in turn will increase urine output. However, if urine output does not increase, intravascular volume overload may result, manifesting as respiratory compromise and hypertension. Volume overload may respond to diuretics, but dialysis may be necessary in some patients.

Prophylactic treatment for infections is started postoperatively. Perioperative antibiotics are usually given to prevent wound infection. *P. jiroveci* prophylaxis, usually with trimethoprim-sulfamethoxazole, may also decrease the incidence of urinary tract infection (UTI). Antiviral medication is given to prevent CMV disease, usually oral valganciclovir, the duration of therapy depending upon pretransplantation donor and recipient serologic status and on whether lymphocyte-depleting induction immunosuppression was given.[263,264] Some centers prescribe antifungal prophylaxis, especially in patients with prolonged intensive care unit stay or antibiotic treatment. Low-molecular-weight heparin or aspirin is often given after transplantation to prevent graft thrombosis.[265]

EARLY COMPLICATIONS OF KIDNEY TRANSPLANTATION

DELAYED GRAFT FUNCTION

Delayed graft function (DGF) is usually defined as the need for dialysis during the first week after renal transplantation.[266] The most common cause of DGF is postischemic acute injury of the graft, which is associated with deceased-donor kidney, prolonged ischemic time, and hemodynamic factors during and immediately after transplantation.[159] Laparoscopic donor nephrectomy may have been associated with a higher risk for recipient DGF,[267] but later data showed no difference in adverse outcomes for kidneys procured by laparoscopy.[268] Deceased-donor kidneys are associated with a higher risk for DGF, particularly from donors after cardiac death.[269] DGF adversely affects long-term graft survival and function, reducing 5-year survival by approximately 20%, both in living- and deceased-donor kidney transplants.[159,270] Other causes of DGF include graft thrombosis, which can be diagnosed by ultrasonography or radionuclide scan, and may require surgical revision. Thrombosis can be prevented by meticulous surgical technique and attention to fluid balance, as well as identifying and treating patients with thrombophilic risk factors. Use of antibody induction may decrease the incidence both of postischemic DGF and graft thrombosis in pediatric renal transplantation,[271,272] though the reasons for this are not clear.

Urologic complications such as urinary leak or obstruction may also cause DGF or acute decrease in urine output; diagnosis is aided by ultrasonography and radionuclide scan. Ureteral stents are sometimes placed at transplantation for 4 to 6 weeks to prevent obstruction, but their use is controversial and may be associated with increased risk for UTI.[273]

Hyperacute rejection or accelerated acute rejection superimposed upon postoperative ATN may also present as DGF. Hyperacute rejection is usually due to preformed anti–donor ABO or HLA antibodies, manifesting as irreversible rapid destruction of the graft within minutes to hours of transplantation. Because blood type and HLA matching have been routinely performed, these reactions are exceedingly rare. Pretreatment of recipients with grafts mismatched for ABO antigens or with DSA with desensitization protocols generally prevents this disastrous outcome.[200,212-214] Graft nephrectomy is usually the only therapeutic option.

FSGS recurrence can manifest as primary nonfunction and requires a graft biopsy for diagnosis, particularly if presenting as oligoanuria.[274,275]

ACUTE REJECTION

Acute renal allograft rejection is a common complication of pediatric renal transplantation, though its frequency has decreased significantly from over 70% in 1987 to 1990, to 13% since 2007.[159] This is thought to be due to newer, more potent immunosuppressive medications now used. The highest risk for acute rejection is in the first few weeks to months; however, it may occur at any time, even years after transplantation. It is more frequent after deceased-donor transplantation compared to living donor (15% versus 10% in 2007 to 2010),[159] suggesting susceptibility of the graft with longer ischemic time, for example, due to exposure of antigens promoting an immune reaction. It is also more common in African Americans[159] and in non-European immigrant children compared to native Western Europeans, adjusted for donor source.[276] Graft tenderness and fever as manifestations of acute rejection are unusual in the present era of immunosuppression, and acute decrease in GFR may be the only sign. Even a small increase in serum creatinine level, particularly when baseline creatinine level is normal, may indicate a significant decrease in GFR and should prompt investigation. This will include urinalysis and urine culture to rule out infection and glomerular disease, BK virus polymerase chain reaction (PCR), and ultrasonography to look for obstruction, fluid collection, or vascular compromise. Biopsy should be performed whenever possible to confirm the diagnosis, because other causes of graft dysfunction, such as drug toxicity, particularly calcineurin inhibitor, or viral infection including BK virus–associated nephropathy (BKVAN), may be difficult to distinguish from acute rejection on clinical grounds alone. Graft biopsy is safely performed under ultrasonographic guidance, and light general anesthesia or conscious sedation is helpful in reducing anxiety and pain. The Banff criteria are used to grade acute rejection.[277] Acute cellular rejection is characterized by lymphocyte infiltration of tubules (tubulitis) and interstitium, with involvement of arterial walls in more severe cases. In acute AMR there is acute tissue injury, including findings of ATN, capillary endothelial swelling, arteriolar fibrinoid necrosis, or fibrin thrombi in glomerular capillaries. In addition, there is evidence of an antibody-mediated complement activation—C4d deposition in the peritubular capillaries of the allograft, together with circulating DSA. The two types of acute rejection may coexist.

The cornerstone of therapy for acute cellular rejection is high-dose corticosteroids, most often pulse intravenous methylprednisolone. In steroid-resistant rejection, lymphocyte-depleting agents, particularly rabbit ATG, may be administered. Premedication with methylprednisolone and antihistamine usually prevents a cytokine release syndrome, which may be seen, particularly with the first dose of rabbit ATG. Approximately 50% to 60% of children treated for acute rejection will have a complete response, with GFR returning to baseline, and another 30% to 40% will have a partial response.[159] When acute rejection is diagnosed, the possibility of underimmunosuppression must be addressed. This may be due to underdosing of medications, or more commonly, particularly in teenage patients, nonadherence to immunosuppressive drugs.[278,279] Attention must be given to maintenance immunosuppression, considering adding prednisone to a steroid-free protocol, substituting cyclosporine for tacrolimus, or increasing the antimetabolite dose, in order to improve response to therapy and reduce the incidence of recurrent acute rejection.[280] Acute AMR is often refractory to conventional antirejection therapy and has a high rate of graft loss. Intensification of maintenance immunosuppression and plasmapheresis, with or without intravenous immune globulin, have been used with some success in children.[281,282] Therapies aimed at depleting B cells (rituximab), plasma cells (bortezomib), and inhibition of complement (eculizumab) have also been described in pediatric patients, with mixed results.[283-285] Acute rejection is a predictor for tubular atrophy and interstitial fibrosis and adversely affects long-term graft survival and function.[286-288]

Close monitoring is imperative to avoid early acute rejection and enable its prompt detection and treatment. Serum creatinine level is monitored daily in the first few days after transplantation, followed by at least twice weekly for 2 to 3 months, together with drug concentration monitoring. Later, if there are no complications, the frequency of testing is decreased to once a month after the first 6 to 12 months. Even stable children and adolescents require regular follow-up at the pediatric transplant clinic, to help prevent nonadherence and the resulting graft rejection, as well as for long-term management of the many other aspects of their health.

INFECTIONS

As more-potent immunosuppressive agents were introduced into the treatment of renal transplantation, the frequency of acute rejection decreased, as did hospitalizations for rejection episodes. In the pediatric population in particular, the price for this has been a higher rate of infections, particularly CMV and EBV, and the emergence of new infection-related complications—PTLD and BKVAN. The use of antibody induction and the presence of indwelling vascular or urinary catheters increase the risk for infection.[226,289]

Hospitalization for infection was higher in children after kidney transplantation in the first 3 years compared to adults (47.4% vs. 39.8%).[290] In the immediate posttransplantation period, the most frequent infections are surgical, UTI, and pneumonia. Subsequently, in the early months after transplantation, viral infections are common, cause significant morbidity, and may adversely affect graft function.

URINARY TRACT INFECTION

UTI is a common complication in children who have undergone renal transplantation, with an overall frequency of 30% to 40% over the first 3 years. Risk factors include a pretransplantation diagnosis of obstructive uropathy or VUR, bladder abnormalities, and pretransplantation UTI.[291] Ureteral stents placed during transplantation may also increase the risk for UTI.[273] Although graft dysfunction may occur during allograft pyelonephritis, long-term graft function may not be affected.[291-293] Trimethoprim-sulfamethoxazole prophylaxis for *Pneumocystis* infection may reduce the incidence of UTI, but bacterial susceptibilities vary between medical centers and may render this strategy ineffective. Many clinics routinely culture urine from patients who have undergone transplantation at every visit, and the indication for treatment of asymptomatic bacteriuria without pyuria remains unclear, because resistant organisms may emerge.[294] The association between VUR to the kidney graft and UTI is not clear, though preexisting reflux to the native kidneys is a risk factor for UTI after transplantation. A study in adults found early VUR to the graft in 40.7% of patients, despite using extravesical mucosal tunneling technique to prevent reflux. There was no increased incidence of UTI or impact on graft function.[295] Nonetheless, in children with recurrent UTI after transplantation and documented VUR, small case series have shown successful endoscopic correction, particularly in patients without underlying lower urinary tract abnormalities.[296]

CYTOMEGALOVIRUS

Despite widespread use of antiviral prophylactic treatment, CMV infection continues to be a common, and occasionally severe, complication of pediatric renal transplantation.[264] The most vulnerable group is children who are seronegative for CMV before transplantation, receive a kidney from a seropositive donor, and then develop a primary infection.[297] Children who receive rabbit ATG induction are also at a higher risk for CMV infection.[226,264] According to OPTN data, 64% of children undergoing kidney transplantation in 2007 to 2011 had negative CMV serologic results, whereas donors were more likely to have positive results (60.6% of deceased donors and 50.7% of live donors in the United States).[160] Secondary infection may also occur, either as reactivation of the host strain or infection from the donor strain, and may be less severe clinically. Valganciclovir has been shown to be at least as effective as oral ganciclovir in children for CMV prevention and has better bioavailability and easier once-daily dosing.[263] Dosing should be based on body surface area and corrected for renal function.[298] The main adverse effect of prophylaxis is hematologic toxicity, occasionally necessitating dose reduction or discontinuation of treatment.[264,299] The duration of treatment is usually 3 to 6 months, depending on the state of seroconversion. Most cases of CMV infection occur after cessation of prophylaxis, in 25% to 40% of pediatric kidney transplant recipients.[264,297,299] Infection is generally defined as positive CMV PCR results (viremia) and may be asymptomatic. CMV disease is defined as viremia with clinical symptoms, most commonly fever and malaise, with tissue-invasive disease in some cases, involving the respiratory, hepatic, and gastrointestinal tracts. Allograft dysfunction, leukopenia, and thrombocytopenia are frequently observed laboratory findings. In invasive disease, treatment is usually started with intravenous ganciclovir, followed by oral valganciclovir when clinical improvement and reduction in viral load are seen. Although the VICTOR study demonstrated equivalent efficacy of oral valganciclovir and intravenous ganciclovir in adult transplant recipients, it is not clear if these findings can be extrapolated to the pediatric population.[300] Immunosuppression should be reduced, usually by discontinuation of the antimetabolite drug—azathioprine or mycophenolate.[300] Hyperimmune CMV globulin preparation may be given to the most severe cases, though its efficacy is questionable.[297] Although CMV infection is usually an indicator of overimmunosuppression, there have been studies linking CMV with acute rejection.[301] Subclinical CMV, as well as EBV infection, which may occur despite prophylactic treatment, is associated with chronic allograft injury in children.[302] Treatment is continued until after viral eradication is demonstrated, followed by a prophylactic dose for several weeks. Relapse may occur after the end of therapy[299]; therefore viral monitoring should be continued for several weeks after treatment cessation, and after reintroduction of the antimetabolite, which is usually at a lower dose than before CMV infection. Failure to respond to therapy, either clinically or virologically, may be due to viral ganciclovir resistance, usually due to viral UL97 mutations. Treatment options include high-dose ganciclovir or switching to foscarnet, which is nephrotoxic, though studies in children are lacking.[300,303]

EPSTEIN-BARR VIRUS INFECTION

Similar to the situation with CMV serologic results, approximately half of the pediatric patients undergoing renal transplantation are seronegative for EBV, whereas only 10% of donors are EBV naive.[160] Seronegative patients receiving grafts from EBV-positive patients are at a higher risk for infection; therefore EBV disease is more common in younger children. EBV infection may be asymptomatic, it can present as an acute viral syndrome, or it may be associated with PTLD. Of the patients with primary EBV infection, adolescents may be more likely to develop PTLD and have a poorer prognosis.[304]

Monitoring viral load in peripheral blood by quantitative PCR, particularly in high-risk patients in the first year after transplantation, is important to identify infection and enable early intervention. A prospective study in Germany found that primary infection occurred in 63% of seronegative pediatric patients and reactivation or reinfection in 44% of seropositive patients, though many of the infections were asymptomatic.[305] More intensive immunosuppression is associated with a higher rate of symptomatic EBV infection. Prophylaxis with ganciclovir or valganciclovir in high-risk patients was shown to reduce the incidence of EBV viremia and also to decrease the viral load in those who were infected.[306] Clinical disease usually presents with protracted fever, lymphadenopathy, tonsillitis, and hepatosplenomegaly. Laboratory findings may include leukopenia, atypical lymphocytes, elevated liver enzyme levels, and IgM antibodies for EBV, and allograft dysfunction may occur. Diagnosis is confirmed by EBV viral load, which is also used to monitor the course of the disease and response to therapy. PTLD appears to be due to B cell proliferation induced by infection with EBV, and there is a continuum of EBV-associated diseases from mononucleosis to full-blown monomorphic lymphoma. Imaging will help in detecting lymphoid masses, which might require biopsy to rule out malignant PTLD. The cornerstone of therapy and prevention of PTLD is immunosuppression reduction when there is a significant EBV viral load, specifically, decreasing the dose of the antimetabolite or discontinuing the antimetabolite and lowering the target levels of tacrolimus. Antiviral therapy for persistent EBV viremia with valganciclovir has been shown to be effective in reducing viral loads in pediatric liver transplant recipients, but its use in treatment of EBV infection after renal transplantation is controversial. Some children after renal transplantation may have persistent high EBV viral load without ever developing PTLD.[305,307] Adolescents with primary EBV infection are more likely to develop PTLD and have a poorer prognosis.[304]

BK VIRUS INFECTION

BK polyomavirus infection emerged as an important clinical entity in patients undergoing renal transplantation in the late 1990s, coinciding with the introduction of more potent immunosuppression regimens. BK virus infection may result in BKVAN, manifesting as tubulointerstitial nephritis with graft dysfunction and potential graft loss, as well as ureteral stenosis and hemorrhagic cystitis. Although previously thought to be rare in children, data from NAPRTCS showed a prevalence of 4.6%, similar to that in adults.[308] BK transmission occurs in childhood, when the virus remains latent in the tubular epithelial cells. Immunosuppression after transplantation may cause reactivation and high-rate viral replication in the kidney graft and is therefore considered a consequence of immunosuppression. Young recipients may develop primary BK infection transmitted from the donor kidney. Risk factors for BKVAN include antibody induction, DR mismatch, and treatment for rejection.[308]

The virus appears first in the urine and if progression occurs, is detected in the blood by quantitative PCR for viral DNA. Histologic changes are observed in patients with persistent or increasing plasma viral loads.[309] Surveillance is recommended to enable early diagnosis and intervention. Detection of viruria has questionable clinical implications, because it is not correlated with graft damage, but it does identify patients at risk for subsequent viremia. Monitoring plasma quantitative PCR periodically, particularly in the early months after transplantation, after acute rejection, and at any time when there is an unexplained elevation of the serum creatinine level, is the accepted strategy for diagnosis in children.[309,310] Kidney biopsy is performed if there is graft dysfunction. Typical findings include cytopathic changes and tubulointerstitial nephritis, which can be difficult to differentiate from other viral infections or acute cellular rejection and may even coexist with other conditions in some cases. Immunohistochemical staining for SV40 viral antigen is highly specific for BKVAN. Relevant histologic findings in association with high BK viral load in the blood are diagnostic.

Initial treatment of BK viremia is reduction of immunosuppression, usually discontinuation of the antimetabolite or decrease in the target levels of the calcineurin inhibitor. This is best done when persistent viremia or increasing viral load is observed and can prevent progression to overt nephropathy.[309-312] The reduction of immunosuppression enables the patient's immune system to clear viremia more effectively by expanding BK virus–specific cell immunity and specific immunoglobulins.[309] Treatment of established BKVAN is often less successful. Several medications with antiviral activity have been used to treat patients with BKVAN unresponsive to immunosuppression minimization, with varying degrees of success, but no randomized controlled studies have been performed.[313] These medications include intravenous γ-globulin, quinolone antibiotics, cidofovir, and leflunomide.[314,315]

VARICELLA

Immunization against varicella-zoster virus is recommended before transplantation, because the use of live attenuated viral vaccine is controversial in immunocompromised patients.[185] Varicella infection in an unimmunized renal transplant recipient may result in severe disease, with visceral involvement in some cases. Postexposure prophylaxis of nonimmunized patients with varicella-zoster immunoglobulin should be administered as early as possible, and if clinical disease develops, treatment with intravenous acyclovir is initiated. Temporary discontinuation of the antimetabolite, or dose reduction, is usually recommended.[316]

OTHER INFECTIONS

Respiratory Viruses

Respiratory viruses, in particular influenza virus infection, may be associated with severe morbidity in the immunosuppressed host. Disease severity may be related to the degree of immunosuppression, and clinical presentation may be atypical. Pretransplantation vaccination is recommended, as well as yearly seasonal inactivated influenza vaccine after transplantation. Young children (<9 years) receiving the vaccine for the first time should receive two doses, 4 weeks apart. Vaccine immunogenicity is variable, but data suggest that immunization reduces mortality and clinical severity as well as infection-related acute rejection.[317]

Cutaneous Warts

Cutaneous warts, usually due to infection with human papillomavirus, are common in children after renal transplantation. Although malignant potential is low, these lesions can be numerous and cause distress due to cosmetic issues. Lesions may be refractory to treatment or recurrent.[318]

Pneumocystis jiroveci Pneumonia

P. jiroveci pneumonia is a classic example of an opportunistic infection, which is very rare in the immunocompetent host. With the widespread use of prophylaxis, usually with trimethoprim-sulfamethoxazole, the true incidence of posttransplantation infection is unknown. Antipneumocystis prophylaxis is usually given for 6 to 12 months after kidney transplantation, after which net immunosuppression is lower. *Pneumocystis* infection may coexist with CMV or respiratory viruses and should be considered in the immunosuppressed child with unexplained respiratory symptoms.[319,320]

RECURRENCE OF PRIMARY KIDNEY DISEASE

According to NAPRTCS data, 7.8% of grafts in children are lost to disease recurrence.[159] The most common recurring kidney disease is FSGS, but MPGN (type II in particular), atypical HUS, primary hyperoxaluria type 1, and others can recur in the graft. It is important to identify patients at risk for recurrence to enable early diagnosis and therapeutic intervention.

FSGS is responsible for approximately 10% of ESKD in children in the United States, presenting as steroid-resistant nephrotic syndrome, and carries an overall risk of 30% for recurrent nephrotic syndrome. It is, however, a histologic finding that may be caused by different underlying pathogenetic mechanisms, for example, genetic mutations in genes responsible for components of the glomerular barrier such as podocin. This group of genetic structural abnormalities causing FSGS has a low rate of recurrence post-transplantation. In idiopathic FSGS the risk for recurrence is higher in children than in adults, in patients with rapidly progressive disease, and in those who already had recurrence in a previous graft.[274] Native kidney nephrectomy before or during transplantation surgery should be considered in children with FSGS who have residual urine output, to enable prompt diagnosis of recurrence. Recurrent FSGS is thought to be due to humoral factors that cause damage to the glomerular barrier, which is the rationale for treatment strategies aimed at removal of such a factor. Serum soluble urokinase-type plasminogen activator receptor has been identified as a possible permeability factor responsible for recurrent FSGS, though this has not been supported in pediatric studies.[321,322] Preemptive and therapeutic plasmapheresis for disease recurrence, as well as treatment with anti-CD20 antibody rituximab, have shown some efficacy in achieving remission of proteinuria. Recurrent FSGS in the graft, particularly if unresponsive to therapy, is associated with a high rate of graft failure.[275]

MPGN type I is the underlying diagnosis in 1.7% of children receiving their initial kidney transplant and may recur in 20% to 30% after transplantation. MPGN type II is rarer, but the recurrence rate is higher at 45% and is a cause of graft failure in many of the patients. There is no evidence of any successful treatment for either of these conditions. Recurrence in a subsequent graft is almost universal.[195]

Atypical HUS causes ESKD in more than half of patients. It may be due to various disorders of complement regulation, including mutations in complement factor H or I, membrane cofactor protein, and others. The specific cause of the disease should be investigated before considering transplantation, to assess the risk for recurrence. Renal transplantation without specific intervention is associated with a very high rate of recurrence and of graft loss. Eculizumab, an anti–complement factor 5 monoclonal antibody aimed at stopping uncontrolled complement activation, has been used both to prevent and to treat recurrence of atypical HUS after transplantation with excellent results, as shown in a case series from France.[198] Three patients in whom treatment was discontinued experienced a relapse, suggesting that long-term therapy is needed.

In primary hyperoxaluria type 1, abnormal massive oxalate production by the liver causes ESKD, and this process continues after isolated kidney transplantation, causing graft failure. Combined liver-kidney transplantation corrects the underlying enzymatic defect and enables long-term graft survival.[197]

Other diseases that may recur and may cause graft dysfunction or failure include lupus nephritis, IgA nephropathy, Henoch-Schönlein nephritis, membranous nephropathy, and diabetic nephropathy.

CHRONIC ALLOGRAFT NEPHROPATHY

The most common cause of graft loss after the first year is CAN, accounting for approximately 35% of failed kidney grafts, according to several pediatric databases worldwide.[3,160] CAN is also known as chronic rejection, transplant nephropathy, and chronic renal allograft dysfunction or injury. There are no universally accepted diagnostic criteria, and the pathogenesis is not completely understood. On biopsy, the revised 2005 Banff classification system changed the terminology to grading of interstitial fibrosis and tubular atrophy, without evidence of any specific cause, although pathologic involvement also typically includes the blood vessels and glomeruli.[277] Clinically, CAN is suspected when there is a slow deterioration in allograft function beyond the first 3 months after transplantation with no evidence of acute rejection, drug toxicity, infection, or other pathologic process. There may also be increasing proteinuria and worsening hypertension. The etiology of CAN is multifactorial and includes immunologic and nonimmunologic factors. Adequate long-term immunosuppression is important in prevention of immunologically mediated CAN, although chronic calcineurin inhibitor toxicity may be difficult to distinguish from CAN in some cases. Changes in immunosuppression may occasionally ameliorate CAN, for example, treatment with mycophenolate in children with CAN may improve graft function.[243] Optimal control of hypertension and treatment of hyperlipidemia are also important. Nonadherence to medical therapy in pediatric renal transplant recipients is associated with a higher rate of chronic rejection and graft loss.[323]

PATIENT SURVIVAL

Survival of children after kidney transplantation improved in 1996 to 2007 compared to the previous decade and was 96.3% for recipients of deceased-donor allografts and 97% for recipients of living-donor allografts, at 5 years. Survival was lower in infants younger than 24 months at transplantation. The most common cause of death was infection (28.5%), followed by cardiopulmonary causes (14.7%) and malignancy (11.3%). Overall, death was more likely in patients with failed grafts, though 47.5% of patients who died had a functioning allograft.[159] Survival after renal transplantation is higher than in children remaining on chronic dialysis. Adjusted all-cause mortality is approximately fourfold higher in children undergoing dialysis than in children after renal transplantation.[2]

GRAFT SURVIVAL

A similar improvement in graft survival is seen over time, with 5-year deceased-donor graft survival of 78.4% in the cohort of 1996 to 2010 compared to 62.4% in patients undergoing transplantation in 1986 to 1995. In living-donor kidney allografts the increase in 5-year graft survival is more modest: 85.7% in the cohort of 1996 to 2010 compared to 78.9% in patients undergoing transplantation in 1986 to 1995.[159] Data from Australia, pooling living- and deceased-donor renal transplantation in children, demonstrates 5-year graft survival of approximately 80% since 2002.[3] Reports from several developing countries that have a pediatric kidney transplantation program (some with the living-donor option only) have shown 5-year graft survival of 65% to 92%.[324] Graft failure is defined by return to dialysis, repeat transplantation, or death. The most common cause of graft failure is CAN or chronic rejection (35%), with various types of acute rejection responsible for 15% of graft loss. In comparison to adults, death with functioning graft is less common in children (9%), whereas vascular thrombosis or technical difficulties are more frequent (approximately 11%).[159] This is due to better general health in pediatric kidney recipients on the one hand, and smaller blood vessels, which make vascular anastomoses technically challenging on the other. Children who receive a living-donor kidney have a graft half-life of 15 years, compared to 11 years in those who receive a deceased-donor allograft.[160] Prognostic factors associated with shorter graft survival include race (black vs. nonblack), prior transplantations, HLA mismatching, and blood transfusions. A study showed that patients receiving their graft at age 14 to 16 years were at risk for graft failure, in particular if they were black or did not have private insurance.[325] It is difficult to evaluate the association of antibody induction therapy with graft outcome because of patient selection bias.[159] Delayed graft function due to ATN is associated with a 20% reduction in 5-year graft survival in living- and deceased-donor kidney recipients.[159] GFR, estimated by a serum creatinine–based formula, has also improved over the last decade, with approximately 70% of patients in 2010 discharged from the hospital after renal transplantation with eGFR greater than 60 mL/min/1.73 m^2, which is essentially unchanged 1 year later.[160]

Graft failure may be associated with an inflammatory reaction, which may be severe enough to necessitate graft nephrectomy. This is more common in early graft loss or high-grade rejection by biopsy. However, graft nephrectomy is associated with higher circulating HLA antibodies, which may affect future retransplantation outcomes.[326]

LONG-TERM FOLLOW-UP OF CHILDREN WITH KIDNEY TRANSPLANT

HYPERTENSION

Blood pressure monitoring is an integral part of regular follow-up of pediatric kidney transplant recipients. The appropriate-sized cuff should be used, and at least two or three measurements should be performed when the child is calm. Blood pressure measurements are compared to normal value for gender, age, and height percentile, as published in "The Fourth Report on the Diagnosis, Evaluation, and Treatment of High Blood Pressure in Children and Adolescents,"[327] which provides ninetieth and ninety-fifth percentiles. The vast majority of children reaching ESKD have hypertension, defined as values above the ninety-fifth percentile, and it remains a problem for many patients after renal transplantation. In a European study reporting data from 10 countries, approximately two-thirds of children receiving RRT had hypertension, but uncontrolled hypertension was more common in children undergoing dialysis than in patients who have undergone transplantation.[47]

In the early period after transplantation the causes of hypertension include volume overload, acute rejection, and therapy with corticosteroids and calcineurin inhibitors, which are given at higher doses at this time. Hypertension may appear months or even years after transplantation, as shown in a cohort of pediatric renal transplant recipients in the United Kingdom.[328] Ambulatory 24-hour blood pressure monitoring is a useful tool in diagnosing masked or nocturnal hypertension, which may be quite common.[329,330]

Hypertension is often associated with graft dysfunction from any cause but may also be due to renal allograft artery stenosis, or end-stage native kidneys even with a well-functioning graft. Obesity that predates transplantation or develops subsequently is also associated with hypertension and metabolic syndrome.[331]

New-onset hypertension, occasionally associated with a murmur audible over the graft, should be investigated with imaging to rule out renal artery stenosis. Allograft artery stenosis can in some cases be corrected by angioplasty, with improvement in hypertension. Antihypertensive medication is prescribed as necessary, with target blood pressure measurements under the ninetieth percentile for age and height, as in other high-risk pediatric groups.[327] Choice of therapeutic agent depends on the underlying cause; angiotensin-converting enzyme (ACE) inhibitors and angiotensin receptor blockers may be appropriate in patients with hypertension, particularly associated with proteinuria, but possibly hazardous in uncorrected allograft artery stenosis. Diuretics are helpful in treatment of early volume overload–associated hypertension, whereas calcium channel blockers may minimize calcineurin inhibitor–related renal vasoconstriction.[332,333] Uncontrolled hypertension may affect graft function, as shown in adults in the Collaborative Transplant Study, which demonstrated that lowering systolic blood pressure was associated with improved graft function.[334]

CARDIOVASCULAR DISEASE

LVH is the most frequent cardiac abnormality in children after renal transplantation, with a prevalence of 10% to 50% in various studies.[335-338] LVH is correlated to hypertension and also to the presence of metabolic syndrome.[339] In most children with LVH it appears before transplantation, and some studies have shown improvement in left ventricular mass index after transplantation.[337]

Cardiovascular mortality is much higher in children with CKD compared to the general pediatric population.

Although mortality is lower in children after kidney transplantation than in children undergoing dialysis, it remains unacceptably high. According to the NAPRTCS database, 14.7% of mortality is due to cardiopulmonary causes, second only to infection and ahead of malignancy.[159] Traditional risk factors such as hypertension, dyslipidemia, diabetes mellitus, and obesity are more frequent due to impaired renal function and the adverse effects of immunosuppressive medications. Nontraditional risk factors such as abnormalities in calcium-phosphorus metabolism, anemia, hyperuricemia, and hyperhomocysteinemia are frequent in children with CKD and are correlated with arterial stiffness and carotid intimal-medial thickness.[48] Some of these risk factors may persist after transplantation, particularly if graft function is impaired. Whereas vascular lesions progress in children with CKD, abolition of the uremic state by transplantation resulted in stabilization or partial regression of CKD-associated arteriolopathy in one study.[340]

Interventions to reduce premature cardiovascular disease after renal transplantation include optimization of graft function and treatment of hypertension. Corticosteroid minimization or avoidance protocols reduce blood pressure and blood cholesterol levels,[246] as does changing from cyclosporine- to tacrolimus-based immunosuppression.[234,236] Dietary interventions should be offered to all children, in particular to those with obesity and dyslipidemia. Encouraging physical activity is important, as is education to prevent smoking in young transplant recipients. Treatment with 3-hydroxy-3-methylglutaryl–coenzyme A reductase inhibitors has been shown to be effective and safe in reducing total and LDL cholesterol levels in children.[341] Although the Assessment of LEscol in Renal Transplantation (ALERT) study showed a reduction in cardiac deaths and nonfatal myocardial infarctions in adults,[342] this has not been shown in other studies, and there are data beginning in the pediatric age-group with subsequent end points for cardiovascular events.

METABOLIC SYNDROME AND DIABETES MELLITUS

Metabolic syndrome, a combination of abdominal obesity, hypertension, dyslipidemia, and insulin resistance, is increasingly common, and its frequency correlates with age. It is estimated to be approximately 9% in children older than 12 years in the United States.[343] Screening and prevention of metabolic syndrome in childhood is important, because it continues into adulthood and carries an increased risk for cardiovascular disease, and even in childhood, there is evidence of significant atherosclerotic changes. In a study of children undergoing renal transplantation in six centers in the United States, 18.8% were diagnosed with metabolic syndrome at the time of transplant, which increased to 37% 1 year later.[339] Dietary intervention and physical activity are the mainstay of prevention and treatment. In patients treated with corticosteroids, late steroid withdrawal has been shown to improve metabolic parameters and decrease the frequency of metabolic syndrome from 39% to 6% 2 years later.[249]

New-onset diabetes mellitus after transplantation is less common in children than in adult patients, with an incidence of 7.1% at 3 years. However, its frequency may be increasing. It is associated with older age (adolescents versus younger children), higher BMI, and treatment with tacrolimus.[344] Fasting blood glucose level should be monitored regularly in the first months after transplantation; hemoglobin A_{1c} is also helpful in diagnosing insidious-onset diabetes. Corticosteroid dose is reduced if possible, and usually a combination of dietary modification and pharmacologic therapy is needed.

CANCER

Immunosuppressive therapy for prevention of rejection after solid organ transplantation carries a risk for malignancy. In children, 2.4% of kidney transplant recipients develop a malignancy,[159] of which 84% were classified as lymphoproliferative cancers. The 3-year incidence of malignancy increased from 1.05% in 1987 to 1990 to 2.96% in 1999 to 2002; however, in the latest cohort an improvement has been noted, 1.13% in 2003 to 2010. This trend mirrors the introduction of newer, more potent immunosuppressive agents such as tacrolimus in the early 1990s, followed by the use of lower doses and immunosuppression minimization protocols in subsequent years. A study that collected data from nine centers in France reported a 6% rate of malignancies in all pediatric solid organ transplant recipients, most of which were PTLD.[345]

PTLD is an uncontrolled proliferation of B cells in the constellation of posttransplantation immunosuppression, most often associated with EBV infection. The cumulative incidence of PTLD in children in the United States is 2% at 5 years following transplantation but is 4.5% in children who are EBV seronegative at the time of kidney transplantation.[160] On the other hand, PTLD in children infected with EBV who were previously seronegative is associated with better survival.[346] Diagnosis is made by histologic examination of involved tissue and is classified by the World Health Organization into four categories: early lesions, polymorphic PTLD, monomorphic PTLD, and Hodgkin's lymphoma. Early lesions are usually managed by immunosuppression reduction to restore the host's virus-specific immunity and by monitoring of viral loads to assess response. In CD20-positive B cell polymorphic disease, rituximab, an anti-CD20 antibody, is often effective together with immunosuppression reduction. Monomorphic disease is most frequently large B cell lymphoma and may also respond to rituximab therapy, but many patients require the addition of chemotherapy. Hodgkin's lymphoma PTLD is very rare. In a retrospective study of 45 consecutive patients with PTLD younger than 25 years, 80% of tumors expressed EBV and 70% were CD20 positive. Both of these presented earlier after transplantation, and CD20-positive PTLD was associated with a higher 5-year survival.[347] Patients with PTLD are at risk for graft dysfunction and loss, due to acute rejection or CAN.[304,346]

Other types of cancer in children after renal transplantation include the urinary tract, primarily renal cell or urothelial cell carcinoma, which may arise from the native kidneys or the allograft.[348] Nonmelanoma skin cancer is common in transplant recipients, though more frequently diagnosed in young adults than in children.[349] Regular use of high protection factor sunscreen can reduce the incidence of skin cancer, and referral for an annual

ANEMIA

Anemia is usually defined in children as hemoglobin concentration more than 2 standard deviation (SD) below mean for age, or dependency on ESA therapy. It is common in children after renal transplantation; in one study 25% of children were anemic 1 year after transplant with a higher frequency in recent years compared to previous decades.[352] The authors suggest this is related to newer immunosuppressive medications such as tacrolimus and mycophenolate. Another study found the frequency of anemia peaked at 1 month after transplantation, reaching 84%, and remained above 60% up to 5 years later. Iron deficiency, as well as suboptimal production of erythropoietin, is frequently found.[353] Both studies found that in the long term, anemia was correlated with creatinine clearance level, reflecting the fact that anemia is a marker of allograft dysfunction due to impaired erythropoietin production. Immunosuppressive agents with a direct antiproliferative action on the bone marrow, in particular azathioprine and mycophenolate, are associated with anemia, as well as leukopenia and neutropenia. Other causes of anemia include nutritional deficiencies and blood loss, particularly in the perioperative period, viral infections, chronic inflammation, severe hyperparathyroidism, and treatment with ACE inhibitors. CMV infection is associated with anemia, as well as leukopenia and thrombocytopenia, in some patients, and the anemia resolves with antiviral treatment. Parvovirus B19 infection has been described in pediatric kidney transplant recipients, presenting as severe anemia with reticulocytopenia and bone marrow findings compatible with pure red cell aplasia.[354] Parvovirus B19 infection can be confirmed by bone marrow and sometimes peripheral blood PCR, and treatment with intravenous immunoglobulin is successful in viral eradication and correction of anemia.[355]

Posttransplantation anemia should be treated to optimize oxygen delivery to organs and improve patient well-being. It is important to avoid unnecessary blood transfusions, which may cause alloantigen sensitization.[356] An iron-rich diet is insufficient, and oral iron supplementation is usually required, with or without ESAs. In some patients, parenteral iron sucrose or sodium ferric gluconate may be beneficial, because it results in faster repletion of iron stores and is not dependent on patient compliance.[357] Complete blood count and iron stores parameters should be monitored, and other causes of anemia, including vitamin B_{12} and folate deficiencies, occult infection, inflammation, or blood loss must always be considered in the differential diagnosis.

Leukopenia or neutropenia may also be seen in renal transplant recipients, though the frequency in children is not known.[358] It is usually noted in the first few months after transplantation and is associated with immunosuppressive medications, most frequently mycophenolate, though both viral infections and antiviral prophylactic therapy may also induce neutropenia. Drug withdrawal may increase the risk for rejection or viral infection, respectively, and granulocyte colony-stimulating factor therapy may accelerate recovery in severe cases.[359]

BONE HEALTH AND GROWTH

One of the issues that are unique to renal transplantation in children is that of linear growth, which is closely related to bone health and mineral metabolism, as well as hormonal factors. Preexisting renal osteodystrophy at the time of transplantation, impaired graft function, and the effects of medications, particularly corticosteroids, are the main causes of bone disease and growth retardation. Successful kidney transplantation corrects many of the metabolic abnormalities that characterize CKD; however, some may persist, particularly in cases of decreased allograft function. New mineral disturbances may appear such as hypophosphatemia, which is enhanced by residual hyperparathyroidism and hypomagnesemia due to calcineurin inhibitor treatment. Vitamin D deficiency is common among children with CKD and does not improve significantly after transplantation, whereas PTH levels decrease in most patients and are inversely correlated with 25-hydroxyvitamin D concentrations.[360,361] Bone mineral density is usually measured by dual energy x-ray absorptiometry, which has limitations in children with CKD because it underestimates bone mass in children with poor growth. After adjusting for height and age, bone mineral density is still significantly lower among patients who have received a transplant compared with controls.[362] Peripheral quantitative computed tomography is another modality to assess bone mineralization that may overcome these limitations.[363] Therapeutic strategies include steroid minimization, promoting good nutrition, regular physical activity, and correction of metabolic abnormalities and vitamin D deficiency.[364]

At the time of transplantation, most children have linear growth retardation, with a mean height deficit of −1.75 SDs according to NAPRTCS data.[159] After transplantation, reversal of the uremic milieu should allow normal GF/IGF-1 secretion and function; however, catch-up growth is not seen in all patients. Improved height deficit is observed in children younger than 6 years at transplantation, whereas other age-groups tend to maintain a relatively normal growth rate without improvement in z scores (Figure 76.5).

A large study compared children treated with RRT enrolled in the EDTA registry between 1985 and 1988 with a later cohort of German children followed between 1998 and 2009; most of the patients in both groups underwent transplantation. The mean height SDS improved significantly over the time period studied, with overall score increasing from −3.03 to −1.8; the improvement was mainly noted in adolescents.[365]

Corticosteroid treatment and impaired allograft function are associated with decreased linear growth. Steroid avoidance or early steroid withdrawal protocols have shown improved linear growth particularly in younger children.[246,366] Interestingly, one retrospective study found greater growth velocity in children who received a living related donor graft compared with deceased-donor graft, despite similar GFR.[367] Although recombinant human GH (rhGH) is not approved for use in pediatric renal transplant recipients with growth retardation in Europe or North America, several studies have demonstrated its efficacy. A NAPRTCS randomized controlled study showed improved growth velocity at 1 year with no increase in adverse effects such as acute rejection.[368] A meta-analysis found that five

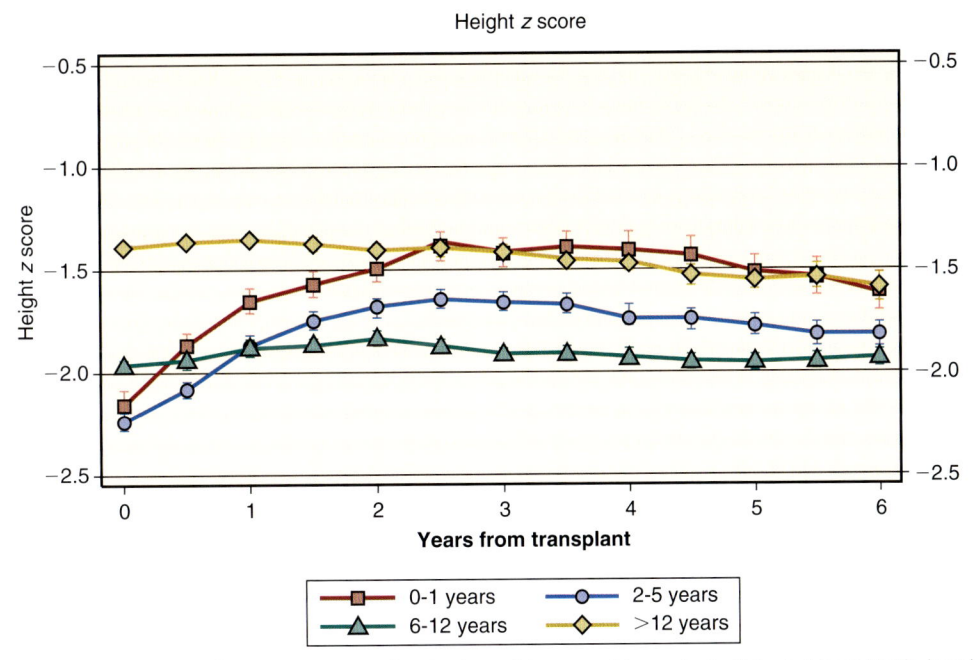

Figure 76.5 Standardized height score (z score; mean ± standard error) by age at transplant. (Adapted from North American Pediatric Renal Trials and Collaborative Studies: *NAPRTCS 2010 annual transplant report*. Available at: https://web.emmes.com/study/ped/annlrept/2010Report.pdf. Accessed July 10, 2013, p 6-4, Exhibit 6.2.)

randomized controlled trials with a total of over 400 patients demonstrated an increase of 0.52 height SDS in the treatment groups compared to controls. Acute rejection and GFR were not significantly different between the groups.[369] Treatment with rhGH improves final adult height without affecting graft function.[370] Analysis of NAPRTCS data from the past 20 years demonstrates an increase in height z score at the time of transplantation over time, from 1987 to 2010, which has a major impact on final height. Final adult height in pediatric renal transplant recipients has improved over time also as a result of steroid minimization protocols, a lower incidence of acute rejection and consequent steroid use, and broader use of rhGH in transplant recipients.[371]

UROLOGIC ISSUES

Early urologic complications include urinary leak or obstruction, discussed earlier. Ureteral obstruction may occur later after renal transplantation, though approximately half of the cases are in the first 3 months. Children with ESKD due to posterior urethral valves are at the highest risk for ureteral stenosis, most likely due to an abnormal bladder wall.[372] BK virus infection has been reported to be associated with ureteral stenosis; however, a causal relationship has not been established. In fact, a retrospective study of 67 adult kidney transplant recipients with BK infection found the incidence of ureteral stenosis to be 8.9%, which was similar to the control group.[373]

Vesicoureteral reflux to the allograft is quite common (40%), though its clinical impact on most patients may not be significant, because no change in frequency of UTI or graft function was observed in adults.[295] In children after transplantation, on the other hand, VUR was found in 58% and was associated with an increased risk for pyelonephritis. Antibiotic prophylaxis prevented recurrent infection in these patients.[374] Allograft VUR was associated with renal failure in children whose primary cause of CKD was posterior urethral valves, suggesting that abnormal bladder function was the cause of both VUR and of graft dysfunction.[375] In patients who do experience recurrent febrile UTI associated with documented allograft VUR, endoscopic correction is a feasible option and less invasive than open surgery.[376,377]

Boys who undergo renal transplantation due to posterior urethral valves may have ongoing bladder dysfunction. Small defunctionalized bladders can increase in capacity and compliance after transplantation, but meticulous care must be taken to ensure good drainage in the initial posttransplantation period.[187,378] Bladder dysfunction may manifest as increased postvoiding volume; daytime frequency, urgency, or incontinence; and nighttime incontinence. Some children may require intermittent catheterization, particularly if they have undergone bladder augmentation.[379]

PUBERTY AND REPRODUCTION

Delayed onset of puberty, menstrual irregularity, and infertility are common in patients with CKD, particularly ESKD. After transplantation many of the hormonal disturbances resolve, and fertility is usually restored. Pubertal development was found to be normal in females and most males after renal transplantation in childhood.[380] Pregnancy after renal transplantation is high risk both to the mother and the fetus; planned pregnancy and close monitoring of the patient and fetus are crucial to achieve good outcomes. However, 71% to 76% of pregnancies produce a live birth; the percentage is higher with meticulous prenatal care in patients with stable graft function and well-controlled hypertension.[241] Changes in medications, including immunosuppressive regimen, may be necessary before considering pregnancy, to avoid teratogenic effects of medications, such as mycophenolate, sirolimus, ACE inhibitors, and others.[247] Adolescent patients in particular need counseling regarding contraception to avoid unplanned pregnancy. The form of contraception used must take into account safety and efficacy of the method and patient adherence.

NONADHERENCE

Patient adherence to the medical regimen, or in the case of children, parental or caregiver adherence, is crucial to maximize good clinical outcomes in organ transplantation. Adherence can be measured by missed appointments, prescription-filling patterns, self-report or patient questionnaires, variance in immunosuppressive drug levels, or various electronic monitoring systems.[279,381] The prevalence of drug nonadherence in pediatric renal transplant recipients varies in studies between 6% and 45% depending on the group and the method used to assess adherence.[182,278] Adolescents are at high risk for nonadherence and have shorter graft survival.[159,182] In fact, between the ages of 17 and 24 years the adjusted hazard ratio of graft loss was 1.61 compared to age 3 to 17 years and 1.28 compared to young adults older than 24 years.[183] Other risk factors for nonadherence include family conflicts, poor communication between family and medical staff, lack of supervision in taking medications, and deceased-donor graft.[382]

Persistent nonadherence is associated with acute rejection, graft loss, and death, as well as increased medical costs.[279,323,383,384] It is important to develop strategies to improve patient and family adherence to the medical regimen, using a multidisciplinary approach aimed at improving communication between the medical team and the family, as well as between the patient and caregivers. Attention to adverse effects and trying to minimize them, as well as simplifying the medication regimen, may help improve patient adherence.

TRANSITION

The transition of adolescents or young adults from the pediatric to adult nephrology or transplant unit is a challenging process, which may potentially be associated with nonadherence and graft loss.[385] Although some clinics may use chronologic age alone to guide timing, other measures such as medical adherence, patient competency, and responsibility for care should be taken into account. Use of specialized transition clinics may assist in a smoother transition, less medication changes, and higher patient satisfaction.[386] Assessment of an adolescent's readiness to take on responsibility for his or her care should be performed, and adolescents need to take an active part in preparing for transition.[381,387] Some studies have shown no increase in acute rejection or graft loss after planned patient transfer to adult care.[388,389]

REHABILITATION AND QUALITY OF LIFE

Optimizing kidney transplantation in children cannot be defined only by excellent patient and graft survival rates. Studies measuring overall health, general well-being, and psychosocial adjustment, including school attendance, level of education, neurodevelopmental outcome, psychologic morbidity, and other parameters, using various questionnaires and scales have reported good long-term psychosocial outcomes after transplantation. Although health-related quality of life is higher in pediatric kidney transplant recipients compared with those remaining on dialysis, it is still lower than in healthy controls.[390] Many issues remain pertinent, for example, distress arising from physical symptoms and body image, adverse effects of medications, nonadherence, and psychologic problems such as anxiety and depression. School function is affected by prolonged absences for medical reasons, which affects academic achievements and peer relationships.[391] This is in addition to the higher frequency of learning disabilities, specifically in the areas of memory and executive functions in children with CKD,[72] although studies have shown improvement in specific neurocognitive functions in children after transplantation.[90]

Kidney transplantation in childhood has a long-term influence on socioeconomic rehabilitation in adulthood. Two studies report on adult outcomes of children who underwent transplantation in an earlier era (1970s and early 1980s) and reached adulthood. One study found a lower level of education than in the general population and a lower rate of independent living, marriage, and parenthood, although most of the patients were employed.[392] A significant correlation was found between education level, employment, marriage, independent living, and final height. A similar study from the United States also demonstrated a high rate of employment, as well as education levels and overall satisfaction equivalent to the general population, despite significant physical morbidity.[349] Of note, in both these studies a large percentage of the patients were severely short and therefore different from other cohorts who are treated with rhGH. A later study from Portugal followed adolescent renal transplant recipients into adulthood and reported similar levels of education to the general population, though lower rates of employment, particularly among those whose allograft had failed.[393]

Complete reference list available at ExpertConsult.com.

KEY REFERENCES

2. Pediatric ESRD. In U.S. Renal Data System: 2012, *Annual data report: atlas of chronic kidney disease and end-stage renal disease in the United States.* National Institutes of Health, National Institute of Diabetes and Digestive and Kidney Diseases, Bethesda, MD. Available at: http://www.usrds.org/2012/view/v2_08.aspx. Accessed July 14, 2013.
3. Paediatric report. In Australia and New Zealand Dialysis and Transplant Registry: *2012 Annual report,* ed 35, pp 1–10, 2012. Available at: http://www.anzdata.org.au/anzdata/AnzdataReport/35thReport/2012c11_paediatric_v1.9.pdf. Accessed July 5, 2013.
4. ESPN/ERA-EDTA Registry: *ESPN/ERA-EDTA registry annual report 2010,* 2012. Available at: http://www.espn-reg.org/files/ESPN%20ERAEDTA%20AR2010.pdf. Accessed July 4, 2013.
11. Lewis MA, Shaw J, Sinha MD, et al: UK Renal Registry 12th annual report (December 2009): chapter 14: demography of the UK paediatric renal replacement therapy population in 2008. *Nephron Clin Pract* 115:c279–c288, 2010.
19. Pruthi R, O'Brien C, Casula A, et al: UK Renal Registry 15th annual report: chapter 4: demography of the UK paediatric renal replacement therapy population in 2011. *Nephron Clin Pract* 123(Suppl 1):81–92, 2013.
20. Bone mineral and vitamin D requirements and therapy. National Kidney Foundation: K/DOQI clinical practice guidelines for

28. Hodson EM, Willis NS, Craig JC: Growth hormone for children with chronic kidney disease. *Cochrane Database Syst Rev* (2): CD003264, 2012.
29. North American Pediatric Renal Trials and Collaborative Studies: *NAPRTCS 2011 annual dialysis report.* Available at: http://www.emmes.com/study/ped/annlrept/annualrept2011.pdf. Accessed on June 1, 2013.
33. Goodman WG, Goldin J, Kuizon BD, et al: Coronary-artery calcification in young adults with end-stage renal disease who are undergoing dialysis. *N Engl J Med* 342:1478–1483, 2000.
39. K/DOQI clinical practice guidelines for bone metabolism and disease in children with chronic kidney disease. *Am J Kidney Dis* 46(Suppl 1):S8–S100, 2005.
47. Kramer AM, van Stralen KJ, Jager KJ, et al: Demographics of blood pressure and hypertension in children on renal replacement therapy in Europe. *Kidney Int* 80:1092–1098, 2011.
53. Shroff RC, Donald AE, Hiorns MP, et al: Mineral metabolism and vascular damage in children on dialysis. *J Am Soc Nephrol* 18:2996–3003, 2007.
54. Groothoff JW, Gruppen MP, Offringa M, et al: Increased arterial stiffness in young adults with end-stage renal disease since childhood. *J Am Soc Nephrol* 13:2953–2961, 2002.
67. Hooper SR, Gerson AC, Butler RW, et al: Neurocognitive functioning of children and adolescents with mild-to-moderate chronic kidney disease. *Clin J Am Soc Nephrol* 6:1824, 2011.
72. Gipson DS, Hooper SR, Duquette PJ, et al: Memory and executive functions in pediatric chronic kidney disease. *Child Neuropsychol* 12:391–405, 2006.
79. McDonald SP, Craig JC, Australian and New Zealand Paediatric Nephrology Association: Long-term survival of children with end-stage renal disease. *N Engl J Med* 350:2654–2662, 2004.
81. Kramer A, Stel VS, Tizard J, et al: Characteristics and survival of young adults who started renal replacement therapy during childhood. *Nephrol Dial Transplant* 24:926–933, 2009.
83. Groothoff JW, Gruppen MP, Offringa M, et al: Mortality and causes of death of end-stage renal disease in children: a Dutch cohort study. *Kidney Int* 61:621–629, 2002.
84. Gillen DL, Stehman-Breen CO, Smith JM, et al: Survival advantage of pediatric recipients of a first kidney transplant among children awaiting kidney transplantation. *Am J Transplant* 8:2600–2606, 2008.
95. Tangeraas T, Bjerre A, Lien B, et al: Long-term outcome of pediatric renal transplantation: the Norwegian experience in three eras 1970-2006. *Pediatr Transplant* 19:769–768, 2008.
101. Hayes WN, Watson AR, Callaghan N, et al: Vascular access: choice and complications in European paediatric haemodialysis units. *Pediatr Nephrol* 27:999–1004, 2012.
120. Fischbach M, Terzic J, Menouer S, et al: Intensified and daily hemodialysis in children might improve statural growth. *Pediatr Nephrol* 21:1746–1752, 2006.
131. Schmitt CP, Nau B, Gemulla G, et al: Effect of the dialysis fluid buffer on peritoneal membrane function in children. *Clin J Am Soc Nephrol* 8:108–115, 2013.
135. Warady BA, Feneberg R, Verrina E, et al: Peritonitis in children who receive long-term peritoneal dialysis: a prospective evaluation of therapeutic guidelines. *J Am Soc Nephrol* 18:2172–2179, 2007.
139. Chua AN, Warady BA: Adherence of pediatric patients to automated peritoneal dialysis. *Pediatr Nephrol* 26:789–793, 2011.
159. North American Pediatric Renal Trials and Collaborative Studies: *NAPRTCS 2010 annual transplant report.* Available at: https://web.emmes.com/study/ped/annlrept/2010_Report.pdf. Accessed July 10, 2013.
160. Pediatric transplant. In Scientific Registry of Transplant Recipients: *OPTN/SRTR 2011 annual data report: kidney.* pp 37-44. Available at: http://srtr.transplant.hrsa.gov/annual_reports/2011/pdf/01_kidney_12.pdf. Accessed June 29, 2013.
163. Axelrod DA, McCullough KP, Brewer ED, et al: Kidney and pancreas transplantation in the United States, 1999-2008: the changing face of living donation. *Am J Transplant* 10:987–1002, 2010.
171. Bar-Dayan A, Bar-Nathan N, Shaharabani E, et al: Kidney transplantation from pediatric donors: size-match-based allocation. *Pediatr Transplant* 12:469–473, 2008.
174. Samuel SM, Tonelli MA, Foster BJ, et al: Survival in pediatric dialysis and transplant patients. *Clin J Am Soc Nephrol* 6:1094–1099, 2011.
179. Chavers B, Najarian JS, Humar A: Kidney transplantation in infants and small children. *Pediatr Transplant* 11:702–708, 2007.
187. Alexopoulos S, Lightner A, Concepcion W, et al: Pediatric kidney recipients with small capacity, defunctionalized urinary bladders receiving adult-sized kidney without prior bladder augmentation. *Transplantation* 91:452–456, 2011.
196. Van Stralen KJ, Verrina E, Belingheri M, et al: Impact of graft loss among kidney diseases with a high risk of post-transplant recurrence in the paediatric population. *Nephrol Dial Transplant* 28:1031–1038, 2013.
199. Shishido S, Hyodo YY, Aoki Y, et al: Outcomes of pediatric ABO-incompatible kidney transplantation are equivalent to ABO compatible controls. *Transplant Proc* 44:214–216, 2012.
208. Gloor JM: The clinical utility of comprehensive assessment of donor specific anti-HLA antibodies in the clinical management of pediatric kidney transplant recipients. *Pediatr Transplant* 15:557–563, 2010.
214. Pradhan M, Raffaelli RM, Lind C, et al: Successful deceased donor renal transplant in a sensitized pediatric recipient with the use of plasmapheresis. *Pediatr Transplant* 12:711–716, 2008.
242. Jungraithmayr TC, Wiesmayr S, Staskewitz A, et al: Five-year outcome in pediatric patients with mycophenolate mofetil-based renal transplantation. *Transplantation* 83:900–905, 2007.
246. Sarwal MM, Ettenger RB, Dharnidharka V, et al: Complete steroid avoidance is effective and safe in children with renal transplants: a multicenter randomized trial with three-year follow-up. *Am J Transplant* 12:2719–2729, 2012.
249. Höcker B, Weber LT, Feneberg R, et al: Improved growth and cardiovascular risk after late steroid withdrawal: 2-year results of a prospective, randomised trial in paediatric renal transplantation. *Nephrol Dial Transplant* 25:617–624, 2010.
262. Salvatierra O, Jr, Millan M, Concepcion W: Pediatric renal transplantation with considerations for successful outcomes. *Semin Pediatr Surg* 15:208–217, 2006.
264. Camacho-Gonzalez AF, Gutman J, Hymes LC, et al: 24 weeks of valganciclovir prophylaxis in children after renal transplantation: a 4-year experience. *Transplantation* 91:245–250, 2011.
275. Fine RN: Recurrence of nephrotic syndrome/focal segmental glomerulosclerosis following renal transplantation in children. *Pediatr Nephrol* 22:496–502, 2007.
282. Kranz B, Kelsch R, Kuwertz-Bröking E, et al: Acute antibody-mediated rejection in paediatric renal transplant recipients. *Pediatr Nephrol* 26:1149–1156, 2011.
290. Chavers BM, Solid CA, Gilbertson DT, et al: Infection-related hospitalization rates in pediatric versus adult patients with end-stage renal disease in the United States. *J Am Soc Nephrol* 18:952–959, 2007.
305. Höcker B, Fickenscher H, Delecluse HJ, et al: Epidemiology and morbidity of Epstein-Barr virus infection in pediatric renal transplant recipients: a multicenter, prospective study. *Clin Infect Dis* 56:84–92, 2013.
334. Opelz G, Döhler B, Collaborative Transplant Study: Improved long-term outcomes after renal transplantation associated with blood pressure control. *Am J Transplant* 5:2725–2731, 2005.
349. Bartosh SM, Leverson G, Robillard D, et al: Long-term outcomes in pediatric renal transplant recipients who survive into adulthood. *Transplantation* 76:1195–1200, 2003.
366. Grenda R, Watson A, Trompeter R, et al: A randomized trial to assess the impact of early steroid withdrawal on growth in pediatric renal transplantation: the TWIST study. *Am J Transplant* 10:828–836, 2010.
384. Chisholm-Burns MA, Spivey CA, Rehfeld R, et al: Immunosuppressant therapy adherence and graft failure among pediatric renal transplant recipients. *Am J Transplant* 9:2497–2504, 2009.

SECTION XIII

GLOBAL CONSIDERATIONS IN KIDNEY DISEASE

77 Latin America

Leonardo V. Riella | Miquel C. Riella

CHAPTER OUTLINE

TROPICAL DISEASES AND KIDNEY INJURY, 2440
Dengue Fever, 2440
Yellow Fever, 2441
Malaria, 2442
Leptospirosis, 2443
NEPHROTOXICITY DUE TO VENOMS, 2444
Spiders, 2444
Lonomia Caterpillars, 2445
Snakes, 2446

CHRONIC KIDNEY DISEASE IN LATIN AMERICA, 2447
Prevalence of Chronic Kidney Disease, 2448
Risk Factors for Chronic Kidney Disease, 2448
Mesoamerican Nephropathy, 2448
END-STAGE KIDNEY DISEASE IN LATIN AMERICA, 2449
TRANSPLANTATION, 2451
TRENDS AND THE FUTURE, 2451

Two hundred years after achieving political independence from European colonizers, Latin America became an area of rapid growth and great economic opportunity. Despite the unifying term, this region is very heterogenous, consisting of 20 different countries with different languages and degrees of economic as well as social development. Even within a single country such as Brazil, different regions may have diverse levels of development and medical needs.

The total population of Latin America is estimated at 595 million people. Brazil, Mexico, Chile, Colombia, and Peru represent more than 70% of the population and account for three-quarters of its gross domestic product (GDP). Poverty and extreme poverty are present in 29% and 11% of the population, respectively, with a predominance in rural areas.[1] Average life expectancy in Latin America is 74 years, though differences of more than 10 years can be seen between countries. Similar differences are observed in infant mortality rate, ranging from 7.8 deaths per 1000 live births in Chile to 50 in Bolivia (average 15.5). Other problems, such as maternal mortality, malnutrition, and the lack of access to safe water and sanitation, tend to be obscured by regional averages.[1] High prevalence of certain infectious diseases, such as tuberculosis, malaria, dengue fever, and cholera, is also characteristic. Total health expenditure in Latin America rose to 7.3% of GDP in 2010, though this figure is still inferior to that of the United States (14%) and Europe (8.5%), and almost half of Latin America's population lack health insurance (46%).[1]

On the basis of its geographic location, diverse ethnic backgrounds, and socioeconomic status, Latin America is the setting for a number of unique diseases that may affect kidney function and are reviewed in this chapter. Infections such as dengue fever, malaria, yellow fever, leptospirosis, schistosomiasis, and leprosy are prevalent, and nephrotoxicity from the venom of spiders, caterpillars, or snakes has become more frequent with changes in the environment. In addition, chronic kidney disease (CKD) has become a major health concern with the epidemic of western metabolic syndrome and unique obscure cases of progressive kidney disease in sugarcane agricultural workers. This chapter attempts to summarize the current status of care of patients with kidney disease in Latin America and to describe some leading priorities necessary for the improvement and progress of kidney health in the region.

TROPICAL DISEASES AND KIDNEY INJURY

DENGUE FEVER

Dengue fever (DF) is a mosquito-borne infection that causes a severe flulike illness and, sometimes, a potentially lethal complication called *dengue hemorrhagic fever* (DHF). The main dengue vector is the female of the *Aedes aegypti* mosquito. Male mosquitoes do not transmit the disease because they feed on plant juices. DF and DHF are primarily diseases of tropical and subtropical areas, and the four different dengue serotypes are maintained in a cycle that involves humans and the *Aedes* mosquito. Global incidence of dengue has grown dramatically in recent decades.

Approximately half the world's population lives in areas potentially at risk for dengue and 50 to 100 million cases are estimated to occur annually.[2,3] Brazil has the highest absolute number of cases and the highest incidence of the disease in Latin America.[2] The principal method for prevention of dengue virus transmission is to directly combat the disease-carrying mosquitoes. The higher incidence of dengue in Latin America has been ascribed to global warming and ecosystem modifications, facilitating the dissemination of pathogens and vectors of the disease. In addition, demographic factors, including uncontrolled migration of people and unplanned urbanization, have facilitated the increase in occurrence of dengue in urban areas and large cities.

Dengue is caused by one of four closely related, but antigenically distinct, virus serotypes (DEN-1, DEN-2, DEN-3, and DEN-4) of the genus *Flavivirus*. Infection with one of these serotypes provides immunity to only that serotype for life; therefore, persons living in a dengue-endemic area can have more than one dengue infection during their lifetimes.

Dengue virus infection may manifest clinically as an undifferentiated fever, DF, DHF, or dengue shock syndrome (DSS). DHF usually occurs in patients who have previously been infected with other serotypes of dengue virus ("secondary infection"), although it may follow primary infections, particularly in infants.[3] Classic dengue fever is an acute febrile illness accompanied by headache, retroorbital pain, and muscle and joint pains that lasts approximately 5 days but that has no specific physical findings except a maculopapular rash in about 50% of cases. DHF is a severe form of the disease and it manifests with fever, hemorrhagic phenomena, thrombocytopenia, and evidence of plasma leakage (high hematocrit, pleural effusion, ascites, and hypoalbuminemia). Malaria, leptospirosis, hantavirus infection, typhoid fever, human immunodeficiency virus (HIV) infection, enterovirus infection, influenza, and sepsis must be ruled out in the differential diagnosis. The diagnosis of acute dengue virus infection is mainly a clinical one, but serologic tests are available in specialized reference laboratories, including hemagglutination inhibition (HI) assay (considered the gold standard), immunoglobulin (Ig) G or IgM enzyme immunoassays, and reverse transcription polymerase chain reaction (RT-PCR) analysis for dengue virus RNA.

KIDNEY INVOLVEMENT IN DENGUE FEVER

Renal injury, composed of acute tubular injury, glomerulonephritis, or hemolytic uremic syndrome, has been reported in patients with dengue fever. Clinical presentation is variable, ranging from an elevation in creatinine, proteinuria, and active urinary sediment to thrombotic microangiopathy. The possible pathogenesis of renal involvement includes ischemic or hemoglobin-associated tubular injury, glomerular injury, secondary immune complex deposition, and thrombotic microangiopathy.[4] Lima and colleagues described a case of DHF-induced acute kidney injury (AKI), in which renal injury occurred without hemodynamic instability, hemolysis, rhabdomyolysis, or use of nephrotoxic drugs.[2]

The prevalence of AKI in dengue infection is variable, ranging from 0.3% to as high as 15%.[4] In a series from Thailand, 51 deaths were reported among 6154 cases of DHF with an overall incidence of AKI of 0.3%, but an incidence of 33.3% among the fatal cases. Kidney biopsies performed in patients with DHF and proteinuria, hematuria, or both revealed glomerular changes characterized by hypertrophy and hyperplasia of mesangial and endothelial cells, presence of monocyte-like cells in some of the glomerular capillary lumens, and focal thickening of the glomerular basement membrane. Immune complexes (IgG, IgM or both, and C3) were found in glomeruli and arterioles in biopsy specimens from 10 cases that were collected 2 weeks after the onset of symptoms. Dense, spherical particles were found in the 12 cases in which electron microscopy was carried out. The researchers in this series hypothesized that the particles might be nucleocapsid cores of dengue virions.[5]

Experimental studies with inoculation of the virus in mice suggest that the dengue virus can induce glomerulopathy. In one study in which the dengue virus type 2 was inoculated in mice, diffuse proliferative glomerular injury was seen 14 days after the inoculation, and in another study, enlarged glomerular volume, increased endocapillary and mesangial cellularity, and glomerular IgM deposition were observed 48 hours after virus inoculation.[6] In a case report from Brazil, the presence of proteinuria, hematuria, generalized edema, and hypertension associated with low levels of C3 and C4 suggested an immune-mediated acute glomerular injury.[4]

There is no specific treatment for dengue fever, so management consists of supportive care, including controlling fever (acetaminophen), preventing dehydration (oral [PO] or intravenous [IV] fluids), and managing complications such as bleeding. Aspirin and nonsteroidal antiinflammatory drugs (NSAIDS) should be avoided. There are no vaccines available, and the only mode of prevention is to protect against the mosquito bite by covering exposed skin areas and using an effective mosquito repellent, such as *N,N*-diethyl-meta-toluamide (DEET).

YELLOW FEVER

Yellow fever (YF) is a viral hemorrhagic fever transmitted by infected mosquitoes. There are three types of transmission cycle: sylvatic, intermediate, and urban. All three cycles exist in Africa, but in South America, only sylvatic and urban yellow fever occur.[7] *Sylvatic* (or jungle) yellow fever occurs in tropical rainforests, where monkeys, infected by sylvatic mosquitoes, pass the virus onto other mosquitoes that feed on them; these mosquitoes, in turn, bite and thus infect humans entering the rainforest. This type of transmission produces sporadic cases, the majority of which affect young men working in the forest (e.g., logging). The *intermediate* cycle of yellow fever transmission, which occurs in humid or semihumid savannahs of Africa, can produce small-scale epidemics in rural villages. Semidomestic mosquitoes infect both monkey and human hosts, and increased contact between human and infected mosquito leads to disease. This is the most common type of outbreak seen lately in Africa. *Urban yellow fever* results in large, explosive epidemics when travelers from rural areas introduce the virus into areas with high human population density. Domestic mosquitoes, most notably *Aedes aegypti*, carry the virus from person to person. These outbreaks tend to spread outward from one source to cover a wide area. Since October 2008, an intense increase in circulation of the jungle yellow fever virus has been observed in the Americas, affecting Argentina and Brazil in the southern part of the continent, Colombia and Venezuela in the Andean region, and Trinidad and Tobago in the Caribbean (Figure 77.1).[7]

Yellow fever transmission in the Americas continues to follow the jungle cycle. However, in order to avoid the

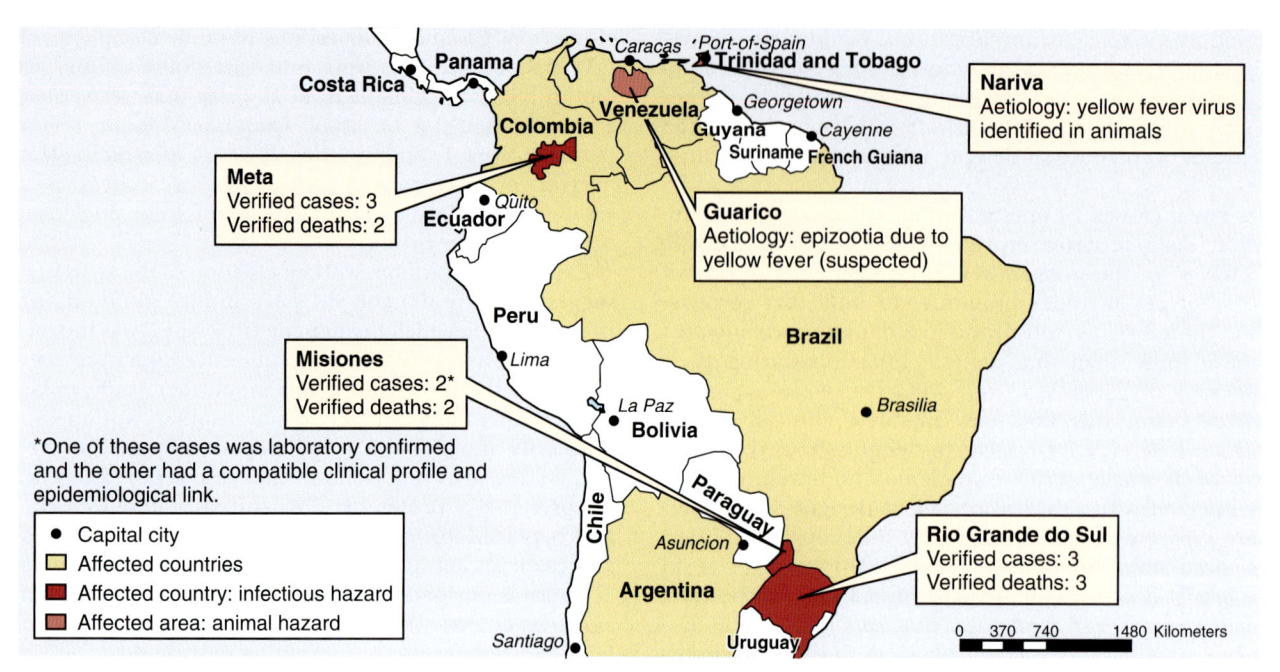

Figure 77.1 Yellow fever events in South America and Caribbean by first administrative level, January 2009. (Data from Pan American Health Organization: *Control of yellow fever: field guide,* 2005 [Scientific and Technical Publication No. 603]. Available at www.paho.org/english/ad/fch/im/fieldguide_yellowfever.pdf. Accessed January 24, 2011.)

reurbanization of this disease—there has already been an outbreak, confirmed at the beginning of 2008 and successfully controlled—*A. aegypti* control measures are critical, mainly in cities and in localities bordering affected areas. These measures also facilitate the prevention of dengue outbreaks.

One of the most important mechanisms for preventing yellow fever is vaccination. The live attenuated vaccine against yellow fever yields protective immunity in about 90% of individuals within 10 days of receiving the 0.5-mL subcutaneous dose, and in nearly 100% of individuals within 3 to 4 weeks after vaccination. A booster dose is recommended every 10 years. The World Health Organization (WHO) recommends vaccination for travelers to yellow fever–endemic areas of Africa and South America as well as for residents of those areas. The vaccine is contraindicated in persons who have known egg allergy or are immunosuppressed (e.g. transplant recipients). Yellow fever causes epidemics that can affect 20% of the population. When epidemics occur in unvaccinated populations, case-fatality rates may exceed 50%. Clinical presentation is characterized by three stages: infection, remission, and intoxication. The period of infection consists of viremia with nonspecific symptoms and signs including fever, malaise, headache, joint pain, nausea, and vomiting. This is followed by a period of remission with resolution of symptoms for up to 2 days. The subsequent period of intoxication is characterized by hepatic dysfunction, AKI, coagulopathy (low platelets), and shock. Diagnosis is confirmed by serologic testing such as IgM enzyme immunoassays or RT-PCR analysis for the yellow fever virus genome.

RENAL INVOLVEMENT IN YELLOW FEVER

Renal complications occur most often in the severe form of the disease between the fifth and seventh days, with reduction in urine volume and albuminuria. The mechanism of kidney involvement is poorly understood, although multiple etiologies are possible, including ischemic tubular injury due to shock, rhabdomyolysis, glomerulonephritis, and acute interstitial nephritis.[8,9] In experimental kidney injury, during the first 24 hours it appears to be related to hypovolemia, and later, oliguria, metabolic acidosis, albuminuria, and cylindruria occur. Viral antigen has been found in glomeruli and tubules. No treatment beyond supportive care is currently available.[7]

MALARIA

Cases of malaria declined 32% in Latin America and the Caribbean between 2000 and 2010, and deaths dropped nearly 40%. Yet more than 140 million people in the region (16% of the population) remain at risk of the disease.[7] The progress so far is largely due to improved treatment of the most deadly form of the disease along with more effective mosquito control.

Malaria is caused by *Plasmodium* parasites, which are carried by mosquitoes and transmitted to people through their bites. In Latin America and the Caribbean, 75% of malaria infections are caused by *Plasmodium vivax* and are rarely fatal, while 25% are caused by the more lethal *Plasmodium falciparum*, the dominant malaria parasite in Africa. Out of a total 775,500 malaria cases in 2007 in Latin America and the Caribbean, 212 deaths were reported.[7]

The clinical manifestations of malaria vary according to geography and prior immunity. Following the bite of an infected female *Anopheles* mosquito, the inoculated sporozoites go to the liver within 1 hour. Individuals are asymptomatic for 2 to 3 weeks (depending on parasite species), until the erythrocytic stage of the parasite life cycle. Release of merozoites from infected red blood cells when they rupture causes fever, malaise, headache, nausea, vomiting, and myalgias. Severe cases of hyperparasitemia may be associated with shock, acute respiratory distress syndrome (ARDS), AKI, coagulopathy, and hepatic failure. Physical findings include pallor, petechiae, jaundice, hepatomegaly, and splenomegaly. Clinical suspicion should prompt a confirmatory test for the parasite, which may involve light microscopy (visualization of parasites in stained blood samples), a rapid diagnostic test (detecting antigen or antibody), or a molecular technique for detecting parasite genetic material.

RENAL INVOLVEMENT IN MALARIA

AKI is one of the most dreaded complications of severe malaria. According to WHO criteria, AKI (serum creatinine level ≥ 3 mg/dL or ≥ 265 µmol/L) occurs as a complication of *P. falciparum* malaria in less than 1% of cases, but the mortality rate in these cases may be up to 45%. It is more common in adults than children. Renal involvement varies from mild proteinuria to severe azotemia associated with metabolic acidosis. It may be oliguric or nonoliguric. AKI may occur as a component of multiorgan dysfunction or as a lone complication. AKI is seen mostly in *P. falciparum* infections, but can occasionally occur with *P. vivax* and *P. malariae*. Malarial AKI is commonly found in nonimmune adults and older children with falciparum malaria.

Several hypotheses have been proposed to explain the pathogenesis, including mechanical obstruction of glomerular capillaries by infected erythrocytes, immune-mediated glomerular injury, and acute tubular necrosis secondary to shock and/or free hemoglobin tubular toxicity.[10] Possibly more than one of these mechanisms may occur simultaneously to produce the clinical manifestation. The predominant lesions on biopsy are acute tubular necrosis and mild proliferative glomerulopathy. Patients with these findings tend not to progress to chronic kidney disease. Excessive fluid administration, oxygen toxicity, and yet unidentified factors may contribute to pulmonary edema, acute respiratory distress syndrome (ARDS), multiorgan failure, and death.[11]

The management of malaria-induced AKI includes appropriate antimalarials (parenteral artesunate or quinine), fluid and electrolyte management, and early renal replacement therapy. Currently, high-quality intensive care, early institution of RRT, and avoidance of nephrotoxic drugs are standard practice for the prevention and management of AKI. Preliminary data suggest that albumin infusion for volume expansion may reduce mortality rates.[12]

LEPTOSPIROSIS

Leptospirosis is a zoonosis with protean manifestations caused by the spirochete, *Leptospira interrogans*. The genus *Leptospira* consists of two species, *L. interrogans* and *L. biflexa*, only the former of which is known to cause human disease. More than 200 serovars of *L. interrogans* have been identified.

Leptospirosis is distributed worldwide except for the polar regions. However, the majority of clinical cases occur in the tropics. Leptospirosis presents a greater problem in humid tropical and subtropical areas, where most developing countries are found, than in areas with temperate climates. The magnitude of the problem in tropical and subtropical regions can be largely attributed not only to climatic and environmental conditions but also to the greater likelihood of contact with a *Leptospira*-contaminated environment caused by, for example, local agricultural practices as well as poor housing and waste disposal, all of which give rise to many sources of infection.[1]

Human leptospirosis is endemic in Latin America and usually reaches epidemic levels after either higher rainfall periods with flooding or natural disasters such as hurricanes. In Brazil, 23,574 cases were reported from 1997 through 2008 with a mortality rate of 11.2% (Figure 77.2).

The natural hosts for the organism are various mammals, including rodents, dogs, pigs, cattle, and horses; humans are only incidentally infected, typically after exposure to the environment contaminated by animal urine, contaminated water or soil, or infected animal tissue. Portals of entry include cuts and abraded skin, mucous membranes, or conjunctiva. The infection is rarely caused by ingestion of food contaminated with urine or via aerosols. Controversy exists as to whether *Leptospira* can penetrate the intact skin.

Leptospirosis is a potentially serious but treatable disease. It can provoke a broad range of manifestations, from benign infection (characterized by nonspecific symptoms) to Weil's disease, a severe form of the disease that causes jaundice,

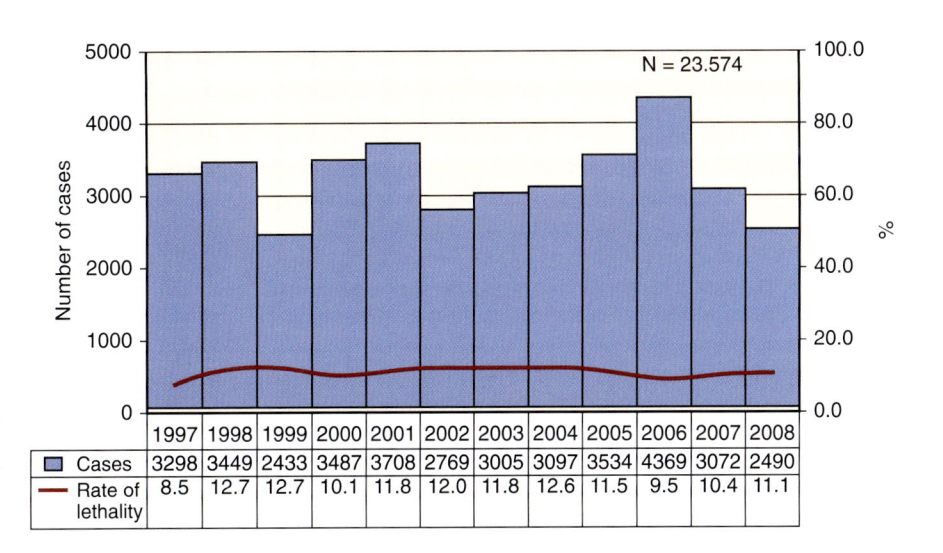

Figure 77.2 Cases and lethality of leptospirosis in Brazil, 1997 to 2008. (Brazilian Health Ministry. Epidemiological situation of leptospirosis. Available at: http://portalsaude.saude.gov.br/index.php/situacao-epidemiologica-dados. Accessed on 02/10/2014.)

	1997	1998	1999	2000	2001	2002	2003	2004	2005	2006	2007	2008
Cases	3298	3449	2433	3487	3708	2769	3005	3097	3534	4369	3072	2490
Rate of lethality	8.5	12.7	12.7	10.1	11.8	12.0	11.8	12.6	11.5	9.5	10.4	11.1

N = 23.574

hemorrhagic events, and AKI. Its symptoms may mimic those of a number of other unrelated infections, such as influenza, meningitis, hepatitis, dengue, and viral hemorrhagic fever.

Leptospirosis manifests as an abrupt onset of fever, rigors, myalgias, and headache in 75% to 100% of patients, after an incubation period of 2 to 26 days (average 10 days). After the acute septicemic stage, hyperbilirubinemia occurs in 85% of cases.[13] On physical examination conjunctival suffusion is an important sign. Most patients have muscle tenderness, splenomegaly, lymphadenopathy, pharyngitis, hepatomegaly, muscle rigidity, abnormal respiratory auscultation, or rash.

The most widely used method for diagnosing leptospirosis is the microscopic agglutination test (MAT), which is performed using two blood samples collected 2 weeks apart. The MAT results are considered positive when the antibody titers are four times higher than the reference value.[14] Available in some laboratories, detection of antigens by PCR offers the possibility of earlier diagnosis.

RENAL INVOLVEMENT IN LEPTOSPIROSIS

Renal involvement is common in leptospirosis. Clinical manifestations vary from urinary sediment changes to AKI, which is observed in 44% to 67% of patients.[13,15] Leptospirosis manifesting as AKI is a severe disease frequently leading to multiorgan failure and death. Leptospirosis-induced AKI typically is nonoliguric and often includes hypokalemia.[14]

The renal pathologic findings in leptospirosis are characterized by acute interstitial nephritis that may be associated with acute tubular necrosis.[16] The tubular injury may reflect a direct toxic effect of leptospiral compounds on tubular epithelial cells or indirect effects of dehydration, hypovolemia, and ischemia due to ionic wasting defects and the inability to concentrate urine.[13,17] Vasculitis is also observed in the acute phase of the disease. A cellular infiltrate consisting primarily of mononuclear cells can be diffuse or can be focused around the glomeruli and venules.[14] There are data suggesting that inflammation is most likely a secondary feature following acute epithelial damage and is observed only in patients who survive long enough for this feature to develop.[18]

Silver and other immunohistochemical staining reveals large numbers of intact leptospires throughout the tubular basement membrane, among tubular cells, and within the tubular lumens and the interstitium with associated interstitial nephritis. In some cases organisms are seen in limited numbers within glomeruli, but glomerular changes in general are not remarkable.

An experience of leptospirosis-associated AKI in Thailand showed that the use of hemodialysis or hemofiltration was associated with lower mortality (0 vs. 10%), shorter recovery time (8 vs. 16 days) and faster reduction in serum levels of bilirubin, urea, and creatinine in comparison with standard peritoneal dialysis.[19] There is, however, no data from randomized clinical trials evaluating different methods of RRT in patients with leptospirosis.[17]

The vast majority of infections with *Leptospira* are self-limiting. Two small, randomized, placebo-controlled trials showed a benefit of antimicrobial therapy. In one of these trials, in which doxycycline (100 mg PO twice daily) was compared with placebo, doxycycline shortened the illness by an average of 2 days and prevented shedding of the organism in the urine. In a second trial, patients with severe leptospirosis who were treated with penicillin had fewer days of fever, more rapid resolution of serum creatinine elevations, and shorter hospital stays; penicillin therapy also prevented urinary shedding. Therefore, symptomatic patients should receive antimicrobial therapy to shorten the duration of illness and reduce shedding of organisms in the urine. For patients with mild leptospirosis a course of doxycycline, amoxicillin, or azithromycin is recommended. Severe leptospirosis is usually treated with intravenous penicillin (1,500,000 U every 6 hours). Intravenous ceftriaxone (1 g once daily) or cefotaxime (1 g every 6 hours) has efficacy equivalent to that of penicillin. Treatment must be maintained for 7 days.

Doxycycline prophylaxis appears to be protective, reducing morbidity and mortality during outbreaks.[14] Control of reservoirs is difficult and no vaccines are available. China and Brazil, countries in which leptospirosis is a major health problem, have completed the sequence of the *L. interrogans* genome. Together with new genetic tools and proteomics, new insights have been made into the biology of *Leptospira* and the mechanisms used to adapt to host and external environments. Surface-exposed proteins and putative virulence determinants have been identified that may serve as subunit vaccine candidates.[20]

NEPHROTOXICITY DUE TO VENOMS

SPIDERS

Spiders of the genus *Loxosceles* are known colloquially as recluse spiders, violin spiders, fiddleback spiders, and, in South America, by the nonspecific name "brown spiders." In South America, *Loxosceles* spiders of medical importance are found in Brazil and Chile. The most common species involved in envenomations are *Loxosceles laeta, Loxosceles intermedia,* and *Loxosceles gaucho. L. laeta* is often considered the most dangerous of the recluse spiders, in part because it is the species that attains the largest body size.

Recluses are found mostly inside homes, in basements, in attics, behind bookshelves and dressers, and in cupboards. As their name implies, these spiders prefer dark, quiet areas that are rarely disturbed. Out of doors, they are found under objects, such as rocks and the bark of dead trees.

Loxosceles spider bites are the leading cause of spider envenomation and necrotic arachnidism in humans. The venom of the spiders is inoculated to paralyze and digest their prey. *Loxoscelism,* the term used to describe lesions and reactions induced by bites from spiders of the genus *Loxosceles,* causes skin necrosis, rhabdomyolysis, hemolysis, coagulopathy, AKI, and systemic inflammatory response syndrome (SIRS) in humans (Figure 77.3). Loxoscelism is currently considered a serious public health problem in southern Brazil. There are 3000 reports of *Loxosceles* bites annually and it constitutes the third leading cause of accidents involving venomous animals in Brazil.[20a]

The venom can trigger a powerful host of inflammatory responses characterized by local and systemic production of cytokines and chemokines as well as activation of complement and nitric oxide production, together with inflammatory cell migration and platelet aggregation.[21] The venom

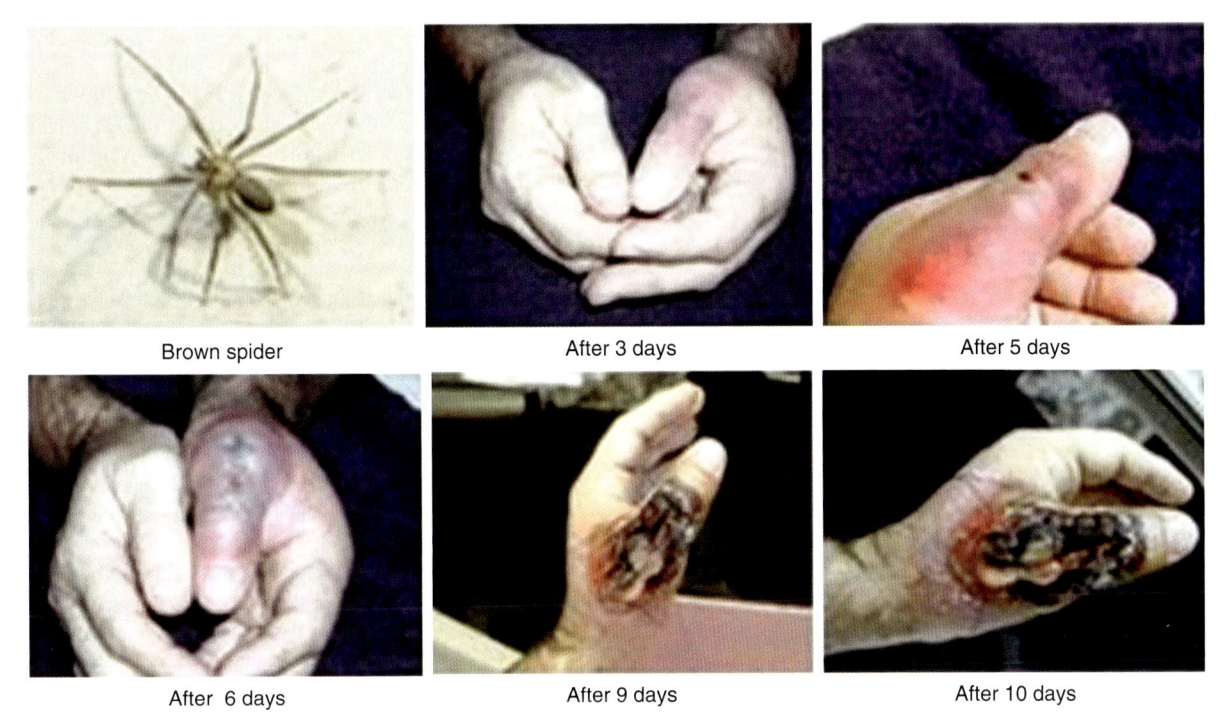

Figure 77.3 Evolution of skin lesions after brown spider bite.

also has a direct hemolytic effect on red blood cells and damages the membranes of endothelial cells in blood vessel walls.[22]

RENAL INVOLVEMENT IN LOXOSCELISM

Rhabdomyolysis and hemolysis are recognized co-factors involved in the genesis of AKI[22] and there is also evidence of a direct nephrotoxic action. The nephrotoxic effect of the *Loxosceles* spider venom is demonstrated experimentally in mice exposed to whole venom. Light microscopic analysis of kidney biopsy specimens showed alterations including hyalinization of proximal and distal tubules, erythrocytes in Bowman's space, glomerular collapse, tubule epithelial cell blebs and vacuoles, interstitial edema, and deposition of eosinophilic material in the tubule lumen.[23] Electron microscopic findings indicated changes including glomerular epithelial and endothelial cell cytotoxicity as well as disorders of the basement membrane. Tubule alterations include epithelial cell cytotoxicity with cytoplasmic membrane blebs, mitochondrial changes, increase in smooth endoplasmic reticulum, presence of autophagosomes, and deposits of amorphous material in the tubules. In the same study, confocal microscopy with antibodies against venom proteins showed direct binding of toxins to renal structures, confirmed by competition assays.[23]

The treatment of a recluse spider bite involves local wound care, pain management, and tetanus prophylaxis if indicated. Dapsone may be administered in some cases, both to prevent progression to necrosis, and to reduce pain. Antivenoms for the treatment of recluse spider bites are available in Brazil, Mexico, and Peru, although not in the United States. The bites of South American *Loxosceles* species (e.g., *L. gaucho*) are more severe than those of recluse spiders found in the United States.

The results of studies involving animal models suggest that specific antivenom decreases the lesion size and limits systemic illness even when its administration is delayed. To date, the most extensive use of antivenin treatment has been in Brazil, and the Brazilian Ministry of Health has developed guidelines for its use in extensive cutaneous lesions or severe systemic illness.[22] South American recluse antivenoms may help reduce the risk of dermonecrosis as well as systemic envenomation and its severe complications (e.g., hemolysis, AKI, and disseminated intravascular coagulation [DIC]). The data regarding efficacy of antivenom treatment is largely based on animal studies and the benefit in humans is not well established.

LONOMIA CATERPILLARS

Caterpillars are the larval stage of moths and butterflies and are found worldwide.[24] *Lonomia* caterpillars (family: Saturniidae) are found in South America and their venom affects mainly the coagulation system.[25] Accidental poisoning by caterpillars has become increasingly frequent in southern Brazil, partly owing to deforestation and elimination of natural predators.[24] Accidental contact with caterpillars' bristles induces allergic and toxic signs and symptoms that range from mild cutaneous reaction to severe systemic reactions, depending mainly on the number and species of the caterpillar involved. Symptoms include local irritation, urticarial dermatitis, allergy, ocular injuries, osteochondritis, hemorrhage, secondary coagulopathy, and AKI. Hemorrhagic complications including intracerebral hemorrhage can result in death.[14,24]

Caterpillars cluster in large numbers on tree barks and blend in very well (Figure 77.4). Contact with large numbers of caterpillars can occur, exposing the individual to large,

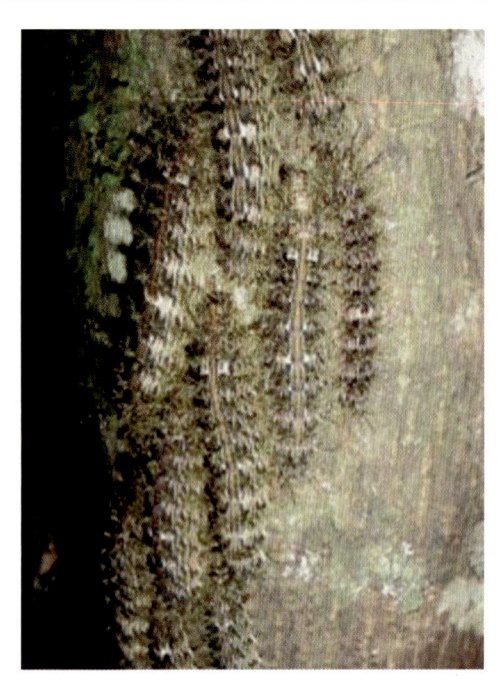

Figure 77.4 Cluster of caterpillars on the trunk of a tree. (Photo by M. Vennegoor.)

dangerous doses of venom. Two species of *Lonomia*, the Brazilian caterpillar *Lonomia obliqua* and the Venezuelan caterpillar *Lonomia achelous*, provoke activation of the coagulation cascade through the action of several compounds that are the subject of toxicology research.[24] In *L. obliqua* bristle extract, toxins were identified, including a factor X activator named Losac and a prothrombin activator named Lopap. Zannin and colleagues reported a series of 105 patients poisoned by *L. obliqua* and found coagulation factor depletion and enhanced levels of fibrin degradation in keeping with a DIC, although platelet counts were typically preserved.[26]

Mortality in Brazil secondary to these toxins peaked at 20% before falling to less than 2% following the introduction of the anti-*Lonomia* horse serum (in Brazil) in 1995 and educational campaigns. Since 1989 the southern Brazilian States have reported accidental poisoning by *L. obliqua* in 2067 individuals. AKI developed in 1.9% of patients, and of these, 32% required dialysis, with 10.3% going on to have CKD.[27] Our group has reported an event with a successful outcome due to early recognition and treatment with the antivenom serum.[28]

RENAL INVOLVEMENT IN *LONOMIA* ACCIDENTS

Even with anti-*Lonomia* serum, AKI can still occur.[29] Coagulation factors tend to be more profoundly altered in all patients with AKI, in keeping with their having more severe cases. The renal lesion appears to be secondary to massive deposition of fibrin in the glomeruli leading to ischemia. Some of the toxin components also cause direct toxicity to endothelium and tubular cells. The histology is poorly characterized because the coagulopathy prevents biopsies in the acute phase of the illness.

When travelling to endemic zones in Central and South America, travelers should be aware of poisonous caterpillars and avoid direct contact. Accidental poisoning should be reported immediately to the health authorities nearest the site where the poisoning took place, because they are more likely to have immediate access to anti-*Lonomia* serum. Most countries do not stock this product, so timely administration and supportive measures are critical.

SNAKES

Envenomation resulting from snakebites is a particularly important public health problem in rural areas of tropical and subtropical countries situated in Africa, Asia, Oceania, and Latin America. One study estimates that at least 421,000 envenomations and 20,000 deaths occur worldwide from snakebite each year but warns that these figures may be as high as 1,841,000 envenomations and 94,000 deaths. The highest burdens of snakebites are in South Asia, Southeast Asia, and sub-Saharan Africa.[30]

There are approximately 3000 species of snakes, of which approximately 19% are venomous. Most snakebites occur in tropical regions, where they represent a serious public health burden because of the resulting morbidity and mortality. Latin America is the third most affected area after Asia and Africa. Snakebites are more common in the rainy seasons and are related to the increase in human activity in rural areas. The most affected group is 25- to 49-year-old men. Lower limbs are the most frequently injured sites.

Epidemiologic data on snakebite envenomation in Latin America are scarce. In Brazil, there are 20,000 accidents involving venomous snakes per year, an incidence of 13.5 accidents per 100,000 inhabitants, and a mortality rate of about 0.45%. AKI is one of the main complications after snakebite envenomation and it is an important cause of death in affected patients. Snakebite-induced renal injury has been reported with almost all venomous snakes; however, AKI is more frequent with *Vipera russelli* in Asia as well as *Bothrops* and *Crotalus* in South America.[31]

CROTALUS SNAKES

The South American rattlesnake, which belongs to the Viperidae family, Crotalinae subfamily, *Crotalus* genus, is represented in Brazil by a single species, *Crotalus durissus*, distributed into 5 subspecies, of which *Crotalus durissus terrificus* and *Crotalus durissus collilineatus* are the most important. *Crotalus* venom effects are multiple and the most important clinical manifestations are neurotoxicity, myotoxicity, nephrotoxicity, and coagulopathy.

Crotalus venom induces clinical manifestations that can vary from mild local to severe systemic manifestations. Neurotoxicity may manifest as eyelid ptosis, blurred and/or double vision, ophthalmoplegia, and facial paralysis. Myotoxicity is revealed by generalized myalgia and myoglobinuria due to the rhabdomyolysis. The coagulopathy caused by the thrombin-like enzyme produces blood incoagulability and afibrinogenemia in 40% to 50% of patients, although bleeding is a rare manifestation.[32]

Renal Involvement in *Crotalus* Bites

The prevalence of AKI associated with *Crotalus* envenomation ranges from 10% to 29% and occurs within the first 24 to 48 hours after the bite. Experimental and clinical studies suggest that the pathogenesis of *Crotalus* venom–

induced AKI likely is related to rhabdomyolysis, renal vasoconstriction, and direct tubular cell toxicity.

Crotalus venom and probably *crotoxin*, the most important component of the venom, have direct and indirect actions on renal cells. Histologic injury usually found in *Crotalus* snakebite victims is acute tubular necrosis, although cases of interstitial nephritis have also been reported. Shock, hypotension, hemolysis, sepsis, or nephrotoxic drugs can contribute to the AKI. In one report dialysis was necessary in 24% of cases.[33] Mortality rates reported for AKI after *Crotalus* envenomation range from 8% to 17%.

BOTHROPS SNAKES

In Latin America, the vast majority of snakebite envenomations are inflicted by species of the genus *Bothrops*. *Bothrops asper*, a species widely distributed in southern Mexico, Central America, and the northern areas of South America, is responsible for the majority of cases in these regions.

Snakes of the *Bothrops* genus belong to the Viperidae family and Crotalinae subfamily. There are more than 30 species distributed from southern Mexico to Argentina and Brazil. The most important species are *Bothrops asper* in Central America and *Bothrops atrox*, *Bothrops erythromelas*, *Bothrops neuwiedi*, *Bothrops moojeni*, *Bothrops jararaca*, *Bothrops jararacussu*, and *Bothrops alternatus* in Brazil.[32] These species are found in rural areas and on the outskirts of large cities and prefer humid environments such as forests, plantation areas, and structures (e.g., barns, silos, and wood deposits) that are thought to contribute to the proliferation of snakes and rodents. These animals have nocturnal or crepuscular habits and an aggressive defensive behavior.[32]

Bothrops venom has proteolytic, coagulant, and hemorrhagic activity. A direct nephrotoxic action of the venom has also been shown. Local manifestations at the bite site such as edema, blisters, and necrosis are caused by the venom's proteolytic action. Lesions result from the activity of proteases, esterases, hyaluronidases, and phospholipases (phospholipase A_2 [PLA_2]), release of inflammatory mediators, action of hemorrhagins on the vascular endothelium, and the procoagulant action of the venom.[32,34]

The pathogenesis of these pathologic alterations has been investigated in experimental models. The observed effects result mostly from the combined action of Zn^{2+}-dependent metalloproteinases (SVMPs) and myotoxic PLA_2.[34] SVMPs are able to degrade extracellular matrix components, such as those present in the basement membrane of microvessels and at the dermal-epidermal junction, whereas myotoxic PLA_2 disrupts the integrity of the plasma membrane of skeletal muscle fibers. In addition, a prominent inflammatory reaction of multifactorial origin develops, resulting in a pronounced edema and an inflammatory cell infiltrate. The edema, in turn, contributes to hypovolemia and may promote increments in intracompartmental pressures in some muscle compartments, thus inducing further ischemia and tissue damage.

Bothrops venoms activate factor X and prothrombin, either alone or simultaneously. They also have thrombin-like activity, converting fibrinogen into fibrin. These actions may lead to DIC. *Bothrops* venom may induce platelet function abnormalities as well as a low platelet count.

Hemorrhagic manifestations result from the action of hemorrhagins, the metalloproteinases containing zinc described previously, in association with low platelet count and coagulation abnormalities. Moreover, hemorrhagins are potent inhibitors of platelet aggregation.[32,34]

Early and progressive pain and edema, bruises, blisters, and bleeding are frequently observed at the venom inoculation area. In most severe cases, there is necrosis of soft tissues with abscess formation and the development of compartment syndrome, which may result in functional or anatomic loss of the affected limb.[32] Systemic manifestations include bleeding (preexisting skin injuries, gingival bleeding, epistaxis, hematemesis, and hematuria), nausea, vomiting, sudoresis, and hypotension. The most severe systemic complications are shock, AKI, septicemia, and a DIC-like syndrome.[32]

Renal Involvement in *Bothrops* Bites

AKI associated with *Bothrops* envenomation has been attributed to hemodynamic changes, myoglobinuria, hemoglobinuria, coagulation abnormalities, and direct venom nephrotoxicity.[31] Myoglobinuria is unlikely to be an important factor in the pathogenesis of renal injury because *Bothrops* venom may cause localized muscular injury but does not have a systemic myotoxic effect like *Crotalus* venom and does not induce significant increase in creatine kinase.

The development of hypotension or shock is a rare event after a *Bothrops* snakebite. Venom may cause hemodynamic abnormalities as a result of sequestration of fluids at the bite site, bleeding, and release of vasoactive substances. *Bothrops* venom is considered hemolytic in vitro and there are clinical reports of anemia and hemolysis after *Bothrops* envenomation as well as reports of hemoglobinuria after administration of *Bothrops* venom to rats. Hemoglobinuria might contribute to renal injury, worsening renal vasoconstriction, glomerular coagulation, and tubular nephrotoxicity.

Renal dysfunction after *Bothrops* poisoning occurs early, is usually severe and oliguric, and presents the need for dialysis in 33% to 75% of cases. The most frequent renal structural injury found is acute tubular necrosis, although cases of bilateral cortical necrosis, interstitial nephritis, and acute glomerulonephritis with mesangial proliferation have also been reported. The mortality rate of *Bothrops* venom–induced AKI ranges from 13% to 19%.

Management of snakebites involves immobilizing the injured part of the body in order to reduce the spread of venom and expediting transfer to an appropriate medical center. Tourniquets are not indicated because of the risk of significant ischemic damage. Expert consultation with a clinical toxicologist/poison control center is necessary for timely administration of the appropriate antivenom.

CHRONIC KIDNEY DISEASE IN LATIN AMERICA

Latin America has undergone tremendous demographic and socioeconomic development in the past few decades. Improvement in sanitation, access to clean water, and expansion of health care programs have contributed to a significant reduction in infant mortality as well as death due to malnutrition and infectious diseases, resulting in an improvement in life expectancy. However, urbanization and assimilation of western lifestyle have resulted in an increase in noncommunicable diseases such as diabetes, obesity, and hypertension, leading to a significant rise in kidney disease prevalence.[35,36] Currently, cardiovascular disease, diabetes, and malignancies are the leading causes of death in Latin America. This section discusses the prevalence of, risk factors for, and treatment strategies for CKD in various Latin American countries as well as the importance of the development of health programs for earlier detection and prevention of CKD in this population.

PREVALENCE OF CHRONIC KIDNEY DISEASE

The prevalence of CKD in Latin America is difficult to assess owing to the lack of reliable and systematically recorded information in the region. Most of the data comes from voluntary registries so may be skewed or incomplete, creating an inaccurate picture. In addition, these records are confounded by heterogeneity in the population screened as well as in the methods used to determine glomerular filtration rate and proteinuria. If we extrapolate the values published in the Third National Health and Nutrition Examination Survey (NHANES III) for the population of Latin America in comparable age groups, there may be 47,000,000 patients with CKD in the region. In a Mexican population-based study, the prevalence rate of creatinine clearance (C_{cr}) less than 15 mL/min was 1142 per million population, and that of C_{cr} less than 60 mL/min was 80,788 per million population.[37] Most of the data available are based on advanced stages of CKD (end-stage kidney disease [ESKD]), showing that the prevalence has been growing by 7% annually during the past 10 years in Latin America. As an example, the prevalence of RRT has risen from 131 patients per million people (pmp) in 1993 to a projected rate of 630 pmp in 2010.[38] The improvement in life expectancy has also further enlarged the burden of chronic noncommunicable diseases such as diabetes and hypertension and as a consequence, of CKD. Coping with this growth in noncommunicable diseases may be unsustainable and unaffordable for most countries, urging interventions to halt the trend. In order to achieve this goal, better characterization of the problem through data collection is critical.

RISK FACTORS FOR CHRONIC KIDNEY DISEASE

Following the universal trend, the major risk factors for CKD in Latin America are hypertension and diabetes. Diabetic nephropathy is responsible for more than 30% of all cases of CKD in the region, though variation occurs (Mexico 40% vs. Argentina 20%).[36,38] The epidemic of diabetes is expected to continue worldwide, and an increase of more than 248% is forecast for the region from 2000 to 2030. Hypertension also is a silent cause of CKD, with prevalence as high as 30% in the Mexican population. An evaluation of 8883 individuals in Southern Brazil showed that 16% of the population screened had a history of hypertension. A family history of hypertension or diabetes was present in 42%.[39] In addition, 30% of patients evaluated in this screening program had signs of hematuria, 6% had proteinuria, and 3% had hematuria and proteinuria.[39] In a Mexican screening study, 9.2% of participants had proteinuria, which was strongly associated with hypertension, diabetes, obesity, and age.[40] Sedentary lifestyle, smoking, and unhealthy dietary habits that include high fat and high carbohydrate consumption adopted in Latin America have contributed to the described comorbidities and expansion of obesity.

Other important risk factors for CKD in the region include infectious complications, glomerulonephritis, and interstitial nephritis of unclear etiology (the last is discussed later as Mesoamerican nephropathy).

In summary, it is clear that the rising incidence of CKD is a major public health concern in Latin America, and diligent assessment of its prevalence, geographic distribution, and risk factors will be critical to establishing appropriate prevention programs for early screening and intervention. Uruguay has initiated a prevention program enrolling patients with CKD, and preliminary results showed a significant improvement in blood pressure and glycemic control in association with a reduction in the rate of deterioration of renal function (from 3.1 mL/min/year to −0.13 mL/min/year in patients with CKD stages 2 to 3).[41] In Southern Brazil, the Pro-Renal Foundation has taken a leading role in raising awareness of chronic kidney disease in the community.[39] It has completed a study on 6000 individuals randomly selected in the community and found a prevalence of CKD of 11.4% (unpublished data, MCR). Pro-Renal Foundation has also been a local pioneer in providing multiprofessional care for patients with CKD with teams of nephrologists, nurses, social workers, dentists, podiatrists, psychologists, and dietitians.[42]

These successes demonstrate that it is possible to modify health trends in Latin America with the help of the local community. Even basic interventions, such as encouraging lifestyle changes through exercise and dietary substitutions, in combination with augmenting the awareness of blood pressure and blood glucose control may yield significant reductions in occurrence and progression of kidney disease.

MESOAMERICAN NEPHROPATHY

Over the last decade we have seen numerous reports from Central America regarding a rising prevalence of CKD, particularly among agricultural workers. CKD in this region seems to have a higher prevalence in men, favoring regions with lower altitudes and in particular affects workers involved with sugarcane plantations.[37,43-48] The World Health Organization had demonstrated a high prevalence of CKD in regions of Nicaragua, Costa Rica, and El Salvador, with the highest mortality in the latter country.[1]

These early reports described a clinical presentation characterized by an elevation of serum creatinine and nonnephrotic proteinuria in young men without evidence of any known risk factors for CKD, raising the possibility of an interstitial disease due to an unknown environmental or occupational hazard. Another hypothesis raised was an ischemic injury as a result of the heavy workload in a hot climate leading to chronic dehydration and hypovolemia. The significance of heat stress was suggested by the male preponderance and high prevalence in low-altitude farming villages close to the Pacific Ocean, where it is hotter. The combination of repeated episodes of dehydration during heavy manual work and perhaps the concomitant use of nonsteroidal antiinflammatory drugs may explain the renal lesion. Nonetheless, it is clear that a second "hit" would be necessary for significant kidney injury to develop in such healthy young men. This endemic form of chronic kidney disease of unknown etiology was named Mesoamerican nephropathy (MeN) and seemed to be endemic to Pacific coastal communities in Central America.[46]

Wijkström and colleagues presented the first study on the correlation of clinical data with biochemical and morphologic findings in patients with MeN. The investigators analyzed renal biopsy samples from eight male sugarcane workers (aged 22-57 years) from a rural area of El Salvador who had presented with impaired renal function (estimated glomerular filtration rate 27-77 mL/min/1.73 m^2), inactive urinary sediment, and nonnephrotic proteinuria.[43] The morphologic picture was similar in biopsy specimens of all included patients. Chronic tubulointerstitial damage with tubular atrophy and interstitial fibrosis was found in combination with chronic glomerular changes. The most striking and surprising finding was the presence of relatively extensive global sclerosis, involving 29% to 78% of glomeruli analyzed.[43] These biopsies confirmed the suspicion of a primary tubulointerstitial disease. Immunofluorescence and electron microscopy did not show immune complex deposits, so an immune complex disease seems unlikely.[43]

In one study, recurrent dehydration has been shown to raise serum osmolarity and activate the polyol pathway in the kidney, leading to increased conversion of glucose to sorbitol and fructose. Fructose in turn can be metabolized by the fructokinase that is constitutively present, resulting in the generation of uric acid, oxidants, and chemokines that can cause local tubulointerstitial injury.[49,50] The same group has also shown that repeated dehydration can cause chronic kidney injury in mice and that this injury is fructokinase-dependent, because mice with knockout of fructokinase are protected.[49] Thus, it is possible that Mesoamerican nephropathy may be a kidney disease due to chronic dehydration and that recurrent dehydration is almost certainly a component of its pathogenesis leading to tubulointerstitial injury. However, toxins or heavy metals might contribute as a second factor in the development of the disease. Though originally reported in Central American, MeN could represent a larger entity, explaining CKD epidemics seen in countries such as Sri Lanka, Bangladesh, and central Australia (Table 77.1).[45]

END-STAGE KIDNEY DISEASE IN LATIN AMERICA

The prevalence of ESKD in Latin America is extrapolated from data provided about RRT in the region. However, due to the heterogeneous availability of RRT according to the nations' health care coverage and budget, these numbers do not clearly represent the true prevalence. The best available information comes from the Latin American Dialysis and Kidney Transplant Registry (LADKTR), a committee of the Latin American Society of Nephrology and Hypertension (SLANH), that has been collecting data since 1991 (Table 77.2). These data show a growth of more than 200% in the prevalence of ESKD in Latin America over the past 13 years (Figure 77.5). Data collected in 2010 from the 20 SLANH countries show that 189,137 patients were undergoing long-term hemodialysis (44% in Brazil), 65,824 were undergoing long-tem peritoneal dialysis (65% in Mexico), and more than 58,000 were living with a functioning kidney graft[51] (see Table 77.1).

Although RRT is provided to all patients with a diagnosis of ESKD in Argentina, Brazil, Chile, Cuba, Puerto Rico, Uruguay, and Venezuela, some countries may provide RRT for as little as 20% of such patients and others, such as Bolivia, may pay for only twice-weekly dialysis.[51] The consequence of this heterogeneous coverage is that the prevalence rate of RRT may vary enormously among countries (see Table 77.2). Thus, the prevalence rate is more than 600 pmp in Puerto Rico, Chile, Uruguay, and Argentina; between 300 and 600 pmp in Colombia, Brazil, Mexico, Panama, and Venezuela; and significantly lower, perhaps less than 100 pmp, in the remaining countries. The leading cause of ESKD in Latin America is diabetes, with the highest incidence reported in Puerto Rico (65%), Mexico (51%), Venezuela (42%), and Colombia (35%).[51]

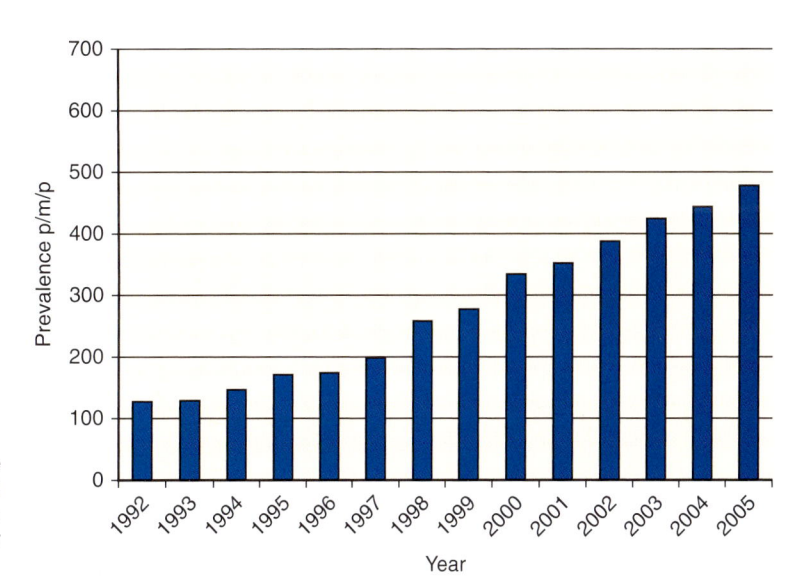

Figure 77.5 End-stage kidney disease (ESKD) prevalence rate (all modalities) in Latin America between 1992 and 2005. p/m/p, Patients per million population. (From Latin American Dialysis and Transplant Registry. Available at: http://www.nature.com/kisup/journal/v3/n2/full/kisup20132a.html.)

Table 77.1 Population, Socioeconomic Indices, Prevalence and Incidence of Hemodialysis, Peritoneal Dialysis, and Transplantation in 2008 in Latin American Countries

Country (Year of Data)	Population (In Millions)	% >65 Years	Health Expenditure (in Constant Dollars (2007)	Gross National Income	Life Expectancy at Birth (yr)	% Urban Population	Prevalence Rates (pmp) HD	PD	LKG	Total RRT	Incidence Rate	No. Kidney Tx	% Dead Donor Kidneys	Kidney Tx Rate
Argentina	39,939	10.51	1322	7160	75	92	595	25	132	752	142	998	SO	25
Bolivia (2007)	9,694	4.66	219	1450	66	65.58	98	18	17	133	NR	79	48	8
Brazil	192,004	6.44	799	7440	72	85.58	404	42	182	629	144	3780	54	20
Chile	16,804	8.76	768	9510	79	88.44	811	41	184	1036	172	282	73	16.8
Colombia (2007)	45,011	5.25	516	4610	73	74.2	265	125	45	435	143	715	91	16
Costa Rica	4,518	6.06	878	6060	79	62.74	26	11	257	294	NR	114	39	25
Cuba	11,202	11.21	1001	5550	79	75.64	206	12	93	311	87	144	94	13
Ecuador	13,485	6.36	434	3730	75	64.92	263	37	10	291	38	57	39	4
El Salvador	6,133	7.04	402	3460	71	60.7	121	347	63	531	NR	28	0	5
Guatemala	13,689	4.36	336	2670	70	48.58	109	130	34	273	NR	85	16	6
Honduras	7,326	4.24	260	1780	72	47.88	165	16	2	183	195	18	0	2
Mexico	108,468	6.23	823	10,000	75	77.2	269	384	56	709	431	2259	25	21
Nicaragua (2005)	5,675	4.43	258	1050	73	56.74	10	22	3	35	NR	4	0	1
Panama	3,399	6.38	773	6280	76	73.2	244	76	43	363	131	25	56	7
Paraguay (2006)	6,238	4.99	253	2130	72	60.3	80	2	9	92	NR	27	19	4
Peru	28,836	5.73	327	3990	73	71.3	189	35	42	266	31	80	0	3
Puerto Rico	3,958	13.34		33,259	79	98.32	997	80	92	1170	338	94	30	24
Dominican Republic	9,638	5.90	411	4340	73	69.02	119	12	15	146	NR	102	7	11
Uruguay	3,350	13.74	994	8020	76	92.3	757	68	254	1079	165	119	94	36
Venezuela (2007)	28,121	5.33	641	9170	74	93.66	292	72	34	399	120	278	64	10
Total no. for all Latin American countries	557,488	6.63	718	7012	73	78.57	342	119	106	568	208	9288	53	17

HD, hemodialysis; LKG, living with a kidney functioning graft; NR, not reported; PD, peritoneal dialysis; pmp, per million people; RRT, renal replacement therapy; Tx, transplant.
From Cusumano AM, Gonzalez Bedat MC, García-García G, et al: Latin American Dialysis and Transplant Registry: 2008 report (data 2006). Clin Nephrol 74[Suppl 1]:S3-S8, 2010.

Table 77.2 Potential Causes of Mesoamerican Nephropathy

Toxins	Pesticides and agricultural chemicals
	Heavy metals
	Herbal toxins
Drugs	Nonsteroidal anti-inflammatory drugs
Infections	Leptospirosis
	Pyelonephritis
Genetic/developmental susceptibility	Low birth weight
	Specific genetic predisposition of unclear origin (*APOL1*-like)
Heat-related volume depletion	Ischemia
	Repeated rhabdomyolysis
	Fructose-mediated injury

The low prevalence of ESKD in some regions should raise the suspicion of underdiagnosis and/or lack of available resources to offer RRT. The direct correlation of the degree of development of a country with the prevalence of RRT suggests that access to ESKD care is an important component. One report has confirmed this relationship by showing that RRT prevalence and kidney transplantation rates correlated significantly with gross domestic product, health expenditure, proportion of the population older than 65 years, life expectancy at birth, and proportion of the population living in urban settings.[51] Owing to the substantial economic burden of providing dialysis in many countries that still lack essentials such as sanitation, prevention strategies to halt kidney disease progression are critical.

TRANSPLANTATION

Renal transplantation has also developed significantly in Latin America, with more than 20 countries having active programs and more than 9500 kidney transplantations performed in 2009. The kidney transplantation rate increased from 3.7 pmp in 1987 to 6.9 pmp in 1991 and to 17.1 in 2008, although there were remarkable geographic variations in that year, from 36 pmp in Uruguay to 3 pmp in Peru. These rates are still remarkably lower than those in other developed countries, such as the United States (46 pmp) and Sweden (41 pmp). About 52% of these transplants are from deceased donors, though some countries, such as Nicaragua, Peru, and El Salvador, performed solely living-donor kidney transplantation. Brazil and Mexico account for 63% of renal transplantations in Latin America (3780 and 2259, respectively).[51]

Brazil has been one of the countries with the greatest expansion in kidney transplantation numbers, in part because of its free universal health coverage system, which includes full ambulatory and hospital medical care along with provision of all immunosuppressive drugs for patients undergoing transplantation. A single city in Brazil (São Paulo) has developed the largest kidney transplantation program in the world, through which 7833 procedures were performed in a 12-year period.[52] The annual number of kidney transplantations increased from 428 in 1999 to 1048 in 2010 in association with a significant improvement in organ procurement (35% donor success rate; 22.5 pmp effective donations). In addition to increased efficiency in organ procurement, several other factors have contributed to this expansion, including the development of a dedicated hospital for kidney transplantations and a system for rapid workups of recipient and donor. This program has approximately 5011 patients on the waiting list, and the recipient selection is based on HLA matching. A significant proportion of the recipients was of black ethnicity and had been on dialysis for a long time. More than 700 first consultations for living donation are done every year, and the majority of patients are followed locally after transplantation, with more than 200 appointments per day. Transplant outcomes among living-donor recipients are comparable to those reported in large registries but inferior outcomes have been observed among recipients of deceased-donor organs, likely due to prolonged ischemia time.

The criteria for brain death are well established and culturally accepted in all Latin American countries, and family consent is required for organ donation.[52] The regulations for living donors are also well defined, with restrictions against unrelated donors and prohibition of any kind of commerce. Access to transplantation is limited by the health care models of individual countries. In addition, lack of an organized organ procurement system leads to significant limitation in the number of organs available in many countries. One of the greatest challenges is to reduce the regional disparities related to access to transplantation. Furthermore, improvements and resources could be better used, with the development of a Latin American registry of outcomes of transplanted patients and living donors. Lastly, clinical and experimental studies to better understand the transplantation-related immune response of the ethnically diverse Latin American population would be critical to further advance the transplantation field in this region.

TRENDS AND THE FUTURE

The greatest challenge for the nephrology community in Latin America in the coming years will be dealing with the growing number of patients with ESKD, the lack or incompleteness of health care coverage for RRT in some countries, late referrals, shortage of trained personnel, small kidney transplantation programs, and lack of registries. In addition, early identification and aggressive treatment of infectious diseases complicated by AKI may minimize long-term renal sequelae. In spite of the worldwide concern about the increasing number of patients with ESKD and efforts to identify risk groups as well as development of strategies for prevention of chronic kidney disease, there is little activity in Latin America. Dialogue between the nephrology community and government authorities in the region has to be based on data, which are lacking. Only a few countries have reliable registries of ESKD and transplantation programs. The lack of universal health care coverage in some countries and, in many cases, a restrictive renal replacement program poses a much greater challenge because it reflects the public health agenda of a particular country and is a difficult scenario to modify. It is to be hoped that the combined efforts of scientific nephrology and transplantation societies, kidney foundations, and patient organizations will develop screening and prevention programs for CKD, educate the community, establish registries and more active kidney transplantation programs, and persuade public health authorities of the importance of kidney disease prevention and treatment.

Complete reference list available at ExpertConsult.com.

KEY REFERENCES

1. Health Situation in the Americas: Basic Indicators 2012 of the Pan American Health Organization/World Health Organization (PAHO/WHO) 2012.
2. Lima EQ, Gorayeb FS, Zanon JR, et al: Dengue haemorrhagic fever-induced acute kidney injury without hypotension, haemolysis or rhabdomyolysis. *Nephrol Dial Transplant* 22(11):3322–3326, 2007.
3. Malavige GN, Fernando S, Fernando DJ, et al: Dengue viral infections. *Postgrad Med J* 80(948):588–601, 2004.
4. Khalil MAM, Sarwar S, Chaudry MA, et al: Acute kidney injury in dengue virus infection. *Clin Kidney J (2012)* 5:390–394, 2012.
5. Boonpucknavig V, Bhamarapravati N, Boonpucknavig S, et al: Glomerular changes in dengue hemorrhagic fever. *Arch Pathol Lab Med* 100(4):206–212, 1976.
6. Boonpucknavig S, Vuttiviroj O, Boonpucknavig V: Infection of young adult mice with dengue virus type 2. *Trans R Soc Trop Med Hyg* 75(5):647–653, 1981.
7. Pan American Health Organization/World Health Organization: Update: situation of yellow fever in the Americas (30 January 2009; last updated June 16, 2010). Available at http://www.paho.org/hq/index.php?option=com_content&view=article&id=568:update-situation-yellow-fever-americas-30-january-2009&Itemid=40266&lang=en. Accessed January 24, 2011.
8. Monath TP: Yellow fever: a medically neglected disease. Report on a seminar. *Rev Infect Dis* 9(1):165–175, 1987.
9. Lima EQ, Nogueira ML: Viral hemorrhagic fever-induced acute kidney injury. *Semin Nephrol* 28(4):409–415, 2008.
10. Barsoum RS: Malarial acute renal failure. *J Am Soc Nephrol* 11(11):2147–2154, 2000. PMID: 11053494.
11. Mishra SK, Das BS: Malaria and acute kidney injury. *Semin Nephrol* 28(4):395–408, 2008.
12. Maitland K, Pamba A, English M, et al: Randomized trial of volume expansion with albumin or saline in children with severe malaria: preliminary evidence of albumin benefit. *Clin Infect Dis* 40(4):538–545, 2005.
13. Cetin BD, Harmankaya O, Hasman H, et al: Acute renal failure: a common manifestation of leptospirosis. *Ren Fail* 26(6):655–661, 2004.
14. Andrade L, de Francesco Daher E, Seguro AC: Leptospiral nephropathy. *Semin Nephrol* 28(4):383–394, 2008.
15. Sitprija V, Losuwanrak K, Kanjanabuch T: Leptospiral nephropathy. *Semin Nephrol* 23(1):42–48, 2003.
16. Covic A, Goldsmith DJ, Gusbeth-Tatomir P, et al: A retrospective 5-year study in Moldova of acute renal failure due to leptospirosis: 58 cases and a review of the literature. *Nephrol Dial Transplant* 18(6):1128–1134, 2003.
17. Cerqueira TB, Athanazio DA, Spichler AS, et al: Renal involvement in leptospirosis—new insights into pathophysiology and treatment. *Braz J Infect Dis* 12(3):248–252, 2008.
18. Arean VM: The pathologic anatomy and pathogenesis of fatal human leptospirosis (Weil's disease). *Am J Pathol* 40:393–423, 1962.
19. Wiwanitkit V: Comparison between blood exchange and classical therapy for acute renal failure in Weil's disease: appraisal on Thai reports. *Nephrology (Carlton)* 11(5):481, 2006.
20. McBride AJ, Athanazio DA, Reis MG, et al: Leptospirosis. *Curr Opin Infect Dis* 18(5):376–386, 2005.
21. de Souza AL, Malaque CM, Sztajnbok J, et al: Loxosceles venom-induced cytokine activation, hemolysis, and acute kidney injury. *Toxicon* 51(1):151–156, 2008.
22. Hogan CJ, Barbaro KC, Winkel K: Loxoscelism: old obstacles, new directions. *Ann Emerg Med* 44(6):608–624, 2004.
23. Luciano MN, da Silva PH, Chaim OM, et al: Experimental evidence for a direct cytotoxicity of *Loxosceles intermedia* (brown spider) venom in renal tissue. *J Histochem Cytochem* 52(4):455–467, 2004.
24. Carrijo-Carvalho LC, Chudzinski-Tavassi AM: The venom of the *Lonomia* caterpillar: an overview. *Toxicon* 49(6):741–757, 2007.
25. Arocha-Pinango CL, Guerrero B: [Hemorrhagic syndrome induced by caterpillars. Clinical and experimental studies. Review]. *Invest Clin* 44(2):155–163, 2003.
26. Zannin M, Lourenco DM, Motta G, et al: Blood coagulation and fibrinolytic factors in 105 patients with hemorrhagic syndrome caused by accidental contact with *Lonomia obliqua* caterpillar in Santa Catarina, southern Brazil. *Thromb Haemost* 89(2):355–364, 2003.
27. Gamborgi GP, Metcalf EB, Barros EJ: Acute renal failure provoked by toxin from caterpillars of the species *Lonomia obliqua*. *Toxicon* 47(1):68–74, 2006.
28. Riella M, Chula D, de Freitas S, et al: Acute renal failure and haemorrhagic syndrome secondary to toxin of caterpillars (*Lonomia obliqua*). *NDT Plus* 1:445–446, 2008.
29. Burdmann EA, Antunes I, Saldanha LB, et al: Severe acute renal failure induced by the venom of *Lonomia* caterpillars. *Clin Nephrol* 46(5):337–339, 1996.
30. Kasturiratne A, Wickremasinghe AR, de Silva N, et al: The global burden of snakebite: a literature analysis and modelling based on regional estimates of envenoming and deaths. *PLoS Med* 5(11):e218, 2008.
31. Chugh KS: Snake-bite-induced acute renal failure in India. *Kidney Int* 35(3):891–907, 1989.
32. Amaral CFS, Bucaretchi F, Araújo FAA, et al: *Manual de diagnóstico e tratamento de acidentes por animais peçonhentos*, ed 2, 2001, Fundação Nacional de Saúde.
33. Pinho FM, Zanetta DM, Burdmann EA: Acute renal failure after *Crotalus durissus* snakebite: a prospective survey on 100 patients. *Kidney Int* 67(2):659–667, 2005.
34. Machado Braga MD, Costa Martins AM, Alves CD, et al: Purification and renal effects of phospholipase A(2) isolated from *Bothrops insularis* venom. *Toxicon* 51(2):181–190, 2008.
35. Cusumano AM, Gonzalez Bedat MC: Chronic kidney disease in Latin America: time to improve screening and detection. *Clin J Am Soc Nephrol* 3(2):594–600, 2008.
36. Jha V, Garcia-Garcia G, Iseki K, et al: Chronic kidney disease: global dimension and perspectives. *Lancet* 382(9888):260–272, 2013.
37. Amato D, Alvarez-Aguilar C, Castaneda-Limones R, et al: Prevalence of chronic kidney disease in an urban Mexican population. *Kidney Int Suppl* 97:S11–S17, 2005.
38. Correa-Rotter R, Cusumano AM: Present, prevention, and management of chronic kidney disease in Latin America. *Blood Purif* 26(1):90–94, 2008.
39. Mazza Nascimento M, Riella MC: Raising awareness of chronic kidney disease in a Brazilian urban population. *Braz J Med Biol Res* 42(8):750–755, 2009.
40. Rosas M, Attie F, Pastelin G, et al: Prevalence of proteinuria in Mexico: a conjunctive consolidation approach with other cardiovascular risk factors: the Mexican Health Survey, 2000. *Kidney Int Suppl* 97:S112–S119, 2005.
41. Rodriguez-Iturbe B: Progress in the prevention of chronic kidney disease in Latin America. *Nat Clin Pract Nephrol* 4(5):233, 2008.
42. Riella MC: Nephrologists Sans Frontieres: a kidney foundation—advancing research and helping patients meet their needs. *Kidney Int* 69(8):1285–1287, 2006.
43. Wijkstrom J, Leiva R, Elinder CG, et al: Clinical and pathological characterization of Mesoamerican nephropathy: a new kidney disease in Central America. *Am J Kidney Dis* 62(5):908–918, 2013.
44. Ramirez-Rubio O, McClean MD, Amador JJ, et al: An epidemic of chronic kidney disease in Central America: an overview. *J Epidemiol Community Health* 67(1):1–3, 2013.
45. Johnson RJ, Sanchez-Lozada LG: Chronic kidney disease: Mesoamerican nephropathy—new clues to the cause. *Nat Rev Nephrol* 9(10):560–561, 2013.

46. Peraza S, Wesseling C, Aragon A, et al: Decreased kidney function among agricultural workers in El Salvador. *Am J Kidney Dis* 59(4):531–540, 2012.
47. Torres C, Aragon A, Gonzalez M, et al: Decreased kidney function of unknown cause in Nicaragua: a community-based survey. *Am J Kidney Dis* 55(3):485–496, 2010.
48. Cerdas M: Chronic kidney disease in Costa Rica. *Kidney Int Suppl* 97:S31–S33, 2005.
49. Cirillo P, Gersch MS, Mu W, et al: Ketohexokinase-dependent metabolism of fructose induces proinflammatory mediators in proximal tubular cells. *J Am Soc Nephrol* 20(3):545–553, 2009.
50. Nakayama T, Kosugi T, Gersch M, et al: Dietary fructose causes tubulointerstitial injury in the normal rat kidney. *Am J Physiol Renal Physiol* 298(3):F712–F720, 2010.

78 Africa

Saraladevi Naicker | Sagren Naidoo

CHAPTER OUTLINE

FLUID AND ELECTROLYTE
ABNORMALITIES, 2455
ACUTE KIDNEY INJURY, 2457
  Major Causes of Acute Kidney Injury,
  by Region, 2457
  Acute Kidney Injury in Human
  Immunodeficiency Virus Infection, 2457
  Acute Kidney Injury and Toxins, 2458
  Pregnancy-Related Acute Kidney Injury, 2458
  Acute Kidney Injury in the Intensive
  Care Unit, 2458
  Therapy for Acute Kidney Injury, 2459
CHRONIC KIDNEY DISEASE, 2459
  Glomerular Filtration Rate Estimation, 2459
  Prevalence of Chronic Kidney Disease, 2459

Causes of Chronic Kidney Disease, 2459
  Hypertension, 2459
  Glomerulonephritis, 2461
  Diabetic Nephropathy, 2463
  Renal Disease Due to Sickle Cell
  Anemia, 2463
  Renal Replacement Therapy, 2463
  Prevention Strategies, 2465
CHALLENGES FOR NEPHROLOGY
PRACTICE IN AFRICA, 2465
CONCLUSION, 2465

Africa, the second largest and second most populous continent, with a land mass of 30.2 million km^2 (11.7 million square miles) and 54 countries, including adjacent islands, was home to a population of 1.1 billion as of 2013. This continent of people, of diverse ethnic origins, religions, and languages, is expected to grow to 2.4 billion by the year 2050.[1] The mortality due to human immunodeficiency virus (HIV)–acquired immunodeficiency syndrome (AIDS) has been decreasing since about 2005 with the increasing availability of antiretroviral therapy (ART), allowing average life expectancy at birth to increase again in Africa from 50 years in 2000 to 56 years in 2011.[2]

Rapid urbanization, which is occurring in many parts of the continent, contributes to overcrowding and poverty. Millions of Africans live in overcrowded and unhygienic conditions, in which lack of clean water and inadequate sanitation foster breeding grounds for infectious diseases. This milieu of infectious disease is conducive to the development of acute and chronic kidney diseases. Diseases that had seemed to be under control, such as tuberculosis and malaria, have become major health problems, and resistance to therapy has developed. HIV and AIDS have reached epidemic proportions; 25 million people live with HIV infection or AIDS in sub-Saharan Africa.[3]

Although infections and parasitic diseases are still the leading cause of death in Africa—with more than 5.5 million deaths in 2005 and more than 2 million deaths caused by HIV infection or AIDS—noncommunicable diseases are coming to the forefront, having caused more than 2.4 million deaths in 2005.[4] Africa has a double burden of disease; although infectious disease remains the major health problem, the incidence of noncommunicable diseases such as hypertension and diabetes mellitus is increasing. Heart disease, diabetes, and stroke together constitute the second most important cause of death in adult South Africans, with kidney disease in fifth place (Figure 78.1).[5] This dual pattern of disease is responsible for the burden of acute kidney injury (AKI, resulting from infectious disease) and chronic kidney disease (CKD, in the form of glomerular disorders mediated by infectious diseases, as well as chronic disorders such as hypertension and diabetes mellitus). AKI caused by infections such as malaria and HIV predominate in many parts of sub-Saharan Africa. Hypertension is common in the populations of sub-Saharan Africa, with a reported prevalence of 21% to 25% in South Africa, and has been reported to be a major cause of end-stage kidney disease (ESKD) in this region.

Approximately 70% of the least industrialized countries of the world are in sub-Saharan Africa, with an annual gross domestic product per capita of less than $1500; half the population live on less than $1 per day. Annual per capita expenditure on health care ranges from US$9 to US$158, in comparison with more than US$2000 in Europe. Those in low-income countries have a decreased life expectancy, probably as a result of an increased burden of disease (especially infectious disease), inadequate financial resources,

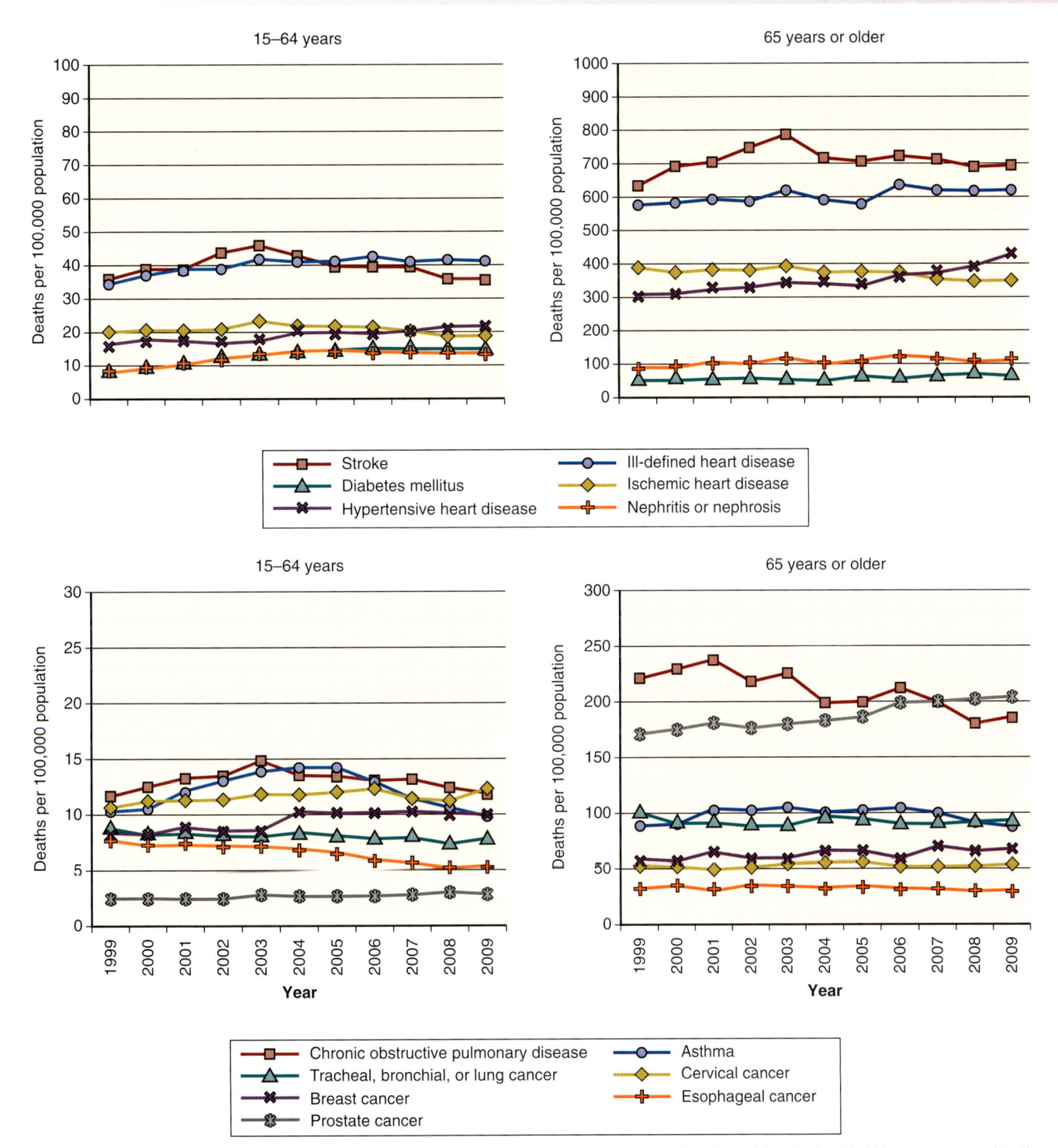

Figure 78.1 Deaths caused by different diseases/100,000 population in 15- to 64-year-old male and female South Africans compared to the population aged 65 years and older.

and limited access to health care.[6] Health care workers from Africa continue to emigrate to more affluent regions.[7] Large rural areas of Africa have no health professionals to serve these populations. Table 78.1 shows the distribution of physicians and nephrologists in a spectrum of African countries compared with industrialized nations and their corresponding rates of renal replacement therapy (RRT).[8] Most of Africa, consisting of low-income countries, has the lowest numbers of physicians and nurses to serve its population.

There are no nephrologists in many parts of Africa; elsewhere, the numbers vary.[8,9]

FLUID AND ELECTROLYTE ABNORMALITIES

Diarrheal diseases are major causes of death in Africa; much of the morbidity and mortality is probably caused by dehydration and electrolyte abnormalities. The cholera

Table 78.1 Global Health Work Force and Delivery of Renal Replacement Therapy in Africa and Non-African Countries

Country	Year	Population	GNI (Per Capita)	Physicians (Per 10,000 Population)	Nephrologists (pmp)	Prevalence of HD (pmp)	Prevalence of CAPD (pmp)	Renal Transplantations/Year
North Africa								
Egypt	2008	81,121,000	6,060	179,900 (24)	500 (6.5)	421	45	500
Morocco	2008	31,951,000	4,600	1,303 (<1)	135 (4.5)	162	30	13
Tunisia	2008	10,549,000	9,060	2,245 (<1)	70 (<1)	650	20	70
West Africa								
Cameroon	2004	19,598,000	2,270	3,124 (1.6)	6 (0.3)	3.6	ND	ND
Cote d'Ivoire	2008	19,737,000	1,800	2,746 (1.4)	ND	6	ND	ND
Ghana	2009	24,391,000	1,620	2,033 (0.8)	2 (0.1)	6.4	0	0
Mali	2008	15,369,000	1,030	729 (0.5)	ND	1.3	ND	ND
Nigeria	2008	158,423,000	2,240	55,376 (3.5)	70 (0.3)	6.3	0	70
Senegal	2008	12,433,000	1,910	741 (0.6)	2 (0.2)	4	2	0
East and Central Africa								
DRC	2004	65,965,000	320	5,827 (0.9)	7 (0.1)	ND	0.2	ND
Ethiopia	2007	82,949,000	1,040	1,806 (0.2)	2 (<0.1)	ND	ND	ND
Kenya	2002	40,512,000	1,640	4,506 (1.1)	15 (0.5)	6.4	0.7	10
Southern Africa								
Mauritius	2004	1,280,000	13,980	1,303 (10.2)	10 (8.3)	ND	ND	ND
South Africa	2011	50,586,000	10,360	38,236 (7.6)	108 (2.1)	41.4	21.2	250
Non-African Countries								
SLANH region	2006	544,233,000	4,756	ND	ND	280.6	96.7	8224
UK	2008	63,047,000	35,840	ND	ND	342	69	2,230
United States	2010	313,847,000	47,310	ND	ND	1,132.5	89.6	179,361

CAPD, Continuous ambulatory peritoneal dialysis; DRC, Democratic Republic of Congo; GNI, gross national income; HD, hemodialysis; ND, no data; SLANH, Sociedad Latinoamericana de Nefrología e Hipertensión.
From Swanepoel CR, Wearne N, Okpechi IG. Nephrology in Africa—not yet Uhuru. Nat Rev Nephrol 9:610-622, 2013.)

epidemics in Zimbabwe in 2008 to 2009 highlighted this problem, which coincided with significant deterioration in the social services and infrastructure of the country, with deteriorating food and water supplies after economic and political crises. Health care provision was hampered and, consequently, more than 3000 people died. Refugees from this cholera epidemic ensured that the epidemic spread regionally, although the health care system in South Africa limited deaths in that country.[10] Diarrhea-causing rotavirus has been identified as a leading cause of preventable mortality and morbidity in children in Africa.[11] HIV-infected patients also frequently present with gastrointestinal disease, which results in marked fluid loss. In a case-control study, Moshabela and colleagues found that the clinical and social determinants of diarrheal illness in a rural HIV/AIDS clinic in South Africa were related to female gender, older age, limited access to water, and pre-ART status.[12] A study of 400 consecutive patients with HIV infection in Nigeria revealed that hyponatremia occurred in 74%, hypokalemia in 11%, and hyperkalemia in 5.6%.[13] Hyponatremia, hypokalemia, hyperkalemia, and acidosis were the major abnormalities in HIV-infected individuals who had never received ART.[14] This pattern persists in Africa. In the era of highly active antiretroviral therapy (HAART), the most frequent abnormalities reported were hyperuricemia (41.3%), hypophosphatemia (17.2%), and low bicarbonate levels (13.6%); hypocalcemia was present in 9.2% of those with a CD4 count below $200/mm^3$.

Protease inhibitor therapy was a significant risk factor for hyperuricemia, whereas non-nucleoside reverse transcriptase inhibitors were associated with less hyperuricemia.[15] In a randomized trial and longitudinal study of first-line therapy in HIV-infected adults in South Africa in 2011, female gender, increased body mass index (BMI), and use of stavudine (d4T) were confirmed as contributing to and increased risk of developing lactic acidosis.[16,17] In a longitudinal study of 9040 HIV-infected individuals, stavudine was demonstrated to be associated with lactic acidosis.[17] Fanconi's syndrome, presence of a hyperchloremic nonanion gap metabolic acidosis, hypokalemia, hypophosphatemia, glucosuria, and proteinuria have been described in a patient secondary to the use of tenofovir.[18] Functional adrenal insufficiency resulting in hyponatremia, hyperkalemia, acidosis, and hypotension has also been described in African patients with advanced HIV disease.[19] Hyperkalemia related to trimethoprim-sulfamethoxazole (cotrimoxazole) has been widely described and is frequently seen in HIV-positive patients, but its prevalence in Africa has not been reported.

Although the spectrum of electrolyte, acid-base, and water balance disorders is wide, the limitations or absence of laboratory services, especially in rural areas, make diagnosis difficult. Self-prepared oral solutions may be all the therapy that is available in many areas.[20] Nathoo and associates[21] described a range of electrolyte abnormalities—particularly hypokalemia and acidosis—in Zimbabwean children treated for dehydration with a simple, self-prepared, salt-sugar solution. They recommended potassium-containing World Health Organization (WHO) oral rehydration solution as the preferred rehydration solution. Changes to oral rehydration solutions to make them hypo-osmolar have been promoted. A reduced-osmolarity WHO oral rehydration solution has been associated with less vomiting, less stool output, and reduced need for unscheduled intravenous infusions in comparison with standard oral rehydration solution in infants and children with noncholera diarrhea.[22]

ACUTE KIDNEY INJURY

Treatment of acute kidney injury (AKI) is challenging in Africa because of the burden of disease (especially HIV-related AKI in sub-Saharan Africa, diarrheal disease, malaria, and nephrotoxins), late presentation of patients to health care facilities, and lack of resources in many countries to support patients with established AKI. The causes of AKI in Africa differ from those in more industrialized countries; nephrotoxins, infections, and obstetric and surgical complications are major causes of AKI in most parts of Africa.[23] On the basis of sporadic regional publications, the annual incidence has been estimated as 150 per million population (pmp).[24]

MAJOR CAUSES OF ACUTE KIDNEY INJURY, BY REGION

The major causes of AKI in Africa were determined from a survey of colleagues in nephrologic practice in different regions in Africa and are presented in Table 78.2.[23] Infections (e.g., malaria, HIV, diarrheal diseases), nephrotoxins, obstetric complications, and surgical complications were reported as the major causes in all regions. This pattern has not changed substantially from published literature of the previous 4 decades.[24] Medical causes were the dominant cause of AKI, occurring in 65% of patients in Durban, South Africa, followed by gynecologic (17%), surgical (10%), and obstetric (7.3%) causes; the overall mortality rate was 35%.[25] The most common cause was nephrotoxins, mainly herbal remedies. A subsequent study in the period from 1986 to 1988 from the same region revealed that sepsis replaced nephrotoxins as the predominant cause of AKI.[26] In a 5-year audit of 45 patients, Okunola and colleagues described sepsis (35.5%), pregnancy-related events (22.2%), and toxin nephropathy as the major causes of AKI in Nigeria.[27] Factors limiting the outcomes of AKI are late referral, severity of AKI, and financial constraints[28]

ACUTE KIDNEY INJURY IN HUMAN IMMUNODEFICIENCY VIRUS INFECTION

AKI is a common complication in ambulatory HIV-infected patients compared with uninfected patients, with an odds ratio of 2.82 for those treated with ART and 4.62 in the pre-HAART era.[29] Patients hospitalized with complications of HIV may be at increased risk of AKI that develops in relation to volume depletion, hemodynamic stress, infections, malignancy, and administration of nephrotoxic medication or radiocontrast material. HIV-related renal disease can manifest as AKI or CKD or as AKI superimposed on CKD. AKI in hospitalized HIV-infected patients who have never received ART is associated with a sixfold higher risk of in-hospital mortality. The most important risk factors include severe levels of immunosuppression (CD4 count < 200 cells/mm^3) and opportunistic infection. The most common causes are acute tubular necrosis and thrombotic microangiopathy. After initiation of ART, HIV-infected patients with AKI still have an increased risk of in-hospital mortality, and episodes of AKI seem to be more frequent in the first year of ART. In such patients, AKI has been associated with infection, antibiotics, and antifungal agents. Risk factors are low CD4 count, co-infection with hepatitis C, acute or chronic liver injury, diabetes mellitus, and underlying CKD. Kidney injury related to ART occurs in less than 10% of patients.[29]

Data on AKI with HIV infection in developing countries are emerging. According to a survey of patients referred to the acute renal service at Johannesburg Hospital, Johannesburg, South Africa, over a 1-year period from November 2005 to October 2006, 101 of 700 patients (14.8%) were HIV-positive, with a mean age of 38 years. Sepsis was the cause of AKI in 60% of the HIV-positive patients. Mortality occurred in 44% of the HIV-positive patients and 47% of a control group of HIV-negative patients. Hyponatremia ($P = 0.018$), acidosis ($P = 0.018$), anemia ($P = 0.019$), and

Table 78.2 Most Common Causes of Acute Kidney Injury in Africa, by Region*

Region	Country	Causes
North Africa	Algeria, Egypt, Morocco	Toxins, surgery, obstruction, infection
West Africa	Cameroon, Cote d'Ivoire, Nigeria, Senegal, Democratic Republic of Congo	Infection or malaria, toxins, obstetric complications
East Africa	Burundi, Rwanda, Ethiopia, Eritrea, Sudan	Infection or malaria, toxins, surgery or trauma
Southern Africa	South Africa, Mozambique, Zambia, Zimbabwe, Malawi	Infection or malaria, toxins, obstetric complications

*We thank our colleagues who contributed information reported in Table 78.2: Dr. M. Soliman (Egypt), Dr. F. Haddoum (Algeria), Dr. G. Ashuntantang (Cameroon), Dr. D. Gnionsahe (Cote d'Ivoire), Dr. E. Bamgboye (Nigeria), Dr. A. Niang (Senegal), Dr. M. Ntseka (Democratic Republic of Congo), Dr. A. Twahir (Kenya), Dr. J. Ntarindwa (Rwanda), Dr. R. Nkurunziza (Burundi and Mozambique), Dr. D. Windus (Eritrea), Dr. C. E. Ndhlovu (Zimbabwe), Dr. J. Chabu (Zambia), and Dr. D. Namarika (Malawi).

hyperphosphatemia ($P = 0.003$) were predictors of mortality in HIV-positive patients with AKI.[30] A 5-year study of 117 HIV-positive patients with AKI in Cape Town showed that sepsis was present in over 50% of patients at presentation. Acute tubular necrosis was diagnosed in 58%; mortality occurred in 41%.[31] In our experience, hospitalized patients in South Africa are at advanced stages of immunosuppression; many cases of AKI are prerenal due to volume loss, which implies that with aggressive and appropriate management, the AKI is potentially reversible, even if patients have an underlying chronic component. This concept is critical for physicians who manage patients in regions where access to intensive or high-care units and acute dialysis is limited or unavailable.

Glomerular disease in HIV-infected patients can also manifest as AKI and may be the underlying condition on which an additional acute insult has precipitated a decline in kidney function. Herbal toxin ingestion, sepsis, or severe gastroenteritis with dehydration commonly results in AKI in our experience.

ACUTE KIDNEY INJURY AND TOXINS

Among the nephrotoxic agents encountered in some African countries, especially in East Africa and the Maghreb, are some hair dye preparations that contain paraphenylenediamine. Some of these hair dyes are added to henna, which is a traditional cosmetic agent applied to the upper and lower limbs to increase its skin staining effect. Paraphenylenediamine can be absorbed through the skin, but more severe intoxication is produced by ingestion of the hair dye, mostly in suicide attempts.[32] In addition to acute tubular necrosis, AKI can be caused by rhabdomyolysis and hemoglobinuria, which occur with paraphenylenediamine poisoning. A cohort study of 315 patients was reported in 2006[33]; the mean age was 23 ± 9 years, with a clear female predominance. In 93.3% of cases, the intoxication was caused by a suicide attempt. Mortality occurred in 47% and resulted from other manifestations of the poisoning—namely, angioedema, which occurs early, and arrhythmias caused by direct cardiotoxicity of the chemical.[32] There is no known antidote. Accordingly, immediate dialysis is recommended to remove the toxin.

Plant toxins may cause AKI when they are used as traditional medicines. A common nephrotoxic plant is impila (ox-eye daisy; *Callilepis laureola*), found in South Africa, Democratic Republic of Congo, Zimbabwe, and Zambia.[34,35] Other identified plant toxins are fava beans, poisonous mushrooms, and *Euphorbia matabelensis*, a shrub. Nephrotoxicity can occur because of direct renal injury with acute tubular necrosis and acute interstitial nephritis or by indirect mechanisms, such as intravascular hemolysis and dehydration that results from diarrhea.

Animal toxins are a major cause of AKI in Africa. Snakebites cause AKI secondary to systemic manifestations, which include intravascular hemolysis, hypotension, blood hyperviscosity, myoglobinuria, and hemorrhage. Snake venom can produce various renal lesions such as acute tubular necrosis, cortical necrosis, acute interstitial nephritis, and diffuse proliferative glomerulonephritis (GN). Scorpion stings cause AKI in some patients as a result of disseminated intravascular coagulation and hemorrhage.

PREGNANCY-RELATED ACUTE KIDNEY INJURY

Obstetric AKI has become rare in industrialized countries, whereas it continues to be a frequent clinical problem in many African countries, mainly secondary to preeclampsia and eclampsia (74.5%), septic conditions (11%), and obstetric hemorrhage (7.2%).[36] Dialysis was required for this clinical condition in 75% of patients. In Morocco, pregnancy-related AKI occurred in the third trimester in 66.6% and postpartum in 25% of patients. Preeclampsia and hemorrhagic shock (25%) were reported as the major causes of AKI.[37] Hemodialysis was required in 16.2% of the patients. Poor prognosis was related to age older than 38 years and advanced stage, according to the RIFLE criteria (*r*isk, *i*njury, *f*ailure, *l*oss, *e*nd-stage kidney disease). In a retrospective study of patients admitted to an ICU for eclampsia in Nigeria over a 42-month period from 2001 to 2005, Okafor and Efetie found a case-fatality rate of 29%, with 9.1% deaths related to AKI.[38] The incidence of eclampsia was inversely related to good antenatal care, standard of living, and literacy rate. During a prospective study of 178 consecutive women with eclampsia in Morocco, Mjahed and associates[39] found that the incidence of AKI (serum creatinine concentration >140 µmol/L) was 25.8%. Dialysis was needed in one third of patients, and mortality rates were higher among patients with AKI than those without AKI (32.6% vs. 9.1%). Randeree and coworkers found that pregnancy-related disorders were responsible for 16% of all cases of AKI that necessitated dialysis from 1990 to 1992 in South Africa, with the major causes being preeclampsia or eclampsia, septic abortion, and herbal toxins; maternal mortality was reported to be 5%.[40]

ACUTE KIDNEY INJURY IN THE INTENSIVE CARE UNIT

There are no prospective studies available that compare the outcomes of AKI in HIV-infected patients to those of uninfected patients admitted to an intensive care unit (ICU). Meyers and Bonegio reported on risk factors and mortality in patients who required dialysis for AKI in an ICU in Johannesburg, South Africa, in three cohorts—1968 to 1972 (110 patients), 1975 to 1984 (520 patients), and 1998 to 1999 (335 patients).[41] Incidence of AKI was calculated as 48 pmp/year. Mortality rates were 32% among medical patients, 84% among surgical patients, and 36% among obstetric patients; among patients with septic abortions, the mortality rate was 75%. The overall mortality rate among ICU patients was 73%, in comparison with 27% among non-ICU patients with AKI. Ezekiel and associates[42] reported on outcomes of 174 patients undergoing dialysis for AKI in the ICU in Johannesburg from January 2003 to December 2004; 53% of patients supported by continuous venovenous hemodialysis died, in comparison with 38% of those treated with intermittent hemodialysis. This outcome likely reflects the greater severity of illness in the former group. In a single-center cohort study over 12 months at Tygerberg hospital in Cape Town, AKI was associated with a high mortality and longer duration of stay in ICU, higher APACHE (Acute Physiology and Chronic Health Evaluation) score, and need for mechanical ventilation.[43] The need for dialysis and multiorgan failure were indicators of a higher mortality rate. In a modern, single-center trauma unit in Johannesburg, a retrospective study of 64 patients with severe trauma (burns, penetrating and blunt trauma) requiring dialysis has shown that mortality in trauma patients with AKI was high, with the highest being in burn patients (84%). This study showed that survival was not related to any of the published risk factors (e.g., trauma scores [Revised Trauma Score, Injury Severity Score], APACHE II, age, duration of dialysis) in patients requiring hemodialysis for AKI.[44]

THERAPY FOR ACUTE KIDNEY INJURY

Prevention of AKI is vital because many countries in Africa are not able to provide RRT. Education regarding the avoidance of nephrotoxins, prompt treatment of infections, and fluid replacement are important facets of therapy. If basic health care services are underdeveloped, treatment of reversible AKI may be delayed. Such a delay often leads to severe kidney injury and death. Most patients who are supported with dialysis undergo hemodialysis; acute peritoneal dialysis is provided in a few countries, especially for children, currently the focus of the International Society of Nephrology (ISN) *Saving Young Lives* project. Continuous RRT (when available) and sustained low-efficiency dialysis (SLED) are provided for ICU patients who are hemodynamically unstable. Many dialysis technologies are, however, not available in most countries, and only a few people in Africa can afford RRT. Mortality caused by AKI is therefore very high, ranging from 13.3% to 79.8% (compared with 12.1% for hospitalized AKI patients in the United States).[8]

CHRONIC KIDNEY DISEASE

GLOMERULAR FILTRATION RATE ESTIMATION

There are no reliable statistics in most African countries because of the lack of renal registries. The lack of reporting is further complicated by the controversies in the tools used to diagnose CKD. One study found that the CKD-EPI (Epidemiology Collaboration) equation with the correction factor for ethnicity was more accurate than the Cockcroft-Gault and Modification of Diet in Renal Disease (MDRD) equations in estimating the prevalence of CKD in a population of mixed ancestry.[45] Van Deventer and coworkers have reported that the MDRD formula without the ethnicity factor and the Cockcroft-Gault with correction for bias can be used to assess CKD prevalence in black African patients.[46] Similarly, MDRD-eGFR (estimated glomerular filtration rate) calculated without the African American correction factor improved GFR prediction in African CKD patients in Durban, South Africa.[47]

PREVALENCE OF CHRONIC KIDNEY DISEASE

There is a general impression that CKD is at least three to four times more frequent in Africa than in more industrialized countries; this is substantiated by analysis of the causes of death, which revealed that uremia accounted for 1% to 1.5% of total annual deaths among Egyptians, both in the predialysis era and for 2 decades thereafter.[48] It has been estimated that death from renal disease is in the range of 200 pmp.[49] Figure 78.2 shows the incidence and prevalence of ESKD globally and in some sub-Saharan countries.[50]

CAUSES OF CHRONIC KIDNEY DISEASE

In the North African countries of Morocco, Libya, Tunisia, Egypt, and Algeria, which share similar sociodemographic features, Barsoum, in direct contact with nephrologists from these countries, has found that glomerulonephritis, diabetes, hypertensive nephrosclerosis, chronic interstitial nephritis, and polycystic kidney disease accounted for 9% to 20%, 11% to 18%, 10% to 35%, 7% to 17%%, and 2% to 3%, respectively, of the causes of CKD. Diabetes has become more common than the glomerulonephritides.[51] In a cross-sectional study in the Democratic Republic of the Congo, one in three at-risk persons was reported as having CKD.[52] In a single center in Sudan, the vast majority of ESKD patients on dialysis had an unknown cause for their renal failure. It was speculated that the cause in patients younger than 40 years was glomerular disease; patients between the ages of 40 and 60 years had hypertension listed as the cause, and in patients older than 60 years, the cause was most likely obstructive uropathy. However, in 53.6% of patients, the cause of ESKD was listed as unknown.[53]

A South African study of 1126 patients described the main clinical presentations as chronic renal failure in 37.9%, nephrotic syndrome in 16.7%, hypertension in 13.2%, and abnormal urinary findings in 10.5%. Renal biopsy revealed focal segmental glomerulosclerosis in 3.8%, minimal change in 1.9%, membranoproliferative disease in 3%, and membranous glomerular disease in 2.3%. Hypertension was suspected to be the cause in 51.2% of patients with CKD.[54]

Even though adult polycystic kidney disease has been described in West and East Africa, it is grossly underreported in Africa. In Senegal, the prevalence of autosomal dominant polycystic kidney disease (ADPKD) has been reported to be as high as 1 in 250. Age and GFR were identified as the major risk factors for hypertension in these patients.[55,56] A new *PKD1* mutation has been described in Senegal, a deletion-insertion mutation. Molecular testing found a deletion of two nucleotides, A and C, at positions 7290 and 7291, followed by the insertion of five base pairs (CTGCA) located on exon 18 of the *PKD1* gene.[57]

The reported annual incidence of new patients with CKD ranges between 34 and 200 pmp in North Africa.[58] CKD is prevalent in Nigeria, accounting for 8% to 12% of hospital admissions.[59] CKD affects mainly adults aged 20 to 50 years in sub-Saharan Africa and is primarily secondary to hypertension and glomerular diseases. In industrialized countries, in contrast, CKD manifests in middle-aged and older patients and is predominantly secondary to diabetes mellitus and hypertension.[60-64]

HYPERTENSION

The South African Demographic Health Survey of more than 13,000 adults in 1998 showed that the prevalence of hypertension was 21.3% among adults of both genders, according to WHO/International Society of Hypertension criteria. In addition, hypertension in South Africans was characterized by poor rates of awareness of the diagnosis and

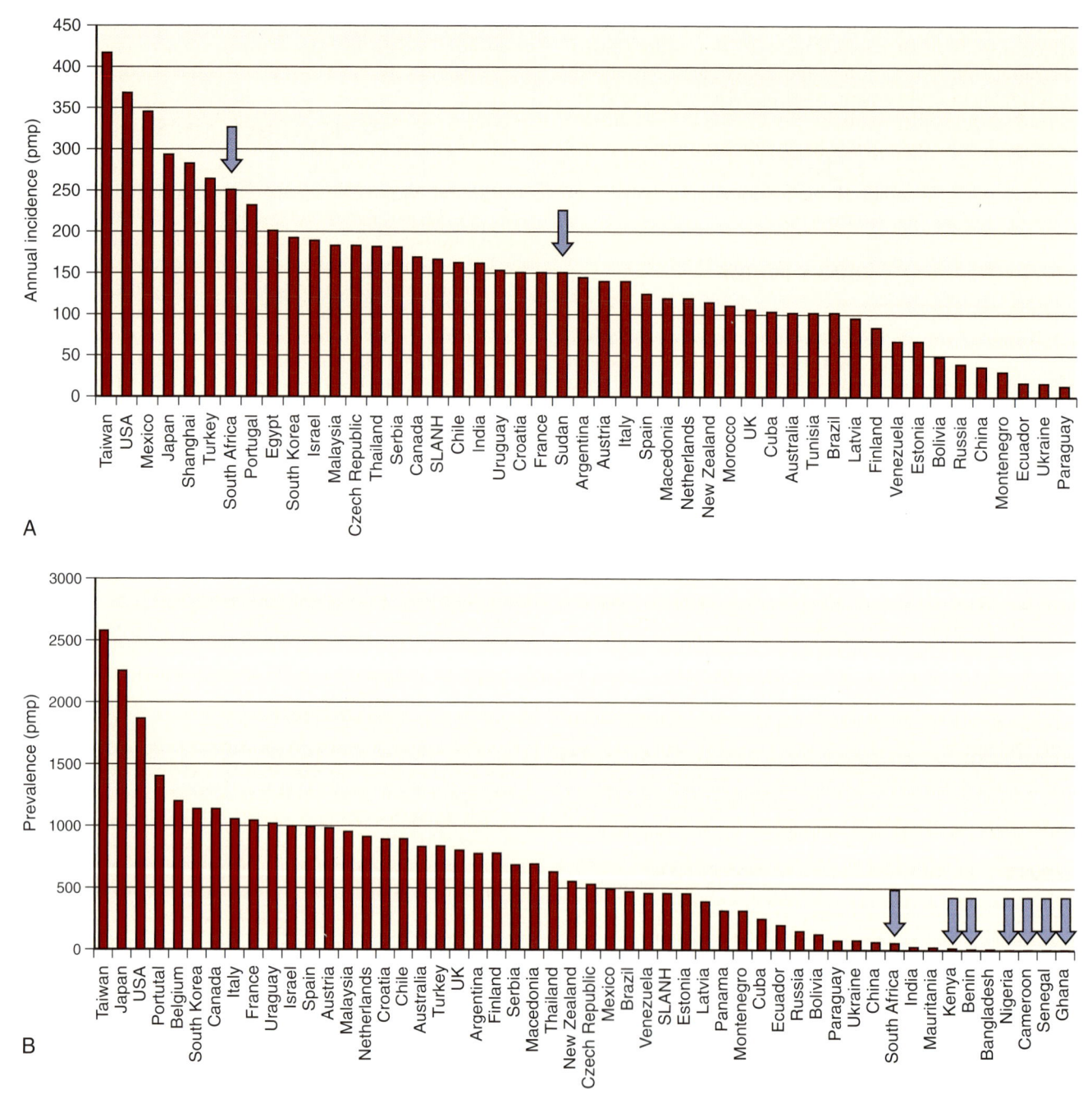

Figure 78.2 A, B, Incidence and prevalence of end-stage kidney disease worldwide.

even poorer rates of adequate blood pressure control; fewer than 50% of patients were receiving treatment, and fewer than one third of those were achieving adequate control.[65] Edwards[66] reported on blood pressure (BP) control of about 12,000 patients with hypertension who consulted with 3503 private practice physicians in South Africa. All patients were covered by medical health insurance. The proportion with adequate BP control (BP < 140/90 mm Hg) was only 34.7%. Connor and colleagues[67] reported on 9731 persons, 30 years of age or older, who sought private sector primary health care services; the overall hypertension prevalence rate was 55%—59% in black Africans, 55% in Indians, and 50% in whites. Uncontrolled hypertension (>140/90 mm Hg) was present in 47%. Hendricks and associates[68] carried out four cross-sectional household surveys in Kwara State, Nigeria; Nandi district, Kenya; Dar es Salaam, Tanzania; and Greater Windhoek, Namibia, between 2009 and 2011. They sampled 5500 households and 7568 individuals older than 18 years. The prevalence of hypertension was 19.3% in rural Nigeria, 21.4% in rural Kenya, 23.7% in urban Tanzania, and 38.0% in urban Namibia. Control of hypertension ranged from 2.6% in Kenya to 17.8% in Namibia. Obesity prevalence (BMI > 30) ranged from 6.1% (Nigeria) to 17.4% (Tanzania).

The Birth-to-Ten study (a birth cohort study that was initiated in Johannesburg, Soweto, in 1990) reported that 11.6% of children aged 5 years had significant hypertension (BP ≥ 115/74 mm Hg but <124/84 mm Hg), with substantial variation among ethnic groups: 12.5% black; 10.5% Indian, and 0% white. Severe hypertension (≥124/84 mm Hg) was observed in 10.7%. Levitt and coworkers[69] showed that the systolic BP of the children at age 5 years was inversely related to birth weight independent of current weight, height, gestational age, or socioeconomic status. The highest level of systolic BP at 5 years was found in children who had a low birth weight and who had gained the most weight since birth.

The Kenyan Luo migration study of Poulter and colleagues[70] was the first to show that migration of people living in traditional rural villages on the northern shores of Lake Victoria to the urban settings of Nairobi was associated with an increase in BP. The urban migrants had higher body weight, pulse rate, and urinary sodium/potassium ratio than those who remained in the rural areas, implying that weight gain and increased dietary sodium are important factors in the pathogenesis of hypertension associated with urbanization.

Hypertension is an important association with CKD in Africa; it has been listed as the cause of CKD in 25% of ESKD cases in Senegal, 29.8% in Nigeria, 45.6% in South Africa, and 48.7% in Ghana, especially in black patients.[71] Prevalence studies in the adult black population of Natal, South Africa, have shown that hypertension is present in 25% of urban Zulus (a black South African ethnic group), 17.2% of whites, and 14% of Indians.[72] The clinical pattern of severe uncontrolled hypertension in hospitalized patients takes a rapid course, with uremia and death, frequently from cerebral hemorrhage. Malignant hypertension is an important cause of morbidity and mortality among urban black South Africans; hypertension accounts for 16% of all hospital admissions and, untreated, they had a 5-year survival of about 1%. Hypertension affects about 25% of the adult population and is listed as the cause of ESKD in 21% of patients receiving RRT in the South African registry report.[73] Hypertension was the most common reported cause of ESKD, accounting for 34.6% of cases of ESKD in black South Africans. In a study to determine the pathologic basis of ESKD in black South Africans, Gold and colleagues[74] reported that essential malignant hypertension was the most common cause, occurring in 49% of patients with ESKD. In a 6-year study of 3632 patients with ESKD, based on statistics from the South African Dialysis and Transplantation Registry, hypertension was reported to be the cause of ESKD in 4.3% of white patients, 34.6% of black patients, 20.9% of patients of mixed ancestry, and 13.8% of Indians. Among patients with essential hypertension, 15.9% developed ESKD and, in 57% of these, it was associated with malignant hypertension.[75]

Hypertensive nephropathy is viewed as the major cause of ESKD in many other parts of Africa. In a 10-year study of 368 patients with CKD in Nigeria, the cause was undetermined in 62%. Of the remaining patients for whom the cause was ascertained, hypertension accounted for 61%, diabetes mellitus for 11%, and chronic GN for 5.9%.[76] CKD accounted for 10% of all medical admissions in that study. ESKD accounted for 24% of medical admissions in most major referral hospitals in Nigeria; hypertension and chronic GN were the leading causes of CKD in all centers, and diabetic nephropathy was the third most common cause.

GLOMERULONEPHRITIS

Glomerular disease is common in Africa and is a significant cause of ESKD, according to reports from North Africa[77] and sub-Saharan Africa.[78-80] Reports from different areas of Africa have elaborated differences in the prevalence of patterns of glomerular injury. For example, in Nigerian children with nephrotic syndrome, membranoproliferative patterns predominate, whereas in series from South Africa, focal segmental glomerulosclerosis (FSGS) seems to be most common.[81,82] Similarly, the incidence of several infections known to be associated with glomerular disease varies across Africa. Quartan malaria in association with nephrotic syndrome has been reported primarily in children from areas in West Africa, where infection with *Plasmodium malariae* is endemic.[83,84] Although epidemiologic data from many regions in Africa are sparse, the incidence of glomerular disease, particularly nephrotic syndrome, seems to be many times higher in Africa than elsewhere in the world.[85] Furthermore, Africans, even after they have left the continent, seem to have more aggressive disease, with poor outcomes. The most common glomerular diseases in Africa reflect the high burden of infectious diseases on the continent. From north to south, biopsy series results are dominated by diseases such as schistosomiasis, hepatitis B and C, malaria, HIV infection and, perhaps most common, poststreptococcal GN.[86-89]

POSTSTREPTOCOCCAL GLOMERULONEPHRITIS

Poststreptococcal GN (PSGN) remains common in several parts of Africa. Although the exact incidence is unknown, it was overwhelmingly the most common cause of acute nephritis in sub-Saharan Africa in series from the middle to late twentieth century.[87-92] Poststreptococcal GN occurs in areas in which infection with *Streptococcus* organisms remains epidemic. This situation is closely linked to socioeconomic factors such as poverty, poor living conditions, and poor access to health care. The association of PSGN with socioeconomic and racial circumstances has been demonstrated starkly in data from apartheid era South Africa.[90,93] During the apartheid era, hospitals were racially segregated; socioeconomic and living conditions of black South Africans were in dire contrast to those of most white communities. Poststreptococcal GN accounted for only 2.5/1000 pediatric admissions to a white hospital versus 10.7/100 pediatric admissions to a black hospital. Today, in contrast, the frequency of PSGN seems to be decreasing in North Africa[91,92,94,95], possibly in relation to general improvements in socioeconomic and health conditions in this area, but PSGN has increased in sub-Saharan Africa in association with the HIV epidemic.

HEPATITIS B VIRUS NEPHROPATHY

Hepatitis B is endemic in many areas of Africa. Glomerular involvement tends to follow the geographic distribution of the virus. Infection acquired perinatally or in childhood may manifest with chronic glomerular disease, often without features of overt liver disease.[91,94] Hepatitis B–related membranous GN was a feature in biopsy series from children in South Africa and Zimbabwe.[96-100] In Nigeria, however, an association with membranoproliferative GN has been described epidemiologically, with few reports of membranous GN.[101] The hepatitis B vaccination program in South Africa has, fortunately, decreased the incidence of this condition.[102]

MALARIA

Malaria is endemic in many areas of Africa. Nephrotic syndrome in association with quartan malaria was reported mostly from Nigeria in the 1970s. However, questions have been raised about the role of malaria in the pathogenesis of this condition, and biopsy series from Nigeria have revealed a decreased prevalence.[103-106] *Plasmodium falciparum* malaria is largely associated with AKI, although glomerular damage may also occur.

SCHISTOSOMIASIS

Schistosomal disease with *Schistosoma haematobium* or *Schistosoma mansoni* is endemic to Egypt and Sudan in particular, but also to several areas of sub-Saharan Africa. Renal failure results predominantly from deposition of ova in the genitourinary system, which causes obstruction. However, these organisms can also cause immune-mediated glomerular disease. Immune complexes containing *S. haematobium* or *S. mansoni* worm antigens may become deposited in the glomeruli, which leads to different patterns of GN, including mesangioproliferative, exudative, and membranoproliferative types, focal segmental sclerosing lesions, or amyloidosis. Exudative lesions occur in the presence of *Salmonella* co-infection. The development of membranoproliferative GN and focal segmental sclerosis correlates with the degree of associated hepatic fibrosis; immunoglobulin A (IgA) appears to play a major role in the pathogenesis of the liver and kidney lesions.[107]

HUMAN IMMUNODEFICIENCY VIRUS–ASSOCIATED RENAL DISEASE

HIV infection is epidemic in sub-Saharan Africa. Although HIV causes renal disease in various ways, HIV-associated glomerular disease is the most common mechanism for ESKD in infected patients. HIV-related glomerular disease has been described in association with various histologic patterns. Gerntholtz and associates[108] described their findings in a retrospective review of biopsy findings in HIV-positive patients obtained over 2 years. Only 27% of the 99 biopsy samples showed classic, HIV-associated nephropathy (HIVAN), and 21% had various forms of immune complex disease without evidence of other infections. A typical ball in cup pattern of basement membrane reaction to immune complexes was described. Of note, in more than half the biopsies, other diagnoses were made, including IgA nephropathy, postinfectious GN, and membranous nephropathy. This adds to the description of the variation in the pattern of HIV-associated GN described previously.[109,110] Wearne and coworkers[111] have described a series of 192 biopsies in HIV-positive individuals in Cape Town; HIVAN was the most common finding, present in 110 biopsies and in combination with immune complex disease in a further 42 biopsies. The authors also described a fetal variant of FSGS in this biopsy series.

Data on the prevalence of HIV-related glomerular disease in Africa are scarce because, in Africa, patients with the disease present late, often requiring dialysis at presentation, and biopsy is not performed. In a study of 615 ART-naive, HIV-positive patients in Durban, South Africa, Han and colleagues[112] prospectively screened for proteinuria, including microalbuminuria, and found that only 6% had persistent proteinuria. Of these patients, 30 consented to renal biopsy, and 25 were found to have HIVAN on histology. In contrast, Emem and associates[13] found evidence of kidney disease as manifested by proteinuria or abnormal serum creatinine level in 38% of 400 consecutive HIV-positive patients. However, biopsies were performed in only 10 patients. Peters and coworkers[113] reported on the effect of ART on renal outcomes in 508 Ugandans over 2 years of follow-up. Baseline data showed that 8% had a serum creatinine concentration higher than 133 µmol/L, and 20% had reduced renal function (creatinine clearance rate = 25 to 50 mL/min). After 2 years of ART, the median serum creatinine concentration decreased by 16%, and the median creatinine clearance rate increased by 21%. The authors suggested that in resource-constrained settings, in which the ability to monitor renal function may be limited, ART could be initiated at standard weight-based dosing regimens and doses adjusted thereafter if kidney function did not improve. Outcomes of ART for 4 to 5 years in 3316 HIV-infected individuals in Zimbabwe and Uganda showed that CKD stage 4 or 5 was present in 2.8% of patients after 4 years.[114]

In a study from Johannesburg, initiation of ART produced rapid and sustained immunologic, clinical, and renal responses, irrespective of histology. The histologic patterns were highly variable, ranging from nonspecific lesions such as mesangial hyperplasia and interstitial nephritis to HIV immune complex disease (HIV-ICD), with or without features of HIVAN; the histologic response to treatment was variable, including no change, progression, and regression of lesions.[115]

The predilection for HIVAN in individuals of African descent has suggested a genetic predisposition; initial studies indicated an association with polymorphisms of *MYH9*, encoding nonmuscle myosin IIA heavy-chain protein on chromosome 22.[116] The identification of a *MYH9* genetic variation as a risk factor for FSGS (both idiopathic and HIV-related) and hypertensive ESKD has suggested a strong genetic link with these conditions in those of African origin. Subsequent studies confirmed that variants of a gene closely associated with *MYH9*, *APOL1*, may contribute to the risk of FSGS and presumed hypertension-related CKD in people of African descent.[117-119] Kopp and colleagues[119] have reported that African Americans carrying two *APOL1* risk alleles had a greatly increased risk for glomerular disease, and *APOL1*-associated FSGS (both related to HIV and idiopathic) occurred earlier and progressed to ESKD more rapidly. A study recently completed in Johannesburg has, for the first time in a South African black population, confirmed the genetics of HIV CKD. *MYH9* risk alleles (E1 haplotypes rs4821480, rs4821481, and rs3752462) were associated with an odds ratio of 2.1 for HIVAN (95% confidence interval [CI], 0.07 to 60.99; $P = 0.67$), whereas in a recessive model, individuals carrying any combination of two *APOL1* risk alleles G1 and G2 had 89-fold higher odds (95% CI, 17.7 to 911.7; $P_{FET} = 1.2 \times 10^{-14}$) of developing HIVAN.[120] Several studies have been published and some are underway surveying the potential contribution of the *APOL1* risk variant to CKD in other regions of Africa as well.[121-123] The relationship between HIVAN and *APOL1*-mediated risk is further highlighted by combined findings of low levels of *APOL1* kidney disease risk alleles and of HIVAN in certain regions of Africa, such as Ethiopia.[123]

NEPHROTIC SYNDROME IN CHILDREN

The incidence of FSGS has been rising globally, particularly in Africa.[82,124-127] The lack of quality pathology services in many parts of Africa also makes assessment of the prevalence of glomerular injury difficult. In two large series, Bhimma and associates[82,128] reviewed the records of 636 children with nephrotic syndrome in Durban, South Africa. They noted striking differences in the patterns of glomerular disease in children of different races in the same area. These patterns included a predominance of steroid-sensitive, minimal change disease in children of Indian origin and a predominance of FSGS lesions in black children. In the few cases of minimal change disease in black children, more than 50% (18 of 32) had steroid-resistant disease. This has led to the practice of treating nephrotic syndrome in Indian and white children with steroids empirically while reserving biopsy for all black children or other children with steroid resistance. Also in this study, 81 of 236 (34.3%) black children had hepatitis B–related disease, but no cases occurred in any other population group. The prevalence of this disease has now regressed following the introduction of hepatitis B vaccination. Thomson[93] reported a similar pattern of biopsy findings in Johannesburg, in which FSGS predominated. Patterns of steroid resistance among black patients are consistent in several areas of the world.[128-130] Although reports of association with steroid resistance and various mutations in podocyte proteins are available from Europe, Asia, the Middle East, and North America (where African American patients are included), there are few data from Africa.[29,130] However, Thomson did confirm the presence of congenital nephrotic syndrome in African infants.[93]

OTHER DISORDERS RELATED TO GLOMERULONEPHRITIS

Although previously thought to be uncommon, several more recent reports have indicated that lupus nephritis occurs more commonly than previously reported throughout Africa.[131-135] Lupus nephritis occurred in 13% of all patients with GN in Tunisia[134] and in 39% of all patients with secondary GN in Cape Town.[35] Among people with proliferative lupus nephritis, cumulative event-free survival rates (with a composite end point of doubling of serum creatinine level, ESKD, or death) were 54%, 34%, and 27% at 1, 10, and 15 years, respectively.[135] Reports of IgA nephropathy, however, remain uncommon in sub-Saharan Africa.[136-138]

DIABETIC NEPHROPATHY

Diabetes mellitus represents one of the most daunting health care challenges today. The number of patients with diabetes mellitus worldwide is currently estimated to be about 135 million; this number is expected to rise to about 300 million by 2025. The main reasons for this increase are population aging, unhealthy diets, obesity, and sedentary lifestyle. Although the increase in cases will exceed 40% in industrialized countries, it is anticipated to be about 170% in developing countries.[139] The prevalence of diabetes mellitus in Africa is anticipated to rise to 12.7 million by 2025, an increase of 140%.[140]

Diabetes mellitus currently affects 9.4 million people in Africa. The prevalence of diabetic nephropathy in diabetic populations is estimated to be 14% to 16% in South Africa[141], 23.8% in Zambia, 12.4% in Egypt, 9% in Sudan, and 6.1% in Ethiopia. Diabetes accounts for 11% of patients with ESKD in Nigeria[76] and 9% to 15% in Kenya.[142] Only a minority of these patients are offered RRT in public sector dialysis programs in South Africa because of associated comorbid conditions. Most will therefore die from ESKD unless they are able to fund RRT themselves or have health insurance. Afifi and coworkers[143] have described increasing numbers of diabetic patients in ESKD in the Egyptian renal data system. The prevalence of patients with diabetic nephropathy undergoing dialysis increased from 8.9% to 14.5% between 1996 and 2001. This study and others have confirmed the poor rates of survival in Africa among diabetic patients undergoing dialysis.[144]

RENAL DISEASE DUE TO SICKLE CELL ANEMIA
(see also Chapter 33)

The prevalence of sickle cell disease is 2% in West Africa. Renal manifestations of sickle cell disease include renal papillary necrosis, glomerulonephritis, hypertension, and ESKD. U.S. studies have shown that sickle cell disease accounts for less than 1% of patients initiating RRT. A study of adults with sickle cell disease in Nigeria has found that 41.7% had stage 2 CKD and 2.7% had stage 3 CKD; no patients were reported with stage 4 or 5 CKD.[145]

RENAL REPLACEMENT THERAPY

RRT places an unaffordable financial burden on poor countries. The availability of RRT is very limited in much of sub-Saharan Africa because of high costs and shortage of skilled personnel, and these limitations are responsible for the high rates of morbidity and mortality associated with ESKD (Figures 78.3 and 78.4). Most dialysis centers are situated in cities, which places a further burden on many patients who have to travel long distances to a dialysis center. Because of technical and human resource limitations, dialysis is often inefficient; the availability of essential therapy such as erythropoietin is erratic, which results in only partial rehabilitation of patients undergoing chronic dialysis.

In 2011, RRT was accessed by approximately 2,164,000 patients globally but only 19,550 in sub-Saharan Africa; less than 1% of the population of dialysis recipients was from sub-Saharan Africa (Figure 78.5).[146] Most African countries, because they have low-income regions, have a correspondingly poor availability of RRT. The current rate of dialysis treatment ranges from 421 pmp in Egypt to fewer than 20 pmp for most of the rest of Africa (and is zero in many countries of sub-Saharan Africa). The corresponding statistics in industrialized countries are as follows, according to the U.S. Renal Data System report for 2013: 2309 pmp in Japan; 1924 pmp in the United States; 1382 pmp in Mexico; and 871 pmp in the United Kingdom.[147] In-center hemodialysis is the modality for RRT in most African countries. Many patients are undertreated with dialysis; only 20% of

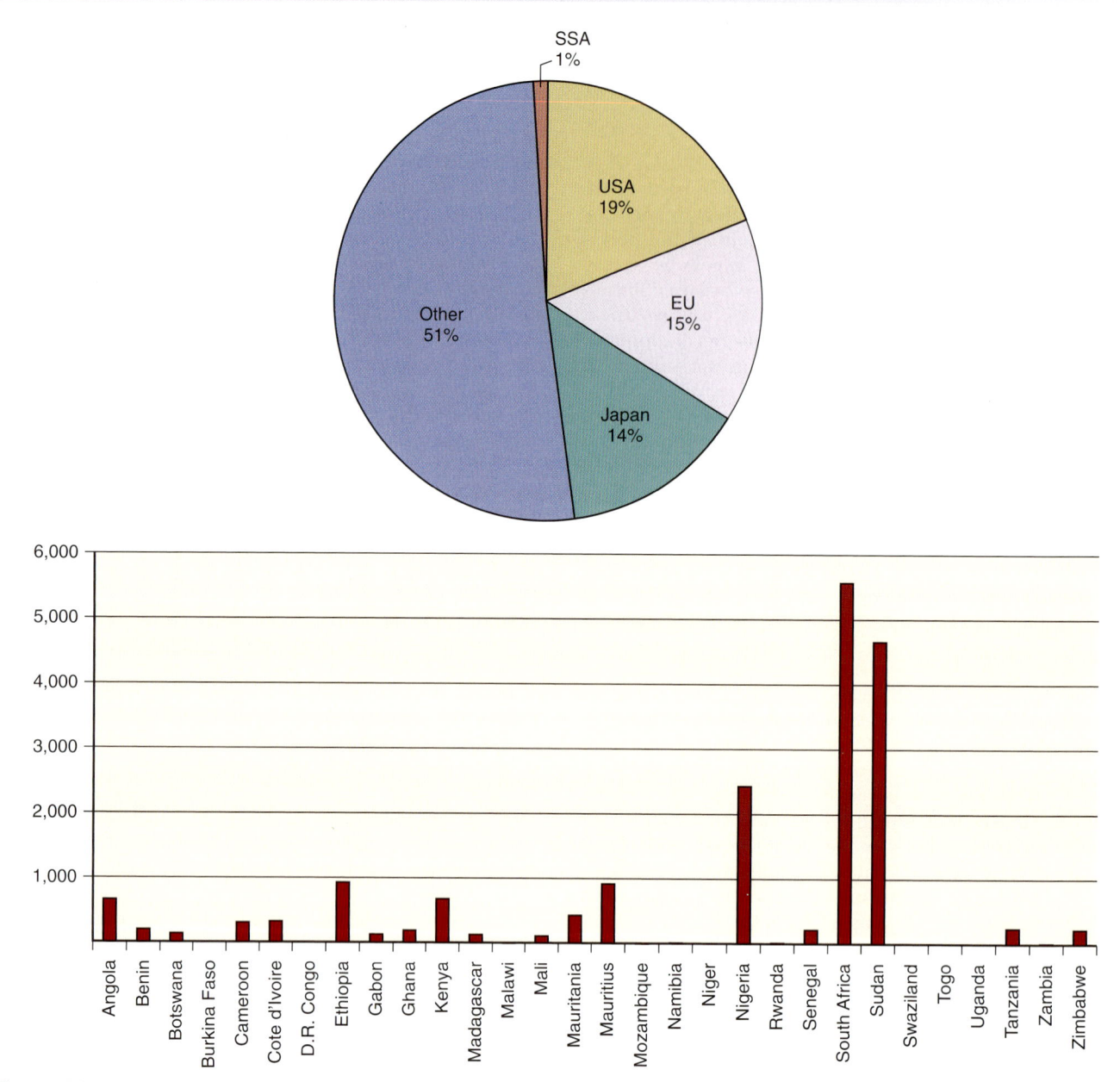

Figure 78.3 **Top panel,** Proportion of reported dialysis patients worldwide by country or geographic region. **Bottom panel,** Reported numbers of dialysis patients by country (or region) in Africa. EU, European Union; SSA, Sub-Saharan Africa.

patients in a Nigerian center could afford to have dialysis three times weekly, and 70% could afford it only once weekly.[148,149]

Rates of patients undergoing dialysis were 133 pmp in South Africa in 2012—two thirds on hemodialysis and one third for continuous ambulatory peritoneal dialysis (CAPD)[150] in comparison with 421 pmp for hemodialysis and 45 pmp for CAPD in Egypt and 650 pmp for hemodialysis and 20 pmp for CAPD in Tunisia.[9] The availability of CAPD is limited in sub-Saharan Africa because of the high cost of dialysis fluids and the perception of a high rate of peritonitis. The average cost of hemodialysis in Africa is US$100/session. The annual cost of CAPD is equivalent to that of in-center hemodialysis.

Transplantation is performed in only a few African countries—South Africa, Kenya, Nigeria, Tunisia, Morocco, and Egypt. Most of the transplants are from living donors, except in South Africa, where deceased donor kidneys are transplanted to a greater extent (80% from deceased donors and 20% from living donors). Deceased donation is hampered in many countries by lack of a legal framework governing brain death and by religious and social constraints; as a result, opportunities for commercial transplantation abound. Thus, transplantation is limited by cost, donor shortages, and lack of a brain death law in most of sub-Saharan Africa. The transplantation rate averages 4 pmp in Africa and 9.2 pmp in South Africa.[9] Funding for RRT is primarily private in much of Africa; the governments of only a few countries (e.g., Mali, Mauritius, South Africa) provide RRT for small numbers of patients. Indigent South Africans are able to access government-provided chronic dialysis only if they are eligible for transplantation. In many African countries, chronic dialysis is not sustainable because patients are unable to afford dialysis beyond the first 2 to 3 months.

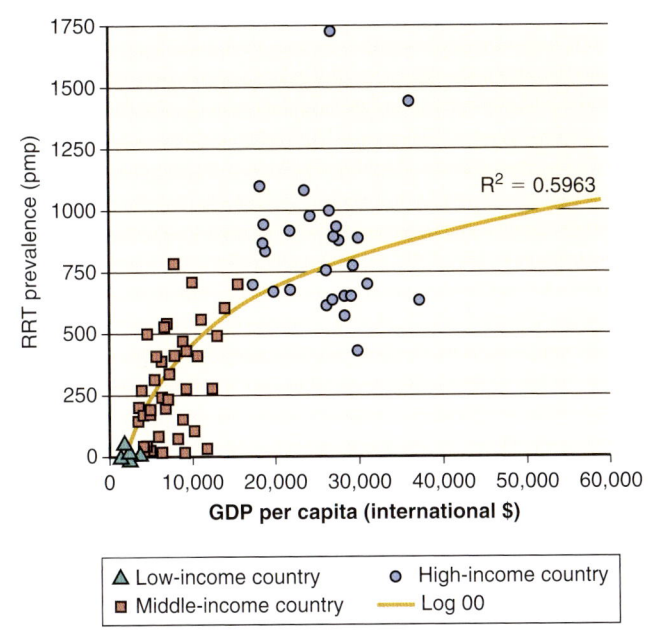

Figure 78.4 RRT prevalence according to gross domestic product (GDP) in different countries. R-squared or coefficient of determination.

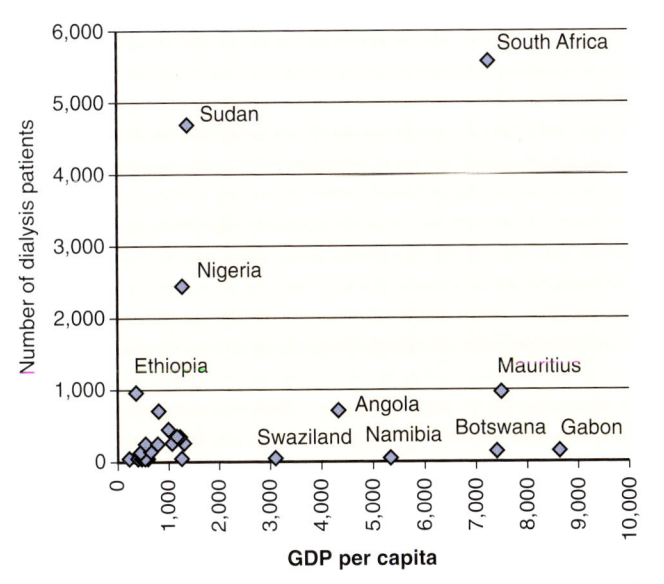

Figure 78.5 Number of dialysis patients versus gross domestic product (GDP) per capita by country.

The reality is that not enough money is available for health care in developing countries, and the provision of RRT is especially challenging in sub-Saharan Africa. The primary goal should be promotion of prevention strategies at all levels of health care in Africa. In countries with a national program for RRT and with appropriate use of donor aid, the goal should be a circumscribed chronic dialysis program, with as short a time on dialysis as possible and increased availability of transplantation (from living related and deceased donors). Patients with renal disease should be referred to a nephrologist at an early stage so that measures to retard progression of disease and plan timely transplantation or dialysis may be instituted; this is particularly important when related donors may be available.

PREVENTION STRATEGIES

Screening programs have been developed in most of Africa. One of the largest is the MaReMar project; 10,524 individuals were screened for CKD and will be followed up over 5 years under the aegis of the Ministry of Health in Morocco, together with the Moroccan Society of Nephrology, WHO, and International Society of Nephrology (ISN). Shortage of health care workers and lack of availability of pharmaceutical agents on a sustained basis to retard progression of CKD are impediments in many African countries. Screening for CKD in populations at high risk (e.g., patients with hypertension, diabetes mellitus, HIV infection, and family history of renal disease) should probably be instituted as the first step in CKD prevention in developing countries, such as those in Africa.[9,71,151] Education of patients and health care workers with regard to hypertension, diabetes, obesity, proteinuria, and health promotion (e.g., prudent diet, cessation of smoking, exercise) is essential. The programs of the ISN and World Kidney Day have heightened awareness of renal disease among medical professionals and the public in developing countries. Efforts should be made to optimize therapy for hypertension, diabetes mellitus, and renal disease. Implementation of recommended targets for control of hypertension and diabetes is essential. In areas with insufficient numbers of physicians, nurses and other health care workers could be trained to manage these conditions at a local level, with clearly defined criteria for referral of patients. Even though there are active screening programs in a few countries in sub-Saharan Africa, which have detected a CKD prevalence of 5% to 33%, based on proteinuria and increased serum creatinine levels, data on the prevention and treatment arms of these programs are not available.

CHALLENGES FOR NEPHROLOGY PRACTICE IN AFRICA

Lack of resources (finances and health care workers) is a major constraint on optimal renal care in many parts of Africa. Although RRT may be available, it is not sustainable for many patients because of lack of funding. Transplantation is not available in many African countries, which also contributes to morbidity in CKD patients. Rationing of services is practiced in many parts of Africa, including South Africa; as a result, only small numbers of patients are selected for RRT.[152] Reliable statistics are not available because renal registries are just beginning to be developed in African countries. Appropriate training and retention of health care workers is a challenge for many African countries. The health status of Africans is intricately woven into their sociopolitical and economic milieu. Ensuring stable societies is crucial to the goal of improved health for all.

CONCLUSION

ESKD is challenging for the physician and a death sentence for most patients in Africa. Provision of RRT is especially daunting in sub-Saharan Africa. Nephrologists and physicians are faced with large numbers of patients with ESKD and inadequate facilities, funding, and support. Increasing disease burdens are predicted as the dual epidemics of HIV and diabetes with hypertension reach their peak in Africa.

Support from the ISN and its global outreach programs have gradually improved the capability of physicians in many African countries to provide renal care. Although prevention strategies are recognized as optimal therapy in managing CKD, they are still underdeveloped in much of Africa, mainly because of the lack of health care workers and funding.

Complete reference list available at ExpertConsult.com.

KEY REFERENCES

1. Population Reference Bureau: *World population data sheet 2013.* Available at: http://www.prb.org/Publications/Datasheets/2013/2013-world-population-data-sheet/data-sheet.aspx. Accessed November 5, 2013.
2. World Health Organization: *Global health observatory, world health statistics, 2013.* Available at: http://www.who.int/gho/mortality_burden_disease/life_tables/situation_trends_text/en. Accessed November 5, 2013.
3. UNAIDS: *Report on the global AIDS epidemic 2013, global fact sheet.* Available at: http://www.unaids.org/en/resources/campaigns/globalreport2013/factsheet. Accessed November 5, 2013.
5. Mayosi BM, Flisher A, Lalloo UG, et al: The burden of non-communicable diseases in South Africa. *Lancet* 374:935–947, 2009.
9. Naicker S: Burden of end-stage renal disease in sub-Saharan Africa. *Clin Nephrol* 74(Suppl 1):13–16, 2010.
19. Meya DB, Katabira E, Otim M, et al: Functional adrenal insufficiency among critically ill patients with human immunodeficiency virus in a resource-limited setting. *Afr Health Sci* 7:101–107, 2007.
22. Hahn S, Kim Y, Garner P: Reduced osmolarity oral rehydration solution for treating dehydration due to diarrhoea in children: systematic review. *BMJ* 323:81–85, 2001.
23. Naicker S, Aboud O, Gharbi MB: Epidemiology of acute kidney injury in Africa. *Semin Nephrol* 28:348–353, 2008.
29. Wyatt CM, Arons RR, Klotman PE, et al: Acute renal failure in hospitalized patients with HIV: risk factors and impact on in-hospital mortality. *AIDS* 20:561–565, 2006.
30. Vachiat AI, Musenge E, Wadee S, et al: Renal failure in HIV-positive patients—a South African experience. *Clin Kidney J* 1–6, 2013.
31. Arendse C, Okpechi I, Swanepoel C: Acute dialysis in HIV-positive patients in Cape Town, South Africa. *Nephrology* 16:39–44, 2011.
37. Arryhani M, El Youbi R, Sqalli T: Pregnancy-related acute kidney injury: experience of the nephrology unit at the University Hospital of Fez, Morocco. *ISRN Nephrol* 2013:109034, 2012.
38. Okafor UV, Efetie RE: Critical care of eclamptics: challenges in an African setting. *Trop Doct* 38:11–13, 2008.
39. Mjahed K, Alaoui SY, Barrou L: Acute renal failure during eclampsia: incidence, risk factors and outcome in intensive care unit. *Ren Fail* 26:215–221, 2004.
43. Friederickson DV, Van der Merwe L, Hattingh L, et al: Acute renal failure in the medical ICU still predictive of high mortality. *S Afr Med J* 99:873–875, 2009.
45. Matsha TE, Yako Y, Rensburg MA, et al: Chronic kidney disease in mixed ancestry population: prevalence, determinants and concordance between kidney function estimators. *BMC Nephrol* 14:75, 2013.
46. Van Deventer HE, George JA, Paiker JE, et al: Estimating glomerular filtration rate in black South Africans by use of the Modification of Diet in Renal Disease and Cockcroft-Gault equations. *Clin Chem* 54:1197–1202, 2008.
47. Madala ND, Nkwanyana N, Dubula T, et al: Predictive performance of eGFR equations in South Africans of African and Indian ancestry compared with ^{99m}Tc-DTPA imaging. *Int Urol Nephrol* 44:847–855, 2012.
50. Jha V, Garcia-Garcia G, Iseki K, et al: Chronic kidney disease: global dimension and perspectives. *Lancet* 382:260–272, 2013.
52. Sumaili EK, Cohen EP, Zinga CV, et al: High prevalence of undiagnosed kidney disease among at-risk populations in Kinshasa, the Democratic Republic of Congo. *BMC Nephrol* 10:18, 2009.
54. van Rensburg BW, van Staden AM, Rossouw GJ, et al: The profile of adult nephrology patients admitted to the Renal Unit of the Universitas Tertiary Hospital in Bloemfontein, South Africa from 1997 to 2006. *Nephrol Dial Transplant* 25:820–824, 2010.
55. Ka EF, Seck SM, Niang A, et al: Patterns of autosomal dominant kidney disease in black Africans. *Saudi J Kidney Dis Transpl* 21:81–86, 2010.
56. Fary Ka E, Seck SM, Niang A, et al: Patterns of autosomal dominant polycystic kidney diseases in black Africans. *Saudi J Kidney Dis Transpl* 21:81–86, 2010.
57. Seck SM, Gueye S, Diouf B: A new PKD-1 mutation discovered in a black African woman with autosomal polycystic kidney disease. *Nephrourol Mon* 5:769–772, 2013.
68. Hendricks ME, Wit FW, Roos MT, et al: Hypertension in sub-Saharan Africa: cross-sectional surveys in four rural and urban communities. *PLoS One* 7:e32638, 2012.
70. Poulter N, Khaw KT, Hopwood BE, et al: The Kenyan Luo migration study: observations on the initiation of a rise in blood pressure. *BMJ* 300:967–972, 1990.
71. Arogundade FA, Barsoum RS: CKD prevention in sub-Saharan Africa: a call for governmental, nongovernmental, and community support. *Am J Kidney Dis* 51:515–523, 2008.
102. Bhimma R, Coovadia HM, Adhikari M, et al: The impact of the hepatitis B virus vaccine on the incidence of hepatitis B virus–associated membranous nephropathy. *Arch Pediatr Adolesc Med* 157:1025–1030, 2003.
107. Barsoum RS: Schistosomiasis and the kidney. *Semin Nephrol* 23:34–41, 2003.
108. Gerntholtz TE, Goetsch SJ, Katz I: HIV-related nephropathy: a South African perspective. *Kidney Int* 69:1885–1891, 2006.
109. D'Agati V, Appel GB: Renal pathology of human immunodeficiency virus infection. *Semin Nephrol* 18:406–421, 1998.
110. Haas M, Kaul S, Eustace JA: HIV-associated immune complex glomerulonephritis with "lupus-like" features: a clinicopathologic study of 14 cases. *Kidney Int* 67:1381–1390, 2005.
111. Wearne N, Swanepoel CR, Boulle A, et al: The spectrum of renal histologies seen in HIV with outcomes, prognostic indicators and clinical correlations. *Nephrol Dial Transplant* 27:4109–4118, 2012.
112. Han TM, Naicker S, Ramdial PK, et al: A cross-sectional study of HIV-seropositive patients with varying degrees of proteinuria in South Africa. *Kidney Int* 69:2243–2250, 2006.
113. Peters PJ, Moore DM, Mermin J, et al: Antiretroviral therapy improves renal function among HIV-infected Ugandans. *Kidney Int* 74:925–929, 2008.
114. Stöhr W, Reid A, Walker AS, et al: Glomerular dysfunction and associated risk factors over 4-5 years following antiretroviral therapy initiation in Africa. *Antivir Ther* 16:1011–1020, 2011.
115. Fabian J, Naicker S, Goetsch S, et al: The clinical and histological response of HIV-associated kidney disease to antiretroviral therapy in South Africans. *Nephrol Dial Transplant* 28:1543–1554, 2013.
116. Kopp JB, Smith MW, Nelson GW, et al: MYH9 is a major-effect risk gene for focal segmental glomerulosclerosis. *Nat Genet* 40:1175–1184, 2008.
117. Genovese G, Friedman DJ, Ross MD, et al: Association of trypanolytic ApoL1 variants with kidney disease in African Americans. *Science* 329:841–845, 2010.
118. Tzur S, Rosset S, Shemer R, et al: Missense mutations in the APOL1 gene are highly associated with end-stage kidney disease risk previously attributed to the MYH9 gene. *Hum Genet* 128:345–350, 2010.
119. Kopp JB, Nelson GW, Sampath K, et al: APOL1 genetic variants in focal segmental glomerulosclerosis and HIV-associated nephropathy. *J Am Soc Nephrol* 2:2129–2137, 2011.
120. Kasembeli AN, Duarte R, Ramsay M, et al: Risk variants are strongly associated with HIV-sssociated nephropathy in black South Africans. *J Am Soc Nephrol* 2015 Mar 18. pii: ASN.2014050469. [Epub ahead of print.]
121. Thomson R, Genovese G, Canon C, et al: Evolution of the primate trypanolytic factor APOL1. *Proc Natl Acad Sci U S A* 111:E2130–E2139, 2014.

122. Ulasi II, Tzur S, Wasser WG, et al: High population frequencies of APOL1 risk variants are associated with increased prevalence of non-diabetic chronic kidney disease in the Igbo people from south-eastern Nigeria. *Nephron Clin Pract* 123:123–128, 2013.
123. Behar DM, Kedem E, Rosset S, et al: Absence of APOL1 risk variants protects against HIV-associated nephropathy in the Ethiopian population. *Am J Nephrol* 34:452–459, 2011.
135. Ayodele OE, Okpechi IG, Swanepoel CR: Long-term renal outcome and complications in South Africans with proliferative lupus nephritis. *Int Urol Nephrol* 45:1289–1300, 2013.
152. Moosa MR, Kidd M: The dangers of rationing dialysis treatment: the dilemma facing a developing country. *Kidney Int* 70:1107–1114, 2006.

79 Near and Middle East

Suheir Assady | Rawi Ramadan | Dvora Rubinger

CHAPTER OUTLINE

ACUTE KIDNEY INJURY, 2469
CHRONIC KIDNEY DISEASE, 2472
Epidemiology, 2472
Causes of Chronic Kidney Disease, 2476
Genetic Disorders, 2476
MANAGEMENT OF END-STAGE KIDNEY DISEASE IN THE MIDDLE EAST, 2486
Dialysis, 2487
Kidney Transplantation, 2489
SUMMARY, 2492

This chapter is a discussion of the epidemiology, causes, predisposing factors, management, and prevention of kidney diseases, and future strategies for dealing with kidney diseases in the Near and Middle East are proposed. The term *Near and Middle East* is a historical, Eurocentric, and Western term that was used to describe a geographic region whose boundary is imprecise and whose internal borders are constantly changing because of political and historical evolution.[1] Therefore the Near and Middle East, hereafter called the *Middle East*, is defined for the purpose of this chapter as the region that encompasses the following 20 countries (in alphabetical order): Algeria, Bahrain, Egypt, Iran, Iraq, Israel, Jordan, Kuwait, Lebanon, Libya, Morocco, Oman, Palestinian Authority, Qatar, Saudi Arabia, Syria, Tunisia, Turkey, the United Arab Emirates (UAE), and Yemen (Figure 79.1).

The Middle East (ME) has always been important for (1) its strategic location as a tricontinental hub that links Asia, Africa, and Europe; (2) its economic resources; and (3) its spiritual significance as the birthplace of the world's three major monotheistic religions: Judaism, Christianity, and Islam. Of the adherents to the three religions, Muslims constitute the largest religious population in the ME; the sizes of the Christian and Jewish populations are smaller and vary from country to country in the ME.[1] Although the ME has several cultural, linguistic, and geographic associations, considerable disparity exists between the different countries in terms of economy, resources, political systems, health care systems and expenditure, and disease incidence and prevalence.

According to data from the World Health Organization (WHO),[2] the estimated population in the 20 ME countries in 2012 was 468,470,000, and the median ages ranged between 19 and 31.5 years (Table 79-1). The gross national income (GNI) per capita varies for each ME country. According to the classification system of the World Bank,[3,4] most ME countries are considered "developing countries." Egypt, Morocco, Syria, Palestinian Authority, and Yemen are considered lower-middle-income countries because the GNI per capita of each is between $1046 and $4125 (USD) per annum, whereas Algeria, Iran, Iraq, Jordan, Lebanon, Libya, Tunisia, and Turkey are considered upper-middle-income countries because the GNI per capita of each is between $4126 and $12,745 per annum. The following countries are considered high-income countries because the GNI per capita of each is more than $12,746 per annum: Bahrain, Israel, Kuwait, Oman, Qatar, Saudi Arabia, and UAE (Figure 79.2). Inevitably, disease incidence, prevalence, course, and outcomes are affected by the different socioeconomic factors and health policies in each country[5-7] (see Figure 79.2). For example, the life expectancy and infant mortality rate in each ME country are concordant with the socioeconomic, political, and health status of that country. The median life expectancy in the 20 ME countries ranges from 58 to 83 years for men and from 66 to 84 years for women. The life expectancy for men is lowest in the low-income ME countries and in countries affected by man-made conflicts (see Table 79.1).

The mortality rate before the age of 5 years in Yemen, the poorest country in the ME, is at least five times higher (60 per 1000 live births) than that in industrialized high-income ME countries (4 to 12 per 1000 live births; see Table 79.1). Also, a health disparity exists among minority populations who live in industrialized ME countries and individuals of ME origin who live in countries that are not in the ME.[7-13] Many developing ME countries have been affected by various types of natural disasters (such as earthquakes, floods, and droughts) and other disasters (such as military conflicts). Casualties, displacement, and migration are significant consequences of such disasters and adversely affect the socioeconomic stratum and health status of a country.[14,15] Therefore many ME countries and their communities need help in upgrading their existing health structures to improve their ability to cope with any future disasters. Consequently, the WHO and national and international nephrology societies, such as the International Society of Nephrology (ISN), have pooled their resources to enhance the resilience of nations to the effects and consequences of disasters.[14,16-19]

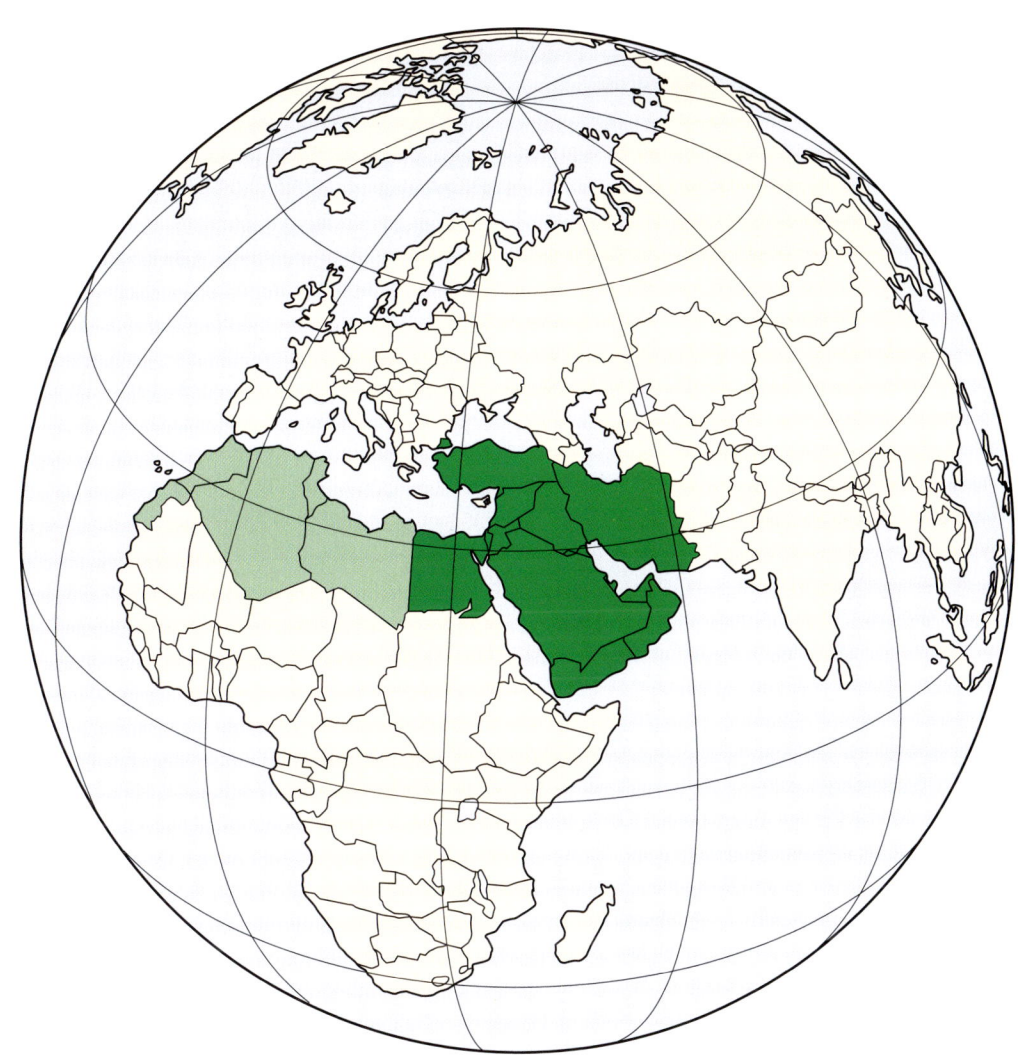

Figure 79.1 Map of Middle Eastern countries. Countries illustrated in *light green* also known as "El Maghreb"; those in *dark green*, as "El Mashreq."[1] (Adapted and modified from a public domain image available at http://en.wikipedia.org/wiki/Middle_East.)

ACUTE KIDNEY INJURY

As in many countries worldwide, data on the incidence and prevalence of acute kidney injury (AKI) in many ME countries are scarce and imprecise because of an inconsistent definition of AKI in medical reports, underreporting, seasonal dependency on the occurrence of AKI, and the frequency and location of natural and human-engendered disasters.[17,20,21] There are large knowledge gaps about the age, number, natural history, and outcome of patients with AKI in either the community or hospitals and about the use of preventive measures in each ME country. Most published reports on AKI in ME countries have concerned a short-term study in a tertiary-level hospital or a single-center study, and of these studies, only a few were of the prospective type. Moreover, the definition of AKI is not consistent in these reports.[22-27] Al-Homrany reported that the incidence of AKI among hospitalized patients was 0.6% in a 2-year prospective study in one hospital in southern Saudi Arabia.[24] Of these cases of AKI, 62% were hospital acquired and 38% were community acquired. In a 1-year retrospective cohort study from a single center in northern Israel, Shema and associates reported that the annual incidence rate of AKI among hospitalized adult patients was 1% to 5.1%, depending on the AKI definition that was used.[25] In a case series study of the ME respiratory syndrome coronavirus outbreak, AKI requiring renal replacement therapy (RRT) was reported in 58% of critically ill patients.[28] This percentage is high, compared to that reported in equivalent critically ill patients who were treated during the severe acute respiratory syndrome epidemic in Canada (5%).[29]

The causes of AKI have changed over time in ME countries. A nationwide prospective study, conducted by the Turkish Society of Pediatric Nephrology Acute Kidney Injury Study Group,[30] demonstrated that the cause of AKI in Turkish pediatric patients has greatly evolved during the last 2 decades. Acute gastroenteritis and acute poststreptococcal glomerulonephritis have decreased significantly as causes of AKI, and prematurity, malignancy, and congenital heart disease have increased. In adults, obstructive uropathy, unspecified postsurgical complications, and crush injury were the most prevalent causes of AKI in Syria during the 1980s, according to Hadidy and colleagues.[22] In contrast,

Table 79.1 Demographics, Health Indicators, and Human Development Index in Middle Eastern Countries and Western Industrialized Countries

Country	Total Population	Median Age (years)	Life Expectancy at Birth (years) Male	Life Expectancy at Birth (years) Female	Rate of Mortality before Age 5 Years (per 1000 Live Births)	Country Ranking in Human Development Index (of 185 Countries)*
Middle Eastern Countries						
Algeria	38,482,000	26.62	71	74	20	93
Bahrain	1,318,000	30.07	78	80	10	48
Egypt	80,722,000	24.93	71	75	21	112
Iran	76,424,000	27.99	72	75	18	76
Iraq	32,778,000	19.5	65	72	34	131
Israel	7,644,000	30.1	80	84	4	16
Jordan	7,009,000	23.6	72	75	19	100
Kuwait	3,250,000	28.95	80	80	11	54
Lebanon	4,647,000	29.4	72	76	9	72
Libya	6,155,000	26.25	58	74	15	64
Morocco	32,521,000	26.7	70	74	31	130
Oman	3,314,000	25.88	70	76	12	84
Palestinian Authority†	4,046,901	NA	71	75	23	110
Qatar	2,051,000	31.64	83	81	7	36
Saudi Arabia	28,288,000	27.03	74	80	9	57
Syria	21,890,000	22.21	73	77	15	116
Tunisia	10,875,000	29.89	74	78	16	94
Turkey	73,997,000	29.04	73	73	14	90
United Arab Emirates	9,206,000	29.37	75	77	8	41
Yemen	23,852,000	18.78	63	66	60	160
Western Countries Industrialized Countries						
Australia	23,050,000	37.08	80	84	5	2
Canada	34,838,000	39.99	80	84	5	11
France	63,937,000	40.43	78	85	4	20
Germany	82,800,000	45.09	78	83	4	5
Italy	60,885,000	43.99	80	85	4	25
Japan	127,000,000	45.53	79	86	3	10
United Kingdom	62,783,000	40.7	79	82	5	26
United States	318,000,000	37.3	76	81	7	3

*Data from the 2013 Human Development Report published for the United Nation Development Programme. Available at: http://hdr.undp.org/sites/default/files/reports/14/hdr2013_en_complete.pdf. Accessed April 5, 2014.
†Data from World Bank: Indicators. Available at: http://data.worldbank.org/indicator. Accessed April 5, 2014.
NA, Not available.
Source data for country profiles from the World Health Organization: Countries. Available at: http://www.who.int/countries/en/. Accessed April 5, 2014.

Said reported findings similar to those from industrialized countries in 215 patients with AKI, whose ages ranged between 12 and 90 years, in three Jordanian hospitals over an 18-month study period.[31] Renal parenchymal disease was the most common cause of AKI (58%), and acute tubular necrosis (ATN) and contrast-induced nephropathy were the two most prevalent causes of renal parenchymal disease. Prerenal causes (28%) and postrenal causes (14%) accounted for the remaining causes of AKI.[31] Of note, obstructive uropathy was a common cause of AKI as a result of the high prevalence of nephrolithiasis in the study patients who originally came from Yemen and Sudan. In another study from one center in Qatar, ATN was reported in 83% of all patients with AKI, who were referred mainly from intensive care units.[32] Al-Homrany[24] reported that ATN resulting from sepsis, ischemia, and rhabdomyolysis, as well as distinctive causes, such as malaria and snakebites (4.6% of all cases), were the major causes of AKI in tropical southern Saudi Arabia.

Malaria is rarely reported as a primary cause of AKI in most ME countries, except for Yemen.[33,34] In the Hajjah and Sanaa regions of Yemen, malaria caused by *Plasmodium falciparum* was the cause of 29% of all cases of AKI.[34] However, prerenal disorders, such as infectious diarrheal diseases, are still the predominant cause of AKI in Yemen because of the tropical climate and poor hygiene. Malarial kidney injury is often a consequence of several hemodynamic, immune, and metabolic disturbances, which may also be accompanied by central nervous system sequelae and by fluid and electrolyte alterations.[35,36] Malarial kidney disease can manifest as AKI in the form of (1) ATN that accompanies or occurs as a complication of severe hemolysis,

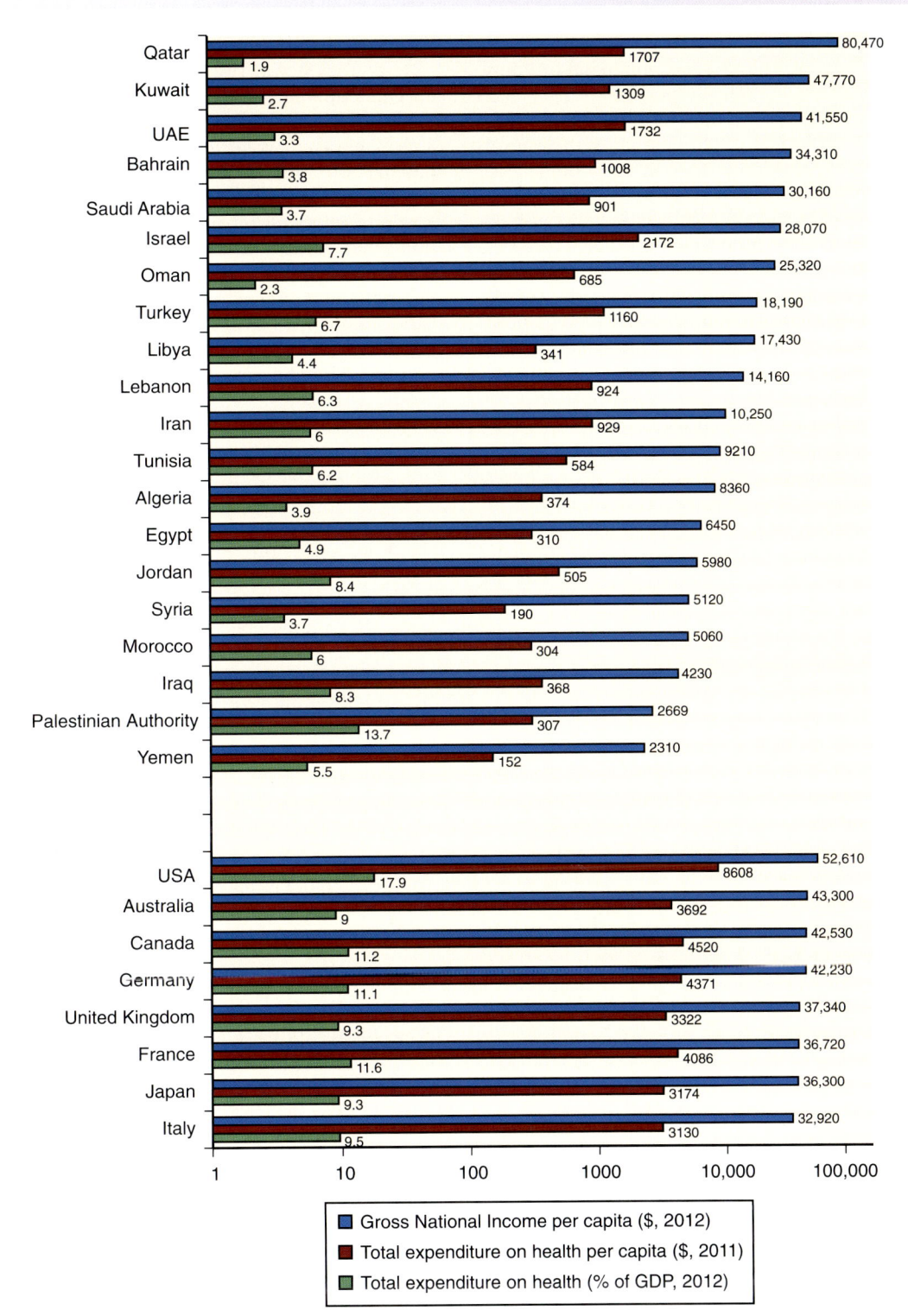

Figure 79.2 Indices of wealth and health care expenditure in the 20 Middle Eastern and selected Western and industrialized countries in 2012. For each country, three indices are presented: gross national income per capita, on a purchasing power parity, expressed in international dollars (*blue bars*); total expenditure on health per capita, expressed in international dollars (*red bars*); and total expenditure on health, expressed as percentages of gross domestic product (GDP) (*green bars*). The upper seven countries are the wealthy high-income Middle East nations. UAE, United Arab Emirates; USA, United States of America. (Data from the World Health Organization: *Countries*. Available at http://www.who.int/countries/en/. Accessed April 5, 2014.)

hemodynamic derangements, and tissue hypoxemia; (2) interstitial nephritis; or (3) glomerular mesangial proliferative lesions with immune complex deposits.[35]

Reporting of the cause of AKI may, however, be biased by the type of referral hospital that documents the various causes. In a retrospective 18-month study from one cancer hospital in the UAE, sepsis and drug-induced nephrotoxicity were the leading causes of AKI because 30% of the patients were immunocompromised and were receiving chemotherapy.[37] Preexisting comorbid conditions, such as diabetes, hypertension, and chronic kidney disease (CKD), were documented in approximately one-third of all patients with AKI in Jordan and the UAE[23,37] and in as many as 87% of all such patients in Qatar.[32] AKI-associated mortality rates range between 18% and 77% in ME countries.[22-25,31,32,37,38] Al-Homrany[24] reported that uncontrolled sepsis and multiorgan failure were the leading causes of death in southern Saudi Arabia. In his study, mortality was associated with advanced age, oliguria, hospital-acquired AKI, the need for dialysis, and hepatic failure.[24]

Devastating earthquakes have struck some ME countries and are a constant threat because their territory encompasses the Great African Rift Valley. In several publications, investigators have described and analyzed the factors that have had major implications for kidney involvement and outcomes in survivors who sustained crush syndrome in catastrophic earthquakes in Turkey and Iran. Crush syndrome often causes profound hypovolemic shock that (1) is complicated and aggravated by gross disorders of acid-base balance and electrolytes, of which hyperkalemia is life-threatening, and (2) increases susceptibility to myoglobinuric AKI. These complications can occur within hours of the initial injury and can lead to early loss of limb or life.[16,39,40] According to data that were collected after the 1999 Marmara earthquake in Turkey and the 2003 Bam earthquake in Iran, the number of casualties, the incidence of crush injury, and the incidence of myoglobinuric AKI are related to several variables, including the following:

1. The intensity of the earthquake and the magnitude of the aftermath.
2. The time of the day that the earthquake happened: The Turkish earthquake occurred during the night and was associated with more crush injuries than earthquakes that have occurred during the day, because the victims were in the supine position.
3. The population density and the type of residential area at the site of the earthquake: The population density in rural areas, where the buildings are single storied and made from light construction materials, is less than that in urban areas, where the buildings may be multistoried and made of heavy construction materials.
4. The climate: Earthquake survivors suffer more volume depletion and dehydration in hot weather than in cold weather.
5. The time to rescue, because it reflects both the amount of time under the rubble and the magnitude of imposed pressure in a given time.
6. The extent of destruction of health care facilities at the site of the earthquake and the distance from referral hospitals.
7. The availability of medical support and the availability and efficiency of rescue teams.
8. The availability of RRT.[16,19,40-42]

An important issue in such disasters is the selection of patients with AKI who need early referral to specialized nephrology facilities. The ISN Renal Disaster Relief Task Force in cooperation with European Renal Best Practice published comprehensive clinical practice guidelines for the management of crush victims in mass disasters.[19] These recommendations included both medical and logistic principles and were based on lessons that have been learned from the activities of the Renal Disaster Relief Task Force in disaster-affected areas during the past 2 decades.[16,19,40-43] Of note, vigorous fluid resuscitation and the use of mannitol are now proven therapies for saving limbs and preventing the development of compartment syndrome in crush injuries, which is the second leading cause of death after disasters (Figure 79.3). These therapies can also reduce the need to perform fasciotomies, which are associated with severe bleeding, sepsis, and amputations.[19,39,40,44,45]

In summary, it is difficult to draw general conclusions about the epidemiology, causes, and outcomes of AKI in many ME countries because of regional variation and methodologic differences in the few studies that have been performed in the region. Well-conducted studies in which the published definition of AKI[46] is used are needed to clarify the actual occurrence of AKI. Accordingly, the results of these studies can then be used to identify the needed infrastructure and evaluate treatment strategies to improve the clinical outcomes.

CHRONIC KIDNEY DISEASE

EPIDEMIOLOGY

The incidence and prevalence of noncommunicable diseases are changing rapidly as a result of demographic transition, and the burden of disease has consequently shifted from the pediatric population to the adult population in many ME countries.[8,47-50] This demographic shift in the burden of disease is exemplified by the emerging epidemic of diabetes mellitus that is occurring globally and affects Arab and Chaldean Americans. In 2013 the International Diabetes Federation ranked Saudi Arabia (24%), Kuwait (23.1%), and Qatar (22.9%) as having the seventh, ninth, and tenth highest estimated prevalence of diabetes mellitus, respectively, in the world.[51] The International Diabetes Federation also predicts that the prevalence of diabetes mellitus in ME countries will increase by 2035. These alarming statistics for ME countries have been attributed to a combination of increasing urbanization, aging populations, increasing obesity, and falling levels of physical activity.[7,8,47,48,52-60] Accordingly, the direct and indirect medical expenditures that are associated with diabetes mellitus will become a profound economic burden. As a result, ME countries with limited or scarce resources (see Figure 79.2) will be unable to cope with the social, economic, and public health consequences of complications of diabetes mellitus, one of which is CKD.

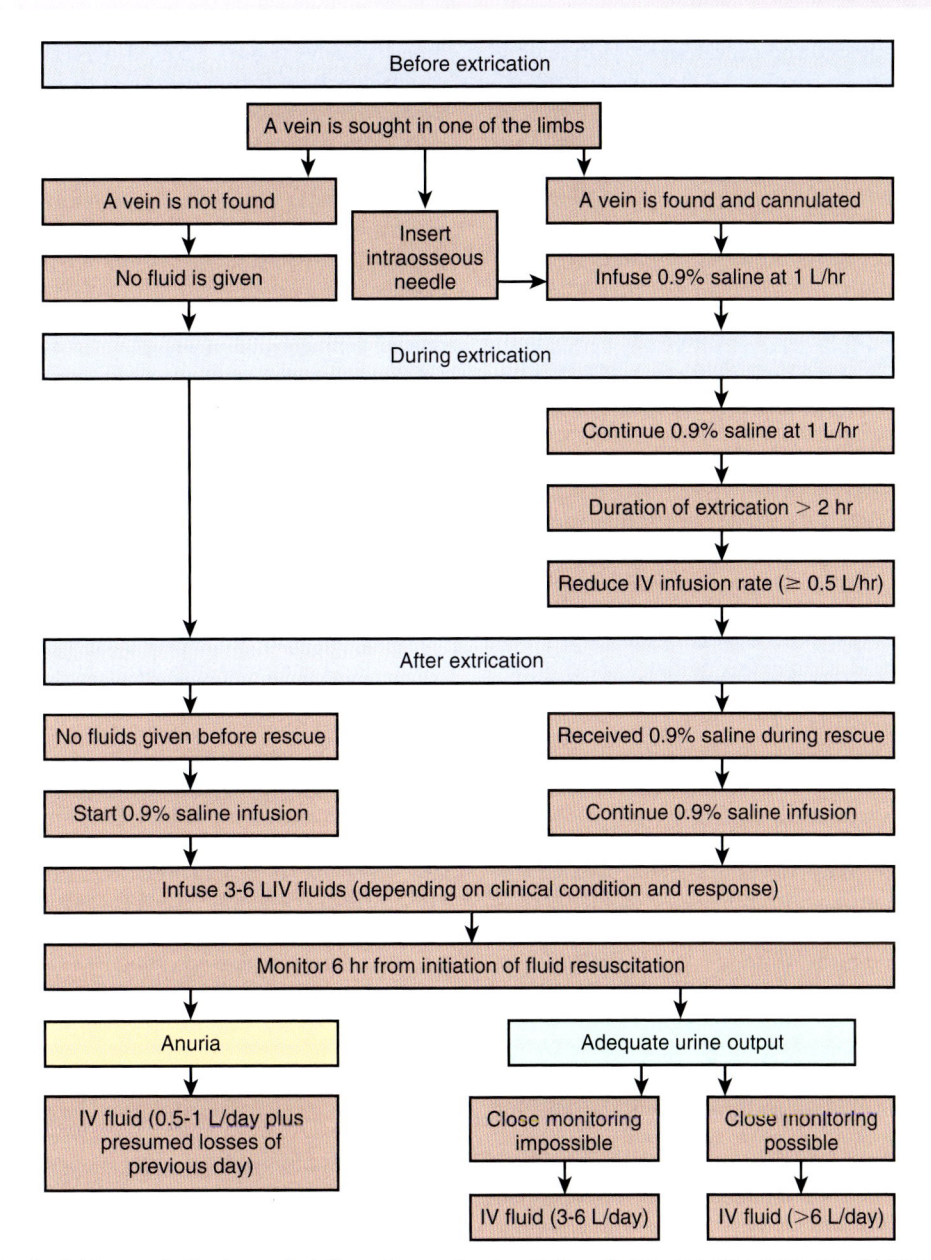

```
┌─────────────────────────────────────┐
│         Before extrication          │
└─────────────────────────────────────┘
              │
   ┌──────────────────────────┐
   │ A vein is sought in one of the limbs │
   └──────────────────────────┘
      │         │         │
      ▼         ▼         ▼
 ┌─────────┐ ┌────────┐ ┌──────────────┐
 │A vein is│ │ Insert │ │A vein is found│
 │not found│ │intraos-│ │and cannulated │
 │         │ │seous   │ │               │
 │         │ │needle  │ │               │
 └─────────┘ └────────┘ └──────────────┘
      │         │         │
      ▼         └────────►▼
 ┌─────────┐            ┌──────────────────┐
 │No fluid │            │Infuse 0.9% saline│
 │is given │            │at 1 L/hr         │
 └─────────┘            └──────────────────┘
```

Figure 79.3 Algorithm for fluid resuscitation in crush victims of mass disasters before, during, and after extrication. IV, Intravenous. (Modified from Sever MS, Vanholder R: Management of crush victims in mass disasters: highlights from recently published recommendations. *Clin J Am Soc Nephrol* 8:328-335, 2013; and adapted from Gibney RT, Sever MS, Vanholder RC: Disaster nephrology: crush injury and beyond. *Kidney Int* 85:1049-1057, 2014.)

In addition, the common practice of consanguineous marriages in ME countries has led to a high incidence of genetic disorders, some of which may lead to CKD and end-stage kidney disease (ESKD), especially in children, and possibly alter the pattern of renal disease in these countries.[7,61-66] Genetic renal diseases and their complications in the ME are discussed further later in this chapter.

It is difficult to estimate the incidence and prevalence of CKD in most ME countries. Obtaining the epidemiologic statistics concerning CKD, ESKD, and RRT is a work in progress that is hampered by the lack of well-conducted cross-sectional and longitudinal cohort studies and a lack of reliable registries that incorporate data on comorbid conditions. Furthermore, additional research is required to establish the best, cost-effective approach for screening for CKD.[67]

Hence the creation of a reliable and easily accessible medical registry is urgently needed in the ME countries where one is lacking, unreliable, or difficult to access. The information in these registries is essential for planning health policies and the allocation of funds. Community-based screening programs for CKD and risk factors, such as diabetes mellitus, obesity, proteinuria, and hypertension, have been launched in developing countries worldwide under the auspices of the Research and Prevention Committee of the ISN. This initiative includes ongoing programs in Egypt and Morocco.[68,69] These programs are expected to detect CKD in populations in which the people are unaware of such chronic diseases.

The Egypt Information, Prevention, and Treatment of Chronic Kidney Diseases program was the first to report interim results. It investigated the prevalence of microalbuminuria among first-degree relatives of people with ESKD in the city of Damanhour and the surrounding towns in Al-Buhayrah governorate, in Lower Egypt.[70] Microalbuminuria was detected in 10.6% of participants. In an adjusted logistic regression analysis, smoking and personal history of cardiovascular disease were strongly associated with microalbuminuria. In long-term, nationwide, population-based, retrospective cohort studies, overweight, obesity, or persistent asymptomatic isolated hematuria detected in Israeli adolescents and young adults were strongly associated with an increased cumulative incidence of treated ESKD, with crude hazard ratios of 3, 6.89, and 18.5, respectively.[71,72] Therefore, although not proven yet, it is hoped that early detection of CKD and its risk factors will increase health awareness and early intervention, which in turn may modify disease course, complexity, and costs of overall therapy.[67,68,73]

Similarly, the International Federation of Kidney Foundations is attempting to raise awareness of CKD by creating educational programs in industrialized and developing countries.[74] In addition, many ME countries are involved in the activities of the World Kidney Day initiative of the ISN to enhance public and governmental awareness of the burden of and risk factors for CKD.

The actual or estimated number of patients with CKD at each stage of the classification developed by Kidney Disease: Improving Global Outcomes (KDIGO),[75] in each ME country, is unclear.[76] In 2007 a study involving 31,999 taxi drivers in Tehran, mostly males, showed that 6.5% of drivers had an estimated glomerular filtration rate (eGFR) of less than 60 mL/min/1.73 m^2.[77] However, community-based studies revealed considerable differences in CKD prevalence between counties of Iran (10.2% to 18.9%).[58,78] In a pioneering work, Tohidi and colleagues[79] examined the incidence of CKD among a subgroup, 20 years or older, of the Tehran Lipid and Glucose Study, which is a long-term community-based prospective study. During 10-year follow-up, the cumulative incidence of CKD stages 3 to 5 among women and men was 27.8% and 14.2%, respectively. Age, hypertension, and diabetes were found to be independent predictors of CKD stages 3 to 5 in both genders, with greater relative risks among men than women. In addition, for males, high-normal blood pressure and, for females, current smoking and being single or divorced/widowed were significant risk factors of CKD.[79]

According to the Chronic REnal Disease In Turkey (CREDIT) study,[57] the population-based estimated prevalence rates for CKD stages 1, 2, 3, 4, and 5 among Turkish adults were 5.4%, 5.2%, 4.7%, 0.3%, and 0.2%, respectively, with overall prevalence of 15.8%. Moreover, the frequency of concomitant cardiovascular risk factors such as diabetes, hypertension, dyslipidemia, and obesity was increased in patients with CKD, and odds ratios versus non-CKD population were 3.22, 2.86, 1.60, and 1.65, respectively. Based on analysis of one spot urine specimen per participant, 10.2% of the cohort subjects had microalbuminuria and 2% had macroalbuminuria.[57] The causes of CKD were not detailed, but the study cohort continues to be followed longitudinally. A small pilot study, which is part of the Global SEEK Project, demonstrated the feasibility of screening and early detection of CKD in a Saudi population. Using standardized GFR prediction equations, the prevalence of CKD stages 1, 2, and 3 was relatively low, 3.5%, 1.6%, and 0.6%, respectively, which may be attributed to the low mean age of the participants (37.4 ± 11.3 years).[80]

In Kuwait a 4-year prospective study from one referral center by El-Reshaid and associates[81] reported a high incidence of CKD among Kuwaiti nationals. Specifically, they reported an average annual incidence of 366 per million population (pmp), with a higher incidence among the elderly population (aged 60 years or older) of 913 pmp. Of patients with CKD who were admitted to the center, 6% presented with uremic syndrome, and 40% experienced acute deterioration of their kidney function that resulted mainly from drugs (mostly over-the-counter nonsteroidal antiinflammatory drugs), infection, and volume depletion. Yet the authors did not report categories of eGFR or proteinuria in their patients.

Although the number of patients who underwent preemptive kidney transplantation might not be included, estimates of the prevalence and incidence of ESKD are more reliable in countries that have a national database in which each patient who has received RRT is registered. Nevertheless, patient numbers in a national registry in ME countries may be underestimated for two additional reasons: (1) The treatment of ESKD may be beyond the reach of the average citizen in low-income ME countries, such as Yemen, and (2) a high number of expatriates live in some ME countries that may not be included. Tables 79.2 and 79.3 summarize the available data on ESKD from published articles, registries, and abstracts of proceedings of international symposia in ME countries. Of note, most investigators relied mainly on the results of limited retrospective studies and answers to questionnaires that were sent to leading nephrologists in each country and not on accurate documented statistics, registries, or results of epidemiologic studies.

Israel and Turkey report their ESKD data to the European Renal Association–European Dialysis and Transplantation Association registry,[82] and the United States Renal Data System.[83] The registry in Turkey was established in 1990.[84,85] In 2011[83] the prevalence of ESKD was 868 per million Turkish population (50% of the reported U.S. prevalence), and the incidence rate for new RRT patients was 238 pmp (66% of the U.S. incidence). Diabetic nephropathy and hypertension were the two main causes of ESKD in Turkey.[82,83,85,86]

Data from the report of the Israeli Center for Disease Control (ICDC) indicated that the incidence of ESKD increased by 65.5% during the past 2 decades, from 113 to 187 pmp. The average annual increase was highest in the years 1996 to 1999, but it has stabilized since 2003. The increase in ESKD was observed mainly in the elderly population (aged 65 years or older). Likewise, a 2.7-fold increase in the prevalence of ESKD was observed, from 416 pmp in 1990 to 1109 pmp in 2010. Of note, diabetes mellitus was the cause of ESKD in 11.5% of prevalent patients in 1990 and increased to 42.7% in 2010.[87,88] The Tunisian registry was started in 1990 and has also reported an increase in the incidence and prevalence of ESKD.[89] The incidence of ESKD increased from 81.6 pmp in the period 1992 to 1993 to 158.8 pmp in 2000 to 2001; the average annual increase was 9.6%. The incidence of ESKD in elderly persons, women, and individuals with diabetic nephropathy has risen steeply. However, regional variations were noted among urban and rural districts.[89,90]

Table 79.2 Epidemiology of Renal Replacement Therapy in Middle Eastern Countries

Country	Dialysis				Kidney Transplantation	
	First Hemodialysis*	No. of Hemodialysis Centers	Incidence[†]	Prevalence[†]	Date of Country's First Transplantation	Incidence[†]
Algeria	1962	281	104	482	1986	3.9
Bahrain	1971	NA	120	428	1995	35
Egypt	1958	1050	NA	412	1976	13.8
Iran	1965	316	63.8	507	1967	31.6
Iraq	1967	27	NA	83	1973	12.2
Israel	1948	76	184	771	1964	34.5
Jordan	1968	75	111	607	1972	29.2
Kuwait	1976	4	72	240	1979	20
Lebanon	1960	66	NA	700	1972	17.2
Libya	1972	53	282	624	1989	8.6
Morocco	1980	197	42	415	1990	0.56
Oman	1983	12	NA	189	1988	6.2
Palestinian Authority	NA	13	NA	240.3	2011	NA
Qatar	1981	5	202	536	1986	3.3
Saudi Arabia	1971	182	129	499	1979	22
Syria	1974	66	111	228	1976	16.2
Tunisia	1963	146	142	812	1986	13.2
Turkey	1965	834	198.7	773	1975	39.3
United Arab Emirates	1975	17	NA	329	1985	2.3
Yemen	1982	13	64	91	1998	1.4

*For acute kidney injury or end-stage kidney disease.
[†]Per million population.
NA, Not available

Data from Abomelha[301]; Aghighi et al[99]; Al Arrayed[300]; Erek et al[84]; Batieha et al[102]; Erlik et al[347]; Saeed et al[298]; Saeed[341]; Mahdavi-Mazdeh[366]; Najafi et al[100]; Al Sayyari[303]; Soliman et al[112]; Barsoum et al[394]; Khader et al[395]; Shaheen et al[352,353]; Shigidi et al[308]; Masri and Haberal[345]; Alashek et al[96]; the 2012 report by the Saudi Center for Organ Transplantation[91]; the 2013 report by the Israeli Center for Disease Control; the 2011 report of the European Renal Association–European Dialysis and Transplantation Association[82]; the 2012 report of the Lebanese kidney registry[92]; the Hashemite Kingdom of Jordan Ministry of Health, Non-Communicable Diseases Directorate: National Registry of End Stage Renal Disease (ESRD) annual report 2012. Available at: www.moh.gov.jo/Documents/annual%20report-2012.pdf; El Matri[356]; El Matri A: Economic challenge of renal replacement therapy in the Arab world (poster session). Presented at the 2009 World Congress of Nephrology, Satellite Conference: 7th Conference on Kidney Disease in Disadvantaged Populations; Milan, May 26-28, 2009; and Benghanem Gharbi M: Epidemiology of ESRD in the Maghreb (lecture). Presented at the 5th Maghrebian Congress of Nephrology, March 19-22, 2014, Djerba Island, Tunisia.

Table 79.3 Modalities of Renal Replacement Therapy for Treating End-Stage Kidney Disease in Selected Middle Eastern Countries

Country	Transplantation (%)	Peritoneal Dialysis (%)	Hemodialysis (%)
Algeria	7.8	2.1	90.1
Iran	44.7	4.1	51.2
Israel	36.2	6.2	57.6
Jordan	13.9	2.4	83.6
Kuwait	5	12.5	82.5
Lebanon	18	4	78
Libya	19.4	0.7	79.9
Morocco	2.6	0.4	97
Oman	39.1	1.8	59.1
Qatar	48.4	6.5	45.2
Saudi Arabia	34	6	60
Tunisia	9.3	2.4	88.3
Turkey	11	7.3	81.7
United Arab Emirates	34.2	4.6	61.2

Data from Najafi et al[100]; Najafi[302]; the 2012 report by the Saudi Center for Organ Transplantation[91]; the 2013 report by the Israeli Center for Disease Control; the 2011 report of the European Renal Association–European Dialysis and Transplantation Association[82]; the 2012 report of the Lebanese kidney registry[92]; and Benghanem Gharbi M: Epidemiology of ESRD in the Maghreb (lecture). Presented at the 5th Maghrebian Congress of Nephrology, March 19-22, 2014, Djerba Island, Tunisia.

The Saudi Center for Organ Transplantation (SCOT) has established an open-access RRT registry that provides annual information on the epidemiology and treatment of ESKD in Saudi Arabia. In 2012 the incidence and prevalence of RRT were 151 pmp and 751 pmp, respectively.[91]

In March 2011, Lebanon launched its national kidney registry,[92] aiming to report reliable data on prevalence, incidence, patient management, practice patterns, clinical outcomes, and survival among CKD patients. In the first annual report of the registry in 2012, the incidence of ESKD and patient survival could not be accurately calculated because of incomplete data. However, the prevalence was estimated to be 855 pmp.[92]

A comprehensive 1-year observational study, conducted by Alashek and colleagues,[60,93-96] shed light on the epidemiology of ESKD and RRT practices in Libya before the conflict. The prevalence and incidence of dialysis-treated ESKD from mid-2009 until August 2010 were 624 pmp and 282 pmp, respectively.[60]

In Iran a treatment program for ESKD was introduced in 1975. The reported number of Iranians with ESKD has also increased, and this increase is mirrored in the growing number of dialysis centers and renal transplantation programs. The incidence and prevalence of ESKD were 49.9 pmp and 238 pmp, respectively, in 2000 and increased to 63.8 pmp and 357 pmp, respectively, in 2006.[97-99] By the end of 2009, 38,060 adult patients were receiving RRT in Iran, giving a prevalence of 507 pmp.[100]

In the ME countries for which detailed data are available, there is a male predominance among patients with ESKD, similar to that reported worldwide.[83,101] The mean age of patients undergoing dialysis in each ME country varies between 42 and 68 years. Interestingly, the youngest patients with ESKD on dialysis are in the developing ME countries, and the oldest patients with ESKD on dialysis are in Israel.[86,88,97,102-104] Of note, kidney diseases and risk factors or therapy in expatriates—who may make up as much as 50% of the population, especially in the wealthy Gulf countries—have not been carefully investigated. This population needs to be distinguished from the resident population and may require special attention because of their different ethnic, socioeconomic, and environmental backgrounds.[10,12,97,105]

CAUSES OF CHRONIC KIDNEY DISEASE

The causes of CKD in ME countries are highly influenced by the bioecology of a particular region, and the ethnic and socioeconomic background of its population. Accordingly, the various causes of CKD are ranked differently in ME countries. The populations of the five ME countries in North Africa—Morocco, Algeria, Tunisia, Libya, and Egypt—have similar ethnicity and socioeconomic backgrounds, in that they are of African descent that has been intermixed with Berber, Arab, and Mediterranean population streams.[106] In the 1990s, interstitial nephritis and glomerulonephritis each accounted for approximately 20% of all cases of CKD in these countires.[106] The number of individuals with interstitial nephritis increased during the 2000s, possibly as a result of environmental pollution and abuse of over-the-counter drugs.[107] Most cases of glomerulonephritis are of the proliferative type, whereas immunoglobulin A (IgA) nephropathy is rare. The high prevalence of proliferative glomerulonephritis in these ME countries reflects postinfectious glomerulonephritis caused by viruses, bacteria, and parasites. In Egypt, Libya, and southern Algeria, approximately 7% of patients with CKD suffered from obstructive uropathy as a result of urinary schistosomiasis caused by *Schistosoma haematobium* or *Schistosoma mansoni*. It is noteworthy that tuberculosis, other bacterial infections, and familial Mediterranean fever (FMF) are the main causes of renal (type AA) amyloidosis in many ME countries.[106,108]

However, the frequency of causes of ESKD has changed. All ME countries except Algeria and Yemen report diabetes mellitus as the most frequent cause of ESKD (20% to 48%) in incident patients receiving RRT, followed by hypertension (11% to 30%) and glomerulonephritis (11% to 24%).[10,50,60,82,88,91,92,97,98,100,109-112]

GENETIC DISORDERS

Genetic kidney diseases have received much attention in pediatric and adult nephrology because the underlying molecular defects in many of these diseases have been elucidated as a result of advances in genetics and molecular biology. The ME population is ethnically and genetically diverse.[113] The primary demographic features of Arab Muslim and Druze communities in the ME include large families, rapid population growth, and high rates of consanguinity. Among Palestinian Arabs, more than 40% of marriages are between relatives, and of these, 50% are between first cousins.[113,114] In Bedouin society, 40% of women of childbearing age are married to first cousins.[115] In contrast, the consanguinity rate among Israeli Jews is reported to be 2.3%, and of these, first-cousin marriages account for 0.8%. The highest consanguinity rate among Israeli Jews (7.1%) is found among Eastern (i.e., Asian non-Sephardic) Jews.[116]

High consanguinity rates have also been reported in the Saudi Arabian, Kuwaiti, Lebanese, and Moroccan populations.[61,63-65,117-119] The results of an epidemiologic survey from Lebanon revealed that 26% of patients receiving chronic hemodialysis were the children of consanguineous parents.[61] In addition, Barbari and colleagues[61] reported that the risk for a family history of kidney disease was particularly high among patients from consanguineous families who were receiving hemodialysis. Populations with a high rate of consanguinity also have an increased prevalence of adulthood diseases that are associated with renal insufficiency, such as hypertension, metabolic syndrome, and diabetes mellitus.[62,120] A study of kidney biopsies from three pathology centers in Lebanon showed that mesangioproliferative glomerulonephritis was significantly more frequent among Muslims and offspring of consanguineous unions, whereas focal segmental glomerulosclerosis was most prevalent in Christians.[66]

A significant proportion of genetic kidney diseases are inherited in an autosomal recessive manner. It is therefore not surprising that these diseases occur most frequently in communities with high consanguinity rates.[121] Consanguineous populations are not expected to have a different mutation rate. Consanguinity, however, may enhance allelic and locus heterogeneity.[62,120-122] Seventy-one different autosomal recessive kidney diseases were reported in Palestinian Arabs (reviewed by Zlotogora)[114]; these include primary renal diseases (congenital nephritic syndrome and nephronophthisis), metabolic and tubular defects (cystinuria, Bartter's syndrome, renal tubular acidosis, and oxalosis), and FMF (discussed in detail later in this chapter). The influence of genetic factors is very evident in pediatric patients with kidney diseases, particularly in Saudi Arabia and Syria, where increased numbers of congenital and hereditary kidney and urologic diseases are now being reported.[113,123] The results of an extensive study of both Jewish and Bedouin populations in southern Israel showed that genetic kidney diseases are overrepresented in the pediatric population (Table 79.4).[64]

CYSTIC KIDNEY DISEASES

Autosomal dominant polycystic kidney disease is one of the most common genetic renal diseases in adults and occurs in 3% to 10% of ESKD patients in several ME communities.[88,124-126] Autosomal recessive polycystic disease (ARPKD, Online Mendelian Inheritance in Man [OMIM] catalog number 263200) occurs with a proposed incidence of 1 per 20,000 to 1 per 40,000. In most cases the mortality is very high in the first month of life. Its principal manifestations include fusiform dilation of the renal collecting ducts and distal tubules, and dysgenesis of the hepatic portal triad. ARPKD is associated with mutations in the *PKHD1* gene on chromosome 6p12, encoding fibrocystin, a membrane protein located on the primary cilium.[127] At least 300 mutations in *PKHD1* gene have been reported. Several mutations were reported in Turkish and Israeli children who participated in a large international study.[128,129] Likewise, other ciliopathies, including juvenile nephronophthisis, infantile nephronophthisis, and Joubert's syndrome with mutations in *NPHP1*, *NPHP2 (INVS)*, and *NPHP3*, encoding nephrocystin 1, inversin, and nephrocystin 3, respectively, have been reported in several ME countries[130-132] (see also Table 79.5).

GENETIC GLOMERULAR DISEASES

A substantial number of patients in the ME with renal disease have familial glomerular diseases whose spectrum includes familial hematuria, Alport's syndrome, IgA nephropathy, and familial focal glomerulosclerosis.[64,123,133] A recessive form of steroid-resistant nephrotic syndrome has been shown to be associated with mutations in the *NPHS2* gene, which encodes the glomerular protein podocin.[134] The most common phenotype is of a nephrotic syndrome that is resistant to immunosuppressive treatment in early childhood, and most patients with this disease develop ESKD after 5 to 20 years. In a group of children from two consanguineous families of Israeli Arab descent, mutation analysis of the *NPHS2* gene revealed homozygosity for the C412T nonsense mutation (R138X).[135] The same mutation was also found in Israeli Arab patients with nonfamilial steroid-resistant nephrotic syndrome, but not in Jewish children or in children from both ethnic groups with steroid-sensitive nephrotic syndrome.[135] Interestingly, cardiac anomalies, especially left ventricular hypertrophy,

Table 79.4 Genetic Kidney Diseases in Southern Israel, 1994 to 2010

Type of Disease	Disease	OMIM No.	No. of Patients	No. of Families	No. of Bedouin Patients	No. of Jewish Patients
Glomerular	Alport's syndrome	301050	5	3	0	5
	Benign familial hematuria	141200	3	2	2	1
Tubular	Familial hyperkalemic hypertension	145260	1	1	0	1
	Cystinuria	220100	14	7	14	0
	Distal RTA	602722	4	3	2	2
	Nephrogenic diabetes insipidus	125800	18	11	17	1
	Type 2 Bartter's syndrome	241200	10	6	3	7
	Type 4 Bartter's syndrome	602522	20	13	20	0
	Unclassified Bartter's syndrome		3	3	1	2
	Familial hypomagnesemia	602014	21	15	21	0
	Gitelman's syndrome	263800	3	3	1	2
	Hypophosphatemic rickets	307800	4	2	3	1
Cystic/NPHP	ADPKD	173900	14	13	0	14
	ARPKD	263200	16	12	13	3
	Bardet-Biedl syndrome	209900	5	4	5	0
	Juvenile nephronophthisis	256100	3	3	2	1
	Infantile nephronophthisis	602088	5	4	5	0
Metabolic	Fanconi-Bickel syndrome	227810	2	2	2	0
	Xanthinuria	278300	5	2	5	0
	Lowe's syndrome	309000	1	1	0	1
	Cystinosis	219800	3	3	0	3
Other	Atypical HUS	134370	8	4	8	0
	Renal tubular dysgenesis	267430	5	5	4	1
Total			173	122	128	45

ADPKD, Autosomal dominant polycystic kidney disease; ARPKD, autosomal recessive polycystic kidney disease; CKD, chronic kidney disease; HUS, hemolytic uremic syndrome; NPHP, nephronophthisis; OMIM, Online Mendelian Inheritance in Man catalog (http://www.ncbi.nlm.nih.gov/omim); RTA, renal tubular acidosis.
Modified from Landau D, Shalev H: Childhood genetic renal diseases in southern Israel. Harefuah 149:180-185, 2010.

pulmonary stenosis, and discrete subaortic stenosis, were detected in a high proportion of the children with *NPHS2* mutations.[136] Frishberg and associates[136] speculated that podocin may have a role in normal cardiac development because podocin messenger RNA is reported to be expressed in the human fetal heart.

At least 53 *NPHS2* mutations have also been found in Turkish children with familial and sporadic steroid-resistant nephrotic syndrome.[137,138] Among Turkish patients with these mutations, the proportion of patients with CKD or ESKD was significantly higher (19 of 73) than that of patients without these mutations (28 of 222). Furthermore, the mean time for progression to ESKD was significantly shorter in patients with these mutations than in those without these mutations.[138]

The *NPHS1* gene encodes nephrin, an essential protein for maintaining the normal structure and function of the slit diaphragm of the visceral glomerular epithelial cell. Three mutations in the *NPHS1* gene were reported in 12 children with congenital nephrotic syndrome from a large consanguineous Israeli Arab family.[122] Steroid-sensitive nephrotic syndrome is rarely reported to have a familial pattern. However, a familial pattern associated with this condition has been reported in Israeli Bedouin families with a high rate of consanguinity, and the authors of the report proposed that the increased incidence of steroid-sensitive nephrotic syndrome resulted from selective enrichment of susceptibility genes in this population.[139]

A study evaluated causative mutations related to childhood nephrotic syndrome in 49 families from Saudi Arabia.[140] Sixty-two patients were screened for mutations in genes associated with congenital, infantile, or childhood nephrotic syndrome, such as *NPHS1*, *NPHS2*, *LAMB2* (laminin-β_2), *PLCE1* (phospholipase Cε_1), *CD2AP* (CD2-associated protein), *MYO1E* (myosin 1E), *WT1* (Wilms' tumor 1), *PTPRO* (protein tyrosine phosphatase receptor type O), and *NEIL1* (Nei endonuclease VII-like 1).[140] A homozygous mutation in the *NPHS2* gene was found in 11 (22%) families, and was the most common cause of nephrotic syndrome. Other mutations were found in *NPHS1* (12%), *PLCE1* (8%), and *MYO1E* (6%) genes. Focal segmental glomerulosclerosis was the most common pattern of histopathologic injury, and a significant proportion of patients developed ESKD requiring RRT.[140]

The Rho family of small GTPases (Rho GTPases) is associated with actin remodeling, and podocyte migratory ability. Alterations in Rho GTPases signaling interfere with podocyte mobility and cause proteinuria.[141] Rho GDP-dissociation inhibitor 1, a regulator of Rho GTPases, is a protein that in humans is encoded by the *ARHGDIA* gene and is also expressed in podocytes. *ARHADIA* mutations, associated with steroid-resistant nephrotic syndrome and early death due to ESKD, were reported in three siblings from a family of Ashkenazi Jews and in a Moroccan infant.[142]

GENETIC METABOLIC DISEASES AND INHERITED TUBULAR DISORDERS

Primary hyperoxaluria type 1 and type 2 are relatively rare autosomal recessive inborn errors of glyoxylate metabolism. Types 1 and 2 are characterized by overproduction of oxalate in the liver, and type 2 by oxalate overproduction in other tissues.[143,144] The more frequent primary hyperoxaluria type 1 (OMIM number 604285) is caused by a deficiency of the liver-specific peroxisomal enzyme alanine-glyoxylate aminotransferase (AGT), which catalyzes the conversion of glyoxylate to glycine. Primary hyperoxaluria type 2 (OMIM numbers 260000 and 604296) is caused by a deficiency of the cytosolic enzyme glyoxylate reductase (glyoxylate hydroxypyruvate reductase), which catalyzes the reduction of glyoxylate and hydroxypyruvate. When AGT activity is absent, glyoxylate is converted to oxalate, which forms insoluble calcium oxalate, which in turn is deposited in the kidneys and causes progressive renal insufficiency (nephrolithiasis, nephrocalcinosis, and progressive inflammation with interstitial fibrosis). Deposition of calcium oxalate also occurs in extrarenal tissues, including the retina, myocardium, blood vessels, bone, and central nervous system.[143,144]

Cases of primary hyperoxaluria type 1 and isolated cases of type 2 have been reported in Israeli families.[145-147] In 22 Israeli Arab families with type 1 hyperoxaluria at least 15 different mutations in the AGT-encoding *AGXT* gene have been detected.[145,147] Marked intrafamilial phenotypic heterogeneity with no definite genotype-phenotype correlation was noted in these families, and the prevalent phenotype was one of early onset of disease with progression to ESKD in the first decade of life.[147] A large European study of 155 patients from 129 families with type 1 hyperoxaluria, including a large proportion of ME individuals, showed that the most common mutation was p.GLY170Arg (allelic frequency 21.5%). This mutation was associated with a better long-term prognosis.[148]

In 2010, primary hyperoxaluria type 3 (OMIM number 613597) was described in Ashkenazi Jews with calcium oxalate nephrolithiasis.[149] In affected members of nine unrelated families without type 1 or type 2 hyperoxaluria, Belostotsky and colleagues found loss-of-function mutations in *HOGA1*, formerly *DHDPSL*, which encodes a mitochondrial 4-hydroxy-2-oxoglutarate aldolase that catalyzes the fourth step in the hydroxyproline pathway.[149,150]

Primary hyperoxaluria is a common cause of nephrolithiasis, nephrocalcinosis, and kidney failure in children from the ME countries in western North Africa, from Saudi Arabia, and from Kuwait.[106,151,152] Primary hyperoxaluria is probably underdiagnosed because by the time of diagnosis, advanced CKD has usually developed, or it is diagnosed on biopsy of kidney transplant recipients with early graft dysfunction resulting from oxalate deposition.[144]

Cystinuria is another common cause of nephrolithiasis in various ethnic groups in ME countries.[106,151,153] This autosomal recessive kidney disease is caused by a mutation in either one or both of two genes: the *SLC3A1* gene on chromosome 2p16.3, which encodes the solute carrier family 3 (cystine, dibasic, and neutral amino acid transporters), member 1 (also known as rBAT, ab$^{o,+}$, AT transporter related protein); and the *SLC7A9* gene on chromosome 19q13.1, which encodes the solute carrier family 7 (cationic amino acid transporter, y+ system), member 9 (also known as BAT1, b$^{o,+}$, AD transporter protein). The disease manifestations caused by either mutation are similar.[111,154,155] Mutations in *SCL3A1* have been detected in Turks, Muslim Arabs, Druze, and Ashkenazi and Sephardic Jews of Persian and Yemenite origin. The disease is also common among Libyan Jews, in whom the estimated prevalence is 1 per 2500 and the carrier rate is 1 per 25. In this population the disease is caused by a single founder mutation, V170M, in the *SLC7A9* gene.[111,155-159]

Fabry's disease is a rare X-linked sphingolipidosis caused by deficiency of α-galactosidase A (ceramide trihexosidase). A mutation in the gene that encodes this enzyme results in insufficient breakdown of lipids, which accumulate to harmful levels in the eyes, kidneys, autonomic nervous system, and cardiovascular system. In untreated patients the accumulation of globotriaosylceramide in lysosomes may result in multiple organ damage that includes the development of ESKD between the fourth and fifth decades of life. Histologic evidence of Fabry's disease has been detected in graft biopsy samples many years after successful kidney transplantation.[160,161] Although most disease features have been reported in adults, a pediatric disease phenotype that includes acroparesthesia, skin manifestations, and glomerular alterations has been described.[161-163] Fabry's disease has been diagnosed in families in Israel and Turkey.[160,161,163-165] However, Fabry's disease is probably underdiagnosed in other ME countries because of limited screening or awareness.

Bartter's syndrome and Gitelman's syndrome belong to a group of inherited salt-losing tubulopathies with distinct phenotypes; they are caused by inherited defects in ion transporters in the loop of Henle and distal convoluted tubule, respectively. Most cases of the variants of Bartter's syndrome in the ME are reported in Israeli Arabs, in large Bedouin communities living in southern and northern Israel, and in Kuwaiti children.[64,166,167]

Renal hypodysplasia is the most common congenital anomaly of the kidney and urinary tract. To better understand its pathologic basis, Vivante and associates identified 20 Israeli pedigrees with isolated nonsyndromic renal hypodysplasia and screened for mutations in genes known to be involved in kidney development.[168] Two brothers were found to have a heterozygous *PAX2* nonsense mutation, responsible for renal-coloboma syndrome, which includes kidney dysplasia, eye coloboma, and hearing impairment. Nine affected subjects from two unrelated families were found to harbor heterozygous *HNF1B* mutations. These mutations associated with variable renal phenotypes and hyperuricemia. In one family, two affected brothers were heterozygous for a missense mutation in *WNT4*. Functional analysis of this variant in different cell lines revealed both agonistic and antagonistic canonical WNT stimuli. In primary cultures of human fetal kidney cells, this mutation caused loss of function, resulting in diminished canonical WNT/β-catenin signaling. These findings were interpreted as suggestive of a role for heterozygous *WNT4* variants in renal hypodysplasia.[168]

Some rare genetic kidney diseases that have been reported in ME communities are listed in Table 79.5.[156,169-187] Other nonrenal genetic diseases may cause glomerular and tubulointerstitial complications; an example is sickle cell anemia, a hemoglobinopathy that is prevalent in the ME countries in western North Africa and the Arabian Peninsula.[106,113,154,188,189]

FAMILIAL MEDITERRANEAN FEVER

FMF is the most common of the hereditary periodic fever syndromes and a common genetic disease in the ME. FMF is an autoinflammatory autosomal recessive inherited disease that is characterized by recurrent attacks of fever, serositis, arthritis, and erysipelas-like skin lesions. The disease affects several ethnic groups in the ME, including Sephardic Jews, Armenians, Turks, and Arabs.[190] The most significant complication of FMF is renal amyloidosis that progresses to nephrotic syndrome and ESKD. Renal amyloidosis is occasionally diagnosed in patients without a typical history of FMF attacks.

In the 1990s two groups identified the *MEFV* gene by positional cloning as the underlying genetic cause of FMF.[191,192] At least 296 mutations in the *MEFV* gene have been reported, and more than 150 of these mutations have been found to be associated with FMF.[193] The *MEFV* gene encodes the protein pyrin (or marenostrin). The gene is located on the short arm of chromosome 16 (16p13.3) and includes 10 exons that encode 781 amino acids. The *MEFV* gene is expressed predominantly in polymorphonuclear cells (PMNCs), eosinophils, and monocytes but not in lymphocytes. It is also expressed in dendritic cells and fibroblasts from the synovium, peritoneum, and skin.[194,195] Pyrin is thought to be involved in the regulation of cellular processes that are associated with the synthesis, processing, and release of inflammatory proteins by PMNCs and with cell death.[196]

The carrier frequency of mutant alleles is high, as much as 1 in 3 to 1 in 5 in certain populations in ME countries (Armenians, Jews, and Turks), and the most common reported mutations are in M694V, V726A, M680I, M694I in exon 10 and E148Q in exon 2.[197,198] The first four mutations are believed to be pathogenic, with the M694V homozygotes having the most severe phenotype. Although the E1489Q homozygotes are asymptomatic in 50% of cases, this variant may be associated with other systemic inflammatory diseases, including Behçet's disease, vasculitis, ulcerative colitis, rheumatoid arthritis, and multiple sclerosis.[199] The most frequent *MEFV* mutations in the ME populations are listed in Table 79.6.[199-227] Mutations in the *MEFV* gene have also been reported in Spanish, Italian, Greek, Portuguese, Indian, Chinese, and Japanese populations.[228,229] Most *MEFV* mutations are single–amino acid substitutions (missense), and many patients with FMF have a single *MEFV* mutation.

The clinical spectrum of FMF and the elucidation of the molecular biology, structure, and regulation of pyrin and its role during inflammation have been reviewed.[196,230-232] Five different domains have been identified within pyrin: a PYRIN domain, a bZIP transcription factor basic domain, a B-box zinc finger domain, an α-helical (coiled-coil) domain, and a B30.2 domain (Figure 79.4). The B30.2. domain is present in primate and human pyrin but not in rodent pyrin.[232] It includes a SPRY domain that is located in front of the C-terminal region, and a PRY extension at the N terminus (not shown in Figure 79.4). The SPRY domain is a protein interaction module, which is implicated in several biologic pathways, including those that regulate innate and adaptive immunity.[233]

Each pyrin domain has a distinct role in protein-protein interactions during inflammation that results in cytokine activation, transcriptional regulation, cytoskeleton signaling, and apoptosis. The PYRIN domain had been found in more than 20 inflammatory and apoptotic proteins. Through homotypic domain interactions, the PYRIN domain can bind to the common adaptor apoptosis–associated specklike

Table 79.5 Rare Genetic Diseases with Renal Involvement Reported in Middle Eastern Communities

Country/Community	Disease	OMIM No.	Phenotype	Defect/Mutation	References
Saudi Arabs, Turks	Alström's syndrome*	203800	Retinal degeneration, obesity, cardiomyopathy, sensorineural hearing loss, insulin resistance, renal impairment	ALMS1 gene, ubiquitously expressed, encodes a protein of unknown function	156, 176
Israeli Jews of Iraqi origin	Renal hypouricemia type I	220150	Hypouricemia, hyperuricosuria, nephrolithiasis, exercise-induced acute kidney injury	SLC22A12 gene, encodes uric acid transporter URAT1	180
Israeli Arabs	Renal hypouricemia type II	612076	Increased renal clearance of uric acid, hypouricemia, nephrolithiasis, exercise-induced acute kidney injury	SLC2A9 gene, encodes glucose transporter 9 (GLUT9)	169, 173, 181
Israeli Jews, Turks	Dent's disease*	300009	Low-molecular-weight proteinuria, hypercalciuria, nephrocalcinosis, nephrolithiasis, rickets, renal failure, hypokalemic metabolic alkalosis, focal glomerulosclerosis	CLCN5, encodes the chloride/proton ClC-5 antiporter	170, 172, 182
Egyptian and Saudi Arabs, Turks, Iranians	Cystinosis	219750 (adult) 219900 (juvenile) 219800 (infantile)	Failure to thrive, polydipsia, polyuria, Fanconi-like syndrome; corneal, conjunctival, and retinal deposition	CTNS, encodes the lysosomal cystine carrier protein	177, 178, 185, 186
Israeli Druze	Autosomal recessive proximal tubulopathy with hypercalciuria		Proximal tubulopathy, hypercalciuria, normal or slightly elevated urinary phosphate excretion	SLC2A2 (GLUT2), encodes the glucose transporter 2†	184
Israeli Arabs	Autosomal recessive Fanconi's syndrome and hypophosphatemic rickets	613388	Proximal tubulopathy, renal phosphate wasting, normocalciuria, bone mineral deficiency, decreased glomerular filtration rate	SLC34A1, encodes the renal sodium phosphate cotransporter IIa	183
Israeli Arabs	Familial renal glycosuria and aminoaciduria‡	233100 and 182381	Glycosuria, aminoaciduria	SLC5A2, encodes the kidney-specific Na+/glucose cotransporter	175
Israeli Jews	Proximal renal tubular acidosis and glaucoma	604278 and 603345	Short stature, deformed teeth, bilateral glaucoma, blindness, metabolic acidosis	SLC4A4, encodes the sodium bicarbonate cotransporter (NBCe1)	171
Israeli Arabs and Jews	Familial autosomal recessive renal tubular acidosis	267300	Distal renal tubular acidosis, deafness	ATP6V1B1, encodes the B1-subunit of H+-ATPase	187
Israeli Arabs	Familial autosomal recessive renal tubular acidosis	259730	Proximal and distal renal tubular acidosis, osteopetrosis, mental retardation	CA2, encoding carbonic anhydrase	187
Egyptian Arabs	Familial hypomagnesemia with hypercalciuria and nephrocalcinosis	248250	Hypocalcemia, hypomagnesemia, hypercalciuria, nephrocalcinosis, congenital cataracts	CLDN16, the claudin-16 gene	179
Iranians	Familial lecithin-cholesterol acyltransferase deficiency§	245900	Lower extremity edema, proteinuria, corneal opacities, hypercholesterolemia, hemolytic anemia	Lecithin-cholesterol acyltransferase (LCAT) gene	174

*X-linked.
†Homozygous mutations in GLUT2 also cause Fanconi-Bickel syndrome.
‡Autosomal recessive.
§Diagnosis made on the basis of family history and electron microscopic findings on kidney biopsy.
OMIM, Online Mendelian Inheritance in Man catalog (http://www.ncbi.nlm.nih.gov/omim).

Table 79.6 Genotype-Phenotype Correlations in Several Patient Populations with Familial Mediterranean Fever

Population/ Community	Frequent Mutations	Phenotype	Amyloidosis (% Patients)	Associated Syndromes and Diseases	Reference
Israeli Jews and Arabs	M680I, M694V, M694I, V726A	Arthritis, fever, serositis, vasculitis	1.4% (associated with mutation in M694V)	NR	Brik et al[213]
Israeli Jews and Arabs	M694V (very common in Jews), M694I (exclusive in Arabs), M680I, V726A, E148Q	Arthritis, fever, serositis, vasculitis	NR	NR	Ben-Chetrit et al[212]
Israeli Arabs	M694V (associated with severe disease), V726A (most common)	Arthritis, fever, serositis, vasculitis	NR	NR	Shinawi et al[223]
Israeli Jews of North African origin and Arabs*	M694I, M694V (very common in North African Jews), E148Q	Synovitis, pleuritis, abdominal pain, skin rash	95%*	Focal glomerulosclerosis	Ben-Chetrit and Backenroth[211]
Israeli Jews of North African origin, Ashkenazi Jews, Jews of Iraqi origin, Israeli Arabs, and Druze	E148Q, M694V (very common in North African Jews), V726A	FMF criteria[217]	4.6% (most common in M694V homozygous)	NR	Zaks et al[226]
Israeli Jews (Ashkenazi and non-Ashkenazi), Arabs, and Druze	M694V (very common in Jews), E148Q, M694V, V726A (equally common in Arabs), E148Q (most common in Druze)	Fever, serositis	NR	NR	Sharkia et al[227]
Turks	M680I, M694V, M694I, V726A, E148Q	Abdominal pain, fever, arthralgia, chest pain, skin rash	3% (mostly associated with M694V)	NR	Solak et al[224]
Turks	M680I, M694V, V726A	Abdominal pain, fever, arthralgia, pleuritis, muscle pain, skin rash	12.9%; 0.9% as the main disease manifestation (phenotype II, associated with M694V)	Nonamyloid renal disease, Henoch-Schönlein purpura, polyarteritis nodosa, Behçet's syndrome, rheumatic fever, uveitis, inflammatory bowel disease	Tunca et al[225]
Turks†	M680I, M694V (most common), V726A, E148Q	Abdominal pain, fever, arthralgia, chest pain, erysipelas-like lesion, vomiting, family history of renal failure	0%	NR	Caglayan et al[205]
Turks	M680I, M694V (most common), M694I, V726A E148Q (common)	Abdominal pain, fever, arthritis, pleuritis, erysipelas-like erythema, peritonitis	NR	NR	Ozdemir et al[200]
Turks	M680I, M694V (most common), V726A, E148Q	Fever, arthritis, pleuritis, erysipelas-like erythema, peritonitis, vasculitis	8.6% (most common in M694V homozygous)	NR	Kasifoglu et al[202]
Azeri Turks	M680I, M694V (most common), M694I, V726A E148Q	Fever, serositis, synovitis, kidney failure	NR	NR	Mohammadnejad et al[201]

Continued on following page

Table 79.6 Genotype-Phenotype Correlations in Several Patient Populations with Familial Mediterranean Fever (Continued)

Population/ Community	Frequent Mutations	Phenotype	Amyloidosis (% Patients)	Associated Syndromes and Diseases	Reference
Jordanian Arabs Palestinian Arabs	M680I, M694V, M694I, V726A, E148Q	Abdominal pain, fever, arthralgia, myalgia, skin rash	1% (associated with M694V)	Protracted fever, myalgia syndrome; 42% homozygous for M694V	Langevitz et al,[216] Majeed et al[218]
Jordanian Arabs	M680I, M694V, V726A, E148Q	Abdominal pain, fever, arthralgia	9% (M694V in 1 patient, V726A/M680I in 2 patients)	Celiac disease, folliculitis	Medlej-Hashim et al[220]
Palestinian Arabs	M680I, M694V, V726A, E148Q	NR	NR	NR	Ayesh et al[209]
Arabs from Jordan, Egypt, Syria, Iraq, and Saudi Arabia	M694V, V726A, E148Q	NR	NR	NR	Al-Alami et al[208]
Iranian Azeris who live in Turkey	M680I, M694V, M694I, V726A, E148Q	Abdominal pain, fever, arthralgia, pleuritis, skin rash	7%	NR	Esmaeili et al[215]
Iranians (72% Azeri)	M680I (most common), M694V, V726A	Fever, peritonitis, arthralgia, pleuritis, skin rash	5.6%	NR	Bidari A et al[207]
Egyptian Arabs	M680I, M694V, V726A	Abdominal pain, chest pain, fever, arthritis, myalgia	NR	NR	Settin et al[222]
Egyptian Arabs	M680I, M694I (most common), M694V, V726A, E148Q	Fever, serositis	Mostly associated with M694V	NR	El Gezery et al[204]
Egyptian Arabs	V726A (most common), M694V (common), M680I, M694I, E148Q	Abdominal pain, fever, arthralgia, pleuritis, skin rash, myalgia	2.9% (associated with M694V)	NR	El-Garf et al[203]
Syrian Arabs	M680I, M694V, M694I, V726A, E148Q, A744S, R761H	Serositis, fever, arthritis, pleuritis	5%	NR	Mattit et al[219]
Lebanese Arabs	M680I, M694V (very frequent), M694I, V726A, E148Q (very frequent); minor alleles also detected	Serositis, fever, arthritis, chest pain	NR	NR	Sabbagh et al[221]
Algerian, Moroccan, and Tunisian Arabs	M694V and M694I (most common), M680I, M680I, A744S, V726A, E148Q	Serositis, fever, arthritis, chest pain	NR	NR	Belmahi et al[210]
Algerians	M694I (most common), M694V, E148Q, A744S, M680I	Abdominal pain, fever, arthritis, chest pain, erythema	8%	NR	Ait-Idir et al[206]
Tunisian Arabs	M680I (most common), M694V, M694I, V726A, E148Q, A744S, R761H, 1692del	FMF criteria[217]	3.5%	NR	Chaabouni et al[214]

*Study performed in patients with end-stage kidney disease.
†Study performed in compound heterozygous patients.
FMF, Familial Mediterranean fever; NR, not reported.

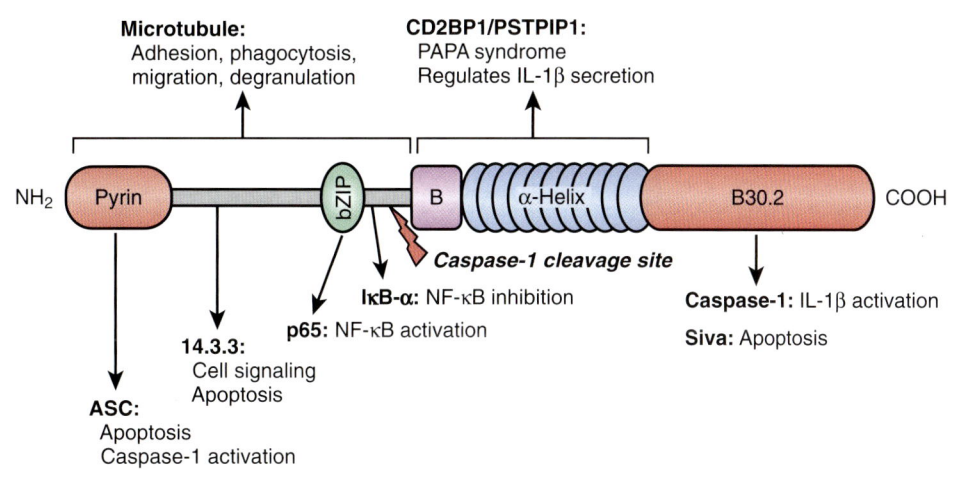

Figure 79.4 The structure of pyrin and its interacting proteins. Pyrin comprises five domains, each of which has specific protein-protein interactions: a PYRIN domain, a bZIP transcription factor basic domain, a B-box zinc finger domain, an α-helical (coiled-coil) domain, and a B30.2 domain. B30.2 includes a SPRY domain, located in front of the C-terminal region, and a PRY extension at the N terminus (not shown in figure). The entire N terminus of pyrin is necessary to bind pyrin to microtubules, and three serine residues, which are located between the PYRIN and the bZIP domains, are essential for the 14.3.3 protein–PYRIN interaction. The PYRIN domain interacts with common adaptor apoptosis–associated specklike protein (ASC); the bZIP basic domain and adjacent sequences interact with p65 and IκB kinase α (IκB-α); the B-box zinc finger and α-helical (coiled-coil) domains interact with PAPA protein (PSTPIP1), which is also known as CD2BP1; and the B30.2 domain interacts with caspase-1. The caspase-1–mediated cleavage site of pyrin is located between the bZIP basic domain and the B-box zinc finger domain. (Adapted from Chae JJ, Aksentijevich I, Kramer DL: Advances in understanding of familial Mediterranean fever and possibilities for targeted therapy, *Br J Haematol* 146:467-478, 2009.)

protein (ASC), which has an N-terminal PYRIN domain and a C-terminal CARD domain, participates in the proteolytic activation of caspase-1 in cytoplasmic protein complexes (inflammasomes), and regulates the maturation and secretion of the proinflammatory cytokines interleukin (IL)–1β, IL-18, and IL-33.[234] Inflammasomes contain members of the nucleotide-binding oligomerization domain, leucine-rich repeat, and PYRIN domain–containing subfamily of proteins, now known as NLRP proteins. Mutations in the gene expression of the NLRP protein, *NLRP3* (cryopyrin), are associated with monogenic autoinflammatory diseases (cryopyrin-associated periodic syndromes).[235,236]

The presence of the bZIP transcription factor basic domain, the B-box zinc finger domain, and two universal nuclear localization signals in the N terminus of pyrin suggests that pyrin may act as a nuclear factor. Several studies have shown that pyrin is cleaved by caspase-1, and the N-terminal cleaved fragment (330 amino acids) localizes to the nucleus and potentiates activation of nuclear factor κ light-chain enhancer of activated B cells (NF-κB).[237] The N terminus of pyrin is also needed for pyrin to bind to the microtubules. The three serine residues 208, 209, and 242 that are located between the PYRIN and bZIP domains are critical for the interactions with 14.3.3 proteins, which are potent antiapoptotic factors and play an important role in the subcellular compartmentalization of pyrin.[238]

The effects of pyrin on IL-1β are complex. Pyrin competitively binds with the ASC adaptor protein through the PYRIN domain (see Figure 79.4), an action that prevents ASC binding to caspase-1 and the formation of the inflammasome. Pyrin also binds to caspase-1 through the B30.2 domain. The overall result of these two actions is suppression of IL-1β release. Under certain circumstances, however, the interaction of pyrin with ASC adaptor protein modulates the arrangement of pyroptosome, a protein that activates caspase-1 and promotes the release of IL-1β.[239] The B30.2 domain of pyrin is the target of most *MEFV* mutations. This domain, which is located at the C-terminal domain of the protein, is a site of ligand binding and signal transduction. Thus mutations in the B30.2 domain may lead to an excessive inflammatory response as a result of the decreased ability of pyrin to control IL-1β activation.

The putative role of pyrin in the pathogenesis of FMF is depicted in Figure 79.5. According to this model, the active caspase-1 subunits p10 and p20 are produced in the inflammasome by inducing proximity-mediated autocatalysis. The wild-type B30.2 domain of pyrin interacts with the p20 and p10 subunits and consequently prevents the formation of an active p20/p10 heterodimer. In FMF, FMF-associated pyrin B30.2 mutants interact with the p20 and p10 subunits but to a lesser extent than does the wild-type B30.2 domain, therefore enabling assembly of the p20/p10 heterodimer, activation of IL-1β, and the induction of inflammation. The active p20/p10 heterodimer then cleaves pyrin at Asp330, which is located between the bZIP basic domain and the B-box zinc finger domain. The N-terminal–cleaved fragment then interacts with the p65 subunit of NF-κB and the inhibitor protein IκB kinase α through the bZIP basic domain and adjacent sequences to activate NF-κB and induce the expression of inflammatory genes.[196] An alternative hypothesis of pyrin stimulation has been proposed.[235,240] According to this hypothesis, under stimulation, pyrin forms its own inflammasome with ASC and caspase-1 that is able to activate IL-1.[235] Another study showed that a severe autoinflammatory phenotype occurs independently of *NLRP3*, in homozygous but not in heterozygous knock-in mice carrying the mutated human pyrin. This study also suggested that missense PYRIN mutations are gain-of-function mutations with a dosage effect.[240]

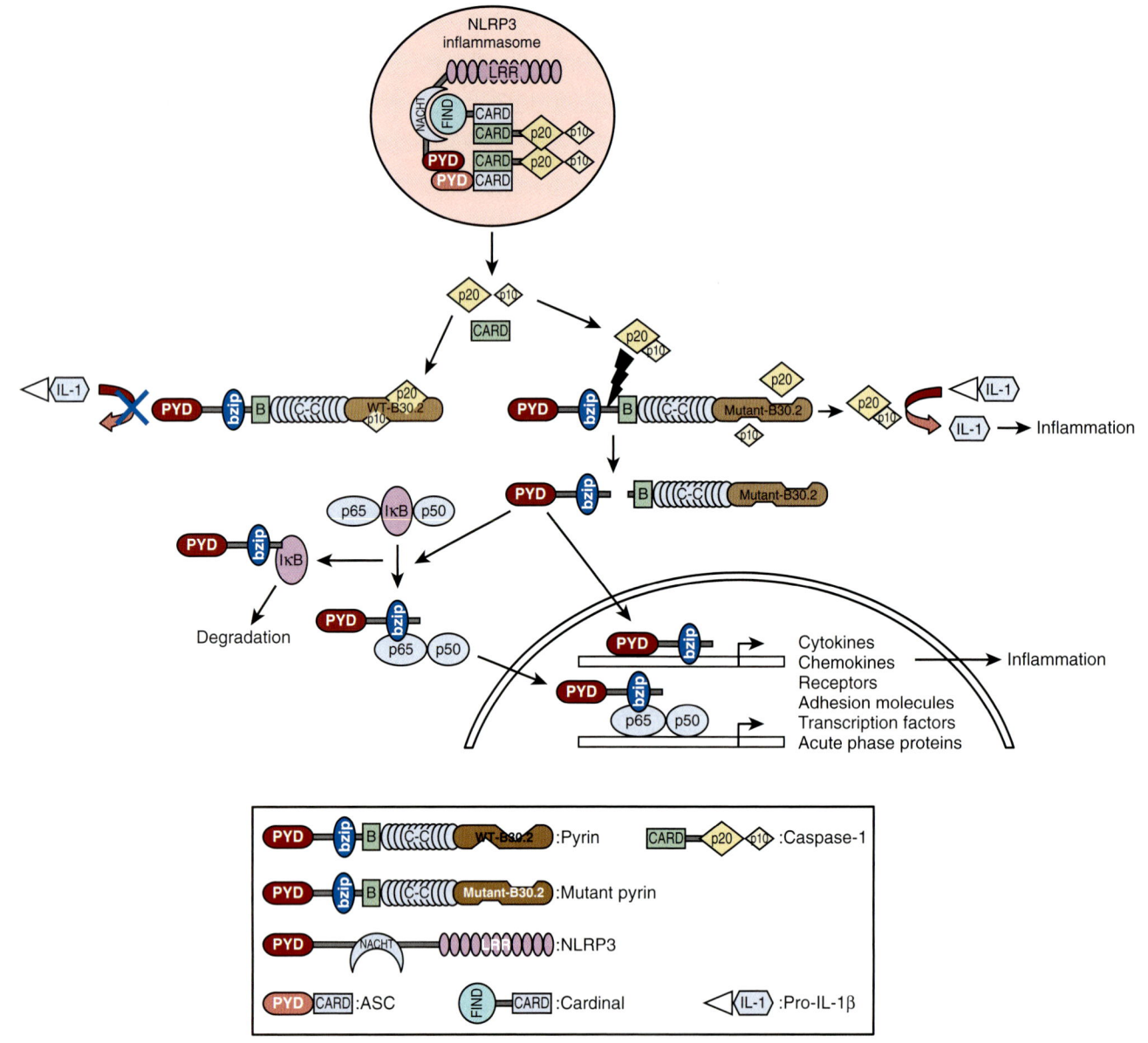

Figure 79.5 **Proposed role of pyrin in the pathogenesis of familial Mediterranean fever (FMF).** The structural organization of a representative inflammasome (NLRP3) is shown. The active caspase-1 subunits p10 and p20 are produced in the inflammasome by inducing proximity-mediated autocatalysis. The wild-type B30.2 domain of pyrin interacts with the p20 and p10 subunits and, as a consequence, prevents formation of an active p20/p10 heterodimer. FMF-associated pyrin B30.2 mutants interact with p20 and p10 but to a lesser extent than does the wild-type B30.2 domain, therefore enabling p20/p10 heterodimer assembly, IL-1β activation, and induction of inflammation. The active p20/p10 heterodimer cleaves pyrin at Asp330 (located between the bZIP basic domain and the B-box zinc finger domain). The N-terminal–cleaved fragment interacts with p65 and IκB kinase α (IκB-α) through the bZIP basic domain and adjacent sequences, by which NF-κB is activated with induction of inflammatory genes expression. IL-1β, Interleukin-1β; NF-κB, nuclear factor κ light-chain enhancer of activated B cells. (Adapted with permission from Chae JJ, Aksentijevich I, Kramer DL: Advances in understanding of familial Mediterranean fever and possibilities for targeted therapy, *Br J Haematol* 146:467-478, 2009.)

Clinical Spectrum and Renal Disease

The wide clinical spectrum and the genotype-phenotype correlations in FMF are influenced by genotype (extent and position of the *MEFV* mutation), ethnicity, and environmental factors. In Arab patients with FMF, the worst disease severity is associated with alleles carrying the mutations M694V/M694V and M694V/M726A, whereas the M694I/M694I mutation is associated with a mild form of the disease.[241] In Turkish patients with FMF, the common M694V mutation is associated with more severe disease but not with amyloidosis.[225,231] In contrast, the homozygous M694V mutation was reported to be associated with amyloidosis in Jews from North Africa, in Arabs, in Turks, and also with the protracted febrile myalgia syndrome, which is a type of myalgia that is associated with FMF in Arabs.[212,213,218,220,225,226,241]

FMF has traditionally been considered an autosomal recessive genetic disease, but as many as 25% of patients with clinical FMF have only one *MEFV* mutation.[224,225,230] This finding could explain the vertical transmission of the disease in some families. In patients with FMF who have a single *MEFV* mutation, an additional but less common mutation may account for the disease, but this has not yet been confirmed in carefully performed studies. A dominant segregation of a heterozygous *MEFV* mutation was reported in some families. Therefore it was suggested that complex alleles can lead to a more severe form of disease.[242] One study reported that heterozygous mutations at amino acid position 577 of pyrin (T577) can induce autosomal dominant autoinflammatory disease. The T577 is located in front of the C-terminal B30.2/SPRY domain and is crucial for pyrin function.[243,244] The T577 mutations were found in a family of Turkish descent with autosomal dominant FMF phenotype and also in European patients with other periodic syndromes. The impact of *MEFV* mutations has been shown in other inflammatory diseases, such as Henoch-Schönlein purpura, polyarteritis nodosa, Behçet's disease, rheumatic heart disease, and rheumatoid arthritis (reviewed by Guz and associates).[231] Of interest is that individuals who carry a single mutated allele in the *MEFV* gene can also suffer from the syndrome of *p*eriodic *f*ever, *a*phthosis, *p*haryngitis, and *a*denitis (PFAPA); ankylosing spondylitis; and Crohn's disease.[245]

Secondary or reactive AA amyloidosis is the most severe complication of FMF. Before the advent of colchicine treatment, amyloidosis was reported to occur in approximately 75% of patients with FMF who were older than 40 years.[246] The disease is caused by the extracellular deposition of amyloid A fibrils. These fibrils consist of β-pleated sheet polymers of the N-terminal fragments, the products of incomplete proteolytic digestion of the acute-phase precursor serum amyloid A (SAA) protein, whose production is markedly increased in chronic inflammatory processes.[247] Amyloidosis is frequently found in Jews from North African countries in the ME, in Turks, and in Armenians. As mentioned earlier, a positive association of amyloidosis with the M694V mutation has been reported in patients from several ethnic groups.[211,213,218,220,224,225,248] The M694V mutation has also been found in patients with FMF phenotype II, in which amyloidosis is detected before the onset of clinical symptoms of FMF.[225] Phenotype III is defined as the presence of two *MEFV* mutations (homozygous or compound heterozygote state) without clinical manifestation of FMF or amyloidosis. This condition, however, like phenotype II, could predispose to development of amyloidosis in families in which one sibling is afflicted with FMF.[249] A screening study of patients with FMF from 14 countries worldwide—which included Israel, Turkey, Qatar, Jordan, and Lebanon—revealed that amyloid nephropathy was present in 11.4% of patients with FMF.[250] In this study, however, the country of recruitment, rather than *MEFV* genotype, was found to be the leading risk factor for amyloidosis.[250] These findings underscore the relative contribution of environmental factors to the genetic background in defining the phenotypic variation and severity of the disease.[251]

Male gender, a positive family history of amyloidosis, pain flares in joints, and the SAA1 α/α genotype have been suggested as additional risk factors for amyloidosis.[242] Albuminuria is usually the first manifestation of renal involvement in patients with FMF and amyloidosis, and in untreated patients it may appear early in the course of FMF.[252] In one study, serum cystatin C level was found to be significantly increased in patients with FMF and secondary amyloidosis. It was suggested that cystatin C serum level may be an early marker of renal impairment even before the onset of albuminuria.[253] Proteinuria, mostly represented by albumin, can reach the nephrotic range with urinary protein excretion rates higher than 20 g/day. If untreated, AA amyloidosis progresses to ESKD that ultimately necessitates RRT. Renal disease due to amyloidosis accounts for 35% and 60% of deaths in men and women, respectively, with FMF.[254] Extrarenal deposits of AA amyloid can be found in liver, spleen, lung, thyroid, heart, adrenal glands, stomach, and testes. These deposits can be clinically significant and are associated with intestinal malabsorption and adrenal insufficiency that are often diagnosed after the initiation of chronic hemodialysis or after kidney transplantation.[252,255,256]

The diagnosis of amyloidosis can be confirmed by tissue biopsy; the sensitivities of the rectal or bone marrow biopsy and renal biopsy are 79.5% and 88%, respectively, whereas the sensitivity of biopsy of abdominal fat is lower.[257-259] The presence of amyloid deposits is demonstrated histologically with Congo red staining of the biopsy tissue sample. Congo red–stained amyloid has an orange appearance when viewed under a light microscope and an apple-green birefringence when viewed under polarized light. Another amyloid-specific stain, thioflavin T, is used less frequently than Congo red. Amyloidosis is diagnosed definitively on electron microscopy by the demonstration of characteristic amyloid fibrils. The AA protein in tissue can also be detected with antibodies against AA protein.[259]

In addition to AA amyloidosis, other kidney diseases have been diagnosed in patients with FMF. It is worthwhile mentioning that many of the reports of systemic and inflammatory diseases in patients with FMF contain descriptions of kidney involvement.[225] In fact, the frequency of the reported nonamyloid glomerular lesions reflects the number of kidney biopsies that are performed in patients with abnormal findings on urinalysis or on kidney function tests. Recurrent focal and proliferative glomerulonephritis and polyarteritis nodosa were described in an early report of the disease.[260] Rapidly progressive glomerulonephritis, mesangial proliferative glomerulonephritis, IgA nephropathy, and membranous nephropathy have also been reported.[225,230,261-264]

Treatment of Familial Mediterranean Fever

Daily oral colchicine is the most effective therapy for patients with FMF, and its use since the 1980s has dramatically changed the course of the disease. Colchicine prevents both acute attacks of FMF and SAA amyloidosis.[265,266] The mechanism of colchicine action is not well understood. It is believed that one of its major actions is to interact with cytoskeletal structures, such as microtubules. It has been shown that colchicine accumulates in PMNCs, where it depolymerizes the microtubules and suppresses microtubule dynamics. Pyrin is also expressed in PMNCs and associates with microtubules.[267] Because colchicine also has an inhibitory effect on chemotaxis and reduces serum levels of IL-6, IL-8, and tumor necrosis factor-α,[268] its antiinflammatory action is thought to be related to its ability to suppress NF-κB activation by attenuating calpain-mediated IκB kinase α degradation, which is enhanced by N-terminal cleaved pyrin.[237] Suppression of caspase-1 expression in PMNCs was also suggested to be a potential mechanism of action of colchicine.[269]

In vitro, colchicine was shown to have a specific effect on pyrin and pyrin-interacting protein such as proline-serine-threonine phosphatase interacting protein 1 (PSTPIP1) and ASC. In THP-1 cells, colchicine reorganized cytoskeleton and downregulated MEFV expression. This effect, which may result in a reduction of level of a proinflammatory mutant pyrin, may explain the suppressive mechanism of colchicine on FMF attacks.[270]

The most common adverse effects of colchicine are gastrointestinal, especially abdominal pain and diarrhea. Colchicine toxicity from overdosing is associated with hepatic, renal, muscle, and cerebral effects.[271] Nonresponsiveness to colchicine has been reported in 5% to 10% of patients. The reasons for nonresponsiveness are complex and include noncompliance, socioeconomic factors, and clinical factors. In M694V homozygotes, a significant proportion of patients show partial or minimal response to colchicine despite being treated with appropriate doses.[272] In contrast, prolonged colchicine-free remission was noted in some individuals, none of whom was homozygous for this mutation.[273]

One study revealed the existence of an association between polymorphism of adenosine triphosphate–binding cassette, subfamily B, member 1 (*ABCB1*) gene and the response to colchicine in Turkish patients with FMF. The *ABCB1* gene encodes p170 (also known as multidrug resistance 1 [MDR1]), a glycoprotein that functions as a drug transport pump, which can cause a variety of drugs, including colchicine, to become extruded from cells. In this study, patients with FMF who had the TT genotype for the 3435C→T variant of *ABCB1* responded better to colchicine in terms of treatment efficacy and lower dose requirements in comparison with patients who had the CT and CC genotypes.[274] These results warrant validation in further studies in patients with FMF from different ethnic populations.

Thalidomide, nonsteroidal antiinflammatory drugs, corticosteroids, azathioprine, prazosin, and eprodisate disodium, an inhibitor of fibril formation, are occasionally used to treat patients with FMF whose disease is refractory to colchicine.[259,275-277] Interferon-α was one of the first drugs that was used to treat patients with FMF who were refractory to colchicine.[278] Two studies of patients with FMF who were treated with interferon-α showed that the duration and pain intensity of the majority of the attacks were reduced by more than 50%.[279,280] In addition, clinical improvement has been reported in patients with FMF who were treated with the tumor necrosis factor-α antagonists etanercept or infliximab.[276,281,282] Because most inflammatory manifestations of FMF are believed to be associated with the induction of IL-1β production by mutations in the C-terminal B30.2 domain of pyrin (see Figure 79.4), it has been proposed that IL-1β antagonists may be an effective therapy for FMF. The IL-1β receptor antagonist anakinra has been shown to have a beneficial effect in patients with FMF and with cryopyrin-associated periodic syndromes.[275,277] Indeed, significant improvement and resolution of FMF symptoms have been reported in patients with colchicine-resistant FMF who were treated with anakinra.[275,283,284] Anakinra elicited a beneficial therapeutic response in individuals with FMF and chronic kidney disease, and even in a patient on maintenance hemodialysis and after kidney transplantation.[284,285] The main limitation of anakinra treatment in patients with FMF is probably the need for daily subcutaneous injections. Administration of either the long-acting IL-1 decoy receptor rilonacept (IL-1 Trap) every week or the administration of canakinumab, a human monoclonal antibody against IL-1β, every 8 weeks has also been associated with rapid remission of symptoms in FMF and cryopyrin-associated periodic syndromes.[233,286,287] Therefore these antibodies seem to be promising therapeutic options in patients with refractory FMF or who are resistant to colchicine.

Familial Mediterranean Fever and End-Stage Kidney Disease

In contrast to the poor prognosis of patients with primary (AL) amyloidosis who require RRT, most patients with FMF and secondary (AA) amyloidosis do relatively well with chronic dialysis.[288] However, the issue of which dialysis modality is the ideal for the treatment of FMF-associated ESKD is still unresolved,[65] and prospective studies that compare the different modalities are still needed. Of the dialysis modalities, hemodialysis is more widely used in patients with FMF. Continuous ambulatory peritoneal dialysis (CAPD), however, has been performed successfully in selected patients. The effects of CAPD on azotemia and overall survival are similar in patients with nonamyloid diseases and patients with FMF. However, the serum albumin levels are reported to be lower and the rate of peritonitis and requirements for erythropoietin-stimulating agents (ESAs) were higher in patients with FMF who received CAPD than in patients with FMF who received hemodialysis.[289,290]

A considerable number of patients with FMF and ESKD have undergone kidney transplantation in the last few decades. The rates of survival of patients and allografts are reported to be worse or similar to those in the general population of kidney transplant recipients.[65,225,291-294] Maintenance colchicine therapy is obligatory after kidney transplantation because it may prevent the recurrence both of FMF symptoms and of amyloidosis. However, recurrence of AA amyloidosis has been frequently reported 8 to 10 years after kidney transplantation,[295] and the rate of recurrence may be as high as 71%.[294] Adverse drug effects are seen in kidney transplant recipients with FMF who are taking cyclosporine. In addition, increased gastrointestinal complications can be observed in patients who are treated with a combination of mycophenolate mofetil and colchicine.[296]

MANAGEMENT OF END-STAGE KIDNEY DISEASE IN THE MIDDLE EAST

Dialysis and kidney transplantation are available in all ME countries. In all industrialized and many developing ME countries, RRT is accessible to every patient with ESKD, regardless of the patient's socioeconomic status or whether the patient has health insurance.[10,12,33,89,97,102,103,106,110,162,297-301] On the other hand, the number of patients offered RRT in other developing ME countries may be affected by late diagnosis and referral, the presence of comorbid conditions, the country's health system, reimbursement, and the availability of dialysis facilities.[106]

DIALYSIS

PERITONEAL DIALYSIS

Throughout the ME, hemodialysis is the preferred treatment modality for ESKD (see Table 79.3). Peritoneal dialysis is an underused treatment modality for ESKD, although its use is increasing in Tunisia, Kuwait, Iran, Saudi Arabia, Qatar, and Turkey.[302-304] Several medical and nonmedical factors play an important role in inhibiting the widespread use of peritoneal dialysis throughout the ME: (1) Health providers generally offer low or no reimbursement for peritoneal dialysis; (2) the numbers of peritoneal dialysis training programs, qualified nephrologists, and skilled dialysis nurses are limited, and the salaries of attending physicians for peritoneal dialysis are low; (3) many patients have poor education and poor hygiene practices; and (4) patients and caregivers have concerns about high rates of peritonitis.

At the end of 2006, 38,824 patients were treated with dialysis (87.4% with hemodialysis, 12.6% with peritoneal dialysis) in Turkey, and 99.7% of all patients receiving dialysis were covered by the social security system.[162] The Turkish experience in establishing a peritoneal dialysis program has been outstanding and could be used as an example by other ME countries. The Turkish Multicenter Peritoneal Dialysis Study Group (TULIP) has established a platform for organizing peritoneal dialysis facilities and units. The group helped standardize patient records and various peritoneal dialysis treatments and maximized the number of patients with ESKD who can benefit from this treatment modality. This group has published clinical research that has affected peritoneal dialysis practice locally and worldwide.[162] The Turkish peritoneal dialysis program has good rates of survival of patients and technique efficacy, which are comparable with those in Western industrialized countries.[109] The peritoneal dialysis dropout rate was 21%, and the incidence of peritonitis was one episode per 35.5 patient-months in 2007. Dyslipidemia was the most common noninfectious complication[86]; cardiovascular diseases (42.3%), followed by infections (19.9%) and cerebrovascular events (13.6%), were the major causes of death among Turkish patients undergoing peritoneal dialysis.[86,109] Moreover, peritoneal dialysis has been suggested as a means of reducing the seroconversion rate for hepatitis C virus (HCV) in populations with ESKD and a high prevalence of infection[305]; such treatment thereby confers an advantage to kidney transplant candidates.[306]

Peritoneal dialysis was started in Iran in 1978 and in Saudi Arabia and Kuwait during the 1980s with imported peritoneal dialysis solutions. The costs of this treatment are low in Turkey and Iran because peritoneal dialysis solutions began to be produced locally in Turkey in 1994 and in Iran in 1995.[302] Establishment of a peritoneal dialysis registry and a multidisciplinary approach has dramatically increased the numbers of patients undergoing peritoneal dialysis in Iran since 2001.[100] The peritonitis rate in these patients is reported to be one episode per 19.4 patient-months, and the dropout rate is 11%; dropout is caused mainly by infectious complications.[302] In 2010 the 1-year, 3-year, and 5-year patient survival rates in Iran were reported as 89%, 64%, and 49%, respectively, whereas technique survival rates were 90%, 73%, and 58%.[100] The peritonitis rate was one episode in 25 patient-months, and the main causes of death among Iranian patients undergoing peritoneal dialysis were cardiac events (46%), cerebral stroke (10%), and infection (8%).[100] Interestingly, use of peritoneal dialysis is growing in Qatar since its introduction in 1997, and peritoneal dialysis is offered to approximately 23% of ESKD patients. Most of these patients are non-Qatari male expatriates, a group that favors a mode of dialysis that can be self-administered, secures the ability to work or travel, requires less dietary restrictions, and potentially decreases the hospital and medical cost.[304]

These advantages of peritoneal dialysis, which provides flexibility and ease of adjustment for lifestyle and daily schedule, encouraged some clinically stable Moslem patients on peritoneal dialysis to fast during the holy month of Ramadan.[307] However, patients who intend to fast need to be comprehensively educated and followed up by their peritoneal dialysis units.[307]

HEMODIALYSIS

There are limited published data on hemodialysis in the ME with regard to practice patterns and outcomes, such as the quality of dialysis, survival of patients per technique, type of vascular access, standard dialysate solutions and dialyzers, medical complications and their management, comorbid conditions, and other measures of quality assurance.[94,96,103,299,300,308-313] In general, quality is ensured according to best medical practice guidelines in industrialized ME countries with more resources, easily accessible health care systems, and advanced medical supplies, such as in Israel and the Gulf Cooperation Council countries. In ME countries that lack resources, prescription of hemodialysis is minimal, and the quality of dialysis is dictated by nonmedical financial considerations. In these countries, dialysis may be offered only once or twice weekly because of lack of skilled personnel, the distance of the dialysis centers from the patient's residence, and inability of the patient to pay for more frequent treatment. On this last point, the number of patients who withdraw from hemodialysis therapy because of financial problems has not been documented. Nonetheless, a small number of patients do seek pre-ESKD care in most ME countries.[5,103]

Practice guidelines for hemodialysis have been developed in Egypt. These included five main domains: personnel, patient care practices, infection prevention and control, facility, and documentation or records. Before distribution of the guidelines, one study disclosed flawed compliance and variability in adoption of evidence-based hemodialysis guidelines among 16 Egyptian facilities affiliated with the Ministry of Health and Population.[309] Therefore it is mandatory to distribute these guidelines to all hemodialysis facilities in Egypt, along with organization of workshops to educate staff and follow-up to ensure implementation of the guidelines. In Libya the provision of dialysis was adequate in 2010. Yet several areas for improvement have been identified by Alashek and associates,[96] such as lack of national dialysis practice guidelines and few clinical practitioners were familiar with KDOQI guidelines. Because of continuous drought, many dialysis centers were obliged to dig their own wells to maintain water supply. However, testing of water quality was not regularly practiced. In addition, wide discrepancy in methods applied to manage and monitor patients was observed between centers.[94,96]

According to the 2012 SCOT report,[311] 12,844 patients receiving hemodialysis were treated in 182 centers in Saudi

Arabia. Of these patients, approximately 24% are on the waiting list for kidney transplantation. Bicarbonate dialysis solutions were used in all centers, and only a few centers (6.3%) still use acetate dialysis solutions. The predominant type of vascular access for hemodialysis is arteriovenous fistulas (71.2% of all patients), followed by jugular catheters (12.6%), and arteriovenous grafts (7.6%). In comparison, the prevalent types of vascular access in Israel in 2013 were arteriovenous fistulas (60%), arteriovenous grafts (10%), and permanent catheters (30%; E. Golan, April 2014, personal communication). In Tehran, arteriovenous fistula is the type of vascular access used most in patients receiving hemodialysis (91%); only 3% of such patients have arteriovenous grafts, and 4% have permanent catheters.[97] Arteriovenous fistula is also preferred in Turkey: in 2008, arteriovenous fistula were used in 85.4% of Turkish patients receiving hemodialysis, grafts were used in 2.9%, permanent tunneled catheters were used in 7.7%, and temporary catheters were used in 4%.[312]

Reuse of dialyzers is not practiced in Saudi Arabia, Libya, and Iran[96,314] and is prohibited by law in Egypt.[103] Approximately 87% of Saudi patients receiving hemodialysis are treated with ESAs, and of these patients, approximately 23% have hemoglobin levels lower than 10 g/dL. In Turkey, ESAs are administered to 61.8% of patients receiving hemodialysis. In comparison, 48.2% of patients receiving hemodialysis in Tehran have anemia as a result of low-dose treatment with ESAs, and dialysis may be inadequate because the mean measured treatment adequacy for these patients was 0.97 ± 0.25.[97] Thus common clinical practice for hemodialysis in Iran does not meet all the targets recommended by international guidelines.[97,313]

No adequate studies have been conducted to describe the patterns, prevalence, or therapy of CKD-associated mineral bone disorders (CKD-MBDs) in patients undergoing dialysis in any of the 20 ME countries. In developing ME countries, the use of aluminum-based phosphate binders, presence of high amounts of strontium in the soil, and the use of dialysis acetate concentrates that are contaminated with strontium have been implicated as causes of osteomalacia in adult patients receiving hemodialysis and rickets in pediatric patients receiving hemodialysis.[315,316] Hyperphosphatemia and increased serum level of calcium-phosphorus product are serious problems in dialysis recipients in developing ME countries, and their occurrence is correlated with poor patient knowledge of appropriate diet. In a large cross-sectional multicenter study that included 1005 patients in Egypt who were undergoing hemodialysis, two-thirds of the patients had hyperphosphatemia, and one-third had an elevated serum level of calcium-phosphorus product. The patients used mainly calcium-based phosphate binders.[317] In most developing ME countries, economic considerations hinder the use of the newer non–calcium-based phosphate binders, calcium-sensing receptor agonists (calcimimetics), or vitamin D receptor agonists. Therefore prolonged or additional dialysis sessions are frequently prescribed to control hyperphosphatemia in patients receiving hemodialysis.[97,317]

The results of one survey suggested that practicing Saudi nephrologists have an adequate perception of the morbidity in patients with CKD-MBDs.[318] However, the results of this survey also identified a need for creating national guidelines because the physicians' assessment of the prevalence, patterns, and results of therapeutic interventions in patients with CKD-MBDs was relatively inadequate. Approximately 25% of their patients had hyperphosphatemia (serum phosphorus levels > 6 mg/dL), and 20% had hypocalcemia (serum calcium levels < 8.4 mg/dL), although vitamin D was administered orally to most patients. In view of the current status of CKD-MBD in the ME countries and the associated economic and logistic constraints, a committee of experienced nephrologists from the region was constituted. Its members examined the KDIGO guidelines and formulated recommendations that can be implemented practically for the management of CKD-MBD in the ME.[319]

MANAGEMENT OF END-STAGE KIDNEY DISEASE WITH VIRAL HEPATITIS

Available global data indicate that the prevalence of chronic infection with hepatitis B virus (HBV) and HCV is high in populations of the African and ME regions.[320,321] These two viral infections have considerable effects on morbidity and mortality among patients with ESKD, as well as on graft survival in kidney transplant recipients.[103,322-325] However, surveys are still needed to correctly estimate the incidence and prevalence of these infections in patients with CKD and ESKD in each ME country. In addition, screening will identify patients who would benefit from a number of highly efficacious, new oral therapies.[326-328] The HCV epidemic is particularly devastating in Egypt, where its prevalence in the general population is estimated to be more than 18%. The start of the HCV epidemic in Egypt is attributed to the use of unsterilized needles and syringes during the mass antischistosomiasis treatment programs that were conducted during the 1960s and 1970s.[329] Several studies reported a dismal prevalence of anti-HCV serologic findings among Egyptian patients undergoing hemodialysis and kidney transplant recipients that ranged between 46% and 100%.[103,329-332] Implementation of an infection control program by 60 Egyptian dialysis facilities resulted in improvements in infection control practices among health care workers and a subsequent decrease in the annual incidence of HCV infection among patients undergoing dialysis from 28% to 6%, 3 years later.[330]

Among Saudi patients receiving hemodialysis, according to the 2012 SCOT report,[311] the prevalence of HBV positivity is 3.8%, whereas HCV infection continued to be problematic (18.7%). Nonetheless, it has decreased compared with previous reports.[311] However, there is considerable variability in the prevalence of HCV infection between the various regions of Saudi Arabia (11% to 23%).[311,333] This variability is important to consider when patients receiving hemodialysis travel to other units and emphasizes the importance of screening them for seroconversion after their return. The annual rate of HCV seroconversion in Saudi patients receiving hemodialysis is between 7% and 9%. The most common variant of the virus is HCV genotype 4[334] (which is also prevalent in North African countries in the ME[103,322,330,335]), followed by HCV genotype 1a and HCV genotype 1b. Implementation of strict measures of infection control and isolation of HCV-positive patients and dialysis machines resulted in a significant drop in the annual incidence of HCV infections from 2.4% to 0.2% in one Saudi hemodialysis center.[333]

In Iran, where genotypes 3a and 1a are the common variants, impressive drops in the rates of HCV and hepatitis B surface antigen (HBsAg) positivity have been reported in patients receiving hemodialysis. These decreases (14.4% in 1999 to 4.5% in 2006 for HCV and 3.8% in 1999 to 2.6% in 2006 for HBV) have been attributed to the introduction of several measures, such as strict isolation policies, no reuse of dialyzers, compulsory HBV vaccination in patients, and early kidney transplantation.[314] Implementation of routine virologic testing, strict isolation measures, HBV vaccination, and ESA administration with few blood product transfusion requirements have resulted in a low prevalence of both HBV (1.7% to 2%) and HCV (3.7% to 5.7%) infection among Israeli patients receiving dialysis between 2005 and 2010, according to the 2012 ICDC report.[88]

Using second-generation immunoassays to detect HCV infection in 30 Turkish dialysis centers, Köhler found that the prevalence of HCV was 49.9% in 1995.[323] Sayiner and colleagues reported that the duration of dialysis, kidney transplantation history, and history of blood products transfusion were all related to HCV transmission and high prevalence of HCV among Turkish patients receiving hemodialysis.[336] Turkey is also endemic for HBV infection. Ten percent of patients receiving hemodialysis and 2.9% of blood donors are HBsAg positive. Of note is that the 2008 registry of the Turkish Society of Nephrology[312] reported a decline in the prevalence of HBV infection (4.5%), HCV infection (12.7%), and both infections (0.9%) in Turkish patients receiving hemodialysis. The results of a survey that was conducted among Jordanian patients receiving hemodialysis during 2003 revealed HBV positivity in 4% and HCV positivity in 21%, with annual seroconversion rates of 0.34% for HBV and 2.6% for HCV.[102] In 2007, high seropositivity for HBV (8%) and HCV (22%) was also detected in Palestinian patients undergoing hemodialysis who were residing in the Gaza Strip.[337]

Alashek and colleagues found a remarkably high prevalence of seropositivity for HCV among Libyan patients undergoing hemodialysis (31.1%), which is 25-fold higher than the general population.[95] The overall incidence of seroconversion during this 1-year prospective study was 7.1%, with wide variation between hemodialysis units. Conversely, the prevalence of HBsAg positivity was low (2.6%) with seroconversion incidence of 0.6%. Factors that were associated with seroconversions, such as duration of dialysis, history of receiving dialysis in another center in Libya, and prior kidney transplant, possibly suggest nosocomial transmission.[95] In comparison, the adjusted prevalence of HBV is 4.6% among patients in Germany who are undergoing hemodialysis, 4.3% in Italy, 3.7% in France, 2.1% in Spain, 2.1% in Japan, and 2.4% in the United States, and adjusted seroconversion rates range from 0.4 to 1.8 per 100 patient-years.[338] The adjusted prevalence of HCV also varies among these countries: 22.9% in Spain, 20.5% in Italy, 10.4% in France, 3.8% in Germany, 2.6% in the United Kingdom, 14.8% in Japan, and 14% in the United States. The adjusted seroconversion rates range from 1.2 to 3.9 per 100 patient-years and are highest in Italy and Spain.[339]

DIALYSIS-RELATED OUTCOMES

With regard to other dialysis-related outcomes, reports from Egypt have revealed significant center-specific effects (which were not defined) on the survival and quality of life of patients receiving dialysis; these effects were dependent largely on funding.[103] In Syria, the 3-year survival rate among patients receiving hemodialysis was unsatisfactory, ranging from 26% to 64% in different hemodialysis centers.[298] In Jordan, the 1-year mortality rate among patients receiving hemodialysis is approximately 20%.[102] In Libya, the 1-year mortality was similar to Jordan and many other countries (21.2%). However, this is a poor outcome when taking into consideration the young mean age of patients undergoing hemodialysis. Although not reported, it is expected that the survival of Libyan ESKD patients was aggravated by the conflicts in their country.[93] According to the 2012 ICDC report,[88] the unadjusted 1-year, 2-year, 3-year, and 10-year survival rates among Israeli patients receiving dialysis were 80%, 66.6%, 54.9%, and 10%, respectively, from 1990 to 2010. Of note, there appears to be a survival advantage for Arab patients over Jewish patients on maintenance dialysis in Israel, in contrast to the life expectancy of Arabs in the general population which is 3 to 4 years lower than that of the Jewish population.[87] The survival of patients undergoing hemodialysis was high in Qatar, with 1-year and 5-year survival rates of 84% and 53%, respectively.[308]

It is of interest that a health disparity exists for both legal and illegal immigrants from ME countries with CKD who live and work in Western industrialized countries and may need RRT. The ethnic and educational backgrounds of these patients are different from those of the local population. Accordingly, they face potential problems with communication, health insurance, and care.[9] Fogazzi and Castelnovo reported their experience with such patients who were treated in an Italian dialysis unit.[340] Although the number of patients was small, they reported that those receiving hemodialysis who came from developing countries, which included some ME countries, were younger at the initiation of dialysis (38.2 ± 7.9 years versus 63 ± 12.6 years), were referred at a later stage of their disease, and had more infections, such as tuberculosis and viral hepatitis, than did patients from the local population who were undergoing hemodialysis. Furthermore, they also reported that a visit to their native countries was usually associated with medical complications, such as worsening of anemia.

KIDNEY TRANSPLANTATION

In ME countries, as in all other countries, kidney transplantation is recognized as the treatment of choice for ESKD. The beneficial effects of kidney transplantation on life expectancy, quality of life, and medical expenses are greater than those associated with maintenance dialysis. However, legislative obstacles, an underdeveloped and poorly funded health infrastructure, poor public awareness of the importance of organ donation, lack of effective kidney transplantation programs, cultural and religious barriers, and lack of trained multidisciplinary medical teams are some of the obstacles that prevent the promotion of kidney transplantation in some ME countries.[341-346]

Most ME countries are members of the Middle East Society for Organ Transplantation (MESOT). MESOT includes Iran, Turkey, and all of the Arab countries in the ME, as well as Pakistan, Cyprus, and some countries of central Asia.[342,345] There are very few organ procurement centers in the MESOT member countries for overseeing the activities of organ donation, sharing, and transplantation at a national level.

Israel is not a member of MESOT; it has its own national center for organ transplantation. The first successful living- and deceased-donor kidney transplants in the ME were performed in Israel (1964 and 1966, respectively)[347] and were reported to have been performed in Iran in 1967 and 2003, respectively.[345,348] The first successful kidney transplantation in an Arab country in the ME was performed with a kidney from a deceased donor with no heartbeat in Jordan in 1972. Most other ME countries, such as Lebanon and Turkey, started their kidney transplantation programs during the early 1970s, and Egypt and Saudi Arabia commenced their programs in 1976 and 1979, respectively. Since then, the remaining ME countries have established their own kidney transplantation programs; Libya did so in 2004. Currently, kidney transplantation programs are active in most ME countries but are relatively limited in Algeria, Yemen, the UAE, and Bahrain (see Table 79.2).[303,341,345,349-353]

Most kidneys for transplantation are obtained from living donors. An important milestone that paved the way for organ donation for transplantation from deceased donors in the Arab countries in the ME was the Amman declaration in 1986. In this declaration, Islamic theologians recognized that brain death was irreversible and could be used to declare a person legally dead, thereby making it permissible to disconnect that person from mechanical life-support systems. This declaration was preceded in 1982 by a resolution of the Islamic Council in Saudi Arabia that permitted the use for transplantation of organs from both living and deceased donors.[303,354,355] Similar declarations have since been made by religious authorities in Egypt, Turkey, and Iran.[303,355] As a result of these declarations, most Arab countries in the ME, including Egypt, have now enacted laws for regulated organ donation for transplantation from both living and cadaveric donors, and transplantation programs for kidneys and other organs are beginning to expand.[298,356,357] Yet programs for donation after cardiac death are limited in many Arab countries because of religious, legal, ethical, and social issues.[358]

In his code of Jewish law, the Mishneh Torah (Laws of Sanhedrin, 12:3), the twelfth century philosopher and physician Maimonides interpreted the Talmud as saying that someone who saves the life of one person is considered to have saved the entire world. This is similar to what is written in the Koran, Chapter 5, verse 32: "… if any one saved a life, it would be as if he saved the life of all mankind." Therefore organ donation that saves life is considered in Islam and Judaism to be a good deed. With regard to living related donors, Bulka argued that organ donation is permissible, because the danger to the donor is minimal, but it is not obligatory.[359] Likewise, Christians believe that organ donation is an act of love and nobility (e.g., as interpreted from Corinthians and from the parable of the Good Samaritan in Luke, Chapter 10, verses 25 to 37).[360]

Active deceased-donor kidney transplantation programs exist in Iran, Israel, Turkey, and eight Arab countries: Algeria, Kuwait, Lebanon, Morocco, Oman, Qatar, Saudi Arabia, and Tunisia.[341,361] However, deceased-donor kidney transplantation is inadequate to address the current need for allografts, and the number of patients on kidney transplantation waiting lists in these ME countries is progressively increasing. The use of kidneys from living related donors is increasing, but the gap between demand and supply is continuously widening in all ME countries. To meet the growing demand for kidneys and the shortfall in donors, some countries have initiated kidney transplantation programs involving organs from living unrelated donors. Using emotionally related donors extends donor eligibility to include individuals who are not genetically related to recipients.

Although kidney transplantation involving organs from deceased donors is increasing in the ME, it accounts for less than 21% of kidney transplantations in most ME countries, with large national variations.[345] In 2011, of the kidneys that were used for the 5934 kidney transplantations that were performed in Turkey, 27% were from deceased donors, according to the European Renal Association–European Dialysis and Transplant Association registry.[82] In Saudi Arabia, kidney transplantation from living unrelated donors is forbidden. SCOT reported that 624 kidney transplantations were performed in 2012, and 19% (118) of the kidneys were obtained from deceased donors[362]; the rest were obtained from living related donors. In fact, in 2006 Saudi Arabia had the highest reported rate of living-donor kidney transplantation worldwide at 32 procedures pmp, followed by Jordan (29 procedures pmp), Iceland (26 procedures pmp), Iran (23 procedures pmp), and the United States (21 procedures pmp).[297] However, the quoted Saudi statistic should be interpreted cautiously because the rate of living related donor kidney transplantations is 10.1 pmp. According to Nöel, the report by Horvat and colleagues probably included "transplant tourism" activity because it incorporated data on kidney transplantation in Saudi patients from living unrelated donors that was performed in other countries.[297,363]

In Egypt approximately 7% of Egyptian patients with ESKD are offered kidney transplantation in the year of diagnosis, and no kidneys are obtained from deceased donors: 80% of the kidneys are obtained from living unrelated donors, and 20% are obtained from living related donors. In 2013, 264 kidney transplantations were performed in Israel; of the transplanted kidneys, 43.5% were obtained from deceased donors and 54.5% from living related and living unrelated donors. However, the ratio of deceased donors to living donors is not constant, according to the annual reports of the Israeli National Transplant Center. Kidney transplantation in Syria commenced in 1976 with exclusive reliance on kidneys from living related donors. Since 2003, transplantation of kidneys from deceased donors has been allowed. As of 2010, 13.2 pmp kidney transplantations were performed, of which 22% were from deceased donors.[298,341]

In Iran the living unrelated donor transplantation program operates under the close supervision and scrutiny of the Ministry of Health and Medical Education, the Iranian Scientific Society of Organ Transplantation, the Foundation for Patients with Special Diseases, and the Dialysis and Transplant Patients Association (DATPA).[364] In the "Iranian model," patients who need kidney transplantation are referred to the DATPA, a charity founded in 1978 by Iranian patients with ESKD, which acts as a liaison agency between patients and potential donors. The altruistic volunteers are also registered by the DATPA and undergo evaluation in the foundation's clinics. Several important features characterize the "Iranian model" of living unrelated donors for kidney transplantation: No coercion is allowed; written consent is obtained from the donor and the donor's parents or spouse; donors are rewarded with gifts from the government; no commercialism is allowed; the medical teams receive no financial benefit; recipients and donors must be Iranian citizens; and time on the waiting list is minimal.[350,365] Consequently, the annual number of kidney transplantations has substantially increased in Iran, from 1421 in 2000 to 2285 in 2010.[350,366] However, the 86% share of living unrelated kidney donation in 2000 (20.1 pmp) decreased to 75% in 2006 (23 pmp) and 69% in 2010 (21.8 pmp). This change was mainly due to a substantial parallel increase in brain-dead kidney donation (2.2% in 2000, equivalent to 0.4 pmp, increasing to 26% and 7.9 pmp in 2010), after the Organ Transplantation and Brain Death Act in 2000, which legalized brain-dead organ donation.[366] Of note, 10 years after the introduction of the controlled living unrelated donor kidney transplantation program in Iran, the national waiting list for renal transplants was eliminated.[302,367]

Simforoosh and associates reported that patient and graft survival of 2155 Iranian recipients of kidneys from living unrelated donors after 15 years were 76.4%, and 53.2%, respectively.[368] These results are comparable with survival data in the 2003 annual report of the United States Renal Data System on living donor kidney transplantations.[369] However, the Iranian model has been criticized for ethical reasons because 85% of the vendors are very poor, a fact that may increase the risk that potential donors will withhold relevant medical information.[370] A study from the Shiraz Transplant Center revealed that Iranian paid unrelated donors have a lower quality of life and a higher incidence of microalbuminuria compared with related donors.[371] Hence the lack of long-term donor follow-up and the direct financial connection between donor and recipient are major weak points that should be ethically reviewed.[366,372-374]

COMMERCIAL KIDNEY TRANSPLANTATION

The lack of deceased donors for kidney allograft transplantation, combined with other medical factors (prolonged graft survival and improved surgical techniques, including laparoscopic nephrectomy) and nonmedical factors (economic and cultural), have motivated a large number of patients with ESKD to seek kidney transplants from living unrelated donors outside their home countries. This practice is often called "commercial kidney transplantation" or "organ tourism" because the donor sells his or her kidney for a certain amount of money. These kidney transplantations are performed in many countries around the world, such as the Philippines, Russia, India, China, Pakistan, and South Africa, as well as some ME countries, such as Turkey, Iraq, and Egypt.[343,375-378] The surgery is commonly performed in substandard conditions under the cover of secrecy. Many transplant recipients return to their homelands 1 to 2 weeks after transplantation without crucial information (a complete medical report; important information about the donor; HLA typing; and details of the medical treatment, surgery, and postoperative care). In addition, the recipients are exposed to potential risk for infection, such as HBV, HCV, or human immunodeficiency virus infection, as well as tuberculosis from inadequately evaluated donors. Thus the results of such commercial kidney transplantations are reported to be substandard.[376-378]

To undermine the practice of global commercial kidney transplantation, the Transplantation Society and the ISN convened an international summit meeting in Istanbul, Turkey, in April 2008. The outcome of this meeting was the "Declaration of Istanbul on Organ Trafficking and Transplant Tourism," which suggested that strategies to increase the donor pool and encourage legitimate, lifesaving transplantation programs be developed by countries to prevent organ trafficking, transplant commercialism, and transplant tourism. In addition, strategies should be aimed at stopping and prohibiting unethical activities, as well as encouraging safe and accountable practices that both meet the needs of transplant recipients and protect donors.[375,379,380] Many ME countries need to develop national self-sufficiency in organ donation to combat organ tourism and achieve global justice in transplantation.[375,379]

In 2008, two laws were approved by the Israeli parliament: the Brain-Respiratory Death Law and the Organ Transplantation Law. As a result, health insurance reimbursement for transplantation performed abroad that contravenes local Israeli laws was prohibited, and criminal penalties for brokering organ sales were introduced. Consequently, Israel has both increased organ donations from living and deceased sources and has reduced the number of transplant candidates seeking transplantation abroad (from 150 in 2006 to 41 in 2013).[361,381] In Egypt, however, in spite of the April 2010 organ transplantation law, which prohibits and penalizes organ trafficking and permits deceased donation in accord with the WHO Guiding Principles and the Declaration of Istanbul, little enforcement has been evident, and the problem of a black market in organs from living donors has increased.[343,357,375,382]

PHARMACOLOGIC TREATMENT OF KIDNEY TRANSPLANT RECIPIENTS

In general, all approved medications that are used worldwide to treat kidney transplant recipients are also used in the ME.[349,366] In all ME countries with kidney transplantation programs, induction therapy with methylprednisolone, lymphocyte-depleting agents, or IL-2 receptor antagonists is widely used. In most of the commercial transplantation programs, induction therapy is routinely given to reduce the frequency of acute graft rejection so that the recipient can be discharged early after the transplantation surgery. No reports have yet been published on the long-term complications of this routine treatment, such as bone marrow suppression, cytomegalovirus infections, and posttransplantation lymphoproliferative disorder.

Maintenance treatment after kidney transplantation in most ME countries consists of triple therapy with corticosteroids, azathioprine or mycophenolate mofetil, and calcineurin inhibitors. For economic reasons, several countries prefer to prescribe azathioprine and the cheap generic forms of cyclosporine instead of mycophenolate mofetil and tacrolimus. A small number of kidney transplantation centers have started prescribing rapamycin, a drug that inhibits a serine/threonine kinase called the mammalian target of rapamycin (mTOR), to prevent transplant rejection.[355,366] Treatment of acute rejection in most ME countries consists mainly of methylprednisolone (Solu-Medrol) and rabbit antithymocyte globulin (Thymoglobulin). Hyperimmune globulins and plasmapheresis are rarely used because both are expensive.

POSTTRANSPLANTATION COMPLICATIONS

There are only a few reports in the literature on the outcomes, as well as patient and graft survival rates, after kidney transplantation in ME countries. In general, these reports claim that outcomes in Saudi Arabia, Kuwait, Egypt, and North African countries in the ME are in line with international standards, although infections remain the main reason for morbidity and mortality.[10,106,368,377,383] Distinctive infections are of special concern in some ME countries. Tuberculosis is prevalent among dialysis recipients in some countries such as Saudi Arabia, Yemen, Turkey, and the North African countries in the ME.[346,384-388] Patients in these countries are at increased risk for developing active tuberculosis after kidney transplantation, and approximately 30% have symptoms of tuberculosis in extrapulmonary organs, particularly the lymph nodes, gastrointestinal tract, and peritoneal cavity. The Mantoux test often yields negative results in kidney transplant recipients, possibly because of the suppression of cellular immunity. Tuberculosis in the graft kidney tends to manifest as granulomatous interstitial nephritis. Urinalysis results are often negative for bacilli. The diagnosis is usually made on kidney biopsy or after nephrectomy in recipients, who often present with fever of unknown origin and deteriorating graft function.

Prophylactic treatment with isoniazid or rifampin for patients at high risk (Mantoux skin test reaction of >10 mm) has decreased the development of active tuberculosis. An important sequela of this treatment is the induction of cytochrome P450 enzymes by the antituberculous drugs, which results in a severe drop in the circulating therapeutic levels of calcineurin inhibitors and, consequently, severe acute rejection. Therefore increasing the dose of calcineurin inhibitors and frequent monitoring of their circulating levels are mandatory in such cases.[346,386,387]

Viral hepatitis, as discussed previously, is also common in the ME, especially among patients receiving dialysis. Eligible patients with HBV and HCV infections are offered transplantation in many ME kidney transplantation centers after appropriate presurgical workup and management.[331,387]

The most common types of neoplasia among kidney transplant recipients are skin malignancies, lymphoproliferative disorders, and Kaposi's sarcoma. The incidence of some uncommon tumors in the general population (e.g., Kaposi's sarcoma) can be 400- to 500-fold higher among kidney transplant recipients. Kaposi's sarcoma is most often seen in transplant recipients of Mediterranean, Jewish, and Arabic descent. Its reported incidence is 0.5% in most Western industrialized countries and as high as 5.3% in Saudi Arabia.[387,389-392] The preponderance of cases of Kaposi's sarcoma in certain ethnic groups appears to be linked to the geographic distribution of human herpesvirus 8 infection, inasmuch as more than 80% of transplant recipients with Kaposi's sarcoma are seropositive for human herpesvirus 8 before undergoing transplantation.[392]

SUMMARY

The ME has a strategic global location. Its fascinating geography is combined with rich national histories, cultures, and resources. In addition, the countries of the ME differ in their economics, political systems, culture, and bioecology, all of which eventually translate into disparities in their health systems, as well as in disease epidemiologic features, causes, management, and outcomes. The burden of kidney diseases is high in all ME countries and is compounded by many risk factors in the region, although data from developing countries are possibly underestimates. Practicing nephrologists in the ME are familiar with the genetic background, social habits, and culture of their patients. However, this is not so for many individuals of ME origin who now live in non-ME countries. Nephrologists in those countries need to take these considerations into account when diagnosing or treating the kidney diseases and comorbid conditions of their patients of ME origin. Therefore the emerging epidemic of diabetes mellitus in many ME countries is pertinent, and the prevailing genetic kidney diseases in the various population groups who live in the ME have been reviewed in this chapter.

Moreover, the ME has experience in management of mass disasters and consequent kidney complications, which can be implemented in regions outside of the ME. However, several issues still need to be addressed and hurdles must be overcome to improve the overall management of kidney diseases in the ME. Well-conducted epidemiologic cohort studies are urgently needed, and regional and national registries must be established as sources of transparent and accurate data. The results of the studies should provide accurate estimates of the public health burden of AKI, CKD, and ESKD; their risk factors; and comorbid conditions. This information should also improve the quality of therapy provided to patients. In addition, these efforts should also focus on the special needs of refugees in countries where human-engendered and natural disasters have occurred.

The entire international nephrology community agrees that improving existing diagnostic methods and establishing preventive strategies for the detection and treatment of kidney diseases at the earliest possible stage is of utmost importance, especially in countries with limited resources or health expenditures. Therefore, to achieve these goals, ME countries need to invest in (1) training qualified nephrologists and medical personnel; (2) public education and campaigns for lifestyle modification to combat obesity and diabetes mellitus and for proper use of over-the-counter drugs; (3) premarital genetic counseling to decrease the burden of genetic diseases; (4) vigorous treatment of comorbid conditions, which include infectious diseases, and strategies for preventing dehydration in tropical ME countries; and (5) use of low-cost, generic medication.

Because transplantation is the most cost-effective treatment for ESKD, ME countries also need to create a societal environment that motivates and encourages its population to support organ donation for transplantation in patients with ESKD. Encouraging organ donation through deceased donors, living related donors, and paired-exchange kidney transplantation programs, as well as organ sharing among the MESOT member states, will enable ME countries to reach national sufficiency for organ transplantation. The establishment of such programs will then help to reduce the long waiting lists in each ME country and combat unethical commercial kidney transplantation.[342,345,393]

Complete reference list available at ExpertConsult.com.

KEY REFERENCES

1. Held CC, Cummings JT: *Middle East patterns: places, peoples, and politics*, ed 5, Boulder, CO, 2011, Westview Press.
18. Zimmerman C, Kiss L, Hossain M: Migration and health: a framework for 21st century policy-making. *PLoS Med* 8:e1001034, 2011.
19. Sever MS, Vanholder R: Recommendation for the management of crush victims in mass disasters. *Nephrol Dial Transplant* 27(Suppl 1):i1–i67, 2012.
21. Lameire NH, Bagga A, Cruz D, et al: Acute kidney injury: an increasing global concern. *Lancet* 382:170–179, 2013.
30. Duzova A, Bakkaloglu A, Kalyoncu M, et al: Etiology and outcome of acute kidney injury in children. *Pediatr Nephrol* 25:1453–1461, 2010.
35. Barsoum RS: Malarial acute renal failure. *J Am Soc Nephrol* 11:2147–2154, 2000.
50. Farag YM, Kari JA, Singh AK: Chronic kidney disease in the Arab world: a call for action. *Nephron Clin Pract* 121:c120–c123, 2012.
52. Alhyas L, McKay A, Majeed A: Prevalence of type 2 diabetes in the states of the Co-operation Council for the Arab States of the Gulf: a systematic review. *PLoS One* 7:e40948, 2012.
57. Süleymanlar G, Utaş C, Arinsoy T, et al: A population-based survey of chronic renal disease in Turkey—the CREDIT study. *Nephrol Dial Transplant* 26:1862–1871, 2011.
60. Alashek WA, McIntyre CW, Taal MW: Epidemiology and aetiology of dialysis-treated end-stage kidney disease in Libya. *BMC Nephrol* 13:33, 2012.
66. Karnib HH, Gharavi AG, Aftimos G, et al: A 5-year survey of biopsy proven kidney diseases in Lebanon: significant variation in prevalence of primary glomerular diseases by age, population structure and consanguinity. *Nephrol Dial Transplant* 25:3962–3969, 2010.
68. Perico N, Bravo RF, De Leon FR, et al: Screening for chronic kidney disease in emerging countries: feasibility and hurdles. *Nephrol Dial Transplant* 24:1355–1358, 2009.
70. Gouda Z, Mashaal G, Bello AK, et al: Egypt Information, Prevention, and Treatment of Chronic Kidney Disease (EGIPT-CKD) programme: prevalence and risk factors for microalbuminuria among the relatives of patients with CKD in Egypt. *Saudi J Kidney Dis Transpl* 22:1055–1063, 2011.
71. Vivante A, Golan E, Tzur D, et al: Body mass index in 1.2 million adolescents and risk for end-stage renal disease. *Arch Intern Med* 172:1644–1650, 2012.
79. Tohidi M, Hasheminia M, Mohebi R, et al: Incidence of chronic kidney disease and its risk factors: results of over 10 year follow up in an Iranian cohort. *PLoS One* 7:e45304, 2012.
85. Süleymanlar G, Serdengeçti K, Altiparmak MR, et al: Trends in renal replacement therapy in Turkey, 1996-2008. *Am J Kidney Dis* 57:456–465, 2011.
86. Utaş C: The development of PD in Turkey. *Perit Dial Int* 28:217–219, 2008.
87. Kalantar-Zadeh K, Golan E, Shohat T, et al: Survival disparities within American and Israeli dialysis populations: learning from similarities and distinctions across race and ethnicity. *Semin Dial* 23:586–594, 2010.
89. Counil É, Cherni N, Kharrat M, et al: Trends of incident dialysis patients in Tunisia between 1992 and 2001. *Am J Kidney Dis* 51:463–470, 2008.
96. Alashek WA, McIntyre CW, Taal MW: Provision and quality of dialysis services in Libya. *Hemodial Int* 15:444–452, 2011.
97. Mahdavi-Mazdeh M, Zamyadi M, Nafar M: Assessment of management and treatment responses in haemodialysis patients from Tehran province, Iran. *Nephrol Dial Transplant* 23:288–293, 2008.
100. Najafi I, Alatab S, Atabak S, et al: Seventeen years' experience of peritoneal dialysis in Iran: first official report of the Iranian Peritoneal Dialysis Registry. *Perit Dial Int* 34:636–642, 2014.
110. Calderon-Margalit R, Gordon ES, Hoshen M, et al: Dialysis in Israel, 1989-2005—time trends and international comparisons. *Nephrol Dial Transplant* 23:659–664, 2008.
112. Soliman AR, Fathy A, Roshd D: The growing burden of end-stage renal disease in Egypt. *Ren Fail* 34:425–428, 2012.
113. Teebi AS, Teebi SA: Genetic diversity among the Arabs. *Community Genet* 8:21–26, 2005.
142. Gee HY, Saisawat P, Ashraf S, et al: ARHGDIA mutations cause nephrotic syndrome via defective RHO GTPase signaling. *J Clin Invest* 123:3243–3253, 2013.
144. Hoppe B: An update on primary hyperoxaluria. *Nat Rev Nephrol* 8:467–475, 2012.
149. Belostotsky R, Seboun E, Idelson GH, et al: Mutations in DHDPSL are responsible for primary hyperoxaluria type III. *Am J Hum Genet* 87:392–399, 2010.
173. Dinour D, Gray NK, Campbell S, et al: Homozygous SLC2A9 mutations cause severe renal hypouricemia. *J Am Soc Nephrol* 21:64–72, 2010.
183. Magen D, Berger L, Coady MJ, et al: A loss-of-function mutation in NaPi-IIa and renal Fanconi's syndrome. *N Engl J Med* 362:1102–1109, 2010.
194. Centola M, Wood G, Frucht DM, et al: The gene for familial Mediterranean fever, MEFV, is expressed in early leukocyte development and is regulated in response to inflammatory mediators. *Blood* 95:3223–3231, 2000.
195. Matzner Y, Abedat S, Shapiro E, et al: Expression of the familial Mediterranean fever gene and activity of the C5a inhibitor in human primary fibroblast cultures. *Blood* 96:727–731, 2000.
217. Livneh A, Langevitz P, Zemer D, et al: Criteria for the diagnosis of familial Mediterranean fever. *Arthritis Rheum* 40:1879–1885, 1997.
251. Ben-Zvi I, Brandt B, Berkun Y, et al: The relative contribution of environmental and genetic factors to phenotypic variation in familial Mediterranean fever (FMF). *Gene* 491:260–263, 2012.
269. Manukyan G, Petrek M, Tomankova T, et al: Colchicine modulates expression of pro-inflammatory genes in neutrophils from patients with familial Mediterranean fever and healthy subjects. *J Biol Regul Homeost Agents* 27:329–336, 2013.
275. Ter Haar N, Lachmann H, Ozen S, et al: Treatment of autoinflammatory diseases: results from the Eurofever Registry and a literature review. *Ann Rheum Dis* 72:678–685, 2013.
290. Sahin S, Sahin GM, Ergin H, et al: The effect of dialytic modalities on clinical outcomes in ESRD patients with familial Mediterranean fever. *Ren Fail* 29:315–319, 2007.
302. Najafi I: Peritoneal dialysis in Iran and the Middle East. *Perit Dial Int* 29(Suppl 2):S217–S221, 2009.
304. Shigidi MM, Fituri OM, Chandy SK, et al: Peritoneal dialysis, an expanding mode of renal replacement therapy in Qatar. *Saudi J Kidney Dis Transpl* 22:587–593, 2011.
309. Ahmed AM, Allam MF, Habil ES, et al: Compliance with haemodialysis practice guidelines in Egypt. *East Mediterr Health J* 19:4–9, 2013.
311. Dialysis in the Kingdom of Saudi Arabia. *Saudi J Kidney Dis Transpl* 24:853–861, 2013.
328. Liang TJ, Ghany MG: Current and future therapies for hepatitis C virus infection. *N Engl J Med* 368:1907–1917, 2013.
329. Frank C, Mohamed MK, Strickland GT, et al: The role of parenteral antischistosomal therapy in the spread of hepatitis C virus in Egypt. *Lancet* 355:887–891, 2000.
341. Saeed B: Pediatric versus adult kidney transplantation activity in Arab countries. *Saudi J Kidney Dis Transpl* 24:1031–1038, 2013.
345. Masri M, Haberal M: Solid-organ transplant activity in MESOT countries. *Exp Clin Transplant* 11:93–98, 2013.
356. El Matri A: History of nephrology in Mediterranean Arab countries. *J Nephrol* 26:170–174, 2013.
362. Organ transplantation in Saudi Arabia—2012. *Saudi J Kidney Dis Transpl* 24:1298–1308, 2013.
366. Mahdavi-Mazdeh M: The Iranian model of living renal transplantation. *Kidney Int* 82:627–634, 2012.
371. Fallahzadeh MK, Jafari L, Roozbeh J, et al: Comparison of health status and quality of life of related versus paid unrelated living kidney donors. *Am J Transplant* 13:3210–3214, 2013.
375. Danovitch GM, Chapman J, Capron AM, et al: Organ trafficking and transplant tourism: the role of global professional ethical standards—the 2008 Declaration of Istanbul. *Transplantation* 95:1306–1312, 2013.

80 Indian Subcontinent

Vinay Sakhuja | Harbir Singh Kohli

CHAPTER OUTLINE

ACUTE KIDNEY INJURY, 2495
Acute Kidney Injury Due to Infections, 2496
Acute Kidney Injury Due to Snakebite and Insect Stings, 2499
Acute Kidney Injury Due to Chemical Toxins, 2500
Acute Kidney Injury Due to Intravascular Hemolysis and Glucose-6-Phosphate Dehydrogenase Deficiency, 2501
Acute Cortical Necrosis, 2501
CHRONIC KIDNEY DISEASE, 2502
Incidence and Prevalence, 2502

Demographics of End-Stage Kidney Disease, 2502
Financial and Reimbursement Issues, 2503
Hemodialysis, 2503
Peritoneal Dialysis, 2504
Kidney Transplantation, 2504
Glomerulonephritis, 2506
Renovascular Hypertension, 2506
Renal Calculi, 2507
Indigenous Therapies, 2507
SUMMARY, 2508

The Indian subcontinent occupies the southern portion of the Asian continent and includes India, Pakistan, Bangladesh, Sri Lanka, Nepal, Bhutan, and the Maldives. The subcontinent is home to well over one fifth of the world's population, making it the most densely populated region in the world. These countries are all approximately at the same stage of economic development and are considered emerging and developing economies according to the International Monetary Fund's *World Economic Outlook* report.[1,2] Most of the population of the region lives in rural areas, relies on agriculture for its livelihood, and has limited access to health care. The countries of the subcontinent fall into the category of "medium" human development[3] as measured by the human development index, which takes into account not only the standard of living as determined by purchasing power parity but also the literacy rate and life expectancy.

India is the largest country in the subcontinent, with a population of more than 1 billion, and is also the largest economy in the region. It has enjoyed impressive economic growth, as a result of which India has been put into the category of "newly industrialized countries," a classification between "industrialized" countries and "developing" countries. The mean per capita gross national product has grown, but 0.7 billion people still continue to live on less than one U.S. dollar a day. Economic and development indicators of major countries of the region are shown in Table 80.1.[2,3] This combination of underdevelopment plus a rapidly growing economy is reflected in the disease spectrum. On the one hand, countries of the subcontinent are challenged with epidemics of infectious disease, and on the other hand, diabetes mellitus, the so-called disease of the affluent, has reached epidemic proportions. Health care in the public sector in these countries is organized in the shape of a pyramid, with primary health centers at the bottom, followed by intermediate-level hospitals, and referral hospitals at the top. Specialized care for disease is usually available only at the major referral hospitals. There are only about 900 nephrologists in India. There is a thriving private sector health care industry, but treatment costs are quite high, and only the rich or patients whose expenses are covered by their employers can afford treatment in these hospitals.

The differences in living standards and availability of health care determine the variations in disease patterns, management practices, and disease outcome. The spectrum of kidney diseases in this region is characterized by a mix of conditions that are globally encountered and those specific to the subcontinent. The latter can be secondary to a genetic predisposition in specific ethnic groups or related to exposure to environmental factors like climatic conditions, infectious agents, envenomation, and chemical toxins. A high prevalence of nephrolithiasis in some areas, aggravated by dehydration caused by a combination of exposure to high ambient temperatures and a high prevalence of diarrheal diseases, is an example. Genetic factors that predispose to kidney disease in the tropics include glucose-6-phosphate dehydrogenase (G6PD) deficiency, which gives rise to intravascular hemolysis and pigment-induced acute kidney injury (AKI). Indigenous health care systems are still popular in rural areas, and patients are frequently treated with herbs and potions that could add to the burden of kidney disease.

Table 80.1 Economic and Development Indicators on the Indian Subcontinent

	India	Pakistan	Bangladesh	Sri Lanka
Population (billions)	1.22	0.193	0.163	0.021
Population growth rate (%)	1.31	1.55	1.58	0.91
Life expectancy at birth (yr)	67.48	66.7	70.36	76.15
Median age (yr)	26.7	22.2	23.9	31.4
Percentage of total population that is elderly (>65 yr)	5	4	5	8
Literacy rate (%)	64.84 (year 2011)	55 (year 2009)	57.7 (year 2011)	92.5 (year 2010)
Infant mortality rate (per 1000 live births, year 2013)	44.6	59.35	47.30	9.24
Per capita gross domestic product purchasing power parity (U.S.$) (year 2012)	3800	3100	2000	6000
Percentage living below national poverty line	29.8	22.3	31.5	8.9
Human development index	0.554	0.515	0.515	0.715
Country ranking by human development index (of 179 countries)	136	146	146	92

Table 80.2 Causes of Acute Kidney Injury in a Tertiary Referral Center on the Indian Subcontinent (Percentage)

	1965-1974*	1975-1980*	1981-1986*	2001-2006†
Medical causes	67	55	61	65
Diarrheal diseases	23	12	10	7.3
Intravascular hemolysis due to glucose-6-phosphate dehydrogenase deficiency	12	12	6	1
Glomerulonephritis	11	9	9.5	11
Copper sulfate poisoning	12	12	6	1
Chemical and drug exposure	4	5	7	7.2
Snakebites and insect stings	3	3	2.5	6.5
Sepsis	0	3	4	17.8
Miscellaneous	7	11	17	13.2
Obstetric causes	22	21	9	5
Surgical causes	11	24	30	30

*Data from Chugh KS, Sakhuja V, Malhotra HS, et al: Changing trends in acute renal failure in third world countries-Chandigarh study. Q J Med 73:1117-1123, 1989.
†Authors' unpublished data.

ACUTE KIDNEY INJURY

Reliable statistics on the patterns and prevalence of AKI in this region are not available, but it is the most commonly encountered renal emergency.[4-6] About 0.1% to 0.25% of all hospital admissions are for AKI. Most of the causes of AKI described elsewhere in the world are encountered in the Indian subcontinent as well. Several causes, however, either are unique or are seen with increased frequency in this part of the world. Compared with industrialized countries, in which AKI is mainly a disease of the elderly and is seen primarily in hospitalized patients, community-acquired AKI in otherwise healthy individuals is common in countries in this region, a characteristic they share with other developing countries.[7] Patients with AKI are younger in this region than their counterparts in the West. The median age of patients with AKI in the West increased from 41.2 years in the 1950s to 60.5 years in the 1980s[8]; the average age of patients with AKI in India is 37.1 years.[7] Hospital-acquired AKI is more common in the elderly population than in the young.[9]

Over the years there has been a change in the spectrum of AKI (Table 80.2). Improvements in obstetric care have led to a virtual disappearance of pregnancy-related AKI in the industrialized world. The rate of obstetric AKI in India also has declined from 22% to 5% of all cases of AKI in the last four decades. The frequency distribution of AKI is bimodal in terms of the duration of gestation. The first peak, seen between 8 and 16 weeks of gestation, is associated chiefly with induced septic abortions. The abortion practices include the use of sticks; the insertion of abortifacient chemicals, pastes, and soap solutions; and dilation and curettage performed under unhygienic conditions and by untrained personnel.[10] The incidence of AKI has decreased since the legalization and regulation of abortions and the wider availability of medical facilities.[10,11] The second peak, after 34 weeks of gestation, is related to preeclampsia, eclampsia, abruptio placentae, postpartum hemorrhage, and puerperal sepsis. Acute cortical necrosis has been observed in about 25% of patients with obstetric AKI in parts of India.[10]

The proportion of AKI from surgical causes has increased from 11% to 30%. Obstructive nephropathy constitutes a major cause of surgical AKI.[12] The high incidence of nephrolithiasis contributes and is related to inherited metabolic disorders, dietary factors, and fluid losses. Faith in the efficacy of indigenous medicines to dissolve stones causes delay in surgical intervention and hastens the development of renal failure. In urban areas, the causes of AKI are similar to those in the industrialized world, but in rural areas, AKI is mainly the result of diarrheal illnesses, chemicals, snakebite, and insect stings.[13] Renal failure after the suicidal ingestion of copper sulfate has shown a significant decline,[14,15] possibly because of the easy availability of other poisons, such as organophosphorus insecticides.[16] Data from a large tertiary care referral institute in India has shown that sepsis as a cause of AKI has increased almost seven times from just 1.57% from 1983 through 1995 to 11.43% from 1996 to 2008.[17]

Finally, treatment facilities are grossly inadequate. Patients are referred late, only after renal failure becomes severe and complications set in. They often require immediate dialysis, and, therefore, the mortality rate is high. Intermittent peritoneal dialysis is still used in several areas[18-20] because hemodialysis (HD) facilities are limited to bigger cities. The outcome of AKI is worse in the elderly than in the younger population.[21] Conditions causing AKI that are specific to the Indian subcontinent are discussed in the following sections.

ACUTE KIDNEY INJURY DUE TO INFECTIONS

DIARRHEAL DISEASES

AKI secondary to diarrhea is encountered not only in children but also in adults. In adults diarrheal diseases cause 30% of all AKI,[7] whereas 35% to 50% of all children undergoing dialysis for AKI have preceding diarrhea and dehydration.[12,22,23] This problem is common in rural areas and urban slums inhabited by poverty-stricken individuals, where sanitation is poor and potable water is not available. The incidence increases during summer and the rainy season. Associated vomiting is an early feature of rotavirus infection. Loose watery stools indicate infection with enterotoxigenic *Escherichia coli* or *Vibrio cholerae*. Fever, cramps, tenesmus, and blood and mucus in stools suggest *Shigella, Salmonella,* or enteroinvasive *E. coli* infection. The diagnosis of cholera can be confirmed by microscopic demonstration of the highly motile *V. cholerae* organisms in a hanging drop preparation; culture is necessary to confirm the presence of other organisms.

Early and adequate fluid replacement is the cornerstone of therapy. Widespread use of the oral rehydration solution recommended by the World Health Organization has led to a significant decline in the mortality rate from this condition. Intravenous rehydration with lactated Ringer's solution may be required in patients with severe dehydration, persistent vomiting, or paralytic ileus. Hypokalemia may worsen as the metabolic acidosis is corrected, and large amounts of potassium may be required to prevent life-threatening cardiac arrhythmias. Because peritoneal dialysis fluid is potassium free, potassium should be replaced through an intravenous or intraperitoneal route in patients treated with this modality. Volume depletion secondary to acute gastroenteritis is presumed to be the most common cause of kidney injury' occasionally, acute cortical necrosis can also occur.[23a]

HEMOLYTIC UREMIC SYNDROME

Hemolytic uremic syndrome is responsible for 25% to 55% of all cases of pediatric AKI in some parts of the subcontinent.[24-26] This condition is seen mainly in preschool-aged children and is less common in adults. The main feature is oliguric renal failure, preceded by a diarrheal prodrome in about 70% of cases. Neurologic involvement is seen in 30% to 50% of cases. Examination shows pallor and mild icterus. Renal failure is severe and requires prolonged dialysis. Diagnosis is confirmed by demonstration of fragmented erythrocytes on blood smear as well as of thrombocytopenia. Supportive evidence includes unconjugated hyperbilirubinemia and increased plasma lactate dehydrogenase levels. The etiologic organism in the Indian subcontinent is usually *Shigella* and not *E. coli*.[27,28] The histologic hallmark of this condition is thrombotic microangiopathy in the renal vasculature. Histologic examination shows frequent involvement of arterioles and small arteries with severe intimal proliferation and luminal stenosis. Patchy or diffuse renal cortical necrosis develops in up to 40% of patients.[24] The treatment is mainly supportive. Plasma infusions or plasma exchange is used infrequently; the outcome is poor, with a mortality rate of 60%.[29] Of those who recover, a significant proportion are left with residual renal dysfunction and eventually progress to end-stage kidney disease (ESKD).

MALARIA

Malaria is caused by the protozoan *Plasmodium* and is transmitted by the *Anopheles* mosquito. Of the four *Plasmodium* species, AKI is seen most frequently with *Plasmodium falciparum* infection. A few reports have described an association of AKI with *Plasmodium vivax* infection.[30,31] Multiple organ dysfunctions have been also associated with vivax malaria.[32]

These forms of malaria predominate in warmer regions closer to the equator in the subcontinent (parts of India, Pakistan, Bangladesh, and Sri Lanka) and are associated with intense year-round transmission. In addition to being a burden to the native communities, malaria is a danger to nonimmune travelers to endemic areas.

The contribution of malaria to overall hospital admissions for AKI varies from 2% to 39%.[33] The incidence of malarial AKI among those living in endemic areas is 2% to 5%, but 25% to 30% of nonimmune visitors with malaria experience renal failure.[34] Among those with severe parasitemia, as many as 60% have AKI.[35] In Pakistan, malaria-induced AKI also contributes significantly to the total AKI burden.[36]

Clinical Features

Malaria causes classic paroxysms of spiking fever along with malaise, myalgia, headache, and chills, and the disease can be confused with a viral illness. Nausea, vomiting, and hypotension are common in nonimmune individuals. Severe infection may involve several vital organs, including the central nervous system, manifesting as deep coma and seizures, noncardiogenic pulmonary edema, shock, and disseminated intravascular coagulation (DIC). AKI usually is seen by the end of the first week and is nonoliguric in 50% to 75% of cases.[34] In more than 75%, AKI is associated with cholestatic jaundice. It is usually associated with a hypercatabolic state, with a rapid increase in creatinine levels. In a study from India, of a total of 101 patients with malarial AKI over a 1-year period, about 37% required dialytic support, and hospital mortality was around 10%.[37] Other manifestations include nonnephrotic proteinuria, microscopic hematuria, hemoglobinuria, and electrolyte abnormalities.

Diagnosis can be established by the demonstration of asexual forms of the parasite in peripheral blood smears stained with Giemsa stain. Staining with the fluorescent dye acridine orange allows more rapid diagnosis. Also, simple but specific antibody-based card tests that detect *P. falciparum*–specific histidine-rich protein 2 or lactate dehydrogenase antigens in finger-stick blood samples have been introduced. They allow differentiation of falciparum from non-falciparum malarias, but results can remain positive for several weeks after acute infection. A scoring system based on the number of organ systems involved has been suggested for judging the severity and predicting outcomes in falciparum malaria.[38]

Histologic Features

Acute tubular necrosis is the most common lesion found on histologic analysis. Pigment casts may be seen in tubular lumina in patients with intravascular hemolysis. Varying degrees of interstitial edema and mononuclear cell infiltrate are common accompaniments.[38]

Pathogenesis

Disease severity is related to the intensity of infection. The most important pathogenetic factor is the hemodynamic change caused by altered erythrocyte rheology. The infected cell becomes more spherical and less deformable as a result of the formation of membrane protuberances or knobs on the cell surface. These knobs extrude a strain-specific adhesive variant protein of high molecular weight that mediates attachment to receptors on venular and capillary endothelium, causing a phenomenon called *cytoadherence*. The major adhesive protein family is known as *P. falciparum erythrocyte membrane protein*. The cell surface receptors for these knobs include complement receptor 1, glycosaminoglycans, intercellular adhesion molecule-1, chondroitin sulfate B, CD36, platelet endothelial cell adhesion molecule 1/CD31, thrombomodulin, E- and P-selectins, and vascular cell adhesion molecule-1. Some of these receptors are expressed constitutively, whereas others are induced by inflammatory mediators released in severe disease. Infected erythrocytes also adhere to uninfected red cells, platelets, monocytes, and lymphocytes. These aggregated and sequestered red blood cells interfere with microcirculatory flow in the kidneys and other organs.[39] This phenomenon is unique to *P. falciparum* infection and has not been observed in infection with other species.

Treatment

Mortality from malarial AKI varies between 15% and 50%.[35] Severe falciparum malaria requires intensive nursing and close multidisciplinary care.[35] Prompt assessment of volume status, blood glucose level, and acid-base status is essential. All patients with *P. falciparum* infection should be presumed to have chloroquine-resistant infection. The cinchona alkaloids (quinine or quinidine) are the mainstay of treatment because of their activity against chloroquine-resistant strains. Quinine often causes hyperinsulinemia and hypoglycemia, and many centers recommend administration of a continuous infusion of 5% to 10% dextrose to all patients.[40] Compounds derived from artemisinin (isolated from the Chinese herb *Artemisia annua*) such as artesunate, artemether, and arteether are particularly valuable in areas with quinine resistance and in patients with recurrent quinine-induced hypoglycemia. All patients should also receive gametocidal therapy (tetracycline or pyrimethamine/sulfadoxine). Mefloquine, halofantrine, atovaquone, artemisinin, and pyrimethamine/sulfadoxine (Fansidar) derivatives are possible alternatives for resistant falciparum malaria. Patients with evidence of hemolysis should receive adequate hydration and parenteral sodium bicarbonate to alkalinize the urine to a pH of more than 7.0. AKI is usually associated with a hypercatabolic state, and frequent dialysis may be needed.[41] Hyperkalemia should be watched for and adequately treated. The peritoneal microcirculation is impaired as a result of clogging with infected erythrocytes and vasoconstriction, reducing the efficacy of peritoneal dialysis. Despite these limitations peritoneal dialysis has been shown to improve survival by 16% with early institution of manual immediate PD in AKI due to falciparum malaria.[42] Exchange transfusion has also been tried in patients with severe parasitemia.

LEPTOSPIROSIS

Leptospirosis, the most widespread zoonosis in the world,[43] is particularly prevalent in parts of southern and western India.[44,45] The animal hosts include rats, mice, gerbils, hedgehogs, foxes, dogs, cattle, sheep, pigs, and rabbits. Even asymptomatic animals carry a high number of organisms ($>10^{10}$/g) in their kidneys and shed leptospira in urine for years. Human infection occurs incidentally either directly through contact with the urine or tissue of an infected animal or indirectly through contaminated water, soil, or vegetation. The usual portals of entry are abraded skin and exposed mucosae. Leptospirosis is an occupational hazard for coal miners and sewage, abattoir, and farm workers as well as workers in the aquaculture industry. The genus *Leptospira* includes the pathogenic *Leptospira interrogans* strains and the saprophytic *Leptospira biflexa*. The disease occurs throughout the year, with an increase in incidence during or soon after the rainy season, especially after floods. Adult men are affected most frequently.

Clinical Features

The manifestation of leptospirosis varies from subclinical infection or a self-limited anicteric febrile illness to severe and potentially fatal disease.[43,44] Symptoms appear 1 to 2 weeks after exposure and are typically biphasic in character. The leptospiremic phase is characterized by high fever with chills, headache, and severe muscle aches and tenderness. Renal failure develops in the second, immune phase, when patients also have progressive jaundice, epistaxis, hemoptysis, gastrointestinal bleeding, hemorrhagic pneumonia, and bleeding into the adrenal glands. The triad of renal failure, cholestatic jaundice, and bleeding constitutes *Weil's syndrome*. AKI occurs in 20% to 85% of cases.[45-47] In about half the cases of AKI, renal failure is associated with polyuria and hypokalemia along with increased fractional excretion of potassium. Renal failure is mild and nonoliguric in patients without icterus. Hypotension is noted in more than 60% of cases and is often unresponsive to volume expansion and inotropic support. Hypotensive patients are also more likely to have adult respiratory distress syndrome.

Diagnosis is based on either culture or serologic testing. Organisms can be isolated in blood cultures during the first phase and later from urine. However, growth takes up to 4 weeks in Fletcher's or Stuart's semisolid medium. The macroscopic agglutination test can be used as a screening test but is not specific. The benchmark is the microscopic agglutination test, but this is a complex procedure that requires maintenance of live *Leptospira* cultures. An immunoglobulin M (IgM)–specific dot enzyme-linked immunosorbent assay has been found to be specific in diagnosing leptospirosis in endemic areas. Urinalysis during the leptospiremic phase reveals mild proteinuria as well as hyaline and granular casts.

Histologic Features

The kidneys typically are swollen and may be bile stained. The main lesions seen on light microscopy are interstitial edema and infiltration with mononuclear cells and eosinophils. Mild and transient mesangioproliferative glomerulonephritis with C3 and IgM deposition may sometimes be observed.[48]

Pathogenesis

Renal involvement results from direct invasion of the renal tissue by the organism, which leads to liberation of enzymes, metabolites, and endotoxins as well as complement activation. Ultrastructural studies after inoculation of *Leptospira pomona* into mice showed the organism infiltrating the glomerular capillary lumen at day 2, the interstitium at days 4 to 8, the proximal tubular cells by day 10, and the tubular lumen by day 14.[48a] Several leptospiral outer membrane proteins have been localized to the proximal tubules and interstitium of infected animals. The addition of *Leptospira* endotoxin to human macrophages induces tumor necrosis factor-α. The glycoprotein component of endotoxin could inhibit renal Na^+-K^+–adenosine triphosphatase (Na^+-K^+-ATPase), in turn affecting the apical Na-K-2Cl cotransporter and leading to potassium wasting. An upregulation of nuclear factor-kappaB binding to DNA was noted on addition of outer membrane extracts from pathogenic serovars to cultured medullary thick ascending limb cells; it was accompanied by an increase in inducible nitric oxide synthase, monocyte chemoattractant protein-1, and tumor necrosis factor-α. Alterations in intravascular volume, hemoglobinuria, and myoglobinuria also contribute.[48] The tubules become insensitive to the action of antidiuretic hormone.

Treatment

Leptospirosis is a self-limiting disease, and patients with mild cases recover spontaneously. The emphasis is on symptomatic measures, together with correction of hypotension and fluid and electrolyte imbalances. Administration of crystalline penicillin or doxycycline shortens the duration of fever and hospital stay and may hasten amelioration of leptospiruria. In a meta-analysis of controlled trials the role of various antibiotics in treatment of leptospirosis was found to be uncertain; this finding could be attributed to lack of adequate clinical trials. The role of penicillin in the treatment of leptospirosis can be debated.[49] Patients with renal failure need close monitoring and dialysis when necessary. Poor prognostic indicators include increasing age and the presence of jaundice, pulmonary complications, hyperbilirubinemia, diarrhea, hyperkalemia, pulmonary rales, or hypotension on admission. Internal hemorrhage and myocarditis are common causes of death.

ZYGOMYCOSIS

Zygomycosis is a rare opportunistic infection caused by fungi of the order *Mucorales* and genera *Rhizopus*, *Absidia*, and *Rhizomucor*. Organ involvement occurs through vascular invasion, which leads to thrombosis of large and small arteries and infarction and necrosis of the affected organ. The major presentations have rhinocerebral, pulmonary, gastrointestinal, and disseminated forms. Renal mucormycosis involving the major renal vessels has been reported primarily in northern India in the last decade and may occur as isolated renal involvement or as part of disseminated disease.[50] The administration of intravenous fluids contaminated with fungus may be responsible in some patients. Bilateral involvement leads to oliguric AKI. The condition usually develops in otherwise immunocompetent individuals; presentation is with fever, lumbar pain, pyuria, and oliguria. Computed tomography (CT) reveals enlarged nonenhancing kidneys with perirenal collections and/or intrarenal abscesses (Figure 80.1).[51] The diagnosis can be confirmed by demonstration of hyphae in the material obtained by aspiration or percutaneous biopsy. The only definitive treatment is extensive debridement of affected tissue, which may include bilateral nephrectomy, and systemic antifungal therapy with amphotericin B. Bilateral renal mucormycosis carries an extremely poor prognosis.[50]

DENGUE FEVER

Dengue fever is the most prevalent mosquito-borne viral disease. There are four closely related, but serologically distinct dengue viruses, called DENV-1, DENV-2, DENV-3, and DENV-4, of the genus *Flavivirus*. The infection is primarily

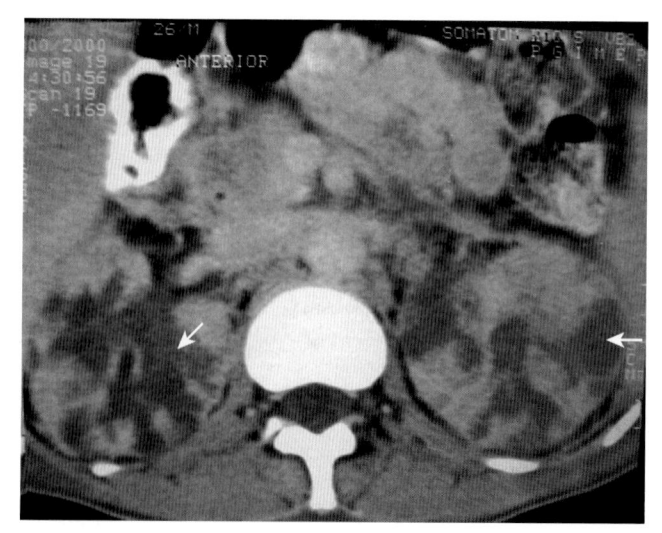

Figure 80.1 Renal mucormycosis. Contrast-enhanced computed tomography scan showing bulky kidneys with large nonenhancing areas (*arrows*) involving the cortex and medulla and with no contrast in the pelvicalyceal system.

transmitted by *Aedes* mosquitoes, particularly *Aedes aegypti*. Dengue fever is self-limiting illness with symptoms including fever, headache and muscle and joint pain. However, a life-threatening dengue hemorrhagic fever (DHF) develops in a small minority of patients, with low platelet count, bleeding, and capillary plasma leakage. In severe cases patients may have dengue shock syndrome. The cardinal features of DHF are increased vascular permeability (plasma leakage syndrome), marked thrombocytopenia, hemorrhagic tendency (as demonstrated by a positive tourniquet test result), and spontaneous bleeding.

In a study from South India AKI was seen in 10.8% of patients with dengue fever. Of these, 12 (5.4%) had mild AKI; 7 (3.1%) had moderate AKI, and 5 (2.2%) had severe AKI according to Acute Kidney Injury Network (AKIN) criteria.[52] Proposed mechanisms for AKI are capillary leak, shock resulting in hypoperfusion, and acute tubular necrosis. Additionally, hemolysis or rhabdomyolysis contribute to AKI. Of 198 patients with dengue admitted to an intensive care unit 15 (7.6%) required dialytic support.[53] Presence of dengue hemorrhagic and dengue shock syndrome, neurologic involvement, and prolonged activated partial thromboplastin time have been found to be independent predictors of AKI. Mortality is about 6% to 9% in patients with dengue fever and AKI. AKI during hospitalization for dengue fever is a predictor of death.[54]

ACUTE KIDNEY INJURY DUE TO SNAKEBITE AND INSECT STINGS

SNAKEBITE

Snakebite is an occupational hazard and occurs when people are working barefoot in the fields. On the Indian subcontinent, AKI develops after bites by snakes of the viper family such as Russell's viper, the saw-scaled viper *(Echis carinatus)*, and pit vipers. The incidence of AKI varies from 13% to 32% in India after Russell's viper or *E. carinatus* bites[55-57] and is 27% in Sri Lanka after bites of unidentified vipers.[58]

Clinical Features

The severity of the symptoms and signs is related to the type of venom as well as to the dose injected during the bite. Severely envenomed patients experience DIC, which frequently results in spontaneous bleeding and coagulopathy. The latter features often dominate the clinical course until coagulation returns to normal.[59] Many viper-envenomed patients have hypotensive shock as a consequence of hypovolemia from significant blood loss. Blood can ooze continuously from the fang marks, and severe hemorrhage may manifest as hematemesis, melena, hemoptysis, or bleeding into the muscles, fascial compartments, serous cavities, and subarachnoid space.[60] Pain and swelling of the bitten part are generally the earliest symptoms, appearing within a few minutes. The swelling may spread to involve the whole limb and is due to exudation of plasma or extravasation of blood into the subcutaneous tissues. Blistering or local necrosis is observed in one third to one half of patients.

In patients with AKI, oliguria often develops rapidly, within the first 24 hours, but it may be delayed until 2 to 3 days after the bite. Some patients become anuric, whereas occasional patients remain nonoliguric. Urine may show gross or microscopic hematuria. Some patients complain of pain in the renal angle preceding oliguria, which may be a useful clue to impending renal failure. Jaundice and hemoglobinuria resulting from intravascular hemolysis are not infrequent after Russell's viper or *E. carinatus* bites and have been reported in India and Sri Lanka.[57]

Laboratory investigations reveal varying degrees of anemia, resulting from a combination of intravascular hemolysis and blood loss. Hemolysis results in unconjugated hyperbilirubinemia, reticulocytosis, elevated plasma free hemoglobin level, and hemoglobinuria. In some patients, the peripheral blood smear may show fragmented erythrocytes, suggesting microangiopathic hemolysis. The blood fails to coagulate normally, and features of DIC are often present.[60] Thrombocytopenia may occur, however, even in the absence of a consumptive coagulopathy.

The mortality rate for snakebitten patients with AKI varies with the nature of the renal lesion. According to one report, although only 16% of those with acute tubular necrosis died, as many as 80% of those with cortical necrosis had a fatal outcome.[57]

Histologic Features

Renal histologic examination shows either acute tubular or cortical necrosis. Glomerular changes have been described in rare cases, but their significance is not known.

Acute Tubular Necrosis. Acute tubular necrosis is the predominant lesion seen in 70% to 80% of snakebitten patients with AKI. On light microscopy, the tubules appear dilated and lined by flattened epithelium. Severe cases exhibit cell necrosis and desquamation of necrotic cells from the basement membrane. Hyaline, granular, or pigment casts are seen in tubular lumina. Varying degrees of interstitial edema, hemorrhage, and inflammatory cell infiltration are present. Later biopsy specimens reveal regenerating tubular epithelium. Intrarenal blood vessels are usually unaffected.

On ultrastructural examination, proximal tubules show dense intracytoplasmic bodies that represent degenerating organelles or protein resorption droplets.[61] Small areas of basement membrane are denuded. Distal tubular cells have a dilated endoplasmic reticulum and many degenerating organelles. Apoptosis, a prominent feature in the distal tubules, indicates a high cell turnover. In the interstitium, fibroblasts appear active, with increased numbers of organelles and cytoplasmic processes. Mast cells and eosinophils show both granulated and partially degranulated forms.

Acute Cortical Necrosis. Bilateral diffuse or patchy cortical necrosis has been observed in 20% of patients with snakebite-induced AKI.[57] The presence of fibrin thrombi in the arterioles is a prominent feature in these patients. A narrow subcapsular rim of cortex often escapes necrosis. The area underlying this rim, however, shows necrosis of glomerular as well as tubular elements. The necrotic zone is often bordered by an area of hyperemia and leukocytic infiltration.

Pathogenesis

The exact pathogenesis of AKI following snakebite is not well established because of the lack of a reproducible animal model. However, a number of factors may contribute, including bleeding, hypotension, circulatory collapse, intravascular hemolysis, DIC, microangiopathic hemolytic anemia, and also the direct nephrotoxicity of the venom. Bleeding either into tissues or externally and loss of plasma into the bitten extremity can produce hypotension and circulatory collapse. These effects are caused by venom metalloproteinases that degrade basement membrane proteins surrounding the vessel wall, leading to loss of integrity. Hemorrhagic toxins have been isolated from the venom of many snakes of the Viperidae and Crotalidae families.[59] In addition, vasodilation and increased capillary permeability can aggravate the circulatory disturbances of shock. Hemolysis results from the action of phospholipase A_2, which is present in almost all snake venoms. Phospholipase A_2 causes hemolysis directly by hydrolysis of red blood cell membrane phospholipids or indirectly via production of the strongly hemolytic lysolecithin from plasma lecithin. The human hemostatic system is regulated through a number of critical interactions involving blood proteins, platelets, endothelial cells, and subendothelial structures. Snake venoms, particularly those from the viper and pit viper families, contain many proteins that interact with members of the coagulation cascade and the fibrinolytic pathway.

Treatment

The therapeutic approach to renal failure after snakebite is the same as that to AKI from any other cause. Early administration of antivenom is vital; delay results in a steep increase in the dose requirements. Indications include prolonged coagulation time or failure of blood coagulation, spontaneous systemic bleeding, intravascular hemolysis, local swelling involving more than two segments of the bitten limb, and a serum concentration of fibrin degradation products greater than 80 μg/mL. Knowledge of the offending snake species allows administration of monovalent antivenom if available. Immunodiagnostic techniques are helpful in identification of the venom antigen. Enzyme-linked immunosorbent assay has been used extensively in rural Thailand for this purpose.[62] The currently available test, however, is not quick enough for clinical application. Because only polyvalent antivenom is available in most parts of Asia, precise identification of the snake is not essential for management.

Indian studies recommend initial administration of 20 to 100 mL of antivenom, followed by repeated dose of 25 to 50 mL every 4 to 6 hours until the effects of systemic envenomation disappear.[60,63] A simple way to monitor antivenom treatment efficacy is by monitoring whole-blood clotting time three or four times daily. Coagulability is generally restored within 6 hours of an adequate dose. The test must be performed for at least 3 more days, because delayed absorption of the venom can lead to recurrence of the coagulopathy. Immunoassays permit serial estimation of venom levels and are useful in guiding antivenom therapy.

Other therapeutic measures include replacement of lost blood with fresh blood or plasma, maintenance of electrolyte balance, administration of tetanus immunoglobulin, and treatment of pyogenic infection with antibiotics. The prognosis is good in patients who receive adequate doses of antivenom. One study showed the outcome for venom-induced AKI to be better after HD than after peritoneal dialysis.[64] The overall mortality rate is about 30%.[57]

BEE, WASP, AND HORNET STINGS

Honeybees, yellow jackets, hornets, and paper wasps are stinging insects belonging to the order Hymenoptera. An isolated sting causes just a local allergic reaction, but attack by a swarm of insects introduces a large dose of the venom sufficient to cause systemic symptoms.[65-67] These include vomiting, diarrhea, hypotension, loss of consciousness, and AKI. Patients with AKI have been reported to have received from 22 to more than 1000 stings. AKI is secondary to hemolysis and/or rhabdomyolysis. Hemolysis results from the action of a basic protein fraction as well as melittin and phospholipase A present in the venom. Rhabdomyolysis has been attributed to polypeptides, histamine, serotonin, and acetylcholine. A direct nephrotoxic role for these venoms has also been suggested. Renal biopsy specimens reveal acute tubular necrosis.

ACUTE KIDNEY INJURY DUE TO CHEMICAL TOXINS

COPPER SULFATE POISONING

Copper sulfate is a strong corrosive that produces symptoms within minutes of ingestion. Metallic taste, excessive salivation, burning retrosternal and epigastric pain, nausea, and repeated vomiting are the initial features. The vomitus is blue-green and turns deep blue on the addition of ammonium hydroxide, which allows it to be differentiated from bile. Diarrhea, hematemesis, and melena follow. Jaundice, hypotension, convulsions, and coma may develop in severe cases. Acute pancreatitis, myoglobinuria, and methemoglobinemia have also been reported. AKI is seen in 20% to 25% of cases and is invariably oliguric. Hemoglobinuria may be seen in about 40% of cases. Diuresis ensues after 7 to 10 days and is usually followed by complete renal recovery.[14]

Copper can produce considerable oxidative stress and interferes with the activity of several key enzymes such as Na^+-K^+-ATPase, G6PD, glutathione reductase, and catalase. Direct nephrotoxicity, severe hemolysis, and hypovolemia secondary to fluid loss are the main factors responsible for kidney injury. In experimental animals, copper sulfate causes toxic damage to the proximal tubules. Histologic examination usually shows acute tubular necrosis, with predominant involvement of the proximal tubules. Hemoglobin casts may be seen in patients with intravascular hemolysis. Acute cortical necrosis has been seen rarely.

Management entails gastric lavage using 1% potassium ferrocyanide, which leads to the formation of insoluble cupric ferrocyanide. Egg whites or milk can be administered as an antidote. Emesis should not be induced. Any volume deficit should be corrected quickly. Hyperkalemia may be severe and sustained because of the ongoing hemolysis and requires early and frequent dialysis.

ETHYLENE GLYCOL POISONING

Diethylene and polyethylene glycols have been used as cheap substitutes for propylene glycol as vehicles in pediatric syrup preparations. Epidemics of diethylene glycol–induced AKI have been reported in India and Bangladesh.[68-70] In one large study, 236 deaths were recorded among 339 children with unexplained AKI in a children's hospital in Dhaka, Bangladesh. A total of 51 children had ingested a brand of acetaminophen (paracetamol) known to contain diethylene glycol, whereas 85% of the remaining patients had ingested an unknown elixir for fever.[68] In another report, 14 patients died of AKI after administration of glycerol to decrease intracranial or intraocular pressures.[69]

Analysis of this preparation showed it to be 70% ethylene glycol. Autopsy revealed acute cortical necrosis as the most frequent lesion.

ETHYLENE DIBROMIDE POISONING

Ethylene dibromide (EDB), a pesticide fumigant, is absorbed from the skin, gastrointestinal tract, and intestinal mucosa. Both accidental and suicidal poisonings with EDB have been reported. AKI and hepatocellular injury are the chief manifestations.[71,72] The mortality remains very high despite all supportive measures.[73] EDB is postulated to lead to generation of free oxygen radicals through the cytochrome P450 pathway, causing lipid peroxidation and membrane damage. Dimercaprol has been suggested as an antidote on the basis of the structural similarities of the two compounds.

CHROMIC ACID POISONING

Chromic acid (H_2CrO_7) and its salts (chromates and dichromates) are used in the electroplating, leather tanning, and anticorrosive metal treatment industries. Renal lesions have been reported after acute ingestion of large quantities of these substances.[74,75] Ingestion is followed by severe abdominal pain, vomiting, gastrointestinal bleeding, and circulatory collapse. Renal damage manifests as acute tubular necrosis. Dichromate is directly nephrotoxic and causes extensive proximal tubular necrosis. Hypotension and hemolysis also contribute to tubular damage. Management entails gastric lavage with alkaline solutions such as sodium bicarbonate to prevent absorption and intravenous fluids to combat hypotension. Forced diuresis enhances renal excretion of the compound. Reducing agents such as vitamin C have been shown to prevent chromic acid–induced acute tubular necrosis in experimental animals.

HAIR DYE–RELATED AKI

Hair dye and its constituent paraphenylenediamine (PPD) have been reported as an accidental and intentional cause of poisoning on the Indian subcontinent. Acute poisoning with PPD due to accidental or intentional consumption causes edema of face and neck, resulting in severe respiratory distress that requires tracheostomy. The preceding manifestations are followed by rhabdomyolysis and AKI. In one study, AKI was seen in 32% of patients consuming hair dye. The mean nephrotoxic dose was 79 mL.[76] Mechanisms of AKI are direct nephrotoxicity, myoglobinuria, hemoglobinuria, hypovolemia, and hypotension. The renal lesions are usually found to be acute tubular necrosis or acute interstitial nephritis in patients undergoing biopsy. Renal replacement therapy is required in 82% of patients in whom AKI develops.[76] The overall mortality rate is about 26%, and death is attributed mainly to acute respiratory distress, cardiac arrhythmias, and shock.[77]

ACUTE KIDNEY INJURY DUE TO INTRAVASCULAR HEMOLYSIS AND GLUCOSE-6-PHOSPHATE DEHYDROGENASE DEFICIENCY

G6PD is a key enzyme that protects erythrocytes from oxidative stresses. Deficiency caused by mutations in the *G6PD* gene causes intravascular hemolysis. The gene is located on the X chromosome, and hence males carrying the affected gene have more severe hemolysis. The severity also depends on the nature of the genetic defect. The G6PD variant (Mediterranean) in parts of India and Pakistan leads to hemolysis only in response to oxidative stress.[78] Individuals deficient in the enzyme cannot maintain an adequate level of reduced glutathione, leading to precipitation of oxidized hemoglobin in red blood cells, which are then sequestered and lysed. Hemolytic crisis develops within hours of exposure to the stress, most commonly in the form of drugs, toxins, or infections. Specific causes include pharmacologic agents such as primaquine, sulfonamides, acetylsalicylic acid, nitrofurantoin, nalidixic acid, furazolidone, niridazole, doxorubicin, and phenazopyridine; toxic compounds such as naphthalene balls; infections such as viral hepatitis, rickettsiosis, typhoid fever, and urinary tract infections; and severe metabolic acidosis of any cause. Passage of dark urine followed by oliguria is the most common presentation.[79] Of all causes of AKI, G6PD deficiency may contribute to 5% to 10% of cases in certain regions.[6] Estimation of G6PD level in the erythrocytes by the fluorescent spot test confirms the deficiency. Normally the enzyme activity decreases as the cells age, and older cells with the lowest enzyme activity are destroyed first in a crisis. This process can result in a false-negative test result during a hemolytic episode when the surviving red blood cell population consists of younger erythrocytes, especially in an individual with mild deficiency. The test should therefore be repeated after the patient has recovered from the acute episode to confirm the diagnosis.

ACUTE CORTICAL NECROSIS

Acute renal cortical necrosis is the most catastrophic of all types of AKI. Of more than 2900 patients with AKI treated with dialysis over 28 years in a study in northern India, 3.8% were found to have acute cortical necrosis.[80] It can develop after a variety of conditions, the most common being obstetric complications and snakebite. Obstetric complications were responsible in 56% of all cases of acute cortical necrosis, whereas snakebite accounted for 14%. In children, the most common cause is hemolytic uremic syndrome. The most striking feature of this condition is prolonged oliguria or anuria. This phase may extend for weeks to months, and patients with diffuse cortical necrosis may never enter a diuretic phase.[81,82]

Renal recovery depends on the amount of viable cortical tissue and can be slow and incomplete as the surviving nephrons hypertrophy to compensate for the lost nephron mass. In the study in northern India, only 17% of patients could discontinue dialysis by the end of 3 months. Kidney function deteriorates with time in patients who have achieved partial functional recovery. The longest recorded dialysis-free survival has been 12 years.[80]

The gold standard for establishing the diagnosis is renal biopsy, although CT has emerged as a reliable noninvasive imaging modality for early diagnosis of acute cortical necrosis.[83,84] The characteristic findings include a lack of enhancement of renal cortex except for the subcapsular rim after injection of a contrast agent, medullary enhancement, and absence of pelvicalyceal excretion. Cortical tram-track or eggshell calcification develops later and may be detected on a plain radiograph, ultrasonogram, or CT scan. Histologic examination shows a variable degree of necrosis of all elements of the renal parenchyma, especially the cortical region. Some cortical tissue in the subcapsular and juxtamedullary regions may be spared, and its hypertrophy is responsible for partial recovery of renal function. Other findings include fibrin thrombi in the glomerular capillaries, fibrinoid necrosis of vessel walls, calcification of the necrotic areas, and cortical hemorrhages. The lesions may be classified into patchy and diffuse types, depending on whether the entire parenchyma or only a part of the renal tissue examined shows features of acute cortical necrosis.[80] Needle biopsy can at best give only an approximate idea of the extent of the lesions and can underestimate or overestimate the extent of lesions because of sampling error.

The pathogenesis of acute cortical necrosis remains unclear. The main hypotheses are vasospasm of small vessels and toxic capillary endothelial damage. Prolonged vasospasm of both cortical and medullary vessels induces cortical necrosis in experimental animals. The reasons for increased propensity for renal cortical necrosis during pregnancy are not clear. Renal vasculature in pregnancy may be more prone to vasoconstriction secondary to the effect of sex hormones. Similarities between acute cortical necrosis and the generalized Shwartzman reaction induced in experimental animals by injection of endotoxin have also been noted. Unlike in nonpregnant animals, in which two small doses administered 24 hours apart cause this phenomenon, only one injection is sufficient in pregnant rabbits.

The presence of fibrin thrombi in the vasculature of patients with acute cortical necrosis has led to consideration of intravascular coagulation as the initial event. A role for endothelium-derived vasoactive substances in the genesis of acute cortical necrosis has also been proposed.[81] The increased endothelin-1 levels in women with preeclampsia could contribute to renal ischemia, and a potential role for polymorphisms in the endothelin-1 gene has been suggested. However, more studies are needed to establish the exact role of endothelin in the pathogenesis of acute cortical necrosis.

equation) in a cohort of 3398 otherwise healthy adults.[88] Studies from Pakistan,[89] Nepal,[90] and Bangladesh[91] have reported CKD prevalences of 25.3%, 10.7%, and 13.1% to 16%, respectively, in the general population. These figures must be interpreted with caution because of the wide variations in the definition of CKD, study methodology, and sampled population. Despite a high prevalence of CKD, there is a low awareness of the disease; only 7.9% and 2.3% of subjects were aware of the disease in the studies from India[87] and Pakistan,[89] respectively. Lack of both health care resources and education is possibly responsible for the low awareness of disease.

Commonly used formulas for estimation of glomerular filtration rate (GFR) such as the MDRD equation have been validated only in small population-based studies in the Indian subcontinent.[92,93] Differences in body habitus and dietary habits make it likely that these formulas may require further validation and possibly correction factors for accurate assessment of GFR in this population.[93] Two of the later studies showed the mean measured GFR in healthy Indian adults (kidney donors) to be only 81 mL/min, substantially lower than values reported in the West.[94,95] This finding raises the question of whether the thresholds used to define CKD should be modified. The crude and age-adjusted incidences of ESKD in India have been estimated to be 151 and 232 per million population, respectively.[96] This means that 250,000 to 300,000 new patients need RRT every year. Data on the prevalence of ESKD are not available.

DEMOGRAPHICS OF END-STAGE KIDNEY DISEASE

In the past, glomerulonephritis was reported to be the most common cause of ESKD in the Indian subcontinent.[97] The high prevalence of glomerular diseases was linked to the prevalence of bacterial and viral infections. The etiologic spectrum, however, has been changing in the past decade (Table 80.3).

CHRONIC KIDNEY DISEASE

INCIDENCE AND PREVALENCE

An accurate estimate of the number of patients on the Indian subcontinent who have chronic kidney disease (CKD) or need renal replacement therapy (RRT) is not available owing to the lack of nationwide registry data. In India, Mani reported a prevalence of CKD of 1.1% among a rural population of 25,000 who were subjects of a universal screening program in which serum creatinine concentration was measured only in those with hypertension or proteinuria.[85] Agarwal and colleagues screened 4700 adults in an urban community and found a point prevalence of 7852 per million individuals with a serum creatinine level greater than 1.8 mg/dL.[86] Another cross-sectional study that screened 5588 adults from different parts of India reported a CKD prevalence of 17.2% with about 6% having CKD stage 3 or worse.[87] Prevalence of early stages of CKD (stage 1-3) was reported to be about 13.1% to 15% (with use of the Chronic Kidney Disease Epidemiology Collaboration [CKD-EPI] or Modification of Diet in Renal Disease study [MDRD]

Table 80.3 Causes of Chronic Kidney Disease/End-Stage Kidney Disease in India and Pakistan (Percentage)

	India (N = 57,273)*	Pakistan (N = 6127)†
Diabetic nephropathy	31.3	40.35
Hypertension	12.9	28.89
Chronic glomerulonephritis	13.8	11.57
Chronic interstitial nephritis/calculus disease/obstructive nephropathy	10.4	7.6
Other/unknown	31.8	11.48

*Data from Rajapurkar MM, John GT, Kirpalani AL, et al: What do we know about chronic kidney disease in India: first report of the Indian CKD registry. BMC Nephrol 13:10, 2012.
†Data from Dialysis registry of Pakistan 2007-2008, Karachi, 2008, The Kidney Foundation.

Diabetic nephropathy, previously restricted to high-income urban residents and older individuals, has now emerged as the most important cause of CKD in this region. According to Indian CKD Registry, which has information on more than 57,000 patients, diabetes was listed as the primary diagnosis in 31% of cases of the CKD.[98] The frequency increased to 40% in incident ESKD cases.[96] In the elderly (>60 years) diabetic nephropathy accounted for around 58% of all cases of CKD[99]; however, this is not a nationwide registry. According to the Dialysis Registry of Pakistan, more than 40% of ESKD is due to diabetic nephropathy.[100] In Sri Lanka and Bangladesh too, diabetic nephropathy is an important cause of CKD.[101,102] This change has paralleled the increase in the prevalence of type 2 diabetes in the general population, especially in the areas undergoing rapid urbanization.[103] The projected increase in the prevalence of diabetes in the region suggests that these numbers will rise further over the next 15 years.[103a]

Certain diseases have been shown to predominate in specified geographic locations. Obstructive nephropathy due to urolithiasis is common in Pakistan and contiguous parts of northern India, which constitute a "renal stone belt."

A large proportion of Indian patients with ESKD come for treatment with a relatively short history of kidney problems and advanced renal failure with no previous health records. This makes the task of determining the primary disease difficult. Thus there is a large proportion of patients with ESKD of unknown etiology, which accounts for over one third of all patients at our center. Reports of CKD of uncertain etiology also emerged from the north central provinces of Sri Lanka. Most of the affected individuals were male paddy farmers of low socioeconomic status who had progressive nonproteinuric CKD.[104,105] Biopsy specimens showed tubulointerstitial nephritis with minimal inflammation and extensive fibrosis. The disease bears a strong resemblance to Balkan nephropathy and Chinese herbal nephropathy. It has been suggested that this could be a result of exposure to environmental toxins: residual pesticides, fluoride, aluminium, and cadmium that contaminate drinking water, rice, and edible fish.

The role of the intrauterine environment in the development of chronic disease in adults, particularly systemic arterial hypertension and CKD, has come to the fore and could explain the link between poverty and malnutrition in the mother and subsequent development of CKD in the offspring. Low birth weight and early malnutrition followed by overnutrition in adult life have been shown to be associated with the development of metabolic syndrome, diabetes, and diabetic nephropathy in an Indian cohort.[106] Whether nephrogenesis is influenced by intrauterine malnutrition and/or any adverse intrauterine environment is a matter of ongoing investigation (see discussion of nephron endowment and developmental programming of blood pressure and renal function in Chapter 23). The finding of a high prevalence of proteinuria and high blood pressure in southern Asian children could be part of this jigsaw puzzle.[107,108] Also not investigated is the role of dietary habits and indigenous medicines. Whether any of these factors has an adverse effect on kidney function remains unknown.

The mean age of patients with CKD, including those requiring RRT, is generally lower in this region than in other parts of the world. The mean age of Indian patients with CKD is 50.1 ± 14.6 years; 70.3% are males and 29.7% females according to the Indian CKD registry.[98] This lower mean age is likely related to unique environmental exposures at a younger age and poor availability of health care, which delays diagnosis and leads to a loss of opportunities to institute timely preventive measures, culminating in faster progression to ESKD.

FINANCIAL AND REIMBURSEMENT ISSUES

Unlike in Western nations, the concept of health insurance (both government funded and private) is in a primitive stage on the Indian subcontinent. The costs of RRT, therefore, have to be borne by most patients out of their own funds.[109] Some government and private organizations cover the cost of treatment of employees and their dependents as part of employment benefits. The overall cost of RRT is less in dollar terms than in the industrialized countries because of the lower staff salaries and the low cost of drugs. Nevertheless, it is still several times higher than the per capita gross national product and remains out of reach for the majority of the population.

One Indian study reported that about two thirds of patients who needed RRT obtained financial assistance from employers or accepted charity, one third sold property or family valuables, and a quarter took out loans to cover the cost.[85] Many patients raised funds in more than one way. Only 4% were able to cover the cost using their family resources.

According to the Indian CKD Registry, about 57% of patients with ESKD are not receiving any replacement therapy. The situation is even worse in the elderly; one study reported that of those elderly patients who started HD, only 18% were still receiving dialytic support at the end of 1 year.[99] The cost is also influenced by late presentation, with resulting poor clinical status that necessitates hospitalization. Poor hygiene, hot and humid climate, and overcrowding predispose to a variety of life-threatening infections. It is reported that 12% to 18% of all patients undergoing dialysis eventually have tuberculosis.[110]

HEMODIALYSIS

There are about 5500 dialysis centers in India, over 90% in the private sector. Pakistan had 140 dialysis centers in 2004, which increased to 175 in 2009. They are spread over 53 cities; about 30% are government funded, and 45% are under private management. The rest are run by community support or charitable agencies. In both countries, a large number of dialysis units are small minimal care facilities, owned and looked after by non-nephrologists or even technicians.[110a]

Decisions on the frequency and duration of HD sessions are based on patient symptomatology, financial considerations, and the availability of dialysis slots. Most patients receive one or two 4-hour sessions every week. Dialyzer reuse is practically universal, and reprocessing is often performed manually. The absence of regulation by the government or professional societies has prevented standardization of dialysis procedures, including establishment of minimum standards for dialysis machines, water quality, type of dialyzers, and reuse policies.[109]

Viral hepatitis is among the most common viral infections encountered in patients undergoing dialysis. Hepatitis B vaccination, despite low seroconversion rates, has reduced the prevalence from 32% to 4.7% among patients in India.[111] Hepatitis C virus (HCV) has emerged as the predominant cause of viral hepatitis in patients undergoing maintenance HD. The annual incidence of HCV infection as detected by anti-HCV antibodies among patients at an Indian HD center was reported to be as high as 18%, compared with around 2% in patients receiving continuous ambulatory peritoneal dialysis.[112] Prevalence of HCV was found to be 27.7% when HCV RNA was tested in patients receiving HD at a tertiary care hospital.[113] The high incidence of HCV in HD units could be related to the high prevalence of HCV seropositivity in patients undergoing HD, total transfused blood volume, lack of enforcement of universal precautions, high comorbid illness burden, and greater frequency of intervention. It has been shown that isolation of HCV-infected patients during HD significantly decreases the HCV seroconversion rate, from 36.2% to 2.7%.[114]

Malnutrition affects most patients receiving dialysis in this region; the reported frequency is 44% to 77%.[115] The imposition of protein restriction in patients who are already consuming a calorie-deficient diet, delay in initiation of dialysis, and delivery of inadequate dialysis contribute to this problem. In fact, in one study, protein malnutrition was found to increase in as many as 86% of Indian patients after initiation of dialysis.[116]

PERITONEAL DIALYSIS

Facilities for HD are available only in the larger cities. Because peritoneal dialysis (PD) can be done at home, it could be regarded as the preferred form of dialysis for the majority of patients who live in rural areas and small towns. Despite this advantage, PD continues to be grossly underutilized. The major reason is its higher cost in comparison with HD on the subcontinent. Other reasons include delayed presentation to dialysis units, which gives insufficient time for patient education and preparation, and the fact that many nephrologists are not adequately trained to provide PD. Concerns are often raised on the grounds that poorly educated patients are likely to be nonadherent with therapy and would be at greater risk of peritonitis owing to the hot, humid climate and poor hygienic conditions.

Although PD has been available for close to 25 years in India, this modality is used in fewer than 20% of all patients. In 2008, the number of patients treated with long-term PD in India and Pakistan was only around 6500 and 100, respectively.[117] Patients are assigned to PD not as a matter of choice but mainly because they are unfit for other modalities of RRT. In one large hospital, only 8% of PD recipients were started on PD directly; 92% were shifted after receiving HD for a mean duration of about 6 months. Of those, two thirds were switched because they tolerated HD poorly, 30% because of comorbid conditions and vascular access problems, and 3% because of lifestyle issues.[118] Patients who initially received PD were more likely to have diabetes mellitus and coronary artery disease. Their average age was 63 years, compared with 34 years for the HD population.

The patient's economic status also determines the PD prescription. The most common practice is to start patients on three 2-L exchanges daily.[119] It is not uncommon for patients to reduce the number of exchanges as their financial resources dwindle and eventually to die of the complications of underdialysis. Cycler-assisted PD and the use of newer solutions remain the exclusive privilege of the rich.

In addition to factors directly related to PD, cardiovascular disease is an important killer. Patients often do not undergo cardiovascular evaluation, having already exhausted their resources on PD. This scenario is similar to that seen in the early years of PD practice in Mexico, where aggressive marketing led non-nephrologists to start PD without attention to quality.[120]

Peritonitis remains the major problem associated with PD on the Indian subcontinent. The initial rate of peritonitis was one episode every 5 to 6 patient-months,[121] but this declined significantly as training improved and patients switched to the double-bag system. Some programs reported a higher incidence of infections in the summer months.[121] Peritonitis rates are now around 0.39 to 0.41 episodes per patient year.[122-125] Two unique features of PD-related infections in Indian patients are a high rate of culture-negative cases and a predominance of gram-negative peritonitis mainly in northern India. Culture-positive peritonitis was found in only 63% to 72% of episodes.[122,123]

Gram-negative bacteria constitute 60% to 66% of all organisms found on culture of patients undergoing PD.[126-129] *E. coli* is most commonly found. Other organisms are *Klebsiella pneumoniae*, *Acinetobacter calcoaceticus*, *Pseudomonas aeruginosa*, and *Enterobacter* species. Overall, organisms of fecal origin are more common than those of skin origin. This finding could be related to the unique habit of ablution after defecation in the region, which facilitates the transfer of fecal organisms to the hand. Patients with gram-negative peritonitis require more frequent hospitalization and have higher risks of catheter loss, switch to HD, and death.[123]

In southern India, Pakistan, and Nepal, gram-positive infections are predominant, in contrast to the pattern of infections seen in North India.[126,129] Fungal peritonitis is noted in about 10% to 14% of all peritonitis episodes.[127] More than 90% of these are *Candida* infections. Most episodes are preceded by bacterial peritonitis. Prompt catheter removal improves outcomes. Despite the high frequency of mycobacterial infections in the community, tuberculous peritonitis has not emerged as a significant problem in the Indian PD population.

Malnutrition is a major problem in these patients. Prasad and associates showed that nutritional status at the time of PD initiation was predictive of peritonitis rates. Malnourished patients experienced significantly more peritonitis episodes than patients with normal nutritional status (1.0 vs. 0.2 annually).[130]

KIDNEY TRANSPLANTATION

Constraints in operating an effective maintenance dialysis program leave renal transplantation as the only viable option for patients with ESKD. However, transplantation activity falls woefully short of demand: lack of finances, lack of an organized cadaver-donor transplant program, and social issues are the major stumbling blocks.

Cadaver donors are seldom used because of absence or ineffectiveness of an organ procurement network, lack of facilities for taking care of potential donors, and poor public education. The process depends on the initiative of individual transplant physicians, surgeons, and cooperating intensive care units. Even though more than 70,000 road fatalities are recorded annually in India, lack of prompt transport and unavailability of life-support services preclude organ donation, even in situations in which the families could be approached for consent.[131] Of around 4000 renal transplantations performed annually in India, only 2% use organs from cadaveric donors. For transplantations involving living related donors in India, the proportion of spousal donors (mainly wives) has increased over the last decade and they constitute around 40% of all donors.[132]

Affordability is another major barrier. Even though patients do not have to bear hospitalization costs in state-subsidized hospitals, the cost of immunosuppressive therapy is not reimbursed. In a prospective analysis of 50 kidney transplant recipients in India, direct expenses for kidney transplantation—physician fees, cost of drugs and disposables, dialysis, and costs of laboratory investigations and hospitalization—were estimated to range from $2,151 to $23,792 and indirect expenses—travel, food, stay, and loss of income—from $226 to $15,283 (all in U.S. dollars). Overall, about 54%, 8%, and 10% of families suffered from severe, moderate, and some financial crisis, respectively.[133] Antibody induction therapy and prophylaxis for cytomegalovirus infection are therefore rarely used. Pretransplantation HCV infections also often go untreated. Patients are non-adherent with regimens of expensive drugs like calcineurin inhibitors, leading to high rates of graft loss. The cost of treating steroid-resistant rejections is prohibitive. Cost reduction strategies that are frequently used include limiting induction therapy to high-risk patients, using cytochrome P450 inhibitors (ketoconazole/non-dihydropyridine calcium channel blocker), using azathioprine instead of mycophenolate mofetil, continuing prednisolone long term, and using bioequivalent generic drugs.

The worldwide shortage of organs for transplantation gave rise to the practice of the purchase of kidneys from poor donors by affluent persons in India in the 1980s and early 1990s.[134] The buyers came from both within and outside the country; hence the term *transplant tourism*. The exploitation of donors and substandard medical care provided to recipients were widely condemned and prompted the enactment of a law by the Indian Parliament in 1994 officially banning this practice. Since then, it has been carried out only clandestinely in India; it is more common in some parts of Pakistan, although exact numbers are not known.[135,136] The Human Organ and Tissue Transplantation Ordinance, which was passed in September 2007 in Pakistan, explicitly and unambiguously makes buying and selling of human organs a crime and prohibits transplantation of organs from Pakistanis into foreigners.[137] Of late, more transplants from unrelated living donors are being done in Sri Lanka, as reported in the lay press.

Infections complicate the course in 50% to 75% of kidney transplant recipients in the region, with mortality ranging from 20% to 60%.[115] Rubin categorized these infections into those occurring within the first month after transplantation, those occurring within 2 to 6 months, and those occurring thereafter.[138] The reported 6-month milestone of a decrease in the susceptibility to infections after stepdown of immunosuppression is not seen in these patients. This lack reflects an altered susceptibility pattern caused by coexisting infections in immunosuppressed patients in the region together with a higher prevalence of endemic infections.[139]

Tuberculosis affects 10% to 13% of renal transplant recipients in India[140-142] and results from reactivation of a quiescent focus. It manifests in the first year after transplantation in more than 50% of patients. Although pleuropulmonary involvement is the most common, disseminated disease occurs in about 30% of patients. Unusual sites of involvement include the skin, tonsils, vocal cords, and prostate.

Renal transplant recipients with tuberculosis present numerous diagnostic difficulties. The Mantoux test is generally unhelpful, classical radiologic findings are seen only in a minority, examination of a sputum smear for acid-fast bacilli has a low yield, and culture takes 4 to 6 weeks. Bronchoalveolar lavage, bone marrow biopsy, and liver biopsy must be used to make a diagnosis of tuberculosis.

There are also problems with treatment of tuberculosis in transplant recipients, specifically in selecting antituberculous drugs and determining duration of therapy. Rifampicin is a well-known hepatic P450 microsomal enzyme inducer that increases the clearance of both prednisolone and calcineurin inhibitors. The dosage of calcineurin inhibitors needs to be increased threefold to fourfold to maintain therapeutic blood levels. This change raises the cost of therapy and is unacceptable to the vast majority of patients. The alternative regimen that has been successfully utilized consists of a combination of isoniazid, ethambutol, pyrazinamide, and ofloxacin or ciprofloxacin.[143] The optimal duration of therapy is a matter of debate. For combinations using rifampicin and isoniazid, 9 months of treatment has been recommended.[143] However, the duration is increased to 18 months for patients who are not receiving rifampicin.[140] Initiation of isoniazid chemoprophylaxis during dialysis prevents the development of tuberculosis after transplantation. However, isoniazid can cause hepatic dysfunction, for which it often must be discontinued.[144] Drug-resistant mycobacterial strains are also of concern, and the incidence of primary isoniazid resistance is increasing steadily.[145] The role of isoniazid prophylaxis thus remains controversial.[146]

Other common infections in transplant recipients are hepatitis B and hepatitis C, both of which are highly prevalent in patients undergoing dialysis. Hepatitis B is encountered in about 5%, whereas hepatitis C is seen in 15% to 20%. The cost of interferon therapy and indirect expenses (including dialysis) during therapy for HCV infection are so prohibitive that the majority (≈75%) of HCV-positive patients undergo kidney transplantation without receiving anti-HCV treatment.[147] Although patient and graft survivals at 5 years were reported to be similar in HCV-positive and HCV-negative patients, serious bacterial infections were significantly more common in HCV-positive patients.[148,149] The rate of cytomegalovirus infection was found to increase from 4% in the years before calcineurin inhibitors were widely used to 17% in the calcineurin inhibitor era in one autopsy series. Primary infection is seldom seen because the vast majority of both donors and recipients are seropositive.[110] Opportunistic fungal infections occur in 4% to

7% of recipients, but these carry a high mortality rate, more than 65%.[150,151] Malaria and leishmaniasis are also encountered.[152]

GLOMERULONEPHRITIS

In the absence of a biopsy registry, the exact spectrum of glomerulonephritis cannot be known. However, a large study of more than 5400 kidney biopsy specimens at a south Indian tertiary care center that treats not only patients from India but also those from neighboring countries provides an insight into the range of glomerulonephritis in the region.[153] Primary glomerulonephritis was diagnosed in 71% of all biopsy specimens. Mesangioproliferative glomerulonephritis without IgA was the most common lesion (20.2%), followed by idiopathic focal segmental glomerulosclerosis (FSGS) (17%), minimal change disease (11.6%), membranous nephropathy (9.8%), IgA nephropathy (8.6%), and membranoproliferative glomerulonephritis (3.7%). Postinfectious glomerulonephritis accounted for 12.3% of all lesions.

To ascertain changing trends, biopsy data collected between 1971 and 1985 were compared with later data in the same study. The later data showed significant increases in FSGS (17% vs. 8.6%) and membranous glomerulonephritis (9.8% vs. 6.4%) during the period 1986 to 2002, whereas minimal change disease (11.6% vs. 16.5%) and membranoproliferative glomerulonephritis (3.7% vs. 7.2%) decreased significantly during the same period. Thus, in comparison with other registries, the prevalence of IgA nephropathy is much lower than that in East Asians, whereas FSGS is more common. Similar trends have been reported in another study from the northern region of the subcontinent.[154] Analysis of data for adults presenting with nephrotic syndrome due to primary glomerular disease reveals that FSGS is the most common lesion in both India and Pakistan. The frequency of occurrence of other primary glomerular diseases in these patients is shown in Table 80.4.[154-156] The morphologic categories of FSGS in the Indian population have been described and are different from those in the West.[157] There is a lower prevalence of the perihilar and collapsing variants and a higher prevalence of tip and cellular variants. Secondary amyloidosis is an important cause of glomerular disease on the subcontinent and is much more common than primary amyloidosis. Tuberculosis is the main cause of secondary amyloidosis in India, accounting for two thirds of cases, whereas rheumatoid arthritis is responsible in only 6% of cases.[158,159]

RENOVASCULAR HYPERTENSION

The most common causes of renovascular hypertension worldwide are fibromuscular dysplasia in the young and atherosclerosis in the elderly. On the Indian subcontinent, however, Takayasu's arteritis or nonspecific aortoarteritis is the main cause of renovascular hypertension in young adults as well as in children, accounting for 59% to 80% of all cases in these groups.[160,161] In the elderly, as elsewhere, atherosclerosis is the most common cause.

Takayasu's arteritis is an inflammatory vascular disease of unknown etiology predominantly affecting young females in the second and third decades. It involves the large elastic arteries and results in occlusive or ectatic changes mainly in the aorta and its major branches. The average age of Indian patients is between 25 and 30 years.[162]

Aortoarteritis has been classified into the following types according to the sites of involvement: type I affects the branches of the aortic arch; type IIa affects the ascending aorta, aortic arch, and its branches; type IIb affects the ascending aorta, aortic arch, and its branches and the descending thoracic aorta; type III affects the thoracic aorta, abdominal aorta, and/or renal arteries; type IV affects the abdominal aorta and/or renal arteries; type V is a combination of types IIb and IV. Involvement of a coronary or pulmonary artery is indicated by appending the suffix $C(+)$ or $P(+)$ to any of the types.[163] Involvement of the abdominal aorta and/or renal arteries is more common in India and other Southeast Asian countries and South America than in Japan, where the aortic arch and its branches are more commonly involved. In Indian and Bangladeshi patients, type III

Table 80.4 Spectrum of Primary Glomerular Lesions Causing Nephrotic Syndrome on the Indian Subcontinent*

	India (N = 324)†	Pakistan (N = 316)‡	Nepal (N = 137)§
Focal segmental glomerulosclerosis	99 (30.6)	126 (39.9)	11 (8.0)
Membranous nephropathy	79 (24.4)	84 (26.6)	58 (42.3)
Membranoproliferative glomerulonephritis	58 (17.9)	14 (4.4)	30 (21.9)
Minimal change disease	48 (14.8)	50 (15.8)	14 (10.2)
Postinfectious glomerulonephritis	9 (2.8)	9 (2.8)	4 (2.9)
Immunoglobulin A nephropathy	6 (1.8)	8 (2.5)	3 (2.2)
Other	25 (7.7)	25 (8.0)	17 (12.4)

*Numbers in parentheses are percentages.
†Data from Rathi M, Bhagat RL, Mukhopadhyay P, et al: Changing histologic spectrum of adult nephritic syndrome over five decades in Northern India: a single center experience. *Ind J Nephrol* 24:13-18, 2014.
‡Data from Kazi JI, Mubarak M, Ahmed E, et al: Spectrum of glomerulonephritides in adults with nephrotic syndrome in Pakistan. *Clin Exp Nephrol* 13:38-43, 2009.
§Data from Garyal, Kafle RK: Histopathological spectrum of glomerular disease in Nepal: a seven-year retrospective study. *Nepal Med Coll J* 10:126-128, 2008.

disease is the most common, accounting for 53% to 76% of all cases.[164]

In a large study of 650 cases in India, clinical manifestations of aortoarteritis included unequal pulses (96%), hypertension (72%), oliguria due to renal failure (30%), intermittent claudication (25%), neurologic symptoms (amaurosis fugax, syncope, transient ischemic attacks) (22.5%), eye changes (8.1%), and skin manifestations (erythema nodosum, Raynaud's phenomenon, leg ulcers) (3.8%).[164] It is important to record blood pressure in all four limbs, because arteries supplying the upper limbs are often involved in the disease process.

The renal artery is narrowed at its ostium and in the proximal third. Bilateral renal artery stenosis is seen in about half of all patients (Figure 80.2). Histologic findings in affected vessels vary according to the stage of the disease. In the early stages, granulomatous inflammation and infiltration with polymorphs, mononuclear cells, and multinucleated giant cells are seen in all the layers but are more marked in the adventitia than in the media or intima.[165] These features may also be seen around the vasa vasorum, which show endothelial proliferation and obliteration of the vessel lumen. In more advanced disease, the inflammatory process is less evident, but adventitial fibrosis and intimal smooth muscle proliferation and fibrosis result in marked luminal narrowing.

Nonspecific ischemic glomerular lesions resulting from arterial narrowing and hypertension are frequently observed in patients with renal artery involvement. Rarely, glomerular lesions such as mesangioproliferative, focal proliferative, membranoproliferative, and crescentic forms of glomerulonephritis have been reported. Renal amyloidosis in association with Takayasu's arteritis has also been reported in rare instances.[166]

Prednisolone, at a dosage of 1 mg per kg body weight per day tapered to 15 mg/day by 3 months,[166a] often dramatically improves the constitutional symptoms, halts disease progression in patients with inflammatory stage disease, and lowers the erythrocyte sedimentation rate (ESR) toward normal. However, even the ESR is not a reliable marker of disease activity. If progression of disease is seen in patients undergoing steroid therapy, cytotoxic drugs such as cyclophosphamide or azathioprine may be used. Alternatively, low-dose methotrexate may enhance the efficacy of steroid therapy and facilitate steroid sparing. The results of balloon angioplasty with stent placement in narrowed arteries are highly encouraging. In patients in whom stents cannot be implanted, surgical reconstruction may be carried out after the disease becomes inactive.

RENAL CALCULI

Parts of northern India and Pakistan compose an important part of the "renal stone belt," where nephrolithiasis is responsible for 5% of all cases of ESKD.

The available literature on urinary calculi shows a different stone pattern across the world, highlighting different geographic and etiologic factors. Studies in northern India have shown that the vast majority (>90%) of calculi are calcium oxalate stones, predominantly calcium oxalate monohydrate (80%).[167] Apatite, struvite, and uric acid stones account for less than 2% each. This incidence of calcium oxalate monohydrate stones is significantly higher than that in Western countries, where such stones constitute up to 55% of the total.[168] Classically, staghorn calculi are composed of calcium magnesium ammonium phosphate. However, in Indian studies, even staghorn calculi are made up predominantly of calcium oxalate. Reasons for the high incidence of calcium oxalate calculi in this region could include the oxalate-rich vegetarian diet along with its high carbohydrate content and the high mineral and fluoride content of drinking water. Fluoride is thought to promote stone formation by increasing oxaluria and insoluble calcium fluoride in urine.[169]

INDIGENOUS THERAPIES

HERBAL MEDICINE TOXICITY

On the subcontinent a combination of ignorance, poverty, nonavailability of health facilities, high cost of modern medicines, and the widespread belief in indigenous systems drives people to turn to indigenous drugs. It is commonly believed that that these remedies are gentler and without any side effects. Herbal remedies are often classified as dietary supplements for regulatory and marketing purposes and hence are exempt from rigorous safety testing. However, adulteration of herbal medicines is common in many countries. A state government report cited the finding of undeclared pharmaceuticals or heavy metals in 32% of Asian patent medicines sold in California.[170] The high heavy metal content of indigenous herbal drugs could be due to heavily polluted soil or irrigation water. Dwivedi and Dey found

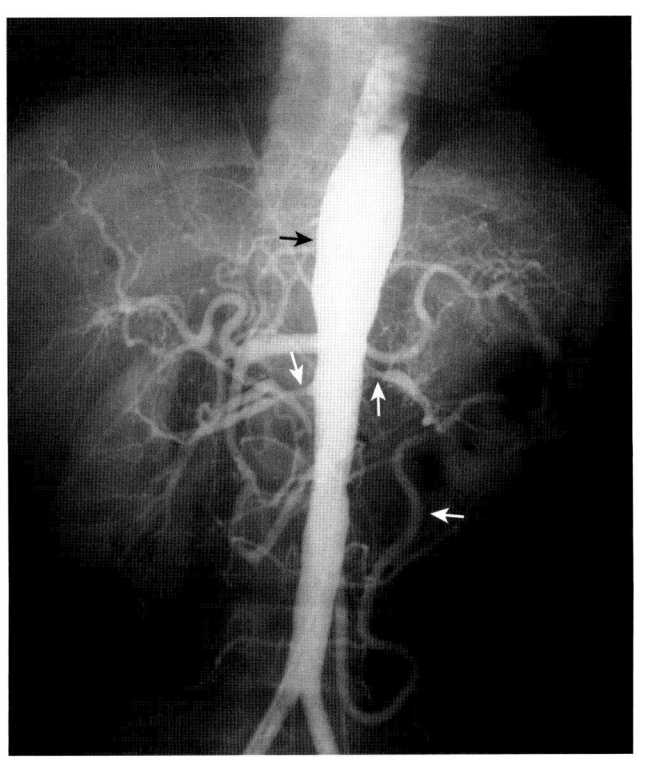

Figure 80.2 Takayasu's arteritis. Bilateral renal artery narrowing (*vertical arrows*) with post-stenotic dilation on the left side, dilation and irregularity of the abdominal aorta (*black arrow*), and a large collateral vessel (*horizontal arrow*) arising from the inferior mesenteric artery.

high lead and cadmium levels in the leaves of medicinal plants from India.[171]

The medical community has increasingly recognized the potential role of these remedies in causing harm to various organ systems, including the kidneys. Indigenous therapies may cause AKI as well as CKD. In AKI the cause-and-effect relationship is easier to establish because there is a temporal relation between intake of the agents and injury. However, physicians often do not seek the history of intake of natural medicines. Moreover, a chemical analysis of such drugs is seldom carried out. Recently Prakash and colleagues described the case of a 60-year-old man who had unexplained kidney failure.[172] Investigation revealed that he had been taking an herbal medicine from India containing a large amount of lead. After discontinuation of the herbal medicine and several sessions of lead chelation therapy, his creatinine level declined. This case highlights the need for clinicians to consider lead intoxication due to indigenous medicinal therapy in the differential diagnosis of patients with AKI or CKD.

TOXICITY OF NATURAL MEDICINES FROM ANIMAL SOURCES

The raw gallbladder or bile of freshwater and grass carp is used in parts of eastern India to reduce fever, treat cough, decrease hypertension, improve visual acuity, treat rheumatism, and promote general health.[173] A syndrome of acute hepatic and renal failure has been reported in exposed patients. Symptoms appear minutes to hours after ingestion and include abdominal pain, nausea, vomiting, and watery diarrhea. Hepatocellular jaundice is observed in more than 60% of patients. AKI sets in within 48 hours and is oliguric in the majority of patients. More than 75% also show microscopic hematuria. The duration of AKI ranges from 2 to 3 weeks. The variation in symptomatology is likely to be related to differences in the varieties of fish or amount of bile ingested as well as in individual susceptibility. Renal histologic examination reveals tubular necrosis and interstitial edema.

The mechanism by which AKI develops is not well understood and may include bradycardia and hypotension owing to the cardiotoxic effect of the bile salts. Bile salts also inhibit intestinal Na^+-K^+-ATPase, which increases mucosal permeability and leads to diarrhea. Bile produces diuresis, excessive salt loss, and cardiac depression in rats. Hypotension and hemolysis may also contribute to renal failure. Recovery has been universal among patients who have sought medical attention in a timely manner, and death has occurred only in those who reported late and had multiorgan failure.

SUMMARY

The spectrum of both acute and chronic kidney disease on the Indian subcontinent differs significantly from that encountered both in the industrialized world and in other developing countries. Community-acquired AKI in otherwise healthy individuals continues to be common in the region. Although glomerulonephritis has been the most common cause of ESKD, it is being replaced by diabetic nephropathy. The lack of an adequate number of nephrologists and the high cost of treatment pose the biggest challenges to the management of patients with kidney disease in this region of the world.

Complete reference list available at ExpertConsult.com.

KEY REFERENCES

7. Jayakumar M, Prabahar MR, Fernando EM, et al: Epidemiologic trend changes in acute renal failure—a tertiary center experience from south India. *Ren Fail* 28:405–410, 2006.
9. Kohli HS, Madhu C, Muthu Kumar T, et al: Treatment related acute renal failure in the elderly: a hospital based prospective study. *Nephrol Dial Transplant* 15:212–217, 2000.
11. Prakash J, Kumar H, Sinha DK, et al: Acute renal failure in pregnancy in a developing country: twenty years of experience. *Ren Fail* 28:309–313, 2006.
13. Cerda J, Bagga A, Kher V, et al: The contrasting characteristics of acute kidney injury in developed and developing countries. *Nat Clin Pract Nephrol* 4(3):138–153, 2008.
16. Murali R, Bhalla A, Singh D, et al: Acute pesticide poisoning: 15 years experience of a large north-west Indian hospital. *Clin Toxicol (Phila)* 47:35–38, 2009.
21. Kohli HS, Bhat A, Aravindan AN, et al: Predictors of mortality in elderly patients with acute renal failure in a developing country. *Int Urol Nephrol* 39(1):339–344, 2007.
26. Jamal A, Ramzan A: Renal and post-renal causes of acute renal failure in children. *J Coll Physicians Surg Pak* 14:411–415, 2004.
32. Mehndiratta S, Rajeshwari K, Dubey AP: Multiple-organ dysfunction in a case of *Plasmodium vivax* malaria. *J Vector Borne Dis Mar* 50(1):71–73, 2013.
37. Shukla VS, Singh RG, Rathore SS, et al: Outcome of malaria-associated acute kidney injury: a prospective study from a single center. *Ren Fail* 35(6):801–805, 2013.
38. Mishra SK, Mohanty S, Satpathy SK, et al: Cerebral malaria in adults—a description of 526 cases admitted to Ispat General Hospital in Rourkela, India. *Ann Trop Med Parasitol* 101:187–193, 2007.
45. Ittyachen AM, Krishnapillai TV, Nair MC, et al: Retrospective study of severe cases of leptospirosis admitted in the intensive care unit. *J Postgrad Med* 53:232–235, 2007.
50. Gupta KL, Joshi K, Sud K, et al: Renal zygomycosis: an under-diagnosed cause of acute renal failure. *Nephrol Dial Transplant* 14:2720–2725, 1999.
52. Mehra N, Patel A, Abraham G, et al: Acute kidney injury in dengue fever using Acute Kidney Injury Network criteria: incidence and risk factors. *Trop Doct* 42(3):160–162, 2012.
56. Sharma N, Chauhan S, Faruqi S, et al: Snake envenomation in a north Indian hospital. *Emerg Med J* 22:118–120, 2005.
59. Kohli HS, Sakhuja V: Snake bite and acute renal failure. *Saudi J Nephrology* 14(2):165–176, 2003.
65. Vikrant S, Patial RK: Acute renal failure following multiple honeybee stings. *Indian J Med Sci* 60:202–204, 2006.
73. Singh N, Jatav OP, Gupta RK, et al: Outcome of sixty four cases of ethylene dibromide ingestion treated in tertiary care hospital. *J Assoc Physicians India* 55:842–845, 2007.
76. Sandeep Reddy Y, Abbdul Nabi S, Apparao C, et al: Hair dye related acute kidney injury—a clinical and experimental study. *Ren Fail* 34(7):880–884, 2012.
78. Khan M: Glucose 6 phosphate dehydrogenase deficiency in adults. *J Coll Physicians Surg Pak* 14:400–403, 2004.
80. Chugh KS, Jha V, Sakhuja V, et al: Acute renal cortical necrosis—a study of 113 patients. *Ren Fail* 16:37–47, 1994.
84. Jha V, Sakhuja V: Postpartum renal cortical necrosis. *Nephrol Dial Transplant* 20:1010, 2005.
87. Singh AK, Farag YM, Mittal BV, et al: Epidemiology and risk factors of chronic kidney disease in India—results from the SEEK (Screening and Early Evaluation of Kidney Disease) study. *BMC Nephrol* 14:114, 2013.
88. Varma PP, Raman DK, Ramakrishnan TS, et al: Prevalence of early stages of chronic kidney disease in apparently healthy central government employees in India. *Nephrol Dial Transplant* 25(9):3011–3017, 2010.
89. Saeed ZI, Hussain SA: Chronic kidney disease in Pakistan: an under-recognized public health problem. *Kidney Int* 81(11):1151, 2012.

90. Sharma SK, Dhakal S, Thapa L, et al: Community-based screening for chronic kidney disease, hypertension and diabetes in Dhahran. *JNMA J Nepal Med Assoc* 52(189):205–212, 2013.
91. Huda MN, Alam KS, Harun-Ur R: Prevalence of chronic kidney disease and its association with risk factors in disadvantageous population. *Int J Nephrol* 267–329, 2012.
93. Jessani S, Levey AS, Bux R, et al: Estimation of GFR in South Asians: A study from the general population in Pakistan. *Am J Kidney Dis* 63:49–58, 2014.
94. Barai S, Bandopadhayaya GP, Patel CD, et al: Do healthy potential kidney donors in India have an average glomerular filtration rate of 81.4 ml/min? *Nephrol Physiol* 101:21–26, 2005.
96. Modi GK, Jha V: The incidence of end-stage renal disease in India: a population-based study. *Kidney Int* 70:2131–2133, 2006.
98. Rajapurkar MM, John GT, Kirpalani AL, et al: What do we know about chronic kidney disease in India: first report of the Indian CKD registry. *BMC Nephrol* 13:10, 2012.
99. Kohli HS, Bhat A, Aravindan AN, et al: Spectrum of renal failure in elderly patients. *Int Urol Nephrol* 38(3–4):759–765, 2006.
100. *Dialysis registry of Pakistan 2007-2008*, Karachi, 2008, The Kidney Foundation.
105. Wanigasuriya KP, Peiris-John RJ, Wickremasinghe R, et al: Chronic renal failure in north central province of Sri Lanka: an environmentally induced disease. *Trans R Soc Trop Med Hyg* 101:1013–1017, 2007.
109. Jha V: Current status of end-stage renal disease care in India and Pakistan. *Kidney Int Suppl* 3:157–160, 2013.
112. Johnson DW, Hannah D, Qiang Y, et al: Frequencies of hepatitis B and C infections among haemodialysis and peritoneal dialysis patients in Asia-Pacific countries: analysis of registry data. *Nephrol Dial Transplant* 24:1598–1603, 2009.
113. Jasuja S, Gupta AK, Choudhry R, et al: Prevalence and association of hepatitis C viremia in hemodialysis patient at a tertiary care hospital. *Indian J Nephrol* 19:62–67, 2009.
114. Agarwal SK, Dash SC, Gupta S, et al: Hepatitis C virus infection in haemodialysis: the "no-isolation" policy should not be generalized. *Nephron Clin Pract* 111:133–140, 2009.
118. Mahajan S, Tiwari SC, Kalra V, et al: Factors affecting the use of peritoneal dialysis among the ESRD population in India: a single-center study. *Perit Dial Int* 24:538–541, 2004.
123. Prasad KN, Singh K, Rizwan A, et al: Microbiology and outcomes of peritonitis in northern India. *Perit Dial Int* 34:188–194, 2014.
126. Abraham G, Pratap B, Sankarasubbaiyan S, et al: Chronic peritoneal dialysis in South Asia-challenges and future. *Perit Dial Int* 28:13–19, 2008.
132. Mittal T, Ramachandran R, Kumar V, et al: Outcomes of spousal versus related donor kidney transplants: A comparative study. *Indian J Nephrol* 24:58–63, 2014.
133. Ramachandran R, Jha V: Kidney transplantation is associated with catastrophic out of pocket expenditure in India. *PLoS ONE* 4;8(7):e67812, 2013.
137. Akhtar F: Organ transplantation law in Pakistan to curb kidney trade: chance for global reflection. *NDT Plus* 1(2):128–129, 2008.
139. John GT: Infections after renal transplantation in India. *Indian J Nephrol* 13:14–19, 2003.
147. Duseja A, Choudhary NS, Gupta S, et al: Treatment of chronic hepatitis C in end stage renal disease: experience at a tertiary care centre. *Trop Gastroenterol* 33(3):189–192, 2012.
153. Narasimhan B, Chacko B, John GT, et al: Characterization of kidney lesions in Indian adults: towards a renal biopsy registry. *J Nephrol* 19:205–210, 2006.
154. Rathi M, Bhagat RL, Mukhopadhyay P, et al: Changing histologic spectrum of adult nephritic syndrome over five decades in Northern India: A single center experience. *Ind J Nephrol* 24:13–18, 2014.
157. Nada R, Kharbanda JK, Bhatti A, et al: Primary focal segmental glomerulosclerosis in adults: is the Indian cohort different? *Nephrol Dial Transplant* 24(12):3701–3707, 2009.
164. Panja M, Mondal PC: Current status of aortoarteritis in India. *J Assoc Physicians India* 52:48–52, 2004.
172. Prakash S, Hernande GT, Dujaili I, et al: Lead poisoning from an Ayurvedic herbal medicine in a patient with chronic kidney disease. *Nat Rev Nephrol* 41:297–300, 2009.

81 The Far East

Chuan-Ming Hao | Fan-Fan Hou | Walter G. Wasser

CHAPTER OUTLINE

ACUTE KIDNEY INJURY, 2510
Acute Kidney Injury due to Infections, 2511
Acute Kidney Injury due to Toxins and Chemicals, 2523
CHRONIC KIDNEY DISEASE, 2526
Chronic Kidney Disease After Infection, 2527
Diabetes Mellitus, 2529
Glomerulonephritis, 2529
ANCA-Associated Vasculitides, 2532
Hepatitis B/Hepatitis C Virus–Associated Nephritis, 2532
Human Immunodeficiency Virus Infection, 2533
Distal Renal Tubular Acidosis, 2533
Herbal Medicines, 2533
Betel Nut Chewing, 2534

RENAL REPLACEMENT THERAPY, 2534
Taiwan, 2534
Japan, 2534
Hong Kong, 2535
China, 2535
Korea, 2535
Thailand, 2535
Malaysia, 2535
Singapore, 2536
Indonesia, 2536
Vietnam, 2536
The Philippines, 2536
SCIENTIFIC PUBLICATIONS, 2536

The Far East consists of East Asia (including Northeast Asia), Southeast Asia, and the Russian Far East (part of North Asia, Siberia), with South Asia sometimes also included for economic and cultural reasons. Geographically, this area covers approximately 12,000,000 km^2, or approximately 28% of the Asian continent. More than 1.5 billion people, approximately 38% of the population of Asia and 22% of all people in the world, live in geographic East Asia. The territories and regions that are conventionally included under the term Far East are East Asia: China (with Hong Kong and Macau), Japan, Mongolia, North Korea, South Korea, and Taiwan; Southeast Asia: Brunei, Cambodia, Timor-Leste (East Timor), Indonesia, Laos, Malaysia, Myanmar, Papua New Guinea (PNG), the Philippines, Singapore, Thailand, Vietnam; and North Asian Russia.

The Far East is an area with extreme heterogeneity in ethnic composition, environment, and socioeconomic conditions. Thus, differences in living standards, environments, cultural practices, availability of health care, and genetic susceptibility determine the variations in disease patterns and management practices. In general, this area has the following characteristics: (1) high incidence of infections (bacterial, viral, and parasitic) and their associated kidney complications, including community-acquired acute kidney injury (AKI), particularly in tropical areas; (2) high incidence of toxic injury, including snakebites and bee stings, and high rate of herbal medication use, which may lead to kidney damage; (3) diabetic nephropathy as the most common cause of chronic kidney disease (CKD) and end-stage kidney disease (ESKD) in some countries and regions, with glomerulonephritis as the major cause of CKD/ESKD in other countries, particularly in developing countries; and (4) different genetic susceptibilities to certain kidney diseases and treatment responses, such as immunoglobulin A (IgA) nephropathy.

ACUTE KIDNEY INJURY

AKI is a common renal emergency in the Far East. The causes of AKI vary with socioeconomic status, climate, and cultures.

In developed, large, urban areas, the pattern of AKI is very similar to that found in developed countries and regions in other areas of the world; it is predominantly a hospital-acquired disease occurring mostly in older, critically ill patients with multiorgan failure and complex medical or surgical conditions. The main cause of AKI in this population is renal ischemia, principally due to sepsis, which is often associated with nephrotoxic drugs. In contrast, in rural areas or smaller cities in the countryside, particularly in developing tropical regions, AKI is usually a community-acquired disease, affecting younger and previously healthy individuals. In this population, the specific causes of AKI include diarrheal diseases with dehydration, infectious diseases, animal venoms (snakes and bees), and natural medicines.

ACUTE KIDNEY INJURY DUE TO INFECTIONS

Tropical infections can cause AKI in four major ways: (1) direct invasion of the renal parenchyma by microbial agents; (2) induction of an immune response that leads to renal inflammation; (3) induction of hemodynamic disturbances that lead to tubular necrosis; and (4) intrinsic renal injury associated with pigment nephropathy.

Typical causes of AKI that are epidemic to Far East are zoonoses such as leptospirosis, scrub typhus, hantavirus, dengue, and malaria. Leptospirosis and hantavirus are rodent-borne diseases; the vector for scrub typhus is a chigger-mite, an ectoparasite that is isolated from wild rodents[1]; and mosquitoes are the vector for malaria and dengue. Bunyaviridae is a newly described virus emanating from Chinese domestic animals that is spread by ticks. The clinical characteristics of AKI due to these infections can be similar,[2] co-infection has been demonstrated,[2,3] and serologic identification is necessary to guide antibiotic therapy.

LEPTOSPIROSIS

Leptospirosis, the most widespread zoonosis, is caused by a microorganism of the genus *Leptospira*, a spirochetal infection.[4] This disease is caused by infected mammals (especially rodents, cattle, swine, dogs, horses, sheep, and goats), the natural hosts, which shed spirochetes through urine into water or soil that in turn infect humans via skin or the gastrointestinal route. The most common exposure routes are occupational, recreational, and household contacts with animals and exposure from episodes of flooding.

Leptospira outer membrane proteins (OMPs) elicit inflammation and tubular injury through a Toll-like receptor (TLR)–dependent pathway, followed by activation of nuclear transcription factor kappaB and mitogen-activated protein kinases with differential induction of chemokines and cytokines that are relevant to tubular inflammation.[5,6] Leptospira OMPs may activate the transforming growth factor-β/SMAD-associated fibrosis pathway, leading to extracellular matrix accumulation.[6,7] One study showed that Leptospira OMP extract induces an increase in fibronectin production through a TLR2-mediated pathway.[8] In Taiwan, a genomic analysis of *Leptospira santarosai* serovar shermani, the most frequently encountered serovar, is presently underway to categorize those sequences associated with virulence.[9] Genomic sequencing should permit studies of pathogenesis and development of leptospiral vaccines.

Leptospirosis can provoke a broad range of manifestations, from benign infection (characterized by nonspecific symptoms) to Weil's disease, a severe form of the disease that causes jaundice, myocarditis, and pulmonary hemorrhage. The early phase of leptospirosis manifestation lasts 3 to 7 days and includes fever, headaches, myalgia (especially in the calves), nausea, vomiting, malaise, and conjunctival hyperemia. In this phase, it is possible to isolate leptospires from blood samples. Eighty percent to 90% of patients are symptom free after this initial phase. Only 10% progress to the second phase, Weil's disease. In this phase, which may last from 4 to 30 days, more severe symptoms, such as jaundice, meningitis, pulmonary hemorrhage, and AKI, can occur[6] (Tables 81.1 through 81.3).

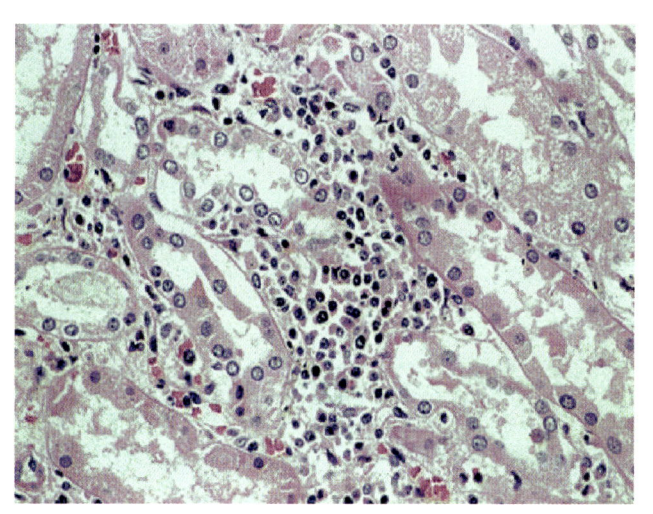

Figure 81.1 The renal pathology from a patient who died of leptospirosis. Kidney histopathology of a patient who died of leptospirosis. The micrograph shows focal interstitial nephritis and moderate acute tubular necrosis. (From Abdulkader RC, Silva MV: The kidney in leptospirosis. *Pediatr Nephrol.* 23:2111, 2008.)

The kidney is one of the principal target organs of *Leptospira*. The reported incidence of AKI in severe leptospirosis varies from 40% to 60%.[10] A presentation of fever, jaundice, and AKI in acutely ill patients should alert the clinician to consider leptospirosis.[11] A case-control study was conducted in patients with multiorgan dysfunction to differentiate leptospirosis from other infections.[12] Twenty-two confirmed cases of leptospirosis were identified from 169 suspected cases, and 21 cases were excluded. The confirmed leptospirosis group most commonly presented with fever (95.5%, 21/22), AKI (86.4%, 19/22), myalgia (72.7%, 16/22), and jaundice (63.6%, 14/22). The following presenting signs and symptoms were more common in the confirmed leptospirosis group: hemorrhagic diathesis, myalgia, enlarged kidneys, sterile pyuria, and thrombocytopenia. Penicillin treatment in the confirmed leptospirosis group, even in a group with multiorgan dysfunction, was associated with a low fatality rate, 4.5% (1/22). Thrombocytopenia appears to be closely related to the occurrence of AKI, seems to be independent of disseminated intravascular coagulopathy (DIC), and was present in all cases of AKI without icterus.[13]

Tubulointerstitial nephritis is the main cause of AKI in leptospirosis.[14,15] Glomerular manifestations, when present, are of a mild, nonspecific, reactive nature (Figures 81.1 and 81.2). Tubular functional alterations precede a decrease in the glomerular filtration rate. Both humans and experimental animals demonstrate increased urinary fractional excretion of potassium and sodium, which suggests increased distal potassium secretion caused by increased distal sodium delivery consequent to proximal tubule damage and the impairment of sodium reabsorption.[16] The characteristic laboratory finding is hypokalemia in the setting of nonoliguric AKI. Proximal tubular dysfunction (bicarbonaturia,

Table 81.1 Differences in Clinical Manifestations Between Confirmed and Excluded Cases of Suspected Leptospirosis*

Value	Confirmed Cases (%)	Excluded Cases (%)	P Value
Acute renal failure	86.4	76.2	0.46
Thrombocytopenia	86.4	57.1	0.045
Pancreatitis[†]	43.8	12.5	0.19
Rhabdomyolysis[‡]	23.6	15.4	0.69
Jarisch-Herxheimer reaction[§]	22.2	0	0.037
Respiratory failure[ǁ]	13.6	0	0.24

*Values are means ± (min-max) or frequency of presentation (%). Leptospirosis surveillance was performed at Chang Gung Memorial Hospital, Taiwan, between September 2000 and December 2001 after flooding caused by Typhoon Nali, which had occurred 1 month previously, and the number of leptospirosis cases peaked to seven. *Leptospira shermani,* the most common serovar, was identified in 86.4% (n = 19) of the confirmed cases, followed by *Leptospira bratislava* in 13.6 % (n = 3). Suspected clinical cases were included in the sample and investigated. Diagnosis was confirmed with fourfold or greater increase in microscopic agglutination test (MAT) titer in paired sera; positive immunoglobulin M (IgM) dipstick with single MAT titer ≥400; or isolation of Leptospira. Cases were classified as excluded on basis of confirmed etiology other than leptospirosis or negative paired serologic titers.

Twenty-two confirmed cases and 21 excluded cases of leptospirosis were identified from among 169 suspected cases. The most common presentations in the confirmed group were fever (95.5%), acute renal failure (86.4%), myalgia (72.7%), and jaundice (63.6%). The prevalences of myalgia (72.7% vs. 25%; $P = 0.022$) and hemorrhagic diathesis (45.5% vs. 7.7%; $P = 0.027$) were significantly higher in confirmed cases than excluded cases. The Jarisch-Herxheimer reaction is thought to be associated with endotoxin-related cytokine release and was found to be specific for leptospirosis ($P = 0.037$).

[†]Pancreatitis: acute abdominal pain with serum lipase 3× normal upper limit.
[‡]Rhabdomyolysis: myalgia, muscle tenderness with elevated creatine kinase.
[§]See text for description.
[ǁ]Respiratory failure: mechanical ventilation support for hypercapnia or hypoxia.
Modified from Yang H, Hsu P, Pan M, et al: Clinical distinction and evaluation of leptospirosis in Taiwan: a case-control study. J Nephrol 18:45-53, 2005.

Table 81.2 Differences in Renal Manifestation Between Confirmed and Excluded Cases of Suspected Leptospirosis*

Value	Confirmed Cases (n = 22)	Excluded Cases	P Value
Kidney size (cm): left	12.8 ± 0.8 (11.2-13.9)	10.9 ± 1.2 (8.4-12.9)	0.002
Kidney size (cm): right	12.5 ± 0.8 (11.0-13.6)	10.8 ± 1.3 (8.3-12.5)	0.009
K + (mEq/L):			
Hypokalemia (<3.5 mEq/L (%)	50	16.7	0.045
Hyperkalemia (>5.0 mEq/L) (%)	5	22.2	0.16
Na (mEq//L)	135.5 ± 4.8 (126-145)	137.5 ± 5.4 (127-144)	0.24
Significant hyponatremia (< 130 mEq/L (%)	40	26.7	0.49
Proteinuria (%)[†]	86	74	0.44
Hematuria (%)[‡]	45	42	>0.99
Pyuria (%)[§]	52.4	15	0.02
Specific gravity	1.012 ± 0.007 (1.00-1.03)	1.015 ± 0.006 (1.005-1.025)	0.16
Oliguria (%)[ǁ]	13.3	35.7	0.21

*Values are means ± SD (min-max) or frequency of presentation (%). In confirmed cases, ARF developed in 86.4% of patients and oliguria in 13.3% of patients. Hemodialysis (HD) was administered to two patients with renal failure. In comparison with excluded cases, the confirmed cases had a significantly higher percentages of presentations including pyuria (52.4% vs. 15%; $P = 0.02$) and hypokalemia (50% vs. 16.7%; $P = 0.045$). Ultrasonography revealed that renal size in the confirmed cases was significantly larger than in the excluded cases. Renal biopsy was performed in four of the confirmed cases. All of the lesions revealed acute tubulointerstitial nephritis.

[†]Proteinuria: urinary protein excretion >300 mg/day.
[‡]Hematuria: >5 red blood cells per high-power microscopic field.
[§]Pyuria: >5 white blood cells per high-power microscopic field.
[ǁ]Oliguria: a 24-hr urine volume <500 mL.
Modified from Yang H, Hsu P, Pan M, et al: Clinical distinction and evaluation of leptospirosis in Taiwan: a case-control study. J Nephrol 18:45-53, 2005.

Table 81.3 Clinical Presentations and Odds Ratios Associated with Leptospirosis*

Feature	Odds Ratio	95% Confidence Interval	P Value
Hemorrhagic diathesis	10.0	1.1-90.8	0.04
Myalgia	8.0	1.4-45.8	0.02
Nephromegaly	7.5	2.5-22.7	0.0004
Risk factor exposure	6.9	1.8-26.4	0.005
Sterile pyuria	6.2	1.4-27.8	0.017
Hypokalemia	5.0	1.1-22.3	0.035
Thrombocytopenia	4.8	1.1-21.1	0.04

*Myalgia, hemorrhagic diathesis, and thrombocytopenia were the most distinct presentations of leptospirosis in comparison with the excluded cases in this study. However, the comparison of excluded and confirmed leptospirosis cases revealed that differences in the more common presentations, such as fever, acute renal failure, and jaundice, were not statistically significant and can also be caused by overwhelming sepsis.

From Yang H, Hsu P, Pan M, et al: Clinical distinction and evaluation of leptospirosis in Taiwan: a case-control study. J Nephrol 18:45-53, 2005.

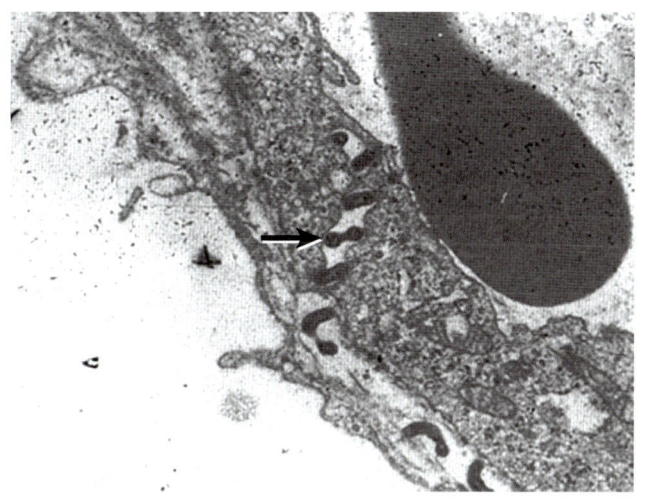

Figure 81.2 Electron micrograph of the kidney biopsy specimen from the same patient as in Figure 81.1 showing a leptospire *(arrow)* between two endothelial cells. (From Abdulkader RC, Silva MV: The kidney in leptospirosis. *Pediatr Nephrol.* 23:2111, 2008.)

glycosuria, decreased proximal sodium reabsorption, phosphaturia, magnesuria, and uricosuria) can occur even in the absence of AKI.[14,17,18] Rhabdomyolysis is often part of the clinical picture.[17] In one study, defective Na-K-2Cl cotransporter (NKCC2) was identified in *L. santarosai* serovar shermani–infected patients with polyuria and hypokalemia.[19] In another, OMP extract downregulated NKCC2 messenger RNA (mRNA) expression and inhibited NKCC2 cotransport activity in medullary thick ascending limb cells in vitro.[20]

The diagnosis of leptospirosis most commonly depends on the serologic detection of leptospiral antibodies using the microscopic agglutination test (MAT). Other tests include polymerase chain reaction (PCR), leptospiral culture, and enzyme-linked immunosorbent assay (ELISA) tests for IgM.[21,22]

The effectiveness of early antibiotic treatment has been demonstrated in leptospira infection, improvement in serum creatinine being observed within days of intravenous penicillin treatment (Figure 81.3).[12] Outpatients with mild disease should receive treatment with doxycycline (adults: 100 mg orally twice daily) or azithromycin (adults: 500 mg orally once daily for 3 days). Pregnant women should be treated with either azithromycin or amoxicillin. Hospitalized adults with severe disease should receive either penicillin (1.5 million units intravenously [IV] every 6 hours), doxycycline (100 mg IV twice daily), ceftriaxone (1 to 2 g IV once daily), or cefotaxime (1 g IV every 6 hours) for a duration of at least 7 days. Pregnant women with severe leptospirosis may be treated with intravenous penicillin, ceftriaxone, cefotaxime, or azithromycin, but not doxycycline.

SCRUB TYPHUS (TSUTSUGAMUSHI DISEASE)

Scrub typhus is a potentially fatal infectious disease that is caused by the organism *Orientia tsutsugamushi*, an obligate intracellular bacterium that belongs to the family Rickettsiaceae in the order Rickettsiales.[23,24] This typhus is a zoonosis that is transmitted by infected larval trombiculid mites (also known as chiggers) and is widespread in the Asia-Pacific region, including Afghanistan, China, Korea, the islands of the southwestern Pacific, and northern Australia.[25] The first six cases of scrub typhus were reported among United Nations military personnel during the Korean War in 1951.[26] Typical signs include eschar formation, typically at the site of the chigger bite, and an acute febrile illness with symptoms that include abrupt fever, chills, severe headache, rash, lymphadenopathy, abdominal pain, and myalgia.[26] The clinical manifestations and complications of scrub typhus vary; most symptoms are mild, but severe complications have been reported, including acute respiratory distress syndrome (ARDS), encephalitis, interstitial pneumonia leading potentially to ARDS, myocarditis and pericarditis, rhabdomyolysis, AKI, and acute hepatic failure.[23] Multiorgan failure generally occurs in a small percentage of patients.[26] AKI after tsutsugamushi disease has been reported to range from 8% to 40% of patients in association with septic shock, DIC, vasculitis, and volume depletion.[27-29]

Reports have demonstrated a risk of AKI of about 20% in groups of older individuals. Older age as defined in these studies (>65 years and 70 years) and previous CKD

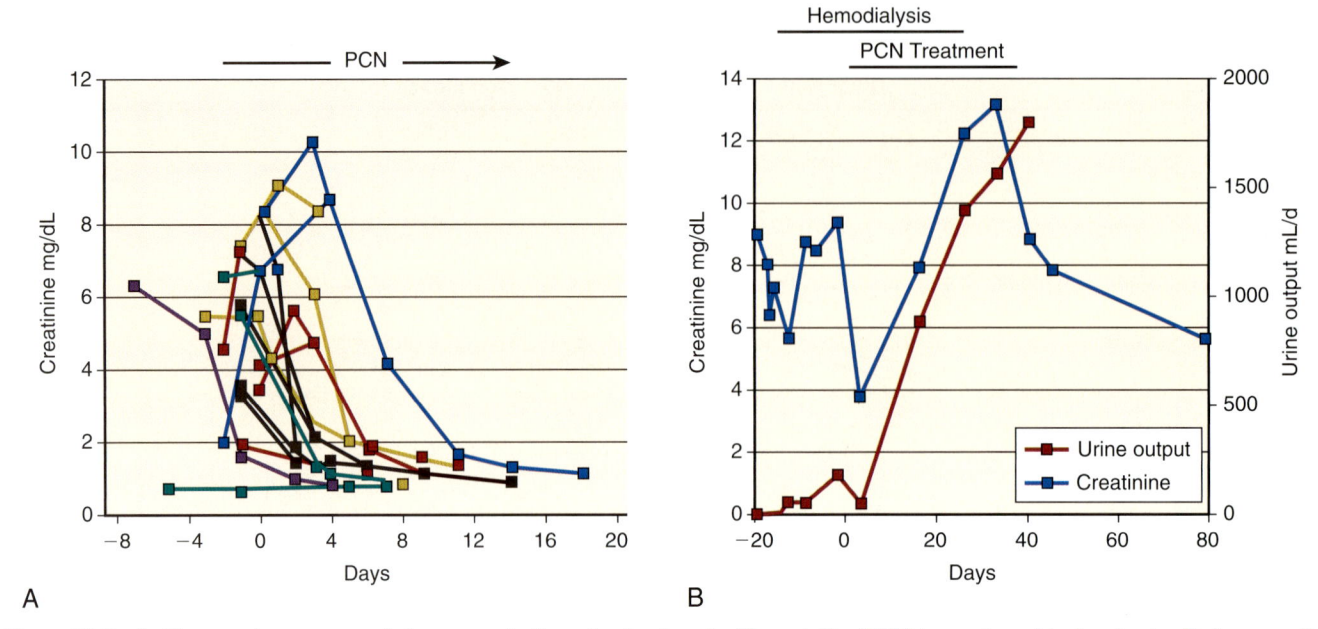

Figure 81.3 A, Changes in serum creatinine concentration after treatment with penicillin (PCN) in confirmed leptospirosis. **B,** A case with anuric acute kidney injury and a delay in penicillin treatment. (From Yang H, Hsu P, Pan M, et al: Clinical distinction and evaluation of leptospirosis in Taiwan: a case-control study. *J Nephrol.* 18:45-53, 2005.)

Table 81.4 Differences in the Clinical Presentation and Frequency of Complications Between Elderly and Non-Elderly Patients with Scrub Typhus[*]

	No. of Patients (%)		
	Elderly (n = 328)	**Non-elderly (n = 287)**	***P* Value**
No complication	177 (54.0)	221 (77.0)	
Complications:	151 (46.0)	66 (23.0)	<0.001
Acute kidney injury	75 (22.9)	22 (7.7)	<0.001
Pneumonia	70 (21.3)	32 (11.1)	0.001
Septic shock	46 (14.0)	13 (4.5)	<0.001
Meningoencephalitis	31 (9.5)	12 (4.2)	0.011
Acute respiratory distress syndrome	11 (3.4)	5 (1.7)	0.208
Peptic ulcer	6 (1.8)	7 (2.4)	0.600
Gastrointestinal bleeding	4 (1.2)	1 (0.3)	0.379
Cholecystitis	3 (0.9)	2 (0.7)	0.100
Death or hopeless discharge	10 (3.0)	1 (0.3)	0.013

[*]A retrospective study to examine differences between elderly and non-elderly patients with scrub typhus and to identify risk factors predictive of disease outcomes was performed. A total of 615 Korean patients admitted to a tertiary care hospital with scrub typhus between 2001 and 2011 were enrolled in the study, 328 of whom were >65 years of age. Of the elderly patients, 46.0% (151/328) experienced at least one complication compared with only 23.0% (66/287) of younger patients. A linear trend was observed between age and complication rates (*P* = 0.002). The most common complication in elderly patients was acute kidney injury (75/328, 22.9%).
Modifed from Jang M, Kim J, Kim U, et al: Differences in the clinical presentation and the frequency of complications between elderly and non-elderly scrub typhus patients. *Arch Gerontol Geriatr* 58:196-200, 2014.

(estimated glomerular filtration rate [eGFR] <60 mL/min) were risk factors for the development of AKI and a generally more severe clinical course (Table 81.4).

Sun and colleagues evaluated the incidence, clinical characteristics, and severity of AKI associated with scrub typhus on the basis of the Risk, Injury, Failure, Loss and End-stage kidney disease (RIFLE) classification. A total of 223 Korean patients with scrub typhus were monitored until renal recovery or for at least 3 months. The incidence of AKI was 21.1%, of which 10.7% of the cases were classified as "Risk," 9.4% as "Injury," and 1% as "Failure." In comparison with patients in whom AKI did not develop, those in the AKI group were older (70 ± 9 vs. 61 ± 14 years of age, *P* = 0.01) and had one or more comorbidities, such as hypertension, diabetes, and CKD (77% vs. 22%, *P* = 0.01). Age and comorbidity were significant independent predictors of AKI. After treatment with antibiotics and supportive care all patients recovered baseline renal function without renal replacement therapy (RRT).[30]

A retrospective study from a single Korean medical center evaluated 615 individuals with scrub typhus who were older than 16 years.[31] Forty-six percent of patients who were older than 65 years of age had one or more complications, compared with 23% of younger patients. AKI was the most common complication, occurring in 23% of elderly individuals. Mental confusion and dyspnea were more common in older patients, whereas the frequencies of fever, rash, and eschars were similar in the two groups. Delays in therapy were also associated with a higher risk of complications. The average time from onset of illness to effective therapy was modestly greater in patients with complications than in those without complications (approximately 7 versus 6 days). CKD was a risk factor for severe disease in the elderly, as was hypoalbuminemia.

Kidney biopsies have been reported in only small numbers of patients (4), and their findings have been indicative of tubulointerstitial nephritis (3) or mesangial hyperplasia (1).[27-29] In one report, a patient who presented with nephrotic syndrome had membranous nephropathy that responded to antibiotics.[32] Another interesting report described the direct invasion of *Orientia tsutsugamushi* on electron microscopy in a kidney biopsy specimen from a patient with scrub typhus; histologic examination showed chronic interstitial nephritis and acute tubular necrosis (ATN).[33]

Serologic diagnosis may be performed by the indirect fluorescent antibody (IFA) test. Among patients living in endemic areas, the serologic diagnosis of acute infection must be differentiated from immunity against a scrub typhus background. When using the IFA test,[34] a diagnosis of acute scrub typhus infection should be based on at least a fourfold increase in titer in paired samples that are drawn at least 14 days apart. A single measurement should only be used when there is sufficient locally validated evidence for a positive test result. A common cutoff titer is 1:50 (range 1:10 to 1:400). Serum PCR technology can diagnose scrub typhus.[35] In addition to serum PCR, eschar PCR also appears to be a sensitive and specific assay for scrub typhus despite prior antibiotic treatment.[36] The latter two assays are not generally available outside of specific centers. Treatment should be initiated with doxycycline 100 mg orally or IV twice daily.[37] Alternatively, chloramphenicol in doses of 250 to 500 mg orally or IV every 6 hours is similarly effective. Because the delayed administration of doxycycline was independently associated with major organ dysfunction, including AKI, early empiric doxycycline therapy should be considered.[37]

AKI associated with scrub typhus infection is not rare. The possibility of scrub typhus should be considered when a patient presents with fever and AKI, particularly if an eschar is detected, as well as in the patient with a history of environmental exposure in areas where scrub typhus is endemic. Even in the setting of AKI, most patients show response to antibiotics. One unusual patient is described, age 71, in whom kidney biopsy demonstrated tubulointerstitial nephritis requiring maintenance hemodialysis.[38] Prompt diagnosis and the use of appropriate antibiotics can rapidly alter the clinical course of the disease and prevent the development of serious or even fatal complications, including dialysis dependence.

HANTAVIRUS

Hantaviruses are single-stranded, enveloped, negative-sense RNA viruses in the Bunyaviridae family.[39] Hantaviruses infect rodents but do not cause disease in these hosts. Hantavirus infection is acquired by the inhalation of aerosolized virus-containing particles or by contact with the feces, urine, or secretions of infected rodents. Some strains of hantavirus cause potentially fatal diseases in humans, such as hantavirus hemorrhagic fever with renal syndrome (HFRS) and hantavirus pulmonary syndrome (HPS), and others have not been associated with human disease.

In HFRS, the clinical picture is characterized by AKI, often with massive proteinuria due to tubular and glomerular involvement.[39] The viruses that cause HFRS include Hantaan, Dobrava, Saaremaa, Seoul, and Puumala. Hantaan virus is widely distributed in eastern Asia, particularly in China, Russia, and Korea.[40,41] Puumala virus is found in Scandinavia, Western Europe, and western Russia. Dobrava virus is found primarily in the Balkans, and Seoul virus is found worldwide. Saaremaa is found in central Europe and Scandinavia. Infection with hantavirus is associated with significant morbidity and mortality worldwide. It has been estimated that hantaviruses cause hemorrhagic fever with renal syndrome in more than 150,000 people annually in China, far western Russia, and Korea. Generally, only approximately a quarter of patients have a severe course; however, the mortality reported from Korea is 5% to 10%, whereas European forms of the disease show 0.5% mortality.[39]

Symptoms of HFRS usually develop within 1 to 2 weeks after exposure to infectious material, but in rare cases, they may take up to 8 weeks to develop. Initial symptoms begin suddenly and include intense headaches, back and abdominal pain, fever, chills, nausea, and blurred vision. Individuals may have flushing of the face, inflammation or redness of the eyes, or a rash. Later symptoms can include low blood pressure, acute shock, vascular leakage, and AKI.

HFRS follows a typical clinical course, as follows[39]:

Febrile phase: Symptoms include redness of cheeks and nose; fever; chills; sweaty palms; diarrhea; malaise; headaches; nausea; abdominal and back pain; respiratory symptoms, such as the ones common in the influenza virus; and gastrointestinal symptoms. These symptoms normally occur for 3 to 7 days and arise approximately 2 to 3 weeks after exposure.

Hypotensive and hemorrhagic phase: This phase occurs often with thrombocytopenia (Figure 81.4). Hypotension is due to increased vascular permeability, which can lead to tachycardia and hypoxemia. Laboratory values show leukocytosis and elevations of lactate dehydrogenase and C-reactive protein. This phase can last for approximately 2 days.

Kidney phase: This phase lasts for 3 to 7 days and is characterized by the onset of AKI with frequent oliguria, hematuria, proteinuria, and hypoalbuminemia. The oliguric phase is followed by a diuresis of 3 to 6 L per day that can last for days.

Serology is the primary method of diagnosis: When symptoms are present, patients predictably exhibit both hantavirus IgM and even IgG.[42] Diagnostic hantavirus assays

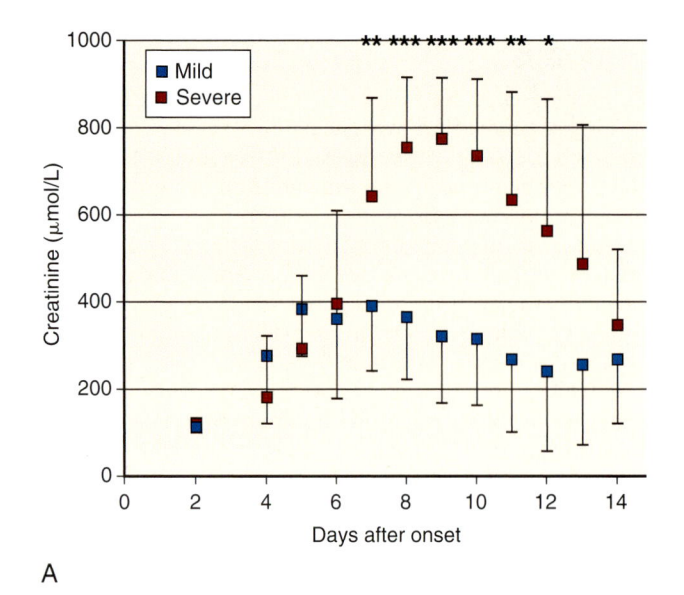

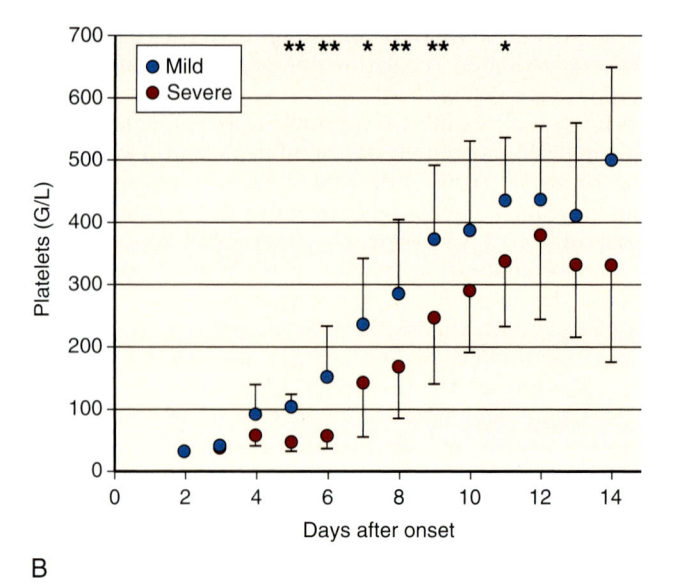

Figure 81.4 Course of serum creatinine levels **(A)** and platelet counts **(B)** in patients with milder or severe acute renal failure during infection with European hantavirus, nephropathica epidemica (NE). Nadir in platelet count is predictive of severe renal failure. Mean values and S.D. are shown. Mean values in mild cases were compared with those in severe cases using Student t-test (*$P<0.05$, **$P<0.01$, ***$P<0.0001$). Levels of platelets rose significantly faster in milder than in severe cases of NE. In milder cases, platelets reached values of the lower limit of the reference range (150-440 gigaparticles per liter [G/L]) within the first week after illness onset, whereas in severe cases platelet counts at day 5 and 6 were still very low. Interestingly, creatinine levels up to day 6 after the onset of symptoms were equal, and although milder cases then showed a continuous decrease, creatinine levels increased suddenly at day 7 in severe cases. (From Krautkrämer E, Zeier M, Plyusnin A: Hantavirus infection: an emerging infectious disease causing acute renal failure. *Kidney Int* 83:23-27, 2013.)

include ELISA, strip immunoblot assay (SIA), Western blot, IFA, complement fixation, hemagglutinin inhibition, and focus or plaque reduction neutralization tests. Hantaan virus and Seoul virus infections are often diagnosed in centers in the Far East with the use of bead agglutination (HantaDia), ELISA, and IFA formats.[43] Reverse transcription PCR (RT-PCR) is often used as a confirmatory diagnostic test because serology has a high diagnostic accuracy. A study from China describes centers without hantavirus testing available at the time of diagnosis of hemorrhagic fever, making accurate diagnosis challenging.[44]

The basic mechanisms underlying HFRS pathogenesis relate to increased vascular permeability suggested by an increase in hematocrit, a decrease in serum protein levels, and a vascular leak as demonstrated by tracer studies.[45] HFRS pathogenesis appears to be immune mediated, involving immune complexes, the B cell response, the T cell response, and hantavirus-induced cytokine production. The complement system is activated in hantavirus infections via both classical and alternate pathways, and the findings are similar to those of septic shock.[46] The causative agents appear to infect endothelial cells without cytopathic effects, suggesting that viral replication together with the immune response are involved in tissue injury.[39] Hantaviral entry in target cells is mediated by integrins and CD55. Upon cell entry, viral replication takes place. Studies of biopy samples and *in vitro* cellular studies demonstrate a disruption of cell-to-cell contact, which correlates with the clinical picture (Figure 81.5).[47]

Supportive therapy is the mainstay of care for patients with hantavirus infections. Care includes careful management of the patient's fluid (hydration) and electrolyte (e.g., sodium, potassium, and chloride) levels, maintenance of the correct oxygen and blood pressure levels, and appropriate treatment of any secondary infections. Dialysis may be required to treat uremia and fluid overload. Intravenous administration of ribavirin, an antiviral drug, has been shown to decrease illness and death associated with HFRS if used early in the disease,[48] although this outcome has not been uniform.[49] The severity of the disease varies according to the virus causing the infection. Hantaan and Dobrava virus infections are commonly observed in the Far East and usually cause severe symptoms, whereas Seoul, Saaremaa, and Puumala virus infections are usually more moderate. The Hantaan virus RNA load also correlates with disease severity.[50] Studies of acute infection have been published from Korea[43,51] and China.[52] In a report of HFRS due to hantavirus (11 patients with detectable hantavirus RNA by RT-PCR) from Korea, 35 patients were seen over a 10-year period; 77% had AKI and 34% required ICU admission to intensive care units. Complete recovery can require weeks or months.[51] Although the long-term kidney prognosis for hantaviruses in Europe has been described as favorable, hypertension is a reported consequence of infection, and follow-up has not extended beyond 10 years.[53] Long-term follow-up data for hantaviruses in the Far East are not available.

SEVERE FEVER WITH THROMBOCYTOPENIA SYNDROME VIRUS

Patients with severe fever with thrombocytopenia syndrome (SFTS) virus, which was initially recognized in the Henan and Hubei Provinces of China between 2007 and 2010, present with respiratory and gastrointestinal symptoms, chills, joint pain, myalgia, thrombocytopenia, leukopenia, and some hemorrhagic manifestations. SFTS results in multiorgan dysfunction and AKI in about 20% of cases and has

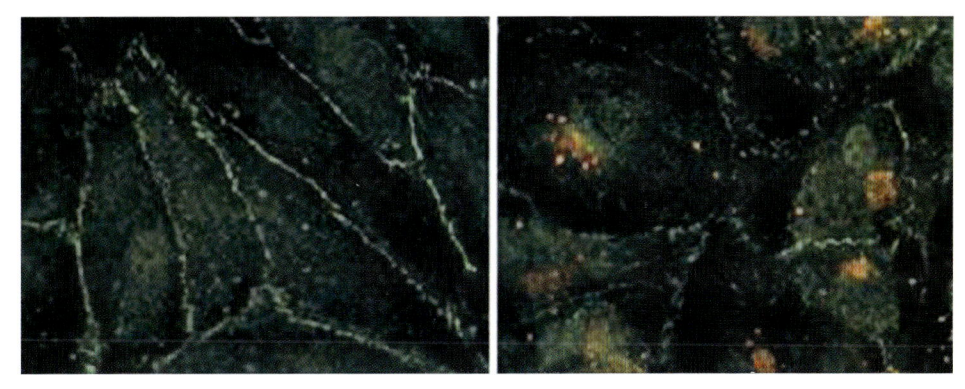

Figure 81.5 Hantavirus infection disrupts cell-to-cell contacts. Human renal glomerular endothelial cells were infected with European hantavirus, Puumala, and analyzed for the expression of hantaviral N antigen *(red)* and localization of the tight junction marker protein ZO-1 *(green)* by immunofluorescence. **Left,** Uninfected human renal glomerular endothelial cells with well-organized cell-to-cell contacts forming an intact monolayer. **Right,** Infected cells display hantavirus-induced changes at their margins, with a discontinuous staining of ZO-1 and breakdown of the endothelial barrier function. (From Krautkrämer E, Zeier M, Plyusnin A: Hantavirus infection: an emerging infectious disease causing acute renal failure. *Kidney Int* 83:23-27, 2013.)

a case-fatality rate of 12% to 30%[54] (Figure 81.6). Genetic analysis shows that this virus is a novel member of the Bunyaviridae family of the viral genus *Phlebovirus*. Both SFTS virus and viral DNA have been isolated from *Haemaphysalis longicornis* ticks, and viral RNA has been detected in *Rhipicephalus microplus* ticks from domestic animals in China.[54] A subsequent report of 48 cases of SFTS indicated that within a few days of onset, patients exhibited coagulation defects, hematuria, and ecchymoses—gastrointestinal bleeding was seen in 10%, proteinuria in 98%, azotemia (creatinine >150 mmol/L) in 64%, and hepatic dysfunction in 95%—leading to encephalopathy (48%) and coma (8%). Dialysis was required in 23% of the patients; 27% of the patients died.[55]

Since then, 2500 cases of SFTS have been reported from 11 provinces of China with an average case-fatality rate of 7.3%.[56] This disease has been reported from Japan[57] and elsewhere,[56] and a genetically related virus has been reported from the United States.[58]

A study from Dandong, China, showed the similarity in presentation between SFTS (*Phlebovirus*) and HFRS (Hantaan virus and Seoul virus) and the need for serologic diagnosis (IgM and IgG for hantavirus) and PCR for the detection of SFTS.[44] Notably, enlarged lymph nodes were observed only in the SFTS cases (44%). AKI was more prominent in the hantavirus cases than in the SFTS virus cases (85% vs. 23%).[44]

The immune response to SFTS shows that $CD3^+$ and $CD4^+$ T lymphocyte counts are lower than normal and that natural killer (NK) cell counts are increased.[59] NK cells produce interferon, tumor necrosis factor α (TNF-α), interleukin-10 (IL-10), and granulocyte-colony stimulating factor (G-CSF).[60] Serum from patients contains nearly undetectable levels of interferon-β, one of the defense mechanisms of the host's innate immune system.[61] Several proinflammatory cytokines that are associated with the severity of SFTS are abnormally expressed in a cytokine storm.[62]

Specific antibodies to the SFTS virus are detectable after 7 days and are usually detected by ELISA; IgM becomes undetectable at 4 months, and IgG is detectable for up to 4 years.[56] A fourfold rise in antibody titer indicates infection.

Because PCR is a highly specific, sensitive, and rapid diagnostic method for laboratory SFTS virus diagnosis, the multiplex RT-PCR assay, which can detect four hemorrhagic fever pathogens (SFTS virus, Hantaan virus, Seoul virus, and Dengue virus), is clinically useful when available.[63]

Therapy at present is mostly supportive with the use of intravenous fluids and blood. G-CSF and broad-spectrum antibiotics are given as needed.[56] In the event of AKI, RRT should be initiated.

MALARIA

Malaria is the most widespread parasitic disease worldwide: in 2013, 200 million people worldwide were infected, causing 584,000 deaths.[64,64a] Malaria is caused by parasites of the genus *Plasmodium*, which are transmitted via the bites of infected female *Anopheles* mosquitoes, inoculating microscopic mobile sporozoites that seek out and invade hepatocytes, where they multiply (Figure 81.7).[61] The sporozoites multiply in the liver, producing merozoites at a factor of 10^5, which then burst and invade red blood cells (RBCs). Illness begins when parasite numbers in the circulation reach more than 10^8.[64] Five species of *Plasmodium* can infect and can be transmitted by humans. The vast majority of deaths are caused by *Plasmodium falciparum* and *Plasmodium vivax*, whereas *Plasmodium ovale* and *Plasmodium malariae* cause a generally milder form of malaria that is rarely fatal. The zoonotic species *Plasmodium knowlesi*, which is prevalent in Southeast Asia, causes malaria in macaques but can also cause severe infections in humans.[65] Malaria is common in tropical and subtropical regions because rainfall, warm temperatures, and stagnant waters provide an environment that is ideal for mosquito larvae. In the Far East, malaria is common in rural China, Cambodia, Indonesia, Laos, Malaysia, Myanmar, and the Philippines.

In *P. falciparum* malaria, protuberances emerge on the infected erythrocyte 15 hours after invasion, promoting adherence to the vascular endothelium. The parasitic proteins include ring surface proteins 1 and 2 and *P. falciparum* erythrocyte membrane protein-1 (PfEMP-1), and they promote adherence using the endothelial cell receptors CD36, thrombospondin (TSP), and intracellular adhesion molecule-1 (ICAM-1) or chondroitin sulfate A.[66]

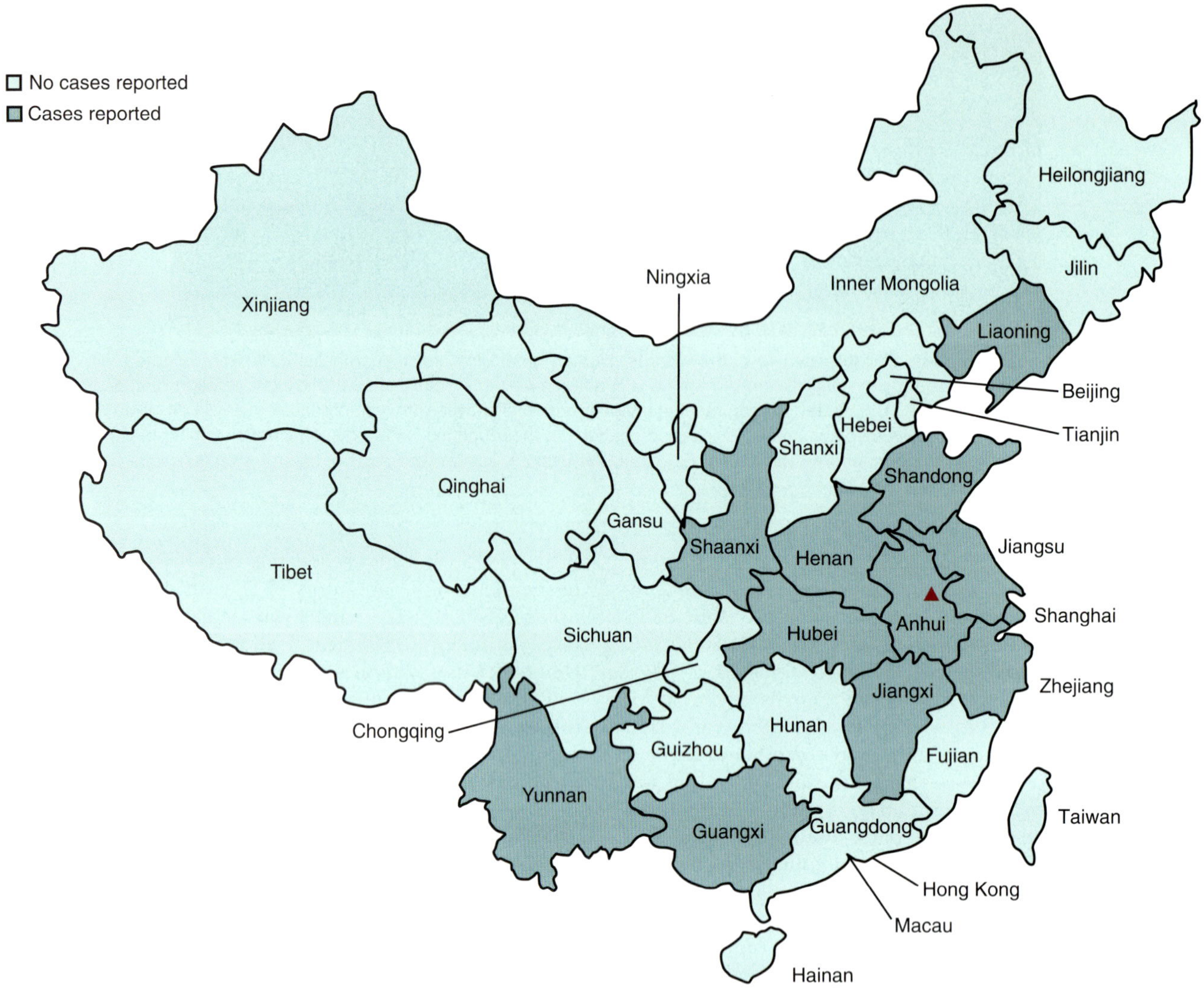

Figure 81.6 Geographic distribution of cases of severe fever with thrombocytopenia syndrome (SFTS) in mainland China in 2012. The *red triangle* represents the first SFTS case, in Dingyuan county, Chuzhou city, Anhui province, in September 2006. (From Liu Q, He B, Huang S, et al: Severe fever with thrombocytopenia syndrome, an emerging tick-borne zoonosis. *Lancet Infect Dis* 14:763-772, 2014.)

Parasite-infected erythrocytes are less pliable, contributing to capillary plugging and decreased tissue perfusion.[67] Pro-inflammatory cytokines, such as IL-1β and tumor necrosis factor-α (TNF-α), upregulate adhesion molecules. Adherence causes sequestration of parasite-infected RBCs into vital organs and allows parasites to interfere with tissue perfusion, metabolism, and endothelial function. In experimental models, *P. falciparum* merozoite proteins have been shown to use a Scr-family-kinase–dependent kinase to disrupt endothelial barrier function, causing vascular permeability.[68] The geographic distributions of sickle cell disease and many other hemoglobinopathies are roughly similar to the distribution of malaria, suggesting that these disorders confer a survival advantage against the disease. Similarly, a role for complement receptor 1 has been postulated in which individuals with polymorphisms in the *CR1* gene are protected against severe disease.

Symptoms of malaria include fever, headache, shivering, and vomiting. Malaria appears between 10 and 15 days after the malaria-containing mosquito bite. If not treated, malaria can quickly become life-threatening by disrupting the blood supply to vital organs. The classic symptom of malaria is a paroxysm—a cyclic occurrence of sudden coldness followed by shivering and then fever and sweating, occurring every 2 days (tertian fever) in *P. vivax* and *P. ovale* infections and every 3 days (quartan fever) for *P. malariae*. *P. falciparum* infection can cause recurrent fever every 36 to 48 hours or a less pronounced and almost continuous fever.

Severe disease results from cytoadherence of erythrocytes (many parasitized), causing organ damage, altered consciousness, ARDS, hypotension, metabolic acidosis, hepatic failure, hypoglycemia, coagulopathy, severe anemia or massive intravascular hemolysis, hemoglobinuria, and AKI. AKI is a feature of blackwater fever, in which hemoglobin from lysed RBCs appears in the urine. AKI is one of the most dreaded complications of severe malaria.

Malarial AKI is found in up to 4.5% of the native patients of endemic areas, whereas in nonimmune individuals, usually of European ancestry, AKI occurs in as many as 30% of cases.[69] According to a study by Kanodia and associates of 100 hospitalized patients with malarial AKI from India,

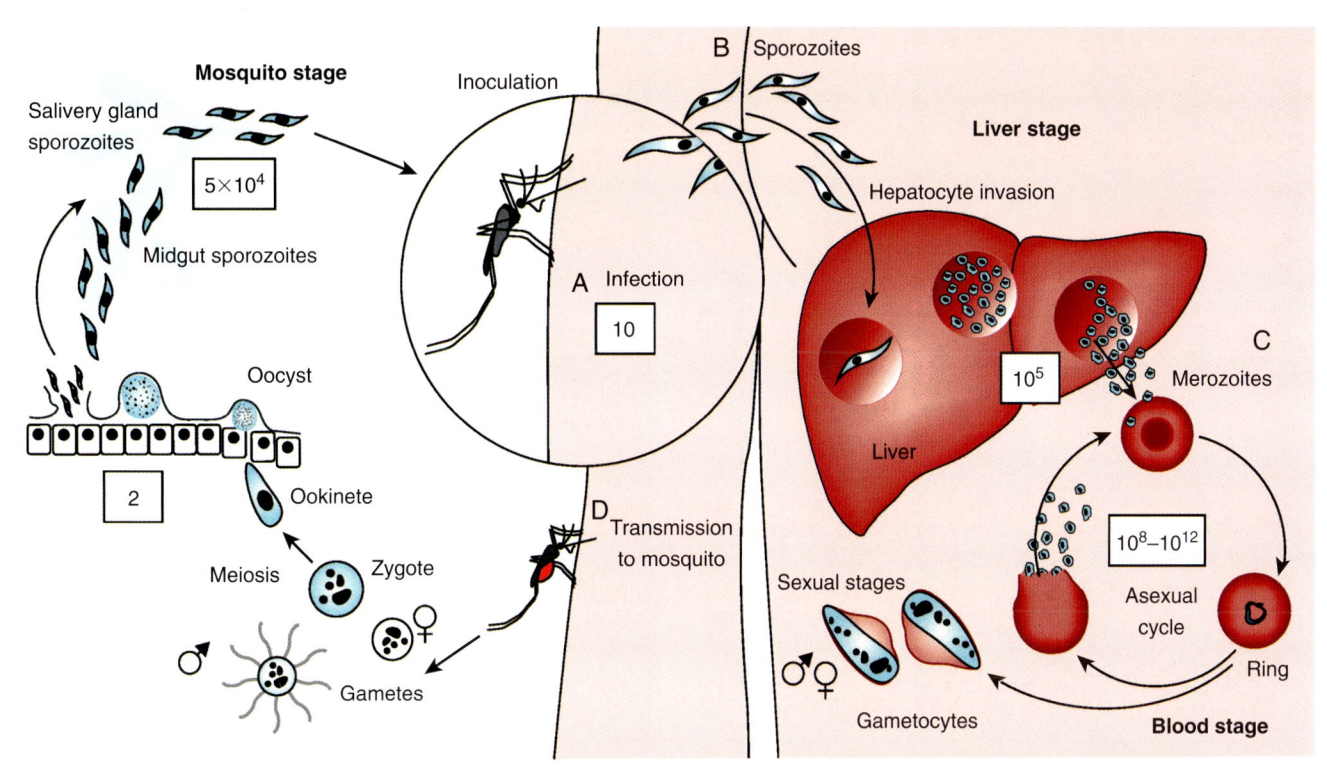

Figure 81.7 Life cycle of *Plasmodium falciparum* in the human body and the anopheline mosquito. The cycle begins with inoculation of motile sporozoites into the dermis (**A**; magnified), which then travel to the liver (**B**); each sporozoite invades a hepatocyte and then multiplies. After about a week, the liver schizonts burst, releasing into the bloodstream thousands of merozoites, which invade red blood cells and begin the asexual cycle (**C**). Illness starts when total asexual parasite numbers in the circulation reach roughly 100 million. Some parasites develop into sexual forms (gametocytes). Gametocytes are taken up by a feeding anopheline mosquito (**D**) and reproduce sexually, forming an ookinete and then an oocyst in the mosquito gut. The oocyst bursts and liberates sporozoites, which migrate to the salivary glands to await inoculation at the next blood feed. The entire cycle can take roughly 1 month. Estimated numbers of parasites are shown in *boxes*—a total body parasite burden of 10^{12} corresponds to roughly 2% parasitemia in an adult. (From White NJ: Malaria. *Lancet* 383:723-735, 2014.)

P. falciparum was the causative organism in 85% of the patients, *P. vivax* in 2%, and both in 13%.[70] Patients with AKI required dialysis (78%). Sixty-four percent of patients with AKI recovered completely, 10% recovered incompletely, and 5% experienced ESKD; death occurred in 21% of the patients.[70] Predictors of mortality were low hemoglobin, oligoanuria on admission, increased lactic dehydrogenase (LDH), hyperbilirubinemia, increased aspartate transaminases, elevated alanine transaminases, cerebral malaria, DIC, and high serum creatinine.[70] Using the RIFLE criteria, Thanachartwet and coworkers evaluated 257 medical records of adult hospitalized patients with severe falciparum malaria and found that 73.9% (190 patients) had AKI. RRT was required in 11.6% (5 patients) of patients with RIFLE-I disease and 44.9% (48 patients) of patients with RIFLE-F disease. The in-hospital mortality gradually increased with the severity of AKI. Therefore, the RIFLE criteria can be used to diagnose AKI and predict outcomes in patients with severe malaria.[71]

The clinical features of malarial AKI consist of jaundice (75%); anemia (70%); thrombocytopenia (70%), which may progress to frank DIC; hypotension due to reduced peripheral vascular resistance (20%); proteinuria, usually less than 1 gram per 24 hours (60%); hyponatremia (55%) and hyperkalemia; lactic acidosis, hemolysis, and rhabdomyolysis[69,72] (Figure 81.8). Various histologic lesions have been associated with malarial AKI, including interstitial nephritis and proliferative and segmental necrotizing glomerulonephritis[69]; however, ATN is the most consistent histologic finding.[69,73] Glomerular lesions of mesangial proliferation are observed at autopsy in the kidneys of 20% of patients with falciparum malaria (Figures 81.9 and 81.10).[69]

Diagnosis is made by thick and thin blood film microscopy, but sensitive and specific antibody-based rapid diagnostic tests that detect *P. falciparum* histidine-rich protein 2 (PfHRP2) antigens in finger-stick blood specimens are now performed widely.[64]

In Asia, parenteral artesunate treatment significantly reduces mortality of malarial AKI to 14.7% from the 22.4% seen with quinine treatment.[64] Resistance to artemisin in *P. falciparum* has emerged in Western Cambodia and on the Thailand-Myanmar border.

Severe falciparum malaria is a medical emergency and requires intensive care: treatment of fever, seizure control, hypoglycemia monitoring, correction of acidosis and hyperkalemia, treatment of bacterial confection with broad-spectrum antibiotics, treatment of hypotension with volume expansion and pressors, and mechanical ventilation for deterioration of respiratory status with the early use of positive-pressure ventilation.[74] AKI should be monitored and treated with an RRT, such as hemofiltration, especially in the setting of hypotension.[75] The use of exchange transfusions has been suggested in the setting of severe parasitemia to prompt a reduction of the parasite load, correct anemia, and eliminate cytokines, but this approach remains controversial.[76] Despite optimal treatment, the mortality in patients with greater than 10% parasitemia ranges from 20% to 40% in the context of impaired cerebral or kidney function and approaches 80% in the presence of ARDS.[76]

DENGUE VIRAL INFECTION

Dengue, a systemic viral infection that is transmitted between humans by *Aedes* mosquitoes, is a leading cause of illness and death in the tropics and subtropics, with a large burden in many of the countries in the Far East.[77] As many as 400 million people are infected yearly. Dengue is caused by four viral serotypes of the genus flavivirus (DENV-1 to DENV-4).[78]

After an incubation period of up to 8 days after a mosquito bite, symptoms may appear that include fever, headache, muscle and joint pain, and a characteristic rash that is similar to measles, lasting up to 7 days. In a small proportion of cases, the disease develops into the life-threatening dengue hemorrhagic fever (DHF), resulting in bleeding, thrombocytopenia, DIC, and blood plasma leakage, as evidenced by hemoconcentration, hypoproteinemia, pleural effusions, and ascites, or into dengue shock syndrome (DSS), in which systemic vascular leaks and severe hypotension occur and fluid resuscitation is required.[79] Patients with dengue infection may also experience hepatitis, neurologic disorders, and myocarditis. If this infection is left untreated, the mortality rate may reach 20%; intravenous hydration may reduce the rate to less than 1%[78] (Table 81.5). Since 2009, a revised World Health Organization (WHO) classification has replaced the previous designations with just two categories: dengue with and without warning signs, and severe dengue.[78]

Dengue is transmitted by several species of mosquito within the genus *Aedes,* principally *Aedes aegypti.*[78] The virus has four different types; infection with one type usually confers lifelong immunity to that type but only short-term immunity to the others. Subsequent infection with a different type increases the risk of severe complications. Because there is no commercially available vaccine and no specific antimicrobial therapy, prevention aims at reducing the habitat and the number of mosquitoes and limiting exposure to bites.

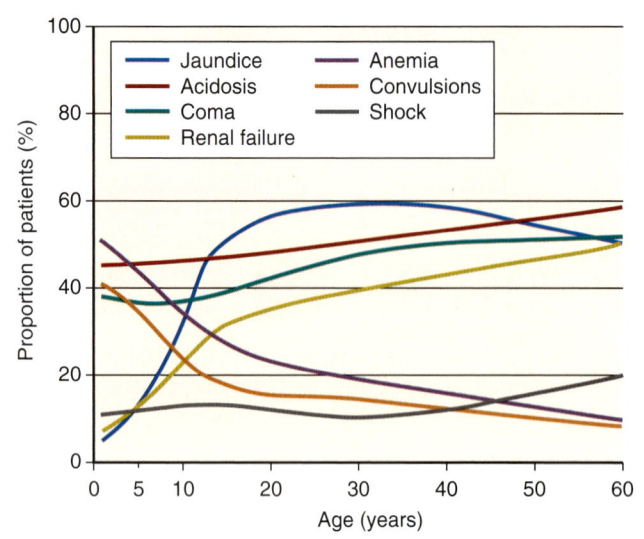

Figure 81.8 **Manifestations of severe falciparum malaria by age in children associated with central nervous system involvement, acidosis, and uremia.** Data from 3228 prospectively studied African children with severe falciparum malaria. Uremia here is defined as a blood urea nitrogen level higher than 7.14 mmol/L. The percentages denote the observed mortality associated with the presenting signs. (From White NJ: Malaria. *Lancet* 383:723-735, 2014; data from von Seidlein L, Olaosebikan R, Hendriksen IC, et al: Predicting the clinical outcome of severe falciparum malaria in African children: findings from a large randomized trial. *Clin Infect Dis* 54:1080-1090, 2012.)

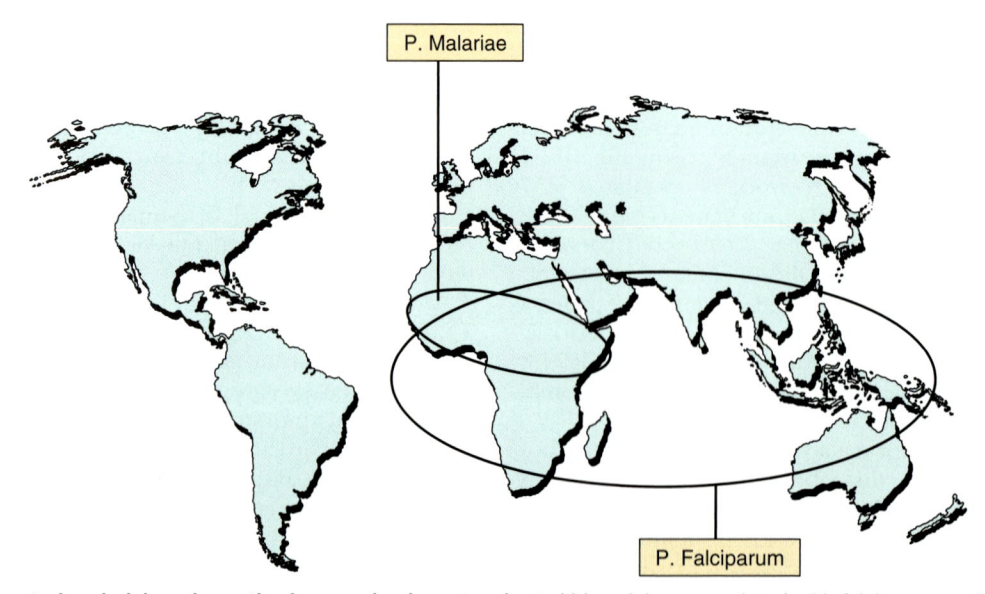

Figure 81.9 **Reported malarial nephropathy from endemic areas.** Acute kidney injury associated with falciparum malaria (*P. falciparum*) has been reported from Southeast Asia, India, and sub-Saharan Africa. (From Barsoum RS: Malarial acute renal failure. *J Am Soc Nephrol* 11:2147-2154, 2000.)

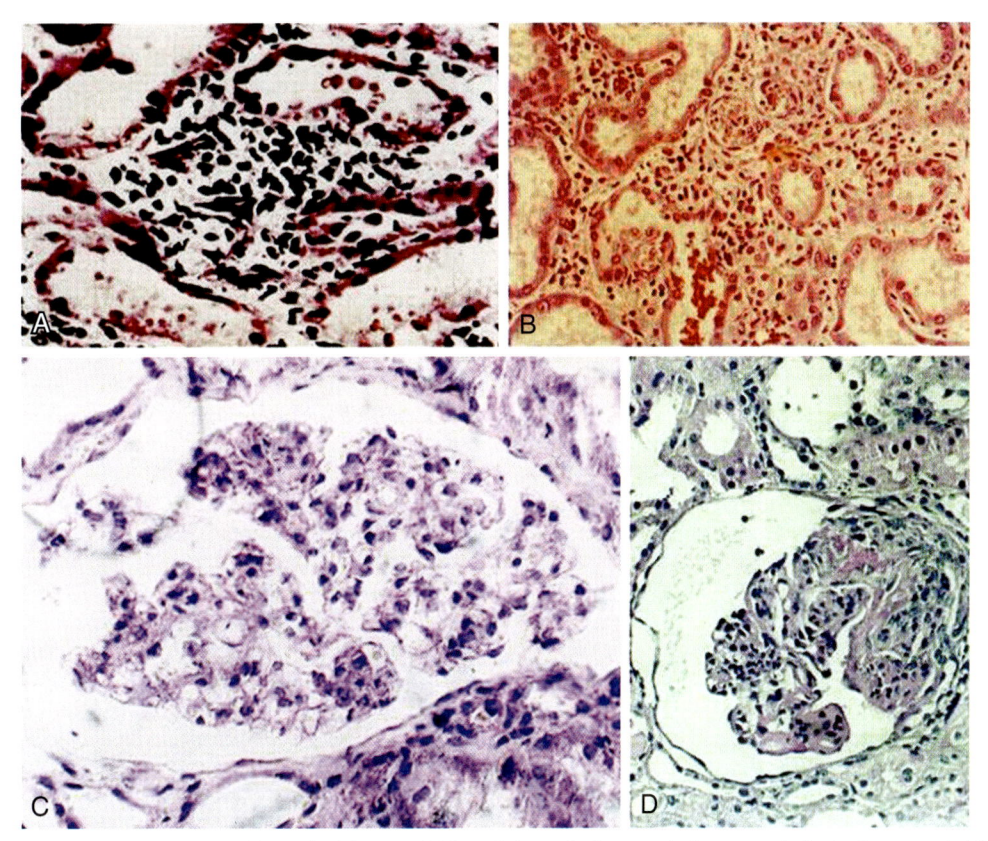

Figure 81.10 Renal lesions associated with malarial acute kidney injury. A, Acute tubular necrosis (note the remarkable epithelial disruption, red blood cells in the tubular lumen and interstitial edema, and cellular infiltration). B, Acute interstitial nephritis. C, Proliferative glomerulonephritis. D, Segmental necrotizing glomerulonephritis. (From Barsoum RS: Malarial acute renal failure. *J Am Soc Nephrol* 11:2147-2154. 2000.)

Dengue infection has been associated with a variety of kidney disorders. Proteinuria has been detected in as many as 74% of patients with severe dengue infection.[80] Hematuria has been reported in up to 12.5% of patients.[81] Various types of glomerulonephritis have been reported during or shortly after dengue infection in humans and in mouse models of dengue infection. Mesangial proliferation and immune complex deposition are the dominant histologic features of dengue-associated glomerulonephritis.[82] On rare occasions, dengue infection is associated with IgA nephropathy and lupus nephritis, and one patient has been reported to have anti–glomerular basement membrane (anti-GBM) antibody disease with antineutrophil cytoplasmic antibody (ANCA) and myeloperoxidase (MPO) specificity.[83] Severe dengue infection, particularly DHF and DSS, may give rise to multiorgan failure. AKI is a potential complication of severe dengue infection and is typically associated with hypotension, rhabdomyolysis, or hemolysis.[84] The prevalence of AKI varies, reported to be 0.9% in Thai children, 1.6% among 617 children with DHF in Colombia, 3.3% in hospitalized adults with DHF, 4.9% in 81 Chinese patients with DHF/DSS, and 5% in patients with DHF in Qatar.[85-87]

The development of AKI in patients with dengue infection is associated with increased mortality. In Thailand, the prevalence of AKI in fatal DHF was 33.3%, compared with 0.3% in all cases of DHF.[88] In a retrospective study, 60% of hospitalized patients with DHF and AKI died[88]; these patients were predominantly male and elderly and had other comorbid conditions.[88] A multivariable analysis showed that DSS was an independent risk factor for the development of AKI in patients with DHF.[85,88]

The diagnosis of acute dengue virus infection is most frequently accomplished serologically. For an acute-phase serum specimen that is obtained 3 days or more after the onset of illness, an IgM immunoassay (IgM antibody capture ELISA [MAC-ELISA] or equivalent) is the procedure of choice for rapid diagnosis. If the acute-phase sample that was obtained within the first 3 days after the onset of illness has a negative IgM assay result, testing for the presence of the dengue viral RNA or NS1 antigen is performed. To confirm a positive IgM result or if the result of initial testing is negative in a patient with suspected dengue virus infection, a convalescent-phase serum sample should be obtained at least 10 to 14 days after acute-phase serum collection. The acute and convalescent specimens should be analyzed together with a hemagglutination inhibition (HI) assay or enzyme immunoassay for definitive serologic testing.[78]

SEVERE ACUTE RESPIRATORY SYNDROME

Severe acute respiratory syndrome (SARS) began as a highly infectious atypical pneumonia caused by the SARS coronavirus (SARS-CoV) between November 2002 and July 2003 (Figure 81.11).[89,90] The SARS outbreak emerged in southern China but eventually caused 8273 cases and 775 deaths in multiple countries, with the majority of cases in Hong Kong.[91] In the initial months, many of the affected

Table 81.5 Clinical Manifestations and Laboratory Confirmation of Dengue Infection

Dengue Fever (DF)	Acute febrile illness with ≥ 2 of the following: • Headache • Retro-orbital pain • Myalgia • Rash • Hemorrhagic manifestations • Leukopenia

Dengue Hemorrhagic Fever (DHF)	All of the following must be present:
	1. Fever, lasting 2 to 7 days, occasionally biphasic
	2. Hemorrhagic manifestations with at least one of the following:
	  • Positive tourniquet test result
	  • Petechiae, ecchymoses, or purpura
	  • Bleeding from mucosa, gastrointestinal tract, injection sites, or other locations
	  • Hematemesis or melena
	3. Thrombocytopenia (≤100,000 red blood cells/mm^3)
	4. Evidence of plasma leakage manifested as at least one of the following:
	  • Increase in the hematocrit level 20% for age, sex, and population
	  • Decrease in the hematocrit after volume replacement ≥ 20% of baseline
	  • Signs of plasma leakage, such as pleural effusion, ascites, and hypoproteinemia

Dengue Shock Syndrome (DSS)	Criteria for DHF associated with: • Tachycardia • Pulse pressure < 20 mm Hg • Hypotension for age • Cold skin • Restlessness
Laboratory Criteria Confirmation	At least one of the following: • Isolation of dengue virus from serum or autopsy samples • ≥Fourfold change in immunoglobulin G or M antibody specific to dengue virus • Detection of dengue virus in tissue, serum, or cerebrospinal fluid by immunohistochemistry, immunofluorescence, or enzyme-linked immunosorbent assay

From Lizarraga KJ, Nayer A: Dengue-associated kidney disease. J Nephropathol 3:57-62, 2014.

---

yielded a SARS-CoV–like virus with 99% homology to the human SARS-CoV–like virus;[94] workers who handled the animals in these wet markets had antibodies to the animal SARS–like virus, although they did not have SARS disease, making it likely that these wet markets provide an interface for the transmission of the virus to humans.[95] Evidently, the animal precursor SARS-CoV–like virus adapted to more efficient human-to-human transmission, and SARS arose.[95] The major routes for the transmission of SARS are droplet infection, aerosolization, and fomites.[89] The initial symptoms are flulike and include lower respiratory tract symptoms such as fever, myalgia, lethargy, cough, and a sore throat.[96] The only symptom common to all patients appears to be a fever above 38°C (100°F). Some patients have presented with diarrhea and hepatic dysfunction.[97] Laboratory evaluation shows decreased platelet counts, profound lymphopenia (T cell with decreased CD4$^+$ and CD8$^+$ cells), liver function abnormalities, and prolonged coagulation profile (DIC).[89] Chest radiography shows infiltrates or a ground-glass appearance. Thirty percent of individuals with SARS require ICU management; the overall fatality rate is 15%, progressively increasing with age, with patients older than 65 years showing a mortality rate of more than 50%.[89]

The WHO and CDC issued criteria for the definition of SARS.[96,97a] The case definition consists of a history of fever or documented fever, one or more symptoms of lower respiratory tract illness (cough, difficulty breathing, and shortness of breath), and radiographic evidence of lung infiltrates consistent with pneumonia or ARDS or autopsy findings consistent with the pathology of pneumonia or ARDS without an identifiable cause and no alternative diagnosis fully explaining the illness. The required laboratory diagnostic tests include one or both of the following: detection of the virus (RT-PCR) by an assay for viral RNA present in two separate samples and virus culture from any clinical specimen. The detection of antibody (an increase in antibody titer, either from negative to positive or at least a fourfold increase) is performed by ELISA and/or IFA.

Chu and colleagues examined the records of 536 individuals who were diagnosed with SARS using the case definition and admitted to a Hong Kong hospital.[98] Among these 536 patients with SARS, 36 (6.7%) had AKI, which occurred for a median duration of 20 days (range 5-48 days) after the onset of viral infection, despite a normal plasma creatinine concentration at presentation, and in the context of multiorgan failure and ARDS. A total of 92% of those with AKI died. Death due to SARS occurred more often in patients with AKI than in those without (92% vs. 9%; $P < 0.0001$). Kidney pathology evaluation in 7 patients with SARS (who underwent postmortem examination) showed ATN in 6 (86%) patients. SARS-CoV has never been successfully isolated from the postmortem kidney tissue of infected patients.[99] With these findings considered, the etiology of SARS AKI seems more likely related to the systemic inflammatory response in the context of multiorgan failure than to kidney viral infection per se.[100]

OPISTHORCHIASIS

Opisthorchiasis is a parasitic disease caused by species of liver flukes in the genus *Opisthorchis* (specifically, *Opisthorchis viverrini* and *Opisthorchis felineus*). Opisthorchiasis is prevalent in geographic regions in which raw cyprinid fishes

---

individuals had had contact with the live animal game trade.[92] The etiologic agent of SARS was identified as a coronavirus that was not previously observed to cause disease in humans.[93] Specimens that were collected from apparently healthy animals in the wild game market in Guangdong

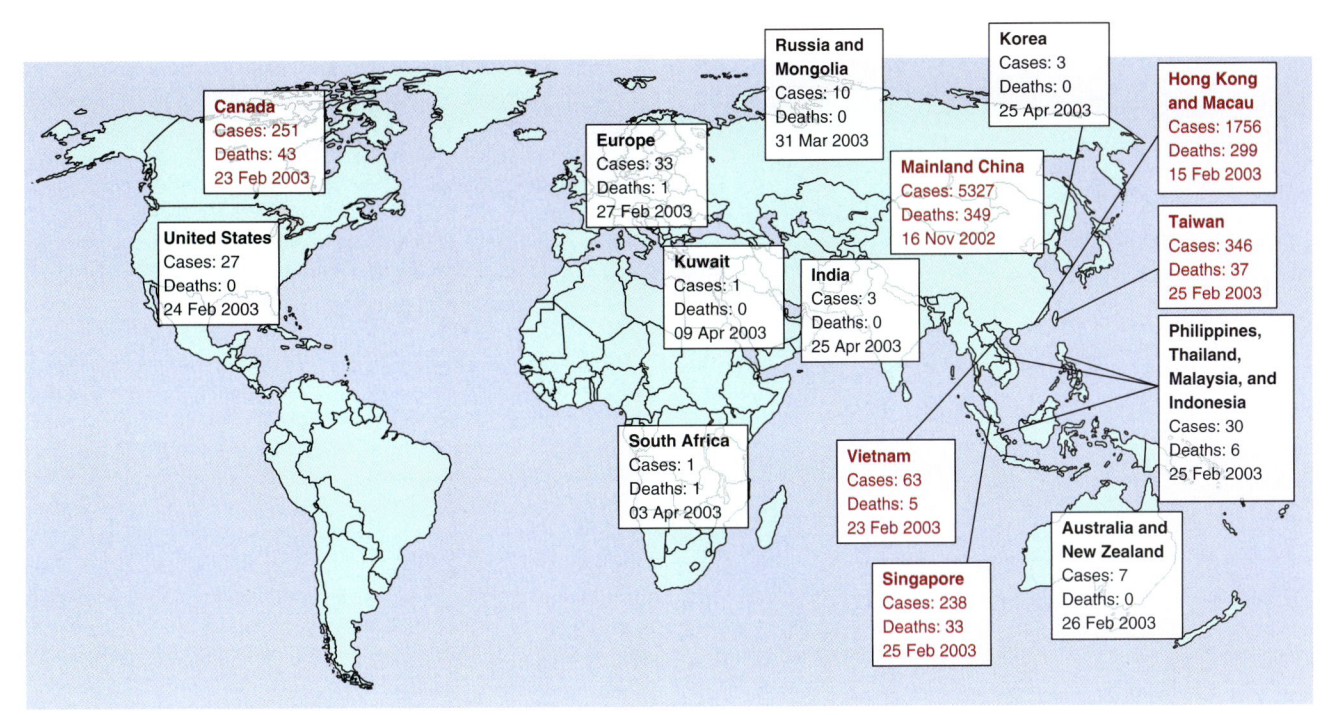

Figure 81.11 The global spread of severe acute respiratory syndrome (SARS). The number of probable cases of SARS and the date of onset of the first case in each country (or group of countries) is denoted. The countries with notes in *red* are those where substantial local transmission occurred. The data are based on World Health Organization table "Summary of probable SARS cases with onset of illness from 1 November 2002 to 31 July 2003" (available at http://www.who.int/csr/sars/country/table2004_04_21/en_21/en/print.html). (From Peiris JS, Guan Y, Yuen KY: Severe acute respiratory syndrome. *Nat Med* 10:S88-S97, 2004; and Christian MD, Poutanen SM, Loufty MR, et al: Severe acute respiratory syndrome. *Clin Infect Dis* 38:1420-1427, 2004.)

are a staple of the human diet.[101-103] These parasites cause immense suffering to tens of millions of people; more than 600 million in total are at risk of infection. The prevalence of human infection can be as high as 70% in some regions, for example, in Khon Kaen Province in Thailand.[104] In the Lao People's Democratic Republic, the prevalence of opisthorchiasis was 40% in 1992, with infection of approximately 1,744,000 people. *O. felineus* is prevalent in Vietnam, the Philippines, and India, whereas *O. viverrini* is common in Thailand, Laos, and Cambodia. Humans become infected by consuming raw or undercooked fish. This infection can be eliminated by the drug praziquantel; however, despite efforts at mass drug administration in northeast Thailand, opisthorchiasis prevalence remains high.[105]

This parasite establishes itself in the bile ducts of the liver as well as the extrahepatic ducts and the gallbladder of the mammalian (definitive) host.[104] The liver is the affected organ, with parasites lodging in the biliary tract. Experimental and epidemiologic evidence links these opisthorchis infections to the etiology of cholangiocarcinoma and advanced periductal (bile duct) fibrosis.[106-108] In the setting of obstructive jaundice due to cholangiocarcinoma, AKI frequently occurs.[109] AKI is observed in 49% of patients with cholangiocarcinoma and severe jaundice. Multiple factors are responsible for the development of AKI, including hypovolemia, endotoxemia, cardiac dysfunction, hypotension, hyperbilirubinemia, and hyperuricosuria. Hyponatremia and hypokalemia secondary to natriuresis and kaliuresis are frequently observed.

Although renal disease has not been considered a critical pathology of chronic opisthorchiasis, hamster models of opisthorchiasis do show development of mesangiocapillary glomerulonephritis that is characterized by immune complex deposition and IgG and C3 deposition with opisthorchiasis antigen.[110] A corollary to the findings in the hamster model system has been reported after the examination of individuals in seven villages with high opisthorchiasis transmission along the Chi River Basin in Khon Kaen, Thailand. Urinary IgG to opisthorcis antigen is an effective biomarker for ultrasonography-detected advanced periductal fibrosis (adjusted odds ratio [OR], 6.69; 95% confidence interval [CI], 2.87 to 15.58) and cholangiocarcinoma (adjusted OR, 71.13; 95% CI, 15.13 to 334.0), providing an inexpensive screening method for the pathologic detection of affected individuals.[111]

ACUTE KIDNEY INJURY DUE TO TOXINS AND CHEMICALS

SNAKEBITE

The number of snakebites that occur globally each year may be as high as 5 million, with the majority in South Asia, Southeast Asia, and Sub-Saharan Africa, resulting in as many as 94,000 deaths.[112] The affected regions often include rural areas lacking medical facilities. Kidney involvement has been observed in victims of bites from snakes belonging to three families, Elapidae, Viperidae, and Colubridae (Table 81.6).[113] In tropical Asia, bites of Russell's viper and the saw-scaled viper are most common. The other snakes that have been reported to cause kidney toxicity include sea snakes, green pit vipers, and hump-nosed pit vipers.[114]

Table 81.6 Distribution of Nephrotoxic Snakes in Asian Countries

	Cambodia	China	India	Indonesia	Japan	Laos	Malaysia	Myanmar	Nepal	Pakistan	Philippines	Sri Lanka	Taiwan	Thailand	Vietnam
Saw-scaled viper (Echis carinatus)			+*							+*		+*			
Russell's viper (Daboia russellii)	+	+	+*	+				+*	+	+		+*	+	+	+
Green pit viper (Crypelytrops, Trimeresurus, Protobothrops)	+	+	+	+	+*	+	+	+	+		+	+	+	+	+
Hump-nosed pit viper (Hypnale hypnale)			+*									+*			
Sea-snake (Hydrophinae)	+	+	+	+	+		+*	+		+		+	+	+	+

*Represents published report.
From Kanjanabuch T, Sitprija V: Snakebite nephrotoxicity in Asia. Sem Nephrol 28:363-372, 2008.

Proteinuria, hematuria, and AKI are among the common clinical renal manifestations of snakebites.[114] Cobra venom causes proteinuria in rats following intrarenal injection.[115] The geographic variation and the species of snake are important factors; proteinuria generally disappears as patients recover. Nephrotic syndrome has been described.[116] Hematuria may occur as a result of coagulation defects and vascular injury; extracapillary proliferative glomerulonephritis has been reported.[117,118] AKI occurs in 5% to 29% of snakebites.[119,120] The pathogenesis of AKI following snakebites includes bleeding, hypotension, circulatory collapse, intravascular hemolysis, DIC, microangiopathic hemolytic anemia, hemolytic uremic syndrome, rhabdomyolysis, and the direct nephrotoxicity of venom. Monospecific antivenin administration is the treatment of choice; plasmapheresis and plasma exchange can be used when antivenin is not available.[121,122] Dialysis has been used successfully to treat snakebite AKI.[123] Death can occur in 1% to 20% of cases.[113]

INSECT STINGS

Wasps and bees are venomous arthropods belonging to the order Hymenoptera.[124] The order consists of three families: Apidae (bees), Vespidae (wasps), and Formicidae (ants). Most wasp or bee sting victims do not seek medical attention owing to the minor, self-limiting, and localized nature of symptoms. Wasp and bee stings are associated with a wide variety of reactions, ranging from mild local reactions (such as edema, erythema, and urticaria) to fatal systemic complications (such as anaphylactic shock, hemolysis, rhabdomyolysis, AKI, myocardial infarction, acute hepatic failure, and encephalitis). AKI is among the rare but important life-threatening complications of insect stings that forces patients to seek medical care. AKI usually develops only after multiple stings, often in relation to rhabdomyolysis and hemolysis.[125] The usual underlying lesion is ATN[125] occasionally with interstitial nephritis,[126] and the course is generally characterized by recovery.

Xuan and colleagues reported a study from Vietnam of 65 patients who were attacked by swarming hornets, in 38 (59%) of whom AKI developed, 29 (76%) requiring dialysis.[127] These investigators reported that the patients who experienced more than 50 stings had a high mortality (19%), 90% had AKI, and 22% had shock. Shock, which appeared to develop 2 to 3 days after the wasp stings, had a particularly poor prognosis (4/7 patients, or 57%, died). In contrast, Zhang and associates reported a retrospective analysis of 103 patients from China who were admitted with multiple wasp stings (>50 stings), in 81 (79%) of whom oliguric AKI developed. Of the 75 patients with AKI available for follow-up, only 7 (9.3%) died, and 8 (10.7%) went on to have CKD.[128]

A host of kidney injury effects due to animal toxins from scorpions, spiders, jellyfish, and centipedes has been reported; they have been reviewed by Sitprija and coworkers.[129]

RAW CARP BILE

The raw bile of carp from the family Cyprinidae, which includes the grass carp *(Ctenopharyngodon idellus),* the common carp *(Cyprinus carpio),* the silver carp *(Hypophthalmichthys molitrix),* the black carp *(Mylopharyngodon piceus),* and the bighead carp *(Aristichthys nobilis),* is nephrotoxic. In East Asia, the ingestion of raw carp bile is traditionally believed to improve visual acuity, stop coughing, and decrease fever. The amount of bile that is ingested, ranging from 15 to 30 mL, can cause toxicity. Poisoning symptoms, which occur 10 minutes to 12 hours after ingestion, include abdominal pain, nausea, vomiting, and diarrhea, followed by jaundice in 62% and AKI in 54% of patients.[130] Bradycardia and convulsions may be observed. Hematuria is observed in 77% of patients. Oliguria can occur 2 to 48 hours after ingestion, and the duration of renal failure is 2 to 3 weeks. AKI is attributed to the nephrotoxicity of cyprinol, a bile alcohol in the bile and bile acid.[131] Volume depletion from diarrhea may be a contributing factor.

DJENKOL BEANS

Djenkol beans *(Pithecellobium lobatum* and *Pithecellobium jiringa)* are consumed by people in Southeast Asian countries, especially Indonesians, Malaysians, and Thais.[132] These beans are considered a delicacy and are eaten raw, fried, boiled, or roasted. AKI due to djenkolic acid in the bean occurs after the ingestion of the raw beans (often more than five beans) with a low fluid intake. However, susceptibility varies among individuals. Toxicity may be caused by a single bean for some individuals but by 20 beans in others. There is also variation in the djenkolic acid content in beans from various sources. The consumption of boiled beans does not cause toxicity because djenkolic acid is removed by this process. Poisoning symptoms occur 2 to 6 hours after the beans are ingested and include abdominal discomfort, nausea, vomiting, loin pain with colic, dysuria, gross hematuria, and oliguria.[133] Hypertension may be present. In one report of 22 patients with djenkol bean poisoning, dysuria was noted in 77%, hematuria in 68%, proteinuria in 45%, hypertension in 36%, and AKI in 55%.[134] Needle-like crystals of djenkolic acid are observed in the urine; kidney biopsy reveals focal areas of ATN.[134] AKI is attributed to mechanical irritation and to the obstruction of renal tubules and the urinary tract by djenkolic acid crystals. Urolithiasis can occur. Treatment requires hydration and urine alkalinization with sodium bicarbonate to increase djenkolic acid solubility.[134] Most patients recover within a few days.

STAR FRUIT

The ingestion of star fruit *(Averrhoa carambola)* as a cause of oxalate nephropathy was first described in Taiwan.[135] Drinking a large quantity of pure fresh star fruit juice can cause nausea, vomiting, abdominal pain, backache, and oliguric AKI. The development of renal failure is determined by the content of oxalate in each fruit and the state of hydration of the individual. The high oxalate content of the star fruit and renal pathologic changes showing diffuse calcium oxalate deposition suggest oxalate nephropathy. One study indicated that apoptosis is the mode of renal tubular cell death.[136] Patients with CKD should be warned against ingestion of even small amounts of star fruit, which may result in AKI.[137]

TOXIC MUSHROOMS

Amanita, Cortinarius, and *Galerina* mushrooms are nephrotoxic. Amatoxin, phallotoxin, and orellanine are among the toxic substances that have been implicated.[138-140] Amatoxin inhibits DNA-dependent RNA polymerase II. Phallotoxin binds to F-actin and polymerizes G-actin. Orellanine is toxic to proximal tubular cells. Clinical presentations of mushroom toxicity begins with gastrointestinal symptoms, consisting of abdominal pain, nausea, vomiting, and diarrhea 10 to 14 hours after ingestion, followed by jaundice and renal failure. AKI and hepatic injury are severe, with a mortality rate of more than 50%. Kidney manifestations may be delayed by 1 to 4 days.[140] Treatment with acetylcysteine,[141] plasmapheresis, charcoal hemoperfusion, hemodiafiltration, and dialysis with the Molecular Absorbent Regenerating System should be performed within 48 hours of ingestion.[142]

Recommendations for patients with amatoxin-containing mushroom poisoning include performing gastrointestinal decontamination with activated charcoal, aggressively managing fluid losses due to vomiting and diarrhea, disrupting the hepatocellular uptake of amatoxins with silibinin dihemisuccinate or, if silibinin is not available, high-dose intravenous penicillin G, providing antioxidant therapy with intravenous N-acetylcysteine, and anticipating and providing supportive care for fulminant hepatic failure, including intensive care in an institution with liver transplantation capability.[143]

MELAMINE

An epidemic of melamine contamination of baby formula was reported to be associated with the development of urinary tract stones in 2008 in China.[144] More than 250,000 children in China were exposed to the tainted infant formula, more than 50,000 were hospitalized, and at least 6 died.[145] Children from other Asian countries, including Taiwan, Singapore, and Vietnam, were reportedly exposed as well. Melamine was apparently added to milk to falsely elevate the protein content determination by the Kjeldahl method because this method detects not only the nitrogen in protein but also the nitrogen in organic nitrogenous compounds such as melamine.[146] Infants who were exposed to high-melamine formula were 7.0 times as likely to have stones as those who were exposed to non-melamine formula. Unlike typical urinary tract stones, most of the melamine-associated stones were not characterized by shadowing on ultrasonography.[144] An analysis of the stone composition demonstrated melamine and uric acid.[146]

Melamine is an organic base and a trimer of cyanamide with a 1,3,5-triazine skeleton containing 66% nitrogen by mass.[146] Melamine combines with cyanuric acid to form melamine cyanurate, which is absorbed into the bloodstream and excreted by the kidney, provoking tubular damage and obstruction. Long-term toxic exposure in animals leads to granulomatous tubulointerstitial changes and fibrosis.[147]

CHRONIC KIDNEY DISEASE

As in the rest of the world, CKD is a growing problem in the Far East, partly because of the increasing prevalence of noncommunicable diseases, such as hypertension and diabetes, and partly because the population is aging. In Far East countries, the causes of CKD, the risk factors for and complications of CKD, and the availability of medical help vary greatly because of differences in genetics, environment, cultures, and socioeconomics. The early identification of CKD and the control of its risk factors are critical to preventing rapid progression and to reducing the risk of cardiovascular morbidity and mortality.

Serum creatinine-based GFR estimation (eGFR) is widely used to assess kidney function in clinical practice and for epidemiologic studies. The method that is used for eGFR calculation was first developed by the Modification of Diet in Renal Disease (MDRD) Study Group in a North American sample. This equation includes a coefficient for people of African ethnicity. Several studies have tested the validity of the MDRD equation in the Asian population. Zuo and colleagues reported that in Chinese patients, the GFR that was estimated by the MDRD study equation was significantly lower than the measured GFR in CKD stages 1 and 2 and significantly higher than the measured GFR in CKD stages 3, 4, and 5.[148] In healthy Korean subjects, the MDRD equation was also found to underestimate the measured GFR.[149] Modifying the racial coefficient for the MDRD equation has been attempted to improve the estimation of the GFR in Chinese[150] and Japanese[151] populations. However, a 30% difference in the reported coefficients between Chinese and Japanese population has been observed.[152] Although the GFR that is calculated by the MDRD equation has limitations with respect to the accuracy of serum creatinine determination and patient ethnicity, it is a practical index and is widely used in staging CKD.

According to available data, the prevalence of CKD in Far East countries and regions varies from 8% to 17% of the population. These differences may come from the heterogeneity in the populations that are screened, the methods that are used to determine the glomerular filtration rate, and proteinuria assays.

Zhang and associates reported a cross-sectional survey of a nationally representative sample of Chinese adults with 47,204 participants.[153] CKD was defined by either an eGFR less than 60 mL/min/1.73 m^2 using the adjusted MDRD equation or the presence of albuminuria.[150] The adjusted prevalence of eGFR less than 60 mL/min/1.73 m^2 was 1.7% (95% CI, 1.5 to 1.9), and that of albuminuria (>30 mg/g creatinine) was 9.4% (95% CI, 8.9 to 10.0). The overall prevalence of CKD was 10.8% (95% CI, 10.2 to 11.3)[154] On the basis of these data, the estimated number of people with CKD in China is 119.5 million (95% CI, 112.9 to 125.0)[153] (Table 81.7). The prevalence of CKD was higher in the north (16.9%) and southwest (18.3%) regions than in the other regions in China. In Japan, a survey of 574,024 participants from the general adult population in 2005 showed the following prevalences of CKD by stage: 1 (0.6%), 2 (1.7%), 3 (10.5%), and 4 and 5 (0.2%) (total 12.9%).[155] In a study from Taiwan, a nationally representative cohort of 200,000 individuals who were randomly sampled from National Health Insurance enrollees was followed from 1996 to 2003. The prevalence of clinically recognized CKD (defined as having a diagnostic code for CKD present in either an inpatient or outpatient service claim form among those who have not reached ESKD requiring RRT) increased from 1.99% in 1996 to 9.83% in 2003. The overall incidence rate from 1997 to 2003 was 1.35 per 100 person-years.[156]

Table 81.7 Chronic Kidney Disease (CKD) Epidemics in the United States and China

	United States	China
Number of people with CKD (% of population)	26.3 million (13.1%)	119.5 million (10.8%)
Prevalence of CKD types (%):		
1	1.78	5.70
2	3.24	3.40
3 (a and b)	7.69	1.60
4	0.35	0.10
5		0.03
5d	0.18	
Incidence of end-stage kidney disease	362.4 cases per 1 million people per year; rate of increase slowing	80 cases or more per 1 million people per year, with likely exponential acceleration
Renal replacement therapy	Third highest prevalence of CKD stage 5/dialysis or transplantation worldwide	Disproportionately rare, but frequency rapidly increasing
Cost of end-stage kidney disease	US$39.46 billion per year in public and private spending[7]	
Main cause	Diabetes mellitus (roughly 50%) and hypertension (roughly 25%)[7]	Unknown; diabetes mellitus is probably a major contributor
Number of kidney transplantations[7]	17,413 per year	
Timing of start of dialysis	Tends to be early (eGFR 10-15 mL/min/1.73 m^2). Low-protein diets or keto-analogs used much less to slow CKD progression	Tends to be late (eGFR <10 mL/min/1.73 m^2). Replacement renal therapy alternatives more likely than in U.S. (e.g., dietary intervention or uremic toxin modulation)

eGFR, Estimated glomerular filtration rate.
Adapted from Kovesdy CP, Kalantar-Zadeh K: Enter the dragon: a Chinese epidemic of chronic kidney disease? Lancet 379:783-785, 2012.

The etiology of CKD in the Far East area varies in different regions. Data from the Chinese Renal Data System, a national registry system for patients undergoing dialysis, revealed that glomerular disease was the most common cause of ESKD (57.4%), followed by diabetic nephropathy (16.4%), hypertension (10.5%), and cystic kidney disease (3.5%).[157] A shift in the epidemiology of kidney disease has been observed in China. Among elderly Chinese patients, the leading causes of CKD are diabetes mellitus and hypertension.[158] Moreover, it is possible that the prevalence of diabetic nephropathy in China will continue to increase, given the rapid increase in the prevalence of diabetes mellitus.[159] Diabetic nephropathy now accounts for 46.2% and 43.2% of cases of ESKD in the more developed regions of Hong Kong and Taiwan, respectively.[160]

CHRONIC KIDNEY DISEASE AFTER INFECTION

Throughout the industrialized and developing world, the incidence of infection-related glomerulonephritis (IRGN) has decreased in the past five decades.[161,162] These trends relate to early and effective antibiotic use; the increasing improvements in living conditions, nutrition, and general sanitation; and the practice of water fluoridation, which has been shown to attenuate the expression of *Streptococcus pyogenes* virulence factors.[163] Carapetis and associates estimated the incidence of poststreptococcal glomerulonephritis in less developed countries and more developed countries, respectively, at 24.3 cases and 6 cases per 10^5 person-years in children and at 2 and 0.3 cases per 10^5 person-years in adults. These values represent a total of about a half million new cases worldwide annually, with a 1% death rate (5000 patients), 97% of these occurring in less developed countries. Additionally, these calculations represent only symptomatic poststreptococcal glomerulonephritis, which is a fraction of the total number.

Hass reported in 2003 from the United States a rate of 18% for ultrastructural evidence of IRGN among kidney biopsies of patients with diabetic nephropathy.[164] Nasr and colleagues also reported from the United States on the changing clinical picture of IRGN; 109 cases of IRGN in patients 65 years or older and diagnosed by kidney biopsy, of whom 61% had diabetes mellitus or malignancy.[165] The sites of infection were skin, pneumonia, and urinary tract; the organisms were staphylococci (46%), streptococci (16%), gram-negative organisms (12%), and the rest unknown. Hypocomplementemia was present in 72% of patients, the mean peak creatinine was 5.1 mg/dL, and 46% of patients required acute dialysis. Of the 72 patients with more than 3 months of follow-up, only 22% achieved complete recovery, 44% had persistent CKD, and 33% progressed to ESKD. Three reports from the Far East corroborate the U.S. findings, describing 36 patients from Thailand,[166] 20 patients from Taiwan,[167] and 64 patients from China[168] (Table 81.8). The average age was 47, 61, and 29 years, respectively; the organisms were both streptococcus and non-streptococcus; and a total of 29%, 40%, and 12% of patients had CKD, 13%, 20%, and 4% with ESKD, respectively. These findings confirm that IRGN in the Far East occurs in adults as well as children; manifests with more heterogeneous organisms and sites of infection; and results in persistent CKD for many individuals.

Yang and coworkers demonstrated, among 3045 participants of a Taiwan survey, that individuals with previous

Table 81.8 Clinical Spectrum of Non-epidemic Infection-Related Glomerulonephritis in Adults

	Study		
	Srisawat et al[166]	Wen et al[167]	Luo et al[168]
Period of study	1998-2005	2000-2008	2000-2009
Country	Thailand	Taiwan	China
No. of pts	36	20	64
Biopsy incidence (%)	NA	NA	NA
Median age (years)	47	NA (mean 61)	29
Male:Female	1:1.3	2.3:1	1.5:1
Percentage of pts with alcoholism	NA	NA	2
Percentage of pts with diabetes	NA	NA	2
Most common sites of infection	NA	Skin (20%) Endocarditis (20%) Lung (15%) Bone/joint (15%) Urinary tract (15%)	Upper respiratory tract (67%) Skin (20%)
Most common bacteria	Streptococcus (22%)* Non-streptococcus† (78%)	Staphylococcus (60%)* Streptococcus (15%)	Streptococcus (67%)* Non-streptococcus† (33%)
Percentage of pts without clinical evidence of infection	NA	5	NA
Duration of follow-up in months (mean)	NA	27	12-118 (42)
Normal renal function (compete recovery) (%)	71	30	86
Persistent renal dysfunction (%)	16	20	8
End-stage kidney disease (%)	13	20	4
Death (%)	NA	30	0
Correlates of renal outcome by multivariate analysis	NA	NA	Underlying disease

NA, Not applicable; pts, patients.
*Determined by elevated anti–streptolysin O titers and/or culture.
†Type of nonstreptococcal infection not known.
From Nasr SH, Radhakrishnan J, D'Agati VD: Bacterial infection related glomerulonephritis in adults. Kidney Int 83:792-803, 2013.

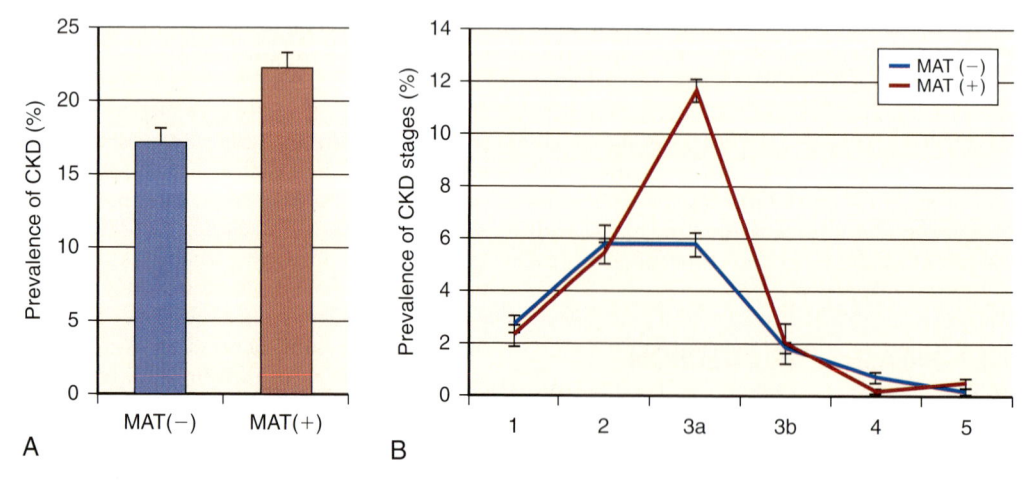

Figure 81.12 Chronic kidney disease (CKD) and leptospirosis in Taiwan. A, Prevalence of CKD according to positive (+; ≥100) or negative (−; 0) results of the microscopic agglutination test in a 2007 population-based survey (n = 3045). B, Prevalence of CKD stages according to MAT results. **$P < 0.001$. Higher CKD prevalence was found in patients with previous exposure to Leptospira infection, as indicated by positive MAT result. (From Dr. Chih-Wei Yang, personal communication, April 2015.)

Leptospira exposure (as measured by a MAT titer of ≥100) had a lower eGFR (98 ± 0.4 vs. 100.8 ± 0.6 mL/min/1.73 m²; $P < 0.001$) and a higher percentage of CKD stages 3a to 5 (14.4% vs. 8.5%) than those without Leptospira exposure (Dr. Chih Wei Yang, personal communication April 2015) (Figure 81.12). These findings are consistent with those from a long-term study of individuals with AKI due to leptospirosis in Sri Lanka, in which 4 of 44 patients (9%) had persistently abnormal kidney function after 1 year consistent with CKD stage 3.[169] It is unclear, at present, whether the nature of the kidney injury in these individuals with leptospirosis infection is related to AKI or to interstitial

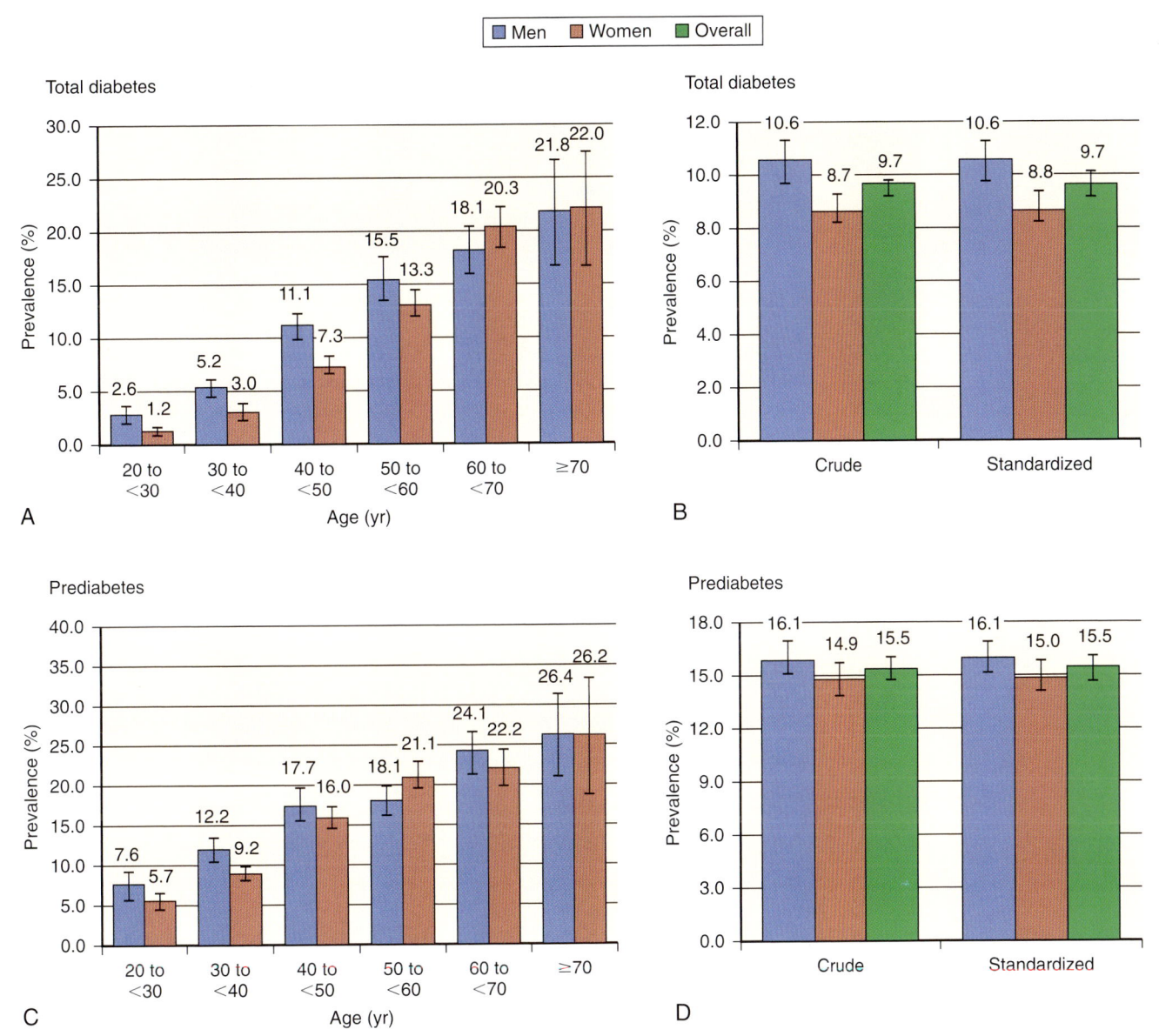

Figure 81.13 Age-specific prevalences of diabetes and prediabetes among Chinese adults 20 years or older. The prevalences of total diabetes (A) and prediabetes (C) among men and women are shown, according to age. The crude and age-standardized prevalences of total diabetes and prediabetes among men and women are shown in B and D, respectively. Total diabetes includes both previously diagnosed diabetes and previously undiagnosed diabetes. Prediabetes was defined as impaired fasting glucose or impaired glucose tolerance test result. Error bars indicate 95% confidence intervals. (From Yang W, Lu J, Weng J, et al: Prevalence of diabetes among men and women in China. N Engl J Med 362:1090-1101, 2010.)

nephritis. These data, however, underscore the role of infection in the burden of CKD in the Far East as well as worldwide.

DIABETES MELLITUS

According to the WHO, as of 2010, an estimated 285 million people worldwide had diabetes, 90% of whom had type 2 diabetes mellitus. This incidence is increasing rapidly worldwide, and by 2030, the prevalence is projected to be 439 million.[170] In China, studies have reported a prevalence of type 2 diabetes of 9.7% to 11.6% of the adult population, with an estimated 92 to 113.9 million affected individuals (Figure 81.13).[159] Importantly, the epidemic of diabetes and prediabetes in China shows no sign of abating.[171] The high prevalence of diabetes may also translate into a major epidemic of diabetes-related complications, including CKD.

GLOMERULONEPHRITIS

PRIMARY GLOMERULONEPHRITIS

Primary glomerular diseases (PGDs) are the most common renal diseases in Far East countries. According to data from a single center in China, among 8909 kidney biopsy specimens from 1997 to 2011, 6337 (71.13%) were diagnosed as showing primary glomerular disease. IgA nephropathy (IgAN) was the most common PGD (36.66%). The frequency of membranous nephropathy (MN) increased

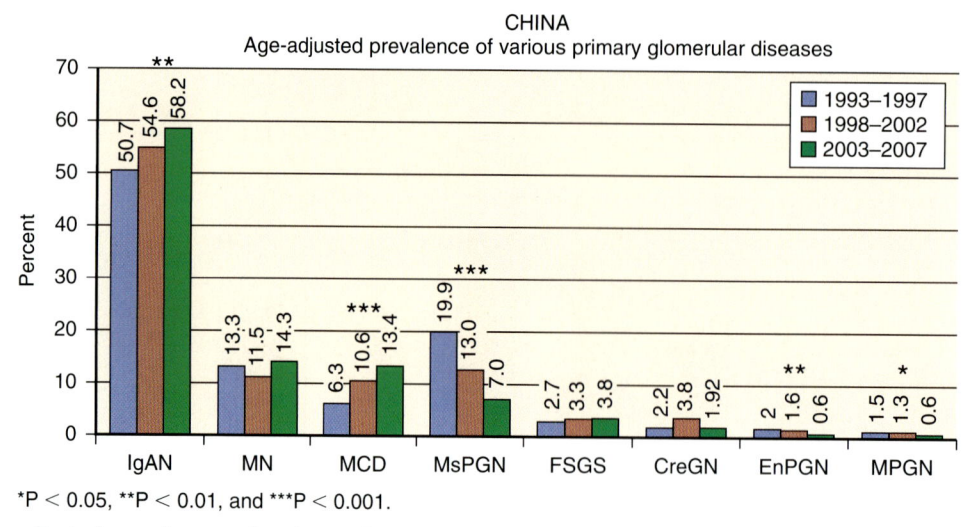

Figure 81.14 Age-adjusted prevalences of various primary glomerular diseases in China. *P < 0.05; **P < 0.01; ***P < 0.001. CreGN, Crescentic glomerulonephritis; EnPGN, endocapillary proliferative glomerulonephritis; FSGS, focal segmental glomerulosclerosis; IgAN, immunoglobulin A (IgA) nephropathy; MCD, minimal change disease; MN, membranous nephropathy; MPGN, membranoproliferative glomerulonephritis; MsPGN, non-IgA mesangioproliferative glomerulonephritis. (From Zhou FD, Zhao MH, Zou WZ, et al: The changing spectrum of primary glomerular diseases within 15 years: a survey of 3331 patients in a single Chinese centre. *Nephrol Dial Transplant* 24:870-876, 2009.)

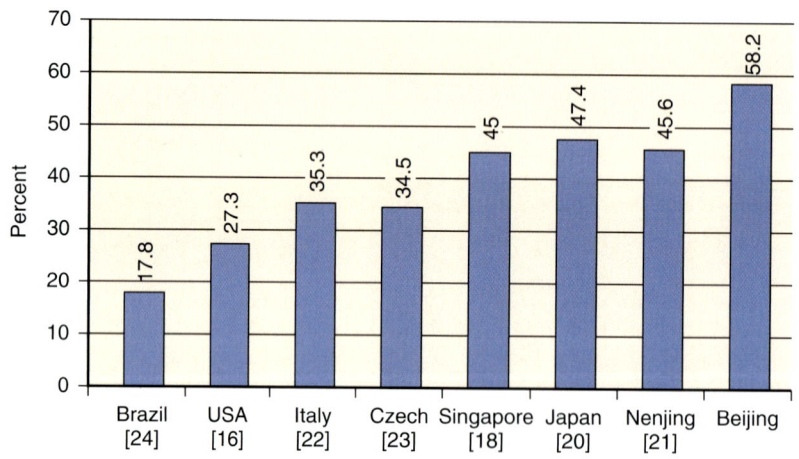

Figure 81.15 Frequency of IgA nephropathy in primary glomerular diseases in different countries. (From Zhou FD, Zhao MH, Zou WZ, et al: The changing spectrum of primary glomerular diseases within 15 years: a survey of 3331 patients in a single Chinese centre. *Nephrol Dial Transplant* 24:870-876, 2009.)

significantly from 6.48% in the period 1997 to 1999 to 22.79% in the period 2009 to 2011. MN was the most frequently found PGD in patients 60 years or older (39.64%)[172,173] (Figures 81.14 and 81.15).

IgA nephropathy is the most common PGD in Asians, is moderately prevalent in Europeans, and is rare in Africans. In a geospatial analysis of 85 populations, a genetic risk score based on the replicated genome-wide associated study (GWAS) loci is highest in Asians, intermediate in Europeans, and lowest in Africans, accounting for the known differences in prevalence of IgAN among world populations.[174-176]

The Oxford classification of IgAN has been validated in Asian countries. In a study of 410 patients with IgAN from one center in China, the performance of the Oxford classification to predict ESKD was evaluated. Segmental glomerulosclerosis, tubular atrophy, and interstitial fibrosis were independent predictive factors of ESKD. Patients in whom more than 25% of glomeruli had endocapillary hypercellularity also had higher proteinuria, lower eGFR value, and higher mean blood pressure than those whose glomeruli had less endocapillary hypercellularity. Mesangial hypercellularity and tubular atrophy and interstitial fibrosis were independent predictors of the lack of therapeutic efficacy of renin angiotensin aldosterone system (RAAS) blockade alone. Crescents were not significant in predicting prognosis or in therapeutic efficacy.[177] Tanaka and colleagues from Japan reported that proteinuria (hazard ratio [HR], 1.30, for every 1 g/24 hours), eGFR (HR, 0.84, for every 10 mL/min), mesangial proliferation (HR, 1.85), segmental sclerosis (HR, 3.21), and interstitial fibrosis/tubular atrophy (Oxford classification T1: HR, 5.30; T2: HR, 20.5) were independent risk factors for development of ESKD in people with IgAN.[178] Another study with 69 adult Korean patients with IgAN showed that in the Oxford classification, endocapillary hypercellularity (E) and tubular atrophy/interstitial fibrosis (T) lesions predicted the renal outcome after clinical variables were considered.[179] These studies suggest that the Oxford classification may aid in predicting the prognosis and providing a therapeutic strategy in patients with IgAN in Asia.

Long-term renal survival and related risk factors in patients with IgA nephropathy have been analyzed from a cohort of 1155 cases from the Nanjing Glomerulonephritis Registry database.[180] Thirty-six percent of Chinese adult patients with IgAN progress to ESKD within 20 years. Higher proteinuria, hypertension, reduced GFR, hypoproteinemia and hyperuricemia are independent predictors of an unfavorable renal outcome. Patients with time-average proteinuria (TA-P) values more than 1.0 g/day evidenced a 9.4-fold greater risk of ESKD than patients with TA-P values less than 1.0 g/day and a 46.5-fold greater risk than those with TA-P values less than 0.5 g/day. Patients in whom therapy achieved TA-P values less than 0.5 g/day benefited much more than did those in whom therapy achieved TA-P values between 0.5 and 1.0 g/day (HR, 13.1 for ESKD). Ninety percent of these patients were treated with a RAAS inhibitor for at least 12 months, and 19% were treated with immunosuppression.

Moriyama and associates reported a 30-year analysis of 1012 patients with IgA nephropathy at a single center in Japan.[181] The 10-, 20-, and 30-year renal survival rates were 84.3%, 66.6%, and 50.3%, respectively. The initial treatment consisted of corticosteroids in 26.9% of the patients, RAAS inhibitors in 28.9%, and tonsillectomy plus steroids in 11.7% (Figure 81.16).

Six months of steroid treatment is renal protective in Asian patients with IgA nephropathy,[182] a finding consistent with the results from other regions.[183] Tonsillectomy combined with steroid pulses is a frequently used protocol in the treatment of active IgAN in Japan,[184] on the basis of retrospective studies showing that tonsillectomy plus steroids improves renal outcomes.[181,185] A multicenter randomized controlled trial was conducted to evaluate the effect of tonsillectomy in patients with IgAN.[186] Within 12 months of the time of baseline measurements, the percentage decrease in urinary protein excretion was significantly larger in the tonsillectomy plus steroids group than that in the steroids alone group. However, the frequency of the disappearance of proteinuria, hematuria, or both (clinical remission) at 12 months was not significantly different between the groups. The impact of tonsillectomy on renal function outcomes remains to be clarified.

The effects of mycophenolate mofetil (MMF) on IgAN from the available data from randomized controlled trials are variable. Patients with IgAN from Asia seem to have a better response to MMF. A study of 40 patients from Hong Kong found a significant reduction in proteinuria at 18 months with MMF given for 6 months in comparison with controls.[187] A 6-year follow-up of the same cohort demonstrated a kidney survival benefit.[188] A favorable effect of MMF on IgAN nephropathy was also observed in another study from China.[189] However, in a study from Belgium, no difference in proteinuria reduction or preservation of GFR was observed.[190] Similarly, a North American study found no benefits over a period 24 months of a 1-year regimen of MMF at 2 g/day in comparison with placebo in 32 patients.[191] The reasons for this heterogeneity of outcomes requires further investigation, but different ethnicities or differences in drug levels may be contributory factors.

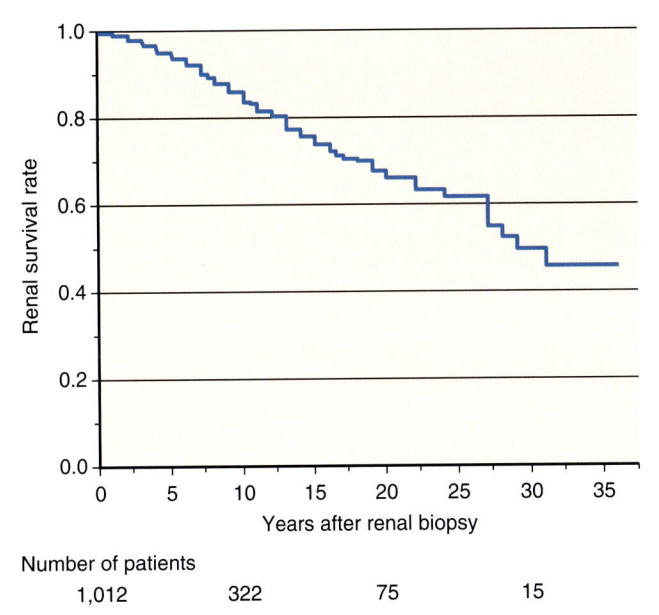

Figure 81.16 Prognosis in immunoglobulin A (IgA) nephropathy: 30-year analysis of 1012 patients at a single center in Japan. Little is known about the long-term prognosis of patients with IgA nephropathy (IgAN). Initially, the disease was regarded as benign. In this retrospective cohort study reporting the long-term outcome of IgAN, spanning from 1974 to 2011, 1012 patients at Tokyo Women's Medical University were diagnosed with primary IgAN by kidney biopsy. IgAN was diagnosed by light microscopic findings of mesangial proliferative changes, immunofluorescence findings of mesangial IgA and C3 deposition, and electron microscopic findings of electron-dense deposits in the mesangial area. Patients were observed for a mean 7.9 ± 7.1 years (maximum 36 years); 4 patients died during the observation period. A retrospective analysis showed that the 10-, 20-, 30-, and 36-year cumulative renal survival rates were 84.3%, 66.6%, 50.3%, and 46.4%, respectively. IgAN is *not* a benign disease, with approximately 50% of patients progressing to end-stage kidney disease within 30 years despite treatment. (From Moriyama T, Tanaka K, Iwasaki C, et al: Prognosis in IgA nephropathy: 30-year analysis of 1,012 patients at a single center in Japan. *PLoS ONE* 9:e91756, 2014.)

The incidence of idiopathic membranous nephropathy has increased significantly in the past 10 years in China. The reason for this increase in not known. Qin and coworkers examined the prevalence of serum PLA2R autoantibody in Chinese patients with idiopathic membranous nephropathy, showing that 82% of these patients had the PLA2R antibody,[192] a value that is comparable to data from Western countries.

SECONDARY GLOMERULONEPHRITIS

Lupus Nephritis

Systemic lupus erythematosus (SLE) is a common disease in Asian populations and is associated with more renal complications than in white populations. A systematic review of SLE in Asia has shown higher rates of renal involvement in Asian patients (21% to 65% at diagnosis and 40% to 82% at follow-up) than in Caucasian patients.[193] Of all of the secondary glomerular diseases that are diagnosed by renal biopsy, lupus nephritis (LN) is the most common in Asian countries, including China, Japan, Korea, Malaysia, and

Thailand. LN accounts for 60% to 90% of cases of secondary glomerulonephritis in Asian countries.[194-196] In females, LN accounts for more than 80% of cases of secondary glomerulonephritis in these countries. Asian patients with SLE may also present with more severe nephritis than other ethnic groups, and lupus nephritis is an major cause of ESKD in Asia.[197] Genetic susceptibility to SLE among Asian populations is responsible for the high incidence of organ damage.

The management of lupus nephritis has evolved considerably, and the outcome of treatment has improved over the past three decades. There is evidence that treatment outcomes following cyclophosphamide (CYC) or MMF therapy vary according to race and ethnicity.[198] In a report of Chinese patients with proliferative LN, treatment with either intravenous or oral CYC resulted in favorable long-term outcomes, with 5- and 10-year renal survival rates of 88.7% and 82.8%, respectively.[199] MMF combined with prednisolone for 6 months showed an efficacy comparable to that of oral CYC in Chinese patients, and MMF treatment was associated with lower rates of severe infection, alopecia, and amenorrhea.[200] Equivalence of efficacy between MMF and intravenous pulse CYC, both combined with corticosteroids, as induction therapy has also been demonstrated in Malaysian patients with proliferative LN.[201] Regarding the MMF dose for the induction treatment of proliferative LN, the target dose is mostly within the range of 1.5 to 2 g/day in Chinese studies, but there are few data on the optimal dosage in other Asian populations.[202] Higher targeted doses, 3 g/day, seem to raise the risk of severe infection.[203] With prompt diagnosis and treatment, the long-term outcome in Asian patients with LN appears more favorable than in patients of African or Hispanic descent.[202]

Over the past few decades, the survival of patients with LN has improved significantly because of advances in immunosuppressive and supportive treatments and earlier diagnosis. Data from a single center in Hong Kong showed 5-, 10-, and 20-year survival rates of patients with LN to be 98.6%, 98.25%, and 90.5%, respectively.[204] Infection is a leading complication of immunosuppressive treatment and is the cause of death in 50% of patients.[204] The management of patients should consider infections that are prevalent or endemic in Asian countries, such as hepatitis B and tuberculosis, because prophylaxis or preemptive treatment may be indicated.

ANCA-ASSOCIATED VASCULITIDES

ANCA-associated vasculitides (AAVs) are characterized by the necrotizing inflammation of small vessels in conjunction with ANCAs directed to either proteinase 3 (PR3) or MPO. According to one report from Japan, the annual incidence of AAV was 22.6 per million,[205] similar to that reported in Europe, 10 to 20 per million.[206] However, the incidence of microscopic polyangiitis (MPA) is much higher in Asian countries, as reported from China and Japan, relative to northern Europe, where granulomatosis with polyangiitis (GPA) is predominant.[205,207,208] MPA constitutes approximately 80% to 83% of cases of AAV in China and Japan.[205,209] In terms of antigenicity, sera from approximately 80% Chinese patients with AAV showed MPO.[209] Even in patients with a clinical picture of GPA, approximately 60% have ANCAs associated with MPO antibodies. This geographic difference may reflect different genetic backgrounds. A genomewide association study supports genetic differences in MPA and GPA.[210]

MPA or GPA mostly occurs in older adults, although it has been reported at all ages. According to a series of 234 cases from China, more than 40% of patients with AAVs are elderly (>65 years old at diagnosis), and 94.9% of the elderly patients have MPO-ANCAs.[211] The annual incidence of MPA was approximately 10 times higher in seniors than in younger adults (15 to 64 years old).[205] Compared with younger patients, older patients had more severe pulmonary involvement and a higher risk of secondary pulmonary infection after the initiation of immunosuppressive therapy.[211]

Patients with AAVs typically present with constitutional symptoms, including fever, migratory arthralgias, malaise, anorexia, and weight loss. Prodromal symptoms may last for weeks to months without evidence of specific organ involvement. Such organs as the ears, nose, and throat (ENT), lung, and kidney are mostly involved. In a study comparing the organ involvement of new-onset of AAVs between Japan and the United Kingdom, ENT and respiratory involvements were more common in the United Kingdom than in Japan. Of patients with MPA in Japan, 93% had renal involvement, and 7% ENT involvement; in patients with GPA, 100% had ENT involvement, and 38% renal involvement.[205]

The survival of patients with AAV has improved substantially over the past 10 years, although the mortality is still relatively high. In a cohort study of 398 patients who were followed up for an average of 25.5 months, 135 out of 398 patients (33.9%) died. Secondary infection was the leading cause of death (53/153, or 39.3%) during the first year after diagnosis, whereas cardiovascular events were the leading cause of death (15/53, or 28.8%) 12 months after diagnosis.[212]

HEPATITIS B/HEPATITIS C VIRUS–ASSOCIATED NEPHRITIS

According to the WHO, East Asia is one of the regions in the world with the highest hepatitis B prevalence. Five percent to 10% of the adult population in these areas are chronically infected with HBV. In contrast, less than 1% of the population in Western Europe and North America are chronically infected.[213] Glomerulonephritis is an important extrahepatic manifestation of chronic hepatitis B virus (HBV) infection. Hepatitis B virus–associated glomerulonephritis (HBV-GN) is one of the most common forms of secondary glomerulonephritis in countries such as China, although its incidence decreased after the popularization of HBV vaccination.[214]

The diagnosis of HBV-GN is usually established by serologic evidence of persistent HBV infection, serologic evidence of circulating hepatitis B surface antigen (HBsAg) and hepatitis B e antigen (HBeAg), or by the presence of glomerular deposits containing one or more HBV-related antigens in an immunohistochemical study.[215,216] The most common pattern of renal involvement in renal biopsy is membranous nephropathy, followed by membranoproliferative glomerulonephritis, IgAN, and focal segmental glomerulosclerosis.[217]

Many of the data on the treatment of HBV-related glomerular diseases are derived from patients with membranous nephropathy, whereas data on membranoproliferative glomerulonephritis (MPGN) and focal segmental glomerulosclerosis remain largely anecdotal.[217] Treatment with interferon or nucleoside analogues has been reported to lead to a reduction of proteinuria in patients with HBV-related membranous nephropathy. Interferon treatment given for 4 to 12 months was associated with the sustained remission of proteinuria in 20% to 100% of patients and with the clearance of HBeAg in 20% to 80%. The resolution of proteinuria was often associated with the clearance of HBeAg and/or HBsAg and usually occurred within 6 months of seroconversion.[217,218] HBeAg is considered to be a marker of HBV replication and infectivity: HBeAg seroconversion (disappearance of HBeAg and appearance of anti-HBe antibodies) is usually associated with a decrease in HBV DNA and remission. In patients who are initially HBeAg negative, monitoring of HBV DNA levels is required, documenting hepatitis B viremia suppression, to ensure that therapy is effective.

Nucleoside analogs, such as lamivudine, telbivudine, adefovir, entecavir, and tenofovir, suppress HBV replication through their inhibitory effect on viral DNA polymerase.[217] In comparison with interferon, nucleoside analogs offer the advantages of convenient administration and high tolerability but may lead to the selection of drug-resistant HBV strains or mutations. Some nucleoside analogs may have nephrotoxic effects. Lamivudine is effective in the treatment of HBV-GN; however, the emergence of resistance mutations in the reverse transcriptase domain of HBV polymerase frequently results in overt viral rebound and disease progression. Resistance to entecavir is rare.[219] Entecavir also appears to be safe in patients with kidney disease, but the dose must be adjusted in patients with impaired kidney function.[219] The long-term use of adefovir or tenofovir has been associated with dose-dependent renal toxicity. The inhibition of mitochondrial DNA replication may result in the disruption of normal mitochondrial respiratory function in proximal renal tubular epithelial cells, leading to abnormal phosphorus absorption. Qi and colleagues, evaluating the prolonged effect of different nucleosides on eGFR, found that adefovir treatment was associated with a decrease in eGFR, lamivudine and entecavir did not significantly influence eGFR, and telbivudine treatment increased eGFR.[220] The mechanism by which telbivudine increases eGFR remains unknown.

East Asia is also a region with high prevalence of hepatitis C virus (HCV) infection, with a seroprevalence of 3.7%.[221] In China, the reported incidence of HCV infection increased from 0.7 cases per 100,000 in 1997 to 15.0 cases per 100,000 in 2012.[222] MPGN is the most common renal manifestation of HCV infection,[223] although other nephropathies, such as MN and IgAN, have also been detected.[224]

HUMAN IMMUNODEFICIENCY VIRUS INFECTION

Human immunodeficiency virus (HIV) infection is a common infectious disease. By the end of 2013, approximately 35 million people worldwide were infected with HIV. There are approximately 3.4 million patients with HIV infection in Southeast Asia; the prevalence is substantially higher in Thailand and Papua New Guinea. Although numerous studies have reported demographic data for kidney disease in HIV-infected patients in Western countries, only a few studies have investigated kidney disease in Asian populations with HIV.[225] A study from Japan showed that the presence of albuminuria presents a potentially significant risk for renal dysfunction in Japanese patients with HIV,[226] consistent with findings in Western populations.[227] In Hong Kong, CKD is prevalent in Chinese patients with HIV, but those with CKD are more likely to be older, to use indinavir, and to have a CD4+ lymphocyte count nadir of less than 100 cells/μL.[228] In one study in Thai patients with HIV who exhibited proteinuria, the most common renal pathologic change was mesangial proliferative glomerulonephritis.[229] Of special note is that none of the cases in this series demonstrated a pathologic finding of HIV-associated nephropathy.[229] This result suggests that ethnic and genetic differences exist in susceptibility to the development of HIV-associated nephropathy.[230,231]

DISTAL RENAL TUBULAR ACIDOSIS

In some tropical countries, particularly Thailand, Malaysia, the Philippines, and Papua New Guinea, distal renal tubular acidosis (dRTA), caused by mutations of the *SLC4A1* gene encoding the erythroid and kidney isoforms of anion exchanger 1 (AE1 or band 3), has a high prevalence. Here, the disease is almost invariably recessive and can result from either homozygous or compound heterozygous *SLC4A1* mutations.[232] The high prevalence of recessive dRTA in the tropics suggests the existence of an environmental factor that has favored the local evolution of these *SLC4A1* mutations.[232] In a study by Khositseth and associates, the majority of patients were young children, with an average age of 4 years old at clinical presentation.[232] Males and females were approximately equally represented. At presentation, the most conspicuous feature was failure to thrive, with body weights usually less than the third percentile. Rickets was present in 74% of patients. Medullary nephrocalcinosis was found in at least 80% of patients. On initial presentation, patients had the characteristic blood and urine biochemistry of dRTA, with hyperchloremic acidosis and urine pH values that were inappropriately alkaline in the presence of acidosis. Hypokalemia was present in the majority. The plasma creatinine values were usually in the normal range.[232]

HERBAL MEDICINES

The use of herbs as supplementary or alternative medicines is common in China and many other Asian countries.[233] Traditional Chinese herbal medicines are used for the treatment of kidney and other diseases. Triptolides, extracts of *Tripterygium wilfordii* Hook F, have been used to treat glomerulonephritis for more than 30 years in China, with antiproteinuric effects.[234] *Astragalus* and *Rheum palmatum L* are frequently used to treat chronic kidney disease. Chen and associates reported results of a randomized trial comparing Shenqi particle, a specific mixture of 13 traditional Chinese medicine remedies, to conventional immunosuppression with cyclophosphamide-prednisone in 190 patients with biopsy-confirmed idiopathic membranous nephropathy.[235] After 48 weeks, the primary outcomes of complete or partial remission occurred at a similar rate in the two groups (Shenqi 73.1% vs. standard 78.3%). Fewer serious adverse events were reported in the Shenqi particle group than in the standard therapy group.[235]

However, some herbal medicines are known to cause nephrotoxicity. Approximately 10% of ESKD incidents in Taiwan are due to Chinese herb nephropathy.[236] The best-described renal toxicity associated with traditional Chinese herbal medication is aristolochic acid-induced nephropathy (AAN).[237,238] Aristolochic acid is also responsible for the Balkan endemic nephropathy. Despite the awareness of the toxicity of aristolochic acid, some Chinese herbal preparations may still contain traces of this compound. The pathology of AAN is characterized by extensive renal interstitial fibrosis and tubular atrophy without obvious glomerular injury. Uroepithelial malignancies are commonly observed in long-term associations with AAN.[233] In one cohort of 300 patients with AAN, 13 presented with AKI, 7 with abrupt tubular dysfunction but normal serum creatinine concentration, and 280 with chronic tubulointerstitial nephropathy and decreased eGFR.[237]

Taxus celebica, which is used in traditional Chinese medicine to treat diabetes mellitus, can cause fever, gastrointestinal upset, hemolysis, and AKI.[239,240] Toxicity is due to the flavonoid sciadopitysin. The long-term use of ma huang *(Ephedra sinica),* an ancient Chinese stimulant, can cause ephedrine renal stone formation.[241] The consumption of rhubarb *(Rheum)* leaves can induce oxalate renal stones owing to the high oxalic acid content.[242]

BETEL NUT CHEWING

Betel nut is the fourth most widely used addictive substance in the world, particularly in Southeast Asia countries and areas. In addition to its association with oral cancer, cardiovascular disorders, metabolic syndrome, type 2 diabetes mellitus and liver cirrhosis, betel nut chewing has been reported to be associated with CKD. The association between betel nut use and CKD is independent of age, body mass index (BMI), smoking, alcohol consumption, hypertension, diabetes, and hyperlipidemia.[243]

RENAL REPLACEMENT THERAPY

The incidence and prevalence of RRT in ESKD patients in the Far East varies from the highest to the lowest globally. The low incidence and prevalence in some areas are caused by the lack of universal insurance or cost coverage for RRT and the lack of nephrologists.

Taiwan and Japan are the countries with the highest incidence and prevalence of RRT in the world and show a constant increase year by year.[243a] In Japan, the prevalence of ESKD reached 2309 per million in 2011.[243a] Preferences of RRT modality differ among the Far East countries. The overall proportional utilization of PD by patients currently undergoing dialysis in the Far East region is lower than the utilization of hemodialysis, and the growth in PD use remains modest except in Hong Kong. In Hong Kong, more than 80% of patients undergoing RRT receive PD, the highest reported rate worldwide, which results from a "PD first" government policy.

Renal transplantation rates reflect not only the countries' health care systems but also cultural diversity. In some countries, deceased-donor kidney transplantation is not accepted by the community. Despite the high number of dialysis recipients in Japan, only a small number are registered with Japan's Organ Transplant Network for organ allocation. There is cultural resistance to mutilation of the body, and the concept of brain death has not been widely accepted by some communities.

Although the average age of patients with ESKD or on dialysis in China is 10 years younger than in Western countries, and the average body mass index is lower, the cause of ESKD is primarily glomerulonephritis instead of diabetes or hypertension, and the main cause of death is still cardiovascular disease (CVD).[244] According to a 2013 report, there are currently more than 40,000 prevalent PD recipients in China, representing approximately 20% of the total dialysis population.[245]

TAIWAN

Taiwan has the highest incidence and prevalence rates of ESKD.[243a] The incidence and prevalence rates of ESKD in Taiwan in 2010 were 361 and 2580 per million population, respectively.[243a] Almost 90% of the patients with ESKD were on hemodialysis. There are several possible explanations for the high incidence and prevalence of ESKD in Taiwan. First, the launching of the National Health Insurance (NHI) program in 1995 began to provide free cost coverage for dialysis therapy without copayment. Second, the better health care system may improve the survival rate of patients with chronic diseases and increase the overall life expectancy. Third, the low transplantation rate and low mortality rate in dialysis recipients further increase the numbers of people requiring dialysis.[160] Diabetes mellitus (43.2%), chronic glomerulonephritis (25.1%), hypertension (8.3%), and chronic interstitial nephritis (2.8%) are major underlying renal diseases causing ESKD. Older age, diabetes, hypertension, smoking, obesity, regular use of herbal medicine, long-term lead exposure, and hepatitis C are associated with higher risk for CKD.[160]

JAPAN

In Japan, the prevalence of ESKD reached 2309 per million in 2011.[243a] According to the 2011 report from The Japanese Society for Dialysis Therapy (JSDT),[246] the total number of prevalent dialysis patients was 2383 per million population. There were a total of 36,590 dialysis recipients in 2012,[247] and the leading cause of ESKD was diabetes (44.2%). The number of patients in Japan with chronic glomerulonephritis has decreased linearly since 1998. The survival among Japanese dialysis recipients is better than that among recipients in Europe and the United States; the reasons for this difference remain to be determined. Patient compliance with a dialysis regimen among Japanese patients is good. The most common vascular access is an arteriovenous fistula. A relatively small body size, with a mean BMI of approximately 21 kg/m^2, might be advantageous for receiving adequate dialysis.[246] Renal transplantation is performed in approximately only 1200 patients per year, and transplantation from deceased donors is uncommon, being approximately 200 annually for a total Japanese population of 128 million people.[246]

HONG KONG

In Hong Kong, peritoneal dialysis was used by 74% of patients in 2011.[243a] The establishment of a "PD first" policy in Hong Kong has contributed significantly to the development of a successful RRT program. A cost analysis indicates that the yearly expenditure for a patient receiving PD is approximately 40% of that for a patient receiving hemodialysis. Several retrospective studies showed a significant association between survival advantage and receiving PD in the initial period of dialysis treatment.[248] PD is also associated with better residual kidney function preservation, lower infection risk, and greater patient satisfaction while reducing financial stress to governments by addressing the burden of managing the growing number of patients with ESKD.[248] Despite successes in improving patient survival, PD treatment has limitations, notably the shortcoming of technique failure. In nearly 40% of all new dialysis recipients, diabetic nephropathy was the underlying disease, whereas in 21% it was glomerulonephritis.

CHINA

A survey by the Chinese Society of Blood Purification estimated that the point prevalence of patients with ESKD on maintenance hemodialysis or peritoneal dialysis was 71.9 per million population in mainland China in 2008.[157] The estimated prevalence of ESKD in China is ~250 cases per million population.[245] The lower rate of dialysis in China may stem from unaffordable health care, major financial risks associated with out-of-pocket medical expenses, and inequalities in access to health care and in health status across populations with different socioeconomic status and across urban and rural regions.[157] These issues are now being tackled under the new Chinese health reform strategy. As of 2014, basic medical insurance covered more than 95% of urban and rural residents with a high reimbursement policy for ESKD.[245]

Although hemodialysis is the major dialysis modality in China, by 2014, the use of PD was increasing. The major advantages of PD as a RRT for China include it being home based, which is especially important for patients in China's vast rural areas, allowing greater independence freedom of movement. PD has been shown to slow decreases in residual kidney function and has generally stable hemodynamics and good middle molecule clearance. In addition, the annual cost of PD is ~CN Y93,520 (USD $14,380) whereas HD costs CN Y103,416 (US $15,910).[245] As of 2014, approximately 1024 hospitals offered PD to more than 40,000 patients with ESKD accounting for ~20% of the dialysis patients in China. Most supplies were produced by Baxter China and a few local Chinese companies. A few (0.2%) PD patients were treated with automated PD; newer solutions such as icodextrin, low-glucose-degradation-product-solutions were made available. The quality and utilization of PD vary tremendously. Although major centers in large cities had excellent patient survival rates (Shanghai 97%, 79%, 71%, 64% at 1, 2, 3, 5 years, respectively; death-censored survival rates of 97%, 93%, 90%, 88%, respectively, and a peritonitis incidence rate of 0.198 per patient-year); the results from underdeveloped regions in northwest and southwest China were less encouraging.[245]

Data from the Chinese Renal Data System, a national registry system for patients undergoing dialysis, revealed that glomerular disease was the most common cause of end-stage renal disease (ESKD; 57.4%), followed by diabetic nephropathy (16.4%), hypertension (10.5%), and cystic kidney disease (3.5%).[157] The main causes of death for patients on hemodialysis in China were cardiovascular (31.0%), stroke (20.3%), infection (19.9%), and other causes (28.8%). No large cohort study on dialysis outcomes in Chinese populations has been published.

KOREA

The incidence and prevalence of ESKD in Korea in 2011 were 205 per million population and 1225 per million population, respectively.[243a] According to the statistics of the National Health Insurance Service (NHIC) on medical aid, the number of hemodialysis recipients in Korea increased by 31.9% from 44,136 in 2006 to 58,232 in 2010.[249] According to data from the ESKD Registry Committee of the Korean Society of Nephrology, in 2009, the proportion of patients undergoing RRT was 66.3% on HD, 13.5% on PD, and 20.2% with a kidney transplant.[250] The most common primary causes of ESKD were diabetic nephropathy (45.4%), hypertensive nephrosclerosis (18.3%), and chronic glomerulonephritis (11.1%).[250] The overall 5-year survival rate of male patients undergoing dialysis was 65.4%, and that of female patients was 67.4%.[250]

THAILAND

In Thailand, the incidence rate of reported ESKD in 2011 was 227 per million population. The prevalence of ESKD in Thailand reached 750 per million population in 2011.[243a] Of affected patients, 72.6% were receiving hemodialysis, 19.8% were on PD, and 7.4% had a functioning renal transplant. As reported by Thailand Renal Replacement Therapy (TRT) registry data, the total yearly prevalence of RRT increased by an average of 14.8% after the implementation of national health insurance and the "PD First" policy from 2007 to 2009.[251] The incidence of all RRT modalities rose by an average of 34.8% from 2007 to 2009. The yearly incidence of HD modestly increased (8.1%), and the total yearly incidence of PD increased remarkably by 157.8%. Diabetic nephropathy was the cause of ESKD in 34.6% of patients receiving RRT in 2007. In the Thai registry, patients with ESKD related to high blood pressure (hypertensive nephropathy) for whom there was no other clinical information, such as renal biopsy results, accounted for 47% of cases. Patients with primary glomerulonephritis accounted for 5.8% of prevalent cases.

MALAYSIA

Malaysia has seen a remarkable growth in the number of patients receiving RRT, most of whom are on hemodialysis. Data from the National Renal Registry (NRR) showed that in 2010, a total of 24,773 patients were receiving RRT, of whom nearly 80% were on HD.[252] Patients older than 65 years constitute the fastest-growing group of HD recipients. Diabetes mellitus is the most common cause of ESKD in the country.[252]

SINGAPORE

The incidence of reported ESKD in Singapore in 2011 was 279 per million population, and the prevalence was 1661 per million population.[243a] Hemodialysis accounted for 87% and PD for 13% of dialysis therapy. The prevalence of patients with a kidney transplant was 353, 360, and 369 per million population in 2009, 2010, and 2011, respectively. More than 60% received a kidney from a deceased donor. The proportion of incident patients with ESKD due to diabetes in 2011 was 60%.

INDONESIA

The prevalences of patients with ESKD and patients receiving RRT in Indonesia have not been reported. A questionnaire survey from 13 nephrology centers in Indonesia showed that the prevalence of ESKD had risen, and the results of this study support previous data. A national registry of ESKD has just been developed for Indonesia. Although hemodialysis facilities have been developed rapidly, further development is still required. Continuous ambulatory peritoneal dialysis as an alternative RRT is only now being introduced. Kidney transplantation programs are expanding very slowly.[253] RRT still imposes a high cost of treatment for ESKD; therefore, these treatments are unaffordable for most patients. Government health insurance has begun to cover financially strained families requiring RRT.[253] A questionnaire survey in Java showed an increasing prevalence and incidence of RRT. The prevalence of RRT (HD, CAPD, and transplantation) in Indonesians increased from 1517 in 2002 to 3549 in 2006, with a rise in the prevalence rate from 10.2 to 23.4 per million population.[253] Health insurance is limited primarily to government officials. Most of the cost of dialysis must be covered by patients. The provision of RRT is therefore limited because the average gross domestic product per capita is far less than the cost of dialysis. Renal transplantation is performed in a few centers in major cities. Kidney donors are living relatives because deceased donors are not accepted.[253]

VIETNAM

The data available to public about the RRT in Vietnam are limited. According to a preliminary study, the prevalence of treated ESKD in Vietnam is approximately 120 per million population,[254] and the most common causes of the disease are glomerulonephritis, hypertension, and diabetes mellitus. PD was first performed in 1968, and hemodialysis in 1983. The first kidney transplant procedure was performed in 1992. In 2007, approximately 4000 patients with ESKD were treated with hemodialysis. Hemodialysis facilities are located in major cities. The total number of dialysis units has risen from 20 in 2001 to more than 60 in 2009. During the 10-year period 1992 to 2002, only 200 patients received a kidney transplant in Vietnam.

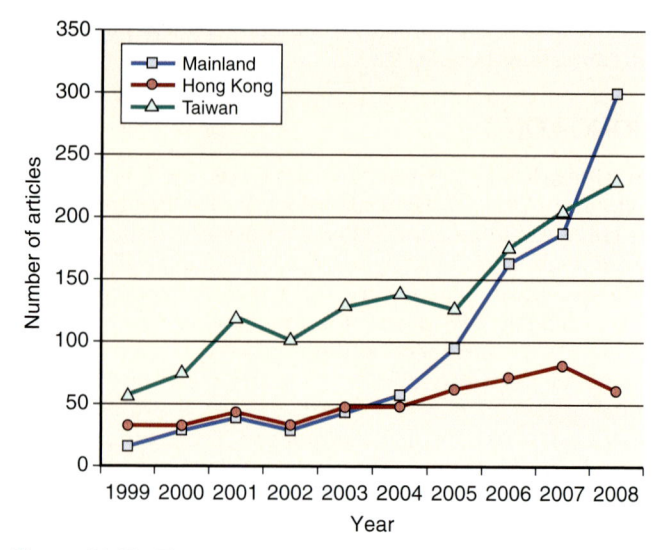

Figure 81.17 Trends in annual numbers of articles published by researchers from mainland China, Hong Kong, and Taiwan from 1999 to 2008. (From Xu J, Mao ZG, Kong M, et al: Scientific publications in nephrology and urology journals from Chinese authors in East Asia: a 10-year survey of the literature. *PLoS ONE* 6:e14781, 2011.)

THE PHILIPPINES

The incidence and prevalence of ESKD in the Philippines in 2011 were 103 and 159 per million population, respectively.[243a] Hemodialysis was the modality in 96.4% of all dialysis recipients in the same year. The transplantation rate was 3.8 per million population. The leading cause of ESKD in the Philippines is diabetic nephropathy occurring in ~45% of patients.

SCIENTIFIC PUBLICATIONS

Nephrology and urology have been practiced in China, Hong Kong, and Taiwan since the 1950s and have developed significantly in mainland China since China's integration with the international community in the 1980s. A 2011 report assessed the contribution of Chinese writers from the different regions to kidney research.[255] A total of 101,632 articles were published in 61 journals from 1999 to 2008 (Figure 81.17). The number of articles from the mainland has exceeded that from Hong Kong since 2004 and surpassed that from Taiwan in 2008. The total number of randomized control trials did not differ among the three regions. According to the *ISI Journal Citation Report*, the cumulative impact factor (after exclusion of those publications for which this information was not available) of articles from Taiwan (3620.7) was much higher than that of articles from mainland China (2272.9) and Hong Kong (1589.2; $P = 0.008$). However, articles from Hong Kong had the highest impact factor (3.2), followed by those from Taiwan (2.7) and mainland China (2.3; $P < 0.001$).

Complete reference list available at ExpertConsult.com.

KEY REFERENCES

6. Yang CW: Leptospirosis renal disease: understanding the initiation by Toll-like receptors. *Kidney Int* 72:918–925, 2007.

12. Yang HY, Hsu PY, Pan MJ, et al: Clinical distinction and evaluation of leptospirosis in Taiwan—a case-control study. *J Nephrol* 18:45–53, 2005.
22. Yang HY, Yen TH, Lin CY, et al: Early identification of leptospirosis as an ignored cause of multiple organ dysfunction syndrome. *Shock* 38:24–29, 2012.
27. Yen TH, Chang CT, Lin JL, et al: Scrub typhus: a frequently overlooked cause of acute renal failure. *Ren Fail* 25:397–410, 2003.
31. Jang MO, Kim JE, Kim UJ, et al: Differences in the clinical presentation and the frequency of complications between elderly and non-elderly scrub typhus patients. *Arch Gerontol Geriatr* 58:196–200, 2014.
38. Kim DPH: A case of scrub typhus requiring maintenance hemodialysis. *Kidney Res Clin Pract* 32:190–193, 2013.
44. Chen ZH, Qin XC, Song R, et al: Co-circulation of multiple hemorrhagic fever diseases with distinct clinical characteristics in Dandong, China. *PLoS ONE* 9:e89896, 2014.
55. Li W, He YW: Infection with a novel virus causes hemorrhagic fever in China. *Int J Infect Dis* 17:e556–e561, 2013.
64. White NJ, Pukrittayakamee S, Hien TT, et al: Malaria. *Lancet* 383:723–735, 2014.
69. Barsoum RS: Malarial acute renal failure. *J Am Soc Nephrol* 11:2147–2154, 2000.
71. Thanachartwet V, Desakorn V, Sahassananda D, et al: Acute renal failure in patients with severe falciparum malaria: using the WHO 2006 and RIFLE criteria. *Int J Nephrol* 2013:841518, 2013.
78. Guzman MG, Harris E: Dengue. *Lancet* 385:453–465, 2015.
96. Peiris JS, Yuen KY, Osterhaus AD, et al: The severe acute respiratory syndrome. *N Engl J Med* 349:2431–2441, 2003.
98. Chu KH, Tsang WK, Tang CS, et al: Acute renal impairment in coronavirus-associated severe acute respiratory syndrome. *Kidney Int* 67:698–705, 2005.
113. Kanjanabuch T, Sitprija V: Snakebite nephrotoxicity in Asia. *Semin Nephrol* 28:363–372, 2008.
127. Xuan BH, Mai HL, Thi TX, et al: Swarming hornet attacks: shock and acute kidney injury—a large case series from Vietnam. *Nephrol Dial Transplant* 25:1146–1150, 2010.
128. Zhang L, Yang Y, Tang Y, et al: Recovery from AKI following multiple wasp stings: a case series. *Clin J Am Soc Nephrol* 8:1850–1856, 2013.
137. Niticharoenpong K, Chalermsanyakorn P, Panvichian R, et al: Acute deterioration of renal function induced by star fruit ingestion in a patient with chronic kidney disease. *J Nephrol* 19:682–686, 2006.
138. Frank H, Zilker T, Kirchmair M, et al: Acute renal failure by ingestion of *Cortinarius* species confounded with psychoactive mushrooms: a case series and literature survey. *Clin Nephrol* 71:557–562, 2009.
144. Guan N, Fan Q, Ding J, et al: Melamine-contaminated powdered formula and urolithiasis in young children. *N Engl J Med* 360:1067–1074, 2009.
145. Ingelfinger JR: Melamine and the global implications of food contamination. *N Engl J Med* 359:2745–2748, 2008.
148. Zuo L, Ma YC, Zhou YH, et al: Application of GFR-estimating equations in Chinese patients with chronic kidney disease. *Am J Kidney Dis* 45:463–472, 2005.
151. Matsuo S, Imai E, Horio M, et al: Revised equations for estimated GFR from serum creatinine in Japan. *Am J Kidney Dis* 53:982–992, 2009.
152. Rule AD, Teo BW: GFR estimation in Japan and China: what accounts for the difference? *Am J Kidney Dis* 53:932–935, 2009.
153. Zhang L, Wang F, Wang L, et al: Prevalence of chronic kidney disease in China: a cross-sectional survey. *Lancet* 379:815–822, 2012.
162. Nasr SH, Radhakrishnan J, D'Agati VD: Bacterial infection-related glomerulonephritis in adults. *Kidney Int* 83:792–803, 2013.
165. Nasr SH, Fidler ME, Valeri AM, et al: Postinfectious glomerulonephritis in the elderly. *J Am Soc Nephrol* 22:187–195, 2011.
171. Xu Y, Wang L, He J, et al: Prevalence and control of diabetes in Chinese adults. *JAMA* 310:948–959, 2013.
172. Zhou FD, Zhao MH, Zou WZ, et al: The changing spectrum of primary glomerular diseases within 15 years: a survey of 3331 patients in a single Chinese centre. *Nephrol Dial Transplant* 24:870–876, 2009.
175. Yu XQ, Li M, Zhang H, et al: A genome-wide association study in Han Chinese identifies multiple susceptibility loci for IgA nephropathy. *Nat Genet* 44:178–182, 2012.
176. Gharavi AG, Kiryluk K, Choi M, et al: Genome-wide association study identifies susceptibility loci for IgA nephropathy. *Nat Genet* 43:321–327, 2011.
177. Shi SF, Wang SX, Jiang L, et al: Pathologic predictors of renal outcome and therapeutic efficacy in IgA nephropathy: validation of the Oxford classification. *Clin J Am Soc Nephrol* 6:2175–2184, 2011.
178. Tanaka S, Ninomiya T, Katafuchi R, et al: Development and validation of a prediction rule using the Oxford classification in IgA nephropathy. *Clin J Am Soc Nephrol* 8:2082–2090, 2013.
179. Lee H, Yi SH, Seo MS, et al: Validation of the Oxford classification of IgA nephropathy: a single-center study in Korean adults. *Korean J Intern Med* 27:293–300, 2012.
180. Le W, Liang S, Hu Y, et al: Long-term renal survival and related risk factors in patients with IgA nephropathy: results from a cohort of 1155 cases in a Chinese adult population. *Nephrol Dial Transplant* 27:1479–1485, 2012.
181. Moriyama T, Tanaka K, Iwasaki C, et al: Prognosis in IgA nephropathy: 30-year analysis of 1,012 patients at a single center in Japan. *PLoS ONE* 9:e91756, 2014.
184. Matsuzaki K, Suzuki Y, Nakata J, et al: Nationwide survey on current treatments for IgA nephropathy in Japan. *Clin Exp Nephrol* 17:827–833, 2013.
186. Kawamura T, Yoshimura M, Miyazaki Y, et al: A multicenter randomized controlled trial of tonsillectomy combined with steroid pulse therapy in patients with immunoglobulin A nephropathy. *Nephrol Dial Transplant* 29:1546–1553, 2014.
192. Qin W, Beck LH, Jr, Zeng C, et al: Anti-phospholipase A2 receptor antibody in membranous nephropathy. *J Am Soc Nephrol* 22:1137–1143, 2011.
200. Chan TM, Li FK, Tang CS, et al: Efficacy of mycophenolate mofetil in patients with diffuse proliferative lupus nephritis. Hong Kong-Guangzhou Nephrology Study Group. *N Engl J Med* 343:1156–1162, 2000.
212. Lai QY, Ma TT, Li ZY, et al: Predictors for mortality in patients with antineutrophil cytoplasmic autoantibody-associated vasculitis: a study of 398 Chinese patients. *J Rheumatol* 41:1849–1855, 2014.
215. Johnson RJ, Couser WG: Hepatitis B infection and renal disease: clinical, immunopathogenetic and therapeutic considerations. *Kidney Int* 37:663–676, 1990.
217. Chan TM: Hepatitis B and renal disease. *Curr Hepat Rep* 9:99–105, 2010.
226. Ando M, Yanagisawa N, Ajisawa A, et al: Urinary albumin excretion within the normal range is an independent risk for near-term development of kidney disease in HIV-infected patients. *Nephrol Dial Transplant* 26:3923–3929, 2011.
233. Zhong Y, Deng Y, Chen Y, et al: Therapeutic use of traditional Chinese herbal medications for chronic kidney diseases. *Kidney Int* 84:1108–1118, 2013.
236. Wu FL, Chen YM, Lai TS, et al: Does Chinese herb nephropathy account for the high incidence of end-stage renal disease in Taiwan? *Nephron Clin Pract* 120:c215–c222, 2012.
237. Yang L, Su T, Li XM, et al: Aristolochic acid nephropathy: variation in presentation and prognosis. *Nephrol Dial Transplant* 27:292–298, 2012.
245. Yu X, Yang X: Peritoneal dialysis in China: meeting the challenge of chronic kidney failure. *Am J Kidney Dis* 65:147–151, 2015.
254. Van Bui P: How peritoneal dialysis has developed in Vietnam. *Perit Dial Int* 28(Suppl 3):S63–S66, 2008.
255. Xu J, Mao ZG, Kong M, et al: Scientific publications in nephrology and urology journals from Chinese authors in East Asia: a 10-year survey of the literature. *PLoS ONE* 6:e14781, 2011.

82 Oceania Region

Gavin J. Becker | John F. Collins | David C.H. Harris

CHAPTER OUTLINE

AUSTRALIA, 2539
Access to Health Care in Australia, 2539
Renal Replacement Therapy in Australia, 2540
Renal Supportive Care, 2544
Chronic Kidney Disease in Australia, 2544
Analgesic Nephropathy in Australia, 2544
Renal Disease in Indigenous Australians, 2546
NEW ZEALAND, 2549
Access to Health Care in New Zealand, 2549
Health Status of the Indigenous Population, 2549

Ethnic Differences in Microalbuminuria, Diabetes, Hypertension, and Glomerulonephritis, 2550
Chronic Kidney Disease and Diabetes, 2550
Renal Replacement Therapy, 2551
End-Stage Kidney Disease in Maori and Pacific Peoples, 2552
Reasons for Differences in Incidence of End-Stage Kidney Disease and Outcomes for Indigenous Maori and Pacific Populations, 2553
PACIFIC ISLANDS, 2553
CONCLUDING REMARKS, 2554

Oceania is a term coined by the French explorer Dumont d'Urville (1790-1842) that is now generally used to encompass a group of about 14 nations, mainly in the South Pacific (Figure 82.1). It includes Australia (population, 23.3 million), New Zealand (4.5 million), Papua New Guinea (7.1 million), and many other island nations with populations ranging from 858,000 to less than 2000 (Table 82.1). There are also great variations in economy, ethnicity, geography, and climate. The per capita income (gross domestic product [GDP] nominal per capita) does not account for cost of living, and purchasing power ranges from among the world's highest (Australia, $67,039; New Zealand, $38,674), to under $10,000 in many island nations (see Table 82.1). The combination of small population and low income means that renal care services are limited or absent in most of these small Pacific islands, as are accurate data on the incidence of renal disease. Exceptions to this are the Pacific Island groups, including French Polynesia, New Caledonia, and American Samoa, which are managed as dependent territories and thus have access to more substantial renal services.

This chapter discusses renal disease in Australia, New Zealand, and the island nations of Oceania, but not in the dependent territories. Because of the limited services in and data for the small island nations in Oceania, most of the focus will be on Australia and New Zealand.

The population mix of Oceania nations has important implications for the incidence of chronic kidney disease (CKD). Not only do Australia and New Zealand have large white communities of European heritage, but both have significant indigenous and Asian populations. In Australia, the indigenous Australians (sometimes termed *Aboriginal Australians*) are the descendants of the original human inhabitants of Australia who arrived on the continent over 40,000 years ago during the last Ice Age; they were separated from the rest of the world until the arrival of British settlers (mainly convicts) in 1788. The Aboriginal Australians and Torres Strait Islanders represent about 2.5% of Australians[1] and have been clearly demonstrated to have a very high risk of CKD.[2] In New Zealand, the Maori are the indigenous people of Polynesian origin, probably arriving from about 1200 AD, following a long period during which sea-borne Polynesians and Melanesians colonized the South Pacific Islands. Maori people also have a very high incidence of CKD.[2]

Throughout the rest of the Pacific Islands are the descendants of Melanesian (particularly in Papua New Guinea and the Solomon Islands), Micronesian (mainly in northern Oceania), and Polynesian (mainly in the Solomons and western Oceania) settlers, with a considerable intermixture and influences of Asian and white populations. Again, these island people, as far as can be ascertained, are particularly prone to CKD.

Australia and New Zealand have developed a number of valuable resources for monitoring and recommending management approaches for patients with renal disease (Table 82.2). They are fortunate in having maintained, since 1965, a comprehensive database of all patients beginning renal

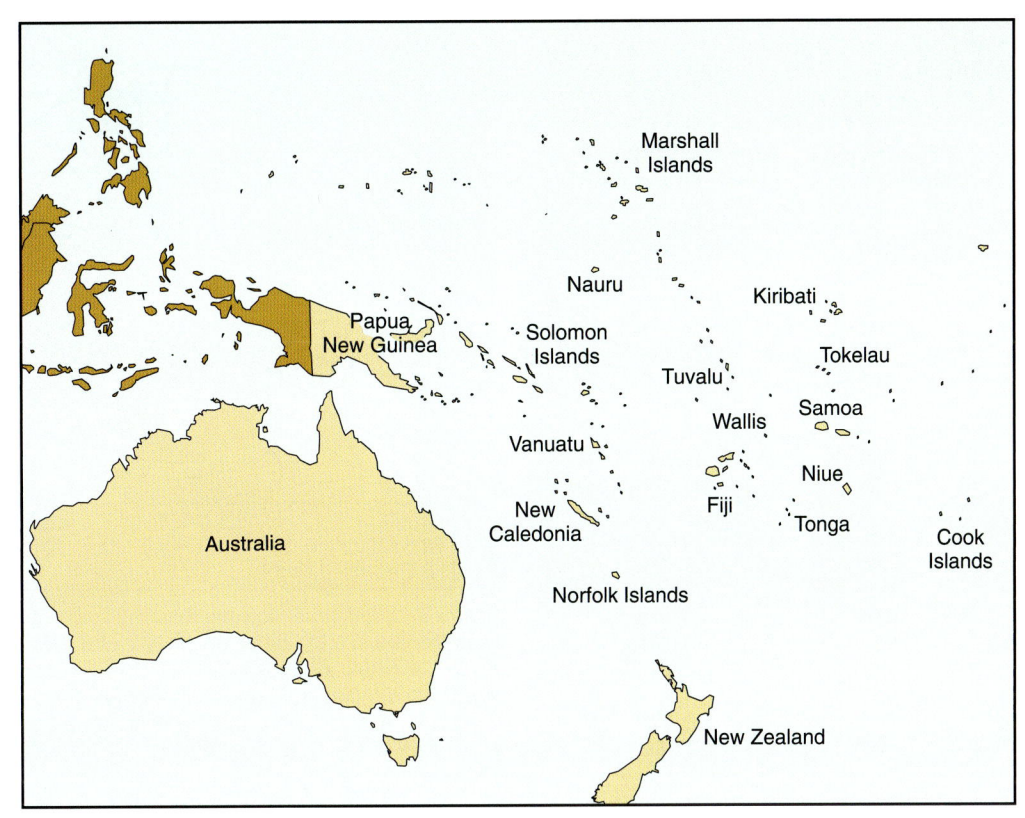

Figure 82.1 Oceania region, an area mainly in the South Pacific, comprising Australia, New Zealand, Papua New Guinea, and a number of island states. (Modified from Geography World: Available at: http://www.geographyworldonline.com. Accessed December 2013.)

replacement therapy (RRT)—the Australia and New Zealand Dialysis and Transplant Registry (ANZDATA). The past and most recent annual reports, including by regular and occasional chapters of items of interest, can be accessed online (http://www.anzdata.org.au).[3] This registry has provided an invaluable resource for health care surveillance, clinical care planning, research into renal diseases, and descriptions of outcomes of RRT. From ANZDATA reports and associated papers comes information essential to this chapter. There is also a registry of living renal transplant donors (Australia and New Zealand Organ Donation Registry [ANZOD], which can also be accessed through the ANZDATA website).[3] There are no accessible registries of renal disease for the rest of Oceania.

The Australian and New Zealand Society of Nephrology (ANZSN; http://www.nephrology.edu.au) and Kidney Health Australia (KHA; http://www.kidney.org.au; previously the Australian Kidney Foundation) combined in 1999 to set up an ongoing, evidence-based, clinical practice guideline (CPG) project titled *Caring for Australasians with Renal Impairment* (CARI, http://www.cari.org.au). Since then, a large number of CPGs have been produced that can be accessed through this website. A valuable resource for evidence from clinical trials for such CPGs is the Cochrane Renal Group, based in Sydney, Australia (http://www.cochrane-renal.org). The KHA has developed a number of other valuable initiatives and resources, such as the health professional education program Kidney Check Australia Taskforce (KCAT), which can be accessed via the KHA website. In addition, ANZSN and KHA jointly sponsor a biannual Dialysis, Nephrology, and Transplantation workshop that examines important contemporary issues in nephrology practice, including the CARI CPGs. Australia and New Zealand have a strong tradition of basic and clinical renal disease research. Coordination of multicenter clinical trials investigating renal disease is being facilitated by the Australasian Kidney Trials Network (http://www.uq.edu.au/aktn).

AUSTRALIA

ACCESS TO HEALTH CARE IN AUSTRALIA

Australia has a taxpayer-funded medical care provision system (Australian Medicare) that provides health care to all Australians at minimal or no direct cost to the patient, as well as an active private health system underpinned by private health insurance. Accordingly, at least theoretically, all forms of renal care are available to all Australians. However, there are many areas of Australia that are sparsely populated, particularly those where indigenous Australians commonly live and, although health care costs are low for the patient, they are by no means negligible, because transport, a proportion of medication expenses, and accommodation costs when away from home are not covered under the Medicare arrangement. Accordingly, strategies to deal with geographic distance (e.g., transplantation, home and satellite dialysis) and to minimize cost to Australia and the patient are an ongoing reality of nephrology practice. Poor

Table 82.1 Population and Gross Domestic Product per capita of Oceania Nations

Nation	Population (in thousands)*	GDP per Capita ($ per person/year)†
American Samoa	56	3,629
Australia	23,168	67,039
Cook Islands	15	13,478
Fiji	858	4,391
Kiribati	106	1,813
Marshall Islands	56	3,448
Federated States of Micronesia	101	2,855
Nauru	10	6,954
New Caledonia	259	38,690
New Zealand	4,474	38,674
Niue	2	4,700
Palau	21	11,096
Papua New Guinea	7,060	1,794
Samoa	189	6,300
Solomon Islands	561	1,518
Tokelau Islands	1.4	Not available
Tonga	103	4,335
Tuvalu	11	3,713
Vanuatu	265	3,168

*Data from Wikipedia: List of countries by population. Available at: http://www.wikipedia.org/wiki/list_of_countries_by_population. Accessed December 2013.
†Data from National Accounts Main Aggregates Database, December 2012, United Nations Statistics Division; Nuie data from The World Factbook, Central Intelligence Agency, October 2013. Available at: http://en.wikipedia.org/wiki/List_of_countries_by_GDP_(nominal_PPP)_per_capita. Accessed December 2013.

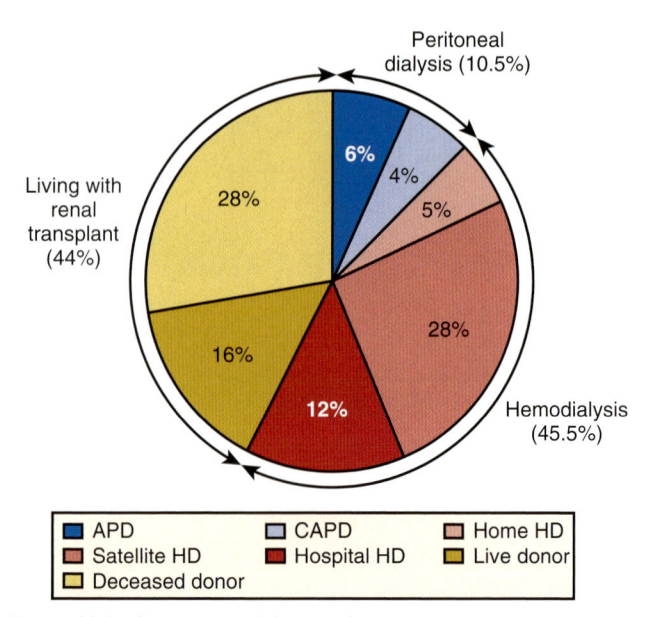

Figure 82.2 Patients receiving renal replacement therapy in Australia in December 2011 (total, 19,751 patients; 88,597 patients pmp). APD, Automated peritoneal dialysis; CAPD, continuous ambulatory peritoneal dialysis; HD, home hemodialysis. (Data from McDonald S, Clayton P, Hurst K [editors]: ANZDATA registry report, thirty-fifth report, Adelaide, Australia, 2012, Australia and New Zealand Dialysis and Transplant Registry.)

access to nephrology services by those in rural and remote communities has been compounded by a relative deficit in the number of nephrologists who service these communities. It is doubtful that all Australians who should have renal care are recognized and treated, and isolated indigenous communities and the socioeconomically underprivileged are particularly vulnerable to remaining unnoticed. This concern is underscored by marked variation in the standardized incidence of patients beginning RRT in the various capital cities of Australia.[4] In areas where socioeconomic disadvantage is more common, the incidence of RRT is higher,[5] yet late referral is more frequent, which suggests less access to care before end-stage kidney disease (ESKD) has developed.[4,6]

RENAL REPLACEMENT THERAPY IN AUSTRALIA

The 2012 ANZDATA Registry report[7] showed that on December 31, 2011, there were 19,751 Australians (885 patients per million population [pmp]) receiving RRT, 392 pmp with a functioning renal transplant, and 493 pmp undergoing dialysis (Figure 82.2). In 2011, 2453 Australians commenced RRT, an incidence rate of 110 persons pmp, similar to that of New Zealand (108 pmp)[7] and the United Kingdom (UK; 108 pmp),[8] but markedly lower than in the other predominantly white populations in the United States (348 pmp in 2010),[9] Canada (159 pmp),[10] and Europe as a whole, UK included (123 pmp).[11] The explanation for these discrepancies is unclear, but the prevalence and treatment of causes of progressive CKD, as well as acceptance criteria for RRT, are suspected to be two contributing factors.[12] Even among various regions or states of Australia, the incidence rates vary widely, influenced partly by the proportion of the population made up of indigenous Australians, who have a

Table 82.2 Valuable Australia and New Zealand Websites Relevant to Renal Disease*

Website	URL
Australian and New Zealand Dialysis and Transplant Registry (ANZDATA)	http://www.anzdata.org.au
Australian and New Zealand Organ Donor Registry (ANZOD)	
Australasian Kidney Trials Network (AKTN)	http://www.uq.edu.au/aktn
Australian and New Zealand Society of Nephrology	http://www.nephrology.edu.au
Caring for Australasians with Renal Impairment (CARI)	www.cari.org.au
Cochrane Renal Group	www.cochrane-renal.org
Kidney Health Australia (KHA)	www.kidney.org.au
Transplantation Society of Australia and New Zealand	www.tsanz.com.au

*Accessed December 2013.

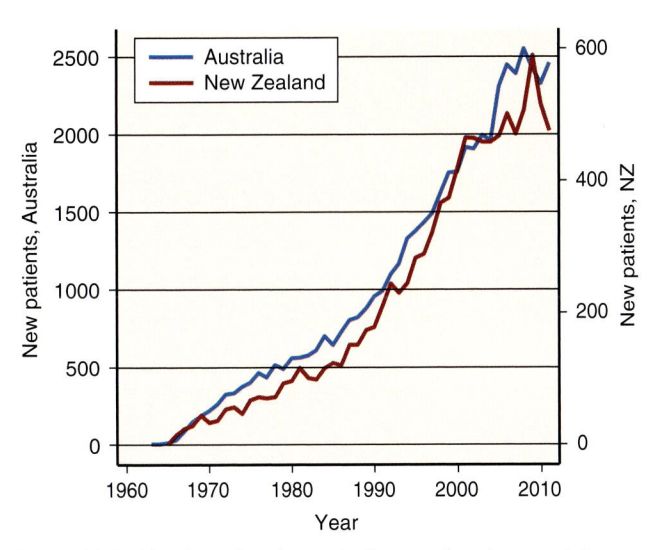

Figure 82.3 Number of patients starting renal replacement therapy in Australia and New Zealand. (From McDonald S, Clayton P, Hurst K [editors]: *ANZDATA registry report, thirty-fifth report,* Adelaide, Australia, 2012, Australia and New Zealand Dialysis and Transplant Registry.)

Table 82.3 Age, Gender, and Coded Causes of End-Stage Kidney Disease in Patients Beginning Renal Replacement Therapy

Parameter	United States (2010 figures)*	Australia (2011 figures)[†]
Number (% male)	114,281 (56.9%)	2453 (59.6%)
Incidence rate (pmp)	348	110
% of cases > 75 yr	25.1	20.8
Coded causes of ESKD (%)		
• Diabetes	44	35
• Hypertension	29	15
• Glomerulonephritis	6	23
• Polycystic disease	2	6
• Other (including unknown)	—	21

*Data from Collins AJ, Foley RN, Herzog C, et al: US Renal Data System 2012 annual data report. *Am J Kidney Dis* 61(Suppl 1):A7, e1-e476. 2013.
[†]Data from McDonald S, Clayton S, Hurst K (editors): *ANZDATA registry report, thirty-fifth report,* Adelaide, Australia, 2012, Australia and New Zealand Dialysis and Transplant Registry.

particularly high incidence rate of RRT when compared with nonindigenous Australians.[2,7,13,14] Nonindigenous rural Australians have a lower incidence of RRT; whether this reflects lower disease rates or differential uptake or access to RRT is not known.[15]

There was an almost continuous growth in the number of Australians commencing RRT each year from 1965 until about 2005; since then, the number has stabilized at about 2500 new RRT patients (110 pmp)/year (Figure 82.3).[3,7] The age and coded causes of renal failure for patients commencing RRT in 2010 in the United States[9] and 2011 in Australia[7] are summarized in Table 82.3. The mean age in the United States was slightly higher, at 63.0 years, compared with 60.0 years in Australia. Of U.S. incident RRT patients, 25% were 75 years of age or older, whereas in Australia only about 21% were in this age group (Figure 82.4), confirming a greater tendency for older patients to begin RRT in the United States. In addition, there is a great discrepancy in the coded causes of ESKD, with the United States reporting more cases than Australia as being due to diabetes (43% vs. 35%) and hypertension (28% vs. 15%); Australia had a much higher proportion coded as glomerulonephritis (23% vs. 6%). The higher proportion caused by diabetes could account for some of the higher incidence rates of RRT in the United States. The higher proportion of cases due to hypertension in the United States is balanced by the higher proportion due to glomerulonephritis in Australia, a discrepancy that may be real or may be related to coding and renal biopsy practices.

The pressures of remote geography, cost, and a belief that home therapies offer a better lifestyle, with less morbidity and mortality, have led Australia to encourage home dialysis and renal transplantation. Accordingly, the 2012 ANZDATA report[7] showed that at the end of 2011, 27.7% of the 10,998 Australian dialysis patients were receiving some form of home treatment; of these, 18.8% were

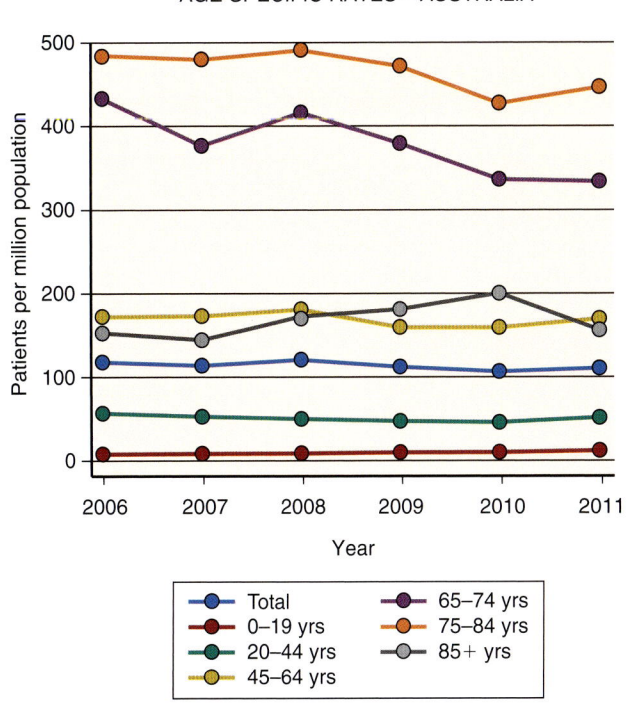

Figure 82.4 Acceptance of new patients for renal replacement therapy in 2006 to 2011—age-specific rates for Australia. (From McDonald S, Clayton P, Hurst K [editors]: *ANZDATA registry report, thirty-fifth report,* Adelaide, Australia, 2012, Australia and New Zealand Dialysis and Transplant Registry.)

undergoing peritoneal dialysis [PD] and 7.9% home hemodialysis [HD]. Of RRT patients, 44.3% were alive with a functioning renal transplant, meaning that overall nearly 60% of all 19,751 prevalent RRT Australians were treated at home (see Figure 82.2).

The economic issues of RRT in Australia have been analyzed in depth. In 2006, a report on the economic impact of ESKD in Australia showed the potential savings to be made by increasing the number of ESKD patients treated by renal transplantation or home dialysis rather than hospital-based dialysis.[16] This was followed by further analyses, which indicated that from 2005 to 2010, increasing renal transplantations by 10% to 50% would have saved between A$5.8 to $26.2 million in cumulative costs, and switching all new RRT patients from hospital HD to home HD or home PD would have saved A$46.6 million or A$122.1 million, respectively.[17] Government policy in Australia therefore strongly encourages renal transplantation over dialysis and home dialysis over hospital dialysis.

DIALYSIS

In December 2011, 10,998 persons (493 pmp) were undergoing dialysis treatment in Australia. Of these, 8.8% received home HD, 18.8% received PD (virtually all at home), and 72.3% were on hospital- or satellite unit–based HD[18] (see Figure 82.2). The distinction between hospital and satellite unit is blurred, because many satellite units are positioned in or near smaller metropolitan and rural hospitals.

Home Hemodialysis

Home HD began in Australia in 1967, after a patient traveling in the United States became uremic and was treated with HD in Seattle. He was then sent to the Royal Melbourne Hospital and was taught to perform dialysis, which he then did at home in Sydney (see George[19] for a review of the history of home HD in Australia). In 1968, the advisory body to the government on health and science, the National Health and Medical Research Committee (NHMRC), suggested that if renal transplantation were unlikely or impossible, the preferred alternative should be HD for financial and medical reasons. Since then, there has been ongoing encouragement of home HD throughout Australia, with observational evidence suggesting a survival benefit[20] (Figure 82.5). This has not been matched, however, by a rise in the proportion of Australian dialysis patients performing home HD, which peaked at 52% in 1977 and is now only 8.8%, with stable, actual patient numbers around 950 to 980 since around 2010.[7] Many clinicians hope that an evidence-based change in technology (simpler machines) or practice (extended hours or increased frequency) would be required to increase home HD numbers and proportions.[21-23] There are marked regional variations in home HD rates,[18] from the lowest proportion in South Australia (2.5% of all dialysis patients) to the highest in New South Wales/Australian Capital Territory (NSW/ACT; 12.8%), suggesting that geography, demographics, and local attitudes all play a role.

Nocturnal home HD has been enthusiastically promoted and implemented by many HD services as a method of increasing dialysis hours, frequency, or dose, as well as increasing the adoption of home HD.[21,24-26] Usually, with conventional HD machines and consumables, patients undergo dialysis for 8 to 10 hours at home overnight on alternate nights or on 6 nights a week. A variety of clinical advantages and cost savings over satellite or center HD have been suggested.[24,25] In many cases, however, the change has only meant that patients who would previously have performed more conventional home HD are now performing nocturnal home HD because the same technologic barriers of machine complexity, vascular access, and environmental constraints still exist. Accordingly, this has not yet resulted in any increase in the proportion of HD patients performing home HD.

Consistent with data suggesting an increased mortality associated with the use of central venous catheters (CVCs) and arteriovenous grafts (AVGs),[27] great attention has been paid to vascular access modalities in Australia.[28-30] Despite this, and despite evidence showing that an early referral and access program could reduce CVC usage,[31] in 2011 54% of Australians began HD with a CVC (42% tunneled, 12% nontunneled), with great center to center variation from a reported 0 to about 80% of patients in each of 45 centers commencing HD with an arteriovenous fistula (AVF) or AVG.[7] A previous review of HD access trends from 2000 to 2005 found an increase in the use of CVCs and AVGs.[30] Multivariate analyses were performed to examine the effects of age, gender, race, body mass index (BMI), time of referral, smoking status, cause of ESKD, comorbid conditions, and duration of dialysis on the type of access in each cohort year from 2000 to 2005. However, adjustment for these factors did not alter the trend, which was then attributed to

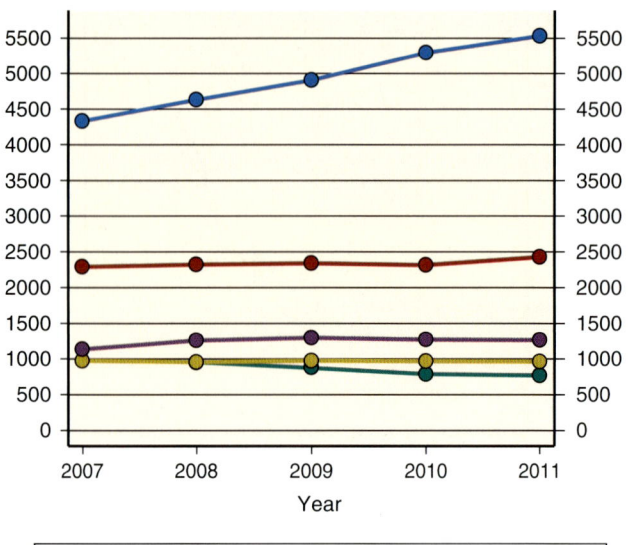

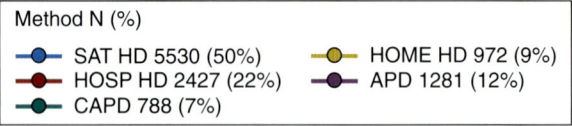

Figure 82.5 Method and location of dialysis in Australia (December 2007 to 2011). APD, Automated peritoneal dialysis; CAPD, continuous automated peritoneal dialysis; HD, home hemodialysis; SAT satellite. (From McDonald S, Clayton P, Hurst K [editors]: *ANZDATA registry report, thirty-fifth report,* Adelaide, Australia, 2012, Australia and New Zealand Dialysis and Transplant Registry.)

unidentified practice patterns, attitudes, or preferences. No systematic approach to changing this situation is currently in place.

Recent prominent randomized clinical trials (RCTs) involving dialysis practices in Australia and New Zealand have included the IDEAL study, comparing early with late initiation of dialysis,[32] and the balANZ study, comparing the effects of peritoneal dialysis with low levels of glucose degradation products with conventional solutions.[33] It is too early to determine whether these RCTs will have any effect on Australian dialysis practices. The death rate among patients receiving dialysis in Australia in 2011 was 13.7/100 patient-years, with some indication of a steady improvement over the last decade.[7] Comparisons are, however, confounded by factors such as age, comorbidities, and withdrawal of transplanted patients.

RENAL TRANSPLANTATION

The renal transplantation rate for Australians in 2011 was 37 pmp, just over one third of the rate of patients beginning RRT (110 pmp).[7] Renal transplant rates have increased slowly but reasonably steadily over the decades[3] (374 in 1981, 470 in 1991, 541 in 2001, and 825 cases/year in 2011). Deceased donor transplant numbers increased from 344 to 570/year from 2007 to 2011. Live donor transplantation has become a very important part of RRT in Australia, increasing from 78 in 1991 to 255 cases/year in 2011.[3] The peak was in 2008, when 354 live donor transplants resulted in 43.5% of all renal transplantations. Since then, this has steadily declined toward 2011, both in number (255/year) and proportion (30.9% of renal transplantations). Some of this decrease may be attributable to a previous catch-up period in which, as confidence in live donor transplantation increased, a backlog of dialysis patients previously languishing on dialysis were transplanted, but research is required to ascertain what barriers still exist. There is considerable variation in these rates among regions, states, and individual hospitals, which suggests variations in local practices and attitudes to living donation. The proportion of live donor transplantations performed before dialysis (preemptive) has increased from 26% in 2007 to 37% in 2011.[3]

Many other factors have contributed to the overall increase in transplantation rates, including a federal government–funded organ donor recruitment program, reintroduction of nonbeating heart organ donors, introduction of ABO incompatible donations, and a nationwide, paired, kidney exchange program. Concurrent with this, the deceased renal donor kidney waiting list in Australia has been decreasing, from 1380 on the active waiting list on December 31, 2007 to 1190 on December 31, 2010.[7] The death rate for transplant patients with functioning grafts in 2011 was 2.3% (the major causes being cardiovascular and malignancy); the graft failure rate was 2.2% (mainly due to chronic allograft nephropathy), giving a total annual graft loss rate of 4.5%.[7]

The benefits of a system in Australia whereby renal dialysis and renal transplantation units were integrated to facilitate patient movement between these modalities of RRT were outlined over 30 years ago.[34] However, the trend toward the establishment of free-standing, publicly funded and private dialysis units has gradually decreased such integration over that period. The effect on transplantation rates has not been assessed, but a comparison of transplantation activity and waiting times in free-standing and integrated programs will be of interest in the future.

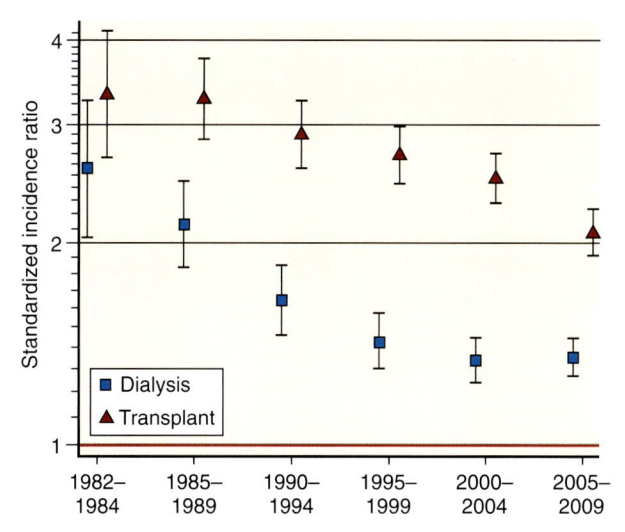

Figure 82.6 Risk of cancer after transplantation, 1982 to 2009. (Date from McDonald S, Clayton P, Hurst K [editors]: *ANZDATA registry report, thirty-fifth report,* Adelaide, Australia, 2012, Australia and New Zealand Dialysis and Transplant Registry.)

Cancer in Renal Transplant Recipients

Because of the combination of a large population of people of northern European heritage (fair skin), intense summer sunlight, and an outdoor culture, Australia and New Zealand became a focus for data on renal transplantation–related skin and other cancers from the very early days of renal transplantation.[36-44] Australia has the highest community rate of skin cancer in the world, almost four times that in the United States, UK, and Europe. Nearly two of every three Australians will have one or more skin cancers by the age of 70 years.[45] It should not be surprising, therefore, that as early as 1977 high cancer rates in renal transplant recipients in Australia and New Zealand were being reported[35] and, by 1981 the ANZDATA report began an annual review of cancers in renal transplant recipients, which is still ongoing. By 1982, these reviews showed that by 10 years after transplantation, over 30% of recipients had some form of skin cancer, and a further 10% had a non–skin cancer.[44] By 30 years after transplantation, 80% of Australian and New Zealand recipients had contracted some form of cancer, with 75% being skin cancers[36] (Figure 82.6).

If skin cancers and cancers known to cause renal failure are excluded, the risk of cancer in Australian and New Zealand transplant recipients is still over three times that in the general population, with a standardized incidence ratio (SIR) of 3.27, whereas the dialysis population has only a slightly increased risk (SIR = 1.35).[46] The 2012 ANDATA registry indicated an SIR after kidney transplantation for all cancers of 2.51.[7] This risk of cancer of two to three times that of the general community is not dissimilar to the rate found in renal transplant recipients in the United States,[47] with a similar but not identical pattern dominated by virus-associated conditions, (e.g., those linked to human papillomavirus [genitourinary and nasopharyngeal cancers], Epstein-Barr virus [lymphoproliferative diseases, nasopharyngeal cancer], and human herpesvirus type 8 [Kaposi's sarcoma, lymphoma]).[37,46] The relative risk decreases with increasing age and is lower for those with diabetic kidney disease, perhaps due to competing cardiovascular risk.[42]

Attention has thus been focused on the health and economic impact of screening programs for nonskin cancer in renal patients.[42,48] Although economic analyses have suggested that annual cervical cancer screening by the Papanicolaou (Pap) test of female renal transplant recipients aged 18 years or older is cost-effective,[43] and fecal occult blood testing or even regular surveillance colonoscopy for bowel cancer has been suggested,[40,41] doubts are raised when all physical, psychologic, and economic costs and benefits are considered. This has led to recommendations for an individualized approach and for further research, including prospective randomized trials.[48]

RENAL SUPPORTIVE CARE

As is happening globally, in recent years in Australia, there has been a steady increase in the age of patients presenting or dying with advanced kidney failure,[49] with estimates that about 50%, especially older persons, do not receive RRT.[50,51] Many of these older patients are frail and have considerable comorbidity. Dialysis may not be in their best interest. The ANZDATA 2012 report indicated that the presence of one to three or more comorbidities (e.g., chronic heart disease, peripheral vascular disease, cerebrovascular disease, chronic lung disease, diabetes mellitus) at the time of commencing dialysis in older ANZ patients was associated with an increased hazard ratio (HR) for death of 1.43, 1.61, and 2.00, respectively, when compared with patients without any comorbidity.[7] In older patients with high comorbidity, survival may be no better with dialysis than with conservative nondialysis care.[52] Moreover, any increase in survival time in patients with comparable comorbidity may be consumed mainly by days on dialysis, and the quality of life may be no better with dialysis than with conservative care.[53] Accordingly, in Australia, as elsewhere, there has been a renewed interest in offering a supportive alternative to dialysis.[54] In conjunction with palliative care experts, comprehensive ANZSN guidelines focusing especially on symptom control have now been developed for renal supportive and palliative care.[55] Many of the details of clinical care in these recommendations are equally applicable to patients on dialysis, since they often suffer the same symptoms. Of the 1476 Australian dialysis patients who died in 2011 (nearly 40%), 485 were reported to have withdrawn from dialysis therapy for a wide variety of reasons, with the most being coded as "psychosocial."[7] The palliative care and symptom control requirements of this group of patients also warrant formal addressing.

CHRONIC KIDNEY DISEASE IN AUSTRALIA

The prevalence of CKD in Australia was first systematically estimated in the AusDiab Kidney Study.[56,57] Over 11,000 noninstitutionalized Australian adults aged 25 years or older were interviewed in 1999 and 2000 and tested for proteinuria (defined as a spot urine protein/creatinine ratio > 0.20 mg/mg), hematuria (dipstick testing confirmed by microscopy), and reduced estimated creatinine clearance adjusted for body size (defined as <60 mL/min/1.73 m^2 by the Cockcroft-Gault equation). Approximately 16% had at least one such indicator of damage, a prevalence of CKD similar to that seen in screening projects conducted elsewhere in the West. The most common finding was a reduced estimated creatinine clearance, which was present in 9.7% of those screened, mostly in subjects 65 years of age or older, particularly women. As elsewhere, much of this reduction in renal function seemed to be age-related, whereas proteinuria (2.4%) was associated more closely with diabetes.[57] When the Modification of Diet in Renal Disease (MDRD) and Chronic Kidney Disease Epidemiology Collaboration (CKD-EPI) formulas were used to define estimated creatinine clearance, the prevalence of CKD was reduced to 13.4% and 11.5%, respectively.[58] Most of those reclassified in this way as having no CKD were at low risk for cardiovascular disease. The causes of renal failure requiring RRT have changed considerably over the last 3 decades, with a decrease in the proportion and number of cases due to analgesic nephropathy and an increase in those coded as diabetic nephropathy or nephropathy due to hypertension. The latter could include a variety of conditions, such as various forms of nephrosclerosis, and probably reflects an aging population beginning RRT. The mean age at RRT commencement was 43 years in 1978 and increased to 60 years in 2011 (Table 82.4).[3,7]

The pattern of renal biopsy–proven glomerulonephritis in the state of Victoria in southern Australia was studied in a retrospective review examining all native kidney biopsy reports from hospitals in 1995 and 1997.[59] The biopsy rate for native kidneys was 21.5 individuals undergoing biopsy/year/100,000 population. The most common forms of glomerulonephritis found were immunoglobulin A (IgA) disease, focal segmental glomerulosclerosis (FSGS; of all types), vasculitis, and lupus glomerulonephritis. A similar study was performed and reported for the white population of Minnesota.[60] Biopsy rates were similar in the two studies; it is interesting to note that reasonably similar proportions of the same types of glomerular abnormality were found.

In the Victorian biopsy study, the calculated incidence and proportions of lupus nephritis, membranous nephropathy, IgA disease, and FSGS differed in patients who were beginning RRT, most likely reflecting the differing relative likelihood that patients with these diseases will progress to ESKD and RRT.[59] In all of Australia in 2011, of patients beginning and coded as having ESKD due to glomerulonephritis, 26% had biopsy-proven IgA disease, 14% glomerulosclerosis, 11% various forms of vasculitis, 7% membranous glomerulonephritis, and 5% lupus. Correctly or not, 15% were coded as having presumed glomerulonephritis without a renal biopsy having been performed.[7]

ANALGESIC NEPHROPATHY IN AUSTRALIA

A feature of Australian nephrology, not devoid of an element of Australian embarrassment, is the history of analgesic nephropathy (see detailed reviews by Kincaid-Smith,[61] Burry,[62] and Nanra[63,64]). Within about a decade of the first description in Swiss watch factory workers of an association between intake of phenacetin-containing analgesics, renal papillary necrosis, and chronic interstitial nephritis, the

Table 82.4 Changing Patterns in Renal Replacement Therapy (RRT) in Australia*

	Year				
	1977	1987	1997	2007	2011
No. of patients beginning RRT (pmp)	28	46	79	110	110
New transplants (pmp)	20	25	27	29	37
Total number with ESKD (pmp)	135	311	430	802	885
Mean age of new RRT patients (yr)	43	Not available	55.2	60.2	60.0
Cause of renal failure (%)					
• Glomerulonephritis	34	33	34	25	23
• Analgesic nephropathy	22	13	5	2	1
• Diabetic nephropathy	5	8	21	31	42
• Hypertension	5	5	12	16	11
• Polycystic kidney disease	2	8	6	6	5
• Other (including unknown)	34	41	28	26	18

*Over 34 years.
Data from ANZDATA registry reports 1979 to 2012, Adelaide, Australia, Australia and New Zealand Transplant Registry.

disease was widely recognized in Australia. An added association, that of peptic ulceration, was attributed to the aspirin contained in the compound analgesics regularly consumed in Australia.[65]

The social trend leading to this phenomenon could be seen to be particularly Australian. Although men could relieve their stress by enjoying "a few beers with their mates," women were left at home, where "a cup of tea, a Bex, and a good lie down" was the recommended solace. Bex and Vincent's brands of powders and pills were the most common compound analgesics freely available over the counter in general stores and milk bars throughout Australia. These contained aspirin, phenacetin, and caffeine (APC); encouraged by solid advertising campaigns, some women (and occasionally men) took 8 to 20 compound analgesic pills and powders every day for headaches, dysmenorrhea, other aches and pains, and even fatigue. The APC powders and pills combined the nephrotoxicity of phenacetin with the addictive properties of caffeine, and aspirin might have altered papillary microcirculation. The powders were especially troublesome, because they could be taken in large amounts without water and hence without dilution. Attempts to reduce intake were frustrated by caffeine withdrawal headache.

The virtual eradication of this disorder has been a triumph of investigative clinical research combined with laboratory science and applied public health measures. The descriptions of strong epidemiologic associations between phenacetin or compound analgesic intake and renal papillary necrosis were followed by experimental demonstrations of renal papillary necrosis and chronic tubulointerstitial nephritis induced in animals by various analgesics and nonsteroidal antiinflammatory drugs (NSAIDs).[63,64]

A determined effort by a group of Australian nephrologists led to the banning of the sale of compound analgesics in milk bars and grocery stores, as well as limitation of their availability from pharmacies from 1979 to the present. The age distribution of patients beginning maintenance dialysis for ESKD coded as being due to analgesic nephropathy quickly began to rise. As an indicator of just how long it takes for such a health measure to travel through all age groups in a community, aging patients with this disease continued to enter dialysis programs for many years, concurrent with an increase in the acceptance of older patients into RRT programs. Accordingly, the highest actual number of patients (not population-adjusted) beginning dialysis in Australia and coded as having analgesic nephropathy was in 1991, with 118 such patients (12% of all incident patients), 13 years after the banning of the APC compounds.[3,66] Since then, the number has declined steadily, to 42 patients in 2007 (2%) and only 2 to 5 patients (0 to 1%) per year since then (Figure 82.7). It seems likely that most patients with analgesic nephropathy now entering RRT programs in Australia are the very old survivors of the group, who were ingesting large amounts of compound analgesics before 1979 and are now 30 years older.[66]

It has been noticed that renal papillary necrosis, the hallmark of the phenacetin-associated analgesic syndrome, has

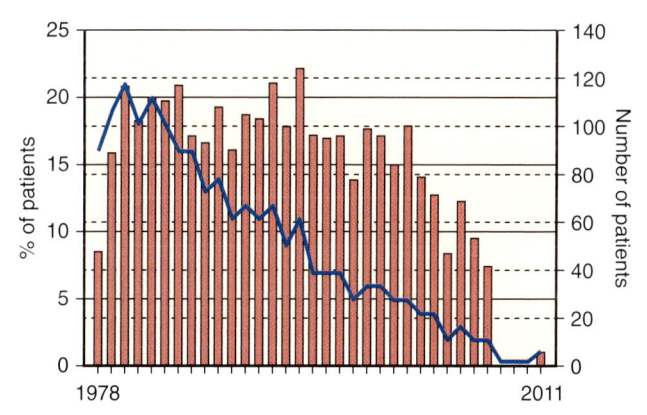

Figure 82.7 Number and proportion of Australian patients beginning renal replacement therapy (RRT) for whom analgesic nephropathy was coded as the cause of end-stage kidney disease (ESKD). *Bars* indicate the absolute numbers of patients/year; *blue line* represents the proportion of new RRT patients. (Data from *ANZDATA registry reports 1979 to 2012,* Adelaide, Australia, Australia and New Zealand Transplant Registry.)

become less common than the finding of tubulointerstitial nephritis on renal biopsy.[63] Similarly, transitional cell carcinoma of the uroepithelium, a common finding in cases of analgesic nephropathy due to APC abuse, is not often seen in the more recently diagnosed cases, in which NSAIDs have been implicated as the cause of chronic tubulointerstitial nephritis.

In Switzerland, where analgesic nephropathy was also common, changes typical of analgesic disease were found in 3% to 4% of autopsy cases during 1978 to 1980.[67] Phenacetin was banned from mixed analgesics in 1981 and was not available after 1983. An autopsy study conducted in 2000 found only one clear case of analgesic nephropathy in 616 consecutive autopsies, and that was in a patient who had had transplantation for ESKD due to analgesic nephropathy 14 years previously.[67] No new cases of classic analgesic nephropathy were found, although other patients had papillary necrosis or chronic interstitial fibrosis thought not to be due to analgesic abuse.

From 1971 to 2005, 10.2% of the 31,654 incident RRT patients in Australia were coded as having analgesic nephropathy.[66] Compared with nondiabetic patients receiving RRT, these patients had more vascular and pulmonary comorbid conditions and a higher all-cause, cardiovascular, infection, and cancer mortality.

RENAL DISEASE IN INDIGENOUS AUSTRALIANS

The indigenous Australian people had lived a mainly nomadic isolated existence for about 50,000 years before the white invasion, commencing with the arrival of the First Fleet in Sydney Cove in 1788. Their descendants now number about 549,370, or 2.5% of the overall Australian population.[1] They are irregularly distributed throughout Australia, with the highest numbers in NSW and Queensland, but the highest population proportion is in the Northern Territory, where they represent over 25% of the population. The incidence of ESKD in these indigenous Australians (as in indigenous New Zealanders) far exceeds that in the nonindigenous population.[14,68-72] In 2011, 250 indigenous persons began RRT in Australia, an incidence rate of over 450 pmp for Aboriginal and Torres Strait Island people,[72] about four times the incidence rate for Australians overall (110 pmp).[7] This incidence varies considerably in different states; it is lowest (140 pmp of Aboriginal and Torres Strait Island people) in Victoria/Tasmania and highest in the Northern Territory and Western Australia (980 and 630 pmp of Aboriginal and Torres Strait Island people, respectively). In the remote regions of the Northern Territory and Western Australia, the incidence can be as high as 30 times the national incidence for all Australians.[14] The average age of indigenous persons beginning RRT is about 10 years younger than the age for nonindigenous people,[63] with a particularly high relative incidence rate among those aged 35 to 64 years (Figure 82.8).

The reasons for the excessive burden of kidney disease among indigenous Australians have been the subject of much concern, investigation, and speculation for many years. Because indigenous Australians have been an isolated race for over 50,000 years, it seems possible that genetic influences could play a role. There are no good scientific data to support this notion, and it would not explain the

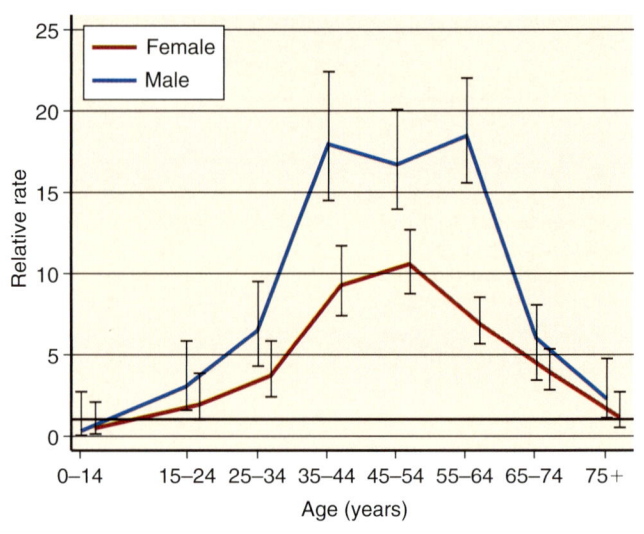

Figure 82.8 Relative incidence rate of renal replacement therapy for aboriginal versus nonaboriginal Australians. (From McDonald S, Jose M, Hurst K: End-stage kidney disease among indigenous peoples of Australia and New Zealand. In McDonald S, Clayton P, Hurst K, editors: *ANZDATA registry report, thirty-fifth report*, Adelaide, Australia, 2012, Australia and New Zealand Dialysis and Transplant Registry.)

vast geographic differences in incidence within indigenous Australians. However, worldwide, wherever adequate RRT is generally available, incidence rates are higher in nonwhite populations.

In the United States, rates among African Americans and Native Americans are 3.6 and 1.8 times higher, respectively, than the rates among whites.[12] In northern California, white persons have a much lower incidence of ESKD than African Americans or Asians living in the same area.[73] The ESKD Incidence Study Group reported that in Europe, Canada, and the Asia-Pacific region, all nonwhite populations had excess ESKD compared with their white counterparts.[6] In Asia, Japan and Taiwan, two nonwhite nations in which RRT is generally available, have the world's highest incidence of RRT for ESKD.[74,75] In Australia, immigrants from the British Isles and the rest of Europe have been shown to have a lower incidence of RRT than Australian-born citizens, whereas those from Asia, the Middle East, and southern Europe have a higher incidence.[76]

In all transitional non-Hispanic, nonwhite races studied, a higher incidence of type 2 diabetic ESKD has been found than in whites.[77] This might have a genetic basis, which has been suggested by familial clustering of diabetic nephropathy in type 2 diabetes in white and nonwhite families, but gene linkage studies to determine possible underlying genetic factors are at this stage very much in their infancy.[77] Hypertension is also more common in indigenous Australians.[78]

It is currently impossible to dissociate genetic or racial associations from geographic and socioeconomic considerations, and the latter are more amenable to intervention. One accepted framework links socioeconomic deprivation to low birth weight, fewer pancreatic islets, and fewer nephrons, and hence a propensity to the development of type 2 diabetes and progression of CKD[79,80] (see also Chapter 23). This would be consistent with the high rates of RRT in indigenous Australians and the regional variations, with much higher rates in the more disadvantaged remote areas of Australia.[14] It could also perhaps contribute to the high rates in Asia, where the years surrounding World War II were characterized by social and dietary deprivation.[81] Glomerulomegaly has been reported in renal biopsy specimens from Aboriginal patients with renal disease,[82-85] but a very small autopsy study ($n = 10$) of Aboriginal Australians without renal disease did not show any evidence that the glomeruli were larger than those in Australian whites ($n = 17$). However, the kidneys were much smaller, as was the body size of the Aboriginal individuals, which was proportionately reduced.[85]

Socioeconomic deprivation and isolation bring continuing health risks after birth. These include exposure to infections and toxins, reduced access to health care facilities, and often inadequate education about lifestyle risks, such as smoking and obesity, all of which can contribute to the risk of renal disease. In indigenous Australians, excessive incidences of ESKD due to type 2 diabetes and glomerulonephritis have been noted; in addition, type 1 diabetes, hypertensive renal disease, and analgesic nephropathy occur more frequently than in the nonindigenous population.[70]

The global problem of increasing ESKD in disadvantaged and developing populations is an ongoing concern, and the focus of efforts is to differentiate the influences of ethnicity from those of the environment.[73,86-89] In indigenous Australians, particularly those in remote regions, a wide range of risk factors for CKD has been identified. In 1998, Hoy and colleagues published the results of a community-wide screening program conducted in an isolated Northern Territory Aboriginal island community, where the ESKD incidence rate was 2700 pmp/year.[90] The results were truly shocking. Among the 71% for whom birth weight was known, 27.6% of individuals had been low-birth-weight babies (<2.5 kg). Many children had infections (e.g., skin sores, 67%; chronic middle ear disease, 80%; productive cough, 10%). Episodes of poststreptococcal glomerulonephritis had been experienced by 28.4% of those younger than 30 years and in 86% of them before 10 years of age. An association between childhood poststreptococcal glomerulonephritis and later albuminuria or proteinuria was demonstrated in later reports.[91]

Of the adults, 75% smoked, and many drank alcohol to excess; 20% had skin sores, 33% were overweight (BMI > 25 kg/m^2), 24% were hypertensive (systolic blood pressure ≥ 140 mm Hg or diastolic blood pressure ≥ 90 mm Hg, usually untreated), 19% had diabetes, and a further 12% had impaired glucose tolerance. Perhaps not surprisingly in this context, microalbuminuria or overt albuminuria was found in 5% of children aged 5 to 9 years, and this rose progressively with age, so in those individuals aged 50 years or older, 38% had microalbuminuria and 47% had overt albuminuria. Of all participants, 25% had hematuria by dipstick testing. Even after adjustment for all confounders, the following were found to be risk factors for an elevated albumin/creatinine ratio: in those between 5 and 17 years, low birth weight and scabies; in those between 5 and 29 years, a history of poststreptococcal glomerulonephritis; and in those 18 years and older, scabies, obesity, hypertension, diabetes, and hyperlipidemia.

The message from this study was the multifaceted nature of the associations between environmental and clinical risk factors, all of which could be attributed to "poverty, disadvantage and accelerated lifestyle change." Most importantly, it was the authors' view that this situation was amenable to intervention.[90] Studies in which individuals were followed over the next 1 to 6 years (mean = 3.9 years) showed increasing albuminuria and decreasing glomerular filtration rate (GFR).[92] In the same community, a study of 825 adults followed from 1.0 to 9.8 years (mean = 5.8 years) showed that for each 10-fold increase in the urine albumin/creatinine ratio, the risk of renal death was increased by more than 400-fold, the risk of cardiovascular death by fourfold, and all-cause mortality by 3.7-fold.[93]

The obvious challenge was to establish an intervention program. This was achieved using screening for hypertension, diabetes, and microalbuminuria and then treating the patients for 1 month to 4.56 years.[94] Treatment included health education, use of an angiotensin-converting enzyme inhibitor, and control of blood pressure, glucose and lipid levels. The outcomes of treated patients were compared with those of a cohort of historical controls matched for disease severity who had received no treatment or inconsistent treatment. In the treated cohort, the natural death rate was 50% that of the control cohort, and the renal death rate was 47% that of the control rate. It was estimated that treatment of as few as 11.6 persons was needed to prevent one natural death.[94] The program was unfortunately interrupted, which allowed a resurgence of deaths and ESKD in this population.[95] With aggressive political pressure brought to bear, and armed with these data, this program has now been reestablished, funded, and expanded in connection with a government policy to enhance the outlook for indigenous Australians; however, positive outcomes have yet to be published.

There are many types of renal disease found in indigenous Australian communities. In the 1998 study reported by Hoy and colleagues,[90] 88 renal biopsies were performed and, even among diabetic individuals, only 28% showed features of diabetic nephropathy. Glomerulomegaly was common in conjunction with variable degrees of focal or global glomerulosclerosis. In analyses comparing the findings of renal biopsies performed on Aboriginal Australian patients and on white patients in South Australia and the Northern Territory, glomerular hypertrophy, mesangial proliferation—including IgA disease, mesangiocapillary glomerulonephritis, and diabetic nephropathy—were more common in indigenous Australians, as were other proliferative forms of glomerular abnormality, which perhaps represented atypical postinfectious glomerulonephritis.[82,96] Obviously, the indications for renal biopsy would have influenced these findings. For example, in a type 2 diabetic patient with clinically typical diabetic nephropathy, renal biopsy might rarely have been performed, whereas in a patient with hematuria and acute deterioration in function, renal biopsy might have been more commonly performed.

The demonstration of various forms of proliferative glomerular changes suggests a causative role for the chronic infections found in this population. Even illnesses not directly related to lifestyle or infections may be more common and/or more severe in indigenous Australians. For example, it has been reported that systemic lupus erythematosus is more prevalent and severe in Northern Territory Aboriginal people.[97]

Clarifying the relationship between genes and the environment is an expectation of twenty-first-century medical science. In the meantime, there are ample opportunities for intervention, irrespective of genetic influences. The isolated nature of many indigenous Australian communities, particularly in the north and west of the continent, and their greater need for treatment has raised particular issues in relationship to RRT. Special programs have evolved. Satellite HD units in remote regions[14] have been followed by home dialysis programs directed at remote areas, with ongoing close cooperation among staff, tribal elders, patients, and their communities.[98-100] PD is often considered the first choice for ESKD patients living in remote areas.[98,99] Poor housing and hygiene are at least partially responsible for higher rates of peritonitis, technique failure, and mortality with PD.[100] Isolation, language barriers (many indigenous Australians in remote areas speak little English), recruitment and retention of support staff, and problems such as delivery of supplies, particularly during the tropical wet season, are ongoing difficulties in providing care.[101]

As with white Australians, renal transplantation is a preferred option compared with dialysis; however, there are significant barriers resulting in transplantation rates for indigenous Australians that are only about one third those in nonindigenous patients.[102-104] Live donors are uncommon, partly for cultural and socioeconomic reasons and also because of the very high prevalence of hypertension, diabetes, renal diseases, and other comorbidities in related prospective donors. Between 1990 and 2011, of patients younger than 18 years starting RRT in Australia, indigenous patients were least likely to receive a live donor transplant.[105]

Since Aboriginal patients may be undergoing dialysis hundreds or in some cases 1000 miles from the nearest transplantation center, geography is an obvious barrier to workup for transplantation, listing, and even timely access to the patient when a deceased donor graft becomes available. Cultural issues are protean. Adequately counseling the patient and obtaining consent to undergo an operation involving risk and insertion of another person's body part can be difficult, even when language barriers are not a factor. Donation of organs from deceased indigenous Australians often is not possible due to strict cultural views regarding the dignity of the dead.

Deceased organ allocation in Australia is controlled by a national organ-matching system that is heavily weighted toward HLA matching. Because HLA antigens are distributed variably in different populations, and few deceased donors are indigenous, this works against indigenous populations receiving deceased donor grafts.[102] The outcome is that indigenous patients are less likely to be listed for transplantation or are delayed in listings for deceased donor transplantation. Even when listed, they are likely to wait about twice as long as nonindigenous patients[106] and to receive poorly matched grafts, allocated more because of waiting time than HLA match.

Graft survival is also poorer among indigenous than nonindigenous Australians (Figure 82.9).[50,51,77,106] Among first deceased donor organ recipients, the risk ratios for graft loss and for patient death have been reported to be 3.1 (95% confidence interval [CI], 2.2 to 4.2) and 3.6 (95% CI, 2.5 to 5.1) for indigenous recipients compared with their nonindigenous counterparts.[106] As expected, the number of HLA mismatches was significantly greater in Aboriginal recipients (mean = 4.11 mismatches) than in nonindigenous recipients (mean = 2.95 mismatches), and more Aboriginal recipients were presensitized against HLA antigens.[106]

TRANSPLANT OUTCOMES

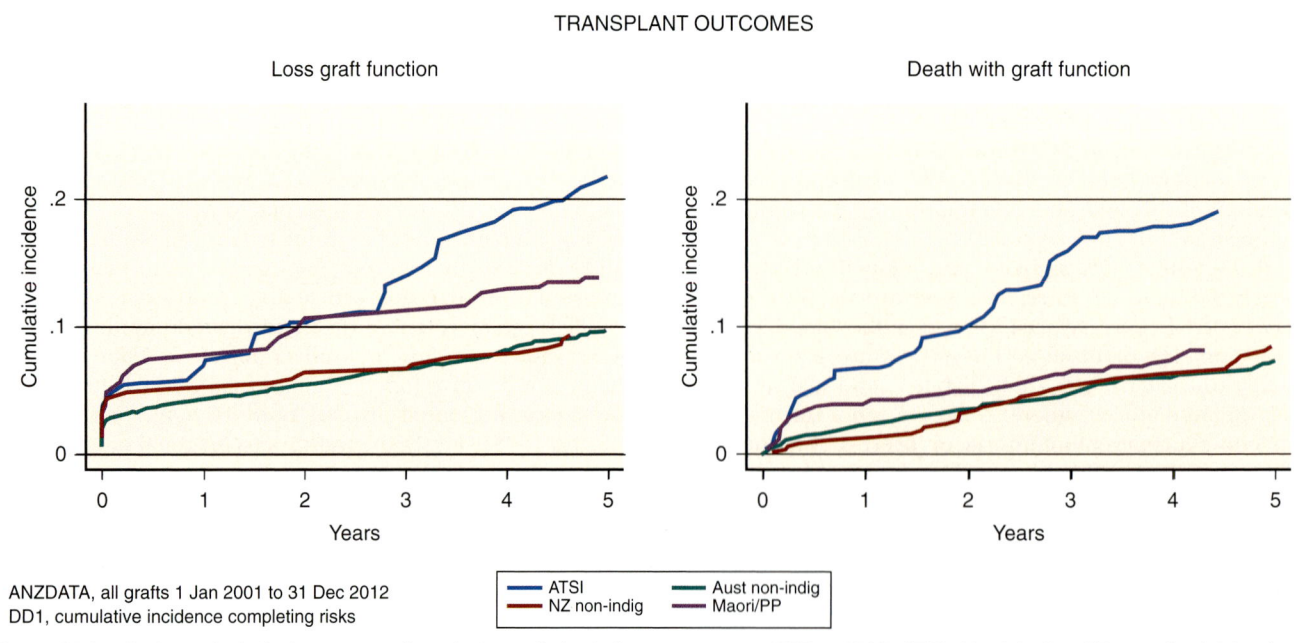

ANZDATA, all grafts 1 Jan 2001 to 31 Dec 2012
DD1, cumulative incidence completing risks

ATSI — Aust non-indig
NZ non-indig — Maori/PP

Figure 82.9 Graft survival of primary transplants in Australia by indigenous status, 1977 to 2003. ATSI, Aboriginal and Torres Strait Islanders; PP, Pacific Island People. (Redrawn from McDonald S: Indigenous transplant outcomes in Australia: what the ANZDATA Registry tells us. *Nephrology* 9:s138-s143, 2004.)

Worldwide, the issues surrounding CKD in indigenous populations and in developing societies continue to vex nephrologists and, more recently, governments. A continuing effort to stimulate global cooperation, as through the Global Outreach program of the International Society of Nephrology (ISN-GO; www.theisn.org) and the Kidney Disease: Improving Global Outcomes (KDIGO) initiatives, hopefully will force the World Health Organization and other global health interests to focus on this ongoing tragedy.

NEW ZEALAND

The land mass that is now called New Zealand consists of two major islands and many smaller islands, which broke away from what is now Australia about 70 million years ago.[107] New Zealand is situated approximately 1240 miles (2000 km) east and south of Australia and has a very large coastline around two major islands, with a total size of 165,000 square miles (see Figure 82.1). The first New Zealanders traveled thousands of miles from the tiny islands of East Polynesia in a vast tropical ocean to the temperate New Zealand islands. They transformed their East Polynesian way of life into a distinctively Maori culture.[107] This Maori settlement began about 800 years ago, probably over a period of several hundred years.

By the time of the first contact with European explorers (1642), the Maori population had reached about 100,000 people. Further contact with Europeans occurred, steady immigration of European settlers commenced around 1840, and by 1900 there were 17 settlers for every Maori New Zealander. A second wave of Polynesian immigration to New Zealand started in 1950 and was driven by New Zealand's need for workers and the promise of high wages. This led to a substantial population of Pacific peoples in New Zealand, many living within the region of Auckland, New Zealand's largest city (population >1,400,000). In New Zealand in 2013 there were 4.47 million people.[108] For the purposes of this chapter, Maori and Pacific peoples are both labelled as *indigenous*, although this is not strictly correct for the latter group.

ACCESS TO HEALTH CARE IN NEW ZEALAND

New Zealand has a taxpayer-funded public health system. Most of the daily business of New Zealand's health system, and around 75% of the funds, are administered by 20 district health boards (DHBs), which plan, manage, provide, and purchase services for the populations of their districts.[109] This includes funding for primary care, public health services, care for the aged, and secondary and tertiary care, as well as services provided by other nongovernmental health providers, including Maori and Pacific providers. New Zealand citizens and permanent residents are provided with government-funded health care. This includes free access to all modalities of RRT. The New Zealand Ministry of Health is responsible for directing policy and ensuring that DHBs provide a fully comprehensive range of preventive and health management services to their populations. It focuses on strategy, policy, and system performance, providing advice on improvement of health outcomes, reduction of inequalities and increase in participation, nationwide planning, and coordination and collaboration across the sectors.

There is a comprehensive private primary health care system substantially but not fully funded by the DHBs. It coordinates the management of patient care and is the first medical contact for all patients. Over the last decade, there has been a strong government focus on increasing the roles of and funding for primary health care, particularly in the area of chronic disease screening and management. Primary health care plays a central role in the diagnosis and management of patients with stages 1 to 3 CKD. The Ministry of Health Renal Advisory Board recommends referral to nephrology services for all patients with stage 4 CKD, and earlier for those with signs of active kidney diseases, such as proteinuria and hematuria.

There are relatively low partial charges that most patients pay for primary care and for outpatient pharmaceuticals. This, along with transportation costs, constitutes a barrier to health care, particularly for those in the lowest socioeconomic groups, many of whom are Maori or Pacific people, among whom the incidence of diabetes and kidney disease is high.[110]

HEALTH STATUS OF THE INDIGENOUS POPULATION

In New Zealand census data, ethnicity is self-identified. The resident population in New Zealand in 2013 was 4.47 million, of whom 74% identified themselves as being of European origin, 14.9% of Maori origin, 7.4% of Pacific origin, and 11.8% of Asian origin, as well as other ethnicities. The total adds up to more than 100% because some people identify with more than one ethnic group.[111]

The Maori population has, on average, the poorest health status of any ethnic group in New Zealand.[112,113] This has been recognized for some time, and the government, through the Ministry of Health, has made it a key priority to reduce the health inequalities that affect the Maori. For both Maori and non-Maori populations, the major causes of death are chronic diseases. Ischemic heart disease is the leading cause of death for both populations; lung cancer is the second leading cause of death in Maori, and diabetes is the third leading cause in Maori males and the fifth leading cause in Maori females. Diabetes is not one of the top five causes of death for non-Maori of either gender.

Life expectancy at birth of non-Maori exceeded that of Maori by 8.6 years for males and 7.9 for females in 2005 to 2007.[113] Approximately 75% of this difference is due to higher death rates at age 40 to 79 years for Maori males and higher death rates at age 50 to 84 years for Maori females. The Maori/non-Maori differential partly reflects different rates of diabetes and smoking. The cause of death statistics for 2005 show that age-standardized death rates from diabetes were four times higher for male Maori than for male non-Maori and five times higher for female Maori than for female non-Maori. The 2006 census reported that 42% of Maori aged 15 years and older were regular smokers compared with 18% of non-Maori.[108]

The gap between Maori and non-Maori life expectancy has narrowed.[113] In 1995 to 1997, it was 9.1 years, but by 2000 to 2002 it had dropped to about 8.5 years and in 2005 to 2007 the gap was 8.2 years. Detailed statistics are not available for the Pacific population, but the age-standardized death rates can be compared. (The standardized death rate indicates the overall death rate defined as deaths/1000 population if the observed age- and gender-specific death rates are applied to a standard population.) In 2005 to 2007, there was an age-standardized death rate by ethnic group of 9.9 for Maori, 8.8 for Pacific peoples, and 5.4 for European and other ethnic groups. The overall standardized death rate for the New Zealand population was 5.8.[113] There are still major disparities in New Zealand between Pacific peoples and others across a range of socioeconomic indicators, including unemployment, occupational and industrial distribution, self-employment, personal and household incomes, housing tenure, and access to household amenities.[114]

ETHNIC DIFFERENCES IN MICROALBUMINURIA, DIABETES, HYPERTENSION, AND GLOMERULONEPHRITIS

In New Zealand, cross-sectional studies of particular groups have addressed the prevalence of microalbuminuria, diabetes, and hypertension. In a study of 3960 nondiabetic, nonhyperlipidemic, nonproteinuric middle-aged working men and women aged 40 years and older, microalbuminuria was found to be five times more common in Maori and Pacific people than in Europeans.[115] The Diabetic Heart and Health Study was a population-based survey of 1011 Pacific people and 1745 European people.[116] In this study the prevalence of diabetes was 26.2% in Samoan men, 35.8% in Tongan women, and 17.8% in Tongan men. Approximately one in three Maori and Pacific individuals had hypertension (blood pressure > 140/90 mm Hg) compared with one in five of others. In a New Zealand workforce study of 5651 employed people aged 40 to 64 years, mean systolic and diastolic blood pressures were higher in Maori (by 5 to 6 mm Hg) and Pacific people (by 4 to 6 mm Hg) than in Europeans.[117] The odds ratio for treatment of hypertension in those with hypertension was 0.33 (95% CI, 0.19 to 0.58) for Maori and 0.27 (95% CI, 0.16 to 0.47) for Pacific people compared with Europeans.

The first nationally representative study on nutrition and blood pressure was published in 2013.[118] The overall prevalence of hypertension was 31%, with 15% reporting taking antihypertensive medications. Rates increased from 18.6% in those aged 30 to 39 years to 59.9% in those aged 60 to 69 years. For men, Maori had a statistically significant higher prevalence of hypertension ($P = 0.024$) compared with people of European origin. For women, both Maori and Pacific people had a significantly higher prevalence of hypertension ($P = 0.001$ for both).

Glomerulonephritis has also been shown to be more common among Maori and Pacific people than Europeans. The New Zealand Glomerulonephritis Survey (NZGS) included all 803 patients in four of the five nephrology centers in New Zealand who were older than 14 years and had biopsy-proven glomerulonephritis during the years 1972 to 1983.[119] Polynesian people (mostly Maori) were found to have a higher incidence of postinfectious glomerulonephritis, mesangiocapillary glomerulonephritis, and focal glomerulosclerosis, but a lower incidence of IgA nephropathy.[119] Poststreptococcal glomerulonephritis is reported to be the most common cause of severe acute glomerulonephritis in New Zealand children, with most patients (85%) being of Maori or Pacific ethnicity.[120] In a recently published nationwide study, the annual incidence was reported at 9.7 episodes/100,000 (Pacific, 45.5; Maori, 15.7; Asian, 2.1; European or Other, 2.6/100,000).[121]

In a small study, Maori and Pacific people with systemic lupus erythematosus were shown to have a significantly higher risk of developing lupus nephritis.[122]

Long-term outcome data were recently presented for patients enrolled in the NZGS.[123] After a median follow-up of 30.1 years (range, 1 to 42.3 years), 264 of the study population (34.5%) progressed to ESKD, of whom 181 (62%) were transplanted; 401 (47.2%) have died, with the highest mortality rate in patients with rapidly progressive glomerulonephritis (RPGN; 88%), those with dense deposit disease (83%), and those with ESKD at the time of biopsy (86%). This is the longest reported follow-up series of patients with glomerulonephritis.

CHRONIC KIDNEY DISEASE AND DIABETES

Diabetes mellitus is the most common cause of ESKD in New Zealand, accounting for 40% of new ESKD cases, a rate similar to that reported in the United States.[7] Diabetes is diagnosed more than 10 years earlier in Maori and Pacific people compared with Europeans and is associated with a higher incidence of renal complications.[124]

The Diabetes Cohort Study, based on primary health care data collected prospectively from the year 2000 onward, includes approximately 60% of all those diagnosed with diabetes in New Zealand (Pacific people, 90%; Maori, 38%).[125] In the years 2000 to 2006,[125] 75,529 people had at least one medical checkup; 0.3% were undergoing dialysis and were excluded from further analysis. For 65,171 (86%), the urine albumin/creatinine ratio was recorded.

Important findings are that the average age at diagnosis of diabetes was 50 years for Maori and Pacific people as opposed to 61 years for those of European ancestry. Maori and Pacific people were overrepresented in the lowest socioeconomic quintile (56.8% of Maori and 65% of Pacific people vs. 23% of Europeans), and BMIs were much higher in the Maori and Pacific population than in the European population (34, 33, and 29 kg/m^2, respectively). There was also a much higher incidence of smoking in Maori and Pacific diabetic populations. Abnormal albuminuria of any degree occurred in 28% of European, 50% of Maori, and 49% of Pacific people. Those with severe macroalbuminuria (albumin level > 100 mg/mmol or 880 mg/g creatinine) were much more likely to be Maori or Pacific (8.11% and 7.8% of cases, respectively) than European (1.7% of cases). Based on Cox regression analysis, the adjusted proportional odds ratio for an elevated urine albumin/creatinine ratio was associated with a higher hemoglobin A_{1C} level, higher systolic blood pressure, higher BMI, lower socioeconomic quintile, current smoker status, and Maori and Pacific ethnicity.

The Diabetes Cohort Study group has recently developed and validated a risk stratification tool using multiple factors (e.g., age, gender, ethnicity, duration of diabetes, smoking status, presence of cardiovascular disease, HbA_{1C}, serum creatinine level, albuminuria) to predict fatal or nonfatal ESKD. This tool provides more accurate risk

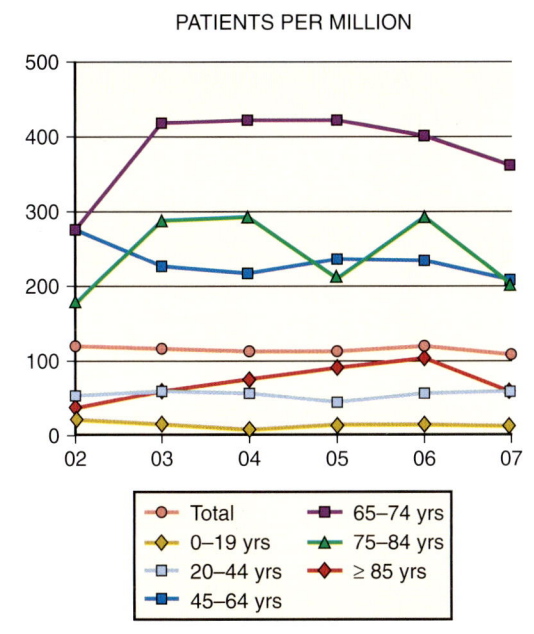

Figure 82.10 Acceptance of new patients for renal replacement therapy in 2002 to 2007—age-specific rates for New Zealand. (From McDonald S, Excell L, Livingston B [editors]: *ANZDATA registry report, thirty-first report,* Adelaide, Australia, 2008, Australia and New Zealand Dialysis and Transplant Registry.)

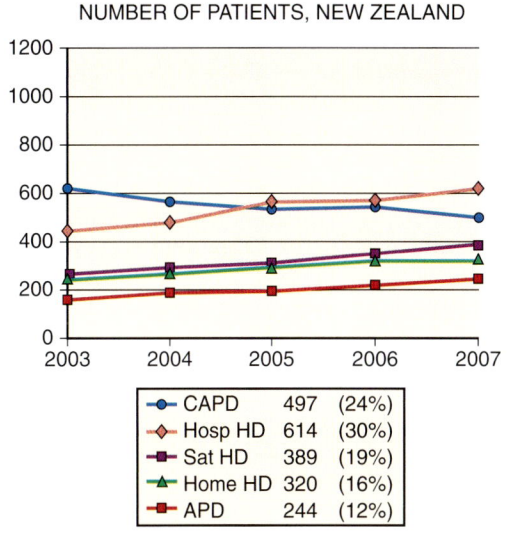

Figure 82.11 Method and location of dialysis in New Zealand (December 2003 to 2007). APD, Automated peritoneal dialysis; CAPD, continuous ambulatory peritoneal dialysis; HD, home hemodialysis. (From McDonald S, Excell L, Livingston B [editors]: *ANZDATA registry report, thirty-first report,* Adelaide, Australia, 2008, Australia and New Zealand Dialysis and Transplant Registry.)

RENAL REPLACEMENT THERAPY

Dialysis and kidney transplantation first became available in New Zealand in the 1960s. As in other countries, the number of patients beginning dialysis had steadily increased but has plateaued over the last 5 years, ranging from 108 to 135 patients per million (ppm), which is comparable to the rates in Australia[7] (Figure 82.10).

In New Zealand, there is a very strong focus on home therapies. New Zealand has the highest utilization of home HD of any reported population.[12] Ten years ago,[16] 80% of all New Zealand dialysis patients were undergoing some form of home dialysis, with 56% receiving PD and 24% receiving home HD. More recently, these percentages have decreased, although the total numbers receiving home therapies have increased. The most recent ANZDATA report,[13] based on December 2012 data, listed 2469 patients undergoing dialysis therapy and 1520 with functioning renal transplants. Of the dialysis patients, 19% were undergoing home HD and 31% were undergoing PD (47% by automated PD[7]; Figure 82.11). There is a particularly high utilization of PD by those older than 65 years. In the age group 75 to 84 years, 33% of all New Zealand patients were undergoing PD, compared with 17% of Australian patients in this age group.

There are many reasons for the high utilization of home therapies. New Zealand renal services have always provided home therapies as the standard of care for all new dialysis patients. There has been strong support for this approach from health funders and providers of renal services, and there is a firmly held consensus among nephrologists that this is the best way to optimize outcomes and limit expenditure. In addition, because of New Zealand's small, thinly spread population, home therapies allow widespread access to treatment. Thus, there has been limited availability of hospital and satellite HD facilities until relatively recently. In some parts of New Zealand, home therapy is used by more than 90% of dialysis patients,[127] and access to hospital dialysis is minimal. This home-focused strategy has been an important determinant of the slower growth of dialysis use by the older population compared with that in Australia.

Concerns about the possibility of inequitable access to dialysis led to a 2-year audit in 1997 and 1998 of the outcome for all patients with ESKD ($n = 823$) who came for assessment and evaluation at all New Zealand renal services. Of those who were assessed and evaluated, 86% with ESKD were offered dialysis therapy; of that group, 5% chose not to have dialysis, and the remainder began RRT. Compared with those who started dialysis, those not offered treatment were older (mean, 67.4 vs. 53.3 years), had much higher rates of comorbid conditions and had reduced ability to perform the activities of daily living.[128]

In New Zealand, the numbers commencing dialysis peaked in 2009 at 135/million population (pmp) and have since eased back; most recently, it was 111 pmp in 2012.[13] The rate of dialysis commencement for new patients aged 65 to 74 years averaged 400 pmp/year between 2003 and 2006 but has since declined and most recently was 309 pmp in 2012. This compares to a current rate of 233 pmp for those aged 45 to 64 years, which has not changed significantly over the last decade. The number of patients beginning dialysis among those aged 75 to 84 years was 213 pmp in 2012, which is less than half that reported for the same age group in Australia. These differences reflect the different approaches to RRT undertaken in Australia and New Zealand, most particularly the emphasis that New Zealand places on home HD therapy, with limited access to facility dialysis in many centers. As at December 31, 2012, there were 552 pmp managed on dialysis, and prevalent patient numbers have increased by 3.8%/year over the last 6 years. The most common comorbid condition in patients beginning RRT is coronary artery disease, with 20% of new patients with definite disease in 2012 and another 10% suspected of having coronary artery disease.[7] New Zealand has had a high incidence of diabetic nephropathy as a cause of renal failure, particularly among the indigenous population. In 2012, 50% of all new patients starting RRT had diabetes, and 95% of these had type 2 diabetes. Glomerulonephritis accounted for 20% of causes of ESKD; the most common forms of glomerulonephritis were focal sclerosing glomerulonephritis, primary and secondary, and IgA nephropathy. Renal transplantation commenced in 1965 in New Zealand[129] and is currently performed in three units across the country.

Transplantation rates in New Zealand have changed little over the last decade. In 2010 and 2011, 4.0% of all dialysis patients underwent transplantation, and the transplant rate was 27 pmp/year in 2011 compared with 37 pmp/year in Australia. Over the last decade, the proportion of patients receiving kidney transplants from living donors has risen; in 2011, it was 48%. This is a reflection of the shortage of deceased donors and the introduction of donor laparoscopic nephrectomy, which is associated with lower morbidity and shorter recovery time.[130] The rates of loss of grafts and death with a functioning graft have improved over the 5 years from 2006 to 2011, from 6% to 4.6% annually. Since 1999, there has been a national kidney allocation system for all deceased donor kidneys based on an agreed-on algorithm, which allocates organs on the basis of the number of HLA mismatches and recipient waiting time.[131] This has ensured improved equality of access for all patients on the waiting list.[132]

END-STAGE KIDNEY DISEASE IN MAORI AND PACIFIC POPULATIONS

Overall, the incidence rates (pmp) for ESKD in indigenous peoples in New Zealand are considerably higher than those for nonindigenous people. Direct comparisons are confounded by different age distributions—the indigenous population is considerably younger than the nonindigenous population (Figure 82.12).

In the years 2003 to 2007, the incidence of RRT initiation among Maori people was 262 pmp, among Pacific people, 283 pmp, and among people of European ancestry, 77 pmp (according to ANZDATA information).[13] Thus, there is an overall 3.5-fold higher incidence of treated ESKD in Maori and Pacific peoples. Maori and Pacific patients accounted for 57% of the total dialysis population but only 16% of those with functioning transplants in 2012.

Diabetes is the primary cause of new ESKD in 63% of Maori patients and 65% of Pacific patients, but in only 17% of patients of European ancestry. Thus, the incidence of ESKD secondary to diabetes is 13.6-fold higher for Maori than for Europeans and the incidence for Pacific people is 14.7-fold higher than for Europeans.[7,76] In addition, Maori patients have been shown to progress at a significantly faster rate from their first kidney-related hospital admission to a requirement for RRT compared with New Zealand Europeans.[133] There is also an increased incidence of glomerulonephritis as a cause of ESKD in the indigenous population, with Maori having a 1.9-fold higher incidence of glomerulonephritis (particularly lupus nephritis) and Pacific people a 2.3-fold higher incidence than Europeans. The incidence of ESKD secondary to hypertension is also higher in the indigenous group.[76]

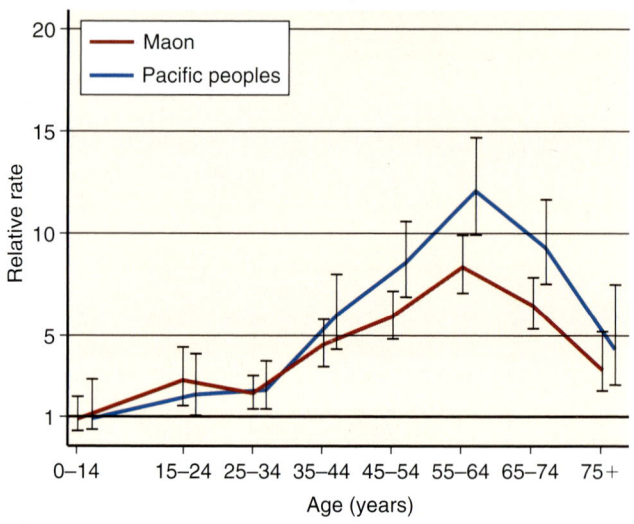

OUTCOME OF RENAL REPLACEMENT THERAPY

Maori and nonindigenous people have similar rates of survival on dialysis when survival is adjusted for age, presence of diabetes, gender, select comorbid conditions, and exclusion from transplantation. In contrast, Pacific peoples have a significantly better survival—70% at 5 years compared with 50% to 60% for the Maori and nonindigenous population. The explanation for this difference is yet to be determined. It may be related to an increased incidence of cardiovascular events in the Maori population.

A recent analysis looked at the association between ethnicity and cardiovascular outcomes in people with type 2 diabetes in New Zealand.[125] Data were collected for 48,044 patients with type 2 diabetes, with a median follow-up of 2.5 years. The HR for first cardiovascular event, defined as first recorded fatal or nonfatal cardiovascular event (ischemic heart disease, cerebrovascular accident, transient ischemic attack, or peripheral vascular disease) were 1.3 (95% CI, 1.19 to 1.41) for Maori and 1.04 (95% CI, 0.95 to 1.13) for Pacific people compared with people of European ancestry.

Figure 82.12 Overall, the incidence rates (pmp) for ESKD in indigenous peoples in New Zealand are considerably higher than those for nonindigenous peoples. Direct comparisons are confounded by the different age distributions; the indigenous population is considerably younger than the nonindigenous population. (From McDonald S, Jose M, Hurst K. End-stage kidney disease among indigenous peoples of Australia and New Zealand. In McDonald S, Clayton P, Hurst K, editors: *ANZDATA Registry report, thirty-fifth report*, Adelaide, Australia, 2012, Australia and New Zealand Dialysis and Transplant Registry.)

TRANSPLANTATION

Transplantation rates for Maori and Pacific people are approximately 25% of those for Europeans. The adjusted likelihood of receiving a transplant was significantly lower in these groups in the years 1995 to 2003, with an HR of 0.23 compared with Europeans.[134] This trend of unequal access to renal transplantation is not unique to New Zealand. Compared with white patients, the adjusted likelihood of receiving a transplant for indigenous patients has been found to be significantly lower in most countries with multiple ethnic groups (e.g., Australia, HR = 0.23; Canada, HR = 0.34; United States, HR = 0.44). A recent analysis of this situation[7] has indicated that it is partly related to a reduced listing rate of about 50% and a reduced transplantation rate of about 50% among those recorded as being of Maori and Pacific extraction. The causes of reduced listing are likely to be multifactorial, relating to increased rates of morbid obesity, comorbid conditions associated with diabetes, and probably to other factors involving socioeconomic status and access to health care. For Maori and Pacific patients who undergo transplantation, graft survival is reduced compared with nonindigenous patients. Among recipients of a deceased donor graft, there is a 50% 8-year graft survival among Maori and Pacific patients, compared with a 50% 14-year graft survival among nonindigenous patients. Part of the reason for reduced graft survival in Maori patients is their increased mortality. At 8 years, patient survival is 75% for the Maori population versus 90% for the nonindigenous population and a similar rate for the Pacific population.

REASONS FOR DIFFERENCES IN INCIDENCE OF END-STAGE KIDNEY DISEASE AND OUTCOMES FOR INDIGENOUS MAORI AND PACIFIC POPULATIONS

The reasons for the marked differences in ESKD cause, incidence rates, and outcome of therapies in Maori and Pacific patients compared with nonindigenous patients could relate to a number of factors. Low birth weight has been shown to be a significant predictor of subsequent kidney disease.[85] Birth weights of 2.5 kg and below were recorded in 7.3% of Maori, 4.9% of Pacific, and 5.7% of European live births in New Zealand in 2005.[135] Genetic factors may play a role, such as the amylin gene mutations found in 7% of Maori, which are associated with a fivefold higher incidence of diabetes.[136] Differences in cultural practices are also likely to be important and include consumption of high-fat, high-protein diets and a tendency to minimize the personal significance of asymptomatic chronic disease.[137] The documented higher rates of smoking, obesity, and lower socioeconomic status are factors associated with CKD progression. In addition, novel risk factors for CKD such as hyperuricemia[138] and periodontitis[139] are also more common in Polynesian populations.[140,141]

Disparity in health care outcomes can be defined as differences in appropriate treatment leading to poorer outcomes not attributable to patients' clinical or demographic characterisics.[142] Based on this definition, a higher frequency of adverse events and poorer outcomes has been documented for Maori in obstetric care.[143] Additional studies using indicators such as disease-specific mortality, avoidable hospitalization, and avoidable mortality have each consistently shown evidence for health care outcome disparity.[143] Although there have been no robust assessments of disparity in the health care of Maori and Pacific patients with kidney disease, it is possible that similar issues occur in these populations and account for some of the differences in outcome. To this end, since 2000, a growing number of government and DHB-funded initiatives have been in place to detect and prevent diabetes and its complications.[144]

PACIFIC ISLANDS

There is considerable evidence for a high rate of kidney disease in many Pacific Island populations, which is worsening with westernization and urbanization. Based on ANZDATA studies, in which self-reported ethnicity is recorded for Maori and Pacific peoples according to nation of origin, and on data retrieved for persons normally resident in Australia or New Zealand, the rates of ESKD (treated by RRT) in Maori and Pacific adults were two to ten times higher than those of "other" New Zealanders and nonindigenous Australians.[76] This was still only a little more than half the rate seen in indigenous Australians. The excess in Maori and Pacific people was attributed to type 2 diabetes and diabetic nephropathy, hypertensive renal disease, and glomerulonephritis, particularly lupus and membranoproliferative glomerulonephritis. Diabetes and other cardiovascular risk factors have been shown to be common in Pacific Island immigrants in New Zealand.[116] Similarly, in Hawaii, the native population is of Polynesian ancestry and has a significantly higher prevalence rate of diabetes compared with other ethnic groups, as well as a higher rate of ESKD secondary to diabetes.[145]

The high incidence of diabetic nephropathy secondary to type 2 diabetes is not surprising, because the latter disease is prevalent in many Pacific Island nations. Over 25 years ago, very high rates of type 2 diabetes were reported in Nauru and the Republic of Kiribati.[146,147] In the tiny island of Nauru in the central Pacific, which then had a population of about 4000, the prevalence rate of diabetes was over 25% by age 44 years, 40% by 54 years, and 54% by 64 years.[146] At that time, this made the Nauruan incidence of diabetes among the highest known in the world, second only to that of the Pima Indians of North America, who had rates among adults older than 25 years about twice that of Nauruans. Since then, it has become obvious that most of those in the Pacific Island nations have high incidence rates of diabetes and, as a consequence, high but poorly documented rates of diabetic kidney disease.[148-152]

The provision of renal services in island nations correlates with the level of dependence, with fully independent Pacific countries having limited availability of renal services. French Polynesia and New Caledonia are protectorates of France, and American Samoa is a protectorate of the United States; as a consequence, their populations have access to renal services similar to that in the mother countries. The Cook Islands, Niue, and Tokelau Islands were previously New Zealand dependencies, and their populations are entitled to access renal services in New Zealand. Samoa (formerly Western Samoa) has established dialysis for some of its population, as have Fiji, Nauru, and Palau. Other countries have no access to dialysis and limited or no renal care for their populations. Because the problems of economy and geography are unlikely to be resolved in the near future, most efforts should be aimed at primary prevention, such as early detection and appropriate treatment of diabetes.[153,154]

CONCLUDING REMARKS

Kidney disease in the Oceania region offers unique opportunities and challenges. The small population and high GDP per capita in Australia and New Zealand have allowed for the development of integrated systems to provide publicly funded RRT for their citizens, as well as resources such as the ANZDATA Registry to supply data for benchmarking. An unexplained issue is the low rate of RRT compared with the United States and Canada. Historically, analgesic nephropathy has been a disease for which identification, research, and public health measures allowed the virtual eradication of a major cause of ESKD in the past. The low population density has encouraged a high proportion of home-based therapies, both transplantation and dialysis. Unfortunately, with transplantation has come a very high incidence of skin cancer. The situation for the indigenous populations, the Aboriginal people in Australia and the Maori and Pacific Island people in New Zealand, is not so impressive. Very high rates of ESKD requiring RRT are seen in these populations. Lifestyle issues are a very important part of the modifiable risk factors, which must be addressed to reduce this disease burden. Whether there are additional ethnic or social predispositions to CKD remains to be clarified.

Complete reference list available at ExpertConsult.com.

KEY REFERENCES

5. Grace BS, Clayton P, Cass A, et al: Socio-economic status and incidence of renal replacement therapy: a regional study of Australian patients. *Nephrol Dial Transplant* 27:4173–4180, 2012.
6. Cass A, Cunningham J, Wang Z, et al: Social disadvantage and variation in the incidence of end-stage renal disease in Australian capital cities. *Aust N Z J Public Health* 25:322–326, 2001.
7. McDonald S, Clayton P, Hurst K, editors: *ANZDATA registry report, thirty-fifth report*. Available at: <www.anzdata.org.au>. Accessed November 2013.
12. ESKD Incidence Study Group: Geographic, ethnic, age-related and temporal variation in the incidence of end-stage renal disease in Europe, Canada and the Asia-Pacific region, 1998-2002. *Nephrol Dial Transplant* 21:2178–2183, 2006.
13. McDonald S, Jose M, Hurst K: End-stage kidney disease among indigenous peoples of Australia and New Zealand. In McDonald S, Clayton P, Hurst K, editors: *ANZDATA registry report, thirty-fifth report*. Available at: <www.anzdata.org.au>. Accessed November 2013.
14. Cass A, Cunningham J, Wang Z, et al: Regional variation in the incidence of end-stage renal disease in indigenous Australians. *Med J Aust* 175:24–27, 2001.
15. Gray NA, Dent H, McDonald SP: Renal replacement therapy in rural and urban Australia. *Nephrol Dial Transplant* 27:2069–2076, 2012.
17. Howard K, Salkeld G, White S, et al: The cost-effectiveness of increasing kidney transplantation and home-based dialysis. *Nephrology (Carlton)* 14:123–132, 2009.
18. Briggs N, McDonald S, Hurst K: Method and location of dialysis. In McDonald S, Clayton P, Hurst K, editors: *ANZDATA registry report, thirty-fifth report*. Available at: <www.anzdata.org.au>. Accessed November 2013.
20. Marshall MR, Hawley CM, Kerr PG, et al: Home hemodialysis and mortality risk in Australian and New Zealand populations. *Am J Kidney Dis* 58:782–793, 2011.
21. Agar JW: International variations and trends in home hemodialysis. *Adv Chronic Kidney Dis* 16:205–214, 2009.
22. Agar JW, Hawley CM, George CR, et al: Home haemodialysis in Australia—is the wheel turning full circle? *Med J Aust* 192:403–406, 2010.
25. Jun M, Jardine MJ, Gray N, et al: Outcomes of extended hours hemodialysis performed predominantly at home. *Am J Kidney Dis* 61:247–253, 2013.
28. Polkinghorne KR, McDonald SP, Atkins RC, et al: Epidemiology of vascular access in the Australian hemodialysis population. *Kidney Int* 64:1893–1902, 2003.
32. Cooper BA, Branley P, Bulfone L, et al: A randomized, controlled trial of early versus late intiation of dialysis. *N Eng L Med* 363:609–619, 2010.
33. Johnson DW, Brown FG, Clarke M, et al: Effects of biocompatible versus standard fluid on peritoneal dialysis outcomes. *J Am Soc Nephrol* 23:1097–1107, 2012.
41. Collins MG, Teo E, Cole SR, et al: Screening for colorectal cancer and advanced colorectal neoplasia in kidney transplant recipients: cross-sectional prevalence and diagnostic accuracy study of fecal immunochemical testing for haemoglobin and colonoscopy. *BMJ* 25(345):e4657, 2012.
42. Webster AC, Craig JC, Simpson JM, et al: Identifying high-risk groups and quantifying absolute risk of cancer after kidney transplantation: a cohort study of 15,183 recipients. *Am J Transplant* 7:2140–2151, 2007.
43. Webster A, Wong G: Cancer report. In McDonald S, Excell L, Livingston B, editors: *ANZDATA Registry report, thirty-first report*, Adelaide, Australia, 2008, Australia and New Zealand Dialysis and Transplant Registry, pp 10.1–10.6.
46. Vajdic CM, McDonald SP, McCredie MR, et al: Cancer incidence before and after kidney transplantation. *JAMA* 296:2823–2831, 2006.
51. Sparke C, Moon L, Green F, et al: Estimating the total incidence of kidney failure in Australia including individuals who are not treated by dialysis or transplantation. *Am J Kidney Dis* 61:413–419, 2013.
52. Chandna SM, Da Silva-Gane M, Marshall C, et al: Survival of elderly patients with stage 5 CKD: comparison of conservative management and renal replacement therapy. *Nephrol Dial Transplant* 26:1608–1614, 2011.
53. Da Silva-Gane M, Wellsted D, Greenshields H, et al: Quality of life and survival in patients with advanced kidney failure managed conservatively or by dialysis. *Clin J Am Soc Nephrol* 7:2002–2009, 2012.
54. Crail S, Walker R, Brown M: Renal Supportive Care working group. Renal supportive and palliative care: position statement. *Nephrol* 18:393–400, 2013.
58. White SL, Polkinghorne KR, Atkins RC, et al: Comparison of the prevalence and mortality risk of CKD in Australia using the CKD Epidemiology Collaboration (CKD-EPI) and Modification of Diet in Renal Disease (MDRD) Study GFR estimating equations: the AusDiab (Australian Diabetes, Obesity and Lifestyle) Study. *Am J Kid Dis* 55:660–670, 2010.
66. Chang SH, Mathew TH, McDonald SP: Analgesic nephropathy and renal replacement therapy in Australia: trends, comorbidities and outcomes. *Clin J Am Soc Nephrol* 3:768–776, 2008.
67. Mihatsch MJ, Khanlari B, Brunner FP: Obituary to analgesic nephropathy—an autopsy study. *Nephrol Dial Transplant* 21:3139–3145, 2006.
70. Stewart JH, McCredie MR, McDonald SP: The incidence of treated end-stage renal disease in New Zealand Maori and Pacific Island people and in indigenous Australians. *Nephrol Dial Transplant* 19:678–685, 2004.
72. McDonald S, Jose M, Hurst K: End-stage kidney disease among indigenous peoples of Australia and New Zealand. In McDonald S, Clayton P, Hurst K, editors: *ANZDATA registry report, thirty-fifth report*, Adelaide, Australia, 2012, Australia and New Zealand Dialysis and Transplant Registry.
78. Stewart JH, McCredie MR, Williams SM, et al: The enigma of hypertensive ESKD: observations on incidence and trends in 18 European, Canadian, and Asian-Pacific populations, 1998 to 2002. *Am J Kidney Dis* 48:183–191, 2006.

79. Hoy WE, Rees M, Kile E, et al: A new dimension to the Barker hypothesis: low birth weight and susceptibility to renal disease. *Kidney Int* 56:1072–1077, 1999.
84. Young RJ, Hoy WE, Kincaid-Smith P, et al: Glomerular size and glomerulosclerosis in Australian Aborigines. *Am J Kidney Dis* 36:481–489, 2000.
86. Feehally J: Ethnicity and renal disease. *Kidney Int* 68:414–424, 2005.
88. Hossain MP, Goyder EC, Rigby JE, et al: CKD and poverty: a growing global challenge. *Am J Kidney Dis* 53:166–174, 2009.
89. El Nahas AM: Kidney diseases in the developing world and ethnic minorities. *N Engl J Med* 354:2628–2629, 2006.
90. Hoy WE, Mathews JD, McCredie DA, et al: The multidimensional nature of renal disease: rates and associations of albuminuria in an Australian Aboriginal community. *Kidney Int* 54:1296–1304, 1998.
92. Hoy WE, Wang Z, Van Buynder P, et al: The natural history of renal disease in Australian Aborigines. Part 1. Changes in albuminuria and glomerular filtration rate over time. *Kidney Int* 60:243–248, 2001.
93. Hoy WE, Wang Z, Van Buynder P, et al: The natural history of renal disease in Australian Aborigines. Part 2. Albuminuria predicts natural death and renal failure. *Kidney Int* 60:249–256, 2001.
100. Lim WH, Boudville N, McDonald SP, et al: Remote indigenous peritoneal dialysis patients have a higher risk of peritonitis, technique failure, all-cause and peritonitis-related mortality. *Nephrol Dial Transplant* 26:3366–3372, 2011.
116. Sundborn G, Metcalf PA, Gentles D, et al: Ethnic differences in cardiovascular disease risk factors and diabetes status for Pacific ethnic groups and Europeans in the Diabetes Heart and Health Survey (DHAH) 2002-2003, Auckland New Zealand. *N Z Med J* 121:28–39, 2008.
117. Gentles D, Metcalf P, Dyall L, et al: Blood pressure prevalences and levels for a multicultural population in Auckland, New Zealand: results from the Diabetes, Heart and Health Survey 2002/2003. *N Z Med J* 119:U2318, 2006.
118. McLean RM, Williams S, Mann J, et al: Blood pressure and hypertension in New Zealand: results from the 2008/2009 Adult Nutrition Survey. *N Z Med J* 126:66–79, 2013.
120. Wong W, Morris MC, Zwi J: Outcome of severe acute post-streptococcal glomerulonephritis in New Zealand children. *Pediatr Nephrol* 24:1021–1026, 2009.
121. Wong W, Lennon D, Crone DR, et al: Prospective population-based study on the burden of disease from post-streptococcal glomerulonephritis of hospitalized children in New Zealand: epidemiology, clinical features and complications. *J Paediatr Child Health* 49:850–855, 2013.
123. Chembo C, Pilmore H, Walker R, et al: New Zealand survey of glomerulonephritis. *Nephrology* 18(Suppl 1):15–77, 2013.
126. Elley CR, Robinson T, Moyes SA, et al: Derivation and validation of a renal risk score for people with type 2 diabetes. *Diabetes Care* 36:3113–3120, 2013.
133. Joshy G, Dunn P, Fisher M, et al: Ethnic differences in the natural progression of nephropathy among diabetes patients in New Zealand: hospital admission rate for renal complications, and incidence of end-stage renal disease and renal death. *Diabetologia* 52:1474–1478, 2009.
134. Yeates KE, Cass A, Sequist TD, et al: Indigenous people in Australia, Canada, New Zealand and the United States are less likely to receive renal transplantation. *Kidney Int* 76:659–664, 2009.
136. Poa NR, Cooper GJ, Edgar PF: Amylin gene promoter mutations predispose to type 2 diabetes in New Zealand Maori. *Diabetologia* 46:574–578, 2003.
144. Joshy G, Simmons D: Epidemiology of diabetes in New Zealand: revisit to a changing landscape. *N Z Med J* 119:U1999, 2006.

CHALLENGES IN NEPHROLOGY

SECTION XIV

83 Ethical Dilemmas Facing Nephrology: Past, Present, and Future

Alvin H. Moss

CHAPTER OUTLINE

PAST, 2558
Nephrology's Contribution to the Birth of Bioethics, 2558
Patient Selection Criteria and the Overt Rationing of Dialysis, 2559
Advance Directives and Patients Undergoing Dialysis, 2561
Effect of Reimbursement, 2562
Conflicts of Interest, 2562
PRESENT, 2562
Clinical Practice Guideline on Withholding and Withdrawing Dialysis, 2562
End-of-Life Care, 2567
The "Difficult" Patient Undergoing Dialysis, 2567
FUTURE, 2568
Dialysis of the Older Patient, 2568
Treatment of Chronic Pain, 2569
Palliative Care and Referral to Hospice, 2569
Access to Renal Transplantation, 2570
The Coming Fiscal Crisis in Nephrology and the Prospect of the Return of Rationing, 2572
CONCLUSION, 2572

PAST

NEPHROLOGY'S CONTRIBUTION TO THE BIRTH OF BIOETHICS

A chapter about the ethical issues facing nephrology needs to start with an acknowledgment of the key role that nephrology played in the development of the field of bioethics. Nephrology has this unique position because its life-sustaining therapies, kidney dialysis and renal transplantation, predate other life-sustaining therapies. In his 1964 presidential address to the American Society of Artificial Internal Organs, Dr. Belding Scribner, one of the early fathers of nephrology, identified four major ethical problems that he and his nephrology colleagues were facing: (1) patient selection for dialysis; (2) termination of dialysis, which he called "dialysis suicide" but which has since been referred to as "stopping" or "withdrawing" dialysis; (3) "death with dignity," which involved the treatment of patients with end-stage kidney disease (ESKD) who were having dialysis withheld or withdrawn; and (4) donor selection for transplantation.[1]

In 1945 in the Netherlands, Dr. Willem Kolff first used hemodialysis to save the lives of patients with acute kidney injury (AKI) from trauma or poisoning. In 1954, the first successful renal transplantation was performed between identical twins, and the recipient lived 8 years.[2] In 1960, Dr. Scribner invented the arteriovenous shunt, which enabled patients with ESKD to undergo long-term hemodialysis. In 1962 the Seattle Artificial Kidney Center opened and faced the unprecedented ethical problem of determining which patients should be given access to long-term hemodialysis in its nine-bed capacity dialysis center. There were many more patients seeking treatment than there were trained staff and machines available to provide dialysis to them. Journalist Shana Alexander called national attention to this ethical problem in her Life magazine article, "They Decide Who Lives, Who Dies: Medical Miracle Puts Moral Burden on Small Committee."[3] In 1968, a Harvard Medical School committee defined brain death as a new criterion for death.[4] The legal recognition of brain death as death enabled cadaveric kidney transplantation.

In 1972, the U.S. Congress included ESKD in the Social Security Amendments to the Medicare bill, Public Law 92-603 (HR 1), which established the End-Stage Renal Disease Program. One of the sponsors of the ESRD Amendment, Senator Russell Long of Louisiana, was, in retrospect, overly optimistic about the benefits of dialysis. He said at the time of passage of the bill, "We are the greatest nation in the world, the wealthiest per capita. Are we so hard pressed that we cannot pay for…a life extended for 10-15 years?"[5] The ESRD Amendment, Section 299I of Public Law 92-603, provided financial support for kidney dialysis and transplantation to all persons eligible for Social Security coverage. The number of persons who would need to be supported by the program and the cost of the program were greatly underestimated. At the time it was thought that perhaps 11,000 patients per year might need to receive dialysis at a cost of approximately $250 million. The fact that not all could receive dialysis who might benefit from it created the first ethical problem alluded to in Dr. Scribner's American Society of Artificial Internal Organs presidential address.

PATIENT SELECTION CRITERIA AND THE OVERT RATIONING OF DIALYSIS

The problem of selecting patients for dialysis had major ramifications, because the patients denied access would die. The solution of the physicians of the Seattle dialysis center was to ask the county medical society to appoint a committee of seven laypersons to make the selection decisions for them from among persons they had identified as being medically appropriate. The physicians recognized that the selection decision went beyond medicine and would entail value judgments about who should have access to dialysis and be granted the privilege of continued life. Historian David Rothman says that their decision to have laypersons engaged in life-and-death decision making was the historic event that signaled the entrance of bioethics into medicine.[6] Bioethics scholar Albert Jonsen believes that the field of bioethics emerged in response to these events in Seattle because they caused a nationwide controversy that stimulated the reflection of scholars regarding a radically new problem at the time, the allocation of scarce life-saving resources.[7]

The physicians regarded children and patients older than 45 years as medically unsuitable for dialysis, but they gave the committee members no other guidelines with which to work. At first the committee members considered choosing patients by lottery, but they rejected this idea because they believed that difficult ethical decisions *could* be made about who should live and who should die. In the first few meetings, the committee members agreed on factors they would weigh in making their decisions: age and sex of the patient, marital status and number of dependents, income, net worth, emotional stability, educational background, occupation, and future potential. They also decided to limit potential candidates to residents of the state of Washington. As the selection process evolved, a pattern emerged of the values the committee was using to reach its decisions. The committee weighed very heavily a person's character and contribution to society.[3]

Once it became public, the Seattle patient selection process for dialysis was subjected to harsh criticism. The committee was castigated for using middle-class American values and social-worth criteria to make decisions.[8] The selection process was believed to have been unfair and to have undermined American society's view of equality and the value of human life. Critics of the Seattle patient selection committee criteria wrote, "The prejudices and mindless clichés that pollute the committee's deliberations ... [rule out] creative non-conformists, who rub the bourgeoisie the wrong way but who historically have contributed so much to the making of America. The Pacific Northwest is no place for a Henry David Thoreau with bad kidneys."[9]

In 1972, the passage of the ESRD Amendment to Public Law 92-603 virtually eliminated the need to ration dialysis. This legislation classified patients with a diagnosis of ESKD as disabled, authorized Medicare entitlement for them, and provided the financial resources to pay for their dialysis. The only requirement for this entitlement was that the patients or their spouses or (if dependent children) parents be insured or entitled to monthly benefits under Social Security. When Congress passed this legislation, its members believed that money should not be an obstacle to providing life-saving therapy.[10] Although the legislation stated that patients should be screened for "appropriateness" for dialysis and transplantation, the primary concern was to make dialysis available to those who needed it. Neither Congress nor physicians thought it necessary or proper for the government to determine patient selection criteria.

By 1978, many U.S. physicians believed that it was morally unjustified to deny dialysis treatment to any patient with ESKD.[8] As a consequence, patients who would not previously have been accepted as dialysis candidates were started on treatment. A decade later, the first report of the U.S. Renal Data System documented the progressively greater acceptance rate of patients for dialysis treatment,[11] and subsequent reports have shown that the sharp rise in the number of patients undergoing dialysis could be explained in part by the inclusion of patients who had poor prognoses, especially the elderly and those with diabetic nephropathy.[12] By 2000, of the new patients starting dialysis, 48% were 65 years or older and 45% had diabetes as the cause of ESKD. Observers raised concerns about the appropriateness of treating patients with a limited life expectancy and quality of life.[13,14] Specifically, questions were raised about the appropriateness of providing dialysis to two groups of patients: those with a limited life expectancy despite the use of dialysis, and those with severe neurologic disease. The first group included patients with kidney failure and other life-threatening illnesses, such as atherosclerotic cardiovascular disease, cancer, chronic pulmonary disease, and acquired immunodeficiency syndrome (AIDS). The second group included patients whose neurologic disease rendered them unable to relate to others, such as those in a persistent vegetative state and those with severe dementia or cerebrovascular disease.[15]

The Institute of Medicine Committee for the Study of the Medicare End-Stage Renal Disease Program, which issued its report in 1991, acknowledged that the existence of the public entitlement for treatment of ESKD does not obligate physicians to treat all patients who have kidney failure with dialysis or transplantation.[14] For some patients with kidney failure, the burdens of dialysis may substantially outweigh the benefits; the provision of dialysis to these patients would violate the medical maxim, "Be of benefit and do no harm." This committee recommended that guidelines be developed for identifying such patients and that the guidelines allow physicians discretion in assessing individual patients. The committee thought that such guidelines might help nephrologists make dialysis decisions more uniformly, with greater ease, and in a way that promoted patient benefit and the appropriate use of dialysis resources. Subsequent studies confirmed the committee's concerns and demonstrated that nephrologists differed in how they made decisions to start or stop dialysis for patients.[16,17]

ACCESS TO DIALYSIS AND THE JUST ALLOCATION OF SCARCE RESOURCES

The numbers of patients undergoing dialysis steadily grew each year, resulting in an ever-increasing cost of the Medicare ESRD Program. In the 1980s, the United States experienced record-breaking budget deficits, and questions began to be raised about continued federal funding of the ESRD Program. Observers wondered whether the money was well spent or whether more good could be done by using the same resources for other patients.[18] Critics of the ESRD Program observed that it satisfied neither of the first principles of distributive justice: equality and utility. On neither a macroallocation nor a microallocation level did the ESRD Program provide equality of access. On the macroallocation level, observers asked, as a matter of fairness and equality, why the federal government should provide almost total support for one group of patients with end-stage disease—those with ESKD—and deny such support to those whose failing organs happened to be hearts, lungs, or livers.[10,18] On a microallocation level, only 93% of patients with ESKD had been eligible for Medicare ESKD benefits. The poor and ethnic minorities were thought to constitute most of the ineligible. The Institute of Medicine Committee for the Study of the Medicare End-Stage Renal Disease Program recommended that the U.S. Congress extend Medicare entitlement to all citizens and resident aliens with ESKD.[15]

From a utilitarian perspective, the ESRD Program could not be argued to be maximizing the good for the greatest number. In the 1980s, more than 5% of the total Medicare budget was being spent on patients undergoing dialysis or kidney transplantation, who represented fewer than 0.2% of the active Medicare patient population. Furthermore, although in 2000 more than 40 million Americans were without basic health insurance, the cost to treat one patient with ESKD receiving dialysis—of whom there were more than 300,000—exceeded $50,000 per year. Despite the high cost, the unadjusted 1-year mortality for patients with ESKD approached 25%; for many, life on dialysis was synonymous with physical incapacitation, dependency, chronic depression, and disrupted family functioning.[19]

CESSATION OF AND WITHDRAWAL FROM DIALYSIS

In the 1960s patients were fortunate to be chosen by dialysis selection committees to receive dialysis. No one considered that patients might want to stop dialysis and die. Faced with patients' requests to "turn off the machine," physicians and ethicists grappled with whether stopping dialysis was "dialysis suicide" and a form of psychopathology or whether, given the unprecedented nature of the life-sustaining therapy, requests to stop dialysis should be analyzed differently. To reason about this issue, ethicists and theologians drew on Catholic moral theology and the distinction between ordinary and extraordinary means. They concluded that patients may refuse or stop life-sustaining interventions such as dialysis, which they regarded as extraordinary.[20]

In its report *Deciding to Forego Life-Sustaining Treatment*, the President's Commission for the Study of Ethical Problems in Medicine and Biomedical and Behavioral Research considered the ethical and legal issues raised by the use of life-sustaining treatments such as dialysis. The commission understood that "biomedical developments of the past several decades ... have made death more a matter of deliberate decision. Matters once the province of fate have now become a matter of human choice" (pp. 1-2).[21] The President's Commission reached two major conclusions that provide justification for withholding and withdrawing dialysis: "the voluntary choice of a competent and informed patient should determine whether or not life-sustaining therapy will be undertaken; and health care professionals serve patients best by maintaining a presumption in favor of sustaining life, while recognizing that competent patients are entitled to choose to forgo any treatments, including those that sustain life" (p. 3).[21]

Similarly, in its 1993 annual report the End-Stage Renal Disease Data Advisory Committee to the U.S. Renal Data System articulated ethical justifications and general and specific principles to be used in making decisions about withholding or withdrawing dialysis. This report reflected the deliberations of an ad hoc committee gathered to examine bioethical issues related to ESKD. The ad hoc committee was composed of nephrologists, ethicists, and health policy experts. The Data Advisory Committee endorsed the recommendations of this ad hoc committee. The report described two ethical justifications for forgoing dialysis: (1) the right of patients to refuse dialysis based on the ethical principle of respect for autonomy and the legal right of self-determination; and (2) a judgment that dialysis does not offer a reasonable expectation of medical benefit based on the ethical principles of beneficence and nonmaleficence.[22]

Withdrawal from dialysis has long been known to be the third most common cause of death in patients undergoing dialysis, after cardiovascular diseases and infections. In the earliest major study calling attention to the frequency of dialysis withdrawal, researchers in one large dialysis program noted that dialysis withdrawal accounted for 22% of deaths.[23] Subsequent research found that older patients and those with diabetes were the most likely to stop dialysis. Over time, as the percentage of diabetic and older patients (those 65 years or older) receiving dialysis rose, withdrawal from dialysis became more common. According to a survey of dialysis units performed in 1990, most dialysis units had withdrawn one or more patients from dialysis in the preceding year, with the mean number being three.[16]

Because of the greater frequency of decisions to withhold and withdraw dialysis in the 1980s and 1990s, the clinical practices of nephrologists in reaching these decisions with patients and families generated heightened interest. Discussions of the ethics and process of withholding or withdrawing dialysis became more frequent.[24] In this later analysis, the two ethical justifications that were given for withholding or withdrawing dialysis essentially agreed with earlier formulations: (1) the patient's right to refuse dialysis, which was based on the right of self-determination; and (2) an unfavorable balance of benefits to burdens for the patient that continued life with dialysis would entail.

Nephrologists and ethicists recommended that decisions to start or stop dialysis be made on a case-by-case basis, because individual patients evaluate benefits and burdens differently. These authorities noted that such decisions should result from a process of shared decision making between the nephrologist and the patient with decision-making capacity. If the patient lacked decision-making capacity, the decisions were to be made on the basis of the patient's expressed wishes (given either verbally or in a written advance directive) or, if these were unknown, the patient's best interests. They also advised that in cases in which patients lacked decision-making capacity, a surrogate be selected to participate with the physician in making decisions for the patient. Questions were identified to help nephrologists evaluate a patient's request to stop dialysis (see Table 83.1). If, after patient evaluation based on the questions in Table 83.1, the patient still requested discontinuation of dialysis, nephrologists were counseled to honor the competent patient's request.

In several studies, 9 out of 10 nephrologists indicated that they would stop dialysis at the request of a patient with decision-making capacity.[16,17] In half or more of the cases in which decisions were made to withdraw dialysis, patients lacked decision-making capacity. Nephrologists expressed a willingness to stop dialysis of "irreversibly incompetent" patients who had clearly said they would not want dialysis if they were in such a condition, but they disagreed about stopping dialysis of patients without clear advance directives.[17] Consistent with the President's Commission report, from the beginning of the availability of dialysis, there has been a presumption in favor of continued dialysis for patients who cannot or have not expressed their wishes. In the absence of an advance directive a patient's right to forgo dialysis was therefore usually difficult to exercise.

ADVANCE DIRECTIVES AND PATIENTS UNDERGOING DIALYSIS

The Patient Self-Determination Act, which applied to institutions participating in Medicare and Medicaid and became effective December 1, 1991, was intended to educate health care professionals and patients about advance directives and to encourage patients to complete them. Although the ESRD Program was almost entirely funded by Medicare, dialysis units were inadvertently left out of the act. The completion of advance directives as part of the process of advance care planning has been recognized as particularly important for patients undergoing dialysis for four reasons[25]: (1) about half of the dialysis population is elderly, and the elderly have the shortest life expectancy with dialysis and are the most likely to withdraw or be withdrawn from dialysis; (2) prior discussion of advance directives has been shown to help such patients and their families approach death in a reconciled fashion[26]; (3) patients who discuss and complete written advance directives are significantly more likely to have their wish to die at home respected; and (4) unless a specific directive to withhold cardiopulmonary resuscitation is obtained—which can be done in the framework of advance care planning—it will be automatically provided, although it rarely leads to extended survival in patients undergoing dialysis.[27]

For these reasons, nephrologists have been encouraged to discuss the circumstances under which patients would want to discontinue dialysis and forgo cardiopulmonary resuscitation and to urge patients to complete written advance directives.[28] When patients lack decision-making capacity and have not completed advance directives, ethically complex issues often arise in making the decision whether to start or stop dialysis. In these situations, many

Table 83.1 Systematic Evaluation of a Patient or Family Request to Stop Dialysis[35]

1. Determine the reasons or conditions underlying the patient/surrogate desires regarding withdrawal of dialysis. Such assessment should include specific medical, physical, spiritual, and psychological issues, as well as interventions that could be appropriate. Some of the potentially treatable factors that might be included in the assessment are as follows:
    (a) Underlying medical disorders, including the prognosis for short- or long-term survival on dialysis
    (b) Difficulties with dialysis treatments
    (c) The patient's assessment of his or her quality of life and ability to function
    (d) The patient's short- and long-terms goals
    (e) The burden that costs of continued treatment/medications/diet/transportation may have on the patient/family/others
    (f) The patient's psychological condition, including depression and conditions or symptoms that may be caused by uremia
    (g) Undue influence or pressure from outside sources, including the patient's family
    (h) Conflict between the patient and others
    (i) Dissatisfaction with the dialysis modality, the time, or the setting of treatment
2. If the patient wishes to withdraw from dialysis, did he or she consent to referral to a counseling professional (e.g., social worker, spiritual advisor, psychologist, or psychiatrist)?
3. If the patient wishes to withdraw from dialysis, are there interventions that could alter the patient's circumstances that might result in his or her considering it reasonable to continue dialysis?
    (a) Describe possible interventions.
    (b) Does the patient desire the proposed intervention(s)?
4. In cases in which the surrogate has made the decision to either continue or withdraw dialysis, has it been determined that the judgment of the surrogate is consistent with the stated desires of the patient?
5. Questions to consider when a patient asks to stop dialysis:
    (a) Is the patient's decision-making capacity diminished by depression, encephalopathy, or other disorder?
    (b) Why does the patient want to stop dialysis?
    (c) Are the patient's perceptions about the technical or quality-of-life aspects of dialysis accurate?
    (d) Does the patient really mean what he or she says or is the decision to stop dialysis made to get attention, help, or control?
    (e) Can any changes be made that might improve life on dialysis for the patient?
    (f) Would the patient be willing to continue dialysis while the factors responsible for the patient's request are addressed?
    (g) Has the patient discussed his or her desire to stop dialysis with significant others such as family, friends, or spiritual advisors? What do they think about the patient's request?

nephrologists indicate that they would consult an ethics committee, if available, for assistance in making decisions in different cases.[16]

EFFECT OF REIMBURSEMENT

Reimbursement affects both dialysis techniques and the quality of care provided to patients undergoing dialysis.[15] There has been concern on the part of dialysis providers that their ethical obligation to provide competent, quality care to their patients is being compromised by insufficient funding of the Medicare ESRD Program. In the 1980s, cost was the federal policy makers' primary concern about the program, and federal reimbursement rates for dialysis were reduced twice. By 1989, the average reimbursement rate for freestanding dialysis units, adjusted for inflation, was 61% lower than it had been when the program began.[15] When the U.S. Congress established the Medicare ESRD Program, the highest estimate for cost of the program by 1977 was $250 million; the actual cost in 1977 was approximately $1 billion.[8] At least two major reasons were held to be responsible for the higher cost: the growing number of patients being started on dialysis, for some of whom dialysis would have been "unthinkable" 10 years earlier, and the growth of in-center dialysis while the use of less costly home dialysis declined.

Despite inflation and increases in the costs of salaries, equipment, and supplies, there were only two modest increases in the Medicare reimbursement to dialysis providers in the 1990s. By the end of the twentieth century, the rate of reimbursement for dialysis by Medicare adjusted for inflation was only one third of the amount in 1973. A longtime historian of the ESRD Program, Richard Rettig, observed, "No other part of Medicare has been subjected to this severe, even punitive, economic discipline."[29] Meanwhile, the incidence of ESKD in the United States had tripled over the previous 20 years. Almost 100,000 new patients were starting dialysis each year.

CONFLICTS OF INTEREST

A conflict of interest occurs when there is a clash between a physician's personal financial gain and the welfare of his or her patients. Although a conflict of interest generally exists for all physicians who practice fee-for-service medicine, there is a potentially greater conflict of interest for physicians who share in the ownership of for-profit dialysis units in which they treat patients. Physicians who receive a share of the profits are financially rewarded for reducing costs. Although measures to reduce costs may simply lead to greater efficiency, they may also compromise patient welfare if they entail reducing dialysis time; purchasing cheaper, possibly less effective dialyzers and dialysis machines; and hiring fewer registered nurses, social workers, and dietitians.

In the past, for-profit dialysis companies were quite open about their policy of giving physicians a financial stake in their companies. Such companies flourished under the ESRD Program.[30] Since the inception of the program, physicians and dialysis units have been paid on a per-patient and per-treatment basis, respectively, and the acceptance rate of patients to dialysis in the United States is higher than anywhere else in the world.[12] This higher rate has been at least partly attributed to the acceptance for dialysis in the United States of a much higher number of patients with poor prognoses. Some have argued that this high acceptance rate is a sign that nephrologists and dialysis units are seeking to maximize their incomes, whereas others have commented that many physicians believe they are obligated to provide dialysis to all patients with ESKD who want it.[13]

In the 1990s, the concerns about conflicts of interest heightened. Two thirds of patients with ESKD were undergoing dialysis in for-profit units. Short dialysis times were found disproportionately in for-profit units and were associated with higher mortality. Patients treated in for-profit dialysis units were noted to have a 20% higher mortality rate and a referral rate for renal transplantation 26% lower than that for patients treated in not-for-profit units.[31] The nephrologist who owned all or a share of a for-profit unit was confronted with a clear conflict of interest. In responding to financial pressures created by a dialysis reimbursement rate that failed to keep up with inflation and in instituting cost-cutting measures, he or she was believed to be treading a very fine line between maintaining adequate profit to keep the dialysis unit open and compromising patient care.

A decade earlier, nephrologist and then *New England Journal of Medicine* editor Arnold Relman had anticipated the predicament that nephrologist owners of dialysis units would face. He had warned that the private enterprise system—the so-called new medical-industrial complex—had a particularly striking effect on the practice of dialysis, and he urged physicians to separate themselves totally from any financial participation so as to maintain their integrity as professionals.[32] Education of nephrologists about these issues, both in training and in continuing education courses, was advocated to help them to identify present and potential conflicts of interest and resolve them in a way that placed patients' interests first.

To hold dialysis units, both for-profit and nonprofit, accountable for the quality of care they provided, the Medicare ESRD Program, through the 18 ESRD Networks, established quality indicators to measure the performance of individual dialysis units and all the dialysis units within a region. These measures monitored adequacy of dialysis, anemia management, vascular access placement, and standardized mortality ratios as well as other indicators.

PRESENT

CLINICAL PRACTICE GUIDELINE ON WITHHOLDING AND WITHDRAWING DIALYSIS

In 1991, the Institute of Medicine Committee for the Study of the Medicare End-Stage Renal Disease Program recommended development of a clinical practice guideline "for evaluating patients for whom the burdens of renal replacement therapy may substantially outweigh the benefits."[15] After that time, nephrologists reported being increasingly asked to provide dialysis to patients for whom they perceived dialysis to be of marginal benefit. Not surprisingly, in a 1997 survey of the Renal Physicians Association and the American Society of Nephrology leadership, the topic of who should receive dialysis and how that decision should be made was given highest priority for guideline development, because the renal professional community recognized that the incident and prevalent ESRD population had changed substantially. A growing number of patients who were initiating renal replacement therapy were elderly and had substantial numbers of comorbid conditions, which in turn adversely affected the patients' health-related quality of life. On the basis of currently available data, from the U.S. Renal Data System for 1993 to 1995, the incident treatment rate per million population per year was found to have increased for all age categories.[33] For Americans 55 years or older, the highest incident treatment rates in descending order were for 75- to 79-year-old, 70- to 74-year-old, and 80- to 84-year-old patients. Older patients were noted to have the most comorbid conditions and to be at the greatest risk for development of illnesses during their subsequent course of dialysis.

In 2000, the Renal Physicians Association and the American Society of Nephrology published the clinical practice guideline *Shared Decision-Making in the Appropriate Initiation of and Withdrawal from Dialysis*.[34] Since then, researchers have extensively investigated dialysis decision making and have found a substantial body of new evidence with regard to (1) the poor prognosis of some elderly patients with stage 4 and stage 5 chronic kidney disease (CKD), many of whom are likely to die prior to initiation of dialysis or for whom dialysis may not provide a survival advantage over medical management without dialysis; (2) the prevalence of cognitive impairment in patients undergoing dialysis and the need to periodically assess them for decision-making capacity; (3) the underrecognition and undertreatment of pain and other symptoms in patients undergoing dialysis; (4) the underutilization of hospice in patients undergoing dialysis; and (5) the distinctly different treatment goals of patients with ESRD that are based on their overall condition and personal preferences. In 2010, the Renal Physicians Association developed a second edition of the guideline to provide clinicians, patients, and families with (1) the most current evidence about the benefits and burdens of dialysis for patients with diverse conditions, (2) recommendations for quality in decision making about treatment of patients with AKI, CKD, and ESKD, and (3) practical strategies to help clinicians implement the guideline recommendations.[35]

In this second edition, the Renal Physicians Association made explicit recommendations to integrate palliative care into the treatment of patients with CKD and ESKD and to develop quality metrics for patients undergoing dialysis whose goals of care are mainly comfort distinct from those whose goals are aggressive, life-prolonging therapy with optimization of function. The association also noted that good communication improves patients' adjustment to illness, increases adherence to treatment, and results in higher patient and family satisfaction with care. The new guideline calls on nephrologists and other members of the interdisciplinary team to communicate information, including prognosis, that patients and families can use to reach informed decisions about dialysis and transplantation options, and urges nephrology fellowship programs to incorporate training in effective, empathetic communication skills so that patients' decisions can be based on an accurate understanding of their overall condition and the pros and cons of treatment options.[35]

The objectives for both editions of this guideline are listed in Table 83.2. The second edition provides ten recommendations with regard to decision making about withholding or withdrawing dialysis and the care of patients who forgo dialysis (Table 83.3). The guideline recommends shared decision making, which it defines as the process by which physicians and patients agree on a specific course of action based on a common understanding of the treatment goals and the risks and benefits of the chosen course in comparison with reasonable alternatives. The association acknowledges, however, that there are limits to the shared decision-making process that protect the rights of patients and the professional integrity of health care professionals. The guideline states that the patient has the right to refuse dialysis even if the renal care team disagrees with the patient's decision and wants the patient to undergo dialysis. Similarly, the renal care team has the right to refuse to offer dialysis when the expected benefits do not justify the risks.

The most difficult ethical quandaries for nephrologists have lately been how to address conflicts when the family of a dying patient undergoing dialysis who lacks decision-making capacity requests that "everything possible be done" when the nephrologist believes that such treatment would be nonbeneficial. The guideline provides recommendations for how to resolve such conflicts.

The target audience for the guideline was health care providers involved in the care of patients with either AKI or ESRD: nephrologists, intensivists, primary care physicians, nephrology nurses, advanced practice nurses, and nephrology social workers. The writers thought it might also be useful to patients and their families, renal dietitians, dialysis technicians, renal administrators, clergy, and policy makers. This guideline has been widely quoted in the nephrology and palliative care literature, and studies have documented the effectiveness of the guideline in managing patient care.[36,37]

In a study to determine whether nephrologists' attitudes and reported practices in dialysis decision making had changed over time, survey responses from 296 nephrologists

---

Table 83.2 Objectives of the Clinical Practice Guideline *Shared Decision Making in the Appropriate Initiation of and Withdrawal from Dialysis*

- Synthesize available research evidence regarding patients with acute kidney injury and end-stage renal disease (ESRD) as a basis for making recommendations about withholding and withdrawing dialysis.
- Enhance understanding of the principles and processes useful for and involved in making decisions to withhold or withdraw dialysis.
- Promote ethically as well as medically sound decision making in individual cases.
- Recommend tools that can be used to promote shared decision making in the care of patients with acute kidney injury or ESRD.
- Offer a publicly understandable and acceptable ethical framework for shared decision making among health care providers, patients, and their families.

From Renal Physicians Association: Shared decision-making in the appropriate initiation of and withdrawal from dialysis, ed 2, Rockville, MD, 2010, Renal Physicians Association.

Table 83.3 *Clinical Practice Guideline* **Recommendations for Shared Dialysis Decision Making**

Establishing a Shared Decision-Making Relationship	RECOMMENDATION NO. 1: Develop a Physician-Patient Relationship for Shared Decision Making.
	Shared decision making is the recognized preferred model for medical decision making because it addresses the ethical need to fully inform patients about the risks and benefits of treatments, as well as the need to ensure that patients' values and preferences play a prominent role. Because of the number and complexity of decisions involved in treating kidney failure, a shared decision-making relationship is particularly important for patients with acute kidney injury (AKI); stage 4 and 5 chronic kidney disease (CKD); and stage 5 CKD requiring dialysis or end-stage kidney disease (ESKD). Participants in shared decision making should involve at a minimum the patient and the physician. In addition, patients should identify and include a person who could serve as their decision maker in the event they lose decision-making capacity. If a patient lacks decision-making capacity, decisions should involve the person legally authorized to make health care decisions on behalf of the incapacitated patient. This person is often (though not always) a family member and will be called "the legal agent" in the remainder of this document. With the patient's consent, shared decision making may include family members or friends and other members of the health care team.
Informing Patients	RECOMMENDATION NO. 2: Fully Inform AKI, Stage 4 and 5 CKD, and ESRD Patients About Their Diagnosis, Prognosis, and All Treatment Options.
	In the setting of critical illness many patients with CKD will require urgent dialysis and the vast majority of patients with AKI will have multiple medical problems, in addition to kidney failure. The concept of shared decision making necessitates a multidisciplinary approach including nephrologists, intensivists, and others as appropriate and decisions about acute renal replacement therapy should be made in the context of other life-sustaining treatments. For example, a decision to withhold dialysis in a patient agreeing to and receiving multiple other forms of life-sustaining therapy could represent discordant treatment in the same way that offering dialysis to a patient who has decided to forgo other forms of life-sustaining therapy might be inappropriate. Intensive care physicians need to be included in shared decision making for kidney patients in the intensive care unit (ICU). For ESRD patients, the shared decision-making options include: 1) available dialysis modalities and kidney transplantation if applicable; 2) not starting dialysis and continuing medical management; 3) a time-limited trial of dialysis; and 4) stopping dialysis and receiving end-of-life care. Choices among options should be made by patients or, if patients lack decision-making capacity, their designated legal agents. Their decisions should be informed and voluntary. The renal care team, in conjunction with the primary care physician, should ensure that the patient or legal agent understands the benefits and burdens of dialysis and the consequences of not starting or stopping dialysis. Research studies have identified a population of chronic kidney disease patients for whom the prognosis is particularly poor. This population has been found to include patients with two or more of the following characteristics: 1) elderly (defined by research studies identifying poor outcomes in patients who are age 75 years and older); 2) patients with high comorbidity scores (e.g., modified Charlson Comorbidity Index score of 8 or greater); 3) marked functional impairment (e.g., Karnofsky Performance Status Scale score of less than 40); and 4) severe chronic malnutrition (e.g., serum albumin level less than 2.5 g/dL using the bromcresol green method). Patients in this population should be informed that dialysis may not confer a survival advantage or improve functional status over medical management without dialysis and that dialysis entails significant burdens that may detract from their quality of life.
	RECOMMENDATION NO. 3: Give All Patients with AKI, Stage 5 CKD, or ESRD an Estimate of Prognosis Specific to Their Overall Condition.
	To facilitate informed decisions about starting dialysis for AKI, stage 5 CKD, or ESRD, all patients should have their prognosis estimated and discussed, with the realization that the ability to predict survival in the individual patient is limited. Depending on the setting, a primary care physician, intensivist, or nephrologist who is familiar with estimating and communicating prognosis should conduct these discussions (see RECOMMENDATION NO. 10 for communication strategies). For patients with ESRD, the "surprise" question, "Would I be surprised if this patient died in the next year?," can be used together with known risk factors for poor prognosis: age, comorbidities, severe malnutrition, and poor functional status. For patients with stage 5 CKD pre-dialysis, the estimate of prognosis should be discussed with the patient or legal agent, patient's family, and among the medical team members to develop a consensus on the goals of care and whether dialysis or active medical management without dialysis should be used to best achieve these goals. These discussions should occur as early as possible in the course of the patient's kidney disease and continue as the kidney disease progresses. For ESRD patients on dialysis who experience major complications that may substantially reduce survival or quality of life, it is appropriate to reassess treatment goals, including consideration of withdrawal from dialysis.

Table 83.3 *Clinical Practice Guideline* Recommendations for Shared Dialysis Decision Making (Continued)

Facilitating Advance Care Planning	RECOMMENDATION NO. 4: Institute Advance Care Planning.
	The purpose of advance care planning is to help the patient understand his/her condition, identify his/her goals for care, and prepare for the decisions that may have to be made as the condition progresses over time. For chronic dialysis patients, the interdisciplinary renal care team should encourage patient-family discussion and advance care planning and include advance care planning in the overall plan of care for each individual patient. The renal care team should designate a person to be primarily responsible for ensuring that advance care planning is offered to each patient. Patients with decision-making capacity should be *strongly* encouraged while they have capacity to talk to their legal agents to ensure that the legal agent knows the patient's wishes and agrees to make decisions according to these wishes.
	The renal care team should attempt to obtain written advance directives from all dialysis patients. Where legally accepted, Physician Orders for Life-Sustaining Treatment (POLST) or similar state-specific forms, also should be completed as part of the advance care planning process. At a minimum, each dialysis patient should be asked to designate a legal agent in a state-specific advance directive. Advance directives should be honored by dialysis centers, nephrologists, and other nephrology clinicians except possibly in situations in which the advance directive requests treatment contrary to the standard of care (see RECOMMENDATION NO. 8 on conflict resolution).
Making a Decision to Not Initiate or to Discontinue Dialysis	RECOMMENDATION NO. 5*: If Appropriate, Forgo (Withhold Initiating or Withdraw Ongoing) Dialysis for Patients with AKI, CKD, or ESRT in Certain, Well-Defined Situations.
	These situations include the following: • Patients with decision-making capacity, who being fully informed and making voluntary choices, refuse dialysis or request that dialysis be discontinued. • Patients who no longer possess decision-making capacity who have previously indicated refusal of dialysis in an oral or written advance directive. • Patients who no longer possess decision-making capacity and whose properly appointed legal agents/surrogates refuse dialysis or request that it be discontinued. • Patients with irreversible, profound neurological impairment such that they lack signs of thought, sensation, purposeful behavior, and awareness of self and environment.
	RECOMMENDATION NO. 6: Consider Forgoing Dialysis for AKI, CKD, or ESRD Patients Who Have a Very Poor Prognosis or for Whom Dialysis Cannot Be Provided Safely.
	Included in these categories of patients are the following: • Those whose medical condition precludes the technical process of dialysis because the patient is unable to cooperate (e.g., advanced dementia patient who pulls out dialysis needles) or because the patient's condition is too unstable (e.g., profound hypotension). • Those who have a terminal illness from nonrenal causes (acknowledging that some in this condition may perceive benefit from and choose to undergo dialysis). • Those with stage 5 CKD older than age 75 years who meet two or more of the following statistically significant very poor prognosis criteria (see RECOMMENDATIONS No. 2 and 3): 1) clinicians' response of "No, I would not be surprised" to the surprise question; 2) high comorbidity score; 3) significantly impaired functional status (e.g., Karnofsky Performance Status score less than 40); and 4) severe chronic malnutrition (i.e., serum albumin less than 2.5 g/dL using the bromcresol green method).
Resolving Conflicts About What Dialysis Decisions to Make	RECOMMENDATION NO. 7: Consider a Time-Limited Trial of Dialysis for Patients Requiring Dialysis, but Who Have an Uncertain Prognosis, or for Whom a Consensus Cannot Be Reached About Providing Dialysis.
	If a time-limited trial of dialysis is conducted, the nephrologist, the patient, the patient's legal agent, and the patient's family (with the patient's permission to participate in decision making) should agree in advance on the length of the trial and parameters to be assessed during and at the completion of the time-limited trial to determine whether dialysis has benefited the patient and whether dialysis should be continued.
	RECOMMENDATION NO. 8: Establish a Systematic Due Process Approach for Conflict Resolution If There Is Disagreement About What Decision Should Be Made with Regard to Dialysis.
	Conflicts may occur between the patient/legal agent and the renal care team about whether dialysis will benefit the patient. Conflicts also may occur within the renal care team or between the renal care team and other health care providers. In sitting down and talking with the patient/legal agent, the nephrologist should try to understand their views, provide data to support his/her recommendation, and correct misunderstandings. In the process of shared decision making, the following potential sources of conflict have been recognized: 1) miscommunication or misunderstanding about prognosis; 2) intrapersonal or interpersonal issues; or 3) special values. If dialysis is indicated emergently, it should be provided while pursuing conflict resolution, provided the patient or legal agent requests it.

Continued on following page

Table 83.3	*Clinical Practice Guideline* **Recommendations for Shared Dialysis Decision Making** (Continued)

Providing Effective Palliative Care	**RECOMMENDATION NO. 9:** To Improve Patient-Centered Outcomes, Offer Palliative Care Services and Interventions to All AKI, CKD, and ESRD Patients Who Suffer from Burdens of Their Disease.
	Palliative care services are appropriate for people who choose to undergo or remain on dialysis and for those who choose not to start or to discontinue dialysis. With the patient's consent, a multi-professional team with expertise in renal palliative care, including nephrology professionals, family or community-based professionals, and specialist hospice or palliative care providers, should be involved in managing the physical, psychological, social, and spiritual aspects of treatment for these patients, including end-of-life care. Physical and psychological symptoms should be routinely and regularly assessed and actively managed. The professionals providing treatment should be trained in assessing and managing symptoms and in advanced communication skills. Patients should be offered the option of dying where they prefer, including at home with hospice care, provided there is sufficient and appropriate support to enable this option. Support also should be offered to patients' families, including bereavement support where appropriate. Dialysis patients for whom the goals of care are primarily comfort should have quality measures distinct from patients for whom the goals are aggressive therapy with optimization of functional capacity.
	RECOMMENDATION NO. 10: Use a Systematic Approach to Communicate About Diagnosis, Prognosis, Treatment Options, and Goals of Care.
	Good communication improves patients' adjustment to illness, increases adherence to treatment, and results in higher patient and family satisfaction with care. Patients appreciate sensitive delivery of information about their prognosis and the ability to balance reality while maintaining hope. In communicating with patients, the critical task for clinicians is to integrate complicated biomedical facts and conditions with emotional, social, and spiritual realities that are equally complex but not well described in the language of medicine. This information must be communicated in a way that patients, legal agents, and families can understand and use to reach informed decisions about dialysis and transplantation options. Patients' decisions should be based on an accurate understanding of their condition and the pros and cons of treatment options. To facilitate effective communication, reliance upon a multidisciplinary approach including nephrologists, intensivists, and others as appropriate is warranted. Decisions about acute renal replacement therapy in AKI should be made in the context of other life-sustaining treatments. Intensive care physicians should be included in shared decision making for kidney patients in the ICU to facilitate discussions on global disease or injury prognosis. Fellowship programs should incorporate training to help nephrologists develop effective, empathetic communication skills, which are essential in caring for this patient population.

From Renal Physicians Association: Shared decision-making in the appropriate initiation of and withdrawal from dialysis, 2nd ed, Rockville, MD, 2010, Renal Physicians Association.

*Medical management incorporating palliative care is an integral part of the decision to forgo dialysis in AKI, CKD, or ESRD, and attention to patient comfort and quality of life while dying should be addressed directly or managed by palliative care consultation and referral to a hospice program (see RECOMMENDATION NO. 9 on palliative care services).

who completed an online survey in 2005 were compared with those from 318 nephrologists who completed a similar mailed survey in 1990. More than half of the respondents indicated awareness of and use of the guideline.

In 2005, less variability was noted in reported practices to withhold dialysis from a permanently unconscious patient (90% would withhold in 2005 vs. 83% in 1990, $P < 0.001$) and to stop dialysis in a severely demented patient (53% in 2005 would stop vs. 39% in 1990, $P < 0.00001$). In 2005, significantly more dialysis units were reported to have written policies on cardiopulmonary resuscitation (86% in 2005 vs. 31% in 1990, $P < 0.0001$) and withdrawal of dialysis (30% in 2005 vs. 15% in 1990, $P < 0.0002$). Nephrologists were also more likely to honor a do-not-resuscitate order for a patient undergoing dialysis (83% in 2005 vs. 66% in 1990, $P < 0.0002$) and to consider consulting an ESRD network ethics committee (52% in 2005 vs. 39% in 1990, $P < 0.001$). The study concluded that nephrologists' reported practices in end-of-life care had changed significantly over the 15 years separating the two surveys, suggesting that the development of the clinical practice guideline was worthwhile.[37]

In another study of the guideline's effectiveness, nephrologist members of the Renal Physicians Association and the Canadian Society of Nephrology were invited to participate in an online survey of their end-of-life decision-making practices. The purpose of the study was to determine nephrologists' perceived preparedness to make end-of-life decisions and factors associated with the highest level of preparedness. A total of 39% of 360 respondents perceived themselves as very well prepared to make end-of-life decisions. In multivariate analysis, very well-prepared nephrologists had completed their fellowships before 1992 and were more aware of the Renal Physicians Association and American Society of Nephrology guideline on dialysis decision making ($P < 0.001$ for all). These very well-prepared nephrologists had stopped dialysis of more patients in the previous year (odds ratio [OR] 2.39; $P = 0.002$), used time-limited trials more often (OR 2.38; $P = 0.003$), and referred more patients to hospice (OR 1.84; $P = 0.024$).

The study concluded that nephrologists who have been in practice longer and are knowledgeable about the Renal Physicians Association and American Society of Nephrology guideline report greater preparedness to make end-of-life decisions and report doing so more often in accordance with guideline recommendations. The investigators recommended that nephrology fellowship programs teach the recommendations in the guideline.[36] Earlier research had shown that nephrology fellows were not prepared to manage pain and address decision making at the end of life. The majority of fellows had reported not knowing how to respond to a patient's request to stop dialysis or when to refer a patient undergoing dialysis to hospice.[38]

END-OF-LIFE CARE

In the wake of public dissatisfaction with end-of-life care and efforts to legalize physician-assisted suicide in several states, physician groups, including the Renal Physicians Association and American Society of Nephrology, recognized their ethical responsibility to improve end-of-life care for their patients. In 1997, in a joint position statement titled "Quality Care at the End of Life," these two organizations urged nephrologists and others involved in the care of patients with ESKD to obtain education and skills in palliative care.[39] They noted that such knowledge and skills were especially important for nephrologists because they treat patients with ESKD who die from complications despite the continuation of dialysis or after withholding or withdrawal of dialysis. For example, in 2011, 92,000 patients undergoing dialysis died, and withdrawal from dialysis was second only to cardiovascular disease as the second most common cause of death in this group.

In 1999, the Robert Wood Johnson Foundation convened a series of work groups to evaluate how end-of-life care could be improved for special populations of patients. The Foundation included the ESRD population because it perceived a readiness to address end-of-life care issues among the health care professionals treating patients with ESKD. In its report issued in 2002, the Foundation's ESRD Workgroup noted that "most patients with ESRD, especially those who are not candidates for renal transplantation, have a significantly shortened life expectancy."[40] In the United States, patients undergoing dialysis live about one-quarter as long as patients of the same age and gender not undergoing dialysis. The adjusted 1-year probability of survival for ESKD patients newly starting dialysis is 78%; and the 10-year survival probability for such patients is only 19 percent. The report also noted that life expectancy is also shortened by comorbid conditions. Forty-five percent of patients newly diagnosed with ESKD have diabetes, and many have other comorbid conditions, including hypertension, congestive heart failure, ischemic heart disease, and peripheral vascular disease. The report observed that the care of patients with ESKD requires expertise not only in the medical and technical aspects of maintaining patients on dialysis but also in palliative care—encompassing pain and symptom management, advance care planning, and attention to ethical, psychosocial, and spiritual issues related to starting, continuing, withholding, and stopping" (p. 5).[40]

The Robert Wood Johnson Foundation ESRD Workgroup also noted the following with regard to the unresolved issue of cardiopulmonary resuscitation in the dialysis unit: (1) research studies of cardiopulmonary resuscitation have indicated that the outcomes for patients with ESKD are poor; (2) most patients undergoing dialysis express a preference for undergoing cardiopulmonary resuscitation, but more than 90% believe that the wish of a patient undergoing dialysis not to undergo cardiopulmonary resuscitation should be respected by dialysis unit personnel[41]; and (3) it is necessary for nephrologists and other members of the renal team to educate patients undergoing dialysis about the likely outcome of cardiopulmonary resuscitation based on patients' particular medical conditions. The group recommended that "dialysis units should adopt policies regarding cardiopulmonary resuscitation in the dialysis unit that respect patients' rights of self-determination, including the right to refuse cardiopulmonary resuscitation and to have a do-not-resuscitate order issued and honored"[40] (p. 11). The Renal Physicians Association and the American Society of Nephrology accepted this recommendation and revised their position statement in "Quality Care at the End of Life" in 2002 to include this and other recommendations of the ESRD Workgroup.

THE "DIFFICULT" PATIENT UNDERGOING DIALYSIS

As early as 1990, the "difficult" patient undergoing dialysis was identified as one of the top three ethical challenges facing nephrologists.[42] In 1998, when the Renal Physicians Association and the American Society of Nephrology were first developing their *Shared Decision-Making* clinical practice guideline, the Centers for Medicare and Medicaid Services (CMS) asked them to devote a chapter to such patients.[34] Dialysis units are facing an increasing number of patients who are disruptive or difficult to treat. These patients pose ethical challenges to dialysis personnel because they disrupt the smooth functioning of a dialysis unit, interfering with the ability of dialysis staff to promote the benefit and maintain the welfare of the difficult patients, other patients, and the staff.[43]

Verbal and physical abuse, nonadherence to medical advice, and substance abuse are considered the defining features of a disruptive or difficult patient undergoing dialysis.[44] In a survey completed by dialysis unit caregivers, approximately 69% of the respondents indicated that their facilities had witnessed an increase in disruptive-difficult patient situations within the 5 years preceding the survey. Forty-nine percent of the survey participants said that they were not adequately trained to deal with disruptive-difficult patient situations. Forty percent of dialysis facilities where these participants worked lacked written policies addressing a disruptive-difficult patient situation.[44]

The ESKD community collaborated in the Decreasing Dialysis Patient-Provider Conflict (DPC) project to develop resources to promote understanding, education, and ability to cope with patient-provider conflict. This project was funded by the CMS and coordinated by the Forum of ESRD Networks. The goal was to increase awareness of conflict and improve skills to decrease conflict. The project also created a common language to describe conflict. These efforts were undertaken to improve staff-patient relationships and to create safer dialysis facilities.[43]

The spectrum of disruptive-difficult patients undergoing dialysis ranges from the patient whose behavior harms only himself or herself to the patient whose behavior endangers other patients and staff in the dialysis unit.[45] Nephrologists and other dialysis personnel have a moral obligation to deal with the difficult-disruptive patient in the broader context of protecting and promoting patient rights and well-being. Mere nonadherence should not usually lead to denial of treatment by a physician or to discharge from the dialysis unit. In the case of a patient undergoing dialysis, the nephrologist or other nephrology clinician should consider the ethical and legal obligations to the patient who requires dialysis, a life-sustaining treatment. At the same time, the caregiver has to safeguard the interests of other patients and staff in the unit. The ethical principles of respect for patient autonomy, beneficence, nonmaleficence, and justice apply as much to the other patients as to the disruptive-difficult patient. Nephrologists and other dialysis personnel must use their judgment to balance the implementation of these principles while dealing with disruptive-difficult patients. Discharge of a disruptive-difficult patient from a dialysis unit should be undertaken only as a last resort, after the other strategies presented in Table 83.4 have been exhausted.[46] Commentators noted that the application of ethical principles can help dialysis staff (1) balance their ethical obligations to disruptive and difficult patients with those to other patients and staff and (2) establish policies and strategies for the treatment of challenging patients. This approach allows health care professionals to identify the limited situations in which involuntary patient discharge from a dialysis unit is ethically justified.[46]

FUTURE

DIALYSIS OF THE OLDER PATIENT

Old age is no longer seen as a contraindication to dialysis, and patients starting dialysis who are older than 85 years have become common. The number of very elderly patients with stage 5 CKD has been projected to rise considerably in coming years.[47] This increase in the very elderly receiving dialysis has been attributed to the aging of the population, the increasing prevalence of type 2 diabetes mellitus, the initiation of dialysis in patients with higher glomerular filtration rates, and a more liberal acceptance approach to providing dialysis to the very elderly. Deciding whether or not to provide dialysis to the very elderly is challenging, because it includes consideration of comorbid conditions, reduced overall life span, and the impact of the dialysis treatment itself on the patient's quality of life.[47]

Between 1996 and 2003, rates of dialysis initiation among octogenarians and nonagenarians in the United States increased by 57%. The incidence of dialysis initiation increased for each 5-year age group from 65 to 69 years and up, with the most dramatic increase among patients between 75 and 84 years of age.[48] This increase translated into a near doubling of the number of patients starting dialysis who were older than 80 years in the United States. The survival of these very elderly patients undergoing dialysis was modest. Although median survival for patients beginning dialysis at 65 to 70 years of age was 24.9 months, median survival for patients 85 to 89 years of age was only 8.4 months. Clinical characteristics associated with these very elderly patients who were likely to live the shortest on dialysis were older age, nonambulatory status, and presence of comorbid conditions. Geriatric researchers proposed that more discussions of prognosis and advance care planning, as recommended by the Renal Physicians Association and American Society of Nephrology clinical practice guideline,[34] would be needed with elderly patients and their families to determine the relative benefits and goals of care.[48]

In a study to compare the survival of 129 patients who had stage 5 CKD and were older than 75 years who were managed either with dialysis or conservatively without dialysis, the researchers found that those who opted for dialysis had a 2.9-fold greater survival.[47] The researchers underscored that conservative management in their study was not

Table 83.4 Strategies for Dealing with the Disruptive or Difficult Patient Undergoing Dialysis[46]

Strategies for Working with the Patient

1. Learn the patient's story and seek to understand his or her perspective.
2. Identify the patient's goal for treatment.
3. Share control and responsibility for treatment with the patient.
   - Educate the patient so that he or she can make informed decisions.
   - Involve the patient in the treatment as much as possible.
   - Negotiate a behavioral contract.
4. Appoint a patient advocate.

Strategies for Preparing the Staff

1. Teach the staff not to criticize patients or call them names.
2. Have the staff use "reflective listening" to show that the patient has been heard.
3. Deal directly with problem behavior; involve the patient, build on the patient's strength, and be clear about who is to do what and when.
4. Take a nonjudgmental approach.
5. Focus on the issue that started the disagreement.
6. Detail the consequences of aberrant behavior in terms that are comprehensible.
7. Prepare a behavior contract that specifies what is to be done by the patient and the renal team.
8. Prepare in advance to manage anger.
9. Be patient and persistent.
10. Do not tolerate verbal abuse.
11. Outline for the staff step by step the means of coping with agitated and disruptive patients.
12. Establish and publicize a grievance procedure.
13. After effective resolution of a conflict, follow up with the patient to monitor the patient's progress and demonstrate to the patient the commitment to resolve a conflict.
14. Contact law enforcement officials when physical abuse is threatened or occurs.
15. As a last resort consider transfer of the patient to another facility or discharge.
16. Consult with legal counsel before proceeding with plans for discharge, and do not discharge the patient without advance notice and disclosure of future treatment options.
17. Contact the end-stage renal disease network if satisfactory resolution has not occurred with the use of these strategies.

simply the absence of dialysis but entailed active disease management with treatment of anemia and other complications of CKD. In a Cox proportional hazards regression analysis, modality choice (to treat with dialysis or not), age, and comorbidity were most strongly associated with survival. In multivariate analysis there was no survival advantage for patients with ischemic heart disease who chose dialysis ($P = 0.27$). There was also no survival advantage for those patients with the highest comorbidity score when those who chose dialysis were compared with those who chose conservative management.

In this study, the researchers were surprised to note that the presence of comorbid conditions had no effect on the decision whether or not to initiate dialysis. The researchers concluded that comorbid conditions, and especially ischemic heart disease, substantially reduced the survival advantage for elderly patients who chose dialysis. They urged that comorbid conditions be one of the main considerations in shared decision making with elderly patients about whether or not to initiate dialysis. Others have also noted that the presence of comorbid conditions is an independent prognostic factor in predicting survival of patients who are managed conservatively without dialysis.[49,50]

A study of 209,622 U.S. veterans with CKD stages 3 to 5 examined outcomes by stage of CKD and age. The researchers noted that older members of the cohort, especially those 75 years or older, were far more likely to die than to have ESKD and start dialysis. They cautioned against "age-neutral" approaches to the management of CKD, observing that because such a small number of elderly patients initiate dialysis, there is a need for prognostic tools that will enable clinicians to identify the subgroup of older patients who are most likely to benefit from dialysis.[51] Pointing out that the rates of dialysis withdrawal are highest among the oldest patients, one writer raised the possibility that the standard content of informed consent for dialysis warrants an age-sensitive approach that is attuned to very different balances of pros and cons of dialysis between older patients with multiple comorbid conditions and younger patients with limited or no comorbid conditions.[52] An integrated prognostic tool to estimate 6-month mortality in patients undergoing dialysis was developed and validated, with a C-statistic of 0.80. It takes account of age, serum albumin, dementia, peripheral vascular disease, and the nephrologist's response to the "surprise question"—"Would I be surprised if this patient died in the next six months?"[53] The accuracy of this tool in the stage 5 CKD population remains to be studied.

TREATMENT OF CHRONIC PAIN

As early as 1990 the World Health Organization identified the treatment of pain as an ethical issue. It declared that freedom from pain should be seen as a right of patients and that treatment of pain is the measure of the respect for this right.[54] Judged by this standard, the right to be free from pain is not being respected for most patients undergoing dialysis. In the first decade of the twenty-first century, three studies of chronic pain in patients undergoing dialysis reached the same conclusion: The pain of three quarters of these patients is undertreated or untreated.[55-57]

Several studies have found that 50% or more of patients undergoing dialysis experience chronic pain and that it is one of the most common and severe symptoms that such patients report.[55,58] Using the World Health Organization three-step analgesic ladder, researchers have documented that in the vast majority of patients undergoing dialysis this pain can be managed successfully.[56] Like other patient populations, most patients undergoing dialysis do not report pain unless they are explicitly asked about it.[56] Nephrologists are largely unaware of their patients' symptoms.[58]

For the pain of patients undergoing dialysis to be adequately managed, it needs to be assessed for intensity and quality. Pain intensity is assessed on a 0 to 10 scale in which 0 equals no pain at all and 10 equals the worst pain imaginable.[55] Pain that is described as aching, dull, throbbing, or sharp is nociceptive pain. Pain that is described as burning, tingling, stabbing, or numb is neuropathic pain. Depending on the intensity of the pain, nociceptive pain is usually responsive to step I pain medications such as acetaminophen, step II pain medications such as tramadol, or step III pain medications such as hydromorphone, fentanyl, and methadone. Neuropathic pain most often responds best to medications for peripheral neuropathy or seizures, such as gabapentin, pregabalin, desipramine, nortriptyline, and valproic acid. Because of an improved understanding of the metabolism of opioids, it is now known that drugs that have renally excreted metabolites are more likely to cause opioid neurotoxicity in patients with CKD. For that reason, codeine, meperidine, morphine, and propoxyphene are not recommended for use in patients with CKD.[59]

Researchers have recommended that nephrologists implement a standardized symptom assessment protocol to improve clinicians' recognition of symptoms as well as their utilization of symptom-alleviating treatments.[58] Not only do objective studies demonstrate an inverse relationship between the number of symptoms (including pain) that patients undergoing dialysis experience and their self-reported quality of life[60,61]; qualitative focus group studies of patients undergoing dialysis have identified adequate pain and symptom management as a vital component of quality end-of-life care.[62] Treatment of pain has been associated with improved quality of life for such patients.[56]

PALLIATIVE CARE AND REFERRAL TO HOSPICE

Palliative care is especially appropriate for patients undergoing dialysis because of their advanced age, significantly shortened life expectancy, high symptom burden, and multiple comorbid illnesses. In addition, there is a greater need for advance care planning for these patients because of their dependence on life-sustaining treatment for their continued existence and because a decision to stop dialysis is the second most common reason for death.[63] The "surprise question"—"Would I be surprised if this patient died in the next year?"—has been determined to identify patients undergoing dialysis at high risk for early death. The odds of dying within a year for patients in the "No, I would not be surprised" group were 3.5 times higher than for patients in the "Yes" group (OR 3.507, 95% confidence interval 1.356 to 9.067; $P = 0.01$). Nephrologists have been encouraged to implement the surprise question monthly on dialysis rounds to screen patients and identify those for whom referral for palliative care consultation is appropriate.[64]

Although in 2000 the Renal Physicians Association and the American Society of Nephrology included a recommendation for palliative care in their guideline, there is still a need for significant improvement in palliative care for patients undergoing dialysis and for greater collaboration between nephrologists and palliative care clinicians.[65,66] One particular area in which palliative care has been found to be deficient for patients undergoing dialysis is referral to hospice. In 2001 and 2002, patients undergoing dialysis who were dying were found to use hospice roughly half as often as dying patients in the nation as a whole (13.5% vs. >22%). Even among patients who withdrew from dialysis, only a minority (41.9%) used hospice. This low percentage was of particular concern, because death after dialysis withdrawal is much more predictable than death in patients with cancer. After dialysis withdrawal, 96% of patients die within 30 days.[67]

To encourage consideration of hospice, in 2004 the CMS added a question about hospice use prior to death to the CMS-2746 ESRD Death Notification form. The U.S. Renal Data System *2008 Annual Data Report* noted that hospice use after dialysis withdrawal in the 2005 to 2006 cohort had increased significantly, to 54.8%, and attributed the increase in hospice use to the educational efforts of the Renal Physicians Association and the American Society of Nephrology.[68]

Patients undergoing dialysis may receive both the Medicare ESRD benefit and the Medicare hospice benefit, but many dialysis units and hospice programs have been unaware of this eligibility. To continue dialysis under the Medicare dialysis benefit and also qualify for the Medicare hospice benefit, a patient must be certified by his or her attending physician to (1) have a life expectancy of 6 months or less if the disease takes its normal course and (2) have a terminal diagnosis for hospice other than kidney disease, such as cancer or end-stage heart disease.[67]

ACCESS TO RENAL TRANSPLANTATION

In 1964, Dr. Scribner was prescient when he identified donor selection for transplantation as one of the major ethical problems faced by nephrologists. At the time of Dr. Scribner's 1964 American Society of Artificial Internal Organs presidential address, a huge demand for donor kidneys in the twenty-first century was unthinkable. In its *2008 Annual Data Report,* the U.S. Renal Data System indicated that 68,576 persons were on the kidney transplant waiting list. Because the growth in the number of transplantations has not kept pace with the growth in the incidence of ESKD, the number of transplantations per 100 dialysis patient–years actually fell by 29% between 1991 and 2006.[68] In many parts of the country the average waiting time on the list for a kidney transplant is longer than 5 years. Organ shortage has replaced immunologic barriers as the major hurdle to transplantation.[69]

There is little disagreement that (1) the quality of life for patients with ESKD is better after successful transplantation or that (2) most patients prefer renal transplantation to continuing on dialysis.[70] Research has shown that, compared with dialysis, kidney transplantation leads to a longer life, a better quality of life, and lower costs for the health care system. Furthermore, transplantation of a kidney from a living donor leads to better patient and graft survival than transplantation of an organ from a deceased donor. Research has also shown that unrelated living-donor transplants can be associated with survival results equivalent to those for related living-donor transplants.[69]

The "profound organ shortage" has created the ethical challenge of trying to help patients in need of transplants to gain access to them more expeditiously while maintaining the integrity of the overall allocation system. Since 2000, the number of live donors has exceeded that of deceased donors, but because two kidneys are usually available from cadaveric donors, most kidney transplants are still of cadaveric kidneys.[71] Alternative sources of organs to attempt to address the shortage include elderly brain-dead donors (using extended criteria for donation), living donors, and donors without a heartbeat (what has been called *donation after cardiac death*). It has been estimated that even if all potential deceased donors became actual deceased donors, there would still be a shortage of organs.[72] Because of the shortfall in potential deceased donors, the use of unrelated living donors has been said to hold the greatest potential for increasing the number of organ donors in the future.[69]

Organ donation by a living donor presents a unique ethical dilemma in that the physician risks the health and sometimes even the life of a healthy person to save or improve the life of a patient. This practice is also of concern because no national organization or allocation policies regulate it.[73]

There are three categories of organ donation by living persons: (1) directed donation to a loved one or a friend, (2) nondirected donation to a general pool in which the organ goes to the person at the top of the waiting list, and (3) directed donation to a stranger. Each category raises ethical concerns. In directed donation, there is the concern that pressure can be put on the family member or friend to donate. Directed donation to a stranger raises concerns about the motivation of the person making the donation. There are often psychologically suspect motivations such as trying to compensate for depression, seeking media attention, and hoping to become involved in the life of the recipient. Directed donation to a stranger may occur when a patient advertises for an organ publicly, whether on television, billboards, or an Internet site. Matchingdonors.com is one such Internet site, and the number of individuals registering as potential donors on the site increased from more than 2000 donors in 2005 to more than 6000 donors in 2009.

Ethicists have called for higher standards of responsibility and accountability for solicitation of organs over the Internet.[74] Directed donations to strangers potentially violate standards of fairness. In one case the family of a brain-dead Florida man who was known to be a racist insisted that the man's organs be donated only to recipients who were white. In another case, a Jewish man in New York who wanted to help someone of his own faith donated one of his kidneys to a Jewish child in Los Angeles who needed a kidney transplant.[74] These two cases are contrary to the United Network for Organ Sharing policies, which bar directed donation to patients based on race, sex, religion, and national origin.[73]

The scarcity of kidneys for organ donation has led transplant programs to seek creative ways to obtain organs for their patients. A variant of directed donation is "paired exchange." Two couples with reciprocal blood type and cross-match incompatibilities have the donor from each couple donate to the recipient in the other couple. Paired exchanges have occasionally even been expanded to "triple swaps" or even much larger exchanges.[75]

Because of the potential harm to living donors, a consensus statement was developed to guide organ transplantation from living donors. This consensus statement included the following requirements for the living organ donor: the person must be competent, willing to donate, free from coercion, medically and psychosocially suitable, fully informed of the risks and benefits of being a donor, and fully informed of the risks, benefits, and alternative treatment options for the recipient. The statement also indicated that the benefits to both the donor and recipient must outweigh the risks associated with the donation and transplantation of the living-donor organ.[76]

Over the years there has been an undercurrent suggesting that living donors or families of deceased donors should be compensated for agreeing to donate. Proponents of an approach that would permit the sale of organs for transplantation have argued that it would resolve the scarcity of organs and the life-or-death situations that occur with it.[77] At times it is not always clear what approach is being advocated in a proposal to allow donor kidneys to be sold. It could entail compensating families for the removal of a cadaveric organ, allowing the purchase of a kidney from a living donor, creating an open market in organs with supply and demand setting the price, establishing a regulated market with an official body fixing the price of organs, or setting up a futures market with a donor agreeing to give an organ after death in exchange for immediate compensation or for compensation that would go to his or her estate.[77] Others have questioned whether a market in organs would increase the supply by providing an incentive to donate or decrease the supply by countering the prevailing ethos of altruism that motivates donations.[78]

An appealing argument that has been made for organ sale is that it may provide a means for indigent people to escape from poverty. At least two studies in India quashed this idea by showing that donors' health and financial status were worse after the sale of organs.[77] An international summit reached a consensus that transplant commercialism (defined as a practice in which an organ is treated as a commodity, including being bought or sold), transplant tourism, and organ trafficking should be prohibited.[79]

Another ethically troubling aspect of renal transplantation in the United States is the racial disparity. Studies have found that blacks are less likely than whites to be deemed appropriate candidates for transplantation, to be referred for transplant evaluation, to complete a transplant evaluation, to be added to a transplant waiting list, and to receive a kidney transplant.[80] There are multiple factors at play, including clinical characteristics such as body mass index greater than 35 and social characteristics such as level of education. The transplant community has addressed racial disparity in part by removing the HLA-B match as a priority for allocation of organs, which has resulted in more transplants for blacks. To promote equality in treatment of patients, efforts continue to be undertaken to eliminate system-wide disparities in renal transplantation.[81]

In 2006, an Institute of Medicine committee released a report on how to raise the rates of postmortem (deceased-donor) organ donation. The committee concluded that four proposed approaches to increase deceased-donor organ donations were unwise and might even be counterproductive and recommended five other approaches instead (Table 83.5).[82] The committee noted that even if its five recommended approaches were effective, it still doubted that they would close the gap between demand and supply for kidney organ donors.

The committee identified as another potential source of organ donors the estimated 22,000 people who die suddenly of cardiac arrest outside the hospital. It proposed demonstration projects in cities with sophisticated trauma and emergency response systems to determine whether it is feasible to increase organ donations after cardiac death in these circumstances. The committee realized that this approach is controversial because it would necessitate inserting a vascular access device and beginning organ preservation techniques while seeking to locate the family and obtain their consent for donation. The report called for organ procurement organizations to "work with relevant stakeholders to obtain community authorization" for such an approach. It noted that education and efforts to gain public trust would be key to the success of this approach.[83]

Although not charged with studying living-donor organ donation, the Institute of Medicine committee did express

Table 83.5	Institute of Medicine (IOM) Recommendations with Regard to Increasing Postmortem Organ Donations
IOM recommended against the following approaches	• Provision of financial incentives • Assignment of priority to persons who registered for postmortem organ donation if they ever need an organ transplant • Requirement for mandated choice forcing people to commit with regard to their willingness to be a postmortem organ donor • Presumption of consent to postmortem organ donation with an opt-out provision
IOM recommended in favor of the following approaches	• Enhanced public education about organ donation • Influencing of the sociocultural atmosphere to support an expectation of donation • Simplification of ways for people to register to be organ donors • Expansion of the efforts of state donor registries • Improvement in organ procurement organizations' systems so that best practices result in a higher percentage of families giving consent for organ donation

Data from Childress JF, Liverman CT (editors): Organ donation: opportunities for action, Washington, DC, 2006, National Academies Press.

concern about it and stated that the practice of organ donation by living donors "needs a careful review and assessment on its own."[83] In particular, the committee cited the need for additional scientific evidence about long-term risks to donors (some studies have suggested a significant risk of hypertension 5 to 10 years after donation), disclosure of these potential risks to prospective donors, and more attention to the consent process to ensure that it is informed and voluntary.

Commentators have been aware of the role of the media in influencing the public's attitudes toward organ donation. They have criticized the media's focus on the more controversial proposals such as buying and selling organs to the neglect of less headline-grabbing but still potentially effective approaches such as donation after circulatory death.[82] The Institute of Medicine committee recognized that for its recommendations on increasing postmortem organ donations to succeed, the media will need to play a major role in public education and trust building.

THE COMING FISCAL CRISIS IN NEPHROLOGY AND THE PROSPECT OF THE RETURN OF RATIONING

Commentators on the Medicare ESRD Program have warned that nephrologists and the Program face a harsh economic future. They point to the looming financial insolvency of Medicare and to the Patient Protection and Affordable Care Act of 2010 as an effort, in part, to remedy the health care economic crisis. They note that the Medicare ESRD Program is "low-hanging fruit" because it is disproportionately expensive, with roughly 6% of Medicare dollars each year being used to pay for services to patients with ESKD, who constitute only about 1% of Medicare beneficiaries. No other chronic disease program is so generously funded by the U.S. government. Among the scenarios the commentators predict on the basis of Medicare's need to control costs is age-based rationing of dialysis. They note that elderly patients undergoing hemodialysis are likely targets for several reasons: Those 75 years of age and older are the fastest-growing segment of the dialysis population and constitute more than 25% of incident patients starting dialysis; the elderly undergoing dialysis are more expensive than younger patients—average annual costs for one elderly patient receiving dialysis exceed $100,000 (compared to average annual cost per patient of $88,000)—and there is increasing evidence for shorter survival with dialysis in the elderly than in younger patients, especially if the elderly have significant comorbid conditions.[84]

Discrimination based on age alone—age-based rationing—is controversial and is not supported as ethically justifiable by most ethicists.[85] Equal regard for persons regardless of their age has been said to appropriately focus on a person as a whole rather than as an accumulation of life years. Age discrimination imposes on older people the judgment that, relatively speaking, their lives are not worth living, even if they disagree.[85] The movement in medicine is toward patient-centered care, and the height of patient-centered care is shared decision making.[86] As previously noted in the *Shared Decision-Making* clinical practice guideline, with rare exceptions the nephrologist and the patient decide together whether dialysis is something the patient wants to undertake given the patient-specific estimate of prognosis and the likelihood of benefits and burdens of a course of dialysis for a patient based on the patient's overall condition.[35] Covert age rationing of dialysis by the British National Health Service in the 1980s raised the ire of the British people and caused the Service to raise the level of dialysis services provided to the elderly to be more consistent with those in neighboring European countries. Because the use of age as a criterion for dialysis was discredited in debates in Britain, researchers doubt that Britain will return to it.[87]

In line with the commentators' predictions regarding the Medicare ESRD Program, on July 1, 2013, CMS released a proposed rule that would cut 12% from the prospective payment system (PPS) "bundle" that became effective in 2011 to pay dialysis facilities for the provision of dialysis services to patients with ESKD. Section 153(b) of the Medicare Improvements for Patients and Providers Act of 2008 (MIPPA) amended the Social Security Act to require CMS to implement a fully bundled PPS for renal dialysis services furnished to Medicare beneficiaries for the treatment of ESKD effective January 1, 2011.[88]

On November 22, 2013, the CMS issued a final rule that updated payment policies and rates under the ESRD PPS for renal dialysis services furnished to beneficiaries on or after January 1, 2014. This final rule implements a provision in the American Taxpayer Relief Act of 2012 that reduces payments to account for changes in the utilization of ESKD-related drugs and biologicals. The final rule provides for a 3- to 4-year phase-in of this 12% decrease to mitigate its impact on providers and is likely to take effect in 2016 or 2017.[89] The nephrology community has yet to respond to how it will continue dialysis after a 12% cut in reimbursement for each treatment is fully implemented.

CONCLUSION

The ethical issues facing nephrologists in the 1950s and 1960s were said to have ushered in the field of bioethics. Despite being decades old, the ESRD Program is still confronted with ethical challenges about who should receive dialysis, what the appropriate ethical response to difficult patients is, the amount of federal funding the program should receive, and how systems of care should be improved to best treat patients with ESKD at the end of life. Because of the use of paired exchanges, triple swaps, directed donation to strangers, and organ donation after circulatory death outside the hospital as methods to help overcome the large and growing organ shortage, nephrologists know that new ethical issues arise with every advance in renal transplantation. With the growth in the ESKD population, the changes in its demographics, and the economic challenges being presented by a federal government that is increasingly unwilling to fund the current level of dialysis services for patients with ESKD, there is every expectation that in the future, nephrologists will continue to be at the forefront of those facing ethical issues in medicine.

Complete reference list available at ExpertConsult.com.

KEY REFERENCES

1. Scribner B: Ethical problems of using artificial organs to sustain human life. *Trans Am Soc Artif Intern Organs* 10:209–212, 1964.

2. Merrill JP, Murray JE, Harrison JH, et al: Successful homotransplantations of the human kidney between identical twins. *JAMA* 106:277–282, 1956.
3. Alexander S: They decide who lives, who dies. *Life* 53:102–125, 1962.
4. Report of the Ad Hoc Committee at Harvard Medical School to examine the definition of brain death: A definition of irreversible coma. *JAMA* 205:337–340, 1968.
5. Rettig RA: The policy debate on patient care financing for victims of end-stage renal disease. *Law Contemp Probl* 40:196–206, 1976.
6. Rothman DJ: *Strangers at the bedside: a history of how law and bioethics transformed medical decision making*, New York, 1991, Basic Books.
7. Jonsen AR: *The new medicine and the old ethics*, Cambridge, MA, 1990, Harvard University Press.
8. Fox RC, Swazey JP: *The courage to fail: a social view of organ transplants and dialysis*, ed 2 rev, Chicago, 1978, University of Chicago Press.
9. Sanders D, Dukeminier J: Medical advances and legal lag: hemodialysis and kidney transplantation. *UCLA Law Rev* 15:366–380, 1968.
10. Rettig RA: Origins of the Medicare kidney disease entitlement: the Social Security Amendments of 1972. In Hanna KE, editor: *Biomedical politics*, Washington, DC, 1991, National Academies Press, pp 176–208.
11. National Institute of Diabetes and Digestive and Kidney Diseases: *United States Renal Data System: USRDS 1989 annual data report*, Bethesda, MD, 1989, National Institutes of Health, National Institute of Diabetes and Digestive and Kidney Diseases.
12. Hull AR, Parker TF, III: Proceedings from the Morbidity, Mortality and Prescription of Dialysis Symposium, Dallas TX, September 15 to 17. *Am J Kidney Dis* 15:375–383, 1989.
13. Fox RC: Exclusion from dialysis: a sociologic and legal perspective. *Kidney Int* 19:739–751, 1981.
14. Levinsky NG, Rettig RA: The Medicare end-stage renal disease program: a report from the Institute of Medicine. *N Engl J Med* 324:1143–1148, 1991.
15. Rettig RA, Levinsky NG: *Kidney failure and the federal government*, Washington, DC, 1991, National Academies Press.
16. Moss AH, Stocking CB, Sachs GA, et al: Variation in the attitudes of dialysis unit medical directors toward reported decisions to withhold and withdraw dialysis. *J Am Soc Nephrol* 4:229–234, 1993.
17. Singer PA: Nephrologists' experience with and attitudes towards decisions to forego dialysis: the End-Stage Renal Disease Network of New England. *J Am Soc Nephrol* 2:1235–1240, 1992.
18. Moskop JC: The moral limits to federal funding for kidney disease. *Hastings Cent Rep* 17:11–15, 1987.
19. Dottes AL: Should all individuals with end-stage renal disease be dialyzed? *Contemp Dial Nephrol* 12.19–30, 1991.
20. Jonsen AR: *The birth of bioethics*, New York, 1998, Oxford University Press.
21. President's Commission for the Study of Ethical Problems in Medicine and Biomedical and Behavioral Research: *Deciding to forego life-sustaining treatment*, Washington, DC, 1983, US Government Printing Office.
22. ESRD Data Advisory Committee: *1993 annual report*, Washington, DC, 1993, US Department of Health and Human Services, pp 29–33.
23. Neu S, Kjellstrand CM: Stopping long-term dialysis: an empirical study of withdrawal of life-supporting treatment. *N Engl J Med* 314:14–20, 1986.
24. Hastings Center: *Guidelines on the termination of life-sustaining treatment and the care of the dying*, Bloomington, 1987, Indiana University Press.
25. Moss AH: Dialysis decisions and the elderly. *Clin Geriatr Med* 10:463–473, 1994.
26. Swartz RD, Perry E: Advance directives are associated with "good deaths" in chronic dialysis patients. *J Am Soc Nephrol* 3:1623–1630, 1993.
27. Lehrich RW, Pun PH, Tanenbaum ND, et al: Automated external defibrillators and survival from cardiac arrest in the outpatient hemodialysis clinic. *J Am Soc Nephrol* 18:312–320, 2007.
28. Moss AH, Holley JL, Upton MB: Outcomes of cardiopulmonary resuscitation in dialysis patients. *J Am Soc Nephrol* 3:1238–1243, 1992.
29. Rettig RA: Historical perspective. In Levinsky NG, editor: *Ethics and the kidney*, New York, 2001, Oxford University Press, p 16.
30. Kolata GB: NMC thrives selling dialysis. *Science* 208:379–382, 1980.
31. Levinsky NG: Quality and equity in dialysis and renal transplantation. *N Engl J Med* 341:1691–1693, 1999.
32. Relman AS: The new medical-industrial complex. *N Engl J Med* 303:963–970, 1980.
35. Renal Physicians Association: *Shared decision-making in the appropriate initiation of and withdrawal from dialysis*, ed 2, Rockville, MD, 2010, Renal Physicians Association.
36. Davison SN, Jhangri GS, Holley JL, et al: Nephrologists' reported preparedness for end-of-life decision-making. *Clin J Am Soc Nephrol* 1:1256–1262, 2006.
37. Holley JL, Davison SN, Moss AH: Nephrologists' changing practices in reported end-of-life decision-making. *Clin J Am Soc Nephrol* 2:107–111, 2007.
38. Holley JL, Carmody SS, Moss AH, et al: The need for end-of-life care training in nephrology: National survey results of nephrology fellows. *Am J Kidney Dis* 42:813–820, 2003.
40. Robert Wood Johnson Foundation: *Promoting Excellence in End-of-Life Care program, End-Stage Renal Disease Workgroup: Recommendations to the field*, Princeton, NJ, 2002, Robert Wood Johnson Foundation. Available at http://www.promotingexcellence.org/esrd. Accessed May 5, 2011.
41. Moss AH, Hozayen O, King K, et al: Attitudes of patients toward cardiopulmonary resuscitation in the dialysis unit. *Am J Kidney Dis* 38:847–852, 2001.
43. Schwartz P, Rudavsky S, Christakis A: *Report of the Dialysis Patient-Provider Conflict (DPPC)—a consensus project with the participation of the community of stakeholders*. Available at http://esrdncc.org/professionals/decreasing-dialysis-patient-provider-conflict/. Accessed March 14, 2015.
46. Hashmi A, Moss AH: Treating disruptive and difficult dialysis patients: practical strategies based on ethical principles. *Nat Clin Pract Nephrol* 4:515–520, 2008.
47. Murtagh FEM, Marsh JE, Donohoe P, et al: Dialysis or not? A comparative study of survival of patients over 75 years with chronic kidney disease stage V. *Nephrol Dial Transplant* 22:1955–1962, 2007.
48. Kurella M, Covinsky KE, Collins AJ, et al: Octogenarians and nonagenarians starting dialysis in the United States. *Ann Intern Med* 146:177–183, 2007.
51. O'Hare AM, Choi AI, Bertenthal D, et al: Age affects outcomes in chronic kidney disease. *J Am Soc Nephrol* 18:2758–2765, 2007.
53. Cohen LM, Ruthazer R, Moss AH, et al: Predicting six-month mortality in patients maintained with hemodialysis. *Clin J Am Soc Nephrol* 5(1):72–79, 2010.
55. Davison SN: Pain in hemodialysis patients: prevalence, cause, severity, and management. *Am J Kidney Dis* 42:1239–1247, 2003.
64. Moss AH, Ganjoo J, Sharma S, et al: Utility of the "surprise" question to identify dialysis patients with high mortality. *Clin J Am Soc Nephrol* 3:1379–1384, 2008.
66. Davison SN: The ethics of end-of-life care for patients with ESRD. *Clin J Am Soc Nephrol* 7:2049–2057, 2012.
69. Matas AJ, Southerland DER: The importance of innovative efforts to increase organ donation. *JAMA* 294:1691–1693, 2005.
79. The Declaration of Istanbul on Organ Trafficking and Transplant Tourism: *Clin J Am Soc Nephrol* 3:1227–1231, 2008.
84. Andersen MJ, Friedman AN: The coming fiscal crisis: Nephrology in the line of fire. *Clin J Am Soc Nephrol* 8:1252–1257, 2013.

84 Health Disparities in Nephrology

Yoshio N. Hall | Glenn M. Chertow

CHAPTER OUTLINE

DISPARITY, 2574
HEALTH JUSTICE, 2575
SOCIAL ORIGINS OF DISPARITIES IN NEPHROLOGY, 2575
Prenatal Environment and Disparities in Kidney Disease Risk, 2575
Postnatal Environment and Disparities in Kidney Disease Risk, 2576
Race, Social Conditions, and Disparities in Kidney Disease Risk, 2577
BIOLOGIC ORIGINS OF DISPARITIES IN NEPHROLOGY, 2578

HEALTH SYSTEM AND DISPARITIES IN NEPHROLOGY, 2578
Unequal Health System Access and Surveillance, 2578
Importance of Health System Structure, 2579
DISPARITIES IN THE TREATMENT OF KIDNEY DISEASE, 2580
Chronic Kidney Disease, 2580
End-Stage Kidney Disease, 2580
MOVING TOWARD MORE EQUITABLE CARE, 2582
INITIATIVES TO REDUCE DISPARITIES, 2583

Disparities in the incidence, progression, and treatment of kidney disease according to socioeconomic status, race-ethnicity, and geographic location have been documented for many years. These relative differences arise and are sustained via multiple intermediaries, including biologic susceptibility, differential access to high-quality health care, and contextual impediments to healthy living. This chapter provides a framework for evaluating systematic differences in health, describes what is known about root causes of disparities in nephrology and nephrology care, and highlights broad strategies for addressing key determinants of these inequities.

DISPARITY

The term "health disparity" often refers to suboptimal health processes or outcomes experienced by demographically defined groups that occur in the context of social or economic inequality. The U.S. National Library of Medicine defines a *health status disparity* as variation in rates of disease occurrence and disabilities between (among) socioeconomic and/or geographically defined population groups.[1] On the other hand, a *health care disparity* refers to a difference in access to or availability of health care facilities and services.[1] Health status and health care disparities relate to systematic inequalities in health among social groups that are deemed to be avoidable by reasonable means.

This chapter covers four broad areas of health status and health care disparities in nephrology observed in socially disadvantaged groups: (1) disparities in the incidence and prevalence of risk factors for chronic kidney disease (CKD); (2) disparities in the progression and treatment of CKD; (3) disparities in the incidence of end-stage kidney disease (ESKD); and (4) disparities in the treatment of ESKD.

Worldwide estimates of ESKD incidence vary widely and are strongly influenced by the availability of funding for the treatment of kidney disease and its risk factors.[2] In fact, prior to passage of U.S. Public Law 92-603 in 1972, access to maintenance dialysis in the United States was often based on the candidate's financial health and social worth criteria such as occupation.[3] Such biases remain operative in many countries, where people of low socioeconomic status and members of socially disadvantaged minority groups experience higher incidence of ESKD.[4-8] In the United States, for example, black Americans compose approximately 13% of the general adult population but constitute over one third of persons receiving maintenance dialysis.[2,9] Paradoxically, despite this higher burden of ESKD, black Americans receive proportionately far fewer living and deceased donor kidney transplants than white counterparts.[2,9,10] Although much less is known about non–dialysis requiring CKD, reports suggest that compared with U.S. adults with earlier stages of CKD, those with more advanced CKD are younger and more likely to be nonwhite, poor, and uninsured.[2,11] The magnitude and persistence of these disparities have led some governments to prioritize elimination of the disparities while also attempting to reduce the overall burden and costs of CKD.[12,13]

HEALTH JUSTICE

In 1966, Dr. Martin Luther King, Jr. proclaimed, "Of all the forms of inequality, injustice in health care is the most shocking and inhumane." The pursuit of equal health outcomes or equal access to health care plays a prominent role in contemporary debates on health care.[14,15] Examples of equal access and equal outcomes with respect to health care reflect the Aristotelian principles of horizontal and vertical equity.[16] However, such debates in health care often include conflicting views of justice. For example, a medical model of justice focuses attention at a point in time when someone who is already ill seeks access to scarce and/or an expensive service such as dialysis or kidney transplantation. (Many credit the birth of bioethics in the United States to the introduction of the arteriovenous shunt by Belding Scribner in 1960 which allowed for long-term hemodialysis to treat patients with ESKD.) In contrast, a social model of justice highlights how social determinants such as access to education, employment, preventative care, safe neighborhoods, and nutritional foods affect the health of a population.[15,17] In other words, the social model focuses on how a person's need for health care arose in the first place. Although inequities in distributive justice (e.g., in kidney transplantation) persist in many areas of medicine, health status and health care disparities in nephrology have focused growing attention on the social conditions that place people at risk for kidney disease as well as some of its determinants (e.g., obesity, type 2 diabetes mellitus, and hypertension).[14,18]

SOCIAL ORIGINS OF DISPARITIES IN NEPHROLOGY

Link and Phelan originally referred to social conditions, including social class, race, income, and education level, as "fundamental causes of disease because these conditions govern access to resources that influence health and disease."[19] Prior studies have reported that the incidence of progressive CKD and ESKD is highest among persons living in the most impoverished neighborhoods.[4,8,20] Additional U.S.-based studies have reported lack of health insurance coverage and residence in a high-poverty area as exposures linked with worse CKD-related biochemical abnormalities at dialysis initiation and marked delays in receipt of a kidney transplant.[21-23] Although these disparities arise from a variety of mechanisms, including biologic susceptibility and economic vulnerability, environmental exposures such as contextual impediments to healthy living likely play a central role. Discussion of the hypothesized influences of social conditions on disparities in nephrology through various life stages uses the framework shown in Figure 84.1.

PRENATAL ENVIRONMENT AND DISPARITIES IN KIDNEY DISEASE RISK

In 1990, Barker noted, "The womb may be more important than the home" in terms of the origins of adult disease.[24] Much debate surrounds the influence of early fetal programming on subsequent risk of chronic diseases such as CKD. The "critical periods" model is one of three models that have been proposed to explain how socioeconomic position over the life course may influence subsequent health.[25] Intrauterine growth retardation and low birth weight are invariably linked with measures of maternal poverty.[26-28] The "fetal programming" hypothesis is based on the critical periods model and states that intrauterine growth retardation results in permanent alterations in fetal physiology that become deleterious later in adult life.[24] Brenner hypothesized that retardation of renal development as occurs in individuals of low birth weight both increases postnatal risks for systemic and glomerular hypertension and predisposes an individual to further nephron

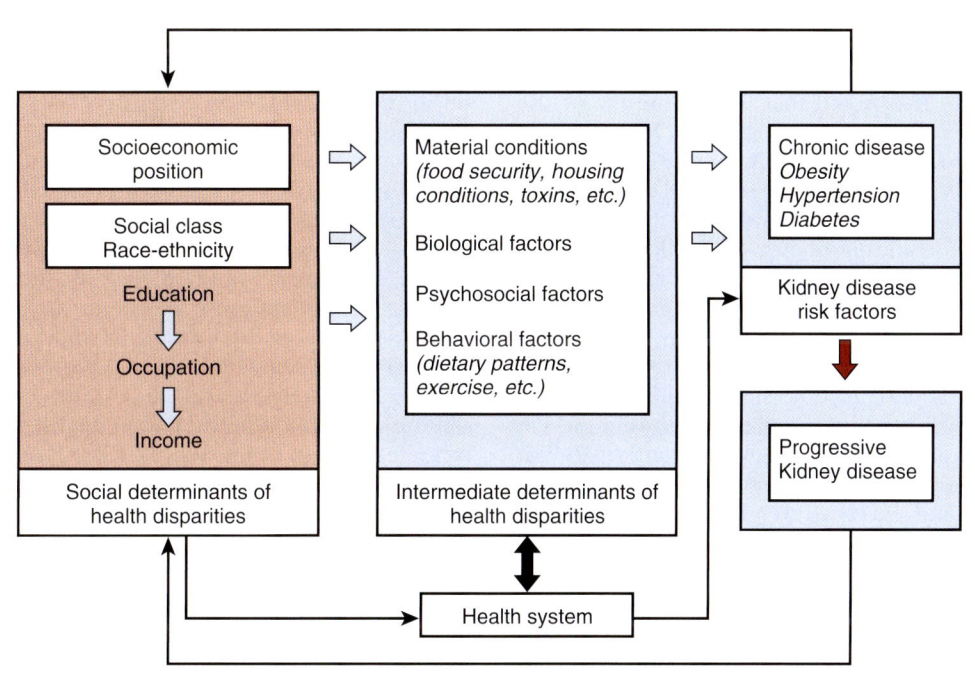

Figure 84.1 Social determinants of health disparities framework.

loss and the development of progressive kidney disease.[29-31] This hypothesis draws support from reports of (1) a direct relationship between birth weight and nephron number,[32] (2) an inverse relation between birth weight and hypertension later in life,[24,33-36] and (3) an inverse relation between nephron number and blood pressure.[37]

In addition to hypertension, low birth weight has been variably linked with CKD risk factors such as diabetes and obesity and has been directly associated with later-life onset of microalbuminuria, reduced kidney function, and ESKD.[38-41] One study conducted on a cohort of term singletons born around the time of the 1944-1945 Dutch famine found that midgestational exposure to famine was associated with microalbuminuria and that late gestational exposure was associated with glucose intolerance.[39] Notably, a rapid increase in nephron number occurs in midgestation, which is a critical period for determining nephron endowment at birth.[39] Moreover, rapid growth and weight gain during infancy and childhood that occur after intrauterine growth restriction (and/or low birth weight) are associated with increased risks of insulin resistance, obesity, diabetes, and hypertension.[29,41,42]

Because low birth weight is strongly linked to indices of parental poverty and occurs more commonly among some racial-ethnic minority groups, researchers have posited that low birth weight may partly account for socioeconomic and racial-ethnic disparities in kidney disease.[43,44] For example, Australian Aboriginals experience higher rates of poverty and an approximate tenfold higher risk of ESKD than nonindigenous Australians.[45] One study conducted in a remote Australian Aboriginal community (where low-birth-weight infants compose approximately 25% of live births) observed that low as compared with high birth weight was significantly associated with lower kidney volumes, higher blood pressure, and later in life, higher levels of urinary albumin excretion.[37] In the Bogalusa Heart Study, a biracial prospective cohort study of cardiovascular risk factors in children and adolescents in the Southern United States, the prevalence of low birth weight was higher among black than white infants.[46] Subsequent reports have linked lower birth weight in this cohort with higher blood pressure levels later in life. These reports have also noted that the magnitude of the association between lower birth weight and higher blood pressure appears to increase with advancing age.[35,36,46]

Globally, many high- and medium-income countries are now faced with a rising incidence of maternal overnutrition.[47-49] In some countries, maternal obesity has replaced tobacco smoking as the most important preventable risk factor for adverse pregnancy outcomes including preterm births.[47,49] In addition to preterm delivery, excessive weight gain during pregnancy is associated with increased risk for development of obesity, diabetes, and hypertension in the offspring.[47] Less is known, however, about the pathways through which excessive weight gain during pregnancy and maternal obesity affect later-life CKD risk factors. The degree to which maternal obesity and excessive weight gain during pregnancy contribute to socioeconomic and racial-ethnic disparities in kidney disease incidence is likewise unknown. The trend toward increasing survival of low-birth-weight infants further underlines the importance of intrauterine fetal environment and timing of insults in future risk for development of precursors to progressive kidney disease.[44]

POSTNATAL ENVIRONMENT AND DISPARITIES IN KIDNEY DISEASE RISK

Over the past two decades, the nephrology community has paid increasing attention to how a person's living environment may influence his or her downstream risk of chronic disease. This heightened attention is evidenced by the growing body of literature examining the associations of individual-level socioeconomic status, area-level characteristics, and kidney disease processes and outcomes.[4,20,50,51] Persons residing in impoverished neighborhoods experience more crime, less access to high-quality educational and employment opportunities, and poorer health outcomes in comparison with persons from less distressed areas.[17,52] Several contemporary studies have described higher incidence of ESKD as well as higher prevalence of CKD in areas of high residential poverty than in areas of low residential poverty.[4,20,50] However, much debate surrounds how and how much adverse social conditions in childhood and early adult life influence a person's subsequent risk of developing kidney disease.[18] Many writers posit that social conditions act through a host of intermediaries such as housing, diet, and social networks, thereby molding health-related behaviors, which in turn influence CKD risk.[19,51,53] The social distribution of important CKD risk factors, including the higher prevalence of type 2 diabetes mellitus, hypertension, and obesity within poor as compared with less impoverished areas, lends evidence to these claims.[14,18] This unequal distribution of intermediary exposures linked to kidney disease is further compounded by the vulnerability of certain groups (i.e., persons of low socioeconomic position) to health-compromising illnesses such as ESKD. Poor health then exerts potent feedback on an individual's socioeconomic position through lost income or medical costs associated with a major illness (see Figure 84.1).[53]

The concept of *allostatic load*, the accumulation of physiologic insults due to repeated insults or chronic stressors experienced in daily life, has gained increasing interest as a model for explaining socioeconomic (and racial-ethnic) disparities in the processes and outcomes of chronic diseases.[54,55] Specific measures of allostatic load include levels of hormones secreted in response to stress and biomarkers that reflect the effects of these hormones on the body.[54,56] This concept, which is based on the cumulative exposures theory, posits that stress may accumulate from early life and manifest as an accumulation of physiologic dysregulation.[54,57] Chronic stressors such as food insecurity, discrimination, living in substandard housing, inadequate access to health care, and exposure to violence are more pronounced among persons of lower than of intermediate or higher socioeconomic status.[55,56] Such psychosocial stressors may lead to hypertension and autonomic dysregulation (e.g., diminished heart rate variability), which in turn are linked to increased risk of incident ESKD.[56,58] Accordingly, higher levels of exposure and adaptation to life stressors experienced more commonly by the poor or members of some racial-ethnic minority groups may put them at greater risk for kidney disease through the aforementioned pathways than their less impoverished or white counterparts.[59-61]

Similarly, contemporary debates in many industrialized countries have increasingly focused on the role of nutrition and childhood obesity on later-life risks for development of chronic disease.[62,63] Estimates suggest that more than a third of children in North America and Europe, and approximately a quarter in the western Pacific and southeast Asia, are overweight or obese.[64] Public health policy and nutrition experts attribute the marked growth in childhood obesity to the widespread availability of energy-dense, inexpensive foods and the low energy requirements of modern daily life.[64] In the United States, the prevalence of childhood obesity is markedly higher among black and Hispanic children than among non-Hispanic white children.[62]

Several studies have also linked residence in impoverished areas with higher levels of processed food consumption (rich in sodium and phosphorus), lower levels of physical activity, and increased risk for chronic diseases such as cardiovascular disease, diabetes, and hypertension in comparison with residence in more affluent areas.[51,65-67] In addition to offering fewer options for affordable, nutritious foods, poorer neighborhoods tend to have fewer (or less attractive) areas to promote physical activity such as parks and community centers.[67] The undue influence of crime, poor housing quality, and suboptimal educational and medical infrastructure may also render poor communities less supportive of healthy lifestyles than less distressed neighborhoods.[17,51] One study linked racial-ethnic disparities in childhood obesity to differential exposure to risk factors during early life, such as gestational diabetes, rapid infant weight gain, excessive television viewing, and high intake of sugar-sweetened beverages or fast food.[63] The strong relation between childhood obesity and later-life antecedents of kidney disease (obesity, hypertension, metabolic syndrome, type 2 diabetes mellitus) suggests that interventions targeting the early life period may contribute substantially to reducing socioeconomic and racial-ethnic disparities in kidney and other chronic diseases.[68]

Perhaps the strongest evidence that neighborhood socioeconomic distress may influence downstream CKD risk factors and lead to health status disparities emanates from the Moving to Opportunity Study.[69,70] During the period 1994-1998, the U.S. Department of Housing and Urban Development conducted this "randomized social experiment" in five cities (Baltimore, Boston, Chicago, Los Angeles, and New York City) to examine the extent to which relocating from a more to a less distressed neighborhood might influence downstream health outcomes. Collectively, 4498 women (90% were either black or Hispanic) with children from high-poverty neighborhoods were randomly assigned to one of three groups: 1788 were assigned to receive housing vouchers that were redeemable only if they relocated to a low-poverty area; 1312 received unrestricted vouchers, and 1398 were assigned to a control group that offered neither of these opportunities. In terms of CKD risk factors, the study found that participants who received a voucher to relocate to a low-poverty neighborhood experienced absolute risk reductions of 5% and 4% for extreme obesity and diabetes, respectively, 10 to 15 years later in comparison with controls.[69] Notably, the effects of relocation occurred without detectable effects on individual-level income.[71] In other words, an individual may experience substantial benefits by moving from a more to a less impoverished neighborhood in terms of reducing long-term risk for development of progressive CKD. However, the strong correlation between neighborhood characteristics (e.g., crime, educational and employment opportunities, recreation, social norms renders the evaluation of specific pathways to these outcomes elusive.[17] Although provocative, the results of the Moving to Opportunity Study highlight the challenges faced by policymakers and clinicians in addressing more proximal mediators of socioeconomic disparities in important CKD risk factors. These findings also raise questions about how we might improve a person's or family's health through altering social support via simple, low-cost means, such as text messaging and Web-based networks.

RACE, SOCIAL CONDITIONS, AND DISPARITIES IN INCIDENT KIDNEY DISEASE

Regrettably in many parts of the world, race is highly correlated with socioeconomic conditions. Link and Phelan emphasize that race is itself so closely tied to social and economic resources that it should also be considered a fundamental cause of health inequality.[19] Insight into the origins of racial-ethnic disparities in kidney disease, however, requires a firm understanding of the social context in which the inequities occur. For example, the United States has witnessed substantially higher incidence rates of ESKD among members of racial-ethnic minority groups, most prominently among black Americans, than among white Americans.[2,5,72] Black Americans are also much more likely than white Americans to be members of the urban "underclass" (residing in areas of intensely concentrated poverty) and to lack health insurance coverage and access to a usual source of care.[73] These data led to claims that social disadvantage largely explains the disparity in kidney disease risk between black and white Americans through pathways previously described.[72] In fact, nearly three quarters of the excess risk of incident CKD among blacks in comparison with whites in the Atherosclerosis Risk in Communities Study was attributable to measures of socioeconomic status and health care access.[74,75] However, studies in other U.S. health care settings indicate that a substantial fraction of the excess risk of incident ESKD among black and white Americans remains unexplained even after one has accounted for differences in the distribution of ESKD risk factors, measures of socioeconomic status, and access to health care.[72,76-78] The persistence of marked racial disparities in ESKD risk within settings where socioeconomic gradients are theoretically reduced, along with emerging genetic data (see later) linking African ancestry to certain forms of progressive kidney disease, further highlights the complex influences of gene-environment interactions on these disparities.[77-80]

Our understanding of disparities in kidney disease among other racial-ethnic groups is less well developed, but the origins of these disparities have common social constructs. In North America, for example, the prevalence of ESKD is substantially higher among Native Americans (primarily among American Indians and Aboriginal Canadians) than among non-Hispanic whites.[81,82] This situation is mirrored in the indigenous people (Aboriginals, Maori, and other Pacific Islanders) of Australia and New Zealand.[45] Differences in social circumstances and prevalent CKD risk factors may account for substantial fractions of this excess risk of ESKD among indigenous people.[45,83] In addition to encountering higher rates of poverty than their white counterparts, indigenous people from North America, Australia, and New

Zealand also experience a higher prevalence of CKD risk factors such as diabetes, hypertension, and obesity.[45,82,84] In fact, long-term cohort studies of Aboriginal Australians suggest that the lifetime risk of ESKD among people with diabetes may be as high as 41% in this group.[85] Moreover, the remote location of many indigenous communities combined with cultural differences in their approach to illness often hinders the implementation of interventions to adequately address these risk factors.[84,86,87] Notably, the U.S. Indian Health Services began systematic efforts in the 1990s to identify, screen for, and address CKD risk factors, including diabetes, among American Indians.[83,88] These efforts have been widely touted as the primary reason for the steady decline in ESKD incidence among American Indians over the ensuing two decades.[2,89] Lastly, detection of racial-ethnic disparities in nephrology strongly depends on the manner in which health statistics are collected and organized. Unlike in many European countries, where health statistics are commonly organized according to occupational or class hierarchies, health data in North America, Australia, and New Zealand have historically included race or ethnicity.

BIOLOGIC ORIGINS OF DISPARITIES IN NEPHROLOGY

Although differences in the built environment undoubtedly play a central role in promoting racial-ethnic disparities in the incidence and treatment of kidney diseases, epidemiologic and genetic studies support the presence of strong biologic influences as well.[79,80] Notably, the higher ESKD incidence experienced by members of racial-ethnic minority groups in comparison with non-Hispanic whites exists even within integrated health systems (with theoretically equal care access) and among socioeconomically disadvantaged populations (in which socioeconomic gradients are attenuated).[77,78,90] The persistence of racial-ethnic differences in ESKD risk in these studies suggests that factors other than socioeconomic status and health care access play a more influential role in determining disease progression than previously inferred.[79,80]

Like many chronic diseases, kidney disease is hypothesized to occur among susceptible individuals through a complex interaction of genetic predisposition and environmental exposures.[80] In the United States, blacks have a twofold higher likelihood than whites of having a first-degree relative with ESKD.[91] Shared exposures from the familial environment such as poverty, nutrition, and health-related behaviors may contribute to these associations, but further studies have linked *APOL1* gene mutations with certain types of progressive nondiabetic kidney disease including focal segmental glomerulosclerosis and human immunodeficiency virus (HIV) nephropathy.[79,92] Owing partly to the protective effects conferred by *APOL1* mutations against trypanosomal disease and other pathogens, *APOL1* mutations appear to be relatively common among individuals of West African descent but virtually absent among persons from Europe, East Africa, and other regions.[92] It has been estimated that as much as 40% of the increased burden of progressive nondiabetic CKD in Sub-Saharan African ancestry populations could be eliminated if the injury mechanism for APOL1 risk variants could be overcome.[93-95] However, the detailed mechanisms whereby APOL1 variants induce kidney injury are yet to be fully elucidated.[96] Furthermore, the relative contributions of biology and built environment to black-white disparities in glomerular disease have yet to be clarified. Similar observations linking *APOL1* mutations with progressive CKD or ESKD among other ancestral groups have not been described and specific *genetic* causes for the substantially higher risk of ESKD in these groups relative to European whites remain unclear.[80] Please refer to Chapter 43 for further discussion of the complex relations among ancestry, genes, and various forms of kidney disease.

HEALTH SYSTEM AND DISPARITIES IN NEPHROLOGY

More than 30 years ago, Donabedian proposed a model for assessing the quality of medical care based on structure, process, and outcome. According to Donabedian's model, "process—the method by which health care is provided— is limited by the structure or environment in which it operates."[97] The health system plays an important role in mediating disparities in nephrology. Health systems are responsible for promoting and implementing interventions to improve health by altering exposure to key intermediaries. However, in many countries, differential access to the health system and differential access to high-quality health care often lead to relative differences in the receipt of key interventions to promote and maintain health.

UNEQUAL HEALTH SYSTEM ACCESS AND SURVEILLANCE

Disparities in the surveillance and treatment of CKD risk factors may contribute to the higher incidence of more advanced CKD in persons of low socioeconomic status than in those of intermediate or high socioeconomic status. In the United States, more than a third of patients with incident ESKD are persons of severely limited economic means (enrolled in Medicaid, the U.S. joint federal and state health insurance program for the poor, or uninsured at ESKD onset).[2] However, persons with CKD from impoverished communities are difficult to identify because there is no national system for tracking the care of poor or uninsured patients in most countries.[2] In other words, disadvantaged patients with non–dialysis-dependent CKD are essentially "invisible" to much of the health care system until they actually have ESKD. In many instances, CKD can be slowed or prevented. Interventions such as blood pressure lowering, angiotensin inhibitor use, and avoidance of nephrotoxins are effective in reducing morbidity and slowing CKD progression.[98-102] Because of differences in health system access according to socioeconomic position, however, the time and resources needed to effectively implement these interventions in patients with CKD from socially disadvantaged groups are limited, as evidenced by underutilization of these therapies among the poor and uninsured.[11,103]

Using national data, we previously reported that in comparison with U.S. adults with earlier stages of CKD, those with more advanced CKD were younger and more likely to be nonwhite, poor, and uninsured (Figure 84.2).[11]

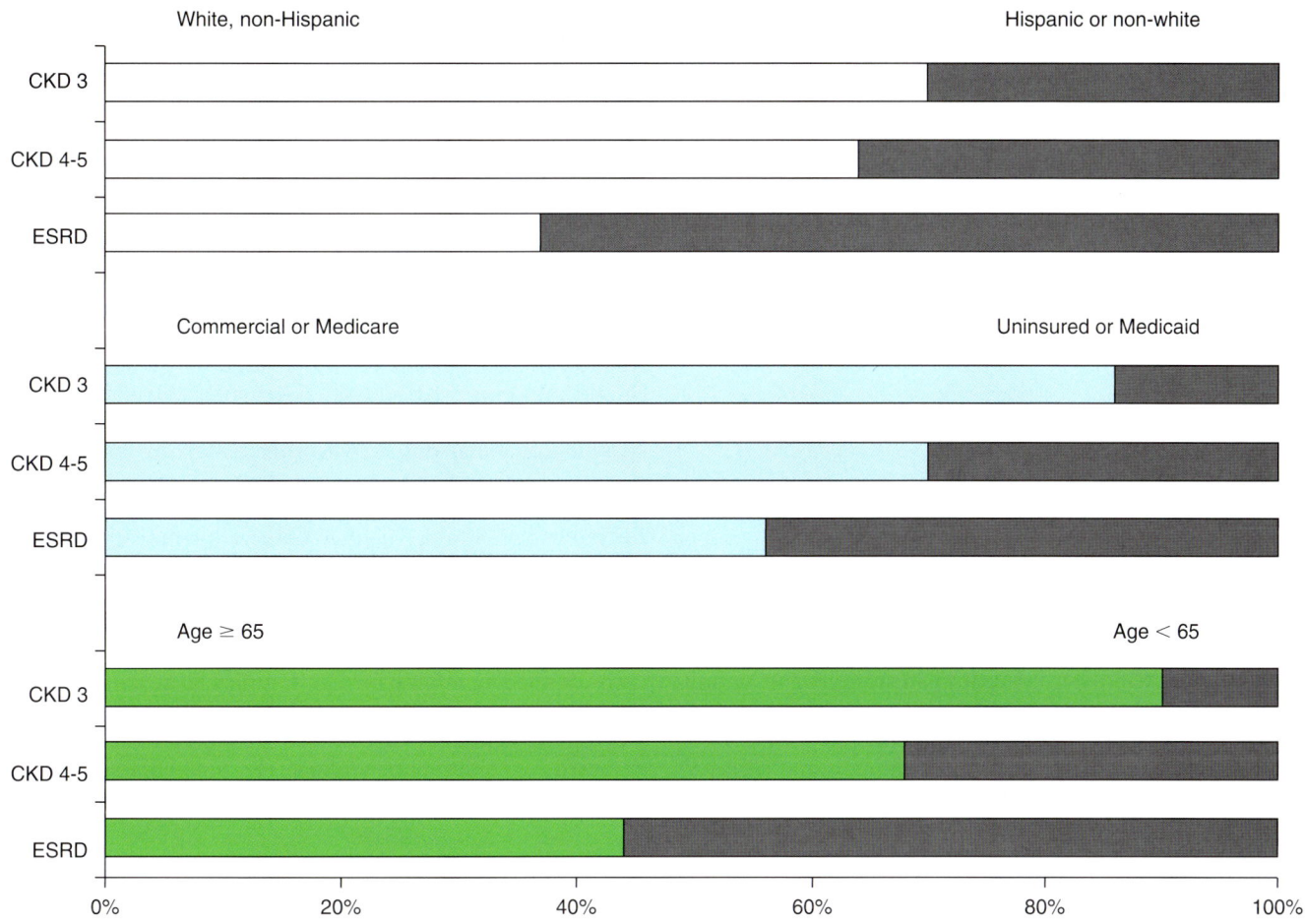

Figure 84.2 Demographic composition of U.S. adults with chronic kidney disease (CKD) by disease stage (CKD_3 through CKD_5). ESRD, End-stage renal (kidney) disease.

Consistent with the differential exposure framework from Figure 84.1, uninsured adults with CKD had a higher prevalence of risk factors for progression to ESRD than their insured counterparts but were far less likely to receive interventions based on and recommended by clinical practice guidelines to slow disease progression.[11]

As noted earlier, prior studies showed that lack of health insurance coverage, residential poverty, and nonwhite race-ethnicity were independently associated with worse CKD-related laboratory abnormalities at dialysis initiation, including more severe hypoalbuminemia, azotemia, and anemia, and with marked delays in accessing the transplant waiting list and in receiving a kidney transplant.[21,22,104] These reports suggest that socially disadvantaged groups may receive less and perhaps substandard care in earlier stages of CKD.[51,105] Although differences in individual-level factors such as adherence to screening and treatment recommendations may partly contribute to these disparities, it is likely that differential access to the health system plays a central role in determining which groups receive these interventions, particularly at earlier stages of CKD.[106] Yet to a certain degree, such disparities in ESRD incidence by socioeconomic status appear to exist even within developed countries with universal access to care.[107,108]

IMPORTANCE OF HEALTH SYSTEM STRUCTURE

The medical care of most poor and underserved populations is concentrated in the hands of relatively few providers.[109] For example, owing to their relatively limited options for ongoing ambulatory care, many of America's poor and underinsured seek ambulatory care from public hospitals and safety net health care clinics.[110,111] Even within universal health care systems, the isolated nature of some minority communities strongly influences the frequency and quality of care received.[84,86] Several United States–based studies have now demonstrated that socioeconomic and racial-ethnic disparities in care may be partly explained by differences in where and by whom patients are treated, leading to systematic differences in the care environment, provider quality, and access to care.[112-114] For example, Bach and associates found that black and white Medicare beneficiaries were treated for the most part by different physicians. Strikingly, 80% of all outpatient primary care visits by black patients in this study were accounted for by only 22% of physicians.[112] Moreover, the primary care physicians who cared primarily for black patients were less likely to be board certified, more likely to be in training, and more likely to report encountering system barriers to providing high-quality care to their patients (e.g., securing referrals to specialists).[112] Varkey and colleagues further found that clinics serving higher proportions of patients from racial-ethnic minority groups were more chaotic than and had different organizational characteristics from those of other clinics.[113] In short, several key factors linked to the provision of high-quality medical care, such as provider experience and subspecialist access, differ markedly according to the health system. Such health system–level determinants may delay or restrict the access of poor and underserved patients to receiving adequate management of kidney disease and its antecedent risk factors.

DISPARITIES IN THE TREATMENT OF KIDNEY DISEASE

CHRONIC KIDNEY DISEASE

Blood pressure control is a central target to reduce morbidity and mortality in CKD.[98] Hypertension as a contributing cause of ESKD is blamed for more than a quarter of incident cases in the United States.[2] Hypertension is also the most common modifiable risk factor for CKD progression among uninsured American adults with CKD, affecting approximately 57% of this population as compared with obesity (40%), diabetes (22%), and overt albuminuria (13%).[11] However, several United States–based studies have described marked disparities in blood pressure control in CKD according to measures of socioeconomic status and health system access. For example, data from the U.S. National Health and Nutrition Examination Surveys indicated that hypertensive adults with CKD who lacked health insurance were far less likely to be receiving treatment for their hypertension than insured counterparts.[11] Moreover, among hypertensive adults with CKD, those who lacked health insurance coverage were 55% less likely to be receiving treatment with an angiotensin inhibitor than insured adults (Table 84.1).[11]

Similarly, Olomu and associates reported that only 38% of hypertensive patients achieved target blood pressure control in a federally qualified health clinic in Michigan[103]; the national average is 50%.[115] Even fewer (31%) hypertensive patients with diabetes achieved target blood pressure control in the same clinic.[103]

In addition to experiencing reduced access to high-quality care, low-income and racial-ethnic minority groups may harbor risk factors that heighten their risk for CKD morbidity and mortality. While observing a high (10%-35%) prevalence of moderate-to-advanced CKD among ambulatory users of a large safety net health system, we found that the prevalence of "socially determined" risk factors that might influence CKD outcomes—such as chronic viral diseases, substance abuse, homelessness, and mental illness—was far higher than observed in other health care settings.[78,116] In one safety net setting, more than 7% of persons with moderate-to-advanced CKD progressed to ESKD and 16% died during follow-up (median observation time 6.6 years).[78] Notably, nearly 30% of patients were never assessed for proteinuria, and fewer than 20% were ever seen by nephrology specialists during follow-up.[78] The elusive nature of this population, their frequent loss to follow-up, and limited provider accountability further complicate patient-provider interactions, highlighting a critical need for more effective strategies to enhance CKD risk factor surveillance and management in traditionally underserved populations in order to mitigate health status and health care disparities.

END-STAGE KIDNEY DISEASE

ESKD now affects an estimated 2.5 million individuals worldwide and at considerable cost to society.[2] In some high-income countries with universal access to ESKD treatment, there are persistent racial-ethnic and socioeconomic disparities in access to certain types of renal replacement therapies.[2] In most medium- and low-income nations, access to ESKD treatment remains limited and is governed predominantly by socioeconomic position and occupation.[117]

DIALYSIS: PROCESS AND OUTCOME

In terms of access to maintenance dialysis, socioeconomic disparities are evident at several levels, from the country's health system to the individual patient. Regular access to maintenance dialysis remains, for the most part, limited to patients receiving care in high-income nations.[2,118] In many low-income and in some middle-income countries, most patients who initiate dialysis either die or stop treatment within the first 3 months because of cost restraints.[13,118] The numbers who do not receive treatment for ESKD is unknown. Within high-income nations, an increasing number of studies have focused on differences in dialysis process measures as indicators of the quality of dialysis care received.[119-122] A large fraction of these studies emanate from the United States, likely reflecting incorporation of specific measures for anemia management and dialysis adequacy into facility performance assessment and care reimbursement.[120,121]

As noted previously, there are prominent and persistent racial-ethnic disparities in process measures at dialysis initiation that largely reflect the presence and quality of care leading up to ESKD.[104,123] However, data from the U.S.

Table 84.1	Odds Ratio (OR) of Hypertension Treatment and Renin-Angiotensin Antagonist Use Among Uninsured as Compared with Insured U.S. Adults with Chronic Kidney Disease and Hypertension

Outcome	Unadjusted OR (95% CI)	Adjusted OR (95% CI)
Hypertension treatment*	0.44 (0.31-0.62)	0.59 (0.40-0.85)
Renin-angiotensin-aldosterone inhibitor use†	0.34 (0.20-0.59)	0.45 (0.26-0.77)

*Treated: We considered participants with hypertension to be "treated" if they reported that they were currently taking medications to lower blood pressure.
†Adjusted for age, sex, race-ethnicity, health insurance status, CKD stage, diabetes, obesity, and overt albuminuria.
CI, Confidence interval.

Centers for Medicare and Medicaid Services (CMS) suggest that these disparities attenuate and may even reverse for some racial-ethnic groups over time.[124,125] In two studies from the CMS's ESRD Clinical Performance Measures Project, Frankenfield and associates reported that Hispanic and Asian patients undergoing hemodialysis experienced process measures (e.g., arteriovenous fistula use and serum albumin, hemoglobin, and dialysis adequacy targets) that were equivalent, and in some cases superior, to those of non-Hispanic whites 1 year after dialysis initiation; and that black patients receiving hemodialysis continued to experience the worst process measures of all racial-ethnic groups surveyed.[125,126] While the first study did not elucidate specific mechanisms by which racial-ethnic differences in process measures abated, it seems plausible that the establishment of a regular site of care with access to wraparound services (i.e., social work, dietician, primary nephrology care) may have offset the lack of, or variation in, medical care received prior to ESKD onset. Whether achievement of specified targets for these measures actually reflects dialysis-related quality of care remains a source of substantial debate.[119,120,122] Regardless, in the setting of universal access to dialysis services, more research is needed to determine how quality improvement methods can be effectively targeted to reduce health disparities without misprioritizing low-value care and creating unwarranted and wasteful incentives that might also exclude vulnerable patients.[122,127]

KIDNEY TRANSPLANTATION: PROCESS

In terms of survival and quality of life, kidney transplantation is the optimal treatment for most patients who progress to ESKD. However, significant disparities in receiving a transplant according to socioeconomic status, race-ethnicity, and geography persist worldwide.[2,23,128-130] In the United States, transplantation rates are significantly lower among the poor and among most racial-ethnic minority groups than among disadvantaged groups and whites, respectively.[2] Racial-ethnic disparities are also present in Canada, where kidney transplantation rates in Aboriginal, African, Indo Asian, and East Asian Canadians range from one half to two thirds those of white Canadians.[129] In Australia, transplantation rates in Aboriginal Australians experience are 77% lower than those in non-indigenous Australians, and in New Zealand, Maori/Pacific Islanders are similarly disadvantaged.[45] Although key mediators of, and their relative contributions to, racial-ethnic disparities in transplant access vary by population and health system, many are directly linked to social conditions described previously.

For example, in the United States, American Indian and black patients encounter delays in accessing the kidney transplant waiting list that are partly attributable to lower socioeconomic status and a higher prevalence of diabetes in comparison with white patients.[23,130,131] Similarly, contextual poverty and health insurance coverage account for the largest fraction of the disparity in live-donor kidney transplantations among American Indians, Alaska Natives, and black and Hispanic Americans in comparison with white Americans.[132] On the other hand, geographic differences (primarily attributed to organ availability) account for substantial fractions of the disparity in receiving a deceased donor kidney from the waiting list among U.S. Hispanics, Pacific Islanders, and American Indians/Alaska Natives.[23]

Additional studies have identified differences in attitudes and knowledge about kidney transplantation among black and Hispanic Americans in comparison with white Americans.[133] Providers may also be less likely to recommend kidney transplantation to minority patients owing to impaired communication and misconceptions regarding its benefits relative to prolonged dialysis.[9,134] The influence of cultural and/or linguistic isolation on delays in accessing the transplant waiting list or in receiving a kidney transplant remains understudied.[23]

Specific mechanisms by which socioeconomic status influence access to transplantation include low educational attainment, suboptimal health insurance coverage, and contextual impediments to healthy living. Poor or uninsured patients appear to encounter more difficulty than less disadvantaged patients in navigating the complex steps required to successfully receive a kidney transplant.[130,135] This may be a direct effect of low educational attainment, inadequate insurance coverage, and suboptimal patient-provider communication, all of which have been linked with delays in accessing the transplant waiting list, in completing the transplant evaluation, and in successful receipt of a transplant.[87,130,131,134,136] Nephrology providers also appear reticent to refer poor patients for transplant because of concerns about inadequate coverage for prescription and procedural costs.[134,137] In a national survey of U.S. transplant programs, more than 70% responded that they frequently or occasionally exclude patients from the kidney transplant waiting list owing to concerns that the patients will not be able to afford the immunosuppressive medications.[138]

Although socioeconomic status and contextual poverty are linked with disparities in transplantation rates in the United States,[63,130,139] the magnitude of such disparities is markedly higher in middle-income nations such as in Mexico, where transplantation rates are more than tenfold higher among insured patients than among uninsured patients.[140] As concerning is the unethical practice of organ trafficking and exploitation of disadvantaged populations for profit that occur in many low- and middle-income nations.[117] This pervasive commercialization of live donor transplantation is supported by reports of affluent foreigners undergoing large fractions of the kidney transplantations performed in some low- and middle-income countries.[141] Although some writers justify paying persons to donate a kidney as mutually benefitting recipient and donor, one study conducted in India showed that such transactions do not lead to long-term economic benefit and may be associated with a decline in health for the donor.[142]

Historically, racial-ethnic differences in the distribution of ABO blood type and antibodies to human leukocyte antigens (HLA) have been linked with disparities in receiving a deceased donor kidney transplant among patients who have successfully accessed the waiting list.[23,143,144] In particular, black candidates have encountered marked delays in receiving a deceased donor kidney owing partly to their higher frequencies of ABO types that are associated with longer waits.[9,144-146] However, the influence of biologic perpetrators of racial-ethnic disparities in transplantation access, such as the distribution of blood type and HLA, has progressively declined as a result of changes in the deceased donor allocation policy. Recognizing the contribution of HLA matching to racial disparities in receiving a deceased donor kidney,

U.S. policymakers eliminated the HLA-B locus as a priority for the allocation of deceased kidney donors on May 7, 2003.[147] This change led to an increase in the proportion of deceased donor organs directed to minority candidates on the waiting list. Specifically, in the 6 years after the policy change, deceased donor transplantation in minority recipients rose 40%, compared with an 8% rise for non-Hispanic whites and a 23% increase overall.[148] Moreover, this improved access to transplantation for minority groups has not been accompanied by declines in short-term graft survival during the initial period after the policy change.[148]

In 2013, the U.S. Organ Procurement and Transplantation Network approved additional amendments to the kidney allocation policy that included changes to promote greater equity in accessing deceased donor kidneys.[149] In particular, two amendments, one that allows for blood type B recipients to receive kidney offers from donors with certain subtypes of blood type A and another that calculates waiting time from the start of dialysis (or qualifying estimated glomerular filtration rate [eGFR] ≤ 20 mL/min), will likely lead to further reductions of the racial-ethnic gap in transplantation rates in the United States.[149,150] Additional measures to promote greater racial-ethnic and social equity in rates of assigning patients to the waiting list and in living donor kidney transplantation remain areas of heightened investigation.

KIDNEY TRANSPLANTATION: OUTCOMES

Socioeconomic and racial-ethnic disparities in kidney transplantation extend to outcomes after receipt of a functional allograft. Similar to transplant access, specific causes of these disparities in allograft survival may differ by population and health system, but the root causes commonly reflect differential social conditions and access to high-quality health care. For example, adherence to posttransplantation immunosuppressive therapy remains a critical determinant of long-term allograft survival. Regrettably, the inability to afford immunosuppressive medications appears to be a primary mechanism that restricts disadvantaged patients from not only receiving a kidney transplant but also in maintaining one.[151,152] In the United States, for example, federal prescription drug coverage for immunosuppressive medications extends to only 36 months after kidney transplantation, with few exceptions.[151] For this reason, disadvantaged patients are particularly vulnerable to the long-term financial burden of maintaining a functional allograft.[153] In one study, more than 40% of transplant recipients reported financial difficulty after transplantation, with health-related out-of-pocket expenses averaging approximately $475 per month.[152] Socioeconomic disparities in maintaining a transplant are magnified in medium-income countries such as Mexico and Pakistan, where excellent long-term results for allograft survival are offset by the prohibitive cost of immunosuppressive and antiviral medications. In these countries, transplant access and allograft maintenance for the average citizen often require a state-sponsored model.[36,117,140]

Racial differences in biologic factors such as age at transplantation, HLA mismatching, and APOL1 genotype status may account to some degree for the disparity in allograft survival between some racial-ethnic groups, such as between black and white Americans.[9,145,154] Although prevailing beliefs attribute reduced graft survival among black recipients to heightened immune responsiveness and poorer immunologic matching, remarkably few reports have actually linked better HLA matching with improved graft survival in this racial group.[9,143,155] In addition, Asian recipients enjoy the longest graft survival of all racial-ethnic groups despite the presence of suboptimal HLA matching comparable to that observed in black recipients.[9,156] Alternatively, pharmacokinetic studies report greater clearance and/or lower bioavailability of certain immunosuppressive agents among black than among white transplant recipients.[157-159] However, the influence of these biologic factors on racial disparities in allograft survival is likely mediated at least in part through differences in immunosuppressive medication regimens and nonadherence.[151,160-162] In the United States, nonadherence strongly correlates in turn with social factors such as household income, presence and type of health insurance coverage, and history of drug abuse.[9,151,163,164]

Lastly, studies have raised concerns regarding inequities in the quality of transplanted organs based on recipient socioeconomic status and race-ethnicity.[165] Emerging data on provision of comparatively "lower quality organs" to black, low-income, or less educated recipients than to white, more affluent or college-educated counterparts has cast additional light on the complex nuances that underlie this social gap in allograft access and survival.[165,166]

MOVING TOWARD MORE EQUITABLE CARE

Currently, global cost estimates of treating CKD remain elusive. In the United States alone, treatment of CKD costs the federal government more than $56 billion annually, including $26 billion for ESKD. Hence, there is an urgent need to identify cost-effective strategies to address CKD risk factors, particularly among populations that bear a disproportionate burden of disease.[1] Strategies to reduce disparities in chronic diseases include three general approaches: (1) targeted programs, (2) gap programs, and (3) gradient programs.[53,167] *Targeted programs* comprise strategies aimed at improving the health of groups that are particularly disadvantaged in terms of disease burden or treatment access. Such targeted programs are advantageous in that they focus on a well-defined, often small segment of the population. This aspect provides for ease in monitoring and assessing results. However, the targeted approach is similarly weakened by its narrow focus and its lack of commitment to reduce the disparity between the most and least disadvantaged groups. In some instances, health gains in the targeted groups may still lag behind those observed in less disadvantaged groups, leading to widening of the disparities.[53] An example is programs that attempt to promote live-donor kidney transplantation among patients of low socioeconomic status. Although such programs may increase live-donor kidney transplantation rates among the poor, the disparity between patients of lower and those of intermediate or higher socioeconomic status may actually increase owing to the differential effects of other programs (e.g., paired donation) or resource-mediated advances (e.g., Internet use and social networking).

Strategies that aim to target the health gap address the issue of disparities, but these programs are more challenging than those that seek to improve the health status of targeted groups. In order to succeed, *gap programs* must achieve absolute improvements in health status among, for example, persons in the lowest socioeconomic position at a rate of improvement that exceeds that observed in the comparison group. Like targeted programs, gap programs often focus solely on the most disadvantaged groups and largely ignore gradients in health and the health status of those in the intermediary groups.[53] For example, over the past decade, collective efforts to increase kidney donation in the United States among black Americans have yielded a near doubling of the donation rate of deceased donor kidneys (from 15.1 per million population [pmp] in 2000 to 28.1 pmp in 2010) from this racial group. However, donation rates from deceased donors of American Indian (7.7 pmp) and Asian (8.5 pmp) descent have seen only modest gains during the same period, and they remain far below those of white donors (21.4 pmp) in 2010.[2]

Addressing socioeconomic gradients in health relies on comprehensive strategies that involve the entire population. In contrast to targeted and gap programs, *gradient strategies* address the effect of socioeconomic inequality on health across the socioeconomic hierarchy. In other words, a gradients model addresses not only intermediaries of health disparities among the disadvantaged but also systematic inequities in life course exposures (educational and occupational opportunities, nutrition, living standards, and health care access) that strongly influence an individual's position in the socioeconomic hierarchy.[53] Needless to say, gradient strategies must often contend with conflicting political agendas, major logistical challenges, and prohibitive costs.[168] Moreover, such strategies commonly yield results only in a prolonged timeframe. These three strategies (targeted, gap, and gradient) for reducing disparities are intended to complement one another and can often provide sequential layers for addressing socioeconomic (and racial-ethnic) inequities.[53]

On the basis of the framework shown in Figure 84.1, researchers have identified four major intervention areas for addressing socioeconomic and racial-ethnic disparities in kidney disease.[53] First, reducing inequalities in the distribution of structural determinants such as education, occupation, and income may alter social stratification and mitigate its effects on health outcomes. Second, addressing specific intermediary determinants that mediate the effects of socioeconomic position on health (e.g., consumption of high-calorie foods and beverages, lack of physical exercise, unhealthy living conditions, and cigarette smoking) may reduce specific health-damaging exposures that disproportionately affect disadvantaged groups; in other words, changing the distribution of risk factors related to socioeconomic position may attenuate long-term health consequences for underprivileged groups.[18] Third, reversing the effect of health status on socioeconomic position may lessen the vulnerability of disadvantaged groups to the health-damaging conditions they face[14]; examples include programs to keep persons with chronic diseases such as diabetes and CKD within the workforce.[153] Lastly, targeting the delivery of health care to socially disadvantaged groups may reduce the unequal consequences of illness and prevent further disease progression and economic loss; such strategies might offer additional care or health coverage to members of disadvantaged groups who have conditions (obesity, diabetes, hypertension, homelessness) that are linked to the excess burden of progressive CKD in these groups.[53]

INITIATIVES TO REDUCE DISPARITIES

Successful initiatives to reduce socioeconomic and racial-ethnic disparities in CKD risk factors might reference the U.S. government–sponsored Vaccines for Children Program, the Standards of Care for Diabetes and Kidney Disease Programs administered by the U.S. Indian Health Services, and the U.S. National Health Service Corps' scholarship and loan repayment programs. A generation ago, fatal outbreaks of measles in predominantly poor, minority communities in several U.S. cities underscored marked disparities in vaccination coverage that placed disadvantaged children at increased risk for disease. In direct response to these disparities, the U.S. government initiated the Vaccines for Children Program, which now purchases and provides vaccines for children who are particularly vulnerable to lapses in vaccination coverage (i.e., those who were uninsured, on Medicaid, or of American Indian or Alaska Native ancestry, or who had health insurance that did not cover universally recommended vaccines). From 2000 to 2010, racial-ethnic disparities in vaccination series completion rates in the United States decreased from 6% to 4% (for minority groups vs. non-Hispanic white children), and poverty-related inequalities from 8% to 3%.[169]

Several decades ago, in response to rising concerns over the burden of ESKD due to diabetes in many American Indian communities, the Indian Health Service established the Standards of Care for Diabetes Program (followed later by the Kidney Disease Program) in order to improve the screening of and the management of patients with diabetes and CKD.[89] Based on the Chronic Care Model, these two programs implemented routine reporting of estimated glomerular filtration rate, annual monitoring of protein excretion, utilization of renin-angiotensin system antagonists, and aggressive control of blood pressure in association with enhanced patient and provider education.[89,170] By 2001, age-adjusted ESKD incidence among American Indians with diabetes had decreased by 31% from that in 1990. By 2006, 82% of American Indians with hypertension and diabetes were receiving a renin-angiotensin-aldosterone system inhibitor. Perhaps without coincidence, American Indians are the only U.S. racial or ethnic group in which ESKD incidence has consistently declined over the past decade.[2,89] A similar gap initiative by the Australian government, the Medical Outreach–Indigenous Chronic Disease Program, aims to close the disparity in life expectancy between indigenous and non-indigenous Australians by improving access of indigenous people to best-practice chronic disease management.[13] Notably, the five areas of highest priority include diabetes and chronic kidney disease.

In 1970, the U.S. government established the National Health Service Corps to help underserved communities across the nation receive critically needed primary medical, oral, and mental and behavioral health care. Through the National Health Service Corps, clinicians receive scholarships and loan repayment in return for committing to practice in underserved areas for a defined period. More than 40,000 primary care clinicians have participated in this program since its inception. Later reports suggest that 82% of clinicians continue to practice in underserved communities 1 year after their service completion and that 55% remain for 10 years. Notably, long-term retention rates are higher for those who serve in rural as opposed to urban communities.[171]

Many U.S. policymakers and health care providers lauded passage of the Affordable Care Act as a fundamental step toward achieving equitable access to health care for all Americans. However, as Schrag noted in 1983, the ability to pay for health services does not necessarily guarantee their availability.[172] In order to address socioeconomic and racial-ethnic disparities in treatment of kidney disease and its antecedent risk factors, U.S. policymakers will need to work with health systems to tackle the unequal distribution of experienced health care providers situated in areas of low and high poverty. In terms of kidney transplant access, efforts to reduce economic vulnerability by providing medication prescription benefits to disadvantaged groups at risk for nonadherence to posttransplantation regimens may partially address socioeconomic and racial-ethnic inequities in transplant access as well as in long-term allograft survival.[151] To date, lobbying efforts have failed to convince the U.S. Congress to extend support for immunosuppressive medications beyond 3 years after transplantation.

SUMMARY

Socioeconomic and racial-ethnic disparities in the incidence and treatment of kidney disease and its risk factors occur worldwide. They occur within and between countries, and the reader is referred to the Global Considerations in Kidney Disease section of this edition (Chapters 77 through 82) for consideration of particular constituencies. Despite widespread recognition of these disparities for more than two decades, negligible progress has been made in reducing the gaps between persons of low socioeconomic status and their less impoverished counterparts, and between racial-ethnic minority groups and white majority groups. Although we have more in-depth knowledge of the root causes and consequences of these disparities, including their social determinants, we have done little to address the structural elements that allow these disparities to persist. Marked differences in education, living conditions, and employment opportunities combined with inequitable access to high-quality health care and genetic susceptibility act in tandem to promote and maintain disparate milieus for chronic diseases. In the setting of such widespread inequities, we should anticipate that disparities in health outcomes such as kidney disease will continue to plague the nephrology community for the foreseeable future. The persistence of socioeconomic and racial-ethnic disparities in nephrology marks our field as one that remains in crisis.

Fortunately, several countries including the United States have now prioritized initiatives aimed to reduce socioeconomic gaps in health insurance coverage, maternal prenatal care, smoking, nutrition, and childhood obesity in order to improve the overall quality of health care to, and mitigate the effects of social conditions that disproportionately affect, disadvantaged populations. Reducing disparities based on social factors may improve health care quality more than would marginal improvements in overall medical care.[169] The social distribution of diabetes, hypertension, and obesity and their indelible link to kidney disease provides further evidence in favor of this approach to address disparities in nephrology.[18] Unfortunately, many high- and medium-income countries continue to witness stagnant or reduced social mobility, increased social unrest, and widening inequities in living conditions. Needless to say, even in the presence of astute public policies aimed to address marked differences in social conditions, reducing long-standing disparities in nephrology will remain a major challenge for the foreseeable future.

Complete reference list available at ExpertConsult.com.

KEY REFERENCES

3. Alexander S: They decide who lives, and who dies. *Life* 53:102–125, 1962.
4. Volkova N, McClellan W, Klein M, et al: Neighborhood poverty and racial differences in ESRD incidence. *J Am Soc Nephrol* 19(2):356–364, 2008.
5. Klag MJ, Whelton PK, Randall BL, et al: End-stage renal disease in African-American and white men. 16-year MRFIT findings. *JAMA* 277(16):1293–1298, 1997.
9. Young CJ, Gaston RS: Renal transplantation in black Americans. *N Engl J Med* 343(21):1545–1552, 2000.
10. Eggers PW: Racial disparities in access to transplantation: a tough nut to crack. *Kidney Int* 76(6):589–590, 2009.
15. Jecker NS: A broader view of justice. *Am J Bioeth* 8(10):2–10, 2008.
17. Macintyre SA, Ellaway A: *Neighborhoods and health*, New York, NY, 2003, Oxford Univ. Press.
18. Braveman PA, Cubbin C, Egerter S, et al: Socioeconomic disparities in health in the United States: what the patterns tell us. *Am J Public Health* 100(Suppl 1):S186–S196, 2010.
19. Link BG, Phelan J: Social conditions as fundamental causes of disease. *J Health Soc Behav* Spec No:80–94, 1995.
21. Kausz AT, Obrador GT, Arora P, et al: Late initiation of dialysis among women and ethnic minorities in the United States. *J Am Soc Nephrol* 11(12):2351–2357, 2000.
23. Hall YN, Choi AI, Xu P, et al: Racial ethnic differences in rates and determinants of deceased donor kidney transplantation. *J Am Soc Nephrol* 22(4):743–751, 2011.
24. Barker DJ: The fetal and infant origins of adult disease. *BMJ* 301(6761):259–262, 1990.
32. Hughson M, Farris AB, 3rd, Douglas-Denton R, et al: Glomerular number and size in autopsy kidneys: the relationship to birth weight. *Kidney Int* 63(6):2113–2122, 2003.
37. Hoy WE, Hughson MD, Bertram JF, et al: Nephron number, hypertension, renal disease, and renal failure. *J Am Soc Nephrol* 16(9):2557–2564, 2005.
38. Luyckx VA, Bertram JF, Brenner BM, et al: Effect of fetal and child health on kidney development and long-term risk of hypertension and kidney disease. *Lancet* 382(9888):273–283, 2013.
43. Luyckx VA, Brenner BM: The clinical importance of nephron mass. *J Am Soc Nephrol* 21(6):898–910, 2010.
51. Diez Roux AV, Merkin SS, Arnett D, et al: Neighborhood of residence and incidence of coronary heart disease. *N Engl J Med* 345(2):99–106, 2001.
52. Sampson RJ, Raudenbush SW, Earls F: Neighborhoods and violent crime: a multilevel study of collective efficacy. *Science* 277(5328):918–924, 1997.
53. Solar O, Irwin A: *A conceptual framework for action on the social determinants of health, social determinants of health discussion paper 2 (policy and practice)*, Geneva, 2010, WHO Press.
55. Lynch JW, Kaplan GA, Shema SJ: Cumulative impact of sustained economic hardship on physical, cognitive, psychological, and social functioning. *N Engl J Med* 337(26):1889–1895, 1997.

63. Taveras EM, Gillman MW, Kleinman KP, et al: Reducing racial/ethnic disparities in childhood obesity: the role of early life risk factors. *JAMA Pediatrics* 167(8):731–738, 2013.
67. Auchincloss AH, Diez Roux AV, Mujahid MS, et al: Neighborhood resources for physical activity and healthy foods and incidence of type 2 diabetes mellitus: the multi-ethnic study of atherosclerosis. *Arch Intern Med* 169(18):1698–1704, 2009.
69. Ludwig J, Sanbonmatsu L, Gennetian L, et al: Neighborhoods, obesity, and diabetes—a randomized social experiment. *N Engl J Med* 365(16):1509–1519, 2011.
70. Ludwig J, Duncan GJ, Gennetian LA, et al: Neighborhood effects on the long-term well-being of low-income adults. *Science* 337(6101):1505–1510, 2012.
73. Wilson WJ: *The truly disadvantaged: the inner city, the underclass, and public policy*, Chicago, IL, 1987, University of Chicago Press.
76. Brancati FL, Whittle JC, Whelton PK, et al: The excess incidence of diabetic end-stage renal disease among blacks. A population-based study of potential explanatory factors. *JAMA* 268(21):3079–3084, 1992.
78. Hall YN, Choi AI, Chertow GM, et al: Chronic kidney disease in the urban poor. *Clin J Am Soc Nephrol* 5(5):828–835, 2010.
79. Genovese G, Friedman DJ, Ross MD, et al: Association of trypanolytic ApoL1 variants with kidney disease in African Americans. *Science* 329(5993):841–845, 2010.
80. Rosset S, Tzur S, Behar DM, et al: The population genetics of chronic kidney disease: insights from the MYH9-APOL1 locus. *Nat Rev Nephrol* 7(6):313–326, 2011.
85. Wang Z, Hoy WE: Diabetes and lifetime risk of ESRD in high-risk remote-dwelling Australian Aboriginal people: a 20-year cohort study. *Am J Kidney Dis* 62(4):845–846, 2013.
88. Shah VO, Scavini M, Stidley CA, et al: Epidemic of diabetic and nondiabetic renal disease among the Zuni Indians: the Zuni Kidney Project. *J Am Soc Nephrol* 14(5):1320–1329, 2003.
89. Narva AS, Sequist TD: Reducing health disparities in American Indians with chronic kidney disease. *Semin Nephrol* 30(1):19–25, 2010.
97. Donabedian A: The quality of medical care. *Science* 200(4344):856–864, 1978.
99. Ruggenenti P, Perna A, Mosconi L, et al: Randomised placebo-controlled trial of effect of ramipril on decline in glomerular filtration rate and risk of terminal renal failure in proteinuric, non-diabetic nephropathy. *Lancet* 349(9069):1857–1863, 1997.
101. Brenner BM, Cooper ME, de Zeeuw D, et al: Effects of losartan on renal and cardiovascular outcomes in patients with type 2 diabetes and nephropathy. *N Engl J Med* 345(12):861–869, 2001.
102. Jafar TH, Stark PC, Schmid CH, et al: Progression of chronic kidney disease: the role of blood pressure control, proteinuria, and angiotensin-converting enzyme inhibition: a patient-level meta-analysis. *Ann Intern Med* 139(4):244–252, 2003.
105. Williams DR, Collins C: Racial residential segregation: a fundamental cause of racial disparities in health. *Public Health Rep* 116(5):404–416, 2001.
112. Bach PB, Pham HH, Schrag D, et al: Primary care physicians who treat blacks and whites. *N Engl J Med* 351(6):575–584, 2004.
113. Varkey AB, Manwell LB, Williams ES, et al: Separate and unequal: clinics where minority and nonminority patients receive primary care. *Arch Intern Med* 169(3):243–250, 2009.
13. Jha V, Garcia-Garcia G, Iseki K, et al: Chronic kidney disease: global dimension and perspectives. *Lancet* 382(9888):260–272, 2013.
120. Himmelfarb J, Berns A, Szczech L, et al: Cost, quality, and value: the changing political economy of dialysis care. *J Am Soc Nephrol* 18(7):2021–2027, 2007.
124. Sehgal AR: Impact of quality improvement efforts on race and sex disparities in hemodialysis. *JAMA* 289(8):996–1000, 2003.
128. Epstein AM, Ayanian JZ, Keogh JH, et al: Racial disparities in access to renal transplantation—clinically appropriate or due to underuse or overuse? *N Engl J Med* 343(21):1537–1544, 2000.
130. Alexander GC, Sehgal AR: Barriers to cadaveric renal transplantation among blacks, women, and the poor. *JAMA* 280(13):1148–1152, 1998.
142. Goyal M, Mehta RL, Schneiderman LJ, et al: Economic and health consequences of selling a kidney in India. *JAMA* 288(13):1589–1593, 2002.
147. Roberts JP, Wolfe RA, Bragg-Gresham JL, et al: Effect of changing the priority for HLA matching on the rates and outcomes of kidney transplantation in minority groups. *N Engl J Med* 350(6):545–551, 2004.
151. Kasiske BL, Cohen D, Lucey MR, et al: Payment for immunosuppression after organ transplantation. American Society of Transplantation. *JAMA* 283(18):2445–2450, 2000.
165. Mohandas R, Casey MJ, Cook RL, et al: Racial and socioeconomic disparities in the allocation of expanded criteria donor kidneys. *Clin J Am Soc Nephrol* 8(12):2158–2164, 2013.
169. Woolf SH, Johnson RE, Phillips RL, Jr, et al: Giving everyone the health of the educated: an examination of whether social change would save more lives than medical advances. *Am J Public Health* 97(4):679–683, 2007.

85

Care of the Older Adult with Chronic Kidney Disease

Meghan J. Elliott | Ann M. O'Hare | Brenda R. Hemmelgarn

CHAPTER OUTLINE

BACKGROUND, 2586
Prevalence of Chronic Kidney Disease and Age-Related Changes in Estimated Glomerular Filtration Rate, 2586
Estimated Glomerular Filtration Rate, 2587
Prevalence and Implications of Albuminuria, 2587
Screening for Chronic Kidney Disease, 2587
Adverse Outcomes Associated with Reduced Estimated Glomerular Filtration Rate, 2588
TREATMENT CONSIDERATIONS, 2590

Management of Common Comorbidities, 2590
Special Considerations Regarding Medication Use, 2594
Tools to Aid Medication Use, 2594
CARE FOR OLDER ADULTS WITH END-STAGE KIDNEY DISEASE, 2596
Dialysis Initiation, 2596
Kidney Transplantation, 2598
Advanced Care Planning, 2599
CONCLUSION, 2600

BACKGROUND

Although chronic kidney disease (CKD) is a significant public health issue for patients of all ages, there is a limited body of literature addressing the management of CKD in older adults. However, most health care practitioners would agree that caring for older adults with CKD presents unique challenges because of the substantial differences between older and younger patients with this condition. In this chapter, we will provide an overview of care for the older adult with CKD. We begin by presenting background on the prevalence and outcomes associated with CKD in older adults. We then focus on treatment and common comorbid conditions (hypertension, diabetes, dyslipidemia and anemia), followed by considerations when caring for older adults with more severe CKD, including the options of kidney replacement therapy, as well as management strategies including shared decision making and advanced care planning.

PREVALENCE OF CHRONIC KIDNEY DISEASE AND AGE-RELATED CHANGES IN ESTIMATED GLOMERULAR FILTRATION RATE

CKD, defined as an estimated glomerular filtration rate (eGFR) of less than 60 mL/min/1.73 m² for longer than 3 months, is common, with prevalence in the adult population of 8%. This rate increases substantially to almost 45% among individuals 70 years of age and older.[1] Contemporary guidelines for the care of patients with CKD generally recommend that the same definition and approach to staging of CKD be applied to both older and younger adults. However, there is considerable debate in the literature as to whether differences in eGFR among patients of different ages, and the resultant increased prevalence of CKD among older adults, represents the course of "natural" aging, or whether these changes reflect the presence of underlying kidney disease.[2] In an evaluation of 365 healthy potential kidney donors, Rule and colleagues[3] have described marked increases in the prevalence of renal fibrosis and a linear reduction in GFR (using the gold standard for assessing kidney function—iothalamate clearance) of 4.6 mL/min/decade in men and 7.1 mL/min/decade in women with increasing age. However, the level of the GFR did not correlate perfectly with degree of fibrosis, and there was substantial heterogeneity in GFR among patients of the same age with similar degrees of fibrosis. It has been argued that this decline in GFR with age is natural and not a pathologic phenomenon, and that these reductions begin from about the age of 30 years.[4] At the same time, multiple studies have shown that older and younger patients with lower levels of eGFR and proteinuria are at increased risk for death, progression of kidney disease, and other adverse health outcomes, although the magnitude of relative and absolute risks for some outcomes vary systematically with age.

ESTIMATED GLOMERULAR FILTRATION RATE

In most cases, kidney function in routine clinical practice is estimated based on serum creatinine concentration, rather than determined using exogenous filtration markers such as inulin, iothalamate, or other radiocontrast clearance measures. Use of serum creatinine concentration alone to estimate kidney function, however, may underestimate the prevalence of chronic kidney disease, especially among those with low muscle mass, including women and older adults. Over the last 10 to 15 years, there have been major advances in the approach to estimating GFR through the use of estimating equations. Nevertheless, commonly used formulas may overestimate or underestimate true GFR in older adults. This has been shown using data from the Third National Health and Nutrition Examination Survey (NHANES III; Figure 85.1). In general, however, the Modification of Diet in Renal Disease equation[5] and the Chronic Kidney Disease Epidemiology Collaboration (CKD-EPI)[6] provide a closer approximation than the Cockcroft-Gault equation[7] to the true GFR, including among older adults. For further discussion of methods for estimating GFR, see Chapter 26.

In estimating kidney function using a creatinine-based equation, it is important to recognize that the loss of muscle mass that may occur with aging may result in a decrease in serum creatinine level and an overestimation of eGFR, particularly among patients with more severe underlying comorbid conditions. There is considerable interest in determining whether other clearance markers, and in particular serum cystatin C, are more accurate in estimating GFR in older adults.[8,9] Cystatin C is a cysteine proteinase with endogenous and constant production that is freely filtered, catabolized, and reabsorbed, but not secreted, by the kidney tubules.

The Kidney Disease Improving Global Outcomes (KDIGO) 2012 Clinical Practice Guideline for Evaluation and Management of CKD[10] has recommend reporting eGFR using the 2009 CKD-EPI creatinine-based equation, with the use of additional tests such as cystatin C or a clearance measurement for confirmatory testing in specific circumstances. For example, use of cystatin C may be especially useful in confirming the presence of CKD in patients with an eGFR of 45 to 59 mL/min/1.73 m² based on creatinine-based equations. Exogenous filtration markers may be used to measure kidney function when the results may affect treatment decisions, such as acceptance for kidney donation or dose adaptation of toxic drugs. Contemporary clinical practice guidelines for CKD do not comment on the potential implications of age in the use of these equations to estimate the GFR.

PREVALENCE AND IMPLICATIONS OF ALBUMINURIA

Albuminuria is now recognized as an important risk factor for adverse outcomes and is independently associated with mortality, vascular events, and progression to end-stage kidney disease (ESKD), independent of the eGFR.[11,12] The prognostic value of albuminuria appears to be relevant for the older adult population as well. Although an earlier study ($N = 13,177$; age ≥ 75 years) in the United Kingdom suggested that albuminuria was associated with a modest increase in risk of death, this association was not present at all levels of eGFR.[13] In contrast, a more recent study of 94,934 U.S. veterans with diabetes demonstrated an association between the albumin-to-creatinine ratio (ACR) and increased mortality risk.[14] Importantly, this increased risk was not attenuated with age and was also present at all levels of eGFR, with mortality rates increasing with higher levels of albuminuria (Figure 85.2). A large meta-analysis of 46 cohorts worldwide, the CKD Prognosis Consortium,[15] has provided the strongest evidence to date of a graded and independent risk of albuminuria on the risk of mortality and ESKD outcomes, across all ages. Together this evidence supports the important prognostic value of albuminuria for adverse outcomes in adults of all ages.

SCREENING FOR CHRONIC KIDNEY DISEASE

Screening for CKD in the general population has been advocated, although this is an area of considerable controversy.[16,17] Although population-based screening does have potential benefits through early identification and treatment of affected patients, it also carries with it certain risks, such as identification of patients with only mild disease for whom additional treatment might not be warranted.[18] The earlier National Kidney Foundation/Kidney Disease

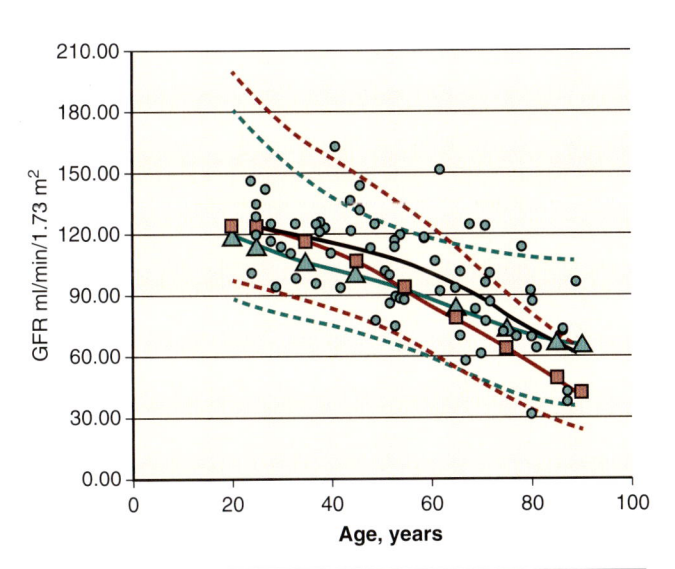

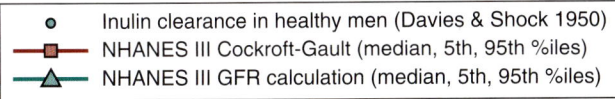

Figure 85.1 Percentiles of GFR, Cockcroft-Gault creatinine clearance by age, and inulin clearance in healthy men. Percentiles are calculated using a fourth-order polynomial weighted quantile regression. The solid line shows a polynomial regression to the inulin data. Dashed lines without symbols show the 5th and 95th percentiles for GFR estimates. (Reprinted with permission from Coresh J, Astor BC, Greene T, et al: Prevalence of chronic kidney disease and decreased kidney function in the adult US population: Third National Health and Nutrition Examination Survey. *Am J Kidney Dis* 41(1):1-12, 2003.)

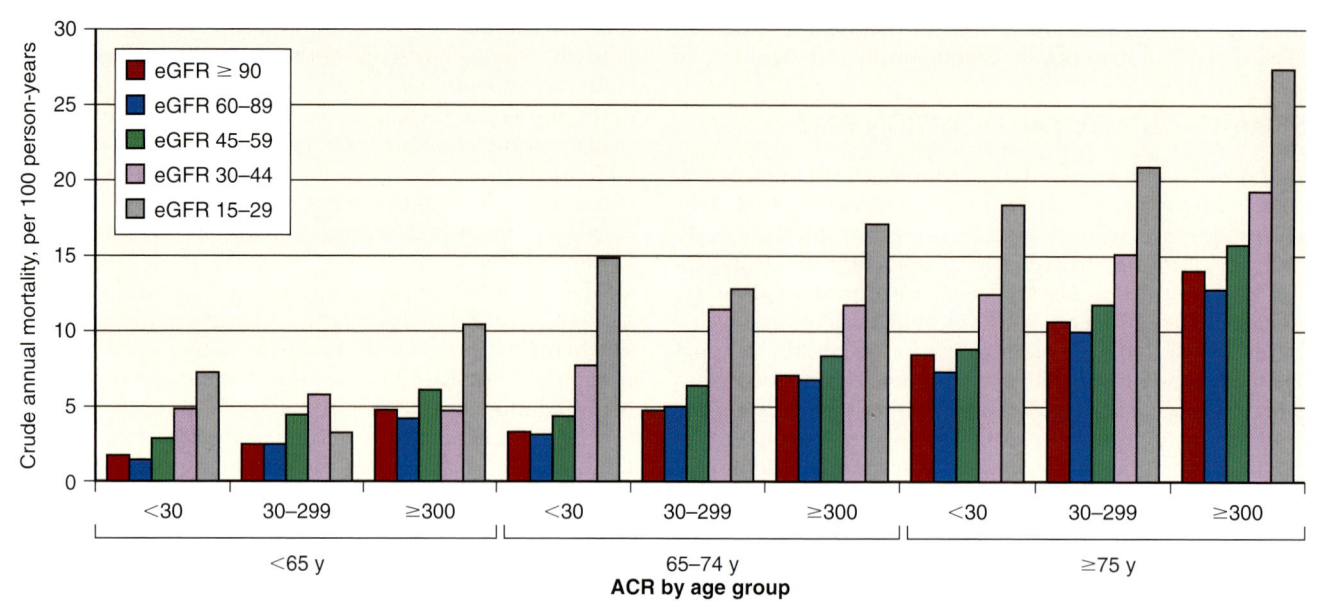

Figure 85.2 Crude annual mortality rates by albumin-to-creatinine ratio (ACR, in mg/g), estimated glomerular filtration rate (eGFR, in mL/min/1.73m^2), and age group. (Reprinted with permission from O'Hare AM, Hailpern SM, Pavkov ME, et al: Prognostic implications of the urinary albumin to creatinine ratio in veterans of different ages with diabetes. *Arch Intern Med* 170:930-936, 2010.)

Outcomes Quality Initiative[19] clinical practice guidelines for CKD have recommended targeted screening of high-risk patients, including those with diabetes or hypertension and older than 60 years, whereas the more recent KDIGO CKD guidelines[10] do not address the issue of screening.

Evidence to support screening for CKD in the general population is limited. Hallan and associates[20] used data from a large-scale (N = 65,604) health survey in Norway to evaluate screening strategies for CKD in the general population, with the outcomes of ESKD and cardiovascular mortality. The authors reported that screening people with hypertension, diabetes, or age 55 and older was the most effective screening strategy; they detected over 90% of all cases of CKD, with the number needed to screen to find one case of 8.7. A cohort study in the Netherlands (N = 6879), with 6 years of follow-up for the primary outcome of kidney replacement therapy, reported that screening for albuminuria was effective in identifying patients at increased risk for progressive kidney disease, including 40% of those who were previously not known to have kidney disease.[21] They were unable to determine whether the benefits of screening for albuminuria to prevent ESKD were sufficient to outweigh the costs and effort. Using a population-based cohort from Alberta, Canada, Manns and coworkers[22] reported that population-based screening for CKD using eGFR was not cost-effective for the overall population, older adults, or those with hypertension. However, they did find that targeted screening of people with diabetes was associated with a cost per quality-adjusted life year was similar to that accepted in other publically funded interventions.

These studies, suggesting that the overall benefit of detecting and treating asymptomatic CKD among people without diabetes is low and not cost-effective, seem to provide evidence for a targeted case-finding approach, rather than a general screening strategy for adults of all ages. The purpose of screening is to identify people at an early stage to prevent disease progression. The potential benefits of screening to identify CKD in older adults, among whom both life expectancy and the risk of progression may be lower, are uncertain.

ADVERSE OUTCOMES ASSOCIATED WITH REDUCED ESTIMATED GLOMERULAR FILTRATION RATE

MORTALITY

Older adults with mild reductions in eGFR (e.g., 45 to 59 mL/min/1.73 m^2) have a similar risk of death compared with those of similar age, but with higher levels of eGFR.[23] However, more severe reductions in eGFR have consistently been shown to be associated with worse outcomes. Raymond and colleagues[24] have shown that although the relative mortality risk may be attenuated, the absolute mortality risk increases with declining eGFR for all ages (Figure 85.3).

The age-dependent effects of CKD on the competing risks of ESKD and death are evident in Figure 85.4.[23] As shown in this figure, among patients with a comparable level of eGFR, the relative frequency of these outcomes (death and ESKD) varies substantially by age. Older individuals, especially those older than 75 years, are much more likely to die than develop ESKD, even when their eGFR is severely reduced. A recent study from the CKD Prognosis Consortium[15] has provided further evidence of the importance on adverse outcomes and mortality risk of CKD in older adults. In this large collaborative meta-analysis, including more than 2 million participants from 46 cohorts, CKD was associated with excess mortality risks among older adults that were as high as, or higher than, the excess risk observed among middle-aged adults. Similar to prior studies, the relative risk of death at each level of eGFR was generally lower at older ages, with the result that the threshold level of eGFR at which the absolute risk of death increased above the referent was lower in older compared with younger patients.

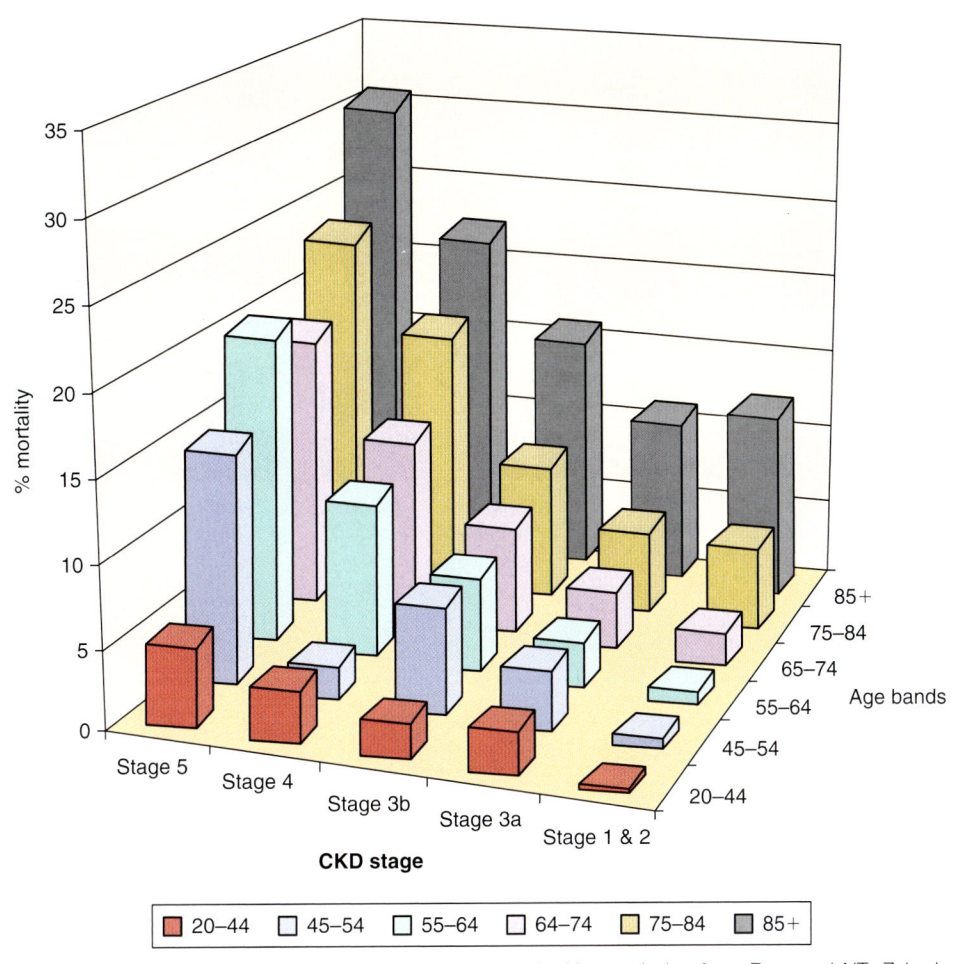

Figure 85.3 Average annual mortality by age and eGFR bands. (Reprinted with permission from Raymond NT, Zehnder D, Smith SC, et al: Elevated relative mortality risk with mild-to-moderate chronic kidney disease decreases with age. *Nephrol Dial Transplant* 22:3214-3220, 2007.)

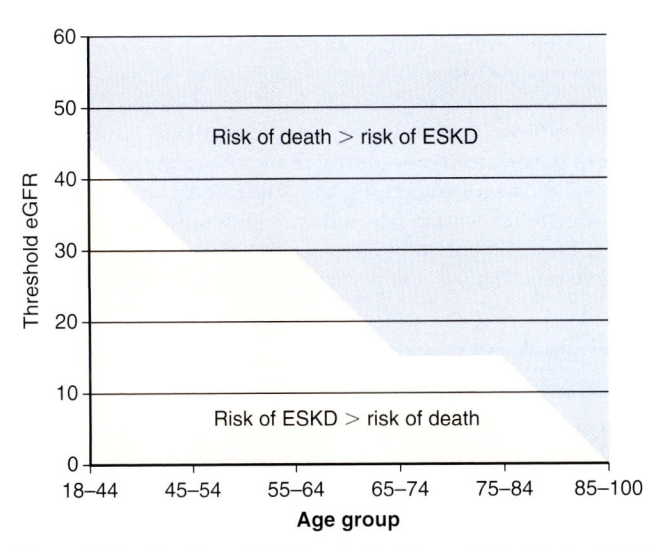

Figure 85.4 Baseline eGFR threshold below which risk for ESKD exceeded risk for death for each age group. (Reprinted with permission from O'Hare AM, Choi AI, Bertenthal D, et al. Age affects outcomes in chronic kidney disease. *J Am Soc Nephrol* 18:2758-2765, 2007.)

END-STAGE KIDNEY DISEASE

As noted, the age-dependent effects of CKD on the risk of ESKD have been demonstrated (see Figure 85.4),[23] with older individuals much more likely to die than progress to ESKD that requires dialysis. In defining the progression of CKD in older adults, most studies have focused on the development of ESKD requiring long-term dialysis as the outcome, a definition that reflects disease progression and a treatment decision. Using a population-based cohort of more than 1.8 million adults from the province of Alberta, Canada, we found that the rate of progression to treated kidney failure (defined as the initiation of long-term dialysis or receipt of a kidney transplant) and untreated kidney failure (defined as progression to a sustained eGFR < 15 mL/min/1.73 m^2) varied substantially by age.[25] Among younger participants, the absolute and relative risks of treated kidney failure were highest. However, the rate of progression to untreated kidney failure was considerably higher among older participants (Figure 85.5). What these results suggest is that kidney disease does progress in older adults, and that the actual prevalence of advanced kidney disease and incidence of progressive CKD may be underestimated when defined by receipt of kidney replacement therapy alone.

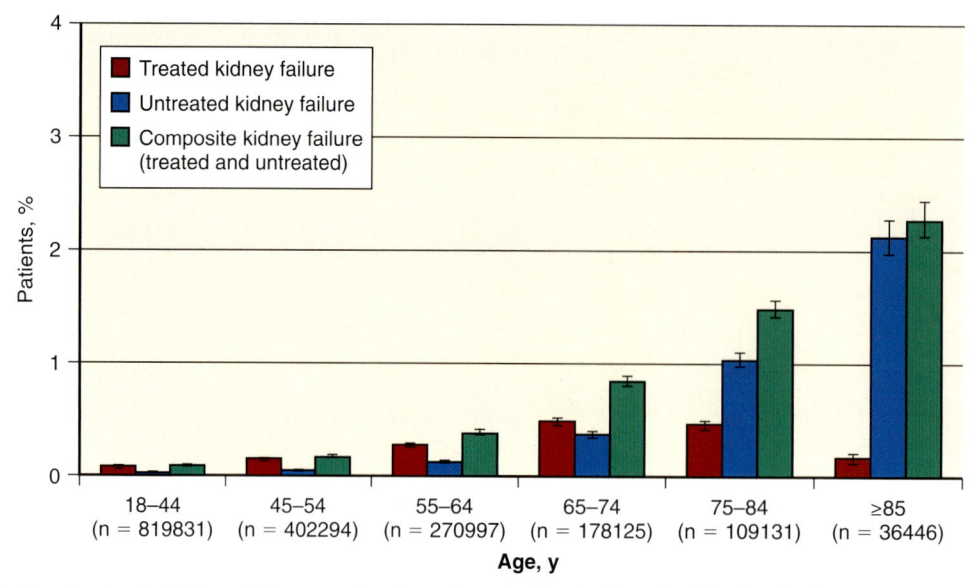

Figure 85.5 Treated and untreated kidney failure as a function of age in Alberta, Canada. (Reprinted with permission from Hemmelgarn BR, James MT, Manns BJ, et al: Rates of treated and untreated kidney failure in older vs younger adults. *JAMA* 307:2507-2515, 2012.)

CARDIOVASCULAR DISEASE, STROKE, DIABETES, AND CONGESTIVE HEART FAILURE

CKD has been associated with an increased risk of cardiovascular disease events in multiple populations,[11,26] including older adults.[27,28] In the Cardiovascular Health Study, a community-based cohort of U.S. adults aged 65 years and older, those with CKD had more than twice the prevalence of coronary artery disease compared with those without CKD, and they were more than 50% more likely to have hypertension.[29,30] Stevens and associates[28] also reported the prevalence of CKD and comorbid illness in U.S. individuals aged 65 and older using three large data sources—the Kidney Early Evaluation Program (KEEP; $N = 27,017$), the National Health and Nutrition Examination Survey (NHANES), 1999 to 2006 ($N = 5,538$) and the Medicare 5% sample ($N = 1,236,946$). Among members of these cohorts with CKD, the prevalence of diabetes ranged from 21.4% to 46.2%, whereas the prevalence of hypertension was 90% or higher in all three cohorts. The prevalence of high cholesterol, coronary artery disease, congestive heart failure, cardiovascular disease, and cancer for the KEEP and NHANES cohorts are presented in Figure 85.6. These data, from multiple sources, clearly demonstrate the high burden of chronic conditions in older adults with CKD. Management of these common chronic conditions among older adults with CKD will be discussed later in this chapter.

FUNCTIONAL AND COGNITIVE IMPAIRMENT AND FRAILTY

Unfortunately, most of the evidence regarding functional and cognitive impairment and frailty in older adults with kidney disease has been limited to those with ESKD on dialysis. However, there is evidence that advanced CKD is also associated with a high prevalence of cognitive and functional impairment,[31] and that albuminuria is an independent risk factor for cognitive impairment.[32] Cognitive impairment in patients with CKD seems to follow a pattern most consistent with vascular disease and primarily affects attention and executive function. With respect to physical function, individuals with CKD have evidence of reduced physical function based on tests of balance and gait speed,[27,33] as well as lower levels of physical activity overall.[27,33,34]

Following the initiation of dialysis, there is evidence that there can be significant decline in functional status among older adults. Among nursing home residents, decline in functional status after dialysis initiation was independent of age, gender, race, and functional status trajectory before starting dialysis.[35] Overall, only 13% of patients maintained their predialysis functional status at 1 year (Figure 85.7). Even among older adults living independently in the community at the time of dialysis initiation, a large proportion lose independence and transition to nursing homes or related care facilities following initiation of dialysis. A retrospective study reported that although most patients 80 years of age and older were living independently at home at the time of dialysis initiation, more than 30% experienced functional loss requiring caregiver support or transfer to a nursing home within 6 months.[36] Outcomes after dialysis initiation are discussed in greater detail in a later section of this chapter.

TREATMENT CONSIDERATIONS

MANAGEMENT OF COMMON COMORBIDITIES

These include hypertension, diabetes, dyslipidemia, and anemia.

HYPERTENSION

Multiple chronic conditions, including hypertension and diabetes, among others, are common in older adults with CKD, particularly among the very old (>85 years).[37,38] The relationship between CKD and hypertension is complex, with CKD contributing to the pathophysiology

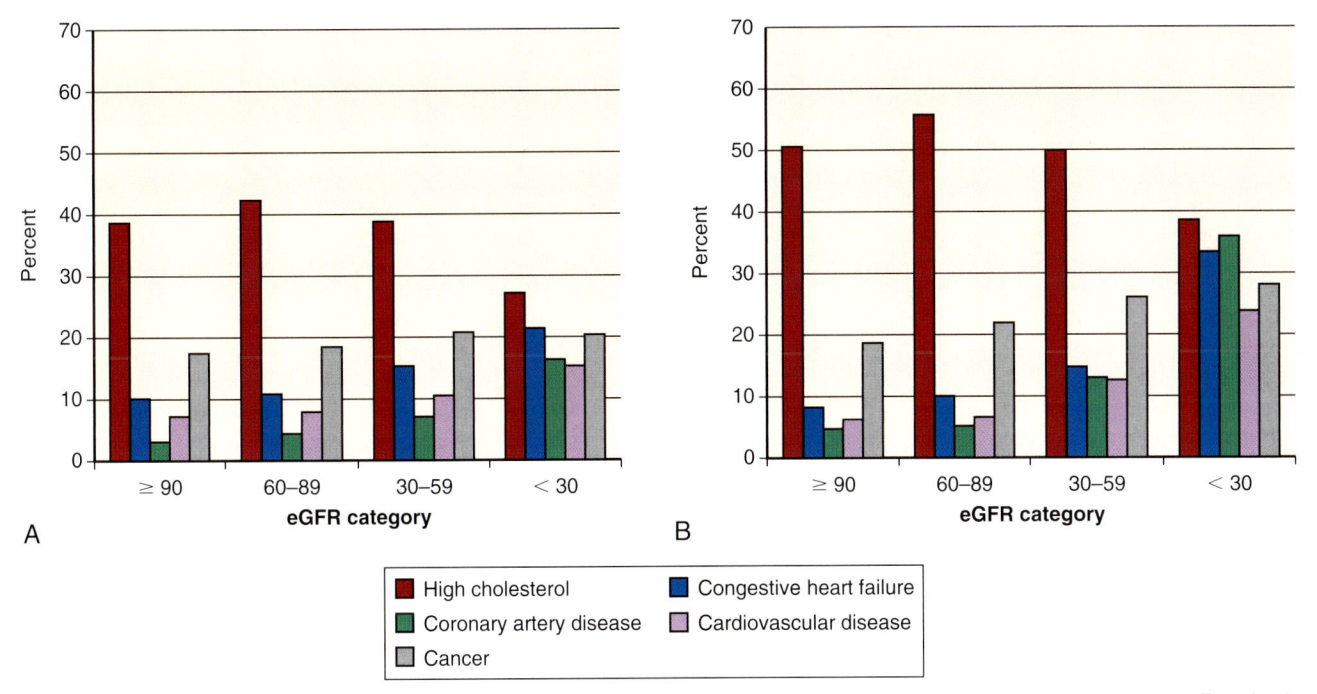

Figure 85.6 Comorbid conditions by level of eGFR in Kidney Early Evaluation Program **(A)** and National Health and Nutrition Examination Survey **(B)**. (Reprinted with permission from Stevens LA, Li S, Wang C, et al: Prevalence of CKD and comorbid illness in elderly patients in the United States: results from the Kidney Early Evaluation Program (KEEP). *Am J Kidney Dis* 55(Suppl 2):S23-S33, 2010.)

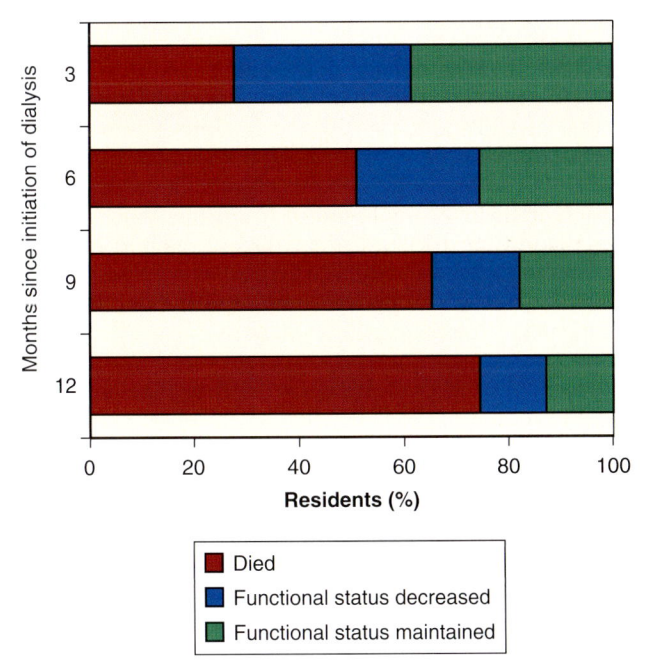

Figure 85.7 Survival and functional status after initiation of dialysis among nursing home residents. (Reprinted with permission from Kurella Tamura M, Covinsky KE, Chertow GM, et al: Functional status of elderly adults before and after initiation of dialysis. *N Engl J Med* 361:1539-1547, 2009.)

of hypertension and blood pressure influencing the progression of underlying CKD. Large population-based studies have observed that CKD is commonly seen among older individuals with hypertension, and hypertension is commonly observed among older persons with CKD.[39-41]

There is variability in the recommended target blood pressure for patients with CKD across guidelines. The Canadian Hypertension Education Program recommends targeting a blood pressure less than 140/90 mm Hg, regardless of age, for patients with nondiabetic CKD.[42] However, guidelines from KDIGO[43] recommend a lower target of less than 130/80 mm Hg for those with proteinuria and less than 140/90 mm Hg for all others with CKD; guidelines from the National Institute for Health and Care Excellence[44] recommend a target of less than 150/90 mm Hg in people aged 80 years and older.

Treatment decisions for older adults with hypertension and CKD should take several factors into consideration, including goals of therapy (e.g., slowing CKD progression, cardiovascular protection, and/or reducing mortality), treatment targets, potential adverse consequences of therapy, and patient-specific factors, such as comorbidities and preferences. In contrast to younger individuals, arterial stiffening that commonly occurs with advancing age predisposes older adults with or without CKD to isolated systolic hypertension, with diastolic blood pressures that generally decline with age.[45,46] Advanced age and elevated systolic blood pressure are risk factors for orthostatic hypotension, which is observed in up to 30% of older adults and can complicate blood pressure reduction strategies.[47,48]

Most data describing the benefits of treating elevated blood pressure in older adults have been extrapolated from observational studies and randomized controlled trials (RCTs) in older adults with hypertension, irrespective of underlying kidney function. Several large trials of older adults with hypertension (with most having isolated systolic hypertension) have reported that hypertension treatment versus placebo reduces cardiovascular end points, most notably stroke, even among the very old (≥80 years).[49-51] A

2009 Cochrane systematic review of RCTs including patients 60 years of age and older with baseline systolic blood pressure (BP) 140 mm Hg or higher and/or diastolic BP 90 mm Hg or higher found that treatment to lower BP reduced overall mortality (relative risk [RR] 0.90; 95% confidence interval [CI], 0.84 to 0.97) and cardiovascular morbidity and mortality (RR, 0.72; 95% CI, 0.68 to 0.77), with similar results observed among patients with isolated systolic hypertension.[52] However, among the very old (≥80 years), total mortality risk was not reduced with treatment of hypertension, despite a similar benefit on cardiovascular morbidity and mortality. It should be noted that the targeted and achieved systolic BPs in these studies were well above the 130-mm Hg targets currently recommended in certain CKD guidelines. Furthermore, these trials excluded patients with varying degrees of kidney impairment at baseline on the basis of serum creatinine measurements, precluding widespread application of the results to older persons with more advanced CKD.

Data comparing different pharmacologic agents for reducing BP and/or slowing progression of CKD in older adults are sparse. Angiotensin-converting enzyme (ACE) inhibitors or angiotensin receptor blockers (ARBs) have established benefits in patients with diabetic and/or proteinuric CKD, and thus are recommended as first-line therapy in these settings by several clinical practice guidelines, irrespective of underlying hypertension.[43] It is less clear whether these agents should be used as initial treatment of hypertension in all older adults with CKD. Most trials guiding these recommendations excluded patients older than 70 years and selected for those with proteinuria and for those with diabetes, whereas most older adults with CKD do not have proteinuria or diabetes.[53] Also, limited safety data exist on the use of these and other agents in older individuals with or without CKD.[52,54] In the Cochrane meta-analysis described above, a significantly greater number of older adults treated for hypertension withdrew from the trials due to adverse drug effects than controls (RR, 1.71; 95% CI, 1.45 to 2.00), although only three trials reported these data.[52] An ongoing randomized trial, SPRINT (Systolic Blood Pressure Intervention Trial), assessing systolic BP targets of less than 120 or 140 mmHg in patients without diabetes or significant proteinuria, has included both older and CKD patients and is likely to provide additional evidence to guide hypertension treatment in this population.[55,56]

The 2012 KDIGO hypertension guidelines do not make specific recommendations regarding BP treatment targets or specific antihypertensive agents for older adults with CKD due to lack of available evidence. However, they suggested that cautiously targeting a BP of less than 140/90 mm Hg is reasonable in the absence of adverse effects, such as orthostatic hypotension.[43] Because current hypertension guidelines for CKD patients do not make specific recommendations based on patient age, it is reasonable to individualize treatment for the older patient with CKD, with consideration given to comorbidities or indications for a specific therapy, risk of adverse events from therapy, concurrent medications prescribed, quality of life, and patient preference. It is reasonable to begin therapy at a low dose, titrate gradually, and monitor closely for clinical response and adverse effects.

DIABETES

As with hypertension, the prevalence of type 2 diabetes mellitus increases with advancing age and frequently coexists with comorbidities such as CKD and cardiovascular disease.[57] Furthermore, diabetic nephropathy is the leading cause of CKD and ESKD worldwide, particularly among the rapidly growing North American older population.[1] Diabetic kidney disease is responsible for at least one third of incident ESKD cases in individuals older than 75 years, rates that have almost doubled between 1996 and 2006.[58,59] Among these older individuals with diabetic ESKD, life expectancy is at least 25% lower than similarly aged persons without diabetes and is largely attributable to the substantial cardiovascular disease burden in this population.[59]

Despite the tremendous morbidity and impact on health care resources, care of the older individual with diabetic kidney disease remains underemphasized and underrepresented in current practice guidelines. Most diagnostic and treatment considerations for this population are extrapolated from data on younger persons with diabetic kidney disease or older diabetic patients, without specific reference to the presence of nephropathy. Screening for kidney disease in people with type 2 diabetes should begin at the time of diagnosis, with assessment of both a random albumin-to-creatinine ratio and serum creatinine level (for estimation of GFR), repeated annually if normal.[60,61] The diagnostic criteria for diabetic kidney disease are the same, regardless of patient age, and require persistent albuminuria more than 30 mg/day and/or depressed eGFR, generally defined as less than 60 mL/min/1.73 m^2. However, the decline in GFR that typically accompanies advancing age does not necessarily indicate progressive kidney disease and should be interpreted in light of the expected natural history of diabetic nephropathy.[3,4] Furthermore, atypical presentations of diabetic kidney disease, such as impaired GFR in the absence of albuminuria and albuminuria related to nondiabetic kidney disease, are more commonly observed in older than younger diabetic patients.[62,63]

Strict metabolic control (hemoglobin A_{1c} less than 6.5% to 7.0%) has been shown to delay the onset of albuminuria and progression of CKD but not macrovascular outcomes in patients with type 2 diabetes.[64-66] However, no RCTs have addressed the impact of intense glycemic control on microvascular or macrovascular complications in patients with diabetes older than 65 years with or without CKD. Although those treated with an intensive glycemic control strategy in the ADVANCE (Action in Diabetes and Vascular Disease: Preterax and Diamicron Modified Release Controlled Evaluation)[66a] and ACCORD (Action to Control Cardiovascular Risk in Diabetes)[66b] trials demonstrated renoprotective benefits (mean age of participants, 66 and 62 years, respectively), they were largely at the expense of increased risk of severe hypoglycemic episodes, which occurred two to three times more frequently in the intensive groups than in controls. This complication is concerning because older individuals are already at increased risk for severe hypoglycemia due to age-related reduction in counterregulatory hormonal responses, hypoglycemia unawareness, and physical and cognitive barriers impairing prompt treatment of hypoglycemia.[67,68] The altered pharmacokinetic properties of medications used to treat diabetes with advancing age and/

or CKD can further predispose these patients to unintended adverse effects. Because hypoglycemia in older adults, even when mild, can impair cognitive function, increase falls risk, and predispose to cardiovascular events and dementia,[69,70] avoidance of hypoglycemia is one of the main principles of diabetes management in this population, with or without underlying CKD.

Clinical practice guidelines recommend targeting a hemoglobin A_{1c} value of less than 7.0% to prevent or delay the progression of microvascular complications in adult diabetics with or without CKD, which includes albuminuria or depressed GFR.[10,60,61,71] In otherwise healthy older adults with diabetes, the same glycemic targets are reasonable when the risk of hypoglycemia is low. However, in frail older individuals at risk for hypoglycemia or with limited life expectancy, glycemic targets should be extended above this to a hemoglobin A_{1c} level of 8.5% or lower, or fasting plasma glucose level of 5.0 to 12.0 mmol/L, because the risks of hypoglycemia outweigh the benefits of tight glycemic control.[10,60,72] Hemoglobin A_{1c} may not accurately reflect glycemic control in older patients with diabetes and CKD who have shortened red cell survival, even if receiving iron or erythropoiesis-stimulating agents, and should be interpreted with caution.[73,74] In these individuals, pre- and postprandial home blood glucose readings may provide a more accurate estimate of true glycemic control.

Oral hypoglycemic agents are typically first-line therapies for treatment of diabetes in older patients, although some should be administered cautiously at a reduced dose or avoided altogether in the setting of more advanced kidney impairment due to concerns regarding adverse events. Metformin is an effective agent that should be given in a reduced dose in older patients with stage 3 CKD and discontinued when the GFR falls below 30 mL/min/1.73m^2 due to the potential for lactic acidosis with accumulation.[75] The sulfonylureas and thiazolidinediones should also be used cautiously in older adults because of concerns regarding severe hypoglycemia and exacerbating symptomatic heart failure, respectively.[76,77] Of the sulfonylureas, glyburide appears to portend the highest risk of hypoglycemia, particularly in the setting of kidney impairment,[77] whereas others such as glipizide and gliclazide are metabolized through hepatic mechanisms and could be continued cautiously without dose adjustment until advanced renal impairment develops.[78,79] Repaglinide, a short-acting meglitinide, can be used in those with advanced CKD without dose adjustment and has a lower risk of hypoglycemia in older adults than the sulfonylureas.[71,80] Although newer agents, such as the dipeptidyl peptidase (DPP)-4 inhibitors and glucagon-like peptide (GLP)-1 analogues, are effective agents that cause minimal hypoglycemia in young and old patients, many require a reduced dose or discontinuation in the setting of impaired kidney function.[81-83] Insulin therapy may be required to achieve adequate and stable glycemic control in advanced CKD or in those with poor control, despite oral hypoglycemic agents. In this case, a dosage reduction of 25% to 50% and careful titration are recommended for patients with an eGFR of 10 to 50 mL/min/1.73 m^2 due to less predictable responses and hypoglycemia risks.[84] Pharmacologic therapy for older diabetic patients with CKD should be individualized according to patient profile, preferences, and response to treatment, with careful adjustment as needed to attain treatment targets without hypoglycemia or other significant side effects.

DYSLIPIDEMIA

CKD is associated with an increased risk of major cardiovascular events and mortality, independent of hypertension and diabetes.[26] In fact, the rate of coronary death or myocardial infarction among patients with CKD is similar to that of patients with diabetes, and thus may be considered a coronary risk equivalent.[85] This risk, associated with CKD, appears to be age-dependent, with those older than 50 years at greatest risk. Although dyslipidemia is an important modifiable risk factor for cardiovascular disease in the general population, its role and relevance in the CKD population, and in particular older adults with CKD, is less clear. Some evidence exists to guide pharmacologic treatment of dyslipidemia in the predialysis CKD population,[86-89] but no trials have specifically addressed persons of advanced age with CKD.

In the PROSPER (PROspective Study of Pravastatin in the Elderly at Risk) trial of older individuals aged 70 to 82 years, treatment with 40 mg of pravastatin as compared with placebo reduced the risk of fatal or nonfatal myocardial infarction or stroke by 15%.[90] However, those with advanced kidney disease (serum creatinine level > 200 µmol/L) were excluded from this study. A post hoc analysis of three pravastatin trials (mean age, 65.7 years) has found that pravastatin significantly reduces cardiovascular outcomes in patients with moderate CKD (eGFR = 30 to 59.99 mL/min/1.73 m^2) to a similar extent as in those with normal kidney function.[91] More recently, the SHARP (Study of Heart and Renal Protection) trial reported a lower incidence of major atherosclerotic events in patients with CKD treated with low-dose simvastatin plus ezetimibe compared with placebo, with similar benefits seen among the subgroup of those 70 years and older at randomization.[86] Since the publication of SHARP, two meta-analyses of lipid-lowering therapies in patients with CKD have found similar cardiovascular benefits in the nondialysis CKD population, although neither specifically addressed the role of age.[87,88]

The most recent KDIGO guidelines have recommended initiation of statin therapy, with or without ezetimibe in combination, for all nondialysis patients older than 50 years with eGFR less than 60 mL/min/1.73 m^2, irrespective of baseline lipid profile, because these patients are at significantly increased risk for cardiovascular events and are most likely to benefit from treatment.[89] However, no guidelines for evaluating and treating dyslipidemia specific to older persons with CKD currently exist, so these recommendations are often applied similarly to this older population. Given the propensity for polypharmacy and adverse medication reactions in older adults with CKD, initiation of lipid therapy should be carefully considered, weighing the potential benefits and risks (as discussed in a later section of this chapter).

ANEMIA

Anemia associated with CKD may be seen once the eGFR declines below 60 mL/min/1.73 m^2, but it is more common at an eGFR less than 30 mL/min/1.73 m^2. At this point, approximately half of patients with stage 4 CKD and nearly all patients with stage 5 CKD develop anemia.[92] Among older adults, the prevalence of anemia is also significantly greater than in the general population, with 10% of individuals older than 65 years being anemic.[93] Therefore, determining the underlying cause of the anemia and appropriate investigations and treatment in older adults with CKD and anemia can be challenging, particularly in the earlier stages of CKD.

According to NHANES III data, the anemia in older individuals (≥65 years) was attributable to CKD in approximately 8% of cases,[93] highlighting the importance of considering other causes of anemia in this population. Numerous factors may contribute to the anemia seen in older adults with CKD, including nutritional deficiencies (e.g., iron, vitamin B_{12}, or folate deficiency), malignancies (particularly hematologic and gastrointestinal malignancies), medication use, and other comorbidities, in addition to the erythropoietin deficiency seen in the anemia of CKD.[94] Furthermore, using eGFR criteria alone to establish the likelihood of anemia being attributable to CKD in older persons may not be appropriate, given the potential for misclassification of true kidney function using GFR estimating equations in older individuals. Therefore, a reasonable approach to diagnosing the cause of anemia in this population would include initial evaluation of a complete blood count and red cell parameters, reticulocyte count, iron studies, and kidney function.[95] Abnormalities in these test results or other clinical indices may guide additional testing, including, for example, serum and urine protein electrophoresis, peripheral blood smear, hematology consultation, or referral for colonoscopy, as indicated.

Any reversible causes of anemia identified in older adults with CKD should be treated accordingly. If the anemia is thought to be secondary to underlying CKD, iron supplementation to replete the iron deficiency commonly seen in CKD, as well as erythropoietin-stimulating agents (ESAs), are the principal therapies. A full review and guidelines for hemoglobin targets and available therapies for anemia in the general CKD and ESKD populations are available. However, it is important to note that current CKD guidelines do not make anemia treatment recommendations specifically for older adults with CKD.[95-98] Instead, the guidelines for the general CKD population are often similarly applied to older individuals, despite the relative lack of clinical trials in this age group. Although most of these studies include persons older than 65 years, none have been designed to assess this population specifically. For example, the landmark TREAT (Trial to Reduce Cardiovascular Events with Aranesp Therapy) study (median age of participants, 68 years) found that in patients with CKD and diabetes, a higher hemoglobin target (13 g/dL in the darbepoetin group vs. 9 g/dL in the control group) did not reduce the risk of cardiovascular or kidney events and was associated with an increased risk of stroke.[99] Similar results were noted in the different age subgroups. Given the prevalent comorbidities in older adults with CKD, such as vascular disease, malignancy, atrial fibrillation, and hypertension, the increased risk of stroke or other adverse events with higher hemoglobin targets is particularly concerning. Therefore, the general CKD recommendations to initiate ESA at a hemoglobin concentration between 9.0 and 10.0 g/dL[95] may be reasonably applied to older adults with CKD and anemia, although individual patient concerns and preferences should also be taken into consideration.

SPECIAL CONSIDERATIONS REGARDING MEDICATION USE

Given the high burden of comorbidities among older individuals, it is not surprising that they take, on average, five prescription and nonprescription medications daily.[100] Safe medication prescribing in older adults with CKD is complicated not only by the number of medications and presence of comorbidities, but by the altered pharmacokinetics and pharmacodynamics in the setting of advancing age and presence of CKD. The combined age-related changes and CKD may increase the risk of drug accumulation and potential for adverse drug effects.[101,102] Evidence to guide prescribing is severely limited in this segment of the population because a large proportion of clinical trials has excluded those older than 65 years[103]; therefore, treatment decisions are often based on evidence extrapolated from patient groups with fewer physiologic deficits.[104] Relatively little research has been done to define the safety and effectiveness of medications in older adults with kidney disease.[100] Factors to consider when assessing medications in the older CKD population include individual-specific factors (e.g., eGFR, alterations in body composition and weight, overall health, and the indications for each medication) and drug factors (Table 85.1). Drugs that have a narrow therapeutic index, are primarily eliminated by the kidneys, or have active metabolites that are primarily eliminated by the kidneys should be assessed for adjustments of dose, interval, or both, depending on pharmacokinetic and pharmacodynamic parameters.[105] Individuals should be monitored carefully for the intended drug response and appearance of any adverse effects that might indicate toxicity, and the drug dosing regimen should be altered as required.

TOOLS TO AID MEDICATION USE

Several tools have been developed to identify medications for which the risks of use in older adults outweigh the benefits and to identify medications that have been omitted but are indicated and likely to benefit. These tools include the following: the Beers Criteria[106]; Screening Tool to Alert doctors to the Right Treatment (START)[107]; and Screening Tool of Older Person's potentially inappropriate Prescriptions (STOPP).[108] START has focused on ensuring that medications that are indicated and likely to provide benefit are not omitted in older adults, whereas the Beers Criteria and STOPP have aimed to minimize exposure to medications for which risks in older adults outweigh potential benefits. The Beers criteria are divided into three sections—potentially inappropriate medications (PIMs) for all older adults, PIMs used for drug-disease or drug-syndrome interactions, and PIMs to be used with caution in older adults. The STOPP list is arranged by physiologic system and provides a concise explanation as to why a medication may be considered inappropriate. The medications of concern are those that have anticholinergic or extrapyramidal side effects or may cause sedation, orthostatic hypotension, constipation or delirium or increased risk of bleeding. Prescribing multiple medications, regardless of indication, is a risk factor for reduced adherence, falls, weight loss, and other adverse outcomes, so reducing the overall number of medications is an important strategy to reduce risk.[100]

Table 85.1 Key Elements in Considering Risks and Benefits When Prescribing for Older Adults with Kidney Disease

Risk Considerations

Medication-Associated Risk

- Is the medication cleared in whole or in part by the kidney? Does the medication have a narrow therapeutic window?
- Is the medication thought to be of high risk in the general older population or in individuals with similar comorbidities to the patient in question?
- Does the medication have potential central nervous system effects?
- Are data available to guide dosing in patients with kidney disease (pharmacokinetic studies, drug level monitoring)?

Patient-Associated Risk

- Is the patient already taking multiple medications?
- Does the patient have cognitive dysfunction, poor vision, frailty? Risk of additional medications may be higher in this group.
- Does the patient have a history of adherence problems, and what would the consequences be of patient-related erratic dosing?

Benefit Considerations

- What is the population in which this medication has been studied? Does it include older adults or those with kidney disease? Is there observational or clinical trial evidence that benefits extend to those with kidney disease?
- If patients with kidney disease have not been studied, does the medication have a "track record" of safety in postapproval studies?
- Would benefits of the medication be due to improvement in symptoms or in decrease in risk from asymptomatic disease? What are the patient's preferences in adding new medications?
- Does the medication address a problem for which the patient is at significant risk (e.g., cardiovascular disease in patients with kidney disease)? Is the patient likely to accrue significant absolute risk reduction from the new medication?

From Rifkin DE, et al: Medication issues in older individuals with CKD. Adv Chronic Kidney Disease 17:320-328, 2010.

USE OF ANALGESICS, SEDATIVES, AND PSYCHOTROPICS

Analgesics are among the most commonly used medications in older adults.[100] Older adults should not be denied access to pain medications, but initial therapy should start with low doses and include careful upward titration and frequent assessments to ensure effectiveness and avoid adverse effects.[109] Opiates increase the risk of severe constipation without concurrent use of laxatives, may exacerbate cognitive impairment when used in older adults with dementia, and can have sedative effects, which may increase the risk of falls.[108] Morphine, codeine, and meperidine are not recommended for use in CKD because of the accumulation of neurotoxic metabolites that are excreted by the kidney system.[106] Hydromorphone, tramadol (with dose and interval adjustments), and oxycodone are the preferred opioids for initial therapy in CKD.[110] Methadone and fentanyl are also safe for use in those with CKD, but should not be used in opioid-naive persons.[111] Long-acting benzodiazepines (e.g., chlordiazepoxide, flurazepam, nitrazepam), benzodiazepines with long-acting metabolites (e.g., diazepam), and any benzodiazepine use for longer than 1 month are associated with increased risk of cognitive impairment, delirium, falls, fractures, and motor vehicle accidents in older adults.[106,108] All benzodiazepines should be avoided for the treatment of insomnia, agitation, or delirium; however, appropriate use in older adults includes treatment of withdrawal and severe anxiety disorder and end-of-life care.[106] Nonbenzodiazepine sedatives, such as zopiclone, have similar adverse event rates as benzodiazepines and are not recommended to be used for longer than 90 days.[106]

Psychotropic medications such as tricyclic antidepressants and antipsychotics should generally be avoided due to sedation, anticholinergic side effects, orthostatic hypotension, and potential to cause delirium.[108] However, low-dose amitriptyline and nortriptyline have been effective in persistent pain syndromes.[108]

REFERRAL TO NEPHROLOGISTS AND STRATEGIES FOR OPTIMIZING CARE

Late referral to nephrologists is common and has been reported to be associated with increased morbidity and mortality. However, not everyone with CKD needs to be seen by a nephrologist, which may be particularly true for older individuals with multiple comorbidities who are more likely to die than progress to ESKD. Although observational data from the general population suggest that earlier nephrology consultations result in better access to peritoneal dialysis and kidney transplantation,[112] as well as better preparation for the chosen modality and overall survival,[113,114] much less is known about the role that nephrologists play in the decision about whether to initiate dialysis or choose conservative management for older adults with kidney failure.[115]

Furthermore, a U.S.-based study of 323,977 adults 67 years of age and older who initiated dialysis reported that despite trends toward earlier use of nephrology consultation in older patients approaching dialysis, there was no improvement in 1-year survival rates after dialysis initiation.[116] The KDIGO Clinical Practice Guidelines for CKD[10] have outlined indications for which referral to specialist kidney care services be considered, including an eGFR less than 30 mL/min/1.73 m^2, persistent albuminuria (ACR > 30 mg/mmol), and other factors, such as rapid progression of CKD, refractory hypertension, and abnormalities of serum potassium levels. These indications, however, are for the general population and do not take into account the presence of advanced age or comorbidities. Further evidence is required to provide clear indications for referral for older adults with CKD.

Given the complexity of care for older individuals with CKD, a standardized multidisciplinary treatment approach may improve management and outcomes in this population. Observational studies have consistently shown that patients with CKD are generally undertreated with respect to receipt of indicated cardiovascular medications and, of those treated, a large proportion do not achieve optimal treatment targets for their conditions[117,118] Chronic disease management programs, with a coordinated multidisciplinary team that includes medicine, nursing, pharmacy, and nutrition, have been proposed as a strategy for optimizing care for patients with CKD.[119] A longitudinal cohort study of 6978 older outpatients with CKD in Alberta, Canada, has shown that participation in a multidisciplinary care program reduces the risk of death by approximately 50% compared to older adults with CKD and a similar comorbidity and eGFR who were not managed in a multidisciplinary care clinic.[120] Although the observational data appears promising, results from RCTs regarding the effect of multidisciplinary care are less convincing. Barrett and coworkers[121] have reported no difference in targeted outcomes (blood pressure or low-density lipoprotein cholesterol levels) among 474 patients with CKD who were randomly assigned to a nurse-coordinated team versus standard care. However, the mean eGFR in this study was 42 mL/min/1.73 m^2 and was not limited to older individuals. Considering the complexity of care required for these patients, an organized and standardized approach targeting the highest risk individuals would appear to be reasonable, particularly given the evidence to support such care delivery to patients with other chronic conditions, including diabetes.[122]

CARE FOR OLDER ADULTS WITH END-STAGE KIDNEY DISEASE

DIALYSIS INITIATION

Approximately one in four patients treated with long-term dialysis in the United States is older than 75 years. These older patients currently represent one of the fastest growing demographic groups within the ESKD population. Several lines of indirect evidence suggest that criteria for dialysis initiation in the United States have become more inclusive over time. First, the incidence of ESKD defined as treatment with long-term dialysis or kidney transplantation has increased over the last decade, particularly in older adults. This trend does not appear to be completely explained by a rising prevalence of CKD and/or associated risk factors, such as diabetes and hypertension.[123,124] Second, patients are initiating long-term dialysis at progressively higher levels of kidney function, as reflected in eGFR measures. This trend also does not appear to reflect changes in the composition of the ESKD population because the same pattern is present across a wide range of different subgroups.[125] Rather, secular trends toward initiation of dialysis at higher levels of eGFR most likely reflect changes in clinical practice, whereby dialysis is now initiated earlier in the course of advanced kidney disease compared with earlier years.[125]

Almost nothing is known about how often U.S. patients with advanced stages of CKD choose not to be treated with dialysis. Recent evidence from Alberta, Canada, has suggested that the burden of advanced kidney disease among older adults may be more substantial than previously recognized.[25] This study demonstrated that older adults with advanced kidney disease are less likely to be treated with dialysis than their younger counterparts, and that there is probably a relatively large "reservoir" of older adults with very low levels of eGFR who do not undergo chronic dialysis (see Figure 85.5). These findings are consistent with single-center studies from Europe and Australia demonstrating that a substantial number of older patients with advanced kidney disease are treated conservatively and do not receive dialysis.[126-131] Almost nothing is known about dialysis treatment practices in the United States, and what is known comes from registry data that do not include patients with advanced kidney disease who are not treated with dialysis or transplantation. Nevertheless, several lines of indirect evidence support the possibility that in the United States, a substantial number of older adults with advanced kidney disease are not treated with dialysis. Based on registry data, the incidence of treated ESKD per million population peaks in the 75- to 79-year age group and decreases thereafter, despite a linear increase in the overall prevalence of CKD with increasing age.[124] Similar patterns have been reported for the incidence of hospitalized patients with acute kidney injury (AKI) treated with dialysis.[132] There is also marked variation across U.S. hospital referral regions in the incidence of treated ESKD in older adults[133]; the highest incidence is observed in regions with the highest levels of health care spending, with the most pronounced regional differences in incidence observed in much older patients (Figure 85.8). However, these studies provide only indirect information about U.S. treatment practices for advanced kidney disease.

OUTCOMES

Although it is often assumed that treatment with dialysis will extend life and alleviate the signs and symptoms of advanced kidney disease, there is growing evidence that these benefits may not always accrue in older adults. Median life expectancy after the initiation of chronic dialysis in the United States is less than 2 years for patients aged 75 years or older.[127,128,130,134-140] Quartiles of life expectancy for U.S. patients aged 65 years and older are presented in Figure 85.9. Limited observational data have suggested that in much older patients with a high burden of comorbidity and/or disability, survival may be no better for those who initiate dialysis than for those managed without dialysis (often referred to as supportive or conservative care).[130] As noted above, several studies have reported that in older adults, level of disability and functional impairment may actually increase rather than decrease after dialysis is initiated.[35,36] There is often substantial escalation of care after dialysis is initiated, with many patients experiencing high rates of hospitalization and use of life-prolonging procedures, such as intubation, feeding tube placement, and cardiopulmonary resuscitation, compared with older adults with other chronic conditions.[141] It is possible that for some of these patients, any survival benefit afforded by dialysis may be outweighed by the additional treatment burden.

Although registry data serve as a valuable source of information about outcomes in older adults with ESKD who are treated with dialysis, almost nothing is known about outcomes among those who are not treated with dialysis. What little is known about this group comes from a handful of small, single-center studies that have examined outcomes among patients with advanced kidney disease who were managed conservatively.[127,128,130] Survival generally appears to be better for patients who initiate dialysis as compared with those managed conservatively, but some studies have suggested that there may be a subgroup of older patients with a high burden of comorbidity who do not experience a meaningful gain in life expectancy after dialysis

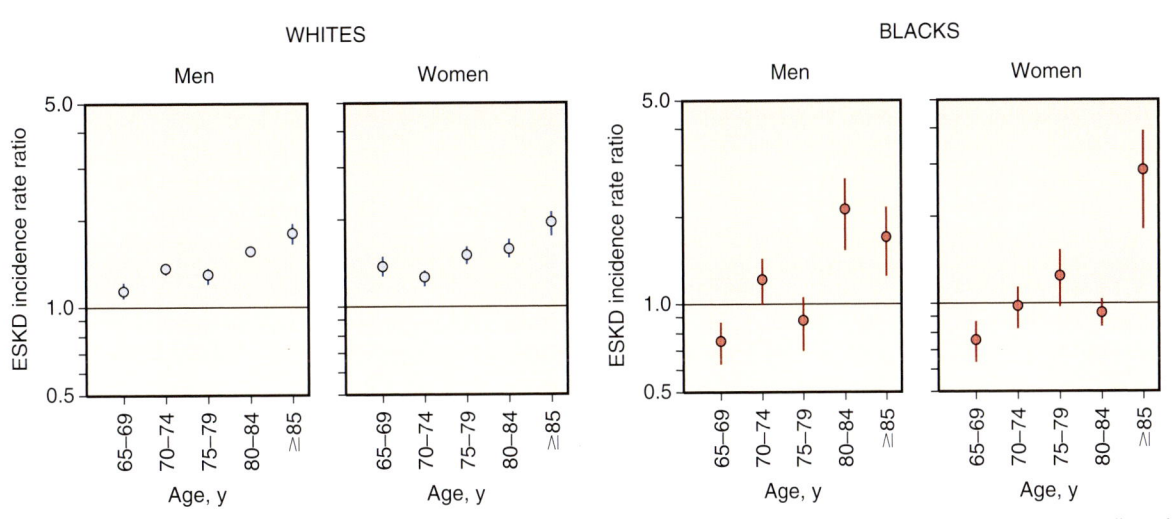

Figure 85.8 Regional variation in the incidence rate ratio of ESKD in regions with the highest versus lowest end-of-life expenditure index by age, gender, and race. (Reprinted with permission from O'Hare AM, Rodriguez RA, Hailpern SM, et al: Regional variation in health care intensity and treatment practices for end-stage renal disease in older adults. *JAMA* 304:180-186, 2010.)

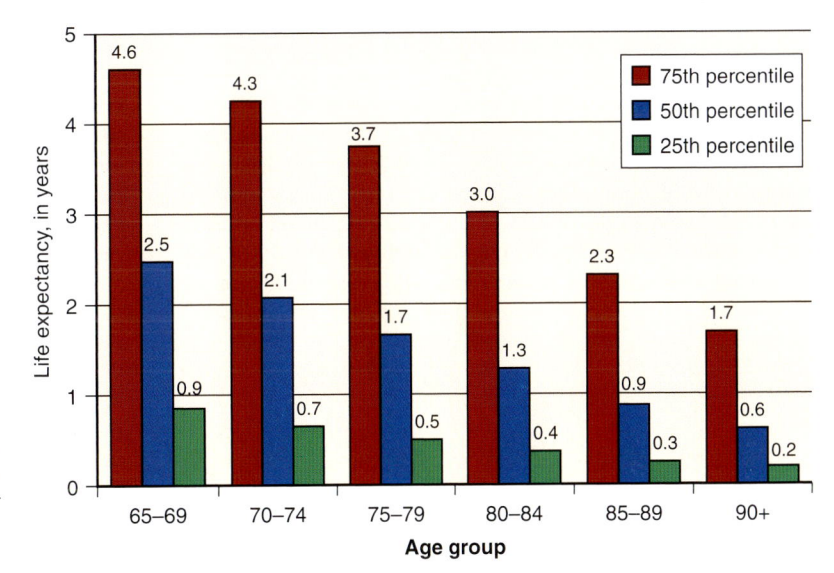

Figure 85.9 Quartiles of life expectancy after dialysis initiation by age group. (Reprinted with permission from Tamura MK, Tan JC, O'Hare AM: Optimizing renal replacement therapy in older adults: a framework for making individualized decisions. *Kidney Int* 82:261-269, 2012.)

initiation.[127,128,130] To our knowledge, comparative outcome data based on treatment assignment are lacking for older adults with advanced kidney disease, nor are we aware of studies that have reported other outcomes that might matter to patients and their families, such as quality of life and independence.

SHARED DECISION MAKING ABOUT DIALYSIS INITIATION

Most contemporary clinical practice guidelines recommend that patients, their families, and providers engage in a process of shared decision making around dialysis initiation.[142-144] The American Board of Internal Medicine's Choosing Wisely Campaign recently highlighted shared decision making around dialysis initiation as one of "five things" that should be prioritized in patients with kidney disease.[145] However, it is important to recognize that for many patients, treatment decisions about dialysis are best viewed as a process, rather than as a discrete decision occurring at single point in time.[146,147] Available data have suggested that there may be ample opportunity to enhance this process to ensure that treatment decisions are optimally aligned with patient values and preferences. Many older patients with advanced kidney disease face a singularly complex set of treatment decisions toward the end of their lives, often in the setting of great uncertainty about the relative benefits and harms of recommended interventions.[148,149] Approximately one third ultimately discontinue this therapy before death.[149] Many patients with ESKD are not aware of their prognosis, and many have unrealistic expectations about their expected disease course and appropriate treatment options.[150] Qualitative studies conducted among older patients followed in nephrology clinics seem to suggest that dialysis is more often presented as a necessity than as a true treatment choice.[148]

KIDNEY REPLACEMENT THERAPY: DIALYSIS MODALITY SELECTION

Ideally, discussions about dialysis versus more conservative approaches should be integrated with decisions about dialysis modality because there are large differences in treatment models for center hemodialysis, home hemodialysis, and peritoneal dialysis, and the experiences of patients receiving each modality may be quite distinct. The decision regarding treatment options for advanced kidney disease among older adults must take into account their higher burden of illness, increased comorbidities, and life expectancy, as discussed earlier. Although discussion regarding prognosis may be difficult for care providers, most patients referred to nephrologists report wanting to know this prognostic information.[151] Among patients 65 years of age and older initiating dialysis in the United States, most of them (93% to 98%) will start in-center hemodialysis as their initial modality choice, followed by peritoneal dialysis (2% to 5%) and preemptive transplantation (0% to 2%), as shown in Figure 85.10.[152]

Survival in general is reported to be comparable for patients initiating hemodialysis or peritoneal dialysis, but there has been some suggestion that for the subgroup of patients aged 65 and older with diabetes, survival with peritoneal dialysis is lower than for hemodialysis.[153] However, selection bias, rather than the effect of treatment itself, may explain the lower reported survival rates for patients initiating dialysis on peritoneal dialysis.[154] Among older adults, there are other reported advantages to peritoneal dialysis over hemodialysis. A recent review of kidney replacement therapy for older adults[152] has clearly demonstrated that compared with hemodialysis using a central venous catheter (a common form of vascular access among older adults), peritoneal dialysis is associated with reduced rates of hospitalization for sepsis, a serious infection-related morbidity common among hemodialysis patients with a central venous catheter. There are also other advantages to choosing peritoneal dialysis, including fewer invasive interventions[155] and greater preservation of residual kidney function. The extent to which protein loss and resultant malnutrition may attenuate the treatment advantages of peritoneal dialysis in older adults remains to be determined.

VASCULAR ACCESS

Currently, in the United States and elsewhere in developed countries, arteriovenous fistulas are viewed as the preferred form of vascular access for hemodialysis.[156,157] However, some studies have questioned the appropriateness of this approach for all older adults, for whom reduction in life expectancy and increased risk of failed fistula maturation may negate any potential survival benefits of fistulas over grafts as a dialysis access choice.[152,158] DeSilva and colleagues[159] analyzed data from 115,425 incident U.S. patients on hemodialysis aged 67 years and older for mortality outcomes based on first vascular access placed; they found no difference in mortality for patients with a graft as the first access compared with a fistula. Importantly, the authors also reported that only 50.7% of these older patients who had a fistula placed as their first access actually used the fistula at the time of dialysis initiation. Delayed maturation of fistulas in older adults is not uncommon. Given the complexity of their care, a more practical approach has been proposed to guide the choice of vascular access for older adults initiating hemodialysis.[160] Further factors are important to consider in making decisions regarding vascular access, including patient preferences and goals and the prognosis and circumstances of the individual patient,[161] to ensure a more patient-centered approach to vascular access planning.

KIDNEY TRANSPLANTATION

There has been a large increase in the number of older adults who have received a kidney transplant over the past decade, with a doubling of the proportion of newly transplanted patients aged 65 years and older in the United States.[162] The decision to pursue kidney transplantation does not rely on age alone because there is no specific chronologic age beyond which transplantation would not be considered. However, the decision to undergo transplantation in older adults involves a careful assessment of the potential benefits and harms, including an assessment of comorbidity and time spent on dialysis (an important risk factor for patient and graft survival).[163] Although there are benefits of transplantation for younger and older patients,[164] the survival advantage of deceased donor kidney transplantation is not recognized for approximately 8 months postsurgery due to the increased mortality risk during the perioperative and early posttransplantation period.[165] The length of time it takes to achieve a survival advantage with transplantation is longer for older patients because of their higher postoperative mortality risk. One study ($N = 25,468$) has confirmed earlier reports of an early risk of transplantation from different sources, with living donor transplantation being the safest decision for older patients.[164] However, kidney transplantation in those deemed eligible does have acceptable results. In a study using national registry data,

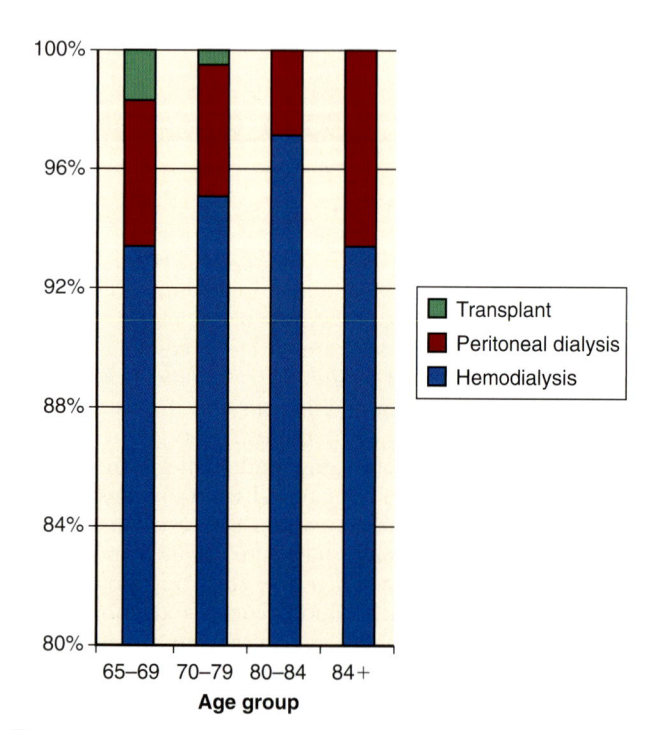

Figure 85.10 Initial kidney replacement therapy modality in the United States in 2008, according to age group. (Reprinted with permission from Tamura MK, Tan JC, O'Hare AM: Optimizing renal replacement therapy in older adults: a framework for making individualized decisions. *Kidney Int* 82:261-269, 2012.)

Rao and associates[166] have reported that even patients aged 70 years and older demonstrate a survival benefit with transplantation. There is considerable lack of evidence to guide decisions regarding transplant referral and eligibility in older adults; there is a need to develop more selective criteria for determining which older adults would benefit from transplantation to reduce the number of patients on the waiting list with little potential gain from transplantation.

ADVANCED CARE PLANNING

Advanced care planning (ACP) is the process whereby patients engage in discussions with their families and providers about their preferences for treatment should they develop a serious, life-threatening illness (especially one that leaves them unable to communicate these preferences). This process can provide an important opportunity to ensure that patients receive care at the end of life that is congruent with their preferences. Integration of ACP into the care of older adults with advanced kidney disease prior to initiation of chronic dialysis may provide a useful context for disease-related treatment decisions (e.g., dialysis initiation, preparation for dialysis, choice of dialysis modality, referral for transplantation). This approach may also strengthen the process of ACP by grounding theoretical discussions about future health states and treatment preferences in the reality of a patient's evolving experience of illness. In the next section, we provide a brief summary of approaches to ACP and summarize available literature about patients with kidney disease.

ADVANCE DIRECTIVES

Advance directives represent the cornerstone of the ACP process. Advance directives usually address the question of who will serve as the patient's surrogate decision maker and/or information about the patient's preference for life-sustaining interventions in the event of a serious illness.[167] Although advance directives may be a useful tool for promoting ACP, there is growing evidence that completion of advance directives alone may not be sufficient to ensure that patients receive care at the end of life that is congruent with their preferences.[168-172] It can be impossible to predict the myriad circumstances and treatment decisions that arise in the clinical setting, and the wording in advance directives is often too vague and inflexible to be helpful in supporting real-world clinical decisions.[173] In addition, surrogate decision makers are often poorly educated and prepared for their role, particularly if they have not participated in the ACP process with the patient.[174-182]

BROADER CONCEPTUALIZATIONS OF ADVANCED CARE PLANNING

ACP is increasingly conceptualized more broadly as a process in which advance directives represent one of several supportive tools. Pearlman and coworkers and others[183-186] have argued that similar to other preventive and health promotion interventions, completion of advance directives and ACP can be conceptualized as a process of behavior change with discrete stages, including precontemplation, contemplation, preparation, action, and reflection. This approach is appealing because it explicitly recognizes the complexity and time-dependent nature of ACP and acknowledges that patients may be at different stages along the continuum of behavior change at any given time.

Beyond documenting preferences, key elements of ACP include providing patients and their families with information about their prognosis and the expected course of their underlying illness, eliciting their values, goals, and preferences for care in the event of known complications of the underlying illness, communicating these preferences with family and providers, and periodically reviewing and updating these preferences in light of changes in health status or life events. Patient-centered, process-oriented approaches to ACP have shown some success in promoting end-of-life care that is more congruent with patient preferences.[170] Detering and colleagues tested a facilitated ACP intervention using the "Respecting Choices" framework—a comprehensive program to help instruct medical professionals on how best to honor end-of-life choices of their patients.[187] The study was conducted in 309 older medical inpatients in Australia; it found that of the 56 patients who died within 6 months, end-of-life wishes were much more likely to be known and followed in the intervention group compared with the control group. In the intervention group, family members of patients who died had significantly less stress, anxiety, and depression than those of the control patients. Patient and family satisfaction was also higher in the intervention group.

DISEASE-SPECIFIC ADVANCED CARE PLANNING

Building on the basic Respecting Choices model of facilitated patient-centered ACP, Briggs and associates have developed a disease-specific process to facilitate ACP in chronically and terminally ill patients tailored to the specific treatment decisions that tend to arise in patients with specific advanced disease states.[188-191] The disease-specific ACP model recognizes that patients with specific advanced disease states may face unique treatment decisions and incorporates condition-specific treatment scenarios into the ACP process. A disease-specific approach to ACP has been tested in small randomized trials for advanced conditions such as congestive heart failure and patients undergoing chronic dialysis.[188-191] Trials using this approach have demonstrated that patients and proxies are receptive to the intervention, and that the disease-specific model results in an improved understanding of patient goals among intervention group surrogates. When patients were followed longitudinally to the time of death, end-of-life wishes were fulfilled more frequently among patients in the intervention group, and family members experienced less stress, anxiety, and depression.[188,190]

ADVANCED CARE PLANNING IN PATIENTS WITH KIDNEY DISEASE

Most prior studies of ACP in patients with kidney disease focused on advance directives rather than on the broader process of ACP.[192-197] Most have also been cross-sectional in nature and have not provided information on outcomes associated with ACP. In general, these studies reported relatively low rates of completion of advance directives among dialysis patients and the failure of advance directives to address uniquely kidney issues, such as dialysis withdrawal. Most were conducted at the level of the dialysis facility and thus focused exclusively on patients already receiving chronic dialysis rather than patients with earlier stages of CKD. Only one single-center study has described patterns of ACP in patients with advanced kidney disease who had not yet initiated chronic dialysis. This study demonstrated that among approximately 500 patients in a predialysis clinic at a single center in Canada, less than 10% of patients reported having a discussion about end-of-life care issues with their nephrologist during the previous year.[198] Most patients reported that they would welcome the opportunity to discuss prognosis and treatment preferences with their nephrologist, but expected physicians to initiate these discussions.[199]

There have been very few interventional studies of ACP in patients with CKD. The aforementioned trial using the Respecting Choices framework included patients receiving chronic dialysis. It was found that the program led to greater understanding of preferences between patients and their surrogates and resulted in end-of-life care that was more congruent with patient preferences.[188,190] Davison and coworkers implemented a disease-specific, patient-centered ACP model in dialysis units in Northern Alberta, Canada, and provided a detailed description of their process, including detailed examples of open-ended questions that were used in semistructured interviews to promote ACP.[200] We are not aware of prior efforts to adapt and test a patient-centered approach to ACP in patients with advanced CKD who are not yet on dialysis.

CONCLUSION

CKD is common among older adults, but caring for these patients presents unique challenges because there are considerable differences between older and younger patients with CKD. In particular, equations for estimating GFR to diagnose and monitor CKD perform less well in older adults. Treatment strategies must often address multiple comorbid conditions, including hypertension, diabetes, dyslipidemia, anemia, and cognitive impairment. In many cases, evidence to guide therapy is extrapolated from younger patients with CKD, although important differences regarding treatment targets and drug dosing considerations have been noted. Finally, there are unique issues to consider when caring for older adults with more severe CKD, including options of renal replacement therapy, shared decision making, and advanced care planning.

Complete reference list available at ExpertConsult.com.

KEY REFERENCES

1. Coresh J, Selvin E, Stevens LA, et al: Prevalence of chronic kidney disease in the United States. *JAMA* 298:2038–2047, 2007.
2. Glassock RJ, Rule AD: The implications of anatomical and functional changes of the aging kidney: with an emphasis on the glomeruli. *Kidney Int* 82:270–277, 2012.
3. Rule AD, Gussak HM, Pond GR, et al: Measured and estimated GFR in healthy potential kidney donors. *Am J Kidney Dis* 43:112–119, 2004.
4. Winearls CG, Glassock RJ: Dissecting and refining the staging of chronic kidney disease. *Kidney Int* 75:1009–1014, 2009.
10. Kidney Disease: Improving Global Outcomes (KDIGO): 2012 clinical practice guidelines for the evaluation and management of chronic kidney disease. *Kidney Int Suppl* 3:1–163, 2013.
11. Hemmelgarn BR, Manns BJ, Lloyd A, et al: Relation between kidney function, proteinuria, and adverse outcomes. *JAMA* 303:423–429, 2010.
12. Hallan S, Astor B, Romundstad S, et al: Association of kidney function and albuminuria with cardiovascular mortality in older vs younger individuals: The HUNT II Study. *Arch Intern Med* 167:2490–2496, 2007.
13. Roderick PJ, Atkins RJ, Smeeth L, et al: CKD and mortality risk in older people: a community-based population study in the United Kingdom. *Am J Kidney Dis* 53:950–960, 2009.
14. O'Hare AM, Hailpern SM, Pavkov ME, et al: Prognostic implications of the urinary albumin to creatinine ratio in veterans of different ages with diabetes. *Arch Intern Med* 170:930–936, 2010.
15. Hallan SI, Matsushita K, Sang Y, et al: Age and association of kidney measures with mortality and end-stage renal disease. *JAMA* 308:2349–2360, 2012.
22. Manns B, Hemmelgarn B, Tonelli M, et al: Population-based screening for chronic kidney disease: cost effectiveness study. *BMJ* 341:c5869, 2010.
23. O'Hare AM, Choi AI, Bertenthal D, et al: Age affects outcomes in chronic kidney disease. *J Am Soc Nephrol* 18:2758–2765, 2007.
25. Hemmelgarn BR, James MT, Manns BJ, et al: Rates of treated and untreated kidney failure in older vs younger adults. *JAMA* 307:2507–2515, 2012.
26. Go AS, Chertow GM, Fan D, et al: Chronic kidney disease and the risks of death, cardiovascular events, and hospitalization. *N Engl J Med* 351:1296–1305, 2004.
27. Shlipak MG, Stehman-Breen C, Fried LF, et al: The presence of frailty in elderly persons with chronic renal insufficiency. *Am J Kidney Dis* 43:861–867, 2004.
28. Stevens LA, Li S, Wang C, et al: Prevalence of CKD and comorbid illness in elderly patients in the United States: results from the Kidney Early Evaluation Program (KEEP). *Am J Kidney Dis* 55(Suppl 2):S23–S33, 2010.
35. Kurella Tamura M, Covinsky KE, Chertow GM, et al: Functional status of elderly adults before and after initiation of dialysis. *N Engl J Med* 361:1539–1547, 2009.
36. Jassal SV, Chiu E, Hladunewich M: Loss of independence in patients starting dialysis at 80 years of age or older. *N Engl J Med* 361:1612–1613, 2009.
43. Kidney Disease: Improving Global Outcomes (KDIGO): *KDIGO clinical practice guideline for the management of blood pressure in chronic kidney disease*. Available at: <http://www.kdigo.org/clinical_practice_guidelines/pdf/KDIGO_BP_GL.pdf>. Accessed August 16, 2013.
53. O'Hare AM, Kaufman JS, Covinsky KE, et al: Current guidelines for using angiotensin-converting enzyme inhibitors and angiotensin II-receptor antagonists in chronic kidney disease: is the evidence base relevant to older adults? *Ann Intern Med* 150:717–724, 2009.
54. Turgut F, Balogun RA, Abdel-Rahman EM: Renin-angiotensin-aldosterone system blockade effects on the kidney in the elderly: benefits and limitations. *Clin J Am Soc Nephrol* 5:1330–1339, 2010.
85. Tonelli M, Muntner P, Lloyd A, et al: Risk of coronary events in people with chronic kidney disease compared with those with diabetes: a population-level cohort study. *Lancet* 380:807–814, 2012.
87. Upadhyay A, Earley A, Lamont JL, et al: Lipid-lowering therapy in persons with chronic kidney disease: a systematic review and meta-analysis. *Ann Intern Med* 157:251–262, 2012.
88. Palmer SC, Craig JC, Navaneethan SD, et al: Benefits and harms of statin therapy for persons with chronic kidney disease: a systematic review and meta-analysis. *Ann Intern Med* 157:263–275, 2012.
89. Kidney Disease: Improving Global Outcomes (KDIGO): KDIGO 2013 Clinical Practice Guidelines for lipid management in chronic kidney disease. *Kidney Int Suppl* 3:259–305, 2013.
100. Rifkin DE, Winkelmayer WC: Medication issues in older individuals with CKD. *Adv Chronic Kidney Dis* 17:320–328, 2010.
101. McLean AJ, Le Couteur DG: Aging biology and geriatric clinical pharmacology. *Pharmacol Rev* 56:163–184, 2004.
102. Lassiter J, Bennett WM, Olyaei AJ: Drug dosing in elderly patients with chronic kidney disease. *Clin Geriatr Med* 29:657–705, 2013.
104. Hubbard RE, O'Mahony MS, Woodhouse KW: Medication prescribing in frail older people. *Eur J Clin Pharmacol* 69:319–326, 2013.

105. Verbeeck RK, Musuamba FT: Pharmacokinetics and dosage adjustment in patients with renal dysfunction. *Eur J Clin Pharmacol* 65:757–773, 2009.
106. American Geriatrics Society Beers Criteria Update Expert Panel: American Geriatrics Society updated Beers Criteria for potentially inappropriate medication use in older adults. *J Am Geriatr Soc* 60:616–631, 2012.
107. Barry PJ, Gallagher P, Ryan C, et al: START (Screening Tool to Alert doctors to the Right Treatment)—an evidence-based screening tool to detect prescribing omissions in elderly patients. *Age Ageing* 36:632–638, 2007.
108. Gallagher P, O'Mahony D: STOPP (Screening Tool of Older Persons' potentially inappropriate Prescriptions): application to acutely ill elderly patients and comparison with Beers' criteria. *Age Ageing* 37:673–679, 2008.
109. Fine PG: Treatment guidelines for the pharmacological management of pain in older persons. *Pain Med* 13(Suppl 2):S57–S66, 2012.
110. Murtagh FE, Chai MO, Donohoe P, et al: The use of opioid analgesia in end-stage renal disease patients managed without dialysis: recommendations for practice. *J Pain Pall Care Pharmacother* 21:5–16, 2007.
115. Winkelmayer WC, Kurella Tamura M: Predialyis nephrology care of older individuals approaching end-stage renal disease. *Semin Dial* 25:628–632, 2012.
119. Ronksley PE, Hemmelgarn BR: Optimizing care for patients with CKD. *Am J Kidney Dis* 60:133–138, 2012.
120. Hemmelgarn BR, Manns BJ, Zhang J, et al: Association between multidisciplinary care and survival for elderly patients with chronic kidney disease. *J Am Soc Nephrol* 18:993–999, 2007.
121. Barrett BJ, Garg AX, Goeree R, et al: A nurse-coordinated model of care versus usual care for stage 3/4 chronic kidney disease in the community: a randomized controlled trial. *Clin J Am Soc Nephrol* 6:1241–1247, 2011.
124. Kurella Tamura M, Covinsky KE, Collins AJ, et al: Octogenarians and nonagenarians starting dialysis in the United States. *Ann Intern Med* 146:177–183, 2007.
125. O'Hare AM, Choi AI, Boscardin WJ, et al: Trends in timing of initiation of chronic dialysis in the United States. *Arch Intern Med* 171:1663–1669, 2011.
130. Murtagh FE, Marsh JE, Donohoe P, et al: Dialysis or not? A comparative survival study of patients over 75 years with chronic kidney disease stage 5. *Nephrol Dial Transplant* 22:1955–1962, 2007.
152. Tamura MK, Tan JC, O'Hare AM: Optimizing renal replacement therapy in older adults: a framework for making individualized decisions. *Kidney Int* 82:261–269, 2012.
160. O'Hare AM: Vascular access for hemodialysis in older adults: a "patient first" approach. *J Am Soc Nephrol* 24:1187–1190, 2013.
161. O'Hare AM, Allon M, Kaufman JS: Whether and when to refer patients for predialysis AV fistula creation: complex decision making in the face of uncertainty. *Semin Dial* 23:452–455, 2010.
173. Sudore RL, Fried TR: Redefining the "planning" in advance care planning: preparing for end-of-life decision making. *Ann Intern Med* 153:256–261, 2010.
187. Detering KM, Hancock AD, Reade MC, et al: The impact of advance care planning on end of life care in elderly patients: randomised controlled trial. *BMJ* 340:c1345, 2010.
197. Kurella Tamura M, Goldstein MK, Perez-Stable EJ: Preferences for dialysis withdrawal and engagement in advance care planning within a diverse sample of dialysis patients. *Nephrol Dial Transplant* 25:237–242, 2010.
198. Davison SN: End-of-life care preferences and needs: perceptions of patients with chronic kidney disease. *Clin J Am Soc Nephro* 5:195–204, 2010.

86
Tissue Engineering, Stem Cells, and Cell Therapy in Nephrology

L. Spencer Krane | Anthony Atala

CHAPTER OUTLINE

SOURCES OF CELLS FOR THERAPY, 2603
Stem Cells, 2603
Embryonic Stem Cells, 2603
Stem Cells Derived from Amniotic Fluid and Placenta, 2607
Adult Stem Cells, 2607
INTRARENAL PROGENITOR CELLS, 2608
BIOMATERIALS, 2609
Design and Selection of Biomaterials, 2609
CELL-BASED THERAPIES FOR TREATMENT OF KIDNEY DISEASE, 2610

Mesenchymal Stem Cells in Acute Kidney Injury, 2611
Developmental Approaches to Renal Regeneration, 2613
Immunogenicity of Renal Anlagen, 2613
Functional Transplantation of Metanephroi, 2614
Xenotransplantation of Renal Anlagen, 2615
Preservation of Renal Anlagen, 2616
In Situ Development of Renal Units, 2616
Summary, 2617

Patients with kidney disease were the first to benefit from transplantation, as the kidney was the first entire human organ to be replaced in 1955.[1] In the early 1960s, Murray performed a nonrelated kidney transplantation from one non–genetically identical patient into another. This transplant, which overcame the immunologic barrier, marked a new era in medical therapy and opened the door for use of transplantation as a means of therapy for different organ systems. However, the complications of those initial procedures still exist. For example, combating the side effects of immunosuppressive medications while monitoring and controlling graft rejection remains a significant clinical concern. Donor organ shortages exist throughout the world and many patients sit for years, waiting for transplants. To meet these challenges, new technologies for renal replacement therapy have been developed.

With technical and manufacturing advances, synthetic materials were introduced to replace or rebuild diseased tissues or parts in the human body. The advent of new synthetic materials, such as tetrafluoroethylene (Teflon) and silicone, led to the development of a wide array of devices that could be applied for human use. These early devices were based on structural support, and they have particular clinical utility in orthopedics as hip or knee replacements. The functional capacity of human tissue composition and architecture has been much more difficult to achieve.

Simultaneous with the development of new biomaterials for structural support in the body, scientists were rapidly adding to the body of knowledge in the biologic sciences, and new techniques for cell harvesting, culture, and expansion were developed. The areas of cell biology, molecular biology, and biochemistry were advancing rapidly. In addition, studies of the extracellular matrix and its interaction with cells, and with growth factors and their ligands, led to a better understanding of cell and tissue growth and differentiation. The concept of cell transplantation took hold in the research arena and culminated with the first human bone marrow cell transplant in the 1970s.

At this time, a natural evolution occurred wherein researchers began to combine the field of devices and materials sciences with techniques from cell biology, in effect starting a new field, called *tissue engineering*. As more scientists from different fields came together with the common goal of tissue replacement, the field of tissue engineering became more formally established. Tissue engineering was defined as "an interdisciplinary field which applies the principles of engineering and life sciences towards the development of biologic substitutes that aim to maintain, restore or improve tissue function." The first use of the term *tissue engineering* in the literature can be traced to a reference dealing with corneal tissue in 1985.[2]

Since the inception of tissue engineering, its goal has been the successful replacement or repair of diseased organs. In patients with end-stage kidney disease (ESKD), this is a daunting task. The difficulty in applying regenerative medicine techniques to the kidney is inherent in the complexity of the organ. Clinically, not only is the kidney responsible for secretion and filtration, but it has endocrine properties as well. The kidney produces erythropoietin and renin and secretes active vitamin D by converting circulating 25-hydroxycholecalciferol into 1,25-dihydroxycholecalciferol. In addition, the kidney releases prostaglandins into the circulation. Complete renal tissue regeneration or replacement must provide for these functions in addition to strict replacement of filtration.

Embryologically, the kidney is derived from the integration of several anlagen (see Chapter 1). While the metanephros is responsible for the development of the proximal section of the nephrons, the ureteric bud forms the collecting ducts and distal structures. The large vessels of the kidney are induced from extrarenal tissues. Divergent embryologic origin converges to produce at least 26 distinct functional cells in the kidney.[3] The heterogeneity of the kidney produces hurdles with in vitro culture and in identifying potential renal stem or progenitor cells.

This chapter summarizes the current strategies in tissue engineering aimed at improving renal function and includes a discussion of the identification of various types of stem cells, including renal progenitor cells, and their potential role in future therapeutics. Developmental approaches for renal replacement therapy are also reviewed.

SOURCES OF CELLS FOR THERAPY

STEM CELLS

The cells used in regenerative medicine techniques can be autologous or heterologous in origin, and they can be either native cells or stem cells. Stem cells are defined as having three important properties: the ability to self-renew, the ability to differentiate into a number of different cell types, and the ability to easily form clonal populations (populations of cells derived from a single stem cell). In general, there are three broad categories of stem cells obtained from living tissue that are used for cell therapies. Embryonic stem (ES) cells are obtained through the aspiration of the inner cell mass of a blastocyst or, more recently, a single cell from this mass. Fetal and neonatal amniotic fluid and placenta may contain multipotent cells that may be useful in cell therapy applications. Adult stem cells, on the other hand, are usually isolated from organ or bone marrow biopsies and have a progressively more limited repertoire of differentiation capacity.

Many techniques for generating stem cells have been studied over the past few decades. Some of these techniques have yielded promising results, but others require further research.

EMBRYONIC STEM CELLS

In 1981, pluripotent cells were found in the inner cell mass of the human embryo, and the term *human embryonic stem cell* was coined.[4] These cells are able to differentiate into all cells of the human body, excluding placental cells (only cells from the morula are totipotent, that is, able to develop into all cells of the human body). These cells have great therapeutic potential, but their use is limited by both biologic and ethical factors. The societal controversy surrounding stem cells began in 1998 with the creation of human embryonic stem (hES) cells derived from discarded products of in vitro fertilization. hES cells were isolated from the inner cell mass of a blastocyst (an embryo 5 days after in vitro fertilization) using an immunosurgical technique. Given that some cells cannot be expanded ex vivo, hES cells could be an ideal resource for regenerative medicine because of their fundamental properties: the ability to self-renew indefinitely and the capacity to differentiate into cells from all three embryonic germ layers. Skin and neurons have been formed, indicating ectodermal differentiation.[5-7] Blood, cardiac cells, cartilage, endothelial cells, and muscle have been formed, indicating mesodermal differentiation.[8-10] Pancreatic cells have been formed, indicating endodermal differentiation.[11] In addition, as further evidence of their pluripotency, ES cells can form embryoid bodies, which are cell aggregations that contain all three embryonic germ layers while in culture, and can form teratomas in vivo.[12] These cells have demonstrated longevity in culture and can maintain their undifferentiated state for at least 80 passages when grown using current published protocols.[13,14]

Various researchers have shown that ES cells may be useful in renal regenerative medicine. Schuldiner and colleagues were able to induce differentiation of hES into cells that produce the renal-specific products renin and Wilms' tumor 1 (WT1) using culture media, including activin A and hepatocyte growth factor.[15] Kim and Dressler have evaluated whether murine ES cells could be cultured in vitro to renal precursor cells and mesoderm. By culturing the ES cells in activin A, retinoic acid, and bone morphogenic protein 7 (Bmp7), they were able to induce genetic expression of paired box gene 2 (Pax-2, a marker of intermediate mesoderm, from which the renal epithelial cells arise), WT1 (seen in high levels in podocytes), cadherin 6 (an early marker for proximal tubules), and Lim1 (seen in intermediate mesoderm). These cells also formed tubule-like structures when introduced in vivo to cultured kidney rudiments from 12.5-day embryonic mice.[16]

Vigneau and colleagues showed that ES expressing brachyury, an embryonic nuclear transcription factor that possibly denotes mesoderm, may differentiate into renal progenitor cells in the presence of activin A. When these cells were injected into a developing metanephros, they were incorporated into the blastemal cells of the nephrogenic zone. Additionally, after only a single injection into the kidneys of live newborn mice, the cells were capable of integration into proximal tubules. At 7 months, there was no evidence of teratoma formation, and the cellular morphology and polarization appeared normal.[17] Narayanan and colleagues found ES could be induced in vitro to produce tight junctions and have a polarized morphology with apical microvilli and tubular structure. When placed in a bioreactor and stimulated with parathyroid hormone, they noted significant increase in intracellular cyclic adenosine monophosphate.[18]

Recently, Morizane and coworkers, using activin to stimulate kidney-specific protein (KSP) expression, have been able to use anti-KSP antibodies to identify a population of murine ES cells that had the capacity to grow as tubular structures in vitro and incorporate into murine embryonic kidneys. These cells had expression profiles characteristic of metanephric mesenchyme but without tubule-specific genes. After in vitro stimulation with WNT4, they expressed segment-specific genes for the proximal and distal tubule, loops of Henle, podocytes, collecting duct, and Bowman's capsule.[19]

In addition to the societal and ethical dilemma surrounding the use of hES cells, their clinical application is limited because they represent an allogenic resource and thus have the potential to evoke an immune response. New stem cell technologies (such as somatic cell nuclear transfer and reprogramming) promise to overcome this limitation.

SINGLE-CELL EMBRYO BIOPSY

One major objection to hES cell research is that it results in the destruction of embryos. Thus, a method of isolating these cells without destroying the embryo would be advantageous. In 2006, Chung and colleagues[20] were the first authors to report the generation of mouse ES cell lines in this manner. Their method was based on a technique used to obtain a single-cell embryo biopsy for preimplantation genetic diagnosis. Cells were taken from eight-cell blastomeres rather than from blastocysts. The cells differentiated into derivatives of all three embryonic germ layers in vitro as well as into teratomas in vivo. In addition, the mouse embryos that resulted from the biopsied blastomeres developed to term without a reduction in their developmental potential.

OBTAINING CELLS FROM ARRESTED EMBRYOS

hES cell lines can also be derived from arrested embryos.[21] During in vitro fertilization, only a small proportion of zygotes produced will develop successfully to the morula and blastocyst stages. Over half the embryos stop dividing[22,23] and are, therefore, considered dead embryos.[24] Such embryos have unequal or fragmented cells and blastomeres and are usually discarded. Not all the cells within these arrested embryos, however, are abnormal,[21,25] and these embryos might be a source of hES cells. More studies are needed to characterize the full proliferation and differentiation potential of ES cells derived from arrested embryos.

THERAPEUTIC CLONING (SOMATIC CELL NUCLEAR TRANSFER)

Somatic cell nuclear transfer (SCNT), or therapeutic cloning, entails the removal of an oocyte nucleus in culture, followed by its replacement with a nucleus derived from a somatic cell obtained from a patient. After nuclear transfer, the gene expression pattern of the transferred nucleus must be reprogrammed to that similar to an early embryo. This is accomplished through DNA modifications, including histone protein modification, cytosine methylation, chromatin remodeling, and reengineering the framework of the normal methylation patterns. This is accomplished in vitro through a series of chemical signals or introduction of electric potentials.

At this point, it is extremely important to differentiate between the two types of cloning that exist—reproductive cloning and therapeutic cloning. Both involve the insertion of donor DNA into an enucleated oocyte to generate an embryo that has identical genetic material to its DNA source. After this point, however, there are important differences in the ethical and scientific implications of the techniques. In reproductive cloning, the embryo that is produced using SCNT is implanted into the uterus of a pseudopregnant female to produce an infant that is a clone of the donor. A world-famous example of this type of cloning resulted in the birth of a sheep named Dolly in 1997.[26] However, there are many ethical concerns surrounding such practices, and as a result, human reproductive cloning has been banned in most countries.

While therapeutic cloning also produces an embryo that is genetically identical to the donor, this process is used to generate blastocysts that are explanted and grown in culture, rather than in utero. ES cell lines can then be derived from these blastocysts, which are only allowed to grow up to a 100-cell stage. At this time, the inner cell mass is isolated and cultured, resulting in ES cells that are genetically identical to the patient. This process is detailed in Figure 86.1. It has been shown that nuclear transferred ES cells derived from fibroblasts, lymphocytes, and olfactory neurons are pluripotent and can generate live pups after injection into blastocysts. This shows that the embryos generated from cells produced by SCNT have the same developmental potential as blastocysts that are fertilized and produced naturally.[27-29] In addition, the ES cells generated by SCNT are perfectly matched to the patient's immune system, and no immunosuppressants would be required to prevent rejection should these cells be used in regenerative medicine applications.

Although ES cells derived from SCNT contain the nuclear genome of the donor cells, mitochondrial DNA (mtDNA) contained in the oocyte could lead to immunogenicity after transplantation. To assess the histocompatibility of tissue generated using SCNT, Lanza and coworkers microinjected the nucleus of a bovine skin fibroblast into an enucleated oocyte.[30] Although the blastocyst was implanted (reproductive cloning), the purpose was to generate kidney, cardiac, and skeletal muscle cells, which were then harvested, expanded in vitro, and seeded onto biodegradable scaffolds. These scaffolds were then implanted into the donor steer from which the cells were cloned to determine if cells were histocompatible. Analysis revealed that cloned renal cells showed no evidence of T cell response, suggesting that rejection will not necessarily occur in the presence of oocyte-derived mtDNA. This finding represents a step forward in overcoming the histocompatibility problem of stem cell therapy.

To determine whether renal tissue could be formed using an alternative cell source, SCNT was performed to generate histocompatible tissues, and the feasibility of engineering syngeneic renal tissues in vivo using these cloned cells was investigated (Figure 86.2). Renal cells from the cloned embryos were harvested, expanded in vitro, and seeded onto three-dimensional renal devices. The devices were implanted into the back of the same steer from which the cells were cloned and were retrieved 12 weeks later. This process produced functioning renal units. Urine production and viability were demonstrated after transplantation back into the nuclear donor animal. Chemical analysis suggested unidirectional secretion and concentration of urea nitrogen and creatinine. Microscopic analysis revealed formation of organized glomeruli and tubular structures. Immunohistochemical and reverse transcriptase polymerase chain reaction (RT-PCR) analysis confirmed the expression

CHAPTER 86 — TISSUE ENGINEERING, STEM CELLS, AND CELL THERAPY IN NEPHROLOGY   2605

THERAPEUTIC CLONING STRATEGIES

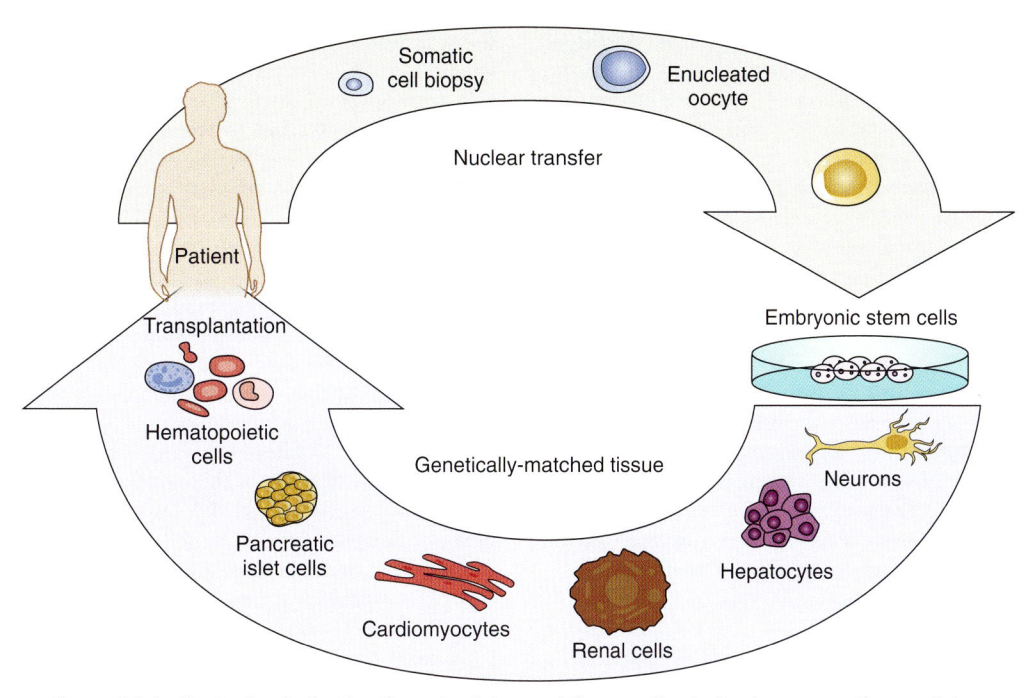

Figure 86.1 Illustration indicating the potential use of therapeutic cloning in regenerative medicine.

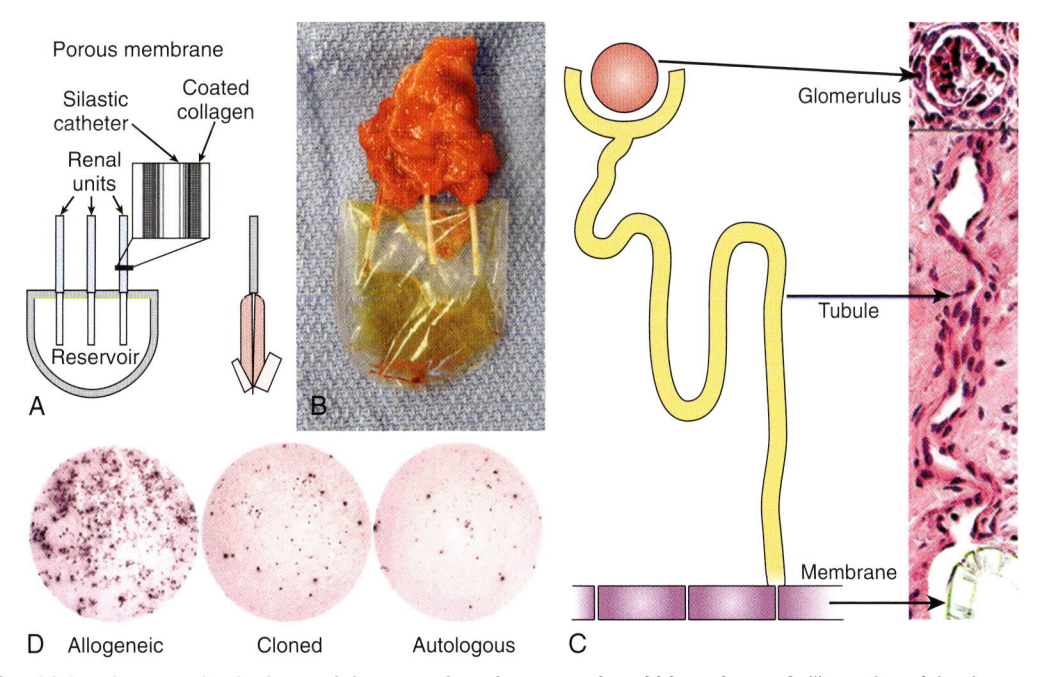

Figure 86.2 Combining therapeutic cloning and tissue engineering to produce kidney tissue. **A,** Illustration of the tissue-engineered renal unit. **B,** Renal unit seeded with cloned cells, 3 months after implantation, showing the accumulation of urine-like fluid. **C,** Clear unidirectional continuity between the mature glomeruli, their tubules, and Silastic catheter. **D,** Enzyme-linked immunosorbent spot (ELISpot) analyses of the frequencies of T cells that secrete interferon-γ (IFNγ) after stimulation with allogeneic renal cells, cloned renal cells, or nuclear donor fibroblasts. Cloned renal cells produce fewer IFNγ spots than the allogeneic cells, indicating that the rejection response to cloned cells is diminished. The presented wells are single representatives of duplicate wells.

of renal messenger RNA (mRNA) and proteins. These studies demonstrated that cells derived from nuclear transfer can be successfully harvested, expanded in culture, and transplanted in vivo with the use of biodegradable scaffolds on which the single suspended cells can organize into tissue structures that are genetically identical to that of the host. These studies were the first demonstration of the use of therapeutic cloning for regeneration of tissues in vivo.

However, although promising, SCNT has certain limitations that require further improvement before its clinical application in addition to the ethical considerations regarding the potential of the resulting embryos to develop into clones if implanted into a uterus. In addition, this technique has not been shown to work in humans to date. The initial failures and fraudulent reports of nuclear transfer in humans reduced enthusiasm for human applications,[31-33] although it was recently reported that nonhuman primate ES cell lines were generated by SCNT of nuclei from adult skin fibroblasts.[34,35] In addition, before SCNT-derived ES cells can be used as clinical therapy, careful assessment of quality of the lines must be determined. For example, some cell lines generated by SCNT have contained chromosomal translocations, and it is not known whether these abnormalities originated from aneuploid embryos or if they occurred during ES cell isolation and culture. In addition, the low efficiency of SNCT (0.7%) and the inadequate supply of human oocytes further hinder the therapeutic potential of this technique. Still, these studies renew the hope that ES cell lines could one day be generated from human cells to produce patient-specific stem cells with the potential to cure many human diseases that are currently untreatable.

ALTERED NUCLEAR TRANSFER

Altered nuclear transfer is a variation of SCNT in which a genetically modified nucleus from a somatic cell is transferred into a human oocyte. This embryo, which contains a deliberate genetic defect, is capable of developing into a blastocyst, but the induced defect prevents the blastocyst from implanting in the uterus. This process has the potential to generate customized hES cells from the blastocyst stage.[36] Human embryos with this genetic defect might lack the capacity to develop into viable fetuses, as a result of their inability to implant, thus providing a source of stem cells without destroying viable embryos. Proof of concept was obtained in mice by Meissner and Jaenisch[37] in 2006 using embryos lacking the *Cdx2* homeobox gene.

The viability of human embryos lacking the *CDX2* gene is unclear, as is whether this mutation restricts human developmental potential into certain lineages. While much research must be done before therapeutic strategies based on this technique can ever enter the clinic, at this time hES cells derived from altered nuclear transfer can provide opportunities to study pluripotency in hES cells, without the need for destruction of viable embryos. The exact effects of *CDX2* gene knockout on the development of human embryos are not well known. The effects of this gene however, have been thoroughly investigated in the gastric and intestinal epithelium.[38,39]

REPROGRAMMING (INDUCED PLURIPOTENT STEM CELLS)

Reports of the successful transformation of adult cells into pluripotent stem cells through a type of genetic "reprogramming" have been published. Reprogramming is a technique that involves dedifferentiation of adult somatic cells to produce patient-specific pluripotent stem cells. The advantage of this technique is that it obviates the need for creation of embryos. Cells generated by reprogramming would be genetically identical to the somatic cells (and thus, the patient who donated these cells) and would not be rejected. Takahashi and Yamanaka initially discovered that mouse embryonic fibroblasts and adult mouse fibroblasts could be reprogrammed into an "induced pluripotent state (iPS)."[40] These iPS cells were capable of immortal growth similar to the self-renewing characteristics of ES cells, expressed genes specific for ES cells, and generated embryoid bodies in vitro and teratomas in vivo. When iPS cells were injected into mouse blastocysts, they differentiated into several cell types. This discovery earned the Nobel Prize in Medicine in 2012. While iPS cells selected in this way were pluripotent, they were not identical to ES cells. Unlike ES cells, chimeras made from iPS cells did not result in full-term pregnancies. Gene expression profiles of the iPS cells showed that they possessed a distinct gene expression signature that was different from that of ES cells. In addition, the epigenetic state of the iPS cells was somewhere between that found in somatic cells and that found in ES cells, suggesting that the reprogramming was incomplete.

Wernig and colleagues significantly improved these results in July 2007.[41] In this study, DNA methylation, gene expression profiles, and the chromatin state of the reprogrammed cells were similar to those of ES cells. Teratomas induced by these cells contained differentiated cell types representing all mesoderm, ectoderm, and endoderm. Most importantly, the reprogrammed cells from this experiment were able to form viable chimeras and contribute to the germ line like ES cells, suggesting that these iPS cells were completely reprogrammed.

It has been shown that reprogramming of human cells is possible.[42,43] Yamanaka generated human iPS cells that are similar to hES cells in terms of morphology, proliferation, gene expression, surface markers, and teratoma formation. Thompson's group showed that retroviral transduction of the stem cell markers *OCT4, SOX2, NANOG*, and *LIN28* could generate pluripotent stem cells. However, in both studies, the human iPS cells were similar but not identical to hES cells. Recent efforts by several researchers have demonstrated successful creation of iPS in a porcine model. They each published retroviral transfection of cells with expression of stem cell markers. Due to the similarities with human and porcine kidneys, these are exciting potential preclinical models for future therapeutic directions.[44]

The reprogramming of somatic cells to iPS has led to debate as to the most suitable somatic cells to be used as the source. Song and associates have used renal mesangial cells for iPS creation. Human mesangial cells were obtained from an 18-year-old male. These were virally transfected with Oct3/4, Sox-2, c-Myc, and Klf4. These iPS cells demonstrated normal karyotypes and had downregulation of mesangial-specific proteins, including megsin; Thy-1; desmin, a smooth muscle actin; and RUNX1. RT-PCR confirmed expression of ES cell markers, including nanog, Sox-2, Oct3/4, and fibroblast growth factor 4. After 18 days, these cells had differentiated into embryoid bodies and showed gene expression of endoderm, mesoderm, and ectoderm.[45] These studies confirm that mesangial cells are a potential source for iPS cells; however, obtaining these cells in vivo would be prohibitively invasive on a routine basis because they would require kidney biopsy.

Zhou and colleagues have proposed using renal tubular cells found in the urine as an ideal population of cells for reprogramming. They grew CD13 (a renal tubular marker) positive cells from urine from healthy individuals on enriched medium. At passage two, these cells were transfected with Oct4, Sox2, c-Myc, and Klf4 and confirmed with green fluorescent protein. These cells, obtained from 12 healthy volunteers up to age 65, had DNA microarray global gene expression similar to that of ES cells with normal karyotypes. They were able to induce teratoma, hepatocyte, cardiomyocyte, and neural differentiation in these cells.[46]

The iPS cells have also been used to generate podocytes, which previously were very difficult to create due to their specialized function, terminal differentiation, and complex cytoarchitecture. Song and colleagues describe a 10-day specific culture regimen that generates iPS-derived cells that have similar morphologic appearance to human podocytes following nephrectomy. In addition, they demonstrate increased expression of WT1, synaptopodin, nephrin, and Pax-2 while downregulating OCT3/4 and integrating into embryonic kidneys appropriately.[47]

STEM CELLS DERIVED FROM AMNIOTIC FLUID AND PLACENTA

The amniotic fluid and placental membrane contain a heterogeneous population of cell types derived from the developing fetus.[48,49] Cells found in this heterogeneous population include mesenchymal stem cells (MSCs).[50,51] In addition, the isolation of multipotent human and mouse amniotic fluid- and placental-derived stem (AFPS) cells that are capable of extensive self-renewal and give rise to cells from all three germ layers was reported in 2007.[52] AFPS cells represent approximately 1% of the cells found in the amniotic fluid and placenta. The undifferentiated stem cells expand extensively without a feeder cell layer and double every 36 hours. Unlike hES cells, the AFPS cells do not form tumors in vivo. Lines maintained for over 250 population doublings retained long telomeres and a normal complement of chromosomes. AFPS cell lines can be induced to differentiate into cells representing each embryonic germ layer, including cells of adipogenic, osteogenic, myogenic, endothelial, neural-like, and hepatic lineages. In addition to the differentiated AFPS cells expressing lineage-specific markers, such cells can have specialized functions. Cells of the hepatic lineage secreted urea and α-fetoprotein, while osteogenic cells produced mineralized calcium. In this respect, they meet a commonly accepted criterion for multipotent stem cells, without implying that they can generate every adult tissue.

AFPS cells represent a new class of stem cells with properties somewhere between those of embryonic and adult stem cell types, probably more agile than adult stem cells, but less so than ES cells. Unlike embryonic and induced pluripotent stem cells, however, AFPS cells do not form teratomas and, if preserved for self-use, avoid the problems of rejection. The cells could be obtained either from amniocentesis or chorionic villous sampling in the developing fetus, or from the placenta at the time of birth. They could be preserved for self-use and used without rejection, or they could be banked. A bank of 100,000 specimens could potentially supply 99 percent of the U.S. population with a perfect genetic match for transplantation. Such a bank may be easier to create than with other cell sources, since there are approximately 4.5 million births per year in the United States.

Since the discovery of the AFPS cells, other groups have published on the potential of the cells to differentiate to other lineages, such as cartilage[53] and lung.[54] Perin and colleagues investigated if AFPS cells could differentiate into renal structures by labeling human cells and injecting them into murine embryologic renal tissues. The anlagen were cultured in vitro using a novel method to allow embryologic survival through 10 days in culture. The AFPS cells integrated in renal structures including C and S bodies. RT-PCRs demonstrated zonula occludens 1, claudin, and glial-derived neurotrophic factor, all of which are early markers for renal differentiation and were not seen in AFPS cells not injected into the anlagen.[55] This study demonstrates that AFPS cells can differentiate into renal lineage when cultured in vitro with renal precursors.

AFPS cells derived from humans can be combined with disassociated murine kidneys to produce chimeric renal structures. When CellTracker-labeled hAFPS were grown with the disaggregated E11.5 murine kidneys, expression of WT1, Pax-2, and laminin was noted in the CellTracker-labeled cells. This effect was noted to be mammalian target of rapamycin (mTOR) dependent, and p70S6K-mediated phosphorylation of endogenous S6 protein could be reduced using small interfering RNA (siRNA) targeted at mTOR.[56]

A potential application for AFPS could be delaying progression of renal tubular fibrosis and progressive glomerulopathy. Using a murine Col4a5-/- model that develops abnormal glomerular morphology and tubular fibrosis, Sedrakyan and colleagues noted a 20% improvement in overall survival with the infusion AFPS at 1.5 months. One theory is that this effect was due to an antifibrotic role with downregulation of transforming growth factor-β (TGF-β) transcription factors in the AFPS mice. An immunosuppressive effect was noted with decreased local M-1 macrophage recruitment and reduced tumor necrosis factor (TNF-α), C-X-C motif ligand 2 (CXCL2), macrophage colony-stimulating factor (M-CSF), and CC motif chemokine ligand 2 (CCL2) expression locally.[57] Renoprotection by AFPS was noted in the glycerol-induced renal dysfunction model as well. In this case, the effect was more persistent than the effect found using MSCs.[58] Although this approach is promising, further in vivo studies and functional assays are required prior to clinical applications with AFPS.

ADULT STEM CELLS

Adult stem cells, especially hematopoietic stem cells (HSCs), are the best understood cell type in stem cell biology.[59] However, adult stem cell research remains an area of intense study, as the potential of these cells for therapy may be applicable to myriad degenerative disorders. Within the past decade, adult stem cell populations have been found in many adult tissues other than the bone marrow and the gastrointestinal tract, including the brain,[60,61] skin,[62] and muscle.[63] Many other types of adult stem cells have been identified in organs all over the body and are thought to serve as the primary repair entities for their corresponding organs.[64] The discovery of such tissue-specific progenitors has opened up new avenues for research.

Although almost all adult stem cells are tissue specific, a notable exception is the MSC, also known as the multipotent adult progenitor cell. This cell type is derived from bone marrow stroma.[65,66] Such cells can differentiate in vitro into numerous tissue types[67,68] and can also differentiate developmentally if injected into a blastocyst. Multipotent adult progenitor cells can develop into a variety of tissues, including neuronal,[69] adipose,[63] muscle,[63,70] liver,[71,72] lung,[73] spleen,[74] and gut tissue,[66] but notably not bone marrow or gonads. There has been considerable research into the identification, characterization, and expansion of renal multipotent progenitor cell.

INTRARENAL PROGENITOR CELLS

The kidney possesses the ability to perform endogenous repair following acute injury. This is made evident by the fact that most patients with acute kidney injury (AKI) do not progress to chronic kidney disease (CKD) or ESKD, but instead they regain function (see Chapter 31). Understanding the cellular responses that permit regeneration of renal tissue can help investigators identify mechanisms associated with endogenous repair and provide guidance for developing future therapeutics. Recent evidence suggests that within the renal parenchyma, a progenitor cell that is able to differentiate into the various cells of the nephron may exist. Using a zebrafish model, progenitor cells have been identified which can form new functional nephrons during growth or following injury and repair. In this study, the integration of cells required a previous aggregation and not single cell transplantation. The "community effect" with cells responding to signals within their environment is not novel,[75] and these insights may help to translate to mammalian progenitor cell identification.

One functional definition of a stem cell in the skin or stomach would be the ability to retain bromodeoxyuridine (BrdU) over long chase periods. BrdU is a synthetic nucleoside analog of thymidine, which is incorporated into the DNA during replication. Retention of this compound for extended periods of time suggests that a cell has a very long cell cycle time, and this is one characteristic of stem cells. Maeshima and colleagues were able to identify such label-retaining cells localized in renal tubular epithelial cells of normal adult rats 2 weeks after intraperitoneal BrdU injections.[76] Following ischemic insult in these rats, a high proportion of cells positive for BrdU and proliferating cell nuclear antigen (PCNA) were found in the tubules; this suggests that the cells responsible for regeneration of tubular epithelium are derived from the BrdU+ population. The authors subsequently characterized in vitro properties of the label-retaining cells. These Hoechst^{Low}BrdU+ cells identified by fluorescence-activated cell sorter (FACS) demonstrated significant plasticity. Additionally, when injected into day 15 rat metanephros, a proportion of the labeled cells stained positive for proximal tubule (*Lotus tetragonolobus* lectin) and ureteric bud (*Dolichos biflorus* lectin) markers.[77] Following unilateral ureteral obstruction, the BrdU label-retaining cells were found to replicate at high numbers based on PCNA staining. Also, these cells appeared to cross the tubular basement membrane and contribute to fibrosis of the kidney as they had an epithelial to mesenchymal transition. The BrdU+ cells were noted to lose staining for E-cadherin (an epithelial marker) and develop positivity for α-smooth muscle action and vimentin.[77]

Oliver and associates injected BrdU subcutaneously in 3.5-day rats and harvested their kidneys beginning at 2 months. They found the label-retaining cells were localized in the renal papillae in the region closest to the urinary space. Co-staining with von Willebrand factor ruled out the possibility that these cells were of vascular origin. They were able to isolate and culture the BrdU cells in vitro and when cultured appropriately could produce epithelial or mesenchymal proteins.[78] The authors subsequently induced an ischemic insult and this caused a decrease in the population of papillary BrdU cells, with a concomitant rise in Ki-67 (a marker for cellular proliferation) positive cells localized in the outer renal papillae adjacent to the urinary space. The authors concluded that this population of cells was associated with renal repair following AKI.[78] Kim and associates injected BrdU into pregnant rats between embryonic days 17 and 19 and histologically examined the resulting kidneys at 2 and 6 months after birth. They found these label-retaining cells were localized to the corticomedullary junction as tubular cells or to the papilla as epithelial, endothelial, or interstitial cells.[79]

While it has been demonstrated that these BrdU-retaining cells respond to renal insult with propagation, others have challenged whether these are in fact renal progenitor cells. Vogetseder and colleagues evaluated kidneys of rats following 2 weeks of BrdU administration for label retention or cyclin D1 (a protein heavily expressed in early G_1 and required for cell cycle progression). They described BrdU retention in tubular epithelial cells based on proportions of Ki-67 or cyclin D1.[80] Their findings suggested that the BrdU population may in fact be a quiescent differentiated cell rather than a true renal stem cell.

Other methods for identifying stem cells include the recognition of specific cell surface markers. Bussolati and colleagues chose to evaluate if CD133+ cells reside in the human renal parenchyma.[81,82] CD133 is expressed in hematopoietic and progenitor cells, and also in the embryonic kidney. The observed CD133 population was approximately 0.8% of the total cell population within the renal cortex. These cells expressed Pax-2 but not CD45 (a marker of hematopoietic lineage) or c-Kit or CD90 (stem cell markers).[82] In vivo these cells formed tubule-like structures after implantation into immunocompromised mice.[82] Following enzymatic digestion of rat kidneys, Plotkin and associates identified a single clone that expressed Sca-1, CD44, CD34; transcription factors Pod-1 and BF-2; and receptors for sonic hedgehog, bone morphogenic protein, and retinoic acid. When these cells were injected subcapsularly following ischemia/reperfusion injury, the isolated cells integrated into the peritubular capillaries and periphery of the papillae.[83] Gupta and coworkers enzymatically digested 4-week-old rat kidneys and grew the cellular suspension in culture methods similar to those used for bone marrow–derived cells. They identified a population of cells that were capable of more than 200 population doublings without senescence and expressed vimentin, octamer-binding transcription factor 4 (Oct-4), and Pax-2 without any markers of either major histocompatibility complex (MHC) class or other markers of differentiated cells. When labeled cells from this study were reintroduced in vivo, they demonstrated integration into the renal architecture but did not improve kidney function following ischemia-reperfusion injury.[81] The identification of renal cells that can integrate into the renal parenchyma could have future implications for therapy and nephron replacement. Integration of nephrons is especially promising in patients with CKD to prevent progression to ESKD (see Chapter 52).

The CD133+ cells have demonstrated the ability to produce erythropoietin upon stimulation. This is restricted to CD133+ cells that are also CD73+. When these cells undergo epithelial transition, they are no longer capable of producing erythropoietin. This is a mesenchymal population that resides in the inner medulla.[84]

Podocytes present a novel model for understanding and identifying potential renal progenitor cells (see Chapter 4). Podocytes are postmitotic cells lacking proliferative capacity, yet are routinely found in the urine in even healthy individuals.[85] The number of cells lost in the urine exceeds that which would be expected for kidney survival of 80 years. Therefore, it has been hypothesized that an inherent population of progenitor cells may reside in the kidney and is capable of regenerating podocytes. Several groups have investigated the role of progenitor cells as they are involved in podocyte regeneration. Sagrinati and colleagues found a population of CD133CD24+ cells that were localized opposite the vascular pole of Bowman's capsule. These parietal epithelial cells (PECs) were between 0.5% and 4% of the total cellular population, were maintained up to 90 population doublings, and expressed Oct-4 and BmI-1. When introduced in vitro following glycerol-induced rhabdomyolysis-associated AKI, these cells attenuated renal injury as measured by lower blood urea nitrogen levels 7 to 10 days after injection.[86]

In further investigations of the PECs, this group identified three subpopulations of these cells. A subset of undifferentiated cells, only CD133/24+ was located at the urinary pole. A second transitional population of cells expressing CD133/24 but also nestin, complement receptor 1 (CR1), and podocalyxin (PDX) (all podocyte markers) were located between the urinary and vascular pole. Contiguous with the podocytes was a subset of cells that no longer expressed CD133/24 but were positive for nestin, CR1, and PDX.[87] In vitro, the only cells capable of differentiating into tubular cells were those which were CD133/24+ but not PDX+. To evaluate in vivo properties of these cells, a focal segmental glomerulosclerosis (FSGS) model of renal dysfunction was created with doxorubicin (Adriamycin) infusion. The CD133/24+PDX− cells reduced albuminuria and decreased glomerular and tubular quantitative injury.[87] In a series of experiments, Appel and associates evaluated the CD133+ PECs and concluded that the PECs were capable of migration along the glomerular tuft to replace podocyte populations. They examined the cells at the base of the vascular pole adjacent to the podocytes and noted that only these cells were able to be stained with both PEC markers (claudin-1) and podocyte-specific markers (nestin, dipeptidyl peptidase IV, aminopeptidase A). A PEC-specific promotor (podocalyxin) was identified which could trace the migration of cells and pointed to recruitment of PECs by podocytes.[88]

Another possible source for podocyte regeneration is from renin-producing cells. In fate mapping, renin lineage cells (RLCs) following creation of an FSGS model of renal insufficiency, it was found that 14% of glomeruli had labeled RLCs. These cells, which had presumably migrated from the juxtaglomerular apparatus, had up to 50% coexpression of WT1 and 30% coexpression of nephrin or podocin. These RLCs also served as progenitor cells for the PECs. In these cells, which migrate, expression of claudin-1 and Pax-2, indicative of PECs, was noted.[89]

Identification of renal progenitor cells is a substantial step toward understanding the inherent regenerative capacity of the kidney. The ability to identify the subset(s) of cells responsible for endogenous kidney repair and expansion of these cells in vitro could provide future therapeutic implications. Care must be taken in referring to these identified cells as renal stem cells. No group has yet demonstrated a population of cells that satisfy the strict definition of stem cell, including the ability to form clonal populations in vitro. However, this technology still needs refinement prior to clinical usage.

BIOMATERIALS

For renal regenerative therapy and development of an implantable renal unit, it is mandatory that biocompatible materials be developed that can assist in function and provide the structural and architectural parameters needed for solute excretion. Biomaterials in renal regenerative medicine function as an artificial extracellular matrix (ECM) and elicit biologic and mechanical functions of native ECM found in tissues in the body. Native ECM brings cells together into tissue, controls the tissue structure, and regulates the cell phenotype.[90] Biomaterials facilitate the localization and delivery of cells and/or bioactive factors (e.g., cell adhesion peptides, growth factors) to desired sites in the body; define a three-dimensional space for the formation of new tissues with appropriate structure; and guide the development of new tissues with appropriate function.[91] Direct injection of cell suspensions without biomaterial matrices has been used in some cases,[92,93] but it is difficult to control the localization of transplanted cells. Localization of transplanted renal cells can be performed with subcapsular injection or direct injection into the renal artery. However, most mammalian cell types are anchorage dependent and will die if not provided with a cell-adhesion substrate.

DESIGN AND SELECTION OF BIOMATERIALS

The design and selection of biomaterials in renal regenerative therapy must provide structural integrity for implantation and adhesion capabilities for cellular attachment. The selected biomaterial should be biodegradable and bioresorbable to support the reconstruction of a completely normal tissue without inflammation. Such behavior of the biomaterials avoids the risk of inflammatory or foreign-body responses that may be associated with the permanent presence of a foreign material in the body. The degradation rate and the concentration of degradation products in the tissues surrounding the implant must be at a tolerable level.[94]

The biomaterials should provide an appropriate regulation of cell behavior (e.g., adhesion, proliferation, migration, differentiation) in order to promote the development of functional new tissue. Cell behavior in engineered tissues is regulated by multiple interactions with the microenvironment, including interactions with cell-adhesion ligands[95] and with soluble growth factors.[96] Cell adhesion–promoting factors (e.g., arginine–glycine–aspartic acid [RGD]) can be presented by the biomaterial itself or incorporated into the biomaterial in order to control cell behavior through ligand-induced cell receptor signaling processes.[97,98] The biomaterials provide temporary mechanical support sufficient to withstand in vivo forces exerted by the surrounding tissue and maintain a potential space for tissue development. The mechanical support of the biomaterials should be maintained until the engineered tissue has sufficient mechanical integrity to support itself.[99] This potentially can be achieved by an appropriate choice of mechanical and degradative properties of the biomaterials.[91]

Generally, three classes of biomaterials have been used for tissue engineering: naturally derived materials, such as collagen and alginate; acellular tissue matrices, such as bladder submucosa and small-intestinal submucosa; and synthetic polymers, such as polyglycolic acid (PGA), polylactic acid (PLA), and poly(lactic-co-glycolic acid) (PLGA). Naturally derived materials and acellular tissue matrices have the potential advantage of biologic recognition. Synthetic polymers can be produced reproducibly on a large scale with controlled properties of strength, degradation rate, and microstructure.

Collagen is the most abundant and ubiquitous structural protein in the body, and it may be readily purified from both animal and human tissues with an enzyme treatment and salt/acid extraction.[100] Collagen has long been known to elicit minimal inflammatory and antigenic responses,[101] and it has been approved by the U.S. Food and Drug Administration (FDA) for many types of medical applications, including wound dressings and artificial skin.[102] Intermolecular cross-linking reduces the degradation rate by making the collagen molecules less susceptible to an enzymatic attack. Intermolecular cross-linking can be accomplished by various physical (e.g., ultraviolet radiation, dehydrothermal treatment) or chemical (e.g., glutaraldehyde, formaldehyde, carbodiimides) techniques.[100] Collagen contains cell-adhesion domain sequences (e.g., RGD) that exhibit specific cellular interactions. This may help to retain the phenotype and activity of many types of cells, including fibroblasts[103] and chondrocytes.[104] This material can be processed into a wide variety of structures such as sponges, fibers, and films.[105-107] In vitro cultures of heterogeneous renal cell populations on collagen have demonstrated tubular development.[108]

Alginate, a polysaccharide isolated from seaweed, has been used as an injectable cell delivery vehicle[109] and a cell immobilization matrix owing to its gentle gelling properties in the presence of divalent ions such as calcium. Alginate is a family of copolymers of D-mannuronate and L-guluronate. The physical and mechanical properties of alginate gel are strongly correlated with the proportion and length of the polyguluronate block in the alginate chains.[109] Efforts have been made to synthesize biodegradable alginate hydrogels with mechanical properties that are controllable in a wide range by intermolecular covalent cross-linking and with cell-adhesion peptides coupled to their backbones.[110] Alginate has been used in developmental approaches to renal regeneration, although it was not found to support ureteric bud branching in vitro.[111]

Acellular tissue matrices are collagen-rich matrices prepared by removing cellular components from tissues. For kidney regeneration, matrices are often prepared by mechanical and chemical manipulation of functional kidneys. Following decellularization of the kidney, the extracellular matrix may provide structural support for cellular seeding. Due to the complex interaction between kidney structure and function, a structural equivalent would be difficult to create de novo, and therefore efforts have been made to produce decellularized kidneys for cell seeding. This process has been completed successfully in rats seeded with ES cells.[112]

The most recent developments in biomaterials are creation of decellularized native kidneys. By using combinations of detergents, research studies have demonstrated successful maintenance of kidney ultrastructure. In porcine models, which are very similar to human kidneys in terms of size and complexity,[113] Orlando and colleagues have taken discarded human kidneys and used a sodium dodecyl sulfate solution to decellularize the kidneys. Subsequently, with histologic and electron microscopic analysis, only the acellular matrix remains. The delicate structure of the glomerulus and tubules remains intact. Immunostains have demonstrated removal of antigenic markers.[114]

Implantation of these decellularized models has been successful using a small animal model. In rats, Song and colleagues have successfully decellularized the kidneys using similar detergents. Subsequently, they perfused human umbilical venous endothelial cells into the renal artery and suspended rat neonatal kidney cells into the ureter. Both in vitro and in vivo, they were able to demonstrate improved glucosuria and albuminuria as compared to decellularized controls.[115]

CELL-BASED THERAPIES FOR TREATMENT OF KIDNEY DISEASE

The functional heterogeneity and complex cellular architecture within the kidney present many challenges to cellular therapies. There are several hurdles to overcome in providing successful cellular therapy. These include ensuring delivery of the cells allows for homing to the necessary location and the type of cell delivered. While some groups have evaluated the possibility of using stem cells from various lineages, others have focused on the usage of differentiated renal cells to improve function.

Isolation of a single cell type for reintroduction in to the kidney may be an initial step in providing cellular therapies for renal dysfunction. Anemia associated with CKD requires recombinant erythropoietin injection for patients with ESKD and presents as a platform for future clinical applications of cellular therapy. Isolation and culture of erythropoietin-producing renal cells has been described by Aboushwareb and coworkers.[116] The cells demonstrate increased erythropoietin expression when exposed to hypoxic environments.[117] These cells represent a potential lineage for future treatment of renal dysfunction–associated anemia. Bartholomew and colleagues transfected baboon MSCs with human erythropoietin vectors and evaluated whether these cells were capable of in vivo erythropoietin production. These cells could successfully produce erythropoietin for up to 28 days in severe combined immunodeficient mice and 137 days in baboons.[118] Targeting of anemia associated with renal dysfunction or other singular functions of the kidney may provide pathways to introduce cellular therapies for renal dysfunction.

Targeting specific cells in the nephron could provide disease-specific cellular therapy. Patients may have tubular dysfunction versus podocyte dysfunction and require specific therapy based on pathology. Han and associates described how primary rabbit proximal tubule cells could produce functional tubular units. Following enzymatic digestion of the cortex and removal of glomeruli, tubules were formed in vitro with luminal formation. Function was demonstrated with lucifer yellow, a fluorescent substrate of the p-aminohippurate transport system.[119] In patients with tubular dysfunction, introduction of cultured tubules could direct therapy at the pathologic cause.

Development of heterogeneous populations of renal cells could also represent a potentially viable option for cellular therapy of kidney disease. Joraku and coworkers developed an in vitro method for cultivation of renal cells which allowed for development of tubular structures. This technique involves digestion of the entire murine kidney followed by cultivation on rat-tail type 1 collagen. Upon histologic examination, cells from thick ascending loop of Henle stained positive for Tamm-Horsfall protein.[108] As of yet, the published reports of reintroduced adult renal cells have not demonstrated improvements in renal function, and the barrier of immune recognition has not been overcome either.[120]

MESENCHYMAL STEM CELLS IN ACUTE KIDNEY INJURY

AKI is a significant cause of morbidity and mortality. However, it is clear that not all patients who experience AKI will develop CKD. Therefore, the body exhibits some regenerative properties that improve renal function following acute insult. Several researchers have demonstrated that MSCs can ameliorate renal injury.

DIFFERENTIATION OF MESENCHYMAL STEM CELLS INTO RENAL TISSUE

Several studies have investigated the role of MSCs in direct integration into kidney tissue. These findings were initially described in transplant recipients. Poulsom and colleagues analyzed biopsies of transplanted kidneys from female donors of male recipients. They found that in the tubular epithelium (identified by positive staining for cell adhesion molecule 5.2), 0.6% to 6.8% of the cells contained Y chromosomes.[121] Gupta and associates reported that approximately 1% of renal tubular epithelium was Y chromosome positive in similar patients. They ruled out likelihood of these being inflammatory cells by co-staining with CD45, a protein tyrosine phosphatase present on all differentiated hematopoietic cells except plasma cells and erythrocytes. They did not find the Y-positive population of cells in patients without acute tubular necrosis in the transplanted kidney, indicating the role of the MSCs is likely regenerative after injury.[122] In female mice undergoing bone marrow transplantation from males, Poulsom and coworkers demonstrated 7.9% of renal epithelial cells contained Y chromosomes.[121] Lin and colleagues also reported the presence of *SRY* gene and Y chromosome in renal tubules of female mice undergoing bone marrow transplant from male donors.[123]

Following bone marrow depletion in wild-type rats, Ito and colleagues transfused bone marrow–derived mesenchymal stem cells (BMSCs) from rats labeled with enhanced green florescence protein (EGFP). They found mesangial cell integration in vivo following induction of glomerulonephritis with anti–Thy-1 antibodies.[124] Rookmaker and colleagues also tracked transplanted BMSCs in the glomerular interstitium of rats using MHC-1 as a label. They found that increasing BMSCs were recruited to mesangial integration following anti-Thy1 antibody administration, which once again indicated the role of BMSC in repairing AKI.[125] Cornacchia and associated induced glomerulosclerosis in normal mice following bone marrow transplant from nonobese diabetic transgenic mice prone to glomerular dysfunction.[126]

Despite these initial studies, further studies evaluating the role of MSCs in integration into the proliferating tubular epithelium have raised some controversy.[127] In a follow-up study from Poulsom's group, they transplanted BMSCs derived from male donors to irradiated females and induced acute renal injury with supraphysiologic doses of folic acid. While there was integration into the tubules of the cells containing Y chromosomes, this was estimated at only 10% of the S phase cells following injury, and, thus, the authors concluded that the role of BMSCs in tubule integration is likely limited.[128] Lin and coworkers in 2005 examined BrdU uptake in renal tissues following ischemia injury in EGFP transgenic female mice who had received bone marrow transplants from male donors. They found only 11% of the BrdU+ cells to be donor derived, indicating that most of the regenerative effort was completed by the host. Additionally, they found that vimentin, a marker of dedifferentiated tubule cells, was only positive in the EGFP cells, demonstrating host origin.[129] Duffield and colleagues injected both β-galactosidase– and green florescence protein (GFP)–labeled bone marrow, derived from male donors, into female mice. Despite improvement in renal function in the chimeric mice after ischemic injury, the only GFP-labeled cells detected in the kidney were leukocytes. All the β-galactosidase expression in the renal tubules was endogenous, and due to the high PCNA staining, the regenerating tubules appeared to be derived from the host and not the donor marrow.[130]

Using a study of transgenic mice, Humphreys and colleagues concluded that the repair of injured nephrons was accomplished by the intrinsic surviving tubular epithelial cells with minimal if any contribution from extrarenal cells. By using genetic fate-mapping techniques, they successfully labeled the tubular cells but not the interstitial cells in transgenic mice. These kidneys were then subjected to an ischemia-reperfusion injury. They found that replicating cells expressing Ki-67 also expressed the red fluorescent protein used to label the kidneys. They could not detect cells not expressing fluorescent labels in the injured or uninjured kidneys.[131] Summarized together, the evidence no longer points to MSCs directly associated with tubulogenesis. However, the improvements in renal function with MSC administration are compelling, and this points to a role in contributing to the microenvironment of repair and the immunomodulatory effects of MSCs.

RECRUITMENT OF MESENCHYMAL STEM CELLS TO RENAL TISSUE FOLLOWING ACUTE INJURY

While the majority of tubular regeneration is completed by tubular epithelial cells, MSCs appear to play a renoprotective role when administered at the time of kidney injury. The functions fulfilled by MSCs must therefore be paracrine in nature. By improving the microenvironment of the regenerating tissue, they promote healing and return of renal function. In order to achieve local effect, MSCs must be present following injury. Kale and associates demonstrated significant increase in Lin-Sca-1$^+$ cells (BMSCs) in the peripheral circulation 24 hours following ischemia-reperfusion injury in mice.[132] Togel and colleagues discovered a mobilization of CD34$^+$ cells following ischemia-reperfusion injury in mice. The mechanism of chemotaxis has not been fully elucidated, but it may involve stromal cell–derived factor-1 (SDF-1), CD44, chemokine signaling, or other mechanisms.[133] Ponte and colleagues have demonstrated with in vitro migration assays that MSCs are recruited in higher numbers following response to growth factors as compared to chemokines. They respond especially well to insulin-like growth factor-1 (IGF-1),[134] known to be associated with stem cell–mediated renal repair.[135] Lange and coworkers preloaded MSCs with iron oxide nanoparticles prior to administration in an ischemia-reperfusion rat model. They found a significant improvement in serum creatinine values in days 2 and 3 following MSC administration and using magnetic resonance imaging could identify these cells in the kidney.[136] Immediately and 24 hours after MSC infusion, Togel and associates found labeled donor cells on the endothelial basement membrane by using two-photon laser in vivo microscopy.[137] As evidenced by their attraction to the kidney following injury, despite the fact that they are not incorporated into the renal tubules, MSCs may supplement the endogenous regenerative capacities of the kidney.

Several animal studies have demonstrated that infusion of MSCs following kidney injury is renoprotective and can improve outcomes in these animals. Following cisplatin-induced kidney injury in C57/B6 mice, Morigi and colleagues found that injection of MSCs, but not HSCs, significantly reduced serum urea concentration 4 and 5 days following injection. The MSC-treated mice also demonstrated reduced tubular loss and an increase in tubular differentiation as measured by Ki-67 staining.[138] Kunter and colleagues evaluated whether MSCs could improve renal function in a rat model of glomerulonephritis induced by anti–Thy-1.1 antibody administration. Two days following injury, MSCs were infused into the renal artery. At 10 days, a significant improvement in creatinine clearance (0.43 ± 0.1) was seen as compared to those rats given injection of just medium (0.29 ± 0.1). At 30 and 60 days, proteinuria and serum urea nitrogen were significantly reduced in the MSC-treated rats. However, these researchers also found that the glomeruli of the kidneys following MSC therapy contained single, or clusters of, adipocytes, which appeared to be derived from the MSCs.[139] The exact mechanism of the improvement in renal function has not been elucidated, but these studies clearly show promise that MSCs may play a role in preventing renal dysfunction following acute injury.

There has been a single case report of using CD34$^+$ HSCs in the treatment of kidney disease. A 1-year-old male with bilateral multicystic kidney disease was given an allogenic transplantation of HSCs into the aorta proximal to the branching of the renal arteries. The only clinical improvement noted was a decrease in medication requirement; however, the child succumbed to his disease 5 months following the injection.[140] Such single reports are reminders that the current status of these therapies is experimental and that only in rare clinical situations can these therapies possess clinical applicability.

In patients with fibrotic kidneys, there is concern that MSC treatment may promote fibrogenesis-associated tubulointerstitial disease, as has been seen in models of ureteral obstruction.[141] However, the renoprotective role of MSCs may apply to CKD as well. Ninichuk and colleagues evaluated the effect of MSCs that were injected into mice deficient for the α3-chain of type IV collagen (COL4A3). These mice are characterized by an abnormal assembly of glomerular basement membranes and present with renal dysfunction similar to human Alport's disease. MSC injection was initiated at 4 weeks of age and continued weekly for a total of four injections. At the conclusion of this period, the kidneys were histologically examined and there was a reduction of interstitial fibrosis and preservation of the peritubular capillaries. These histologic differences were not translated to objective measurements of renal function as serum urea nitrogen and creatinine were similar between the controls and the MSC group.[142]

Using a rat 5/6 nephrectomy model for CKD, Choi and coworkers investigated whether MSCs could improve renal dysfunction. They found at 30 days, the total protein-to-creatinine ratio was significantly lower in the MSC-treated rats.[143] Also using the 5/6 nephrectomy rat model, Cavaglieri and colleagues found significant improvement in blood pressure, proteinuria, albuminuria, and serum creatinine at 30 days following therapy. They also found improvements in glomerulosclerosis and interstitial fibrosis on histologic examination.[144] This study used subcapsular injection of MSCs, establishing this as a viable method for introducing MSCs in vivo. This may explain the differences in results seen between this study and others.

Recent studies have demonstrated that it is possible that these cells are capable of inducing angiogenesis. Chen and associates isolated MSCs from rat kidneys and placed these on Matrigel-filled angioreactors. Fifteen days following implantation the MSCs, angioreactors demonstrated neovessels that were apparently patent and functional, as they stained positive for *Lycopersicon esculentum* lectin.[145]

While the exact role of MSC therapy in providing support to the kidney is still being evaluated, there is clearly a renoprotective effect of MSCs on the kidney following acute injury.

Another possible explanation for the improvements seen with MSC administration could be associated with the immunosuppressive capabilities of MSCs.[146,147] Following ischemia-reperfusion injury, cellular necrosis and apoptosis initiate a proinflammatory cascade. Immunomodulation has been shown to reduce consequences of ischemia. MSCs lack MHC-2 and have reduced MHC-1 expression. By definition, they also lack the costimulatory molecules CD80 and CD86.[147] This likely indicates that they can escape natural killer cell activation and lack the necessary antigen presentation pathway for T cell stimulation. MSCs also can keep dendritic cells in an immature state, may reduce interleukin-2 (IL-2) production, and increase CD4CD25+ regulatory T cells.[146] Semedo and associates reported that IL-4 mRNA is upregulated and IL-1β mRNA is downregulated following MSC infusion in rats undergoing ischemia-reperfusion injury.[148] This group also used the 5/6 nephrectomy remnant kidney model to elucidate the immunomodulatory effect of MSCs. On histologic examination, decreased collagen and fibrosis were noted in the MSC-treated rats. Furthermore, expression of IL-10 was increased and interferon-γ (IFN-γ), TGF-β, and TNF-α were significantly decreased in the treated rats.[149] As sustained inflammatory reaction is associated with renal dysfunction, the role of MSCs in improving the microenvironment of the kidney and promoting regeneration may be derived from their antiinflammatory and immunomodulatory properties.

More recent developments have been aimed at improving the homing and migration. This could produce important paracrine effects locally. Chemotaxis of MSCs to the kidney following ischemia-reperfusion injury is obviously complex; however, SDF-1 and C-X-C motif receptor 4 (CXCR4) may play an important role. In a murine model of ischemia-reperfusion injury, both SDF-1 and its receptor CXCR4 were upregulated. Injected BMSCs had reduced homing with antibodies targeted at CXCR4.[133] Using a glycerol-induced murine injury, Herrera and colleagues noted that homing of MSCs was inhibited by either preincubation of the MSCs with anti-CD44 antibodies or MSCs derived from CD44 knockout mice. This highlights the role of CD44 and hyaluronan for which CD44 is the principal cell surface receptor.[150]

Improving efficacy of MSCs in the treatment of AKI has been explored as well. Preconditioning murine MSCs with IGF-1 was shown to improve cisplatin-induced renal injury as compared to non-preconditioned cells. Likely this was due to improved chemotaxis associated with a twofold increased expression of CXCR4 on the MSCs when assessed with flow cytometry.[151] Transfection of human MSCs with VEGF demonstrated both in vitro (using TMCK-1 epithelial cells) and in vivo protective effects as compared to nontransfected MSCs in a cisplatin-induced renal injury. MSCs transfected[152] with an adenovirus containing human tissue kallikrein have been shown to inhibit apoptosis as compared to nontransfected cells in an ischemia-reperfusion assessment.[153] The ability to introduce MSCs in the context of AKI and potentially improving their effects through either preconditioning or genetic modifications remains another source of cell therapy for renal regeneration.

Human studies evaluating the role of MSCs as immunoregulatory have been mixed. Initial reports of MSC therapy for 8 patients with grade III/IV acute graft-versus-host disease (GVHD) demonstrated survival at latest follow-up in 63%, with improved survival as compared to a matched cohort with steroid-resistant GVHD.[154] In a phase II trial of patients with steroid-resistant GVHD, 55 patients were treated with infusion of MSCs expanded in vitro. Of these patients receiving therapy, 30 had a complete response, and 9 had a partial response following infusion. There were no serious toxicities associated with therapy, and at a median follow-up of 1.3 years, complete responders had significantly improved survival as compared to nonresponders.[155] These results represent promise for the immunomodulatory effect of infused MSCs, and further studies are under way to define the role of these cells in future therapies.

The initial phase I trials evaluating the usage of MSCs for prevention of AKI are currently ongoing. The first of these studies is recruiting patients who are undergoing pump coronary bypass or cardiac valve surgery who have a high risk of postoperative kidney injury. Another study currently being performed involves usage of MSCs in a phase I trial for patients with AKI following cisplatin chemotherapy.[156] In patients undergoing living donor transplantation, autologous MSCs given as induction therapy was associated with a significant decrease in acute rejection episodes and in opportunistic infections at 1 year as compared to those receiving the anti–IL-2 antibody basiliximab. These MSC patients also had improved early graft function as determined by 1-month values of estimated glomerular filtration rate.[157] While these may be promising technologies in selected patients, much more work needs to be done with MSCs prior to widespread clinical applications. At the minimum, a well-regulated and heavily ethically scrutinized system for ensuring reliability and predictability of manufactured cells must be in place.[158]

DEVELOPMENTAL APPROACHES TO RENAL REGENERATION

In mammalian embryonic kidney development, there are two successive steps leading to development of the metanephros. Initially the ureteric buds are formed at the caudal end of the wolffian ducts; subsequently, the metanephric mesenchyme induced by the ureteric buds and the ureteric buds themselves interact to produce the metanephros. The metanephros becomes the permanent kidney. In mice they originate during day 11 of embryonic development (E11), during E12 in rats, between E21 and E28 in pigs, and during the fifth week in humans. Outgrowths arising from the distal end of the ureteric bud push radially into the surrounding metanephric mesenchyme. The metanephric mesenchyme differentiates into all tubular structures of the adult nephron, with the exception of the collecting system, which is derived from the ureteric bud.

To develop viable renal tissue for clinical application and tissue regeneration, transplantation of metanephroi has been attempted. Transplantation of metanephroi appears to have two significant promising features promoting its future clinical usage. First is the decreased immunogenicity that has been attributed to metanephric tissue. Extensive literature has documented the lack of antigenicity and cotransmitters in metanephric tissue. Second, transplanted metanephroi have been successful in developing complex vascularization induced from the host. This would promote survival in the host or allow development of tissues in vivo.

IMMUNOGENICITY OF RENAL ANLAGEN

The age of the developing metanephros is related to successful transplantation. Metanephric tissues develop in rats on E12. Valasco and Hegre performed a series of transplantations from the fetal kidneys of E15 to E19 rats. Following subcapsular implantation, they noted complete rejection of the E19 transplants at 10 days following transplantation. Complete rejection in the E15 transplants took 40 days.[159]

In immunocompetent Sprague-Dawley rats, Foglia and colleagues transplanted metanephroi from E15 to E21 outbred Sprague-Dawley rats underneath the renal capsule. In evaluating the tissues on posttransplantation day 10, the transplants from E15 and E16 had proliferation of glomeruli and tubules as compared to the E20 and E21 transplants. Additionally, the researchers noted a significantly decreased lymphocytic infiltration in the E15 and E16 transplants as compared to the E20 and E21 transplants.[160] Under similar transplantations with adult renal tissue, acute rejection is apparent by posttransplantation day 10.[160] Dekel and colleagues found similar immune responses to human embryonic tissue transplanted in immunodeficient mice. As the age of the metanephroi increased from 7 weeks to 14 weeks, growth of transplanted tissue diminished, while lymphocyte-mediated tissue destruction and rate of necrosis increased.[161]

Primordium kidney transplantation produces a reduced immune response in comparison to human tissue transplanted into rats. Dekel and coworkers evaluated the expression on inflammatory cytokines in chimeric rats following subcapsular implantation of either adult or fetal human renal tissue. Rats had been given body irradiation and randomized to undergo allogenic human peripheral blood mononuclear cell (PBMC) adoptive transfer. There was substantially reduced rejection and apoptosis among the fetal transplants. Levels of helper T cell subtype 1 cytokines, IL-2, and IFN-γ decreased in the fetal transplants, particularly in the first two weeks following PBMC infusion, whereas IL-4 mRNA expression increased. Among the β-chemokines MIP-1 and RANTES (regulated on activation, normal T expressed, and secreted) and their receptor CCR5, mRNA expression was reduced following PBMC transfusion. Fas ligand expression was also inhibited in the fetal tissues. This study and others provide evidence that the immune response to transplanted renal tissue is clearly dampened in fetal tissues as compared to adults.[162]

Rogers and colleagues evaluated whether a mismatch in MHC locus RT1 in rats plays a role in metanephroi transplantation in rats. Using PVG rats (RT1c) as donors and PVG-RT1-AVL hosts, they performed E15 metanephroi omental transplantations. While renal function of the transplanted metanephroi in both RT1-matched and nonmatched hosts was less than 1% of normal renal function, they found no difference in function between the two.[163] They detailed that one reason for this lack of immune reaction against the mismatched embryonic donors is that at the metanephros stage, there are no mature dendritic cells present, and therefore the costimulatory molecules are not present in these tissues. Recent publications have brought into doubt whether immunosuppressive regimens with tacrolimus or fingolimod (FTY720) are required for successful transplantation across the MHC.[164]

The development of renal vasculature is a complex process, and the studies evaluating the origins of the renal circulatory system are conflicting. Branches of the abdominal aorta terminate in a plexus of arteries that supply the major vessels of the kidney. This is initiated by the renal anlagen during development as it attracts the developing aorta. By definition, this makes the kidney a chimeric organ in that its blood supply is derived from elsewhere. The ability of the metanephroi to attract its own blood supply is being exploited by researchers to find improved methods of vasculogenesis for transplanted tissues. All implanted metanephroi are capable of inducing angiogenesis, as evidenced by implantation survival and often function. However, quantification of the blood flow has been described in only one study. Dilworth and associates measured effective renal blood flow (EBRF) in transplanted E15 rat metanephroi. They found that the EBRF was approximately 5% that of the native kidney, and this translated to a higher vascular resistance and decreased glomerular filtration rate (GFR) in the transplanted metanephroi.[165] While transplanted metanephroi are capable of attracting arterial inflow, future directions will be to increase this capability to provide for development of physiologic GFR.

FUNCTIONAL TRANSPLANTATION OF METANEPHROI

Renal anlagen transplanted into a host have demonstrated functional capabilities with differentiation into renal tissue, production of urine, and improved survival in anephric rodents. Initial studies demonstrating the feasibility of metanephroi transplantation were conducted by Woolf and coworkers, who implanted pieces of E13 to E16 metanephroi into cortical tunnels fashioned in newborn mice.[166] Abrahamson and colleagues also were able to demonstrate survival and function of metanephroi transplanted subcapsularly in rats.[167] Rogers and colleagues not only implanted metanephroi outside the renal capsule in the omentum but also performed a ureteroureterostomy allowing for quantification of urine production.[168] Rogers and colleagues were the first to demonstrate improved survival associated with metanephros transplantation. They implanted E15 rat metanephroi into the omentum of rats at the same time as unilateral nephrectomy. Three weeks following transplantation they performed ureteroureterostomy between the host ureter and the transplanted metanephroi in some of the rats. At 20 weeks following initial transplantation, they performed contralateral nephrectomy, forcing animals into ESKD. They demonstrated a significant prolongation of life in the animals with intact excretory urinary tract versus controls or transplants without ureteroureterostomy.[169] Marshall and colleagues successfully transplanted rat metanephroi into the omentum and patches of retroperitoneal fat in the renal bed, adjacent to the circumflex iliac vessels, and adjacent to the aorta and vena cava. They were able to demonstrate presence of urinary cysts in all locations at 21 days posttransplantation. In renal units with urinary cysts, ureteroureterostomy was performed at this time point. When they measured inulin clearance 130 days after ureteroureterostomy, they demonstrated the transplanted unit contributed up to 11% of the total GFR as measured by inulin clearance.[170]

Integration of new nephrons into a diseased kidney has promise in sparing patients from renal replacement therapy. Investigations into this possibility in an animal model have been promising. Woolf and colleagues implanted embryonic tissue into the renal cortex of newborn mice. They found that the donor tissue integrated into new nephrons and the glomeruli of the donated tissue was vascularized by the host. They found mature tubules and tubular extension into the medulla, but they could not confirm that these nephrons connected to a collecting duct.[166] Rogers and colleagues performed a similar experiment placing E15 rat metanephroi in adult male mice. They, too, found that nephron development and creation of a chimeric kidney occurred.[168] However, like Woolf, they could not verify that the nephron connected to the collecting duct despite transplantation of a portion of the ureteric bud.[166,168]

Instead of transplanting metanephroi, Kim and colleagues digested E17.5 rat metanephroi into a single-cell suspension and then introduced these cells into a 5/6 remnant rat kidney model. The fetal cells had stem cell lineage noted on FACS as they were positive for c-kit, Oct-4, CD34, CD133 as compared to digested adult rat kidneys. The authors noted that 10 weeks following subcapsular injection, the rats receiving E17.5 cells had improved survival, serum creatinine, and proteinuria as compared to rats receiving adult renal cell suspensions.[120] Cells derived from the metanephric mesenchyme have been demonstrated to have organotypic arrangement without or with an intact ureteric bud. Ganava and colleagues created disassociated E11.5 murine metanephroi cellular suspensions and, when cultured with intact ureteric buds, as expected, they created developing nephrons with a singular collecting duct tree. When these E11.5 metanephroi were cultured with disaggregated ureteric bud suspensions, which had been re-aggregated into ureteric bud cysts, anatomy similar to an intact developing kidney was observed.[171] Potential for self-organization creates promise in creating de novo organs from these developmental tissues.

Using E11.5 murine cells, Xinaris and associates created a single-cell suspension containing both ureteric bud and metanephric mesenchymal cells. After demonstrating tubular creation in vivo, the investigators implanted the cells under the renal capsule in athymic mice. Harvest at 3 weeks demonstrated primarily proximal tubular maturation noted with aquaporin-1 expression, although thick ascending limbs and distal tubular areas were also noted. However, WT1, nephrin, CD2AP, and synaptopodin stains were negative, demonstrating lack of glomerulogenesis. With the use of stimulation by VEGF, morphologic glomerulogenesis could be improved.[172]

Blastocyte complementation is another approach that has been used for whole organ reconstruction. This technique obviates the need for creation of the complex environment of organogenesis in vitro. Successful adaptation of this in the pancreas[173] and liver[174] has motivated experimentation in renal models. Sall1 is expressed in the metanephric mesenchyme and renal stroma in the embryonic and newborn kidney. It is essential for ureteric bud attraction to the mesenchyme, and mice deficient in this die shortly after birth due to renal agenesis or severe dysgenesis. Usui and coworkers injected iPS cells, labeled with EGFP into the blastocytes of Sall1−/− mice. Morphologically normal renal units developed in these animals. Histologically, they confirmed that the majority of the renal stroma was labeled with EGFP, confirming iPS cell lineage. The collecting duct epithelia and kidney stromal elements such as vessels and nerves were composites of host and iPS-derived cells.[175]

XENOTRANSPLANTATION OF RENAL ANLAGEN

Xenotransplantation of renal anlagen has been found to lead to successful differentiation of renal tissues with demonstration of renal function. Rogers and Hammerman transplanted E15 rat metanephroi into 10-week-old C57Bl/6J mice. They found that only in mice receiving tolerance-inducing agents human CTLA4IG, anti-CD45RB, and anti-CD154 did the metanephroi develop into renal structures. Glomerular epithelium demonstrated positivity for mouse anti-CD31, demonstrating murine origin.[176] In light of the shortage of donor kidneys available for transplantation, animal kidney xenografts are an attractive option. The porcine model represents an ideal candidate because pigs are plentiful and they have a similar-size kidney, with comparable architecture and physiologic parameters. Unfortunately, the transplantation of vascularized organs of porcine origin is challenging due to preformed antigens against pig epithelium.[177] Pigs and other nonprimate mammals possess Galα1-3Gal, a saccharide present on epithelial cells, which up to 85% of primate antibodies are directed against.[178] However, as demonstrated in previous studies, renal vasculature appears host derived following metanephroi transplantation; therefore, this could provide a mechanism for circumventing this difficulty.

Rogers and colleagues implanted E28 porcine metanephroi into Lewis rats. In the rats treated with tacrolimus and anti-CD45, the metanephroi demonstrated differentiation and growth. However, in nonimmunosuppressed rats, no trace of transplanted renal anlagen could be detected beginning at 4 weeks following transplantation.[179] Dekel and colleagues transplanted E27 to E28 porcine metanephroi into immunodeficient mice. This age was superior to earlier precursors as those produced nonrenal differentiation. They demonstrated functionality 6 weeks following transplantation by determining urea and creatinine concentrations in urine cysts that were significantly higher than the sera but more dilute than in urine collected from the bladder.[179]

In immunocompromised rats undergoing human metanephroi transplantation with concurrent unilateral nephrectomy, Dekel and associates demonstrated functional renal tissue in rats using dimercaptosuccinic acid scans.[180] Further studies by this group evaluated cluster analysis of cDNA expression profiles at serial time points of transplanted human metanephroi, occurring every 4 weeks beginning at 12 weeks. This expression was compared with time-controlled nontransplanted fetal renal tissues. They found exceptional similarity in expression profiles, with slight changes seen in markers for ischemia and oxidative stress in the transplanted metanephroi.[180]

Yokoo and colleagues used a chimeric model of injecting human MSCs into a developing rodent metanephros to investigate another potential mechanism for kidney development. They followed these cells in vitro by labeling them with LacZ. Histologic examination determined integration and nephron formation by human MSCs. RT-PCR showed the human MSCs expressed both podocyte and tubular epithelial cell specific genes. They assessed function by measuring α-galactosidase A activity in the chimeric mouse kidneys as compared to wild-type kidneys because mice do not possess α-galactosidase A enzyme.[181]

Further investigations from this group have demonstrated in vivo growth of the chimeric kidneys created in vitro previously. These rat renal anlagen seeded with human MSCs were implanted onto the omentum of host rats. At 2 weeks, the rats were sacrificed and histologic examination determined differentiated mesangial cells with desmin staining and podocytes with synaptopodin and WT1 positivity. In transplants that were left in place for 4 weeks, the metanephroi appeared hydronephrotic, with the appearance of fluid-filled cyst. Cyst fluid had creatinine and urea levels that were more than 20 times higher than those found in the serum and comparable to that in native urine.[182] Recent publications from Yokoo and associates have addressed endocrine function in developing chimeric kidneys. Using the same model of in vivo culture of rat metanephroi following human MSC implantation, erythropoietin expression was evaluated. Immunostaining and RT-PCR confirmed both human and rat erythropoietin-producing cells within the transplanted tissue. By inducing anemia, human erythropoietin production in these rats significantly increased, demonstrating appropriate physiologic responses to anemia.[183] Development of functional kidneys from transplanted MSCs would produce individualized kidneys for recipients overcoming both a donor shortage and need for immunosuppression.

Transplanted metanephroi may also be able to recruit erythropoietin-producing MSCs to allow endogenous hormonal production. In a xenotransplanted rat-to-mouse or pig-to-cat model, Matsumoto and colleagues found metanephroi transplanted could recruit host cells to differentiate into erythropoietin-producing tissues. This was confirmed with species-specific PCR. They then activated a suicide gene in the ER-E2F1 mouse model and found production of erythropoietin from endogenous non-xenotransplanted cells after 2 weeks.[184] By activating the suicide gene, they provide a potential model for transplantation without need for immunosuppression due to lack of remaining foreign antigen.

PRESERVATION OF RENAL ANLAGEN

Inevitably, if metanephroi have future clinical applicability, it is presumed that a safe method for transporting the primordium needs to be developed. While theoretically, immediate transference could occur, dependable methods for storage and transportation would provide flexibility in timing and allow sites of excellence in metanephroi harvesting to exist and export the renal anlagen. In human allogeneic kidney transplantation, the renal unit is flushed with University of Wisconsin (UW) solution and then stored in ice cold UW solution until implantation is possible. Rogers and Hammerman compared metanephroi transplanted immediately with those preserved in UW solution for 3 days. They found that with the addition of recombinant human growth factors to the UW solution, renal function in the preserved metanephroi was similar to that of the immediately transplanted units.[185] Unfortunately, efforts to bank metanephroi through cryopreservation have been unsuccessful thus far.[186] Recent efforts to create mesoderm from iPS cells have been described, but further differentiation of these cells has yet to be characterized.[187]

Steer and colleagues evaluated the possibility of producing renal units in vitro through the combination of separately cultured metanephric mesenchyme and ureteric buds. They isolated rat ureteric buds on E13.5, cultured them for 8 days, and subsequently divided the culture into thirds, repeating the process with the cultured ureteric bud cultures. At this point, these cultures were introduced to mesenchymal cultures and the interaction was evaluated for renal markers. Using immunofluorescence staining for occluden and *Dolicus biflorus,* they found that the cultured ureteric bud and mesenchymal combinations produced renal primordia which were identical to renal anlagen formed from fresh mesenchyme and ureteric buds.[188] Osafune and associates were able to induce both glomerular and tubule differentiation from a single clone derived from E11.5 mice. This clone strongly expressed Sall-1, a zinc-finger nuclear factor essential for kidney development.[189] Rosines and colleagues have described a technique for in vitro three-dimensional development of renal tissue through inducing an epithelial tubule or Wolffian duct to undergo budding in a stepwise fashion.

The initial step utilizes culture techniques with specific cytokine concentrations to initiate the outgrowth of the ureteric bud from the Wolffian duct. They found that a single bud was capable of branching in vitro, and, therefore, this isolate bud was co-cultured with metanephric mesenchyme. Co-culture created nephron-like structures that demonstrated uptake of 6-carboxyfluorescein, an organic anion that is taken up by specific tubular transporters. At this point the recombined tissue was implanted under the renal capsule of host rats. The implanted tissue had multiple glomeruli, and the cells of the glomerulus expressed the endothelial marker platelet endothelial cell adhesion molecule 1 (PECAM-1). Erythrocytes were also noted within the glomeruli, indicating blood flow to the implanted tissue.[190] Taken together, these studies demonstrate that rather than being preserved, large quantities of renal anlagen could be expanded in vitro and retain the intrinsic ability to induce renal differentiation.

IN SITU DEVELOPMENT OF RENAL UNITS

An attractive potential renal regenerative therapy would be the combination of many of the previously noted individual approaches. A kidney that could be created in vitro and subsequently implanted into a patient with renal dysfunction would obviate the need for finding a suitable donor or lifelong dialysis. If this construct were seeded with autologous cells, there would be no need for immunosuppression. Previous studies have demonstrated that a bladder scaffold seeded with autologous cells can be transplanted in vivo with excellent results with up to 5 years of follow-up. While the kidney represents a more ambitious endeavor in terms of architecture and function, the promising results of this previous organ regeneration create an open door for using this therapy.

Potentially, heterogeneous cell populations seeded on an implantable biomaterial could provide one avenue for treatment. Autologous cell populations could be obtained with a kidney biopsy, grown in vitro, and seeded onto scaffold for future implantation. Atala and associates plated donor rabbit kidney cells, including distal tubules, glomeruli, and proximal tubules, in vitro, and after expansion, these were seeded onto biodegradable polyglycolic acid scaffolds and implanted subcutaneously into athymic mice.[191] The implants consisted of individual cell types and a mixture of all three. Histologic examination showed progressive formation and organization of the nephron segments within the polymer fibers. Additionally, BrdU incorporation into the renal cell DNA was confirmed. It was unclear if the tubular structures found on the scaffolds were de novo from the implanted cells or if they merely represented fragments of donor tubules that had survived the original dissociation and culture process intact. To further investigate, mouse renal cells were harvested and expanded in culture. Subsequently, the single isolated cells were seeded on biodegradable polymers and immune-competent syngeneic hosts. Here, renal epithelial cells reconstituted tubular structures in vivo. The analyses of the retrieved implants demonstrated renal epithelial cells first organized into a structure with a solid center. Subsequently, canalization into a hollow tube could be seen at 2 weeks. Histologic examination with nephron-specific lectins revealed successful reconstitution of proximal tubules, distal tubules, loops of Henle, collecting tubules, and collecting ducts. These results clearly showed that single-cell suspensions grown in vitro are capable of reconstituting into tubule structures. The tubules contained homogeneous cell types within each tubule.

Yoo and colleagues evaluated murine renal cells grown in vitro.[192] They harvested the cells, expanded them in culture, and seeded them onto a tubular device constructed from polycarbonate. At one end of the tubular device was a Silastic catheter that terminated into a reservoir. The device was subcutaneously implanted into athymic mice. The implanted device demonstrated extensive vascularization in addition to glomerular formation and highly organized tubular architecture. Immunohistochemistry staining for alkaline phosphatase showed positivity in the proximal tubule–like structures. Osteopontin, which is secreted by the proximal and distal tubular cells and the cells of the thin loop of Henle, was found on immunocytochemical staining of the tubular sections. The extracellular matrix of the newly formed tubules stained uniformly positive for fibronectin. The fluid collected from the reservoir was yellow and the uric acid concentration was 66 mg/dL (as compared to 2 mg/dL in plasma). The creatinine concentration of the fluid (27.91 ± 7.56 mg/dL) was 8.2 times higher than that found in the serum (4.49 ± 0.08 mg/dl). This demonstrates that single cells can form multicellular structures, become organized into functional renal units, and are capable of unidirectional excretion of solutes through a urine-like fluid.

Ross and colleagues have used a combination of renal scaffold and ES cells to induce in vitro formation of a kidney. Using a series of detergents following an intricate protocol to preserve physiologic pressure, they successfully decellularized a rat kidney as evidenced by histologic examination. At this point, ES cells from a GFP-labeled mouse were injected through either the ureter or renal artery, and the tissue was cultured in vitro. Without the use of differentiation agents, immunostains and RT-PCR demonstrated Pax-2 (a critical factor in branching morphogenesis and expressed in both the ureteric bud and induced metanephric mesenchyme) and kidney-specific cadherin (an adhesion protein expressed by distal nephron tubular cells at later developmental stages).[112] Here the decellularized extracellular matrix induced the differentiation of ES cells and raises the possibility for using decellularized porcine kidneys, with similar renal architecture, as a possible future clinical intervention in humans.

Development of a renal tubular assist device (RAD) to attenuate hemofiltration has been another avenue of cellular therapy investigated. Humes and colleagues have designed an extracorporeal device that works in concert with hemofiltration units. Here, proximal tubule cells are seeded in confluent monolayers in a multifiber bioreactor. When used for dialysis, blood is pumped through a conventional hemofilter. Following processing through a conventional hemofilter, the ultrafiltrate is again processed through the RAD. The filtered blood exiting the hemofilter enters the RAD through the extracapillary space port and then disperses throughout the fibers of the device. The hollow fiber membrane protects the cells lining the inner surface of the hollow fibers from immune-related attack. The purpose of these devices is to supplement hemofiltration and improve the physiologic functions of the kidney not addressed with hemofiltration. Initial studies using porcine tubular cells demonstrated significantly improved ammonia excretion and elevated plasma levels of 1,25 dihydroxyvitamin D3 in dogs with acute uremia. Cells on the RAD demonstrated replicative capacity as they returned to baseline function 2 weeks following usage.[193]

A phase I/II trial of the RAD was performed in 10 ICU patients with AKI. Proximal tubules cells for the RAD were derived from human kidney tissue that was intended for transplantation but discarded due to anatomic or fibrotic concerns. These patients had significant other comorbidities with multiple concomitant illness and multiple organ failures. The most common adverse effects were hypovolemia, thrombocytopenia, and hyperglycemia. The RAD did appear to have an immunomodulatory effect as there was a significant decline in IL-6, IL-10, and granulocyte colony-stimulating factor. Despite high predicted 30-day mortality rates, 60% of patients survived at 30 days.[194] It is difficult to interpret efficacy from a phase I/II trial, so the results from the phase III, multicenter, randomized controlled open label trial were reported recently. Here, 58 patients were randomized to 40 with RAD and hemofiltration versus 18 with hemofiltration alone. With a median treatment duration of 35.9 hours, there was only one malfunction of an RAD. Patients receiving RAD renal supplementation were found to have an earlier recovery of kidney function, although this was not statistically significant. Survival was significantly improved at 180 days in patients with RAD support. Using subgroup analysis, higher survival rates were noted for RAD patients for all sets of organ failure.[195] It is important to recognize that the patients enrolled in these studies are critically ill patients in the intensive care unit. Despite this, a substantive effect on survival and renal recovery was noted, paving the way for future investigations.

SUMMARY

The kidney is an incredibly diverse and complex organ. Not only is it responsible for excretion, but it provides resorptive, homeostatic, metabolic, and endocrine functions as well. Current methods of supplementing renal dysfunction have been well established and improve mortality. However, transplantation and hemodialysis are not without significant morbidity. Additionally, for patients with CKD, recovery of renal function is not currently possible. Identification of stem cells, including renal progenitor cells, has improved our understanding of the endogenous regenerative capacity of the kidney. These cells may provide clues in the future to understanding how to supplement kidney functional capacity and prevent patients from progressing to ESKD.

Developmental approaches to renal dysfunction hold significant promise with the potential for an unlimited supply of donor organs. Organs would be tailor matched for the recipient and there would not be a need for immunosuppression. The course of treatment for patients with ESKD could be drastically changed. Bioengineering and regenerative medicine are reaching toward a future that will significantly change the way renal dysfunction is managed, and, as a result, patient outcomes will be improved.

Complete reference list available at ExpertConsult.com.

KEY REFERENCES

7. Zhang SC, Wernig M, Duncan ID, et al: In vitro differentiation of transplantable neural precursors from human embryonic stem cells [see comment]. *Nat Biotechnol* 19:1129–1133, 2001.
17. Vigneau C, Polgar K, Striker G, et al: Mouse embryonic stem cell-derived embryoid bodies generate progenitors that integrate long term into renal proximal tubules in vivo. *J Am Soc Nephrol* 18:1709–1720, 2007.
19. Morizane R, Monkawa T, Fujii S, et al: Kidney specific protein-positive cells derived from embryonic stem cells reproduce tubular structures in vitro and differentiate into renal tubular cells. *PLoS ONE* 8:e64843, 2013.
20. Chung Y, Klimanskaya I, Becker S, et al: Embryonic and extraembryonic stem cell lines derived from single mouse blastomeres. *Nature* 439:216–219, 2006.
30. Lanza RP, Chung HY, Yoo JJ, et al: Generation of histocompatible tissues using nuclear transplantation [see comment]. *Nat Biotechnol* 20:689–696, 2002.
33. Hwang WS, Ryu YJ, Park JH, et al: Evidence of a pluripotent human embryonic stem cell line derived from a cloned blastocyst. *Science* 303:1669–1674, 2004.
40. Takahashi K, Yamanaka S: Induction of pluripotent stem cells from mouse embryonic and adult fibroblast cultures by defined factors. *Cell* 126:663–676, 2006.
45. Song B, Niclis JC, Alikhan MA, et al: Generation of induced pluripotent stem cells from human kidney mesangial cells. *J Am Soc Nephrol* 22:1213–1220, 2011.
46. Zhou T, Benda C, Duzinger S, et al: Generation of induced pluripotent stem cells from urine. *J Am Soc Nephrol* 22:1221–1228, 2011.
47. Song B, Smink AM, Jones CV, et al: The directed differentiation of human iPS cells into kidney podocytes. *PLoS ONE* 7:e46453, 2012.
53. Kolambkar YM, Peister A, Soker S, et al: Chondrogenic differentiation of amniotic fluid-derived stem cells. *J Mol Histol* 38:405–413, 2007.
55. Perin L, Giuliani S, Jin D, et al: Renal differentiation of amniotic fluid stem cells. *Cell Prolif* 40:936–948, 2007.
57. Sedrakyan S, Da Sacco S, Milanesi A, et al: Injection of amniotic fluid stem cells delays progression of renal fibrosis. *J Am Soc Nephrol* 23:661–673, 2012.
58. Hauser PV, De Fazio R, Bruno S, et al: Stem cells derived from human amniotic fluid contribute to acute kidney injury recovery. *Am J Pathol* 177:21–2010, 2011.
66. Jiang Y, Jahagirdar BN, Reinhardt RL, et al: Pluripotency of mesenchymal stem cells derived from adult marrow [see comment] [erratum appears in *Nature* 447(7146):879-80]. *Nature* 418:41–49, 2002.
76. Maeshima A, Yamashita S, Nojima Y: Identification of renal progenitor-like tubular cells that participate in the regeneration processes of the kidney. *J Am Soc Nephrol* 14:3138–3146, 2003.
77. Maeshima A, Sakurai H, Nigam SK: Adult kidney tubular cell population showing phenotypic plasticity, tubulogenic capacity, and integration capability into developing kidney. *J Am Soc Nephrol* 17:188–198, 2006.
82. Bussolati B, Bruno S, Grange C, et al: Isolation of renal progenitor cells from adult human kidney. *Am J Pathol* 166:545–555, 2005.
83. Plotkin MD, Goligorsky MS: Mesenchymal cells from adult kidney support angiogenesis and differentiate into multiple interstitial cell types including erythropoietin-producing fibroblasts. *Am J Physiol Renal Physiol* 291:F902–F912, 2006.
86. Sagrinati C, Netti GS, Mazzinghi B, et al: Isolation and characterization of multipotent progenitor cells from the Bowman's capsule of adult human kidneys. *J Am Soc Nephrol* 17:2443–2456, 2006.
88. Appel D, Kershaw DB, Smeets B, et al: Recruitment of podocytes from glomerular parietal epithelial cells. *J Am Soc Nephrol* 20:333–343, 2009.
108. Joraku A, Stern KA, Atala A, et al: In vitro generation of three-dimensional renal structures. *Methods* 47:129–133, 2009.
112. Ross EA, Williams MJ, Hamazaki T, et al: Embryonic stem cells proliferate and differentiate when seeded into kidney scaffolds. *J Am Soc Nephrol* 20:2338–2347, 2009.
113. Sullivan DC, Mirmalek-Sani SH, Deegan DB, et al: Decellularization methods of porcine kidneys for whole organ engineering using a high-throughput system. *Biomaterials* 33:7756–7764, 2012.
114. Orlando G, Booth C, Wang Z, et al: Discarded human kidneys as a source of ECM scaffold for kidney regeneration technologies. *Biomaterials* 34:5915–5925, 2013.
116. Aboushwareb T, Egydio F, Straker L, et al: Erythropoietin producing cells for potential cell therapy. *World J Urol* 26:295–300, 2008.
117. Gyabaah K, Aboushwareb T, Guimaraes Souza N, et al: Controlled regulation of erythropoietin by primary cultured renal cells for renal failure induced anemia. *J Urol* 188:2000–2006, 2012.
123. Lin F, Cordes K, Li L, et al: Hematopoietic stem cells contribute to the regeneration of renal tubules after renal ischemia-reperfusion injury in mice. *J Am Soc Nephrol* 14:1188–1199, 2003.
128. Fang TC, Alison MR, Cook HT, et al: Proliferation of bone marrow-derived cells contributes to regeneration after folic acid-induced acute tubular injury. *J Am Soc Nephrol* 16:1723–1732, 2005.
132. Kale S, Karihaloo A, Clark PR, et al: Bone marrow stem cells contribute to repair of the ischemically injured renal tubule. *J Clin Invest* 112:42–49, 2003.
137. Togel F, Hu Z, Weiss K, et al: Administered mesenchymal stem cells protect against ischemic acute renal failure through differentiation-independent mechanisms. *Am J Physiol Renal Physiol* 289:F31–F42, 2005.
138. Morigi M, Imberti B, Zoja C, et al: Mesenchymal stem cells are renotropic, helping to repair the kidney and improve function in acute renal failure. *J Am Soc Nephrol* 15:1794–1804, 2004.
139. Kunter U, Rong S, Boor P, et al: Mesenchymal stem cells prevent progressive experimental renal failure but maldifferentiate into glomerular adipocytes. *J Am Soc Nephrol* 18:1754–1764, 2007.
144. Cavaglieri RC, Martini D, Sogayar MC, et al: Mesenchymal stem cells delivered at the subcapsule of the kidney ameliorate renal disease in the rat remnant kidney model. *Transplant Proc* 41:947–951, 2009.
151. Xinaris C, Morigi M, Benedetti V, et al: A novel strategy to enhance mesenchymal stem cell migration capacity and promote tissue repair in an injury specific fashion. *Cell Transplant* 22:423–436, 2013.
157. Tan J, Wu W, Xu X, et al: Induction therapy with autologous mesenchymal stem cells in living-related kidney transplants: a randomized controlled trial. *JAMA* 307:1169–1177, 2012.
161. Dekel B, Burakova T, Arditti FD, et al: Human and porcine early kidney precursors as a new source for transplantation. *Nat Med* 9:53–60, 2003.
168. Rogers SA, Lowell JA, Hammerman NA, et al: Transplantation of developing metanephroi into adult rats. *Kidney Int* 54:27–37, 1998.
171. Ganeva V, Unbekandt M, Davies JA: An improved kidney dissociation and reaggregation culture system results in nephrons arranged organotypically around a single collecting duct system. *Organogenesis* 7:83–87, 2011.
172. Xinaris C, Benedetti V, Rizzo P, et al: In vivo maturation of functional renal organoids formed from embryonic cell suspensions. *J Am Soc Nephrol* 23:1857–1868, 2012.
175. Usui J, Kobayashi T, Yamaguchi T, et al: Generation of kidney from pluripotent stem cells via blastocyst complementation. *Am J Pathol* 180:2417–2426, 2012.

181. Yokoo T, Ohashi T, Shen JS, et al: Human mesenchymal stem cells in rodent whole-embryo culture are reprogrammed to contribute to kidney tissues. *Proc Natl Acad Sci U S A* 102:3296–3300, 2005.
182. Yokoo T, Fukui A, Ohashi T, et al: Xenobiotic kidney organogenesis from human mesenchymal stem cells using a growing rodent embryo. *J Am Soc Nephrol* 17:1026–1034, 2006.
183. Yokoo T, Fukui A, Matsumoto K, et al: Generation of a transplantable erythropoietin-producer derived from human mesenchymal stem cells. *Transplantation* 85:1654–1658, 2008.
191. Atala A, Schlussel RN, Retik AB: Renal cell growth in vivo after attachment to biodegradable polymer scaffolds. *J Urol* 153:4, 1995.
192. Yoo JJ, Ashkar S, Atala A: Creation of functional kidney structures with excretion of kidney-like fluid in vivo. *Pediatrics* 98(Suppl):605, 1996.
195. Tumlin J, Wali R, Williams W, et al: Efficacy and safety of renal tubule cell therapy for acute renal failure. *J Am Soc Nephrol* 19:1034–1040, 2008.

87 Quality Improvement Initiatives in Kidney Disease

Sandeep S. Soman | Jerry Yee | Kevin Ho

CHAPTER OUTLINE

QUALITY IMPROVEMENT AND QUALITY IMPROVEMENT TOOLS, 2620
History of Quality and Quality Improvement in Health Care, 2621
Assessing Quality in Chronic Diseases and Kidney Disease, 2621
Quality Improvement Tools, 2622
Quality Improvement in Nephrology, 2625
QUALITY IMPROVEMENT INITIATIVES IN END-STAGE KIDNEY DISEASE, 2625
Emerging Quality Improvements in Kidney Disease, 2625
Role of Erythropoiesis-Stimulating Agents in Catalyzing Quality Improvement, 2626
Bundled Prospective Payment System and Quality Incentive Program, 2628
Vascular Access Practice, Fistula First Breakthrough Initiative, and Quality Improvement, 2629
A View to the Future, 2631
QUALITY INITIATIVES IN CHRONIC KIDNEY DISEASE, 2632

QUALITY IMPROVEMENT AND QUALITY IMPROVEMENT TOOLS

Quality is a concept that describes those features of a product or service to which value is ascribed. Consequently, the nature of quality varies among products and services, individuals, and organizations. Here, quality is discussed in relation to its significance in health care. Quality does not incorporate any idea of relative cost. Although it may be used in conjunction with cost, allowing consideration of value, the implementation of quality should not be seen as a cost-cutting exercise.[1] The Institute of Medicine (IOM) has defined quality as "the degree to which health services for individuals and populations increase the likelihood of desired health outcomes and are consistent with current professional knowledge."[2] Batalden and colleagues have proposed defining quality as the combined and unceasing efforts of everyone involved—health care professionals, patients and their families, researchers, payers, planners, and educators—to make the changes that will lead to better patient outcomes (health), better system performance (care), and better professional development (learning).[3] However, to define quality by the development of expectations or standards, it is necessary to describe dimensions of quality, also known as elements or domains.

The IOM has proposed a national statement of purpose for the health care system as a whole, wherein all involved parties (in health care) would accept as their explicit purpose "to continually reduce the burden of illness, injury, and disability, and to improve the health and functioning of the people of the United States." Also, the parties would adopt a shared vision of six specific aims for improvement. These aims are built around the core need for health care to be the following[2]:

- Safe—avoiding injuries to patients from the care that is intended to help them
- Effective—providing services based on scientific knowledge to all who could benefit and refraining from providing services to those not likely to benefit
- Patient-centered—providing care that is respectful of and responsive to individual patient preferences, needs, and values, and ensuring that patient values guide all clinical decisions
- Timely—reducing waits and sometimes harmful delays for those who receive and those who give care
- Efficient—avoiding waste, including waste of equipment, supplies, ideas, and energy
- Equitable—providing care that does not vary in quality because of personal characteristics such as gender, ethnicity, geographic location, and socioeconomic status

HISTORY OF QUALITY AND QUALITY IMPROVEMENT IN HEALTH CARE

Over the past decade, the health care industry has moved away from being an industry based on trust and partnership between patients and their physicians to one of gentle (and, at times, less gentle) tension among those who provide care, those who receive it, and those who pay for it. Whenever society begins to lose confidence in an institution, there is typically demand for greater oversight of the institution and the related push for more data about the institution and the products or services it provides.[4]

The roots of the quality improvement movement can be traced back to the work of epic figures such as Ignaz Semmelweis, the nineteenth century Hungarian obstetrician who championed the importance of handwashing in medical care. In addition, Florence Nightingale, the English nurse, identified the association between poor living conditions and high death rates among soldiers treated at army hospitals. Florence Nightingale was an extraordinary woman who is popularly known for her work in the Crimean War and her subsequent influence on nursing as a profession. Her contributions to statistical science are less well appreciated, although several commentaries exist.[5-7] In the early nineteenth century, American medicine was disorganized and of poor quality, with the control of medical education in the hands of proprietary and for-profit institutions. Several organizations and individuals undertook extensive efforts to correct this. Founded in part for this reason in 1847 as a confederation of state and local societies, the American Medical Association (AMA) encouraged Abraham Flexner's research, which by 1910 led to his *Report to the Carnegie Foundation,* which documented the deplorable state of U.S. medical schools and major hospitals. In the same year, Codman noted the need to improve hospital conditions and track patients to verify that their care had been effective. Ernest Codman, a U.S. surgeon, pioneered the creation of hospital standards and emphasized and implemented strategies to assess health care outcomes.[7] Although few followed Codman's lead, his efforts contributed to the American College of Surgeons' establishment of the Hospital Standardization Program in 1917.[8,9] The modern quality movement has since transformed to include a wide variety of stakeholders, a range of unique and modified approaches, and an evolving set of goals.[10]

ASSESSING QUALITY IN CHRONIC DISEASES AND KIDNEY DISEASE

Assessing quality of care for chronic conditions tends to be complex because management of these conditions require multiple processes, stratification by severity may be necessary, the need for clinical detail from health records is greater, the need to tailor delivery of this care to the individual is important, and the settings of care are varied. However, failure to receive high-quality care for chronic conditions may have the most significant potential consequences for the health and functioning of the population.

Chronic illness has replaced infectious diseases as the leading cause of death worldwide. Approaches for treating chronic conditions are growing from high-tech treatments such as coronary artery bypass graft surgery, angioplasty, left-right ventricular assist devices, and orthotopic heart transplantation to low-tech solutions, such as home care and assistive devices. However, knowledge about the quality of care for chronic illness or the efficacy of many treatments for producing desirable outcomes is in its infancy. For example, hip fractures and strokes, the two most common disabling conditions in older persons, often result in profound functional decline. Among patients who have suffered hip fracture, between 55% and 75% experience loss of their ability to perform basic activities of daily living. Among stroke survivors, nearly 40% continue to manifest moderate functional impairments 6 months later, and 10% to 15% remain severely disabled. Despite this, the effectiveness of different rehabilitation options for restoring function and preventing long-term nursing home placement is largely unknown.[11]

In other cases, even when knowledge of the most efficacious treatment of chronic conditions exists, treatment approaches are unevenly applied. There has been some improvement in this over the past 2 decades. Diabetes care represents one example. In 1989, 49% of persons with diabetes mellitus in the United States had received a dilated eye examination in the past year; in 2012, this figure had improved to 62.8%.[2,13] A study of Medicare beneficiaries for claims submitted between July 1, 1990, and June 30, 1991 in the states of Alabama, Iowa, and Maryland, reported that only 46% of participants had undergone an eye examination and only 16% a glycosylated hemoglobin test, a marker of glucose control in diabetes.[13] The Centers for Disease Control and Prevention (CDC) has reported that 69% of adult patients with diabetes mellitus had a glycosylated hemoglobin test during the period 2009 to 2010.[12]

Similar findings have been demonstrated for mental health conditions. One study found that only 20% to 30% of general medicine patients with depression were prescribed antidepressant medications. Among persons prescribed medication, 30% were prescribed a subtherapeutic dose.[14] A consensus panel on the undertreatment of depression concluded that "there is overwhelming evidence that individuals with depression are being seriously undertreated."[15]

Assessing quality and developing benchmarks in the diagnosis and management of kidney diseases has been challenging for numerous reasons, some of which are addressed in more detail below. The lineage of kidney disease as a subject of study generally is traced to 1827, when Richard Bright (1789-1858) described his eponymous disease of the kidneys in albuminuric, dropsical patients who died from kidney failure. Shortly thereafter, Pierre Rayer (1793-1867) published his monumental three-volume *Traité des Maladies des Reins* in 1840 and, 2 years later, William Bowman (1816-1892) demonstrated the connection of the glomerulus to the tubule, arguably the first contribution of morphology to kidney function.[16] More than 150 years later, the initial set of clinical practice guidelines for dialysis care was published in 1997 by the Dialysis Outcomes Quality Initiative (DOQI).

While DOQI guideline development was underway, it became evident to all those involved in the process that the care of patients with chronic kidney disease (CKD) should begin earlier, well before the ravages of failing kidneys had occurred, at a time when early detection and intervention could delay or prevent the need for kidney replacement therapy and improve outcomes of those progressing to dialysis. To reflect this change, the name of the guideline initiative was changed to KDOQI (Kidney Disease Outcomes Quality Initiative) at the beginning of the millennium. In 2002, KDOQI published the clinical practice guidelines for CKD, which for the first time in history provided a uniform definition for and staging of CKD based on its severity. The paradigm shift the guidelines that produced marks a significant moment in the advancement of nephrology. Nephrology reverted to its roots as the study of chronic disease that Bright had described, but was now refined and polished by lessons learned over the preceding decades.[17]

However, the development of these guidelines was also constrained by the available level of evidence-based data. A study was undertaken by Lopez-Vargas and associates[19] to compare the scope, content, and consistency of published guidelines on CKD stages 1 to 3. Analyzing the level of evidence presented in the KDOQI, the authors reported that the grade of evidence in the studies used to generate the guidelines ranged from grade C (studies of lower level evidence, such as case-control studies or case series, expert opinion, composition of original articles), grade S (analysis of individual patient data from a single large, generalizable study of high methodologic quality), grade R (review of reviews and selected original articles) to grade O (opinion). None of the evidence presented was grade A or B—namely, based on scientific evidence that had been established by trials of high level evidence, randomized controlled trials (RCTs) with a high degree of power with freedom from major biases, and/or meta-analyses of RCTs (decision analyses based on properly conducted studies or based on scientific evidence from studies of intermediate-level evidence, RCTs of low-power, well-conducted non-RCTs, or cohort studies, respectively).[18,19] This is not surprising, given how few clinical trials have been conducted in kidney disease.[20]

Coca and coworkers[21] have studied RCTs of treatments for chronic congestive heart failure and acute myocardial infarction currently listed (at the time of the study) as class I or II recommendations in the current American College of Cardiology/American Heart Association guidelines. A total of 153 trials were reviewed. Patients with kidney disease were reported as excluded in 86 trials (56%). Patients with CKD were more likely to be excluded from trials that were multicenter, of moderate enrollment size, North American, that tested renin angiotensin aldosterone system antagonists and anticoagulants, and that tested chronic congestive heart failure. Only eight original articles (5%) reported the proportion of enrolled patients with CKD, and only 15 (10%) reported mean baseline kidney function. While 81 trials (53%) performed subgroup analyses of some baseline characteristic in the original article, just four subgroup analyses of treatments stratified by kidney disease were performed (3%). It was concluded that major cardiovascular disease trials frequently excluded patients with CKD and did not provide adequate information on the kidney function of enrollees or the effect of interventions on patients with kidney disease.[21]

The lack of information on the safety and efficacy of therapeutic interventions in CKD has been further hampered by the lack of awareness of CKD among affected individuals as well as primary care providers. In a recent study to assess CKD awareness among individuals with clinical markers of impaired kidney function, CKD awareness was assessed in 1852 adults with an estimated glomerular filtration rate (GFR) less than 60 mL/min/1.73 m^2 using 1999 to 2008 National Health and Nutrition Examination Survey (NHANES) data. The answer for CKD awareness was a binary response (yes/no) to the question: "Have you ever been told you have weak or failing kidneys?" Participants were grouped by distribution of the following abnormal markers of CKD: hyperkalemia, acidosis, hyperphosphatemia, elevated blood urea nitrogen, anemia, albuminuria, and uncontrolled hypertension. Odds of CKD awareness associated with each abnormal marker and groupings of markers were estimated by multivariable logistic regression. Surprisingly, 90% of individuals with two to four markers of CKD and 84% of individuals with five markers of CKD were unaware of their disease.[22]

Estimates of primary care provider recognition of CKD remain alarmingly low. Reported physician documentation of CKD with International Classification of Diseases, Ninth Revision, Clinical Modification (ICD-9-CM) codes in a large managed care cohort with more than 10,000 individuals with CKD stages 3 to 5 was only 14.4%.[23] Early referral of patients to nephrologists is optimal, but given the relatively small number of practicing nephrologists nationwide, nephrologists cannot manage all patients with CKD exclusively. The burden of CKD management thus falls largely on primary care providers. Although current data are limited, the general consensus is that awareness of CKD by all types of primary care providers is unacceptably low, and knowledge of CKD management is particularly poor among family practice physicians.[24] Boulware and colleagues used several clinical scenarios to ascertain knowledge surrounding basic CKD awareness and management; 40% of U.S. family physicians failed to recognize progressive CKD in a patient with a serum creatinine level of 2.0 mg/dL and gross proteinuria.[25]

Agrawal and associates have demonstrated similar rates of awareness among internal medicine residents (physicians in training) across the United States.[26] Again using a clinical vignette describing a patient with persistent proteinuria and estimated GFR (eGFR) of 76 mL/min/1.73 m^2, only 54% of responders correctly identified proteinuria as a marker of CKD. However, 65% of residents correctly identified CKD stage 3 with an eGFR range of 30 to 59 mL/min/1.73 m^2, and nearly 87% and 73% noted that eGFR and a random urine albumin/creatinine ratio, respectively, should be used to evaluate a patient at high risk of CKD.[25] Examination of medical records to ascertain primary care physician recognition of CKD has yielded similar results. In one academic, outpatient, family medicine practice, only 13.9% of physicians documented awareness of CKD stage 3, defined by any written evidence of CKD recognition in the medical chart; this included CKD in the problem list, ordering of diagnostic investigations for impaired kidney function, and referral to a nephrologist.[27] However, it was important to note that CKD recognition increased dramatically after an educational curriculum to 85.1%, suggesting that provider identification of CKD could be improved through targeted interventions.[27]

QUALITY IMPROVEMENT TOOLS

Errors are caused by system or process failures, so it is important to adopt various process improvement techniques to identify inefficiencies, ineffective care, and preventable errors that could then influence changes associated with systems.[28] Efforts to improve quality need to be measured to demonstrate "whether improvement efforts (1) lead to change in the primary endpoint in the desired direction, (2) contribute to unintended results in different parts of the system, and (3) require additional efforts to bring a process back into acceptable ranges."[29] Health care systems are complex entities, and the uniquely differing models of delivery of services available, unpredictable nature of health care, and occupational differentiation and interdependence among clinicians and systems make measuring quality difficult.[30-32] One of the challenges in using measures in health care is the attribution variability associated with high-level cognitive reasoning, discretionary decision making, problem solving, and experiential knowledge.[33-35]

The rationale for measuring quality improvement is the belief that good performance reflects good-quality practice, and that comparing performance among providers and organizations will encourage better performance. There has been a surge in measuring and reporting the performance of health care systems and processes.[29,36,37] While public reporting of quality performance can be used to identify areas needing improvement and ascribe national, state, or other level benchmarks, some providers have been sensitive to the publication of comparative performance data.[38,39] Another audience for public reporting—consumers—has had problems interpreting the data in reports and has consequently not used the reports to the extent hoped to make informed decisions for higher quality care.[29,40]

The complexity of health care systems and delivery of services, unpredictable nature of health care, and occupational differentiation and interdependence among clinicians and systems makes measuring quality difficult. One of the challenges in using measures in health care is the variability in attribution associated with high-level cognitive reasoning, discretionary decision making, problem solving, and experiential knowledge.[36] Another measurement challenge is whether a near-miss could have resulted in harm or whether an adverse event represented a rare aberration or one likely to recur.[36]

In our complex medical environment, physicians have relied primarily on paper tools, memory, and hard work to improve the care given to patients. However, creation of reliable and sustained improvement in health care is difficult with the use of traditional methods. Improvement often requires deliberate redesign of processes based on knowledge of human factors—how people interact with products and processes and tools known to assist improvement. The clear ethical imperative to enhance the quality and safety of care, while fulfilling external accreditation requirements and consumer expectations, requires physicians to address quality of care issues systematically.[41,42]

Continuous quality improvement (CQI) subscribes to the principle that opportunity for improvement exists in every process on every occasion. Within an organization, it requires a commitment to improve operations, processes, and activities constantly to meet patient needs in an efficient, consistent, and cost-effective manner. The CQI model emphasizes the view of health care as a process and focuses on the system rather than on the individual when considering improvement opportunities.[43]

Table 87.1 Summary of Commonly Used Methodologies in Health Care Quality Improvement

Methodology	Approach to Improvement	Process Overview
PDSA (PDCA)	Develop hypothesis, test by conducting experiments and testing improvements iteratively on a local basis; scale based on results	Plan. Do. Study (or check). Act.
Lean	Eliminate waste, improve flow, maximizing value added and minimizing non–value-added activities	Identify value. Identify value stream. Flow. Pull. Perfection.
Six Sigma	Reducing variation and eliminating deviation in processes	Define. Measure. Analyze. Improve. Control.

A host of methodologies are available for achieving quality improvement and include Plan-Do-Study-Act (PDSA), Six Sigma, lean production strategies, root cause analysis, failure modes and effects analysis, and a number of techniques used in different stages of these methodologies (e.g., flow diagrams or charts, cause and effect diagrams, Pareto diagrams, histograms, run charts, control charts among others).[10] The most common quality improvement (QI) methodologies used in health care are PDSA, Six Sigma, and lean strategies. The choice of methodology depends on the nature of the improvement project. Within most methodologies, users will find similar techniques. Most of them typically include iterative testing of ideas and redesign of process or technology based on lessons learned. More recently, experts have been using principles from different methodologies for the same project (i.e., use of lean-sigma methodology), thus making distinctions less relevant.[43] Three of the most commonly used methodologies in health care quality improvement are briefly discussed here and are summarized in Table 87.1.

PLAN-DO-STUDY-ACT

The PDSA, also known as the Plan-Do-Check-Act (PDCA), is a common approach for improving processes in health care (as well as in other industries). The basic premise of this approach (Figure 87.1) is to develop (Plan) a hypothesis (Change), experiment with this change in process (Do), study the results (Study), and take action depending on the results (Act). This approach is considered a staple of health care and is a central tenet of the United Kingdom's National Health Service QI framework.

LEAN

The lean principle has been defined as a set of concepts, principles, and tools used to create and deliver the most value from the customer's perspective while consuming the fewest resources and fully using the knowledge and skills of the people performing the work (Figure 87.2). Lean is based on the principle that the purpose of any organization is to create value for the people it serves (its users or customers). Value is created by satisfying a need or solving a problem for the customer (in the case of laboratory medicine, the customers are usually clinicians and patients). All value is delivered by processes—predictable sequences of actions linked together to deliver a desired outcome. Lean refers to the end to end process, extending from the customer request to delivery of the service back to the customer. This is termed the *value stream.* Lean management systems focus on understanding what the customer needs and then redesigning and continuously improving the value stream by removing the waste (*muda,* Japanese term for waste) that prevents value being delivered to service users. Waste is best defined as anything that consumes resources but does not contribute to creating value for the customer. Lean thinking subdivides waste into a number of categories, but the most important type of waste to eliminate is error or defects that occur as a result of problems in the process. In addition to waste, lean identifies and targets two other signs of an unproductive process; (1) unevenness of workflow, which is often created by a poorly designed process in which capacity and demand are not matched at each step, resulting in queues with excessive work in progress; (2) overburdening of staff or equipment by creating unreasonable expectations of what can be done at any point in time given the current state of the process. Lean is about helping people work smarter, not driving them to work harder.[44] The eight common so-called wastes of health care are as follows:

1. Unnecessary motion—the many physical steps needed to gather equipment, move patients, and confirm instructions or orders
2. Unnecessary transportation
3. Defects and errors—Time spent doing something incorrectly and then inspecting for and correcting errors
4. Waiting—time spent waiting for the next event or step in the process to occur
5. Inventory—any supply in excess of the bare minimum needed to meet customer demand
6. Processing waste—extra effort that provides no value from patient perspective, such as repeatedly asking the same questions
7. Overproduction—doing more than what is needed or sooner than when it is needed
8. Unused human potential—any situation in which people are not used to the maximum of their potential to add value to processes[44a]

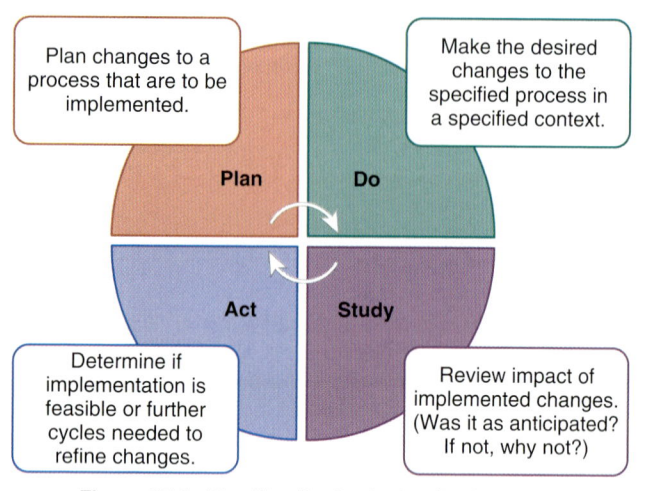

Figure 87.1 The Plan-Do-Study-Act (PDSA) Cycle.

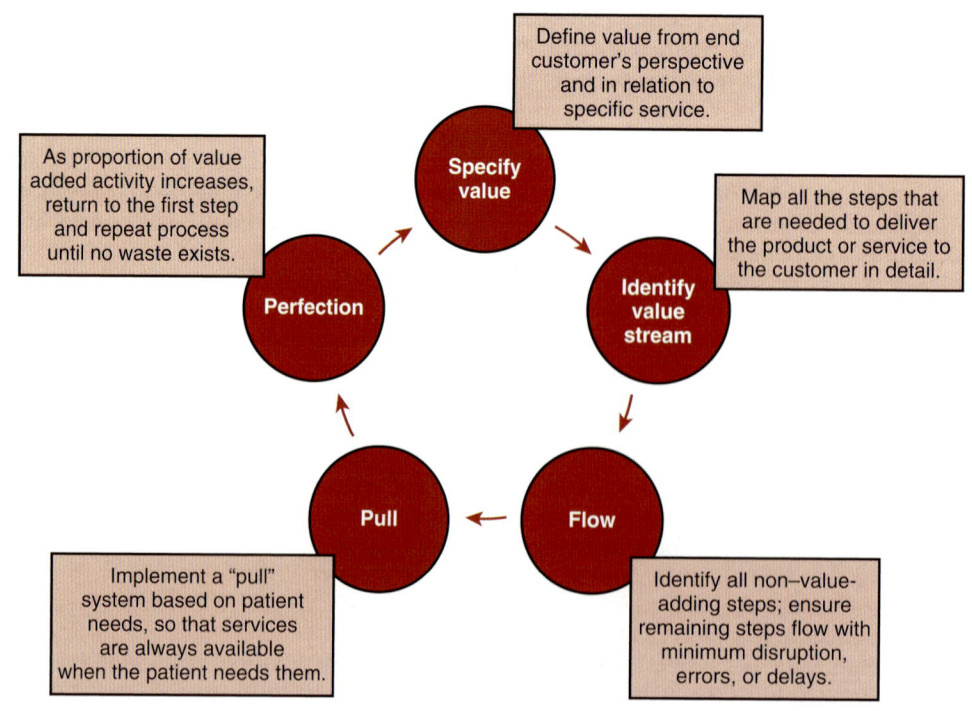

Figure 87.2 Lean principles.

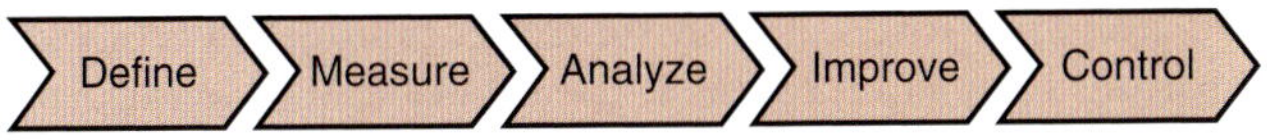

Figure 87.3 Six Sigma DMAIC (Define-Measure-Analyze-Improve-Control) process.

SIX SIGMA

Six Sigma was originally developed as a set of tools and strategies by Motorola in 1986 to improve processes. It was subsequently made famous by General Electric after it won the Malcolm Baldrige National Quality Award in 1988. As its premise, Six Sigma emphasizes the use of information and statistical analyses to rigorously and routinely measure and improve an organization's performance, practices, and systems. The goal of Six Sigma is to reduce the occurrence of defects or errors from their current level within a health care organization (HCO) to the Six Sigma standard of 3.4 defects or errors per million opportunities (DPMO). Although Six Sigma may vary in how it is used in an organization, it has several defining factors that all implementations should have in common. These five elements are as follows:

1. Intent—Six Sigma initiatives are undertaken with the intent to achieve significant improvement.
2. Strategy—This is applied throughout an HCO as a corporate strategy or where appropriate at the tactical level on individual projects.
3. Methodology—Numerous methodologies are available; the one most commonly used in health care is the DMAIC (Define, Measure, Analyze, Improve, and Control; Figure 87.3).
4. Tools—Numerous tools can be used; some are specific to Six Sigma (requirements gathering, Kano's model, statistical analysis, and experimentation), while others (most statistical methods) have been adopted into the methodology.
5. Measurements—Three of the most common measurements used in Six Sigma are DPU (defects/errors per unit), DPMO, and Sigma level (one sigma level is ≈690,000 DPMO, while a Six Sigma level is ≈3.4 DPMO).[44a]

QUALITY IMPROVEMENT IN NEPHROLOGY

In 1965, Medicare was enacted to provide health insurance for persons 65 years of age and older, thereby decreasing age-based health disparities and attempting to create a social safety net for this age group. In 1972, this benefit was extended to all who were disabled, regardless of age. This Social Security Amendment, signed by President Richard M. Nixon on October 30, 1972, included Medicare coverage for those "disabled" with end-stage kidney disease (ESKD) and resulted in expanded access to dialytic therapies and transplantation, beginning on July 1, 1973.[45,46] It remains the only disease-specific entitlement program with coverage for all modalities of renal replacement therapy (RRT, as any form of dialysis or kidney transplantation) and non–renal-related services, regardless of age. The immediate impact in 1973 was the provision of the option of RRT for over 90% of U.S. citizens who required it. Unfortunately, although allowing payment for RRT, it did not address other barriers to accessing care or the numerous socioeconomic variables that were subsequently confirmed to influence patient outcomes.

To understand the consequences of this entitlement funding, the Health Care Finance Administration in 1977 established a data system requiring annual reports from dialysis providers. This system was succeeded by the U.S. Renal Data System (USRDS), an independently contracted entity charged with monitoring RRT practices and outcomes.[47,48] The objective was to establish best practices and initiate studies to improve care via the analysis of ESKD treatment data. The 1991 IOM report, *Kidney Failure and the Federal Government*, outlined the quality of ESKD care, driving the focus toward care processes and patient-centered outcomes, including health-related quality of life (QOL) and functional status.[49] This report imposed shared responsibility among providers, payers, and patients. To achieve this goal, the distribution and sharing of large volumes of CKD data among engaged stakeholders would be required. It is anticipated that critical analyses of such data would yield greater understanding and future education regarding health disparity, inhomogeneity of practice, quality of care and, conceivably, cost. Furthermore, such analyses have the potential to inform and identify targeted interventions for enhanced care.

QUALITY IMPROVEMENT INITIATIVES IN END-STAGE KIDNEY DISEASE

EMERGING QUALITY IMPROVEMENTS IN KIDNEY DISEASE

These include the National End-Stage Renal Disease Program, ESKD networks, ESKD quality initiative, and Three-Part Aim. Quality improvement initiatives in nephrology are robust and are largely attributable to the advent of the National End-Stage Renal Disease Program, Section 299I of Public Law 92-603 under Medicare, passed by Congress on October 30, 1972. The National End-Stage Renal Disease Program is Medicare's only disease-specific program that guarantees coverage to all individuals based on diagnosis, which in 2011 applied to 615,899 prevalent patients with ESKD and 6009 dialysis facilities across the United States.[49a] The subsequent establishment of 32 coordinating ESKD network organizations in 1976 fostered the aim of delivering high-quality service to ESKD patients in a safe, effective, patient-centered, timely, efficient, and equitable fashion.[50,51] In 1978, Congress amended Title XVIII of the Social Security Act to improve cost-effectiveness and quality of care to ESKD patients, encouraging accountability as well as kidney transplantation and home dialysis.[52] Multiple stakeholders involved in the provision of ESKD services were linked together into Network Coordinating Councils. The Centers for Medicare & Medicaid Services (CMS) reduced the number of ESKD Networks in 1998, awarding contracts to 18 geographically designated organizations. These networks are expected to support and cooperate with each other and with Quality Improvement Organizations (QIOs), Medicare Advantage organizations, state survey agencies, professional and patient organizations, and ESKD facilities and providers. Individually, each network must ensure that patients "get the right care at the right time" by adhering to the following principles[51]:

- Ensuring the effective and efficient administration of benefits
- Improving quality of care for ESKD patients
- Collecting data to measure quality of care
- Providing assistance to ESKD patients and providers
- Evaluating and resolving patient grievances

CMS later solicited competitive contract and award proposals from nine networks in June 2012. These challenged awardees with the task of achieving national improvement goals in alignment with the Health and Human Services National Quality Strategy[53] and the CMS Three-Part Aim (so-called Triple Aim by the IOM) of improved care, lower per capita cost, and enhancement of population-based health care, among other priorities.[54]

The CMS Quality Initiative launched in 2002 was expanded in 2004 to include dialysis facilities that provide services for patients with ESKD, leading to the ESKD Quality Initiative. The objective of the initiative was to stimulate and support significant improvement in the quality of dialysis care, which varied widely. Goals of the initiative included compliance with governmentally designed Conditions for Coverage (CfCs) and the standardization and refinement of dialysis care measures, the results of which would be electronically available to lay personnel and patients. These would enable more informed decisions to be made via Dialysis Facility Compare, hosted by the official Medicare website, Medicare.gov.[55] The provision and maintenance of health care quality was an explicit goal that would be achieved by strategic partnerships among all involved stakeholders. Components of the Initiative were several. The CfCs were revised and published in 2005 as a notice of proposed rule making.[56] An In-Center Hemodialysis Patient Consumer Assessment of Healthcare Providers and Systems (ICH CAHPS) survey was developed in partnership with the Agency for Healthcare Research and Quality (AHRQ) to evaluate patients' experiences. An agency-wide initiative, the Fistula First Breakthrough Initiative (FFBI),[57] would promote a major shift in vascular access practice using the goal of a graduated increase in prevalence rates for arteriovenous fistulas. A standard battery of Clinical Performance Measures was conceived to measure dialysis adequacy, anemia management, and vascular access practice to identify areas for quality improvement based on the National Kidney Foundation Kidney Disease Outcomes Quality Initiative (NKF KDOQI) clinical practice guidelines, with the latter complementing the FFBI. In addition, standardization of data elements and their transmission to CMS by an ESKD information system, Consolidated Renal Operations in a Web-based Network (CROWN), would facilitate data entry and analysis.

Quality improvement in ESKD at the legislative level has been interdependent, with a confluence of initiatives occurring at multiple levels, including renal physician, nursing and patient-based advocacy organizations, dialysis providers and facilities, state survey agencies, and health systems. The high costs of ESKD have provided legislative impetus, with an emphasis on cost-effectiveness. With an increasing annual prevalence of dialysis patients (+3.2% in 2011), the cost of dialysis has escalated in parallel with combined Medicare and non-Medicare expenses of $49.3 billion.[58] Initial high priorities for CMS have been the QI issues and health care costs associated with anemia management and vascular access practice. Both areas have directly catalyzed implementation of the 2011 bundled ESKD Prospective Payment System (PPS) and pay-for-performance Quality Incentive Program (QIP), thus foreshadowing the creation of accountable care organizations with quality measure–based monitoring to incentivize improvements in the quality of care while containing overall costs.[59]

ROLE OF ERYTHROPOIESIS-STIMULATING AGENTS IN CATALYZING QUALITY IMPROVEMENT

Likely the single most important driving factor initially leading to the development of the 2011 bundled ESKD PPS and QIP has been the use of erythropoiesis-stimulating agents (ESAs) to manage anemia in ESKD. Approaching 10% of the total Medicare cost for dialysis has been the cost of ESAs, which represent the highest drug class expenditure in Medicare Part B and the major, modifiable hemodialysis treatment cost.[60] Decisions regarding optimal anemia management using ESAs to achieve hemoglobin and hematocrit targets have been directly tied to cost-effective dialysis care and optimal patient outcomes as reflections of quality of care. This has been a governmental priority leading to multiple CMS reimbursement policy changes against a backdrop of U.S. Food and Drug Administration (FDA)–issued public advisories, as well as the institution of the Quality Incentive Program in January 1, 2012.[61] Studying the use of ESAs in ESKD provides important insight into the interactions among clinical study data, evidence-based scientific guidelines, health care economics, and national policies aiming to improve patient care.[59,62]

Anemia of chronic kidney disease is a well-established ESKD complication, with a prevalence of 44% in CKD stage 4 patients to more than 90% in CKD stage 5 patients on hemodialysis.[63-66] The introduction of the first ESA, epoetin alfa, in 1989[67] represented a clinical breakthrough by dramatically improving hemoglobin levels in ESKD patients and their QOL while reducing frequent blood transfusions, particularly those on hemodialysis. With FDA approval based on such benefits, ESA use (epoetin alfa, darbepoetin alfa) in hemodialysis patients became widespread, not only throughout the United States (93.6% of U.S. patients as of 2011) but worldwide.[68] Total expenditures for ESAs alone rose from $246 million in 1991 to almost $1.9 billion by 2006, representing approximately 10% of total Medicare dialysis costs, with peak expenditures occurring in 2004 (Figure 87.4).

It is noteworthy that in the period leading up to 2004, the threefold increase in weekly administered epoetin dose (Figure 87.5) originated as a product of observational study data, changes in clinical practice guidelines and clinical practice, and financial incentives for dialysis providers based on Medicare payments for ESAs outside of the bundled payment system composite rate. The initial target hematocrit approved by the FDA in 1989 was 30% to 33%, based in part on data regarding optimal cerebral oxygen transport[69] and, by 1991, the mean monthly hemoglobin level in the United States was 9.6 g/dL, with 28% of patients having a hemoglobin level less than 9 g/dL.[58] However, evidence supported improved clinical parameters associated with higher hematocrit levels (cardiac function, exercise tolerance, muscle strength, cognitive function, QOL),[70,71] while increased risks of hospitalization and mortality were associated with hemoglobin levels less than 10 to 11 g/dL in large observational studies.[72-77] Anemia management practice in ESKD was initially driven by such observational data, the results of which were translated into clinical practice guidelines (Table 87.2). Both the NKF KDOQI clinical practice guidelines published in 1997[78] and subsequent 2001 NKF KDOQI update[79] accordingly recommended a hemoglobin target of 11 to 12 g/dL. Within several years, observational studies suggested a further survival benefit with even higher hemoglobin levels, 12 to 13 g/dL.[72,74,76,77] Revised KDOQI guidelines in 2006, supported by a new CMS epoetin coverage reimbursement policy, further raised the target upper limit to 13 g/dL,[80] with the effect that by the end of 2006, only 18.6% of U.S. hemodialysis patients had a hemoglobin level less than 11 g/dL, with 53.4% having a hemoglobin level higher than 12 g/dL, in striking contrast to 15 years prior.

Following 2006, however, clinical practice and FDA guidelines, and the payment and target criteria of the CMS bundled Prospective Payment System and Quality Incentive Program, respectively, underwent dramatic change in response to a number of randomized control studies (see Table 87.2). These linked hemoglobin targets and ESA dosing to concerns over cardiovascular mortality and all-cause mortality. ESA administration to achieve higher (≥ 13 g/dL) and lower (≤ 11.5 g/dL) hemoglobin targets was examined in RCTs of hemodialysis patients (Normal Hematocrit Cardiac Trial) and in late-stage G3B-G4 chronic kidney disease patients (CHOIR, CREATE, and TREAT studies). The Normal Hematocrit Cardiac Trial was prematurely halted given a higher occurrence of the primary end point (time to death, first nonfatal myocardial infarction [MI]) in the higher hemoglobin group.[81] Similarly, in CHOIR (Correction of Hemoglobin and Outcomes in Renal Insufficiency[82]) and, to a lesser extent in CREATE (Cardiovascular Risk Reduction by Early Anemia Treatment with Epoetin Beta[83]), higher hemoglobin targets were associated with worse composite cardiovascular outcomes and death compared to lower hemoglobin targets. No differences in the composite end points of cardiovascular/all-cause death or ESKD/all-cause death were observed in TREAT (Trial to Reduce Cardiovascular Events with Aranesp Therapy), with the exception of a small increased stroke risk.[84] In a meta-analysis of 27 RCTs of ESA treatment in CKD patients, Palmer and colleagues[85] found no increased risks for

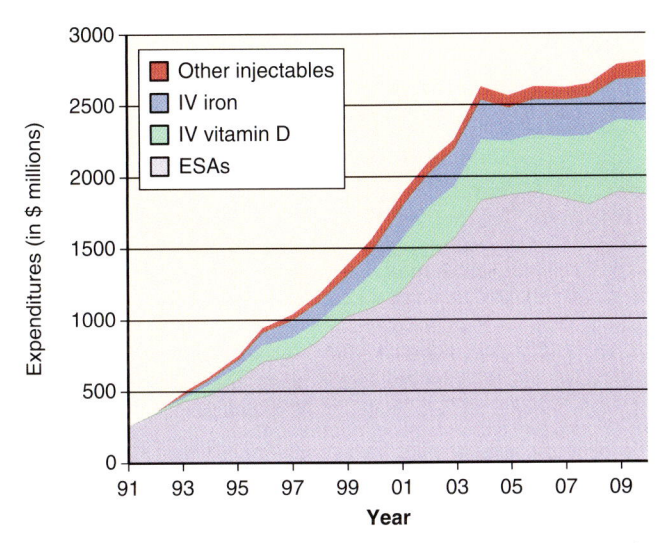

Figure 87.4 Yearly Medicare costs for injectable medications for dialysis patients. Erythropoiesis-stimulating agents (ESAs) accounted for $1.87 billion of the total $28 billion spent in 2010, followed by $519 million for vitamin D analogues and $304 million for intravenous (IV) iron. (Adapted from U.S. Renal Data System: *USRDS 2012 annual data report: atlas of chronic kidney disease and end-stage renal disease in the United States,* Bethesda, Md, 2012, National Institutes of Health, National Institute of Diabetes and Digestive and Kidney Disease.)

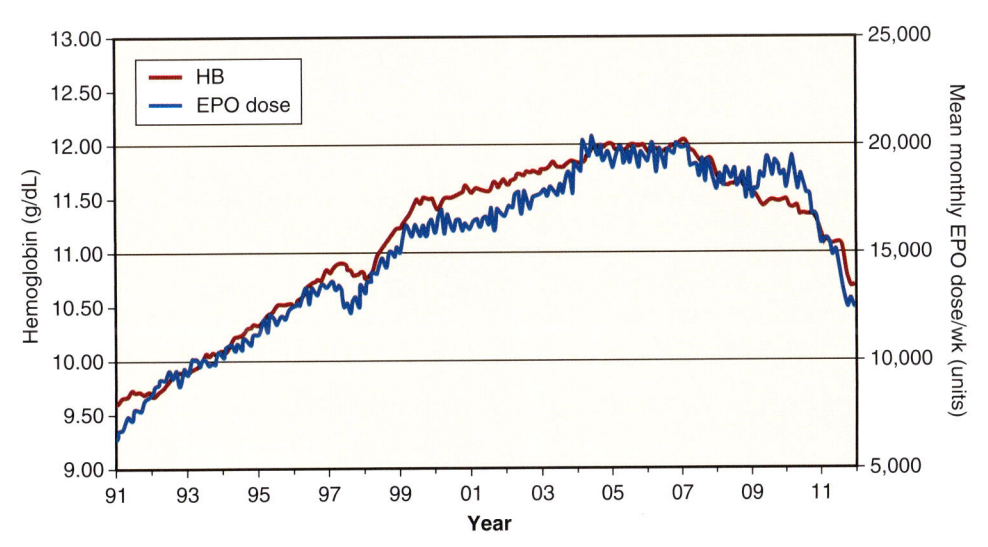

Figure 87.5 Mean monthly hemoglobin (HB) and monthly erythropoietin alfa (EPO) dose per week for prevalent hemodialysis patients. EPO doses consistently declined, beginning in 2006 from a peak monthly dose per week and mean monthly Hb of 20,128 U and 12.0 g/dL, respectively, to 12,460 U and 10.7 g/dL by the end of 2011. (Adapted from U.S. Renal Data System: *USRDS 2013 annual data report: atlas of chronic kidney disease and end-stage renal disease in the United States,* Bethesda, Md, 2013, National Institutes of Health, National Institute of Diabetes and Digestive and Kidney Disease.)

Table 87.2 Changes in Hemoglobin (Hb) and Hematocrit (Hct) Target Guidelines in End-Stage Kidney Disease Over Time

Month, Year	Organization	Hemoglobin, Hematocrit Targets
June 1989	FDA	Hct 30%-33%
1989	HCFA	Hct ≤ 36%
June 1994	FDA	Hct 30%-36%
1995	NKF—Dialysis Outcomes Quality Initiative established	
1997	NKF DOQI	Hb 11 to 12 g/dL
Feb 1997	HCFA	Hct ≤ 36.5%
Aug 1998	Normal HCT study published	
1999	EBPG established	
2001	NKF-KDOQI	Hb 11-12 g/dL
2004	EBPG	Hb >11 g/dL; Hb >14 g/dL not recommended
Apr 2006	CMS EMP	Hb 10-12 g/dL; 25% ESA dose reduction for Hb >13 g/dL
May 2006	NKF-KDOQI	Hb ≥ 11 g/dL; Hb ≥ 13 g/dL not recommended
November 2006	CHOIR and CREATE studies published	
November 2006	FDA	Hb 10-12 g/dL; avoid Hb >12 g/dL; black box warning
March 2007	FDA	Hb ≤ 12 g/dL; hold ESAs if Hb > 12 g/dL; use lowest dose to avoid blood transfusions.
September 2007	NKF-KDOQI	Revision, Hb 11-12 g/dL; Hb ≥ 13 g/dL not recommended
January 2008	CMS EMP	50% dose reduction for Hb >13 g/dL × 3 consecutive months; maximum monthly epoetin 400,000 U/mo or darbepoetin 1200 µg/mo
November 2009	TREAT study published	
2011	FDA	Post-6/24/11: Hb 10 to ≤11 g/dL; use lowest dose to avoid blood transfusions; warning of increased risks if Hb > 11 g/dL (death, adverse cardiovascular outcomes, stroke, venous thromboembolism, vascular access thrombosis, tumor progression)
January 2011	CMS	Prospective Payment System: inclusion of ESAs, IV iron, and IV vitamin D sterols
November 2011	CMS ESKD QIP (PY 2012)	Hb 10-12 g/dL
2012	KDIGO	Hb ≥ 9-11.5 g/dL; Hb ≥ 13 g/dL not recommended
November 2012	CMS ESKD QIP (PY 2013)	Hb ≤ 12 g/dL; avoid Hb > 12 g/dL (Hb < 10 g/dL retired; no Hb lower threshold)

CMS EMP, CMS erythropoiesis-stimulating agent monitoring program; CMS, Centers for Medicare & Medicaid Services; EBPG, European Best Practice Guidelines; FDA, U.S. Food and Drug Administration; HCFA, Health Care Financing Administration; IV, intravenous; KDIGO, Kidney Disease Improving Global Outcomes; NKF DOQI/KDOQI, National Kidney Foundation Dialysis/Kidney Disease Outcomes Quality Initiative; QIP, Quality Incentive Program.

See text for Normal HCT, CHOIR (Correction of Hemoglobin and Outcomes in Renal Insufficiency), CREATE (Cardiovascular Risk Reduction by Early Anemia Treatment with Epoetin Beta), and TREAT (Trial to Reduce Cardiovascular Events with Aranesp Therapy) studies.

all-cause mortality or significant cardiovascular events between higher and lower hemoglobin targets, but there were increased risks for progressive hypertension, stroke, and vascular access thrombosis. The end result was a reversal in ESA use, mean hemoglobin levels, and Medicare expenditures, in part through mandated (CMS ESA Monitoring Program, FDA) guidelines (see Table 87.2).[86,87] By the end of 2011, the use of ESKD agents, primarily ESAs, had decreased by one third when compared to 2007, thus lowering Medicare expenditures by an estimated $750 million.[88] The mean hemoglobin level in hemodialysis patients at the end of 2011 was 10.7 g/dL compared to 12.1 g/dL in 2007 (see Figure 87.5), while lower ESA use would also translate to an increased transfusion rate in hemodialysis patients.[58]

BUNDLED PROSPECTIVE PAYMENT SYSTEM AND QUALITY INCENTIVE PROGRAM

To reduce total expenditures for ESKD by shifting financial risk from payer to dialysis provider in the wake of events related to ESA use and cost, a bundled PPS for outpatient dialysis treatment costs was implemented in January 2011 under the aegis of the Medicare Improvement for Patients and Providers Act of 2008 (MIPPA).[89] Under this act, dialysis services were to be reimbursed by fixed compensation, the composite rate, in a bundled payment system that encompassed all costs, including prior separately billed items such as ESAs and vitamin D analogues, thus disincentivizing ESA use for potential financial gain by dialysis providers.[90] In the United States and Japan, the primary cost end point was to contain ESA payments.[91] A similar bundled payment system in Japan (2006) targeted an overall reduction of 4% in expenditures compared to the mandated MIPPA reduction of 2%. The effect was a decrease in hemodialysis ESA dose by 11.8%.[92] While the largest source of dialysis facility income was the composite rate in the United States, the second largest source, approximately 20% of all payments to facilities, consisted of Medicare ESA payments.[93] Effective January 1, 2012, CMS also instituted the QIP, its first system-wide, pay-for-performance system. This consisted of three quality metrics, again with the emphasis on measuring ESA use in ESKD anemia management (hemoglobin < 10 g/dL, hemoglobin > 12 g/dL; urea reduction ratio ≥ 65%). Both the PPS and QIP encourage dialysis facilities to maximize Medicare payment reimbursement based on performance.[89] The net effect was a continued decline in ESA prescribing, mean weekly dose of epoetin alfa administered to ESKD patients,[88] as well as a concomitant lower use of intravenous iron and vitamin D analogues (see Figure 87.5).[87]

Highlighting the balance between health care quality improvement and cost containment, commentary from patient organizations (e.g., Kidney Care Partners,[94] American Kidney Fund[95]), physician organizations (e.g., Renal Physicians Association,[96] National Kidney Foundation, American Society of Nephrology), and nursing organizations (e.g., American Nephrology Nurses Association[97]) during the planning and implementation period of the MIPPA voiced the need to avoid juxtaposing health care quality improvement against financial disincentive. While there have been real economic incentives to reduce ESA use, the health benefits resulting from a reduction are not as clear cut. Subsequent to the Normal Hematocrit Cardiac Trial and CHOIR, analyses have suggested that ESA hyporesponsiveness, and not simply a high hemoglobin target, achieved hemoglobin level, or absolute ESA dose, may play a role in mortality risk by indicating coexisting disease burden.[66,77,98-100] An optimal hemoglobin range is yet to be determined beyond previously studied and currently mandated targets.[62,101,102]

Under the bundled payment system, quality improvement initiatives based on anemia management strategies, which optimize cost-effectiveness by limiting total ESA dose while at the same time achieving stable target hemoglobin levels and minimizing variation,[103-107] will be strongly favored. Anemia management algorithms, which were initially paper based and facility centered or later computer assisted and dialysis provider–wide, have been credited for increasing the percentage of patients achieving hemoglobin targets,[106] reducing hemoglobin standard deviations from target levels,[86] and improving efficiency in anemia management.[108] Computer-assisted algorithms based on pharmacodynamic modeling or artificial neural network strategies promise further reductions in hemoglobin level variability (cycling) and improved patient safety.[109-114]

VASCULAR ACCESS PRACTICE, FISTULA FIRST BREAKTHROUGH INITIATIVE, AND QUALITY IMPROVEMENT

Increasing the early creation and use of permanent vascular access, optimally an arteriovenous fistula (AVF)[115] or arteriovenous graft (AVG), as opposed to a tunneled dialysis catheter (TDC) in hemodialysis patients, has been a major goal and an established standard of care for incident and prevalent hemodialysis patients to improve survival and reduce morbidity and hospitalization.[116] Optimally, a CKD stage 5 patient begins outpatient hemodialysis after 6 months or more of vascular access planning by a nephrologist using a vascular access, surgeon-constructed AVF, which is associated with the lowest rates of thrombosis and infection. However, the vast majority of U.S. hemodialysis patients initiate dialysis using a TDC, which is associated not only with the highest complication rate but also the worst survival outcomes, principally from cardiac death. Cardiac death has remained the most important cause of mortality in incident dialysis patients, accounting for 35% of deaths, with two thirds of these due to cardiac sudden death.[58,117]

Early on, USRDS Dialysis Morbidity and Mortality Study Wave 1 data in 5507 prevalent hemodialysis patients showed that patients with TDCs had a higher mortality risk than patients dialyzed using an AVF. TDCs were associated with higher infection-related and cardiac-related deaths; overall, 45% of deaths were cardiac deaths.[118] The association of increased mortality and morbidity with TDC use in hemodialysis patients has been well established in multiple studies with an especially high risk in incident patients.[119-123] The greatest mortality risk occurs during the initial 90 to 120 days (27.5 deaths/100 person-years), accounting for 50% of deaths during the first year and coinciding with the period during which over 80% of U.S. hemodialysis patients initiated dialysis using a TDC.[58,123,124] Patients initiating dialysis using a TDC have an increased mortality risk during their first 3 months of hemodialysis compared to those initiating dialysis using an AVF, likely related to bacteremia, central venous stenosis, chronic inflammation, ESA resistance, hospitalization, and, most significantly, cardiovascular events.[120,125] In 4802 incident hemodialysis patients from the Dialysis Outcomes and Practice Patterns Study (DOPPS), dialysis catheters accounted for the largest attributable fraction of mortality risk during this early period and represented the primary modifiable mortality risk factor.[123] The higher mortality risk of hemodialysis patients in the United States compared to that in Europe and Japan (36% to 40% and 3.6-fold greater, respectively), in whom TDC use is substantially lower (0% to 5% in >90% facilities in Japan), is attributable in large part to differences in vascular access practice.[102,122]

Studies of incident and prevalent hemodialysis patient populations have demonstrated a significant reduction in mortality and hospitalization following vascular access conversion from TDC to permanent vascular access, in particular for AVFs.[120,121,123,126] In 3904 incident hemodialysis patients, conversion of a TDC to permanent access within a 4-month period was associated with a reduction in mortality risk over the subsequent 8 months.[120] Similarly, conversion of TDCs to AVFs in incident hemodialysis patients from DOPPS I and II also decreased the risk of death during the first year on hemodialysis. In contrast, failure of permanent vascular access and conversion to TDC was associated with an 81% increase in mortality.[126]

In 2011, over 80% of U.S. incident hemodialysis patients began dialysis as an outpatient using a TDC, while only 15.8% and 2.9% of incident patients used an AVF or AVG, respectively. Overall, 37% of patients had a permanent vascular access in use or maturing. These figures attest to the importance of pre-ESKD nephrology care prior to dialysis initiation, given that 42% of patients initiating therapy had not seen a nephrologist. Initiation using an AVF occurred in only 10.5% of those without prior nephrology care in contrast to 50.2% of those with prior care.[58] In keeping with other studies,[127,128] Bradbury concluded that pre-ESKD nephrology care is associated with a lower risk of death within the first year of hemodialysis,[123] especially within the first 4-month period, but not afterward. This might have

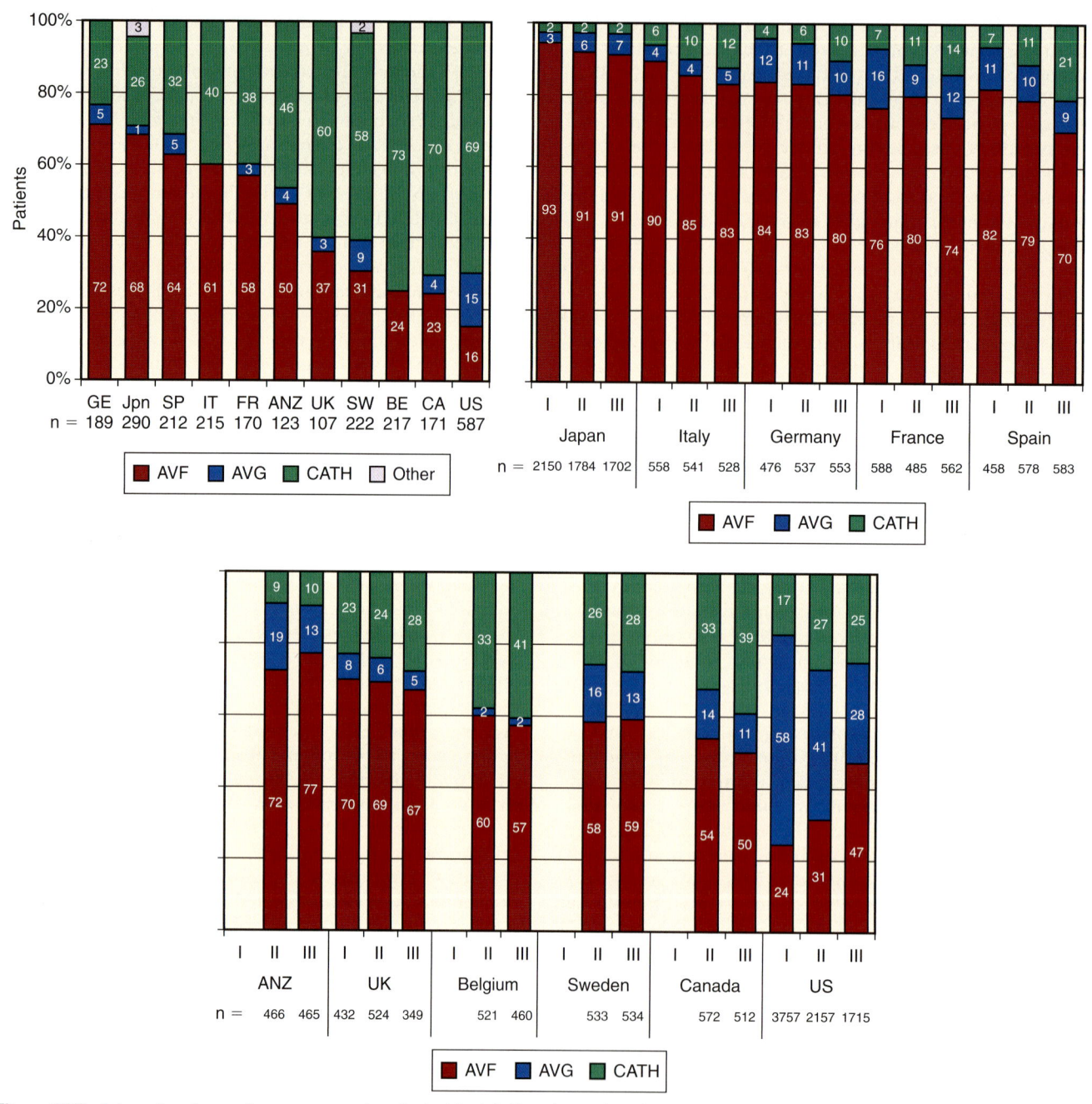

Figure 87.6 International vascular access use trends. Incident (*left*) and prevalent (*right*) hemodialysis patients (N ≥ 35,000) are indicated by country in DOPPS I, II, and III (1996 to 2007). ANZ, Australia-New Zealand; AVF, arteriovenous fistula; AVG, arteriovenous graft; BE, Belgium; CA, Canada; CATH, hemodialysis catheter; FR, France; GE, Germany; IT, Italy; Jpn, Japan; SP, Spain; SW, Sweden; UK, United Kingdom; US, United States. (From Ethier J, Mendelssohn DC, Elder SJ, et al: Vascular access use and outcomes: an international perspective from the dialysis outcomes and practice patterns study. *Nephrol Dial Transplant* 23:3219-3226, 2008.)

been anticipated if there were a role for vascular access planning in modifying mortality risk. In some regions, 73% of patients were reported hospitalized for initiation of hemodialysis therapy and almost invariably with dialysis catheter placement.[129] When ESKD occurs as a result of inpatient acute kidney injury superimposed on preexistent CKD, the proportion of patients initiating dialysis with a TDC will be higher and will have had inadequate prior nephrology care.

The median conversion time from TDC to AVF is 105 days, and fewer than 50% of incident U.S. hemodialysis patients have a functioning AVF in use by the end of the first year. By comparison, the rate of AVF use in other parts of the world is significantly greater, from 69% in the United Kingdom to 85% in Italy to 91% in Japan (Figure 87.6).[130] Multiple obstacles exist that impede the conversion of TDCs in incident hemodialysis patients to an AVF, mainly because of late patient referrals to a nephrologist and vascular access surgeon, insufficient patient education and vessel preservation, late vascular access planning and construction, suboptimal vascular access monitoring, and vascular access choice in older patients. Fortunately, several solutions based on multidisciplinary care have been detailed.[102,131,132] Finally, the maturation of AVFs is important because failure of maturation leads to repeated TDC use, an issue well illustrated in octogenarians.[133] Therefore, the option of initiating hemodialysis with an AVG must be strongly considered when the prediction of AVF maturation is dubious.[134]

Recognition of these patient outcomes has led to mutually reinforcing national quality improvement initiatives. Initial vascular access guidelines were published by NKF DOQI in 1997 and later updated by NKF KDOQI in 2006 to include a target of 10% or less of patients using TDCs for 90 days or longer.[129] The National Vascular Access Improvement Initiative (NVAII), formed in 2003, was recognized as a breakthrough initiative by CMS in 2005, with subsequent establishment of the FFBI coalition, comprised of CMS and all 18 national ESKD networks and with assistance from the Institute for Healthcare Improvement.[131,132] FFBI initially targeted AVF placement and use rates of 50% and 40% in incident and prevalent hemodialysis patients, respectively, as advocated by NKF DOQI with a revised use rate of 66% by 2009. To promote and facilitate implementation of these guidelines, the Renal Physicians Association joined efforts at the national level with dialysis providers, QI organizations, FFBI, and ESKD networks to create the collaborative Vascular Access Initiative (VAI) in 2010. Moreover, Medicare CKD Education Benefits, implemented in 2010, advocated early evaluation and placement of permanent vascular access to reduce dialysis catheter use for incident hemodialysis patients. In 2011, additional vascular access measures were added to the CMS QIP, including the percentage of hemodialysis patients using AVFs, percentage of hemodialysis patients using a TDC for 90 days or longer, and reporting of dialysis-related infections to the National Healthcare Safety Network of the CDC as of 2014.[104]

Viewed from the perspective of the FFBI, TDC use in prevalent hemodialysis patients stabilized and then declined in concert with a greater than 16% decline in first-year mortality rates from 2003 to 2010, compared to minimal change from 1993 to 2003.[58] Progress in achieving FFBI goals has been clearly evident in prevalent patients but much less so in incident patients.[58,131] AVF use in prevalent patients rose from 32% in 2003 to 56% in 2010, along with an increasing percentage of dialysis facilities achieving the 66% AVF use target (6.4% in 2007 and 19% in 2010), while TDC use decreased from 27% to 24%.[135] Importantly this improvement in vascular access practice benefits hemodialysis adequacy outcomes as currently measured by the CMS ESKD QIP (urea reduction rate [URR] $\geq$ 65%; later single-pool [sp] Kt/V $\geq$ 1.2, where Kt/V is the product of dialyzer blood water urea clearance [K] and dialysis treatment time [t] divided by distribution volume of urea [V], a number used to quantify dialysis treatment adequacy). In over 35,000 hemodialysis patients enrolled in DOPPS, a significantly higher fraction of those using TDCs were found to have inadequate clearances (spKt/V < 1.2) when compared to patients using permanent vascular accesses.[130] However, one unintended consequence of the FFBI was to magnify a substantial maturation failure rate of newly created AVFs, thereby leading to increased numbers of hemodialysis catheters being placed.[120] An increased TDC prevalence with increased risks of inadequate dialysis clearance and catheter-related bacteremia has promulgated transformation from a fistula first initiative to one of catheter last. Furthermore, with the CMS PPS and QIP, it became evident that the clinical and economic costs of TDCs greatly outweighed those of AVFs. Overall, vascular access complications account for frequent hospitalizations and 14% of all ESKD expenses.[136,137]

A VIEW TO THE FUTURE

With the ESKD Quality Initiative of 2004, a 4-year ESKD Disease Management Demonstration (DMD) project was launched with an aim of providing more opportunity for Medicare beneficiaries to join integrated care management systems. The financially capitated DMD undertaking tested the effectiveness of various disease management models in cost containment and delivery of quality care by eligible organizations, which included Disease Management Organizations (DMOs), dialysis providers, Medicare Advantage plans, and integrated health systems. The DMD trial began in 2006 in anticipation of the construction of accountable care organizations (ACOs) and three participating DMOs that would receive CMS-capitated payments for assuming the risk of the total cost of care per patient enrollee.[138] Patient self-management was encouraged, and education regarding diabetes and cardiovascular disease was provided to patients. DMOs separately developed and implemented coordinated care systems for a common set of elements and those specifically chosen. DMD success was gauged by the DMO's ability to improve hospitalization and mortality outcomes, patient satisfaction, and cost efficiency compared to a fee-for-service control group. Payment was based on an expanded bundle of dialysis services, with additional items or services reimbursed on a fee-for-service basis above the Medicare composite rate. Included in the DMD was a 5% payment schedule incentivizing quality based on measures of dialysis adequacy, anemia management, vascular access practice, serum albumin level, and CKD mineral-bone disorder. Protocols to drive more homogeneous responses for clinical problems were designed and deployed. Ascertainment of responses and analyses were conducted by two independent groups. Multiple interventions were required to achieve these ends, including employment of additional personnel for care coordination among physicians, nurses, and ancillary care partners. Notably, protocol changes and process of care enhancements were permissible and malleable. Namely, changes were predicated on protocol successes in any DMO-prespecified areas.

Thus, following analysis, the program was considered significant and successful.[139] One DMO reported less cardiovascular disease–related hospitalization compared to fee-for-service plans. Another that had designed an oral nutritional supplementation regimen demonstrated a reduction in 1-year mortality. In the USRDS 2007 Annual Data Report, the DMO hemodialysis catheter insertion rates were statistically decreased compared to the fee-for-service group, 8% versus 18%. Medication adherence and diabetes care were also improved in DMOs. Notably, DMO patients reported greater satisfaction with their health care delivery systems.[140] However, the disease management programs did not improve QOL, and this result may have reflected an inability to determine a statistically significant outcome within the time constraints imposed by the DMD project.

The Patient Protection and Affordable Care Act of 2010 and CMS regulations currently preclude nephrology-specific

ACOs. The ACO program, initiated April 1, 2012 subsequent to the 2011 ESKD PPS and in parallel to the 2012 ESKD QIP, shares similarities with these programs, including an incentivized approach to quality improvement.[9] As directed by the Medicare Shared Savings Program, which facilitates coordination and cooperation among providers to improve quality of care, ACOs are health care organizations that aim to control costs while delivering quality care for a minimum census of 5000 Medicare fee-for-service beneficiaries.[141] However, the following providers and suppliers of services are permitted to form ACOs: physicians, physician assistants, nurse practitioners, and clinical nurse specialists in group practices; individual practices of ACO professionals in the same network; partnerships or joint venture arrangements between hospitals and ACO professionals; hospitals employing ACO professionals; critical access hospitals that bill under method II (Optional Payment Method with billing of the Medicare Administrative Contractor for facility and professional services furnished to its outpatients by physicians/practitioners who have reassigned billing rights to the facility); and recognized providers or suppliers. Unlike the ESKD PPS, which does not cover costs external to the dialysis treatment, ACOs seek to improve quality and reduce costs through improved coordination of outpatient and inpatient care in a global fashion and to provide the full continuum of care.

As of 2014, the Comprehensive ESKD Care (CEC) Initiative developed by the Center for Medicare and Medicaid Innovation under the Affordable Care Act (Section 3021) aimed to partner with providers and suppliers through the creation of ESKD Seamless Care Organizations (ESCOs), consisting of dialysis units, nephrology practices, and Medicare-enrolled providers or suppliers in an effort to provide enhanced integrated care coordination with goals that included reducing hospitalizations and readmissions, reducing TDC use, and increasing access to home dialysis modalities and renal transplantation while reducing total per capita expenditures. To be eligible for shared cost savings with CMS through a number of incentivized payment arrangements, depending on whether a large dialysis organization facility is involved, these organizations will be responsible for all care offered to a group of 500 or more matched ESKD beneficiaries under a new Medicare-covered payment and service delivery model while meeting a minimum level of measured quality performance.[142] CEC quality measures are intended to include and align with ESKD QIP measures, which have emphasized dialysis adequacy, anemia management, and vascular access practice, as well as additional measures of preventive health, chronic disease management, care coordination and hospitalization and readmission, patient safety, patient and caregiver experience, and QOL.

QUALITY INITIATIVES IN CHRONIC KIDNEY DISEASE

Although the federal government has gradually achieved improvements in ESKD care, particularly in relation to improvements in AVF prevalence, with a concomitant reduction in hemodialysis catheters through the FFBI, the management of patients with non–dialysis-dependent CKD is noticeably absent of organizational involvement by the government.

Recently, The Joint Commission (TJC) delineated eligibility requirements for certification of CKD clinics under the rubric of the Advanced Chronic Kidney Disease Certification process. The objective of this process was to ensure that eligible programs possessed the critical elements for long-term success in improving outcomes, which had been demonstrated.[143] Qualifying clinics would directly provide or facilitate coordinated care of patients with CKD stages 1 to 4 and would have the following characteristics: (1) standard method of delivering or facilitating coordinated care from diagnosis to management, based on the NKF KDOQI evidence-based clinical practice guidelines; (2) secure and timely system for sharing information across settings and providers, with safeguards of patient rights and privacy; (3) comprehensive performance improvement programs that used outcomes data to continually enhance existing treatment plans and clinical practices; and (4) clinical practices that enabled tailored treatment plans and interventions and supported participant self-management activities. Qualifying clinics would be awarded a Certificate of Distinction for Chronic Kidney Disease if the criteria of TJC were fulfilled, as specified in the CKD section of the *Organization Review Process Guide 2014: Disease-Specific Care Certification*.

Within the CKD sphere, multiple iterations of multidisciplinary (also known as interdisciplinary) clinics have been implemented, with the premise of providing well-coordinated, integrated, high-quality, and safe care for patients with CKD.[144,145] The overarching guiding principle behind interdisciplinary CKD clinics is that of the chronic disease management model, advocated by Wagner and associates and others.[146-148] This framework model has been suitably adapted to multiple disease entities, including chronic obstructive pulmonary disease, heart failure, and diabetes mellitus, and is adaptable to a patient-centered health care approach.[149] Similarly, it would be anticipated that interdisciplinary CKD clinics would reduce hospitalization rates of patients with advanced CKD, which represents a significant cost containment for this group of patients.[150,151]

In alignment with the chronic disease management model of Wagner and colleagues' and TJC's specifications, homogeneity of practice among clinic health care providers, along accepted guidelines, represents a major objective of CKD clinics. In this fashion, metricized data outcomes are feasible, preferably in an electronic health record, and serve as a resource for practice improvement.[146,152] Ostensibly, CKD clinics would identify at-risk patients for progressive CKD and then, at a minimum, ensure a smooth transition to a form of RRT. Participation in peritoneal dialysis or preemptive kidney transplantation would thereby be facilitated. Commensurately, those patients who would ultimately undergo hemodialysis and require vascular access would experience a reduction in hemodialysis catheter placements and a reciprocal increase in vascular accesses, either a preferred AVF or an AVG.[153] In addition, interdisciplinary CKD clinics would provide targeted, educational material for patients to inform patients more fully about their disease processes.[154,155] Finally, in incident hemodialysis patients, the occurrence of pre-ESKD nephrology CKD visits[127] and an increased frequency of these visits, with improved management of modifiable risk factors prior to dialysis initiation,[128] have been associated with improved survival during the first year on dialysis.

For patients with high levels of comorbidity, critical, patient-centered decision making regarding the appropriateness of initiating long-term RRT would also be most suitably advanced in the CKD clinic environment to which a patient had become accustomed. In addition, leaders in a particular CKD clinic would provide local and regional educational support to family practitioners and internists who might not have been appropriately screening and identifying patients with CKD, either because of unawareness or inappropriate application of screening guidelines.[156,157] Late referral to a nephrologist of an advanced-stage CKD patient, with an estimated GFR of approximately 15 mL/min/1.73 m^2, may result in substantially higher costs and comorbidities. It is presumed that rapid access to a CKD clinic will avoid these costs and, in particular, costs associated with urgent or emergent inpatient initiation of dialysis.[158,159]

Typically, interdisciplinary CKD clinics involve combinations of a nephrologist, renal dietitian, social worker, and advanced practice registered nurse (APRN) or physician assistant (PA). In some models, a pharmacist and diabetes educator represent integrated components of the clinic.[160] The intensity of care provided by an APRN or PA also varies; this is locally determined by the prevailing clinic's operational model—namely, what types and how much follow-up care would the supervising nephrologist provide in comparison to APRNs and PAs (Figure 87.7). In some clinics, a newly presenting patient with CKD would always be evaluated by a nephrologist, whereas in others, the initial contact might be with an APRN or nurse practitioner (NP). Follow-up could be solely with an advanced health care provider or physician, or might be dependent on the complexity of a case. For example, follow-up evaluations of individuals with advancing CKD from diabetes mellitus or hypertension would generally be carried out by advanced practitioners, while cases of severe glomerulonephritis or other rarer forms of kidney disease with specific comorbidities might be primarily cared for by the nephrologist.

The functionality of an interdisciplinary CKD clinic is predicated by the scope of practice intended and contingent on personnel and resource availability (Table 87.3). Some clinics may offer intravenous drug administrations, medication infusion therapy, and blood transfusions, while others may have point-of-care laboratory services. Nearly all CKD clinics manage the anemia of CKD within their clinic space, which requires careful and close collaboration with pharmacy services as well as data management. To this end, efficient and cost-effective incorporation of an algorithmic and standardized computerized anemia management program (CAMP) has been developed and validated

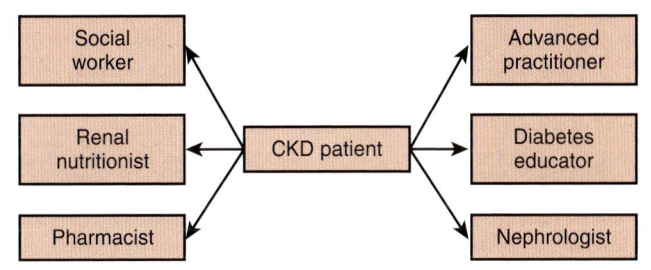

Figure 87.7 Proposed patient-centered model for an interdisciplinary chronic kidney disease (CKD) clinic. An interdisciplinary CKD clinic that is patient centered has the patient at the nexus of interactions among various health care providers, each with a particular specialty. Interactions flow through the patient to ensure that processes of care and transitions of care continually involve the patient.

Table 87.3 Potential Components of Interdisciplinary Chronic Kidney Disease Clinic

Function	Requirements	Implementation Personnel	Ancillary Requirements
Clinical evaluation	Clinic space	Nurse, advanced practitioner, physician, medical assistant	Kidney ultrasound
Anemia management—parenteral iron and ESA delivery	Pharmacy stockage of iron and ESA prescribing entity	Nursing	Infusion, transfusion area Medication disposal area
Blood transfusion			
Immunization, vaccination	Clinic space Pharmacy stockage of vaccinations	Dependent on specific regulations governing this activity	
Infusion therapy—medications, electrolyte(s), glucose	Infusion area	Nursing	Physician oversight
Point-of-care laboratory testing	Dedicated laboratory space and equipment	Laboratory technician, medical assistant	Medication disposal area
Urinalysis	Laboratory space, microscope	Laboratory technician, physician	Urine reflectance spectrophotometer, phase contrast module, polarizing filters
Nutritional therapy	Clinic space	Renal dietitian	
Social work	Office space	Social worker	Translator(s)
Patient education	Clinic space	Advanced practitioner, physician, diabetes educator	

ESA, Erythropoiesis-stimulating agent.

in real-world practice in a large academic CKD clinic.[161] Immunizations are also administered within interdisciplinary CKD clinics, attenuating in part the immunization gap in advanced CKD.[162] Immunization with recombinant hepatitis B vaccine generates a higher titer in the pre-ESKD patient in comparison to those who were immunized after commencement of dialysis.[163,164] This so-called vaccination-forward strategy, when successful, also provides a measure of protection to health care personnel by reducing hepatitis B transmissibility. Finally, patients should undergo vaccinations with any live attenuated viruses prior to the administration of any immunosuppression medication administration, whether for specific causes of CKD or following transplantation.

Renal-specific care by these clinics is often rendered along guidelines established by the NKF. The product of four chronic renal failure work groups—hemodialysis, peritoneal dialysis, vascular access, and anemia—the first NKF DOQI guidelines were published in 1997 as an improvement initiative. Changes to the original guidelines were provided by NKF KDOQI after a three-stage review process by a dedicated steering committee, advisory board, and experts in the field.[165] KDOQI established clinical practice guidelines (CPGs) for all stages of CKD and related complications, as defined by the IOM as "systematically developed statements to assist practitioner and patient decisions about appropriate health care for specific clinical circumstances."[166] Through a contractual agreement signed in 2004, the NKF assisted in the founding and initial management of Kidney Disease: Improving Global Outcomes (KDIGO), which was established in 2003 and incorporated in Brussels as a Foundation in the Public Interest in 2006, an entity distinct from KDOQI.[167] Its mission was to fulfill the need for international cooperation and consolidation in the development and implementation of clinical practice guidelines of CKD. To date, KDIGO has developed nine sets of evidence-based guideline and has participation by 86 countries (Table 87.4).[168] These guidelines include many of the aspects of comprehensive kidney care, and quality and safety issues are generally embedded within the guidelines.

Overall, interdisciplinary CKD clinics have rapidly evolved into small, kidney-specific entities that deliver care based on the prevailing evidence base as much as possible. Multiple iterations are based on needs and resources. Operational success has been examined from generally a cost-only standpoint, a flawed approach,[169-171] to ensure that a level of high-quality, seamless, and integrated care, personnel, equipment, and information technology will be attained. However, this is offset by a reduction in the number of complications suffered by patients with CKD. A single-year delay of RRT in a patient with advanced CKD allows sufficient time for kidney transplantation evaluation, patient education, and truly informed consent. Recently, the results of the Multifactorial Approach and Superior Treatment Efficacy in Renal Patients with the Aid of Nurse Practitioners (MASTERPLAN) study,[172] a CKD intervention trial of 788 participants with median follow-up of 5.7 years designed in 2005, has demonstrated that NP care versus conventional physician care improves renal end points. In patients with a mean eGFR of 35 mL/min/1.73 m² at the outset, the trajectory of eGFR decline was significantly less steep in the group whose care was guided by NPs. Notably, cost savings were also noted with NP-directed care. Cardiovascular events were not reduced by the interventional group.

A separate, prospective, 3-year cohort study from Taiwan, which included 1056 patients with an eGFR less than 60 mL/

Table 87.4	Kidney Disease: Improving Global Outcomes (KDIGO) Clinical Practice Guideline Publications	
Date of Issue	Clinical Practice Guideline	Source (URL)
April 2008	Prevention, Diagnosis, Evaluation and Treatment of HCV in CKD	http://www.kdigo.org/pdf/KI%20Hep%20C%20GL%20Apr%202008.pdf
August 2009	Diagnosis, Evaluation, Prevention and Treatment of CKD-MBD	http://www.kdigo.org/clinical_practice_guidelines/pdf/CKD/KDIGO%20CKD-MBD%20GL%20KI%20Suppl%20113.pdf
October 2009	Care of Kidney Transplant Recipients	http://www.kdigo.org/clinical_practice_guidelines/pdf/TxpGL_publVersion.pdf
March 2012	Acute Kidney Injury	http://www.kdigo.org/clinical_practice_guidelines/pdf/KDIGO%20AKI%20Guideline.pdf
June 2012	Glomerulonephritis	http://www.kdigo.org/clinical_practice_guidelines/pdf/KDIGO-GN-Guideline.pdf
August 2012	Anemia in CKD	http://www.kdigo.org/clinical_practice_guidelines/pdf/KDIGO-Anemia%20GL.pdf
December 2012	Blood Pressure in CKD	http://www.kdigo.org/clinical_practice_guidelines/pdf/KDIGO_BP_GL.pdf
January 2013	CKD Evaluation and Management	http://www.kdigo.org/clinical_practice_guidelines/pdf/CKD/KDIGO_2012_CKD_GL.pdf
November 2013	Lipid Management in CKD	http://www.kdigo.org/clinical_practice_guidelines/Lipids/KDIGO%20Lipid%20Management%20Guideline%202013.pdf

CKD, Chronic kidney disease; HCV, hepatitis C virus; MBD, mineral and bone disorder.
Adapted from Kasiske BL, Wheeler DC. Kidney Disease: Improving Global Outcomes—an update. Nephrol Dial Transplant 29:763-769, 2014.

min/1.73 m², has also demonstrated superior outcomes in its multidisciplinary group.[173] The decline of eGFR in CKD stages 4 and 5 was slower (−5.1 vs. −7.1 mL/min/year; $P =$ 0.01) after 33.1 months of mean follow-up, and hospitalizations were reduced by 40%. Mortality was reduced by 51% in the multidisciplinary cohort, and there was instead a 68% increase in the likelihood of dialysis initiation. By contrast, in the 2-year, cost-effectiveness Canadian Prevention of Renal and Cardiovascular Endpoints Trial (CanPREVENT), nursing- or nephrologist-supported (intervention group) versus usual care (controls) did not result in a superior outcome for eGFR decline. However, the intervention group demonstrated a higher QOL and fewer resources.[174,175] The cost savings was dominated by fewer hospitalization days for the intervention group. Finally, the patient population differed from MASTERPLAN subjects and had a shorter follow-up period of only 2 years.

Complete reference list available at ExpertConsult.com.

KEY REFERENCES

1. Atkinson S, Ingham J, Cheshire M, et al: Defining quality and quality improvement. *Clin Med* 10:537–539, 2010.
2. Committee on Quality of Health Care in America; Institute of Medicine: *Crossing the quality chasm: a new health system for the 21st century*, Washington, DC, 2001, The National Academies Press.
3. Batalden PB, Davidoff F: What is "quality improvement" and how can it transform healthcare? *Qual Saf Health Care* 16:2–3, 2007.
6. Grier B, Grier M: Contributions of the passionate statistician (Florence Nightingale). *Res Nurs Health* 1:103–109, 1978.
8. Luce JM, Bindman AB, Lee PR: A brief history of health care quality assessment and improvement in the United States. *West J Med* 160:263–268, 1994.
10. Colton D: Quality improvement in health care. Conceptual and historical foundations. *Eval Health Prof* 23:7–42, 2000.
16. Eknoyan G: A decade after the KDOQI CKD guidelines: a historical perspective. *Am J Kidney Dis* 60:686–688, 2012.
18. National Kidney Foundation: K/DOQI clinical practice guidelines for chronic kidney disease: evaluation, classification, and stratification. *Am J Kidney Dis* 39(Suppl 1):S1–S266, 2002.
19. Lopez-Vargas PA, Tong A, Sureshkumar P, et al: Prevention, detection and management of early chronic kidney disease: a systematic review of clinical practice guidelines. *Nephrology* 18:592–604, 2013.
21. Coca SG, Krumholz HM, Garg AX, et al: Underrepresentation of renal disease in randomized controlled trials of cardiovascular disease. *JAMA* 296:1377–1384, 2006.
22. Tuot DS, Plantinga LC, Hsu C-Y: Chronic kidney disease awareness among individuals with clinical markers of kidney dysfunction. *Clin J Am Soc Nephrol* 6:1838–1844, 2011.
24. Plantinga LC, Tuot DS, Powe NR: Awareness of chronic kidney disease among patients and providers. *Adv Chronic Kidney Dis* 17:225–236, 2010.
25. Boulware LE, Troll MU, Jaar BG, et al: Identification and referral of patients with progressive CKD: a national study. *Am J Kidney Dis* 48:192–204, 2006.
26. Agrawal V, Ghosh AK, Barnes MA, et al: Perception of indications for nephrology referral among internal medicine residents: a national online survey. *Clin J Am Soc Nephrol* 4:323–328, 2009.
29. Marshall MN, Shekelle PG, Davies HTO, et al: Public reporting on quality in the United States and the United Kingdom. *Health Aff (Millwood)* 22:134–148, 2003.
36. Hughes RG: Tools and strategies for quality improvement and patient safety. In Hughes RG, editor: *Patient safety and quality: an evidence-based handbook for nurses*, Rockville, Md, 2008, Agency for Healthcare Research and Quality.
37. Loeb JM: The current state of performance measurement in health care. *Int J Qual Health Care* 16(Suppl 1):5–9, 2004.
38. Schoen C, Davis K, How SK, et al: U.S. health system performance: a national scorecard. *Health Aff (Millwood)* 25:w457–w475, 2006.
41. Hibbard JH, Stockard J, Tusler M: Does publicizing hospital performance stimulate quality improvement efforts? *Health Aff (Millwood)* 22:84–94, 2003.
42. Shine KI: Health care quality and how to achieve it. *Acad Med* 77:91–99, 2002.
43. Varkey P, Reller MK, Resar RK: Basics of quality improvement in health care. *Mayo Clinic Proc* 82:735–739, 2007.
49. Rettig RA, Sadler JH, Meyer KB, et al: Assessing health and quality of life outcomes in dialysis: a report on an Institute of Medicine workshop. *Am J Kidney Dis* 30:140–155, 1997.
54. Berwick DM, Nolan TW, Whittington J: The triple aim: care, health, and cost. *Health Aff (Millwood)* 27:759–769, 2008.
72. Collins AJ, Li S, St Peter W, et al: Death, hospitalization, and economic associations among incident hemodialysis patients with hematocrit values of 36% to 39%. *J Am Soc Nephrol* 12:2465–2473, 2001.
67. Eschbach JW, Abdulhadi MH, Browne JK, et al: Recombinant human erythropoietin in anemic patients with end-stage renal disease. Results of a phase III multicenter clinical trial. *Ann Intern Med* 111:992–1000, 1989.
71. Moreno F, Sanz-Guajardo D, Lopez-Gomez JM, et al: Increasing the hematocrit has a beneficial effect on quality of life and is safe in selected hemodialysis patients. Spanish Cooperative Renal Patients Quality of Life Study Group of the Spanish Society of Nephrology. *J Am Soc Nephrol* 11:335–342, 2000.
73. Ma JZ, Ebben J, Xia H, et al: Hematocrit level and associated mortality in hemodialysis patients. *J Am Soc Nephrol* 10:610–619, 1999.
75. Madore F, Lowrie EG, Brugnara C, et al: Anemia in hemodialysis patients: variables affecting this outcome predictor. *J Am Soc Nephrol* 8:1921–1929, 1997.
81. Besarab A, Bolton WK, Browne JK, et al: The effects of normal as compared with low hematocrit values in patients with cardiac disease who are receiving hemodialysis and epoetin. *N Engl J Med* 339:584–590, 1998.
82. Singh AK, Szczech L, Tang KL, et al: Correction of anemia with epoetin alfa in chronic kidney disease. *N Engl J Med* 355:2085–2098, 2006.
83. Drüeke TB, Locatelli F, Clyne N, et al: Normalization of hemoglobin level in patients with chronic kidney disease and anemia. *N Engl J Med* 355:2071–2084, 2006.
84. Pfeffer MA, Burdmann EA, Chen CY, et al: A trial of darbepoetin alfa in type 2 diabetes and chronic kidney disease. *N Engl J Med* 361:2019–2032, 2009.
85. Palmer SC, Navaneethan SD, Craig JC, et al: Meta-analysis: erythropoiesis-stimulating agents in patients with chronic kidney disease. *Ann Intern Med* 153:23–33, 2010.
90. Thamer M, Zhang Y, Kaufman J, et al: Dialysis facility ownership and epoetin dosing in patients receiving hemodialysis. *JAMA* 297:1667–1674, 2007.
99. Solomon SD, Uno H, Lewis EF, et al: Erythropoietic response and outcomes in kidney disease and type 2 diabetes. *N Engl J Med* 363:1146–1155, 2010.
123. Bradbury BD, Fissell RB, Albert JM, et al: Predictors of early mortality among incident US hemodialysis patients in the Dialysis Outcomes and Practice Patterns Study (DOPPS). *Clin J Am Soc Nephrol* 2:89–99, 2007.
134. Lok CE, Allon M, Moist L, et al: Risk equation determining unsuccessful cannulation events and failure to maturation in arteriovenous fistulas (REDUCE FTM I). *J Am Soc Nephrol* 17:3204–3212, 2006.
135. Lynch JR, Wasse H, Armistead NC, et al: Achieving the goal of the Fistula First breakthrough initiative for prevalent maintenance hemodialysis patients. *Am J Kidney Dis* 57:78–89, 2011.
141. Nissenson AR, Maddux FW, Velez RL, et al: Accountable care organizations and ESKD: the time has come. *Am J Kidney Dis* 59:724–733, 2012.
148. Von Korff M, Gruman J, Schaefer J, et al: Collaborative management of chronic illness. *Ann Intern Med* 127:1097–1102, 1997.
153. Lorenzo V, Martin M, Rufino M, et al: Predialysis nephrologic care and a functioning arteriovenous fistula at entry are associated with better survival in incident hemodialysis patients: an observational cohort study. *Am J Kidney Dis* 43:999–1007, 2004.
159. St Peter WL, Khan SS, Ebben JP, et al: Chronic kidney disease: the distribution of health care dollars. *Kidney Int* 66:313–321, 2004.

161. Yessayan L, Sandhu A, Besarab A, et al: Intravenous iron dextran as a component of anemia management in chronic kidney disease: a report of safety and efficacy. *Int J Nephrol* 2013:703038, 2013.
164. Dinits-Pensy M, Forrest GN, Cross AS, et al: The use of vaccines in adult patients with renal disease. *Am J Kidney Dis* 46:997–1011, 2005.
172. Peeters MJ, van Zuilen AD, van den Brand JA, et al: Nurse practitioner care improves renal outcome in patients with CKD. *J Am Soc Nephrol* 25:390–398, 2014.
173. Chen Y-R, Yang Y, Wang S-C, et al: Effectiveness of multidisciplinary care for chronic kidney disease in Taiwan: a 3-year prospective cohort study. *Nephrol Dial Transplant* 28:671–682, 2013.
174. Hopkins RB, Garg AX, Levin A, et al: Cost-effectiveness analysis of a randomized trial comparing care models for chronic kidney disease. *Clin J Am Soc Nephrol* 6:1248–1257, 2011.
175. Barrett BJ, Garg AX, Goeree R, et al: A nurse-coordinated model of care versus usual care for stage 3/4 chronic kidney disease in the community: a randomized controlled trial. *Clin J Am Soc Nephrol* 6:1241–1247, 2011.

Index

A

AA amyloidosis, 1128-1132, 1157, 2485
Abatacept, 1104-1105
ABCG2, 221, 221*t*
Abdomen, plain radiograph of, 846, 847*f*, 873
Abdominal aortic aneurysm, 1261
Abdominal compartment syndrome, 999, 2138
ABO blood group antigens, 2236-2237, 2581-2582
ABO-incompatible renal transplantation, 2156-2157, 2423
Aboriginal Australians. *See* Australia, indigenous (Aboriginals) population of
Abscess, renal. *See* Renal abscess
Absolute hypovolemia. *See* Hypovolemia, absolute
Acanthocytes, 756, 756*f*
Accountable care organizations, 2631-2632
Accuracy, of estimating glomerular filtration rate equations, 785
Acebutolol, 1656*t*-1657*t*, 1658
Acellular tissue matrices, 2610
Acetaminophen poisoning, 2187-2188
Acetazolamide, 450, 541, 629, 1704
Acetoacetic acid, in ketoacidosis, 247
Acetylcholine, 101-102, 110
Acetylcholine receptor, 587-588
N-Acetyl-seryl-lysyl-proline, 1887-1888
Acid(s)
　dietary sources of, 517
　excretion of, diurnal variation in, 256
　production of, 514-515
　protein catabolism for generation of, 517
　renal excretion of, 518-519
Acid/alkali-sensing receptors, 256
Acid-base balance
　age-related changes in, 740-741, 740*f*
　in children, 2382-2383, 2382*t*
　in elderly, 740-741, 740*f*
　hyperkalemia and, 537
　renal regulation of, 514-515
Acid-base disorders. *See also specific disorder*
　cellular adaptations to, 245-246
　compensatory mechanisms for, 513-514, 516, 517*f*
　diagnosis of, 511, 521-525, 521*t*, 524*t*
　management of, 511
　mixed, 521-523, 525, 550-552
　urinary tract infection and, 778
Acid-base homeostasis, 512-514
　buffer systems in, 512-514
　citrate excretion in, 247-248
　description of, 5, 512
　hepatic role in, 517

Page numbers followed by "*f*" indicate figures, and "*t*" indicate tables.

Acid-base homeostasis *(Continued)*
　organic anion excretion in, 247-248
　pulmonary involvement in, 512
　renal role in, 517
　sensors involved in, 256
　soluble adenylyl cyclase in, 256
　type B intercalated cell in, 241
Acid-base nomogram, 522, 522*f*
Acid-base regulation, 331, 1749
Acid-base status, 237, 563, 1336-1337
Acid-base transport, 244
Acid-base transporters, 238, 1454-1457
Acidemia, 518, 522, 2177
Acidosis
　adverse effects of, 1758-1759
　causes of, 526*t*
　of chronic kidney disease, 549-550, 684-685, 1758-1759
　collecting duct's response to, 244
　in elderly, 740
　high anion gap. *See* High anion gap acidosis
　hyperkalemic, 572
　insulin resistance and, 1816-1817
　lactic. *See* Lactic acidosis
　metabolic. *See* Metabolic acidosis
　normal anion gap, 525*t*
　of progressive renal failure, 541-543
　respiratory. *See* Respiratory acidosis
　uremic, 549-550
Acquired immunodeficiency syndrome, 883
Acquired perforating dermatosis, 1944, 1944*f*
Acromegaly, 609, 627, 1550
Actin cytoskeleton, 294
Actin-associated proteins, 294-295
Actinin-4, 113
α-Actinin-4, 113, 1430
Action myoclonus-renal failure syndrome, 1432
Activating protein-1, 1787
Activity product ratio, 1327-1328
ACTN4 mutations, 1028
ActRIIB, 1967
Acute allergic interstitial nephritis, 2270
Acute coronary syndrome, 1721-1722
Acute cortical necrosis, 2499, 2501-2502
Acute decompensated heart failure, 997-998, 1719-1722, 2139, 2140*f*
Acute Dialysis Quality Initiative, 960
Acute fatty liver of pregnancy, 992, 1617*t*, 1632
Acute glomerular disease, 1002
Acute interstitial nephritis
　causes of, 1218-1219, 1218*t*
　clinical features of, 1219-1220
　definition of, 1218
　description of, 964-965, 1002
　drugs that cause, 1218-1220, 1218*t*

Acute interstitial nephritis *(Continued)*
　infections associated with, 1219
　kidney biopsy of, 1220
　management of, 1220-1221
　pathology of, 1219
　prognosis for, 1220-1221
　proteinuria and, 1219
　after renal transplantation, 2270
　serum creatinine levels in, 1219-1220
　after thiazide diuretic therapy, 1732
　ultrasonography of, 1220
Acute kidney injury (AKI)
　in acute respiratory distress syndrome, 2138-2139
　in Africa. *See* Africa, acute kidney injury in
　anemia associated with, 983
　animal model for, 299
　atheroembolic, 744
　bee stings as cause of, 2500, 2525
　biologic agent and, 1398
　biomarkers for
　　cystatin C, 935, 989
　　description of, 930-932, 931*t*
　　glutathione S-transferase, 938-939
　　hepcidin-25, 939
　　insulin-like growth factor-binding protein-7, 989
　　interleukin-18, 939, 989
　　kidney injury molecule-1, 941, 989
　　liver-type fatty acid-binding protein, 942-943, 989
　　β_1-microglobulin, 937-938
　　β_2-microglobulin, 938
　　multiple, 953
　　N-acetyl-β-D-glucosaminidase, 947
　　netrin-1, 943
　　neutrophil gelatinase-associated lipocalin, 943-946, 989
　　performance data on, 952*t*
　　tissue inhibitor of metalloproteinase 2, 989
　after bone marrow transplantation, 991*t*, 992-993
　in *Bothrops* envenomations, 2447
　in cancer, 990, 991*t*, 1390
　cardiac arrest as cause of, 970
　cardiac surgery-related, 991*t*, 992
　cardiac tissues affected by, 982
　causes of, 770, 770*t*, 959, 959*t*-960*t*, 963-968
　characteristics of, 1390
　chronic kidney disease secondary to, 678, 691, 747, 926-927, 1777-1778, 1778*f*
　cold ischemia–warm reperfusion model of, 970
　complications of, 994-997, 995*t*
　　acid-base homeostasis, 995
　　cardiac, 996
　　extracellular volume overload, 996

Acute kidney injury (AKI) (Continued)
gastrointestinal, 996
hematologic, 996
hyperkalemia, 994-995, 2140
hypermagnesemia, 995
hyperphosphatemia, 995
hypocalcemia, 995
hypokalemia, 995
hypomagnesemia, 995
infectious, 996
malnutrition, 996
nutritional, 996
potassium homeostasis, 994-995
recovery-related, 996-997
uremic syndrome, 996
volume overload, 996
conceptual model of, 962f
continuous renal replacement therapy for, 2417-2418
contrast media-induced nephropathy as cause of, 853, 964-966, 1000
after coronary angiography, 1009
after coronary artery bypass grafting, 992
COX metabolites in, 377
critical illness-related, 941
in *Crotalus* envenomations, 2446-2447
cytochrome P450 in, 385
definition of, 648, 649t, 769-770, 958-962
dengue fever as cause of, 2441, 2498-2499
in diabetic nephropathy, 1315
diagnostic approach, 771-773, 772t, 961
dialysis for, 652f, 744, 990-992
distant organs affected by, 982-983
diuretics for, 1725-1726
drug disposition affected by, 2035-2040
drug dosing in, 2046, 2051t-2054t, 2145-2146
in elderly, 742-744, 2513-2514
end-stage kidney disease as risk factor for, 744, 1009, 1777-1778
epidemiology of, 647-648
evaluation of
biomarkers. *See* Acute kidney injury, biomarkers for
blood urea nitrogen, 988
clinical assessment, 983-986, 984t-985t
imaging, 989-990
kidney biopsy, 772-773, 990
laboratory tests, 988
magnetic resonance angiography, 989-990
radiologic, 989-990
ultrasonography, 989-990
urine assessments, 986-988, 987t-988t
experimental models of, 968-983, 969t
in Far East. *See* Far East, acute kidney injury in
glomerular filtration rate in, 788, 932, 947-948, 963, 2043, 2145
hantavirus as cause of, 2515-2516, 2517f
health resource utilization for, 1010
hematopoietic stem cell transplantation and, 1394
hepatorenal syndrome and, 993-994, 994t, 998-999
hornet stings as cause of, 2500
hospital-acquired, 744
hospitalization costs for, 1010
hyperphosphatemia caused by, 627
imaging of, 863f-864f, 866-871, 866f-871f
incidence of, 648, 650t, 652f, 770, 926-927, 962-963, 1390, 2495
in Indian subcontinent. *See* Indian subcontinent, acute kidney injury in
insect stings as cause of, 2525

Acute kidney injury (AKI) (Continued)
in intensive care unit patients, 2137, 2458-2459
intermittent hemodialysis for, 1006-1007, 1315, 2141t
intrinsic
acute glomerular disease as cause of, 1002
acute phosphate nephropathy as cause of, 966-967
acute tubular necrosis as cause of, 964
acute vasculitis as cause of, 1002
aminoglycoside nephrotoxicity as cause of, 966
causes of, 960t, 964-968
cisplatin nephrotoxicity as cause of, 966, 968t, 990
contrast media-induced nephropathy as cause of, 853, 964-966, 965t, 1000
description of, 744, 771, 772t
early-goal directed therapy for, 999
endogenous nephrotoxins that cause, 967-968
general principles of, 999-1000
hypotension and, 999
interstitial disease as cause of, 964-965
iron chelators as cause of, 967
mortality rates for, 1008
myoglobin as cause of, 967
nephrotoxins that cause, 965-968
prevention of, 999-1002
renal artery occlusion as cause of, 964
tubulointerstitial diseases as cause of, 964-968
uric acid as cause of, 967-968
kidney function in, 994
in Latin America, 2440-2444
in leptospirosis, 2444, 2497-2498
liver disease and, 991t, 993-994
loading drug dose in, 2046
Lonomia caterpillar stings as cause of, 2446
in loxoscelism, 2445
maintenance drug dose in, 2046
malaria as cause of, 2443, 2470-2472, 2496-2497, 2517-2520, 2519f-2521f
mesenchymal stem cells in, 2611-2613
in Middle East, 2469-2472
mortality rates for, 742, 1008-1009, 1390
multifactorial causes of, 771
in multiple myeloma, 990, 1002, 2152
nephrolithiasis and, 1632-1633
nephrotic syndrome and, 991t, 994
neutrophil gelatinase-associated lipocalin levels in, 772
nondialytic supportive management of, 1002-1004, 1003t
hypermagnesemia, 1003t, 1004
hypernatremia, 1003-1004, 1003t
hyperuricemia, 1003t, 1004
hypocalcemia, 1003t, 1004
hyponatremia, 1003, 1003t
intravascular volume, 1003
metabolic acidosis, 1003t, 1004
nonsteroidal antiinflammatory drugs as cause of, 362-363, 743-744
nutrition management in, 1003t, 1004
obstruction as cause of, 968
obstructive nephropathy as cause of, 2496
obstructive uropathy and, 1632-1633
oliguric, 959, 995, 1001-1002
outcomes of, 1008-1010
pathophysiology of, 769-770, 1396
acute tubular necrosis, 970-983
algorithm for, 971f
apoptosis in, 974-975
coagulation, 980-981

Acute kidney injury (AKI) (Continued)
cytoskeleton, 971-974, 979
endothelial dysfunction, 979
endothelial progenitor cells, 982
epithelial cell injury, 970-983
experimental models, 968-983, 969t
heat shock proteins, 977-978
heme oxygenase, 977-978
inflammation, 981
intracellular skeletal changes, 971-974
necrosis in, 974-975
parenchymal inflammation, 975-977
reactive oxygen species, 977-978
stem cells, 978-979
T_{reg} cells, 977
vascular tone, 979
peritoneal dialysis for, 2120
polyuria in, 299
porphyria cutanea tarda in, 1946, 1946f
postrenal
asymptomatic presentation of, 986
causes of, 960t, 968
clinical features of, 984t-985t
diagnosis of, 984t-985t
management of, 1002-1003
prevention of, 1002-1003
urine sediment evaluations, 986-987
in pregnancy, 990-992, 991t, 1631-1633
prematurity as risk factor for, 711-712
prerenal
in abdominal compartment syndrome, 999
in acute decompensated heart failure, 997-998
in cancer, 990
causes of, 959t, 963-964
clinical assessment, 983-985
clinical features of, 984t-985t
definition of, 997
description of, 959
diagnosis of, 983-985
in heart failure, 997-998
hepatorenal syndrome and, 998
hypovolemia in, 963
in liver failure, 998-999
management of, 997-999
prevention of, 997-999
renal replacement therapy for, 997
urine sediment evaluations, 986-987
prerenal azotemia as cause of, 963
prevalence of, 648
pulmonary disease and, 991t, 993
recovery from, complications during, 996-997
renal function assessments in, 2043-2044
renal replacement therapy for, 962-963
continuous, 1007-1008
in critically ill patients, 2137, 2139-2140
definition of, 1004-1005
duration of, 1005-1006
indications for, 1005-1006, 1005t, 2140
in intensive care unit, 2139-2140
intermittent hemodialysis, 1006-1007, 1315
modalities of, 1006-1008
peritoneal dialysis, 1008
prolonged intermittent, 1008
in renal transplantation, 2271t
RIFLE criteria for, 648, 770, 770t, 930-931, 960, 961t, 2138
risk factor for, 959
scleroderma associated with, 1002
in sepsis, 338, 999, 2137-2138
severe fever with thrombocytopenia syndrome virus as cause of, 2516-2517, 2518f

Acute kidney injury (AKI) *(Continued)*
  snakebites as cause of, 2499-2500
  after solid organ transplantation, 991*t*, 992-993
  sphingosine-1 phosphate receptor, 979
  staging of, 961, 2043
  toxins that cause, 965-968, 2458
  tumor lysis syndrome and, 990, 992*t*, 1395-1397
  ultrasonography of, 866-867
  urinary microscopy evaluations, 937, 937*t*
  urine output in, 959
  wasp stings as cause of, 2500, 2525
  zygomycosis as cause of, 2498, 2498*f*
Acute Kidney Injury Network, 930-931
Acute liver failure, 2139
Acute mountain sickness, 1704
Acute myelogenous leukemia, 1390
Acute myocardial infarction, 623, 1721
Acute phase reactant proteins, 1970
Acute phosphate nephropathy, 966-967
Acute poststreptococcal glomerulonephritis
  in children, 1054, 2331-2333
  clinical features of, 1057, 2332
  coagulation abnormalities in, 1058
  complement levels in, 1058
  cryoglobulins in, 1058
  in developing communities, 1054
  diagnosis of, 2332
  differential diagnosis of, 1057, 2332-2333
  in elderly, 1057
  electron microscopy findings, 1055-1056, 1056*f*
  epidemic, 1054
  epidemiology of, 1054, 2331-2332
  hematuria in, 1057
  hypertension in, 1057
  immunofluorescence microscopy findings, 1055, 1055*f*
  incidence of, 1054
  infectious agents associated with, 1057
  laboratory findings in, 1057-1058
  light microscopy findings, 1054-1055, 1055*f*
  natural history of, 1057
  nephrotic syndrome caused by, 1054-1059
  pathogenesis of, 1056-1057, 2332
  pathology of, 1054-1056, 1055*f*-1056*f*
  prognosis for, 1058-1059, 2333
  pyoderma and, 2331-2332
  streptococcal proteins in, 1056-1057
  streptozyme test for, 1058
  treatment of, 1058-1059, 2333
  ultrastructural features of, 1056*f*
Acute pyelonephritis. *See* Pyelonephritis, acute
Acute radiation nephropathy, 1193
Acute renal failure, 1021. *See also* Acute kidney injury
Acute renal ischemia, 141-142
Acute respiratory distress syndrome, 2138-2139
Acute thrombotic microangiopathy, after renal transplantation, 2269
Acute tubular necrosis (ATN), 2139
  atrial natriuretic peptide for, 1001
  clinical features of, 984*t*-985*t*
  description of, 744
  diagnosis of, 984*t*-985*t*
  dopamine for, 1001
  fenoldopam for, 1001
  intravascular volume depletion as risk factor for, 999
  intrinsic acute kidney injury and, 999

Acute tubular necrosis (ATN) *(Continued)*
  ischemic, 984*t*-985*t*, 985, 2263-2264, 2263*t*
  loop diuretics for, 1001-1002
  magnetic resonance imaging of, 870*f*
  mannitol for, 1002
  morphologic changes in, 971, 972*f*
  natriuretic peptides for, 1001
  nephrotoxic medications as cause of, 999-1000
  pathophysiology of, 970-983
  pharmacologic therapy for, 1001-1002
  pigment-induced, 985
  in pregnancy, 1631-1632
  renal transplantation with, 910*f*
  risk factors for, 999
  snakebite as cause of, 2499
  urinary protein excretion in, 987
Acute tubulointerstitial nephritis, 1209
Acute vasculitis, 1002
ADAM17, 360-361
ADAMTS1, 977
ADAMTS13, 1154, 1175, 1188-1189, 2356
  deficiency of, thrombotic thrombocytopenia purpura associated with, 1188-1191, 2154-2155
Adamts1, 30
Adamts4, 30
Addison's disease, 315, 538, 588-589
Adenine nucleotide translocase, 126-127
Adenine phosphoribosyl transferase deficiency, 1347
Adenohypophysitis, 475-476
Adenosine, 108-109, 135, 136*f*
Adenosine diphosphate, 124
Adenosine monophosphate-activated protein kinase (AMPK), 140-142, 141*f*, 732-733
Adenosine triphosphatases, 124
Adenosine triphosphate, 124, 129, 130*f*
Adenosine triphosphate-binding cassette, subfamily B, 2486
Adenosine type 1 receptor antagonists, 1714
Adenovirus infection, 1404
Adhesion proteins, 25
AdiC, 230*t*
Adiponectin, 1300, 1770-1771
Adipsic hypernatremia, 477-478
Adjuvant therapy, 1381-1382
ADMTS13, 1299
Adrenal adenomas, 575-576, 576*f*
Adrenal cortex, 305
Adrenal glands, 2-3, 852-853, 1919-1920
Adrenal hypoplasia congenita, 588
Adrenal insufficiency, 493, 495, 588-589
α2-Adrenergic agonist, 1629
α-Adrenergic antagonists, 456, 562, 1698
β-Adrenergic antagonists
  airway disease and, 1661
  calcium channel blockers and, 1669, 1691
  central adrenergic agonists and, 1692
  central nervous system effects of, 1661
  in coronary artery disease patients, 1660
  description of, 1564-1565, 1629
  dosing of, 1649*t*-1650*t*
  efficacy of, 1660-1661
  in elderly, 1685
  hyperkalemia treated with, 594-595
  hypertensive urgencies and emergencies treated with, 1698
  indications for, 1660
  lipid levels affected by, 1661
  mechanism of action, 1656-1659
  nonselective, 1656-1659, 1657*t*, 1661

β-Adrenergic antagonists *(Continued)*
  pharmacodynamic properties of, 1657*t*
  pharmacokinetics properties of, 1657*t*
  pharmacologic properties of, 1656*t*
  plasma renin activity affected by, 1659-1660
  potassium concentration affected by, 563*t*
  renal effects of, 1659-1660
  in renal insufficiency patients, 1649*t*-1650*t*
  renin-angiotensin-aldosterone inhibitors and, 1692
  safety of, 1660-1661
  selective, 1656, 1658
  sympathoadrenal drive affected by, 1688
  with vasodilatory properties, 1658-1659, 1658*t*-1659*t*
  withdrawal of, 1661
α$_2$-Adrenergic receptors, 1673
β$_1$-Adrenergic receptors, 1656, 1661
β$_2$-Adrenergic receptors, 1656, 1661
Adrenocorticotropic hormone (ACTH)
  aldosterone levels affected by, 575
  in chronic kidney disease, 1919
  deficiency of, 474
  ectopic, 577
  glomerular disease treated with, 1171-1172
  membranous nephropathy treated with, 1044
  secretion of, 463
  vasopressin 3 receptor's role in release of, 410
Adrenomedullin, 418, 437
Advance directives, 2561-2562, 2599
Advanced care planning, 2599-2600
Advanced glycosylation end products, 730-732, 1318, 1815, 2126-2127
Advanced glycosylation end receptor 1, 730-731, 731*f*
Advanced oxidation protein products, 1909
Adynamic bone disease, 1843
Aedes aegypti, 2441, 2520
Afferent arterioles, 85*f*, 138
Affordable Care Act, 2584, 2631-2632
Africa
  acute kidney injury in, 2457-2459, 2457*t*
  autosomal dominant polycystic kidney disease in, 2459
  children in, nephrotic syndrome in, 2463
  cholera in, 2455-2456
  chronic kidney disease in, 2459-2461, 2465
  diabetes mellitus in, 2463
  diabetic nephropathy in, 2463
  dialysis in, 2463-2464, 2464*f*-2465*f*
  diarrheal diseases in, 2455-2456
  end-stage kidney disease in, 2460*f*, 2461-2462, 2465-2466
  fluid and electrolyte abnormalities in, 2455-2457
  glomerular diseases in
    description of, 2461
    focal segmental glomerulosclerosis, 2463
    hepatitis B virus nephropathy as cause of, 2461-2462
    HIV-associated, 2462-2463
    malaria as cause of, 2462
    poststreptococcal glomerulonephritis, 2461
    schistosomiasis as cause of, 2462
  glomerular filtration rate estimations in, 2459

Africa *(Continued)*
  hemodialysis in, 2463-2464
  hepatitis B virus nephropathy in, 2461-2462
  human immunodeficiency virus in, 2455-2458, 2462-2463
  hypertension in, 2459-2461
  leading causes of death in, 2454, 2455*f*
  malaria in, 2462
  nephrology-specific challenges for, 2465
  nephrotoxic agents in, 2458
  population of, 2454
  renal replacement therapy in, 2456*t*, 2463-2465, 2464*f*
  renal transplantation in, 2464
  sickle cell anemia in, 2463
  snakebites in, 2458
  sub-Saharan, 2454-2455
  urbanization of, 2454
African American Study of Kidney Disease and Hypertension, 679, 1553, 1553*f*
African Americans
  antihypertensive drug therapy in, 1686, 1686*t*
  chronic kidney disease in, 666, 674
  end-stage kidney disease in, 663, 665-666, 674, 1028-1029, 1770
  focal segmental glomerulosclerosis in, 1028, 1769-1770
  thiazide diuretics in, 1686
Agalsidase alfa, 1145
Agalsidase beta, 1145
Age/aging. *See also* Elderly
  acid-base balance affected by, 740-741, 740*f*
  aldosterone levels affected by, 738
  ammonia excretion affected by, 740
  atrial natriuretic peptide levels affected by, 738-739
  calcium balance affected by, 741-742
  coronary heart disease and systolic blood pressure by, 1527*f*
  creatinine levels affected by, 737
  glomerular filtration rate affected by, 736-737, 737*f*, 2586-2587
    estimated, 2586-2587
  hypertension and, 1525
  membrane cholesterol in, 742
  phosphate balance affected by, 742
  potassium balance affected by, 741, 741*f*
  renal function affected by, 1878
  renal plasma flow affected by, 735-736, 736*f*
  sodium conservation in, 737-738
  sodium excretion affected by, 738-739
  urinary concentration affected by, 739-740
  urinary dilution affected by, 740
Agonistic Ang II type I receptor autoantibody, 1623
AGT1, 229
Agtr1a, 35
Agtr1b, 35
Air embolism, in hemodialysis, 2075
A-kinase anchoring proteins, 292-293
AL amyloidosis, 1128-1132
Alagille syndrome, 2297*t*
Albright's hereditary osteodystrophy, 616
Albumin
  catabolism of, in hypoalbuminemia, 1796
  excretion rate for, 1288, 1291, 1296-1297
  fragments of, 794
  free fatty acids binding to, 1761
  hepatic synthesis of, 1796

Albumin *(Continued)*
  loop diuretic binding to, 1707-1708
  normal levels of, 791, 1796
  plasma, 602, 791, 1798
  as plasmapheresis replacement fluid, 2162
  podocyte function for, 112-113
  in proximal tubule, 1784-1785, 1785*f*
  reabsorption of, by proximal tubular cells, 1791
  serum, 683, 1969-1970, 2099
  urinary
    acute kidney injury and, 948
    albumin-to-creatinine ratios, 792, 795-796
    excretion of, 1288, 1291, 1296-1297
    high-performance liquid chromatography measurement of, 794
    hypoalbuminemia secondary to loss of, 1796
    laboratory methods for measurement of, 794-795
    low-protein diet effects on, 1312
    measurement of, 793-795
    in minimal change disease, 1022
    timed versus random collection of, 795
Albumin dialysis, 2171, 2172*t*
Albumin-to-creatinine ratio, 792, 795-796, 2587, 2588*f*
Albuminuria, 1556-1557. *See also* Hypoalbuminemia
  angiotensin receptor blockers for, 1308
  angiotensin-converting enzyme inhibitors for, 1308
  cannabinoid receptor 1 blockade as cause of, 120
  cardiovascular disease and, 1860-1861
  chronic kidney disease progression, 948
  in diabetic nephropathy, 1283
  hypertension as risk factor for, 1765
  metabolic control for, 2592-2593
  mortality risks associated with, 673
  in older adults, 2587
  thromboxane A_2's role in, 378
Albuterol, 594-595
Alcohol consumption, 685-686
Alcoholic ketoacidosis, 547
Alcoholism, 633
Aldh1a2, 23
Aldolase B deficiency, 1445
Aldosterone
  action of, 310-311
  adrenal cortex synthesis of, 305
  adrenal release of, 569
  age-related changes in, 738
  angiotensin II in production of, 305-306, 408-409, 2366-2367
  apical sodium channels affected by, 179
  basolateral membrane effects of, 312
  calcium channel blockers effect on, 1662
  chemical structure of, 304*f*
  in chronic kidney disease, 1919-1920
  collagen synthesis stimulated by, 1757
  collecting duct bicarbonate reabsorption regulated by, 244
  colon and, 316-317
  in congestive heart failure, 322
  diuretic-induced secretion of, 1728
  epithelial sodium channels affected by, 172-173, 311-312, 409, 565-566, 1800, 2366-2367
  glomerulus secretion of, 305
  heart failure and, 431
  hyperkalemia effects on, 182, 2366-2367
  ion transport effects of, 321

Aldosterone *(Continued)*
  kaliuresis affected by, 588
  lung and, 317
  mineralocorticoid receptor binding of, 310
  nonepithelial actions of, 322-323
  nongenomic effects of, 321
  potassium chloride effects on, 741*f*
  potassium loading affected by, 179-180
  potassium secretion regulation by, 312-314, 317, 564-566
  in primary aldosteronism, 321-322
  in principal cells, 567
  production of, 408-409
  renin effects on secretion of, 568, 568*f*
  renovascular effects of, 101
  serum- and glucocorticoid-regulated kinase induction by, 317-318
  SGK-1 induction by, 173
  sodium absorption regulation by, 310-315
  sodium chloride transport affected by, 171-173
  sodium-retaining effect of, 409
  synthesis of, 304*f*-305*f*, 305-306, 588
  systemic effects of, 1309
Aldosterone antagonists
  chronic kidney disease progression affected by, 2003
  description of, 1564
  epithelial sodium channel inhibitors and, 1692
  indications for, 451
  selective aldosterone receptor antagonists, 1678-1679
Aldosterone receptors, 304-305
Aldosterone-producing adenomas, 575
Aldosterone/renin ratio, 1529*f*
Aldosterone-sensitive distal nephron, 311*f*, 314-315, 316*f*, 318-320
Alemtuzumab, 2248, 2255-2256
Alfacalcidol, 2026, 2032
Alginate, 2610
Aliphatic amines, 1812-1813
Aliskiren
  characteristics of, 1677
  combination therapy using, 1678
  efficacy of, 1678
  immunoglobulin A nephropathy treated with, 1068
  proteinuria caused by, 1678
  renal effects of, 1677-1678
  renin-angiotensin-aldosterone system blockade using, 1309
  safety of, 1678
Alkalemia, 186, 523
Alkali gain, 519-520
Alkali therapy, 535-536, 542, 546, 1362-1364, 1363*t*
Alkalosis
  causes of, 526*t*
  metabolic. *See* Metabolic alkalosis
  respiratory. *See* Respiratory alkalosis
Alkylating agents
  adverse effects of, 1168-1169
  bone marrow suppression caused by, 1169
  glomerular disease treated with, 1168-1170
  malignancy risks, 1169
  ovarian failure caused by, 1168-1169
  steroid-sensitive nephrotic syndrome treated with, 2329
  toxicity of, 1169-1170
Allergic interstitial nephritis, 984*t*-985*t*, 1158
Alloantibodies, 1903

Allograft rejection, 378
Allopurinol, 1363t, 1364
Allostatic load, 2576
Alpert syndrome, 2297t
Alport's syndrome, 1421-1424
  clinical features of, 1138-1139
  course of, 1141
  definition of, 1138
  description of, 755, 761, 872
  diagnosis of, 1423-1424
  electron microscopy of, 1139-1140, 1140f
  end-stage kidney disease secondary to, 1138
  genetics of, 1140-1141, 1421-1422, 1782
  high-frequency sensorineural deafness in, 1139
  immunofluorescence microscopy of, 1139
  light microscopy of, 1139
  manifestations of, 1423
  ocular abnormalities in, 1139
  pathogenesis of, 1140-1141, 1421-1422
  pathology of, 1139-1140, 1140f, 1423-1424
  proteinuria in, 1141
  skin manifestations of, 1953
  treatment of, 1141
  variants of, 1139
Alström's syndrome, 1509
Altered nuclear transfer, 2606
Almandine, 333
Aluminum, 1843, 1844f, 1887, 1935
Aluminum-containing binders, 2022
Amatoxin, 2525-2526
Ambulatory blood pressure monitoring. See Blood pressure, ambulatory monitoring of
American Joint Committee on Cancer staging system, 1378
Amifostine, for cisplatin nephrotoxicity, 1001
Amiloride, 489, 590, 1712-1713, 1726
Amiloride-sensitive sodium channel, 125
Amino acid(s)
  anionic, 228-229
  branched-chain, 1971
  catabolism of, 1963-1964, 2084
  in chronic kidney disease, 1972
  D–, 1809-1810
  essential, 1971-1972
  metabolism of, uremia effects on, 1817
  metabolites of, 1972
  neutral, 224-226
  in peritoneal dialysis solutions, 2125
  plasma, 1971-1973, 1972f
  reabsorption of, 222, 223f
  transepithelial flux of, 222
Amino acid decarboxylase, 152-153
Amino acid reabsorption, 1445, 1446f
Amino acid transport, 222-229, 1445-1450
Amino acid transporters
  anionic, 228-229
  apical, 222-228
  basolateral, 228
  cationic, 226-228
  5 + 5 inverted repeat fold of, 229
  heteromeric, 225-227, 226f, 231-232
  neutral, 222-226
  SLC6 transporters, 229-230
  structure of, 229-232
Aminoaciduria, 223t, 1436-1437, 1445, 1612
ε-Aminocaproic acid, 587
Aminoglycosides, 621-622, 966, 1235t-1236t
Aminophylline, 1714

Amlodipine besylate, 1665
Ammonia
  assessment of, 840f
  bicarbonate reabsorption affected by, 245
  blood levels of, 1962
  chemistry of, 248
  collecting duct secretion of, 252, 252f
  formation of, 2036
  hyperkalemia effects on, 537-538, 537t, 571
  impaired excretion of, 1344, 1344f
  interstitial, sulfatide binding of, 251-253
  molecular forms of, 248
  production of, 248-249, 250f, 515f, 517, 1344-1345
  secretion of, 1344-1345
  synthesis of, 537f, 1749
  transport of, 251-253, 1706
  urinary concentrations of, 529
Ammonia excretion
  age-related changes in, 740
  hyperkalemia effects on, 537t
  impaired, 538
  in metabolic acidosis response, 246f
  pathways of, 537f
  Rhbg's role in, 255
  Rhcg's role in, 255
  urinary, 528-529, 538, 840
Ammonia metabolism
  aquaporins in, 254
  in bicarbonate generation, 248-255
  carbonic anhydrase in, 254-255
  description of, 248
  glutamate dehydrogenase in, 253
  H^+-K^+-ATPase in, 254
  Na^+-K^+-ATPase in, 254
  Na^+-K^+-$2Cl^-$ cotransport in, 254
  phosphate-dependent glutaminase in, 253
  potassium channels in, 254
  proteins involved in, 253-255
  Rh glycoproteins in, 255
  schematic diagram of, 249f
  sulfatides in, 255-256
Ammoniagenesis, 248-251, 251f, 840
Amniotic fluid- and placental-derived stem cells, 2607
Amphotericin B, 621, 2131
Amphotericin B deoxycholate, 1254, 1254t
Amyloid light-chain amyloidosis, 1392
Amyloidosis
  AA, 1128-1132, 1157, 2485
  AL, 1128-1132
  characteristics of, 1128
  course of, 1131-1132
  diagnosis of, 1129
  dialysis-related, 1949
  in elderly, 746-747
  end-stage kidney disease progression of, 1131-1132
  hereditary, 1129-1131
  immunofluorescence microscopy of, 1130f
  melphalan for, 1131-1132
  multiple myeloma in, 1128
  nephrotic syndrome in, 1129
  pathology of, 1129-1131, 1130f-1131f
  prognosis for, 1131-1132
  renal disease in, 1129
  renal transplantation in, 1132
  serum amyloid A in, 1128-1129, 1130f
  serum amyloid P in, 1128
  treatment of, 1131-1132

Anabolic hormones, for anorexia, 2125
Anabolic steroids, 1159
Anakinra, 1913, 2486
Analgesic nephropathy, 686, 1221-1223, 1223f-1224f, 2544-2546
Analgesics, 686, 1222t, 2595
Anasarca, 1798
Andersen's syndrome, 573
Androgen deprivation therapy, 1923
Androgens, 152
Anemia
  adverse outcomes of, 1888
  in autosomal dominant polycystic kidney disease, 1888
  blood transfusion for, 1004
  in children, 2405-2406, 2434
  of chronic disease, 1885-1887
  in chronic kidney disease
    adverse outcomes of, 1888, 2013
    algorithm for, 1900f
    causes of
      aluminum overload, 1887
      blood loss, 1885, 1962
      drugs, 1887-1888
      erythropoietin production, 1884, 2013, 2089
      folic acid deficiency, 1887
      inflammation, 1887
      iron metabolism abnormalities, 1885-1887
      shortened red blood cell survival, 1884-1885, 2013
      uremic erythropoiesis inhibitors, 1885
      vitamin D deficiency, 1887
      zinc deficiency, 1887
    definition of, 1875-1878
    description of, 683, 983, 1299-1300, 1776, 1863-1864, 1871-1872, 2593-2594
    in elderly, 2593-2594
    flowchart for, 1900f
    management of, 2013-2014, 2610-2611
    menses associated with, 1921
    pathobiology of, 1878-1884
    prevalence of, 1875-1878, 1876f-1877f, 2626
    red blood cell transfusion for, 1902-1904, 1903f
    stroke risks, 1930
  definition of, 1875-1878
  in diabetes mellitus, 1877-1878
  in diabetic nephropathy, 1299-1300, 1316
  diabetic retinopathy and, 1888
  drugs that affect, 1887-1888
  in elderly, 2593-2594
  in end-stage kidney disease, 1875-1876, 1879f, 2405-2406
  erythropoietin response to, 1316, 1871
  in maintenance hemodialysis, 2097-2098
  megaloblastic, 1883
  pathobiology of, 1878-1884
  prevalence of, 1875-1878, 1876f-1877f
  racial predilection of, 1876-1877
  after renal transplantation, 2434
  stroke risks associated with, 1930
  treatment of, 1871-1872
    erythropoiesis-stimulating agents, 1889-1892, 1900-1902, 2405-2406, 2626-2628
    iron in, 1892-1904, 2098
      intravenous, 1896-1900, 1897t
      markers of, 1893-1896

Anemia (Continued)
    parenteral, 1898
        safety of, 1900-1902
    recombinant human erythropoietin, 1906, 2097
    red blood cell transfusion, 1902-1904, 1903f
    trials of, 1901-1902
    uremic platelet dysfunction and, 1905, 1907f
    in women, 1876-1877
Aneurysmectomy, for renal artery aneurysms, 1203-1204
Angioedema, 1648
Angiogenesis, 6, 32, 34
Angiogenic imbalance, 1621-1623
Angiography
    central vein stenosis, 2212f-2213f
    magnetic resonance. See Magnetic resonance angiography
    renal artery, 1202
Angioimmunoblastic lymphadenopathy, 1159
Angiokeratoma corporis diffusum universale. See Fabry's disease
Angiolymphoid hyperplasia with eosinophilia, 1159
Angiomyolipomas, 891, 893f, 1368-1369, 1375-1376, 1500
Angioplasty, 2198-2202, 2198t, 2200f, 2208-2210, 2209t
Angiopoietin 1, 34-35
Angiopoietin 2, 34-35
Angiopoietin-like 4, 1021
Angiotensin, 1568-1569
Angiotensin-(1-7), 333, 408, 445, 1644
Angiotensin-(1-12), 333
Angiotensin-(2-10), 333
Angiotensin A, 333
Angiotensin I, 35, 326, 1530-1531
Angiotensin II, 35, 139, 183, 1580
    AT_1 receptors for, 152
    acid-base regulation and, 331
    in aldosterone production, 305-306, 408-409, 2366-2367
    angiotensin receptor blockers effect on, 1653-1654
    apelin and, 420
    atrial natriuretic peptide inhibition of, 154
    bicarbonate reabsorption affected by, 237-238, 408
    blockade of, 1598f
    blood pressure levels affected by, 1532f, 1640-1641
    calcium channel blockers effect on, 1662
    chloride absorption activated by, 174
    in chronic kidney disease progression, 1764-1765
    collecting ducts affected by, 244-245
    efferent arterioles affected by, 99
    epidermal growth factor receptor transactivation by, 329f
    formation of, 1530-1531
    functions of, 333
    glomerular capillary hypertension and, 1738
    glomerular filtration rate affected by, 408
    hemodynamic effects of, 331
    juxtaglomerular granular cell expression of, 53
    juxtaglomerular nephrons affected by, 99, 100f
    K_f affected by, 99
    mediation of, 407

Angiotensin II (Continued)
    medullary blood flow affected by, 90
    mesangial cells affected by, 99
    in nephron injury after renal mass ablation, 1756-1757
    nitric oxide release stimulated by, 99
    nonhemodynamic effects of, 1763-1764
    norepinephrine effects on, 110
    nuclear factor-κB activation by, 334
    oxidative stress and, 982
    as paracrine agent, 407
    peritubular carbon dioxide effects on, 237
    physiologic effects of, 330-331, 409
    podocytes affected by, 1788
    potassium intake effects on, 567-568
    pregnancy and, 1613f
    profibrotic effects of, 729
    proximal sodium chloride reabsorption affected by, 152, 153f
    proximal tubule bicarbonate reabsorption affected by, 237
    proximal tubule synthesis and secretion of, 152
    proximal tubule transport affected by, 408
    in renal artery stenosis, 907
    renal fibrosis in aging kidneys, 728-729
    renal hemodynamics affected by, 407-408
    renal hypoperfusion, role in, 1577-1578
    in renal metabolism, 139
    renal vascular responses to, 384
    ROMK activity affected by, 566-567
    sodium chloride absorption affected by, 155
    sodium reabsorption affected by, 407-408
    sodium transport affected by, 331
    transforming growth factor-β expression induced by, 334
    in tubuloglomerular feedback, 399
    urinary tract obstruction effects on expression of, 1278f
    vasoconstrictive effects of, 99-100, 409, 963, 1270, 1645
Angiotensin II inhibitors, 1067-1068
Angiotensin II receptors, 1530-1531, 1623-1624, 1652t, 1653, 2236
Angiotensin III, 332
Angiotensin IV, 332-333
Angiotensin peptides, 332-333
Angiotensin receptor(s), 35, 1569-1570
Angiotensin receptor blockers
    acute kidney injury after initiation of therapy with, 2006t
    adverse effects of, 1655
    albuminuria treated with, 1308
    angiotensin II affected by, 1653-1654
    angiotensin-converting enzyme inhibitors and, 1654, 1764-1765, 2002-2003
    biphenyl tetrazoles, 1651-1653
    cancer risks and, 1655-1656
    in children, 2362
    chlorthalidone and, 1681
    in chronic kidney disease patients, 1654
    description of, 1563-1564, 1598f
    direct renin inhibitors and, 1764-1765
    dosing of, 1649t-1650t, 1654-1655
    drug interactions with, 1656
    efficacy of, 1654-1656
    focal segmental glomerulosclerosis treated with, 1031
    in hypertensive patients, 1653-1654
    mechanism of action, 1651
    metabolic effects of, 1655
    neutral endopeptidase inhibitors and, combination therapy using, 345-346
    nonbiphenyl tetrazoles, 1653
    nonheterocyclic derivatives, 1653

Angiotensin receptor blockers (Continued)
    nonsteroidal anti-inflammatory drugs effect on, 1656
    in pregnancy, 1647, 1655
    renal effects of, 1653-1654
    renal function affected by, 1655
    in renal insufficiency patients, 1649t-1650t
    renin-angiotensin-aldosterone system inhibition by, 591f, 1642f, 1651, 2000-2003, 2001f
    renoprotection using, 729, 1757, 1764-1765, 1995, 1998t, 2000-2003, 2001f
    safety of, 1654-1656
    thiazide diuretics and, 1655
    urinary protein excretion affected by, 1654
Angiotensin receptor–neprilysin inhibitor, 345-346
Angiotensin type 1 receptor, 328-330, 1277
    angiotensin II effects mediated by, 328-329
    dimerization of, 330
    expression of, 328-329
    G protein-mediated signaling and, 329
    internalization of, 330
    ligand-independent activation of, 330
    reactive oxygen species and, 329
    regulation of, 330f
    tyrosine kinases and, 329-330
Angiotensin type 2 receptor, 331, 1277
Angiotensin type 1 receptor-associated protein 1, 330, 330f
Angiotensin-(2-B), 332
Angiotensin-(3-B), 332
Angiotensin-converting enzyme, 27, 100-101, 328, 1308
Angiotensin-converting enzyme 2, 332
Angiotensin-converting enzyme escape, 1644
Angiotensin-converting enzyme inhibitors, 1563, 1569-1570, 1598f, 1630. See also specific drug
    acute kidney injury after initiation of therapy with, 2006t
    adverse effects of, 1648
    albuminuria treated with, 1308
    anaphylactoid reactions caused by, 1650
    angioedema caused by, 1648
    angiotensin peptide levels affected by, 1644
    angiotensin receptor blockers and, 1654, 1764-1765, 2002-2003
    antiproteinuric effects of, 1308
    blood pressure control using, 1303-1305, 1928-1929
    calcium channel blockers and, 1669, 1681-1682, 1684f
    carboxyl, 1641-1644, 1643t
    in children, 2362
    cough caused by, 1648, 1685
    cutaneous reactions to, 1650
    diabetic nephropathy treated with, 1308, 1998-1999
    dosing of, 1649t-1650t
    drug interactions with, 1650
    efficacy of, 1646-1650
    focal segmental glomerulosclerosis treated with, 1031
    glomerular filtration rate affected by, 1299, 1645
    glucose metabolism affected by, 1648
    hyperkalemia caused by, 591-592, 1650
    hypertension treated with, 2592
    hypertensive urgencies and emergencies treated with, 1697t, 1698
    hyponatremia and, 497

Angiotensin-converting enzyme inhibitors (Continued)
  hypotension caused by, 1648
  indications for, 1647
  leukopenia caused by, 1650
  mechanism of action, 1640-1641, 1641t, 1642f
  metabolic effects of, 1647-1648
  microalbuminuria treated with, 1305-1306, 1999
  pharmacodynamics of, 1643t
  pharmacokinetics of, 1643t
  phosphinyl, 1644
  plasmapheresis in patients receiving, 2164
  in pregnancy, 1647, 1685
  renal artery stenosis treated with, 907
  renal effects of, 1644-1646, 1644t
  renal function affected by, 1645-1646
  in renal insufficiency patients, 1649t-1650t
  renal protective effects of, 729
  renin-angiotensin-aldosterone system inhibition by, 591f, 1642f, 1998-2000
  renograms enhanced with, 908
  renoprotection using, 1995, 1998, 1998t
  safety of, 1646-1650
  scleroderma renal crises treated with, 1197-1198
  stroke risk reduction using, 1928-1929
  sulfhydryl, 1641, 1643t
  tissue specificity of, 1645
Angiotensinogen, 35, 326
Angpt1, 34
Anion exchanger(s), 238, 243, 1339, 1339f
Anion gap, 523-524, 524t, 837
Anionic amino acids, 228-229
Annexin II, 1836-1837
Anorexia, 2099, 2125, 2357
Antegrade pyelography, 1268, 1268f
Anthropometrics, 1971
Antiangiogenic therapy, 1382
Anti–B cell therapy, 119
Antibacterial agents, 1235t-1236t
Antibiotics, 1218, 1365
Antibodies
  anti-ADAMTS13, 1189
  anti-glomerular basement membrane, 1124
  anti-glomerular basement membrane glomerulonephritis, 1079
  anti-MPO, 1083-1085
  antineutrophil cytoplasmic. See Antineutrophil cytoplasmic antibodies
  antinuclear, 1098-1099
  antiphospholipid, 1106-1107
  anti-Ro/SSA, 1099
  anti-U1RNP, 1108
Antibody-mediated rejection, 2423
Anti-CD20 monoclonal antibody, 2256
Anticoagulation
  antiphospholipid syndrome treated with, 1107-1108
  atrial fibrillation treated with, 1932
  extracorporeal dialysis circuit patency maintained using, 1007
  during hemodialysis, 2091-2092, 2092t
  in membranous nephropathy, 1041-1042
  plasmapheresis use of, 2162
  regional, 2092
  in renal replacement therapy, 2144
  renal vein thrombosis treated with, 1206

Antidiuretic hormone. See Arginine vasopressin
Antifungal agents, 1235t-1236t
Antigens
  human leukocyte. See Human leukocyte antigens
  tubulointerstitial, 1214-1215, 1228-1229
Anti-glomerular basement membrane antibodies, 1124
Anti-glomerular basement membrane autoantibodies, 1124-1125
Anti-glomerular basement membrane disease. See also Goodpasture's syndrome
  clinical features of, 1125
  corticosteroids for, 1126-1127
  course of, 1126-1127
  electron microscopy of, 1126
  etiology of, 1124
  immunofluorescence microscopy of, 1126, 1126f
  kallikrein-kinin system in, 350
  laboratory findings in, 1125
  methylprednisolone for, 1126-1127
  pathogenesis of, 1124-1125
  pathology of, 1125-1126, 1126f
  plasmapheresis for, 1126-1127, 2149-2150, 2149t-2150t
  prognosis for, 1126-1127
  recurrence of, in renal allograft, 1127, 2270
  renal transplantation after, 2150
  rituximab for, 1126-1127
  treatment of, 1126-1127
Anti-glomerular basement membrane glomerulonephritis, 746
  animal models of, 1079-1080
  antibodies in, 1079
  antigens in, 1078-1079
  autoantibodies in, 1079
  characteristics of, 1076
  clinical features of, 1080-1081
  complement in, 1080
  electron microscopy of, 1078, 1078f
  end-stage kidney disease progression of, 1080-1081
  epidemiology of, 1076
  genetic susceptibility to, 1076
  immunofluorescence microscopy of, 1077, 1077f
  laboratory findings in, 1081
  light microscopy of, 1077-1078
  mouse models of, 1076
  natural history of, 1080-1081
  pathogenesis of, 1078-1080
  pathology of, 1077-1078, 1077f-1078f, 1077t
  plasmapheresis for, 1081
  prednisone for, 1081
  T cells in, 1079-1080
  treatment of, 1081
  tubulointerstitial changes in, 1078
Antihypertensive drug therapy, 1563-1565, 1563t
  β-adrenergic antagonists. See β-Adrenergic antagonists
  in African Americans, 1686, 1686t
  angiotensin receptor blockers. See Angiotensin receptor blockers
  angiotensin-converting enzyme inhibitors. See Angiotensin-converting enzyme inhibitors
  bedtime dosing of, 1692
  blood pressure goals, 1680-1681

Antihypertensive drug therapy (Continued)
  during breastfeeding, 1631
  calcium channel blockers. See Calcium channel blockers
  cardiovascular protection using, 2009-2011
  central adrenergic agonists. See Central adrenergic agonists
  central and peripheral adrenergic neuronal blocking agents, 1673
  combination therapies, 1681-1682, 1683t, 1689-1692, 1690f
  direct-acting vasodilators, 1673-1674, 1674t
  dosing of, 1692
  drug interactions, 1694
  in elderly, 1682-1685, 1684t
  endothelin receptor antagonists, 1675
  gender-based, 1685, 1686t
  history of changes to, 1587
  hypotension risks during hemodialysis secondary to, 2106
  morning dosing of, 1692
  new types of, 1696f
  nonadherence to, 1695
  in obese patients, 1686-1688, 1688t
  in older adults, 1682-1685
  peripheral α$_1$-adrenergic antagonists. See Peripheral α$_1$-adrenergic antagonists
  in pregnancy, 1629f, 1630t, 1685, 1687f
  rapid-acting oral drugs, 1699
  in renal insufficiency patients, 1649t-1650t
  in renal transplantation recipients, 2284t
  renin inhibitors, 1677-1678
  selective aldosterone receptor antagonists, 1678-1679
  for slowing chronic kidney disease progression, 1995-1998
  therapeutic effect with, 1684f
  tyrosine hydroxylase inhibitor, 1679-1680
Anti–IL-2R antibodies, 2248
Antimicrobial agents, 1234, 1235t-1236t, 1238-1239, 1238t, 1243-1244, 1247
Anti-MPO antibodies, 1083-1085
Antimycin A, 133
Antineoplastic drugs, 497
Antineutrophil cytoplasmic antibodies
  in anti-glomerular basement membrane glomerulonephritis, 1079
  crescentic glomerulonephritis induced by, 2150-2151
  cytoplasmic, 1086, 1111-1112, 1120
  in eosinophilic granulomatosis with polyangiitis, 1117
  in granulomatous with polyangiitis, 1111-1112
  in immunoglobulin A nephropathy, 1064
  laboratory tests for, 1115
  in microscopic polyangiitis, 1114-1115
  in pauci-immune crescentic glomerulonephritis, 1082
  perinuclear, 1086, 1111-1112, 1120
  in systemic lupus erythematosus, 1093-1094
  in temporal arteritis, 1120
Antineutrophil cytoplasmic antibody-associated vasculitides, 2351-2352, 2532
Antineutrophil cytoplasmic antibody-associated vasculitis, 350, 1084, 1086, 2150-2151
Antinuclear antibodies, in systemic lupus erythematosus, 1098-1099
Antioxidants, 1626

Antiphospholipid syndrome, 1106-1108, 1107f
Anti-phospholipase A_2 receptor antibodies, 746-747
Antiphospholipid antibodies, 1106-1107
Antiphospholipid nephropathy, 1106-1107
Antiphospholipid syndrome
   bilateral adrenal hemorrhage caused by, 588-589
   catastrophic, plasmapheresis for, 2158-2159
   clinical features of, 1200-1201
   definition of, 1200
   mechanisms of, 1201
   pathology of, 1201
   thrombotic microangiopathy caused by, 1200-1201
   treatment of, 1201
Antiplatelet therapy, 1625, 1625f, 1873, 1931-1932, 2012-2013
Anti-rheumatoid arthritis therapy-induced glomerulopathy, 1158-1159
Anti-Ro/SSA antibodies, 1099
Antisense oligonucleotides, 7-9
Anti-thin basement membrane nephritis, 1228-1229
Antithrombin III, 1206, 1803
Antithymocyte globulins, 1637t, 2247-2248, 2255, 2423-2424
Anti-U1RNP antibodies, 1108
Aorta, coarctation of, 1550, 1571f
Aortic baroceptors, 396
Aortic valve calcification, 1859, 2408
Aortoarteritis, 2506-2507
ApcT, 230t
Apelin, 419-420, 438, 446-447
Apical organic anion transporters, 219
Apical potassium channels, 159-160, 176-177, 564
Apical sodium channels, 179
Apical sodium hydrogen exchange, 154-155
Aplasia, 2294
Apnea, sleep, 1939-1940
Apo calbindin D28K, 192
APOL1, 674-676, 1153, 1165, 1429, 1770
Apolipoprotein-1, 693-694
Apolipoprotein A-1, 1801
Apolipoprotein B100, 2159
Apolipoprotein C, 1801
Apolipoprotein L-1, 1029
Apolipoprotein(a), 2100
Apoptosis
   in acute kidney injury pathophysiology, 974-975
   description of, 718
   of endothelial cells, 4-5, 1789
   erythropoietin suppression of, 1882-1883, 1882f
   of podocytes, 1788
   of proximal tubular cells, 1212, 1791
   tumor necrosis factor-like weak inducer of, 743
   in vascular calcification, 1836-1837
Apparent mineralocorticoid excess syndrome, 577-578, 1463
Appetite, loss of, 1819
Aquaporin(s)
   in ammonia metabolism, 254
   description of, 1468
   in nonepithelial cells, 288
   permeability properties of, 286
   in principal cells, 289, 289f
   in *Xenopus* oocytes, 288
Aquaporin-1, 147-148, 234, 254, 260-261, 273-276, 299, 805, 805f

Aquaporin-2
   basolateral, in cell migration and tubule morphogenesis, 290
   in cirrhosis, 300
   in cirrhosis-related water retention, 446
   clathrin-coated pits' role in recycling of, 291
   connecting tubule expression of, 69
   definition of, 286
   description of, 805, 805f, 1275
   in elderly, 739
   endocytosis of, phosphorylation's role in, 293
   endocytotic proteins and, 293-294
   endogenous, 289
   in endosomes, 287-288
   exocytosis of, phosphorylation's role in, 293
   exogenous, 288-289
   expression of, 286, 287f, 481f, 498, 1712
   in hypercalcemia, 299, 481
   in hypokalemia, 299
   in hyponatremia, 299-300
   impermeability of, 286
   in intracellular compartments, 291
   knockout mice model of, 276, 290f
   lithium effects on, 297-299, 298f
   membrane topology of, 286f
   methyl-β-cyclodextrin effects on, 292f
   nephrogenic diabetes insipidus and, 285, 298f, 481-482, 2338
   phosphorylation of, 293-294
   physiologic and pathophysiologic conditions associated with, 297t
   plasma membrane accumulation of, S256 residue's role in, 293
   plasma membrane expression of, 286, 287f
   in polyuria, 297
   in principal cells, 173, 289
   as recycling membrane protein, 291
   recycling of, 291
   S256 and, 293-294
   statins effect on, 301
   vasopressin effects on, 410, 805
Aquaporin-2 protein, 1472f
Aquaporin-2 trafficking
   actin cytoskeleton's role in, 294
   actin-associated proteins involved in, 294-295
   collecting duct used to examine, 289
   intracellular pathways of, 291
   kidney tissue slices used to examine, 289
   microtubules and, 295
   regulation of, 283f, 291-296, 296f
   SNARE proteins and, 295-296
   vasopressin-regulated, 287-288
Aquaporin-3, 254, 276, 289
Aquaporin-4, 276, 289, 299
Aquaporin-8, 254
Arachidonic acid
   cytochrome P450 metabolism of, 382, 382f-383f
   de-esterification of, 355
   definition of, 355
   epoxygenase metabolites of, 383
   esterification of, 355
   lipoxygenase metabolism of, 379f
   metabolism of, 355, 356f, 375, 382, 382f-383f
   metabolites of, 355
Arachnoid membrane cyst, 1491
ARAP1. *See* Angiotensin type 1 receptor-associated protein 1
Arcuate arteries, 84
Area cribrosa, 43, 44f

Arginine vasopressin receptor antagonists, 504-506, 509
Aristolochic acid, 755
Aristolochic acid nephropathy, 1223-1226, 2534
β-Arrestin, 282-284
Arrestin-receptor complexes, 283-284
Arrhythmias, 569-571, 598, 2107
Artemisinin, 2497
Arterial blood gas measurement, 521, 521t
Arterial calcification
   bone calcification and, 1836
   in chronic kidney disease, 1856-1857, 1857f, 1864, 1866
   clinical manifestations of, 1850
   detection of, 1847
   histology of, 1835f
Arterial stiffness, 1535, 1856
Arterial tone, 1856
Arterial wall thickening, in chronic kidney disease, 1855-1856
Arteriohyalinosis, 728f
Arteriosclerosis, 1315, 1855
Arteriovenous fistulas
   accessory vein ligation in, 2208-2209, 2209f
   angioplasty of, 2208-2210, 2209t
   blood flow rate, 2413
   digital subtraction angiography of, 2210f
   in elderly, 747-748, 2598
   failure of, 2206-2207
   hemodialysis vascular access using, 2064-2065, 2065f
   immature, 2206-2209, 2207t, 2209f
   maturation of, 2207, 2208f
   native, 2207
   neointimal hyperplasia in, 2194, 2195f
   preoperative vascular mapping of, 2203-2206, 2206f, 2206t
   quality improvement and, 2629-2631
   after renal transplantation, 911
   side-to-side, 2064-2065
   sonographic vascular mapping of, 2205-2206, 2206f
   stenotic lesions, angioplasty of, 2208, 2209f
   thrombosis of, 2210-2212
   tunneled catheters versus, 2629-2631
   vascular access stenosis in, 2194
   vascular mapping of, 2203-2206, 2206f, 2206t
Arteriovenous grafts
   failure of, 2194-2195
   hemodialysis using, 2065-2067, 2066f
   mortality associated with, 2542-2543
   percutaneous thrombectomy of, 2199-2202, 2199t, 2201f-2202f
   primary patency of, 2198, 2198t
   stenosis of
     angioplasty for, 2198-2202, 2198t, 2200f
     detection methods, 2195, 2196t
     monitoring of, 2196t
     pathophysiology of, 2197-2198
     stent deployment for, 2202-2203, 2204f-2205f
     surveillance for, 2194-2198, 2196t-2198t
     thrombosis secondary to, 2194-2195, 2196t, 2197
   thrombectomy of, 2199-2202, 2199t, 2201f-2202f
   thrombosis of, 2194-2195, 2196t, 2197
   vascular access stenosis, 2194
Arteriovenous shunt, 1949, 2558
Ascites, cirrhotic, 449, 1712, 1723
Ascorbic acid, 1361
ASCT2, 225

ASKP1240, 2259
Aspergillosis, 1150
Aspirin, 380, 2012
Aspirin, phenacetin, and caffeine, 2545
Asymmetric dimethylarginine, 443, 735
    as chronic kidney disease biomarker, 685, 950, 1811, 1934-1935
    endothelial dysfunction in chronic kidney disease and, 1856
    plasma levels of, 950
Asymptomatic bacteriuria, 1633
    antimicrobial treatment of, 1247
    biofilm formation as cause of, 1246
    description of, 749, 777
    diagnosis of, 1246
    epidemiology of, 1245-1246, 1245t
    Escherichia coli as cause of, 1246
    host factors associated with, 1246
    in men, 1245t
    microbiology of, 1246
    pathogenesis of, 1246
    in pregnancy, 1245-1247
    prevalence of, 1245
    pyuria associated with, 1246
    in renal transplantation recipients, 1248
    risk factors for, 1246
    treatment of, 1246-1247
Asymptomatic microscopic hematuria, 754-755
AT_1 receptor, 382, 407
AT_2 receptor, 407
Atenolol, 1656t-1657t, 1658
Atheroembolic acute kidney injury, 744
Atheroembolic renal disease, 1191-1193, 1192f
    cholesterol-lowering agents for, 1193
    clinical features of, 1191-1192
    differential diagnosis of, 1191
    distal protection devices for, 1193
    hypertension in, 1191
    hypocomplementemia in, 1192
    laboratory findings, 1192
    mechanisms of, 1192-1193
    outcomes of, 1191-1192
    pathology of, 1192, 1192f
    in renal allografts, 1191
    renal artery stenosis and, 1192-1193
    treatment of, 1193
Atherosclerosis
    calcifications associated with, 1833-1835, 1855
    in children, 2407-2408
    description of, 1855, 1859-1860
    fibromuscular disease versus, 1581-1582
    malnutrition and, 1930
    natural history of, 1802
    progression of, 1585, 1598-1599
    renal artery aneurysms caused by, 1203
    risk factor for, 1201
Atherosclerotic plaque, 1604
Atherosclerotic renal artery stenosis, 1580, 1583-1584
    angioplasty and stenting for, 1600-1602
    concurrent diseases associated with, 1587
    hypertension and, 1595-1596
    medical versus interventional therapy trials for, 1596t
    percutaneous transluminal renal angioplasty for, 1602-1603
    prevalence of, 1581t
    progression of, 1586f
    stenting and, 1600-1602
Atherosclerotic renovascular disease, 1568f, 1582f

ATPase, H^+ transporting, lysosomal accessory protein 2, 332
ATPases. *See* Adenosine triphosphatases
ATP6V1B1, 2385
Atrial fibrillation
    anticoagulation for, 1932
    in chronic kidney disease, 1859, 1908
    in end-stage kidney disease, 1929-1930
    in hemodialysis, 2107
    stroke risks associated with, 1928t, 1929-1930, 1932
    valvular heart disease and, 1929-1930
Atrial natriuretic peptide (ANP)
    acute tubular necrosis treated with, 1001
    age-related changes in, 738-739
    aldosterone levels affected by, 305-306
    angiotensin II inhibition by, 154
    atrial pressure effects on, 395
    blood pressure affected by, 342
    brain natriuretic peptide versus, 340
    cardiovascular effects of, 342
    in cirrhosis-related sodium retention, 447, 448f
    description of, 339, 413
    as disease biomarkers, 343
    in effective arterial blood volume regulation, 413-414
    furosemide effects on, 1717
    growth regulatory properties of, 414
    half-life of, 340
    in heart failure, 433
    natriuretic action of, 1799
    natriuretic effects of dopamine modulated by, 154
    plasma levels of, 414
    in portal hypertension, 447
    proANP, 340
    prostaglandins effect on, 436-437
    recombinant, 344
    renal effects of, 342
    smooth muscle affected by, 413-414
    sodium retention and, 447, 448f
    structure of, 339-340, 339f, 413
    synthesis of, 339-340
    therapeutic uses of, 344
    volume expansion effects on, 589
Atrial sensors, 394-395
Atrium, 395
Atypical hemolytic-uremic syndrome. *See* Hemolytic-uremic syndrome, atypical
Australia
    analgesic nephropathy in, 2544-2546
    chronic kidney disease in, 2544
    dialysis in, 2540f, 2542-2544
    end-stage kidney disease in, 2539-2540, 2541t
    health care access in, 2539-2540
    hemodialysis in, 2540f, 2542-2543
    indigenous (Aboriginals) population of
        chronic kidney disease in, 2549
        description of, 2538
        end-stage kidney disease in, 2547
        renal disease in, 2546-2549
        renal replacement therapy in, 2546
        renal transplantation in, 2548, 2548f
    peritoneal dialysis in, 2540f
    population of, 2540t
    renal replacement therapy in, 2540-2544, 2540f-2543f, 2545f, 2545t
    renal supportive care in, 2544
    renal transplantation in, 2540f, 2543-2544, 2543f
    Torres Strait Islanders, 2538, 2546

Australia and New Zealand Dialysis and Transplant Registry, 2538-2539
Australian and New Zealand Society of Nephrology, 2539, 2541-2542
Autacoids, 52
Autoantibodies, 1064, 1093, 1099, 1124-1125
Autoimmune chronic active hepatitis, 1156
Autoimmune diseases, 1228-1229
Autoimmune hypoparathyroidism, 617
Autonephrectomy, 882
Autonomic diabetic polyneuropathy, 1320
Autonomic nervous system, 54-55
Autonomic neuropathy, 1939
Autophagy, 734-735, 735f, 1837
Autoregulation, renal, 104-110, 396, 1740-1741
Autosomal diabetes insipidus, 1473
Autosomal dominant distal renal tubular acidosis, 1456f
Autosomal dominant early-onset hypertension with severe exacerbation during pregnancy, 1463
Autosomal dominant hypocalcemia with hypercalciuria, 2345
Autosomal dominant hypomagnesemia, 2388-2389
Autosomal dominant hypophosphatemic rickets, 630-631, 1452
Autosomal dominant polycystic kidney disease, 1371, 1416
    in Africa, 2459
    anemia in, 1888
    in children, 2319-2321
    computed tomography of, 869f, 1486f, 1491f
    cyst in, 1484f
    description of, 885
    diagnosis of, 1485-1487
    diverticular disease and, 1492
    epidemiology of, 1479
    gender differences in, 658
    genetics of, 1479-1480, 1486f
    genotype-phenotype correlations for, 1417
    glomerular filtration rate and, 1490f
    hypertension and, 1487-1489
    imaging of, 885-888, 888f-889f, 1486f
    magnetic resonance imaging of, 1486f
    manifestations of, 1487-1492
    in Middle East, 2477
    pain in, 1489, 1493
    pathogenesis of, 1480-1483
    progression of, 658, 1488f
    renal cyst infection associated with, 1250-1251
    renal failure and, 1489-1491
    tolvaptan for, 505
    treatment of, 1492-1496
    ultrasound of, 1485f, 1485t
Autosomal dominant polycystic kidney disease in situ, 1483f
Autosomal dominant tubulointerstitial kidney disease, 1504-1505
Autosomal recessive Alport's syndrome, 1423
Autosomal recessive ciliopathies with interstitial nephritis and renal cystic disease, 1505-1509, 1507t
Autosomal recessive distal renal tubular acidosis, 1456f
Autosomal recessive hypercholesterolemia, 179-180
Autosomal recessive hypophosphatemic rickets, 631, 1452, 1830

Autosomal recessive polycystic kidney disease, 1416-1417, 1496-1500, 1497f-1498f, 2319-2321
Autosomal recessive pseudohypoaldosteronism type I, 539, 539f
Avosentan, 338
Axial osmolality gradient, 265
Axitinib, 1383-1384, 1383f
Azathioprine
  adverse effects of, 1170, 2425
  in children, 2425
  definition of, 1170
  immunoglobulin A nephropathy treated with, 1068
  immunosuppressive uses of, 2245, 2254t, 2257, 2425
  lupus nephritis treated with, 1169-1170
  membranous nephropathy treated with, 1045
  prednisone and, 2257
  during pregnancy, 1637, 1637t
  toxicity of, 1170
Azilsartan medoxomil, 1651, 1652t
Azotemia, 1727. See also Prerenal azotemia
Azotemic renovascular disease, 1567-1568, 1577-1579

B

B7-1, 116
B cells, 1793
Bacille de Calmette-Guérin, 1254
Bacteremia, 1240, 2220
Bacterial peritonitis, 2128
Bacterial prostatitis, 750, 1247-1248
Bacteriuria
  asymptomatic. See Asymptomatic bacteriuria
  definition of, 1231-1232
  in elderly, 1243
Bad, 1791
Balkan endemic nephropathy, 1224-1226, 1225f
Bangladesh. See Indian subcontinent
Barbiturates, 2183
Bardet-Biedl syndrome, 1417, 1509, 2322, 2322t
Bardoxolone methyl, 1313
Bariatric surgery, 1342f
Baroreceptors, 396, 468
Bartonella henselae, 1149-1150
Bartter's syndrome, 176, 189-190, 554, 1417-1418, 1457-1459
  antenatal, 578, 2334-2335, 2336f
  in children, 2333-2335, 2344, 2376-2378, 2377f, 2377t
  classic, 578, 2334, 2378
  clinical manifestations of, 578, 2377-2378
  clinical presentation of, 1458-1459, 2333-2334
  hypocalcemia with, 2335
  metabolic alkalosis caused by, 551-552, 554
  in Middle East, 2479
  pathogenesis of, 1457-1458
  prevalence of, 2333
  pseudo-, 579-583
  renal magnesium wasting in, 622
  thick ascending limb and, 579f
  treatment of, 1459, 2335, 2377-2378
  types of, 578-579, 2334-2335, 2377f, 2377t
Barttin, 157, 161
Base, 517
Basement membrane. See also Glomerular basement membrane
  of Bowman's capsule, 52-53

Basement membrane (Continued)
  epithelial, 25
  of peritubular capillaries, 89-90
  plasma protein passage across, 1013
  proximal tubule, 1284f
  of thin limbs of loop of Henle, 62
Basolateral intercellular space, 55-56
Basolateral organic anion transporters, 219
B^0AT1, 222-225
B^0AT3, 224-225
Beckwith-Wiedemann syndrome, 2297t
Bee stings, 2500, 2525
Beer potomania, 496
Beers criteria, 2594
Belatacept, 2248, 2254t, 2258-2259
Belimumab, 1104-1105
Benazepril hydrochloride, 1641-1642, 1643t
Bence Jones proteins, 990
Benidipine, 1665
Benign cystic neoplasm, 1369-1370
Benign epithelial tumor, 1368
Benign mesenchymal tumor, 1368-1369
Benign neoplasm, 1368-1370
Benign prostatic hyperplasia, 1261, 1280
β-trace protein, 935-936
Betaxolol, 1656t-1657t, 1658
Betel nut chewing, 2534
Bevacizumab, 1383f, 1384, 1398
BGT1, 226
Bias, of estimating glomerular filtration rate equations, 785
Bicarbonate
  cytosolic, 234-235
  diarrhea effects on, 528-529
  excretion of, 551
  in extracellular fluid, 514, 519, 830f
  gain of, systemic response to, 519-520
  gastrointestinal loss of, 529, 529t
  generation of
    ammonia metabolism in, 248-255
    carbon dioxide retention effects on, 516
    citrate excretion in, 247-248
    organic anion excretion in, 247-248
    titratable acid excretion in, 246-247
  in hemodialysis dialysate, 2094-2095
  hydrogen removal by, 835
  luminal, 234, 241
  metabolic alkalosis caused by, 552-553
  in paracellular sodium chloride transport, 147
  in peritoneal dialysis solutions, 2119, 2125
  plasma concentration of
    arterial blood gas values and, 521
    chloride repletion for, 520
    description of, 513-514
    in high anion gap acidosis, 524-525
    increase in, renal response to, 520
  proximal tubule excretion of, 519
  regeneration of, 515
  secretion of, 244-245
  serum, 684-685
  supplementation of, 684-685, 2004
  urine, 2382
Bicarbonate reabsorption
  ammonia effects on, 245
  angiotensin II effects on, 408
  carbonic anhydrase for, 1703-1704
  carbonic anhydrase inhibitors effect on, 136
  in chronic kidney disease, 1749
  in collecting ducts
    aldosterone regulation of, 244
    anion exchangers in, 243
    carbonic anhydrase's role in, 243
    cells involved in, 239-241, 239f-241f
    chloride channel's role in, 243

Bicarbonate reabsorption (Continued)
  cortical, 242
  H^+-ATPase's role in, 242
  H^+-K^+-ATPase's role in, 242-243
  hormonal regulation of, 244-245
  inner medullary, 242
  intercalated cells involved in, 239-241, 239f-241f
  kidney anion exchanger 1's role in, 243
  outer medullary, 242
  paracrine regulation, 245
  principal cells involved in, 241
  proteins involved in, 242-244
  segments of, 239
  sodium-bicarbonate cotransporters in, 243-244
  in connecting tubules, 241-242
  in distal convoluted tubule, 238-239
  diuretics effect on, 1703-1704
  intercalated cells involved in, 239-241, 239f-241f
  in loop of Henle, 238
  metabolic acidosis effects on, 236-238, 244
  metabolic alkalosis effects on, 244
  osmotic gradient caused by, 147-148
  proximal, 151
  in proximal tubule
    acid-base effects on, 237
    angiotensin II effects on, 237
    calcium-sensing receptor effects on, 238
    carbonic anhydrase in, 237
    description of, 530
    electroneutral sodium-bicarbonate cotransporter in, 236-237
    endothelin effects on, 237
    general mechanisms of, 234-235
    H^+-ATPase in, 235-236
    luminal flow rate effects on, 237
    metabolic acidosis effects on, 236-237
    Na^+-H^+ exchangers in, 235
    parathyroid hormone effects on, 237-238
    potassium effects on, 237
    regulation of, 237-238
    schematic diagram of, 236f, 2384f
  sites of, 234, 235f
  in thick ascending limb, 238
Bikunin, 1330-1331
Bilateral cortical necrosis, 1631-1632
Bilateral disease, 1570t
Bilateral renal artery stenosis, 1595
Bilateral ureteral obstruction, 299
Bile acid metabolism, 734
Bile salts, 2508
Bilirubin, 790
Biochemical hypoparathyroidism, 1453
Bioelectrical impedance analysis, 2079, 2096, 2099
Bioethics, 2558-2562
Biofilms, catheter-related bacteremia caused by, 2220
Bioflavonoids, 2036
Biomarkers
  acute kidney injury, 930-932, 931t
  candidate markers, 927
  chronic kidney disease. See Chronic kidney disease, biomarkers for
  chronic kidney disease–mineral bone disorder, 1840t
  clinical utility of, retrospective studies of, 928
  Critical Path Initiative for, 953
  definition of, 927, 927t
  development of, 927-930

Biomarkers (Continued)
  diabetic nephropathy, 1294t
  discovery of, 927-930
  exploratory studies for, 927-928
  future of, 954
  glomerular filtration, 932-936
  ideal, 930, 930t
  Integrated Discrimination Improvement Index for, 929-930
  Kidney Health Initiative on, 953-954
  multiple, combination of, 952-953, 953t
  natriuretic peptides as, 343-344
  Net Reclassification Index for, 929-930
  performance analysis of, 929-930, 929f
  pharmacodynamic, 927t
  predictive, 927t
  prognostic, 927t
  prospective screening studies for, 928-929
  qualification process for, 928-929
  receiver operator characteristic curve for, 929, 929f
  serum, 931
  surrogate endpoint, 927t
  urinary
    albuminuria as, 948
    cystatin C, 948-949
    description of, 931
    glomerular cell injury, 936-937
    glutathione S-transferase, 938-939
    hepcidin-25, 939
    insulin-like growth factor-binding protein-7, 949
    interleukin-18, 939-941
    kidney injury molecule-1, 941-942
    liver-type fatty acid-binding protein, 942-943
    β_1-microglobulin, 937-938, 1041
    β_2-microglobulin, 938
    N-acetyl-β-D-glucosaminidase, 947
    nephrin, 936-937
    netrin-1, 943
    neutrophil gelatinase-associated lipocalin, 943-947
    podocalyxin, 936
    podocyte count, 936
    proteinuria as, 947-948
    for renal fibrosis, 951-952
    tissue inhibitor metalloproteinase-2, 949
    tubular injury, 937-949
  urinary tract obstruction, 1263
  validation process for, 928
Biomaterials, 2602, 2609-2610
Biopsy
  bone, 1842-1846, 1845t
  kidney. See Kidney biopsy
Biotin, 1983-1984
Biphenyl tetrazoles, 1651-1653
Birth weight
  blood pressure affected by, 706-709, 707f-708f
  categories of, 694t
  chronic kidney disease and, 712
  end-stage kidney disease and, 712, 713f
  fetal drug exposure effects on, 719
  gestational hyperglycemia effects on, 717-718
  glomerular characteristics by, 696t
  glomerular filtration rate affected by, 709-710
  low. See Low birth weight
  nephron number and, 703-705
  proteinuria and, 710-711
  renal function affected by, 709-712

Birt-Hogg-Dube syndrome, 1374, 1951-1952, 1952f, 1952t
Bisoprolol, 1656t-1657t, 1658
Bisphosphonates, 611, 627, 1399, 2396
BK channels, 179, 564, 574
BK virus, 1404-1405, 2272, 2428, 2430
Bladder cancer, 755, 1261
Bladder dysfunction, 1320, 2314
Bladder tumors, 862f
Blood
  arterial, pH of, 2382
  loss of, 1885, 1962
  phosphorus in, 196, 197t, 626
Blood pressure. See also High blood pressure; Hypertension
  ambulatory monitoring of, 1538, 1540-1542, 1541t-1542t, 1693, 1694f
  angiotensin II and, 1532f, 1640-1641
  atrial natriuretic peptide effects on, 342
  birth weight effects on, 706-709, 707f-708f
  catch-up growth effects on, 721-722
  in children, 2360
  chronic kidney disease and, 679, 1563f
  classification of, 765, 765t
  control of, 1527-1528, 1552-1553
    angiotensin-converting enzyme inhibitors for, 1303-1305, 1317, 1928-1929
    antihypertensive drug therapy goals for, 1680-1681. See also Antihypertensive drug therapy
    cardiovascular disease risk prevention through, 1867-1868, 2009
    in chronic kidney disease management, 1867, 1975, 2009, 2283
    in diabetic nephropathy, 1303-1312
    dietary modifications for, 1931
    during hemodialysis, 1316, 2103
    intravenous agents, 1630-1631
    in kidney disease patients, 1689, 1689t
    kidney's role in, 1861
    nighttime ventilation techniques for, 1694
    renoprotection through, 1765-1767
  developmental programming of, 709, 709f
  diastolic, 1524, 1524t, 1526f, 1681
  in elderly, 745, 745f, 2010f, 2592
  endothelium and, 1534-1535
  EP4 receptor's role in regulation of, 372
  glomerular volume and, 709, 709f
  goals for, 1680-1681
  hepatocyte growth factor effects on, 1741
  homeostasis of, 393f
  kidney function decline and, 1562f
  left ventricular hypertrophy and, 1688-1689
  low birth weight effects on, 707, 1627f
  magnesium and, 623
  measurement of, 766, 1525t, 1538-1542, 1539f
  metabolic capacity and, 722f
  metabolic load and, 722f
  mortality in veterans with chronic kidney disease, 1559f
  nephron number and, 697t-698t, 709, 709f
  in patients undergoing dialysis, 1561-1562
  physiology of, 1528
  plasmapheresis effects on, 2163
  preeclampsia prevention and, 1626
  prematurity effects on, 706-709, 707f-708f
  rapid reduction of, 1699-1700

Blood pressure (Continued)
  soluble epoxide hydrolase in regulation of, 385
  stroke risks and, 1929f
  sudden reduction in, 1700
Blood urea nitrogen, 123, 933-934, 988, 1808, 1959, 1968-1969
BMAL1 gene, 256
Bmp4, 31
BMP4, 2297-2298
Bmp1ra, 27
Body fluids, 391f-392f, 460-462, 461f, 486, 2365, 2414
Body lead burden, 686-687
Body mass index, 1323f, 1343f, 1771
Bohr effect, 527
BOLD magnetic resonance imaging, 864, 1271
Bone
  biology of, 1831-1833
  calcification of, 1836
  calcium-sensing receptor's role in, 1826
  cellular components of, 1832
  composition of, 1831-1832
  histology of, 1844f
  hyperparathyroid, 1844f
  immunosuppressive agents effect on, 1851-1852
  magnesium in, 193, 193t
  mineralization of, 1845
  phosphorus in, 196
  postrenal transplantation changes in, 1851-1852
  remodeling of, 1830, 1832, 1833f-1834f, 1845, 1849
  resorption of, 611-612
  trabecular, 1831-1832, 1842
  turnover of, 1845-1846, 1845t
  volume of, 1845
Bone disease, 1352-1355, 1437, 1843
Bone formation rate, 1845
Bone marrow transplantation (BMT), 991t, 992-993, 1193, 2249-2250
Bone marrow-derived fibrocytes, 1793
Bone marrow-derived mesenchymal progenitor cells, 1197
Bone marrow-derived mesenchymal stem cells, 2611
Bone mineral density (BMT)
  fractures and, 1852, 2283
  minimal change disease effects on, 1022
  posttransplantation reductions in, 2282-2283
  stone formers and, 1353t
  thiazide diuretics effect on, 1726-1727
Bone morphogenetic proteins (BMPs), 28-29, 34, 1217, 1757-1758, 1843
Bone pain, 2282
Bone-specific alkaline phosphatase, 1842
Bortezomib, 1105, 2248-2249
Bosniak renal cyst classification, 1375, 1376t
Bothrops snakebites, 2447
Bouin's fixative, 919
Bowel dysfunction, 2314
Bowman's capsule, 4-5, 45-46, 52-53
Bowman's space, 45-46, 47f, 94-96, 95f, 1789
BQ-123, 338
Brachyury, 2603
Bradford-Hill criteria, of causality, 670, 670t
Bradykinin, 417, 1740
Bradykinin receptors, 347, 350
Brain herniation, 503

Brain natriuretic peptide (BNP)
  antifibrotic effects of, 342
  atrial natriuretic peptide versus, 340
  as biomarker, 343-344
  in cirrhosis, 447
  description of, 339
  in effective arterial blood volume regulation, 414
  half-life of, 340
  in heart failure, 433-434
  nephrectomy effects on levels of, 1739
  NT-proBNP, 343, 433-434, 453
  plasma levels of, 414, 434
  preproBNP, 340
  pro-, 1800
  recombinant, 344
  renal effects of, 342
  secretion of, 414
  structure of, 339f, 340, 413
  synthesis of, 340
  therapeutic uses of, 344
Branched-chain amino acids, 1971
Branching morphogenesis, 5
Branchio-oto-renal syndrome, 2297t, 2299, 2318
Brazil, 2451. See also Latin America
Breast cancer, 607-608, 1670
Breastfeeding, 1631, 1638
Brescia-Cimino procedure, 2064
Bright's disease, 1855
Bromodeoxyuridine, 2608
Bronchiectasias, 1492
Bronchogenic carcinoma, 499-500
Brugada sign, 570-571
Brush border
  of pars convoluta cells, 56-59
  of proximal tubule, 55, 57f
Brush border membrane vesicles, 211
Brushite, 1323, 1328, 1342f
Buckley's syndrome, 1050
Bufadienolide, 419
Buffer systems
  in acid-base homeostasis, 512-514
  open, 513
    physicochemical, chemical equilibria of, 512-513
  regulation of, 513-514
Buffering, 512, 519
Bumetanide, 1707
Bundled prospective payment system, 2628-2629
Burst-forming units–erythroid, 1882-1883
bZIP transcription factor, 2483

C

C fibers, 1942
C3, 1761, 1792
C3 convertases, 1183-1184
C5 convertase, 1183-1184
C3 glomerulonephritis, 1046, 1046f-1047f, 1050, 1053
C3 glomerulopathies
  algorithm for, 1054f
  classification of, 1046, 1046f
  dense deposit disease. See Dense deposit disease
  description of, 1045-1046
  diagnosis of, 1054f
  eculizumab for, 1159
  epidemiology of, 1050
  immunofluorescence microscopy findings, 1051
  nephrotic syndrome caused by, 1045-1046
  pathogenesis of, 1052, 1052f
  pathology of, 1050-1052, 1051f

C3 nephritic factor, 1146-1147
Cadmium nephropathy, 1227
Caenorhabditis elegans, 19
Cairo-Bishop criteria, 990, 992t
Calbindin, 2390-2391
Calbindin-D28K, 66-67, 192
Calcidiol, 1828, 1841, 1848
Calcific uremic arteriolopathy. See Calciphylaxis
Calcifications
  aortic valve, 1859
  arterial. See Arterial calcification
  in atherosclerosis, 1855
  extraskeletal, 1850
  metastatic, 1945-1946
  mitral valve, 1859
  renal, 871-878
  renal parenchymal, 1775
  vascular. See Vascular calcification
Calcimimetics
  for chronic kidney disease–mineral bone disorder, 1873, 2026-2028
  definition of, 2026
  for secondary hyperparathyroidism, 2032
Calcineurin, 189
Calcineurin inhibitors, 1398-1399
  adverse effects of, 1167-1168
  bone pain caused by, 2282
  glomerular disease treated with, 1167-1168
  hyperkalemia associated with, 541, 2281
  hypertension caused by, 1167-1168
  hypomagnesemia caused by, 622
  immunosuppressive uses of, 2256, 2271, 2424-2425
  lupus nephritis treated with, 1104
  malignancies induced by, 1168
  membranous nephropathy treated with, 1043-1044
  nephrotoxicity caused by, 378, 1167, 2259, 2268-2269, 2272-2275
  podocytes affected by, 119
  renal transplantation uses of, 2256, 2271
  steroid-resistant nephrotic syndrome treated with, 2330-2331
  steroid-sensitive nephrotic syndrome treated with, 2329-2330
  toxicity of, 1168
  vasoconstriction caused by, 2265
Calciphylaxis, 1944-1945, 1945f, 2103
Calcitonin, 1400
  bicarbonate reabsorption stimulated by, 245
  bone resorption inhibition using, 612
  in children, 2390-2391
  nephrogenic diabetes insipidus treated with, 301
Calcitonin gene-related peptide, 110
Calcitriol, 1830, 1872-1873, 1923-1924, 2025, 2089
Calcium
  absorption of, 185-187, 1824-1825
  blood forms of, 602
  bound form of, 186
  calcimimetics effect on, 1873, 2027
  in cellular processes, 185-186
  in children. See Children, calcium in
  in chronic kidney disease–mineral bone disorder, 1847
  citrate association with, 219
  components of, 186f
  daily ingestion of, 601-602
  dosage of, 1361
  excretion of, 1334f
    in Bartter's syndrome, 578
    in chronic kidney disease, 2031

Calcium *(Continued)*
  diuretics effect on, 1726
  hypocalcemia prevention goals for, 2393
  in proximal renal tubular acidosis, 533
  fibroblast growth factor-23 effects on levels of, 2019-2020
  filtered, 188f
  forms of, 186
  fractional excretion of, 1706, 1749-1750
  free, 186, 602
  globulin binding of, 602
  glomerulus filtration of, 187
  in hemodialysis dialysate, 2094, 2106
  homeostasis of
    age-related changes in, 741-742
    description of, 1824-1825
    disorders of. See Hypercalcemia; Hypocalcemia
    hormones involved in, 1838-1839
    modulation of, 601
    parathyroid hormone effects on, 601, 1826-1827, 1923-1924
    parathyroid hormone–vitamin D endocrine system regulation of, 187, 187f
    schematic diagram of, 186f
    whole-body, 601-602
  hyperkalemia treated with, 593-594
  insulin effects on deposition of, 1914
  intestinal hyperabsorption of, 1331-1333
  intracellular, 306
  ionized, 1824
  kidney stones and, 1324
  measurement of, 2028-2029
  monitoring of, 2014
  nephron loss-specific adaptations in metabolism of, 1749-1750
  oxalate concentration versus, 1325-1327
  parathyroid hormone and, 606f, 1827f, 2023
  preeclampsia prevention use of, 1626
  protein-bound, 186, 187f, 602
  reabsorption of, 187-189
    in distal tubule, 189, 190f
    intestinal, 741-742
    in loop of Henle, 188-189
    metabolic acidosis effects on, 191
    metabolic alkalosis effects on, 191
    parathyroid hormone effects on, 1828
    in proximal tubule, 188, 188f
    in thick ascending limb, 188
  renal parenchymal deposits of, 1775
  serum, 186, 186f, 1822, 1824, 1851
  transport of. See Calcium transport
  whole-body amount of, 601-602
Calcium acetate, 2022
Calcium antagonist, 1560
Calcium carbonate, 2022
Calcium channel blockers (CCBs), 1564, 1629, 1995
  adverse effects of, 1668
  angiotensin II affected by, 1662
  angiotensin-converting enzyme inhibitors and, 1669, 1681-1682, 1684f
  antiproteinuric effects of, 1667
  atherogenesis inhibition by, 1669
  benzothiazepines, 1663-1664
  β-blockers and, 1669, 1691
  breast cancer and, 1670
  contraindications for, 1668
  dihydropyridines, 1662, 1664-1670, 1668t, 1699
  diphenylalkylamine, 1664
  diuresis caused by, 1662

INDEX

Calcium channel blockers (CCBs) (Continued)
  diuretics and, 1691
  dosing of, 1649t-1650t
  drug interactions with, 1669-1670, 1670t
  dual therapy using, 1691
  efficacy of, 1668-1671
  in elderly, 1685
  hemodynamic effects of, 1666-1667, 1668t
  hypertensive urgencies and emergencies treated with, 1697t, 1698-1699
  indications for, 1662
  long-term effects of, 1667
  mechanism of action, 1662
  nondihydropyridines, 1662
  nonhemodynamic effects of, 1667
  pharmacodynamics of, 1663t
  pharmacokinetics of, 1663t
  renal autoregulation blockade by, 105
  renal effects of, 1666-1667, 1667t
  in renal insufficiency patients, 1649t-1650t
  in renal transplantation recipients, 1667
  renin-angiotensin-aldosterone inhibitors and, combination therapy using, 1690-1691
  safety of, 1668-1671
  side effects of, 1689-1690
  types of, 1662-1666, 1663t
  vasodilatory properties of, 1662, 1685
Calcium channels, 1662
Calcium chloride, 593-594
Calcium citrate, 1758-1759
Calcium gluconate, 593-594, 618
Calcium oxalate, 1324-1325, 1328, 1338f. See also Oxalate
Calcium oxalate stones, 873, 1260, 1323, 1323f, 1325, 1326f, 1633, 2507
Calcium phosphate stones, 873, 1323f, 1325, 1326f, 1633
Calcium stone, 1323, 1323f, 1331-1341, 1352-1355, 1633
Calcium transport
  in distal nephron, 190f
  in distal tubule, 192f
  epithelial, 1826f
  parathyroid hormone effects on, 187
  proteins involved in, 191-193
  regulation of, 189-191
    calcium-regulating hormones involved in, 189
    diuretics in, 189-191
    estrogens in, 191
    extracellular calcium in, 189
    Klotho in, 191
    metabolic acidosis effects on, 191
    novel proteins involved in, 191
    proteins involved in, 191
    sclerostin in, 191
  renal, 1825
  transcellular, 188
  transepithelial, 1706
Calcium-binding protein 39, 163
Calcium-containing binders, 2022, 2031, 2094
Calcium/magnesium-sensing receptor–associated disorder, 1466
Calcium–parathyroid hormone–fibroblast growth factor-23 loop, 1839
Calcium-phosphate deposition, in end-stage kidney disease, 1775
Calcium-regulating hormones, 189

Calcium-sensing receptor (CaSR)
  activation of
    in hypercalcemia, 609-610
    parathyroid hormone secretion affected by, 2026
    phospholipase C stimulation secondary to, 1827f
  apical, 574
  bicarbonate reabsorption affected by, 238, 245
  in bone, 1826
  calcimimetic agent interaction with, 2020
  calcimimetic targeting of, 2026-2027
  description of, 164, 164f, 189, 448, 601-602, 1825
  expression of, 1825-1826
  gain-of-function mutations in, 614-616
  gene expression, 1334
  mutations of, 579, 2378
  in vascular calcification, 1826
Calculated panel reactive antibody, 2260
Caloric intake, in chronic kidney disease, 1973
Calorie restriction, 732-733
Calyceal cyst, 1518
Calyceal diverticulum, 889
Camptomelic dysplasia, 2297t
Cancer
  acute kidney injury and, 990, 991t, 1390
  angiotensin receptor blockers and, 1655-1656
  renal failure and, 1390t
  in renal transplantation recipients, 2284-2286, 2285t, 2543-2544
  viral infections associated with, 2285t
Candesartan cilexetil, 1651-1652, 1652t
Candida species, 1254, 1404, 2129
Candidate gene, 1348
Candiduria, 1254, 1254t
Cannabinoid receptor 1 blockade, albuminuria caused by, 120
Cannabinoid receptors, in cirrhosis, 443-444
Capillarization of sinusoids, 441
Capillary hydraulic pressure, 426
Captopril
  adverse effects of, 1648
  characteristics of, 1641
  dosage of, 1641
  hypertensive urgencies and emergencies treated with, 1697t
  proteinuria associated with, 1159, 1645
  renography enhanced with, 908
  sodium excretion affected by, 444-445
Captopril challenge test, 1546
Captopril trial, 1555
Carbamazepine, 471, 497, 2182-2183
Carbapenems, 1235t-1236t
Carbenoxolone, 577
Carbohydrates, 128f, 1816
Carbon dioxide, 255, 513-514
Carbon dioxide load, 512
Carbon dioxide tension, 515-516
Carbon dioxide–bicarbonate system, 513
Carbon monoxide poisoning, 545
Carbonic acid, 234
Carbonic anhydrase
  in ammonia secretion, 253-255
  in bicarbonate reabsorption, 237, 243
  collecting duct ammonia secretion affected by, 253
  deficiency of, 531-532
  description of, 1702

Carbonic anhydrase (Continued)
  II, 237
  intercalated cell levels of, 71-72
  IV, 237, 243, 254-255
  metabolic acidosis effects on, 244
  in proximal tubule bicarbonate reabsorption, 237
  XII, 243
Carbonic anhydrase II, 530-532, 1455
Carbonic anhydrase inhibitors
  adverse effects of, 1704
  bicarbonate reabsorption affected by, 136
  bicarbonate wasting caused by, 532
  in elderly, 1704
  indications for, 1704
  long-term administration of, 1703-1704
  mechanism of action, 1702-1704
  metabolic acidosis caused by, 1730
  pharmacokinetics of, 1704
  site of action, 1702-1704
  urine alkalization using, 2168
Carboxyl angiotensin-converting enzyme inhibitors, 1641-1644, 1643t
3-Carboxy-4-methyl-5-propyl-2-furanpropionic acid, 2037
Carboxypeptidase G_2, 2188
Cardenolide, 419
Cardiac arrest, 970, 2107
Cardiac dysfunction, 2139
Cardiac filling sensors, 394-396
Cardiac output, 83, 85, 133, 393-394, 396
Cardiac remodeling, 342
Cardiac surgery, 991t, 992
Cardioembolic stroke, 1927
Cardiorenal syndrome, 2139
Cardiovascular calcification index, 1847
Cardiovascular disease
  albuminuria and, 1860-1861
  antihypertensive drug therapy for, 1688-1689
  in children, 2406-2409, 2421-2422, 2432-2433
  in chronic kidney disease. *See* Chronic kidney disease, cardiovascular disease associated with
  clinical manifestations of, 1859-1860
  in diabetes nephropathy, 1295, 1316-1317
  diagnosis of, 2101-2102
  in elderly, 2590
  estimated glomerular filtration rate and, 1855, 1866, 2008
  hyperlipidemia and, 1802
  in kidney disease, 1166
  kidney function and, 1860
  microalbuminuria and, 1295
  mortality caused by, 2409
  occlusive, antiplatelet therapy for, 1873
  in peritoneal dialysis, 2127-2128
  preeclampsia and, 1618, 1618f
  premature, 1855
  in renal transplantation recipients, 2283-2284
  risk factors for, 1201
    anemia, 1863-1864, 1930
    chronic kidney disease–mineral bone disorder, 1864-1865, 1872-1873
    coagulation defects, 1863
    congestive heart failure, 1862t
    diabetes mellitus, 1865
    dyslipidemia, 1863, 2011
    fibroblast growth factor-23, 2101
    in hemodialysis patients, 2100-2101

Cardiovascular disease (Continued)
  homocysteine, 1864, 1970
  hypertension, 1861, 1862t, 1873, 2127, 2421-2422
  inflammation, 1865, 2100
  left ventricular hypertrophy, 1295-1296, 1857-1858, 2101-2102, 2421-2422
  list of, 1862t
  obesity, 1865-1866
  oxidative stress, 1865, 2100-2101
  phosphate retention, 1978-1979
  stroke, 1862t
  vitamin D levels, 1864-1865
  treatment of, 2101-2102
  in type 1 diabetes mellitus, 1295
  urolithiasis and, 1351, 1351f
Cardiovascular system
  bradykinin effects on, 417
  COX-2 inhibitor effects on, 363-364
  hypermagnesemia manifestations of, 625
  hypomagnesemia manifestations of, 622-623
  natriuretic peptides effect on, 342
Caribbean, 2442f
Caroli's disease, 1496-1497
Carotid baroceptors, 396
Carotid endarterectomy, 1932
Carotid-femoral pulse wave velocity, 1535
Carp bile, raw, 2525
Carperitide, 344
Carteolol, 1656t-1657t, 1657
Carvedilol, 1658t-1659t, 1659
Case-control studies, 671
Casein kinase 2, 154
CASK, 29
Caspase-1, 2485-2486
Caspase-3, 1817, 1965
Cast nephropathy, 1391-1393
Castleman's disease, 1159
Casts, in urine, 800, 800t, 801f
Cat scratch disease, 1149-1150
Catabolism
  amino acid, 1963-1964
  fats, 128f
  muscle, 1967
  myostatin activation caused by, 1967
  protein, 128f, 517, 1959-1960
Catastrophic antiphospholipid antibody syndrome, 2158-2159
Catch-up growth, 721-723
Catecholamines
  arginine vasopressin effects on, 1717
  hypokalemic effect of, 562
  myocardial infarction effects on, 1729
  phosphate transport affected by, 200-201
  thermogenic effect of, 137
Catecholamine-secreting tumor, 1548
β-Catenin, 28-29, 1832-1833, 1834f
Caterpillar stings, 2445-2446, 2446f
Catestatin, 438, 1533
Catheters
  bacteremia associated with, 2220
  hemodialysis. See Hemodialysis, catheters for
  infection of, 2068f
  peritoneal dialysis. See Peritoneal dialysis, catheters used in
  subclavian, 2145
  tunneled. See Tunneled catheters
Cation exchange resins, 596-597
Causality, Bradford-Hill criteria of, 670, 670t
ClC-K1 channel, 156-157, 157f, 161, 278
CD28, 2240-2241

CD133+ cells, 2609
CD4+ T cells, 1216, 1795
Cd2ap, 38
CD2AP disease, 1430
CD2-associated protein, 113
Cdc42, 38, 39f
CDX2 gene, 2606
CE45, 2611
Cefotaxime, 1241t
Ceftazidime, 2041
Ceftriaxone, 1241, 1241t
Celiprolol, 1658t-1659t, 1659
Cell membrane, 125
Cell-mediated immunity, 1233
Central α$_2$-adrenergic agonist, 1698
Central adrenergic agonists
  dosing of, 1649t-1650t
  efficacy of, 1672
  mechanism of action, 1671
  pharmacodynamics of, 1671, 1672t
  pharmacokinetics of, 1671, 1671t
  receptor binding of, 1671t
  renal effects of, 1672
  in renal insufficiency patients, 1649t-1650t
  safety of, 1672
  types of, 1671-1672
Central and peripheral adrenergic neuronal blocking agents, 1673
Central diabetes insipidus. See Diabetes insipidus, central
Central hypervolemia, 394-395
Central nervous system, 342, 419, 501-502
Central vein stenosis, 2212-2214, 2212f-2214f
Central venous catheters, 2412-2413, 2542-2543
Centrifugation, 2160, 2161f
Cephalosporins, 1235t-1236t
Cerebral blood flow, 1700
Cerebral edema, 813, 1619-1620, 1705
Cerebral hypoperfusion, 1930
Cerebral salt wasting, 493
Cetuximab, 575, 1398
CHADS$_2$ score, 1932
Channel-activating protease-1, 565-566
Charcot-Marie Tooth neuropathy-associated glomerulopathy, 1429
CHARGE syndrome, 2300
CHD7, 2300
Chemokine(s), 1794, 2241, 2243
Chemokine C-C motif receptor 1, 1754-1755
Chemokine ligand 2, 976
Chemokine ligand 8, 1233
Chemotherapy, 1385
  cast nephropathy and, 1392
  hyperuricemia and, 1396
  nephrotoxic injury and, 1397
  tumor cell necrosis after, 968
  volume expansion before, 628
  for Wilms' tumor, 1387
Childbirth, 1617
Children. See also Infants
  acid-base equilibrium in, 2382-2383, 2382t
  acute postinfectious glomerulonephritis in, 2331-2333
  Bardet-Biedl syndrome in, 2322, 2322t
  Bartter's syndrome in, 2333-2335, 2344, 2376-2378, 2377f, 2377t
  blood pressure screening in, 2360
  calcitonin in, 2390-2391
  calcium in
    balance of, 2389-2390, 2389f-2390f
    disorders of, 2391-2396
    distribution of, 2389, 2389f
    intestinal absorption of, 2390
    regulation of, 2389

Children (Continued)
  chronic kidney disease in
    angiotensin receptor blockers for, 2362
    angiotensin-converting enzyme inhibitors for, 2362
    cardiovascular comorbidities, 2359-2361
    demographics of, 2309
    description of, 2308
    development effects of, 2357-2359
    glomerular filtration rate assessments, 2309
    growth failure secondary to, 1918, 2357-2359, 2358f-2359f
    hypertension caused by, 2360, 2421-2422
    intima-media thickness changes associated with, 2361, 2361f
    left ventricular hypertrophy with, 2360-2361, 2421-2422, 2432
    metabolic acidosis with, 2359
    neurodevelopment dysfunctions secondary to, 2309
    nutrition effects of, 2357-2359
    progression of, 2361-2362, 2362f
    pubertal delay caused by, 2357, 2435-2436
    recombinant growth hormone therapy for, 2359, 2359f
    renal function changes, 2361
    renal transplantation for, 2422
    vitamin D deficiency associated with, 2434
  chronic kidney disease–mineral bone disorder in, 2361, 2406
  congenital anomalies of the kidney and urinary tract in. See Congenital anomalies of the kidney and urinary tract (CAKUT)
  continuous renal replacement therapy in, 2417-2418
  creatinine concentration in, 2341f
  cystinosis in, 2339-2340, 2341f
  cystinuria in, 2345-2346, 2346f
  dehydration in, 2367-2368, 2373-2374, 2373t
  Dent's disease in, 2344-2345
  dialysis in
    hemodialysis. See Children, hemodialysis in
    long-term, renal transplantation advantages over, 2410-2411, 2410f
    modality changes, 2417
    peritoneal. See Children, peritoneal dialysis in
  diuretic renography in, 1266-1267
  EAST syndrome in, 167, 2379
  end-stage kidney disease in, 2308-2309, 2321
    anemia secondary to, 2405-2406
    arrhythmias associated with, 2408
    atherosclerosis associated with, 2407-2408
    cardiovascular diseases associated with, 2406-2409, 2421-2422
    chronic kidney disease–mineral bone disorder associated with, 2406
    clinical consequences of, 2404-2409
    congenital anomalies of the kidney and urinary tract as cause of, 2361, 2404, 2421
    description of, 2308-2309, 2321
    diastolic dysfunction associated with, 2408
    electrolyte imbalance secondary to, 2405
    epidemiology of, 2403, 2419t

Children (Continued)
  etiology of, 2404, 2404t
  growth effects, 2405
  hyperkalemia associated with, 2405
  hypertension secondary to, 2406-2407
  left ventricular hypertrophy associated with, 2408, 2421-2422
  life expectancy of, 2404
  linear growth effects, 2405
  metabolic acidosis secondary to, 2405
  mortality rate for, 2409
  neurodevelopment effects of, 2408-2410, 2408f
  nutrition effects, 2404-2405
  renal osteodystrophy associated with, 2407f
  renal replacement affected by, 2409
  renal replacement therapy for. See Children, renal replacement therapy in
  valvular disease associated with, 2408
  vascular calcification associated with, 2407-2408
  weight effects, 2404-2405
 extracellular fluid in, 2365-2366, 2368, 2414
 familial hypomagnesemia with hypercalciuria and nephrocalcinosis in, 2345
 fibroblast growth factor-23 in, 2390-2391, 2400
 focal segmental glomerulosclerosis in, 1030, 1032
 Gitelman's syndrome in, 2335, 2378-2379
 glomerular diseases in, 2322-2340
 glomerular filtration rate in, 787, 787t, 2309-2310
 growth in
  end-stage kidney disease effects on, 2405
  failure of, chronic kidney disease as cause of, 2357-2359, 2358f-2359f
 hematuria in, 1014-1015
 hemodialysis in
  apparatus for, 2413-2414
  blood flow, 2413-2414
  complications of, 2414-2415
  continuous renal replacement therapy versus, 2418
  costs of, 2411
  dialyzer for, 2413
  dose of, 2414
  fluid removal, 2414
  machine for, 2413
  peritoneal dialysis versus, 2411, 2412t, 2417
  renal transplantation versus, 2410
  tubing for, 2413
  vascular access for, 2412-2414
 hemolytic-uremic syndrome in
  atypical, 2354t, 2355-2362
  clinical features of, 2354t
  cobalamin C synthase deficiency as cause of, 2356-2357
  complement disorders as cause of, 2355-2356, 2355f
  definition of, 2352
  diacyl glycerol kinase ε mutations as cause of, 2356
  diagnosis of, 2353
  epidemiology of, 2352-2353
  pathogenesis of, 2353
  prognosis for, 2354-2355
  Shiga toxin-associated, 2352-2357

Children (Continued)
  Streptococcus pneumoniae-associated, 2355
  treatment of, 2353-2354
  von Willebrand factor-cleaving protease deficiency as cause of, 2356
 hereditary hypophosphatemic rickets with hypercalciuria in, 2345
 hospitalized, hyponatremia in, 2372
 hypercalcemia in, 608, 2393-2396, 2394t, 2396f, 2397t
 hypercalciuria in, 2340, 2344, 2344f
 hyperkalemia in, 2380-2382, 2380t-2381t
 hypernatremia in, 2367-2370
 hypernatremic dehydration in, 2367-2368, 2374
 hyperosmolality in, 2367-2370, 2367t
 hyperphosphatemia in, 2398-2400, 2399f, 2399t
 hypertension in, 2329, 2421-2422
 hypocalcemia in
  citrate blood product infusions as cause of, 2391
  diagnostic workup for, 2392
  early neonatal, 2391
  late neonatal, 2391
  lipid infusions as cause of, 2391
  monitoring of, 2393
  respiratory alkalosis as cause of, 2392
  treatment of, 2392-2393, 2394t
 hypokalemia in, 2375-2379, 2375t, 2376f-2378f, 2377t
 hypomagnesemia in
  autosomal dominant, 2388-2389
  causes of, 2387t
  description of, 2387
  familial
   with hypercalciuria and nephrocalcinosis, 2387-2388
   with secondary hypocalcemia, 2388, 2388f
  isolated autosomal recessive, with normocalciuria, 2389
 hyponatremia in, 2370-2372, 2371t
 hypo-osmolality in, 2370-2371, 2371t
 hypophosphatemia in, 2396-2398, 2397t-2398t, 2398f
 immune complex-mediated crescentic glomerulonephritis in, 1073
 inborn errors of metabolism in, renal replacement therapy in, 2417
 intracellular fluid in, 2365-2366
 intrinsic renal failure in, 2368t
 Joubert's syndrome in, 2322, 2322t
 kidney malformation in, 2294-2295, 2295f
 kidney stones in, 2340-2342
 left ventricular hypertrophy in, 2360-2361, 2421-2422, 2432
 Liddle's syndrome in, 2379
 linear growth in, 2405, 2434-2435
 lower urinary tract abnormalities in, 2296
 magnesium in
  disorders involving, 2386-2389
  metabolism of, 2386-2389
 Meckel-Gruber syndrome in, 2322, 2322t
 medications in, 2409-2410
 membranoproliferative glomerulonephritis type I in, 1049
 membranous nephropathy in, 1041
 metabolic acidosis in, 2382-2383, 2382t
 minimal change disease in, 1021
 nephritic syndrome in, 2331-2333
 nephrocalcinosis in, 2340

Children (Continued)
 nephrogenic diabetes insipidus in, 2338-2339, 2368-2370, 2370t
 nephrogenic syndrome of inappropriate diuresis in, 2372-2373
 nephrolithiasis in
  clinical features of, 2342-2343
  diagnosis of, 2343
  genetic, 2344-2348
  hypercalciuria in, 2340, 2344-2345, 2344f
  hyperoxaluria in, 2340, 2346-2348, 2422
  hyperuricosuria in, 2342, 2343t
  hypocitraturia in, 2340-2342
  interventional treatment of, 2343-2344
  nonhypercalciuric, 2345-2348
  risk factors for, 2340-2342
  treatment of, 2343-2344
  urinary tract infections associated with, 2342
 nephronophthisis in, 2321-2322
 nephronophthisis-related ciliopathies in, 2321
 nephrotic syndrome in, 2322-2333
  in Africa, 2463
  classification of, 2323
  congenital, 1414, 2324t, 2325-2326
  definition of, 2323
  early-onset, 2324t, 2325-2326
  hereditary, 2323-2327, 2324t, 2325f
  idiopathic
   allergic responses associated with, 2327
   classification of, 2328-2329
   clinical features of, 2328
   definition of, 2327
   epidemiology of, 2327
   glucocorticoids for, 2329
   incidence of, 2327
   mesangioproliferative glomerulonephritis with, 2327-2328
   microscopic hematuria in, 2328
   pathogenesis of, 2327-2328
   proteinuria in, 2327
   renal biopsy for, 2328-2329
   treatment of, 2329-2331
  infantile and childhood, 2324t, 2326-2327
  juvenile, 2324t, 2327
  late-onset, 2324t, 2327
  pathogenesis of, 2323
  plasma exchange for, 2331
  steroid-resistant
   calcineurin inhibitors for, 2330-2331
   description of, 2323
   focal segmental glomerulosclerosis in, 2328
   molecular genetic screening for, 2326f
   mycophenolate mofetil for, 2331
   renin-angiotensin-aldosterone antagonists for, 2331
   rituximab, 2331
   syndromic forms of, 2323
   treatment of, 2330-2331
  steroid-sensitive, 2329-2330
 neurodevelopment of, 2408-2410, 2408f
 nutrition in, 2357-2359, 2404-2405
 obesity in, 2576-2577
 obstructive uropathy in, 1279
 oculocerebrorenal syndrome in, 2345
 parathyroid hormone in, 2390-2391

Children (Continued)
  peritoneal dialysis in
    access for, 2415
    adequacy of, 2416
    adherence to, 2417
    automated, 2415
    complications of, 2416-2417
    continuous ambulatory, 2415
    continuous renal replacement therapy versus, 2418
    contraindications, 2415
    dwell time for, 2416
    exchange volume of, 2416
    global disparities in, 2417
    hemodialysis versus, 2411, 2412t, 2417
    Kt/V assessments, 2416
    nocturnal intermittent, 2415
    prescription for, 2415-2416
    renal transplantation versus, 2410
    solutions for, 2415-2416
    termination of, 2417
    tidal, 2415
  phosphate in
    balance of, 2389-2390, 2389f-2390f
    dietary intake of, 2390
    disorders of, 2396-2399, 2397t-2400t, 2398f-2399f
    distribution of, 2389, 2390f
    fractional excretion of, 2397
    homeostasis of, 2391f
    regulation of, 2389
  polycystic kidney disease in, 2319-2321, 2320f
  polydipsia in, 2369, 2370t
  polyuria in, 2369, 2370t
  potassium in
    disorders involving, 2374-2382
    metabolism of, 2374-2382
  prerenal failure in, 2368t
  proteinuria in, 798, 2310-2311
  pseudohypoaldosteronism in, 2380-2382
  racial-ethnic disparities, 2583
  recurrent focal segmental glomerulosclerosis in, 2156
  renal disorders in, 2308-2309, 2309f
  renal function in, 2309-2311, 2361
  renal replacement therapy in
    continuous, 2417-2418
    costs of, 2411
    inborn errors of metabolism, 2417
    quality of life effects of, 2409-2410
    renal transplantation versus, 2410-2411, 2410f
  renal transplantation in
    ABO compatibility in, 2423
    acute rejection of, 2428
    advantages of, over long-term dialysis, 2410-2411, 2410f
    allocation of, 2419-2420
    allografts
      artery stenosis, 2432
      delayed function of, 2427-2428
      failure of, 2432
      loss of, 2427
      survival of, 2432
      vesicoureteral reflux to, 2435
    anemia after, 2434
    blood pressure monitoring after, 2432
    bone health and growth after, 2434-2435, 2435f
    cancer after, 2433-2434
    cardiovascular disease after, 2432-2433
    chronic allograft nephropathy after, 2431
    in chronic kidney disease patients, 2422

Children (Continued)
  complications of
    acute rejection, 2428
    BK virus infection, 2430
    cutaneous warts, 2430
    cytomegalovirus infection, 2429
    delayed graft function, 2427-2428
    Epstein-Barr virus infection, 2429-2430
    infections, 2428-2431
    Pneumocystis jiroveci pneumonia, 2430-2431
    primary kidney disease recurrence, 2431
    respiratory viruses, 2430
    ureteral obstruction, 2435
    urinary tract infection, 2429
    urologic, 2435
    varicella infection, 2430
  contraindications, 2420
  cost-effectiveness of, 2411
  demographics of, 2419, 2419t
  HLA matching and sensitization for, 2422-2423
  hypertension after, 2432
  immunosuppression for
    antimetabolites, 2425-2426
    azathioprine, 2425
    calcineurin inhibitors, 2424-2425
    combination therapies, 2426-2427
    corticosteroids, 2426
    cyclosporine, 2424-2425
    induction, 2423-2424
    maintenance, 2424-2427, 2424f
    mammalian target of rapamycin inhibitors, 2426
    mycophenolate mofetil, 2425-2426
    sirolimus, 2426
    tacrolimus, 2425
  incidence of, 2419-2420
  metabolic syndrome after, 2433
  patient nonadherence after, 2436
  postoperative period, 2427
  posttransplantation lymphoproliferative disorder after, 2433
  preoperative management of, 2427
  prevalence of, 2419-2420
  puberty after, 2435-2436
  quality of life after, 2410, 2436
  recipient preparation, 2420-2422, 2421t
  rehabilitation after, 2436
  rejection of, 2428
  reproduction effects of, 2435-2436
  survival benefits of, 2410, 2431-2432
  timing of, 2420
  transition after, 2436
  urologic complications of, 2435
  renal tubular acidosis in, 2335-2338, 2337t, 2383-2386
  socioeconomic disparities, 2583
  sodium in
    disorders involving, 2365-2374
    metabolism of, 2365-2367
  solute urinary excretion rates in, 2343t
  statural growth in
    chronic kidney disease effects on, 2357-2359, 2358f-2359f
    end-stage kidney disease effects on, 2405
  syndrome of inappropriate antidiuretic hormone secretion in, 2372
  thirst in, 2366
  thrombosis in, 1805
  total body water in, 2365, 2414
  urinary calculi in, 2340
  urinary protein excretion in, 2310-2311

Children (Continued)
  urinary tract disorders in
    posterior urethral valves, 2316, 2317f, 2435
    primary megaureter, 2315-2316
    spectrum of, 2308-2309, 2309f
    ureteropelvic junction obstruction, 2311, 2314-2315, 2315f
    vesicoureteral reflux, 2311, 2313-2314, 2314f
  urinary tract infection in, 2313-2314
  urinary tract obstruction in, 1258
  urolithiasis in, 2340-2348
  vascular calcification in, 2407-2408
  vasculitides in
    antineutrophil cytoplasmic antibody-associated, 2351-2352
    eosinophilic granulomatosis with polyangiitis, 2351
    granulomatosis with polyangiitis, 2351
    Henoch-Schönlein purpura, 2348-2350
    microscopic polyangiitis, 2351
    polyarteritis nodosa, 2350-2351
    Takayasu's arteritis, 2352
  vitamin D in, 2390-2391
  water metabolism in, 2365-2367
Chimerism, 2249
China
  diabetes mellitus in, 2529, 2529f
  end-stage kidney disease in, 2535
  hemodialysis in, 2535
  idiopathic membranous nephropathy in, 2531
  peritoneal dialysis in, 2535
  primary glomerular diseases in, 2529-2531, 2530f
  renal replacement therapy in, 2535
  scientific publications in, 2536
Chinese herb nephropathy, 1223-1224, 1225f, 2534
Chlorambucil, for membranous nephropathy, 1042-1043, 1169
Chloride
  deficiency of, in metabolic alkalosis, 520
  fractional excretion of, 814-815
  in urine, 816
Chloride channels, 161-162, 243
Chloride formate exchange, 148
Chloride oxalate exchange, 148
Chloride transport, 156-158, 157f, 163, 314
Chloride-bicarbonate exchanger mutation, 1457
Chlorine, 144
Chlorpropamide, 487, 497
Chlorthalidone, 1681, 1685, 1710
Chloruresis, 553
CHOIR study, 1901-1902
Cholecalciferol, 1923, 2025, 2390
Cholera, 2455-2456
Cholesterol, 1801, 1828
Cholesterol embolization syndrome, 1192-1193
Cholesterol ester transfer protein, 1802
Cholesterol feeding, 1578
Cholinesterase inhibitors, 1938
Chondrocalcinosis, 580, 2379
Chromodomain helicase DNA binding protein 1-like protein, 2300
Chromophilic carcinoma, 1371, 1371t
Chromophobe tumors, 892
Chromophobic carcinoma, 1371, 1371t, 1372f
Chronic allograft glomerulopathy, 923

Chronic allograft nephropathy, 2244, 2273, 2425, 2431
Chronic antibody-mediated rejection, 2274
Chronic bacterial prostatitis, 750, 1247-1248
Chronic heart failure, 1722
Chronic hypertension, 1627-1631, 1629f
Chronic hyponatremia, 502-504, 815
Chronic hypoxia, in interstitial fibrosis, 1217-1218
Chronic inflammatory demyelinating polyneuropathy, 2158
Chronic ischemia, 1794
Chronic kidney disease (CKD)
   acidosis of, 549-550, 1758-1759
   acute kidney injury as cause of, 652, 678, 691, 747, 926-927, 1777-1778, 1778f
   acute phase reactant proteins in, 1970
   adrenal androgens in, 1920
   adrenal glands in, 1919-1920
   adrenocorticotropic hormone in, 1919
   advanced care planning in, 2599-2600
   in Africa. See Africa, chronic kidney disease in
   in African Americans, 666, 2577
   aldosterone in, 1919-1920
   alkali therapy for, 542
   amino acids in, 1972
   ammonia synthesis, 1749
   anemia associated with. See Anemia, in chronic kidney disease
   animal models of, 1835-1836
   anthropometrics in, 1971
   atrial fibrillation in, 1859, 1908
   in Australia, 2544, 2549
   bicarbonate reabsorption in, 1749
   biomarkers for
     anemia, 683, 1299-1300, 1776, 1863-1864, 2594
     asymmetric dimethylarginine, 685, 950, 1811
     bicarbonate, 684-685
     creatinine, 933
     cystatin C, 934-935, 2043
     dyslipidemia, 683-684, 1863, 2011
     fibroblast growth factor-23, 950, 1864
     interleukin-18, 940-941
     kidney injury molecule-1, 942
     liver-type fatty acid-binding protein, 943
     β_1-microglobulin, 938
     β_2-microglobulin, 938
     monocyte chemoattractant protein-1, 950-951
     N-acetyl-β-D-glucosaminidase, 947
     neutrophil gelatinase-associated lipocalin, 946-947
     performance data on, 952t
     phosphate, 685
     serum albumin, 683
     serum bicarbonate, 684-685
     serum phosphate, 685
     serum uric acid, 684
     symmetric dimethylarginine, 1811
     uric acid, 684
     urinary protein excretion, 682-683, 947
   birth weight and, 712
   bleeding in, 1885
     desmopressin for, 1906
     diagnosis of, 1906
     pathophysiology of, 1904-1906
     risk factors for, 1905f
     treatment of, 1906
   blood pressure and, 1559f, 1563f, 1867-1868, 1975, 2283
   blood urea nitrogen in, 1959

Chronic kidney disease (CKD) (Continued)
   bradykinin receptors in, 350
   caloric requirements in, 1973
   cardiovascular disease associated with, 681-682
     antihypertensive agents for, 2010
     antiplatelet therapy for, 2012-2013
     arterial calcification, 1856-1857, 1857f, 1864, 1866
     arterial disease, 1855-1857, 1855t
     arterial stiffening, 1856
     arterial wall thickening, 1855-1856
     arteriosclerosis, 1855
     atrial fibrillation, 1859, 1908
     cardiac disease, 1857-1859
     characteristics of, 1855t
     clinical manifestations of, 1859-1860
     congenital heart disease, 2421-2422
     description of, 681-682, 2008-2009
     dietary factors, 1970
     dysrhythmias, 1859
     in elderly, 2593
     endothelial dysfunction, 1856, 2407
     epidemiology of, 1860-1861, 1860f
     interventions for, 2008-2013
     left ventricular function changes, 1859
     left ventricular hypertrophy, 1295-1296, 1857-1858
     myocardial disease, 1858f
     myocardial fibrosis, 1858-1859
     overview of, 1854-1855
     relationship between, 1861-1865
     risk factors for
       anemia, 1863-1864
       chronic kidney disease–mineral bone disorder, 1864-1865, 1872-1873
       coagulation defects, 1863
       congestive heart failure, 1862t
       diabetes mellitus, 1865
       dyslipidemia, 1863, 2011
       homocysteine, 1864, 1970
       hypertension, 1861, 1862t, 1873, 2421-2422, 2461
       inflammation, 1865
       list of, 1862t
       obesity, 1865-1866
       oxidative stress, 1865, 2100-2101
       phosphate retention, 1978-1979
       stroke, 1862t
       vitamin D levels, 1864-1865
     risk prediction, 1866-1867
     risk prevention in
       anemia correction, 1871-1872
       antiplatelet therapy, 1873
       blood pressure reductions, 1867-1868, 2009
       glycemic control, 1871
       homocysteine levels, 1872
       low-density lipoprotein cholesterol reductions, 1868-1871, 1869f-1870f
       smoking cessation, 1867, 1991
       uncertainties regarding, 1855
     summary of, 1873-1874
     valvular diseases, 1859
   cardiovascular events and, 670
   carotid endarterectomy in, 1932
   causes of, 1414t, 1415-1416
   in children. See Children, chronic kidney disease in
   chronic cognitive impairment in, 1936-1938, 1937f-1938f
   chronic kidney disease–mineral bone disorder in, 2030f

Chronic kidney disease (CKD) (Continued)
   classification of, 1989f
   clinics for, 2632, 2633f, 2633t
   cognitive impairment in, 1818-1819
   computed tomography of, 869, 869f
   cortisol in, 1919-1920
   costovertebral tenderness in, 776
   creatinine excretion in, 1961
   cytochrome P450 in, 385, 2038-2039
   deep vein thrombosis in, 1906-1907, 1908f
   definition of, 773, 1927, 1987
   dehydroepiandrosterone in, 1920
   dehydroepiandrosterone sulfate in, 1920
   demographics of, 2578-2579
     age, 673-674
     ethnicity, 660-662, 674
     gender, 655-660, 673-674
     race, 660-663, 666
   description of, 652
   diagnostic approach, 774-776, 2621
   dialysis for, 1971, 2016
   dietary modifications in, 1982-1983
   dietary support during
     justification for, 1956-1959
     low-protein diet, 1977, 1981-1982, 1994
     modified diets, 1982-1983
     potassium intake, 1975
     randomized controlled trials of, 1979-1981
     salt intake, 1974-1975
     summary of, 1984-1985
   1,25-Dihydroxyvitamin D levels in, 1913, 2014
   disordered mineral metabolism in, 2019-2023
   disparities in treatment of, 2580
   drug disposition affected by, 2035-2040
   drug dosing in, 2044-2046, 2045t, 2051t-2054t
   dyslipidemia in, 683-684, 1863, 2011
   early-stage, 669-670
   economic costs of treating, 2134, 2582
   in elderly, 747, 2568-2569, 2594-2596
   electrolyte balance alterations in, 1968
   endometrial hyperplasia in, 1921
   endothelin in, 337
   endothelin-1 in, 337-338
   endothelin-A receptors in, 337-338
   endothelin-B receptors in, 337-338
   end-stage kidney disease progression of, 671, 776, 962, 1737, 2007-2008
   energy intake in, 1973
   energy requirements in, 1973
   environmental exposures as cause of, 665
   epidemiology of, 643-647
   erectile dysfunction in, 1921-1922
   estimated glomerular filtration rate in, 1989-1990
   ethnicity and, 660-662, 674, 1769-1770
   extracellular fluid in, 775-776, 1747-1748
   in Far East. See Far East, chronic kidney disease in
   fibrinogen levels in, 1863, 1905-1906
   fibroblast growth factor-23 concentrations in, 950, 1749-1750, 1775, 1831, 1864, 2019
   follicle-stimulating hormone in, 1920-1921
   gender differences in, 655-660, 673-674
   genetic factors, 674-675
   genomewide association studies, 676
   global incidence of, 655, 656f
   glomerular filtration rate in, 681, 773, 932, 1749

Chronic kidney disease (CKD) *(Continued)*
  glomerulonephritis as cause of, 775
  gonadal dysfunction in, 1920-1923
  gonadotropic hormone axis in, 2358
  graft-versus-host disease-related, 1395
  growth hormone in, 1916-1919
  health-related quality of life in patients with, 1818
  hematopoietic stem cell transplantation and, 1394
  hemodynamic factors, 676-681
    acquired nephron deficit, 676-678
    blood pressure, 679
    nephron endowment, 676
    nephron loss, 676-678
    nephron number, 676-678
  hepatocyte growth factor in, 1757
  hepcidin concentrations in, 1886
  hereditary factors, 674-676
  high-density lipoprotein cholesterol in, 1863
  1α-hydroxylase deficiency in, 617
  hyperaldosteronism in, 1919
  hyperammonemia in, 1962
  hypercholesterolemia in, 1970
  hypercoagulability in, 1906-1909, 1908f
  hypercortisolism in, 1919
  hyperkalemia in, 585
  hyperphosphatemia caused by, 627, 1774-1775
  hyperprolactinemia in, 1919
  hypertension and, 1544-1545, 1559-1560
  hypoactive sexual desire disorder in, 1921
  hypocalciuria in, 1749-1750
  hypogonadism in, 1921-1922
  hypothalamic-pituitary-gonadal axis disturbances in, 1920
  hypothyroidism in, 1916
  hypoxia in, 139
  imaging of, 863f-864f, 866-871, 866f-871f
  incidence of, 645, 926-927
    in Africa, 2459
    disparities in, 2575, 2578
    ethnicity-based, 660-662
    gender-based, 655, 656f
    in Indian subcontinent, 2502
    in Middle East, 2474
    race-based, 660-662, 2584
    socioeconomic factors, 664-665, 664f, 2578, 2584
  inflammation and, 1865, 1909, 1969-1970
  inflammatory cell infiltration in, 334
  insulin resistance in, 1315, 1912-1916, 1913t
  interdisciplinary clinics for, 2632-2634, 2633f
  international comparisons of, 647
  intraarterial volume status assessments in, 775-776
  intrauterine growth restriction and, 665
  iodide retention in, 1915
  iron balance in, 1893
  iron therapy in, 1898-1900, 1899t
  kallikrein-kinin system in, 350
  Kidney Disease Improving Global Outcomes classification of, 773, 774t
  Kidney Disease Outcomes Quality Initiative for, 773, 773t
  kidney stones and, 1352
  klotho in, 1831, 1832t
  in Latin America, 2447-2449
  leukocytes in, 1909
  low birth weight and, 712, 2576
  luteinizing hormone in, 1920-1921
  malnutrition in, 1971

Chronic kidney disease (CKD) *(Continued)*
  metabolic acidosis in, 542, 1913, 2004, 2357, 2359
  micronutrients in, 1983
  in Middle East patients. *See* Middle East, chronic kidney disease in
  mineralocorticoid receptor blockade in, 322
  monitoring of, 2005-2006
  mortality rates in, 773
  muscle mass losses in, 1968
  musculoskeletal complications of, 775
  mutation analysis for, 1412
  National Kidney Foundation classification system for, 773, 773t, 1736, 1957-1958, 1958t
  nephron losses in, 676-678, 1991f
  neurologic aspects of
    cerebrovascular disease, 1926
    cognitive function disorders. *See* Cognitive function disorders
    description of, 1926
    neuropathy, 1939
    sleep apnea, 1939-1940
    stroke, 1926-1934. *See also* Stroke
  in New Zealand, 2550-2551
  nitrogenous products turnover in
    ammonia, 1962
    creatinine, 1961
    fecal nitrogen, 1962
    nonurea nitrogen, 1962-1963
    overview of, 1959
    urea, 1959-1961
    uric acid, 1961-1962
  nonurea nitrogen levels in, 1962
  nutritional counseling in, 1985f
  obesity in, 679-680, 1770-1771, 1992
  25(OH)D levels and, 2031-2032
  in older adults, 747, 2568-2569, 2586-2588
  ophthalmic complications of, 775
  orthostatic hypotension and, 776
  outcome of, by stages, 645
  oxidative stress and, 1758, 1865
  palliative care for, 2563
  parathyroid hormone in, 2014, 2019
  phosphate in, 1977-1979, 2019
  phosphorus retention in, 1977-1978
  plasma protein binding in, 2037
  potassium intake in, 1975
  preeclampsia effects on, 680-681
  pregnancy effects on, 680-681, 1633-1638
  prematurity and, 712
  prevalence of, 645, 655, 656f, 669-670, 2108-2109
    in Africa, 2459
    age-based, 673, 747
    ethnicity-based, 661-662
    in Far East, 2526, 2527t
    income-based, 665
    in Indian subcontinent, 2502
    in Latin America, 2448
    in Middle East, 2474
    race-based, 661-662
    socioeconomic factors, 665
    trends in, 646t
  primary care provider recognition of, 2622
  primary hypertension and, 1562-1565
  prognosis for, 1972-1973
  progression of, 1552-1553
    acidosis effects on, 684-685, 1963-1964, 2004
    acute kidney injury effects on, 678, 1777-1778
    in African Americans, 674
    albuminuria as risk factor for, 948

Chronic kidney disease (CKD) *(Continued)*
  anemia as predictor of, 683, 1776, 2013
  angiotensin II in, 1764-1765
  asymmetric dimethylarginine as risk factor for, 685
  biomarkers of, 949-950
  blood pressure in, 679, 2009
  body mass index and, 1771
  calcium channel blockers effect on, 1995
  calcium metabolism and, 1774-1775
  in children, 2361-2362, 2362f
  description of, 671, 776
  diabetic nephropathy effects on, 681
  dietary protein intake and, 1767-1768
  dihydropyridine calcium channel blockers effect on, 1995-1996
  dyslipidemia as predictor of, 683-684, 1772-1774
  to end-stage kidney disease, 671, 776, 962, 1737, 2007-2008
  ethnic differences in, 662
  fibroblast growth factor-23 in, 1775
  gender differences in, 657, 1768-1769
  hyperlipidemia in, 1802-1803
  hyperparathyroidism and, 1775
  hypertension effects on, 673, 679, 1765-1767
  hyperuricemia in, 684, 1228, 2004
  low-protein diet effects on, 1981-1982, 1994
  male sex hormones in, 1923
  mechanism of, 1990
  metabolic syndrome effects on, 679-680, 1770-1771, 1992
  obesity effects on, 679-680, 1770-1771, 1992
  phosphate metabolism and, 1774-1775
  podocyte injury in, 1753-1754
  preeclampsia effects on, 680-681
  in pregnancy, 680-681
  primary renal disease effects on, 681
  proteinuria as predictor of, 2361-2362
  racial differences in, 662
  renal calcium deposition and, 1775
  renal risk scores for, 691
  renin-angiotensin-aldosterone system inhibition, 1764-1765
  risk factors for, 673, 1990, 2361-2362
  slowing of. *See* Chronic kidney disease, slowing progression of
  smoking effects on, 685, 1776-1777
  socioeconomic factors, 665-666
  sympathetic nervous system overactivity in, 1771-1772
  total protein measurements used in, 793
  unified hypothesis of, 1763-1764, 1764f
  uric acid-lowering therapy effects on, 684
  prolactin in, 1919
  prolactinemia in, 1919
  protein in
    intake of, 1975-1976
    losses of, 1965, 1967
    low-protein diet, 1977, 1994
    randomized controlled trials of, 1979-1980
    requirements for, 1976, 1976t
  protein stores in, assessment of
    anthropometrics for, 1971
    complement, 1970-1971
    insulin-like growth factor-1, 1970-1971
    nitrogen balance for, 1968-1969, 1975

Chronic kidney disease (CKD) *(Continued)*
- overview of, 1968
  - plasma amino acids, 1971-1973, 1972f
  - prealbumin, 1970-1971
  - serum albumin, 1969-1970
  - serum transferrin, 1970-1971
  - urea nitrogen appearance rate, 1969
- protein-energy wasting in, 1817, 1913, 1994-1995
- proteinuria associated with, 682-683, 947-948, 2361-2362
- pulmonary embolism in, 1906-1907
- quality initiatives in, 2632-2635, 2633f, 2633t-2634t
- race and, 660-663, 666
- recombinant human growth factor in, 1918
- renal replacement therapy for, in stage 5 patients, 2016
- renal risk scores, 687-691, 688t-689t
- renal transplantation for, 2016
- renoprotection in
  - angiotensin receptor blockers for, 2000-2003, 2001f
  - angiotensin-converting enzyme inhibitors for, 1995, 1998-2000, 1998t
  - strategies for, 2006-2008, 2008t
- risk factors for, 773, 774t, 1849
  - alcohol consumption, 685-686
  - analgesics, 686
  - asymmetric dimethylarginine, 685
  - cadmium, 687
  - childhood obesity, 679-680
  - cocaine use, 686
  - epidemiologic studies for identifying, 670-671
  - heavy metal exposure, 686-687
  - high dietary protein intake, 680
  - hypertension, 679, 1861, 1868, 1873, 1974-1975, 2461, 2590-2591
  - hyperuricemia, 684, 1228, 2004
  - initiation, 673
  - in Latin America, 2448
  - lead exposure, 686-687
  - list of, 672t
  - maternal, 2576
  - nephron number, 676-678
  - nephrotoxins, 685-687
  - obesity, 679-680, 1771
  - postnatal environment, 2576
  - prenatal environment, 2575-2576
  - protein intake, high dietary, 680
  - racial-ethnic disparities in, 2583
  - recreational drug use, 686
  - serum bicarbonate levels, 684-685
  - serum phosphate levels, 685
  - serum uric acid levels, 684
  - smoking, 685, 1776-1777, 1867
  - social contribution of, 2576
  - socioeconomic conditions, 2576-2577
  - susceptibility, 671-673
- risk stratification for, 786, 1990
- in scleroderma, 1196-1197
- screening for, 669-670, 2587-2588
- secondary hyperparathyroidism in, 2024f
- sex hormones in, 1921, 1923
- sexual function in, 1920-1921
- sleep disorders in
  - periodic limb movements of sleep, 1939-1940
  - prevalence of, 1939
  - restless legs syndrome, 1940, 1940t
  - sleep apnea, 1939-1940

Chronic kidney disease (CKD) *(Continued)*
- slowing progression of
  - antihypertensive therapy for, 1995-1998
  - bicarbonate supplementation for, 684-685, 2004
  - blood pressure lowering for, 1996-1998, 2009
  - dietary protein restriction for, 1767-1768, 1994-1995
  - glycemic control for, 1995
  - hyperuricemia correction, 2004
  - initiation of therapies for, 2006-2007
  - lifestyle interventions for, 1990-1995
  - metabolic acidosis treatment for, 2004
  - monitoring for, 2005-2006
  - proteinuria treatment for, 2004-2005
  - rationale for, 1990
  - renin-angiotensin-aldosterone system inhibition for, 1764-1765, 1998-2004, 2127
  - smoking cessation for, 1776-1777, 1991-1992
  - sodium restriction for, 1993-1994, 1993f
  - strategies for, 2006-2008, 2008t
  - weight loss for, 1992-1993
- socioeconomic factors, 663-666, 664f, 2576
- somatotropic axis in, 1917f
- stage 1 and 2
  - abdominal ultrasonography in, 2015
  - diagnosis of, 2014
  - glomerular filtration rate reductions in, 2029-2031
  - management of, 1988t
  - monitoring guidelines in, 2015t
  - phosphate restriction in, 2031
  - stepped care approach in, 2014-2015
  - treatment of, 2029-2031
- stage 3
  - calcium monitoring in, 2014
  - glomerular filtration rate in, 2015
  - glomerular filtration rate reductions in, 2029-2031
  - management of, 1988t
  - monitoring guidelines in, 2015t
  - parathyroid hormone monitoring in, 2014
  - phosphate restriction in, 2031
  - phosphorus monitoring in, 2014
  - stepped care approach in, 2015
  - vitamin D analogues in, 2031-2032
- stage 4
  - cardiovascular events in, 2015
  - dialysis preparations in, 2016
  - glomerular filtration rate in, 2015-2016, 2029-2031
  - hepatitis B vaccination in, 2016
  - management of, 1988t
  - monitoring guidelines in, 2015t
  - preemptive renal transplantation indications in, 2016
  - stepped care approach to, 2015-2016
  - vitamin D analogues in, 2031-2032
- stage 5
  - glomerular filtration rate in, 2016
  - hyperphosphatemia in, 2020
  - hypocalcemia in, 2020
  - management of, 1988t
  - monitoring guidelines in, 2015t
  - pericarditis in, 2107-2108
  - renal replacement therapy in, 2016
  - stepped care approach to, 2016
  - transition from, to end-stage kidney disease, 2063-2064

Chronic kidney disease (CKD) *(Continued)*
- systemic complications of, 773-774
- targeted programs for, 2582
- testosterone deficiency in, 1921
- thyroid hormone disturbances in, 1915-1916, 1915t
- thyrotropin levels in, 1915-1916
- trace elements in, 1983-1984
- treatment of, 2013, 2580
- trials in nondiabetic, 1553
- ubiquitin-protease system in, 1964-1965
- urea in, 1959-1961, 1968-1969
- uric acid excretion in, 1813, 1961
- vascular calcifications in, 1850, 2102-2103
- vitamin D in
  - actions of, 1923-1924
  - deficiency of, 1775, 1849, 1912, 1924
  - metabolism of, 1923-1924
  - supplementation of, 1924, 2406
- vitamins in, 1983-1984
- volume overload in, 776
- white cell function in, 1909-1910

Chronic Kidney Disease Epidemiology Collaboration, 645, 677-678, 759, 784t, 785-786, 2005

Chronic Kidney Disease Hard Point Trials in Diabetes, 1555-1556

Chronic kidney disease–mineral bone disorder (CKD–MBD)
- biochemical abnormalities in
  - bone-specific alkaline phosphatase, 1842
  - calcium, 1847-1848
  - clinical consequences of, 1847-1850
  - collagen-based bone biomarkers, 1842
  - fibroblast growth factor-23, 1841, 1848
  - fracture secondary to, 1849
  - klotho, 1841-1842
  - parathyroid hormone, 1839-1841, 1840f, 1848
  - phosphorus, 1847-1848
  - sclerostin, 1842
  - tartrate-resistant acid phosphatase 5B, 1842
  - vitamin D, 1841, 1848-1849
- biomarkers for, 1840t
- bone assessments in
  - bone biopsy for, 1842-1846, 1845t
  - dual-energy x-ray absorptiometry for, 1846
  - high-resolution peripheral computerized tomography for, 1846
  - histomorphometry for, 1842-1845, 1844f
  - micro-computed tomography for, 1846-1847
  - micro-magnetic resonance imaging for, 1846-1847
  - noninvasive, 1846-1847
  - quantitative computed tomography for, 1846
- bone formation in, 1843, 1845t
- calcimimetics for, 1873, 2026-2028
- calcium-sensing receptor in, 1825-1826
- cardiovascular disease and, 1864-1865, 1872-1873
- in children, 2361, 2406
- in chronic kidney disease, 2030f
- clinical management of, 2028-2029
- definition of, 2020
- 1,25-dihydroxycholecalciferol, 2024f, 2025
- in end-stage kidney disease, 2029

Chronic kidney disease–mineral bone disorder (CKD–MBD) (Continued)
　fracture in, 1849
　hormonal regulation of
　　fibroblast growth factor-23, 1830-1831
　　Klotho, 1830-1831
　　parathyroid hormone, 1826-1828
　　vitamin D, 1828-1830
　hyperphosphatemia and, 1977, 2021
　management of, 2013-2014
　in Middle East, 2488
　pathophysiology of, 1822-1839
　phosphate concentrations in, 1864, 1872, 1923
　in renal transplantation recipients, 1850-1852
　treatment of, 2028-2029
　　cinacalcet and vitamin D analogues for, 2029
　　overview of, 2021t
　　phosphate-binding agents, 2020-2023
　　principles of, 2020-2021
　　vitamin D analogues, 2020
　vitamin D metabolism abnormalities in, 2025
　vitamin D sterols for, 2026
Chronic pain, 2569
Chronic radiation nephropathy, 1194
Chronic renal injury, polyuria in, 299
Chronic tubulointerstitial nephritis
　Balkan endemic nephropathy, 1224-1226, 1225f
　causes of
　　analgesics, 1221-1223, 1222t
　　aristolochic acid, 1223-1226
　　autoimmune diseases, 1228-1229
　　cadmium, 1227
　　Chinese herbs, 1223-1224
　　hyperuricemia, 1227-1228
　　lead, 1226-1227
　　lithium, 1226, 1226f
　　overview of, 1222t
　　sarcoidosis, 1228
　　urate nephropathy, 1227-1228
　clinical features of, 1221
　pathology of, 1221
Churg-Strauss syndrome. See Eosinophilic granulomatosis with polyangiitis
Chvostek's sign, 612-613, 623, 995
Chylomicrons, 1801-1802
Chyluria, 1255
Cicaprost, 377
Cigarette smoking. See Smoking
Cilazapril, 1642, 1643t
Ciliopathies, 2319-2322, 2320f, 2322t
Cilioprotein, 1506f
Cinacalcet, 612, 631, 1873, 2026-2027, 2029, 2032
Ciprofloxacin, 1405
　crystalluria caused by, 1259-1260
　for pyelonephritis, 1241-1242, 1241t
　for urinary tract infection, 1244
Cirrhosis
　apelin in, 446-447
　aquaporin-2 protein abundance in, 300
　ascites with, 449, 1712, 1723
　brain natriuretic peptide in, 447
　carbon tetrachloride-induced, 494
　COX metabolites in, 378
　C-type natriuretic peptide in, 447
　diuretics for, 1722-1724
　extracellular fluid expansion associated with, 299-300
　fluid retention in, 1724f
　glomerulonephritis caused by, 1156

Cirrhosis (Continued)
　hyponatremia associated with, 494
　intrahepatic vascular pressure in, 439
　norepinephrine levels in, 445
　prostaglandins in, 378
　renal biopsy of, 1156-1157
　sinusoidal pressure in, 439
　sodium retention in
　　apelin in, 446-447
　　arginine vasopressin in, 446
　　atrial natriuretic peptide in, 447, 448f
　　brain natriuretic peptide in, 447
　　C-type natriuretic peptide in, 447
　　Dendroaspis natriuretic peptides in, 447
　　effector mechanisms, 444-449
　　endothelin in, 446
　　natriuretic peptides in, 447-449
　　overflow hypothesis, 449
　　pathogenesis of, 449
　　prostaglandins in, 448-449
　　renin-angiotensin-aldosterone system in, 444-445, 452
　　sympathetic nervous system in, 445-446
　treatment of
　　α-adrenergic agonists, 456
　　liver transplantation, 458
　　midodrine, 456
　　pharmacologic, 455-457
　　PROMETHEUS, 458
　　renal replacement therapy, 457-458
　　somatostatin analogues, 456
　　systemic vasoconstrictors, 455-456
　　terlipressin, 455-456
　　transjugular intrahepatic portosystemic shunt, 457
　　vasoconstrictor antagonists, 455
　　vasodilators, 455
　　vasopressin 2 receptor antagonists, 456-457
　　vasopressin-1 receptor analogues, 455-456
　tubular sodium reabsorption and, 444
　underfilling hypothesis of, 449
　volume-sensing abnormalities as cause of, 439-444, 447
　sympathetic nervous system in, 445-446
　vasopressin levels in, 446
　water retention in, 439, 446
Cirrhotic cardiomyopathy, 441
Cisplatin, 621, 966, 968t, 990, 1001, 1397
Cited1, 29
Cited1-EGFP transgene, 19
Citrate
　acid-base homeostasis role of, 247-248
　actions of, 1337
　basolateral transport of, 248
　bicarbonate generation secondary to excretion of, 247-248
　calcium affinity for, 219
　excretion of, 247-248, 841, 2385
　functions of, 219
　as kidney stone inhibitor, 1330, 1337f
　proximal tubule absorption and metabolism of, 217f, 248
Citrate transport disorders, 219
Citric acid cycle, 126
Class I HLA molecules, 2231-2233, 2232f
Class II HLA molecules, 2233
Classical congenital adrenal hyperplasia, 1547
Clathrin, 56-59
Clathrin-coated pits, 291

Claudins
　-2, 55-56
　-10, 55-56
　-14, 189
　-16, 160, 161f, 195-196, 195f
　-19, 160, 194-196, 195f
　description of, 147, 188-189
CLC-K2, 161, 243
CLDN19, 2388
Clear cell carcinoma, 890f, 1371-1374, 1371t, 1372f, 1377
Clevidipine, 1665, 1695t, 1698-1699
Clinical endpoint, 927t
CLINITEK system, 797
Clock gene, 256
CL⁻-OH exchange, 148
Clonidine
　with diuretics, 445-446
　hypertensive urgencies and emergencies treated with, 1697t
　indications for, 1629, 1671-1672, 1671t-1672t
Clopidogrel, 1932, 2012
c-Met, 1757
Coagulation, 980-981, 1863
Coagulation factors, 1018t, 1803
Coated pits, 56-59
Cobalamin C deficiency, 1188, 2356-2357
Cocaine, 686
Cockcroft-Gault equation, 784t, 786, 2042-2044, 2064, 2587f
Cognitive function disorders
　delirium syndromes. See Delirium syndromes
　dialysis dementia, 1935-1936
　uremic encephalopathy, 1934-1935
Cognitive impairment, 1935-1938, 1937f 1938f, 2590
Cohort studies, 671
Col3A1, 1213
COL4A3, 1141-1142
COL4A4, 1141-1142
Colchicine
　adverse effects of, 2486
　familial Mediterranean fever treated with, 2485-2486
　gout treated with, 2282
　polymorphonuclear cell accumulation of, 2485-2486
Cold ischemia time, 2265, 2278
Collagen, 1757, 2610
Collagen IV, 951-952, 1139
Collapsing focal segmental glomerulosclerosis, 1026, 1029-1031, 1159, 2328
Collapsing glomerulopathy, 1153
Collecting duct (CD)
　acid secretion, 1276
　acid-base transport in, 244-245
　alkalosis and, 244
　ammonia secretion by, 252, 252f
　anatomy of, 44-45, 45f, 69-75, 262, 263f, 269f
　angiotensin II effects on, 244-245
　carbonic anhydrase in, 243
　cells of, 30, 69-70, 239-241, 239f-241f, 282
　cortical. See Cortical collecting duct
　EETs in, 385
　elongation of, 25-26
　embryology of, 5, 6f
　endothelin-1 synthesis by, 245
　EP3 receptor mRNA in, 371
　HKα expression in, 242-243
　HKα₂ expression in, 242-243
　HKβ expression in, 242-243

Collecting duct (CD) *(Continued)*
  hydrogen in, 242, 1276
  initial, 239
  inner medullary, 44-45, 45f, 69-70, 74-75
  intercalated cells involved in, 239-241, 239f-241f
  lithium in, 297-298
  metabolic acidosis and, 244
  metabolic alkalosis and, 244
  outer medullary, 44-45, 45f, 69-70, 73-74
  papillary, 27, 75f
  potassium in, 178, 540-541, 1729f
  regions of, 69-70
  respiratory acidosis and, 244
  segments of, 239, 262
  sodium absorption in, 73
  sodium transport in, 374
  tubulopathy of, 1417-1418
  tumor of, 1371, 1371t
  urea accumulation, 268-269, 268f
  vasopressin effects on, 296-297
  water absorption in, 269f, 270-271
  water impermeability of, 491
  water permeability in, prostaglandins' effect on, 301
Collecting system
  composition of, 5
  duplicated, 864f, 2296, 2303, 2303f, 2313
  formation of, 25-27
  water absorption in, 271
Colloid osmotic pressure, 94-96, 95f, 98
Colloid solutions, for hypovolemia, 425
Colon, 316-317
Colonic isoform, 242
Columns of Bertin, 850
"Comet tail" sign, 874-876
Complement
  activation of, 1183f, 1213-1214
  in acute poststreptococcal glomerulonephritis, 1058
  in anti-glomerular basement membrane glomerulonephritis, 1080
  in atypical hemolytic-uremic syndrome, 1183-1185
  genetic abnormalities in, 1184
  hemolytic-uremic syndrome caused by disorders of, 2355-2356, 2355f
  in membranoproliferative glomerulonephritis, 1049
  in membranous nephropathy, 1041
  nephritic syndrome levels of, 759-760, 759t
Complement factor 1, 1185
Complement factor B, 1185
Complement factor D, 1788
Complement factor H, 1184-1185, 2355-2357
Complement factor H-related proteins, 1184
Complement inhibitors, 1186
Complement protein D, 1810
Computed tomography angiography, 853f, 904, 904f-905f
Computed tomography angiography (CTA), 853f, 904, 904f-905f
Computed tomography (CT), 851-856
  anatomy on, 852-853, 852f-855f
  angiomyolipomas on, 891, 893f
  autosomal dominant polycystic kidney disease on, 869f, 885-888, 888f, 1486f
  chronic kidney disease on, 869, 869f
  contrast-enhanced
    acute pyelonephritis on, 878-880, 880f
    description of, 851

Computed tomography (CT) *(Continued)*
  emphysematous pyelonephritis on, 882f
  hydronephrosis on, 872f
  nephropathy caused by, 853-856
  obstructive urography evaluations, 871, 873f
  pyelonephritis on, 882f, 1241
  renal abscess on, 880, 881f
  renal cysts on, 883-885, 886f-887f, 891f
  renal masses on, 883-885, 886f, 890, 892f
  after renal transplantation, 910
  renal tuberculosis on, 884f
  renal vein thrombosis on, 909, 1205
  xanthogranulomatous pyelonephritis on, 881, 883f
  corticomedullary phase on, 853f
  definition of, 851
  description of, 851
  dual-energy, 852f
  excretory phase on, 854f
  helical, 1265-1266
  history of, 851
  kidney stones on, 873, 875f, 1359
  multidetector, 851
  nephrographic phase on, 854f
  polycystic kidney disease on, 869f
  renal cell carcinoma on, 894f, 898f
  renal colic on, 873
  renal cysts on, 883-885, 886f-887f
  renal mucormycosis on, 2498f
  renal parenchymal disease on, 880-881
  ureteral stone on, 875f-876f
  urinary tract obstruction on, 1265-1266, 1266f
  xanthogranulomatous pyelonephritis on, 1252
Computed tomography scanners, 851
Computed tomography urography
  intravenous urography versus, 852
  normal findings on, 855f
  technique for, 851-852
Conception, 1635
Conflicts of interest, 2562
Congenital adrenal hyperplasia, 1461, 1547
Congenital anomalies of the kidney and urinary tract (CAKUT), 713, 1415-1416
  branchio-oto-renal syndrome, 2297t, 2299, 2318
  ciliopathies, 2319-2322, 2320f, 2322t
  clinical management of, 2304-2305
  clinical presentation of, 2302-2304
  copy number variants in, 2300
  definitions, 2311
  description of, 2294
  DSTYK in, 2300
  ectopic kidney, 2295, 2295f, 2305, 2311
  end-stage kidney disease progression of, 2361, 2404, 2421
  epidemiology of, 2296, 2311
  fetal presentation of, 2302
  functional consequences of, 2301-2302
  genetics of, 2296, 2297t
  genotype-phenotype correlations for, 1416
  GLI3 repressor, 2299
  hedgehog signaling, 2299
  horseshoe kidney, 2295, 2296f, 2303-2304, 2311
  in utero environment effects on, 2300-2301, 2301t
  in utero management of, 2304-2305
  Kallmann's syndrome, 2297t, 2318
  long-term outcomes of, 2305

Congenital anomalies of the kidney and urinary tract (CAKUT) *(Continued)*
  molecular pathogenesis of, 2297-2300
  multicystic dysplastic kidney, 889, 2294-2296, 2295f, 2303, 2305, 2312-2313
  mutant alleles associated with, 2297
  neuropsychiatric disorders and, 2300
  outcomes of, 2305
  pathogenesis of, 1416, 2296-2302
  posterior urethral valves, 2316, 2317f, 2435
  postnatal management of, 2304-2305
  primary megaureter, 2315-2316
  prune-belly syndrome, 2318-2319
  renal agenesis, 2302, 2311-2312
  renal collecting system duplication, 2296, 2303, 2303f, 2313
  renal coloboma syndrome, 2297t, 2317-2318
  renal cyst and diabetes syndrome, 2316-2317
  renal dysplasia. *See* Renal dysplasia
  renal ectopy, 2295, 2295f, 2303, 2305, 2311
  renal fusion, 2303-2305, 2311
  sporadic forms of, 2299-2300
  syndromic forms of, 2316-2322
  Townes-Brocks syndrome, 2318
  ureteric budding, 2297-2298
  ureteropelvic junction obstruction, 2314-2315, 2315f
  VACTERL association, 2318
  VATER association, 2318
  vesicoureteral reflux, 2311, 2313-2314, 2314f
Congenital chloridorrhea, 553
Congenital heart disease, 2421-2422
Congenital hydronephrosis, 1259
Congenital lipoid adrenal hypoplasia, 588
Congenital nephrotic syndrome of the Finnish, 1426-1428
Congestive heart failure. *See* Heart failure
Conivaptan, 504, 1713-1714
Connecting segment cell, 239
Connecting tubules
  anatomy of, 68-69
  aquaporin-2 expression by, 69
  bicarbonate reabsorption in, 241-242
  cells of, 68-69
  chloride absorption in, 170
  functional role of, 241-242
  intercalated cells in, 68-69
  potassium secretion by, 176-178
  in rat, 68-69
  sodium chloride transport in, 169-171
  in sodium reabsorption, 69
  water absorption in, 271
Connective tissue growth factor, 951, 1300
Connexin 40, 400
Connexins, 55-56
Conn's syndrome, 321
Continuous ambulatory peritoneal dialysis (CAPD)
  antibiotic administration in, 2130t
  azotemia treated with, 2486
  in children, 2415
  description of, 1318, 1963-1964, 2049, 2117, 2119-2120
  frequency of exchanges, 2122
  residual kidney function affected by, 2126
Continuous cyclic peritoneal dialysis, 2119
Continuous flow centrifugation, 2160

Continuous hemodiafiltration, 598
Continuous positive airway pressure, for sleep apnea, 1940
Continuous quality improvement, 2623
Continuous renal replacement therapy (CRRT)
    acute kidney injury treated with, 1007-1008
    administration of, 2141
    in children, 2417-2418
    critically ill patients treated with, 2141, 2141t
    drug dosing in, 2048-2049
    hepatorenal syndrome treated with, 457
    metformin clearance during, 2185
    poison removal using, 2171
    renal function estimations in, 2044
Continuous venovenous hemodiafiltration, 1007, 2142
Continuous venovenous hemodialysis, 1007-1008
Continuous venovenous hemofiltration, 1007, 2142
Contrast media
    computed tomography enhanced with. See Computed tomography (CT), contrast-enhanced
    in elevated creatinine patients, 854-856
    estimated glomerular filtration rate and, 854-856
    high osmolar, 847-848
    intravenous, 849, 854
    iodinated, 847-848
    low osmolar, 847-848, 855-856
    magnetic resonance angiography using, 859-861, 862f
    magnetic resonance urography using, 861-863, 862f
    nephropathy caused by, 853-854, 964-966, 1000
    nephrotoxicity of, 1000, 2273
Convection, 2068-2069, 2068f, 2078, 2112
Cooperative Study of Renovascular Hypertension, 1569
Copper, 1444
Copper sulfate poisoning, 2500
Copy number variants, 2300
Core binding factor α-1, 1835
Cori cycle, 132
Corin, 340, 1800
Coronary artery bypass grafting, acute kidney injury after, 992
Coronary artery calcification, 1850
Coronary artery disease, 1660
Coronary heart disease, 1527f
Cortical blood flow, 87
Cortical collecting duct (CCD)
    AE1 immunoreactivity in, 72-73
    apical potassium channels in, 564
    autosomal recessive type I pseudohypoaldosteronism in, 539
    bicarbonate reabsorption in, 242, 245
    cells of, 70, 70f
    characteristics of, 44-45, 45f, 69-70
    chloride absorption in, 170
    initial collecting tubule/duct, 65-66, 68, 69f, 70
    intercalated cells of, 70-71, 72f, 239, 239f
    luminal surface of, 71f
    medullary ray collecting duct, 70
    metabolism, 133
    parts of, 70
    potassium secretion by, 73, 176-178, 563-564, 1748-1749
    principal cells of, 70, 70f, 74
    prostaglandin synthesis in, 365

Cortical collecting duct (CCD) (Continued)
    SK channels in, 180f
    sodium chloride transport in, 169-171
    vasopressin effects on, 819
    voltage defects in, 539f
    water absorption in, 569
Cortical interstitium, 77-78
Cortical labyrinth, 261-262
Cortical nephrons, 45
Cortical stromal cells, 5-6
Cortical tubules, 89, 90f
Cortical-medullary junction, 91
Corticomedullary arcades, 6
Corticosteroids. See also specific drug
    acute interstitial nephritis treated with, 1002
    adverse effects of, 1166-1167, 2426
    anti-glomerular basement membrane disease treated with, 1126-1127
    in children, 2426
    eosinophilic granulomatosis with polyangiitis treated with, 1117-1118
    fracture risks, 1167
    glomerulonephritis treated with, 1166-1167
    gout treated with, 2282
    Henoch-Schönlein purpura treated with, 1124
    immunosuppressive uses of, in renal transplantation, 2245, 2254t, 2259, 2426
    linear growth affected by, 2434-2435
    membranous nephropathy treated with, 1042
    minimal change disease treated with, 1022-1023, 1023t
    mixed connective tissue disease treated with, 1109
    osteopenia caused by, 1166-1167
    perinatal exposure to, 717
    polyarteritis nodosa treated with, 1119-1120
    during pregnancy, 1637
    pruritus treated with, 1943
    Takayasu arteritis treated with, 1121
    temporal arteritis treated with, 1120
    toxicity of, 1167
Corticosterone, 309
Cortisol, 305, 309, 1919-1920
Costimulatory signal blockers, 2258-2259
Costovertebral angle pain, 1240, 1250
Coulomb's law, 124
Countercurrent multiplication paradigm, 266, 267f
COX-1, 355, 360f361f, 361, 411-412
COX-2
    description of, 355
    expression of, 357-361
        acute ischemic injury effects on, 377
        in cirrhosis, 448
        cyclosporine A effects on, 378
        in developing kidney, 363
        in diabetes mellitus, 378
        glomerular, 376
        in loop of Henle, 373-374
        in macula densa, 357-358, 359f, 360
        in medullary interstitial cells, 360-361
        in renal cortex, 357-361
        in renal medulla, 360-361, 360f
    glucocorticoids effect on, 357
    immunohistochemistry for, 1274f
    knockout mice model of, 358-360
    prostaglandin synthesis in renomedullary interstitial cells mediated by, 80
    prostanoids from, 357-358

COX-2 (Continued)
    reactive oxygen species as mediator of, 379
    renin release and, 568
    sodium intake effects on, 412
COX-2 inhibitors
    acute kidney injury caused by, 362-363
    cardiovascular effects of, 363-364
    heart failure and, 437
    hyperkalemia caused by, 590
    nephrogenesis affected by, 719
    proteinuria treated with, 377-378
    renin production affected by, 360
    thrombotic events and, 363-364
    vascular tone affected by, 363
C1q nephropathy, 1034-1035
C-reactive protein, 1910, 1969-1970, 2100
CREATE trial, 1901
Creatine phosphate, 1961
Creatine–creatine phosphate, 1961
Creatinine
    in children, 2341f
    contrast media administration in patients with elevated levels of, 854-856
    cystatin C and, 934-935
    degradation of, 1961
    excretion of
        age of patient and, 1961
        in chronic kidney disease, 1961
        factors that affect, 1961
        fractional, 1199
        variability in, 796
    formation of, 1961
    glomerular filtration rate and, 678, 782-783, 933, 2309-2310, 2587, 2587f
    Jaffe method for measuring, 782, 787
    measurement of, 782-783
    plasma
        glomerular filtration rate estimations using, 782-783, 783f
        in hypovolemia diagnosis, 423
        trimethoprim-sulfamethoxazole effects on, 2273
    secretion of, 782
    serum
        acute interstitial nephritis levels of, 1219-1220
        age-related changes in, 737
        angiotensin receptor blockers effect on, 2006
        angiotensin-converting enzyme inhibitors effect on, 2006
        degradation and, 1961
        as glomerular filtration rate biomarker, 933
        glomerular filtration rate effects on, 782, 933
        renal function assessments using, 783
        storage of, 933
    in titratable acid excretion, 247
    in uremia, 1808
Creatinine clearance, 736, 783, 2544
    estimated, 2042, 2042t, 2044
    peritoneal dialysis dosage based on, 2120-2121
Creatol, 1811
Crescentic glomerulonephritis
    definition of, 1072-1073
    diagnostic classification of, 1074f
    immune complex-mediated
        in children, 1073
        electron microscopy findings, 1075
        epidemiology of, 1075
        immunofluorescence microscopy findings, 1075

Crescentic glomerulonephritis *(Continued)*
   light microscopy findings, 1075
   methylprednisolone for, 1076
   pathogenesis of, 1075-1076
   pathology of, 1075
   treatment of, 1076
   immunopathologic categories of, 1073t-1074t
   pauci-immune
     anti-MPO antibodies in, 1083-1085
     antineutrophil cytoplasmic autoantibodies in, 1082-1084, 1086-1087
     anti-PR3 autoantibodies in, 1083
     clinical features of, 1085-1086
     crescent formation in, 1082
     cyclophosphamide for, 1087-1088
     electron microscopy of, 1083
     end-stage kidney disease progression of, 1086
     epidemiology of, 1081-1082
     immunofluorescence microscopy of, 1082-1083
     laboratory findings in, 1086-1087
     light microscopy of, 1082, 1082f
     methylprednisolone for, 1087-1089
     natural history of, 1085-1086
     pathogenesis of, 1083-1085
     pathology of, 1082-1083, 1082f
     plasmapheresis for, 1088
     PR3 in, 1083
     prognostic factors for, 1086
     relapse prevention in, 1089
     after renal transplantation, 1086
     rituximab for, 1088-1089
     segmental fibrinoid necrosis in, 1082f
     T cells in, 1084
     treatment of, 1087-1089
     urinalysis findings in, 1086-1087
Crescentic immunoglobulin A nephropathy, 1068
c-ret receptor, 719
Critical care nephrology. *See* Critically ill patients
Critical Path Initiative, 953
Critically ill patients
   acute kidney injury in, 2137-2139
   acute respiratory distress syndrome, 2138-2139
   cardiac dysfunction, 2139
   cardiorenal syndrome, 2139
   drug dosing in, 2145-2146
   fluid management for, 2138
   hemodialysis in, 2142
   hypocalcemia caused by, 618
   liver dysfunction, 2139
   outcomes in, 2142
   pulmonary dysfunction, 2138-2139
   renal replacement therapy in
     anticoagulation during, 2144
     continuous renal replacement therapy, 2141-2142, 2141t
     drug dosing considerations, 2145
     euvolemia, 2144
     fluid balance, 2144
     hemodynamic stability, 2144
     intensity of, 2142-2144
     intermittent hemodialysis, 2140-2142, 2141t
     subclavian catheters used in, 2145
     sustained low-efficiency dialysis, 2141t, 2142, 2145-2146
     ultrafiltration, 2144
     vascular access, 2145

Critically ill patients *(Continued)*
   sepsis, 2137-2138
   volume overload in, 2144
Crossed renal ectopy, 2295, 2295f, 2304
Cross-reactive groups, 2236
Cross-sectional studies, 670
Crotalus snakebites, 2446-2447
Crotoxin, 2447
Cryoglobulin(s), 1058, 1137, 2152
Cryoglobulinemia, 1071, 2152
Cryoglobulinemic glomerulonephritis, 1137-1138, 1137f, 1138f
Cryoplasty balloon, for stenotic lesions, 2212
Cryoprecipitate, 1906
Crystals, 1327
   agglomeration of, 1329
   aggregation assessments, 1329
   growth of, 1327f, 1329
   nucleation of, 1327f, 1328-1329
   in urine, 800-802, 801t
CTLA-4-Ig, 1034, 1104-1105, 2248
C-type natriuretic peptide (CNP)
   in cirrhosis, 447
   description of, 339
   in effective arterial blood volume regulation, 414-415
   functions of, 340
   in heart failure, 342, 434-435
   knockout mouse models of, 343
   plasma concentrations of, 340
   preproCNP, 340
   structure of, 339f, 340
   synthesis of, 340
Cullin 3, 168
Cushing's disease, 556
Cushing's syndrome, 766, 1549
Cutaneous metastases, 1949
Cutting balloons, for stenotic lesions, 2212
CXCL13, 1793
CXCR4, 34
CXCR7, 34
Cyclic adenosine monophosphate (cAMP)
   apical sodium hydrogen exchange affected by, 154-155
   description of, 463
   hormones that stimulate, 1706
   soluble adenylyl cyclase production of, 256
   vasopressin effects on, 282-283
Cyclic GMP, 101, 398
Cyclical pulsatile load, 1535
Cyclin-dependent kinase, 1745
Cyclooxygenases (COX), 355, 357
   -1. *See* COX-1
   -2. *See* COX-2
   in arachidonic acid metabolism, 355, 356f
   description of, 355
   enzymatic chemistry of, 357
   expression of, antiinflammatory steroids' regulation of, 357
   gene expression, 357
   metabolites
     in acute kidney injury, 377
     in cirrhosis, 378
     in diabetes mellitus, 378
     in glomerular inflammatory injury, 375-376
     in glomerular noninflammatory injury, 376-377
     in hepatorenal syndrome, 378
     in sodium transport, 373-374
     in urinary tract obstruction, 377-378
     in water transport, 373-374

Cyclooxygenases (COX) *(Continued)*
   molecular biology of, 355
   nephronal distribution of, 364-366
   reactive oxygen species generated by, 379
   sources of, 364-366
Cyclophosphamide, 1397-1398
   adverse effects of, 1168-1169
   focal segmental glomerulosclerosis treated with, 1032
   glomerular disease treated with, 1168-1170
   granulomatous with polyangiitis treated with, 1112-1114
   lupus nephritis treated with, 1102-1103
   malignancy risks, 1169
   membranous nephropathy treated with, 1042-1043
   microscopic polyangiitis treated with, 1112-1113, 1115-1116
   minimal change disease treated with, 1023
   ovarian failure caused by, 1168-1169
   pauci-immune crescentic glomerulonephritis treated with, 1087-1088
   polyarteritis nodosa treated with, 1119-1120
   side effects of, 1113-1114
   steroid-sensitive nephrotic syndrome treated with, 2329
   toxicity of, 1169-1170
Cyclosporin A, 378, 1398-1399, 1637, 1637t. *See also* Cyclosporine
Cyclosporine
   adverse effects of, 2330
   in children, 2424-2425
   fibrillary glomerulonephritis treated with, 1134
   focal segmental glomerulosclerosis treated with, 1033
   glomerular disease treated with, 1167-1168
   hyperkalemia caused by, 590
   hypomagnesemia caused by, 622
   immunosuppressive uses of, 2246-2247, 2254t, 2256-2257
   lupus nephritis treated with, 1104
   membranous nephropathy treated with, 1043
   minimal change disease treated with, 1023-1024
   nephrogenesis affected by, 719
   nephrotoxicity of, 2264
   renal transplantation uses of, 2246-2247, 2254t, 2256-2257, 2269
   side effects of, 1023
   steroid-sensitive nephrotic syndrome treated with, 2329-2330
CYP24A1, 2390
CYP11B2, 305
CYP27B1, 1830, 2390
Cyst. *See* Renal cyst
Cyst hemorrhage, 1493
Cystatin C
   as acute kidney injury biomarker, 935, 989
   as chronic kidney disease biomarker, 934-935, 2043
   Chronic Kidney Disease Epidemiology Collaboration equation for measuring, 786
   clearance of, 1810
   creatinine and, 934-935

Cystatin C *(Continued)*
  description of, 678, 737
  glomerular filtration rate estimations using, 783-784, 934-935, 2310
  urinary, 948-949
Cysteamine, 1441f, 2339
Cysteine, 1346f
Cysteinyl leukotriene receptors, 380
Cystic disease of renal sinus, 1517
Cystic fibrosis transmembrane regulator protein, 160
Cystic kidney disease, 1416, 1514-1516, 1515f-1516f
Cystic neoplasm, 1516-1517
Cystic nephroma, 1517
Cystic partially differentiated nephroblastoma, 1517
Cystic renal cell carcinoma, 1515f, 1516
Cystic renal mass, 1375. *See also* Bosniak renal cyst classification
Cystine, 1346f, 1441f, 1817
Cystine chelation therapy, 1365
Cystine stone, 1345-1346, 1448
Cystinosis, 1439-1441, 1440t, 2339-2340, 2341f
Cystinuria, 1445
  characteristics of, 223t, 227
  in children, 2345-2346, 2346f
  classification of, 228, 1448
  dietary intervention in, 1361-1362
  in Middle East, 2478-2479
  mutations in, 227
  rBAT/b$^{0,+}$AT in, 227-228
Cystitis, 1633
  antimicrobial agents for, 1238-1239, 1238t
  description of, 1231-1232
  diagnosis of, 1237-1238
  emphysematous, 1251
  epidemiology of, 1236
  Escherichia coli as cause of, 749-750, 778, 1233
  host factors, 1237
  microbiology of, 1236-1237
  pathogenesis of, 1236-1237
  prophylaxis for, 1239
  pyuria associated with, 1238
  recurrence of, 1237, 1239-1240
  reinfection of, 1237
  sexual intercourse as cause of, 1237
  spermicides and, 1237, 1239-1240
  Staphylococcus saprophyticus as cause of, 1237
  treatment of, 1238-1239, 1238t
  urine culture for, 1237-1238
Cytapheresis, 2160-2161
Cytochrome P450
  4A2 gene, 385
  in acute kidney disease, 385, 2038-2039
  alterations in, 2038-2039
  in chronic kidney disease, 385, 2038-2039
  CYP3A4, 2039
  description of, 355
  metabolites of, from arachidonic acid metabolism
    description of, 382, 382f-383f
    in hypertension, 385
    in renal blood flow autoregulation, 384
    as second messengers, 383-384
    in tubuloglomerular feedback, 384
  monooxygenases, 382-383
  parathyroid hormone effects on, 2019
  in proximal tubule, 384
  vasculature affected by, 383-384
Cytofolds, 47

Cytokines
  bicarbonate transport regulation by, 238
  macrophage production of, 976
  prostaglandin E$_2$ synthesis stimulated by, 376
  renal transplantation and, 2241
  in scleroderma, 1197
  suppressors of cytokine signaling, 1913
  therapeutic uses of, 1382
  tubular epithelial cell release of, 1215
  in tubulointerstitial injury, 1212-1213
Cytology, urine, 799
Cytomegalovirus, 1255, 2278, 2287-2288, 2429
Cytoplasmic antineutrophil cytoplasmic antibody, 759-760, 1109-1110
Cytoreductive nephrectomy, 1381
Cytotoxic lymphocyte activation antigen 4, 2240
Cytotoxic nephropathy, 1402-1403

D

Daclizumab, 2256
D–amino acids, 1809-1810
Dark cells, 70, 72f
Dcn, 31
Dead in bed syndrome, 572-573
Decorin, 31
Deep vein thrombosis (DVT)
  in chronic kidney disease, 1906-1907, 1908f
  in membranous nephropathy, 1041
  in nephrotic syndrome, 1804
  risk of, factors that affect, 1908f
Dehydration, 2367-2368
  description of, 2367-2368
  fluid therapy for, 2373-2374, 2373t
  hypernatremic, 2367-2368, 2374
  hypertonic, 478-480
  urinary concentrating ability affected by, 296-297
7-Dehydrocholesterol, 1828
Dehydroepiandrosterone, 1920
Dehydroepiandrosterone sulfate, 1920
Delirium syndromes
  definition of, 1934
  depression and, 1937-1938
  dialysis dysequilibrium, 1935
  differential diagnosis of, 1934t
  uremic encephalopathy, 1934-1935
Delta1, 30
Delta gap, 837
Dementia, 1935-1936, 1938
Dendritic cells, 976-977, 1792-1793
Dendroaspis natriuretic peptide, 339-341, 339f, 415, 447
Dengue fever
  acute kidney injury caused by, 2498-2499, 2520-2521, 2522t
  in Far East, 2520-2521, 2522t
  in Indian subcontinent, 2498-2499
  in Latin America, 2440-2441
Dengue hemorrhagic fever, 2520-2521
Dengue shock syndrome, 2520-2521
Denosumab, 612
Dense deposit disease
  classification of, 1046f
  clinical features of, 1052
  description of, 1046
  epidemiology of, 1050
  genetics of, 1052
  hypocomplementemia in, 1052-1053
  light microscopy findings in, 1051, 1051f
  lipodystrophy associated with, 1053

Dense deposit disease *(Continued)*
  microhematuria in, 1052
  pathogenesis of, 1052
  pathology of, 1050-1051
  retinal deposits associated with, 1053
  treatment of, 1053
Dentin matrix protein, 1830
Dent's disease, 1437-1438, 2344-2345
Denys-Drash syndrome, 1431, 2325
Deoxycorticosterone, 304f
Depletional hyponatremia, 503-504
Depression, 1937-1938, 2063
Dermatitis, arteriovenous shunt, 1949
Dermatosis, acquired perforating, 1944, 1944f
Desferrioxamine, 1887
Desmopressin
  central diabetes insipidus treated with, 487-488
  description of, 162-163, 175, 279, 282
  hyponatremia caused by, 488, 496-497
  kidney biopsy-related bleeding complications treated with, 915-917
  nephrogenic diabetes insipidus applications of, 484, 487, 2338
  renal response to, 808-809
  uremic bleeding treated with, 1906
  urine flow rate affected by, 806, 810-811
  vasopressin deficiency treated with, 285
Developmental origins of health and disease, 694
Developmental programming
  birth weight and, 694, 694t
  of blood pressure, 709, 709f
  definition of, 694
  mechanisms of, 713-723, 715t, 725f
    apoptosis, 718
    catch-up growth, 721-723
    congenital urinary tract obstruction, 719-720
    c-ret receptor function, 719
    fetal exposures
      to drugs, 719
      to glucocorticoids, 717
      to hyperglycemia, 717-718
    gender, 720
    glial cell line-derived neurotrophic factor, 719
    maternal nutrient restriction, 715-717
  nephron endowment, 696-701
  nephron number, 695-696, 695t
  prematurity and, 694, 694t
  of renal function and disease, 703-712
  renin-angiotensin-aldosterone system and, 703, 704t-705t
  transgenerational effects of, 722-723
Dexamethasone, 696-699
D1g1, 29
DHA (2,8-dihydroxyadenine) stone, 1347
Diabetes Control and Complications Trial, 1301-1302
Diabetes insipidus (DI), 1467-1473
  acquired, 285
  acute traumatic, 488-489
  calcium stones and uric acid stones, 1343f
  causes of, 808-809
  central
    adenohypophisitis and, 475-476
    arginine vasopressin for, 488
    causes of, 473-476, 473t
    clinical manifestations of, 483
    description of, 285, 809, 2369-2370
    desmopressin for, 487-488
    familial, 474-475, 475f
    idiopathic, 475-476

Diabetes insipidus (DI) (Continued)
    partial, 809-810, 810f
    pathophysiology of, 476-477, 478f
    polyuria in, 810-811
    treatment of, 487-489
  characteristics of, 285
  clinical manifestations of, 483
  definition of, 282
  dipsogenic, 482
  familial, 285
  fluid deprivation test for diagnosis of, 485, 485t
  magnetic resonance imaging of, 485-486
  nephrogenic. See Nephrogenic diabetes insipidus
  partial, 477
  postsurgical, 488
  of pregnancy, 1612
  thiazide diuretics for, 1727
  thirst mechanisms in, 484
  treatment of
    arginine vasopressin, 486
    chlorpropamide, 487
    desmopressin, 487
    goals for, 486
    natriuretic agents, 487
    options for, 486t
    prostaglandin synthase inhibitors, 487
    thiazide diuretics, 487
Diabetes mellitus (DM)
  in Africa, 2463
  anemia in, 1877-1878
  in China, 2529, 2529f
  chronic kidney disease progression affected by, 681, 1865
  COX-2 in, 378
  Diabetes Outcome Clinical Trial, blood pressure levels achieved in, 1554t
  dipeptidyl peptidase-4 inhibitors for, 2593
  in elderly, 2590, 2592-2593
  end-stage kidney disease caused by, 2060, 2280
  in Far East, 2529
  glucagon-like peptide-1 analogues for, 2593
  glyburide for, 2593
  glycemic control in, 1301-1303, 1995
  hemoglobin A_{1c} in, 2593
  hyperkalemia in, 586-587
  hypoglycemic agents for, 2593
  hypomagnesemia in, 620
  malnutrition associated with, 1315
  maternal, 2301
  maturity-onset diabetes type 5, 2299-2300
  mesangial expansion in, 1288, 1292
  in Middle East, 2472
  in New Zealand, 2550-2551
  new-onset, after transplantation, 1320
  oral hypoglycemic agents for, 2593
  osmotic diuresis in, 812-813
  plasma renin levels in, 334-335
  posttransplantation, 1320, 2283
  pregnancy and, 1634
  prevalence of, 1865
  renal disorders in, 1291-1292, 2592
  renal failure in, 1314-1318, 1314t
    after renal transplantation, 2433
    renal transplantation in patients with, 1318-1319, 2288-2289
  repaglinide for, 2593
  stroke risks associated with, 1928t, 1929, 1931
  telmisartan versus losartan trial, 1557

Diabetes mellitus (DM) (Continued)
  thiazide diuretics and, 1730
  transplantation for
    islet cell, 1319-1320
    new-onset diabetes after, 1320
    renal, 1318-1319, 2288-2289
    renal-pancreas, 1319
  type 1
    blood pressure in, 1297-1298
    cardiovascular disease in, 1295
    chronic kidney disease in, 1981
    diabetic nephropathy in, 1285, 1293, 1294t, 1299, 1312
    end-stage kidney disease in, 1295
    glomerular filtration rate in, 1296
    glomerular structure in, 1291
    glomeruli in, 1287f
    hypertension in, 1297-1298
    mesangial expansion in, 1288, 1292
    microalbuminuria in, 1283, 1292-1294
    nephropathy in, 1290-1291
    peripheral capillary filtration surface in, 1288-1289
    podocyte number in, 1287-1288
    proteinuria in, 1292-1293, 1300
    structural-functional relationships in, 1288-1289, 1289f
    urinary kallikrein excretion in, 350
  type 2
    blood pressure in, 1298
    cardiovascular morbidity in, 1306-1308
    diabetic nephropathy in, 1293, 1294t
    glomerular structure in, 1291
    glucose-lowering therapies for, 1313
    metformin for, 1315
    microalbuminuria in, 1283, 1292-1293
    nephropathy in, 1290-1291
    podocyte number in, 1287-1288
    structural-functional relationships in, 1291
    telmisartan versus losartan trial, 1557
  urinary tract infections in, 1320
  urolithiasis and, 1350-1351
Diabetic ketoacidosis (DKA), 525, 546-547, 570, 628, 633, 2398
Diabetic nephropathy, 1556-1557
  acute kidney injury in, 1315
  "acute-on-chronic" renal failure in, 1315
  in Africa, 2463
  albuminuria in, 1283
  amputations in patients with, 1318
  anemia in, 1299-1300, 1316
  biomarkers for, 1294t
  bladder dysfunction in, 1320
  cardiovascular disease in, 1295, 1316-1317
  characteristics of, 1298
  chronic kidney disease caused by, 2503, 2592
  complications of, 1300, 1313t
  course of, 1296-1300
  description of, 112, 378
  diabetic retinopathy associated with, 1300
  electron microscopy of, 1284f
  endothelin system in, 337-338
  end-stage kidney disease caused by, 681, 1295, 1313-1314, 2592
  extracellular matrix accumulation in, 1286
  extrarenal complications in, 1300
  fluid retention in, 1298f
  genes associated with, 1299
  glycemic control in, 1301-1303
  hemodialysis for, 1316-1318
  hypertension in, 1314-1315, 1667

Diabetic nephropathy (Continued)
  kallikrein-kinin system in, 349-350
  light microscopy of, 1285f
  malnutrition associated with, 1315
  mesangial matrix fraction in, 1285-1286, 1285f
  microalbuminuria in, 1289-1290, 1292t, 1294-1298, 1301-1302
  mortality rates for, 1295
  natural history of, 1298
  normoalbuminuria, 1293-1294, 1296
  in Pacific Islands, 2553
  pathology of, 1284t
  pathophysiology of, 1298-1300, 1865
  peripheral neuropathy associated with, 1300
  podocytes in, 115t, 116-117, 120
  pregnancy in patients with, 1300, 1634
  prognosis for, 1295-1296, 1311-1312
  progression of, 658-659, 1298-1299, 1298f
  proteinuria in, 1295, 2004-2005
  reactive oxygen species in, 337
  recurrence of, after renal transplantation, 2275-2276
  renal replacement therapy for
    hemodialysis, 1316-1318
    initiation of, 1316
    peritoneal dialysis, 1318
  reversibility of, 1292
  risk factors for, 1290, 1294t, 1299
  transplantation for
    islet cell, 1319-1320
    new-onset diabetes after, 1320
    renal, 1318-1319
    renal-pancreas, 1319
  treatment of
    angiotensin receptor blockers, 2002
    angiotensin-converting enzyme inhibitors, 1308, 1998-1999, 2002
    blood pressure control, 1303-1312
    description of, 1300-1301
    dietary protein restriction, 1312
    glycemic control, 1301-1303
    lipid-lowering therapy, 1312
    new modalities for, 1312-1313, 1314t
    vitamin D, 1312-1313
  type 1, 1288-1289, 1289f
  type 2, 1291, 1999
  in type 1 diabetes mellitus, 1290-1291, 1312
  in type 2 diabetes mellitus, 1290-1291
  urinary proteomic profiles for, 1300
  urinary tract infections in, 1320
  urotensin II levels in, 352
  vascular access in, 1315
Diabetic retinopathy, 1300, 1318, 1888
Diacylglycerol, 355
Dialysance, 2071
Dialysate pump, 2078
Dialysis
  acute kidney injury treated with, 744
  advance directives and, 2561-2562
  in Africa, 2463-2464, 2464f,2465f
  albumin, 2171
  amyloidosis associated with, 1949
  in Australia, 2540f, 2542-2544
  blood pressure management in patients undergoing, 1561-1562
  cardioembolic stroke in, 1927
  cessation of, 2560-2561, 2561t
  chronic inflammation in, 1969-1970
  chronic kidney disease treated with, 1971
  "difficult" patients undergoing, 2567-2568, 2568t

Dialysis (Continued)
  drug clearance during, 2047
  early initiation of, 1971
  in elderly, 744, 2568-2569, 2590, 2591f, 2596-2598
  energy expenditure during, 1973
  epidemiology of, 2191-2192
  ethical dilemmas
    access, 2560
    advance directives, 2561-2562
    age-based rationing, 2572
    cessation of treatment, 2560-2561, 2561t
    conflicts of interest, 2562
    denial of treatment, 2559
    "difficult" patients, 2567-2568, 2568t
    older patients, 2568-2569
    patient selection, 2559-2561
    rationing, 2559-2561, 2572
    reimbursement, 2562
    shared decision-making, 2563t-2566t
    withdrawal of treatment, 2560-2567, 2561t, 2563t
    withholding of treatment, 2562-2567
  folate deficiency associated with, 1887
  goals of, 2069
  health disparities in, 2580-2581
  hemodialysis. See Hemodialysis
  history of, 2059
  hyperkalemia treated with, 598-599
  hypermagnesemia treated with, 626
  hypoalbuminemia in patients receiving, 1969-1970
  isothermic, 2095
  life expectancy after initiation of, in elderly, 2596, 2597f
  lupus nephritis treated with, 1100
  Medicare costs for, 2627f
  in Middle East, 2487-2489
  muscle wasting in, 1817
  in New Zealand, 2551-2552
  in older adults, 2596-2598
  payment for, 1902
  peritoneal. See Peritoneal dialysis
  physical functioning in patients receiving, 1818
  potassium removal with, 598-599
  pregnancy and, 1635-1636
  protein intake after, 1983
  reimbursement for, 2562
  renal function assessments in, 2044
  shared decision-making, 2563t-2566t, 2597
  skin manifestations of, 1944
  steal syndrome associated with, 1948
  stroke risks associated with, 1927-1928, 1930
  sustained low-efficiency, 2141t, 2142, 2145-2146, 2171, 2459
  taste acuity reductions secondary to, 1819
  uremia treated with, 2083
  uremic platelet dysfunction affected by, 1905
  vascular access for, 2191-2192
  vascular calcification in, 1850
  withdrawal of, 2560-2561, 2561t
Dialysis dementia, 1935-1936
Dialysis disequilibrium syndrome, 1935, 2106-2107, 2414
Dialysis Outcomes and Practice Patterns Study, 643
Dialysis Outcomes Quality Initiative, 2621-2622, 2631
Diarrhea
  acute kidney injury in Indian subcontinent patients caused by, 2496
  bicarbonate levels affected by, 528-529

Diarrhea (Continued)
  fluid therapy for, 2496
  magnesium deficiency caused by, 620
Diastolic blood pressure, 1524, 1524t, 1526f
Diastolic dysfunction, 1688t, 2408
Diazoxide, 1696-1697
Dibasic aminoaciduria, 226-227
Dicarboxylate-sulfate transporters. See NaDC transporters
Dicarboxylic aminoaciduria, 223t, 229, 1450
Dicer1, 39
Dichloroacetate, for lactic acidosis, 546
Diet
  low-protein. See Low-protein diet
  phosphorus-restricted, 2031
  sodium-restricted, 450
  uremic solutes affected by, 1814-1815
Dietary potassium, 559-560, 566, 584t, 1975
Dietary reference intake, 2405
Dietary sodium. See Sodium, dietary
Diffuse diabetic glomerulosclerosis, 1285-1286, 1287f
Diffusion, 2068-2069, 2068f, 2078, 2112
Diffusion-weighted imaging, 863-864, 871f
Digitalis-like factors, 419
Digoxin, 587, 2073
Dihydropyridine calcium channel blockers, 1662, 1664-1667, 1699, 1995-1996
1,25-Dihydroxycholecalciferol, 2024f, 2025, 2032
Dihydroxyeicosatrienoic acids, 382-383
1,25-Dihydroxyvitamin D
  absorptive hypercalciuria independent of, 1332-1333
  calcitriol as replacement for, 2089
  catabolism of, 2390
  chronic kidney disease levels of, 1913, 2014
  dependence, 1331-1332
  description of, 1864-1865
  fibroblast growth factor-23 suppression of, 2031-2032
  functions of, 2023-2024
  hemodialysis replacement of, 2089
1,25-Dihydroxyvitamin D3, 1632-1633
1α25-Dihydroxyvitamin D
  description of, 187f
  humoral hypercalcemia of malignancy and, 607
  osteoclastic bone resorption caused by, 603
  phosphate transport regulation by, 200
Diltiazem hydrochloride, 1663-1664, 1663t, 1668t, 1697t
Dilutional acidosis, 529-530
Dimethylamine, 1812-1813
Dimethylarginine dimethylaminohydrolase, 443, 685
Dipeptidyl peptidase-4 inhibitors, 2593
Dipsogenic diabetes insipidus, 482
Direct renin inhibitors, 1564, 1764-1765, 2003-2004
Direct-acting vasodilators
  combination therapies using, 1692
  dosing of, 1649t-1650t
  efficacy of, 1674
  hypertensive urgencies and emergencies treated with, 1695t, 1696-1699
  indications for, 1565
  mechanism of action, 1673
  renal effects of, 1674
  in renal insufficiency patients, 1649t-1650t
  safety of, 1674
  types of, 1673-1674, 1674t

Disasters, 2472, 2473f
Discoid lupus erythematosus, 1950, 1950f
Disease management organizations, 2631
Disequilibrium pH, 253
Dissecting renal artery aneurysms, 1204
Disseminated histoplasmosis, 1405
Dissolution therapy, 1365
Distal calcium, 1334f
Distal convoluted tubule (DCT)
  anatomy of, 65-68, 165, 261-262
  bicarbonate reabsorption in, 238-239
  cells of, 65-66, 67f, 167, 238-239
  11-β-hydroxysteroid dehydrogenase in, 66-67
  loop diuretics effect on, 1715
  luminal surface of, 68f
  magnesium reabsorption in, 194
  magnesium transport in, 195f
  microprojections on, 65-66
  mineralocorticoid receptor expression in, 315
  Na^+K^+-ATPase activity in, 66
  NCC expression by, 165-166
  pars convoluta of, 68f
  potassium secretion by, 176-178
  sodium absorption in, 566-568
  sodium pump activity in, 129
  thiazide and thiazide-like diuretics action on, 1710, 1711f
  water impermeability of, 67-68
  water transport pathways in, 274f
Distal potassium-sparing diuretics
  adverse effects of, 1713
  drug interactions, 1713
  hyperkalemia caused by, 1713, 1732
  indications for, 1713
  loop diuretics and, 1719
  magnesium excretion affected by, 1730
  mechanism of action, 1712
  pharmacokinetics of, 1712-1713
  sites of action, 1712
  thiazide diuretics and, 1719
Distal protection devices, 1193
Distal renal tubular acidosis, 1456f, 1457
  alkali therapy for, 535-536
  classical, 534, 534t-535t
  clinical spectrum of, 534-535, 535t
  in Far East, 2533
  features of, 534-535
  generalized, 534t
  H^+K^+-ATPase's involvement in, 534
  hyperkalemic, 540, 589
  hypokalemic, 534, 581
  pathophysiology of, 533-534
  pyelonephritis caused by, 534-535
  treatment of, 535-536, 536t
  type A intercalated defects, 534
Distal tubule
  adaptations of, to nephron loss, 1746
  ammonia secretion in, 252
  anatomy of, 63
  calcium in, 189, 190f, 192f
  embryology of, 5
  macula densa of, 54
  potassium secretion measurements, 569
  segments of, 63
  water absorption in, 271
Diuresis, postobstructive, 1281
Diuretic renography, 1266-1267
Diuretics, 1564, 1629-1630
  acute kidney injury treated with, 1725-1726
  adenosine type 1 receptor antagonists, 1714
  adverse drug interactions, 1732

Diuretics (Continued)
　adverse effects of
　　azotemia, 1727
　　drug allergy, 1732
　　extracellular volume depletion, 1727
　　hypercalcemia, 1730
　　hyperglycemia, 1730-1731
　　hyperkalemia, 1730
　　hyperlipidemia, 1731
　　hyperuricemia, 1731
　　hypokalemia, 1728-1730, 1729f
　　hypomagnesemia, 1730
　　hyponatremia, 492-493, 1727-1728, 1727f
　　impotence, 1731-1732
　　malignancies, 1732
　　metabolic alkalosis, 1730
　　ototoxicity, 1732
　　skin-related, 1732
　　vitamin B deficiency, 1732
　bicarbonate reabsorption affected by, 1703-1704
　β-blockers and, combination therapy using, 1691
　braking phenomenon, 1714-1716, 1715f-1716f, 1716t
　breast milk transmission of, 1732
　calcium channel blockers and, combination therapy using, 1691
　calcium excretion affected by, 1726
　calcium transport regulation by, 189-191
　carbonic anhydrase inhibitors. See Carbonic anhydrase inhibitors
　chloruresis induced by, 553
　clonidine added to, 445-446
　combination therapies, 1719
　distal potassium-sparing. See Distal potassium-sparing diuretics
　dopaminergic agents as, 1713
　edematous conditions treated with, 1719-1725
　heart failure treated with, 1719-1722
　hypercalcemia treated with, 1726
　hypervolemia treated with, 450-451
　hypokalemia caused by, 574
　hypovolemia caused by, 502
　idiopathic edema treated with, 1725
　liver cirrhosis treated with, 1722-1724
　loop. See Loop diuretics
　mechanism of action, 1703f
　metabolic alkalosis caused by, 553, 1704
　modulators of response to
　　arginine vasopressin, 1717
　　atrial natriuretic peptide, 1717
　　catecholamines, 1717
　　eicosanoids, 1716-1717
　　renin angiotensin aldosterone system, 1716
　nephrolithiasis treated with, 1726
　nephrotic syndrome treated with, 1723f, 1724-1725
　neprilysin inhibitors, 1714
　nesiritide, 1714
　osmotic. See Osmotic diuretics
　osteoporosis treated with, 1726-1727
　pharmacokinetics of, 1720
　potassium excretion affected by, 595
　potassium-sparing. See Potassium-sparing diuretics
　proximal tubule, for hypervolemia, 450
　renal tubular acidosis treated with, 1726
　renin-angiotensin-aldosterone inhibitors and, combination therapy using, 1691

Diuretics (Continued)
　resistance to, 451, 1717-1719, 1718f, 1724, 1797
　sites of action, 1703f
　thiazide. See Thiazide diuretics
　thiazide-like. See Thiazide-like diuretics
　urea channel inhibitors, 1714
　vasopressin receptor antagonists, 1713-1714
　volume depletion caused by, 422
Diverticular disease, 1492
Djenkol beans, 2525
DNA microarrays, 2249
Dominant inheritant disease, 1411-1412, 1411t
Donor-specific anti-HLA antibody, 2260, 2422
Dopamine
　acute tubular necrosis treated with, 1001
　natriuretic effects of, 152-154
　phosphate transport affected by, 201
　renal toxicity prevention using, 1398
Dopamine D_1-like receptor agonist, 1699
Doppler color-flow ultrasonography, 848-849, 850f
Doppler ultrasonography
　description of, 848-849, 850f
　renal artery stenosis evaluations, 903-904
　renal transplantation assessments using, 910
　renal vein thrombosis evaluations, 1204
　urinary tract obstruction evaluations, 1265
Double-antibody radioimmunoassay, for urinary albumin measurement, 794
Double-filtration plasmapheresis, 2160
Doxazosin, 1676, 1676t
Doxercalciferol, 2032
Doxycycline, for leptospirosis prophylaxis, 2444
DP receptors, 369
D-Penicillamine, 1158-1159, 1445
Drosophila, 20
Drug(s). See also specific drug
　absorption of, 2035-2036
　acute interstitial nephritis caused by, 1218-1220, 1218t
　clearance of, 2039, 2039t
　distribution of, 2036-2037
　in elderly patients, 2594-2596, 2595t
　high anion gap acidosis caused by, 543, 547-550
　hypercalcemia caused by, 609
　hyperkalemia caused by, 540, 540t, 590-592
　hypocalcemia caused by, 617-618
　hypophosphatemia caused by, 632
　intraperitoneal administration of, 2049
　lactic acidosis caused by, 545
　malabsorption of, 2036
　metabolism of, 2037-2039
　metabolites of, 2038t
　potassium loss caused by, 574-575
　renal excretion of, 2039, 2039t
　systemic lupus erythematosus caused by, 1099-1100
　tubulointerstitial diseases caused by, 1218-1219, 1218t
　urinary tract obstruction caused by, 1260
Drug disposition
　absorption, 2035-2036
　distribution, 2036-2037, 2036t
　intravenous administration effects on, 2035, 2035f
　metabolism, 2037-2039

Drug dosing
　in acute kidney injury, 2046, 2051t-2054t, 2145-2146
　in chronic kidney disease, 2044-2046, 2045t, 2051t-2054t
　Cockcroft-Gault equation for, 2042-2044
　in continuous renal replacement therapy, 2048-2049
　in hemodialysis, 2046-2048, 2048t
　intravenous administration, 2035, 2035f
　in peritoneal dialysis, 2049
　pharmacodynamics, 2040-2041
　pharmacogenomics, 2039-2040
　pharmacokinetic considerations, 2035-2039, 2036t
　recommendations for, 2051t-2054t
　renal function assessments, 2041-2044
　renal replacement therapy considerations for, 2145
Drug resistance transporters, 211
Dry weight, 2095-2096
DSTYK, 2300
Dual energy x-ray absorptiometry (DEXA), 1846, 2099
Duane-radial ray syndrome, 2297t
Ducts of Bellini, 43, 44f, 74, 264
Dutch Renal Artery Stenosis Intervention Cooperative (DRASTIC), 1596t, 1602-1603
Dynactin, 295
Dyneins, 295
Dyslipidemia, 1442
　chronic kidney disease and, 683-684, 1772-1774, 1863, 2011
　in elderly, 2593
　renal injury and, 1772-1773
　statins for, 1773-1774, 1931, 2011, 2593
　treatment of, 1773-1774, 2011
Dysnatremias, 2137
Dyspigmentation, 1943f
Dysplasia, renal. See Renal dysplasia
Dyspnea, 434
Dysrhythmias, 1859

E

EAAT3, 228-229
Eagle-Barrett syndrome. See Prune-belly syndrome
Early endosomal antigen 1, 1275
EAST syndrome, 167, 2379
Eating disorders, 581-583
E-Cadherin, 36
Echinococcus granulosus, 1255
Echocardiography, 1866
Eclampsia, 1616-1617
Ectonucleotide pyrophosphatase/phosphodiesterase 1, 631
Ectopic adrenocorticotropic hormone, 577
Ectopic kidneys, 850-851, 2295, 2295f, 2305, 2311
Eculizumab
　antiphospholipid-associated thrombotic microangiopathy treated with, 1201
　atypical hemolytic-uremic syndrome treated with, 1186, 2356
　C3 glomerulopathies treated with, 1159
　description of, 1045, 2269
　glomerular diseases treated with, 1171
Edema
　blood volume alterations and, 1798-1799
　cerebral, 813, 1619-1620, 1705
　formation of, 1798-1800, 1798f-1799f

Edema (Continued)
  in hypervolemia, 426
  hyponatremia with, 495
  interstitial pressure effects on, 761
  intrarenal mechanisms of, 1799-1800, 1799f
  metabolic alkalosis caused by, 553
  in nephrotic syndrome, 761, 1798-1800, 1798f-1799f
  nonsteroidal antiinflammatory drugs as cause of, 361-362
  "overfill" mechanism of, 1799f
  plasma oncotic pressure and, 1798
  preeclampsia and, 1616
  "underfill" hypothesis of, 1798f
Effective arterial blood volume, 393-394
  assessment of, 815-818
  cardiac output and, 393-394
  conditions that affect, 422
  decreased, 813-818
  definition of, 393
  expansion of, 402-403
  extracellular fluid volume and, 393, 813
  hydrogen buffering in, 836f
  low, 814, 816
  regulation of, 394-421
    adrenomedullin in, 418
    afferent limb in, 394-398
    apelin in, 419-420
    atrial natriuretic peptide in, 413-414
    atrial sensors in, 394-395
    brain natriuretic peptide in, 413-414
    cardiac filling sensors in, 394-396
    cardiac output sensors in, 396
    central nervous system sensors, 397
    C-type natriuretic peptide in, 414-415
    Dendroaspis natriuretic peptide, 415
    digitalis-like factors in, 419
    effector mechanisms for, 398
    efferent limb for, 398
    endothelin in, 415-416
    endothelium-derived factors in, 415-420
    gastrointestinal tract sensors, 397-398
    glomerular filtration rate in, 398-421
    glomerulotubular balance, 400-407
    glucagon-like peptide-1 in, 420
    guanylin peptides in, 397-398
    hepatoportal receptors in, 397
    humoral mechanisms involved in, 407-420
    kinins in, 417-418
    natriuretic peptides in, 413-415
    neural mechanisms involved in, 405-407
    neuropeptide Y in, 419
    nitric oxide in, 416-417
    novel factors in, 420-421
    organ perfusion sensors in, 396-398
    pressure natriuresis in, 403
    prostaglandins in, 411-413
    pulmonary sensors in, 395-396
    renal nerves in, 405-407
    renin-angiotensin-aldosterone system in, 407-409
    sympathetic nervous system in, 405-407, 407f
    tubular reabsorption in, 398-421
    tubuloglomerular feedback in, 399-400
    urotensin in, 418-419
    vasopressin in, 415
    ventricular sensors in, 395-396
  renal nerves and, 405-407
  sodium retention secondary to reductions in, 426-427
Effective osmolality, 461
Effective renal plasma flow (ERPF), 1575f

Egypt. *See* Middle East
EHHADH, 60-61
Eicosanoid(s)
  cellular origin of, 355
  diuretic therapy response affected by, 1716-1717
  in glomerular hyperfiltration, 1740
  hydroxyeicosatetraenoic acids. *See* Hydroxyeicosatetraenoic acids
  nephron loss adaptations and, 1740
  in pressure natriuresis, 404
Eicosanoid receptor, 366-367
Elastography, 849
Elderly
  acid-base balance in, 740-741, 740f
  acidosis in, 740
  acute kidney injury in, 742-744, 2513-2514, 2514t
  acute poststreptococcal glomerulonephritis in, 1057
  β-adrenergic antagonists in, 1685
  advance directives in, 2599
  advanced care planning in, 2599-2600
  albuminuria in, 2587
  aldosterone levels in, 738
  amyloidosis in, 746
  analgesics in, 2595
  anemia in, 2593-2594
  antihypertensive drug therapy in, 1682-1685, 1684t
  arteriovenous fistula in, 747-748
  atrial natriuretic peptide in, 738-739
  bacteriuria in, 1243
  benzodiazepines in, 2595
  blood pressure measurement in, 745, 745f, 2010f, 2592
  calcium balance in, 741-742
  calcium channel blockers in, 1685
  carbonic anhydrase inhibitors in, 1704
  cardiovascular disease in, 2590
  chronic bacterial prostatitis in, 750
  chronic kidney disease in, 747, 2568-2569, 2594-2596
  cognitive impairment in, 2590
  congestive heart failure in, 2590
  creatinine levels in, 737
  diabetes mellitus in, 2590, 2592-2593
  dialysis in
    for acute kidney injury, 744
    ethical dilemmas, 2568-2569
    functional declines after initiation of, 2590, 2591f
    vascular access for, 2598
  drug prescribing in, 2594-2596, 2595t
  dyslipidemia in, 2593
  end-stage kidney disease in, 2589, 2596-2598
  estimated glomerular filtration rate in
    comorbidities based on, 2591f
    end-stage kidney disease and, 2589
    measurement of, 2587
    mortality and, 2588, 2589f
    reduced, adverse outcomes associated with, 2588-2590, 2589f
  filtration fraction in, 738f
  frailty in, 2590
  functional impairment in, 2590
  glomerular disease in, 746-747
  glomerular filtration rate affected by, 736-737, 737f
  glomerulonephritis in, 746
  hematuria in, 1014-1015
  hemodialysis in, 747-748, 2598
  hypernatremia in, 742
  hypertension in, 744-746, 745f, 2590-2592
  hypodipsia in, 480

Elderly (Continued)
  hyponatremia in, 497, 501, 742
  immunosuppressive agents in, 749
  kidney of, structural changes in, 727-728
  medication use in, 2594-2596, 2595t
  minimal change disease in, 746
  multiple myeloma in, 746
  nephrologist referral for, 2595-2596
  nephrotic syndrome in, 746-747
  opioids in, 2595
  osmoregulation disorders in, 742
  paraproteinemia in, 746
  peritoneal dialysis in, 747
  phosphate balance in, 742
  potassium balance in, 741, 741f
  psychotropics in, 2595
  pyuria in, 1246
  renal clearance in, 744
  renal cysts in, 750
  renal diluting capacity in, 740
  renal fibrosis in
    advanced glycosylation end products, 730-732
    angiotensin II, 728-729
    autophagy, 734-735
    bile acid metabolism, 734
    calorie restriction, 732-733
    description of, 728
    farnesoid X receptor, 734
    Klotho, 734
    lipid metabolism, 733-734
    nitric oxide, 730
    oxidative stress, 732
    transforming growth factor-β, 729-730
  renal plasma flow in, 735-736, 736f
  renal replacement therapy in, 747-748
  renal transplantation in, 748-749, 748t, 2598-2599
  renin levels in, 737-738
  renovascular disease in, 746
  scrub typhus in, 2514t
  sedatives in, 2595
  sodium in, 737-739, 738f
  stroke in, 2590
  thiazide diuretics in, 1682-1685
  urinary concentration in, 739-740
  urinary dilution in, 740
  urinary tract infection in, 749-750
  water diuresis in, 743, 743f
Electrocortin, 304-305. *See also* Aldosterone
Electrolyte-free water balance, 807
Electrolytes, 393f, 1968, 2117-2118. *See also specific electrolyte*
Electron microscopy
  acute poststreptococcal glomerulonephritis findings, 1055-1056, 1056f
  Alport's syndrome findings, 1139-1140, 1140f
  anti-glomerular basement membrane disease findings, 1126
  anti-glomerular basement membrane glomerulonephritis findings, 1078, 1078f
  biopsy analysis using, 922, 923t
  chronic allograft glomerulopathy diagnosis using, 923
  diabetic nephropathy findings, 1284f
  Fabry's disease findings, 1144, 1144f
  fibrillary glomerulonephritis findings, 1070-1071, 1070f, 1133f
  focal segmental glomerulosclerosis findings, 1026-1027
  human immunodeficiency virus nephropathy findings, 1152f

Electron microscopy (Continued)
  immune complex-mediated crescentic glomerulonephritis findings, 1075
  immunotactoid glomerulopathy findings, 1070f, 1071, 1133f
  lupus nephritis findings, 1095f-1096f, 1097
  membranoproliferative glomerulonephritis findings, 1047-1048, 1048f
  membranous nephropathy findings, 1035-1037, 1036f-1037f, 1037t
  microscopic polyangiitis findings, 1115
  minimal change disease findings, 1019, 1019f-1020f
  nail-patella syndrome findings, 1143f
  pauci-immune crescentic glomerulonephritis findings, 1083
  thrombotic microangiopathy findings, 1178f
Electron transport chain, 127
Electroneutral chloride-bicarbonate exchanger, 243
Electroneutral sodium-bicarbonate cotransporter, 236-237
Electroneutral sodium-bicarbonate transporter 1, 238
Embolectomy, for renal artery thromboembolism, 1202
Embolic disease, 907f
Embryonic stem cells, 2603-2607
Emphysematous cystitis, 1251
Emphysematous pyelonephritis, 881, 882f, 1251
Enalapril maleate, 1642-1643, 1643t, 1697t
Enalaprilat, 1695t, 1698
Encapsulating peritoneal sclerosis, 2133, 2416-2417
Encephalopathy, 500-501, 2139
Endocytosis, 49
End-of-life care, 2567
Endogenous acids, 514-517, 542, 740
Endometrial hyperplasia, 1921
Endometriosis, 1261
Endosomes, 287-288
Endothelial cells
  activation of, 980f
  apoptosis of, 4-5, 1789
  in coagulation, 980-981
  cytoskeletal structure of, 979
  endothelin-1 secretion by, 335
  functions of, 979
  glomerular, 46-48, 46f
    apoptosis of, 1789
    description of, 1781-1782
    glycocalyx of, 47
    injury to, 1789
    intermediate filaments in, 47
    maturation of, 39-40
    vascular endothelial growth factor receptor expression by, 47-48
  inflammation mediated by, 981
  injury to, 980f, 981-982, 1175
  migration of, 4-5
  nucleus of, 47
  permeability of, 979-980
  plasticity of, 1217
  receptors of, 1753
Endothelial dysfunction, in chronic kidney disease, 1856, 1860-1861, 2407
Endothelial nitric oxide, 1578
Endothelial nitric oxide synthases, 442-443, 728, 730, 979
Endothelial progenitor cells, 982, 1752-1753

Endothelin, 335-339
  in chronic kidney disease, 337-338
  cirrhosis levels of, 446
  collecting duct acid-base transport affected by, 245
  definition of, 335
  in diabetic nephropathy, 337-338
  in effective arterial blood volume regulation, 415-416
  in essential hypertension, 336-337
  factors that stimulate production of, 103
  genes for, 103
  glucose effects on synthesis of, 337
  isoforms of, 335, 335f
  medullary blood flow affected by, 90
  nephron loss adaptations and, 1739
  physiologic actions of, 336
  portal hypertension and, 446
  production of, 416
  proximal tubule bicarbonate reabsorption affected by, 237
  receptors for, 103-104
  renal blood flow affected by, 336
  renal effects of, 336
  in renal injury, 337
  secretion of, 335-336
  structure of, 335-336, 335f
  synthesis of, 335-336
  transmural pressure effects on, 110
  vasodilatory prostaglandin production affected by, 104
Endothelin-1, 103-104, 417
  in chronic kidney disease, 337-338
  cirrhosis levels of, 446
  collecting duct synthesis of, 245
  description of, 415
  diuretic actions of, 416
  in endotoxemia, 338
  in essential hypertension, 336
  in hepatorenal syndrome, 338, 446
  natriuretic actions of, 416
  in preeclampsia, 338
  renal effects of, 336, 415
  secretion of, 335-336
  in systemic lupus erythematosus, 338
  systemic vascular resistance affected by, 453
  in vascular disease, 1197
Endothelin-2, 415
Endothelin antagonists, for heart failure, 452-453
Endothelin peptide, 1578-1579
Endothelin receptors, 335-339, 1198
Endothelin-A receptors
  antagonists of, 338-339, 415, 1313
  in chronic kidney disease, 337-338
  description of, 335, 415, 1739
  expression of, 336
  location of, 336
Endothelin-B receptors
  antagonists of, 338-339
  in chronic kidney disease, 337-338
  description of, 335, 415, 1739
  expression of, 336
  location of, 336
Endothelin-converting enzymes, 335
Endothelium, 1534-1535, 1752-1753
Endothelium-dependent vasodilation, 436
Endothelium-dependent vasorelaxation, 1619
Endothelium-derived nitric oxide, 404
Endothelium-derived relaxation factor (EDRF), 99-100, 102f
Endotoxemia, 338

Endovascular renal angioplasty and stenting, 1599-1602
End-stage kidney disease (ESKD)
  in Aboriginal Australians, 2547, 2577-2578
  acute kidney injury as risk factor for, 652, 744, 1009, 1777-1778
  in Africa, 2460f, 2461-2462, 2465-2466
  in African Americans, 663, 665-666, 1028-1029, 1770
  age as risk factor for, 673, 2060f
  alcohol consumption and, 686
  Alport's syndrome progression to, 1138
  in American Indians, 2583
  in amyloidosis, 1131-1132
  anemia in, 1875-1876, 1879f, 2626
  anti-glomerular basement membrane glomerulonephritis progression to, 1080-1081
  APOL1 gene and, 674-676
  arterial calcification in, 1856
  atrial fibrillation in, 1908
  atypical hemolytic-uremic syndrome as cause of, 2431
  in Australia, 2539-2540, 2541t
  birth weight and, 712, 713f
  bone disease in, 2281-2282
  C3 glomerulonephritis in, 1053-1054
  calcium measurements in, 2028-2029
  calcium-phosphate deposition in, 1775
  causes of, 1421, 2060, 2061f, 2061t, 2404, 2404t
  characteristics of, 1635
  in China, 2535
  chronic kidney disease progression to, 652, 674, 776, 962, 2007-2008, 2063-2064
  chronic kidney disease–mineral bone disorder treatment in, 2029
  congenital abnormalities of the kidney and urinary tract, 713, 2361, 2405
  cystinosis progression to, 2339
  delirium syndromes in
    definition of, 1934
    dialysis dysequilibrium, 1935
    differential diagnosis of, 1934t
    uremic encephalopathy, 1934-1935
  diabetes mellitus as cause of, 2060, 2280
  diabetic nephropathy as cause of, 681, 1295, 2592
  dialysis for. See also Dialysis
    chronic kidney disease–mineral bone disorder treatment in patients on, 2029
    in elderly, 2596-2598
    maintenance, 2113
    peritoneal, 2133-2134
  Disease Management Demonstration, 2631
  epidemiology of, 638-647, 639f-640f, 642f-643f, 2403
  erectile dysfunction in, 1921-1922
  estimated glomerular filtration rate and, 675f
  ethnicity and, 1769
  etiology of, 639, 2404, 2404t
  in Far East, 2534-2536
  fibrillary glomerulonephritis progression to, 1072, 1134
  focal segmental glomerulosclerosis progression to, 2155, 2404
  gastrointestinal symptoms in, 2036
  gender differences, 656-657, 659
  genetic factors, 674-675

End-stage kidney disease (ESKD) *(Continued)*
　global prevalence of, 643, 644f, 2060, 2574
　glomerulonephritis progression to, 1161
　glycemic control in, 1315
　granulomatous with polyangiitis progression to, 1114
　hazard ratios for, 675f
　health disparities in, 2577-2578
　hematocrit target for, 2628t
　hemodialysis for, 2097
　hemoglobin target for, 2098, 2628t
　Henoch-Schönlein purpura progression to, 1123-1124
　heroin nephropathy progression to, 1157-1158
　historical description of, 2403
　in Hong Kong, 2535
　human immunodeficiency virus nephropathy as cause of, 1153
　hyperkalemia in, 585, 2405
　hyperprolactinemia in, 1919
　hypertension in, 1765, 1770, 2406-2407
　hypogonadism in, 1921-1922
　immunoglobulin A nephropathy progression to, 1065
　immunotactoid glomerulopathy progression to, 1072
　incidence of, 638-641, 639f-640f, 656, 926-927, 1479, 2007-2008, 2059-2060, 2059f-2060f, 2575, 2577, 2597f
　in Indonesia, 2536
　insulin resistance in, 1816
　international comparisons of, 643, 644f
　interstitial fibrosis as cause of, 1216-1217
　in Japan, 2534-2535
　kidney stones and, 1352
　in Korea, 2535
　in Latin America, 2449-2451, 2449f, 2450t
　lead exposure and, 1226-1227
　lupus nephritis progression to, 1100
　magnetic resonance imaging of, 889f
　in Malaysia, 2535-2536
　in Maori population, 2552-2553
　Medicare costs and, 1524
　Medicare program, 2558-2559, 2562, 2572, 2625
　in microalbuminuria, 1303f
　in Middle East, 2473-2474, 2476
　mortality rates for, 641, 642f, 645, 773, 2061-2063, 2062f
　in Native Americans, 2583
　in New Zealand, 2550, 2552-2553
　obesity as risk factor for, 679, 1300
　obstructive uropathy progression to, 764
　25(OH)D levels and, 1872-1873
　palliative care for, 2563
　parathyroid hormone levels in, 2023-2026
　pauci-immune crescentic glomerulonephritis progression to, 1086
　pericardial disease secondary to, 2107-2108
　in Philippines, 2536
　phosphorus measurements in, 2028-2029
　potassium in, 174-175, 2093
　poverty and, 666
　preeclampsia as risk factor for, 681
　prevalence of, 641-642, 2059-2060, 2574
　quality improvement in, 2625-2626
　Quality Initiative for, 2626
　race and, 1769f, 2577, 2597f
　rapidly progressive glomerulonephritis progression to, 2150
　renal risk scores for, 690-691, 690f

End-stage kidney disease (ESKD) *(Continued)*
　renal transplantation for, 1181-1182
　scleroderma renal crisis progression to, 1198
　sickle cell disease progression to, 1200
　in Singapore, 2536
　skin manifestations of, 1942-1945, 1943f, 1945f
　smoking and, 1992
　in Social Security Amendments to Medicare bill, 2558-2559, 2562
　stroke in, risk factors for, 1928-1933
　in Taiwan, 2534
　testosterone supplementation in, 1922-1923
　in Thailand, 2535
　treatment of, 1424, 1493-1494
　　dialysis. See Dialysis
　　disparities in, 2580-2582
　　economic considerations in, 2025-2026
　　renal transplantation. See Renal transplantation
　　vitamin D sterols, 2026
　trends in, 639f
　ultrasonography of, 868, 868f
　vascular calcification in, 2128
　in Vietnam, 2536
　X-linked Alport's syndrome and, 1424
End-stage liver disease, 610
End-stage renal disease. See End-stage kidney disease
Energy-based tissue ablation, 1380
Enteric hyperoxaluria, 1325, 1340, 2340
Enterohemorrhagic *Escherichia coli*, 2154
Eosinophil(s), 799-800
Eosinophilia, 988
Eosinophilic granulomatosis with polyangiitis (EGPA), 1012-1013
　antineutrophil cytoplasmic antibodies in, 1117
　in children, 2351
　clinical features of, 1117
　corticosteroids for, 1117-1118
　course of, 1117-1118
　description of, 1116-1118
　laboratory features of, 1117
　pathogenesis of, 1117
　pathology of, 1116, 1116f
　prognosis for, 1117-1118
　symptoms of, 1117
　treatment of, 1117-1118
Eosinophiluria, 799-800, 986-987
EP receptors
　EP1 receptors, 370, 379
　EP2 receptors, 370-371, 373
　EP3 receptors, 371-372
　EP4 receptors, 372-373
　renal cortical hemodynamics affected by, 372
　renal function regulated by, 372-373
Epac, 294-295
Ephedrine, 1347
Ephrin-Eph family, 34
Ephrins, 34
Epidermal basement membranes, 1142t
Epidermal growth factor, 24-25, 1217
Epidermal growth factor receptor, 329f, 621
Epistaxis, 1328-1329
Epithelial angiomyolipoma, 1501
Epithelial basement membranes, 25
Epithelial calcium channel, 580
Epithelial cells
　injury to, 970-983
　parietal, 4-5, 52-53, 52f-53f, 1789-1790
　plasticity of, 1217

Epithelial sodium channel(s)
　aldosterone effects on, 172-173, 311-312, 409, 565-566, 1800, 2366-2367
　amiloride effects on, 565, 590, 1712
　composition of, 1462f
　description of, 166-167, 169
　inhibitors of, 590-591, 1692
　knockout mice model, 278
　lithium and, 297-298
　localization of, 278
　pentamidine effects on, 591
　potassium secretion affected by, 313
　proteolytic cleavage activation of, 312
　serum- and glucocorticoid-regulated kinase stimulation of, 318, 319f
　SGK-1 effects on, 172-173
　sodium absorption via, 175
　sodium reabsorption via, 169-170, 310-311, 314-317, 319-320
　tissue kallikrein effects on, 349
　triamterene effects on, 1712
　vasopressin activation of, 173-174
Epithelial-to-mesenchymal transition, 1217, 1793-1794
Epithelioid angiomyolipoma, 1368-1369
Eplerenone, 322, 540-541, 1678-1679, 1692
Epoetin, 1890, 2626-2627
Epoxides, 383-384
Epoxygenases, 383
Epratuzumab, 1104
Eprosartan, 1652, 1652t
Epstein-Barr virus, 1151, 1404, 2429-2430
Epstein's syndrome, 1140t
Equilibrative nucleoside transporter 1, 399
Equilibrium solubility product, 1325-1327
Erectile dysfunction, 1921-1922
Ergocalciferol, 1923, 2025, 2032, 2390
ERK1/2, 1217
Eruptive xanthomas, 1946-1947, 1946f
Erythrocytes. See also Red blood cell(s)
　dysmorphic, 798
　erythropoietin production by, 1878
　ferritin concentration, 1894
　uremic, 1884-1885
　in urine, 798-799, 799f
　zinc protoporphyrin concentration, 1894
Erythrocytosis, 1375
　definition of, 1888
　in hemodialysis, 1888
　polycystic kidney disease as cause of, 1888
　posttransplantation, 1888-1889
　in renal artery stenosis, 1889
　in renal tumors, 1889
Erythroferrone, 1885
Erythropoiesis
　burst-forming units–erythroid, 1882-1883
　description of, 1878-1884
　erythropoietin regulation of, 1875, 1878-1883
　folate in, 1883-1884
　hypoxia-inducible factors, 1880-1881, 1880f
　inefficient, in megaloblastic anemia, 1883
　inflammation effects on, 1887
　iron in, 1883-1884, 1893
　model of, 1882f
　parathyroid hormone effects on, 1887
　testosterone effects on, 1922
　uremic inhibitors of, 1885
　vitamin B_{12} in, 1883-1884
Erythropoiesis-stimulating agents (ESA)
　anemia treated with, 1889-1892, 2405-2406, 2626
　ascorbic acid added to, 1900
　darbepoetin alfa, 1890-1892

Erythropoiesis-stimulating agents (ESA) (Continued)
  epoetin, 1890
  during hemodialysis, 2098
  hemoglobin concentration affected by, 1892, 1902
  hypoxia-inducible factor stabilizers, 1892
  initiation of, 1892
  maintenance of, 1892
  methoxypolyethylene glycol epoetin beta, 1892
  prolactin levels affected by, 1919
  resistance to, 2098
  risk/benefit relationship for, 1902
  route of administration, 2098
  trials of, 1901-1902
Erythropoietin
  anemia in chronic kidney disease and, 1884, 2013, 2089, 2097-2098, 2610-2611
  apoptosis suppression by, 1882-1883, 1882f
  bone marrow clearance of, 1881
  carbohydrate chains of, 1881
  clearance of, 1881
  definition of, 1878
  description of, 1316, 1871
  endogenous production of, 1887-1888
  erythropoiesis regulation by, 1875, 1878-1883
  hyperparathyroidism and, 1887
  hypoxia-inducible factor stabilizers effect on, 1892
  identification of, 1881
  liver production of, 1881
  in posttransplantation erythrocytosis, 1889
  production of, 1884, 1887-1888, 2602-2603
  protein intake effects on, 1980
  purification of, 1881
  recombinant human, 1888-1890, 1895, 1906, 1922, 2097
  serum levels of, 1883
  stroke risk prevention using, 1932-1933
Erythropoietin receptors, 1881, 1887
Escherichia coli
  asymptomatic bacteriuria caused by, 1246
  enterohemorrhagic, 2154
  0157:H7, 1179, 2154
  prostatitis caused by, 1247
  urinary tract infection caused by, 749-750, 778, 1233, 1236-1237, 1240
  uropathogenic, 1236-1237, 1239
Esmolol hydrochloride, 1695t, 1698
ESRD Amendment to Public Law, 2559
Essential amino acids, 1971-1972
Essential fatty acid deficiency, 355, 375
Essential hypertension, 336-337
Estimated creatinine clearance, 2042, 2044
Estimated glomerular filtration rate. *See* Glomerular filtration rate, estimated
Estradiol, 191
Estrogens, 191, 1906
Et-B receptor, 256
Ethacrynic acid, 1732
Ethanol-induced high anion gap acidosis, 548
Ethical dilemmas
  bioethics, 2558-2562
  chronic pain, 2569
  conflicts of interest, 2562
  dialysis-related. *See* Dialysis, ethical dilemmas

Ethical dilemmas (Continued)
  end-of-life care, 2567
  fiscal crisis in nephrology, 2572
  hospice referral, 2569-2570
  palliative care, 2569-2570
  reimbursement, 2562, 2572
  renal transplantation access, 2570-2572
Ethnicity
  chronic kidney disease and, 660-662, 1769-1770
  definition of, 660
  end-stage kidney disease and, 1769
  hypertension and, 693-694, 1526-1527
  kidney stones and, 1348
Ethylene dibromide poisoning, 2501
Ethylene glycol
  acute kidney injury caused by, 2500-2501
  extracorporeal treatments for, 2173-2178, 2174t, 2176t
  fomepizole for, 548
  high anion gap acidosis caused by, 548
Eukaryotes, 36
Euvolemia, 2141, 2144
Euvolemic hyponatremia, 504-505, 507f
Everolimus, 1383f, 1384, 2247, 2258, 2426
Excitation, 856
Expanded polytetrafluoroethylene, 2064-2066
Experimental atherosclerosis, 1578f
Explant cultures, 8f, 9
Extended-spectrum β-lactamase, 1239
External magnetic field, 856
Extracapillary proliferation, 921t
Extracellular fluid (ECF)
  bicarbonate in, 514, 519, 830f
  calcium concentration in, 601
  in children, 2365-2366, 2368, 2414
  chlorine in, 144
  description of, 390-391
  homeostasis of, 1748
  mannitol distribution in, 1704
  osmotic pressure of, 461
  potassium in, 174-175
  sodium in, 144
  solute composition of, 461
  total body water in, 460
Extracellular fluid volume (ECFV)
  assessment of, 835
  depletion of, 492-493, 1727
  description of, 391-393
  effective arterial blood volume and, 393, 813
  expansion of, 621
  in heart failure, 431f
  hematocrit for estimating of, 814t
  nephron loss-specific adaptations in, 1747-1748
Extracellular matrix 1, 31-32
Extracellular matrix (ECM)
  biomaterials as substitute for, 2609-2610
  connective tissue growth factor in production of, 1300
  diabetic nephropathy accumulation of, 1286
  myofibroblast production of, 1763
Extracorporeal shock wave lithotripsy, for urinary calculi, 1279-1280
Extracorporeal ultrafiltration, 451, 2139
Extraglomerular mesangium, 53-54
Extraskeletal calcifications, 1850
Extrauterine pregnancy, preeclampsia and, 1618
Eya1, 21
EYA1, 22, 2298-2299, 2318

Ezetimibe, 1869, 1869f, 2593
Ezrin, 155

F

Fabry's disease, 1143-1145, 1144f, 1952, 2479
F-actin, 972
Factitious hyperkalemia, 585
Factitious hyponatremia, 490
Factor VIII, 1803
Familial clustering, 1348
Familial diffuse mesangial sclerosis, 1429-1430
Familial hyperaldosteronism, 575, 1464
Familial hypercholesterolemia, 2159
Familial hypertension with hyperkalemia, 179-180, 183, 589-590, 2381-2382
Familial hypocalcemia with hypercalciuria, 614-616
Familial hypocalciuric hypercalcemia, 608, 622, 2391, 2395
Familial hypokalemic alkalosis, 578-580
Familial hypomagnesemia
  description of, 193-194
  with hypercalciuria and nephrocalcinosis, 1466, 2345, 2387-2388
  with secondary hypocalcemia, 2388, 2388f
  with secondary hypocalcemia, 1466
Familial iminoglycinuria, 1450
Familial Mediterranean fever (FMF)
  AA amyloidosis associated with, 2485-2486
  clinical spectrum of, 2479, 2484-2485
  colchicine for, 2485-2486
  description of, 1132, 2479
  end-stage kidney disease and, 2486
  genetics of, 2479, 2481t-2482t
  genotype-phenotype correlations, 2481t-2482t
  interferon-α for, 2486
  MEFV mutation in, 2479, 2484-2485
  pyrin's role in, 2479-2483, 2483f-2484f, 2486
  renal diseases associated with, 2484-2485
  treatment of, 2485-2486
Familial neurohypophyseal diabetes insipidus, 1469
Familial renal glucosuria, 1454
Familial renal hamartomas associated with hyperparathyroidism-jaw tumor syndrome, 1503
Familial renal hypouricemia, 1453
Familial tumoral calcinosis, 627, 1453
Fanconi syndrome, 530-531
  acquired versus inherited, 1435, 1435t
  causes of, 1439
  characteristics of, 580-581, 1435
  clinical presentation of, 1436-1437
  description of, 209
  GLUT2 mutations in, 207
  hypophosphatemia caused by, 632
Fanconi-Bickel syndrome, 209
Far East
  acute kidney injury in
    dengue fever as cause of, 2520-2521, 2522t
    djenkol beans as cause of, 2525
    hantavirus as cause of, 2515-2516, 2517f
    infections as cause of, 2511-2523, 2511f, 2512t
    insect stings as cause of, 2525
    leptospirosis as cause of, 2511-2513, 2511f, 2512t

Far East (Continued)
  malaria as cause of, 2517-2520, 2519f-2520f
  melamine as cause of, 2526
  mushrooms as cause of, 2525-2526
  opisthorchiasis as cause of, 2522-2523
  raw carp bile as cause of, 2525
  scrub typhus as cause of, 2513-2515
  severe acute respiratory syndrome as cause of, 2521-2522, 2523f
  severe fever with thrombocytopenia syndrome virus as cause of, 2516-2517, 2518f
  snakebites as cause of, 2523-2525, 2524t
  star fruit as cause of, 2525
 ANCA-associated vasculitides in, 2532
 betel nut chewing in, 2534
 China. See China
 chronic kidney disease in
  description of, 2526
  diabetes mellitus as cause of, 2529
  diagnostic criteria for, 2526
  etiology of, 2527
  infectious causes of, 2527-2529
  leptospirosis as cause of, 2528f
  prevalence of, 2526, 2527t
 countries of, 2510
 demographics of, 2510
 diabetes mellitus in, 2529
 distal renal tubular acidosis in, 2533
 end-stage kidney disease in, 2534-2536
 glomerulonephritis in, 2527-2532, 2528t, 2530f
 granulomatous with polyangiitis in, 2532
 hepatitis B/hepatitis C virus-associated glomerulonephritis in, 2532-2533
 herbal medicines in, 2533-2534
 Hong Kong, 2535
 human immunodeficiency virus infection in, 2533
 immunoglobulin A nephropathy in, 2530-2531, 2530f-2531f
 Indonesia, 2536
 Japan. See Japan
 Korea, 2535
 lupus nephritis in, 2531-2532
 Malaysia, 2535-2536
 microscopic polyangiitis in, 2532
 Philippines, 2536
 renal replacement therapy in, 2534-2536
 scientific publications in, 2536
 Singapore, 2536
 systemic lupus erythematosus in, 2531-2532
 Taiwan, 2534
 Thailand, 2535
 Vietnam, 2536
Farnesoid X receptor, 728, 733-734
Fat catabolism, 128f
Fat malabsorption syndromes, 617
Fat-soluble vitamins, 1984
Fatty acid-binding protein 1, 942
Fatty acids, 1967
Febuxostat, 1363t, 1364-1365, 2282
Fecal elimination enhancement techniques, for poison removal, 2168-2169
Fecal nitrogen, 1962
Fechtner's syndrome, 1140t
Felodipine, 1665
Female sex hormones, 1921
Fenoldopam mesylate, 1001, 1695t, 1699, 1713
Ferric carboxymaltose, 1896, 1897t
Ferric citrate, 1896, 2023
Ferric gluconate, 1896, 1897t, 1898-1899
Ferritin, 50f, 1893-1894

Fertility, 1635
Ferumoxytol, 1896-1898, 1897t
"Fetal programming" hypothesis, 2575-2576
Fetuin-A, 1836-1838
Fetus
 congenital anomalies of the kidney and urinary tract in, 2302
 exposures in
  to drugs, 719
  to glucocorticoids, 717
  to hyperglycemia, 717-718
 hydronephrosis in, 2314-2315
 loss of, in systemic lupus erythematosus, 1100
 sodium transport maturation in, 2302
 urinary tract obstruction in, 1258-1259, 1279
FGF9, 29
FGF20, 29
FHHt, 589-590
Fibrillary glomerulonephritis
 characteristics of, 1069-1070, 1132
 clinical features of, 1072
 cyclosporine for, 1134
 electron microscopy findings, 1070-1071, 1070f, 1133f
 end-stage kidney disease progression of, 1072, 1134
 epidemiology of, 1072
 fibrils in, 1132
 hematuria in, 1072
 immunofluorescence microscopy findings, 1071, 1071f, 1134f
 immunotactoid glomerulopathy versus, 1069-1070
 light microscopy findings, 1071
 monoclonal gammopathy and, 1071
 nephrotic syndrome caused by, 1069-1072
 pathogenesis of, 1071
 pathology of, 1070-1071, 1070f, 1133f
 pulmonary hemorrhage associated with, 1072
 recurrence of, after renal transplantation, 1072
 renal biopsy for, 1132-1134
 treatment of, 1072, 1134
Fibrinogen, 1863, 1905-1906, 2163
Fibroblast growth factor-7, 202
Fibroblast growth factor-23
 assays for, 1841f
 calcium levels affected by, 2019-2020
 cardiovascular disease and, 2101
 in children, 2390-2391, 2400
 in chronic kidney disease, 950, 1749-1750, 1775, 1831, 1864, 1977-1979, 2019
 in chronic kidney disease–mineral bone disorder, 1830-1831, 1841, 1841f, 1848
 definition of, 1830
 description of, 191, 197-198, 198f, 201, 627, 631
 1,25-dihydroxyvitamin D, 2031-2032
 phosphate concentration affected by, 1749-1750, 1775, 1776f, 1872, 1978, 2281, 2390-2391
 postrenal transplantation levels of, 1851
 receptors for, 1749-1750
 vitamin D activation affected by, 1774, 1864-1865
Fibroblastic growth factor signaling pathways, 24-25
Fibroblast-specific protein 1, 1067, 1217
Fibrocytes, bone marrow-derived, 1793
Fibrofolliculoma, 1374
Fibromuscular disease, 1580-1582, 1599-1600

Fibromuscular dysplasia, 907, 907f, 1580-1581
Fibronectin glomerulopathy, 1134
Fibrosarcoma, 1386
Fibrosis
 definition of, 921t
 renal. See Renal fibrosis
 renin-angiotensin-aldosterone system in, 334
 tubulointerstitial, 729f, 1754-1755, 1763, 1793
Fibrous intimal thickening, 728f
Fick's law, 2112
Filariasis, 1150-1151
Filtration barrier, 5
Filtration fraction, 138-139, 415-416, 738f
Filtration slit, 49-51, 1782-1783, 1783f
Filtration slit membrane, 51. See also Slit diaphragm
Fish oil, 376, 1069, 1803
Fistula
 arteriovenous. See Arteriovenous fistulas
 dialysis-associated steal syndrome secondary to, 1948
Fixatives, for light microscopy, 919
FK506-binding proteins, 2247
FKHRL1, 730-731
Flexner, Abraham, 2621
Flow cytometric cross-match, 2260
Flt1, 39
Fluconazole, 1254, 1254t
5-Flucytosine, 1254, 1254t
Fludrocortisone, 539
Fludrocortisone suppression test, 1546
Fluid deprivation test, 485
Fluid overload, 1726, 2138, 2144
Fluid restriction, for hyponatremia, 504, 504t
Fluid therapy, 1361, 2138
Fluorine 18 2-fluoro-2-deoxy-D-glucose, 865, 900, 1377
Fluoroquinolones, 1235t-1236t
Focal adhesion kinase, 120
Focal necrotizing glomerulonephritis, 2151
Focal segmental glomerulonephritis (FSGN), 657
Focal segmental glomerulosclerosis (FSGS), 1429
 ACTN4 mutations in, 1028
 in Africa, 2463
 in African Americans, 1028, 1769-1770
 APOL1 gene and, 1429
 APOL1 in, 1028-1029
 in Australia, 2544
 cause of, 1430
 cellular variant of, 1026
 in children, 1030, 1032
 classification of, 1025t
 clinical features of, 1024-1025, 1030-1031
 collapsing, 1026, 1029-1031, 1159, 2328
 electron microscopy findings, 1026-1027
 end-stage kidney disease progression from, 2155, 2404
 epidemiology of, 1025
 gene mutations associated with, 1027t
 glomerular enlargement associated with, 1030
 glomerular scarring in, 1025-1026
 glomerular tip lesion variant of, 1026, 1030-1031
 glomerulomegaly associated with, 1146, 1146f
 HIV-associated, 1028, 1030
 immunofluorescence microscopy findings, 1026, 1026f
 infections that cause, 1030

Focal segmental glomerulosclerosis (FSGS) (Continued)
  laboratory findings in, 1031, 1050t
  light microscopy findings, 1024f, 1025-1026
  malignant conditions associated with, 1030
  mechanism of action, 116
  medications associated with, 1030
  natural history of, 1030-1031
  nephron loss as cause of, 1029
  nephrotic syndrome caused by, 1024-1035
  NPHS2 mutations in, 1027-1028
  pamidronate and, 1030
  parietal epithelial cell activation in, 1789-1790
  pathogenesis of, 1027-1030, 1027t
  pathology of, 1024f, 1025-1027, 1026f, 1027t
  perihilar, 1026, 1030
  permeability factor associated with, 1029-1030
  podocytes in, 115t, 116, 118-119, 1027, 1029
  prednisone for, 1167
  primary, 1025, 1025t
  prognostic indicators for, 1031
  proteinuria in, 1024-1025, 1030-1031, 1164, 1750-1752
  recurrent
    in children, 2156, 2422, 2431
    description of, 1034, 2270
    immunosuppressive drugs for, 2155-2156
    plasmapheresis for, 2155-2157
    risk factors for, 2155, 2270
  renal fibrosis secondary to, 1034
  after renal transplantation, 1034
  secondary, 1025, 1025t
  in sickle cell disease, 1199
  in steroid-resistant nephrotic syndrome, 2328
  treatment of
    angiotensin II receptor blockers, 1031
    angiotensin inhibitors, 1031-1032
    angiotensin-converting enzyme inhibitors, 1031
    CTLA-4-Ig, 1034
    cyclophosphamide, 1032
    cyclosporine, 1033
    glucocorticoids, 1032
    mycophenolate mofetil, 1033
    prednisone, 1032
    sirolimus, 1033-1034
  tubulointerstitial injury in, 1026, 1763
  variants of, 1026, 1029-1031
Folate, 1883-1884
Folic acid, 1887, 1983
Follicle-stimulating hormone, 1920-1921
Folliculin gene, 1374
Fomepizole, 548, 2177-2178
Food allergy, 1021
Foot processes, of podocytes. See Podocyte(s), foot processes of
Forced diuresis, 2167
Forearm loop graft, 2065-2066, 2066f
Formic acid, 2174
Forward genetics, 9
Foscarnet, 618
Fosinopril sodium, 1644
4F2hc/LAT2, 225-226, 231
4F2hc/y⁺LAT1, 228
Foxc1, 27

Foxd1, 31
FOXO3, 733
FP receptors, 369-370
Fractional excretion
  of calcium, 1749-1750
  of chloride, 814-815
  of creatinine, 1199
  of magnesium, 619-621
  of organic anions, 216
  of potassium, 2375-2376
  of sodium, 814-815, 987, 1659, 1708-1710, 1747
Fracture
  bone mineral density reductions associated with, 1852
  in chronic kidney disease–mineral bone disorder, 1849
  hip, 1849
  after renal transplantation, 1851
  risks of, 1846
Frailty, 2590
Fras1, 22-23
Fraser's syndrome, 22-23, 26f, 1431, 2297t, 2325
Free calcium, 602
Free fatty acids, 1761
Free ionized calcium, 1325-1327
Free light chains, 1391-1393
Fresh-frozen plasma (FFP), 1185, 2155, 2162
Frizzled receptor, 28-29
Fructose intolerance, 531
Fuhrman grading system, 1378
Fumarate hydratase gene, 1373-1374
Fumarylacetoacetate hydrolase, 1443
Fungal peritonitis, 2129
Fungal urinary tract infection, 1254
Fungemia, 1805
Furin, 340
Furosemide
  albumin and, 1708
  arginine vasopressin levels affected by, 1717
  atrial natriuretic peptide affected by, 1717
  bioavailability of, 1720
  in cirrhosis patients, 1723
  description of, 871, 1706
  hyponatremia treated with, 506
  left ventricular hypertrophy treated with, 1721-1722
  metabolism of, 1709f
  natriuretic response to, 1715-1717, 1723-1724
  pharmacokinetics of, 1709f
  plasma protein binding of, 1724-1725
  potassium loss caused by, 1716
  proximal secretion of, 1708
  renin-angiotensin-aldosterone system activation by, 1714
  sodium excretion and, 1710f
  thick ascending limb receptor for, 1725
FXYD2, 2388-2389

G

G protein-coupled receptor kinases, 283
G protein-coupled receptors
  4, 256
  illustration of, 367f
  vasopressin 2 receptor as. See Vasopressin 2 receptor
G protein-mediated signaling, 329
GadC, 230t

Gadolinium-chelate contrast media, for magnetic resonance imaging. See Magnetic resonance imaging, gadolinium-chelate contrast media
Galactose-deficient IgA1, 1064
Galactosemia, 1444
α-Galactosidase A, 1145, 2479
Gallium nitrate, 612
Galloway-Mowat syndrome, 1431
GALNT3, 627
Gamble phenomenon, 277-278
Ganglionic blocking agent, 1698
Gap junctions, 53-54, 56
Gap programs, 2583
Gastric aspiration, 553
Gastrointestinal fistula, 620
Gastrointestinal therapeutic system, 1665
Gastroparesis, 2125
Gender differences
  antihypertensive drug therapy, 1685, 1686t
  autosomal dominant polycystic kidney disease progression and, 658
  chronic kidney disease, 655-660, 673-674, 1768-1769
  developmental programming and, 720
  diabetic nephropathy progression and, 658-659
  end-stage kidney disease, 656-657, 659, 2060f
  focal segmental glomerulonephritis and, 657
  glomerular disease and, 657
  glomerular filtration rate and, 655, 736
  glomerulonephritis and, 657
  hormone replacement therapy and, 659-660
  hypertension and, 1525
  immunoglobulin A nephropathy and, 657
  lupus nephritis and, 658
  membranous nephropathy and, 657
  oral contraceptives and, 659-660
  primary glomerular disease progression and, 657
Gene panel, 1413
Generalized lipodystrophy, 1146-1147
Genetic hypercalciuric stone-forming rat, 1333
Genetic mapping, 1410, 1412
Genetic testing, for autosomal dominant polycystic kidney disease, 1486f
Genetics
  of Alport's syndrome, 1140-1141, 1421-1422, 1782
  of autosomal dominant polycystic kidney disease, 1479-1480, 1486f
  of hypertension, 1529-1530
  of kidney stones, 1348-1350
  of nephrocalcinosis, 1349f
  of urolithiasis, 1349f
  of Wilms' tumor, 1387
Genitourinary tract. See Urinary tract
Genitourinary tuberculosis, 1252-1254, 1260
Genodermatoses, 1951-1953, 1952f, 1952t
Genomewide association study, 1348-1349
Genomics, 2249
Genotyping, 2039-2040
Gentamicin
  acute pyelonephritis treated with, 1241, 1241t
  nephrogenesis affected by, 719
  nephrotoxicity of, 966, 967f
Geophagia, 586
Gerota's fascia, 852-853

Gestational diabetes insipidus, 471, 480, 489
Gestational hypertension, 1627-1631
Ghrelin, 420, 2125
Giant cell arteritis, 1120
Gibbs-Donnan effect, 391-392
Gitelman's syndrome, 67-68, 1417-1418, 1457-1459, 1459f, 2379
  characteristics of, 580, 2333
  in children, 2335, 2378-2379
  chondrocalcinosis in, 2379
  clinical presentation of, 1459
  hypocalciuria in, 580
  management of, 2379
  metabolic alkalosis caused by, 551-552, 554-555
  in Middle East, 2479
  pathogenesis of, 1459
  plasma renin levels in, 580
  potassium-sparing diuretics for, 1727
  prevalence of, 2333
  prognosis for, 2335
  renal magnesium wasting in, 622
  treatment of, 1459
GLEPP1 disease, 1431
Glial-derived neurotrophic factor (GDNF), 22-23, 701-702, 719
Globotriaosylceramide, 1143-1144
Globulin, calcium binding to, 602
Glomerular basement membrane (GBM)
  anatomy of, 48-49
  anionic sites in, 48-49
  anti-GBM disease. See Anti-glomerular basement membrane disease
  composition of, 48
  electron microscopy analysis of, 922
  embryology of, 4-5, 118
  glomerular filtration barrier and, 48-49, 50f
  histology of, 48f
  hydraulic connectivity of, 98
  inherited disorders affecting, 1421-1426
  layers of, 48, 48f
  maturation of, 39-40
  morphologic nature of, 1424f
  organization of, 1782
  permeability of, 48-49
  podocytes effect on, 118
  proteinuria and, 2323
  in rat models, 48, 48f
  surface area of, 2301-2302
  thickness of, 922, 1285, 1293f
Glomerular capillaries
  description of, 46, 84
  function of, 1780
  histology of, 93f
  hydraulic pressures in, 94-96, 95f
  loss of, 1790
  mesangial cells and, 1753
  pressures of, 94, 95f
  scanning electron microscopy of, 1751f
  ultrafiltration coefficient of, 98
  wall of, 46, 1781
Glomerular capillary membrane
  endothelial cell layer of, 1781-1782
  epithelial filtration slits, 1782-1783, 1783f
  filtering surface of, 1781
  organization of, 1781
  ultrastructure of, 1781-1783
Glomerular diseases, 1404
  acute, 1002
  bacterial infections associated with, 1149-1150
  categorization of, 1012-1013
  cause of, 1421
  crescent formation in, 1077t

Glomerular diseases *(Continued)*
  drugs associated with, 1157-1158
  in elderly, 746-747
  filariasis and, 1150-1151
  gender differences in, 657
  global, 920
  heroin nephropathy and, 1157-1158
  interstitial damage in, 1211f
  leishmaniasis and, 1150-1151
  miscellaneous diseases associated with, 1159
  neoplasia associated with, 1157
  nephritic features of, 1013t
  nephrotic features of, 1013t
  parasitic diseases associated with, 1150-1151
  pathogenesis of, 1012
  podocytes involved in, 113, 115t
  primary
    algorithm for, 1070f
    C3 glomerulopathies. See C3 glomerulopathies
    categorization of, 1070f
    crescent formation in, 1077t
    definition of, 1012-1013
    in elderly, 746
    in Far East, 2529-2531, 2530f
    focal segmental glomerulosclerosis. See Focal segmental glomerulosclerosis
    hematuria in, 1014-1016, 1015t
    immune complex-mediated crescentic glomerulonephritis. See Immune complex-mediated crescentic glomerulonephritis
    membranoproliferative glomerulonephritis. See Membranoproliferative glomerulonephritis
    membranous nephropathy. See Membranous nephropathy
    minimal change disease. See Minimal change disease
    nephrotic syndrome caused by. See Nephrotic syndrome, glomerular diseases that cause
    proteinuria in, 1013-1014
    serologic findings in, 1050t
  schistosomiasis and, 1150
  secondary
    antiphospholipid syndrome, 1106-1108, 1107f
    definition of, 1012-1013
    in elderly, 746
    Fabry's disease, 1143-1145, 1144f
    fibrillary glomerulonephritis. See Fibrillary glomerulonephritis
    granulomatous with polyangiitis. See Granulomatous with polyangiitis
    heavy-chain deposition disease, 1134-1136, 1135f
    Henoch-Schönlein purpura, 1121-1124
    immunotactoid glomerulopathy. See Immunotactoid glomerulopathy
    lecithin-cholesterol acyltransferase deficiency, 1147-1148, 1147f
    light-chain deposition disease, 1134-1136, 1135f
    lipodystrophy, 1146-1147
    lipoprotein glomerulopathy, 1148
    lupus nephritis. See Lupus nephritis
    mixed connective tissue disease, 1108-1109
    mixed cryoglobulinemia, 1137-1138
    monoclonal immunoglobulin deposition disease, 1134-1136, 1135f

Glomerular diseases *(Continued)*
    nail-patella syndrome, 1142-1143, 1143f
    polyarteritis nodosa, 1118-1120
    sarcoidosis, 1127-1128
    sickle cell nephropathy, 1145-1146, 1145f
    Sjögren's disease, 1127
    systemic lupus erythematosus. See Systemic lupus erythematosus
    Takayasu arteritis, 1120-1121
    temporal arteritis, 1120
    Waldenström's macroglobulinemia, 1136, 1136f-1137f
  segmental, 920
  terminology used to describe, 920, 921t
  treatment of
    adrenocorticotropic hormone, 1171-1172
    algorithms for, 1172-1173
    alkylating agents, 1168-1170
    azathioprine, 1170
    calcineurin inhibitors, 1167-1168
    considerations for, 1172-1173
    corticosteroids, 1166-1167
    cyclophosphamide, 1168-1170
    cyclosporine, 1167-1168
    eculizumab, 1171
    mycophenolate mofetil, 1170
    ocrelizumab, 1171
    rituximab, 1171
    tacrolimus, 1167-1168
  trypanosomiasis and, 1150-1151
  tubulointerstitial injury caused by, 1210
  ultrafiltration capacity affected by, 1797
  visceral infections associated with, 1149
Glomerular endothelial cells, 46-48, 46f
  apoptosis of, 1789
  description of, 1781-1782
  glycocalyx of, 47
  injury to, 1789
  intermediate filaments in, 47
  maturation of, 39-40
  vascular endothelial growth factor receptor expression by, 47-48
Glomerular endotheliosis, preeclampsia and, 1619, 1621f
Glomerular filtration
  determinants of, 94-98
    alterations in, 97-98
    colloid osmotic pressure, 98
    glomerular plasma flow rate, 97
    transcapillary hydraulic pressure difference, 97-98
  obstructive nephropathy effects on, 1269-1271
  regulation of, 98-110
  urinary tract obstruction effects on, 1269-1271
Glomerular filtration barriers, 1436f
  anatomy of, 791
  functional properties of, 1780
  glomerular basement membrane and, 48-49, 50f
  illustration of, 50f
  schematic of three layers of, 1427f
  vascular endothelial growth factor-A for, 32-34, 33f
Glomerular filtration coefficient, 96-97
Glomerular filtration rate (GFR), 1575f, 1576f, 1598f
  in acute kidney injury, 788, 932, 1390, 2043, 2145
  age-related changes in, 736-739, 737f
  angiotensin II effects on, 408
  angiotensin-converting enzyme inhibitors effect on, 1299, 1645

Glomerular filtration rate (GFR) *(Continued)*
 autoregulation of, 105
 autosomal dominant polycystic kidney disease and, 1490*f*
 biomarkers for, 781-787
  blood urea nitrogen, 933-934
  creatinine, 782-783, 933
  creatinin clearance, 783
  cystatin C, 783-784, 934-935, 2310
  EDTA, 786-787
  endogenous, 782-786
  exogenous, 786-787, 932
  inulin, 786
  radiolabeled markers, 786-787
  serum, 932-936
  β-trace protein, 935-936
  unlabeled radiocontrast agents, 787
  urea, 782, 933-934
 birth weight effects on, 709-710
 calculation of, 781
 in children, 787, 787*t*, 2309-2310
 in chronic kidney disease, 681, 773, 932, 1749, 2029-2031
 creatinine as marker of, 678, 2309-2310
 decline in
  hypothyroidism associated with, 496
  polycystic kidney disease as cause of, 681
  renal risk scores to predict, 690-691
 definition of, 781, 1797
 description of, 780-781
 drug dosing considerations, 788
 in effective arterial blood volume regulation, 398-421
 endogenous markers of, 737
 estimated
  in acute kidney injury, 788, 947-948, 963
  in adolescents, 787, 787*t*
  in Africa, 2459
  age-related changes in, 2586-2587
  biomarkers for. *See* Glomerular filtration rate, biomarkers for
  cardiovascular disease and, 1855, 1866, 2008
  in children, 787, 787*t*, 2043
  in chronic kidney disease, 1989-1990
  Chronic Kidney Disease Epidemiology Collaboration equation for, 784*t*, 785-786
  Cockcroft-Gault equation for, 784*t*, 786, 2587*f*
  contrast media risks and, 854-856
  creatinine as biomarker for, 932-933, 2309-2310
  cystatin C as biomarker of, 783-784, 934-935, 2310
  description of, 677-678
  in drug dosing, 788
  equations for, 784-786, 784*t*, 2042*t*, 2310, 2502
  hemoglobin affected by, 2405-2406
  MDRD equation for, 645, 677-678, 782, 784*t*, 785-786, 788, 2526
  measurement of, 2587
  in pediatrics, 2043
  in pregnancy, 788
  reduced, adverse outcomes associated with, 2588-2590
 expression of, 781
 filtration-reabsorption system, 204
 gender differences in, 655, 736
 homocysteine levels and, 1864
 hyperphosphatemia caused by reductions in, 627

Glomerular filtration rate (GFR) *(Continued)*
 leukotriene A₄ effects on, 380
 liver transplantation effects on, 458
 in low birth weight, 710
 measurement of, 677-678, 781, 2041-2042, 2042*t*
 neural regulation of, 110
 normal, 781
 oxygen consumption rate and, 134-135
 parathyroid hormone levels affected by, 1865
 physiology of, 781
 polycystic kidney disease effects on, 681
 during pregnancy, 1611-1612, 1612*f*
 prematurity effects on, 709-710
 reduction of, 1582-1583
 regulation of
  factors involved in, 1296
  glomerular transcapillary hydraulic pressure difference in, 1296
  glomerular ultrafiltration coefficient in, 1296
  oncotic pressure in, 1296
  renal plasma flow in, 1296
  in urinary tract obstruction setting, 1270-1271
 renal blood flow and, 134, 138, 401-402
 renal function assessments using, 2041-2042
 renal plasma flow effects on, 1296
 renin-angiotensin system's role in control of, 99
 single-nephron, 1269, 1271, 1737-1738, 1743, 1746-1747, 1785
 size of, 1819-1820
 sodium chloride reabsorption affected by, 150
 technetium 99m-labeled diethylenetriaminepentaacetic assessments of, 865
 total, for single nephron, 94, 96
 tubuloglomerular feedback control of, 108-109, 209-210
 in type 1 diabetes mellitus, 1296
 in uremia, 1819-1820
Glomerular hematuria, 756-757, 757*t*, 798, 1015
Glomerular hyperfiltration, 1737-1738
Glomerular hypertension, 1737-1738
Glomerular injury
 biomarkers for
  blood urea nitrogen, 933-934
  cystatin C, 934-935
  description of, 932-936
  podocalyxin, 936
  podocyte count, 936
  β-trace protein, 935-936
 cyclooxygenase metabolites in, 375-377
 progressive, 1787*f*
Glomerular permselectivity, 1783-1784
Glomerular plasma flow rate, 97
Glomerular proteinuria, 791
Glomerular sclerosis, 1578
Glomerular ultrafiltrate, 1784
Glomerular volume, 696, 709, 709*f*
Glomerulogenesis, 699
Glomerulomegaly, 705, 1146, 1146*f*
Glomerulonephritis, 1403-1404
 acute poststreptococcal. *See* Acute poststreptococcal glomerulonephritis
 anti-glomerular basement membrane, 746
 C3, 1046, 1046*f*-1047*f*
 calcineurin inhibitors for, 1167-1168
 cardiovascular mortality in, 1165

Glomerulonephritis *(Continued)*
 chronic kidney disease caused by, 775
 cirrhosis as cause of, 1156
 clinical trials in, 1163
 corticosteroids for, 1166-1167
 crescentic. *See* Crescentic glomerulonephritis
 cryoglobulinemic, 1137-1138, 1137*f*-1138*f*
 diagnostic classification of, 1074*f*
 diseases that cause, 1059*t*
 in elderly, 746
 end-stage kidney disease caused by, 1161
 fibrillary. *See* Fibrillary glomerulonephritis
 gender differences in, 657
 global impact of, 1161-1163, 1162*t*
 in granulomatous with polyangiitis, 1112
 IgA, 2275, 2544
 immunopathologic categories of, 1073*t*-1074*t*
 immunotactoid. *See* Immunotactoid glomerulopathy
 incidence of, 1161-1162
 in Indian subcontinent, 2506, 2506*t*
 infection-related, 2527, 2528*t*
 kidney biopsy for, 2544
 malignancy and, 1403*t*
 mesangiocapillary, 1047-1048
 in New Zealand, 2550
 outcome measures in, 1163
 pauci-immune necrotizing, 1084-1085
 poststreptococcal, 757
 proliferative glomerulonephritis with monoclonal IgG deposits, 1136
 rapidly progressive. *See* Rapidly progressive glomerulonephritis
 societal burden of, 1161
 in Takayasu arteritis, 1120-1121
Glomerulopathy
 anti-rheumatoid arthritis therapy-induced, 1158-1159
 collapsing, 1153
 fibronectin, 1134
 hepatic, 1156*f*
 HIV-associated, 1151
 lipoprotein, 1148
 nondiabetic, 1300
 obesity as cause of, 679-680, 1770-1771
 sickle, 1146, 1146*f*
 sickle cell, 1200
Glomerulosclerosis
 age-related decreases in, 728-729
 in Balkan endemic nephropathy, 1225
 characteristics of, 1786-1787
 focal segmental. *See* Focal segmental glomerulosclerosis
 glomerular hypertrophy and, 1759
 illustration of, 728*f*
 nodular, 1285-1286, 1287*f*
Glomerulotubular balance
 description of, 150, 1736-1737
 in effective arterial blood volume regulation, 400-407
 illustration of, 152*f*
 luminal composition in, 402
 maintenance of, 1747
 nephron loss adaptations, 1746
 peritubular capillary Starling forces in, 400-402
 peritubular factors in, 151-152
 in proximal tubule sodium chloride transport, 150-152, 151*f*
Glomerulotubular junction abnormalities, 1286*f*

Glomerulus
  aldosterone secretion by, 305
  anatomy of, 46f-47f, 107f
  calcium filtration by, 187
  capillary loops of, 46f, 92-93, 92f, 1019f
  capillary wall of, 1020f
  cells of, 4-5, 46-53, 46f, 52f. See also
    Podocyte(s)
  classification of, 84
  cross-section of, 107f
  development of, 4-5, 33f, 36-39, 37f
  function of, 46
  histology of, 47f
  hypertrophy of, after nephron loss,
    1742-1743, 1759
  inherited systemic syndromes affecting,
    1431-1432
  juxtamedullary, 45-46
  low-glycotoxin diet effects on, 732f
  magnesium filtration by, 194
  mesangium of, 98-99
  microcirculation of, 92-94, 92f
  mineralocorticoid receptor expression in,
    315
  murine model of, 36f
  nephrectomy-related changes in, 1751f
  nephron loss responses by, 1737-1741
  nephron number and, 696
  permselective dysfunction, 1786
  proteinuria-induced damage to, 1786-
    1790, 1787f
  variations in, 45-46
  vascular pathways in, 93, 93f
  volume of, 45-46
GlpT, 213-214, 230t
GltPh, 230t
Glucagon, 1767
Glucagon-like peptide-1, 420
Glucocorticoid(s)
  adverse effects of, 1166
  angiotensin II inhibitors and, for IgA
    nephropathy, 1068
  bicarbonate reabsorption affected by, 238
  COX-2 expression regulated by, 357
  deficiency of, 495
  description of, 1400
  fetal exposure to, 717
  focal segmental glomerulosclerosis treated
    with, 1032
  glomerulonephritis treated with, 1166
  hypercalcemia treated with, 612
  idiopathic nephrotic syndrome treated
    with, 2329
  immunoglobulin A nephropathy treated
    with, 1067-1068
  membranoproliferative
    glomerulonephritis type I treated
    with, 1049-1050
  musculoskeletal effects of, 1166-1167
  podocytes affected by, 119
Glucocorticoid-remediable
  hyperaldosteronism, 555-556, 575,
  1463-1464
Gluconeogenesis, 130-132
Glucose
  absorption of, 206f, 1730
  endothelin synthesis affected by, 337
  insulin and, 594
  lactate conversion to, 132
  metabolism of, angiotensin-converting
    enzyme inhibitors effect on, 1648
  in peritoneal dialysis solutions, 2117-2119
  plasma concentration of, 204-205
  reabsorption of, in proximal tubule,
    129-130, 205
  renal handling of, 205

Glucose (Continued)
  sources of, 812
  transport of. See Glucose transport
  urinary excretion of, 205f
  in urine, 790
Glucose degradation products, 2117-2119,
  2126-2127
Glucose transport, 204-215
  characteristics of, 206f
  inherited disorders of, 1453-1454
  maximal rate of, 205
  monogenic defects of, 207-210
  physiology of, 204-205
  proteins involved in
    cell model of, 205-207
    GLUT1, 207
    GLUT2, 207
    SGLT1, 205-206
    SGLT2, 206-207
  proximal tubule, 205-207
Glucose transporter diseases, 209
Glucose-galactose malabsorption, 206-207,
  1454
Glucose-6-phosphate dehydrogenase
  deficiency, 2494, 2501
Glucosuria, 206-207, 1437, 1454, 1454t, 1612
GLUT1, 207, 208t
GLUT2, 207, 208t
GLUT4, 207, 208t
GLUT9, 221, 221t
Glutamate, 253, 623
Glutamate dehydrogenase, 248, 253
Glutamine, 129-130, 249-251, 517
τ-Glutamyl transpeptidase, 253
Glutathione, 549
Glutathione S-transferase, 938-939, 1898,
  1909
Glyburide, 2593
Glycemic control
  cardiovascular disease risk prevention
    through, 1871
  in chronic kidney disease, 1871, 1995
  in diabetic nephropathy, 1301-1303
  in end-stage kidney disease, 1315
  during hemodialysis, 1317
Glycinuria, 223t
Glycogen, 1442f
Glycogen storage disease type 1, 1442
Glycogenosis (von Gierke's disease),
  1442-1443
Glycolysis, 132
β_2-glycoprotein I-specific antiphospholipid
  antibody IgG, 1201
Glycosaminoglycan, 1331
Glycosuria, 205, 207-209, 790
Glycosylated hemoglobin, 1931
Glycyrrhetinic acid, 556, 596
Glycyrrhizinic acid, 577
Glyoxylate reductase/hydroxypyruvate
  reductase (GRHPR), 1337-1338,
  2347-2348
Glypican-3, 2299
Gold salts, 1158
Goldblatt hypertension, 1568-1569
Goldmann voltage equation, 124-125
Golgi apparatus, 56
Gonadal dysfunction
  in chronic kidney disease, 1920-1923
  in men, 1921-1923
  in women, 1920-1921
Gonadal dysgenesis, 2-3
Gonadotropin-releasing hormone, 2318
Goodpasture's syndrome. See also Anti-
  glomerular basement membrane
  disease
  clinical features of, 1125

Goodpasture's syndrome (Continued)
  components of, 1124
  course of, 1126-1127
  description of, 759-760, 1076, 1080-1081
  laboratory findings in, 1125
  pathogenesis of, 1124-1125
  prognosis for, 1126-1127
  treatment of, 1126-1127
Gordon's syndrome, 179-180, 539-540,
  589-590, 827, 2381-2382. See also
  Pseudohypoaldosteronism
Gout, 1442, 1731, 2282
Graft-versus-host disease (GVHD)
  chronic kidney disease related to, 1395
  description of, 2249-2250
  glomerulonephritis associated with,
    1404
  nephrotic syndrome after, 1021
  transplantation-associated thrombotic
    microangiography and, 1395
Granular casts, 800, 800t, 801f
Granular cells, juxtaglomerular, 53, 54f, 55
Granulomatous disease, 610
Granulomatous interstitial nephritis, 1228
Granulomatous with polyangiitis (GPA)
  antineutrophil cytoplasmic antibodies in,
    1111-1112
  in children, 2351
  clinical features of, 1111-1112
  course of, 1112-1114
  cyclophosphamide for, 1112-1114
  definition of, 1109
  end-stage kidney disease progression of,
    1114
  eosinophilic, 1116-1118, 2351
  in Far East, 2532
  glomerulonephritis in, 1112
  immunosuppressive agents for, 1112
  incidence of, 1109
  laboratory features of, 1111-1112
  lower respiratory tract disease associated
    with, 1111
  methotrexate for, 1113
  mycophenolate mofetil for, 1113-1114
  organ involvement in, 1111
  papillary necrosis in, 1110
  pathogenesis of, 1110-1111
  pathology of, 1109-1110, 1109f-1110f
  plasmapheresis for, 1113
  recurrence of, after renal transplantation,
    2275
  relapse of, 1113
  renal findings in, 1112
  rituximab for, 1113
  survival rates in, 1112
  tissue injury in, 1110-1111
  treatment of, 1088-1089, 1112-1114
Greater splanchnic nerve, 80-81
Grip1, 25
Growth arrest-specific gene 6, 1932
Growth differentiating factor 8. See
  Myostatin
Growth differentiation factor 15, 1887
Growth factors, 1212-1213, 1744, 1792
Growth hormone
  in chronic kidney disease, 1916-1919
  definition of, 1917-1918
  functions of, 1916-1917
  hypercalcemia caused by, 609
  phosphate excretion affected by, 200
  recombinant, for pediatric chronic kidney
    disease, 2359, 2359f
  uninephrectomy effects on, 1744
Guaifenesin, 1347
Guanabenz, 1671t-1672t, 1672
Guanfacine, 1671t-1672t, 1672

Guanidinoacetic acid, 1810-1811
Guanidinosuccinic acid, 1904
Guanylate cyclase A, 395
Guanylin peptides, 397-398
Guillain-Barré syndrome, 2158
Gynecomastia, 1713

H

Haber-Weiss-Fenton reaction, 1892-1893
Hairy cell leukemia, 1118-1120
Half-and-half nails, 1949-1950, 1949f
Half-maximum effect, 2040, 2040f
HANAC syndrome, 1425
Hand ischemia, vascular access-induced, 2214
Hantavirus, 2515-2516, 2517f
Hartnup's disorder, 222-224, 223t, 1449-1450
H^+-ATPase, 331
  acquired defects in, 534
  in bicarbonate reabsorption, 235-236, 242
  genetic defects in, 242
  in hydrogen secretion, 239
  in proximal tubule bicarbonate reabsorption, 235-236
  P-type, 239
  vacuolar, 242
Health care
  in Australia, 2539-2540
  equitable, 2582-2583
  gap programs, 2583
  in Latin America, 2451-2452
  in Middle East, 2471f
  in New Zealand, 2549
  socioeconomic gradients in, 2583-2584
  targeted programs, 2582
  wastes in, 2623-2624
Health disparities
  biologic origins of, 2578
  in chronic kidney disease treatment, 2580
  definition of, 2574
  in end-stage kidney disease, 2577-2578
  health system access and surveillance, 2578-2579
  health system structure, 2579-2580
  in nephrology, 2578-2580
  postnatal environment, 2576
  prenatal environment, 2575-2576
  race and, 2577-2578
  social determinants of, 2575f
  social origins of, 2575-2578, 2584
  strategies to reduce, 2582-2584
Health justice, 2575
Health status disparity, 2574
Heart failure (HF)
  acute decompensated, 997-998, 1719-1722, 2139, 2140f
  adrenomedullin in, 437
  aldosterone and, 322, 431
  antinatriuretic systems in, 429-433
  apelin in, 438
  atrial natriuretic peptide in, 433
  baroreceptor reflex impairment in, 427
  brain natriuretic peptide in, 343, 433-434
  cardiac output decrease in, 393
  cardiopulmonary reflex impairment in, 427
  catestatin in, 438
  chronic, 1722
  COX-2 inhibitors and, 437
  C-type natriuretic peptide in, 342, 434-435

Heart failure (HF) (Continued)
  diuretics for, 1719-1722, 1720f
  dyspnea caused by, 434
  extracellular fluid, 299-300, 431f
  glomerular hemodynamic alterations in, 429
  high blood pressure and, 1522-1524
  hypertension and, 1660-1661
  hyponatremia in, 432, 493-494
  natriuretic peptide receptors in, 435
  natriuretic peptides in, 433-435, 453
  nesiritide for, 453, 1720-1721
  neuropeptides in, 438
  nitric oxide in, 435-436
  norepinephrine levels in, 432
  NT-proBNP as biomarker of, 343
  peroxisome proliferator-activated receptors in, 438-444
  prerenal acute kidney injury in, 97-998
  progression of, 1722
  prostaglandins in, 436-437
  renal blood flow decreases in, 429-430
  renin-angiotensin-aldosterone system in, 429-431, 451-452
  sodium balance in, 435
  sodium reabsorption in, 429, 431
  sodium retention in, 427-429, 428f, 431
  sympathetic nervous system in, 432, 435
  treatment of
    β-blockers, 452
    endothelin antagonists, 452-453
    natriuretic peptide blockers, 453
    nesiritide, 453
    neutral endopeptidase inhibitors, 453-454
    nitric oxide donor, 452
    omapatrilat, 453-454
    reactive oxygen species, 452
    renin-angiotensin-aldosterone system inhibition, 451-454
    vaptans, 454
    vasopeptidase inhibitors, 453-454
    vasopressin receptor antagonists, 454-455
  urotensin in, 437-438
  vasoconstrictor systems in, 429-433
  vasopressin in, 432-433
Heat shock protein 70, 977
Heat shock protein 90, 301-302, 977-978
Heavy-chain deposition disease, 1134-1136, 1135f
Hedgehog signaling, 2299
HELLP syndrome, 480, 990-992, 1182, 1613-1627, 1617t
Hemangioma, 1369
Hemangiopericytoma, 1369
Hematomas
  magnetic resonance imaging of, 876-878, 878f-879f
  perirenal, 2253
  renal transplantation with, 911f
  subcapsular, 878f-879f, 910, 911f
Hematopoietic stem cell transplantation (HSCT), 1392
  acute kidney injury after, 993
  cast nephropathy and, 1392
  chronic kidney disease and, 1394
  complications of, 1393
  purpose of, 1393-1394
  renal syndromes associated with, 1393t, 1394
  total-body irradiation and, 1400-1401
  types of, 993

Hematuria
  in acute poststreptococcal glomerulonephritis, 1057
  algorithm for, 758f
  causes of, 800t
  in children, 1014-1015
  definition of, 754-755, 798, 1014
  diagnostic approach, 755-757, 756f, 758f
  in elderly, 1014-1015
  familial
    Alport's syndrome. See Alport's syndrome
    differential diagnosis of, 1142
    renal replacement therapy for, 1141
    thin basement membrane nephropathy, 1141-1142
  in fibrillary glomerulonephritis, 1072
  glomerular, 756-757, 757t, 798, 1015
  glomerular disease in, 1014-1016, 1015t
  gross, 754-756
  history-taking, 755-756
  in immunoglobulin A nephropathy, 1065
  kidney biopsy evaluations, 1016
  macroscopic, 1065
  malignancy risks in, 759f
  microscopic, 754-755, 799, 1022, 1065, 1198-1199
  proteinuria and, 758-759
  pyuria and, 756
  in sickle cell disease, 1198-1200
  transient, 798, 1015
  urinary tract infection as cause of, 755
Hematuria-associated deafness, 1421-1422
Heme oxygenase, 977-978
Heme oxygenase 1, 2194
Hemodialysis (HD)
  acute coronary syndromes in patients receiving, 2102
  acute kidney injury treated with, 1006-1007, 1315
  adequacy of
    blood urea nitrogen measurements, 2084
    clearance monitoring as indicator of, 2079
    historical perspectives on, 2082-2083
    measurements of, 2083-2087, 2109
    urea reduction ratio, 2085-2087, 2087f
  advances in, 2109
  in Africa, 2463-2464
  air embolism prevention in, 2075
  anticoagulation during, 2091-2092, 2092t
  antiphospholipid antibodies in patients receiving, 1107
  in Australia, 2540f, 2542-2543
  barbiturate poisoning treated with, 2183
  blood clotting during, 2091-2092
  blood flow in, 2080, 2091
  blood leaks during, 2108
  blood loss caused by, 1885
  blood pressure management in, 1316, 2103
  blood urea nitrogen measurements, 2084
  cardiovascular disease in patients receiving, 2101-2102
  cardiovascular problems during, 1316-1317
  catheters for
    description of, 2067-2068
    nontunneled temporary, 2214-2216
    temporary, 2214-2216
    tunneled
      bacteremia of, 2220
      complications of, 2217, 2217f-2218f

Hemodialysis (HD) *(Continued)*
  description of, 2216
  dysfunction of, 2219-2220
  exchange of, 2219-2220
  femoral, 2218
  insertion of, 2216-2217, 2217f-2218f
  less common locations for, 2218-2219, 2219f
  prevalence of use, 2629-2630
  transhepatic, 2219
  translumbar, 2218-2219, 2219f
 cerebral hypoperfusion associated with, 1930
 in China, 2535
 cognitive impairment in, 1937f
 comorbid conditions associated with, 2063
 complications of
  arrhythmias, 598, 2107
  atrial fibrillation, 2107
  cardiac arrest, 2107
  central vein stenosis, 2212-2214, 2212f-2214f
  disequilibrium syndrome, 2106-2107, 2414
  hemolysis, 2108
  hemorrhage, 2108
  hypoglycemia, 2108, 2415
  hypophosphatemia, 2415
  hypotension, 2105-2106, 2170, 2414
  hypothermia, 2414
  muscle cramps, 2107
  myocardial stunning, 2107
  pericardial disease, 2107-2108
  pulmonary hypertension, 2413
  ventricular arrhythmias, 2107
 conductivity clearance in, 2087
 coronary artery calcification associated with, 1850
 coronary artery disease in patients receiving, 2102
 in critically ill patients, 2142
 depression in patients receiving, 2063
 diabetic nephropathy treated with, 1316-1318
 dialysance, 2071
 dialysate
  bicarbonate concentration of, 2094-2095
  calcium concentration in, 2094, 2106
  composition of, 2092-2095
  computer controls for, 2079-2080
  delivery system for, 2075, 2078
  flow rate for, 2091
  glucose concentration in, 2092, 2095
  hypotension concerns, 2105-2106
  magnesium concentration in, 2094
  potassium concentration in, 2093
  sodium concentration in, 2092-2093
  sodium ramping of, 2079-2080, 2092-2093
  solutes in, 2080t
  temperature of, 2095
  ultrapure, 2082
 dialysate pump, 2078
 dialyzers
  biofeedback systems used with, 2080
  clearance by, 2072-2074
  definition of, 2075
  description of, 2413
  functions of, 2076-2077
  high-efficiency, 2077-2078
  high-flux, 2077-2078, 2092-2093
  hollow-fiber, 2075-2076
  membranes, 2076-2077, 2091, 2108
  monitoring by, 2079-2080
  reactions to, 2108

Hemodialysis (HD) *(Continued)*
  reuse of, 2096-2097
  selection of, 2090-2091
  ultrafiltration coefficient, 2091
  values for, 2077t
 discomforts during, 2085
 dose of, 2087, 2414, 2627f
 drugs during, 2046-2048, 2048t
 dry weight, 2095-2096
 duration of, 2085, 2088-2090
 in elderly, 747-748, 2598
 end-stage kidney disease treated with, 2097
 erythrocytosis in, 1888
 erythropoiesis-stimulating agents during, 2098
 ethical dilemmas. *See* Dialysis, ethical dilemmas
 ethylene glycol poisoning treated with, 2178
 extracorporeal circuit
  air detector, 2075
  arterial pressure monitor, 2075
  blood circuit, 2075
  components of, 2074-2082
  dialysate circuit, 2078-2079
  monitoring by, 2079-2080
  pressure monitors, 2075
  venous air trap, 2075
  venous pressure monitor, 2075
 frequency of, 2090
 future of, 2108-2109
 glycemic control during, 1317
 goals of, 2069, 2089-2090
 hematocrit monitoring during, 2079
 hepatitis B vaccination in, 2016, 2104
 hepatitis C in, 2504
 history of, 2059, 2074-2075, 2082-2083, 2558
 home-based, 2542-2543
 homocysteine levels in, 2100
 hormone replacement uses of, 2089
 hypermagnesemia treated with, 626
 hyperpigmentation associated with, 1944
 hypokalemia during, 2093
 hypophosphatemia during, 2074, 2415
 incidence of, 2059-2060
 in Indian subcontinent, 2503-2504
 infections in patients receiving, 2061, 2104-2105
 inflammation in, 1913
 insulin resistance affected by, 1317
 intermittent, 1006-1007, 2140-2141, 2181
 intravenous iron in, 1891f
 isopropanol poisoning treated with, 2178
 KT/V for, 2088, 2109
 in Latin America, 2450t
 left ventricular hypertrophy, 2100-2102
 lipid abnormalities in, 2100
 maintenance
  anemia during, 2097-2098
  anorexia associated with, 2099
  cardiovascular disease risks, 2100-2102
  end-stage kidney disease during, 2097
  hepatitis B management during, 2104
  hepatitis C management during, 2104
  hypertension management during, 2103-2104
  immune disorders in patients receiving, 2104-2105
  nutrition during, 2098-2100
  primary care management during, 2105
  protein-energy wasting in, 2099
  vascular access for, 2066-2067, 2192
  vitamin supplementation during, 2099-2100

Hemodialysis (HD) *(Continued)*
 in Malaysia, 2535-2536
 malnutrition during, 1317-1318, 2089-2090, 2098t, 2504
 metabolic acidosis correction during, 2094-2095
 methanol poisoning treated with, 2178
 in Middle East, 2475t, 2487-2488
 mineral metabolism-related issues in patients receiving, 2102-2103
 mortality caused by, 2060-2063, 2062f, 2063t, 2085f-2086f
 native kidney in, 2069, 2089
 nephrologist referral in, 2063
 nocturnal, 1936, 2088, 2542
 nutrition during, 1817-1818, 2089-2090
 outcome determinants, 2109
 paraquat poisoning treated with, 2186
 peritoneal dialysis versus, 2087, 2134-2135, 2411
 pneumonia in patients receiving, 2105
 poison removal using, 2169-2170, 2170t, 2172t
 pressure monitors used in, 2075
 prevalence of, 2059-2060
 principles of, 2068-2074, 2068f
 protein binding effects, 2073f
 protein-energy wasting in, 1317-1318, 2098-2099
 psychologic support during, 2063
 pyrogenic reactions during, 2082
 rebound after, 2093
 short daily, 2088-2089
 skin manifestations of, 1944
 sleep apnea in patients receiving, 2101
 solute clearance in
  description of, 2069-2070
  determinants of, 2072, 2072t
  dialyzer, 2072-2074
  dose increase effects on, 2089f
  factors that affect, 2070-2071
  flow-limited, 2071f, 2073f
  membrane-limited, 2072f-2073f
  mode of, 2142
  monitoring of, 2079
  removal rate versus, 2070
  standard, 2088
  urea, 2070
  whole body, 2072-2074
 solute sequestration, 2072-2073, 2074f
 sudden death risks in, 2093, 2101
 survival rates for, 2060-2061, 2062f
 theophylline poisoning treated with, 2187
 toxin removal by, 2069
 treatment time for, 2085, 2088-2090
 tubing used in, 2413
 ultrafiltration, 2068-2069, 2080, 2095, 2105
 ultrafiltration rate, 2095-2096
 urea in, 2083-2087, 2083f-2084f
 uremia treated with, 2083
 vaccination recommendations, 2105
 vascular access for
  arteriovenous fistulas, 2064-2065, 2065f, 2075, 2412-2413, 2598
  arteriovenous grafts, 2065-2067, 2066f, 2075, 2412-2413, 2542-2543
  background on, 2064
  catheters, 2067-2068, 2075, 2412-2413
  central venous catheters, 2412-2413, 2542-2543
  in children, 2412-2413
  in elderly, 2598
  expanded polytetrafluoroethylene materials used in, 2064-2066
  health care costs based on, 2064, 2072t

Hemodialysis (HD) (Continued)
 ideal characteristics of, 2064t
 infection risks, 2104
 loss of, 2067
 maintenance of, 2066-2067
 monitoring of, 2066-2067
 prophylactic therapy for, 2067
 surveillance of, 2066-2067
 top-ladder technique, 2066
 in Vietnam, 2536
 water used in
  bacteria in, 2081-2082
  endotoxins in, 2081-2082
  hazards associated with, 2080-2081
  microbiology of, 2081-2082
  quality monitoring of, 2082
  treatment systems for, 2080-2082, 2081f
 zinc deficiency in, 1887
Hemofiltration, 2142, 2170, 2172t
Hemoglobin
 end-stage kidney disease levels of, 2098
 erythropoiesis-stimulating agents effect on, 1892, 1902
 glycosylated, 1931
 health-related quality of life affected by, 1902
 in hypovolemia, 423
 recombinant human erythropoietin effects on, 2097
 reticulocyte, 1895
 in urine, 790
Hemoglobin A_{1c}, 2593
Hemoglobin SC disease, 1198-1199
Hemoglobin SS, 1145-1146, 1199
Hemolytic disease of the fetus and newborn, 2159
Hemolytic-uremic syndrome (HUS)
 acute kidney injury in Indian subcontinent patients, 2496
 atypical, 1175
  C3 convertases in, 1183-1185
  characteristics of, 2154
  cobalamin C synthase deficiency as cause of, 1188, 2356-2357
  complement abnormalities in, 1183-1185, 2355-2356, 2355f
  complement factor B in, 1185
  complement factor H in, 1184-1185, 2154, 2355-2357
  complement inhibitors for, 1186
  course of, 1185
  diacylglycerol kinase-ε in, 1185, 2356
  eculizumab for, 1186, 2356
  end-stage kidney disease caused by, 2431
  fresh-frozen plasma for, 1185-1186
  genetic forms of, 2422
  genetic screening in, 1187f
  liver transplantation for, 1186-1188
  mechanisms of, 1183-1185
  membrane cofactor protein in, 1184-1185
  outcomes of, 1184t, 1185
  plasmapheresis for, 2154, 2354
  in pregnancy, 1182
  prognosis for, 2356-2357
  renal transplantation for, 1186, 2357
  sporadic, 1182
  thrombomodulin in, 1185
  treatment of, 1185-1188, 2356-2357
  von Willebrand factor-cleaving protease deficiency as cause of, 2356
 in children. See Children, hemolytic-uremic syndrome in

Hemolytic-uremic syndrome (HUS) (Continued)
 classification of, 1176t
 clinical features of, 1175-1176, 2154
 cobalamin C metabolism abnormality associated with, 1188
 de novo posttransplantation, 1182
 description of, 990-992, 1157
 laboratory findings, 1176-1178
 mechanism of action, 1179-1191
 plasmapheresis for, 2154-2155
 postpartum, 1182
 prognosis for, 2354-2355
 recurrence of, after renal transplantation, 2270
 Shiga toxin-associated, 1179-1182, 2352-2357
 Shiga-like toxin, 1175-1176
 Streptococcus pneumoniae-associated, 1182, 2355
Hemolytic-uremic syndrome/thrombotic thrombocytopenic purpura, 1617t, 1632
Hemoperfusion, 2169-2170, 2172t, 2183
Hemopexin, 1020
Hemophagocytic syndrome, 1159, 1402-1403
Hemorrhage
 cyst, 1493
 during hemodialysis, 2108
 intracerebral, 1927
 pulmonary, 1072
Hemorrhagic cystitis, 1405
Hemorrhagic fever with renal syndrome, 2515-2516
Hemorrhagic stroke, 1927, 1931
Hemostasis, 1804
Henderson equation, 521-522
Henderson-Hasselbalch equation, 521-522, 2382
Henoch-Schönlein purpura (HSP)
 in children, 2348-2350
 clinical findings in, 1121
 corticosteroids for, 1124
 course of, 1123-1124
 end-stage kidney disease progression of, 1123-1124
 epidemiology of, 2348
 gender predilection of, 1121
 histopathologic features of, 2348, 2349f
 imaging of, 2349f
 immunoglobulin A nephropathy and, 1122-1123
 immunoglobulins in, 1122-1123
 laboratory findings in, 1121-1122
 pathogenesis of, 1123, 1951
 pathology of, 1122-1123, 1122f
 prognosis for, 1123-1124, 2350
 renal manifestations of, 1121, 2348-2350
 skin manifestations of, 1951, 1951f
 symptoms of, 1121
 treatment of, 1123-1124, 1951, 2350
Henry's law, 513
Heparan sulfate, 1288
Heparin, 2091-2092, 2144, 2162
Heparinase, 1013
Heparin-induced thrombocytopenia, 1909
Hepatic glomerulopathy, 1156f
Hepatitis B
 in Africa, 2461-2462
 cryoglobulinemia associated with, 1137
 in dialysis patients, 2504
 end-stage kidney disease and, 2488
 in Far East, 2532-2533
 glomerular manifestations of, 1154-1157

Hepatitis B (Continued)
 glomerulonephritis associated with, in Far East patients, 2532-2533
 nephropathy associated with, 1154-1155, 2461-2462
 nucleoside analogs for, 1155
 in polyarteritis nodosa, 1118-1120
 proteinuria in, 1154
 treatment of, 1155
 vaccination for, 2016, 2104
Hepatitis B antigenemia, 1154
Hepatitis B surface antigen, 2532
Hepatitis C
 clinical features of, 1155-1156
 cryoglobulinemia associated with, 1138
 end-stage kidney disease and, 2488
 in Far East, 2533
 glomerulonephritis associated with, in Far East patients, 2532-2533
 in hemodialysis patients, 2104, 2504
 immunosuppressive therapy for, 1156
 membranoproliferative glomerulonephritis associated with, 1155f, 2273
 membranous nephropathy associated with, 1155
 mixed cryoglobulinemia associated with, 1155
 pathogenesis of, 1155
 pathologic features of, 1155-1156, 1155f
 pegylated interferon for, 1156
 proteinuria in, 1156
 renal allograft dysfunction caused by, 2273, 2280
 renal disease associated with, 1155-1156
 ribavirin for, 1156
Hepatocellular jaundice, 2508
Hepatocyte growth factor (HGF), 120, 1212, 1741, 1757
Hepatocyte nuclear factor-1β, 1503-1504, 2316-2317
Hepatointestinal reflexes, 397
Hepatoportal receptors, 397
Hepatopulmonary syndrome, 442
Hepatorenal reflexes, 397, 440
Hepatorenal syndrome (HRS), 2139
 acute kidney injury and, 993-994, 994t, 998-999
 COX metabolites in, 378
 endothelin-1 in, 338, 446
 mortality rate for, 455
 peripheral arterial vasodilation and, 442
 prerenal acute kidney injury and, 998
 prognosis for, 455
 sodium retention in, 378
 treatment of, 998-999
  α-adrenergic agonists, 456
  liver transplantation, 458
  midodrine, 456
  peritoneovenous shunting, 998-999
  pharmacologic, 455-457
  PROMETHEUS, 458
  renal replacement therapy, 457-458
  somatostatin analogues, 456
  systemic vasoconstrictors, 455-456
  terlipressin, 455-456, 998-999
  transjugular intrahepatic portosystemic shunt, 457, 998-999
  vasoconstrictor antagonists, 455
  vasodilators, 455
  vasopressin 1 receptor analogues, 455-456
  vasopressin 2 receptor antagonists, 456-457

Hepatorenal syndrome (HRS) (Continued)
  type 1, 449, 455
  type 2, 449, 455
Hepcidin, 1885-1886, 1886f
Hepcidin-25, 939
Herbal medicine, 2507-2508, 2533-2534
Hereditary angiopathy nephropathy, aneurysm and muscle cramp (HANAC syndrome), 1425
Hereditary cystic kidney disorder, 1479-1505
Hereditary fructose intolerance, 1445
Hereditary hypokalemic salt-losing tubulopathy, 1473
Hereditary hypophosphatemic rickets with hypercalciuria, 631-632, 1453, 2345
Hereditary leiomyomatosis and renal cell carcinoma syndrome, 1373-1374, 1952, 1952f, 1952t
Hereditary nephritis, 1140-1141. See also Alport's syndrome
Hereditary osteo-onychodysplasia. See Nail-patella syndrome
Hereditary polycystic kidney disease, 1371
hERG, 569
Hernia, 2132
Heroin nephropathy, 686, 1157-1158
Herpes zoster vaccination, 2105
Heteromeric amino acid transporters, 225-227, 226f, 231-232
Heterotrimeric G proteins, 282-284
Hexokinase, 790
High anion gap acidosis, 543, 2382t
  causes of, 524, 525t, 543, 543t
  definition of, 523
  description of, 528
  drugs as cause of, 543, 547-550
  ethanol as cause of, 548
  ethylene glycol as cause of, 548
  features of, 524-525
  isopropyl alcohol as cause of, 549
  ketoacidosis as cause of, 543, 546-547
  lactic acidosis as cause of, 543t, 544-546
  methanol as cause of, 548-549
  paraldehyde as cause of, 549
  propylene glycol acid as cause of, 549
  pyroglutamic acid as cause of, 549
  salicylate as cause of, 547-548
  screening of, 543
  toxins as cause of, 543, 548-550, 2181
  uremia as cause of, 549-550
  uremic acidosis as cause of, 543
High blood pressure, 1522-1524, 1527f. See also Blood pressure; Hypertension
High osmolar contrast media, 847-848
High-cutoff dialyzers, 2153
High-cutoff hemodialysis, 1393
High-density lipoprotein, 1761, 1863, 2100
High-efficiency dialyzers, 2077-2078
High-flux dialyzers, 2077-2078, 2092-2093
Highly active antiretroviral therapy, 1153, 2455-2456
High-molecular-weight plasma proteins, 791
High-resolution peripheral computerized tomography, 1846
Hill coefficient, 2040-2041
Hill equation, 2040
Hilus cyst, 1517
Hip fractures, 1849, 2282-2283
Hippurate, 1809f, 1811-1812
Histomorphometry, in chronic kidney disease–mineral bone disorder, 1842-1843, 1844f
HKα, 242
HKβ, 242
H^+-K^+-ATPase, 178, 254, 534
HLA-DR, 2233

HLA-DR3, 1040
HMG-CoA reductase inhibitors, for dyslipidemia, 1931
HO-1, 978
hOCT2A, 212
Hodgkin's disease, 1021, 1157
Hodgkin's lymphoma, 1404
Hollow-fiber dialyzers, 2075-2076
Home blood pressure monitoring, 1538, 1540-1542, 1541t-1542t
Homeostasis model assessment, 1912, 1914f
Homocysteine, 1817, 1864, 1872, 1930, 1938, 1970, 2100
Homocystinuria, 1864
Homogeneous population, 1163
Hong Kong, 2535
Hopewell hypothesis, 1470-1471
Hormone(s). See also specific hormone
  replacement therapy, 659-660
  sodium reabsorption regulation by, 126
Hornet stings, 2500
Horseshoe kidney, 2295, 2296f, 2303-2304, 2311
Hospice referral, 2569-2570
Hounsfield unit, 851
Hox11, 22
Hoxa11, 22
HoxB7-EGFP, 19, 20f
Hoxc11, 22
H.P. Acthar Gel, 1172
Human antichimeric antibodies, 1171
Human Development Index, 2470t
Human embryonic stem cells, 2603-2607
Human immunodeficiency virus (HIV)
  in Africa. See Africa, human immunodeficiency virus in
  in Far East, 2533
  focal segmental glomerulosclerosis associated with, 1028, 1030
  glomerular lesions in, 1153-1154
  glomerulopathies associated with, 1151
  in hemodialysis patients, 2104-2105
  immunoglobulin A nephropathy in, 1154
  renal transplantation in patients with, 2289
Human immunodeficiency virus nephropathy
  in Africa, 2462
  clinical features of, 1151-1152
  course of, 1153
  electron microscopy of, 1152f
  end-stage kidney disease caused by, 1153
  pathogenesis of, 1152-1153
  pathology of, 1152, 1152f-1153f
  podocytes in, 116
  treatment of, 1153
Human leukocyte antigens (HLA)
  class I, 2231-2233, 2232f
  class II, 2233
  inheritance of, 2233-2234, 2234f
  loci strengths, 2235-2236
  racial differences in, 2582
  sensitization, 1903, 2422-2423
  typing of, 2234-2235
Human polyomavirus infection, 2272-2273
Humoral hypercalcemia of malignancy, 603, 607-608
Hungry bone syndrome, 616, 620
Hyaline casts, 800, 800t
Hyalinosis, 921t
Hyaluronidase, 1013
Hyaluronan, 273
Hydralazine, 1673-1674, 1674t, 1695t
Hydration, 854-855

Hydraulic pressure, 94-96, 95f
Hydraulic pressure gradient, 94
Hydraulic pressure profile, 85, 85f
Hydrogen, 835, 841, 844, 1758-1759
Hydrogen gradient, 126-127
Hydronephrosis
  bilateral, 862f
  calyces in, 867-868
  congenital, 1259
  contrast-enhanced computed tomography of, 872f
  definition of, 764, 1257
  fetal, 2314-2315
  grading of, 867-868
  mild, 867-868, 867f
  moderate, 867-868, 867f
  morbidity of, 1264-1265
  nonobstructive, 765, 868
  renal cystic disease versus, 868
  severe, 867-868, 868f
  in transplanted kidney, 911
  ultrasonography of, 867-869, 867f-868f, 1263
  unilateral, 1259
Hydrostatic pressure, 813
Hydroureter, 764-765
Hydroxyapatite, 196
β-Hydroxybutyric acid, 247
Hydroxyeicosatetraenoic acids
  12(S)-, 380, 382
  15-, 380-381
  19-, 382-384
  20-, 382-384
  description of, 355, 380
1α-Hydroxylase, 1829f
11β-Hydroxylase deficiency, 1461
17α-Hydroxylase deficiency, 1461
11β-Hydroxysteroid dehydrogenase, 66-67, 577, 1919-1920
11β-Hydroxysteroid dehydrogenase type 2
  in blood vessels, 320-321
  defective, 320
  description of, 304-305, 717
  expression of, 320
  mineralocorticoid receptor activity affected by, 320
  mineralocorticoid specificity and, 320
  pharmacologic inhibition of, 577, 596
  roles of, 321
25-Hydroxyvitamin D, 1924, 2014, 2390
25-Hydroxyvitamin D 1α-hydroxylase, 187
Hyperaldosteronism
  in chronic kidney disease, 1919
  glucocorticoid-remediable, 555-556
  idiopathic, 575-577
  kaliuresis in, 576-577
  potassium loss caused by, 575-577, 576f
  primary, 575, 576f, 1545-1547
  sleep-disordered breathing and, 1547
  sodium reabsorption reinforced by, 1724-1725
Hyperammonemia, 1962, 2181
Hyperbicarbonatemia, 520
Hypercalcemia, 1375
  algorithm for, 605f
  aquaporin-2 membrane targeting affected by, 299, 481
  bisphosphonates for, 611, 2396
  bone resorption inhibition in, 611-612
  calcium-sensing receptor activation by, 609-610
  causes of, 602-603, 603t
    1,25 $(OH)_2$ vitamin D, 608
    acromegaly, 609
    acute kidney disease, 610
    breast cancer, 607-608

Hypercalcemia (Continued)
  chronic kidney disease, 610
  estrogens, 609
  familial primary hyperparathyroidism syndromes, 608
  granulomatous disease, 610
  growth hormone, 609
  immobilization, 610
  lithium, 609
  liver disease, 610
  malignancy, 603-604, 607-608
  medications, 609
  milk-alkali syndrome, 609-610
  nonparathyroid endocrinopathies, 608-609
  pheochromocytoma, 609
  primary hyperparathyroidism, 604-607
  selective estrogen receptor modifiers, 609
  thiazide diuretics, 609, 1730
  vitamin A, 609
  vitamin D, 609
  in children. See Children, hypercalcemia in
  clinical features of, 604t, 2393-2394
  description of, 185-186
  diagnosis of, 604-605, 605f, 2396, 2396f
  familial hypocalciuric, 608, 2391, 2395
  glucocorticoids for, 612
  humoral hypercalcemia of malignancy, 603, 607-608
  hypercalciuria induced by, 604
  hypertension and, 1549
  idiopathic infantile, 2394
  incidence of, 602
  laboratory findings in, 604
  loop diuretics for, 610-611
  of malignancy, 1399-1400, 1399t
  management of, 610-612, 611t
  mild, 608-609
  neonatal, 2394t
  pathophysiology of, 602-603
  in peritoneal dialysis patients, 2132
  pharmacologic therapy for, 611t
  in renal transplantation recipients, 2281
  sarcoidosis and, 1228
  signs and symptoms of, 603-604
  treatment of, 2396, 2397t
  vitamin D-mediated, 609
  volume repletion for, 610-611
  Williams-Beuren syndrome as cause of, 2394-2395
Hypercalcemia-hypercalciuria of malignancy, 767-768
Hypercalciuria, 1331-1335, 1437
  absorptive, 1331-1333, 1333f
  autosomal dominant hypocalcemia with, 2345
  in children, 2340, 2344, 2344f
  familial hypomagnesemia with, 1466
  familial hypomagnesemia with hypercalciuria and nephrocalcinosis, 2345, 2387-2388
  genetic hypercalciuric rat model of, 1333-1334
  hereditary hypophosphatemic rickets with, 631-632, 2345
  hypercalcemia-induced, 604
  in hypophosphatemia, 629
  metabolic acidosis associated with, 191
  in nephrolithiasis, 2340, 2344, 2344f
Hypercalciuric calcium nephrolithiasis, 1364t

Hypercapnia
  acute, 526-527
  arginine vasopressin secretion affected by, 470
  chronic, 516
  metabolic alkalosis secondary to, 553-554
  positive end-expiratory pressure as cause of, 526
Hyperchloremic metabolic acidosis, 1437, 2382-2383
  algorithm for, 842f
  assessment of, 840-841
  case study of, 840-844
  clinical approach to, 841-844, 842f, 842t
  description of, 528-530, 529t, 764, 768
  toluene metabolism as cause of, 843f
Hypercholesterolemia, 301, 1129, 1970
Hypercoagulability
  in chronic kidney disease, 1906-1909, 1908f
  clinical consequence of, 1804-1805
  in membranous nephropathy, 1041
  in nephrotic syndrome, 1803-1805, 1803f
  pathogenesis of, 1803-1804
Hypercortisolism, 1549, 1919
Hyperdibasic aminoaciduria, 223t
Hyperglycemia, 1454t
  diuretics as cause of, 1730, 1731f
  fetal exposure to, 717-718
  gestational, 717-718
  glycosuria caused by, 790
  maternal, 717f
  in peritoneal dialysis patients, 2132
  thiazide diuretics as cause of, 1730, 1731f
Hyperhomocysteinemia, 2284
Hyperkalemia
  acid-base balance and, 537
  in acute kidney injury, 994-995, 2140
  in Addison's disease, 589
  aldosterone affected by, 182, 2366-2367
  algorithm for, 593f, 826f
  ammonia production and excretion affected by, 537-538, 537t
  angiotensin-converting enzyme inhibitors as cause of, 591-592, 1650
  Brugada sign associated with, 570-571
  calcineurin inhibitors associated with, 541, 2281
  cardiac arrhythmias associated with, 570-571
  cardiac effects of, 570-571, 593-594
  causes of, 825-827, 826t
  in children, 2380-2382, 2380t-2381t
  chronic, 828-830, 829f
  in chronic kidney disease, 585
  clinical approach to, 592, 825-828
  clinical sequelae of, 592
  consequences of, 570-572
  COX-2 inhibitors as cause of, 590
  cyclosporine as cause of, 590
  definition of, 585, 2380
  description of, 818
  in diabetes mellitus, 586-587
  distal potassium-sparing diuretics as cause of, 1713, 1732
  diuretics as cause of, 1730, 1732
  drug-induced, 540, 540t
  electrocardiographic abnormality associated with, 571, 571t
  in end-stage kidney disease, 585, 2405
  epidemiology of, 585
  epithelial sodium channel inhibition as cause of, 590-591, 591f

Hyperkalemia (Continued)
  excessive potassium intake as cause of, 586
  factitious, 585
  familial hypertension with, 179-180, 183, 2381-2382
  hereditary tubular defects as cause of, 589-590
  hospitalization for, 592
  hyperphosphatemia and, 1003-1004
  hyperuricemia and, 994-995
  hyporeninemic hypoaldosteronism and, 589
  impaired net acid excretion disorders with, 536-541
  medications that cause, 590-592
  mineralocorticoid antagonists as cause of, 591-592
  mortality rate for, 585
  muscle effects of, 570-571
  non-anion gap metabolic acidosis and, 536
  nonsteroidal antiinflammatory drugs as cause of, 362
  potassium excretion in, 827
  potassium redistribution as cause of, 586-588
  potassium shift out of cells as cause of, 825-827, 826t
  potassium-sparing diuretics as cause of, 451
  of primary mineralocorticoid deficiency, 538
  proximal tubule bicarbonate reabsorption affected by, 237
  pseudohyperkalemia, 585-586, 827, 829, 2380
  red cell transfusion as cause of, 586
  renal consequences of, 571-572
  in renal transplantation recipients, 2281
  renin and, 814t
  renin-angiotensin-aldosterone system inhibitors as cause of, 591-592, 741, 2005-2006
  tacrolimus as cause of, 590
  tissue necrosis as cause of, 586
  treatment of, 1003-1004, 2381t
    β_2-adrenergic agonists, 594-595
    albuterol, 594-595
    algorithm for, 593f
    calcium, 593-594
    cation exchange resins, 596-597
    dialysis, 598-599
    insulin in, 594
    mineralocorticoids in, 595-596
    potassium binders, 597-598
    potassium redistribution in, 594-595
    potassium removal agents in, 595-596
    sodium bicarbonate, 595, 595f
    sodium polystyrene sulfonate, 596-597
  trimethoprim as cause of, 590, 828
Hyperkalemic acidosis, 572
Hyperkalemic hyperchloremic metabolic acidosis, 536t, 538, 541
Hyperkalemic periodic paralysis, 567f, 571
Hyperkalemic renal tubular acidosis, 540, 1726, 2337t, 2338
Hyperlactatemia, 545
Hyperlipidemia
  cardiovascular disease and, 1802
  causes of, 2284
  clinical consequences of, 1802-1803
  description of, 2127

Hyperlipidemia (*Continued*)
  nephrotic, 1801-1803, 1801f, 1803f, 1816-1817
  in peritoneal dialysis patients, 2132
  renal injury secondary to, 1773
  in renal transplantation recipients, 2284
  thiazide diuretics as cause of, 1731
Hypermagnesemia
  in acute kidney injury, 995, 1003t, 1004
  cardiovascular system manifestations of, 625
  causes of, 625
  in chronic renal failure, 616
  clinical manifestations of, 625-626
  description of, 193
  dialysis for, 626
  hemodialysis for, 626
  nervous system manifestations of, 625
  progressive, 625
  renal insufficiency and, 625
  treatment of, 625
Hypermineralocorticoidism, 551
Hypernatremia
  in acute kidney injury, 1003-1004, 1003t
  adipsic, 477-478
  in children, 2367-2370
  in elderly, 742
  osmoreceptor dysfunction as cause of, 489
  prevention of, in nephrogenic diabetes insipidus, 2338
Hyperosmolality, 478-479, 483, 2367-2370, 2367t
Hyperoxaluria, 1337-1340, 1338f, 1342f, 2340, 2346-2348, 2422, 2431, 2478
Hyperparathyroidism, 603
  in chronic kidney disease, 1912
  erythropoietin and, 1887
  hypertension and, 1549
  hypophosphatemia caused by, 630
  hypophosphaturia caused by, 630
  left ventricular hypertrophy and, 1924
  lithium and, 1226
  maternal, 2391
  neonatal severe, 608, 2395-2396
  posttransplantation, 2282
  primary, 603-604
  in renal transplantation recipients, 2282
  secondary, 1797-1798, 1827-1828, 1835-1836, 1887, 2023, 2026, 2031-2032
Hyperparathyroidism–jaw tumor syndrome, 608
Hyperphosphatemia
  in acute kidney injury, 1004
  causes of, 626-627, 627t, 2399, 2399t
    acromegaly, 627
    acute kidney injury, 627, 995
    bisphosphonates, 627
    chronic kidney disease, 627, 1774-1775
    exogenous phosphate load, 627-628
    familial tumoral calcinosis, 627
    glomerular filtration rate reductions, 627
    hypoparathyroidism, 627
    metabolic acidosis, 628
    pseudohypoparathyroidism, 627
    respiratory acidosis, 628
    rhabdomyolysis, 628
    tumor lysis syndrome, 628
  in children, 2398-2400, 2399f, 2399t
  in chronic kidney disease stage 5, 2020
  chronic kidney disease–mineral bone disorder secondary to, 1977, 2021
  clinical manifestations of, 628-629
  definition of, 626
  diagnosis of, 2399, 2399f

Hyperphosphatemia (*Continued*)
  hyperkalemia and, 1003-1004
  imaging of, 2399
  in intensive care unit settings, 628
  neonatal, 2389
  phosphate-binding agents for, 2029. *See also* Phosphate-binding agents
  pseudo-, 628
  treatment of, 628-629, 2021, 2399, 2400t
  tumor lysis syndrome and, 1396
Hyperprolactinemia, 1919
Hyperprostaglandin E syndrome, 2376-2377
Hypertension, 1549. *See also* Blood pressure; High blood pressure; Secondary hypertension
  in acute poststreptococcal glomerulonephritis, 1057
  in Africa, 2459-2461
  African American study of kidney disease and hypertension, 1553
  age and, 1525
  albuminuria risks, 1765
  angiotensin II-dependent mouse model of, 369
  antihypertensive treatment, 1563t
  in antiphospholipid syndrome, 1200
  arterial stiffness and, 1535
  in atheroembolic renal disease, 1191
  atherosclerotic renal artery stenosis and, 1595-1596
  autosomal dominant early-onset hypertension with severe exacerbation during pregnancy, 1463
  autosomal dominant polycystic kidney disease and, 1487-1489, 1492-1493
  bevacizumab causing, 1398
  blood pressure measurement and, 1539f
  calcineurin inhibitors as cause of, 1167-1168
  cardiovascular disease and, 1688-1689, 1861, 1868, 2127
  in children, 2329, 2360, 2406-2407, 2421-2422
  chronic kidney disease and, 673, 679, 1544-1545, 1765-1767, 1861, 1868, 1873, 1974-1975, 2360, 2421-2422, 2590-2591
  clinical outcome trials for, 1552-1562
  congenital adrenal hyperplasia and, 1547
  definition of, 1680
  in diabetic nephropathy, 1314-1315
  diagnostic approach, 765-767
  drug-resistant, 1974-1975
  economics of, 1528
  effects of, 1522, 1523f
  in elderly, 744-746, 745f, 1557-1560, 1558t, 2590-2592
  endothelin's role in, 336-337
  in end-stage kidney disease, 1765, 1770, 2406-2407
  epidemiology of, 1524-1527
  ethnicity and, 662f, 693-694, 1526-1527
  evaluation of, 1536-1543, 1537t
  familial, with hyperkalemia, 179-180, 183
  fractional excretion of sodium affected by, 1747-1748
  gender and, 662f, 1525
  genetics of, 1529-1530
  gestational, 1627-1631
  glomerular, 1737-1738
  glomerular hematuria and, 758
  heart failure and, 1660-1661
  in hemodialysis patients, 2103-2104
  immune system and, 1535-1536
  inherited disorders with, 1459-1464
  intraabdominal, 2138

Hypertension (*Continued*)
  intrahepatic, 441
  isolated systolic, 1685
  kallikrein-kinin system in, 349
  laboratory tests for, 1542-1543, 1543t
  lifestyle factors, 693-694, 745-746
  malignant, 758, 1194-1195, 1765
  masked, 2360
  medical versus interventional therapy trials for, 1596t
  metabolic acidosis caused by, 555
  in New Zealand, 2550
  nonsteroidal antiinflammatory drugs as cause of, 361-362
  obesity and, 766, 1533-1534, 1694
  peripheral vasoconstriction and, 1572
  in polyarteritis nodosa, 1119
  potassium intake and, 1542
  preeclampsia and, 1615-1618, 1615t
  in pregnancy, 681
  pressure-natriuresis curve in, 701
  prevalence of, 765, 1487, 1528f
  pseudohypertension, 766
  race and, 662f, 1526-1527
  after radiation nephropathy, 1194-1195
  refractory, 1695
  renal artery stenosis and, 1582
  in renal transplantation recipients, 911, 1637, 2283-2284, 2284t, 2432
  resistant, 1691t, 1693-1695
  salt-sensitive, 1974-1975
  in scleroderma renal crisis, 1196
  secondary, 766t, 1694
  sleep-disordered breathing and, 766
  sodium intake and, 1542, 1993
  stroke risks associated with, 1522, 1928-1931, 1928t, 1933-1934
  sympathetic nervous system activation effect on, 1533f
  symptoms of, 766
  systemic hemodynamics and extracellular fluid volume, 1543
  telmisartan versus losartan trial, 1557
  thyroid dysfunction and, 1549
  traditional cut points of blood pressure for, 1524t
  treatment of
    β-adrenergic antagonists, 1660. *See also* β-Adrenergic antagonists
    angiotensin receptor blockers, 1654, 2592
    angiotensin-converting enzyme inhibitors, 2592
    description of, 1195, 1314-1315, 1930-1931, 2283-2284
    in elderly, 2591-2592
    intravenous agents, 1630-1631
    in older adults with chronic kidney disease, 1559-1560
    during pregnancy, 1629
  treatment-resistant, 1580
  in type 1 diabetes mellitus, 1297-1298
  urolithiasis and, 1351-1352
  volume overload as cause of, 2127
  weight loss benefits for, 1992
  in Williams-Beuren syndrome, 2395
Hypertensive emergencies, 1550-1552
  definition of, 1695
  diazoxide for, 1696-1697
  direct-acting vasodilators for, 1695t, 1696-1699
  drug treatment of, 1695-1700, 1697t
  parenteral drugs for, 1695t, 1696-1699
  treatment of, 1551t
  types of, 1551t, 1693t
Hypertensive nephropathy, 2459

Hypertensive nephrosclerosis, 639-641, 775, 1765
Hypertensive urgencies
 definition of, 1695
 direct-acting vasodilators for, 1695t, 1696-1699
 drug treatment of, 1695-1700
Hypertonic dehydration, 478-480
Hypertonic saline, 503
Hypertriglyceridemia, 2284
Hyperuricemia, 994-995, 1396, 1962
 in acute kidney injury, 1003t, 1004
 cause of, 1442
 chronic kidney disease progression affected by, 684, 1228, 2004
 chronic tubulointerstitial nephritis caused by, 1227-1228
 protease inhibitors as cause of, 2456-2457
Hyperuricosuria, 1335-1336, 1336f, 1342-1343, 2342, 2343t
Hyperventilation, 527
Hypervolemia
 arterial volume overload in, 449
 clinical manifestations of, 449
 definition of, 425
 diagnosis of, 449-450
 edema in, 426
 etiology of, 425-426
 interstitial fluid accumulation in, 449
 pathophysiology of, 426-429
 prerenal azotemia and, 450
 sodium retention in. *See also* Sodium retention
  effective arterial blood volume reductions and, 426-427
  pathophysiology of, 426
  primary, 425-426, 449
  secondary, 426, 449
  systemic factors that stimulate, 426-433
  treatment of, 450-451
 treatment of, 450-451
  collecting duct diuretics, 451
  distal tubule diuretics, 451
  diuretics, 450-451
  extracorporeal ultrafiltration, 451
  loop diuretics, 450-451
  proximal tubule diuretics, 450
Hypoactive sexual desire disorder, 1921
Hypoalbuminemia
 consequences of, 1797-1798
 description of, 1041, 1969-1970, 2169
 drug toxicity risks secondary to, 1797
 in nephrotic-range proteinuria, 1796-1798, 1796f
 pathogenesis of, 1796-1797, 1796f
 venous thromboembolism and, 1805
Hypoaldosteronism
 hyporeninemic, 538, 538t, 588-589, 1057
 isolated, in critically ill patients, 538-539, 539t
 primary, 588
Hypocalcemia
 in acute kidney injury, 1003t, 1004
 algorithm for, 614f
 autosomal dominant hypocalcemia with hypercalciuria, 2345
 Bartter's syndrome and, 2335
 calcium gluconate for, 618
 cataracts secondary to, 613
 causes of, 613t, 2392t
  acute kidney injury, 995
  acute pancreatitis, 618
  alcohol consumption, 616

Hypocalcemia *(Continued)*
 critical illness, 618
 drugs, 617-618
 foscarnet, 618
 hypoparathyroidism, 614-617
 magnesium disorders, 616-617
 medications, 617-618
 regional citrate anticoagulation, 617
 vitamin D, 617
 in children. *See* Children, hypocalcemia in
 chronic, 618
 in chronic kidney disease stage 5, 2020
 Chvostek's sign in, 612-613
 cinacalcet dosing and, 2027
 clinical features of, 612t
 definition of, 612
 diagnosis of, 613-614, 2392, 2393f
 familial, with hypercalciuria, 614-616
 familial hypomagnesemia with secondary hypocalcemia, 2388, 2388f
 hypomagnesemia and, 624
 laboratory findings, 613
 management of, 618
 monitoring of, 2393
 neonatal, 2391-2393, 2392t, 2394t
 in nephrotic syndrome, 1797-1798
 in plasmapheresis, 2163
 signs and symptoms of, 612-613
 treatment of, 2163, 2392-2393, 2394t
 Trousseau's sign in, 612-613
 tumor lysis syndrome and, 1396
 workup for, 2392, 2393f
Hypocalciuria
 in chronic kidney disease, 1749-1750
 in Gitelman's syndrome, 580
 isolated dominant hypomagnesemia with, 1466
 thiazide diuretics as cause of, 190-191
Hypocapnia, 516, 527
Hypochromic red blood cells, 1894-1895
Hypocitraturia, 1336-1337, 1337t, 2340-2342
Hypocomplementemia, 1052-1053, 1137, 1148-1149, 1192
Hypodipsia, 480
Hypogastric plexus, 80-81
Hypoglycemia
 arginine vasopressin secretion affected by, 470
 cause of, 1442
 during glucose treatment of hyperkalemia, 594
 during hemodialysis, 2108, 2415
 in renal insufficiency, 1816
Hypogonadism, 1920-1923
Hypokalemia
 in acute kidney injury, 995
 adverse effects of, 1729
 aquaporin-2 and, 299
 arrhythmias secondary to, 569
 cardiovascular consequences of, 570
 causes of, 822t
  Bartter's syndrome, 578-580
  Gitelman's syndrome, 580
  magnesium deficiency, 581
  nonrenal, 574
  renal tubular acidosis, 580-581
 in children, 2375-2379, 2375t, 2376f-2378f, 2377t
 citrate excretion in, 247
 clinical approach to, 581-583, 582f, 821-825
 description of, 299, 818
 diagnostic algorithm for, 2376f
 diuretics as cause of, 1728-1730, 1729f

Hypokalemia *(Continued)*
 in eating disorders, 581-583
 emergencies associated with, 821
 epidemiology of, 572
 during hemodialysis, 2093
 high potassium excretion and, 825
 hyperpolarization caused by, 570
 in hypomagnesemia, 624
 hypovolemia and, 424-425
 inherited disorders with, 1459-1464
 low potassium excretion and, 823-825
 magnesium deficiency and, 823
 metabolic acidosis and, 821, 1723
 in metabolic alkalosis, 550-551, 821-823
 in peritoneal dialysis patients, 2132
 polyuria in, 570
 potassium shift into cells as cause of, 821, 824
 in primary hyperaldosteronism, 576-577
 proximal tubule bicarbonate reabsorption affected by, 237
 rebound hyperkalemia in, 583
 redistribution and, 572-573
 refeeding syndrome and, 572-573
 renal consequences of, 570
 renin and, 814t
 rhabdomyolysis associated with, 586
 sodium polystyrene sulfonate for, 2168-2169
 spurious, 572
 in thyrotoxic periodic paralysis, 573-574
 transtubular potassium concentration gradient in, 569
 treatment of, 583-585, 824-825
 ventricular arrhythmia risks, 569
 volume expansion in, 584
Hypokalemic alkalosis, familial, 578-580
Hypokalemic nephropathy, 2375
Hypokalemic periodic paralysis, 569, 571, 573-574, 1704
Hypomagnesemia, 1465-1466
 in acute kidney injury, 995
 aminoglycosides as cause of, 621-622
 amphotericin B as cause of, 621
 autosomal dominant, 2388-2389
 calcineurin inhibitors as cause of, 622
 calcium-sensing disorders as cause of, 622
 cardiovascular manifestations of, 622-623
 causes of, 2387t
 in children, 2387-2389, 2387t
 clinical manifestations of, 622-624
 cutaneous losses as cause of, 620
 description of, 618-625, 2387
 in diabetes mellitus, 620
 diuretics as cause of, 1730
 electrolyte homeostasis and, 624
 epidermal growth factor receptor blockers as cause of, 621
 familial
  description of, 193-194
  with hypercalciuria and nephrocalcinosis, 2387-2388
  with secondary hypocalcemia, 2388, 2388f
 hypocalcemia and, 624
 hypokalemia in, 624
 incidence of, 619
 intestinal malabsorption as cause of, 620
 intravenous magnesium replacement for, 624
 isolated autosomal recessive, with normocalciuria, 2389
 loop diuretics as cause of, 621

Volume 1 pp. 1-1321 • Volume 2 pp. 1322-2636

Hypomagnesemia (Continued)
  neuromuscular system manifestations of, 623
  oral magnesium replacement for, 624-625
  parathyroid hormone resistance caused by, 617
  in parenteral nutrition patients, 620
  pentamidine as cause of, 622
  potassium-sparing diuretics for, 625
  proton pump inhibitors as cause of, 620
  refeeding syndrome as cause of, 620
  renal magnesium wasting as cause of, 620-622
  in renal transplantation recipients, 2281
  skeletal system manifestations of, 623-624
  tetany of, 193
  treatment of, 624-625
  tubule nephrotoxins as cause of, 621
Hyponatremia
  in acute kidney injury, 1003, 1003t
  acute symptomatic, 501
  aquaporin-2 in, 299-300
  brain herniation caused by, 503
  case studies of, 816-817
  causes and pathogenesis of
    angiotensin-converting enzyme inhibitors, 497
    antineoplastic drugs, 497
    carbamazepine, 497
    chlorpropamide, 497
    congestive heart failure, 493-494
    desmopressin, 488, 496-497
    diuretics, 492-493, 1727-1728, 1727f
    drugs, 496-497
    endurance exercise, 496
    extracellular fluid volume depletion, 492-493
    extracellular fluid volume excess, 493-495
    glucocorticoid deficiency, 495
    heart failure, 432, 493-494
    hepatic failure, 494
    hypothyroidism, 495-496
    narcotics, 497
    nephrotic syndrome, 494-495
    oxcarbazepine, 497
    primary polydipsia, 496
    psychotropic drugs, 497
    renal failure, 495
  central nervous system symptoms in, 501-502
  in children, 2370-2372, 2371t
  chronic, 502-504, 508, 815, 817
  cirrhosis and, 494
  classification of, 501t, 815
  clinical manifestations of, 500-501
  definition of, 815
  depletional, 503-504
  diagnosis of, 492f
  edema and, 495
  in elderly, 497, 501, 742
  euvolemic, 504-505, 507f
  factitious, 490
  hospital-acquired, 496
  in hospitalized children, 2372
  hypo-osmolality and, 490-491
  hypovolemic, 492-493
  incidence of, 490
  laboratory tests for, 816
  morbidity and mortality associated with, 500-503
  in osmoreceptor dysfunction, 480
  in peritoneal dialysis patients, 2132
  postoperative, 496
  prevalence of, 490
  in psychosis, 496

Hyponatremia (Continued)
  sodium concentration monitoring in, 508
  spontaneous correction of, 507-508
  symptoms of, 500-503, 506-508
  syndrome of inappropriate antidiuretic hormone secretion as cause of, 497-498
  thiazide diuretics and, 817-818
  transient, 477
  translocational, 491
  treatment of
    arginine vasopressin receptor antagonists, 504-506, 509
    fluid restriction, 504, 504t
    furosemide, 506
    future of, 508-509
    guidelines for, 506-508
    hypertonic saline, 503
    isotonic saline, 503-504
    neurologic outcomes secondary to, 503
    urea, 506
Hyponatremic encephalopathy, 500-501, 2371
Hyponatremic hypertensive syndrome, 575
Hypo-osmolality, 490-491, 2370-2371, 2371t
Hypoparathyroidism
  acquired, 616-617
  algorithm for, 614f
  autoimmune, 617
  in children, 613
  genetic causes of, 614-616
  genetic syndromes with, 615t
  hyperphosphatemia caused by, 627
  hypocalcemia caused by, 614-617
  incidence of, 614
  after thyroid surgery, 616
Hypoparathyroidism, sensorineural deafness, and renal anomalies syndrome, 2297t
Hypophosphatemia
  in acute leukemia, 633
  causes of, 629-633, 2397, 2397t
    alcoholism, 633
    autosomal dominant hypophosphatemic rickets, 630-631
    autosomal recessive hypophosphatemic rickets, 631
    description of, 629-630
    diabetic ketoacidosis, 633, 2398
    drugs, 632
    Fanconi's syndrome, 632
    hereditary hypophosphatemic rickets with hypercalciuria, 631-632
    hyperparathyroidism, 630
    kidney transplantation, 632
    malabsorption, 632-633
    malnutrition, 632
    phosphate redistribution, 633
    phosphatonins, 630-631
    refeeding syndrome, 633
    respiratory alkalosis, 633
    tumor-induced osteomalacia, 631
    vitamin D, 633
    X-linked hypophosphatemia, 630
  in children, 2396-2398, 2415
  chronic, 629
  clinical manifestations of, 629
  definition of, 629
  diagnosis of, 629
  drug-induced, 632
  hematologic effects of, 629
  in heat stroke, 633
  in hemodialysis, 2074, 2415
  1α-hydroxylase system stimulated by, 2390
  25-hydroxyvitamin D_3 1α-hydroxylase induced by, 200

Hypophosphatemia (Continued)
  hypercalciuria in, 629
  imaging of, 2398
  intravenous phosphorus for, 634
  isoproterenol and, 200-201
  metabolic consequences of, 629
  mild, 2396-2397
  moderate, 629
  neuromuscular abnormalities secondary to, 629
  phosphate replacement therapy for, 633-634
  in renal transplantation recipients, 2281
  skeletal abnormalities secondary to, 629
  in toxic shock syndrome, 633
  treatment of, 633-634, 2398, 2398t
Hypophosphatemic rickets, 630-632
Hypophosphaturia, 630
Hypopituitarism, 495
Hypoplasia, 10t-17t
Hyporeninemic hypoaldosteronism, 538, 538t, 586, 588-589, 1057
Hypotension
  angiotensin-converting enzyme inhibitors as cause of, 1648
  during hemodialysis, 2105-2106, 2170
  orthostatic, 1538-1539
Hypothalamic gonadotropin-releasing hormone, 1635
Hypothermia, 2414
Hypothyroidism, 495-496, 1916
Hypotonic polyuria, 473t, 482-484
Hypouricemia, 498
Hypovolemia, 963
  absolute, 421-422, 424-425
  arginine vasopressin secretion by, 467-468
  clinical manifestations of, 423
  colloid solutions for, 425
  definition of, 421
  diagnosis of, 423-425
  diuretic-induced, 502
  etiology of, 421
  hemoglobin findings in, 423
  hypoalbuminemia and, 441
  hypokalemia and, 424-425
  laboratory findings in, 423-424
  metabolic acidosis and, 424
  in nephrotic syndrome, 422-423
  plasma potassium concentration in, 423
  plasma sodium concentration in, 423
  potassium chloride for, 424-425
  relative, 422-423, 425, 439
  renal allograft dysfunction caused by, 2265-2266
  renal vein thrombosis caused by, 1206
  replacement fluids for, 424-425
  signs and symptoms of, 423
  treatment of, 424-425
  urea levels in, 423
  urine biochemical parameters for, 423-424
Hypovolemic thirst, 472
Hypoxia
  arginine vasopressin secretion affected by, 470
  in chronic kidney disease, 139
  intrarenal, 139-140
  postglomerular, 1790
Hypoxia-inducible factors, 1373
  -1α, 1888
  -2α, 1888
  anemia and, 1880-1881, 1880f
  description of, 140, 970
  in postglomerular hypoxia, 1790
  preeclampsia and, 1619
  stabilizers, 1892
  von Hippel-Lindau gene and, 1373f

INDEX

I

Ibandronate, 611-612
I-BOP, 367-368
Ichthyosis, 1943-1944
Icodextrin peritoneal dialysis solution, 2118, 2415-2416
Idiopathic calcium oxalate intake, 1325
Idiopathic hypercalciuria, 1331
Idiopathic infantile hypercalcemia, 2394
Idiopathic rapidly progressive glomerulonephritis, 2151
Ifosfamide, 1397
IgA glomerulonephritis, 2275, 2544
IgA nephropathy. *See* Immunoglobulin A nephropathy
Imaging
  acute kidney injury, 863*f*-864*f*, 866-871, 866*f*-871*f*
  acute pyelonephritis, 878-880
  angiography. *See* Angiography
  angiomyolipomas, 891, 893*f*
  autosomal dominant polycystic kidney disease, 885-888, 888*f*-889*f*
  captopril-enhanced renography, 908
  chronic kidney disease, 863*f*-864*f*, 866-871, 866*f*-871*f*
  computed tomography. *See* Computed tomography
  fibromuscular dysplasia, 907, 907*f*
  iodinated contrast media used in, 847-848
  kidney development studies using, 19
  lymphoma, 899, 902*f*
  magnetic resonance imaging. *See* Magnetic resonance imaging
  malacoplakia, 881-882
  medullary sponge kidney, 888-889
  metastases, 899, 902*f*
  multicystic dysplastic kidney, 889
  obstructive urography evaluations, 871
  pyelonephritis, 1241
    acute, 878-880
    chronic, 882-883
    emphysematous, 881, 882*f*
    xanthogranulomatous, 881, 883*f*
  renal abscess, 880, 881*f*-882*f*
  renal calcifications, 871-878
  renal cell carcinoma, 892, 894*f*-899*f*
  renal function evaluations, 865-866, 866*f*
  renal hamartomas, 891, 893*f*
  renal masses, 883-899, 884*f*-899*f*
  renal neoplasms, 891
  renal transplantation assessments, 909-910, 909*f*-913*f*
  renal tuberculosis, 882, 884*f*
  renal tubular ectasia, 888-889
  renal vascular disease, 903-907, 904*f*-907*f*
  renal vein thrombosis, 908-909
  transitional cell carcinoma, 898-899, 900*f*-901*f*
  ultrasonography. *See* Ultrasonography
Imidapril, 1643, 1643*t*
Imidazole receptor agonists, 1649*t*-1650*t*
IMINO^B, 224-225
Iminoglycinuria, 223*t*, 224, 1450
Immobilization, hypercalcemia caused by, 610
Immune complex-mediated crescentic glomerulonephritis
  aspergillosis associated with, 1150
  in children, 1073
  electron microscopy findings, 1075
  epidemiology of, 1075
  in HIV-infected patients, 1154

Immune complex-mediated crescentic glomerulonephritis *(Continued)*
  immunofluorescence microscopy findings, 1075
  light microscopy findings, 1075
  methylprednisolone for, 1076
  pathogenesis of, 1075-1076
  pathology of, 1075
  treatment of, 1076
Immune disorders, 2104-2105
Immune system, 1535-1536
Immune tolerance, 2229-2230
Immunity, 334, 1233
Immunofluorescence microscopy
  acute poststreptococcal glomerulonephritis findings, 1055, 1055*f*
  Alport's syndrome findings, 1139
  amyloidosis findings, 1130*f*
  anti-glomerular basement membrane disease findings, 1126, 1126*f*
  anti-glomerular basement membrane glomerulonephritis findings, 1077, 1077*f*
  C3 glomerulonephritis findings, 1051-1052
  dense deposit disease findings, 1051, 1051*f*
  fibrillary glomerulonephritis findings, 1071, 1071*f*, 1134*f*
  focal segmental glomerulosclerosis findings, 1026, 1026*f*
  immune complex-mediated crescentic glomerulonephritis findings, 1075
  immunoglobulin A nephropathy findings, 1060-1061
  immunotactoid glomerulopathy findings, 1071
  lupus nephritis findings, 1095*f*-1096*f*, 1097
  membranoproliferative glomerulonephritis findings, 1046-1047, 1048*f*
  membranous nephropathy findings, 1037-1038, 1037*t*, 1038*f*
  microscopic polyangiitis findings, 1115
  minimal change disease findings, 1019
  nail-patella syndrome findings, 1143
  pauci-immune crescentic glomerulonephritis findings, 1082-1083
  sickle cell nephropathy findings, 1145-1146, 1145*f*
  Waldenström's macroglobulinemia findings, 1136
Immunoglobulin A, 1233. *See also* Henoch-Schönlein purpura
Immunoglobulin A nephropathy
  antineutrophil cytoplasmic autoantibodies in, 1064
  autoantibodies in, 1064
  in children, 1059
  classification of, 920, 1059*t*
  clinical features of, 1065-1066
  crescentic, 1068
  description of, 355
  end-stage kidney disease secondary to, 1065
  familial, 1060
  in Far East, 2530-2531, 2530*f*-2531*f*
  galactose-deficient IgA1 in, 1064
  gender differences in progression of, 657
  genetics of, 1060
  genomewide association studies of, 1060
  geographic distribution of, 1059-1060

Immunoglobulin A nephropathy *(Continued)*
  hematuria in, 758, 1065
  Henoch-Schönlein purpura and, 1122-1123
  in HIV-infected patients, 1154
  idiopathic, 1065
  IgA1 in, 1063-1064
  IgA levels in, 1066-1067
  immunofluorescence microscopy findings, 1060-1061
  in Japan, 2531*f*
  laboratory findings in, 1066-1067
  linkage studies of, 1060
  macroscopic hematuria in, 1065
  magnetic resonance imaging of, 870*f*
  microscopic hematuria in, 1065, 1067
  minimal change disease and, 1404
  mycophenolate mofetil for, 1068, 2531
  natural history of, 1065-1066
  nephrotic syndrome caused by, 1059-1069
  outcomes of, 1063, 1066
  Oxford-MEST score, 1063
  pathogenesis of, 1063-1064, 1431
  pathology of, 1060-1063
  podocyte injury in, 1064
  in pregnancy, 1066
  prognostic factors, 1065-1066
  progression of, 1063, 1065-1066, 1068
  proteinuria in, 1065-1066, 1069, 1164-1165
  after renal transplantation, 1069
  secondary, 1065
  treatment of
    aliskiren, 1068
    angiotensin II inhibitors, 1067-1068
    azathioprine, 1068
    cyclophosphamide, dipyridamole, and warfarin combination therapy, 1068
    fish oil, 1069
    glucocorticoids, 1067-1068
    mycophenolate mofetil, 1068
    omega-3 fatty acids, 1069
    prednisone, 1067
    summary of, 1069
    tonsillectomy, 1068-1069
  upper respiratory tract infection and, 755
Immunoglobulins
  G, in membranous nephropathy, 1037-1039, 1038*f*
  in Henoch-Schönlein purpura, 1122-1123
  light chains, 967-968
  M, in minimal change disease, 1018*t*, 1019
Immunohistochemical assay, 921-922
Immunologic intolerance, 1620-1621
Immunophilins, 2247
Immunosuppression
  allograft survival rates with, 2236
  breastfeeding and, 1638
  cancer risks secondary to, 2284, 2433
  future of, 2290
  history of, 2229
  during pregnancy, 1637-1638, 1637*t*
Immunosuppressive agents
  alemtuzumab, 2248, 2255-2256
  allograft survival rates with, 2236
  anti-CD20 monoclonal antibody, 2256
  antiproliferative, 2257-2258
  antithymocyte globulins, 2255
  azathioprine, 2245, 2254*t*, 2257
  belatacept, 2248, 2254*t*, 2258-2259
  bone histology affected by, 1851-1852
  calcineurin inhibitors, 2256
  cessation of, 2290
  corticosteroids, 2245, 2254*t*, 2259

Immunosuppressive agents (Continued)
  costimulatory signal blockers, 2258-2259
  cyclosporine, 2246-2247, 2254t, 2256-2257
  daclizumab, 2256
  in elderly, 749
  everolimus, 2247, 2258
  genomics for, 2249
  granulomatous with polyangiitis treated with, 1112
  hepatitis C treated with, 1156
  history of, 2229
  interleukin-2 receptor antagonist, 2256
  JAK3 inhibitor, 2258
  lupus nephritis treated with, 1103, 1105
  maintenance types of, 2256-2257
  mammalian target of rapamycin inhibitors, 2247, 2258
  mechanism of action, 2246f, 2253-2255, 2254f
  monoclonal antibodies, 2248-2249, 2255-2256
  muromonab-CD3, 2255-2256
  mycophenolate mofetil, 2245-2246, 2246f, 2254t, 2257-2258
  mycophenolic acid, 2245-2246, 2246f
  overview of, 2253-2255, 2254t
  polyclonal immune globulins, 2247-2248, 2255
  proteomics, 2249
  protocols for, 2259
  rapamycin, 2247
  rituximab, 2256
  sirolimus, 2254t, 2258
  tacrolimus, 2247, 2254t, 2257-2258
  tofacitinib, 2258
  voclosporin, 2257
Immunotactoid glomerulopathy
  characteristics of, 1069-1070, 1132
  clinical features of, 1072
  cryoglobulinemia and, 1071
  electron microscopy findings, 1070f, 1071, 1133f
  end-stage kidney disease progression of, 1072, 1134
  epidemiology of, 1072
  fibrillary glomerulonephritis versus, 1069-1070
  immunofluorescence findings, 1071
  light microscopy findings, 1071
  nephrotic syndrome caused by, 1069-1072
  pathogenesis of, 1071
  pathology of, 1070f, 1071, 1133f
  proteinuria in, 1072, 1132
  renal insufficiency in, 1072
  treatment of, 1072
Immunotherapy, 1385
Immunoturbidimetric technique, 794
Impetigo, 1953
Importin-α, 306-307
Impotence, 1731-1732
Inborn errors of metabolism, 2417
Incidentaloma, 766-767
India. See Indian subcontinent
Indian subcontinent
  acute kidney injury in
    acute cortical necrosis as cause of, 2501-2502
    bee stings as cause of, 2500
    causes of, 2495, 2495t
    chemical toxins as cause of, 2500-2501
    chromic acid poisoning as cause of, 2501
    copper sulfate poisoning as cause of, 2500
    demographics of, 2495
    dengue fever as cause of, 2498-2499

Indian subcontinent (Continued)
    diarrheal diseases as cause of, 2496
    ethylene dibromide poisoning as cause of, 2501
    ethylene glycol poisoning as cause of, 2500-2501
    glucose-6-phosphate dehydrogenase deficiency as cause of, 2501
    hair dye as cause of, 2501
    hemolytic uremic syndrome as cause of, 2496
    hornet stings as cause of, 2500
    infections as cause of, 2496-2499
    intravascular hemolysis as cause of, 2501
    leptospirosis as cause of, 2497-2498
    malaria as cause of, 2496-2497
    snakebites as cause of, 2499-2500
    surgical causes of, 2496
    wasp stings as cause of, 2500
    zygomycosis as cause of, 2498, 2498f
  aortoarteritis in, 2506-2507
  chronic kidney disease in
    causes of, 2502-2503, 2502t
    demographics of, 2502-2503
    diabetic nephropathy as cause of, 2503
    financial issues, 2503
    hemodialysis for, 2503-2504
    incidence of, 2502
    peritoneal dialysis for, 2504
    prevalence of, 2502
    reimbursement issues, 2503
  development indicators in, 2495t
  economic indicators in, 2495t
  end-stage kidney disease in, 2503
  geography of, 2494
  glomerulonephritis in, 2506, 2506t
  hemodialysis in, 2503-2504
  herbal medicine toxicity in, 2507-2508
  indigenous therapies of, 2507-2508
  nephrolithiasis in, 2507
  nephrotic syndrome in, 2506t
  renal calculi in, 2507
  renal replacement therapy in, 2503-2504
  renal transplantation in, 2504-2506
  renovascular hypertension in, 2506-2507
  Takayasu arteritis in, 2506
Indoles, 1812
Indomethacin, 1269
Indonesia, 2536
Indoxyl sulfate, 1812
Induced pluripotent stem cells, 2606-2607
Inducible nitric oxide synthases, 416, 979, 1739
INF2 disease, 1429
INF2 protein, 1429
Infants. See also Children
  hypocalcemic, 2392
  renal transplantation in, 2420
  syndrome of inappropriate antidiuretic hormone secretion in, 499
Infection(s)
  acute interstitial nephritis caused by, 1219
  in acute kidney injury, 996
  acute kidney injury caused by
    in Far East, 2511-2523, 2511f, 2512t
    in Indian subcontinent, 2496-2499
  catheter-related, 2068f, 2128, 2131
  focal segmental glomerulosclerosis caused by, 1030
  glomerulonephritis caused by, 2527, 2528t
  in hemodialysis patients, 2061, 2104-2105
  renal transplantation complicated by, 2286-2288, 2287t, 2420-2421, 2505-2506
  susceptibility to, in nephrotic syndrome, 1805

Infection stone, 1323f, 1346-1347, 1365-1366
Infectious endocarditis, 1148-1149
Inferior vena cava occlusion, 440
Inferior venacavography, 1204-1205
Inflammation
  in acute kidney injury pathophysiology, 981
  anemia of chronic disease and, 1887
  cardiovascular disease risks, 1865, 2100
  in chronic kidney disease, 1865, 1909, 1969-1970
  erythropoiesis affected by, 1887
  in hemodialysis, 1913
  markers of, 1942
  oxidative stress affected by, 1758
  in peritoneal dialysis, 2125-2126
  protein wasting and, 1817
  in proteinuria, 1792-1794
  renal parenchymal, 975-977
  renin-angiotensin-aldosterone system and, 334
  tubulointerstitial, 1215
Inflammatory bowel disease, hyperoxaluria in, 1342f
Informed consent, for kidney biopsy, 917-919
Infusion equilibrium technique, 1332
Inherited Fanconi's syndrome, 1435, 1435t
Inherited primary glomerular disorder of unknown cause, 1431
Inherited renal tubulopathy, 1417-1418
Inhibition of crystal agglomeration, 1329
Inhibitory factor 1, 140
Initial collecting tubules, 65-66, 68, 69f, 70, 241-242
Innate inflammatory immune response, 1791-1792
Inner medulla
  concentrating mechanism of, 271-273
  description of, 45, 45f, 91-92, 91f
  sodium chloride concentration in, 271-273
  urea accumulation in, 268-270
Inner medullary collecting duct (IMCD)
  anatomy of, 44-45, 45f, 74, 75f, 166, 239, 262
  bicarbonate reabsorption in, 242
  cell of, 241
  eNOS activation in, 417
  Na^+-K^+-ATPase in, 254
  portions of, 74, 77f
  potassium transport in, 133
  principal cells of, 75, 76f
  terminal portion of, 77f
Inositol 1,4,5-triphosphate, 1825
Insect stings, 2525
Institute of Medicine, 2620
Insulin
  diabetic ketoacidosis treated with, 547
  glucose and, 594
  hypokalemic effect of, 562, 570
  Na^+-H^+ exchanger activation by, 818
  phosphate excretion affected by, 200
  potassium distribution affected by, 562, 587, 594
Insulin receptor substrate 1, 1913
Insulin receptor-related receptor, 256
Insulin resistance
  adverse effects of, 1816
  cardiovascular risk and, 1914
  causes of, 1913, 1913t
  in chronic kidney disease, 1315, 1912-1916, 1913t
  definition of, 1912
  in end-stage kidney disease, 1816

Insulin resistance *(Continued)*
  hemodialysis effects on, 1317
  homeostasis model assessment-estimated, 1912, 1914f
  in peritoneal dialysis, 1913
  thiazolidinediones for modulating of, 2127
  treatment of, 1914-1915
  uremic, 1816, 1913-1915
  vitamin D in, 1913
Insulin-like growth factor-binding proteins
  -1, 718
  -7, 949, 989
  description of, 1917-1918
Insulin-like growth factors
  -1, 181, 197-198, 200, 1212, 1967, 1970-1971, 2099, 2612
  -2, 1744
  description of, 718
Intact nephron hypothesis, 1736-1737
Integrated Discrimination Improvement Index, 929-930
$\alpha_8\beta_1$-Integrin, 25
β-Integrin receptors, on mesangial cells, 51-52
Intensive care unit, 628, 2137, 2139-2140, 2458-2459
Intercalated cells
  acid-base perturbations and, 245-246
  basolateral anion exchanger in, 243
  bicarbonate secretion by, 519
  carbonic anhydrase levels in, 71-72
  collecting ducts
    bicarbonate reabsorption, 239-241, 239f-241f
    description of, 30, 69-71, 72f
  in connecting tubules, 68-69
  of cortical collecting duct, 70-71, 72f
  of distal convoluted tubule, 238-239
  of inner medullary collecting duct, 75
  kidney anion exchanger 1 in, 243
  mineralocorticoid receptor, 314
  non-A, non-B, 241
  of outer medullary collecting duct, 74f
  transcellular chloride absorption across, 171
  type A, 70-72, 72f, 239-241, 240f-241f, 533-534
  type B, 70-72, 72f, 240f-241f, 241, 519
  type C, 241
Intercellular adhesion molecule-1, 1097, 1215
Intercellular junctions, 4-5
Interdisciplinary clinics, 2632-2634, 2633f
Interferon, 1385
Interferon-α, 1159, 1398, 2486
Interleukin-2, 1385, 1398, 2248
Interleukin-2 receptor antagonist, 2256
Interleukin-6, 1197, 1233, 2100
Interleukin-8, 1233
Interleukin-13, 1020
Interleukin-18, 939-941, 989
Interlobar arteries, 84
Interlobular arteries, 84, 84f
Intermesenteric plexus, 80-81
Intermittent centrifugation, 2160
Intermittent hemodialysis, 1006-1007
International Verapamil-Trandolapril Study (INVEST), 1553-1554
Internist's tumor, 1374
Interpodocyte space, 1781
Interstitial calcium plaque, 1325
Interstitial cells, 77-80, 78f

Interstitial fibrosis, 728f. *See also* Renal fibrosis
  chronic hypoxia in, 1217-1218
  end-stage kidney disease caused by, 1216-1217
  epithelial-mesenchymal transitions in, 1217
  pathophysiology of, 1277
  tubulointerstitial injury caused by, 1216-1218
Interstitial fibrosis and tubular atrophy, 2244
Interstitial nephritis, 363, 1158, 1505-1509, 1507t, 2476
Interstitial pressure, 761
Interventional nephrologists, 2193, 2193t
Interventional nephrology
  access-induced hand ischemia, 2214
  arteriovenous fistulas. *See* Arteriovenous fistulas
  arteriovenous grafts. *See* Arteriovenous grafts
  central vein stenosis treated with, 2212-2214, 2212f-2214f
  hemodialysis catheters. *See* Hemodialysis, catheters for
  percutaneous kidney biopsy, 2222-2224, 2223t, 2224f
  peritoneal dialysis catheters, 2220-2222
  personal safety in, 2194
  procedures performed in, 2193t
  radiation safety in, 2194
  rationale for, 2192-2194
  stenotic lesions treated with, 2212
Intestine
  calcium absorption in, 185-187, 1824-1825
  magnesium homeostasis by, 193-194, 193f
  phosphorus secretion into, 196
  potassium loss in, 574
Intraabdominal hypertension, 2138
Intracellular adhesion molecule-1, 728
Intracellular fluid
  in children, 2365-2366
  description of, 390-391
  osmotic pressure of, 461
  potassium in, 174
  solute composition of, 461
  total body water in, 460
Intracerebral hemorrhage, 1619-1620, 1927
Intracranial aneurysm, 1494-1495
Intracranial pressure, 2139
Intradialytic hypotension, 1007
Intrahepatic hypertension, 441
Intrarenal progenitor cells, 2608-2609
Intrauterine growth restriction, 665, 700f, 2300
Intravenous immune globulin, 1105, 2157
Intravenous pyelography, 1253, 1253f, 1265, 1265f, 1359
Intravenous urography
  computed tomography urography versus, 852
  description of, 846-847
  excretory phase of, 847f
  kidney stone disease evaluations, 873
  medullary sponge kidney on, 888-889
  nephrogram, 846-847, 847f
  renal masses on, 883
  transitional cell carcinoma evaluations, 898-899, 900f
Intrinsic acute kidney injury. *See* Acute kidney injury (AKI), intrinsic
Intrinsic kidney disease, 1544-1550
Inulin, 786
Iodide, 1915

Iodinated contrast media, 847-848
Iodine 131-labeled ortho-iodohippurate, 865
Iodocholesterol scintigraphy, 1546
Iododerma, 1947, 1947f
Iohexol, 736, 787, 2310
Ion exchange resins, 596
Ion trapping, 2168
Ionized calcium, 1824
Iothalamate, 787
IP receptors, 369
IQGAP1, 113
Iran. *See* Middle East
Irbesartan, 1305-1306, 1652, 1652t
Iron
  anemia treated with, 1892-1904, 2098
    intravenous iron, 1896-1900, 1897t
    markers of, 1893-1896
    parenteral administration, 1898
    safety of, 1900-1902
  balance of, 1896
  bone marrow, 1895
  chronic kidney disease treated with, 1898-1900, 1899t
  deficiency of, 1887, 1893, 1940
  description of, 1892-1900
  in erythropoiesis, 1883-1884, 1893
  intravenous, for anemia, 1891f, 1896-1900, 2098
  liver magnetic resonance imaging of, 1895
  markers of, 1893-1896
    bone marrow, 1895
    erythrocyte ferritin concentration, 1894
    erythrocyte zinc protoporphyrin concentration, 1894
    hypochromic red cells, 1894-1895
    reticulocyte hemoglobin content, 1895
    serum ferritin, 1893
    serum transferrin receptor, 1893-1894
  maternal restriction from, 716
  metabolism of, 1885-1887, 1886f
  parenteral administration of, 1898
  serum, 1893
Iron chelators, 967
Iron dextran, 1896, 1897t
Iron isomaltoside 1000, 1897t, 1898
Iron sucrose, 1896, 1897t
Ischemia-reperfusion injury, 1786
Ischemic nephropathy, 1567-1568
  diagnosis and evaluation of, 1588-1594, 1588t
  endovascular renal angioplasty and stenting, 1599
  management of, 1608f
  mechanism of, 1574-1575
  pathophysiology of, 1570-1580
  surgical treatment of, 1604-1607
  therapy goals for, 1588
Ischemic renal injury, 350
Ischemic stroke, 1927
Islet cell transplantation, 1319-1320
Isolated dominant hypomagnesemia with hypocalciuria, 1466
Isolated hypoaldosteronism, 538-539, 539t
Isolated office hypertension, 1540
Isolated proteinuria, 1013-1014
Isolated recessive hypomagnesemia, 1466-1467
Isolated renal hypoplasia, 2297t
Isolated systolic hypertension, 1685
Isopropanol, 2173-2178, 2174t, 2176t
Isopropyl alcohol-induced high anion gap acidosis, 549
Isoproterenol, 200-201, 245
Isosmotic sodium storage, 1530

Isosthenuria, 986
Isothermic dialysis, 2095
Isotonic saline, 503-504
Isotopic renography, 1266-1267, 1280
Isradipine, 1665, 1669-1670
Israel, 2477t

J

Jaffe method, 782, 787
JAK3 inhibitor, 2258
Janus tyrosine kinases-2, 1881-1882
Japan, 2531f, 2534-2535
Joubert's syndrome, 1508-1509, 2322, 2322t
Juxtaglomerular apparatus (JGA)
  anatomy of, 53
  angiotensin I secretion by, 326
  autonomic innervation of, 54-55
  composition of, 35
  definition of, 106
  description of, 35-36
  histology of, 54f
  noradrenergic nerve endings in, 327
  renin secretion by, 334-335, 360, 568
  vascular component of, 53
Juxtaglomerular cell tumor, 1369
Juxtaglomerular granular cells, 53, 54f, 55
Juxtaglomerular nephrons, 99, 100f
Juxtamedullary arterioles, 88f

K

Kaliuresis, 181-182, 574-577, 588
Kallikrein, 245, 346-350
Kallikrein-kinin system
  in anti-glomerular basement membrane disease, 350
  in antineutrophil cytoplasmic antibody-associated vasculitis, 350
  bradykinin receptors, 347
  in chronic kidney disease, 350
  components of, 346-347
  definition of, 346
  description of, 417
  in diabetic nephropathy, 349-350
  discovery of, 346
  enzymatic cascade of, 348f
  genetic mutations of, 349
  in hypertension, 349
  in ischemic renal injury, 350
  kallikrein, 346-347
  kallistatin, 347
  kininases, 347
  kininogen, 346
  in lupus nephritis, 350
  plasma, 347-348
  renal, 348-349
  renal blood flow regulation by, 348
  renin-angiotensin-aldosterone system and, 418
  tissue, 347-348
Kallistatin, 347
Kallmann's syndrome, 2297t, 2318
Kaposi's sarcoma, 2285, 2492
Kayser-Fleisher ring, 1444-1445
KCC4, 243
KCC proteins, 150
KCNJ5, 568-569, 575
KCNJ1, 2334
KCNQ1, 177
Ketoacidosis
  acetoacetic acid excretion in, 247
  alcoholic, 547
  diabetic, 525, 546-547, 628, 633, 2398
  high anion gap acidosis caused by, 543, 546-547

Ketoacidosis (Continued)
  β-hydroxybutyric acid excretion in, 247
  starvation, 547
  treatment of, metabolic acidosis after, 555
Ketoconazole, 1332-1333
15-Ketodehydrogenase, 374
α-Ketoglutarate, 218-219, 517
Ketones, 790
K_f, 99
Kidney
  afferent nerve supply to, 81
  agenesis of, 2302
  anatomy of, 42-82, 260f, 849f. See also specific anatomy
  in animals, 43
  arteries of, 83-85
  bisected, 43f-44f
  blood flow to. See Renal blood flow
  congenital anomalies of. See Congenital anomalies of the kidney and urinary tract
  dysplasia of. See Renal dysplasia
  efferent nerve supply to, 80-81
  embryology of, 2603
  function of. See Renal function
  gluconeogenesis by, 130-132
  gross features of, 42-43
  horseshoe, 2295, 2296f, 2303-2304, 2311
  in utero development of, 2302
  innervation of, 80-81
  length of, 42-43
  lymphatic system of, 80, 80f
  malformation of, in children, 2294-2295, 2295f, 2311. See also Congenital anomalies of the kidney and urinary tract
  microcirculations of. See Microcirculations
  outer cortical region of, 5
  peptide clearance by, 1810
  regeneration of, developmental approaches to, 2613
  regions of, 43
  size of, 850
  ultrasonography of, 850-851, 850f
  vascular-tubule relations in, 87
  vasculature of, 42, 43f
  veins of, 83-85
  weight of, 42
Kidney anion exchanger, 239-241
Kidney anion exchanger 1, 243
Kidney biopsy
  acute cortical necrosis diagnosis using, 2501-2502
  acute interstitial nephritis evaluations, 1220
  acute kidney injury diagnosis using, 772-773, 990
  algorithm for, 918f
  bleeding complications of, 915-917, 2223
  cirrhosis evaluations, 1156-1157
  complications of, 915-917, 2223
  contraindications for, 917, 917t, 2223
  description of, 915
  diagnoses obtained from, 916f
  electron microscopy analysis, 922, 923t
  fetal, 1280
  for fibrillary glomerulonephritis, 1132-1134
  flowchart for, 918f
  glomerular disease on, 920
  glomerulonephritis evaluations, 2544
  hematuria evaluations, 1016
  history of, 915
  idiopathic nephrotic syndrome, 2328-2329
  immunohistochemical assay, 921-922
  indications for, 915-917, 916t

Kidney biopsy (Continued)
  informed consent for, 917-919
  laparoscopic, 917, 917t
  light microscopy in
    biopsy report details about, 924
    fixative for, 919
    specimen examination, 920, 920t
    staining for, 919-920
    thin sections for, 919
  nephritic syndrome evaluations, 760
  nephrotic syndrome evaluations, 763-764
  open approach, 917, 917t
  percutaneous, 2222-2224, 2223t, 2224f
  performing of, 918-919
  real-time ultrasound guidance during, 2223-2224, 2223t, 2224f
  report from, 924
  risks of, 917t
  safety of, 915-917
  specimens, 919-920, 920t, 923-924
  transjugular, 917, 917t
  ultrasonography uses during, 850
Kidney development
  adhesion proteins in, 25
  collecting system, 5
  fetal, maternal single kidney effects on, 721
  genetic analysis of, 21-40, 22f
    adhesion proteins, 25
    collecting system, 25-27
    juxtaglomerular apparatus, 35-36
    nephron development, 30-31
    non-GDNF pathways in metanephric mesenchyme, 23
    stromal cell lineage, 31-32
    tubulogenesis, 30-31
    ureteric bud and metanephric mesenchyme interaction, 21-25
    ureteric bud positioning, 27-28
    vascular formation, 32-35, 33f
  imaging studies of, 19
  interstitial cells, 5-6
  lineage tracing studies of, 19
  metanephros, 3, 3f-4f
  model systems for studying
    antisense oligonucleotides, 7-9
    Caenorhabditis elegans, 19
    conditional mouse lines, 18t
    Drosophila, 20
    knockout mouse models, 9-19, 10t-17t
    mutant phenotypic analyses, 7
    nonmammalian, 19-21
    organ culture, 6-9
    transgenic mouse models, 9-19, 10t-17t
    Xenopus laevis, 21
    zebrafish, 20-21
  nephrogenic zone, 5
  nephron, 4-5
  overview of, 4f
  programming of, 713-723, 715t
  renal stroma, 5-6
  stages of, 2-3, 3f
  urogenital system, 2-3
  vasculature, 6, 7f
Kidney disease
  acute. See Acute kidney injury
  advanced care planning for, 2599-2600
  African American study of kidney disease and hypertension, 1553
  cardiovascular disease in, 1166
  causes of, 1410-1411
  chronic. See Chronic kidney disease
  genetic approaches to, 1410
  lymphoma and, 1401-1402
  preeclampsia and, 1617-1618
  uromodulin-associated, 165

Kidney Disease: Improving Global Outcomes, 669-670, 773, 774t, 792t, 930-931, 931t, 960-961, 1005, 1839-1841, 1846, 1868-1871, 1902, 1989-1990, 1989f, 2025, 2028, 2191-2192, 2404-2405, 2474, 2587, 2621-2622, 2632, 2634t
Kidney Disease Outcomes Quality Initiative, 643-645, 669-670, 773, 773t
Kidney donor profile index, 2279
Kidney Health Australia, 2539
Kidney Health Initiative, 953-954
Kidney injury molecule-1, 941-942, 989
Kidney size, 700-701, 700f, 713-715
Kidney stones. *See also* Calcium oxalate stones; Calcium stone; Urolithiasis
　analysis of, 1359
　calcium oxalate, 1260
　causes of
　　calcium intake, 1324
　　dietary factors, 1354
　　melamine, 1348
　　over-the-counter drugs, 1347
　　protein consumption, 1324
　in children, 2340-2342
　chronic kidney disease and, 1352
　diagnostic approach
　　computed tomography, 873, 875f-876f
　　history-taking, 767-768
　　imaging, 768-769, 871-878, 874f-878f
　　intravenous urography, 873
　　laboratory tests, 768
　　magnetic resonance imaging, 876, 876f
　　magnetic resonance urography, 876-878, 877f
　　physical examination, 768
　　plain radiographs, 874f
　　review of systems, 767-768
　　ultrasonography, 873, 875f
　　urine studies, 768
　differential diagnosis of, 769, 769t
　enteric hyperoxaluria and, 1325
　environment, lifestyle, and medical history for, 1355
　epidemiology of, 1322-1324
　family history of, 1355-1356
　genetics and, 1348-1350
　histopathology of, 1325
　imaging studies of, 1359-1360
　incidence of, 1324
　inhibitors of, 1329-1331, 1329t, 1337f
　interstitial calcium plaque and, 1325
　laboratory evaluation for, 1356-1360
　management of, 1360-1366, 1360f
　medications associated with, 767
　nonsteroidal anti-inflammatory drugs for, 769
　occurrence of, 1323f
　pharmacotherapeutic trial for, 1363t
　predisposing medical conditions for, 767-768
　prevalence of, 767, 1260, 1322-1323
　in renal fusion, 2304
　risk factors for, 767
　risk of, 1327f
　Roux-en-Y gastric bypass and, 1340, 1341t
　in sarcoidosis, 1228
　signs and symptoms of, 767, 1355
　treatment of, 769
　types of, 1323f
　ureteral obstruction caused by, 1260
　urinary tract cancer and, 1352
　vertebral bone loss and, 1354-1355

Kidney transplantation. *See* Renal transplantation
Kidneys, ureters, and bladder x-ray, 846, 847f, 1359
Kidney-specific chloride channel 1 knockout mice model, 278
Kidney-specific protein, 2603-2604
Kif26b, 22-23
Killer inhibitory receptors, 2243
Kimmelstiel-Wilson nodular lesions, 1285-1286
Kimura's disease, 1159
Kinases, in aquaporin-2 trafficking, 292-293
Kindlin-2, 1217
Kininases, 347
Kininogen, 346
Kinins, 346-347, 417-418
Kir1.1, 278
Kir3.4, 306
KIR4.1 protein, 167
KIR4.2 protein, 167
Klotho, 191, 1822, 1830-1831, 1832t, 1841-1842, 1978-1979, 2390
KLOTHO, 627, 632, 732, 734
Knockout mice models
　aquaporin-1, 273-276
　aquaporin-2, 276
　aquaporin-3, 276
　aquaporin-4, 276
　epithelial sodium channel, 278
　kidney development studies using, 9-19, 10t-17t
　kidney-specific chloride channel 1, 278
　Na$^+$-H$^+$-exchanger isoform 3, 278
　Na$^+$-K$^+$-2Cl cotransporter type 2, 278
　prostanoid receptors, 368f
　renal outer medullary potassium, 278
　type 2 vasopressin receptor, 278-279
　UT-A1/3 urea transporter, 276-278
Korea, 2535
Korotkoff phase V disappearance of sound, 1524
Kussmaul's sign, 761-762

L

Labetalol, 1629, 1630t, 1658, 1658t, 1695t, 1697t
Lacidipine, 1666
Lacis, 53
β-Lactams, 719, 1234, 1239
Lactate
　handling of, 130-132
　L-lactic acidosis and, 544-545
　metabolism of, 544
　in peritoneal dialysis solutions, 2117
　in renal metabolism, 131f
Lactic acid, 544
Lactic acidosis, 543t, 544-546
　alkali therapy for, 546
　carbon monoxide poisoning as cause of, 545
　case study of, 839-840
　clinical features of, 545
　clinical spectrum of, 545
　D-, 544
　diagnosis of, 545
　dichloroacetate for, 546
　drugs that cause, 545
　hyperphosphatemia caused by, 628
　inborn errors of metabolism as cause of, 545
　L-, 544-546
　medical conditions associated with, 545

Lactic acidosis *(Continued)*
　metformin-associated, 2184-2185
　physiology of, 544-545
　toxins that cause, 545
　treatment of, 545-546, 555
Lactobacillus crispatus probiotic, 1239-1240
LacY, 213-214
Lama5, 25
Lamb2, 25
LAMB2 gene, 1426
Lamc1, 25
Laminin disease. *See* Pierson's syndrome
Lanthanum carbonate, 2021-2022
Laparoscopic kidney biopsy, 917, 917t
Large vessel renovascular disease, 1578f
L-arginine, 979
Latency-associated protein, 1212-1213
Latin America
　acute kidney injury in, 2440-2444
　brain death criteria in, 2451
　chronic kidney disease in, 2447-2449
　demographic changes in, 2447-2448
　dengue fever, 2440-2441
　end-stage kidney disease in, 2449-2451, 2449f, 2450t
　health care coverage in, 2451-2452
　hemodialysis in, 2450t
　leptospirosis, 2443-2444, 2443f
　life expectancy in, 2440
　Lonomia caterpillar stings, 2445-2446, 2446f
　malaria, 2442-2443
　nephropathy in, 2448-2449
　peritoneal dialysis in, 2450t
　population of, 2440
　renal replacement therapy in, 2449, 2450t
　renal transplantation in, 2451
　snakebites, 2446-2447
　spider bites, 2445-2446, 2445f
　trends in, 2451-2452
　yellow fever, 2441-2442, 2442f
Laws of thermodynamics, 123
L-Carnitine, 2107, 2125
LCAT gene, 1148
LCZ696, 345-346
Lead
　chronic kidney disease risks, 686-687
　chronic tubulointerstitial nephritis caused by, 1226-1227
　end-stage kidney disease secondary to exposure to, 1226-1227
Lead nephropathy, 686-687, 1227
Lean principles, 2623-2624, 2623t, 2624f
Lecithin-cholesterol acyltransferase (LCAT), 1147-1148, 1147f, 1802
Lecticans, 30
Left ventricle, 434, 1857, 1859
Left ventricular ejection fraction, 434
Left ventricular hypertrophy (LVH)
　blood pressure and, 1688-1689
　as cardiovascular disease risk factor, 1295-1296, 1857-1858, 1924, 1978-1979, 2100-2102, 2421-2422
　in children, 2360-2361, 2421-2422, 2432
　in chronic kidney disease, 2360-2361
　description of, 1295-1296, 1857-1858
　furosemide for, 1721-1722
　in pediatric end-stage kidney disease, 2408, 2421-2422, 2432
　treatment of, 1721
Leiomyoma, 1369
Leishmaniasis, 1150-1151
Leptin, 1819

Leptospira spp., 2443, 2497-2498, 2511
Leptospirosis
  acute kidney injury caused by, 2443-2444, 2443f, 2497-2498, 2511-2513, 2511f, 2512t
  clinical features of, 2497-2498
  clinical manifestations of, 2511, 2512t-2513t
  diagnosis of, 2498, 2513
  in Far East, 2511-2513, 2511f, 2512t, 2528f
  histologic features of, 2498
  in Indian subcontinent, 2497-2498
  pathogenesis of, 2498
  pathology of, 2511f, 2513f
  penicillin for, 2513, 2514f
  treatment of, 2498, 2513, 2514f
Lercanidipine, 1666
Lesch-Nyhan syndrome, 1347
Leucovorin, 2188
Leukemia, 1401-1403
Leukocyte(s)
  activation of, 1909-1910
  functional impairment of, 1909
  in urine, 799-800
  vascular endothelium adherence of, 981
Leukocyte esterase, 790
Leukocytoclastic angiitis, 1154
Leukocytoclastic vasculitis, 1950-1951, 1951f
Leukopenia, 1650, 2434
Leukotriene A_4, 379-381
Leukotriene B_4, 381-382
Leukotriene B_4 receptor, 380
Leukotriene C_4, 381
LeuT fold, 229, 230t, 231f
Levamisole, 2330
Levodopa, 1940
Levofloxacin, 1241t
Lgr5-EGFP transgene, 19
Lhx1, 23
Licorice, 556
Liddle's syndrome, 311-312, 556, 565, 578, 1462-1463, 1463t, 2379
Lifestyle modifications
  chronic kidney disease progression affected by, 1990-1995
  hypertension treated with, 745-746
  restless legs syndrome managed with, 1940
Light- and heavy-chain deposition disease, 1134-1136
Light microscopy
  acute poststreptococcal glomerulonephritis findings, 1054-1055, 1055f
  Alport's syndrome findings, 1139
  anti-glomerular basement membrane glomerulonephritis findings, 1077-1078
  biopsy analysis using, 919-920, 920t, 924
  dense deposit disease findings, 1051
  diabetic nephropathy findings, 1285f
  Fabry's disease findings, 1144, 1144f
  fibrillary glomerulonephritis findings, 1071
  focal segmental glomerulosclerosis findings, 1024f, 1025-1026
  immune complex-mediated crescentic glomerulonephritis findings, 1075
  immunotactoid glomerulopathy findings, 1071
  membranoproliferative glomerulonephritis findings, 1046, 1047f
  membranous nephropathy findings, 1038, 1038f

Light microscopy *(Continued)*
  microscopic polyangiitis findings, 1114-1115, 1114f
  minimal change disease findings, 1015t, 1016-1019
  pauci-immune crescentic glomerulonephritis findings, 1082, 1082f
Light-chain deposition disease, 1134-1136, 1135f, 1391-1393
LIM homeobox transcription factor 1 beta, 1431
Limulus amoebocyte lysate assay, 2082
Lincosamides, 1235t-1236t
Lindsay's nail, 1949-1950, 1949f
Lineage tracing, kidney development studies using, 19
Lip cancer, 2285
Lipid(s)
  β-adrenergic antagonist therapy effects on, 1661
  glomerular-filtered, 1213
  metabolism of, 733-734, 1816-1817
  peroxidation of, 375
  in renal disease, 1773
  uremia effects on metabolism of, 1816-1817
Lipid rafts, 37-38
Lipid-lowering therapy, 1312
Lipiduria, 762-763, 763f
Lipocalin 2. *See* Neutrophil gelatinase-associated lipocalin
Lipodystrophy, 1053, 1146-1147
Lipofuscin, 728f
Lipoid nephrosis, 1016, 1019
Lipoma, 1369
Lipopolysaccharides, 238
Lipoprotein
  high-density, 1761, 1863, 2100
  low-density. *See* Low-density lipoprotein
  in nephrotic syndrome, 1802
  synthesis of, 1801
  very-low-density, 1801-1802
Lipoprotein glomerulopathy, 1148
Lipoprotein lipase, 1802
Lipoprotein(a), 1863, 2100
Lipoprotein-X, 1148
Lipotoxicity, 1344-1345, 1345f
Lipoxins, 380
Lipoxygenases
  5-, 379-380
  10-, 379-380
  15-, 379-380
  arachidonic acid metabolism by, 379f
  biologic activities of, 381
  description of, 355, 379-380
  enzymes, 379-380
  in renal pathophysiology, 381-382
Lisinopril, 1643, 1643t
Lithium
  aquaporin-2 expression affected by, 297-299, 298f
  chronic tubulointerstitial nephropathy caused by, 1226, 1226f
  hypercalcemia caused by, 609
  hyperparathyroidism associated with, 1226
  loop diuretics effect on, 1732
  minimal change disease caused by, 1159
  nephrogenic diabetes insipidus caused by, 297-299, 298f, 379, 482, 1226
  nephrotoxicity of, 379
  overdose of, 2180-2181
  polyuria caused by, 379
  renal cysts caused by, 889, 890f
  toxicokinetics of, 2180

Lithogenesis, 1325-1329
Lithotripsy, 878f
Live donor nephrectomy, 2252
Live donor renal transplantation, 2252, 2278, 2582
Liver
  cancer of, acute kidney injury and, 1390
  dysfunction of, 2139
  tyrosinemia and, 1443
  Wilson's disease and, 1444
Liver cyst, 1484
Liver disease, 991t, 993-994, 998-999
Liver flukes, 2522-2523
Liver transplantation
  atypical hemolytic-uremic syndrome treated with, 1186-1188
  glomerular filtration rate after, 458
  hepatorenal syndrome treated with, 458
  Model of End-stage Liver Disease scores, 458
Liver-type fatty acid-binding protein, 942-943, 989, 1213
Lixivaptan, 454, 456-457
LLC-PK1 cells, 160, 161f
Localized renal cystic disease, 1512-1513
Long QT syndrome, 569
Lonomia caterpillars, 2445-2446, 2446f
Loop diuretics
  absorption of, 1707
  acute kidney injury treated with, 1725-1726
  acute tubular necrosis treated with, 1001-1002
  adverse effects of, 1710
  calcium transport regulation by, 189-190
  ceiling doses of, 1726t
  distal convoluted tubule hypertrophy caused by, 1715
  distal potassium-sparing diuretics and, 1719
  dose-response curve for, 1721f
  drug interactions, 1732
  hypercalcemia treated with, 610-611
  hyperlipidemia caused by, 1731
  hypervolemia treated with, 450-451
  hypokalemia caused by, 1728
  hypomagnesemia caused by, 621
  idiopathic nephrotic syndrome treated with, 2329
  indications for, 1710
  lithium plasma concentrations affected by, 1732
  magnesium reabsorption affected by, 1730
  mechanism of action, 1705-1707, 1705f
  metabolic alkalosis caused by, 1704, 1730
  metabolism of, 1707-1708
  in nephrotic syndrome, 1725
  ototoxicity caused by, 1732
  pharmacokinetics of, 1707-1710
  proximal fluid reabsorption affected by, 1706
  renin secretion stimulation by, 1706-1707
  resistance to, 1718f, 1797
  sites of action, 1705-1707
  thiazide diuretics and, 1712-1713
  thromboxane A_2 excretion affected by, 1717
Loop of Henle, 1458f
  adaptations of, to nephron loss, 1746
  anatomy of, 45, 259-261
  bicarbonate reabsorption in, 238
  calcium reabsorption in, 188-189
  computer-assisted reconstruction of, 261f
  descending portion of, 259-260, 260f
  description of, 2302
  diuretic action on, 1705f

Loop of Henle *(Continued)*
  length of, 45
  potassium transport in, 175-176, 563-564
  sodium reabsorption by, 1747
  thick ascending limb of. *See* Thick ascending limb
  thin limbs of, 61-63, 63f-64f
Losartan potassium, 1309, 1652-1653, 1652t
Loss of appetite, 1819
Low birth weight
  acute kidney injury in, 711-712
  blood pressure in patients with, 707
  catch-up growth, 721
  chronic kidney disease in, 712, 2576
  congenital anomalies of the kidney and urinary tract and, 2300
  description of, 694, 694t
  dexamethasone and, 696-699
  glomerular filtration rate in, 710
  preeclampsia and, 1617-1618
  proteinuria and, 710-711
  risk factors for, 722
  treatment-induced decrease in blood pressure and, 1627f
Low osmolar contrast media, 847-848, 855-856
Low-density lipoprotein
  apheresis, 2159
  catabolism of, 1802
  description of, 1213, 1863
  mesangial cells affected by, 1761-1762
  in nephrotic syndrome, 1761, 1801
  normalization of, 1970
  oxidized, 1773
  reductions in, for cardiovascular disease prevention, 1868-1871, 1869f-1870f
  statins for reduction of, 1868-1869
Low-density lipoprotein receptor-related proteins 5 and 6, 1832-1833
Lower urinary tract abnormalities, 2296, 2311
Lower-molecular-weight iron dextran, 1896
Lowe's syndrome, 1438-1439, 2345
Low-molecular-weight proteins, 791, 1810t
Low-protein diet
  chronic kidney disease progression affected by, 1977, 1981-1982, 1994
  meta-analyses of, 1981-1982, 1982f
  after renal transplantation, 1977
  serum albumin affected by, 1312
  transforming growth factor-β affected by, 1958
Loxosceles spider bites, 2444, 2445f
Loxoscelism, 2444
LP1, 223t
L-type calcium channels, 1662
Luminal carbonic acid, 234
Luminal flow rate, 237
Lung, 317
Lupus erythematosus
  discoid, 1950, 1950f
  systemic. *See* Systemic lupus erythematosus
Lupus glomerulonephritis, 920
Lupus nephritis
  activity and chronicity, 1097
  azathioprine for, 1169-1170
  bortezomib for, 1105
  calcineurin inhibitors for, 1104
  classification of, 1094, 1094f-1096f, 1094t
  clinical manifestations of, 1098
  course of, 1100-1102
  cyclophosphamide for, 1102-1103
  cyclosporine, 1104
  description of, 1092

Lupus nephritis *(Continued)*
  dialysis for, 1100
  diffuse proliferative, 1098, 1102
  electron microscopy of, 1095f-1096f, 1097
  end-stage, 1098
  epidemiology of, 1092-1093
  in Far East, 2531-2532
  focal proliferative, 1098
  gender differences in, 658
  immunofluorescence microscopy of, 1095f-1096f, 1097
  immunosuppressive agents for, 1103, 1105
  intravenous immune globulin for, 1105
  kallikrein-kinin system in, 350
  membranous, 1098, 1101-1102, 1105
  methylprednisolone for, 1102-1103
  mycophenolate mofetil for, 1103-1104, 1169-1170
  natural history of, 1101-1102
  neutrophil extracellular traps in, 1093-1094
  ocrelizumab for, 1104
  pathogenesis of, 1093-1094
  pathology of, 1094-1097, 1094f-1096f, 1094t
  plasmapheresis for, 1105, 2151-2152
  prednisone for, 1102
  pregnancy and, 1100, 1634-1635
  prognosis for, 1100-1102
  proteinuria remission in, 1165-1166
  recurrence of, after renal transplantation, 2275
  renal transplantation for, 1100
  rituximab for, 1104
  serologic tests for, 1098-1099
  silent, 1098
  survival rates, 2532
  T cell activation therapies for, 1104-1105
  tacrolimus for, 1104-1105
  treatment of, 1102-1106, 2532
Lupus podocytopathy, 1097-1098
Luteinizing hormone, 1920-1921
Lymph node dissection, 1380-1381
Lymphangioleiomyomatosis, 1368-1369
Lymphatic capillaries, 80
Lymphatic system, 80, 80f
Lymphoceles, 910-911
Lymphocytes, 1793
Lymphoma, 899, 902f, 1401-1402
Lysinuric protein intolerance, 228, 1449
Lysosomal associated membrane protein 2, 1110
Lysosomes, 59-60, 61f, 284-285

M

Macroalbuminuria, 791-792
Macrolides, 1235t-1236t
Macromolecule, 1330-1331
Macrophages
  B cells and, 1216
  cytokines production by, 976, 1215-1216
  infiltrating, 1754-1755
  in proteinuria, 1793-1795
  T cells and, 1216
  in tubulointerstitial injury, 1794
Macrovascular diseases, 1201-1204
Macula densa
  anatomy of, 53-54
  basement membrane of, 54
  cells of, 106
  COX-2 expression in, 357-358, 359f, 360
  neuronal nitric oxide synthases in, 109
  nitric oxide production by, 108-109

Macula densa *(Continued)*
  renin release regulated by, 358-360, 359f
  in renin secretion, 1706
Magnesium
  absorption of, 2387
  blood pressure and, 623
  in bone, 193, 193t
  in cellular processes, 193
  in children, 2386-2389
  concentrations of, 186t, 193, 193t
  cytoplasmic, 581
  dietary intake of, 193-194
  disorders of
    hypermagnesemia. *See* Hypermagnesemia
    hypocalcemia caused by, 616-617
    hypomagnesemia. *See* Hypomagnesemia
  fractional excretion of, 619-621, 1706
  functions of, 193
  glomerulus filtration of, 194
  in hemodialysis dialysate, 2094
  homeostasis of, 193-194, 193f
  inherited disorders of processing of, 1465-1467
  intravenous replacement of, 624
  as kidney stone inhibitor, 1329-1330
  oral replacement of, 624-625
  in plasma, 193
  preeclampsia prevention and, 1626-1627
  reabsorption of, 194, 194f, 1468f, 1730
  recommended daily allowance of, 624
  regulation of, 2387
  renal wasting of, 620-622
  role of, 1465-1466
  serum, 193, 619, 2387
  serum concentration of, 193, 619, 2387
  tissue concentrations of, 193t
  transport of, 195-196, 195f, 195t, 1467t
  uptake of, factors that affect, 195t
  urinary excretion of, 194
Magnesium deficiency
  in acute myocardial infarction, 623
  bone compartment redistribution as cause of, 620
  bone mass decreases in, 623-624
  causes of, 619-622, 619f
  description of, 618-625
  diarrhea as cause of, 620
  dietary causes of, 620
  electrolyte homeostasis and, 624
  extrarenal causes of, 620
  hypokalemia and, 581, 823
  intravenous magnesium replacement for, 624
  metabolic acidosis caused by, 555
  migraine headache and, 624
  oral magnesium replacement for, 624-625
  potassium-sparing diuretics for, 625
  prevention of, 624
  treatment of, 624-625
Magnesium tolerance test, 618-619
Magnetic resonance angiography (MRA)
  acute kidney injury evaluations, 989-990
  contrast-enhanced, 859-861, 862f, 904-905, 906f, 1202
  fibromuscular dysplasia on, 907, 907f
  limitations of, 905-906
  motion artifacts associated with, 905-906
  phase-contrast, 859-861, 906
  renal artery stenosis on, 904-906
  renal artery stents on, 906-907, 906f
  renal transplantation applications of, 911, 912f

Magnetic resonance imaging (MRI), 856-864
  acute pyelonephritis on, 880
  acute tubular necrosis on, 870f
  autosomal dominant polycystic kidney disease on, 885-888, 889f, 1486f
  BOLD, 864, 1271
  clear cell carcinoma in von Hippel–Lindau disease, 890f
  contraindications for, 857
  corticomedullary differentiation on, 860f
  definition of, 856
  description of, 846
  diabetes insipidus diagnosis using, 485-486
  diffusion-weighted imaging, 863-864, 871f
  end-stage kidney disease on, 889f
  external magnetic field, 856
  gadolinium-chelate contrast media, 857-859, 878
    acute tubular necrosis imaging using, 870f
    adverse reactions to, 857
    applications of, 857
    chemical structure of, 858f
    description of, 857
    in nephrogenic systemic fibrosis, 858-859
    paramagnetic effects of, 858f
    recommendations for, 859
    in renal disease, 858-859
    technique for, 859, 861f
  hematoma evaluations, 876-878, 878f-879f
  immunoglobulin A nephropathy on, 870f
  implanted medical devices as contraindication for, 857
  kidney stone evaluations, 876, 876f, 1359-1360
  liver, for iron deposition evaluations, 1895
  lymphoma, 899, 902f
  principles of, 856
  pulse repetition time, 856-857
  pulse sequences, 856-857
  pyelonephritis on, 880, 882-883, 883f
  renal abscess on, 880, 882f
  renal cell carcinoma on, 892, 895f-897f
  renal cysts on, 883-885, 886f-887f, 889f
  renal function evaluations using, 863-864
  renal parenchymal disease on, 869, 870f, 880-881
  after renal transplantation, 910
  renal transplantation applications of, 870f, 911, 912f
  renal tuberculosis on, 884f
  renal vein thrombosis on, 909, 1205
  signal characteristics, 857f
  T1 weighting, 856-857
  T2 weighting, 856-857, 860f
  technique for, 859-863, 860f-863f
  tissue signal intensity, 856
  transitional cell carcinoma on, 898-899, 902f
  ureteral stone evaluations, 877f
  urinary tract obstruction on, 1267-1268, 1267f
  urine on, 857f-858f
  xanthogranulomatous pyelonephritis on, 883f
Magnetic resonance renography, 863
Magnetic resonance urography
  applications of, 863, 864f
  contrast media-enhanced, 861-863, 862f
  kidney stone evaluations, 876-878, 877f
  technique for, 861-863
  T2-weighted, 863
  ureteropelvic junction obstruction findings, 2315, 2315f
  urinary tract obstruction on, 1267-1268

Magnetic resonance urography *(Continued)*
MAGUK, 29
Major histocompatibility complex, 2230-2231, 2230f
Malabsorption syndromes, 620, 632-633
Malacoplakia, 881-882, 1262
Malaria, 1150. *See also Plasmodium falciparum*
  acute kidney injury caused by, 2496-2497, 2517-2520, 2519f-2521f
  in Africa, 2462
  clinical features of, 2496-2497
  clinical manifestations of, 2520f
  diagnosis of, 2497, 2519
  in Far East, 2517-2520, 2519f-2521f
  histologic features of, 2497
  in Indian subcontinent, 2496-2497
  in Latin America, 2442-2443
  in Middle East, 2470-2472
  nephropathy caused by, 2520f
  pathogenesis of, 2497
  renal lesions associated with, 2521f
  symptoms of, 2518
  treatment of, 2497, 2519-2520
Malaysia, 2535-2536
Malignancies
  alkylating agents and, 1169
  calcineurin inhibitors as cause of, 1168
  cyclophosphamide and, 1169
  diuretics as cause of, 1732
  glomerulonephritis associated with, 1403t
  hematuria and, 759f
  humoral hypercalcemia of, 603, 607-608
  hypercalcemia of, 1399-1400, 1399t
  membranous nephropathy, 1035, 1157
  pelvic, obstructive uropathy caused by, 1261
  syndrome of inappropriate antidiuretic hormone secretion associated with, 499
Malignant hypertension, 758, 1194-1195, 1765
Malignant neoplasm, 1370-1387
Malnutrition
  in acute kidney injury, 996
  atherosclerosis and, 1930
  in chronic kidney disease, 1971
  definition of, 1969
  in diabetes mellitus, 1315
  in hemodialysis, 1317-1318, 2089-2090, 2098t, 2504
  hypophosphatemia caused by, 632
  maternal. *See* Maternal malnutrition
  in peritoneal dialysis, 2504
  serum albumin levels used to diagnose, 1969
Malnutrition, inflammation, and atherosclerosis syndrome, 1970
Mammalian target of rapamycin, 1374
  description of, 238, 732-733
  inhibitors of, 2247, 2258, 2426. *See also* Everolimus; Sirolimus
Mammary-ulnar syndrome, 2297t
Manidipine, 1665
Mannitol, 1002, 1704, 1717
Maori. *See* New Zealand
Marrow infusion syndrome, 1394
Masked hypertension, 1540, 1540f
Mass transfer area coefficient, 2070-2071, 2112-2113
Masson's trichrome stain, 919-920
MATE1, 212t, 214-215
MATE2-K, 212t, 214-215
Maternal endothelial dysfunction, 1619
Maternal malnutrition, 715-717
Maternal obesity, 2576
Maternal overnutrition, 2576

Matrix extracellular phosphoglycoprotein, 201-202
Matrix gamma-carboxyglutamate protein, 1838
Matrix metalloproteinases, 977, 1794
Matrix vesicles, 1836-1837
Matrix-Gla protein, as kidney stone inhibitor, 1331
Maturity-onset diabetes type 5, 2299-2300, 2317
May-Hegglin anomaly, 1141
MDR1, 211, 212t
MDRD equation, 645, 677-678, 782, 784t, 785-786, 788, 2042-2043, 2526, 2544
MDRD study, 1553, 1979-1980, 1982-1983, 1994
Mechanical ventilation, 526
Meckel-Gruber syndrome, 1417, 1509, 2322, 2322t
Medial calcification, 1850
Medial fibroplasia, 1580-1581, 1580f
Medical expulsive therapy, 1360, 1360f
Medicare coverage, for end-stage kidney disease, 1524, 2558-2559, 2562, 2572, 2625, 2627f
Medicare Improvement for Patients and Providers Act of 2008, 2628-2629
Mediterranean diet, 1957
Medullary blood flow, 90, 362f
Medullary capillaries, 92
Medullary circulation, 105
Medullary collecting ducts
  functions of, 73-74
  inner, 44-45, 45f, 69-70, 74-75
  outer, 44-45, 45f, 69-70, 73-74, 133
  prostaglandin synthesis in, 365
  sodium absorption modulation by, 314
  solute transport in, 133
  water absorption in, 569
Medullary cystic kidney disease, 1504, 1504f
Medullary fibroma, 1369
Medullary interstitial cells, COX-2 expression in, 360-361
Medullary interstitium, 78-80, 79f, 262-264, 269f, 273
Medullary microcirculation, 86f, 90-92
Medullary osmotic gradient, 238
Medullary plasma flow, 403-404
Medullary potassium recycling, 175-176
Medullary ray collecting duct, 70
Medullary rays of Ferrein, 43
Medullary renal cell carcinoma, 1372
Medullary sponge kidney, 888-889, 1513-1514, 1513f
Medullary stromal cells, 5-6
Megalin, 56-59, 1791
Megalin-25, 2390
Megaloblastic anemia, 1883
Megaureter, primary, 2315-2316
Megestrol acetate, 1920
Melamine, 1348, 2526
Melphalan, 1131-1132
Membrane cofactor protein, 1184-1185, 2356
Membrane permeability constant, 2070-2071
Membrane-associated C-terminal fragment, 1791
Membranoproliferative glomerulonephritis
  algorithm for, 1046f
  C3 glomerulopathy variant of, 1047. *See also* C3 glomerulopathies; Dense deposit disease
  characteristics of, 2328-2329
  classification of, 1045-1046, 1046f
  complement alterations in, 1049
  complement-mediated, 1045-1046, 1046f

Membranoproliferative glomerulonephritis (Continued)
  hepatitis C-associated, 1155f, 2273
  immune complex-mediated, 1045-1046, 1046f, 1048-1049
  neoplasia associated with, 1157
  nephrotic syndrome caused by, 1045-1050
  primary, 1045
  recurrence of, after renal transplantation, 1155-1156, 2275, 2422, 2431
  respiratory tract infections associated with, 1053
  secondary causes of, 1049t
  subtypes of, 1045
  type I
    in children, 1049
    clinical features of, 1049
    electron microscopy findings of, 1047-1048, 1048f
    epidemiology of, 1049
    glomerular capillary wall findings in, 1048f
    glucocorticoids for, 1049-1050
    hyaline thrombi associated with, 1046, 1048
    immunofluorescence findings, 1046-1047, 1048f
    laboratory findings in, 1050t
    light microscopy findings, 1046, 1047f
    mesangial dense deposits in, 1047-1048
    mycophenolate mofetil for, 1050
    pathogenesis of, 1048-1049, 1049t
    pathology of, 1046-1048, 1047f·1048f, 1051f
    prognosis for, 1049
    treatment of, 1049-1050
    ultrastructural findings of, 1047-1048, 1047f
  type II, 1050t, 1051. See also Dense deposit disease
  type III, 1047-1048, 1050
  types of, 2328-2329
Membranous glomerulonephritis, 1164
Membranous nephropathy
  anticoagulation prophylaxis in, 1041-1042
  carcinoma associated with, 1157
  in children, 1041
  chlorambucil for, 1042-1043, 1169
  clinical features of, 1040-1041
  complement in, 1041
  deep vein thrombosis in, 1041
  electron microscopy findings, 1035-1037, 1036f·1037f, 1037t
  epidemiology of, 1035
  gender differences in, 657
  geographic variations in, 1035
  glomerular capillary wall findings in, 1037-1038, 1038f
  hepatitis C associated with, 1155
  HLA-DR3 and, 1040
  hypercoagulability associated with, 1041
  immune complex deposits in, 1039
  immunofluorescence microscopy findings, 1037-1038, 1037t, 1038f
  immunoglobulin G in, 1037-1039, 1038f
  interstitial disease in, 1039-1040
  laboratory findings in, 1041-1042, 1050t
  light microscopy findings, 1038, 1038f
  malignancies associated with, 1035, 1157
  mesangial dense deposits in, 1037, 1037t
  mesangial hypercellularity in, 1038
  natural history of, 1040-1041
  nephritogenic antigens in, 1038-1039
  nephrotic syndrome caused by, 1035-1045

Membranous nephropathy (Continued)
  pathogenesis of, 1038-1040
  pathology of, 1035-1038, 1036f·1038f, 1037t
  phospholipase A_2 receptors in, 1035, 1039
  podocytes in, 115t, 116
  progression of, 1038, 1040-1041, 1045
  proteinuria in, 1035, 1039-1041, 1158-1159
  recurrence of, 2275
  renal failure progression of, 1040-1041
  renal insufficiency associated with, 1040
  renal vein thrombosis in, 1041
  survival estimations in, 1040
  in systemic lupus erythematosus, 1037
  treatment of
    adrenocorticotropic hormone, 1044
    azathioprine, 1045
    calcineurin inhibitors, 1043-1044
    chlorambucil, 1042-1043
    corticosteroids, 1042
    cyclophosphamide, 1042-1043
    cyclosporine, 1043
    eculizumab, 1045
    methylprednisolone, 1042
    mycophenolate mofetil, 1044
    prednisolone, 1043
    rituximab, 1044-1045
    summary of, 1045
    tacrolimus, 1043-1044
  ultrastructural stages of, 1036-1037, 1036f
Mendelian disease, 1411
Mendelian randomization, 671
Mental health conditions, 2621
Meperidine, 2038, 2038t
Mercaptopropionylglycine, 1159
α-Mercaptopropionylglycine, 2346
6-Mercaptopurine, 2425
Mesangial advanced glycosylation end receptor 1, 730-731
Mesangial cells
  angiotensin II effects on, 99
  autacoid generation by, 52
  COX-1 localization to, 361f
  description of, 5
  extraglomerular, 53-54
  glomerular, 46f, 51-52
  glomerular function role of, 1744-1745, 1788
  β-integrin receptors on, 51-52
  low-density lipoprotein effects on, 1761-1762
  matrix of, 51-52
  microfilaments of, 51
  morphology of, 51
  in nephron development, 36
  nephron loss-related hemodynamic injury, 1753
  phagocytic properties of, 52
  platelet-derived growth factor-B effects on, 1789
  prostanoids effect on, 377
  proteinuria effects on, 1788-1789
  in renal hypertrophy, 1744-1745
  survival factors for, 1788
Mesangiocapillary glomerulonephritis, 1047-1048
Mesangioproliferative glomerulonephritis, 2327-2328
Mesenchymal stem cells (MSC)
  acute kidney injury applications of, 2611-2613
  in amniotic fluid and placenta, 2607
  bone marrow-derived, 2611

Mesenchymal stem cells (MSC) (Continued)
  description of, 2607
  differentiation of, into renal tissue, 2611
  immunosuppressive capabilities of, 2612-2613
Mesoamerican nephropathy, 2448-2449, 2451t
Mesonephros, 2-3, 3f, 20-21
Messenger RNA, 1738-1739, 2604-2605
Metabolic acidosis
  in acute kidney injury, 1003t, 1004
  added acids as cause of, 835-841
  ammonia excretion in, 246f
  anion gap in, 528
  anorexia caused by, 2125
  assessment of, 835-837, 836t
  bicarbonate reabsorption affected by, 238, 830
  calcium reabsorption affected by, 191
  carbonic anhydrase inhibitors as cause of, 1730
  causes of, 834t-835t
  characteristics of, 522
  in children, 2382-2383, 2382t, 2405
  in chronic heart failure patients, 556-557
  in chronic kidney disease, 542, 1913, 2004, 2357, 2359
  citrate excretion in, 247
  clinical approach to, 833-841
  collecting duct's response to, 244
  compensatory responses for, 518t
  Cushing's disease as cause of, 556
  definition of, 833
  distal renal tubular acidosis. See Distal renal tubular acidosis
  drugs that cause, 547-548
  extracellular volume expansion as cause of, 555
  glucocorticoid-remediable hyperaldosteronism as cause of, 555-556
  glutamate dehydrogenase activity affected by, 253
  glutamine transport affected by, 251
  hemodialysis for correction of, 2094-2095
  high anion gap. See High anion gap acidosis
  high-protein diet and, 1971
  hypercalciuria associated with, 191
  hyperchloremic, 528-530, 529t, 764, 768, 2382-2383
  hyperkalemic hyperchloremic, 536t, 538, 541
  hyperphosphatemia caused by, 628
  hypertension as cause of, 555
  hypokalemia and, 821, 1723
  hypovolemia with, 424
  after ketoacidosis treatment, 555
  after lactic acidosis treatment, 555
  licorice ingestion as cause of, 556
  Liddle's syndrome as cause of, 556
  magnesium ion deficiency as cause of, 555
  non-anion gap, 528-530, 529t, 532, 536
  nonreabsorbable anions as cause of, 555
  pathophysiology of, 528
  peritoneal dialysis for correction of, 2125
  phosphate excretion increases in, 247
  potassium ion deficiency as cause of, 555
  primary aldosteronism as cause of, 555
  proximal tubule bicarbonate reabsorption affected by, 236-237
  proximal tubule phosphate-dependent glutaminase activity affected by, 253
  in renal transplantation recipients, 2281

Metabolic acidosis (Continued)
  renin levels and, 555-556
  salicylates as cause of, 547-548
  symptoms of, 556
  titratable acid in, 246f
  toluene metabolism as cause of, 843f
  treatment of, 556-557, 2004
Metabolic alkalosis
  acid-base transport changes secondary to, 244
  assessment of, 831
  Bartter's syndrome as cause of, 551-552, 554
  bicarbonate administration as cause of, 552-553
  calcium reabsorption affected by, 191
  case studies of, 831-833
  causes of, 551-552, 551t, 832t
  characteristics of, 522
  chloride deficiency in, 520
  citrate administration as cause of, 2163
  citrate excretion in, 247
  clinical approach to, 831
  compensatory responses for, 518t
  congenital chloridorrhea as cause of, 553
  diagnosis of, 550-552, 552f, 552t
  diuretics as cause of, 553, 1704
  edematous states as cause of, 553
  gastric aspiration as cause of, 553
  gastrointestinal causes of, 553
  Gitelman's syndrome as cause of, 551-552, 554-555
  hypercapnic response to, 519
  hypokalemia in, 550-551, 821-823
  hypoventilation caused by, 519
  after ketoacidosis treatment, 555
  after lactic acidosis treatment, 555
  loop diuretics as cause of, 1704, 1730
  milk-alkali syndrome as cause of, 553
  mixed, 550-552
  pathophysiology of, 550f
  posthypercapnia as cause of, 553-554
  potassium deficiency in, 520
  respiratory compensation for, 550
  simple, 550-552
  villous adenoma as cause of, 553
  vomiting as cause of, 525, 553
Metabolic evaluation, 1356, 1357t-1358t
Metabolic substrates, 126-132
Metabolic syndrome, 679-680, 1350-1351, 1770-1771, 1992, 2284, 2433
Metabolism
  angiotensin II's role in, 139
  basics of, 126-127
  cortical collecting duct, 133
  definition of, 122
  natriuretic peptides effect on, 342-343
  renal autoregulation mediation by, 109-110
  thermodynamic approach to, 123
Metal-binding proteins, 1018t
Metanephric adenoma, 1368
Metanephric blastema, 44-45
Metanephric mesenchyme
  bone morphogenetic protein-7 expression in, 29
  cell populations in, 7f
  condensing, 29, 31
  description of, 3
  early lineage determination of, 21
  endothelial progenitors within, 6
  gene expression in, 2298-2299
  non-GDNF pathways in, 23
  stromal cells from, 5-6
  ureteric bud and, 4f, 5-6, 21-25

Metanephros, 2-3, 3f, 6-7, 7f-8f, 22f, 2603, 2613-2615
Metastases
  cutaneous, 1949
  imaging of, 899, 902f
  recurrence rate of, 1381
  renal cell carcinoma, 896f, 1949
  resection of, 1381
  treatment of, 1385
Metastatic calcifications, 1945-1946
Metformin, 1315, 1915, 2184-2185
Methanol, 548-549, 2173-2178, 2174f, 2176t
Methotrexate, 990, 1113, 1398, 2188-2189
Methoxypolyethylene glycol epoetin beta, 1892
Methylcobalamin, 2100
Methyl-β-cyclodextrin, 292f
Methyldopa, 1629, 1630t, 1671-1672, 1671t-1672t, 1695t, 1698
Methylguanidine, 1810-1811
Methylprednisolone
  anti-glomerular basement membrane disease treated with, 1126-1127
  immune complex-mediated crescentic glomerulonephritis treated with, 1076
  lupus nephritis treated with, 1102-1103
  membranous nephropathy treated with, 1042
  pauci-immune crescentic glomerulonephritis treated with, 1087-1089
Metolazone, 450
Metoprolol, 1656t-1657t, 1658, 1660-1661
Metyrosine, 1679-1680
Microalbuminuria, 1556
  angiotensin-converting enzyme inhibitors for, 1305-1306, 1999
  as biomarker, 948
  cardiovascular disease and, 1295
  course of, 1296-1298
  criteria for, 1785-1786
  definition of, 791-792, 1296-1297, 1785-1786
  in diabetic nephropathy, 1289-1290, 1292t
  end-stage kidney disease in, 1303f
  hormone replacement therapy and, 659-660
  as hyperfiltration sign, 710
  incidence of, 1292-1294, 1292t
  microvascular complications in, 1302f
  in New Zealand, 2550
  oral contraceptives and, 659-660
  pathophysiology of, 1296-1298
  prevalence of, 1292-1294, 1292t
  primary prevention of, 1301-1302
  prognosis for, 1294-1295
  renin-angiotensin-aldosterone system blockade for prevention of, 1304
  secondary prevention of, 1302
  smoking and, 1777, 1991-1992
Microcirculations
  description of, 6
  glomerular, 92-94, 92f
  medullary. See Medullary microcirculation
  types of, 83
  vasomotor properties of, 98-99
Micro-computed tomography, 1846-1847
β_1-microglobulin, 937-938, 1041
β_2-microglobulin, 938, 1810, 1949
Micro-magnetic resonance imaging, for bone assessments, 1846-1847
Micronutrients, 1983
Microorganisms, in urine, 802
MicroRNA-21, 729-730

Microscopic agglutination test, for leptospirosis, 2444
Microscopic hematuria, 754-755, 799, 1022, 1065, 1198-1199
Microscopic polyangiitis
  antineutrophil cytoplasmic antibodies in, 1114-1115
  in children, 2351
  clinical features of, 1115
  cyclophosphamide for, 1112-1113, 1115-1116
  electron microscopy of, 1115
  in Far East, 2532
  immunofluorescence microscopy of, 1115
  laboratory tests for, 1115
  light microscopy of, 1114-1115, 1114f
  pathogenesis of, 1110, 1115
  pathology of, 1114-1115, 1114f
  prognosis for, 1115-1116
  proteinuria in, 1115
  recurrence of, after renal transplantation, 2275
  renal findings in, 1115
  treatment of, 1115-1116
Microtubules, 295, 296f
Microvascular diseases
  antiphospholipid syndrome. See Antiphospholipid syndrome
  atheroembolic renal disease, 1191-1193, 1192f
  chronic cognitive impairment secondary to, 1936
  endothelial cell injury in, 1175
  glycemic control for, 1871
  hemolytic-uremic syndrome. See Hemolytic-uremic syndrome
  overview of, 1175-1201
  radiation nephropathy, 1193-1195
  scleroderma. See Scleroderma
  sickle cell disease. See Sickle cell disease
  thrombotic microangiopathies. See Thrombotic microangiopathies
  thrombotic thrombocytopenia purpura. See Thrombotic thrombocytopenia purpura
Microvascular injury, 1197
Microvascular rarefaction, 1578f
Microvascular thrombosis, 1179f
Microvilli, 56-59, 2111
Micturition cystourethrography, 2313
Middle East
  acute kidney injury in, 2469-2472
  Bartter's syndrome in, 2479
  chronic kidney disease in, 2472-2486, 2477t, 2480t-2482t, 2483f
  chronic kidney disease–mineral bone disorder in, 2488
  consanguinity rates in, 2476
  countries of, 2468, 2469f
  cystinuria in, 2478-2479
  definition of, 2468
  demographics of, 2470t
  diabetes mellitus in, 2472, 2476
  dialysis in, 2487-2489
  disasters in, 2472, 2473f
  earthquakes in, 2472
  end-stage kidney disease in
    diabetes mellitus as cause of, 2476
    familial Mediterranean fever and, 2486
    hemodialysis for, 2487-2488
    hepatitis with, 2488-2489
    management of, 2486-2492
    peritoneal dialysis for, 2487
    statistics regarding, 2473-2474

Middle East (Continued)
  Fabry's disease in, 2479
  familial Mediterranean fever in. See Familial Mediterranean fever
  genetic kidney diseases in, 2476-2486, 2477t, 2480t-2482t, 2483f
  Gitelman's syndrome in, 2479
  health care expenditures in, 2471f
  health indicators in, 2470t
  hemodialysis in, 2475t, 2487-2488
  Human Development Index in, 2470t
  life expectancy in, 2468, 2470t
  malaria in, 2470-2472
  map of, 2469f
  mortality rate in, 2468, 2470t
  nephrolithiasis in, 2478-2479
  peritoneal dialysis in, 2475t, 2487
  population of, 2468
  primary hyperoxaluria type 1 and 2 in, 2478
  renal hypoplasia in, 2479
  renal parenchymal disease in, 2469-2470
  renal replacement therapy in
    hemodialysis, 2475t, 2487-2488
    peritoneal dialysis, 2475t, 2487
    statistics regarding, 2475t
  renal transplantation in, 2475t, 2489-2492
  summary of, 2492
  wealth in, 2471f
Midodrine and octreotide, for hepatorenal syndrome, 456
Milk-alkali syndrome, 553, 609-610
Mineral metabolism, 2102-2103
  disordered, 1850-1851, 2019-2023
  in peritoneal dialysis patients, 2132
Mineralocorticoid(s)
  antagonists of, 591-592
  bicarbonate reabsorption affected by, 238
  excess of, 320, 1547
  hyperkalemia treated with, 595-596
  resistance, 540
Mineralocorticoid receptors
  aldosterone action and, 306f
  aldosterone binding to, 310
  cortisol binding by, 309
  description of, 304-305, 1679
  distal convoluted tubule expression of, 315
  DNA-binding domain of, 307-308, 308f
  domain structure of, 307-310, 308f-309f
  expression sites for, 315
  functioning of, 306-310
  glomerulus expression of, 315
  as hormone-regulated transcription factor, 306-307
  11β-hydroxysteroid dehydrogenase type 2 effects on, 320
  intercalated cell, 314
  ligand/hormone-binding domain of, 307-309, 309f
  N-terminal domain of, 310
  nuclear translocation of, 307f
  preinitiation complex, 310
  proximal convoluted tubule expression of, 315
  thick ascending limb expression of, 315
  transcription initiation, 310
Minimal change disease
  acute renal failure associated with, 1021
  bone mineral density reductions in, 1022
  in children, 1021, 1023
  clinical features of, 1021-1022, 1021t
  conditions associated with, 1021, 1021t
  corticosteroids for, 1022-1023, 1023t

Minimal change disease (Continued)
  cyclophosphamide for, 1023
  cyclosporine for, 1023-1024
  in elderly, 746
  electron microscopy findings in, 1019, 1019f-1020f
  epidemiology of, 1016-1024
  food allergy and, 1021
  genetic findings in, 1020
  hemopexin in, 1020
  in Hodgkin's disease, 1021, 1157
  Hodgkin's lymphoma and, 1404
  IgA nephropathy and, 1404
  immunofluorescence microscopy findings in, 1019
  incidence of, 1016
  interleukin-13 in, 1020
  laboratory findings in, 1022, 1050t
  light microscopy findings in, 1015t, 1016-1019
  lithium as cause of, 1159
  mesangial dense deposits in, 1019
  natural history of, 1021-1022
  nephrotic syndrome caused by, 1016-1034, 1158
  nonsteroidal anti-inflammatory drugs that cause, 1021, 1021t
  pathogenesis of, 1019-1021
  pathology of, 1016-1019
  podocyte foot process effacement in, 1019, 1020f
  prednisone for, 1022-1024, 1167
  proteinuria in, 1022
  steroid-resistant, 1023-1024
  T cell abnormalities in, 1019-1020
  treatment of, 1022-1024
  tumor necrosis factor-related apoptosis-induced ligand alterations in, 1020
Minimal change nephropathy, 114-116, 115t
Minimal inhibitory concentrations, 2041
Mini-Mental State Examination, 1936-1937
Minoxidil, 1674, 1674t, 1692
Minute ventilation, 1612
miRNAs, 36
Mithramycin, 1400
Mitochondria, 142
Mitochondrial diseases, 142
Mitochondrial disorder, 1432
Mitral valve calcification, 1859
Mitral valve prolapse, 1492
Mixed acid-base disorders, 521-523, 525, 550-552
Mixed chimerism, 2249
Mixed connective tissue disease, 1108-1109
Mixed cryoglobulinemia, 1137-1138, 1155, 2152
Mixed epithelial stromal tumor, 1369-1370, 1517
Mixed lymphocyte reaction, 2235
Mixed metabolic-respiratory disturbance, 522
Mixed uremic osteodystrophy, 1843, 1844f
Mixed-bed ion-exchange system, 2081
Mixing entropy, 122
Model of End-stage Liver Disease, 458
Modification of Diet in Renal Disease study. See MDRD study
Moexipril hydrochloride, 1643, 1643t
Molecular Adsorbent Recirculating System, 457-458, 2171
Mönckeberg's calcification, 1833-1835
Mönckeberg's sclerosis, 1855-1856
Moncrief-Popovich catheter, 2115-2116

Monoclonal antibodies, 2248-2249, 2255-2256
Monoclonal gammopathies, 1030, 1071
Monoclonal immunoglobulin deposition disease, 1134-1136, 1135f
Monocyte chemoattractant protein-1, 729, 950-951, 967-968, 1148, 1215-1216
Monocytes, 1792-1793
Monogenic disease, 1411, 1411t
Monogenic hypercalciuria, rodent models for, 1350t
Monomethylamine, 1812-1813
Mononeuropathy, 1939
Moxonidine, 1671-1672, 1671t-1672t
Mucormycosis, 1405
Muehrcke's lines, 762
Muir-Torre syndrome, 1952-1953, 1952t
Multicystic dysplastic kidney, 889, 1510-1511, 2294-2296, 2295f, 2303, 2305, 2312-2313, 2312f
Multidetector computed tomography, 851
Multidrug resistance protein, 375
Multilocular cystic nephroma, 1369-1370, 1517
Multimedia depth filters, for hemodialysis water treatment, 2081
Multiple cutaneous and uterine leiomyoma, 1373-1374
Multiple endocrine neoplasia, 608, 1548
Multiple myeloma
  acute kidney injury and, 990, 1002, 1390, 2152
  cast nephropathy and, 1391
  diagnosis of, 1391
  in elderly, 746
  free light chains in, 2152, 2153f
  incidence of, 1390-1391
  kidney involvement and, 1391
  manifestations of, 1392
  plasmapheresis for, 2153t
  presentation of, 1391
  treatment of, 1392-1393
Multiple-dose activated charcoal, 2168, 2183
Multipotent adult progenitor cell, 2607-2608
Multivesicular bodies, 59-60
Muromonab-CD3, 1637t, 2248, 2255, 2423
Muscle
  atrophy of, 1965-1968
  catabolism of, 1967
  potassium depletion in, 1968
  protein losses, 1965, 1966f, 1970
Muscle cramps, 2107
Muscle wasting, 1817
Mushrooms, 2525-2526
Myasthenia gravis, 2158
Mycobacterium tuberculosis, 1150, 1252-1253
Mycophenolate mofetil (MMF)
  adverse effects of, 1170, 2257-2258, 2330
  in children, 2425-2426
  focal segmental glomerulosclerosis treated with, 1033
  glomerular disease treated with, 1170
  granulomatous with polyangiitis treated with, 1113-1114
  hematologic complications of, 1170
  immunoglobulin A nephropathy treated with, 1068, 2531
  immunosuppressive uses of, 2245-2246, 2246f, 2254t, 2257-2258, 2425-2426
  lupus nephritis treated with, 1103-1104, 1169-1170
  membranoproliferative glomerulonephritis type I treated with, 1050

Mycophenolate mofetil (MMF) *(Continued)*
   membranous nephropathy treated with, 1044
   during pregnancy, 1637-1638, 1637t
   steroid-resistant nephrotic syndrome treated with, 2331
   steroid-sensitive nephrotic syndrome treated with, 2330
   toxicity of, 1170
Mycophenolate sodium, 2258
Mycophenolic acid, 2245-2246, 2246f, 2426
Mycophenolic acid glucuronide, 2245-2246
Myeloma cast nephropathy, 990, 1002. *See also* Cast nephropathy
Myeloma cells, 603
Myeloperoxidase, 1910
MYH9, 1028
Myocardial disease, 1858f
Myocardial fibrosis, 1858-1859
Myocardial infarction, 1351f
Myocardial stunning, 2079, 2107
MYO1E, 2326
MYO1E disease, 1430-1431
Myoepithelial cells, 53
Myofibrillar proteins, 1965
Myofibroblasts, 977, 1763
Myogenic mechanism, for renal autoregulation, 105-106
Myoglobin, 790, 967
Myoinositol, 1813
Myosin I, 294-295
Myosin light-chain kinase, 294-295
Myostatin, 1967-1968

N

N-Acetylcysteine, 856, 1000
N-acetyl-β-D-glucosaminidase, 947
NaDC transporters, 217-218, 217f-218f, 218t
NADH, 132
Nadolol, 1656t-1657t, 1657
Na^+-H^+ exchangers
   ammonia metabolism and, 253
   insulin effects on, 818
   isoform 3, 136, 1273
   knockout mice model of, 278
   in proximal tubule bicarbonate reabsorption, 235
Nail-patella syndrome, 762, 1142-1143, 1143f, 1431
Na^+-K^+-ATPase. *See* Sodium pump
Na^+-K^+-ATPase enzyme, 560
Na^+-K^+-$2Cl^-$ cotransporter, 254, 278, 299
Nandrolone decanoate, 1922
National Cooperative Dialysis Study, 2082-2083
National Health Service Corps, 2583-2584
National Institutes of Health prostatitis classification, 1247, 1247t
National Kidney Foundation Kidney Disease Outcomes Quality Initiative, 773, 773t, 1736, 1818, 1957-1958, 1958t
Native kidney, 2069, 2089, 2610
Natriuresis, 342, 410-411
Natriuretic hormones, 152-153
Natriuretic peptide(s), 1534
   actions of, 342-343
   acute tubular necrosis treated with, 1001
   antifibrotic effects of, 342
   atrial. *See* Atrial natriuretic peptide
   brain. *See* Brain natriuretic peptide
   in cardiac remodeling, 342
   cardiovascular effects of, 342
   central nervous system effects of, 342
   in cirrhosis, 447-449
   C-type. *See* C-type natriuretic peptide

Natriuretic peptide(s) *(Continued)*
   definition of, 339
   Dendroaspis. *See Dendroaspis* natriuretic peptide
   as disease biomarkers, 343-344
   in effective arterial blood volume regulation, 413-415
   in heart failure, 433-435, 453
   metabolism mediation by, 342-343
   nephron loss adaptations and, 1739
   neutral endopeptidase, 341-342, 345, 413
   as renal disease biomarkers, 343-344
   renal effects of, 342
   in sodium retention, 447-449
   structure of, 339-341, 339f
   synthesis of, 339-341
   therapeutic uses of, 344-345
   types of, 339
   urodilatin. *See* Urodilatin
Natriuretic peptide precursor type A, 339-341
Natriuretic peptide precursor type C, 340-341
Natriuretic peptide receptors
   -A, 341
   -B, 341-342
   biologic effects of, 341
   -C, 341
   description of, 341
   kinase homology domain of, 341
Nausea, 469-470, 469f
NBC3, 243-244
NBCe.1, 530
NBCe1-A, 234-237
NCC, 66-68, 580
Nck1, 38
Nck2, 38
Near and Middle East. *See* Middle East
Nebivolol, 1658t-1659t, 1659
Necrosis, 586, 921t, 974-975
Necrotizing pancreatitis, 1732
Nedd4-2, 172-173, 312, 318-319, 565
Neoadjuvant therapy, 1382
Neointimal hyperplasia, 2194, 2195f, 2202
Neonatal severe hyperparathyroidism, 608, 2395-2396
Neonates
   hypercalcemia in, 2394t
   hyperphosphatemia in, 2389
   renal vein thrombosis in, 1206
Neoplasia, 1157
Neoplasms
   angiomyolipomas, 891, 893f
   benign, 1368-1370
   benign cystic, 1369-1370
   cystic, 1516-1517
   imaging of, 891
   malignant, 1370-1387
   oncocytoma, 891-892
   after renal transplantation, 911
Neph1, 38
Nephelometry, 794-795
Nephrectomy, 1379. *See also* Partial nephrectomy
   adjuvant therapy after, 1381
   allograft, 2290
   cytoreductive, 1381
   for emphysematous pyelonephritis, 1251
   glomerulus changes after, 1751f
   inferior vena caval involvement with tumor thrombus and, 1381
   proteinuria after, 1752f
   renal hypertrophy after, 1742
   whole-kidney responses to, 1741-1742, 1742f

Nephrin, 37-38, 113, 936-937, 1413-1414, 1414t, 1426, 2323
Nephrin disease, 1426-1428
Nephritic syndrome
   characteristics of, 757
   in children, 2331-2333
   complement levels in, 759-760, 759t
   diagnostic approach, 757-760, 759t-760t
   glomerular hematuria associated with, 758-759
Nephritis
   acute interstitial. *See* Acute interstitial nephritis
   allergic interstitial, 984t-985t, 1158
   anti-thin basement membrane, 1228-1229
   granulomatous interstitial, 1228
   interstitial, 1158
   shunt, 1149
   tubulointerstitial, 1220-1221
Nephroblastoma, 1386-1387
Nephrocalcinosis, 1417
   in children, 2340
   description of, 534-535, 871-873, 2385
   familial hypomagnesemia with, 1466
   familial hypomagnesemia with hypercalciuria and, 2387-2388
   genetic causes of, 1349f
   hypercalcemia and dehydration as cause of, 2393-2394
Nephrogenesis
   COX-2 inhibitors effect on, 719
   cyclosporine effects on, 719
   gentamicin effects on, 719
   β-lactam effects on, 719
   onset of, 699
   penicillin effects on, 719
   tripartite inductive interactions regulating, 28f
Nephrogenic diabetes insipidus (NDI), 1470
   acquired causes of, 285, 297
   amiloride for, 489
   aquaporin-2 and, 285, 298f, 481-482, 2338
   calcitonin for, 301
   causes of, 285, 297, 480-482
   in children, 2338-2339, 2368-2370, 2370t
   congenital, 285, 480-481, 2338, 2369-2370
   definition of, 2338, 2368
   description of, 285
   desmopressin test for, 484, 2338
   diagnosis of, 809, 2338
   heat shock protein 90 for, 301-302
   hereditary, 285, 297
   history of, 480-481
   hypernatremia prevention in, 2338
   knockout mouse models of, 282
   lithium as cause of, 297-299, 298f, 379, 482, 1226
   molecular therapies for, 2338-2339
   pathophysiology of, 482
   phosphodiesterase inhibitors for, 300-301
   prostaglandins for, 301
   secretin for, 301
   statins for, 301
   treatment of, 285, 300-302, 489-490, 2338-2339
   type II, 285
   X-linked, 278-279, 300, 1470-1473, 2338
Nephrogenic syndrome of inappropriate antidiuresis, 499
Nephrogenic syndrome of inappropriate diuresis, 2372-2373
Nephrogenic systemic fibrosis, 858-859, 1947-1948, 1948f-1949f
Nephrogenic zone, 4f-5f, 5, 28-29
Nephrogram, 847f

Nephrolithiasis, 1417, 1419
  acetazolamide as risk factor for, 1704
  in children. See Children, nephrolithiasis in
  diagnostic approach, 767-769
  differential diagnosis of, 769, 769t
  diuretics for, 1726
  hypercalciuric, 2340, 2344-2345, 2344f
  in Indian subcontinent, 2507
  medications associated with, 767
  metabolic syndrome and, 1350-1351
  in Middle East, 2478-2479
  nonsteroidal anti-inflammatory drugs for, 769
  obesity and, 1351f
  predisposing medical conditions for, 767-768
  prevalence of, 767, 1260
  risk factors for, 767
  risk of developing, 873
  in sarcoidosis, 1228
  symptoms of, 767
  treatment of, 769, 1493
  ureteral obstruction caused by, 1260
Nephrologist referral, 2063, 2595-2596
Nephromegaly, 2320f
Nephron, 44-69
  active transport along, 126-132
  anatomy of, 44-69, 45f
  autonomic innervation of, 54-55
  components of, 44-45
  cortical, 45
  development of, 4-5, 30-31, 36-39, 44-45, 2309
  distal
    aldosterone-sensitive, 311f, 314-315, 316f, 319-320
    calcium transport mechanisms in, 190f
    cortical, potassium secretion in, 819
    development of, 30
    intercalated cells in, 166
    potassium in, 563-564
    potassium secretion by, vasopressin effects on, 182
    sodium chloride and potassium transport in, 182-183
  diuretics site of action in, 1703f
  generalized dysfunction of, 541t
  gluconeogenic enzymes along, 131f
  high-affinity adrenergic receptors in, 405
  juxtaglomerular, angiotensin II effects on, 99, 100f
  juxtamedullary, 45, 45f, 85, 89f, 90-91, 93
  lactate production along, 130-132
  long-looped, 259
  low mass, knockout and transgenic models for studying, 10t-17t
  maturation of, 5
  number of, 44-45
  phosphorus reabsorption along, 198-199, 199f
  secretory nature of, 204
  short-looped, 259
  sodium pump activity along, 142, 146f
  substrates along, 131f
  tight junctions in, 147f
  types of, 259
Nephron endowment
  chronic kidney disease risks, 676, 1769
  development programming of, 696-701
  kidney transplantation affected by, 723-724
  low, 1769

Nephron loss
  chronic kidney disease risks, 676-678, 1991f
  focal segmental glomerulosclerosis caused by, 1029
  glomerular hemodynamic adaptations to
    bradykinin, 1740
    description of, 1737-1738
    eicosanoids in, 1740
    endothelins in, 1739
    mediators of, 1738-1741
    natriuretic peptides in, 1739
    nitric oxide in, 1740
    renin angiotensin aldosterone system in, 1738-1739
    urotensin II, 1740
  injury after
    acidosis, 1758-1759
    aldosterone, 1757
    angiotensin II, 1756-1757
    bone morphogenetic protein-7, 1757-1758
    cellular infiltration in remnant kidneys, 1754-1755
    description of, 1755
    endothelial cells in, 1752-1753
    hepatocyte growth factor, 1757
    hypertrophy, 1759
    mechanical stress in, 1752
    mesangial cells in, 1753
    microRNAs, 1758
    oxidative stress, 1758
    podocytes, 1753-1754
    proteinuria, 1760-1763
    transforming growth factor-β, 1755-1756
  long-term adverse consequences of adaptations to, 1750-1752, 1751f-1752f
  mesangial cell response to, 1744-1745
  renal autoregulatory mechanism adjustments to, 1740-1741
  renal hypertrophic responses to
    algorithm for, 1745f
    description of, 1741
    endocrine effects, 1744
    glomerular enlargement, 1742-1743
    growth factors, 1744
    mechanisms involved in, 1745f
    mechanisms of, 1743-1745
    mesangial cells, 1744-1745
    renotropic factors, 1743-1744
    solute load, 1743
    tubular cell responses, 1745
    whole-kidney, 1741-1742, 1742f
  tubule function adaptations to
    acid-base regulation, 1749
    calcium metabolism, 1749-1750
    description of, 1745
    distal nephron, 1746
    glomerulotubular balance, 1746-1747
    loop of Henle, 1746
    phosphate metabolism, 1749-1750
    potassium excretion, 1748-1749
    proximal tubule solute handling, 1745-1746
    sodium excretion, 1747-1748
    urinary concentration and dilution, 1748
Nephron mass, 724, 2278
Nephron number
  birth weight and, 703-705
  blood pressure and, 697t-698t, 709, 709f
  congenital deficit in, 701
  genetic variants associated with, 713-715
  glomerular volume and, 696

Nephron number (Continued)
  glomerulomegaly associated with, 705
  intrauterine growth restriction effects on, 700f
  kidney size as correlate of, 700-701, 700f
  low, 705, 705t, 721
  maternal hyperglycemia effects on, 717f
  maternal nutrient restrictions that affect, 716
  maternal vitamin A restriction effects on, 716
  plausibility of, 695-696
  postnatal augmentation of, 701
  prematurity and, 703-705
  programming of, in humans, 699-701
  renal size and, 697t-698t
  rescue of, 720-721
  variability of, 676, 695t, 699, 724
  vitamin A deficiency effects on, 716, 721
Nephronectin gene, 25
Nephronophthisis, 1508-1509, 2321-2322
Nephronophthisis-related ciliopathies, 1416-1417, 2321
Nephron-sparing surgery, 1379-1380
Nephropathy
  acute phosphate, 966-967
  analgesic, 686, 1221-1223, 1223f-1224f, 2544-2546
  antiphospholipid, 1106-1107
  aristolochic acid, 1223-1226, 2534
  Balkan endemic, 1224-1226, 1225f
  BK virus-associated, 2428-2429
  bone marrow transplantation, 1193-1194
  cadmium, 1227
  Chinese herb, 1223-1224, 1225f, 2534
  chronic allograft, 2244, 2273, 2425, 2431
  contrast media-induced, 853-856
  C1q, 1034-1035
  hepatitis B-associated, 1154-1155
  heroin, 1157-1158
  hypertensive, 2459
  hypokalemic, 2375
  in Latin America, 2448-2449
  lead, 686-687, 1227
  malarial, 2520f
  Mesoamerican, 2448-2449, 2451t
  myeloma cast, 990, 1002
  nonsteroidal antiinflammatory drug-induced, 1158
  obstructive. See Obstructive nephropathy
  salt-losing, 493
  sickle cell, 1145-1146, 1145f
  urate, 1227-1228
  warfarin-related, 1068
Nephrotic syndrome, 1435
  acute kidney injury in, 991t, 994
  albumin stores in, 1796-1797
  in amyloidosis, 1129
  anticoagulant abnormalities in, 1803-1804
  anticoagulation prophylaxis in, 1206-1207
  anticonvulsants that cause, 1159
  antithrombin III deficiency in, 1206, 1803
  biochemical findings in, 760
  characteristics of, 1016
  in children. See Children, nephrotic syndrome in
  coagulation factors in, 1018t
  deep vein thrombosis in, 1804
  diagnostic approach, 761-764
  diuretics for, 1723f, 1724-1725
  edema associated with, 761, 1798-1800, 1798f/1799f
  in elderly, 746-747
  in Epstein-Barr virus infection, 1151

Nephrotic syndrome (Continued)
  etiology of, 1016
  glomerular diseases that cause
    acute poststreptococcal glomerulonephritis, 1054-1059
    C3 glomerulopathies, 1045-1046, 1050-1054
    C1q nephropathy, 1034-1035
    fibrillary glomerulonephritis, 1069-1072
    focal segmental glomerulosclerosis, 1024-1035
    immunoglobulin A nephropathy, 1059-1069
    immunotactoid glomerulopathy, 1069-1072
    list of, 1017t-1018t
    membranoproliferative glomerulonephritis, 1045-1050
    membranous nephropathy, 1035-1045
    minimal change disease, 1016-1034
  gold salts and, 1158
  after graft-versus-host disease, 1021
  high-density lipoprotein in, 1801
  hypercoagulability in, 1803-1805, 1803f
  hyperlipidemia associated with, 1801-1803, 1801f, 1803f, 1816-1817
  hypoalbuminemia caused by, 1796-1798, 1796f
  hypocalcemia in, 1797-1798
  hyponatremia in, 494-495
  hypovolemia in, 422-423
  in Indian subcontinent, 2506t
  infection susceptibility in, 1805
  intrarenal sodium retention in, 1801
  lipiduria associated with, 762-763, 763f
  lipoprotein in, 1802
  loop diuretics in, 1725
  low-density lipoprotein in, 1761, 1801
  mechanisms of, 761
  nail-patella syndrome with, 762
  nonsteroidal antiinflammatory drugs as cause of, 363, 1158
  plasma protein alterations in, 1018t
  plasmin-induced fibrinolysis reduction in, 1804
  platelet aggregation in, 1804
  protein requirements in, 1976-1977
  in proteinuria, 1796
  pulmonary embolism in, 1805
  renal artery stenosis associated with, 1159
  renal vein thrombosis in, 1204-1206, 1804
  renal water handling defects associated with, 1800
  renin-angiotensin-aldosterone system inhibition in, 1799
  secondary, 760, 760t
  skin findings, 762
  steroid-resistant, 1413-1415, 1414t
    calcineurin inhibitors for, 2330-2331
    characteristics of, 1428-1429
    description of, 2323
    focal segmental glomerulosclerosis in, 2328
    genetics of, 1428
    GLEPP1 disease and, 1431
    manifestations of, 1428-1429
    molecular genetic screening for, 2326f
    monogenic causation of, 1413-1414
    mutations causing, 1414
    mycophenolate mofetil for, 2331
    pathogenesis of, 1415, 1428
    renin-angiotensin-aldosterone antagonists for, 2331
    rituximab, 2331
    single-gene causes of, 1415, 1415f

Nephrotic syndrome (Continued)
    syndromic forms of, 2323
      treatment of, 1429, 2330-2331
    steroid-sensitive, 2329-2330
    thromboembolism risks in, 1804
    venous thromboembolism in, 1805
    vitamin D-binding protein loss in, 1797
Nephrotoxic medications, 999-1000
Nephrotoxins, 685-687, 965-968
Neprilysin inhibitors, 1714
Nernst equation, 569-570
Nesiritide, 344, 453, 1714, 1720-1721
Net acid excretion, 1344f
Net Reclassification Index, 929-930
N-Ethyl-N-nitrosourea, 9-17
Netrin-1, 943
Neurogenic bladder, urinary tract obstruction in, 1280
Neurohypophyseal neurons, 477
Neurohypophysis, 463, 467, 467f, 474
Neuromuscular system, 623
Neuronal nitric oxide synthases, 109-110, 399
Neuronal Wiskott-Aldrich syndrome protein, 38
Neuropathy, 1939
Neuropeptides
  in heart failure, 438
  Y, 81, 419, 429, 438
Neutral endopeptidase, 341-342, 345, 413
Neutral endopeptidase inhibitors, 345-346, 453-454
Neutropenia, 2434
Neutrophil extracellular traps, 1093-1094
Neutrophil gelatinase-associated lipocalin, 772, 943-947, 989, 1263
New Zealand
  chronic kidney disease in, 2550-2551
  diabetes mellitus in, 2550-2551
  dialysis in, 2551-2552
  end-stage kidney disease in, 2550, 2552-2553
  geography of, 2549
  glomerulonephritis in, 2550
  health care access in, 2549
  hypertension in, 2550
  life expectancy in, 2549
  Maori population of
    description of, 2538
    end-stage kidney disease in, 2552-2553
    health status of, 2549-2550
    leading causes of death in, 2549
    life expectancy in, 2549
    renal replacement therapy in, 2552
    renal transplantation in, 2553
    statistics regarding, 2549
  microalbuminuria in, 2550
  population of, 2540t
  renal replacement therapy in, 2541f, 2551-2552, 2551f
  renal transplantation in, 2552
New-onset diabetes mellitus after transplantation, 1320, 2283
Next-generation sequencing technique, 1412
NH_3, 248, 249f, 252-253, 384, 570
NH_4^+, 248, 249f, 253
NHE2, 238-239
NHE3, 154-155, 159, 235, 251, 254, 2302
NHE8, 235
NHE proteins, 148-150
NHERF, 155f
NHERF-1, 155
NHERF-2, 155
Niacin, 1872
Nicardipine hydrochloride, 1663t, 1665-1666, 1695t, 1698

Nicotinamide adenine dinucleotide phosphate-oxidase, 1758
Nicotinamide mononucleotide, 1788
Nicotinic acetylcholine receptor, 2158
Nifedipine, 1663t, 1664-1665, 1669-1670
Nisoldipine, 1663t, 1666
Nitric oxide, 1578
  acetylcholine effects on, 101-102
  angiotensin II-induced release of, 99
  cyclic guanosine monophosphate mediation of, 139
  in effective arterial blood volume regulation, 416-417
  endothelial production of, 1856
  glomerular filtration regulation by, 101-102
  in heart failure, 435-436
  inhibitors of, 101-102, 1740
  macula densa production of, 108-109
  nephron loss adaptations and, 1740
  platelet-activating factor effects on production of, 1741
  renal fibrosis in aging kidney, 730
  in renal hemodynamics, 416-417
  renal hemodynamics regulation by, 101-102
  in sodium balance, 417
  soluble guanylate cyclase effects on, 416
  vasodilatory effects of, 417
Nitric oxide synthases
  description of, 101, 138-139
  endothelial, 442-443, 728, 730, 979
  inducible, 416, 979
  isoforms of, 416
  neuronal, 109-110, 399, 416
  nitric oxide inhibition by, 400
Nitrites, 790
Nitroflurbiprofen, 377
Nitrofurantoin, 750, 1238t, 1244
Nitrogen, 1962-1963
Nitrogen balance, 1959, 1960f, 1968-1969, 1975
Nitroglycerin, 1695t, 1697
NKCC1, 177, 254, 562
NKCC2, 64, 125, 141, 158, 162-163, 188, 251, 254, 278, 396-397, 399, 450-451, 560, 702-703, 1705
NKCC2A, 55
NKCC2B, 55
NLRP3, 1193
Nodular glomerulosclerosis, 1285-1286, 1287f
Non-A, non-B intercalated cell, 241
Non-anion gap metabolic acidosis, 528-530, 529t, 536
Nonbiphenyl tetrazoles, 1653
Noncaseating granulomas, 1228
Noncontrast computed tomography, 1359
Nondiabetic chronic kidney disease, 1553
Nondiabetic glomerulopathy, 1300
Nonequilibrium thermodynamics, 123
Nonobstructive hydronephrosis, 765, 868
Nonobstructive intrahepatic bile duct dilatation, 1496-1497
Nonosmotic sodium storage, 1530
Nonreabsorbable anions, 555
Nonspecular reflectors, 848
Nonsteroidal antiinflammatory drugs (NSAIDs)
  acute kidney injury caused by, 362-363, 743-744
  angiotensin receptor blocker natriuretic effects affected by, 1656
  Bartter's syndrome treated with, 2335
  complications of, 361-363
  edema caused by, 361-362

Nonsteroidal antiinflammatory drugs (NSAIDs) *(Continued)*
  hyperkalemia caused by, 362
  hypertension caused by, 361-362
  interstitial nephritis caused by, 363
  minimal change disease caused by, 1021, 1021t
  nephrolithiasis analgesia using, 769
  nephropathy caused by, 1158
  nephrotic syndrome caused by, 363, 1158
  nephrotoxic syndromes caused by, 1218-1219
  papillary necrosis caused by, 362
  prostaglandin E_2 blockade by, 371
  renal dysgenesis caused by, 363
  renal insufficiency associated with, 362-363
  sodium retention caused by, 361-362
Nonurea nitrogen, 1962-1963
Nordihydroguaiaretic acid, 385
Norepinephrine, 432, 445
Normeperidine, 2038, 2038t
Normoalbuminuria, 1293-1294, 1296
North American Pediatric Renal Trials and Collaborative Studies, 2403, 2419, 2434-2435
Norverapamil, 1664
Notch group, 30
Notch3 receptors, 1215-1216
Notch signaling pathway, 36
Novel erythropoiesis-stimulating protein, 1881
NPHP1, 2321
NPHS1, 1413-1414, 1414t, 1419, 1786, 2325, 2478
NPHS2, 118, 1027-1028, 1413-1414, 1414t, 2422, 2477-2478
NT-proBNP, 343-344
Nuclear factor of activated T cells, 2239
Nuclear factor-κB, 334, 603, 730, 974
Nuclear medicine. *See also* Radiopharmaceuticals
  acute pyelonephritis evaluations, 880
  description of, 864-865
  obstructive urography evaluations, 871
  renal cell carcinoma imaging using, 900-901
  after renal transplantation, 911-912
Nutrition. *See also* Malnutrition
  disease affected by, 1957
  health affected by, 1957
  during hemodialysis, 1817-1818, 2089-2090, 2098-2100
  during peritoneal dialysis, 1817-1818, 2124-2126
  preeclampsia prevention through, 1626
  status markers for, 2099
  uremia effects on, 1817-1818

O

OAT1, 1712
OAT3, 1712
OATPs, 218t, 219
Obesity
  antihypertensive drug therapy in patients with, 1686-1688, 1688t
  cardiovascular disease risks, 1865-1866
  childhood, 2576-2577
  chronic kidney disease progression affected by, 679-680, 1770-1771, 1865-1866, 1992-1993
  end-stage kidney disease risks, 679, 1300

Obesity *(Continued)*
  glomerulopathy caused by, 679-680, 1770-1771
  hypertension and, 766, 1533-1534, 1694
  maternal, 2576
  mortality risks, 1866
  nephrolithiasis and, 1351f
  renal plasma flow increases secondary to, 1771
  urolithiasis and, 1350-1351
Obstructive nephropathy
  acute kidney injury caused by, 2496
  description of, 1257
  glomerular filtration affected by, 1269-1271
  isolated perfused tubules in, 1273t
  pathophysiology of, 1268-1277
  renal blood flow affected by, 1269-1271
  urine concentration affected by, 1275-1276
  urine dilution affected by, 1275-1276
Obstructive uropathy
  acute kidney injury and, 1632-1633
  in children, 1279
  contrast-enhanced computed tomography of, 871
  definition of, 764, 1257
  diagnostic approach, 764-765, 871
  end-stage kidney disease progression from, 764
  extrinsic causes of, 1260-1261
  gastrointestinal processes that cause, 1261
  imaging of, 871
  in men, 1261
  nuclear medicine of, 871
  pain in, 1262
  pelvic malignancies as cause of, 1261
Occlusive, 1598-1599
Oceania
  Australia. *See* Australia
  demographics of, 2538
  history of, 2538
  map of, 2539f
  New Zealand. *See* New Zealand
  Pacific Islands, 2538, 2540t, 2553-2554
  population of, 2540t
  summary of, 2554
Ocrelizumab, 1104, 1171
OCT1, 211-214, 212t
OCT2, 211-214, 212t, 213f
OCT3, 211-214, 212t
Octreotide, 456
Oculocerebrorenal dystrophy, 1438-1439
Oculocerebrorenal syndrome, 2345
Ogilvie's syndrome, 574
1,25(OH)D, 617, 742, 1829-1830
1,25(OH)$_2$D, 1830, 1841, 1848
Older adults. *See* Elderly
Oligomeganephronia, 1759
Oliguric renal failure, 425-426
Olive oil, 1957
Olmesartan medoxomil, 1309, 1652t, 1653, 1655
Omapatrilat, 345, 453-454
Omega-3 fatty acids, 1069
Oncocytic carcinoma, 1371, 1371t, 1372f
Oncocytoma, 891-892, 1368, 1501
Oncotic pressure, plasma, 1798
One-kidney renal clip hypertension, 1568-1569, 1570t, 1573f
One-kidney renovascular hypertension, 1571-1572
OPC 31260, 299-300
Opioids, 1942-1943, 2595

Opisthorchiasis, 2522-2523
Oral contraceptives, 659-660
Oral glucose tolerance test, 1912
Orellanine, 2525-2526
Organ perfusion sensors, 396-398
Organic acids, 516-517
Organic anion(s)
  classes of, 216t
  definition of, 216
  description of, 215-216
  excretion of, 247-248
    in acid-base homeostasis, 247-248
    in bicarbonate generation, 247-248
  fractional excretion of, 216
  proximal tubule secretion of, 216
  transport of, 215-219, 216t
Organic anion transporters
  characteristics of, 218t
  clinical relevance of, 219
  description of, 125
  NaDC family of, 217-218, 218f, 218t
  OAT family of, 218-219, 218t
  OATP family of, 218t, 219
  types of, 218t
Organic anion transporting polypeptide, 211
Organic cation(s)
  apical exit of, 211
  peritubular uptake of, 210
  reabsorption of, 211
  secretion of, 210, 210f
  transport of, 210-215, 210f
  type I, 210
  type II, 210
Organic cation transporters
  apical, 212t, 214-215
  basolateral, 211-214
  MATE1, 212t, 214-215
  MATE2-K, 212t, 214-215
  OCT1, 211-214, 212t
  OCT2, 211-214, 212t, 213f
  OCT3, 211-214, 212t
  regulation of, 214
  single-nucleotide polymorphisms in, 214
  structure of, 213-214
Organum vasculosum of the lamina terminalis, 464-465
Orientia tsutsugamushi, 2513
Ornipressin, 455
Oro-facial-digital syndrome type 1, 1504
Orthostatic hypotension, 776, 1538-1539, 1677, 1939
Orthostatic proteinuria, 1014
Osmolal gap, 840
Osmolality
  definition of, 461, 2366
  effective, 461
  plasma, 461, 466f, 468f, 2366
  total, 461
  urine, 465, 789, 1748
Osmolar gap, 490-491
Osmole excretion rate, 807-808, 811-812
Osmolytes, 502, 502f
Osmoreceptor dysfunction
  causes of, 477-478
  clinical manifestations of, 483
  hypernatremia caused by, 489
  hyponatremia in, 480
  pathophysiology of, 478-480
  patterns of, 478
  treatment of, 489
Osmoreceptor neuron, 466-467
Osmotic demyelination syndrome, 504-505, 505f, 505t

Osmotic diuresis
    case studies of, 812-813
    clinical approach to, 812
    description of, 811-813
    in diabetes mellitus patient, 812-813
    evaluation of, 811-812
Osmotic diuretics
    adverse effects of, 1705
    dosage of, 1704
    indications for, 1705
    mechanism of action, 1704
    pharmacokinetics of, 1704
    sites of action, 1704
    sodium reabsorption affected by, 422
Osmotic pressure, 461, 464-467
Osmotic thirst, 471-472
OSR1, 163, 714-715
Osr1, 21
Osteitis fibrosa cystica, 606, 2020-2021
Osteoblasts, 1832, 1842
Osteocalcin, 1726-1727
Osteocytes, 1832
Osteodystrophy
    mixed uremic, 1843, 1844*f*
    renal, 1842, 1845, 1845*t*, 2407*f*, 2434
Osteomalacia, aluminum-induced, 1843, 1844*f*
Osteonecrosis, 2282
Osteopenia, 2282
Osteopontin, 1330
Osteoporosis, 1352, 1726-1727, 2282-2283
Osteoprotegerin, 1300, 1832, 1833*f*, 1838
Ouabain, 721
Outer medulla
    anatomy of, 45, 45*f*, 65*f*, 91, 91*f*
    axial sodium chloride gradient in, 265-268
    concentrating mechanism in, 268
    osmolality gradient of, 266, 267*f*
Outer medullary collecting duct (OMCD), 44-45, 45*f*, 73-74, 133, 166, 178, 242
Ovarian cyst, 1491
Ovarian dysfunction, 1920
Overflow hypothesis, 494
Overflow proteinuria, 791
Overt nephropathy, 1557
Oxalate, 1813. *See also* Calcium oxalate
    absorption of, 1339, 1339*f*
    calcium concentration versus, 1325-1327
    hepatic metabolism and, 1337-1338
    homeostasis of, 1340
    kidney stones and, 1324, 1337-1340
    recommended dosage of, 1361
    role of, 1339
Oxaloacetic acid, 248-249
Oxalobacter formigenes, 1339-1340, 2347
Oxalosis, 985-986
Oxcarbazepine, 497
Oxford-MEST score, 1063
Oxidant stress, 1815, 1817
Oxidative stress, 1579
    angiotensin II and, 982
    cardiovascular disease risks, 2100-2101
    chronic kidney disease and, 1758, 1865
    definition of, 1865
    preeclampsia and, 1620
2-Oxoglutarate, 245, 248-249
Oxygen, 126, 131*f*
Oxygen consumption, 133-135, 137*f*
Oxygen consumption rate, 134-135
Oxygen transport, 134
Oxytocin, 463

P

p53, 974
Pacific Islands, 2538, 2540*t*, 2553-2554
Pain, 1262, 1489, 1493, 2569
Pakistan. *See* Indian subcontinent
Palliative care, 2563, 2569-2570
Pallister-Hall syndrome, 2297*t*, 2299
Pamidronate, 1030
p-Aminohippurate, 216, 216*f*
p-Aminohippuric acid, 86
Pancreas-kidney transplantation, 1319, 2289
Pancreatic cyst, 1491
Panel reactive antibody, 2157
Pantothenic acid, 1983-1984
Papillary collecting ducts, 27, 75*f*
Papillary necrosis
    in granulomatous with polyangiitis, 1110
    nephrolithiasis versus, 769
    nonsteroidal antiinflammatory drugs as cause of, 362
    in sickle cell disease, 1198-1199, 1199*f*
Papillary renal cell carcinoma, 892, 897*f*, 1372*f*, 1373
Paracellin-1, 160
Paraldehyde-induced high anion gap acidosis, 549
Paramembranous cisternal system, 56
Paraneoplastic glomerular disease, 1403-1404
Paraoxonase, 2101
Parapelvic cyst, 1517
Paraphenylenediamine, 2501
Paraproteinemia, 628, 746, 1435
Paraquat, 2185-2186
Parasitic diseases, 1150-1151, 1255
Parathormone, 1453
Parathyroid carcinoma, 607
Parathyroid gland disease, 2019-2020
Parathyroid hormone. *See also* Hyperparathyroidism
    assays for, 1839-1841, 1840*f*
    bone remodeling and, 1834*f*, 1849, 2020-2021
    calcimimetics effect on, 1873
    calcium and
        description of, 606*f*, 1827*f*
        homeostasis, 601, 1826-1827, 1923
        transport, 187
    calcium-sensing receptor activation effects on, 2026
    in children, 2390-2391
    in chronic kidney disease–mineral bone disorder, 1826-1828, 1839-1841, 1840*f*, 1848
    cinacalcet effects on, 2027, 2032
    cleavage of, 1827
    cytochrome P450 enzymes affected by, 2019
    deficiency of, 601
    erythropoiesis affected by, 1887
    functions of, 1826-1827, 1923
    glomerular filtration rate effects on, 1865
    magnesium depletion effects on, 2387
    monitoring of, in stage 3 chronic kidney disease, 2014
    mortality and, 2020
    net acid excretion and, 740-741
    NH3 activity affected by, 235
    phosphate excretion affected by, 197-198, 1838-1839, 1977-1978
    phosphate wasting and, 199*f*
    phosphate-binding agents effect on, 2031
    phosphorus homeostasis affected by, 197-198
    proximal tubule bicarbonate reabsorption affected by, 237-238
    systemic effects of, 1847
    TRPV5 channels affected by, 189
    urea production affected by, 1968

Parathyroid hormone *(Continued)*
    urinary phosphate excretion increased by, 200
    vitamin D analogues effect on, 2027-2029
Parathyroid hormone(1-34), 618
Parathyroid hormone(1-84), 1839
Parathyroid hormone receptors, 603, 1749-1750, 1775, 1827, 1833
Parathyroid hormone-dependent resorptive hypercalciuria, 1335
Parathyroid hormone–fibroblast growth factor-23–1,25(OH)2D loop, 1838-1839
Parathyroid hormone-independent resorptive hypercalciuria, 1335
Parathyroid hormone-related protein, 607, 1399
Parathyroidectomy, 607, 2282
Paraventricular nuclei, 463
Parenteral nutrition, 620
Paricalcitol, 1312-1313, 2025-2026, 2029, 2032
Parietal epithelial cells, 4-5, 52-53, 52*f*53*f*, 1789-1790
Parinaud oculoglandular syndrome, 1149-1150
Pars convoluta
    anatomy of, 55-60, 58*f*
    basolateral intercellular space of, 55-56
    cells of, 55-56
    illustration of, 59*f*
    lateral cell processes of, 56, 58*f*
    vacuolar-lysosomal system in, 59-60
Pars recta, 60-61, 62*f*
Partial lipodystrophy, 1146-1147
Partial nephrectomy, 1380, 1380*t*
Partial pressure of carbon dioxide, 515-516
Parvovirus B19 infection, 1255
Passive countercurrent multiplier mechanism, 272
Passive Heymann nephritis, 377
PAT2, 224
Patient Self-Determination Act, 2561
Patiromer, 597
Pauci-immune crescentic glomerulonephritis
    anti-MPO antibodies in, 1083-1085
    antineutrophil cytoplasmic autoantibodies in, 1082-1084, 1086-1087
    anti-PR3 autoantibodies in, 1083
    clinical features of, 1085-1086
    crescent formation in, 1082
    cyclophosphamide for, 1087-1088
    electron microscopy of, 1083
    end-stage kidney disease progression of, 1086
    epidemiology of, 1081-1082
    immunofluorescence microscopy of, 1082-1083
    laboratory findings in, 1086-1087
    light microscopy of, 1082, 1082*f*
    methylprednisolone for, 1087-1089
    natural history of, 1085-1086
    pathogenesis of, 1083-1085
    pathology of, 1082-1083, 1082*f*
    plasmapheresis for, 1088
    PR3 in, 1083
    prognostic factors for, 1086
    relapse prevention in, 1089
    after renal transplantation, 1086
    rituximab for, 1088-1089
    segmental fibrinoid necrosis in, 1082*f*
    T cells in, 1084
    treatment of, 1087-1089
    urinalysis findings in, 1086-1087
Pauci-immune necrotizing glomerulonephritis, 1084-1085

PAX2, 2298
Pax2, 23, 27
Pax8, 23
Pazopanib, 1383, 1383f
p-cresol, 1812
p-cresyl sulfate, 1963, 2097
PDGF-B, 36
Pediatrics. See Children; Infants
Pegylated interferon, 1156
Pelvic malignancies, 1261
Pelvic neurofibromas, 1262
Penbutolol, 1656t-1657t, 1657-1658
Pendrin, 243-244
Penicillamine, 1448
Penicillin(s), 719, 1235t-1236t, 2513, 2514f
Pentamidine, 540-541, 591, 622
Pentoxifylline, 1313
Peptides, 1810
Peptidyl leukotrienes, 380
Percutaneous angioplasty/stent, 1569-1570
Percutaneous kidney biopsy, 2222-2224, 2223t, 2224f
Percutaneous mechanical thrombectomy
  of arteriovenous fistulas, 2210-2212
  of arteriovenous graft, 2199-2202, 2199t, 2201f-2202f
Percutaneous transluminal renal angioplasty, 1600
  arteriovenous fistulas treated with, 2208-2210, 2209t
  atherosclerosis renal artery stenosis treated with, 1602-1603
  central vein stenosis treated with, 2213-2214
  complications after, 1603t
Pericardial disease, 2107-2108
Pericytes, 5-6, 1777-1778, 1794
Perihilar focal segmental glomerulosclerosis, 1026
Perindopril, 1643-1644, 1643t
Perinephritic abscess, 1250
Perinuclear antineutrophil cytoplasmic antibody, 759-760
Periodic limb movements of sleep, 1939-1940
Peripheral α_1-adrenergic antagonists
  combination therapies using, 1692
  efficacy of, 1677
  mechanism of action, 1676
  moderately selective, 1675-1676, 1676t
  orthostatic hypotension caused by, 1677
  pharmacodynamics of, 1676t
  pharmacokinetics of, 1676t
  renal effects of, 1677
  safety of, 1677
  types of, 1676-1677, 1676t
Peripheral adrenergic neuronal blocking agents, 1649t-1650t
Peripheral arterial vasodilation, 439
Peripheral neuropathy, 1300
Peripolar cells, 53
Perirenal hematomas, 2253
Perirenal lymphangioma, 1517
Perirenal urinoma, 1517
Peritoneal dialysis (PD)
  access for, 2114-2116, 2415
  acute kidney injury treated with, 1008, 2120
  adequacy of
    in children, 2416
    clearance targets, 2122-2124, 2123t
    considerations for, 2120t
    definition of, 2120
    indicators for evaluating, 2120-2121

Peritoneal dialysis (PD) (Continued)
  solute clearance determinants used in, 2121-2122
  targets, 2122-2124, 2123t
  urea clearance as indicator of, 2120
anorexia secondary to, 2125
automated, 2049, 2114, 2117, 2119, 2130t, 2415
cardiovascular disease in, 2127-2128
catheters used in
  bowel perforation during placement of, 2221
  complications associated with, 2116-2117
  description of, 2114-2116
  diaphragmatic leaks, 2132
  entrapment of, 2116-2117
  fluoroscopic insertion of, 2220-2221
  impaired drainage of, 2116
  infections associated with, 2116, 2128, 2131
  insertion of, 2220-2221
  leaks from, 2132, 2416
  Moncrief-Popovich, 2115-2116
  nonrigid, 2116
  peritoneoscopic insertion technique for, 2221-2222
  presternal, 2115, 2222
  removal of, 2131
  rigid, 2116
  segments of, 2114-2115
  surgical placement of, 2116
  swan-neck, 2115, 2115f, 2221
  Tenckhoff, 2114-2115, 2115f, 2221, 2415
in China, 2535
complications of
  catheter-related, 2116-2117, 2416
  encapsulating peritoneal sclerosis, 2133, 2416-2417
  fluid leaks, 2416
  hernia, 2132
  hypercalcemia, 2132
  hyperglycemia, 2132
  hyperlipidemia, 2132
  hypokalemia, 572, 2132
  hyponatremia, 2132
  infections, 2116, 2128, 2131, 2416
  intraabdominal pressure, 2131
  intraperitoneal pressure increases, 2131
  mechanical, 2131-2132
  metabolic, 2132
  noninfectious, 2131-2133
  peritonitis. See Peritonitis
  ultrafiltration failure, 2416
continuous ambulatory. See Continuous ambulatory peritoneal dialysis (CAPD)
continuous cyclic, 2119
cost-effectiveness of, 2134-2135
definition of, 2220-2221
in developing countries, 2135
diabetic nephropathy treated with, 1318
dialysate, 2117, 2121
dose of, 2087, 2120-2121, 2121t
drug dosing in, 2049
economics of, 2134-2135
ethical dilemmas. See Dialysis, ethical dilemmas
exchanges, frequency of, 2122
fluid removal in, 2121-2122
gastroparesis associated with, 2125
hemodialysis versus, 2087, 2134-2135, 2411
in Hong Kong, 2535
in Indian subcontinent, 2504

Peritoneal dialysis (PD) (Continued)
  inflammation during, 2125-2126
  insulin resistance in, 1913
  intraabdominal pressure in, 2112
  intravenous iron in, 1891f
  Kt/V assessments, 2416
  in Latin America, 2450t
  L-carnitine and, 2125
  malnutrition in, 2504
  mass transfer area coefficient, 2112-2113
  in Middle East, 2475t, 2487
  mineral metabolism abnormalities in patients receiving, 2132
  modalities for, 2119-2120
  nocturnal intermittent, 2119, 2122, 2415
  nutrition during, 1817-1818, 2124-2126
  outcomes of, 2122-2124, 2133-2134
  peritonitis associated with. See Peritonitis
  poison removal using, 2171, 2172t
  prescription for, 2119, 2122, 2415-2416, 2504
  protein-energy wasting in, 2124, 2124t
  reasons for reduced use of, 2134-2135
  residual kidney function after, 2126-2127
  in Singapore, 2536
  solutes, 2112-2114, 2121-2122
  solutions
    amino acids in, 2125
    bicarbonate-based, 2119, 2125
    biocompatible, 2126-2127
    composition of, 2117-2118, 2117t
    dextrose in, 2117
    dosage calculations, 2121t
    electrolytes in, 2117-2118
    glucose-containing, 2117-2119, 2127, 2132
    glucose-sparing, 2119
    icodextrin, 2118, 2415-2416
    lactate as buffer in, 2117
    osmolality of, 2122
    pediatric, 2415-2416
  survival rates affected by, 2134
  in Thailand, 2535
  tidal, 2415
  volume exchange, 2122
  water transport during, 2113-2114
Peritoneal equilibration test, 2113-2114
Peritoneal membrane, 2111-2112, 2113t, 2133, 2416-2417
Peritoneovenous shunting, 998-999
Peritoneum
  capillaries of, 2111-2112
  definition of, 2111
  interstitium of, 2112
  mesothelial cells of, 2111-2112
  microvessels of, 2111
  surface area of, 2111
Peritonitis
  bacterial, 2128-2129
  catheter removal in patients with, 2131
  in children, 2416
  clinical course of, 2128-2129
  definition of, 2128-2129
  diagnosis of, 2128-2129
  fungal, 2129, 2131
  gram-negative bacteria that cause, 2128-2131, 2504
  gram-positive bacteria that cause, 2128-2130, 2504
  in Indian subcontinent, 2504
  mycobacterial, 2129, 2131
  polymicrobial, 2131
  prevention of, 2131
  Pseudomonas aeruginosa, 2128-2131

Peritonitis (Continued)
  refractory, 2131
  relapsing, 2131
  Staphylococcus aureus, 2128, 2130
  treatment of, 2129-2131, 2130t
Peritubular capillaries
  anatomy of, 88f
  basement membrane of, 89-90
  density, 727-728
  dynamics of, 89-90
  efferent vessels as source of, 90
  fenestrations, 89
  surface of, 89
Peritubular capillary Starling forces, 400-402
Peritubular interstitial cells, 5-6
Peritubular protein, 151-152
Perivascular matrix, 980
Permeability factor, 1029-1030
Permissive hypercapnia, 2138-2139
Peroxisome proliferator-activated receptor τ
  angiotensin receptor blockers effect on, 733
  description of, 174
  fatty acid oxidation affected by, 733, 1761
  fluid retention induced by, 438-439
Peroxisome proliferator-activated receptors, 374-375, 438-444
Peroxisomes, in pars recta, 60-61
Peroxynitrite scavengers, 452
PGI. *See* Prostacyclin
pH
  buffering, 512
  description of, 512
  disequilibrium, 253
  NH_3 affected by, 249f
  NH_4^+ affected by, 249f
  plasma potassium levels affected by, 563
  urine. *See* Urinary pH
Phallotoxin, 2525-2526
Pharmacodynamic biomarker, 927t
Pharmacodynamics, 2040-2041
Pharmacogenomics, 2039-2040
Pharmacokinetics, 2035-2037, 2036t
Pharmacotherapeutic trial, 1363t
Phase-contrast magnetic resonance angiography, 859-861
Phenformin-induced lactic acidosis, 545
Phenobarbital, 2183
Phenols, 1811-1812
Phenoxybenzamine, 1675-1676
Phentolamine mesylate, 1675-1676, 1695t, 1698
Phenytoin, 2183-2184
Pheochromocytoma, 1547-1549
Philippines, 2536
Phleboliths, 874-876
Phlorizin, 206-207
Phosphate. *See also* Hyperphosphatemia; Hypophosphatemia
  additives, 1979
  age-related changes in, 742
  in blood, 196, 197t, 626
  in bone, 196
  in cellular processes, 196
  in children
    balance of, 2389-2390, 2389f-2390f
    dietary intake of, 2390
    disorders of, 2396-2399, 2397t-2400t, 2398f-2399f
    distribution of, 2389, 2390f
    fractional excretion of, 2397
    homeostasis of, 2391f
    regulation of, 2389
  in chronic kidney disease, 1977-1979, 2019
  in chronic kidney disease–mineral bone disorder, 1864, 1872

Phosphate (Continued)
  concentrations of, 197t
  dietary
    fibroblast growth factor-23 affected by, 1978
    intake of, 196, 2390
    parathyroid hormone affected by, 1978
    phosphate-binding agents for, 2021-2022
    restriction of, 1774-1775
  dietary protein intake and, 1977
  distribution of, 197t
  excretion of, 1450-1451
    acetazolamide effects on, 629
    insulin effects on, 200
    in metabolic acidosis, 247
    parathyroid hormone effects on, 197-198, 1977-1978
    urinary, 199-200
    urinary tract obstruction relief effects on, 1276-1277
  fibroblast growth factor-23 effects on concentration of, 1749-1750, 1775, 1776f, 1872, 1978, 2281, 2390-2391
  filtered, 246-247
  homeostasis of, 196-198, 196f-197f, 1924
  intestinal absorption of, 2021
  metabolism of, 626, 1749-1750, 1774-1775
  niacin effects on, 1872
  redistribution of, 633
  replacement therapy, 633-634
  serum, 685, 1978-1979
  as titratable acid, 246-247
  transport of, 1450-1451
    catecholamines effect on, 200-201
    dietary, 199-200
    dopamine effects on, 201
    growth hormone effects on, 200
    inherited disorders of, 1450-1453
    insulin effects on, 200
    insulin-like growth factor-1 effects on, 200
    intestinal, 1824f
    parathyroid hormone effects on, 200
    phosphatonins effect on, 201-202
    regulation of, 199-202
    renal nerves and, 200-201
    serotonin effects on, 201
    sodium-mediated, 1749-1750
    transporters involved in, 247
    vitamin D metabolites, 200
  urinary excretion of, 199-201
Phosphate binders, 1872, 1945
Phosphate wasting
  Fanconi's syndrome and, 1437
  matrix extracellular phosphoglycoprotein and, 201-202
  renal, 631
  tumors associated with, 201-202
  urinary, inherited disorders of, 631f
Phosphate-binding agents
  aluminum-containing binders, 2022
  calcium-containing binders, 2022, 2031, 2094
  chronic kidney disease–mineral bone disorder treated with, 2020-2023, 2031
  lanthanum carbonate, 2021-2022
  magnesium, 2023
  parathyroid hormone levels affected by, 2031
Phosphate-binding resins, 2022-2023
Phosphate-dependent glutaminase, 248, 251f, 253
Phosphate–parathyroid hormone–fibroblast growth factor-23 loop, 1839

Phosphatidylinositol-3-kinase, 312, 1964
Phosphatonins, 197-198, 1830
  fibroblast growth factor-23, 191, 197-198, 198f, 201
  hypophosphatemia as cause of increased production or activity of, 630-631
  phosphate transport affected by, 201-202
Phosphaturia, 1437
Phosphinyl angiotensin-converting enzyme inhibitors, 1644
Phosphocreatine, 782
Phosphodiesterase inhibitors, 300-301
Phosphoenolpyruvate, 248-249
Phospho*enol*pyruvate carboxykinase, 248-249, 253
Phosphofructokinase, 514
Phospholipase A_2, 164, 355
Phospholipase A_2 receptor, 1035, 1039, 1155
Phospholipase C, 399, 1827f
Phospholipase Cε1, 1413-1414, 1414t
Phospholipase Cε1 disease, 1429-1430
Phosphoric acid, 247, 517
Phosphorus
  absorption of, 1823
  balance of, 1823-1824
  in blood, 196, 197t, 626
  in bone, 196
  in cellular processes, 196
  in chronic kidney disease, 1977-1978
  in chronic kidney disease–mineral bone disorder, 1847
  concentrations of, 197t
  daily intake of, 626
  dietary intake of, 196
  distribution of, 197t
  in end-stage kidney disease, 2028-2029
  homeostasis of, 196-198, 196f-197f, 1822-1824, 1838-1839
  hormonal feedback systems that regulate, 197, 197f
  in hydroxyapatite, 196
  inorganic, 1822-1823
  intravenous repletion of, for hypophosphatemia, 634
  metabolism of, 1979
  monitoring of, 2014
  in plasma, 196
  reabsorption of, 198-199, 199f
  secretion of, 196
  serum, 196, 1822, 1839f
  sodium-phosphate cotransporters and, 198-199
  transport of, proteins involved in, 202
Phospho-specific antibodies, 154-155
Physiologic hydronephritis, 1633
Pierson's syndrome, 1426, 1782, 2325
Pindolol, 1656t-1657t, 1658
Pirfenidone, 1034
Pivmecillinam, 1238t
Placenta, 1618, 2607
Placental growth factor, 1623f
Placental protein 13, 1624
Placental vascular remodeling, 1618-1619
Placentation, 1614f
Plain radiographs, 846, 873, 874f
Planar cell polarity, 30-31
Plan-Do-Study-Act, 2623, 2623t, 2624f
Plant toxins, 2458
Plasma
  albumin concentrations in, 602, 791
  arginine vasopressin concentrations in, 466f
  atrial natriuretic peptide levels in, 414
  bicarbonate concentration in, 513-514, 520
  brain natriuretic peptide levels, 414

Plasma (Continued)
  filtration of, 781
  growth factors in, 1212
  kallikrein, 346
  kallikrein-kinin system, 347-348
  magnesium in, 193
  neutrophil gelatinase-associated lipocalin, 945-946
  phosphorus in, 196
  renin concentration in, 328
  urotensin II levels, 352
  vasoactive hormones effect on, 1799
  vasopressin levels in, 282
Plasma aldosterone concentration/plasma renin activity, 576
Plasma amino acids, 1971-1973, 1972f
Plasma cells, 1135-1136, 1233
Plasma membrane, 286, 287f
Plasma membrane calcium pump A1, 192-193, 192f
Plasma oncotic pressure, 1798
Plasma osmolality
  description of, 461, 468f, 2366
  measurement of, 484, 490
  plasma vasopressin and, 500f
  reduction in, 486
  thirst and, 471-472
Plasma proteins
  abnormal filtration of, 1786
  basement membrane passage of, 1013
  bicarbonate reabsorption affected by, 238
  binding of, in chronic kidney disease, 2037
  description of, 89
  furosemide binding to, 1724-1725
  glomerular ultrafiltration of, 1790
  high-molecular-weight, 791
  in nephrotic syndrome, 1018t
  podocytes effect on, 118
  poison binding to, 2169
  in proteinuria, 1013-1014
Plasma renin concentration assay, 328
Plasma renin concentration immunologic assay, 328
Plasmapheresis
  adverse events during, 2162-2163
  albumin as replacement fluid for, 2162
  angiotensin-converting enzyme inhibitors and, 2164
  anticoagulation for, 2162
  anti-glomerular basement membrane disease treated with, 1126-1127, 2149-2150, 2149t-2150t
  anti-glomerular basement membrane glomerulonephritis treated with, 1081
  antineutrophil cytoplasmic antibody-associated vasculitis treated with, 2150-2151
  atypical hemolytic-uremic syndrome treated with, 2154, 2354
  blood pressure reductions caused by, 2163
  catastrophic antiphospholipid antibody syndrome treated with, 2158-2159
  chronic inflammatory demyelinating polyneuropathy treated with, 2158
  clotting factor decreases after, 2164t
  colloidal starch as replacement fluid for, 2162
  complications of, 2162-2164, 2163t
  cryoglobulinemia treated with, 2152
  definition of, 2148
  double-filtration, 2160
  familial hypercholesterolemia treated with, 2159

Plasmapheresis (Continued)
  fibrinogen levels affected by, 2163
  fresh frozen plasma for, 2155
  general principles of, 2148-2149
  granulomatous with polyangiitis treated with, 1113
  Guillain-Barré syndrome treated with, 2158
  hematologic disorders treated with, 2152-2154
  hemolytic uremic syndrome treated with, 2154-2155
  history of, 2148
  hypocalcemia during, 2163
  idiopathic rapidly progressive glomerulonephritis treated with, 2151
  intravenous immunoglobulin and, 2157
  lupus nephritis treated with, 1105, 2151-2152
  mixed cryoglobulinemia treated with, 2152
  multiple myeloma treated with, 2153t
  myasthenia gravis treated with, 2158
  myeloma cast nephropathy treated with, 1002
  pathologic factors removed using, 2149, 2149t
  pauci-immune crescentic glomerulonephritis treated with, 1088
  poison removal using, 2171
  in pregnancy, 2159
  premature delivery secondary to, 2159
  rapidly progressive glomerulonephritis treated with, 2150-2151
  renal transplantation applications of, 2155-2157
  replacement fluids for, 2162
  techniques of, 2159-2162, 2161f
  thrombotic thrombocytopenic purpura treated with, 2154-2155
  toxin removal using, 2159
  venous access for, 2161-2162
Plasminogen activator inhibitor-1, 378, 729, 1212-1213
Plasmodium falciparum, 1150, 2442-2443, 2470-2472, 2496, 2517-2518, 2519f. See also Malaria
Platelet(s)
  aggregation of, 1189f, 1804
  hyperaggregability of, hypoalbuminemia's role in, 1798, 1804
  thromboxane modulation of, 368
  in uremia, 1904-1905
  uremic, 1905, 1907f
Platelet-activating factor, 1741
Platelet-derived growth factor receptor, 330
Platelet-derived growth factor-B, 1789
PLCE1, 1413-1414, 1414t
PLCE1 disease, 1429-1430
Plicamycin, 612, 1400
PMCA. See Plasma membrane calcium pump A1
Pneumocystis jiroveci pneumonia, 2430-2431
Pneumocystosis, 2288
Pneumonia, 2105
Podocalyxin, 118, 936
Podocin, 37-38, 1413-1414, 1414t
Podocin disease. See Nephrotic syndrome, steroid-resistant
Podocyte(s)
  albumin passage affected by, 112-113
  angiopoietin-like 4 overproduction in, 1021
  angiotensin II effects on, 1788

Podocyte(s) (Continued)
  anti–B cell therapy effects on, 119
  apoptosis of, 1788
  biologic functions of, 112-113
  calcineurin inhibitors effect on, 119
  Cdc42 inactivation in, 38, 39f
  characteristics of, 49
  COX-2 overexpression in, 376
  cytoskeleton of, 113
  definition of, 791, 2609
  depletion of, 118-119
  in diabetic nephropathy, 115t, 116-117, 120
  disease-induced injury of, 117-119
  endocytosis by, 49
  filtration slit, 49-51, 1782-1783, 1783f
  in focal segmental glomerulosclerosis, 115t, 116, 118-119
  foot processes of
    description of, 36, 38, 49, 51f, 113
    effacement of
      in congenital nephrotic syndrome, 2325
      in Fabry's disease, 1144
      in focal segmental glomerulosclerosis, 1027, 1029
      in membranous nephropathy, 1036-1037
      in minimal change disease, 1016, 1019, 1020f
    function of, 2325f
    maintenance of, 2325f
  future therapeutic approaches for, 120
  glomerular basement membrane and, 4-5, 118
  in glomerular diseases, 113, 115t
  glucocorticoids effect on, 119
  in human immunodeficiency virus nephropathy, 116
  hypertrophy of, 1754
  in immunoglobulin A nephropathy, 1064
  inherited disorders affecting, 1426-1431
  injury of
    in chronic kidney disease progression, 1753-1754
    effacement after, 117-118, 117f
    glomerulosclerosis secondary to, 118-119
    hepatocyte growth factor effects on, 120
    after nephron loss, 1753-1754
    proteinuria affected by, 118
  in membranous nephropathy, 115t, 116
  in minimal change nephropathy, 114-116, 115t
  molecular anatomy of, 113, 115f
  morphologic features of, 36
  parathyroid hormone receptor expression by, 1775
  plasma protein passage affected by, 118
  protein uptake by, 1787
  proteinuria effects on, 1787-1788
  regeneration of, 2609
  renin-angiotensin-aldosterone inhibitors effect on, 119-120
  slit diaphragm in, 38-39, 51, 118, 1782-1783, 1782f
  structure of, 113, 114f
  summary of, 120
  transcription factors expressed by, 36-37
  ultrastructure of, 38f, 113, 114f, 1788
  vascular endothelial growth factor expression by, 1752-1753
  vascular endothelial growth factor-A, 32
Podocyte count, 936

Podocytopathy, 114-116
Poison removal/poisonings
  chromic acid, 2501
  copper sulfate, 2500
  corporeal treatments for, 2167-2169, 2168t
  description of, 2166-2167
  elimination enhancement techniques for, 2166-2167, 2167f
  ethylene dibromide, 2501
  extracorporeal treatments for
    acetaminophen, 2187-2188
    albumin dialysis, 2171, 2172t
    barbiturates, 2183
    carbamazepine, 2182-2183
    combination therapies, 2171
    continuous renal replacement therapy, 2171
    criteria for, 2169
    duration of, 2173
    endogenous clearance effects on, 2169
    ethylene glycol, 2173-2178, 2174t, 2176t
    exchange transfusion, 2171, 2172t
    extraction ratio, 2169
    factors that affect, 2169
    hemodialysis, 2169-2170, 2170t, 2172t
    hemofiltration, 2170, 2172t
    hemoperfusion, 2169-2170, 2172t
    heparinization, 2173
    indications for, 2172-2173
    isopropanol, 2173-2178, 2174t, 2176t
    lithium, 2180-2181
    metformin, 2184-2185
    methanol, 2173-2178, 2174t, 2176t
    methotrexate, 2188-2189
    paraquat, 2185-2186
    peritoneal dialysis, 2171, 2172t
    phenytoin, 2183-2184
    plasmapheresis, 2171
    poison-related factors that affect, 2169
    rebound after discontinuation of, 2173
    salicylic acid, 2178-2180
    technical considerations, 2173
    theophylline, 2186-2187
    therapeutic plasma exchange, 2171
    toxic alcohols, 2173-2178, 2174t, 2176t
    valproic acid, 2181-2182
    vascular access for, 2173
  hair dye, 2501
  multiple-dose activated charcoal for, 2168
  rebound after extracorporeal treatment discontinuation, 2173
  statistics regarding, 2167t
Polar cushion, 53
Polyarteritis nodosa
  angiographic findings in, 1119
  in children, 2350-2351
  classic, 1118-1119
  clinical features of, 1119, 2350
  corticosteroids for, 1119-1120
  cyclophosphamide for, 1119-1120
  diagnosis of, 2350
  gender predilection of, 1118
  hairy cell leukemia associated with, 1118-1120
  hepatitis B virus associated with, 1118-1120
  hypertension in, 1119
  incidence of, 1118
  laboratory tests, 1119, 2350
  microscopic, 1118
  pathogenesis of, 1118-1119, 2350
  pathology of, 1118
  prognosis for, 1119-1120
  renal findings in, 1119
  survival rate for, 1119-1120
  treatment of, 1119-1120, 2350-2351

Polychronotropism, 1385
Polyclonal immune globulins, 2247-2248, 2255
Polycystic kidney disease, 1416, 1479
  adult-acquired, 888, 889f
  in children. See Children, polycystic kidney disease in
  classification of, 885
  computed tomography of, 869f, 1489f, 1491f
  extrarenal manifestations of, 775
  glomerular filtration rate declines secondary to, 681
  hypothetical pathways upregulated and downregulated in, 1482f, 1483
  infantile, 885
  organomegaly associated with, 885
Polycystic liver disease, 1491, 1491f, 1494
Polycystin, 1477-1478, 1478f
Polycystin protein, 1481f
Polydipsia
  in children, 2369, 2370t
  primary. See Primary polydipsia
  psychogenic, 482
Polygenic disease, 1411t, 1412, 1419
Polygenic hypercalciuria, 1349-1350
Polygenic kidney disease, 1410
Polyols, 1813
Polyomavirus infection, 1404-1405, 2272-2273
Polyuria, 1437
  in acute renal injury, 299
  aquaporin-2 dysregulation in, 297
  in children, 2369, 2370t
  in chronic renal injury, 299
  classification of, 804
  definition of, 804
  differential diagnosis of, 483-486
  effects of, 1473
  in hereditary hypokalemic salt-losing tubulopathy, 1473
  in hypokalemia, 570
  hypotonic, 473t, 483-484
  lithium-induced, 379
Poorly differentiated renal cell carcinoma, 899f
Porphyria cutanea tarda, 1946, 1946f
Portal hypertension, 446-447
Port-wine stain, 1952
Positron emission tomography, 899-903
Positron emission tomography–computed tomography, 899-903
Posterior urethral valves, 2316, 2317f, 2435
Postglomerular hypoxia, 1790
Postobstructive diuresis, 1281
Postpartum recovery, 1617
Postrenal azotemia, 968
Postrenal failure, 770
Postrenal proteinuria, 791
Poststenotic renal perfusion pressure (iliac), 1570-1571, 1571f
Poststreptococcal glomerulonephritis
  acute. See Acute poststreptococcal glomerulonephritis
  in Africa, 2461
  description of, 757
  in New Zealand, 2550
Posttransplantation diabetes mellitus, 1320, 2283
Posttransplantation lymphoproliferative disorder (PTLD), 2285-2286, 2286t, 2423-2424, 2426, 2429, 2433
Potassium
  adrenal sensing, 568-569
  assessment of, 820-821
  balance of, 174, 741, 741f

Potassium (Continued)
  cell membrane permeability to, 125
  in children, 2374-2382
  connecting tubule secretion of, 176-178
  cortical collecting duct secretion of, 176-178
  deficiency of, 481, 520
  depletion of, 547, 1968
  deprivation of, 180-182
  dietary intake of, 559-560, 566, 584t, 1975
  distal convoluted tubule secretion of, 176-178
  distal nephron secretion of, vasopressin effects on, 182
  distribution of
    acid-base status effects on, 563
    factors that affect, 562-563, 562t-563t, 563f
    hyperkalemia caused by, 586-588
    illustration of, 560f
    insulin effects on, 562, 587, 594
    sympathetic nervous system effects on, 562
  diuretics effect on, 1728
  efflux of, 560-562
  in end-stage kidney disease, 174-175, 2093
  excessive intake of, 586
  excretion of
    abnormal rate of, 821
    in acquired tubular defects, 589
    diuretics effect on, 595, 1711-1712
    fractional, 2375-2376
    in hereditary tubular defects, 589-590
    high, 825
    in hyporeninemic hypoaldosteronism, 589
    low, 823-825
    nephron loss-specific adaptations in, 1748-1749
    reductions in, 588-590
    regulation of, 536-537
    thiazide diuretics effect on, 1711-1712
    urinary, 564f, 569, 595, 820
    urinary tract obstruction relief effects on, 1276
  extracellular, 174-175, 568f
  fractional excretion of, 2375-2376
  in hemodialysis dialysate, 2093
  hemodialysis effects on, 599
  homeostasis of, 565-567, 579, 587, 1748-1749
  intracellular, 174, 560
  loading of, 179-180
  loss of
    apparent mineralocorticoid excess, 577-578
    Bartter's syndrome and, 578-580
    diuretics as cause of, 574-575
    drugs as cause of, 574-575
    familial hypokalemic alkalosis as cause of, 578-580
    fecal, 574
    gastric, 574
    Gitelman's syndrome and, 580
    hyperaldosteronism as cause of, 575-577, 576f
    intestinal, 574
    Liddle's syndrome as cause of, 578
    minimization strategies for, 585
    nonrenal causes of, 574
    renal tubular acidosis as cause of, 580-581
  medullary recycling of, 175-176
  monocarboxylic acids effect on, 818f
  normal levels of, 559-563
  oral supplementation of, 583-585

Potassium (Continued)
  parenteral administration of, 583-584
  plasma, in hypovolemia, 423
  proximal tubule bicarbonate reabsorption affected by, 237
  reabsorption of
    by collecting duct, 178
    in distal nephron, 564
    in loop of Henle, 563-564
    in proximal tubule, 175, 563-564
  redistribution of, 586-588, 594-595
  renal excretion of, 818-819
  secretion of
    aldosterone in, 312-314, 317, 565-566
    in aldosterone-sensitive distal nephron, 319-320
    arginine vasopressin effects on, 1717
    connecting tubule's role in, 69
    cortical connecting tubule's role in, 73, 563-564, 1748-1749
    in cortical distal nephron, 819
    in distal colon, 174-175
    distal sodium absorption and, 566-568
    epithelial sodium channel activity effects on, 313
    pathways of, 563f
    potassium intake effects on, 566
  serum, 564f, 596, 1728
  in skeletal muscle, 174-175, 560
  sodium polystyrene sulfonate effects on, 596
  succinylcholine-induced efflux of, 587-588, 587f
  transcellular distribution of, 818-830
  transtubular potassium concentration gradient, 569, 573-574, 820-821, 2380
  urinary excretion of, 180, 564f, 2302
Potassium binders, 597-598
Potassium channels
  in ammonia metabolism, 254
  apical, 159-160, 313
  drugs that affect, 588
Potassium chloride
  description of, 424-425, 583
  oral preparations of, 584-585, 585t
  transport of, 162, 178
Potassium ion deficiency, 555
Potassium transport
  aldosterone effects on, 179-180, 564
  distal, 179-182
  in distal nephron, 563-564
  in inner medullary collecting duct, 133
  in loop of Henle, 175-176
  mechanisms of, 560-563, 561f
  in proximal tubule, 175, 175f
  sodium chloride transport and, in distal nephron, 182-183
  transepithelial, 175-176
Potassium wasting, 569, 1437
Potassium-chloride cotransporter, 150, 564
Potassium-sparing diuretics
  distal. See Distal potassium-sparing diuretics
  Gitelman's syndrome treated with, 1727
  hypervolemia treated with, 451
  hypomagnesemia treated with, 625
  mechanism of action, 451
  side effects of, 451
Potting compound, 2075-2076
POU domain-containing transcription factor, 30
Pou3f3, 30
Poverty, 666
Power Doppler ultrasonography, 850f

Pramipexole, 1940
Praziquantel, 1255
Prazosin, 1676t, 1677, 1697t, 1714
Prealbumin, 1970-1971
Predictive biomarker, 927t
Predictive Safety Testing Consortium, 953
Prednisolone, 1043, 2329
Prednisone
  anti-glomerular basement membrane glomerulonephritis treated with, 1081
  azathioprine and, 2257
  focal segmental glomerulosclerosis treated with, 1032, 1167
  immunoglobulin A nephropathy treated with, 1067
  lupus nephritis treated with, 1102
  minimal change disease treated with, 1022-1024, 1167
  during pregnancy, 1637, 1637t
Preeclampsia. See also Pregnancy
  acute kidney injury and, 1632
  angiogenic imbalance and, 1621-1623
  cardiovascular disease and, 1618, 1618f
  cerebral changes with, 1619-1620
  characteristics and effect of, 1613-1627
  chronic kidney disease progression affected by, 680-681
  clinical features of, 1616
  diabetes and, 1634
  diagnosis of, 1615t
  edema and, 1616
  endothelin-1 in, 338
  extrauterine pregnancy and, 1618
  glomerular endotheliosis and, 1619, 1621f
  hemodynamic and vascular changes with, 1619
  hypertension and, 1615-1618, 1615t
  hypoxia-inducible factor and, 1619
  immunologic intolerance and, 1620-1621
  incidence of, 1613
  intracerebral parenchymal hemorrhage and, 1619-1620
  kidney disease and, 1617-1618
  long-term cardiovascular and renal outcomes from, 1617-1618
  low birth weight and, 1617-1618
  management and treatment of, 1626-1627
  maternal and neonatal mortality during, 1617
  maternal endothelial dysfunction and, 1619
  medical conditions associated with, 1614
  oxidative stress and, 1620
  pathogenesis of, 1618-1624, 1620f
  placenta role in, 1618
  placental growth factor and, 1623f
  placentation in, 1614f
  plasma renin levels in, 1623-1624
  postpartum recovery and, 1617
  prevention of, 1625-1626
  proteinuria in, 798, 1615t, 1616, 1618
  renal changes with, 1619
  risk factors for, 1614-1615, 1615t
  screening for, 1624-1625
  seizures and, 1616
  sickle cell disease and, 1618
  soluble fms-like tyrosine kinase-1 and, 1621, 1622f
  uric acid levels and, 1616
  vascular endothelial growth factor and, 1619, 1621-1623
  vascular endothelial growth factor receptor 1 and, 1621

Pregnancy, 1617-1618. See also Preeclampsia
  acute fatty liver of, 992, 1632
  acute kidney injury in, 990-992, 991t, 1631-1633, 2458
  acute tubular and bilateral cortical necrosis in, 1631-1632
  angiotensin II and, 1613f
  angiotensin receptor blockers in, 1647, 1655
  angiotensin-converting enzyme inhibitors during, 1647, 1685
  antihypertensive treatment during, 1629f, 1630t, 1685, 1687f
  asymptomatic bacteriuria in, 1245-1247
  atypical hemolytic-uremic syndrome in, 1182
  characteristics of, 1610
  chronic kidney disease and, 680-681, 1633-1638
  diabetes insipidus of, 1612
  in diabetic nephropathy patients, 1300, 1634
  1,25-dihydroxyvitamin d3 levels during, 1632-1633
  drug classification for, 1637
  glomerular filtration rate estimations in, 788
  hemodynamic and vascular changes during, 1610-1611, 1611f
  hypertension in, 681, 1627-1631
  immunoglobulin A nephropathy during, 1066
  immunosuppressive therapy during, 1637-1638, 1637t
  kidney stones during, 1633
  long-term dialysis and, 1635-1636
  lupus nephritis and, 1100, 1634-1635
  maternal and neonatal mortality, 1617
  maternal nutrient restriction in, 715-717
  mean arterial pressure changes during, 1611f
  mechanism of vasodilation in, 1612-1613
  mycophenolic acid exposure during, 2426
  physiologic changes during, 1611t
  plasmapheresis in, 2159
  preeclampsia in, 680-681
  prostaglandin synthesis in, 378-379
  proteinuria in, 798
  pyelonephritis in, 1245-1246
  renal adaptation to, 1611-1612
  renal allograft function effect on, 1636-1637
  renal donation and, 1638
  renal transplantation in, 2289-2290
  in renal transplantation recipient, 1636-1638, 1636f, 2435-2436
  respiratory alkalosis of, 1612
  soluble fms-like tyrosine kinase-1 levels in, 1623
  systemic lupus erythematosus and, 1100
  thiazide diuretics during, 1732
  thrombotic microangiopathy during, 1632
  uric acid levels and, 1612, 1616
Prehypertension, 2360
Prematurity
  acute kidney injury risks, 711-712
  blood pressure affected by, 706-709, 707f-708f
  categories of, 694t
  chronic kidney disease and, 712
  glomerular filtration rate affected by, 709-710
  nephron number and, 703-705
  risk factors for, 722

PreproBNP, 340
PreproCNP, 340
Prepro-urotensin II, 418-419
Prerenal azotemia, 450, 770
　acute kidney injury caused by, 963
　in liver disease, 998
　radiocontrast media-induced acute kidney injury, 964
　renal sympathetic nerve activity in, 963
　volume-nonresponsive, 963
　volume-responsive, 963
Pressor kidney, 1568-1569
Pressure monitors, 2075
Pressure natriuresis, 373, 402-405, 1528-1529, 1529f
Presternal catheter, 2115
Preterm infants, sodium retention in, 2366-2367
Pretubular aggregates, 3, 28, 30
Primary aldosteronism, 322-323, 555, 1546
Primary cilium, 1477-1478, 1478f, 1505-1506, 1506f
Primary hyperaldosteronism, 575, 576f, 1545-1547
Primary hyperoxaluria, 1337-1338, 2346-2348, 2422, 2431, 2478
Primary hyperparathyroidism
　age of onset, 606
　clinical presentation of, 606
　diagnosis of, 606
　familial syndromes, 608
　hypercalcemia caused by, 604-607
　osteitis fibrosa cystica in, 606
　parathyroid carcinoma as cause of, 607
　parathyroidectomy for, 607
　surgery for, 606-607
Primary hypertension, 1562-1565
Primary hypoaldosteronism, 588
Primary megaureter, 2315-2316
Primary mineralocorticoid deficiency, 538
Primary polydipsia
　causes of, 482, 497-498
　definition of, 482
　hyponatremia in, 496
　pathophysiology of, 482-483
　treatment of, 490
Principal cells
　aldosterone in, 567
　aquaporin expression in, 289, 289f
　bicarbonate reabsorption affected by, 241
　in collecting ducts, 30, 69-70, 241
　in cortical collecting duct, 70, 70f, 74
　in inner medullary collecting duct, 75, 76f
　in outer medullary collecting duct, 73-74
ProANP, 340
Pro-brain natriuretic peptide, 1800
Progenitor cells, 1795, 2608-2609
Prognostic biomarker, 927t
Programmed death 1, 1215, 2240-2241
Progressive hypermagnesemia, 625
Progressive renal failure, acidosis of, 541-543
Progressive vascular occlusion, 1585-1587, 1598
PROK2, 2318
Prolactin, 1919
Prolactinemia, in chronic kidney disease, 1919
Proliferative glomerulonephritis, 1136, 1159
Prolonged intermittent renal replacement therapy, 1008
Prolyl-4-hydroxylase domains, 140
PROMETHEUS, 458
Pronephric duct, 2-3
Pronephric tubules, 2-3
Pronephros, 2-3, 3f, 20-21
Propranolol, 1656t-1657t, 1657

Propylene glycol-induced high anion gap acidosis, 549
Prorenin, 327-328, 327f
(Pro)renin receptor, 331-332
Prospective payment system, 2628-2629
Prostacyclin
　age-related changes in, 735-736
　description of, 364-365
　metabolism of, 374
　renal epithelial effects of, 369
　vasodilator role of, 369
Prostacyclin synthase, 364-365
Prostaglandin(s)
　angiotensin II effects on production of, 99
　aspirin effects on, 380
　atrial natriuretic peptide and, 436-437
　in cirrhosis, 378, 448-449
　classification of, 375
　COX-2–derived, 568
　cyclopentenone, 374-375
　description of, 1579
　in effective arterial blood volume regulation, 411-413
　as fatty acids, 375
　half-life of, 374
　in heart failure, 436-437
　metabolism of, 374-375
　nephrogenic diabetes insipidus treated with, 301
　PGD$_2$, 99
　in pregnancy, 378-379
　sodium retention and, 448-449
　synthesis of, 80, 360, 742
　transport of, 375
　as vasodilators, 411-412
　vasodilatory, 359f
　in volume homeostasis, 411
　w/w-1 hydroxylation of, 374
Prostaglandin A$_2$, 374
Prostaglandin D$_2$, 365
Prostaglandin D synthase, 365
Prostaglandin E$_2$, 412
　cytokines that stimulate synthesis of, 376
　hydroxylation of, 374
　medullary blood flow affected by, 362f
　metabolism of, 374
　nonsteroidal anti-inflammatory drug-induced blockade of, 371
　prohypertensive effects of, 372
　proximal tubule effects of, 373
　renal function by, 372
　salt excretion and, 362f
　sodium absorption affected by, 361-362
　sodium reabsorption affected by, 1716-1717
　vasoconstrictive effects of, 372
　water excretion and, 362f
Prostaglandin E synthases, 366
Prostaglandin F$_{2\alpha}$, 365, 374
Prostaglandin F$_{2\alpha}$ receptor, 369-370
Prostaglandin H$_2$, 364, 364f
Prostaglandin 9-ketoreductase, 365-366
Prostaglandin receptors, 367f
Prostaglandin synthase inhibitors, 487
Prostaglandin synthases, 357, 358f, 364f
Prostaglandin transporter, 375
Prostanoid receptors
　DP receptors, 369
　EP1 receptors, 370
　EP2 receptors, 370-371
　EP3 receptors, 371-372
　EP4 receptors, 372
　FP receptors, 369-370
　intrarenal distribution of, 367f
　IP receptors, 369

Prostanoid receptors *(Continued)*
　knockout mice models of, 368f
　mRNA, 366f
　tissue distribution of, 366f
　TP receptors, 366-369
Prostanoids
　cyclooxygenase-2–derived, 357-358
　degradation of, 411
　glomerular damage mediated by, 376
　mesangial cells affected by, 377
　transport of, 375
　vasodilatory, 376-377
Prostate cancer, 1261
Prostate gland, 1234, 1677
Prostatitis
　acute bacterial, 1247
　bacille de Calmette-Guérin as cause of, 1254
　chronic bacterial, in elderly, 750
　Escherichia coli as cause of, 1247
　National Institutes of Health classification of, 1247, 1247t
Protease inhibitors, 2456-2457
Protein
　catabolism of, 128f, 517, 1959-1960
　dietary
　　albumin synthesis affected by, 1796
　　caspase-3 effects on, 1965
　　in chronic kidney disease, 1767-1768, 1975-1977, 1976t
　　in diabetic kidney disease, 1981
　　hemodynamic responses to changes in, 1958
　　high intake of, chronic kidney disease risks associated with, 680
　　hypermetabolism and, 1958
　　low-protein diet, 1312, 1970, 1976-1977
　　maternal, restriction of, 723
　　metabolic acidosis effects on, 1963-1964
　　myostatin effects, 1967-1968
　　in nephrotic syndrome, 1976-1977
　　oxidative stress and, 1958
　　phosphates and, 1977
　　proteinuria increases associated with, 1962
　　renal function affected by, 1767-1768, 1958-1959, 1981
　　requirements for, factors that affect, 1963-1968
　　restriction of, 1312, 1767-1768, 1980-1981, 1994-1995
　　transforming growth factor-β affected by, 1958
　　transforming growth factor-β levels affected by, 1958
　　ubiquitin-protease system effects on, 1964-1965
　　urinary albumin affected by, 1312
　DNA variation, 1435t
　external losses of, 1968
　high-molecular-weight, 791
　kidney stones and, 1324, 1354
　low-molecular-weight, 791, 1810t
　metabolism of, uremia effects on, 1817
　muscle, 1965, 1966f, 1970
　normal levels of, 791
　physiology of, 791
　podocyte uptake of, 1787
　proximal tubule reabsorption of, 1784-1786
　slit diaphragm, 113
　Tamm-Horsfall, 791, 947
　tissue, loss of, 1817
　total, 793, 794t
　as uremic solute, 1810

Protein (Continued)
　urinary
　　in acute tubular necrosis, 987
　　in children, 2310-2311
　　description of, 112, 682-683
　　diurnal variation in excretion of, 796
　　excretion of, 682-683, 947, 1654, 1784
　　factors that affect, 792t
　　fluctuations in excretion of, 796
　　postural effects on excretion of, 796
　　protein-to-creatinine ratios, 792, 795-796
　　reagent strip testing for, 797
　　timed versus random collection of, 795
　　24-hour testing of, 795-796
　water homeostasis and, 1468
　in Western diets, 740-741
Protein C, 980-981
Protein kinase A, 154-155, 214, 292-293
Protein kinase C, 292-293
Protein kinase G, 292-293
Protein overload, 1212, 1792
Protein-bound calcium, 602
Protein-bound solutes, 1814
Protein-energy wasting
　in chronic kidney disease, 1817, 1913, 1994-1995
　during hemodialysis, 1317-1318, 2098-2099
　insulin-like growth factor-1 as biomarker of, 2099
　megestrol acetate for, 1920
　in peritoneal dialysis, 2124, 2124t
Protein-restricted diet, 1984
Protein-to-creatinine ratios, 792, 795-796
Proteinuria, 1398
　acute interstitial nephritis and, 1219
　aliskiren as cause of, 1678
　bevacizumab causing, 1398
　birth weight and, 710-711
　bone marrow-derived fibrocytes in, 1793
　captopril and, 1159, 1645
　categorization of, 791-792
　causes of, 1013-1014
　changes after long-term treatment, 1556t
　in children, 798, 2310-2311
　in chronic kidney disease, 682-683, 947-948, 2004-2005, 2361-2362
　COX-2 inhibitors effect on, 377-378
　C1q nephropathy as cause of, 1034-1035
　criteria for, 1785-1786
　definition of, 1785-1786
　dendritic cells in, 1792-1793
　description of, 790
　in diabetic nephropathy, 1295, 2004-2005
　diagnosis of, 947
　dietary proteins and, 1959, 1994-1995
　experimental models of, 1761-1762
　Fanconi's syndrome and, 1437
　fixed, 1014
　in focal segmental glomerulosclerosis, 1024-1025, 1030-1031, 1164, 1750-1752
　glomerular, 791, 1780, 1785-1786
　glomerular basement membrane and, 2323
　glomerular damage caused by, 1786-1790, 1787f
　as glomerular disease, 1013-1014
　as glomerular injury marker, 1760-1761
　gold salts and, 1158
　hematuria and, 758-759
　in hepatitis B, 1154
　in hepatitis C, 1156
　hereditary syndromes, 2323-2325

Proteinuria (Continued)
　in immunoglobulin A nephropathy, 1065-1066, 1069, 1164-1165
　in immunotactoid glomerulopathy, 1072, 1132
　interstitial inflammation and injury in, 1792-1794
　in ischemia-reperfusion injury, 1786
　isolated, 1013-1014, 2311
　Kidney Disease Improving Global Outcomes categories of, 792t
　in kidney transplantation, 798
　kidney-derived progenitor cells in, 1795
　lipid-lowering therapy effects on, 1774
　low birth weight and, 710-711
　in lupus nephritis, 1165-1166
　lymphocytes in, 1793
　macrophages in, 1793-1795
　measurement of, 792-793, 792t, 794t
　mechanisms of
　　glomerular capillary wall, 1780-1784
　　glomerular permselectivity, 1783-1784
　in membranous glomerulonephritis, 1164
　in membranous nephropathy, 1035, 1039-1041, 1158-1159
　mesangial cells affected by, 1788-1789
　in microscopic polyangiitis, 1115
　in minimal change disease, 1022
　monocytes in, 1792-1793
　after nephrectomy, 1752f
　nephrotic syndrome in, 1796
　nephrotic-range
　　description of, 1796
　　edema caused by, 1798-1800, 1798f, 1799f
　　hypercoagulability associated with, 1803-1805, 1803f
　　hyperlipidemia associated with, 1801-1803, 1801f, 1803f, 1816-1817
　　hypoalbuminemia caused by, 1796-1798, 1796f
　　infection susceptibility, 1805
　orthostatic, 1014
　overflow, 791
　parietal epithelial cells in, 1789-1790
　plasma proteins in, 1013-1014
　podocytes affected by, 118, 1787-1788
　postglomerular hypoxia in, 1790
　postrenal, 791
　posttransplantation recurrence of, 1427-1428
　preeclampsia and, 798, 1615t, 1616, 1618
　proximal tubular cells in, 1791-1792
　reagent strip testing for, 797
　reduced, benefits of, 2010f
　regulatory T cells in, 1795
　renal allograft survival affected by, 2280
　renal artery stenosis and, 1584
　renal damage and, 1762-1763
　renal function affected by, 1645
　renin-angiotensin-aldosterone system in, 334
　serum albumin levels affected by, 683
　in sickle cell disease, 1199
　smoking and, 1991-1992
　statins effect on, 2011
　stroke risks associated with, 1928t, 1930
　in temporal arteritis, 1120
　treatment of, 1141, 1163-1166, 1429, 2004-2005
　tubular, 791, 793
　tubular cell activation and damage induced by, 1211-1212

Proteinuria (Continued)
　tubular damage caused by, 1790-1792, 1790f
　tubuloglomerular disconnection in, 1791
　in type 1 diabetes mellitus, 1292-1293, 1300
　types of, 791
　urinary cystatin C associated with, 949
　urinary protein in
　　description of, 112, 682-683
　　diurnal variation in excretion of, 796
　　excretion of, as chronic kidney disease biomarker, 682-683
　　factors that affect, 792t
　　fluctuations in excretion of, 796
　　postural effects on excretion of, 796
　　protein-to-creatinine ratios, 792, 795-796
　　reagent strip testing for, 797
　　timed versus random collection of, 795
　　24-hour testing of, 795-796
　urine studies for, 762-763
Proteomics, 2249
Proteus infections, 778
Proton ATPase subunit mutation, 1457
Proton pump inhibitors, 620
Proximal convoluted tubule (PCT)
　cells of, 59-60
　embryology of, 5
　filtered glutamine reabsorption in, 249
　fractional reabsorption of sodium in, 816
　illustration of, 58f
　mineralocorticoid receptor expression in, 315
Proximal renal tubular acidosis, 1455, 1456t
　acquired, 530-532
　calcium excretion in, 533
　carbonic anhydrase deficiency, 531-532
　clinical spectrum of, 532, 532t
　diagnosis of, 532-533, 533f
　features of, 532-533, 532t
　inherited, 530-532
　model of, 531-532
　pathogenesis of, 530-532
　physiology of, 530
　vitamin D deficiency and, 531
Proximal tubular cells
　activation of, 1791-1792
　albumin reabsorption by, 1791
　apoptosis of, 1212, 1791
　gene upregulation in, 1762
　histology of, 1784f
　megalin effects on, 1791
　protein filtration effects on, 1786
　protein overload of, 1790f
　in proteinuria, 1791-1792
Proximal tubule, 1440f, 1447f
　albumin degradation in, 1784, 1785f
　amino acid reabsorption in, 223f
　ammonia reabsorption in, 251
　ammoniagenesis in, 248
　anatomy of, 55
　angiotensin II in, 152, 384
　basement membrane, 1284f
　bicarbonate in
　　excretion of, 519
　　reabsorption of. See Bicarbonate reabsorption, in proximal tubule
　brush border of, 55, 57f
　calcium reabsorption in, 188, 188f
　citrate absorption and metabolism in, 217f, 248
　claudin expression in, 147
　cytochrome P450 in, 384

Proximal tubule (Continued)
  diuretics mechanism of action in, 1703f
  dopamine in, natriuretic effects of, 154
  electrolyte reabsorption functions of, 61
  enlargement of, 1745-1746
  filtered protein handling by, 1786
  fluid delivery from, 491
  functions of, 61, 144-145
  gap junctions in, 56
  glucose in, 129-130, 205, 206f
  glutamine synthetase expression by, 251
  as glyconeogenic organ, 204-205
  inherited disorders associated with dysfunction of, 1435-1445
  lateral cell processes of, 58f
  length of, 55
  lysosomes from, 59-60, 61f
  magnesium reabsorption in, 194, 194f
  microvilli of, 1784, 1784f
  natriuretic hormone targeting of, 152-153
  organic anion in, 216, 216t
  organic cation transport by, 210-211, 210f
  pars convoluta of. See Pars convoluta
  pathogenesis of, 1435-1436
  phosphate reabsorption in, 199f, 247
  phosphate-dependent glutaminase activity in, 253
  potassium channels in, 254
  potassium in, 175, 175f
  prostaglandin E_2 effects on, 373
  protein reabsorption by, 1784-1786
  in rat, 55, 56f-57f
  segments of, 55, 56f-57f, 145f. See also Pars convoluta; Pars recta
  serotonin synthesis in, 201
  sodium in, 132, 430f
  solutes, 132, 145f, 403f, 1745-1746
  ultrafiltered protein receptors in, 1792
  uric acid transport by, 220f
  water transport pathways in, 274f
Proximal tubule defect, 1417-1418
Proximal tubulopathy, GLUT2 mutation in, 209
Prune-belly syndrome, 2318-2319
Pruritus, 1942-1943, 1943f
Prussian blue, 2168-2169
Psen1, 30
Psen2, 30
Pseudoaneurysm, 2253
Pseudohyperkalemia, 585-586, 827, 829, 2380
Pseudohyperphosphatemia, 628
Pseudohypertension, 766, 1685, 1693
Pseudohypoaldosteronism, 179-180, 827, 2377-2378
  in children, 2380-2382
  type I, 539, 539f, 589, 1464, 2380-2381
  type II, 539-540, 589-590, 1464, 1465f, 2381-2382
Pseudohypocalcemia, 617
Pseudohyponatremia, 490, 816
Pseudohypoparathyroidism, 627, 1453
Pseudo-Kaposi's sarcoma, 1947
Pseudomonas aeruginosa peritonitis, 2128-2131
Pseudo-obstruction, 574
Pseudoporphyria, 1946
Pseudopseudohypoparathyroidism, 616
Psychogenic polydipsia, 482
Psychosis, 496
Psychotropic drugs, 497
Pubertal delay, 2357, 2435-2436
Pulmonary dysfunction, 2138-2139
Pulmonary embolism, 1805, 1906-1907
Pulmonary hemorrhage, 1072
Pulmonary hypertension, 2413
Pulmonary sensors, 395-396

Pulse pressure, 1681
Pulse repetition time, 856-857
Pulsus paradoxus, 761-762
Pure red cell aplasia, 2097
Pyelocalyceal cyst, 1518
Pyelocalyceal diverticula, 1518
Pyelonephritis
  acute, 1240-1242
    ciprofloxacin for, 1241-1242, 1241t
    clinical presentation of, 1241
    contrast-enhanced computed tomography of, 878-880, 880f, 1241
    imaging of, 878-880
    magnetic resonance imaging of, 880
    nuclear medicine of, 880
    treatment of, 1241-1242, 1241t
    ultrasonography of, 878, 880f
    vesicoureteral reflux associated with, 878
  bacille de Calmette-Guérin, 1254
  chronic, 882-883
  emergent interventions for, 778
  emphysematous, 881, 1251
  in pregnancy, 1245-1246
  xanthogranulomatous, 881, 883f, 1251-1252
Pyelorenal cyst, 1518
Pyk2, 256
Pyocystis, 1252
Pyoderma, 2331-2332
Pyrin, 2479-2483, 2483f, 2486
Pyrogenic reactions, 2082
Pyroglutamic acid-induced high anion gap acidosis, 549
Pyrophosphate, 1330, 1838
Pyuria, 756, 1238, 1246

Q

Quality, 2620-2622
Quality improvement
  arteriovenous fistulas and, 2629-2631
  continuous, 2623
  in end-stage kidney disease, 2625-2626
  erythropoiesis-stimulating agents in catalyzing, 2626-2628
  history of, 2621
  in kidney disease, 2625-2626
  lean principles, 2623-2624, 2623t, 2624f
  in nephrology, 2625
  overview of, 2620-2625
  Plan-Do-Study-Act, 2623, 2623t, 2624f
  prospective payment system, 2628-2629
  rationale for measuring, 2623
  Six Sigma, 2625, 2625f
  vascular access and, 2629-2631
Quality incentive program, 2628-2629
Quality of life, 2410, 2436, 2570
Quinapril hydrochloride, 1643t, 1644
Quinton-Scribner shunt, 2064

R

Race. See also specific race
  chronic kidney disease and, 660-663, 666
  definition of, 660
  end-stage kidney disease and, 1769f, 2577, 2597f
  health disparities and, 2577-2578
  hypertension and, 1526-1527
  renal function differences based on, 661t
Radiation, 2194
Radiation nephropathy
  acute, 1193
  chronic, 1194
  clinical features of, 1193

Radiation nephropathy (Continued)
  definition of, 1193
  malignant hypertension after, 1194-1195
  mechanisms of, 1194
  pathogenesis of, 1194
  pathology of, 1194
  renin-angiotensin-aldosterone system activation in, 1194
  treatment of, 1194-1195
  types of, 1193-1194
Radiation-associated kidney injury, 1400-1401
  clinical presentation of, 1401
  diagnosis of, 1401
  epidemiology of, 1400
  laboratory findings, 1401
  pathogenesis of, 1400
  prognosis for, 1401
  treatment of, 1401
Radiologist's tumor, 1374
Radiopharmaceuticals, 864-865
  fluorine 18 2-fluoro-2-deoxy-D-glucose, 865, 900
  iodine 131-labeled ortho-iodohippurate, 865
  technetium 99m-labeled diethylenetriaminepentaacetic acid, 864-866
  technetium 99m-labeled dimercaptosuccinic acid, 865, 880
  technetium 99m-labeled mercaptoacetyltriglycine, 865, 866f, 869-871, 874f, 913f
Ramipril, 1553, 1643t, 1644, 1650, 2362
Randall's plaque, 873-874, 1325, 1326f, 1329
Randomized controlled trials, 671
RANK, 1832, 1833f
RANKL, 603, 607, 1832, 1833f
RANTES, 729, 976-977, 1791
Rapalog, 1496
Rapamycin, 2247
Rapidly progressive glomerulonephritis (RPGN)
  categorization of, 1072-1073, 2150
  characteristics of, 2150
  definition of, 1072-1073
  end-stage kidney disease secondary to, 2150
  idiopathic, 2151
  neoplasia associated with, 1157
  nomenclature of, 1072-1073
  plasmapheresis for, 2150-2151
Ras-related C3 botulinum toxin substrate 1, 1753-1754
Raw carp bile, 2525
Rayer, Pierre, 2621
Raynaud's phenomenon, 1195
rBAT/b$^{0,+}$AT, 227-228
Rbpj, 35
Reactive oxygen species (ROS)
  in acute kidney injury, 977-978
  angiotensin type 1 receptor and, 329
  COX-2 actions mediated by, 379
  in diabetic nephropathy, 337
  in heart failure treatment, 452
  mitochondrial generation of, 732
Recalcification syndrome, 616
Receiver operator characteristic curve, 929, 929f
Receptor tyrosine kinase, 256
Receptor-mediated endocytosis, 341, 1791
Recessive disease, 1411, 1411t
Recluse spider bites, 2444-2445, 2445f
Recombinant atrial natriuretic peptide, 344
Recombinant growth hormone, 2125

Recombinant human erythropoietin, 1888-1890, 1895, 1906, 1922, 2097
Recombinant human growth factor, 1918
Recombinant tissue plasminogen activator, 1933
Recreational drugs, 686
Red blood cell(s). *See also* Erythrocytes
  in dialyzer, 2074
  erythropoiesis-stimulating agents effect on, 1892
  hypochromic, 1894-1895
  shortened survival of, anemia in chronic kidney disease secondary to, 1884-1885, 2013
  transfusion of, 586, 1902-1904, 1903f
  uremic, 1884-1885
Red blood cell casts, 756, 756f
Refeeding syndrome, 572-573, 620, 633
Refractory hypertension, 1695
Regional anticoagulation, 2092
Regional citrate anticoagulation, 2092, 2144
Regulated intramembrane proteolysis, 1791
Regulatory T cells, 1795, 2240, 2250
Reimbursement, 2503, 2562, 2572
Relative density of urine, 789
Relaxin, 465-466, 729-730
Remediable hypertension. *See* Secondary hypertension
Renal abscess
  contrast-enhanced computed tomography of, 880, 881f
  imaging of, 880, 881f-882f
  magnetic resonance imaging of, 880, 882f
  management of, 1250
  in transplanted kidney, 911
  urinary tract involvement of, 1250
Renal acidification, 1455f
Renal amyloidosis, 588-589
Renal anlagen, 2613-2616
Renal aplasia, 10t-17t
Renal artery
  angiography of, 1202
  description of, 42
  occlusion of, 964, 1201-1204
  stenosis of. *See* Renal artery stenosis
  stents in, magnetic resonance angiography of, 906-907, 906f
  thromboembolism of, 1201-1202
  thrombosis of, 964, 1202-1203, 2253, 2266
Renal artery aneurysms
  atherosclerosis as cause of, 1203
  classification of, 1203
  clinical features of, 1203
  dissecting, 1204
  incidence of, 1203
  mechanisms of, 1203
  rupture of, 1203
  saccular, 1203
  treatment of, 1203-1204
Renal artery angioplasty, 1595t, 1604
Renal artery stenosis, 1547
  acute kidney injury caused by, 964
  angiotensin II in, 907
  angiotensin-converting enzyme inhibitors for, 907
  arterial pressure and blood flow, 1570f
  atheroembolic renal disease and, 1192-1193
  atherosclerotic. *See* Atherosclerotic renal artery stenosis
  clinical features of, 1584f
  computed tomography angiography of, 904, 904f-905f
  Doppler ultrasonography of, 903-904

Renal artery stenosis *(Continued)*
  endovascular revascularization of, 1202
  epidemiology of, 1580-1581
  erythrocytosis associated with, 1889
  in Indian subcontinent, 2507, 2507f
  Kaplan-Meier survival for, 1585f
  magnetic resonance angiography of, 904-906, 906f
  management of, 1586t
  nephrotic syndrome associated with, 1159
  noninvasive assessment of, 1589t
  progression of, 1598-1599
  proteinuria and, 1584
  renin-angiotensin-aldosterone system activation in, 1574f
  renovascular hypertension and, 903, 1570-1571
  tissue hypoxia and, 139-140
  transplantation, 2272
Renal autoregulation, 104-110, 104f
  cellular mechanisms involved in, 105
  factors involved in, 110
  metabolic mechanisms that mediate, 109-110
  myogenic mechanism for, 105-106
  tubuloglomerular feedback mediation of, 106-109
Renal baroreceptor, 327
Renal biopsy. *See* Kidney biopsy
Renal blood flow
  adrenomedullin effects on, 418
  angiotensin II effects on, 407-408
  autoregulation of, 104-110, 104f, 384, 396-397
  calculation of, 85-86
  as cardiac output, 83, 85, 133
  characteristics of, 440f
  cortical, 87
  effective, 2614
  endothelin effects on, 336
  epoxygenase metabolites effect on, 383
  formula for calculating, 85
  glomerular filtration rate determination by, 134, 138, 401-402
  heart failure-related decreases in, 429-430
  intrarenal distribution of, 87-98
  kallikrein-kinin system regulation of, 348
  leukotriene A_4 effects on, 380
  medullary, 90
  obstructive nephropathy effects on, 1269-1271
  oxygen consumption and, 133-135
  oxygen delivery by, 126
  prostaglandins effect on, 436
  rate of, 83
  renal plasma flow used to estimate, 86
  renin-angiotensin system's role in control of, 99-101
  total, 85-87
  tubuloglomerular feedback control of, 108-109
  urinary tract obstruction effects on, 1269-1271
  urine formation from, 83
  vasomotor properties of, 98
  vasopressin effects on, 410
Renal calcifications, 871-878
Renal calcium excretion, 1334f
Renal candidiasis, 1404
Renal cell carcinoma, 1370
  acquired cystic kidney disease and, 1515f
  biologic pathways in, 1383f
  calcifications associated with, 871-872
  classification of, 1371, 1371t

Renal cell carcinoma *(Continued)*
  clear cell, 892, 895f-896f
  clinical features of, 1374-1375
  computed tomography of, 1376f-1377f
  epidemiology of, 1370-1371
  Fuhrman grading system for, 1378
  hormones produced by, 1375
  imaging of, 892, 894f-899f
    computed tomography, 894f, 898f
    magnetic resonance imaging, 892, 895f-897f
    positron emission tomography, 899-903
    positron emission tomography–computed tomography, 899-903
  laboratory features of, 1374-1375
  metastasis of, 896f, 1377-1378, 1377t, 1381
  molecular biology and hereditary disorders, 1372-1374
  nuclear medicine of, 900-901
  oncocytic, 891-892
  papillary, 892, 897f
  pathology for, 1371-1372, 1371t
  poorly differentiated, 899f
  prognosis for, 1375
  pseudocapsule with, 897f
  radiologic diagnosis of, 1375-1377
  staging of, 892-898, 895f, 1377-1379
    American Joint Committee on Cancer staging system, 1378
    survival rate and, 1378t
    TNM staging system, 1378, 1378t
  survival rate for, 1378-1379, 1379f
  symptoms of, 1374
  treatment of, 1375
    chemotherapy, 1385
    immunotherapy, 1385
    surgical, 1379-1381
    systemic therapy, 1381-1385
    vaccine, 1384-1385
  vascular thrombosis in, 898, 899f
Renal colic, 769, 873, 1360
Renal collecting system. *See* Collecting system
Renal coloboma syndrome, 2297t, 2317-2318
Renal corpuscle, 45-46, 46f-47f, 89f
Renal cortex
  anatomy of, 43, 43f
  calcification of, 872
  COX-2 expression in, 357-361
  cysts of, 889, 890f
  direct tubule innervation in, 81
  hemodynamics of, EP receptor regulation of, 372
  infarction of, in sickle cell disease, 1199
  interstitial cells in, 77-78, 78f
  medullary rays of, 90-91
  necrosis of, 2499, 2501-2502
  reabsorption in, 87
  ultrasonography of, 850
  venous drainage of, 93-94
Renal cortical adenoma, 1368
Renal crisis, scleroderma, 1195-1198, 1195f-1196f
Renal cyst(s), 1490f
  in autosomal dominant polycystic kidney disease, 1484f
  category I, 890
  category II, 890, 891f
  category III, 890
  category IV, 890, 891f-892f
  complex, 883-885, 887f
  contrast-enhanced computed tomography of, 883-885, 886f, 891f
  cortical, 889, 890f

Renal cyst(s) (Continued)
  in elderly, 750
  evolution of, 1477f
  hydronephrosis versus, 868
  imaging of, 883-885, 885f-887f
  infected, 1250-1251
  knockout and transgenic models for studying, 10t-17t
  lithium as cause of, 889, 890f
  magnetic resonance imaging of, 883-885, 887f, 889f
  nontubular origin, 1517-1518
  occurrence of, 1501
  in other organs, 1491
  simple, 886f, 1511-1512, 1512f
  treatment of, 1493
  ultrasonography of, 883, 885f
Renal cyst and diabetes syndrome, 2316-2317, 2389
Renal cystic ciliopathy, 1416-1417
Renal cystic disease. *See also* Cystic kidney disease
  autosomal recessive ciliopathies with, 1505-1509, 1507t
  classification of, 1475, 1476t
  evolution of cyst in renal tubules, 1477f
  localized or unilateral, 1512-1513
  pathogenesis of, 1417
Renal cystic dysplasia, 1510-1511, 1510f-1511f
Renal cystic neoplasm, 1516-1517
Renal dysgenesis, 363
Renal dysplasia
  clinical features of, 2302
  clinical presentation of, 2303
  definition of, 2294-2295
  description of, 2312
  diagnosis of, 2312
  histology of, 2295f
  management of, 2305
  multicystic, 889, 2294-2296, 2295f, 2303, 2305, 2312-2313
  prognosis for, 2305
Renal ectopy, 2295, 2295f, 2303, 2305, 2311
Renal epithelial cells, 128
Renal epithelial cyst, 1475-1479
Renal epithelium, 126, 137f
Renal fibrosis. *See also* Interstitial fibrosis
  biologic mediators and modulators of, in elderly
    advanced glycosylation end products, 730-732
    angiotensin II, 728-729
    autophagy, 734-735
    bile acid metabolism, 734
    calorie restriction, 732-733
    description of, 728
    farnesoid X receptor, 734
    Klotho, 734
    lipid metabolism, 733-734
    nitric oxide, 730
    oxidative stress, 732
    transforming growth factor-β, 729-730
  biomarkers for, 951-952
  focal segmental glomerulosclerosis progression to, 1034
  microRNAs in, 1758
  microvascular rarefaction and, 1578f
  pathogenesis of, 1278
  urinary biomarkers for, 951-952
Renal function
  in acute kidney injury, 2043-2044
  age-related changes in, 1878, 2034
  angiotensin receptor blockers effect on, 1655

Renal function (Continued)
  angiotensin-converting enzyme inhibitors effect on, 1645-1646
  assessment of, 2005, 2034
  birth weight effects on, 709-712
  cardiovascular disease and, 1860
  in children, 2309-2311
  in continuous renal replacement therapy, 2044
  creatinine clearance in, 2042t
  developmental programming of, 703-712
  in dialysis, 2044
  dietary modification effects on, 1957
  dietary protein influences on, 1767-1768, 1958-1959, 1981
  in drug dosing, 2041-2044
  early growth effects on, 722
  glomerular filtration rate as indicator of, 2041-2042
  imaging of, 865-866, 866f
  magnetic resonance imaging evaluation of, 863-864
  in nephrotic hypoalbuminemia, 1797
  thermodynamic analysis of, 123
  tubulointerstitial disease effects on, 1210
  after urinary tract obstruction, 1280-1281
Renal fusion, 2303-2305, 2311
Renal gluconeogenesis, 130-132
Renal glucosuria, 1454. *See also* Glucosuria
Renal hamartomas, 891, 893f
Renal hemodynamics, 101-104
Renal hilum, 42
Renal hypercalciuria, 1334-1335
Renal hypoperfusion, 436, 1570t, 1577-1578
Renal hypoplasia
  definition of, 2311
  description of, 2311-2312
  isolated, 2297t
  maternal diabetes and, 2301
  in Middle East, 2479
Renal infection, 878-883, 880f-885f, 1404-1405. *See also specific type of infection*
Renal insufficiency
  angiotensin-converting enzyme inhibitor dosing in, 1649t-1650t
  hypermagnesemia caused by, 625
  hypoglycemia secondary to, 1816
  in immunotactoid glomerulopathy, 1072
  in membranous nephropathy, 1040
  salt-losing nephropathy associated with, 493
  stents for, 1603-1604
  urinary concentration affected by, 1748
Renal interstitium
  anatomy of, 75-80
  composition of, 75-77
  cortical, 77-78
  inflammation and injury to, in proteinuria, 1792-1794
  medullary, 78-80, 79f
Renal ischemia, acute, 141-142
Renal kallikrein-kinin system, 348-349
Renal lobus, 43
Renal lymphangioma, 1369
Renal masses
  ablation of, 1741t, 1755-1757. *See also* Nephron loss
  contrast-enhanced computed tomography of, 883-885, 886f
  cystic, 890, 891f
  imaging of, 883-899, 884f-899f
  intravenous urography of, 883
Renal medulla
  adenosine effects on, 136f
  anatomy of, 43
  axial osmolality gradient in, 265

Renal medulla (Continued)
  blood supply of, 91
  calcifications in, 872
  countercurrent multiplication paradigm of, 266, 267f
  COX-2 expression in, 360-361, 360f
  glypican-3 and, 2299
  growth of, 2301-2302
  inner, 45, 45f, 91-92, 91f
  interstitium of, 75-77, 262-264
  lactate concentrations in, 132
  outer, 45, 45f, 65f, 91, 91f
  prostaglandin synthesis in, 360
  in tubular reabsorption of sodium, 404f
  urea accumulation in, 269, 269f
  urea recycling in, 270, 270f
  uric acid deposits in, 1961
  vascular-tubule relations, 92
  zones of, 45
Renal metabolism, 131f
Renal neoplasms
  angiomyolipomas, 891, 893f
  imaging of, 891
  oncocytoma, 891-892
  after renal transplantation, 911
Renal nerve stimulation, 110
Renal osteodystrophy, 1842, 1845, 1845t, 2407f, 2434
Renal outer medullary potassium. *See* ROMK
Renal oxygenation, 133-137, 134f
Renal papilla, 43, 44f
Renal parenchyma
  calcifications in, 1775
  calcium deposits in, 1775
  dendritic cell accumulation in, 1792
  inflammation of, 975-977
Renal parenchymal disease, 868-869, 870f, 880-881, 2469-2470
Renal pelvis
  anatomy of, 44f, 264
  description of, 42
  transitional epithelium of, 43
  tumors of, 1352, 1385-1386
Renal perfusion injury, 1579-1580
Renal perfusion pressure, 396, 402-405, 1570-1571, 1571f, 1575-1576
Renal phosphate excretion, 1450-1451
Renal phosphate transport, 1450-1453
Renal plasma flow
  age-related changes in, 735-736, 736f
  "effective", 86, 87f
  glomerular filtration rate affected by, 1296
  hypothyroidism and, 496
  obesity effects on, 1771
  rate of, 86
  renal blood flow estimated using, 86
  technetium 99m-labeled diethylenetriaminepentaacetic assessments of, 865-866
Renal proximal tubule. *See* Proximal tubule
Renal pyramids, 43, 872-873
Renal replacement therapy (RRT)
  acute kidney injury treated with. *See* Acute kidney injury (AKI), renal replacement therapy for
  in Africa, 2456t, 2463-2465, 2464f
  in Australia, 2540-2544, 2540f-2543f, 2545f, 2545t
  in China, 2535
  chronic kidney disease stage 5 treated with, 2016
  continuous. *See* Continuous renal replacement therapy
  in elderly, 747-748, 2597-2598
  familial hematuria treated with, 1141
  in Far East, 2534-2536

Renal replacement therapy (RRT) (Continued)
    future of, 2108-2109
    global uses of, 643
    hemodialysis. See Hemodialysis
    hepatorenal syndrome treated with, 457-458
    in Hong Kong, 2535
    hybrid, 2048-2049
    in Indian subcontinent, 2503-2504
    in Indonesia, 2536
    intensity of, 2142-2144
    in intensive care unit, 2139-2140
    intermittent hemodialysis, 2140-2141
    in Japan, 2534-2535
    in Korea, 2535
    in Latin America, 2449, 2450t
    in Malaysia, 2535-2536
    metformin poisoning treated with, 2185
    in Middle East, 2475t
    modalities, 2140-2142
    in New Zealand, 2541f, 2551-2552, 2551f
    in older adults, 2544
    in Philippines, 2536
    in Singapore, 2536
    sustained low-efficiency dialysis, 2141t, 2142, 2145-2146
    in Taiwan, 2534
    in Thailand, 2535
    uremic solute removal using, 1813-1814
    uremic syndrome caused by, 1926
    in Vietnam, 2536
Renal revascularization. See Revascularization
Renal risk scores
    for chronic kidney disease, 687-691, 688t-689t
    for end-stage kidney disease, 690-691, 690f
Renal salt wasting, 828
Renal sarcoma, 1386
Renal scarring, 1240
Renal sensors, 396-397
Renal sinus, 84, 1517
Renal stones. See Kidney stones; Nephrolithiasis
Renal transplantation
    ABO-incompatible, 2156-2157, 2423
    in Aboriginal Australians, 2548, 2548f
    abscess after, 911
    access to, 2570-2572
    acute tubular necrosis after, 910f, 2263-2264, 2263t
    in African Americans, 2581
    allogenic immune response in
        antigen recognition, 2229
        characteristics of, 2228-2230
        definition of, 2228-2229
        description of, 2253-2255
        immune tolerance, 2229-2230
        self–nonself discrimination, 2229
        self-tolerance, 2230
    allografts
        alloantibody response against, 2243
        biopsies of, 2267t, 2272
        delayed function of
            algorithm for, 2263f
            allograft survival affected by, 2277
            causes of, 2263-2264, 2427-2428
            in children, 2427-2428
            cold ischemia time and, 2265, 2278
            cyclosporine nephrotoxicity as cause of, 2264
            definition of, 2427-2428
            diagnosis of, 2262
            hyperacute rejection as cause of, 2264

Renal transplantation (Continued)
        incidence of, 2262
        induction regimens effect on, 2265t
        ischemic acute tubular necrosis as cause of, 2263-2264, 2263t
        outcome of, 2264-2265
        patient survival affected by, 2277
        risk factors for, 2262, 2263t
        significance of, 2264-2265
        tacrolimus nephrotoxicity as cause of, 2264
    dysfunction of
        biopsy diagnosis of, 2267t, 2269
        calcineurin inhibitor nephrotoxicity as cause of, 2268-2269, 2272, 2274-2275
        chronic antibody-mediated rejection as cause of, 2274
        description of, 2244-2245
        drug-related nephrotoxicity as cause of, 2273
        in early posttransplantation period, 2265-2271, 2266f
        hepatitis C virus as cause of, 2273
        human polyomavirus infection as cause of, 2272-2273
        hypovolemia as cause of, 2265-2266
        in immediate posttransplantation period, 2261-2265
        intrarenal, 2266-2271
        late, 2271-2276
        in late posttransplantation period, 2271-2273
        postrenal, 2270-2271
        radiocontrast nephrotoxicity as cause of, 2273
        renal vessel thrombosis as cause of, 2266
        sclerosing/chronic allograft nephropathy, 2273, 2274t
    failure of, 2432
    human leukocyte antigen matching effects on, 2277-2278
    immune response to, 2237
    late loss of, 2273-2276
    nephrectomy of, 2290
    placement of, 2251-2252, 2252f
    in pregnant patients, 2289-2290
    proteinuria effects on survival of, 2280
    rejection of. See Renal transplantation, rejection of
    renal artery thrombosis of, 2253
    survival of, 2235-2236, 2235f, 2276-2280, 2432
allorecognition in, 2237, 2238f
in amyloidosis, 1132
anatomy of, 2251-2252, 2252f
antigen(s)
    ABO blood group, 2236-2237
    blood transfusion effects on, 2237
    human leukocyte antigens (HLA)
        class I, 2231-2233, 2232f
        class II, 2233
        inheritance of, 2233-2234, 2234f
        loci strengths, 2235-2236
        typing of, 2234-2235
    major histocompatibility complex, 2230-2231, 2230f
    non-human leukocyte antigens, 2236
    nonself, 2230
    recognition of, 2229
antigen-presenting cells
    description of, 2229, 2253-2255

Renal transplantation (Continued)
    T cells and, interactions between, 2237-2241, 2253-2255
anti-glomerular basement membrane disease, 1127, 2150, 2270
arteriovenous fistulas after, 911
atheroembolic renal disease after, 1191
atypical hemolytic-uremic syndrome treated with, 1186, 2357
in Australia, 2540f, 2543-2544, 2543f
B cells, 2229, 2242-2243
biochemical changes after, 1851
biomarkers after, 939-940
biopsy specimens after, 923
bone changes after, 1851-1852
brain death effects on, 983
calcium monitoring after, 2283
chemokines, 2241, 2243
in children. See Children, renal transplantation in
in chronic kidney disease, 2016
commercial, in Middle East, 2491
complications of
    acute allergic interstitial nephritis, 2270
    acute pyelonephritis, 2269-2270
    acute thrombotic microangiopathy, 2269
    BK virus infection, 2430
    bone mineral density reductions, 2282-2283
    cutaneous warts, 2430
    cytomegalovirus, 2287-2288, 2288t, 2429
    hemorrhagic, 2253
    infectious, 2286-2288, 2287t, 2505-2506
    lymphocele, 2253
    in Middle East patients, 2492
    opportunistic infections, 2287, 2505-2506
    parvovirus B19 infection, 1255
    perirenal hematomas, 2253
    Pneumocystis jiroveci pneumonia, 2430-2431
    renal artery stenosis, 2272
    renal artery thrombosis, 2253
    renal vein thrombosis, 2253
    respiratory viruses, 2430
    surgical, 2253
    tuberculosis, 2505
    urinary tract infections, 2269-2270, 2429
    urinary tract obstruction, 2271
    urine leaks, 2270-2271
    varicella infection, 2430
    vascular, 2253
contrast-enhanced computed tomography after, 910
cost-effectiveness of, 2411
cytokines, 2241
diabetes mellitus after, 1320, 2283, 2433
in diabetes mellitus patients, 2288-2289
diabetic nephropathy treated with, 1318-1319, 2275-2276
donor kidney
    age of donor, 2278
    allograft survival affected by, 2278-2279
    from cardiac death donor, 2279, 2571
    cold storage preservation of, 2252
    from deceased donors, 2278, 2490, 2571, 2571t
    directed donation, 2570
    ethical dilemmas, 2570
    gender of donor, 2278
    handling of, 2252-2253
    imaging assessment of, 909-910
    kidney donor profile index, 2279

Renal transplantation (Continued)
  live, 2252, 2278, 2582
    in Middle East patients, 2490
    multidetector computed tomography of, 909-910
    nephron endowment effects on, 723
    nephron mass in, 2278
    nondirected donation, 2570
    pregnancy and, 1638
    preservation of, 2252-2253
    race and ethnicity of donor, 2278
    radiologic assessment of, 909
    solicitation of, 2570
  Doppler ultrasonography evaluations, 910
  in Egypt, 2490
  in elderly, 748-749, 748t, 2598-2599
  end-stage kidney disease treated with, 1181-1182, 2581-2582
  erythrocytosis after, 1888-1889
  ethical dilemmas, 2570-2572
  in failing kidney patients, 2290
  failure of, 723, 2277f
  fetal and neonatal outcomes in, 1636
  fibrillary glomerulonephritis recurrence after, 1072
  fibrosis after, 2245
  focal segmental glomerulosclerosis recurrence after
    in children, 2156, 2422, 2431
    description of, 1034, 2270
    immunosuppressive drugs for, 2155-2156
    plasmapheresis for, 2155-2157
    risk factors for, 2155, 2270
  fractures after, 1851
  future of, 2290
  granulomatous with polyangiitis recurrence after, 2275
  health disparities in, 2581-2582
  hematoma after, 911f
  hemolytic-uremic syndrome recurrence after, 2270
  history of, 2229, 2602
  in HIV-infected patients, 2289
  hydronephrosis after, 911
  hypophosphatemia caused by, 632
  IgA glomerulonephritis recurrence after, 2275
  imaging assessments before, 909-910, 909f-913f
  immune monitoring in, 2269
  immune tolerance in, 2229-2230, 2249
  immunoglobulin A nephropathy after, 1069
  immunosuppressive agents used in. See Immunosuppressive agents
  in Indian subcontinent, 2504-2506
  in infants, 2420
  infectious complications of, 2286-2288, 2287t
  in Iran, 2490-2491
  ischemic acute tubular necrosis after, 2263-2264, 2263t
  laboratory testing after, 2260t
  in Latin America, 2451
  live donor nephrectomy, 2252
  low-protein diet after, 1977
  lupus nephritis treated with, 1100, 2275
  lymphoceles after, 910-911
  magnetic resonance angiography after, 911, 912f
  magnetic resonance imaging of, 870f, 910
  in Maori population, 2553
  membranoproliferative glomerulonephritis recurrence after, 1155-1156, 2275, 2422, 2431

Renal transplantation (Continued)
  membranous nephropathy recurrence after, 2275
  metabolic syndrome after, 2284, 2433
  metanephros, 2614-2615
  microscopic polyangiitis recurrence after, 2275
  in Middle East, 2475t, 2489-2492
  mineral metabolism changes after, 1851
  neoplasms after, 911
  nephron endowment effects on, 723-724
  in New Zealand, 2552-2553
  nuclear medicine after, 911-912
  outcomes of
    allograft survival, 2276
    disparities in, 2582
    fetal, 1636
    improvements in, 2280-2281
    neonatal, 1636
    patient survival, 2276
    racial-ethnic disparities in, 2582
    short-term, 2276
  pancreas transplantation and. See Renal-pancreas transplantation
  parathyroid hormone monitoring after, 2283
  pauci-immune crescentic glomerulonephritis recurrence after, 1086
  phosphate monitoring after, 2283
  plasma cells, 2242
  positive T cell cross-match, 2157
  preemptive, in stage 4 chronic kidney disease, 2016
  pregnancy and, 1636-1638, 1636f, 2435-2436
  prevalence of, 642-643
  procedure for, 2251-2253
  quality of life after, 2410, 2436, 2570
  racial-ethnic disparities in, 2581-2582
  recipients
    acute kidney injury in, 2271t
    age of, 2279
    allograft survival affected by, 2279-2280
    anogenital cancers in, 2285
    antihypertensive agents in, 2284t
    body size of, 2280
    bone disorders in, 2281-2283
    calcidiol levels in, 1851
    calcineurin inhibitor-associated bone pain in, 2282
    calcium channel blockers in, 1667
    calcium levels in, 1851
    cancer in, 2284-2286, 2285t, 2433-2434, 2543-2544
    cardiovascular disease in, 2283-2284
    chronic kidney disease–mineral bone disorder in, 1850-1852
    cinacalcet use in, 2032
    compliance by, 2280
    cross-match of, 2260-2261
    cytomegalovirus disease in, 2287-2288, 2288t
    desensitization of, 2261
    diabetes mellitus in, 2283
    electrolyte disorders in, 2281
    ethnicity of, 2279
    flow cytometric cross-match of, 2260
    gender of, 2279-2280
    α-glutathione S-transferase levels in, 939
    gout in, 2282
    hip fractures in, 2282-2283
    hospitalization of, 2290
    hypercalcemia in, 2281
    hyperhomocysteinemia in, 2284
    hyperkalemia in, 2281

Renal transplantation (Continued)
    hyperlipidemia in, 2284
    hyperparathyroidism in, 2282
    hypertension in, 911, 2280, 2283-2284, 2284t
    hypertriglyceridemia in, 2284
    hypomagnesemia in, 2281
    hypophosphatemia in, 2281
    immunizations in, 2288, 2288t
    immunologic status of, 2260-2261
    immunosuppression of, 2280. See also Immunosuppressive agents
    Kaposi's sarcoma in, 2285, 2492
    leukopenia in, 2434
    lip cancer in, 2285
    medical status of, 2259-2260
    metabolic acidosis in, 2281
    metabolic syndrome in, 2284
    in Middle East, 2491
    neoplasia in, 2492
    nephron endowment effects on, 723-724
    neutropenia in, 2434
    osteonecrosis in, 2282
    osteoporosis in, 2282-2283
    pediatric, 2420-2422, 2421t
    pneumocystosis in, 2288
    posttransplant care of, 2261
    posttransplantation lymphoproliferative disorder, 2285-2286, 2286t
    pregnant, 2289-2290
    proteinuria measurement in, 798
    race of, 2279
    rejection risk factors in, 2260t
    sensitization of, 2280
    skin cancer in, 2285, 2285t, 2433-2434, 2492, 2543-2544
    surgery in, 2290, 2290t
    urinary tract infection in, 1248-1249
    vaccinations in, 2288, 2288t
    vascular calcification in, 1852
  rejection of
    accelerated, 2264
    acute
      allograft loss risks, 2280
      antibody-mediated, 2268
      cellular, 2244, 2266-2268, 2267t, 2276f, 2428
      in children, 2428
      humoral, 2157, 2244, 2266-2268, 2267t, 2276f
    acute calcineurin inhibitor nephrotoxicity versus, 2268-2269, 2272, 2274-2275
    chronic, 2244-2245, 2244f, 2268
    chronic antibody-mediated, 2274
    corticosteroids for, 2268
    effector mechanisms of, 2242-2244
    hyperacute, 912-913, 2264
    immune monitoring for prevention of, 2269
    immunosuppression for prevention of. See Immunosuppressive agents
    immunosuppressive agent cessation as precipitate of, 2290
    late acute, 2271-2272
    magnetic resonance imaging of, 911, 912f
    plasmapheresis for, 2157
    risk factors for, 2260t
  scintigraphy after, 913
  skin conditions after, 1947t
  small vessel vasculitis recurrence after, 1086
  socioeconomic factors and, 2581
  stroke in, 1927-1928

Renal transplantation (Continued)
  survival rates, 2410
  T cell(s)
    activation of, 2254f
    adhesion molecules on, 2239-2240
    allorecognition, 2237, 2238f
    anergic, 2240
    antigen-presenting cells and, interactions between, 2237-2241, 2253-2255
    CD4+, 2239, 2242
    CD8+, 2239, 2243f
    costimulatory molecules, 2240-2241
    cross-match, 2157
    cytotoxic CD8+, 2239
    description of, 2229
    helper, 2241-2242
    immune response, 2253-2255
    interleukin-17–producing lineage of, 2243-2244
    receptor complex of, 2237-2239
    regulatory, 2240, 2250
  thrombotic thrombocytopenia purpura recurrence after, 2270
  timing of, 2278
  tissue remodeling after, 2245
  tolerogenic protocols in, 2249-2250
  tumor necrosis factor, 2241
  ultrasonography evaluations, 910
  urinary tract infection after, 1248-1249
  urine extravasation after, 913
  urinoma after, 910, 911f
  vascular calcification after, 1852
Renal tuberculosis, 882, 884f, 1253f
Renal tubular acidosis, 1437
  characteristics of, 2335
  in children, 2335-2338, 2337t, 2383-2386, 2383t
  distal
    alkali therapy for, 535-536
    autosomal recessive, 2335
    causes of, 2335
    in children, 2384-2386
    classical, 534, 534t-535t
    clinical spectrum of, 534-535, 535t
    in Far East, 2599
    features of, 534-535
    generalized, 534t
    H^+-ATPase defects in, 242
    H^+-K^+-ATPase's involvement in, 534
    hyperkalemic, 540, 589
    hypokalemic, 534, 581
    pathophysiology of, 533-534
    primary type 1, 2384-2386
    pyelonephritis caused by, 534-535
    treatment of, 535-536, 536t
    type A intercalated defects, 534
  diuretics for, 1726
  hyperkalemic, 1726, 2337t, 2338
  inherited, 1456t
  mixed, 2338
  nephrocalcinosis in, 872
  proximal, 1455, 1456t
    acquired, 530-532
    autosomal dominant, 2383
    calcium excretion in, 533
    carbonic anhydrase deficiency, 531-532
    causes of, 2335-2336
    characteristics of, 580-581
    in children, 2383-2384
    clinical spectrum of, 532, 532t
    diagnosis of, 532-533, 533f
    features of, 532-533, 532t
    inherited, 530-532

Renal tubular acidosis (Continued)
    model of, 531-532
    NBCe1 defects as cause of, 236-237
    pathogenesis of, 530-532
    physiology of, 530
    vitamin D deficiency and, 531
  treatment of, 2338
  type 1, 2386t
  type 2, 2386t
  type 4, 2386, 2386t
  types of, 542t, 2337t
Renal tubular assist device, 2617
Renal tubular dysgenesis, 2294-2295, 2297t, 2300
Renal tubular ectasia, 888-889
Renal tumors
  erythrocytosis in, 1889
  pelvic, 1352, 1385-1386
Renal ultrasonography
  acute kidney injury diagnosis using, 772
  chronic kidney disease diagnosis using, 776
  obstructive uropathy diagnosis using, 765
  urinary tract infection evaluations, 778
Renal vascular disease, 903-907, 904f-907f
Renal vein thrombosis
  acute, 1204, 1206, 1804
  anticoagulation for, 1206
  chronic, 1204, 1804
  clinical features of, 1204
  contrast-enhanced computed tomography of, 1205
  description of, 994
  diagnosis of, 1204-1205
  Doppler ultrasonography of, 1204
  hypovolemia as cause of, 1206
  imaging of, 908-909
  inferior venacavography of, 1204-1205
  magnetic resonance imaging of, 1205
  manifestations of, 1804
  mechanisms of, 1205-1206
  in membranous nephropathy, 1041
  in neonates, 1206
  in nephrotic syndrome, 1204-1206, 1804
  predisposing factors, 1205f, 1206
  renal allograft dysfunction caused by, 2266
  in renal transplantation allograft, 2253
  risk factors for, 1206t
  thrombolysis for, 1206
  treatment of, 1206-1207
  warfarin for, 1206
Renalase, 1533
Renal-pancreas transplantation, 1319, 2289
Renin
  age-related changes in, 737-738
  aldosterone secretion affected by, 568, 568f
  COX-2 inhibitors effect on production of, 360
  description of, 326-327
  drug-induced impairments in, 540
  EP4 receptor effects on release of, 372-373
  expression of, 53, 55, 370
  glucocorticoid-remediable hyperaldosteronism effects on, 555-556
  hyperkalemia and, 814t
  hypokalemia and, 814t
  juxtaglomerular apparatus secretion of, 334-335, 360, 568
  juxtaglomerular granular cell expression of, 53, 55
  loop diuretics effect on, 1706-1707

Renin (Continued)
  macula densa's role in release of, 358-360, 359f
  metabolic acidosis and, 555-556
  metabolic control of, 327-328
  neural control of, 327
  plasma
    β-adrenergic antagonist therapy effects on, 1659-1660
    age-related changes in, 737-738
    description of, 328
    in diabetes mellitus, 334-335
    diuretic therapy effects on, 1716
    edema formation and, 1798-1799
    in Gitelman's syndrome, 580
    in hyporeninemic hypoaldosteronism, 592
    plasma aldosterone concentration/plasma renin activity, 576
    primary aldosteronism effects on, 555
  regulation of, 568-569
  secretion of, 327-328, 1706, 2603
  structure of, 326
  tubular control of, 327-328
Renin inhibitors, 568, 1677-1678, 1764-1765
Renin lineage cells, 2609
Renin profiling, 1542-1543
Renin-angiotensin system, 99-102, 139
Renin-angiotensin-aldosterone system (RAAS), 1401
  activation beyond renal artery stenotic lesion, 1574f
  activation of, 1716
  aliskiren for blockade of, 1309
  almandine, 333
  angiotensin-(1-7), 333, 408, 445
  angiotensin-(1-12), 333
  angiotensin-(2-10), 333
  angiotensin A, 333
  angiotensin III, 332
  angiotensin IV, 332-333
  angiotensin peptides, 332-333
  angiotensin type 1 receptor. See Angiotensin type 1 receptor
  angiotensin type 2 receptor, 331
  angiotensin-(2-B), 332
  angiotensin-(3-B), 332
  angiotensin-converting enzyme, 328
  angiotensin-converting enzyme 2, 332
  angiotensinogen, 326
  arginine vasopressin secretion affected by, 470
  blockade of, 1180, 1304, 1309, 1311, 1889
  blood pressure regulation and, 1530-1532
  in cirrhosis-related sodium retention, 444-445
  components of, 326f
  description of, 27, 35-36, 100-101, 325
  in developing kidney, 703
  developmental programming of, 703, 704t-705t
  in diabetic nephropathy progression, 1298
  disordered regulation of, 1645
  diuretic therapy affected by, 1716
  in effective arterial blood volume regulation, 407-409
  elements of, 1531f
  in fibrosis, 334
  furosemide effects on, 1714
  in heart failure, 429-431, 451-454
  identification of, 1568-1569

Renin-angiotensin-aldosterone system (RAAS) *(Continued)*
　immunity and, 334
　inflammation and, 334
　inhibition of
　　acute kidney injury secondary to, 2006, 2006t
　　dual, 1691-1692
　　inflammation managed with, 2126
　　in nephrotic syndrome, 1799
　　renoprotective effects of, 639, 1752
　　for slowing chronic kidney disease progression, 1646, 1998-2004, 2127
　inhibitors of
　　aldosterone antagonism, 2003
　　angiotensin receptor blockers, 591f, 1642f, 1651, 1681, 1689, 1764-1765, 2000-2003, 2001f
　　angiotensin-converting enzyme inhibitors, 591f, 1642f, 1681, 1689, 1764-1765, 1998-2000
　　β-blockers and, 1692
　　calcium channel blockers and, 1681-1682, 1690-1691
　　description of, 1778
　　direct renin inhibitors, 2003-2004
　　diuretics and, 1691
　　heart failure treated with, 451-454
　　hyperkalemia caused by, 591-592, 741, 2005-2006
　　podocytes affected by, 119-120
　　steroid-resistant nephrotic syndrome in children treated with, 2331
　　thiazide diuretics with, 1681
　intracrine, 333-334
　intrarenal, 333-334
　kallikrein-kinin system and, 418
　mutations of, 2300
　nephron loss and, 1738-1739
　in one-kidney and two-kidney renovascular hypertension, 1571-1572
　physiologic and functional studies of, 1588-1589, 1589t
　potassium homeostasis affected by, 568
　prorenin in, 327-328, 327f
　(pro)renin receptor, 331-332
　in proteinuria, 334
　in radiation nephropathy, 1194
　renin, 326-328
　schematic diagram of, 326f
　in sodium retention, 444-445, 452
　sympathetic nervous system and, 703, 1533f
　in tubuloglomerular feedback, 400
　in urinary tract obstruction, 1279
Reninoma, 1369
Renomedullary interstitial cells, 78-80, 1369
Renoprotection
　aldosterone antagonists for, 2003
　amniotic fluid- and placental-derived stem cells for, 2607
　angiotensin receptor blockers for, 1764-1765, 1995, 1998t
　angiotensin-converting enzyme inhibitors for, 1757, 1995, 1998-2000, 1998t
　after nephrectomy, 1763-1764
　rationale for interventions for, 1990
　renin-angiotensin-aldosterone system inhibition for, 1752, 1998-2004
　spironolactone for, 2003
　strategies for, 2006-2008, 2008t
　weight loss for, 1992-1993
Renorenal reflex, 1269
Renovascular disease, 1567-1568. *See also* Renovascular hypertension
　in elderly, 746

Renovascular disease *(Continued)*
　medical therapy for, 1595-1599
　milestones in, timeline for, 1569f
　progressive vascular occlusion with, 1598
　reconstructed views of, 1592f
　secondary hypertension and, 1568-1569
　treatment of, 746
Renovascular hypertension, 1547, 1568-1569, 1595t. *See also* One-kidney renal clip hypertension; Renovascular disease; Two-kidney renal clip hypertension
　clinical features of, 1581-1582, 1583t
　development of, phases of, 1574, 1574f
　diagnosis and evaluation of, 1588-1594, 1588f
　endovascular renal angioplasty and stenting, 1599
　epidemiology of, 1580-1581
　in Indian subcontinent, 2506-2507
　management of, 1608f
　mechanism sustaining, 1572-1574
　pathophysiology of, 1570-1580
　prospective trials for, 1602-1603
　renal artery aneurysms associated with, 1203
　renal artery stenosis and, 903, 1570-1571
　renin-angiotensin-aldosterone system's role in, 1571-1572
　surgical treatment of, 1604-1607, 1605t
　syndromes associated with, 1583t
　therapy goals for, 1588
　vascular lesions producing, 1570t
Repaglinide, 2593
Reproductive cloning, 2604
Reserpine, 1673
Residual bodies, 59-60
Residual syndrome, 1807-1808
Resistant hypertension, 1691t, 1693-1695
Resistin, 1816
Resistive index, 849-850
Resorptive hypercalciuria, 1335
Respiratory acidosis
　carbon dioxide tension changes and, 515-516
　causes of, 525-526, 526t
　chronic, 527
　clinical features of, 526
　collecting duct's response to, 244
　compensatory responses for, 518t
　diagnosis of, 527
　hyperphosphatemia caused by, 628
　mechanical ventilation as cause of, 526
　proximal tubule bicarbonate reabsorption affected by, 237
　treatment of, 527
Respiratory alkalosis
　in alcoholics, 633
　carbon dioxide tension changes and, 515-516
　causes of, 526t, 527-528
　compensatory responses for, 518t
　description of, 527
　diagnosis of, 528
　effects of, 527
　hypocalcemia caused by, 2392
　hypophosphatemia caused by, 633
　plasma potassium affected by, 563
　of pregnancy, 1612
　treatment of, 528
Respiratory center depression, 526
Restenosis, 1603-1604
Resting energy expenditure (REE), 1815-1816, 1973
Resting membrane potential, 569-570, 818
Restless legs syndrome, 1818-1819, 1939-1940, 1940t

Ret, 23-24, 24f
RET, 2297-2298
Ret-GFRα1, 22
Reticulocyte hemoglobin content, 1895
Retinitis pigmentosa, 2321
Retinoic acid response element, 1795
Retinoids, 31-32
Retinol binding protein, 1816
Retrograde pyelography, 1268
Retroperitoneal fibrosis, 1261-1262
Revascularization, 1585f, 1586t, 1607t
　atheroembolism risks, 746
　benefits of, 1607
　of kidneys, 1599
　renal artery stenosis and, 1592f
　renal functional outcomes after, 1606f
Reverse causality, 1861
Reverse osmosis water treatment system, 2081f
Reversible posterior leukoencephalopathy, 1619-1620
Rh glycoproteins
　in ammonia metabolism, 255
　carbon dioxide transport by, 255
　RhAG/Rhag, 255
　RhBG/Rhbg, 255
　RhCG/Rhcg, 255
Rhabdomyolysis, 586, 628
Rh-associated glycoprotein, 586
Rheumatoid arthritis, 1168
Rhpj, 30
Ribavirin, 1156
Riboflavin, 1983
Ribosomal protein S6 kinase 1A, 732-733
Rickets, 630-631
RIFLE criteria, 770, 770t, 930-931, 960, 961t, 1390, 2138
Right ventricular failure, 1722
Rilmenidine, 1671-1672, 1671t-1672t
Rilonacept, 2486
Risk factors
　Bradford-Hill causality criteria, 670, 670t
　definition of, 670
　identification of, 670-671
Rituximab
　adverse effects of, 1171
　anti-glomerular basement membrane disease treated with, 1126-1127
　glomerular disease treated with, 1171
　granulomatous with polyangiitis treated with, 1113
　immunosuppressive uses of, 2256
　lupus nephritis treated with, 1104
　membranous nephropathy treated with, 1044-1045
　nephrotic syndrome treated with, 2330-2331
　pauci-immune crescentic glomerulonephritis treated with, 1088-1089
　podocytes affected by, 119
　toxicity of, 1171
Robo2, 27
ROBO2, 2297-2298
Rofecoxib, 437
Rolipram, 300-301
ROMK, 159-160, 163, 176, 179-181, 278, 310-311, 541, 564, 566, 578-579, 581, 1728, 2334
Ropinirole, 1940
Roux-en-Y gastric bypass, 1340, 1341t
Rubinstein-Taybi syndrome, 2297t
Rumack-Matthew nomogram, 2187-2188
Runx-2, 1835

INDEX

S

S256, 293
Salicylates
    high anion gap acidosis caused by, 547-548
        metabolic acidosis caused by, 547-548
    poisoning, 2178-2180
Saline, 855-856
Sall1, 22-23
SALL1, 2298-2299
Salt, 258-259, 1354. *See also* Sodium
Salt sensitivity, 1528-1529, 1533-1534
Salt substitutes, 584-585
Salt-induced hypercalciuria, 1354
Salt-losing nephropathy, 493
Salt-losing tubulopathies, 1460f, 2334t. *See also* Bartter's syndrome; Gitelman's syndrome
Salt-sensitive hypertension, 1974-1975
Samoa, 2553-2554
Saponification, 620
Sarcoidosis, 762, 1127-1128, 1228
Sarcopenia, 1922
Satavaptan, 457
Saudia Arabia. *See* Middle East
Scar collagen, 1286
SCARB2 disease, 1432
Schimke's immuno-osseous dysplasia, 1432
Schistosoma haematobium, 755, 1255, 1260, 2462
Schistosomiasis, 1150, 1260, 2462
Schwartz equation, 2043, 2310
Scintigraphy, 913, 1266
Scleroderma
    acute kidney injury associated with, 1002
    chronic kidney disease in, 1196-1197
    clinical features of, 1195
    collagen production in, 1197
    cytokines in, 1197
    definition of, 1195
    immunologic mediators in, 1197
    laboratory findings in, 1196
    microvascular injury in, 1197
    pathogenesis of, 1197
    pathology of, 1196-1197
    Raynaud's phenomenon, 1195
    renal crisis, 1195-1198, 1195f-1196f
    renal involvement in, 1195-1196
    treatment of, 1197-1198, 1198t
Sclerosing/chronic allograft nephropathy, 2273
Sclerosis, 921t
Sclerosteosis, 191
Sclerostin, 191, 610, 1842
Scriber, Belding, 2558
Scrub typhus, 2513-2515
Sebastian's syndrome, 1141
Secondary hyperparathyroidism, 1827-1828, 1835-1836, 1887, 2023, 2026, 2031-2032
Secondary hypertension, 766t, 1543-1550, 1568-1569, 1628
Secondary tubulopathy, 1417-1418
γ-Secretase inhibitor, 30
Secreted procollagen type 1C propeptide, 1842
Secretin, for nephrogenic diabetes insipidus, 301
Sedatives, 2595
Seizure, 1616, 1626-1627
Selective aldosterone receptor antagonists, 1678-1679
Selenium supplementation, 2099-2100
Self-tolerance, 2230
Seminal vesicle cyst, 1491

Senior-Loken syndrome, 2321
Sensorimotor neuropathy, 1819
Sepsis, 2137-2138
Sequestered solutes, 1814
Serine 552, 235
Serine-threonine kinase, 565
Serotonin, 201
Serum amyloid A, 1128-1129, 1130f, 1969-1970, 2485
Serum amyloid P, 1128
Serum- and glucocorticoid-regulated kinase
    aldosterone induction of, 317-318
    in aldosterone-sensitive distal nephron, 318
    epithelial sodium channel stimulation by, 318, 319f
    molecular mechanisms of action, 318-320
    Nedd4-2 inhibition by, 318-319
    in sodium transport, 319
Serum chemistry, 1356
Serum frizzled-related protein 4, 197-198, 198f, 201
SeSAME syndrome, 167
Sevelamer hydrochloride, 563, 627, 2031
Seventh sickly cell nephrology, 1372
Severe acute respiratory syndrome, 2521-2522, 2523f
Severe fever with thrombocytopenia syndrome virus, 2516-2517, 2518f
Sex hormones, 400, 1921, 1923
Sexual intercourse, 1237
sFlt1, 39
SGK-1, 172-173, 567
SGLT1, 205-206
SGLT2, 206-207
SGLT3, 207
SGLT2, 207-209
Shear stress, 1578
Shh, 27
Shiga toxin-associated hemolytic-uremic syndrome, 1179-1182, 2352-2357
Shunt nephritis, 1149
Shwartzman reaction, 2502
Sickle cell disease
    in Africa, 2463
    clinical features of, 1198-1199
    cortical infarction in, 1199
    end-stage kidney disease secondary to, 1200
    focal segmental glomerulosclerosis in, 1199
    hematuria in, 1198-1200
    hemoglobin SS in, 1199
    mechanisms of, 1199-1200
    medullary lesions in, 1199
    pathogenesis of, 1199-1200
    pathology of, 1199
    preeclampsia and, 1618
    proteinuria in, 1199
    renal papillary necrosis in, 1198-1199, 1199f
    treatment of, 1200
    tubular dysfunction in, 1199
    vasoocclusion mediated by, 1199
Sickle cell glomerulopathy, 1146, 1146f, 1200
Sickle cell nephropathy, 1145-1146, 1145f
Sieving coefficient, 2170
Signal transducers and activators of transcription, 1760-1761, 1882
Signal-induced proliferation-associated gene 1, 295
Sildenafil citrate, 300-301
Silicosis, 1159

Simple cyst, 1511-1512, 1512f
Simple hypoplasia, 2294
Simpson-Golabi Behmel syndrome, 2297t
Simultaneous pancreas-kidney transplantation, 1319
Singapore, 2536
Single-gene kidney disorder, 1411-1412, 1413t, 1418
Single-nephron glomerular filtration rate, 1269, 1271, 1737-1738, 1743, 1746-1747, 1785
Single-pass albumin dialysis, 2171
Sinusoidal occlusion syndrome, 1394-1395
Sinusoidal pressure, 439-440
Sir2, 733
siRNA, 7-9
Sirolimus
    adverse effects of, 2426
    in children, 2426
    focal segmental glomerulosclerosis treated with, 1033-1034
    immunosuppressive uses of, 2254t, 2258, 2426
    during pregnancy, 1637, 1637t
SIRT1, 733
Sirtuins, 732-733, 1788
SITS, 146-147
Six1, 21
Six2, 29
SIX1, 2298-2299
Six Sigma, 2625, 2625f
Six2-EGFP transgene, 19
Size-exclusion high-performance liquid chromatography, 795
Sjögren's disease, 1127
S6K1, 733
SK channels, 180f, 564-565
Skeletal ciliopathy, 1509
Skeletal muscle, 174-175, 560, 1967
Skeletal system, 623-624
Skin
    cancer of, 2285, 2285t, 2433-2434, 2492, 2543-2544
    diuretics-related adverse effects of, 1732
    nitrogen losses from, 1963
Skin conditions and disorders, 1943t, 1947t, 1949t-1950t, 1952t-1953t
    acquired perforating dermatosis, 1944, 1944f
    in Alport's syndrome, 1953
    arteriovenous shunt dermatitis, 1949
    in Birt-Hogg-Dube syndrome, 1951-1952, 1952f, 1952t
    calciphylaxis, 1944-1945, 1945f
    cutaneous metastases, 1949
    dialysis-associated steal syndrome, 1948
    dyspigmentation, 1943f
    eruptive xanthomas, 1946-1947, 1946f
    in Fabry's disease, 1952
    genodermatoses, 1951-1953, 1952f, 1952t
    in Henoch-Schönlein purpura, 1951, 1951f
    in hereditary leiomyomatosis and renal cell carcinoma syndrome, 1952, 1952f, 1952t
    ichthyosis, 1943-1944
    impetigo, 1953
    iododerma, 1947, 1947f
    leukocytoclastic vasculitis, 1950-1951, 1951f
    Lindsay's nail, 1949-1950, 1949f
    metastatic calcification, 1945-1946
    in metastatic renal cell carcinoma, 1949
    in Muir-Torre syndrome, 1952-1953, 1952t

Skin conditions and disorders (Continued)
  nails, 1949-1950, 1949f
  in nephrogenic systemic fibrosis, 1947-1948, 1948f-1949f
  porphyria cutanea tarda, 1946, 1946f
  port-wine stain, 1952
  post-renal transplantation, 1947t
  pruritus, 1942-1943, 1943f
  pseudo-Kaposi's sarcoma, 1947
  pseudoporphyria, 1946
  streptococcal skin infection, 1953
  in systemic lupus erythematosus, 1950, 1950f
  in tuberous sclerosis, 1952
  in von Hippel–Lindau disease, 1952, 1952t
  xerosis, 1943, 1943f
SLC6 transporters, 229-230
SLC22, 375
SLC1A1, 228-229
SLC1A5, 225
SLC3A1/SLC7A9, 227-228
SLC3A2/SLC7A7, 228
SLC3A2/SLC7A9, 225-226
SLC5A1, 205-206
SLC6A6, 224-225
SLC6A18, 224
SLC6A19, 222-224
SLC6A20, 224
SLC7A13, 229
SLC16A10, 225
Slc26A6, 148-149
Slc26A7, 243
SLC36A2, 224
SLC3A1, 2345
SLC7A9, 2345
SLC12A1, 158-159
SLC12A3, 2378-2379
SLC22A, 218-219
Sleep apnea, 1533f, 1939-1940, 2101
Sleep disorders
  periodic limb movements of sleep, 1939-1940
  prevalence of, 1939
  restless legs syndrome, 1940, 1940t
  sleep apnea, 1939-1940
Sleep-disordered breathing, 766
Slit2, 27
Slit diaphragm
  definition of, 4-5, 51, 791
  in podocytes, 38-39, 51, 118, 791, 1782-1783, 1782f
  proteins, 113
  studies of, 51
  topologic organization of, 38
Slit pote, 49-51
SMAD1, 27
Small vessel vasculitis
  eosinophilic granulomatosis with polyangiitis, 1116-1118
  granulomatous with polyangiitis. See Granulomatous with polyangiitis
  microscopic polyangiitis. See Microscopic polyangiitis
  after renal transplantation, 1086
Smith, Homer, 1568-1569
Smith-Lemli-Opitz syndrome, 2297t
Smoking
  cessation of, 1867, 1991-1992, 2102
  chronic kidney disease risks, 685, 1776-1777, 1867
  fibromuscular dysplasia and, 1580-1581
  renal allograft survival affected by, 2283
  sympathetic nervous system affected by, 1776-1777
Smooth muscle, 371, 413-414

Snakebites
  acute kidney injury caused by, 2499-2500, 2523-2525, 2524t
  in Africa, 2458
  Bothrops, 2447
  Crotalus, 2446-2447
  in Far East, 2523-2525, 2524t
  in Indian subcontinent, 2499-2500
  in Latin America, 2446-2447
SNARE hypothesis, 295-296, 311
SNARE proteins, 295-296
SNAT3, 251
Sodium
  absorption of
    aldosterone-sensitive distal nephron and, 313-314
    in collecting ducts, 73
    distal, 566-568
    electrogenic, 316-317
    epithelial sodium channels, 175
    medullary collecting ducts in regulation of, 314
    prostaglandin E_2 effects on, 361-362
    regulation of, 310-315
  altered handling of, by kidney, 701-703
  balance of, 2366-2367
  in children, 2365-2374
  daily filtration of, 422
  deficit of, 323, 2374
  dietary
    in chronic kidney disease, 1974-1975
    diuretic braking phenomenon affected by, 1714, 1715f
    in edematous patients, 1719, 1725
    renal hypertrophy inhibition of, 1759
    restriction of, 566, 1716, 1725, 1993-1994
    stroke risks associated with, 1928t, 1930
    thromboxane A_2 expression regulated by, 365
  excretion of
    age-related changes in, 738-739, 738f
    captopril effects on, 444-445
    description of, 391, 395
    in elderly, 738-739, 738f
    endothelin effects on, 416
    furosemide and, 1710f
    interstitial pressure in control of, 402-405
    intrarenal control of, 402
    nephron loss-specific adaptations in, 1747-1748
    prostaglandin synthesis inhibition effects on, 412
    sympathetic nervous system in, 405, 432
  in extracellular fluid, 144
  fractional excretion of, 814-815, 987, 1659, 1708-1710, 1747
  in hemodialysis dialysate, 2092-2093
  metabolism of, 2365-2367
  monitoring of, 508
  nonsteroidal antiinflammatory drug-induced retention of, 361-362
  plasma, 423, 816, 2371
  restriction of, 1993-1994
  serum concentration of, 491, 523
  transport of
    angiotensin II effects on, 331
    in collecting duct, 374
    COX-1 metabolite effects on, 373-374
    COX-2 metabolite effects on, 373-374
    maturation of, in fetus and infant, 2302
    metabolic cost of, 135-136
    in proximal tubule, 132
    serum- and glucocorticoid-regulated kinase in, 319

Sodium (Continued)
    in thick ascending limb, 132-133
    transepithelial, 420
    urinary tract obstruction effects on, 1274
  in urine, 492, 816
Sodium balance, 1530
  arginine vasopressin effects on, 498
  central nervous system sensors of, 397
  disorders of
    hypernatremia. See Hypernatremia
    hyponatremia. See Hyponatremia
  nitric oxide in, 417
  physiology of, 390-421
  two-compartmental model of, 391f
Sodium bicarbonate, 595, 595f, 855-856, 1364, 2168
Sodium chloride
  absorption of
    angiotensin II effects on, 155
    description of, 144
    neurohumoral influences on, 152, 153f
    paracellular, 145-146
  dietary, 1993-1994
  hyponatremia treated with, 506
  in inner medulla, 271-273
  reabsorption of
    angiotensin II effects on, 152, 153f
    by thick ascending limb, 158
    description of, 145f, 146-147
    epithelial sodium channels' role in, 169-170
    glomerular filtration rate effects on, 150
    proximal, 152
Sodium chloride transport
  aldosterone effects on, 171-173
  apical, 158-159, 169-170
  in connecting tubules
    aldosterone effects on, 171-173
    arachidonic acid metabolites effects on, 174
    mechanisms of, 169-171
    regulation of, 171-174
  in cortical connecting duct
    aldosterone effects on, 171-173
    arachidonic acid metabolites effects on, 174
    mechanisms of, 169-171
    regulation of, 171-174
    vasopressin effects on, 173
  in cortical connecting tubules, 566
  in distal convoluted tubule
    description of, 148, 165-174
    mechanisms of, 166-167, 167f
    NCC expression, 165-166
    regulation of, 167-169
  electroneutral, 171
  in loop of Henle, 156-165
    thin ascending limb, 156-158, 157f
    thin descending limb, 156
  overview of, 144-174
  paracellular, 147-148, 160
  potassium transport and, in distal nephron, 182-183
  in proximal tubule, 144-156
    glomerulotubular balance in, 150-152, 151f
    neurohumoral influences on, 152-154, 153f
    paracellular, 147-148
    regulation of, 150-156
    transporters, regulation of, 154-156
  thiazide-sensitive electroneutral, 182-183
  in thick ascending limb
    activating influences on, 162-164
    apical mechanisms of, 158-160

Sodium chloride transport *(Continued)*
    basolateral mechanisms of, 160-162
    calcium-sensing receptor effects on, 164-165
    inhibitory influences on, 164-165, 164f
    paracellular mechanisms of, 160
    regulation of, 162-165
    ROMK protein effects on, 159-160
    transepithelial, 162
  in thin ascending limb, 156-158, 157f
  in thin descending limb, 156
  transcellular, 148-150
  transepithelial
    apical potassium channels for, 159
    by intercalated cells, 170f
    by principal cells, 170f
    calcium-sensing receptor inhibitory effects on, 164f
    cAMP-generating hormone stimulation of, 164
    description of, 148-149
    in proximal tubule, 149f
    stimulation of, 164
    in thick ascending limb, 158f, 162-164
  vasopressin effects on, 162-163
Sodium cotransporter, 69
Sodium hydrogen exchange, 148, 154, 154f
Sodium intake, 1528-1529
Sodium nitroprusside, 1575f, 1695t, 1697
Sodium phosphate-IIa transporter, 202f
Sodium polystyrene sulfonate, 596-597, 2168-2169
Sodium potential, 124-125
Sodium pump, 1729
  abundance of, 128-129
  adenosine triphosphatases, 124
  adenosine triphosphate and, 124
  in ammonia metabolism, 254
  basolateral, 150, 154-156, 160-161, 1800
  in bicarbonate reabsorption, 242-243
  bile salts and, 2508
  in collecting duct bicarbonate reabsorption, 242-243
  description of, 123, 1277
  digoxin effects on, 587
  in distal convoluted tubule, 129
  electrochemical gradients created using, 310
  energy and, 124-126
  kinetics of, 126
  metabolic substrates, 129
  nephron distribution of, 146f
  in nephron segments, 129, 129f
  ouabain inhibition of, 132
  physiologic conditions that affect, 243
  potassium uptake activated by, 573
  protein expression and activity, 129
  pump-leak processes, 124-125
  renal sodium transport effects on, 135
  sodium reabsorption and, 142
  structure of, 124, 124f
  in transcellular calcium transport, 188
  transport activity of, 1800
  in uremia patients, 1819
Sodium reabsorption
  age-related changes in, 737
  aldosterone-stimulated, 318
  angiotensin II effects on, 407-408
  connecting tubule's role in, 69
  efficiency of, 136
  electrogenic, 313
  electroneutral, 313
  fractional, 1726
  in heart failure, 429, 431

Sodium reabsorption *(Continued)*
  hormones that regulate, 126
  hyperaldosteronism effects on, 1724-1725
  hypocalciuria and, 190-191
  loop of Henle, 1747
  metabolic cost of, 135-137
  osmotic diuretics effect on, 422
  prostaglandin E_2 effects on, 1716-1717
  proximal tubule, 430f
  regulation of, 1800
  sodium pump and, 142
  in thick ascending limb, 135, 137
  transport systems in, 2378f
  tubular
    in cirrhosis, 444
    renal medulla's role in, 404f
    ureteral obstruction effects on, 1272
    urinary tract obstruction effects on, 1272-1275
  tubular disorders that affect, 422
  vasopressin effects on, 282
Sodium retention
  in cirrhosis. *See* Cirrhosis, sodium retention in
  in heart failure. *See* Heart failure, sodium retention in
  in hepatorenal syndrome, 378
  renin-angiotensin-aldosterone system in, 444-445, 452
Sodium wasting, 1437
Sodium-bicarbonate cotransporters, 243-244
Sodium-bicarbonate symporter mutation, 1455
Sodium-glucose cotransport, 205
Sodium-glucose-linked cotransporters, 209-210
Sodium-hydrogen exchanger regulatory factor, 155f
Sodium-hydrogen exchanger regulatory factor 1, 632
Sodium-phosphate cotransporters, 198-199, 626, 1450-1451, 1451f
Sodium-restricted diet, 450
Solid organ transplantation, 991t, 992-993
Solitary fibrous tumor, 1369
Soluble adenylyl cyclase, 256, 1348-1349
Soluble epoxide hydrolase, 385
Soluble fms-like tyrosine kinase-1, 1621, 1622f, 1623
Soluble guanylate cyclase, 416
Soluble urokinase receptor, 2327-2328
Solute disequilibrium, 2072-2073
Solute load hypothesis, 1743
Solute sequestration, 2072-2073
Solute transport
  active transport along nephron, 126-132
  cell polarity, 126
  in medullary collecting ducts, 133
  metabolic efficiency regulation during, 138-142
  in proximal tubule, 132
  sodium potential for, 124-125
  sodium pump for. *See* Sodium pump
  in thick ascending limb, 132-133
  vectorial, 126
Somatic cell nuclear transfer, 2604-2606
Somatostatin, 1916-1917
Somatostatin analogues, 456, 1495-1496
Somatotropic axis, 1917
Sorafenib, 1382-1383, 1383f
Sorbitol, 596-597
SOST gene, 191, 1832-1833
South America. *See* Latin America
Sox17, 35

Sox18, 35
SPAK, 163, 168-169
Specific gravity of urine, 789
Specimens
  kidney biopsy, 919-920, 920t, 923-924
  urine, 788
Specular reflectors, 848
Spermicides, 1237, 1239-1240
Sphingomyelin phosphodiesterase acid-like 3b, 119, 1171
Sphingosine-1 phosphate receptor, 979
Spider venom, 2445-2446, 2445f
Spinal meningeal diverticula, 1491
Spironolactone
  adverse effects of, 1713
  Gitelman's syndrome treated with, 1727
  indications for, 1713
  magnesium excretion affected by, 1730
  pharmacokinetics of, 1713
  potassium secretion in collecting duct inhibited using, 540-541
  renoprotection using, 2003
Splanchnic vasodilation, 442
Spot urinalysis, 1356
Sprouty, 24-25
Spry1, 24-25, 27
Spurious hypokalemia, 572
SQSTM1, 734-735
Squamous cells, 800
Sri Lanka. *See* Indian subcontinent
SRY gene, 2611
SSIGN scoring system, 1379
Staghorn calculus, 877f, 879f, 883f, 2507
Staphylococcus aureus, 1148, 2128, 2351
Staphylococcus epidermidis, 2128
Staphylococcus saprophyticus, 1237
Star fruit, 2525
STAR trial, 1590, 1597t
Starling equation, 94, 400
Starling forces, 89, 426, 1799
Starvation ketoacidosis, 547
Statins
  dyslipidemia treated with, 1773-1774, 1931, 2011, 2593
  nephrogenic diabetes insipidus treated with, 301
  proteinuria effects, 2011
Steal syndrome, dialysis-associated, 1948, 2216f
Steatosis, 1344-1345, 1345f
Stem cells
  in acute kidney injury pathophysiology, 978-979
  adult, 2607-2608
  amniotic fluid- and placental-derived, 2607
  bromodeoxyuridine retention by, 2608
  description of, 2603
  embryonic, 2603-2607
  identification of, 2608-2609
  induced pluripotent, 2606-2607
  mesenchymal. *See* Mesenchymal stem cells
  transplantation. *See* Hematopoietic stem cell transplantation
  in tubular epithelial cell injury, 978-979
Stent/stenting
  angioplasty and, 1602-1604
  for arteriovenous graft stenosis, 2202-2203
  atherosclerotic renal artery stenosis and, 1600-1602
  complications after, 1603t
  endovascular renal angioplasty and, 1599-1602
  for renal insufficiency, 1603-1604

Steroid biosynthesis pathway, 1461, 1461f
Steroidogenic acute regulatory protein, 306
Steroidogenic factor-1, 588
Steroid-resistant minimal change disease, 1023-1024
Sterol regulatory element binding protein-1, 733
Stokes-Einstein radius, 791
Stone former, 1328, 1344f, 1351f-1352f, 1353t-1354t
Streptococcal skin infection, 1953
Streptococcus pneumoniae, 1175-1176, 1182, 2355
Streptococcus viridans, 1148
Streptozyme test, 1058
Stress, 470
Stroke
    antiplatelet therapy for prevention of, 1931-1932
    characteristics of, 1926-1927
    in chronic kidney disease, 1926-1934
    classification of, 1927
    in dialysis, 1927-1928
    in elderly, 2590
    epidemiology of, 1927-1928, 1927t
    erythropoietin for, 1932-1933
    hemorrhagic, 1927, 1931
    hospitalization for, 1927f
    hypertension and, 1522
    intracranial stenosis as cause of, 2395
    ischemic, 1927
    management of, 1933-1934
    prevention of, 1930-1933
    recombinant tissue plasminogen activator effects on, 1933
    in renal transplantation, 1927-1928
    risk factors for
        anemia, 1928t, 1930
        atrial fibrillation, 1928t, 1929-1930, 1932
        diabetes mellitus, 1928t, 1929, 1931
        dialysis-associated factors, 1930
        homocysteine, 1930
        hypertension, 1928-1931, 1928t, 1929f, 1933-1934
        modifiable, 1928t
        nutrition, 1928t, 1930
        proteinuria, 1928t, 1930
    subtypes of, 1927t
    symptoms of, 1926-1927
    thrombolytic therapy for, 1933
    transient ischemic attack versus, 1926-1927
    vitamin B supplementation for, 1932
Stroma, 5-6, 31-32
Stromal cell-derived factor 1, 2353
Stromal cells, 5-6, 31-32
Struvite, 768
Struvite stones, 1249
Subcapsular hematoma, 878f-879f, 910, 911f
Subcapsular urinoma, 1517
Subclavian artery stenosis, 2214, 2215f
Subclavian catheters, 2145
Subclinical hypothyroidism, 1916, 2395
Subfornical organ, 470
Subpodocyte space, 1781
Substance P, 110
Succinate, 328
Succinate dehydrogenase complex, 139
Succinylcholine, 587-588, 587f
Sucroferric oxyhydroxide, 2023
Sudden death, 2093, 2101
Sulfadiazine, 1259-1260
Sulfatides, 252, 255-256
Sulfhydryl angiotensin-converting enzyme inhibitors, 1641, 1643t

Sulfuric acid, 516
Sulodexide, 1313
Sunitinib, 1382, 1383f
Superior vena cava occlusion, 2214f
Superoxide dismutase, 732, 1758
Suppressors of cytokine signaling, 1913, 2357-2358
Surgery, 606-607, 1366
Surgical revascularization, 1203
Surrogate endpoint biomarker, 927t
Surveillance, 1380
Sylvatic yellow fever, 2441
Symmetric dimethylarginine, 1811
Sympathetic nervous system, 1532-1533
    in cirrhosis, 445-446
    in effective arterial blood volume regulation, 405-407, 407f
    functions of, 703
    in heart failure, 432, 435
    hyperactivity, 1532-1533
    overactivity of, in chronic kidney disease progression, 1771-1772
    potassium distribution affected by, 562
    renin-angiotensin-aldosterone system regulation by, 703
    smoking effects on, 1776-1777
    in sodium excretion, 405, 432
    vasopressin and, 406
Syndrome of inappropriate antidiuretic hormone (SIADH) secretion
    clinical settings of, 498-500
    description of, 816, 2372
    disorders associated with, 499t
    hyponatremia caused by, 497-498
    hypouricemia associated with, 498
    in infants, 499
    long-term treatment of, 509f
    malignancy-associated, 499
    pathophysiology of, 498
    urea for, 506
Syngeneic, 2228-2229
Synpaptopodin, 113
Synpharyngitis nephritis, 1065
Syntaxin 4, 295-296
Syphilis, 1149
Systemic arterial pressure (carotid), 1570-1571, 1571f
Systemic inflammatory response syndrome, 2444
Systemic lupus erythematosus (SLE)
    anti-DNA antibodies in, 1098-1099, 1107-1108
    anti-dsDNA antibodies in, 1099
    antineutrophil cytoplasmic antibodies in, 1093-1094
    anti-nRNP antibodies in, 1099
    antinuclear antibodies in, 1098-1099
    antiphospholipid antibodies in, 1106-1107
    antiphospholipid syndrome in, 1200
    anti-Ro/SSA antibodies in, 1099
    atherogenesis in, 1105-1106
    autoantibodies in, 1093, 1099
    clinical manifestations of, 1098
    diagnosis of, 1093
    drug-induced, 1099-1100
    endothelin-1 in, 338
    epidemiology of, 1092-1093
    factors that affect, 1093
    in Far East, 2531-2532
    fetal loss in, 1100
    gender predilection of, 1092-1093, 1098
    genetic predisposition to, 1093
    hemolytic complement in, 1099
    incidence of, 1092-1093
    lupus nephritis. *See* Lupus nephritis
    lupus podocytopathy in, 1097-1098

Systemic lupus erythematosus (SLE) *(Continued)*
    malar rash associated with, 1950
    medications that cause, 1099-1100
    membranous nephropathy in, 1037
    monitoring of, 1099
    pathogenesis of, 1093-1094
    pregnancy and, 1100
    renal flares, 1101
    serologic tests of, 1098-1099
    skin manifestations of, 1950, 1950f
    T cells in, 1093
    tubulointerstitial disease in, 1097-1098
    vascular lesions in, 1097-1098
    in women, 1092-1093, 1098
Systemic therapy, 1381-1385
Systemic vasculitis, 1088
Systolic blood pressure, 1680-1681
    before and after two-kidney renal clip hypertension placement, 1572f
    before and after two-kidney renal clip placement for hypertension, 1572f
    coronary heart disease and, 1527f
    hypertension and, 1524, 1524t
    importance of, 1524
    Joint National Committee classifications for, 1526f
Systolic hypertension, 1554f

T

T cell(s)
    adhesion molecules on, 2239-2240
    allorecognition, 2237, 2238f
    anergic, 2240
    antigen recognition by, 1215
    antigen-presenting cells and, 2237-2241
    in anti-glomerular basement membrane glomerulonephritis, 1079-1080
    CD4+, 1216, 1795, 2239, 2242
    CD8+, 2239, 2243f
    costimulatory molecules, 2240-2241
    cytotoxic CD8+, 2239
    description of, 2229
    helper, 2241-2242
    interleukin-2 activation of, 2247
    interleukin-17–producing lineage of, 2243-2244
    macrophages and, 1216
    in minimal change disease, 1019-1020
    monoclonal antibody activation of, 2247
    in pauci-immune crescentic glomerulonephritis, 1084
    receptor complex of, 2237-2239
    regulatory, 1795, 2240, 2250
    in systemic lupus erythematosus, 1093
    in tubulointerstitial infiltrate, 1793
T cell cross-match, 2157
T cell immunoglobulin and mucin domains-containing protein-1, 941
T cell immunoglobulin mucin-1, 2243-2244
Tacrolimus, 1398-1399
    in children, 2425
    glomerular disease treated with, 1167-1168
    hyperkalemia caused by, 590
    hypomagnesemia caused by, 622
    immunosuppressive uses of, 2247, 2254t, 2257-2258, 2425
    lupus nephritis treated with, 1104-1105
    membranous nephropathy treated with, 1043-1044
    nephrotic syndrome treated with, 2329-2330
    nephrotoxicity of, 2264
    during pregnancy, 1637, 1637t

INDEX

Taiwan, 2534
Takayasu arteritis, 1120-1121, 2352, 2506
Tamm-Horsfall protein, 791, 800, 947, 967, 1214-1215, 1232, 1259-1260, 1330, 1391
Tamoxifen, 2133
Targeted agent, 1382
Tartrate-resistant acid phosphatase 5B, 1842
TASK-1, 568
TASK-3, 568
TAT1, 225
TauT, 224-225
Taxus celebica, 2534
T-box transcription factor, 34-35
Tbx18, 34-35
Tcf21, 31
TCF2, 2299-2300, 2317
Technetium 99m-labeled diethylenetriaminepentaacetic acid, 864-865
Technetium 99m-labeled dimercaptosuccinic acid, 865, 880
Technetium 99m-labeled mercaptoacetyltriglycine, 865, 866*f*, 869-871, 874*f*, 913*f*
Telmisartan, 1652*t*, 1653
Tempol, 732
Temporal arteritis, 1120
Temsirolimus, 1383*f*, 1384
Tenckhoff catheters, 2114-2115, 2115*f*, 2221, 2415
Terazosin, 1676*t*, 1677
Teriparatide, 618
Terlipressin, 455-456, 998-999
Terminal web, 56-59
Terry's nails, 762
TERT, 1153
Testosterone deficiency, 1921
Tetany, 523, 554
Tezosentan, 338
Thailand, 2444, 2535
The Joint Commission, 2632-2633
Theophylline poisoning, 2186-2187
Therapeutic cloning, 2604-2606, 2605*f*
Therapeutic plasma exchange, 1393, 2171. *See also* Plasmapheresis
Thermofiltration, 2160-2161
Thiazide diuretics
  absorption of, 1712
  acute interstitial nephritis after initiation of, 1732
  adverse effects of, 1712
    hypercalcemia, 609, 1730
    hyperglycemia, 1730
    hyperlipidemia, 1731
    hyperuricemia, 1731
    hypocalciuria, 190-191
    hypokalemia, 1728
    impotence, 1731-1732
  in African Americans, 1686
  angiotensin receptor blockers and, 1655
  bone mineral density affected by, 1726-1727
  central diabetes insipidus treated with, 487
  description of, 1362, 1363*t*, 1560, 1564
  diabetes insipidus treated with, 487, 1727
  diabetes mellitus and, 1730
  differences among, 1712
  distal convoluted tubule action of, 1710, 1711*f*
  distal potassium-sparing diuretics and, 1719
  in elderly, 1682-1685, 1684*t*

Thiazide diuretics (Continued)
  extracellular fluid volume affected by, 190-191
  hypercalcemia caused by, 609, 1730
  hyperglycemia caused by, 1730, 1731*f*
  hyperlipidemia caused by, 1731
  hyperuricemia caused by, 1731
  hypervolemia treated with, 451
  hypocalciuria caused by, 190-191
  hypokalemia caused by, 1728
  hyponatremia and, 817-818
  indications for, 1712
  loop diuretics and, 1712-1713
  mechanism of action, 451, 1710-1712
  nephrogenic diabetes insipidus treated with, 2370
  osteocalcin inhibition by, 1726-1727
  pharmacokinetics of, 1712
  potassium excretion affected by, 1711-1712
  in pregnancy, 1732
  side effects of, 1689-1690
  sites of action, 1710-1712
  vasodilation using, 1685
  water clearance affected by, 1728, 1728*f*
Thiazide-like diuretics, 1710-1712, 1711*f*
Thiazolidinediones, 174, 2127
Thick ascending limb. *See also* Loop of Henle
  acid-base transporters in, 238
  ammonia in, 245, 251
  anatomy of, 45, 61, 63-65, 158
  apical potassium channels in, 159-160
  Bartter's syndrome and, 579*f*
  bicarbonate reabsorption in, 238
  calcium reabsorption in, 188
  cells of, 63-64, 158, 164-165, 1273
  chloride channels in, 161-162
  claudins expressed in, 160
  defect in, hypokalemia as indication of, 815
  EP3 receptor mRNA in, 371
  20-HETE and, 385
  innervation of, 81
  luminal surface of, 66*f*
  magnesium in, 194, 194*f*
  mineralocorticoid receptor expression in, 315
  mitochondria of, 63-64
  NKCC2 function in, 163
  reabsorptive processes in, 64-65
  sodium chloride transport in
    activating influences on, 162-164
    apical mechanisms of, 158-160
    basolateral mechanisms of, 160-162
    calcium-sensing receptor effects on, 164-165
    inhibitory influences on, 164-165, 164*f*
    paracellular mechanisms of, 160
    regulation of, 162-165
    ROMK protein effects on, 159-160
    transepithelial, 162
  sodium reabsorption in, 135, 137, 1272-1273
  sodium transport in, 132-133
  solute transport in, 132-133
  transepithelial resistance in, 160
  tumor necrosis factor-α expression in, 164
  urea recycling in, 270
Thin ascending limb
  apical chloride transport in, 156-157
  basolateral chloride transport in, 156-157
  osmolality in, 272

Thin ascending limb (Continued)
  passive countercurrent multiplier mechanism, 272
  sodium chloride transport in, 156-158, 157*f*
Thin basement membrane nephropathy, 1141-1142, 1424-1425
Thin descending limb, 156, 263*f*
Thin limbs of loop of Henle
  anatomy of, 61-63, 63*f*-64*f*
  early descending, 64*f*
  epithelium of, 65*f*
  types of, 61-62, 64*f*
Thiopurine methyltransferase, 2257, 2425
Thirst, 471-473, 2366
Thomsen-Friedenreich antigen, 1182
Thrombectomy, 2199-2202, 2199*t*, 2201*f*-2202*f*
Thrombin, 1904, 1907
Thrombin-activable fibrinolysis inhibitor, 1803-1804
Thromboembolism
  in nephrotic syndrome, 1804
  renal artery, 1201-1202
  venous, hypoalbuminemia and, 1805
Thrombolytic therapy, 1206, 1933
Thrombomodulin, 1185
Thrombosis
  arteriovenous fistula, 2210-2212
  arteriovenous graft, 2194-2195, 2196*t*
  in children, 1805
  deep vein. *See* Deep vein thrombosis
  renal artery, 964, 1202-1203, 2253, 2266
  renal vein. *See* Renal vein thrombosis
Thrombospondin-1, 1752-1753
Thrombotic events, COX-2 inhibitors and, 363-364
Thrombotic microangiopathies, 1405-1406
  acute, 2269
  antiphospholipid syndrome as cause of, 1200-1201
  causes of, 1405*t*
  description of, 1175
  electron microscopy of, 1178*f*
  hemolytic-uremic syndrome. *See* Hemolytic-uremic syndrome
  pathology of, 1178-1179, 1178*f*
  during pregnancy, 1632
  thrombotic thrombocytopenia purpura. *See* Thrombotic thrombocytopenia purpura
  treatment of, 1181*t*
Thrombotic thrombocytopenia purpura (TTP)
  ADAMTS13 deficiency associated with, 1188-1191, 2154-2155
  classification of, 1176*t*
  clinical features of, 1176, 2154
  description of, 990-992, 1157
  hematopoietic stem cell transplantation and, 1188
  laboratory findings, 1176-1178
  pathogenesis of, 2154-2155
  pathology of, 1179
  plasmapheresis for, 2154-2155
  platelet aggregation in, 1189*f*
  recurrence of, after renal transplantation, 2270
Thromboxane A_2, 364-365, 367-368, 1579
  in albuminuria, 378
  allograft rejection and, 378
  biosynthesis of, 376
  half-life of, 374
  loop diuretics effect on, 1717

Thromboxane A₂ *(Continued)*
  synthesis of, 1270
  vasoconstriction induced by, 377, 411, 1270
Thromboxane A₂ receptor, 368
Thromboxane A₂ synthase, 378-379
Thromboxane synthase, 364-365
Thrombus, 1177f
Thyroid dysfunction, 1549
Thyroid hormone disturbances, 1915-1916, 1915t
Thyroid hormone-binding globulin, 1915-1916
Thyroid surgery, 616
Thyroid-stimulating hormone, 1915-1916
Thyrotoxic periodic paralysis, 573
Thyrotropin, 1915-1916
Thyroxine, 1915-1916
Ticlopidine, 1189
Tie2 receptor, 34
Tight junctions, 147f, 188-189
Timolol, 1656t-1657t, 1657
TINU syndrome, 1229
Tiopronin, 1365
Tissue engineering
  definition of, 2602
  goal of, 2602-2603
  intrarenal progenitor cells, 2608-2609
  renal anlagen, 2613-2616
  renal units, 2616-2617
  stem cells used in
    adult, 2607-2608
    amniotic fluid- and placental-derived, 2607
    bromodeoxyuridine retention by, 2608
    description of, 2603
    embryonic, 2603-2607
    identification of, 2608-2609
    induced pluripotent, 2606-2607
    mesenchymal
      acute kidney injury applications of, 2611-2613
      bone marrow-derived, 2611
      description of, 2607
      differentiation of, into renal tissue, 2611
  therapeutic cloning, 2604-2606, 2605f
Tissue factor pathway inhibitor, 1803-1804, 1904
Tissue inhibitors of metalloproteinases (TIMP), 949, 989, 1757, 1794
Tissue ischemia, 1579
Tissue kallikrein, 181-182
Tissue kallikrein-kinin system, 347-348
Tissue necrosis, 586
Tissue plasminogen activator, 1804
Tissue-nonspecific alkaline phosphatase, 1838
Titratable acid excretion, 246-247
  buffers involved in, 246, 246f
  creatinine in, 247
  as phosphate, 246-247
  as phosphoric acid, 247
  uric acid in, 247
  urinary buffers involved in, 246-247, 246f
TMP, 540-541
TNM staging system, 1378, 1378t
Tobacco smoking. *See* Smoking
Tofacitinib, 2258
Toll-like receptor-2, 976, 1201
Toll-like receptor-4, 238, 976, 1201
Toluene-induced metabolic acidosis, 843f
Tolvaptan, 454, 504-505, 508, 1495, 1713-1714
Tonicity balance, 807-808, 808f

Tonicity-responsive enhancer-binding protein, 392
Tonsillectomy, 1068-1069
Topiramate-induced non-anion gap metabolic acidosis, 532
Torres Strait Islanders, 2538, 2546
Torsades de pointes, 569
Torsemide, 1707
Total body water, 460, 486, 2365, 2414
Total iron binding capacity, 1893
Total osmolality, 461
Total-body irradiation, 1400
Townes-Brock syndrome, 2297t, 2298-2299, 2318
Toxic alcohols, 839
Toxic gain of function, 1469-1470
Toxins. *See also* Poison removal/poisonings
  acidosis caused by, 543, 548-550
  acute kidney injury caused by, 2500-2501
  plasmapheresis for removal of, 2159
TP receptors, 366-369
Trabecular bone, 1831-1832, 1842
Trace elements, 1983-1984, 2099-2100
Trandolapril, 1643t, 1644
Tranexamic acid, 1906
Transcapillary hydraulic pressure difference, 97-98
Transcapillary hydrostatic pressure difference, 1760f
Transcription factor, 7
Transcription factor 3, 1372
Transepithelial potassium transport, 175-176
Transepithelial potential difference, 145-146
Transepithelial sodium chloride transport
  apical potassium channels for, 159
  by intercalated cells, 170f
  by principal cells, 170f
  calcium-sensing receptor inhibitory effects on, 164f
  cAMP-generating hormone stimulation of, 164
  description of, 148-149
  in proximal tubule, 149f
  stimulation of, 164
  in thick ascending limb, 158f, 162-164
Transferrin, serum, 1970-1971
Transferrin receptor, serum, 1893-1894
Transferrin saturation, 1893, 1894f
Transforming growth factor-β
  angiotensin II's role in expression of, 334
  definition of, 1212-1213
  low-protein diet effects on, 1958
  α₂-macroglobulin and, 1212-1213
  in nephron injury after renal mass ablation, 1755-1756
  renal fibrosis in aging kidney, 729-730
  role of, 1579
  stimulation of, 729-730
Transforming growth factor-β₁, 951
Transgenic mouse models, kidney development studies using, 9-19, 10t-17t
Transient hematuria, 1015
Transient hyponatremia, 477
Transient ischemic attack, 1926-1927
Transient receptor potential cation channel, 113, 1753-1754
Transient receptor potential channel melastatin 6, 1711-1712
Transient receptor potential vanilloid channels, 467, 1825
Transitional cell carcinoma, 898-899, 900f-902f
Transjugular intrahepatic portosystemic shunt, 457, 998-999
Translocation carcinoma, 1372
Translocational hyponatremia, 491

Transmembrane domains, of LeuT fold, 229
Transmembrane serine protease 6, 1887
Transmural pressure, 110
Transplant tourism, 2505
Transplantation
  hematopoietic stem cell, 1392
    acute kidney injury after, 993
    chronic kidney disease and, 1394
    complications of, 1393
    purpose of, 1393-1394
    renal syndromes associated with, 1393t
      acute kidney injury and, 1394
    total-body irradiation and, 1400-1401
    types of, 993
  islet cell, 1319-1320
  renal. *See* Renal transplantation
  renal-pancreas. *See* Renal-pancreas transplantation
Transplantation renal artery stenosis, 2272
Transplantation-associated thrombotic microangiography, 1395
Transtubular potassium concentration gradient, 569, 573-574, 820-821, 2380
Transtubular potassium gradient, 536-537
Treatment-resistant hypertension, 1580
Triamterene, 1712-1713
Tribonat, 546
Tricarboxylic acid cycle, 328
Trichomonas vaginalis, 1255
Trichorhinophalangeal syndrome, 29
Trichrome stain, 919-920
Triiodothyronine, 1915-1916
Trimethaphan camsylate, 1695t, 1698
Trimethoprim-sulfamethoxazole, 590, 750, 1238t, 2456-2457
Trimethylamine, 1812-1813
Triple phosphate, 768
Triple-helical type IV collagen molecule, 1421
TROP2, 25
Tropical diseases
  dengue fever. *See* Dengue fever
  leptospirosis. *See* Leptospirosis
  malaria. *See* Malaria
  yellow fever, 2441-2442, 2442f
Troponin I, 2101
Troponin T, 2101
Trousseau's sign, 612-613, 623, 995
Trpc6, 39
TRPC6 disease, 1430
TRPM6 channel, 196, 620
Trpm6 protein, 193-194
TRPV5, 189, 190f, 191-192, 741
Trypanosome spp., 1150-1151
Trypanosomiasis, 1150-1151
Tryptophan, 1812, 1983-1984
Tsutsugamushi disease, 2513-2515
T-type calcium channels, 1662
Tuberculosis, 882, 884f, 1252-1254, 1253f, 1260, 2505
Tuberous sclerosis, 1952, 1952t
Tuberous sclerosis complex, 1368-1369, 1374, 1500-1502
Tubular atrophy, 728f
Tubular epithelial cells, 1215, 1274, 1277-1279
Tubular proteinuria, 791, 793
Tubular stretch, 1278
Tubule fluid, 265-273
Tubuloglomerular feedback, 55, 135, 209-210, 1269
  adenosine's role in mediation of, 108-109, 135
  angiotensin II antagonists effect on, 109
  angiotensin II in, 399
  definition of, 106

INDEX

Tubuloglomerular feedback *(Continued)*
  in effective arterial blood volume regulation, 399-400
  mechanism of action, 108f
  renal autoregulation mediation by, 106-109
  renal blood flow controlled by, 108-109
  renin-angiotensin-aldosterone system in, 400
  responses of, 109
  sex hormones that regulate, 400
Tubulointerstitial antigens, 1214-1215, 1228-1229
Tubulointerstitial diseases
  acute interstitial nephritis. *See* Acute interstitial nephritis
  chronic tubulointerstitial nephritis. *See* Chronic tubulointerstitial nephritis
  drugs that cause, 1218-1219, 1218t
  in HIV-related nephropathy, 1152
  renal function affected by, 1210
  structure-function relationships in, 1209-1210
  in systemic lupus erythematosus, 1097-1098
Tubulointerstitial fibrosis, 729f, 1754-1755, 1763, 1793
Tubulointerstitial inflammation, 1215
Tubulointerstitial injury
  antigens in, 1214-1215
  cellular infiltrates in, 1215-1216
  complement components in, 1213-1214
  cytokines associated with, 1212-1213
  description of, 1209
  in focal segmental glomerulosclerosis, 1026
  genetic diseases that cause, 1210
  glomerular diseases that cause, 1210
  glomerular-filtered lipids associated with, 1213
  growth factors associated with, 1212-1213
  interstitial fibrosis, 1216-1218
  macrophages in, 1794
  mechanisms of, 1210-1218
  tubulointerstitial antigens in, 1214-1215
Tubulointerstitial nephritis, 622, 1209, 1220-1221, 2511-2513
Tumor lysis syndrome, 990, 992t
  characteristics of, 1395-1397
  classification of, 1396, 1396t
  definition of, 628
  hyperphosphatemia caused by, 628
  prevention of, 628
  risk factors for, 1396t
  treatment of, 1396-1397
Tumor necrosis factor, 2241
Tumor necrosis factor-α-converting enzyme, 329
Tumor necrosis factor-like weak inducer of apoptosis, 743
Tumor necrosis factor-related apoptosis-induced ligand, 1020
Tumor vaccine, 1384-1385
Tumor-induced osteomalacia, 197-198, 631
Tunneled catheters
  arteriovenous fistulas versus, 2629-2631
  bacteremia of, 2220
  complications of, 2217, 2217f-2218f
  description of, 2216
  dysfunction of, 2219-2220
  exchange of, 2219-2220
  femoral, 2218
  insertion of, 2216-2217, 2217f-2218f

Tunneled catheters *(Continued)*
  less common locations for, 2218-2219, 2219f
  transhepatic, 2219
  translumbar, 2218-2219, 2219f
Turkey. *See* Middle East
Turnover, mineralization, and volume classification system, 1845, 1845t
Twin study, 1348
Two-kidney renal clip hypertension, 1568-1569, 1570t, 1571-1572, 1572f-1573f
Type 1 diabetes mellitus. *See* Diabetes mellitus, type 1
Type 2 diabetes mellitus. *See* Diabetes mellitus, type 2
Type 2 vasopressin receptor, 278-279
Type A intercalated cells, 70-72, 72f
Type AB cystinuria, 1448
Type B cystinuria, 1448
Type B intercalated cells, 70-72, 72f
Type IV collagen, 1421
Type IV collagen disease, 1421-1425
Type IV collagen gene, 1422f
Tyrosine hydroxylase inhibitor, 1679-1680
Tyrosine kinases, 329-330
Tyrosinemia, 1443-1444

U

Ub-activating enzyme, 1964
Ubiquitin-protease system, 1964-1965, 1970
UFP-803, 352
Ularitide, 344-345, 1001
Ulnar-mammary syndrome, 2297t
Ultrafiltration
  convection during, 2112
  extracorporeal, 2139
  failure of, 2416
  in hemodialysis, 2068-2069, 2080, 2095, 2105
Ultrafiltration coefficient, 1797
Ultrafiltration rate, 2095-2096
Ultrasonography, 848-851
  acute interstitial nephritis evaluations, 1220
  acute kidney injury evaluations, 866-867, 989-990
  acute pyelonephritis evaluations, 878, 880f
  anatomy on, 849f, 850-851
  angiomyolipomas on, 891
  antenatal, 1264-1265
  arteriovenous fistula vascular mapping using, 2205-2206, 2206f
  autosomal dominant polycystic kidney disease, 1485f, 1485t
  contrast-enhanced, 849-850
  description of, 848
  diagnostic, 848
  end-stage kidney disease diagnosis using, 868, 868f, 888
  equipment used in, 848
  fetal, for urinary tract obstruction diagnosis, 1258-1259
  hydronephrosis diagnosis using, 867-869, 867f-868f, 1263
  increased through-transmission, 848
  intravenous contrast agents used with, 849
  kidney biopsy uses of, 850, 2223-2224, 2223t, 2224f
  for kidney stones, 1359
  lymphoceles on, 910-911
  nonspecular reflectors, 848
  obstruction evaluations, 871

Ultrasonography *(Continued)*
  power Doppler, 850f
  pyelonephritis evaluations, 878, 880f, 881-883
  renal colic on, 873
  renal cysts on, 883, 885f
  renal parenchymal disease on, 868
  renal transplantation assessments using, 910
  resistive index, 849
  specular reflectors, 848
  ureteropelvic junction obstruction findings, 2315
  urinary tract obstruction findings, 1263-1265, 1264f, 1267f
  urinoma after renal transplantation on, 910, 911f
Uncoupling protein isoforms, 127
Unilateral renal artery stenosis, 1595-1598
Unilateral renal cystic disease, 1512-1513, 1570t
Upper limit of metastability, 1327
Upper tract urothelial carcinoma, 1386
Urantide, 352
URAT1, 221, 221t
Urate, 816, 1453
Urate nephropathy, 1227-1228
Urate-induced calcium oxalate stone, 1336f
Urban yellow fever, 2441
Urea
  blood urea nitrogen, 123, 933-934, 988, 1808, 1959, 1968-1969
  in chronic kidney disease, 1959-1961, 1968-1969
  clearance of, 2070
  degradation of, 1960-1961
  excretion of, 1808
  fractional clearance of, 2120
  glomerular filtration rate estimations using, 782
  hemodialysis generation of, 2083-2084, 2083f-2084f
  hyponatremia treated with, 506
  in inner medulla, 268-270
  intrarenal recycling of, 820f
  osmotic diuresis evaluations, 811-812
  parathyroid hormone effects on production of, 1968
  peritoneal dialysis clearance of, 2120
  plasma, 423, 816, 2036
  production of, 1960-1961, 1968
  recycling of, in renal medulla, 270, 270f
  serum concentration of, 2070
Urea channel inhibitors, 1714
Urea nitrogen
  blood, 123, 933-934, 988, 1959, 1968-1969
  serum, 2072
Urea nitrogen appearance rate, 1969
Urea reduction ratio, 2085-2087, 2087f
Urea transporters, 276-278, 277f, 410, 740
Ureaplasma urealyticum, 1242
Urease inhibitor, 1365
Uremia, 1421-1422
  amino acid metabolism affected by, 1817
  carbohydrate metabolism affected by, 1816
  chronic, nitrogenous product turnover in
    ammonia, 1962
    creatinine, 1961
    fecal nitrogen, 1962
    nonurea nitrogen, 1962-1963
    overview of, 1959
    urea, 1959-1961
    uric acid, 1961-1962

Uremia *(Continued)*
  clinical features of, 1807
  creatinine accumulation in, 1808
  glomerular filtration rate in, 1819-1820
  growth failure in children caused by, 2358-2359
  hemodialysis for, 2083
  high anion gap acidosis caused by, 549-550
  immune disorder induced by, 2104
  insulin resistance in, 1816, 1914-1915
  lipid metabolism affected by, 1816-1817
  loss of appetite associated with, 1819
  metabolic effects of, 1808t, 1815-1818
  neurologic function in, 1818-1819
  nutrition affected by, 1817-1818
  platelets in, 1904
  protein metabolism affected by, 1817
  protein-binding defect in, 2037f
  resting energy expenditure affected by, 1815-1816
  sensorimotor neuropathy in, 1819
  signs and symptoms of, 1808t, 1818-1820
  sleep-wake cycle disruptions in, 1939
  sodium pump inhibition in, 1819
  solutes retained in. *See* Uremic solutes
Uremic acidosis, 549-550
Uremic cardiomyopathy, 1858-1859
Uremic encephalopathy, 1934-1935
Uremic platelet dysfunction, 1905, 1907f
Uremic polyneuropathy, 1939
Uremic solutes, 1808t
  aliphatic amines, 1812-1813
  aromatic compounds, 1811-1812
  chemical structure of, 1809f
  D–amino acids, 1809-1810
  description of, 1807
  dietary effects on, 1814-1815
  gastrointestinal function effects on, 1814-1815
  guanidines, 1810-1811
  hippurate, 1809f, 1811-1812
  indoles, 1812
  organic transport systems for clearance of, 1815
  oxalate, 1813
  peptides, 1810
  phenols, 1811-1812
  polyols, 1813
  protein-bound, 1814
  proteins, 1810
  renal replacement therapy for removal of, 1813-1814
  sequestered, 1814
  tryptophan metabolites, 1812
  urea, 1808-1809
  uric acid, 1813
Uremic syndrome, 773, 996, 1926, 1969
Ureter(s), 43, 2303f, 2313
Ureteral jets, 850, 850f
Ureteral mesenchyme, 34-35
Ureteral obstruction
  causes of, 1260
  endometriosis as cause of, 1261
  glomerular hemodynamics in, 1270t
  nephrolithiasis as cause of, 1260
  after pediatric renal transplantation, 2435
  sodium reabsorption affected by, 1275
  tubular sodium reabsorption affected by, 1272
  urinary calculi as cause of, 1280
Ureteral stents, 1246, 2429
Ureteral stones, 873, 875f-877f
Ureteral strictures, 1260

Ureteric bud
  BMP7 expression in, 29
  branching of, 5, 25, 28f, 2298
  collecting duct from, 44-45
  congenital anomalies of the kidney and urinary tract and, 2297-2298
  ectopic, 10t-17t
  epithelial, 3
  epithelial cells, 25
  genes required by, 23-25
  glial-derived neurotrophic factor transcriptional regulation and, 22-23
  induction of, 22-23
  metanephric mesenchyme and, 4f, 5-6, 21-25
  outgrowth of, 2297-2298
  positioning of, 27-28
  Spry1 deficiency effects on, 24-25
Ureteric stones, 873
Ureteropelvic junction, 43, 1258-1259, 1262, 2298, 2311, 2314-2315, 2315f
Uric acid
  in chronic kidney disease, 1813, 1961
  drugs that affect, 221
  fractional clearance of, 1961
  functions of, 1228
  glomerular filtration of, 220
  metabolism of, 996
  nephrotoxicity of, 967-968
  physiochemistry of, 1341-1342
  pregnancy and, 1612, 1616
  reabsorption of, 221
  renal handling of, 220-221, 220f
  secretion of, 221
  serum levels of, 1962
  in titratable acid excretion, 247
  transport of, 220-221, 220f, 221t
  in uremia, 1813
Uric acid nephropathy, 1259-1260
Uric acid stones, 1227, 1323f-1324f, 1324, 1341-1345, 1342t, 1351
Uric acid transporters, 220-221, 220f, 221t
Uricase deficiency, 1341
Uricosuria, 1653
Uricosuric drugs, 220f, 221
Uridine triphosphate, 174
Urinalysis
  chronic kidney disease evaluations, 776
  ethylene glycol exposure determined with, 2177
  hematuria evaluations, 756
  pauci-immune crescentic glomerulonephritis findings, 1086-1087
  renal tuberculosis findings, 1253
  urinary tract infection evaluations, 777-778
  urine properties on, 788-790, 789t
  urine specimen for, 788
Urinary buffers, 246-247, 246f
Urinary calculi
  characteristics of, 1279-1280
  in children, 2340
  composition of, 873
  extracorporeal shock wave lithotripsy for, 1279-1280
  obstruction caused by, 1279-1280. *See also* Urinary tract obstruction
  passage of, 873
Urinary dilution, 740
Urinary microscopy, 937, 937t
Urinary pH, 789-790, 841f, 1327, 1341-1344, 2168
Urinary pole, 89f
Urinary prothrombin fragment 1, 1330
Urinary space. *See* Bowman's space

Urinary supersaturation estimation, 1357-1359
Urinary tract
  congenital anomalies of. *See* Congenital anomalies of the kidney and urinary tract
  emphysematous cystitis, 1251
  emphysematous pyelonephritis of, 1251
  host defenses of, 1232, 1232t
  infected renal cyst involvement of, 1250-1251
  obstruction of. *See* Urinary tract obstruction
  perinephric abscess involvement of, 1250
  pyocystis of, 1252
  renal abscess involvement of, 1250
  xanthogranulomatous pyelonephritis of, 1251-1252
Urinary tract cancer, 1352
Urinary tract infection (UTI)
  acid-base disorders associated with, 778
  acute pyelonephritis and, 1633
  acute uncomplicated
    antimicrobial agents for, 1238-1239, 1238t
    description of, 1231-1232
    diagnosis of, 1237-1238
    epidemiology of, 1236
    Escherichia coli as cause of, 749-750, 778, 1233
    host factors, 1237
    microbiology of, 1236-1237
    pathogenesis of, 1236-1237
    prophylaxis for, 1239
    pyelonephritis in, 1240
    pyuria associated with, 1238
    recurrence of, 1237, 1239-1240
    reinfection of, 1237
    sexual intercourse as cause of, 1237
    spermicides and, 1237, 1239-1240
    Staphylococcus saprophyticus as cause of, 1237
    treatment of, 1238-1239, 1238t
    urine culture for, 1237-1238
  in AIDS patients, 883
  anatomic abnormalities associated with, 777
  asymptomatic, 1231-1232
  asymptomatic bacteriuria. *See* Asymptomatic bacteriuria
  as autonomic diabetic polyneuropathy sequelae, 1320
  bacteria that cause, 777-778
  bacteriuria, 1231-1232
  Candida albicans, 1254
  in children, 2313-2314, 2429
  clinical presentation of, 777
  complicated
    antimicrobial treatment of, 1243-1244
    clinical presentation of, 1243
    description of, 1231-1232
    epidemiology of, 1242
    Escherichia coli as cause of, 1242
    hospitalization for, 1242
    host factors associated with, 1242-1243
    imaging of, 1244
    laboratory diagnosis of, 1243
    microbiology of, 1242
    pathogenesis of, 1242-1243
    recurrent, 1244-1245
    sequelae of, 1242
    supportive care for, 1244
    treatment of, 1243-1244
    urinary tract abnormalities associated with, 1232t, 1242-1243

Urinary tract infection (UTI) *(Continued)*
  cystitis. *See* Urinary tract infection, acute uncomplicated
  definition of, 1231-1232
  description of, 1231
  in diabetes mellitus, 1320
  diagnosis of, 777-778, 1233-1234, 1234*t*
  in elderly, 749-750
  Escherichia coli as cause of, 749-750, 778, 1233, 1240, 1242
  fungal, 1254
  hematuria caused by, 755
  immune responses to, 1232-1233
  inflammatory responses to, 1232-1233
  in men, 777
  nephrolithiasis and, 2342
  parasitic infestations as cause of, 1255
  prevalence of, 777
  pyelonephritis
    acute nonobstructive, 1240-1242
    bacteremia in, 1240
    ciprofloxacin for, 1241*t*
    costovertebral angle pain or tenderness associated with, 1240
    description of, 1231-1232
    diagnosis of, 1240-1241
    epidemiology of, 1240
    imaging of, 1241
    pathogenesis of, 1240
    renal scarring caused by, 1240
  recurrent, 777, 1239-1240
  reinfection, 1232, 1237
  relapse of, 1232
  in renal failure patients, 1249
  renal function assessments in, 778
  in renal transplant recipients, 1248-1249, 2269-2270, 2429
  risk factors for, 777, 1248, 2269-2270
  signs and symptoms of, 749
  stones associated with, 1249
  symptomatic, 1231-1232
  treatment of
    antimicrobial agents, 1234, 1235*t*-1236*t*, 1238-1239, 1238*t*
    β-lactams, 1239
    nitrofurantoin, 750, 1238*t*
    pharmacokinetic and pharmacodynamic considerations for, 1234
    pivmecillinam, 1238*t*
    trimethoprim-sulfamethoxazole, 750, 1238*t*
  urinary frequency associated with, 777
  urinary tract abnormalities associated with, 1232*t*
  urine culture of, 1233-1234, 1234*t*, 1237-1238
  uroepithelial cells, 1232-1233
  in urolithiasis patients, 1249-1250
  vaginitis and, 777
  viral causes of, 1255
  voiding symptoms associated with, 777
Urinary tract obstruction
  abdominal aortic aneurysm as cause of, 1261
  acquired causes of, 1259-1262, 1259*t*
  acute, 1258
  angiotensin II expression in, 1278*f*
  benign prostatic hyperplasia as cause of, 1261, 1280
  biomarkers of, 1263
  bladder cancer as cause of, 1261
  in children, 1258
  chronic, 1258
  classification of, 1258

Urinary tract obstruction *(Continued)*
  clinical aspects of, 1262
  congenital, 719-720, 1258-1259, 1258*t*
  COX metabolites in, 377-378
  description of, 299
  diagnosis of, 1262-1268, 1264*f*-1268*f*
  diuresis after, 1281
  divalent cations excretion affected by relief of, 1276-1277
  drugs that cause, 1260
  etiology of, 1258-1262, 1258*t*, 1264
  extrinsic causes of, 1260-1262
  fetal, 1258-1259, 1279-1280
  glomerular filtration affected by, 1269-1271
  glomerular filtration rate regulation during, 1270-1271
  hematologic abnormalities that cause, 1262
  imaging of
    antegrade pyelography, 1268, 1268*f*
    antenatal ultrasonography, 1264-1265
    computed tomography, 1265-1266, 1266*f*
    Doppler ultrasonography, 1265
    intravenous pyelography, 1265, 1265*f*
    isotopic renography, 1266-1267, 1280
    magnetic resonance imaging, 1267-1268, 1267*f*
    magnetic resonance urography, 1267-1268
    retrograde pyelography, 1268
    ultrasonography, 1263-1265, 1264*f*, 1267*f*
    Whitaker test, 1268
  incidence of, 1257-1258
  intrinsic causes of, 1259-1260, 1259*t*
  malignant neoplasms as cause of, 1262
  in neurogenic bladder, 1280
  partial, 1280
  pathophysiology of, 1268-1277
  pelvic neurofibromas as cause of, 1262
  phosphate excretion affected by relief of, 1276-1277
  potassium excretion affected by relief of, 1276
  prenatal, 1258-1259, 1279-1280
  prevalence of, 1257-1258
  in prostate cancer, 1261
  relief of
    diuresis after, 1281
    divalent cations excretion affected by, 1276-1277
    kidney biopsy after, 1280-1281
    phosphate excretion affected by, 1276-1277
    potassium excretion affected by, 1276
    renal function after, 1280-1281
    urine acidification affected by, 1276
  renal blood flow affected by, 1269-1271
  renal damage caused by, 1280
  renal enzymes affected by, 1277*t*
  renal function recovery after, 1280-1281
  renal gene expression affected by, 1277*t*
  in renal transplantation recipients, 2271
  renin-angiotensin-aldosterone system in, 1279
  retroperitoneal processes that cause, 1261-1262
  signs and symptoms of, 1262
  sodium reabsorption affected by, 1272-1275
  sodium transport affected by, 1274
  terms associated with, 1257

Urinary tract obstruction *(Continued)*
  treatment of, 1279-1281
  tubular epithelial cells after resolution of, 1277-1279
  tubular function affected by, 1271-1277
  unilateral, 1281
  ureteropelvic junction, 1258-1259
  uric acid nephropathy as cause of, 1259-1260
  urine acidification affected by relief of, 1276
  urine concentration affected by, 1275-1276
  urine dilution affected by, 1275-1276
  urine flow affected by, 1274-1275
  urine output affected by, 1262
Urinary trefoil factor 1, 1331
Urine
  acidification of, 74, 1276, 1365-1366
  alkalinization of, 2168, 2180
  ammonia excretion in, 528-529, 538, 840, 841*f*
  assessment of, in acute kidney injury evaluations, 986-988, 987*t*-988*t*
  bilirubin in, 790
  casts in, 800, 800*t*, 801*f*
  cells in, 798-800
  chloride concentration in, 816
  citrate excretion in, 219
  cloudy, 788-789
  color of, 788-789, 789*t*
  crystals in, 800-802, 801*t*, 1329
  cytology of, 799
  daily volume of, 1257
  eosinophils in, 799-800
  erythrocytes in, 798-799, 799*f*
  extravasation of, after renal transplantation, 913
  fetal, 2302
  fluorine 18 2-fluoro-2-deoxy-D-glucose excretion in, 865
  formation of, 83, 94, 122
  gadolinium effects on, 858*f*
  glucose in, 205*f*, 790
  hemoglobin in, 790
  ketones in, 790
  leukocyte esterase in, 790
  leukocytes in, 799-800
  lipids in, 800
  low volume and uric acid stones, 1343
  magnesium excretion in, 194
  magnetic resonance imaging of, 857*f*-858*f*
  microorganisms in, 802
  microscopy evaluation of, 798-802, 799*f*, 800*t*-801*t*, 801*f*
  myoglobin in, 790
  neutrophil gelatinase-associated lipocalin, 944-945
  nitrites in, 790
  nitrogenous compounds in, 1962
  odor of, 789
  osmolality of, 789, 807
  phosphate excretion in, 199-200
  potassium excretion in, 180, 569, 820
  protein in, 112, 793, 947
  relative density of, 789
  sodium concentration in, 816
  specific gravity of, 789
  squamous cells in, 800
  sterility of, 1232, 1232*t*
  Tamm-Horsfall protein in, 1232
  urobilinogen in, 790
  urothelial cells in, 800

Urine chemistry, 1356-1359
Urine concentration
　ability, 271
　age-related changes in, 739-740
　aquaporins in, 274f
　assessment of, 789
　in elderly, 739-740
　knockout mice models of, 273-279
　loop of Henle in, 259-261
　mechanisms of, 92, 270
　nephron loss-specific adaptations in, 1748
　renal insufficiency effects on, 1748
　sites of, 264-265
　specific gravity, 789
　statins effect on, 301f
　urinary tract obstruction effects on, 1275-1276
　vasopressin in, 282
　water reabsorption effects on, 1748
Urine culture, 1233-1234, 1234t, 1237-1238
Urine dilution, 264-265, 1275-1276, 1748
Urine dipstick tests, 762-763, 777-778
Urine flow rate, 806, 810-811
Urine formation product ratio, 1328-1329
Urine leaks, 2270-2271
Urine osmolality, 465, 476, 479f
Urine osmoles, 811-812
Urine output, 959, 1262
Urine saturation, 1327
　factors influencing, 1327
　measurement of, 1327
　oxalate and calcium role in, 1340
　in stone formers, 1328
Urine sediment, 986-987, 987t
Urine specimen, 788
Urine studies, 762-763, 768
Urine volume, 476
Uriniferous pseudocyst, 1517
Urinoma, 910, 911f
Urobilinogen, 790
Urodilatin, 339, 339f, 341, 344-345
Uroepithelial cells, 1232-1233
Urogenital ridge, 2-3
Urogenital system, 2-3
Uroguanylin, 398
Urolithiasis. See also Kidney stone
　body mass index and, 1323f
　cardiovascular disease and, 1351, 1351f
　causes of, 1349, 1349f
　definition of, 1322
　diabetes mellitus and, 1350-1351
　differential diagnosis of, 769t
　epidemiology of, 1322-1324
　hypertension and, 1351-1352
　obesity and, 1350-1351
　polygenic animal model for, 1349-1350, 1350t
　prevalence by gender and weight, 1323f
　risk factors for, 1350-1351
　as systemic disorder, 1350-1355
　urinary tract infection in, 1249-1250
Uromodulin, 165, 800, 1214-1215, 1348-1349
Uromodulin-associated kidney disease, 165
Uropathogenic *Escherichia coli*, 1236-1237, 1239
Urotensin, 437-438
Urotensin I, 351
Urotensin II
　definition of, 351
　in diabetic nephropathy, 352
　in effective arterial blood volume regulation, 418-419
　in heart failure, 437-438
　interventional studies of, 352
　in kidney, 352

Urotensin II (Continued)
　nephron loss adaptations and, 1740
　physiologic role of, 351-352
　plasma levels of, 352
　prepro–U-11 mRNA, 351
　in renal disease, 352
　secretion of, 351
　synthesis of, 351, 351f
　urinary concentrations of, 352
　urine levels of, 352
　vasoconstrictive properties of, 351-352, 419
Urotensin II receptor, 352, 418-419
Urothelial cells, in urine, 800
Urothelial tumor, 1385
UT-A1/3 urea transporter knockout mice, 276-278
Uteroplacental insufficiency, 696-699

V

Vaccinations
　in hemodialysis patients, 2105
　in renal transplantation recipients, 2288, 2288t
　yellow fever, 2442
Vaccine, 1384-1385
VACTERL association, 2318
Vaginitis, 777
Valganciclovir, 2429-2430
Valproic acid, 2181-2182
Valsalva maneuver, 1204
Valsartan, 1652t, 1653
Valvular heart disease, 1859, 1929-1930, 2408
VAMP-2, 295-296
Vaptans
　adverse effects of, 455
　heart failure treated with, 454
　hyponatremia treated with, 504-505, 508
　loop diuretic-sparing effect of, 454-455
Vasa recta
　ascending, 92, 267, 269-270
　counterflow arrangement of, 262
　definition of, 262
　descending, 92, 269-270
　description of, 6, 87
　oxygen shunting, 133
　urea recycling through, 270
Vascular access
　in critically ill patients, for renal replacement therapy, 2145
　in diabetic nephropathy, 1315
　dialysis, 2191-2192
　for extracorporeal treatments for poisoning, 2173
　hand ischemia induced by, 2214
　hemodialysis. See Hemodialysis, vascular access for
　international trends in, 2630f
　quality improvement and, 2629-2631
Vascular calcification
　in adults, 2102-2103, 2128
　apoptosis in, 1836-1837
　assessment of, 1847
　atherosclerotic disease in, 1833-1835
　calcium-sensing receptor in, 1826
　cellular transformation in, 1835-1836
　in children, 2407-2408
　in chronic kidney disease, 1850, 2102-2103
　coronary artery, 1850
　in dialysis patients, 1850
　inhibitors of
　　fetuin-A, 1837-1838
　　matrix gamma-carboxyglutamate protein, 1838

Vascular calcification (Continued)
　　osteoprotegerin, 1838
　　pyrophosphate, 1838
　matrix vesicles in, 1836-1837
　pathophysiology of, 1833-1839, 1836f
　pathways in, 1837f
　prevalence of, 1837
　after renal transplantation, 1852
Vascular dementia, 1938
Vascular endothelial growth factor receptor 1, 1621
Vascular endothelial growth factor (VEGF)
　COX-2 inhibition effects on, 378
　downregulation of, 1794
　endothelial cell expression of, 47-48
　insulin-like growth factor-1 effects on production of, 1744
　podocyte expression of, 1752-1753
　preeclampsia and, 1619, 1621-1623
Vascular endothelial growth factor-A, 32-34, 33f
Vascular endothelial growth factor-C, 392
Vascular endothelium, 1752-1753
Vascular smooth muscle cells, 1835, 2102-2103
Vascular thrombosis, 898, 899f
Vascular tone, 363, 383f, 979
Vasculature, renal
　arteries, 83-85
　description of, 262
　development of, 6, 32-35, 33f
　EP2 receptor effects on, 373
　hydraulic pressure profile of, 85, 85f
　illustration of, 7f
　innervation of, 110
　molecular genetics of, 32-35, 33f
　vasoconstrictors that affect, 99
　veins, 83-85
Vasculitis, 1165-1166, 1950-1951, 1951f
Vasculogenesis, 6, 32
Vasodilation, 422, 1612-1613
Vasodilators
　direct-acting. See Direct-acting vasodilators
　parenteral, 1695t, 1696-1699
Vasohibin-1, 120
Vasopeptidase inhibitors, 345, 453-454
Vasopressin
　apical chloride transport affected by, 163
　aquaporin-2 phosphorylation sites modified by, 293, 805
　aquaporin-2 trafficking in collecting duct principal cells regulated by, 287-288
　bicarbonate reabsorption affected by, 238
　in bronchogenic carcinoma, 499
　cardiac function effects of, 432-433
　central diabetes insipidus treated with, 285, 488
　chloride transport affected by, 157-158
　cirrhosis-related water retention affected by, 446
　clearance of, 471
　copeptin fragment of, 463
　cortical collecting duct affected by, 819
　deficiency of, 474-477
　description of, 409-410, 2366
　diabetes insipidus treated with, 486
　distal nephron potassium secretion affected by, 182
　distribution of, 471
　diuretic therapy response affected by, 1717
　in effective arterial blood volume regulation, 415
　epithelial sodium channel activation by, 173-174

Vasopressin (Continued)
  fluid deprivation test for, 485, 485t
  functions of, 410
  furosemide levels affected by, 1717
  gene, 463, 465f
  in gestational diabetes insipidus, 471
  in heart failure, 432-433
  hemodynamic stimuli that affect, 467-468
  hypothalamic pathways that regulate, 464f
  inactivation of, 471
  natriuresis effects of, 410-411
  nephrogenic diabetes insipidus and, 285
  neurohypophysis production of, 463, 474
  neurophysin peptide fragment of, 463
  nonosmotic regulation of, 467-471
  osmotic regulation of, 464-467, 478
  plasma levels of, 282, 466f, 479f
  precursors of, 463
  prostaglandin E_2 effects on, 373-374
  renal blood flow affected by, 410
  renal response to, 808-809
  secretion of, 282
    baroreceptor mechanisms involved in, 468, 469t
    blood volume effects on, 468
    description of, 462-471
    drinking effects on, 468-469
    drugs that affect, 469t, 471
    hormones that affect, 469t
    hypercapnia effects on, 470
    hypoglycemia effects on, 470
    hypovolemia effects on, 467-468
    hypoxia effects on, 470
    nausea effects on, 469-470, 469f
    opioid inhibition of, 471
    renin-angiotensin-aldosterone system effects on, 470
    stress effects on, 470
    thirst and, 472-473
  sodium balance affected by, 498
  sodium chloride transport affected by, 162-163, 173
  sodium reabsorption affected by, 278, 282
  structure of, 463-464
  sympathetic nervous system and, 406
  synthesis of, 462-471, 474
  transepithelial sodium chloride transport affected by, 163-164
  in urinary concentration, 282
  water balance affected by, 498
  in water excretion, 258-259, 259f, 270-271
  water permeability effect on, 1469f
  water retention affected by, 446
  water transport regulation by, 374
Vasopressin 1A receptor, 245, 410
Vasopressin 1 receptor, 282, 455-456
Vasopressin 2 receptor, 282-285
  antagonists, for hepatorenal syndrome, 456-457
  arginine vasopressin activation of, 2366
  β-arrestin and, 282-284
  description of, 282
  downregulation, accessory proteins involved in, 282-283
  heterotrimeric G proteins and, 282-284
  internalization effects on, 284-285, 291
  lysosome degradation of, 284-285
  messenger RNA, 282-283
  trafficking of, 284f
  in urine concentration, 282
Vasopressin 3 receptor, 410
Vasopressin disorders
  description of, 473
  diabetes insipidus. See Diabetes insipidus

Vasopressin disorders (Continued)
  hyponatremia. See Hyponatremia
  hypotonic polyuria, 473t
  pathophysiology of, 473
Vasopressin receptor, 1471f
Vasopressin receptor antagonists, 454-455, 504-506, 509, 1713-1714
Vasopressin-vasopressin receptor antagonist, 1495
Vasopressin-vasopressin receptor mutation, 1471f
Vasopressin-vasopressin receptor shuttle pathway, 1468-1470
VATER association, 2318
Vectorial transport, 126
Venacavography, 1204-1205
Venoocclusive disease, 993, 1394-1395
Venous thromboembolism, 1805
Ventricular sensors, 395-396
Ventriculoperitoneal shunts, 1149
Verapamil hydrochloride, 1663t, 1664, 1668-1669, 1668t, 1697t
Vertebral fracture, 1352f
Vertical nystagmus, 623
Very-low-density lipoprotein, 1801-1802
Vesicoureteral reflux
  antibiotic prophylaxis in, 2314
  bladder and bowel dysfunction as risk factor for, 2314
  in children, 2311, 2313-2314, 2314f, 2435
  definition of, 2313
  diagnosis of, 2313
  epidemiology of, 2313
  grading of, 2313, 2314f
  management of, 2314
  prognosis for, 2313-2314
  in pyelonephritis, 878, 882-883
  in renal agenesis, 2302
  in renal ectopy, 2311
Vibrio sodium-galactose symporter, 207, 208f
Vietnam, 2536
Villous adenoma, 553
Viral urinary tract infection, 1255
Visceral epithelial cells, 49-51, 52f. See also Podocyte(s)
Visceral infections, 1149
Vitamin A
  hypercalcemia caused by, 609
  maternal restriction of, nephron number affected by, 716
  nephron number affected by, 721
  teratogenicity of, 716-717
Vitamin B, 1732, 1932, 1938
Vitamin B_6, 1983
Vitamin B_{12}, 1883-1884, 1983
Vitamin C, 1983
Vitamin D
  absorptive hypercalciuria and, 1331
  in children, 2390-2391
  in chronic kidney disease, 1912, 1923-1924
  in chronic kidney disease–mineral bone disorder, 1828-1830, 1841, 1848-1849
  deficiency of
    acquired, 1775
    anemia in chronic kidney disease and, 1887
    calcitriol for, 1872-1873, 1923-1924
    cardiovascular mortality risks, 2099-2100
    in chronic kidney disease, 1775, 1849, 1912, 1924, 2434
    in chronic kidney disease–mineral bone disorder, 1848-1849

Vitamin D (Continued)
    diseases and disorders associated with, 1848-1849, 1923-1924
    hypophosphatemia caused by, 633
    1,25(OH)D levels, 617, 1872-1873
    populations with, 617
    proximal renal tubular acidosis and, 531
  description of, 617
  diabetic nephropathy treated with, 1312-1313
  dietary supplementation of, 617
  forms of, 2390
  health benefits of, 1848-1849
  hypercalcemia caused by, 609, 2132
  hypertension and, 1549
  hypocalcemia caused by, 617
  in insulin resistance, 1913
  metabolism of, 1828f
  parenteral, 2026
  renal 1-hydroxylation of, 1749-1750
  rickets prevention using, 2394
  supplementation of, 1849, 1924, 2406
  types of, 1923
Vitamin D_2, 2390
Vitamin D_3, 2390
Vitamin D analogues
  in chronic kidney disease, 2032
  cinacalcet and, 2029, 2032
  description of, 2023-2026
  parathyroid hormone affected by, 2027-2029
Vitamin D receptor, 1333, 1831f
Vitamin D receptor mutant mice, 200-201
Vitamin D response elements, 2023-2025
Vitamin D sterols, 2026, 2029
Vitamin D-binding protein, 1797, 1828-1829, 1923-1924, 2390
Vitamin D-dependent rickets type 1, 617
Vitamin E, 1984
Vitamin K_2, 1838
Voclosporin, 2257
Voiding cystourethrogram, 2317f
Voltage-dependent calcium channels, 108
Volume overload
  clinical manifestations of, 776
  in critically ill patients, 2144
  extracorporeal ultrafiltration for, 2139
  in hypervolemia, 449
  resistant hypertension caused by, 1693
Volume repletion, 610-611
Voluntary exploratory data submissions, 928
Vomiting, 553
von Gierke's disease, 1442-1443
von Hippel–Lindau disease, 889, 890f, 1952, 1952t
von Hippel-Lindau disease type 2, 1548
von Hippel-Lindau gene, 1372-1373, 1373f
von Hippel–Lindau protein, 1881
von Hippel-Lindau syndrome, 1373, 1380, 1502-1503
von Willebrand factor, 1179, 1188, 1904-1906
von Willebrand factor-cleaving protease deficiency, 2356
V_2R. See Vasopressin 2 receptor
V_2R gene, 279

W

WAGR syndrome, 1387
Waldenström's macroglobulinemia, 1136, 1136f-1137f, 2153-2154

Warfarin, 1068, 1206, 1908, 2040
Wasp stings, 2500, 2525
Water
  collecting duct absorption sites, 269f, 270-271
  evaporative loss of, 462
  excretion of
    arginine vasopressin's role in, 270-271
    decreases in, 815
    endothelin effects on, 416
    factors that affect, 491
    free, 462-463
    insensible loss, 462
    regulation of, 258-259
  homeostasis of, 1468
  insensible loss of, 462
  metabolism of, 462-473, 2365-2367
  permeability of, vasopressin effect on, 1469f
Water balance
  acquired disorders of, 297
  arginine vasopressin effects on, 498
  calculation of, 811
  electrolyte-free, 807
  long-term regulation of, 296-302
Water channels, 805
Water deprivation, 110
Water diuresis, 805-813
  assessment of
    electrolyte-free water balance, 807
    osmole excretion rate, 807-808
    tonicity balance, 807-808, 808f
    urine flow rate for, 806
    urine osmolality, 807
  clinical approach to, 808-809
  desalination of luminal fluid, 806
  description of, 271
  driving force for, 805
  in elderly, 743, 743f
  filtrate, distal delivery of, 805-806
  urine volume during, 805
  water channels, 805
  water permeability, residual, 806

Water retention
  aquaporin-2 in, 446
  in cirrhosis. See Cirrhosis, water retention in
Water softener, 2081
Water transport, 373-374
Water-soluble vitamins, 1983-1984
Weak acid, 512
Weak base, 512
Wegener's type antineutrophil cytoplasmic antibody-associated vasculitis, 350
Weigert-Meyer rule, 2313
Weight loss, 1992-1993
Weil's disease, 2443-2444
Whitaker test, 1268
White cell function, 1909-1910
White coat hypertension, 1540, 1540f
Whittam model, 127-128, 127f
Whole-exome sequencing technique, 1410, 1418
Williams-Beuren syndrome, 2394-2395
Wilms' tumor, 1386-1387
Wilms' tumor 1, 2603
Wilms' tumor-1 gene, 7-9, 1413-1414, 1414t
Wilms' tumor oncogene, 1431
Wilson's disease, 1444-1445
With-no-lysine kinases, 819
WNK1, 179-180, 590, 1712
WNK4, 163, 183, 313, 539-540, 590
WNK kinases, 168, 180, 566
WNK-dependent signaling, 183
WNK-SPAK/OSR1 signaling cascade, 181f
Wnt4, 28
Wnt11, 28
Wnt9b, 28
Wolffian duct, 2-3
Wolframin, 475
Wolfram's syndrome, 475
WT1, 36-37
WT1, 2326

X

Xanthelasma palpebrarum, 762
Xanthine dehydrogenase, 1347

Xanthine oxidase inhibitors, 1364-1365, 2425
Xanthine stone, 1347
Xanthinuria, 1347
Xanthogranulomatous pyelonephritis, 881, 883f, 1251-1252
Xanthomas, eruptive, 1946-1947, 1946f
Xenogeneic, 2228-2229
Xenopus oocytes, 21, 288
Xerosis, 1943, 1943f
X-linked Alport's syndrome, 1423-1424
X-linked diabetes insipidus, 1473
X-linked hypophosphatemia, 630
X-linked hypophosphatemic rickets, 201-202, 1437, 1451-1452, 1830
X-linked nephrogenic diabetes insipidus, 278-279, 300, 1470-1473
X-linked recessive nephrolithiasis, 1437
Xp11.2 translocation carcinoma, 1372
X-ray, 1359

Y

Yellow fever, 2441-2442, 2442f

Z

Zebrafish, 20-21
Zellweger's syndrome, 2297t
Zenker's fixative, 919
Zero-order processes, 2069
Zinc
  deficiency of, 1887, 2099-2100
  supplementation of, 1984
Zinc-dependent metalloproteinases, 2447
Zoledronate, 611
Zonula adherens, 55-56
Zonula occludens, 972-973
Zonula occludens 1, 113
ZS-9, 597-598
Zucker diabetic fatty rat, 1344-1345, 1345f
Zygomatosis, 1405
Zygomycosis, 2498, 2498f